Unit V Psychosocial Basis for Nursing Practice

Unit VI Scientific Basis for Nursing Practice

Unit VII Basic Human Needs

Unit VIII Clients With Special Needs

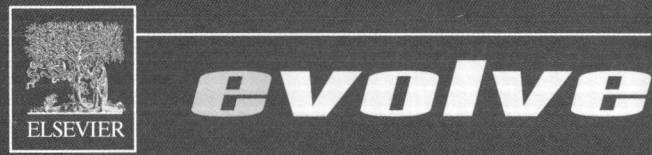

Evolve provides online access to free learning resources and activities designed specifically for the textbook you are using in your class. The resources will provide you with information that enhances the material covered in the book and much more.

Visit the Web address listed below to start your learning evolution today!

http://evolve.elsevier.com/Potter/fundamentals/

Evolve® Student Learning Resources for Potter & Perry: *Fundamentals of Nursing,* **7th Edition,** offer the following features:

Student Resources

- **Audio Summaries** for each chapter are downloadable to an mp3 device or CD.

- **Student Learning Activities** include Hangman, Match Its, and Drag and Drops.

- **Animations** include exciting images related to various chapters in the textbook.

- **Video Clips** demonstrate important steps in various nursing skills throughout the textbook.

- **WebLinks** are an exciting resource that lets you link to hundreds of websites carefully chosen to supplement the content of the textbook.

- **Content Updates** include the latest information from the authors of the textbook to help keep you current with recent developments in this area of study.

Fundamentals of Nursing

Fundamentals of Nursing

7th EDITION

Patricia A. POTTER RN, MSN, PhD, FAAN
Research Scientist
Barnes-Jewish Hospital
Siteman Cancer Center at Washington
   University School of Medicine
St. Louis, Missouri

Anne Griffin PERRY RN, EdD, FAAN
Professor and Chair
Department of Primary Care and Health
   Systems Nursing
School of Nursing
Southern Illinois University
Edwardsville, Illinois

Section Editors

Amy Hall, RN, BSN, MS, PhD
Chair
Department of Nursing and
   Health Sciences
Associate Professor of Nursing
University of Evansville
Evansville, Indiana

Patricia A. Stockert, RN, BSN,
   MS, PhD
Professor and Associate Dean
Undergraduate Program
Saint Francis Medical Center
   College of Nursing
Peoria, Illinois

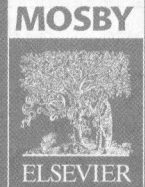

With over 1100 illustrations

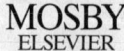

MOSBY
ELSEVIER

11830 Westline Industrial Drive
St. Louis, Missouri 63146

Fundamentals of Nursing, 7th Edition   ISBN: 978-0-323-06784-3

Copyright © 2009, 2005, 2001, 1997, 1993, 1989, 1985 by Mosby, Inc., an affiliate of Elsevier Inc.

All rights reserved. No part of this publication may be reproduced or transmitted in any form or by any means, electronic or mechanical, including photocopying, recording, or any information storage and retrieval system, without permission in writing from the publisher.

Permissions may be sought directly from Elsevier's Rights Department: phone: (+1) 215 239 3804 (US) or (+44) 1865 843830 (UK); fax: (+44) 1865 853333; e-mail: healthpermissions@elsevier.com. You may also complete your request on-line via the Elsevier website at http://www.elsevier.com/permissions.

NOTICE

Knowledge and best practice in this field are constantly changing. As new research and experience broaden our knowledge, changes in practice, treatment and drug therapy may become necessary or appropriate. Readers are advised to check the most current information provided (i) on procedures featured or (ii) by the manufacturer of each product to be administered, to verify the recommended dose or formula, the method and duration of administration, and contraindications. It is the responsibility of the practitioner, relying on their own experience and knowledge of the patient, to make diagnoses, to determine dosages and the best treatment for each individual patient, and to take all appropriate safety precautions. To the fullest extent of the law, neither the Publisher nor the Authors assumes any liability for any injury and/or damage to persons or property arising out of or related to any use of the material contained in this book.

The Publisher

International Standard Book Number: 978-0-323-06784-3

Executive Editor: Susan Epstein
Developmental Editor: Lynda Huenefeld
Publishing Services Manager: John Rogers
Project Manager: Beth Hayes
Design Direction: Amy Buxton

Printed in Canada

Last digit is the print number: 9 8 7 6 5 4 3 2

Working together to grow libraries in developing countries

www.elsevier.com | www.bookaid.org | www.sabre.org

ELSEVIER   BOOK AID International   Sabre Foundation

Contributors

Marjorie Baier, RN, PhD
Associate Professor
School of Nursing
Southern Illinois University
Edwardsville, Illinois

Sylvia K. Baird, RN, BSN, MM
Manager of Nursing Quality
Spectrum Health
Grand Rapids, Michigan

Karen Balakas, RN, PhD, CNE
Associate Professor
Goldfarb School of Nursing at Barnes-Jewish College
St. Louis, Missouri

Lois Bentler-Lampe, RN, MS
Instructor
Saint Francis Medical Center College of Nursing
Peoria, Illinois

Sheryl Buckner, RN-BC, MS, CNE
Academic and Staff Developer, Clinical Instructor
College of Nursing
University of Oklahoma
Oklahoma City, Oklahoma

Jeri Burger, RN, PhD
Assistant Professor
College of Nursing and Health Professions
University of Southern Indiana
Evansville, Indiana

Janice C. Colwell, RN, MS, CWOCN, FAAN
Clinical Nurse Specialist
University of Chicago Hospitals
Chicago, Illinois

Eileen Costantinou, RN, MSN, BC
Consultant
Center for Practice Excellence
Barnes-Jewish Hospital
St. Louis, Missouri

Margaret Ecker, RN, MS
Director, Nursing Quality
Kaiser Permanente Los Angeles Medical Center
Los Angeles, California

Susan J. Fetzer, RN, PA, BSN, MSN, MBA, PhD
Associate Professor
College of Health and Human Services
University of New Hampshire
Durham, New Hampshire

Victoria N. Folse, APRN, BC, LCPC, PhD
Assistant Professor
School of Nursing, Illinois Wesleyan University
Bloomington, Illinois

Steve Kilkus, RN, MSN
Faculty
Edgewood College School of Nursing
Madison, Wisconsin

Judith Ann Kilpatrick, RN, MSN, DNSc
Assistant Professor
Widener University School of Nursing
Chester, Pennsylvania

Lori Klingman, RN, MSN
Faculty, School of Nursing
Ohio Valley General Hospital
McKees Rocks, Pennsylvania

Anahid Kulwicki, RN, DNS, FAAN
Deputy Director
Wayne County Department of Health and Human Services
Professor
Oakland University
School of Nursing
Rochester, Michigan

Annette Lueckenotte, RN, MS, BC, GNP, GCNS
Gerontologic Clinical Nurse Specialist
Barnes-Jewish West County Hospital
Creve Coeur, Missouri

Barbara Maxwell, RN, BSN, MS, MSN, CNS
Associate Professor of Nursing
Ulster Department of Nursing
The State University New York
Stone Ridge, New York

Elaine Neel, RN, BSN, MSN
Nursing Instructor
Graham Hospital School of Nursing
Canton, Illinois

Wendy Ostendorf, BSN, MS, EdD
Associate Professor
Neumann College
Aston, Pennsylvania

Patsy Ruchala, RN, DNSc
Director and Professor
Orvis School of Nursing
University of Nevada–Reno
Reno, Nevada

Lynn Schallom, MSN, CCRN, CCNS
Clinical Nurse Specialist
Surgical Critical Care
Barnes-Jewish Hospital
St. Louis, Missouri

Ann Tritak, BS, MS, EdD
Dean of Nursing
School of Nursing
Saint Peters College
Jersey City, New Jersey

Janis Waite, RN, MSN, EdD
Professor of Nursing
Saint Francis Medical Center College of Nursing
Peoria, Illinois

Jill Weberski, RN, MSN, PCCN, CNS
Instructor
Saint Francis Medical Center College of Nursing
Peoria, Illinois

Mary Ann Wehmer, RN, MSN, CNOR
Nursing Faculty
College of Nursing and Health Professions
University of Southern Indiana
Evansville, Indiana

Joan Wentz, RN, MSN
(Retired) Assistant Professor of Nursing
Goldfarb School of Nursing at Barnes-Jewish College
St. Louis, Missouri

Katherine West, BSN, MSEd, CIC
Infection Control Consultant
Infection Control/Emerging Concepts, Inc.
Manassas, Virginia

Rita Wunderlich, RN, MSN(R), PhD
Chair, Baccalaureate Nursing Program
St. Louis University School of Nursing
St. Louis, Missouri

Valerie Yancey, RN, PhD
Associate Professor
Southern Illinois University
Edwardsville, Illinois

Reviewers

JoAnn Acierno, RN, BSN
Assistant Professor
Clarkson College
Omaha, Nebraska

Marianne Adam, RN, MSN, CRNP
Assistant Professor
Moravian College
Bethlehem, Pennsylvania

Joni Adams, RN, BSN, MSN
Assistant Professor
Ivy Tech Community College of Indiana
Evansville, Indiana

Pamela Adamshick, BSN, MSN, PhD(c), APRN-BC
Assistant Professor of Nursing
St. Luke's School of Nursing at Moravian College
Bethlehem, Pennsylvania

Rebecca L. Alexander, RN, MN
Nursing Faculty
Florence-Darlington Technical College
Florence, South Carolina

Colleen Andreoni, APRN, BC-NP
Certified Nurse Practitioner
Rife & Associates Family Medicine
Orland Park, Illinois

Suzanne L. Bailey, BC, MSN, APRN
Associate Professor
University of Evansville
Evansville, Indiana

Martha C. Baker, RN, PhD, APRN-BC
Director, Bachelor of Science in Nursing Program
Southwest Baptist University
Springfield, Missouri

Doris Bartlett, RN, MS
Adjunct Faculty
Bethel College
Mishawaka, Indiana

Julie Baylor, PhD, RN
Assistant Professor
Bradley University
Peoria, Illinois

Terry Bichsel, RN, BSN
Practical Nursing Coordinator
Moberly Area Community College
Moberly, Missouri

Joanne Bonesteel, RN, MSN
Nursing Faculty
Excelsior College School of Nursing
Albany, New York

Therese M. Bower, EdD, MSN, RN, CNS, CNE
Nursing Instructor
Firelands Regional Medical Center School of Nursing
Sandusky, Ohio

Sally B. Boyster, RN-C, MS, CNE-NLN
Professor of Nursing Science
Rose State College
Midwest City, Oklahoma

Jeanie Burt, RN, MSN, MA
Assistant Professor
Harding University College of Nursing
Searcy, Arkansas

Nathania Bush, RN MSN
Assistant Professor of Nursing
Morehead State University
Morehead, Kentucky

Darlene Nebel Cantu, RNC, MSN, BSN
Faculty
San Antonio College
San Antonio, Texas
Online Faculty
University of Phoenix

Susan Carlson, RN, MS, APRN, BC, NPP
Assistant Professor
Monroe Community College
Rochester, New York

Linda M. Cason, MSN, RN, CCRN, CNRN, BC
Adjunct Faculty
University of Evansville
Evansville, Indiana

Barbara Caton, RN, BSN, MSN
Assistant Professor
Southwest Missouri State University–West Plains
West Plains, Missouri

Shari L. Clarke, APRN, MSN
Family Nurse Practitioner
Kennesaw State University
Kennesaw, Georgia

Kim Clevenger, RN,C, MSN
Assistant Professor of Nursing
Morehead State University
Morehead, Kentucky

Suzanne M. Costello, RN, BSN, MSN
Professional Nurse Educator
Educational Specialist–Allied Health Education
Jameson Hospital School of Nursing
New Castle, Pennsylvania

Carol DeBlois, RN, BSN, MA, CNOR
Director
Bridgeport Hospital School of Nursing
Bridgeport, Connecticut

Lynn M. Derickson, APRN, P/MH, MS
Instructor of Nursing
Wor-Wic Community College
Salisbury, Maryland

Susan Droske, RN, MN, CPNP
Professor, Health Occupations Department
Texarkana College
Texarkana, Texas

Catherine Eddy, RN, MSN
Director/Assistant Professor of Nursing
University of South Dakota–Rapid City Campus
Rapid City, South Dakota

Sandra Baran Englert, MSN, RN
Assistant Professor
D'Youville College
Buffalo, New York

Susan Erue, RN, BSN, MS, PhDc, Ed
Associate Professor and Chair Division of Nursing
Iowa Weslayan College
Mt. Pleasant, Iowa

Linda Fluharty, BSN, MSN, RNC
Associate Professor
Ivy Tech Community College of Indiana
Indianapolis, Indiana

Patricia Freed, RN, EdD, EINEC
Associate Professor
Saint Louis University
St. Louis, Missouri

Margaret Freel, RN, MSN, CNRN, APN/CS
Professor Emerita
Niehoff School of Nursing Loyola University of Chicago
Chicago, Illinois

John P. Harper, RN, MSN, BC
QM & I Reviewer, Clinical Instructor
Taylor Hospital
Ridley Park, Pennsylvania

Monica Hentemann, RN, BSN, OCN
Oncology Nursing Department
Spectrum Health
Grand Rapids, Michigan

Deborah Himes, MSN, RN, APRN-BC
Instructor of Nursing
Brigham Young University
Provo, Utah

Janice Hoffman, RN, PhD
Faculty
John Hopkins School of Nursing
Baltimore, Maryland

Phyllis Howard, RN, BSN
Practical Nursing Program Coordinator
Ashland Community & Technical College
Ashland, Kentucky

Susie Huyer, RN, MSN, CHPN
Hospice Administrator
Heartland Hospice
Fairfax, Virginia

Penny Killian, RN, MSN, PNP
Assistant Professor
College of Nursing & Health Professions
Drexel University
Philadelphia, Pennsylvania

Linda L. Kerby, RN-C-R, BSN, MA, BA
Educational Consultant
Mastery Educational Consultants
Leawood, Kansas

Robin Lockhart, RN, MSN
Assistant Professor
Midwestern State University
Wichita Falls, Texas

Laura Logan, CNS, MSN, RN
Faculty for School of Nursing
Stephen F. Austin State University
Nacogdoches, Texas

Rosemary Macy, BS, MS, PhD
Associate Professor
Boise State University
Boise, Idaho

Rosanna Marker-Faour, MSN, BSN, CSN
Nursing Instructor
Coastal Education Institute
Carnegie, Pennsylvania

B. Gail Marshall, RN, BSN, MSN
Associate Professor
Luzerne County Community College
Nanticoke, Pennsylvania

Barbara Maxwell, BSN, MS, MSN, CNS
Associate Professor of Nursing
SUNY Ulster Department of Nursing
Stone Ridge, New York

Patricia C. McCahan, MSN, RN
Nursing Faculty
Cabarrus College of Health Sciences
Concord, North Carolina

Tammy McConnell, MSN, RN, APRN-BC (FNP)
Admissions and Progression Coordinator, Clinical Coordinator,
    Nursing Instructor
Greenville Technical College
Greenville, South Carolina

Linda J. Minyard, RN, BSN, MN, CPR
Nursing Department
Glendale Community College
Glendale, Arizona

Claudia Mitchell, RN, MSN
Associate Director BSN Program-Clermont
University of Cincinnati College of Nursing
Cincinnati, Ohio

Susan A. Moore, PhD, RN
Assistant Professor
University of Memphis
Memphis, Tennessee

Bernadette O'Halloran, RN, MSN
Clinical Instructor
University of Connecticut
Storrs, Connecticut
Nangatuck Valley Community College
Waterbury, Connecticut

Wendy Petro, RN, BSN, MPH
Registered Nurse
Sentara Home Health and Hospice
Chesapeake, Virginia

Beth Hogan-Quigley, RN, MSN, CRNP
Associate Course Director
University of Pennsylvania School of Nursing
Philadelphia, Pennsylvania

Cherie Rebar, RN, MSN, MBA, FNP-S, ND
Assistant Professor of Nursing
Kettering College of Medical Arts
Kettering, Ohio

Anita K. Reed, RN, MSN
Instructor of Nursing
St. Elizabeth School of Nursing
Lafayette, Indiana

Kathleen Rizzo, RN, MSN
Assistant Professor of Nursing
St. Louis Community College–Forest Park
St. Louis, Missouri

Diane Saleska, RN, MSN
Assistant Clinical Professor
Coordinator Nursing Skills Center
College of Nursing
University of Missouri–St. Louis
St. Louis, Missouri

Susan Scholtz, RN, BSN, DNSc
Associate Professor of Nursing
Moravian College
Associate Professor of Nursing
Bethlehem, Pennsylvania

Ruth E. Schumacher, BSN, MSN
Nursing Instructor
University of Illinois at Chicago
Chicago, Illinois

Katie Selle, RN,C, MA
Associate Professor of Nursing
Clarke College
Dubuque, Iowa

Gale Sewell, RN, MSN, CNE
Assistant Professor of Nursing
Indiana Wesleyan University
Marion, Illinois

Ruth A. Shearer, RN, MS, MSN
Associate Professor of Nursing
Bethel College
Mishawaka, Indiana

Patti C. Simmons, RN, MN, CHPN
Assistant Professor of Nursing
North Georgia College and State University
Dahlonega, Georgia

Fernisa Sison, RN, MSN, FNP-BC
Instructor–Family Nurse Practitioner
San Joaquin Delta College
Stockton, California

Mary W. Surman, BSN, RN, CWOCN
Certified Wound, Ostomy, Incontinence Nurse
Our Lady of the Lake Regional Medical Center
Baton Rouge, Louisiana

Marianne Fasano Swihart, RN, MEd, MSN, CRNI, CETN, PCCN
Assistant Director of Nursing
Pasco-Hernando Community College
New Port Richey, Florida

Tracy Szirony, RNC, PhD, CHPN
Associate Professor of Nursing
College of Nursing
University of Toledo
Toledo, Ohio

Rowena Tessman, APRN, PhD
Vice President of Medical Services
Sweetser
Saco, Maine

Scott C. Thigpen RN, MSN, CCRN, CEN
Assistant Professor of Nursing
South Georgia College
Douglas, Georgia

Donna L. Thompson, MSN, CRNP, CCCN
Assistant Professor
Neumann College
Aston, Pennsylvania
Continence Specialist
Fair Acres Geriatric Center
Lima, Pennsylvania

Linda Turchin, RN, MSN
Assistant Professor of Nursing
Fairmont State University
Fairmont, West Virginia

Lynda Frances Turner, RN, BC, EdD, MSN
Associate Professor
Marshall University School of Nursing
Huntington, West Virginia

Josie Veal, MSN, RN, APRN-BC
Family Nurse Practitioner and Nurse Educator
Milwaukee Area Technical College
Milwaukee, Wisconsin

Michelle Hand Villegas, RN, MSN
Assistant Professor
Midwestern State University School of Nursing
Wichita Falls, Texas

Sandra L. Walker, PhD, RN
ADN Instructor and Program Coordinator
Southwest Georgia Technical College
Thomasville, Georgia

Kim Webb, MN, RN
Nursing Chair
Northern Oklahoma College
Tonkawa, Oklahoma

Eileen Bagatti Whitwam, MSN, ARNP
Professor of Nursing
Daytona Beach Community College
Daytona Beach, Florida

Laura B. Williams, MSN, CRNP
Retired Nursing Faculty
University of Alabama at Birmingham School of Nursing
Birmingham, Alabama

Ginia Wilson, RN, MS
Professor of Nursing
Rose State College
Midwest City, Oklahoma

Rosemary H. Wittstadt, RN, EdD
Assistant Professor of Nursing
Towson University
Towson, Maryland

Janice Womack, RN
Associate Nurse Executive
Northwest Georgia Regional Hospital
Rome, Georgia

Toni C. Wortham, RN, BSN, MSN
Professor
Madisonville Community College
Madisonville, Kentucky

Jeanne Zack, RN, PhD(c), CIC
Manager Infection Prevention and Control
Missouri Baptist Medical Center
St. Louis, Missouri

Contributors to Previous Edition

Jeanette Adams, APRN, MSN, PhD, CRNI
Nursing Consultant
Coconut Grove, Florida

Myra. A. Aud, RN, PhD
Assistant Professor
Sinclair School of Nursing
University of Missouri–Columbia
Columbia, Missouri

Marjorie Baier, PhD, APRN, BC
Associate Professor
School of Nursing
Southern Illinois University
Edwardsville, Illinois

Janice Boundy, RN, PhD
Professor, Director of Graduate Program
Saint Francis College of Nursing
Peoria, Illinois

Anna Brock, BSN, MSN, PhD, MEd
Professor
College of Nursing
University of Southern Mississippi
Hattiesburg, Mississippi

Pamela L. Cherry, RN, BSN, MSN, DNSc
Associate Professor of Nursing
Humboldt State University
Arcata, California

Janice C. Colwell, RN, MS, CWOCN
Clinical Nurse Specialist, Wound, Ostomy & Skin Care
University of Chicago Hospitals
Chicago, Illinois

Eileen Costantinou, RN, MSN
Professional Practice Consultant
Barnes-Jewish Hospital
St. Louis, Missouri

Christine Durbin, RN, MSN, JD, PhDc
Instructor, School of Nursing
Southern Illinois University
Edwardsville, Illinois

Margaret Ecker, RN, MS, PNP
Director of Education
Saint John's Health Center
Santa Monica, California

Martha Keene Elkin, RN, MS, IBCLC
Nursing Educator for Associate Degree Nursing
Private Practice Lactation Consultant
Mother Care of Maine
Sumner, Maine

Susan Jane Fetzer, RN, BA, BSN, MSN, MBA, PhD
Associate Professor
University New Hampshire
Durham, New Hampshire

Victoria N. Folse, APRN, PhD, CS, LCPC
Assistant Professor
Illinois Wesleyan University
Bloomington, Illinois

Leah W. Frederick, RN, MS, CIC
Infection Control Consultant
Infection Control Consultants
Scottsdale, Arizona

Amy Hall, RN, BSN, MS, PhD
Associate Professor
Saint Francis Medical Center College of Nursing
Peoria, Illinois

Mimi Hirshberg, RN, MSN
Clinical Assistant Professor
Barnes College of Nursing and Health Studies
University of Missouri–St. Louis
St. Louis, Missouri
IV Therapist
Vascular Access Service
Barnes-Jewish Hospital
St. Louis, Missouri

Steve Kilkus, RN, MSN
Nursing Faculty
Edgewood College
Madison, Wisconsin

Judith Ann Kilpatrick, RN, DNSc
Assistant Professor
Widener University School of Nursing
Chester, Pennsylvania

Kristine M. L'Ecuyer, RN, MSN, CCNS
Adjunct Assistant Professor
Saint Louis University School of Nursing
St. Louis, Missouri

Annette G. Lueckenotte, RN, MS, BC, GNP, GCNS
Gerontologic Nurse Practitioner & Educator
Barnes-Jewish West County Hospital
St. Louis, Missouri

Joyce Larson, RN, MS, PhD
President, Founder Culture and Counts
Adjunct Hillsborough Community College
Tampa, Florida

Ruth Ludwick, BSN, MSN, PhD, RNC
Professor
Kent State University, College of Nursing
Kent, Ohio

Elaine K. Neel, BSN, MSN
Nursing Instructor
Graham Hospital School of Nursing
Canton, Illinois

Dula Pacquiao, BSN, MA, EdD
Professor, Director of Transcultural Nursing Institute and
    Coordinator of Graduate Program
Kean University
Union, New Jersey

Nancy C. Panthofer, RN, MSN
Lecturer
Kent State University College of Nursing
Kent, Ohio

Elaine U. Polan, RNC, BSN, MS
Nursing Program Supervisor
Vocational Education & Extension Board Practical Nursing
    Program
Uniondale, New York

Patsy L. Ruchala, RN, DNSc
Associate Director for Graduate Nursing Programs
Georgia State University, Byrdine F. Lewis School of Nursing
Atlanta, Georgia

Debbie Sanazaro, RN, MSN, GNP
Assistant Professor
St. Louis University School of Nursing
St. Louis, Missouri

Marilyn Schallom, RN, MSN, CCRN, CCNS
Clinical Nurse Specialist
Surgical Critical Care
Barnes-Jewish Hospital
St. Louis, Missouri

Patricia A. Stockert, RN, BSN, MS, PhD
Associate Professor, Coordinator
Saint Francis Medical Center College of Nursing
Peoria, Illinois

Marshelle Thobaben, RN, MS, PHN, APNP, FNP
Chair and Professor
Humboldt State University
Arcata, California

Pamela Becker Weilitz, RN, MSN(R), BC, ANP, M-SCNS
Adult Nurse Practitioner
Private Practice
St. Louis, Missouri

Joan Domigan Wentz, BSN, MSN
Assistant Professor (Retired)
Jewish Hospital College of Nursing and Allied Health
St. Louis, Missouri

Rita Wunderlich, BSN, MSN(r), PhD
Assistant Professor, Med/Surg Nursing
St. Louis University
St. Louis, Missouri

This book is dedicated to William N. Potter and Grace L. Potter.
They surrounded me with love and embodied me with a strong work ethic.
I will always hold them in my heart.
PATRICIA A. POTTER

The book is dedicated to all nurses. To those nurses who are at the bedside and who are educators, researchers, and administrators. To those nurses who attain certification in their areas of specialization. Nursing would not be where it is without all of us working together.

This book is also dedicated to a long and wonderful friendship with my co-author, Dr. Patricia A. Potter.
ANNE G. PERRY

Preface to the Student

Fundamentals of Nursing provides you with all of the fundamental nursing concepts and skills you will need as a beginning nurse in a visually appealing, easy-to-use format. We know how busy you are and how precious your time is. As you begin your nursing education, it is very important that you have a resource that includes all the information you need to prepare for lectures, classroom activities, clinical assignments, and exams—and nothing more. We've designed this text to meet all of those needs. This book was designed to help you succeed in this course and prepare you for more advanced study. In addition to the readable writing style and abundance of full-color photographs and drawings, we've incorporated numerous features to help you study and learn. With this text, you will also receive a Companion CD-ROM that includes NCLEX®-Style chapter review questions and interactive learning activities, access to the Evolve course website that includes all of the resources from the Companion CD, as well as access to clips from Mosby's Nursing Skills DVDs; and access to Nursing Skills Online.

Check out the following special learning aids featured in Fundamentals of Nursing:

---

38 | Client Safety

Learning Objectives begin each chapter to help you focus on the key information that follows.

✳ OBJECTIVES

Mastery of the content in this chapter will enable the student to:

- Describe how unmet basic physiological needs of oxygen, nutrition, temperature, and humidity threaten clients' safety.
- Discuss the purpose of the National Patient Safety Goals.
- Discuss the specific risks to safety related to developmental age.
- Identify factors to assess when it becomes necessary to physically restrain a client.
- Describe the four categories of risks in a health care agency.
- Describe assessment activities designed to identify clients' physical, psychosocial, and cognitive status as it pertains to their safety status.

- Identify nursing diagnoses associated with risks to safety.
- Develop care plans for clients whose safety is threatened.
- Describe nursing interventions specific to clients' age for reducing risk of falls, fires, poisonings, and electrical hazards.
- Describe methods to evaluate interventions designed to maintain or promote safety.

✳ MEDIA RESOURCES

Companion CD
- NCLEX®-Style Review Questions
- Audio Glossary
- Interactive Learning Activities
- English/Spanish Glossary

***evolve* Website**
- NCLEX®-Style Review Questions
- Audio Glossary
- English/Spanish Glossary
- Interactive Learning Activities
- Weblinks
- Audio Summaries

✳ KEY TERMS

Air pollution, p. 814
Ambularm, p. 838
Aura, p. 817
Bed-Check, p. 838
Bioterrorism, p. 814
Carbon monoxide, p. 812
Environment, p. 812
Food and Drug Administration (FDA), p. 812
Food poisoning, p. 812
Hypothermia, p. 812
Immunization, p. 813

Land pollution, p. 814
Noise pollution, p. 814
Pathogen, p. 813
Poison, p. 840
Pollutant, p. 814
Relative humidity, p. 812
Restraint, p. 829
Seizure, p. 817
Seizure precautions, p. 842
Status epilepticus, p. 845
Water pollution, p. 814

Media Resources boxes detail what electronic resources are available to you for every chapter.

Key Terms are listed at the beginning of each chapter and are boldfaced and defined in the text. Page numbers help you quickly find where each term is defined.

811

842   Unit 7   Basic Human Needs

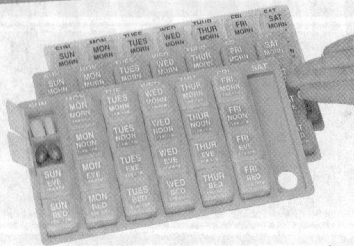

Figure 38-17 One-Day-At-A-Time medicine organizer. (Courtesy Apothecary Products, Inc, Burnsville, Minn.)

✴ BOX 38-13   PROCEDURAL GUIDELINES

Interventions for Accidental Poisoning in the Home Setting

1. Assess for airway patency, breathing, and circulation (ABCs) in all clients in whom accidental poisoning is suspected.
2. Remove any visible materials from areas such as the mouth and eyes to terminate exposure.
3. Identify the type and amount of substance ingested, if possible. This helps to determine the antidote.
4. Call the poison control center before attempting any interventions. The universal phone number for poison control is (800) 222-1222.
5. If directed by a physician, give oral fluids to assist vomiting.
6. If directed, save vomitus for laboratory analysis, which will assist with further treatment.
7. Position the victim with the head to the side to prevent aspiration of vomitus, and assist in keeping the airway open.
8. Never induce vomiting in an unconscious victim or in a client experiencing convulsions, because aspiration will occur.
9. Never induce vomiting if any of the following substances have been ingested: lye, household cleaners, hair care products, grease or petroleum products, or furniture polish. Vomiting increases internal burns.
10. If instructed to take the victim to the emergency department, call an ambulance. Emergency equipment is sometimes en route.
11. In the case of convulsions, cessation of breathing, or unconsciousness, call 911.
12. Do not administer syrup of ipecac to induce vomiting. It has not been proven effective in preventing poisoning.

American Academy of Pediatrics: News release—don't treat swallowed poison with syrup of ipecac, 2004, www.aap.org/advocacy/releases/novpoison.htm.

✴ BOX 38-14   CLIENT TEACHING

Prevention of Electrical Hazards

Objective
- Client will recognize electrical hazards in the home and eliminate them.

Teaching Strategies
- Discuss grounding appliances and other equipment.
- Provide examples of common hazards: frayed cords, damaged equipment, and overloaded outlets.
- Discuss guidelines to prevent electrical shocks:
  - Use extension cords only when necessary, and use electrical tape to secure the cord to the floor where it will not be stepped on.
  - Do not run wires under carpeting.
  - Grasp the plug, not the cord, when unplugging items.
  - Keep electrical items away from water.
  - Do not operate unfamiliar equipment.
  - Disconnect items before cleaning.

Evaluation
- Have client list electrical hazards existing in the home.
- Review steps the client will take to eliminate these hazards.
- Check the home after the client has had an opportunity to eliminate hazards.

Client Teaching boxes present an important patient education topic and tell you what and how to teach clients and how to evaluate learning.

on the telephone in homes with young children. In all cases of suspected poisoning, clients should call this number immediately (Box 38-13).

Electrical Hazards. Electrical equipment needs to be in good working order and grounded. The third (longer) prong in an electrical plug is the ground. Theoretically, the ground prong carries any stray electrical current back to the ground, hence its name. The other two prongs carry the power to the piece of electrical equipment. Improperly grounded or malfunctioning electrical equipment increases the risk of electrical injury and fire. Educating both the client and the family reduces the risk for electrical hazards in the home environment (Box 38-14).

If a client receives an electrical shock in a health care setting, immediately determine whether the client has a pulse. If the client has no pulse, initiate cardiopulmonary resuscitation (CPR) and notify emergency personnel (see Chapter 40). If the client has a pulse and remains alert and oriented, quickly obtain vital signs and assess the skin for signs of thermal injury. Make sure to notify the client's physician. If an electrical shock occurs in the home, follow the same procedure but have the client go to the emergency department and then notify the client's physician.

Seizures. Clients who have experienced some form of neurological injury or metabolic disturbance are at risk for a seizure. A seizure involves a hyperexcitation of neurons in the brain leading to a sudden, violent, involuntary series of contractions of a group of muscles. The client often loses consciousness. **Seizure precautions** encompass all nursing interventions to protect the client from traumatic injury, positioning for adequate ventilation and drainage of oral secretions, and providing privacy and support following the seizure (Skill 38-2).

During a seizure a client's jaw muscles become tense. Research has found that significant injury to the client's oral cavity is rare, even during the most violent seizures. Injury instead occurs from a caregiver forcing an object into the client's mouth and from the teeth biting down on a hard object. Soft objects will possibly break in the mouth during a seizure and be aspirated. The Epilepsy Foundation (2006), in its recommendations for seizure first aid,

Chapter 38   Client Safety   831

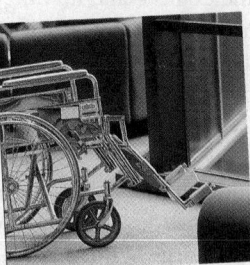

10 Safety locks on wheelchairs.

Procedural Guidelines provide streamlined, step-by-step guidelines to apply when performing basic skills.

✴ BOX 38-9   EVIDENCE-BASED PRACTICE

Effects of Nursing Rounds

Evidence Summary

Hospitalized clients often require assistance with basic activities of daily living such as eating, toileting, and ambulating. Clients usually communicate their needs by use of the call light. Not meeting client needs in a timely fashion decreases client satisfaction and places clients at greater risk for injury. Researchers wanted to know if nursing rounds every 1 or 2 hours would reduce call light usage, increase client satisfaction, and reduce frequency of client falls. During rounding the following items were performed for each client: pain management, toileting, positioning, and items such as call light, telephone, TV remote, bed light switch, tissue, and water placed within reach and garbage can next to bed. In addition, before leaving the room, the nurse asked, "Is there anything else I can do for you before I leave? I have time while I'm here in the room." The client was also told someone would be back in 1 (or 2) hours to round again. A 6-week nationwide quasi-experimental study was conducted on 27 nurs-

ing units in 14 hospitals. Researchers took baseline data on call light usage during the initial 2 weeks. Rounding at set intervals, including specific nursing actions, was associated with statistically significant reduced client call light usage, increased client satisfaction, and in the 1-hour rounding group, client falls.

Application to Nursing Practice
- Nursing rounds performed at set intervals will positively affect client satisfaction and safety and lead to fewer distractions for staff
- The nurse's ability to meet the client's needs affects the client's perception of the quality of nursing care.
- Anticipate client needs by performing rounds, including specific actions, at 1-hour intervals.

Reference
Meade CM and others: Effects of nursing rounds on patients' call light use, satisfaction and safety, *Am J Nurs* 106(9):58, 2006.

Evidence-Based Practice boxes provide a summary of nursing research evidence on a specific topic and explains its implications for nursing practice.

Whenever a client is restrained, there is a natural tendency for the client to try to remove the restraint. When this occurs, client injury is common. Restrained clients easily become entangled in a restraint device in attempts to get out of the device. In some cases, death has resulted because of strangulation or asphyxiation. As a result, nursing homes and many health care facilities have banned the use of the jacket (vest) restraint because of this risk. The use of any restraint is also associated with serious complications, including pressure ulcers, constipation, pneumonia, urinary and fecal incontinence, and urinary retention (see Chapter 47). Contractures, nerve damage, and circulatory impairment are also potential hazards. In addition, restrained clients experience a loss of self-esteem, humiliation, fear, and anger.

SAFETY ALERT Routine assessment of a client in restraints is critical to prevent injury. Because of the risk of injury from restraints, regulatory agencies such as TJC and the Centers for Medicaid and Medicare Services (CMS) enforce standards for the safe use of restraints and define clients' rights and choices regarding their use. Under these guidelines, reasons for use of a physical restraint are to be clearly stated. The use of restraints must be part of the client's medical treatment, all less restrictive interventions must be tried first, other disciplines must be consulted, and supporting documentation must be provided (CMS, 2006).

The movement is for health care organizations to become restraint-free environments. Restraints do not prevent falls or injury. In fact, clients incur less severe injuries if left unrestrained (Capezuti and others, 1998; Strumpf and others, 1998). A multi-

Safety Alerts indicate techniques you can use to ensure client and nurse safety.

※ TABLE 38-2 Interventions to Promote Safety for Children and Adolescents—cont'd

INTERVENTION	RATIONALE
Adolescents	
Encourage enrollment in driver's education classes.	Many injuries in this age-group are related to motor vehicle accidents.
Provide information about the effects of using alcohol and drugs.	Adolescents are prone to risk-taking behaviors and are subject to peer pressures.
Provide sex education, emphasizing safe sex practices, including abstinence.	Many adolescents begin sexual relationships. Pregnancy and sexually transmitted diseases sometimes result.
Refer adolescents to community and school-sponsored activities.	The adolescent needs to socialize with peers, yet needs some supervision.
Encourage mentoring relationships between adults and adolescents.	Adolescents are in need of role models after whom they can pattern their behavior.
Teach them safe use of the Internet.	Avoids overuse and possible exposure to inappropriate websites.

Modified from Hockenberry M, Wilson D: *Wong's nursing care of infants and children*, ed 8, St. Louis, 2007, Mosby.

Focus on Older Adults boxes prepare you to address the special needs of older adults.

※ BOX 38-8

FOCUS ON OLDER ADULTS

Physiological Changes of Aging and Their Impact on Client Safety

- Older adults experience alterations in vision and hearing. Encourage yearly vision and hearing examinations and frequent cleansing of glasses and hearing aids as a means of preventing falls and burns.
- Some older adults have slowed reaction time. Teach clients safety tips for avoiding automobile accidents. Sometimes driving needs to be restricted to daylight hours or suspended.
- Range of motion, flexibility, and strength decrease. Encourage supervised exercise classes for older adults, and teach them to seek assistance with household tasks as needed. Safety features, such as grab bars in the bathroom, are often necessary.
- Reflexes are slowed, and the ability to respond to multiple stimuli is reduced. Provide adequate, meaningful stimuli but prevent sensory overload.
- Nocturia and incontinence are more frequent in older adults. Institute a regular toileting schedule for the client. A recommended frequency is every 3 hours. Give diuretics in the morning. Provide assistance, along with adequate lighting, to clients who need to go to the bathroom at night.
- Memory is sometimes impaired. Clients need to use medication organizers, which can be purchased at any drugstore at a

very reasonable cost. These dispensers can be filled once a week with the proper medications to be taken at a specific time during the day.
- The family plays a significant role in the care of older adults. One in five caregivers reported providing more than 40 hours of care per week (National Alliance for Caregiving, Association for the Advancement of Retired Persons, 2004). Encourage the family to allow the older adult to remain as independent as possible and provide help only for those things that are especially stressful or depleted.
- The high prevalence of chronic conditions in older adults results in the use of a high number of prescription and over-the-counter medications. Coupled with age-related changes in pharmacokinetics, there is a greater risk of serious adverse effects. Medications typically prescribed for older adults include anticholinergics, diuretics, anxiolytic and hypnotic agents, antidepressants, antihypertensives, vasodilators, analgesics, and laxatives, all of which may themselves pose risks or may interact to increase the risk for falls. Review the client's drug profile to ensure that any of the above-noted drugs are used cautiously, and assess the client regularly for any adverse effects that increase fall risk.

to older adults involve falls, automobile accide
lated to burns or f
Control, 2(
changes in
ability to m
(see Chapte
tiple medica
age-related s
iar environm
Leuckenotte,
adults, such
chances of inj

CULTURAL ASPECTS OF CARE

※ BOX 38-7

Environment of Care

Cultural phenomena affecting health and safety include personal space, social organizations, communication, and environmental control. While conducting a home assessment for risks to safety, nurses need to realize that they have entered the client's territory and that the client's attitude toward his or her residence and belongings must be appreciated. For example, clients from Western Europe and the British Isles may be considered aloof and distant in terms of space. It is sometimes very difficult for them to have an outsider in their home who is suggesting changes with regard to their personal belongings. It is particularly difficult to determine a client's attitude toward his or her home environment when the client speaks another language.

Another culturally sensitive issue is the client's sense of environmental control. Be aware of health beliefs and practices that will affect the outcome of interventions. For example, reliance on family and religious organizations, as opposed to community resources, will possibly affect the client's compliance with nursing interventions and referrals.

Nurses and health care providers need to learn to be sensitive when asking questions and showing respect for different cultural beliefs. Adapting to different cultural beliefs and practices requires flexibility and a respect for others' viewpoints. Respect for the belief systems of others and the effects of those beliefs on the client's well-being are critically important to competent care. Nurses need to have the ability and knowledge to communicate and to understand health behaviors influenced by culture.

Implications for Practice

- Resistance to changing long-standing habits interferes with a cultural group's acceptance of injury prevention practices. Include family members who have a strong influence, such as a dominant male or older woman, when providing safety education.
- Evaluate the use of traditional ethnic remedies or foods that contain lead because they increase a client's risk for lead poisoning.
- Living in rural areas and in manufactured housing places the client at greater risk for fire-related injuries and death. Stress the importance of having working smoke detectors and a multipurpose fire extinguisher.
- Assess the client's smoking and drinking habits. Residential fire deaths are often attributed to the use of cigarettes and alcohol.
- Clients who live in poverty and have low educational levels are at greater risk for injury and disease. Assist the client and family in identifying community resources such as the local health office or clinic.
- Be aware of family patterns and how the client and family interact with each other. Family disruption and weak intergenerational ties increase a client's risk for injury due to violent behavior.

Modified from Giger JN, Davidhizar R: The Giger and Davidhizar transcultural assessment model, *J Transcult Nurs* 13:185, 2002.

Cultural Aspects of Care boxes prepare you to care for clients of diverse populations.

(e.g., wearing seat belts or installing outdoor lighting) and participation in wellness programs.

Nurses participate by supporting legislation and working in community-based settings. Because environmental and community values have the greatest influence on health promotion, community and home health nurses are able to assess and recommend safety measures in the home, school, neighborhood, and workplace.

Developmental Interventions

Infant, Toddler, and Preschooler Infants, toddlers, and preschoolers depend on adults to protect them from injury. Growing children are curious and completely trusting of their environment and do not perceive themselves to be in danger. Nurses are frequently in a position to educate parents or guardians about reducing risks of injuries for young children (see Chapter 12). Nurses working in prenatal and postpartum settings can easily incorporate safety into the care plan of the childbearing family. Community health nurses are able to assess the home and show parents how to promote safety in their homes (Table 38-2). Educate parents that children under 5 years are also more susceptible to diseases such as measles, mumps, and chickenpox. Immunizations, given before the age of 2 years and at recommended intervals,

Adolescent Risks to the safety of adolescents involve many factors outside the home environment, particularly their almost constant involvement with members of their peer group (see Chapter 12). Adults serve as role models for adolescents and, through providing examples, setting expectations, and providing education, can help adolescents minimize risks to their safety. This age-group has a high incidence of suicide because of feelings of decreased self-worth and hopelessness. Be aware of the risks posed at this time, and be prepared to teach adolescents and their parents measures to prevent accidents and injury.

Adult Risks to young and middle-age adults frequently result from lifestyle factors such as child rearing, high stress levels, inadequate nutrition, use of firearms, excessive alcohol intake, and substance abuse (see Chapter 13). In this fast-paced society there also appears to be more expression of anger, which will possibly quickly precipitate accidents (e.g., "road rage"). Adults need to have the opportunity to discuss the choices they have made in their lifestyle and the types of threats to safety that exist. Given information about threats to their well-being, some adults will make necessary modifications in lifestyle practices. Useful resources are stress management centers (see Chapter 31), employee assistance programs, and health promotion activities, which are in

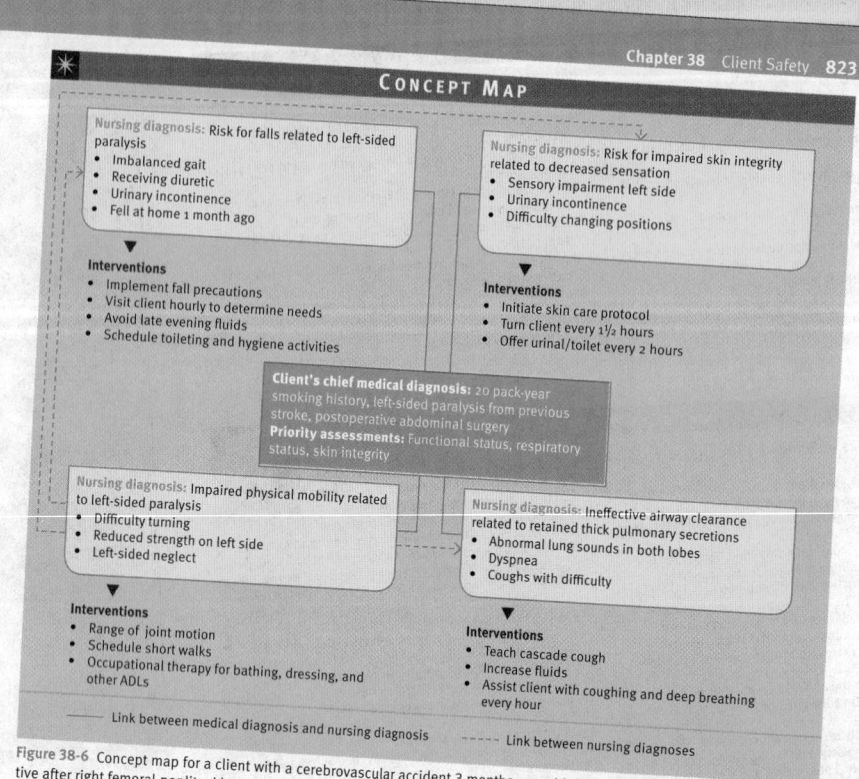

Chapter 38   Client Safety   823

CONCEPT MAP

Nursing diagnosis: Risk for falls related to left-sided paralysis
- Imbalanced gait
- Receiving diuretic
- Urinary incontinence
- Fell at home 1 month ago

Interventions
- Implement fall precautions
- Visit client hourly to determine needs
- Avoid late evening fluids
- Schedule toileting and hygiene activities

Nursing diagnosis: Risk for impaired skin integrity related to decreased sensation
- Sensory impairment left side
- Urinary incontinence
- Difficulty changing positions

Interventions
- Initiate skin care protocol
- Turn client every 1½ hours
- Offer urinal/toilet every 2 hours

Client's chief medical diagnosis: 20 pack-year smoking history, left-sided paralysis from previous stroke, postoperative abdominal surgery
Priority assessments: Functional status, respiratory status, skin integrity

Nursing diagnosis: Impaired physical mobility related to left-sided paralysis
- Difficulty turning
- Reduced strength on left side
- Left-sided neglect

Interventions
- Range of joint motion
- Schedule short walks
- Occupational therapy for bathing, dressing, and other ADLs

Nursing diagnosis: Ineffective airway clearance related to retained thick pulmonary secretions
- Abnormal lung sounds in both lobes
- Dyspnea
- Coughs with difficulty

Interventions
- Teach cascade cough
- Increase fluids
- Assist client with coughing and deep breathing every hour

——— Link between medical diagnosis and nursing diagnosis
- - - - Link between nursing diagnoses

Figure 38-6 Concept map for a client with a cerebrovascular accident 3 months ago with left-sided paralysis, 2 days postoperative after right femoral-popliteal bypass.

Concept Maps show you the association between multiple nursing diagnoses for a client with a selected medical diagnosis and the relationship between nursing interventions.

Collaborate to establish wa[...] involvement within the hom[...] cation of the client and fam[...] to reduce safety risks over th[...]

Collaborative Care. Clie[...] select resources within their c[...] neighborhood block homes, lo[...] bors willing to check on a clie[...] the client and family and other[...] occupational and physical ther[...] the nurse's plan of care. For ex[...] to go to a rehabilitation facility[...] before being discharged home.[...] understand the need for resource[...] that will promote their safety.

818   Unit 7   Basic Human Needs

Knowledge
- Basic human needs
- Potential risks to client safety from physical hazards, lifestyle, risks associated with health care environment, environmental risks, and biohazards
- Influence of developmental stage on safety needs
- Influence of illness/medications on client safety

Experience
- Caring for clients whose mobility or sensory impairments increase threats to safety
- Personal experience in caring for younger siblings or children

ASSESSMENT
- Identify actual and potential threats to the client's safety
- Determine impact of the underlying illness on the client's safety
- Identify the presence of risks for the client's developmental stage and client's environment
- Determine impact of environmental influence of the client's safety

Standards
- Apply intellectual standards such as accuracy, significance, and completeness when assessing for threats to the client's safety
- Apply ANA standards for nursing practice
- Apply agency practice standards (e.g., fall prevention or restraint protocols)
- Review and apply the most TJC patient safety goals

Attitudes
- Demonstrate perserverance when necessary to identify all safety threats
- Be responsible for collecting unbiased, accurate data regarding threats to the client's safety
- Show discipline in conducting a thorough review of the client's home environment

Figure 38-4 Critical thinking model for safety assessment.

The unique **Critical Thinking Model** clearly shows the components of critical thinking to apply during steps of the nursing process to help you provide the best care for your clients.

BOX 38-3   NURSING ASSESSMENT QUESTIONS

Activity and Exercise
- Do you use any assistive devices such as a wheelchair, walker, or cane to help you move or get around? Did someone show you how to use them safely?
- Do you have any difficulty bathing? Dressing? Eating? Using the bathroom? Transferring out of the bed or chair?
- What type of exercise or physical activity do you get? How often?
- How many meals do you eat in a typical day? How do you handle meal preparation?
- Do you do your own laundry? How do you do this, and where are these appliances located?
- Do you drive an automobile? When do you normally drive? How far?
- How often do you wear a safety belt when in the car?
- Have you recently been involved in a motor vehicle accident?

Medication History
- What medications do you take?
- Has your doctor or pharmacist reviewed your medicines with you?
- Do any medications make your dizzy or light-headed?

History of Falls
- Have you ever fallen or tripped over anything in your home?
- Have you ever suffered an injury from a fall? What was it, and how did it happen?
- Did you have any symptoms right before you fell? What were they?
- What activity were you performing before the fall?

Home Maintenance and Safety
- Who does your simple home maintenance or minor home repairs?
- Who shovels your snow? Tends to your lawn?
- Do you feel safe in your home? What things in your environment make you feel unsafe?
- Do you have someone to call in case of an emergency?
- How do you feel about making modifications to your home to make it safer? Do you need help finding resources to help you do this?

Nursing Assessment Questions boxes help you learn how to properly pose assessment questions when you interview clients.

The five-step Nursing Process provides a consistent framework for presentation of content in clinical chapters.

Safety and the Nursing Process

◆ Assessment

To conduct a thorough client assessment, consider possible threats to the client's safety, including the client's immediate environment, as well as any individual risk factors. Ask the client specific questions related to safety (Box 38-3).

such as perseverance, and any standards of practice that are applicable. For example, the American Nurses Association (ANA) standards for nursing practice address the nurse's responsibility in maintaining client safety. TJC (2006) also provides standards for safety (e.g., in the administration of medications, use of restraints, and use of medical devices). You refer to all of this information and experience as you conduct a detailed assessment of a specific client. For example, while assessing a specific client's home environment, the nurse will consider knowledge regarding typical locations within the home where dangers commonly exist. If a client has a visual impairment, you will apply previous experiences in caring for clients with visual [...] how to thoroughly assess the client's needs.

Nursing History. A nursing history includes data about the client's level of wellness to determine if any underlying conditions exist that pose threats to safety. For example, give special attention to assessing the client's gait, muscle strength and coordination, balance, and vision. Consider a review of the client's developmental status as you analyze assessment information. Also review if the client is taking any medications or undergoing any procedures [...] use of diuretics increases the fre-

Nursing Skills are presented in a clear, two-column format that includes Steps and Rationales to help you learn *how* and *why* a skill is performed.

Video Icons indicate video clips associated with specific skills that are available on the free CD-Companion and Evolve Student Learning Resources.

Delegation Considerations guide you in delegating skills to nursing assistive personnel.

Critical Decision Points alert you to critical steps within a skill to ensure safe and effective client care.

Video

APPLYING RESTRAINTS

❋ SKILL 38-1

Delegation Considerations

The skill of applying restraints can be delegated. However, the nurse is always responsible for assessment of client's safety needs, selection of appropriate alternative interventions, evaluation of effectiveness of restraint, and ongoing assessment to prevent complications of restraint use. The nurse directs nursing assistive personnel to:

• Inform the nurse of any redness, excoriation, or constriction of circulation under the restraint.

• Ask for assistance if the client has any mobility restrictions that will affect how to remove or reapply a restraint.

• Change client's position; provide range of motion, skin care, toileting, and opportunities for socialization.

Equipment

• Proper restraint: mitten, belt, extremity

• Padding (if needed)

STEPS

1. Assess whether client needs a restraint. Does the client continually try to interrupt needed therapy? Is the client repeatedly trying to ambulate independently, creating a serious risk of injury?

2. Assess client's behavior, such as confusion, disorientation, agitation, restlessness, combativeness, or inability to follow directions. Consult with gerontological nurse specialist if available.

3. Review agency policies regarding restraints. Check physician's order versus licensed independent practitioner's order for purpose, type, location, and duration of restraint. Check agency policy to determine if a signed consent is needed for use of restraint.

RATIONALE

Use restraints only when other measures have failed to prevent interruption of therapy such as traction, IV infusions, or nasogastric tube feedings; to prevent a confused or combative client from self-injury by falling out of bed or a wheelchair; to prevent a client from removing a urinary catheter, surgical drain, or life support equipment; and to reduce risk of injury to others by the client.

If client's behavior continues despite attempts to eliminate cause of behavior, use of physical restraint will possibly be necessary.

An order by a licensed independent practitioner is necessary to apply restraints. The least restrictive type of restraint should be ordered.

Critical Decision Point: Because restraints limit the client's ability to move freely, the nurse must make clinical judgments appropriate to the client's condition and agency policy. If the nurse restrains a client in an emergency situation because of violent or self-destructive behavior that presents an immediate danger, a face-to-face physician assessment within 1 hour is necessary (CMS, 2006).

4. Review manufacturer's instructions before entering client's room. Determine the most appropriate size restraint.

5. Gather equipment, and perform hand hygiene upon entering room.

6. Introduce self to client and family. Assess their feelings about restraint use. Explain that restraint is temporary and designed to protect client from injury.

7. Inspect placement area of restraint. Assess condition of skin underlying area where restraint will be.

8. Approach client in a calm, confident manner. Explain what you plan to do.

9. Adjust bed to proper height, and lower side rail on side of client contact.

10. Provide privacy. Make sure client is comfortable and in proper body alignment. Drape client as needed.

11. Pad skin and bony prominences (if necessary) before applying restraints.

12. Apply appropriate-size restraint, making sure it is not over an IV line or other device (e.g., dialysis shunt).

   A. **Belt restraint:** Device that secures client to bed or stretcher. Apply over clothes or gown. Remove wrinkles from front and back of restraint while placing it around client's waist. Bring ties through slots in belt. Avoid placing belt across the chest or too tightly across the abdomen (see illustration).

The nurse should be familiar with all devices used for client care and protection. Incorrect application of a restraining device will possibly result in client injury or death.

Promotes organization and reduces transmission of microorganisms.

Helps minimize client anxiety during application of the device and helps minimize family concern during maintenance of restraint.

Restraints compress and interfere with functioning of devices or tubes. Provides baseline assessment data regarding skin integrity.

Reduces client anxiety and promotes cooperation.

Allows nurse to use proper body mechanics and prevent injury.

Privacy prevents lowering of self-esteem. Proper body alignment promotes comfort, prevents contractures and neurovascular injury.

Padding reduces friction and pressure on skin and underlying tissue.

IV lines and other therapeutic devices sometimes become occluded.

Restrains center of gravity and prevents client from rolling off stretcher or sitting up while on stretcher or from falling out of bed. Tight application interferes with ventilation.

844 Unit 7 Basic Human Needs

✳ **SKILL 38-2**

SEIZURE PRECAUTIONS—CONT'D

STEPS

7. If possible, turn client on side, with head flexed slightly forward.
8. Do not restrain client. Loosen clothing.
9. Do not put anything into the client's mouth such as fingers, tongue depressor, or medicine.

RATIONALE

Prevents tongue and dentures from blocking the airway and promotes drainage of secretions, thus reducing risk of aspiration. Prevents musculoskeletal injury.

Critical Decision Point: Putting something in the client's mouth will possibly result in injury to the jaw, tongue, or teeth and cause stimulation of the gag reflex, causing vomiting, aspiration, and respiratory distress.

10. Stay with client, observing the sequence and timing of seizure activity.

Continued observation is necessary to ensure adequate ventilation during and following seizure activity. Accurate, specific observations will assist in documentation, diagnosis, and treatment of the seizure disorder.

11. After the seizure is over, explain what happened and answer client's questions. Foster an atmosphere of acceptance and respect.

Informing clients of the type of seizure activity experienced will assist them in participating knowledgeably in their care.

12. Following seizure, perform hand hygiene and assist client to position of comfort in bed with padded side rails up and bed in low position. Place call light within reach, and provide a quiet, nonstimulating environment.

Provides for continued safety. Clients are often confused and sleepy following a seizure.

Status Epilepticus

13. For a client experiencing status epilepticus, put on clean gloves and insert an oral airway when the jaw is relaxed between seizure activity. Hold airway with curved side up, insert downward until airway reaches back of throat, then rotate and follow natural curve of the tongue. Do not place fingers near or in client's mouth.

Prevents transmission of infection. Client is in continual seizure state and requires oral airway to ensure airway patency. Client will possibly inadvertently bite nurse's fingers during a seizure if nurse does not use caution.

14. Access oxygen and suction equipment. Prepare for IV insertion.

Intensive monitoring and treatment are required for this medical emergency.

15. Use pillows/pads to protect client from injuring self.

Helps avoid traumatic injury.

Recording and Reporting

- Record the timing of seizure activity and sequence of events. Record presence of aura (if any), level of consciousness, posture, color, movements of extremities, incontinence, and patterns of sleep following the seizure.
- Document client's response and expected or unexpected outcomes.
- Report to health care provider immediately as seizure begins. Status epilepticus is an emergency situation requiring immediate medical management.

Unexpected Outcomes and Related Interventions

1. Client suffers traumatic injury.
   a. Continue to protect client from further injury.
   b. Notify the health care provider immediately.
   c. Ensure environment is free of safety hazards.
2. Client verbalizes feelings of embarrassment
   a. Offer support, and allow client to verbalize
   b. Encourage client and family to participate ing and planning care.

Home Care Considerations

- Communicate with client and family to identify precipitating factors.
- Teach family to care for the client during a seizure.
- Assess client's home for environmental hazards in light of seizure condition.
- Provide family with guidelines to detect status epilepticus.
- Until a seizure condition is well controlled (usually for at least 1 year), the client should not take a tub bath or engage in activities such as swimming unless a knowledgeable family member is present. Driving may also be restricted during this time.
- Client needs to wear a medical alert bracelet or tag and have an ID card noting the presence of a seizure disorder and listing the medications taken.

Recording and Reporting provides guidelines for what to chart and report with each skill.

Home Care Considerations explain how to adapt skills for the home setting.

Unexpected Outcomes and Related Interventions alert you to what might go wrong as you perform a skill and provide guidelines for appropriate responses.

Chapter 38 Client Safety **837**

✳ **SKILL 38-1**

APPLYING RESTRAINTS—CONT'D

STEPS

13. Attach restraints to movable part of the bed frame, which moves when the head of bed is raised or lowered (see illustration).

RATIONALE

Client will possibly be injured if restraint is secured to side rail and it is lowered.

Critical Decision Point: Do not attach end of restraint to side rails.

14. Secure restraints with a quick-release tie (see illustration). Do not tie in a knot.

Allows for quick release in an emergency.

15. Insert two fingers under the secured restraint (see illustration).

16. Assess proper placement of restraint, skin integrity, pulses, temperature, color, and sensation of the restrained body part at least every 2 hours (TJC, 2006) or according to agency policy.

A tight restraint will possibly cause constriction and impede circulation. Checking for constriction prevents neurovascular injury. Frequent assessment prevents complications, such as suffocation, skin breakdown, and impaired circulation.

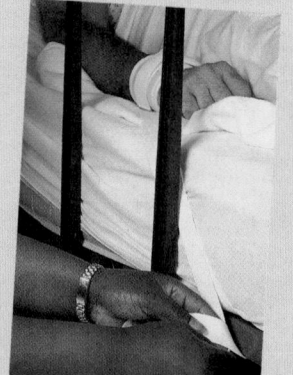

STEP 13 Tie restraint strap to bed frame or hook under bed.

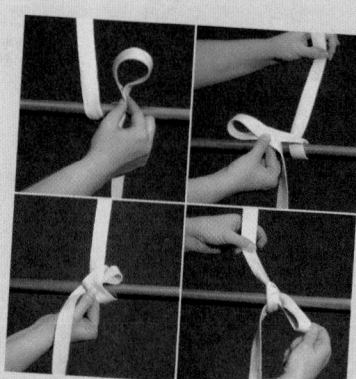

STEP 14 The Posey quick-release tie. (Courtesy JT Posey Co, Arcadia, Calif.)

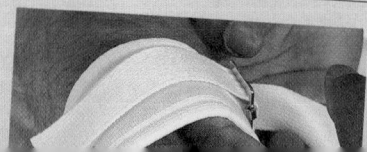

Clear, close-up **photos** and **illustrations** show you how to perform important skill procedures.

Nursing Care Plans demonstrate how comprehensive a plan of care should be for a client. Each plan helps you understand the process of assessment, the association of assessment findings with defining characteristics in the formation of nursing diagnoses, the identification of goals and outcomes, the selection of nursing interventions and the process for evaluating care.

NURSING CARE PLAN
Risk for Injury

Assessment

Mr. Key, a visiting nurse, is seeing Ms. Cohen, an 85-year-old woman, at her home. The client is recovering from a mild stroke affecting her left side. Ms. Cohen lives alone but receives regular assistance from her daughter Peggy and son Michael, who both live within 10 miles. Mr. Key's assessment included a discussion of Ms. Cohen's health problem and how the stroke has affected her, as well as a pertinent physical examination.

Assessment Activities*
Ask Ms. Cohen how the stroke has affected her mobility.
Conduct a home hazard assessment.

Observe Ms. Cohen's gait and posture.

Assess Ms. Cohen's muscle strength.
Assess visual acuity with corrective lenses.

Findings/Defining Characteristics
She responds, "I **bump into things, and I'm afraid I'm going to fall.**"
Cabinets in kitchen are **disorganized and full of breakable items** that could fall out. **Throw rugs are on floors;** bathroom **lighting is poor** (40-watt bulbs); **bathtub lacks safety strips or grab bars;** home cluttered with furniture and small objects.
Ms. Cohen has kyphosis and has a **hesitant, uncoordinated gait.** She frequently **holds walls for support.**
Left arm and leg weaker than right.
Ms. Cohen has **trouble reading and seeing** familiar objects at a distance while wearing current glasses.

*****Defining characteristics** are shown in bold type.

Nursing Diagnosis: Risk for injury related to impaired mobility, decreased visual acuity, and physical environmental hazards.

Planning
Goal

Home will be free of hazards within 1 month.

Ms. Cohen and family will be knowledgeable of potential hazards for Ms. Cohen's age-group within 1 week.

Ms. Cohen will express greater sense of feeling safe from falls in 1 month.
Ms. Cohen will be free of injury within 2 weeks.

Expected Outcomes (NOC)†
Risk Control
Modifiable hazards in kitchen and hallway will be reduced in the home within 1 week. Revisions to bathroom completed in 1 month.
Knowledge: Personal Safety
Ms. Cohen and daughter will identify risks and the steps to avoid them in the home at the conclusion of a teaching session next week.
Fall Prevention Behavior
Ms. Cohen will report improved vision with the aid of new eyeglasses.
Ms. Cohen will be able to safely ambulate throughout the home and perform personal care activities within 2 weeks.

†Outcome classification labels from Moorhead S and others: *Nursing outcomes classification (NOC)*, ed 4, St. Louis, 2008, Mosby.

Nursing Interventions Classification (NIC) and Nursing Outcomes Classification (NOC) terminologies are used in the care plans to build your knowledge of nursing concepts.

Interventions (NIC)†
Fall Prevention
- Review findings from home hazard assessment with Ms. Cohen and daughter.

- Establish a list of priorities to modify, and have Ms. Cohen's son assist in installing bathroom safety devices.
- Install lighting (75-watt bulbs, nonglare) throughout the home. Have son install blinds over kitchen windows.

- Discuss with Ms. Cohen and daughter the normal changes of aging, effects of recent stroke, associated risks for injury, and how to reduce risks.
- Encourage daughter to schedule vision testing for new prescription ~~within~~ ~~weeks~~ ~~tive de-~~
- Refer to a ~~vices for~~

†Intervention

Rationale

Fall risks for homebound older adults include visual disturbances, unsteady gait, and postural changes (Meiner and Leuckenotte, 2006). Home hazard evaluation will highlight extrinsic factors that lead to falls.
Modification of environment reduces fall risk (McCullagh, 2006).

With aging, the pupil loses the ability to adjust to light, causing sensitivity to glare. Glare makes it difficult to clearly see a walking path (Meiner and Lueckenotte, 2006).
Education regarding hazards reduces fear of falling (American Geriatrics Society, 2001).

Improved visual acuity reduces incidence of falls (Edelman and Mandle, 2006).
Exercise often improves gait, balance, and flexibility. Modifying ~~problems~~ by increasing lower extremity strength reduces

Rationales for each of the interventions in the care plans demonstrate the evidence to support nursing care approaches.

NURSING CARE PLAN
Risk for Injury—cont'd

Evaluation section explains how to evaluate and determine whether client outcomes have been achieved.

Evaluation
Nursing Actions
Ask Ms. Cohen and family to identify risks.

Observe environment for elimination of hazards.

Reassess Ms. Cohen's visual acuity.

Observe Ms. Cohen's gait and posture.

Client Response/Finding
Ms. Cohen and daughter able to identify risks during a walk through the home and expressed a greater sense of safety as a result of changes made.
Throw rugs have been removed. Lighting has increased to 75 watts except in bathroom and bedroom.
Ms. Cohen has new glasses and says she is able to read better, as well as see distant objects more clearly.
Ms. Cohen's gait remains hesitant and uncoordinated; she reports that her daughter has not had time to take her to the physical therapist.

Achievement of Outcome
Ms. Cohen and daughter are more knowledgeable of potential hazards.

Environmental hazards have been partially reduced.

Ms. Cohen's vision has improved, enabling her to ambulate more safely.

Outcome of safe ambulation has not been totally achieved; continue to encourage Ms. Cohen and daughter to go to physical therapy appointment.

✳ TABLE 38-2 Interventions to Promote Safety for Children and Adolescents

INTERVENTION	RATIONALE
Infants and Toddlers	
Have infants sleep on their backs or sides. Teach parents the mnemonic "back to sleep."	Sleeping on the stomach with the mouth and nose in close proximity to the mattress is associated with sudden infant death syndrome (SIDS) (Hauck and others, 2003).
Do not fill cribs with pillows, large stuffed toys, or comforters. Sheets should fit snugly.	Possibility for infants to become entwined in sheets and other bedding and suffocate.
Pacifiers should not be attached to string or ribbon and placed around a child's neck.	Reduces risk for choking.
All instructions for preparing and storing formula must be followed.	Proper formula preparation and storage prevents contamination. A formula comes in a concentrated form, or is already premixed with water and ready to use. Following directions ensures proper concentration of the formula. Undiluted formula causes fluid and electrolyte disturbances; very diluted formula will not provide sufficient nutrients.
Use large, soft toys without small parts, such as buttons.	Small parts become dislodged, and choking and aspiration will possibly occur.
Playpens with mesh sides should not be left with a side down; spaces between crib slats should be less than 2⅜ inches (6 cm) apart.	Possibility for a child's head becoming wedged in the lowered mesh side or in between crib slats, and asphyxiation may occur.
Never leave crib sides down or leave babies unattended ~~~~	

846 Unit 7 Basic Human Needs

◆ Evaluation

You apply the components of critical thinking to the evaluation step of the nursing process (Figure 38-18). You evaluate the actual care delivered by the health care team based on the expected outcomes. If you have met the client's goals, you consider the nursing interventions effective and appropriate. If not, you determine whether new risks to the client have developed or whether previous risks remain. The client and family need to participate to find permanent ways to reduce risks to safety. The nurse continually assesses the client's and family's need for additional support services such as home care, physical therapy, counseling, and further teaching.

When you have developed a good relationship with a client and the client feels safe and secure in the relationship, as well as in the environment, the client will most likely demonstrate less anxiety and verbalize satisfaction with the surroundings. You need to determine, however, if client expectations have been met. If outcomes are not met, these are questions to ask: Are you satisfied with changes made to the environment? Do you believe that your safety is ensured? If client expectations have not been met, you reassess not only the client and the environment but also the client's expressed desires.

• • •

A safe environment is essential to promoting, maintaining, and restoring health. Incorporating critical thinking skills in the application of the nursing process, the nurse assesses the client and the environment to determine risk factors for injury; clusters risk factors; formulates a nursing diagnosis; and plans specific interventions, including client education. The expected outcomes include a safe physical environment, a client whose expectations have been met, a client who is knowledgeable about safety factors and precautions, and a client free of injury.

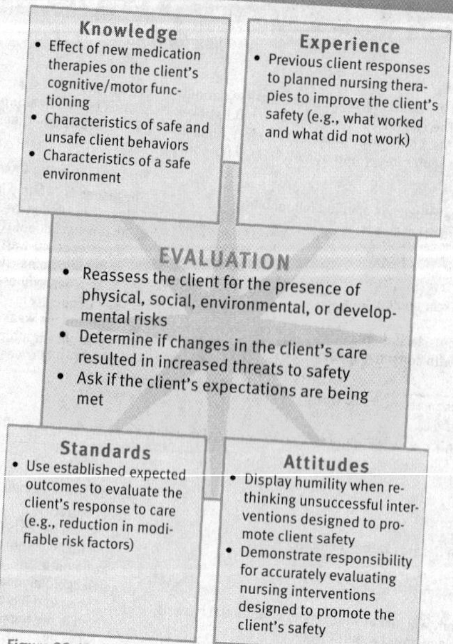

Knowledge
• Effect of new medication therapies on the client's cognitive/motor functioning
• Characteristics of safe and unsafe client behaviors
• Characteristics of a safe environment

Experience
• Previous client responses to planned nursing therapies to improve the client's safety (e.g., what worked and what did not work)

EVALUATION
• Reassess the client for the presence of physical, social, environmental, or developmental risks
• Determine if changes in the client's care resulted in increased threats to safety
• Ask if the client's expectations are being met

Standards
• Use established expected outcomes to evaluate the client's response to care (e.g., reduction in modifiable risk factors)

Attitudes
• Display humility when rethinking unsuccessful interventions designed to promote client safety
• Demonstrate responsibility for accurately evaluating nursing interventions designed to promote the client's safety

Figure 38-18 Critical thinking model for safety evaluation.

Chapters end with **Key Concepts** to help you review. These are also available on the Evolve course website in audio format for download to CD or Mp3.

■ Key Concepts

• In the community a safe environment means basic needs are achievable, reducing physical hazards and the transmission of pathogens, controlling pollution, and maintaining sanitation.
• In a health care agency a safe environment is one that minimizes falls, client-inherent accidents, procedure-inherent accidents, and equipment-related accidents.
• A factor that reduces atmospheric oxygen is the presence of high carbon monoxide levels, which results from an improperly functioning furnace.
• Prolonged exposure to extreme environmental temperatures causes client injury or even death.
• Reduction of physical hazards in the environment includes providing adequate lighting, decreasing clutter, and securing the home.
• Reduce the transmission of pathogens through medical and surgical asepsis, immunization, adequate food sanitation, insect and rodent control, and appropriate disposal of human waste.

• Children less than 5 years of age are at greatest risk for home accidents that result in severe injury and death.
• The school-age child is at risk for injury at home, at school,

Chapter 38 Client Safety 847

■ Critical Thinking Exercises

While making a routine visit, Peggy, Ms. Cohen's daughter, finds Ms. Cohen at the bottom of her porch steps. Ms. Cohen is complaining of hip pain and cannot get up. Peggy calls 911. A few hours later, Ms. Cohen is hospitalized for repair of her right hip fracture.

1. List three environmental interventions to promote Ms. Cohen's safety in her room.
2. Ms. Cohen's bed has four side rails. What position would you put the rails in and why?
3. What are Ms. Cohen's intrinsic factors that make her at higher risk for falls while in the hospital?

Ms. Cohen requires IV antibiotics to be delivered postoperatively. Shortly after the first dose, she became restless and started picking at her IV.

1. What might be precipitating Ms. Cohen's behavior?
2. Why should the nurse avoid using physical restraints on Ms. Cohen?
3. List two interventions that can be utilized to prevent the use of restraints on Ms. Cohen.

Several restraint alternatives were attempted, but due to Ms. Cohen's restlessness she was successful at pulling out her IV. It becomes necessary to restrain Ms. Cohen temporarily during IV antibiotic therapy.

1. You know that a physician's or health care provider's order is required for the restraint. What are essential components of the restraint order?
2. What assessment is performed on Ms. Cohen's upper extremity while she is restrained?
3. The physician orders bilateral upper limb restraints. Your assessment of Ms. Cohen reveals that during the day only her left arm needs to be restrained in order to maintain her IV. Can you remove the right limb restraint?

Critical Thinking Exercises at the end of each chapter provide questions that require you to apply content you have learned in the chapter to simple case studies and clinical scenarios.

■ NCLEX®-Style Review Questions

1. The physiological changes that occur during the aging process increase the older client's risk for:
   1. Poisoning
   2. Alcoholism
   3. Falls and burns
   4. Medication errors
2. You discover an electrical fire in a client's room. Your first action would be to:
   1. Activate the fire alarm
   2. Confine the fire by closing all doors and windows
   3. Evacuate any clients or visitors in immediate danger
   4. Extinguish the fire by using the nearest fire extinguisher

3. A parent calls the pediatrician's office frantic about the bottle of cleaner that her 2-year-old son drank. Which of the following is the most important instruction you can give to this parent?
   1. Give the child milk.
   2. Give the child syrup of ipecac.
   3. Call the poison control center.
   4. Take the child to the emergency department.
4. A couple is with their adolescent daughter for a school physical. The parents tell you that they are worried about all the safety risks affecting this age. As you plan to teach the parents about these risks, you remember that adolescents are at a greater risk for injury from:
   1. Home accidents
   2. Physiological changes of aging
   3. Poisoning and child abduction
   4. Automobile accidents, suicide, and substance abuse
5. During the night shift a client is found wandering the hospital halls looking for a bathroom. The nurse's initial intervention would be to:
   1. Insert a urinary catheter
   2. Ask the physician to order a restraint
   3. Assign a staff member to stay with the client
   4. Provide scheduled toileting during the night shift
6. Lisa, a nurse assistant, is working with you during your shift. One of your clients has upper limb restraints. In delegating care of this client to the Lisa, you would tell her to:
   1. Move the client to a room closer to the nurses' station
   2. Check to see if the client can have a medication for sleep
   3. Call the physician if the client becomes more agitated with the restraint
   4. Report any signs of redness, excoriation, or constriction of circulation under the restraint
7. The family of your confused, ambulatory client insists that all four side rails be up when the client is alone. The best way to handle this situation would be to:
   1. Ask them to stay with the client at all times
   2. Inform them of the risks associated with side rail use
   3. Thank them for being conscientious and put the four rails up
   4. Provide the client a one-to-one sitter while the side rails are up
8. During your assessment of a 56-year-old man, he reports increased alcohol consumption due to stress at work. One of your expected outcomes for this client will be to:
   1. Decrease stress in his life
   2. Teach him ways to promote sleep
   3. Decrease his alcohol intake during stress
   4. Provide the client with resources for al

NCLEX®-Style Review Questions at the end of each chapter, with the answer key included in the text, help you review and evaluate what you have learned.

Preface to the Instructor

The nursing profession is always responding to dynamic change and continual challenges. Today, nurses need a broad knowledge base from which to provide care. More importantly, nurses require the ability to know how to apply best evidence in practice to ensure the best outcomes for their clients. The role of the nurse includes assuming the lead in preserving nursing practice and demonstrating its contribution to the health care of our nation. Nurses of tomorrow, therefore, need to become critical thinkers, client advocates, clinical decision makers, and client educators within a broad spectrum of care services.

The seventh edition of *Fundamentals of Nursing* was revised to prepare today's students for the challenges of tomorrow. This textbook is designed for beginning students in all types of professional nursing programs. The comprehensive coverage provides fundamental nursing concepts, skills, and techniques of nursing practice and a firm foundation for more advanced areas of study.

To address the needs of all levels of learners, as well as those students whose native language is not English, this revision of *Fundamentals of Nursing* was edited by an English-as-a-Second-Language/Readability specialist to streamline the text, improve readability, and enhance comprehension.

Fundamentals of Nursing provides a contemporary approach to nursing practice, discussing the entire scope of primary, acute, and restorative care. This new edition addresses a number of key current practice issues, including safe patient handling and informatics in nursing. A new, cutting-edge chapter on *Caring for the Cancer Survivor* helps prepare students to address the unique health care needs of patients who have survived cancer, but still face the physical and emotional after-effects of the illness and its therapy. A new chapter on *Evidence-Based Practice* helps students understand how to translate nursing research and use findings at the bedside for best nursing practice. Evidence-based practice is one of the most important initiatives in health care today. The increased focus on applying current evidence in skills and client care plans helps students understand how the latest research findings should guide their clinical decision making.

We are indebted to the many educators and students who have shared their thoughts, visions, and ideas with us, and we credit each of them as valuable collaborators for this revision.

Features

We have carefully developed this seventh edition with the student in mind. We have designed this text to welcome the new student to nursing, communicate our own love for the profession, and promote learning and understanding. Key features of the text include the following:

Classic Features

- **Comprehensive** coverage and readability of all fundamental nursing content.
- **Full-color** text to enhance visual appeal and instructional value.
- **Nursing process** format provides a consistent organizational framework for clinical chapters.
- Covers **health promotion and acute and continuing care** to address today's practice in various settings.
- A **health promotion/wellness** thread is used consistently throughout the text.
- **Cultural diversity** is presented in Chapter 9, stressed in clinical examples throughout the text, and highlighted in special boxes.
- **Client education** is presented in Chapter 25 and stressed in boxes that list teaching objectives, strategies, and evaluation for clinical topics throughout the text.
- **Gerontologic nursing** principles are addressed in Chapter 14, as well as in special Focus on Older Adults boxes throughout the text.
- **Diverse clinical settings** are addressed throughout the text, describing practice examples in clinics, extended care facilities, and the home, as well as acute care settings.
- A **critical thinking model** provides a framework for clinical chapters, showing how elements of critical thinking, including knowledge, critical thinking attitudes, intellectual and professional standards, and experience, are integrated throughout the nursing process for making clinical decisions.
- Important **nursing skills** are presented in a clear, two-column format with a rationale for all steps; whenever possible, rationales are based on the most current research evidence.

- **Unexpected Outcomes and Related Interventions** are highlighted within nursing skills to help students anticipate and appropriately respond to possible problems faced while performing skills.
- **Procedural Guidelines** boxes provide more streamlined, step-by-step instructions for performing very basic skills.
- **Concept Maps** show you the association between multiple nursing diagnoses for a client with a selected medical diagnosis and the relationship between nursing interventions.
- **Nursing Care Plans** guide students on how to conduct an assessment and analyze the defining characteristics that indicate nursing diagnoses. The plans include NIC and NOC classifications to familiarize students with this important nomenclature. The evaluation sections of the plans show students how to evaluate and then determine the outcomes of care.
- **Evidence-Based Practice** boxes provide a summary of nursing research evidence on a specific topic and explains its implications for nursing practice, helping students to understand how research can be translated to the beside.
- **Safety Alerts** indicate techniques students can use to ensure client and nurse safety.
- **Media Resources** boxes detail what electronic resources are available for the student every chapter.
- **Video Icons** indicate video clips associated with specific skills that are available on the free CD-Companion and Evolve Student Learning Resources.

New Features

- New chapters and expanded content:
  - *Caring for the Cancer Survivor* chapter addresses the unique physical and emotional needs of cancer survivors dealing with the after-effects of their illness and treatment. With 10,000,000 cancer survivors in the United States, nurses in all settings need to understand their common types of health problems.
  - *Evidence-Based Practice* chapter teaches students a six-step process for asking clinical questions and learning how to analyze and apply the best scientific evidence in practice. The chapter offers skills on how to conduct literature searches and tips for applying evidence in real practice situations.
  - *Documentation and Informatics* chapter incorporates basic concepts of nursing informatics in health care.
  - Safe patient handling guidelines include the latest 2006 guidelines for transfer and ambulation techniques.
  - New 2007 IV guidelines from the Infusion Nurses Society.
  - New 2006 Pressure Ulcer Staging guidelines from National Pressure Ulcer Advisory Panel.
  - Assessment Questions boxes help students learn how to clearly and effectively conduct a client assessment.

Ancillaries
For the Student
Companion CD-ROM Free Companion CD-ROM in each text includes Test Taking Skills and NCLEX®-Style Review Questions in addition to Butterfield's Fluids and Electrolytes program, interactive learning activities, and an English/Spanish Audio Glossary.

Evolve Course Website Students can access downloadable audio and video clips for on-the-go learning with portable media

devices, plus NCLEX®-Style review questions, Mosby's Nursing Skills video clips, audio chapter summaries, a searchable Spanish/English audio glossary, *Butterfield's Fluids & Electrolytes Tutorial*, test-taking tips, and chapter-specific web links.

Study Guide and Skills Performance Checklists
- Provide an ideal supplement to help students understand and apply the content of the text. Each chapter includes multiple sections:
  - Preliminary Reading includes a chapter assignment from the text.
  - Comprehensive Understanding provides a variety of activities to reinforce the topics and main ideas from the text.
  - Review Questions are NCLEX®-Style multiple-choice questions that require students to provide rationales for their answers. Answers and rationales are provided in the answer key.
  - Clinical chapters include an Application of Critical Thinking Synthesis Model that expands the case study from the chapter's Care Plan and asks students to develop a step in the synthesis model based on the nurse and client in the scenario. This helps students learn to apply both content learned and the critical thinking synthesis model.
  - Procedure Performance Checklists are included so that students can evaluate skill competency.

Clinical Companion Equip your students with a concise, portable guide to all the facts and figures they'll need to know in their early clinical experiences.

Virtual Clinical Excursions This workbook/CD-ROM package provides a hands-on learning experience that lets students care for a variety of clients on a multifloor virtual hospital.

Nursing Skills Online Focusing on the skills that are most difficult to teach and/or that pose the greatest risk to client safety, this one-of-a-kind, interactive, and evaluative online course engages students in media-rich learning modules with realistic, case-based lessons to help students review and evaluate their competency before performing skills in the clinical setting.

For the Instructor
Instructor's Electronic Resource CD-ROM Access unparalleled support with new *Integrated Lesson Plans* that tie together every chapter resource you need for the most effective class presentations, plus an ExamView test bank with more than 1800 NCLEX®-Style questions accompanied by rationales and page references, and over 100 audience response system questions for use with i>Clicker and other systems.

- *Integrated Lesson Plans* give you everything you need to deliver effective lectures and provide engaging student learning and application opportunities, including live links to teaching resources and classroom teaching strategies.

EVOLVE Online Courseware Includes secure access to all content from the Instructor's Electronic Resource, including Integrated Lesson Plans, ExamView Computerized Test Bank, Electronic Image Collection, PowerPoint Slides, and all student online resources.

Mosby's Nursing Video Skills on DVD Show your students how to safely perform nursing skills. Version 3.0 includes all-new footage and an exciting, interactive format on basic, intermediate, and advanced DVDs. Sold separately.

We are pleased to note the growing number of men currently involved in the practice of nursing, and we acknowledge their dedication, skill, and professionalism. We have therefore made every effort to eliminate any gender-specific pronouns. In a very few instances, we have used she to refer to the nurse and he to refer to the client in order to clearly communicate to the reader.

The development of this textbook resulted from the combined efforts of many talented professionals committed to excellence. We appreciate their dedication and enthusiasm. Throughout the text we have attempted to acknowledge the contributions of our professional nurse colleagues who make a difference in the lives of their clients and the communities they serve. We are very proud to be associated with such fine individuals.

Acknowledgments

- We wish to acknowledge Suzi Epstein, Executive Editor, for her vision, organization, creativity, and support to develop a text that offers a state-of-the-art approach to the design, organization, and presentation of *Fundamentals of Nursing*. Her skill as an editor enables us to be innovative; her skillful and thoughtful editing provided needed attention to detail in designing such a comprehensive text.
- Lynda Huenefeld and Robyn Brinks, Developmental Editors, whose organization skills and attention to detail are the best in the business. Their patience and gracious manner skillfully tracked manuscript, authors, and deadlines, all the while maintaining their cool and a wonderful sense of humor.
- Amy Hall and Patricia Stockert, section editors, whose talents help to take this text to the next level. Their attention to detail, knowledge of the nursing literature, and commitment to excellence were integral components of this text from planning to publication. Amy and Patti, thank you for a wonderful partnership.
- Beth Hayes, Project Manager, who is an accomplished production editor. Beth juggles multiple aspects of the book, while keeping the book and the authors on deadline. She is talented and calm under pressure, and through her sense of humor and commitment to excellence guided this text to completion.
- Tricia Kinman, readability specialist, whose editing and knowledge helped us to create a text that is informative and maintains a consistent reading level for our students.
- Mike Defilippo, St. Louis, Missouri, for his excellent photography.
- Deaconess Gateway Hospital, Newburgh, Indiana, for their assistance with the photographs to help bring the text to life.
- Graphic World Illustration Studio, for the computer expertise that provides clear, detailed illustrations to enhance and complement the textbook.

Contents

Unit IV Professional Standards in Nursing Practice

Unit VI Scientific Basis for Nursing Practice

Unit VII Basic Human Needs

Unit VIII Clients With Special Needs

1 | Nursing Today

✳ OBJECTIVES

Mastery of content in this chapter will enable the student to:
- Discuss the historical development of professional nursing roles.
- Describe educational programs available for professional registered nurse education.
- Describe the roles and career opportunities for nurses.
- Discuss the influence of social and economic changes on nursing practices.

✳ MEDIA RESOURCES   ✳ KEY TERMS

 Companion CD
- NCLEX®-Style Review Questions
- Audio Glossary
- Interactive Learning Activities
- English/Spanish Glossary

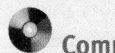 **Website**
- NCLEX®-Style Review Questions
- Audio Glossary
- English/Spanish Glossary
- Interactive Learning Activities
- Weblinks
- Audio Summaries

Nursing is an art and a science. As a professional nurse, you will learn to deliver care artfully with compassion, caring, and a respect for each client's dignity and personhood. As a science, nursing is based on a body of knowledge that is continually changing with new discoveries and innovations. When you integrate the science and art of nursing into your practice, the quality of care you provide to your clients is at a level of excellence that benefits clients and their families.

The opportunities for a nursing career are limitless. You may choose from any number of career paths, including clinical practice, education, research, management, administration, and even entrepreneurship. As a student, it is important for you to understand the scope of nursing practice and how nursing influences the lives of your clients.

The client is the center of your practice. The client includes the individual, family, and/or community. Clients have a wide variety of health care needs, experiences, vulnerabilities, and expectations. But this is what makes nursing both challenging and rewarding. Making a difference in your client's life is fulfilling: for example, helping a dying client find relief from pain, helping a young mother learn parenting skills, and finding ways for older adults to remain independent in their homes. Nursing offers personal and professional rewards every day. This chapter presents a contemporary view of the evolution of nursing and nursing practice and the historical, practical, social, and political influences on the discipline of nursing.

When giving care, it is essential to provide a specified service according to standards of practice and to follow a code of ethics (American Nurses Association [ANA], 2000, 2004). Professional practice includes knowledge from social and behavioral sciences, biological and physiological sciences, and nursing theories. In addition, nursing practice incorporates social values, professional autonomy, a sense of commitment and community, and a code of ethics (ANA, 2003). The **American Nurses Association (ANA)** defined **nursing** as

> the protection, promotion, and optimization of health and abilities, prevention of illness and injury, alleviation of suffering through the diagnosis and treatment of human response, and advocacy in the care of individuals, families, communities, and populations (ANA, 2003, p. 6).

This definition asserts the prominence and importance nursing holds in providing health care to our global community.

Expert clinical nursing practice is a commitment to the application of knowledge and clinical experience. Your ability to interpret clinical situations and make complex decisions is the foundation for your nursing care and is the basis for the advancement of nursing practice and the development of nursing science (Benner, 1984; Benner, Tanner and Chesla, 1997). Critical thinking skills are essential to nursing (see Chapter 15). When providing nursing care, you must make clinical judgments about your clients' health care needs based on fact, experience, and standards of care. You gain knowledge, expertise, and lifelong learning through the continual process of critical thinking and reflection (Benner and others, 1997; Domino, 2005).

Historical Perspective Highlights

Nursing has and always will respond to the needs of its clients. In times of war, nursing's response was to meet the needs of the wounded in combat zones and military hospitals in the United States and abroad. When communities face health care crises, such as disease outbreaks or insufficient health care resources, nurses establish community-based immunization and screening programs, treatment clinics, and health promotion activities.

Our clients are most vulnerable when they are injured, sick, or dying. Historically nursing has made it a priority to meet the needs of clients and their communities. This commitment still continues today.

Nurses are active in social policy and political arenas. Nurses and their professional organizations lobby for health care legislation to meet the needs of clients, particularly the medically underserved. For example, nurses in communities provide home visits to newborns of high-risk mothers (e.g., adolescent, poorly educated mothers or medically underserved). These visits result in fewer emergency department visits, fewer newborn infections, and reduced infant mortality (Lesser and others, 2005; Schneiderman, 2006).

Nurses study and test new and better ways to help their clients. Nurse researchers are leaders in expanding knowledge in nursing and other health care disciplines. Early in nursing's history during the Crimean War, Florence Nightingale studied and implemented methods to improve battlefield sanitation, which ultimately reduced illness, infection, and mortality (Cohen, 1984). Today nurses are active in determining the best practices for skin care management, pain control, nutritional management, and care of older adults, to cite just a few examples.

Nursing continuously responds and adapts to new challenges. The evolution of nursing brings the profession to one of the most challenging and exciting times in history. Nurses are in a unique position to refine and shape the future of health care (Grindel, 2006). Nursing is a combination of knowledge from the physical sciences, humanities, and social sciences, along with clinical competencies needed to meet the individual needs of clients and their families.

Knowledge of our profession's history increases your ability to understand the social and intellectual origins of the discipline. Although it is not practical to describe all of the historical aspects of professional nursing, some of the more significant milestones since the late 1800s are described in Box 1-1.

Florence Nightingale

In *Notes on Nursing: What It Is and What It Is Not,* Florence Nightingale established the first nursing philosophy based on health maintenance and restoration (Nightingale, 1860). Her views on nursing came from a spiritual philosophy, developed in her adolescence and adulthood (Macrae, 1995), and reflected the changing needs of society. She saw the role of nursing as having "charge of somebody's health" based on the knowledge of "how to put the body in such a state to be free of disease or to recover

---

✳ BOX 1-1 Selected Milestones in Nursing History Since the Late 1800s

1860	Nightingale Training School for Nurses was established at St. Thomas' Hospital in London, England. This was the first organized program for training nurses.
1874	First nurses' training school in Canada was founded in St. Catherine's, Ontario.
1882	United States ratified the American Red Cross, founded by Clara Barton.
1883	Mary Agnes Snively assumed directorship of Toronto General Hospital and began to form the Canadian National Association of Trained Nurses, which was to become the Canadian Nurses Association (CNA).
1896	Nurses' Associated Alumnae of the United States and Canada (NAAUSC) was established. This group was an initial nursing professional group. It later became the American Nurses Association.
1893	Henry Street Settlement opened by Lillian Wald and Harriet Brewster.
1901	First university-affiliated nursing program. The Army Nurse Corps was established.
1908	Navy Nurse Corps was established; Canadian National Association of Trained Nurses (later changed to the Canadian Nurses Association, 1924) was founded.
1911	NAAUSC became the American Nurses Association (ANA).
1922	Sigma Theta Tau, National Honor Society of Nursing, was formed by six student nurses from Indiana University.
1923	Goldmark Report: Rockefeller Foundation–funded survey identified need for increased financial support to university-based schools of nursing; as a result the Yale School of Nursing was developed.
1948	Brown Report: Dr. Esther Lucille Brown concluded that all nursing education programs should be affiliated with universities and have their own budgets. She recommended a broad academic education within a university and 2 years of nursing education focused on technical skills.

1952	Dr. Mildred Montag established the first associate degree nursing program. *Nursing Research* was established.
1953	National League for Nursing (NLN), in collaboration with universities, developed graduate nursing education.
1960	Yale University School of Nursing defined nursing as a profession, interaction, and relationship between two human beings.
1964	Nurses Training Act was passed, bringing almost $300 million into nursing education.
1965	Jerome Lysaught directed the National Commission on Nursing and Nursing Education Report, which recommended that nursing roles and responsibilities be clarified in relation to other health care professionals. Also recommended increased financial support and career opportunities to attract and retain nurses; ANA position paper defined nursing.
1975	NLN required theory-based curriculum for accreditation.
1985	ANA published *Code for Nurses With Interpretive Statements*.
1994	Health care reform.
1996	The Pew Report: Looking at future nursing needs and shortages. Institute of Medicine (IOM) Report: parallel to the Pew Report.

Data from Donahue MP: *Nursing: the finest art—an illustrated history*, ed 2, St. Louis, 1996, Mosby.

---

from disease" (Nightingale, 1860). During the same year, she developed the first organized program for training nurses, the Nightingale Training School for Nurses at St. Thomas' Hospital in London.

Nightingale was the first practicing nurse epidemiologist (Cohen, 1984). Her statistical analyses connected poor sanitation with cholera and dysentery. She viewed nursing as a search for truth in finding answers to health care questions or discovering and using God's laws of healing in nursing practice (Macrae, 1995).

In 1853 Nightingale went to Paris to study with the Sisters of Charity and was later appointed superintendent of the English General Hospitals in Turkey. During this period she brought about major reforms in hygiene, sanitation, and nursing practice. She volunteered during the Crimean War in 1853 and traveled the battlefield hospitals at night carrying her lamp; she thus was known as the "lady with the lamp." The sanitary, nutrition, and basic facilities in the battlefield hospitals were poor at best. Eventually she was given the task to organize and improve the quality of the sanitation facilities. As a result, the mortality rate at the Barracks Hospital in Scutari, Turkey, was reduced from 42.7% to 2.2% in 6 months (Donahue, 1996; Woodham-Smith, 1983).

The Civil War to the Beginning of the Twentieth Century

The Civil War (1860 to 1865) stimulated the growth of nursing in the United States. Clara Barton, founder of the American Red Cross, tended soldiers on the battlefields, cleansing their wounds, meeting their basic needs, and comforting them in death. The U.S. Congress ratified the American Red Cross in 1882 after 10 years of lobbying by Barton. Dorothea Lynde Dix, Mary Ann Ball (Mother Bickerdyke), and Harriet Tubman also influenced nursing during the Civil War (Donahue, 1996). As superintendent of the female nurses of the Union Army, Dix organized hospitals, appointed nurses, and oversaw and regulated supplies to the troops. Mother Bickerdyke organized ambulance services, supervised nurses, and walked abandoned battlefields at night, looking for wounded soldiers. Harriet Tubman was active in the Underground Railroad movement and assisted in leading over 300 slaves to freedom (Donahue, 1996).

The first professionally trained African American nurse was Mary Mahoney. She was concerned with relationships between cultures and races, and as a noted nursing leader, she brought forth an awareness of cultural diversity and respect for the individual, regardless of background, race, color, or religion.

Isabel Hampton Robb helped found the Nurses' Associated Alumnae of the United States and Canada in 1896. This organization became the American Nurses Association in 1911. She authored many nursing textbooks, including *Nursing: Its Principles and Practice for Hospital and Private Use* (1894), *Nursing Ethics* (1900), and *Educational Standards for Nurses* (1907), and was one of the original founders of the *American Journal of Nursing* (AJN) (Donahue, 1996).

Nursing in hospitals expanded in the late nineteenth century. However, nursing in the community did not increase significantly until 1893, when Lillian Wald and Mary Brewster opened the Henry Street Settlement, which focused on the health needs of poor people who lived in tenements in New York City (Donahue, 1996). Nurses working in this settlement were some of the first to demonstrate autonomy in practice because they frequently encountered situations that required quick and innovative problem solving and critical thinking without the supervision or direction of a health care provider. The poor people also needed nursing therapies aimed at maintaining wellness through proper nutrition, hygiene, and shelter. Wald described her activities with the Henry Street Settlement in the textbook *The House on Henry Street* (1915).

Twentieth Century

In the early twentieth century a movement toward a scientific, research-based defined body of nursing knowledge and practice was evolving. Nurses began to assume expanded and advanced practice roles. Mary Adelaide Nutting was instrumental in the affiliation of nursing education with universities. She became the first professor of nursing at Columbia University Teachers College in 1906 (Donahue, 1996). In addition, the Goldmark Report concluded that nursing education needed increased financial support and suggested that university schools of nursing receive the money.

As nursing education developed, nursing practice also expanded. In 1901 the Army Nurse Corps was established, followed in 1908 by the Navy Nurse Corps. By the 1920s nursing specialization was developing. Graduate nurse-midwifery programs began, and in the late 1940s and early 1950s specialty-nursing organizations, such as the Association of Operating Room Nurses, American Association of Critical Care Nurses, and Oncology Nursing Society, were formed. By 1970 the Emergency Room Nurses Organization had formed, which was changed to the Emergency Nurses Association in 1995.

Twenty-First Century

Nursing practice and education continue to evolve to meet the needs of society. In 1990 the American Nurses Association established the Center for Ethics and Human Rights. The Center provides a forum to address the complex ethical and human rights issues confronting nurses and designs activities and programs to increase ethical competence in nurses (ANA, 2001). Nursing's code of ethics was revised in 2001 to reflect current ethical issues affecting health care and nursing practice (see Chapter 22).

Today the profession faces multiple challenges. Nurses and nurse educators are revising nursing practice and school curricula to meet the ever-changing needs of society, including bioterrorism, emerging infections, and disaster management. Advances in technology and informatics (see Chapter 26), the high acuity level of care of hospitalized clients, and early discharge from health care institutions require nurses in all settings to have a strong and current knowledge base from which to practice. In addition, nursing and the Robert Wood Johnson Foundation are taking a leadership role in developing standards and policies for end-of-life care through the *Last Acts Campaign* (see Chapter 30). The End-of-Life Nursing Education Consortium (ELNEC) offered collaboratively by the American Association of Colleges of Nursing (AACN) and the City of Hope Medical Center has brought end-of-life care and practices into nursing curricula.

Nursing practice occurs in multiple care settings, including health care institutions and foundations, the community, and the home. In addition, nurses are active in political and lobbying groups, social and not-for-profit agencies, and work to establish social health care policies. These activities increase nursing's public visibility and, at the same time, increase the public's awareness of professional nursing. The challenge now is to prepare professional nurses to deliver complex, multifaceted care in multiple care settings.

Societal Influences on Nursing

Multiple external forces affect nursing. These include demographic changes of the population, human rights, increasing numbers of medically underserved, and the threat of bioterrorism.

Demographic Changes

Demographic changes affect the population. Changes influencing health care in recent decades include the population shift from rural areas to urban centers; the increased life span; the higher incidence of chronic, long-term illness; and the increased incidence of diseases such as alcoholism and lung cancer. Nursing responds to such changes by exploring new methods to provide care, by changing nursing education, and by establishing practice standards.

Women's Health Care Issues

The women's movement brought about many changes in society as women increasingly demanded economic, political, occupational, and educational equality. As a result, there is greater sensitivity to the health care needs of women and the role of women in health care research. There are emerging health care specialties dealing with the needs of women. These new specialties expand from the traditional obstetrical specialty and address issues ranging from well women's examinations to oncological subspecialties and management of menopause. Because of the prior lack of female subjects in biomedical research, the federal government now requires studies to routinely include women in research, unless specific exception criteria are met. For example, research focusing on management of prostatic cancer is an exception.

Human Rights Movement

The human rights movement changed the way society viewed the rights of all of its members, including minorities, clients with terminal illness, pregnant women, and older adults. Many groups have special health care needs, and nursing responds by respecting the human rights of all clients and their right to quality care. Nurses advocate the rights of all clients, but they also recognize the special needs of some groups. Thus nurses created bills of rights for dying, hospitalized, and pregnant clients, as well as other groups, to ensure that clients' rights are protected while receiving quality care.

Medically Underserved

The rising rates of underemployment and low-paying jobs, mental illness, and homelessness and rising health care costs all contribute to an increase in the medically underserved population. Some of the medically underserved population are poor and on Medicaid. Others are part of the working poor in that they cannot afford their own insurance, but they make too much money to qualify for Medicaid. In addition, there is an increase in the mentally ill population who have little or no access to health care. Today, nurses work in many health care settings providing health promotion and disease prevention to the homeless, mentally ill, and others who have limited access to health care or who lack health care insurance (Cunningham, McKenzie, and Taylor, 2006).

Threat of Bioterrorism

The world is a changing place; the threats of bioterrorism are continuous. Many health care agencies, schools, and communities have educational programs to prepare for nuclear, chemical, or biological attack. Nurses are active in disaster preparedness. For example, nurses work with community disaster preparedness groups and hospitals to determine what specific nursing activities are needed. This activity sometimes ranges from participating in vaccine research, decontamination in the event of biological attack, triage for mass casualty, to crisis response units. If a disaster were to occur, nurses would be essential in evaluating the strengths and weaknesses of any disaster plan.

Needs of the Consumer

The consumers' movement increased public awareness of the value and costs of products and services. It influenced health care by appealing for new kinds of health care agencies, such as health maintenance organizations, demanding culturally sensitive care, creating new forms of health insurance, and voicing concern about the rising costs of health care (see Chapter 2). Consumers are more knowledgeable about health and illness and are becoming more vocal in their desire for high-quality care. Because nurses generally interact with clients more than other health care professionals do, you may be called on to answer questions about the quality and costs of health care.

Cultural Diversity

Because the world's population is more mobile, you will care for clients from many different cultures. You need an awareness of how different cultures view health and illness (see Chapter 9). You are continually challenged to be culturally aware and competent. Care that is not culturally competent may be more costly and ineffective (Sullivan, 1999). *Healthy People 2010,* a federal document that outlines health care goals for the public, is one example of meeting the health of multiple cultures by defining goals and

objectives for health (U.S. Department of Health and Human Services [USDHHS], 2006).

Safety

Client safety is a priority in health care. You need to protect clients from physical and emotional injury by continually assessing for and eliminating safety hazards (see Chapter 38). The Joint Commission (TJC) annually updates and publishes *National Patient Safety Goals* on its website (http://www.jointcommission. org/PatientSafety/).

Examples of threats to client safety include medication errors, improper client transfers, client falls, and incorrect procedures. You reduce medication errors by consciously adhering to the six rights of medication administration and avoiding abbreviations on the "do not use" abbreviations list, which is posted on the National Patient Safety Goals website listed above (see Chapter 35).

Injuries to both caregiver and client occur during client transfer. The caregiver is at risk for musculoskeletal injuries. The client is at risk for falls, as well as musculoskeletal injuries. There is a shift from ineffective, injury-prone client transfer techniques to evidence-based practices for safe client handling (see Chapters 37 and 47). Examples of these evidence-based practices include using the proper equipment for clients transfer and the use of client lift teams (Nelson and Baptiste, 2004).

Clients fall due to many factors, such as improper transfer techniques, client age, side effects of medications, impaired mobility, or confusion (see Chapter 38). Learn your agency's fall prevention program for reducing client falls. Programs that use a multidimensional approach in designing fall prevention strategies have the greatest reduction in fall rates (Centers for Disease Control and Prevention [CDC], 2006).

In the operating room, surgery centers, or invasive diagnostic centers, there are specific guidelines, such as "time out" and "read back" procedures specifically designed for client safety (see Chapter 50). These procedures ensure that it is the right client and right procedure and are designed to promote client safety.

Health Promotion and Wellness

Today there is a greater emphasis on health promotion, health maintenance, and illness prevention (see Chapter 6). Exercise, nutrition, and healthy lifestyles interest many people. Nursing responds to this greater concern for health promotion by providing programs in the community such as health fairs and wellness programs; educational programs for specific diseases; and client and family teaching activities in hospitals, clinics, primary care facilities, and other health care settings.

Influence of Today's Health Care Delivery System

Today's health care delivery system is a complex and highly regulated system (see Chapter 2). When you work in the health care system, you must be aware of methods to contain health care costs, provide evidence-based care, and participate in nursing and biomedical research. In addition, the nursing shortage will further challenge your practice.

Rising Health Care Costs

Skyrocketing health care costs present challenges to the profession, consumer, and the health care delivery system as well (see Chapter 2). You are responsible for providing the client with the best-quality care in an efficient and economically sound manner. The challenge is to use health care and client resources wisely. For example, your client needs to learn how to perform self-intermittent urinary catheterization at home. The question to raise is whether the procedure should be performed with clean versus sterile equipment. Choosing the more cost-effective, clean technique does not compromise care because your client is in the home environment, which is cleaner and without the risks for health care-associated infections. However, you use your critical thinking skills to clinically evaluate each client to determine which clients perform procedures safely using clean technique. You also play a role in managing health care costs by participating in product evaluation. Most health care institutions invite their nurses to participate in product review committees to select the most clinically and cost-effective items for clinical use.

Evidence-Based Practice

All clients need the most current, effective, state-of-the-art care in a rapidly changing health care system. As a health care provider, you face the challenge of providing the most appropriate and effective nursing interventions for improving client outcomes. One way to achieve this is to practice from an evidence-based practice framework. Evidence-based practice is a problem-solving approach to clinical practice that uses the best available evidence along with your expertise and client preferences and values in making decisions about care (Sackett and others, 2000). Evidence-based nursing practice requires you to actively pursue the best scientific evidence when making decisions (see Chapters 2 and 5).

Nursing and Biomedical Research

Nursing and scientific knowledge continue to expand. When nurses participate in nursing research, they share a "commitment to the advancement of nursing science and the ethical conduct of nursing science" (ANA, 1997). Research findings add to advancement of nursing science and professional practice. For example, researchers concluded that the nursing intervention of massaging the reddened skin on pressure points actually caused more tissue damage, and now massage on pressure points is contraindicated (see Chapter 48). Other researchers noted the technique of auscultation for verifying feeding tube placement was inaccurate and should not be used (see Chapter 44). When you use research findings in your nursing practice, you base your nursing care on science, rather than tradition (see Chapter 5). The beneficiary of this care is your client. Through research, nursing knowledge advances and nurses are able to provide the highest-quality state-of-the-art nursing care (Engelke and Marshburn, 2006).

Nursing Shortage

There is an ongoing global nursing shortage. This shortage affects all aspects of nursing, but it also represents challenges and opportunities for the profession (Rosenkoetter and Nardi, 2006). Many health care dollars are invested in strategies aimed at recruiting a well-educated, critically thinking, motivated, and dedicated nursing workforce (Boychuk, 2001). There is a direct link between nursing care and positive client outcomes, reduced complication rates, and a more rapid return of the client to the preillness state (Aiken and others, 2003; Blendon, DesRoches, Brodie, and others, 2002).

Like it or not, the nursing shortage affects the needs of the consumer (Block and Sredl, 2006). With fewer nurses in the workplace, it is important for you to learn to use your client contact time efficiently and professionally. Time management, therapeutic communication, client education, and compassionate implementation of psychomotor skills are just a few of the essential skills you need. For example, using a well-organized approach to prepare your client to self-administer blood pressure medication at home can help your client to understand the importance of taking the medication as ordered. Most importantly your clients leave the health care setting with a positive image of nursing and a feeling that they received quality care. Your client should never feel rushed or that he or she was one of your many clients or tasks. If a certain aspect of client care requires 15 minutes of contact, it will take the same time to deliver the care in an organized manner as it would in a rushed, harried manner. However, the impression you leave with your client will be far different. You have the opportunity and obligation to present our profession and practice in the best possible manner.

Nursing as a Profession

Nursing is not simply a collection of specific skills, and you are not simply a person trained to perform specific tasks. Nursing is a profession. No one factor absolutely differentiates a job from a profession, but the difference is important in terms of how you practice. To act professionally you administer care in a conscientious and knowledgeable manner, and you are responsible to yourself and others. A profession has the following primary characteristics:

- A profession requires an extended education of its members, as well as a basic liberal foundation.
- A profession has a theoretical body of knowledge leading to defined skills, abilities, and norms.
- A profession provides a specific service.
- Members of a profession have autonomy in decision making and practice.
- The profession as a whole has a code of ethics for practice.

Scope and Standards of Practice

Since 1960, the American Nurses Association has engaged in documenting the scope of nursing and developing standards of practice. In 2004, the ANA reviewed and completely updated *Nursing: Scope and Standards of Practice* (ANA, 2004). Within this document are the Standards of Practice and Standards of Professional Performance. It is important that you know and apply these standards in your practice. The document is usually available in most schools of nursing and practice settings. The goal of this document is to improve the health and well-being of all individuals, communities, and populations through the significant and

✳ BOX 1-2 ANA Standards of Nursing Practice

1. **Assessment:** The registered nurse collects comprehensive data pertinent to the patient's health or the situation.
2. **Diagnosis:** The registered nurse analyzes the assessment data to determine the diagnoses or issues.
3. **Outcomes Identification:** The registered nurse identifies expected outcomes for a plan individualized to the patient or the situation.
4. **Planning:** The registered nurse develops a plan that prescribes strategies and alternatives to attain expected outcomes.
5. **Implementation:** The registered nurse implements the identified plan.
6. **Evaluation:** The registered nurse evaluates progress toward attainment of outcomes.

Reprinted with permission from American Nurses Association: *Nursing: scope and standards of practice,* © 2004, Nursesbooks.org, Silver Spring, Md.

✳ BOX 1-3 ANA Standards of Professional Performance

7. **Quality of Practice:** The registered nurse systematically enhances the quality and effectiveness of nursing practice.
8. **Education:** The registered nurse attains knowledge and competency that reflects current nursing practice.
9. **Professional Practice Evaluation:** The registered nurse evaluates one's own nursing practice in relation to professional practice standards and guidelines, relevant statutes, rules, and regulations.
10. **Collegiality:** The registered nurse interacts with and contributes to the professional development of peers and colleagues.
11. **Collaboration:** The registered nurse collaborates with patient, family, and others in the conduct of nursing practice.
12. **Ethics:** The registered nurse integrates ethical provisions in all areas of practice.
13. **Research:** The registered nurse integrates research findings into practice.
14. **Resource Utilization:** The registered nurse considers factors related to safety, effectiveness, cost, and impact on practice in the planning and delivery of nursing services.
15. **Leadership:** The registered nurse provides leadership in the professional practice setting and the profession.

Reprinted with permission from American Nurses Association: *Nursing: scope and standards of practice,* © 2004, Nursesbooks.org, Silver Spring, Md.

visible contributions of registered nursing using standard-based practice (ANA, 2004).

Standards of Practice. The six Standards of Practice describe a competent level of nursing care (Box 1-2). The levels of care are demonstrated by the critical thinking model known as the nursing process: assessment, diagnosis, outcomes identification and planning, implementation, and evaluation (ANA, 2004). The nursing process is the foundation of clinical decision making and includes all significant actions taken by nurses in providing care to clients (see Chapters 15 to 20).

Standards of Professional Performance. The nine ANA Standards of Professional Performance (Box 1-3) describe a competent level of behavior in the professional role (ANA, 2004). These standards provide objective guidelines for nurses to be accountable for their actions, their clients, and their peers. The standards provide a method to assure clients that they are receiving high-quality care, that the nurses know exactly what is necessary to provide nursing care, and that measures are in place to determine whether care meets the standards.

Code of Ethics. The **code of ethics** is the philosophical ideals of right and wrong that define the principles you will use to provide care to your clients. It is important for you to also incorporate your own values and ethics into your practice. As you incorporate these values, you explore what type of nurse you will be and how you will function within the discipline (Mathes, 2005). Ask yourself, how do your ethics, values, and practice compare with established standards? The ANA has a number of publications that address ethics and human rights in nursing. The *Code of Ethics for Nurses With Interpretive Statements* is a guide for carrying out nursing responsibilities that provide quality nursing care and provides for the ethical obligations of the profession (ANA, 2001). In addition, the ANA established the Center for Ethics and Human Rights to address the complex and ethical human rights issues confronting nursing (ANA, 2002). Chapter 22 gives several examples of specific statements of nursing's code of ethics and how nurses apply ethics in their everyday practice.

Nursing Education

To become a nurse you require a significant amount of formal education. The issue of standardization of nursing education and entry into practice remains a major controversy. In 1965 the ANA published a position paper on nursing education that emphasizes the role of education for the advancement of the science of the profession (ANA, 1965). Most nurses agree that nursing education is important to practice and that education needs to respond to changes in health care created by scientific and technological advances. There are various education preparations for the registered nurse. In addition, there is graduate nurse education and continuing and in-service education for practicing nurses.

Professional Registered Nurse Education

Currently in the United States the most frequent way to become a **registered nurse (RN)** is either through completion of an associate degree or baccalaureate degree program. Graduates of both programs are eligible to take the National Council Licensure Examination for Registered Nurses (NCLEX-RN®) to become registered nurses in the state in which they will practice.

The associate degree program in the United States is a 2-year program that is usually offered by a university or community college. This program focuses on the basic sciences and theoretical and clinical courses related to the practice of nursing.

The baccalaureate degree program usually includes 4 years of study in a college or university. The program focuses on the basic sciences and on theoretical and clinical courses, as well as courses in the social sciences, arts, and humanities to support nursing theory. In Canada the degree of Bachelor of Science in Nursing (BScN) or Bachelor in Nursing (BN) is equivalent to the degree of Bachelor of Science in Nursing (BSN) in the United States. The American Association of Colleges of Nursing (AACN) published the *Essentials of Baccalaureate Education for Professional Nursing: A Final Report* (1998). This document delineated essential knowledge, practice and values, attitudes, personal qualities, and professional behavior for the baccalaureate-prepared nurse and guides faculty on the structure and evaluation of the curriculum and the performance of the graduate (AACN, 1998).

The National League for Nursing Accreditation Council (NLNAC) published the *NLNAC Interpretive Guidelines*. This document identifies core competencies for the professional nurse and supports the Pew Health Commission and the Institute of Medicine's competencies for health professionals (NLNAC, 2005).

Graduate Education

After obtaining a baccalaureate degree in nursing, you can pursue graduate education leading to a master's or doctoral degree in any number of graduate fields, including nursing. A nurse completing a graduate program can receive a master's degree in nursing. The graduate degree provides the advanced clinician with strong skills in nursing science and theory with emphasis on the basic sciences and research-based clinical practice. A master's degree in nursing is valuable for the roles of nurse educator, nurse administrator, or advanced practice nurse.

Doctoral Preparation. Professional doctoral programs in nursing (DSN or DNSc) prepare graduates to apply research findings to clinical nursing. Other doctoral programs emphasize more basic research and theory and award the research-oriented Doctor of Philosophy (PhD) in nursing. Recently the American Association of Colleges of Nursing recommended the Doctor of Nursing Practice (DNP) as the terminal practice degree and required preparation for all advanced practice nurses by 2015 (Chase and Pruitt, 2005; Dracup and others, 2005). The DNP is a practice doctorate preparing advanced practice nurses, such as nurse practitioners and certified registered nurse anesthetists (Magyary and others, 2006).

The need for nurses with doctoral degrees is increasing. Expanding clinical roles, continuing demand for well-educated nursing faculty and new areas of nursing specialties, such as nursing informatics, are just a few reasons for increasing the number of doctorally prepared nurses. It is important to continue to do research in areas such as nursing theory, basic science, and clinical practice to expand nursing knowledge. Doctorally prepared nurses are needed to educate the beginning nurse and those seeking advanced academic and clinical preparation.

Continuing and In-Service Education

Nursing is a knowledge-based profession, and technological expertise and clinical decision making are qualities that our health care consumers demand and expect (Levett-Jones, 2005). Continuing education programs are one way to help you remain current in nursing skills, knowledge, and theory. **Continuing education** involves formal, organized educational programs offered by universities, hospitals, state nurses associations, professional nursing organizations, and educational and health care institutions. An example is a program on caring for older adults with dementia

offered by a university or a program on safe medication practices offered by a hospital. Continuing education updates your knowledge about the latest research and practice developments, helps you to specialize in a particular area of practice, and teaches you new skills and techniques (Levett-Jones, 2005).

In-service education programs are instruction or training provided by a health care agency or institution. An in-service program is held in the institution and is designed to increase the knowledge, skills, and competencies of nurses and other health care professionals employed by the institution. For example, a hospital might offer an in-service program to inform nurses about primary nursing before it is implemented at the hospital or a program on the newest safety syringes for administering parenteral medications.

Continuing and in-service education are important as you enter your practice, whether your practice setting focuses on the adult or child, the chronically or acutely ill, or the home or hospital. These programs help you to implement new knowledge and skills and gain information about newer roles in nursing. Ongoing education provides information about multiple career paths and opportunities.

Nursing Practice

You will have an opportunity to practice in a variety of settings, in many roles within those settings, and with other caregivers in other related health professions. Administrators in hospitals and other health care agencies and institutions guide the practice of nursing only in part. State and provincial Nurse Practice Acts establish specific legal regulations for practice, and professional organizations establish standards of practice as criteria for nursing care.

The ANA is concerned with legal aspects of nursing practice, public recognition of the significance of nursing practice to health care, and implications for nursing practice regarding trends in health care. Nursing protects, promotes, and optimizes our clients' health, prevents illness and injury, alleviates suffering through the diagnosis and treatment of human responses, and advocates for the care of our clients (ANA, 2003). This definition illustrates the consistent orientation of nurses to the provision of care to promote the well-being of their clients. Today the nursing profession remains committed to the care and nurturing of both healthy and ill people, individually or in groups and communities (ANA, 2003).

Nurse Practice Acts

In the United States, the State Boards of Nursing oversee Nurse Practice Acts (NPAs). NPAs regulate the scope of nursing practice and protect public health, safety, and welfare. This protection includes shielding the public from unqualified and unsafe nurses. Although each state defines for itself the scope of nursing practice, most have similar practice acts. The definition of nursing practice published by the ANA is representative of the scope of nursing practice as defined in most states. In the last decade, however, many states have revised their Nurse Practice Acts to reflect nursing's growing autonomy and the expanded roles of nurses in

---

✳ BOX 1-4 Benner: From Novice to Expert

Novice: Beginning nursing student, or any nurse entering a situation in which there is no previous level of experience, for example, an experienced operating room nurse chooses to now practice in home health. The learner learns via a specific set of rules or procedures, which are usually stepwise and linear.

Advanced Beginner: A nurse who has had some level of experience with the situation. This experience may only be observational in nature, but the nurse is able to identify meaningful aspects or principles of nursing care.

Competent: A nurse who has been in the same clinical position for 2 to 3 years. This nurse understands the organization and the specific care required by the type of clients, for example, surgical, oncology, or orthopedic clients. This nurse is a competent practitioner who is able to anticipate nursing care and establish long-range goals. In this phase, the nurse has usually had experience with all types of psychomotor skills required by this specific group of clients.

Proficient: A nurse with greater than 2 to 3 years of experience in the same clinical position. This nurse perceives a client's clinical situation as a whole, is able to assess an entire situation, and can readily transfer knowledge gained from multiple previous experiences to a situation. This nurse focuses on managing care as opposed to managing and performing skills.

Expert: A nurse with diverse experience who has an intuitive grasp of an existing or potential clinical problem. This nurse is able to zero in on the problem and focus on multiple dimensions of the situation. This nurse is skilled at identifying client-centered problems, as well as problems related to the health care system or perhaps the needs of the novice nurse.

Data from Benner P: *From novice to expert: excellence and power in clinical nursing practice,* Menlo Park, Calif, 1984, Addison-Wesley.

---

practice. For example, Nurse Practice Acts expanded their scope to include the minimum education, required certifications, and practice guidelines for advanced practice nursing, such as nurse practitioners and certified registered nurse anesthetists. A nurse practitioner must have a master's degree in an advanced nursing specialty and have current certification from an appropriate body, such as the American Nurses Credentialing Center or the National Certification Board for Pediatric Nurse Practitioners. The expansion of scope of practice includes skills unique to the advanced practice role, for example, advanced assessment, prescriptive authority for certain medications and diagnostic procedures, and some invasive procedures.

Licensure and Certification

Licensure. In the United States, RN candidates must pass the NCLEX-RN® the individual State Boards of Nursing administer. Regardless of educational preparation, the examination for RN licensure is exactly the same in every state in the United States. This provides a standardized minimum knowledge base for nurses.

Certification. Beyond the NCLEX-RN®, the nurse may choose to work toward certification in a specific area of nursing practice. Minimum practice requirements are set, based on the

certification the nurse is seeking. National nursing organizations, such as the ANA, have many types of certification for you to work toward, such as certification in medical surgical nursing or geriatric nursing. After passing the initial examination, you maintain your certification by ongoing continuing education and clinical or administrative practice.

Science and Art of Nursing Practice

Because nursing is both an art and a science, nursing practice requires a blend of the most current knowledge and practice standards with an insightful and humane approach to client care. Your clients' health care needs are multidimensional. Thus your care will reflect the needs and values of society and professional standards of care and performance, meet the needs of each client, and integrate evidence-based findings to provide the highest level of care. Although nursing has a specific body of knowledge, your socialization into the profession and practice are essential components of the discipline. Clinical expertise takes time and commitment. According to Benner (1984), an expert nurse passes through five levels of proficiency when acquiring and developing generalist or specialized nursing skills (Box 1-4).

Use the competencies of critical thinking to integrate information from the scientific and nursing knowledge bases, derive knowledge from past and present experiences, apply critical thinking attitudes to a clinical situation, and implement intellectual and professional standards (see Chapter 15). When you provide well thought out care with compassion and caring, you provide each of your clients the best of the science and art of nursing care (see Chapter 8).

Professional Responsibilities and Roles

As a nurse, you are responsible for obtaining and maintaining specific knowledge and skills for a variety of professional roles and responsibilities. In the past, a nurse's principal role was to provide care and comfort when completing specific nursing functions. However, changes in nursing have expanded the professional nursing role to include increased emphasis on health promotion and illness prevention, as well as concern for the client as a whole.

Autonomy and Accountability

Autonomy is an essential element of professional nursing. There are independent nursing interventions you will initiate without medical orders. For example, you implement coughing and deep breathing exercises for a new postoperative client. You actively collaborate with other health professionals to pursue the best treatment plan for a client. For example, you consult with a wound care specialist when your client has a complex wound that is difficult to heal. With increased autonomy comes greater responsibility and accountability. Accountability means that you are responsible, professionally and legally, for the type and quality of nursing care provided. You need to keep current and competent in nursing and scientific knowledge and technical skills. The nursing profession also regulates accountability through nursing audits and standards of practice.

Caregiver

As **caregiver,** you help the client regain health and a maximal level of independent function through the healing process. Healing involves more than achieving improved physical well-being. You need to meet all health care needs of the client, including measures to restore emotional, spiritual, and social well-being. As a caregiver, you help the client and family set goals and assist them with meeting these goals with minimal financial cost, time, and energy.

Advocate

As a **client advocate,** you protect your client's human and legal rights and provide assistance in asserting those rights if the need arises. For example, you may provide additional information to help a client decide whether or not to accept a treatment, or you find an interpreter to help family members communicate their concerns. You may sometimes need to defend clients' rights in a general way by speaking out against policies or actions that put clients in danger or conflict with their rights. In advocating for the client, you need to be aware of the client's religion and culture.

Educator

Through client education, you explain concepts and facts about health, demonstrate procedures such as self-care activities, reinforce learning or client behavior, and evaluate the client's progress in learning. Some of your client teaching is unplanned and informal. For example, during a casual conversation you respond to questions about a health issue, such as smoking cessation, immunizations, or lifestyle habits. Other teaching activities are planned and more formal, such as when you teach your client to self-administer insulin injections. You need to use teaching methods that match your client's capabilities and needs and incorporate other resources, such as the family, in teaching plans (see Chapter 25).

Communicator

Communication is central to the nurse-client relationship. The nurse-client relationship helps you to know your clients, their strengths and weaknesses, their needs, and their fears. Communication is essential for all nursing roles and activities. You will routinely communicate with clients and families, other nurses and health care professionals, resource persons, and the community. Without clear communication, it is impossible to give comfort and emotional support, give care effectively, make decisions with clients and families, protect clients from threats to well-being, coordinate and manage client care, assist the client in rehabilitation, or provide client education. The quality of communication is a critical factor in meeting the needs of individuals, families, and communities (see Chapter 24).

Manager

Today's health care environment is fast paced and complex; managers need to establish an environment for collaborative care to provide quality care and good client outcomes (Figure 1-1). A

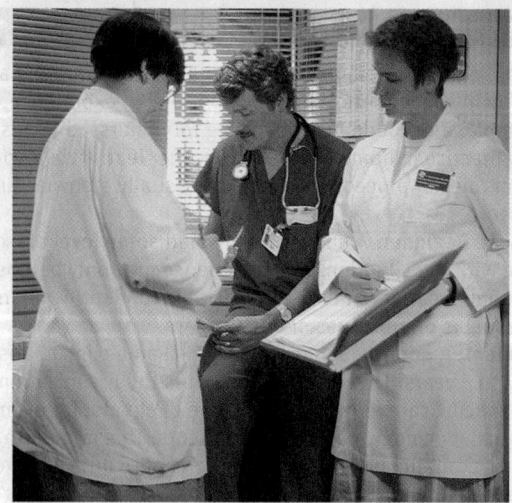

Figure 1-1 Collaboration facilitates quality care.

manager coordinates the activities of members of the nursing staff in delivering nursing care and has personnel, policy, and budgetary responsibility for a specific nursing unit or agency. The manager performs many activities, which may include helping to establish and evaluate performance goals for the unit, monitoring professional nursing standards of practice, recruiting and hiring new employees, determining the staff development and continuing education needs, and evaluating employees. A manager also establishes and implements quality improvement plans for the unit. For example, if the incidence of pressure ulcers increases, the manager implements a plan consisting of an in-service program on pressure ulcer risk assessment and a skin care protocol. Part of the plan also includes evaluation methods to determine the effectiveness of the quality improvement plan on pressure ulcer incidence.

Career Development

Innovations in health care, expanding health care systems and practice settings, and the increasing needs of clients have been a stimulus for new nursing roles. Today the majority of nurses practice in hospital settings, followed by community-based care, ambulatory care, and nursing homes/extended care settings.

Nursing provides an opportunity for you to commit to lifelong learning and career development in order to provide clients with the state-of-the-art care they need. Career roles are specific employment positions or paths. Because of increasing educational opportunities for nurses, the growth of nursing as a profession, and a greater concern for job enrichment, the nursing profession offers expanded roles and different kinds of career opportunities. Your career path is limitless. You will probably switch career roles more than once, moving from clinical practice to an administrative role and then to an educator position. Other examples of career roles include advanced practice nurses, nurse researchers, nurse risk managers, quality improvement nurses, consultants, and even business owners.

Clinician. Most nurses provide direct client care in an acute care setting. As health care returns to the home care setting, there are increased opportunities for you to provide direct care in the client's home as well as in a hospital setting. You will use the nursing process and critical thinking skills to provide care that is both restorative and curative. You will also educate clients and families to promote health maintenance and self-care. In collaboration with other health care team members, you focus your care on returning the client to his or her home and usual state of health.

In the hospital, you may choose to practice in a medical-surgical setting or concentrate on a specific area of practice, such as critical care or emergency care. Most specialty care areas require some experience as a medical-surgical nurse and additional continuing or in-service education. Many intensive care unit (ICU) and emergency department nurses are required to have certification in advanced cardiac life support and critical care, emergency nursing, or trauma nursing. Hospital-based nurses sometimes choose to practice in specialty areas such as transplantation, rehabilitation, or oncology. Larger medical centers offer more opportunity to concentrate practice in a single area.

Advanced Practice Nurses.
The **advanced practice nurse** (**APN**) is generally the most independently functioning nurse. An APN has a master's degree in nursing, advanced education in pharmacology and physical assessment, and certification and expertise in a specialized area of practice (ANA, 2002a). The APN works in primary, acute, or restorative care settings. The APN functions as a clinician, educator, case manager, consultant, and researcher within his or her area of practice to plan or improve the quality of nursing care for the client and family. For example, a nurse practitioner in a community clinic manages the health care of a group of clients by monitoring their chronic health problems and diagnosing and treating any new developing problems. *Advanced practice nurse* is an umbrella term for an advanced clinical nurse that includes nurse practitioners, clinical nurse specialists, certified registered nurse anesthetists, and nurse-midwives.

Clinical Nurse Specialist.
The **clinical nurse specialist** (**CNS**) is an APN who is an expert clinician in a specialized area of nursing practice. The specialty may be identified by a population (e.g., geriatrics), a setting (e.g., critical care), a disease specialty (e.g., diabetes), a type of care (e.g., rehab), or a type of problem (e.g., pain) (National Association of Clinical Nurse Specialists, 2008) CNS practice in a wide variety of settings. They function as clinicians, educators, consultants, and researchers to improve the quality of care to clients and family (Figure 1-2).

Nurse Practitioner.
The **nurse practitioner** provides health care to a group of clients, usually in an outpatient, ambulatory care, or community-based setting. Nurse practitioners provide care for clients with complex problems and provide a more holistic approach than physicians, attending to symptoms of non-pathological conditions, comfort, and comprehensiveness of care. A significant percentage of primary care visits by clients extend beyond the boundaries of medicine and demand the expertise of the nurse. The nurse practitioner is able to establish a collaborative provider-client relationship. A nurse practitioner may work with a specific group of clients or with clients of all ages and health care needs. The major nurse practitioner categories are acute care, adult, family, pediatric, women's, and geriatric. A nurse practitioner has the knowledge and skills necessary to detect and

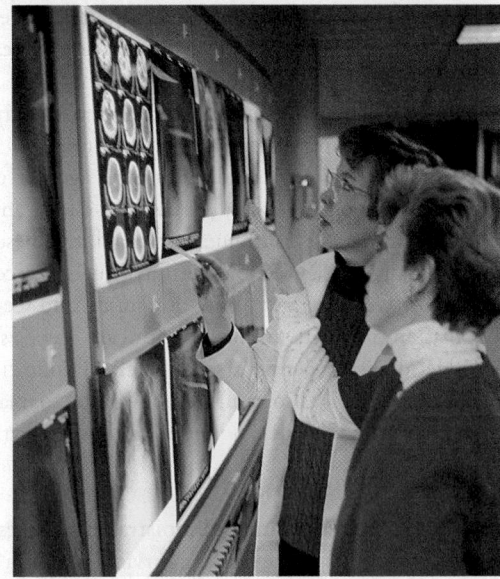

Figure 1-2 Nurse specialist consults on a difficult client case.

manage self-limiting acute and chronic stable medical conditions, such as asthma, diabetes mellitus, and hypertension.

Certified Nurse-Midwife.
A **certified nurse-midwife** (**CNM**) is an RN who is also educated in midwifery and is certified by the American College of Nurse-Midwives. The practice of nurse-midwifery involves providing independent care for women during normal pregnancy, labor, and delivery, as well as care for the newborn. It includes some gynecological services such as routine Papanicolaou (Pap) smears, family planning, and treatment for minor vaginal infections. A CNM practices with a health care agency that provides medical consultation, collaborative management, and referral.

Certified Registered Nurse Anesthetist.
A **certified registered nurse anesthetist** (**CRNA**) is an RN with advanced education in a nurse anesthesia accredited program. Nurse anesthetists provide surgical anesthesia under the guidance and supervision of an anesthesiologist, who is a physician with advanced knowledge of surgical anesthesia.

Nurse Educator.
A **nurse educator** works primarily in schools of nursing, staff development departments of health care agencies, and client education departments. Nurse educators need experience in clinical practice to provide them with practical skills and theoretical knowledge. A faculty member in a school of nursing educates students to become professional nurses. Nursing faculty members are responsible for teaching current nursing practice, trends, theory, and necessary skills in laboratories and clinical settings. Nurse educators in schools of nursing usually have graduate degrees in nursing and additional education. Many hold doctorate or advanced degrees in nursing, education, or administration, such as a master's degree in business administration (MBA). Generally they have a specific clinical, administrative, or research specialty and advanced clinical experience.

Nurse educators in staff development departments of health care institutions provide educational programs for nurses within their institution. These programs include orientation of new personnel, critical care nursing courses, assisting with clinical skill competency, safety training, and instruction about new equipment or procedures. These nursing educators often participate in the development of nursing policies and procedures.

The primary focus of the nurse educator in an agency's department of client education is to teach ill or disabled clients and their families how to self-manage their illness or disability. These nurse educators are usually specialized and certified, such as a certified diabetic educator (CDE) or an ostomy care nurse, and see only a specific population of clients. In most health care agencies, however, the budget does not permit a separate client education department. Therefore it is also your responsibility to plan and provide client and family education during hospitalization or clinic or home care visits.

Nurse Administrator.

A **nurse administrator** manages client care and the delivery of specific nursing services within a health care agency. Nursing administration begins with positions such as the assistant nurse manager. Experience and additional education sometimes lead to a middle-management position, such as nurse manager of a specific client care area or house supervisor, or to an upper-management position, such as assistant or associate director or director of nursing services.

Nurse manager positions usually require at least a baccalaureate degree in nursing, and director and nurse executive positions generally require a master's degree. Chief nurse executive and vice president positions in large health care organizations often require preparation at the doctoral level. Nurse administrators often have advanced degrees such as a master's degree in business administration (MBA), hospital administration (MHA), public health (MPH), or health service administration.

In today's health care organizations, directors may have responsibility for more than nursing personnel. Responsibilities often include a particular service or product line, such as medicine or cardiology, and include supportive functions and personnel such as medicine clinics, cardiac diagnostics, or outpatient services such as cardiac catheterization. In addition, the director is responsible for ancillary personnel such as cardiology technicians, respiratory therapists, social workers, and dietitians.

Vice presidents of nursing or chief nurse executives often have responsibilities for all clinical functions within the hospital. This may include all ancillary personnel who provide and support client care services. The nursing administrator needs to be skilled in business and management, as well as understand all aspects of nursing and client care. Functions of administrators include budgeting, staffing, strategic planning of programs and services, employee evaluation, and employee development (Marriner Toomey, 2004).

Nurse Researcher.

The **nurse researcher** investigates problems to improve nursing care and to further define and expand the scope of nursing practice (see Chapter 5). The nurse researcher often works in an academic setting, hospital, or independent professional or community service agency. The preferred educational requirement is a doctoral degree, with at least a master's degree in nursing.

Professional Nursing Organizations

A **professional organization** deals with issues of concern to those practicing in the profession. In North America the major professional nursing organizations are the **National League for Nursing (NLN)** and the ANA. The NLN advances excellence in nursing education to prepare nurses to meet the needs of a diverse population in a changing healthcare environment. The NLN (2007) sets standards for excellence and innovation in nursing education.

ANA's purpose is to improve standards of health and the availability of health care, to foster high standards for nursing, and to promote the professional development and general and economic welfare of nurses. The ANA is part of the **International Council of Nurses (ICN)**. The objectives of the ICN parallel those of the ANA: promoting national associations of nurses, improving standards of nursing practice, seeking a higher status for nurses, and providing an international power base for nurses.

The ANA is active in political, professional, and financial issues affecting health care and the nursing profession. ANA is a strong lobbyist in professional practice issues, such as limits of overtime hours. For example, ANA extensively lobbied state legislatures to restrict the length of overtime any one nurse's shift can be extended. When nurses' shifts last longer than 12 to 16 hours, both the client's and nurse's safety are at risk. There is an increased risk of treatment errors and nurse injury when the nurse's workday is extended.

Nursing students take part in organizations such as the National Student Nurses Association (NSNA) in the United States and the Canadian Student Nurses Association (CSNA) in Canada. These organizations consider issues of importance to nursing students, such as career development and preparation for licensing. NSNA often cooperates in activities and programs with the professional organizations.

Some professional organizations focus on specific areas such as critical care, nursing administration, nursing research, or nurse-midwifery. These organizations seek to improve the standards of practice, expand nursing roles, and foster the welfare of nurses within the specialty areas. In addition, professional organizations present educational programs and publish journals.

Future Trends in Nursing

Nursing is not a static, unchanging profession but is continuously growing and evolving as society changes, as health care emphases and methods change, as lifestyles change—and as nurses themselves change. To speak of nursing at all is to speak of nursing as it is at a given time, and in this sense, this chapter is about trends in nursing.

The current philosophies and definitions of nursing demonstrate the holistic trend in nursing—to address the whole person in all dimensions, in health and illness, and in interaction with the family and community. Nursing continues to draw on the social sciences and other fields as the focus of nursing care expands.

Expansion of Employment Opportunities

Nursing practice trends include a growing variety of employment settings in which you have an opportunity for greater independence, autonomy, and respect as a member of the health care team. Nursing roles continue to expand and develop, broadening the focus of nursing care. For example, you may find your interests focus on complementary and alternative medicine and look for a position in settings using alternative therapies (see Chapter 36). Or you might choose to practice in a free-standing birthing center. It is important to remember that the opportunities are limitless for caring, compassionate, and competent nursing care; there is an area of nursing for every interest.

Nursing's Public Perception

Consumers of health care are more informed than ever, and with the Internet, consumers have access to more health care and treatment information. Recently the media highlighted preventable medical errors, such as medication errors and surgical errors. Publications like *To Err Is Human* (Institute of Medicine [IOM], 2000) describes strategies for government, health care providers, industry, and consumers to reduce preventable medical errors. The safety section in this chapter (see p. 5), and Chapter 38 expand the discussion on client safety.

If you, or a friend or member of your family, have become ill or hospitalized or have visited an emergency department, you have received nursing care; as an ANA campaign noted, "Everybody needs a *Nurse.*" The Johnson and Johnson Foundation developed a compelling, attention-getting media campaign on the nursing profession. These media clips show nursing practice, and the nurses featured in the advertisements describe their satisfaction with the profession.

Nursing is a pivotal health care profession; as frontline health care providers, nurses practice in all health care settings and constitute the largest number of professionals. Nurses are essential to providing skilled, specialized, knowledgeable care; to improving the health status of the public; and to ensuring safe, effective quality care (ANA, 2002a). In addition, the American public rated nurses high in honesty and ethics in their professional role (Gallup Organization, 1999-2001).

Nursing's Impact on Politics and Health Policy

Political power or influence is known as the ability to influence or persuade an individual holding a government office to exert the power of that office to affect a desired outcome. Nurses' involvement in politics is receiving greater emphasis in nursing curricula, professional organizations, and health care settings. Professional nursing organizations have employed lobbyists to urge state legislatures and the U.S. Congress to improve the quality of health care.

The ANA works for the improvement of health standards and the availability of health care services for all people, fosters high standards of nursing, stimulates and promotes the professional development of nurses, and advances their economic and general welfare. The purposes are unrestricted by considerations of nationality, race, creed, lifestyle, color, gender, or age. The ANA employs RNs as lobbyists at the federal level. State nursing orga-

nizations also hire lobbyists and legislative specialists to work on state nursing issues and assist with federal efforts. Finally, lobbyists working on behalf of nursing are employed in Washington, DC, by professional organizations such as the American Federation of Teachers, NLN, American College of Nurse-Midwives, American Public Health Association, and AACN. These groups aim to remove financial barriers to health care, increase the quality of nursing care available, increase economic rewards to nurses, and expand professional nursing roles.

You can influence policy decisions at all governmental levels. One way to get involved is by participating in ANA's national efforts, such as *Nursing's Agenda for the Future: A Call to the Nation* (ANA, 2002a). This effort is critical to exerting nurses' influence early in the political process. If nurses become serious students of social needs, activists in influencing policy to meet those needs, and generous contributors of time and money to nursing organizations and to candidates working for universal good health care, then the future is bright indeed.

Political activism and commitment are a part of professionalism and are an important aspect of the delivery of health care. You need to view politics as a reality that includes the arts of influence, compromise, and social interaction. Nurses have been involved in a different sort of politics in schools of nursing and in health care settings when seeking additional resources, more self-direction, and accountability with authority. The skills you learn in such experiences can be transferred to the politics of health care policy making.

As long as nurses stay involved in health care policy and practice, misinformed outsiders cannot impose their will on nursing and nursing practice. Nonnursing groups, often led by other health care providers, make attempts to impose institutional licensure, mandatory continuing education, and curtailment of advanced nursing practice and try to place other limits on the nursing profession. Nursing has its own voice in decisions made in these and numerous other areas affecting the practice and quality of nursing care. Although nurses have often successfully prevented infringement on the profession's self-governance, the future of nursing requires that nurses individually and collectively seek a greater influence on health care policies affecting nursing practice.

Key Concepts

- Nursing responds to the health care needs of society, which are influenced by economic, social, and cultural variables of a specific era.
- Changes in society, such as increased technology, new demographic patterns, consumerism, health promotion, and the women's and human rights movements, lead to changes in nursing.
- Nursing definitions reflect changes in the practice of nursing and help bring about changes by identifying the domain of nursing practice and guiding research, practice, and education.
- Nursing standards provide the guidelines for implementing and evaluating nursing care.
- The multiple roles and functions of the nurse include caregiver, client advocate, manager, communicator, and educator.

- Specific career roles include caregiver, nurse educator, advanced practice nurse, administrator, and researcher.
- Professional nursing organizations deal with issues of concern to specialist groups within the nursing profession.
- Nurses are becoming more politically sophisticated and, as a result, are able to increase nursing's influence on health care policy and practice.

Critical Thinking Exercises

1. Observe various levels of nursing practice, such as a staff nurse, advanced practice nurse, and nurse educator. Identify similarities and differences in their roles and educational preparation.

2. Look at a local newspaper or local employment website and see what nursing employment opportunities exist in your community.

3. Outline some career objectives for yourself over the next 5 years. Obviously the first would be to complete your nursing program. But decide what you want to do as a professional nurse, and then outline strategies to achieve these goals.

NCLEX®-Style Review Questions

1. You practice using nursing's code of ethics for professional registered nurses. This code:
   1. Improves self–health care
   2. Protects the client from harm
   3. Ensures identical care to all clients
   4. Defines the principles by which nurses provide care to their clients

2. Lacey Conrad, an 18-year-old woman, is in the emergency department with fever and cough. The physician asks you to obtain her vital signs, auscultate her lung sounds, listen to her heart sounds, determine her level of comfort, and collect blood and sputum samples for analysis. Which standard of practice are you performing?
   1. Diagnosis
   2. Evaluation
   3. Assessment
   4. Implementation

3. Lacey Conrad remains in the emergency department and has developed wheezing and shortness of breath. The physician orders a medicated nebulizer treatment now and in 4 hours. Which standard of care are you performing?
   1. Planning
   2. Evaluation
   3. Assessment
   4. Implementation

4. You are caring for a client with end-stage lung disease. The client wants to go home on oxygen and be comfortable. The family wants the client to have a new surgical procedure. You explain the risk and benefits of the surgery to the family and discuss the client's wishes with the family. You are acting as the client's:
   1. Educator
   2. Advocate
   3. Caregiver
   4. Case manager

5. Evidence-based practice is defined as:
   1. Nursing care based on tradition
   2. Scholarly inquiry of nursing and biomedical research literature
   3. A problem-solving approach to clinical practice based on best practices
   4. Quality nursing care provided in an efficient and economically sound manner

6. The examination for RN licensure is exactly the same in every state in the United States. This examination:
   1. Guarantees safe nursing care for all clients
   2. Ensures standard nursing care for all clients
   3. Ensures that honest and ethical care is provided
   4. Provides a minimal standard of knowledge for practice

7. Contemporary nursing requires that the nurse possess knowledge and skills for a variety of professional roles and responsibilities. Which of the following are examples? (Choose all that apply.)
   1. Providing bedside care
   2. Autonomy and accountability
   3. Following health care provider orders
   4. Increased emphasis on health promotion and illness prevention

8. Advanced practice nurses generally:
   1. Function independently
   2. Function as unit directors
   3. Work in acute care settings
   4. Work in the university setting

2 | The Health Care Delivery System

✳ OBJECTIVES

Mastery of content in this chapter will enable the student to:

- Compare the various methods for financing health care.
- Explain the advantages and disadvantages of managed health care.
- Explain the relationship between population-based managed care and disease prevention.
- Discuss the types of settings that provide various health care services.
- Discuss the role of nurses in different health care delivery settings.
- Differentiate primary care from primary health care.
- Discuss the implications that changes in the health care system have on nursing.
- Discuss opportunities for nursing within the changing health care delivery system.

✳ MEDIA RESOURCES ✳ KEY TERMS

Companion CD
- NCLEX®-Style Review Questions
- Audio Glossary
- English/Spanish Glossary
- Interactive Learning Activities

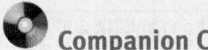 **Website**
- NCLEX®-Style Review Questions
- Audio Glossary
- English/Spanish Glossary
- Interactive Learning Activities
- WebLinks
- Audio Summaries

Acute care, p. 20
Adult day care centers, p. 26
Assisted living, p. 25
Capitation, p. 16
Case management, p. 21
Client-centered care, p. 28
Critical pathway, p. 21
Diagnosis-related groups (DRGs), p. 16
Discharge planning, p. 21
Extended care facility, p. 24
Globalization, p. 29
Home care, p. 23
Hospice, p. 26
Independent practice association (IPA), p. 18
Integrated delivery networks (IDNs), p. 17
Managed care, p. 17
Medicaid, p. 23
Medicare, p. 23

Minimum Data Set (MDS), p. 25
Nursing informatics, p. 29
Nursing-sensitive outcomes, p. 27
Primary care, p. 19
Professional standards review organizations (PSROs), p. 16
Prospective payment system (PPS), p. 16
Rehabilitation, p. 23
Resource utilization groups (RUGs), p. 16
Respite care, p. 26
Restorative care, p. 23
Skilled nursing facility, p. 24
Utilization review (UR) committees, p. 16
Vulnerable populations, p. 30
Work redesign, p. 21

The U.S. health care system is very complex and is constantly changing. A broad variety of services are available from different disciplines of health professionals, but gaining access to services is often very difficult for those with limited health care insurance. Those who are uninsured often seek heath care services when they are sicker, thus requiring more costly services. The continuing development of new technologies and medications, which shortens length of stay (LOS), also causes health care costs to increase. As a result, health care institutions are managing health care more as businesses than as service organizations. The challenge to health care providers is to reduce health care costs while maintaining high-quality care for clients. Health care providers are discharging clients sooner from hospitals, resulting in more clients needing nursing homes or home care. Often families provide care for their loved ones in the home setting. Nurses also face significant challenges to prevent gaps in health care across many health care settings so that individuals remain healthy and well within their own homes and communities.

Nursing is a caring discipline. Values of the nursing profession are rooted in helping persons to regain, maintain, or improve health; prevent illness; and find comfort and dignity. The health care system of the new millennium is less service oriented and more business oriented because of cost-saving initiatives. Nursing continues to lead the way in change and to retain values for client care while meeting the challenges of new roles and new responsibilities.

Health Care Regulation and Competition

Through most of the twentieth century, few incentives existed for controlling health care costs. There were few obstacles to stop a client from staying in the hospital. Insurers or third-party payers paid for whatever the health care providers ordered for a client's care and treatment. However, as health care costs continued to rise out of control, regulatory and competitive approaches had to control health care spending. The federal government, the biggest consumer of health care which paid for Medicare and Medicaid, created **professional standards review organizations (PSROs)** to review the quality, quantity, and cost of hospital care (Sultz and Young, 2004). Medicare-qualified hospitals had physician-supervised **utilization review (UR) committees** to review the admissions, diagnostic testing, and treatments provided by physicians who cared for clients receiving Medicare. The intent of URs was to identify and eliminate overuse of diagnostic and treatment services. Many hospitals added nursing case managers to meet the guidelines established by Medicare, Medicaid, and other payers.

One of the most significant factors that influenced payment for health care was the **prospective payment system (PPS)**. Established by Congress in 1983, the PPS eliminated cost-based reimbursement. Hospitals serving clients who received Medicare benefits were no longer able to charge whatever the client's care cost. Instead, the PPS grouped inpatient hospital services for Medicare clients into 468 **diagnosis-related groups (DRGs)**. Each group had a fixed reimbursement amount with adjustments based on

---

✳ BOX 2-1 Clinical Scenario of a DRG Example

Mr. Truman, a 70-year-old man, went to his cardiologist because he was experiencing chest pain and shortness of breath. He had cardiac surgery almost 10 years before but was beginning to have recurrent chest pain, even at rest. He has a history of hypertension and emphysema. Mr. Truman has smoked 1 pack of cigarettes a day for 54 years and has had difficulty following a low-fat diet. He has been counseled to quit smoking, but he has been unwilling to stop. He was hospitalized late in the afternoon on November 1 after having a chest x-ray examination and laboratory work at an outpatient testing center. He had an echocardiogram on November 2. Early in the morning on November 3, Mr. Truman had a cardiac catheterization, and the cardiologist determined he did not need surgery. He was discharged on the evening of November 3. During his hospital stay, Mr. Truman received usual and customary care and experienced no complications.

Principal diagnosis: Chest pain, not otherwise specified (NOS)
Secondary diagnosis: Hypertension NOS, hyperlipidemia, tobacco use disorder, other lung disease, history of past noncompliance
Principal procedure: Left heart cardiac catheterization
DRG assigned: DRG 125: Circulatory disorders except acute myocardial infarction with cardiac catheterization without complex diagnosis
Average length of stay: 2.8 days
Actual length of stay: 2 days
Expected payment from Medicare (based on 2.8 days): estimated national average hospital base rate × relative weight for DRG = $4430 × 1.146 = $5077
Actual hospital charges for Mr. Truman: $11,700
Actual reimbursement from Medicare: $5300
Loss for hospital: $6400

Data from Ingenix and others: *DRG expert,* ed 21, Clifton Park, NY, 2005, Thomson Delmar Learning.

DRG, Diagnosis-related group.

---

case severity, rural/urban/regional costs, and teaching costs. Hospitals receive a set dollar amount for each client based on the assigned DRG, regardless of the client's length of stay or use of services in the hospital. Box 2-1 provides a hypothetical scenario showing how the DRG PPS is used to determine reimbursement for a client's care. Most health care providers (e.g., health care networks or managed care organizations) now receive capitated payments. **Capitation** means the providers received a fixed amount per client or enrollee of a health care plan (Gosden and others, 2005). The aim of capitation is to build a payment plan for select diagnoses or surgical procedures that consists of the best standards of care, including essential diagnostic and treatment procedures at the lowest cost.

Capitation and prospective payment have influenced the way health care providers deliver care in all types of settings. Many now use DRGs in the rehabilitation setting, and **resource utilization groups (RUGs)** in long-term care. In all settings, health care providers make efforts to manage costs so that the organizations remain profitable. For example, when clients are hospitalized for lengthy periods, hospitals have to absorb the portion of costs that are not reimbursed. This simply adds more pressure to ensure that clients are managed effectively and discharged as soon as is reasonably possible. Soon after prospective payment began, hospitals started to increase discharge planning activities, and hospital lengths of stay began to shorten. Because clients are discharged home as soon as possible, home care agencies now provide complex technological care, including intravenous therapy, mechanical ventilation, and long-term parenteral nutrition.

The term **managed care** describes health care systems in which there is administrative control over primary health care services for a defined client population. The provider or health care system receives a predetermined capitated payment for each client enrolled in the program. In this case, the managed care organization assumes financial risk in addition to providing client care. The organization's focus of care shifts from individual illness care to concern for the health of its covered population. If people stay healthy, the cost of medical care declines. Systems of managed care focus on containing or reducing costs, increasing client satisfaction, and improving the health or functional status of the individual (Sultz and Young, 2004).

Although the goal of managed care is to increase access to health care while decreasing costs, health care spending continues to rise. The National Health Statistics Group reported that health care spending increased from $888 billion, or 13.4% of the Gross Domestic Product (GDP), in 1993 to $1.679 trillion, or 15.3% of the GDP, in 2003. Heffler and others (2005) project an increase to $3.586 trillion, or 18.7% of the GDP, in the year 2014. Some factors that increase health care spending include increases in health care wages and costs of prescription drugs, higher insurance premiums for employees, and increased consumers' demand for improved technology. Table 2-1 summarizes the most common types of health care insurance plans.

Emphasis on Population Wellness

The United States health care delivery system faces many issues such as rising cost of health care, increased access to services, a growing population, improved quality of outcomes, and threats of bioterrorism. As a result, the emphasis of the health care industry today is shifting from managing illness to managing health of a community and the environment.

The Health Services Pyramid developed by the Core Functions Project (U.S. Public Health Service, 1994/2000) serves as a model for improving the health care of U.S. citizens (Figure 2-1). The pyramid shows that population-based health care services provide the basis for preventive services. These services include primary, secondary, and tertiary health care (Box 2-2). Achievements in the lower tiers of the pyramid contribute to the improvement of health care delivered by the higher tiers. The emphasis on wellness, as well as the health of populations and the environment, has enhanced quality of life (Merzel and D'Afflitti, 2003). Americans have experienced an increase in life expectancy by 22 years over the past century, a 50% decrease in adult deaths related to coronary heart disease and stroke, and a 50% decrease in deaths of children (U.S. Department Health and Human Services, 2002). The improvement in mortality rates has been credited to advancements in sanitation and infectious diseases (e.g., water, sewage, immunization, and crowded living conditions); client teaching (e.g., dietary habits, decrease in tobacco use, and blood

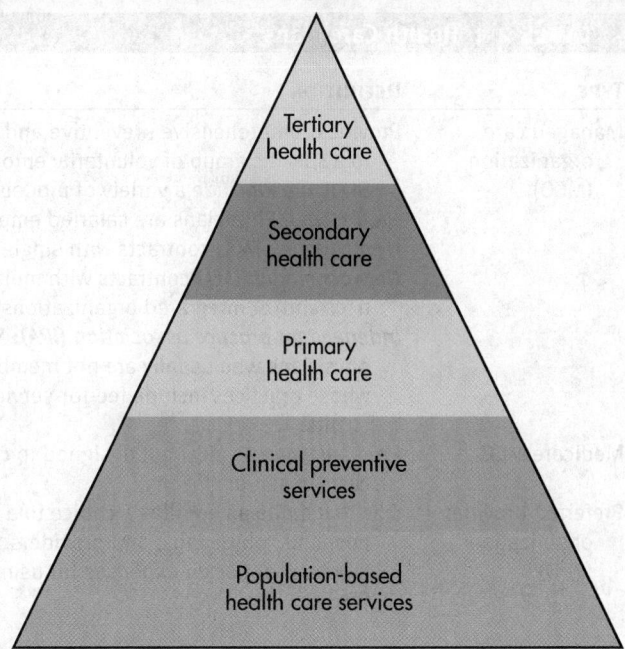

Figure 2-1 Health services pyramid. (U.S. Public Health Service: *The core functions project*, Washington, DC, 1994/update 2000, Office of Disease Prevention and Health Promotion. From Stanhope M, Lancaster J: *Community and public health nursing*, ed 6, St. Louis, 2004, Mosby.)

pressure control); and injury prevention programs (e.g., seat belt restraints, child seats, and helmet laws).

Health Care Settings and Services

Currently the U.S. health care system has six levels of care settings in which health care providers offer services. Health care providers offer disease prevention, health promotion, and primary, secondary, and tertiary health care services in a variety of heath care settings. The health care settings or levels of health care are preventive, primary, secondary, tertiary, restorative, and continuing care settings. Larger health care systems have developed **integrated delivery networks (IDNs)** that include a set of providers and services organized to deliver a continuum of care to a population of clients at a capitated cost in a particular setting (Oodyke, 2004). An integrated system reduces duplication of services across levels or settings of care to ensure that clients receive care in the most appropriate settings.

Changes unique to each setting of care have developed because of health care reform. For example, many health care providers now place greater emphasis on wellness, directing more resources toward primary and preventive care services. Nurses are especially important as client advocates in maintaining continuity of care throughout the levels of care. Nurses have the opportunity to provide leadership to communities and health care systems (Box 2-3). The ability to find strategies that better address client needs at all levels of care is critical to the success of improving the health care delivery system.

✳ TABLE 2-1 Health Care Plans

TYPE	DEFINITION	CHARACTERISTICS
Managed care organization (MCO)	Provides comprehensive preventive and treatment services to a specific group of voluntarily enrolled persons. Structures include a variety of models: *Staff model:* Physicians are salaried employees of the MCO. *Group model:* MCO contracts with single group practice *Network model:* MCO contracts with multiple group practices and/or integrated organizations. *Independent practice association (IPA):* MCO contracts with physicians who usually are not members of groups and whose practices include fee-for-service and capitated clients.	Focus on health maintenance, primary care. All care provided by a primary care physician. Referral needed for access to specialist and hospitalization.
Medicare MCO	Program same as MCO but designed to cover health care costs of senior citizens.	Premium generally less than supplemental plans.
Preferred provider organization (PPO)	One that limits an enrollee's choice to a list of "preferred" hospitals, physicians, and providers. An enrollee pays more out-of-pocket expenses for using a provider not on the list.	Contractual agreement exists between a set of providers and one or more purchasers (self-insured employers or insurance plans). Comprehensive health services at a discount to companies under contract. Focus on health maintenance.
Exclusive provider organization (EPO)	One that limits an enrollee's choice to providers belonging to one organization. Sometimes able to use outside providers at additional expense.	Limited contractual agreement. Less access to select specialists.
Medicare	A federally administered program by the Commonwealth Fund or the Centers for Medicare and Medicaid Services (CMS); a financially funded national health insurance program in the United States for people 65 years and older. Part A provides basic protection for medical, surgical, and psychiatric care costs based on diagnosis-related groups (DRGs). Part B is a voluntary medical insurance; covers physician and certain outpatient services. Part C is a managed care provision that provides a choice of three insurance plans. Part D is a Prescription Drug Improvement (Berkowitz, 2005-2006).	Payment for plan deducted from monthly individual Social Security check. Covers services of nurse practitioners. Does not pay full cost of certain services. Supplemental insurance encouraged.
Medicaid	Federally funded, state-operated program that provides: (1) health insurance to low-income families; (2) health assistance to low-income people with long-term care (LTC) disabilities; and (3) supplemental coverage and LTC assistance to older adults and Medicare beneficiaries in nursing homes. Individual states determine eligibility and benefits.	Finances a large portion of maternal and child care for the poor. Reimburses for nurse-midwifery and other advanced practice nurses (varies by state). Reimburses nursing home funding.
Private insurance	Traditional fee-for-service plan. Payment computed after client receives services on basis of number of services used.	Policies typically expensive. Most policies have deductibles that clients have to meet before insurance pays.
Long-term care insurance	Supplemental insurance for coverage of long-term care services. Policies provide a set amount of dollars for an unlimited time or for as little as 2 years.	Very expensive. Good policy has a minimum waiting period for eligibility; payment for skilled nursing, intermediate, or custodial care and home care.

✳ BOX 2-2   Common Health Care Definitions

Disease prevention: Activities that protect people from becoming ill because of actual or potential health threats

Health promotion: Activities that develop human attitudes and behaviors to maintain or enhance well-being

Managed care organization: Organization that provides or contracts for specific health care services (e.g., hospital care, prescription medications)

Primary care: Provision of integrated, accessible health care services by health care professionals who address a majority of personal health care needs, develop partnerships with clients, and care for families and communities

Primary health care: Combination of primary and public health care that is accessible to individuals and families in a community and provided at an affordable cost

Primary prevention: Health-promoting behaviors or activities that reduce the occurrence of an illness

Public health: Community and interdisciplinary care aimed at preventing disease and promoting health

Secondary prevention: Early diagnosis and treatment of illness (e.g., screening for hypertension)

Tertiary prevention: Care that prevents further progression of disease

Data from Stanhope M, Lancaster J: *Community and public health nursing,* ed 6, St. Louis, 2004, Mosby.

✳ BOX 2-3   Examples of Health Care Services

Primary Care (Health Promotion)
Prenatal care
Well-baby care
Nutrition counseling
Family planning
Exercise classes

Preventive Care
Blood pressure and cancer screening
Immunizations
Poison control information
Mental health counseling and crisis prevention
Community legislation (seat belts, air bags, bike helmets)

Secondary Acute Care
Emergency care
Acute medical-surgical care
Radiological procedures

Tertiary Care
Intensive care
Subacute care

Restorative Care
Cardiovascular and pulmonary rehabilitation
Sports medicine
Spinal cord injury programs
Home care

Continuing Care
Assisted living
Psychiatric and older adult day care

Preventive and Primary Health Care

In settings where clients receive preventive and **primary care,** such as schools, physician offices, occupational health clinics, and nursing centers, health promotion is a major theme (Table 2-2). Health promotion is a key to quality health care. Successful programs help clients acquire healthier lifestyles and achieve a decent standard of living. The focus of health promotion is to keep people healthy through personal hygiene, good nutrition, clean living environments, regular exercise, rest, and the adoption of positive health attitudes. Health promotion programs lower the overall costs of health care by reducing the incidence of disease, minimizing complications, and thus reducing the need to use more expensive health care resources. In contrast, preventive care is more disease oriented and focused on reducing and controlling risk factors for disease through activities such as immunization and occupational health programs.

Primary care focuses on health services provided on an individual basis, whereas *primary health care* focuses on improved health outcomes for an entire population. Primary health care includes primary care as well as health education, proper nutrition, maternal/child health care, family planning, immunizations, and control of diseases. The primary health care model (Figure 2-2) requires collaboration between health professionals and community members. This model emphasizes health promotion, the development of health polices, and the prevention of diseases within communities. The parts of the model are linked with each other and affect each other either positively or negatively. Success-

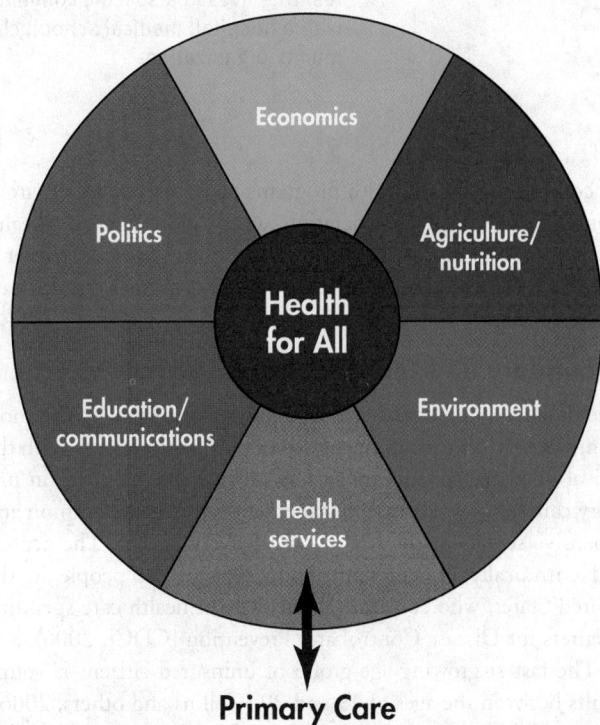

Figure 2-2 Primary health care model: a multisectoral or intersectoral approach. (© 1996 by P. Hatcher, J. Shoultz, W. Patrick; from Shoultz J, Hatcher PA: Looking beyond primary care to primary health care: an approach to community-based action, *Nurs Outlook* 45[1]:23, 1997.)

✴ TABLE 2-2 Preventive and Primary Care Services

TYPE OF SERVICE	PURPOSE	AVAILABLE PROGRAMS/SERVICES
School health	Comprehensive programs that include health promotion principles throughout a school's curriculum. Emphasizes program management, interdisciplinary collaboration, and community health principles.	Positive life skills Nutritional planning Health screening Counseling Communicable disease prevention Crisis intervention
Occupational health	A comprehensive program designed for health promotion and accident or illness prevention. Aim is to increase worker productivity, decrease absenteeism, and reduce use of expensive medical care.	Environmental surveillance Physical assessment Health screening Health education Communicable disease control Counseling
Physicians' offices	Provide primary health care (diagnosis and treatment). Many focus on health promotion practices. Nurse practitioners often partner with a physician in managing client population.	Routine physical examination Health screening Diagnostics Treatment of acute and chronic ailments
Nursing centers	Nurse-managed clinics provide nursing services with a focus on health promotion and health education, chronic disease assessment management, and support for self-care and caregivers.	Day care Health risk appraisal Wellness counseling Employment readiness Acute and chronic care management
Block and parish nursing	Nurses living within a neighborhood provide services to older clients or those unable to leave their home. Fills in gaps not available in traditional health care system.	Running errands Transportation Respite care Homemaker aides Spiritual health
Community centers	Outpatient clinics that provide primary care to a specific client population (e.g., well-baby, mental health, diabetes) that lives in a specific community. Often associated with a hospital, medical school, church, or other community organization.	Physical assessment Health screening Disease management Health education Counseling

ful community-based health programs take societal and environmental factors into consideration when addressing the health needs of communities (Merzel and D'Afflitti, 2003). Chapter 3 provides a more comprehensive discussion of primary health care in the community.

Secondary and Tertiary Care

The diagnosis and treatment of illness are traditionally the most common services used in the health care delivery system. With the arrival of managed care, many now deliver these services in primary care settings. Disease management is the most common and expensive service of the health care delivery system. The acutely and chronically ill represent about 20% of the people in the United States, who consume about 80% of health care spending (Centers for Disease Control and Prevention [CDC], 2006).

The fastest growing age-group of uninsured citizens is young adults between the ages of 19 and 29 (Collins and others, 2006). Young adults turning 19 years of age from low-income families are especially in danger of being uninsured due to the inability to attend college and find employment with health care benefits. Coverage for young adults is important for various reasons. This age-group has a high incidence of obesity, pregnancy, and HIV. People in this age-group are also less likely to see a doctor on a regular basis and to follow up on a problem if they do not have health insurance.

People who do not have health care insurance often wait longer before presenting for treatment; thus they are usually sicker and need more health care. As a result, secondary and tertiary care (also called **acute care**) is more costly. With the arrival of more advanced technology and managed care, physicians now perform simple surgeries in office surgical suites instead of in the hospital. Cost to the client is lower in the office because the general overhead cost of the facility is lower.

Hospitals. Hospital emergency departments, urgent care centers, critical care units, and inpatient medical-surgical units are sites that provide secondary and tertiary levels of care. Nurses in these settings communicate closely with all members of the health care team. The ability to think critically and to identify clients' changing problems quickly and accurately is essential. Planning and coordination of care are necessary to deliver services in a competent and timely manner. Nurses need to apply evidence-based information when selecting nursing interventions to improve client outcomes. Nurses continually include the client in the evaluation of care and modify interventions appropriately until the best outcomes occur.

Satisfaction with health care services is important to acute care organizations. Client satisfaction becomes a priority in a busy, stressful location such as the inpatient nursing unit. Clients expect to receive courteous and respectful treatment, and they want to be involved in daily care decisions. Acute care nurses need to be responsive to learning client needs and expectations early to form effective partnerships that ultimately enhance the level of nursing care given.

Because of managed care, the number of days clients can expect to be hospitalized is limited based on their DRGs upon admission. Therefore nurses need to use resources efficiently to help clients successfully recover and return home (Box 2-4). To contain costs, many hospitals have redesigned nursing units. Because of **work redesign,** more services are available on nursing units, thus minimizing the need to transfer and transport clients across multiple diagnostic and treatment areas.

Hospitalized clients are acutely ill and need comprehensive and specialized tertiary health care. The services provided by hospitals vary considerably. Some small rural hospitals offer only limited emergency and diagnostic services, as well as general inpatient services. In comparison, large urban medical centers offer comprehensive, up-to-date diagnostic services, trauma and emergency care, surgical intervention, intensive care units, inpatient services, and rehabilitation facilities. Larger hospitals also offer professional staff from a variety of specialties such as social service, respiratory therapy, physical and occupational therapy, and speech therapy. The focus in hospitals is to provide the highest quality of care possible so that clients are discharged early but safely to the home or another health care facility that will adequately manage remaining health care needs.

Because of the need to contain costs, many hospitals use a **case management** model of care. In this model, a case manager, who is usually a nurse or a social worker, coordinates the efforts of all disciplines to achieve the most efficient and appropriate plan of care for the client. Case management focuses particularly on discharge planning. The case manager advises nursing staff on specific nursing care issues, coordinates the referral of clients to services provided by other disciplines, ensures that staff implements client education, and monitors the client's progress through discharge. In many settings, a case manager continues caring for clients after discharge from acute care facilities.

Discharge planning begins the moment a client is admitted to a health care facility. Nurses play a large role in **discharge planning** in the hospital where continuity of care is important. To achieve continuity of care, nurses use critical thinking skills and apply the nursing process (see Unit III). To anticipate and identify the client's needs, nurses work with all members of the multidisciplinary health care team. Nurses take the lead to develop a plan of care that moves the client from the hospital to another level of health care, such as the client's home or a nursing home. Discharge planning is a centralized, coordinated, multidisciplinary process that ensures that the client has a plan for continuing care after leaving a health care agency.

One tool nurses use in an acute care setting to coordinate client care is a critical pathway. A **critical pathway** is a multidisciplinary treatment plan that outlines the treatments or interventions clients need to have while in the hospital for a specific condition or procedure. For example, there are critical pathways

---

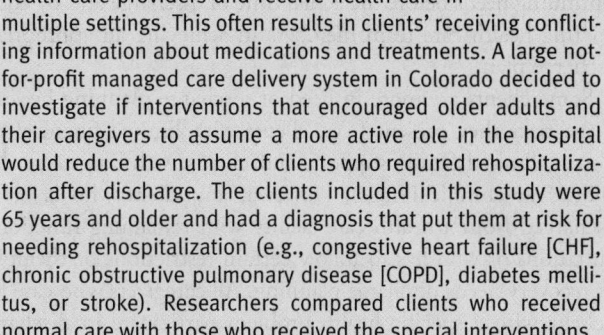

✳ BOX 2-4 **EVIDENCE-BASED PRACTICE**

Preparing Clients and Caregivers to Participate in Care

Evidence Summary

Older adults often experience fragmentation of health care because they see many different health care providers and receive health care in multiple settings. This often results in clients' receiving conflicting information about medications and treatments. A large not-for-profit managed care delivery system in Colorado decided to investigate if interventions that encouraged older adults and their caregivers to assume a more active role in the hospital would reduce the number of clients who required rehospitalization after discharge. The clients included in this study were 65 years and older and had a diagnosis that put them at risk for needing rehospitalization (e.g., congestive heart failure [CHF], chronic obstructive pulmonary disease [COPD], diabetes mellitus, or stroke). Researchers compared clients who received normal care with those who received the special interventions.

A transition coach who was a nurse practitioner (NP) instructed and provided interventions for the client. The NP encouraged self-management of the illness and directed communication between the client and other health care providers during and after the hospital stay. The NP maintained a personal health record for each client. After discharge from the hospital, the transition coach called or visited clients who went to a skilled nursing facility at least once a week. For the client who was discharged to home, the transition coach scheduled a home visit within 24 to 72 hours of discharge. During the home visits the NP reviewed medications with the client and reconciled discrepancies. The transition coaches provided encouragement and support to facilitate management of the illness at home. The coaches also provided medication education and information on warning symptoms that indicated a need to call a health care provider.

The clients who received the client-centered interventions were half as likely to require further hospitalizations for their illnesses. Clients in this group also reported a high level of confidence in getting information needed to manage their illnesses. They felt more comfortable communicating with their health care provider and better understood their medications.

Application to Nursing Practice

The results from this study support the benefits associated with following clients closely in all levels of health care. Although the managed care organization had to employ an NP, the reduction in hospitalizations probably outweighed the costs associated with this program. Nurses at the bedside are often able to help clients avoid rehospitalizations by providing education about disease management and medications. Nurses also support and help clients maintain open, honest communication with all their health care providers. Empowering clients to better manage their illnesses will help reduce health care costs and enhance client satisfaction.

Coleman EA and others: Preparing patients and caregivers to participate in care delivered across settings: the care transitions intervention, *J Am Geriatr Soc* 52(11):1817, 2004.

for clients who have pneumonia, or congestive heart failure or undergo cardiac catheterization. The critical pathway helps ensure collaboration among different members of the health care team, which enables the client to be discharged in an appropriate length of time.

Because clients leave hospitals as soon as their physical conditions allow, they often have continuing health care needs when they go home or to another facility. For example, a surgical client requires wound care at home after surgery. A client who has had a stroke still requires ambulation training. Clients and families worry about how they will care for unmet needs and manage over the long term. Nurses help by anticipating and identifying clients' continuing needs before the actual time of discharge and by coordinating health care team members in achieving an appropriate discharge plan.

Some clients are more in need of discharge planning because of the risks they present (e.g., clients with limited financial resources, limited family support, and clients with long-term disabilities or chronic illness). However, any client who is being discharged from a health care facility with remaining functional limitations or who has to follow certain restrictions or therapies for recovery needs discharge planning. All caregivers who care for a client with a specific health problem participate in discharge planning. The process is truly multidisciplinary. For example, the client with diabetes visiting a diabetes management center requires the group effort of a diabetes nurse educator, dietitian, and physician to ensure that the client returns home with the right information to manage the condition. A client who has experienced a stroke will not be discharged from a hospital until the team has established plans with physical and occupational therapists to begin a program of rehabilitation.

Effective discharge planning often requires referrals to various health care disciplines. In many agencies a health care provider's order is necessary for a referral, especially when planning specific therapies (e.g., physical therapy). It is best to have clients and families participate in referral processes so that they are involved early in any necessary decision making. Some tips on making the referral process successful include the following:

- Make a referral as soon as possible.
- Inform the care provider receiving the referral of as much information about the client as possible. This avoids duplication of effort and exclusion of important information.
- Involve the client and family in the referral process, including selecting the necessary referral. Explain the service the referral will provide, the reason for the referral, and what to expect from the referral's services.
- Determine what the referral discipline recommends for the client's care, and include this in the treatment plan as soon as possible.

The nurse provides resources to meet a client's limitations to improve long-term outcomes. Discharge planning depends on comprehensive client and family education (see Chapter 25). Clients need to know what to do when they get home, how to do it, and what to observe for when problems develop. Clients require the following instruction before they leave health care facilities:

- Safe and effective use of medications and medical equipment
- Instruction in potential food-drug interactions and counseling on nutrition and modified diets
- Rehabilitation techniques to support adaptation to and/or functional independence in the environment

- Access to available and appropriate community resources
- When and how to obtain further treatment
- The client's and family's responsibilities in the client's ongoing health care needs and the knowledge and skills needed to carry out those responsibilities

Intensive Care. An intensive care unit (ICU) or critical care unit is a hospital unit in which clients receive close monitoring and intensive medical care. ICUs have advanced technologies, such as computerized cardiac monitors and mechanical ventilators. Although many of these devices are on regular nursing units, the clients hospitalized within ICUs are monitored and maintained on multiple devices. Nursing and medical staff within an ICU have special knowledge about critical care principles and techniques. An ICU is the most expensive delivery site for medical care because each nurse usually cares for only one or two clients at a time and because of all the treatments and procedures the clients in the ICU require.

Psychiatric Facilities. Clients who suffer emotional and behavioral problems such as depression, violent behavior, and eating disorders often require special counseling and treatment in psychiatric facilities. Located in hospitals, independent outpatient clinics, or private mental health hospitals, psychiatric facilities offer inpatient and outpatient services, depending on the seriousness of the problem. Clients enter these facilities voluntarily or involuntarily. Hospitalization involves relatively short stays with the purpose of stabilizing clients before transfer to outpatient treatment centers. Clients with psychiatric problems receive a comprehensive multidisciplinary treatment plan that involves them and their families. Medicine, nursing, social work, and activity therapy work together to develop a plan of care that enables clients to return to functional states within the community. At discharge from inpatient facilities, clients usually receive a referral for follow-up care at clinics or with counselors.

Rural Hospitals. Access to health care in rural areas has been a serious problem. Most rural hospitals have experienced a severe shortage of primary care providers. Many have closed because of economic failure. In 1989 the Omnibus Budget Reconciliation Act (OBRA) directed the U.S. Department of Health and Human Services (USDHHS) to create a new health care organization, the rural primary care hospital (RPCH). An RPCH provides 24-hour emergency care, with no more than six inpatient beds for providing temporary care for 72 hours or less to clients needing stabilization before transfer to a larger hospital. Physicians, nurse practitioners, or physician assistants staff the RPCH. The RPCH provides inpatient care to acutely ill or injured persons before transferring them to better-equipped facilities. Basic radiological and laboratory services are also available.

With health care reform, more big-city health care systems are branching out and establishing connections or mergers with rural hospitals. The rural hospitals provide a referral base to the larger tertiary care medical centers. Nurses who work in rural hospitals or clinics often function independently in the absence of a physician. Competence in physical assessment, clinical decision making, and emergency care are essential. Advanced practice nurses (e.g., nurse practitioners and clinical nurse specialists) use medical protocols and establish collaborative agreements with staff physicians.

Restorative Care

Clients recovering from an acute or chronic illness or disability often require additional services to return to their previous level of function or reach a new level of function limited by their illness or disability. The goal of **restorative care** is to help individuals regain maximal functional status and to enhance quality of life through promotion of independence and self-care. With the emphasis on early discharge from hospitals, clients usually require some level of restorative care. For example, some surgical clients require ongoing wound care and activity and exercise management until they have recovered enough to independently resume normal activities of daily living.

The intensity of care has increased in restorative care settings, because clients leave hospitals earlier. Clients receive intravenous fluids (see Chapter 41), enteral nutrition (see Chapter 44), and pain control (see Chapter 43) in a home or rehabilitation setting. The restorative health care team is an interdisciplinary group of health professionals that includes the client and family or significant others. In restorative settings, nurses recognize that success is dependent on effective and early collaboration with clients and their families. Clients and families require a clear understanding of goals for physical recovery, the rationale for any physical limitations, and the purpose and potential risks associated with therapies. Clients and families are more likely to follow treatment plans and achieve optimal functioning when they are involved in restorative care.

Home Health Care (Home Care). **Home care** is the provision of medically related professional and paraprofessional services and equipment to clients and families in their homes for health maintenance, education, illness prevention, diagnosis and treatment of disease, palliation, and rehabilitation (Box 2-5). Nursing is one service most clients use in home care. However, home care sometimes also includes medical and social services; physical, occupational, speech, and respiratory therapy; and nutritional therapy. These services usually occur once or twice a day, up to 7 days a week. A home care service also coordinates the access to and delivery of home health equipment, or durable medical equipment (DME), which is any medical product adapted for home use.

Home care agencies provide almost every type of health care service in the client's home. Health promotion and education are traditionally the primary objectives of home care, yet at present, most clients receive home care because they have a need for nursing or medical care. The focus is on client and family independence. Nurses address recovery and stabilization of illness in the home and identify problems related to lifestyle, safety, environment, family dynamics, and health care practices.

Approved home care agencies usually receive reimbursement for services from the government (such as **Medicare** and **Medicaid** in the United States), private insurance, and private pay. The government has strict regulations that govern reimbursement for home care services. An agency cannot simply charge whatever it

---

✳ BOX 2-5 Home Care Services

Wound Care
Sterile dressing changes, debridement, irrigations, packing, and instructing clients and families in wound care techniques

Respiratory Care
Oxygen therapy, mechanical ventilation, suctioning, and care of tracheostomies

Vital Signs
Monitoring blood pressure and cardiopulmonary status; instructing clients and families in vital sign measurement

Elimination
Ostomy care, appliance application, skin care, and irrigation; insertion of urinary catheters, irrigation, and instructing families in catheter management; home dialysis

Nutrition
Administration of tube feedings and enteral feedings; assessment of nutrition and hydration status; instructing clients and families in tube feedings

Rehabilitation
Ambulation training, use of assistive devices, range-of-motion exercises, and instructing clients and families in transfer techniques

Medications
Monitoring compliance; administering injections; and instructing clients and families in drug information, medication preparation, and steps to take in the event of side effects

Intravenous Therapy
Administration of blood products, analgesic and chemotherapeutic agents, and long-term hydration; instructing clients and families in use of intravenous devices, steps to take in the event of disconnection of accidental fluid infusion, and side effects

Laboratory Studies
Blood glucose monitoring (including client and family instruction) and drawing blood for specific diagnostic purposes

---

wants for a service and expect to receive full reimbursement. Government programs set the cost of reimbursement of most professional services.

Nurses in home care provide individualized care. They have a caseload and assist clients in adapting to permanent or temporary physical limitations so they are able to assume a more normal daily home routine. Home care requires a strong knowledge base in many areas, such as family dynamics (see Chapter 10), cultural practices (see Chapter 9), spiritual values (see Chapter 29), and communication principles (see Chapter 24).

Rehabilitation. **Rehabilitation** restores a person to the fullest physical, mental, social, vocational, and economic potential possible (Clemen-Stone and others, 2002). Clients require rehabilitation after a physical or mental illness, injury, or chemical addiction. Specialized rehabilitation services, such as cardiovascular, neurological, musculoskeletal, and pulmonary rehabilitation programs, help clients and families adjust to necessary changes in lifestyle and learn to function with the limitations of their disease. Drug rehabilitation centers help clients become free from drug dependence and return to the community.

Rehabilitation services include physical, occupational, and speech therapy and social services. Ideally rehabilitation begins the moment a client enters a health care setting for treatment. For example, some orthopedic programs now have clients perform physical therapy exercises before major joint repair to enhance their recovery postoperatively. Initially rehabilitation usually focuses on the prevention of complications related to the illness or injury. As the condition stabilizes, rehabilitation helps to maximize the client's functioning and level of independence.

Rehabilitation occurs in many health care settings, including special rehabilitation agencies, outpatient settings, and the home. Frequently clients needing long-term rehabilitation (e.g., clients who have had strokes and spinal cord injuries) have severe disabilities affecting their ability to carry out the activities of daily living. When rehabilitation services occur in outpatient settings, clients receive treatment at specified times during the week but remain at home the rest of the time. Health care providers apply specific rehabilitation strategies to the home environment so that clients will achieve the highest levels of function and independence. Nurses and other members of the health care team visit homes and help clients and families learn to adapt to illness or injury.

Extended Care Facilities.

An **extended care facility** provides intermediate medical, nursing, or custodial care for clients recovering from acute illness or clients with chronic illnesses or disabilities. Extended care facilities include intermediate care and skilled nursing facilities. Some include long-term care and assisted living facilities. At one point, extended care facilities primarily cared for older adults. However, because hospitals discharge their clients sooner, there is a greater need for intermediate care settings for clients of all ages. For example, health care providers transfer a young client who has experienced a traumatic brain injury resulting from a car accident to an extended care facility for rehabilitative or supportive care until discharge to the home becomes a safe option. The growth of extended care facilities will increase as the number of older adults grows.

An intermediate care or **skilled nursing facility** offers skilled care from a licensed nursing staff. This often includes administration of intravenous fluids, wound care, long-term ventilator management, and physical rehabilitation. Clients receive extensive supportive care until they are able to move back into the community or into residential care. Extended care facilities provide around-the-clock nursing coverage. Nurses who work in a skilled nursing facility need nursing expertise similar to that of nurses working in acute care inpatient settings along with a background in gerontological nursing principles (see Chapter 14).

Continuing Care

Continuing care describes a variety of health, personal, and social services provided over a prolonged period. These services are for persons who are disabled, who never were functionally independent, or who suffer a terminal disease. The need for continuing health care services is growing in the United States. People are living longer, and many of those with continuing health care needs have no immediate family members to care for them. A decline in the number of children families choose to have, the aging of care providers, and the increasing rates of divorce and remarriage com-

---

✳ **BOX 2-6**   **FOCUS ON OLDER ADULTS**

Meeting Holistic Needs in the Health Care Delivery System

Enhancing Access to Care
- Refer older adult clients to parish nurses for close monitoring and early identification of problems.
- Provide health counseling to help clients acknowledge their need for help and to work through fears associated with health care (e.g., costs, life changes, loss of autonomy).

Education Needs
- Thoroughly assess clients' learning needs.
- Provide education to older adult clients about management of chronic illnesses and symptoms that require assistance from a health care provider.

Advocacy
- Make appropriate referrals to optimize independence; older adult clients often need help with medication administration, home maintenance, dental care, and transportation.
- Help clients interpret medical bills and apply for free or reduced-cost medication programs.

Integrating Health and Faith
- Help clients and caregivers manage anxiety, despair, and anger.
- Use variety of holistic interventions (e.g., prayer, establishing presence, reading scripture, providing anticipatory guidance) to help clients cope with concerns.

Data from Rydholm L: Documenting the value of faith community nursing. I. Saving hundreds, making cents: a study of current realities, *Creat Nurs* 12(2):10, 2006.

plicate this problem. Continuing care is available within institutional settings (e.g., nursing centers or nursing homes, group homes, and retirement communities), communities (e.g., adult day care and senior centers), or the home (e.g., home care, home-delivered meals, and hospice) (Meiner and Lueckenotte, 2006). Nurses need to be creative in meeting the needs of clients, especially older adult clients, who need continuing care (Box 2-6).

Nursing Centers or Facilities.

The language of long-term care is confusing and constantly changing. The nursing home has been the dominant setting for long-term care (Meiner and Lueckenotte, 2006). With the Omnibus Budget Reconciliation Act of 1987 the term *nursing facility* became the term for nursing homes and other facilities that provide long-term care. Now *nursing center* is the most appropriate term. A nursing center typically provides 24-hour intermediate and custodial care such as nursing, rehabilitation, dietary, recreational, social, and religious services for residents of any age with chronic or debilitating illnesses. In some cases clients stay in nursing centers for room, food, and laundry services only. The majority of persons living in nursing centers are older adults. A nursing center is a resident's temporary or permanent home with surroundings made as homelike as possible (Sorrentino, 2003). The philosophy of care is to provide a planned, systematic, and interdisciplinary approach to nursing care to help residents reach and maintain their highest level of function (Resnick and Fleishell, 2002).

BOX 2-7 Major Regulatory Requirements Defined by OBRA 1987

- Resident rights
- Admission, transfer, and discharge rights
- Resident behavior and facility practices
- Quality of life
- Resident assessment
- Quality of care
- Nursing services
- Dietary services
- Physician services
- Specialized rehabilitative services
- Dental services
- Pharmacy services
- Infection control
- Physical environment
- Administration

From Health Care Financing Administration, Department of Health and Human Services: Requirements for states and long term care facilities, 42 CFR 483 Subpart B (483.1-75), October 1, 2004, http://a257.g.akamaitech.net/7/257/2422/12feb20041500/edocket.access.gpo.gov/cfr_2004/octqtr/42cfr483.1.htm.

OBRA, Omnibus Budget Reconciliation Act.

BOX 2-8 Minimum Data Set and Examples of Resident Assessment Protocols

Minimum Data Set
Resident's background
Cognitive, communication/hearing, and vision patterns
Physical functioning and structural problems
Mood, behavior, and activity patterns
Psychosocial well-being
Bowel and bladder continence
Health conditions
Disease diagnoses
Oral/nutritional and dental status
Skin condition
Medication use
Special treatments and procedures

Resident Assessment Protocols (Examples)
Delirium
Falls
Pressure ulcers
Psychotropic drug use

According to the U.S. Bureau of the Census, just over 5% of people 65 years and older live in nursing centers and other facilities (MissouriFamilies, 2005). Nursing centers have been under attack for years because of claims regarding inadequate care and abuse. Many of the claims have been true (Fleck, 2002). As a result, the nursing center industry has become one of the most highly regulated industries in the United States. These regulations have raised the standard of services provided (Box 2-7). One regulatory area that deserves special mention is that of resident rights. Nursing facilities have to recognize residents as active participants and decision makers in their care and life in institutional settings (Meiner and Lueckenotte, 2006). This also means that

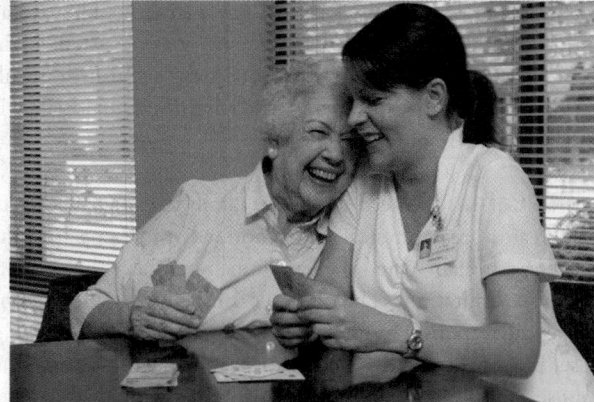

Figure 2-3 Providing nursing services in assisted living facilities promotes physical and psychosocial health.

family members are active partners in the planning of residents' care.

Interdisciplinary functional assessment of residents is the cornerstone of clinical practice within nursing centers (Meiner and Lueckenotte, 2006). Government regulations require that staff comprehensively assess each resident and that they make care planning decisions within a prescribed period. A resident's functional ability (e.g., ability to perform activities of daily living) and long-term physical and psychosocial well-being are the focus. Staff must complete the Resident Assessment Instrument (RAI) on all residents. The RAI consists of the **Minimum Data Set (MDS)** (Box 2-8), Resident Assessment Protocols (RAPs), and utilization guidelines of each state. The RAI ultimately provides a national database for nursing facilities so that policy makers will better understand the health care needs of the long-term care population. In addition, the MDS is a rich resource for nurses in determining the best type of interventions to support the health care needs of this growing population.

Assisted Living. Assisted living is one of the fastest growing industries within the United States. There are approximately 36,000 assisted living facilities that house more than 900,000 people in the United States (NCAL, 2006). **Assisted living** offers an attractive long-term care setting with a homier environment and greater resident autonomy. Clients require some assistance with activities of daily living but remain relatively independent within a partially protective setting. A group of residents live together, but each resident has his or her own room and shares dining and social activity areas. Usually people keep all of their personal possessions in their residences. Facilities range from hotel-like buildings with hundreds of units to modest group homes that house a handful of seniors. Assisted living provides independence, security, and privacy all at the same time (Ebersole and others, 2004). These facilities promote physical and psychosocial health (Figure 2-3) Services in an assisted living facility include laundry, assistance with meals and personal care, 24-hour oversight, and housekeeping (Sorrentino, 2003). Some facilities provide assistance with medication administration. Nursing care services are not directly available, although a home care nurse can visit a client in an assisted living facility. Unfortunately, most residents of assisted living facilities pay privately. The average monthly fee is $2627 (National Center for Assisted Living [NCAL], 2006). With no government fee caps and little regulation, assisted living is not always an option for individuals with limited financial resources.

Respite Care. The need to care for family members within the home creates great physical and emotional problems for adult caregivers, especially when the family member has either physical or cognitive limitations. The caregiver is usually an adult who not only has the responsibility for providing care to a loved one (e.g., spouse, parent, or sibling) but often has to maintain a full-time job, raise a family, and manage the routines of daily living as well. **Respite care** is a service that provides short-term relief or time off for persons providing home care to an ill, disabled, or frail older adult (Meiner and Lueckenotte, 2006). Trained volunteers in the home also provide respite care. The family caregiver is able to leave the home for errands or some social time while a responsible person stays in the home to care for the loved one.

Adult Day Care Centers. **Adult day care centers** provide a variety of health and social services to specific client populations who live alone or with family in the community. Services offered during the day allow family members to maintain their lifestyles and employment and still provide home care for their relatives (Meiner and Lueckenotte, 2006). Day care centers are usually associated with a hospital or nursing home or exist as independent centers. Frequently the clients need continuous health care services (e.g., physical therapy or counseling) while their families or support persons work. The centers usually operate 5 days per week during typical business hours and usually charge on a per diem (daily) basis. Adult day care centers allow clients to retain more independence by living at home, thus potentially reducing the costs of health care by avoiding or delaying an older adult's admission to a nursing center. Nurses working in day care centers provide continuity between care delivered in the home and in the center. For example, nurses ensure that clients continue to take prescribed medication and administer specific treatments. Knowledge of community needs and resources is essential in providing adequate support of clients (Ebersole and others, 2004).

Hospice. A **hospice** is a system of family-centered care that allows clients to live and remain at home with comfort, independence, and dignity while easing the pains of terminal illness. The focus of hospice care is palliative care, not curative treatment (see Chapter 43). A hospice benefits a client in the terminal phases of any disease, such as cardiomyopathy, multiple sclerosis, acquired immunodeficiency disease (AIDS), or cancer. The client, family, and health care provider agree that further treatment will not reverse the disease process. Staff works together to provide care that ensures death with dignity in the client's home. Hospice care is available 24 hours a day, 7 days a week, and services continue without interruption if the client's care setting changes. Occasionally a client is admitted to a hospice unit within a hospital. The client and family have to accept the fact that the hospice will not use emergency measures such as cardiopulmonary resuscitation to prolong life. The focus is on symptom management and ensuring the client's comfort. The hospice's multidisciplinary team works

continuously with the client's health care provider to develop and maintain a client-directed individualized plan of care. Hospice nurses provide care and support for the client and family during the illness and at the time of death; they continue to offer counseling to the family after the client's death. Many hospice programs provide respite care, which is important in maintaining the health of the primary caregiver and family.

Issues in Health Care Delivery

The climate in health care today influences health care professionals as well as consumers. Because those who provide client care are the most qualified to make changes in the health care delivery system, nurses need to participate fully and effectively within all aspects of health care. As nursing faces issues of how to maintain health care quality while reducing costs, nurses need to acquire the knowledge, skills, and values necessary to practice competently and effectively. It will also become more important than ever before to collaborate with other health care professionals to design new approaches for client care delivery.

Competency

The 1998 Pew Health Professions Commission recommended 21 competencies for health care professionals in the twenty-first century. The competencies emphasize the importance of public service, caring for the health of communities, and developing ethically responsible behaviors (Box 2-9). A consumer of health care expects that the standards of nursing care and practice in any health care setting are appropriate, safe, and efficacious. Health care organizations ensure quality care by establishing policies, procedures, and protocols that are scientifically sound and follow national accrediting standards. A nurse's responsibility is to follow policies and procedures and to know the most current practice standards. Ongoing competency is a nurse's responsibility. It is also the nurse's responsibility to obtain necessary continuing education and certifications.

Evidence-Based Practice

As professionals, nurses are challenged to stay familiar with new information in order to provide the highest quality of client care. Nursing practice is dynamic and always changing because of new information coming from research studies, practice trends, technological development, and social issues affecting clients. Nurses need to analyze new knowledge to make sound and informed decisions about client care (Barnsteiner and Prevost, 2002).

Evidence-based practice is a problem-solving approach to clinical practice that involves the concientious use of current best evidence, along with clinical expertise and client preferences and values in making decisions about client care (Melayk and Fineout-Overholt, 2005). Evidence-based practice, research-based practice, and best practice are terms that are often used interchangeably. However, research-based practice refers to the use of knowledge based on the results of research studies, where evidence-based practice adds a nurse's clinical experience, practice trends, and client preferences (Melnyk and Fineout-Overholt, 2004).

The goal of evidence-based practice is to provide nurses with evidence-based data to provide effective client care (see Chapter 5).

✴ **BOX 2-9 Pew Health Professions Commission Twenty-One Competencies for the Twenty-First Century**

1. Embrace a personal ethic of social responsibility and service
2. Exhibit ethical behavior in all professional activities
3. Provide evidence-based, clinically competent care
4. Incorporate the multiple determinants of health in clinical care
5. Apply knowledge of the new sciences
6. Demonstrate critical thinking, reflection, and problem-solving skills
7. Understand the role of primary care
8. Rigorously practice preventive health care
9. Integrate population-based care and services into practice
10. Improve access to health care for those with unmet health needs
11. Practice relationship-centered care with individuals and families
12. Provide culturally sensitive care to a diverse society
13. Partner with communities in health care decisions
14. Use communication and information technology effectively and appropriately
15. Work in interdisciplinary teams
16. Ensure care that balances individual, professional, system, and societal needs
17. Practice leadership
18. Take responsibility for quality of care and health outcomes at all levels
19. Contribute to continuous improvement of the health care system
20. Advocate for public policy that promotes and protects the health of the public
21. Continue to learn and help others learn

From the Pew Health Professions Commission, The Fourth Report of the Pew Health Professions Commission: *Recreating health professional practice for a new century*, 1998, The Commission.

Evidence-based practice assists nurses in resolving problems that occur in the clinical setting. It also helps nurses provide innovative health care that exceeds quality standards and helps nurses provide consistent client care using effective and efficient decision-making processes (Spector, 2005).

Quality Health Care

Initially the Centers for Medicaid and Medicare Services (CMS, formerly the Health Care Financing Administration [HCFA]) created ways for Medicare and Medicaid to make sure that health care providers used only medically needed services. Later CMS created quality standards for health care facilities, as well as health care providers. Quality health care is difficult to define. What clients define as quality health care is not necessarily the same as what health professionals define as quality. Quality improvement (QI) focuses on improving the performance of all providers (Milgate and Hackbarth, 2005-2006). QI is a continuous process, not a one-time statistic reported in isolation. With QI, providers receive outcome feedback and make corrections accordingly.

Health plans throughout the United States rely on the Health Plan Employer Data and Information Set (HEDIS) as a quality measure. The National Committee for Quality Assurance (NCQA) created HEDIS to collect various data to measure the quality of care and services provided by different health plans. It is the database of choice for CMS. HEDIS compares how well health plans perform in three key areas: quality of care, access to care, and client satisfaction with the health plan and doctors (HEDIS, 2004). For accreditation purposes, The Joint Commission requires health care organizations to determine how well an organization meets client needs and expectations. Organizations are using outcomes such as client satisfaction to redesign how they manage and deliver care in hopes of improving quality in the long term.

Nursing-Sensitive Outcomes. Nursing-sensitive outcomes are client outcomes that are directly related to nursing care. They have a major effect on client safety and quality of care (Stanton, 2004). Nurses assume accountability and responsibility for the consequences of these outcomes. Recently in health care and research a greater emphasis has been placed on nursing-sensitive outcomes. The evaluation of client outcomes remains important to nursing and the health care delivery system. However, nurses are just beginning to overcome the challenges associated with measuring the impact of these outcomes.

Nurses assume responsibility for a variety of outcomes that include individuals, family caregivers, the family, and the community. Moorhead and others (2008) have developed a research-based outcomes classification system, the Nursing Outcomes Classification (NOC), to help nurses better define and measure the impact of their interventions. NOC emphasizes outcomes that nursing interventions most affect. However, all health care disciplines can use this system.

The American Nurses Credentialing Center (ANCC) has established a Magnet Recognition Program to recognize health care organizations that achieve excellence in nursing practice (ANCC, 2007). Health care organizations that decide to apply for Magnet Status have to demonstrate leadership in nursing. Nurses are also required to collect data on specific nursing-sensitive quality indicators or outcomes and to compare their outcomes against a national, state, or regional database to demonstrate quality of care.

There are many nursing-sensitive outcomes that nurses measure. Examples of nursing-sensitive outcomes include the incidence of hospital-acquired pneumonia, deep vein thrombosis, urinary tract infections, pressure ulcers, falls, failure to rescue, and 30-day mortality (Stanton, 2004). Because of the importance of nursing-sensitive outcomes, the AHRQ recently funded several nursing research studies that looked at the relationship of nurse staffing levels to adverse client outcomes. These studies found a connection between higher levels of staffing by registered nurses (RNs) in hospitals and fewer negative client outcomes. For example, the incidence of hospital-acquired pneumonia was highly sensitive to RN staffing levels. Adding just 30 minutes of RN staffing per client day greatly reduced the incidence of pneumonia in clients following surgery. These studies also found that increased levels of nurse staffing positively impacted nurse satisfaction. Other studies are investigating how nurses' workloads affect client safety and how nurses' working conditions affect medication safety. Measuring and monitoring nursing-sensitive outcomes reveal the interventions that improve clients' outcomes. Nurses and health care facilities use nursing-sensitive outcomes to improve

✳ BOX 2-10   The Dimensions of Client-Centered Care

Respect Values, Preferences, and Expressed Needs

Clients expect to be treated with dignity and respect.

Clients want to be informed and involved in decisions about their care.

Clients' perceptions of needs should not be completely different from those identified by a care provider.

Coordination and Integration of Care

A competent and caring staff reduces feelings of powerlessness.

Clients look for someone to be in charge of care and to communicate clearly with other health care team members.

Clients expect to have services and procedures well coordinated.

Clients need to know at all times whom to call for help.

Information, Communication, and Education

Clients expect to receive accurate and timely information about their clinical status, progress, or prognosis.

Clients and families need to be informed of major changes in therapies or status.

Clients need tests and procedures explained clearly in language they understand.

Clients and family members want to know how to manage care on their own.

Physical Comfort

Physical care that provides comfort is one of the most elemental services caregivers provide.

Nurses need to respond in a timely and effective way to any request for pain medication, explain the extent of pain clients can expect, and offer alternatives for pain management.

Clients expect privacy and to have their cultural values respected.

The health care setting environment needs to be clean and comfortable.

Emotional Support and Relief of Fear and Anxiety

Clients look to care providers to share their fears and concerns.

Clients need to understand the impact illness will have on their ability to care for themselves and their family.

Clients worry about their ability to pay for their medical care. Identify staff that will help alleviate this worry.

Involvement of Family and Friends

Care providers need to recognize and respect the family and friends on whom clients rely for support.

Clients have the right to determine if family members are to be involved in decisions about their care.

Clients expect those family or friends who will provide physical support and care after discharge to be properly informed.

Transition and Continuity

Clients want information about medications to take, dietary or treatment plans to follow, and danger signals to look for after hospitalization or treatment.

Clients expect to have their continuing health care needs met after discharge with well-coordinated services.

Clients and family members expect access to necessary health care resources after discharge.

Data from Gerteis M and others: *Through the patient's eyes,* San Francisco, 1993, Jossey-Bass.

---

nurses' workloads, enhance client safety, and develop sound policies related to nursing practice and health care.

Client Satisfaction.   Almost every major health care organization measures certain aspects of client satisfaction. The Picker/Commonwealth Program for Patient-Centered Care has identified seven dimensions of **client-centered care** (Box 2-10) that most affect clients' experiences with health care (Gerteis and others, 1993). The seven dimensions cover most of the scope of nursing practice. This is not a surprise, because nurses are involved in almost every aspect of a client's care in a hospital. A close look shows that most of the aspects reflected in client satisfaction are applicable to almost any health care setting.

The Picker/Commonwealth Program has a survey tool that measures client satisfaction along the seven dimensions. The survey looks globally at client perceptions of care in an attempt to understand how all hospital departments influence client satisfaction. The program conducts the survey through telephone interviews after the client leaves the health care setting. Many other companies have developed similar client satisfaction surveys that are distributed in the mail to clients. Staff involved in client care receives the satisfaction scores as feedback regarding their success in meeting client expectations. The nursing staff is responsible for identifying unique issues that influence client satisfaction on their unit. For example, nurses working on an oncology unit will have different client satisfaction issues around physical comfort than nurses caring for new mothers. Client satisfaction findings become the basis for many quality improvement studies.

It is important for nurses to recognize the need to identify client expectations. The seven dimensions of care provide a useful guide. By learning early what a client expects with regard to information, comfort, and availability of family and friends, nurses are able to better plan client care. Nurses routinely ask about a client's expectations when the client first enters a health care setting, while care continues, and when a client is discharged. Client expectations are an important measure of the evaluation of nursing care.

Technological Advancements and Nursing Informatics

Advances in technology are constantly evolving. People work, play, and view the world much differently because of these advances. Technological advancements also influence where and how nurses provide care to clients. Sophisticated equipment such as electronic intravenous (IV) infusion devices, cardiac telemetry (a device that monitors a client's heart rate wherever the client is on a nursing unit), and computerized medication dispensation systems (see Chapter 35) are just a few examples that have changed health care. In many ways, technology makes the nurse's work easier, but it does not replace the nurse's judgment. For example, it is the nurse's responsibility when managing a client's intravenous therapy to monitor the infusion to be sure it infuses on time and without complications. An electronic infusion device provides a constant rate of infusion, but nurses need to be sure that they calculate the rate correctly. The device will set off an alarm if the infusion slows, making it important for the nurse to respond to the alarm and to troubleshoot the problem. Technology does not replace a nurse's critical eye and clinical judgment.

Technology also affects the way we communicate with others. Personal computers, cell phones, personal digital assistants (PDAs), and television allow us to communicate and share information or data with others in a variety of formats around the world. People expect accurate information to be delivered to them as it develops. Managing communication, information, and data is challenging in health care. Health care agencies use data to measure their outcomes and to improve client care. Accrediting bodies, insurance companies, and Medicare/Medicaid all require collection and reporting of accurate data. Furthermore, nurses need accurate, up-to-date information to make the best decisions about client care. Therefore it is crucial that nurses help health care agencies develop an effective way to manage the collection, interpretation, and distribution of information.

Nursing informatics combines the best of computer science and information science with nursing science. It supports nursing practice and the delivery of nursing care by providing nurses with a way to manage and process nursing data, information, and knowledge (Huber, 2006). **Data** are individually distinct pieces of reality. Examples of data nurses collect and use include a client's blood pressure or the measurement of a client's wound. Nurses gain or use **information** when they organize, structure, or interpret data. A nurse uses information when looking at trends in a client's blood pressure readings over the past 24 hours or when evaluating the changes in a wound's size over the past 3 weeks. **Knowledge** develops when nurses combine and identify relationships between different pieces of information. For example, nurses know that diet plays an important role in blood pressure control and wound healing. They use this knowledge to teach clients at risk for developing high blood pressure to limit their salt intake and to teach clients who have wounds the importance of eating a well-rounded diet that includes adequate protein, vitamins, and minerals. The focus of nursing informatics is not on the technology or the computer; rather, the focus of informatics is on the organization, analysis, and dissemination of information (American Nurses Association, 2007).

Nursing informatics improves the way nurses provide health care and enhances client outcomes. For example, many health care agencies now use an **electronic health record (EHR)**. The EHR is replacing the traditional printed medical record and provides a comprehensive electronic record of a client's medical problems, treatment, diagnostic procedures, and nursing care. Nurses and other health care providers electronically document data about clients, as well as care provided, in one place, which enhances communication among the health care team, resulting in better client care (see Chapter 26). An EHR also provides valuable information for research and quality improvement activities. For example, a nurse researcher who wishes to track a nursing staff's progress in timely assessment of clients' pain will examine a computerized database to review actual client assessments and the time they occurred.

Documentation on a clinical information system minimizes free text entries and allows nurses to enter information quickly on specially designed flow sheets, pop-up screens, and nursing care plans. The computer displays important data in a way that allows nurses to follow their clients' progress and course easily. An elec-

tronic system does not reduce the responsibility for documenting clinical information accurately and completely in a timely manner. All members of the health care team usually have access to the electronic record; thus nurses have to make the information accessible as soon as possible. Many hospitals have placed computers at the client's bedside so nurses are able to document care as soon as it is provided. It is important to remember not to depersonalize care when using a bedside computer system. When entering data, it is often easy to avoid interacting with the client, who is usually interested in the information being recorded. The use of electronic information systems also requires strict confidentiality protocols. It is now easier for an individual to visit a nursing unit and try to gain access to a computer to obtain client information. Therefore nurses help ensure that information is accessible only to those directly involved in a client's care.

Nurses need to play a role in evaluating and implementing new technological advances. They use technology and informatics to improve the effectiveness of nursing care, enhance safety, and improve client outcomes. Most importantly, it is essential for nurses to remember that the focus of nursing care is not the machine or the technology. Rather, the focus of nursing care is the client. Therefore nurses need to constantly attend to and connect with their clients and ensure that their clients' dignity and rights are preserved at all levels of care.

Globalization of Health Care

In today's society, many forces continuously affect and reshape the health care delivery system. Advances in communication, primarily through the Internet, allow nurses, clients, and other health care providers to talk with others worldwide about health care issues. However, despite advances in technology and communication, the poorest areas in the world are still underserved (Simpson, 2004).

Nurses need to understand how worldwide communication and globalization of health care influences nursing practice. Health care consumers demand quality and service and have become more knowledgeable. They often have searched the Internet about their health concerns and medical conditions. They also use the Internet to select their health care providers. As a result of **globalization**, physicians and health care providers have to make their services more accessible. Because of advances in communication, nurses and other health care providers practice across state and national boundaries. Furthermore, health care institutions in the United States are currently experiencing a nursing shortage. In an effort to provide quality care, health care institutions are recruiting nurses from around the world to work in the United States. The hiring of nurses from other nations has forced American hospitals to better understand and work with nurses from different cultures who have different needs (Nash and Gremillion, 2004).

Many problems affect the health status of people around the world. For example, poverty is still deadlier than any disease and is the most frequent reason for death in the world today. Nations and communities that experience poverty have limited access to vaccines, clean water, and standard medical care. The growth of urbanization also currently is affecting the world's health. As cities become more densely populated, problems with pollution, noise, crowding, inadequate water, improper waste disposal, and other environmental hazards become more apparent. Children, women, and older adults are **vulnerable populations** most threatened by urbanization. Although globalization of trade, travel, and culture improves the availability of health care services, the spread of communicable diseases such as tuberculosis and severe acute respiratory syndrome (SARS) has become more common. Finally, the results of global environmental changes and disasters affect health. Changes in climate and natural disasters threaten food supplies and often allow infectious diseases to spread more rapidly (Simpson, 2004).

As a leader in health care, remain aware of what is happening in the community, nation, and around the world. There are more than 5 million nurses worldwide (Simpson, 2004). Nursing's unique focus on caring helps nurses address the issues presented by globalization. Nurses and the nursing profession are able to help overcome these issues by working together to improve nursing education throughout the world, by retaining nurses and recruiting people to be nurses, and by being an advocate for changes that will improve the delivery of health care (Simpson, 2004). Be prepared for future health care issues. Globalization has influenced many other industries, and it is affecting the health care delivery system today. As a leader, nursing has to take control and be proactive in developing solutions before someone outside of nursing takes control (Nash and Gremillion, 2004).

The Future of Health Care

This discussion on the health care delivery system began with the issue of change. Change threatens many, but it also opens up opportunities for improvement. The ultimate issue in designing and delivering health care is ensuring the health and welfare of the population. Health care in the United States and around the world is not perfect. Many clients do not receive continuity of care when they see multiple health care providers. Many clients are uninsured or underinsured and do not have access to necessary services. However, health care organizations are trying to become better prepared to deal with the challenges in health care. Many health care organizations are changing how they provide their services, reducing unnecessary costs, improving access to care and trying to provide high-quality client care. Professional nursing is an important player in the future of health care delivery. The solutions necessary to improve the quality of health care depend largely on the active participation of nurses.

✳ Key Concepts

- Increasing costs and decreasing reimbursement are forcing health care institutions to deliver care more efficiently without sacrificing quality.
- In a managed care system the provider of care receives a predetermined capitated payment regardless of the services a client uses.
- The Medicare prospective reimbursement system is based on payment calculated on the basis of DRG assignment.
- Levels of health care describe the range of services and settings where health care is available to clients in all stages of health and illness.
- Health promotion occurs in home, work, and community settings.

- Nurses are facing the challenge of keeping populations healthy and well within their own homes and communities.
- Successful community-based health programs involve building relationships with the community and incorporating cultural and environmental factors.
- Hospitalized clients are acutely ill, requiring better coordination of services before discharge.
- Rehabilitation allows an individual to return to a level of normal or near-normal function after a physical or mental illness, injury, or chemical dependency.
- Home care agencies provide almost every type of health care service with an emphasis on client and family independence.
- Discharge planning begins at admission and helps in the transition of a client's care from one environment to another.
- Health care organizations are being evaluated on the basis of outcomes such as prevention of complications, clients' functional outcomes, and client satisfaction.
- Nurses need to remain knowledgeable and proactive about issues in the health care delivery system to provide quality client care and positively affect health.

✳ Critical Thinking Exercises

Jackie is a 22-year-old nursing student with a 3-year-old son and a 1-year-old daughter; she has silently suffered verbal abuse from her husband for the past year. Now her husband has separated from her and is threatening divorce because he is intimidated by her potential to be independent of him if she becomes a nurse. She is worried about being left without health insurance and a financial income. Due to the stress of home life, school, finances, and multiple role responsibilities, Jackie has developed stress-related anxiety. She came to the emergency department with symptoms of heart palpitations, shortness of breath, diarrhea, nausea, and vomiting.

1. What type of services does Jackie need at this time? (Select all that apply.)
   1. Disease prevention
   2. Health promotion
   3. Health protection
   4. Primary care
   5. Secondary care
   6. Tertiary care

2. Jackie is admitted to a general medical unit for dehydration and exhaustion. She is receiving an intravenous infusion of 5% dextrose with normal saline to replace the fluids she has lost, a mild sedative to calm her, and an upper and lower gastrointestinal (GI) x-ray series. If these x-ray films are normal, Jackie will be discharged in the morning.
   a. What type of care does Jackie need right now?
   b. What discharge planning can be started for Jackie at this time? (Think about what you would need if you were in Jackie's shoes.)
   c. What type of care or support will Jackie need if her husband comes to visit her?

3. The results of Jackie's x-ray films are normal at this time, so she is discharged to home. You are the nurse responsible for completing an assessment of community resources available to assist Jackie. Use the Internet or your personal knowledge to find resources available in your community that can help Jackie.

✳ NCLEX®-Style Review Questions

1. Which of the following is the biggest consumer of health care?
   1. Hospitals
   2. Businesses
   3. Federal government
   4. Private insurance companies

2. Which of the following was most significant in influencing competition in health care costs?
   1. Medicare and Medicaid
   2. Diagnosis-related groups
   3. Managed care organizations
   4. Prospective payment system

3. A nurse is working in an acute care hospital that uses a case management model. Which of the following activities should the nurse communicate with the case manager? (Select all that apply.)
   1. Management of a client transfer to the x-ray department
   2. Coordination of a client transfer to the step-down rehabilitation unit
   3. Obtaining permission to bring in special food to a client by the family
   4. Follow-up after a client's discharge to evaluate whether needs have been met

4. Which of the following clients need to be in an extended care facility with skilled nursing? (Select all that apply.)
   1. A client who had a stroke, can talk, and has lost bowel and bladder control
   2. A severely brain injured client on a ventilator with intravenous medications

3. A client with Alzheimer's disease who is abusive, combative, and a threat to self and others
4. A young child who recently had a spinal cord injury and is living with quadriplegia and needs to learn a new way of life

5. Which of the following statements is true about evidence-based practice? (Select all that apply.) Evidence-based practice:
   1. Is based only on the results of research
   2. Assists nurses with meeting standards of practice
   3. Helps nurses solve dilemmas in the clinical setting
   4. Requires nurses to review and critique research and practice findings

6. Which of the following are population-based interventions for hypertension? (Select all that apply.)
   1. Providing education to five clients to prevent hypertension
   2. Obtaining a medication prescription and follow-up appointment
   3. Identifying the prevalence of hypertension by age, race, and sex
   4. Discovering the subpopulation with the highest rate of untreated hypertension

7. A client is receiving health care by a health care provider who is a salaried employee. Which type of managed care organization (MCO) does the client belong to? (Select all that apply.)
   1. Staff model
   2. Group model
   3. Network model
   4. Independent practice association

3 | Community-Based Nursing Practice

✳ OBJECTIVES

Mastery of content in this chapter will enable the student to:

- Explain the relationship between public health and community health nursing.
- Differentiate community health nursing from community-based nursing.
- Discuss the role of the community health nurse.
- Discuss the role of the nurse in community-based practice.
- Identify characteristics of clients from vulnerable populations that influence the community-based nurse's approach to care.
- Describe the competencies important for success in community-based nursing practice.
- Describe elements of a community assessment.

✳ MEDIA RESOURCES ✳ KEY TERMS

 Companion CD
- NCLEX®-Style Review Questions
- Audio Glossary
- English/Spanish Glossary
- Interactive Learning Activities

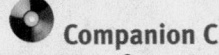 **Website**
- NCLEX®-Style Review Questions
- Audio Glossary
- English/Spanish Glossary
- Interactive Learning Activities
- WebLinks
- Audio Summaries

Community-based nursing, p. 35
Community health nursing, p. 34
Incident rates, p. 33

Population, p. 34
Public health nursing, p. 34
Vulnerable populations, p. 35

The rapid pace of today's health care climate results in clients moving from acute care, hospital-based settings to community-based care that focuses on health promotion, disease prevention, and restorative care. Organized health care services need to be where people live, work, and learn. Contemporary community-based nursing practice is a collaborative, evidenced practice model designed to meet the health care needs of the community (Downie, Ogilve and Wichmann, 2005). A healthy community includes elements that enable people to maintain a high quality of life and productivity. For example, safety and access to health care services are elements that enable people to function productively in the community (U.S. Department of Health and Human Services [USDHHS], 2001). As community health care partnerships develop, nursing is in a strategic position to play an important role in health care delivery and to improve the health of the community.

The focus of health promotion and disease prevention continues to be essential for the holistic practice of professional nursing. Nursing's history documents the roles of nurses in establishing and meeting the public health goals of their clients. Within community health settings, nurses are leaders in assessing, diagnosing, planning, implementing, and evaluating the types of public and community health services needed. Community health nursing and community-based nursing are components of a health care delivery system that improve the health of the general public.

Community-Based Health Care

It is important to understand the importance of community-based health care. Community-based health care is a model of care that reaches everyone in the community (including the poor and underinsured), focuses on primary rather than institutional or acute care, and provides knowledge about health and health promotion and models of care to the community (National Library of Medicine, 1993). Community-based health care occurs outside traditional health care institutions, such as hospitals. It provides services for acute and chronic conditions to individuals and families within the community (Stanhope and Lancaster, 2006).

Today the challenges in community-based health care are many. Social lifestyles, political policy, and economic initiatives all influence public health problems. Some of these problems include an increase in homeless and immigrant populations, an increase in sexually transmitted diseases, underimmunization of infants and children, and life-threatening diseases (e.g., clients living with human immunodeficiency virus [HIV] and other emerging infections). More than ever before, health care reform is necessary to bring attention to the health care needs of all communities.

Achieving Healthy Populations and Communities

The U.S. Department of Health and Human Services Public Health Service designed a program to improve the overall health status of people living in this country. The *Healthy People Initiative* was created to establish ongoing health care goals (see Chapter 6). The overall goals of *Healthy People 2010* are to increase life expectancy and quality of life and to eliminate health disparities through an improved delivery of health care services (USDHHS, 2000).

Improved delivery of health care occurs through the assessment of health care needs of individuals, families, and communities; development and implementation of public health policies; and improved access to care. For example, assessment includes systematic data collection on the population, monitoring of the population's health status, and accessing available information about the health of the community (Stanhope and Lancaster, 2006). A comprehensive community assessment can lead to community health programs, such as adolescent smoking prevention, sex education, and proper nutrition. Examples of assessment include, but are not limited to, gathering information on **incident rates** for identifying and reporting of new infections or diseases, determining adolescent pregnancy rates, and reporting the number of motor vehicle accidents by teenage drivers.

Health professionals provide leadership in developing public policies to support the population's health (Stanhope and Lancaster, 2006). Strong policies are driven by community assessment. For example, when assessing the frequency of human immunodeficiency virus (HIV) cases, the findings could lead to an evidence-based HIV prevention program to reduce the incidence of risky behaviors in inner-city adolescent parents (Koniak-Griffin and others, 2003; Lesser and others, 2005) (Box 3-1).

Improved access to care ensures that essential community-wide health services are available and accessible to the total community (Stanhope and Lancaster, 2006). Examples include prenatal care programs for the uninsured and educational programs to ensure the competency of public health professionals. Population-based public health programs focus on disease prevention, health protection, and health promotion. This focus provides the foundation for health care services at all levels (see Chapter 2).

The five-level health services pyramid is an example of how to provide community-based services within existing health care services in a community (see Figure 2-1, p. 17). In this population-focused health care services model the goals of disease prevention, health protection, and health promotion provide a foundation for primary, secondary, and tertiary health care services.

A rural community often has a hospital to meet the acute care needs of its citizens. However, a community assessment might reveal that there are minimal services to meet the needs of expectant mothers, reduce teenage smoking, or provide nutritional support for older adults. Community-based programs are able to provide these services and are effective in improving the health of the community. When the lower-level services are accessible and effective, there is a greater likelihood that the higher levels will contribute to the total health of the community (U.S. Public Health Service, 1995/2000). For example, if there is inadequate mosquito control in a community, it becomes more difficult to enforce health promotion efforts and to prevent the occurrence of mosquito-borne diseases. On the other hand, when a community has the resources for providing childhood immunizations, primary preventive care services are able to focus on child developmental problems and child safety.

The principles of public health practice aim at achieving a healthy environment for all individuals. Health care providers apply these principles for individuals, families, and the communities in which they live. Nursing plays a role in all levels of the health services pyramid. By using public health principles you are better able to understand the types of environments in which clients live

---

> **BOX 3-1   EVIDENCE-BASED PRACTICE**
>
> ## HIV Prevention in Community Settings
>
> ### Evidence Summary
> Inner-city adolescent mothers and fathers are at risk for HIV due to the impact of childhood poverty and lack of resources, social oppression, community violence, and social isolation. All of these factors lead to high-risk behaviors, such as early unprotected sexual activity. In addition, alcohol and substance abuse, abusive relationships, and multiple sexual partners increase the risk of HIV for adolescent parents living in the community. Adolescent mothers alter and reduce their HIV risk factors; however, the fathers are behind in changing their risk factors. There is evidence that shows the effectiveness of a culturally sensitive community-based educational program directed toward adolescent mothers and fathers to help reduce their HIV risk factors. The educational program was culturally sensitive, appropriate for adolescent parents, and recognized the resources and difficulties within the community.
>
> ### Application to Nursing Practice
> - Teach adolescent parents how to cope with growth and development as well as new-parenting stressors and issues. For example, let them know that there will be times when they want to go out with their friends but do not have child care. A solution might be to have a child-appropriate activity, such as a pizza dinner.
> - Resources available to inner-city parents are few and difficult to access.
> - Educational programs that are developmentally and culturally appropriate and in a convenient location, such as a school or community center, are successful with this age-group.
> - The curriculum needs input from the community, the target population, and health care experts in order to be effective.
> - Successful participants are valuable resources for subsequent educational programs and mentoring for other adolescent parents.
>
> ---
>
> Lesser J and others: Respecting and protecting our relationships: a community research HIV prevention program for teen fathers and mothers, *AIDS Educ Prev* 17(4):347, 2005.
>
> *HIV,* Human immunodeficiency virus.

and the types of interventions necessary to help keep clients healthy.

Community Health Nursing

Frequently the terms *community health nursing* and *public health nursing* are used interchangeably. There are similarities. A **public health nursing** focus requires understanding the needs of a **population,** or a collection of individuals who have in common one or more personal or environmental characteristics (Stanhope and Lancaster, 2006). Examples of populations include high-risk infants, older adults, or a cultural group such as Native Americans. A public health nurse understands factors that influence health promotion and health maintenance, the trends and patterns influencing the incidence of disease within populations, environmen-

tal factors contributing to health and illness, and the political processes used to affect public policy. For example, the nurse uses data on increased incidents of playground injuries to lobby for a policy to use shock-absorbing material rather than concrete for new public playgrounds.

Public health nursing requires preparation at the basic entry level and sometimes requires a baccalaureate degree in nursing that includes educational preparation and clinical practice in public health nursing. A specialist in public health has a graduate level education with a focus in the public health sciences (American Nurses Association [ANA], 1999).

Community health nursing is a nursing practice in the community, with the primary focus on the health care of individuals, families, and groups in a community. The goal is to preserve, protect, promote, or maintain health (Stanhope and Lancaster, 2006). The emphasis of such nursing care is to improve the quality of health and life within that community. In addition, the community health nurse provides direct care services to subpopulations within a community. These subpopulations are often a clinical focus in which the nurse has expertise. For example, a case manager follows older adults recovering from stroke and sees the need for community rehabilitation services or a nurse practitioner gives immunizations to clients with the objective of managing communicable disease within the community. By focusing on subpopulations, the community health nurse cares for the community as a whole and considers the individual or family as only one member of a group at risk.

Competence as a community health nurse requires the ability to use interventions that include the broad social and political context of the community (Stanhope and Lancaster, 2006). The educational requirements for entry-level nurses practicing in community health nursing roles are not as clear as those for public health nurses. Not all hiring agencies require an advanced degree. However, nurses with a graduate degree in nursing who practice in community settings are considered community health nurse specialists, regardless of their public health experience (Stanhope and Lancaster, 2006).

Nursing Practice in Community Health

Community-focused nursing practice requires a unique set of skills and knowledge. In the health care delivery system, nurses who become expert in community health practice usually have advanced nursing degrees, yet the baccalaureate-prepared generalist is also quite competent in formulating and applying population-focused assessments and interventions (Diekemper, Smith Battle, and Drake, 1999). The expert community health nurse understands the needs of a population or community through experience with individual families and working through their social and health care issues. Critical thinking is important in applying knowledge of public health principles, community health nursing, family theory, and communication in finding the best approaches in partnering with families.

Successful community health nursing practice involves building relationships with the community and being responsive to changes within the community (Diekemper and others, 1999). For example, when there is an increase in the incidence of grandparents' assuming child care responsibilities, establishing an instructional program in cooperation with local schools assists and supports grandparents in this caregiving role. The community health nurse becomes an active part of a community. This nurse knows the community members, needs, and resources and then works in collaboration with the community leaders to establish effective health promotion and disease prevention programs. This requires working with highly resistant systems (e.g., welfare system) and trying to encourage them to be more responsive to the needs of a population. Skills of client advocacy, communicating people's concerns, and designing new systems in cooperation with existing systems help to make community-nursing practice effective.

Community-Based Nursing

Community-based nursing care takes place in community settings such as the home or a clinic, where the focus is on the needs of the individual or family. It involves the acute and chronic care of individuals and families and enhances their capacity for self-care and promotes autonomy in decision making (Stanhope and Lancaster, 2004). You use critical thinking and decision making for the individual client and family—assessing health status, diagnosing health problems, planning care, implementing interventions, and evaluating outcomes of care. Because nurses provide direct care services where clients live, work, and play, it is important that your nursing care remains focused on the individual and family and that you respect and incorporate the values of a community (Newman, 2005).

Community-based nursing centers function as the first level of contact between members of a community and the health care delivery system. The ideal is to provide health care services close to where clients live. This approach helps to lessen the cost of health care for the client as well as the stress associated with the financial burdens of care. In addition, these centers offer direct access to nurses and client-centered health services and readily incorporate the client and the client's family or friends into a plan of care (Pastor, 2005).

The social interaction units of the human ecology model are represented by four circles: the inner circle of the client and the immediate family, the second circle of people and settings that have frequent contact with the client and family, the third circle of the local community and its values and policies, and the outer circle of larger social systems such as government and church (Figure 3-1). In community-based practice you need to understand the interaction of all of the units while caring for the client and family in their environment. Typically you will interact within the first three circles when providing health care. For example, a home care nurse working with a newly diagnosed client with diabetes works closely with the client and family to establish a comprehensive plan for the client's health. You learn the habits or lifestyle patterns when the client is with friends and co-workers and anticipate ways to plan the client's exercise schedule and meal routines. Knowing the resources available in the community (e.g., medical supply shops for glucose monitoring supplies and local diabetes association support groups) assists you in providing comprehensive support for the client's needs.

With the individual and family as the clients, the context of community-based nursing is family-centered care within the

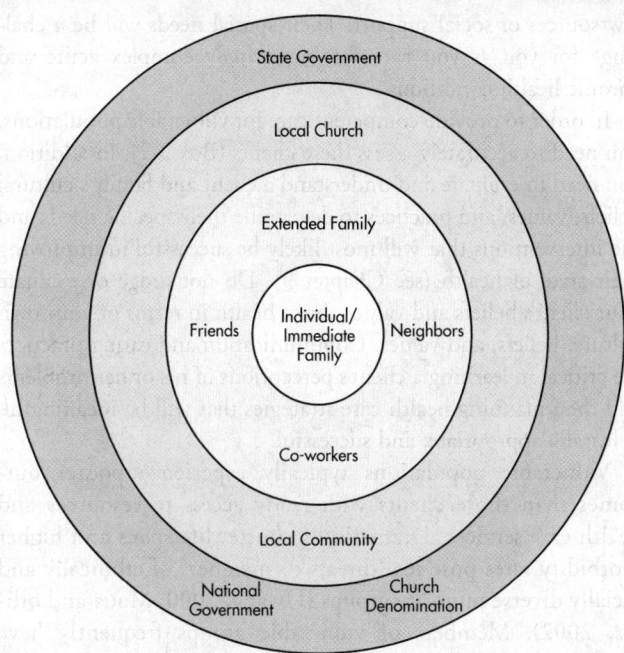

Figure 3-1 These concentric circles represent the social interaction units of the human ecology model. (From Ayers M, Bruno AA, Langford RW: *Community-based nursing care: making the transition,* St. Louis, 1999, Mosby.)

community. This focus requires a strong knowledge base in family theory (see Chapter 10), principles of communication (see Chapter 24), group dynamics, and cultural diversity (see Chapter 9). You learn to partner with your clients and families so that ultimately the client and family assume responsibility for their health care decisions. The family becomes involved in planning, decision making, implementation, and evaluation of health care approaches.

Vulnerable Populations

In a community setting nurses care for clients from diverse cultures and backgrounds and with various health conditions. However, changes in the health care delivery system have made high-risk groups the principal clients. For example, you are not likely to visit low-risk mothers and babies. Instead, adolescent mothers or mothers with drug addiction are more likely to receive home care services. **Vulnerable populations** are those clients who are more likely to develop health problems as a result of excess risks, who have limits in access to health care services, or who are dependent on others for care. Individuals living in poverty, older adults, homeless persons, immigrant populations, individuals in abusive relationships, substance abusers, and severely mentally ill persons are examples of vulnerable populations (Hwang, 2000; Moua and others, 2002). Vulnerable individuals and their families often belong to more than one of these groups. In addition, health care vulnerability affects all age-groups (Sebastian, 2006). Vulnerable individuals are also a specific population with a unique health care problem.

Vulnerable clients come from varied cultures, have different beliefs and values, face language and literacy barriers, and have few sources of social support. Their special needs will be a challenge for you as you care for increasingly complex acute and chronic health conditions.

In order to provide competent care for vulnerable populations, you need to accurately assess these clients (Box 3-2). In addition, you need to evaluate and understand a client and family's cultural beliefs, values, and practices to determine their specific needs and the interventions that will most likely be successful in improving their state of health (see Chapter 9). Do not judge or evaluate your client's beliefs and values about health in terms of your own culture, beliefs, and values. Communication and caring practices are critical in learning a client's perceptions of his or her problems and then planning health care strategies that will be meaningful, culturally appropriate, and successful.

Vulnerable populations typically experience poorer outcomes than those clients with ready access to resources and health care services. Dramatically shorter life spans and higher morbidity rates pose real threats to members of ethnically and racially diverse minority groups (Hwang, 2000; Moua and others, 2002). Members of vulnerable groups frequently have many risks or combinations of risk factors that make them more sensitive to the negative effects of individual risk factors (Rew and others, 2001). It is essential for community-based nurses to assess members of vulnerable populations by taking into account the multiple stressors that affect their clients' lives. It is also important to learn the clients' strengths and resources for coping with stressors.

Immigrant Population. Researchers predict that the immigrant population will grow by 1 million people each year (Moua and others, 2002; U.S. Census Bureau, 2007). Immigrant populations face multiple diverse health issues that cities, counties, and states need to address. These health care needs pose significant legal and policy issues. For some immigrants access to health care is limited because of language barriers and lack of benefits, resources, and transportation. In addition, some immigrant populations have specific health care risks such as hepatitis B; tuberculosis; intestinal parasites; and visual, hearing, and dental problems (Stanhope and Lancaster, 2006).

Frequently the immigrant population practices nontraditional healing practices (see Chapter 9). Although many of these healing practices are effective and complement traditional therapies, it is important that you know and understand all of your client's health care practices.

Certain immigrant populations left their homes as a result of oppression, war, or natural disaster (e.g., Bosnians and Somalis). It is important for you to be sensitive to both these physical and psychological stressors and consequences and to identify the ap-

---

✳ BOX 3-2 Guidelines for Assessing Members of Vulnerable Population Groups

Setting the Stage

Create a comfortable, nonthreatening environment.

Learn as much as you can about the culture of the clients you work with so that you will understand cultural practices and values that influence their health care practices.

Provide culturally competent assessment by understanding the meaning of language and nonverbal behavior in the client's culture.

Be sensitive to the fact that the individual or family you are assessing has other priorities that are more important to them. These include financial or legal problems. You will sometimes need to give them some help with their most urgent priority before you are able to address traditional health concerns.

Collaborate with others as appropriate; do not provide financial or legal advice. However, make sure to connect the client with someone who will help them.

Nursing History of an Individual or Family

You often have only one opportunity to work with a vulnerable person or family. Try to complete a history that provides all the essential information you need to help the individual or family on that day. This means that you have to organize in your mind exactly what you need to ask and why the data are necessary.

Use a modified comprehensive assessment form to focus on the special needs of the vulnerable population group. However, be flexible. With some clients, it is both impractical and unethical to cover all questions on a comprehensive form. If you know that you are likely to see the client again, ask the less urgent questions at the next visit.

Include questions about social support, economic status, resources for health care, developmental issues, current health problems, medication, and how the person or family manages their health status. Your goal is to obtain information that will enable you to provide family-centered care.

Determine if the individual has any condition that compromises his or her immune status, such as HIV/AIDS. Is the individual undergoing therapy that results in immunodeficiency, such as cancer chemotherapy?

Physical Examination or Home Assessment

Complete a thorough physical examination (on an individual) or home assessment. Collect only useful data.

Be alert for indications of mental and physical abuse, changes from normal physical examination findings (see Chapter 33), or substance use (e.g., underweight, being inadequately clothed).

Observe a family's living environment. Does the family live in an insect- or rat-infested environment? Do they have running water, functioning plumbing, electricity, and a telephone? Is perishable food (e.g., mayonnaise) left sitting out on tables and countertops? Are bed linens reasonably clean? Is paint peeling on the walls and ceilings? Is ventilation adequate? Is the temperature of the home adequate? Is the family exposed to raw sewage or animal waste? Is the home next to a busy highway, possibly exposing the family to high noise levels and automobile exhaust?

From Sebastian JG: Vulnerability and vulnerable populations: an overview. In Stanhope M, Lancaster J: *Foundations of nursing in the community: community-oriented practice,* ed 2, St. Louis, 2006, Mosby.

AIDS, Acquired immunodeficiency syndrome.

propriate resources to help understand your clients and their health care needs (Stanhope and Lancaster, 2006).

Poor and Homeless Persons. People who live in poverty are more likely to live in hazardous environments, work at high-risk jobs, eat less nutritious diets, and have multiple stressors in their life. When researchers compared the life expectancies of European Americans and African Americans, the causes of the differences were related to low socioeconomic status rather than ethnicity (Decker and others, 2006; Hwang, 2000). Clients with low income levels not only lack financial resources, but also live in poor environments and face practical problems such as poor or unavailable transportation. Homeless clients have even fewer resources than the poor. They are usually jobless and do not have the advantage of shelter and cope with finding a place to sleep at night and finding food (Table 3-1). Nurses help homeless people identify available resources such as mobile health clinics and soup kitchens (Figure 3-2).

Abused Clients. Physical, emotional, and sexual abuse, as well as neglect, are major public health problems affecting older adults, women, and children (Rew and others, 2001; Sebastian,

---

✳ TABLE 3-1 Nursing Interventions for Care of the Homeless

Level of Prevention		
PRIMARY INTERVENTION	**SECONDARY INTERVENTION**	**TERTIARY INTERVENTION**
Stage 1: Prevent or Reduce Frequency of Homeless Experiences		
Improvement of physical environment (community, home)	Health screening	Control of spread of disease
Provision of adequate housing	Referral programs	Treatment of tuberculosis and acquired immunodeficiency syndrome (AIDS)
Health education	Case management	
Sex education	Case finding	Drug and alcohol treatment programs
Drug and alcohol education	Screening for iron, tuberculosis, human immunodeficiency virus (HIV), hemoglobin, substance use	Treatment of mental illnesses
Good nutrition		Strengthening of support systems
Pregnancy and nutrition	Diagnostic services	
Advocacy	Treatment of acute illnesses	
Support of legislation that helps the poor	Treatment of potentially life-threatening illnesses (e.g., rehydration of young children)	
Increased minimum wage		
Child day care		
Access to health care		
Stage 2: Assist Homeless in Reducing Factors That Keep Them Homeless and in Gaining Skills to Move Into Higher Level of Functioning		
Teaching regarding effective coping behaviors	Screen for chronic illnesses	Treatment for major mental illnesses
Teaching regarding avoidance of potentially violent situations	Screen for leg ulcers	Treatment for major illnesses and injuries
	Screen for drug abuse	
Advocacy	Screen for trauma	Detoxification programs
Health education	Screen for hypertension	Management of chronic illnesses
Interpersonal skills training	Screen for cancer	Management of AIDS symptoms
Development of interrelationships with service providers	Provide immunizations	
Recommendations regarding food and handling and exposure to infectious diseases	Monitoring of psychiatric status and compliance with medical plan	
Teaching regarding importance of good nutrition	Monitoring for status of infectious diseases	
Referrals for legal assistance	Provision of on-site care in shelters and service centers	
Stage 3: Increase Amount of Interaction With Service Providers and Acceptance of Resources		
Advocacy	Case management	Protection from violence
Outreach program	Mobile treatment programs	Promotion of wet and dry detoxification
Promotion of legislation regarding homeless mentally ill	Monitoring for changes in health status	Treatment for major illnesses
Promotion of legislation for care to homeless	Provision of access to basic nutritional needs	Help for persons in getting into mental health programs
Location of homeless through outreach programs		Supervised housing
Multiservice programs in service sites		Promotion of increased independence

Data from Sebastian JG: Vulnerability and vulnerable populations: an overview. In Stanhope M, Lancaster J: *Foundations of nursing in the community: community-oriented practice,* ed 2, St. Louis, 2006, Mosby; Decker S and others: From the streets to assisted living: perceptions of vulnerable population, *J Psychosoc Nurs Ment Health Serv* 44(6):18, 2006; Hwang SW: Mortality among men using homeless shelters in Toronto, Ontario, *JAMA,* 283(16):2152, 2000; Hwang SW, Bugeja AL: Barriers to appropriate diabetes management among homeless people in Toronto, *Can Med Assoc J* 163(2):161, 2000; and Rew L and others: Correlates of resilience in homeless adolescents, *J Nurs Scholarsh* 33(1):33, 2001.

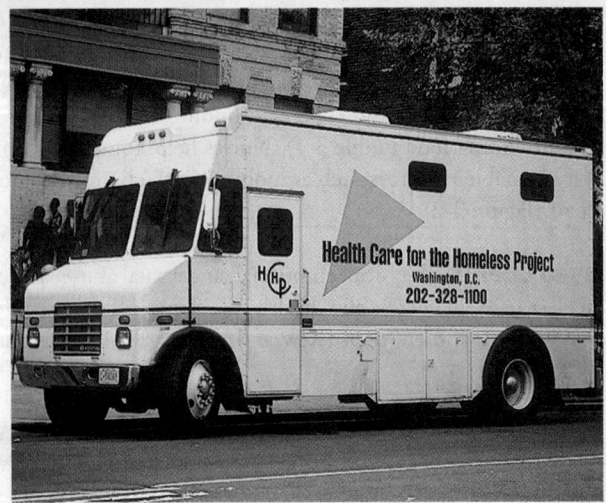

Figure 3-2 The homeless population has unique health care needs.

2006). Risk factors for abusive relationships include mental health problems, substance abuse, socioeconomic stressors, and dysfunctional family relationships. For some, there are not any risk factors present. When dealing with clients at risk for or who have suffered abuse it is important to provide protection. Interview your client at a time when the client has privacy and the individual suspected of being the abuser is not present. Clients who are abused fear retribution if they discuss their problems with a health care provider. Most states have abuse hot lines that nurses and other health care providers must notify when they identify an individual as being at risk.

Clients Who Abuse Substances.

Substance abuse is a term that describes more than the use of illegal drugs. This term also includes the abuse of alcohol and prescribed medications such as antianxiety agents and opioid analgesics. A client with substance abuse has health and socioeconomic problems. The socioeconomic problems result from the financial strain of the cost of drugs, criminal convictions from illegal activities used to obtain drugs, communicable disease from sharing drug paraphernalia, and family breakdown. For example, health problems for cocaine users often include nasal and sinus disorders and cardiac alterations that are sometimes fatal (Decker and others, 2006; Sebastian, 2006). Objectively assess your client's substance use in terms of the amount, frequency, and type of use in order to gain useful information to assist the client. Frequently these clients avoid health care for fear of judgmental attitudes and concerns over being arrested by the police.

Severely Mentally Ill Persons.

When a client has a severe mental illness such as schizophrenia or severe personality disorders such as bipolar disorder, there are multiple health and socioeconomic problems you will need to explore. Many clients with severe mental illnesses are homeless or live in poverty. Others lack the ability to maintain employment or to even care for themselves on a daily basis. Clients suffering from mental illness often require medication therapy, counseling, housing, and vocational assis-

tance. In addition, mentally ill clients are at greater risk of abuse and assault.

The mentally ill are no longer routinely hospitalized in long-term psychiatric institutions. Instead, the goal is to offer community resources within their community. Although comprehensive service networks are in every community, many clients with mental illnesses still go untreated. In addition, because of their mental illness many are unable to maintain employment and obtain adequate housing, and they become homeless (Cunningham, McKenzie, and Taylor, 2006). Many clients are left with fewer and more fragmented services, with little skill in surviving and functioning within the community. Collaboration with multiple community resources is a key to helping clients with severe mental illness to obtain adequate health care.

Older Adults.

With the increasing older adult population, there are simultaneous increases in the number of clients suffering from chronic diseases and a greater demand for health care services. View health promotion in the older adult from a broad context. You need to understand what health means to older adult clients and the steps they take to maintain their own health and improve their level of function (Meiner and Leuckenotte, 2006). Thorough assessment and appropriate community-based interventions provide an opportunity to improve the lifestyle and quality of life of older adults (Table 3-2).

Competency in Community-Based Nursing

Nurses in community-based practices have a variety of skills and talents to successfully assist clients with meeting their health care needs. To be successful in this setting you will be a caregiver, case manager, collaborator, educator, counselor, client advocate, change agent, and epidemiologist (Teeley and others, 2006).

Caregiver

First and foremost is the role of caregiver. In the community setting you manage and care for the community's health. You apply the nursing process (see Unit III) in a critical thinking approach to ensure appropriate, individualized nursing care for specific clients and their families. In addition, you individualize care within the context of the client's community so that long-term success is more likely. Together with the client and family you develop a caring partnership to recognize actual and potential health care needs and identify needed community resources. As a caregiver, you also help to build a healthy community, which is one that is safe and includes elements to enable people to achieve and maintain a high quality of life and function.

Case Manager

In community-based practice, case management is an important competency (see Chapter 2). It is the ability to establish an appropriate plan of care based on assessment of clients and families and to coordinate needed resources and services for the client's well-being across a continuum of care. Generally a community-

✳ TABLE 3-2 Common Health Problems in Community-Dwelling Older Adults

PROBLEM	COMMUNITY HEALTH NURSING ROLES AND INTERVENTIONS
Hypertension	Monitor blood pressure and weight; educate about nutrition and antihypertensive drugs; teach stress management techniques; promote an optimal balance between rest and activity; establish blood pressure screening programs; assess client's current lifestyle and promote lifestyle changes; promote dietary modifications by using techniques such as a diet diary.
Cancer	Obtain health history; promote monthly breast self-examinations and yearly Pap smears and mammograms for older women; promote regular physical examinations; encourage smokers to stop smoking; correct mistaken beliefs about processes of aging; provide emotional support and quality of care during diagnostic and treatment procedures.
Arthritis	Educate adult about management of activities, correct body mechanics, availability of mechanical appliances, and adequate rest; promote stress management; counsel and assist the family in improving communication, role negotiation, and use of community resources; teach adult to be cautious of false advertisements that promise a cure for arthritis.
Visual impairment (e.g., loss of visual acuity, eyelid disorders, opacity of the lens)	Assist in making arrangements for eye care, such as outpatient cataract surgery, and vision examinations; help client and family safely adapt the home environment for the visually impaired client.
Hearing impairment (e.g., presbycusis)	Assist in making arrangements for hearing examination and obtain necessary prostheses; identify reputable resources in the community, and teach adult to be cautious of false advertisements.
Confusional states	Provide for a protective environment; promote activities that reinforce reality; assist with adequate personal hygiene, nutrition, and hydration; provide emotional support to the family; recommend applicable community resources such as adult day care, home care aides, and homemaker services.
Alzheimer's disease	Maintain the best possible functioning, protection, and safety; foster human dignity; demonstrate to the primary family caregiver techniques to dress, feed, and toilet adult; provide frequent encouragement and emotional support to caregiver; act as an advocate for client when dealing with respite care and support groups; protect the clients' rights; provide support to maintain family members' physical and mental health; maintain family stability; recommend financial services if needed.
Dental problems	Perform oral assessment, and refer as necessary; emphasize regular brushing and flossing, proper nutrition, and dental examinations; encourage clients with dentures to wear and take care of them; calm fears about dentist; help provide access to financial services (if necessary) and access to dental care facilities.
Medication use and abuse	Obtain drug history; educate adult about safe medication storage, the danger of polypharmacy, the risks of drug-drug and drug-food interactions, and general information about drug (e.g., drug name, purpose, side effects, dosage); instruct adult about presorting techniques (using small containers with one dose of drug that are labeled with specific administration times).
Substance abuse	Arrange and monitor detoxification if appropriate; counsel adults about substance abuse; promote stress management to avoid need for drugs or alcohol; encourage adult to use self-help groups such as Alcoholics Anonymous and Al-Anon; educate public about dangers of substance abuse.

Data from Stanhope M, Lancaster J: *Foundations of nursing in the community: community-oriented practice*, ed 2, St. Louis, 2006, Mosby; and Meiner S, Leuckenotte AG: *Gerontologic nursing*, ed 3, St. Louis, 2006, Mosby.

based case manager assumes responsibility for the case management of multiple clients. This usually involves clients who are at greatest risk for needing extensive coordination of health care services (e.g., clients with neurological disease, trauma victims, and clients with complex medical or psychiatric conditions). The greatest challenge is coordinating the activities of multiple providers and payers, in different settings, throughout a client's continuum of care. An effective case manager eventually learns the obstacles, limits, and even the opportunities that exist within the

community that influence the ability to find solutions for clients' health care needs. Case management with individual clients and families reveals the big picture of health services and the health status of a community.

Change Agent

A community-based nurse is also a change agent. This involves identifying and implementing new and more effective approaches to problems. Act as a change agent within a family system or act

BOX 3-3 Factors That Support Adoption of Change

- Client must perceive the innovation or change as more advantageous than other alternatives. The nature of the innovation determines what specific type of relative advantage (e.g., social, economic, community good) is important to those who adopt the change.
- The innovation or change must be compatible with existing values, past experiences, and needs of potential adopters. A change agent will determine needs of clients and recommend changes that fulfill those needs.
- Let clients try the innovation or change on a limited basis. New ideas that clients are able to experiment with are usually adopted more quickly. Clients trying out a new technology are able to find out how it works in their own situation.
- Clients adopt simple innovations or changes more readily than those that are complex. An innovation must be easy to understand and use.
- Clients adopt an innovation more quickly when you clearly communicate the results and when the results are visible.

Data from Rogers EM: *Diffusion of innovations*, ed 5, New York, 2003, Free Press.

as mediator on problems within the client's community. You will identify any number of problems (e.g., quality of community child care services, availability of older adult day care services, or the status of neighborhood violence). As a change agent, empower individuals and their families to creatively solve problems or become instrumental in creating change within a health care agency.

To effect change you gather and analyze facts and implement programs. This requires you to be very familiar with the community itself. Many communities are resistant to change, preferring to provide services in the established manner. Before analyzing necessary facts, it is often necessary to manage conflict between the health care providers, clarify their roles, and clearly identify the needs of the clients. If the community has a history of poor problem solving, you will have to focus on developing problem-solving capabilities (Stanhope and Lancaster, 2006). Box 3-3 describes the factors that increase the likelihood that change will be accepted and adopted. Consider each factor as having potential in helping the change process. For example, if a nurse is trying to improve a client's adherence to routine health care visits, it is useful to offer an alternative site, such as a nursing clinic, that is closer and has more convenient hours for the client to visit.

Client Advocate

Client advocacy perhaps is more important today in community-based practice because of the confusion surrounding access to health care services. Your clients often need someone to help them walk through the system, identify where to go for services, how to reach individuals with the appropriate authority, what services to request, and how to follow through with the information they received. In the community setting you are often the one who presents the client's point of view to obtain appropriate resources. It is important to provide the information necessary for clients to make informed decisions in choosing and using services appropriately. In addition, it is important for you to support and, at times, defend your clients' decisions.

Collaborator

In a community-based nursing practice you need to be competent in working not only with individuals and their families, but also with other related health care disciplines. Collaboration, or working in a combined effort with all those involved in care delivery, is necessary to develop a mutually acceptable plan that will achieve common goals (Stanhope and Lancaster, 2006). For example, when your client is discharged home with terminal cancer, you collaborate with hospice staff, social workers, and pastoral care to initiate a plan to support the client and family. For collaboration to be effective, you will need mutual trust and respect for each professional's abilities and contributions. Similarly, clients need to trust in the health care providers. Teamwork is essential for exploring client issues, knowing the contributions each professional offers, clarifying roles, and developing a plan of care that client and health care providers will accept and support.

Counselor

A counselor helps clients identify and clarify health problems and choose appropriate courses of action to solve those problems. For example, in employee assistance programs or women's shelters, a major amount of nurse-client interaction is through counseling. As a counselor, you are responsible for providing information, listening objectively, and being supportive, caring, and trustworthy. You do not make decisions but rather help your clients reach decisions that are best for them (Stanhope and Lancaster, 2006). Clients and families often require assistance in first identifying and clarifying health problems. For example, a client who repeatedly reports a problem in following a prescribed diet is actually unable to afford nutritious foods or has family members who do not support good eating habits. You need to discuss with your client factors that block or aid problem resolution, identify a range of solutions, and then discuss which solutions are most likely to be successful. You also encourage your client to make decisions and encourage confidence in the choice the client makes.

An important factor in becoming an effective counselor is knowing what a community has to offer your clients. Frequently clients have to go outside their own family to obtain the support that is necessary to improve their health status. Directing clients to appropriate resources requires that you know those resources well. What services do agencies provide, which staff members are usually available quickly, what reimbursement limitations affect access, and is there coordination between agencies within the community?

Educator

In a community-based setting you have an opportunity to work with single individuals and groups of clients. Establishing relationships with community service organizations offers educational support to a wide range of client groups. Prenatal classes, infant care, child safety, and cancer screening are just some of the health education programs provided in a community practice setting (Corrarino and others, 2000).

When the goal is to help your clients assume responsibility for their own health care, your role as an educator takes on greater importance (Stanhope and Lancaster, 2006). Clients and families have to gain the skills and knowledge needed to learn how to give care themselves. Assess your client's learning needs and readiness to learn within the context of the individual, the systems the individual interacts with (e.g., family, business, and school), and the resources available for support. Adapt your teaching skills so you can instruct the client within the home setting and make the learning process meaningful. In this practice setting you have the opportunity to follow clients over time. Planning for return demonstration of skills, using follow-up phone calls, and referring to community support and self-help groups give you an opportunity to provide continuity of instruction and to reinforce important instructional topics (see Chapter 25).

Epidemiologist

As a community health nurse, you will also apply principles of epidemiology. Your contacts with families, community groups such as schools and industries, and health care agencies place you in a unique position to initiate epidemiological activities. You may be involved in case finding, health teaching, and tracking incident rates of an illness. For example, a cafeteria worker in the local high school is diagnosed with active tuberculosis (TB). As a community health nurse, you are involved in finding new TB exposures or active disease within the worker's home, employment network, and community. Your skills are also used for noninfectious health problems, such as tracking the incidence of elevated lead levels in children in a particular community.

You may decide to focus on epidemiology as a primary role in your community health setting. To do this effectively advanced education in a master's degree program in epidemiology is usually necessary. Nurse epidemiologists are responsible for community surveillance for risk factors; for example, identifying increased fetal and infant mortality rates, increases in adolescent pregnancy, presence of infectious and communicable diseases, and outbreaks of head lice. Nurse epidemiologists protect the community's level of health, develop sensitivity to changes in the health status of the community, and help identify the cause of these changes.

Community Assessment

When practicing in a community setting, you need to learn how to assess the community at large. Community assessment is the systematic data collection on the population, monitoring the population's health status, and making information available about the health of the community (Stanhope and Lancaster, 2006). This is the environment where clients live and work. Without an adequate understanding of that environment, any effort to promote the client's health and to institute necessary change is unlikely to be successful. The community has three components: structure or locale, the people, and the social systems. To develop a complete community assessment you need to take a careful look at each of the three components to begin to identify needs for health policy, health programs, and needed health services (Box 3-4).

When assessing the structure or locale, travel around the neighborhood or community and observe its design, the location of services, and the locations where residents meet. Obtain the demographics of the population by accessing statistics on the

---

✳ BOX 3-4 Community Assessment

Structure
Name of community or neighborhood
Geographical boundaries
Emergency services
Water and sanitation
Housing
Economic status (e.g., average household income, number of residents on public assistance)
Transportation

Population
Age distribution
Sex distribution
Growth trends
Density
Education level
Predominant ethnic groups
Predominant religious groups

Social System
Education system
Government
Communication system
Welfare system
Volunteer programs
Health system

---

community from a local public health department or public library. Acquire information about existing social systems, such as schools or health care facilities, by visiting various sites and learning about their services.

Once you have a good understanding of the community, perform all individual client assessments against that background. For example, when assessing a client's home for safety, consider the following: does the client have secure locks on doors? Are windows secure and intact? Is lighting along walkways and entryways operational? As you conduct the client assessment, know the level of community violence and the available resources when help is necessary. Always assess an individual in the context of the community.

Changing Clients' Health

In a community-based practice nurses care for clients from diverse backgrounds and in diverse settings. It is relatively easy over time to become familiar with the available resources within a particular community practice setting. Likewise, with practice you learn how to identify the unique needs of individual clients. However, the challenge is promoting and protecting a client's health within the context of the community. For example, can a client with lung disease have the quality of life necessary when a community has a serious environmental pollution problem? Similarly, nurses bring together the resources necessary to improve the continuity of care that clients receive. You are a key figure in reducing the duplication of health care services and locating the best services for a client's needs.

Perhaps the most important theme to consider is how well you understand your clients' lives. This begins by establishing strong, caring relationships with clients and their families (see Chapter 8). As you gain experience, you are able to advise, counsel, and teach effectively after being accepted by the client's family and by understanding what truly makes the client unique. The day-to-day activities of family life are the variables that influence how you will adapt nursing interventions. The time of day a client goes to work, the availability of the spouse and client's parents to provide child care, and the family values that shape views about health are just a few examples of the many factors you will consider in community-based practice. Once you acquire a picture of a client's life, you then design interventions to promote health and prevent disease within the community-based practice setting.

Key Concepts

- Principles of public health nursing practice focus on assisting individuals and communities with achieving a healthy living environment.
- Essential public health functions include community assessment, policy development, and access to resources.
- When population-based health care services are effective, there is a greater likelihood that the higher levels of services will contribute efficiently to health improvement of the population.
- The community health nurse cares for the community as a whole and considers the individual or family only one member of a group at risk.
- Successful community health nursing practice involves building relationships with the community and being responsive to changes within the community.
- The community-based nurse's competence is based on decision making at the level of the individual client.
- The special needs of vulnerable populations are a challenge that nurses face in caring for these clients' increasingly complex acute and chronic health conditions.
- An important principle in dealing with clients at risk for or who have suffered abuse is protection of the client.
- Clients who abuse substances often avoid health care for fear of being arrested.
- In community-based practice it is important to understand what health means to older adults and the steps they need take to maintain their own health.
- A community-based nurse is competent as a caregiver, collaborator, educator, counselor, change agent, client advocate, case manager, and epidemiologist.
- Clients are more likely to accept a change if it is more advantageous, compatible, realistic, and easy to adopt.
- Assessment of a community includes three elements: structure or locale, the people, and the social systems.

Critical Thinking Exercises

You are managing community care for Katie, age 17, who has cerebral palsy and is severely disabled. Because of the impact of this adolescent's disability you are also providing care to Monica, age 50, who is a single parent. Katie is the youngest of three children. Her siblings are Josh, age 22, and Marilyn, age 19. Katie attends the local school district's special education program, and Monica works as a teachers' aide in another school in the district. Katie will remain in the special educa-

tion program until she is 21. Monica does not know what will happen when Katie is 21, and she has not investigated any other community resources for Katie in the last 10 years. Both siblings are in college and live in the home and are helpful in Katie's care. Josh will graduate from college, and his mother is encouraging him to move from the home.

1. What would you assess in the community to identify resources that provide family support in the care of a disabled child?

2. What resources do you think you need to identify for the family to assist Katie's siblings in moving from the home and beginning their careers?

3. How would your role as a change agent help the family begin to envision the new family structure as Josh and Marilyn move out of the home?

NCLEX®-Style Review Questions

1. The overall goal of *Healthy People 2010* is to:
   1. Assess the health care needs of individuals, families, or communities
   2. Develop and implement public health policies and improve access to care
   3. Gather information on incident rates of certain diseases and social problems
   4. Increase life expectancy and quality of life and to eliminate health disparities

2. Community health nursing is a nursing approach that merges knowledge from which of the following professional nursing theories? (Select all that apply.)
   1. Population sciences
   2. Public health sciences
   3. Mental health sciences
   4. Environmental sciences

3. You are caring for a Bosnian community. You identify that the children are undervaccinated and the community is unaware of resources. As you assess the community, you determine that there is a health clinic with a 5-mile radius. You meet with the community leaders and explain the need for immunizations, the location of the clinic, and the process of accessing health care resources. Which of the following practices are you providing? (Select all that apply.)
   1. Educating about community resources
   2. Teaching the community about illnesses
   3. Promoting autonomy in decision-making
   4. Improving the health care of the community's children

4. Vulnerable populations of clients are those who are more likely to develop health problems as a result of:
   1. Chronic diseases, homelessness, and poverty
   2. Poverty and limits in access to health care services
   3. Lack of transportation, dependence on others for care, and homelessness
   4. Excess risks, limits in access to health care services, and dependency on others for care

5. Which of the following are major public health problems commonly affecting older adults? (Select all that apply.)
   1. Substance abuse
   2. Confusional states
   3. Financial limitations
   4. Communicable diseases
   5. Acute and chronic physical illnesses

6. The local health department received information from the Centers for Disease Control and Prevention that the flu was expected to be very contagious this season. You are asked to set up flu vaccine clinics in local churches and senior citizen centers. This activity is an example of which level of prevention?
   1. Tertiary intervention
   2. Primary intervention
   3. Nursing intervention
   4. Secondary intervention

7. The local school has an increasing number of adolescent parents, and you work with the school district to design and teach classes about infant care, child safety, and time management. These are examples of which nursing role?
   1. Educator
   2. Advocate
   3. Consultant
   4. Case manager

8. You are practicing in an occupational health setting. There are a large number of employees who smoke, and you design an employee assistance program for smoking cessation. This is an example of which nursing role:
   1. Educator
   2. Counselor
   3. Collaborator
   4. Case manager

9. In your community clinic you care for Lisa, a 40-year-old woman who takes insulin to manage her diabetes. She is having increased difficulty in managing her disease, and you want her to try a new insulin pump to help her control the disease. Which of the following change factors increase the likelihood that she will accept this new insulin pump? (Select all that apply.)
   1. Lisa tries the insulin pump on a limited basis.
   2. Lisa views use of the insulin pump as a simpler way to control her blood sugars.
   3. The insulin pump is compatible with Lisa's existing needs, values, and past experiences.
   4. Lisa perceives the insulin pump as more advantageous than other alternatives to insulin administration.

10. What are the three elements that are included in a community assessment?
    1. Environment, families, and social systems
    2. People, neighborhoods, and social systems
    3. Structure or locale, people, and social systems
    4. Health care systems, geographic boundaries, and people

4 | Theoretical Foundations of Nursing Practice

✳ OBJECTIVES

Mastery of content in this chapter will enable the student to:

- Explain the influence of nursing theory on a nurse's approach to practice
- Describe types of nursing theories.
- Describe the relationship between theory, the nursing process, and client needs.

- Discuss selected theories from other disciplines.
- Discuss selected nursing theories.
- Describe the value of nursing theory to nursing practice.

✳ MEDIA RESOURCES   ✳ KEY TERMS

 Companion CD

- NCLEX®-Style Review Questions
- Audio Glossary
- English/Spanish Glossary
- Interactive Learning Activities

evolve Website

- NCLEX®-Style Review Questions
- Audio Glossary
- English/Spanish Glossary
- Interactive Learning Activities
- WebLinks
- Audio Summaries

Assumptions, p. 46
Concepts, p. 46
Content, 47
Descriptive theory, p. 47
Domain, p. 45
Environment/situation, p. 45
Feedback, p. 47
Grand theories, p. 46
Health, p. 45
Input, p. 47
Interdisciplinary theory, p. 47

Middle-range theories, p. 46
Nursing, p. 45
Nursing theory, p. 45
Nursing's paradigm, p. 45
Output, p. 47
Paradigm, p. 45
Person, p. 45
Phenomenon, p. 46
Prescriptive theories, p. 47
Theory, p. 46

Providing excellent, evidence-based nursing care is an expectation for all nurses. You will learn to apply knowledge from nursing science, basic social sciences, physical sciences, biobehavioral sciences, ethics, and health policy. To address individual and family responses to health problems, theory-based nursing practice is necessary to design and implement nursing interventions to meet your client's needs. Initially you might find nursing theory difficult to understand or appreciate. However, as you increase your knowledge about theories you will find that these theories help to describe, explain, predict, and/or prescribe nursing care measures. For example, a theory about caring gives you a way to communicate with your clients and their families. The scientific work used in developing theories expands the scientific knowledge of the profession. Theories offer well-grounded rationales or reasons for how and why nurses perform specific interventions.

Expertise in nursing is a result of knowledge and clinical experience. The expertise required to interpret clinical situations and make clinical judgments is the essence of nursing care and is the basis for advancing nursing practice and nursing science (Benner and Tanner, 1987; Carnevali and Thomas, 1993). You will learn from experience and grow professionally by being familiar with nursing theory and applying theory to your practice. Well-developed theories are an important basis for your approach to client care.

The Domain of Nursing

The **domain** is the perspective of a profession. It provides the subject, central concepts, values and beliefs, phenomena of interest, and the central problems of a discipline. The domain of nursing provides both the practical and theoretical aspects for the discipline. It is the knowledge of nursing practice, including nursing history, nursing theory, education, practice, and research. It provides a means to identify and treat clients' health care needs at all levels of health and in all health care settings.

A paradigm is useful in describing the domain of a discipline. A **paradigm** links science, philosophy, and theories accepted and applied by the discipline. Nursing's paradigm includes four linkages: the person, health, environment/situation, and nursing (Figure 4-1). The elements of **nursing's paradigm** direct the activity of the nursing profession, including knowledge development, philosophy, theory, educational experience, research, and practice (Tomey and Alligood, 2006).

Person is the recipient of nursing care, including individual clients, families, and communities. The person is central to the nursing care you provide. Because the person's needs are often

complex, it is important to provide individualized client-centered care.

Health has different meanings for each client, the clinical setting, and the health care profession (see Chapter 6). Health is dynamic and continuously changing. Your challenge is to provide the best possible care based on the client's level of health and health care needs at the time of care delivery.

Environment/situation includes all possible conditions affecting the client and the setting in which health care needs occur. There is a continuous interaction between the client and the environment. This interaction has positive and negative effects on the person's level of health and health care needs. In addition, factors in the home, school, workplace, or community all influence a client's level of health and health care needs. For example, an adolescent girl with type 1 diabetes needs to adapt her treatment plan to physical activities of school, to the demands of a part-time job, and to the timing of social events, such as her prom.

In medicine, physicians diagnose and treat disease. In contrast, **Nursing** is the ". . . diagnosis and treatment of human responses to actual or potential health problems . . ." (ANA, 2003). The scope of nursing is broad. For example, a nurse does not medically diagnose the client's heart condition but instead assesses the client's response to the disease and may develop nursing diagnoses of fatigue, change in body image, and altered coping. From these nursing diagnoses, the nurse creates an individualized plan of care for each of the client's health problems (see Unit III). You will use critical thinking skills to integrate knowledge, experience, attitudes, and standards into the individualized plan of care for each client. Theory is one aspect of knowledge that allows you to successfully care for clients.

Theory

Theories are designed to explain a phenomenon, such as self-care or caring (Fawcett, 2005). For example, the nurse using Orem's self-care deficit theory helps clients meet their own therapeutic self-care demands. In this theory, nursing assists clients by acting for, doing, or guiding physical and/or psychological support (Fawcett, 2005). Orem's theory contains a detailed framework of self-care concepts that are linked in such a way as to explain, describe, or predict the type of nursing care that assists clients with achieving a better level of health (McEwen and Willis, 2007). A theory is a way of seeing through a "set of relatively concrete and specific concepts and the propositions that describe or link the concepts" (Fawcett, 2005).

A **nursing theory** is a conceptualization of some aspect of nursing communicated for the purpose of describing, explaining, predicting, and/or prescribing nursing care (Meleis, 2006). For example, Orem's theory (2001) explains the factors within a client's living situation that support or interfere with the client's self-care ability. As a result, a nurse who practices by this theory can anticipate such factors when designing an education plan for the client. This theory has value in helping nursing design interventions to promote the client's self-care in managing an illness, such as diabetes or arthritis.

Theories constitute much of the knowledge of a discipline, and theory and inquiry are vital linkages to each other (Fawcett

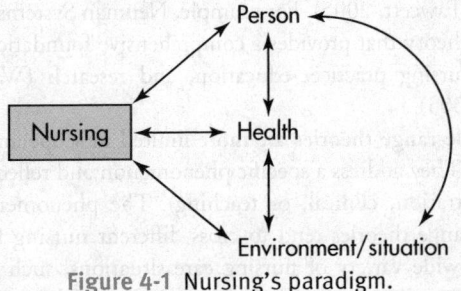

Figure 4-1 Nursing's paradigm.

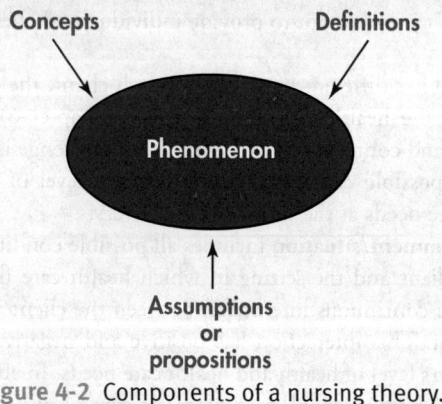

Figure 4-2 Components of a nursing theory.

and others, 2001). Nursing theories provide nurses with a perspective to view client situations, a way to organize data, and a method to analyze and interpret information. If a nurse uses Orem's theory in practice, the nurse assesses and interprets the data to determine the client's self-care needs, self-care deficits, and self-care abilities in the management of a disease. The theory then guides the design of individualized nursing interventions. Application of nursing theory in practice depends on the nurse's knowledge of nursing and other theoretical models, how these models relate to each other, and the use of these models in designing nursing interventions.

Nursing is a learned profession, a science, and an art. Nurses need a theoretical base to demonstrate the science and art of the profession when they promote health and wellness for their clients, whether the client is an individual, a family, or a community.

Components of a Theory

A **theory** is a set of concepts, definitions, and assumptions or propositions to explain a phenomenon (Figure 4-2). The theory explains how these elements are uniquely related in the phenomenon. Researchers test the theories, and as a result, the researcher sees a clearer perspective of all parts of a phenomenon. For example, Kristin Swanson studied the phenomenon of caring by conducting extensive interviews with clients and their professional caregivers (Swanson, 1991). Swanson's theory of caring defines five components of caring: knowing, being with, doing for, enabling, and maintaining belief (see Chapter 8). These components provide a foundation of knowledge for the direction and delivery of caring nursing practice. This theory provides a basis for identifying and testing nurse caring behaviors to determine if caring improves client health outcomes.

Phenomenon. Nursing theories focus on the phenomena of nursing and nursing care. A **phenomenon** is an aspect of reality that people consciously sense or experience (Meleis, 2006). Examples of phenomena of nursing include caring, self-care, and client responses to stress. In Neuman Systems Model (1995), phenomena include all client responses, environmental factors, and nursing actions.

Concepts. A theory consists of interrelated concepts. These **concepts** can be simple or complex and relate to an object or

event that comes from individual perceptual experiences (Tomey and Alligood, 2006). They are ideas and mental images. Concepts help to describe or label phenomena. Using Neuman Systems Model (1995) as an example, there are concepts that affect the client system. The client system is an open structure that includes internal and external environmental factors (Tomey and Alligood, 2002). These factors are physiological, psychological, sociocultural, and environmental and may relate to health and wellness, prevention, stressors, and defense mechanisms (Meleis, 2006).

Definitions. The definitions within a theory communicate the general meaning of the concepts. These definitions describe the activity necessary to measure the concepts, relationships, or variables within a theory (Chinn and Kramer, 2004; Tomey and Alligood, 2006). For example, Neuman Systems Model uses a system approach to describe how clients deal with stressors in their internal or external environments. Nurses using Neuman's theory in practice focus their care on client responses to the stressors (Meleis, 2006). For example, when clients take on a new role within their employment, they may react to the stress by eating an improper diet. In this situation the nurse focuses on the client response to the stressors and designs interventions related to improving nutritional intake.

Assumptions. **Assumptions** are the "taken for granted" statements that explain the nature of the concepts, definitions, purpose, relationships, and structure of a theory (Chinn and Kramer, 2004; Meleis, 2006). For example, in Neuman Systems Model the assumptions include the following: clients are dynamic; the relationships between the theory's concepts influence a client's protective mechanisms and determine a client's response; clients have a normal range of responses; stressors attack flexible lines of defense followed by the normal lines of defense; and the nurse's actions focus on primary, secondary, and tertiary prevention (Neuman, 1995).

Types of Theory

The general purpose of a theory is important because it specifies the context and situation in which the theory applies (Chinn and Kramer, 2004). Theories have different purposes and are sometimes classified by levels of abstraction (grand theories versus middle-range theories) or the goals of the theory (descriptive or prescriptive). Theories describe, predict, or prescribe activities for the phenomena of interest (Box 4-1).

Grand theories are broad in scope, complex, and therefore require further specification through research. A grand theory does not provide guidance for specific nursing interventions but provides the structural framework for broad, abstract ideas about nursing (Fawcett, 2005). For example, Neuman Systems Model is a grand theory that provides a comprehensive foundation for scientific nursing practice, education, and research (Walker and Avant, 2005).

Middle-range theories are more limited in scope and are less abstract. They address a specific phenomenon and reflect practice (administration, clinical, or teaching). The phenomena within middle-range theories tend to cross different nursing fields and reflect a wide variety of nursing care situations, such as uncertainty, incontinence, social support, quality of life, and caring

✳ **BOX 4-1 Goals of Theoretical Nursing Models**

- Identify domain and goals of nursing.
- Provide knowledge to improve nursing administration, practice, education, and research.
- Guide research and expand nursing's knowledge base.
- Identify research techniques and tools used to validate nursing interventions.
- Formulate legislation governing nursing practice, research, and education.
- Formulate regulations interpreting nurse practice acts.
- Develop curriculum plans for nursing education.
- Establish criteria for measuring quality of nursing care, education, and research.
- Guide development of nursing care delivery system.
- Provide systematic structure and rationale for nursing activities.

(Meleis, 2006). For example, Mishel's theory of uncertainty in illness (1988, 1990) focuses on clients' experiences with cancer while living with continual uncertainty. The theory provides a basis to assist clients in coping with the uncertainty and the illness response.

Descriptive theories are the first level of theory development. They describe phenomena, speculate on why phenomena occur, and describe the consequences of phenomena. These theories explain, relate, and in some situations predict nursing phenomena (Meleis, 2006). For example, theories of growth and development describe the maturation processes of an individual at various ages (see Chapter 11). Descriptive theories do not direct specific nursing activities but help to explain client assessments.

Prescriptive theories address nursing interventions for a phenomenon and predict the consequence of a specific nursing intervention. In nursing, a prescriptive theory designates the prescription (i.e., nursing interventions), the conditions under which the prescription occurs, and the consequences (Meleis, 2006). Prescriptive theories are action oriented and test the validity and predictability of a nursing intervention. These theories guide nursing research to develop and test specific nursing interventions (Fawcett, 2005). For example, Mishel's theory of uncertainty predicts that increasing the coping skills of clients with gynecological cancer assists their ability to deal with the uncertainty of the cancer diagnosis and treatment (Mishel, 1997; Mishel and Sorenson, 1991). Thus the theory provides a framework to design interventions that support and strengthen clients' coping resources.

Relationship of Theory to Nursing Practice

As nursing continues to grow as a profession, knowledge is needed to prescribe specific interventions to improve client outcomes. Nursing theories and related concepts continue to evolve. Florence Nightingale spoke with firm conviction about the "nature of nursing as a profession that requires knowledge distinct from medical knowledge" (Nightingale, 1860). The overall goal of nursing knowledge is to explain the practice of nursing as different and distinct from the practice of medicine, psychology, and social work (Chinn and Kramer, 2004).

Theory generates nursing knowledge for use in practice. The integration of theory into practice is the basis for professional nursing (McEwen and Wills, 2007). The nursing process is used in clinical settings to determine the individual client needs (see Unit III). Although the nursing process is central to nursing, it is not a theory. It provides a systematic process for the delivery of nursing care, not the knowledge component of the discipline. However, a theory can direct how a nurse uses the nursing process. For example, a theory of caring influences what to assess, how to determine client needs, how to plan care, how to select individualized nursing interventions, and how to evaluate client outcomes. Useful theories are adaptable to different clients and all care settings.

Interdisciplinary Theories

To practice in today's health care systems, nurses need a strong scientific knowledge base from nursing and other disciplines, such as the physical, social, and behavioral sciences. Knowledge from these other disciplines includes relevant theories that explain phenomena. An **interdisciplinary theory** explains a systematic view of a phenomenon specific to the discipline of inquiry. For example, Piaget's theory of cognitive development helps to explain how children think, reason, and perceive the world (see Chapter 12).

Systems Theory

A system is made up of separate components. The components are interrelated and share a common purpose to form a whole. There are two types of systems, open and closed. An open system, such as a human organism or processes like the nursing process, interacts with the environment, exchanging information between the system and the environment. Factors that change the environment also affect the system. A closed system, such as a chemical reaction within a test tube, does not interact with the environment.

Like all systems, the nursing process has a specific purpose or goal. The goal of the nursing process is to organize and deliver an individualized approach to nursing care. As a system, the nursing process has the following components: input, output, feedback, and content (Figure 4-3). **Input** for the nursing process is the data or information that comes from a client's assessment (e.g., how the client interacts with the environment and the client's physiological function). **Output** is the end product of a system and in the case of the nursing process it is whether the client's health status improves or remains stable as a result of nursing care.

Feedback serves to inform a system about how it functions. For example, in the nursing process the outcomes reflect the client's responses to nursing interventions. The **content** is the product and information obtained from the system. Again, using the nursing process as a example, the content is the information about the nursing care for clients with specific health care problems. For example, clients with impaired mobility have common skin care needs and interventions (e.g., hygiene and scheduled positioning changes) that are very successful in reducing the risk for pressure ulcers.

Some nursing theories use a systems theory as a base. For example, Neuman (1995) defines a total-person model of wholism

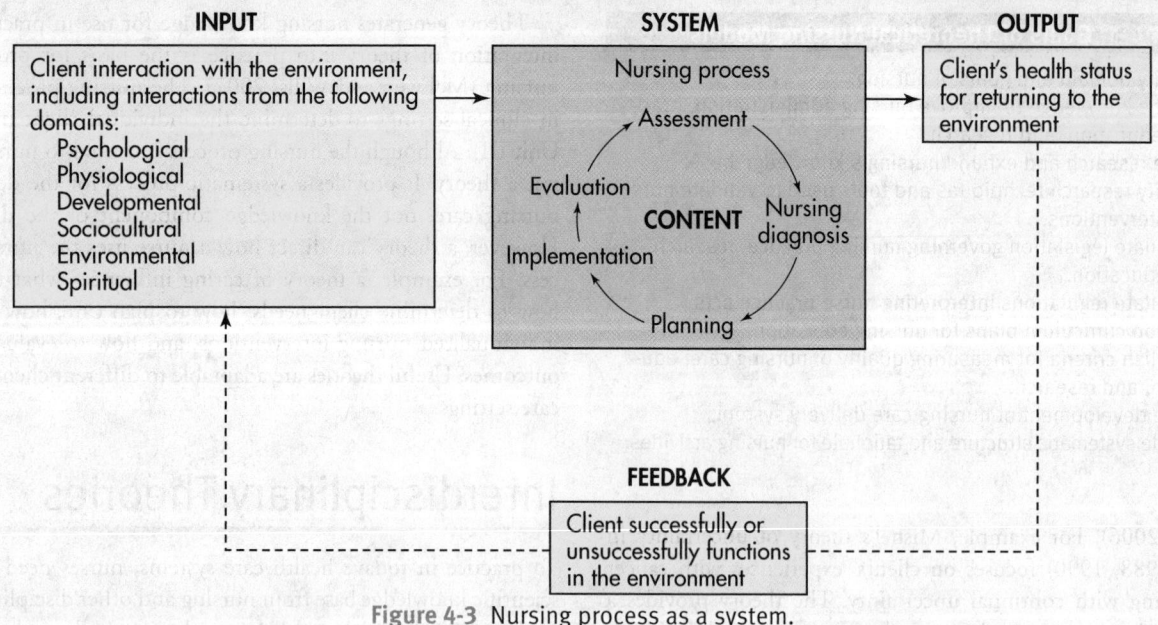

Figure 4-3 Nursing process as a system.

and an open-systems approach. As an open system, a person interacts with the environment. The environment is both external and internal, and the person interacts with stressors from the environment, which may affect the well-being of the client.

Basic Human Needs

Maslow's hierarchy of needs is an interdisciplinary theory that is useful for designating priorities of nursing care. The hierarchy of basic human needs includes five levels of priority. The most basic, or first level, includes physiological needs, such as air, water, and food. The second level includes safety and security needs, which involve physical and psychological security. The third level contains love and belonging needs, including friendship, social relationships, and sexual love. The fourth level encompasses esteem and self-esteem needs, which involve self-confidence, usefulness, achievement, and self-worth. The final level is the need for self-actualization, the state of fully achieving potential and having the ability to solve problems and cope realistically with life's situations. Maslow's hierarchy is useful in setting client priorities. Basic physiological and safety needs are usually the first priority, especially when a client is severely dependent physically. However, you will encounter situations in which a client has no emergent physical or safety needs. Instead, you will give high priority to the psychological, sociocultural, developmental, or spiritual needs of the client.

Clients entering the health care system generally have unmet needs. For example, a person brought to an emergency department experiencing acute pneumonia has an unmet need for oxygen, the most basic physiological need. An older woman in a high-crime area is concerned about physical safety and, while hospitalized, has a need for psychological security because of fear that her home will be burglarized. A widowed homemaker whose children have moved away feels that she does not belong or is not loved. Nurses in all practice settings try hard to help clients and their families meet these needs. The hierarchy of needs is a way to plan for individualized care. One need will take priority over an-

other, such as improving oxygen status before the nurse implements stress management techniques.

Developmental Theories

Human growth and development is an orderly predictive process that begins with conception and continues through death. There are a variety of well-tested theoretical models that describe and predict behavior and development at various phases of the life continuum. Chapter 11 details these developmental theories, and Chapters 12 through 14 demonstrate changes in growth and development in various age-groups.

Psychosocial Theories

Nursing is a diverse discipline that strives to meet the physiological, psychological, sociocultural, developmental, and spiritual needs of clients. There are theoretical models to explain and/or predict client responses in each of these domains. For example, Chapter 9 discusses models for understanding cultural diversity and implementing care to meet the diverse needs of the client. Chapter 10 describes family theory and how to meet the needs of the family when the family is the client or when the family is the caregiver. Chapter 30 discusses several models of grieving and demonstrates how to assist clients through loss, death, and grief.

Selected Nursing Theories

Definitions and theories of nursing can help you understand the practice of nursing. The following sections describe, in chronological order of theory development, selected theories and their concepts (Table 4-1).

Nightingale's Theory

Florence Nightingale's work was an initial model for nursing. Meleis (2006) notes that Nightingale's concept of the environment was the focus of nursing care and her suggestion that nurses

✳ TABLE 4-1 Summary of Nursing Theories

THEORIST	GOAL OF NURSING	FRAMEWORK FOR PRACTICE
Nightingale—1860	Facilitate "the body's reparative processes" by manipulating client's environment	Nurse manipulates client's environment to include appropriate noise, nutrition, hygiene, light, comfort, socialization, and hope.
Peplau—1952	Develop interaction between nurse and client (Peplau, 1952)	Nursing is a significant, therapeutic, interpersonal process (Peplau, 1952). Nurses participate in structuring health care systems to facilitate interpersonal relationships (Tomey and Alligood, 2006).
Henderson—1955	Work independently with other health care workers (Tomey and Alligood, 2006), assisting client in gaining independence as quickly as possible (Henderson, 1966); to help client gain lacking strength	Nurses help client to perform Henderson's 14 basic needs (Henderson, 1966).
Abdellah—1960	Provide service to individuals, families, and society; to be kind and caring but also intelligent, competent, and technically well prepared to provide this service (Tomey and Alligood, 2006)	This theory involves Abdellah's 21 nursing problems (Abdellah and others, 1960).
Rogers—1970	Maintain and promote health, prevent illness, and care for and rehabilitate ill and disabled client through "humanistic science of nursing" (Rogers 1970, 1990)	"Unitary man" evolves along life process. Client continuously changes and coexists with the environment.
Orem—1971	Care for and help client attain total self-care	Nursing care is necessary when the client is unable to fulfill biological, psychological, developmental, or social needs (Orem, 2001).
King—1971	Use communication to help client reestablish positive adaptation to environment	Nursing is a dynamic interpersonal process between nurse, client, and health care system (King, 1981).
Neuman—1972	Assist individuals, families, and groups in attaining and maintaining maximal level of total wellness by purposeful interventions	Stress reduction is goal of systems model of nursing practice. Nursing actions are in primary, secondary, or tertiary level of prevention (Neuman, 1995).
Leininger—1978	Provide care consistent with nursing's emerging science and knowledge with caring as central focus (Chinn and Kramer, 2004)	With this transcultural care theory, caring is the central and unifying domain for nursing knowledge and practice.
Roy—1979	Identify types of demands placed on client, assess adaptation to demands, and help client adapt	This adaptation model is based on the physiological, psychological, sociological, and dependence-independence adaptive modes (Roy, 1980).
Watson—1979	Promote health, restore client to health, and prevent illness (Tomey and Alligood, 2006)	Involves the philosophy and science of caring. Caring is an interpersonal process comprising interventions to meet human needs (Watson, 1979, 1985).
Brenner and Wrubel—1989	Focus on client's need for caring as a means of coping with stressors of illness (Chinn and Kramer, 2004)	Caring is central to the essence of nursing. Caring creates the possibilities for coping and enables possibilities for connecting with and concern for others (Benner and Wrubel, 1989).

Modified from Chinn PL, Kramer ML: *Integrated knowledge development in nursing,* ed 6, St. Louis, 2004, Mosby.

need not know all about the disease process were early attempts to differentiate between nursing and medicine.

Nightingale did not view nursing as limited to the administration of medications and treatments but rather as oriented toward providing fresh air, light, warmth, cleanliness, quiet, and adequate nutrition (Nightingale, 1860). Through observation and data collection, she linked the client's health status with environmental factors and initiated improved hygiene and sanitary conditions during the Crimean War.

Nightingale's "descriptive theory" provides nurses with a way to think about clients and their environments. Nightingale's letters and writings direct the nurse to act on behalf of the client.

Her visionary principles included the areas of practice, research, and education. Most important, her concepts and principles shaped and defined nursing practice (Tomey and Alligood, 2006). Nightingale taught and used the nursing process, noting that "vital observation [assessment] . . . is not for the sake of piling up miscellaneous information or curious facts, but for the sake of saving life and increasing health and comfort."

Peplau's Theory

Hildegard Peplau's theory (1952) focuses on the individual, the nurse, and the interactive process. The result is the nurse-client relationship. The client is an individual with a need, and nursing is an interpersonal and therapeutic process. Nursing's goal is to educate the client and family and to help the client reach mature personality development (Chinn and Kramer, 2004).

In developing a nurse-client relationship, the nurse can serve as a resource person, counselor, and surrogate. For example, when the client seeks help, the nurse and client first discuss the nature of the problem and the nurse explains the services available. As the nurse-client relationship develops, the nurse and client mutually define the problem and potential solutions. The client gains from this relationship by using available services to meet needs, and the nurse assists the client in reducing anxiety related to the health care problem.

Peplau's theory is unique: the collaborative nurse-client relationship creates a "maturing force" through which interpersonal effectiveness meets the client's needs. When the client's original needs are resolved, new needs sometimes emerge. The following phases characterize the nurse-client interpersonal relationship: orientation, identification, explanation, and resolution (Chinn and Kramer, 2004).

Henderson's Theory

Virginia Henderson defines nursing as "assisting the individual, sick or well, in the performance of those activities that will contribute to health, recovery, or a peaceful death and that the individual would perform unaided if he or she had the necessary strength, will, or knowledge" (Harmer and Henderson, 1955; Henderson, 1966). The process of nursing strives to do this as rapidly as possible, and the goal is independence. Henderson organized the theory into 14 basic needs of the whole person and includes phenomena from the following domains of the client: physiological, psychological, sociocultural, spiritual, and developmental. Together the nurse and client work together to meet these needs and attain client-centered goals.

Rogers' Theory

Martha Rogers (1970) considers the individual (unitary human being) as an energy field coexisting within the universe. The individual is a unified whole, continuously interacting with the environment, possessing personal integrity and manifesting characteristics that are more than the sum of the parts (Rogers, 1970, 1990). The unitary human being is a "four dimensional energy field identified by pattern and manifesting characteristics that are specific to the whole and which cannot be predicted from the knowledge of parts" (Tomey and Alligood, 2006). The four dimensions of Rogers' theory—energy fields, openness, pattern and organization, and dimensionality—aid in the development of principles related to human development.

Orem's Theory

Dorothea Orem's self-care deficit theory (1971) focuses on the client's self-care needs. Orem defines self-care as a learned, goal-oriented activity directed toward the self in the interest of maintaining life, health, development, and well-being. The goal of Orem's theory is to help the client perform self-care. Nursing care is necessary when the client is unable to fulfill biological, psychological, developmental, or social needs. The nurse determines why a client is unable to meet these needs, what needs to be done to enable the client to meet them, and how much self-care the client

is able to perform. The goal of nursing is to increase the client's ability to independently meet these needs (Orem, 2001).

Leininger's Theory

Leininger's cultural care diversity and universality theory (1991) states that care is the essence of nursing and the dominant, distinctive, and unifying feature of nursing. Human caring varies among cultures in its expressions, processes, and patterns. Social structure factors, such as the client's religion, politics, culture, and traditions are significant forces affecting care and influencing the client's health and illness patterns. The goal of Leininger's theory is to provide the client with culturally specific nursing care. To provide care to clients of unique cultures the nurse safely integrates the client's cultural traditions, values, and beliefs into the plan of care. For example, some cultures believe that the leader in the community needs to be present during health care decisions. As a result, the health care team may need to reschedule when rounds occur in order to include the community leader. In addition, symptom expression also differs among cultures. For example, a person with an Irish background might be stoic and not complain about pain. In contrast, a person from a Middle Eastern culture might be very vocal about pain. In both examples, the nurse needs to be skillful in incorporating the client's cultural practices in assessing the client's level of pain (e.g., is the pain getting worse or remaining the same?).

Roy's Theory

Sister Callista Roy's adaptation theory (Roy, 1980, 1989; Roy and Obloy, 1979) views the client as an adaptive system. According to Roy's model, the goal of nursing is to help the person adapt to changes in physiological needs, self-concept, role function, and interdependent relations during health and illness (Tomey and Alligood, 2006). The need for nursing care occurs when the client cannot adapt to internal and external environmental demands. All individuals must adapt to the following demands:

1. Meeting basic physiological needs
2. Developing a positive self-concept
3. Performing social roles
4. Achieving a balance between dependence and independence

The nurse determines what demands are causing problems for a client and assesses how well the client is adapting to them. Nurses direct care at helping the client adapt. For example, a postoperative client who has a significant blood loss and now has a low hematocrit value needs nursing interventions to assist in adapting to the associated fatigue. The nurse designs interventions to allow sufficient rest periods.

Watson's Theory

Jean Watson's philosophy of transpersonal caring (1979, 1985, 1987) defines the outcome of nursing activity in regard to the humanistic aspects of life (Tomey and Alligood, 2006). Nursing action's purpose is to understand the interrelationship between health, illness, and human behavior. Thus nursing is concerned with promoting and restoring health and preventing illness.

Watson designed the model around the caring process, assisting clients in attaining or maintaining health or dying peacefully. This caring process requires the nurse to be knowledgeable about human behavior and human responses to actual or potential health problems. The nurse also needs to know individual needs, how to respond to others, and strengths and limitations of the client and family, as well as those of the nurse. In addition, the nurse comforts and offers compassion and empathy to clients and their families. Caring represents all factors the nurse uses to deliver care to the client (Watson, 1987).

Benner and Wrubel's Theory

The primacy of caring is a model proposed by Patricia Benner and Judith Wrubel (1989). Caring is central. Caring creates possibilities for coping, enables possibilities for connecting with and concern for others, and allows for the giving and receiving of help (Chinn and Kramer, 2004). Caring means that persons, events, projects, and things matter to people. Caring presents a connection and represents a wide range of involvement (e.g., caring about one's family, caring about one's friendships, and caring about one's clients). Benner and Wrubel see the personal concern as an inherent feature of nursing practice. In caring for one's clients, nurses help clients recover by noticing those interventions that are successful and guide future caregiving (Edwards, 2001).

•••

Application of nursing theory in practice depends on nurses having knowledge of the theories, as well as an understanding of how the theories relate to one another. Theories are the organizing frameworks for the science of nursing and the substantive approaches for nursing care. They provide critical thinking structures to guide clinical reasoning and problem solving.

The Link Between Theory and Knowledge Development in Nursing

Nursing has its own body of knowledge that is both theoretical and practical. Theoretical knowledge includes and "reflects on the basic values, guiding principles, elements, and phases of a conception of nursing" (Meleis, 2006). The goals of theoretical knowledge stimulate thinking and create a broad understanding of the "science" and practices of the nursing discipline.

Practical knowledge is not organized in the same manner as theoretical knowledge. Practical knowledge or the "art" of nursing is based on nurses' experience in providing care to clients. You achieve this through personal knowing gained through reflection on care experiences, synthesis, and integration of the art and science of nursing.

An earlier discussion in this chapter indicated that theories provided direction to nursing research. The relationships of components in a theory help drive the research questions for understanding nursing phenomena. For example, the relationship of components within Orem's self-care deficit theory led nurse researchers to test approaches for improving self-care. Older hospitalized adults were able to learn their medication schedules and improve their activities of daily living before discharge and were discharged earlier and had fewer complications (Glasson and others, 2006).

The relationship between nursing theory and nursing research helps to build the discipline's knowledge base. As more research is conducted, the discipline learns to what extent a given theory is useful in providing knowledge that improves client care.

Theory-generating research tries to discover and describe relationships of phenomena without imposing preconceived notions (e.g., hypotheses) of what the phenomena under study mean (Chinn and Kramer, 2004). In theory-generating research, the investigator makes observations in order to view a phenomenon in a new way. For example, a researcher wants to understand end-of-life surrogate decision making. In this example, the researcher interviews surrogate decision makers. From these interviews the researcher makes objective observations about the surrogate decision-making process, resulting in an initial theory of surrogate decision making.

Theory-testing research determines how accurately a theory describes a nursing phenomenon. The investigator has some preconceived idea as to how the client describes the phenomenon, and the researcher generates research questions or hypotheses to test the assumptions of the theory. No one study tests all components of a theory; researchers test the theory through a variety of research activities. Using the previous example of surrogate decision making, the researcher tests elements of the theory. For example, interviews of decision makers indicated that there was a need for more knowledge about end-of-life care expectations. The researcher then designs and tests an educational program that incorporates end-of-life expectation with one that does not to determine which is most effective for groups of surrogate caregivers.

Theory-generating or theory-testing research increases nursing's knowledge base. As a result, nurses incorporate research-based interventions into practice (King and Fawcett, 1997). As research activities continue, not only does the knowledge and science of nursing increase, but also clients are the recipients of the best evidence-based nursing practice (see Chapter 5).

As an art, nursing relies on knowledge gained from practice and reflection on past experiences. As a science, nursing draws on scientifically tested knowledge applied in the practice setting (Kikuchi, Simmons, and Romyn, 1996). But it is the "expert nurse" who transports the art and science of nursing into the scientific realm of creative caring.

✳ Key Concepts

- Theoretical nursing models provide knowledge to improve practice, guide research and nursing curricula, and identify the domain and goals of nursing practice.
- A nursing theory is a conceptualization of some aspect of nursing communicated for the purpose of describing, explaining, predicting, and/or prescribing nursing care.
- Grand theories are the complex structural framework for broad, abstract ideas.
- Middle-range theories are more limited in scope and less abstract. These theories address specific phenomena or concepts and reflect practice.
- Nursing's paradigm identifies four links of interest to the profession: the person, health, environment/situation, and nursing. Nurse theorists agree that these four components are essential to the development of theory.

- Theory is the generation of nursing knowledge used for practice. Nursing process is the method for applying the theory or knowledge. The integration of theory and nursing process is the basis for professional nursing.
- Theories from nursing and other disciplines help explain how the roles and actions of nurses fit together in nursing.
- Theory-generating research tries to discover and describe relationships without imposing preconceived notions (e.g., hypotheses) of what the phenomenon under study means.
- Theory-testing research determines how accurately a theory describes nursing phenomena.

✳ Critical Thinking Exercises

1. Part of your education includes experiences in different types of health care settings. Taking Orem's theory, explain how it might apply in different health care settings.
   a. Acute care
   b. Community based

2. The following are examples of theory-generating or theory-testing research. Determine whether they are theory- or research-generating and explain.
   a. Do clients who receive a prescribed exercise program wean more quickly from the mechanical ventilator?
   b. What are the perspectives of clients about weaning from mechanical ventilation?
   c. How does a family member affected by divorce perceive his or her family hardiness?
   d. How does a family member in a divorced family measure his or her own level of hardiness?

✳ NCLEX®-Style Review Questions

1. Nursing's paradigm includes:
   1. Health, person, environment, and theory
   2. Concepts, theory, health, and environment
   3. Nurses, physicians, models, and client needs
   4. The person, health, environment/situation, and nursing

2. Which of the following statements about prescriptive theories is accurate? Prescriptive theories:
   1. Describe phenomena
   2. Have the ability to explain nursing phenomena
   3. Reflect practice and address specific phenomena
   4. Provide a structural framework for broad abstract ideas

3. A theory is a set of concepts, definitions, relationships, and assumptions that:
   1. Formulate legislation
   2. Explain a phenomenon
   3. Measure nursing functions
   4. Reflect the domain of nursing practice

4. There is a contemporary move toward nursing as a science, or evidence-based practice. This suggests:
   1. One theory will guide nursing practice
   2. Scientists will decide nursing decisions
   3. Nursing will base client care on the practice of other sciences
   4. Theories will be tested to describe or predict client outcomes

5. To practice in today's health care environment, nurses need a strong scientific knowledge base from nursing and other disciplines, such as the physical, social, and behavioral sciences. This is an example of which of the following?
   1. Systems theories
   2. Developmental theories
   3. Interdisciplinary theories
   4. Health and wellness models

6. Knowledge of which of the following assist nurses in understanding and predicting the client's health behaviors, including use of health care services and adherence to recommended therapies?
   1. Systems theories
   2. Interdisciplinary theories
   3. Health-and-wellness models
   4. Stress and adaptation models

7. Which theories begin with conception and continue through death in an orderly process?
   1. Systems theories
   2. Developmental theories
   3. Interdisciplinary theories
   4. Stress and adaptation theories

8. Maslow's hierarchy of needs is useful to nurses, who continually prioritize a client's nursing care needs. The most basic or first-level needs include:
   1. Self-actualization
   2. Air, water, and food
   3. Love and belonging
   4. Esteem and self-esteem needs

9. Leininger's theory of cultural care diversity and universality specifically addresses:
   1. Caring for clients from unique cultures
   2. Understanding of the humanistic aspects of life
   3. Variables affecting a client's response to a stressor
   4. Caring for clients who cannot adapt to internal and external environmental demands

10. As an art, nursing relies on knowledge gained from practice and reflection on past experiences. As a science, nursing relies on:
    1. Experimental research
    2. Nonexperimental research
    3. Physician-generated research
    4. Scientifically tested knowledge

5 | Evidence-Based Practice

✳ OBJECTIVES

Mastery of content in this chapter will enable the student to:

- Discuss the benefits of evidence-based practice.
- Describe the five steps of evidence-based practice.
- Develop a PICO question.
- Explain the levels of evidence in the literature.
- Discuss ways to apply evidence in practice.
- Explain how nursing research improves nursing practice.

- Discuss the steps of the research process.
- Discuss priorities for nursing research.
- Explain the relationship between evidence-based practice and quality improvement.
- Describe the components of a quality improvement program.

✳ MEDIA RESOURCES ✳ KEY TERMS

 Companion CD

- NCLEX®-Style Review Questions
- Audio Glossary
- English/Spanish Glossary
- Interactive Learning Activities

 Website

- NCLEX®-Style Review Questions
- Audio Glossary
- English/Spanish Glossary
- Interactive Learning Activities
- WebLinks
- Audio Summaries

Rick has been a registered nurse (RN) in the emergency department for over 5 years. During that time the nurses have followed a policy of restricting family visitation when clients experience critical events requiring emergency resuscitation. The policy allows nurses to attend to the client and administer life-saving care without family interference. The nurses have assumed that the experience of watching a loved one be resuscitated is too traumatic for family members. However, Rick has noticed for some time that the families of resuscitated clients experience significant stress when they are unable to stay with a loved one. Later, after the resuscitation, the staff may face anger or resentment from families. Rick raises the question with the other RNs in the department, "What are the benefits of family visitation during resuscitation? Is it possible that family presence during resuscitation will improve outcomes for our families?"

Most nurses like Rick practice nursing according to what they learn in nursing school, their experiences in practice, and the policies and procedures of their institution. Such an approach to practice does not mean that nursing practice is based on up-to-date information. It may mean that nursing practice is based on tradition and not on current evidence. If Rick went to the scientific literature for articles about family presence during resuscitation, he would find evidence that shows the benefits of such an approach (Meyers and others, 2000; Clark and others, 2005). The evidence from research studies and the opinions of critical care experts provide a basis for Rick and his colleagues to make evidence-based changes to their visitation policy. The use of evidence in practice enables clinicians like Rick to provide the highest quality of care to their clients and families.

A Case for Evidence

Nurses practice in an "age of accountability" where quality and cost issues drive the direction of health care (Kizer and others, 2000; Newhouse and others, 2005). The general public is more informed about their own health, the health care issues affecting society, and the incidence of medical errors within health care institutions across the country. Greater scrutiny is being given to why certain health care approaches are used, which ones work and which ones do not. As a result, evidence-based practice (EBP) is a response to the broad societal forces that nurses and other health professionals must contend with (Newhouse and others, 2005). EBP is a guide for nurses to structure how to make accurate, timely, and appropriate clinical decisions.

Nurse clinicians regularly face many important clinical decisions when caring for clients (e.g., what to assess in a client, what interventions are necessary, and which interventions are best). It is very important to translate best evidence into best practices at a client's bedside. Using a sliding board to transfer a client from bed to stretcher instead of lifting and using the research-based Braden scale to routinely assess a client's risk for skin breakdown are ways nurses use evidence at the bedside. **Evidence-based practice (EBP)** is a problem-solving approach to clinical practice that integrates the conscientious use of best evidence in combination with a clinician's expertise and client preferences and values in making decisions about client care (Figure 5-1) (Melnyk and Fineout-Overholt, 2005; Sackett and others, 2000).

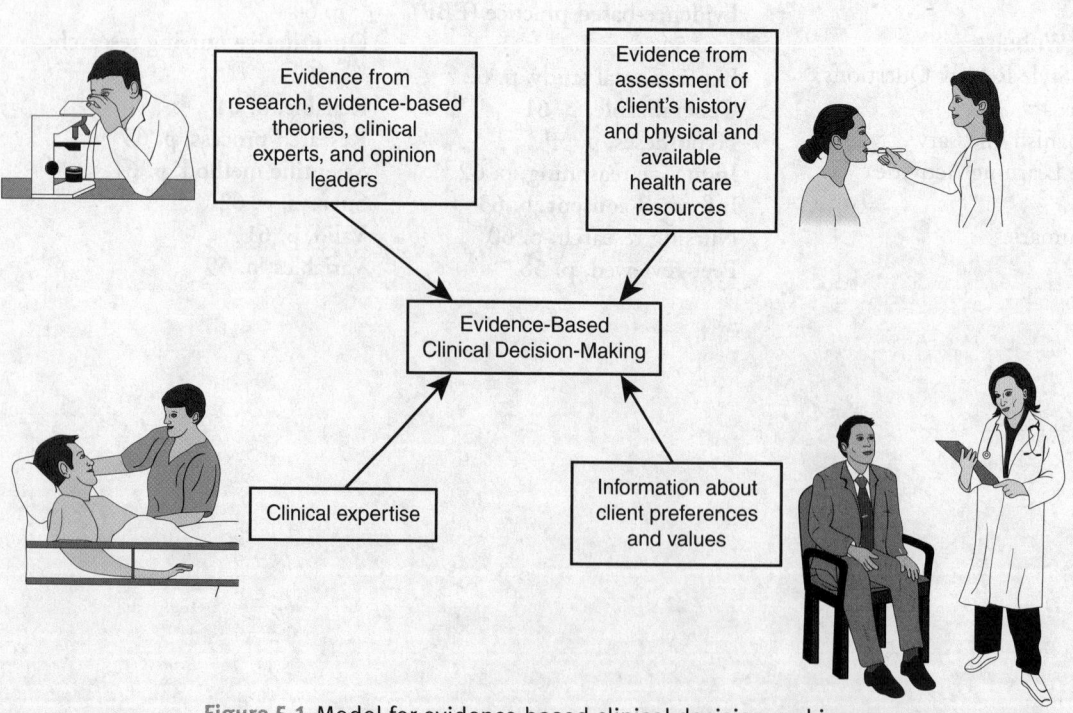

Figure 5-1 Model for evidence-based clinical decision making.

As a professional nurse, you need to stay informed and be aware of the most current evidence. Typically, new students will diligently read their textbooks and assigned scientific articles. A good textbook incorporates evidence into the practice guidelines and procedures it describes. However, a textbook relies on the scientific literature, which is often outdated by the time the book is published. Articles from nursing and the health care literature are available on almost any topic involving nursing practice. However, although the scientific basis of nursing practice has grown, some practices are not "research based" (based on findings from well-designed research studies), because findings are inconclusive or the practices have not yet been studied (Titler and others, 2001). The challenge is to be able to obtain the very best, most current information at the right time, when you need it for client care.

The best information is the evidence that comes from well-designed, systematically conducted research studies, mostly found in scientific journals. Unfortunately, much of that evidence never reaches the bedside. Nurses in practice settings, unlike educational settings, often do not have easy access to databases for scientific literature. Instead, nurses often care for clients on the basis of tradition, convenience, or the standard, "It has always been done this way."

Another source of information comes from nonresearch evidence. This includes quality improvement and risk management data; international, national, and local standards; infection control data, benchmarking, retrospective, or concurrent chart reviews; and clinicians' expertise. It is important for you to learn to rely more on research evidence rather than solely on nonresearch evidence. When you face a clinical problem, always ask yourself where the best evidence is to help you find the best solution in caring for clients.

Even when you use the best evidence available, application and outcomes will differ based upon your clients' values, preferences, concerns, and/or expectations (Oncology Nursing Society [ONS], 2005). EBP is not finding research evidence and blindly applying it without using good judgment. As a nurse, you will develop critical thinking skills to determine whether evidence is relevant and appropriate to your clients and to a clinical situation. For example, a single research article suggests that the use of therapeutic touch is consistently effective in reducing abdominal incision pain. However, if your clients' cultural beliefs prevent the use of touch, you will likely need to search for a better evidence-based therapy that clients will accept. Using your clinical expertise and considering clients' values and preferences ensures that you will apply the evidence available in practice both safely and appropriately. Research shows that clients who receive care based on the most recent and best evidence from well-designed research studies experience 28% better outcomes (Heater and others, 1988).

Steps of Evidence-Based Practice

EBP is a systematic approach to rational decision making that facilitates achievement of best practices (Newhouse and others, 2005). Using a step-by-step approach ensures that you will obtain the strongest available evidence to apply in client care. There are five steps of EBP (Melnyk and Fineout-Overholt, 2005):

1. Ask a clinical question.
2. Collect the most relevant and best evidence.
3. Critically appraise the evidence you gather.
4. Integrate all evidence with one's clinical expertise and client preferences and values in making a practice decision or change.
5. Evaluate the practice decision or change.

Ask the Clinical Question. Always think about your practice when caring for clients. Question what does not make sense to you and question what needs clarification. Think about a problem or area of interest that is time consuming, costly, or not logical (Callister and others, 2005). If you keep a clinical journal, your entries will be a rich source for clinical questions. Titler and others (2001) suggest using problem- and knowledge-focused triggers to think critically about clinical and operational nursing unit issues. A problem-focused trigger is one you face while caring for a client or a trend you see on a nursing unit. For example, while caring for an unconscious client, you think, What is the best solution to use when giving mouth care to this client? Examples of problem-focused trends include the increasing number of client falls or incidence of urinary tract infections on a nursing unit. Such trends lead you to ask, "How can I reduce falls on my unit?" or "What is the best way to prevent urinary tract infections in postoperative clients?"

A knowledge-focused trigger is a question regarding new information available on a topic. For example, "What is the current evidence to improve pain management in clients with migraine headaches?" Important sources of this type of information are standards and practice guidelines available from national agencies such as the Agency for Healthcare Research and Quality (AHRQ), the American Pain Society (APS), or the American Association of Critical Care Nurses (AACN). Other sources of knowledge-focused triggers include recent research publications and nurse experts within an organization (Titler and others, 1994).

The questions you ask will eventually lead you to the evidence for an answer. When you ask a question and then go to the scientific literature, you do not want to read 100 articles in order to find the handful that are most helpful. You want to be able to read the best four to six articles that specifically address your practice question. Melnyk and Fineout-Overholt (2005) suggest using a PICO format to state your question. The four elements of a **PICO question** are summarized in Box 5-1. The more focused a question you ask, the easier it will become to search for evidence in the scientific literature. For example, a well-designed PICO question is, *Does the use of therapeutic distraction (I) compared with standard reorientation to the environment (C) reduce the incidence of wandering (O) in clients with dementia (P)?* Another example is, *Is a client's (P) blood pressure more accurate (O) while measuring with the client's legs crossed (I) versus the client's feet flat on the floor (C)?* Note that a well-designed PICO question does not have to follow the sequence of P, I, C, and O. The aim is to ask a question that contains as many of the PICO elements as possible.

Inappropriately formed questions (e.g., What is the best way to reduce wandering? What is the best way to measure blood pressure?) will likely lead to many irrelevant sources of information, making it difficult to find the best evidence. The PICO format allows you to ask questions that are intervention focused. For questions that are not intervention focused, the meaning of the letter *I* can be "interest area" (Melnyk and Fineout-Overholt, 2005). For example, *What is the difference in retention (O) of new*

✳ BOX 5-1   Developing a PICO Question

P = Patient population of interest
Identify patients by age, gender, ethnicity, and disease or health problem.
I = Intervention of interest
What is the intervention that is worthwhile to use in practice (e.g., a treatment, diagnostic test, prognostic factor)?
C = Comparison of interest
What is the usual standard of care or current intervention used now in practice?
O = Outcome
What result do you wish to achieve or observe as a result of an intervention (e.g., change in client behavior, physical finding, client perception)?

✳ TABLE 5-1   Searchable Scientific Literature Databases and Sources

DATABASES	SOURCES
AHRQ	Agency for Healthcare Research and Quality. Includes clinical guidelines and evidence summaries http://www.ahrq.gov
CINAHL	Cumulative Index of Nursing and Allied Health Literature. Includes studies in nursing, allied health, and biomedicine. http://www.cinahl.com
MEDLINE	Includes studies in medicine, nursing, dentistry, psychiatry, veterinary medicine, and allied health. http://www.ncbi.nim.nih.gov
EMBASE	Biomedical and pharmaceutical studies. http://www.embase.com
PsycINFO	Psychology and related health care disciplines. http://www.apa.org/psycinfo/
Cochrane Database of Systematic Reviews	Full text of regularly updated systematic reviews prepared by the Cochrane Collaboration. Includes completed reviews and protocols. http://www.cochrane.org/reviews
National Guidelines Clearinghouse	Repository for structured abstracts (summaries) about clinical guidelines and their development. Also includes condensed version of guideline for viewing. http://www.guideline.gov
PubMed	Health science library at the National Library of Medicine. Offers free access to journal articles. http://www.nlm.nih.gov
On-Line Journal of Knowledge Synthesis for Nursing	Electronic journal containing articles that provide a synthesis of research and an annotated bibliography for selected references.

---

nursing graduates (P) who have previous experience as nurse assistants (I) versus those who do not(C)? Some questions do not always contain all of the PICO elements. An example is a meaning question, *How do clients with cystic fibrosis (P) rate their quality of life (O)?* which contains only a **P** and an **O**.

The questions you raise using a PICO format help to identify knowledge gaps within a clinical situation. When you raise well thought-out questions, the type of evidence you do not have for clinical practice becomes more clear. Examples of different knowledge gaps include the following (ONS, 2005):

- *Diagnosis:* Questions about the selection and interpretation of diagnostic tests. Example: Does the use of a disposable oral thermometer compared with an electronic oral thermometer measure body temperature accurately in a client with a endotracheal tube?
- *Prognosis:* Questions about the client's likely clinical outcome. Example: Is there a difference in the incidence of deep vein thrombosis in surgical clients receiving subcutaneous heparin administration compared to subcutaneous low-molecular-weight heparin?
- *Therapy:* Questions about the selection of the most beneficial treatments. Example: What bowel regimen is most effective in relieving constipation caused by the administration of opioid therapy in clients with chronic pain?
- *Prevention:* Questions about screening and prevention methods to reduce the risk of disease. Example: Does performance of a prostate-specific-antigen (PSA) test in an older adult who is asymptomatic of prostate disease decrease his risk of mortality from prostate cancer?
- *Education:* Questions about best teaching strategies for colleagues, clients, or family members. Example: Is the use of visual aids compared with low-literacy teaching booklets a more effective teaching strategy to educate low-literacy adults about therapeutic diets?

Remember, do not be satisfied with clinical routines. Always question and use critical thinking to consider better ways to provide client care.

Collect the Best Evidence.   Once you have a clear and concise PICO question, you are ready to search for evidence. You will find the evidence you need in a variety of sources: agency policy and procedure manuals, quality improvement data, existing clinical practice guidelines, or computerized bibliographical databases. Do not hesitate to ask for help to find appropriate evidence. Your faculty will of course always be a key resource. When you are assigned to a health care setting, consider using experts such as advanced practice nurses, staff educators, risk managers, and infection control nurses.

When you go to the scientific literature for evidence, it is wise to seek the assistance of a medical librarian. A medical librarian knows the various databases that are available to you (Table 5-1). The databases are a repository of published scientific studies, including peer-reviewed research. A **peer-reviewed** article means that a panel of experts familiar with the article's topic or subject matter has reviewed the article. The librarian is available to help translate your PICO question into the language or key words that will yield the best evidence search. When conducting a search, it is necessary to enter and manipulate different key words until you get the combination that gives you the key articles you want to read about your question. When you enter a word to search into a database, be prepared for some confusion with the evidence you obtain. The vocabulary within published articles is often vague. The word you select sometimes has one meaning to one author and a very different meaning to another. A medical librarian helps you learn how to choose alternative words or terms that identify your PICO question and to thus obtain relevant evidence.

MEDLINE and CINAHL are among the best-known comprehensive databases and represent the scientific knowledge base of health care (Melnyk and Fineout-Overholt, 2005). Among the many databases, some are available through vendors at a cost, some are free of charge, and some offer both options. As a student, you will have access to an institutional subscription through a vendor purchased by your school. One of the more common vendors is OVID, which offers several different databases. There are also databases available free on the Internet. The Cochrane Database of Systematic Reviews is a valuable source of synthesized evidence (i.e., preappraised evidence). The Cochrane database includes the full text of regularly updated systematic reviews and protocols for reviews currently under way. Collaborative review groups prepare and maintain the reviews. The protocols provide the background, objectives, and methods for reviews in progress (Melnyk and Fineout-Overholt, 2005). The National Guidelines Clearinghouse (NGC) is a database supported by the AHRQ. It contains **clinical guidelines**, systematically developed statements about a plan of care for a specific set of clinical circumstances involving a specific client population. Examples of clinical guidelines on NCG include care of children and adolescents with type 1 diabetes and practice guidelines for the treatment of adults with low back pain. The NGC is invaluable when developing a plan of care for a client (see Chapter 18).

The pyramid in Figure 5-2 represents the hierarchy of available evidence. At this point in your nursing career, you cannot be an expert on all aspects of the types of studies conducted. But you can learn enough about the types of studies to help you know which ones have the best scientific evidence. At the top of the pyramid are systematic reviews or meta-analyses. These reviews are at the heart of EBP (Stevens, 2001). A panel of experts reviews the evidence about a specific clinical question or issue and summarizes the state of the science. A systematic review or meta-analysis reviews only those studies that are randomized controlled trials (RCTs).

An RCT is the highest level of experimental research, when researchers test an intervention (e.g., new drug, therapy or an education method) against the usual standard of care (Box 5-2). Researchers assign subjects to either a control or treatment group through random assignment. In other words, all subjects in a study have equal chance to be in either group. The treatment group receives the experimental intervention, and the control group receives the usual standard of care. The researchers measure both groups for the same outcomes to see if there is a difference. When an RCT is completed, the researcher will know if the intervention leads to better outcomes than the standard of care.

In a systematic review or meta-analysis an independent researcher reviews all of the RCTs conducted on the same clinical question or issue and reports on whether the evidence is conclusive and in favor of the intervention or whether further study is necessary and why. A systematic review is the perfect answer to a

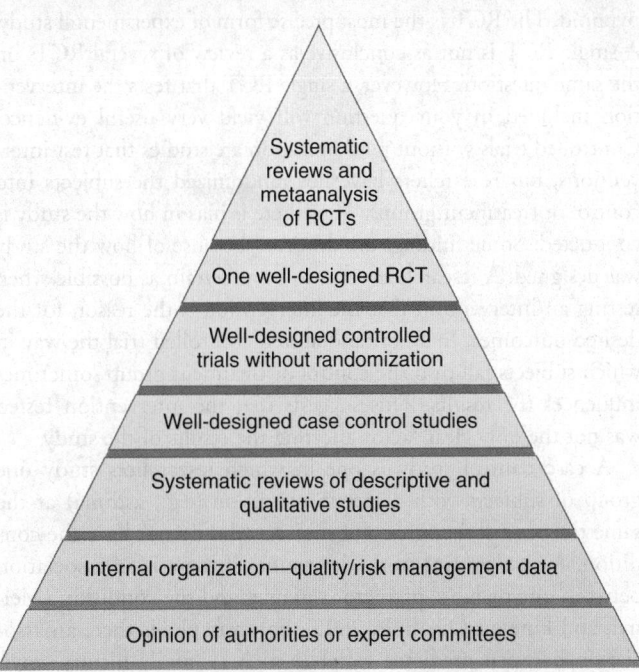

Figure 5-2 Hierarchy of evidence. *RCIs,* Randomized controlled trials. (Modified from Guyatt G, Rennie D: *User's guide to the medical literature,* Chicago, 2002, American Medical Association; Melnyk BM, Fineout-Overholt E: *Evidence-based practice in nursing and healthcare: A guide to best practice,* Philadelphia, 2005, Lippincott Williams & Wilkins.)

✳ **BOX 5-2 Example of a Randomized Controlled Trial (RCT)**

Research Question: Will the use of a formal education program for clients at risk for diabetes compared with a traditional educational pamphlet improve client's blood glucose level and weight control?

Subjects: 130 adult clients with risk factors for diabetes who visit a local medicine clinic.

Randomization: Clients were randomly assigned to one of two groups using a random numbers table.

Treatment Group: 65 clients attend an 8-hour class on diabetes prevention, with group discussion, lecture, and interactive computer program use.

Control Group: 65 clients receive a printed pamphlet outlining risks for diabetes and health promotion strategies.

Outcome Measure: Both groups have blood glucose levels and weight measured before receiving education and every month for 3 months after receiving education.

Analysis: Statistical tests comparing the blood glucose levels and weight for the two groups will show if the treatment has the predicted effect.

PICO question. It will explain if the evidence that you are searching for exists. In the Cochrane Library all entries include information on systematic reviews. If you use MEDLINE or CINAHL, enter a textword "systematic review" or the MeSH heading of *evidence-based medicine* to obtain systematic reviews.

As you look at the hierarchy pyramid in Figure 5-2, the level of rigor or exactness in how a study is conducted moves down the pyramid. The RCT is the most precise form of experimental study. A single RCT is not as conclusive as a review of several RCTs on the same question. However, a single RCT that tests the intervention included in your question will yield very useful evidence. Controlled trials without randomization are studies that test interventions, but researchers have not randomized the subjects into control or treatment groups. Thus there is **bias** in how the study is conducted. Some findings are distorted because of how the study was designed. A researcher wants to be as certain as possible when testing an intervention that the intervention is the reason for the desired outcomes. In a nonrandomized controlled trial the way in which subjects fall into the control or treatment group sometimes influences the results. This suggests that the intervention tested was not the only clear factor affecting the results of the study.

A case control study is one in which researchers study one group of subjects with a certain condition (e.g., asthma) at the same time as another group of subjects who do not have the condition. A case control study determines if there is an association between one or more predictor variables and the condition (Melnyk and Fineout-Overholt, 2005). For example, is there an association between predictor variables such as family history, environmental exposure to dust, or nutrition and the incidence of asthma? Often a case control study is conducted retrospectively, or after the fact. Researchers look back in time and review available data about their two groups of subjects to understand what variables explain the condition. These studies are done with a small number of subjects, but there is again a risk of bias. Sometimes the subjects in the two groups differ on certain other variables (e.g., amount of stress or history of contact allergies) that also influence the incidence of the condition, more so than the variables being studied.

Individual RCTs are the gold standard for research. Other forms of research have lesser value in guiding practice (Titler and others, 2001). RCTs establish cause and effect and are excellent for testing drug therapies or medical treatments. However, this approach is not always the best for testing nursing interventions. The nature of nursing causes researchers to ask questions that are not always answered best by an RCT or even a controlled trial without randomization. Nurses care for clients' responses to a disease or health problem. For example, nurses assist clients with problems such as knowledge deficits, symptom management, and coping with psychological distress. Learning to understand how clients experience health problems cannot always be addressed through an RCT.

Qualitative research (see p. 62) offers answers when trying to understand clients' experiences with health problems and the contexts in which the experiences occur. Clients have the opportunity to tell their stories and share their experiences in qualitative studies. The findings are in-depth because clients are usually very descriptive in what they choose to share. Examples of qualitative studies include "Client's perceptions of nurses' caring in a palliative care unit" and "The perceptions of stress by family members of critically ill clients." Qualitative research is valuable in identifying information about how clients cope or manage various health problems and their perceptions of illness.

The data from a health care setting is valuable in telling you about trends in clinical practice. Most hospitals, for example, keep monthly records on key quality of care or performance indicators such as medication errors or infection rates. All Magnet-designated hospitals maintain the National Data Base for Nursing Quality Improvement (NDNQI). The database includes information on falls, pressure ulcer incidence, and nurse satisfaction. Typically quality and risk management data will not give you evidence in finding a solution to a problem, but the data will inform you about the nature or severity of problems occurring within the health care setting. With the use of quality data you may choose to refine or redirect your PICO question. The use of clinical experts may be at the bottom of the evidence pyramid, but do not consider clinical experts as a poor source of evidence. Expert clinicians use evidence frequently as they build their own practice, and they are rich sources of information for clinical problems.

Critique the Evidence. Perhaps the most difficult step in the EBP process is critiquing or analyzing the available evidence. The critiquing of evidence involves its evaluation, which includes determining the value, feasibility, and utility of evidence for making a practice change (ONS, 2005). When critiquing evidence, first evaluate the scientific merit and clinical applicability of each study's findings. Then with a group of studies and expert opinion determine what findings have a strong enough basis for use in practice. After critiquing the evidence you will be able to answer the questions, Do the articles together offer evidence to explain or answer my PICO question? Do the articles show the evidence is true and reliable? Can I use the evidence in practice?

As a student new to nursing, it will take time to acquire the skills to critique evidence like an expert. When you read an article from the literature, do not let the statistics or technical wording cause you to put the article down and walk away. Know the elements of an article, and use a careful approach when reviewing each one. Evidence-based articles include the following elements:

- *Abstract.* An abstract is a brief summary of the article that quickly tells you if the article is research or clinically based. An abstract summarizes the purpose of the study or clinical query, the major themes or findings, and the implications for nursing practice.
- *Introduction.* The introduction contains information about its purpose and the importance of the topic for the audience who reads the article. There is usually brief supporting evidence as to why the topic is important from the author's point of view.

Together, the abstract and introduction tell you if you want to continue to read the entire article. You will know if the topic of the article is similar to your PICO question or related closely enough to provide you useful information. Continue to read the next elements of the article:

- *Literature review or background.* A good author offers a detailed background of the level of science or clinical information that exists about the topic of the article. Therefore it offers an argument about what led the author to conduct a study or report on a clinical topic. This section of an article is very valuable. Perhaps the article itself does not address your PICO question the way you desire, but it will possibly lead you to other, more useful articles. Once you have read a literature review of a research article, you should have a good idea of how past research led to the researcher's question. For example, a study designed to test an educational intervention for older adult family caregivers will review literature that describes characteristics of caregivers, the type of factors influencing caregivers' ability to cope with stressors of caregiving, and any previous educational interventions used with families.

- *Manuscript narrative.* The "middle section" or narrative of a manuscript will differ according to the type of evidence-based article it is (Melnyk and Fineout-Overholt, 2005). A clinical article will describe a clinical topic, which often includes a description of a client population, the nature of a certain disease or health alteration, how clients are affected, and the appropriate nursing therapies. An author sometimes writes a clinical article to explain how to use a therapy or new technology. A research article will contain several subsections within the narrative, including the following:
  - *Purpose statement:* Explains the focus or intent of a study. It identifies what concepts will be researched. This includes research questions or **hypotheses**—predictions made about the relationship or difference between study **variables** (concepts, characteristics, or traits that vary within subjects). An example of a research question is, What characteristics are common among older adults who have annual breast screening?
  - *Methods or design:* Explains how a research study is organized and conducted in order to answer the research question or to test the hypothesis. This is where you learn the type of study to be conducted (e.g., RCT, case control study, or qualitative study). You also learn how many subjects or persons are in a study. In health care studies, subjects may include clients, family members, or health care staff. The language in the methods section is sometimes confusing, because it explains details about how the researcher designs the study to minimize bias so as to obtain the most accurate results possible. Use your faculty member as a resource to help interpret this section.
- *Results or conclusions.* Clinical and research articles will have a summary section. In a clinical article, the author explains the clinical implications for the topic presented. In a research article, the author details the results of the study and explains whether a hypothesis is supported or how a research question is answered. This section will include a statistical analysis if it is a quantitative study (see p. 62). A qualitative study will present a very thorough summary of the descriptive themes and ideas that arise from the researcher's analysis of data. Do not let the statistical analysis in an article stump you. Read carefully, and ask these questions, Does the researcher describe the results? Were the results significant? Have a faculty member assist you in interpreting statistical results. A good author will also discuss any limitations to a study in the results section. This information on limitations will be valuable in helping you decide if you want to use the evidence with your clients.
- *Clinical implications.* A research article will include a section that explains if the findings from the study have clinical implications. The researcher will explain how to apply findings in a practice setting for the type of subjects studied.

After you have critiqued each article for your PICO question, synthesize or combine the findings from all of the articles to determine the state of the evidence. Use critical thinking to consider the scientific rigor of the evidence and how well it answers your area of interest. Consider the evidence in light of your clients' concerns and preferences. Your review of articles offers a snapshot conclusion based on combined evidence about one focused topical area. As a clinician, judge whether to use the evidence for a particular client or group of clients, who usually have complex medical histories and patterns of responses (Melnyk and Fineout-Overholt, 2005). Ethically it is important to consider evidence that will benefit clients and do no harm. Decide if the evidence is relevant, easily applicable in your setting of practice, and has the potential for improving client outcomes.

Integrate the Evidence. Once you decide that the evidence is strong and applicable to your clients and clinical situation, incorporate the recommended evidence into practice. Your first step is to simply apply the research in your plan of care for a client (see Chapter 18). Use the evidence you find as a rationale for an intervention you plan to try. For instance, you learned about an approach to bathe older adults who are restless and decide to use the technique during your next clinical assignment. You use the bathing technique with your own assigned clients, or you work with a group of other students or nurses in revising a policy and procedure or developing a new clinical protocol. Another example, after being concerned about the rate of intravenous (IV) catheter dislodgment, you go to the evidence to compare the efficacy of gauze dressings versus transparent dressings. The literature suggests that transparent dressings on peripheral IV sites result in fewer catheter dislodgments than gauze dressings with no increase in phlebitis or infiltration rates (Melnyk and Fineout-Overholt, 2005; Trepepi-Bova and others, 1997). As a result of your findings you meet with the policy and procedure committee to recommend the use of transparent dressings routinely. You then implement the use of transparent dressings in the routine care of peripheral IV catheters.

Evidence is useful in a variety of ways through teaching tools, clinical practice guidelines, policies and procedures, and new assessment or documentation tools. Depending on the amount of change needed to apply evidence in practice, it becomes necessary to involve a number of staff from a given nursing unit. It is important to consider the setting where you want to apply the evidence. Is there support from all staff, does the practice change(s) fit with the scope of practice in the clinical setting, and are there resources (time, secretarial support, and staff) available to make a change? When evidence is not strong enough to apply in practice, your next option is to conduct a pilot study to investigate your PICO question. A pilot study is a small-scale research study or one that includes a quality or performance improvement project.

As a nursing student integrating evidence, your focus will begin with searching for and applying best evidence to improve the care you directly provide your clients. The evidence available within nursing gives you an almost unlimited access to innovative and effective nursing interventions. Using an evidence-based practice approach will improve your skills and knowledge as a nurse and improve your clients' outcomes.

Evaluate the Practice Decision or Change. After applying evidence in your practice, your next step is to evaluate the effect. How does the intervention work? How effective was the clinical decision for your client or practice setting? Sometimes your evaluation is as simple as determining if the expected outcomes you set for an intervention are met (see Chapters 18 and 20). For example, after the use of a transparent IV dressing, does the IV dislodge or does the client develop the complication of phlebitis? When using a new approach to preoperative teaching, does the client learn what to expect after surgery?

When an evidence-based practice change occurs on a larger scale, an evaluation will be more formal. For example, evidence showing factors that contribute to pressure ulcers might lead a nursing unit to adopt a new skin care protocol. To evaluate the protocol, the nurses will track the incidence of pressure ulcers over a course of time (e.g., 6 months to a year). In addition, the nurses will collect data to describe both the clients who develop ulcers and those that do not. This comparative information is valuable in determining the effects of the protocol and whether modifications are necessary.

Nursing Research

Research means to search again or to examine carefully (Langford, 2001). It is a systematic process that asks and answers questions that generate knowledge. The knowledge then provides a scientific basis for nursing practice and validates the effectiveness of nursing interventions. Dr. Norma Metheny has spent many years asking questions about how to prevent the aspiration of tube feeding in clients who receive feeding through nasogastric tubes (Metheny and others, 1988, 1989, 1990, 1994, 2000). Through her research she identified factors that increase the risk of aspiration and approaches to use in determining tube feeding placement. Dr. Metheny's findings are incorporated into this textbook and have changed the way nurses administer tube feedings to clients. Through research, Dr. Metheny has contributed to the scientific body of knowledge that has saved clients' lives and helped to prevent the serious complication of aspiration.

The International Council of Nurses (ICN) (1986) supports the need for nursing research as a means for improving the health and welfare of people. **Nursing research** is a way to identify new knowledge, improve professional education and practice, and use resources effectively. The National Institute of Nursing Research (NINR) and the ICN regularly update the broad priorities for nursing research (Box 5-3). The NINR (2006) supports clinical and basic research to establish a scientific basis for the care of individuals across the life span. Research priorities for the nursing profession guide the research efforts of nurse scientists in those health care areas with the greatest need.

Nursing research has the support of professional and specialty organizations. In 2003 the ANA revised the *Standards of Nursing Practice*. Within this document are the Standards of Professional Performance (see Chapter 1). Standard 13 recommends that the professional nurse use research findings in practice (ANA, 2003). In addition to the ANA, nursing specialty organizations such as the AACN, the Oncology Nursing Society (ONS), and Sigma Theta Tau International (STTI) actively support the conduct of research for advancing nursing science.

✳ BOX 5-3 Key Areas of Health Care Research

- Chronic illness
- Quality and cost-effective care
- Health promotion and disease prevention
- Management of symptoms
- Adaptation to new technologies
- Health disparities
- Palliative care at end of life

Data from National Institute of Nursing Research: *About NINR: mission statement,* http://ninr.nih.gov/ninr/, accessed July 10, 2006.

Outcomes Management Research

Outcomes management is an area of research that has recently received a great deal of attention. The management of care delivery outcomes is a growing concern for nurse clinicians and researchers (Melnyk and Fineout-Overholt, 2005). Outcomes research is research designed to assess and document the effectiveness of health care services and interventions (Polit and Beck, 2004). For example, studying the effects of an outpatient education program on the ability of older adult clients to follow a nutrition and exercise program is an outcome study. This type of research is a response of the health care industry to the increased demand from policy makers, insurers, and the public to justify care practices and systems in terms of improved client outcomes and costs (Hinshaw, Feetham, and Shaver, 1999; Polit and Beck, 2004).

Care delivery outcomes are the observable or measurable effects of some intervention or action (Melnyk and Fineout-Overholt, 2005). As is the case with the expected outcomes you develop in a plan of care (see Chapter 18), a care delivery outcome focuses on the recipient of service (e.g., client, family, or community) and not the provider (e.g., nurse or physician). For example, an outcome of a diabetes education program is that clients are able to self-administer insulin, not the nurses' success in instructing all clients newly diagnosed with diabetes.

A problem in outcomes research is the clear definition or selection of measurable outcomes. Many researchers fail to consider all components of outcome measurement. Components of an outcome include the outcome itself, how it is observed (the indicator), its critical characteristics (how it is measured), and its range of parameters (Melnyk and Fineout-Overholt, 2005). For example, health care settings commonly measure the outcome of client satisfaction when they introduce new services (e.g., new care delivery model or outpatient clinic). The outcome is client satisfaction, observed through clients' responses to a client satisfaction instrument including characteristics such as nursing care, physician care, support services, and the health setting environment. Clients complete the instrument, responding to a scale (parameter) designed to measure their degree of satisfaction (e.g., scale of 1 to 5). The combined score on the instrument yields a measure of satisfaction, an outcome that the facility can track over time.

Frequently researchers choose outcomes that do not measure a true impact of care delivery, particularly nursing care delivery. For example, common outcome measures include morbidity, mortality, readmission rate, or length of stay. Although important outcomes to understand, they do not always measure the true effect

BOX 5-4 Examples of Nursing-Sensitive Outcome Measures

- Central line bacteremia rate
- Compliance/adherence to actions (e.g., diet, medication regimen, activity restrictions)
- Failure to rescue
- Fall rate
- Functional status
- Nosocomial (health care–associated) infection rate
- Nosocomial (health care–associated) pressure ulcer rate
- Symptom reduction

Modified from Ingersoll G: Generating evidence through outcomes management. In Melnyk BM, Fineout-Overholt E, editors: *Evidence based practice in nursing and healthcare,* Philadelphia, 2005, Lippincott Williams & Wilkins.

of a specific intervention on care delivery. For example, if a nurse researcher intends to measure the success of a nurse-initiated protocol to manage blood glucose levels in critically ill clients, the researcher will not likely measure mortality. The outcome is very broad and susceptible to many factors other than the nurse-initiated protocol (e.g., the selection of medical therapies, the clients' acuity of illness, or the onset of medical complications). Instead, the nurse researcher will have a better idea of the effects of the protocol by measuring the outcome of blood glucose range. The nurse researcher obtains the blood glucose level of clients placed on the protocol and compares blood glucose levels to a desired range that represents good blood glucose control. The nursing literature now addresses the identification of "nursing-sensitive outcomes," or outcomes that are sensitive to nursing practice (Ingersoll and others, 2000). Box 5-4 summarizes some recently proposed nursing-sensitive outcome indicators that have not yet been fully tested and validated.

Scientific Method

The **scientific method** is the foundation of research and the most reliable and objective of all methods of gaining knowledge. This method is an advanced, objective means of acquiring and testing knowledge. It guides you in applying research evidence in practice, as well as in conducting research. When using research findings to add to or change practice, you need to understand the process a researcher uses to guide a study. For example, when you consider whether to change the procedure for how to insert a feeding tube, you need to know if a newly recommended procedure was tested on similar clients and what were the outcomes or results. The scientific method is a systematic step-by-step process that provides support that the findings from a study are **valid, reliable,** and **generalizable** to subjects similar to those researched.

Researchers use the scientific method to understand, explain, predict, or control a nursing phenomenon (Polit and Beck, 2004). Systematic, orderly procedures characterize this method in order to limit the possibility for error, although it is not without fault. The scientific method minimizes the chance that bias or opinion by the researcher will influence the results of research and thus the

knowledge gained. Polit and Beck (2004) describe the characteristics of scientific research as follows:

- The problem area or what the researcher chooses to study is identified.
- The steps of planning and conducting an investigation occur in a systematic and orderly way.
- Researchers try to control external factors that are not under study but can influence a relationship between phenomena they are studying. For example, if a nurse is studying the relationship between diet and heart disease, the nurse has to control other characteristics among subjects such as stress or smoking history, because they are contributing factors to this disease. Clients on an investigational diet and clients on a regular diet would both have to have similar levels of stress and smoking histories to test the true effect of the diet.
- Evidence that is part of experience (**empirical data**) is gathered directly or indirectly through the use of observations and assessments and is the basis for discovering new knowledge.
- The goal is to understand phenomena in order to apply the knowledge generally, to a broad group of clients.

Nursing and the Scientific Approach

In the past, much of the information used in nursing practice was borrowed from other disciplines such as biology, physiology, psychology, and sociology. Often this information was applied to nursing without testing it. For example, nurses use several methods to help clients sleep. Interventions such as giving a client a back rub, making sure that the bed is clean and comfortable, preparing the environment by dimming the lights, and talking to a worried or anxious client are frequently used nursing measures and, in general, are logical, commonsense approaches. However, when these measures are considered in greater depth, questions arise about their applications. For example, are they the best methods to promote sleep? Do different clients in different situations require other interventions to promote sleep?

Research provides a way for nursing questions and problems to be studied in greater depth within the context of nursing. If nurses do not use an evidence-based approach to practice, they often rely on personal experience or the statements of nursing experts alone. If an intervention works for most clients, you may become satisfied with this success without questioning whether there might be a better way for other clients. If the intervention is not successful, you might use an approach practiced by a colleague or try a different sequence of accepted measures. Even if an intervention discovered with this approach is effective for one or more clients, it is not always appropriate for other clients in other settings. Nursing interventions must be tested through research to determine the measures that work best with specific clients.

Nursing research addresses issues important to the discipline of nursing. Some of these issues relate to the profession itself, education of nurses, client and family needs, and issues within the health care delivery system. Once research is completed, it is important to disseminate or communicate the findings. One method of dissemination is through publication of the findings in professional journals. As a nurse, you will acquire knowledge about a wide range of human needs and responses to health problems.

✳ BOX 5-5　Types of Research

Historical Research: Studies designed to establish facts and relationships concerning past events. Example: A study examining the societal factors that led to the acceptance of advanced practice nurses by clients.

Exploratory Research: Initial study designed to develop or refine the dimensions of phenomena or to develop or refine a hypothesis about the relationships among phenomena. Example: a pilot study testing the benefits of a new exercise program for older adults with dementia.

Evaluation Research: Study that tests how well a program, practice, or policy is working. Example: A study measuring the outcomes of an informational campaign designed to improve parents' ability to follow immunization schedules for their children.

Descriptive Research: Study that measures characteristics of persons, situations, or groups and the frequency with which certain events or characteristics occur. Example: a study to examine RNs' biases toward caring for obese clients.

Experimental Research: Study in which the investigator controls the study variable and randomly assigns subjects to different conditions to test the variable. Example: An RCT comparing chlorhexidine with Betadine in reducing the incidence of IV site phlebitis.

Correlational Research: Study that explores the interrelationships among variables of interest without any active intervention by the researcher. Example: A study examining the relationship between RNs' educational levels and their satisfaction in the nursing role.

RNs, Registered nurses; *RCT*, randomized controlled trial; *IV*, intravenous.

Nursing research uses many methods to study clinical problems (Box 5-5). There are two broad approaches to research: quantitative and qualitative methods.

Quantitative Research.

Quantitative nursing research is the study of nursing phenomena that offers precise measurement and quantification. For example, you can quantitatively measure pain severity, extent of wound healing, and body temperature. Quantitative research is the precise, systematic, objective examination of specific concepts. Quantitative research focuses on numerical data, statistical analysis, and controls to eliminate bias in findings (Polit and Beck, 2004). Although there are many quantitative methods, the following sections briefly describe experimental, survey, and evaluation research.

Experimental Research.

As discussed previously, an RCT is the hallmark of scientific research. In a true experimental study the conditions are tightly controlled to eliminate bias and to ensure that findings can be generalizable to similar groups of subjects.

Surveys.

Surveys are common in quantitative research. Surveys obtain information from populations regarding the frequency, distribution, and interrelation of variables among subjects in the study (Polit and Beck, 2004). An example is a survey designed to measure nurses' perceptions of physicians' willingness to collaborate in practice. Surveys obtain information about practices, education, experience, opinions, and other characteristics of people. The most basic function of a survey is description. Surveys gather a large amount of data to describe the population as well as the topic of study. It is important in survey research that the population sampled is large enough to keep sampling error at a minimum. Researchers must carefully construct and pretest the survey items used in questionnaires and interviews to determine correctness in style, ease of use, and appropriateness for the research question.

Evaluation Research.

Evaluation research is a form of quantitative research that involves finding out how well a program, practice, procedure, or policy is working (Polit and Beck, 2004). An example is outcomes management research. Ultimately, the purpose of evaluation research is to determine the success of a program. Evaluation research determines why a program or some components of the program were successful or unsuccessful. When programs are unsuccessful, evaluation research identifies problems with the program and opportunities for change, why the program was unsuccessful, or even barriers to program implementation.

Qualitative Research.

Qualitative nursing research is the study of phenomena that are difficult to quantify or categorize. This method describes information obtained in a nonnumerical form (e.g., data in the form of written transcripts from a series of interviews). Qualitative research involves **inductive reasoning** to develop generalizations or theories from specific observations or interviews (Polit and Beck, 2004). For example, a nurse conducts extensive interviews with individual cancer survivors and then summarizes the common themes from all of the interviews to inductively determine the characteristics of cancer survivors' quality of life. Qualitative research involves the discovery and understanding of important behavioral characteristics or phenomena. An example is a qualitative research study conducted by Sheldon and others (2006) that described difficult communication in nurse-client interactions from nurses' perspectives.

There are a number of different qualitative research methods. Ethnography involves the description and interpretation of cultural behavior (Polit and Beck, 2004). For example, a researcher will study the behaviors of residents suffering from Alzheimer's disease within a nursing home. This type of research is closely associated with the field of anthropology, which focuses on the culture of a study population.

Phenomenology is a research method with roots in philosophy (Polit and Beck, 2004) and a focus on what people experience in regard to daily practices or experiences and how they interpret those experiences. Typically, phenomenologic researchers have study participants tell their stories about the phenomena in question. For example, Wongvatunyu and Porter (2005) studied women's experiences of helping young adults with traumatic brain injury (TBI). The researchers studied women's perceptions, actions, and intentions relevant to helping young adults with TBI.

Grounded theory is a method of collecting and analyzing qualitative data with the aim of developing theories and theoretical propositions that are grounded in real-world observations (Polit and Beck, 2004). For example, in studying difficult communication in nurse-client interactions, Sheldon and others (2006) held focus groups with nurses to explore their perceptions of difficult communication. The results of the focus groups yielded five themes describing difficult communication. Further study of the same topic might eventually develop those themes into a meaningful communication theory.

Research Process

The **research process** is an orderly series of steps that allow a researcher to move from asking the research question to finding the answer (Figure 5-3) (Langford, 2001). Usually the answer to the initial research question leads to new questions and other areas of study. The research process builds knowledge for use in other, similar situations. Nurses seek knowledge about the reason why a particular event happens or the best way to provide care for clients with a certain health problem. The research process gives knowledge that a nurse can repeatedly apply to a whole group or class of clients.

The research process usually consists of the following: problem identification, study design, conducting the study, data analysis, and use of the findings (Table 5-2). Initially the researcher identifies an area of inquiry (identifying a problem), which often results from clinical practice. For example, a nurse notices that many clients have difficulty sleeping the night before discharge following open-heart surgery. Based on work with these clients, the nurse determines that most of them have concerns about their activity tolerance and pain once they return home. The nurse reviews the relevant literature to determine what is known about postoperative activity level and pain immediately following open-heart surgery. After reviewing the literature, the researcher notes that many clients report poor activity tolerance and pain control. However, there is limited research on nursing interventions to improve these areas.

Following identification of the problem and review of the literature, the researcher designs the study protocol. In this example, the nurse designs a study in which some of the clients receive the standard discharge planning and others receive an additional discharge planning intervention for activity tolerance and pain control. In this study the sample will include all first-time open-heart surgical clients who are having an aortic valve repair. Subjects will be excluded if they were on preoperative pain medication for arthritis, cancer, or other chronic painful conditions. The researcher will choose each subject for one of the two groups (experimental or control) randomly. The control group will receive standard discharge planning, whereas the experimental or treatment group will receive the standard discharge planning plus the additional intervention for activity tolerance and pain control. Each subject will have a 50-50 chance of being in each group. The researcher will also select appropriate instruments to measure postoperative pain and activity tolerance. In addition, the researcher will follow all subjects in the same manner with regard to postoperative home care, follow-up appointments, and physical examinations.

Before conducting any study with human subjects, the researcher obtains approvals from the agency's human subjects committee or institutional review board (IRB). An IRB includes scientists and laypersons who review all studies conducted in the institution to ensure that ethical principles, including the rights of human subjects, are followed. For example, researchers must protect the confidentiality of those who participate in the study, provide informed consent, minimize risks to subjects, identify

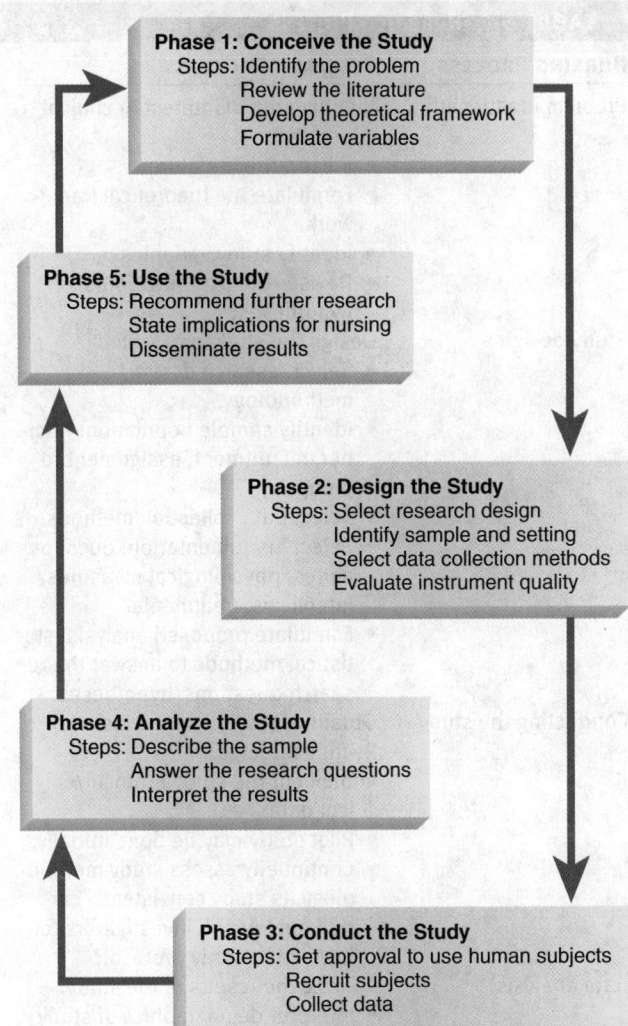

Figure 5-3 The phases and steps of the research process. (From Langford RW: *Navigating the maze of nursing research,* St. Louis, 2001, Mosby.)

risks and benefits of participating, ensure that participation in the study is voluntary, and allow subjects to withdraw from studies at any time. **Informed consent** means that research subjects (1) are given full and complete information about the purpose of the study, procedures, data collection, potential harm and benefits, and alternative methods of treatment; (2) are capable of fully understanding the research and the implications of participation; (3) have the power of free choice to voluntarily consent or decline participation in the research; and (4) understand how the researcher maintains confidentiality or anonymity. **Confidentiality** guarantees that any information the subject provides will not be reported in any manner that identifies the subject and will not be accessible to people outside the research team (Polit and Beck, 2004). **Anonymity** occurs when even the researcher cannot link the subject to the data (Polit and Beck, 2004).

Once a study begins, the researcher collects all data from the subjects as indicated in the study design protocol. In the example, each subject will receive the designated discharge planning and all other postoperative care. The researcher analyzes the data from

✳ **TABLE 5-2** Research Process

NURSING PROCESS	RESEARCH PROCESS
Problem identification	Identify area of interest or clinical problem: • Review the literature. • Formulate the theoretical framework. • Identify study variables. • Devise research question(s)/hypotheses.
Study design	Design the study protocol: • Select research design/methodology. • Identify sample population: number, recruitment, assignment to groups. • Select data collection methods. • Select instrumentation: questionnaires, physiological measures, interviews, treatments. • Formulate proposed analysis: statistical methods to answer the research questions/hypotheses.
Conducting the study	Obtain necessary approvals. Recruit subjects. Implement the study protocol/collect data: • Pilot study may be done initially. • Continually assess study methodology. Is study consistently carried out? Are all investigators following the study protocol?
Data analysis	Analyze the results of the study: • Interpret demographics of study population. • Analyze each research question/hypothesis. • Interpret the results, including conclusions, limitations.
Use of the findings	Formulate recommendations for further research. Determine implications for nursing. Disseminate the findings: presentations, publications, research utilization.

the pain and activity tolerance instruments from the two groups studied. A statistical comparison of the results will determine whether clients who received the new discharge interventions had improved activity levels and pain control when compared with clients receiving only standard discharge planning. If the clients receiving the new care slept better, had better pain control, and reported adequate activity tolerance, the nurse researcher has acquired new knowledge about how generally to help first-time postoperative open-heart clients with an aortic valve repair.

In any study a researcher addresses the study limitations. Limitations might include a small sample size, a unique setting where the study was conducted, or the failure of the study to include representative cultural groups or age-groups. In our example

this is a first-time study and the results are not ready for use for all clients discharged after an aortic valve repair. In addition, perhaps there was a limitation with the sample size, because there were subjects who did not complete the discharge intervention. Limitations help a researcher to decide how to refine or adapt a study for further investigation in the future.

A researcher also addresses the implications for nursing practice. This is critical to ultimately help fellow researchers, clinicians, educators, and administrators know how to apply findings from a study in practice. In this study the researcher recommends that after open-heart surgery all clients receive the expanded discharge planning instruction because of better pain control and improved activity tolerance after discharge. The researcher further explains how to introduce the intervention into a practice setting to be effective.

• • •

Nursing research improves nursing practice and raises the standards for the profession. Promoting evidence-based practice and research increases the scientific knowledge base for practice. The recipients of these improvements to practice are clients, their families, and the communities in which they live.

Quality and Performance Improvement

Quality data is near the bottom of the evidence pyramid (Figure 5-2). Every health care organization gathers data on a number of health outcome measures as a way to gauge its quality of care. This is the focus of outcomes management (see p. 60). Examples of quality data include fall rates, number of medication errors, incidence of pressure ulcers, and infection rates. Health care organizations actively promote efforts for improving client care and outcomes, particularly with respect to reducing medical errors and enhancing client safety. Quality data is the outcome of both quality improvement (QI) and performance improvement (PI) initiatives. The Joint Commission (TJC) defines **quality improvement (QI)** as an approach to the continuous study and improvement of the processes of providing health care services to meet the needs of clients and others (TJC, 2005). An institution's QI program focuses on improvement of health care–related processes (e.g., medication delivery or fall prevention). Performance measurement means what an institution does and how well it does it. In **performance improvement (PI)** an organization analyzes and evaluates current performance to use results to develop focused improvement actions. PI activities are typically clinical projects conceived in response to identified clinical problems and designed to use research findings to improve clinical practice (Melnyk and Fineout-Overholt, 2005).

Evidence-based practice and quality improvement go hand in hand. When implementing an EBP project, it is important to review available QI data. The information is invaluable for understanding the extent of a problem within your organization. QI data offer information about how to focus EBP efforts. For example, if a nursing unit has experienced an increase in the number of client falls over the last several months, the QI data can potentially be valuable in identifying the type of clients who fall, time of day of falls, and possible precipitating factors (e.g., efforts to reach the bathroom, multiple medications, or client confusion). A thorough analysis of QI data then leads clinicians to identify the best evidence available for correcting quality problems. Once the staff apply the evidence in a fall prevention protocol, they will implement the protocol (in this case, focusing efforts on care approaches during evening hours) and evaluate its results. Reliable quality data improves the relevance and scope of an EBP project.

Quality Improvement Programs

A well-organized QI program focuses on processes or systems that significantly contribute to outcomes. Facilities need a systematic approach organizationally to ensure that everyone supports a continuous QI philosophy. This begins with the organizational culture, where all staff members understand their responsibility toward maintaining and improving quality. Typically in health care, many individuals are involved in single processes of care. For example, medication delivery involves the nurse who prepares and administers the drugs, the health care provider who prescribes medications, the pharmacist who prepares the dosage, the secretary who communicates about new orders being written, and the transporter who delivers medications. Thus all members of the health care team collaborate together in QI activities. As a member of the nursing team, you will participate in recognizing trends in practice, identifying when recurrent problems develop, and initiating opportunities to improve the quality of care.

The QI process begins at the staff level, where problems are defined. This requires staff members to know the practice standards or guidelines that define quality. Unit QI committees review activities or services considered to be most important in providing quality care to clients. To identify the greatest opportunity for improving quality, the committees consider those activities that are high volume (greater than 50% of a unit's activity), high risk (potential for trauma or death), and problem areas (potential for client, staff, or institution). For example, on an orthopedic nursing unit, hip surgery volume is high, older adults over age 80 have more postoperative complications, and family members are dissatisfied with clients' pain control. TJC's annual National Patient Safety Goals provide another focus for QI committees to explore and identify problem areas (TJC, 2006) (see Chapter 38). Sometimes the problem is presented to a committee in the form of a sentinel event, an unexpected occurrence involving death or serious physical or psychological injury. Once a committee defines the problem, it applies a formal model for exploring and resolving quality concerns. There are many models for QI and PI. One model is the PDSA cycle: plan, do, study, and act:

Plan—Review available data to understand existing practice conditions or problems in order to identify the need for change.
Do—Select an intervention on the basis of the data reviewed, and implement the change.
Study—Study (evaluate) the results of the change
Act—If the process change is successful with positive outcomes, act on the practices by incorporating them into daily unit performance.

In the following example, a QI committee applies the PDSA model for addressing a practice problem:

On the 32-bed medicine oncology unit there has been an increased incidence of client falls. The number of falls has progressively increased over the last 6 months. Added to the problem is the fact that the oncology clients receive chemotherapy, which lowers their platelet counts and increases their susceptibility to injury (bruising and serious bleeding internally) when they fall. One of TJC's client safety goals is reducing the risk of client harm from falls (TJC, 2006). The nurse manager on the oncology unit brings together a QI committee consisting of nurses, pharmacists, physicians, advanced practice nurses, and risk management staff. The QI committee decides to conduct a root cause analysis in their planning. They review all available data to find the real cause of the problem and then work on dealing with it. The committee learns that the majority of falls involved adults under the age of 60. The clients fell in attempts to go to the bathroom or when they tried to get up to a chair. Many clients have received IV Benadryl, a medication administered before blood transfusions.

The committee members conduct a literature review for the problems, focusing on the effects of Benadryl, toileting and falls, and interventions used to reduce falls. Based on the scientific evidence, the committee selects an intervention, an hourly nursing rounds protocol. The plan is to have RNs check on clients on the even hours and assistive personnel check routinely on odd hours. During rounds the staff apply approaches to focus on key fall risk factors: offering clients the chance to use the toilet, offering timely comfort measures, explaining the effects of Benadryl (causes dizziness), and removing barriers around the client's bedside. Once the protocol is implemented, the nursing unit gathers data on the number and characteristics of successive falls. After 3 months the evaluation data shows that falls have generally declined. The staff have complied with the rounds protocol except on shifts when their staffing numbers were low. On one of those shifts a client was found after falling. The committee reviews the data carefully and recommends permanent implementation of the nursing rounds protocol. Discussion also involves how to ensure rounds are conducted even when staffing is low.

Quality improvement combined with evidence-based practice is the foundation for excellent client care and outcomes. Once a QI committee makes a practice change, it is important to communicate results to staff in all appropriate organizational departments. Practice changes will likely not last when QI committees fail to report findings and results of interventions. Regular discussions of QI activities through staff meetings, newsletters, and memos are good communication strategies. Often a QI study reveals information that will prompt organization-wide change. An organization must be responsible for responding to the problem with the appropriate resources. Revision of policies and procedures, modification of standards of care, and implementation of new support services are examples of ways an organization responds.

✳ Key Concepts

- A challenge in evidence-based practice is to be able to obtain the very best, most current information at the right time, when you need it for client care.
- Using your clinical expertise and considering clients' values and preferences ensures that you will apply the evidence in practice both safely and appropriately.
- The five steps of evidence-based practice provide a systematic approach to rational clinical decision making.
- The more focused a PICO question is, the easier it will become to search for evidence in the scientific literature.
- The hierarchy of available evidence offers a guide about the types of literature or information that offer the best scientific evidence.
- A randomized controlled trial is the highest level of experimental research, in which a researcher measures a control group and experimental group for the same outcomes to see if there is a difference.
- Expert clinicians are a rich source of evidence because they use evidence frequently to build their own practice and solve clinical problems.
- The critiquing of evidence involves its evaluation, which includes determining the value, feasibility, and utility of evidence for making a practice change.
- After critiquing all articles for a PICO question, synthesize or combine the findings to consider the scientific rigor of the evidence and whether it has application in practice.
- When you decide to apply evidence, consider the setting and whether there is support from staff and available resources.
- Research is a systematic process that asks and answers questions that generate knowledge, which provides a scientific basis for nursing practice.
- Outcomes research is designed to assess and document the effectiveness of health care services and interventions.
- Nursing research involves two broad approaches for conducting studies: quantitative and qualitative methods.
- The research process usually consists of the following steps: problem identification, study design, conducting the study, data analysis, and use of the findings.
- A thorough analysis of QI data leads clinicians to identify the best evidence available for correcting quality problems.

✳ Critical Thinking Exercises

1. The nursing staff on a medical unit have been reviewing their quality data on the incidence of pressure ulcers. They are concerned about the increase in incidence over the last 3 months. One nurse recently talked with the wound care specialist about the treatment of incontinence in the care of pressure ulcers. The specialist recommended a new product called "Fanny Wipes," which contains an emollient and is effective in cleansing and reducing skin irritation and inflammation. Traditionally the nurses have used soap and water to cleanse clients after an episode of incontinence. What would be a PICO question for this group to ask?

2. A nurse conducts a literature search and obtains articles about a PICO question: Does the use of toileting rounds compared with routine client observation reduce the incidence of falls in clients at risk for falls? The nurse obtains an article that contains a literature review about the problem of falls within medical centers, characteristics of clients who are at risk for falling, the special risk of older adults, and the association of falls with clients' attempts to toilet independently. The majority of clients cared for by the unit where the nurse works are middle-age adults. How will this article prove useful to the nurse?

✳ NCLEX®-Style Review Questions

1. A nurse researcher interviews senior oncology nurses, asking them to describe how they deal with the loss of a client. The analysis of the interviews yields common themes describing the nurses' grief. This is an example of a(n):
   1. Historical study
   2. Qualitative study
   3. Correlational study
   4. Experimental study

2. An operating room nurse is talking with colleagues during a meeting and asks, "I wonder if we would see fewer wound infections if we used chlorhexidine instead of povidone-iodine to clean the skin of our surgical clients?" In this example of a PICO question, the *P* is:
   1. Betadine use
   2. Surgical clients
   3. Chlorhexidine use
   4. Operating room nurse

3. A nurse researcher is designing an exercise study that involves 100 clients who attend a wellness clinic. As the clients come to the clinic, they have a choice as to whether they want to be in the new exercise program or remain in the traditional program. The nurse plans to measure the clients' self-report of exercise before and 6 months after the program begins. What factor might influence the results of this study in an unfavorable way?
   1. Bias
   2. Anonymity
   3. Sample size
   4. Random sampling

4. The foundation of research is based on which of the following:
   1. Evidence
   2. Experience
   3. Critical thinking
   4. Scientific method

5 Number the following steps of evidence-based practice in the appropriate order:
   ___ Integrate the evidence.
   ___ Ask the burning clinical question.
   ___ Evaluate the practice decision or change.
   ___ Critically appraise the evidence you gather.
   ___ Collect the most relevant and best evidence.

6. When a researcher gives a subject full and complete information about the purpose of a study, this is an example of:
   1. Bias
   2. Anonymity
   3. Confidentiality
   4. Informed consent

7. A new nurse on an orthopedic unit is assigned to a client on skeletal traction. The nurse asks a colleague, "What is the best practice for cleaning pin sites in skeletal traction?" This question is an example of a:
   1. Hypothesis
   2. PICO question
   3. Problem-focused trigger
   4. Knowledge-focused trigger

8. The nurses on a medical unit have seen an increase in the number of pressure ulcers that develop in their clients. The nurses decide to initiate a quality improvement project using the PDSA model. Which of the following is an example of "Do" from that model?
   1. Implement the new skin care protocol on all medicine units.
   2. Review the data collected on clients cared for using the protocol.
   3. Review the QI reports on the six clients who developed ulcers over the last 3 months.
   4. Based on findings from clients who developed ulcers, implement an evidence-based skin care protocol.

6 | Health and Wellness

✳ OBJECTIVES

Mastery of content in this chapter will enable the student to:

- List the two general *Healthy People 2010* public health goals for Americans.
- Discuss the definition of health.
- Discuss the health belief, health promotion, basic human needs, and holistic health models to understand the relationship between the client's attitudes toward health and health practices.
- Describe variables influencing health beliefs and practices.

- Describe health promotion, wellness, and illness prevention activities.
- Discuss the three levels of preventive care.
- Describe four types of risk factors.
- Discuss risk factor modification and changing health behaviors.
- Describe variables influencing illness behavior.
- Describe the impact of illness on the client and family.
- Discuss the nurse's role in health and illness.

✳ MEDIA RESOURCES   ✳ KEY TERMS

 Companion CD
- NCLEX®-Style Review Questions
- Audio Glossary
- English/Spanish Glossary
- Interactive Learning Activities

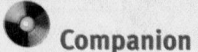 **Website**
- NCLEX®-Style Review Questions
- Audio Glossary
- English/Spanish Glossary
- Interactive Learning Activities
- WebLinks
- Audio Summaries

Active strategies of health promotion, p. 75
Acute illness, p. 79
Chronic illness, p. 79
Health, p. 69
Health behavior change, p. 78
Health behaviors, p. 70
Health belief model, p. 70
Health promotion, p. 75
Holistic health model, p. 72

Illness, p. 78
Illness behavior, p. 79
Illness prevention, p. 75
Passive strategies of health promotion, p. 75
Primary prevention, p. 75
Risk factor, p. 77
Secondary prevention, p. 75
Tertiary prevention, p. 75
Wellness, p. 75

In the past, most individuals and societies viewed good health, or wellness, as the opposite or absence of disease. This simple attitude ignores states of health between disease and good health. Health is a multidimensional concept and must be viewed from a broader perspective. An assessment of the client's state of health is an important aspect of nursing.

Models of health offer a perspective to understand the relationships between the concepts of health, wellness, and illness. Nurses are in a unique position to assist clients in achieving and maintaining optimal levels of health. Nurses understand the challenges of today's health care system and embrace the opportunity to use wellness activities to promote health and wellness and prevent illness. In an era of cost containment and advanced technology, nurses can be a vital link to the improved health of individuals and society. Nurses can identify actual and potential risk factors that predispose a person or a group to illness. In addition, the nurse may use risk factor modification strategies to promote health and wellness and prevent illness.

When illness does occur, different attitudes about illness cause people to react in different ways to illness or the illness of a family member. Medical sociologists call the reaction to illness, illness behavior. Nurses who understand how clients react to illness can minimize the effects of illness and assist clients and their families in maintaining or returning to the highest level of functioning.

Healthy People Documents

In 1979 an influential document, *Healthy People: The Surgeon General's Report on Health Promotion and Disease Prevention,* was published. This report introduced national goals for improving the health of Americans by 1990. It outlined priority objectives for preventive services, health protection, and health promotion that addressed improvements in health status, risk reduction, public and professional awareness of prevention, health services and protective measures, and surveillance and evaluation. The report served as a framework for the 1990s as the United States began to focus more on health promotion and disease prevention instead of illness care. The strategy announced by the Secretary of Health and Human Services required a cooperative effort by government, voluntary and professional organizations, businesses, and individuals. Widely cited by popular media, in professional journals, and at health conferences, it has inspired health promotion programs throughout the country.

The next document, published in 1990, *Healthy People 2000: National Health Promotion and Disease Prevention Objectives,* identified health improvement goals and objectives to be reached by the year 2000 (U.S. Department of Health and Human Services [USDHHS], 1990). Research has shown dramatic progress in improving the nation's health (Burggraf and Barry, 2000). For example, since the 2000 initiatives, infant mortality has declined, childhood vaccinations have risen to an all-time high, and the death rate from coronary heart disease and stroke have declined.

Healthy People 2010 is the latest document and serves as a road map for improving the health of all people in the United States for the first decade of the twenty-first century (USDHHS, 2000). This newest edition emphasizes the link between individual health and community health and the premise that the health of communities determines overall health status of the nation. The two overarching goals for *Healthy People 2010* are (1) to increase quality and years of healthy life and (2) to eliminate health disparities (USDHHS, 2000). The 2010 document includes 28 focus areas with 467 objectives (http://www.health.gov/healthypeople). The document includes four areas: (1) promoting healthy behaviors, (2) promoting healthy and safe communities, (3) improving systems for personal and public health, and (4) preventing and reducing diseases and disorders.

Definition of Health

Defining health is difficult. The World Health Organization (WHO) defines **health** as a "state of complete physical, mental and social well-being, not merely the absence of disease or infirmity" (WHO, 1947). Many other aspects of health need to be considered. Health is a state of being that people define in relation to their own values, personality, and lifestyle. Each person has a personal concept of health. Pender, Murdaugh, and Parsons (2006) define health as the actualization of inherent and acquired human potential through goal-directed behavior, competent self-care, and satisfying relationships with others, while adjustments are made as needed to maintain structural integrity and harmony with the environment.

Individuals' views of health vary among different age-groups, genders, races, and cultures (Pender, 1996; Pender and others, 2006). Pender (1996) explains that "all people free of disease are not equally healthy." Pender and others (2006) note that views of health have broadened to include mental, social, and spiritual well-being, as well as a focus on health at the family and community levels.

To help clients identify and reach health goals, the nurse must discover and use information about their concepts of health. Pender and others (2006) suggest that for many people, conditions of life rather than pathological states are what define health. Life conditions can have positive or negative effects on health long before an illness is evident (Pender and others, 2006). Life conditions may include socioeconomic variables such as environment, diet, and lifestyle practices or choices, as well as many other physiological and psychological variables.

Health and illness must be defined in terms of the individual. Health can include conditions previously considered to be illness. For example, a person with epilepsy who has learned to control seizures with medication and who functions at home and at work may no longer consider himself or herself ill. Nurses' attitudes toward health and illness should consider the total person, as well as the environment in which the person lives, to individualize nursing care and enhance meaningfulness of the client's future health status.

Models of Health and Illness

A model is a theoretical way of understanding a concept or idea. Models represent different ways of approaching complex issues. Because health and illness are complex concepts, models are used to understand the relationships between these concepts and the client's attitudes toward health and **health behaviors.**

Health beliefs are a person's ideas, convictions, and attitudes about health and illness. They may be based on factual information or misinformation, common sense or myths, or reality or false expectations. Because health beliefs usually influence health behavior, they can positively or negatively affect a client's level of health. Positive health behaviors are activities related to maintaining, attaining, or regaining good health and preventing illness. Common positive health behaviors include immunizations, proper sleep patterns, adequate exercise, and nutrition. Negative health behaviors include practices actually or potentially harmful to health, such as smoking, drug or alcohol abuse, poor diet, and refusal to take necessary medications.

Nurses have developed the following health models to understand clients' attitudes and values about health and illness and to provide effective health care. These nursing models allow nurses to understand and predict clients' health behavior, including how they use health services and adhere to recommended therapy.

Health Belief Model

Rosenstoch's (1974) and Becker and Maiman's (1975) **health belief model** (Figure 6-1) addresses the relationship between a person's beliefs and behaviors. It provides a way of understanding and predicting how clients will behave in relation to their health and how they will comply with health care therapies.

The first component of this model involves the individual's perception of susceptibility to an illness. For example, a client needs to recognize the familial link for coronary artery disease. After this link is recognized, particularly when one parent and two siblings have died in their fourth decade from myocardial infarction, the client may perceive the personal risk of heart disease.

The second component is the individual's perception of the seriousness of the illness. This perception is influenced and modified by demographic and sociopsychological variables, perceived threats of the illness, and cues to action (e.g., mass media campaigns and advice from family, friends, and medical professionals). For example, a client may not perceive his heart disease as serious, which may affect the way he takes care of himself.

The third component—the likelihood that a person will take preventive action—results from the person's perception of the benefits of and barriers to taking action. Preventive action may include lifestyle changes, increased adherence to medical therapies, or a search for medical advice or treatment. A client's perception of susceptibility to disease, as well as his or her perception of the seriousness of an illness, helps to determine the likelihood that the client will or will not partake in healthy behaviors.

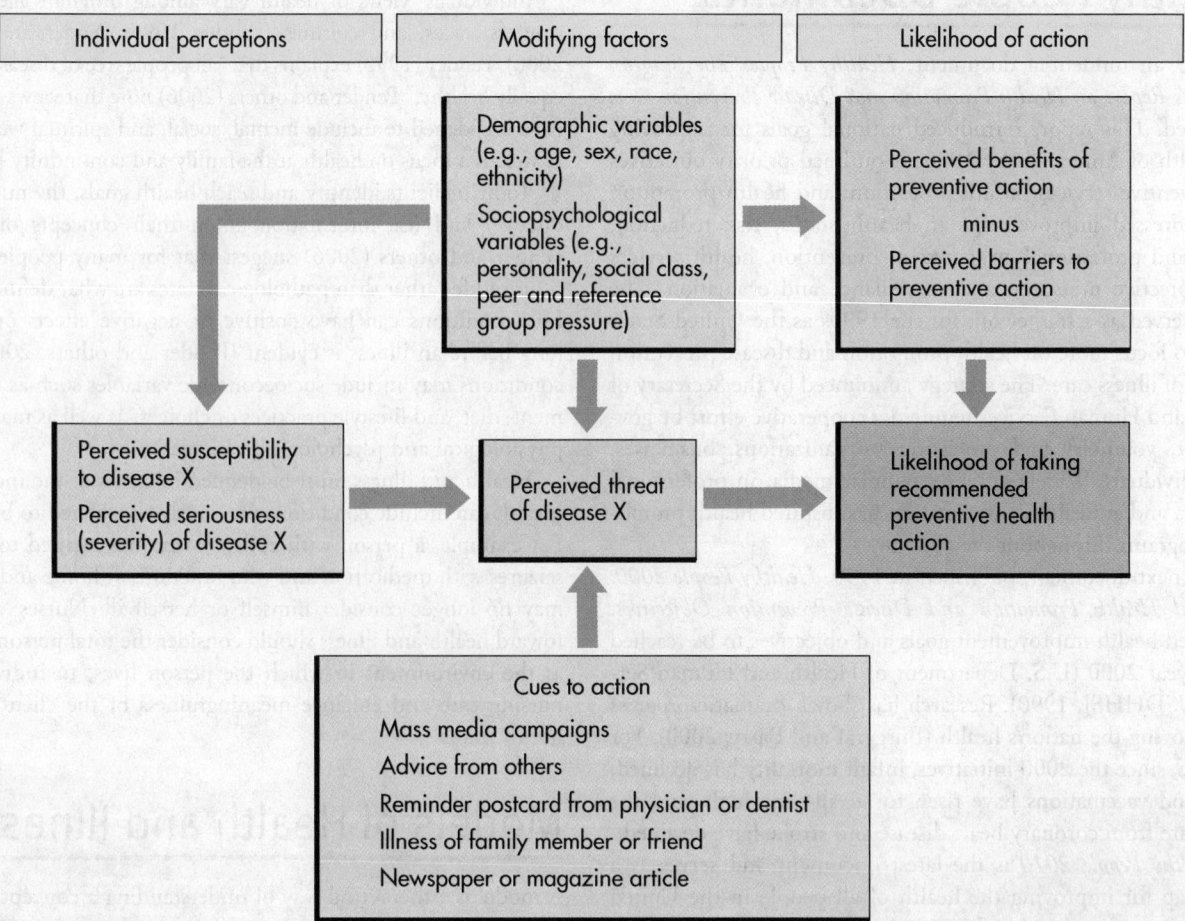

Figure 6-1 Health belief model. (Data from Becker M, Maiman L: Sociobehavioral determinants of compliance with health and medical care recommendations, *Med Care* 13[1]:10, 1975.)

The health belief model helps nurses understand factors influencing clients' perceptions, beliefs, and behavior in order to plan care that will most effectively assist clients in maintaining or restoring health and preventing illness.

Health Promotion Model

The health promotion model (HPM) proposed by Pender (1982; revised, 1996) was designed to be a "complementary counterpart to models of health protection" (Figure 6-2). It defines health as a positive, dynamic state, not merely the absence of disease (Pender and others, 2002). Health promotion is directed at increasing a client's level of well-being. The health promotion model describes the multidimensional nature of persons as they interact within their environment to pursue health (Pender, 1993, 1996; Pender and others, 2002). The model focuses on the following three areas: (1) individual characteristics and experiences, (2) behavior-specific knowledge and affect, and (3) behavioral outcomes. The HPM notes that each person has unique personal characteristics and experiences that affect subsequent actions. The set of variables for behavioral-specific knowledge and affect have important motiva-

tional significance. These variables can be modified through nursing actions. Health-promoting behavior is the desired behavioral outcome and is the end point in the HPM. Health-promoting behaviors should result in improved health, enhanced functional ability, and better quality of life at all stages of development (Pender and others, 2002) (Box 6-1).

Basic Human Needs Model

Basic human needs are elements that are necessary for human survival and health (e.g., food, water, safety, and love). Although each person has other unique needs, all people share the basic human needs, and the extent to which basic needs are met is a major factor in determining a person's level of health.

Maslow's hierarchy of needs is a model that nurses use to understand the interrelationships of basic human needs (Figure 6-3). According to this model, certain human needs are more basic than others; that is, some needs must be met before other needs (e.g., fulfilling the physiological needs before the needs of love and belonging). Self-actualization is the highest expression of one's individual potential and allows for continual discovery of self. Maslow's

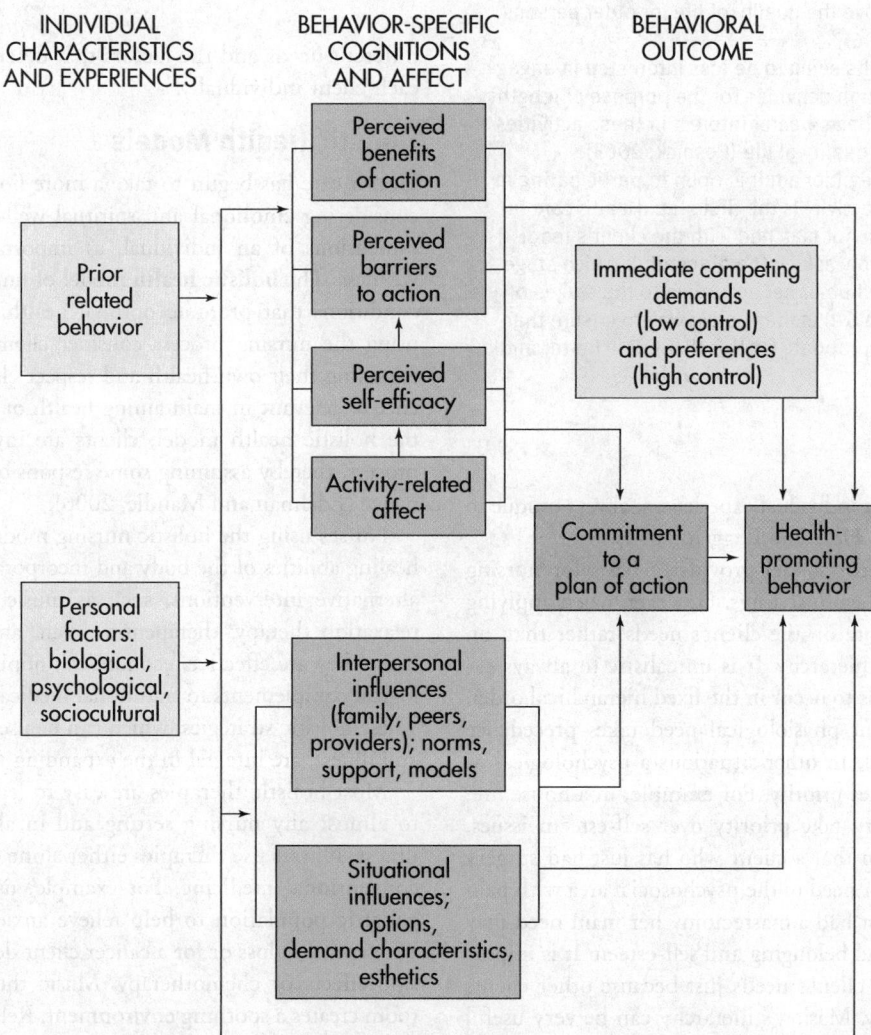

Figure 6-2 Health promotion model (revised). (Redrawn from Pender NJ, Murdaugh CL, Parsons MA: *Health promotion in nursing practice,* ed 4, Upper Saddle River, NJ, 2002, Prentice Hall.)

✳ BOX 6-1   FOCUS ON OLDER ADULTS

Health Promotion

- Because the population of the world is getting older and individuals are living longer, health promotion activities are important to help maintain function and independence and improve quality of life (Resnick, 2003).

- Focusing on self-care abilities and practices that foster health while aging are important nursing interventions (Pender and others, 2002).

- Factors that have been reported to affect older adults' willingness to engage in health promotion activities may include socioeconomic factors, beliefs and attitudes for clients and providers, encouragement by a health care professional, specific motivation based on efficacy beliefs, access to resources, age, number of chronic illnesses, mental and physical health, marital status, and cognitive status (Resnick, 2003).

- There is an increasing prevalence of high blood pressure, obesity, and diabetes among persons 75 and older, and this is the population age that is increasing (Mokdad and others, 2004).

- Scientific evidence increasingly indicates that physical activity can extend years of active independent life, reduce disability, and improve the quality of life for older persons (Chodzko-Zajko, 2006).

- Generally, older adults seem to be less interested in engaging in health promotion activities for the purpose of lengthening lives but may have greater interest in these activities only if they improve quality of life (Resnick, 2003).

- Knowing whether the older adult is open to participating in a health promotion activity is the first step. Health care interventions are often not matched with the client's readiness to change. Simply asking the older adult which stage would best describe him or her according to the stages of change model (Table 6-1) is the easiest way to ensure that interventions are appropriate for the client (Reicherter and Green, 2005).

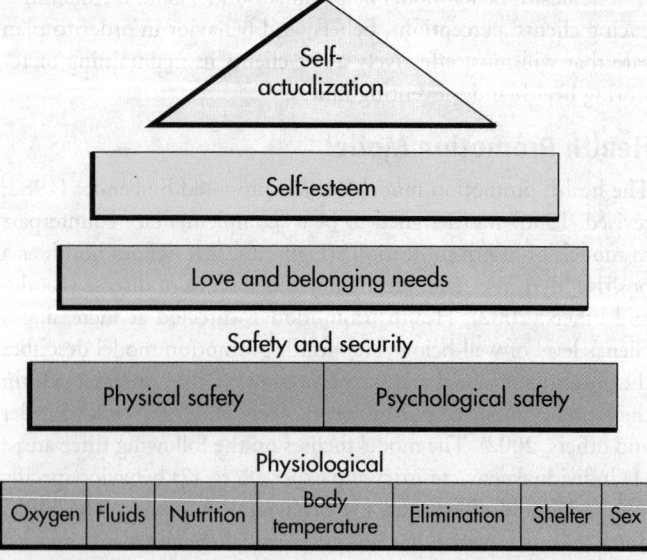

Figure 6-3 Maslow's hierarchy of needs. (Redrawn from Maslow AH: *Motivation and personality*, ed 3, Upper Saddle River NJ, 1970, Prentice Hall.)

model takes into account individual experiences, always unique to the individual (Ebersole, Hess, and Luggen, 2004).

The hierarchy of needs model provides a basis for nursing clients of all ages in all health settings. However, when applying the model, the focus care on the client's needs rather than on strict adherence to the hierarchy. It is unrealistic to always expect a client's basic needs to occur in the fixed hierarchical order. In all cases an emergent physiological need takes precedence over a higher-level need. In other situations a psychological or physical safety need takes priority. For example, in a house fire, fear of death and injury take priority over self-esteem issues. Although it would seem that a client who has just had surgery might have the strongest need in the psychosocial area with pain control, if the client just had a mastectomy her main need may be in the area of love and belonging and self-esteem It is important not to assume the client's needs just because other clients reacted in a certain way. Maslow's hierarchy can be very useful when applied to each client individually. To provide the most effective care, the nurse needs to understand the relationships of

different needs and the factors that determine the priorities for each client individually.

Holistic Health Models

Health care has begun to take a more holistic view of health by considering emotional and spiritual well-being, as well as other dimensions of an individual, as important aspects of physical wellness. The **holistic health model** of nursing attempts to create conditions that promote optimal health. In this model, nurses using the nursing process consider clients the ultimate experts regarding their own health and respect clients' subjective experience as relevant in maintaining health or assisting in healing. In the holistic health model, clients are involved in their healing process, thereby assuming some responsibility for health maintenance (Edelman and Mandle, 2006).

Nurses using the holistic nursing model recognize the natural healing abilities of the body and incorporate complementary and alternative interventions, such as music therapy, reminiscence, relaxation therapy, therapeutic touch, and guided imagery, because they are effective, economical, noninvasive, nonpharmacological complements to traditional medical care (see Chapter 36). These holistic strategies, which can be used in all stages of health and illness, are integral in the expanding role of nursing.

Most holistic therapies are easy to learn and can be applied to almost any nursing setting and in all stages of health and illness. Nurses use therapies either alone or in conjunction with conventional medicine. For example, use reminiscence in the geriatric population to help relieve anxiety for a client dealing with memory loss or for a cancer client dealing with the difficult side effects of chemotherapy. Music therapy in the operating room creates a soothing environment. Relaxation therapy may be useful in any setting to distract a client during a painful procedure, such as a dressing change. Breathing exercises are com-

❋ **TABLE 6-1** Stages of Health Behavior Change

STAGE	DEFINITION	NURSING IMPLICATIONS
Precontemplation	Not intending to make changes within the next 6 months.	Client will not be interested in information about the behavior and may be defensive when confronted with the information.
Contemplation	Considering a change within the next 6 months.	Ambivalence may be present, but clients will more likely accept information as they are developing more belief in the value of change.
Preparation	Making small changes in preparation for a change in the next month.	Client believes advantages outweigh disadvantages of behavior change. May need assistance in planning for the change.
Action	Actively engaged in strategies to change behavior. This stage may last up to 6 months.	Be aware of previous habits that may prevent action on new behaviors. Identify barriers and facilitators of change.
Maintenance stage	Sustained change over time. This stage begins 6 months after action has started and continues indefinitely.	Changes need to be integrated into the client's lifestyle.

Data from Prochaska JO, DiClemente CC: Stages of change in the modification of problem behaviors, *Prog Behav Modif* 28:184, 1992; and Conn VS: A staged-based approach to helping people change health behaviors, *Clin Nurs Spec* 8(4):187, 1994.

monly taught to help clients deal with the pain associated with labor and delivery.

Recently there has been an increase in the number of people using alternative and complementary medical therapies. Nurses should be aware that their clients may have previous knowledge or experience with alternative and complementary therapies and may therefore be accepting of holistic nursing interventions. Nurses can help all clients recognize the many options available and assist them in making choices to enhance health.

Variables Influencing Health and Health Beliefs and Practices

There are many variables that influence a client's health beliefs and practices. Internal and external variables influence how a person thinks and acts. As previously stated, health beliefs usually influence health behavior, or health practices, and likewise positively or negatively affect a client's level of health. Therefore understanding the effects of these variables allows the nurse to plan and deliver individualized care.

Internal Variables

Internal variables include a person's developmental stage, intellectual background, perception of functioning, and emotional and spiritual factors.

Developmental Stage. A person's thought and behavior patterns change throughout life. The nurse must consider the client's level of growth and development when using his or her health beliefs and practices as a basis for planning care. The study of development involves finding patterns or general principles that apply to most people most of the time (Murray and Zentner, 2001). The concept of illness for a child, adolescent, or adult depends on the individual's developmental stage. Fear and anxiety are common

among ill children, especially if thoughts about illness, hospitalization, or procedures are based on lack of information or lack of clarity of information. Emotional development may also influence personal beliefs about health-related matters. For example, the nurse uses different techniques for teaching about contraception to an adolescent than would be used for an adult. Knowledge of the stages of growth and development helps the nurse predict the client's response to the present illness or the threat of future illness. The nurse then adapts the planning of nursing care to these expectations, as well as to the client's abilities to participate in self-care.

Intellectual Background. A person's beliefs about health are shaped in part by the person's knowledge, lack of knowledge, or incorrect information about body functions and illnesses, educational background, and past experiences. These variables influence how a client thinks about health. In addition, cognitive abilities shape the *way* a person thinks, including the ability to understand factors involved in illness and to apply knowledge of health and illness to personal health practices. Cognitive abilities also relate to a person's developmental stage. A nurse considers intellectual background so that these variables can be incorporated into nursing care (Edelman and Mandle, 2002).

Perception of Functioning. The way people perceive their physical functioning affects health beliefs and practices. When nurses assess a client's level of health, they gather subjective data about the way the client perceives physical functioning, such as level of fatigue, shortness of breath, or pain. They also obtain objective data about actual functioning, such as blood pressure, height measurements, and lung sound assessment. This information allows nurses to more successfully plan and implement individualized care.

Emotional Factors. The client's degree of stress, depression, or fear, for example, can influence health beliefs and practices. The manner in which a person handles stress throughout each phase of life will influence the way the person reacts to illness. A person who generally is very calm may have little emotional response during illness, whereas an individual unable to cope emotionally with the threat of illness may either overreact to illness and assume it is life threatening or deny the presence of symptoms and not take therapeutic action (see Chapter 31).

Spiritual Factors. Spirituality is reflected in how a person lives his or her life, including the values and beliefs exercised, the relationships established with family and friends, and the ability to find hope and meaning in life. Spirituality serves as an integrating theme in people's lives (see Chapter 29). Religious practices are one way that people exercise spirituality. There are some religions that restrict the use of certain forms of medical treatment. Nurses must understand clients' spiritual dimensions to involve them effectively in nursing care.

External Variables

External variables influencing a person's health beliefs and practices include family practices, socioeconomic factors, and cultural background.

Family Practices. The way that clients' families use health care services generally affects their health practices. Their perceptions of the seriousness of diseases and their history of preventive care behaviors (or lack of them) influence how clients will think about health. For example, if a young woman's mother never had annual gynecological examinations or Pap smears, it is unlikely the daughter will follow such practices.

Socioeconomic Factors. Social and psychosocial factors increase the risk for illness and influence the way that a person defines and reacts to illness. Psychosocial variables include the stability of the person's marital or intimate relationship, lifestyle habits, and occupational environment. A person generally seeks approval and support from social networks (neighbors, peers, and co-workers), and this desire for approval and support affects health beliefs and practices.

Social variables partly determine how the health care system provides medical care. Because the health care system is organized in certain ways, it determines how clients can obtain care, the treatment method, the economic cost to the client, and potential reimbursement to the health care agency or client.

Like social variables, economic variables may affect a client's level of health by increasing the risk for disease and influencing how or at what point the client enters the health care system. A person's compliance with the treatment that is designed to maintain or improve health is also affected by economic status. A person who has high utility bills, a large family, and a low income tends to give a higher priority to food and shelter than to costly drugs or treatment or expensive foods for special diets. A client may decide to take medication every other day, rather than every day as prescribed, to save money. This could greatly affect effectiveness of the medication.

Cultural Background. Cultural background influences beliefs, values, and customs. It influences the approach to the health care system, personal health practices, and the nurse-client rela-

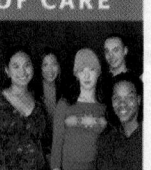

✳ BOX 6-2   CULTURAL ASPECTS OF CARE

Cultural Health Beliefs

The cultural and ethnic backgrounds of clients shape their views of health, wellness, and illness. Cultural understanding of illness may affect the way a client reports symptoms. For example, because clinical depression is stigmatized in some cultures, a client with depression may report only physical symptoms such as fatigue and weight loss. Culture can also affect clients' perceptions of illness causation and treatment. For example, some cultures have been found to attribute breast cancer to "sinful" behaviors, and other cultures have been found to believe that surgical treatment of breast cancer would cause it to metastasize. Differences in beliefs, values, and traditional health care practices are also relevant when planning end-of-life care. In addition, many cultures incorporate spiritual practices, and therefore spirituality overlaps with culture. When exploring information about culture, nurses should consider beliefs, values, daily practices, spirituality, and their implications for the way a client understands illness, perceives treatment plans, and makes health care decisions.

Implications for Practice
- Be aware of the impact of culture on a client's view and understanding of illness.
- When teaching clients about their illness and treatment regimens, it is important for nurses to understand that unique cultural perceptions exist regarding the cause of an illness and its treatment.
- Focus on understanding the client's traditions, values, and beliefs and how these dimensions may affect health, wellness, and illness.

Data from Kundhal KK: Cultural diversity: an evolving challenge to physician-patient communication, *JAMA* 289(1):94, 2003; McEvoy M: Culture and spirituality as an integrated concept in pediatric care, *MCN Am J Matern Child Nurs* 28(1):39, 2003; and Crawley L and others: Strategies for culturally effective end-of-life care, *Ann Intern Med* 136(9):673, 2002.

tionship. Cultural background may also influence an individual's beliefs about causes of illness, as well as remedies or practices to restore health (Box 6-2). If nurses are not aware of their own and other cultural patterns of behavior and language, they may not be able to recognize and understand a client's behavior and beliefs and may have difficulty interacting with the client. As with family and socioeconomic variables, cultural variables must be incorporated into a client's care plan (see Chapter 9).

Health Promotion, Wellness, and Illness Prevention

Health care has become increasingly focused on health promotion, wellness, and illness prevention. The rapid rise of health care costs has motivated people to seek ways of decreasing the incidence and minimizing the results of illness or disability.

The concepts of health promotion, wellness, and illness prevention are closely related and, in practice, overlap to some extent.

All are focused on the future; the difference between them involves motivations and goals. **Health promotion** activities, such as routine exercise and good nutrition, help clients maintain or enhance their present levels of health. Health promotion activities motivate people to act positively to reach more stable levels of health. **Wellness** education teaches people how to care for themselves in a healthy way and includes topics such as physical awareness, stress management, and self-responsibility. Wellness strategies help persons achieve new understanding and control of their lives. **Illness prevention** activities such as immunization programs protect clients from actual or potential threats to health. Illness prevention activities motivate people to avoid declines in health or functional levels.

Nurses emphasize health promotion, wellness-enhancing strategies, and illness prevention activities as important forms of health care because they assist clients in maintaining and improving health. The goal of a total health program is to improve a client's level of well-being in all dimensions, not just physical health. Total health programs are based on the belief that many factors can affect a person's level of health.

The leading health indicators as defined by *Healthy People 2010* are physical activity, overweight and obesity, tobacco use, substance abuse, responsible sexual behavior, mental health, injury and violence, environmental quality, immunization, and access to health care (USDHHS, 2000). These indicators show the importance of health promotion and illness prevention and encourage all to participate in the improvement of health (USDHHS, 2000).

Health can be influenced by individual practices, such as poor eating habits and little or no exercise. It can also be affected by physical stressors, such as a poor living environment, exposure to air pollutants, and an unsafe environment. Hereditary and psychological stressors, such as emotional, intellectual, social, developmental, and spiritual factors, also influence one's level of health. Total health programs are directed at individuals' changing their lifestyle by developing habits that improve their level of health.

Other programs are aimed at specific health care problems. For example, support groups exist to help people with human immunodeficiency virus (HIV) infection. Exercise programs encourage participants to exercise regularly to reduce their risk of cardiac disease. Stress reduction programs teach participants to cope with stressors and reduce their risks for multiple illnesses, such as infections, gastrointestinal disease, and cardiac disease.

Some health promotion, wellness education, and illness prevention programs are operated by health care agencies; others are independently operated. Many corporations have developed on-site health promotion activities for employees. Likewise, colleges and community centers offer health promotion and illness prevention programs. Nurses may be actively involved in these programs or may be consultants or give referrals. The goal of these activities is to improve the client's level of health through preventive health services, environmental protection, and health education.

Health care professionals who work in the field of health promotion use proactive attempts to prevent illness or disease. Health promotion activities can be passive or active. With **passive strategies of health promotion,** individuals gain from the activities of others without acting themselves. The fluoridation of municipal drinking water and the fortification of homogenized milk with vitamin D are examples of passive health promotion strategies. With **active strategies of health promotion,** individuals are motivated to adopt specific health programs. Weight reduction and smoking cessation programs require clients to be actively involved in measures to improve their present and future levels of wellness while decreasing the risk of disease.

Health promotion, as outlined in the *American Journal of Health Promotion,* is the science and art of helping people change their lifestyle to move toward a state of optimal health. This definition suggests that health and illness are affected by choices made by individuals (Raphael, 2002). An individual takes responsibility for health and wellness by making appropriate lifestyle choices. Lifestyle choices are important in that they affect a person's quality of life. Positive lifestyle choices and the avoidance of negative lifestyle choices may also play a role in the prevention of illness. As well as improving quality of life, prevention of illness also has an economic impact in that it decreases health care costs.

Levels of Preventive Care

Nursing care oriented to health promotion, wellness, and illness prevention can be understood in terms of health activities on primary, secondary, and tertiary levels (Figure 6-4).

Primary Prevention. **Primary prevention** is true prevention; it precedes disease or dysfunction and is applied to clients considered physically and emotionally healthy. Primary prevention aimed at health promotion includes health education programs, immunizations, and physical and nutritional fitness activities. It can be provided to an individual or to a general population, or it can focus on individuals at risk for developing specific diseases. Primary prevention includes all health promotion efforts, as well as wellness education activities that focus on maintaining or improving the general health of individuals, families, and communities (Edelman and Mandle, 2002). Primary prevention includes specific protection such as immunization for influenza and hearing protection in occupational settings.

Secondary Prevention. **Secondary prevention** focuses on individuals who are experiencing health problems or illnesses and who are at risk for developing complications or worsening conditions. Activities are directed at diagnosis and prompt intervention, thereby reducing severity and enabling the client to return to a normal level of health as early as possible (Edelman and Mandle, 2006; Pender, 1993). A large portion of nursing care related to secondary prevention is delivered in homes, hospitals, or skilled nursing facilities. It includes screening techniques and treating early stages of disease to limit disability by averting or delaying the consequences of advanced disease. Screening activities also become a key opportunity for health teaching as a primary prevention intervention (Edelman and Mandle, 2006).

Tertiary Prevention. **Tertiary prevention** occurs when a defect or disability is permanent and irreversible. It involves minimizing the effects of long-term disease or disability by interventions directed at preventing complications and deterioration (Edelman and Mandle, 2006). Activities are directed at rehabilita-

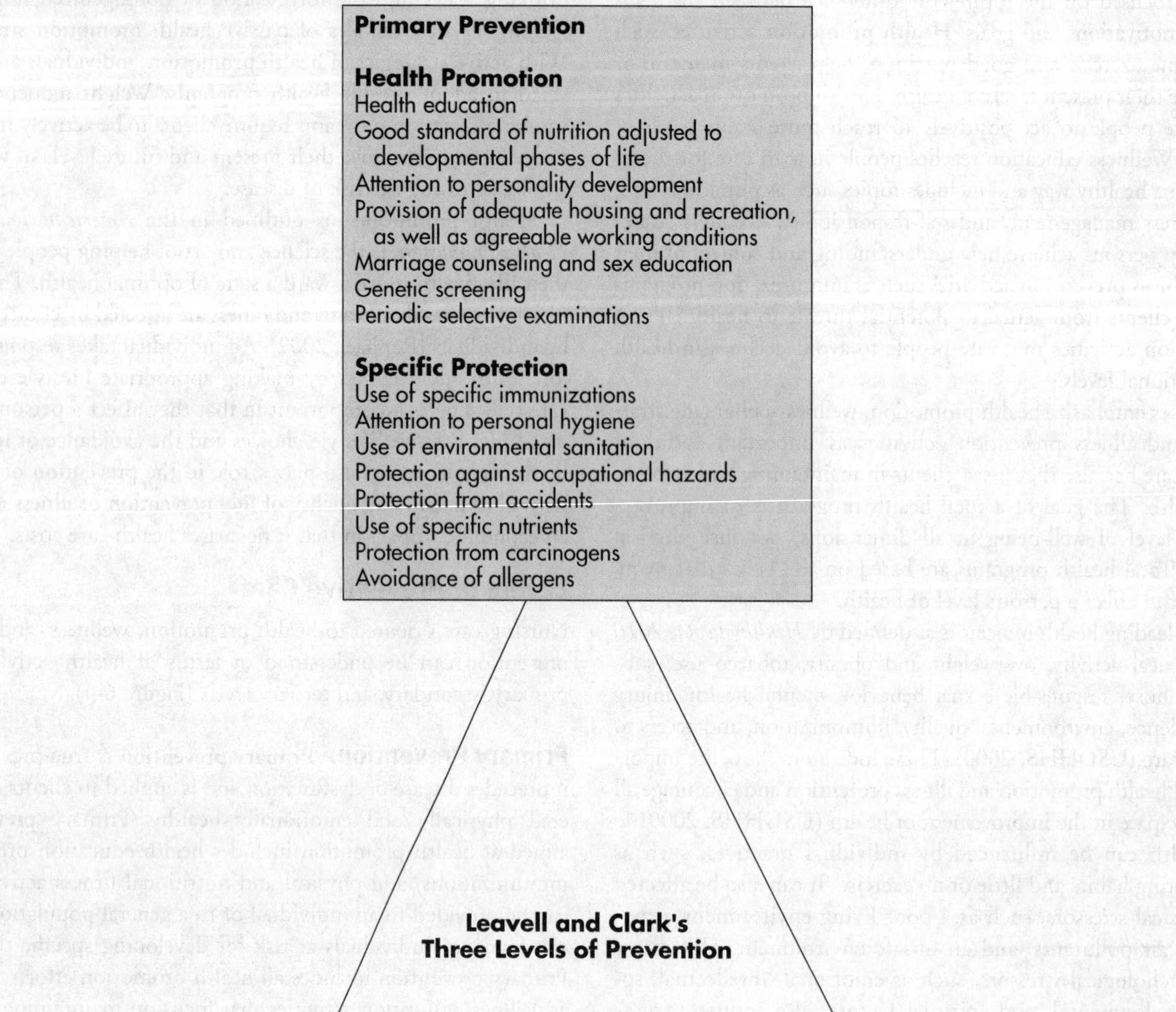

Primary Prevention

Health Promotion
Health education
Good standard of nutrition adjusted to
    developmental phases of life
Attention to personality development
Provision of adequate housing and recreation,
    as well as agreeable working conditions
Marriage counseling and sex education
Genetic screening
Periodic selective examinations

Specific Protection
Use of specific immunizations
Attention to personal hygiene
Use of environmental sanitation
Protection against occupational hazards
Protection from accidents
Use of specific nutrients
Protection from carcinogens
Avoidance of allergens

**Leavell and Clark's
Three Levels of Prevention**

Secondary Prevention

Early Diagnosis and Prompt Treatment
Case-finding measures: individual and mass
    screening surveys
Selective examinations to
    Cure and prevent disease process
    Prevent spread of communicable disease
    Prevent complications and sequelae
    Shorten period of disability

Disability Limitations
Adequate treatment to arrest disease process and
    prevent further complications and sequelae
Provision of facilities to limit disability and
    prevent death

Tertiary Prevention

Restoration and Rehabilitation
Provision of hospital and community facilities for
    retraining and education to maximize use of
    remaining capacities
Education of public and industry to use rehabilitated
    persons to fullest possible extent
Selective placement
Work therapy in hospitals
Use of sheltered colony

Figure 6-4 The three levels of prevention developed by Leavell and Clark. (Data from Leavell H, Clark AE: *Preventive medicine for the doctors in his community,* ed 3, New York, 1965, McGraw-Hill; and modified from Edelman CL, Mandle CL: *Health promotion throughout the life span,* ed 5, St. Louis, 2002, Mosby.)

✳ TABLE 6-2 Actual Causes of Death in the United States in 1990 and 2000

ACTUAL CAUSE	No. (%) IN 1990*	No. (%) IN 2000
Tobacco	400000 (19)	435000 (18.1)
Poor diet and physical inactivity	300000 (14)	400000 (16.6)
Alcohol consumption	100000 (5)	85000 (3.6)
Microbial agents	90000 (4)	75000 (3.1)
Toxic agents	60000 (3)	55000 (2.3)
Motor vehicle	25000 (1)	43000 (1.8)
Firearms	35000 (2)	29000 (1.2)
Sexual behavior	30000 (1)	20000 (0.8)
Illicit drug use	20000 (<1)	17000 (0.7)
Total	1060000 (50)	1159000 (48.2)

*Data are from McGinnis JM and Foege WH: Actual causes of death in the United States, *JAMA* 270:2207, 1993. The percentages are for all deaths.
From Mokdad AH and others: Actual causes of death in the United States, 2000. *JAMA* 291(10):1238, 2004.

tion rather than diagnosis and treatment. Care at this level aims to help clients achieve as high a level of functioning as possible, despite the limitations caused by illness or impairment. This level of care is called preventive care because it involves preventing further disability or reduced functioning.

Risk Factors

A **risk factor** is any situation, habit, social or environmental condition, physiological or psychological condition, developmental or intellectual condition, or spiritual or other variable that increases the vulnerability of an individual or group to an illness or accident. An understanding of risk factors, behavior, risk factor modification, and behavior modification are integral components of health promotion, wellness, and illness prevention activities. Nurses in all areas of practice often have opportunities to assist clients in adopting activities to promote health and decrease risks of illness.

The presence of risk factors does not mean that a disease will develop, but risk factors increase the chances that the individual will experience a particular disease or dysfunction. Nurses and other health care professionals are concerned with risk factors, sometimes called health hazards, for several reasons. Risk factors play a major role in how a nurse identifies a client's health status. They can also influence health beliefs and practices if a person is aware of their presence. Risk factors can be placed in the following interrelated categories: genetic and physiological factors, age, physical environment, and lifestyle.

Genetic and Physiological Factors

Physiological risk factors involve the physical functioning of the body. Certain physical conditions, such as being pregnant or overweight, place increased stress on physiological systems (e.g., the circulatory system), increasing susceptibility to illness in these areas. Heredity, or genetic predisposition to specific illness, is a major physical risk factor. For example, a person with a family history of diabetes mellitus is at risk for developing the disease later in life. Other documented genetic risk factors include family histories of cancer, heart disease, kidney disease, or mental illness.

Age

Age increases or decreases susceptibility to certain illnesses. For example, an infant born prematurely and all neonates are more susceptible to infections. The risk of heart disease increases with age for both sexes. Also, many kinds of cancer pose a greater risk for persons over age 45 than for younger persons. Age risk factors are often closely associated with other risk factors such as family history and personal habits. Nurses need to educate their clients about the importance of regularly scheduled checkups for their age-group. U.S. authorities have identified a schedule of recommendations for health screenings, immunizations, and counseling. Access to scientific evidence, recommendations on clinical prevention services and information on how to implement recommended preventative services into practice can be found at www.ahrq.gov/clinic/prevenix.htm.

Environment

Where we live and the condition of that area (its air, water, and soil) determine how we live, what we eat, the disease agents to which we are exposed, our state of health, and our ability to adapt (Murray and Zentner, 2001). The physical environment in which a person works or lives can increase the likelihood that certain illnesses will occur. For example, some kinds of cancer and other diseases are more likely to develop when industrial workers are exposed to certain chemicals or when people live near toxic waste disposal sites. Nursing assessments extend from the individual to the family and the community in which they live (Murray and Zentner, 2001).

Lifestyle

Many activities, habits, and practices involve risk factors. Lifestyle practices and behaviors can have positive or negative effects on health. Practices with potential negative effects are risk factors. Some habits are risk factors for specific diseases. For example, excessive sunbathing increases the risk of skin cancer, and being overweight increases the risk of cardiovascular disease. Mokdad and others (2004) identified modifiable behavioral risk factors that are leading causes of mortality in the United States (Table 6-2). Their analysis showed that although smoking remains the leading cause of mortality, poor diet and physical inactivity may soon rise to the top as the leading cause of death. These data highlight the importance of an emphasis on preventive care. This information also represents a huge impact on the economics of the health care system. Therefore it is important to understand the impact of lifestyle behaviors on health status. Nurses educate their clients and the public on wellness-promoting lifestyle behaviors.

Stress is a lifestyle risk factor if it is severe or prolonged or if the person is unable to cope with life events adequately. Stress threatens mental health (emotional stress), as well as physical well-being (physiological stress). Both may play a part in the development of an illness and affect the ability to adapt to potential changes associated with an illness, as well as the ability to survive a life-threatening illness. Stress also interferes with health promotion activities and the ability to implement needed lifestyle modifications. Emotional stressors may result from life events such as divorce, pregnancy, death of a spouse or family member, and financial instabilities. Job-related stressors, for example, may overtax a person's cognitive skills and decision-making ability, leading to "mental overload" or "burnout" (see Chapter 31). Stress also threatens physical well-being and has been associated with illnesses such as heart disease, cancer, and gastrointestinal disorders (Pender and others, 2006). Always review life stressors as part of a comprehensive risk factor analysis.

The goal of risk factor identification is to merely assist clients in visualizing those areas in their life that can be modified or even eliminated to promote wellness and prevent illness. More comprehensive health risk appraisals, using a variety of available health risk appraisal forms, can be done to estimate a person's specific health threats based on the presence of various risk factors (Edelman and Mandle, 2002). It is important to understand that implementation of a health risk appraisal must be linked with educational programs and other community resources in order to result in necessary lifestyle changes and in risk reduction (Pender and others, 2002).

Risk Factor Modification and Changing Health Behaviors

Identifying risk factors is the first step in health promotion, wellness education, and illness prevention activities. Discuss health hazards with the client following a comprehensive nursing assessment; then the client can decide if he or she wants to maintain or improve his or her health status by taking risk reduction actions (Edelman and Mandle, 2006). Risk factor modification, health promotion or illness prevention activities, or any program that attempts to change unhealthy lifestyle behaviors can be considered a wellness strategy. Emphasize wellness strategies that teach clients to care for themselves in a healthier way because they have the ability to increase the quality of life, as well as decrease the potential high costs of unmanaged health problems.

Attempts to change may be aimed at the cessation of a health-damaging behavior (e.g., tobacco use or alcohol misuse) or at the adoption of a healthy behavior (e.g., healthy diet or exercise) (Pender and others, 2006). Changing health behavior is difficult, especially those behaviors that people ingrain in their lifestyle pat-

terns. The role of nurses' using a health promotion model for identification of risky behaviors and implementation of the change process cannot be overemphasized, because it is the nurse who spends the greatest amount of time in direct contact with clients. In addition, leading causes of death continue to relate to health behaviors that require a change, and nurses are challenged to motivate and facilitate health behavior change in working with individuals, families, and communities (Edelman and Mandle, 2006).

An understanding of the process of changing behaviors can help nurses support difficult **health behavior change** in their clients. It is believed that change involves movement through a series of stages. The stages of change are described by DiClemente and Prochaska (1998) in the transtheoretical model of change (see Table 6-1, p. 73). These stages range from no intention to change (precontemplation), considering a change within the next 6 months (contemplation), making small changes (preparation), actively engaging in strategies to change behavior (action), to maintaining a changed behavior (maintenance stage). As individuals attempt a change in behavior, relapse followed by recycling through the stages occurs frequently. When relapse occurs, the person will return to the contemplation or precontemplation stage before attempting the change again. Relapse is a learning process, and what is learned from relapse can be applied to the next attempt to change. It is important to understand what occurs at the various stages of the change process in order to time the implementation of interventions (wellness strategies) adequately and to provide appropriate care at each stage.

Once a stage of change has been identified, the processes of change facilitate movement through the stages. The processes of change, or nursing interventions, should be appropriately chosen to match the stage of change (DiClemente and Prochaska, 1998). Most behavior change programs are designed (and have a chance of success) for those people who are ready to take action regarding their health behavior problems. Only a minority of people are actually in this action stage (Prochaska, 1991). Further work needs to be done to design interventions and wellness strategies for people in all stages of health behavior change. Changes will be maintained over time only if they are integrated into an individual's overall lifestyle (Box 6-3). Maintenance of healthy lifestyles can prevent hospitalizations and potentially lower the cost of health care.

Illness

Illness is a state in which a person's physical, emotional, intellectual, social, developmental, or spiritual functioning is diminished or impaired compared with previous experience. Cancer is a disease process, but one client with leukemia who is responding to treatment may continue to function as usual, whereas another client with breast cancer who is preparing for surgery may be affected in dimensions other than the physical.

Illness therefore is not synonymous with disease. Although nurses must be familiar with different kinds of diseases and their treatments, they are concerned more with illness, which may include disease but also includes the effects on functioning and well-being in all dimensions.

✳ BOX 6-3   CLIENT TEACHING

Lifestyle Changes

Objective
- Health risks related to poor lifestyle habits (e.g., high-fat diet, sedentary lifestyle) will be reduced through behavior change.

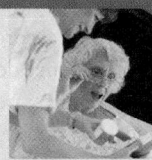

Teaching Strategies
- Practice active listening, and ask the client how he or she prefers to learn (Vanderhoff, 2005).
- Begin with determining what information the client has regarding health risks related to poor lifestyle.
- Ask the client what barriers and benefits he or she perceives with the planned lifestyle change (Vanderhoff, 2005).
- Assist the client in establishing goals for change.
- In collaboration with the client, establish time lines for modification of eating and exercise lifestyle habits.
- Reinforce the process of change with the client.
- Use written resources at an appropriate reading level (Vanderhoff, 2005).
- Include family members to support the lifestyle change.

Evaluation
- Have the client maintain an exercise and eating calendar to track adherence and provide positive reinforcement.
- Ask the client to discuss success with lifestyle changes, such as minutes spent in activity or actual number of fruits and vegetables eaten.
- Have the client identify community resources used in making change.

✳ BOX 6-4   EVIDENCE-BASED PRACTICE

Changes in Diabetes Self-Care Behaviors

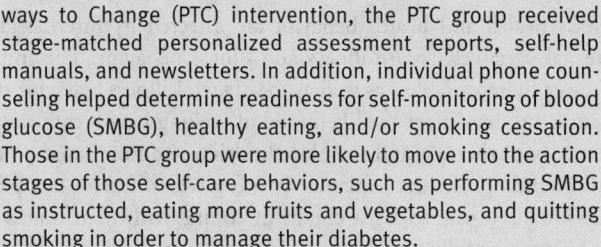

Evidence Summary

Diabetes self-management is critical, complex, and demanding. In a comparison between diabetes Treatment as Usual (TAU) with the Pathways to Change (PTC) intervention, the PTC group received stage-matched personalized assessment reports, self-help manuals, and newsletters. In addition, individual phone counseling helped determine readiness for self-monitoring of blood glucose (SMBG), healthy eating, and/or smoking cessation. Those in the PTC group were more likely to move into the action stages of those self-care behaviors, such as performing SMBG as instructed, eating more fruits and vegetables, and quitting smoking in order to manage their diabetes.

Application to Nursing Practice

As health care professionals, we need to help clients move through the stages of behavior change. It is important to assess and determine the client's readiness for change and target messages appropriately. When a client is not even beginning to think about eating more fruits and vegetables in his or her diet, it is unrealistic to tell the client to eat at least five fruits and vegetables every day. It would be more appropriate to inform the client why this is important, have the client identify a favorite fruit or vegetable, and give one or two simple suggestions as to how to incorporate the fruits or vegetables in their diet. By helping clients through the change process, we can reduce long-term complications of diabetes.

Reference

Jones H and others: Changes in diabetes self-care behaviors make a difference in glycemic control: the Diabetes Stages of Change (DiSC) study, *Diabetes Care* 26(3):732, 2003.

Acute Illness and Chronic Illness

Acute illness and chronic illness are two general classifications of illness used in this chapter. Both acute and chronic illnesses have the potential to be life threatening. An **acute illness** usually has a short duration and is severe. The symptoms appear abruptly, are intense, and often subside after a relatively short period. An acute illness may affect functioning in any dimension. A **chronic illness** persists, usually longer than 6 months, and can also affect functioning in any dimension. The client may fluctuate between maximal functioning and serious health relapses that may be life threatening. A person with a chronic illness is similar to a person with a disability in that both have limitations (of varying degrees) in function resulting from either a pathological process or an injury. Mechanic (1995) notes that "a chronic disabling disease interferes with ongoing life adaptations by making the performance of routine tasks more challenging." In addition, the social surroundings and physical environment in which the individual lives can affect the abilities, motivation, and psychological maintenance of the disabled person.

Chronic illnesses and disabilities remain a leading health problem in North America for older adults and children. Issues of coping and living with a chronic illness can be complex and overwhelming. A major role for nursing is to provide client education aimed at helping clients manage their illness or disability. The goal of managing a chronic illness is to reduce the occurrence of symptoms or to improve the tolerance of symptoms. By enhancing wellness, nurses may help improve the quality of life for clients living with chronic illnesses or disabilities.

It is important to understand that clients with chronic diseases and their families are faced with a process called normalization, in which they adapt to the disease. Studies of families with children facing illness challenges have found that over time, family members come to view both the child and their life as normal (Knafl and Deatrick, 2002). There is a relationship between family members' beliefs about their illness experiences and their illness management behaviors that affects the process of normalization (Knafl and Deatrick, 2002).

Illness Behavior

People who are ill generally act in a way that medical sociologists call **illness behavior.** It involves how people monitor their bodies, define and interpret their symptoms, take remedial actions, and use the health care system (Mechanic, 1982) (Box 6-4). Personal history, social situations, social norms, and the opportunities and constraints of community institutions can all affect illness behavior (Mechanic, 1995). Although there is a large variability in the way people react to an illness, illness behavior displayed in sickness can be used to manage life adversities (Mechanic, 1995). In other words, if people perceive themselves to be ill, illness behaviors can be coping mechanisms. For example, illness behavior can result in clients' being released from roles, social expectations, or responsibilities. For a homemaker, for example, the "flu" may be viewed as an added stressor, or it may be a temporary release from child care and household responsibilities.

Variables Influencing Illness and Illness Behavior

Just as health and health behavior are affected by internal and external variables, so are illness and illness behavior. The influences of these variables, as well as the stage of illness behavior the client is in, may affect the likelihood of seeking health care, compliance with therapy, and therefore health outcomes. Based on an understanding of these variables and behaviors, nurses can plan individualized care to assist clients in coping with their illness at various stages of illness. The goal of nursing is to promote optimal functioning in all dimensions throughout an illness.

Internal Variables. Internal variables influencing the way clients behave when they are ill are their perceptions of symptoms and the nature of the illness. If clients believe that the symptoms of their illnesses disrupt their normal routine, they are more likely to seek health care assistance than if they do not perceive the symptoms to be disruptive. If clients believe that the symptoms are serious or perhaps life threatening, they are also more likely to seek assistance. Persons awakened by crushing chest pains in the middle of the night generally view this symptom as potentially serious and life threatening, and they will probably be motivated to seek assistance. However, such a perception can also have the opposite effect. Individuals may fear serious illness, react by denying it, and not seek medical assistance.

The nature of the illness, either acute or chronic, also affects a client's illness behavior. Clients with acute illnesses are likely to seek health care and comply readily with therapy. On the other hand, a client with a chronic illness, in which the symptoms may not be cured, but only partially relieved, may not be motivated to comply with the therapy plan. Chronically ill clients may become less actively involved in their care, may experience greater frustration, and may comply less readily with care. Because nurses generally spend more time than other health care professionals with chronically ill clients, they are in the unique position of being able to assist these clients in overcoming problems related to illness behavior. A client's coping skills, as well as his or her locus of control, are other internal variables that affect the way the client behaves when ill (see Chapter 31).

External Variables. External variables influencing a client's illness behavior include the visibility of symptoms, social group, cultural background, economic variables, accessibility of the health care system, and social support. The visibility of the symptoms of an illness affects body image and illness behavior. A client with a visible symptom may be more likely to seek assistance than a client without such a visible symptom.

Clients' social groups may assist them in recognizing the threat of illness or support the denial of potential illness. Families, friends, and co-workers all may influence clients' illness behavior. Clients often react positively to social support while practicing positive health behaviors. A person's cultural and ethnic back-

ground teaches the person how to be healthy, how to recognize illness, and how to be ill. The effects of disease and its interpretation vary according to cultural circumstances. Ethnic differences can influence decisions about health care and the use of diagnostic and health care services (Murray and Zentner, 2001). Dietary practices among ethnic groups, occupations held by certain cultural groups, and cultural beliefs are other factors that contribute to illness and the distribution of disease (Murray and Zentner, 2001).

Economic variables influence the way a client reacts to illness. Because of economic constraints, a client may delay treatment and in many cases may continue to carry out daily activities. Clients' access to the health care system is closely related to economic factors. The health care system is a socioeconomic system that clients must enter, interact within, and exit. For many clients, entry into the system is complex or confusing, and some clients may seek nonemergency medical care in an emergency department because they do not know how otherwise to obtain health services. The physical proximity of clients to a health care agency often influences how soon they enter the system after deciding to seek care.

Impact of Illness on the Client and Family

Illness is never an isolated life event. The client and family must deal with changes resulting from illness and treatment. Each client responds uniquely to illness, requiring nurses to individualize nursing interventions. The client and family commonly experience behavioral and emotional changes, as well as changes in roles, body image and self-concept, and family dynamics.

Behavioral and Emotional Changes

People react differently to illness or the threat of illness. Individual behavioral and emotional reactions depend on the nature of the illness, the client's attitude toward it, the reaction of others to it, and the variables of illness behavior.

Short-term, non–life-threatening illnesses evoke few behavioral changes in the functioning of the client or family. A husband and father who has a cold, for example, may lack the energy and patience to spend time in family activities and may be irritable and prefer not to interact with his family. This is a behavioral change, but the change is subtle and does not last long. Some may even consider such a change a normal response to illness.

Severe illness, particularly one that is life threatening, can lead to more extensive emotional and behavioral changes, such as anxiety, shock, denial, anger, and withdrawal. These are common responses to the stress of illness. The nurse can develop interventions to assist the client and the family in coping with and adapting to this stress because the stressor itself cannot usually be changed.

Impact on Body Image

Body image is the subjective concept of physical appearance (see Chapter 27). Some illnesses result in changes in physical appearance, and clients and families react differently to these changes. Reactions of clients and families to changes in body image depend on the type of changes (e.g., loss of a limb or an organ), their adaptive capacity, the rate at which changes takes place, and the support services available.

When a change in body image occurs, such as results from a leg amputation, the client generally adjusts in the following phases: shock, withdrawal, acknowledgment, acceptance, and re-habilitation. Initially the client may be shocked by the change or impending change and may depersonalize it and talk about it as though it were happening to someone else. As the client and family recognize the reality of the change, they become anxious and may withdraw, refusing to discuss it. Withdrawal is an adaptive coping mechanism that assists the client in making the adjustment. As the client and family acknowledge the change, they move through a period of grieving. At the end of the acknowledgment phase, they accept the loss. During rehabilitation the client is ready to learn how to adapt to the change in body image through use of a prosthesis or changing lifestyles and goals.

Impact on Self-Concept

Self-concept is a mental self-image of strengths and weaknesses in all aspects of personality. Self-concept depends in part on body image and roles but also includes other aspects of psychology and spirituality (see Chapters 27 and 29). The impact of illness on the self-concepts of clients and family members may be more complex and less readily observed than role changes.

Self-concept is important in relationships with other family members. A client whose self-concept changes because of illness may no longer meet family expectations, leading to tension or conflict. As a result, family members may change their interactions with the client. In the course of providing care, a nurse is able to observe changes in the client's self-concept (or in the self-concepts of family members) and develop a care plan to help them adjust to the changes resulting from the illness.

Impact on Family Roles

People have many roles in life, such as wage earner, decision maker, professional, child, sibling, or parent. When an illness occurs, parents and children try to adapt to major changes resulting from a family member's illness. Role reversal is common (see Chapter 10). If a parent of an adult becomes ill and cannot carry out usual activities, the adult child often assumes many of the parent's responsibilities and in essence becomes a parent to the parent. Such a reversal of the usual situation can lead to stress, conflicting responsibilities for the adult child, or direct conflict over decision making.

Such a change may be subtle and short term or drastic and long term. An individual and family generally adjust more easily to subtle, short-term changes. In most cases they know that the role change is only temporary and will not require prolonged adjustment phases. Long-term changes, however, require an adjustment process similar to the grief process (see Chapter 30). The client and family often require specific counseling and guidance to assist them in coping with the role changes.

Impact on Family Dynamics

Because of the effects of illness on the client and family, family dynamics often change. Family dynamics is the process by which the family functions, makes decisions, gives support to individual members, and copes with everyday changes and challenges. If a parent in a family becomes ill, family activities and decision making often come to a halt as the other family members wait for the illness to pass, or they delay action because they are reluctant to assume the ill person's roles or responsibilities. Because of the effects of illness, family dynamics often change. The nurse must view the whole family as a client under stress, planning care to help the family regain the maximal level of functioning and well-being (see Chapter 10).

▓ Key Concepts

- Health and wellness are not merely the absence of disease and illness.
- A person's state of health, wellness, or illness depends on individual values, personality, and lifestyle.
- The health belief model considers the relationship between a person's health beliefs and health behaviors.
- The health promotion model highlights factors that increase individual well-being and self-actualization.
- Maslow's hierarchy of needs model emphasizes identification of clients' individual needs, prioritizing the needs, and encouraging the client's individual discovery of self (self-actualization).
- Holistic health models of nursing promote optimal health by incorporating active participation of clients in improving their health state.
- Health beliefs and practices are influenced by internal and external variables and should be considered when planning care.
- Health promotion activities help maintain or enhance health.
- Wellness education teaches clients how to care for themselves.
- Illness prevention activities protect against health threats and thus maintain an optimal level of health.
- Nursing incorporates health promotion, wellness, and illness prevention activities rather than simply treating illness.
- The three levels of preventive care are primary, secondary, and tertiary.
- Risk factors threaten health, influence health practices, and are important considerations in illness prevention activities.
- Improvement in health may involve a change in health behaviors.
- The transtheoretical model of change describes a series of changes that are progressed through for successful behavior change rather than simply assuming all clients are in an "action" stage.
- Illness behavior, like health practices, is influenced by many variables and must be considered by the nurse when planning care.
- Illness can have many effects on the client and family, including changes in behavior and emotions, family roles and dynamics, body image, and self-concept.

▓ Critical Thinking Exercises

1. Mrs. Campbell is a 62-year-old African American widow. Her daughter and her daughter's two children, ages 10 and 12, live with her. Mrs. Campbell is a retired housekeeper

from the hospital. Her daughter works second shift managing a local restaurant. Mrs. Campbell's eyesight is failing from diabetes (diagnosed 15 years ago), and she was just discharged from the hospital with complications from her diabetes and she now needs insulin injections. Mrs. Campbell is overweight and previously did not routinely make her health care provider appointments. You are a home care nurse, and her physician ordered home care visits upon discharge to monitor her insulin.

a. Using the health belief model, identify two individual health perceptions that may be influencing Mrs. Campbell.

b. Identify two ways you could use the health promotion model as you plan your care for Mrs. Campbell.

c. Using Maslow's hierarchy, what needs can you identify that are important for Mrs. Campbell?

d. What is the impact of Mrs. Campbell's disease on her family?

2. Ms. Barlett is a 20-year-old single white woman with a 6-week-old boy and an 18-month-old girl. She currently does not have a job. She smokes one pack of cigarettes per day. The father of the children is involved in their care and gives her money when he can. Her mother lives 500 miles away, but her father lives close by. He occasionally stops by to see her.

a. Identify internal and external variables that are impacting Ms. Barlett's ability to care for herself.

b. What primary intervention activities are important for her and her family?

c. Using the transtheoretical model of change, what question could you ask her to determine how to target smoking cessation? What plan will you make?

✳ NCLEX®-Style Review Questions

1. Abby Smith is a parish nurse for her Catholic church. The first Sunday of every month she has a free blood pressure screening. She is providing what level of prevention?
   1. Tertiary prevention
   2. Primary prevention
   3. Secondary prevention
   4. Quaternary prevention

2. Mr. Jones is 72 years old and was diagnosed with chronic obstructive pulmonary disease 5 years ago. For the last 2 years, he has been participating in a pulmonary rehabilitation exercise class offered by the local hospital at a fitness facility. This is what level of prevention?
   1. Tertiary prevention
   2. Primary prevention
   3. Secondary prevention
   4. Quaternary prevention

3. Based on the transtheoretical model of change, what is the most appropriate response to a client, Ms. Johnson, who states: "Me, exercise? I haven't done that since junior high gym class, and I hated it then!"
   1. "That's fine. Exercise is bad for you anyway."
   2. "OK. I want you to walk 3 miles 4 times a week, and I'll see you in one month."
   3. "I understand. Can you think of one reason why being more active would be helpful for you?"
   4. "I'd like you to ride your bike 3 times this week and eat at least four fruits and vegetables every day."

4. The previous client, Ms. Johnson, returns to your clinic the next month and states: "I have noticed how many people are out walking in my neighborhood. Is walking good for you?" What is the best response to help Ms. Johnson through the stages of change for exercise?
   1. "Walking is OK. I really think running is better."
   2. "Yes, walking is great exercise. Do you think you could go for a 5-minute walk this next week?"
   3. "Yes, I want you to begin walking. Walk for 30 minutes every day, and start eating more fruits and vegetables, too."
   4. "They probably aren't walking fast enough or far enough. You need to spend at least 45 minutes if you are going to do any good."

5. Mr. Brown has been laid off from his construction job and has many bills needing to be paid. He is going through a divorce from his marriage of 15 years and has been seeing his pastor to help him with this difficult time. He does not have a primary health care provider because he has never really been sick and his parents never took him to the physician when he was growing up. Which of the following are internal variables influencing Mr. Brown's health practices?
   1. Difficulty paying his bills
   2. Seeing his pastor as a means of support
   3. Family practice of not routinely seeing a health care provider
   4. Increased stress in his life with the divorce and the loss of a job
   5. Both 1 and 3
   6. Both 3 and 4

6. The previous client, Mr. Brown, is being seen in the clinic today with concerns regarding weight loss and a frequent burning sensation in his throat. Rob Miller is the nurse today. In his care of Mr. Brown, after Rob's initial assessment, he would tell the primary health care provider:
   1. "Mr. Brown is fine. You'll be in and out in no time."
   2. "Mr. Brown is having gastroesophageal reflux and needs medication."
   3. "Mr. Brown is feeling sorry for himself because he is going through some tough times. I'm not sure there is much you can do for him."
   4. "I think Mr. Brown is struggling with his loss of income and his loss of his role as husband. It will be important to refer him for guidance with his losses."

7. When taking care of clients, nurse Olson routinely asks clients if they take any vitamins or herbal medications. She encourages family members to bring in music that the client likes to help the client relax. She also frequently prays with her clients if that is important to them. Nurse Olson is using which model?
   1. Holistic
   2. Health belief
   3. Transtheoretical
   4. Health promotion

8. When illness does occur, different attitudes about illness cause people to react in different ways. Medical sociologists call the reaction to illness:
   1. Health belief
   2. Illness behavior
   3. Health promotion
   4. Illness prevention

9. The health belief model addresses the relationship between a person's belief and behaviors, thus:
   1. A person who smokes does not practice the model
   2. This model provides a basis for caring for clients of all ages
   3. A person who does not take necessary medications does not practice the model
   4. It provides a way of understanding and predicting how clients will behave in relation to their health and how they will comply with health care therapies

10. Karen Smith works in a special care unit in Denver, Colorado, for children with severe immunology problems. Today she is caring for a 3-year-old boy from Greece. The boy's father is with him, while his mother and sister are back in Greece. Karen is having difficulty communicating with the father. What should she do?
    1. Care for the boy as she would any other client.
    2. Ask the manager to talk with the father and keep him out of the unit.
    3. Have another nurse care for the boy because maybe that nurse will do better with the father.
    4. Search for help with interpretation and understanding of the cultural differences by contacting someone from the Greek community in Denver.

7 | Caring for the Cancer Survivor

OBJECTIVES

Mastery of content in this chapter will enable the student to:
- Discuss the concept of cancer survivorship.
- Describe the influence of cancer survivorship on clients' quality of life.
- Discuss the effects cancer has on the family.
- Explain the nursing implications related to cancer survivorship.
- Discuss the essential components of survivorship care.

 MEDIA RESOURCES   **KEY TERMS**

 Companion CD
- NCLEX®-Style Review Questions
- Audio Glossary
- Interactive Learning Activities
- English/Spanish Glossary

evolve Website
- NCLEX®-Style Review Questions
- Audio Glossary
- English/Spanish Glossary
- Interactive Learning Activities
- WebLinks
- Audio Summaries

Biological response modifiers (biotherapy). p. 87
Cancer-related fatigue (CRF), p. 86
Cancer survivor, p. 85
Chemotherapy, p. 85
Hormone therapy, p. 85
Lumpectomy, p. 87

Mastectomy, p. 87
Neuropathy, p. 86
Oncology, p. 92
Paresthesias, p. 86
Posttraumatic stress disorder (PTSD), p. 87
Radiation therapy, p. 85

There is a population of clients that has not been recognized for the extent and nature of health problems that it experiences. Currently there are 10 million cancer survivors in the United States (Institute of Medicine [IOM], 2006). The number of survivors will continue to grow as more than 1 million new cases of cancer are diagnosed each year (American Cancer Society [ACS], 2006). Cancer survivors' health care problems have largely been ignored or misunderstood because of the belief that for those who receive treatment, survive, and are given a "clean bill of health," their health problems are over. Such is not the case. There are many different trajectories or courses for cancer survival (Box 7-1). With the advances made in diagnosis and treatment, more clients are becoming long-term survivors of cancer, whereas others with cancers such as lymphoma control their disease with ongoing or periodic treatment. The major forms of cancer therapy—surgery, **chemotherapy, hormone therapy, biotherapy,** and **radiation therapy**—often create unwanted, long-term effects on tissues and organ systems that impair a person's health and quality of life in small and large ways (IOM, 2006). Thus cancer survivorship has enormous implications for the way these individuals monitor and manage their health throughout their lives. As a nurse, you will care for these clients when they seek care for their cancer as well as when they seek care for other medical conditions.

The National Cancer Institute (2004) offers a definition of a **cancer survivor:** "An individual is considered a cancer survivor from the time of diagnosis, through the balance of his or her life." Consider that family members and friends are also survivors, because they experience the effects cancer has on their loved ones. Cancer truly is a life-changing event. Evidence shows that there is a neglected phase of cancer care, the period following first diagnosis and initial treatment and before the development of a recurrence of the initial cancer or death (IOM, 2006). In this phase of their disease, survivors do not have consistent health care follow-up. Frequent contact with a cancer care provider often suddenly stops, and survivors' unique psychosocial needs often go unnoticed or untreated. Despite the incredible advances made in cancer care, there are many long-term survivors who suffer unnecessarily and die from delayed cancer diagnoses or treatment-related chronic disease.

As nurses, we have the responsibility to better understand the needs of cancer survivors and to provide the most current evidence-based approaches for managing late and long-term effects of cancer and cancer treatment. Up to 75% of survivors have serious health deficits, both physical and psychological, that are related to their treatment (Aziz and Rowland, 2003). There is also evidence to suggest that survivors among racial and ethnic minority and other underserved populations have more posttreatment symptoms and poorer treatment outcomes than whites (Centers for Disease Control and Prevention [CDC], 2004). The disparities in health among ethnic groups are related to a complex interplay of economic, social, and cultural factors, with poverty being a key factor (IOM, 2006). Being able to provide comprehensive care to a cancer survivor begins with recognizing the effects of cancer and its treatment and learning about the survivor's own meaning of health.

The Effects of Cancer on Quality of Life

As people live longer after diagnosis and treatment for cancer, it becomes important to understand the types of distress many survivors experience and how it affects their quality of life (Figure 7-1). Evidence shows that cancer survivors have poorer health

✳ BOX 7-1 The Seasons of Cancer Survival

Acute Survival: Starts with the diagnosis of cancer. Diagnostic and therapeutic efforts dominate. Fear and anxiety are constant elements of this phase.

Extended Survival: Period during which a client goes into remission or has ended the basic, rigorous course of treatment and enters a phase of watchful waiting. Client will undergo periodic examinations and/or intermittent therapy. Psychologically, the fear of recurrence is common. This is usually a period of physical limitations. Diminished strength, fatigue, pain, nausea, reduced tolerance for exercise, or hair loss often occur in the acute phase, but clients now have to deal with cancer in the home, community, and workplace.

Permanent Survival: This phase is roughly equated with "cure," but the experience permanently affects the survivor. Problems with employment and insurance are common. The long-term secondary effects of cancer treatment on health represent an area in which permanent survivors are at risk.

Modified from Mullan F: Seasons of survival: reflections of a physician with cancer, *N Engl J Med* 313(4):270, 1985; and Institute of Medicine and National Research Council, Hewitt M, Greenfield S, Stovall E, editors: *From cancer client to cancer survivor: lost in transition*, Washington, DC, 2006, National Academies Press.

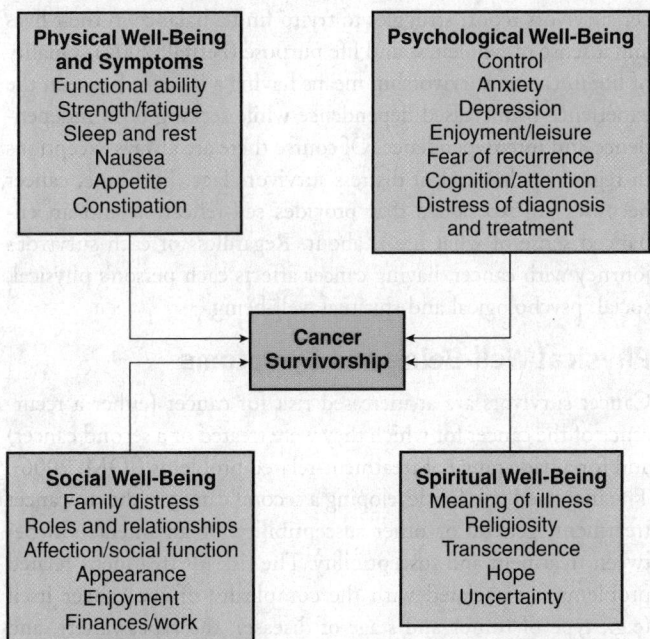

Figure 7-1 Dimensions of quality of life affected by cancer. (From Ferrell B: *Introduction to cancer survivorship strategies for success, survivorship education for quality cancer care,* Pasadena, Calif, 2006, City of Hope National Medical Center.)

✳ BOX 7-2 EVIDENCE-BASED PRACTICE

The Burden of Illness for Cancer Survivors

Evidence Summary

A group of researchers wanted to learn about the burden of illness among cancer survivors. They studied more than 1,800 cancer survivors, as well as individuals without cancer (control group) who were matched with cancer survivors by age, sex, and educational attainment. The study examined several measures of burden or stress, including a person's sense of utility or feeling useful, a perception of overall health, and days lost from work. The results of the study showed that cancer survivors had poorer outcomes across all measures: lower utility, higher levels of lost productivity, and more likely to report their health as fair or poor when matched with control subjects.

Application to Nursing Practice

As a nurse, learn to assess the many ways in which cancer affects the lives of clients who are survivors. Because cancer causes long-term effects, spend time assessing clients' symptoms, the effects of symptoms on lifestyle and self-care ability, the effects on client relationships, the clients' ability to remain productive and successful in their jobs, their economic security, and their physical well-being. Clients' self-perceptions are also important to understand when you attempt any intervention that requires the client to be motivated and involved.

Reference

Yabroff KR and others: Burden of illness in cancer survivors: findings from a population-based national sample, *J Natl Cancer Inst* 96(17):1322, 2004.

✳ TABLE 7-1 Examples of Late Effects of Surgery Among Adult Cancer Survivors

PROCEDURE	LATE EFFECT
Any procedure	Pain, psychosocial distress, impaired wound healing
Surgery involving brain or spinal cord	Impaired cognitive function, motor sensory alterations, altered vision, swallowing, language, bowel and bladder control
Head and neck surgery	Difficulties with communication, swallowing, and breathing
Abdominal surgery	Risk of intestinal obstruction, hernia, altered bowel function
Lung resection	Difficulty breathing, fatigue, generalized weakness
Prostatectomy	Urinary incontinence, sexual dysfunction, poor body image

Modified from Institute of Medicine and National Research Council, Hewitt M, Greenfield S, Stovall E, editors: *From cancer client to cancer survivor: lost in transition*, Washington, DC, 2006, National Academies Press.

Susan was an Army nurse, who learned 7 months after discharge from the Army that she had Hodgkin's disease. Hodgkin's is a malignancy of lymphoid tissue. Susan received an aggressive course of treatment, including surgery, 6 months of chemotherapy, and 3 months of total lymph node irradiation. It took many months for her bone marrow to heal and blood values to return to normal. After a few years she had bilateral mastectomies for treatment-related breast cancer. She also received 3 years of immunotherapy for cancer in situ (tumor not metastasized) of the bladder. She continues to experience many noncancer conditions: premature menopause, early osteoporosis, hypothyroidism, lung fibrosis, and atrophy of neck and upper chest muscles (Leigh, 2006).

outcomes than similar individuals without cancer (Box 7-2). Cancer survivors report struggles to try to find a balance in their lives and a sense of wholeness and life purpose (Ferrell, 2004). Quality of life in cancer survivorship means having a balance between the experience of increased dependence while seeking both independence and interdependence. Of course there are always exceptions in regard to the level of distress survivors face. For some, cancer becomes an experience that provides self-reflection and an enhanced sense of what life is about. Regardless of each survivor's journey with cancer, having cancer affects each person's physical, social, psychological and spiritual well-being.

Physical Well-Being and Symptoms

Cancer survivors are at increased risk for cancer (either a recurrence of the cancer for which they were treated or a second cancer) and for a wide range of treatment-related problems (IOM, 2006). The increased risk for developing a second cancer is due to cancer treatment, genetic or other susceptibility, or an interaction between treatment and susceptibility. The risk for treatment-related problems is associated with the complexity of the cancer itself (e.g., type of tumor and stage of disease); the type, variety, and intensity of treatments used; and the age and underlying health status of the client.

The following description offers an example of how a cancer survivor's physical health problems can be so complex and burdensome.

Such a story like the one above is not unusual among survivors but highlights the long disease course many cancer survivors face. There are a number of tissues and body systems that are impaired as a result of cancer and its treatment (Table 7-1). Late effects of chemotherapy include osteoporosis, congestive heart failure, diabetes, amenorrhea in women, sterility in men and women, gastrointestinal motility problems, abnormal liver function, impaired immune function, **paresthesias**, hearing loss, and problems with thinking and memory (IOM, 2006). Treatment for cancer or the cancer itself often induces pain and **neuropathy** (Polomano and Farrar, 2006). **Cancer-related fatigue (CRF)** and associated sleep disturbances are the most frequent and disturbing complaints of people with cancer (Barton-Burke, 2006). Certain conditions resolve over time, but irreversible tissue damage causes conditions to progress and persist indefinitely. Health care professionals do not always recognize these conditions as delayed problems. Often conditions such as osteoporosis, hearing loss, or change in memory are instead considered as age related. The problem is that for many survivors, these conditions go undiagnosed and are never treated.

Cognitive changes are a set of physical symptoms very common in survivors that develop from their disease, treatment, the complications of treatment, underlying medical conditions, and psychological responses to the diagnosis of cancer (Nail, 2006).

Cognitive changes can occur during all phases of the cancer experience, from small deficits in information processing to acute delirium. Often the cognitive impairments survivors experience are not evident to someone else but are apparent to the person experiencing them, especially in relation to work performance with high cognitive demands (Anderson-Hanley and others, 2003). For example, clients report attention problems, loss of memory, and difficulty in recognizing and solving problems. Studies show that when clients receive systemic cancer treatment, including chemotherapy or **biological response modifiers (biotherapy)**, there is a generalized, subtle effect on cognitive function. In addition, systemic treatment causes both short-term and persistent cognitive impairment in a variety of cognitive domains. Researchers do not yet understand the effects of specific cognitive changes on survivors' daily lives (Nail, 2006).

Most cancer survivors (61%) are over the age of 65 (IOM, 2006). The most common cancers for this age-group include cancer of the colon, pancreas, prostate, lung, and bladder. Often health care providers wrongly attribute the symptoms of cancer or the symptoms from the side effects of treatment to aging. This often leads to late diagnosis or a failure to provide aggressive and effective treatment of symptoms.

Cancer is a chronic disease, because of the serious consequences and the persistent nature of some of cancer's late effects (IOM, 2006). There is great diversity in the range of effects clients suffer. For example, a 46-year-old woman with early stage melanoma on the right arm undergoes successful surgery and only has the effect of an inconspicuous scar. In contrast, Susan, the Army nurse diagnosed with Hodgkin's disease, underwent intensive chemotherapy followed by an extended course of radiation. She faced serious and substantial long-term health problems from her treatment. Cancer clients present significant variations in the type of conditions they develop and the length of time the conditions persist.

There are numerous factors that contribute to survivors' not receiving timely and appropriate treatment for the effects of their disease or treatment. Survivors are often reluctant to report symptoms because of a fear of being perceived as ungrateful for being disease-free or a fear of cancer recurrence (Polomano and Farrar, 2006). Survivors are not always aware that painful conditions or syndromes are common and frequently believe that pain relief is not possible (see Chapter 43) (Box 7-3). Health care providers have limited awareness of the prevalence and incidence of pain and other symptoms among survivors and frequently have limited education in symptom management. In the case of pain management, health care providers do not acknowledge the potential for chronic pain following curative cancer therapies or they fail to inform clients about potential long-term consequences of cancer treatment (Polomano and Farrar, 2006). There are few health care settings that track the health-related quality of life and symptomatology of clients over time. Thus there is limited evidence about the long-term patterns of symptoms most commonly associated with certain forms of cancer and its treatment.

Research involving breast cancer survivors is extensive. Women with a history of breast cancer are the largest group of cancer survivors (IOM, 2006). After their primary treatment for breast cancer, women generally report decreased physical functioning but good emotional functioning, especially those who undergo

---

✳ BOX 7-3   Examples of Chronic Pain Syndromes Associated With Cancer Treatments

Postoperative Pain Syndromes
Postmastectomy syndrome
Post–radical neck dissection pain
Postamputation pain
Fistula formation

Postradiation Pain Syndromes
Myelopathy
Enteritis or proctitis
Lymphedema
Brachial or lumbosacral plexopathy

Postchemotherapy Pain Syndromes
Peripheral neuropathy
Avascular necrosis of femur or humerus

Modified from Polomano RC, Farrar JT: Pain and neuropathy in cancer survivors, *Am J Nurs* 106(3 suppl):39, 2006.

---

mastectomy or receive chemotherapy (Ganz and others, 2004). Persistent symptoms 1 year after either **lumpectomy** or **mastectomy** to treat early-stage breast cancer often include numbness in the chest wall or axilla, tightness, pulling in the arm or axilla, fatigue, difficulty sleeping, and hot flashes (Shimozuma and others, 1999). By 2 to 3 years after surgery, breast cancer survivors report a quality of life more favorable than that reported by clients with other common medical conditions (Ganz and others, 1996). However, these same clients reported problems with sexual function, body image, and physical function after 3 years.

Psychological Well-Being

The physical effects of cancer and its treatment sometimes extend to cause serious psychological distress (see Chapter 31). In the context of cancer, distress is defined as a multifactorial unpleasant emotional experience of a psychological, social, and or spiritual nature (see Chapter 29) that interferes with the ability to cope effectively with cancer, its symptoms, and its treatment (Wilkes, 2003). Survivors' feelings of distress range along a continuum from sadness to disabling depression (Vachon, 2006). The long-term presence of fatigue and sleep disturbances, for example, is often associated with anxiety and depression in many cancer survivors (Barton-Burke, 2006). Research has associated depression with decreased cancer survivorship. A study conducted by Brown and others (2003) suggested that a cancer diagnosis and its effects predispose people to distress, which if maintained over time will enhance disease progression.

Another common psychological problem for survivors is **posttraumatic stress disorder (PTSD)**. PTSD is a psychiatric disorder characterized by an acute emotional response to a traumatic event or situation. Cancer survivors experience symptoms of PTSD (e.g., grief, nightmares, panic attacks, or fear) at a rate of 4% to 19%, as a result of their diagnosis, treatment, or a past traumatic episode (Kwekkeboom and Seng, 2002). Being female, younger, less educated, and having a lower income and less social and emotional support increases the risk for PTSD. Studies of clients with PTSD suggest that the stress response of the hypothalamus-pituitary-adrenal system is abnormal (see Chapter 31). This same

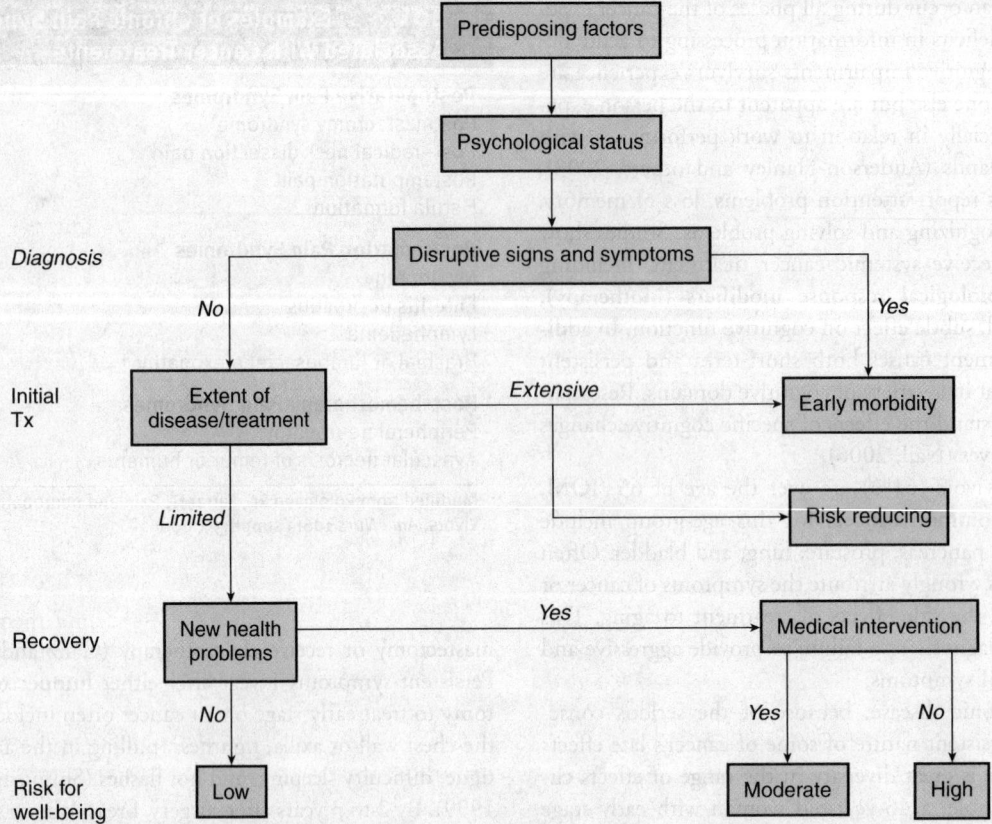

Figure 7-2 Predicting psychological well-being. (Modified from Andersen BL: Predicting sexual and psychologic morbidity and improving the quality of life for women with gynecologic cancer, *Cancer* 71[4 suppl]:1678, 1993. © 1996 American Cancer Society. This material is reproduced with permission of Wiley-Liss, Inc., a subsidiary of John Wiley & Sons, Inc.)

negative feedback inhibition of cortisol resulting in cortisol alterations also occurs in cancer (Yehuda, 2003).

The disabling effects of chronic cancer symptoms disrupt family and personal relationships, impair individuals' work performance, and often isolate survivors from normal social activities. Such changes in lifestyle create serious implications for a survivor's psychological well-being. When cancer changes a client's body image or alters sexual function, the survivor frequently experiences significant anxiety and depression in interpersonal relationships. In the case of breast cancer survivors, studies show that poorer self-ratings of quality of life are associated with poor body image, coping strategies, and a lack of social support (IOM, 2006).

The risk for a cancer survivor having psychological problems is high because of a complex set of factors. Anderson and others (1993) developed a model for predicting the psychological well-being in women with gynecological cancer (Figure 7-2). The model has applications for other client groups as well. How well a survivor adapts to the cancer experience depends upon predisposing factors (e.g., age, gender, race, income, prior psychiatric disorder, marital status, coping style, and social support), their current psychological status, and the presence of disruptive signs and symptoms. When a client has few disruptive signs and symptoms and the cancer is less extensive, the risk of poor psychological well-being is low. In contrast, the risk of psychological distress is high in a client who has numerous disruptive signs and symptoms, an advanced stage of cancer, and other health problems.

There are factors that help ease the psychological stress associated with having cancer. A survivor's appraisal of the cancer experience makes a difference. A survivor who sees cancer as a challenging experience and a controllable threat will have less stress (Jacobsen, 2006). Clients who use problem-oriented, active, and emotionally expressive coping processes also manage stress well (see Chapter 31). Survivors who have social and emotional support systems and maintain open communication with their treatment providers will also likely have less psychological distress (Jacobsen, 2006).

Social Well-Being

Cancer affects any age-group (Figure 7-3). The developmental effects of cancer are perhaps best seen in the social impact that occurs across the life span. For adolescents and young adults, cancer seriously alters a young person's social skills, sexual development, body image, and the ability to think about and plan for the future (see Chapter 11). Cancer interrupts their lives, causing young survivors to either feel out of touch with the interests of their peers or to perceive interests as superficial (Blum, 2006). In addition, because cancer makes them feel different, young survivors, out of fear of rejection, have problems with dating and developing new relationships. Often the course of cancer or its treatment causes young adults to delay leaving their parents. The natural separation that occurs when young adults finish school and look to start their careers is postponed or stopped. Often a young adult then feels ill equipped to take on the real world.

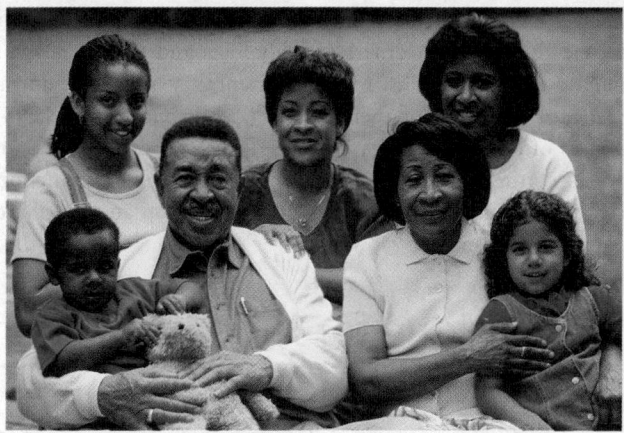

Figure 7-3 A family representing young and old.

TABLE 7-2 Limitations Imposed by Cancer and Its Treatment as Reported by Survivors	
AREA OF LIMITATION	**PERCENT OF SURVEY (%)**
Physical tasks	18
Lift heavy loads	26
Stoop, kneel, crouch	14
Concentrate for long periods	12
Analyze data	11
Keep pace with others	22
Learn new things	14

Modified from Bradley CJ, Bednarek HL: Employment patterns of long-term cancer survivors, *Psycho-Oncology* 11:188, 2002.

Adults (ages 30 to 59) who have cancer experience significant changes in their families. Once a member of the family is diagnosed with cancer, every family member's role, plans, and abilities change (Blum, 2006). The healthy spouse often takes on added job responsibilities to provide additional income for the family. A spouse, sibling, grandparent, or child often has to assume caregiving responsibilities for the cancer client. Clients who experience changes in sexuality, intimacy, and fertility will see their marriages affected, too often resulting in divorce.

A history of cancer significantly affects employment opportunities and the ability of a survivor to obtain and retain health and life insurance (IOM, 2006). Often a survivor experiences health-related work limitations (Table 7-2) that require a reduced work schedule or a complete change in employment. However, most cancer survivors who worked before their diagnosis return to work following their treatment (Spelten and others, 2002). The problem is that employers and supervisors often assume that persons with cancer are not able to perform job responsibilities as well as they did before their diagnosis; thus job discrimination is common. Cancer survivors report problems in the workplace, including dismissal, failure to hire, demotion, and denial of promotion. Many survivors also experience "job lock." A survivor will stay in an undesirable job or one that has become difficult to perform in order not to lose insurance benefits.

The economic burden of cancer is enormous. If a survivor's illness affects his or her ability to work, less income goes to the individual and family. Also, there is usually an increase in high out-of-pocket expenses for prescription drugs, medical devices and supplies, and expenses for coinsurance and copayments (IOM, 2006). For low-income survivors, the problems are even greater if they are uninsured or underinsured. Most Americans have health insurance that provides insurance coverage for most cancer-related care. However, approximately 42 million Americans have no health insurance at all. The uninsured do not receive the care they need, they suffer from a poorer state of health, and they are more likely to die earlier than those who have insurance (IOM, 2006). There have been many studies linking a lack of health insurance with poor cancer outcomes.

Older adults face numerous social concerns as a result of cancer. Often the disease will cause a survivor to retire prematurely.

The older adult faces a fixed income and the limitations of Medicare reimbursement. Many cancer survivors see their retirement pensions erode away quickly. They often have to use their income for basic expenses and cancer care costs, thus limiting opportunities for any social activities. Many older adults have moved to retirement residences in other states and find themselves isolated from the social support of family once cancer is diagnosed. Older adults also face a high level of disability as a result of cancer and cancer treatment. Older adults with cancer report a higher incidence of limitations in activities of daily living (ADLs) than older adults without cancer (IOM, 2006). As a result, many older cancer survivors require ongoing caregiving support either from family members or professional caregivers.

Spiritual Well-Being

The experience of cancer challenges a person's spiritual well-being (see Chapter 29). Key features of spiritual well-being include a harmonious interconnectedness, creative energy, and a faith in a higher power or life force (Brown-Saltzman, 2006). Cancer and its treatment create physical and psychological changes that cause survivors to question "Why me?" and to wonder if perhaps their disease is some form of punishment. Survivors often experience a level of spiritual distress, a disruption in a person's spirit or life principle. Survivors most at risk for spiritual distress are those with energy-consuming anxiety, an inability to forgive, low self-esteem, maturational losses, and mental illness (Brown-Saltzman, 2006). Additional risk factors include poor relationships and situational losses (see Chapter 29).

Relationships are critical for cancer survivors, relationships with a God, a higher power, nature, family, or community. Cancer threatens relationships because it makes it difficult for survivors to maintain a connection and a sense of belonging with what is important to them. Cancer isolates survivors from meaningful interaction and support, which then threatens their ability to maintain hope. The long courses of treatment, the reoccurrence of cancer, and the lingering side effects of treatment all create a level of uncertainty for survivors.

Cancer and Families

A survivor's family takes different forms: the traditional nuclear family, extended family, single-parent family, close friends, and blended families (see Chapter 10). Once cancer affects a member of the family, it affects all other members as well. It is usually a member of the family who becomes the client's caregiver. Family caregiving is a stressful experience, depending on the relationship between client and caregiver and the nature and extent of the client's disease. For members of the "sandwich generation," caregivers who are 30 to 50 years old are often caught in the middle of caring for their own immediate family as well as a parent with cancer. The demands are many, from providing ongoing encouragement and support and assisting with household chores to providing hands-on physical care (e.g., bathing, assisting with toileting, or changing a dressing) when cancer is advanced. Caregiving also involves the psychological demands of communicating, problem solving, and decision making; social demands of remaining active in the community and work; and economic demands of meeting financial obligations.

Family Distress

Relationships between cancer survivors and family members become difficult to maintain because family members often do not know, do not understand, or report not having the skills or confidence to support the survivor's reactions to cancer. There is evidence to suggest that changes in family roles and the burden on family caregivers negatively affect the quality of life and well-being of caregivers and cancer survivors (Stetz and Brown, 2004; Strang and Koop, 2003). Mellon and others (2006) interviewed cancer survivors and their family caregivers, finding that one of the strongest predictors for cancer survivors' quality of life were family stressors and social support. In their study, family caregivers reported a lower quality of life than that of their family members. The researchers also noted that ongoing concerns and problems facing survivors and their family are important determinants of adjustment and quality of life. Families generally find themselves ill prepared to deal with cancer. Cancer survivorship has not yet become a distinct phase of cancer care; thus professional caregivers often fail to inform and educate clients and their families about what to expect during the cancer experience. Professional caregivers do not usually address the psychosocial needs of cancer clients and their families.

Couples who experience the acute phase of breast cancer treatment often function in a survival mode, during which time competing demands from job or other family members distract them from attending to each other's needs, thoughts, and feelings (Lewis, 2006). Often a couple struggles with interpersonal problem solving, because they do not have the communication or problem-solving skills to understand one another's views, concerns, or fears. We know less about what happens to family relationships in long-term survivorship. Lewis (2006) suggests two possible outcomes: benefit-finding behavior (identifying positive aspects in the cancer experience) or heightened interpersonal tension.

Families struggle to maintain core functions when one of their members is a cancer survivor. Core family functions include maintaining an emotionally and physically safe environment, interpreting and reducing the threat of stressful events (including the cancer) for family members, and nurturing and supporting the development of individual family members (Lewis, 2006). In child-rearing families, this means providing an attentive parenting environment for children and providing information and support to children when their sense of well-being becomes threatened.

When a member of the family has cancer, these core functions become threatened. Mothers of school-age and adolescent children reported the inability to be the parent they want to be during the treatment phase of their disease (Zahlis and Lewis, 1998). Spouses often do not know what to do to support the survivor, and they struggle with how to help. In the end, family functions become fragmented and family members develop an uncertainty about their roles.

Implications for Nursing

Cancer survivorship creates many implications for nursing. As a profession, nursing has to take a lead in helping survivors plan for optimal lifelong health. Much needs to be done in conducting nursing research to find appropriate interventions for the effects of cancer and its treatment. Nurses are in a strong position to take the lead in improving public health efforts to manage the long-term consequences of cancer. Improvement is also necessary in the education of nurses and survivors about the phenomenon of survivorship. As a nursing student, you too can make a difference. This section will address approaches to incorporate cancer survivorship into your nursing practice.

Survivor Assessment

Knowing that there are many cancer survivors in the health care system, consider how to assess those clients who report a history of cancer. It is important to make assessment of cancer survivor's needs a standard part of your practice. When you are collecting a nursing history (see Chapter 33), explore with your clients their history of cancer, including the diagnosis and type of treatment they either are undergoing or have received in the past. Be aware that some clients do not always report they have had cancer. So, when a client tells you he or she has had surgery, ask if it was cancer related. When a client reveals a history of chemotherapy, radiation, biotherapy, or hormone therapy, you need to refer to resources to help you understand how those therapies typically affect clients in both the short and long term. Once you do so, extend your assessment to determine if these treatment effects exist for your client. Remember, you need to consider not only the effects of the cancer and its treatment but how it will affect any other medical condition. For example, if a client also has heart disease, how will the fatigue related to chemotherapy affect this individual?

Understanding the cancer experience comes from a client's own story. Asking a general question about the client being a cancer survivor will coach the client into revealing his or her story. For example, you might ask, "Having cancer is a journey for many. How does the disease most affect you right now? or "What is the biggest problem that you are experiencing from cancer?" This type of question will help you focus on the area that is most important to the client. Communicate to clients your interest in their situation. Show a caring approach so that clients know their story will be accepted (see Chapter 8). You might further ask, "What can I do to help you at this point?"

Symptom management is an ongoing problem for many cancer survivors. If cancer is their primary diagnosis, it will be natural for you to explore any presenting symptoms. Be sure to learn

TABLE 7-3	Assessment Questions for Cancer Survivors	
CATEGORY	**EXAMPLES OF QUESTIONS**	
Symptoms	• Have you had any pain or discomfort in the area where you had surgery or radiation; discomfort, pain, or unusual sensations in your hands or feet; weakness in your legs or arms; or problems moving around? • Are you experiencing fatigue, sleeplessness, shortness of breath? If so, please describe. • Sometimes people feel as if they are starting to have problems after chemotherapy such as paying attention, remembering things, or finding words. Have you noticed any changes like these?	
Psychosocial problems	• How distressed are you feeling at this point on a scale of 0 to 10 with 10 being the worst distress that you could imagine? • How do you think your family is doing with your cancer? • What do you see in your family members' responses to your cancer that is a concern for you?	
Sexuality problems	• If you have had sexual changes, what strategies have you tried to make things better? Have these strategies worked? • Would you be open to a health care provider who knows how to help you? • Since your cancer, do you see yourself differently as a person?	

specifically how any symptoms are affecting the client. For example, is pain also causing fatigue, or is a neuropathy causing the client to walk with an abnormal gait? If cancer is secondary, you do not want important symptoms to go unrecognized. Ask the client, "Since your diagnosis and treatment of cancer, what physical changes or symptoms have you had?" "Tell me how these changes affect you now." Depending on the symptoms a client identifies, you will explore each one in order to gain a complete picture of the client's health status (Table 7-3). Remember, some clients are reluctant to report or discuss their symptoms. Be patient, and once you identify a symptom, explore the extent to which the symptom is currently affecting the client.

Because you know that cancer affects a client's quality of life in many ways, be sure to explore the client's psychological, social, and spiritual needs and resources. Sometimes you will not be able to conduct a thorough assessment when you perform an initial nursing history. If this is the case, incorporate your assessment into your ongoing client care. Observe your client's interactions with family members and friends. When you are administering care to clients, talk about their daily lives and determine the extent to which cancer has changed their lifestyle.

One area that is often difficult for nurses to assess well is a client's sexuality. Sexuality is more than simply the physical ability to perform a sex act or conceive a child. It also includes a person's body image, sexual response (e.g., interest and satisfaction), and

sexual roles and relationships (see Chapter 28). Surgery for many cancers is disfiguring, and chemotherapy and radiation often alter a client's sexual response. Cancer therapies have the potential to cause fatigue, apathy, nausea, vomiting, malaise, and sleep disturbances, all of which interfere with a client's libido (Pelusi, 2006). It is important to simply realize that cancer often does influence the client's sexuality. It helps to develop a comfort level in acknowledging with clients that sexual changes are common at any age level. Ask a client, "Since your diagnosis and treatment of cancer, has your ability or interest in sexual activity changed? If so, how?" Clients will appreciate your sensitivity and interest in their well-being. When clients begin to discuss their sexual problems, know the expert resources in your institution (e.g., psychologist or social worker) available for client referral.

Client Education

It is nursing's responsibility to educate survivors and their families about the consequences of cancer and cancer treatment. This means that when you care for a cancer survivor, you need to understand the nature of the client's particular disease and know the effects of each therapy a client receives and the short- and long-term consequences. You will play a key role in preparing a cancer survivor with the knowledge and resources needed for ongoing self-management. Lorig (2003) defines the purpose of self-management education as the provision of skills for clients to live an active and meaningful life with chronic disease. In designing education that promotes self-management in caregiving, plan activities on the basis of the caregiver's and cancer survivor's perceived disease-related problems and assist them with problem solving and gaining the self-efficacy or confidence to deal with these problems. Client education will help survivors assume more healthy lifestyle behaviors that will then give them control of some aspects of their health and improve outcomes from cancer and chronic illness.

When caring for clients with an initial diagnosis of cancer, reinforce their health care provider's explanations of the risks related to their cancer and treatment, what they need to self-monitor (e.g., appetite and weight and effects of fatigue and sleeplessness), and what to discuss with health care providers in the future. If you teach clients about the potential for treatment effects such as pain, neuropathy, or cognitive change, they are more likely to report their symptoms. Survivors need to learn how to manage problems related to persistent symptoms. For example, survivors with neuropathy need to learn how to protect the hands and feet, prevent falls, and avoid accidental burns.

Because survivors have an increased risk for developing a second cancer and/or chronic illness, it is important to educate them about lifestyle behaviors that will improve the quality of their lives. Health promotion education is timely after an initial cancer diagnosis, when many survivors become motivated to change their behavior (Satia and others, 2004). Many survivors become interested in learning more about dietary supplements and nutritional complementary therapies to manage disease symptoms (IOM, 2006). Scientific evidence shows there are several health promotion areas of interest to cancer survivors: smoking cessation, physical activity, diet and nutrition (see Chapter 44), and the use of complementary and alternative medicine (see Chapter 36). You teach clients useful strategies to promote their health.

For example, behavioral interventions for increasing physical activity among cancer survivors have shown positive and consistent effects on vigor, cardiorespiratory fitness, quality of life, fatigue, and depression (Holtzman and others, 2004).

Providing Resources

Numerous organizations and agencies provide resources to cancer survivors. The problem is that many survivors do not receive timely and appropriate referral to these resources. As a nurse, you will find that many people (e.g., friends, neighbors, and family members) come to you for advice about health care before they actually become a client. It is important to know that cancer-related hospital and ambulatory care are not standardized. For example, when a client with cancer is hospitalized, the availability of ancillary services for long-term care will vary by care setting. Hospital-based oncologists are usually in larger hospitals and not smaller ones. A National Cancer Institute (NCI)–designated cancer center offers the most comprehensive and up-to-date clinical care. NCI-designated centers also conduct important clinical trials to investigate the most up-to-date cancer therapies. Many clients benefit when they have the opportunity to be in these trials. Your role is to tell clients about the different resources available so that clients are able to make informed choices. For example, some clients choose to travel to a different state in order to go to an NCI cancer center. You can refer clients to the NCI website, http://www.cancer.gov/, where there is a current list of NCI-designated comprehensive cancer centers.

There is a wealth of cancer-related community support services available to survivors through voluntary organizations (Table 7-4). Most offer their services at no cost. Many supportive services offer call centers and web-based information and discussion boards in addition to direct service delivery (IOM, 2006). Health care professionals are not consistent in referring clients to these valuable services. In addition, although community-based services help most survivors, there are gaps in service provision for assistance with transportation, home care, child care, and financial assistance. Become knowledgeable about the services within your community. There are several national agencies across the country, including the American Cancer Society, the Wellness Community (http://www.twcw.org), and agencies targeted to racial groups such as the Sisters Network (http://www.sistersnetworkinc.org) and the Witness Program (http://www.acrc.uams.edu/patients/witness_project).

Components of Survivorship Care

Once a cancer client's primary treatment ends, health care professionals need to develop an organized plan for survivorship care. This does not always occur because of inadequacies in the health care system, including a lack of any one health care provider's assuming responsibility for coordinating care, fragmentation of care between specialists and general practitioners, and a lack of guidance on how survivors can improve their health outcomes (IOM, 2006). Cancer clients often do not receive noncancer care (e.g., care for diabetes or heart conditions) when their cancer diagnosis

✳ TABLE 7-4 Selected Community-Based Survivor Resources

PROGRAM NAME	SERVICES
Cancer Care http://www.cancercare.org	One-to-one counseling; group therapy; information and education
I Can Cope (American Cancer Society) http://www.cancer.org	Series of classes taught by physicians, nurses, social workers, and others Information, peer support
ACOR (Association of Cancer Online Resources) http://www.acor.org	Group discussion and peer support Information and education Includes Internet discussion group LTS (Long-term survivors)
LIVESTRONG Lance Armstrong Foundation and Centers for Disease Control and Prevention http://www.livestrong.org	Information and education
Disease-Specific Support Services	
Reach to Recovery http://www.cancer.org	Breast cancer
Man to Man http://www.cancer.org	Prostate cancer
Colon Cancer Alliance http://www.ccalliance.org	Colon cancer

shifts attention away from care that is routine but necessary. There is also poor follow-up of cancer care even though recommended guidelines exist. For example, some women with a history of breast cancer do not get annual mammograms, and some clients with colorectal cancer do not have regular colorectal exams. The Institute of Medicine (IOM) (2006) has made recommendations for four essential components of survivorship care: (1) prevention and detection of new cancers and recurrent cancer; (2) surveillance for cancer spread, recurrence, or second cancers; (3) intervention for consequences of cancer and its treatment (e.g., medical problems, symptoms, and psychological distress); and (4) coordination between specialists and primary care providers.

Survivorship Care Plan

If health care professionals succeed in improving cancer survivorship care, a strategy is needed for survivors' ongoing clinical care. The IOM (2006) made several recommendations for improving survivorship care within the United States. One recommendation was the provision of a "survivorship care plan" written by the principal provider that coordinated the client's **oncology** treatment. The IOM also recommended that the time and effort to develop such care plans be included in coverage by health insurance companies. Ideally, you would review a survivorship care plan with a client at the time he or she is formally discharged from a treatment program. The plan would become a guide for any future cancer or cancer-related care. Health care providers would

---

✳ BOX 7-4   A Survivorship Care Plan

Upon discharge from cancer treatment, every client and his or her primary health care provider should receive a record of all care received and a follow-up plan incorporating available evidence-based standards of care.

Care Summary
Diagnostic tests performed and results
Tumor characteristics (e.g., site, stage, and grade)
Dates when treatment started and stopped
Surgery, chemotherapy, radiotherapy, transplant, hormonal therapy, or gene therapy provided, including the specific agents used
Psychosocial, nutritional, and other supportive services provided
Full contact information on treating institutions and key providers
Identification of a key point of contact and coordinator of care

Follow-up Plan
Likely course of recovery
Description of recommended cancer screening and other periodic testing/examinations
Information on possible late and long-term effects of treatment and symptoms of such effects
Information on possible signs of recurrence and second tumors
Information on the possible effects of cancer on marital/partner relationship, sexual functioning, work, and parenting
Information on the potential insurance, employment and financial consequences of cancer and, as necessary, referral to counseling, legal aid, and financial assistance
Specific recommendations for healthy behaviors
Information on genetic counseling and testing as appropriate
Information on known effective chemoprevention strategies for secondary prevention
Referrals to specific follow-up care providers
A listing of cancer-related resources and information

Modified from the President's Cancer Panel (2004) and Institute of Medicine and National Research Council, Hewitt M, Greenfield S, Stovall E, editors: *From cancer client to cancer survivor: lost in transition*, Washington, DC, 2006, National Academies Press.

---

use the plan as a guide for client education. Survivors would use the plan to raise questions with physicians to prompt appropriate care during follow-up visits. Box 7-4 highlights the components of a survivorship care plan.

Few health care agencies provide survivorship care plans at this time. Those that do are usually children's hospitals. Thus nurses and other health care providers need to become more vigilant in recognizing cancer survivors and attempting to link them with the support and resources they require. Nurses can make a difference in considering the long-term issues cancer survivors face after their time of diagnosis and in contributing to solutions to manage or relieve cancer-associated health problems. A strong multidisciplinary approach that includes nurses, oncology specialists, dietitians, social workers, pastoral care, and rehabilitation professionals is necessary. Together, an interdisciplinary team will provide a plan of care that addresses treatment-related problems and future health risks and offers a wellness focus to give clients a sense of hope as they enter their survivor experience.

✳ Key Concepts

- The health care system has largely ignored or misunderstood cancer survivors' health care problems.
- The definition of cancer survivor also includes family members, friends, and caregivers who are also affected by survivorship.
- The majority of cancer survivors have serious health deficits that are related to their treatments.
- Evidence shows that cancer survivors have poorer health outcomes than similar individuals without cancer.
- Survivors are often reluctant to report symptoms because of a fear of being perceived as ungrateful for being disease-free or a fear of cancer recurrence.
- How well a survivor adapts to the cancer experience psychologically depends upon predisposing factors, the person's current psychological status, the extent of his or her disease, and the presence of disruptive signs and symptoms.
- The developmental effects of cancer have a social impact that occurs across the life span.
- Relationships between cancer survivors and family members become difficult to maintain because family members often do not know, understand and report not having the skills or confidence to support the survivor's reactions to cancer.
- As a nursing student, incorporate cancer survivorship care into your nursing practice through client assessment, education, and referral of clients to available resources.
- Because survivors are at an increased risk for developing a second cancer and/or chronic illness, it is important to educate them about lifestyle behaviors that will improve the quality of their lives.
- Once a cancer client's primary treatment ends, health care professionals should develop an organized plan for survivorship care.
- A client's principal health care provider should write a survivorship care plan that coordinates the client's oncology treatment.
- Ideally, you would review a survivorship care plan with a client at the time he or she is formally discharged from a treatment program, and it would become a guide for any future cancer or cancer-related care.

✳ Critical Thinking Exercises

1. Do you have a friend or family member who has cancer and is willing to talk about it? If so, ask the individual to tell you what the experience has been like and what he or she would recommend to help you provide better care for survivors.

2. Ms. Ritter is a 32-year-old woman who visits the medical outpatient clinic for her final course of chemotherapy to treat breast cancer. She is married and has one child, a daughter, who is 6 years old. She and her husband have hoped to have another child in the near future but now wonder if that will be possible. She has shared with the nursing staff her concerns about the future and how cancer will affect her and her family. Her case manager talks with her about a survivorship care plan before discharge

from the clinic. Identify two follow-up care plan components that would be important when considering Ms. Ritter's role as a wife and parent.

3. Ms. Ritter tells her nurse, "This chemotherapy has made me feel so tired, and there are many nights I cannot sleep very well. I am looking forward to this going away." What is an appropriate response the nurse might give Ms. Ritter?

✳ NCLEX®-Style Review Questions

1. Cancer survivors are at risk for treatment-related problems. Which of the clients listed below has the greatest risk for developing such a problem?
   1. An 80-year-old woman undergoing surgery for removal of a basal cell carcinoma on the face
   2. A 71-year-old man receiving chemotherapy and radiation for an advanced-stage lymphoma
   3. A 26-year-old man receiving chemotherapy for testicular cancer that is localized to the testicle
   4. A 48-year-old woman receiving radiation for Hodgkin's disease that involves lymph nodes extending above and below the diaphragm

2. Wallace is a 34-year-old who has been a survivor of Hodgkin's disease for 5 years. He continues to have symptoms related to his chemotherapy treatment. Wallace is a computer whiz and enjoys Internet discussion groups. What resource might a nurse refer him to in order to share information with other cancer survivors?
   1. ACOR
   2. I Can Cope
   3. Cancer Care
   4. LIVESTRONG

3. The nurse reviews the medical record of a new client admitted to her nursing unit. She notices that the client had a history of bladder cancer 3 years ago. Which of the following factors should she consider when conducting an assessment of this client? (Select all that apply.)
   1. The number and type of cancer therapies given to the client
   2. The presence of other medical conditions affecting the client
   3. Use of an approach that results in the client telling his or her story
   4. Cancer survivors readily report the symptoms they are experiencing
   5. Assessment of sexuality focuses on whether the client can perform a sexual act

4. A nurse working in a medicine clinic knows it is important to recognize cancer survivors who are most at risk for posttreatment symptoms. Which of the following clients will likely be at greatest risk for posttreatment symptoms?
   1. A 50-year-old mother of three who was diagnosed with breast cancer at a late stage
   2. A 20-year-old male college student diagnosed with leukemia whose father had lung cancer
   3. A 32-year-old Hispanic woman who has been diagnosed with cervical cancer and receives Medicaid
   4. A 72-year-old African American retired Air Force captain who had surgical removal of his colon for cancer and now also is receiving radiation

5. A 41-year-old man who underwent a craniotomy for the removal of a brain tumor 2 years ago comes to the clinic for his 6-month follow-up visit. In planning your assessment, you will anticipate that the client may possibly experience which of the following late effects of surgery? (Select all that apply.)
   1. Pain
   2. Fatigue
   3. Blurred vision
   4. Difficulty breathing
   5. Poor attention span

6. In order to successfully assess if a client is experiencing cognitive changes as a result of cancer treatment or complications of treatment, which of the following will likely be most relevant?
   1. Describe for me your medication schedule.
   2. How distressed are you feeling right now on a scale of 0 to 10?
   3. Tell me about when you first noticed symptoms from your chemotherapy.
   4. Tell me what you notice differently in your ability to get work done at your office.

8 | Caring in Nursing Practice

OBJECTIVES

Mastery of the content in this chapter will enable the student to:

- Discuss the role that caring plays in building a nurse-client relationship.
- Compare and contrast theories on caring.
- Discuss the potential implications when nurses' perceptions of caring differ from the clients' perception of caring.
- Explain how an ethic of care influences nurses' decision making.

- Describe ways to express caring through presence and touch.
- Describe the therapeutic benefit of listening to clients.
- Explain the relationship between knowing a client and clinical decision making.

MEDIA RESOURCES   KEY TERMS

Companion CD

- NCLEX®-Style Review Questions
- Audio Glossary
- Interactive Learning Activities
- English/Spanish Glossary

evolve Website

- NCLEX®-Style Review Questions
- Audio Glossary
- English/Spanish Glossary
- Interactive Learning Activities
- WebLinks
- Audio Summaries

Caring, p. 96
Comforting, p. 101
Ethic of care, p. 100

Presence, p. 100
Transcultural, p. 96
Transformative, p. 97

Caring is central to nursing practice, but it is even more important in today's hectic health care environment. The demands, pressure, and time constraints in the health care environment leave little room for caring practice, which results in nurses and other health professionals becoming cold and indifferent to client needs (Watson, 2006a). Increasing use of technological advances for rapid diagnosis and treatment often causes nurses and other health care providers to perceive the client relationship as less important. Technological advances become dangerous without a context of skillful and compassionate care. It is time to value and embrace caring practices and expert knowledge that are the heart of competent nursing practice (Brenner and Wrubel, 1989; Lesniak, 2005). When you engage clients in a caring and compassionate manner, you learn that the therapeutic gain in caring makes enormous contributions to the health and well-being of your clients.

Have you ever been ill or experienced a problem requiring health care intervention? Think about that experience. Then consider the following two scenarios and select the situation that you believe most successfully demonstrates a sense of caring.

A nurse enters a client's room, greets the client warmly while touching the client lightly on the shoulder, makes eye contact, sits down for a few minutes and asks about the client's thoughts and concerns, listens to the client's story, looks at the intravenous (IV) solution hanging in the room, briefly examines the client, and then checks the vital sign summary on the bedside computer screen before departing the room.

A second nurse enters the client's room, looks at the IV solution hanging in the room, checks the vital sign summary sheet on the bedside computer screen, and acknowledges the client but never sits down or touches the client. The nurse makes eye contact from above while the client is in the vulnerable horizontal position. The nurse asks a few brief questions about the client's symptoms and then leaves.

There is little doubt that the first scenario presents the nurse in specific acts of caring. The nurse's calm presence, parallel eye contact, attention to the client's concerns, and physical closeness all express a person-centered, comforting approach. In contrast, the second scenario is task-oriented and expresses a sense of indifference to client concerns. During times of illness or when a person seeks the professional guidance of a nurse, caring is essential in helping the individual reach positive outcomes.

Theoretical Views on Caring

Caring is a universal phenomenon influencing the ways in which people think, feel, and behave in relation to one another. Since Florence Nightingale, nurses have studied caring from a variety of philosophical and ethical perspectives. A number of nursing scholars developed theories on caring because of its importance to the practice of nursing. This chapter does not detail all of the theoretical positions on caring, but it helps you understand how caring is at the heart of a nurse's ability to work with all clients in a respectful and therapeutic way.

Caring Is Primary

Patricia Benner (1984) and Benner and Wrubel (1989) offer nurses a rich, holistic understanding of nursing practice and caring through the interpretation of expert nurses' stories. After listening to nurses'

stories and analyzing their meaning, Benner described the essence of excellent nursing practice, which is caring. The stories revealed the nurses' behaviors and decisions that express caring. Caring means that persons, events, projects, and things matter to people (Benner and Wrubel, 1989). It is a word for being connected.

Caring determines what matters to a person; it describes a wide range of involvements, from parental love to friendship, from caring for one's work to caring for one's pet, to caring for and about one's clients. Benner and Wrubel (1989) note: "Caring creates possibility." Personal concern for another person, an event, or thing provides motivation and direction for people to care. Caring as a framework has practical implications for transforming nursing practice (Boykin and others, 2003). Caring is an inherent feature of nursing practice whereby nurses help clients recover in the face of illness, give meaning to that illness, and maintain or reestablish connection. Caring helps nurses identify successful interventions, and this concern then guides future caregiving.

Clients are not all the same. Each individual brings a unique background of experiences, values, and cultural perspectives to a health care encounter. Caring is always specific and relational for each nurse-client encounter. As nurses acquire more experience, they typically learn that caring helps them to focus on the clients for whom they care. Caring facilitates a nurse's ability to know a client, allowing the nurse to recognize a client's problems and to find and implement individualized solutions.

In addition to their work in understanding caring, Benner and Wrubel (1989) describe the relationship between health, illness, and disease. Health is not the absence of illness, nor is illness identical with disease (see Chapter 6). Health is a state of being that people define in relation to their own values, personality, and lifestyle. Health exists along a continuum. Illness is the experience of loss or dysfunction, whereas disease is the manifestation of an abnormality at the cellular, tissue, or organ level. Some clients have a disease (e.g., arthritis or diabetes) but do not experience the sense of being ill or decrease in function. Some individuals do not seek health care until there is a disruption, loss, or concern. For example, a client has had diabetes for a number of years but does not sense being ill until the disease causes serious visual impairment, threatening the ability to work. Illness therefore has meaning only within the context of the person's life.

Because illness is the human experience of loss or dysfunction, any treatment or intervention given without consideration of its meaning to an individual is likely to be worthless. Expert nurses understand the difference between health, illness, and disease. Through caring relationships, nurses learn to listen to clients' stories about their illness so that they obtain an understanding of the meaning of illness. With this understanding, they provide therapeutic, client-centered care.

The Essence of Nursing and Health

From a **transcultural** perspective, Madeleine Leininger (1978) describes the concept of care as the essence and central, unifying, and dominant domain that distinguishes nursing from other health disciplines. Care is an essential human need, necessary for the health and survival of all individuals. Care, unlike cure, assists an individual or group in improving a human condition. Acts of caring refer to the nurturant and skillful activities, processes, and decisions to assist people in ways that are empathetic, compas-

★ **BOX 8-1** **CULTURAL ASPECTS OF CARE**

Nurse Caring Behaviors

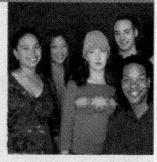

Nurses must provide caring behaviors based on clients' cultural values and beliefs. Although the need for human caring is universal, its application is based on cultural norms. For example, providing time for family presence is often more valuable to traditional Asian families than nursing presence. Using touch to convey caring sometimes crosses cultural norms. Sometimes gender-congruent caregivers or the client's family need to provide caring touch. When listening to the client, some cultures view eye contact as disrespectful.

Implications for Practice

- Know the client's cultural norms for caring practices.
- Know the client's cultural practices regarding end-of-life care. In some cultures it is considered insensitive to tell the client he or she is dying.
- Determine if a member of the client's family or cultural group is the best resource to use for caring practices of providing presence or touching.
- Determine the need for gender-congruent caregivers.
- Avoid the use of idioms because they can often create misunderstanding between client/family and caregiver.
- Know the client's cultural practices regarding the removal of life support.

Data from Galanti GA: *Caring for patients from different cultures*, ed 3, Philadelphia, 2004, University of Pennsylvania Press; and Watson J: Caring theory as an ethical guide to administrative and clinical practices, *Nurs Adm Q* 30(1):48, 2006.

sionate, and supportive. An act of caring is dependent on the needs, problems, and values of the client. Leininger's studies of numerous cultures around the world found that care helps protect, develop, nurture, and provide survival to people. Care is vital to recovery from illness and to the maintenance of healthy life practices in all cultures.

Leininger (1988) stresses the importance of nurses' understanding cultural caring behaviors. Even though human caring is a universal phenomenon, the expressions, processes, and patterns of caring vary among cultures (Box 8-1). Caring is very personal, and thus expression of caring differs for each client. For caring to achieve cure, nurses need to learn culturally specific behaviors and words that reflect human caring in different cultures to identify and meet the needs of all clients (see Chapter 9).

Transpersonal Caring

Clients and their families expect a high quality of human interaction from nurses. Unfortunately, many of the conversations occurring between clients and their nurses are very brief and disconnected. Watson's theory of caring (1979, 1988) is a holistic model for nursing that suggests that a conscious intention to care promotes healing and wholeness (Hoover, 2002). It is complementary to conventional science and modern nursing practices. The theory integrates human caring processes with healing environments, incorporating the life-generating and life-receiving processes of human caring and healing for nurses and their clients (Watson, 2006b). The theory describes a consciousness that al-

lows nurses to raise new questions about what it means to be a nurse, to be ill, and to be caring and healing. Transpersonal caring theory rejects the disease orientation to health care and places care before cure (Watson, 1988). The practitioner looks beyond the client's disease and its treatment by conventional means. Instead, transpersonal caring looks for deeper sources of inner healing to protect, enhance, and preserve a person's dignity, humanity, wholeness, and inner harmony.

In Watson's view, caring becomes almost spiritual. Caring preserves human dignity in the technological, cure-dominated health care system (Watson, 2006b). The emphasis is on the nurse-client relationship. The focus is on the persons behind the client and nurse, as well as the caring relationship (Table 8-1). A nurse communicates caring-healing to the client through the consciousness of the nurse. This takes place during a single caring moment between nurse and client. A connection forms between the one cared for and the one caring. The model is **transformative,** because the relationship influences both the nurse and the client, for better or for worse (Hoover, 2002; Watson, 2006b). The caring-healing consciousness promotes healing. Application of Watson's caring model in practice enhances nurses' caring practices (Box 8-2).

Swanson's Theory of Caring

Kristen Swanson (1991) studied clients and professional caregivers in an effort to develop a theory of caring for nursing practice. Three different groups were interviewed: women who miscarried, parents and health care professionals in a newborn intensive care unit, and socially at-risk mothers who received long-term, public health intervention. All groups were in a perinatal (before, during, or after the birth of a child) setting or context and experienced the phenomenon of caring. Researchers asked each group questions regarding how they experienced or expressed caring in their situation. After analyzing the stories and descriptions of the three groups, Swanson developed a theory of caring. The theory describes caring as consisting of five categories or processes (Table 8-2). Swanson (1991) defines caring as a nurturing way of relating to a valued other, toward whom one feels a personal sense of commitment and responsibility. This theory supports the claim that caring is a central nursing phenomenon but not necessarily unique to nursing practice.

Swanson's contributions (1991) are valuable in providing direction for how to develop useful and effective caring strategies. Each of the caring processes has definitions and subdimensions that serve as the basis for nursing interventions. Nursing care and caring are crucial in making positive differences in clients' health and well-being outcomes (Swanson, 1999a). Thus research findings used to develop the theory are useful to guide clinical nursing practice. For example, Swanson (1999b) tested the effects of caring-based counseling on women's emotional well-being in the first year after miscarrying. Caring-based counseling was significant in reducing women's depression and anger, particularly for women in the first 4 months following miscarriage.

Summary of Theoretical Views

Nursing caring theories have common themes. Caring is highly relational. Caregiving relationships open up possibilities or close them down (Benner, 2004). The nurse and the client enter into a

✳ TABLE 8-1 Watson's 10 Carative Factors

CARATIVE FACTOR	EXAMPLE IN PRACTICE
Forming a human-altruistic value system	Use loving-kindness to extend yourself. You use self-disclosure appropriately to promote a therapeutic alliance with your client.
Instilling faith-hope	Provide a connectedness with the client that offers purpose and direction when trying to find the meaning of an illness.
Cultivating a sensitivity to one's self and to others	Learn to accept yourself and others for their full potential. A caring nurse matures into becoming a self-actualized nurse.
Developing a helping-trusting, human caring relationship	Learn to develop and sustain helping-trusting, authentic caring relationship through effective communication with your clients.
Promoting and expressing positive and negative feelings	Support and accept your clients' feelings. In connecting with your clients you show a willingness to take risks in what you share with one another.
Using a creative problem-solving caring processes	Apply the nursing process in systematic, scientific problem-solving decision making in providing client-centered care.
Promoting transpersonal teaching-learning	Learn together while educating the client to acquire self-care skills. The client assumes responsibility for learning.
Providing for a supportive, protective, and/or corrective mental, physical, societal, and spiritual environment	Create a healing environment at all levels, physical and nonphysical. This promotes wholeness, beauty, comfort, dignity, and peace.
Meeting human needs	Assist clients with basic needs with an intentional care and caring consciousness.
Allowing for existential-phenomenological-spiritual forces	Allow spiritual forces to provide a better understanding of yourself and your client.

✳ BOX 8-2   **EVIDENCE-BASED PRACTICE**

Enhancing Caring

Evidence Summary

Caring facilitates healing and improves client satisfaction with nursing care. However, does the instructional process influence human caring? Do nurse educators present instructional methods that improve students' caring practices? Undergraduate nursing students received a 15-week educational module on nursing as human caring. The purpose of the module was to improve students' understanding of caring practices and to thus make them more caring practitioners. Researchers interviewed the students before and after completing the module to understand the effect of this module on their caring practices. For example, they asked students about factors that facilitated and impeded their caring practices. The students reported an increased self-awareness in regard to (1) connecting in relationships with self and others, (2) finding purpose and meaning in life, and (3) clarifying values. Several students spoke of becoming more tolerant of others, recognizing persons' uniqueness and appreciating their perspectives. By recognizing themselves as caring persons, the students gained meaning in their lives. Many were able to relate a great deal of satisfaction in recognizing that

they were caring persons and how nursing allowed them to express that. Students worked through the emotional issues and practical constraints, which allowed them to grow spiritually and connect with clients at a deeper level. Finally, students also expressed an enhanced appreciation of what they valued.

Application to Nursing Practice

- Increasing knowledge and understanding of caring helps nurses begin to understand a client's world and to change their approach to nursing care.
- The use of caring in nursing practice encourages a more holistic approach to nursing care.
- As nurses use caring, they get to know their clients and therefore better meet their needs.
- The caring model involves a closeness, commitment, and involvement in the nurse-client relationship.

Reference

Hoover J: The personal and professional impact of undertaking an educational module on human caring, *J Adv Nurs* 37(1):79, 2002.

---

relationship that is much more than one person simply "doing tasks for" another. There is a mutual give-and-take that develops as nurse and client begin to know and care for one another. Frank (1998) described a personal situation when he was suffering from cancer: "What I wanted when I was ill, was a mutual relationship of *persons* who were also clinician and client." It was important for Frank to be seen as one of two fellow human beings, not the dependent client being cared for by the expert technical clinician.

Caring seems highly invisible at times, when a nurse and client enter a relationship of respect, concern, and support. The nurse's

empathy and compassion become a natural part of every client encounter. However, when caring is absent, it becomes very obvious. For example, if the nurse shows disinterest or chooses to avoid a client's request for help, the nurse's inaction quickly conveys an uncaring attitude. Benner and Wrubel (1989) relate the story of a clinical nurse specialist who learned from a client what caring is all about: "I felt that I was teaching him a lot, but actually he taught me. One day he said to me (probably after I had delivered some well-meaning technical information about his disease), 'You are doing an OK job, but I can tell that every time

✳ TABLE 8-2 Swanson's Theory of Caring

CARING PROCESS	DEFINITIONS	SUBDIMENSIONS
Knowing	Striving to understand an event as it has meaning in the life of the other	Avoiding assumptions Centering on the one cared for Assessing thoroughly Seeking cues Engaging the self or both
Being with	Being emotionally present to the other	Being there Conveying ability Sharing feelings Not burdening
Doing for	Doing for the other as he or she would do for the self if it were at all possible	Comforting Anticipating Performing skillfully Protecting Preserving dignity
Enabling	Facilitating the other's passage through life transitions (e.g., birth, death) and unfamiliar events	Informing/explaining Supporting/allowing Focusing Generating alternatives Validating/giving feedback
Maintaining belief	Sustaining faith in the other's capacity to get through an event or transition and face a future with meaning	Believing in/holding in esteem Maintaining a hope-filled attitude Offering realistic optimism "Going the distance"

From Swanson K: Empirical development of a middle-range theory of caring, *Nurs Res* 40(3):161, 1991.

you walk in that door you are walking out.'" In this nurse's story, the client perceived that the nurse was simply going through the motions of teaching and showed little caring toward the client. Clients quickly know when nurses fail to relate to them.

As the nurse practices caring, the client senses a commitment on the part of the nurse and is willing to enter into a relationship allowing the nurse to gain an understanding of the client's experience of illness. In a study of oncology clients, one client described a nurse's caring as "putting the heart in it" and "having an investment" that makes "clients feel that you are with them" (Radwin, 2000). Thus the nurse becomes a coach and partner rather than a detached provider of care.

A nurse is working with a client recently diagnosed with diabetes mellitus who must also learn to administer daily insulin injections. In this scenario the nurse's caring behavior might be enabling. When a nurse practices enabling, the client and nurse work together to identify alternatives and resources. As the nurse enables the client, diabetes management is explained and the nurse supports the client in progressing through self-care activities.

Another common theme is to understand the context of the person's life and illness. It is difficult to show caring to another individual without gaining an understanding of who they are and their perception of their illness. Exploring the following questions with your client will assist you in understanding your client's perception of illness: How was your illness first recognized? How do you feel about the illness? How does the illness affect your daily life practices? Knowing the context of a client's illness helps you choose and individualize interventions that will actually help

the client. This approach is more successful than simply selecting interventions on the basis of your client's symptoms or disease process.

Clients' Perceptions of Caring

Swanson's theory of caring (1991) provides an excellent beginning to understand the behaviors and processes that characterize caring. Other researchers studied caring from clients' perceptions (Table 8-3). Identifying nurse behaviors that clients perceive as caring emphasizes what clients expect from their caregivers. Clients continue to value nurses' effectiveness in performing tasks; but clearly clients value the affective dimension of nursing care (Williams, 1997). Establishing a reassuring presence, recognizing an individual as unique, and keeping a close, attentive eye on the client are recurrent caring behaviors that clients value. All clients are unique; however, understanding common behaviors that clients associate with caring helps you learn to express caring in practice.

The study of clients' perceptions is important because health care is placing greater emphasis on client satisfaction (see Chapter 2). What clients experience in their interactions with institutional services and health care professionals, and what they think of that experience, determines how clients use the health care system and how they can benefit from it (Gerteis and others, 1993; Mayer, 1986). When clients sense that health care providers are sensitive, sympathetic, compassionate, and interested in them as people,

✳ TABLE 8-3 A Comparison of Research Studies Exploring Nurse Caring Behaviors (as Perceived by Clients)

WOLF (2003) PERCEPTIONS OF CARDIAC CLIENTS	ATTREE (2001) GENERAL MEDICAL CLIENTS' AND FAMILIES' PERCEPTIONS	CHANG AND OTHERS (2005) PERCEPTIONS OF CANCER CLIENTS
Managing equipment skillfully	Checking up on clients	Being accessible to client and family
Being perceptive and compassionate	Being compassionate and pa- tient	Providing comfort
Being physically present	Demonstrating sensitivity and sympathy	Trusting relationship between client and nurse
Using a soft, gentle voice		Monitoring symptoms and following through with
Returning to client voluntarily without being asked	Using a calm, gentle, and kind approach	interventions
Providing comfort and security		Anticipating client and family needs
Helping to reduce pain		

they usually become active partners in the plan of care (Attree, 2001). Williams (1997) studied the relationship between clients' perceptions of four dimensions of caring and their satisfaction with nursing care. Clients in the study indicated that they were more satisfied when they perceived nurses to be caring. Radwin (2000) found that oncology clients associated excellent nursing care with attentiveness, partnership, individualization, rapport, and caring. As institutions look to improve client satisfaction, creating an environment of caring is a necessary and worthwhile goal. Clients' satisfaction with nursing care is an important factor in their decision to return to a hospital.

As you begin clinical practice, it is important to consider how clients perceive caring and what are the best approaches to providing care. Behaviors associated with caring offer an excellent starting point. It is also important to determine an individual client's perceptions and unique expectations. Frequently clients and nurses differ in their perceptions of caring (Mayer, 1987; Wolf, Miller, and Devine, 2003). For that reason, focus on building a relationship that allows you to learn what is important to your clients. For example, you have a client who is fearful of having an intravenous catheter inserted, and you are still a novice at catheter insertion. Instead of giving a lengthy description of the procedure to relieve anxiety, you decide the client will benefit more by obtaining assistance from a skilled staff member. Knowing who clients are helps you select caring approaches that are most appropriate to the clients' needs.

Ethic of Care

Caring is a moral imperative. Through caring for other human beings, ultimately human dignity is protected, enhanced, and preserved. Watson (1988) suggests that caring, as a moral ideal, provides the stance from which one intervenes as a nurse. This stance is critical for ensuring that nurses practice ethical standards for good conduct, character, and motives. Chapter 22 explores the importance of ethics in professional nursing. The term *ethics* refers to the ideals of right and wrong behavior. In any client encounter, a nurse needs know what behavior is ethically appropriate. An ethic of care is unique so that professional nurses do not

make professional decisions based solely on intellectual or analytical principles. Instead, an ethic of care places caring at the center of decision making. What resources should be used to care for an indigent client? Is it caring to place a disabled relative in a long-term care facility?

An **ethic of care** is concerned with relationships between people and with a nurse's character and attitude toward others. Nurses who function from an ethic of care are sensitive to unequal relationships that lead to an abuse of one person's power over another—intentional or otherwise. In health care settings clients and families are often on unequal footing with professionals because of the client's illness, lack of information, regression caused by pain and suffering, and unfamiliar circumstances. An ethic of care places the nurse as the client's advocate, solving ethical dilemmas by attending to relationships and by giving priority to each client's unique personhood.

Caring in Nursing Practice

It is impossible to prescribe ways that will guarantee whether or when a nurse becomes a caring professional. Experts disagree as to whether caring is teachable or more fundamentally a way of being in the world. For those who find caring a normal part of their life, caring is a product of their culture, values, experiences, and relationships with others. Persons who do not experience care in their lives often find it difficult to act in caring ways. As nurses deal with health and illness in their practice, they grow in the ability to care. Nursing behaviors related to caring include providing presence, a caring touch, and listening. Nurses who demonstrate caring use a caring approach in each encounter with clients.

Providing Presence

Providing **presence** is a person-to-person encounter conveying a closeness and a sense of caring. Fredriksson (1999) explains that presence involves "being there" and "being with." "Being there" is not only a physical presence, but also includes communication and understanding. The interpersonal relationship of "being there" seems to depend on the fact that a nurse is attentive to the client (Cohen and others, 1994). This type of presence is something the nurse offers to the client with the purpose of achieving some goal, such as support, comfort, or encouragement, to diminish the intensity of unwanted feelings, or for reassurance (Fareed, 1996; Pederson, 1993).

"Being with" is also interpersonal. The nurse gives himself or herself, which means being available and at a client's disposal (Pederson, 1993). If clients accept the nurse, they will invite him or her to see, share, and touch their vulnerability and suffering. One's human presence never leaves one unaffected (Watson, 2003). The nurse then enters the client's world. In this presence, the client is able to put words to feelings and to understand himself or herself in a way that leads to identifying solutions, seeing new directions, and making choices (Gilje, 1997).

When a nurse establishes presence, eye contact, body language, voice tone, listening, and having a positive and encouraging attitude act together to create an openness and understanding. The message conveyed is that the other's experience matters to the one caring (Swanson, 1991). Establishing presence with a client enhances the nurse's ability to learn from the client. This strengthens the nurse's ability to provide adequate and appropriate nursing care.

It is especially important to establish presence when clients are experiencing stressful events or situations. Awaiting a physician's report of test results, preparing for an unfamiliar procedure, and planning for a return home after serious illness are just a few examples of events in the course of a person's illness that can create unpredictability and dependency on care providers. The nurse's presence helps to calm anxiety and fear related to stressful situations. Giving reassurance and thorough explanations about a procedure, remaining at the client's side, and coaching the client through the experience all convey a presence that is invaluable to the client's well-being.

Touch

Clients face situations that are embarrassing, frightening, and painful. Whatever the feeling or symptom, clients look to nurses to provide comfort. The use of touch is one **comforting** approach where the nurse reaches out to clients to communicate concern and support.

Touch is relational and leads to a connection between nurse and client. Touch involves contact and noncontact touch (Fredriksson, 1999). Contact touch involves obvious skin-to-skin contact, whereas noncontact touch refers to eye contact. It is difficult to separate the two. Both in turn are described within three categories: task-orientated touch, caring touch, and protective touch (Fredriksson, 1999).

Nurses use task-orientated touch when performing a task or procedure. The skillful and gentle performance of a nursing procedure conveys security and a sense of competence. An expert nurse learns that any procedure is more effective when administered carefully and in consideration of any client concern. For example, if a client is anxious about having a procedure, such as the insertion of a nasogastric tube, the nurse offers comfort through a full explanation of the procedure and what the client will feel. The nurse then expresses that the procedure will be performed safely, skillfully, and successfully. This is done in the way that supplies are prepared, the client is positioned, and the naso-

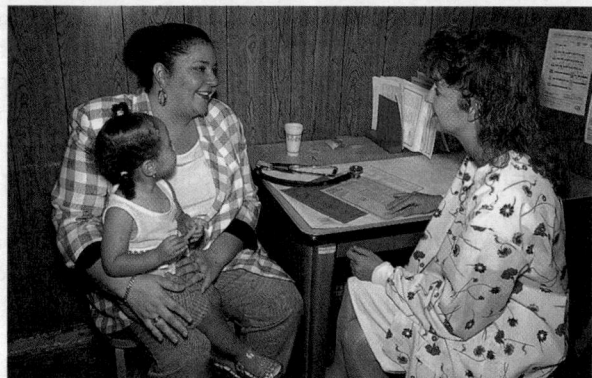

Figure 8-1 Nurse listening to client.

gastric tube is gently manipulated and inserted. Throughout a procedure the nurse talks quietly with the client to provide reassurance and support.

Caring touch is a form of nonverbal communication, which successfully influences a client's comfort and security, enhances self-esteem, and improves reality orientation (Boyek and Watson, 1994). You express this in the way you hold a client's hand, give a back massage, gently position a client, or participate in a conversation. When using a caring touch, the nurse is making a connection with the client and showing acceptance of the individual (Tommasini, 1990).

Protective touch is a form of touch used to protect the nurse and/or client (Fredriksson, 1999). The client views it either positively or negatively. The most obvious form of protective touch is preventing an accident, for example, holding and bracing the client to avoid a fall. Protective touch is also a kind of touch that protects the nurse emotionally. A nurse withdraws or distances herself or himself from a client when the nurse is unable to tolerate suffering or needs to escape from a situation that is causing tension. When used in this way, protective touch elicits negative feelings in a client (Fredriksson, 1999).

Because touch conveys many messages, use it with discretion. Touch itself is a concern when crossing cultural boundaries of either the client or the nurse (Benner, 2004). The client generally permits task-orientated touch, because most individuals give nurses and physicians a license to enter their personal space to provide care (see Box 8-1). Know and understand if clients are accepting of touch and how they interpret the nurse's intentions.

Listening

Caring involves an interpersonal interaction that is much more than two persons simply talking back and forth. In a caring relationship the nurse establishes trust, opens lines of communication, and listens to what the client has to say (Figure 8-1). Listening is key, because it conveys the nurse's full attention and interest. Listening includes "taking in" what a client says, as well as an interpretation and understanding of what the client is saying and giving back that understanding to the person talking (Kemper, 1992). Listening to the meaning of what a client says helps create a mutual relationship. True listening leads to truly knowing and responding to what really matters to the client and family (Boykin and others, 2003).

When an individual becomes ill, he or she usually has a story to tell about the meaning of their illness. Any critical or chronic illness affects all of a client's life choices and decisions, sometimes affecting the individual's identity. Being able to tell that story helps the client break the distress of illness. Thus a story needs a listener. Frank (1998) described his own feelings during his experience with cancer: "I needed a [health care professional's] gift of listening in order to make my suffering a relationship between *us,* instead of an iron cage around *me.*" He needed to be able to express what he needed when he was ill. The personal concerns that are part of a client's illness story determine what is at stake for the client. Caring through listening enables the nurse to be a participant in the client's life.

To listen effectively, listeners need to silence themselves to listen with openness (Fredriksson, 1999). Fredriksson describes silencing one's mouth and also the mind. It is important to remain intentionally silent and to concentrate on what the client has to say. A nurse needs to be able to give clients his or her full, focused attention as they tell their stories.

When an ill person chooses to tell his or her story, it involves reaching out to another human being. Telling the story implies a relationship that develops only if the clinician exchanges his or her stories as well. Frank (1998) argues that professionals do not routinely take seriously their own need to be known as part of a clinical relationship. Yet, unless the professional acknowledges this need, there is no reciprocal relationship, only an interaction (Campo, 1997). There is pressure on the clinician to know as much as possible about the client, but it isolates the clinician from the client. By contrast, in knowing and being known, each supports the other (Frank, 1998).

Through active listening, you begin to truly know your clients and what is important to them (Bernick, 2004). Learning to listen to a client is sometimes difficult. It is easy to become distracted by tasks at hand, colleagues shouting instructions, or other clients waiting to have their needs met. However, the time you take to listen effectively is worthwhile both in the information gained and in the strengthening of the nurse-client relationship. Listening involves paying attention to the individual's words and tone of voice and entering his or her frame of reference (see Chapter 24). By observing the expressions and body language of the client, you will find cues to help assist the client in exploring ways to achieve greater peace.

Knowing the Client

One of the five caring processes described by Swanson (1991) is knowing the client. The concept comprises both the nurse's understanding of a specific client and the nurse's subsequent selection of interventions (Radwin, 1995). Knowing develops over time as a nurse learns the clinical conditions within a specialty and the behaviors and physiological responses of clients. Intimate knowing helps the nurse respond to what really matters to the client (Bulfin, 2005). To know a client means that the nurse avoids assumptions, focuses on the client, and engages in a caring relationship with the client that reveals information and cues that facilitate critical thinking and clinical judgments (see Chapter 15). Knowing the client is at the core of the process nurses use to make clinical decisions. By establishing a caring relationship, the understanding that develops helps the nurse to better know the client as a unique individual and choose the most appropriate and efficacious nursing therapies.

The caring relationships that a nurse develops over time, coupled with the nurse's growing knowledge and experience, provide a rich source of meaning when changes in a client's clinical status occur. Expert nurses develop the ability to detect changes in clients' conditions almost effortlessly. Clinical decision making, perhaps the most important responsibility of the professional nurse, involves various aspects of knowing the client: responses to therapies, routines and habits, coping resources, physical capacities and endurance, and body typology and characteristics (Tanner and others, 1993). The experienced nurse knows additional facts about his or her clients such as their experiences, behaviors, feelings, and perceptions (Radwin, 1995). When you make clinical decisions accurately in the context of knowing a client well, improved client outcomes will result. Swanson (1999b) notes that when nurses base care on knowing the client, the clients perceive care as personalized, comforting, supportive, and healing.

The most important thing for a beginning nurse to recognize is that knowing a client is more than simply gathering data about the client's clinical signs and condition. Success in knowing the client lies in the relationship you establish. To know a client is to enter into a caring, social process that results in a "bonding" whereby the client comes to feel known by the nurse (Lamb and Stempel, 1994). The bonding then sets the stage for the relationship to evolve into "working" and "changing" phases so that you help the client become involved in his or her care and accept help when needed (Bulfin, 2005).

Spiritual Caring

Spiritual health occurs when a person finds a balance between his or her own life values, goals, and belief systems and those of others (see Chapter 29). Research shows a link between spirit, mind, and body. An individual's beliefs and expectations do have effects on the person's physical well-being.

Establishing a caring relationship with a client involves an interconnectedness between the nurse and the client. This interconnectedness is why Watson (1979, 2006a, 2006b) describes the caring relationship in a spiritual sense. Spirituality offers a sense of connectedness as well, intrapersonally (connected with oneself), interpersonally (connected with others and the environment), and transpersonally (connected with the unseen, God, or a higher power). In a caring relationship, the client and the nurse come to know one another so that both move toward a healing relationship by doing the following (Watson, 2003):

- Mobilizing hope for the client and for the nurse
- Finding an interpretation or understanding of illness, symptoms, or emotions that is acceptable to the client
- Assisting the client in using social, emotional, or spiritual resources
- Recognizing that caring relationships connect us human to human, spirit to spirit.

Family Care

People live in their worlds in an involved way. Each individual experiences life through relationships with others. Thus caring for an individual cannot occur in isolation from that person's family.

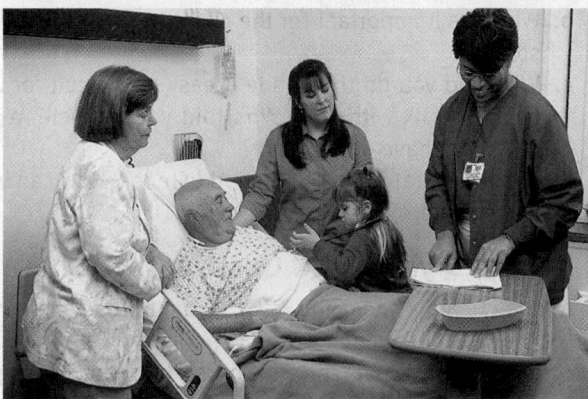

Figure 8-2 Nurse discusses client's health care needs with the family.

※ **BOX 8-3   Nurse Caring Behaviors as Perceived by Families**

- Being honest
- Advocating for client's care preferences
- Giving clear explanations
- Keeping family members informed
- Trying to make the client comfortable
- Showing interest in answering questions and answering them honestly
- Providing necessary emergency care
- Providing for and maintaining client privacy
- Assuring the client that nursing services will be available
- Helping clients to do as much for themselves as possible
- Teaching the family how to keep the relative physically comfortable

Data from Brown CL and others: Caring in action: the patient care facilitator role, *Int J Hum Caring* 9(3):51, 2005; Mayer DK: Cancer patients' and families' perceptions of nurse caring behaviors, *Top Clin Nurs* 8(2):63, 1986; and Radwin L: Oncology patients' perceptions of quality nursing care, *Res Nurs Health* 23(3):179, 2000.

As a nurse, it is important to know the family almost as thoroughly as one knows a client (Figure 8-2). The family is an important resource. Success with nursing interventions often depends on the family's willingness to share information about the client, the family's acceptance and understanding of therapies, whether the interventions fit with the family's daily practices, and whether the family supports and delivers the therapies recommended.

There are many nurse caring behaviors that families of clients with cancer perceived most helpful (Box 8-3). Ensuring the client's well-being and helping the family to be active participants are critical for family members. Although specific to families of clients with cancer, these behaviors offer useful guidelines for developing a caring relationship with all families. Begin a relationship by learning who makes up the client's family and what their roles are in the client's life. Showing the family care and concern for the client creates an openness that then enables a relationship to form with the family. Caring for the family takes into consideration the context of the client's illness and the stress it imposes on all members (see Chapter 10).

The Challenge of Caring

Assisting individuals during a time of need is the reason many enter nursing. When nurses are able to affirm themselves as caring individuals, they achieve a meaning and purpose to their lives (Benner, 2004; Hoover, 2002). Caring is a motivating force for people to become nurses, and it becomes the source of satisfaction when nurses know they have made a difference in their clients' lives.

It is becoming more of a challenge to care in today's health care system. Being a part of the helping professions is difficult and demanding. Nurses are torn between the human caring model and the task-oriented biomedical model and institutional demands that consume their practice (Watson and Foster, 2003). Nurses have increasingly less time to spend with clients, making it much harder to know who they are. A reliance on technology and cost-effective health care strategies and efforts to standardize and refine work processes all undermine the nature of caring. Too often clients become just a number, with their real needs either overlooked or ignored.

The American Nurses Association (ANA), National League for Nursing (NLN), American Organization of Nurse Executives (AONE), and American Association of Colleges of Nursing (AACN), recommend strategies to reverse the current nursing shortage. A number of the strategies have potential for creating work environments that enable nurses to demonstrate more caring behaviors. The strategies include introducing greater flexibility into the work environment structure, rewarding experienced nurse mentors, improving nurse staffing, and providing nurses with autonomy over their practice (Brown and others 2005; Watson and Foster, 2003).

If health care is to make a positive difference in their lives, human beings cannot be treated like machines or robots. Instead, health care has to become more humanizing. Nurses play an important role in making care an integral part of health care delivery. This begins by nurses' making caring a part of the philosophy and environment in the workplace. Incorporating care concepts into standards of nursing care establishes the guidelines for professional conduct. Finally, during day-to-day practice with clients and families, nurses need to be committed to caring and be willing to establish the relationships necessary for personal, competent, compassionate, and meaningful nursing care.

※ Key Concepts

- Caring is the heart of a nurse's ability to work with people in a respectful and therapeutic way.
- Caring is specific and relational for each nurse-client encounter.
- For caring to achieve cure, nurses need to learn those culturally specific behaviors and words that reflect human caring in different cultures.
- Because illness is the human experience of loss or dysfunction, any treatment or intervention given without consideration of its meaning to the individual is likely to be worthless.

- Swanson's theory of caring includes five caring processes: knowing, being with, doing for, enabling, and maintaining belief.
- Caring involves a mutual give and take that develops as nurse and client begin to know and care for one another.
- It is difficult to show caring to individuals without gaining an understanding of who they are and their perception of their illness.
- Presence involves a person-to-person encounter that conveys a closeness and a sense of caring that involves "being there" and "being with" clients.
- Research shows that touch, both contact and noncontact, includes task-orientated touch, caring touch, and protective touch.
- The skillful and gentle performance of a nursing procedure conveys security and a sense of competence in the nurse.
- Listening is not only "taking in" what a client says, it also includes interpretation and understanding of what the client is saying and giving back that understanding to the person talking.
- Knowing the client is at the core of the process nurses use to make clinical decisions.
- Nurses demonstrate caring by helping family members become active participants in a client's care.

✳ Critical Thinking Exercises

1. Mrs. Lowe is a 52-year-old client being treated for lymphoma (cancer of the lymph nodes) that occurred 6 years following a lung transplant. Mrs. Lowe is discouraged about her current health status and has a lot of what she describes as muscle pain. The unit where Mrs. Lowe is receiving care has a number of very sick clients and is short staffed.
   a. You enter her room to do a morning assessment and find Mrs. Lowe crying. How are you going to use caring practices to help Mrs. Lowe, knowing that your day has just begun and you have many nursing interventions to complete?
   b. When you listened to Mrs. Lowe, she explained that her muscle pain was very bothersome and it was particularly worse when she was alone. Both you and Mrs. Lowe determine that an injection for her pain would be beneficial. In what way can you show caring in the way you administer the injection to Mrs. Lowe?
   c. Mrs. Lowe's day is getting better. She seems more comfortable and is crying less. You find that your day is more controlled. What can you do for Mrs. Lowe?

2. During your next clinical practicum, select a client to talk with for at least 15 to 20 minutes. Ask the client to tell you about his or her illness. Review the skills of listening in this chapter and in Chapter 24. Immediately after your discussion, reflect on the discussion with the client and determine if you have enough information about your client to answer the following questions:
   a. What do you believe the client was trying to tell you about his or her illness?

   b. Why was it important for the client to share his or her story?
   c. What did you do that made it easy or difficult for the client to talk with you? What did you do well? What could you have done better?
   d. Would you rate yourself a good listener? How can you listen better?

✳ NCLEX®-Style Review Questions

1. A nurse hears a colleague tell a student nurse she never touches the clients unless she is performing a procedure or doing an assessment. The nurse tells the colleague that:
   1. She does not touch the clients either
   2. Touch is a type of verbal communication
   3. There is never a problem with using touch
   4. Touch forms a connection between nurse and client

2. Of the five caring processes, which describes "knowing" the client?
   1. Anticipating the client's cultural preferences
   2. Determining the client's physician preference
   3. Gathering task-oriented information during assessment
   4. Establishing an enhanced understanding of the client's needs

3. Helping a new mother through the birthing experience demonstrates which of the five caring behaviors?
   1. Knowing
   2. Enabling
   3. Doing for
   4. Being with
   5. Maintaining belief

4. Mr. Kline is fearful of upcoming surgery and a possible cancer diagnosis. He discusses his love for the bible with Jada, his nurse, and she recommends a favorite Bible verse. Another nurse tells Jada that there is no place in nursing for spiritual caring. Jada replies:
   1. Spiritual care should be left to a professional
   2. You are correct, religion is a personal decision
   3. Nurses should not force their religious beliefs on clients
   4. Spiritual, mind, and body connections can affect health

5. A number of strategies have potential for creating work environments that enable nurses to demonstrate more caring behaviors. Some of these include:
   1. Increasing working hours
   2. Increases in monetary gain
   3. Flexibility, autonomy, and improved staffing
   4. Increased input concerning nursing functions from physicians

6. A nurse demonstrates caring by helping family members:
   1. Become active participants in care
   2. Provide activities of daily living (ADLs)
   3. Remove themselves from personal care
   4. Make health care decisions for the client

7. Listening is not only "taking in" what a client says; it also includes:
   1. Incorporating the views of the physician
   2. Correcting any errors in the client's understanding
   3. Injecting the nurse's personal views and statements
   4. Interpreting and understanding what the client means

8. Presence involves a person-to-person encounter that:
   1. Enables clients to care for self
   2. Provides personal care to a client
   3. Conveys a closeness and a sense of caring
   4. Describes being in close contact with a client

9. Clients' perceptions are important because health care:
   1. Always acts in the best interest of the client
   2. Is placing greater emphasis on client satisfaction
   3. Is under investigation for misappropriation of funds
   4. Is carefully watched and regulated by the federal government

9 | Culture and Ethnicity

OBJECTIVES

Mastery of the content in this chapter will enable the student to:

- Describe social and cultural influences in health, illness, and caring patterns.
- Differentiate culturally congruent from culturally competent care.
- Describe steps toward developing cultural competence.
- Identify major components of cultural assessment.
- Use cultural assessment to identify significant values, beliefs, and practices critical to nursing care of individuals experiencing life transitions.
- Demonstrate nursing interventions that achieve culturally congruent care.
- Analyze outcomes of culturally congruent care.
- Apply research findings in culturally congruent care.

MEDIA RESOURCES   ## KEY TERMS

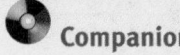
Companion CD
- NCLEX®-Style Review Questions
- Audio Glossary
- Interactive Learning Activities
- English/Spanish Glossary

 Website
- NCLEX®-Style Review Questions
- Audio Glossary
- English/Spanish Glossary
- Interactive Learning Activities
- WebLinks
- Audio Summaries

Acculturation, p. 108
Assimilation, p. 108
Biculturalism, p. 108
Bilineal, p. 116
Confianza, p. 118
Cultural backlash, p. 108
Cultural care accommodation or negotiation, p. 119
Cultural care preservation or maintenance, p. 119
Cultural care repatterning or restructuring, p. 119
Cultural imposition, p. 109
Culturally competant care, p. 108
Culturally congruent care, p. 108
Cultural pain, p. 113
Culture, p. 107
Culture-bound syndrome, p. 110
Emic worldview, p. 108
Enculturation, p. 108
Ethnicity, p. 107
Ethnocentrism, p. 109
Ethnohistory, p. 113
Etic worldview, p. 108

Fictive, p. 116
Halal, p. 117
Haram, p. 117
Hilots, p. 112
Hmong, p. 109
Hwa-Byung, p. 110
Igbos, p. 112
Invisible culture, p. 107
Kosher, p. 117
Matrilineal, p. 116
Naturalistic practitioners, p. 110
Patrilineal, p. 116
Personalismo, p. 118
Personalistic practitioners, p. 110
Rabbi, p. 117
Ramadan, p. 117
Respeto, p. 118
Rites of passage, p. 110
Sabbath, p. 117
Shaman, p. 110
Sikh/Sikhism, p. 107
Simpatia, p. 118
Subcultures, p. 107
Transcultural nursing, p. 108
Visible culture, p. 107

Population Diversity

The demographic profile of the United States is changing dramatically as a result of immigration patterns and significant increases in culturally diverse populations already residing in the country. According to the U.S. Census Bureau (2007), approximately 33% of the population currently belongs to a racial or ethnic minority group (Figure 9-1). The U.S. Census also projects that this percentage will increase to 50% by the year 2050 (U.S. Census Bureau, 2007).

Health Disparities

Despite significant improvements in the overall health status of the U.S. population in the last few decades, the persistence of disparities in health status among ethnic and racial minorities continues to be a serious local and national challenge. Racial and ethnic minorities are more likely than non-Hispanic whites to be poor or near poor. In addition, Hispanics, African Americans, and some Asian subgroups are less likely than non-Hispanic whites to have a high school education. In general, racial and ethnic minorities often experience poorer access to care and lower quality of preventive, primary, and specialty care. Eliminating such disparities in health status of people from diverse racial, ethnic, and cultural backgrounds has become one of the two most important priorities of *Healthy People 2010* (U.S. Department of Health and Human Services [USDHHS], 2000). Health disparity populations are populations that have a significant disparity in the incidence or prevalence of disease or that have a disparity in morbidity, mortality, or survival rates compared to the health status of the general population. The Civil Rights Act states that no person in the United States, regardless of race, color, or national origin, should be excluded from participation, denied benefits, or be subjected to discrimination under any program receiving federal funding. In compliance with these mandates, legislative, regulatory, and accreditation agencies have set standards in support of cultural and linguistic competence in health care.

Understanding Cultural Concepts

The Office of Minority Health (OMH) (n.d.) describes **culture** as the thoughts, communications, actions, customs, beliefs, values, and institutions of racial, ethnic, religious, or social groups. According to Purnell and Paulanka (2003), culture consists of socially transmitted knowledge, behavioral patterns, values, beliefs, norms, and lifestyles of a particular group that guides their worldview and decision making.

Culture has both **visible** (easily seen) and **invisible** (less observable) components. It is important to understand that the invisible value-belief system of a particular culture is often the major driving force behind visible practices. Although a **Sikh** man is easily identified by the visible artifacts that he wears (uncut hair with wooden comb, beard, turban, cotton underwear, steel bracelet, and short sword), nurses cannot appreciate the meanings and beliefs associated with these artifacts without further assessment. These artifacts symbolize his allegiance to the philosophy of Sikhism, and removal of these artifacts without express consent of the individual or his family is sacrilegious and violates the ethnoreligious identity of the person (Jambunathan, 2003). On the other hand, a young Arab woman who wears a veil may not believe in wearing the veil but does so because of her cultural norms.

In any society there is a dominant culture that exists along with other subcultures (Purnell, 2003). Although subcultures have similarities with the dominant culture, they maintain their unique life patterns, values, and norms. In the United States the dominant culture is Anglo-American with origins from Western Europe. **Subcultures** such as the Appalachian and Missouri Ozark cultures represent various ethnic, religious, and other groups with distinct characteristics from the dominant culture. **Ethnicity** refers to a shared identity related to social and cultural heritage such as values, language, geographical space, and racial characteristics. Members of an ethnic group feel a common sense of identity. Some individuals declare their ethnic identity as Irish, Vietnam-

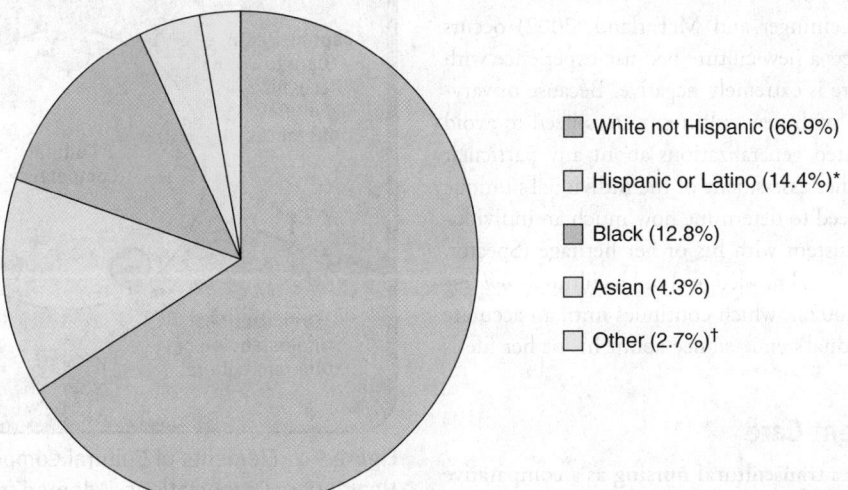

- White not Hispanic (66.9%)
- Hispanic or Latino (14.4%)*
- Black (12.8%)
- Asian (4.3%)
- Other (2.7%)†

Figure 9-1 Summary of U.S. Census Data. (Data from U.S. Census Bureau: *State and county quick facts*, 2007, http://quickfacts.census.gov/qfd/states/00000.html.)

*Hispanics may be of any race, so they also are included in applicable race categories; therefore total percentages reported are greater than 100%.
†Includes Native American, Alaska Native, Native Hawaiian, Pacific Islander, and people reporting two or more races.

ese, or Brazilian. Ethnicity is different from race, which is limited to the common biological attributes shared by a group such as skin color or blood type (Leininger and McFarland, 2002; Purnell and Paulanka, 2003). Examples of racial classifications include blacks and whites.

According to Purnell and Paulanka (2003), significant influences shape an individual's or group's worldview. Primary and secondary characteristics of culture are defined by the degree to which an individual identifies with his or her cultural group. Primary characteristics include nationality, race, gender, age, and religious beliefs. Secondary characteristics include socioeconomic and immigration status, residential patterns, personal beliefs and political orientation.

In any intercultural encounter, there is an insider or native perspective (emic worldview) and an outsider's perspective (etic worldview). For example, a Korean woman requests seaweed soup for her first meal after giving birth. This puzzles the nurse. Although the nurse has an emic view of professional postpartal care, as an outsider to the Korean culture, the nurse is not aware of the significance of the soup to the client. Conversely, the Korean client who has an etic view of American professional care assumes that seaweed soup is available in the hospital because it cleanses the blood and promotes healing and lactation (Korean health beliefs, 2003). Unless the nurse seeks the client's emic view, the nurse is likely to suggest other varieties of soups available from the dietary department, disregarding the cultural meaning of the practice to the client.

The processes of enculturation and acculturation facilitate cultural learning. Socialization into one's primary culture as a child is known as enculturation. The process of adapting to and adopting a new culture is acculturation (Barron and others, 2004; Cowan and Norman, 2006). Acculturation results in varying degrees of affiliation with the dominant culture. Assimilation results when an individual gradually adopts and incorporates the characteristics of the dominant culture (Purnell and Paulanka, 2003). Biculturalism (sometimes known as multiculturalism) occurs when an individual identifies equally with two or more cultures (Purnell and Paulanka, 1998).

Cultural backlash (Leininger and McFarland, 2002) occurs when an individual rejects a new culture because experience with a new or different culture is extremely negative. Because of varying degrees of affiliation with new cultures, nurses need to avoid stereotypes or unwarranted generalizations about any particular group that prevents further assessment of the individual's unique characteristics. Nurses need to determine how much an individual's life patterns are consistent with his or her heritage (Spector, 2002). Maintaining previous knowledge about a culture is *holding* knowledge (Leininger, 2002a), which continues until an accurate assessment of the individual's emic stance about his or her life is obtained.

Culturally Congruent Care

Leininger (2002a) defines transcultural nursing as a comparative study of cultures to understand similarities (culture universal) and differences (culture-specific) across human groups. The goal of transcultural nursing is culturally congruent care, or care that fits the person's valued life patterns and set of meanings. Patterns and meanings are generated from people themselves, rather than pre-

determined criteria. Culturally congruent care is sometimes different from the values and meanings of the professional health care system. Discovering clients' culture care values, meanings, beliefs, and practices as they relate to nursing and health care requires nurses to assume the role of learners and partner with clients and families in defining the characteristics of meaningful and beneficial care (Leininger, 2002b).

Culturally competent care requires specific knowledge, skills, and attitudes in the delivery of culturally congruent care. Pacquiao (2003a) identifies three distinct levels of cultural competence at the individual, organizational, and societal levels. Culturally competent care is the ability of a nurse to bridge cultural gaps in caring, work with cultural differences, and enable clients and families to achieve meaningful and supportive caring. Cultural competence is the synthesis of all three levels. Nurses need system-wide support to implement culturally congruent care. Culturally competent communities and societies are knowledgeable and skilled in using health care services and articulating their rights, as well as needs, to nurses and organizations. For example, a nurse who is aware of Gypsy culture and skilled in dealing with Gypsy families is not able to provide for their need to be present in groups near the bedside of a hospitalized family member. The nurse needs organizational support in adapting space resources to accommodate the volume of visitors who will remain with the client for long periods. Communities of Gypsies need to inform, negotiate, and demand accommodations for their caring patterns from hospital administration and staff.

Cultural Conflicts

Culture provides the context for valuing, evaluating, and categorizing life experiences. Cultural groups transmit their values, morals, and norms from one generation to another, which predisposes

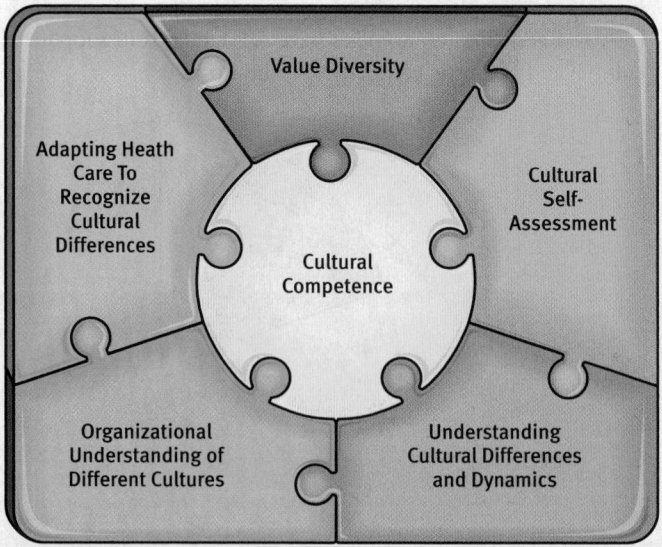

Figure 9-2 Elements of Cultural Competence Required in Health Care Organizations. Adopted from National Center for Cultural Competence: *Definitions of Cultural Competence*, http://www.nccccurricula.info/culturalcompetence.html

members to **ethnocentrism**, a tendency to hold one's own way of life as superior to others. Ethnocentrism is the cause of biases and prejudices that associate negative permanent characteristics with people who are different from the valued group. When a person acts on these prejudices, discrimination occurs. For example, a nurse refuses to give prescribed pain medication to a young African male with sickle cell anemia because of the belief (stereotyped bias) that young male Africans are likely to be drug abusers. Health care practitioners who have cultural ignorance or cultural blindness about differences generally resort to **cultural imposition** and use their own values and lifestyles as the absolute guide in dealing with clients and interpreting their behaviors. Hence, a nurse who believes that people should bear pain quietly as a demonstration of strong moral character will be annoyed when a client insists on having pain medication and will try to deny the client's discomfort.

Cultural Context of Health and Caring

Health, illness, and caring are unique to each culture (Kleinman, 1979; Leininger, 2002a). Culture is the context in which groups of people interpret and define their experiences relevant to life transitions. This includes events such as birth, illness, and dying. It is the system of meanings by which people make sense of their experiences. Culture is how others define social phenomena such as when a person is healthy or requires intervention. For example, in most African groups a thin body is a sign of poor health. In some Hispanic cultures a plump baby is healthy. Traditionally, in Arab culture, pregnancy is not a medical condition but rather a normal life transition; hence, a pregnant woman does not always go to a physician unless she has a problem (Kulwicki, 2003).

Table 9-1 provides a comparison of cultural contexts of health and illness in Western and non-Western cultures. Cultural beliefs highly influence what people believe to be the cause of illness. Many **Hmong** refugees (group of people who originated from the mountainous regions of Laos) believe that epilepsy or seizure disorder is caused by the wandering of the soul; hence treatment includes intervention by a **shaman** who performs the ritual to retrieve the client's soul (Fadiman, 1997; Helsel and others, 2005). Their belief is distinct from the scientifically determined neurological abnormality causing seizures. The biomedical orientation of Western cultures emphasizing scientific investigation and reducing the human body to distinct parts is in conflict with the holistic conceptualization of health and illness in non-Western cultures. Holism is evident in the belief in continuity between humans and nature, and between human events and metaphysical and magico-religious phenomena. Hence, for the Hmong people, epilepsy is connected to the magical and supernatural forces in nature. Establishing a diagnosis of epilepsy in Western cultures requires scientifically proven techniques and confirmed criteria for the abnormality. Such medical criteria are meaningless to the Hmong, who believe in the global causation of the illness that goes beyond the mind and body of the person to forces in nature. Whereas a Hmong will seek a shaman, a Westerner will seek a neurologist. A shaman has an established reputation in the Hmong community, whose qualifications for healing are neither determined by published standardized criteria nor confined to specific bodily systems. A shaman uses rituals symbolizing the supernatural, spiritual, and naturalistic modalities of prayers, herbs, and incense burning.

The dominant value orientation in North American society is individualism and self-reliance in achieving and maintaining health. Caring approaches generally promote the client's independence and ability for self-care. In collectivistic cultures that value group reliance and interdependence such as traditional Asians, Hispanics, and Africans, caring behaviors require actively providing physical and psychosocial support for family or community members. An adult client is not expected to be solely responsible for his or her care and well-being; rather, family and kin are relied

---

✳ TABLE 9-1 Comparative Cultural Contexts of Health and Illness

	WESTERN CULTURES	NON-WESTERN CULTURES
Cause of illness	Biomedical causes	Imbalance between humans and nature Supernatural Magico-religious
Method of diagnosis	Scientific, high-tech Specialty focused Organ-specific manifestations	Naturalistic, magico-religious Holistic Mixed Global, nonspecific symptomatology
Treatment	Specialty specific Pharmacological Surgery	Holistic Mixed (magico-religious, supernatural herbal, biomedical, etc.)
Practitioners/healers	Uniform standards and qualifications for practice	May be learned through apprenticeship Criteria for practice not uniform Reputation established in community
Caring pattern	Self-care Self-determination	Caring provided by others Group reliance and interdependence

Data from Foster G: Disease etiologies in non-Western medical systems, *Am Anthropol* 78:773,1976; Kleinman A: *Patients and healers in the context of culture*, Berkeley, 1979, University of California Press; and Leininger M, McFarland M: *Transcultural nursing: concepts, theories, research and practice*, ed 3, New York, 2002, McGraw-Hill.

upon to make decisions and provide for his or her care (Pacquiao, 2003b). For example, a traditional older Chinese woman refuses to independently perform rehabilitation exercises after hip surgery until her daughter is present. The Western health care provider interprets this as a lack of self-responsibility and motivation for her care. In contrast, the client interprets the nurse's insistence on self-care as uncaring behavior.

Cultural Healing Modalities and Healers

Foster (1976) has identified two distinct categories of healers cross-culturally. **Naturalistic practitioners** attribute illness to natural, impersonal, and biological forces that cause alteration in the equilibrium of the human body. Healing emphasizes use of naturalistic modalities including herbs, chemicals, heat, cold, massage, and surgery. In contrast, **personalistic practitioners** believe that an external agent, which can be human (i.e., sorcerer) or nonhuman (e.g., ghosts, evil, or deity), causes health and illness. Personalistic beliefs emphasize the importance of humans' relationship with others, both living and deceased, and with their deities. For example, a voodoo priest uses modalities that combine supernatural, magical, and religious beliefs through the active facilitation of an external agent or personalistic practitioner. A Haitian woman who believes in voodoo attributes her illness to a curse placed by someone and seeks the services of a voodoo priest to remove the cause. Personalistic approaches also include naturalistic modalities such as massage, aromatherapy, and herbs (see Chapter 36). Some clients seek both types of practitioners and use a combination of modalities to achieve health and treat illness. Different cultural groups in the United States use a variety of cultural healers (Table 9-2).

Because of coexisting and simultaneous use of both healing systems, avoid making rash judgments about clients' practices. Nurses need to gain knowledge and understanding of remedies used by clients to prevent cultural imposition. Many Southeast Asian cultures practice folk remedies such as coining, cupping, pinching, and burning to relieve aches and pains and remove bad wind or noxious elements that cause illness. Other groups, including Eastern Europeans, also use cupping as an acceptable treatment for respiratory ailments. These remedies leave peculiar visible markings on the skin in the form of ecchymosis, superficial burns, strap marks, or local tenderness. Cultural ignorance causes a practitioner to call authorities for suspicion of abuse. Different groups commonly use herbal therapy with some distinct differences from each other. Instead of dismissing the practice as dangerous and incompatible with Western medicine, nurses need to investigate whether the practice needs to be changed. Consultation and collaboration with herbalists and other naturalistic practitioners will prevent unnecessary distress for the client.

Culture-Bound Syndrome

Human groups create their own interpretation and descriptions of biological and psychological malfunctions within their unique social and cultural context (Kleinman, 1980). **Culture-bound syndromes** are illnesses that are specific to one culture. They are used to explain personal and social reactions of the culture's members. *Hwa-byung* is a Korean culture-bound syndrome observed among middle-age, low-income women who are overwhelmed and frustrated by the burden of caregiving for their in-laws, husbands, and children. Symptoms are generally somatic manifestations consist-

ing of insomnia, fatigue, anorexia, indigestion, feelings of an epigastric mass, palpitations, heat, panic, feelings of impending doom, and dyspnea. Women unconsciously avoid expressions of symptoms that counter the cultural ideal of females as the caretaker of elders, husbands, and children. Symptoms reflect the cultural definition of illness as imbalance between heat (yang) and cold (yin) (Purnell and Paulanka, 2003). In the United States these symptoms are defined as depression related to anger and are treated differently (American Psychological Association, 2000).

Culture and Life Transitions

Cultures generally mark transitions to different phases of life by rituals that symbolize cultural values and meanings attached to these life passages. Van Gennep (1960) originated the concept of **rites of passage** as significant social markers of changes in a person's life. Examining the practices surrounding these life events provides a view of the cultural meanings and expressions relevant to these transitions. Sending flowers and get-well greetings to a sick person is a ritual showing love and caring for the client in the Western world. In collectivistic groups such as the Hispanic culture, physical presence of loved ones with the client demonstrates caring. Whereas Americans value individual privacy, most Hispanics value group interdependence.

Pregnancy

All cultures value reproduction because it promotes continuity of the family and community. Pregnancy is generally associated with caring practices that symbolize the significance of this life transition in women. Infertility in a woman is considered grounds for divorce and rejection among Arabs. Pregnancy that occurs outside of accepted societal norms is generally taboo. Among traditional Muslims, pregnancy out of wedlock sometimes results in the family's imposing severe sanctions against the female member (Kulwicki, 2003).

Some cultures that subscribe to hot and cold theory of illness, such as the Hindus, view pregnancy as a hot state, so they encourage cold foods such as milk and milk products, yogurt, sour foods, and vegetables. They believe hot foods such as chilies, ginger, and animal products cause miscarriage and fetal abnormality. Modesty is a strong value among Afghan (Omeri and others, 2006) and Arab women (Kulwicki and others, 2005). These women sometimes avoid or refuse to be examined by male health care providers because of embarrassment. Religious beliefs sometimes interfere with prenatal testing, as in the case of a Filipino couple refusing amniocentesis because they believe that the outcome of pregnancy is God's will.

Childbirth

How individuals express pain and the expectation about how to treat suffering varies cross-culturally. Traditional Puerto Rican and Mexican women often vocalize their pain during labor and avoid breathing through their mouths because this will cause the uterus to rise (Zoucha and Purnell, 2003). Traditional Arab Americans are sometimes physically or verbally more expressive when experiencing pain (Kulwicki, 2003). Fear of drug addiction and the belief that pain is a form of spiritual atonement for one's past deeds motivate most Filipino mothers to tolerate pain without

✳ TABLE 9-2   Cultural Healers

Cultural Group	Healer	Nature of Practice
Chinese and Southeast Asians	Herbalist	Combination of plant, animal, and mineral products in restoring balance based on yin/yang concepts
	Acupuncturist	Yin treatment using needles to restore balance and flow of *qi*; yang treatment using moxibustion or heat with acupuncture may be indicated to restore yin/yang balance
	Fortune teller	Consultation to foretell outcomes of plans and seek spiritual advice to enhance good fortune and deal with misfortune
	Shaman	Combination of prayers, chanting, and herbs to treat illnesses caused by supernatural, psychological, and physical factors
Asian Indians	Ayurvedic practitioner	Combination of dietary, herbal, and other naturalistic therapies to prevent and treat illness
Native American	Shaman	Combination of prayers, chanting, and herbs to treat illnesses caused by supernatural, psychological, and physical factors
African American	Old lady "granny midwife"	Consultation in diagnosing and treating common illnesses and care of women in childbirth and children
	Spiritualist	Spiritual advisement, counseling, and prayers to treat illness or cope with personal and psychosocial problems
	Voodoo practitioners *Hougan* (male) *Mambo* (female)	Combination of herbs, drumming, and symbolic offerings to cure illness, remove curses, and protect a person
Hispanic	*Curandero/a*	Combination of prayers, herbs, and other rituals to treat traditional illnesses, especially in children
	Parteras Lay midwives	Assistance for women in childbirth and newborn care
	Yerbero Herbalist	Consultation for herbal treatment of traditional illnesses
	Sabador Bonesetters	Massage and manipulation of bones and joints used to treat a variety of ailments, including musculoskeletal conditions
	Espiritista Spiritualist	Foretelling of future and interpretation of dreams; combination of prayers, herbs, potions, amulets, and prayers for curing illnesses, including witchcraft
	Santero/a	Combination of prayers, symbolic offerings, herbs, potions, and amulets against witchcraft and curses

Data from Hautman MA: Folk health and illness beliefs, *Nurse Pract* 4(4):23, 1976; Loustaunau MO, Sobo EJ: *The cultural context of health, illness and medicine*, Westport, Conn, 1997, Bergin & Garvey; and Spector RE: *Cultural diversity in health and illness*, ed 6, Englewood Cliffs, NJ, 2004, Prentice Hall.

much complaining or asking for medication (Pacquiao, 2003b). Religious beliefs often prohibit the presence of males, including husbands, from the delivery room. This occurs among devout Muslims, Hindus, and Orthodox Jews (Kulwicki, 2003; Lewis, 2003; Selekman, 2003).

Health care providers other than physicians attend childbirth in some groups, such as *parteras* among Mexicans, grannies and herb doctors among Appalachian and southern African Americans, and *hilots* among Filipinos (Nelms and Gorski, 2006; Pacquiao, 2003b; Purnell, 2003; Shellman, 2004; Zoucher and Purnell, 2003). Known in their communities, these practitioners are affordable and accessible in remote areas. They use a combination of naturalistic, religious, and supernatural modalities combining herbs, massage, and prayers.

Newborn

The age of the child varies in some cultures. Among traditional Vietnamese and Koreans, a newborn is a year old at birth. Once acculturated to the U.S. culture, they assume a bicultural view,

deducting 1 year from the age of the child when speaking to an outsider. In the Yoruba tribes in Nigeria, the baby is named at the official naming ceremony that occurs 8 days after birth and coincides with circumcision. Many cultures around the world greatly celebrate the birth of a son, including Chinese, Asian Indians, Islamic groups, and **Igbos** in West Africa.

The name of the child reflects cultural values of the group. It is typical for a Hispanic baby to have several first names followed by the surnames of the father and mother (e.g., Maria Kristina Lourdes Lopez Vega). The bilineal tracing of descent from both the mother's and father's side in the Hispanic group differs from the patrilineal system, where the last name of the father precedes the child's first name. In the Chinese culture, individuals trace descent only from the paternal side. Hence the name Chen Lu means that Lu is the daughter of Mr. Chen.

Newborns and young children are often considered vulnerable, and many societies use a variety of ways to prevent harm to the child. Among the mostly Catholic Filipinos, parents keep the newborn inside the home until after the baptism to ensure the baby's health and protection. Traditional Arabs and Iranians believe babies are vulnerable to cold and wind; hence they wrap their babies in blankets.

Postpartum Period

In many non-Western cultures the postpartum period is associated with vulnerability of the mother to cold. To restore balance, mothers refuse a shower and prefer a sponge bath. Some groups have special dietary practices to restore balance. Cultural groups have preferences in terms of what types of foods are appropriate to restore balance in women after birth. Some Chinese mothers prefer soups, rice, rice wine, and eggs, whereas rural Iranian families provide pistachio nuts and eggs (Hafizi and Lipson, 2003; Wang, 2003). The length of the postpartum period is generally much longer (30 to 40 days) in non-Western cultures to provide support for the mother and her baby.

Filipino, Mexicans, and Pacific Islanders use an abdominal binder to prevent air from entering the woman's uterus and to promote healing (Purnell, 2003). Among Orthodox Jewish, Islamic, and Hindu cultures, bleeding is associated with pollution. A woman goes into a ritual bath after bleeding stops before she is able to resume relations with her husband (Hafizi and Lipson, 2003; Lewis, 2003). In some African cultures, such as in Ghana and Sierra Leone, some women will not resume sexual relations with their husbands until the baby is weaned.

Grief and Loss

Dying and death bring traditions that are meaningful to groups of people for most of their lives (see Chapter 30). When traditional medical measures fail, cultural beliefs and practices that are religious and spiritual become the focus. Societies assign different meanings to death of a child, a young person, and an older adult (Box 9-1). In Western cultures with strong future time orientation and where a child is expected to survive his or her parents, death of a young person is devastating. However, in other cultures, where infant mortality is very high, the emotional distress over a child's death is tempered by the reality of the commonly observed risks of growing up. Hence, untimely death of an adult is sometimes mourned more deeply.

Societies that believe in the concept of reincarnation, such as devout Hindus and Buddhists, view death as a step toward rebirth. Care of the dying focuses on supporting the client's preparation for a good death. The family will pray and read religious scriptures to the client to improve his or her chances in the next cycle. Buddhists generally believe that life is suffering and suffering ends when a person moves beyond the earthly desires and atones for past misdeeds. A dying Hindu male prepares for a good death by refusing nourishment and medications, concentrating all his energies on the spiritual aspects of the journey to the next cycle (Pacquiao, 2002).

Culture strongly influences pain expression and need for pain medication. Whereas a typical American believes in individual freedom and autonomy as synonymous with freedom from pain and suffering, other groups accept suffering. Do not assume that all people value pain relief equally. Clients suffer **cultural pain** when health care providers disregard their valued way of life (Leininger and McFarland, 2002). Inability of Orthodox Jews to pray in groups at the bedside with the dying client because of

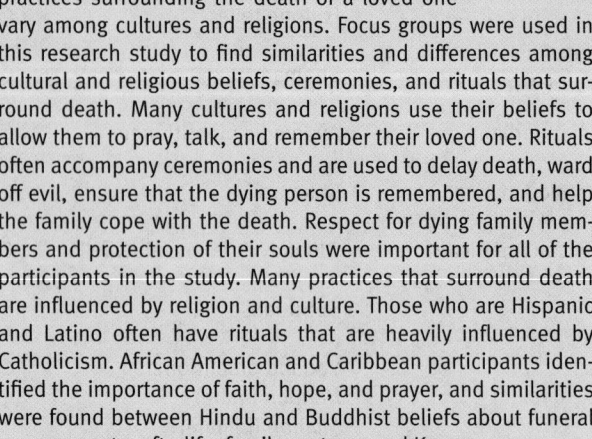

✳ BOX 9-1 **EVIDENCE-BASED PRACTICE**

Cultural Beliefs and Rituals Surrounding Death

Evidence Summary

Although culture and religion are important to people who are dying, as well as their families, practices surrounding the death of a loved one vary among cultures and religions. Focus groups were used in this research study to find similarities and differences among cultural and religious beliefs, ceremonies, and rituals that surround death. Many cultures and religions use their beliefs to allow them to pray, talk, and remember their loved one. Rituals often accompany ceremonies and are used to delay death, ward off evil, ensure that the dying person is remembered, and help the family cope with the death. Respect for dying family members and protection of their souls were important for all of the participants in the study. Many practices that surround death are influenced by religion and culture. Those who are Hispanic and Latino often have rituals that are heavily influenced by Catholicism. African American and Caribbean participants identified the importance of faith, hope, and prayer, and similarities were found between Hindu and Buddhist beliefs about funeral arrangements, afterlife, family customs and Karma.

Application to Nursing Practice

- Be aware of religious and cultural preferences when helping clients and families prepare for death.
- Ask families about the rituals and ceremonies they use to help them cope with the death of a loved one.
- Allow clients and families the ability to participate in planning which rituals will be done at the client's bedside.
- Be sensitive to cultural perceptions regarding organ donation, viewing the body, and preparing for burial.

Reference

Lobar SL and others: Cross-cultural beliefs, ceremonies, and rituals surrounding death of a loved one, *Pediatr Nurs 32*(1):44, 2006.

limitations in the number of visitors allowed causes cultural pain in the client and family. Working with the family and their religious/spiritual leader facilitates culturally congruent care (Pacquiao, 2003a).

Implement organizational policies intended to be sensitive to clients' cultural life patterns. The dominant value in American society of individual autonomy and self-determination is often in direct conflict with diverse groups. Advance directives, informed consent, and consent for hospice are examples of mandates that violate clients' values. Informed consent and advance directives protect the right of the individual to know and make decisions ensuring continuity of these rights even at the time when the individual is incapacitated. However, in other cultures, the group assumes decision making for a family member in these situations and is trusted to make the right decision for the individual. Indeed, some groups such as African Americans, Asian Americans, and Hispanics expect their family to make decisions for them, and family members prefer to protect the individual from unnecessary suffering by knowing the reality of imminent death. These cultures value group interdependence and view individual autonomy as an unnecessary burden for a loved one who is ill (Pacquiao, 2002, 2003a).

The meaning and expressions of grief vary from culture to culture. The color black is not always a symbol of grief. Hindu mourners wear white. Among the usually reserved East Asians, the extent to which mourners publicly express grief reflects the social position and status of the deceased. Korean families sometimes hire people to lead the open grieving. Loud crying and screaming is common.

Religious beliefs also affect attitudes toward cremation, organ donation, and the treatment of body parts. Devout Muslims refuse an autopsy or organ donation for fear of desecrating the dead and because of their belief that one has to be whole to appear in front of the creator. Many prefer burial over cremation (Kulwicki, 2003).

Cultural Assessment

Cultural assessment is a systematic and comprehensive examination of the cultural care values, beliefs, and practices of individuals, families, and communities. The goal of cultural assessment is to gather significant information from the client that will enable the nurse to implement culturally congruent care (Leininger and McFarland, 2002). There are several models for cultural assessment, each involving different levels of skill and knowledge. Leininger's Sunrise Model (2002a) in Figure 9-3 demonstrates the inclusiveness of culture in everyday life and helps to explain why cultural assessment needs to be comprehensive. The model assumes that cultural care values, beliefs, and practices are fixed in the cultural and social structural dimensions of society, which include environmental context, language, and ethnohistory. **Ethnohistory** refers to significant historical experiences of a particular group. For example, the experience with the Great Depression of older Americans has resulted in their tendency to be frugal and to save everything. Encourage clients to share stories about their lives. These stories reveal the broad picture of who they are and the cultural lifestyle they embrace. Leininger's model differentiates folk care, which is caring as defined by the people, from the health care professions, which is based on the scientific, biomedical caring system.

Census Data

A nurse begins cultural assessment by knowing population demographic changes in the community setting of practice. Having background knowledge of a culture assists the nurse in conducting a focused assessment. Gather demographics from the local and regional census data, as well as from the demographic breakdown of clients who come to the health care setting. Population demographics include the distribution of ethnic groups, education, occupations, and incidence of the most common illnesses. Comprehensive cultural assessment requires skill and time; hence preparation and anticipation of need are important.

Asking Questions

One problem in cultural assessment is the lack of ability to assess the insider or emic perspective of the clients and interpret the information during the assessment. It helps to use open-ended, focused, and contrast questions. The aim is to encourage clients to describe values, beliefs, and practices that are significant to their care that health care providers will take for granted unless otherwise uncovered. Culturally oriented questions are by nature broad and require a lot of descriptions (Box 9-2).

Establishing Relationships

In contrast to other types of interviews, cultural assessment is intrusive and time consuming and requires a trusting relationship between participants. Miscommunication commonly occurs in intercultural interactions. This is due to language and communication differences between and among participants, as well as differences in interpreting each other's behaviors. Skill in impression management is essential for nurses. It is based on the nurse's ability to interpret the client's behavior within his or her own context of meanings and to behave in a culturally congruent way. In a sense, it is managing the impression the nurse makes on the client to achieve desired outcomes of communication (Pacquiao, 2000). Impression management requires linguistic skills, culturally congruent interpretation of behaviors of others, listening, and observation skills. In cultural assessment the goal is to generate knowledge about the client's values, beliefs, and practices about nursing and health care. If the nurse's behavior is offensive to the client, he or she will not likely participate in the interaction. Box 9-3 provides the general rules of impression management with specific recommendations for working with interpreters.

Interpreters are more effective when they have knowledge of the dialect spoken by the client. For example, although the Chinese use the same words, people from different regions of China speak the words using different dialects (Purnell and Paulanka, 2003). Upon admission, assess and document language(s) clients speak and write and determine if clients need an interpreter. Federal mandates for culturally competent health care delivery require accommodation for language differences. Nurses need to know their agencies' policies and procedures regarding these mandates. Working with interpreters and clients with little or no fluency in English requires skill development. Try to attend educational programs and practice applications of principles of impression management before an actual client encounter. In hospital settings use an interpreter to communicate information about the client's medical condition. It is not suitable for family members to translate health care information, but they can assist with ongoing interaction during the client's care.

Consider what needs to be discussed with a client when selecting an interpreter. In some Hispanic and Asian groups, a woman's private parts are not generally discussed with members of the opposite sex, including male members of one's family. In societies where adults occupy higher status than the young, a child interpreter is sometimes regarded as disrespectful. With immigrant groups, children learn the English language faster than their parents because of their schooling experience in the new culture when they immigrate at a young age. However, assuming that children are ideal interpreters for their parents is in fact an insult to the authority of the elder who has to take directions from a child.

Compatibility between the ethnic backgrounds of the interpreter and client is another consideration to facilitate trust. An Israeli interpreter will possibly cause much anxiety and distrust in a Palestinian immigrant who experienced violence from these

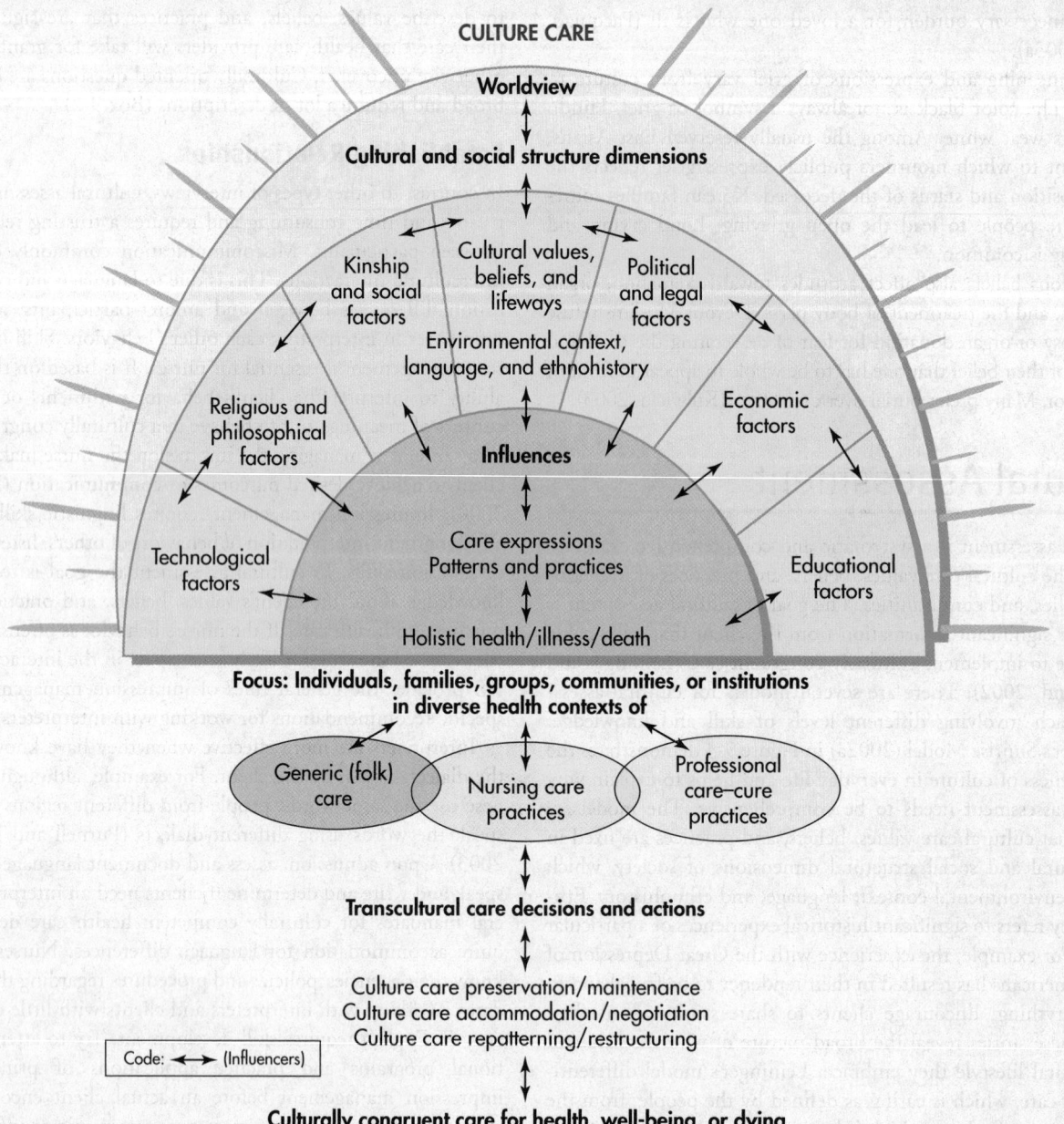

Figure 9-3 Leininger's culture care theory and Sunrise Model. (Reprinted with permission from Leininger MM, McFarland MR: *Transcultural nursing: concepts, theories, research and practice,* ed 3, New York, 2002a, McGraw-Hill.)

groups in the home country. Socioeconomic and educational differences between interpreters and clients sometimes become barriers to effective interpretation. Interpreters need training not only in interpretation but also in knowing their role to repeat back what the client said without making judgment about the content.

Selected Components of Cultural Assessment

Nurses learn various skills needed to gather an accurate and comprehensive cultural assessment over time. The following components of cultural assessment provide insight into the type of information that can be useful in planning and delivering nursing care.

Ethnic Heritage and Ethnohistory. Knowledge of a client's country of origin and its history and ecological contexts are significant to health care. For example, Haitian immigrants have linguistic and communication patterns distinct from those of Jamaicans, though they both come from the Caribbean and have a common history of slavery. Differences come from their colonial history and intermingling with the local indigenous people. Because of cultural differences between India and Jamaica, Hindu immigrants from Jamaica have different cultural characteristics from those originating from India. Hindu immigrants from Jamaica often have nutritional, communication, and health patterns more similar to African Jamaicans than South Asian Hindus. In giving care for an Indian Hindu who grew up in Jamaica, expect

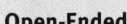

Open-Ended
- What do you think caused your illness?
- How do you want us to help you with your problem?

Focused
- Did you have this problem before?
- Is there someone you want us to talk to about your care?

Contrast
- How different is this problem from the one you had previously?
- What is the difference between what we are doing from what you think we should be doing for you?

Ethnohistory
- How long have you/your parents resided in this country?
- What is your ethnic background or ancestry?
- How strongly does your culture influence you?
- Tell me why you left your homeland.

Social Organization
- Who lives with you?
- Who do you consider members of your family?
- Where do other members of your family live?
- Who makes the decisions for you or your family?
- Who do you go to outside of your family for support?
- What expectations do you have of your family members who are males, females, old, or young?

Socioeconomic Status
- What do you do for a living?
- How different is your life here from back home?

Biocultural Ecology and Health Risks
- What caused your problem?
- How does this problem affect or how has it affected your life and your family?
- How do you treat this problem at home?
- What other problems do you have?

Language and Communication
- What language(s) do you speak at home?
- What language(s) do you use to read and write?
- How should we address or call you?
- What kinds of communication upset or offend you?

Caring Beliefs and Practices
- What do you do to keep yourself well?
- What do you do to show someone you care?
- How do you take care of sick family members?
- Which caregivers do you seek when you are sick?
- How different is what we do from what your family does for you when you are sick?

✳ BOX 9-3   **Rules of Impression Management**

1. Greet clients and their visitors in their own language if possible.
2. Introduce yourself. Tell clients what to call you.
3. Welcome visitors, and request them to introduce themselves and explain how they are related to client.
4. Thank the visitors for coming.
5. Request to talk with client in private, and offer to accompany visitors to the waiting room.
6. Inform visitors that you will get them when you finish with the client.
7. Tell client your purpose.
8. Clarify if client wants someone else, like a family member, to be present.
9. Avoid asking client questions in front of family or spouse that will put him or her at risk with this group.
10. If client needs an interpreter:
    a. Introduce yourself to the interpreter.
    b. Determine qualifications of interpreter.
       (1) Make sure that interpreter can speak the dialect of the client.
       (2) Ensure gender, age, and ethnic compatibility of interpreter with client's preference and topic of discussion.

    (3) Watch for differences in educational and socioeconomic status between client and interpreter.
    (4) Orient interpreter to your purpose and expectation (e.g., assessment of the client's level of pain, intent to explain procedure to client).
  c. Clarify your questions about the interpreter's training, compatibility with the client, and interpreter's understanding of your expectations beforehand.
  d. Introduce the interpreter to the client.
  e. Pace your speech slowly, and allow time for back translation.
  f. Direct your questions to the client.
  g. Request interpreter to ask client for feedback and clarification at regular intervals.
  h. Observe client's nonverbal and verbal behaviors.
  i. Thank both client and interpreter.
11. Ask client whom you will need to consult with for major decisions and how to contact this person.
12. Observe nonverbal behavior, and match degree of distance exhibited by client.

the client to interact more like a Jamaican even though the person looks like he or she is from south India.

People immigrate to another country for various reasons and have different motivations for acculturating to the new country. Refugees are relocated without any choice in their initial resi-

dence, in contrast to immigrants, who have options as to where they go. Refugees experience greater dislocation and deprivation than immigrants who enter a new country with specialized skills and education and have the option to return to their homeland. Age of immigration often determines the level of acculturation, with younger immigrants acculturating faster than older immigrants. Similarities shared by an immigrant group with the dominant culture in society are strong predictors of assimilation. Experiences of white European immigrants differ from those of nonwhite immigrants from Europe and other continents (Svetlana and others, 2006). Although acculturation and length of residence in the new culture are related, other factors such as education, racial characteristics, and familiarity with the language and religion affect the extent of a person's acculturation. Ask clients about the condition or situation that brought them to the United States and how they feel they are adjusting. The nurse needs to understand any problems (such as becoming comfortable with the language or the routines used to set medical appointments) in order to make reasonable and appropriate adjustments to care.

Socioeconomic status in the new society is often not comparable to one's previous status in the country of origin. New immigrants begin with small resources but often keep the values and desires of their previous status. It is important for a nurse to explore the background of the client such as preimmigration and postimmigration status, available resources for medical coverage, health risks in the new environment, and availability of support systems.

Biocultural History. Identify clients' health risks related to sociocultural and biological history on admission. Some distinct health risks are due to the ecological context of the culture. For example, immigrants originating from the region near the Nile River are generally at risk for parasitic infestations that are prevalent in that area. Immigrants from the Third World with poor sanitary conditions and water supply are at risk for infections such as hepatitis. Certain genetic disorders are also linked with specific ethnic groups, such as Tay-Sachs among Ashkenazi Jews and malignant hypertension among African Americans. Lactose intolerance is frequently observed among Asians, Africans, and Hispanics (USDHHS, Office of Minority Health, n.d.).

Social Organization. Cultural groups consist of units of organization defined by kinship, status, and appropriate roles for their members. In the dominant American society the most common unit of social organization is the nuclear family where married children and adults establish separate residences from their parents. Although different configurations of a family exist, the most common is the nuclear household made up of parents and their young children (see Chapter 10). In collectivistic cultures, families are made up of distant blood relatives across three generations and **fictive** or nonblood kin. Kinship extends to both the father's and mother's side of the family (**bilineal**) or is limited to the side of either father (**patrilineal**) or mother (**matrilineal**). Patrilineally extended families exist among Chinese and Hindus, where a woman moves into her husband's clan after marriage and minimizes ties with her own parents and siblings. Consider all options when determining a client's next of kin. This is especially relevant to new immigrants and refugees, who often have not relocated with all members of their family. Collectivistic groups often regard members of their ethnic group as closest kin and want to consult them for health care decisions, as well as permit them to speak on their behalf.

A client's status within the social hierarchy is generally linked with qualities such as age and gender, as well as achieved status such as education and position. The dominant culture in the United States emphasizes achievement as the determinant of status, whereas most collectivistic cultures give higher priority to age and gender. The eldest male is next to his father in terms of authority in many Asian and African cultures. A Korean mother is subject to the authority of her oldest son in the absence of her husband. Sometimes adult Hispanic women will not sign informed consent for surgery or other medical procedures without consulting their husband, oldest son, or brothers. Older adults generally occupy higher status in some societies, resulting in grandparents forcing their decisions over their married children regarding the care of the grandchildren. Nurses determine who has authority for making decisions within the family and how to communicate with the proper individuals.

Culture defines the expected roles of its members. Certain behaviors are acceptable in children but not in adults. Gender also differentiates role expectations. For example, among devout Muslims, females perform the task of caregiving, whereas males are the financial providers and major decision makers. Thus nurses need to anticipate that some Muslim women will insist on staying at the bedside of their children, in-laws, or husbands. However, do not assume that just because the woman is the primary caregiver she will make decisions independently. Determine the family social hierarchy as soon as possible to prevent offending clients and their families. Working with established family hierarchy prevents delays and achieves better client outcomes.

Religious and Spiritual Beliefs. Religious and spiritual beliefs are major influences in the client's worldview about health and illness, pain and suffering, and life and death. Many cultures do not separate religion and spirituality, whereas others have a totally distinct concept of spirituality. Nurses need to understand the emic perspective of their clients. To a Hmong animist, spirits are dead ancestors or forces external to the person. To some Americans, spirituality means an inner, personal relationship with God. Although it is sometimes difficult to find the appropriate time to discuss religion and spirituality in a hospital setting, nurses need to assess what is important to the spiritual well-being of clients and learn as much as possible about clients' spiritual and religious practices (see Chapter 29).

Devout Muslims pray five times daily and undergo an obligatory ritual cleansing of some parts of their body before praying. Nurses need to anticipate the ritual cleansing needs of the client and provide privacy for praying. For example, reschedule diagnostic procedures so that Buddhist clients are able to participate in the festivities of their New Year. Anticipating the needs of Jewish clients during **Sabbath,** when they refrain from using electrical appliances, requires creative accommodations by the staff such as placing articles of care near the client so he or she need not use the call light or telephone to get assistance. Nurses can also send consent for emergency surgeries by facsimile to the **rabbi,** who will then contact the client's next of kin unreachable by telephone during Sabbath.

Religious beliefs are evident in clients' dietary practices (Box 9-4). Devout Hindus avoid beef, and many are vegetarians. Many

Buddhists are vegetarians. *Halal* foods, which include meat, fish, fresh fruit, vegetables, eggs, milk, and cheese, are permissible for Muslims. Halal meat comes from animals slaughtered during a prayer ritual. Prohibited, or *Haram,* foods include non-Halal meat, animals with fangs, pork products, gelatin products, and alcohol (Akhtar, 2002). Muslims fast during the daylight hours for the 28 days of *Ramadan,* which occurs during the ninth lunar month. Although children and sick and frail individuals are exempt from fasting, do not assume that these individuals will eat regular meals during Ramadan. Rescheduling of treatments and medications is often necessary to prevent complications such as hypoglycemia.

Jewish clients who follow a **kosher** diet will avoid meat from carnivores, pork products, and fish without scales or fins. Kosher meat comes from permissible animals that are slaughtered with the least amount of suffering. Kosher foods must not be contaminated by nonkosher foods. Hence meat is served separately from dairy, and dishes used for serving and eating these products are also separated (Selekman, 2003).

The nursing staff needs to have background information available about major holy days and practices for commonly encountered religions. Such information prevents scheduling nonemergency treatments and procedures on major holy days such as the Jewish Yom Kippur, Rosh Hashanah, or Passover. Religious mandates followed by Jehovah's Witnesses require followers to have bloodless surgery and to avoid blood transfusions. Nurses need to identify and contact clients' religious and spiritual leaders before problems occur. Nurses work with these leaders to mediate in times of crisis. On admission, nurses obtain this information from their clients or their clients' families.

Life transitions are often manifested in religious and spiritual beliefs. Several examples follow. Male circumcision occurs among Jewish and Islamic groups. Female circumcision is common among some African and Muslim groups. Anointing of the sick is a Roman Catholic sacrament. Hospitalized Catholic clients often receive daily communion. The family of a critically ill Jewish client will turn his or her head eastward or to the right side. The family of a dying Hindu remains at the bedside to place a drop of the holy water from the River Ganges on the client's lips immediately after death to help his or her soul to the next life. A dying Hispanic client will not be left alone so that a close kin is able to hear the client's wishes, allowing the soul to leave in peace.

Communication Patterns. Different cultural groups have distinct linguistic and communication patterns. These patterns reflect core cultural values of a society. In the dominant American culture that supports individualism, people value assertive communication because it manifests the ideal of individual autonomy and self-determination. In collectivistic cultures the context of relationships among participants shapes communication. Promoting group harmony is a priority, so participants interact based on their expected positions and relationships within the social hierarchy. Individuals are more likely to remain respectful and show deference to older adults or family leaders, even though they disagree on an issue. Differences in status and position, age, gender, and outsider versus insider determine the content and process of communication (Box 9-5). Among Asian cultures, face-saving

---

✳ BOX 9-4   **CLIENT TEACHING**

Cultural Considerations in Healthy Food Choices

Objective
- Client will verbalize healthy foods that are culturally appropriate.

Teaching Strategies
- Refer client to speak with a dietitian who is familiar with cultural food choices.
- Develop a diet plan that includes client's cultural diet preferences.
- Provide culturally sensitive teaching brochures that describe healthy food choices.
- Include people in family who help shop for and prepare food in the home.

Evaluation
- Ask client to keep a food diary for 1 week and evaluate food choices.
- Ask client to describe how cultural food choices will fit within the client's prescribed diet.

---

communication promotes harmony by indirect, ambiguous communication and conflict avoidance. In this culture, messages spoken often have little to do with their meanings. Saying "no" to a superior or older person is not permissible, hence an affirmative response will only mean "I heard you" rather than full agreement. This is likely to happen in a health care setting because a health care provider is perceived as a person of authority to some Asian, African, or Hispanic clients. Observing a client's behavior and clarifying messages heard from a trusted insider will prevent misinterpretation.

In cultural groups with distinct linear hierarchy, negotiation of conflict occurs between persons within the same level of position or authority. Identifying and working with established family hierarchy will prevent miscommunication. In cultures with highly differentiated gender roles, some clients place more value on the advice of a man than a woman. By recognizing and working within this cultural context, nurses become more effective in achieving outcomes.

Culture also shapes nonverbal communication. Culture influences the distance between participants in an interaction, the degree of eye contact, the extent of touching, and how much private information the client will share. Clients use less distance when speaking to trusted insiders and persons of the same age, gender, and position in the social hierarchy. Many ethnic groups tend to speak their own dialect with insiders for ease and privacy and as a marker of insider status. To minimize this distance when communicating with clients, nurses need to establish rapport and behave in a culturally congruent manner through impression management.

Time Orientation

All cultures have past, present, and future time dimensions. It is important for nurses to understand their clients' time orientation. This information is useful in planning a day of care, setting up appointments for procedures, and helping a client plan self-care

✳ BOX 9-5   FOCUS ON OLDER ADULTS

Culturally Sensitive Communication

- Ask older adults how they like to be addressed. If in doubt, address them formally
  (e.g., Mr. Lin).
- Determine client's preferences for touch. For
  example, in the United States, Americans often greet each other with a firm handshake. However, many
  Native Americans see this as a sign of aggression, and
  touch outside of marriage is sometimes forbidden in older
  adults from the Middle East.
- Investigate the client's preferences for silence. Generally,
  Eastern cultures value silence, whereas Western cultures
  are uncomfortable with silence.
- Be aware of the client's beliefs about eye contact during
  conversation. Direct eye contact in European American cultures is a sign of honesty and truthfulness. However, eye
  contact with other groups, such as older Native Americans,
  is not allowed. Older Asian adults sometimes avoid eye
  contact with authority figures because this is considered
  disrespectful, and direct eye contact between genders in
  Middle Eastern cultures is sometimes forbidden except between spouses.

Data from Meiner SE, Leuckenotte AG: *Gerontologic nursing*, ed 3,
St. Louis, 2006, Mosby.

activities in the home. Differences exist in the dimensions of time that cultures emphasize and the manner of expressing time. Communication patterns reflect time orientation. Future time orientation minimizes present time, so communication tends to be direct and focused on task achievement. Business time is separate and distinct from social time. This is the norm in the dominant American culture. In contrast, collectivistic cultures emphasize past and present times to preserve social hierarchy and promote group harmony. Communication is circular and indirect to avoid risks of offending and disrespecting others. These cultures often emphasize social time and mix it with business time. Rushed, hurried, and businesslike communication appears uncaring or disrespectful. This is true with Mexican-Americans, who tend to trust *(confianza)* caregivers who interact with them in a personalistic *(personalismo),* warm, friendly *(simpatia),* and respectful *(respeto)* manner (Zoucha and Purnell, 2003).

Present time orientation is in conflict with the dominant organizational norm in health care that emphasizes punctuality and adherence to appointments. Nurses need to expect conflicts and make adjustments when caring for ethnic groups. Improving a client's access to health services mandates culturally congruent time schedules that accommodate his or her cultural patterns. When making appointments and referrals, explore and manage anticipated barriers to time adherence with the client. For organizational accommodation to occur, nurses need to seek clients' participation and to advocate for clients in recommending changes.

Caring Beliefs and Practices

It is very helpful for nurses to apply clients' and families' concepts of meaningful and supportive care (see Chapter 8) into intervention approaches. Caring expressions integrate the central values of a culture. In collectivistic cultures, caring means active involvement of the group, emphasizing mutual and reciprocal obligations of members to care for each other. When you care for a client, look for ways this type of family can participate in basic care activities. Nurses need to adopt caring practices; work with clients' families as a group, understanding their social hierarchy; and assume a collaborative role with clients and their families.

Many integrate religious and spiritual beliefs in caring practices. For example, African American churches take an active role in caring for their community members. Gender-congruent care is a strong value among Islamics, Orthodox Jews, Hindus, and other groups emphasizing female modesty. Culture differentiates caring roles of males and females. In many cultures, caretaking tasks are the primary responsibility of women, whereas men provide financial support and make major decisions. Age and position in the social hierarchy also influence caring roles and responsibilities. In some cultures, older women are the first group consulted during illness of family members and in the care of women and children.

Obtain information about folk remedies and cultural healers the client uses. Assessment data yields information about the client's beliefs about the illness and the meaning of the signs and symptoms. Focus assessment on the emic perspective of the client. Allowing the client to describe the meanings of care and identify caring behaviors is fundamental to culturally congruent care. Studies conducted with approximately 100 Western and non-Western cultures identified several recurrent caring constructs, which are presented below in priority of dominant rankings in meanings and actions of care (Leininger and McFarland, 2002):

- Respect for and about the client
- Concern for and about the client
- Attention to details/in anticipation of client needs
- Helping/assisting or facilitative acts
- Active listening
- Presence (being physically there)
- Understanding (beliefs, values, lifestyles, and environmental context)
- Connectedness
- Protection (gender related)
- Touching
- Comfort measures

This list represents major care meanings and expressions as defined by the people studied. Use this list to guide behaviors when caring for clients from different cultures.

Experience With Professional Health Care

Understanding the emic perspective of the client about professional health care is valuable in correcting misconceptions and preventing culturally offensive actions. Previous encounters with professional caregivers have enormous implications for adherence to therapies and continuing access of services by clients. For example, if a client has had past problems with male caregivers, be sure female caregivers are the sole provider. If a client perceives a health care resource is inaccessible or not useful, become an intermediary and advocate to find a way the client and resource can connect. Partnership between professionals and the community provides proactive and open feedback from culturally diverse client groups. Use of comparative assessment questions gives nurses insight into clients' perceptions and reactions to different aspects of the health care system. This is an essential step in eventual outcomes evaluation.

Nursing Decisions

Leininger (1991) identified three nursing decision and action modes to achieve culturally congruent care. All three modes of professional decisions and actions assist, support, facilitate, or enable people of particular cultures.

1. **Cultural care preservation or maintenance**—Retain and/or preserve relevant care values so that clients maintain their well-being, recover from illness, or face handicaps and/or death.
2. **Cultural care accommodation or negotiation**—Adapt or negotiate with others for a beneficial or satisfying health outcome.
3. **Cultural care repatterning or restructuring**—Reorder, change, or greatly modify clients' lifestyles for a new, different, and beneficial health care pattern.

Nurses are able to use any or all of these action modes simultaneously. These actions require that nurses have knowledge of clients' culture and have the willingness, commitment, and skills to work with clients and families in decision making. The intended outcome of these actions and decisions is meaningful, supportive, and facilitative care as judged by the client.

Key Concepts

- Culture is the context for interpreting human experiences such as health and illness and provides direction to decisions and actions.
- Culturally congruent care is meaningful, supportive, and facilitative because it fits valued life patterns of clients. Nurses achieve culturally congruent care through cultural assessment and the application of cultural preservation, accommodation, and repatterning.
- Culturally competent care requires knowledge, attitudes, and skills supportive of implementation of culturally congruent care.
- Cultural assessment requires a comprehensive and thorough investigation of a client's cultural values, beliefs, and practices.
- Transcultural nursing is a comparative study and understanding of cultures to identify specific and universal caring constructs across cultures.
- Impression management facilitates culturally congruent communication and intercultural relationships.

Critical Thinking Exercises

A young Mexican mother remains at the bedside of her 3-year-old daughter who has been diagnosed with croup and is inside an oxygen tent. Early in the morning the attending physician, Dr. Lopez, who is also Mexican, calls the nurses' station to tell the mother to keep the baby in the oxygen tent because her oxygen saturation level is dropping. The nurse informs the mother of the physician's instructions and tells her to give plenty of clear liquids to her daughter. Each time the nurse gives the mother a bottle juice for the baby, the mother immediately goes to the bathroom to heat the bottle under running hot water. The mother later communicates to another nurse, who speaks Spanish, that cold is bad for the child's lungs, so at night she takes her daughter out of the oxygen tent.

1. Explain the rationale for the mother's actions.
2. Identify alternative nursing interventions to help the mother to comply with medical instructions.
3. Of the three nursing decisions and action modes described by Leininger, explain which one is the most appropriate for this client.

NCLEX®-Style Review Questions

1. Maria is a 6-year-old child from Mexico. Maria's socialization into the Mexican culture is best described as:
   1. Assimilation
   2. Acculturation
   3. Biculturalism
   4. Enculturation

2. A 46-year-old woman from Bosnia came to the United States 6 years ago. Although she did not celebrate Christmas when she lived in Bosnia, she celebrates Christmas with her family now. This woman has experienced assimilation into the culture of the United States because she:
   1. Choose to be bicultural
   2. Adapted to and adopted the American culture
   3. Had an extremely negative experience with the American culture
   4. Gave up part of her ethnic identity in favor of the American culture

3. Brooke is a nursing student. In order for Brooke to enhance her cultural awareness, she will need to make an in-depth self-examination of her:
   1. Motivation and commitment to caring
   2. Social, cultural, and biophysical factors
   3. Engagement in cross-cultural interactions
   4. Background, recognizing her biases and prejudices

4. Cultural competence is the process of:
   1. Learning about vast cultures
   2. Motivation and commitment to caring
   3. Influencing treatment and care of clients
   4. Acquiring specific knowledge, skills, and attitudes

5. Ken is an RN caring for Mr. DeRosa. Ken has determined Mr. DeRosa is from Russian heritage. Ken has a Russian neighbor who does not keep his property well maintained. Ken tells Mr. DeRosa, "While you are in the rehabilitation center, you will keep your bedside area organized." Ken's statement is an example of:
   1. Assimilation
   2. Ethnocentrism
   3. Personalistic practice
   4. Culture bound syndrome

6. When action is taken on one's prejudices:
   1. Discrimination occurs
   2. Delivery of culturally congruent care is ensured
   3. Effective intercultural communication develops
   4. Sufficient comparative knowledge of diverse groups is obtained

7. Jane is a nursing student who is doing her community health rotation in an inner-city public health department. When she investigates sociodemographic and health data of the people served by the health department, Jane detects disparities in health outcomes between the rich and poor. This is an example of a(n):
   1. Illness attributed to natural and biological forces
   2. Creation of Jane's interpretation and descriptions of the data
   3. Influence of socioeconomic factors in morbidity and mortality
   4. Combination of naturalistic, religious, and supernatural modalities

8. Culture strongly influences pain expression and need for pain medication. However, cultural pain:
   1. Is not expressed verbally or physically
   2. Is expressed only to others of like culture
   3. Is more intense, thus necessitating more medication
   4. May be suffered by a client whose valued way of life is disregarded by practitioners

9. The dominant values in American society on individual autonomy and self-determination:
   1. Do not have an effect on health care
   2. Rarely have an effect on other cultures
   3. May be in direct conflict with diverse groups
   4. May hinder ability to get into hospice programs

10 | Caring for Families

Mastery of the content in this chapter will enable the student to:

- Discuss how the term *family* reflects family diversity.
- Examine current trends in the American family.
- Explain how the relationship between family structure and patterns of functioning affect the health of individuals within the family and the family as a whole.
- Discuss the way family members influence one another's health.

- Discuss the role of families and family members as caregivers.
- Interpret external and internal factors that promote family health.
- Compare family as context to family as client and explain the way these perspectives influence nursing practice.
- Use the nursing process to provide for the health care needs of the family.

MEDIA RESOURCES ✳ KEY TERMS

 Companion CD
- NCLEX®-Style Review Questions
- Audio Glossary
- Interactive Learning Activities
- English/Spanish Glossary

 Website
- NCLEX®-Style Review Questions
- Audio Glossary
- English/Spanish Glossary
- Interactive Learning Activities
- WebLinks
- Audio Summaries

Family, p. 122
Family as client, p. 128
Family as context, p. 128
Family as system, p. 128

Family forms, p. 122
Hardiness, p. 127
Reciprocity, p. 133
Resiliency, p. 127

The Family

The **family** is a central institution in American society; however, the concept, structure, and functioning of the family unit continue to change over time. Although the family is in transition and looks very different from the families of the 1950s, the family unit is here to stay. Families face many challenges, including the effects of health and illness, childbearing and child rearing, changes in family structure and dynamics, and caring for older parents. Family characteristics or attributes, such as durability, resiliency, and diversity, help families adapt to these challenges (Ford-Gilboe, 2002; Hanson and others, 2005).

Family durability is the term for the intrafamilial system of support and structure that extends beyond the walls of the household. For example, the parents may remarry or the children may or may not leave home as adults, but in the end the "family" transcends long periods and inevitable lifestyle changes.

Family resiliency is the ability of the family to cope with expected and unexpected stressors. The family's ability to adapt to role changes, developmental milestones, and crises shows resilience. The goal of the family is not only to survive "the challenge," but also to thrive and to grow as a result of the newly gained knowledge.

Family diversity is the uniqueness of each family unit. For example, some families will experience marriage for the first time and have children in later life, when others are grandparents at the same age. Every person within a family unit has specific needs, strengths, and important developmental considerations.

As you care for clients and their families, you are responsible for understanding family dynamics (e.g., the family makeup [configuration], structure, function, and coping capacity of the family) and then building on the family's relative strengths and resources (Feeley and Gottlieb, 2000). The goal of family-centered nursing care is to promote, support, and provide for the well-being and health of the family and individual family members (Astedt-Kurki and others, 2002; Joronen and Astedt-Kurki, 2005).

Concept of Family

The term *family* brings to mind a visual image of adults and children living together in a satisfying, harmonious manner. For some, this term has the opposite image. Families represent more than a set of individuals, and a family is more than a sum of its individual members (Astedt-Kurki and others, 2001). Families are as diverse as the individuals that compose them, and clients have deeply ingrained values about their families that deserve respect. You need to understand how your clients define their family. Think of the **family** as a set of relationships that the client identifies as family or as a network of individuals who influence each other's lives whether or not there are actual biological or legal ties.

Definition: What Is a Family?

Defining family initially appears to be a simple undertaking. However, different definitions result in heated debates among social scientists and legislators. The definition of family is significant and affects who is included on health insurance policies, who has access to children's school records, who files joint tax returns,

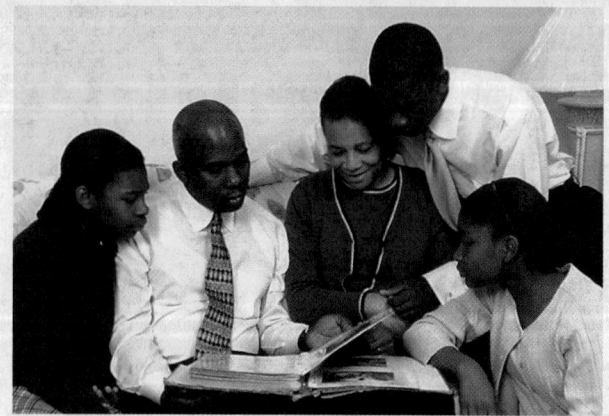

Figure 10-1 Family celebrations and traditions strengthen the role of the family.

and who is eligible for sick-leave benefits or public assistance programs. The family is defined biologically, legally, or as a social network with personally constructed ties and ideologies. For some clients, family includes only persons related by marriage, birth, or adoption. To others, aunts, uncles, close friends, cohabitating persons, and even pets are family. Your personal beliefs do not have to be the same as your client's beliefs. Understand that families take many forms and have diverse cultural and ethnic orientations (Figure 10-1). In addition, no two families are alike. Each has its own strengths, weaknesses, resources, and challenges (Bell and others, 2001).

Current Trends and New Family Forms

Family forms are patterns of people considered by family members to be included in the family. Although all families have some things in common, each family form has unique problems and strengths. Maintain an open mind about what makes up a family so that you do not overlook potential resources and concerns (Box 10-1).

Although the institution of the family remains strong, the family itself is changing. The "typical" family (two biological parents and children) is no longer the norm. People are marrying later, women are delaying childbirth, and couples are choosing to have fewer children or none at all. The number of people living alone is expanding rapidly and represents approximately 26% of all households. Divorce rates have tripled since the 1950s, and although the rate appears to have stabilized, it is now estimated that 55% of marriages will end in divorce (U.S. Census Bureau, 2001). The median interval between divorce and remarriage is about 3 years. Remarriage often results in a blended family with a complex set of relationships among stepparents, stepchildren, half brothers and sisters, and extended family members.

Marital roles are also more complex as families increasingly comprise two wage earners. The majority of women work outside the home, and about 62% of mothers are in the workforce (U.S. Census Bureau, 2001). Balancing employment and family life

✳ BOX 10-1 Family Forms

Nuclear Family
The nuclear family consists of husband and wife (and perhaps one or more children).

Extended Family
The extended family includes relatives (aunts, uncles, grandparents, and cousins) in addition to the nuclear family.

Single-Parent Family
The single-parent family is formed when one parent leaves the nuclear family because of death, divorce, or desertion, or when a single person decides to have or adopt a child.

Blended Family
The blended family is formed when parents bring unrelated children from prior or foster parenting relationships into a new, joint living situation.

Alternative Patterns of Relationships
These relationships include multiadult households, "skip-generation" families (grandparents caring for grandchildren), communal groups with children, "nonfamilies" (adults living alone), cohabitating partners, and homosexual couples.

creates a variety of challenges in terms of child care and household work for both parents. The balance for working parents for child care and household duties is positive when the working parents' job and life satisfactions remain high (Hill, 2005). There is no proof maternal employment is damaging for children (Hill, 2005; Shpancer, Melick, Sayre and others, 2006). However, finding quality child care is a major issue. Managing household tasks is another challenge. Although equal division of labor receives verbal approval, the majority of household tasks remain "women's work." There is some evidence that the fathering role is changing (Hill, 2005). Fathers now participate more fully in day-to-day parenting responsibilities. Twenty-four percent of children (ages 0 to 4) have their fathers as caretakers whether or not the fathers are employed (U.S. Census Bureau, 2001).

The number of single-parent families, which doubled from the 1970s to the 1990s, seems to be stabilizing. Although mothers head the majority of single-parent families, father-only families are on the rise. Forty-one percent of children are living with mothers who have never married; many of these children are a result of an adolescent pregnancy.

Adolescent pregnancy is an ever-increasing concern. The majority of these adolescents continue to live with their families. A teenage pregnancy tends to have long-term consequences for the mother. For example, adolescent mothers quit high school, have inadequate job skills, and have limited health care resources. In addition, the overwhelming task of parenting while still a teenager often severely stresses family relationships and resources. Also, there is an increased risk for continued poverty and poor lifestyles for these families (Black and Ford-Gilboe, 2004; SmithBattle, 2000). Teenage fathers also have stressors placed on them when their partner becomes pregnant. These young men have poorer support systems and fewer resources to teach them how to parent. In addition, adolescent fathers report early adverse family relationships, such as exposure to domestic violence or parental separation or divorce and lack positive fathering role models (Tan and Quinlivan, 2006). As a result, both adolescent parents often struggle with the normal tasks of development and identity but must accept a parenting role that they are not ready for physically, emotionally, socially, and/or financially.

Many homosexual couples define their relationship in family terms. Approximately half of all gay male couples live together, compared with three fourths of lesbian couples. These couples are more open about their sexual preferences and more vocal about their legal rights. Some homosexual families include children, either through adoption or artificial insemination or from prior relationships.

The fastest-growing age-group in America is 65 years of age and over. For the first time in history the average American has more living parents than children, and children are more likely to have living grandparents and even great-grandparents. This "graying" of America continues to affect the family life cycle, particularly the "sandwich generation"—made up of the children of older adults (see section on restorative care). These individuals, who are usually in the middle years, have to meet their own needs along with those of their children and the needs of their aging parents. This balance of needs often occurs at the expense of their own well-being and resources. In addition, many of these caregivers report that support received from professional health professionals is often lacking (Isaksen, Thuen, and Hanestad, 2003). The majority of family caregivers are women; the average age is 46, with 13% being 65 years of age or older, and they frequently provide more than 20 hours of care per week (Schumacher, Beck, and Marren, 2006). Caring for a frail or chronically ill relative is a primary concern for a growing number of families. It is not uncommon for people in their 60s and 70s to be the major caregivers for each other. Box 10-2 provides a list of family nursing gerontological concerns.

More grandparents are raising their grandchildren (U.S. Census Bureau, 2001). This new parenting responsibility is due to a number of societal factors: the increase in the divorce rate, dual-income families, and single parenthood. Most often it is a consequence of legal intervention when parents are unfit or renounce their parental obligations.

Families face many challenges, including changing structures and roles in the changing economic status of society. In addition, there are four further trends that social scientists identify as threats or concerns facing the family: (1) changing economic status (e.g., declining family income and lack of access to health care), (2) homelessness, (3) family violence, and (4) the presence of acute or chronic illnesses.

Changing Economic Status

Making ends meet is a daily concern because of the declining economic status of families. Although two-income families have become the norm, real family income has not increased since 1973. Families at the lower end of the income scale have been particularly affected, and single-parent families are especially vulnerable. The number of American children living below the poverty level continues to rise. In addition, it is estimated that 9 million children are uninsured (Children's Defense Fund [CDF], 2006). A majority of these uninsured children have at least one

✳ **BOX 10-2**   **FOCUS ON OLDER ADULTS**

Caregiver Concerns

- Assess the family for additional caregivers to provide respite care for older adult family members. For example, determine additional roles for members of the family (e.g., providing additional financial support, designating someone to obtain groceries and medications, providing someone to assist with household tasks).
- Assess for caregiver stress, such as tension in relationships with family and care recipient, changes in level of health, changes in mood, and anxiety and depression.
- Caregivers are either spouses, who are sometimes an older adult with declining physical stamina, or middle-age children, who often have other responsibilities.
- Later-life families have a different social network than younger families because friends and same-generation family members often have died or been ill themselves. Look for social support within the community and church affiliation.
- Identify family members, friends, and neighbors who will take the time to socialize with the caregiver to avoid the caregiver's feeling isolated.
- Abuse of older adults in families occurs across all social classes. Spouses are the most frequent abusers. Nurses need to report unexplained bruises and skin trauma to state protective agencies.

parent who works but is unable to afford insurance. When caring for these families, the nurse needs to be sensitive to the family's desire for independence but also help them with obtaining appropriate financial and health care resources. For example, you inform the family where to go within the community to obtain assistance with energy bills, dental and health care, and assistance with school supplies.

Homelessness

Homelessness is a major public health issue. According to public health organizations, "absolute homelessness" describes people without physical shelter who sleep outdoors, in vehicles, abandoned buildings, or other places not intended for human habitation. "Relative homelessness" describes those who have a physical shelter, but one that does not meet the standards of health and safety (Hwang, 2001; National Coalition for the Homeless, 2006).

The fastest growing section of the homeless population is families with children. This includes complete nuclear families and single-parent families. Families with children accounted for 39% of the homeless population (National Coalition for the Homeless, 2006). Poverty, mental and physical illness, and lack of affordable housing are primary causes of homelessness (Folsom and others, 2005). Homelessness severely affects the functioning, health, and well-being of the family and its members. Children of homeless families are often in fair or poor health and have higher rates of asthma, ear infections, stomach problems, and mental illness (see Chapter 3). As a result, usually the only access to health care for these children is through the emergency department (Kushel and others, 2002).

In addition, these children face difficulties such as meeting residency requirements for public schools, inability to obtain previous enrollment records, and enrolling in and attending school. As a result, these children are more likely to drop out of school and become unemployable (National Coalition for the Homeless, 2006). Homeless families and their children are at serious risk for developing long-term health, psychological, and socioeconomic problems. For example, these children are frequently underimmunized and are at risk for childhood illnesses; they may fall behind in school and are at risk of dropping out; or they can develop risky behaviors such as prostitution or substance abuse. Homelessness and its long-term results pose major challenges for our entire society (Kushel and others, 2002; National Coalition for the Homeless, 2006).

Family Violence

The statistics regarding family violence are even more disturbing. Researchers estimate that 3.3 to 10 million children reported being abused or neglected in the period from 1991 to 2004 (Family Violence Prevention Fund, 2006a). Emotional, physical, and sexual abuse occurs toward spouses, children, and older adults and across all social classes. Factors associated with family violence are complex and may include stress, poverty, social isolation, psychopathology, and learned family behavior. In addition, other factors such as alcohol and drug abuse, pregnancy, sexual orientation, and mental illness increase the incidence of abuse within a family (Family Violence Prevention Fund, 2006b). Although abuse sometimes ends when one leaves a specific family environment, negative long-term physical and emotional consequences are often evident. One of these consequences includes moving from one abusive situation to another (Richardson and others, 2002). For example, a child sees marriage as a way to leave an abusive home and in turn marries a person who will continue the abuse within the marriage (Wathen and MacMillan, 2003).

Acute or Chronic Illness

Any acute or chronic illness influences the family economically, socially, and functionally and affects the family's decision-making and coping resources. Hospitalization of a family member is stressful for the whole family. Hospital environments are foreign, physicians and nurses are strangers, the medical language is difficult to understand or interpret, and family members are separated from one another.

During an acute illness, such as a trauma, myocardial infarction, or surgery, family members are often left in waiting rooms anticipating information about their loved one. Communication among family members may be misdirected from fear and worry. In some families, previous family conflicts rise to the surface, while others are suppressed. Provide attentive nursing care to meet the family's need for the frequency and type of communication and support. Understand the family's cultural beliefs and values, and respect the family structure and functioning.

Chronic illnesses pose different challenges for the family. Frequently family patterns and interactions, social activities, work and household schedules, economic resources, and other family needs and functions must be reorganized around the chronic illness or disability. Families also learn how to manage many aspects of their loved one's illness or disability. Astute nursing care helps the family prevent and/or manage medical crises, control symptoms, learn how to provide specific therapies, adjust to changes over the course of the illness, avoid isolation, obtain community resources, and assist in helping the family resolve conflict.

Although it is not the intent of this chapter to provide a complete description of family nursing, examples are used to guide you in an initial understanding of caring for families. The examples of critical trauma, human immunodeficiency virus, and end-of-life care are selected to help you understand the impact of illness on the family.

Trauma.   Trauma is a sudden unplanned event. Family members need to cope with the challenges of a severe, life-threatening event, which can include the stressors associated with an intensive care environment, anxiety and depression, and economic burden, not to mention the impact on the family's functioning and decision making. In caring for these families, answer their questions honestly. When you do not know the answer, find someone who does. Provide realistic assurance; giving false hope breaks the nurse-client trust and also affects how the family can adjust to "bad news." Take time to be sure the family is comfortable. You can bring them something to eat or drink, give them a blanket, or encourage them to get a meal. Sometimes, telling the family that you will stay with their loved one while they are gone is all they need to feel comfortable in leaving. Most family members have a cell phone and can easily be reached if their loved one's condition changes.

Human Immunodeficiency Virus.   During the mid to late 1990s advances in human immunodeficiency virus (HIV) treatment led to declines in acquired immunodeficiency syndrome (AIDS) deaths and slowed the progression from HIV to AIDS (Centers for Disease Control and Prevention [CDC], 2006a). AIDS-related mortality is down, indicating that people with HIV are living longer and better lives. Although the epidemic has slowed, high-risk behaviors, such as unprotected sex, continue to rise, especially with men who have sex with other men (CDC, 2006b). Finding that one is HIV positive is devastating, not only for the individual, but for family and friends as well. As with all serious illnesses, caring for a family member who develops active HIV infection is emotionally and financially devastating, and it affects the entire family.

End-of-Life Care.   You will encounter many families with a terminally ill member. Although people equate terminal illness with cancer, there are many diseases with terminal aspects, for example, congestive heart failure, pulmonary and renal diseases, and neuromuscular diseases. Although some family members may be prepared for their loved-one's death, their need for information, support, assurance, and presence are great (see Chapter 30). The more you know about your client's family, how they interact with one another, their strengths, and their weaknesses, the better. Each family approaches and copes with end-of-life decisions differently. Give the family information about the dying process. Help the family set up home care if they desire and obtain hospice and other appropriate resources, including grief support. Be sure the family knows what to do at the time of death. If you are present at the time of death, be sensitive to the family's needs, for example, provide for privacy and allow sufficient time for saying good-byes.

Theoretical Approaches: An Overview

There are a number of different perspectives to apply when caring for families. It is important that you understand some of the broader perspectives for family nursing. The family health system (FHS) and developmental theories are two perspectives used in this chapter to help you provide nursing care to the family as a whole and the individuals within the family structure. These theoretical perspectives and their concepts provide the foundation for family assessment and interventions.

Family Health System

The FHS is a holistic model that guides the assessment and care for families (Anderson, 2000). The FHS includes five realms/processes of family life: interactive, developmental, coping, integrity, and health. The FHS approach uses family assessment to determine the areas of concern and strengths according to the realms of family life. As a result, you develop a plan of care with family nursing interventions and outcomes. As with all systems, the family system has both unspoken and spoken goals, which vary according to the stage in the family life cycle, family values, and individual concerns of the family members. The goals of the FHS are to improve family health or well-being, assist in family management of illness conditions or transitions, and achieve health outcomes related to the family areas of concern (Anderson, 2000).

Developmental Stages

Families, like individuals, change and grow over time. Although families are far from identical to one another, they tend to go through certain stages. Each developmental stage has its own challenges, needs, and resources and includes tasks that need to be completed before the family is able to successfully move on to the next stage. Societal changes and an aging population have caused changes in the stages and transitions in the family life cycle. For example, adult children are not leaving the nest as predictably or as early as in the past, and many are returning home. In addition, more people are living into their 80s and 90s. Sixty-five is now considered the "backside of middle age," and the length of the midlife stage in the family life cycle has increased, as has the later stage in family life.

McGoldrick and Carter based their 1985 classic model of family life stages on expansion, contraction, and realignment of family relationships that support the entry, exit, and development of the members (Hanson and others, 2005). This model describes the emotional aspects of lifestyle transition and the changes and tasks necessary for the family to proceed developmentally (Table 10-1). Thus a nurse can use this model to promote behaviors to achieve essential tasks and help families prepare for later transitions. For example, helping families prepare for a new baby (see Chapter 13), or how do families cope with the death of a loved one (see Chapter 30).

✳ TABLE 10-1 Stages of the Family Life Cycle

Family Life Cycle Stage	Emotional Process of Transition: Key Principles	Changes in Family Status Required to Proceed Developmentally
Unattached young adult	Accepting parent-offspring separation	• Differentiation of self in relation to family of origin • Development of intimate peer relationships • Establishment of self in work
Joining of families through marriage: newly married couple	Commitment to new system	• Formation of marital system • Realignment of relationships with extended families and friends to include spouse
Family with young children	Accepting new generation of members into system	• Adjusting marital system to make space for children • Taking on parental roles • Realignment of relationships with extended family to include parenting and grandparenting roles
Family with adolescents	Increasing flexibility of family boundaries to include children's independence	• Shifting of parent-child relationships to permit adolescents to move into and out of system • Refocusing on midlife material and career issues • Beginning shift toward concerns for older generation
Launching children and moving on	Accepting multitude of exits from and entries into family system	• Adjusting to the reduction in family size • Developing adult-to-adult relationships between grown children and their parents • Realigning relationships to include in-laws and grandchildren • Dealing with disabilities and death of parents (grandparents)
Family in later life	Accepting shifting of generational roles	• Maintaining own or couple functioning and interests in the face of physiological decline; exploration of new familial and social role options • Making room in system for wisdom and experience of older adults; supporting older generations without overfunctioning for them • Dealing with retirement • Dealing with loss of spouse, siblings, and other peers and preparation for own death; a life review, in which one reviews life experiences and decisions

From Duvall EM, Miller BC: *Marriage and family development*, ed 6, Boston, 2005, Allyn and Bacon. Copyright © 1985 by Pearson Education. Reprinted by permission of the publisher.

Attributes of Families

Structure

Families also have a structure and a way of functioning. Structure and function are closely related and continually interact with one another. Structure is based on the ongoing membership of the family and the pattern of relationships, which are often numerous and complex. For example, a woman's relationships include wife-husband, mother-son, mother-daughter, employee-boss, and colleague-colleague, each with different demands, roles, and expectations. Patterns of relationships form power and role structures within the family. Determine these structures by observing family behavior and interactions.

Structure improves or worsens the family's ability to respond to stressors. Very rigid or very flexible structures impair functioning. A rigid structure specifically dictates who is able to accomplish a task and may limit the number of persons outside the immediate family who assume these tasks. For example, in one family the mother is the only acceptable person to provide emotional support for the children, or the husband is the only one to provide financial support. A change in the health status of the person responsible for a task places a burden on the family be-

cause no other person is available or considered acceptable to assume that task. For example, when a homemaker is ill, the tasks of managing the household (e.g., preparing the meals, maintaining the house, and driving school-age children to appointments and events) need to be shared. The older children may help prepare the meals, and the other parent or a family member drives the children to the events or perhaps the events are rescheduled.

An extremely open structure also presents problems for the family. Consistent patterns of behavior that lead to automatic action do not exist, and enactment of roles is overly flexible. A common example is an inconsistent parenting role. The parent sometimes is a strict authoritarian figure and at other times treats the child as a "best friend and confidant." This type of conduct causes family members to become confused about what behavior is appropriate and who is reliable for support. This creates a general feeling of instability. During a crisis or rapid change, family members do not have a defined structure to "fall back on," and family disintegration is sometimes a result.

Function

Family functioning is what the family does. Specific functional aspects include the way a family reproduces, interacts to socialize its young, cooperates to meet economic needs, and relates to the larger society (Hanson and others, 2005). Family functioning also focuses on the processes used by the family to achieve its goals. These processes include communication among family members, goal setting, conflict resolution, caregiving, nurturing, and use of internal and external resources. Traditional reproductive, sexual, economic, and educational goals that were once universal family goals no longer apply to all families. When the psychological needs of family members are not met, symptoms of family dysfunction are the usual consequence.

Families achieve goals when communication is clear and direct. Clear communication enhances problem solving and conflict resolution, and it facilitates coping with life-changing or life-threatening stressors. Another process to facilitate goal achievement includes the ability to nurture and promote growth. For example, families might have a specific celebration for a good report card, a job well done, or specific milestones. Families also nurture by helping children know right and wrong. In this situation a family might have a specific form of discipline, such as time out or taking away privilege, and the children know when the discipline is given. So when a situation occurs, the child is disciplined and learns not to do that behavior again.

Families need to have multiple resources available. For example, a social network is useful as an excellent resource. Social relationships, such as friends or churches, within the community act as buffers, particularly during times of stress, and reduce a family's vulnerability.

The Family and Health

Many factors influence the health of the family (e.g., its relative position in society, economic resources, and geographical boundaries). Although American families exist within the same culture, they live in very different ways as a result of race, values, social class, and ethnicity. For some minority groups there are multiple generations of single-parent families living together in one home. Class and ethnicity produce differences in the access of families to society's resources and rewards, and this access creates differences in family life, most significantly in different life chances for its members.

Distribution of wealth greatly affects the capacity to maintain health. Low educational preparation, poverty, and decreased amounts of support compound one another, magnifying each other's impact *on* sickness in the family, and magnifying the amount of sickness *in* the family. Economic stability increases a family's access to adequate health care, creates more opportunity for education, increases good nutrition, and decreases stress.

The family is the primary social context in which health promotion and disease prevention take place. The family's beliefs, values, and practices strongly influence health-promoting behaviors of its members (Hartrick, 2000). In turn, the health status of each individual influences how the family unit functions and its ability to achieve goals. When the family satisfactorily functions to meet its goals, its members tend to feel positive about themselves and their family. Conversely, when they do not meet goals, families view themselves as ineffective.

Some families do not place a high value on good health. In fact, some families accept harmful practices. In some cases a family member gives mixed messages about health. For example, a parent continues to smoke while telling children that smoking is bad for them. Family environment is crucial because health behavior reinforced in early life has a strong influence on later health practices. In addition, the family environment is a crucial factor in an individual's adjustment to a crisis. Although relationships are strained when confronted with illness, research indicates that family members have the potential to be a primary force for coping (Bluvol and Ford-Gilboe, 2004).

Attributes of Healthy Families. Ruebin Hill's classic work (1958) noted that it is possible to explain the reactions of crisis-proof and crisis-prone families. The crisis-proof, or effective, family is able to combine the need for stability with the need for growth and change. This type of family has a flexible structure that allows adaptable performance of tasks and acceptance of help from outside the family system. The structure is flexible enough to allow adaptability but not so flexible that the family lacks cohesiveness and a sense of stability. The effective family has control over the environment and influences the immediate environment of home, neighborhood, and school. The ineffective, or crisis-prone, family lacks or believes it lacks control over these environments.

Health promotion research often focuses on the stress-moderating effect of **hardiness** and **resiliency** as factors that contribute to long-term health. Family hardiness is the internal strengths and durability of the family unit. A sense of control over the outcome of life, a view of change as beneficial and growth producing, and an active rather than passive orientation in adapting to stressful events characterize family hardiness (McCubbin, McCubbin, and Thompson, 1996). Resiliency helps to evaluate healthy responses when individuals and families are experiencing stressful events. Resources and techniques a family or individuals within the family use to maintain a balance or level of health assist in understanding a family's level of resiliency.

Family Nursing

To provide compassion and caring for your clients and their families, you need a scientific knowledge base in family theory, as well as an adequate knowledge base in family nursing. A focus on the family is necessary in order to safely discharge clients back to the family or community settings. The members of the family may need to assume the role of primary caregiver. Family caregivers have unique nursing and caregiving needs and too often feel abandoned by the health care system (Reinhard, 2006). When a life-changing illness occurs, the family has to make major adjustments to care for a family member (Bluvol and Ford-Gilboe, 2004).

Family nursing is based on the assumption that all people regardless of age are a member of some type of family form. This family form is the traditional nuclear family, a single-parent family, extended family, or alternate family. The goal of family nursing is to help the family and its individual members reach and maintain maximum health throughout and beyond the illness experience (Box 10-3). Family nursing is the focus of the future across all practice settings and is important in all health care environments.

✳ BOX 10-3   **EVIDENCE-BASED PRACTICE**

Hope, Health, and Quality of Life in Families of Stroke Survivors

Evidence Summary

When a person suffers a stroke, it is often a major life-changing event for the spouse, family, and loved ones. As the client moves through the stroke and rehabilitation phases, families face the financial and emotional burden of the stroke. When the client returns home, any existing disability affects the primary caregiver, usually the spouse, and other members of the family. Families face changes when adjusting to the physical, emotional, and psychological consequences of the stroke. The family's and caregiver's social roles and activities, health-related activities and practices, and family dynamics all change. As a result, family members note changes in their physical and emotional health and a decline in their quality of life.

Application to Nursing Practice

- Focus interventions on the family's strengths (e.g., if some family members are good at helping their loved one exercise, get them involved in physical rehabilitation activities).
- Consider the primary caregiver's experience when designing intervention (e.g., Has the caregiver observed any technical nursing care? Does the caregiver have a health care background? Has he or she provided care to another person?).
- Build on the strengths of the stroke survivor and spouse, including their sense of hope, rather than solely focusing on any weaknesses and challenges.
- Encourage the stroke survivor and caregivers to "tell their story."

Reference

Bluvol A, Ford-Gilboe M: Hope, health work and quality of life in families of stroke survivors, *J Adv Nurs* 48(4):322, 2004.

There are different approaches for family nursing practice. For the purposes of this chapter, family nursing practice has three levels of approaches: (1) **family as context**, (2) **family as client**, and (3) the newest model, called **family as system**, which includes both relational and transactional concepts. If only one family member receives nursing care, it is realistic and practical to view the family as context. When all family members are involved in the daily care of one another, nursing intervention with one individual necessitates some change in the activities of the others, suggesting that family as client is the best approach. All three approaches are useful in providing effective nursing care.

Family as Context

When you view the family as context, the primary focus is on the health and development of an individual member existing within a specific environment (i.e., the client's family). Although the focus is on the individual's health status, assess how much the family provides the individual's basic needs. These needs vary, depending on the individual's developmental level and situation. Because families provide more than just material essentials, you will also need to consider their ability to help the client meet psychological needs. Some family members need direct interventions themselves. For example, consider the following:

You are assigned to care for Patrick Davis, who is newly diagnosed with coronary artery disease. He is recovering following an insertion of a stent to increase coronary blood flow. He is married and has three children, ages 11 to 16, who live at home. The major focus of your care is to modify Patrick's risk factors related to coronary artery disease.

Although you want to care for the whole family, your interactions include only Patrick and his wife. You work with the couple to design interventions and lifestyle changes, such as diet and exercise patterns, to modify Patrick's cardiac risk factors.

Family as Client

When the family as client is the approach, family processes and relationships (e.g., parenting or family caregiving) are the primary focuses of nursing care. Focus your nursing assessment on family patterns versus individual characteristics. Concentrate on patterns and processes that are consistent with reaching and maintaining family and individual health. To illustrate the family as client consider the following:

You are assisting with end-of-life care for David Daniels, who is 35 years old. David and his wife, Lisa, have three school-age children. David expressed a wish to die at home and not in a hospital or extended care facility. Lisa is on family leave from her job to help David though this period. Both Lisa and David are only children. David's parents are no longer living, but Lisa's mother is coming to stay with the family to help Lisa and David and their children as well.

Although David is the primary care recipient, the whole family needs nursing care and support to deal with the stressors of end-of-life care. Therefore you need to plan care to meet not only the client's needs, but also the changing needs of his family during this difficult period. Dealing with very complex family problems often requires an interdisciplinary approach. Always be aware of the limits of nursing practice, and make referrals when appropriate.

Family as System

It is important to understand that although you are able to make theoretical and practical distinctions between the family as context and the family as client, they are not necessarily mutually exclusive. Often, you will use both simultaneously, such as with the perspective of the family as system. A continuation of the previous clinical scenario for David Daniels illustrates the differences:

When you view the family as context, you focus on the client (David) as an individual. You assess and meet David's comfort, hygiene, and nutritional needs. You also meet David's social and emotional needs.

When viewing the family as client, you assess and meet David's family's comfort and nutritional needs. You determine the family's need for rest and their stage of coping. It is important to determine the demands placed on David and the family. In addition, you need to continually evaluate the family's available resources, such as time, finances, coping skills, and energy level, to support David through the end of life.

When viewing the family as system, use elements from both of the above perspectives. Individualize care decisions based on the family assessment and your clinical judgment. For instance, based on your assessment, you determine that the family is not eating adequately. You also determine that Lisa is experiencing more stress, is not sleeping well, and she is trying to "do it all" regarding her children's school and after-school activities. In addition, Lisa does not want to leave David's bedside when members of their church come to help. You recognize that this family is under enormous stress, and basic needs, such as meals, rest, and school activities, are not adequately met. As a result, you determine that (1) the family needs assistance with meals, (2) Lisa needs time to rest, and (3) the family's church is eager to help with David's day-to-day care. Based on these decisions, you work with Lisa, David, and the family to set up a schedule between Lisa, her mother, and two close church members to provide Lisa with some time away from David's bedside. However, David and Lisa determine when this time will be. Because of the church's involvement, members of the church begin to take responsibility for groceries and all meal preparation for the family. In addition, other members of the church help with the children's school and after-school activities.

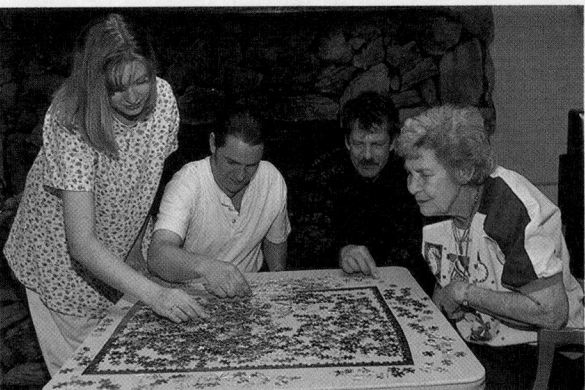

Figure 10-2 Observing family interactions assists in understanding family functioning.

Nursing Process for the Family

Nurses interact with families in a variety of community-based and clinical settings. The nurse uses the nursing process to care for an individual within a family (e.g., the family as context) or the entire family (e.g., the family as client). When initiating the care of families, there are three factors that organize the family approach to the nursing process:

1. That the nurse views all individuals within their family context
2. That families have an impact on individuals
3. That individuals have an impact on families

Assessing the Needs of the Family

Family assessment is a priority when providing adequate family care and support. You have an essential role in helping families adjust to acute and chronic illness, but first you need to understand the family unit, what the illness means to the family members, and what the illness means to family functioning. You also need to understand how the illness has affected the family structure and function, and the support the family requires (Hanson and others, 2005). Although the family as a whole differs from individual members, the measure of family health is more than a summary of the health of all members. The form, structure, function, and health of the family are areas unique to family assessment. Box 10-4 includes the five areas of family life.

Incorporate knowledge of the client's illness, and assess the primary client as well as the family. When focusing on the family, begin the family assessment by determining the client's definition of and attitude toward family and how much you are able to incorporate the family into nursing care. To determine family form and membership, ask who the client considers family or with whom the client shares strong emotional feelings. If the client is unable to express a concept of family, then ask with whom the client lives, spends time, and shares confidences, and then ask whether the client considers them to be family or like family. To

further assess the family structure, you also asks questions that determine the power structure and patterning of roles and tasks (e.g., "Who decides where to go on vacation?" "How are tasks divided in your family?" "Who mows the lawn?" "Who usually prepares the meals?").

You need to assess family functions, such as the ability to provide emotional support for members, the ability to cope with its current health problem or situation, and the appropriateness of its goal setting and progress toward achievement of developmental tasks (Figure 10-2). Also determine whether the family is able to provide and distribute sufficient economic resources and whether its social network is extensive enough to provide support.

You need to recognize and respect the family's cultural background (see Chapter 9). Culture is an important variable when assessing the family because race and ethnicity affect structure, function, health beliefs, values, and the way the family perceives events (Box 10-5). The United States is increasingly more diverse. A large number of immigrants enter the country daily, adding to both the number and the variety of the many ethnic groups that make up the population. American health care institutions tend to operate from a white, middle-class perspective, and immigrant populations have particular difficulty understanding and "fitting into" the system. Cultural assessment educators encourage the use of a "culturagram," which assesses and empowers culturally diverse families and encourages ethnic-sensitive practice. This tool assesses a variety of factors such as language spoken in the home, impact of crisis events, and values regarding family, education, and work.

Drawing conclusions based on cultural backgrounds requires critical thinking and careful consideration. It is imperative to remember that categorical generalizations are misleading (e.g., all Asian Americans are good at math). As many caution, overgeneralizations in terms of racial and ethnic group characteristics do not lead to greater understanding of the culturally diverse family. Culturally different families vary in meaningful and significant ways; however, neglecting to examine similarities will lead to inaccurate assumptions and stereotyping. For example, more similarities than differences exist in parenting behaviors among white, African American, Hispanic, and Asian American parents. In addition, Asian American families use alternative therapies. Other cultures, such as Latino, prefer to stay with their family members during illness (see Chapter 9).

✳ **BOX 10-4** Five Realms of Family Life: Family Health System—Family Assessment Plan

Interactive Processes

Family relationships—Is the family a nuclear or blended family, is it a single-parent family?

Family communication—How do family members share ideas, concerns?

Family nurturing—How are family values set and communicated, how are house rules established?

Intimacy expression—Does the family hug, touch, laugh, or cry together?

Social support—Who in the community, school, or workplace is close to the family?

Conflict resolution—How does conflict resolution occur, who initiates it?

Roles (instrumental and expressive)—What are the formal roles, such as wage earner, disciplinarian, problem solver? What are the informal roles (e.g., peacekeeper)?

Family leisure life—Vacations, what does the family do to relax, do the parents have "date night"?

Developmental Processes

Current family transitions—Recent death, divorces, children leaving/returning home, new births

Family stage task completion or progression—Child-bearing years, empty nesters, grandparenting

Individual developmental issues that affect family development—Individuals in the family with social issues, such as difficulty in school, legal issues, who cannot participate in family development

Development of health issue and family impact—Acute or chronic illnesses, high-risk pregnancies, delayed physical development

Coping Processes

Problem solving—How did the family solve previous problems, is there a single problem solver or family resolution?

Use of resources—Family or individual therapists, Alcoholics Anonymous, conflict resolution resources, anger management resources

Family life stressors and daily hassles—Financial concerns, over-scheduled children, caregiver for older adults

Family coping strategies and effectiveness—How does the family or individuals cope (e.g., exercise, overeating, arguing)?

Past experiences with handling crises—Information about past crisis such as financial stress, illness, legal problems

Family resistance resources—Does the family take measures to avoid stress, such as adhering to a budget, obtaining tutoring resources for their children?

Integrity Processes

Family values—What does the family consider as their important values, which might include health, togetherness?

Family beliefs—For example, beliefs about health/illness, end-of-life care, advance directives

Family meaning—For example, ask what the family means to each member

Family rituals—For example, celebration of holidays, birthdays, weddings; coping with death (e.g., wakes, funerals)

Family spirituality—Ask what spirituality means, how does the family define their spirituality?

Family culture and practices—Identify cultural customs and practice that impact health care

Health Processes

Family health beliefs and beliefs about health concern or problem—Health and illness prevention, wait until a problem occurs

Health behaviors of the family—How does the ill family member react, how does the family react to illness? Does the family react the same way to an ill family member, or does the family react differently when a homemaker is ill versus the wage earner?

Health patterns and health management activities—How does the family manage their health? How do they manage care?

Family care taking responsibilities—When someone is ill, who is the caregiver? Is it always the same person?

Disease conditions, treatments, and consequences for the family—Obtain current disease and treatment history for the family

Family illness stressors—What are these stressors (e.g., worsening of a chronic illness or when "Mom" is sick and cannot run the household)?

Relationship with health care providers and health system access—What type of health care provider does the family have (e.g., primary care, pediatrician)? How often does the family see the providers? Any hospitalizations?

Modified from Anderson KH: The family health system approach to family systems nursing, *J Fam Nurs* 6(2):103, 2000.

A comprehensive, culturally sensitive family assessment is critical to forming an understanding of family life, current changes in family life, and overall goals and expectations. These data provide the foundation for future family-centered nursing care (Anderson, 2000).

Family-Focused Care

Use a family-focused approach to enhance your nursing care. When you establish a relationship with a family, it is important to identify potential and external resources. A complete client and family assessment provides this information. Together with your client and his or her family, develop a plan of care that all members clearly understand and mutually agree on. Whatever goals you establish need to be concrete and realistic, compatible with the family's developmental stage, and acceptable to family members.

Collaboration with family members is essential, whether the family is the client or the context of care (Figure 10-3). Collaborate closely with all appropriate family members when determining what they hope to achieve with regard to the family's health. You base a positive collaborative relationship on mutual respect and trust. The family needs to feel "in control" as much as possible. By offering alternative actions and asking family members for their own ideas and suggestions, you help to reduce the family's feelings of powerlessness. For example, offering options for how to prepare a low-fat diet or how to rearrange the furnishings of a room to accommodate a family member's disability gives the family an opportunity to express their preferences, make choices, and ultimately feel as though they have contributed. Collaborating with other disciplines increases the likelihood of a comprehensive approach to the family's health care needs, and it ensures better continuity of

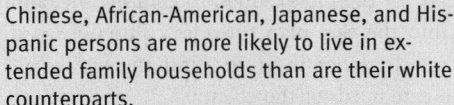
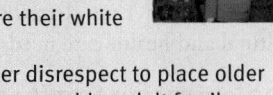

BOX 10-5 — CULTURAL ASPECTS OF CARE

Family Nursing

Families have unique perspectives and characteristics, and they have differences in values, beliefs, and philosophies. Family forms range from traditional nuclear families, to single-parent families, to extended families. The cultural heritage of the family or member of the family affects religious practices, child-rearing practices, recreational activities, and nutritional preferences. You need to be culturally sensitive and respectful when caring for multicultural clients. Incorporate individualized cultural preferences into your plan of care so that it is culturally congruent. Design your care to integrate the personal values, life patterns, and beliefs of the client and family with prescribed therapies.

Implications for Practice

- Whereas the dominant culture in the United States encourages self-care, collectivistic cultures, such as traditional Asians, Hispanics, and Africans, rely on family members to care for the ill.
- In some cultures, including Gypsy, Asian, Middle Eastern, and Hispanic, males are traditionally the authority figures.
- The family structure sometimes includes multiple generations living together. For example, traditional Hispanic and Filipino families include distant blood relatives from the maternal and paternal sides of the family.
- In some cultures, such as traditional Chinese or Japanese cultures, it is the custom for family members to take care of the client's needs.
- Intergenerational support and patterns of living arrangements are related to cultural background. For example, traditional Chinese, African-American, Japanese, and Hispanic persons are more likely to live in extended family households than are their white counterparts.
- In some cultures it is a sign of elder disrespect to place older adults in nursing homes, even when an older adult family member has severe dementia.
- Modesty is a strong value among Arab cultures. Many Arab women bring female family members to health care visits, and a female health care provider must examine the woman.
- In the presence of a critical or terminal illness some cultures, such as Orthodox Jews, come in groups to pray together with the family at the client's bedside.
- Health beliefs differ among various cultures, which affect the decision of a family and its members about when and where to seek help. For example, traditional Asians rarely consider symptoms as psychological and are not likely to go to mental health clinics.

Data from Cox C, Monk A: Strain among caregivers: comparing the experiences of African-American and Hispanic caregivers of Alzheimer's relatives, *Int J Aging Hum Dev* 43(2):93, 1996; Wang Y: People of Chinese heritage. In Purnell LD, Paulanka BJ: *Transcultural health care: a culturally competent approach*, ed 2, Philadelphia, 2003, FA Davis; Bonura D and others: Culturally-congruent end-of-life care for Jewish patients and their families, *J Transcult Nurs* 12(3):211, 2001; Kulwicki AD: People of Arab heritage. In Purnell LD, Paulanka BJ: *Transcultural health care: a culturally competent approach*, ed 2, Philadelphia, 2003, FA Davis; and Galanti GA: *Caring for patients from different cultures*, ed 3, Philadelphia, 2004, University of Pennsylvania Press.

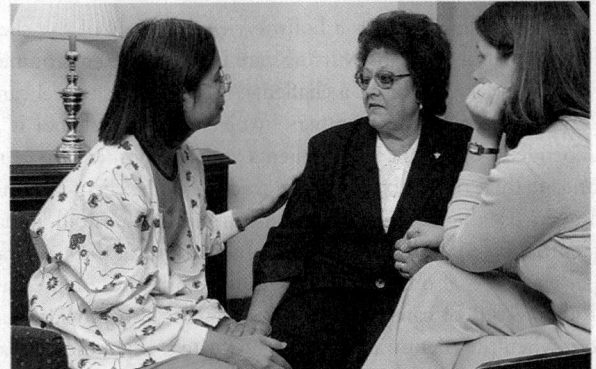

Figure 10-3 Nurse and family members.

care. Using other disciplines is particularly important when discharge planning from a health care facility to home or an extended care facility is necessary (Bluvol and Ford-Gilboe, 2004).

When you view the family as the client, you need to support communication among all family members. This ensures that the family remains informed about the goals and interventions for health care. Often you participate in conflict resolution between family members so that each member is able to confront and resolve problems in a healthy way. Help the family identify and use external and internal resources as necessary. Ultimately, your aim is to help the family reach a point of optimal function, given the family's resources, capacities, and desire to become healthier.

Challenges for Family Nursing

Delegation in the management of nursing care activities is a challenge in family nursing. Often nurses try to enhance family health by delegating duties to family members or to other members of the health care team. For example, you help family members learn how to provide appropriate care for an ill family member. With earlier discharge and more complex family needs at the time of discharge, planning for discharge begins with the initiation of care.

Discharge planning with a family involves an accurate assessment of what will be needed for care at the time of discharge, along with any shortcomings in the home setting. For example, if a postoperative client will be discharged to home and the older adult husband does not feel comfortable with the dressing changes required, you need to find out if there is anyone else in the family or neighborhood who is willing and able to do this. If not, then you will need to arrange for a home care service referral. If the client also needs exercise and strength training, then perhaps a physical therapy referral is necessary.

Cultural sensitivity (see Chapter 9) in family nursing requires recognizing not only the diverse ethnic, cultural, and religious backgrounds of clients, but also the differences and similarities within the same family. When providing family-centered care, recognize and integrate cultural practices, religious ceremonies, and rituals. Using effective and respectful communication techniques enables you to determine the family's cultural practices and collaborate with the family to determine how best to integrate these beliefs and practices within the prescribed health care plan.

For example, traditional Asian and Mexican American cultures frequently want to remain at the bedside around the clock and provide personal care for their loved ones. Integrating the family's values and needs into the care plan provides culturally sensitive and competent care. Together the nurse and the family blend cultural and health care needs of the client.

Implementing Family-Centered Care

Whether caring for a client with the family as context, directing care to the family as client, or providing care to the family as a system, nursing interventions aim to increase family members' abilities in certain areas, to remove barriers to health care, and to do things that the family is not able to do for itself. Assist the family in problem solving, provide practical services, and express a sense of acceptance and caring by listening carefully to family members' concerns and suggestions.

One of the roles you need to adopt is that of educator. Health education is a process by which the nurse and client share information in a two-way fashion (see Chapter 25). Sometimes you will recognize family/client needs for information through direct questioning, but they are generally far more subtle. For example, you recognize that a new father is fearful of cleaning his newborn's umbilical cord or that an older adult woman is not using her cane or walker safely. Respectful communication is necessary. Often you will find the subtle needs for information by saying, "I notice you are trying to not touch the umbilical cord; I see that a lot." Or "You use the cane the way I did before I was shown a way to keep from falling or tripping over it; do you mind if I show you?" When you are confident and skillful instead of coming across as an authority on the subject, your client's defenses will be down, making the client more willing to listen without feeling embarrassed.

However, you need to identify the best time to provide accurate health information about diagnosis, necessary self-care activities, and the projected course of the client's condition. Such information helps the family caregiver to interpret behavior correctly and not to "blame" the client. Caregivers are not born with the knowledge of how to be caregivers, and older adults are not born with the knowledge of how to accept dependency (Schumacher and others, 2006).

Health Promotion. Although the family is the basic social context in which members learn health behaviors, the primary focus on health promotion has traditionally been on individuals. When implementing family nursing, health promotion interventions improve or maintain the physical, social, emotional, and spiritual well-being of the family unit and its members (Ford-Gilboe, 2002). Encourage individual members and the total family to reach their optimal levels of wellness. Identifying qualities that contribute to healthy, resilient families has been a focus of ongoing research for at least three decades. "Strong" families that adapt to expected transitions and unexpected crises and change tend to have clear communication among members, good problem-solving skills, a commitment to each other and to the family unit, and a sense of cohesiveness and spirituality (Schumacher and others, 2006). Health promotion programs aimed at enhancing these attributes are available for families and children in many communities. Be aware of family-oriented services so you are able to refer families as needed. For example, some communities have low-cost fitness ac-

tivities for school-age children designed to reduce the risk for obesity. Encourage health promotion behaviors tied to the developmental stage of the family (e.g., adequate prenatal care for the childbearing family and effective parenting and adherence to immunization schedules for the child-rearing family).

One approach for meeting goals and promoting health is the use of family strengths. Families do not look at their own system as one that has inherent, positive components. Help the family become aware of its own unique strengths, thereby increasing its potential and capabilities. Family strengths include clear communication, adaptability, healthy child-rearing practices, support and nurturing among family members, and the use of crisis for growth. Help the family focus on these strengths instead of its problems and weaknesses. For example, point out that a couple's 10-year marriage has endured many crises and transitions. Therefore they are likely to have the capabilities to adapt to this latest challenge.

Acute Care. Because the family is becoming more of a focus in nursing care, you need to emphasize family needs within the context of today's health care delivery system. Be aware of the implication of early discharge for clients and their families. Remember there are increasing numbers of people within the household now being employed outside the home. These factors are challenges in preparing family members to assist with health care or to locate appropriate community resources. Often when family members assume the role of caregiver, they lose support from significant others and are at risk for caregiver role strain (Schumacher and others, 2006). You need to be sure that families are willing to assume care responsibilities.

Family nursing requires a holistic view not only of the client but of the family as well. Nursing care in the acute environment is very complex, making it a challenge for the client to feel cared for and to keep family members involved. A helpful tool is an independent journal in which clients and family members communicate their thoughts, ideas, and reactions. The client or family members use the journal as an open communication tool, updating entries based on their needs and observations of the acute care experience. It is also helpful for a family member to use the journal as a record of care activities. The journal also provides data about when the client was turned, who visited, when the last pain medication was administered, and any special client requests. This information helps clients and families who are trying to "keep up" with what is happening in the acute care environment.

Restorative and Continuing Care. In restorative and continuing care settings the challenge in family nursing is in trying to maintain clients' functional abilities within the context of the family. This includes having home care nurses help clients remain in their homes following acute injuries or illnesses, surgery, or exacerbation of a chronic illness. It also requires finding ways to better the lives of chronically ill and disabled individuals and their families.

Family Caregiving. One way you provide family care is through support of family caregivers. Family caregiving involves the routine provision of services and personal care activities for a family member by spouses, siblings, or parents. Caregiving activities include personal care (bathing, feeding, or grooming), monitoring for complications or side effects of medications, and providing instrumental activities of daily living (shopping or housekeeping), and the ongoing emotional support and decision making that is necessary. Whenever an individual becomes dependent on another family member for care and assistance, there is significant stress affecting both the caregiver and the care recipient. In addition, the caregiver needs to continue to meet the demands of his or her usual lifestyle (e.g., raising children, working full time, or dealing with personal problems or illness). In many instances adult children are trying to take care of their parents while meeting the needs of their own family. These caregivers are part of the sandwich generation (Box 10-6).

Without adequate preparation and support from health care providers, caregiving puts the family at risk for serious problems, including a decline in the health of the caregiver and that of the care receiver, dysfunctional relationships, and even abusive relationships (Schumacher and other, 2006).

Despite its demands, caregiving is a positive and rewarding experience. Caregiving is more than simply a series of tasks and usually occurs within the context of a family. Whether it is a wife caring for a husband or a daughter caring for a mother, caregiving is an interactional process. The interpersonal dynamics between family members influence the ultimate quality of caregiving. Thus the nurse plays a key role in helping family members develop better communication and problem-solving skills to build the relationships needed for caregiving to be successful (Farran, 2002).

Researchers identified variables, such as caregiver and care recipient expectations of one another, influencing caregiving quality. Carruth (1996) studied the concept of **reciprocity**, acknowledging the importance of the capability of care recipients to share exchanges that contribute to a caregiver's perception of self-worth. When the caregiver knows that the care recipient appreciates his or her efforts and values the assistance provided, a healthier and more satisfying caregiving relationship will exist. When caregiver and client solve problems together, this helps them avoid overprotection or oversolicitous behavior. Clients feel in control of their care and responsible for care decisions. The caregiver also feels very positive and enjoys the caregiving experience (Isaksen and others, 2003).

Providing care and support for family caregivers often involves using available family and community resources (Box 10-7). Establishing a caregiving schedule enabling all family members to participate, having extended family members share any financial burdens posed by caregiving, and having distant relatives send cards and letters communicating their support is very helpful. However, it is imperative for you to understand the relationship between potential caregivers and care recipients. If the relationship is not a supportive one, community services are often a resource for both the client and family.

Use of community resources includes locating a service required by the family or providing respite care so that the family

---

✳ BOX 10-6   Sandwich Generation

- Usually a daughter or daughter-in-law
- Conflicting responsibilities for aging parents, children, spouse, and job
- Frequently tries to "do it all"
- May not recognize need for help or request help
- Potential interventions:
  - Help families establish realistic priorities
  - Suggest that family members use family leave plans or obtain some "flex time" from their employer
  - Explore resources (e.g., deliveries for meals, respite care)

✳ BOX 10-7   **CLIENT TEACHING**

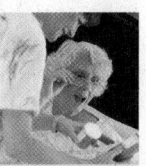

Family Caregiving: Caregiver Role Strain

Objectives
- Client/family will be able to identify three characteristics of caregiver role strain.
- Client/family will design two interventions to reduce caregiver role strain.
- Client/family will describe who/when to call when unable to relieve or reduce caregiver role strain.

Teaching Strategies
- Explain the following to all members of the family involved in caregiving that role strain may be present when the following occur:
  - There is a change in caregiver's appetite/weight, sleeping, or leisure activities. In addition, social withdrawal, irritability, anger, or changes in the caregiver's overall level of health can occur.
  - The caregiver is fearful when learning new therapies or administering new medications to the disabled/ill family member.
  - Caregiver loses interest in his or her personal appearance.
  - Signs of caregiver role strain may intensify if the loved one's health status changes or when institutional care is considered.

- Help family members set up alternating schedules to give primary caregiver some rest.
- Help family members design schedule or other methods to provide groceries, meals, and housekeeping for the caregiver and client.
- Identify community resources for transportation, respite care, and support groups.
- Offer an opportunity to ask questions, and when possible provide a phone number for questions and assistance.
- Provide family members with the caregiver's health care providers contact information, and instruct them to call if the caregiver has health problems, the caregiver seems overly exhausted, or they observe changes in the caregiver's interactions and attention to normal activities.

Evaluation
- Ask the family to identify two to three indicators for caregiver role strain.
- Review with the family their plan to provide groceries, meals, and occasional respite care for the caregiver and client.
- Ask the family where they keep the caregiver's provider's healthcare contact information and when they would call the healthcare provider.

caregiver has time away from the care recipient. Examples of services that are beneficial to families include caregiver support groups, housing and transportation services, food and nutrition services, housecleaning, legal and financial services, home care, hospice, and mental health resources. Before referring a family to a community resource, it is critical that the nurse understands the family's dynamics and knows whether the family wants support. Often a family caregiver will resist help, feeling obligated to be the sole source of support to the care recipient. Be sensitive to family relationships, and help caregivers understand the normalcy of caregiving demands. Given the appropriate resources, caregivers are able to acquire the skills and knowledge necessary to effectively care for their loved ones within the context of the home while maintaining rich and rewarding personal relationships.

Key Concepts

- Family structure and functions influence the lives of its individual members.
- Family members influence one another's health beliefs, practices, and status.
- The concept of family is highly individual; care focuses on the client's attitude toward the family rather than on an inflexible definition of family.
- The family's structure, functioning, and relative position in society significantly influence its health and ability to respond to health problems.
- There are three ways a nurse can view the family: an important context for the individual family member, the client, or a system (simultaneously viewing the family as both client and family in context).
- Measures of family health involve more than a summary of individual members' health.
- Its social class, economic stability, and racial and ethnic background influence the family's health.
- Family members as caregivers are often spouses who are either older adults themselves or adult children trying to work full-time, care for aging parents, and launch teenagers successfully.
- Cultural sensitivity is vital to family nursing. Some members have differing beliefs, traditions, and restrictions even within the same generation.
- Family caregiving is an interactive process that occurs within the context of the relationships among its members.

Critical Thinking Exercises

Kathy is a parish nurse and is working with a family in her church. This is a family of four: Carol, a 45-year-old single mother; her two adolescent sons, Matt and Kent; and Sara, her 76-year-old mother, who is in the last stages of terminal breast cancer. This family has lived together for 10 years, and Sara was a great support to Carol when her husband died 11 years ago. She helped Carol raise Matt and Kent. The family has decided to care for Sara in the home until she dies. Kathy is helping the family care for Sara in the home.

1. What assessments are important?
2. How will Kathy help the family achieve their goal of caring for Sara until she dies?
3. How will Kathy help the family determine their strengths, weaknesses, and resources?

NCLEX®-Style Review Questions

1. The Collins family includes a mother, Jean; stepfather, Adam; two teenage biological daughters of the mother, Lisa and Laura; and a biological daughter of the father, 25-year-old Stacey. Stacey just moved home following the loss of her job in another city. The family is converting a study into Stacey's bedroom and is in the process of distributing household chores. When you talk to members of the family, they all feel that their family can adjust to lifestyle changes. This is an example of family:
   1. Diversity
   2. Durability
   3. Resiliency
   4. Configuration

2. The Collins family (in question 1), which includes a mother, Jean; stepfather, Adam; two teenage biological daughters of the mother, Lisa and Laura; and a biological daughter of the father, 25-year-old Stacey is an example of a(n):
   1. Nuclear family
   2. Blended family
   3. Extended family
   4. Alternative family

3. Karen Johnson is a single mother of a school-age daughter. Linda Brown is also a single mother of two teenage daughters. Karen and Linda are active professionals, have busy social lives, and date occasionally. Three years ago they decided to share a house and share housing costs, living expenses, and child care responsibilities. The children consider one another as their family. This family form is considered a(n):
   1. Diverse family relationship
   2. Blended family relationship
   3. Extended family relationship
   4. Alternative pattern of relationship

4. The most common reason grandparents are called on to raise their grandchildren is due to:
   1. Single parenthood
   2. Legal interventions
   3. Dual-income families
   4. Increased divorce rate

5. Communication among family members is an example of family:
   1. Goals
   2. Function
   3. Structure
   4. Development

6. A family's access to adequate health care, opportunity for education, sound nutrition, and decreased stress is increased by:
   1. Development
   2. Family function
   3. Family structure
   4. Economic stability

7. When nurses view the family as client, their primary focus is on the:
   1. Family within a system
   2. Family process and relationships
   3. Family relational and transactional concepts
   4. Family health and development of an individual member

11 | Developmental Theories

✳ **OBJECTIVES**

Mastery of the content in this chapter will enable the student to:

- Discuss factors influencing growth and development.
- Describe biophysical developmental theories.
- Describe and compare the psychoanalytic/psychosocial theories proposed by Freud and Erikson.
- Describe Piaget's theory of cognitive development.

- Apply developmental theories when planning interventions in the care of clients.
- Discuss nursing implications for the application of developmental principles to client care.

✳ **MEDIA RESOURCES** ✳ **KEY TERMS**

Companion CD
- NCLEX®-Style Review Questions
- Audio Glossary
- Interactive Learning Activities
- English/Spanish Glossary

evolve Website
- NCLEX®-Style Review Questions
- Audio Glossary
- English/Spanish Glossary
- Interactive Learning Activities
- WebLinks
- Audio Summaries

Growth and Development

Understanding normal growth and development helps nurses predict, prevent, and detect any deviations from clients' own expected patterns. Development refers to the patterns of change that begin at conception and continue throughout a lifetime (Santrock, 2007). These patterns include the biological, cognitive, and socioemotional changes that take place during an individual's life span. Development is dynamic and includes progression as well as decline. For example, older adults demonstrate cognitive development resulting in wisdom as they incorporate life experiences into decision making, but they do not perform as well as young adults when speed is required for information processing (Baltes and Kunzmann, 2004; Santrock, 2007). Growth encompasses the physical changes that occur from the prenatal period through older adulthood and also demonstrates both advancement and deterioration. Young children grow more quickly than older children, and by adulthood growth in height ceases. In late adulthood, there is a decline in height with a loss of both muscle and bone (Berger, 2005).

Individuals have unique patterns of growth and development within broad limits. The ability to progress through each developmental phase influences the holistic health of the individual. The success or failure experienced within a phase affects the ability to complete subsequent phases. If individuals experience repeated developmental failures, inadequacies sometimes result. However, when the individual experiences repeated successes, health is promoted. A child not learning to walk by 20 months demonstrates delayed gross motor ability that slows exploration and manipulation of the environment. A child walking by 10 months is able to explore and find stimulation in the environment, thereby enhancing learning.

Today, nurses need to adopt a life span perspective of human development that takes into account all stages of life. Traditionally, development focused on childhood, but a comprehensive view of development also includes the changes that occur during the adult years (Elder and Shanahan, 2006). Nurses also consider the influence of culture and context when assessing the growth and development of a client. An understanding of growth and development throughout the life span assists nurses in planning questions for health screening and health history and in health teaching for clients of all ages.

Developmental Processes

Human growth and development is a complex pattern of movement that involves change in biological, cognitive, and socioemotional processes (Santrock, 2007). An individual's biological inheritance and environmental experiences influence these processes. The nurse applies knowledge of these processes in selecting therapies to promote normal growth and developmental progression. It is important, for example, for you to consider a female client's genetic endowment as well as her health before pregnancy as part of planning for a healthy, positive experience.

Biologic processes produce changes in an individual's physical growth and development. These changes are a result of genetic inheritance that interacts with external influences such as nutrition, exercise, stress, culture, and even climate (Berger, 2005). Height and weight, development of gross and fine motor skills, and sexual maturation resulting from hormonal changes during puberty are examples of changes resulting from biologic processes.

Cognitive processes comprise changes in intelligence, ability to understand and use language, and the development of thinking that shapes an individual's attitudes, beliefs, and behaviors (Berger, 2005; Santrock, 2007). Genes inherited from parents, life experiences, and environmental influences contribute to the changes in cognitive processes. Learning how to take turns during a conversation, playing a board game, and studying for a test all involve cognitive processes.

Socioemotional processes consist of the variations that occur in an individual's personality, emotions, and relationships with others during the individual's lifetime (Santrock, 2007). Genetic endowment and an individual's environmental context play a part in these changes. Temperament or behavioral style can be defined as the biological base of personality development. Most parents realize that their infant has a distinct personality and reacts in a consistent way to changes in routine. Knowledge of infant temperament will help you provide health promotion teaching so that parents are able to better understand their child's behavior (Hockenberry and Wilson, 2008).

Developmental Theories

A theory is a set of interrelated concepts, definitions, and propositions that present an organized view of a subject for the purpose of explaining and making predictions about the subject (see Chapter 4) (LoBiondo-Wood and Haber, 2006). Developmental theories provide a framework for examining, describing, and appreciating human development. For example, knowledge of Erikson's psychosocial theory of development helps caregivers understand the importance of supporting the development of basic trust in the infancy stage. Trust establishes the foundation for all future relationships. Developmental theories are also important in helping nurses assess and treat a person's response to an illness. Understanding the specific task or need of each developmental stage guides caregivers in planning appropriate individualized care for clients.

Human development is a dynamic and complex process that cannot be explained by only one theory. This chapter presents four groups of developmental theory: biophysical, psychoanalytic/psychosocial, cognitive, and moral. Chapters 25 and 29 cover the areas of learning theory and spiritual development.

Biophysical Developmental Theories

Biophysical development is how our physical bodies grow and change. Health care providers are able to quantify and compare the changes that occur as a newborn infant grows into adulthood against established norms. How does the physical body age? What are the triggers that move the body from the physical characteristics of childhood, through adolescence, to the physical changes of adulthood? Biophysical developmental theory describes the process of biological maturation. Gesell described biophysical development and developed a theory based on his observations of children's physical growth. The aging theories covered in Chapter 13 are biophysical developmental theories that define the aging process.

Gesell's Theory of Development.
Arnold Gesell (1880-1961) was a psychologist who also obtained his medical degree to help him explain the physiological processes he was observing in the behavior of children. Through extensive observations in the 1940s, he developed behavior norms that still serve as a primary source of information for childhood development. Today's version of the Gesell test is composed of four behavioral categories: motor, language, adaptive, and personal-social. Health care providers assess each of these subgroups to achieve a developmental quotient (DQ) that distinguishes between normal and abnormal infants (Santrock, 2007).

Fundamental to Gesell's theory of development is that although each child's pattern of growth (development) is unique, this pattern is directed by gene activity. Environmental factors support, change, and modify the pattern, but they do not generate progressions of development (Gesell, 1948). Gesell found the pattern of maturation as a fixed developmental sequence in humans. Sequential development occurs in fetuses, where there is a specified order of organ system development (Crain, 1992). After birth, children grow according to their genetic blueprint and gain skills in an orderly fashion, but at each individual's own pace. For example, most children learn first how to hold a cup with digital grasp at around 15 months of age and handle a cup well, lifting, drinking, and replacing, by 21 months of age. Gesell was clear that not every child develops these skills at the same time. The environment plays a part in child development, but it does not have any part in the sequence of development.

Psychoanalytic/Psychosocial Theory

Theories of **psychoanalytic/psychosocial development** describe human development from the perspectives of personality, thinking, and behavior (Table 11-1). Psychoanalytic theory explains development in terms of inner drives and motives that are primarily unconscious and influence every aspect of an individual's thinking and behavior (Berger, 2005). These drives and motives also occur in stages that every human being experiences in a sequence.

Sigmund Freud.
The first person to provide a formal, structured theory of personality development was Sigmund Freud (1856-1939). Freud constructed his theory of development while working with clients suffering from mental illness. **Freud's psychoanalytic model of personality development states** individuals go through five stages of psychosexual development and that each stage was characterized by sexual pleasure in parts of the body: the mouth, the anus, and the genitals. Freud believed that adult personality is the result of how an individual resolved conflicts between these sources of pleasure and the mandates of reality (Berger, 2005; Santrock, 2007).

Stage 1: Oral (Birth to 12 to 18 Months). Initially, sucking and oral satisfaction are not only vital to life, but also extremely pleasurable in their own rights. Late in this stage, the infant begins to realize that the mother/parent is something separate from self. Disruption in the physical or emotional availability of the parent (e.g., inadequate bonding or chronic illness) could affect an infant's development.

Stage 2: Anal (12 to 18 Months to 3 Years). The focus of pleasure changes to the anal zone. Children become increasingly aware of the pleasurable sensations of this body region with interest in the products of their effort. Through the toilet-training process the child delays gratification in order to meet parental and societal expectations.

✳ TABLE 11-1 Comparison of Major Developmental Theories

DEVELOPMENTAL STAGE/AGE	FREUD (PSYCHOSEXUAL DEVELOPMENT)	ERIKSON (PSYCHOSOCIAL DEVELOPMENT)	PIAGET (COGNITIVE/ MORAL DEVELOPMENT)	KOHLBERG (DEVELOPMENT OF MORAL REASONING)
Infancy (birth to 18 months)	Oral stage	Trust versus mistrust Ability to trust others	Sensorimotor period Progress from reflex activity to simple repetitive actions	
Early childhood/ toddler (18 months to 3 years)	Anal stage	Autonomy versus shame and doubt Self-control and independence	Preoperational period—thinking using symbols; egocentric	Preconventional level Punishment-obedience orientation
Preschool (3-5 years)	Phallic stage	Initiative versus guilt Highly imaginative	Use of symbols; egocentric	Preconventional level Premoral Instrumental orientation
Middle childhood (6-12 years)	Latent stage	Industry versus inferiority Engaged in tasks and activities	Concrete operations period Logical thinking	Conventional level Good boy–nice girl orientation
Adolescence (12-19 years)	Genital stage	Identity versus role confusion Sexual maturity, "Who am I?"	Formal operations period Abstract thinking	Postconventional level Social contract orientation

Stage 3: Phallic or Oedipal (3 to 6 Years). It is during this stage that the genital organs become the focus of pleasure. According to Freud, the boy becomes interested in the penis; the girl becomes aware of the absence of the penis, known as penis envy. This is the time of exploration and imagination as the child fantasizes about the parent of the opposite sex as his or her first love interest, known as the Oedipus or Electra complex. By the end of this stage, the child attempts to reduce this conflict by identifying with the parent of the same sex in a way to win recognition and acceptance.

Stage 4: Latency (6 to 12 Years). This is a stage in which Freud believed that sexual urges, from the earlier oedipal stage, are repressed and channeled into productive activities that are socially acceptable. Within the educational and social worlds of the child, there is much to learn and accomplish. This is where the child places energy and effort.

Stage 5: Genital (Puberty Through Adulthood). This is Freud's final stage. This is a time of turbulence when earlier sexual urges reawaken and are directed to an individual outside the family circle. Unresolved prior conflicts surface during adolescence. Once the individual resolves conflicts, he or she is then capable of having a mature adult sexual relationship.

Components of the human personality develop through Freud's developmental stages. Freud believed that the functions of these components regulate behavior. These components are the id, the ego, and the superego. The id, basic instinctual impulses driven to achieve pleasure, is the most primitive part of the personality and originates in the infant. The ego represents the reality component mediating conflicts between the environment and the forces of the id. The ego helps us judge reality accurately, regulate impulses, and make good decisions. The third component, the superego, performs regulating, restraining, and prohibiting actions. Often referred to as the conscience, the superego is influenced by the standards of outside social forces (e.g., parent or teacher).

The goal in Freud's theory was the development of balance between pleasure-seeking drives and societal pressures. The mature adult has a strong sense of conscience that allows for the experience of pleasure within the boundaries of society. Although many have criticized Freud's theory for gender and cultural biases, it is clear that he gave other theorists a basis for observation of emotion and behavior. Some of Freud's critics contend that he based his analysis of personality development on biological determinants and ignored the influence of culture and experience. Other critics think that Freud's basic assumptions such as the Oedipus complex are not applicable across different cultures. Today's psychoanalysts believe that the role of conscious thought is much greater than Freud imagined (Santrock, 2007).

Erik Erikson. Freud had a strong influence on his psychoanalytic followers, including Erik Erikson, who continued to develop and refine his theory. Erik Erikson constructed a theory of development that differed from Freud's in two major views. Erikson maintained that development occurred throughout the life span and that it focused on psychosocial stages rather than psychosexual stages (Santrock, 2007). Erikson (1902-1994) lived in Germany, Italy, and Austria before coming to the United States and studying college students, children at play, and Native American

culture. These life experiences helped Erikson to understand the importance of culture and the changes that occur throughout adulthood. He used this knowledge in developing a psychoanalytic theory that emphasized developmental change throughout the life span (Berger, 2005).

According to **Erikson's eight stages of development,** individuals need to accomplish a particular task before successfully mastering the stage and progressing to the next one. Each task is framed with opposing conflicts, such as the adolescent's need to develop a sense of personal identity challenged by many confusing choices. These core conflicts remain throughout life.

Each stage builds upon the successful resolution of the previous developmental conflict. Readiness for the task is necessary for success. Tasks once mastered are challenged and tested again during new situations or at times of conflict (Hockenberry and Wilson, 2008). For example, an individual builds trust with an infant through consistent, reliable caregiving; yet the concept of trust is tested when an infant is hospitalized or after the birth of a new baby. Erickson's eight stages of life are described below.

Trust Versus Mistrust (Birth to 1 Year). Establishment of a basic sense of trust is essential for the development of a healthy personality. The infant 's successful resolution of this stage requires a consistent caregiver who is available to meet his needs. From this basic trust in parents, the infant is able to trust in himself, in others, and in the world (Hockenberry and Wilson, 2008). The formation of trust results in faith and optimism. A nurse's use of anticipatory guidance will help parents cope with the hospitalization of an infant and the infant's behaviors when discharged to home. The child's sense of trust may be challenged during hospitalization and may need support from parents when returning home.

Autonomy Versus Sense of Shame and Doubt (1 to 3 Years). By this stage a growing child is more accomplished in some basic self-care activities, including walking, feeding, and toileting. This newfound independence is the result of maturation and imitation. The toddler develops his or her autonomy by making choices. Choices typical for the toddler age-group include activities related to relationships, desires, and playthings. There is also opportunity to learn that parents and society have expectations about these choices. Limiting choices and or harsh punishment lead to feelings of shame and doubt. The toddler who successfully masters this stage achieves self-control and willpower. The nurse is able to model empathetic guidance that offers support for and understanding of the challenges of this stage.

Initiative Versus Guilt (3 to 6 Years). Children like to pretend and try out new roles. Fantasy and imagination allow children to further explore their environment. Also at this time children are developing their superego, or conscience. Conflicts often occur between the child's desire to explore and the limits placed on his or her behavior. These conflicts sometimes lead to feelings of frustration and guilt. Guilt also occurs if the caregiver's responses are too harsh. Preschoolers are learning to maintain a sense of initiative without imposing on the freedoms of others. Successful resolution of this stage results in direction and purpose. Teaching impulse control and cooperative behaviors to the child help the family avoid the risks of altered growth and development.

Industry Versus Inferiority (6 to 11 Years). School-age children are eager to apply themselves to learning socially productive skills and tools. They learn to work and play with their peers.

School-age children thrive on their accomplishments and praise. Without proper support for learning of new skills or if skills are too difficult, children then develop a sense of inadequacy and inferiority. Children at this age need to be able to experience real achievement to develop a sense of competency. Erikson believed that the adult's attitudes toward work are traced to successful achievement of this task (Erikson, 1963).

Identity Versus Role Confusion (Puberty). Dramatic physiological changes associated with sexual maturation mark this stage. There is a marked preoccupation with appearance and body image. This stage in which identity development begins with the goal of achieving some perspective or direction answers the question, "Who am I?" Acquiring a sense of identity is essential for making adult decisions such as choice of vocation or marriage partner. Each adolescent moves in his or her unique way into society as an interdependent member. There are also new social demands, opportunities, and conflicts that relate to the emergent identity and separation from family. Erikson held that successful mastery of this stage resulted in devotion and fidelity to others and to their own ideals (Hockenberry and Wilson, 2008). The nurse provides education and anticipatory guidance for the parent about the changes and challenges to the adolescent. Nurses also assist hospitalized adolescents in dealing with their illness by giving them enough information to allow them to make decisions about their treatment plan.

Intimacy Versus Isolation (Young Adult). Young adults, having developed a sense of identity, deepen their capacity to love others and care for them. They search for meaningful friendships and an intimate relationship with another. Erikson portrayed intimacy as finding the self and then losing the self in another (Santrock, 2007). If the young adult is not able to establish companionship and intimacy, isolation will result because they fear rejection and disappointment (Berger, 2005). You need to understand that during hospitalization young adults will benefit from the support of their partner or significant other because this strengthens their need for intimacy.

Generativity Versus Self-Absorption and Stagnation (Middle Age). Following the development of an intimate relationship, the adult focuses on supporting future generations. The ability to expand one's personal and social involvement is critical to this stage of development. Middle-age adults achieve success in this stage by contributing to future generations through parenthood, teaching, and community involvement. Achievement of generativity results in care as a basic strength. Inability to play a role in the development of the next generation results in stagnation (Santrock, 2007). Nurses assist physically ill adults in choosing creative ways to foster social development. Middle-age persons often find a sense of fulfillment by volunteering some time in a local school, hospital, or church.

Integrity Versus Despair (Old Age). As the aging process creates physical and social losses, some adults also suffer loss of status and function, such as through retirement or illness. These external struggles are also met with internal struggles, such as the search for meaning in life. Meeting these challenges creates the potential for growth and the basic strength of wisdom (Figure 11-1). Many older adults review their lives with a sense of satisfaction even with their inevitable mistakes, whereas others see themselves as failures with their lives marked by despair and re-

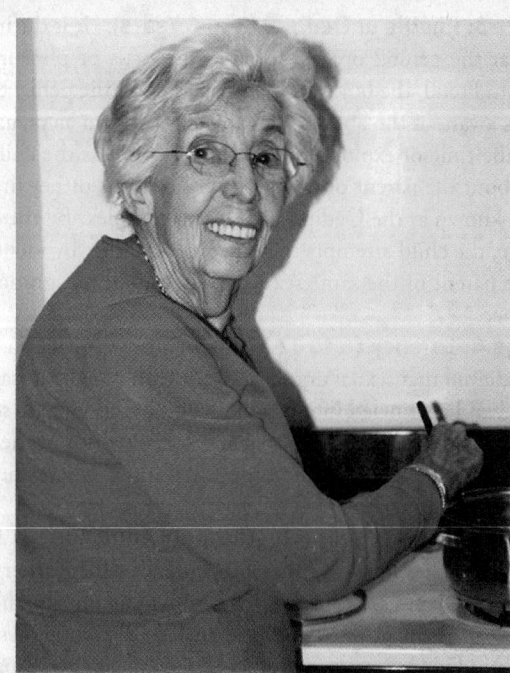

Figure 11-1 Maintaining independence is important to one's self-esteem.

gret. Older adults often engage in a retrospective appraisal of their lives and see it as a meaningful whole or experience regret at goals not achieved (Berger, 2005). Box 11-1 presents research pertaining to the losses experienced by older adults.

Nurses are in positions of influence within their communities and contribute to the valuing of persons at all ages and stages. Persons at all ages and stages need to feel valued, appreciated, and needed. Erikson stated, "Healthy children will not fear life, if their parents have integrity enough not to fear death" (Erikson, 1963). Although, like Freud, Erickson believed that problems in adult life resulted from unsuccessful resolution of earlier stages, his emphasis on family relationships and culture offered a broad, life span view of development.

Theories Related to Temperament. Temperament is a behavioral style that affects the individual's emotional interactions with others (Santrock, 2007). Personality and temperament are often closely linked, and research has shown that individuals possess some enduring characteristics into adulthood. The individual differences children display in responding to their environment significantly influence the way others respond to them and their needs. Knowledge of temperament helps parents to have an understandable perspective of their child and enables health caregivers to guide them appropriately (Hockenberry and Wilson, 2008).

Psychiatrists Stella Chess and Alexander Thomas conducted a 20-year longitudinal study that included children from a wide range of populations, including healthy children of middle-class parents born in the United States and Puerto Rican and American working-class parents with mentally challenged children. The range of data allowed them to look at the behavior of persons

---

❋ **BOX 11-1**   **EVIDENCE-BASED PRACTICE**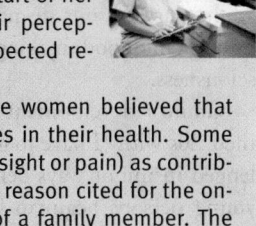

Older Adult Women's Explanation of Depression

Evidence Summary

Many use depression to describe a mood, a symptom, or a syndrome. Its intensity is usually described as mild, moderate, or severe. Examples of depression as a mood include the expression of sadness, hopelessness, and disappointment. The grieving process also expresses the mood of depression. Symptoms of depression appear in three spheres: cognitive (thinking), affective (feeling tone), and psychomotor (action) behaviors. It is not uncommon to see symptoms of depression during chronic illness or as a side effect of many medications. Depression is a common psychiatric condition affecting individuals of all ages. It is important that nurses understand what impact depression and other emotional states have on a person's perceptions about his or her health condition and treatment. As the older adult population increases, the rate of age-related disabilities, chronic illness, and depression will also increase.

This research uses an explanatory model to describe an individual's interpretation of an illness and is based on the individual's general beliefs about health and illness. It provides personal and social meaning to the illness experience. Using this model, clients construct from their beliefs an explanation of the illness and plan their course of treatment. As the nurse, you need to ask questions designed to gain the client's perspective of his or her illness with relationship to its etiology, symptoms, and treatment options.

The researchers interviewed 30 older adult women with depression. Interviews focused on the person's perception of the cause and contributing factors for the start of her illness. The participants identified their perceptions of the severity, duration, and expected results of treatment.

The results showed that most of the women believed that their depression was a result of changes in their health. Some identified loss of function (e.g., poor eyesight or pain) as contributing factors. The second most common reason cited for the onset of depression was due to a death of a family member. The women believe that these deaths contributed to their loneliness. The women did not commonly describe thoughts of suicide; however, they frequently expressed somatic symptoms such as generalized aches and pains.

Application to Nursing Practice

- Understanding the older person's concept of depression assists nurses in explaining complementary and alternative treatment measures.
- Further public education is necessary to prepare for the growing numbers of older persons.
- Treatment centers need to be extended to churches, synagogues, and other social or civic centers.
- Understanding of adult development and its implications for practice is essential in providing nursing care for older adult clients.

Reference
Ugarriza DN: Elderly women's explanation of depression, *J Gerontol Nurs* 28(5):22, 2002.

---

from childhood to early adulthood as they interacted with their environment. Their work introduced the concept of temperament and their belief that an individual's temperament is established by the age of 2 to 3 months (Berger, 2005). Chess and Thomas identified three basic classes of temperament:

- **The easy child**—easygoing and even-tempered. Regular and predictable in his or her habits. An easy child is open and adaptable to change and displays a mild to moderately intense mood that is typically positive.
- **The difficult child**—highly active, irritable, and irregular in habits. Negative withdrawal toward others is typical, and the child requires a more structured environment. A difficult child adapts slowly to new routines, people, or situations. Mood expressions are usually intense and primarily negative.
- **The slow-to-warm-up child**—typically reacts negatively and with mild intensity to new stimuli. The child adapts slowly with repeated contact unless pressured and responds with mild but passive resistance to novelty or changes in routine.

They determined that approximately 50% of the children were "easy," almost 15% were "slow-to-warm-up" children, and just 10% were classified as "difficult." The remaining 25% did not fit into any of their categories (Berger, 2005).

Research on temperament and its stability has continued with an emphasis on the individual's ability to make thoughtful decisions about behavior in demanding situations. Jerome Kagan views temperament in terms of the differences between outgoing,

sociable, bold children and shy, introverted, timid children. He has identified a category he termed "inhibition to the unfamiliar" and found that inhibition is stable throughout early childhood but changes in time with consistent support (Kagan and Fox, 2006).

Knowledge of temperament and how it impacts the parent-child relationship is critical when providing anticipatory guidance for parents. With the birth of a second child, most parents find that the strategies that worked well with the first child no longer work at all. You can individualize counseling to greatly improve the quality of interactions between parents and children (Hockenberry and Wilson, 2008).

Perspectives on Adult Development

Early study of development focused only on childhood because scholars throughout history regarded the aging process as one of inevitable and irreversible decline. However, we now know that although the changes come more slowly, people continue to develop new abilities and adapt to shifting environments. Human development is lifelong. The life span perspective reveals that understanding of adult development requires multiple viewpoints. Two of the ways that researchers have studied adult development are through the stage-crisis view and the life events approach. The most well-known stage theory is the one developed by Erik Erikson that was discussed earlier. Another developmentalist, Roger Gould, also developed a stage theory related to adult development and aging.

Stage-Crisis Theory. Psychiatrist Roger Gould conducted extensive research that supported a set of development themes within stages of adult development. Gould found that over the adult years persons dismantle the protective thinking developed during childhood, making a shift from childhood into adult consciousness.

Gould's development themes start when individuals are in their 20s with "I have to get away from my parents." This is challenged in minor ways before the end of high school but ends as young persons begin to live away from home. The move away from parental influence is gradual as young adults establish themselves as adults.

The second theme occurs during the early 30s and asks, "Is what I am the only way for me to be?" This question occurs when young adults experience the consequences of the decisions of their independence. Everything does not work out magically as expected. There are failures to be overcome. Acceptance for who they are is essential, as is acceptance of their own growing children as being unique and separate.

The third theme occurs in the mid to late 30s and asks, "Have I done the right thing? Is there time to change?" These questions recognize the complexities of adult decisions. The impact of a growing family and aging parents influences this theme. There is a beginning sense of time left to effect wanted results.

The fourth theme, identified in the 40s, "The die is cast," indicates resignation and the belief that possibilities are limited. The personality is set. Individuals believe changes in career are less likely to be successful. Parents are blamed for their lack of choices. Individuals face regret for mistakes made with children.

During the 50s a decrease in negativism occurs. Gould finds a realization of mortality with a concern for one's state of health. There is less responsibility for the welfare of the children and more attachment to the spouse.

Gould believes his research describes a sequential process that takes place between the internal life (personality) of adults and their outer world (e.g., culture and lifestyle). For example, Gould looked at the timing and sequencing of an event, as well as the individual's adjustment and transition into a particular stage. It seemed clear to Gould that events of adulthood are similar in adults; however, the timing and sequencing affect the adjustment and consequences in different individuals. Marriage, for example, occurs before or after pregnancy, the time between the birth of the first and second child sometimes differs, and retirement occurs in the 50s or 60s. Gould's theoretical work will help you appreciate life issues affecting the adult client. You will help adults realistically appreciate their accomplishments and foster their continued development.

Life-Events Approach. The stage theories hold that all individuals experience life in a common progression and focus on a developmental task during a specific age range. The contemporary life-events approach (Santrock, 2007) takes into consideration the variations that occur for each individual. This view considers the individual's personal circumstances (health and family support), how the person views and adjusts to changes, and the current social and historical context in which the individual is living. Researchers have proposed numerous theories related to age, culture, gender, ethnicity, stability, and change to help us appreciate

the dynamic development that occurs throughout the adult years.

Cognitive Developmental Theory

Whereas psychoanalytic/psychosocial theories focus on an individual's unconscious thought and emotions, cognitive theories stress how people learn to think and make sense of their world. As with personality development, cognitive theorists have explored both childhood and adulthood. Some of the theories highlight qualitative changes in thinking, and others expand to include social, cultural, and behavioral dimensions.

Jean Piaget. Jean Piaget (1896-1980), a Swiss biologist and philosopher, was most interested in the development of children's intellectual organization, how they think, reason, and perceive the world. **Piaget's theory of cognitive development** includes four periods that are related to age and demonstrate specific categories of knowing and understanding (Santrock, 2007). He built his theory on years of observing children as they explored, manipulated, and tried to make sense out of the world in which they lived. Piaget believed that individuals move from one stage to the other in seeking cognitive equilibrium or a state of mental balance (Santrock, 2007). Within each of these primary periods of **cognitive development** are specific stages (see Table 11-1).

Period I: Sensorimotor (Birth to 2 Years). During a time of unparalleled changes, the infant develops the schema or action pattern for dealing with the environment (Berk, 2003). These schemas include hitting, looking, grasping, or kicking (Figure 11-2). Schemas become self-initiated activities; for example, the infant learning that sucking achieves a pleasing result generalizes the action to suck fingers, blanket, or clothing. Successful achievement leads to greater exploration.

Period II: Preoperational (2 to 7 Years). This is a time when children learn to think with the use of symbols and mental images. Still egocentric, children see objects and persons from only one point of view, their own. Children believe that everyone experiences the world exactly as they do. Play becomes a primary means by which children foster their cognitive development and learn about the world (Figure 11-3). Nursing interventions during this period will recognize the use of play as the way the child understands the events taking place. You will assist parents in the use of play materials such as thermometers, blood pressure equipment, and syringes that will allow children to communicate feelings about health care procedures they experience.

Language develops and broadens possibilities for thinking about the past or the future. Children can now communicate about events with others. As the language fits into a logical form, it mirrors the thinking process at the time.

Period III: Concrete Operations (7 to 11 Years). Children now achieve the ability to perform mental operations. For example, the child now thinks about an action that before was performed physically. At the earlier stage the child could count to 10, but now he or she counts and understands what each number represents. Children are now able to describe a process without actually performing it. At this time they are able to coordinate two concrete perspectives in social as well as scientific thinking. In other words, they are able to appreciate the difference between their perspective and that of a friend. Reversibility is the primary

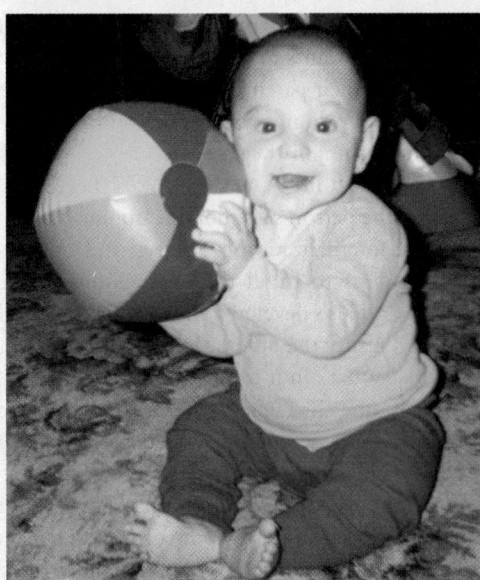

Figure 11-2 Successful achievement of action patterns such as grasping leads to learning and more exploration.

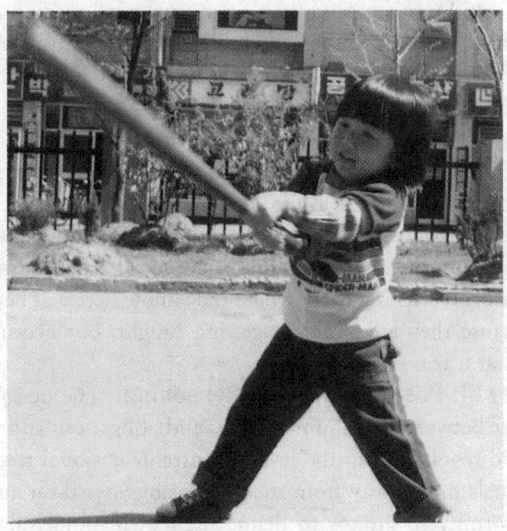

Figure 11-3 Play is important to a child's development.

characteristic of concrete operational thought. Children mentally reverse the direction of their thoughts. Children can now mentally classify objects according to their quantitative dimensions, known as seriation. Another major accomplishment of this stage is conservation, or the ability to see objects or quantities as remaining the same despite a change in their physical appearance (Berk, 2003; Singer and Revenson, 1996). Children begin to cooperate and share new information about the acts they perform. Parents will be able to adjust their approaches to guide the child into helpful activities within the home, such as bargaining about chores in exchange for wishes for privileges (e.g., TV time or playing with friends).

Period IV: Formal Operations (11 Years to Adulthood).
During this stage the individual's thinking moves to abstract and theoretical subjects. Adolescents and young adults begin thinking about such subjects as achieving world peace, finding justice, and

seeking meaning in life. Adolescents are able to organize their thoughts in their minds. They have the capacity to reason with respect to possibilities. New cognitive powers allow the adolescent to do more far-reaching problem solving, including their futures and that of others. This thinking matures, and the depth of understanding increases with experience. For Piaget, this stage marked the end of cognitive development.

Social Cognitive Theory. American psychologist Albert Bandura (1925) pioneered the idea that to understand behavior it was also necessary to understand how people think (Santrock, 2007). Initially Bandura focused on observation of behavior and thought that learning occurred through **modeling.** He did not view modeling as simply imitation. Bandura believed that individuals observe the behaviors of others and then make a deliberate choice whether or not to copy the behavior.

Bandura's current model of development emphasizes interaction among behavior, environment, and personal/cognitive factors. He views learning as active and occurring within a social context. Bandura's social cognitive theory incorporates the personal factors of self-understanding, self-confidence, and self-efficacy in development (Berger, 2005).

Cognitive Changes in Adult Thought. Research into cognitive development in adulthood began in the 1970s and continues today. Piaget had proposed that formal operational thought began in adolescence and that essentially adults use the same type of reasoning. However, research has shown that some individuals do not reach formal operational thought until adulthood, and some adults never develop to the period of formal operations (Santrock, 2007). Other researchers noted that adults do not always come to one answer to a problem but frequently accept several possible solutions. Adults also incorporate emotions, logic, practicality, and flexibility when making decisions (Santrock, 2007). Based on these observations, developmentalists proposed a fifth stage of cognitive development termed postformal thought. Within this stage, adults demonstrate the ability to recognize that answers vary from situation to situation and that solutions need to be sensible. Adults are able to accept contradiction and see the world in shades of gray rather than all black and white.

One of the earliest to develop a theory of adult cognition was William Perry. He studied college students and found that continued cognitive development involved increasing cognitive flexibility. As adolescents were able to move from a position of accepting only one answer to realizing that alternative explanations could be right depending on one's perspective, there was a significant cognitive change (Santrock, 2007).

K. Warner Schaie, a professor of human development at Pennsylvania State University, concluded that we do not develop more sophisticated ways to gain information than proposed by Piaget, but that adults do change *how* they use knowledge. Schaie believes that the emphasis shifts from attaining knowledge or skills to using knowledge for goal achievement.

Moral Developmental Theory

Moral development refers to the changes in a person's thoughts, emotions, and behaviors that influence beliefs about what is right or wrong. It encompasses both *interpersonal* and *intrapersonal* dimensions as it governs how we interact with others (Santrock, 2007). Although various psychosocial and cognitive theorists have addressed moral development within their respective theories, the theories of Piaget and Kohlberg are more widely known (see Table 11-1).

Jean Piaget's Theory of Moral Development.

When Piaget observed and interviewed children, he learned how they thought about rules and moral issues. While watching children play marbles, he questioned them about the rules of the game and asked questions concerning stealing, lying, punishment, and justice (Santrock, 2007). **Piaget's theory of moral development** includes two stages that emerge between the ages of 4 and 10 years. The first stage, **heteronomous morality,** occurs between 4 and 7 years and is characterized by a belief that rules are unchangeable and that when a rule is broken, there is imminent justice. The young child is unable to accept the idea that rules in a game are changeable or that punishment will not automatically follow a transgression (Santrock, 2007). In the second stage, **autonomous morality,** the child understands that people make rules and that they can be changed. At this stage children know that intentions influence the consequences of behaviors. Piaget believed that it was primarily through peer interactions that children were able to develop moral reasoning. In peer groups children are able to disagree and come to a settlement. Parent-child interactions are not equal and thus less likely to foster moral reasoning (Santrock, 2007).

Lawrence Kohlberg's Theory of Moral Development.

Kohlberg's theory of moral development expanded upon Piaget's cognitive theory. He interviewed children, adolescents, and eventually adults, finding that moral reasoning develops in stages (Berger, 2005). From a series of moral dilemmas, he identified six stages of moral development under three levels (Kohlberg, 1981).

Level I: Preconventional Reasoning. At Level I, **preconventional reasoning,** the person reflects on moral reasoning based on personal gain. This closely correlates with Piaget's first stage, in that the person's moral reason for acting, the "why," relates to the consequences the person believes will occur. These consequences come in the form of punishment or reward. It is at this level that children view illness as a punishment for fighting with their siblings or disobeying their parents. Be aware of this thinking and reinforce teaching that the child cannot become ill because of wrongdoing.

Stage 1: Punishment and Obedience Orientation. In this first stage the child's response to a moral dilemma is in terms of absolute obedience to authority and rules. A child in this stage reasons, "I must follow the rules; otherwise I will be punished." The child's avoidance of punishment or the unquestioning deference to authority is characteristic motivation to behave. A child will be home on time for supper because the parents said the child needs to be.

Stage 2: Instrumental Relativist Orientation. In this stage the child recognizes there is more than one right view; a teacher has one view that is different than the child's parent. The decision to do something morally right is based on satisfying one's own needs, and occasionally the needs of others. The child per-

ceives punishment not as proof of being wrong (as in Stage 1), but as something that one wants to avoid (Taffell, 2002). Children at this stage will follow their parent's rule about being home in time for supper because they do not want to be confined to their room for the rest of the evening if they are late.

Level II: Conventional Reasoning. At Level II, **conventional reasoning,** the person sees moral reasoning based on his or her own personal internalization of societal and others' expectations. A person wants to fulfill the expectations of the family, group, or nation and also develop a loyalty to and actively maintain, support, and justify the order. Moral decision making at this level moves from "What's in it for me?" to "How will it affect my relationships with others?" There is emphasis now on social rules and a community-centered approach (Berger, 2005). Nurses observe this when family members make end-of-life decisions for their loved ones. Individual members often struggle with this type of moral dilemma. Grief support will involve an understanding of the level of moral decision making of each family member (see Chapter 30).

Stage 3: Good Boy–Nice Girl Orientation. The individual wants to win approval and maintain the expectations of one's immediate group. "Being good" means having good motives, showing concern for others, and keeping mutual relationships through trust, loyalty, respect, and gratitude. One earns approval by "being nice." For example, a person in this stage stays after school and does odd jobs to win the teacher's approval.

Stage 4: Society-Maintaining Orientation. Individuals expand their focus from a relationship with others to societal concerns during Stage 4. Moral decisions take into account societal perspectives. Right behavior is doing one's duty, showing respect for authority, and maintaining the social order. Adolescents choose not to attend a party where they know beer will be served, not because they are afraid of getting caught, but because they know that it is not right.

Level III: Postconventional Reasoning. The person finds a balance between basic human rights and obligations and societal rules and regulations in the level of **postconventional reasoning.** Individuals move away from moral decisions based on authority or conformity to groups to define their own moral values and principles. Individuals at this stage start to look at what an ideal society would be like. Moral principles and ideals come into prominence at this level (Berger, 2005).

Stage 5: Social Contract Orientation. Having reached Stage 5, an individual follows the societal law but recognizes the possibility of changing the law to improve society. The individual also recognizes that different social groups have different values but believes that all rational people would agree on basic rights, such as liberty and life. Individuals at this stage make more of an independent effort to think out what society should value, not related to what the society as a group would value, as would occur in Stage 4. The United States Constitution is based on this morality.

Stage 6: Universal Ethical Principle Orientation. Stage 6 defines "right" by the decision of conscience in accord with self-chosen ethical principles. These principles are abstract, like the Golden Rule, and appeal to logical comprehensiveness, universality, and consistency (Kohlberg, 1981). For example, the principle of justice requires the individual to treat everyone in an impartial manner, respecting the basic dignity of all people, and

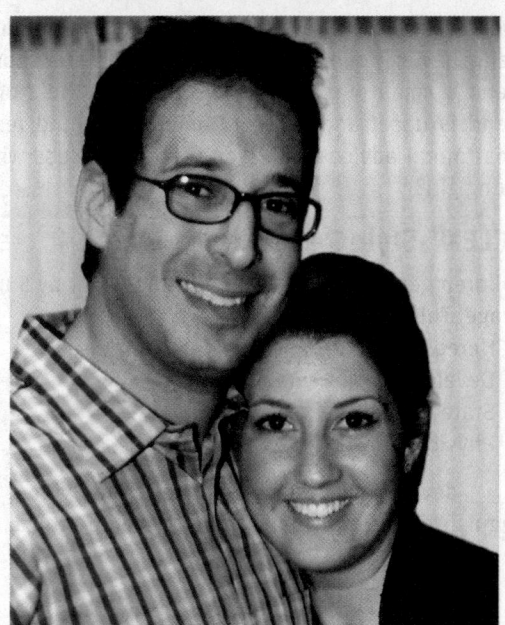

Figure 11-4 Adults need meaningful, close, respectful relationships.

guides the individual to base decisions on an equal respect for all (Figure 11-4). Stage 5 emphasizes the basic rights and the democratic process, whereas Stage 6 defines the principles by which agreements will be most just.

Kohlberg's Critics. Kohlberg constructed a systemized way of looking at moral development. He has been recognized as a leader in moral developmental theory. However, critics of his work raise questions about his choice of research subjects. Most of Kohlberg's subjects were males of the Western philosophical traditions.

Research attempting to support Kohlberg's theory with individuals raised in the Eastern philosophies found that those study participants never rose above Stages 3 or 4 of Kohlberg's model. These findings may suggest that they have not reached higher levels of moral development, as most of the adults raised in the Western traditions did. Or findings may be suggesting that Kohlberg's research design did not allow a way to measure those raised within a different culture.

Kohlberg has also been criticized for age and gender bias. Carol Gilligan, an associate, has criticized Kohlberg for his gender biases (Santrock, 2007). She believes that Kohlberg developed his theory based on a justice perspective that focused on the rights of individuals. In contrast, Gilligan's research looked at moral development from a care perspective that viewed people in their interpersonal communications, relationships, and concern for others (Santrock, 2007). She believes that females are socialized to be nurturing and caring and thus are reluctant to make judgments based solely on justice (Berger, 2005). Other researchers have examined Gilligan's theory in studies with children and have not found evidence to support gender differences (Berger, 2005; Santrock, 2007).

Moral Reasoning and Nursing Practice. Nurses need to know their own moral reasoning level. Recognizing your own moral developmental level is essential in separating your own beliefs from others when helping clients with their moral decision-making process. Recognize the level of moral reasoning used by members of the health care team and its influence on the client's care plan. Ideally all members of the health care team will be on the same level, creating a unified outcome. This is exemplified in the following scenario: The nurse is caring for a homeless person and believes that all clients deserve the same level of care. The case manager, being responsible for resource allocation, complains about the client's length of stay and the amount of resources being expended on this one client. The nurse and the case manager are in conflict because of their different levels of moral decision making within their practices. They decide to hold a health care team conference to discuss their differences and the ethical dilemma of ensuring that the client receives an appropriate level of care.

Conclusion

Developmental theories help nurses to use critical thinking skills when asking how and why people respond as they do. From the diverse set of theories included in this chapter, the complexity of human development is evident. No one theory successfully describes all the intricacies of human growth and development. Today's nurse needs be knowledgeable about several theoretical perspectives when working with clients.

A nurse's assessment of a client requires a thorough analysis and interpretation of data to form accurate conclusions about a client's developmental needs. Accurate identification of nursing diagnoses relies on the nurse's ability to consider developmental theory in data analysis. A nurse compares normal developmental behaviors with those projected by developmental theory. Examples of nursing diagnoses applicable to clients with developmental problems include *risk for delayed development, delayed growth and development,* and *risk for disproportionate growth.* Further detail regarding these diagnoses are in Chapter 12.

Growth and development, as supported by a life span perspective, is multidimensional. The theories included are the basis for a meaningful observation of an individual's pattern of growth and development. They are important guidelines for understanding important human processes that allow nurses to begin to predict human responses and recognize deviations from the norm.

✳ Key Concepts

- Nurses administer care for individuals at various developmental stages. Developmental theory provides a basis for nurses to assess and understand the responses seen in their clients.
- Humans continue to develop throughout their lives. Development does not end at adolescence; persons grow and develop throughout their life span.
- Theory is a way to account for how and why people grow up as they do. Theories provide a framework to clarify and organize existing observations to explain and try to predict human behavior.
- Growth refers to the quantitative changes that nurses measure and compare to norms.

- Development implies a progressive and continuous process of change leading to a state of organized and specialized functional capacity. These changes are quantitatively measurable but are more distinctly measured in qualitative changes.
- Biophysical development theory explores theories of why individuals age from a biological standpoint.
- Cognitive development focuses on the rational-thinking processes that include the changes in how children and adolescents perform intellectual operations.
- Developmental tasks are age-related achievements, the success of which leads to happiness, whereas failure often leads to unhappiness, disapproval, and difficulty in achieving later tasks.
- Developmental crisis occurs when a person is having great difficulty in meeting tasks of the current developmental period.
- Socialization is the outside influence a person receives from family, peers, and society.
- Psychosocial theories describe human development from the perspectives of personality, thinking, and behavior with varying degrees of influence from the internal biological forces and the external societal/cultural forces.
- Temperament is a behavioral pattern that affects the child's interactions with others.
- Moral development theory attempts to define how moral reasoning matures for an individual.

✳ Critical Thinking Exercises

1. A 76-year-old woman has recently been diagnosed with breast cancer. She also has severe cardiovascular disease that limits her choices of treatment. Her oncologist has recommended a series of chemotherapy treatments that her cardiologist believes would be fatal. Her family is urging her to do all that is recommended. The client, who is in good spirits despite her diagnosis, chooses palliative care. Based on her developmental stage, how can you help the family adjust to her choice?

2. A 50-year-old woman expresses dismay that her children ages 20 and 23 are no longer living at home. Her husband is still working full-time but looking to retire in a couple of years. She is concerned that she is not needed and is bored with her life. Identify the developmental task of Erickson's theory that best fits this woman's situation. How will the nurse assist this client in changing her lifestyle while understanding her developmental tasks?

3. Parents of an 18-month-old toddler describe to the nurse during their routine visit to the pediatrician that their child is walking and getting into everything. Using your knowledge of Erikson's developmental theories, what stage is this child in, and what approach would be helpful for these parents?

4. Two 11-year-old girls are spending the day together at the mall. They exit one store, and one of the girls shows her friend a small purse that she stole from the store. Her friend is upset and wonders how she should respond. What moral advice would you want to discuss with this young girl?

✳ NCLEX®-Style Review Questions

1. Children generally double their birth weight by 5 months of age. This is an example of:
   1. Heredity
   2. Development
   3. State of health
   4. Physical growth

2. _____ development is the ability of an individual to distinguish right from wrong and to develop ethical values on which to base his or her actions.
   1. Moral
   2. Cognitive
   3. Psychosocial
   4. Psychoanalytic

3. Freud's _____ developmental stage is a time of turbulence when earlier sexual urges reawaken and are directed to an individual outside the family circle.
   1. Anal
   2. Genital
   3. Latency
   4. Phallic or oedipal

4. The nurse teaches parents how to have their children learn impulse control and cooperative behaviors. This would be during which of Erickson's stages of development?
   1. Trust versus mistrust
   2. Initiative versus guilt
   3. Industry versus inferiority
   4. Autonomy versus sense of shame and doubt

5. A 47-year-old woman expresses dismay to the nurse that her young adult children are unemployed. Her husband is working and near retirement. She is not working and feels bored with her life and unneeded. She is experiencing which of Erickson's stages of development?
   1. Integrity versus despair
   2. Intimacy versus isolation
   3. Identity versus confusion
   4. Generativity versus self-absorption and stagnation

6. The developmental theorist who believes his research describes a sequential process that takes place between the internal life (personality) of adults and their outer world (culture, lifestyle) is:
   1. Freud
   2. Gould
   3. Thomas
   4. Erickson

7. "The die is cast" is consistent with Gould's theme for the:
   1. 30s
   2. 40s
   3. 50s
   4. 70s

8. During this stage of cognitive development, the individual's thinking moves to abstract and theoretical subjects. Thinking can venture into such subjects as achieving world peace, finding justice, and seeking meaning in life.
   1. Sensorimotor
   2. Preoperational
   3. Formal operations
   4. Concrete operations

9. In this level of Kohlberg's moral developmental theory the person reflects on moral reasoning based on personal gain.
   1. Conventional
   2. Preconventional
   3. Postconventional
   4. Instrumental relativist orientation

10. The theorist who believes that girls do not need to separate from their mothers to achieve feminine identity is:
    1. Freud
    2. Gould
    3. Gilligan
    4. Kohlberg

12 | Conception Through Adolescence

OBJECTIVES

Mastery of the content in this chapter will enable the student to:

- Discuss physiological and psychosocial health concerns during the transition of the child from intrauterine to extrauterine life.
- Describe characteristics of physical growth of the unborn child and from birth to adolescence.
- Describe cognitive and psychosocial development from birth to adolescence.
- Describe the interactions that occur between parent and child.
- Describe variables influencing how children learn about and perceive their health status.

- Explain the role of play in the development of the child.
- Identify factors that contribute to self-esteem in youth.
- Describe the influence of the school environment on the development of the child.
- Plan culturally appropriate health promotion activities for children of all backgrounds.
- Discuss ways in which the nurse is able to help parents meet their children's developmental needs.

MEDIA RESOURCES | KEY TERMS

 Companion CD
- NCLEX®-Style Review Questions
- Audio Glossary
- Interactive Learning Activities
- English/Spanish Glossary

 Website
- NCLEX®-Style Review Questions
- Audio Glossary
- English/Spanish Glossary
- Interactive Learning Activities
- WebLinks
- Audio Summaries

Adolescence, p. 168
Apgar score, p. 152
Bonding, p. 154
Embryonic period, p. 150
Embryo, p. 149
Estrogen, p. 168
Fertilization, p. 149
Fetal period, p. 150
Fetus, p. 150
Fontanels, p. 152
Germinal period, p. 149
Hyperbilirubinemia, p. 154
Implantation, p. 150
Inborn errors of metabolism (IEMs), p. 154
Infancy, p. 155

Lanugo, p. 151
Menarche, p. 170
Molding, p. 152
Nagele's rule, p. 149
Neonatal period, p. 152
Placenta, p. 150
Prematurity, p.151
Preschool period, p. 160
Puberty, p. 164
School-age, p. 162
Sexually transmitted disease (STD), p. 173
Teratogens, p. 150
Testosterone, p. 168
Toddlerhood, p. 158
Zygote, p. 149

Stages of Growth and Development

Human growth and development are continuous and complex processes that are typically divided into stages organized by age-groups, such as from conception to adolescence. Although this chronological division is arbitrary, it is based on the timing and sequence of developmental tasks that the child must accomplish to progress to another stage (Box 12-1). Major factors affecting growth and development are in Chapter 11. This chapter focuses on the various physical, psychosocial, and cognitive changes, as well as the health risks and concerns, during the different stages of growth and development.

Selecting a Developmental Framework for Nursing

Providing developmentally appropriate nursing care is easier when you base planning on a theoretical framework (see Chapter 11). An organized, systematic approach ensures that the plan of care assesses and meets the child's and family's needs. If you deliver nursing care only as a series of isolated actions, you will possibly overlook some of the child's developmental needs. A developmental approach encourages organized care directed at the child's current level of functioning to motivate self-direction and health promotion. For example, nurses encourage toddlers to feed themselves to advance their developing independence and thus promote their sense of autonomy. Another example is a nurse's understanding an adolescent's need to be independent, so the nurse establishes a contract about the care plan and its implementation.

Conception

From the moment of conception, human development proceeds at a predictive and rapid rate. During gestation or the prenatal period, the **embryo** grows from a single cell to a complex, physiological being. All major organ systems develop in utero, with some functioning before birth. Development proceeds in a cephalocaudal (head-to-toe) and proximal-distal (central-to-peripheral) pattern (Murray and McKinney, 2006).

Intrauterine Life

Intrauterine life that reaches full term lasts from 36 to 40 weeks of fertilization age or 38 to 42 weeks of gestational age (Murray and McKinney, 2006). You compute the length of pregnancy using **Nagele's rule,** which counts back 3 months from the first day of the last menstrual period (LMP) and then adds 7 days. For example, if the first day of the woman's last menstrual period was on February 15, her due date would be November 22. **Fertilization** occurs when one sperm penetrates the ovum. Fertilization of the ovum takes place in the outer one third of the fallopian tube and occurs within 24 hours of the ovum's release. Once fertilization takes place, the material from both cell nuclei unites. This begins the **germinal period,** which includes the first 2 weeks after conception. The newly formed organism, known as a **zygote,** has its full genetic complement (1 pair of sex chromosomes and 22 pairs of

---

✳ BOX 12-1   Developmental Age Periods

Prenatal Period: Conception to Birth
Germinal: Conception to approximately 2 weeks
Embryonic: 2 to 8 weeks
Fetal: 8 to 40 weeks (birth)

A rapid growth rate and total dependency make this one of the most crucial periods in the developmental process. The relationship between maternal health and certain manifestations in the newborn emphasizes the importance of adequate prenatal care to the health and well-being of the infant.

Infancy Period: Birth to 12 or 18 Months
Neonatal: Birth to 28 days
Infancy: 1 to approximately 12 months

The infancy period is one of rapid motor, cognitive, and social development. Through mutuality with the caregiver (parent), the infant establishes a basic trust in the world and the foundation for future interpersonal relationships. The critical first month of life, although part of the infancy period, is often differentiated from the remainder because of the major physical adjustments to extrauterine existence and the psychologic adjustment of the parent.

Early Childhood: 1 to 6 Years
Toddler: 1 to 3 years
Preschool: 3 to 6 years

Intense activity and discovery occurs during this period, which extends from the time the children attain upright locomotion until they enter school. It is a time of marked physical and personality development. Motor development advances steadily. Children at this age acquire language and wider social relationships, learn role standards, gain self-control and mastery, develop increasing awareness of dependence and independence, and begin to develop a self-concept.

Middle Childhood: 6 to 11 or 12 Years
Frequently referred to as the school age, this period of development is one in which the child moves away from the family group and focuses on the wider world of peer relationships. There is steady advancement in physical, mental, and social development with emphasis on developing skill competencies. Social cooperation and early moral development take on more importance with relevance for later life stages. This is a critical period in the development of a self-concept.

Later Childhood: 11 to 19 Years
Prepubertal: 10 to 13 years
Adolescence: 13 to approximately 18 years

The period of rapid maturation and change known as adolescence is a transitional period that begins at the onset of puberty and extends to the point of entry into the adult world—usually high school graduation. Biologic and personality maturation are accompanied by physical and emotional turmoil, and adolescents often redefine their self-concept. In the late adolescent period the child begins to internalize all previously learned values and to focus on an individual, rather than a group, identity.

From Hockenberry MJ, Wilson D: *Wong's nursing care of infants and children,* ed 8, St. Louis, 2007, Mosby.

autosomal chromosomes). The ovum and the sperm each contribute one chromosome to each pair. It is through this mechanism that genetically programmed diseases (such as Down syndrome) and genetically determined characteristics (such as eye color) are transmitted from parent to child. The zygote moves through the fallopian tube to the uterus within 3 to 4 days.

The **placenta** produces essential hormones that help maintain the pregnancy. Because the placenta is extremely porous, noxious materials such as viruses and drugs also pass from mother to child. The effect of noxious agents on the unborn child depends on the developmental stage in which exposure takes place, with the embryonic stage being the most crucial. The **embryonic period** covers from the beginning of the third week through the eighth week after conception. This is a crucial stage in the development of all organ systems and the main external features. The **fetal period,** which starts with the ninth week after conception, ends with birth. Gestation is commonly divided into equal phases of three months called trimesters.

First Trimester

Physical Changes. During the first trimester, the first 3 calendar months, the uterus continues to be a pelvic organ. After **implantation,** fetal cells continue to differentiate and develop into essential organ systems. These processes of cellular change (differentiation) and staged organ change (development) occur at different rates and times, and each organ is extremely vulnerable to conditions in the environment. Interference with growth sometimes causes the congenital absence of an organ system or extensive structural or functional alterations. Because several organ systems develop at the same time, disruption of one system often occurs with disruption of others. Toward the end of the first trimester, it is possible to detect fetal heart tones (FHTs) and determine gender by the appearance of the external genitalia (Murray and McKinney, 2006). By the twelfth week, the **fetus** has all its body parts, weighs approximately 3 ounces, and is almost 3 inches long. The fetus is able to move all extremities, smile, frown, suck, swallow, and produce urine (Santrock, 2007).

Health Promotion. Several risk factors have an effect on prenatal development: nutrition, stress, infectious disease, drugs, environmental factors, incompatible blood types, maternal age, and paternal factors (Berger, 2005; Murray and McKinney, 2006; Santrock, 2007). These factors capable of producing functional or structural damage to the developing fetus are called **teratogens** (the word comes from the Greek word *tera,* which means "monster"). There are so many teratogens in our environment that nearly every fetus has exposure to some of them. The timing of the exposure, individual genetic susceptibility, and the quantity of the exposure all make the difference as to whether or not a birth defect occurs (Murray and McKinney, 2006; Santrock, 2007). It is important to educate women about avoidable sources of teratogens and assist them in making healthy lifestyle choices before and during pregnancy.

The diet of a woman both before and during pregnancy has a significant effect on the development of the fetus. If a woman does not consume adequate nutrients and calories during pregnancy, she may not be able to meet the nutritional requirements of the fetus. Mothers who eat well have fewer complications of pregnancy and childbirth and bear healthier babies than those with poor nutritional intake (Hilton, 2002; Murray and McKinney, 2006). For women who are at normal weight for height, the recommended weight gain is 25 to 35 pounds (Murray and McKinney, 2006). Nurses are in a key position to provide women with the education they need before conception and throughout an expectant mother's pregnancy.

During the first trimester, many women have conflicting feelings about the pregnancy. Even if it is a welcomed and planned pregnancy, some women feel unprepared and concerned about the added responsibility of parenthood. These feelings are usually resolved by the beginning of the second semester as the ambivalence turns to acceptance (Murray and McKinney, 2006). Women experiencing severe stressors (e.g., marital problems, unwanted pregnancy, or death of a family member) throughout the pregnancy are four times more likely to give birth prematurely. These women are also more vulnerable to engaging in unhealthy behaviors such as smoking, drug use, and poor prenatal care (Santrock, 2007).

Maternal infections such as cytomegalovirus (CMV), rubella (German measles), varicella-zoster (chickenpox), herpes simplex, hepatitis B, and human immunodeficiency virus (HIV) acquired during pregnancy can negatively influence the health of the mother, the fetus, or both. Some infections cross the placental barrier, resulting in severe birth defects, premature labor, or even fetal death. Other infections, such as genital herpes, cause injury during the birth itself.

Some prescription and nonprescription drugs are harmful to the fetus. The United States Food and Drug Administration has established guidelines to help physicians determine whether the benefits of the drug for the mother outweigh the potential effects to the fetus (Murray and McKinney, 2006). Psychoactive drugs, such as alcohol, nicotine, cocaine, marijuana, heroin, and methamphetamine, have all been linked to prenatal damage. Counsel pregnant women to eliminate the use of nonprescription drugs and recreational drugs such as alcohol throughout the entire pregnancy. Also, some complementary and alternative therapies, such as herbal supplements, are harmful during pregnancy. Nurses need to include questions about use of these substances when providing education during pregnancy.

Radiation, chemicals, and environmental pollutants such as carbon monoxide, mercury, and lead are also harmful to the developing fetus. Another potential teratogen is the use of saunas and hot tubs. By raising the mother's body temperature, harm occurs through interference with cell division, resulting in potential birth defects. The critical factor is the maternal temperature and duration of the hyperthermia (Murray and McKinney, 2006; Santrock, 2007).

Incompatibility between the mother's and father's rhesus (Rh) factor presents another risk factor to prenatal development. If the father of the fetus is Rh-positive and the mother is Rh-negative, the developing fetus may be Rh-positive. Individuals who are Rh-positive have an Rh-negative antigen on their red blood cells. Maternal exposure to fetal blood occurs in small amounts during the pregnancy and again during labor. The exposure usually does not cause problems during the first pregnancy because most of the antibodies are formed after the birth. However, future pregnancies with Rh-positive fetuses often result in destruction of the fetal erythrocytes so these mothers are treated with immune globulin to ensure the health of the fetus. (Murray and McKinney, 2006; Santrock, 2007).

The age of the pregnant woman sometimes plays a role in the health of the unborn and the overall pregnancy. Older women are at risk for chromosomal defects and experience more difficulty in becoming pregnant (Santrock, 2007). Studies indicate that pregnant adolescents often seek out less prenatal care than women in their 20s and 30s. Infants of teen mothers are at increased risk for prematurity and low birth weight (Murray and McKinney, 2006).

There are several paternal factors that pose a risk to the fetus. Exposure to lead, radiation, and pesticides have all been implicated in abnormalities in the sperm that cause birth defects. Smoking by the father is shown to result in low birth weight. Some research indicates that a paternal diet low in vitamin C results in increased vulnerability for birth defects and cancer (Santrock, 2007).

Second Trimester

Physical Changes. During the second trimester, the end of month 3 through month 6, the uterus becomes an abdominal organ. Measurement of the height of the uterus above the symphysis pubis is one indicator of fetal growth.

Some organ systems continue basic development, whereas the functional capabilities of others are refined. By the end of the sixth month, most organ systems are complete and able to function. The fetus is therefore considered viable, or capable of life outside the uterus, if given intensive environmental support. The fetus is now about 11 to 14 inches long and weighs almost 1½ pounds. The eyes are now open, and the fetus has a strong grip (Santrock, 2007).

Health Promotion. In the second trimester the fetal heartbeat becomes audible to stethoscope auscultation, and the mother becomes aware of fetal movement. Both events are highly significant to the parents because they provide tangible evidence of the pregnancy and reassure them that the fetus is alive. Changes in maternal behavior during this period include planning for the birth, concern for personal safety, and preoccupation with health and appearance. This is often a good time for education about gestational events and appropriate maternal rest, nutrition, dental care, physical activity, posture, employment, and infant feeding options.

Educate mothers to recognize potential complications and preterm labor, as well as the appropriate actions to take with each. With advances in modern technology, it is possible for 500-g babies of 24 to 26 weeks' gestation to survive; however, there is significant risk of morbidity. **Prematurity** is identified as any infant between 20 and 37 weeks' gestation. Causes for prematurity are poorly understood and are possibly the result of maternal, fetal, or placental problems. Maternal risk factors include physiological stresses such as renal and cardiovascular disease, diabetes mellitus, uterine and cervical abnormalities, obesity, and periodontal disease. History of previous preterm labor and previous pregnancy losses also increase the risk. Research has demonstrated an increased risk among mothers living in poverty, smokers, illicit drug users, adolescents, and mothers receiving poor prenatal care (Murray and McKinney, 2006).

Third Trimester

Physical Changes. During the last 3 months of intrauterine life the fetus grows to approximately 50 cm (19 to 20 inches) in length. Subcutaneous fat is stored, and weight increases to between 3.2 and 3.4 kg (7 pounds to 7 pounds, 8 ounces). The skin thickens, **lanugo** (fine body hair) begins to disappear, and the fetal body becomes rounder and fuller.

A tremendous spurt in brain growth begins during this trimester and lasts well into the first few years of life. At the end of the third trimester the normal fetus is physically able to make the transition from intrauterine to extrauterine life. The cardiac system changes its circulation to end bypassing of the lungs. The lungs are capable of maintaining the inflated state for gas exchange. The primitive temperature maintenance systems, reflexes, and sensory organs are ready for use, and the fetus is gaining immunities from the mother.

Health Promotion. Thoughts of delivering a healthy infant are foremost in the mother's mind as she focuses on preparing her mind and body for the delivery. Parents often seek information regarding the childbirth process and breast-feeding.

Discuss birth-setting choices at this time. Hospitals have been the more traditional setting for childbirth for the past 60 years. Many hospitals have taken a family-centered approach to childbirth. In some areas of the country, freestanding birthing centers are available for those who do not prefer the hospital setting. Women delivering in this setting are required to attend childbirth and parenting classes, and the pregnancy must be low risk. These centers usually have certified midwives who are advanced practice registered nurses specially trained to deliver babies. Mothers need to understand that there is always a possibility of transfer to a hospital if the conditions necessitate it.

A small percentage of mothers choose to deliver at home. Home birth is popular in Sweden and the Netherlands but has a limited following in this country. Control over the birth process seems to be the most attractive factor for mothers who do not believe they have choices in a hospital setting. Another advantage is that the entire family or other persons close to the family are part of the event.

Transition From Intrauterine to Extrauterine Life

The transition from intrauterine to extrauterine life requires profound physiological changes in the newborn. Immediately following birth, the nurse assesses the newborn's cardiorespiratory status, thermoregulation, and the presence of any anomalies that inhibit the infant's adaptation to life outside the womb (Murray and McKinney, 2006). Gestational age and development, exposure to depressant drugs before or during labor, and the newborn's own behavioral style also influence the adjustment to the external environment.

Physical Changes

Perform an immediate assessment of the newborn's condition to determine the physiological functioning of the major organ systems. The most extreme physiological change occurs when the newborn leaves the in utero circulation and develops independent respiratory functioning. Direct nursing care toward maintaining an open airway, stabilizing and maintaining body temperature, and protecting the newborn from infection. The most widely used assessment tool is the **Apgar score.** Heart rate, respiratory effort, muscle tone, reflex irritability, and color are rated to determine overall status. The Apgar assessment is generally conducted at 1 and 5 minutes after birth and is sometimes repeated until the newborn's condition stabilizes.

Psychosocial Changes

After immediate physical evaluation and application of identification bracelets, the nurse promotes the parents and newborn's need for close physical contact. Early parent-child interaction encourages parent-child attachment. Merely placing the family together does not promote closeness. The parents and newborn need to be capable and desirous of exploring and responding to each other. Most healthy newborns are awake and alert for the first half-hour after birth. This is a good time for parent-child interaction to begin. Close body contact, often including breast-feeding, is a satisfying way for most families to start. If immediate contact is not possible, the nurse incorporates it into the care plan as early as possible, which means bringing the newborn to an ill parent or bringing the parents to an ill or premature child.

Health Risks

The removal of nasopharyngeal and oropharyngeal secretions with suction or a bulb syringe ensures airway patency. Newborns are susceptible to heat loss and cold stress (Askin, 2002). Because hypothermia increases oxygen needs, you need to stabilize and maintain the newborn's body temperature. Place the newborn directly on the mother's abdomen and cover him or her in warm blankets, being sure to keep the head well covered; or placed unclothed in an infant warmer with a temperature probe in place. For newborns unable to sustain adequate body temperature, use isolettes and incubators, which supply radiant heat.

Prevention of infection is a major concern in the care of the newborn, whose immune system is immature. Good handwashing technique is the most important factor in protecting the newborn from infection. Nurses help prevent infection by instructing parents and visitors to wash their hands before touching the infant.

Care of the umbilical cord varies according to geographical region and is often based more on institutional policies rather than evidence-based research (Ball and Bindler, 2006). Keeping the umbilical stump clean and dry is the most effective way to prevent infection and promote cord severance. Until the cord dries and falls off, fold the diaper below the umbilicus to prevent accumulation of moisture. Instruct parents to observe for any signs of infection and to sponge bathe the infant until the cord naturally falls off.

Newborn

The **neonatal period** is the first month of life. During this stage the newborn's physical functioning is mostly reflexive, and stabilization of major organ systems is the body's primary task.

Behavior greatly influences interaction between the newborn, the environment, and caregivers. For example, the average 2-week-old smiles spontaneously and is able to look at the mother's face. The impact of these reflexive behaviors is generally a surge of maternal feelings of love that prompt the mother to cuddle the baby.

Nurses apply their knowledge of this stage of growth and development to promote newborn and parental health. If the nurse understands, for example, that the newborn's cry is generally a reflexive response to an unmet need (such as hunger), you assist parents in identifying ways to meet those needs, such as counseling the parents to feed their baby on demand rather than on a rigid schedule.

Physical Changes

A comprehensive nursing assessment is performed as soon as the newborn's physiological functioning is stable, generally within a few hours after birth. At this time the nurse measures height, weight, head circumference, temperature, pulse, and respirations and observes general appearance, body functions, sensory capabilities, reflexes, and responsiveness. Following a comprehensive physical assessment, the nurse assesses gestational age and interactions between infant and parent that indicate successful attachment (Hockenberry and Wilson, 2007).

The average newborn is 2700 to 4000 g (6 to 9 pounds), 48 to 53 cm (19 to 21 inches) in length, and has a head circumference of 33 to 35 cm (13 to 14 inches). Neonates lose up to 10% of birth weight in the first few days of life, primarily through fluid losses by respiration, urination, defecation, and low fluid intake. They usually regain birth weight by the second week of life, and a gradual pattern of increase in weight, height, and head circumference is evident. Accurate measurement as soon as possible after birth provides an index for assessment of potential risk status and future growth (Hockenberry and Wilson, 2007).

Normal physical characteristics include the continued presence of lanugo on the skin of the back; cyanosis of the hands and feet for the first 24 hours; and a soft, protuberant abdomen. Skin color varies according to racial and genetic heritage and gradually changes during infancy. **Molding,** or overlapping of the soft skull bones, allows the fetal head to adjust to various diameters of the maternal pelvis and is a common occurrence with vaginal births. The bones readjust within a few days, producing a rounded appearance. The sutures and **fontanels** are usually palpable at birth. Figure 12-1 shows the diamond shape of the anterior fontanel and the triangular shape of the posterior fontanel between the unfused bones of the skull.

Assess neurological function by observing the newborn's level of activity, alertness, irritability, responsiveness to stimuli, and the presence and strength of reflexes. Normal reflexes include blinking in response to bright lights, startling in response to sudden, loud noises, and sucking, rooting, grasping, yawning, coughing, sneezing, and hiccoughing. Assessment of these reflexes is vital because the newborn depends largely on reflexes for survival and in response to its environment. Figure 12-2 shows the tonic neck reflex in the newborn.

Normal behavioral characteristics of the newborn include periods of sucking, crying, sleeping, and activity. Movements are

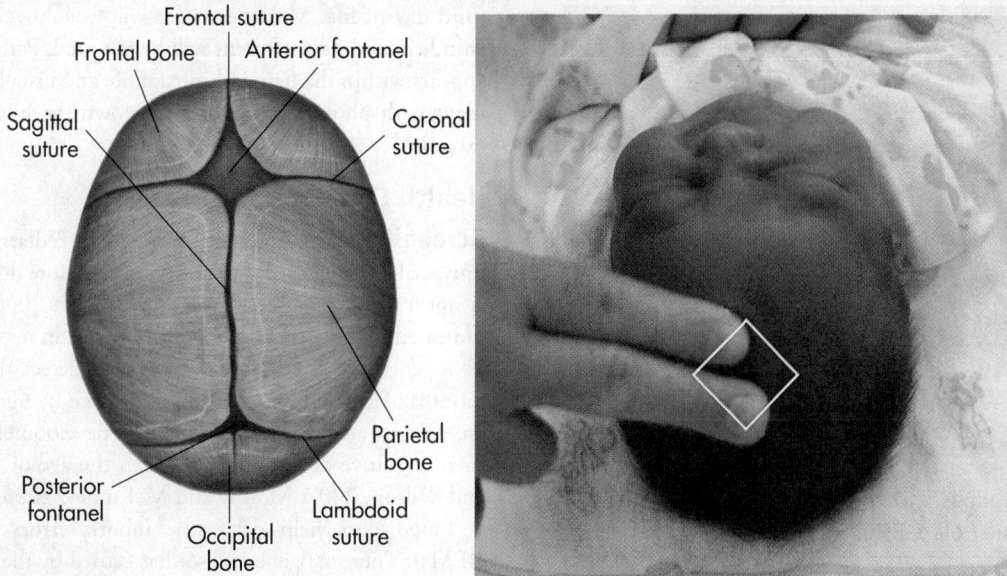

Figure 12-1 Fontanels and suture lines. (From Hockenberry MJ and others: *Wong's nursing care of infants and children,* ed 7, St. Louis, 2003, Mosby.)

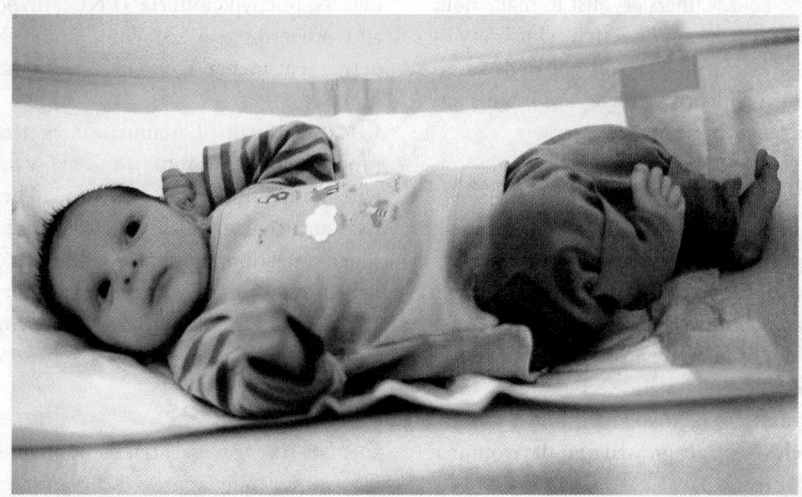

Figure 12-2 Tonic neck reflex. Newborns assume this position while supine. (Courtesy Elaine Polan, RNC, BSN, MS.)

generally sporadic, but they are symmetrical and involve all four extremities. The relatively flexed fetal position of intrauterine life continues as the newborn attempts to maintain an enclosed, secure feeling. Newborns normally watch the caregiver's face, reflexively smile, and respond to sensory stimuli, particularly the primary caregiver's face, voice, and touch.

In accordance with the recommendations of the American Academy of Pediatrics (AAP), position infants for sleep on their back to decrease the risk of sudden infant death syndrome (SIDS) (Hockenberry and Wilson, 2007; Santrock, 2007). Co-sleeping or bed sharing has also been reported to be possibly associated with an increased risk for SIDS (Hockenberry and Wilson, 2007; Santrock, 2007). Safeguards include proper positioning; removing stuffed animals, soft bedding, and pillows; and avoiding overheating of the infant. Individuals should avoid smoking during

pregnancy and around the infant as it places the infant at greater risk for SIDS (Hockenberry and Wilson, 2007).

Cognitive Changes

Early cognitive development begins with innate behavior, reflexes, and sensory functions. Newborns initiate reflex activities, learn behaviors, and learn their desires. For example, newborns learn to turn to the nipple and learn that crying results in parent response of feeding, diapering, and cuddling. At birth, children are able to focus on objects about 8 to 10 inches from their faces and perceive forms. A preference for the human face is apparent. Teach parents about the importance of providing sensory stimulation, such as talking to their babies and holding them to see their faces. This allows infants to seek or take in stimuli, thereby enhancing learning and promoting cognitive development.

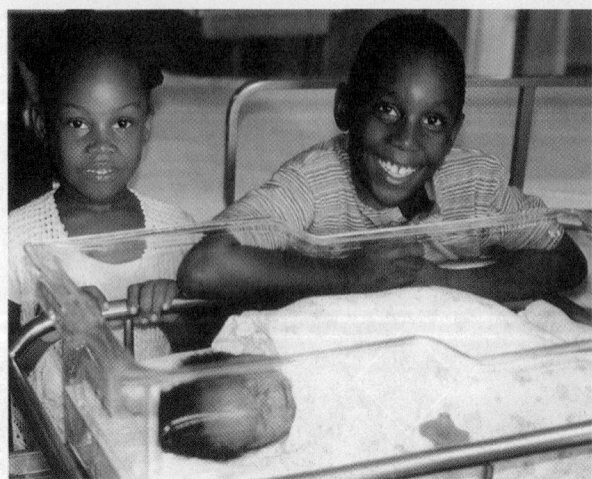

Figure 12-3 Siblings should be involved in newborn care. (Courtesy Elaine Polan, RNC, BSN, MS.)

For newborns, crying is a means of communication to provide cues to parents. Some babies cry because their diapers are wet or they are hungry or want to be held. Others cry just to make noise or because they need a change in position or activity. Their crying will frustrate the parents if they cannot see an apparent cause. With the nurse's help, parents will learn to recognize infants' cry patterns and take appropriate action when necessary.

Psychosocial Changes

During the first month of life, parents and newborns normally develop a strong bond that grows into a deep attachment. Interactions during routine care enhance or detract from the attachment process. Feeding, hygiene, and comfort measures consume much of infants' waking time. These interactive experiences provide a foundation for the formation of deep attachments. Early on, older siblings need to have opportunity to be involved in the newborn's care. Family involvement helps support growth and development and promotes nurturing (Figure 12-3).

If parents or children experience health complications after birth, this will possibly compromise attachment and **bonding**. Infants' behavioral cues are sometimes weak or absent, and care-giving is possibly less mutually satisfying. Some tired or ill parents have difficulty interpreting and responding to their infants. Children with congenital anomalies are often too weak to be responsive to parental cues and require special supportive nursing care. For example, infants born with heart defects tire easily during feedings.

Health Risks

Hyperbilirubinemia refers to an excessive amount of accumulated bilirubin in the blood that causes yellow coloring of the skin, or jaundice. The accumulation occurs when the infant's body is unable to balance the destruction of red blood cells (RBCs) and the use or excretion of by-products. The balance is upset by prematurity, breast-feeding, excess production of bilirubin, certain disease states, or a disturbance in the liver. The most common cause of hyperbilirubinemia is the mild physiological jaundice, or *icterus neonatorum,* that begins on the second or third day of life. Most newborns will not show any evidence of jaundice, and no treatment will be required. Pathologic jaundice appears within the first 24 hours of life and usually requires treatment with phototherapy to break down the bilirubin for easier excretion

Health Concerns

Screening. The American Academy of Pediatrics recommends universal hearing screening of newborns before discharge, but this is not a law in all states (Ball and Bindler, 2006). Studies have indicated that the incidence of hearing loss in newborns is as high as 1 per 1000. If health care providers detect the loss before 3 months of age and intervention is initiated by 6 months, children are able to achieve normal language development that matches their cognitive development through the age of 5 (Hockenberry and Wilson, 2007; Murray and McKinney, 2006).

Blood tests help determine **inborn errors of metabolism (IEMs).** These are genetic disorders caused by the absence or deficiency of a substance, usually an enzyme, essential to cellular metabolism that results in abnormal protein, carbohydrate, or fat metabolism. Although IEMs are rare, they account for a significant proportion of health problems in children. Neonatal screening detects phenylketonuria (PKU), hypothyroidism, galactosemia, and other diseases to allow appropriate treatment that prevent permanent mental retardation and other health problems.

Circumcision. Circumcision is a common and controversial procedure in this country, and many parents have questions about whether to choose it for their son. The controversy surrounds the risks and benefits of the surgical procedure. Risks include hemorrhage, infection, adhesions, and meatal stenosis. Benefits include prevention of penile cancer and urinary tract infections and preservation of male body image to be consistent with peers (Hockenberry and Wilson, 2007).

Safety Concerns

Car Seats. An essential component of discharge teaching is the use of a federally approved car seat for the transport of the infant from the hospital or birthing center to home. Automobile injuries are a leading cause of death in children in the United States. Many of these deaths occur when the child is not properly restrained (Murray and McKinney, 2006). Parents need to learn how to properly fit the restraint to the infant and how to properly install the car seat. The infant should always be in a rear-facing restraint in the backseat of the vehicle. Placing an infant in a rear-facing restraint in the front seat of a vehicle is extremely dangerous in any vehicle with a passenger-side air bag. Parents have many options for car seats, and some infant restraints also convert into a toddler type of restraint.

Cribs. New cribs sold in the United States meet governmental standards for safety, but some older cribs were manufactured before the newer requirements were instituted. Parents need to inspect an older crib to make sure the slats are no more than 6 cm (2.375 inches) apart. The crib mattress should fit snugly, and crib toys or mobiles should be firmly attached with no strings or straps hanging. Instruct parents to remove mobiles as soon as the infant reaches them (Hockenberry and Wilson, 2007).

Infant

During **infancy,** the period from 1 month to 1 year of age, rapid physical growth and change occurs. This is the only period distinguished by such dramatic physical changes and marked development. Psychosocial development advances aided by the progression from reflexive to more purposeful behavior. Interaction between infants and the environment is greater and more meaningful. During this first year of life the nurse easily observes the adaptive potential of infants because changes in growth and development occur so rapidly.

Physical Changes

Steady and proportional growth of the infant is more important than absolute growth values. Charts of normal age- and gender-related growth measurements enable the nurse to compare growth with norms for a child's age. Measurements recorded over time are the best way to monitor growth and identify problems. Size increases rapidly during the first year of life; birth weight doubles in approximately 5 months and triples by 12 months. Height increases an average of 1 inch during each of the first 6 months and about ½ inch each month until 12 months (Hockenberry and Wilson, 2007).

Throughout the first year, the infant's vision and hearing continue to develop. Some infants as young as 3½ months are able to link visual and auditory stimuli (Santrock, 2007). Patterns of body function also stabilize, as evidenced by predictable sleep, elimination, and feeding routines. Motor development proceeds steadily in a cephalocaudal (head-to-toe) direction.

Cognitive Changes

The complex brain development during the first year is demonstrated by the infant's changing behaviors. As the infant receives stimulation through the developing senses of vision, hearing, and touch, the developing brain interprets the stimuli. Thus the infant learns by experiencing and manipulating the environment. Developing motor skills and increasing mobility expand an infant's environment and, with developing visual and auditory skills, enhance cognitive development. For these reasons Piaget (1952) named his first stage of cognitive development, which extends until around the third birthday, the sensorimotor period. Today's researchers have many more methods available to study the cognitive development of infants, and they believe that infants are far more competent than Piaget was able to discern by observation alone (Santrock, 2007).

Infants need opportunities to develop and use their senses. Nurses need to evaluate the appropriateness and adequacy of these opportunities. For example, ill or hospitalized infants sometimes lack the energy to interact with their environments, thereby slowing their cognitive development. Infants need to be stimulated according to their temperament, energy, and age. The nurse uses stimulation strategies that maximize the development of infants while conserving their energy and orientation. An example of this is the nurse's talking to and encouraging an infant to suck on a pacifier while administering the infant's tube feeding.

Language. Speech is an important aspect of cognition that develops during the first year. Infants proceed from crying, coo-

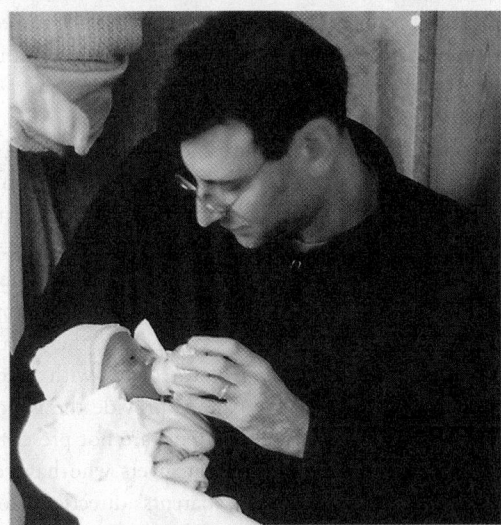

Figure 12-4 Smiling at and talking to an infant encourages bonding. (Courtesy Elaine Polan, RNC, BSN, MS.)

ing, and laughing to imitating sounds, comprehending the meaning of simple commands, and repeating words with knowledge of their meaning. By 1 year, infants not only recognize their own names but are able to say three to five words and understand almost 100 words (Hockenberry and Wilson, 2007). The nurse promotes language development by encouraging parents to name objects on which their infant's attention is focused. The nurse also assesses the infant's language development to identify developmental delays or potential abnormalities.

Psychosocial Changes

Separation and Individuation. During their first year, infants begin to differentiate themselves from others as separate beings capable of acting on their own. Initially, infants are unaware of the boundaries of self, but through repeated experiences with the environment, they learn where the self ends and the external world begins. As infants determine their physical boundaries, they begin to respond to others (Figure 12-4).

Two- and 3-month-old infants begin to smile responsively rather than reflexively. Similarly, they recognize differences in people when their sensory and cognitive capabilities improve. By 8 months, most infants are able to differentiate a stranger from a familiar person and respond differently to the two. Close attachment to the primary caregivers, most often parents, usually occurs by this age. Infants seek out these persons for support and comfort during times of stress. The ability to distinguish self from others allows infants to interact and socialize more within their environments. By 9 months, for example, infants play simple social games such as patty-cake and peek-a-boo. More complex interactive games such as hide-and-seek involving objects are possible by age 1. Erikson (1963) describes the psychosocial developmental crisis for the infant as trust versus mistrust. He explains that the quality of parent-infant interactions determines development of trust or mistrust. The infant learns to trust self, others, and the world through the relationship between the parent and child and the care the child receives (Hockenberry and Wilson, 2007). During infancy the child's temperament or behavioral style becomes apparent and influences the interactions between parent and child. Nurses help parents understand their child's temperament and determine appropriate child-rearing practices (see Chapter 11).

The nurse assesses the availability and appropriateness of experiences contributing to psychosocial development. Hospitalized infants often have difficulty establishing physical boundaries because of repeated bodily intrusions and painful sensations. Limiting these negative experiences and providing pleasurable sensations are interventions that support early psychosocial development. Extended separations from parents complicate the attachment process and increase the number of caregivers with whom the infant must interact. Ideally, the parents provide the majority of care during hospitalization. When parents are not present, make an attempt to limit the number of caregivers who have contact with the infant and to follow the parents' directions for care. These interventions will foster the infant's continuing development of trust.

Play. Play is a meaningful set of activities through which individuals interact with their environment and relate to others. Play provides opportunities for development of cognitive, social, and motor skills. Much of infant play is exploratory as infants use their senses to observe and examine their own bodies and objects of interest in their surroundings. Activities such as infants' placement of their toes in their mouths provide them with pleasure, information about their own body, and help form their early self-concept. Play becomes manipulative as the child learns control of the hands. Adults facilitate infant learning by planning activities that promote the development of milestones and by providing toys that are safe for the infant to explore with the mouth and manipulate with the hands, such as rattles, wooden blocks, plastic stacking rings, squeezable stuffed animals, and busy boxes.

Health Risks

Injury Prevention. Injury due to motor vehicle accidents, aspiration, suffocation, falls, or poisoning are major causes of death in children 6 to 12 months old. An understanding of the major developmental accomplishments during this time period will allow for injury prevention planning. As the child achieves gains in motor development and becomes increasingly curious about the environment, constant watchfulness and supervision is critical for injury prevention.

Child Maltreatment. Child maltreatment includes intentional physical abuse or neglect, emotional abuse or neglect, and sexual abuse (Hockenberry and Wilson, 2007). More children suffer from neglect than any other type of maltreatment. Children of any age can suffer from maltreatment, but the youngest are the most vulnerable. In addition, many children suffer from more than one type of maltreatment. No one profile fits a victim of maltreatment, and the signs and symptoms vary (Box 12-2). The Child Protective Services agencies reported that of the 1 million children suffering from maltreatment, half suffered from some type of neglect, one quarter from physical abuse, and 13% from sexual abuse. More than half, 56%, were under the age of 4 years (U.S. Department of Health and Human Services [USDHHS],

---

BOX 12-2   Warning Signs of Abuse

- Physical evidence of abuse or neglect, including previous injuries
- Conflicting stories about the accident/trauma
- Injury blamed on sibling or another party
- Injury inconsistent with the history, such as a concussion and a broken arm from falling off the bed
- History inconsistent with the child's developmental age, such as a 6-month-old burned by turning on the hot water
- An initial complaint not associated with the signs and symptoms present, for example, bringing the child to the clinic for a cold when there is evidence of physical trauma
- Inappropriate response of the child, especially an older child, such as not wanting to be touched, looking at caregiver before answering any questions
- Previous reports of abuse in the family
- Frequent emergency department or clinic visits

Data from Hockenberry MJ, Wilson D: *Wong's nursing care of infants and children*, ed 8, St. Louis, 2007, Mosby.

2004). All 50 states have a mandatory reporting law for all health professionals to report suspected abuse.

A combination of signs and symptoms or a pattern of injury should arouse suspicion. It is important for the health care provider to be aware of certain disease processes and cultural practices. Lack of awareness of normal variants such as Mongolian spots or cultural practices such as coining will cause the health care provider to assume there is abuse. Children who are hospitalized for maltreatment have the same developmental needs as other children their age, and the nurse will need to support the child's relationship with the parents (Hockenberry and Wilson, 2007).

Health Concerns

Health Perception. The foundation for children's perceptions of their health status is laid early in life. Internal body sensations and experiences with the outside world affect self-perceptions. The nature of this influence and the value of nursing interventions to alter later perceptions are unknown. It is known, however, that parents tend to label children who are ill in early life as more vulnerable than their siblings and that this labeling often affects the children's perceptions of their own health. In addition, because infants and children depend on others for their health care, their experiences with caregivers influence their health attitudes and behavior. The nurse has a responsibility to educate parents and other caregivers about health promotion behavior that will positively affect perception of health and self.

Nutrition. The quality and quantity of nutrition profoundly influences the infant's growth and development. Many women have already selected a feeding method well before the infant's birth, yet others will have questions for the nurse later in the pregnancy. Nurses are in a unique position to help parents select and provide a nutritionally adequate diet for their infant (Box 12-3). Understand that factors such as support, culture, role demands, and previous experiences influence feeding methods (Murray and McKinney, 2006) (Box 12-4).

✳ BOX 12-3 EVIDENCE-BASED PRACTICE

Breast-Feeding

Evidence Summary

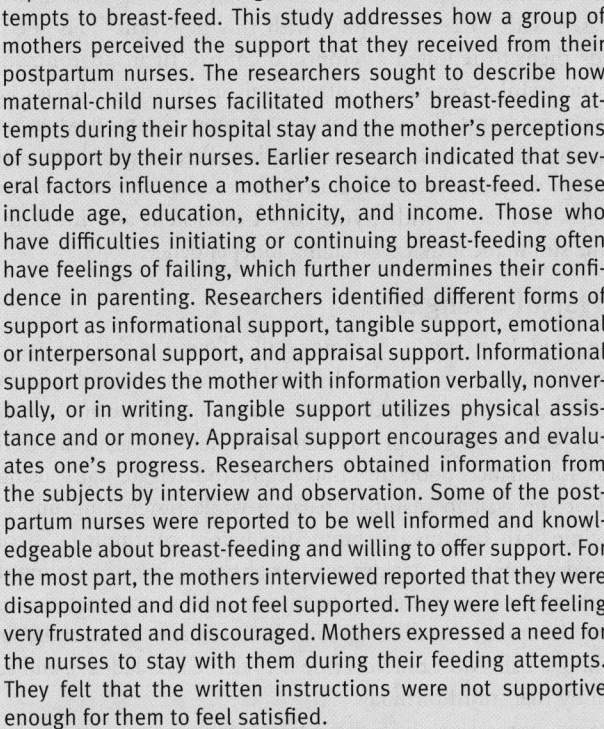

Success in breast-feeding largely depends on the information and support a woman receives during the postpartum period. Nurses play an important role in assisting mothers in their attempts to breast-feed. This study addresses how a group of mothers perceived the support that they received from their postpartum nurses. The researchers sought to describe how maternal-child nurses facilitated mothers' breast-feeding attempts during their hospital stay and the mother's perceptions of support by their nurses. Earlier research indicated that several factors influence a mother's choice to breast-feed. These include age, education, ethnicity, and income. Those who have difficulties initiating or continuing breast-feeding often have feelings of failing, which further undermines their confidence in parenting. Researchers identified different forms of support as informational support, tangible support, emotional or interpersonal support, and appraisal support. Informational support provides the mother with information verbally, nonverbally, or in writing. Tangible support utilizes physical assistance and or money. Appraisal support encourages and evaluates one's progress. Researchers obtained information from the subjects by interview and observation. Some of the postpartum nurses were reported to be well informed and knowledgeable about breast-feeding and willing to offer support. For the most part, the mothers interviewed reported that they were disappointed and did not feel supported. They were left feeling very frustrated and discouraged. Mothers expressed a need for the nurses to stay with them during their feeding attempts. They felt that the written instructions were not supportive enough for them to feel satisfied.

Application to Nursing Practice

- Provide education and support to breast-feeding mothers.
- Anticipate mothers' needs rather than wait for them to be asked for assistance.
- In order to best facilitate breast-feeding, use consistent approaches.
- Provide breast-feeding mothers with verbal support, as well as written information.
- Assess mothers' support system's knowledge of breast-feeding.

Reference

Gill S: The little things: perceptions of breastfeeding support, *J Obstet Gynecol Neonatal Nurs* 30(4):401, 2001.

✳ BOX 12-4 CULTURAL ASPECTS OF CARE

Infant Feeding Methods

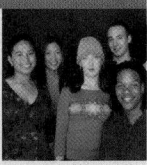

Cultural practices and beliefs have a significant influence on the choice of infant feeding methods. Although cultural norms exist, application of the norms is not always appropriate for all individuals.

Implications for Practice

- Muslim women often breast-feed for the first 2 years, and Mormon women consider breast-feeding a significant component of mothering.
- Immigrants to the United States from countries in which breast-feeding is the usual method of providing infant nutrition may not breast-feed for as long if they do not have the support system they would have had in their country of origin.
- Many cultures choose not to give the infants colostrum. Southeast Asian, Hispanic, and Arab women delay breast-feeding until the milk has come in when they are back home after delivery (Galanti, 2004). Other cultures begin breast-feeding immediately after delivery and offer the breast each time the infant cries.
- Cultural attitudes regarding breast-feeding, modesty, and dietary beliefs are important considerations for the nurse. Some cultures use certain foods that they believe will increase milk production, yet others see bottle-feeding as representing a new way of life.

Data from Murray S, McKinney E: (2006). *Foundations of maternal-newborn nursing*, ed 4, Saunders Elsevier; and Galanti G: *Caring for patients from different cultures*, ed 3, Philadelphia, 2004, University of Pennsylvania Press.

the parent does not desire it, an acceptable alternative is iron-fortified commercially prepared formula. Commercially prepared formulas are manufactured to resemble the nutritional content of human milk. Recent advances in the preparation of infant formula include the addition of nucleotides and long-chain fatty acids, which augment immune function and increase brain development. The use of whole cow's milk, 2% cow's milk, or alternate milk products before the age of 12 months is not recommended. The composition of whole cow's milk will possibly cause intestinal bleeding, anemia, and increased incidence of allergies (Hockenberry and Wilson, 2007).

The average 1-month-old infant takes approximately 18 to 21 ounces of breast milk or formula per day. This amount increases slightly during the first 6 months and decreases after introducing solid foods. The amount of formula per feeding and the number of feedings vary among infants. The addition of solid foods is not recommended before the age of 6 months because the gastrointestinal tract is not sufficiently mature to handle these complex nutrients, and infants are exposed to food antigens that produce food protein allergies. Developmentally, infants are not ready for solid food before 6 months. The extrusion (protrusion) reflex causes food to be pushed out of the mouth. The introduction of cereals, fruits, vegetables, and meats during the second 6 months of life provides iron and additional sources of vitamins. These

Feeding Alternatives. Breast-feeding is recommended for infant nutrition because breast milk contains the essential nutrients of protein, fats, carbohydrates, and immunoglobulins that bolster the ability to resist infection. Studies demonstrate that formula feeding is not equivalent to breast-feeding in providing the best possible nutrition for growth and development. Both the American Academy of Pediatrics and the U.S. Department of Health and Human Services recommend human milk for the first year of life (Hockenberry and Wilson, 2007; Murray and McKinney, 2006). However, if breast-feeding is not possible or if become especially important when children change from breast milk or formula to whole cow's milk after the first birthday. Infants also tolerate well-cooked table foods by 1 year. The amount and frequency of feedings vary among infants, so discuss differing feeding patterns with parents.

Some have used honey to sweeten water and coat pacifiers. Do not use honey in infants less than 1 year of age because of the potential for infant botulism poisoning (Behrman, Kliegman, and Jenson, 2000).

Supplementation. The need for dietary vitamin and mineral supplements depends on the infant's diet. Full-term infants are born with some iron stores. The breast-fed infant absorbs adequate iron from breast milk during the first 4 to 6 months of life. After 6 months, iron-fortified cereal is generally an adequate supplemental source. Because iron in formula is less readily absorbed than that in breast milk, formula-fed infants need to receive iron-fortified formula throughout the first year.

Adequate concentrations of fluoride to protect against dental caries are not available in human milk, and therefore fluoridated water or supplemental fluoride is generally recommended. The presence of fluoride in formula depends on the type of formula and the source of water used in preparing the concentrated forms. Fluoride supplementation is sometimes necessary. A recent concern is the use of complementary and alternative medical therapies in children that may or may not be safe. Inquire about the use of such products to help the parent determine whether or not the product is truly safe for the child (Hockenberry and Wilson, 2007).

Immunizations. The widespread use of immunizations has resulted in the dramatic decline of infectious diseases over the past 50 years and is therefore a most important factor in health promotion during childhood. Although you can give most immunizations to persons of any age, it is recommended that the administration of the primary series begin soon after birth and be completed during early childhood. Vaccines are among the safest and most reliable drugs used. Minor side effects sometimes occur; however, serious reactions are rare. Parents need instructions regarding the importance of immunizations as well as common side effects such as low-grade fever and local tenderness. The recommended schedule for immunizations changes as new vaccines are developed and advances are made in the field of immunology. Stay informed of the current policies, and direct parents to the primary caregiver for their child's schedule. The American Academy of Pediatrics maintains the most current schedule on their Internet website, http://www.aap.org.

Sleep. Sleep patterns vary among infants, with many having their days and nights mixed up until 3 to 4 months of age. Thus it is common for infants to sleep during the day. By 6 months, most infants are nocturnal and sleep between 9 and 11 hours at night. Total daily sleep averages 15 hours. Most infants take one or two naps a day by the end of the first year. Many parents have concerns regarding their infant's sleep patterns, especially if there is difficulty such as sleep refusal or frequent waking during the night. Carefully assesses the individual problem before suggesting interventions to address their concern.

Toddler

Toddlerhood ranges from the time when children begin to walk independently until they walk and run with ease, which is from 12 to 36 months. The toddler has increasing independence bolstered by greater physical mobility and cognitive abilities. Toddlers are increasingly aware of their abilities to control and are pleased with successful efforts with this new skill. This success leads them to repeated attempts to control their environments. Unsuccessful attempts at control result in negative behavior and temper tantrums. These behaviors are most common when parents stop the initial independent action. Parents cite these as the most problematic behaviors during the toddler years and at times express frustration with trying to set consistent and firm limits while simultaneously encouraging independence.

Physical Changes

The rapid development of motor skills allows the child to participate in self-care activities such as feeding, dressing, and toileting. In the beginning the toddler walks in an upright position with a broad-stance and gait, protuberant abdomen, and arms out to the sides for balance. Soon the child begins to navigate stairs, using a rail or the wall to maintain balance while progressing upward, placing both feet on the same step before continuing. Success provides courage to attempt the upright mode for descending the stairs in the same manner. Locomotion skills soon include running, jumping, standing on one foot for several seconds, and kicking a ball. Most toddlers ride tricycles, climb ladders, and run well by their third birthday.

Fine motor capabilities move from scribbling spontaneously to drawing circles and crosses accurately. By 3 years the child draws simple stick people and is usually able to stack a tower of small blocks. Increased locomotion skills, the ability to undress, and development of sphincter control allow toilet training if the toddler has developed the necessary language and cognitive abilities. Parents often consult nurses for an assessment of readiness for toilet training. Recognizing the urge to urinate and or defecate is crucial in determining the child's mental readiness. The toddler must also be motivated to hold on to please the parent rather than letting go to please the self to successfully accomplish toilet training (Hockenberry and Wilson, 2007). The nurse needs to remind parents that patience, consistency, and a nonjudgmental attitude, in addition to the child's readiness, are essential to successful toilet training.

Cognitive Changes

Toddlers increase their ability to remember events and begin to put thoughts into words at about 2 years of age. Toddlers recognize that they are separate beings from their mothers, but they are unable to assume the view of another. Toddlers reason based on their own experience of an event. Toddlers use symbols to represent objects, places, and persons. Children demonstrate this function as they imitate the behavior of another that they viewed earlier (e.g., pretend to shave like daddy), pretend one object is another (use a finger as a gun), and use language to stand for absent objects (e.g., request bottle).

Language. The 18-month-old child uses approximately 10 words. The 24-month-old child has a vocabulary of up to 300 words and is generally able to speak in two-word sentences, although the ability to understand speech is much greater than the number of words acquired (Hockenberry and Wilson, 2007). "Who's that?" and "What's that?" are typical questions children ask during this period. Verbal expressions such as "me do it" and "that's mine" demonstrate the 2-year-old child's use of pronouns and desire for independence and control. By 36 months the child can use simple sentences, follow some grammatical rules, and learn to use five or six new words each day.

Moral Development. Because children's moral development is closely associated with their cognitive abilities, the moral development of toddlers is only beginning. Toddlers do not understand concepts of right and wrong. In the toddler's view, if an action brings punishment it is "bad," and if no punishment results it is "good." However, toddlers do grasp the fact that some behaviors bring pleasant results (positive reinforcement) and others elicit unpleasant results (negative reinforcement). Therefore until toddlers achieve a higher level of cognitive function, they behave simply to avoid the unpleasant and seek out the pleasant (Hockenberry and Wilson, 2007).

Psychosocial Changes

According to Erikson (1963), a sense of autonomy emerges during toddlerhood. Children strive for independence by using their developing muscles to do everything for themselves and become the master of their bodily functions. Their strong wills are frequently exhibited in negative behavior when caregivers attempt to direct their actions. Temper tantrums result when parental restrictions frustrate toddlers. Parents need to provide toddlers with graded independence, allowing them to do things that do not result in harm to themselves or others. For example, young toddlers who want to learn to hold their own cups often benefit from two-handled cups with spouts and plastic bibs with pockets to collect the milk that spills during the learning process. Firm consistent limits, patience, and support allow toddlers to develop socially acceptable behavior and cope with the frustration of learning self-control (Kinservik and Friedhoff, 2000).

Socially, toddlers remain strongly attached to their parents and fear separation from them. In their presence they feel safe, and their curiosity is evident in their exploration of the environment. The child continues to engage in solitary play during toddlerhood but also begins to participate in parallel play, which is playing *beside* rather than *with* another child. Play expands the child's cognitive and psychosocial development. It is always important to consider if toys support development of the child, along with the safety of the toy.

Health Risks

The newly developed locomotion abilities and insatiable curiosity of toddlers make them at risk for injury. Toddlers need close supervision at all times and particularly when in environments that are not childproofed (Figure 12-5).

Poisonings occur frequently because children near 2 years of age are interested in placing any object or substance in their

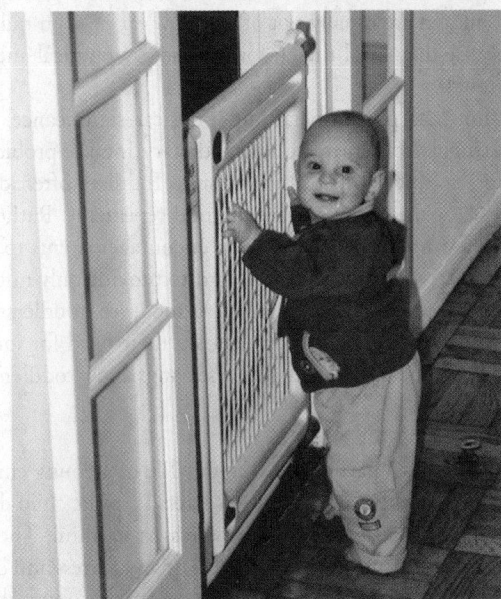

Figure 12-5 Safety precautions should be provided for toddlers. (Courtesy Elaine Polan, RNC, BSN, MS.)

mouths to learn about it. The wise parent removes or locks up all possible poisons, including plants, cleaning materials, and medications. These parental actions create a safer environment for exploratory behavior. Lead poisoning continues to be a serious health hazard in the United States, and children under the age of 6 years are most vulnerable (Hockenberry and Wilson, 2007).

Toddlers' lack of awareness regarding the danger of water and their newly developed walking skills make drowning a major cause of accidental death in this age-group. Limit setting is extremely important for toddlers' safety. Motor vehicle accidents account for half of all accidental deaths in children between the ages of 1 and 4 years. Some of these deaths are the result of unrestrained children, and some are attributed to injuries within the car resulting from not using car seat safety guidelines (Hockenberry and Wilson, 2007). You best accomplish injury prevention by associating various injuries with the attainment of developmental milestones (see Table 12-1, p. 162).

Nutrition. Childhood obesity and the associated chronic disease that results is a source of concern for all health care providers. There have been a number of recommended changes in the diets for both children and adults in the current American Heart Association Dietary Guidelines (2005). Children establish lifetime eating habits in early childhood, and there is increased emphasis on food choices and stress reduction. Children increasingly meet nutritional needs by solid foods. Parents can use the MyPyramid for Kids, introduced by the U.S. Department of Agriculture (2005), as a guide. The healthy toddler requires a balanced daily intake of bread and grains, vegetables, fruit, dairy products, and proteins. Because the consumption of more than a quart of milk per day usually decreases the child's appetite for these essential solid foods and results in inadequate iron intake, advise parents to limit milk intake to 2 to 3 cups per day (Hockenberry and Wilson,

2007). Children are usually not offered low-fat or skim milk until age 2 because they need the fat for satisfactory physical and intellectual growth.

Mealtime has psychosocial and physical significance. If the parents struggle to control toddlers' dietary intake, problem behavior and conflicts will possibly result. Toddlers often develop "food jags," or the desire to eat one food repeatedly. Rather than becoming disturbed by this behavior, encourage parents to offer a variety of nutritious foods at meals and to provide only nutritious snacks between meals. Serving finger foods to toddlers allows them to eat by themselves and to satisfy their need for independence and control. Small, reasonable servings allow toddlers to eat all of their meals.

Stress. Stress is a part of the everyday life of a young child just as it is for an adult. Small amounts of stress help the child develop effective coping skills, but excessive stress is harmful. The nurse assists parents in identifying potential sources of stress and observable behaviors that signal stress beyond the child's coping abilities. Children experience stress with the birth of a sibling, the move into a new home, parental separation and divorce, or serious illness. Observing children playing can often alert the parent to the presence and source of stress. For example, a toddler was observed hitting a doll while saying "Go away!" The parent realized that the recent birth of a new sibling was probably a source of stress for the child (Hockenberry and Wilson, 2007). Frequently children will exhibit *regression* under stressful situations and return to previous patterns of behavior. Encourage parents to ignore the regression and praise the child for age-appropriate behavior.

Preschoolers

The **preschool period** refers to those years between 3 and 5. Children refine the mastery of their bodies and eagerly await the beginning of formal education. Many people consider these the most intriguing years of parenting because children are less negative, more accurately share their thoughts, and more effectively interact and communicate. Physical development occurs at a slower pace than cognitive and psychosocial development.

Physical Changes

Several aspects of physical development continue to stabilize in the preschool years. Children gain about 5 pounds per year; the average weight at 3 years is 32 pounds, at 4 years is 37 pounds, and at 5 years is about 41 pounds. Preschoolers grow 2½ to 3 inches per year, double their birth length around 4 years, and stand an average of 43 inches tall by their fifth birthday. The elongation of the legs results in more slender-appearing children. Little difference exists between the sexes, although boys are slightly larger with more muscle and less fatty tissue. Most children are completely toilet trained by the preschool years (Hockenberry and Wilson, 2007).

Large and fine muscle coordination improves. Preschoolers run well, walk up and down steps with ease, and learn to hop. By 5 years they usually skip on alternate feet, jump rope, and begin to skate and swim. Improving fine motor skills allows intricate ma-

nipulations. They learn to copy crosses and squares. Triangles and diamonds are usually mastered between ages 5 and 6. Scribbling and drawing help to develop fine muscle skills and eye-hand coordination needed for the printing of letters and numbers.

Children need opportunities to learn and practice new physical skills. Nursing care of healthy and ill children includes an assessment of the availability of these opportunities. Although children with acute illnesses benefit from rest and exclusion from usual daily activities, children who have chronic conditions or who have been hospitalized for long periods need ongoing exposure to developmental opportunities. The parents and nurse weave these opportunities into the children's daily experiences, depending on their abilities, needs, and energy level.

Cognitive Changes

Maturation of the brain continues with the most rapid growth occurring in the frontal lobe areas, where planning and organizing new activities and maintaining attention to tasks are paramount. Scientific advances in the use of brain scanning techniques have demonstrated that patterns within the brain change significantly between the ages of 3 to 15 years (Santrock, 2007).

Preschoolers demonstrate their ability to think more complexly by classifying objects according to size or color and by questions such as "Why do they call it the thirty-first day of the month instead of the thirty last?" Children have increased social interaction, as is illustrated by the 5-year-old child who offers a bandage to a child with a cut finger. Children become aware of cause-and-effect relationships, as illustrated by the statement "The sun sets because people want to go to bed." Early causal thinking is also evident in preschoolers. For example, if two events are related in time or space, children link them in a causal fashion. The hospitalized child, for example, reasons, "I cried last night, and that's why the nurse gave me the shot." As children near age 5, they begin to use or learn to use rules to understand causation. They then begin to reason from the general to the particular. This forms the basis for more formal logical thought. The child now reasons, "I get a shot twice a day, and that's why I got one last night." Children in this stage also believe that inanimate objects have lifelike qualities and are capable of action, as seen through comments such as "Trees cry when their branches get broken."

Preschoolers' knowledge of the world remains closely linked to concrete (perceived by the senses) experiences. Even their rich fantasy life is grounded in their perception of reality. The mixing of the two aspects often leads to many childhood fears, and adults sometimes misinterpret it as lying when children are actually presenting reality from their perspective. Preschoolers believe that if a rule is broken punishment will result immediately. During these years they believe that a punishment is automatically connected to an act and do not yet realize that punishment is socially mediated (Santrock, 2007).

The greatest fear of this age-group appears to be that of bodily harm, and this is evident in children's fear of the dark, animals, thunderstorms, and medical personnel. This fear often interferes with their willingness to allow nursing interventions such as measurement of vital signs. Preschoolers cooperate if they are allowed to help the nurse measure the blood pressure of a parent or if they are allowed to manipulate the nurse's equipment.

Moral Development. The preschooler's moral development expands to include a beginning understanding of behaviors considered socially right or wrong. The child continues to be motivated, however, by the wish to avoid punishment or the desire to obtain a reward. The primary difference between this stage of moral development and that of a toddler is that a preschooler is better able to identify behaviors that elicit rewards or punishment and begins to label these behaviors as right or wrong.

Language. Preschoolers' vocabularies continue to increase rapidly, and by the age of 6 children have 8,000 to 14,000 words that they use to define familiar objects, identify colors, and express their desires and frustrations (Santrock, 2007). Language is more social, and questions expand to "Why?" and "How come?" in the quest for information. Phonetically similar words such as *die* and *dye* or *wood* and *would* cause confusion in preschool children. Avoid such words when preparing children for procedures, and assess comprehension of explanations.

Psychosocial Changes

The world of preschoolers expands beyond the family into the neighborhood where children meet other children and adults. Their curiosity and developing initiative lead to the active exploration of the environment, the development of new skills, and the making of new friends. Preschoolers have a surplus of energy that permits them to plan and attempt many activities that are beyond their capabilities, such as pouring milk from a gallon container into their cereal bowls. Guilt arises within children when they overstep the limits of their abilities and feel they have not behaved correctly. Children who in anger wished their sibling were dead experience guilt if that sibling becomes ill. Children need to learn that "wishing" for something to happen does not make it occur. Erikson (1963) recommends that parents help their children strike a healthy balance between initiative and guilt by allowing them to do things on their own while setting firm limits and providing guidance.

Sources of stress for preschoolers can include changes in caregiving arrangements, starting school, the birth of a sibling, parental marital distress, relocation to a new home, or an illness. During these times of stress, preschoolers sometimes revert to bed-wetting or thumb sucking and want the parents to feed, dress, and hold them. These dependent behaviors are often confusing and embarrassing to parents. They will benefit from the nurse's reassurance that these are the child's normal coping behaviors. Provide experiences that these children are able to master. Such successes help children return to their prior level of independent functioning. As language skills develop, encourage children to talk about their feelings. Play is also an excellent way for preschoolers to vent frustration or anger and is a socially acceptable way to deal with stress.

Play. The play of preschool children becomes more social after the third birthday as it shifts from parallel to associative play. Children playing together engage in similar if not identical activity; however, there is no division of labor or rigid organization or rules. Most 3-year-old children are able to play with one other child in a cooperative manner in which they make something or play designated roles such as mother and baby. By age 4, children play in groups of two or three, and by 5 years the group has a temporary leader for each activity.

Pretend play allows children to learn to understand others' points of view, develop skills in solving social problems, and become more creative. Some children have imaginary playmates. These playmates serve many purposes—friends when they are lonely, they accomplish what the child is still attempting and experience what the child wants to forget or remember. Imaginary playmates are a sign of health and allow the child to distinguish between reality and fantasy.

Television, videos, electronic games, and computer programs also help support development and the learning of basic skills. However, these should be only one part of the child's total play activities. The American Academy of Pediatrics recommends that parents schedule limited hours for television viewing so that children spend time in other activities such as reading, physical activity, and socializing with others (Hockenberry and Wilson, 2007).

Health Risks

As fine and gross motor skills develop and the child becomes more coordinated with better balance, falls become much less of a problem. Guidelines for injury prevention in the toddler also apply to the preschooler. Children need to learn about safety in the home, and parents need to continue close supervision of activities. Educating children and their families will help facilitate the *Healthy People 2010* objectives (USDHHS, 2000). Children at this age are great imitators, and so parental example is important. Parental use of a helmet while bicycling will set an appropriate example for the preschooler.

Health Concerns

Little research has explored preschoolers' perceptions of their own health. Parental beliefs about health, children's bodily sensations, and their ability to perform usual daily activities help children develop attitudes about their health. Preschoolers are usually quite independent in washing, dressing, and feeding. Alterations in this independence influence their feelings about their own health.

Nutrition. Nutrition requirements for the preschooler vary little from those of the toddler. The average daily intake is 1800 calories. Oftentimes parents still worry about the amount of food their child is consuming. The quality of the food is more important than quantity in most situations. Preschoolers consume about half of the average adult portions. Finicky eating habits are characteristic of the 4-year-old; however, the 5-year-old is more interested in trying new foods. Some parents express concern about the amount and variety of foods that the child consumes. Suggest to parents that they use the MyPryamid for Children (U.S. Department of Agriculture, Center for Nutrition Policy and Promotion, 2005) and that they record daily food intake for a week so they are able to readily assess their child's diet.

Sleep. Preschoolers average 12 hours of sleep a night and take infrequent naps. Sleep disturbances are common during these years. Disturbances range from trouble getting to sleep to nightmares to prolonging bedtime with extensive rituals. Frequently children have had an overabundance of activity and stimulation.

Helping them to slow down before bedtime usually results in better sleeping habits.

Vision. Vision screening usually begins in the preschool years and needs to occur at regular intervals. One of the most important tests is to determine the presence of nonbinocular vision or strabismus. Early detection and treatment of strabismus is essential by ages 4 to 6 to prevent amblyopia, the resulting blindness from disuse (Hockenberry and Wilson, 2007).

School-Age Children and Adolescents

School-age children and adolescents lead demanding, challenging lives. The developmental changes between ages 6 and 18 are diverse and span all areas of growth and development. Children develop, expand, refine, and synchronize physical, psychosocial, cognitive, and moral skills so that the individual is able to become an accepted and productive member of society. The environment in which the individual develops skills also expands and diversifies. Instead of the boundaries of family and close friends, the environment now includes the school, community, and church. Because of expectations for development, increasing skill and knowledge base, and environmental expansion, the individual experiences new difficulties and dilemmas. With age-specific assessment, the nurse needs to review the appropriate developmental expectations for each age-group. For example, before assessing risk-taking behaviors, the nurse recognizes that adolescents normally strive to achieve a sense of identity while developing a moral code compatible with society.

Direct school-age children and adolescents toward normal developmental behaviors, assisting them in maximizing their abilities and using them to cope (Table 12-1). By helping children and adolescents achieve a necessary developmental balance, the nurse promotes health. School-age children and adolescents need to cope with changes involving other areas of development. For example, 6-year-old children are confronted with new authority figures, teachers, as well as new rules and restrictions. They need to cooperatively work and play with a large group of children of various cultural backgrounds. School-age children have to develop cognitive skills that enhance their reasoning and allow them to learn to read, write, and manipulate numbers. Because of the stress of these changes, some children develop physical and psychosocial health problems (e.g., increased susceptibility to upper respiratory infections, school maladjustment, inadequate peer relationships, or learning disorders). The nurse designs health promotion interventions based on the child's developmental stage.

School-Age Children

During these "middle years" of childhood, the foundation for adult roles in work, recreation, and social interaction is laid. In industrialized countries this school-age period begins when the

TABLE 12-1 Developmental Behaviors of School-Age Children and Adolescents	
SCHOOL-AGE CHILDREN	**ADOLESCENTS**
Relationships With Parents	
Children gradually learn that parents are less than perfect; they are often disillusioned with them and wish that friends' parents were their own. Sometimes they believe that they must be adopted. They rely on parents for unconditional love, security, guidance, and nurturing.	Adolescents' desire for increasing independence and autonomy and continuing need for some dependence and limit setting by parents place strain on their relationship. Effective communication and democratic parenting are best tools for meeting this challenge.
Relationships With Siblings	
Seem to be at odds with one another at home; yet they are each others' best defenders away from home. Younger children often idolize older siblings, and this frequently leads to competition. Older children sometimes envy attention that younger siblings require and are quite bossy and somewhat abusive.	Younger siblings rarely understand their adolescent siblings' need for privacy to think, dream, and talk with peers. Adolescents often enjoy interacting with and guiding younger brothers and sisters when timing is convenient for them and they can remain in control.
Relationships With Peers	
During primary grades (6-7 years), children of both sexes play together, depending on who is available and interested. Around age 8, social groupings of same-sex peers form. These "gangs" allow children to declare their independence from parental rules and establish their own secret codes or languages and rules of membership and behavior. This period is often referred to as *secret society* of childhood. Preadolescents (10-12 years) usually have best friends of same sex. These relationships are often transient, but they are intense and allow discussion of all areas of life. Some interest in heterosexual relationships develops but they usually are not reciprocal.	Peer group is factor of critical influence to adolescents, who have increasing need for recognition and acceptance. Companionship offered by peer groups provides secure environment for individuals to try out new ideas and share similar feelings and attitudes. Adolescents often form cliques with peers from same socioeconomic group with similar interests. Cliques, which are highly exclusive, help their members, who have strong emotional bonds, develop their identities. The crowd, which is more impersonal than the clique, offers opportunities for heterosexual interaction and social activities. The crowd also maintains rigid membership requirements; clique membership is usually a prerequisite for crowd membership.

⁂ TABLE 12-1 Developmental Behaviors of School-Age Children and Adolescents—cont'd

SCHOOL-AGE CHILDREN	ADOLESCENTS
Self-Concept Children's feelings of competence regarding mastery of tasks are key elements in forming self-esteem. Children need to receive positive feedback from teachers and parents regarding their efforts. It is important for children to develop skills in at least one area such as reading, music, or swimming. Pets that require children's care and attention reward them with unconditional love and promote feelings of self-worth.	Formal and informal peer groups are a primary force in shaping self-concept of group members. Popularity and recognition within peer group enhance self-esteem and reinforce self-concept. Total immersion in peer group makes it appear that adolescents have no original thoughts and are incapable of making decisions. Adolescents who withdraw from peers into isolation struggle with developing identity.
Fears There is decline in fears related to body safety such as storms, dogs, darkness, noises, scrapes, and scratches. Fears of supernatural such as ghosts and witches persist and decline slowly. New fears related to school and family occur. They fear ridicule from teachers and friends and disapproval and rejection of parents. They also become frightened about death and items that they hear on news such as war and destruction of environment.	Fears in this age-group center around peer group acceptance, body changes, loss of self-control, and emerging sexual urges. Adolescents constantly examine their bodies for changes and signs of imperfection. Any defect, real or imagined, is cause of endless worry. Adolescents' developing awareness of economic and political problems result in fear of going to war with its resulting death and destruction.
Coping Patterns To deal with stress, school-agers use problem solving and defense mechanisms such as denial and aggression. Several categories of coping behaviors of hospitalized school-agers include inactivity (total silence, lack of activity, and apathy), orientation or precoping (looking and listening, walking around and exploring, and asking questions), cooperation (compliance with care), resistance (attempt to get away from the situation by turning away or making physical or verbal attacks), and controlling (assuming responsibility for self-care and suggesting how things could be done).	Coping behaviors expand with experiences adolescents have gained from life and from developing cognitive maturity. By age 15, most use full range of defense mechanisms, including rationalization and intellectualization. Adolescents' problem-solving abilities have matured, and they are able to reason through philosophical discussions and complex situations that require abstract thinking and proposition of hypotheses. Some adolescents use avoidance coping strategies in which they deny or repress the problem and make an attempt to reduce tension by engaging in substance abuse or avoiding people.
Morals Children learn rules from parents, but their understanding of rules or reasons for them is limited until about 10 years. Before that, they are concerned with own needs first and may cheat to win. After 10, justice is based on "eye for an eye," and punishment should correct situation (e.g., if children break something, they pay to have it fixed).	According to Kohlberg (1964), as youths approach adolescence they reach the conventional level, where internalization of expectations of their family and society begins. Initially there is considerable conformity to rules to win praise or approval from others and to avoid social disapproval or rejection; later, they seek to avoid criticism from persons of authority in institutions.
Diversional Activity School-agers play cooperatively in group activities such as jumping rope, hopscotch, soccer, and baseball. Play becomes competitive, and children often have difficulty learning to lose. Teasing, insults, dares, superstitions, and increased sensitivity are characteristics of this age.	Many teenagers develop special interests in certain sports and concentrate on developing maximal skills therein. Teens often determine recreational activities by what is popular with peers and what provides independence from parents (e.g., computers, cars).
Nutrition Children have definite likes and dislikes. Few nutritional deficiencies occur in this age-group. Children have voracious appetites after school and need quality snacks such as fruit and sandwiches to avoid empty-calorie foods such as chips and candy.	Total nutritional needs become greater during adolescence. Girls' caloric needs decrease, and their need for protein increases slightly. Adolescents need almost twice as much iron as adult men, and growth spurts increase calcium demand.

child starts elementary school around the age of 6 years. **Puberty**, around 12 years of age, signals the end of middle childhood. Children make great developmental strides during these years as they develop competencies in physical, cognitive, and psychosocial skills. During these years children become "better" at things; for example, they run faster and farther as proficiency and endurance develop.

The school or educational experience expands the child's world and is a transition from a life of relatively free play to a life of structured play, learning, and work. The school and home influence growth and development, requiring adjustment by the parents and child. The child learns to cope with rules and expectations presented by the school and peers. Parents have to learn to allow their child to make decisions, accept responsibility, and learn from life's experiences.

Physical Changes

The rate of growth during these early school years is slow and consistent, a relative calm before the growth spurt of adolescence. The school-age child appears slimmer than the preschooler as a result of changes in fat distribution and thickness (Hockenberry and Wilson, 2007). Growth accelerates at different times for different children. The average increase in height is 2 inches per year, and weight, which is more variable, increases by 4 to 7 pounds per year. Many children double their weight during these middle childhood years, and most girls exceed boys in both height and weight by the end of the school years (Hockenberry and Wilson, 2007).

School provides children with the opportunity to compare themselves with large numbers of children of the same age. The physical examination usually required for entrance to formal school is an excellent opportunity to discuss with the child and parents the influences of genetic endowment, nutrition, and exercise on height and weight. Annual measurement of height and weight will reveal alterations in growth that are symptoms of the onset of a variety of childhood diseases.

School-age children become more graceful during the school years because their large muscle coordination improves and their strength doubles. Most children practice the basic gross motor skills of running, jumping, balancing, throwing, and catching during play, resulting in refinement of neuromuscular function and skills. Individual differences in the rate of mastering skills and ultimate skill achievement become apparent during their participation in their many activities and games. Fine motor skills improve, and as children gain control over fingers and wrists, they become proficient in a wide range of activities.

Most 6-year-old children are able to hold a pencil adeptly and print letters and words, but by age 12 the child is able to make detailed drawings and write sentences in script. Painting, drawing, playing computer games, and modeling allow children to practice and improve newly refined skills. Encourage children and have parents encourage them to pursue these activities. The improved fine motor capabilities of youngsters in middle childhood allow them to become very independent in bathing, dressing, and taking care of other personal needs. They develop strong personal preferences in the way these needs are met. Illness and hospitalization threaten children's control in these areas. Therefore it is im-

portant to allow them to participate in care and maintain as much independence as possible. Children whose care demands restriction of fluids cannot be allowed to decide the amount of fluids they will drink in 24 hours, but they can help decide the type of fluids and help keep a record of intake.

Assessment of neurological development is often based on fine motor coordination. This assessment includes penmanship, stacking ability, and performance of sequential, rapid, alternating movements such as touching the finger to the nose and then to the examiner's finger (smooth movement without tremors is the normal response). Fine motor coordination is critical to success in the typical American school, where children have to hold pencils and crayons and use scissors and rulers. The opportunity to practice these skills through schoolwork and play is essential to learning coordinated, complex behaviors.

Other physical changes take place during the school-age years. Dental growth is prominent during the school-age years. The first permanent or secondary teeth erupt at approximately 6 years of age. Development of the permanent teeth has been occurring for some time before eruption. The root is absorbed, leaving the crown, which causes the tooth to become loose and fall out. This makes room for the new permanent teeth. Eruption usually begins with the 6-year molar and follows the same order as with the primary teeth. By 12 years, children have lost all primary teeth, and the majority of permanent teeth have erupted. Infrequent or inadequate dental care remains a persistent problem for many American children.

As skeletal growth progresses, body appearance and posture change. Earlier, the child's posture was a stoop-shouldered, slight lordosis with a prominent abdomen, and this changes to a more erect posture. It is essential to evaluate children, especially girls after the age of 12 years, for scoliosis, the lateral curvature of the spine.

Eye shape alters because of skeletal growth. This improves visual acuity, and normal adult 20/20 vision is achievable. Screening for vision and hearing problems is easier, and results are more reliable because school-age children more fully understand and cooperate with the test directions. The school nurse typically assesses the growth, visual, and auditory status of school-age children and refers those with possible deviations to a health care provider, such as their family practitioner or pediatrician.

Cognitive Changes

Cognitive changes provide the school-age child with the ability to think in a logical manner about the here and now and to understand the relationship between things and ideas. They are now able to use their developed thinking abilities to experience events without having to act them out (Hockenberry and Wilson, 2007). The thoughts of school-age children are no longer dominated by their perceptions, and thus their ability to understand the world greatly expands. Around 7 years of age children are able to use symbols to carry out operations (mental activities) in thought rather than in action. They begin to use logical thought processes with concrete materials (objects, people, and events they can touch and see).

School-age children have the ability to concentrate on more than one aspect of a situation. They begin to understand that others do not always see things as they do and even begin to understand another viewpoint. They now have the ability to recognize that the amount or quantity of a substance remains the same even when its shape or appearance changes. For instance, two balls of clay of equal size remain the same amount of clay even when one is flattened and the other remains in ball shape.

The young child is able to separate objects into groups according to shape or color, whereas the school-age child understands that the same element can exist in two classes at the same time. School-age children are able to reason about the relationships between classes. By 7 or 8 years they develop the ability to place objects in order according to their increasing or decreasing size (Hockenberry and Wilson, 2007; Santrock, 2007). School-age children frequently have collections such as baseball cards or stuffed animals that demonstrate this new cognitive skill.

Middle childhood youngsters use their newly developed cognitive skills to solve problems. Some individuals are better than others at problem solving because of native intelligence, education, and experience, but all children can improve these skills. Middle school-age children who are good problem solvers demonstrate the following characteristics: a positive attitude that the problem can be solved with persistence, a concern for accuracy, the ability to divide the problem into parts for study, and the ability to avoid guessing while searching for facts.

Language Development. Language growth is so rapid during middle childhood that it is no longer possible to match age with language achievements. Children improve their use of language and expand their structural knowledge. They become more aware of the rules of syntax, the rules for linking words into phrases and sentences. They also identify generalizations and exceptions to rules. They accept language as a means for representing the world in a subjective manner and realize that words have arbitrary, rather than absolute, meanings. They use different words for the same object or concept, and they understand that a single word often has many meanings. Children begin to think about language, which enables them to appreciate jokes and riddles. They are not as likely to use a literal interpretation of a word and now reason about its meaning within a context (Hockenberry and Wilson, 2007). Vocabulary development is tied closely to reading. Studies have found that children who enter school with a small vocabulary have more difficulty in learning how to read (Santrock, 2007).

Psychosocial Changes

Erikson (1963) identifies the developmental task for school-age children as industry versus inferiority. During this time, children strive to acquire competence and skills necessary for them to function as adults. School-age children who are positively recognized for success feel a sense of worth. Those faced with failure often feel a sense of mediocrity or unworthiness, which sometimes results in withdrawal from school and peers.

School-age children begin to define themselves based on their internal characteristics more than external characteristics. They begin to define their self-concept and develop self-esteem, an overall self-evaluation. Interaction with peers allows them to define their own accomplishments in relation to others as they work to develop a positive self-image (Santrock, 2007).

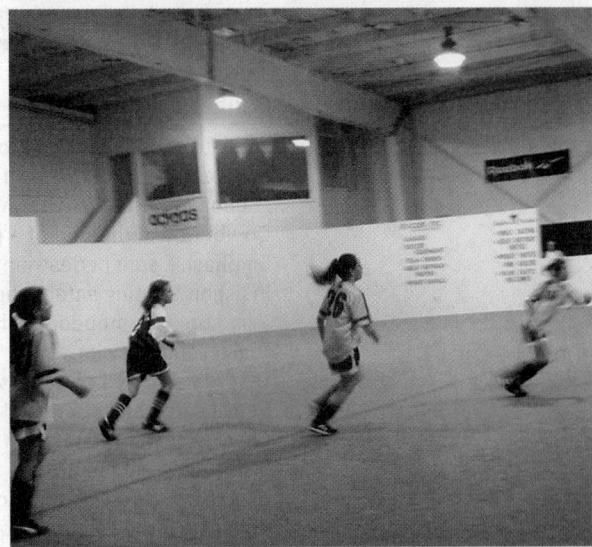

Figure 12-6 School-age children gain a sense of achievement working and playing with peers. (Courtesy Elaine Polan, RNC, BSN, MS.)

Moral Development. The need for a moral code and social rules becomes more evident as school-age children's cognitive abilities and social experiences increase. For example, 12-year-old children are able to consider what society would be like without rules because of their ability to reason logically and their experiences with group play. They view rules as necessary principles of life, not just dictates from authorities. In the early school years, children strictly interpret and adhere to rules. As they develop, they make more flexible judgments and evaluate rules for applicability to a given situation.

Peer Relationships. Group and personal achievements become important to the school-age child. Success is important in physical and cognitive activities. Play involves peers and the pursuit of group goals. Although solitary activities are not eliminated, group play overshadows them. Learning to contribute, collaborate, and work cooperatively toward a common goal becomes a measure of success (Figure 12-6).

The school-age child prefers same-sex peers to opposite-sex peers. In general, girls and boys view the opposite sex negatively. Peer influence becomes quite diverse during this stage of development. Conformity is evident in mannerisms, clothing styles, and speech patterns, which are reinforced and influenced by contact with peers. During this time period, clubs and peer groups become prominent. Group identity increases as the school-age child approaches adolescence.

Sexual Identity. Freud described middle childhood as the latency period because he felt that children of this period had little interest in their sexuality. Today many researchers believe that school-age children have a great deal of curiosity about their sexuality. Some experiment, but this play is usually transitory. Children's curiosity about adult magazines or meanings of sexually explicit words is also an example of their sexual interest. This is

✳ TABLE 12-2 Injury Prevention During School-Age Years

DEVELOPMENTAL ABILITIES RELATED TO RISK FOR INJURY	INJURY PREVENTION
Motor Vehicles	Educate child regarding proper use of seat belts
	Maintain discipline while a passenger in a vehicle (e.g., keep arms inside, do not lean against doors or interfere with driver)
	Do not ride in the bed of a pickup truck
	Emphasize safe pedestrian behavior
	Insist on wearing safety apparel (e.g., helmet) where applicable, such as when riding a bicycle, motorcycle, moped, or all-terrain vehicle
Drowning	Teach child to swim
	Teach basic rules of water safety
	Select safe and supervised places to swim
	Check sufficient water depth for diving
	Swim with a companion
	Use an approved flotation device in water or boat
	Advocate for legislation requiring fencing around pools
	Learn CPR
Burns	Make sure smoke detectors are in homes
	Set hot water temperatures (120°-130° F) to avoid scald burns
	Instruct child in behavior in areas involving contact with potential burn hazards (e.g., gasoline, matches, bonfires or barbecues, lighter fluid, firecrackers, cigarette lighters, cooking utensils, chemistry sets)
	Avoid climbing or flying kites around high-tension wires
	Instruct child in proper behavior in the event of fire (e.g., fire drills at home and school)
	Teach child safe cooking (use low heat, avoid any frying, be careful of steam burns, scalds, or exploding foods, especially from microwaving)
Substance Abuse and Poisoning	Educate child regarding hazards of taking nonprescription drugs and chemicals, including aspirin and alcohol
	Teach child to say "no" if offered illegal or dangerous drugs or alcohol
	Keep potentially dangerous products in properly labeled receptacles—preferably locked and out of reach
Bodily Damage	Help provide facilities for supervised activities
	Encourage playing in safe places
	Keep firearms safely locked up except during adult supervision
	Teach proper care of, use of, and respect for devices with potential danger (e.g., power tools, firecrackers)
	Teach children not to tease or surprise dogs, invade their territory, take dogs' toys, or interfere with dogs' feeding
	Stress eye, ear, or mouth protection when using potentially hazardous objects or devices or when engaged in potentially hazardous sports (e.g., baseball)
	Teach safety regarding use of corrective devices (glasses); if child wears contact lenses, monitor duration of wear to prevent corneal damage
	Stress careful selection, use, and maintenance of sports and recreation equipment such as skateboards and in-line skates
	Emphasize proper conditioning, safe practices, and use of safety equipment for sports or recreational activities
	Use window guards to prevent falls
	Teach stranger safety:
	Caution child to never go with a stranger
	Teach name, address, and phone number and to ask for help from appropriate people (cashier, security guard, policeman) if lost; have identification on child (sewn in clothes, inside shoe)
	Avoid personalized clothing in public places
	Have child tell parents if anyone makes child feel uncomfortable in any way
	Always listen to child's concerns regarding others' behavior
	Teach child to say "no" when confronted with uncomfortable situations

From Hockenberry MJ, Wilson D: *Wong's nursing care of infants and children*, ed 8, St. Louis, 2007, Mosby.

TABLE 12-3 Health Promotion in the School-Age Period

SCHOOL-AGE HEALTH CONCERNS	HEALTH PROMOTION INTERVENTIONS
Nutrition	Provide nutrition education that promotes healthy lifestyle: food guide pyramid; limiting fat intake to 30% of calories, saturated fat to 10% of calories.
Oral hygiene	Provide examples of low cariogenic snacks. Review mechanics of dental hygiene: brushing, flossing. Stress importance of biannual dental checkups.
Infections	Provide immunization information and follow-up. Teach infection prevention practices (hand washing, care of minor skin injuries). Teach concepts of viral and bacterial illness.
Tobacco, alcohol, and drug use	Provide tobacco use prevention programs. Provide information regarding the hazards of drug use.
Human sexuality	Provide information about sexual maturation and reproduction in age-appropriate manner. Encourage parents to view their child's sexual curiosity as part of the developmental process. Discuss with parents the learning needs of their child regarding sexuality. Provide age-appropriate HIV education.

HIV, Human immunodeficiency virus.

the time for children to have exposure to sex education, including sexual maturation, reproduction, and relationships (Hockenberry and Wilson, 2007).

Stress. Today's children experience more stress than children in earlier generations. Stress comes from parental expectations, peer expectations, the school environment, or violence in the family, school, or community. Some school-age children care for themselves before or after school without adult supervision. Latchkey children sometimes feel increased stress and are at greater risk for injury and unsafe behaviors (Hockenberry and Wilson, 2007). The nurse assists the child in coping with stress by helping the parents and child to identify potential stressors and by designing interventions to minimize stress and the child's stress response. Using deep-breathing techniques, positive imagery, and progressive relaxation of muscle groups are interventions that most children can learn. Include the parent, child, and teacher in the intervention for maximal success.

Health Risks

Accidents and injuries are a major health problem affecting school-age children. They now have more exposure to various environments and less supervision, but their developed cognitive and motor skills make them less likely to suffer from unintentional injury. Some school-age children are risk takers and attempt activities that are beyond their abilities (Hockenberry Wilson, 2007). Motor vehicle injuries as a passenger or pedestrian and bicycle injuries are among the most common in this age-group (Table 12-2).

Infections account for the majority of all childhood illnesses; respiratory infections are the most prevalent. The common cold remains the chief illness of childhood. Certain groups of children are more prone to disease and disability, often as a result of barriers to health care. Mental retardation, learning disorders, sensory impairments, and malnutrition are far more prevalent among children living in poverty (USDHHS, 2000).

Poverty and the prevalence of illness are highly correlated. Access to care is often very limited, and health promotion and preventative health care activities are minimal. Infant mortality,

dental problems, poor nutrition, and lack of immunizations continue to be major health concerns for uninsured or impoverished families.

Health Concerns

Perceptions. During the school-age years, identity and self-concept become stronger and more individualized. Perception of wellness is based on readily observable facts such as presence or absence of illness and adequacy of eating or sleeping. Functional ability is the standard by which personal health and the health of others are judged.

Six-year-olds are aware of their body and modest and sensitive about being exposed. Nurses need to provide for privacy and offer explanations of common procedures. This fosters children's self-esteem and lessens their fear of pain and intrusion (Popovich, 2000).

Health Education. The school-age period is a crucial period for the acquisition of behaviors and health practices for a healthy adult life. Because cognition is advancing during the period, effective health education must be developmentally appropriate. Promotion of good health practices is a nursing responsibility. Programs directed at health education are frequently organized and conducted in the school. Effective health education teaches children about their bodies and how the choices they make impact their health (Hockenberry and Wilson, 2007). During these programs, focus on the development of behaviors that positively affect children's health status.

Also instruct parents regarding health promotion appropriate for the school-age child. Parents need to recognize the importance of annual health maintenance visits for immunizations, screenings, and dental care. When their school-age child reaches 10 years of age, parents need to begin discussions in preparation for upcoming pubertal changes. Topics include introductory information regarding menstruation, sexual intercourse, and reproduction. Provide age-appropriate written materials to aid parents in their efforts. Table 12-3 presents a comprehensive list of health promotion topics.

Safety. Because accidents are the leading cause of death and injury in the school-age period, safety is a priority health teaching consideration. Nurses contribute to the general health of children by educating them about safety measures to prevent accidents. At this age, encourage children to take responsibility for their own safety.

Nutrition. Nurses contribute to meeting national policy goals by promoting healthy lifestyle habits, including nutrition. School-age children need to participate in educational programs that enable them to plan, select, and prepare healthy meals and snacks. These foods need to be consistent with the U.S. Department of Agriculture (2005) food guide pyramid nutritional guidelines limiting intake of total and saturated fats and increasing the intake of complex carbohydrates, fruits, and vegetables.

Growth often slows down during the school-age period as compared to infancy and adolescence. School-age children are developing eating patterns that are independent of parental supervision. The school curriculum needs to reinforce the importance of a healthy, balanced diet. The availability of snacks and fast-food restaurants makes it increasingly difficult for children to make healthy choices. Childhood obesity has become a prominent health problem, resulting in increased risk for hypertension, diabetes, coronary heart disease, fatty liver disease, pulmonary complications such as sleep apnea, musculoskeletal problems, dyslipidemia, and potential for psychological problems. Studies have found that overweight children are more often teased, less likely to be chosen as a friend, and more likely to be thought of as lazy and sloppy by their peers (Hockenberry and Wilson, 2007).

Obesity occurs because children often rush into the home after school or play and eat the most easily obtainable and appealing foods. Unfortunately, these foods are often high in calories and low in nutrition. Providing nutritious snacks is often the best way for a parent to ensure good nutritional intake. Caregivers need to provide ready access to fresh fruit, raw vegetables, cheese, popcorn, and high-protein snacks such as skim-milk pudding and hot chocolate. Nurses help families and children prevent obesity through education on proper nutrition and exercise.

Adolescents

Adolescence is the period during which the individual makes the transition from childhood to adulthood, usually between 13 and 20 years. The term *adolescent* usually refers to psychological maturation of the individual, whereas *puberty* refers to the point at which reproduction becomes possible. The hormonal changes of puberty result in changes in the appearance of the young person, and cognitive development results in the ability to hypothesize and deal with abstractions. Adjustments and adaptations are necessary to cope with these simultaneous changes and the attempt to establish a mature sense of identity. In the past, many referred to adolescence as a stormy and stressful period filled with inner turmoil, but today it is recognized that most teenagers successfully meet the challenges of this period. Within adolescence, three subphases exist: early (pre) adolescence (11 to 14 years), middle

adolescence (15 to 17 years), and late adolescence (18 to 20 years). Opportunities, challenges, changes, skills, pressures, and physical, cognitive, and psychosocial development vary widely between the subphases (Table 12-4).

The nurse's understanding of development provides a unique perspective for helping teenagers and parents anticipate and cope with the stresses of adolescence. Nursing activities, particularly education, promote healthy development. These activities occur in a variety of settings, and you can direct them at the adolescent, parents, or both. For example, the nurse conducts seminars in a high school to provide practical suggestions for solving problems of concern to a large group of students, such as treating acne or making responsible decisions about drugs or alcohol use. Similarly, a group education program for parents about how to cope with teenagers would promote parental understanding of adolescent development. These programs are held in the school, clinic, private office, or community center. To learn more about specific topics or problems, identify teenagers' needs and desires. Involvement produces more active, interested learners.

Physical Changes

Physical changes occur rapidly in adolescence. Sexual maturation occurs with the development of primary and secondary sexual characteristics. The following are four main focuses of the physical changes:

1. Increased growth rate of skeleton, muscle, and viscera
2. Sex-specific changes, such as changes in shoulder and hip width
3. Alteration in distribution of muscle and fat
4. Development of the reproductive system and secondary sex characteristics

Wide variation exists in the timing of physical changes associated with puberty between sexes and within the same sex. Girls tend to begin their physical changes approximately 2 years earlier than boys (Santrock, 2007). The rate of height and weight gain are usually proportional, and the sequence of pubertal growth changes is the same in most individuals (see Table 12-4).

Hormonal changes within the body create change when the hypothalamus begins to produce gonadotropin-releasing hormones. This sends the pituitary a signal to secrete gonadotropic hormones. Gonadotropic hormones stimulate ovarian cells to produce **estrogen** and testicular cells to produce **testosterone.** These hormones contribute to the development of secondary sex characteristics such as hair growth and voice changes and play an essential role in reproduction. The changing concentrations of these hormones are also linked to acne and body odor. Understanding these hormonal changes enables the nurse to reassure adolescents and educate them about body care needs.

Boys who mature early are more poised, relaxed, good-natured, skilled in athletic activities, and more likely to be school leaders than boys who mature late. In contrast, girls who mature early are less satisfied with their figures by late adolescence. The reason for this is that early-maturing girls tend to be shorter and somewhat heavier than late-maturing girls who tend to be taller and thinner (Santrock, 2007). The ranges of normal are stressed. As with increases in height and weight, the pattern of sexual

✳ **TABLE 12-4 Growth and Development During Adolescence**

EARLY ADOLESCENCE (11-14 YEARS)	MIDDLE ADOLESCENCE (14-17 YEARS)	LATE ADOLESCENCE (17-20 YEARS)
Growth		
Rapidly accelerating growth reaches peak velocity	Growth decelerating in girls	Physically mature
Secondary sex characteristics appear	Stature reaches 95% of adult height	Structure and reproductive growth almost complete
	Secondary sex characteristics well-advanced	
Cognition		
Explores newfound ability for limited abstract thought	Developing capacity for abstract thinking	Establishes abstract thought
Clumsy groping for new values and energies	Enjoys intellectual powers, often in idealistic terms	Can perceive and act on long-range operations
Comparison of "normality" with peers of same sex	Concern with philosophic, political, and social problems	Able to view problems comprehensively
		Intellectual and functional identity established
Identity		
Preoccupied with rapid body changes	Modifies body image	Body image and gender-role definition nearly secured
Tries out various roles	Very self-centered; increased narcissism	Mature sexual identity
Measurement of attractiveness by acceptance or rejection of peers	Tendency toward inner experience and self-discovery	Phase of consolidation of identity
Conformity to group norms	Has a rich fantasy life	Stability of self-esteem
	Idealistic	Comfortable with physical growth
	Able to perceive future implications of current behavior and decisions; variable application	Social roles defined and articulated
Relationships With Parents		
Defining independence-dependence boundaries	Major conflicts over independence and control	Emotional and physical separation from parents completed
Strong desire to remain dependent on parents while trying to detach	Low point in parent-child relationship	Independence from family with less conflict
No major conflicts over parental control	Greatest push for emancipation; disengagement	Emancipation nearly secured
	Final and irreversible emotional detachment from parents; mourning	
Relationships With Peers		
Seeks peer affiliations to counter instability generated by rapid change	Strong need for identity to affirm self-image	Peer group recedes in importance in favor of individual friendship
Increase of close, idealized friendships with members of the same sex	Behavioral standards set by peer group	Testing of male-female relationships against possibility of permanent alliance
Struggle for mastery takes place within peer group	Acceptance by peers extremely important—fear of rejection	Relationships characterized by giving and sharing
	Exploration of ability to attract the opposite sex	
Sexuality		
Self-exploration and evaluation	Multiple plural relationships	Forms stable relationships and attachment to another
Limited dating, usually socializes with a group	Decisive turn toward heterosexuality (if is homosexual, knows by this time)	Growing capacity for mutuality and reciprocity
Limited intimacy	Exploration of "self-appeal"	Dating as a male-female pair
	Feeling of "being in love"	Intimacy involves commitment rather than exploration and romanticism
	Tentative establishment of relationships	
Psychological Health		
Wide mood swings	Tendency toward inner experiences; more introspective	More constancy of emotion
Intense daydreaming	Tendency to withdraw when upset or feelings are hurt	More likely to conceal anger
Anger outwardly expressed with moodiness, temper outbursts, and verbal insults and name-calling	Changing of emotions in time and range	
	Feelings of inadequacy common; difficulty in asking for help	

From Hockenberry MJ, Wilson D: *Wong's nursing care of infants and children*, ed 8, St. Louis, 2007, Mosby.

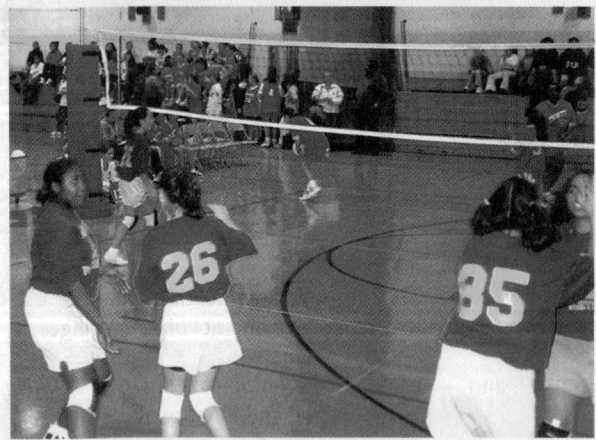

Figure 12-7 Peer interactions help increase self-esteem during puberty. (Courtesy Elaine Polan, RNC, BSN, MS.)

changes is more significant than their time of onset. Large deviations from normal frames require investigation. Being like peers is extremely important for adolescents (Figure 12-7).

Any deviation in the timing of the physical changes is extremely difficult for adolescents to accept. Therefore provide emotional support for those undergoing early or delayed puberty. Even adolescents whose physical changes are occurring at the normal times seek confirmation of and reassurance about their normalcy.

Height and weight increases usually occur during the prepubertal growth spurt, which peaks in girls at about 12 years and in boys at about 14 years. For girls, height increases 2 to 8 inches and weight increases by 15 to 55 pounds. Height for boys increases approximately 4 to 12 inches, and weight increases by 15 to 65 pounds. Adults gain the final 20% to 25% of their height and 50% of their weight during this time period (Hockenberry and Wilson, 2007).

Girls attain 90% to 95% of their adult height by **menarche** (the onset of menstruation) and reach their full height by 16 to 17 years of age, whereas boys continue to grow taller until 18 to 20 years of age. Fat is redistributed into adult proportions as height and weight increase, and gradually the adolescent torso takes on an adult appearance. Although there are individual and sex differences, growth follows a similar pattern for both sexes (see Table 12-4). Growth in the length of the extremities occurs earliest, making the hands and feet appear very large and the legs very long; the individual often appears awkward and clumsy. At the same time the lower jaw and nose become longer and the forehead higher and wider as the baby face of childhood disappears. Next the thighs widen; then the shoulders broaden, and growth of the trunk proceeds. Widening of the female hips and broadening of the male shoulders continue throughout adolescence.

Personal growth curves help the nurse assess physical development. The individual's sustained progression along the curve, however, is more important than a comparison to the norm. The nurse charts growth measurements during routine health assessments to evaluate changes.

Adolescents are sensitive about physical changes that make them different from peers. For this reason they are generally inter-

ested in the normal pattern of growth and their personal growth curves. Consequently, share this information to reassure adolescents that their own patterns are normal.

Cognitive Changes

Changes occurring within the mind and the widening social environment of the adolescent result in the highest level of intellectual development. Without an appropriate educational environment, young persons who possess sufficient neurological development to reach this stage do not always attain it, and those who are guided toward rational thinking sometimes reach this stage early.

The adolescent develops the ability to determine possibilities, rank possibilities, solve problems, and make decisions through logical operations. The teenager thinks abstractly and deals effectively with hypothetical problems. When confronted with a problem, the teenager considers an infinite variety of causes and solutions. For the first time, the young person moves beyond the physical or concrete properties of a situation and uses reasoning powers to understand the abstract. School-age individuals think about what is, whereas adolescents are able to imagine what might be. Adolescents are now able to think in terms of the future rather than just what is currently happening. These newly developed abilities allow the individual to have more insight and skill in playing games such as video games, computer games, and board games that require abstract thinking and deductive reasoning about many possible strategies. A teenager even solves problems requiring simultaneous manipulation of several abstract concepts. Development of this ability is important in the pursuit of an identity. For example, newly acquired cognitive skills allow the teenager to define appropriate, effective, and comfortable sex-role behaviors and to consider their impact on peers, family, and society.

The ability to think logically about these behaviors and their outcomes encourages the adolescent to develop personal thoughts and means of expressing sexual identity. In addition, a higher level of cognitive functioning makes the adolescent receptive to more detailed and diverse information about sexuality and sexual behaviors. For example, sex education includes an explanation of physiological sexual changes and birth control measures.

By midadolescence there is an introspective quality emerging with regard to cognition. At this time adolescents believe that they are unique and the exception, giving rise to their risk-taking behaviors. They often express that they "are able to drive fast and not get into an accident." Other typical adolescent behaviors includes heightened self-consciousness and the desire for privacy.

Adolescents also develop the ability to understand how the ideas or actions of an individual influence others. This complex development of thought leads adolescents to question society and its values. Although adolescents have the capability to think as well as an adult, they do not have experiences on which to build. It is common for teenagers to consider their parents too narrow minded or too materialistic. This results in conflicts between teens and their parents. Cognitive abilities and performance vary greatly among adolescents. In fact, an adolescent performs at different levels in different situations based on past experiences, formal education, and motivation in the use of logic and effective deductive reasoning.

Language Skills. Language development is fairly complete by adolescence, although vocabulary continues to expand. The primary focus becomes communication skills that the adolescent uses effectively in various situations. Adolescents need to communicate thoughts, feelings, and facts to peers, parents, teachers, and other persons of authority. The skills used in these diverse communication situations vary. Adolescents need to select the person with whom to communicate, decide on the exact message, and choose the way to transmit the message. For example, the way teenagers tell parents about failing grades is not the same as the way that they tell friends. Adolescents develop different skills and styles of communication and learn how and when to use them most effectively. Good communication skills are critical for adolescents in overcoming peer pressure and unhealthy behaviors. The following are some hints for communicating with adolescents:

- Do not avoid discussing sensitive issues. Asking questions about sex, drugs, and school opens the channels for further discussion.
- Ask open-ended questions.
- Look for the meaning behind their words or actions.
- Be alert to clues to their emotional state.
- Involve other individuals and resources when necessary.

Psychosocial Changes

The search for personal identity is the major task of adolescent psychosocial development. Teenagers establish close peer relationships or remain socially isolated. Erikson (1963) sees identity (or role) confusion as the prime danger of this stage and suggests that the cliquishness and intolerance of differences seen in adolescent behavior are defenses against identity confusion (Erikson, 1968). Adolescents work at becoming emotionally independent from their parents, while retaining family ties. In addition, they need to develop their own ethical systems based on personal values. They need to make choices about vocation, future education, and lifestyle. The various components of total identity evolve from these tasks and compose adult personal identity that is unique to the individual. Indecisiveness and the inability to make an occupational choice are behaviors indicating negative resolution of the developmental task.

Sexual Identity. Physical changes of puberty enhance achievement of sexual identity. According to Freud these physiological changes of puberty stimulate the libido, the energy source that fuels the sex drive. This is evidenced by the teenager's interest in romantic relationships, as well as their practice of masturbation. The physical evidence of maturity encourages the development of masculine and feminine behaviors. If these physical changes involve deviations, the person has more difficulty developing a comfortable sexual identity. Adolescents depend on these physical clues because they want assurance of maleness or femaleness and because they do not wish to be different from peers.

Without these physical characteristics, achieving sexual identity is difficult. Other influences are cultural attitudes and expectations of sex-role behavior and available role models. Sexual identity involves more than just sexual orientation. It also in-

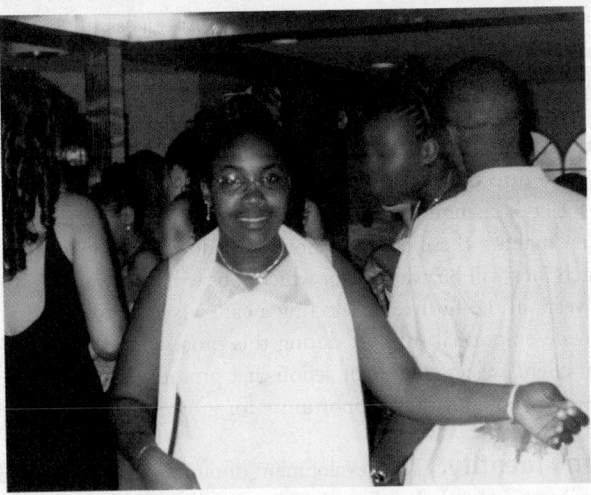

Figure 12-8 Social interactions strengthen a teen's group identity. (Courtesy Elaine Polan, RNC, BSN, MS.)

cludes activities, interests, and behavioral styles (Santrock, 2007). The masculine and feminine behaviors that teenagers see affect the way that they express sexuality.

Group Identity. Adolescents seek a group identity because they need esteem and acceptance (Figure 12-8). Similarity in dress or speech is common in teenage groups. Popularity is a major concern for teens. Peer groups provide the adolescent with a sense of belonging, approval, and the opportunity to learn acceptable behavior. Popularity with opposite-sex and same-sex peers is important. The strong need for group identity seems to conflict at times with the search for personal identity. It is as though adolescents require close bonds with peers so that they later achieve a sense of individuality.

Family Identity. The movement toward stronger peer relationships is contrasted with adolescents' movements away from parents. Although financial independence for adolescents is not the norm in American society, many adolescents work part-time, using their income to bolster independence. When adolescents cannot have a part-time job because of studies, school-related activities, and other factors, parents can provide allowances for clothing and incidentals, which encourage adolescents to develop decision-making and budgeting skills.

Some adolescents and families have more difficulty during these years than others. Adolescents need to make choices, act independently, and experience the consequences of their actions. This testing, however, is best done within a firm, supportive, family foundation. The family needs to allow independence while providing a safe place for adolescents to contemplate actions. Families unable to provide this support complicate movement toward identity formation. Support for the family and adolescent is essential to their success.

Nurses assist families in considering ways that are appropriate for them to foster the independence of their adolescent while maintaining family structure. Many of these discussions often involve curfews, jobs, and participation in family chores. Emancipation from the immediate family is most successful when accomplished gradually and results in a balance between independence and family ties.

Vocational Identity. The selection of an occupation or a vocational direction in life provides a goal for adolescents. Because of society's changing needs, adolescents must be future oriented when making these choices. However, adolescents do not know which jobs will be available or which jobs will be rewarding 10 or 20 years in the future, so selecting a career is a complicated task. Provide emotional support during this process, and help adolescent clients select courses of action that promote self-satisfaction, identity, and continued opportunity for growth.

Moral Identity. The development of moral judgment depends heavily on cognitive and communication skills and peer interaction. Although moral development begins in early childhood, it is consolidated in adolescence because of the presence of certain skills. Adolescents learn to understand that rules are cooperative agreements that they can modify to fit the situation, rather than absolutes. Regarding rules, adolescents learn to use their own judgment rather than use the rules to avoid punishment as in earlier years. Kohlberg (1964) explains moral development in terms of stages (see Chapter 11). At the highest level, morality comes from individual principles of conscience. Adolescents judge themselves by internalized ideals, which often leads to conflict between personal and group values. Group values become less significant in later adolescence.

Not all adolescents attain the same level of moral development. There is, however, a general forward movement through the stages of moral development, and the sequence of the stages is similar for all individuals even when their time of achievement varies. Kohlberg's moral development (1964) has a focus on justice based on reciprocity and equal respect. Females are more likely to give caring responses to moral problems. Males give more justice-oriented responses.

Health Identity. Another component of personal identity is perception of health. This component is of specific interest to health care providers. Healthy adolescents evaluate their own health according to feelings of well-being, ability to function normally, and absence of symptoms (Hockenberry and Wilson, 2007). They also often include health maintenance and health promotion behaviors as important concerns.

Interventions to improve health perception, therefore, concentrate on the adolescent period. The rapid changes during this period make health promotion programs especially crucial. Adolescents try new roles, begin to stabilize their identity, and acquire values and behaviors from which their adult lifestyle will evolve. They are able to identify behaviors such as smoking and substance abuse as threatening to health in general terms but frequently tend to underestimate the effect of potentially negative consequences of their own actions (Hockenberry and Wilson, 2007).

Health Risks
Accidents. Accidents remain the leading cause of death in adolescence. Motor vehicle accidents, which are the most common cause of death, resulted in 74% of all unintentional deaths among

teens 10 to 19 years (Hockenberry and Wilson, 2007). Such accidents are often associated with alcohol intoxication or drug abuse. Bicycling fatalities were 4 to 7 times more likely to occur in males than females. Other frequent causes of accidental death in teenagers are drowning and firearms. Feelings of being indestructible lead to risk-taking behavior. The use of alcohol precedes many injuries (USDHHS, 2000). Youths continue to be both the victims and perpetrators of violence.

Homicide. Homicide is the second leading cause of death in the 15- to 24-year-old age-group and for African American teenagers it is the most likely cause of death. Individuals 12 years of age and older are most likely to be killed by an acquaintance or gang member and most frequently with a firearm. Firearm homicides accounted for 82% of deaths in individuals 13 through 19 years of age in 2002. Because having a gun in the home raises the risk of homicide and suicide for adolescents, include assessment of gun presence in the home when counseling families (Hockenberry and Wilson, 2007).

Suicide. Suicide is the third leading cause of death in adolescents 13 to 19 years of age, and in a recent study by the National Center for Health Statistics, one fifth of high school students indicated that they had contemplated suicide in the previous 12 months (Santrock, 2007). Depression and social isolation commonly precede a suicide attempt, but suicide probably results from a combination of several factors (Box 12-5).

Be able to identify the factors associated with adolescent suicide risk and precipitating events. In addition, be alert to the following warning signs, which often occur for at least a month before suicide is attempted:

- Decrease in school performance
- Withdrawal
- Loss of initiative
- Loneliness, sadness, and crying
- Appetite and sleep disturbances
- Verbalization of suicidal thought

Make immediate referrals to mental health professionals when assessment suggests that adolescents are considering suicide. Guidance will help them focus on the positive aspects of life and strengthen coping abilities.

Substance Abuse. Substance abuse is a concern for all those who work with adolescents. Adolescents often believe that mood-altering substances create a sense of well-being or improve level of performance. All adolescents are at risk for experimental or recreational substance use, but those who have dysfunctional families are more at risk for chronic use and physical dependency. Some adolescents believe that substance use makes them more mature. They further believe that they will look and feel better with drug usage. Current statistics show that by the end of their high school years, 85% of adolescents have used alcohol, 65% have tried smoking, and 49% have experimented with marijuana (Hockenberry and Wilson, 2007). In recent years there has been an increase in the use of the club drug Ecstasy, a methamphetamine having hallucinogenic properties (Santrock, 2007). Tobacco use continues to be a problem among adolescents and, although its

✳ **BOX 12-5 Suicide Risk Assessment**

History
Previous suicide attempt
Suicide attempt by a family member or friend
History of physical or sexual abuse, or neglect
Past psychiatric hospitalization
Death of a parent when child was young

Individual Factors
Hopelessness
Marked, persistent depression
Alcohol or drug abuse
Impulsiveness
Difficulty tolerating frustration
Feelings of self-hatred or excessive guilt, or of humiliation
Thinking disorder (wishing to join a deceased person, hearing voices telling to kill self)
Physical/body image problems and behavioral and developmental problems (delayed puberty, chronic illness, disability, attention deficit hyperactivity disorder, learning disorders)
Gender identity or sexual orientation concerns; gay, lesbian, bisexual, or transgender in an unsupportive environment
Seeing self as totally helpless, a victim of fate
A need to do things perfectly

Family Factors
Difficult home situation; long, bitter parent-child conflict
Hostile parents
Overt rejection by one or both parents
Divorce or separation of parents
Recent or impending move
Family breakup or parental loss
Exposure to unrealistically high parental expectations
Parental indifference with very low expectations

Social/Environmental Factors
Firearms in the home
Incarceration
Lack of effective social support system
Isolation
Exposure to suicide of another
Few social, vocational, educational opportunities

From Hockenberry MJ, Wilson D: *Wong's nursing care of infants and children*, ed 8, St. Louis, 2007, Mosby.

use is declining, 3 out of 10 adolescents are active smokers upon high school graduation.

Eating Disorders. The number of eating disorders is on the rise in adolescent girls, and knowledge of growth progression is a way to discourage radical weight reduction activities. If an adolescent differs drastically from the usual pattern, further assessment is necessary to identify the cause. Areas to include in the assessment are past and present diet history, food records, eating habits, attitudes, health beliefs, and socioeconomic and psychosocial factors (Hockenberry and Wilson, 2007). Weight extremes resulting from excessive or inadequate caloric intake are common during the adolescent years. Allowing the adolescent to see when and how the weight curve changed is a first step in identifying the problem and implementing dietary changes.

Anorexia nervosa and bulimia are two eating disorders that appear in adolescence. Anorexia nervosa is a clinical syndrome with both physical and psychosocial components that involves the pursuit of thinness through starvation. The majority of clients are adolescents and young women who come from well-educated, middle- and upper-class families and are considered competitive and high achievers (Santrock, 2007). Persons with anorexia nervosa have an intense fear of gaining weight and refuse to maintain body weight at the minimal normal weight for their age and height.

Bulimia nervosa is most identified with binge eating and behaviors to prevent weight gain. Behaviors include self-induced vomiting, misuse of laxatives and other medications, and excessive exercise. Unlike anorexia, bulimia occurs within a normal weight range, and so it is much more difficult to detect. Because adolescents rarely volunteer information about behaviors to prevent weight gain, it is important to take a thorough dietary history. Bulimia is a biopsychosocial illness. Society's expectations for thinness have a strong influence on the development of these eating disorders. If left undetected and untreated, these disorders lead to significant morbidity and mortality (Hockenberry and Wilson, 2007; Santrock, 2007).

Sexual Experimentation. Sexual activity among adolescents has declined over the past decade. According to the Centers for Disease Control and Prevention (2004), 46.7% of adolescents between grades 9 and 12 have admitted to having sexual intercourse at least once. Interest in sexual development and sexual practices are normal aspects of adolescent development, and the majority of adolescents do not engage in sexual activities that pose a risk to development (Santrock, 2007). Two prominent consequences of adolescent sexual activity are sexually transmitted disease and pregnancy (Hockenberry and Wilson, 2007).

Sexually Transmitted Disease. Sexually transmitted disease (STD) annually affects 3 million sexually active adolescents. This high degree of incidence makes it imperative that sexually active adolescents be screened for STDs, even when they have no symptoms. The annual physical examination of a sexually active adolescent includes a thorough sexual history and a careful examination of the genitalia so that condylomata acuminata (genital warts), herpes, *Phthirus pubis* (crab lice), primary syphilitic chancres, and other STDs are not missed. Recommended tests for women include Papanicolaou (Pap) smears, cervical cultures for gonorrhea and *Chlamydia* species, and syphilis tests; for men, urethral cultures for gonorrhea and *Chlamydia* species and syphilis tests are recommended. If men have participated in homosexual activities, take rectal and pharyngeal cultures to check for gonorrhea. Be proactive by using the interview process to identify risk factors in the adolescent and provide education to prevent STDs, including HIV, and unwanted pregnancies (Hockenberry and Wilson, 2007).

Pregnancy. Adolescent pregnancy continues to be a major social challenge for our nation. The United States has the highest rate of teenage pregnancy and childbearing yearly as compared to other industrialized nations (Hockenberry and Wilson, 2007; Santrock, 2007). *Healthy People 2010* set as its objectives: (a) reduce teen pregnancy, (b) decrease infant mortality, and (c) encourage prenatal care (USDHHS, 2000). Adolescent pregnancy

✳ **TABLE 12-5** Health Promotion During the Adolescent Period

ADOLESCENT HEALTH CONCERNS	HEALTH PROMOTION INTERVENTION
Unintentional injuries	Advise adolescent to take driver's education course and to wear seat belts.
	Inform the adolescent of risk associated with drinking and driving, use of drugs.
	Promote helmet use by adolescent bicyclists and motorcyclists.
	Ensure adolescent receives proper orientation to the use of all sports equipment.
	Encourage adolescent to swim with a "buddy."
Firearm use and violence	Teach conflict resolution skills.
Tobacco, alcohol, and drug use	Screen for tobacco (including smokeless), alcohol, and drug use and inform of the risks of use.
Suicide	Offer suicide prevention information.
	Teach methods to deal with a suicidal peer.
	Promote suicide alternatives.
Sexually transmitted diseases	Provide adolescent with information regarding disease, mode of transmission, and related symptoms.
	Encourage abstinence from sexual activity; or if sexually active, the use of condoms.
	Provide accurate information about the consequences of sexual activity.

occurs across socioeconomic classes, in public and private schools, among all ethnic and religious backgrounds, and in all parts of the country. Teenage pregnancy with early prenatal supervision is less harmful to both mother and child than earlier believed. Pregnant teens need special attention to nutrition, as well as health supervision and psychological support. Adolescent mothers also need help in planning for the future and in obtaining competent day care for their infants.

Health Concerns

Health Education.
Community and school-based health programs for adolescents focus on health promotion and illness prevention. Nurses are involved in community health through screening and teaching programs (Table 12-5). Through their efforts in the school and community, nurses make a contribution in meeting the *Healthy People 2010* objectives (USDHHS, 2000). Discussions with adolescents need to be private and confidential. Deering and Cody (2002) found that for adolescents to reveal intimate information about their risk-taking behaviors, they first need to feel comfortable and respected as individuals. Large numbers of school-based clinics have been developed and implemented to respond to adolescents' needs. Adolescents are much more likely to use these health care services if they encounter providers who are caring and respectful (Hockenberry and Wilson, 2007).

Nurses play an important role in preventing injuries and accidental deaths. Injury prevention activities and support of organizations that promote responsible behavior, including Mothers Against Drunk Driving (MADD) and Drug Abuse Resistance Education (DARE), and encouraging students to participate in Students Against Drunk Driving (SADD) are types of important activities. Stimulating adolescents to discuss alternatives to driving when under the influence of drugs or alcohol prepares them to consider alternatives when such an occasion arises. The nurse first identifies those adolescents at risk for abuse, provides education to prevent accidents related to substance abuse, and provides counseling to those in rehabilitation.

Extensive educational efforts to prevent the spread of HIV and other STDs in this age-group are a nursing responsibility. Educa-

tion occurs in the school or community and is formal, informal, one-on-one, or in a group setting. Speakers and organizations help in the educational process.

Rural Adolescents.
Fifty percent of adolescents live in the rural South, 27% live in the rural Midwest, and the remaining adolescents are fairly evenly distributed among the two remaining regions of the United States. Areas of concern for these adolescents include limited access to health care, limited health care insurance, limited privacy, lack of transportation to health care, poverty, and farming accidents.

Nurses play an important role in improving the health of the rural adolescent. Decreasing barriers to care, health promotion education, development of coping strategies, efforts to improve the safety of farming equipment and practices, and assessment of health beliefs are important areas for the nurse to address.

Minority Adolescents.
By the next century estimates predict that minorities as a group will become the majority. African American, Hispanic, Latino, Asian, Native American, and Alaska Native American adolescents are the fastest-growing segment in the U.S. population. Minority adolescents experience a greater percentage of health problems and barriers to health care (Hockenberry and Wilson, 2007).

Issues of concern for these adolescents living in a high-risk environment include learning or emotional difficulties, death related to violence, unintentional injuries, increased rate for adolescent pregnancy, STDs, HIV infection, and acquired immunodeficiency syndrome (AIDS). Poverty is a major factor negatively affecting the lives of minority adolescents. Limited access to health services is common. Nurses are able to make a significant contribution to improving access to appropriate health care for adolescents. Base health promotion initiatives on topics of concern for these adolescents.

Nurses working in the community need to adopt culturally sensitive interventions to meet the needs of minority adolescents and their families (Hockenberry and Wilson, 2007). They need to be able to communicate in another language by speaking it or using an interpreter. Teaching materials need to be written in the

13 | Young to Middle Adult

✳ OBJECTIVES

Mastery of the content in this chapter will enable the student to:

- Discuss developmental theories of young and middle adults.
- List and discuss major life events of young and middle adults and the childbearing family.
- Describe developmental tasks of the young adult, the childbearing family, and the middle adult.
- Discuss the significance of family in the life of the adult.

- Describe normal physical changes in young and middle adulthood and in pregnancy.
- Discuss cognitive and psychosocial changes occurring during the adult years.
- Describe health concerns of the young adult, the childbearing family, and the middle adult.

✳ MEDIA RESOURCES   ✳ KEY TERMS

 Companion CD

- NCLEX®-Style Review Questions
- Audio Glossary
- Interactive Learning Activities
- English/Spanish Glossary

 Website

- NCLEX®-Style Review Questions
- Audio Glossary
- English/Spanish Glossary
- Interactive Learning Activities
- WebLinks
- Audio Summaries

Braxton Hicks contractions, p. 183
Climacteric, p. 186
Doula, p. 179
Infertility, p. 182

Lactation, p. 183
Menopause, p. 186
Prenatal care, p. 183
Puerperium, p. 183
Sandwich generation, p. 187

Young and middle adulthood is a period of challenges, rewards, and crises. Challenges may include the demands of working and raising families, although there are many rewards with these as well. Adults also face crises such as caring for their aging parents, the possibility of job loss in a changing economic environment, and dealing with their own developmental needs as well as those of their family members.

Young adulthood is the period between the late teens and the mid to late 30s (Edelman and Mandle, 2002). In 2005, young adults were approximately 27% of the population (U.S. Census Bureau, 2004). Young adults increasingly move away from their families of origin, establish career goals, and decide whether to marry or remain single and whether to begin families. Young adults adapt to new experiences and newly acquired independence.

Middle age occurs between the mid to late 30s and the mid 60s. The transition into middle age occurs when young persons become aware of changes in reproductive and physical abilities that signify the beginning of another stage in life. This is a time of continuing transitions when individuals reassess their life goals and add new goals. In 2005, 39.3% of the population were middle-age adults between the ages of 35 and 64, a slight increase over the 2000 census (U.S. Department of Commerce, 2000)

Classic works by developmental theorists such as Levinson and others (1978), Diekelmann (1976), Erikson (1963, 1982), and Havighurst (1972) attempted to describe the phases of young and middle adulthood and related developmental tasks (see Chapter 11 for an in-depth discussion of developmental theories). Some proposed that intellectual and moral development differ between men and women. According to Gilligan (1993), women struggle with the issues of care and responsibility, and in turn their relationships progress toward a maturity of interdependence. As women progress toward adulthood, the moral dilemma changes from how to exercise their rights without interfering in the rights of others to "how to lead a moral life," which includes obligations to themselves and their families and people in general (Gilligan, 1993).

Traditional masculine roles include providing and protecting. Recently, however, men have been moving into greater disequilibrium. Faced with a societal structure that differs greatly from the norms of 20 or 30 years ago, both men and women are assuming different roles in today's society. Men were traditionally the primary supporter of the family. Today, many women pursue careers and contribute significantly to their families' incomes. In 2004, women constituted 47% of all U.S. workers in the U.S. labor force (Women Employed Institute, 2004). The percentage of working women age 55 years and over also increased from 25.6% in 1999 to 30.5% in 2004 (U.S. Department of Labor, Women's Bureau, 2006). However, according to the American Federation of Labor and Congress of Industrial Organizations (AFL-CIO) (2004) workers' union, women in the United States are paid 76 cents for every dollar men receive for comparable work.

Developmental theories provide nurses with a basis for understanding the life events and developmental tasks of the young and middle adult. Clients present challenges to nurses who themselves are often young or middle adults coping with the demands of their respective developmental period. Nurses need to recognize the needs of their clients even if they are not experiencing the same challenges and events.

Young Adult

Physical Changes

The young adult usually completes physical growth by the age of 20. An exception to this is the pregnant or lactating woman. The physical, cognitive, and psychosocial changes and the health concerns of the pregnant woman and the childbearing family are extensive.

Young adults are usually quite active, experience severe illnesses less commonly than older age-groups, tend to ignore physical symptoms, and often postpone seeking health care. Physical characteristics of young adults begin to change as middle age approaches. Unless clients have illnesses, assessment findings are generally within normal limits.

Cognitive Changes

Critical thinking habits increase steadily through the young and middle adult years. Formal and informal educational experiences, general life experiences, and occupational opportunities dramatically increase the individual's conceptual, problem solving, and motor skills.

Identifying an occupational direction is a major task of young adults. When people know their skills, talents, and personality characteristics, educational preparation and occupational choices are easier and more satisfying. According to the U.S. Department of Labor (2005), a bachelor's or associate's degree is the most significant source of postsecondary education for 12 of the 20 fastest-growing occupations. Many young adults, however, either lack the necessary resources or support systems to facilitate further education or the development of skills necessary for many positions in the workplace. As a result, some young adults have limited occupational choices.

An understanding of how adults learn assists the nurse in developing client education plans (see Chapter 25). Adults enter the teaching-learning situation with a background of unique life experiences, including illness. Therefore, always view adults as individuals. Their adherence to regimens such as medications, treatments, or lifestyle changes such as smoking cessation involves decision-making processes. When determining the amount of information that an individual needs to make decisions about the prescribed course of therapy, consider factors that possibly affect the individual's adherence to the regimen, including educational level, socioeconomic factors, and motivation and desire to learn.

Because young adults are continually evolving and adjusting to changes in the home, workplace, and personal lives, their decision-making processes need to be flexible. The more secure young adults are in their roles, the more flexible and open they are to change. Insecure persons tend to be more rigid in making decisions.

Psychosocial Changes

The emotional health of the young adult is related to the individual's ability to address and resolve personal and social tasks. The young adult is usually caught between wanting to prolong the irresponsibility of adolescence and wanting to assume adult commitments. Certain patterns or trends, however, are relatively predictable. Between the ages of 23 and 28, the person refines self-perception and ability for intimacy. From 29 to 34 the person directs enormous energy toward achievement and mastery of the surrounding world. The years from 35 to 43 are a time of vigorous examination of life goals and relationships. People make changes in personal, social, and occupational areas. Often the stresses of this reexamination results in a "midlife crisis" in which marital partner, lifestyle, and occupation change.

Ethnic and gender factors have a sociological and psychological influence in an adult's life, and these factors pose a distinct challenge for nursing care. Each person holds culture-bound definitions of health and illness. Nurses and other health professionals bring with them distinct practices for the prevention and treatment of illness. Knowing too little about a client's self-perception or beliefs regarding health and illness create conflict between the nurse and the client. Changes in the traditional role expectations of both men and women in young and middle adulthood also lead to greater challenges for nursing care. For example, women often continue to work during the child-rearing years, and many women struggle with the enormity of balancing three careers: wife, mother, and employee. This is a potential source of stress for the adult working woman. Men are more aware of parental and household responsibilities and find themselves having more responsibilities at home while achieving their own career goals (Fortinash and Holoday Worret, 2004). An understanding of ethnicity, race, and gender differences enables the nurse to provide individualized care (see Chapter 9).

Support from the nurse, access to information, and appropriate referrals provide opportunities for achievement of a client's potential. Health is not merely the absence of disease but involves wellness in all human dimensions. The nurse acknowledges the importance of the young adult's psychosocial needs and needs in all other dimensions. The young adult needs to make decisions concerning career, marriage, and parenthood. Although each person makes these decisions based on individual factors, the nurse needs to understand the general principles involved in these aspects of psychosocial development while assessing the young adult's psychosocial status.

Lifestyle. Family history of cardiovascular, renal, endocrine, or neoplastic disease increases a young adult's risk of illness. The nurse's role in health promotion is to identify modifiable factors that increase the young adult's risk for health problems and to provide client education and support to reduce unhealthy lifestyle behaviors (Fager and Melnyk, 2004).

A personal lifestyle assessment (see Chapter 6) helps nurses and clients identify habits that increase the risk for cardiac, malignant, pulmonary, renal, or other chronic diseases. A personal lifestyle assessment of the young adult includes assessment of general life satisfaction, hobbies, and interests; habits such as diet, sleeping, exercise, sexual habits, and use of caffeine, tobacco, alcohol, and illicit drugs; home conditions and pets; economics, including type of health insurance; occupational environment, including type of work and exposure to hazardous substances; and physical or mental stress. Military records, including dates and geographical area of assignments, may also be useful in assessing the young adult for risk factors. Prolonged stress from lifestyle choices increases wear and tear on the body's adaptive capacities. Stress-related diseases such as ulcers, emotional disorders, and infections sometimes occur (see Chapter 31).

Career. A successful vocational adjustment is important in the lives of most men and women. Successful employment not only ensures economic security, but also leads to friendships, social activities, support, and respect from co-workers.

Two-career families are increasing. The two-career family has benefits and liabilities. In addition to increasing the family's financial base, the person who works outside the home is able to expand friendships, activities, and interests. However, there is stress in a two-career family as well. These stressors result from a transfer to a new city; increased expenditures of physical, mental, or emotional energy; child care demands; or household needs. To avoid stress in a two-career family, partners should share all responsibilities. For some families a solution is to limit recreational expenses and instead hire someone to do routine housework. Others set up an equal division of household, shopping, and cooking duties.

Sexuality. The development of secondary sexual characteristics occurs during the adolescent years (see Chapter 12). Physical development is accompanied by the ability to perform sexual acts. The young adult usually has emotional maturity to complement the physical ability and is therefore able to develop mature sexual relationships and establish intimacy. Young adults who have failed to achieve the developmental task of personal integration sometimes develop relationships that are superficial and stereotyped (Fortinash and Holoday Worret, 2004).

Masters and Johnson (1970) contributed important information about the physiological characteristics of the adult sexual response (see Chapter 28). The psychodynamic aspect of sexual activity is as important as the type or frequency of sexual intercourse to young adults. To maintain total wellness, encourage adults to explore various aspects of their sexuality and be aware that their sexual needs and concerns change. As the rate of early initiation of sexual intercourse continues to increase, young adults are at risk for sexually transmitted diseases. Consequently, there is an increased need for education regarding the mode of transmission, prevention, and symptom recognition and management for sexually transmitted diseases.

Childbearing Cycle. Conception, pregnancy, birth, and the puerperium are major phases of the childbearing cycle. The changes during these phases are complex. Education such as Lamaze classes can prepare pregnant women, their partners, and other support persons to participate in the birthing process (Figure 13-1). A current trend in some health care agencies is to provide either professional labor support (Sauls, 2006) or a lay **doula,** a support person to be present during labor to assist women who have no other source of support (Campbell and others, 2006). Stress that many women experience after childbirth has a significant impact on postpartum women's health (Box 13-1).

Types of Families. During young adulthood most individuals experience singlehood and the opportunity to be on their own. Those who eventually marry encounter several changes as they take on new responsibilities. For example, many married couples choose to become parents (Figure 13-2). There are also young adults who choose alternative lifestyles. Chapter 10 reviews forms of families.

Singlehood. Social pressure to get married is not as great as it once was, and many young adults do not marry until their late 20s

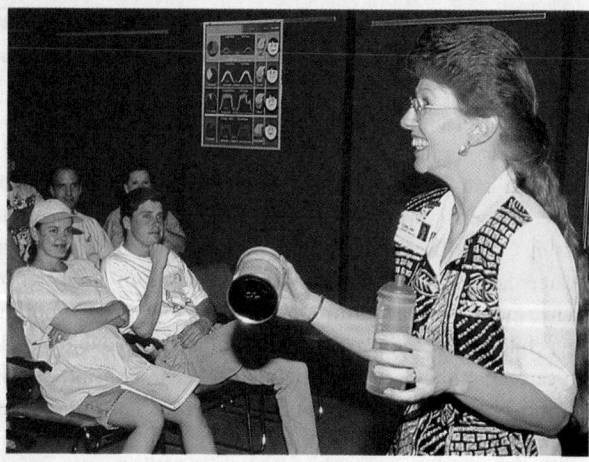

Figure 13-1 Nurse providing Lamaze class for expectant young adults.

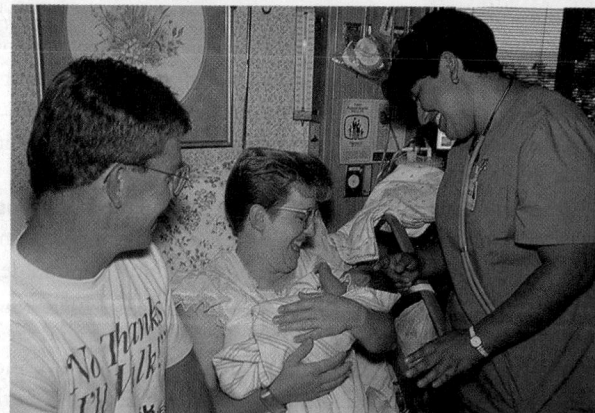

Figure 13-2 Parent-child nurturing is important in adapting to a newborn. (Modified from Stanhope M, Lancaster J: *Community and public health nursing*, ed 5, St. Louis, 2001, Mosby.)

✳ BOX 13-1   EVIDENCE-BASED PRACTICE

Predictors of Postpartum Women's Health Status

Evidence Summary

A woman often experiences dramatic physical and psychosocial changes during the postpartum period that impact health. This research study tried to determine the effects of postpartum stress, depression, and social support on the health of Taiwanese women during their postpartum period. Postpartum stress and depression had significant effects on women's health. In addition, a lack of social support affected women's health adversely.

Application to Nursing Practice

- Assess for potential postpartum stressors, such as fatigue, first-time mother, previous postpartum stress, or feeling of social isolation.
- Identify sources of social support for new mothers after they are discharged from the hospital with their babies, such as new mother visits, young mother groups, and mom's day out activities.
- Create culturally appropriate, primary prevention strategies for stressors that new mothers encounter.
- Educate new mothers and their families on the signs and symptoms of postpartum stress and depression.
- Provide new mothers with information on health care and community resources for use during the postpartum period.

Reference

Hung C: Predictors of postpartum women's health status, *J Nurs Scholarsh* 36(4):345, 2004.

---

or early 30s, or not at all. For young adults who remain single, parents and siblings become the nucleus for a family. Some view close friends and associates as "family." One cause for the increased single population is the expanding career opportunities for women. Women enter the job market with greater career potential and have greater opportunities for financial independence. More single individuals are choosing to live together outside of marriage, as well as to become parents either biologically or through adoption.

Similarly, many married couples choose to separate or divorce if they find their marital situation unsatisfactory.

Parenthood. The availability of contraception makes it easier for today's couples to decide when and if to start a family. One factor influencing this decision is the reason for wanting a child. Social pressures may encourage a couple to have a child or influence them to limit the number of children they have. Economic considerations frequently enter into the decision-making process because having and bringing up children are expensive. General health status and age are also considerations in decisions about parenthood because couples are getting married later and are postponing pregnancies.

Alternative Family Structures and Parenting. Changing norms and values about family life in the United States reveal basic shifts in attitudes in our society. The trend toward greater acceptance of cohabitation without marriage is a factor in the greater numbers of infants being born to unmarried women. Also, approximately 1.5 million parents are gay or lesbian, and up to one third of lesbians are mothers. Many times parents from alternative family structures feel a lack of support and even bias from the health care system (McManus and others, 2006). In recognizing the needs of gay and lesbian parents and their children, the American Academy of Pediatrics (2002) published a policy statement supporting adoption of children and the parenting role by same-sex parents.

Hallmarks of Emotional Health. Most young adults have the physical and emotional resources and support systems to meet the many challenges, tasks, and responsibilities they face. During psychosocial assessment of young adults, assess for 10 hallmarks of emotional health (Box 13-2) that indicate successful maturation in this developmental stage.

Health Risks

Risk Factors. Health risk factors for a young adult originate in the community, lifestyle patterns, and family history. Those lifestyle habits that activate the stress response (see Chapter 31) in-

---

✳ **BOX 13-2 Ten Hallmarks of Emotional Health**

- A sense of meaning and direction in life
- Successful negotiation through transitions
- Absence of feelings of being cheated or disappointed by life
- Attainment of several long-term goals
- Satisfaction with personal growth and development
- When married, feelings of mutual love for partner; when single, satisfaction with social interactions
- Satisfaction with friendships
- Generally cheerful attitude
- No sensitivity to criticism
- No unrealistic fears

---

crease the risk of illness. Smoking is a well-documented risk factor for pulmonary, cardiac, and vascular diseases in smokers and the individuals who receive secondhand smoke. Inhaled cigarette pollutants increase the risk of lung cancer, emphysema, and chronic bronchitis. The nicotine in tobacco is a vasoconstrictor that acts on the coronary arteries, increasing the risk of angina, myocardial infarction, and coronary artery disease. Nicotine also causes peripheral vasoconstriction and leads to vascular problems.

Family History. A family history of a disease puts a young adult at risk for developing it in the middle or older adult years. For example, a young man whose father and paternal grandfather had myocardial infarctions (heart attacks) in their 50s has a risk for a future myocardial infarction. The presence of certain chronic illnesses in the family increases the family member's risk of developing a disease. This family risk is distinct from hereditary disease.

Personal Hygiene Habits. As in all age-groups, personal hygiene habits in the young adult are risk factors. Sharing eating utensils with a person who has a contagious illness increases the risk of illness. Poor dental hygiene increases the risk of periodontal disease. Individuals avoid gingivitis (inflammation of the gums) and periodontitis (loss of tooth support) through oral hygiene (see Chapter 39).

Violent Death and Injury. Violence is the greatest cause of mortality and morbidity in the young adult population. Factors that predispose individuals to violence, injury, or death include poverty, family breakdown, child abuse and neglect, repeated exposure to violence, and ready access to guns. It is important for you to perform a thorough psychosocial assessment, including such factors as behavior patterns, history of physical abuse and substance abuse, education, work history, and social support systems, to detect personal and environmental risk factors for violence. Death and injury occurs from physical assaults, motor vehicle or other accidents, and suicide attempts. In 2002, the death rate (per 100,000 population) for 25- to 34-year-olds in the United States due to homicide was 11.2; the death rate due to accidents was 31.5; and the death rate due to suicide was 12.6 (U.S. Department of Health and Human Services [USDHHS], 2005b).

Substance Abuse. Substance abuse directly or indirectly contributes to mortality and morbidity in young adults. Intoxicated young adults are often severely injured in motor vehicle accidents, resulting in death or permanent disability to other young adults as well.

Dependence on stimulant or depressant drugs sometimes results in death. Overdose of a stimulant drug ("upper") stresses the cardiovascular and nervous systems to the extent that death occurs. The use of depressants ("downers") leads to an accidental or intentional overdose and death.

Caffeine is a naturally occurring legal stimulant that is readily available in carbonated beverages, chocolate-containing foods, coffee and tea, and over-the-counter medications, such as cold tablets, allergy and analgesic preparations, and appetite suppressants. It is the most widely ingested stimulant in North America. Caffeine stimulates catecholamine release, which, in turn, stimulates the central nervous system; it also increases gastric acid secretion, heart rate, and basal metabolic rate. This alters blood pressure, increases diuresis, and relaxes smooth muscle. Consumption of large amounts of caffeine results in restlessness, anxiety, irritability, agitation, muscle tremor, sensory disturbances, heart palpitations, nausea or vomiting, and diarrhea in some individuals.

Substance abuse is not always diagnosable, particularly in its early stages. Nonjudgmental questions about use of legal drugs (prescribed drugs, tobacco, and alcohol), use of soft drugs (marijuana), and use of more problematic drugs (cocaine or heroin) are a routine part of any health assessment. You obtain important information by making specific inquiries about past medical problems, changes in food intake or sleep patterns, or problems of emotional lability. Reports of arrests because of driving while intoxicated, wife or child abuse, or disorderly conduct are reasons for you to investigate the possibility of drug abuse more carefully.

Unplanned Pregnancies. Unplanned pregnancies are a continued source of stress that can result in adverse health outcomes for the mother, infant, and family. Often young adults have educational and career goals that take precedence over family development. Interference with these goals affects future relationships and parent-child relationships.

Determination of situational factors that affect the progress and outcome of an unplanned pregnancy is important. Exploration of problems such as financial, career, and living accommodations; family support systems; potential parenting disorders; depression; and coping mechanisms is important in assessing the woman with an unplanned pregnancy.

Sexually Transmitted Diseases. Sexually transmitted diseases (STDs) are a major health problem in young adults. Examples of STDs include syphilis, chlamydia, gonorrhea, genital herpes, and acquired immunodeficiency syndrome (AIDS). Sexually transmitted diseases have immediate physical effects such as genital discharge, discomfort, and infection. They also lead to chronic disorders, infertility, or even death. Sexually transmitted diseases remain a major public health problem for sexually active persons, with almost half of all new infections occurring in men and women younger than 24 years of age (USDHHS, Centers for Disease Control and Prevention [CDC], 2004).

Environmental or Occupational Factors. A common environmental or occupational risk factor is exposure to work-related hazards or agents that cause diseases and cancer (Table

✳ **TABLE 13-1 Occupational Hazards/Exposures Associated With Diseases and Cancers**

Job Category	Occupational Hazard/Exposure	Work-Related Condition/Cancer
Agricultural workers	Pesticides, infectious agents, gases, sunlight	Pesticide poisoning, "farmer's lung," skin cancer
Anesthetists	Anesthetic gases	Reproductive effects, cancer
Automobile workers	Asbestos, plastics, lead, solvents	Asbestosis, dermatitis
Carpenters	Wood dust, wood preservatives, adhesives	Nasopharyngeal cancer, dermatitis
Cement workers	Cement dust, metals	Dermatitis, bronchitis
Dry cleaners	Solvents	Liver disease, dermatitis
Dye workers	Dyestuffs, metals, solvents	Bladder cancer, dermatitis
Glass workers	Heat, solvents, metal powders	Cataracts
Hospital workers	Infectious agents, cleansers, latex gloves, radiation	Infections, latex allergies, unintentional injuries
Insulators	Asbestos, fibrous glass	Asbestosis, lung cancer, mesothelioma
Jackhammer operators	Vibration	Raynaud's phenomenon
Lathe operators	Metal dusts, cutting oils	Lung disease, cancer
Office computer workers	Repetitive wrist motion on computers and eyestrain	Tendonitis, carpal tunnel syndrome, tenosynovitis

From Stanhope M, Lancaster J: *Community and public health nursing,* ed 6, St. Louis, 2004, Mosby.

13-1). Such lung diseases include silicosis from inhalation of talcum and silicon dust and emphysema from inhalation of smoke. Cancers resulting from occupational exposures may involve the lung, liver, brain, blood, or skin. Questions regarding occupational exposure to hazardous materials should be a routine part of the nurse's assessment.

Health Concerns

Health Promotion. Young adults are generally active and have a minimum of major health problems. However, their lifestyles (e.g., use of tobacco or alcohol) put them at risk for illnesses or disabilities during their middle or older adult years. Young adults are also genetically susceptible to certain chronic diseases such as diabetes mellitus and familial hypercholesterolemia (Huether and McCance, 2004). Crohn's disease, a chronic inflammatory disease of the small intestine, most commonly occurs between 15 and 35 years of age. Many young adults have misconceptions regarding transmission and treatment of STDs. Encourage partners to know one another's sexual history and sexual practices. Be alert for STDs when clients come to clinics with complaints of urological or gynecological problems (see Chapter 33). Assess young adults for knowledge and use of safe-sex practices and genital self-examinations. Provide information on safe sex practices, for example, use of condoms and having only one sex partner.

Infertility. The term **infertility** refers to a prolonged time to conceive. An estimated 10% to 15% of reproductive couples are infertile, and many are young adults. However, about half of the couples evaluated and treated in infertility clinics become pregnant. In about 15% of infertile couples the cause is unknown. Female factors such as ovulatory dysfunction or a pelvic factor is responsible for infertility in 50% of couples, and infertility in 35% of couples is due to a male factor such as sperm and semen abnormalities. For some infertile couples the nurse is the first resource they identify. Nursing assessment of the infertile couple includes comprehensive histories of both the male and female partners to determine factors that have affected fertility as well as pertinent physical findings (Lowdermilk and Perry, 2003).

Exercise. Exercise in young adulthood is increasingly important to prevent or decrease the development of chronic health conditions such as high blood pressure, obesity, and diabetes that develop later in life. Exercise improves cardiopulmonary function by decreasing blood pressure and heart rate; increases the strength and size of muscles; and decreases fatigability, insomnia, tension, and irritability. Conduct a thorough musculoskeletal assessment and exercise history to develop a realistic exercise plan. Encourage regular exercise within the client's daily schedule.

Routine Health Screening. Many of the diseases that appear in later years are avoidable if identified early. Encourage young adults to perform monthly skin, breast, or male genital self-examination (see Chapter 33). Breast cancer is the most common major cancer among women in the United States with a steadily increasing incidence. The nurse's role is extremely important in educating female clients about breast self-examination (BSE) and the current breast screening recommendations. Encourage routine assessment of the skin for recent changes in color or presence of lesions and changes in their appearance. Prolonged exposure to ultraviolet rays of the sun by adolescents and young adults increase the risk for development of skin cancer later in life.

Psychosocial Health. The psychosocial health concerns of the young adult are often related to job and family stressors. As noted in Chapter 31, stress is valuable because it motivates a client to change. However, if the stress is prolonged and the client is unable to adapt to the stressor, health problems will develop.

Job Stress. Job stress occurs every day or from time to time. Most young adults are able to handle day-to-day crises (Figure 13-3). Situational job stress occurs when a new boss enters the workplace, a deadline is approaching, or the worker has new or greater numbers of responsibilities. A recent trend in today's business world and risk factor for job stress is corporate downsizing, leading to increased responsibilities for employees with fewer positions within the corporate structure. Job stress also occurs when a person becomes dissatisfied with a job or the associated responsibilities. Because individuals

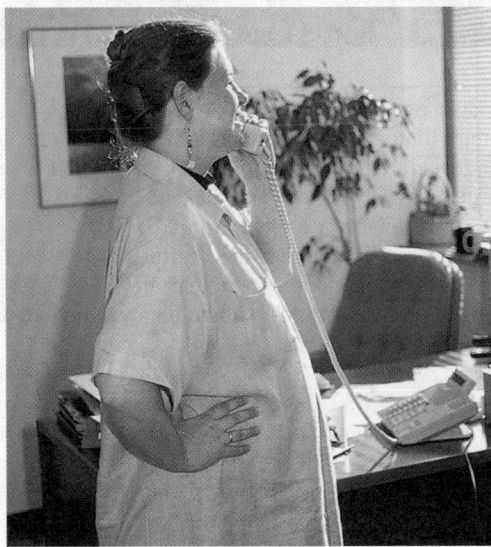

Figure 13-3 The ability to handle day-to-day challenges at work minimizes stress.

perceive jobs differently, the types of job stressors vary from client to client. The nurse's assessment of the young adult includes a description of the usual work performed and present work if different. Job assessment also includes conditions and hours, duration of employment, changes in sleep or eating habits, and evidence of increased irritability or nervousness.

Family Stress. Because of the multiplicity of changing relationships and structures in the emerging young adult family, stress is frequently high (see Chapter 10). Situational stressors occur during events such as births, deaths, illnesses, marriages, and job losses. Stress is often related to a number of variables, including the career paths of both husband and wife, and leads to dysfunction in the young adult family. This is reflected in the fact that the highest divorce rate occurs during the first 3 to 5 years of marriage for young adults under the age of 30. When a client seeks health care and presents stress-related symptoms, you need to assess for the occurrence of a life change event.

Each family has certain predictable roles or jobs for members. These roles enable the family to function and be an effective part of society. When these roles change as a result of illness, a situational crisis often occurs. Assess environmental and familial factors, including support systems and coping mechanisms commonly used by family members.

Pregnant Woman and Childbearing Family. A developmental task for most young adult couples is the decision to begin a family. Although the physiological changes of pregnancy and childbirth occur only in the woman, cognitive and psychosocial changes and health concerns affect the entire childbearing family, including the baby's father, siblings, and grandparents. Single-parent families and young single mothers tend to be particularly vulnerable both economically and socially.

Health Practices. Women who are anticipating pregnancy benefit from good health practices before conception; these include a balanced diet, exercise, dental checkups, avoidance of alcohol, and cessation of smoking.

Prenatal Care. Prenatal care is the routine examination of the pregnant woman by an obstetrician, nurse practitioner, or certified nurse-midwife. Prenatal care includes a thorough physical assessment of the pregnant woman during regularly scheduled intervals; provision of information regarding STDs and other vaginal infections, and urinary infections that will adversely affect the fetus; and counseling about exercise patterns, diet, and child care. Regular prenatal care addresses health concerns that may arise during the pregnancy.

Physiological Changes. The physiological changes and needs of the pregnant woman vary with each trimester. Be familiar with these physiological changes, their causes, and implications for nursing. All women experience some physiological changes in the first trimester. For example, women commonly have morning sickness, breast enlargement and tenderness and fatigue. During the second trimester, growth of the uterus and fetus results in some of the physical signs of pregnancy. During the third trimester increases in **Braxton Hicks contractions** (irregular, short contractions), fatigue, and urinary frequency occur.

Puerperium. The **puerperium** is a period of approximately 6 weeks after delivery. During this time the woman's body reverts to its prepregnant physical status. Determine the woman's knowledge of and ability to care for both herself and for her newborn baby. Assessment of parenting skills and maternal-infant interactions is particularly important. The process of **lactation** or breast-feeding offers many advantages to both the new mother and baby. For the inexperienced mother, breast-feeding can be a source of anxiety and frustration. Be alert for signs that the mother needs information and assistance (Dunn and others, 2006).

Needs for Education. The entire childbearing family needs education about pregnancy, labor, delivery, breast-feeding, and integration of the newborn into the family structure.

Psychosocial Changes. Like the physiological changes of pregnancy, psychosocial changes occur at various times during the 9 months of pregnancy and in the puerperium. Table 13-2 summarizes the major categories of psychosocial changes and implications for nursing intervention.

Health Concerns. The pregnant woman and her partner have many health questions. For example, they wonder whether the pregnancy and baby will be normal. The majority of the health needs related to pregnancy are met with proper prenatal care.

Acute Care. Young adults typically require acute care for accidents, substance abuse, exposure to environmental and occupational hazards, stress-related illnesses, respiratory infections, gastroenteritis, influenza, urinary tract infections, and minor surgery. An acute minor illness causes a disruption in life activities of the young adult and increases stress in an already hectic lifestyle. Dependency and limitations posed by treatment regimens also increase frustration for the young adult. To give young adults a sense of maintaining control of their health care choices, it is important to keep them informed about their health status and involve them in health care decisions.

Restorative and Continuing Care. Chronic conditions are not common in young adulthood, but they sometimes occur. Chronic illnesses such as hypertension, coronary artery disease, and diabetes have their onset in young adulthood without being known

✳ TABLE 13-2 Major Psychosocial Changes During Pregnancy

CATEGORY	IMPLICATIONS FOR NURSING
Body image	Morning sickness and fatigue contribute to poor body image.
	Client feels big, awkward, and unattractive during third trimester when fetus is growing more rapidly.
	Increase in breast size sometimes make the woman feel more feminine and sexually appealing.
	Client takes extra time with hygiene and grooming, trying new hairstyles and makeup.
	Begins to "show" during the second trimester and starts to plan maternity wardrobe.
	General feeling of well-being when woman feels the baby move and hears the heartbeat.
Role changes	Both partners think about and have feelings of uncertainty about impending role changes.
	Clients have feelings of ambivalence about becoming parents and concern about ability to be parents.
Sexuality	Needs reassurance that sexual activity will not harm fetus.
	Desire for sexual activity influenced by body image.
	Desires cuddling and holding rather than sexual intercourse.
Coping mechanisms	Needs reassurance that childbirth and child rearing are natural and positive experiences but are also stressful.
	Often unable to cope with particular stressors such as finding new housing, preparing the nursery, or participating in childbirth classes.
Stresses during puerperium	Returns home from hospital fatigued and unfamiliar with infant care.
	Experiences physical discomfort or feelings of anxiety or depression.
	Necessary for woman to return to work soon after delivery with subsequent feelings of guilt, anxiety, or, possibly, sense of freedom or relief.

to the young adult until later in life. Causes of chronic illness and disability in the young adult include accidents, multiple sclerosis, rheumatoid arthritis, AIDS, and cancer. Chronic illness or disability threatens a young adult's independence and results in the need to change personal, family, and career goals. Nursing interventions for the young adult faced with chronic illness or disability need to focus on problems related to sense of identity, the establishment of independence, reorganization of intimate relationships and family structure, and launching of a chosen career (Santacroce and Lee, 2006).

Middle Adult

In middle adulthood the individual makes lasting contributions through involvement with others. Generally the middle adult years begin around the early to mid 30s and last through the late 60s, corresponding to Levinson's developmental phases of "settling down" and the "payoff years." During this period, personal and career achievements have often already been experienced. Many middle adults find particular joy in assisting their children and other young people in becoming productive and responsible adults (Figure 13-4). They also begin to help aging parents while being responsible for their own children, placing them in the "sandwich generation." Using leisure time in satisfying and creative ways is a challenge that, if met satisfactorily, enables middle adults to prepare for retirement.

Although most middle adults have achieved socioeconomic stability, recent trends in corporate downsizing have left many middle adults either jobless or forced to accept lower-paying jobs. As a result, a greater proportion of the population is currently unable to afford adequate health insurance coverage. Between 2004 and 2005, the number of people in the United States without health insurance coverage increased from 15.6% to 15.9%, and the num-

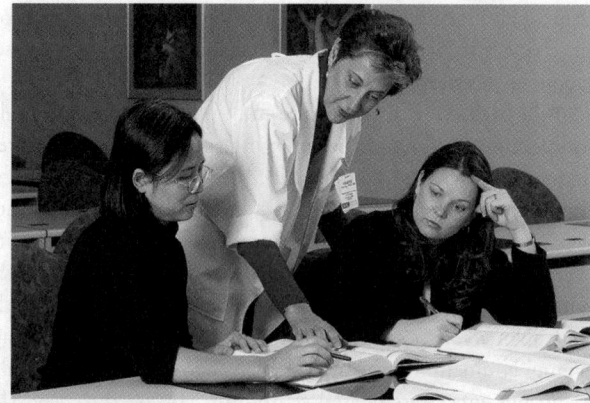

Figure 13-4 Middle adults enjoy assisting young people in becoming productive and responsible adults.

ber of people covered by employment-based health insurance declined from 59.8% to 59.5% (U.S. Census Bureau, 2006).

Men and women need to adjust to inevitable biological changes. As in adolescence, middle adults use considerable energy to adapt self-concept and body image to physiological realities and changes in physical appearance. High self-esteem, a favorable body image, and a positive attitude toward physiological changes occur when adults engage in physical exercise, balanced diets, adequate sleep, and good hygiene practices that promote vigorous, healthy bodies.

Physical Changes

Major physiological changes occur between 40 and 65 years of age. Because of this it is important to assess the middle adult's general health status. A comprehensive assessment offers direction for

✳ **TABLE 13-3   Abnormal Physical Assessment Findings in the Middle Adult**

BODY SYSTEM	ASSESSMENT FINDINGS
Integument	Very thin skin
	Rough, flaky, dry skin
	Lesions
Scalp and hair	Excessive generalized hair loss or patchy hair loss
	Excessive scaliness
Head and neck	Large, thick skull and facial bones
	Asymmetry in movement of head and/or neck
	Drooping of one side of the face
Eyes	Reduced peripheral vision
	Asymmetric position of the light reflex
	Drooping of the upper lid (ptosis)
	Redness or crusting around the eyelids
Ears	Discharge of any kind
	Reddened, swollen ear canals
Nose, sinuses, and throat	Nasal tenderness
	Occlusion of nostril
	Swollen and pale pink or bluish gray nasal mucosa
	Sinuses tender to palpation or upon percussion
	Asymmetric movement or loss of movement of uvula
	Tonsils red or enlarged
Thorax and lungs	Unequal chest expansion
	Unequal fremitus, hyperresonance, diminished or absent breath sounds
	Adventitious lung sounds such as crackles and wheezes
Heart and vascular system	Pulse inequality, weak pulses, bounding pulses, or variations in strength of pulse from beat to beat
	Bradycardia or tachycardia
	Hypertension
	Hypotension
Breasts—female	Recent increase in size of one breast
	Pigskin-like or orange-peel appearance
	Redness or painful breasts
Breasts—male	Soft, fatty enlargement of breast tissue
Abdomen	Bruises, areas of local discoloration, purple discoloration, or pale, taut skin
	Generalized abdominal distention
	Hypoactive, hyperactive, decreased, or absent bowel sounds
Female genitalia	Asymmetric labia
	Swelling, pain, or discharge from Bartholin's glands
	Decreased tone of vaginal musculature
	Cervical enlargement or projection into the vagina
	Reddened areas or lesions in the vagina
Male genitalia	Rashes, lesions, or lumps on skin of shaft of penis
	Discharge from penis
	Enlarged scrotal sac
	Bulges that appear at the external inguinal ring or at the femoral canal when the client bears down
Musculoskeletal system	Uneven weight bearing
	Decreased range of joint motion; swollen, red, or enlarged joint; painful joints
	Decreased strength against resistance
Neurological system	Lethargy
	Inadequate motor responses
	Abnormal sensory system responses: inability to smell certain aromas, loss of visual fields, inability to feel and correctly identify facial stimuli, absent gag reflex

health promotion recommendations, as well as planning and implementing any acutely needed interventions. Table 13-3 summarizes developmental changes to consider when conducting a physical examination (see Chapter 33). The most visible changes are graying of the hair, wrinkling of the skin, and thickening of the

waist. Decreases in hearing and visual acuity are often evident during this period. Often these physiological changes during middle adulthood have an impact on self-concept and body image. The most significant physiological changes during middle age are menopause in women and the climacteric in men.

Perimenopause and Menopause. Menstruation and ovulation occur in a cyclical rhythm in women from adolescence into middle adulthood. Perimenopause is the period during which ovarian function declines, resulting in a diminishing number of ova and irregular menstrual cycles. **Menopause** is the disruption of this cycle, primarily because of the inability of the neurohormonal system to maintain its periodic stimulation of the endocrine system. The ovaries no longer produce estrogen and progesterone, and the blood levels of these hormones drop markedly. Menopause typically occurs between 45 and 60 years of age (see Chapter 28). Approximately 10% of women have no symptoms of menopause other than cessation of menstruation, 70% to 80% are aware of other changes but have no problems, and approximately 10% experience changes severe enough to interfere with activities of daily living.

Climacteric. The **climacteric** occurs in men in their late 40s or early 50s (see Chapter 28). Decreased levels of androgens cause climacteric. Throughout this period and thereafter, a man is still capable of producing fertile sperm and fathering a child. However, penile erection is less firm, ejaculation is less frequent, and the refractory period is longer.

Cognitive Changes

Changes in the cognitive function of middle adults are rare except with illness or trauma. Some middle adults enter educational or vocational programs to prepare themselves with new skills and information for entering the job market or changing jobs.

Psychosocial Changes

The psychosocial changes in the middle adult involves expected events, such as children moving away from home, as well as unexpected events, such as a marital separation or the death of a close friend.

As the nurse, assess major life changes occurring in any middle adult you care for. Also consider the impact that the changes have on that person's state of health. Also include individual psychosocial factors such as coping mechanisms and sources of social support in the assessment.

In the middle adult years, as children depart from the household, the family enters the postparental family stage. Time and financial demands on the parents decrease, and the couple faces the task of redefining their own relationship. As grandchildren arrive, individuals choose grandparenting styles. It is during this period that many middle adults take on healthier lifestyles. Assessment of health promotion needs for the middle adult include adequate rest, leisure activities, regular exercise, good nutrition, reduction or cessation in the use of tobacco or alcohol, and regular screening examinations. Assessment of the middle adult's social environment is also important, including relationship concerns; communication and relationships with children, grandchildren, and aging parents; and caregiver concerns with their own aging or disabled parents.

Career Transition. Career changes occur by choice or as a result of changes in the workplace or society. In recent decades, middle adults more often change occupations for a variety of reasons, including limited upward mobility, decreasing availability of jobs, and seeking an occupation that is more challenging to the individual. In some cases downsizing, technological advances, or other changes force middle adults to seek new jobs. Such changes, particularly when unanticipated, result in stress that affects health, family relationships, self-concept, and other dimensions.

Sexuality. After the departure of their last child from the home, many couples recultivate their relationships and find increased marital and sexual satisfaction during middle age. The onset of menopause and the climacteric affect the sexual health of the middle adult. Some women may desire increased sexual activity because pregnancy is no longer possible. Menopausal women also experience vaginal dryness and dyspareunia or pain during sexual intercourse (see Chapter 28).

During middle age a man may notice changes in the strength of his erection and a decrease in his ability to experience repeated orgasm. Other factors influencing sexuality during this period include work stress, diminished health of one or both partners, and the use of prescription medications. For example, antihypertensive agents have side effects that influence sexual desire or functioning. Sometimes both partners experience stresses related to sexual changes or a conflict between their sexual needs and self-perceptions and social attitudes or expectations (see Chapter 28).

Family Psychosocial Factors. Psychosocial factors involving the family include the stresses of singlehood, marital changes, transition of the family as children leave home, and the care of aging parents.

Singlehood. Many adults over 35 years of age in the United States have never been married. Many of those are college-educated people who have embraced the philosophy of choice and freedom, delayed marriage, and delayed parenthood. Some middle adults chose to remain single, but also opt to become parents either biologically or through adoption. Many single middle adults have no relatives but share a family type of relationship with close friends or work associates. Consequently, some single middle adults feel isolated during traditional "family" holidays such as Thanksgiving or Christmas. In times of illness, middle adults who have chosen to remain single and childless have to rely on other relatives or friends, increasing caregiving demands of those family members who also have other responsibilities. Nursing assessment of single middle adults needs to include a thorough assessment of psychosocial factors, including the individual's definition of family and available support systems.

Marital Changes. Marital changes occurring during middle age include death of a spouse, separation, divorce, and the choice of remarrying or remaining single. A widowed, separated, or divorced client goes through a period of grief and loss in which it is necessary to adapt to the change in marital status. Normal grieving progresses through a series of phases, and resolution of grief often takes a year or more. You need to assess the level of coping of the middle adult to the grief and loss associated with certain life changes (see Chapter 30).

Family Transitions. The departure of the last child from the home is also a stressor. Many parents welcome freedom from child-rearing responsibilities, whereas others feel lonely or without direction because of this change. Eventually parents need to reassess their marriage and try to resolve conflicts and plan for the future. Occasionally this readjustment phase leads to marital conflicts, separation, and divorce (see Chapter 10).

Care of Aging Parents. Increasing life spans in the United States and Canada have led to increased numbers of older adults in the population. Therefore greater numbers of middle adults need to address the personal and social issues confronting their aging parents. Many middle adults find themselves caught between the responsibilities of caring for dependent children and those of caring for aging and ailing parents. These middle adults thus find themselves in the **sandwich generation,** in which the challenges of caregiving can be stressful. The needs of family caregivers is an area that continues to grow.

Housing, employment, health, and economic realities have changed the traditional social expectations between generations in families. The middle adult and the older adult parent often have conflicting priorities related to their relationship while the older adult strives to remain independent. Negotiations and compromises help in defining and resolving problems. Nurses deal with middle and older adults in the community, long-term care facilities, and hospitals. Help identify the health needs of both groups, and assist the multigenerational family in determining the health and community resources available to them as they make decisions and plans. Evaluate family relationships to determine family members' perceptions of responsibility and loyalty in relation to caring for older adult members. Assessment of environmental resources (e.g., number of rooms in the house or stairwells) in relation to the complexity of health care demands for the older adult is also important.

Health Concerns

Health Promotion and Stress Reduction.
Because middle adults are experiencing physiological changes and face certain health realities, their perceptions of health and health behaviors are often important factors in maintaining health. Today's complex world makes individuals more prone to stress-related illnesses such as heart attacks, hypertension, migraine headaches, ulcers, colitis, autoimmune disease, backache, arthritis, and cancer. When adults seek health care, the nurse focuses on the goal of wellness and guides clients to evaluate health behaviors, lifestyle, and environment.

Throughout life, people have many stressors (see Chapter 31). After you identify these stressors, work together with the client to intervene and modify the stress response. Specific interventions for stress reduction fall into three categories. First, minimize the frequency of stress-producing situations. Together with the client identify approaches to prevent stressful situations, such as habituation, change avoidance, time blocking, time management, and environmental modification. Second, increase stress resistance, such as increasing self-esteem, improving assertiveness, redirecting goal alternatives, and reorienting cognitive appraisal. Last, avoid the physiological response to stress. Use relaxation techniques, imagery, and biofeedback to recondition the client's response to stress. Chapters 31 and 36 explain these general interventions in greater detail.

Obesity.
Obesity is a growing health concern for middle adults. In 2005, 23.9% of U.S. adults were obese, and the prevalence of obesity increased between 1995 and 2005 (USDHHS, CDC, 2006). Health consequences of obesity include such ailments as high blood pressure, high blood cholesterol, type 2 (non–insulin dependent) diabetes, coronary heart disease, osteoarthritis, and obstructive sleep apnea. Continued focus on the goal of wellness assists clients in evaluating health behaviors and lifestyle that contribute to obesity during the middle adult years. Counseling related to physical activity and nutrition is an important component of the plan of care for overweight and obese clients.

Forming Positive Health Habits.
A habit is a person's usual practice or manner of behavior. Frequent repetition reinforces this behavior pattern until it becomes the individual's customary way of behaving. Some habits support health, such as exercise and brushing and flossing the teeth each day. Other habits involve risk factors to health, such as smoking or eating foods with little or no nutritional value.

During assessment the nurse frequently obtains data indicating positive and negative health behaviors by the client. Examples of positive health behaviors include regular exercise, adherence to good dietary habits, avoidance of excess consumption of alcohol, participation in routine screening and diagnostic tests (e.g., laboratory screening for serum cholesterol or mammography) for disease prevention and health promotion, and lifestyle changes to reduce stress. The nurse helps the client maintain habits that protect health and offers healthier alternatives to poor habits.

Health teaching and health counseling often focuses on improving health habits (Box 13-3). The more you understand the dynamics of behavior and habits, the more likely your interventions will help the client to achieve or reinforce health-promoting behaviors.

To help clients form positive health habits you become a teacher and facilitator. By providing information about how the body functions and how clients form and change habits, you raise clients' levels of knowledge regarding the potential impact of behavior on health. You cannot change your clients' habits. Clients have control of and are responsible for their own behaviors. Explain psychological principles of changing habits, and offer information about health risks. Offer positive reinforcement (such as praise and rewards) for health-directed behaviors and decisions. Such reinforcement increases the likelihood that the behavior will be repeated. Ultimately, however, the client decides which behaviors will become habits of daily living.

Assist middle adults in considering factors such as prevention of STDs, substance abuse, and accident prevention in relation to decreasing health risks. For example, provide clients with factual information on sexually transmitted disease causes, symptoms, and transmission. Discuss methods of protection during sexual activity with the client in an open and nonjudgmental manner, and reinforce the importance of practicing "safe sex" (see Chapter 28). Provide counseling and support for clients seeking treatment for substance abuse. Assist clients in recognizing and altering unsafe habits and potential health hazards (see Chapter 38). Also, encourage clients to express their feelings to promote problem solving and recognition of risk factors by clients themselves. Barriers to change do exist (Box 13-4). Unless you minimize or eliminate these barriers, it is futile to encourage the client to take action.

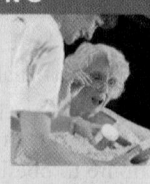

✳ **BOX 13-3** **CLIENT TEACHING**

Positive Health Habits

Objective
- Client will increase exercise patterns to include three 1-mile walks per week to assist in weight loss and improve cardiopulmonary functions.

Teaching Strategies
- Review with client the daily work schedule, identify potential times for exercise, and keep an exercise log.
- Inform client about the effect of exercise on weight control and improved cardiac function.
- Demonstrate how to calculate target heart rate and assess pulse correctly.
- Provide warm-up and cool-down exercises, and demonstrate how to do them.
- Instruct client about support shoes for walking exercises.

Evaluation
- Review client's exercise periods.
- Observe client demonstrate pulse measurement.
- Observe client demonstrate warm-up and cool-down exercises.
- Inspect client's feet for blisters or sores.

✳ **BOX 13-4 Barriers to Change**

External Barriers	**Internal Barriers**
Lack of facilities	Lack of knowledge
Lack of materials	Insufficient skills to effect change in health habits
Lack of social supports	
Lack of motivation	Undefined short- and long-term goals

Psychosocial Health

Anxiety. Anxiety is a critical maturational phenomenon related to change, conflict, and perceived control of the environment. Adults often experience anxiety in response to the physiological and psychosocial changes of middle age. Such anxiety motivates the adult to rethink life goals and stimulates productivity. For some adults, however, this anxiety precipitates psychosomatic illness and preoccupation with death. In this case the middle adult views life as being half or more over and thinks in terms of the time left to live.

Clearly, a life-threatening illness, marital transition, or job stressor increases the anxiety of the client and family. Use crisis intervention or stress management techniques to help the client adapt to the changes of the middle adult years (see Chapter 31).

Depression. Depression is a mood disorder that manifests itself in many ways. Although the most frequent age of onset is between ages 25 and 44, it is common among adults in the middle years and has many causes. The risk factors for depression include being female; disappointments or losses at work, school, or in family relationships; departure of the last child from the home; and family history. In fact, the incidence of depression in women is twice that of men. Persons experiencing mild depression describe themselves as feeling sad, blue, downcast, down in the dumps, and tearful. Other symptoms include alterations in sleep patterns such as difficulty in sleeping (insomnia) or sleeping too much (hypersomnia), irritability, feelings of social disinterest, and decreased alertness. Physical changes such as weight loss or weight gain, headaches, or feelings of fatigue regardless of the amount of rest are also depressive symptoms. Individuals with depression that occurs during the middle years commonly experience moderate-to-high anxiety and have physical complaints. Mood changes and depression are common occurrences during menopause. The abuse of alcohol or other substances makes depression worse. Nursing assessment of the depressed middle adult includes focused data collection regarding individual and family history of depression, mood changes, cognitive changes, behavioral and social changes, and physical changes. Collect assessment data from both the client and the client's family, because family data is often particularly important, depending on the level of depression the middle adult is experiencing.

Community Health Programs. Community health programs offer services to prevent illness, promote health, and detect disease in the early stages. Nurses make valuable contributions to the community's health by taking an active part in the planning of screening and teaching programs and support groups for middle adults.

Family planning, birthing, and parenting skills are program topics in which adults are usually interested. Health screening for diabetes, hypertension, eye disease, and cancer is a good opportunity for the nurse to perform assessment and provide health teaching and health counseling.

Health education programs promote changes in behavior and lifestyle. The nurse as health teacher offers information that enables the client to make decisions about health practices within the context of health promotion for young to middle adults. Be sure that educational programs are culturally appropriate (Box 13-5). Changes to more positive health practices during young and middle adulthood lead to fewer or less complicated health problems as an older adult. During health counseling the nurse and client design a plan of action that addresses the client's health and well-being. Through objective problem solving, the nurse helps the client grow and change.

Acute Care. Acute illnesses and conditions experienced in middle adulthood are similar to those of young adulthood. Injuries and acute illnesses in middle adulthood, however, take a longer recovery period because of the slowing of healing processes. In addition, acute illnesses and injuries experienced in middle adulthood are more likely to become chronic conditions. For those middle adults who are in the sandwich generation, stress levels also increase as the middle adult tries to balance responsibilities related to employment, family life, care of children, and care of aging parents while recovering from an injury or acute illness.

Restorative and Continuing Care. Chronic illnesses such as diabetes mellitus, hypertension, rheumatoid arthritis, or multiple sclerosis affect the roles and responsibilities of the middle adult. Some results of chronic illness are strained family relationships, modifications in family activities, increased health care

✳ BOX 13-5   CULTURAL ASPECTS OF CARE

Culturally Tailored Diabetes Management Program

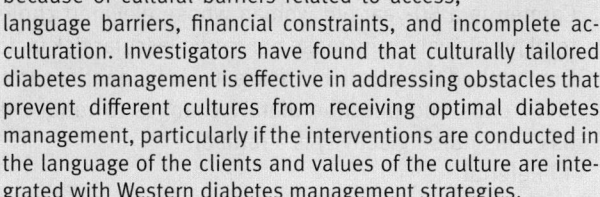

The prevalence of type 2 diabetes in the United States is rising. Not all clients with type 2 diabetes receive appropriate diabetes management because of cultural barriers related to access, language barriers, financial constraints, and incomplete acculturation. Investigators have found that culturally tailored diabetes management is effective in addressing obstacles that prevent different cultures from receiving optimal diabetes management, particularly if the interventions are conducted in the language of the clients and values of the culture are integrated with Western diabetes management strategies.

Implications for Practice
- Be aware of cultural influences that affect participation in diabetes management programs.
- Incorporate cultural values practices into Western diabetes management strategies.
- Emphasize the importance of adequate and appropriate diabetes management.
- To facilitate effective communication, include hands-on activities, culturally relevant videos, and PowerPoint slides.

Modified from Wang CY, Chan SMA: Culturally tailored diabetes education program for Chinese Americans, *Nurs Res* 54(5):347, 2005.

tasks, increased financial stress, the need for housing adaptation, social isolation, medical concerns, and grieving. The degree of disability and the client's perception of both the illness and the disability determine the extent to which lifestyle changes will occur. A few examples of the problems experienced by clients who develop debilitating chronic illness during adulthood include role reversal, changes in sexual behavior, and alterations in self-image. Along with the current health status of the chronically ill middle adult, the nurse needs to assess the knowledge base of both the client and family. This assessment includes the medical course of the illness and the prognosis for the client. In addition, determine the coping mechanisms of the client and family, adherence to treatment and rehabilitation regimens, and the need for community and social services, along with appropriate referrals.

✳ Key Concepts

- Adult development involves orderly and sequential changes in characteristics and attitudes that adults experience over time.
- Many changes experienced by the young adult are related to the natural process of maturation and socialization.
- Young adults are in a stable period of physical development, except for changes related to pregnancy.
- Cognitive development continues throughout the young and middle adult years.
- Emotional health of young adults is correlated with the ability to address and resolve personal and social problems.
- Young adults choose a career and decide whether to remain single or marry and begin a family.

- Pregnant women need to understand physiological changes occurring in each trimester.
- Psychosocial changes and health concerns during pregnancy and the puerperium affect the parents, the siblings, and often the extended family.
- Prenatal care reduces maternal and fetal mortality and morbidity.
- Midlife transition begins when a person becomes aware that physiological and psychosocial changes signify passage to another stage in life.
- Two significant physiological changes of the middle years are menopause in women and the climacteric in men.
- Cognitive changes are rare in middle age except in cases of illness or physical trauma.
- Psychosocial changes for middle adults are often related to career transition, sexuality, marital changes, family transition, and care of aging parents.
- Health concerns of middle adults commonly involve stress-related illnesses, health assessment, and adoption of positive health habits.

✳ Critical Thinking Exercises

Joan K. is a 24-year-old woman who smokes two packs of cigarettes per day. She began smoking when she was 14 years old. Joan complains to the nurse at the clinic, "I just can't seem to kick the habit no matter how hard I try."

1. You know that lifestyle habits such as smoking can have an impact on Joan's health. What information does the nurse need to know to assist Joan in quitting smoking?

2. What nursing interventions would be appropriate for Joan?

Jim D. is a 53-year-old client who is overweight and is being treated for hypertension. His blood pressure is maintained within a normal range with medication. Jim lives with his wife and 19-year-old son. His 85-year-old mother has also just moved in with Jim and his family. The nurse notices that Jim seems very stressed. He tells her that moving his mother into his home is affecting his relationships with his wife and son.

3. How should the nurse react to Jim's statement about the change within his family?

4. Because this is a multigenerational family, what does the nurse need to do to help members of the family remain healthy?

5. What nursing interventions would be appropriate for Jim to reduce his stress?

✳ NCLEX®-Style Review Questions

1. With the exception of pregnant or lactating women, the young adult has usually completed physical growth by the age of:
   1. 18
   2. 20
   3. 25
   4. 30

2. You are completing an assessment on John Weaver, age 24. Following your assessment, you note that his physical and laboratory findings are within normal limits. Because of these findings your interventions are directed toward activities related to:
   1. Instructing him to return in 2 years
   2. Instructing him in secondary prevention
   3. Instructing him in health promotion activities
   4. Implementing primary prevention with vaccines

3. When determining the amount of information that a client needs to make decisions about the prescribed course of therapy, there are many factors affecting the client's compliance with the regimen, including educational level and socioeconomic factors. Which additional factor affects compliance?
   1. Gender
   2. Lifestyle
   3. Motivation
   4. Family history

4. Kathryn Glock is laboring with her first baby, which is coming 2 weeks early. Her husband is in the military and might not get back in time, and both families are unable to be with her during labor. Karen Kline is employed by the birthing area to be a support person who is present during labor to assist Kathryn. This support person is called a(n):
   1. Nurse
   2. Midwife
   3. Assistant
   4. Lay doula

5. Carolyn is a single young adult with a group of close friends from college and work. They celebrate birthdays and holidays together. In addition, they help one another through many stressors. Carolyn views these individuals as:
   1. Family
   2. Siblings
   3. Substitute parents
   4. Alternative family structure

6. Sharing eating utensils with a person who has a contagious illness increases the risk of illness. This type of health risk arises from:
   1. Lifestyle
   2. Community
   3. Family history
   4. Personal hygiene habits

7. Carmen is a 50-year-old woman whose elevated cholesterol profile values increase her cardiovascular risk factor. One method to control this risk factor is to identify current diet trends and describe dietary changes to reduce the risk. This nursing activity is a form of:
   1. Referral
   2. Counseling
   3. Health teaching
   4. Stress management techniques

8. Carmen has a job with frequent deadlines, and she notes that when the deadlines appear she has a tendency to eat high-fat, high-carbohydrate foods. She also explains that she gets frequent headaches and stomach pain during these deadlines. You provide a number of options for Carmen, and she chooses yoga. In this scenario yoga is used as a(n):
   1. Outpatient referral
   2. Counseling technique
   3. Health promotion activity
   4. Stress management technique

14 | Older Adult

✳ OBJECTIVES

Mastery of the content in this chapter will enable the student to:

- Discuss demographic trends related to older adults in the United States.
- Identify common myths and stereotypes about older adults.
- List the types of community-based and institutional health care services available to older adults.
- Identify selected biological and psychosocial theories of aging.
- Discuss common developmental tasks of older adults.

- Describe common physiological changes of aging.
- Differentiate among delirium, dementia, and depression.
- Discuss issues related to psychosocial changes of aging.
- Describe selected health concerns of older adults.
- Identify nursing interventions related to the physiological, cognitive, and psychosocial changes of aging.

✳ MEDIA RESOURCES ✳ KEY TERMS

 Companion CD
- NCLEX®-Style Review Questions
- Audio Glossary
- Interactive Learning Activities
- English/Spanish Glossary

 Website
- NCLEX®-Style Review Questions
- Audio Glossary
- English/Spanish Glossary
- Interactive Learning Activities
- WebLinks
- Audio Summaries

Ageism, p. 193
Alzheimer's disease, p. 202
Delirium, p. 202
Dementia, p. 202
Depression, p. 202
Geriatrics, p. 192
Gerontic nursing, p. 193

Gerontological nursing, p. 192
Gerontology, p. 192
Nonstochastic theories, p. 194
Reality orientation, p. 210
Reminiscence, p. 210
Stochastic theories, p. 194
Validation therapy, p. 210

The identification of age 65 as the start of older adulthood dates back to social reform in Germany in the nineteenth century. Age 65 continues to be the lower boundary for "old age" in demographics and social policy, although many older adults consider themselves to be "middle-age" well into their seventh decade. Chronological age often has little relation to the reality of aging for an older adult. Each person ages in his or her own way according to his or her own schedule and life history. Every older adult is unique, and the nurse needs to approach each one as a unique individual, even though this chapter will make generalizations about the aging process and its effect on individuals.

The number of older adults in the United States is growing, both absolutely and as a proportion of the total population. In 2000 there were 35 million adults over age 65 in the United States, representing 12.4% of the population (Administration on Aging [AOA], 2006). This represents an increase of 3.7 million since 1990. Among those 35 million older adults in 2000, 18.4 million were between ages 65 and 74, 12.4 million were between ages 75 and 85, and 4.2 million were over age 85. According to estimates, the number of older adults will increase to 70 million by 2030. Part of that increase is due to extension of the average life span. Women age 65 in 2003 can expect to live another 19.4 years, and men another 16.4 years.

Two other factors that contribute to the projected increase in the number of older adults are the aging of the baby boom generation and the growth of the population segment over age 85. The baby boomers are the large group of adults born between 1946 and 1964. The first baby boomers will reach age 65 in 2011. As this aging population "bulge" of baby boomers increases the total number of older adults, social and health care programs need to dramatically reform to meet their needs while simultaneously meeting the needs of the group over age 85. The 4.2 million older adults currently over age 85, who are sometimes called the frail elderly, will increase to 8.9 million by 2030. Furthermore, centenarians, those age 100 and over, increased from 37,306 in 1990 to 50,545 in 2000 will continue to increase in number.

The diversity of the group over age 65 will also possibly increase (U.S. Census Bureau, 2005). In 2000, minorities (African Americans, Hispanics, Asians, American Indians/Eskimos/Aleuts, and other Pacific Islanders) made up 18% of the group over age 65. The percentages of older adults from minorities in 2003 were as follows: African-Americans, 8%; Hispanics, 6%; Asian, 3%; American Indians/Eskimos/Aleuts, less than 1%; and other Pacific Islanders, 1%. By 2030 the older adults from these minority groups will account for over 26% of the total group over age 65 (AOA, 2005). Hispanics over age 65 will experience the most dramatic increase.

Nurses need to take the cultural, ethnic, and racial diversity represented by these numbers into account as they care for older adults from these groups. The challenge with these older adults is to gain new knowledge and skills to provide culturally sensitive and linguistically appropriate care. Examples of culturally competent nursing approaches to older adults include respect for preferences in food, music, and religion; appropriate use of the conventions of the handshake, silence, and eye contact; use of interpreters; use of physical assessment norms appropriate for the ethnic group; and asking about personal health practices, family customs, lifestyle preferences, and spiritual resources (Meiner and

Lueckenotte, 2006). Chapter 9 provides further information on culturally competent care.

Variability Among Older Adults

The nursing care of older adults poses special challenges because of great variation in their physiological, cognitive, and psychosocial health. Older adults also vary widely in their levels of functional ability. The majority of older adults are active and involved members of their communities. A smaller number have lost the ability to care for themselves, are confused or withdrawn, and/or are unable to make decisions concerning their needs. Most older adults live in noninstitutional settings. In 2004, 54.7% of older adults in noninstitutional settings lived with a spouse (42% of older women, 71% of older men) (AOA, 2005). However, 31% lived alone (40% of older women, 19% of older men). The remaining 15% lived with family or friends. Only 4.5% of all older adults resided in institutions such as nursing homes. Age influenced living arrangements: the proportion of older adults living with a spouse decreased with age, the proportion living alone increased with age, and the proportion living in an institution increased with age.

Aging does not inevitably lead to disability and dependence. Most older people remain functionally independent despite the increasing prevalence of chronic disease. Nursing assessment, a complex and challenging process, provides valuable clues to the effect of a disease or illness on a client's functional status. Chronic conditions add to the complexity of assessment and care of the older adult. Most older persons have at least one chronic condition, and many have multiple conditions. The most frequently occurring in 2002 to 2003 were hypertension (51%); diagnosed arthritis (48%); all types of heart disease (31%); any cancer (21%); and diabetes (16%) (AOA, 2005). The physical and psychosocial aspects of aging are closely related. For the older person, a reduced ability to respond to stress, the experience of multiple losses, and the physical changes associated with normal aging combine to place the person at high risk for illness and functional deterioration. Although the interaction of these physical and psychosocial factors is sometimes serious, do not assume that all older adults have signs, symptoms, or behaviors representing disease and decline or that these are the only items you need to assess. You also need to identify the older adult's strengths and abilities during the assessment.

Terminology

As the number of older adults increases, gerontological nursing is gaining in importance. Several interchangeable terms describe this specialty (Meiner and Lueckenotte, 2006):

- **Geriatrics** is the branch of medicine dealing with the diagnosis and treatment of diseases and problems affecting older adults.
- **Gerontology** is the study of all aspects of the aging process and its consequences.
- **Gerontological nursing** is concerned with assessment of the health and functional status of older adults; diagnosis, plan-

ning, and implementing health care and services to meet the identified needs; and evaluating the effectiveness of such care. This is the term nurses specializing in this field use most often.
- **Gerontic nursing,** a seldom-used term, considers the nursing care of older adults to be the art and practice of nurturing, caring, and comforting rather than merely the treatment of disease.

Myths and Stereotypes

Despite ongoing research in the field of gerontology, myths and stereotypes about older adults persist. These include false ideas about the physical and psychosocial characteristics and the lifestyles of older adults. However, when health care providers hold negative stereotypes about aging, those stereotypes negatively affect the quality of client care. Nurses, although susceptible to these myths and stereotypes, have the responsibility to replace them with accurate information.

Some stereotype older adults as ill, disabled, and physically unattractive. However, although many experience chronic conditions or have at least one disability that limits their performance of activities of daily living (ADLs), in 2004 37.4% of noninstitutionalized older adults assessed their health as excellent or very good (AARP, 2004). Other common misconceptions are that older adults are not interested in sex and any interest in sexual activities is abnormal. Nurses need to discourage this perception. Older adults do report continued enjoyment of sexual relationships.

Some people believe that older adults are forgetful, confused, rigid, bored, and unfriendly and that they are unable to understand and learn new information. Yet specialists in the field of gerontology view centenarians, the oldest of the old, as having an optimistic outlook on life, good memories, broad social contacts and interests, and tolerance for others. Although changes in vision or hearing and reduced energy and endurance sometimes affect the process of learning, older adults are lifelong learners. Use teaching techniques to compensate for sensory changes, provide additional time for remembering and responding, and present concrete rather than abstract material to facilitate learning by older adults. Other effective teaching techniques draw on the older adult's past experiences and correspond to the identified interests of the older adult rather than to the content areas the health care professional believes are important. Box 14-1 presents additional teaching strategies to address the special learning needs of older adults.

Stereotypes about lifestyles include mistaken ideas about living arrangements and finances. Most older adults live in noninstitutional settings, either with family members or alone. Misconceptions about the financial status of older adults range from beliefs that many are affluent to beliefs that many are poor. According to the Administration on Aging (2005), 9.8% of persons over age 65 had incomes below the poverty level with another 7% classified as near poor. Most older adults (90%) receive Social Security benefits. In the aggregated income of all older adults, Social Security benefits accounted for only 39%, with earnings (27%), assets (14%), and pensions (20%) constituting the remainder of the aggregate income.

BOX 14-1 Older Adult Client's Special Learning Needs

Teaching Strategies
- Make sure the client is ready to learn. Watch for clues that indicate that the client is preoccupied or too anxious to comprehend the material.
- Sit facing the client so that he or she is able to watch your lip movements and facial expressions.
- Speak slowly.
- Keep your tone of voice low; older adults are able to hear low sounds better than high-frequency sounds.
- Present one idea at a time.
- Emphasize concrete rather than abstract material.
- Give the client enough time in which to respond because older adults' reaction times are longer than those of younger persons.
- Focus on a single topic to help the client concentrate.
- Keep environmental distractions to a minimum.
- Defer teaching if the client becomes distracted or tired or cannot concentrate for other reasons.
- Invite another member of the household to join the discussion.
- Use audio, visual, and tactile cues to enhance learning and help the client remember information.
- Ask for feedback to ensure that the client understands the information.
- Use past experience; connect new learning to previous knowledge.
- Compensate for physical discomfort and sensory decrements.
- Support a positive self-image in the learner.
- Use creative teaching strategies.
- Respond to identified interests of learners.
- Emphasize and integrate emotional and personal values in the acquisition of skills and ideas.

Modified from Ebersole P and others: *Geriatric nursing and healthy aging,* ed 2, St. Louis, 2005, Mosby.

In a society that values attractiveness, energy, and youth these myths and stereotypes lead to the undervaluing of older adults. Some people believe that older adults become worthless after they leave the workforce. Others consider the knowledge and experience of older adults too outdated to have any current value. These ideas demonstrate **ageism,** which is discrimination against people because of increasing age, just as people who are racists and sexists discriminate because of skin color and gender. According to experts in the field of gerontology, unopposed ageism has the potential to undermine the self-confidence of older adults, limit their access to care, and distort caregivers' understanding of the uniqueness of each older adult.

Today there are laws banning discrimination on the basis of age. The economic and political power of older adults also challenges ageist views. Older adults are a significant proportion of the consumer economy. As voters and activists in various issues, they have major influence in the formation of public policy. Their participation adds a unique perspective on social, economic, and technological issues because they have experienced almost 100 years of developments. In the past 100 years, we have progressed from riding in horse-drawn carriages to tracking the adventures of the international space station. Gaslights and steam power are replaced by electricity and nuclear power. Computers and copier machines replace typewriters and carbon paper. Older adults lived through the Great Depression. They also experienced two world wars and wars in Korea, Vietnam, the Persian Gulf, and now the war on terror. Older adults saw changes in health care as the era of the family physician gave way to the age of specialization. After witnessing the government initiatives establishing the Social Security system, Medicare, and Medicaid, older adults are currently living with the changes imposed by health care reform. Living through all of these events and changes, older adults have stories and examples of coping with change to share.

Nurses' Attitudes Toward Older Adults

It is important for nurses to assess their own attitudes toward older adults, their own aging, and the aging of their family, friends, and clients. The attitudes of the nurse toward older adults comes from personal experiences with older adults, education, employment experiences, and attitudes of co-workers and employing institutions. The nurse's own age, either as a factor contributing to the amount of experience or as a factor reflecting the nurse's own aging, also contributes to the nurse's attitude toward older adults. Given the increasing number of older adults in health care settings, cultivation of positive attitudes toward older adults and specialized knowledge about aging and the health care needs of older adults are priorities for nurses.

Positive attitudes are based in part on a realistic portrayal of the characteristics and health care needs of older adults. In the past, negative attitudes about aging and older adults contributed to the persistence of stereotypes of older adults as dependent and less attractive than younger clients. Nursing care, under the influence of these attitudes, often ignores the opportunity to respect older adults and actively involve them in care decisions and activities. At times institutional settings, such as hospitals and nursing homes, treated older adults as objects rather than independent, dignified adults. But the time has come for nurses to recognize and address ageism by questioning prevailing negative attitudes and stereotypes and reinforcing the realities of aging as they care for older adults in all care settings.

Theories of Aging

Various theorists have attempted to describe the complex biopsychosocial process of aging. Although there are many theories, there is no single universally accepted theory that predicts and explains the complexities of the aging process. The nurse needs to be aware of the scientific attempts to explain the aging process and the concepts included in the theories. Although the theories are in various stages of development and have limitations, use them to increase understanding of the phenomena affecting the health and well-being of older adults and to guide nursing care. The biological theories of aging are either stochastic theories or nonstochastic theories. **Stochastic theories** view aging as the result of random cellular damage that occurs over time. The accumulated damage

leads to the physical changes that we recognize as characteristic of the aging process. According to the **nonstochastic theories**, genetically programmed physiological mechanisms within the body control the process of aging.

The psychosocial theories of aging explain changes in behavior, roles, and relationships that come with aging. As with biological theories of aging, there is no single universally accepted theory . The theories also reflect the values the theorist and society held at that time. The three classic psychosocial theories of aging are disengagement theory, activity theory, and continuity theory. Disengagement theory, the oldest psychosocial theory, states that aging individuals withdraw from customary roles and engage in more introspective, self-focused activities (Cummings and Henry, 1961). The activity theory, unlike the disengagement theory, considers the continuation of activities performed during middle age as necessary for successful aging (Havighurst, Neugarten, and Tobin, 1963). Continuity theory, or developmental theory (Neugarten, 1964), states that personality remains the same and behavior becomes more predictable as people age. The personality and behavior patterns developed during a lifetime determine the degree of engagement and activity in older adulthood.

Critics suggest that all three psychosocial theories either fail in some measure to consider the many factors that affect an individual's response to the aging process or address those factors in a too simplistic fashion. Although some generalize about aging, biologically and psychosocially each individual ages uniquely.

Developmental Tasks for Older Adults

Theories of aging are closely linked to the concept of developmental tasks appropriate for distinct stages of life. Although no two individuals age in the same way, either biologically or psychosocially, researchers have developed frameworks outlining tasks appropriate developmentally for older adults (Box 14-2). These developmental tasks are common to many older adults and are associated with varying degrees of change and loss. The more common losses are of health, significant others, a sense of being useful, socialization, income, and independent living. The ways that older adults adjust to the changes of aging are highly individualized. For some, adaptation and adjustment are relatively easy. For others, coping with aging changes requires the assistance of family, friends, and health care professionals. Be sensitive to the effect of such losses on older adults and their families, and be prepared to offer support.

✳ BOX 14-2 Developmental Tasks of the Older Adult

- Adjusting to decreasing health and physical strength
- Adjusting to retirement and reduced or fixed income
- Adjusting to death of a spouse
- Accepting self as aging person
- Maintaining satisfactory living arrangements
- Redefining relationships with adult children
- Finding ways to maintain quality of life

Older adults face the necessity of adjustment to the physical changes that accompany aging. The extent and timing of these changes vary from individual to individual, but as body systems age, changes in appearance and functioning occur. These changes are not associated with a disease but are normal changes. The presence of disease sometimes alters the timing of the changes or their impact on daily life. The section on physiological development describes structural and functional changes associated with aging.

Some older adults find it difficult to accept themselves as aging. This is apparent when some older adults, both men and women, understate their ages when asked, adopt younger styles of clothing, or attempt to hide physical evidence of aging with cosmetics. But other older adults deny their own aging in ways that are potentially problematic. For example, some older adults deny functional declines and refuse to ask for assistance with tasks that place their safety at great risk. Others avoid activities designed to benefit older adults, such as senior citizens' centers and senior health promotion activities, and thus do not receive the benefits these programs offer. Acceptance of personal aging does not mean retreat into inactivity, but it does require a realistic review of strengths and limitations.

Older adults retired from employment outside the home have to cope with the loss of that work role. Older adults who worked at home and the spouses of those who worked outside the home also face role changes as they age. Because older adults usually anticipate retirement, they usually plan ahead to make financial plans and consider replacement activities. Many older adults welcome retirement as a time to pursue new interests and hobbies, participate in volunteer activities, continue their education, or start a new business career. Retirement plans for some older adults include changing residence by moving to a different city or state or moving to a different type of housing within the same area.

Reasons other than retirement also lead to changes of residence. For example, physical impairments require relocation to a smaller, single-level home. Severe health problems require the older adult to live with relatives or friends. A change in living arrangements for the older adult usually requires an extended period of adjustment during which assistance and support from health care professionals, friends, and family members are necessary.

The majority of older adults cope with the death of a spouse. In 2004 almost half (43%) of all older women were widows, and 14% of older men were widowers (AOA, 2005). Some older adults must cope with the death of adult children and grandchildren. All experience the deaths of friends. These deaths represent both losses and reminders of personal mortality. Coming to terms with these deaths is often difficult. By assisting older adults through the grieving process, the nurse will help them resolve the issues posed by these deaths.

The redefining of relationships with children that occurred as those children grew up and left home continues as older adults experience the challenges of aging. A variety of issues sometimes occur, including, but not limited to, role reversal, control of decision making, dependence, conflict, guilt, and loss. How these issues surface in situations and how they are resolved depends in part on the past relationship between the older adult and the adult children. All the involved parties have past experiences and powerful emotions. When adult children assist the older adults of their family, they have to find ways to balance the demands of their own children and their careers. Adult children also debate over how much assistance to provide and how much decision-making authority to assume. As adult children and aging parents negotiate the aspects of the changed roles, nurses are able to act as counselors to both the parents and the children. Nurses assist adult children by listening and by helping them distinguish between changes and behaviors related to illness, normal aging changes, and their parents' lifelong preferences and patterns of behavior.

In the face of the changes that come with aging, older adults need to find ways to maintain their quality of life. What defines quality of life varies from person to person. Nurses must listen to what the older adult considers to be most important rather than making assumptions about that individual's priorities. Together the nurse and the older adult work together to maintain or improve the quality of life. Whether quality of life is maintenance of social relationships, continuing to live alone, or continuing activities such as driving or gardening, older adults look to the nurse for assistance.

Community-Based and Institutional Health Care Services

Nurses encounter older adult clients in a wide variety of settings in the community and in institutional health care settings. Outside of the acute care hospital setting, nurses care for older adults in private homes and apartments, retirement communities, adult day care centers, assisted living facilities, and nursing centers or facilities (extended care facilities, intermediate care facilities, skilled nursing facilities). Chapter 2 describes these settings and the services provided in detail.

Nurses assist older adults and their families by providing information and answering questions as they make choices among care options. The assistance of the nurse is especially valuable when older adults and their families are making decisions about moving to a nursing center. Some family caregivers consider nursing center placement when in-home care becomes increasingly difficult or when convalescence (recovery) from hospitalization requires more assistance than the family is able to provide. However, the decision to enter a nursing center needs to come only after the older adult and the family have considered the full range of long-term care choices. Although the decision to enter a nursing center is never final and a nursing center resident is sometimes discharged to home or another less-acute facility, many older adults view the nursing center as their final residence. During the decision-making period, the actual move to the nursing center, and the time after admission, the nurse's role is to provide information about the selection of a good nursing center and to support the older adult and family. Although results of state and federal inspections of nursing centers are available to the public at the nursing centers and at the inspectors' offices, the best way to evaluate the quality of a nursing center is to visit that facility and inspect it personally (Rantz and others, 2001) (Box 14-3).

Assessing the Needs of Older Adults

Gerontological nursing requires creative approaches for maximizing the potential of older adults. With comprehensive assessment information regarding the older adult's strengths, limitations, and resources, the nurse and the older adult identify needs and problems. Together they select interventions to maintain the older adult's physical abilities and create an environment for psychosocial and spiritual well-being. A thorough assessment requires you to actively engage the older adult and provide the older adult enough time to

share important information about his or her health. Assess for changes in physiology, cognition, and psychosocial behavior.

Nursing assessment takes into account five key points to ensure an age-specific approach: (1) the interrelation between physical and psychosocial aspects of aging, (2) the effects of disease and disability on functional status, (3) the decreased efficiency of homeostatic mechanisms, (4) the lack of standards for health and illness norms, and (5) altered presentation and response to specific disease (Meiner and Lueckenotte, 2006). Obtaining a comprehensive assessment of an older adult takes more time than the assessment of a younger adult because of the longer life and medical history and the potential complexity of that history. Plan to spend extra time with the assessment. During the physical examination allow rest periods as needed or conduct the assessment in several sessions because of the reduced energy and limited endurance experienced by some frail older adults.

Sensory changes also affect data gathering. Your choice of communication techniques depend on visual or hearing impairments of the older adult. If older adults are unable to understand your visual or auditory cues, assessment data will possibly be inaccurate or misleading. For example, if older adults have difficulty hearing a nurse's questions, inappropriate responses lead the nurse to believe that they are confused. Communication techniques to use when older adults have visual impairments include the following:

- Sit or stand at eye level, in front of the client in full view.
- Face the older adult while speaking; do not cover your mouth.
- Provide diffuse, bright, nonglare lighting.
- Encourage the older adult to use his or her familiar assistive devices such as glasses or magnifiers.

Techniques to use when older adults are hearing impaired include the following:

- Speak directly to the client; and do not cover your mouth.
- Speak in clear, low-pitched tones at a moderate rate and volume.
- Reduce background noises; move to a quiet, private room.
- Ask if there is a "good ear," and speak toward that ear.
- Encourage the older adult to use assistive devices such as hearing aids or "microphone plus earphones" devices.
- Make sure the hearing aid is working properly (check the battery, check that the hearing aid is turned on, adjust volume controls).
- Check the ear canal for cerumen impaction.

Memory deficits, if present, affect the accuracy and completeness of the data collected. Information contributed by a family member or other caregiver is sometimes necessary to supplement the older adult's recollection of past medical events and information such as allergies and immunizations. Use tact when involving another person in the assessment interview with the older adult. The additional person supplements the answers of the older adult with the consent of the older adult, but the older adult remains the focus of the interview.

During all aspects of the assessment the nurse is responsible for providing culturally congruent care. See Chapter 9 for a detailed description of the components of a cultural assessment. There are

---

✳ BOX 14-3   FOCUS ON OLDER ADULTS

Selection of a Nursing Home: Six Aspects of Quality to Consider

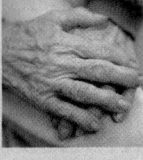

An important step in the process of selecting a nursing home is to visit the nursing home. While looking around the nursing home, consider these aspects of quality.

- **Home:** The nursing home should not feel like a hospital. It is a home, a place where people live. Residents should be encouraged to personalize their rooms. Privacy is respected.
- **Care:** In addition to assistance with basic activities of daily living such as bathing, dressing, eating, oral hygiene, and toileting, staff should assist residents with social and recreational activities. Residents should be out of bed and dressed according to their preferences. Visitors should be able to see the staff actively assisting and interacting socially with residents.
- **Family involvement:** Staff should welcome families when they visit the facility. Whether families wish to provide information, ask questions, participate in care planning, or assist with social activities or physical care, staff should encourage family involvement.
- **Environment:** Residents, their clothing, their belongings, and their surroundings should be clean. The staff should be clean and well groomed. There should be no pervasive odors in the facility. Ample nonglare lighting, minimal noise, plants, comfortable furniture, and pets contribute to a homelike environment.
- **Communication:** Good communication among residents, families, and staff is necessary for quality care. Good communication is respectful and considerate.
- **Staff:** Members of the nursing home staff are attentive to resident requests and actively involved with assisting the residents. They focus on the person, not on the task. The assistance that they provide to residents includes assistance with social or recreational activities, as well as the performance of nursing duties.

Modified from Rantz M, Popejoy L, Zwygart-Stauffacher M: *The new nursing homes: a 20-minute way to find great long-term care,* Minneapolis, 2001, Fairview Press.

ways to provide culturally competent care while communicating with older adults during the assessment process (Box 14-4).

During assessment, exercise caution in the interpretation of the signs and symptoms of diseases and the interpretation of laboratory values. Historically researchers used younger populations to establish the classic signs and symptoms of diseases and the norms for laboratory values. However, the classic signs and symptoms of diseases are sometimes absent, blunted, or atypical in older adults (Meiner and Lueckenotte, 2006). This is possibly due

to age-related changes in organ systems and homeostatic mechanisms, progressive loss of physiological and functional reserves, or coexisting acute or chronic conditions. As a result, the older adult with a urinary tract infection presents with confusion, incontinence, and falls instead of fever, dysuria, frequency, or urgency. Some older adults with pneumonia have tachycardia, tachypnea, and confusion with decreased appetite and functioning, without the more common symptoms of fever and productive cough. Instead of crushing, substernal chest pain and diaphoresis, the older adult with a myocardial infarction experiences a sudden onset of dyspnea often accompanied by anxiety and confusion. Variations from the usual norms for laboratory values are sometimes due to age-related changes in cardiac, pulmonary, renal, and metabolic function (Beers, 2000). Examples of laboratory values that increase during the aging process include alkaline phosphatase, serum cholesterol, triglycerides, serum glucose (postprandial), and serum uric acid. Examples of laboratory values that decrease during the aging process include serum calcium, serum creatine kinase, and creatinine clearance.

It is important to recognize the early indicators of an acute illness in older adults: change in mental status, falls, dehydration, decrease in appetite, loss of function, dizziness, and incontinence (Amella, 2004). A key principle of providing age-appropriate nursing care is timely detection of these cardinal signs of illness so early treatment can begin (Box 14-5). Mental status changes commonly occur as a result of disease and psychological issues, but most often they are drug related. Drug toxicity or adverse drug events are most often linked to mental status changes. A fall is a complex event that needs careful investigation to find out if it was due to environmental causes or the symptom of a new-onset illness. Problems with the cardiac, respiratory, musculoskeletal, neurological, urological, and

---

✳ BOX 14-4   CULTURAL ASPECTS OF CARE

Communication During Assessment

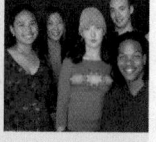

The older adult's cultural values and beliefs about health, illness, and treatment influence the quality of assessment data the nurse collects in an interview. Be knowledgeable about the characteristics of the older adult's cultural group because they affect nurse-client communication during the assessment process (Ebersole and others, 2005).

Implications for Practice
- Use cultural interpreters when necessary.
- Identify how the older adult wishes to be addressed; use culturally appropriate titles.
- Assess the health-related beliefs and practices of the older client's culture group, and adapt questions to obtain information on how the client incorporates them into daily practice.
- Know beliefs and practices of the older client's culture group regarding spatial requirements, eye contact, and touch, and use them to establish rapport.

✳ BOX 14-5   Examples of Altered Presentation of Illnesses in Older Adults Occurring in Various Health Care Settings

Hospital
- Confusion is not inevitable. Look for neurologic events or new medication, or the presence of risk factors for delirium.
- Many hospitalized older adults suffer from chronic dehydration accelerated by acute illness.
- Not all older adults have fevers with infection. Symptoms instead include increased respiratory rate, falls, incontinence, or confusion.

Nursing Center
- Health care providers often under treat pain in older adults, especially those with dementia. Look for nonverbal cues such as grimacing or resistance to care.
- Decline in functional ability (even a minor one, such as the inability to sit upright in a chair) is a signal of new illness.
- Residents with less muscle mass—both the frail and the obese—are at a much higher risk for toxicity from protein-binding drugs such as phenytoin (Dilantin and others) and warfarin (Coumadin and others).
- Urinary and/or fecal incontinence is often a sign of the onset of a new illness.

Ambulatory Care
- Complaints of fatigue or decreased ability to do usual activities are signs of anemia, thyroid problems, depression, or neurologic or cardiac problems.

- Severe gastrointestinal problems in older adults do not always present with the same acute symptoms seen in younger clients. Ask about constipation, cramping sensations, and changes in bowel habits.
- Older adults reporting increased dyspnea and confusion, especially those with a cardiac history, need to go to the ED; these are the most common manifestations of myocardial infarction in this population.
- Depression is common among older adults with chronic illnesses. Watch for lack of interest in former activities, significant personal losses, or changes in role or home life.

Home Care
- Investigate all falls, focusing on balance, gait, and neurologic issues.
- Monitor older adults with late-stage heart disease for loss of appetite as an early symptom of impending failure.
- Drug-drug interactions in older clients who are seeing more than one provider and taking multiple medications are common. Watch for signs.

From Amella EJ: Presentation of illness in older adults, *Am J Nurs* 104(10):40, 2004.

ED, Emergency department.

sensory body systems can present with a fall as a chief symptom of a new-onset condition. Dehydration is common in older adults because of decreased oral intake related to a reduced thirst response and less free water as a consequence of a decrease in muscle mass. With the vomiting and diarrhea that can accompany the onset of an acute illness the older adult is then at risk for further dehydration. Decrease in appetite is a common symptom with the onset of pneumonia, heart failure, and urinary tract infection. Loss of functional ability occurs in a subtle fashion over a period of time, or it occurs suddenly, depending on the underlying cause. Thyroid disease, infection, cardiac or pulmonary conditions, metabolic disturbances, and anemia are common causes of functional decline, so nurses need to identify them early and notify health care providers so proper treatment can be initiated. Dizziness is a commonly occurring sign of a variety of acute illnesses, including anemia, arrhythmia, infection, myocardial infarction, stroke, and brain tumor. New-onset urinary incontinence in the older adult is often associ-

ated with a urinary tract infection, but it is also a symptom of an electrolyte abnormality or an adverse drug event.

Physiological Changes

Perception of well-being defines quality of life. Understanding the older adult's perceptions about health status is essential for accurate assessment and development of clinically relevant interventions. Older adults' concepts of health generally depend on personal perceptions of functional ability. Therefore older adults engaged in activities of daily living usually consider themselves healthy, whereas those who have physical, emotional, or social impairments that limit their activities perceive themselves as ill.

There are frequently observed physiological changes in older adults that are called normal (Table 14-1). These physiological changes are not always pathological processes in themselves, but they make older adults more vulnerable to some common

✳ TABLE 14-1 Common Physiological Changes With Aging

System	Common Changes
Integumentary	Loss of skin elasticity (wrinkles, sagging, dryness, easily tears), pigmentation changes, glandular atrophy (oil, moisture, sweat glands), thinning hair (facial hair: decreased in men, increased in women), slower nail growth, atrophy of epidermal arterioles
Respiratory	Decreased cough reflex; decreased removal of mucus, dust, irritants from airways (decreased cilia); decreased vital capacity (increased anterior-posterior chest diameter); increased chest wall rigidity; fewer alveoli, increased airway resistance; increased risk of respiratory infections
Cardiovascular	Thickening of blood vessel walls; narrowing of vessel lumen; loss of vessel elasticity; lower cardiac output; decreased number of heart muscle fibers; decreased elasticity and calcification of heart valves; decreased baroreceptor sensitivity; decreased efficiency of venous valves; increased pulmonary vascular tension; increased systolic blood pressure; decreased peripheral circulation
Gastrointestinal	Periodontal disease; decrease in saliva, gastric secretions, and pancreatic enzymes; smooth muscle changes with decreased esophageal peristalsis and small intestinal motility
Musculoskeletal	Decreased muscle mass and strength, decalcification of bones, degenerative joint changes, dehydration of intervertebral disks (decreased height)
Neurological	Degeneration of nerve cells, decrease in neurotransmitters, decrease in rate of conduction of impulses
Sensory	
Eyes	Decreased accommodation to near/far (presbyopia), difficulty adjusting to changes from light to dark, yellowing of the lens, altered color perception, increased sensitivity to glare, smaller pupils
Ears	Loss of acuity for high-frequency tones (presbycusis), thickening of tympanic membrane, sclerosis of inner ear, buildup of earwax (cerumen)
Taste	Often diminished, often have fewer taste buds
Smell	Often diminished
Touch	Decreased skin receptors
Proprioception	Decreased awareness of body positioning in space
Genitourinary	Fewer nephrons, 50% decrease in renal blood flow by age 80, decreased bladder capacity
Male	Enlargement of prostate
Female	Reduced sphincter tone
Reproductive	
Male	Sperm count diminishes, smaller testes, erections less firm and slow to develop
Female	Decreased estrogen production, degeneration of ovaries, atrophy of vagina, uterus, breasts
Endocrine	
General	Alteration in hormone production with decreased ability to respond to stress
Thyroid	Decreased secretion
Thymus	Involution of thymus gland
Cortisol, glucocorticoids	Increased anti-inflammatory hormone
Pancreas	Increased fibrosis, decreased secretion of enzymes and hormones

Modified from Ebersole P and others: *Gerontological nursing and healthy aging*, ed 2, St. Louis, 2005, Mosby.

clinical conditions and diseases. Some older adults experience all of these physiological changes, and others experience only a few. The body changes continuously with age, and specific effects on particular older adults depend on health, lifestyle, stressors, and environmental conditions. The nurse needs to know about these normal, more common changes in order to provide appropriate care for older adults and to assist with adaptation to the changes.

General Survey. The general survey begins during the initial nurse-client encounter and includes a quick, but careful, head-to-toe scan of the older adult that the nurse writes in a brief description. An initial inspection of an older adult sometimes reveals eye contact and facial expression appropriate to the situation, as well as common aging changes such as facial wrinkles, gray hair, loss of body mass in the extremities, and an increase of body mass in the trunk.

Integumentary System. With aging, the skin loses resilience and moisture. The epithelial layer thins, and elastic collagen fibers shrink and become rigid. Wrinkles of the face and neck reflect lifelong patterns of muscle activity and facial expressions, the pull of gravity on tissue, and diminished elasticity.

Spots and lesions are often present on the skin. Smooth, brown, irregularly shaped spots (age spots, or senile lentigo) initially appear on the backs of the hands and on forearms. Small, round, red or brown cherry angiomas occur on the trunk. Seborrheic lesions or keratoses appear as irregular, round or oval, brown, watery lesions. Years of sun exposure contribute to the aging of the skin and lead to premalignant and malignant lesions. You need to rule out three malignancies related to sun exposure when examining skin lesions: melanoma, basal cell carcinoma, and squamous cell carcinoma (Beers, 2000) (see Chapter 33).

Head and Neck. The facial features of the older adult become more pronounced from loss of subcutaneous fat and skin elasticity. Facial features appear asymmetrical because of missing teeth or improperly fitting dentures. In addition, common vocal changes include a rise in pitch and a loss of power and range.

Visual acuity declines with age. This is often the result of retinal damage, reduced pupil size, development of opacities in the lens, or loss of lens elasticity. Presbyopia, a progressive decline in the ability of the eyes to accommodate for close, detailed work, is common. There is a reduced ability to see in darkness and to adapt to abrupt changes from dark areas to light areas (and the reverse). More ambient light is necessary for tasks such as reading, as well as for other activities of daily living. However, older adults also have increased sensitivity to the effects of glare, so make sure interventions to increase ambient light do not increase glare. Changes in color vision and discoloration of the lens make it difficult to distinguish between blues and greens and among pastel shades. Dark colors also appear the same.

Auditory changes are often subtle. Most of the time older adults ignore the earlier signs of loss of hearing acuity until friends and family members comment on compensatory attempts such as turning up the volume on televisions and radios. A common age-related change in auditory acuity is presbycusis. Presbycusis affects the ability to hear high-pitched sounds and sibilant consonants such as *s, sh,* and *ch.* Before the nurse assumes presbycusis it is necessary to inspect the external auditory canal for the presence of cerumen. Impacted cerumen, a common cause of diminished hearing acuity, is easy to treat.

Salivary secretion is reduced, and taste buds atrophy and lose sensitivity. The older adult is less able to differentiate among salty, sweet, sour, and bitter tastes. The sense of smell also decreases, further reducing taste.

Thorax and Lungs. Because of changes in the musculoskeletal system, the configuration of the thorax sometimes changes. After age 55 respiratory muscle strength begins to decrease (Beers, 2000). The anteroposterior diameter of the thorax increases. Vertebral changes due to osteoporosis lead to dorsal kyphosis, the curvature of the thoracic spine sometimes called "dowager's hump." Calcification of the costal cartilage causes decreased mobility of the ribs. The chest wall gradually becomes stiffer. Lung expansion decreases. If kyphosis or chronic obstructive lung disease is present, breath sounds are distant.

Heart and Vascular System. Decreased contractile strength of the myocardium results in a decreased cardiac output. The decrease is significant when the older adult experiences anxiety, excitement, illness, or strenuous activity. The body tries to compensate for decreased cardiac output by increasing the heart rate during exercise. However, after exercise, it takes longer for the older adult's rate to return to baseline.

Systolic and/or diastolic blood pressures are sometimes abnormally high. Baroreceptor sensitivity declines, decreasing the ability to produce a compensatory response to hypotensive or hypertensive stimuli (Ebersole, Hess, and Luggen, 2004). More than 50% of older adults have systolic or diastolic hypertension (systolic pressure greater than 140 mm Hg, diastolic pressure greater than 90 mm Hg) (Beers, 2000). Although a common chronic condition, hypertension is not a normal aging change and predisposes older adults to heart failure, stroke, renal failure, coronary heart disease, and peripheral vascular disease.

Peripheral pulses are frequently weaker, although still palpable, in the lower extremities. Older adults sometimes complain that their lower extremities are cold, particularly at night. Changes in the peripheral pulses in the upper extremities are less common.

Breasts. Decreased muscle mass, tone, and elasticity result in smaller breasts in older women. In addition, the breasts sag. Atrophy of glandular tissue, coupled with more fat deposits, results in a slightly smaller, less dense, and less nodular breast. Gynecomastia, enlarged breasts in men, is often due to medication side effects, hormonal changes, or obesity. Both older men and women are at risk of breast cancer.

Gastrointestinal System and Abdomen. Aging leads to an increase in the amount of fatty tissue in the trunk. As a result, the abdomen increases in size. Because muscle tone and elasticity decrease, it also becomes more protuberant. Gastrointestinal function changes include a slowing of peristalsis and alterations in secretions. The older adult experiences these changes as the development of intolerance to certain foods and discomfort due to delayed gastric emptying. Alterations in the lower gastrointestinal tract lead to constipation, flatulence, or diarrhea.

Reproductive System. Changes in the structure and function of the reproductive system occur as the result of hormonal alterations. Female menopause is related to a reduced responsiveness of the ovaries to pituitary hormones and a resultant decrease in estrogen and progesterone levels. In men, there is no definite cessation of fertility associated with aging. Spermatogenesis begins to decline during the fourth decade but continues into the ninth. The changes in reproductive structure and function, however, do not affect libido. Less frequent sexual activity results from illness, death of a sexual partner, decreased socialization, or loss of sexual interest.

Urinary System. Hypertrophy of the prostate gland sometimes develops in older men. This hypertrophy enlarges the gland and displaces pressure on the neck of the bladder. As a result, urinary retention, frequency, incontinence, and urinary tract infections occur. In addition, prostatic hypertrophy results in difficulty initiating voiding and maintaining a urinary stream. Benign prostatic hypertrophy is different from cancer of the prostate. Cancer of the prostate is the second most common cause of cancer death in men over age 50. Approximately 75% of prostate cancers are diagnosed in men over age 65, with 90% of prostate cancer deaths occurring in this age-group (American Cancer Society, 2006).

Urinary incontinence is an abnormal condition for both older men and women, although it affects women more than men (2:1) until age 80, after which they are equally affected (Flaherty, Fulmer, and Mezey, 2003). Older women, particularly those who have had children, experience stress incontinence, an involuntary release of urine that occurs when they cough, sneeze, or lift an object. This is a result of a weakening of the perineal and bladder muscles. Other types of urinary incontinence are urge, overflow, functional, and mixed incontinence. The risk factors for urinary incontinence include age, menopause, diabetes, hysterectomy, stroke, and obesity.

Musculoskeletal System. With aging, muscle fibers become smaller. Muscle strength diminishes in proportion to the decline in muscle mass. Bone mass also declines. Older adults who exercise regularly do not lose as much bone and muscle mass or muscle tone as those who are inactive. Osteoporosis is a major public health threat for an estimated 44 million Americans, or 55% of people age 55 and older. According to estimates, 10 million already have the disease: 8 million are women and 2 million are men. The remaining 34 million have low bone mass, placing them at a higher risk for developing osteoporosis (National Osteoporosis Foundation, 2006). Postmenopausal women experience a greater rate of bone demineralization than older men. Women who maintain calcium intake throughout life and into menopause have less bone demineralization than women with low calcium intake. Older men with poor nutrition and decreased mobility are also at risk for bone demineralization.

Neurological System. There is a decrease in the number and size of neurons in the nervous system that begins in the middle of the second decade. The function of neurotransmitters, chemical substances that enhance or inhibit nerve impulse transmission, also changes with aging due to the decrease in neurons. All voluntary reflexes are slower, and individuals often have less of an ability to respond to multiple stimuli. In addition, older adults frequently report alterations in the quality and the quantity of sleep (see Chapter 42). Reports include difficulty falling asleep, difficulty staying asleep, difficulty falling asleep again after waking during the night, waking too early in the morning, and excessive daytime napping. These problems are due to age-related changes in the sleep-wake cycle.

Functional Changes

Function in older adults includes the physical, psychological, cognitive, and social domains, but the declining function that can occur with aging is usually linked to illness or disease and its degree of chronicity. However, ultimately it is the complex relationship among all of the above areas that influences an older adult's functional abilities and overall well-being.

Keep in mind that it is difficult for the older adult to accept the changes that occur in all the areas of one's life, which in turn have a profound effect on function. Some deny the changes and continue to expect the same performance from themselves regardless of age. Conversely, some overemphasize them and then prematurely limit their activities and involvement in life. Also, the fear of becoming dependent is an overwhelming one for the older adult who is experiencing functional decline as a result of aging. Educate older adults to promote understanding of age-related changes, appropriate lifestyle adjustments, and effective coping. Factors that promote the highest level of function in all the areas include a healthy, well-balanced diet; paced and appropriate activity; regularly scheduled visits with a health care provider; regular participation in meaningful activities; use of stress management techniques; and avoidance of alcohol, tobacco, or illicit drugs.

Ordinarily functional status in older adults refers to the capacity and safe performance of ADLs and is a sensitive indicator of health or illness in the older adult. ADLs are essential to independent living, so carefully assess whether or not the older adult has changed the way he or she completes these tasks. In fact, a sudden change in function, as evidenced by a decline or change in the older adult's ability to perform any one or combination of ADLs often is a sign of the onset of an acute illness or worsening of a chronic problem (Kresevic and Mezey, 2003). Pneumonia, urinary tract infection, dehydration, electrolyte disturbances, and delirium are examples of acute illnesses that may present as a change in function. Worsening of diabetes, cardiovascular disease, or chronic lung disease are examples of chronic conditions that can also present as a change in function.

A variety of health care providers in a range of different settings are able to perform functional assessment. Several standardized functional assessment tools are widely available, and there is an online collection of tools at www.geronurseonline.org for samples of those most commonly used with older adults. When you identify a decline in function, focus nursing interventions on main-

✳ **TABLE 14-2** Comparison of the Clinical Features of Delirium, Dementia, and Depression

Clinical Feature	Delirium	Dementia	Depression
Onset	Sudden/abrupt; depends on cause; often at twilight or in darkness	Insidious/slow and often unrecognized; depends on cause	Happens with major life changes; often abrupt, but can be gradual
Course	Short, daily fluctuations in symptoms; worse at night, in darkness, and on awakening	Long, no diurnal effects; symptoms progressive yet relatively stable over time; some deficits with increased stress	Diurnal effects, typically worse in the morning; situational fluctuations, but less than with delirium
Progression	Abrupt	Slow but uneven	Variable; rapid or slow but even
Duration	Hours to less than 1 month; seldom longer	Months to years	At least 6 weeks; sometimes several months to years
Consciousness	Reduced	Clear	Clear
Alertness	Fluctuates; lethargic or hypervigilant	Generally normal	Normal
Attention	Impaired; fluctuates	Generally normal	Minimal impairment, but is easily distractible
Orientation	Generally impaired; severity varies	Generally normal	Selective disorientation
Memory	Recent and immediate impaired	Recent and remote impaired	Selective or "patchy" impairment; "islands" of intact memory; evaluation often difficult due to low motivation
Thinking	Disorganized, distorted, fragmented; incoherent speech, either slow or accelerated	Difficulty with abstraction; thoughts diminished; judgment impaired; words difficult to find	Intact but with themes of hopelessness, helplessness, or self-deprecation
Perception	Distorted, illusions, delusions, and hallucinations; difficulty distinguishing between reality and misperceptions	Misperceptions usually absent	Intact; delusions and hallucinations absent except in severe cases
Psychomotor behavior	Variable; hypokinetic, hyperkinetic, and mixed	Normal; some have apraxia	Variable; psychomotor retardation or agitation
Sleep/wake cycle	Disturbed; cycle reversed	Fragmented	Disturbed; usually early morning awakening
Associated features	Variable affective changes; symptoms of autonomic hyperarousal; exaggeration of personality type; associated with acute physical illness	Affect tends to be superficial, inappropriate, and labile (changing); attempts to hide deficits in intellect; personality changes, aphasia, agnosia sometimes present; lacks insight	Affect depressed; dysphoric mood; exaggerated and detailed complaints; preoccupied with personal thoughts; insight present; verbal elaboration; somatic complaints, poor hygiene, and neglect of self
Assessment	Distracted from task; numerous errors	Failings highlighted by family, frequent "near miss" answers; struggles with test; great effort to find an appropriate reply; frequent requests for feedback on performance	Failings highlighted by individual, frequent "don't knows"; little effort; frequently gives up; indifferent toward test; does not care or attempt to find answer

From Foreman M and others: Assessing cognitive function. In Mezey M, Fulmer T, Abraham I, editors: *Geriatric nursing protocols for best practice*, ed 2, New York, 2003, Springer. Used by permission of Springer Publishing Company, LLC, New York, New York, 10036.

taining, restoring, and maximizing the older adult's functional status to maintain independence while preserving dignity.

Cognitive Changes

A common misconception about aging is that cognitive impairments are widespread among older adults. Because of this misconception, older adults often fear that they are, or soon will be, cognitively impaired. Younger adults often assume that older adults are confused and no longer able to handle their affairs. Understand that forgetfulness as an expected consequence of aging is a myth. Some structural and physiological changes within the brain associated with cognitive impairment, such as reduction in the number of cells, deposition of lipofuscin and amyloid in cells, and changes in neurotransmitter levels, occur in older adults both with and without cognitive impairment. Symptoms of cognitive impairment, such as disorientation, loss of language skills, loss of the ability to calculate, and poor judgment are not normal aging changes and require you to further investigate the underlying causes.

The three common conditions affecting cognition are **delirium, dementia,** and **depression** (Table 14-2). Distinguishing among these three conditions is challenging, but essential (Foreman and others, 2003). You need to complete a careful and thorough assessment of older adults with cognitive changes in order to distinguish among these three conditions to select appropriate nursing interventions. Appropriate nursing interventions are specific to the cause of the cognitive impairment. The use of techniques such as reality orientation, validation therapy, and reminiscence also depends on the nature of the cognitive impairment.

Delirium. Delirium, or acute confusional state, is a potentially reversible cognitive impairment that is often due to a physiological cause. Physiological causes of delirium can include electrolyte imbalances, cerebral anoxia, hypoglycemia, medications, drug effects, tumors, subdural hematomas, and cerebrovascular infection, infarction, or hemorrhage. Delirium in older adults sometimes accompanies systemic infections and is often the presenting symptom for pneumonia or urinary tract infection. Delirium is also sometimes due to environmental factors such as sensory deprivation or unfamiliar surroundings or psychosocial factors such as emotional distress or pain. Although delirium occurs in any setting, an older adult in the acute care setting is especially at risk because of predisposing factors (physiological, psychosocial, and environmental) in combination with the underlying medical condition. Dementia is an additional risk factor that greatly increases the risk for delirium.

The presence of delirium requires prompt assessment and intervention. The cognitive impairment secondary to delirium usually reverses once providers identify the cause of delirium and begin treatment, unless there has been permanent brain damage.

Dementia. Dementia is a generalized impairment of intellectual functioning that interferes with social and occupational functioning. Cognitive function deterioration leads to a decline in the ability to perform basic and instrumental activities of daily living. Unlike delirium, a gradual, progressive, irreversible cerebral dysfunction characterizes dementia. Because of the close resemblance between delirium and dementia, you need to rule out the presence of delirium whenever you suspect dementia. Bolla and Fille (2000) describe four major types of dementia: **Alzheimer's disease** (50%), diffuse Lewy body disease (DLBD) (15%), frontal-temporal dementia (15%), and vascular dementia (10%). Other causes of dementia, such as infection or trauma, account for another 10% of cases.

Nursing management of older adults with any form of dementia always considers the needs of the older adult and the needs of the family. Those needs change as the progressive nature of dementia leads to increased cognitive deterioration. In addition, you also need to consider the physical, safety, and psychosocial needs of the older adult. The older adult's family needs information and support. To meet the needs of the older adult, individualize nurs-

---

★ **BOX 14-6 Nursing Care Principles for Care of Cognitively Impaired Older Adults**

- Monitor and maintain physical health.
- Assess the person's unique manifestations of the disease as it progresses.
- Adapt method of communication (verbal and nonverbal) based on the abilities of the person.
- Modify the environment to compensate for changes in functional status.
- Facilitate independent performance of activities of daily living.
- Promote social interaction based on abilities.
- Ensure safety at all times.

---

ing care to enhance quality of life and to maximize functional performance by improving cognition, mood, and behavior. General nursing care principles for care of older adults with cognitive changes are in Box 14-6.

Depression. Older adults sometimes experience late-life depression, but it is not a normal part of aging. In fact, it is a treatable medical illness. Various estimates of its prevalence range from 10% to 15% in community-dwelling older adults; 11% to 45% among those requiring inpatient medical care; and up to 50% of nursing home residents (Flaherty and others, 2003). Older adults with dementia also experience depression. When dementia and depression occur together, the distress of the older adult and the family increases.

Psychosocial Changes

The psychosocial changes occurring during aging involve life transitions and loss. The longer people live, the more transitions they have to cope with and the more losses they experience. Life transitions, for which loss is a major component, include retirement and the associated financial changes, changes in roles and relationships, alterations in health and functional ability, changes in one's social network, and relocation. But the universal loss for older adults usually revolves around the loss of relationships through death.

It is important to assess both the nature of the psychosocial changes that occur in older adults as a result of life transitions and loss and the adaptations to the changes. During the assessment, ask how the older adult feels about self, self in relation to others, self as aging, and what coping methods and skills have been beneficial. Areas to address during the assessment include the family, intimate relationships, past and present occupation, finances, housing, social networks, activities, health and wellness, and spirituality. Specific topics related to these areas include retirement, social isolation, sexuality, housing and environment, and death.

Retirement. Many often mistakenly associate retirement with passivity and seclusion. In actuality, it is a stage of life characterized by transitions and role changes. The psychosocial stresses of retirement are usually related to role changes with spouse or within the family and to loss of the work role. There are sometimes problems related to social isolation and finances. The age of retirement varies. Retirement, which is mandatory or voluntary, occurs at a variety of ages. But whether it occurs at age 55, age 65, or age 75, retirement is one of the major turning points in life.

Preretirement planning is an important advisable task for middle-age individuals. People who plan in advance for retirement generally have a smoother transition into retirement. Preretirement planning is more than financial planning, although financial planning is important. Planning begins with consideration of the "style" of retirement desired and includes an inventory of interests, current skills, and general health. Meaningful retirement planning is critical because retirement can last for 30 or more years.

Retirement affects more individuals than the retired person. It affects spouses, adult children, and grandchildren. When the spouse is still working, the retired person faces time alone. For example, the working spouse has new ideas about the amount of participation in housework expected of the retired person. Problems develop when the plans of the retired person conflict with the work responsibilities of the working spouse. The working spouse also has expectations of the retired person that need clarification. For couples, the quality of their communication with each other, their process of decision making about issues such as money or activities, their adherence to either traditional or shared role orientations, and their level of affection and intimacy all affect their adjustment to retirement (Ebersole and others, 2004). Adult children often expect the retired person to become an automatic babysitter for the grandchildren.

Loss of the work role has a major impact on some retired persons. When so much of life has revolved around work and the personal relationships at work, for many the loss of the work role is devastating. Personal identity is often rooted in the work role, and with retirement individuals need to construct a new identity. Individuals also lose the structure imposed on daily life when they no longer have a work schedule. The social exchanges and interpersonal support that occur in the workplace are lost. In the adjustment to retirement the older adult has to develop a personally meaningful schedule and a supportive social network.

The most powerful factors that influence the retired person's satisfaction with life are health status, the option to continue working, and sufficient income (Ebersole and others, 2004). Positive preretirement expectations also contribute to satisfaction in retirement. You are able to help the older adult and family prepare for retirement by discussing with them several key areas. This includes relations with spouse and children, meaningful activities to replace the work role, adjusting or rebuilding social networks, issues related to income and health promotion and maintenance, and long-range planning, including wills and advance directives.

Social Isolation. Many older adults experience social isolation, and the degree of isolation experienced increases with age. There are two forms of isolation. Isolation is sometimes a choice, the result of a desire not to interact with others. Isolation is also sometimes a response to conditions that inhibit the ability or the opportunity to interact with others (Ebersole and others, 2004). Although some older adults choose isolation or a lifelong pattern of reduced interaction with others, other older adults do not choose isolation but are vulnerable to its consequences.

The vulnerability of older adults to isolation increases in the absence of the support of other adults, as occurs with loss of the work role or relocation to unfamiliar surroundings. Impaired hearing, diminished vision, and reduced mobility (e.g., impaired ambulation, inability to use assistive devices independently, or loss of ability to drive) all contribute to reduced interaction with others and thus place the older adult at risk for isolation. The loss of the ability to drive also limits older adults' ability to live independently and can contribute to isolation.

Some older adults withdraw from social interaction because of feelings of rejection (Ebersole and others, 2004). Societal attitudes about aging as unattractive lead to feelings of rejection for some older adults. These older adults see themselves as unattractive and rejected because of changes in their personal appearance due to normal aging changes or because of body image changes following illness or surgery. Society, including health care professionals, also considers some behaviors and situations to be unacceptable. Older adults who are confused or incontinent, who are unable to communicate, who are institutionalized, or who are poor or homeless are examples of older adults who are possibly isolated by society. The societal trend toward the geographic dispersion of families leads to decreased opportunities for interaction among family members. Some older adults consider this rejection by their families.

You can assist lonely older adults with rebuilding social networks and reversing patterns of isolation (Ebersole and others, 2005). Many communities have outreach programs designed to make contact with isolated older adults. Outreach programs sometimes meet nutritional needs, such as Meals on Wheels. Outreach programs also meet socialization needs, such as daily telephone calls by volunteers, or needs for activities, such as outings. Social service agencies in most communities welcome older adults as volunteers and provide the opportunity for older adults to serve while meeting their socialization or other needs. Other organizations within communities such as churches, colleges, community centers, and libraries offer a variety of programs for older adults that increase the opportunity to meet people with similar activities, interests, and needs.

Sexuality. Sexuality is increasingly recognized as an important factor in the care of older adults. All older adults, whether healthy or frail, need to express sexual feelings. Sexuality involves love, warmth, sharing, and touching, not just the act of intercourse. Sexuality is linked with identity and validates the belief that people are able to give to others and have the gift appreciated. Retirement often affects self-esteem, and sexuality plays an important role in helping the older adult maintain self-esteem.

Maintaining sexual health requires integration of somatic, emotional, intellectual, and social aspects of the sexual being. To help the older adult achieve or maintain sexual health, the nurse needs to understand the physical changes in sexual response (see Chapter 28). You need to provide privacy for any discussion of sexuality and maintain a nonjudgmental attitude. Open-ended questions inviting the older adult to explain sexual activities or concerns will elicit more information than a list of closed-ended questions about specific activities or symptoms. Older adults often appreciate information about the typical age-related changes in sexuality. Include information about the prevention of sexually transmitted diseases when appropriate.

The older adult's libido does not decrease, although frequency of sexual activity usually declines. An older woman who does not understand physical changes affecting sexual activity may be concerned that her sex life is nearly over with the onset of menopause. The older man may feel the same when he discovers a change in the firmness of his erection, a decreased need for ejaculation with each orgasm, or a longer recovery period between episodes of intercourse.

In addition to the physical changes that affect sexual functioning, many older adults use prescription medications that depress sexual activity such as antihypertensives, antidepressants, sedatives, or hypnotics. Some drugs increase libido in older adults. For example, phenothiazines increase sexual desire in women, and levodopa has a similar effect in men.

While considering the older adult's need for sexual expression, do not ignore the important need to touch and be touched. Touch is an overt expression with many meanings and is an important part of intimacy. Touch complements traditional sexual methods or serves as an alternative sexual expression when physical intercourse is not desired or possible. Touch serves as an important method of achieving intimacy (Atkinson, 2006). Recognize that knowledge of and comfort with older adults' sexual and intimacy needs will increase with professional growth. Experience in caring for older adults combined with the ability to establish therapeutic connection allows you to learn how to explore clients' sexual concerns. Knowing an older adult's sexual needs allows the nurse to incorporate this information into the nursing care plan.

The sexual preferences of older adults are as diverse as those of the younger population. Clearly, not all older adults are heterosexual, yet little information is available regarding older adult homosexuals and their health care needs. Kanapaux (2003) reported on the barriers and challenges that nurses need to address when treating lesbians and gay men. There is a fear of having to rely for health care on networks and social institutions that have no tolerance for them, and this is particularly difficult for older adults. The discrimination that homosexuals feel keeps them from telling providers their sexual orientation. To be effective caregivers for older homosexuals, be aware of your own beliefs about sexuality and the potential impact of those beliefs on your ability to provide care. Improving communication and creating open and supportive environments of care are necessary to promote successful, healthy aging for this growing population.

Nurses often find that they are called on to help other health care professionals understand the sexual needs of older adults, as well as advise older adults. Not all nurses feel comfortable counseling older adults about sexual health and intimacy-related needs. You need to be prepared to refer older adults to appropriate professional counselors.

Housing and Environment. The extent of the older adult's ability to live independently strongly determines housing choices. Changes in social roles, family responsibilities, and health status influence older adults' living arrangements. Some choose to live with family members. Others prefer their own homes or other housing options near their families. Leisure or retirement communities provide older people with living and social opportunities in a one-generation setting. Federally subsidized housing, where available, offers apartments with communal, social, and, in some cases, food service arrangements.

When assisting older adults with housing needs, assess their activity level, financial status, access to public transportation and community activities, environmental hazards, and support systems. When helping clients consider housing choices anticipate their future needs as much as possible. For example, a housing unit with only one floor and without exterior steps is a prudent choice for the older adult with severe arthritis who has already had lower extremity joint replacement surgery and anticipates the need for future operations.

Housing and environment have a major impact on the health of older adults. The environment either supports or hinders physical and social functioning, enhances or drains energy, and complements or taxes existing physical changes such as vision and hearing. For example, the colors red, orange, and yellow are easiest for older adults to see. In contrast, older adults have difficulty distinguishing between green and blue and among pastel shades. To help older adults in health care settings find their rooms, use pictures or other decorations near their doors as landmarks. Door frames and baseboards in a color that contrasts with the color of the wall improve perception of the boundaries of halls and rooms. Glare from highly polished floors, metallic fixtures, and windows is difficult for the older adult to tolerate.

Furniture needs to be comfortable and designed for the musculoskeletal changes of older adults. Older adults need to examine furniture carefully for size, comfort, and function before purchasing it. Furniture needs to be easy to get into and out of and provide back support. Test dining room chairs for comfort during meals and for height in relation to the table. Older adults often prefer transferring out of a wheelchair to another chair for meals because some styles of wheelchairs do not let older adults sit close enough to the table to eat comfortably. Raising the table to clear the wheelchair arms will bring the table closer to the older adult but will make it too high for comfortable use. To make getting out of bed easier and safer, the height of the bed needs to allow the older adult's feet to be flat on the floor when the older adult is sitting on the side of the bed.

The goal of nursing assessment of the environment is the promotion of independence and functional ability. Assessment of safety, a major component of the older adult's environment, includes risks within the environment and the older adult's ability to recognize and respond to the risks (see Chapter 38). Safety risks include factors leading to injury within the home, such as water heaters set at excessively hot temperatures or throw rugs that could cause a fall, and factors outside of the home, such as deteriorating sidewalks and steps or a high incidence of street crime.

Death.   Part of the life history of an older adult is the experience of loss through the death of relatives and friends (see Chapter 30). This includes the experience of the loss of the older generations of their families and sometimes, sadly, the loss of a child. However, death of a spouse is the loss that affects the lives of most older people. The death of a spouse affects more older women than men, a trend that will probably continue in the future. In spite of these experiences, it is wrong to assume that the older adult is comfortable with the idea of death. A key role of the nurse is supporting older adults in coping with these losses and facilitating adjustment to the life changes imposed by them.

Older people have a wide variety of attitudes and beliefs about death, but fear of their own death is uncommon (Friedman, 2006). The larger concerns of older adults about death concern issues such as fear of being a burden, experiencing suffering, being alone, and the use of life-prolonging measures. The stereotype that the death of an older adult is a blessing does not apply to every older adult. Even as death approaches, many older adults still have unfinished business and are not prepared to die. Families and friends are not always ready to let go of the older adult. The nurse is often the person to whom the older adult and family members or friends turn to for assistance in coping with death and loss. Knowledge of the grieving process, excellent communication skills, understanding of the legal issues, familiarity with community resources, and awareness of one's own feelings, limitations, and strengths as they relate to care of those confronting death is critical.

Addressing the Health Concerns of Older Adults

The three most common causes of death in adults age 65 and over are heart disease, cancer, and cerebrovascular diseases (Centers for Disease Control and Prevention [CDC], 2005). Other frequently reported causes of death are lung disease, accidents/falls, diabetes, kidney disease, and liver disease. All of these causes of death have preventive measures that potentially reduce the frequency of these conditions and delay disability and/or death.

As the population ages and life expectancy increases, there is greater emphasis on health promotion and disease prevention (see Chapter 6). Furthermore, the number of older adults becoming enthusiastic and motivated about these aspects of care is increasing. A number of national programs and projects address preventive practices in the older adult population. One of these, the national initiative *Healthy People 2010,* has two major goals: increase quality and years of healthy life and eliminate health disparity (U.S. Department of Health and Human Services, Public Health Service, 2000). A number of aging-focused organizations are participating in the *Healthy People 2010* initiative by using it as a planning and evaluation tool for older adult health programs and services. For the near future, agencies that serve older adults will continue to collaborate in such efforts to promote health and prevent disease.

The challenges that continue to affect older adults' involvement in these activities are complex and include health care providers as well. For the older adult, previous health care experiences, personal motivation, health beliefs, and culture, as well as non–health-related factors such as transportation and finances, can create barriers to participation. Barriers for providers include beliefs and attitudes about what services and programs to provide and their effectiveness and the lack of consistent guidelines and a coordinated approach (Resnick, 2006).

The nurse's role in health promotion and disease prevention focuses on maintaining and promoting function. Locate where groups of older adults congregate and volunteer to speak about any number of topics, for example, physical fitness, nutrition, safe medication use, home safety, or breast self-examination. Participate in activities such as health screenings and fairs that identify older adults at risk, and advise them about preventive measures (Davidhizar, Eshlernan, and Moody, 2002). Nurses in acute care and long-term care settings also assess the health status of older adults, intervene in acute situations, and, with the older adults, plan strategies to reduce risk and manage chronic conditions. Each contact with an older adult, regardless of setting, offers opportunities to teach and counsel. To be most effective, use an individualized approach to health promotion activities with older adults (Resnick, 2003).

Direct nursing interventions for older adults toward improving or maintaining the older adults' health needs and addressing their concerns. Although various interventions cross all three levels of care, health promotion, acute care, and restorative care, there are approaches unique to each level. When planning interventions, it is important to incorporate the older adult's routines or rituals when possible because the older adult feels more secure with routines. You generally aim the interventions at promoting independence and supporting self-care abilities.

Health Promotion and Maintenance: Physiological Concerns

Older adults, like persons of any age, vary in their desire to participate in health promotion activities, so use an individualized approach, taking into account the person's beliefs about the importance of staying healthy and fit and remaining independent. Researchers have not fully identified the factors that lead to good health in advanced age, but four important factors seem to be genetics, luck, good health habits, and preventive measures. You are unable to do anything about an older adult's genetic heritage or luck, but you will be in a unique position to develop programs that promote older adults' wellness and to recommend preventive measures. Senior citizens' centers, churches, schools, shopping malls, libraries, and hospital lobbies are settings where you will conduct screening tests and present information on health topics. Use creative approaches to incorporate health promotion activities in all health care settings.

Approximately 80% of adults over age 65 have at least one chronic health condition, and 50% have at least two chronic conditions (CDC, 2003). The effect of chronic conditions on the lives of older adults varies widely, but, in general, chronic conditions diminish the well-being and threaten the independence of older adults. Direct nursing interventions at the management of these conditions, but also focus interventions on prevention. General preventive measures for you to recommend to older adults include the following:

- Participation in screening activities (e.g., blood pressure, mammography, depression, vision and hearing testing, colonoscopy)
- Regular exercise
- Weight reduction if overweight
- Eating a low-fat, well-balanced diet

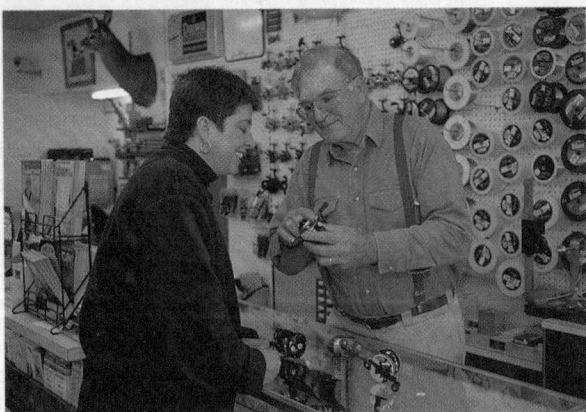

Figure 14-1 This older adult works part-time at a sporting goods store.

- Regular dental visits
- Smoking cessation
- Immunization for influenza, pneumococcal pneumonia, and tetanus

Approximately 95% of the estimated 20,000 to 40,000 deaths per year in the United States from influenza occur among adults age 65 and older (Regan and Fowler, 2002). Providers strongly recommend annual immunization for influenza of all older adults with special emphasis on residents of nursing homes, residential, or long-term care facilities (Reuben and others, 2005). Providers also recommend the pneumococcal pneumonia vaccine for all adults at age 65. The Centers for Disease Control and Prevention recommends persons age 65 years and older receive a second dose of pneumococcal vaccine if they received the vaccine more than 5 years previously and were younger than age 65 at the time of the first dose. For tetanus immunization, providers recommend booster injections every 10 years for adults who have had the primary series for tetanus immunization. However, not all older adults are current with their booster injections and some never received the primary series of injections. Ask older adults about the current status of all three types of immunizations, provide information about the immunizations, and make arrangements for the older adult to receive the immunizations as needed.

Most older adults are interested in their health and are capable of taking charge of their lives. They want to remain independent and to prevent disability (Figure 14-1).

Initial screenings establish baseline data that you will use to determine wellness, identify health needs, and design health maintenance programs. Following initial screening sessions, share with older adults information on nutrition, exercise, medications, and safety precautions. You can also provide information on specific conditions such as hypertension or arthritis or on self-care procedures such as foot and skin care. By providing information about health promotion and self-care, you will significantly improve the health and well-being of older adults.

Heart Disease. Heart disease is the leading cause of death in older adults. Common cardiovascular disorders are hypertension and coronary artery disease. Hypertension is diagnosed when re-

peated blood pressure measurements of 90 mm Hg or greater diastolic and 140 mm Hg or greater systolic are present. Although over 50% of Americans have elevated diastolic and/or systolic pressures, the fact that hypertension is common does not make it normal or harmless. Treatment of systolic pressures 160 mm Hg or higher are linked to reduced incidence of myocardial infarction, stroke, and heart failure (Beers, 2005). In coronary artery disease, partial or complete blockage of one or more coronary arteries leads to myocardial ischemia and myocardial infarction. The risk factors for both hypertension and coronary artery disease include smoking, obesity, lack of exercise, and stress. Additional risk factors for coronary artery disease include hypertension, hyperlipidemia, and diabetes mellitus.

Nursing interventions for hypertension and coronary artery disease address weight reduction, exercise, dietary changes limiting salt and fat, stress management, and smoking cessation. Client teaching includes information about medications, blood pressure monitoring, nutrition, stress reduction techniques, and the symptoms indicating the need for emergency care.

Cancer. Malignant neoplasms are the second most common cause of death among older adults. Nurses participate in programs to educate older adults about early detection, treatment, and risk factors. Examples include smoking cessation, teaching breast self-examination (see Chapter 33), and encouraging all older adults to have annual screening for fecal occult blood. It is also important to educate older adults about the signs of cancer and encourage prompt reporting of nonhealing skin lesions, unexpected bleeding, change in bowel habits, and unexplained weight loss. Cancer is difficult to detect because providers often mistake symptoms as part of the normal aging process. You need to carefully distinguish between signs of normal aging and signs of pathological conditions.

Stroke (Cerebrovascular Accident). Cerebrovascular accidents, the third leading cause of death in the United States, occur as brain ischemia or brain hemorrhage (Beers, 2005). In brain ischemia there is an inadequate supply of blood to areas of the brain due to blockage of blood vessels or general circulatory failure. Brain hemorrhage, either subarachnoid hemorrhage or intracerebral hemorrhage, is less common than brain ischemia. Risk factors for cerebrovascular accidents include hypertension, hyperlipidemia, diabetes mellitus, history of transient ischemic attacks, and family history of cardiovascular disease. Treatment usually includes hospitalization for days or months, depending on the degree of brain damage. Cerebrovascular accidents often impair the functional abilities of older adults and thus limit their ability to live independently. The scope of nursing interventions ranges from teaching older adults about risk reduction strategies to care of the older adult after a cerebrovascular accident and during recovery and rehabilitation.

Smoking. Cigarette smoking is a risk factor in the four most common causes of death: heart disease, cancer, stroke, and lung disease. Smoking cessation is a health promotion strategy for older adults just as it is for younger adults. Older smokers still benefit from smoking cessation (Flaherty and others, 2003). In addition to reducing risk, smoking cessation sometimes stabilizes existing conditions such as chronic obstructive pulmonary disease (COPD) and coronary artery disease. Smoking cessation even contributes to the extension of life or of independent functioning.

There are four sequential approaches to encourage smoking cessation, referred to as the "Four A's" (Flaherty and others, 2003). First, *ask* the older adult about smoking, including the type of tobacco product used, the frequency of smoking, and the number of years smoking. Then, *advise* quitting. It is useful at this time to provide information about the ill effects of smoking and the benefits of quitting. Next, *assist* the older adult with quitting by developing a plan to do so. Suggest various strategies such as the use of gum containing nicotine or nicotine patches and asking family members to reduce smoking. Also consider referral to a local cessation program. If the client rejects smoking cessation, suggest a reduction in smoking. Last, *arrange* with the older adult a quit date and a follow-up visit or contact to discuss the quit attempt. At follow-up visits, offer encouragement and assistance in modifying the plan as necessary. Although some mistakenly believe that older adults do not want to quit smoking or are unable to quit, some older adults do choose to quit smoking and do succeed.

Alcohol Abuse. Community-based epidemiological studies estimate that 10% to 22% of older adults are daily drinkers (Flaherty and others, 2003). Studies of alcohol abuse in older adults report two patterns: a lifelong pattern of heavy drinking that continues and a late-onset pattern when heavy drinking begins late in life. Frequently cited causes of excessive alcohol use are depression, loneliness, and lack of social support.

Many believe that abuse of alcohol is underidentified in older adults (Ebersole and others, 2005). The clues to create suspicion of alcohol abuse are subtle, and coexisting dementia or depression sometimes complicates the assessment of alcohol abuse. Suspicion of alcohol abuse increases when there is a history of repeated falls and accidents, social isolation, recurring episodes of memory loss and confusion, failure to meet home and work obligations, a history of skipping meals or medications, and difficulty managing household tasks and finances. When you suspect abuse of alcohol in the older adult, realize that a variety of treatment needs are present. Treatment includes age-specific approaches that acknowledge the stresses experienced by the older adult and encourage involvement in activities that match the older adult's interests and increase feelings of self-worth. The identification and treatment of coexisting depression is also important. The continuum of interventions range from simple education to formalized treatment programs that include pharmacotherapy, psychotherapy, and rehabilitation.

Nutrition. Lifelong eating habits and situational factors influence how older adults meet their needs for good nutrition. Lifelong eating habits based in tradition, ethnicity, and religion influence the choice of what foods are eaten and how those foods are prepared. Situational factors affecting nutrition include access to grocery stores, finances, the physical and cognitive capability for food preparation, and a place to store food and prepare meals.

Older adults' levels of activity and clinical conditions affect their nutritional needs. Level of activity has implications for the total amount of calories. More sedentary older adults usually need fewer calories than more active older adults. However, activity does not solely determine caloric requirements. Additional calories are often necessary in clinical situations such as recovery from surgery, whereas less calories are necessary when the older adult is diabetic or overweight. Beyond caloric requirements, therapeutic diets restrict fat, sodium, or simple sugars or increase fiber or foods high in calcium, iron, vitamin A, or vitamin C.

Good nutrition for older adults includes appropriate caloric intake and limited intake of fat, salt, refined sugars, and alcohol. Although the nutritional guidelines displayed in the food guide pyramid (see Chapter 44) are the basic recommendations for older adult nutrition, some older adults do not follow these guidelines. Protein intake is sometimes lower than recommended if older adults have reduced financial resources or limited access to grocery stores. Difficulty chewing meat due to poor dentition or poor-fitting dentures also limits protein intake. Fat intake is higher than usual because of the substitution of fast-food restaurant meals for meals prepared at home or because of methods of cooking featuring fried foods and sauces using butter and cream. Some use extra salt and sugar while cooking or at the table to compensate for a diminished sense of taste. Some have reduced vitamin intake because shopping for fresh fruits and vegetables is difficult.

Older adults with dementia have special nutritional needs. As their memory and functional skills decline with the progression of dementia, they lose the ability to remember when to eat, how to prepare food, and eventually how to feed themselves. At the same time their caloric needs increase because of the energy expended in pacing and wandering activities. When caring for older adults with dementia, routinely monitor weight and food intake, serve food that is easy to eat, provide assistance with eating, and offer food supplements as needed to maintain weight (Amella, 2003). Mealtime interventions for older adults with dementia also provide opportunities for socialization and practice with functional skills.

Dental Problems. Dental problems with natural teeth and dentures are common in older adults. Dental caries, gingivitis, broken or missing teeth, and ill-fitting or missing dentures affect nutritional adequacy, cause pain, and lead to infection. Help prevent dental and gum disease through education about routine dental care (see Chapter 39). You will also help older adults find dental services that offer reduced rates and that are accessible to those with impaired mobility.

Exercise. Encourage older adults to maintain physical exercise and activity. The primary benefits of exercise include maintaining and strengthening functional ability and promoting a sense of enhanced well-being. An exercise such as walking builds endurance, increases muscle tone, improves joint flexibility, strengthens bones, reduces stress, and contributes to weight loss. Other benefits of a program of exercise include improvement of cardiovascular function, improved plasma lipoprotein profiles, increased metabolic rate, increased gastrointestinal transit time, reduction of fall-related injuries, prevention of depressive illness, and improved sleep quality. Frail older adults who exercise sometimes experience improved mobility, gait, and balance plus less difficulty getting up from a chair or climbing stairs. Exercise also substantially delays the onset of functional impairment and loss of independence.

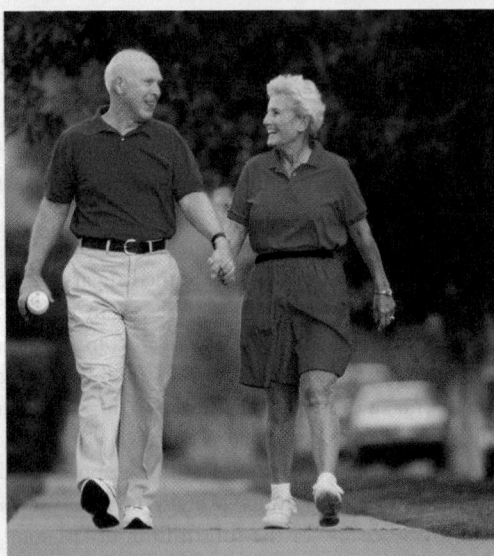

Figure 14-2 This couple enjoys walking together.

Plan an exercise program that meets physical needs while considering physical limitations, and encourage the older adult to stick with the exercise program. Many factors influence an individual's willingness to participate in an exercise program. These include general beliefs about exercise, specific benefits from exercise, past experiences with exercise, personal goals, personality, and any unpleasant sensations associated with exercise.

Walking is the preferred exercise of many older adults (Figure 14-2). Walking and other low-impact exercises such as riding a stationary exercise bicycle or water exercises in a swimming pool protect the musculoskeletal system and joints. There are other exercises you can include in the older adult's activities of daily living. For example, adults can perform arm and leg circles while watching television. But before beginning an exercise program, the older adult needs to have a physical examination. Exercise programs for sedentary older adults who have not been exercising regularly need to begin conservatively and progress slowly. Safety considerations include wearing shoes and clothing appropriate to the exercise, drinking water before and after exercising, avoiding outdoor exercise when the weather is very warm or very cold, and exercising with a partner. Instruct older adults to stop exercising and seek help if they experience chest pain or tightness, shortness of breath, dizziness or light-headedness, joint pain, or palpitations during exercise.

Arthritis. Arthritis, which primarily affects the weight-bearing joints, is a common condition in older adults, especially in women. How much mobility older adults have depends on the extent of the disease and joints affected. The impact of arthritis on the lives of older adults is a combination of the changes in joint range of motion and stability and the amount of pain experienced. Arthritis has no cure, but recently developed pharmacological agents decrease pain and swelling and therefore increase joint motion. Aim your nursing interventions at promoting comfort, functional ability, and safety. Education about self-care techniques, joint protection, and exercises for flexibility and strength is also important.

Falls. Falls are a safety concern of many older adults. Falls lead to fear of additional falls, withdrawal from usual activities, and loss of independence (see Chapters 38 and 47). Hospitalization and placement in a nursing home for rehabilitation or long-term placement is sometimes necessary. Falls increase with advancing age and vary according to the older person's living situation. Researchers estimate that between 30% and 40% of older adults who live independently in their own homes will fall each year (Flaherty and others, 2003).

Among older adults, complications from falls are the leading cause of death. In 2004 nearly 15,000 people age 65 and older died from fall-related injuries; nearly 85% of deaths from falls were among people 75 and older (CDC, 2006). In 2003 more than 1.8 million adults age 65 and older were treated in emergency departments for fall-related injuries, and more than 421,000 were hospitalized (CDC, 2006). Falls are more frequent and more serious for older adults over age 85.

The risk factors leading to falls are a combination of health-related issues and environmental hazards (Tideiksaar, 1998). Health-related issues include the following:

- Impaired vision
- Cardiovascular conditions such as postural hypotension or syncope
- Conditions affecting mobility such as arthritis, muscle weakness, and foot problems
- Conditions affecting balance
- Alterations in bladder function such as frequency or incontinence
- Cognitive impairment
- Adverse medication reactions
  Environmental hazards include the following:
- Poor lighting
- Slippery or wet floors
- Stairs or sidewalks in poor repair
- Shoes in poor repair or with slippery soles
- Household items that are easy to trip over, such as throw rugs, foot stools, and electric extension cords

Direct nursing interventions toward the management of health-related conditions that increase fall risk and the reduction of environmental hazards. Instruct older adults taking medications with adverse effects such as postural hypotension, dizziness, or sedation to be aware of these potential effects and to take precautions such as changing position slowly or ambulating with assistance if unsteady. Simple interventions in the home such as rearranging furniture to provide a clear pathway to the bathroom and providing a night-light in the bathroom reduce falls related to nighttime trips to the toilet. Picking up throw rugs and other items on the floor reduces slipping and tripping. Also, instruct older adults in the safe use of assistive devices such as canes, walkers, and wheelchairs. For those older adults in whom falls cannot be prevented, the goals are fall reduction through modification of risk factors and prevention of serious injury.

Sensory Impairments. The older adult usually has changes in vision, hearing, taste, and smell that are a result of normal aging. Chapter 49 describes in detail the nursing interventions used to maintain and improve sensory function.

Pain. Although pain is not a normal part of healthy aging, persistent physical pain is a significant problem for many older adults. Researchers estimate that 50% of community-dwelling older adults experience pain (Herr, 2002). In nursing homes, 70% to 80% of residents have persistent, untreated pain (American Geriatric Society [AGS], 2002). The causes of pain in older adults include acute (e.g., cancer and surgical procedures) and chronic conditions (e.g., trauma, infection, and neuropathies). The consequences of persistent pain include depression, sleep difficulties, changes in gait and mobility, and decreased socialization. Many factors influence the management of pain, including cultural influences on the meaning and expression of pain for older adults, fears related to the use of analgesic medications, and the problem of pain assessment with cognitively impaired older adults. Nurses caring for older adults have to advocate for appropriate and effective pain management and to use standardized pain tools in their assessments (see Chapter 43). Again, the goal of nursing management of pain in older adults is to maximize function and improve quality of life.

Medication Use. One of the greatest challenges of the nurse caring for older adults is ensuring safe medication use. Approximately two thirds of older adults use prescription and nonprescription drugs, and one third of all prescriptions written are for older adults (Beers, 2000). The most commonly used medications by the community-dwelling are analgesics, diuretics, cardiovascular drugs, and sedative-hypnotics. Drugs most often used by nursing home residents are antipsychotics and sedative-hypnotics, followed by diuretics, antihypertensives, analgesics, cardiovascular drugs, and antibiotics (Beers, 2000). Polypharmacy, the concurrent use of many medications, increases the risk for an adverse drug effect, which is an unintended response to a drug. Although polypharmacy reflects inappropriate prescribing, the concurrent use of multiple medications is necessary in situations where an older adult has multiple acute and chronic conditions. However, periodic and thorough review of all medications is important to restrict the number of medications used to the fewest necessary. The nurse's role with an older adult undergoing drug therapy is to ensure the greatest therapeutic benefit with the least amount of harm.

Older adults are at risk for adverse drug effects because of age-related changes in the absorption, distribution, metabolism, and excretion of drugs, collectively referred to as the process of pharmacokinetics (see Chapter 35). Medications sometimes interact with one another, adding or negating the effect of another drug. Medications also cause confusion; affect balance and mobility; cause dizziness, nausea, and vomiting; or lead to constipation, urinary frequency, or incontinence. Because of these effects, some older adults are unwilling to take medications; others do not adhere to the prescribed dosing schedule.

Managing medications is a very important component of maintaining and promoting good health in old age. For some older adults on large numbers of medications, safely managing medications is a complex activity that easily becomes overwhelming. Complicating the assessment of medication effects and side effects, some older adults take their medications incorrectly because they do not understand the instructions about their medications. You are able to provide valuable assistance to your older adult clients as they carry out this important self-care activity.

Work collaboratively with the older adult to ensure safe and appropriate use of all medications, both prescribed and over-the-counter medications. Teach the older adult the names of all drugs he or she is taking, when and how to take them, and the desirable and undesirable effects of the drugs. Also, teach the older adult how to avoid adverse effects and/or interactions of drugs and how to establish and follow an appropriate self-administration pattern. Strategies for reducing the risk for an adverse medication effects in the older adult include reviewing the medications with the older adult at each visit, examining for potential interactions with food or other drugs, simplifying and individualizing the drug regimen, taking every opportunity to inform the older adult and family about all aspects of medication use, and encouraging the older adult to question the physician, advanced practice nurse, and/or pharmacist about all prescribed drugs and all over-the-counter drugs.

When providers use drugs for the management of confusion, special care is necessary. The sedatives and tranquilizers sometimes prescribed for acutely confused older adults sometimes cause or exacerbate confusion. Carefully administer drugs used to manage confused behaviors, taking into account age-related changes in body systems that affect pharmacokinetic activity. When confusion has a physiological cause (such as an infection), specifically treat that cause, rather than the confused behavior. When confusion varies by time of day or is related to environmental factors, use creative, nonpharmacological measures such as making the environment more meaningful, providing adequate light, encouraging use of assistive devices (glasses and hearing aids), or even making telephone calls to friends or family members to let older adults hear reassuring voices.

Health Promotion and Maintenance: Psychosocial Health Concerns

Interventions supporting the psychosocial health of older adults resemble those for other age-groups. However, some interventions are more crucial for older adults experiencing social isolation, cognitive impairment, or stresses related to retirement, relocation, or approaching death. These interventions include therapeutic communication, touch, reality orientation, validation therapy, reminiscence, and interventions to improve body image.

Therapeutic Communication. The nurse using therapeutic communication perceives and respects the older adult's uniqueness and meets the older adult's expectations. Attentive nurses provide care in a timely fashion, meeting client's expressed or unexpressed needs. A caring nurse expresses attitudes of concern, kindness, and compassion. Knowledgeable nurses not only demonstrate procedural competence but recognize needs and relay information skillfully. Older adult clients also expect nurses to respect their individuality. Clients will accept and respect the nurse who meets these expectations and communicates effectively about concern for the older adult's welfare. However, you cannot simply enter an older adult's environment and immediately establish a therapeutic relationship. First you have to be knowledgeable and skilled in communication techniques (see Chapter 24).

Touch. Throughout life, touch tells us about our environment and the people around us. Gentle touch expresses affection and friendliness. A firm handshake sometimes expresses security. Touch is a therapeutic tool that you will use to help comfort older adults. A pilot study by Wang and Hermann (2006) showed that agitation levels were significantly lower in demented older adults who received a healing touch intervention. Touch provides sensory stimulation, induces relaxation, provides physical and emotional comfort, orients the person to reality, shows warmth, and communicates interest. It is a powerful physical expression of a relationship.

Older adults are often deprived of touching when separated from family or friends. An older adult who is isolated, dependent, or ill; who fears death; or who lacks self-esteem has a greater need for touch. You will recognize touch deprivation by behaviors as simple as an older adult reaching for the nurse's hand or standing close to the nurse. Unfortunately, older men are sometimes wrongly accused of sexual advances when they reach out to touch others. When you use touch, be aware of cultural variations as well as individual preferences (see Chapter 9). Touch should convey respect and sensitivity. Do not use touch in a condescending way such as patting an older adult on the head. When you reach out to an older adult, do not be surprised if the older adult reciprocates.

Reality Orientation. Reality orientation is a communication technique that makes an older adult more aware of time, place, and person. The purposes of reality orientation include restoring a sense of reality, improving the level of awareness, promoting socialization, elevating independent functioning, and minimizing confusion, disorientation, and physical regression.

Although you will use reality orientation techniques in any health care setting, they will be especially useful in the acute care setting. The older adult experiencing a change in environment, surgery, illness, or emotional stress is at risk for becoming disoriented. Environmental changes, such as the bright lights, unfamiliar noises, and lack of windows in specialized units of a hospital, often lead to disorientation and confusion. Absence of familiar caregivers is also disorienting. Using anesthesia, sedatives, tranquilizers, analgesics, and physical restraints with older clients increases disorientation. Anticipate and monitor for disorientation and confusion as possible consequences of hospitalization, relocation, surgery, loss, or illness, and incorporate interventions based on reality orientation into the care plan.

Once used as a therapy with disoriented individuals and groups of cognitively impaired individuals, the principles of reality orientation offer useful guidelines for communicating with acutely confused individuals. The key elements of reality orientation include frequent reminders of person, time, and place; the use of environmental aids such as clocks, calendars, and personal belongings; and stability of environment, routine, and staff. However, do not continue to reorient older adults with chronic cognitive impairment. Communication is always respectful, patient, and calm. You answer questions from the older adult simply and honestly with sensitivity and a caring attitude.

Validation Therapy. Validation therapy is an alternative approach to communication with a confused older adult. Where reality orientation insists that the confused older adult agree with our statements of time, place, and person, validation therapy accepts the description of time and place as stated by the confused older adult. Older adults with dementia are less likely to benefit and more likely to become agitated by the caregiver's insistence on the "correct" time, place, and person.

In validation therapy, you do not challenge or argue with statements and behaviors of the confused older adult. The statements and behaviors represent an inner need or feeling. The appropriate nursing intervention is to recognize and address that inner need or feeling. Validation does not involve reinforcing the confused older adult's misperceptions, but reflects a sensitivity to hidden meanings in statements and behaviors. By listening with sensitivity and validating what the client is expressing, you will convey respect, reassurance, and understanding. Validating or respecting confused older adults' feelings in the time and place that is real to them is more important than insisting on the literally correct time and place (Day, 1997).

Reminiscence. Reminiscence is recalling the past. Many older adults find enjoyment in sharing past experiences. As a therapy, reminiscence uses the recollection of the past to bring meaning and understanding to the present and to resolve current conflicts. Looking back to positive resolutions to problems reminds the older adult of coping strategies used successfully in the past. Reminiscing is also a way to express personal identity. Reflection on past achievements supports self-esteem. For some older adults the process of looking back on past events uncovers new meanings for those events.

During the assessment process, use reminiscence to assess self-esteem, cognitive function, emotional stability, unresolved conflicts, coping ability, and expectations for the future. For example, have a client talk about a previous loss to assess coping. You can also reminisce during direct care activities. Taking time to ask questions about past experiences and listening attentively conveys to an older adult your attitudes of respect and concern.

Although many use reminiscence in a one-on-one situation, it is also used as a group therapy for cognitively impaired or depressed older adults. The nurse organizes the group and selects strategies to start a conversation. For example, the nurse asks the group to discuss families or childhood memories. The nurse adapts the group's size, structure, process, goals, and activities to meet its members' needs.

Body-Image Interventions. The way that older adults present themselves influences body image and feelings of isolation. Some physical characteristics of older adulthood are socially desirable, such as distinguished-looking gray hair. Other features are also impressive, such as a lined face that displays character or wrinkled hands that show a lifetime of hard work. Too often, however, society sees older people as incapacitated, deaf, obese, or shrunken in stature. Consequences of illness and aging that threaten the older adult's body image include invasive diagnostic procedures, pain, surgery, loss of sensation in a body part, skin changes, loss of scalp hair, and incontinence. The use of devices such as dentures, hearing aids, artificial limbs, indwelling catheters, ostomy devices, and enteral feeding tubes also affects body image.

You need to consider the importance to the older adult of presenting a socially acceptable image. When older adults have acute or chronic illnesses, the related physical dependence makes it difficult for them to maintain body image. You influence the older adult's appearance by assisting with grooming and hygiene. It takes little effort to assist the older adult with combing hair, cleaning dentures, shaving, or changing clothing. The older adult does not choose to have an objectionable appearance. You also need to be sensitive to odors in the environment. Odors created by urine and some illnesses are often present. By controlling odors, you will possibly prevent visitors from shortening their stay or not coming at all.

Older Adults and the Acute Care Setting

Older adults in the acute care setting need special attention to help them adjust to the acute care environment and to meet their basic needs for comfort, safety, nutrition/hydration, and skin integrity. The acute care setting poses increased risk for adverse events such as delirium, dehydration, malnutrition, health care agency–acquired infections, urinary incontinence, and falls.

The risk for delirium increases when hospitalized older adults experience immobilization, sleep deprivation, infection, dehydration, pain, sensory impairment, and hypoxia. Medications, especially those that are psychoactive or have anticholinergic properties, are significant risk factors for delirium (Flaherty and others, 2003). Nonmedical causes of delirium include placement in unfamiliar surroundings, bed rest, separation from supportive family members, and stress. Impaired vision or hearing contributes to confusion and interferes with attempts to reorient the older adult. When the prevention of delirium fails, the basis of nursing management begins with identification and treatment of the cause (Box 14-7). Supportive interventions include encouraging family visits, providing memory cues (clocks, calendars, and name tags), and compensating for sensory deficits. Reality orientation techniques are also useful.

Older adults are at greater risk for dehydration and malnutrition during hospitalization because of standard procedures such as limiting food and fluids in preparation for diagnostic tests and medications that decrease appetite. The risk for dehydration and malnutrition also increases when older adults are unable to reach beverages or to feed themselves while in bed or connected to medical equipment. Interventions include getting the client out of bed, providing beverages and snacks frequently, and including favorite foods and beverages in the diet plan.

The increased risk for health care agency–acquired infections in older adults is related to age-related reductions in immune system response. Sixty-five percent of all health care agency–acquired infections occur in hospitalized clients over the age of 60; urinary catheter–related bacteriuria in older adults is the most common type (Beers, 2000). Other health care agency–acquired

---

✳ BOX 14-7   **EVIDENCE-BASED PRACTICE**

Identifying the Needs of Cognitively Impaired Older Adults During and After Hospitalization

Evidence Summary

Cognitive impairment (either delirium or dementia) in older adults hospitalized for medical or surgical conditions adds to the complexity of their care and increases their risk for poor outcomes. However, there is little evidence to guide best practices in the management of these clients and their caregivers. The researchers first wanted to know the prevalence of cognitive impairment in a hospitalized population of older adults. Their findings indicated that family members as well as hospital staff frequently do not recognize symptoms of cognitive impairment. The researchers also wanted to identify the needs of older cognitively impaired clients and those of their caregivers throughout an episode of acute illness and at specific times during and after hospitalization. Researchers interviewed cognitively impaired older clients and their caregivers together four times, and each caregiver was interviewed alone. The three areas of greatest concern to older clients and their caregivers were managing and negotiating care with multiple health care providers, managing illness, and psychosocial support and coping.

Application to Nursing Practice

- Because hospitalized older adults frequently have unrecognized or undiagnosed cognitive impairment, regularly assess older clients on hospital admission and throughout their stay using a screening tool such as the Mini-Mental State Examination (MMSE).
- Know the common risk factors for cognitive impairment in hospitalized older adults (e.g., major surgery, infection, adverse effects of medications, polypharmacy) and implement interventions for prevention and early intervention.
- The effects of cognitive impairment on the course of an acute illness or condition are great. Be aware of how this affects an older client's ability to understand and perform discharge instructions.
- Because cognitive impairment increases older clients' care needs, nurses need to establish collaborative relationships with their caregivers to identify and address the caregivers' needs.
- Referral to appropriate community agencies for postdischarge care is essential.

Reference

Naylor MD and others: Cognitively impaired older adults: from hospital to home, *Am J Nurs* 105(2):52, 2005.

---

infections in this population include surgical site infection, pneumonia, and bloodstream infections. Prevention begins with hand hygiene and measures to minimize the risk of infection from procedures (see Chapter 34). Prevention also includes measures to increase the older adult's resistance to infection.

Older adults in acute care settings are also at risk for becoming incontinent of urine (transient incontinence). Causes of transient urinary incontinence include delirium, untreated urinary tract infection, excessive urine production, medications, depression, restricted mobility, and constipation or stool impaction (Dowling-Castronovo and Bradway, 2003). Design interventions for transient urinary incontinence toward correcting contributing factors. The interventions often include an individualized plan to provide voiding opportunities and modification of the environment to improve access to the toilet. Avoid indwelling urinary catheters if possible. Use measures to prevent skin breakdown as well.

The increased risk for skin breakdown and the development of pressure ulcers is related to changes in aging skin and to situations that occur in the acute care setting such as immobility, incontinence, and malnutrition. The key points in the prevention of skin breakdown are avoiding pressure with proper positioning and the use of a support surface based on risk status, reducing shear forces and friction, providing meticulous skin care and moisture management, and providing nutritional support (see Chapter 48).

Older adults in the acute care setting are at risk for falling and sustaining injuries. Many falls occur as the older adult gets out of bed without assistance, and they are usually associated with toileting. Because falls account for a significant portion of injuries in hospitalized older clients, The Joint Commission (TJC) National Patient Safety Goals for 2007 includes the following as a goal for hospitals: "reduce the risk of patient harm resulting from falls" (TJC, 2007). Requirements for implementation of this important safety goal include establishing a fall reduction program that incorporates interventions to reduce fall risk factors, staff education and training on the fall reduction program, client and family education on the program and individualized fall reduction interventions, and an evaluation of the fall reduction program.

The cause of a fall is typically multifactorial and composed of intrinsic (e.g., gait and balance problems, weakness, or cognitive impairment), or extrinsic (e.g., polypharmacy, poor lighting, or cluttered environment) factors. Sedating medications increase unsteadiness. Medications causing orthostatic hypotension also increase the risk for falls because of the blood pressure drop when the older adult gets out of a bed or chair. The increase in urine output from diuretics increases the risk for falling by increasing the number of attempts to get out of bed to void. Attempts to get out of bed when physically restrained sometimes lead to injury when the older adult becomes entangled in the restraint. Equipment such as wires from monitors, intravenous tubing, urinary catheters, and other medical devices become obstacles to safe ambulation. Impaired vision prevents the older adult from seeing tripping hazards such as trash cans. Confused older adults who try to get out of bed although weak, unsteady, or drowsy benefit from reality orientation or the presence of family members and friends. Interventions to reduce the risk for falling include assistance with ambulation, strengthening exercises, medication monitoring, assistance with toileting, and removal of tripping hazards (see Chapter 38). The goal is to minimize the risk of falling without compromising mobility and functional independence.

Older Adults and Restorative Care

Restorative care refers to two types of ongoing care. The first type of restorative care continues the recovery from acute illness or surgery that began in the acute care setting. The second type of restorative care addresses chronic conditions that affect day-to-day functioning. Both types of restorative care take place in private homes and in long-term care settings.

Direct interventions during convalescence from acute illness or surgery aim at regaining or improving clients' prior level of independence in ADLs. Continue interventions that began in the acute care setting, and later modify them as convalescence progresses. To achieve this continuation, the acute care setting's discharge information needs to include information on the ongoing interventions (e.g., exercise routines, wound care routines, medication schedules, vital sign monitoring, and blood glucose monitoring). Interventions also need to address the restoration of interpersonal relationships and activities at either their previous level or at the level desired by the older adult.

When restorative care addresses chronic conditions, the goals of care include stabilizing the chronic condition, promoting health, and promoting independence in activities of daily living. Interventions to stabilize the chronic condition focus on regulation or prevention. An example of a regulatory intervention is the monitoring of blood glucose levels in diabetes. An example of prevention is a smoking cessation program for the older adult with chronic obstructive pulmonary disease.

Health promotion for older adults, as addressed in this chapter, applies to all older adults. Health promotion interventions occur in all health care settings. For example, nurse-directed programs in long-term care have improved ambulation, reversed urinary incontinence, and reduced confusion.

Interventions to promote independence in ADLs address physical ability, cognitive ability, and safety. The physical ability to perform ADLs requires strength, flexibility, and balance. You need to make accommodation for impairments of vision, hearing, and touch. The cognitive ability to perform ADLs requires the ability to recognize, judge, and remember. Cognitive impairments, such as Alzheimer's disease, interfere with safe performance of ADLs, although the older adult is still physically capable of the activities. Interventions to promote independence in ADLs adapt these requirements to the needs and lifestyle of the older adult. You always consider safety because it is not enough to be able to perform any of the ADLs. The older adult needs to be able to perform the ADLs with only an amount of risk that is acceptable to the older adult.

Beyond the basic activities of daily living, you need to also assess the older adult's ability to perform instrumental activities of daily living (IADLs) and implement appropriate interventions. Instrumental activities of daily living are tasks such as using a telephone, preparing meals, shopping, doing laundry, cleaning the home or apartment, and driving an automobile. To remain living independently at home or in an apartment, older adults need to be able to perform IADLs, purchase services by outside workers, or have a supportive network of family and friends who assist with these tasks.

Restorative care measures focus on activities to prevent, improve, reduce, or eliminate problems. You establish priorities of care and client goals, determine expected outcomes, and select appropriate interventions. You do this with the older adult's participation so that the client understands interventions and to avoid conflicts in approaches or priorities. Consideration of the older adult's lifetime experiences, as well as the values and sociocultural patterns developed, serves as the basis for planning individual care. When the older adult's cognitive status prevents participation in health care decisions, you will need to include the family. Family and friends are rich sources of data because they knew the older adult before the impairment. Frequently, they provide explanations for the older adult's behaviors and suggest methods of management. Thoughtful assessment and planning leads to goals of care that consider the influence of normal aging changes, facilitate an optimal level of comfort and coping, and promote independence in self-care activities.

✳ Key Concepts

- The number of older adults, especially the number of older adults over age 85, is increasing.
- Because nurses' attitudes toward older adults influence the quality of care, nurses need to base nursing care on accurate information about older adults, rather than myths and stereotypes.
- The biological and psychosocial theories of aging offer possible explanations for the changes seen in aging, but every older adult is a unique individual who ages in a unique way.
- The physical changes that accompany aging are normal, not pathological, and often predispose the older adult to disease.
- Cognitive impairment is not normal in older adults and requires assessment and intervention.
- Areas affected by psychosocial changes of aging include retirement, social isolation, change in housing, death, and sexuality.
- Cognitive impairment includes acute, potentially reversible disorders and chronic, irreversible, progressive disorders.
- Nursing interventions for psychosocial concerns include therapeutic communication, touch, reality orientation, validation therapy, reminiscence, and interventions to improve body image.
- The leading causes of death in the older population are heart disease, cancer, stroke, lung disease, accidents/falls, diabetes, kidney disease, and liver disease.
- Health promotion recommendations for older adults include good nutrition, regular exercise, smoking cessation, measures to reduce the risk for falls, and measures to reduce adverse medication effects.
- Acute care settings place older adults at risk for delirium, dehydration, malnutrition, health care agency–acquired infections, urinary incontinence, and falls.
- Restorative nursing interventions, whether accomplished in the older adult's home or in long-term care institutions, stabilize chronic conditions, promote health, and promote independence in basic and instrumental activities of daily living.

✳ Critical Thinking Exercises

Mrs. K. is an 80-year-old woman who is admitted to the hospital postoperatively after an emergency hip replacement secondary to a fall at her home. Her other medical problems are hypertension and anxiety disorder for which she takes a diuretic and a benzodiazepine. She is a retired schoolteacher, lives with her spouse, and is usually very active. She drives, plays bridge weekly with her friends, and participates 2 days a week in a variety of activities at a senior center. She has moderate hearing loss and wears bilateral hearing aids. She wears glasses.

You are assigned to care for her on her first postoperative day. You learn in report that Mrs. K. has been receiving opioids for postoperative pain and intravenous fluids for hydration for the first 24 hours. She has an indwelling urinary catheter. You also hear she was restless all night and slept very little and that she had even tried to get out of bed. You enter Mrs. K.'s room and find her picking at the air and talking to herself. Her hearing aids are in place, and she is wearing her glasses. She is oriented to self only. As you do your shift assessment you recognize that she is delirious.

1. Select the factors that are likely to have contributed to her delirium. Explain how each factor contributes to her delirium.
   1. Analgesic medications
   2. Inactivity
   3. Unfamiliar surroundings
   4. Sensory deficits
   5. Inadequate hydration
   6. Hypertension
   7. Indwelling urinary catheter

2. Mrs. K.'s oxygen saturation and vital signs are within normal limits. Which of the following nursing actions would be the most appropriate for you to take?
   1. Assess for pain, and if present, administer the opioid analgesic ordered.
   2. Obtain a physician order for an additional dose of her benzodiazepine.
   3. Call the physician immediately to inform of your findings.
   4. Remove her hearing aids to blunt out background noises.

3. Select the nursing interventions that would be most appropriate to take with Mrs. K. Provide the rationale for these interventions.
   1. Provide frequent reality orientation and reassurance.
   2. Provide for adequate sleep.
   3. Put hearing aids and glasses in place.
   4. Monitor blood pressure frequently.
   5. Encourage family to assist with orientation.

✳ NCLEX®-Style Review Questions

1. Which two factors contribute to the projected increase in the number of older adults?
   1. Financial success and improved environment
   2. Greater acceptance of older adults and medical problems
   3. Improved medication plan and increase in Medicare funding
   4. The aging of the baby boom generation and the growth of the population segment over age 85

2. Which of the following is true about the theories of aging?
   1. Genetic changes are solely responsible.
   2. The client's environment is the main factor.
   3. There is no single theory that explains aging.
   4. The presence of disease causes a decline in function.

3. The three common conditions affecting cognition in older adults are:
   1. Blindness, hearing loss, and stroke
   2. Delirium, depression, and dementia
   3. Cancer, Alzheimer's disease, stroke
   4. Stroke, heart attack, and cancer of the brain

4. Sexuality is recognized as a factor in the care of older adults, thus:
   1. The need to touch and be touched is decreased
   2. A decrease in an older adult's libido does occur
   3. Any expression of sexuality should be discouraged
   4. All older adults, whether healthy or frail, need to express sexual feelings

5. Older adults experience a change in sexual activity. Which best explains this change?
   1. The need to touch and be touched is decreased.
   2. The sexual preferences of older adults are not as diverse.
   3. Physical changes usually will not affect sexual functioning.
   4. Frequency and opportunities for sexual activity may decline.

6. Visual acuity declines with age. Presbyopia is a progressive decline in:
   1. Ability to see in darkness
   2. Adaptation to abrupt changes from dark areas to light areas
   3. The ability of the eyes to accommodate for close, detailed work
   4. Distinguishing between blues and greens and among pastel shades

7. A common age-related change in auditory acuity is called:
   1. Presbyopia
   2. Presbycusis
   3. Calcification
   4. Hypertrophy

8. Taste buds atrophy and lose sensitivity, and appetite may decrease. The older adult is less able to discern:
   1. Spicy and bland foods
   2. Salty, sour, and bitter tastes
   3. Hot and cold food temperatures
   4. Moist and dry food preparations

9. Kyphosis, a change in the musculoskeletal system, leads to:
   1. Decreased bone density in the vertebrae and hips
   2. Increased risk for pathological stress fractures in the hip and wrist
   3. Changes in the configuration of the spine that affect the lungs and thorax
   4. Calcification of the bony tissues of the long bones, such as in the legs and arm

15 | Critical Thinking in Nursing Practice

Mastery of the content in this chapter will enable the student to:

- Describe characteristics of a critical thinker.
- Discuss the nurse's responsibility in making clinical decisions.
- Discuss how reflection improves a nurse's practice.
- Discuss how journal writing promotes critical thinking.
- Describe the components of a critical thinking model for clinical decision making.
- Discuss critical thinking skills used in nursing practice.
- Explain the relationship between clinical experience and critical thinking.

- Discuss the critical thinking attitudes used in clinical decision making.
- Explain how professional standards influence a nurse's clinical decisions.
- Discuss the relationship of the nursing process to critical thinking.

MEDIA RESOURCES   ## KEY TERMS

 Companion CD
- NCLEX®-Style Review Questions
- Audio Glossary
- Interactive Learning Activities
- English/Spanish Glossary

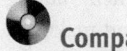 **Website**
- NCLEX®-Style Review Questions
- Audio Glossary
- English/Spanish Glossary
- Interactive Learning Activities
- WebLinks
- Audio Summaries

Clinical decision making, p. 219
Concept map, p. 226
Critical thinking, p. 216
Decision making, p. 219
Diagnostic reasoning, p. 219
Evidence-based knowledge, p. 216

Inference, p. 219
Nursing process, p. 221
Problem solving, p. 219
Prognosis, p. 219
Reflection, p. 226
Scientific method, p. 219

As a nurse, you will face many clinical situations involving clients, family members, health care staff, and peers. In each situation it is important to think smart. To think smart, you have to develop critical thinking skills to face each new experience and problem involving a client's care with open-mindedness, creativity, confidence, and intellectual wisdom. When a client develops a new set of symptoms, asks you to offer comfort, or requires a procedure, it is important to think critically and make sensible judgments so that the client receives the best nursing care possible. Critical thinking is not a simple step-by-step, linear process that you learn overnight. It is a process acquired only through experience, commitment, and an active curiosity toward learning.

Clinical Decisions in Nursing Practice

Nurses are responsible for making accurate and appropriate clinical decisions. Clinical decision making separates professional nurses from technical personnel. It is the professional nurse, for example, who takes immediate action when a client's clinical condition worsens, who decides if a client is having complications that call for notification of a physician or health care provider, or who decides if a teaching plan for a client is ineffective and needs revision. Benner (1984) describes clinical decision making as judgment that includes critical and reflective thinking and action and application of scientific and practical logic. Most clients have health care problems for which there are no clear textbook solutions. Each client's problems are unique, a product of many factors, including the client's physical health, lifestyle, culture, relationship with family and friends, living environment, and experiences. Thus, as a nurse, you do not always have a clear picture of the client's needs and the appropriate actions to take when first meeting a client. Instead, you must learn to question, wonder, and explore different perspectives and interpretations in order to find a solution that benefits the client.

Because no two clients' health problems are the same, you always have to observe each client closely. Search for and examine ideas and inferences about client problems, consider scientific principles relating to the problems, recognize the problems, and develop an approach to nursing care. With experience you will learn to creatively seek new knowledge, act quickly when events change, and make quality decisions for the client's well-being. You will find nursing to be rewarding and fulfilling through the clinical decisions you make. Critical thinking is central to professional nursing practice because it allows you to test and refine nursing approaches, to learn from successes and failures, and to apply new knowledge (e.g., nursing research findings).

Critical Thinking Defined

Thinking and learning are related processes. Over time, your knowledge and clinical experiences expand your ability to make thoughtful observations, judgments, and choices. Most definitions of critical thinking emphasize logic and reasoning (Di Vito-Thomas, 2005). **Critical thinking** is an active, organized, cognitive process used to carefully examine one's thinking and the thinking of others (Chaffee, 2002). It involves recognizing that an issue (e.g., client problem) exists, analyzing information about the issue (e.g., clinical data about a client), evaluating information (reviewing assumptions and evidence) and making conclusions (Settersten and Lauer, 2004). A critical thinker considers what is important in a situation, imagines and explores alternatives, considers ethical principles, and then makes informed decisions. Consider the following case example:

Mr. Jacobs is a 58-year-old client who had a radical prostatectomy for prostate cancer yesterday. His nurse, Tonya, finds the client lying supine in bed with arms extended along his sides, but tensed. When Tonya checks the client's surgical wound and drainage device, she notes the client winces when she gently palpates over the incisional area. She asks Mr. Jacobs when he last turned onto his side, and he responds, "Not since last night some time." Tonya asks Mr. Jacobs if he is having incisional pain, and he nods yes, saying, "It hurts too much to move." Tonya considers the information she has observed and learned from the client to determine he is in pain and has reduced mobility because of it. She decides that she needs to take action to relieve Mr. Jacobs' pain so that she can turn him more frequently and begin to get him out of bed for his recovery.

When you care for a client, critical thinking begins by asking the following questions: What do I really know about this client's situation? How do I know it? What are the options available to me? (Paul and Heaslip, 1995). In Tonya's case, she knew that pain was likely going to be a problem because the client had extensive surgery. Her review of her observations and the client's report of pain confirmed her knowledge that pain was a problem. Her options include giving Mr. Jacobs an analgesic and then waiting until it takes effect so that she is able to reposition and make the client more comfortable. Once he has less acute pain, Tonya might also try teaching Mr. Jacobs some relaxation exercises.

You can begin to learn critical thinking early in your practice. For example, as you learn about administering bed baths and other hygiene measures to your clients, take time to read your textbook and the nursing literature about the concept of comfort. What are the criteria for comfort? How do clients from other cultures perceive comfort? What are the many factors that promote comfort? The use of **evidence-based knowledge,** or knowledge based on research or clinical expertise, makes you an informed critical thinker. Thinking critically and learning about the concept of comfort prepares you to better anticipate your client's needs. You will also identify comfort problems more quickly and offer appropriate care. Critical thinking is a commitment to think clearly, precisely, and accurately and to act on what you know about a situation.

Critical thinking requires not only cognitive skills but a person's habit to ask questions, to remain well informed, to be honest in facing personal biases, and to always be willing to reconsider and think clearly about issues (Facione, 1990). There are core critical thinking skills that, when applied to nursing, show the complex nature of clinical decision making (Table 15-1). Being able to apply all of these skills takes practice. You will also need to have a sound knowledge base and thoughtfully consider the knowledge you get when caring for clients.

✴ TABLE 15-1 Critical Thinking Skills

SKILL	NURSING PRACTICE APPLICATIONS
Interpretation	Be orderly in data collection. Look for patterns to categorize data (e.g., nursing diagnoses [see Chapter 17]). Clarify any data you are uncertain about.
Analysis	Be open-minded as you look at information about a client. Do not make careless assumptions. Do the data reveal what you believe is true, or are there other options?
Inference	Look at the meaning and significance of findings. Are there relationships between findings? Do the data about the client help you see that a problem exists?
Evaluation	Look at all situations objectively. Use criteria (e.g., expected outcomes, pain characteristics, learning objectives) to determine results of nursing actions. Reflect on your own behavior.
Explanation	Support your findings and conclusions. Use knowledge and experience to choose strategies you use in the care of clients.
Self-regulation	Reflect on your experiences. Identify the ways you can improve your own performance. What will make you feel that you have been successful?

Modified from Facione P: *Critical thinking: a statement of expert consensus for purposes of educational assessment and instruction. The Delphi report: research findings and recommendations prepared for the American Philosophical Association,* ERIC Doc No. ED 315-423, Washington, DC, 1990, ERIC.

✴ TABLE 15-2 Concepts for a Critical Thinker

CONCEPT	CRITICAL THINKING BEHAVIOR
Truth seeking	Seek the true meaning of a situation. Be courageous about asking questions; be honest and objective about asking questions.
Open-mindedness	Be tolerant of different views; be sensitive to the possibility of your own prejudices; respect the right of others to have different opinions.
Analyticity	Analyze potentially problematic situations; anticipate possible results or consequences; value reason; use evidence-based knowledge.
Systematicity	Be organized, focused; work hard in any inquiry.
Self-confidence	Trust in your own reasoning processes.
Inquisitiveness	Be eager to acquire knowledge and learn explanations even when applications of the knowledge are not immediately clear. Value learning for learning's sake.
Maturity	Multiple solutions are acceptable. Reflect upon your own judgments; have cognitive maturity.

Modified from Facione N, Facione P: Externalizing the critical thinking in knowledge development and clinical judgment, *Nurs Outlook* 44(3):129, 1996.

Nurses who apply critical thinking in their work focus on options for solving problems and making decisions, rather than quickly and carelessly forming quick solutions (Kataoka-Yahiro and Saylor, 1994). Nurses who work in crisis situations such as the emergency department often act quickly when client problems develop. However, even these nurses exercise discipline in decision making in order to avoid premature and inappropriate decisions. Learning to think critically helps you to care for clients as their advocate, or supporter, and to make better-informed choices about their care. Facione and Facione (1996) identified concepts for thinking critically (Table 15-2). Critical thinking is more than just problem solving. It is an attempt to continually improve how to apply yourself when faced with problems in client care.

Thinking and Learning

Learning is a lifelong process. Your intellectual and emotional growth involves learning new knowledge and refining your ability to think, problem solve, and make judgments. To learn, you have to be flexible and always open to new information. The science of nursing is growing rapidly, and there will always be new information for you to apply in practice. As you have more clinical experiences and apply the knowledge you learn, you will become better able to form assumptions, present ideas, and make valid conclusions.

When you care for a client, always think ahead and ask these questions: What is the client's status now? How might it change and why? What do I know to improve the client's condition? In what way will a specific therapy affect the client? Do not let your thinking become routine or standardized. Instead, learn to look beyond the obvious in any clinical situation, explore the client's unique responses to health alterations, and recognize what actions are needed to benefit the client. Over time your experience with many clients will help you recognize patterns of behavior, see commonalities in signs and symptoms, and anticipate reactions to therapies. Thinking about those experiences will allow you to better anticipate each new client's needs and recognize problems when they develop.

Levels of Critical Thinking in Nursing

Your ability to think critically grows as you gain new knowledge in nursing practice. Kataoka-Yahiro and Saylor (1994) developed a critical thinking model (Figure 15-1) that includes three levels of critical thinking: basic, complex, and commitment. As a begin-

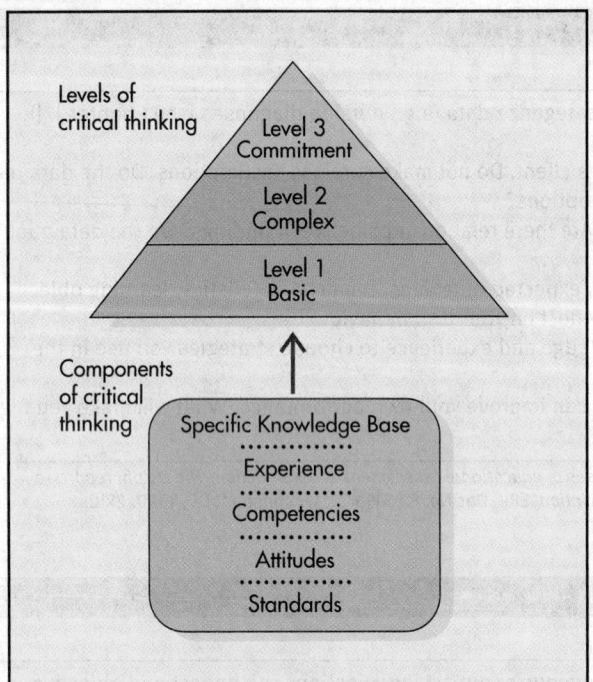

Figure 15-1 Critical thinking model for nursing judgment. (Redrawn from Kataoka-Yahiro M, Saylor C: A critical thinking model for nursing judgment, *J Nurs Educ* 33(8):351, 1994. Modified from Glaser, 1941; Miller and Malcolm, 1990; Paul, 1993; and Perry, 1979.)

ning student you will apply the critical thinking model at the basic level. Then, as you advance in practice, you will adopt complex critical thinking and commitment.

Basic Critical Thinking

At the basic level of critical thinking a learner trusts that experts have the right answers for every problem. Thinking is concrete and based on a set of rules or principles. For example, as a nursing student you use a hospital's procedure manual to confirm how to insert a Foley catheter. You will likely follow the procedure step-by-step without adjusting the procedure to meet a client's unique needs (e.g., positioning to minimize the client's pain or mobility restrictions). You do not have enough experience to anticipate how to individualize the procedure. At this level, answers to complex problems are either right or wrong (e.g., there is too much or not enough air in the Foley catheter balloon), and one right answer usually exists for each problem. Basic critical thinking is an early step in the development of reasoning (Kataoka-Yahiro and Saylor, 1994). A basic critical thinker learns to accept the diverse opinions and values of experts (e.g., instructors and staff nurse role models). However, inexperience, weak competencies, and inflexible attitudes restrict a person's ability to move to the next level of critical thinking.

Complex Critical Thinking

Complex critical thinkers begin to separate themselves from authorities. They analyze and examine choices more independently. The person's thinking abilities and initiative to look beyond ex-

pert opinion begin to change. A nurse learns that alternative, and perhaps conflicting, solutions do exist.

Consider the case of Mr. Rosen, a 36-year-old man who had hip surgery. The client is having pain but is refusing his ordered analgesic. His health care provider is concerned that the client will not progress as planned, delaying rehabilitation. While discussing the importance of rehabilitation with Mr. Rosen, the nurse, Edwin, realizes the client's reason for not taking pain medication. Edwin learns that the client practices meditation at home. As a complex critical thinker, Edwin recognizes that Mr. Rosen has options for pain relief other than accepting analgesics. Edwin decides to discuss meditation and other nonpharmacological interventions with the client as pain control options.

In complex critical thinking each solution has benefits and risks that you learn to weigh before making a final decision. There are options. Thinking becomes more creative and innovative. The complex critical thinker is willing to consider different options aside from routine procedures when complex situations develop. You learn a variety of different approaches for the same therapy.

Commitment

The third level of critical thinking is commitment (Kataoka-Yahiro and Saylor, 1994). At this level a person anticipates the need to make choices without assistance from others. Whatever decision you make, accept accountability for it. As a nurse, you do more than just consider the complex alternatives a problem poses. At the commitment level, you choose an action or belief based on the alternatives available and support it. Sometimes an action is to not take action, or you choose to delay an action until a later time. You choose to delay as a result of your experience and knowledge. Because you take accountability for the decision, you give attention to the results of the decision and determine whether it was appropriate.

Critical Thinking Competencies

Kataoka-Yahiro and Saylor (1994) describe critical thinking competencies as the cognitive processes a nurse uses to make judgments about the clinical care of clients. These include general critical thinking, specific critical thinking in clinical situations, and specific critical thinking in nursing. General critical thinking processes are not unique to nursing. They include the scientific method, problem solving, and decision making. Specific critical thinking competencies in clinical situations include diagnostic reasoning, clinical inference, and clinical decision making. The specific critical thinking competency in nursing involves use of the nursing process.

Scientific Method

The scientific method is a way to solve problems using reasoning. It is a systematic, ordered approach to gathering data and solving problems. The scientific method is used in nursing, medicine, and a variety of other disciplines. It is an approach to looking for the truth or verifying that a set of facts agrees with reality. Nurse researchers use the **scientific method** when testing research questions in nursing practice situations. The scientific method has five steps:

- Problem identification
- Collection of data
- Formulation of a research question or hypothesis
- Testing the question or hypothesis
- Evaluating results of the test or study

Consider the following example of the scientific method in nursing practice.

A nurse caring for clients who receive large doses of chemotherapy for ovarian cancer sees a pattern of clients developing severe inflammation in the mouth (mucositis) (Identifies problem). The nurse reads research articles (Collects data) about mucositis and learns that there is evidence to show that having clients keep ice in their mouths (cryotherapy) during the chemotherapy infusion, reduces severity of mucositis after treatment. The nurse asks (Forms research question), "Do clients with ovarian cancer who receive chemotherapy have less severe mucositis when given cryotherapy versus standard mouthrinse in the oral cavity?" The nurse then designs a study that compares the incidence and severity of mucositis for a group of clients who use cryotherapy versus those who use traditional mouthrinse (Tests the question). The nurse hopes that results from the study will give other oncology nurses a better approach for reducing the frequency and severity of mucositis in clients with ovarian cancer.

Problem Solving

We all face problems every day, such as a computer program that does not function properly or a close friend who has lost a favorite pet. When a problem arises, we obtain information and then use the information plus what we already know to find a solution. Clients routinely present problems in practice. For example, a home care nurse visits a client and learns that the client has difficulty taking her medications regularly. The client is unable to describe what medications she has taken for the last 3 days. The medication bottles are labeled and filled with medications. The nurse has to solve the problem of why the client is not adhering to or following her medication schedule. The nurse knows the client was discharged from the hospital and had five medications ordered. While talking with the client, the nurse learns that the client has two over-the-counter medications she takes regularly as well. When the nurse asks the client to show the medications she takes in the morning, the nurse notices that the client has difficulty reading the medication labels. The client is able to describe the medications she is to take but is uncertain about the times of administration. The nurse recommends having the client's pharmacy relabel the medications in larger lettering. In addition, the nurse shows her some examples of pill organizers that will help her sort her medications by time of day for a period of 7 days.

Effective **problem solving** also involves evaluating the solution over time to make sure that it is effective. It becomes necessary to try different options if a problem recurs. From the example above, during a follow-up visit, the nurse finds that the client has organized her medications correctly and is able to read the labels without difficulty. The nurse obtained information that correctly clarified the cause of the client's problem and tested a solution that proved successful. Having solved a problem in one situation adds to a nurse's experience in practice and allows the nurse to apply that knowledge in future client situations.

Decision Making

When you face a problem or situation and need to choose a course of action from several options, you are making a decision. **Decision making** is a product of critical thinking that focuses on problem resolution. Following a set of criteria helps to make a thorough and thoughtful decision. For example, decision making occurs when a person decides on the choice of a health care provider. To make a decision, an individual has to recognize and define the problem or situation (need for a certain type of health care provider to provide medical care) and assess all options (consider recommended health care providers or choose one whose office is close to home). The person has to weigh each option against a set of criteria (experience, friendliness, and reputation), test possible options (talk directly with the different health care providers), consider the consequences of the decision (examine pros and cons of selecting one health care provider over another), and then make a final decision. Although the set of criteria follows a sequence of steps, decision making involves moving back and forth when considering all criteria. Decision making leads to informed conclusions that are supported by evidence and reason. Examples of decision making in the clinical area include deciding on a choice of dressings for a client with a surgical wound or selecting the best approach for teaching a family how to assist a client who is returning home after a stroke. You will learn to make sound decisions by approaching each clinical situation thoughtfully and by applying each component of the decision-making process mentioned above.

Diagnostic Reasoning and Inference

As soon as you receive information about a client in a clinical situation, **diagnostic reasoning** begins. It is a process of determining a client's health status after you assign meaning to the behaviors, physical signs, and symptoms presented by the client. Diagnostic reasoning begins when you enter into an interaction with a client or when you make physical or behavioral observations. An expert nurse will see the context of a client situation (e.g., recognize that the client who is feeling light-headed with blurred vision and who has a history of diabetes is experiencing a problem with blood glucose levels), observe patterns and themes (e.g., symptoms including weakness, headache, hunger, and visual disturbances that suggest hypoglycemia), and make decisions quickly (e.g., offer a food source containing glucose) (Ferrario, 2004). The information a nurse collects and analyzes leads to a diagnosis of a client's condition. Diagnostic reasoning provides a clear perspective of a client's health status. Nurses do not make medical diagnoses, but they do assess and monitor clients closely and compare the clients' signs and symptoms with those that are common to a medical diagnosis. This type of diagnostic reasoning helps physicians or health care providers pinpoint the nature of a problem more quickly and select proper therapies.

Part of diagnostic reasoning is **inference**, the process of drawing conclusions from related pieces of evidence (Smith Higuchi and Donald, 2002). An inference involves forming patterns of information from data before making a diagnosis. Seeing that a client has lost appetite and experienced a loss in weight over the last month, the nurse infers there is a nutritional problem. An example of diagnostic reasoning is forming a nursing diagnosis such as *imbalanced nutrition, less than body requirements* (see Chapter 17).

In diagnostic reasoning use client data that you gather or collect to logically explain a clinical judgment. For example, after turning a client, you see an area of redness on the right hip. You palpate the area and note that it is warm to the touch and the client complains of tenderness. You push on the area with your finger, and, after you release pressure, the area does not blanch or turn white. You think about what you know about normal skin integrity and the effects of pressure. You form the conclusion the client has a pressure ulcer. As a new student, confirm your judgment with experienced nurses. At times your clinical judgment will be wrong, but consulting with nurse experts will give you feedback to build on future clinical situations.

Often you cannot make a precise diagnosis during your first meeting with a client. You will sometimes sense that a problem exists but not have sufficient data to make a specific diagnosis. Some clients' physical conditions limit their ability to tell you about symptoms. Some clients choose to not share sensitive and important information during your initial assessment. Clients' behaviors and physical responses may become observable only under certain conditions not present during your initial assessment. When uncertain of a diagnosis, continue data collection. As a nurse, you have to critically analyze changing clinical situations until you are able to determine the client's unique situation. Diagnostic reasoning is a continuous behavior in nursing practice. Any diagnostic conclusions that you make will help the physician or health care provider identify the nature of a problem more quickly and select proper medical therapies.

Clinical Decision Making

Clinical decision making is a problem-solving activity that focuses on defining client problems and selecting appropriate treatment (Smith Higuchi and Donald, 2002). When you approach a clinical problem, such as a client who developed an area of redness over the hip, you make a decision that identifies the problem (a pressure ulcer) and then choose the best nursing interventions (skin care and a turning schedule) for that client. Nurses make clinical decisions all the time to improve a client's health or to maintain wellness. This means reducing the severity of the problem or resolving the problem completely. **Clinical decision making** requires careful reasoning so that you choose the options for the best client outcomes on the basis of the client's condition and the priority of the problem.

You improve your clinical decision making by knowing your clients. Nurse researchers found that expert nurses develop a level of knowing that leads to pattern recognition of client symptoms and responses (White, 2003). For example, an expert nurse who worked on a general surgery unit for many years is more likely able to detect signs of internal hemorrhage (e.g., fall in blood pressure, rapid pulse, change in consciousness) than a new nurse. Over time, a combination of experience, time spent in a specific clinical area, and the quality of relationships formed with clients will allow expert nurses to know clinical situations and to quickly

anticipate and select the right course of action (Tanner and others, 1993). Spending more time during initial client assessments to observe client behavior and to measure physical findings are both ways to improve knowing your clients. Also, consistently monitoring clients as problems develop helps you to see how clinical changes develop over time. The selection of nursing therapies is built on both clinical knowledge and client data. It is based on the following:

- The identified status and situation of the client
- Knowledge about the clinical variables (e.g., age, seriousness of problem, pathology of the problem, client's preexisting disease conditions) involved in the situation and how the variables are linked together
- A judgment about the likely course of events and outcome of the diagnosed problem, considering any health risks the client has; includes knowledge about usual patterns of any diagnosed problem or **prognosis**
- Any additional relevant data about requirements in the client's daily living, functional capacity, and social resources
- Knowledge about the nursing therapy options available and the way in which specific interventions will predictably affect the client's situation

Always keep the client your center of focus as you try to solve the client's clinical problems. When you make an accurate clinical decision, this allows you to then set priorities for the interventions to implement first (see Chapter 17). Because different clients bring different variables to a situation, a certain activity is sometimes more of a priority in one situation and less of a priority in another. For example, if a client is physically dependent, unable to eat, and incontinent of urine, you will recognize skin integrity as a greater priority than if the client were immobile but continent of urine and able to eat a normal diet. Do not assume that certain health situations produce automatic priorities. For example, a client who has surgery is anticipated to experience a certain level of postoperative pain, which often becomes a priority of care. However, if the client is experiencing severe anxiety that increases pain perception, it becomes necessary for you to focus on ways to relieve the anxiety before pain relief measures will be effective.

After determining a client's nursing care priorities, select therapies most likely to relieve each problem. A wide range of choices are usually available from nurse-administered to client self-care strategies. Collaborate with the client and then select, test, and evaluate the chosen approaches. You also try to anticipate what might go wrong and consider alternative approaches to minimize or prevent problems.

Nurses make decisions about individual clients and about groups of clients. When you work on a busy hospital unit it is likely you will care for several clients. You use criteria such as the clinical condition of the client, Maslow's hierarchy of needs (see Chapter 6), risks involved in treatment delays, and clients' expectations of care to determine which clients have the greatest priorities for care. For example, a client who is having a sudden drop in blood pressure along with a change in consciousness requires your attention immediately as opposed to the client who needs you to collect a urine specimen or a client who needs your help to walk down the hallway. You visit the client who has had no visitors and has recently been given a diagnosis of cancer before

---

✳ BOX 15-1 Clinical Decision Making for Groups of Clients

- Identify the nursing diagnoses and collaborative problems of each client (see Chapter 17).
- Analyze clients' diagnoses/problems, and decide which are most urgent on the basis of basic needs, the clients' changing or unstable status, and problem complexity (see Chapter 18).
- Consider the time it will take to care for clients whose problems are of high priority (e.g., do you have the time to restart a critical IV when a different client has a medication due?).
- Consider the resources you have to manage each problem, assistive personnel assigned with you, and clients' family members.
- Consider how to involve the clients as decision makers and participants in care.
- Decide how to combine activities to resolve more than one client problem at a time.
- Decide what, if any, nursing care procedures to delegate to assistive personnel so that you are able to spend your time on activities requiring professional nursing knowledge.

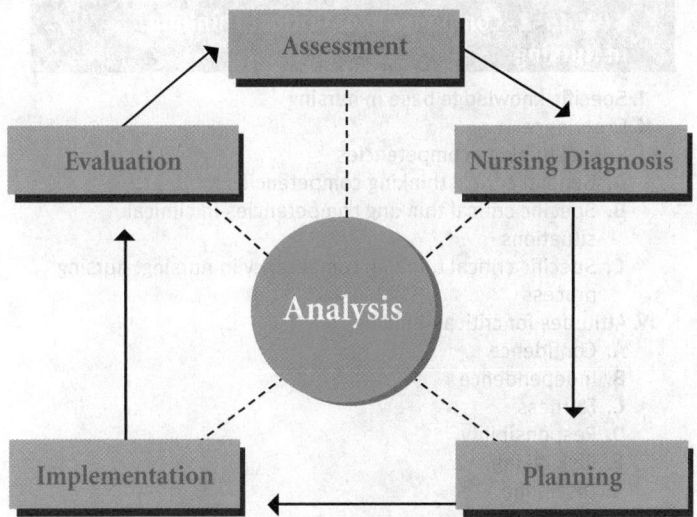

Figure 15-2 Five-step nursing process model.

---

checking on the recovering surgical client whose family has just arrived. In order for you to manage the wide variety of problems associated with groups of clients, skillful, prioritized decision making is critical (Box 15-1).

Nursing Process as a Competency

Nurses apply the **nursing process** as a competency when delivering client care (Kataoka-Yahiro and Saylor, 1994). The nursing process is a five-step clinical decision-making approach that includes assessment, diagnosis, planning, implementation, and evaluation. The purpose of the nursing process is to diagnose and treat human responses to actual or potential health problems (American Nurses Association, 2003). Human responses include client symptoms and physiological reactions to treatment, the need for knowledge when health care providers make a new diagnosis or treatment plan, and a client's ability to cope with loss. Use of the process allows nurses to help clients meet agreed-upon outcomes for better health (Figure 15-2). The nursing process involves the general and specific critical thinking competencies, described earlier, in a way that focuses on a particular client's unique needs. The format for the nursing process is unique to the discipline of nursing and provides a common language and process for nurses to "think through" clients' clinical problems (Kataoka-Yahiro and Saylor, 1994). Unit III describes the nursing process.

The nursing process is often called a blueprint or plan for client cae. It allows flexibility for use in all clinical settings. When you use the nursing process, you identify a client's health care needs, clearly define a nursing diagnosis or collaborative problem, determine priorities of care, and set goals and expected outcomes of care. Then you develop and communicate a client-centered plan of care, deliver nursing interventions, and evaluate the effects of your care. When you become more competent in using the nursing process, you will be able to focus not only on a single client problem or diagnosis but on multiple problems and diagnoses. As a nurse, always be thinking and recognizing what step of the process you are using. Within each step you will apply critical thinking to provide the very best professional care to your clients.

A Critical Thinking Model for Clinical Decision Making

Thinking critically is becoming the benchmark or standard for professional nursing competence. The ability to think critically, improve clinical practice, and decrease errors in clinical judgments is the vision of nursing practice (Di Vito-Thomas, 2005). To help you in the development of critical thinking, this text offers a model for critical thinking. Models help to explain concepts. Because critical thinking in nursing is complex, a model helps explain what is involved as you make clinical decisions and judgments about your clients. Kataoka-Yahiro and Saylor (1994) developed a model of critical thinking for nursing judgment based in part on previous work by Paul (1993), Glaser (1941), Perry (1979) and Miller and Malcolm (1990) (see Figure 15-1). The model defines the outcome of critical thinking: nursing judgment that is relevant to nursing problems in a variety of settings. According to this model, there are five components of critical thinking: knowledge base, experience, critical thinking competencies (with emphasis on the nursing process), attitudes, and standards. The elements of the model combine to explain how nurses make clinical judgments that are necessary for safe, effective nursing care (Box 15-2).

Throughout this text the model will be used for applying critical thinking during the nursing process. Each clinical chapter of the text is initially organized to include both scientific and nursing knowledge. It is your knowledge base (the first critical thinking component) that prepares you to make clinical judgments as a nurse. Then each chapter is organized by the steps of the nursing processes (Chapters 15 through 21). A graphic illustration of the critical thinking model will show you how to apply elements of critical thinking in assessing clients, in planning the interventions you provide, and in evaluating your results. If you learn to apply each element of this model in the way you think about clients, you will become a confident and effective professional.

✷ BOX 15-2   Components of Critical Thinking in Nursing

I. Specific knowledge base in nursing
II. Experience
III. Critical thinking competencies
   A. General critical thinking competencies
   B. Specific critical thinking competencies in clinical situations
   C. Specific critical thinking competency in nursing: nursing process
IV. Attitudes for critical thinking
   A. Confidence
   B. Independence
   C. Fairness
   D. Responsibility
   E. Risk taking
   F. Discipline
   G. Perseverance
   H. Creativity
   I. Curiosity
   J. Integrity
   K. Humility
V. Standards for critical thinking
   A. Intellectual standards
      1. Clear
      2. Precise
      3. Specific
      4. Accurate
      5. Relevant
      6. Plausible
      7. Consistent
      8. Logical
      9. Deep
      10. Broad
      11. Complete
      12. Significant
      13. Adequate (for purpose)
      14. Fair
   B. Professional standards
      1. Ethical criteria for nursing judgment
      2. Criteria for evaluation
      3. Professional responsibility

Modified from Kataoka-Yahiro M, Saylor C: A critical thinking model for nursing judgment, *J Nurs Educ* 33(8):351, 1994. Data from Paul RW: The art of redesigning instruction. In Willsen J, Blinker AJA, editors: *Critical thinking: how to prepare students for a rapidly changing world*, Santa Rosa, Calif, 1993, Foundation for Critical Thinking.

Specific Knowledge Base

The first component of the critical thinking model is a nurse's specific knowledge base. This varies according to a nurse's educational experience, including basic nursing education, continuing education courses, and additional college degrees. In addition, it includes the initiative a nurse shows in reading the nursing literature so as to remain current in nursing science. As a nurse, your knowledge base includes information and theory from the basic sciences, humanities, behavioral sciences, and nursing. Nurses use their knowledge base in a different way from other health care disciplines because they think holistically about client problems. For example, a nurse's broad knowledge base offers a physical, psychological, social, moral, ethical, and cultural view of clients and their health care needs. The depth and extent of knowledge influence your ability to think critically about nursing problems.

Consider this scenario: Robert Perez previously earned a bachelor's degree in education and taught high school for 1 year. He is starting his third year of study in his nursing program. He has successfully completed his required courses in the sciences, health ethics, introduction to nursing concepts, and communication principles. His first clinical course is on health promotion with a clinical assignment on a general medicine clinic. Although he is still new to nursing, his experiences as a teacher and his preparation and knowledge base in nursing will help him know how to interview clients and begin to make clinical decisions about clients' health promotion practices.

Experience

Nursing is a practice discipline. Clinical learning experiences are necessary to acquire clinical decision-making skills (Roche, 2002). In clinical situations, you will learn from observing, sensing, talking with clients and families, and then reflecting actively on all experiences. Clinical experience is the laboratory for testing your nursing knowledge. You will learn that "textbook" approaches form the basis for practice, but you will make safe adaptations or revisions in approaches to accommodate the setting, the unique qualities of the client, and the experiences you have from caring for previous clients. With experience, you begin to understand clinical situations, recognize cues of clients' health patterns, and interpret cues as relevant or irrelevant. Perhaps the best lesson a new nursing student can learn is to value all client experiences, which become stepping-stones for building new knowledge and inspiring innovative thinking.

During the previous summer, Robert worked as a nurse assistant in a nursing home. This experience provided him with valuable time spent in interacting with older adult clients and in giving basic nursing care. As Robert thinks about his clinical experience at the clinic, he recognizes he still has a lot to learn. However, each client has provided him valuable learning experiences. Specifically, he has been able to develop good interviewing skills and understands the importance of the family in an individual's health, and he has learned how nurses are advocates for clients. He has also learned that older adults require more time to perform activities such as eating, bathing, and grooming, so he has adapted these skill techniques. His time in the physical assessment laboratory and the time he worked in the nursing home have helped him begin to be a watchful observer. Robert also knows that his previous experience as a teacher will help him apply educational principles in his nursing role.

You will also learn from personal experiences. The opportunities we have in experiencing different emotions, crises, and successes in our lives and relationships with others builds our experiences as nurses.

The Nursing Process Competency

Competency, specifically the nursing process, is the third component of the critical thinking model. In your practice, you will apply critical thinking components during each step of the nurs-

✳ **TABLE 15-3 Critical Thinking Attitudes and Applications in Nursing Practice**

CRITICAL THINKING ATTITUDE	APPLICATION IN PRACTICE
Confidence	Learn how to introduce yourself to a client; speak with conviction when you begin a treatment or procedure. Do not lead a client to think that you are unable to perform care safely. Always be well prepared before performing a nursing activity. Encourage a client to ask questions.
Thinking independently	Read the nursing literature, especially when there are different views on the same subject. Talk with other nurses and share ideas about nursing interventions.
Fairness	Listen to both sides in any discussion. If a client or family member complains about a co-worker, listen to the story and then speak with the co-worker as well. If a staff member labels a client uncooperative, assume the care of that client with openness and a desire to meet that client's needs.
Responsibility and authority	Ask for help if you are uncertain about how to perform a nursing skill. Refer to a policy and procedure manual to review steps of a skill. Report any problems immediately. Follow standards of practice in your care.
Risk taking	If your knowledge causes you to question a health care provider's order, do so. Be willing to recommend alternative approaches to nursing care when colleagues are having little success with clients.
Discipline	Be thorough in whatever you do. Use known scientific and practice-based criteria for activities such as assessment and evaluation. Take time to be thorough, and manage your time effectively.
Perseverance	Be cautious of an easy answer. If co-workers give you information about a client and some fact seems to be missing, go clarify information or talk to the client directly. If problems of the same type continue to occur on a nursing division, bring co-workers together, look for a pattern, and find a solution.
Creativity	Look for different approaches if interventions are not working for a client. For example, a client in pain may need a different positioning or distraction technique. When appropriate, involve the client's family in adapting your approaches to care methods used at home.
Curiosity	Always ask why. A clinical sign or symptom often indicates a variety of problems. Explore and learn more about the client so as to make appropriate clinical judgments.
Integrity	Recognize when your opinions conflict with those of a client; review your position, and decide how best to proceed to reach outcomes that will satisfy everyone. Do not compromise nursing standards or honesty in delivering nursing care.
Humility	Recognize when you need more information to make a decision. When you are new to a clinical division, ask for an orientation to the area. Ask registered nurses (RNs) regularly assigned to the area for assistance with approaches to care.

ing process. Throughout the clinical chapters of this text, the relationship of critical thinking to the nursing process will be emphasized.

Attitudes for Critical Thinking

The fourth component of the critical thinking model is attitudes. There are 11 attitudes that are central features of a critical thinker (Paul, 1993) (see Box 15-2). These attitudes define how a successful critical thinker approaches a problem. For example, when a client complains of anxiety before having a diagnostic procedure, the curious nurse will explore possible reasons for the client's concerns. The nurse will also show discipline in collecting a thorough assessment to find the source of the client's anxiety. Attitudes of inquiry involve an ability to recognize that problems exist and that there is a need for evidence to support what you suppose is true (Watson and Glaser, 1980). Critical thinking attitudes are guidelines for how to approach a problem or decision-making situation. An important part of critical thinking is interpreting, evaluating, and making judgments about the adequacy of various arguments and available data. Knowing when you need more information, knowing when information is misleading, and recognizing your own knowledge

limits are examples of how critical thinking attitudes guide decision making. Table 15-3 summarizes the use of critical thinking attitudes in nursing practice.

Confidence. When you are confident, you feel certain about accomplishing a task or goal such as performing a nursing procedure or making a diagnostic decision. Confidence grows with experience in recognizing your strengths and limitations. You begin to shift your focus from your own needs (e.g., remembering how to perform a procedure) to the client's needs (White, 2003). When you are not confident in completing a nursing skill, you focus on your feelings of anxiety in not knowing what to do. This will prevent you from giving attention to the client. Always be aware of what you know and what you do not know. When you show confidence, your clients recognize it by how you communicate and the way you perform nursing care. Confidence builds trust between you and your clients.

Thinking Independently. As you gain new knowledge, you learn to consider a wide range of ideas and concepts before forming an opinion or making a judgment. This does not mean you ignore other people's ideas. Instead, you learn to consider all sides of a situation. However, a critical thinker does not accept another person's ideas without question. When thinking independently, you challenge the ways others think and look for rational and logical answers to problems. Begin to raise important questions about your practice. For example, why is one type of surgical dressing ordered over another, why do your clients not get pain relief, and what can you do to help clients with literacy problems learn about their medications? Thinking independently is an important step in evidence-based practice (Chapter 5) when nurses ask questions and look for the evidence behind the clinical problem they identify. Independent thinking and reasoning are essential to the improvement and expansion of nursing practice.

Fairness. A critical thinker deals with situations justly. This means that bias or prejudice does not enter into a decision. For example, regardless of how you feel about obesity, you do not allow personal attitudes to influence the way you care for an overweight client. Look at a situation objectively and analyze all viewpoints to understand the situation completely before making a decision. Having a sense of imagination aids in the development of fairness. Imagining what it is like to be in your client's situation will help you see situations with new eyes and appreciate their complexity.

Responsibility and Accountability. When caring for clients, you are responsible for correctly performing nursing care activities based upon standards of practice. Standards of practice are the minimum level of performance accepted to ensure high-quality care. For example, you do not take shortcuts (e.g., failing to identify a client) when administering medications. A professional nurse is competent in performing nursing therapies and in making clinical decisions about clients. As a nurse, you are also answerable, or accountable for the outcomes of your actions. An accountable nurse is reliable and willing to recognize when nursing care is ineffective. Ultimately, you are accountable for your decisions and the results of your actions made on the client's behalf.

Risk Taking. Persons often associate taking risks with danger. Driving 30 miles an hour over the speed limit is a risk that sometimes results in injury to the driver and an unlucky pedestrian. But risk taking does not always have negative outcomes. Risk taking is desirable, particularly when the result is a positive outcome. A critical thinker is willing to take risks in trying different ways to solve problems. The willingness to take risks comes from experience with similar problems. Risk taking often leads to advances in client care. Nurses in the past have taken risks in trying different approaches to skin and wound care, pulmonary hygiene, and pain management, to name a few. When taking a risk, consider all options, analyze any potential danger to a client, and then act in a well-reasoned, logical, and thoughtful manner.

Discipline. A disciplined thinker misses few details and follows an orderly or systematic approach when making decisions or taking action. For example, you have a client who is in pain. Instead of only asking the client, "How severe is your pain on a scale of 0 to 10?" you ask more specific questions about the character of pain. Your questions thoroughly assess the nature of pain. For example, "What makes the pain worse? Where does it hurt, and how long have you noticed it?" Being disciplined helps identify problems more accurately and to then select the most appropriate interventions.

Perseverance. A critical thinker is determined to find effective solutions to client care problems. This is especially important when problems remain unresolved or when they reoccur. Learn as much as possible about a problem and try various approaches to care. Persevering means to continue to look for more resources until you find a successful approach. For example, a client who is unable to speak following throat surgery poses challenges for the nurse to be able to communicate effectively. Perseverance leads the nurse to try different communication approaches (e.g., message boards or alarm bells) until the nurse finds a method that the client is able to use. A critical thinker who perseveres is not satisfied with minimal effort, but works to achieve the highest level of quality care.

Creativity. Creativity involves original thinking. This means you find solutions outside of the standard routines of care while still keeping standards of practice. Creativity is a motivator that helps you to think of options and unique approaches. A client's clinical problems, social support systems, and living environment are just a few examples of factors that make the simplest nursing procedure more complicated. For example, a home care nurse has to find a way to help an older client with arthritis have greater mobility in the home. The client has difficulty lowering and raising herself in a chair because of pain and limited range of motion in her knees. The nurse uses wooden blocks to elevate the chair legs so that the client is able to sit and stand with little discomfort while making sure the chair is safe to use.

Curiosity. A critical thinker's favorite question is "Why?" In any clinical situation, you will learn a great deal of information about a client. As you analyze client information, data patterns will appear that are not always clear. Having a sense of curiosity motivates you to inquire further (e.g., question family, consult with a physician, or review the scientific literature) and to investigate a clinical situation so that you get all the information you need to make a decision.

Integrity. Critical thinkers question and test their own knowledge and beliefs. Your personal integrity as a nurse builds trust from your co-workers. Nurses face many dilemmas or problems in everyday clinical practice, and everyone makes mistakes at times. A person of integrity is honest and willing to admit to mistakes or inconsistencies in his or her own behavior, ideas, and beliefs. In addition, the professional nurse always tries to follow the highest standards of practice.

Humility. It is important for you to admit to any limitations in your knowledge and skill. Critical thinkers admit what they do not know and try to find the knowledge they need to make proper decisions. It is common for you as a nurse to be an expert in one area of clinical practice but a novice in another. That is because the knowledge in all areas of nursing is unlimited. A client's safety and welfare are at risk if you do not admit your inability to deal with a practice problem. You have to rethink a situation, learn additional knowledge, and then use the new information to form opinions, draw conclusions, and take action.

The first client Robert meets in the clinic is a young man who has signs and symptoms of chlamydia, a sexually transmitted disease. The client has had the symptoms for over 3 weeks and voices concern about what it will mean to have the disease. Robert examines the young man and finds that the client has redness and itching on the penis with a yellowish discharge. He uses discipline to check further and asks if the client has pain on urination. He also checks him for fever. Robert has limited knowledge about chlamydia, so he consults with the clinic nurse practitioner, who explains the nature of the infection, the risks it poses to the client, and the usual course of treatment. Robert returns to the client and speaks confidently with him about chlamydia, the reason for his symptoms, the need to tell sex partners about the infection, and the importance of wearing a condom.

Standards for Critical Thinking

The fifth component of the critical thinking model includes intellectual and professional standards (Kataoka-Yahiro and Saylor, 1994).

Intellectual Standards. Paul (1993) identified 14 intellectual standards (see Box 15-2) universal for critical thinking. An intellectual standard is a guideline or principle for rational thought. You will normally apply these standards when you use the nursing process. When you consider a client problem, apply the intellectual standards such as preciseness, accuracy, and consistency to make sure that all clinical decisions are sound. A thorough use of the intellectual standards in clinical practice makes certain that you do not perform critical thinking haphazardly.

Mrs. Lamar is an 82-year-old client who comes to the medicine clinic for a follow-up following the diagnosis of a diabetic foot ulcer. Robert finds the ulcer on the client's left foot. A quick check of the client's medical record reveals a description of the ulcer by one of the clinic nurses from 2 weeks earlier. The client is receiving a topical medication for the ulcer. Robert uses the same assessment criteria applied during the last clinic visit to examine the client's ulcer (Consistent). He methodically inspects the affected area of the skin, measures the size of the ulcer, and notes the appearance of any drainage (Complete). Robert asks the client to describe how she has been caring for the ulcer to determine if she needs health teaching (Relevant). When the client explains that she washes the ulcer, Robert asks her to describe exactly what she has used to clean the ulcer and how often (Precise). Robert documents the wound location and appearance in the clinic record using specific anatomical terms (Accurate). By applying appropriate intellectual standards, Robert is able to determine that the ulcer is healing and has improved since the last assessment.

Professional Standards. Professional standards for critical thinking refer to ethical criteria for nursing judgments, evidence-based criteria used for evaluation, and criteria for professional responsibility (Paul, 1993). Application of professional standards requires you to use critical thinking for the good of individuals or groups (Kataoka-Yahiro and Saylor, 1994). Professional standards promote the highest level of quality nursing care.

Excellent nursing practice is a reflection of ethical standards. Client care requires more than just the application of scientific knowledge. Being able to focus on a client's values and beliefs helps you to make clinical decisions that are just, faithful to the client's choices, and beneficial to the client's well-being. Critical thinkers maintain a sense of self-awareness through conscious awareness of their beliefs, values, feelings, and the multiple perspectives that clients, family members, and peers present in clinical situations. Chapter 22 summarizes ethical standards to use when clients face ethical dilemmas or problems.

Critical thinking also requires the use of evidence-based criteria for making clinical judgments. These criteria are sometimes scientifically based on research findings (see Chapter 5) or practice based on standards developed by clinical experts and an institution's quality improvement initiatives. An example is the clinical practice guidelines developed by individual clinical agencies and national organizations such as the Agency for Healthcare Research and Quality (AHRQ). A clinical practice guideline includes standards for the treatment of select clinical conditions such as stroke, deep vein thrombosis, and pressure ulcers. Another example is clinical criteria used to categorize clinical conditions, such as the criteria used to stage pressure ulcers (see Chapter 48) and rate phlebitis (see Chapter 41). Evidence-based evaluation criteria set the minimum requirements necessary to ensure appropriate and high-quality care.

Nurses routinely use evidence-based criteria to assess clients' conditions and to determine the efficacy of nursing interventions. For example, accurate assessment of symptoms such as pain or shortness of breath includes use of assessment criteria such as the duration, severity, location, aggravating or relieving factors, and effects on daily lifestyle (see Chapter 33). In this case, assessment criteria allow you to accurately determine the nature of a client's symptom, select appropriate therapies, and then evaluate if the therapies are effective. Another example is the determination of the stage of a pressure ulcer based on scientific criteria, including skin temperature, tissue consistency, and depth of wound (see Chapter 48). The criteria allow you to select the stage of a pressure ulcer and to track how quickly it heals.

The standards of professional responsibility that a nurse tries to achieve are those standards cited in Nurse Practice Acts, institutional practice guidelines, and professional organizations' standards of practice. The American Nurses Association Standards of Professional Performance (see Chapter 1) is an example. These standards "raise the bar" for the responsibilities and accountabilities that a nurse assumes in guaranteeing quality health care to the public.

Developing Critical Thinking Skills

To develop critical thinking skills, it is important to learn how to connect knowledge and theory with practice. Your ability to make sense of what you learn in the classroom, from reading, or from

✳ BOX 15-3   EVIDENCE-BASED PRACTICE

How to "Think Like a Nurse"

Evidence Summary

Faculty use a variety of teaching/learning strate-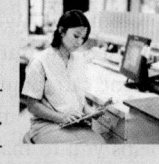
gies in developing critical thinking in students.
This study invited junior and senior nursing students from four different schools of nursing to
answer two questions: (1) How would you describe how you
think when making clinical judgments, and (2) What were the
most important teaching/learning strategies in the development of your clinical judgment? Students described their thinking as a process that developed through experience in practice. Education and practice are combined so that knowledge
gained in the classroom becomes second nature in practice.
Students noted that they learn to think through different options and then to weigh those options when caring for clients.
Then students realized what they need to do first to improve
client outcomes. Clinical experience was the most important
learning strategy in developing clinical judgment. The use of
concept maps to show the interrelatedness of all aspects of
client care was also useful. Case studies allow students to focus, think critically, and tie things together.

Application to Nursing Practice

Teaching and learning strategies that help develop clinical
judgment include the following:
- Case studies displayed on concept maps
- Having in-depth discussion with instructors while observing clinical changes in clients
- Making joint decisions with peers and instructors on client
  care

Reference

Di Vito-Thomas P: Nursing student stories on learning how to
think like a nurse, *Nurse Educ* 30(3):133, 2005.

having dialogue with other students and to then to apply it during
client care is always challenging. There are learning approaches
that will assist you in developing and improving critical thinking
skills (Box 15-3).

Reflective Journaling

How often do you think back on a situation to consider Why did
that occur? How did I act? What could I have done differently?
What knowledge could I have used? **Reflection** is the process of
purposefully thinking back or recalling a situation to discover its
purpose or meaning. Reflection is like rewinding a videotape. It
involves playing back a situation in your head and taking time to
honestly review everything you remember about the situation.
Reflection requires adequate knowledge and is necessary for self-
evaluation.

Reflective journal writing is a tool in developing critical
thought and reflection through clarifying concepts (Bilinski,
2002). Reflective writing gives you as a student the opportunity
to define and express the clinical experience in your own words
(DiVito-Thomas, 2005). By keeping a journal of each of your
clinical experiences, you are able to explore personal perceptions
or understanding of the experience and develop the ability to ap-

ply theory in practice. The use of a journal improves your observation and descriptive skills. Writing skills also improve through
the development of conceptual clarity. The Circle of Meaning
model adapted to nursing encourages concept clarification and a
search for meaning in nursing practice (Bilinski, 2002). The
model uses a series of questions to help you journey through the
clinical experience and find meaning and connections. The questions include the following:

- What experience, situation, or information in your clinical experience seems confusing, difficult, or interesting?
- What is the meaning of the experience? What feelings did you
  have? What feelings did your client have? What influenced the
  experience? What guesses or questions developed with the first
  connection in question one? Give examples.
- Do the feelings, guesses, or questions remind you of any experience from the past or present or something that you think is
  a desirable future experience? How does it relate? What are
  the implications/significance?
- What are the connections between what is being described
  and what you have learned about nursing science, research
  and theory? What are some possible solutions? What approach
  or solution would you choose and why? What is the effectiveness of this approach?

Keeping a journal of your client care experiences will help you
become aware of how you use clinical decision-making skills
(Kessler and Lund, 2004). Begin by recording notes after a clinical experience. Telling a story and drawing a picture are two additional ways to identify the experience you wish to reflect on.
Describe in detail what you felt, thought, and did. Analyze experience by considering feelings, thoughts, and possible meaning.
Challenge any preconceived ideas you have when you look at actual clinical situations. Describe the significance of the experience. Refer to your journal often when you care for clients in
similar situations.

Concept Mapping

As a nurse you will care for clients who have multiple nursing
diagnoses or collaborative problems. A **concept map** is a visual
representation of client problems and interventions that shows
their relationships to one another (Schuster, 2003). The primary
purpose of concept mapping is to synthesize relevant data about a
client, including assessment data, nursing diagnoses, health needs,
nursing interventions, and evaluation measures (Hill, 2006).
Through drawing a concept map, you learn to organize or link
information in a unique way so that the diverse information you
have about a client begins to connect to form meaningful patterns
and concepts. When you see the relationship between the various
client diagnoses and the data that support them, you better understand a client's clinical situation. Over time, concept maps
become more detailed, integrated, and comprehensive as you
learn more about the care of a client and you care for similar clients (Ferrario, 2004). You will see similarities and differences between clients, which helps you build decision-making skills.

Concept maps take many visual forms. However, most students follow a model that makes the concept map a working

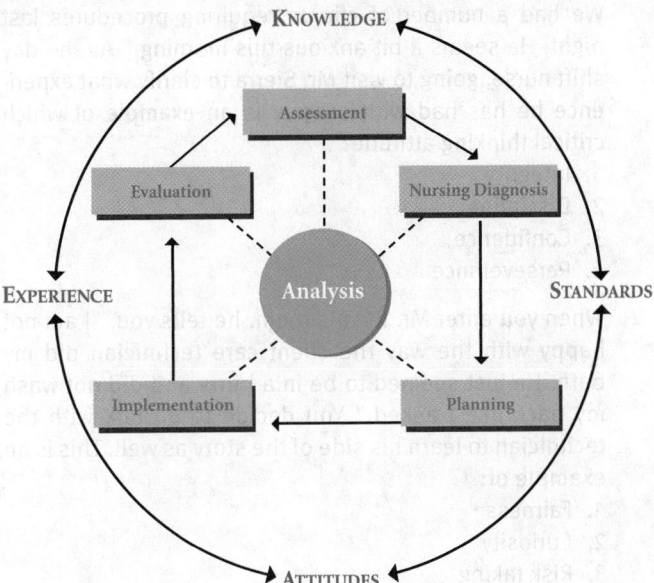

Figure 15-3 Synthesis of critical thinking with the nursing process competency.

document. As a student, you will write and develop the map during your care for the client. You begin by obtaining client data from a variety of sources (e.g., the medical record, pertinent nursing literature, the client's history and physical examination, and other health care providers). Once you gather data, begin to draw components of your map. The client's major medical diagnosis and any comorbidities (unrelated medical conditions) usually form the center of the map. From there you group patterns of assessment data that suggest certain nursing diagnoses. You draw the assessment data along the edges of the map. As you identify the different nursing diagnoses, you draw dotted lines to connect the diagnoses that are related. The links must be accurate to show true clinical relationships. On the map you also list the nursing interventions chosen for the client. Once again you see how any one intervention applies to more than one nursing diagnosis. While caring for a client, you write down the client's responses to your interventions and any clinical impressions you may have.

The final map gives you a broader and more complete understanding of your client's complex health care needs. Chapters 16 through 18 provide diagrams of actual concept maps and more detail on their development. In addition, you will find concept maps within the clinical chapters of this text.

Critical Thinking Synthesis

Critical thinking is a reasoning process by which you reflect on and analyze your own thoughts, actions, and knowledge. To be a good critical thinker requires dedication and a desire to grow intellectually. As a beginning nurse, it is important to learn the steps of the nursing process and to incorporate the elements of critical thinking (Figure 15-3). The two processes go hand-in-hand in making quality decisions about client care. This text provides a model to show you how important critical thinking is in nursing practice. Throughout the clinical chapters of this text, the components of critical thinking are emphasized to help you better understand their relationship to the nursing process.

✳ Key Concepts

- Critical thinking is a process acquired through experience, commitment, and an active curiosity toward learning.
- Clinical decision making involves judgment that includes critical and reflective thinking and action and application of scientific and practical logic.
- Nurses who apply critical thinking in their work focus on options for solving problems and making decisions, rather than rapidly and carelessly forming quick, single solutions.
- Following a procedure step-by-step without adjusting to a client's unique needs is an example of basic critical thinking.
- In complex critical thinking a nurse learns that alternative, and perhaps conflicting, solutions do exist.
- When you face a clinical problem or situation and choose a course of action from several options, you are making a clinical decision.
- In diagnostic reasoning, you collect client data and then logically explain a clinical judgment, such as a nursing diagnosis.
- You improve your clinical decision making by knowing your clients.
- The nursing process is a blueprint for client care that involves both general and specific critical thinking competencies in a way that focuses on a particular client's unique needs.
- The critical thinking model combines a nurse's knowledge base, experience, competence in the nursing process, attitudes, and standards to explain how nurses make clinical judgments that are necessary for safe, effective, nursing care.
- Clinical learning experiences are necessary for you to acquire clinical decision-making skills.
- Reflective journaling gives you the opportunity to define and express the clinical experience in your own words.
- Critical thinking attitudes help you to know when more information is necessary, when information is misleading, and to recognize your own knowledge limits.
- The use of intellectual standards during assessment ensures a complete database of information.
- Professional standards for critical thinking refer to ethical criteria for nursing judgments, evidence-based criteria for evaluation, and criteria for professional responsibility.

✳ Critical Thinking Exercises

1. Josh is a second-year nursing student. He is checking the wound of Mr. Isaac. He notes in the nurses' notes from the last shift that the wound was 3 cm long and when the skin around the wound was palpated, Mr. Isaac verbalized tenderness. When Josh examines the wound, he

measures the length and width in centimeters with a tape measure, observes the character of the tissues and drainage, and palpates around the wound for tenderness and an increase in drainage. He asks Mr. Isaac if he is having discomfort from the wound and if the pain is limiting his activity. Explain which intellectual standards Josh used in the wound assessment, and support your answers.

2. Consider the following statements, and describe which is an example of an inference, problem solving, or diagnostic reasoning. Support your answer with a rationale.
   a. The nurse enters a client's room and observes the intravenous (IV) line is not infusing at the ordered rate. The nurse checks the flow regulator on the tubing, looks to see if the client is lying on the tubing, checks the point of connection between the tubing and the IV catheter, and then checks the condition of the site where the intravenous catheter enters the client's skin. She readjusts the flow rate, and the infusion begins at the correct rate.
   b. The nurse sits down to talk with her client who lost her sister 2 weeks ago. The client reports she is unable to sleep, feels very fatigued during the day, and is having trouble at work. The nurse asks her to clarify the type of trouble, and the client explains she cannot concentrate or even solve simple problems. The nurse records the results of her assessment, describing the client as having ineffective coping.
   c. The nurse reviews a client's medical record and finds that the client has ingested only 600 mL of fluids over the last 24 hours. The client also has a low urinary output. The nurse conducts an assessment and finds the client has poor skin turgor and difficulty concentrating when asked questions about his medical history. The nurse exits the client's room and tells the health care provider that the client is likely becoming dehydrated.

3. Mr. Spicer is a terminally ill client. His wife and son are asking you about his pain control. Mrs. Spicer is asking that the health care provider increase her husband's medication, even if it means he will not be responsive. She does not want her husband to suffer. The son is opposed to too much narcotic, feeling that his father is still able to make decisions for himself. Mr. Spicer remains alert much of the time and is able to talk with you about his feelings regarding death. He seems to appreciate your availability in talking with him. How might you apply the critical thinking attitudes of fairness, responsibility, and creativity in this case study?

✳ NCLEX®-Style Review Questions

1. During change-of-shift report the night nurse states, "Mr. Sierra told me that he has had a bad experience with surgery in the past. I did not get a chance to ask him about it. We had a number of clients requiring procedures last night. He seems a bit anxious this morning." As the day shift nurse, going to visit Mr. Sierra to clarify what experience he has had with surgery is an example of which critical thinking attitude?
   1. Integrity
   2. Discipline
   3. Confidence
   4. Perseverance

2. When you enter Mr. Ryan's room, he tells you, "I am not happy with the way the client care technician did my bath. He just seemed to be in a hurry and did not wash my back like I asked." You decide to go talk with the technician to learn his side of the story as well. This is an example of:
   1. Fairness
   2. Curiosity
   3. Risk taking
   4. Responsibility

3. The surgical unit has initiated the use of a pain rating scale, which is to be used to assess clients' pain severity during their postoperative recovery. Susan, the registered nurse (RN) assigned to Ms. Wills, looks at the pain flow sheet to see Ms. Wills' pain scores over the last 24 hours. Use of the pain scale is an example of which intellectual standard?
   1. Deep
   2. Relevant
   3. Consistent
   4. Significant

4. During the day the nurse spends time instructing a client in how to self-administer insulin. After discussing the techniques and demonstrating an injection, the nurse has the client try it. After two attempts the client obviously does not understand how to prepare the correct dose. When the nurse returns to the medication room, he discusses the situation with the charge nurse, reviewing his approach with the client and asking for her suggestions on his technique. This is an example of:
   1. Reflection
   2. Risk taking
   3. Problem solving
   4. Client assessment

5. A nurse uses an institution's procedure manual to confirm how to insert a Foley catheter. The level of critical thinking the nurse is using is:
   1. Commitment
   2. Scientific method
   3. Basic critical thinking
   4. Complex critical thinking

6. A client had hip surgery 24 hours ago. The nurse refers to the written plan of care, noting that the client has a drainage device collecting wound drainage. The health care provider is to be notified when drainage in the device exceeds 100 mL for the day. When the nurse enters the room, the nurse looks at the device and carefully notes the amount of drainage currently in the device. This is an example of:
   1. Planning
   2. Evaluation
   3. Intervention
   4. Assessment

7. The nurse asks a client how she feels about her impending surgery for breast cancer. Before the discussion the nurse reviewed the description in his textbook of loss and grief in addition to therapeutic communication principles. The critical thinking component involved in the nurse's review of the literature is:
   1. Experience
   2. Problem solving
   3. Knowledge application
   4. Clinical decision making

16 | Nursing Assessment

⁕ **OBJECTIVES**

Mastery of the content in this chapter will enable the student to:
- Discuss the steps of nursing assessment.
- Explain the relationship of critical thinking to assessment.
- Differentiate between subjective and objective data
- Discuss the purposes of a client interview.
- Discuss how the use of interview techniques help clients to tell their health stories.
- Describe the components of a nursing history.
- Describe the relationship between data collection and data analysis.
- Explain the difference between a comprehensive, problem-oriented, and focused assessment.
- Explain the relationship between data interpretation, validation, and clustering.
- Conduct a nursing assessment.

⁕ **MEDIA RESOURCES**   ⁕ **KEY TERMS**

 Companion CD
- NCLEX®-Style Review Questions
- Audio Glossary
- Interactive Learning Activities
- English/Spanish Glossary

 Website
- NCLEX®-Style Review Questions
- Audio Glossary
- English/Spanish Glossary
- Interactive Learning Activities
- WebLinks
- Audio Summaries

The **nursing process** is a professional nurse's approach to identify, diagnose, and treat human responses to health and illness (American Nurses Association, 2003). It is fundamental to how nurses practice. As a nursing student, you will learn the five steps—assessment, diagnosis, planning, implementation, and evaluation—as if they were a linear process (Figure 16-1). However, in fact, the nursing process is continuous, and in practice you will learn to move back and forth between the various steps (Potter and others, 2005). Consider the following scenario:

Lisa, a registered nurse (RN) on an orthopedic nursing unit, enters Ms. Devine's room for the first time at 0730 when her shift begins. Ms. Devine is a 52-year-old woman who had an injury from a fall 2 months ago that caused a ruptured lumbar disk. She is scheduled for a lumbar laminectomy this afternoon. When Lisa first observes Ms. Devine, she notes the client is moving in bed awkwardly and she grimaces when she turns. Ms. Devine looks up and states, "Oh, I am so glad you are here (sighs). The pain in my back seems worse, and I cannot get comfortable. I cannot sit at all, so I will stay in bed for now. I just dread having this surgery, I will be so glad when this is all over (looks away and avoids eye contact)." Lisa observes Ms. Devine's facial grimace and notes her sighing. She responds, "Ms. Devine, you obviously look uncomfortable and a bit upset. Let me ask you a few questions: Show me where the pain is. On a scale of 0 to 10, with 10 the worst pain ever and 0 no pain, how would you rate your pain? Does it become worse when you turn?" As Ms. Devine responds to the questions, Lisa analyzes the data and considers other relevant information, such as the client's medical diagnosis (ruptured lumbar disk) and knowledge of the alterations the condition typically causes (e.g., sciatic pain and change in sensation of the lower extremities). Lisa decides that Ms. Devine has acute pain related to pressure on the spinal nerves. Lisa explains to Ms. Devine a plan to help relieve the discomfort. She then administers an ordered analgesic, repositions Ms. Devine, and discusses how Ms. Devine can practice relaxation exercises. Forty minutes later Lisa returns to Ms. Devine's room to determine if the pain is relieved and if she wants to try the relaxation exercises.

Lisa applied the nursing process while caring for Ms. Devine. Each time you meet a client, you will apply the nursing process to provide appropriate and effective nursing care. The process begins with the first step, assessment, the gathering and analysis of information about the client's health status. You then make clinical judgments about the client's response to health problems in the form of nursing diagnoses. Once you define appropriate nursing diagnoses, you create a plan of care. The plan includes interventions individualized to each of the client's nursing diagnoses. The next step, implementation, involves the actual delivery of planned interventions. After administering interventions, you evaluate the client's response and whether the interventions were effective. The nursing process is central to your ability to provide timely and appropriate care to your clients.

The nursing process is a variation of scientific reasoning that allows you to organize and systematize nursing practice. You will learn to make inferences about the meaning of a client's response to a health problem or generalize about the client's functional state of health. A pattern will begin to form. For example, if Ms. Devine is having acute back pain, the data allows Lisa to infer that the client's mobility is limited. Lisa gathers more informa

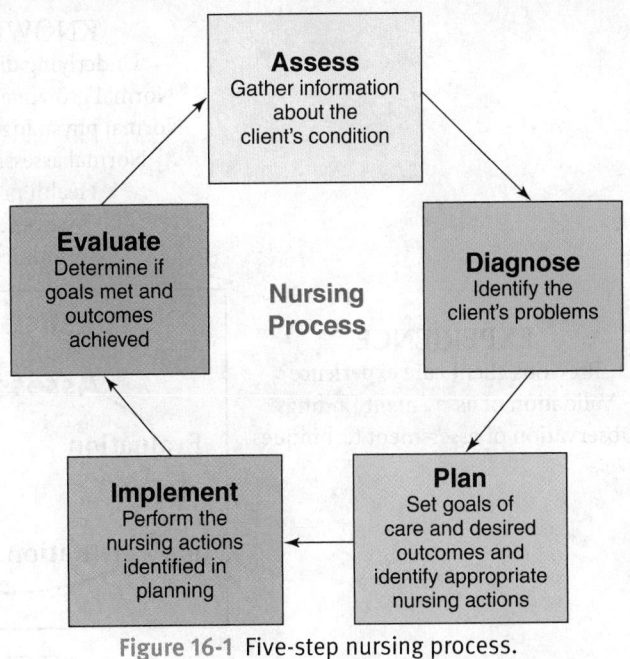

Figure 16-1 Five-step nursing process.

tion (e.g., noting how the client moves and whether the client is able to walk, stand, and sit normally) until an accurate classification of the client's problem is determined, such as the following nursing diagnosis: *impaired physical mobility related to acute back pain.* The clear definition of the client's problems provides the basis for planning and implementing nursing interventions and evaluating the outcomes of care.

Critical Thinking Approach to Assessment

Assessment is the deliberate and systematic collection of data to determine a client's current and past health status and functional status and to determine the client's present and past coping patterns (Carpenito-Moyet, 2005). Nursing **assessment** includes two steps:

- Collection and verification of data from a primary source (the client) and secondary sources (e.g., family, health professionals, and medical record)
- The analysis of all data as a basis for developing nursing diagnoses, identifying collaborative problems, and developing a plan of individualized care

The purpose of assessment is to establish a **database** about the client's perceived needs, health problems, and responses to these problems. In addition, the data reveal related experiences, health practices, goals, values, and expectations about the health care system.

When a plumber comes to your home to repair a problem you describe as a "leaking faucet," the plumber will check the faucet, its attachments to the water line, and the water pressure in the system to determine the real problem. As a nurse, a client will present an initial health problem to you. You will then proceed to observe the client's behaviors, ask questions about the nature of

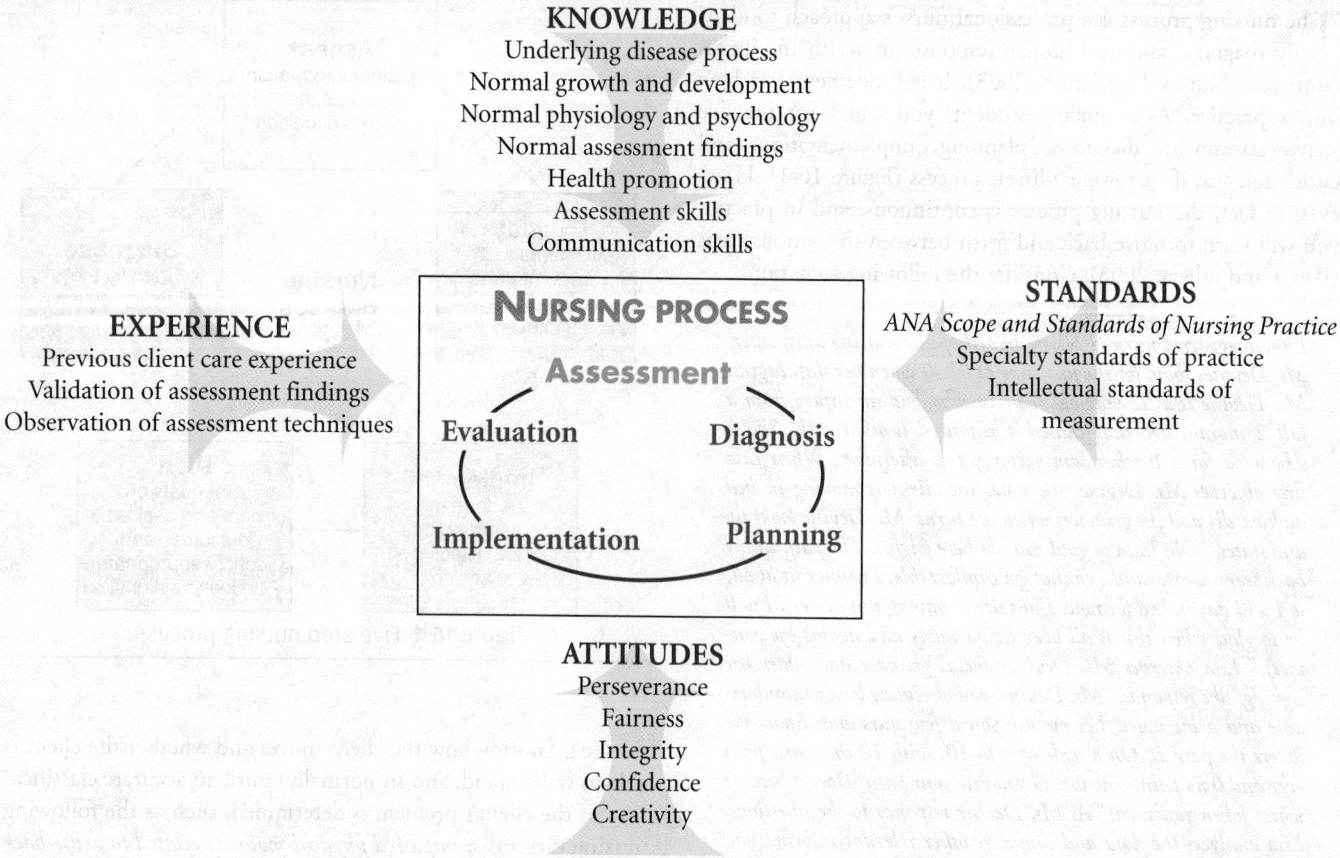

KNOWLEDGE
Underlying disease process
Normal growth and development
Normal physiology and psychology
Normal assessment findings
Health promotion
Assessment skills
Communication skills

EXPERIENCE
Previous client care experience
Validation of assessment findings
Observation of assessment techniques

NURSING PROCESS
Assessment
Evaluation   Diagnosis
Implementation   Planning

STANDARDS
ANA Scope and Standards of Nursing Practice
Specialty standards of practice
Intellectual standards of measurement

ATTITUDES
Perseverance
Fairness
Integrity
Confidence
Creativity

Figure 16-2 Critical thinking and the assessment process.

the problem, listen to the cues the client provides, and conduct a physical examination (see Chapter 33). Sometimes you will also interview family members who are familiar with the client's health problem and review any existing medical record data. All of the data you collect will fall into different sets or patterns of information that point to a diagnostic conclusion. Once a plumber knows the source of the leaking faucet, he is able to repair the faucet. Once you know the nature and source of a client's health problems, you are able to provide interventions that will restore, maintain, or improve the client's health.

Critical thinking is important in the application of assessment (see Chapter 15). Critical thinking allows you to see the big picture when you form conclusions or make decisions about a client's health condition. While gathering data about a client, you will synthesize relevant knowledge, recall prior clinical experiences, apply critical thinking standards and attitudes, and use standards of practice to direct your assessment in a meaningful and purposeful way (Figure 16-2). Your knowledge from the physical, biological, and social sciences allows you to ask relevant questions and collect relevant history and physical assessment data related to the client's presenting health care needs. For example, by knowing that a client has a history of a ruptured lumbar disk, you know to ask if the client has sciatic pain (characteristic pain that radiates or spreads from the buttocks down the leg) and to question how the discomfort affects the client's ability to walk or sit, because these are common symptoms of disk disease. The use of good communication skills and critical thinking intellectual standards enable you to collect complete, accurate, and relevant data.

Prior clinical experience contributes to the skills of assessment. For example, if you cared for a client with back pain in the past, you know the pain is sometimes disabling and limits the client's normal motion. Thus you thoroughly assess the extent to which the pain affects the client's ability to walk normally and to perform daily living activities. Validation of abnormal assessment findings and personal observation of assessments performed by skilled professionals helps you to become competent in assessment. You also learn to apply standards of practice and accepted standards of "normal" for physical assessment data when assessing clients. Use of critical thinking attitudes such as curiosity, perseverance, and confidence ensure you complete a comprehensive database.

Data Collection

As you begin a client assessment, think critically about what to assess. Determine what questions or measurements are appropriate based on your clinical knowledge and experience and your client's health history and responses. When you first meet a client, make a quick observational overview or screening. Usually an overview is based on a treatment situation. For example, a community health nurse assesses the neighborhood and the community of the client; an emergency room nurse uses the ABC (airway-breathing-circulation) approach; and an oncology nurse focuses on the client's symptoms from disease and treatment and grief response. In the case of Ms. Devine, Lisa first focuses on the nature and severity of her client's pain, the risk of limited mobility, and the extent of the client's anxiety. She will later expand her

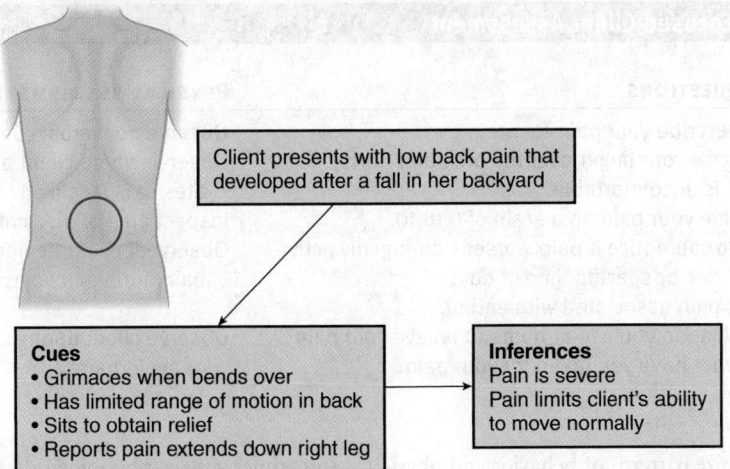

Figure 16-3 Observational overview using cues and forming inferences.

assessment to determine if Ms. Devine has been prepared for her upcoming surgery.

You will learn to differentiate important data from the total data collected. A **cue** is information that you obtain through use of the senses. An **inference** is your judgment or interpretation of those cues (Figure 16-3). For example, a client crying is a cue that possibly implies fear or sadness. You ask the client about any concerns and make known any nonverbal expressions you notice in an effort to direct the client to share his or her feelings. It is possible to miss important cues when you conduct an initial overview. However, always try to interpret cues from the client to know how in-depth to make your assessment. Remember, thinking is human and imperfect. You will acquire appropriate thinking processes in the conduct of assessment, but expect to make mistakes in missing important cues (Lunney, 2006). Assessment is dynamic and allows you to freely explore relevant client problems as you discover them.

After your observational overview, focus on the assessment cues and patterns of information that suggest problem areas. There are two approaches to a comprehensive assessment. One involves use of a structured database format, based upon an accepted theoretical framework or practice standard. Gordon's 11 **functional health patterns** (1994) (Box 16-1), Pender's health promotion model (1996), and the Agency for Healthcare Research and Quality's (AHRQ's) standards for acute pain assessment (1992) are all examples. The theory or practice standard provides categories of information for you to assess. In the example of Gordon's functional health patterns, the model offers a holistic framework for assessment of any health problem. In the case of Ms. Devine, Lisa directs her assessment to the cognitive-perceptual pattern to learn more about what the client knows about the impending surgery and how she prefers to learn and make decisions about her care. Lisa also assesses Ms. Devine's coping–stress tolerance pattern to determine how Ms. Devine is accepting the temporary loss of function and the level of support offered by her husband. A theoretical or standard-based assessment provides for a comprehensive assessment of the client's health care problems.

An assessment moves from the general to the specific. For example, you assess all of Gordon's 11 functional health patterns and then determine if there are patterns or problems. You ask more focused questions about those health patterns that suggest a

---

✳ BOX 16-1 Typology of 11 Functional Health Patterns

Health perception–health management pattern: Describes the client's self-report of health and well-being; how client manages health (e.g., frequency of health care provider visits, adherence to therapies at home); knowledge of preventive health practices.

Nutritional-metabolic pattern: Describes the client's daily/weekly pattern of food and fluid intake (e.g., food preferences or restrictions, special diet, appetite); actual weight, weight loss or gain.

Elimination pattern: Describes patterns of excretory function (bowel, bladder, and skin).

Activity-exercise pattern: Describes patterns of exercise, activity, leisure, and recreation; ability to perform activities of daily living.

Sleep-rest pattern: Describes patterns of sleep, rest, and relaxation.

Cognitive-perceptual pattern: Describes sensory-perceptual patterns; language adequacy, memory, decision-making ability.

Self-perception–self-concept pattern: Describes the client's self-concept pattern and perceptions of self (e.g., self-concept/worth, emotional patterns, body image).

Role-relationship pattern: Describes the client's patterns of role engagements and relationships.

Sexuality-reproductive pattern: Describes the client's patterns of satisfaction and dissatisfaction with sexuality pattern; client's reproductive patterns; premenopausal and postmenopausal problems.

Coping–stress tolerance pattern: Describes the client's ability to manage stress; sources of support; effectiveness of the patterns in terms of stress tolerance.

Value-belief pattern: Describes patterns of values, beliefs (including spiritual practices), and goals that guide the client's choices or decisions.

Data from Gordon M: *Nursing diagnosis: process and application*, ed 3, St. Louis, 1994, Mosby; and Carpenito-Moyet LJ: *Nursing diagnosis: application to clinical practice*, ed 11, Philadelphia, 2005, Lippincott Williams & Wilkins.

✳ TABLE 16-1 Problem-Focused Client Assessment

PROBLEM AND ASSOCIATED FACTORS	QUESTIONS	PHYSICAL ASSESSMENT
Pain	Describe your pain for me.	Observe nonverbal cues.
Nature of pain	Place your finger over the area that hurts/ is uncomfortable.	Observe where client points to pain; note if it radiates or is localized.
	Rate your pain on a scale of 0 to 10.	Inspect area of discomfort, palpate for tenderness.
Precipitating factors	Do you notice if pain worsens during any activities or specific time of day?	Observe if client demonstrates nonverbal signs of pain during movement, positioning, swallowing.
	Is pain associated with eating?	
Relieving factors	What do you use at home to relieve your pain?	Observe client during activities designed to relieve or avoid pain.
	What have you taken for your pain?	

problem exists. You then organize patterns of behavior and physiological responses that relate to a functional health category. The complete assessment of the 11 functional health patterns represents the interaction of the client and the environment, which Gordon calls biopsychosocial integration. According to Gordon (1991), you cannot understand one health pattern without knowledge of the other patterns. Ultimately your assessment identifies functional patterns (client strengths) and dysfunctional patterns (nursing diagnoses), which assist in developing the nursing care plan.

The second approach for conducting a comprehensive assessment is the problem-oriented approach. You focus on the client's presenting situation and begin with problematic areas, such as back pain, difficulty breathing, or apprehension over a procedure. Then ask the client follow-up questions to clarify and expand your assessment. Table 16-1 offers an example of a problem-focused assessment. Once you complete the assessment, thoroughly analyze the extent and nature of the client's problem so that you are able to later develop a care plan.

Whatever approach you use to collect data, you begin to cluster cues, make inferences, and identify emerging patterns and potential problem areas. To do this well, you critically anticipate, which means you try to stay a step ahead of the assessment. Remember to always have supporting cues before you make an inference. Your inferences will direct you to further questions. Once you ask a question of a client or make an observation, the information branches to an additional series of questions or observations (Figure 16-4). You take a risk when you do not anticipate assessment questions. This can cause an incomplete assessment, or you might fail to recognize cues and dismiss relevant problem areas. Knowing how to probe and frame questions is a skill that grows with experience. You will learn to decide which questions are relevant to a situation and to attend to accurate interpretations of data.

Types of Data.
There are two primary sources of data, subjective and objective. **Subjective data** are your clients' verbal descriptions of their health problems. Only clients provide subjective data. For example, Ms. Divine's report of back pain and her expression of dread over having to have surgery are subjective findings. Subjective data usually include feelings, perceptions, and self-report of symptoms. Although only clients provide subjective data relevant to their health condition, be aware that the data

sometimes reflect physiological changes, which you further explore through objective data collection.

Objective data are observations or measurements of a client's health status. Inspection of the condition of a wound, a description of an observed behavior, and the measurement of blood pressure are examples of objective data. The measurement of objective data is based on an accepted standard, such as the Fahrenheit or Celsius measure on a thermometer, centimeters on a measuring tape, or known characteristics of behaviors (e.g., anxiety or fear). When you collect objective data, apply critical thinking intellectual standards (e.g., clear, precise, and consistent) so that you can correctly interpret your findings.

Sources of Data.
As a nurse, you will obtain data from a variety of sources. Each source of data provides information about the client's level of wellness, anticipated prognosis, risk factors, health practices and goals, and patterns of health and illness.

Client. A client is usually your best source of information. Clients who are conscious, alert, and able to answer questions correctly provide the most accurate information about their health care needs, lifestyle patterns, present and past illnesses, perception of symptoms, and changes in activities of daily living. Always consider the setting for your assessment. A client experiencing acute symptoms in an emergency department will not offer as much information as one who comes to an outpatient clinic for a routine checkup. Always be attentive and show a caring presence with the client (see Chapter 8). Let the client know you are interested in what he or she has to say. Clients are less likely to fully reveal the nature of their health care problems when nurses show little interest or are easily distracted by activities around them.

Family and Significant Others. Family members and significant others are primary sources of information for infants or children, critically ill adults, and mentally handicapped, disoriented, or unconscious clients. In cases of severe illness or emergency situations, families are sometimes the only available sources of information for nurses and clients' health care providers. The family and significant others are also important secondary sources of information. They confirm findings a client provides (e.g., whether a client takes medications regularly at home or how well the client sleeps or eats). Include the family when appropriate. Remember, a client does not always wish you to question the family. Often spouses or close friends will sit in during an assessment

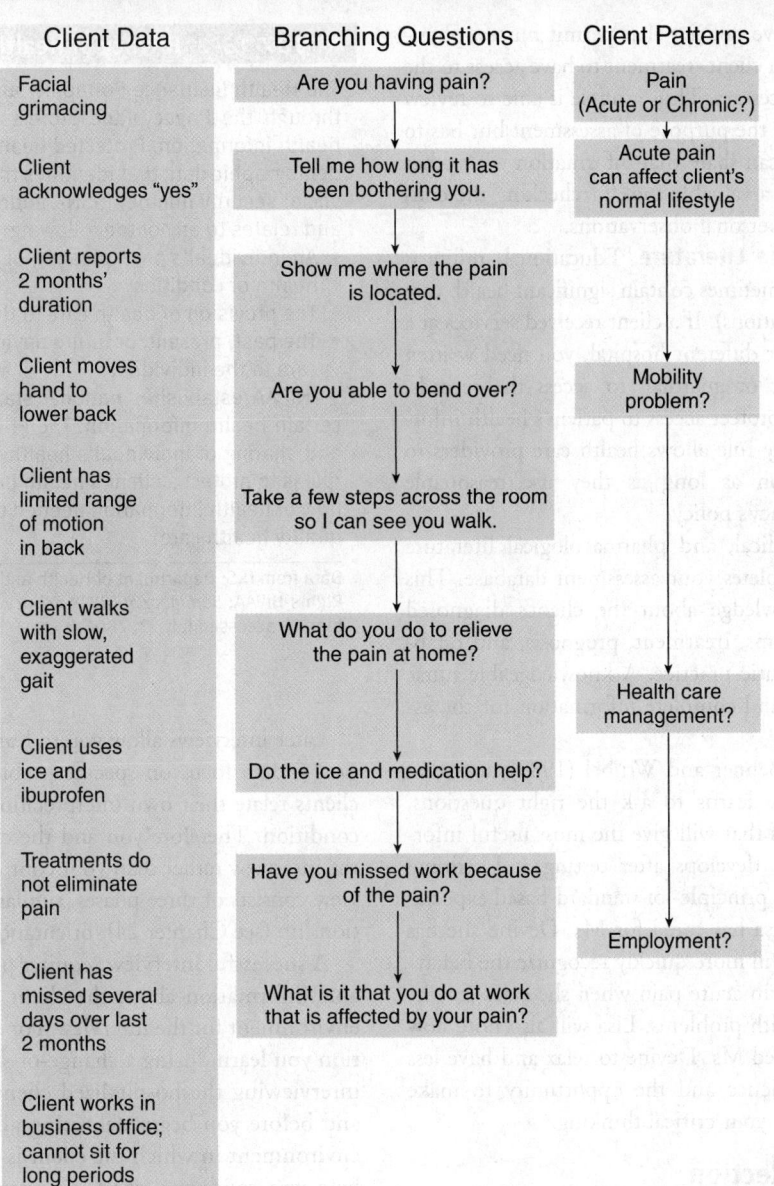

Client Data	Branching Questions	Client Patterns
Facial grimacing	Are you having pain?	Pain (Acute or Chronic?)
Client acknowledges "yes"	Tell me how long it has been bothering you.	Acute pain can affect client's normal lifestyle
Client reports 2 months' duration	Show me where the pain is located.	
Client moves hand to lower back	Are you able to bend over?	Mobility problem?
Client has limited range of motion in back	Take a few steps across the room so I can see you walk.	
Client walks with slow, exaggerated gait	What do you do to relieve the pain at home?	
Client uses ice and ibuprofen	Do the ice and medication help?	Health care management?
Treatments do not eliminate pain	Have you missed work because of the pain?	
Client has missed several days over last 2 months	What is it that you do at work that is affected by your pain?	Employment?
Client works in business office; cannot sit for long periods		

Figure 16-4 Example of branching logic for selecting assessment questions.

and provide their view of the client's health problems or needs. Not only do they supply information about the client's current health status, but they are also able to tell when changes in the client's status occurred. Family members are often very well informed, because of their experiences living with the client and observing how health problems affect daily living activities. Family and friends make important observations about the client's needs that can affect the way care is delivered (e.g., how a client eats a meal or how a client makes choices).

Health Care Team. You frequently communicate with other health care team members in gathering information about clients. In the acute care setting, the change-of-shift report is the way for nurses from one shift to communicate information to nurses on the next shift (see Chapter 26). Typically when nurses, physicians, physical therapists, social workers, or other staff consult on a client's condition, they have information about the client. This in-

cludes how the client is interacting within the health care environment, the client's reactions to treatment, the result of diagnostic procedures or therapies, and how the client responds to visitors. Every member of the team is a source of information for identifying and verifying information about the client.

Medical Records. The medical record is a source for the client's medical history, laboratory and diagnostic test results, current physical findings, and the primary health care provider's treatment plan. Data in the records offer a baseline and ongoing information about the client's response to illness and progress to date. The Health Insurance Portability and Accountability Act (HIPAA) of 1996 has a privacy rule that came into effect on April 14, 2003, to set standards for the protection of health information (HIPAAdvisory, 2003). Information in a client's record is confidential. Each health care agency has policies governing how the information can be shared between health care providers. For example, some hospitals have policies that permit nurses, physicians, and others involved in client treatment to have access to the entire medical record as necessary. Thus a nurse is able to review a client's medical record for the purpose of assessment but has to be aware of how he or she can share that information with other staff. The medical record is a valuable tool for checking the consistency and similarities of personal observations.

Other Records and the Literature. Educational, military, and employment records sometimes contain significant health care information (e.g., immunizations). If a client received services at a community health center or different hospital, you need written permission from the client or guardian to access the records. HIPAA (2006) regulations protect access to patient's health information. The HIPAA privacy rule allows health care providers to share protected information as long as they use reasonable safegaurds. Check your agency's policy.

Reviewing nursing, medical, and pharmacological literature about a client's illness completes your assessment database. This review increases your knowledge about the client's diagnosed problems, expected symptoms, treatment, prognosis, and established standards of therapeutic practice. A knowledgeable nurse obtains relevant, accurate, and complete information for the assessment database.

Nurse's Experience. Benner and Wrubel (1989) note that through experience a nurse learns to ask the right questions, choosing only the questions that will give the most useful information. A nurse's expertise develops after testing and refining propositions, questions, and principle- or standard-based expectations. For example, after Lisa has cared for Ms. Devine she has learned some lessons. Lisa will more quickly recognize the behavior the client showed while in acute pain when she cares for the next client with similar health problems. Lisa will also note how positioning techniques helped Ms. Devine to relax and have less discomfort. Practical experience and the opportunity to make clinical decisions strengthen your critical thinking.

Methods of Data Collection

As a nurse, you will use the client interview, nursing health history, physical examination, and results of laboratory and diagnostic tests to establish a client's assessment database.

Interview and Nursing Health History. The first step in establishing a database is to collect subjective information by interviewing the client. An **interview** is an organized conversation with the client. The initial formal interview involves obtaining the client's health history and information about the current illness. During the initial interview you have the opportunity to do the following:

- Introduce yourself to the client, explain your role, and explain the role of others during care
- Establish a caring therapeutic relationship with the client
- Get insight about the client's concerns and worries
- Determine the client's goals and expectations of the health care system
- Obtain cues about which parts of the data collection phase require further in-depth investigation

---

> ✴ **BOX 16-2 Privacy of Health Information**
>
> The Health Insurance Portability and Accountability Act (HIPAA) through the Privacy Rule protects all individually identifiable health information. Protected health information (PHI) includes demographic data that identifies the individual (e.g., birth date, social security number [SSN], address, medical record number) and relates to any of the following:
>
> - An individual's past, present, or future physical or mental health or condition
> - The provision of health care to the individual
> - The past, present, or future payment for provision of health care to the individual
>
> HIPAA establishes national standards for the protection of certain health information. The Privacy Rule addresses the use and sharing of individual's health information. The goal of this rule is to protect a client's health information while allowing the flow of health information needed to provide and promote high-quality health care.
>
> Data from U.S. Department of Health and Human Services, Office for Civil Rights-HIPAA: *Summary of HIPAA Privacy Rule,* http://www.hhs.gov/ocr/hipaa/, accessed July 23, 2006.

Later interviews allow you to learn more about a client's situation and to focus on specific problem areas. An interview helps clients relate their own interpretation and understanding of their condition. Therefore you and the client become partners during the interview rather than your controlling the interview. An interview consists of three phases, similar to that of a therapeutic relationship (see Chapter 24): orientation, working, and termination.

A successful interview requires preparation. Collect any available information about the client, and then create a favorable environment for the interview. For example, review the information you learn during a change-of-shift report, and then plan on interviewing the hospitalized client as you make client rounds and before you begin delivering any ordered interventions. An environment in which the client is comfortable and relaxed will help you conduct a good interview. Thus in a hospital setting you will often have to intervene with symptom management before the client is able to comfortably talk with you. Some clients interviewed at home prefer that the interview take place in a bedroom away from other family members or in the living room with a spouse present. Remember to let a client decide whether to involve the family. Finally, select a place private enough to allow the client to be comfortable when providing personal information.

Orientation Phase. The orientation phase begins with introducing yourself and your position and explaining the purpose of the interview. Explain to clients why you are collecting data (e.g., for a nursing history or for a focused assessment) and assure them that any information obtained will remain confidential and will be used only by health care professionals who provide their care. HIPAA regulations require clients to sign an authorization before you collect personal health data (HIPAAdvisory, 2003). This usually occurs in admitting and screening areas before you meet the client. Refer to your agency policy for the authorization process. Box 16-2 summarizes protected health information (USDHHS, 2006).

✳ **BOX 16-3**   **FOCUS ON OLDER ADULTS**

Nonverbal Behaviors Conducive to the Nurse-Client Relationship

Nonverbal communication includes all forms of communication that do not involve the spoken word. When older adults have limited hearing or visual deficits, it becomes important for a nurse to use nonverbal communication when establishing nurse-client relationships.

- **Client-directed eye gaze:** Allows the nurse or client who is speaking to check whether information is understood. It is a signal for readiness to initiate interaction with a client. Eye contact shows you are interested in what the other person is saying.
- **Affirmative head nodding:** Has an important social function. It helps to regulate an interaction (especially when people change turns in speaking), it supports spoken language, and it allows for comment upon the interaction concerning the rapport and content of the communication.
- **Smiling:** Smiling is positive and considered as a sign of good humor, warmth, and immediacy. It is most important when a nurse wishes to establish good relationship with clients.
- **Forward leaning:** Shows awareness, attention, and immediacy. During an interaction it also clearly suggests interest in that person.
- **Touch:** Important in building rapport and a relationship with a client. If used appropriately it can also convey affection, care, and comfort.

Modified from Caris-Verhallen WMC and others: Non-verbal behaviour in nurse-elderly patient communication, *J Adv Nurs* 29(4):808, 1999.

During the orientation phase you establish trust and confidence with a client. One important goal for the initial interview is to make the foundation for understanding the client's primary needs. Another is to begin a relationship that allows the client to become an active partner in decisions about care. As the orientation phase proceeds, a client should begin to feel more comfortable speaking with you. Initially you will gather demographic data (e.g., date of birth, gender, race, marital status, religious preference, and occupation), as specified by your facility. Because this information is the least personal, it helps initiate development of the therapeutic relationship and eases transition into the working portion of the interview. While conducting the interview, always be aware that the client is forming an impression about nursing.

The professionalism and the competence you show to clients will improve the nurse-client relationship. Your attitude, professional manner, and appearance encourage a supportive therapeutic relationship with a client. Box 16-3 outlines behaviors important in establishing good relationships, particularly with older adults. Open communication between nurse and client ensures the ongoing identification of the client's health care needs. In an effective interview, you become involved with the client and family and become an advocate, or supporter, for the client.

After making Ms. Devine more comfortable, Lisa decides it is time to get to know her client better. Lisa reviews the interview process

and its objectives, confidentiality, and length. "I want to spend some time better understanding your back pain and then what you know about your surgery. If you are comfortable, I would like to spend about 10 minutes discussing this with you. Everything you share will be confidential." Lisa and Ms. Devine agree mutually on the interview time. Lisa begins by explaining her role.

Lisa: Ms. Devine, as I mentioned earlier, I'm Lisa, the nurse who will be managing your care during your hospital stay and through discharge to your home.

Ms. Devine: Lisa, you may call me Susan. What do you mean by managing my care?

Lisa: I am responsible for coordinating your nursing care with the other nurses while you're here. I will work with them to plan for your discharge back home. Sometimes other nurses will take care of you, but I am the one who plans your care. Once you go home, I'll call you to see how you are doing and if you have any questions.

Ms. Devine: Oh, okay, that sounds great. So whenever you are around, I should ask you questions about what is being planned for me.

Lisa: Absolutely. Now, I want to ask you some questions about your health so we can plan your care together. Before we get started, do you have any questions for me?

Ms. Devine: Yes. I know they plan to remove the disk in my back. It has been hurting so bad. I can't even bend over. Is there a chance I could be paralyzed?

Lisa: Tell me what your doctor has explained about surgery.

Ms. Devine: She has told me that I have a, what was it called, a herniated disk. She said it is pinching nerves in my back. Well, if it pinches nerves, could I not become paralyzed? She did tell me that she has done this procedure many times before.

Lisa: A herniated disk is serious. The disk is normally situated between two vertebrae, but in your case it is now pinching on your spinal nerves. That is why you have so much discomfort. Your surgery is aimed at removing pressure on your nerves. I would suggest you talk with your doctor about your concerns before going into surgery.

Ms. Devine: Okay, that makes me feel a little better. I have some important things going on at my work. My husband and I own our own business. I just want this to be over.

Lisa: Tell me more about your pain.

Working Phase. During the working phase of the interview you gather information about the client's health status. Remember to stay focused, orderly, and unhurried. Use a variety of communication strategies such as active listening, paraphrasing, and summarizing to promote a clear interaction (see Chapter 24). The use of open-ended questions encourages clients to tell their story in detail.

During the working phase, obtain a nursing health history by exploring the client's current illness, health history, and expectations of care. The **nursing health history** includes data about the client's current level of wellness, including a review of body systems, family and health history, sociocultural history, spiritual health, and mental and emotional reactions to illness. The objective for collecting a health history is to identify patterns of health and illness, risk factors for physical and behavioral health problems, changes from normal, and available resources for adaptation

The initial interview is normally the most extensive. Ongoing interviews, which occur each time you interact with your client, do not need to be as extensive. They update the client's status and focus more on changes in previously identified ongoing and new problems. An example of Lisa's interview techniques follows:

Lisa: *Tell me, Susan, about your back pain. (Open-ended question)*
Ms. Devine: *Sometimes it is really sharp, especially when I stand and try to walk.*
Lisa: *On a scale of 0 to 10, with 0 being no pain and 10 being the worst imaginable, how would you rate your pain when it becomes sharp?*
Ms. Devine: *Oh it can be bad, I would rate it an 8 or 9.*
Lisa: *Point to where you notice the pain. (Asking for specificity)*
Ms. Devine: *(points to her lower sacral area) It hurts here, and I also get a deep burning pain in my right buttocks.*
Lisa: *Can you tell me if anything else aggravates the pain?*
Ms. Devine: *This morning I sneezed and thought I was going to faint. Then I could feel the pain go down my right leg.*
Lisa: *Does anything else worsen the pain? (Probes for completeness)*
Ms. Devine: *Well, just about any way I move tends to make my back hurt.*
Lisa: *Any way? (Clarification)*
Ms. Devine: *It hurts when I turn or twist. If I lay flat, it does not bother me.*
Lisa: *In what way has it limited you in your usual activities? (Open-ended question)*
Ms. Devine: *Well, I have not been able to work. I went back about a month ago, but I was miserable when I tried to sit down. I could not tolerate the discomfort.*

Termination Phase. As in the other phases of the interview, termination requires skill on the part of the interviewer. Give your client a clue that the interview is coming to an end. For example, you say, "There are just two more questions I want to ask" or "We'll be finished in about 2 minutes." This helps the client maintain direct attention without being distracted by wondering when the interview will end. This approach also gives the client an opportunity to ask questions. When concluding an interview, summarize the important points and ask the client whether the summary was accurate. End the interview in a friendly manner, telling the client when you will return to provide care. For example, "*Thank you, Susan, You have given me a good picture of your back problem and what you have been told about surgery. I think pain control will be a priority before and after your surgery. Since this is your first time in the hospital, I want to be sure I explain whatever you would like to know. I am going to return in about an hour and talk with you about the surgery and what to expect. Is there anything I can do for you now?*"

A skillful interviewer adapts interview strategies based on the client's responses. You will successfully gather relevant health data when you are prepared for the interview and will be able to carry out each interview phase with minimal interruption.

Interview Techniques. How you conduct the interview is just as important as the questions you ask. Pay attention to the environment, client comfort, and use good communication techniques (see Chapter 24). During the interview you are responsible for directing the flow of the discussion so that you get enough information and your client has the opportunity to contribute freely. Ideally you want clients to tell their stories about their

health problems so that you are able to get as much detailed information as possible.

Some interviews will be focused, whereas others will be comprehensive. Listen and consider the information shared, because this will help you direct the client to give more detail or discuss a topic that will might reveal a possible problem. Because a client's report will include subjective information, validate data from the interview later with objective data. For example, if the client reports difficulty in breathing, you will later assess respiratory rate and lung sounds.

During an interview obtain information about a client's physical, developmental, emotional, intellectual, social, and spiritual dimensions. Physical and developmental information reflects normal functioning and reveals any pathological changes caused by illness, trauma or developmental crisis. Emotional information includes the client's behavioral responses to changes in health and patterns of living. Relevant emotional information includes mood, perceptions, body image, self-concept, and attitudes about sexuality. Intellectual information includes intellectual performance, problem-solving ability, educational level, communication patterns, and attention span. Social information involves environmental, cultural, ethnic, or social patterns that affect the present or future level of wellness. You also collect information about life goals and values and religious practices, part of a client's spirituality.

The interview allows you to observe the client during interactions between the family and the health care environment. Observe nonverbal communication such as use of eye contact, body language, or tone of voice. While observing nonverbal behavior, appearance, and interaction with the environment, determine whether the data you obtain by observation is consistent with what the client states verbally. Your observations will lead you to pursue further objective information to form accurate conclusions.

Clients also obtain information during interviews. If you establish a positive nurse-client relationship, the client will feel comfortable asking you questions about the health care environment, planned treatments, diagnostic testing, and available resources. The client needs this information to make decisions about goals and the plan of care.

A good interview environment is free of distractions, unnecessary noise, and interruptions. The client is more likely to be open and honest if the interview is private, out of earshot of other clients, visitors, and staff. Timing is important in avoiding interruptions. If possible, set aside a 10- to 15-minute period when no other activities are planned. More time is even better, but sometimes difficult to plan when you have multiple clients. Help the client to feel relaxed and unhurried. Before you begin the interview, be sure the client is comfortable. This starts with attending to basic needs such as allowing the client to go to the bathroom or offering pain control. Make the environment comfortable with adequate lighting, warmth, and positioning. If possible, sit facing the client to make eye contact easier. During the interview, observe your client for signs of discomfort or fatigue.

When the interview involves a health history, try to find out, in the client's own words, what the health problem is and what is likely causing it. Remember, clients are usually the best resources in relating their health history. You will begin by asking the client a question to elicit his or her story. For example, say, "So, for what reason did you come to the hospital today?" or "Tell me about the problems you are having." The use of such **open-ended questions** prompts clients to describe a situation in more than one or two words. This technique leads to a discussion in which clients actively describe their health status. The use of open-ended questions strengthens your relationship with a client because it shows that you want to hear the client's thoughts and feelings. Remember to encourage and let the client tell the story all the way through. Reinforce your interest through the use of good eye contact and listening skills. In addition, you may use **back channeling**, which includes active listening prompts such as "all right," "go on," or "uh-huh." These indicate that you have heard what the client says and are attentive to hear the full story. Back channeling encourages a client to give more details.

As the client tells his or her story, encourage a full description without trying to control the direction the story takes. This requires you to probe with further open-ended statements such as, "Is there anything else you can tell me?" or "What else is bothering you?" Ask many questions, probing to exhaustion, until the client has nothing else to say. It also helps to end the client's story by asking the client what might be causing his or her problem. This is called a client's "explanatory model." As a nurse, you are interested in a causal explanation to understand the client's perceptions and responses to any health problems and the meaning the problems have for the client. This information will help you direct the subsequent focused assessment.

Once a client finishes his or her story, use a problem-seeking interview technique. This approach takes the information provided in the client's story and then more fully describes and identifies specific problem areas. For example, a client reports experiencing indigestion over the course of several days and acknowledges having some diarrhea and loss of appetite. The client's explanation for the cause relates to a recent series of trips that changed his eating habits. Focus on the symptoms the client identifies, as well as the general indigestion problem, by asking **closed-ended questions** that limit the client's answers to one or two words such as "yes" or "no" or a number or frequency of a symptom (Box 16-4). For example, you ask, "How often does the diarrhea occur?" or "Do you have pain or cramping?" Closed-ended questions require short answers and clarify previous information or provide additional information. The questions do not encourage the client to volunteer more information than you request. This type of questioning helps you to acquire specific information about health problems such as symptoms, precipitating factors, or relief measures. As you reveal more information, you then have the client give more historical information.

A good interviewer leaves with a complete story that contains enough details for understanding a client's perceptions of his or her health status, as well as the information needed to help identify nursing diagnoses and/or collaborative health problems. Always clarify or validate any information you are unclear about.

Cultural Considerations in Assessment

As a professional nurse, it is important to conduct any assessment with cultural competence. This involves a conscientious understanding of your client's culture so that you can offer better care within differing value systems and act with respect and under-

---

❋ BOX 16-4 Examples of Open- and Closed-Ended Questions

Open-Ended Questions
Tell me how you are feeling.
Your discomfort affects your ability to get around in what way?
Describe how your wife has been helping you.
Give me an example of how you get relief from your pain at home.

Closed-Ended Questions
Do you feel like the medication is helping you?
Who is the person who helps you at home?
Do you understand why you are having the x-ray examination?
Has the warm compress given you relief from your back pain?
Are you having pain now?
On a scale of 0 to 10, how would you rate your pain?

---

standing without imposition of your own attitudes and beliefs (Seidel and others, 2003). You cannot conduct an accurate and complete assessment without considering a client's cultural background. When cultural differences exist between you and a client, be sensitive to them. You must be sure you grasp exactly what a client means and know exactly what a client thinks you mean in words and actions. If you are unsure about what a client is saying, ask for clarification. This avoids making the wrong diagnostic conclusion. Do not make assumptions about a client's cultural beliefs and behaviors without validation from the client (Seidel and others, 2003).

Good communication techniques are important when assessing a client whose culture is different from your own. Communication and culture are interrelated in the way feelings are expressed verbally and nonverbally. If you can learn the variations in how people of different cultures communicate, you will likely be able to gather more accurate information from clients. For example, the Spanish and French use firm eye contact when speaking. However, this is considered rude or immodest by certain Asian or Middle Eastern cultures. Americans often tend to let the eyes wander (Seidel and others, 2003). Using the right approach with eye contact will show respect for your client and likely result in the client sharing more information. It is easier to explore cultural differences if you allow time for thoughtful answers and ask your questions in a comfortable order. Here is an example (Seidel and others, 2003):

When talking about a client's illness:

- What do you think is wrong with you?
- People have told me that there are sicknesses that doctors and nurses don't know about. Have you heard of them? What are they?
- Have you ever know anyone with one of them?
- Have you ever had one of them?
- Do you think you might have it right now?

When you interact to assess any specific client, first know your own cultural self. You need to avoid forming a sense of the client based on prior knowledge of the client's culture. Instead, draw upon the knowledge and then ask questions in a constructive and probing way to allow you to truly know who the client is.

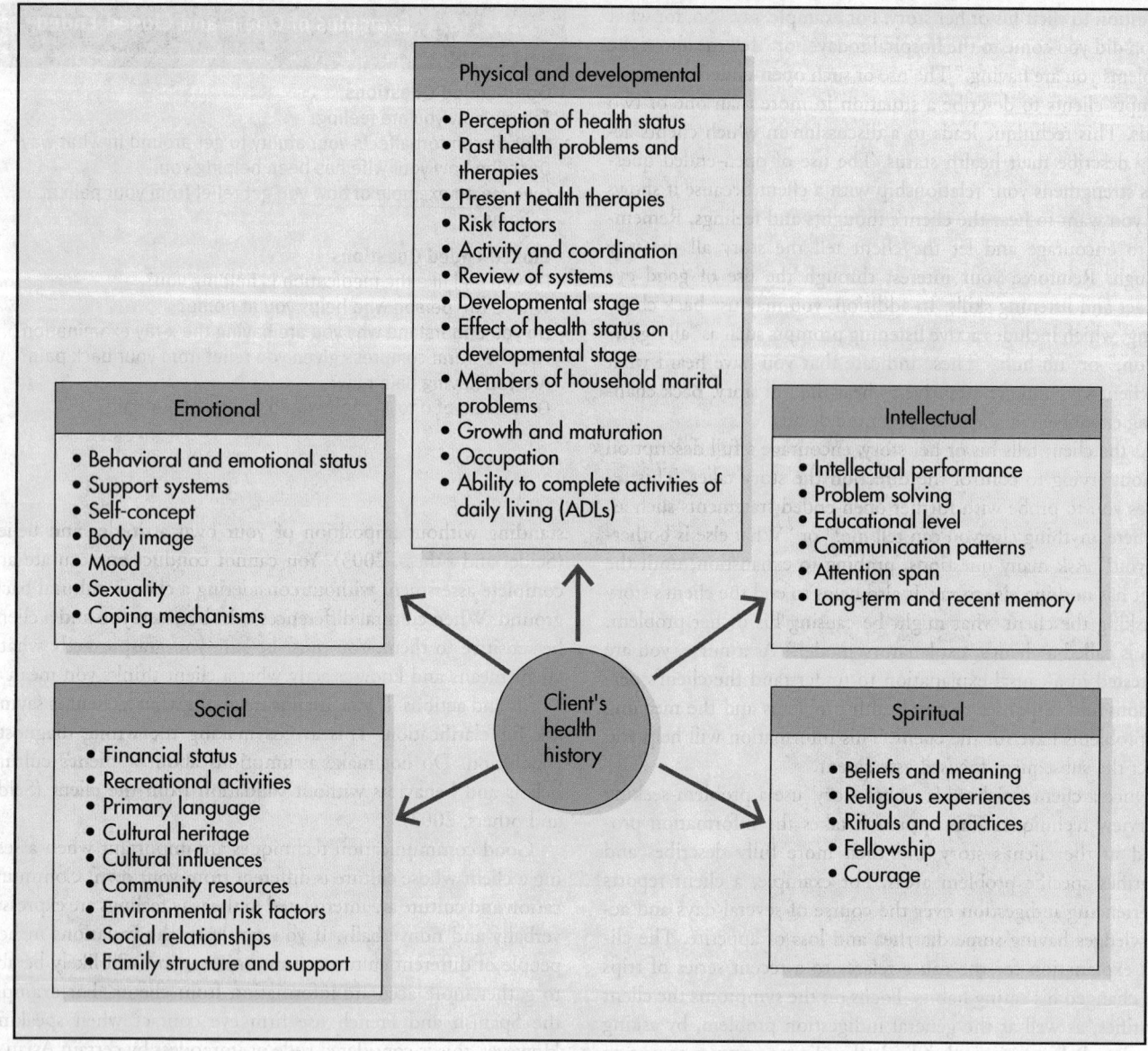

Physical and developmental
- Perception of health status
- Past health problems and therapies
- Present health therapies
- Risk factors
- Activity and coordination
- Review of systems
- Developmental stage
- Effect of health status on developmental stage
- Members of household marital problems
- Growth and maturation
- Occupation
- Ability to complete activities of daily living (ADLs)

Emotional
- Behavioral and emotional status
- Support systems
- Self-concept
- Body image
- Mood
- Sexuality
- Coping mechanisms

Intellectual
- Intellectual performance
- Problem solving
- Educational level
- Communication patterns
- Attention span
- Long-term and recent memory

Social
- Financial status
- Recreational activities
- Primary language
- Cultural heritage
- Cultural influences
- Community resources
- Environmental risk factors
- Social relationships
- Family structure and support

Spiritual
- Beliefs and meaning
- Religious experiences
- Rituals and practices
- Fellowship
- Courage

Client's health history

Figure 16-5 Dimensions for gathering data for a health history.

Nursing Health History

You will gather a nursing health history during either your initial or an early contact with a client. The history is a major component of assessment. Although many health history forms are structured, you learn to use the questions as starting points. A good assessor learns to refine and broaden questions as needed in order to correctly assess the client's unique needs. Time and client priorities determine how complete a history will be. Identify patterns of information about a client's health and illness by collecting data about all health dimensions (Figure 16-5). Incorporating data from all dimensions allows you to develop a complete plan of care. A nursing history usually contains the same basic components.

Biographical Information. Biographical information is factual demographic data about the client. The client's age, address, occupation and working status, marital status, source of health

care, and types of insurance are included. Admitting office staff usually collects this information.

Reason for Seeking Health Care. Ask a client why he or she is seeking health care, because the information contained on the initial admission form sometimes differs from the client's subjective reason for seeking health care. For example, "Tell me, Mr. Lynn, what brought you to the clinic today." You record the client's response in quotations to indicate the subjective response. The client's statement is not diagnostic; instead it is the client's perception of reasons for seeking health care. Clarification of the client's perception identifies potential needs for education, counseling, or referral to community resources.

Client Expectations. The assessment of client expectations is not the same as the reason for seeking medical care, although they are often related. It is important for you to acknowledge what is important to a client seeking health care. Failure to identify a client's expectations of health care providers results in poor client satisfaction. Client satisfaction is a standard measure of quality for all hospitals throughout the country (see Chapter 2). Clients typically have expectations about information for making decisions regarding treatments and a plan of care for returning home, the likely outcome of treatment, cleanliness of the environment, relief of pain and other symptoms, and caring expressed by health care providers. During the initial interview, a client expresses expectations when entering the health care setting. Later, as the client has had interactions with health care providers, it is valuable to assess whether the client's expectations have changed or been met.

Present Illness or Health Concerns. If a client presents with an illness, collect essential and relevant data about the nature and onset of symptoms. Determine when the symptoms began, whether they began suddenly or gradually, and whether they are always present or come and go. Also ask about the duration of symptoms (most recently and over time). Gather information on the location, intensity, and quality of each symptom, as appropriate. For example, when the client describes the presence of fatigue, ask the client to explain if the fatigue is worse before, during or after exercise. Does the fatigue occur more often during a certain time of day? Also assess whether any action precipitates the symptoms, makes them worse, or provides relief.

Health History. The information in a client's health history provides data on the client's health care experiences and current health habits (see Figure 16-5). You want to assess whether the client has ever been hospitalized or injured or had surgery. Include a complete medication history (including herbal and over-the-counter drugs) as well. Also essential are descriptions of allergies, including allergic reactions to food, latex, drugs, or contact agents (e.g., soap). For example, asking clients if they have had problems with medications or food helps to clarify the type and amount of agent, the specific reaction, and whether the client has required treatment. If the client has an allergy, note the specific reaction and treatment on the assessment form.

The history also includes a description of the client's habits and lifestyle patterns. Assessing for the use of alcohol, tobacco, caffeine, or recreational drugs (e.g., methamphetamine or cocaine) determines the client's risk for diseases involving the liver, lungs, heart, or nervous system. Noting the type of habit, as well as the frequency and duration of use, provides essential data.

Assessing patterns of sleep (see Chapter 42), exercise (see Chapter 37), and nutrition (see Chapter 44) are important when planning nursing care. Try to match the plan of care within a health care setting with a client's lifestyle patterns as much as possible. Frequently, you are able to accommodate variations in sleep, activity, and nutritional patterns.

Family History. The purpose of the family history is to obtain data about immediate and blood relatives. The objectives are to determine whether the client is at risk for illnesses of a genetic or familial nature and to identify areas of health promotion and illness prevention (see Chapter 6). The family history also provides information about family structure, interaction, and function that is often useful in planning care (see Chapter 10). For example, a

close, supportive family will help a client adjust to an illness or disability, so you incorporate them into the plan of care. On the other hand, if the client's family is not supportive, it is better to not involve them in care. Stressful family relationships are sometimes a significant barrier when you try to help clients with problems involving loss, self-concept, spiritual health, and personal relationships.

Environmental History. The environmental history provides data about a client's home and working environments with a focus on determining the client's safety. Information about the home environment includes function of utilities, layout of rooms in the house, and the presence of any barriers or risks for injury. The environmental history identifies exposure to pollutants in the workplace, existence of high crime in the client's neighborhood, and available resources that will assist clients in returning to the community.

Psychosocial History. A psychosocial history reveals the client's support system, which often includes spouse, children, other family members, and close friends. The psychosocial history includes information about ways that the client and family typically cope with stress (see Chapter 31). The same behavior, such as walking, reading, or talking with a friend, becomes a nursing intervention if the client experiences stress while receiving health care. You also learn if the client has experienced any recent losses that create a sense of grief (see Chapter 30).

Spiritual Health. Life experiences and events shape a person's spirituality. The spiritual dimension represents the totality of one's being and is difficult to assess quickly (see Chapter 29). Review with clients their beliefs about life, their source for guidance in acting on beliefs, and the relationship they have with family in exercising their faith. Also assess rituals and religious practices clients use to express their spirituality.

Review of Systems. The **review of systems (ROS)** is a systematic method for collecting data on all body systems (see Chapter 33). It is probable that you will not cover all of the questions in each system every time you collect a history (Seidel and others, 2003). Nevertheless, always include some questions about each system in the nursing history, particularly when a client mentions a symptom or sign. The systems you assess depend on the client's condition and the urgency in starting care. During the ROS ask the client about the normal functioning of each body system and any noted changes. Such changes are usually subjective data because they are described as perceived by the client. Findings from the ROS direct assessment during the physical examination.

Documentation of History Findings. As you conduct the nursing health history, record assessment in a clear, concise manner using appropriate terminology. Standardized forms make it easy to enter data as the client responds to questions. In settings that have computerized documentation, entry of assessment data becomes very easy. A clear, concise record is necessary for use by other health care professionals (see Chapter 26). Regardless of the model used in a documentation system, you want a thorough database that provides historical and current information about the client's health. This information then becomes the baseline against which you evaluate any future changes.

Physical Examination

A physical examination is an investigation of the body to determine its state of health. A physical examination involves use of the techniques of inspection, palpation, percussion, auscultation, and smell (see Chapter 33). A complete examination includes a client's height, weight, vital signs, and a head-to-toe examination of all body systems. By performing actual hands-on physical assessment you gather valuable objective information that helps in forming accurate diagnostic conclusions. Always conduct an examination with sensitivity and competence to prevent your client from becoming too anxious.

Observation of Client Behavior

Throughout an interview and physical examination it is important for you to closely observe a client's verbal and nonverbal behaviors. The information adds depth to your objective database. You learn to determine if data obtained by observation matches what the client verbally communicates. For example, if a client expresses no concern about an upcoming diagnostic test but shows poor eye contact, shakiness, and restlessness, all suggesting anxiety, verbal and nonverbal data conflict. Observations direct you to gather additional objective information to form accurate conclusions about the client's condition.

An important aspect of observation includes a client's level of function: the physical, developmental, psychological, and social aspects of everyday living. Observation of the level of function differs from observation you make during an interview. Observation of level of function involves watching what a client does, such as eating or making a decision about preparing a medication, rather than what the client tells you he or she can do. Observation of function can occur in the home or in a health care setting during a return demonstration.

Diagnostic and Laboratory Data

The results of diagnostic and laboratory tests identify or verify alterations questioned or identified during the nursing health history and physical examination. For example, during the history the client reports having a bad cold for 6 days and at present has a productive cough with brown sputum and mild shortness of breath. On physical examination, you notice an elevated temperature, increased respirations, and decreased breath sounds in the right lower lobe. You review the results of a complete blood count (CBC) and note the white blood cell count is elevated (indicating an infection). In addition, the radiologist's report of a chest x-ray examination shows the presence of a right lower lobe infiltrate. Such findings combined suggest the client has the medical diagnosis of pneumonia and the associated nursing diagnosis of *impaired gas exchange*.

Some clients collect and monitor laboratory data in the home. For example, clients with diabetes mellitus often do daily blood glucose monitoring. Ask clients about their routine results to determine their response to illness and information about the effects of treatment measures. Compare laboratory data with the established norms for a particular test, age-group, and gender.

Interpreting Assessment Data and Making Nursing Judgments

The successful analysis and interpretation of assessment data requires critical thinking. When you correctly analyze data, you will see patterns form that lead you to making necessary clinical decisions in your client's care. These decisions are either in the form of nursing diagnoses (see Chapter 17) or collaborative problems that require treatment from several disciplines (Carpenito-Moyet, 2005). When you critically think about interpreting assessment information, you will determine the presence of abnormal findings, what further observations you need to clarify information, and the client's health problems.

Data Validation. Before you begin analyzing and interpreting data, validate the collected information you have to avoid making incorrect inferences (Carpenito-Moyet, 2005). **Validation** of assessment data is the comparison of data with another source to determine data accuracy. For example, you observe a client crying and logically infer it is related to hospitalization or a medical diagnosis. Making such an initial inference is not wrong, but problems result if you do not validate the inference with the client. Instead say, "I notice that you have been crying. Can you tell me about it?" By doing so you will discover the real reason for the crying behavior. Ask your client to validate the information obtained during the interview and history. Validate findings from the physical examination and observation of client behavior by comparing data in the medical record and by consulting with other nurses or health care team members. Often family or friends are able to validate your assessment information.

Validation opens the door for gathering more assessment data because it involves clarifying vague or unclear data. Occasionally you need to reassess previously covered areas of the nursing history or gather further physical examination data. Continually analyze and think about a client's database to make concise, accurate, and meaningful interpretations. Critical thinking applied to assessment enables you to fully understand the client's problems, to judge the extent of the problems carefully, and to discover possible relationships between the problems.

Lisa gathered initial data about the character of Ms. Devine's back pain. She applied critical thinking in her assessment as she considered what she knew about ruptured lumbar disks and the anticipated type of symptoms clients experience. As she assessed Ms. Devine, she applied intellectual standards, being precise (location of pain), consistent and accurate (use of pain rating scale), and complete (probing for factors that worsen pain). Lisa learns additional information about Ms. Devine's concerns about surgery. Ms. Devine tells Lisa, "I hope the surgery goes well. You know, I have a friend who had back surgery, and she took a long time to recover. I want to get back to work without a long absence. If this had just not happened—why did I have to fall?" Lisa could make several inferences from this information, but she applies the critical thinking attitude of discipline and stays focused to ensure her assessment is accurate and comprehensive. She validates her inferences with Ms. Devine, "You sound anxious about having surgery. You know of others who have had difficult outcomes after surgery. Do you think you are uncertain about what to expect?" Ms. Devine confirms Lisa's assessment, "Yes, I am worried. I have never been in a hospital, as you know, and I feel I do not know what that involves. I am a person who likes to have information, so I can make the right decisions and know what to do."

Analysis and Interpretation.

After you collect extensive information about a client, it is time to analyze and interpret the data. Analysis begins by organizing the information into meaningful and usable clusters, keeping in mind your client's response to illness. A data cluster is a set of signs or symptoms that you group together in a logical way. During data clustering, organize data and focus attention on client functions needing support or assistance for recovery. **Data analysis** involves recognizing patterns or trends in the clustered data, comparing them with **standards,** and then coming to a reasoned conclusion about the client's responses to a health problem (Box 16-5). Patterns of meaning begin to form, allowing you to make inferences about client problems.

Through reasoning and judgment you decide what information explains the client's health status. At times this will often direct you to gather additional information for clarification of your interpretation. For example, Ms. Devine tells Lisa she has not been in a hospital and does not know what that involves. Lisa infers or guesses that Ms. Devine has limited knowledge about the laminectomy and the associated nursing care. Instead of making that conclusion, Lisa seeks further information, "Tell me what your doctor has told you about your surgery." Ms. Devine relates, "Well I know the doctor is going to remove something between my vertebrae. She said I will be in the hospital about 2 or 3 days." Lisa asks, "Has anyone talked with you about your care after surgery?" Ms. Devine replies, "No, not really. I have several questions I would like to ask about it." Lisa listens to the additional information provided by Ms. Devine. In looking for patterns of data, Lisa decides Ms. Devine has a knowledge problem because of her limited preparation for the surgery but is interested in learning.

If you are successful in clustering data well in your analysis, you will become proficient in identifying individualized nursing diagnoses and in identifying collaborative problems (Figure 16-6). During clustering, a cue or an individual sign, symptom, or finding will alert your thinking more than others. These cues are especially helpful in identifying nursing diagnoses. In time you will become experienced in recognizing clusters that point to problems such as pain, anxiety, or immobility. Clustering also helps make documentation more concise and focused.

Data Documentation

Data documentation is the last part of a complete assessment. The timely, thorough, and accurate documentation of facts is necessary when recording client data. If you do not record an assessment finding or problem interpretation, it is lost and unavailable to anyone else caring for the client. If there is not specific information, the reader is left with only general impressions. Observation and recording of client status is a legal and professional responsibility. The nurse practice acts in all states and the American Nurses Association Nursing's Social Policy Statement (2003) mandate, or require, accurate data collection and recording as independent functions essential to the role of the professional nurse.

Being factual is easy after it becomes a habit. The basic rule is to record all observations. When recording data, pay attention to facts and make an effort to be as descriptive as possible. Anything

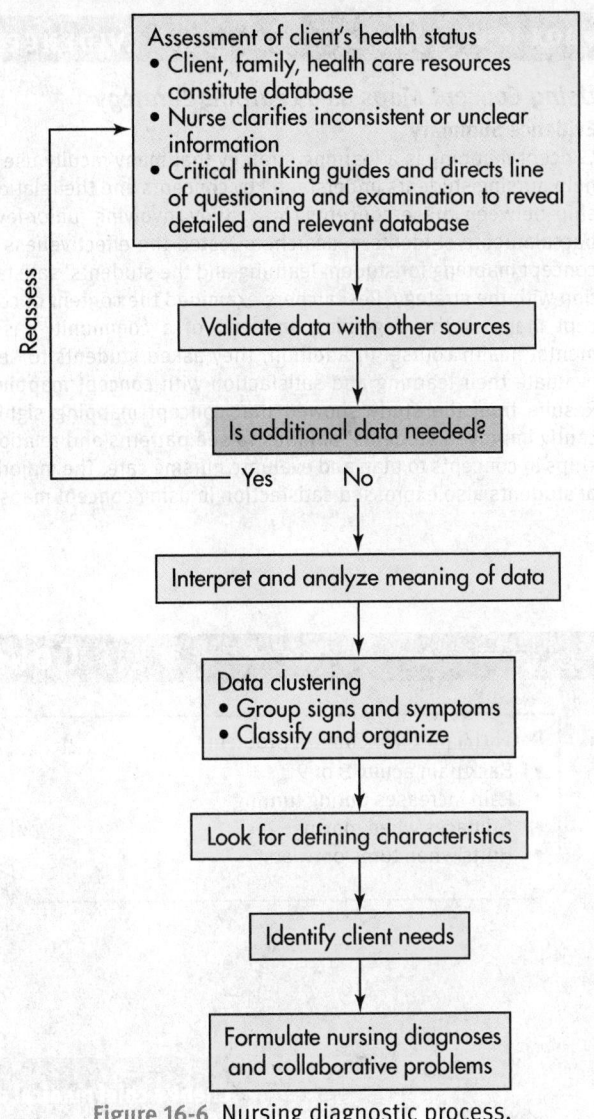

Figure 16-6 Nursing diagnostic process.

⁂ BOX 16-5 Steps of Data Analysis

1. Recognize a pattern or trend.
   Cues: Turns slowly
         Unable to bend over
         Walks with hesitation
2. Compare with normal standards:
   Normal range of motion
   Initiates movement without hesitation
3. Make a reasoned conclusion:
   Mobility limitation
   Reduced activity level

---

heard, seen, felt, or smelled should be reported exactly. Record objective information in accurate terminology (e.g., weighs 170 kg, abdomen is soft and nontender to palpation). Record subjective information from a client in quotation marks. When entering data, do not generalize or form judgments through written communication. Conclusions about such data become nursing diagnoses and thus must be accurate. As you gain experience and become familiar with clusters and patterns of signs and symptoms,

✳ **BOX 16-6**   **EVIDENCE-BASED PRACTICE**

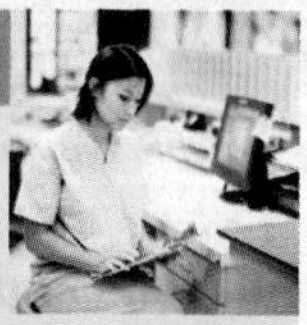

Using Concept Maps as a Learning Strategy

Evidence Summary

Concept mapping is a learning strategy that many faculty use to help nursing students understand key concepts and the relationship between those concepts. In a study involving junior-level baccalaureate students, researchers tested the effectiveness of concept mapping for student learning and the students' satisfaction with the strategy. Researchers examined the content of concept maps at the beginning and end of a community-based mental health course. In addition, they asked students to self-evaluate their learning and satisfaction with concept mapping. Results from the study showed that concept mapping significantly improved students' abilities to see patterns and relationships in concepts to plan and evaluate nursing care. The majority of students also expressed satisfaction in using concept maps.

Application to Nursing Practice

- A concept map allows a student to organize and link information about a client in unique and meaningful ways.
- The relationships seen between multiple nursing diagnoses allow students to plan interventions that are therapeutic for more than one problem area.
- Use of concept maps helps students to reflect and critically think about relationships between clinical information in a way that promotes clinical decision making.

Reference

Hinck SM and others: Student learning with concept mapping of care plans in community-based education, *J Prof Nurs* 22(1):23, 2006.

✳   **CONCEPT MAP**

Potential pattern: Comfort problem?
- Back pain acuity 8 or 9
- Pain increases during turning
- Grimaces when moving
- Hurts when turns or twists

Potential pattern: Not informed?
- No previous experience with surgery
- Reports has not received instruction on post-operative activities
- Asking questions

Client's chief medical diagnosis: Herniated lumbar disk. Scheduled for lumbar laminectomy
Priority assessments: Level of mobility, character of pain, knowledge and perceptions about condition and surgery

Potential pattern: Worried about surgery?
- Reports "dread" over having to have surgery
- Restless
- Uncertain about what to expect after surgery
- Concern over possible paralysis

Potential pattern: Mobility problem?
- Moves in bed awkwardly
- Cannot bend over
- Unable to tolerate sitting

Nursing diagnoses are confirmed after diagnostic process (Chapter 17).

——— Link between medical diagnosis and nursing diagnosis

Figure 16-7 Concept map for Ms. Devine's nursing assessment findings.

you will correctly conclude the existence of a problem. Review Chapter 26 for details on documentation.

Concept Mapping

Most of the clients you care for will present with more than one health problem. A concept map is a visual representation that allows you to graphically show the connections between a client's many health problems. Hinck and others (2006) showed that concept mapping is an effective learning strategy to understand the relationships that exist between client problems (Box 16-6). Your first step in concept mapping is to organize the assessment data you collect for your client. Placing all of the cues together into those clusters that form patterns will lead you to the next step of the nursing process, nursing diagnosis. Through concept mapping you obtain a holistic perspective of your client's health care needs, which ultimately leads you to making better clinical decisions (King and Shell, 2002). Figure 16-7 shows the first step in a concept map that Lisa will develop for Ms. Devine as a result of her nursing assessment. Lisa begins to identify Ms. Devine's problem areas as a result of assessment. The next step (see Chapter 17) will be to identify nursing diagnoses.

✳ Key Concepts

- The nursing process employs critical thinking to identify, diagnose, and treat human responses to health and illness.
- Nursing assessment involves the collection and verification of data and the analysis of all data to establish a database about a client's perceived needs, health problems, and responses to those problems.
- Interpreting the meaning of cues forms an inference, which then leads to identification of meaningful clusters of information.
- The two approaches for conducting a comprehensive assessment are use of a structured database format or use of a problem-oriented approach.
- Once a client provides subjective data, consider exploring the findings further by collecting objective data.
- During assessment critically anticipate and use an appropriate branching set of questions or observations to collect data and cluster cues of assessment information to identify emerging patterns and problems.
- Written data statements are descriptive, to the point, and complete and do not include inferences or interpretative statements.
- Family members and friends sometimes offer observations about the client's needs that will affect the way you deliver care.
- During assessment, encourage clients to tell their stories about their illnesses or health care problems.
- The interview is an organized conversation with a client that begins by establishing a therapeutic relationship with the client and that aids in the investigation and discussion of the client's health care needs.
- Open-ended questions encourage clients to tell their stories in detail, whereas closed-ended questions require brief answers to clarify or provide additional information.
- An interview includes three phases: orientation, working, and termination.

- To form a nursing judgment, you critically assess a client, validate the data, interpret the information gathered, and look for diagnostic cues that will lead you to identify the client's problems.

✳ Critical Thinking Exercises

1. Lisa plans time to talk further about Ms. Devine's knowledge of her surgery: "Ms. Devine, as we talk more about your surgery, I am going to be asking some questions so that we can do a good job planning your nursing care. Before we begin, do you have any questions?" (Client has none.) "Ok, let's begin by my asking you, What do you know about the routine procedures following your surgery?" (Client knows she will be checked often by the nurses.) "Tell me what you mean by checked." (Client says she thinks the nurses will keep a close eye on her). "Does that make you less anxious about surgery?" (Client says it offers her some comfort knowing nurses will be there for her). "Is there anything else your doctor has told you about your recovery?"

   Critique this scenario by answering the following questions:
   a. During the interaction, what questions did Lisa use that were open ended?
   b. Did Lisa probe to exhaustion? If so, what was the purpose?
   c. Critique Lisa's introduction.
   d. What is the advantage of open-ended questions over closed-ended questions?

2. During one of Lisa's visits to Ms. Devine's room, she conducts a more detailed assessment regarding Ms. Devine's concerns about surgery. Ms. Devine states, "I just hope I can go back to doing what I enjoy." Lisa notes Ms. Devine has forgotten what was explained earlier about relaxation exercises. Ms. Devine's eye contact with Lisa is inconsistent, and she moves about frequently in bed. Lisa asks, "What makes you most anxious about surgery?" and Ms. Devine responds, "I am most afraid of injury to my spine." In this interaction describe the subjective versus objective data.

✳ NCLEX®-Style Review Questions

1. The purpose of assessment is to:
   1. Make a diagnostic conclusion
   2. Delegate nursing responsibility
   3. Teach the client about his or her health
   4. Establish a database concerning the client

2. Assessment data must be descriptive, concise, and complete. An assessment should NOT include:
   1. Subjective data from the client
   2. A detailed physical examination
   3. The use of interpersonal and cognitive skills
   4. Inferences or interpretative statements not supported with data

3. A nurse assesses a client who comes to the pulmonary clinic. "Tell me what medications you are on for your breathing problem. I see from your last visit that Dr. Russell recommended routine exercise. Can you also tell me how successful you have been following his plan?" The nurse's assessment covers which of Gordon's functional health patterns?
   1. Value-belief pattern
   2. Cognitive-perceptual pattern
   3. Coping–stress tolerance pattern
   4. Health perception–health management pattern

4. The nurse asks a client, "Ms. Neil, describe for me your typical diet over a 24-hour day. What foods do you prefer? Have you noticed a change in your weight recently?" This series of questions would likely occur during which phase of a client interview?
   1. Working
   2. Orientation
   3. Termination

5. During data clustering a nurse:
   1. Provides documentation of nursing care
   2. Reviews data with other health care providers
   3. Makes inferences about patterns of information
   4. Organizes cues into patterns that lead to identifying nursing diagnoses

6. What type of interview techniques does the nurse use when asking the question, "Do you have pain or cramping?" (Choose all that apply.)
   1. Active listening
   2. Open-ended questioning
   3. Closed-ended questioning
   4. Problem-oriented questioning

7. What techniques encourage a client to tell his or her full story? (Choose all that apply.)
   1. Active listening
   2. Back channeling
   3. Use of open-ended questions
   4. Use of closed-ended questions

8. You gather the following assessment data, which of the following cues form a pattern? (Choose all that apply.)
   1. Client is restless.
   2. Fluid intake for 8 hours is 800 mL.
   3. Client states feels short of breath.
   4. Client has drainage from surgical wound.
   5. Respirations are 24 per minute and irregular.
   6. Client reports loss of appetite for over 2 weeks.

17 | Nursing Diagnosis

✳ OBJECTIVES

Mastery of the content in this chapter will enable the student to:

- Differentiate between a nursing diagnosis, medical diagnosis, and collaborative problem.
- Discuss the relationship of critical thinking to the nursing diagnostic process.
- Describe the steps of the nursing diagnostic process.
- Explain how defining characteristics and the etiological process individualize a nursing diagnosis.

- Explain the benefit of using the NANDA International nursing diagnoses in practice.
- Describe sources of diagnostic errors.
- Identify nursing diagnoses from a nursing assessment.

✳ MEDIA RESOURCES ✳ KEY TERMS

Companion CD

- NCLEX®-Style Review Questions
- Audio Glossary
- Interactive Learning Activities
- English/Spanish Glossary

 Website

- NCLEX®-Style Review Questions
- Audio Glossary
- English/Spanish Glossary
- Interactive Learning Activities
- WebLinks
- Audio Summaries

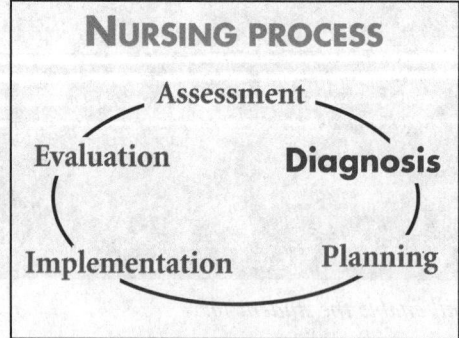

KNOWLEDGE
Underlying disease process
Normal growth and development
Normal pysiology and psychology
Normal assessment findings
Health promotion

EXPERIENCE
Previous client care experience
Validation of assessment findings
Observation of assessment techniques

NURSING PROCESS

Assessment

Evaluation   Diagnosis

Implementation   Planning

STANDARDS
ANA Scope of Nursing Practice
Intellectual standards of
measurement
Client-centered care

ATTITUDES
Critical thinking
(e.g., perseverance, confidence)

Figure 17-1 Critical thinking and the nursing diagnostic process.

After you assess a client thoroughly to gather a database, the next step of the nursing process is to form diagnostic conclusions that determine the nursing care a client receives (Figure 17-1). Some of the conclusions lead to nursing diagnoses, whereas others do not. Diagnostic conclusions include problems treated primarily by nurses (nursing diagnoses) and problems requiring treatment by several disciplines (collaborative problems). Together, nursing diagnoses and collaborative problems represent the range of client conditions that require nursing care (Carpenito-Moyet, 2005).

When physicians refer to commonly accepted medical diagnoses, such as myocardial infarction, diabetes mellitus, or osteoarthritis, they all know the meaning of the diagnoses and the standard approaches for treatment. A **medical diagnosis** is the identification of a disease condition based on a specific evaluation of physical signs, symptoms, the client's medical history, and the results of diagnostic tests and procedures. Physicians are licensed to treat diseases or pathological processes described in medical diagnostic statements.

Nursing has a similar diagnostic language. Nursing diagnosis, the second step of the nursing process, classifies health problems within the domain of nursing. The process of diagnosing is the result of your analysis of data and your resultant identification of specific client responses to health care problems. The term *diagnosis* means "to distinguish" or "to know." A **nursing diagnosis** is a clinical judgment about individual, family, or community responses to actual and potential health problems or life processes (NANDA International, 2007). It is a statement that describes

the client's actual or potential response to a health problem that the nurse is licensed and competent to treat.

A **collaborative problem** is an actual or potential physiological complication that nurses monitor to detect the onset of changes in a client's status (Carpenito-Moyet, 2005). When collaborative problems develop, nurses intervene in collaboration with personnel from other health care disciplines. Nurses manage collaborative problems such as hemorrhage, infection, and cardiac arrhythmia using both physician-prescribed and nursing-prescribed interventions to minimize complications. For example, a client who has a surgical wound is at risk for developing an infection, so a physician prescribes antibiotics. The nurse monitors the client for fever and other signs of infection and implements appropriate wound care measures.

In Chapter 16 you read about Lisa, a registered nurse (RN) on an orthopedic unit, and Ms. Devine, a 52-year-old woman who is scheduled to have a lumbar laminectomy for a herniated disk. Ms. Devine's medical diagnosis is a herniated lumbar disk. Lisa has conducted an assessment of Ms. Devine's health status and needs and has collected information in four different problem areas. Lisa needs to review the clusters and patterns of data she collected to correctly identify the nursing diagnoses that apply to Ms. Devine's situation. One cluster of data includes information about Ms. Devine's inexperience with surgery and her statement that she has not received information about postoperative activities. Lisa decides that the data include defining characteristics for the nursing diagnosis deficient knowledge regarding postoperative routines related to inexperience. Lisa is

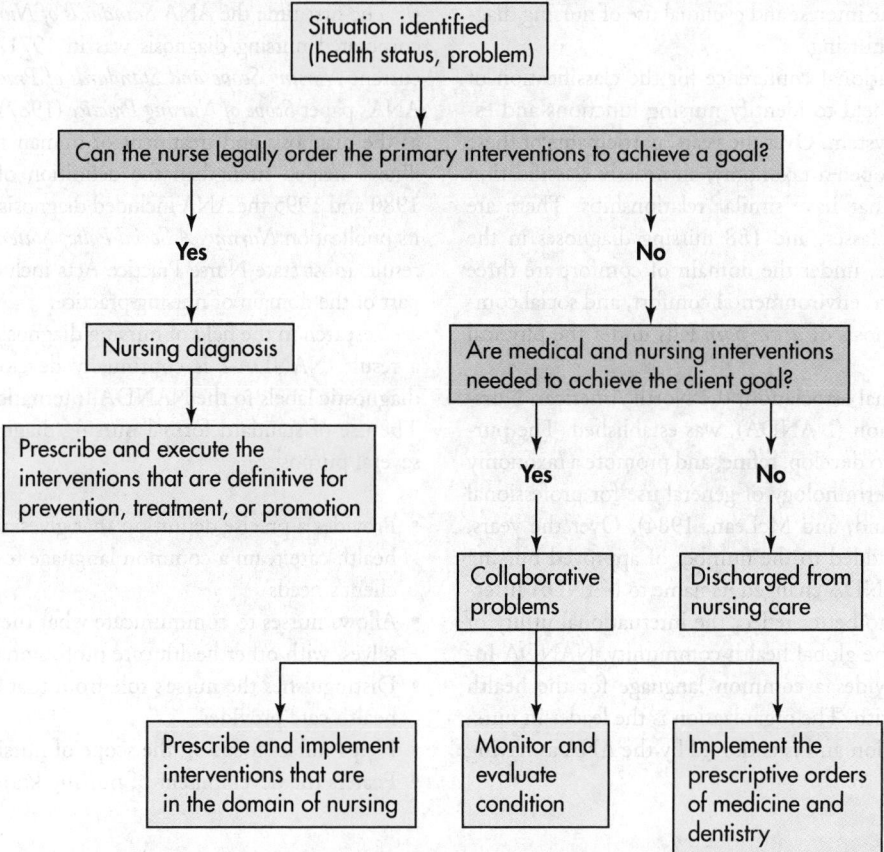

Figure 17-2 Differentiating nursing diagnoses from collaborative problems. (© 1990, 1988, 1985 Lynda Juall Carpenito. Redrawn from Carpenito LJ: *Nursing diagnosis: application to clinical practice,* ed 6, Philadelphia, 1995, JB Lippincott.)

Ms. Devine's primary nurse and will be caring for the client on the following day. Lisa knows from experience that common postoperative collaborative problems include wound infection and acute urinary retention. Lisa will work closely with the physician and other members of the nursing team in an effort to prevent or minimize these problems. Ms. Devine's health care plan will include a combination of interventions directed to resolve or manage nursing and medical diagnoses and any related collaborative problems.

Nursing diagnoses provide the basis for selection of nursing interventions to achieve outcomes for which you, as a nurse, are accountable (NANDA International, 2007). A nursing diagnosis focuses on a client's actual or potential response to a health problem rather than on the physiological event, complication, or disease. In the case of the diagnosis *deficient knowledge regarding postoperative routines,* Lisa will offer instruction to improve Ms. Devine's knowledge of what to expect following surgery and how she is able to participate in her postoperative care.

A nurse cannot independently treat a medical diagnosis such as a herniated disk. However, Lisa will manage Ms. Devine's postoperative laminectomy care, monitoring her postoperative progress and managing wound care, fluid administration, and medication therapy to prevent collaborative problems from developing. Collaborative problems occur or probably will occur in associa-

tion with a specific disease, trauma, or treatment (Carpenito-Moyet, 2005). You will need expert nursing knowledge to assess a client's specific risk for these problems, identify the problems early, and then take preventive action (Figure 17-2). Critical thinking is necessary in identifying nursing diagnoses and collaborative problems so that you appropriately individualize care for your clients.

History of Nursing Diagnosis

Nursing diagnosis was first introduced in the nursing literature in 1950 (McFarland and McFarlane, 1989). Fry (1953) proposed the formulation of nursing diagnoses and an individualized nursing care plan to make nursing more creative. This emphasized the nurse's independent practice (e.g., client education and symptom relief) compared with the dependent practice driven by physicians' orders (e.g., medication administration and intravenous fluids). Initially, professional nursing did not support nursing diagnoses, and in 1955 the *Model Nurse Practice Act* of the American Nurses Association (ANA) (1955) excluded diagnosis or prescriptive therapies. As a result, nurses hesitated to use nursing diagnoses in their practice. However, nursing theorists encouraged defining nursing in terms of client problems. Early theorists, by defining nursing intervention in terms of **client-centered problems,** were partly responsible for the interest and eventual use of nursing diagnosis in contemporary nursing.

In 1973 the first national conference for the classification of nursing diagnosis was held to identify nursing functions and establish a classification system. Over the years, participants of these conferences have developed a taxonomy, an orderly classification system for diagnoses that have similar relationships. There are now 13 domains, 47 classes, and 188 nursing diagnoses in the taxonomy. For example, under the domain of comfort are three classes: physical comfort, environmental comfort, and social comfort. The nursing diagnosis of *acute pain* falls under the physical comfort class.

In 1982 a professional association, the North American Nursing Diagnosis Association (NANDA), was established. The purpose of NANDA was "to develop, refine, and promote a taxonomy of nursing diagnostic terminology of general use for professional nurses" (Kim, McFarland, and McLean, 1984). Over the years, nursing scholars have added to the number of approved nursing diagnoses. In 2003 NANDA changed its name to **NANDA International (NANDA-I)** to better reflect the international utility of nursing diagnosis for the global health community. NANDA International's work provides a common language for the health problems nurses deal with. The organization is the leader in nursing diagnosis classification and is endorsed by the ANA as having the responsibility to do so.

The first time the ANA *Standards of Nursing Practice* (1973) incorporated nursing diagnosis was in 1971, and it remains in the current *Nursing Scope and Standards of Practice* (ANA, 2004). The ANA's paper *Scope of Nursing Practice* (1987), which defines nursing as the diagnosis and treatment of human responses to health and illness, helped strengthen the definition of nursing diagnosis. In 1980 and 1995 the ANA included diagnosis as a separate activity in its publication *Nursing: A Social Policy Statement* (ANA, 2003). As a result, most state Nurse Practice Acts include nursing diagnosis as part of the domain of nursing practice.

Research in the field of nursing diagnosis continues to grow. As a result, NANDA-I is continually developing and adding new diagnostic labels to the NANDA International listing (Box 17-1). The use of standard formal nursing diagnostic statements serves several purposes:

- Provides a precise definition that gives all members of the health care team a common language for understanding the client's needs
- Allows nurses to communicate what they do among themselves, with other health care professionals, and the public
- Distinguishes the nurse's role from that of the physician or health care provider
- Helps nurses focus on the scope of nursing practice
- Fosters the development of nursing knowledge

✳ BOX 17-1 NANDA International Nursing Diagnoses

Activity intolerance
Risk for **Activity** intolerance
Ineffective **Airway** clearance
Latex **Allergy** response
Risk for latex **Allergy** response
Anxiety
Death **Anxiety**
Risk for **Aspiration**
Risk for impaired parent/child **Attachment**
Autonomic dysreflexia
Risk for **Autonomic** dysreflexia
Risk-prone health **Behavior**
Disturbed **Body** image
Risk for imbalanced **Body** temperature
Bowel incontinence
Effective **Breastfeeding**
Ineffective **Breastfeeding**
Interrupted **Breastfeeding**
Ineffective **Breathing** pattern
Decreased **Cardiac** output
Caregiver role strain
Risk for **Caregiver** role strain
Readiness for enhanced **Comfort**
Impaired verbal **Communication**
Readiness for enhanced **Communication**
Decisional **Conflict**
Parental role **Conflict**
Acute **Confusion**
Chronic **Confusion**
Risk for acute **Confusion**
Constipation

Perceived **Constipation**
Risk for **Constipation**
Contamination
Risk for **Contamination**
Compromised family **Coping**
Defensive **Coping**
Disabled family **Coping**
Ineffective **Coping**
Ineffective community **Coping**
Readiness for enhanced **Coping**
Readiness for enhanced community **Coping**
Readiness for enhanced family **Coping**
Risk for sudden infant **Death** syndrome
Readiness for enhanced **Decision making**
Ineffective **Denial**
Impaired **Dentition**
Risk for delayed **Development**
Diarrhea
Risk for compromised human **Dignity**
Moral **Distress**
Risk for **Disuse** syndrome
Deficient **Diversional** activity
Disturbed **Energy** field
Impaired **Environmental** interpretation syndrome
Adult **Failure** to thrive
Risk for **Falls**
Dysfunctional **Family** processes: alcoholism
Interrupted **Family** processes

Used with permission from NANDA International: *NANDA-I nursing diagnoses: definitions and classification 2007-2008*, Philadelphia, 2007, NANDA International.

✳ BOX 17-1   NANDA International Nursing Diagnoses—cont'd

Readiness for enhanced **Family** processes
Fatigue
Fear
Readiness for enhanced **Fluid** balance
Deficient **Fluid** volume
Excess **Fluid** volume
Risk for deficient **Fluid** volume
Risk for imbalanced **Fluid** volume
Impaired **Gas** exchange
Risk for unstable blood **Glucose**
Grieving
Complicated **Grieving**
Risk for complicated **Grieving**
Delayed **Growth** and development
Risk for disproportionate **Growth**
Ineffective **Health** maintenance
Health-seeking behaviors
Impaired **Home** maintenance
Readiness for enhanced **Hope**
Hopelessness
Hyperthermia
Hypothermia
Disturbed personal **Identity**
Readiness for enhanced **Immunization** status
Functional urinary **Incontinence**
Overflow urinary **Incontinence**
Reflex urinary **Incontinence**
Stress urinary **Incontinence**
Total urinary **Incontinence**
Urge urinary **Incontinence**
Risk for urge urinary **Incontinence**
Disorganized **Infant** behavior
Risk for disorganized **Infant** behavior
Readiness for enhanced organized **Infant** behavior
Ineffective **Infant** feeding pattern
Risk for **Infection**
Risk for **Injury**
Risk for perioperative-positioning **Injury**
Insomnia
Decreased **Intracranial** adaptive capacity
Deficient **Knowledge**
Readiness for enhanced **Knowledge**
Sedentary **Lifestyle**
Risk for impaired **Liver** function
Risk for **Loneliness**
Impaired **Memory**
Impaired bed **Mobility**
Impaired physical **Mobility**
Impaired wheelchair **Mobility**
Nausea
Unilateral **Neglect**
Noncompliance
Imbalanced **Nutrition:** less than body requirements
Imbalanced **Nutrition:** more than body requirements
Readiness for enhanced **Nutrition**
Risk for imbalanced **Nutrition:** more than body requirements
Impaired **Oral** mucous membrane
Acute **Pain**
Chronic **Pain**
Readiness for enhanced **Parenting**
Impaired **Parenting**
Risk for impaired **Parenting**
Risk for **Peripheral** neurovascular dysfunction
Risk for **Poisoning**

Post-trauma syndrome
Risk for **Post-trauma** syndrome
Readiness for enhanced **Power**
Powerlessness
Risk for **Powerlessness**
Ineffective **Protection**
Rape-trauma syndrome
Rape-trauma syndrome: compound reaction
Rape-trauma syndrome: silent reaction
Impaired **Religiosity**
Readiness for enhanced **Religiosity**
Risk for impaired **Religiosity**
Relocation stress syndrome
Risk for **Relocation** stress syndrome
Ineffective **Role** performance
Readiness for enhanced **Self-care**
Bathing/hygiene **Self-care** deficit
Dressing/grooming **Self-care** deficit
Feeding **Self-care** deficit
Toileting **Self-care** deficit
Readiness for enhanced **Self-concept**
Chronic low **Self-esteem**
Situational low **Self-esteem**
Risk for situational low **Self-esteem**
Self-mutilation
Risk for **Self-mutilation**
Disturbed **Sensory** perception
Sexual dysfunction
Ineffective **Sexuality** pattern
Impaired **Skin** integrity
Risk for impaired **Skin** integrity
Sleep deprivation
Readiness for enhanced **Sleep**
Impaired **Social** interaction
Social isolation
Chronic **Sorrow**
Spiritual distress
Risk for **Spiritual** distress
Readiness for enhanced **Spiritual** well-being
Stress overload
Risk for **Suffocation**
Risk for **Suicide**
Delayed **Surgical** recovery
Impaired **Swallowing**
Effective **Therapeutic** regimen management
Ineffective **Therapeutic** regimen management
Ineffective community **Therapeutic** regimen management
Ineffective family **Therapeutic** regimen management
Readiness for enhanced **Therapeutic** regimen management
Ineffective **Thermoregulation**
Disturbed **Thought** processes
Impaired **Tissue** integrity
Ineffective **Tissue** perfusion
Impaired **Transfer** ability
Risk for **Trauma**
Impaired **Urinary** elimination
Readiness for enhanced **Urinary** elimination
Wandering
Impaired **Walking**
Risk for self-directed **Violence**
Risk for other-directed **Violence**
Dysfunctional **Ventilatory** weaning response
Impaired spontaneous **Ventilation**
Urinary retention

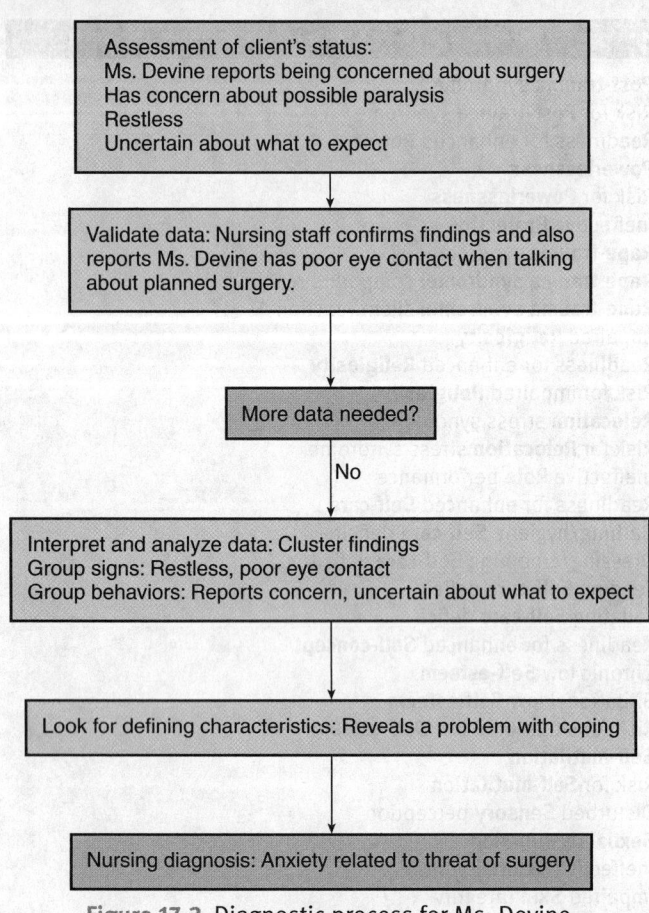

Figure 17-3 Diagnostic process for Ms. Devine.

The flowchart contains the following boxes:

Assessment of client's status:
Ms. Devine reports being concerned about surgery
Has concern about possible paralysis
Restless
Uncertain about what to expect

Validate data: Nursing staff confirms findings and also reports Ms. Devine has poor eye contact when talking about planned surgery.

More data needed?

No

Interpret and analyze data: Cluster findings
Group signs: Restless, poor eye contact
Group behaviors: Reports concern, uncertain about what to expect

Look for defining characteristics: Reveals a problem with coping

Nursing diagnosis: Anxiety related to threat of surgery

✳ BOX 17-2 Examples of NANDA International–Approved Nursing Diagnoses With Defining Characteristics and Related Factors

Diagnosis: Impaired Gas Exchange
Defining Characteristics:
Dyspnea
Abnormal rate, rhythm, depth of breathing
Abnormal arterial pH
Abnormal skin color (pale, dusky)
Hypoxemia
Hypercarbia
Hypoxia
Confusion
Related Factors:
Ventilation perfusion imbalance
Alveolar-capillary membrane changes

Diagnosis: Ineffective Breathing Pattern
Defining Characteristics (Examples):
Dyspnea
Bradypnea: Adults > age 14: ≤11 or >24
Decreased vital capacity
Orthopnea
Altered chest excursion
Use of accessory muscles to breathe
Tachypnea
Pursed-lip breathing
Related Factors:
Hyperventilation
Pain
Chest wall deformity
Anxiety
Musculoskeletal impairment
Body position

Data from NANDA International: *NANDA-I nursing diagnoses: definitions and classification, 2007-2008,* Philadelphia, 2007, NANDA International.

Critical Thinking and the Nursing Diagnostic Process

Diagnostic reasoning is a process of using the assessment data you gather about a client to logically explain a clinical judgment, in this case a nursing diagnosis. The diagnostic process flows from the assessment process and includes decision-making steps (Figure 17-3). These steps include data clustering, identifying client needs, and formulating the diagnosis or problem.

Clusters and patterns of data often contain **defining characteristics,** the clinical criteria or assessment findings that support an actual nursing diagnosis. **Clinical criteria** are objective or subjective signs and symptoms, clusters of signs and symptoms, or risk factors that lead to a diagnostic conclusion. Each NANDA-I approved nursing diagnosis has an identified set of defining characteristics that support identification of a nursing diagnosis (NANDA International, 2007). As a nurse, you will learn to recognize patterns of defining characteristics and then readily select the corresponding diagnosis. Box 17-2 shows two examples of approved nursing diagnoses and their associated defining characteristics. As you analyze clusters of data, begin to consider various diagnoses that might apply to your client. For example, the diagnoses of *impaired gas exchange* and *ineffective breathing pattern* have similar defining characteristics, including dyspnea, abnormal respiratory rate, and abnormal depth of breathing. But when determining a diagnosis, remember that the absence of certain de-

fining characteristics suggests that you reject a diagnosis under consideration. Thus, in the same example, if a client uses accessory muscles to breathe and demonstrates pursed-lip breathing, the diagnosis is not impaired gas exchange. The correct diagnosis is *ineffective breathing pattern*. Always examine the defining characteristics in your database carefully to support or eliminate a nursing diagnosis. To be more accurate, review all characteristics, eliminate irrelevant ones, and confirm the relevant ones.

While focusing on patterns of defining characteristics, you also compare a client's pattern of data with data that are consistent with normal, healthful patterns. Use accepted norms as the basis for comparison and judgment. This includes using laboratory and diagnostic test values, professional standards, and normal anatomical or physiological limits. When comparing patterns, judge whether the grouped signs and symptoms are normal for the client and whether they are within the range of healthful responses. Isolate any defining characteristics not within healthy norms to allow you to identify a problem.

Before finalizing a nursing diagnosis, review the client's general health care needs or problems. Identifying client needs allows you to individualize nursing diagnoses by considering all assessment data and focusing on the more relevant data. For example, after reviewing clusters of data from Ms. Devine's assessment, Lisa was able to recognize that the client had a knowledge problem. However, before Lisa was able to provide appropriate care, it was necessary to define Ms. Devine's problem more specifically. NANDA-I has two nursing diagnoses that apply to knowledge, *deficient knowledge* and *readiness for enhanced knowledge*. A careful review of Ms. Devine's presenting behaviors and self-report of the problem led to the selection of *deficient knowledge* because the client had no previous knowledge of postoperative activities. Her problem was not that she needed knowledge reinforcement, but she had an absence of knowledge. It is critical to select the correct diagnostic label for a client's need. Usually from assessment to diagnosis, you will move from general information to specific. It helps to think of the problem identification phase as the general health care problem and the formulation of the nursing diagnosis as the specific health problem.

Formulation of the Nursing Diagnosis

NANDA-I (2007) has identified four types of nursing diagnoses: actual diagnoses, risk diagnoses, and wellness diagnoses and health promotion nursing diagnoses. An **actual nursing diagnosis** describes human responses to health conditions or life processes that exist in an individual, family, or community. Defining characteristics (manifestations, signs, and symptoms) that cluster in patterns of related cues or inferences support this diagnostic judgment (NANDA International, 2007). The selection of an actual diagnosis indicates that sufficient assessment data are available to establish the nursing diagnosis. In the case of Ms. Devine, Lisa assessed the client to have back pain with a severity rated from 8 to 9 on a 10-point scale. The pain increased with movement. As a result of the pain, Ms. Devine has slept poorly. *Acute pain* is an actual nursing diagnosis.

A **risk nursing diagnosis** describes human responses to health conditions/life processes that will possibly develop in a vulnerable individual, family, or community (NANDA International, 2007). For example, after Ms. Devine has the laminectomy, she will have a surgical incision. The hospital environment poses a risk for nosocomial infection. Thus, after Ms. Devine's surgery, Lisa chooses the nursing diagnosis of *risk for infection*. The key assessment for this type of diagnosis is the presence of data revealing risk factors (incision and hospital environment) that support Ms. Devine's vulnerability. Such data include physiological, psychosocial, familial, lifestyle, and environmental factors that increase the client's vulnerability to, or likelihood of developing, the condition.

A **health promotion nursing diagnosis** is a clinical judgment of a person's, family's, or community's motivation and desire to increase well-being and actualize human health potential as expressed in their readiness to enhance specific health behaviors, such as nutrition and exercise. Health promotion diagnoses can be used in any health state and do not require current levels of wellness (NANDA International, 2007). *Readiness for enhanced comfort* is an example of a health promotion diagnosis.

A **wellness nursing diagnosis** describes human responses to levels of wellness in an individual, family, or community that have a readiness for enhancement (NANDA International, 2007). It is a clinical judgment about an individual, group, or community in transition from a specific level of wellness to a higher level of wellness. You select this type of diagnosis when the client wishes to or has achieved an optimal level of health. For example, *readiness for enhanced coping related to successful cancer treatment* is a wellness diagnosis, and the nurse and the family unit work together to adapt to the stressors associated with cancer survivorship. In doing so, the nurse incorporates the client's strengths and resources into a plan of care, with the outcome directed at improving the level of coping.

Components of a Nursing Diagnosis

The nursing diagnosis flows from the assessment and diagnostic process. Throughout this text, nursing diagnoses are in a two-part format: the diagnostic label followed by a statement of a related

✳ TABLE 17-1 NANDA International Nursing Diagnosis Format

DIAGNOSTIC STATEMENT	RELATED FACTORS
Acute pain	Biological, chemical, physical, or psychological injury agents (e.g., inflammation, edema, burn)
Anxiety	Stress
	Unmet needs
	Interpersonal transmission
	Situational/maturational crises
Impaired skin integrity	Fluid retention
	Excessive secretions
	Immobilization
	Altered circulation

factor (Table 17-1). It is this two-part format that provides a diagnosis meaning and relevance for a particular client. In addition, all NANDA-I approved diagnoses have a definition. Risk factors are a component of all risk nursing diagnoses.

Diagnostic Label. The **diagnostic label** is the name of the nursing diagnosis as approved by NANDA International (see Box 17-1). It describes the essence of a client's response to health conditions in as few words as possible. Diagnostic labels include descriptors used to give additional meaning to the diagnosis. For example, the diagnosis *impaired physical mobility* includes the descriptor *impaired* to describe the nature or change in mobility that best describes the client's response. Examples of other descriptors include *compromised, decreased, deficient, delayed, effective, imbalanced, impaired,* and *increased.*

Related Factors. The **related factor** is a condition or etiology identified from the client's assessment data. It is associated with the client's actual or potential response to the health problem and can change by using nursing interventions. For example, in the case of Ms. Devine, Lisa assessed that Ms. Devine had not received instruction on postoperative activities and she was asking questions. Lisa also learned that Ms. Devine had not had surgery before. The nursing diagnostic statement for Ms. Devine will include the diagnostic label (e.g., *deficient knowledge regarding postoperative routines*) and the related factor (e.g., *related to lack of exposure to instruction*). With the related factor of lack of exposure to instruction, Lisa will implement client instruction on postoperative activities. Related factors for NANDA-I diagnoses include four categories: pathophysiological (biological or psychological), treatment-related, situational (environmental or personal), and maturational (Carpenito-Moyet, 2005). The "related to" phrase is not a cause-and-effect statement; rather, it indicates that the etiology contributes to or is associated with the client's diagnosis (Figure 17-4). The inclusion of the "related to" phrase requires you to use critical thinking skills to individualize the nursing diagnosis and then select nursing interventions (Table 17-2).

The **etiology** of the nursing diagnosis is always within the domain of nursing practice and a condition that responds to nursing interventions. Sometimes health care providers record medical

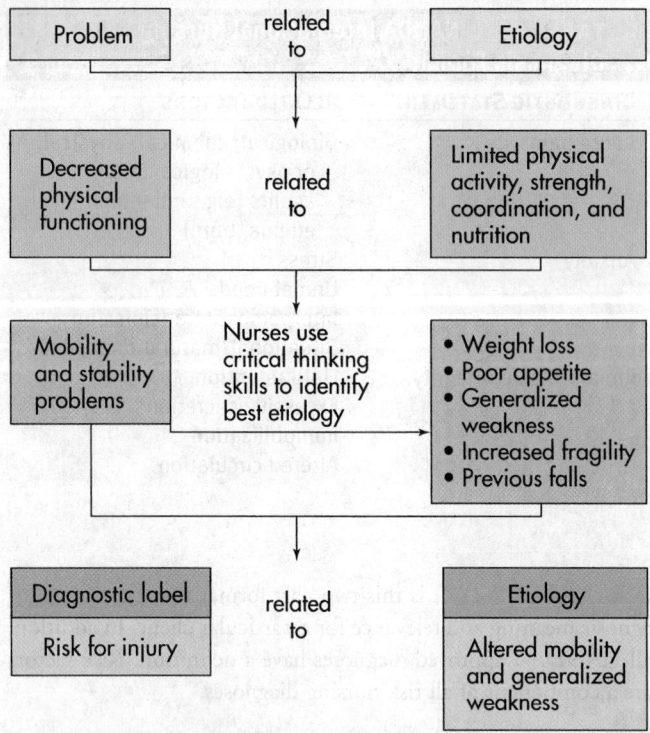

Figure 17-4 Relationship between a diagnostic label and etiology (related factor). (Redrawn from Hickey P: *Nursing process handbook,* St. Louis, 1990, Mosby.)

TABLE 17-2 Comparison of Interventions for Nursing Diagnoses With Different Etiologies

NURSING DIAGNOSES	INTERVENTIONS
Client A	
Anxiety related to uncertainty over surgery	Provide detailed instructions on the surgical procedure, recovery process, and postoperative care activities.
	Plan formal time for client to ask questions.
Impaired physical mobility related to acute pain	Administer analgesics 30 minutes before planned exercise.
	Instruct client in technique to splint painful site during activity.
Client B	
Anxiety related to loss of job	Consult with social work to arrange for job counseling.
	Encourage client to continue health promotion activities (e.g., exercise, routine social activities).
Impaired physical mobility related to musculoskeletal injury	Have client perform active range-of-motion exercises to affected extremity every 2 hours.
	Instruct client on use of three-point crutch gait.

diagnoses as the etiology of the nursing diagnosis. This is incorrect. Nursing interventions do not change a medical diagnosis. However, you direct nursing interventions at behaviors or conditions that you are able to treat or manage. For example, the nursing diagnosis *acute pain related to herniated disk* is incorrect. Nursing actions do not affect the medical diagnosis of a herniated disk. Rewording the diagnosis to read a*cute pain related to pressure on spinal nerves* results in nursing interventions directed at reducing stress on the vertebrae, improving body alignment, and offering nonpharmacological comfort measures.

Table 17-3 demonstrates the association between a nurse's assessment of a client, the clustering of defining characteristics, and formulation of nursing diagnoses. The diagnostic process results in the formation of a total diagnostic label that will allow a nurse to develop an appropriate, client-centered plan of care. The defining characteristics and relevant etiologies are from NANDA International (2007).

Definition. NANDA-I approves a definition for each diagnosis following clinical use and testing. The definition describes the characteristics of the human response identified. For example, the definition of the diagnostic label *impaired physical mobility* is the "limitation in independent, purposeful physical movement of the body or of one or more extremities" (NANDA International, 2007). You will refer to definitions of nursing diagnoses to assist in identifying a client's correct diagnosis.

Risk Factors. Risk factors are environmental, physiological, psychological, genetic, or chemical elements that increase the vulnerability of an individual, family, or community to an unhealth-

ful event (NANDA International, 2007). They are a component of all risk nursing diagnoses. The risk factors are cues to indicate a risk nursing diagnosis is applicable to a client's condition. Examples of risk factors for the nursing diagnosis *risk for infection* include invasive procedures, trauma, malnutrition, immunosuppression, and insufficient knowledge to avoid exposure to pathogens. The risk factors help in selecting the correct risk diagnosis, similar to the manner in which defining characteristics help in the formulation of actual nursing diagnoses. In addition, risk factors are valuable when planning preventive nursing interventions.

Support of the Diagnostic Statement. Nursing assessment data needs to support the diagnostic label, and the related factors need to support the etiology. To collect complete, relevant, and correct assessment data it helps to identify assessment activities that produce specific kinds of data. For example, asking the client about the quality and perception of pain results in subjective data. However, palpating an area, which sometimes elicits a painful facial grimace, provides objective information. Likewise, asking a client to describe the perception of an irregular heartbeat elicits subjective information, and using auscultation to obtain a pulse produces an objective measurement of heart rate and rhythm. When you review assessment data looking for clusters of defining characteristics, consider if you have probed and assessed the client accurately and thoroughly to gather a complete database.

Cultural Relevance of Nursing Diagnoses

When you select nursing diagnoses, it is important to consider your clients' cultural diversity. Similarly, consider your own culture. A client's culture influences the type of health care problems he or she

TABLE 17-3 Defining Characteristics and Etiologies to Support Nursing Diagnoses

Assessment Activities	Defining Characteristics (Clustering Cues)	Nursing Diagnoses	Etiologies ("Related To")
Ask client to rate severity of pain on a scale from 0 to 10.	Verbal report of pain at a level of 8 or 9 when it becomes sharp	Acute pain	Physical pressure on spinal nerves
Observe client's positioning in bed.	Bends knees while on back to lessen pain		
Ask if client has difficulty falling asleep or awakens during night from pain.	Client reports feeling tired, awakens easily		
Observe for any nonverbal signs of discomfort.	Moans and sighs when attempting to find comfortable position in bed		
Observe client's eye contact when talking.	Has poor eye contact when discussing surgery	Anxiety	Threat to health status as a result of surgery
Observe body language.	Restless		
Ask client to describe her feelings about surgery.	Client is uncertain about what to expect following surgery and the outcome of surgery		
Give instruction in topic of interest, and return in 15 minutes to measure retention.	Forgets details of explanation		

faces. Thus, when making a diagnosis, consider how culture influences the related factor for your diagnostic statement. For example, impaired verbal communication related to cultural differences or noncompliance related to client value system reflect diagnostic conclusions that consider a client's unique cultural needs.

Your own culture might influence the cues and defining characteristics you select from your assessment. Wieck (1996) studied how cultural differences among nurses influenced the choice of defining characteristics in making nursing diagnoses. The researchers studied the diagnosis of pain within six different cultural groups of nurses. Generally the nurses were consistent in selecting defining characteristics. However, when diagnosing pain, some of the nurses did not select restlessness or grimace as defining characteristics. The nurses were not familiar with such characteristics because they were not common to how their own culture expressed pain. Being culturally aware and sensitive will improve your accuracy in making nursing diagnoses.

Concept Mapping Nursing Diagnoses

When caring for a client or groups of clients, you need to think critically about client needs and how to prevent problems from developing. Your holistic view of a client heightens the challenge of thinking about all client needs and problems. Few clients have single problems. Often you will care for a client with multiple nursing diagnoses. Therefore a picture of each client usually consists of several interconnections between sets of data all associated with identified client problems (Mueller, Johnston, and Bligh, 2002). Concept mapping is one way to graphically represent the connections between concepts and ideas that are related to a central subject (e.g., the client's health problems).

Hsu and Hsieh (2005) describe a concept map as a scheme that displays visual knowledge in the form of a hierarchical graphic network. By using a concept map as your gather assessment data, you have a visual representation of your client's problems that show their relationships to one another (Schuster, 2003). As you proceed in applying each step of the nursing process, your concept map expands with more detail about planned interventions (see Chapter 18). A concept map promotes critical thinking by causing you to identify, graphically display, and link key concepts by organizing and analyzing information (Hsu and Hsieh, 2005) (Box 17-3).

Figure 17-5 shows the next step in the development of Lisa's concept map for Ms. Devine. Lisa began during the assessment step of the nursing process to gather a database for Ms. Devine. Her assessment included Ms. Devine's perspective of her health problems, as well as the objective and subjective data Lisa collected through observation and examination. Lisa validated findings and added to the database as she learned new information. Data sources include physical, psychological, and sociocultural domains.

Lisa applies clinical reasoning and intuition that reflects her own basic nursing knowledge, her past experiences with clients, patterns seen in similar situations, and reference to institutional standards and procedures (e.g., pain management policies or postoperative teaching protocols) (Ferrario, 2004). As Lisa begins to see patterns of defining characteristics, she places labels to identify the four nursing diagnoses that apply to Ms. Devine. She is also able to see the relationship between the diagnoses and connects them on the care map graphic. If Ms. Devine continues to be anxious, Lisa knows from her experience in caring for clients with pain that Ms. Devine's pain will increase. Likewise, increased pain will heighten anxiety. Anxiety also influences how well Ms. Devine will attend to any instructions, but until she understands what to expect, her anxiety will not diminish. Ms. Devine's pain, if unrelieved, will likely worsen her immobility. Concept mapping organizes and links information to allow you to see new wholes and appreciate the complexity of client care (Ferrario, 2004). Lisa's next step on the care map will be to identify the appropriate nursing interventions for Ms. Devine's care (see Chapter 18).

✳ BOX 17-3

EVIDENCE-BASED PRACTICE

Concept Maps as Assessment Tools

Evidence Summary

Two recent research studies examined the use of concept mapping and its effect on student learning. In one study (Hsu and Hsieh, 2005) the researchers asked 43 students from a 2-year nursing program to participate in concept mapping during a 16-week course. Each student completed six concept maps. All of the first drafts of the maps received low scores, but the third and following drafts progressively showed improvement. Students began with a linear sequence of concepts in their maps to a more highly integrated web of concepts.

In the second study, researchers examined the use of concept maps by 23 junior baccalaureate students (Hinck and others, 2006). The researchers examined the content of the students maps at the beginning and end of a community health course. Results of the study showed that concept mapping significantly improved students' abilities to see patterns and relationships to plan and evaluate nursing care.

Application to Nursing Practice

- Concept mapping is a valuable learning strategy to see the patterns and relationships between clinical information about clients.
- Concept maps promote problem-solving and critical thinking skills by organizing complex client data, analyzing concept relationships, and identifying interventions.

References

Hinck SM and others: Student learning with concept mapping of care plans in community based education, *J Prof Nurs* 22(1):23, 2006.

Hsu L, Hsieh S: Concept maps as an assessment tool in a nursing course, *J Prof Nurs* 21(3):141, 2005.

✳ CONCEPT MAP

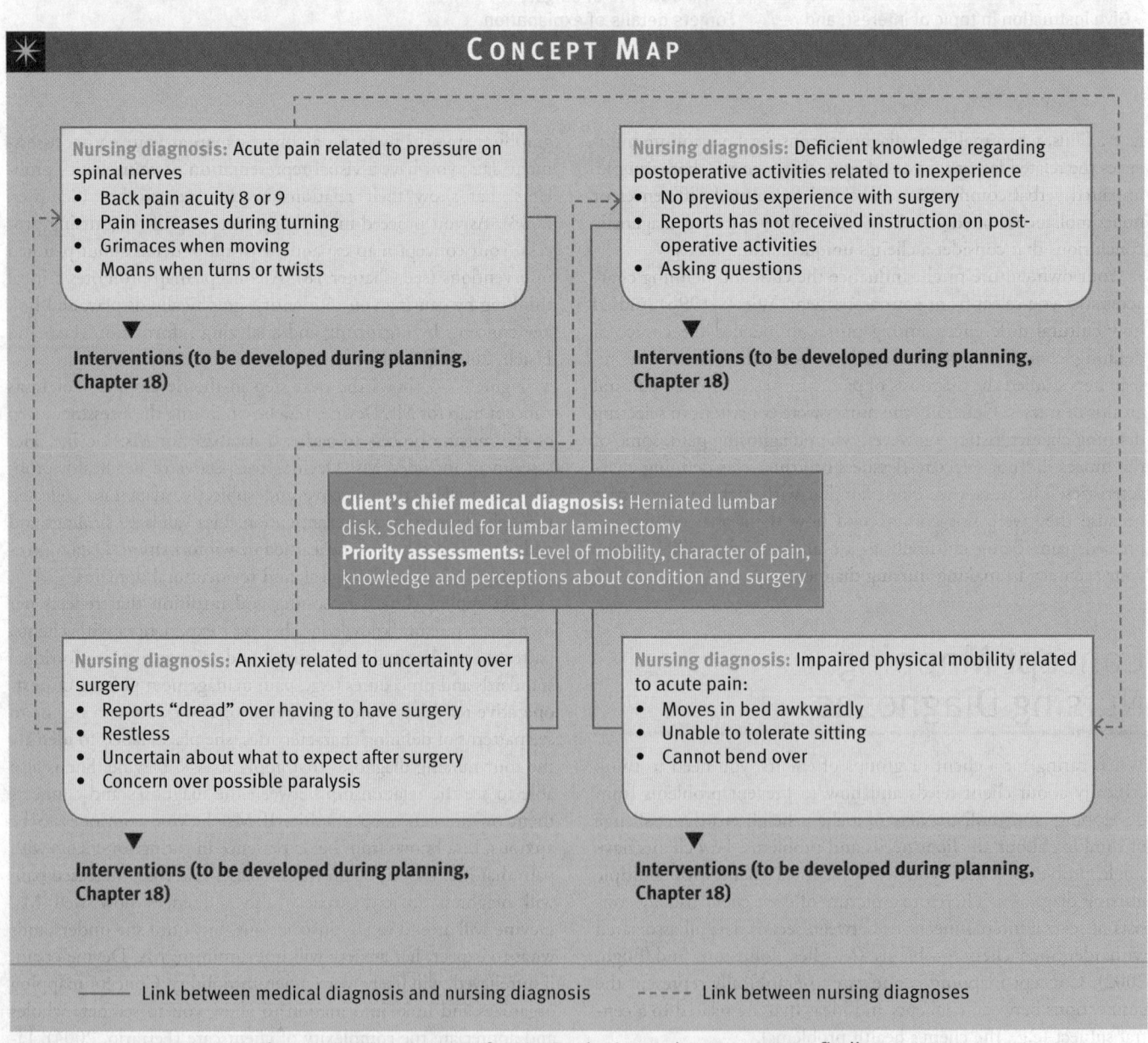

Nursing diagnosis: Acute pain related to pressure on spinal nerves
- Back pain acuity 8 or 9
- Pain increases during turning
- Grimaces when moving
- Moans when turns or twists

▼

Interventions (to be developed during planning, Chapter 18)

Nursing diagnosis: Deficient knowledge regarding postoperative activities related to inexperience
- No previous experience with surgery
- Reports has not received instruction on postoperative activities
- Asking questions

▼

Interventions (to be developed during planning, Chapter 18)

Client's chief medical diagnosis: Herniated lumbar disk. Scheduled for lumbar laminectomy
Priority assessments: Level of mobility, character of pain, knowledge and perceptions about condition and surgery

Nursing diagnosis: Anxiety related to uncertainty over surgery
- Reports "dread" over having to have surgery
- Restless
- Uncertain about what to expect after surgery
- Concern over possible paralysis

▼

Interventions (to be developed during planning, Chapter 18)

Nursing diagnosis: Impaired physical mobility related to acute pain:
- Moves in bed awkwardly
- Unable to tolerate sitting
- Cannot bend over

▼

Interventions (to be developed during planning, Chapter 18)

—— Link between medical diagnosis and nursing diagnosis   - - - - Link between nursing diagnoses

Figure 17-5 Concept map for Ms. Devine's nursing assessment findings.

The advantage of a concept map is its central focus on the client rather than the client's disease or health alteration. This encourages students of nursing to concentrate on clients' specific health problems and nursing diagnoses (Mueller and others, 2002). The focus promotes client participation with the eventual plan of care.

Sources of Diagnostic Errors

Errors occur in the nursing diagnostic process during data collection, clustering, interpretation, and statement of the diagnosis. As a nurse, you need to apply methodical critical thinking for an accurate nursing diagnostic process.

Errors in Data Collection

To avoid errors in data collection be knowledgeable and skilled in all assessment techniques (Box 17-4). Avoid inaccurate or missing data, and collect data in an organized way. The following practice tips are essential to avoid data collection errors:

- Review your level of comfort and competence with interview and physical assessment skills before you begin data collection.
- Approach assessment in steps. Focus on completing a client interview before starting a physical examination. Perhaps focus on only one body system to learn how to gather a complete assessment. Then move to a more complex head-to-toe examination.
- Review your clinical assessments in clinical or classroom settings. They will provide you with a constructive learning opportunity to determine how to revise an assessment or to gather additional information.
- Determine the accuracy of your data. When you auscultate abnormal lung sounds for the first time, be sure of what you hear through the stethoscope. Inaccurate assessment data mean that you will misinterpret data from clients, select inappropriate interventions, and endanger the quality of care (Lunney, 1998). To minimize the risk of inaccuracy, have a more experienced co-worker validate findings or explain why they are incorrect.
- Be organized in any examination. Have the appropriate forms and examination equipment ready to use. Be sure the environment is private, quiet, and comfortable for the client.

Errors in Interpretation and Analysis of Data

Following data collection, review your database to decide if it is accurate and complete. Review data to validate that measurable, objective physical findings support subjective data. For example, when a client reports "difficulty breathing," you want to also listen to lung sounds, assess respiratory rate, and measure the client's chest excursion. When you are not able to validate data, this signals an inaccurate match between clinical cues and the nursing diagnosis (Lunney, 1998). Begin interpretation by identifying and organizing relevant assessment patterns to support the presence of client problems Be careful to consider any conflicting cues or decide if there are insufficient cues to form a diagnosis. Also, it is very important to consider a client's cultural background or developmental stage when you interpret the meaning of cues. For ex-

---

BOX 17-4 Sources of Diagnostic Error

Collecting
Lack of knowledge or skill
Inaccurate data
Missing data
Disorganization

Interpreting
Inaccurate interpretation of cues
Failure to consider conflicting cues
Using an insufficient number of cues
Using unreliable or invalid cues
Failure to consider cultural influences or developmental stage

Clustering
Insufficient cluster of cues
Premature or early closure
Incorrect clustering

Labeling
Wrong diagnostic label selected
Evidence exists that another diagnosis is more likely
Condition is a collaborative problem
Failure to validate nursing diagnosis with client
Failure to seek guidance

---

ample, a client form the Middle East will express pain very differently than an Asian client. Misinterpreting how clients express pain will easily lead to an inaccurate diagnosis.

Errors in Data Clustering

Errors in data clustering occur when data are clustered prematurely, incorrectly, or not at all. Premature closure of clustering occurs when you make the nursing diagnosis before grouping all data. For example, you learn that a client has had urinary incontinence and complains of urgency and nocturia. You cluster the available data and consider that *impaired urinary elimination* is a probable diagnosis. However, incorrect clustering occurs when you try to make the nursing diagnosis fit the signs and symptoms obtained. In this example, further assessment reveals the client has bladder distention and dribbling, and the type of incontinence is likely overflow incontinence. As a result of these findings you are able to make a more accurate diagnosis, *urinary retention*. Always identify the nursing diagnosis from the data, not the reverse. An incorrect nursing diagnosis affects quality of client care.

Errors in the Diagnostic Statement

The correct selection of a diagnostic statement is more likely to result in the appropriate selection of nursing interventions and outcomes (Dochterman and Jones, 2003). To reduce errors, word the diagnostic statement in appropriate, concise, and precise language. Use correct terminology reflecting the client's response to the illness or condition. Use of standardized nursing language from NANDA-I helps ensure accuracy. A diagnostic statement such as "unhappy and worried about health" is not a scientifically based diagnosis, and it will lead to errors. The language needs to be more precise and appropriate, such as *ineffective coping related to fear of medical diagnosis*. Also, the problem and etiology portions of the diagnostic statement need to be within the scope of nursing to diagnose and treat. Additional guidelines to reduce errors in the diagnostic statement follow:

1. Identify the client's response, not the medical diagnosis (Carpenito-Moyet, 2005). Because the medical diagnosis requires medical interventions, it is legally inadvisable to include it in the nursing diagnosis. Change the diagnosis *acute pain related to myocardial infarction* to *acute pain related to physical exertion.*

2. Identify a NANDA-I diagnostic statement rather than the symptom. Identify nursing diagnoses from a cluster of defining characteristics; one symptom is insufficient for problem identification. For example, dyspnea alone does not definitely lead you to a diagnosis. However, the pattern of dyspnea, shortness of breath, pain on inspiration, and productive cough with thick secretions lead you to *ineffective breathing pattern related to increased airway secretions.*

3. Identify a treatable etiology rather than a clinical sign or chronic problem. You will select interventions directed toward correcting the etiology of the problem. A diagnostic test or a chronic dysfunction is not an etiology or a condition that a nursing intervention is able to treat. A client with pneumonia sometimes presents with restlessness, hypoxia, abnormal blood gas levels, and dyspnea. Impaired gas exchange related to altered blood gases is an incorrect diagnostic statement. *Impaired gas exchange related to alveolar capillary membrane changes* is a correct statement.

4. Identify the problem caused by the treatment or diagnostic study rather than the treatment or study itself. Clients experience many responses to diagnostic tests and medical treatment. These responses are the area of nursing concern. The client who has angina and is scheduled for a cardiac catheterization will possibly have a nursing diagnosis of *anxiety related to lack of knowledge about cardiac catheterization.* An incorrect diagnosis is anxiety related to cardiac catheterization.

5. Identify the client response to the equipment rather than the equipment itself. Clients are often unfamiliar with medical technology. The diagnosis of *deficient knowledge regarding the need for cardiac monitoring* is accurate compared with the statement "anxiety related to cardiac monitor."

6. Identify the client's problems rather than your problems with nursing care. Nursing diagnoses are always client centered and form the basis for goal-directed care. "Potential intravenous complications related to poor vascular access" indicates a nursing problem in initiating and maintaining intravenous therapy. The diagnosis *risk for infection related to presence of invasive lines* properly centers attention on client needs.

7. Identify the client problem rather than the nursing intervention. You will plan nursing interventions later after making a diagnosis. The statement "offer bedpan frequently because of altered elimination patterns" changes to *diarrhea related to food intolerance.* This corrects the misstatement and allows proper implementation of the nursing process.

8. Identify the client problem rather than the goal. You always establish goals during the planning step of the nursing process. Goals, based upon accurate identification of a client's

problems, later serve as a basis to determine if you achieve problem resolution. Change the statement "Client needs high-protein diet related to potential alteration in nutrition" to *imbalanced nutrition: less than body requirements related to inadequate protein intake.*

9. Make professional rather than prejudicial judgments. Base nursing diagnoses on subjective and objective client data, and do not include your personal beliefs and values. Remove your judgment from "risk for impaired skin integrity related to poor hygiene habits" by changing the nursing diagnosis to read *risk for impaired skin integrity related to knowledge about perineal care.*

10. Avoid legally inadvisable statements (Carpenito-Moyet, 2005). Statements that imply blame, negligence, or malpractice have the potential to result in a lawsuit. The statement "recurrent angina related to insufficient medication" implies an inadequate prescription by the physician or health care provider. Correct problem identification is *chronic pain related to improper use of medications.*

11. Identify the problem and etiology to avoid a circular statement. Circular statements are vague and give no direction to nursing care. Change the statement "pain related to alteration in comfort" to identify the client problem and cause, *ineffective breathing pattern related to incisional pain.*

12. Identify only one client problem in the diagnostic statement. Every problem has different specific expected outcomes. Confusion during the planning step occurs when you include multiple problems in a nursing diagnosis. Restate "pain and anxiety related to difficulty in ambulating" as two nursing diagnoses, such as *impaired physical mobility related to pain in right knee* and *anxiety related to difficulty in ambulating.* It is permissible to include multiple etiologies contributing to one client problem, as in *complicated grieving related to diagnosed terminal illness and change in family role.*

Documentation

Once you identify a client's nursing diagnoses, list them on the written plan of care. In the clinical facility, list nursing diagnoses chronologically as you identify them. When initiating the original care plan, always place the highest-priority nursing diagnoses first. Thereafter add additional nursing diagnoses to the list. Date a nursing diagnosis at the time of entry. When caring for a client always review the list and identify those nursing diagnoses with the greatest priority, regardless of chronological order.

Nursing Diagnoses: Application to Care Planning

Nursing diagnosis is a mechanism for identifying the domain of nursing. Diagnoses provide direction for the planning process and the selection of nursing interventions to achieve desired outcomes for clients. Just as the medical diagnosis of diabetes leads a physician to prescribe a low-carbohydrate diet and medication for blood glucose control, the nursing diagnosis of *impaired skin integrity* directs a nurse to apply certain support surfaces to a client's bed and to initiate a turning schedule. In Chapter 18 you will learn how unifying the languages of NANDA-I, along with the Nursing Interventions Classification (NIC), and Nursing Outcomes Classification (NOC) facilitate the process of matching nursing diagnoses with accurate and appropriate interventions and outcomes (Dochterman and Jones, 2003). The care plan (see Chapter 18) is a map for nursing care and demonstrates your accountability for client care. By learning to make accurate nursing diagnoses, your subsequent care plan will assist in communicating to other professionals the client's health care problems and ensure that you select relevant and appropriate nursing interventions.

Key Concepts

- Use critical thinking to interpret client assessment data in a meaningful and relevant way to identify nursing diagnoses and provide direction for nursing care.
- Nursing diagnosis is incorporated into the ANA's *Standards of Clinical Nursing Practice,* as well as most state Nurse Practice Acts.
- NANDA-I has developed a common language that allows all members of the health care team to understand a client's needs.
- The diagnostic process includes critical analysis and interpretation of assessment data that reveal a client's response to health care problems, identification of client needs, and formulation of nursing diagnoses.
- The analysis and interpretation of data requires you to validate data, recognize patterns or trends, compare data with healthful standards, and then form diagnostic conclusions.
- Absence of defining characteristics suggests that you reject a proposed diagnosis.
- There are four types of nursing diagnoses: actual, at risk, wellness diagnoses and health promotion diagnoses.
- A nursing diagnosis is written in a two-part format, including a diagnostic label and an etiologic or related factor.
- The "related to" factor of the diagnostic statement assists you in individualizing a client's nursing diagnoses and provides direction for your selection of appropriate interventions.
- Risk factors serve as cues to indicate a risk nursing diagnosis applies to a client's condition.
- Concept mapping offers a visual representation of a client's nursing diagnoses and their relationship with one another.
- Nursing diagnostic errors occur by errors in data collection, interpretation and analysis of data, clustering of data, or in the diagnostic statement.
- Nursing diagnoses improve communication between nurses and other health professionals.

Critical Thinking Exercises

Mr. Wyatt is a 63-year-old man who has been diagnosed for 5 years with chronic bronchitis. He enters the medicine clinic with a verbal report of feeling exhausted and unable to complete normal activities at home. You assess his vital signs and find that after walking down and back from the hallway to the examination room his heart rate stays elevated above his resting rate for 2 minutes. He reports a sense of feeling uncomfortable in breathing (dyspnea). He reports he usually feels good in the morning after sleeping, but by the afternoon he feels worn out whenever he attempts activity. You inform the physician of your initial findings. An electrocardiogram (ECG) ordered by the physician shows some cardiac arrhythmias.

1. What nursing diagnosis would you assign to Mr. Wyatt? (NOTE: complete this question by referring to a reference on NANDA-I nursing diagnoses and defining characteristics.)
2. What other diagnosis might you rule out for Mr. Wyatt?
3. Examine the following two sets of data. Identify normal standards with which to compare the data, and then make a reasoned conclusion about the client need or problem the data tend to support.

Data Set I	Data Set II
Poor oral intake	Awakens 2 to 3 times during
Low white blood	night
cell (WBC) count	Takes about 1 hour to fall
Has a surgical wound	asleep
	Reports becoming tired easily
	at work
	Worried about job security

4. Identify nursing diagnoses that might apply to the data sets in question 3.
5. Review the following nursing diagnoses, and identify those that are stated correctly and those that are stated incorrectly:
   a. Anxiety related to fear of dying
   b. Fatigue related to chronic emphysema
   c. Need for mouth care related to inflamed mucosa
   d. Risk for infection related to reduced immune function

NCLEX®-Style Review Questions

1. A nursing diagnosis is:
   1. The diagnosis and treatment of human responses to health and illness
   2. The advancement of the development, testing, and refinement of a common nursing language
   3. A clinical judgment about individual, family, or community responses to actual and potential health problems or life processes
   4. The identification of a disease condition based on a specific evaluation of physical signs, symptoms, the client's medical history, and the results of diagnostic tests

2. Lisa reviews data she has regarding Ms. Devine's pain symptoms. She compares the defining characteristics for *acute pain* with those for *chronic pain*. In the end she selects *acute pain* as the correct diagnosis. This is an example of Lisa avoiding an error in:
   1. Data collection
   2. Data clustering
   3. Data interpretation
   4. Making a diagnostic statement

3. One of the purposes of the use of standard formal nursing diagnostic statements is to:
   1. Evaluate nursing care
   2. Gather information on client data
   3. Help nurses to focus on the role of nursing in client care
   4. Facilitate understanding of client problems among health care providers

4. The nursing diagnosis *readiness for enhanced communication* is an example of a(n):
   1. Risk nursing diagnosis
   2. Actual nursing diagnosis
   3. Potential nursing diagnosis
   4. Wellness nursing diagnosis

5. The nursing diagnosis *hypothermia* is an example of a(n):
   1. Risk nursing diagnosis
   2. Actual nursing diagnosis
   3. Potential nursing diagnosis
   4. Wellness nursing diagnosis

6. The word *impaired* in the diagnosis *Impaired physical mobility* is an example of a:
   1. Descriptor
   2. Risk factor
   3. Related factor
   4. Nursing diagnosis

7. In the examples listed below, which nurse is acting to avoid a data collection error?
   1. The nurse asks a colleague to chart his or her assessment data.
   2. The nurse considers conflicting cues in deciding the correct nursing diagnosis.
   3. The nurse assessing the edema in a client's lower leg is unsure of its severity and asks a co-worker to check it with him or her.
   4. After doing an assessment the nurse critically reviews his or her level of comfort and competence with interview and physical assessment skills.

8. "Unhappy and worried about health" is not a scientifically based nursing diagnosis, and it can lead to error in:
   1. Data collection
   2. Data clustering
   3. Medical diagnosis
   4. Diagnostic statement

9. Casey is reviewing a client's list of nursing diagnoses in the medical record. The most recent nursing diagnosis is *diarrhea related to intestinal colitis*. This is an incorrectly stated diagnostic statement, best described as:
   1. Identifying the clinical sign instead of an etiology
   2. Identifying a diagnosis based on prejudicial judgment
   3. Identifying the diagnostic study rather than a problem caused by the diagnostic study
   4. Identifying the medical diagnosis instead of the client's response to the diagnosis

10. Which of the following are defining characteristics for the nursing diagnosis *impaired urinary elimination?* (Choose all that apply.)
    1. Nocturia
    2. Frequency
    3. Urine retention
    4. Inadequate urinary output
    5. Receiving intravenous fluids
    6. Sensation of bladder fullness

18 | Planning Nursing Care

✳ OBJECTIVES

Mastery of the content in this chapter will enable the student to:

- Explain the relationship of planning to assessment and nursing diagnosis.
- Discuss the criteria used in priority setting.
- Describe goal setting.
- Discuss the difference between a goal and an expected outcome.
- List the seven guidelines for writing an outcome statement.

- Develop a plan of care from a nursing assessment.
- Discuss the differences between nurse-initiated, physician-initiated, and collaborative interventions.
- Discuss the process of selecting nursing interventions
- Describe the purposes of a written nursing care plan.
- Describe the elements of a concept map.
- Describe the consultation process.

✳ MEDIA RESOURCES   ✳ KEY TERMS

 Companion CD
- NCLEX®-Style Review Questions
- Audio Glossary
- Interactive Learning Activities
- English/Spanish Glossary

 Website
- NCLEX®-Style Review Questions
- Audio Glossary
- English/Spanish Glossary
- Interactive Learning Activities
- WebLinks
- Audio Summaries

Client-centered goal, p. 265
Collaborative interventions, p. 268
Consultation, p. 276
Critical pathways, p. 274
Dependent nursing intervention, p. 268
Expected outcome, p. 264
Goal, p. 264
Independent nursing interventions, p. 267

Kardex, p. 274
Long-term goal, p. 265
Nursing care plan, p. 269
Nursing-sensitive client outcome, p. 266
Planning, p. 262
Priority setting, p. 262
Scientific rationale, p. 271
Short-term goal, p. 265

Lisa is about to begin the planning of nursing care for Ms. Devine. In the diagnostic step of the nursing process, Lisa identified four nursing diagnoses relevant to Ms. Devine's case: acute pain, anxiety, deficient knowledge, and impaired physical mobility. Lisa is responsible for planning Ms. Devine's care from this morning until the time Ms. Devine leaves for surgery. Lisa will not still be working on the unit by the time Ms. Devine returns from surgery, but as her primary nurse, Lisa will provide direction for the staff who will assume Ms. Devine's care. Careful planning involves seeing a relationship between a client's problems, recognizing that certain problems take precedence over others, and proceeding with a safe and efficient approach to care. For each of the diagnoses, Lisa identifies the goals and expected outcomes that she and the client hope to achieve. The goals and outcomes direct Lisa in selecting appropriate therapeutic interventions. Ms. Devine is a client who will partner well with Lisa in selecting interventions suited to her own needs, strengths, and limitations. Lisa knows she needs to move quickly in developing a plan, because Ms. Devine is to go to surgery early in the afternoon.

After you identify a client's nursing diagnoses and strengths, planning nursing care begins. **Planning,** the third step of the nursing process, is a category of nursing behaviors in which a nurse sets client-centered goals and expected outcomes and plans nursing interventions. Select interventions that will resolve the client's problems and achieve the goals and outcomes. Planning requires critical thinking, applied through deliberate decision making and problem solving.

Another aspect of planning is to set priorities for a client. Remember, a single client often has multiple diagnoses and collaborative problems. Eventually you will care for groups of clients. Being able to carefully and wisely set priorities for a single client or group of clients ensures the most timely and appropriate care. Successful planning requires that you collaborate with the client and family, consult with other health care team members, and review related literature. This includes available evidence on the client's health care problems. A plan of care is dynamic and will change as you meet the client's needs or identify new needs.

Establishing Priorities

Priority setting is the ordering of nursing diagnoses or client problems using notions of urgency and/or importance to establish a preferential order for nursing actions (Hendry and Walker, 2004). In other words, as you care for a client or a group of clients, there are certain aspects of care that you need to deal with before others. By ranking nursing diagnoses in order of importance, you attend to the client's most important needs and better organize ongoing care activities. Priorities help you to anticipate and sequence nursing interventions when a client has multiple nursing diagnoses and collaborative problems. Together with your clients, you will select mutually agreed-on priorities based on the urgency of the problems, the client's safety and desires, the nature of the treatment indicated, and the relationship among the diagnoses. Establishing priorities is not merely a matter of numbering the nursing diagnoses on the basis of severity or physiological importance. Fontana (1993) suggests that nurses establish priorities in relation to importance and time. In practice, certain priorities and nursing actions have qualities of both (Hendry and Walker, 2004).

In regard to importance, it helps to classify priorities as high, intermediate, or low. Nursing diagnoses that, if untreated, result in harm to the client or others have the highest priorities. For example, *risk for other-directed violence, impaired gas exchange,* and *decreased cardiac output* are typically high-priority nursing diagnoses that drive the priorities of safety, adequate oxygenation, and adequate circulation. However, it is always important to consider each client's unique situation. High priorities are sometimes both physiological and psychological and may address other basic human needs. Avoid classifying only physiological nursing diagnoses as high priority. Consider Ms. Devine's case. Among Ms. Devine's nursing diagnoses, *acute pain* and *anxiety* are of the highest priority. Lisa knows that she needs to relieve Ms. Devine's acute pain and lessen the client's anxiety so that the client will approach surgery in less distress.

Intermediate priority nursing diagnoses involve the nonemergent, non–life-threatening needs of the client. In Ms. Devine's case, *deficient knowledge* is an intermediate diagnosis. It will be very important for Lisa to be able to properly prepare Ms. Devine for surgery. Focused and individualized instruction will help Ms. Devine understand what to expect during her preoperative preparation and how to participate in postoperative care activities. Attending to the diagnosis of *deficient knowledge* will help to minimize postoperative complications. Once Lisa addresses the higher-priority nursing diagnoses of pain and anxiety, Ms. Devine will more likely be able to learn. Furthermore, once Ms. Devine begins to understand what surgery involves, hopefully her anxiety will lessen.

Low-priority nursing diagnoses are not always directly related to a specific illness or prognosis but affect the client's future well-being. Many low-priority diagnoses focus on the client's long-term health care needs. In Ms. Devine's situation, *impaired physical mobility* is due in part to her pain but also to her medical condition, a herniated disk. Lisa will monitor this diagnosis carefully, especially postoperatively. For now, Lisa will try to make Ms. Devine as comfortable as possible, which may improve her ability to turn and position. However, once surgery is completed, Lisa will reassess her client. If *impaired physical mobility* remains a problem, the diagnosis will be a higher priority because it will become essential for Ms. Devine to achieve more normal mobility for a full recovery and to prevent postoperative complications.

The order of priorities changes as a client's condition changes, sometimes within a matter of minutes. Each time you begin a sequence of care, such as at the beginning of a hospital shift or a client's clinic visit, it is important to reorder priorities. Ongoing client assessment is critical to determine the status of your client's nursing diagnoses. The appropriate ordering of priorities will ensure that you meet a client's needs in a timely and effective way.

When considering time as a factor in setting priorities, White (2003) explains that planning of nursing care occurs in three phases: initial, ongoing, and discharge. Each type of planning contributes to the coordination of the client's nursing care and influences the determination of your priorities. Initial planning involves development of a preliminary plan of care following admission assessment and initial selection of nursing diagnoses. Because of progressively shorter lengths of hospitalization, initial

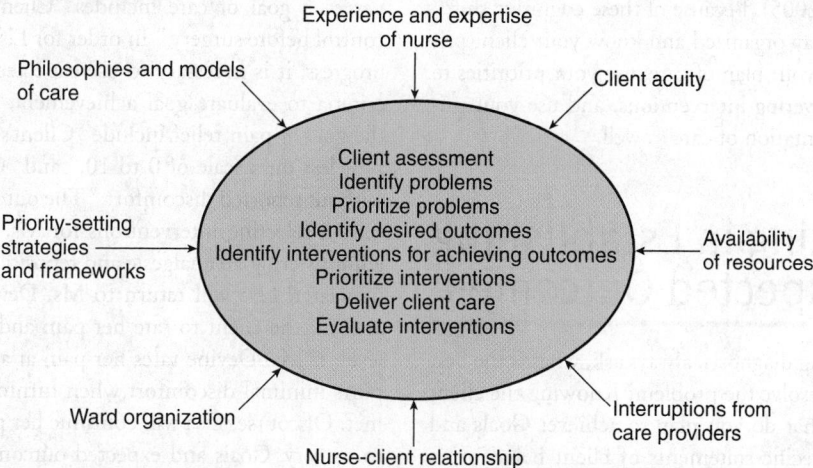

Figure 18-1 A model for priority setting. (Modified from Hendry C, Walker A: Priority setting in clinical nursing practice, *J Adv Nurs* 47[4]: 427, 2004.)

planning is important in addressing nursing diagnoses and collaborative problems to hasten problem resolution. Ongoing planning involves continuous updating of the client's plan of care. As the client's condition changes, you assess new information about the client and evaluate the client's status. During ongoing planning, you sometimes revise the initial plan of care and further individualize your interventions (White, 2003). Finally, discharge planning is the last phase of planning. This involves the critical anticipation and preparation for meeting the client's needs after discharge.

> *Lisa is now involved with the initial planning of Ms. Devine's care. Lisa needs to select interventions to manage each of Ms. Devine's nursing diagnoses before she goes to surgery. Once Ms. Devine returns from surgery, Lisa, or another nurse, will conduct ongoing planning by further assessing Ms. Devine's status and then redefining nursing diagnoses that apply postoperatively. As Ms. Devine recovers from surgery, Lisa and her colleagues will work together in developing a discharge plan that will assist Ms. Devine in returning home in as healthy a condition as possible.*

Priority setting begins at a holistic level when you identify and prioritize a client's main diagnoses or problems (Hendry and Walker, 2004). However, you also need to prioritize the specific interventions or strategies that you will use to help a client achieve desired goals and outcomes. For example, as Lisa considers the high-priority diagnosis of *acute pain* for Ms. Devine, she will decide which among the interventions of administering an analgesic, repositioning, and teaching relaxation exercises, to do first. Critical thinking helps you to prioritize. Lisa knows that a certain degree of pain relief is necessary before a client can attend to relaxation exercises. When she is in the client's room, she will possibly decide to turn and reposition Ms. Devine and then go get her analgesic. However, if Ms. Devine is too uncomfortable to turn, Lisa will choose obtaining and administering the analgesic as her first priority.

Remember to involve the client in priority setting whenever possible. In some situations the client will assign different priorities from what you select. If you both place different values on health care needs and treatments, resolve these differences through open communication, informing the client of all options and consequences. Consulting with and knowing the client's concerns does not relieve you of the responsibility to act in a client's best interests (Nursing and Midwifery Council, 2002). Always assign priorities on the basis of good nursing judgment.

Priorities in Practice

Hendry and Walker (2004) address an important issue regarding priority setting (Figure 18-1). There are many factors within the health care environment that affect your ability to set priorities. For example, in the hospital setting, the model for delivering care (see Chapter 21), the organization of a nursing unit, and interruptions from other care providers affect the minute-by-minute determination of client care priorities. Available resources (e.g., nurse specialists, laboratory technicians, and dietitians), policies and procedures, and supply access will affect priorities as well. Add to this the factor that clients' conditions are always changing, priority setting is a dynamic process as well. For example, Lisa prepared the analgesic for Ms. Devine, takes it to her room, and administers the medication. She plans on letting Ms. Devine relax for about 30 minutes and then returning to begin preoperative teaching for the client's surgery. However, when Lisa returns 30 minutes later, she finds the physician talking with the client and a laboratory technician preparing to obtain a blood specimen for a test that was just ordered. Lisa has to delay her teaching, so she chooses to attend to a different client while Ms. Devine is occupied.

The same factors that influence your minute-by-minute ability to prioritize nursing actions affect the ability to prioritize nursing diagnoses for groups of clients. When you care for more than one client, the nature of nursing work challenges your ability to cognitively attend to a given client's priorities. Nursing care is a nonlinear process (Potter and others, 2005). You will often complete an assessment and identify nursing diagnoses for one client and then leave the room to perform an intervention for a second client. Nurses exercise "cognitive shifts," shifts in attention from one client to another during the conduct of the nursing process. This shifting of attention occurs in response to client needs changing, new procedures being ordered, or environmental processes interacting (Potter and others, 2005). Because of these cognitive shifts, it becomes important to stay organized and know your client priorities. Always work from your plan of care, use your priorities to organize the order for delivering interventions, and use your priorities to organize documentation of care as well.

Critical Thinking in Establishing Goals and Expected Outcomes

Once you identify a nursing diagnosis, always ask, what is the best approach to address and resolve the problem? Knowing the client has a certain diagnosis, what do you plan to achieve? Goals and expected outcomes are specific statements of client behavior or physiological responses that you set to achieve nursing diagnosis or collaborative problem resolution. Goals and outcomes provide a clear focus for the type of interventions necessary to care for your client.

A **goal** is an aim, intent, or end (White, 2003). A goal is a broad statement that describes the desired change in a client's condition or behavior. For example, in the case of Ms. Devine, who has a diagnosis of *acute pain related to pressure on spinal*

nerves, a goal of care includes "Client achieves improved pain control before surgery." In order for Lisa to monitor Ms. Devine's progress, it is necessary to use **expected outcomes** or measurable criteria to evaluate goal achievement. Measurable outcomes for the goal of pain relief include "Client's self-report of pain will be 3 or less on a scale of 0 to 10," and "Client will be able to turn without reported discomfort." The outcomes will gauge Lisa's success in selecting interventions for Ms. Devine's pain relief. After administering an analgesic and repositioning the client a few minutes later, Lisa will return to Ms. Devine's room in 30 minutes and ask the client to rate her pain and to report on her comfort level. If Ms. Devine rates her pain at a 3 or less and similarly reports minimal discomfort when turning, her goal will have been met. Of course, Lisa will continue her plan until Ms. Devine goes to surgery. Goals and expected outcomes serve two purposes: to provide clear direction for the selection and use of nursing interventions and to provide focus for evaluating the effectiveness of the interventions.

Planning nursing care requires critical thinking (Figure 18-2). You need to critically evaluate the identified nursing diagnoses, the urgency of the problems, and the resources of the client and the health care delivery system. You apply knowledge from the medical, sociobehavioral, and nursing sciences to plan client care. The

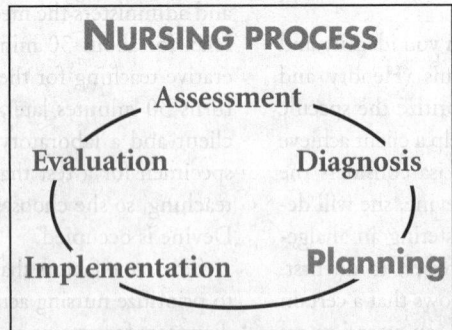

KNOWLEDGE
Client's database and selected nursing diagnoses
Anatomy and physiology
Psychology
Pathophysiology
Normal growth and development
Evidence-based nursing interventions
Role of other health care disciplines
Community resources
Family dynamics
Teaching/learning process
Delegation principles
Priority-setting principles

EXPERIENCE
Previous client care experience
Personal experience in
organizing activities

NURSING PROCESS
Assessment
Evaluation   Diagnosis
Implementation   Planning

STANDARDS
ANA Scope of Nursing Practice
Specialty standards of practice
Client-centered goals and outcomes
Intellectual standards
Agency's policies and procedures

ATTITUDES
Creativity
Responsibility
Perseverance
Discipline

Figure 18-2 Critical thinking and the process of planning care.

selection of goals, expected outcomes, and interventions requires consideration of your previous experience with similar client problems, as well as any established standards for clinical problem management. The goals and outcomes need to meet established intellectual standards by being relevant to client needs, specific, singular, observable, measurable, and time-limited. You will also use critical thinking attitudes in selecting interventions with the greatest likelihood of success. For example, Lisa creatively selects a comfort measure that Ms. Devine practices at home in choosing a plan for managing the client's acute pain. The diagram in Figure 18-3 graphically illustrates the relationships between nursing diagnoses, goals, expected outcomes, and nursing interventions.

Goals of Care

A **client-centered goal** is a specific and measurable behavior or response that reflects a client's highest possible level of wellness and independence in function. Examples include "Client will

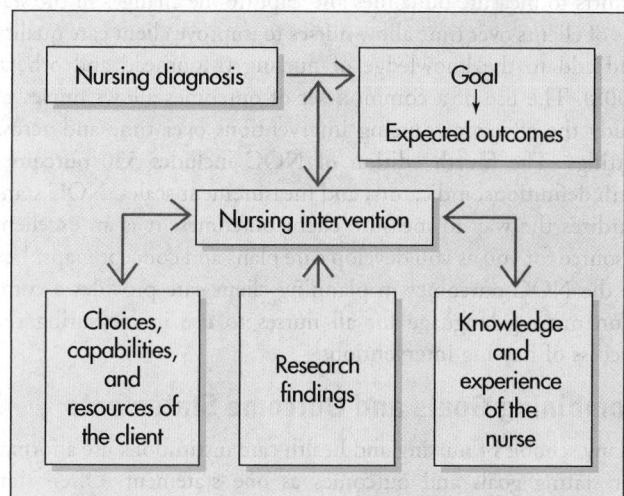

Figure 18-3 From diagnosis to outcome. (Revised and redrawn from Gordon M: *Nursing Diagnosis: process and application,* ed 3, St. Louis, 1994, Mosby.)

perform self-care hygiene independently" and "Client will remain free of infection." A goal is realistic and based on client needs and resources. A client goal represents predicted resolution of a diagnosis or problem, evidence of progress toward resolution, progress toward improved health status, or continued maintenance of good health or function (Carpenito-Moyet, 2005). A goal contains only one behavior or response. The example of "Client will administer a self-injection and demonstrate infection control measures" is incorrect because the statement includes two different behaviors, administer and demonstrate. Instead, word the goal as follows, "Client will administer a self-injection." The specific criteria you use to measure success of the goal are the expected outcomes. For example, "Client will prepare medication dose correctly" and "Client uses medical asepsis when preparing injection site."

Each goal is time-limited so that the health care team has a common time frame for problem resolution. The time frame depends on the nature of the problem, etiology, overall condition of the client, and treatment setting. A **short-term goal** is an objective behavior or response that you expect a client to achieve in a short time, usually less than a week. In an acute care setting, you set goals for over a course of just a few hours. Such was the case when Lisa set the goal for Ms. Devine, "Client's level of comfort will improve before surgery." A **long-term goal** is an objective behavior or response that you expect a client to achieve over a longer period, usually over several days, weeks, or months. For example, "Client will be tobacco-free within 60 days." Goal setting establishes the framework for the nursing care plan. Table 18-1 shows the progression from nursing diagnoses to goals and expected outcomes and the relationship to nursing interventions.

Role of the Client in Goal Setting. Always partner with clients when setting goals. Mutual goal setting is an activity that includes the client and family (when appropriate) in prioritizing the goals of care and in developing a plan of action (McCloskey and Bulechek, 1994). For clients to participate in goal setting, they need to be alert and have some degree of independence in completing activities of daily living, problem solving, and decision making. Unless you set goals mutually and make a clear plan

TABLE 18-1 Examples of Goal Setting With Expected Outcomes for Ms. Devine

NURSING DIAGNOSES	GOALS	EXPECTED OUTCOMES
Acute pain related to pressure on spinal nerves	Ms. Devine's level of comfort will improve before surgery.	Client will be able to turn without reported discomfort in 2 hours. Client's self-report of pain will be 3 or less on a scale of 0 to 10 by time of scheduled surgery.
Anxiety related to uncertainty over surgery	Ms. Devine will accept plan for surgical care before scheduled surgery.	Client will express less uneasiness about surgical experience in next 4 hours. Client will exhibit less facial tension before scheduled surgery.
Deficient knowledge regarding postoperative activities related to inexperience	Ms. Devine will understand treatment procedures planned postoperatively within 4 hours.	Client will describe purpose of postoperative exercises before scheduled surgery. Client will demonstrate use of incentive spirometer and coughing before scheduled surgery. Client will explain purpose of postoperative monitoring activities before scheduled surgery.
Impaired physical mobility related to pain	Ms. Devine will move independently in bed before surgery.	Client will initiate turning without discomfort within 2 hours. Client will position self for care procedures within 2 hours.

for action, clients will not follow the care plan. For example, Lisa and Ms. Devine set the goal "Client will report pain acuity less than 3 on a scale of 0 to 10." Ms. Devine says a level of 3 is a tolerable level of pain for her. If a client or significant other is not able to participate in goal development, you assume responsibility until the client is able to participate (White, 2003). Clients need to understand and see the value of nursing therapies, even though they are oftentimes totally dependent on you as the nurse. When setting goals, advocate for the client by developing nursing interventions that promote the client's return to health or prevent further deterioration.

Expected Outcomes

An expected outcome is a specific measurable change in a client's status that you expect to occur in response to nursing care. Expected outcomes provide a focus or direction for nursing care because they are the desired physiological, psychological, social, developmental, or spiritual responses that indicate resolution of a client's health problems. Taken from both short- and long-term goals, outcomes determine when a specific, client-centered goal has been met.

Usually you develop several expected outcomes for each nursing diagnosis and goal. The reason for the multiple expected outcomes is that sometimes one nursing action is not enough to resolve a client problem. In addition, the listing of the step-by-step expected outcomes gives you practical guidance in planning interventions. Always write expected outcomes sequentially, with time frames (see Table 18-1). Time frames give you progressive steps in which to move a client toward recovery and offer an order for nursing interventions. In addition, time frames set limits for problem resolution. In the case of Ms. Devine, Lisa plans to relieve the client's pain enough so that she is able to turn comfortably in bed within the next 2 hours and to successfully reduce pain severity before surgery.

Always write expected outcome statements in measurable terms. This allows you to note specifically the behavior or physiological response expected for resolution of the client's problem. For example "Client will have less pain" is an inaccurate outcome statement because the phrase "less pain" is nonspecific. The statement "Client will report pain acuity less than 3 on a scale of 0 to 10" is accurate.

Nursing Outcomes Classification. There is much attention in the current health care environment to measuring outcomes sensitive to nursing interventions. This is because it is becoming important for nurses to demonstrate their measurable contributions to client care. Many health care administrators focus on outcomes in determining staffing and other resources for a health care setting. The Iowa Intervention Project has published the Nursing Outcomes Classification (NOC) and has linked the outcomes to NANDA International nursing diagnoses (Moorhead and others, 2008). The Iowa researchers define a **nursing-sensitive client outcome** as an individual, family, or community state, behavior, or perception that is measurable along a continuum in response to a nursing intervention. For any given NANDA International nursing diagnosis there are multiple NOC suggested outcomes. These outcomes have labels for describing the focus of nursing care and include indicators to use in measuring the success with interventions (Table 18-2). The NOC contains outcomes for individuals, family caregivers, the family, and the community for all types of health care settings. Efforts to measure outcomes and capture the changes in the status of clients over time allow nurses to improve client care quality and add to the knowledge of nursing (Moorhead and others, 2008). The use of a common set of outcomes allows nurses to study the effects of nursing interventions over time and across settings. The fourth edition of NOC includes 330 outcomes with definitions, indicators, and measurement scales. NOC standardizes the way to measure client outcomes. It is an excellent resource for you as you develop care plans and concept maps. Use of the NOC outcomes in planning client care provides a common nursing language for all nurses to use in measuring the success of nursing interventions.

Combining Goals and Outcome Statements

Many schools of nursing and health care institutions use a format for stating goals and outcomes as one statement. Often staff within health care settings refer to the terms *goals* and *outcomes* interchangeably. This is acceptable as long as the criteria for writing goals and outcomes are met. For example, the statement "Client will achieve pain control as evidenced by reporting pain acuity less than 3 on a scale of 0 to 10 within 24 hours" is an acceptable statement. The goal portion of the statement broadly describes

✱ TABLE 18-2 Examples of NANDA International Nursing Diagnoses and Suggested NOC Linkages

NURSING DIAGNOSIS	SUGGESTED NOC OUTCOMES (EXAMPLES)	OUTCOME INDICATORS (EXAMPLES)
Deficient knowledge	Knowledge: Treatment Procedures	Description of treatment procedure Description of steps in procedure
	Knowledge: Disease Process	Effects of disease Specific disease process
Activity intolerance	Activity Tolerance	Oxygen saturation with activity Pulse rate with activity Respiratory rate with activity
	Self-Care Status	Bathes self Dresses self Prepares food and fluid for eating

Moorhead S and others: *Nursing outcomes classification*, ed 4, St. Louis, 2008, Mosby.
NOC, Nursing Outcomes Classification.

the desired client status (achieve pain control), and the outcome portion of the statement contains the observable criterion (3 on a pain scale) needed to measure success. The format for the many documentation forms found within health care settings dictates how nurses write goals and outcomes.

Guidelines for Writing Goals and Expected Outcomes

There are seven guidelines for writing goals and expected outcomes. The guidelines are: client-centered, singular, observable, measurable, time-limited, mutual, and realistic.

Client-Centered. Outcomes and goals reflect the client behavior and responses expected as a result of nursing interventions. Write a goal to reflect client behavior, not to reflect your goals or interventions. A correct outcome statement is "Client will ambulate in the hall 3 times a day." A common error is to write "Ambulate client in the hall 3 times a day."

Singular Goal or Outcome. Be precise in evaluating a client response to a nursing action. Each goal and outcome addresses only one behavior or response. If an outcome reads "Client's lungs will be clear to auscultation, and respiratory rate will be 20 breaths per minute by 8/22," consider the outcome when you evaluate that the lungs are clear but the respiratory rate is 28 breaths per minute. You will not know if the client achieved the expected outcome. By splitting the statement into two parts, "Lungs will be clear to auscultation by 8/22" and "Respiratory rate will be 20 breaths per minute by 8/22," you are able to determine if the client achieves each outcome. Singularity allows you to decide if there is a need to modify the plan of care.

Observable. You need to be able to observe if change takes place in a client's status. Observable changes occur in physiological findings and the client's knowledge, perceptions, and behavior. You observe outcomes by directly asking clients about their condition or by using assessment skills. For example, you observe the goal "Client will be able to self-administer insulin" through the outcome of watching "Client prepare insulin dosage correctly by 8/30." For the outcome "Lungs will be clear on auscultation by 8/31," you auscultate the lungs routinely following therapy. The outcome statement "Client will appear less anxious" is not a correct statement because there is no specific behavior observable for "will appear."

Measurable. You will learn to write goals and expected outcomes that set standards against which to measure the client's response to nursing care. Examples such as "Body temperature will remain 98.6° F," and "Apical pulse will remain between 60 and 100 beats per minute" allow you to objectively measure changes in the client's status. Do not use vague qualifiers such as "normal," "acceptable," or "stable" in an expected outcome statement. Vague terms result in guesswork in determining a client's response to care. Terms describing quality, quantity, frequency, length, or weight allow you to evaluate outcomes precisely.

Time-Limited. The time frame for each goal and expected outcome indicates when you expect the response to occur. Time frames assist you and the client in determining if the client is making progress at a reasonable rate. If not, revision to the plan of care becomes necessary. Time frames also promote accountability in the delivery and management of nursing care.

Mutual Factors. Mutually set goals and expected outcomes ensure that the client and nurse agree on the direction and time limits of care. Mutual goal setting increases the client's motivation and cooperation. As a client advocate, apply standards of practice, evidence-based knowledge, safety principles, and basic human needs when assisting clients with setting goals.

Realistic. Set goals and expected outcomes that a client is able to reach. This becomes a challenge when the time allotted for care is limited. Realistic goals provide clients a sense of hope that increases motivation and cooperation. In order to establish realistic goals, you need to assess the resources of the health care facility, family, and client. You also need to be aware of the client's physiological, emotional, cognitive, and sociocultural potential and the economic cost and resources available to reach expected outcomes in a timely manner.

Critical Thinking in Planning Nursing Care

Nursing interventions are treatments or actions, based upon clinical judgment and knowledge, that nurses perform to meet clients' outcomes (Bulechek, Butcher, and Dochterman, 2008). During planning, nurses select interventions designed to assist a client in moving from the present level of health to the level described in the goal and measured by the expected outcomes. The actual implementation of these interventions occurs during the implementation phase of the nursing process (see Chapter 19).

Choosing suitable nursing interventions involves critical thinking applied in decision making. To select interventions, you need to be competent in three areas: (1) knowing the scientific rationale for the intervention, (2) possessing the necessary psychomotor and interpersonal skills, and (3) being able to function within a particular setting to use the available health care resources effectively (Bulechek and others, 2008).

Types of Interventions

There are three categories of nursing interventions: nurse-initiated, physician-initiated, and collaborative interventions. You base the interventions you select on client needs. Some clients require all three categories of interventions, whereas other clients need only nurse- and physician-initiated interventions.

Nurse-initiated interventions are the **independent nursing interventions,** or actions that a nurse initiates. These do not require direction or an order from another health care professional (Wood, 2003). As a nurse, you act independently on a client's behalf. Nurse-initiated interventions are autonomous actions based on scientific rationale. Examples include elevating an edematous extremity, instructing clients in side effects of medications, or directing a client to splint an incision during coughing. Such interventions benefit a client in a predicted way related to nursing diagnoses and client goals (Bulechek and others, 2008). Nurse-initiated interventions require no supervision or direction from others. Each state within the United States has developed Nurse Practice Acts that define the legal scope of nursing practice (see Chapter 23). According to the Nurse Practice Acts in a majority of states, independent nursing interventions pertain to activities of daily living, health education and promotion, and counseling.

Physician-initiated interventions are **dependent nursing interventions,** or actions that require an order from a physician or another health care professional. The interventions are based on the physician's or health care provider's response to treat or manage a medical diagnosis. Nurse practitioners working under collaborative agreements with physicians or who are licensed independently by state practice acts are also able to write such interventions. As the nurse, you intervene by carrying out the independent provider's written and/or verbal orders. Administering a medication, implementing an invasive procedure, changing a dressing, and preparing a client for diagnostic tests are examples of physician-initiated interventions.

Each physician-initiated intervention requires specific nursing responsibilities and technical nursing knowledge. For example, when administering medications, you are responsible for knowing the classification of the drug, its physiological action, normal dosage, side effects, and nursing interventions related to its action or side effects (see Chapter 35). With an invasive procedure, you are responsible for knowing when the procedure is necessary, the clinical skills necessary to complete it, and its expected outcome and possible side effects. You are also responsible for adequate preparation of the client and proper communication of the results. You perform dependent nursing interventions, like all nursing actions, with appropriate knowledge and good clinical judgment (Wood, 2003).

Collaborative interventions, or interdependent nursing interventions, are therapies that require the combined knowledge, skill, and expertise of multiple health care professionals. Typically, when you plan care for a client, you will review the necessary interventions and determine if the collaboration of other health care disciplines is necessary. A client care conference with an interdisciplinary health care team results in selection of interdependent nursing interventions.

In the case study involving Lisa and Ms. Devine, Lisa will initiate independent interventions to help calm Ms. Devine's anxiety and to begin teaching the client about postoperative care activities. In addition, Lisa independently positions Ms. Devine to minimize her discomfort and to promote more normal mobility. Among the dependent interventions Lisa plans to implement are the administration of an analgesic and the completion of any necessary preoperative diagnostic tests. Lisa's collaborative intervention involves consulting with the unit social worker, who will help Ms. Devine with her anxiety over surgery or any other concerns.

When preparing for physician-initiated or collaborative interventions, do not automatically implement the therapy but determine whether it is appropriate for the client. Every nurse faces an inappropriate or incorrect order at some time. The nurse with a strong knowledge base recognizes the error and seeks to correct it. The ability to recognize incorrect therapies is particularly important when administering medications or implementing procedures. Errors occur in writing orders or transcribing them to a documentation form or computer screen. Clarifying an order is competent nursing practice, and it protects the client and members of the health care team. When you carry out an incorrect or inappropriate intervention, it is as much your error as the person who wrote or transcribed the original order. You are legally responsible for any complications resulting from the error (see Chapter 23).

Selection of Interventions

You need to learn to not select interventions randomly. Clients with the diagnosis of *anxiety,* for example, do not always need care in the same way with the same interventions. You treat *anxiety* related to the uncertainty of impending surgery very differently than *anxiety* related to a threat to loss of family role function. When choosing interventions, consider six important factors: (1) characteristics of the nursing diagnosis, (2) goals and expected outcomes, (3) evidence base (e.g., research or proven practice guidelines) for the interventions, (4) feasibility of the intervention, (5) acceptability to the client, and (6) your own competency (Bulechek and others, 2008) (Box 18-1). During deliberation, review resources such as the nursing literature, standard protocols or guidelines, the Nursing Interventions Classification (NIC), critical pathways, policy or procedure manuals, or textbooks. Collaboration with other health professionals is also useful. As you select interventions, review your client's needs, priorities, and previous experiences to select the interventions that have the best potential for achieving the expected outcomes.

Nursing Interventions Classification. The Iowa Intervention Project has developed a set of nursing interventions that provides a level of standardization to enhance communication of nursing care across all health care settings and to compare outcomes (Bulechek and others, 2008; Iowa Intervention Project, 1993). The NIC model includes three levels: domains, classes, and interventions for ease of use. The domains are the highest level (Level 1) of the model, using broad terms (e.g., safety and basic physiological) to organize the more specific classes and interventions (Table 18-3). The second level of the model includes 30 classes, which offer useful clinical categories to refer to when selecting interventions. The third level of the model includes the 542 interventions, defined as any treatment based upon clinical judgment and knowledge that a nurse performs to enhance patient/client outcomes (Bulechek and others, 2008) (Box 18-2). Each intervention then includes a variety of nursing activities from which to choose (Box 18-3). It is the nursing activities that a nurse will commonly use in a plan of care. NIC interventions are also linked with NANDA International nursing diagnoses for ease of use (NANDA International, 2007). For example, if a client has a nursing diagnosis of *acute pain,* there are 21 recommended interventions, including pain management, cutaneous stimulation, and anxiety reduction. Each of the recommended interventions has a variety of activities for nursing care. NIC is a

✳ BOX 18-1   Choosing Nursing Interventions

Characteristics of the Nursing Diagnosis
- Interventions should alter the etiological (related to) factor or signs and symptoms associated with the diagnostic label
- When an etiological factor cannot change, direct the interventions toward treating the signs and symptoms (e.g., NANDA International defining characteristics)
- For potential or high-risk diagnoses, direct interventions at altering or eliminating risk factors for the diagnosis

Expected Outcomes
- Because nurses state outcomes in terms used to evaluate the effect of an intervention, this language assists in selecting the intervention
- Nursing Interventions Classification (NIC) is designed to show the link to Nursing Outcomes Classification (NOC) (Moorhead and others, 2008)

Research Base
- Research evidence in support of a nursing intervention will indicate the effectiveness of using the intervention with certain types of clients
- Refer to the evidence (e.g., research articles or evidence-based practice protocols that describe the utilization of evidence in similar clinical situations and settings)
- When research is not available, use scientific principles (e.g., infection control) or consult a clinical expert about your client population

Feasibility
- A specific intervention has the potential for interacting with other interventions
- Be knowledgeable about the total plan of care
- Consider cost: Is the intervention clinically effective and cost efficient?
- Consider time: Are time and personnel resources available?

Acceptability to the Client
- A treatment plan needs to be acceptable to the client and family and match the client's goals, health care values, and culture
- Promote informed choice; help a client know how to participate in and anticipate the effect of interventions

Capability of the Nurse
- Be prepared to carry out the intervention
- Know the scientific rationale for the intervention
- Have the necessary psychosocial and psychomotor skills to complete the intervention
- Be able to function within the specific setting and effectively and efficiently use health care resources

Modified from Bulechek GM, Butcher HK, and Dochterman JM: *Nursing interventions classification (NIC)*, ed 5, St. Louis, 2008, Mosby.

---

valuable resource for you to select appropriate interventions and activities for your client. NIC is evolving and is practice oriented. The classification is comprehensive, including independent and collaborative interventions. It remains your decision to determine which interventions and activities best suit your client's needs and situation.

Planning Nursing Care

In any health care setting a nurse is responsible for providing a written plan of care for all clients. The plan of care sometimes takes several forms (e.g., nursing Kardex, standardized care plans, and computerized plans). Generally a written nursing care plan includes nursing diagnoses, goals and/or expected outcomes, and specific nursing interventions so that any nurse is able to quickly identify a client's clinical needs and situation. In hospitals and community-based settings, the client often receives care from more than one nurse, physician, or allied health professional. A written nursing care plan makes possible the coordination of nursing care, subspecialty consultations, and scheduling of diagnostic tests.

You design a written plan to direct clinical nursing care and to decrease the risk of incomplete, incorrect, or inaccurate care. As the client's problems and status change, so does the plan. A nursing care plan is a written guideline for coordinating nursing care, promoting continuity of care, and listing outcome criteria to be used in evaluation. The written plan communicates nursing care priorities to other health care professionals. The care plan also

identifies and coordinates resources for delivering nursing care. For example, in a plan you list specific supplies necessary to use in a dressing change.

Written care plans organize information exchanged by nurses in change-of-shift reports (see Chapter 26). You will learn to focus your reports on the nursing care, treatments, and expected outcomes documented in your care plans. At the end of a shift you will discuss care plans and the client's overall progress with the next caregiver. Thus all nurses are able to discuss current and relevant information about the client's plan of care.

The **nursing care plan** enhances the continuity of nursing care by listing specific nursing interventions needed to achieve the goals of care. All nurses who care for a given client will then carry out these nursing interventions throughout a given day during a client's length of stay. A correctly formulated nursing care plan makes it easy to continue care from one nurse to another. The nursing care plan on p. 272 provides an example of a care plan for Ms. Devine, using the format found throughout this text.

When developing an individualized care plan, involve the family and client. The family is a resource to help the client meet health care goals. In addition, meeting some of the family's needs will possibly improve the client's level of wellness.

Most written plans include expected outcome criteria used in the evaluation of care. Proper listing of the criteria provides you with objective statements that help determine whether you have achieved the goals of care. The complete care plan is the blueprint for nursing action. It provides direction for implementation of the plan and a framework for evaluation of the client's response to nursing actions.

✳ TABLE 18-3 Nursing Interventions Classification (NIC) Taxonomy

DOMAIN 1	DOMAIN 2	DOMAIN 3
Level 1 Domains		
1. **Physiological: Basic** Care that supports physical functioning	2. **Physiological: Complex** Care that supports homeostatic regulation	3. **Behavioral** Care that supports psychosocial functioning and facilitates lifestyle changes
Level 2 Classes		
A *Activity and Exercise Management:* Interventions to organize or assist with physical activity and energy conservation and expenditure	G *Electrolyte and Acid-Base Management:* Interventions to regulate electrolyte/acid-base balance and prevent complications	O *Behavior Therapy:* Interventions to reinforce or promote desirable behaviors or alter undesirable behaviors
B *Elimination Management:* Interventions to establish and maintain regular bowel and urinary elimination patterns and manage complications due to altered patterns	H *Drug Management:* Interventions to facilitate desired effects of pharmacological agents	P *Cognitive Therapy:* Interventions to reinforce or promote desirable cognitive functioning or alter undesirable cognitive functioning
C *Immobility Management:* Interventions to manage restricted body movement and the sequelae	I *Neurologic Management:* Interventions to optimize neurologic functions	Q *Communication Enhancement:* Interventions to facilitate delivering and receiving verbal and nonverbal messages
D *Nutrition Support:* Interventions to modify or maintain nutritional status	J *Perioperative Care:* Interventions to provide care before, during, and immediately after surgery	R *Coping Assistance:* Interventions to assist another to build on own strengths, to adapt to a change in function, or to achieve a higher level of function
E *Physical Comfort Promotion:* Interventions to promote comfort using physical techniques	K *Respiratory Management:* Interventions to promote airway patency and gas exchange	S *Patient Education:* Interventions to facilitate learning
F *Self-Care Facilitation:* Interventions to provide or assist with routine activities of daily living	L *Skin/Wound Management:* Interventions to maintain or restore tissue integrity	T *Psychological Comfort Promotion:* Interventions to promote comfort using psychological techniques
	M *Thermoregulation:* Interventions to maintain body temperature within a normal range	
	N *Tissue Perfusion Management:* Interventions to optimize circulation of blood and fluids to the tissue	

From Bulechek GM, Butcher HK, and Dochterman JM: *Nursing interventions classification (NIC)*, ed 5, St. Louis, 2008, Mosby.

✳ BOX 18-2 Example of Interventions for Physical Comfort Promotion

Class: Physical Comfort Promotion
Interventions to promote comfort using physical techniques

Interventions (Examples)
Acupressure
Aromatherapy
Cutaneous Stimulation
Environmental Management: Comfort
Heat/Cold Application
Nausea Management
Pain Management
Progressive Muscle Relaxation
Simple Massage

Examples of Linked Nursing Diagnoses:
Acute Pain
Chronic Pain

From Bulechek GM, Butcher HK, and Dochterman JM: *Nursing interventions classification (NIC)*, ed 5, St. Louis, 2008, Mosby.

✳ BOX 18-3 Example of Interventions and Associated Nursing Activities

Intervention—Environmental Management: Comfort
Examples of Activities:
Create a calm and supportive environment
Provide a safe and clean environment
Adjust room temperature to that most comfortable for the individual
Avoid unnecessary exposure, drafts, overheating or chilling
Prevent unnecessary interruptions and allow for rest period
Monitor skin, especially over bony prominences, for signs of pressure or irritation
Provide prompt attention to call bells which should always be within reach

From Bulechek GM, Butcher HK, and Dochterman JM: *Nursing interventions classification (NIC)*, ed 5, St. Louis, 2008, Mosby.

TABLE 18-3 Nursing Interventions Classification (NIC) Taxonomy—cont'd

DOMAIN 4	DOMAIN 5	DOMAIN 6	DOMAIN 7
4. **Safety** Care that supports protection against harm	5. **Family** Care that supports the family	6. **Health System** Care that supports effective use of the health care delivery system	7. **Community** Care that supports the health of the community
U *Crisis Management:* Interventions to provide immediate short-term help in both psychological and physiological crises V *Risk Management:* Interventions to initiate risk-reduction activities and continue monitoring risks over time	W *Childbearing Care:* Interventions to assist in understanding and coping with the psychological and physiological changes during the childbearing period Z *Childrearing Care:* Interventions to assist in rearing children X *Lifespan Care:* Interventions to facilitate family unit functioning and promote the health and welfare of family members throughout the lifespan	Y *Health System Mediation:* Interventions to facilitate the interface between patient/family and the health care system a *Health System Management:* Interventions to provide and enhance support services for the delivery of care b *Information Management:* Interventions to facilitate communication among health care providers	c *Community Health Promotion:* Interventions that promote the health of the whole community d *Community Risk Management:* Interventions that assist in detecting or preventing health risks to the whole community

Student Care Plans

Student care plans are useful for learning the problem-solving technique, the nursing process, skills of written communication, and organizational skills needed for nursing care. Most important, your use of the nursing care plan helps you apply knowledge gained from the nursing and medical literature and the classroom to a practice situation. Students typically write a care plan for each nursing diagnosis, using a columnar format that includes assessment findings, goals, expected outcomes, nursing interventions with supporting rationales, and evaluative outcome criteria. The student care plan is more elaborate than a care plan used in a hospital or community agency because its purpose is to teach the process of planning care. Each school uses a different format for student care plans. Some schools model the student care plan on what their health care agencies use.

The nursing diagnosis with the highest priority is the beginning point for the nursing care plan, followed by plans for other nursing diagnoses in order of assigned priority. The example in Table 18-4 uses a six-column format. You enter into the assessment column (column 1) all assessment data relevant to the corresponding nursing diagnosis. You then list the goals (column 2) and outcomes (column 3) identified for the client. At this point, you begin to translate the goals and outcomes into an action plan that includes appropriate nursing interventions that offer a coordinated approach to nursing care. You write the action plan in the implementation column (column 4) of the care plan. Write each nursing action to include information necessary to implement nursing care. The following questions will help you in designing a plan:

What is the intervention?
When should each intervention be implemented?
How should the intervention be performed for this specific client?
Who should be involved in each aspect of intervention?

Next, enter a scientific rationale (column 5) for a specific intervention. A **scientific rationale** is the reason that you chose a specific nursing action, based on supporting evidence. Each rationale needs to include a reference, whenever possible, to document the source from the scientific literature. This reinforces the importance of evidence-based nursing practice. It is also important that each intervention be specific and unique to a client's situation. Nonspecific nursing interventions result in incomplete or inac-

NURSING CARE PLAN

Acute Pain

Assessment

Ms. Devine is a 52-year-old woman who had an injury from a fall 2 months ago that caused a ruptured lumbar disk. She is scheduled for a lumbar laminectomy this afternoon. Ms. Devine is the office manager for a realty business she runs with her husband. She has not been able to work regularly over the last month. She has sciatic pain that is sharp and burning, radiating down from her right hip to her right foot. The pain worsens when she sits. Her vital signs are temperature, 99.2° F; blood pressure, 138/82 mm Hg; pulse, 84 beats per minute; and respirations, 24 breaths per minute.

Assessment Activities*	Findings/Defining Characteristics
Observe client's body movements.	Client **limps slightly with right leg. Turns** in bed **slowly.**
Observe client's facial expression.	Client **grimaces** when she attempts to sit down.
Ask client to rate pain at its worst.	Client **rates pain on a scale of 0 to 10 at an 8 or 9 at its worst.**

*Defining characteristics are shown in bold type.

Nursing Diagnosis: Acute pain related to pressure on spinal nerves.

Planning

Goal	Expected Outcomes (NOC)†
	Pain Control
Client achieves improved pain control before surgery.	Client's self-report of pain will be 4 or less on a scale of 0 to 10.
	Client's facial expressions reveal less discomfort when turning and repositioning.

†Outcomes classification labels from Moorhead S and others: *Nursing outcomes classification (NOC),* ed 4, St. Louis, 2008, Mosby.

Interventions (NIC)‡	Rationale
Analgesic Administration	
Set positive expectations regarding effectiveness of analgesics.	Optimizes client's response to medication (Bulechek and Dochterman, 2008).
Give analgesic 30 minutes before turning/positioning and before pain increases in severity.	Medication will exert peak effect when client attempts to increase movement.
Pain Management	
Reduce environmental factors in client's room (e.g., noise, lighting, temperature extremes).	Pleasurable sensory stimuli reduce pain perception.
Offer client information about any procedures and efforts at reducing discomfort.	Information satisfies client interests and enables client to evaluate and communicate pain (McCaffery and Pasero, 1999).
Progressive Muscle Relaxation	
Direct client through progressive muscle relaxation exercise. Coach client through exercise.	Relaxation techniques provide self-control when pain develops, reversing the cognitive and affective-motivational component of pain perception.

‡Intervention classification labels from Bulechek GM, Butcher HK, and Dochterman JM: *Nursing interventions classification (NIC),* ed 5, St. Louis, 2008, Mosby.

Evaluation

Nursing Actions	Client Response/Finding	Achievement of Outcome
Ask client to report severity of pain 30 minutes after analgesic administration.	Ms. Devine reports pain at a level of 5 on a 0 to 10 scale.	Pain is reduced, requires further nonpharmacological intervention to achieve outcome.
Observe client's facial expressions.	Ms. Devine observed to have relaxed facial expression.	Client's level of comfort improving.

curate nursing care, lack of continuity among caregivers, and poor use of resources. Common omissions in writing nursing interventions include action, frequency, quantity, method, or person to perform them. These errors occur when nurses are unfamiliar with the planning process. Table 18-5 illustrates these types of errors by showing incorrect and correct statements of nursing in-

terventions. Finally, column 6 of the care plan includes a section for you to evaluate the plan of care: was each outcome fully met or only partially met? Use the evaluation column to document whether the plan requires revision or when outcomes are met, thus indicating when a particular nursing diagnosis is no longer relevant to the client's plan of care.

✳ **TABLE 18-4 Example of Student Care Plan**

Nursing Diagnosis: Risk for impaired skin integrity related to physical immobility secondary to impaired consciousness

ASSESSMENT	GOALS	EXPECTED OUTCOMES	INTERVENTIONS	RATIONALE	EVALUATION
Fever >102° F for 48 hr causing diaphoresis	Client will achieve fluid intake > output within 24 hr.	Client is afebrile in 24 hr. Fluid intake is 1800 mL/hr.	Turn client every 1½ hr as follows: 8 AM supine 9:30 AM	Turning interval should be based on standard 2-hr turning minus hypoxia time (skin redness	*Student* enters notes to evaluate success of plan in this column:
Changes position on own infrequently	Skin will remain intact through discharge.	Skin over shoulder is free of redness from stage I pressure ulcer.	30-degree left lateral position 11 AM 30-degree right lateral position	usually persists half of time hypoxia occurs) (AHCPR, 1994).	Client has 3-cm circular area of redness over shoulder that blanches well
No skin breakdown noted, 2-cm area of redness over left shoulder lasting 15 min			12:30 PM supine Continue cycle as above. Keep head of bed below 30-degree elevation.	Head of bed below 30-degree angle reduces shear (Bryant and Nix, 2007).	Intake 1800 mL Output 2000 mL Temp 38.1° C Skin dry
Incontinent of urine		Skin remains dry and without breakdown through discharge.	Place client on air-fluidized bed until body fluids are contained.	Excess moisture on intact skin is potential source of skin maceration	
Decreased skin turgor		Skin turgor returns to normal in 48 hr.		Airflow support surface dries skin and prevents pressure ulcers (AHCPR, 1994).	
Braden scale = 10			Offer PO fluids hourly while awake	Reverses hydration.	
			Apply condom urinary catheter.	Catheter provides urinary drainage when clients have spontaneous and complete bladder emptying.	

✳ **TABLE 18-5 Frequent Errors in Writing Nursing Interventions**

TYPE OF ERROR	INCORRECTLY STATED NURSING INTERVENTION	CORRECTLY STATED NURSING INTERVENTION
Failure to precisely or completely indicate nursing actions	Turn client every 2 hours.	Turn client every 2 hours, using the following schedule: 8 AM—supine 10 AM—left side } Repeat at Noon—prone } 4 PM and 2 AM 2 PM—right side
Failure to indicate frequency	Perform blood glucose measurements.	Measure blood glucose before each meal: 7 AM—11 AM—5 PM.
Failure to indicate quantity	Irrigate wound once a shift: 6 AM—2 PM—8 PM.	Irrigate wound with 100 ml normal saline until clear: 6 AM—2 PM—8 PM
Failure to indicate method	Change client's dressing once a shift: 6 AM—2 PM—10 PM.	Replace client's dressing with Neosporin ointment to wound and two dry 4 × 4 dressings secured with hypoallergenic tape, once a shift: 2 PM—10 PM—6 AM.

Institutional Care Plans

Institutional care plans become part of a client's legal medical record. Many hospitals still use a written Kardex nursing care plan. **Kardex** is a trade name for a card-filing system that allows quick reference to the needs of the client for certain aspects of nursing care. Chapter 26 includes a thorough description of a Kardex. The care plan section of a Kardex will have institutional variations. An institutional care plan differs from a student care plan because it lacks a scientific rationale. In practice, it is assumed that professional nurses know the rationales for recommended interventions.

The focus of a nursing care plan will differ by setting and the evolving client situation. For example, the nursing care plan developed for the client returning home is usually based solely on long-term health needs. The plan includes interventions to involve the client, family, and significant others in assuming responsibility for care because the client is to receive nursing care in the home. Same-day surgeries usually have plans focused on clients' short-term needs, (e.g., immediate recovery from surgery and instructions for self-care at home). A long-term care facility will have a plan of care focused on the client's long-term rehabilitation needs.

Computerized Care Plans. A majority of health care facilities now have some type of electronic health record (EHR) and documentation system (Moody and others, 2004). Software programs are available for nursing care plans. In many cases the format is for standardized plans that are based on nursing diagnoses or select problem areas, which nurses are able to individualize for a specific client. Even if a standardized care plan is generally appropriate for a client, you need to add or delete information on the standardized form to individualize it for a client's needs. Failure to do so will result in incomplete and inaccurate care. For example, you select a nursing diagnosis and then individualize the standard care plan by making selections from menus. Each care plan lists generalized nursing diagnoses, goals, outcome criteria, and interventions for specific clients.

Computerized/standardized nursing care plans organize and enhance care planning, and provide documentation for third-party reimbursement. Their design incorporates current evidence-based practice guidelines to achieve the desired client outcomes for a specific group of clients. These plans also encourage nurses to incorporate individual client care needs into the plan of care.

Care Plans for Community-Based Settings. Planning care for clients in community-based settings, for example, clinics, community centers, or clients' homes, involves using the same principles of nursing practice. However, in these settings you need to complete a more comprehensive community, home, and family assessment. Ultimately, the client/family unit must be able to independently provide the majority of health care. You will design a plan to (1) educate the client/family about the necessary care techniques and precautions, (2) teach the client/family how to integrate care within family activities, and (3) guide the client/family on how to assume a greater percentage of care over time. Last, the plan includes nurses' and the client's/family's evaluation of expected outcomes.

Critical Pathways. **Critical pathways** are multidisciplinary treatment plans that outline the treatments or interventions clients need to have while they are in a health care setting for a specific disease or condition. Most pathways are based on medical diagnoses and not nursing, but the related nursing diagnoses common to a medical problem and the associated nursing interventions are incorporated. A critical pathway maps out day to day or even hour to hour the recommended interventions and expected outcomes for a client. For example, a pathway for a surgical procedure such as a colon resection will recommend on a day-by-day basis the client's activities, consults, procedures, and discharge planning activities and educational topics expected for client's progression to discharge. A critical pathway ensures better continuity of care because it maps out clearly the responsibility of each health care discipline. Well-developed pathways incorporate current scientific evidence in the care of the specific condition. Nurses and other health care team members use a pathway to monitor a client's progress and as a documentation tool (see Chapter 26). When using critical pathways to plan care, you eliminate many documentation forms (e.g., the nursing care plan, flow sheets, and nurses' notes) because all of the pertinent components are already on the pathway format.

Concept Maps

Chapter 16 first described concept maps and their use in care planning. Because you care for clients who present with multiple health problems and related nursing diagnoses, it is often not realistic to have a written columnar plan developed for each nursing diagnosis. Plus, the columnar plans do not contain a means to show the association between different nursing diagnoses and different nursing interventions. A concept map is a visual representation of client problems and interventions that shows their relationships to one another (Schuster, 2003). The concept map groups and categorizes nursing concepts to give you a holistic view of your client's health care needs and to help you make better clinical decisions in planning care (King and Shell, 2002).

There are different approaches to writing concept maps. Schuster (2003) suggests some simple steps in preparing for concept mapping and in developing a clinical plan of care:

1. Before you care for a client, gather the clinical assessment database from the client's medical record, including health history, physical assessment data, laboratory and diagnostic data, medication history, and treatment plan.
2. Review all information about the client's health problems, treatments, and medications in the evidence-based literature, course textbooks, pharmacology texts, and other resources.
3. Review on the nursing unit any standardized nursing care plans, critical pathways, clinical protocols, or client education materials appropriate for client care preparation.
4. Prepare the map by first developing a skeleton diagram of the client's chief medical diagnosis and patterns of assessment data you have gathered on your client. Write the client's major medical diagnoses in the middle of the map, then add the assessment patterns like spokes on a wheel (see Chapter 16). Identify and group the related patterns of clinical assessment and medical history data. Remember, sometimes symptoms

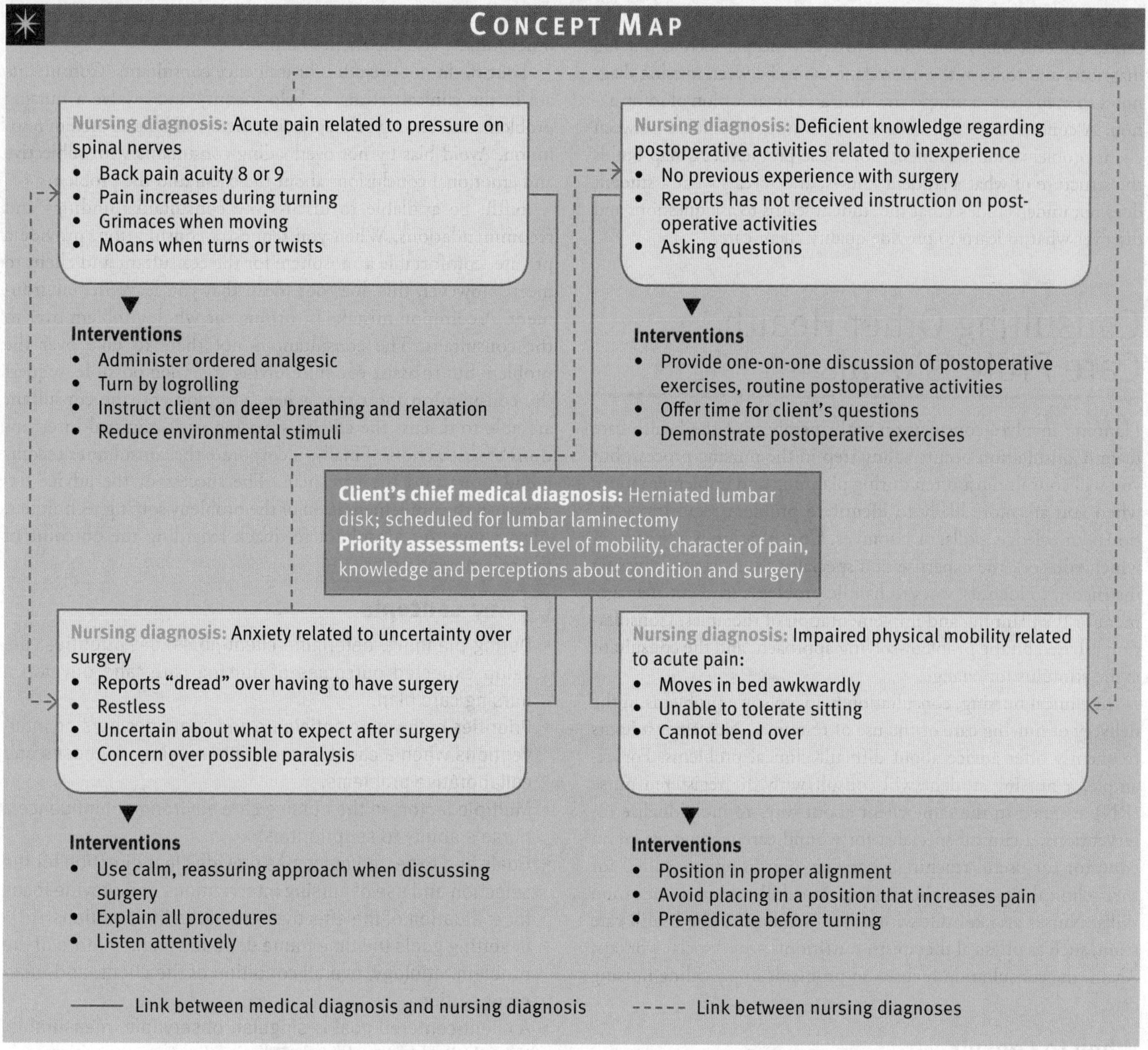

CONCEPT MAP

Nursing diagnosis: Acute pain related to pressure on spinal nerves
- Back pain acuity 8 or 9
- Pain increases during turning
- Grimaces when moving
- Moans when turns or twists

Interventions
- Administer ordered analgesic
- Turn by logrolling
- Instruct client on deep breathing and relaxation
- Reduce environmental stimuli

Nursing diagnosis: Deficient knowledge regarding postoperative activities related to inexperience
- No previous experience with surgery
- Reports has not received instruction on post-operative activities
- Asking questions

Interventions
- Provide one-on-one discussion of postoperative exercises, routine postoperative activities
- Offer time for client's questions
- Demonstrate postoperative exercises

Client's chief medical diagnosis: Herniated lumbar disk; scheduled for lumbar laminectomy
Priority assessments: Level of mobility, character of pain, knowledge and perceptions about condition and surgery

Nursing diagnosis: Anxiety related to uncertainty over surgery
- Reports "dread" over having to have surgery
- Restless
- Uncertain about what to expect after surgery
- Concern over possible paralysis

Interventions
- Use calm, reassuring approach when discussing surgery
- Explain all procedures
- Listen attentively

Nursing diagnosis: Impaired physical mobility related to acute pain:
- Moves in bed awkwardly
- Unable to tolerate sitting
- Cannot bend over

Interventions
- Position in proper alignment
- Avoid placing in a position that increases pain
- Premedicate before turning

——— Link between medical diagnosis and nursing diagnosis   - - - - - Link between nursing diagnoses

Figure 18-4 Concept map for planning Ms. Devine's nursing care.

apply to more than one problem pattern. Repeat symptoms under different categories when appropriate; for example when pain is a symptom for a problem with comfort as well as mobility.

5. Next, review your assessment patterns and identify the nursing diagnoses (see Chapter 17). Do not worry if you have difficulty labeling nursing diagnoses at first. It is important to recognize the major nursing care focus for the client. Add diagnostic labels later if necessary.

6. When planning, analyze relationships among the nursing diagnoses. Draw dotted lines between nursing diagnoses to indicate relationships (Figure 18-4). It is important for you to make meaningful associations between one concept and another concept. The links need to be accurate, meaningful, and complete. You need to be able to explain why nursing di-

agnoses are related. For example, in the case of Ms. Devine, the client's anxiety and acute pain are interrelated; in addition, pain has an influence on the client's reduced mobility.

7. Finally, on a separate sheet of paper or on the map itself, list nursing interventions to attain the outcomes for each nursing diagnosis (see Figure 18-4). This step corresponds to the planning phase of the nursing process.

8. While caring for the client, use the map to write down the client's responses to each nursing activity. Also write your clinical impressions and inferences regarding the client's progress toward expected outcomes and the effectiveness of interventions.

9. Keep the concept map with you throughout the clinical day. As you revise the plan, take notes and add or delete nursing interventions. Use the information recorded on the map for your documentation of client care.

Critical thinkers learn by organizing and relating cognitive concepts. Concept maps help nurses to link concepts such as nursing diagnoses and to learn the interrelationships between nursing diagnoses so as to create a unique meaning and organization of information. A concept map helps students link important ideas between client problems and treatments for those problems. A map builds the structure of what a student knows, and reveals what a student does not understand, so that the student learns to ask questions and discover what to learn to provide quality client care.

Consulting Other Health Care Professionals

Planning involves consultation with members of the health care team. Consultation occurs at any step in the nursing process, but you will consult most often during planning and implementation, when you are more likely to identify a problem requiring additional knowledge, skills, or resources. **Consultation** is a process in which you seek the expertise of a specialist, such as your nursing instructor, to identify ways to handle problems in client management or the planning and implementation of therapies. Consultation is based on the problem-solving approach, and the consultant is the stimulus for change.

In clinical nursing, consultation helps to solve problems in the delivery of nursing care or the use of resources. Nurse consultants frequently offer advice about difficult clinical problems. For example, a nursing student will consult with the registered nurse (RN) assigned to the same client about ways to individualize interventions, a clinical specialist for wound care techniques, or an educator for useful teaching resources. Nurses are consulted for their clinical expertise, client education skills, or staff education skills. Nurses also consult with other members of the health care team, such as physical therapists, nutritionists, and social workers. Again, the consultation focuses on problems in providing nursing care.

When to Consult

Consultation occurs when you identify a problem that you are unable to solve using personal knowledge, skills, and resources. Consultation with other care providers increases your knowledge about the client's problem and helps you to learn skills and obtain resources. A good time to consult with another health care professional is when the exact problem remains unclear. A consultant objectively entering a situation more clearly assesses and identifies the exact nature of the problem, whether it is client, personnel, or equipment oriented. An unbiased consultant often objectively identifies the problem and outlines a method for resolving it.

How to Consult

Begin with your own understanding of a client's clinical problems. The first step in making a consult is to identify the general problem area. Second, direct the consultation to the right professional, such as another nurse or social worker. Third, provide the consultant with relevant information about the problem area. Include a relevant, brief summary of the problem, methods used to resolve the problem so far, and outcomes of those methods. Also share information from the client's medical record, conversations with other nurses, and the client's family.

Fourth, do not prejudice or influence consultants. Consultants are in the clinical setting to help identify and resolve a nursing problem, and biasing or prejudicing them will block problem resolution. Avoid bias by not overloading consultants with subjective and emotional conclusions about the client and the problem.

Fifth, be available to discuss the consultant's findings and recommendations. When you request a consultation, provide a private, comfortable atmosphere for the consultant and client to meet. However, this does not mean that you leave the environment. A common mistake is turning the whole problem over to the consultant. The consultant is not there to take over the problem but to assist you in resolving it. When possible, request the consultation for a time when both you and the consultant are able to discuss the client's situation with minimal interruptions or distractions. Finally, incorporate the consultant's recommendations into the care plan. The success of the advice depends on the implementation of the problem-solving techniques. Always give the consultant feedback regarding the outcome of the recommendations.

✳ Key Concepts

- During planning, determine client goals, set priorities, develop expected outcomes of nursing care, and develop a nursing care plan.
- Priorities help you to anticipate and sequence nursing interventions when a client has multiple nursing diagnoses and collaborative problems.
- Multiple factors in the nursing care environment influence a nurse's ability to set priorities.
- Goals and expected outcomes provide clear direction for the selection and use of nursing interventions and provide focus for evaluation of the effectiveness of the interventions.
- In setting goals the time frame depends on the nature of the problem, etiology, overall condition of the client, and treatment setting.
- A client-centered goal is singular, observable, measurable, time-limited, mutual, and realistic.
- An expected outcome is an objective criterion for goal achievement.
- Nurse-initiated interventions require no supervision or direction from others.
- Physician-initiated interventions require specific nursing responsibilities and technical nursing knowledge.
- Care plans and critical pathways increase communication among nurses and facilitate the continuity of care from one nurse to another and from one health care setting to another.
- A concept map provides a visually graphic way to show the relationship between clients' nursing diagnoses and interventions.
- The Nursing Interventions Classification taxonomy provides a standardization to assist nurses in selecting suitable interventions for clients' problems.
- Correctly written nursing interventions include actions, frequency, quantity, method, and the person to perform them.

- Consultation increases the nurse's knowledge about a client's problem and helps in learning skills and obtaining the resources needed to solve the problem.

✳ Critical Thinking Exercises

Shawn has two different clients. Mr. Gordon is a 52-year-old client who was admitted to the hospital following a motor vehicle accident. He suffered rib fractures and has a laceration along his right thigh. Shawn has identified the following nursing diagnoses: *ineffective breathing pattern related to chest pain, acute pain related to musculoskeletal trauma,* and *risk for infection related to open wound.* Shawn's second client, Ms. Lawrence, is a 63-year-old woman who had surgery yesterday evening for repair of a foot fracture. Her foot is in a cast. Ms. Lawrence's nursing diagnoses include *acute pain related to tissue swelling, impaired mobility related to restricted movement from cast,* and *deficient knowledge regarding cast care related to inexperience.*

1. Among the two clients, which diagnoses are high and which are intermediate priority?

2. Of the two clients, which one has greatest priority regarding pain management?

Ms. Lawrence will likely be discharged in the morning. She lives alone. Shawn begins to plan care by establishing goals and outcomes for the nursing diagnoses.

3. For the nursing diagnosis *deficient knowledge regarding cast care related to inexperience* write one goal and two expected outcomes.

✳ NCLEX®-Style Review Questions

1. Sheila is assigned to a client who has returned from the recovery room following surgery for a colorectal tumor. After an initial assessment Sheila anticipates the need to monitor the client's abdominal dressing, intravenous (IV) infusion, and function of drainage tubes. The client is in pain and will not be able to eat or drink until intestinal function returns. Sheila will have to establish priorities of care in which of the following situations? (Choose all that apply.)
   1. The family comes to visit the client.
   2. The client expresses concern about pain control.
   3. The client's vital signs change, showing a drop in blood pressure.
   4. The charge nurse approaches Sheila and requests a report at end of shift.

2. Sheila's client signals with her call light. Sheila enters the room and finds the drainage tube disconnected, the IV has 100 ml of fluid remaining, and the client has asked to be turned. Which of the following should Sheila perform first?
   1. Reconnect the drainage tubing.
   2. Inspect the condition of the IV dressing.
   3. Improve client's comfort, and turn to her side.
   4. Go to the medication room, and obtain the next IV fluid bag.

3. In her nursing care plan, Sheila enters expected outcomes for her client. Which of the following expected outcomes are written correctly? (Choose all that apply.)
   1. Client will remain afebrile until discharge.
   2. IV site will be without phlebitis by the third postoperative day.
   3. Provide incentive spirometer for deep breathing every 2 hours.
   4. Client will report pain and turn more freely by the first postoperative day.

4. Sheila set a time limit for her outcomes. The time frame serves to:
   1. Indicate which outcome has priority
   2. Indicate the time it takes to complete an intervention
   3. Indicate how long Sheila is scheduled to care for the client
   4. Indicate when the client is expected to respond in the desired manner

5. A client-centered goal is a specific and measurable behavior or response that reflects a:
   1. Physician's goal for the specific client
   2. Client's desire for specified health care interventions
   3. Client's response when compared to another client with a like problem
   4. Client's highest possible level of wellness and independence in function

6. The nurse writes an expected outcome statement in measurable terms. An example is:
   1. Client will be pain free.
   2. Client will have less pain.
   3. Client will take pain medication every 4 hours.
   4. Client will report pain acuity less than 4 on a scale of 0 to 10.

7. Sheila's client is experiencing nausea and abdominal distention postoperatively. Sheila initiates the interventions listed below. Which of the interventions are examples of independent interventions? (Choose all that apply.)
   1. Provide frequent mouth care.
   2. Maintain IV infusion at 100 mL/hr.
   3. Administer Compazine via rectal suppository.
   4. Consult with dietitian on initial foods to offer client.
   5. Control aversive odors or unpleasant visual stimulation that trigger nausea.

8. Collaborative interventions are therapies that require:
   1. Nurse and client intervention
   2. Physician and nurse intervention
   3. Client and physician intervention
   4. Multiple health care professionals

19 | Implementing Nursing Care

✳ OBJECTIVES

Mastery of the content in this chapter will enable the student to:
- Explain the relationship of implementation to the nursing diagnostic process.
- Discuss the differences between protocols and standing orders.
- Describe the association between critical thinking and selecting nursing interventions.
- Identify preparatory activities to use before implementation.
- Discuss steps used to revise a plan of care before performing implementation.
- Define the three implementation skills.
- Describe and compare direct and indirect nursing interventions.
- Select appropriate interventions for an assigned client.

✳ MEDIA RESOURCES   ✳ KEY TERMS

 Companion CD
- NCLEX®-Style Review Questions
- Audio Glossary
- Interactive Learning Activities
- English/Spanish Glossary

 Website
- NCLEX®-Style Review Questions
- Audio Glossary
- English/Spanish Glossary
- Interactive Learning Activities
- WebLinks
- Audio Summaries

Activities of daily living
  (ADLs), p. 285
Adverse reaction, p. 286
Client adherence, p. 288
Clinical guideline, p. 281
Counseling, p. 285
Direct care, p. 279
Implementation, p. 279
Indirect care, p. 279

Instrumental activities of daily
  living (IADLs), p. 285
Interdisciplinary care plans,
  p. 287
Lifesaving measure, p. 285
Nursing intervention, p. 279
Preventive nursing actions,
  p. 286
Standing order, p. 281

You first met Lisa and Ms. Devine in Chapter 16. Lisa is now entering Ms. Devine's room to administer morphine sulfate ordered for her severe back pain. The client is likely not going to surgery for another 4 to 6 hours, so Lisa aims to reduce the client's discomfort before the time Ms. Devine will be going to surgery. Lisa administers the medication, using physical care principles involving safety and infection control. She communicates with Ms. Devine in a calm and reassuring manner to enhance the client's relaxation. Lisa explains that she will return to Ms. Devine's room in about 30 minutes to help her turn and reposition and to offer basic instruction about anticipated postoperative routines. Lisa's interventions are all designed to prepare Ms. Devine for her upcoming surgery.

Implementation, the fourth step of the nursing process, formally begins after the nurse develops a plan of care. With a care plan based on clear and relevant nursing diagnoses, the nurse initiates interventions that are most likely to achieve the goals and expected outcomes needed to support or improve the client's health status. A **nursing intervention** is any treatment, based upon clinical judgment and knowledge, that a nurse performs to enhance client outcomes (Bulechek, Butcher, and Dochterman, 2008). Ideally, the interventions a nurse uses are evidenced based (see Chapter 5), providing the most current, up-to-date, and effective approaches for client problems. Interventions include both direct and indirect care measures, aimed at individuals, families, and/or the community.

Direct care interventions are treatments performed through interactions with clients. For example, a client receives direct intervention in the form of medication administration, insertion of an intravenous infusion, or counseling during a time of grief. **Indirect care** interventions are treatments performed away from the client but on behalf of the client or group of clients (Bulechek and others, 2008). For example, indirect care measures include actions for managing the client's environment (e.g., safety and infection control), documentation, and interdisciplinary collaboration. Both direct and indirect care measures fall under the intervention categories described in Chapter 18: nurse-initiated, physician-initiated, and collaborative. For example, the direct intervention of client education is a nurse-initiated intervention. The indirect intervention of consultation is a collaborative intervention.

Benner (1984) defined the domains of nursing practice, which help to explain the nature and intent of the many ways nurses intervene for clients (Box 19-1). Nursing is both an art and a science. It is not simply a task-based profession. Thus you deliver each intervention within the context of a client's unique situation.

> ✳ **BOX 19-1 Domains of Nursing Practice**
>
> - The Helping Role
> - The Teaching-Coaching Function
> - The Diagnostic and Patient-Monitoring Function
> - Effective Management of Rapidly Changing Situations
> - Administering and Monitoring Therapeutic Interventions and Regimens
> - Monitoring and Ensuring the Quality of Health Care Practices
> - Organizational and Work-Role Competencies
>
> From Benner P: *From novice to expert,* Menlo Park, Calif, 1984, Addison Wesley.

As you learn to intervene for a client, consider the context of his or her clinical situation. Who is the client? What clinical situation is requiring you to intervene? How does the client perceive the interventions you will deliver? In what way do you best support or show caring as you intervene? The answers to these questions enable you to deliver care compassionately and effectively with the best outcomes for your clients.

Critical Thinking in Implementation

The selection of nursing interventions is a complex decision-making process that involves critical thinking. The context in which you deliver care to each client and the many interventions required result in decision-making approaches for each clinical situation (Snyder, 2000). Critical thinking is necessary to consider the complexity of interventions, including the number of alternative approaches and the amount of time available to act.

Before implementing any intervention, use critical thinking to determine whether an intervention is correct and appropriate for a clinical situation. Even though you have planned a set of interventions for a client, you have to exercise good judgment and decision making before actually delivering each intervention. Always think before you act. Clients' conditions sometimes change minute to minute. You also need to consider the scheduling of activities on a nursing unit, which often dictates when and how to complete an intervention. Thus all sorts of factors influence your decision on how and when to intervene. You are responsible for having the necessary knowledge and clinical competency to perform interventions for your clients safely and effectively. Here are some tips to consider when making decisions about implementation:

- Review the set of all possible nursing interventions for the client's problem (e.g., for Ms. Devine's pain, Lisa considers analgesic administration, positioning, relaxation, and any other nonpharmacological approach).
- Review all possible consequences associated with each possible nursing action (e.g., Lisa considers that the analgesic will possibly relieve pain, have little or insufficient effect, or cause an adverse reaction).
- Determine the probability of all possible consequences (e.g., if Ms. Devine's pain has decreased with analgesia and positioning in the past, it is unlikely adverse reactions will occur and the intervention will be successful; however, if the client continues to remain highly anxious, her pain may not be relieved).
- Make a judgment of the value of that consequence to the client (e.g., if the administration of an analgesic is effective, Ms. Devine will likely become less anxious and more responsive to preoperative instruction).

The selection and performance of nursing interventions for a client is part of clinical decision making. The critical thinking model described in Chapter 15 provides a framework for how to make decisions when implementing nursing care (Figure 19-1). You will learn how to implement nursing care using appropriate knowledge. For example, as you proceed with an intervention you will consider what you know about the purpose of the intervention,

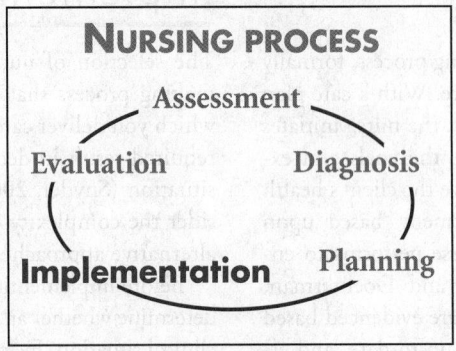

KNOWLEDGE
Expected effects of interventions
Techniques used in performing interventions
Nursing Interventions Classification
Role of other health care disciplines
Health care resources (e.g., equipment, personnel)
Anticipated client responses to care
Interpersonal skills
Counseling theory
Teaching/learning principles
Delegation and supervision principles

EXPERIENCE
Previous client care experience
Knowledge of
successful interventions

NURSING PROCESS
Assessment
Evaluation   Diagnosis
Implementation   Planning

STANDARDS
Standards of practice (e.g., ANA,
subspecialty) and
evidence-based practie guidelines (e.g., AHRQ, APS)
Agency's policies/procedures
for guidelines of nursing
practice and delegation
Intellectual standards
Client's expected outcomes

ATTITUDES
Independent thinking
Responsibility
Authority
Creativity
Discipline

Figure 19-1 Critical thinking and the process of implementing care.

the steps in performing the intervention correctly, the medical condition of the client and his or her expected response. This means it is important that you prepare well before first caring for any client. With experience you will become more proficient in anticipating what to expect in a given clinical situation and how to modify your approach. As you gain clinical experience, you will be able to consider which interventions worked previously, which have not, and why. It also helps to know the clinical standards of practice for your agency. For example, one hospital has a different set of standards for client care in an isolation room compared with another. The standards of practice offer guidelines for selection of interventions, their frequency, and if you are able to delegate the procedures.

As you perform any nursing intervention, apply intellectual standards. Intellectual standards are guidelines for rational thought and responsible action. For example, before you begin teaching a client, consider how to make your instructions relevant, clear, logical, and complete to promote client learning. As a critical thinker, apply critical thinking attitudes when you intervene. For example, show confidence in performing an intervention. When you are unsure of how to perform a procedure, be responsible in seeking assistance from others. Confidence in performing interventions builds trust with clients. Creativity and self-discipline are attitudes that will guide you in reviewing, modifying, and implementing interventions. As a beginning

nursing student, seek out supervision from instructors or experienced nurses to guide you in the decision-making process for implementation.

Standard Nursing Interventions

Health care settings present various ways for nurses to create and individualize a client's plan of care. Each plan of care will be totally unique to that client, with interventions individualized on the basis of the client's specific health problems. In certain situations, a nurse develops that plan on the basis of his or her own knowledge and clinical experience. However, there are systems available that provide standardized interventions for nurses to use in their plan of care. Many clients have common health care problems, and thus standardized interventions for those health problems make it quicker and easier for nurses to intervene. More importantly, if the standards are evidence based, then the nurse is more likely to deliver the most clinically effective interventions to improve client outcomes (see Chapter 5). Standardized interventions, both nurse initiated and physician initiated, are available in the form of clinical guidelines or protocols, preprinted (standing) orders, and Nursing Interventions Classification (NIC) interventions.

Clinical Practice Guidelines and Protocols

A **clinical guideline** or protocol is a document that guides decisions and interventions for specific health care problems or conditions. The guideline or protocol is developed on the basis of an authoritative examination of current scientific evidence and assists nurses, physicians, and other health care providers in making decisions about appropriate health care for specific clinical circumstances (National Guideline Clearinghouse [NGC], 2006). Clinicians within a health care agency sometimes choose to review the scientific literature and their own standard of practice to develop guidelines and protocols in an effort to improve their standard of care. For example, a hospital develops a rapid assessment protocol to improve the identification and early treatment of clients suspected of having a stroke. There are clinical practice guidelines already developed by national health groups, such as the National Institutes of Health and the National Guideline Clearinghouse. These guidelines are readily available to any clinician or health care institution that wishes to adopt evidence-based guidelines in the care of clients with specific health problems. Examples of such guidelines include evidence-based guidelines for cardiovascular disease prevention in women, management of type 2 diabetes, and the prevention, detection, evaluation, and treatment of high blood pressure (NGC, 2006). One valuable source for nursing practice guidelines is the Gerontological Nursing Interventions Research Center (GNIRC) at the University of Iowa. The center has numerous clinical guidelines, including ones for acute confusion and delirium, bathing persons with dementia, elder abuse prevention, and prevention of pressure ulcers (GNIRC, 2006).

Nurses who provide primary care for clients in outpatient settings frequently follow diagnostic and treatment protocols. In such a setting, nurses assess the client and identify abnormalities. The protocol outlines the conditions that nurses are permitted to treat, such as controlled hypertension, and the types of treatment they are permitted to administer, such as antihypertensive medications. In acute care settings it is common to find clinical protocols that outline independent nursing interventions for specific conditions. Examples include protocols for admission and discharge, pressure ulcer care, and incontinence management. Protocols are also used in interdisciplinary settings for diagnostic testing and physical, occupational, and speech therapies.

Standing Orders

A **standing order** is a preprinted document containing orders for the conduct of routine therapies, monitoring guidelines, and/or diagnostic procedures for specific clients with identified clinical problems. The orders direct the conduct of client care in various clinical settings. Licensed, prescribing physicians or health care providers in charge of care at the time of implementation approve and sign standing orders. These orders are common in critical care settings and other specialized practice settings where clients' needs change rapidly and require immediate attention. An example of such a standing order is one specifying certain medications, such as lidocaine or propranolol, for an irregular heart rhythm. After assessing the client and identifying the irregular rhythm, the critical care nurse gives the specified medication without first notifying the physician. The physician's initial standing order covers the nurse's action. Standing orders are also common in the

---

✳ BOX 19-2 Purposes of the Nursing Interventions Classification (NIC)

1. Standardization of the nomenclature (e.g., labeling, describing) of nursing interventions. Standardizes the language nurses use to describe sets of actions in delivering client care.
2. Expansion of nursing knowledge about connections between nursing diagnoses, treatments, and outcomes. These connections will be determined through the study of actual client care using a database that the classification will generate.
3. Development of nursing and health care information systems.
4. Teaching decision making to nursing students. Defining and classifying nursing interventions to teach beginning nurses how to determine a client's need for care and to respond appropriately.
5. Determination of the cost of services provided by nurses.
6. Planning for resources needed in all types of nursing practice settings.
7. Language to communicate the unique functions of nursing.
8. Link with the classification systems of other health care providers.

From Bulechek GM, Butcher HK, and Dochterman JM: *Nursing interventions classification (NIC)*, ed 5, St. Louis, 2008, Mosby.

---

community health setting, where the nurse faces situations that do not permit immediate contact with a physician. Standing orders and clinical protocols give the nurse legal protection to intervene appropriately in the client's best interest.

NIC Interventions

The NIC system developed by the University of Iowa helps to differentiate nursing practice from that of other health care professionals (Box 19-2). The NIC interventions offer a level of standardization to enhance communication of nursing care across settings and to compare outcomes. By using NIC, nurses learn the common interventions recommended for various NANDA International nursing diagnoses. Nurses also learn the numerous care activities for each NIC intervention. Chapter 18 describes the NIC system in more detail.

Implementation Process

Preparation for implementation ensures efficient, safe, and effective nursing care. Five preparatory activities include reassessing the client, reviewing and revising the existing nursing care plan, organizing resources and care delivery, anticipating and preventing complications, and implementing nursing interventions.

Reassessing the Client

Assessment is a continuous process that occurs each time you interact with a client. When you collect new data and identify a new client need, you modify the care plan. You also modify a plan when you resolve a client's health care need. During the initial phase of implementation, reassess the client. This is a partial assessment and sometimes focuses on one dimension of the client, such as level of comfort, or on one system, such as the cardiovascular system. The reassessment helps you decide if the proposed nursing action is still appropriate for the client's level of wellness. For example, Lisa plans to spend a few minutes to talk further with Ms Devine about her concerns over surgery. However, her reassessment reveals Ms. Devine is still a bit uncomfortable and fatigued, requiring Lisa to postpone her discussion. She decides to combine her discussion of Ms. Devine's concerns when she begins preoperative teaching in 30 minutes. When you obtain new data or identify a new client need, modify the nursing care plan.

Reviewing and Revising the Existing Nursing Care Plan

After reassessing a client, review the care plan, compare assessment data to validate the nursing diagnoses, and determine whether the nursing interventions remain the most appropriate for the clinical situation. If the client's status has changed and the nursing diagnosis and related nursing interventions are no longer appropriate, modify the nursing care plan. An out-of-date or incorrect care plan compromises the quality of nursing care. Review and modification enable you to provide timely nursing interventions to best meet the client's needs. Modification of the existing written care plan includes four steps:

1. Revise data in the assessment column to reflect the client's current status. Date any new data to inform other members of the health care team of the time that the change occurred.
2. Revise the nursing diagnoses. Delete nursing diagnoses that are no longer relevant, and add and date any new diagnoses. It is necessary to revise related factors, as well as the client's goals, outcomes, and priorities. Date any revisions.
3. Revise specific interventions that correspond to the new nursing diagnoses and goals. This revision should reflect the client's present status.
4. Determine the method of evaluation for determining if you achieved outcomes.

In the case study involving Lisa and Ms. Devine, it has been 45 minutes since Ms. Devine received an analgesic for her pain. She reports less discomfort, so Lisa initiates preoperative instruction. After about 10 minutes of discussion, Lisa notes that Ms. Devine expresses less concern about surgery and says, "I feel better now that I understand what surgery involves." Ms. Devine's movements are more calm and less restless. Lisa enters her new findings into the care plan. However, she decides not to delete the nursing diagnosis of anxiety as of yet but adds an intervention to her plan: "Encourage verbalization of client's remaining concerns about surgery" (Figure 19-2). Seeing that Ms. Devine responded well to the analgesic, Lisa also adds more nonpharmacological interventions to her plan for pain management.

Organizing Resources and Care Delivery

A facility's resources include equipment and skilled personnel. Organization of equipment and personnel makes timely, efficient, skilled client care possible (see Chapter 21). Preparation for care delivery also involves preparing the environment and client for nursing intervention.

Equipment. Most nursing procedures require some equipment or supplies. Before performing an intervention, decide what supplies you will need and determine their availability. Is equipment in working order to ensure safe use? Place supplies in a convenient location to provide easy access during the procedure. Keep extra supplies available in case of errors or mishaps, but do not open extra supplies unless you need them. This controls costs. After a procedure, return any unopened supplies to storage areas.

Personnel. Nursing care delivery models vary among facilities (see Chapter 21). The system by which nursing is organized determines how nursing personnel are designated for client care delivery. For example, a registered nurse's (RN's) accountabilities differ in a team nursing model compared with a primary nursing model. A primary nurse is accountable for the nursing care a client receives during his or her length of stay. A team nurse is accountable for the care a client receives for a specific shift in which the nurse works. As a nurse, you are responsible for determining whether to perform an intervention or to delegate it to another member of the nursing team. Your assessment of a client directs the decision about delegation and not the intervention alone. For example, you know trained nursing assistive personnel (NAP) are able to competently measure a client's vital signs. However, you learn during change-of-shift report that a male client experienced cardiac irregularities the previous shift. You decide to personally measure the client's vital signs to evaluate his cardiac status. Your judgment is important in this situation to determine the client's status and whether intervention is necessary. In this case, you direct the assistive personnel to provide care to a more stable client.

Nursing staff work together as clients' needs demand it. If a client makes a request, such as use of a bedpan or assistance in feeding, help the client if you have time rather than trying to find the technician who is in a different room. Nursing staff respect colleagues who show initiative, collaborate together, and communicate with one another on an ongoing, reciprocal basis as clients' needs change (Potter and Grant, 2004). When interventions are complex or physically difficult, you will probably need assistance from colleagues. For example, you and a technician will more effectively change a dressing in a large gaping wound when you apply the dressing and the technician assists with client positioning and handing off of supplies.

Environment. A client's care environment needs to be safe and conducive to the implementation of therapies. Client safety is your first concern. If the client has sensory deficits, physical disability, or an alteration in level of consciousness, arrange the environment to prevent injury. As examples, provide assistive devices (e.g., walkers or eyeglasses), rearrange furniture and equipment, and make rooms free of clutter.

The client benefits most from nursing interventions when surroundings are compatible with care activities. When you need to expose a client's body parts, do so privately because the client will then be more relaxed. Reducing distractions enhances a client's learning opportunities. Make sure lighting is adequate to perform procedures correctly.

Client. Before you deliver interventions, be sure the client is as physically and psychologically comfortable as possible. For example, symptoms such as nausea, dizziness, fatigue, or pain frequently interfere with a client's full concentration and ability to

CONCEPT MAP

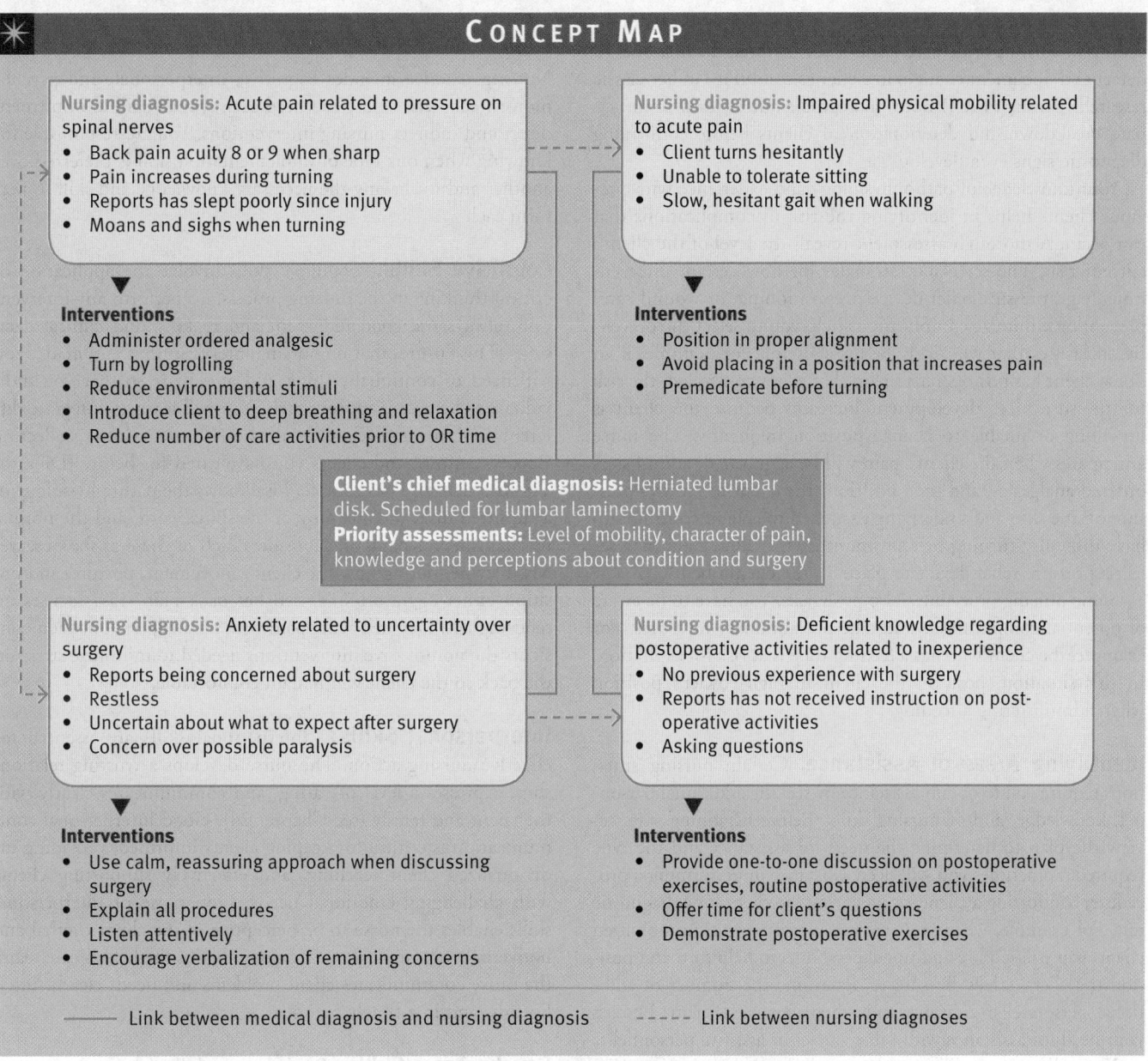

Nursing diagnosis: Acute pain related to pressure on spinal nerves
- Back pain acuity 8 or 9 when sharp
- Pain increases during turning
- Reports has slept poorly since injury
- Moans and sighs when turning

Interventions
- Administer ordered analgesic
- Turn by logrolling
- Reduce environmental stimuli
- Introduce client to deep breathing and relaxation
- Reduce number of care activities prior to OR time

Nursing diagnosis: Impaired physical mobility related to acute pain
- Client turns hesitantly
- Unable to tolerate sitting
- Slow, hesitant gait when walking

Interventions
- Position in proper alignment
- Avoid placing in a position that increases pain
- Premedicate before turning

Client's chief medical diagnosis: Herniated lumbar disk. Scheduled for lumbar laminectomy
Priority assessments: Level of mobility, character of pain, knowledge and perceptions about condition and surgery

Nursing diagnosis: Anxiety related to uncertainty over surgery
- Reports being concerned about surgery
- Restless
- Uncertain about what to expect after surgery
- Concern over possible paralysis

Interventions
- Use calm, reassuring approach when discussing surgery
- Explain all procedures
- Listen attentively
- Encourage verbalization of remaining concerns

Nursing diagnosis: Deficient knowledge regarding postoperative activities related to inexperience
- No previous experience with surgery
- Reports has not received instruction on post-operative activities
- Asking questions

Interventions
- Provide one-to-one discussion on postoperative exercises, routine postoperative activities
- Offer time for client's questions
- Demonstrate postoperative exercises

——— Link between medical diagnosis and nursing diagnosis   - - - - Link between nursing diagnoses

Figure 19-2 Concept map for planning Ms. Devine's nursing care.

cooperate. Offer comfort measures before initiating interventions to help the client participate more fully. If you need a client to be alert, administer a dose of pain medication to relieve discomfort but not to impair mental faculties (e.g., ability to follow instruction, reasoning, and communication). If a client is fatigued, delay ambulation or transfer to a chair until after the client has had a chance to rest.

Even if symptoms are not a factor, make the client physically comfortable during interventions. Start any intervention by controlling environmental factors, taking care of physical needs (e.g., elimination), avoiding interruptions, and positioning the client correctly. Also consider the client's level of endurance, and plan only the amount of activity that the client is able to comfortably tolerate.

Awareness of the client's psychosocial needs helps you create a favorable emotional climate. Some clients feel reassured by having a significant other present to lend encouragement and moral support. Other strategies include planning sufficient time or multiple opportunities for the client to work through and ventilate feelings and anxieties. Adequate preparation allows the client to obtain maximal benefit from each intervention.

Anticipating and Preventing Complications

Risks to clients come from both illness and treatment. As the nurse, be alert for and recognize these risks, adapt your choice of interventions to the situation, evaluate the relative benefit of the treatment versus the risk, and finally initiate risk prevention measures. Many conditions place the client at risk for complications. For example, the client with preexisting left-sided paralysis following a stroke 2 years earlier is at risk for developing a pressure ulcer following orthopedic surgery because it requires traction and bed rest. An obese, diabetic client who has major abdominal surgery is at risk for poor wound healing and developing the complications of a fistula or dehiscence. Nurses are often the first ones to detect and document changes in a client's condition. In her classic research, Benner (1984) notes that expert nurses learn to anticipate breakdown and deterioration of clients before confirming diagnostic signs even develop.

Your knowledge of pathophysiology and experience with previous clients helps in identifying the risk of complications that can occur. A thorough assessment reveals the level of the client's current risk. The scientific rationales for how certain interventions (e.g., pressure relief devices, repositioning, or wound care) prevent or minimize complications help you to select the preventive measures that will likely be most useful. For example, if an obese client has postoperative pain that is not controlled, the risk for pressure ulcer development increases because the client is unwilling or unable to change position frequently. The nurse anticipates when the client's pain will be aggravated, administers ordered analgesics, and then positions the client to remove pressure on the skin and underlying tissues. If the client continues to have difficulty turning or repositioning, the nurse then may select a pressure-relief device to place on the client's bed.

Some nursing procedures also pose risks. You have to be aware of potential complications and take precautionary measures. For example, the client who has a feeding tube is at risk for aspiration. In this situation, position the client in high-Fowler's position when administering a feeding.

Identifying Areas of Assistance.

Certain nursing situations require you to obtain assistance by seeking additional personnel, knowledge, and/or nursing skills. Before beginning care, review the plan to determine the need for assistance and the type required. Sometimes you will need assistance in performing a procedure, comforting a client, or preparing the client for a diagnostic test. For example, when you care for an overweight, immobilized client, you will require additional personnel to help turn and position the client safely. Be sure to determine the number of additional personnel in advance and when you need them. Discuss your need for assistance with other nurses or assistive personnel.

You will require additional knowledge and skills in situations in which you are less familiar or experienced. Because of the continual growth in health care technology, you may lack the skills to perform a procedure. For example, in situations when you are asked to administer a new medication, operate a new piece of equipment, or administer a procedure with which you are unfamiliar, follow these steps:

- Seek necessary knowledge—locate the information you need to be informed about the procedure. Check the scientific literature for evidence-based information, and review resource manuals and the agency's procedure book.
- Collect all equipment necessary for the procedure.
- Have another nurse who has completed the procedure correctly and safely provide assistance and guidance. The assistance can come from another staff nurse, a supervisor, an educator, or a nurse specialist. Requesting assistance occurs frequently in all types of nursing practice and is a learning process that continues throughout educational experiences and into professional development.

Implementation Skills

Nursing practice includes cognitive, interpersonal, and psychomotor (technical) skills. You need each type of skill to implement direct and indirect nursing interventions. You are responsible for knowing when one type of implementation skill is preferred over another and for having the necessary knowledge and skill to perform each.

Cognitive Skills.

Cognitive skills involve the application of critical thinking in the nursing process. To perform any intervention, always use good judgment and make sound clinical decisions. This ensures that no nursing intervention is automatic. You will need to continually think and anticipate so that you individualize client care appropriately. You will learn to integrate different concepts and relate them to each other while recollecting facts, situations, and clients you have cared for before (Di Vito-Thomas, 2005). For example, Lisa knows the pathophysiology of a ruptured disk, the anatomy of the spinal cord, and the normal mechanisms for pain. She considers each of these as she observes Ms. Devine, noting how the client's movement, posture, and position either aggravate or lessen her back pain. Lisa focuses on relieving Ms. Devine's acute pain with an analgesic but then considers the noninvasive interventions needed to minimize stress on the back so the client will remain comfortable.

Interpersonal Skills.

Interpersonal skills are essential for effective nursing action. The nurse develops a trusting relationship, expresses a level of caring, and communicates clearly with the client and family (see Chapter 24). Good interpersonal communication is critical for keeping clients informed, providing individualized client teaching, and effectively supporting clients with challenging emotional needs. Proper use of interpersonal skills enables the nurse to be perceptive of the client's verbal and nonverbal communication. As a member of the health care team, the nurse communicates client problems and needs clearly, intelligently, and in a timely manner.

Psychomotor Skills.

Psychomotor skills require the integration of cognitive and motor activities. For example, when giving an injection you need to understand anatomy and pharmacology (cognitive) and use good coordination and precision to administer the injection correctly (motor). With time and practice you will learn to perform skills correctly, smoothly, and confidently. This is critical in establishing client trust. You are responsible for acquiring necessary psychomotor skills, either through your experience in the nursing laboratory, the use of interactive instructional technology, or through actual hands-on care of clients. In the case of a new skill, always assess your level of competency and obtain the necessary resources to ensure the client receives safe treatment.

Direct Care

Nurses provide a wide variety of direct care measures, those treatments that nurses perform through client interactions. How a nurse interacts affects the success of any direct care activity. Remain sensitive to a client's clinical condition, values and beliefs, expectations, and cultural views. All direct care measures require competent and therefore safe practice. Show a caring approach each time you provide direct care.

Activities of Daily Living

Activities of daily living (ADLs) are activities usually performed in the course of a normal day, including ambulation, eating, dressing, bathing, brushing the teeth, and grooming (see Chapter 39). A client's need for assistance with ADLs is temporary, permanent, or rehabilitative. A client with impaired mobility because of bilateral arm casts has a temporary need for assistance. After the casts are removed, the client will gradually regain the strength and range of motion needed to perform ADLs. A client with an irreversible injury to the cervical spinal cord is paralyzed and thus has a permanent need for assistance. It is unrealistic to plan rehabilitation with the goal of the client's becoming independent with ADLs. Instead, through rehabilitation the client will learn new ways to perform ADLs, becoming more independent. Occupational and physical therapists play a key role in rehabilitation to restore ADL function.

There are clients who will likely require ADL assistance. When your assessment reveals a client is experiencing fatigue, a limitation in mobility, confusion, and pain, assistance with ADLs is likely. For example, a client who experiences shortness of breath avoids eating because of the associated fatigue. Assist the client by setting up meals and offering to cut up food and plan for more frequent, small meals to maintain the client's nutrition. Assistance with ADLs ranges from partial assistance to complete care. Remember to always respect the client's wishes. Most clients want to remain independent in meeting their basic needs. Determine the client's preferences when assisting with ADLs, and let the client participate to the level he or she is able. Involving the client in planning the timing and types of interventions boosts the client's self-esteem and willingness to become more independent.

Instrumental Activities of Daily Living

Illness or disability sometimes alters a client's ability to be independent in society. **Instrumental activities of daily living** (IADLs) include such skills as shopping, preparing meals, writing checks, and taking medications. Nurses within the home care and community health setting frequently assist clients in adapting ways to perform IADLs. Often family and friends are excellent resources for assisting clients. In acute care it is important for you to anticipate how a client's illness will affect the ability to perform IADLs so that you make appropriate referrals. Occupational therapists are very useful in training clients to adapt approaches with IADLs.

Physical Care Techniques

You will routinely perform a variety of physical care techniques when caring for a client. Examples include turning and positioning, performing invasive procedures, administering medications, and providing comfort measures. Physical techniques involve the safe and competent administration of nursing procedures (e.g., urinary catheter insertion, range-of-motion exercises, and administration of injections). The specific knowledge and skills needed to perform these procedures are in subsequent clinical chapters of this text. Common methods for administering physical care techniques appropriately include protecting you and the client from injury, using proper infection control practices, staying organized, and following applicable practice guidelines.

To carry out a procedure, you need to be knowledgeable about the procedure itself, the standard frequency, the steps, and the expected outcomes. In a hospital you will perform many procedures each day. Some of these procedures will be new, so before conducting a new procedure always assess your personal competencies and determine if you need assistance, new knowledge, or new skills. Benner (1984) made an important observation about physical care techniques. There is always variability and thoughtful adaptations that nurses need to make in administering and monitoring client therapies. For example, when you change a complicated dressing, there are many dressing materials to choose from and different cleansing solutions, and the client's size affects how to secure a dressing. Performing any procedure correctly requires critical thinking and thoughtful decision making.

Lifesaving Measures

A **lifesaving measure** is a physical care technique that you use when a client's physiological or psychological state is threatened (see Chapter 40). The purpose of lifesaving measures is to restore physiological or psychological equilibrium. Such measures include administering emergency medications, instituting cardiopulmonary resuscitation, intervening to protect a confused or violent client, and obtaining immediate counseling from a crisis center for a severely anxious client. If an inexperienced nurse faces a situation requiring emergency measures, the proper nursing action is to get an experienced professional.

Counseling

Counseling is a direct care method that helps the client use a problem-solving process to recognize and manage stress and to facilitate interpersonal relationships. As a nurse, you will counsel clients to accept actual or impending changes resulting from stress. Examples include clients facing terminal illness or chronic disease. Counseling involves emotional, intellectual, spiritual, and psychological support. A client and family who need nursing counseling have normal adjustment difficulties and are upset or frustrated, but they are not necessarily psychologically disabled. A good example is the stress a young woman faces when caring for her aging mother. Family caregivers need assistance in adjusting to the physical and emotional demands of caregiving. Likewise, the recipient of care also needs assistance in adjusting to the disability. Clients with psychiatric diagnoses require therapy by nurses specializing in psychiatric nursing or by social workers, psychiatrists, or psychologists.

Many counseling techniques foster cognitive, behavioral, developmental, experiential, and emotional growth in clients. Most of the techniques listed in Box 19-3 require additional knowledge beyond the scope of this text. Counseling encourages individuals to examine available alternatives and decide which choices are useful and appropriate. When clients are able to examine alternatives, they develop a sense of control and are able to better manage stress.

Teaching

Teaching is an important nursing responsibility. Counseling and teaching closely align. Both involve using communication skills to create a change in the client. However, with counseling the change

✳ BOX 19-3 Counseling Strategies and Selected Examples Used by Nurses

Behavior Modification

Client changes from smoking to meditating to cope with stress

Encourage alternative behavior (e.g., introduce exercise as a health promotion activity)

Develop a chart to record and track eating habit changes

Use social skills training (e.g., role playing) to change behaviors (e.g., anger or aggression)

Bereavement Counseling

Assist client in productive reminiscing of loved one

Support client in removing loved one's belongings from home

Biofeedback

Use biological measures (e.g., heart rate, blood pressure) as feedback to modify a body function

Meditation

Relaxation Exercises

Progressive muscle relaxation exercises

Meditation

Crisis Intervention

Therapy designed to assist in coping with crisis

Anticipatory guidance to recognize and avoid modifiable crises

Play Therapy

Assist children through play to cope with loss and grief

Assist children in coping with chronic illness

Assist children in becoming competent in self-care activities

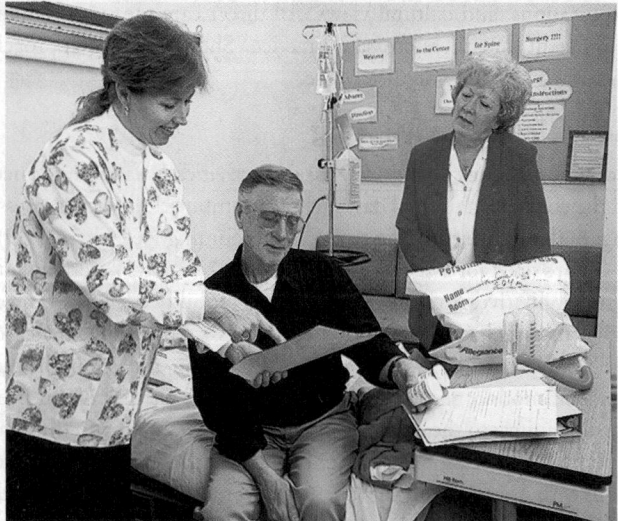

Figure 19-3 Teaching client discharge instructions.

results in the development of new attitudes and feelings, whereas in teaching the focus of change is intellectual growth or the acquisition of new knowledge or psychomotor skills (Redman, 2005).

As a nurse, you teach to present correct principles, procedures, and techniques of health care to clients and to inform clients about their health status. Common examples of teaching topics include medication administration schedules, activity restrictions, health promotion activities (e.g., diet and exercise), and knowledge about disease and related implications. Teaching takes place in all health care settings (Figure 19-3). As a nurse, you are responsible for assessing the learning needs and readiness of clients and you are accountable for the quality of education you deliver. Know your client; be aware of the cultural and social factors that influence a client's willingness and ability to learn. It is also important to know your client's health literacy level. Can he or she read directions or make calculations that sometimes are necessary with self-care skills? The teaching-learning process is an interaction between you and the learner in which you address specific learning objectives (see Chapter 25). The process offers an organizational structure and framework for successful client education.

Controlling for Adverse Reactions

An **adverse reaction** is a harmful or unintended effect of a medication, diagnostic test, or therapeutic intervention. Adverse reactions can possibly follow any nursing intervention, so learn to anticipate and know the adverse reactions to expect. Nursing actions that control for adverse reactions reduce or counteract the reaction. For example, when applying a moist heat com-

press, you want to prevent burning the client's skin. First assess the area requiring the compress. Following application of the compress, inspect the area every 5 minutes for any adverse reaction, such as excessive reddening of the skin from the heat or skin maceration from the moisture of the compress. When completing a physician- or other health care provider–directed intervention, such as medication administration, you need to understand the known and potential side effects of the drug. After administration of the medication, you evaluate the client for any adverse effects. Also, be aware of drugs that counteract the side effects. For example, a client has an unknown hypersensitivity to penicillin and develops hives after three doses. You record the reaction, stop further administration of the drug, and consult with the physician. You then administer an ordered dose of diphenhydramine (Benadryl), an antihistamine and antipruritic medication, to reduce the allergic response and to relieve the itching.

When caring for a client who is undergoing a particular diagnostic test, you need to understand the test and any potential adverse effects. For example, a client has not had a bowel movement in 24 hours after a barium enema. Because bowel impaction is a potential side effect of a barium enema, you increase fluid intake and instruct the client to let nursing personnel know when a bowel movement occurs. Although adverse effects are not common, they do occur. It is important that you recognize the signs and symptoms of an adverse reaction and intervene in a timely manner.

Preventive Measures

Preventive nursing actions promote health and prevent illness to avoid the need for acute or rehabilitative health care. With changes in the health care system, there is and will be greater emphasis on health promotion and illness prevention. Prevention includes assessment and promotion of the client's health potential, application of prescribed measures (e.g., immunizations), health teaching, and identification of risk factors for illness and/or trauma. Consider, for example, the case of Ms. Devine. Lisa learns that her client does not exercise regularly. Ms. Devine is 5 feet 6 inches tall and weighs 160 pounds. Because she is overweight and inactive, once she goes home she is at risk for assuming activities that will place stress on her back. If the client is able to lose some weight and start exercise therapy, she will be less likely to reinjure her back. Lisa plans to consult with the surgeon and physical therapist after surgery to design a plan to help Ms. Devine with weight loss and strengthening of back muscles.

Indirect Care

Indirect care measures are actions that support the effectiveness of direct care interventions (Dochterman and Bulechek, 2004). Many of the measures are managerial in nature, such as emergency cart maintenance and environmental and supply management (Box 19-4). Nurses spend a good amount of time in indirect and unit management activities. Communication of information about clients (e.g., change-of-shift report and consultation) is critical to ensuring that direct care activities are planned, coordinated, and performed with the proper resources. Delegation of care to assistive personnel is another indirect care activity (see Chapter 21). When performed correctly, delegation ensures that the right care provider performs the right tasks so that the nurse and nursing assistive personnel work most efficiently for the client's benefit.

Communicating Nursing Interventions

Any intervention you provide for a client will be communicated in a written and/or oral format. Written interventions are part of the nursing care plan (see Chapter 18) and a client's permanent medical record. Staff in many institutions develop **interdisciplinary care plans,** plans representing the contributions of all disciplines caring for a client. For example, when Ms. Devine begins recovering from lumbar laminectomy, her nursing diagnosis of *impaired physical mobility* will include interventions from nursing (e.g., nonpharmacological pain control and positioning), the surgeon (e.g., activity guidelines and pharmacological pain control), and physical therapy (e.g., ambulation training and exercises).

After completing nursing interventions, you document the treatment and client's response in the appropriate record (see Chapter 26). The record entry usually includes a brief description of pertinent assessment findings, the specific procedure, and the client's response. This information validates the need for the specific nursing intervention. Writing the time and the details of the intervention documents that you performed the procedure.

You will also communicate nursing interventions verbally to other health care professionals. Unless communication is timely and accurate, caregivers can be uninformed, interventions may be needlessly duplicated, procedures may be delayed, or tasks may be left undone. Clients can quickly tell when members of the health care team communicate inconsistent messages, indicating that no one is in charge. Nurses commonly communicate orally when conferring with colleagues, changing shifts, transferring a client to another unit, or discharging a client to another health care agency. Always be clear, concise, and to the point when you communicate nursing interventions.

> ✳ **BOX 19-4 Examples of Indirect Care Activities**
>
> - Documentation
> - Delegation of care activities to unlicensed personnel
> - Medical order transcription
> - Infection control (e.g., proper handling and storage of supplies, use of protective isolation)
> - Environmental safety management (e.g., make client rooms safe, strategically assigning clients in a geographic proximity to a single nurse)
> - Computer data entry
> - Telephone consults with physicians and other health care providers
> - Change-of-shift report
> - Collecting, labeling and transporting specimens
> - Transporting patients to procedural areas and other nursing units
>
> From Bulechek GM, Butcher HK, and Dochterman JM: *Nursing interventions classification (NIC),* ed 5, St. Louis, 2008, Mosby.

Delegating, Supervising, and Evaluating the Work of Other Staff Members

Depending on the system of health care delivery, the nurse who develops the care plan frequently does not perform all of the nursing interventions. Some activities you will coordinate and delegate to other members of the health care team. For example, an RN delegates components of care but not the nursing process itself (American Nurses Association [ANA], 2006). Noninvasive and frequently repetitive interventions such as skin care, ambulation, grooming, vital signs on stable clients, and hygiene measures are examples of care activities that you will assign to assistive personnel such as a nurse assistant. When a nurse delegates aspects of a client's care to another staff member, the nurse assigning tasks is responsible for ensuring that each task is appropriately assigned and is completed according to the standard of care. You are also responsible for delegating direct care interventions to personnel who are competent. Recently the American Nurses Association (ANA) and the National Council of State Boards of Nursing (NCSBN) released a joint statement that lays out 10 principles for delegation (Trossman, 2006). The principles offer a blueprint to help RNs better understand delegation to keep clients safe and to protect their professional practice. Chapter 21 covers the principles of effective delegation in detail.

Achieving Client Goals

Regardless of the type of interventions, you implement nursing care to meet client goals and outcomes. In most clinical situations multiple interventions are necessary to achieve select outcomes. In addition, clients' conditions sometimes change minute by minute. Therefore, as a nurse, it becomes important to be able to apply principles of care coordination such as good time management, organizational skills, and appropriate use of resources to ensure that you deliver interventions effectively and meet desired outcomes (see Chapter 21). Priority setting is also critical in successful implementation. Priorities help you to anticipate and sequence nursing interventions when a client has multiple nursing diagnoses and collaborative problems (see Chapter 18).

Another way to achieve client goals is to assist clients in adhering to their treatment plan. **Client adherence** means that clients and families invest time in carrying out required treatments. To ensure clients a smooth transition across different health care settings (e.g., hospital to home and clinic to home to assisted living), it becomes important to introduce interventions that clients are willing and able to follow. Adequate and timely discharge planning and education of the client and family are the first steps in promoting a smooth transition from one health care setting to another or to the home. To be effective with discharge planning and education, you individualize your care and take into consideration the various factors that influence a client's health beliefs. For example, in order for Lisa to be effective in helping Ms. Devine agree to adopt better exercise habits when she returns home, she will need to know if Ms. Devine understands the threat she faces if she does not exercise. Chapter 6 reviews the principles of the health belief model, which influence how clients adhere to any health care recommendations. You are responsible for delivering interventions in a way that reflects your understanding of a client's health beliefs, culture, lifestyle pattern, and patterns of wellness. In addition, reinforcing successes with the treatment plan encourages the client to follow the care plan.

❋ Key Concepts

- Implementation is the step of the nursing process in which nurses provide direct and indirect nursing care interventions to clients.
- Always think first, and determine if an intervention is correct and appropriate before you implement.
- Clinical guidelines or protocols are evidence-based documents that guide decisions and interventions for specific health care problems.
- When preparing to perform an intervention, reassess the client, review and revise the existing nursing care plan, organize resources and care delivery, anticipate and prevent complications, and implement the intervention.
- During the initial phase of implementation, reassess the client to determine whether the proposed nursing action is still appropriate for the client's level of wellness.
- The implementation of nursing care often requires additional knowledge, nursing skills, and personnel resources.
- Before beginning to perform interventions, be sure the client is as physically and psychologically comfortable as possible.
- To anticipate and prevent complications, a nurse identifies risks to the client, adapts interventions to the situation, evaluates the relative benefit of a treatment versus the risk, and initiates risk prevention measures.
- Successful implementation of nursing interventions requires you to use appropriate cognitive, interpersonal, and psychomotor skills.
- The methods used to ensure that you administer physical care techniques appropriately include protecting the nurse and client from injury, using proper infection control practices, staying organized, and following applicable practice guidelines.

- Counseling is a direct care method that helps clients use problem solving to recognize and manage stress and to facilitate interpersonal relationships.
- Preventive nursing actions include assessment and promotion of the client's health potential, application of prescribed measures (e.g., immunizations), health teaching, and identification of risk factors for illness and/or trauma.
- To complete any nursing procedure, you need to know the procedure, its frequency, the steps, and the expected outcomes.

❋ Critical Thinking Exercises

Sue is a junior nursing student. She is to care for Mr. Nelson, a 63-year-old client who was admitted to the hospital with congestive heart failure and pneumonia. He is receiving medications to improve his heart failure and intravenous (IV) antibiotics to treat his pneumonia. He reports becoming fatigued easily during care activities and states, "I feel short of breath if I try to do too much." Sue notes he has 3+ edema in his lower extremities. Sue has identified nursing diagnoses of *decreased cardiac output* and *activity intolerance*. Sue must still perform hygiene measures, change the client's IV dressing, get him up into a chair, and collect 12 noon vital signs.

1. Before she begins to intervene, how can Sue make Mr. Nelson more comfortable?

2. What type of intervention is vital sign measurement?

3. Sue decides to get assistance from a colleague before trying to get Mr. Nelson up in the chair. Sue decides he may be at risk for falling. This is an example of what type of implementation skill?

When changing Mr. Nelson's IV dressing, Sue cleans the insertion site following clinical practice guidelines and checks the site for signs of phlebitis.

4. These steps are examples of what type of direct care measure?

❋ NCLEX®-Style Review Questions

1. When does implementation begin as the fourth step of the nursing process?
   1. During the assessment phase
   2. Immediately, in some critical situations
   3. After the care plan has been developed
   4. After there is mutual goal setting between nurse and client

2. Mr. Switzer is a 34-year-old client who had a surgical repair of an abdominal hernia this morning. At 12 noon the nurse records Mr. Switzer's vital signs on the recovery room flow sheet. The recording of vital signs is an example of:
   1. Psychomotor skill
   2. Indirect care measure
   3. Physical care technique
   4. Anticipating complications

3. Before beginning insertion of a client's indwelling urinary catheter, the nurse considers the steps to take to avoid the possibility of breaking sterile technique, which could cause a urinary tract infection. This is an example of what type of decision making?
   1. Identifying areas of assistance
   2. Reviewing possible consequences of a nursing action
   3. Reassessing the clinical situation to revise the care plan
   4. Determining the probability of all consequences of the catheterization

4. Interdisciplinary care plans represent:
   1. All nursing personnel having input in the care plan
   2. Contributions of all disciplines caring for the client
   3. The client's expressed wishes and advance directives
   4. Physicians and nurses working together to develop a plan of care

5. Environmental factors heavily affect a client's care. Your first concern for the client includes which of the following?
   1. Safety
   2. Nurse staffing
   3. Confidentiality
   4. Adequate pain relief

6. In which of the following examples is a nurse applying critical thinking attitudes when performing a dressing change?
   1. Following the procedural guideline for a dressing change
   2. Seeking necessary knowledge on the steps of the procedure
   3. Showing confidence in knowing which dressing materials to use
   4. Being sure that the dressing covers the entire wound completely.

7. Which steps do you follow when you are asked to perform a procedure with which you are unfamiliar? (Choose all that apply.)
   1. Seek necessary knowledge.
   2. Reassess the client's condition.
   3. Collect all equipment necessary.
   4. Have an experienced nurse available to assist.
   5. Consider all possible consequences of the procedure.

20 | Evaluation

OBJECTIVES

Mastery of the content in this chapter will enable the student to:

- Discuss the relationship between critical thinking and evaluation.
- Identify the five elements of the evaluation process.
- Explain the relationship between goals of care, expected outcomes, and evaluative measures when evaluating nursing care.
- Give examples of evaluation measures for determining a client's progress toward outcomes.
- Evaluate a set of nursing actions selected for a client.

- Describe how evaluation leads to discontinuation, revision, or modification of a plan of care.
- Explain the association between evaluation and quality improvement (QI).
- Discuss how outcomes management assists an organization in improving the quality of care it delivers.

MEDIA RESOURCES   KEY TERMS

Companion CD
- NCLEX®-Style Review Questions
- Audio Glossary
- Interactive Learning Activities
- English/Spanish Glossary

evolve Website
- NCLEX®-Style Review Questions
- Audio Glossary
- English/Spanish Glossary
- Interactive Learning Activities
- WebLinks
- Audio Summaries

Evaluation, p. 291
Evaluative measures, p. 294
Outcome, p. 298
Outcomes management, p. 298
Performance improvement
  (PI), p. 298

Quality improvement (QI),
  p. 298
Standard of care, p. 297

When a repairman comes to a home to fix a leaking faucet, he turns the faucet on to determine the problem, changes or adjusts parts to the faucet, and then turns the faucet on once again to determine if the leak is fixed. After a client diagnosed with pneumonia completes a 5-day dose pack of antibiotics, the physician often has the client return to the office to have a chest x-ray examination to determine if the pneumonia has cleared. When a nurse delivers an intervention such as applying a warm compress to a wound, several steps are involved. The nurse assesses the appearance of the wound, determines the severity of the wound, applies the appropriate form of compress, and then returns to determine if the condition of the wound has improved. These three scenarios depict what ultimately occurs during the process of evaluation. The repairman rechecks the faucet, the physician orders a chest x-ray film, and the nurse reinspects the client's wound. Evaluation involves two components: an examination of a condition or situation and then a judgment as to whether change has occurred. Ideally, after an intervention takes place, evaluation will reveal an improvement.

The previous chapters on the nursing process describe how you use critical thinking skills to gather client data, form nursing diagnoses, develop a plan of care, and implement the care plan. **Evaluation,** the final step of the nursing process, is crucial to determine whether, after application of the nursing process, the client's condition or well-being improves. You apply all that you know about a client and the client's condition, as well as experience with previous clients, to evaluate whether nursing care was effective. **You conduct evaluative measures to determine if you met expected outcomes, not if nursing interventions were completed**. The expected outcomes are the standards against which the nurse judges if goals have been met and if care is successful.

In the continuing case study, Lisa is now making final preparations to send Ms. Devine off to surgery. Lisa evaluates the interventions she has implemented for the goals to achieve pain control, reduce anxiety, improve mobility, and improve Ms. Devine's knowledge of postoperative activities. Lisa returned to Ms.

Devine's room initially 30 minutes after administering an analgesic. At that time the client reported having pain at a level of a 4. Lisa had set the expected outcome of pain reduced to a level of 3. Lisa then implemented further nonpharmacological interventions. Two hours later she now finds Ms. Devine lying in bed with her eyes closed. The client awakens as Lisa enters and says, "I just had my eyes closed; I am ready to get this over." Lisa asks, "Tell me how you are feeling." Ms. Devine responds, "Okay, really Okay; I feel better, and I am a little less worried than when I first got here." Lisa asks, "On a scale of 0 to 10, tell me how you would rate your pain now." Ms. Devine, "I would say about a 4; it is still there but not as sharp." Lisa continues, "You said you were feeling less worried." Ms. Devine replies, "Yes, I think you have helped me feel less anxious. You know, surgery is nothing anyone wants to have, but I feel better knowing what to expect." Lisa observes Ms. Devine is relaxed and does not show facial grimacing when she turns slightly to her side. Lisa asks, "Can you take just a moment to go over with me what we discussed about your care after surgery?" Ms. Devine responds, "Sure, that would be fine."

Critical Thinking and Evaluation

Evaluation is an ongoing process whenever you have contact with a client. Once you deliver an intervention, gather subjective and objective data from the client, family, and health care team members. You also review knowledge regarding the client's current condition, treatment, resources available for recovery, and the expected outcomes. By referring to previous experiences caring for similar clients, you are in a better position to know how to evaluate your client. Apply critical thinking attitudes and standards to determine whether outcomes of care are achieved (Figure 20-1). If outcomes are met, the overall goals for the client also are met. Compare client behavior and responses that you assessed before delivering nursing interventions with behavior and responses that occur after administering nursing care. Critical thinking directs

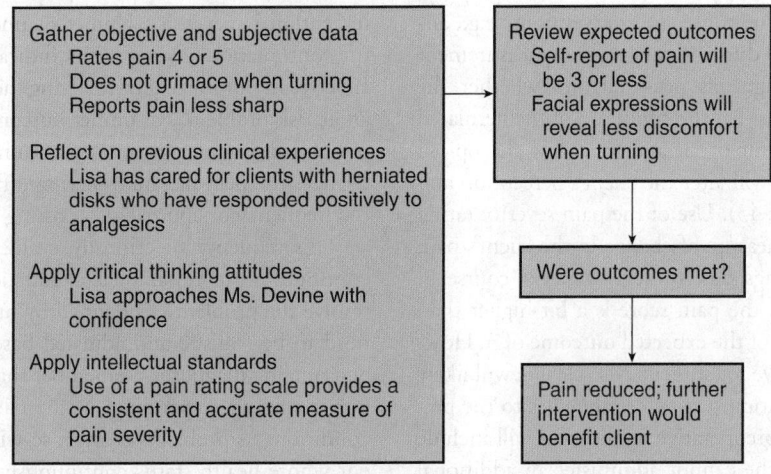

Figure 20-1 Critical thinking and the evaluation process.

KNOWLEDGE

Characteristics of improved phsyiological,
psychological, spiritual, and sociocultural status
Expected outcomes of pharmacological, medical,
nutritional, and other therapies
Unexpected outcomes of pharmacological,
medical, nutritional, and other therapies
Characteristics of improved family and group
dynamics
Community resources

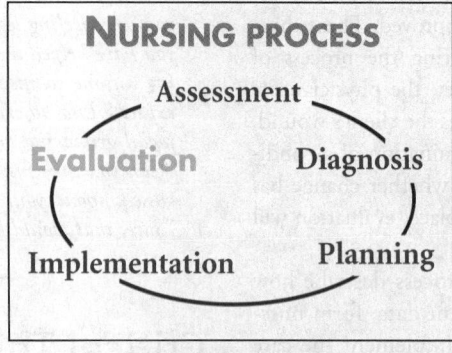

EXPERIENCE
Previous client care experience

NURSING PROCESS
Assessment
Evaluation   Diagnosis
Implementation   Planning

STANDARDS
Expected outcomes of care
Specialty standards of practice
(e.g., American Pain Society;
University of Iowa Evidence-
Based Protocols, Intravenous
Nursing Society)
Intellectual standards

ATTITUDES

Creativity
Responsibility
Perseverance
Humility

Figure 20-2 Critical thinking and evaluation.

you to analyze the findings from evaluation (Figure 20-2). Has the client's condition improved? Is the client able to improve, or are there physical factors preventing recovery? To what degree does this client's motivation or willingness to pursue healthier behavior influence response to therapies?

During evaluation you make clinical decisions and continually redirect nursing care. For example, when Lisa evaluates Ms. Devine for a change in pain severity, she applies knowledge of the disease process, physiological responses to interventions (e.g., analgesics), and the correct procedure for pain severity measurement to interpret whether a change has occurred and whether the change is desirable. Lisa knows that the condition of the herniated disc will not change as a result of an analgesic, but the opioid medication she administered will alter the client's perception and reaction to pain (see Chapter 43). Use of the pain severity rating scale gives Lisa an accurate measure of change in the client's pain perception. Evaluative findings determine Lisa's next course of action. In Ms. Devine's case, the pain score is a bit higher than expected, a score of 4 instead of the expected outcome of 3. However, the client is about to leave for surgery. Ms. Devine will likely receive a preoperative medication just before she goes to the preoperative holding area. The preoperative medication will include an analgesic, so Lisa knows she cannot administer an additional analgesic at this time. She evaluates that Ms. Devine's pain has

been reduced and decides to continue to use basic comfort measures to afford further pain relief.

Positive evaluations occur when you meet desired outcomes, and they lead you to conclude that the nursing intervention(s) effectively met the client's goals. For example, in the case study, Lisa notes that Ms. Devine's pain rating fell from an 8 or 9 to a 4. With an expected outcome of a pain severity of 3, Lisa's interventions showed a successful reduction in pain severity, but continuing intervention is necessary. Unmet or undesirable outcomes, such as the continuation of severe pain, indicate that interventions are not effective in minimizing or resolving the actual problem or avoiding an at-risk problem. An unmet outcome reveals the client has not responded to interventions as planned. As a result, the nurse changes the plan of care by trying different therapies or changing the frequency or approach of existing therapies.

This sequence of critically evaluating and revising therapies continues until you and the client successfully and appropriately resolve the problems, as defined by nursing diagnoses. Outcomes need to be realistic and adjusted based on the client's prognosis and nursing diagnoses. Remember that evaluation is dynamic and ever changing, depending on the client's nursing diagnoses and condition. As problems change, so will expected outcomes. A client whose health status continuously changes requires more frequent evaluation. In addition, you will evaluate priority diagnoses first. For example, Lisa evaluates Ms. Devine's *acute pain* before evaluating the status of the client's *deficient knowledge*.

The Evaluation Process

The purpose of nursing care is to assist the client in resolving actual health problems, preventing the occurrence of potential problems, and maintaining a healthy state. The evaluation process, which determines the effectiveness of nursing care, includes five elements: (1) identifying evaluative criteria and standards, (2) collecting data to determine whether the criteria or standards are met, (3) interpreting and summarizing findings, (4) documenting findings and any clinical judgment, and (5) terminating, continuing, or revising the care plan.

Identifying Criteria and Standards

You evaluate nursing care by knowing what to look for. A client's goals and expected outcomes give you the objective criteria needed to judge a client's response to care.

Goals. A goal is the expected behavior or response that indicates resolution of a nursing diagnosis or maintenance of a healthy state. It is a summary statement of what will be accomplished when the client has met all expected outcomes. In the case of Ms. Devine, in Chapter 18 we described Lisa's plan of care for *acute pain.* Lisa selected the goal "Client achieves improved pain control before surgery." Successful achievement of this goal depends on the success of Lisa's Nursing Interventions Classification (NIC) interventions for analgesic administration, pain management, and progressive muscle relaxation.

Goals often are also based on standards of care or guidelines established for minimal safe practice. For example, the Infusion Nurses Society (INS) has standards of care for prevention of the intravenous (IV) complication phlebitis. When a nurse cares for a client with a peripheral intravenous line, the goal "The IV site will remain free of phlebitis" is established on the basis of sound practice standards. The INS has developed a scale containing physical criteria for determining phlebitis (see Chapter 41).

Expected Outcomes. Outcomes have been broadly defined in the health care literature. Donabedian (1980) defined outcomes as favorable or adverse changes in clients' health states due to prior or concurrent care. When nurses apply the nursing process, expected outcomes are the expected favorable and measurable results of nursing care. A nursing-sensitive client outcome is a measurable client or family state, behavior, or perception largely influenced by and sensitive to nursing interventions (Moorhead and others, 2008). Examples of nursing-sensitive outcomes include reduction in pain severity, incidence of pressure ulcers, and incidence of falls (Box 20-1). In comparison, outcomes largely influenced by medical interventions include client mortality, hospital readmissions, and length of stay. Outcomes are statements of progressive, step-by-step responses or behaviors that the client needs to accomplish to achieve the goals of care. An outcome defines the effectiveness, efficiency, and measurement of the re-

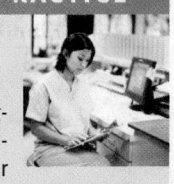

BOX 20-1   EVIDENCE-BASED PRACTICE

Nursing-Sensitive Outcomes
Evidence Summary
Although members of the general public recognize that oncology nurses aim to deliver high-quality care to people with cancer and their families, nurses themselves struggle with ways to measure their influence on client outcomes. The Oncology Nursing Society (ONS) has implemented a project to define and list nursing-sensitive patient outcomes (NSPOs) for the field of oncology. For each outcome the ONS is working to provide references and links to best evidence in the literature, clinical guidelines, a review of existing knowledge, and discussion about measurement of outcomes. Examples of NSPOs include symptom control and management (pain, fatigue, insomnia, nausea, constipation, breathlessness, diarrhea), functional status (activities of daily living [ADLs], instrumental ADLs [IADLs], role functioning, activity tolerance, nutritional status), psychological health status (anxiety, depression, spiritual distress, coping), and economic (home care visits, costs per day per episode of illness).

Application to Nursing Practice
- Establishing NSPOs for clients with cancer helps to provide tools for nurses to use in measuring the impact of nursing care.
- Development of core measures linked to evidence-based practice guidelines will improve nursing practice at the bedside.
- Use of NSPOs helps nursing clearly indicate to consumers the value nursing contributes to health care.

Reference
Given BA, Sherwood PR: Nursing-sensitive patient outcomes—a white paper, *Oncol Nurs Forum* 32(4):773, 2005.

sults of nursing interventions. When you achieve outcomes, the related factors for a nursing diagnosis usually no longer exist. In Ms. Devine's case, the expected outcomes for the goal of achieving improved pain control are *"Client's self-report of pain will be 3 or less on a scale of 0 to 10"* and *"Client's facial expressions reveal less discomfort when turning and repositioning."* When Lisa evaluates Ms. Devine's pain at a level of 4 and notes an absence of facial grimacing during turning, she knows the client's pain has been reduced but further pain relief needs to be achieved. However, the related factor for Ms. Devine's *acute pain* is pressure on spinal nerves, which will not be totally relieved until surgery. The analgesics and noninvasive nursing interventions are designed to reduce the perception of pain from pressure on the nerves, as well as to minimize additional pressure on nerves.

It is important to understand that evaluation is not a description of the achievement of an intervention. Evaluation of Ms. Devine *does not* involve observation of her ability to turn correctly. Evaluation *does* involve observation of the client's behavior (facial expression) during turning.

During the planning phase of the nursing process (see Chapter 18) it is important for you to select an observable client state, behavior, or self-reported perception that will reflect goal achieve-

✳ TABLE 20-1 Linkages Between Nursing Outcomes Classification and Nursing Diagnoses

NURSING DIAGNOSIS	SUGGESTED OUTCOMES	INDICATORS (EXAMPLES)
Pain	Comfort level	Reported physical well-being
		Reported satisfaction with symptom control
		Expressed satisfaction with pain control
	Pain control	Recognizes pain onset
		Uses analgesics appropriately
		Reports pain controlled
	Pain level	Reported pain severity
		Frequency of pain
		Muscle tension
Deficient knowledge	Knowledge: treatment procedures	Description of treatment procedures
	Knowledge: illness care	Description of disease process
		Description of prescribed activity

Modified from Moorhead S and others: *Nursing outcomes classification (NOC)*, ed 4, St. Louis, 2008, Mosby.

ment. One valuable resource is the Nursing Outcomes Classification (NOC), which provides a classification system of nursing-sensitive outcomes. NOC is designed to provide the language for the evaluation step of the nursing process. The purposes of NOC are (1) to identify, label, validate, and classify nursing-sensitive client outcomes; (2) to field test and validate the classification; and (3) to define and test measurement procedures for the outcomes and indicators using clinical data (Moorhead and others, 2008). The NOC project complements the work of NANDA International (NANDA-I) and the NIC project. The NOC classification offers nursing-sensitive outcomes for NANDA-I nursing diagnoses (Table 20-1). For each outcome there are specific recommended evaluation indicators, the client behaviors or responses that are measures of outcome achievement.

Collecting Evaluative Data

Proper evaluation allows you to answer the following questions: What is the client's response to nursing care? Was the therapy effective in improving the client's physical or emotional heath? It is important to evaluate whether each client reaches a level of wellness or recovery that the health care team and client established in the goals of care. In addition, have you met the client's expectations of care? You will ask clients about their perceptions of care, such as "Did you receive the type of pain relief you expected?" "Did you receive enough information to care for your baby at home?" This level of evaluation is important to determine the client's satisfaction with care and to strengthen the partnering between you and the client. Always select appropriate evaluative measures to evaluate client response and expectations.

Evaluating a client's response to nursing care requires the use of **evaluative measures,** which are simply assessment skills and techniques (e.g., auscultation of lung sounds, observation of a client's skill performance, discussion of the client's feelings, and inspection of the skin) (Figure 20-3). In fact, evaluative measures are the same as assessment measures, but you perform them at the point of care when you make decisions about the client's status and progress. The intent of assessment is to identify what if any

problems exist. The intent of evaluation is to determine if the known problems have remained the same, improved, worsened, or otherwise changed.

In many clinical situations it is important to collect evaluative measures over a period of time to determine if a pattern of improvement or change exists. A one-time observation of a pressure ulcer is insufficient to determine that the ulcer is healing. It is important to note a consistency in change. For example, over a period of 2 days is the pressure ulcer gradually decreasing in size, is the amount of drainage declining, is the redness of inflammation resolving? Recognizing a pattern of improvement or deterioration allows you to reason and decide whether the client's problems are resolved.

The primary source of data for evaluation is the client. However, you will also use input from the family and other caregivers. For example, you ask a family member to report on the amount of food the client eats during a meal or how well a client prepared medications in the home. You will sometimes consult with a colleague about how the client responded to pain medication on a previous shift.

Interpreting and Summarizing Findings

A client's clinical condition changes often minute by minute during an acute illness. In contrast, chronic illness results in slow, subtle changes. When you evaluate the effect of interventions, you learn to recognize relevant evidence about a client's condition, even evidence that sometimes does not match clinical expectations. By applying your clinical knowledge and experience, you learn to recognize complications or adverse responses to illness and treatment in addition to expected outcomes.

Using evidence, you make judgments about a client's condition. To develop clinical judgment you learn to match the results of evaluative measures with expected outcomes to determine if a client's status is improving or not. When interpreting findings, you compare the client's behavioral responses and physiological signs and symptoms you expect to see with those actually seen from your evaluation. Comparing expected and actual findings allows you to interpret and judge the client's condition and

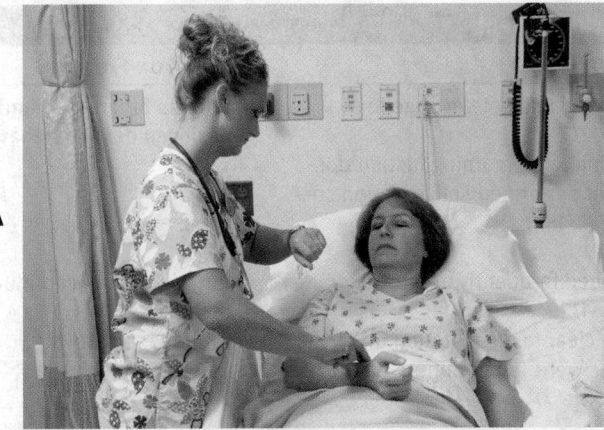

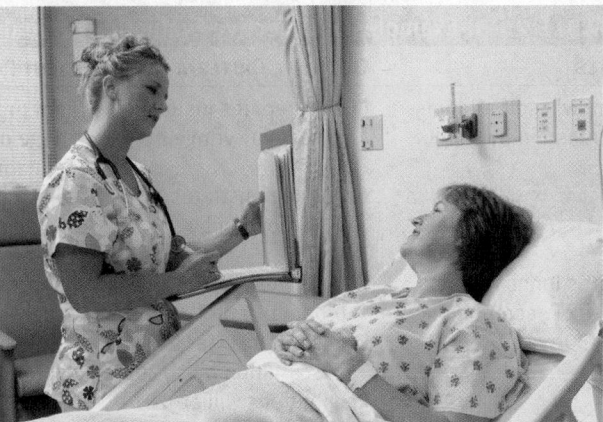

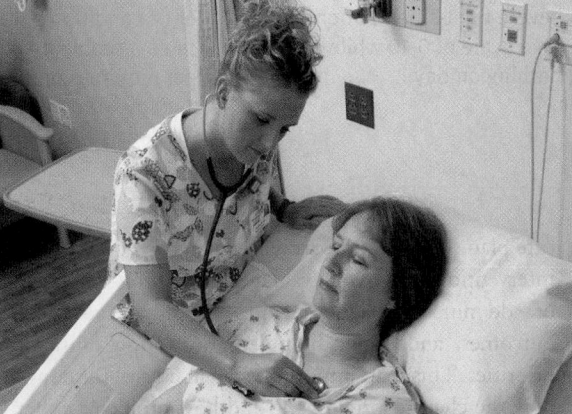

Figure 20-3 Evaluative measures. **A,** Nurse evaluates the client's vital signs. **B,** Nurse confirms the client's medical history. **C,** Nurse evaluates the client's lung sounds.

✳ TABLE 20-2 Evaluative Measures to Determine the Success of Goals and Expected Outcomes

GOALS	EVALUATIVE MEASURES	EXPECTED OUTCOMES
Client's pressure ulcer will heal within 7 days.	Inspect color, condition, and location of pressure ulcer. Measure diameter of ulcer daily. Note odor and color of drainage from ulcer.	Erythema will be reduced in 2 days. Diameter of ulcer will decrease in 5 days. Ulcer will have no drainage in 2 days. Skin overlying ulcer will be closed in 7 days.
Client will tolerate ambulation to end of hall by 11/20.	Palpate client's radial pulse before exercise. Palpate client's radial pulse 10 minutes after exercise. Assess respiratory rate during exercise. Observe client for dyspnea or breathlessness during exercise.	Pulse will remain below 110 beats per minute during exercise. Pulse rate will return to resting baseline within 10 minutes after exercise. Respiratory rate will remain within two breaths of client's baseline rate. Client will deny feeling of breathlessness.
Client will have improved grief resolution by 1/15.	Ask client about frequency of periods of crying, sadness. Review client's sleeping log. Review client's dietary intake.	Client reports decreased frequency of crying, sadness in 2 months. Client has periods of 6-7 hours of sleep without interruption within 10 days. Client has no weight loss in 1 month.

whether predicted changes have occurred (Table 20-2). To objectively evaluate the degree of success in achieving outcomes of care, use the following steps:

1. Examine the outcome criteria to identify the exact desired client behavior or response.
2. Assess the client's actual behavior or response.
3. Compare the established outcome criteria with the actual behavior or response.
4. Judge the degree of agreement between outcome criteria and the actual behavior or response.
5. If there is no agreement (or only partial agreement) between the outcome criteria and the actual behavior or response, what is/are the barriers? Why did they not agree?

Evaluation is easier to perform after you care for a client over a long period. You are then able to make subtle comparisons of client responses and behaviors. When you have not had the

※ **TABLE 20-3 Examples of Objective Evaluation of Goal Achievement**

GOALS	OUTCOME CRITERIA	CLIENT RESPONSE	EVALUATION FINDINGS
Client will self-administer insulin by 12/18.	Client prepares insulin dosage in syringe by 12/17. Client demonstrates self-injection by 12/18.	Client prepared accurate dosage in syringe on 12/17. Client administered morning insulin dosage; client performed self-injection correctly on 12/18.	Client has progressed and achieved desired behavior.
Client's lungs will be free of secretions by 11/30.	Coughing will be nonproductive by 11/29. Lungs will be clear to auscultation by 11/30. Respirations will be 20 per minute by 11/30.	Client coughed frequently and productively on 11/29. Lungs were clear to auscultation on 11/30. Respirations were 18 per minute on 11/29.	Client will require continued therapy. Condition is improving.
Client will be able to perform self-care measures without discomfort in 2 days.	Client will rate pain as 3 on a scale of 0-10 within 2 days. Client will initiate bathing within 2 days.	Client rates severe right-sided abdominal pain as 5 on a scale of 0-10 while attempting bathing on day 2.	Client's condition still indicates a problem. Client requires continued therapy with possibly new care measures

chance to care for a client over an extended time, evaluation improves by referring to previous experiences or asking colleagues who are familiar with the client to confirm evaluation findings. The accuracy of any evaluation improves when you are familiar with the client's behavior and physiological status or have cared for more than one client with a similar problem.

Remember to evaluate each expected outcome and its place in the sequence of care. If not, it will be difficult to determine which outcome in the sequence was not met. Then you cannot revise and redirect the plan of care at the most appropriate time. If the client achieves the expected outcomes, you either continue the care plan to maintain a therapeutic status or discontinue interventions because the goal of care is met. If evaluation determines that the expected outcomes were not met or only partially met, you begin reassessment and revision of the care plan.

There are different degrees of goal achievement. If the client's response matches or exceeds the outcome criteria, the goal is met. If the client's behavior begins to show changes but does not yet meet criteria set, the goal is partially met. If there is no progress, the goal is not met (Table 20-3).

Documenting Findings

Documentation and reporting are an important part of evaluation. Accurate information needs to be present in a client's medical record for nurses to make ongoing clinical decisions. When documenting the client's response to interventions, always describe the same evaluative measures. Your aim is to present a clear argument from the evaluative data as to whether a client is progressing or not. Written nursing progress notes, assessment flow sheets, and information shared between nurses during change-of-shift reports (see Chapter 26) communicate a client's progress toward meeting expected outcomes and goals for the nursing plan of care.

Care Plan Revision

Evaluate expected outcomes and determine if the goals of care have been met. Then decide if you need to adjust the plan of care. If you meet a goal successfully, discontinue that portion of the care plan. Unmet and partially met goals require you to continue intervention. After you evaluate a client, you may want to modify or add nursing diagnoses with appropriate goals and expected outcomes, and establish interventions. You must also redefine priorities. This is an important step in critical thinking—knowing how the client is progressing and how problems either resolve or worsen.

In the case of Ms. Devine, Lisa's initial evaluation at the beginning of this chapter revealed the following: Client reports feeling better, rates pain at a level of 4, is lying in bed relaxed, feels less worried, and does not show facial grimacing when turning. When matching these actual behaviors and responses to expected outcomes, Lisa determines that Ms. Devine's pain and anxiety have lessened. Because the pain is less acute, Ms. Devine's mobility is less restricted. However, Lisa knows that the cause for Ms. Devine's pain has not been corrected. The surgery is still pending, and thus the client's anxiety will possibly increase. Lisa decides to continue the plan of care but makes revisions by adding additional basic comfort measures. The comfort measures will assist in controlling both the pain and anxiety and maintain the client's mobility. She next evaluates whether Ms. Devine remembers the postoperative activities that they discussed earlier: "Ms. Devine, we talked about several things that you will be asked to do following surgery. I want to know if you understand what we discussed. Tell me what to expect about your pain control and activity." Ms. Devine responds, "You said that I would have a device that lets me control how much pain medication I receive. I should not be afraid to use it. I know the doctors will get me up early to move around. You said if I can get control of the pain it will be easier to get up and walk. What I do not remember is something you said about breathing." Lisa, "Good, the device is a PCA. As for breathing, let's practice the incentive spirometer I showed you one more time." Lisa recognizes that Ms. Devine has learned about select postoperative activities but requires further instruction on the incentive spirometer. Deficient knowledge now becomes Lisa's priority until Ms. Devine leaves for surgery.

Careful monitoring and early detection of problems are a client's first line of defense. Always make clinical judgments on your observations of what is occurring with a specific client and not merely on what happens to clients in general. Frequently changes are not obvious. Evaluations are client specific, based on a close familiarity with each client's behavior, physical status, and reaction to caregivers. Critical thinking skills promote accurate evaluation, which leads to the appropriate revision of ineffective care plans and discontinuation of therapy that has successfully resolved a problem.

Discontinuing a Care Plan. After you determine that expected outcomes and goals have been met, you confirm this evaluation with the client when possible. If you and the client agree, then you discontinue that portion of the care plan. Documentation of a discontinued plan ensures that other nurses will not unnecessarily continue interventions for that portion of the plan of care. Continuity of care assumes that care provided to clients is relevant and timely. You will waste much time when you do not communicate achieved goals.

Modifying a Care Plan. When goals are not met, you identify the factors that interfere with goal achievement. Usually a change in the client's condition, needs, or abilities makes alteration of the care plan necessary. For example, when teaching self-administration of insulin, the nurse discovers that the client has developed a new problem, a tremor associated with a side effect of a medication. The client is unable to draw medication from a syringe or inject the needle safely. As a result, the original outcomes "Client will correctly prepare insulin in a syringe" and "Client will administer insulin injection independently" cannot be met. The nurse introduces new interventions (instructing a family member in insulin preparation and administration) and revises outcomes to meet the goal of care.

At times a lack of goal achievement results from an error in nursing judgment or failure to follow each step of the nursing process. Clients often have multiple and complex problems. Always remember the possibility of overlooking or misjudging something. When there is failure to achieve a goal, no matter what the reason, repeat the entire nursing process sequence for that nursing diagnosis to discover changes the plan needs. You then will reassess the client, determine accuracy of the nursing diagnosis, establish new goals and expected outcomes, and select new interventions.

A complete reassessment of all client factors relating to the nursing diagnosis and etiology is necessary when modifying a plan. Reassessment requires critical thinking as you compare new data about the client's condition with previously assessed information. Knowledge from previous experiences helps you direct the reassessment process. Caring for clients and families who have had similar health problems gives you a strong background of knowledge to use for anticipating client needs and knowing what to assess. Reassessment ensures that the database is accurate and current. It will also reveal the missing link (i.e., a critical piece of new information that was overlooked and thus interfered with goal achievement). You sort, validate, and cluster all new data to analyze and interpret differences from the original database. You also document reassessment data to alert other nursing staff to the client's status.

After reassessment, determine what nursing diagnoses are accurate for the situation. Ask whether you selected the correct diagnosis and whether it and the etiological factor are current. Then revise the problem list to reflect the client's changed status. Sometimes you will make a new diagnosis. You base your nursing care on an accurate list of nursing diagnoses. Accuracy is more important than the number of diagnoses selected. As the client's condition changes, the diagnoses also change. For example, a nurse has identified the nursing diagnosis *deficient knowledge related to inexperience* for a newly diagnosed diabetic. The original plan called for the nurse to instruct the client in how to self-administer insulin. After finding that the client has difficulty self-administering insulin because of reduced visual acuity, the nurse reassesses and finds a family member is available as a resource. To develop a plan designed to educate an alternative caregiver about the administration of insulin, the nurse then establishes a new diagnosis: *ineffective health maintenance related to impaired dexterity.*

Goals and Expected Outcomes. When you revise care plans, review the goals and expected outcomes for needed changes. You even need to examine the goals for unchanged nursing diagnoses for appropriateness, because a change in one problem sometimes affects others. Determining that each goal and expected outcome is realistic for the problem, etiology, and time frame is particularly important. Unrealistic expected outcomes and time frames make goal achievement difficult.

Clearly document goals and expected outcomes for new or revised nursing diagnoses so that all team members are aware of the revised care plan. When the goal is still appropriate but has not yet been met, try changing the evaluation data to allow more time. You may also decide at this time to change interventions. For example, when a client's pressure ulcer does not show signs of healing, you choose to use a different support surface or a different type of wound cleanser. All goals and expected outcomes are client centered, with realistic expectations for client achievement.

Interventions. The evaluation of interventions examines two factors: the appropriateness of the interventions selected and the correct application of the intervention. The appropriateness of an intervention is based on the standard of care for a client's health problem. A **standard of care** is the minimum level of care accepted to ensure high quality of care to clients. Standards of care define the types of therapies typically administered to clients with defined problems or needs. If the client who is receiving chemotherapy for leukemia has a specific nursing diagnosis, such as *nausea related to pharyngeal irritation,* the standard of care established by a nursing department for this problem includes pain-control measures for pharyngeal irritation, mouth care guidelines, and diet therapy. The nurse reviews the standard of care to determine whether the right interventions have been chosen or whether additional ones are required.

Increasing or decreasing the frequency of interventions is another approach to ensure appropriate application of an intervention. You adjust interventions on the basis of the client's actual response to therapy, as well as previous experience with similar clients. For example, if a client continues to have congested lung sounds, you increase the frequency of coughing and deep breathing exercises to remove secretions.

During evaluation you find that some planned interventions are designed for an inappropriate level of nursing care. If you need to change the level of care, substitute a different action verb, such as *assist* in place of *provide* or *demonstrate* in place of *instruct.* For example, assisting a client to walk requires a nurse to be at the client's side during ambulation, whereas providing an assistive device suggests the client is more independent. Also, demonstrating requires you to show a client how a skill is performed rather than simply telling the client how to perform it. Sometimes the level of care is appropriate, but the interventions are unsuitable because of a change in the expected outcome. In this case, discontinue the interventions and plan new ones.

Make any changes in the plan of care based on the nature of the client's unfavorable response. Consulting with other nurses often yields suggestions for improving the approach to care delivery. Senior nurses are often excellent resources because of their experience. Simply changing the care plan is not enough. Implement the new plan, and reevaluate the client's response to the nursing actions. *Evaluation is continuous.*

Occasionally during evaluation you will discover unmet client needs. This is normal. The nursing process is a systematic, problem-solving approach to individualized client care, but there are many factors affecting each client with health care problems. Clients with the same health care problem are not treated the same way. As a result, you will sometimes make errors in judgment. The systematic use of evaluation provides a way for you to catch these errors. By consistently incorporating evaluation into practice you will minimize errors and ensure that the client's plan of care is appropriate and relevant.

Quality Improvement

There are many ways to define quality of care. The Institute of Medicine (2002) defines quality as the "degree to which health services for individuals and populations increase the likelihood of desired health outcomes and are consistent with current professional knowledge." Just as each individual nurse is responsible for evaluating the care he or she provides to a client, health care organizations are responsible and accountable for evaluating and improving the quality of client care services provided to all clients. This requires health professionals at all levels to critically evaluate their practices, to incorporate the latest scientific findings into client care, and to measure the success of meeting client outcomes on an ongoing basis.

Quality improvement (QI) and **performance improvement (PI)** are interchangeable terms that describe an approach to the continuous study and improvement of the processes of providing health care services to meet the needs of clients and others (The Joint Commission, 2007). Among the processes that most directly influence clients are those that constitute nursing practice, such as medication administration, fall prevention, skin and wound care, and discharge planning. Progressive organizations are finding ways to merge QI and PI activities with evidence-based practice (see Chapter 5). When an organization reviews its specific outcome data (e.g., fall rates and medication errors), it applies principles of evidence-based practice to find the research-based approaches for resolving performance problems. However, there are still organizations that keep the two programs separate. In these cases QI projects often fail to tap into relevant research evidence, or evidence-based practice projects fail to access available setting-specific outcome data (Brown, 2006). The opportunity to merge QI with evidence-based practice improves the ability to apply the best evidence to practice.

Outcomes Management

Outcomes management is a term for managing the individual clinical outcomes of clients as a result of prescribed treatments. In outcomes management, a hospital, clinic, or physician's office conducts formal measurement of system-level performance and effectiveness (e.g., number of hospital readmissions, infection rates, or number of missed appointments). An **outcome** is the condition to be achieved as a result of care delivery or prescribed treatment. An outcome reveals whether interventions are effective, whether clients progress, how well they are meeting the standards of care, and whether changes in therapy or delivery of care are necessary. In health care today, outcomes management programs exist on individual nursing units or at the level of a health care system or managed care program. The move toward outcomes management has been the result of several national initiatives: client safety, reduction of unnecessary health care costs, identification and use of best practices, and health risk appraisal. Outcomes management has become a priority for all health care organizations because quality is one way to differentiate good and poor performers.

When professional nurses think in terms of outcomes management, their actions become much more purposeful and focused on improving the condition of their clients' health. The purpose of QI and PI is not to identify problems after the fact (although this often occurs) but to identify opportunities prospectively to improve the quality of care or service. A well-organized QI or PI program focuses on processes of care or systems that significantly contribute to outcomes. A systematic approach with everyone in an organization participating creates a culture where all staff understand their responsibility toward maintaining and improving quality. Quality improvement is concerned with exceeding the standard of care, examining ways to be more efficient, improving client satisfaction, and focusing on service (Bower, 2002). Chapter 5 provides more detail on QI and PI processes.

• • •

The evaluation of nursing care is a professional responsibility, and it is a crucial component of nursing care. Evaluation that focuses on a single client's plan of care enables you as a nurse to know the effectiveness of interventions and whether expected outcomes are met. At a system or institutional level, evaluation involves QI and PI activities that focus on the delivery of care provided by an agency or a specific nursing division within an agency. Through the continuous evaluation of care, nurses play a key role in the ongoing improvement of client care.

✳ Key Concepts

• Evaluation is a step of the nursing process that allows nurses to determine whether nursing interventions are successful in improving a client's condition or well-being.

- Evaluation involves two components: an examination of a condition or situation and a judgment as to whether change has occurred.
- During evaluation apply critical thinking to make clinical decisions and redirect nursing care to best meet client needs.
- Positive evaluations occur when you meet desired outcomes, and they lead you to conclude your interventions were effective.
- By comparing the client's actual response (e.g., behaviors and physiological signs and symptoms) to nursing interventions with expected outcomes established during planning, you determine if goals of care are met.
- Evaluative measures are assessment skills or techniques that you use to collect data for evaluation.
- It sometimes becomes necessary to collect evaluative measures over time to determine if a pattern of change exists.
- To interpret evaluative findings, examine the outcome criteria, assess the client's actual behavior or response, compare the outcome criteria with the actual behavior or response, and judge the degree of agreement.
- Documentation of evaluative findings allows all members of the health team to know whether a client is progressing or not.
- As a result of evaluation, a client's nursing diagnoses, priorities, and interventions sometimes change.
- Health care organizations are responsible for evaluating and improving the quality of client care services they provide.
- When professional nurses think in terms of outcomes management, their actions become more purposeful and focused on improving the condition of their client's health.

✳ Critical Thinking Exercises

Mr. Vicar has been visiting the clinic for more than a month. He visits weekly for follow-up care for a chronic venous stasis ulcer of the left leg. The nurse's note at the time of his first visit contained the following information: "Ulcer with irregular margins, 4 cm wide by 5 cm long, approximately 0.5 cm deep, draining foul-smelling purulent yellowish drainage. Only subcutaneous tissue visible. Skin around ulcer, brownish rust in color. Zinc oxide and calamine gauze applied to ulcer; elastic wrap bandage applied to gauze. Client instructed to return in 1 week."

1. As the nurse caring for Mr. Vicar, what expected outcomes would you set for the goal "Wound will demonstrate healing within 4 weeks"?

2. What evaluative measures would you use to determine if the wound shows healing?

Mr. Becker is a 78-year-old man who has been diagnosed with terminal lung cancer. He reports a loss of appetite and a 6-pound weight loss over the last month (152 pounds down to 146 pounds). He is able to chew and swallow food without difficulty. Mr. Becker denies feeling nauseated but states, "I just have no interest in food." His wife reports that he eats only a portion of what is served, "He gets full so quickly." Mrs. Becker also reports that her husband is less active around the house, sleeps poorly, and is unable to talk about his diagnosis. The nurse develops a nursing diagnosis of imbalanced nutrition: less than body requirements related to a decline in food intake.

3. What would be an appropriate goal for Mr. Becker's plan of care?

4. Identify expected outcomes to use in measuring success of the care plan.

5. What evaluative measures would the nurse use to determine Mr. Becker's progress?

Mr. Becker returns to the physician's office 2 weeks later. Mrs. Becker has been serving smaller and more frequent meals as recommended by the nurse. She has also worked hard to select a menu that is appealing to Mr. Becker. He continues to deny feeling nauseated. Mrs. Becker reports, "Some days he seems to eat better, but other days he just won't eat much. I think the smaller portions help." Mr. Becker's weight is now 145 pounds. His food diary shows that there are meals where he has eaten most of his food, but other meals where intake is minimal. He tells the nurse, "I know I should try to eat more, but what is the use?"

6. How would you interpret Mr. Becker's progress?

7. How would you revise the plan of care?

✳ NCLEX®-Style Review Questions

1. A nurse caring for a client with pneumonia sits the client up in bed and suctions the client's airway. After suctioning, the client describes some discomfort in his abdomen. The nurse auscultates the client's lung sounds and provides a glass of water for the client. Which of the following is an evaluative measure used by the nurse?
   1. Suctioning the airway
   2. Sitting client up in bed
   3. Auscultating lung sounds
   4. Asking client to describe type of discomfort

2. A nurse caring for a client with pneumonia sits the client up in bed and suctions the client's airway. After suctioning, the client describes some discomfort in his abdomen. The nurse auscultates the client's lung sounds and provides a glass of water for the client. Which of the following is an appropriate evaluative criterion used by the nurse? (Choose all that apply.)
   1. Client drinks contents of water glass.
   2. Client's lungs are clear to auscultation in bases.
   3. Client reports abdominal pain on scale of 0 to 10.
   4. Client's rate and depth of breathing are normal with head of bed elevated.

3. The evaluation process, which determines the effectiveness of nursing care, includes five elements, one being interpreting findings. Which of the following is an example of interpretation?
   1. Evaluating the client's response to selected nursing interventions
   2. Selecting an observable or measurable state or behavior that will reflect goal achievement
   3. Reviewing the client's nursing diagnoses and establishing goals and outcome statements
   4. Matching the results of evaluative measures with expected outcomes to determine client's status

4. A goal specifies the expected behavior or response that indicates:
   1. The specific nursing action was completed
   2. The validation of the nurse's physical assessment
   3. The nurse has made the correct nursing diagnoses
   4. Resolution of a nursing diagnosis or maintenance of a healthy state

5. A client is recovering from surgery for removal of an ovarian tumor. It is one day after her surgery. Because she has an abdominal incision and dressing, the nurse has selected a nursing diagnosis of *risk for infection*. Which of the following is an appropriate goal statement for the diagnosis?
   1. Client will remain afebrile to discharge.
   2. Client's wound will remain free of infection by discharge.
   3. Client will receive ordered antibiotic on time over next 3 days.
   4. Client's abdominal incision will remain covered with a sterile dressing for 2 days.

6. Unmet and partially met goals require the nurse to do which of the following? (Choose all that apply.)
   1. Redefine priorities
   2. Continue intervention
   3. Discontinue care plan
   4. Gather assessment data on a different nursing diagnosis
   5. Compare the client's response with that of another client

21 | Managing Client Care

✳ OBJECTIVES

Mastery of the content in this chapter will enable the student to:

- Differentiate among the types of nursing care delivery models.
- Describe the elements of decentralized decision making.
- Discuss the ways in which a nurse manager supports staff involvement in a decentralized decision-making model.
- Discuss ways to apply clinical care coordination skills in nursing practice.
- Discuss principles to follow in the appropriate delegation of client care activities.

✳ MEDIA RESOURCES   ✳ KEY TERMS

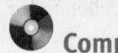

Companion CD

- NCLEX®-Style Review Questions
- Audio Glossary
- Interactive Learning Activities
- English/Spanish Glossary

 Website

- NCLEX®-Style Review Questions
- Audio Glossary
- English/Spanish Glossary
- Interactive Learning Activities
- WebLinks
- Audio Summaries

Accountability, p. 305
Authority, p. 305
Autonomy, p. 305
Case management, p. 304
Decentralized management,
    p. 304

Delegation, p. 309
Primary nursing, p. 303
Responsibility, p. 305
Shared governance, p. 305
Team nursing, p. 303
Total patient care, p. 303

As a nursing student, it is important for you to acquire the necessary knowledge and competencies that ultimately allow you to practice as an entry-level staff nurse (Box 21-1). Regardless of the type of setting you eventually choose to work in as a staff nurse, you will be responsible for using organizational resources, participating in organizational routines while providing direct client care, using time productively, collaborating with all members of the health care team, and using certain leadership characteristics to manage others on the nursing team (Wywialowski, 2004). The delivery of nursing care within the health care system is a challenge because of the changes that are influencing health professionals, clients, and health care organizations (see Chapter 2). However, change offers opportunities. As you develop the knowledge and skills to become a staff nurse, you will learn what it takes to effectively manage the clients you care for and to take the initiative in becoming a leader among your professional colleagues.

Building a Nursing Team

Nurses are self-directed and, with proper leadership and motivation, are able to solve most complex problems. A nurse's education and commitment to practicing within established standards and guidelines ensures a rewarding professional career. As a nurse, it is also important to work in an empowering environment as a member of a solid and strong nursing team. A strong nursing team works together to achieve the best outcomes for clients (Batcheller and others, 2004).

Building an empowered nursing team begins with the nurse executive, who is often vice president or director of nursing. The executive's position within an organization is critical in uniting the strategic direction of an organization with the philosophical values and goals of nursing. The nurse executive is both a clinical and business leader who is concerned with maximizing quality of care and cost-effectiveness while maintaining relationships and professional satisfaction of the staff (Pinkerton, 2001). Perhaps the most important responsibility of the nurse executive is to establish a vision for nursing that enables managers and staff to provide quality nursing care.

It takes an excellent nurse manager and an excellent nursing staff to make an empowering work environment. Together a manager and the nursing staff have to share a vision and philosophy of care for their work unit. A philosophy of care includes the professional nursing staff's values and concerns for the way they view and care for clients. For example, a philosophy addresses the nursing unit's purpose, how staff will work with clients and families, and the standards of care for the work unit (Box 21-2). A philosophy is a vision for how to practice nursing. Selection of a nursing care delivery model and a management structure that supports professional nursing practice is essential to the philosophy of care. The relationship between the nurse and nurse manager contributes to job satisfaction and retention (Ulrich and others, 2005).

Magnet Recognition

One way of creating an empowering work environment is through the Magnet Recognition Program. The American Nurses Credentialing Center Magnet Recognition Program recognizes excellence in nursing service and quality. The Magnet Recognition Program recognizes nursing services that build programs of excellence for the delivery of nursing care, promote quality in environments that support professional nursing practice, and promote achievement of positive client outcomes (American Nurses Credentialing Center, 2006). The 14 Forces of Magnetism provide the structure for the processes that lead to these outcomes. The forces were identified from research that differentiated the organizations that were best able to recruit and retain nurses during the nursing shortages

---

✳ BOX 21-1   Entry-Level Nurse Competencies

- Develop a knowledge base relevant to nursing practice.
- Include a code of conduct in practice that commits the nurse to provide care based on assessed client needs.
- Use the nursing process to make clinical decisions.
- View the client holistically.
- Use oral and written communication skills effectively in interactions with clients, families, nursing staff, and interdisciplinary groups.
- Exhibit a sense of professionalism.
- Accept responsibility to follow an ethical code of conduct.
- Show self-respect and respect for others.
- Interpret legal issues involved in health care.
- Comply with state licensure laws and Nurse Practice Acts, ANA standards of practice, and institutional policies and procedures.
- Defend one's own decisions.
- Participate in lifelong learning to remain competent in a changing practice environment.
- Serve as a role model.
- Show accountability of own nursing actions and actions of subordinates.
- Delegate care activities appropriately.

Modified from Wywialowski EF: *Managing client care,* ed 3, St. Louis, 2004, Mosby.
ANA, American Nurses Association.

✳ BOX 21-2   Developing a Vision for a Nursing Unit

What Is the Nursing Unit's Purpose or Mission?
Why do we exist?
Who are our customers (internal and external)?
What makes us unique?
What is unique about our clients?
How do we accomplish organizational goals or vision?

How Will Staff Work With Clients and Families?
Placing client and family needs first with a client-focused approach
Involving clients and families in all aspects of care
Making communication a priority

What Are the Standards of the Work Unit?
All staff will be competent.
Each staff member is accountable for the care delivered to clients.
Staff will work together with all members of the health care team.

Key Values
Creating an environment of caring
Being self-motivated and self-managed
Supporting a learning environment

of the 1970s and 1980s. The 14 forces are Quality of Nursing Leadership, Organizational Structure, Management Style, Personnel Policies and Programs, Professional Models of Care, Quality of Care, Quality Improvement, Consultation and Resources, Autonomy, Community and the Healthcare Organization, Nurses as Teachers, Image of Nursing, Interdisciplinary Relationships, and Professional Development (ANCC, 2007).

A Magnet hospital has a culture that is dynamic and positive for nurses. Typically a Magnet hospital has clinical promotion systems and research and evidence-based practice programs. The nurses have professional autonomy over their practice and control over the practice environment (Bolton and Goodenough, 2003). A Magnet hospital empowers the nursing team to make changes and be innovative. This culture and empowerment combine to produce a strong collaborative relationship among team members and improve client quality outcomes.

Nursing Care Delivery Models

Since the time of Florence Nightingale there has been a variety of nursing care delivery models, or methods nurses use to provide care for clients. Ideally, the vision and philosophy nurses establish for the quality care of clients guide the selection of a care delivery model. However, too often a lack of nursing resources and business plans from the health care organization influences the final decision. Care delivery has to be effective in helping nurses achieve desirable outcomes for their clients. Some important factors contributing to success are decision-making authority for nurses who provide direct care, autonomy, collaborative practice, and effective methods of communicating with colleagues, physicians, and other health care providers (Ritter-Teitel, 2002; Tiedeman and Lookinland, 2004). In the nursing models, an experienced RN acting as the clinical leader promotes the development of a safe client environment (Batcheller and others, 2004).

Team Nursing. **Team nursing** developed as a care delivery model in response to the severe nursing shortage following World War II (Marriner Tomey, 2004). In team nursing an RN leads a team that is made up of other RNs, licensed practical nurses (LPNs) or licensed vocational nurses (LVNs), and nurse assistants or technicians. The team members provide direct client care to groups of clients under the direction of the RN team leader. In this model, nurse assistants have client assignments rather than being assigned particular nursing tasks.

The team leader, an experienced RN, develops client care plans, coordinates care delivered by the nursing team, and provides care requiring complex nursing skills. The team leader also problem solves with physicians and members of other disciplines and assists the team in evaluating the effectiveness of their care (Wywialowski, 2004). Communication occurs in a hierarchy from charge nurse to charge nurse, charge nurse to team leader, and team leader to team members (Tiedeman and Lookinland, 2004).

One of the limitations of the model is that the team leader does not spend a large amount of time with clients. Depending on the mix of staff members, this sometimes means that clients see an RN infrequently. Risks exist if an RN is unable to make necessary client assessments and be involved in important clinical decision making. The task orientation of the model and the fact that nurses do not always have the same clients each day potentially cause a lack of continuity of care.

An advantage of team nursing is the collaborative style that encourages each member of the team to help the other members. This model has a high level of autonomy for the team leader and is an example of decision making occurring at a clinical level (Marriner Tomey, 2004).

Total Patient Care. **Total patient care** delivery was the original care delivery model developed during Florence Nightingale's time. The model disappeared in the 1930s and became popular during the 1970s and 1980s, when the number of RNs increased (Tiedeman and Lookinland, 2004). An RN is responsible for all aspects of care for one or more clients. The RN may delegate aspects of care to an LPN or unlicensed staff, but the RN is responsible for the care of all assigned clients. The nurse works directly with the client, family, physician, and health care team members. The model typically has a shift-based focus. The same nurse does not necessarily care for the same client over time. Continuity of care from shift to shift or day to day is a problem if staff members do not clearly communicate client needs to one another. Client satisfaction with the model is high, but total patient care is not cost-effective because it requires a high number of RNs to provide care (Tiedeman and Lookinland, 2004).

Primary Nursing. The **primary nursing** model of care delivery was developed to place RNs at the bedside and to improve nursing's accountability for client outcomes and the professional relationships among staff members (Marriner Tomey, 2004). The model became more popular in the 1970s and early 1980s as hospitals began to employ more RNs. Primary nursing supports a philosophy regarding nurse and client relationships.

Primary nursing is a model of care delivery in which the primary nurse assumes responsibility for a caseload of clients over time. Typically the RN selects the clients for his or her caseload and cares for the same clients during their hospitalization or stay in the health care setting. The primary nurse assesses client needs, develops a care plan, and makes sure that appropriate nursing interventions are delivered to the client. The model does not call for an all-RN staff. The model is flexible, and a variety of staffing levels and mixes are used in different health care settings (Tiedeman and Lookinland, 2004).

Primary nursing maintains continuity of care across shifts, days, or visits. The model is applicable in any health care setting. When a primary nurse is off-duty, associate nurses, including LPNs or other RNs, follow through with the developed plan of care. If there are differences in opinion as to client needs, associates and primary nurses work together to redefine the plan as needed. Communication in this model is lateral from nurse to nurse and caregiver to caregiver (Tiedeman and Lookinland, 2004).

Although primary nursing requires the presence of more professional staff members, this does not mean that the model is more costly. Care consistently managed by a single professional minimizes delays in therapies, improves collaboration with other professionals, and helps build the client-nurse relationship. In this model the RN has a high level of clinical autonomy and authority that enhances collaboration with physicians (Marriner Tomey, 2004).

✳ TABLE 21-1 Examples of Organizational Structures

STRUCTURAL APPROACH	CHARACTERISTICS
Centralized management	Single administrator leads organization, with directors overseeing departmental responsibilities. Typically decisions are made by virtue of a person's position in an organization. Decisions are made from top down, with minimal input from staff. Managers tend to have minimal responsibility or accountability for 24-hour operation of nursing unit.
Decentralized management	Structure appears similar to that of centralized organization. Often there are fewer directors. Those staff members who are most knowledgeable about a problem or issue make decisions on basis of knowledge. Managers often have 24-hour accountability and responsibility for staff, budget, and day-to-day management of work unit.
Matrix	Traditional hospital departments become reorganized into business units or specialized work units. Work groups of staff are formed to solve specific problems. Managers with special skills guide staff who often report to another manager.

Case Management. **Case management** is a care management approach that coordinates and links health care services to clients and their families while streamlining costs and maintaining quality (Wywialowski, 2004) (see Chapter 2). The Case Management Society of America (2006) defines case management as "a collaborative process of assessment, planning, facilitation and advocacy for options and services to meet an individual's health needs through communication and available resources to promote quality cost effective outcomes." What is unique about case management is that clinicians, either as individuals or as part of a collaborative group, oversee the management of clients with specific case types (e.g., clients with specific diagnoses presenting complex nursing and medical problems) and are usually held accountable for some standard of cost management and quality.

A case manager coordinates a client's acute care in the hospital, for example, and then follows up with the client after discharge home. Case managers do not always provide direct care but instead they work with and supervise the care delivered by other staff members and actively coordinate client discharge planning. In this situation the case manager helps the client identify health needs, what services and resources are available, and assists the client in determining what is cost-efficient (Kuntz, 2005). The case manager frequently oversees a caseload of clients with complex nursing and medical problems. Often the case manager is an advanced practice nurse who through specific interventions helps to improve client outcomes such as a decrease in readmissions to the hospital and to lower health care costs (Avitall, 2003).

Many organizations use critical pathways or CareMaps in a case management delivery system (see Chapter 18). These are multidisciplinary treatment plans that are for specific cases. The case manager, along with members of the health care team, uses the critical pathways or CareMaps to implement timely interventions in a coordinated plan of care. The plans eliminate the guesswork in client care because all members of the health care team work from the same plan.

Decentralized Decision Making

With a vision for nursing established, it is the manager who directs and supports staff in the realization of that vision. The nurse executive supports managers by establishing a structure that will help to achieve organizational goals and provide appropriate sup-

✳ BOX 21-3 Responsibilities of the Nurse Manager

- Assist staff in establishing annual goals for the unit and systems needed to accomplish goals.
- Monitor professional nursing standards of practice on the unit.
- Develop an ongoing staff development plan, including one for new employees.
- Recruit new employees (interview and hire).
- Conduct routine staff evaluations.
- Establish self as a role model for positive customer service (customers include clients, families, and other health care team members).
- Submit staffing schedules for the unit.
- Conduct regular client rounds and problem solve client or family complaints.
- Establish and implement a unit quality improvement plan.
- Review and recommend new equipment for the unit.
- Conduct regular staff meetings.
- Make rounds with physicians.
- Establish and support staff and interdisciplinary committees.

port to care delivery staff (Table 21-1). It takes a committed nurse executive, an excellent manager, and empowered nursing staff to create an enriching work environment where nursing practice thrives.

Decentralized management, in which decision making is moved down to the level of staff, is very common within health care organizations. This type of management structure has the advantage of creating an environment where managers and staff become more actively involved in shaping a health care organization's identity and determining success. Working in a decentralized structure has the potential for greater collaborative effort, increased competency of staff, increased staff motivation, and ultimately a greater sense of professional accomplishment and satisfaction.

It is clear that progressive organizations achieve more when employees at all levels are actively involved. As a result, the role of a nurse manager has become critical in the management of effective nursing units or groups. Box 21-3 highlights the diverse responsibilities nursing managers assume. To make decentralized decision making work, managers must know how to move decision making down to the lowest level possible. On a nursing unit, it is important for all nursing staff members (RNs, LPNs, and LVNs), nurse assistants, and unit secretaries to become involved. This means that they must be kept well informed and given the opportunity by managers to participate in problem-solving activities. This includes opportunities in direct client care, as well as unit activities such as committee participation. Important elements to the decision-making process are responsibility, autonomy, authority, and accountability (Anders and Hawkins, 2006).

Responsibility refers to the duties and activities that an individual is employed to perform. A professional nurse's responsibilities in a given role are outlined in a position description describing the nurse's duties in client care and in participating as a member of the nursing unit.

Responsibility reflects ownership. The individual who manages the employee has to distribute responsibility, and the employee has to accept it. Managers have to be sure that staff clearly understand their responsibilities, particularly in the face of change. For example, when hospitals participate in work redesign, client care delivery models change significantly. It is the manager's responsibility to clearly define the RN's role within the new care delivery model. If decentralized decision making is in place, professional staff have a voice in identifying the new RN role. Each RN on the work team is responsible for knowing his or her role and how to perform that role on the busy nursing unit. For example, a primary nurse is responsible for completing a nursing assessment of all assigned clients and for developing a plan of care that addresses each of the client's nursing diagnoses (see Unit III). As the staff delivers the plan of care, the primary nurse is responsible for evaluating whether the plan is successful. This responsibility becomes a work ethic for the nurse in delivering excellent client care.

Autonomy is freedom of choice and responsibility for the choices (Marriner Tomey, 2004). Autonomy consistent with the scope of professional nursing practice will maximize your effectiveness as a nurse (Hicks, 2003). With autonomy, a professional nurse makes independent decisions about client care. The nurse plans care for the client within the scope of professional nursing practice and provides the client independent nursing interventions without physician permission (see Chapter 18). Autonomy is not an absolute, but occurs in degrees. Innovation by nurses, increased productivity, higher nurse retention, and greater client satisfaction are results of autonomy in nursing practice (Hicks, 2003). For example, a nurse has the autonomy to develop and implement a discharge teaching plan based on specific client needs for any client who has been hospitalized. The nurse provides nursing care that complements the prescribed medical therapy.

Authority refers to legitimate power to give commands and make final decisions specific to a given position (Anders and Hawkins, 2006; Marriner Tomey, 2004). For example, a primary nurse, managing a caseload of clients, discovers that members of the nursing team did not follow through on a discharge teaching plan for an assigned client. The primary nurse has the authority to consult other nurses to learn why the team did not follow recommendations on the plan of care and to choose appropriate teaching strategies for the client that all members of the team will follow. The primary nurse has the final authority in selecting the best course of action for the client's care.

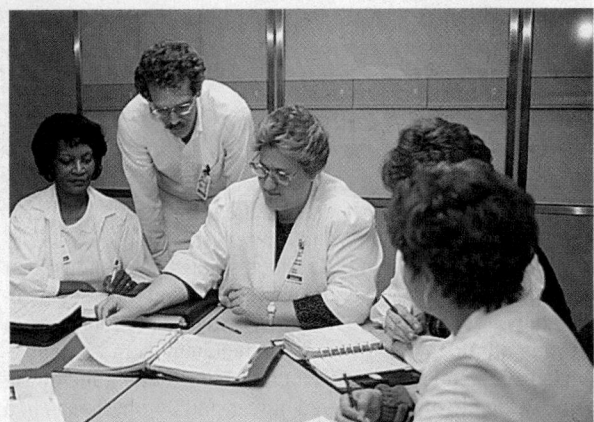

Figure 21-1 Staff collaborating on practice issues.

Accountability refers to individuals being answerable for their actions. It means that as a nurse, you accept the commitment to provide excellent client care and the responsibility for the outcomes of the actions in providing that care (Anders and Hawkins, 2006). A primary nurse is accountable for his or her clients' outcomes and for ensuring that the client learns the information necessary to improve self-care. The nurse demonstrates accountability in checking on the client and family after discharge and in reviewing with the nursing team whether continuity in teaching occurred.

A successful decentralized nursing unit exercises on an ongoing basis the four elements of decision making: responsibility, autonomy, authority, and accountability. An effective manager sets the same expectations for the staff in how decisions are made. Staff routinely meet to discuss and negotiate how to maintain an equality and balance in the elements. Staff members need to feel comfortable in expressing differences of opinion and in challenging ways in which the team functions, while recognizing their own responsibility, autonomy, authority, and accountability. Ultimately, decentralized decision making helps create the unit's vision of professional nursing care.

Staff Involvement. When decentralized decision making exists on a nursing unit, all staff members actively participate in unit activities (Figure 21-1). The influence and control nurses have over their own practice contributes to job satisfaction (Ulrich and others, 2005). Because the work environment promotes participation, all staff members benefit from the knowledge and skills of the entire work group. If the staff learns to value knowledge and the contributions of co-workers, better client care becomes an outcome. Experienced RNs provide leadership and mentoring on a nursing unit while promoting collaborative practice (Batcheller and others, 2004). The nursing manager supports staff involvement through a variety of approaches:

1. *Establishment of nursing practice or problem-solving committees or professional* **shared governance** *councils.* Chaired by senior clinical staff, these groups establish and maintain care standards for nursing practice on their work unit. The committees review and establish standards of care, develop policy and procedures, resolve client satisfaction issues, or develop new

✴ BOX 21-4 EVIDENCE-BASED PRACTICE

Individual Characteristics and Perceptions of Collaboration in the Work Environment

Evidence Summary

Collaboration of health care team members is required to help meet the complex needs of clients in health care settings. Previous studies have shown that nurse-physician collaboration improves client outcomes. In this study, researchers wanted to investigate the relationship between attitudes toward team, commitment to the organization, and perceptions of collaboration among nurses and physicians. A sample of 71 registered nurses and 34 physicians in a Midwest hospital were surveyed using several questionnaires. Results showed that individuals who had stronger orientation to team and commitment to the organization had increased perceptions of collaboration on the unit. It was found that the organization plays an important role in creating an environment and culture that values and promotes collaboration.

Application to Nursing Practice

- Promoting an environment that values teamwork encourages collaborative relationships.
- Open communication between health care team members is critical to the collaboration process.
- Commitment to the organization impacts the nurse-physician collaborative relationship.
- Organizational resources need to be directed toward developing interdisciplinary collaboration.

Reference

Tschannen D: The effect of individual characteristics on perceptions of collaboration in the work environment, *Medsurg Nurs* 13(5):312, 2004.

documentation tools. It is important for the committees to focus on client outcomes rather than only work issues in order to ensure quality care on the unit. Quality of care is further improved when nurses are in control of their own practice (Anders and Hawkins, 2006). The committee establishes methods or systems to ensure that all staff have input or participation on practice issues. Managers do not always sit on a committee, but they receive regular reports of committee progress. The nature of work on the nursing unit determines committee membership. At times, members of other disciplines, for example, pharmacy, respiratory therapy, or clinical nutrition, participate in practice committees or shared governance councils.

2. *Nurse/physician collaborative practice.* Collaboration is a process whereby different perspectives are synthesized to better understand complex problems and an outcome that is a shared solution that could not have been accomplished by a single person or organization (Gardner, 2005). The nursing unit's care delivery model, environment support of teamwork, and organizational values influence how nurses and physicians collaborate (Box 21-4) (Tschannen, 2004). If the unit practices team nursing, it is important for team leaders to regularly participate in physician rounds. If the unit practices primary nursing, the physician communicates either

with each primary nurse or the associate nurse who is assuming care for the client on that day. In a home care or extended care setting, staff members are able to contact physicians with minimal delay and are able to work together on decisions regarding client care. The manager avoids taking care of problems for the staff. Instead, staff members learn to keep physicians informed on what is important regarding their clients. An open communication system that fosters respect, trust, and teamwork between all team members is critical (Hambleton, 2005; Schmalenberg and others, 2005). Physicians sometimes attend practice committees when clinical problems arise and present timely in-service programs on new medical procedures or research findings.

3. *Interdisciplinary collaboration.* The emphasis on efficiency in health care delivery brings all members of the health care team together. Whenever systems or programs are redesigned, interdisciplinary involvement is necessary because most health care processes involve more than one discipline. Mutual respect is a critical part of any collaborative relationship (Ulrich and others, 2005). Gardner (2005) identified essential competencies for collaborative partnerships, including good interpersonal skills, learning to value and manage diversity, developing good conflict resolution skills, learning to create win-win situations, and balancing autonomy and unity in the collaborative relationship. All decisions do not require collaboration (Gardner, 2005). Use your judgment to decide what problems are complex and require a collaborative process. At the client care level, the staff recognizes the importance of prompt referrals and timely communication with other health professionals. Including representatives of the various disciplines together in practice projects, in-service programs, conferences, and staff meetings encourages interdisciplinary collaboration.

4. *Staff communication.* A manager's greatest challenge, especially if a work group is large, is communication with staff. It is difficult to make sure that all staff members receive the same message: the correct message. In the present health care environment, staff quickly become uneasy and distrusting if they fail to hear about planned changes on their work unit. However, a manager cannot assume total responsibility for all communication. Instead, the manager uses a variety of approaches to communicate quickly and accurately to all staff. For example, many managers distribute biweekly or monthly newsletters of ongoing unit or health care agency activities. Minutes of committee meetings are usually in an accessible location for all staff to read. When the team needs to discuss important issues regarding the operations of the unit, the manager conducts staff meetings. When the unit has practice or quality improvement committees, each committee member has the responsibility to communicate directly to a select number of staff. In that way, all staff are contacted and given the opportunity for input.

5. *Staff education.* A professional nursing staff needs to always grow in knowledge. It is impossible to remain knowledgeable of current medical and nursing practice trends without ongoing education. The nurse manager is responsible for making learning opportunities available so that staff members remain competent in their practice. This involves planning in-service programs, sending staff to continuing education classes and

professional conferences, and having staff present case studies or practice issues during staff meetings. Staff members are responsible for pursuing educational opportunities when they know that their competencies are lacking.

Leadership Skills for Nursing Students

It is important that as a nursing student, you prepare yourself for leadership roles. This does not mean that you have to quickly learn how to lead a team of nursing staff. Nursing students first learn to become dependable and competent providers of client care. As a nursing student, you have a responsibility for the care given to your clients and assume accountability for that care. Learn to become a leader by consulting with instructors and nursing staff to get feedback in making good clinical decisions, learning from mistakes and seeking guidance, working closely with professional nurses, and trying to improve your performance during each client interaction. Important leadership skills to learn include clinical care coordination, team communication, delegation, and knowledge building.

Clinical Care Coordination

You will acquire the skills necessary so that you can deliver client care in a timely and effective manner. In the beginning, this often involves only one client but eventually will involve groups of clients. Clinical care coordination includes clinical decision making, priority setting, use of organizational skills and resources, time management, and evaluation.

Clinical Decisions. When you begin an assignment with a client, the first activity involves a focused but complete assessment of the client's condition so you are able to make an accurate clinical decision as to the client's health problems and required nursing therapies. This initial contact is also an important first step in developing a caring relationship with a client. Use a critical thinking approach, applying previous knowledge and experience to the decision-making process (see Chapter 15).

The nursing process offers a framework to determine the level of care a client requires to implement the plan of care and to evaluate its results (see Unit III). If you do not make accurate clinical judgments about a client, undesirable outcomes will probably occur. The client's condition worsens or remains the same when you lose the potential for improvement. An important lesson in organizational skills is to be thorough. Learn to attend and listen to the client, look for any cues (obvious or subtle) that point to a pattern of findings, and direct the assessment to explore the pattern further. Accurate clinical decision making keeps you focused on the proper course of action. Never hesitate to ask for assistance when a client's assessment reveals a changing clinical condition.

Priority Setting. After forming a picture of the client's total needs, you set priorities by deciding on what client needs or problems need to be cared for first (see Chapter 18). It is important to prioritize in all caregiving situations because it allows you to see relationships between client problems and avoid delays in taking action that might cause serious complications for a client (Hendry and Walker, 2004). If a client is experiencing serious physiological or psychological problems, the priority becomes clear. It becomes essential to act immediately to stabilize the client's condition. Hendry and Walker (2004) classify client problems in three priority levels:

- *High priority*—An immediate threat to a client's survival or safety, such as a physiological episode of obstructed airway, loss of consciousness, or a psychological episode of an anxiety attack.
- *Intermediate priority*—Nonemergency, non–life-threatening actual or potential needs that the client and family members are experiencing. Anticipating teaching needs of clients related to a new drug or taking measures to decrease postoperative complications are examples of intermediate priorities.
- *Low priority*—Actual or potential problems that may not be directly related to the client's illness or disease. These problems are often related to the client's developmental needs and or long-term health care needs. An example of a low priority is a client at admission who will eventually be discharged and who needs teaching for self-care in the home.

Many clients have all three types of priorities, requiring a nurse to make careful judgments in choosing a course of action. Obviously high-priority needs demand immediate attention. When a client has diverse priority needs, it helps to focus on the client's basic needs. For example, a client who is in traction reports being uncomfortable from being in the same position. The dietary assistant arrives in the room to deliver a meal tray. Instead of immediately assisting the client with the meal, you reposition the client and offer basic hygiene measures. The client will likely become more interested in eating after he is more comfortable. The client will also then be more receptive to any instruction you want to provide.

Eventually you will be required to meet the priority needs of a group of clients. This means you need to know the priority needs of each client within the group, assessing each client's needs as soon as possible while addressing high priorities first. To identify which clients require assessment first, rely on information from the change-of-shift report, the agency's classification system that identifies client acuity, and information from the medical record. Over time you will learn to spontaneously rank clients' needs by priority or urgency. It is important to think about the resources available, to be flexible in recognizing that priority needs can change, and to consider how to use time wisely.

You also make priorities on the basis of client expectations. Sometimes you will have an excellent plan of care established, but if the client is resistant to certain therapies or disagrees with the approach, you will have very little success. Working closely with the client and showing a caring attitude is important. Share the priorities you have defined with the client to establish a level of agreement and cooperation.

Organizational Skills. Implementing a plan of care requires you to be effective and efficient. Effective use of time means doing the right things, whereas efficient use of time means doing things right (Wywialowski, 2004). Learn to become efficient by combining various nursing activities—in other words, doing more than one thing at a time. For example, during medication administration or while obtaining a specimen, combine therapeutic communication skills, teaching interventions, and assessment and evaluation. Always try to establish and strengthen relationships with clients, and use any client contact as an opportunity to convey important information. Client interaction also provides you an opportunity to show caring and interest in the client. Always attend to the client's behaviors and responses to therapies to assess if any new problems are developing and to evaluate responses to interventions.

As a well-organized nurse, you approach any planned procedures by having all of the necessary equipment available and making sure the client is prepared. Being sure the client is comfortable and well informed will increase the likelihood that the procedure will go smoothly. Sometimes you require the assistance of colleagues to perform or complete a procedure. It is always wise to have the work area organized and preliminary steps completed before asking co-workers for assistance.

As you begin to deliver care based on established priorities, events sometimes occur within the health care setting that can interfere with plans. For example, just as you begin to provide morning hygiene for a hospitalized client, an x-ray technician enters to take a chest film. Once the technician completes the x-ray examination, a phlebotomist arrives to draw a sample of blood. In such a case the nurse's priorities seem to conflict with the priorities of other health care personnel. It is important to always keep the client's needs as the center of attention. The client may have experienced symptoms earlier that required a chest film and laboratory work. In such a case it is important to be sure that the diagnostic tests are completed. In another example, a client is waiting to visit family, and a chest film is a routine order from 2 days earlier. The client's condition has stabilized, and the x-ray technician is willing to return later to shoot the film. In this situation attending to the client's hygiene and comfort so that family members can visit is more of a priority at this time.

Use of Resources. Appropriate use of resources is another important aspect of clinical care coordination. Resources in this case include members of the health care team. In any setting the administration of client care occurs more smoothly when staff members work together. Never hesitate to have staff assist you, especially when there is an opportunity to make a procedure or activity more comfortable and safer for the client. For example, assistance in turning, positioning, and ambulating clients is frequently necessary when clients are unable to move. Having a staff member assist with handling equipment and supplies during more complicated procedures such as catheter insertion or dressing change will help make procedures more efficient. This is an excellent way to learn how to work with assistive personnel. There are also times when you have to recognize personal limitations and use professional resources for assistance. For example, you assess a client and find relevant clinical signs and symptoms but are unfamiliar with the physical condition. Consulting with an RN confirms findings and ensures that you take the proper course of action for the client. Throughout your professional career there are always new experiences. A leader knows his or her limitations and seeks professional colleagues for guidance and support.

Time Management. Changes in health care and increasing complexity of clients creates stress for nurses as they work to meet client needs (Marriner Tomey, 2004). One way to manage this stress is through the use of time management skills. These skills involve learning how, where, and when to use your time. Your attitude and value of time affect time management (Wywialowski, 2004). Because you have a limited amount of time with clients, it is essential to remain goal oriented and to use time wisely. You will quickly learn the importance of using client goals as a way to identify priorities. However, also learn how to establish personal goals and time frames. For example, you are caring for two clients on a busy surgical nursing unit. One had surgery the day before, and the other will be discharged the next day. Clearly, the first client's goals center on restoring physiological function impaired as a result of the stress of surgery. The second client's goals center on adequate preparation to assume self-care at home. In reviewing the therapies required for both clients, you learn how to organize your time so that the activities of care, as well as client goals, are achieved. You need to anticipate when care will be interrupted for medication administration and any diagnostic testing and when is the best time for planned therapies such as dressing changes, client education, and client ambulation.

One useful time management skill involves keeping a to-do list. When you first begin working with a client or clients, it helps to make a list that sequences the nursing activities you need to perform. The change-of-shift report helps in sequencing activities based on what you learn about the client's condition and the care provided before you arrive on the unit. It is helpful to consider activities that have specific time limits in terms of addressing client needs, such as administering a pain medication before a scheduled procedure or instructing clients before their discharge home. You will also analyze the items on the list that are scheduled by agency policies or routines (e.g., medications or intravenous [IV] tubing changes). Note which activities need to be done on time and which activities you can do at your discretion (Wywialowski, 2004). You have to administer medication within a specific schedule, but you are also able to perform other activities while in the client's room. Finally, estimate the amount of time needed to complete the various activities. Activities requiring the assistance of other staff members usually take longer because you have to plan around their schedules.

Good time management also involves completing one task before starting another. If possible, complete the activities started with one client before moving on to the next. Care will then become less fragmented, and you will better able to focus on what you are doing for each client. As a result, it is less likely that you will make errors. Time management requires an ability to anticipate the day's activities, to combine activities when possible, and to avoid interruption by nonessential activities. Box 21-5 summarizes principles of time management.

Evaluation. Evaluation is one of the most important aspects of clinical care coordination (see Chapter 20). It is a mistake to think that evaluation occurs at the end of an activity. Evaluation is an

BOX 21-5 Principles of Time Management

Goal setting: Review the client's goals of care for the day and any goals you have for activities, such as completing documentation, attending a client care conference, giving a staff report, or preparing medications for administration.

Time analysis: Reflect on how you use your time. While working on a clinical area, keep track of how you use your time in different activities. This will provide valuable information to reveal how well organized you really are.

Priority setting: Set the priorities that you have established for clients within set time frames. Determine when is the best time, for example, to have teaching sessions, plan ambulation, and provide rest periods, based on what you know about the client's condition. For example, if a client is nauseated or in pain, it is not a good time for a teaching session.

Interruption control: Everyone needs time to socialize or to discuss issues with colleagues. However, do not let this interrupt important client care activities such as medication administration. Use time during report, mealtime, or team meetings to the best of your advantage. Also, plan time to assist fellow colleagues so that it complements your client care schedule.

Evaluation: At the end of each day, take time to think and reflect about how effectively you used your time. If you are having difficulties, discuss them with an instructor or a more experienced staff member.

ongoing process. Once you assess a client's needs and begin therapies directed at a specific problem area, immediately evaluate if therapies are effective and the client's response. The process of evaluation compares actual client outcomes with expected outcomes. For example, a clinic nurse assesses a foot ulcer of a client who has diabetes to determine if healing has progressed since the last clinic visit. When expected outcomes are not met, evaluation reveals the need to continue current therapies for a longer period, revise approaches to care, or introduce new therapies. As you care for a client throughout the day, it is important to anticipate when to return to the bedside to evaluate care, for example, 30 minutes after a medication was administered, 15 minutes after an IV line has begun infusing, or 60 minutes after discussing discharge instructions with the client and family.

Keeping a focus on evaluation of the client's progress lessens the chance of becoming distracted by the tasks of care. It is common to assume that staying focused on planned activities ensures that you will perform care appropriately. However, task orientation does not ensure good client outcomes. Learn that at the heart of good organizational skills is the constant inquiry into the client's condition and progress toward an improved level of health.

Team Communication

As a part of a nursing team, you are responsible for open, professional communication. Regardless of the setting, an enriching, professional environment is one in which staff members respect one another's ideas, share information, and keep one another informed. On a busy nursing unit this means keeping colleagues informed about clients with emerging problems, physicians who have been called for consultation, and unique approaches that

solved a complex nursing problem. In a clinic setting it may mean sharing unusual diagnostic findings or conveying important information regarding a client's source of family support. One way of fostering good team communication is by setting expectations of one another. A nurse treats colleagues with respect, listens to the ideas of other staff members without interruption, and is honest and direct while communicating. Part of good communication is clarifying what others are saying and building on the merits of coworkers' ideas (Marriner Tomey, 2004). An efficient team knows it is able to count on all members when needs arise. Sharing expectations of what, when, and how to communicate is a step toward establishing a strong work team.

Delegation

The art of effective delegation is a skill you need to observe and practice to improve your own management skills. The American Nurses Association (1995) defines **delegation** as transferring responsibility for the performance of an activity or task while retaining accountability for the outcome. Delegation results in improved efficiency, increased productivity, and development of others (Curtis and Nicholl, 2004; Marriner Tomey, 2004). Asking a staff member to obtain an ordered specimen while you attend to a client's pain medication request effectively prevents a delay in the client gaining pain relief and accomplishes two tasks related to the client. Delegation also provides job enrichment. You show trust in colleagues by delegating tasks to them and showing staff members that they are important players in the delivery of care. Never delegate a task that you dislike doing or would not do independently because this will create negative feelings and poor working relationships. For example, if you are in the room when a client asks to be placed on a bedpan, you should assist the client rather than leave the room to find the nurse assistant. Remember that even though the delegation of a task transfers the responsibility and authority to another person, you retain accountability for the delegated task.

As a nurse, you are responsible and accountable for providing care to clients and will delegate care activities to assistive personnel. Because the steps of the nursing process of assessment, planning, and evaluation require you to use nursing judgment, you will not delegate these activities (American Nurses Association [ANA] and National Council of State Boards of Nursing [NCSBN], 2006). It is important to recognize that when you are delegating to assistive personnel, you delegate tasks, not clients. Do not give assistive personnel sole responsibility for the care of clients. Instead, it is you as the professional nurse in charge of client care who decides what activities assistive personnel may perform independently and what activities the RN and assistant perform in partnership. One way to accomplish this is to have the RN and technician or nurse assistant conduct rounds together. You are able to assess each client as the technician helps to attend to basic client needs. Care is delegated based upon assessment findings and priority setting. As an RN, you will always be responsible for the assessment of a client's ongoing status, but if a client is stable, you delegate vital sign monitoring to the assistive personnel. The RN is the one in most settings who decides when delegation is appropriate. The LPN directs care in many long-term care facilities. The National Council of State Boards of Nursing (1995) has provided some guidelines

---

✳ BOX 21-6 The Five Rights of Delegation

Right Task
The right task is one that is delegable for a specific client, such as tasks that are repetitive, require little supervision, are relatively noninvasive, have results that are predictable, and the potential risk is minimal.

Right Circumstances
The appropriate client setting, available resources, and other relevant factors are considered. In an acute care setting, clients' conditions can change quickly. Good clinical decision making is needed to determine what to delegate.

Right Person
The right person is delegating the right tasks to the right person to be performed on the right person.

Right Direction/Communication
A clear, concise description of the task, including its objective, limits, and expectations, is given. Communication must be ongoing between RN and assistive personnel during a shift of care.

Right Supervision
Appropriate monitoring, evaluation, intervention as needed, and feedback are provided. Assistive personnel should feel comfortable asking questions and seeking assistance.

Modified from National Council of State Boards of Nursing: *Delegation: concepts and decision-making process*, Chicago, 1995, The Council; National Council of State Boards of Nursing, *The five rights of delegation*, Chicago, 1997, The Council; and American Nurses Association (ANA) and National Council of State Boards of Nursing (NCSBN): *Joint statement on delegation*, http://www.ncsbn.org/pdfs/Joint_statement.pdf, 2006.

---

for delegation of tasks in accordance with an RN's legal scope of practice (Box 21-6). As the leader of the health care team, the RN gives clear instructions, effectively prioritizes client needs and therapies, and gives staff timely and meaningful feedback. Assistive personnel respond positively when they are included as part of the nursing team.

As a professional nurse, you cannot simply assign assistive personnel to tasks without considering the implications. Assess a client, and determine a plan of care before identifying which tasks someone else is able to perform. When directing assistive personnel, determine how much supervision is necessary. Is it the first time a staff member performed the task? Does the client present a complicating factor whereby the RN's assistance is necessary? Does the staff member have prior experience with a particular type of client in addition to having received training on skill performance? The final responsibility is to evaluate whether assistive personnel performed a task properly and whether desired outcomes were met.

Appropriate delegation begins with knowing what skills you are able to delegate. This requires you to be familiar with the state's Nurse Practice Act, institutional policies and procedures, and the institution's job description for assistive personnel. These standards help to define the necessary level of competency of assistive personnel.

An institution's policies and procedures and job description for assistive personnel provide specific guidelines in regard to what tasks or activities a nurse is able to delegate. The job description identifies any required education and the types of tasks assistive personnel can perform, either independently or with RN direct supervision. Institutional policy helps in defining the amount of training required of assistive personnel while employed. Procedures detail who is qualified to perform a given nursing procedure, whether supervision is necessary, and the type of reporting required. You need to have a means to easily access policies or have supervisory staff who will inform you about assistive personnel's job duties.

Efficient delegation requires constant communication—sending clear messages and listening so that all participants understand expectations regarding client care. Provide clear instructions when delegating tasks. These instructions initially focus on the procedure itself and what will be accomplished, as well as on the unique needs of a given client. The RN also communicates when and what information to report, such as expected observations and specific client concerns (NCSBN, 2005). Communication is viewed as a two-way process in delegation, so the assistive personnel need to have the chance to ask questions and have your expectations made clear (ANA and NCSBN, 2006). As you become more familiar with a staff member's competency, trust builds and the staff will need fewer instructions, but clarification of clients' specific needs will always be necessary.

Another important step in delegation is evaluation of the staff member's performance, achievement of the client's outcomes, the communication process used, and any problems or concerns that occurred (NCSBN, 2005). When assistive personnel perform the task correctly and do a good job, it is important to provide praise and recognition. If the staff member's performance is not satisfactory, give constructive and appropriate feedback. As a nurse, always give specific feedback in regard to any mistakes that staff members make, explaining how to avoid the mistake or a better way to handle the situation. Giving feedback in private is the professional way and preserves the staff member's dignity. In giving the feedback, make sure to focus on things that are changeable, choose only one issue at a time, and give specific details (Case, 2004). Frequently when the performance of assistive personnel does not meet expectations, the cause is due to inadequate training or assignment to too many tasks. You discover the need to review a procedure with staff and offer demonstration or even recommend that additional training be scheduled with the education department. If too many tasks are being delegated, this might be a nursing practice issue. All staff should discuss the appropriateness of delegation on their unit. Sometimes assistive personnel need help in learning how to prioritize. In some cases, you will need to learn that you are overdelegating.

Here are a few tips on appropriate delegation (Keeling and others, 2000):

- *Assess the knowledge and skills of the delegate:* Determine what the person knows and what he or she is able to do by asking open-ended questions that will elicit conversation and details on he or she knows; for example, "How do you usually put the cuff on when you measure a blood pressure?" or "Tell me how you prepare the tubing before you give an enema."
- *Match tasks to the delegate's skills:* Know what skills are in the training program for assistive personnel at your facility. Determine if personnel have learned critical thinking skills, such as knowing when a client is in harm or knowing the difference

between normal clinical findings and changes to report.

- *Communicate clearly:* Always provide clear directions by describing a task, the desired outcome, and the time period within which assistive personnel should complete the task. Never give instructions through another staff member. Make the person feel as though he or she is part of the team. For example, "I'd like you to help me by getting Mr. Floyd up to ambulate before lunch. Be sure to check his blood pressure before he stands, and write your finding on the graphic sheet. OK?"
- *Listen attentively:* Listen to the response of assistive personnel after you provide directions. Do they feel comfortable in asking questions or requesting clarification? If you encourage a response, listen to what the person has to say. Be especially attentive if the staff member has been given a deadline to meet by another nurse. Help sort out priorities.
- *Provide feedback:* Always give assistive personnel feedback regarding performance, regardless of outcome. Let them know of a job well done. If an outcome is undesirable, find a private place to discuss what occurred, any miscommunication, and how to achieve a better outcome in the future.

Knowledge Building

As a professional nurse, recognize the importance of pursuing knowledge to remain competent. A leader recognizes that there is always something new to learn. Opportunities for learning occur with each client interaction, each encounter with a professional colleague, and each meeting or class session where health care professionals meet to discuss clinical care issues. There is always someone who has had different experiences and knowledge. Inservice programs, workshops, and collegiate courses offer innovative and current information on the rapidly changing world of health care. To become a leader, actively pursue learning opportunities, both formal and informal, and learn to share knowledge with the professional colleagues you encounter.

✳ Key Concepts

- A manager sets a vision or philosophy for a work unit, ensures appropriate staffing, mobilizes staff and institutional resources to achieve objectives, motivates staff members to carry out their work, sets standards of performance, and makes the right decisions to achieve objectives.
- Consideration communicates mutual trust, respect, and rapport between the manager and staff members.
- Empowering staff members brings out the best in a manager and allows him or her to concentrate on effective client care systems, to support risk taking and innovation, and to focus on results and rewards.
- An empowered nursing staff has decision-making authority to change how they practice.
- Nursing care delivery models vary by the responsibility and autonomy of the RN in coordinating care delivery and the roles other staff members play in assisting with care.
- Primary nursing increases nursing autonomy and improves collaboration between nurses and health care providers.

- Critical to the success of decentralized decision making is making staff members aware that they have the responsibility, authority, autonomy, and accountability for the care they give and the decisions they make.
- A nurse manager encourages decentralized decision making by establishing nursing practice committees, supporting nurse-physician and interdisciplinary collaboration, setting and implementing quality improvement plans, and maintaining timely staff communication.
- Clinical care coordination involves accurate clinical decision making, establishing priorities, efficient organizational skills, appropriate use of resources and time management skills, and an ongoing evaluation of care activities.
- To promote an enriching professional environment, each member of a nursing work team is responsible for open, professional communication.
- Effective delegation requires the use of good communication skills.
- When done correctly, delegation improves job efficiency, productivity, and job enrichment.
- An important responsibility for the nurse who delegates nursing care is evaluation of the staff member's performance and client outcomes.

✳ Critical Thinking Exercises

1. You are the nurse on a cardiac step-down unit. You have just received morning shift report on your clients. You have been assigned the following clients. Which client do you need to see first? Explain your answer.
   a. Mr. Dodson, a 52-year-old man who was admitted yesterday with a diagnosis of angina pectoris. He is scheduled for a cardiac stress test at 0900.
   b. Mrs. Wallace, a 60-year old woman who was transferred out of intensive care at 0630 today. She had uncomplicated coronary artery bypass surgery yesterday.
   c. Mr. Workman, a 45-year-old man who experienced a myocardial infarction 2 days ago. He is complaining of chest pain rated as 5 on a scale of 0 to 10.
   d. Mrs. Harris, a 76-year-old woman who had a permanent pacemaker inserted yesterday. She is complaining of incision pain rated as a 6 on a scale of 0 to 10.

2. John, another RN working on your floor, is paired with Tammy, a nursing assistant, to manage care for five clients. John has completed morning assessments and rounds on the assigned clients, and you overhear him giving Tammy directions for what she needs to do in the next hour. John says to Tammy, "Why don't you go to room 415 and see if Mr. Thomas needs anything, and go to room 418 to check if Mrs. Landry is doing all right." Based on what you know about delegation, did John give appropriate or inappropriate directions to Tammy? Provide a rationale for your answer.

3. You are the newly hired nursing care manager on the surgical unit in your hospital. Develop a plan to build an empowered nursing team on your unit.

✷ NCLEX®-Style Review Questions

1. After 0700 shift report the registered nurse (RN), Joan, delegates three tasks to Susan, the nursing assistant. At 1300, Joan tells Susan she would like to talk to her about the first task that was delegated, which was walking Mrs. Taylor in the morning. Joan said to Susan, "You did a good job walking Mrs. Taylor by 0930. I saw that you recorded her pulse before and after the walk. I saw that Mrs. Taylor walked in the hallway barefoot. For safety, the next time you walk a client you need to make sure that the client wears slippers or shoes. Please walk Mrs. Taylor again by 1500." What are the characteristics of good feedback that Joan used when talking to Susan? (Choose all that apply.)
   1. Feedback is given immediately.
   2. Feedback focuses on one issue.
   3. Feedback offers concrete details.
   4. Feedback identifies ways to improve.
   5. Feedback focuses on changeable things.
   6. Feedback is specific about what is incorrectly done only.

2. As the nurse, you need to complete all of the following. Which task do you complete first?
   1. Cough and deep breathe the client who had surgery yesterday.
   2. Make a referral to the home care nurse for a client who is being discharged in 2 days.
   3. Do the teaching on wound care for a client with a wound drain who is being discharged later today.
   4. Notify the health care provider of the decreased level of consciousness in the client who had a stroke yesterday.

3. You are the charge nurse on a surgical unit. You are doing staff assignments for the 3 to 11 shift. Which client do you assign to the licensed practical nurse (LPN)?
   1. Mr. Lilly, who had a total laryngectomy yesterday
   2. Mrs. Amber, who had a mastectomy this morning
   3. Mrs. Ellis, who had a vaginal hysterectomy 2 days ago
   4. Mr. Thielan, who is being discharged this evening following total colectomy

4. The type of care management approach that coordinates and links health care services to clients and their families while streamlining costs and maintaining quality is:
   1. Primary nursing
   2. Total patient care
   3. Functional nursing
   4. Case management

5. While administering medications, the nurse realizes she has given the wrong dose of medication to a client. The nurse acts by completing an incident report and notifying the client's physician. The nurse is exercising:
   1. Authority
   2. Responsibility
   3. Accountability
   4. Decision making

6. Many managers distribute biweekly newsletters of ongoing unit or health care agency activities and post minutes of committee meetings in an accessible location for all staff to read. This is an example of:
   1. Staff communication
   2. Problem-solving committees
   3. Interdisciplinary collaboration
   4. Nurse-physician collaborative practice

7. During the morning rounds a nurse assesses the client's condition. He had major heart surgery 2 days ago. His vital signs are stable, and his incision is clean and healing well. He complains of pain in his lower leg where the vein graft was removed. The nurse finds that the intravenous (IV) infusion is running on time, but only 100 ml remains before the infusion runs out. An order exists for the IV infusion to continue. A second order of priority is:
   1. The need to replace the IV bag with a new one
   2. The need to instruct the client on complications of wound healing
   3. The need to have an analgesic administered to the client for his leg pain
   4. The need for the nurse to determine if the pharmacy has delivered IV solutions ordered for the day

8. A client is experiencing an anxiety attack. This is which priority nursing need for this client?
   1. Low priority
   2. High priority
   3. Intermediate priority
   4. Nonemergency priority

9. The nurse checks on her client who was admitted to the hospital with pneumonia. He has been coughing profusely and has required nasotracheal suctioning. He has an IV infusion of antibiotics. He is febrile. The client asks the nurse if he can have a bath because he has been perspiring profusely. The nurse delegates to the nursing assistant working with her today the task of:
   1. Assessing vital signs
   2. Changing IV dressing
   3. Nasotracheal suctioning
   4. Administering a bed bath

10. Which task is appropriate for an RN to delegate to the nursing assistant?
    1. Explaining to the client about the preparation for an abdominal CT scan
    2. Administering the contrast medium to the client for an abdominal CT scan
    3. Obtaining the intravenous solution that is to be started before the client's CT scan
    4. Assessing vital signs on a client who is having an abdominal computed tomography (CT) scan later in the morning

22 | Ethics and Values

OBJECTIVES

Mastery of the content in this chapter will enable the student to:
- Discuss the role of ethics in professional nursing.
- Discuss the role of values in the study of ethics.
- Examine and clarify personal values.
- Describe general philosophies of health care ethics.

- Explain a nursing perspective in ethics.
- Apply critical thinking to ethical dilemmas.
- Discuss contemporary ethical issues.

MEDIA RESOURCES   KEY TERMS

 Companion CD
- NCLEX®-Style Review Questions
- Audio Glossary
- Interactive Learning Activities
- English/Spanish Glossary

evolve Website
- NCLEX®-Style Review Questions
- Audio Glossary
- English/Spanish Glossary
- Interactive Learning Activities
- WebLinks
- Audio Summaries

Accountability, p. 315
Advocacy, 314
Autonomy, p. 314
Beneficence, p. 314
Code of ethics, p. 314
Confidentiality, p. 315
Consequentialism, p. 317
Deontology, p. 316
Ethic of care, p. 318

Ethics, p. 314
Fidelity, p. 314
Justice, p. 314
Nonmaleficence, p. 314
Responsibility, p. 314
Teleology, p. 318
Value, p. 315
Values clarification, p. 316

Ethics is the study of conduct and character. It is concerned with determining what is good or valuable for individuals, for groups of individuals, and for society at large. Acts that are ethical reflect a commitment to standards beyond personal preferences—standards that individuals, professions, and societies strive to meet. When it comes to decision making in health care, however, differing values between individuals cause intense disagreement about the right thing to do. Understandable conflict occurs between health care providers, families, clients, friends, and people in the community about the right thing to do when ethics, values, and decisions about health care collide. This chapter describes tools for you to use to embrace the role of ethics in your professional life.

Basic Terms in Health Ethics

To discuss ethics, it is helpful to establish a basic vocabulary. Common terms contain specific meanings in the context of health care ethics. Terms include *autonomy, beneficence, nonmaleficence, justice,* and *fidelity.* Your understanding of these special meanings will help you to participate thoughtfully in discussions, and it will help you to shape your own thoughts about ethical issues and situations.

Autonomy

Respect for **autonomy** refers to the commitment to include clients in decisions about all aspects of care. For example, the consent that clients read and sign before surgery illustrates this respect for autonomy. The signed consent ensures that the health care team obtained permission from the client before proceeding with the surgery.

Beneficence

Beneficence refers to taking positive actions to help others. The practice of beneficence encourages the urge to do good for others. The agreement to act with beneficence also requires that the best interests of the client remain more important than self-interest. A child may ask for a pill to be crushed and mixed with a favorite food, even though you know the child is able to swallow pills whole. Your commitment to do good for others guides you to comply with the child's wishes, even if you are having a busy day.

Nonmaleficence

Maleficence refers to harm or hurt; thus **nonmaleficence** is the avoidance of harm or hurt. In health care, ethical practice involves not only the will to do good, but also the equal commitment to do no harm. The health care professional tries to balance the risks and benefits of a plan of care while striving to do the least harm possible. For example, a bone marrow transplant procedure offers a chance at cure but the process involves periods of suffering. Health care providers need to consider the associated discomforts, taking into consideration the suffering that the disease itself causes and the suffering that other treatments will possibly cause. The commitment to provide least harmful interventions illustrates nonmaleficence.

Justice

Justice refers to fairness. Health care providers agree to strive for justice in health care. The term often is used in discussions about health care resources. What constitutes a fair distribution of resources is not always clear. For example, in the United States the number of candidates awaiting liver transplants is around 93,000, far more candidates than donors (United Network for Organ Sharing [UNOS], 2006). What is the fair distribution of this scarce resource? Criteria set by a national multidisciplinary committee make every effort to ensure justice by ranking recipients according to need. This system remains preferable in the United States to the selling of organs for profit, which would favor recipients with the most money, and preferable to a distribution by lottery, which would result in random distribution without regard to justice.

Fidelity

Fidelity refers to the agreement to keep promises. A commitment to fidelity supports the reluctance to abandon clients, even when disagreement occurs about decisions that a client makes. The standard of fidelity also includes an obligation to follow through with care offered to clients. If you assess a client for pain and then offer a plan to manage the pain, the standard of fidelity encourages you to monitor the client's response to the plan. Professional behavior includes revision of the plan as necessary to try to keep the promise to reduce pain.

Professional Nursing Code of Ethics

A **code of ethics** is a set of guiding principles that all members of a profession accept. It is a collective statement about the group's expectations and standards of behavior. Codes serve as guidelines to assist professional groups when questions arise about correct practice or behavior. The American Nurses Association (ANA) established the first code of nursing ethics decades ago. The ANA reviews and revises the code regularly, to reflect changes in practice. Basic principles remain constant, however: responsibility, accountability, advocacy, and confidentiality (Box 22-1).

Advocacy

Advocacy refers to the support of a cause. As a nurse, you advocate for the health, safety, and rights of the client. You safeguard the client's right to physical and auditory privacy. For example, you find a private place for discussion with the client's physician or health care provider about the results of the client's diagnostic testing. As a client advocate, follow institutional policies and procedures to report any occurrence of incompetent, unethical, illegal, or impaired practice by any health care member that has the potential to affect client health or safety.

Responsibility

The word **responsibility** refers to a willingness to respect obligations and to follow through on promises. As a nurse, you are responsible for your actions. You play an active role in shaping your

✳ BOX 22-1 American Nurses Association Code of Ethics

- The nurse, in all professional relationships, practices with compassion and respect for the inherent dignity, worth and uniqueness of every individual, unrestricted by considerations of social or economic status, personal attributes, or the nature of health problems.
- The nurse's primary commitment is to the client, whether an individual, family, group, or community.
- The nurse promotes, advocates for, and strives to protect the health, safety, and rights of the client.
- The nurse is responsible and accountable for individual nursing practice and determines the appropriate delegation of tasks consistent with the nurse's obligation to provide optimum client care.
- The nurse owes the same duties to self as to others, including the responsibility to preserve integrity and safety, to maintain competence, and to continue personal and professional growth.
- The nurse participates in establishing, maintaining, and improving health care environments and conditions of employment conducive to the provision of quality health care and consistent with the values of the profession through individual and collective action.
- The nurse participates in the advancement of the profession through contributions to practice, education, administration, and knowledge development.
- The nurse collaborates with other health professionals and the public in promoting community, national, and international efforts to meet health needs.
- The profession of nursing, as represented by associations and their members, is responsible for articulating nursing values, for maintaining the integrity of the profession and its practice, and for shaping social policy.

Reprinted with permission from American Nurses Association, *Code of Ethics for Nurses with Interpretive Statements,* © 2001 Nursesbooks.org, Silver Spring, MD.

practice, rather than a passive role. You need to remain competent to practice so that you are able to reliably follow through on your responsibilities.

Accountability

Accountability refers to the ability to answer for one's own actions. You will learn to ensure that your professional actions are explainable to your clients and to your employer. Health care institutions also play a role in accountability by monitoring individual and institutional compliance with national standards established by The Joint Commission and the ANA. The following are examples of standards for monitoring and protecting nursing practice:

- National guidelines to ensure client safety and workplace safety through consistent, effective nursing practices
- Monitoring provision of client education about smoking cessation for all client populations
- Establishing national standards for continuing education and curriculum development for nursing schools
- Protection of ethical decision making, by requiring health care institutions to create an accessible multidisciplinary forum for discussion about ethical issues

You will find a compliance officer in most health care institutions. This person is responsible for making sure that the institution remains in compliance with health care standards and regulations. To help monitor compliance, the compliance officer usually maintains a hotline or other easy means of communication. Any employee can use this system to report concerns about noncompliance or ethical issues. For the system to be truly effective, it will ensure protection from retaliation for individuals who make a report.

Confidentiality

The concept of **confidentiality** in health care has widespread acceptance in the United States. Federal legislation known as the Health Insurance Portability and Accountability Act of 1996 (HIPAA) mandates the confidential protection of clients' personal health information. The legislation defines the rights and privileges of clients for protection of privacy without diminishing access to quality care. It establishes fines for violations. For example, you cannot copy or forward medical records without a client's consent. You cannot share health care information, including laboratory results, diagnosis, and prognosis, with others without specific client consent, unless the information is necessary in the course of providing care. When medical records are computerized, computer security measures such as special access codes for all authorized users and computer "firewalls" protect systems from unauthorized access (U.S. Department of Health and Human Services, 2006).

Values

Nursing is a work of intimacy. Nursing practice requires you to be in contact with clients not only physically but also emotionally, psychologically, and spiritually. In most other intimate relationships, you choose to enter the relationship precisely because you anticipate that your values will be shared with the other person. But in the case of nursing, you agree to provide care to your clients solely on the basis of their need for your services. Inevitably, you will work with clients whose values differ from yours. You will work with colleagues whose values differ from yours. To negotiate differences of opinion and value, it is important to have clarity about your own values: what you value, why, and how you respect your own values even as you try to respect those of others whose values differ from yours.

A **value** is a personal belief about the worth of a given idea, attitude, custom, or object that sets standards that influence behavior (Maslow, 1977; Rokeach, 1973). The values that an individual holds reflect cultural and social influences, and these values vary among people and develop and change over time.

Discussions about ethical issues require that you maintain respect for differing values. For example, you may find that your commitment to respect autonomy is challenged by a client's preferences to let others make important health care decisions. In some cultures, decisions about health care flow from group or family-based decisions rather than independent decisions by one person. Your effort to resolve differing opinions and to maintain your cultural competence is the hallmark of an ethical practice (Box 22-2).

✳ BOX 22-2   **CULTURAL ASPECTS OF CARE**

Culturally Competent Care: End-of-Life Decisions

Research about end-of-life care shows that the standard of autonomous decision making is not necessarily a universal standard. Some older adult clients may defer to their children to make decisions for them, as a sign of respect. Still others defer to a group elder to make decisions, even when the client is competent to make decisions. Although respect for autonomy has a strong presence in Western philosophy, especially in health care ethics, other cultures may express a preference for group process in making important decisions. For example, Pottinger, Perivolaris, and Howes (2007) explain that "in some Asian cultures, the family is the smallest unit of identity and value is placed on interdependence as opposed to individualism . . . their strong desire to carry out this responsibility evokes equally strong feelings in Western health care providers who value autonomy in decision making."

Volker (2005) summarizes findings from several surveys of clients from different ethnic backgrounds about preferences at the end of life. The goal of the surveys was to identify cultural differences so that health care providers could provide more culturally sensitive care. One survey showed that European Americans, Mexican Americans, and African Americans agreed with the *concept* of an advance directive. Mexican Americans and African Americans, however, were "less receptive" than European Americans to the need for a *written* advance directive. In another survey, European Americans were less likely than Mexican Americans to want life-sustaining treatments at the end of life. Korean Ameri-

cans were knowledgeable about end-of-life technologies, but would not choose them personally.

Implications for Practice

Volker points out that research that tries to predict behaviors based on ethnicity, however, can be hindered by the lack of uniform definitions for various ethnic groups and by the infinite variety of human beings even if they do seem to come from a particular ethnicity or culture. Culturally competent care therefore requires respect and patience. The American College of Physicians proposes the following ground rules:

1. Acknowledgment of and respect for cultural differences
2. Willingness to negotiate and compromise when world views differ
3. Awareness of one's own values and biases
4. Communication skills that enhance empathy
5. Knowledge of the cultural practices of client groups regularly seen
6. Understanding that all clients are individuals and may not share the same views as others within their own ethnic group

Data from Crawley LM and others: Strategies for culturally effective end of life care, *Ann Intern Med* 136:673, 2002; Pottinger A, Perivolaris A, Howes D: The end of life. In Srivaastava RH, editor: *Guide to clinical cultural competence*, Toronto, 2007, Elsevier Canada; and Volker DL: Control and end of life care: does ethnicity matter? *Am J Hosp Palliat Care* 22(6):442, 2005.

Value Formation

Development of values begins in childhood, shaped by experiences within the family unit. Variations in child rearing result in variations in values and behaviors as the children grow up. The fundamental urge to love and nurture children takes on different expressions within each of the wide variety of cultures in our world.

Schools, governments, religious traditions and other social institutions also play a role in the formation of values, reinforcing or sometimes challenging family values. The nature of the role depends on the nature of the institution. Over time, an individual acquires values by choosing some that the community holds strongly and perhaps discarding or transforming others.

Finally, individual experiences, the unpredictable twists and turns that occur in life, influence value formation. A person who suffers great loss early in life sometimes grows to value things differently than someone whose life has been free of suffering.

Values Clarification

Ethical dilemmas almost always occur in the presence of conflicting values. To resolve ethical dilemmas one needs to distinguish between value, fact, and opinion. Sometimes people have such strong values that they consider these values facts, not opinion. Sometimes people are so passionate about their values that they provoke judgmental attitudes during conflict. Clarifying values—your own, your clients', your co-workers'—is an important and effective part of ethical discourse. In the process of **values clarification**, you need to tolerate differences, which sometimes (although not always) become the key in the search for resolution of ethical dilemmas.

Examine the cultural values exercise in Box 22-3. The values in the exercise conflict are in neutral terms so that you can appreciate how differing values need not indicate "right" or "wrong." For example, for some people it is important to remain silent and stoic in the presence of great pain, and for others it is important to talk about it in order to understand it and control it. Identifying values as something separate from facts can help you find tolerance for others, even when differences between you seem worlds apart (Box 22-4).

Ethics and Philosophy

Philosophical discussion about health care issues has changed over time, just as issues in health care and society itself have changed. Philosophical ideas that shape the ethical discussions have also changed. Ethics began as a standard to which health care professionals referred for the determination of right action. It has grown into a field of study filled with differences of opinion, competing systems of values, and deeply meaningful efforts to understand human interaction. The following discussion will introduce you to a variety of contemporary ethical systems. Ultimately, your personal beliefs, experiences, and values provide the foundation for a philosophy of ethics.

Deontology

A traditional ethical theory, **deontology** proposes a system of ethics that is perhaps most familiar to health care practitioners. Its foundations come from the work of an eighteenth-century philosopher,

✳ BOX 22-3 Cultural Values Exercise

If persons from a variety of cultures were given this questionnaire, some would strongly agree with the beliefs listed on the left and others would strongly agree with the opposite viewpoint listed on the right. Circle 1 if you strongly agree or 2 if you moderately agree with the statement on the left. Circle 3 if you moderately agree or 4 if you strongly agree with the statement on the right.

1. Preparing for the future is an important activity and reflects maturity.	1	2	3	4	Life has a predestined course. The individual should follow that course.
2. Vague answers are dishonest and confusing.	1	2	3	4	Vague answers are sometimes preferred because they avoid embarrassment and confrontation.
3. Punctuality and efficiency are characteristics of a person who is both intelligent and concerned.	1	2	3	4	Punctuality is not as important as maintaining a relaxed atmosphere, enjoying the moment, and being with family and friends.
4. When in severe pain, it is important to remain strong and not to complain too much.	1	2	3	4	When in severe pain, it is better to talk about the discomfort and express frustration.
5. It is self-centered and unwise to accept a gift from someone you do not know well.	1	2	3	4	It is an insult to refuse a gift when it is offered.
6. Addressing someone by his or her first name shows friendliness.	1	2	3	4	Addressing someone by his or her first name is disrespectful.
7. Direct questions are usually the best way to gain information.	1	2	3	4	Direct questioning is rude and could cause embarrassment.
8. Direct eye contact shows interest.	1	2	3	4	Direct eye contact is intrusive.
9. Ultimately, the independence of the individual must come before the needs of the family.	1	2	3	4	The needs of the individual are always less important than the needs of the family.

Modified from Renwick GW, Rhinesmith SH: *An exercise in cultural analysis for managers,* Chicago, 1995, Intercultural Press.

Immanuel Kant (1724-1804). Deontology defines actions as right or wrong based on their "right-making characteristics such as fidelity to promises, truthfulness, and justice" (Beauchamp and Childress, 2001). Deontology specifically does not look to *consequences* of actions to determine rightness or wrongness. Instead, it examines a situation for the *existence of essential rightness or wrongness.* For example, if you try to decide about the ethics of a controversial medical procedure, deontology guides you to focus on how the procedure ensures fidelity to the client, truthfulness, justice, and beneficence. You focus less on the consequences (ethically speaking), such as the greater good. If an act is just, respects autonomy, and provides good, then the act will be right, and it will be ethical, according to this philosophy. Deontology depends on a mutual understanding and acceptance of these principles.

Often in health care ethical dilemmas, people have to choose between conflicting principles. For example, application of the principle of respect for autonomy is sometimes confusing when dealing with children. For example, the health care team recommends a certain course of treatment, but the parent disagrees or even refuses the recommendation. In discussion of the dilemma, participants refer to a guiding principle, such as respect for autonomy. But questions will remain. Whose autonomy should receive the respect? The parent's? Who should speak for the child's best interest? Communities struggle to decide who ultimately is responsible for the well-being of children. A commitment to respect the "rightness" of autonomy is a guiding principle in deontology, but adherence to the principle alone will not necessarily provide answers to ethical dilemmas.

Utilitarianism

A utilitarian system of ethics proposes that the value of something is determined by its usefulness. This philosophy is also known as **consequentialism,** because its main emphasis is on the outcome

✳ BOX 22-4 EVIDENCE-BASED PRACTICE

Can Evidence-Based Practice Eliminate Ethical Dilemmas?

Evidence Summary

Research in health care produces scientific evidence that guides decisions about best practices. Even when the evidence is valid and reliable, however, value judgments and ethics play a role in deciding whether to apply evidence in practice. As Borry, Schotsmans, and Dierickx suggest, health care providers have a "moral obligation" to evaluate clinical research for its honesty, its validity, and its freedom from commercial or professional bias. "Ethical decision making must be informed and legitimated by the best available medical research. Nevertheless, ethical decision making is still primarily a choice based on values and norms." Even when research is well executed, the "right" thing to do may not be clear. Decisions about practice involve value judgments: about outcome, about risks and benefits, about financial implications. Personal values and social standards, as well as scientific evidence, will play a role in decisions about practice standards.

Application to Nursing Practice

Your ability to embrace ethical discourse will serve to support your commitment to evaluate the evidence in evidence-based practice proposals. You will make choices based on content, relevance, reliability, and the ethical implications to your practice whenever you review journal articles and other sources about evidence-based practice.

Reference

Borry P, Schotsmans P, Dierickx K: Evidence-based medicine and its role in ethical decision-making, *J Eval Clin Pract* 12(3):306, 2006.

or consequence of action. A third term associated with this philosophy is **teleology,** from the Greek word *telos,* meaning "end," or the study of ends or final causes. John Stuart Mill (1806-1873), a British philosopher, first proposed its philosophical foundations. The greatest good for the greatest number of people is the guiding principle for determining right action in this system. As with deontology, this theory relies on the application of a certain principle, namely, measures of "good" and "greatest" (Beauchamp and Childress, 2001). The difference between utilitarianism and deontology is in the focus on consequences or outcomes. Utilitarianism measures the effect that an act will have; deontology looks to the presence of principle regardless of outcome.

People have conflicting definitions of "greatest good." For example, research suggests that education about safe sex practices reduces the spread of human immunodeficiency virus (HIV). Reducing incidence of HIV is good for a great number of people. For some, education about sex is best provided within a family setting rather than in school, because it promotes family values. For others, however, the greater good is educating the greatest number of people in the most effective way possible and therefore sex education in the public schools ensures the greatest good. As with deontology, utilitarianism provides guidance, but it does not guarantee agreement.

Feminist Ethics

Feminist ethics critiques conventional ethics such as deontology and utilitarianism. It focuses on inequalities between people (Sherwin, 1993; Wolf, 1996). It looks to the nature of relationships for guidance in the processing of ethical dilemmas. Writers with a feminist perspective concentrate more on practical solutions than on theory.

Feminist ethics proposes that principles distract you from dealing with larger issues of community. Proponents value the role of relationships and the stories about relationships. In fact, they suggest that it is impossible to be unbiased in relationships with people. Feminist ethicists propose that the natural human urge to be influenced by relationships is a positive value (Wolf, 1996). Critics of feminist ethics are concerned about the lack of focus on universal principals. Without guidance from universal principals, they argue, solutions will depend completely on the situation itself.

Ethic of Care

The ethic of care and feminist ethics are closely related. Those who write about **ethic of care** are often nurses or physicians. They promote a philosophy that focuses on understanding relationships, especially personal narratives.

Nel Noddings (1984) uses the term "the one-caring" to identify the individual who provides care, and "the cared-for" to refer to the client or patient. In adopting this language, Noddings hopes to emphasize the role of feelings but not at the expense of principles such as autonomy and beneficence. Edmund Pellegrino (1985), a physician, writes about the moral obligation of physicians, health care providers, and nurses to incorporate notions of care into their professional behavior. His definition of care includes the obligation to appreciate, understand, and even share the pain or condition of a client.

Some authors propose a nursing ethics that sets apart the work of nurses from the work of physicians or health care providers (Boyer and Nelson, 1990; Leininger, 1988; Watson, 1994). As in

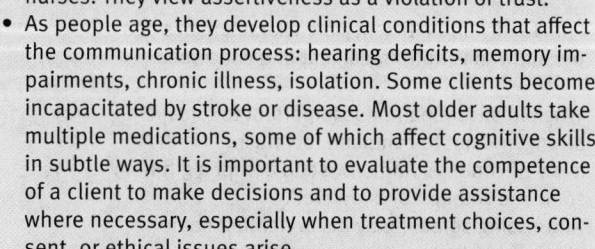

✹ **BOX 22-5** **FOCUS ON OLDER ADULTS**

Ethical Issues and Aging

- Older people are usually not as familiar with the concept of autonomy as people from younger generations. As a result, older adults are sometimes uncomfortable disagreeing with physicians, health care providers, or nurses. They view assertiveness as a violation of trust.
- As people age, they develop clinical conditions that affect the communication process: hearing deficits, memory impairments, chronic illness, isolation. Some clients become incapacitated by stroke or disease. Most older adults take multiple medications, some of which affect cognitive skills in subtle ways. It is important to evaluate the competence of a client to make decisions and to provide assistance where necessary, especially when treatment choices, consent, or ethical issues arise.
- Consensus about medical goals for the older adult is hard to achieve. When is a person so diminished by old age that a treatment plan not only prolongs life, it also prolongs suffering? Working to ensure dignity and comfort is as important as achieving medical success.

Modified from Burke MM, Laramie JA: *Primary care of the older adult: a multidisciplinary approach,* St. Louis, 2003, Mosby.

feminist ethics, these writers propose that you solve ethical dilemmas by attention to relationships and clients' stories. A focus on client stories will lead to clarity about decisions, because individuals often reveal values and moral preferences within clients' personal histories (Box 22-5).

Consensus in Bioethics

You could use each of the above ethical philosophies to justify a position about an issue. None of them, however, guarantees a solution to an ethical dilemma. Bringing different points of view to agreement and harmony, or consensus, requires skill and patience. Building consensus is essentially an act of discovery, where "collective wisdom" guides a group to the best possible decision. It encourages respect for unusual points of view while striving for agreement between all participants (Dressler, 2006). As a strategy for solving dilemmas, consensus building promotes respect and agreement, rather than a particular philosophy or moral system itself. In the example of an ethical dilemma described below, the process is basically one of consensus building.

Nursing Point of View

Professional nurses play a specific role in the management of health care. All clients in the health care system interact with a nurse at some point in ways that are unique to nursing. Nurses generally interact with clients over longer intervals of time than other disciplines. Because nurses are often involved in intimate physical acts such as bathing, feeding, and special procedures, clients and families reveal information not always shared with physicians, health care providers, or others. Details about family life, information about coping styles, personal preferences, and details about fears and insecurities are likely to come out during the course of nursing

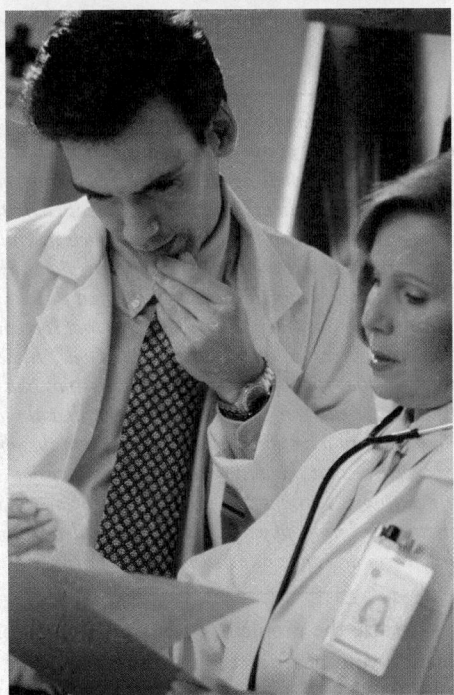

Figure 22-1 Nurses collaborate with other professionals in making ethical decisions. (Copyright 2007 Jupiter Images Corporation.)

✳ BOX 22-6 How to Process an Ethical Dilemma

Step 1. Ask the question, Is this an ethical dilemma? If a review of scientific data does not resolve the question, the question is perplexing, and the answer will have relevance for areas of human concern, then an ethical dilemma probably exists.
Step 2. Gather information relevant to the case. Client, family, institutional, and social perspectives are important sources of relevant information.
Step 3. Clarify values. Distinguish between fact, opinion, and values.
Step 4. Verbalize the problem. A clear, simple statement of the dilemma is not always easy, but it helps to ensure effectiveness in the final plan and facilitates discussion.
Step 5. Identify possible courses of action.
Step 6. Negotiate a plan. Negotiation requires a confidence in one's own point of view and a deep respect for the opinions of others.
Step 7. Evaluate the plan over time.

interventions (Shannon, 1997). Your ability to recognize these aspects of a client's situation, and to express your professional concerns accordingly, will provide critical value to the discussion.

On the other hand, it is important to remember that care of any one client involves many disciplines and thus care often becomes fragmented. The nursing point of view is part of a larger picture that includes all members of the health care team, including other providers of services and even the client and family. Managers and administrators from many different professional backgrounds contribute to ethical discourse with their knowledge of systems, distribution of resources, financial possibilities, or limits (Figure 22-1).

How to Process an Ethical Dilemma

Ethical dilemmas cause distress for both clients and caregivers. Ethical problems often come from controversy and conflict. To overcome controversy, you need to process ethical issues carefully and deliberately. The process needs to promote the free expression of feelings and opinions. However, you do not resolve an ethical dilemma by considering only what people want and feel (Zoloth, 2006).

Resolving an ethical dilemma is in many ways similar to the nursing process. It requires deliberate, systematic discourse (Miller and Babcock, 1996). But it differs from the nursing process because it requires negotiation of differences of opinion. As Zoloth suggests, the resolution of conflicting opinions works best when the following elements are part of the process: the presumption of good will on the part of all participants, strict adherence to confidentiality, client-centered decision making, and the welcome participation of families and primary caregivers (Zoloth, 2006).

Each step in processing an ethical dilemma resembles steps in critical thinking. The process begins with the gathering of all pertinent information, and then the group proceeds through assessment, planning, implementation, and evaluation. To distinguish an ethical problem from other kinds of problems, Curtin (2004) proposes that if the issue is an ethical one, it will entail at least one of the following :

• You are unable to resolve it solely through a review of scientific data. To decide if it is an ethical issue, you need to gather detailed information about the situation. This information comes from medical records, health care literature, consultation with colleagues, or consultation with the client and the client's family.
• It is perplexing. You cannot easily think logically or make a decision about the problem.
• The answer to the problem will have a profound relevance for areas of human concern.

Participants begin the process with a clear statement of the ethical problem. When everyone agrees on the statement of the dilemma, discussion is more likely to remain focused and constructive. Next, a discussion listing possible courses of action helps the group explore options and identify dissent. As a group, you consider and evaluate alternatives with respect for all differences of opinion. Most of the time, persons in an ethical conflict come to resolution and implement a plan. Evaluation of the plan follows (Box 22-6).

How you document the ethical process depends on the institution and on the circumstances. When the process involves a family conference or changes in the management plan, you will document the process in the medical record. Some institutions use a special ethics consultation form to structure documentation. If the ethical concern does not directly affect client care, however, document the discussion in meeting minutes or in a memorandum to those involved in the discussion.

The following case study illustrates the ethical process, step by step.

On your unit, a 35-year-old woman has been hospitalized in the final stages of a struggle with brain cancer. She is a single mother with two children at home. She has received conventional and ex-

perimental treatments. The tumor continues to grow. The medical team agrees that further treatment would be futile. You have cared for this client during past admissions, and during an especially open discussion, she expressed wishes to explore a "do not resuscitate" (DNR) order, but she was discharged before further discussion with her physician took place. During the current admission, her primary physician is out of town. The new attending physician has reviewed the clinical data and agrees that the client is entering the terminal stages of her disease. In his opinion, however, the client is not ready to discuss end-of-life issues. He says that he has asked her about DNR, but she declines to discuss it. You ask him to attend a family conference to discuss DNR orders, but he refuses to do so, because in his opinion the client is not ready to participate.

Step 1. Is this an ethical dilemma? If the question remains perplexing, and the answer will have profound relevance for several areas of human concern, then an ethical dilemma may exist.

The single mother's situation meets the criteria for an ethical dilemma. Review of scientific data will probably not contribute to a resolution of the dilemma, but it is important to review the data carefully to make this determination. The disagreement does not revolve around whether the client is in a terminally ill state, so further clinical information will not change the basic question: Should the client have an opportunity to discuss DNR orders at this time? The question is perplexing. Basically, two professional team members disagree on an assessment of a client's readiness to confront difficult issues related to dying. The answer to the question "Is this client ready to discuss end of life?" has important human implications. If she is not ready, then raising the issues will possibly cause anguish and fear in the client and her family. If she is ready and the team avoids discussion, she will possibly suffer unnecessarily in silence. If she is very close to death, then the lack of a DNR order will necessitate the application of cardiopulmonary resuscitation (CPR) in a futile situation. As a nurse, you know that CPR causes some pain. If applied in a situation where further life is unlikely, then CPR could prolong suffering and reduce dignity. On the other hand, if the client or her loved ones prefer to ensure that all actions to preserve life are taken regardless of the outcome, then a DNR order would violate the client's wishes.

Step 2. Gather as much information as possible that is relevant to the case. Because resolution of dilemmas often comes from unlikely sources, it is helpful to incorporate as much knowledge as possible. Helpful information includes laboratory and test results, the clinical state of the client in question, and current literature about the diagnosis or condition of the client. A client's religious, cultural, and family situation are also part of the assessment.

You obtain all of the clinical information that is relevant to the ethical issue. Because this dilemma exists because two professionals do not agree on a client's state of mind, it is helpful to reassess the client, or even to request an independent assessment of the client's readiness to discuss end-of-life issues. Sometimes family members or significant others in the client's life will hold important clues to a client's state of mind.

Step 3. Examine and determine your own values on the issues. Part of the goal is the accurate identification of one's own opinion.

An equally essential part of the goal is formation of respect for others' opinions.

Reflect on your values. You feel that this client wants a DNR order in place. But does this opinion accurately represent the client's wishes? Your religious beliefs do not prohibit you from getting a DNR if you were in the client's condition. You realize that, unlike the client, you do not have family members such as children or older adult parents who rely on you. Through previous discussion, you learned that the client practices a religion that discourages acts that diminish life in any way, and you realize that she now views a DNR order as giving up or as "acting like God." In addition, you understand that the attending physician has not had time to know this client well. You continue to believe that the client is capable of a discussion, in spite of her statements to the physician. In fact, you believe that she will benefit from a discussion, regardless of the outcome. Perhaps the combination of an unfamiliar caretaker and declining physical health have silenced her even though her fears and concerns persist.

Step 4. Verbalize the problem. After gathering all of the relevant information you then proceed to accurately define the problem. It is helpful to try to state the problem in a few sentences. By agreeing to a statement of the problem, the group is able to have a focused discussion.

Is a DNR order the right thing or the wrong thing for this client? And is she ready to discuss the options?

Step 5. Consider possible courses of action. What options are possible in this situation?

Do you initiate a discussion with the client independent of the physician? Is this outside your professional domain, and is it in the client's best interest for you to facilitate a DNR order from another physician? What if your assessment of the client is incorrect? Do you contribute to the dignity or to the distress of the client? The answers to these questions are sometimes elusive, because they depend on an understanding of client feelings and values that are not necessarily obvious. Even if legally you cannot actually write a DNR order, this fact does not relieve you of troubling questions, because the ability to influence a physician's or client's decision regarding DNR remains.

Step 6. Negotiate the outcome. Negotiations happen informally at the bedside or in a conference room. Sometimes a formal ethics meeting is necessary. Wherever negotiations occur, the nurse has an obligation to articulate a personal point of view.

If an ethics committee meeting occurs, then the discussion will usually involve participants from several disciplines. A facilitator or chairperson will ensure that the group examines all points of view and identifies all relevant issues. A decision or recommendation is the usual outcome of discussion. In the best of circumstances, participants discover a course of action that meets criteria for consensus, or acceptance by all. Occasionally, however, participants leave the discussion disappointed or even opposed to the decision. But in a successful discussion, all members will have agreed on an action or decision.

The discussion focuses on the disagreement between your assessment and the physician's regarding the client's readiness to discuss end-of-life issues. The principles involved during the discussion include beneficence and nonmaleficence: Which plan would provide the most good for this client, a DNR order or no order? A separate question addresses the client's point of view and a respect for autonomy: Would a discussion with the client promote well-being or promote anguish? The commitment to respect a client's autonomy reveals that a troublesome question remains: Does the client want something different from what she is expressing?

With several members of the health care team present, the discussion proceeds. You present your point of view. You continue to sense that the client is ready to discuss DNR orders, but that she is reluctant to trust the circumstances of this admission. But you also respect the attending physician and his analysis and continue to have concerns that the client has changed her mind between the last admission and this one. In the end the team proposes the following: a formal meeting with the client where you, the attending physician, and a supportive family member are present. You support this proposal because you believe that it will maximize support from the client's network of friends and family. In addition, you recognize that in a trusting environment, the client is most likely to express herself most accurately. You suggest that rather than asking if the client wants a DNR order, perhaps the team could wait for her to bring up the issue. In this way, the team would be sure of her consent and willingness to discuss the difficult questions about dying.

Step 7. Evaluate the action.

At the meeting the client in fact opens up. She expresses relief at the chance to explore her options and feelings. You clarify pain management issues with her. She wants to discuss a DNR order but requests a visit from her priest before making a final decision.

Institutional Resources

Health care institutions establish ethics committees to support the processing of ethical dilemmas. Ethics committees are usually multidisciplinary. They serve several purposes: education, policy recommendation, and case consultation. Any person involved in an ethical dilemma, including nurses, physicians, health care providers, clients, and families of clients are able to request access to an ethics committee.

You will also process ethical issues in settings other than in a committee, however. Nurses provide insight about ethical problems at family conferences, staff meetings, or even in meetings one-to-one. Many ethical problems begin when people feel misled or are not aware of their options and do not know when to speak up about their concerns. You address such concerns in a variety of constructive settings. Ethics committees serve to complement relationships and offer a valuable resource for strengthening them.

Issues in Bioethics

You will face professional ethical issues in all kinds of workplaces throughout your career. Issues change as society and technologies change, but common denominators remain: the basic process

used to address the issues and your responsibility to maintain skill and patience in dealing with the issues. The following section describes current issues in which ethical concerns occur.

Quality of Life

Quality of life represents something deeply personal. In health care, researchers have tried to develop quality-of-life measures to define scientifically the value and benefits of certain medical interventions. Social scientists have proposed formulas or other objective measurements for application in individual situations (Fallowfield, 1990; Levine and Ganz, 2002). These formulas take into account the age of the client, the client's ability to live independently, and the client's ability to contribute to society in a gainful way. A quality-of-life measure helps a client and family decide on the merits of a certain risky intervention, such as an organ transplant or experimental drug management. The question of quality of life is central to discussions about futile care, cancer therapy, health care provider–assisted suicide, and DNR discussions.

The population of disabled persons in the United States and elsewhere has redefined quality. The national movement to respect the abilities of the "dis-abled" raised the visibility of quality-of-life issues and forced a reconsideration of the definition of quality. Many school districts, for example, no longer separate physically or mentally challenged children but now integrate these children into "mainstream" classrooms. Public places like restaurants and buses are accessible to people who use wheelchairs (Figure 22-2). Antidiscrimination laws enhance the economic security of people with physical, mental, or emotional challenges. These changes have greatly increased the integration of disabled persons into general society. They remind society in general and health care workers specifically that definitions of quality begin as an individual's definition. Society as a whole benefits from these lessons.

Genetic Screening

Genetic testing alerts a client to a condition that is not yet evident but that is certain to develop in the future. What are the risks and what are the benefits to learning about the presence of disease that has not yet caused symptoms? The gene that indicates the presence of Huntington's disease, for example, is now detectable. Huntington's disease is an inherited degenerative neurological disease, incurable at this time. The disease affects cognitive and

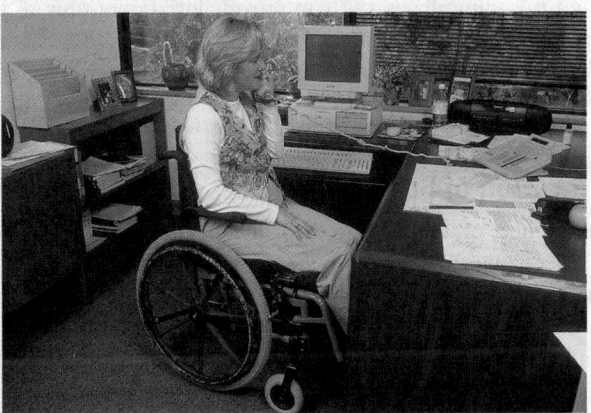

Figure 22-2 Measures can be made to provide accessibility in the work environment.

emotional function, as well as physical function. Symptoms usually do not appear until the third or fourth decade of life. If a parent or grandparent has the disease, offspring are at risk for developing the disease. Some clients are eager to learn if they will develop the disease so that they are able to make decisions about childbearing, career, and retirement planning. Others are reluctant to face the knowledge before symptoms begin, preferring to live life with the uncertainties. As one person whose mother died of Huntington's disease explained, "Cheerful predictions that people could use a positive diagnosis to make rational life choices mystify me ... I doubt if I'd have the confidence to continue. To think that my brain was slowly dying, never to know if thoughts or feelings were artifacts of a diseased brain—how to live with that and keep on working?" (Wexler, 1996).

Futile Care

Futile refers to something that is "useless; hopeless; serving no useful purpose" (Merriam Webster, 2006). In health care discussions, the term refers to interventions unlikely to produce benefit for the client. The term is slippery. Predictions about health are not always accurate. Even when they are, opinions about the value or worth of the outcome differ. For example, a client requests a mastectomy before any symptoms of breast disease have appeared, fearful of a family history, thinking this will prevent future suffering. The physician is reluctant to provide this intervention, based on knowledge of risk factors. In the physician's opinion, the intervention is futile: unlikely to produce benefit that outweighs risk. The client does not agree. In another situation, a physician might urge a client to undergo a liver transplantation for end-stage liver disease. The success of a cure is uncertain, but without the transplant death is inevitable. The client holds the opinion that the transplant is pointless: unlikely to produce benefit that justifies the suffering he anticipates. Agreement on what is best is often elusive.

If the client is dying, in a condition with little or no hope of recovery, then almost any intervention beyond pain management and comfort measures will be seen as futile. In this situation, an agreement to label an intervention as futile helps providers, families, and clients to refrain from prolonging the dying. In other circumstances, the team reasonably and respectfully makes the decision to use certain interventions, such as dialysis for renal failure, even though a cancer has metastasized and is unresponsive to any treatment. This use of an intervention, although technically futile clinically, is a way to provide loved ones time to prepare final farewells, to allow distant relatives to arrive at the bedside, and to resolve personal legal issues such as a will or other financial matters. In this case, the intervention is useless clinically, but it produces benefit in other ways.

Allocation of Scarce Resources: Access to Care

The number of uninsured in the United States grew from 39 million people in 2000 to more than 45.5 million people by 2004. Many of the uninsured are women or children. And although two thirds of the uninsured are poor, over 80% come from working families. In the United States we have tried a variety of strategies to address the issue: managed care, state subsidies for underinsured, and mandated employer health insurance. These all represent efforts to deal with diminishing access to care. And yet the numbers continue to grow (Henry J. Kaiser Family Foundation, 2005).

Although access to care seems larger than your relationship with your job or a client, you will likely discover implications about access in the details of your daily work life. You will care for a client on a plan for discharge from the hospital when you find that the client cannot afford to fill a prescription. Or you admit an uninsured client with advanced disease with no primary physician to oversee the chronic illness. This client will continue to spend time in the hospital until the chronic illness is treated, which further increases health care costs. Dealing with these situations is challenging and will involve a balancing of competing principals and values. Should resources be focused on research for treatment of disease, or is the money better spent understanding prevention of disease? Which activity is more valuable, research or delivery of care? If limited public funds are spent on expensive interventions available only for the few who are able to afford them, will that deplete funds for basic care for many? Resolution of these questions becomes political as well as ethical. Your engagement with the issues will require a commitment to your professional and personal ethics.

Allocation of Scarce Resources: The Nursing Shortage

According to the federal Bureau of Health Professions, the demand for nurses in 2000 was 2 million, and yet we had only 1.89 million available in the United States, a 6% shortfall. When researchers originally made predictions about the shortfall, they did not expect a gap this large until 2007 (Bureau of Health Professions, 2002). The nursing shortage produces difficult working conditions and affects client outcomes. The Institute of Medicine's report on the tremendous magnitude of medication errors points out the role of inadequate staffing as a source of the growth of the problem (Kohn, Corrigan, and Donaldson, 2000).

The shortage is also seen in ethical terms. How does a nurse decide what course to take when the care assignment feels too large to be safe? California is the first state in the United States to pass mandated staffing ratios. Yet some hospitals in California have to cope with a 25% vacancy rate. The law stipulates that if a hospital does not have enough nurses to staff by the law, then the hospital will "close beds." Clients will have to go elsewhere.

Professional issues of advocacy and client abandonment compete with ethical concerns about beneficence, maleficence, and justice. Participation in political solutions plays an important role in the negotiation of personal concerns.

• • •

The courage and intelligence to act, both as an advocate for clients and as a professional member of the health care team, come from a committed effort to learn and to understand ethical principles. As a professional nurse, you provide a unique point of view regarding clients, the health care system that supports clients, and the institutions that make up the health care system. You have a duty and a privilege to articulate that point of view. Learning the language of ethical discourse is a part of the skill necessary to exercise this privilege. Review and consideration of various ethical principles will assist you in forming personal points of view, a necessary factor in the negotiation of difficult ethical situations.

Key Concepts

- Ethics is the study of conduct and character. It is concerned with determining what is good or valuable for individuals and for society at large.
- The American Nurses Association code of ethics provides a foundation for professional nursing.
- Professional nursing promotes accountability, responsibility, advocacy, and confidentiality.
- Standards of ethics in health care include autonomy, beneficence, nonmaleficence, justice, and fidelity.
- The process of values clarification helps you to explore values and feelings and to decide how to act on personal beliefs.
- Ethical problems come from differences in values, changing professional roles, technological advances, and social issues that influence quality of life.
- A standard process for thinking through ethical dilemmas helps health care providers resolve conflict about right actions.
- The nurse's point of view offers a unique voice in the resolution of ethical dilemmas.

Critical Thinking Exercises

1. Complete the "cultural values" exercise on p. 317 with your classmates or with members of another class of professionals. Compare the answers and discuss the differences.

2. You are caring for a 17-year-old client who has been admitted for treatment of sickle cell crisis. She needs fluid management and comfort management. Even though she is receiving opioids around-the-clock, she continues to report acute pain. She also complains about her roommate, the food, and the intravenous line. She comes from a community far from the hospital, and her mother cannot visit every day. She has an older brother who has been convicted of possession of illegal drugs. Discuss your approach to this client. Rank her needs. What is your priority action, based on what you know so far? Examine and describe your opinions about pain, pain management, and addiction.

3. You are a clinic nurse in a small community clinic. A 45-year-old male client has been coming to the clinic for several years for treatment and support of his acquired immunodeficiency syndrome (AIDS). During recent months he has lost his long-term companion to AIDS. In addition, both his parents died many years ago. His clinical condition has deteriorated. His vision is failing, his nutritional status is difficult to maintain, and he has been hospitalized three times in the past 3 months for pneumonia. He asks for your help in planning his suicide. Discuss your response to his request. Begin by an examination of your personal feelings about suicide. Include a discussion about your understanding of AIDS: Where does it come from? Who gets the disease? Why? What are your feelings and opinions about people with AIDS? Construct your response, keeping in mind the ethical principles of fidelity, autonomy, beneficence, and nonmaleficence. Because all of these principles collide in this example, it will be im-

portant to identify each and recognize personal responses to the role that each plays in this narrative. For the sake of this discussion, assume that it is illegal in your state for nurses to prescribe medicines. What are your possible courses of action?

4. You have been assigned the care of a 98-year-old woman who was recently admitted from home with a diagnosis of pneumonia. She has a history of cardiac disease and takes a number of medications. She had been fairly active until the past few days, when her cough worsened and she developed a fever. You note that her pulse has become weak and thready and that her respirations are increasingly labored. The client is now too weak to respond to you. When you mention to the family that you may need to call the physician or health care provider and even "call a code," the son and the daughter become distraught, saying that they do not want their mother to be kept alive on "machines." They report that they have discussed this situation with their mother. You find that documentation of these wishes is not in the chart. The family members have not discussed this situation with their physician or health care provider. What actions would you consider taking at this moment? Take into account the ethical principles of autonomy and beneficence. What are your personal values about interventions at the end of life?

NCLEX®-Style Review Questions

1. In the United States, access to health care usually depends on a client's ability to pay for health care, either through insurance or by paying cash. The client the nurse is caring for needs a liver transplant to survive. This client has been out of work for several months and does not have insurance or enough cash. A discussion about the ethics of this situation would involve predominately the principle of:
   1. Accountability, because you as the nurse are accountable for the well-being of this client
   2. Respect for autonomy, because this client's autonomy will be violated if he does not receive the liver transplant
   3. Ethic of care, because the caring thing that a nurse could provide this client is resources for a liver transplant
   4. Justice, because the first and greatest question in this situation is how to determine the just distribution of resources

2. It may seem redundant that health care providers, including professional nurses, agree to "do no harm" to their clients. The point of this agreement is to reassure the public that in all ways the health care team will not only work to heal clients, they agree to do this in the least painful and harmful way possible. The principle that describes this agreement is called:
   1. Beneficence
   2. Accountability
   3. Nonmaleficence
   4. Respect for autonomy

3. A child's immunization may cause discomfort during administration, but the benefits of protection from disease, both for the individual and for society, outweigh the temporary discomforts. This involves the principle of:
   1. Fidelity
   2. Beneficence
   3. Nonmaleficence
   4. Respect for autonomy

4. If a nurse assesses a client for pain and then offers a plan to manage the pain, the principle that encourages the nurse to monitor the client's response to the plan is:
   1. Fidelity
   2. Beneficence
   3. Nonmaleficence
   4. Respect for autonomy

5. Nurses agree to be advocates for their clients. Practice of advocacy calls for the nurse to:
   1. Seek out the nursing supervisor in conflicting situations
   2. Document all clinical changes in the medical record in a timely manner
   3. Work to understand the law as it applies to the client's clinical condition
   4. Assess the client's point of view and prepare to articulate this point of view

6. Successful ethical discussion depends on people who have a clear sense of personal values. When many people share the same values, it may be possible to identify a philosophy of utilitarianism, which proposes that:
   1. The value of something is determined by its usefulness to society
   2. The value of people is determined solely by leaders in the Unitarian Church
   3. The decision to perform a liver transplant depends on a measure of the moral life that the client has led so far
   4. The best way to determine the solution to an ethical dilemma is to refer the case to the attending physician or health care provider

7. The philosophy sometimes called the ethic of care suggests that ethical dilemmas can best be solved by attention to:
   1. Clients
   2. Relationships
   3. Ethical principles
   4. Code of ethics for nurses

8. In most ethical dilemmas the solution to the dilemma requires negotiation among members of the health care team. The nurse's point of view is valuable because:
   1. The principle of autonomy guides all participants to respect their own self-worth
   2. Nurses have a legal license that encourages their presence during ethical discussions
   3. Nurses develop a relationship to the client that is unique among all professional health care providers
   4. The nurse's code of ethics recommends that a nurse be present at any ethical discussion about client care

9. Ethical dilemmas often arise over a conflict of opinion. Once the nurse has determined that the dilemma is ethical, a critical first step in negotiating the difference of opinion would be to:
   1. Consult a professional ethicist to ensure that the steps of the process occur in full
   2. Gather all relevant information regarding the clinical, social, and spiritual aspects of the dilemma
   3. Ensure that the attending physician or health care provider has written an order for an ethics consultation to support the ethics process
   4. List the ethical principles that inform the dilemma so that negotiations agree on the language of the discussion

23 | Legal Implications in Nursing Practice

✳ OBJECTIVES

Mastery of the content in this chapter will enable the student to:

- Explain the legal concepts of standard of care and informed consent.
- Describe the legal responsibilities and obligations of nurses regarding the following federal statutes: Americans With Disabilities Act (ADA), Emergency Medical Treatment and Active Labor Act (EMTALA), Health Insurance Portability and Accountability Act of 1996 (HIPAA), and the Patient Self-Determination Act (PSDA).

- List sources for standards of care for nurses.
- Describe the nurse's role regarding a "do not resuscitate" (DNR) order.
- Define legal aspects of nurse-client, nurse–health care provider, nurse-nurse, and nurse-employer relationships.
- List the elements needed to prove negligence.
- Describe the nursing implications associated with legal issues that occur in nursing practice.

✳ MEDIA RESOURCES ✳ KEY TERMS

 Companion CD
- NCLEX®-Style Review Questions
- Audio Glossary
- Interactive Learning Activities
- English/Spanish Glossary

***evolve* Website**
- NCLEX®-Style Review Questions
- Audio Glossary
- English/Spanish Glossary
- Interactive Learning Activities
- WebLinks
- Audio Summaries

Administrative law, p. 326
Assault, p. 331
Battery, p. 331
Civil laws, p. 326
Common law, p. 326
Confidentiality, p. 329
Criminal laws, p. 326
Defamation of character, p. 331
Felony, p. 326
Incident report, p. 336
Informed consent, p. 332
Intentional torts, p. 331
Libel, p. 332
Living wills, p. 328

Malice, p. 332
Malpractice, p. 332
Misdemeanor, p. 326
Negligence, p. 332
Nurse Practice Acts, p. 326
Occurrence report, p. 336
Privacy, p. 329
Regulatory law, p. 326
Risk management, p. 336
Slander, p. 332
Standards of care, p. 326
Statutory law, p. 326
Tort, p. 331

Safe nursing practice includes an understanding of the legal boundaries within which nurses practice. As with all aspects of nursing, an understanding of the implications of the law supports critical thinking on the nurse's part. Nurses need to understand the law to protect themselves from liability and to protect their clients' rights. Nurses need not fear the law but rather view the information that follows as the foundation for understanding what our society expects from professional nursing care providers. Society took greater interest in the safe delivery of health care following the 1999 report published by the Institute of Medicine, *To Err Is Human*. This report estimated that between 44,000 and 98,000 Americans die each year due to preventable errors (Kohn, Corrigan, and Donaldson, 2000). The Institute called for legal reform in the area of medical malpractice and tort liability. The laws in our society are fluid and constantly changing. As technology expands the role of the nurse, the ethical dilemmas associated with client care increase and often become legal issues as well. Thus as health care evolves, the legal implications for health care evolve as well.

Legal Limits of Nursing

As a professional nurse, you need to understand the legal limits influencing your practice. This, along with good judgment and sound decision making, ensures your clients receive safe and appropriate nursing care.

Sources of Law

The legal guidelines that nurses follow come from statutory law, regulatory law, and common law. Elected legislative bodies such as state legislatures and the U.S. Congress create **statutory law.** An example of state statutes are the Nurse Practice Acts found in all 50 states (see Chapter 1). These **Nurse Practice Acts** describe and define the legal boundaries of nursing practice within each state. An example of a federal statute enacted by the U.S. Congress is the Americans With Disabilities Act (ADA) (1990). This statute protects the rights of handicapped individuals in the workplace, in educational institutions, and throughout our society. **Regulatory law,** or **administrative law,** reflects decisions made by administrative bodies such as State Boards of Nursing when they pass rules and regulations. An example of regulatory law is the duty to report incompetent or unethical nursing conduct to the State Board of Nursing. **Common law** results from judicial decisions made in courts when individual legal cases are decided. Examples of common law include informed consent and the client's right to refuse treatment. However, the nurse most frequently encounters common laws involving negligence and malpractice.

Statutory law is either civil or criminal. **Criminal laws** prevent harm to society and provide punishment for crimes (Black, 2004). There are two classifications of crimes. A **felony** is a crime of a serious nature that has a penalty of imprisonment for greater than 1 year or even death. A **misdemeanor** is a less serious crime that has a penalty of a fine or imprisonment for less than 1 year. An example of criminal conduct for nurses is misuse of a controlled substance.

Civil laws protect the rights of individual persons within our society and encourage fair and equitable treatment among people (Black, 2004). Generally, violations of civil laws cause harm to an individual or property. The damages for civil laws involve the payment of money, unlike criminal laws, which sometimes result in imprisonment. However, under many federal and state laws, sanctions for violations include both civil and criminal penalties.

Standards of Care

Standards of care are the legal guidelines for nursing practice and provide the minimum acceptable nursing care. Standards reflect values and priorities of the profession (see Chapter 1). The American Nurses Association (ANA) has developed standards for nursing practice, policy statements, and similar resolutions. The standards outline the scope, function, and role of the nurse in practice. Nursing standards of care are set out in every state's Nurse Practice Act, by the federal and state laws regulating hospitals and other health care institutions, by professional and specialty nursing organizations, and by the policies and procedures established by the health care facility where nurses work (Guido, 2006). In a malpractice lawsuit, nursing standards of care measure nursing conduct and determine whether the nurse acted as any reasonably prudent nurse would act under the same or similar circumstances. A breach of the nursing standard of care is one element that must be proven in the tort of nursing negligence or malpractice (Blumenreich, 2005).

The law defines the standards of care for nurses to follow. All state legislatures have passed Nurse Practice Acts that define the scope of nursing practice. With the increased use of assistive personnel (e.g., nurse assistants), some State Boards of Nursing have defined the registered nurse's responsibilities specifically and developed position statements and guidelines to help licensed nurses delegate safely (National Council of State Boards of Nursing [NCSBN], 2005). Nurse Practice Acts establish educational requirements for nurses, distinguish between nursing and medical practice, and generally define the scope of nursing practice. The rules and regulations enacted by a State Board of Nursing define the practice of nursing more specifically. For example, a state board develops a rule regarding intravenous therapy. All nurses are responsible for knowing the provisions of the Nurse Practice Act for the state in which they work, as well as the rules and regulations enacted by the State Board of Nursing and other regulatory administrative bodies.

The Joint Commission (TJC) (2007) requires that accredited hospitals have written nursing policies and procedures. These internal standards of care are quite specific and should be accessible on all nursing units. For example, a policy/procedure outlining the steps to follow when changing a dressing or administering medication provides specific information about how nurses are to perform these tasks. Some hospitals are also now using commercially published procedural textbooks to reference the institution's general policies and procedures. You need to know the policies, procedures, and protocols of your employing institution so that you use the same standard of care as the other nurses in your institution. Institutional policies and procedures need to conform to state and federal laws, as well as community standards, and cannot conflict with legal guidelines that define acceptable standards of care (Ashley, 2004).

In a lawsuit for malpractice or nursing negligence, a nursing expert testifies to the jury about the standards of nursing care as applied to the facts of the case (Box 23-1). The jury uses the stan-

✳ BOX 23-1 Anatomy of a Lawsuit

Pleadings Phase

Petition-elements of the claim: The plaintiff outlines what the defendant nurse did wrong and how as a result of that alleged negligence the plaintiff was injured.

Answer: The nurse admits or denies each allegation in the petition. The prosecutor has to prove anything that the nurse does not admit.

Discovery

Interrogatories: Written questions requiring answers under oath. Usual questions concern witnesses, insurance experts, and which health care providers the plaintiff has seen before and after the incident.

Medical records: The defendant obtains all of the plaintiff's relevant medical records for treatment before and after the incident.

Witnesses' depositions: Questions are posed to the witness under oath to obtain all relevant, nonprivileged information about the case.

Parties' depositions: The plaintiff and defendants (physician, nurse, hospital personnel) are almost always deposed.

Other witnesses: Factual witnesses, both neutral and biased, are deposed to obtain information and their version of the case. This includes family members on the plaintiff's side and other medical personnel (e.g., nurses) on the defendant's side.

Treating physicians' or health care provider's depositions: Before subsequent treating, physicians' or health care provider's depositions are taken to establish issues such as those concerning preexisting conditions, causation, the nature and extent of injuries, and permanency.

Experts: The plaintiff selects experts to establish the essential legal elements of the case against the defendant. The defendant selects experts to establish the appropriateness of the nursing care.

Trial

Following discovery phase of 1 to 3 years or longer, trial may last days to months.

Proof of Negligence

The nurse owed a duty to the client.

The nurse did not carry out the duty or breached the duty (failure to use that degree of skill and learning ordinarily used under the same or similar circumstances by members of his or her profession).

The client was injured.
  Medical bills, lost wages
  Pain and suffering
  Perinatal damages
  Wrongful death damages

The client's injury was caused by the nurse's failure to carry out that duty ("but for" the breach of duty the client would not have been injured).

dards of care to determine whether the nurse acted appropriately. Nurse experts base their opinions on existing standards of practice established by Nurse Practice Acts, professional organizations, institutional policies and procedures, federal and state hospital licensing laws, TJC standards, job descriptions, and current nursing research literature (Guido, 2006).

Usually, general duty nurses are responsible for meeting the same standards as other general duty nurses in similar settings. However,

specialized nurses such as nurse anesthetists, operating room (OR) nurses, intensive care nurses, or certified nurse-midwives have specially defined standards of care and skills. Ignorance of the law or of standards of care is not a defense against malpractice. However, at the time of trial, the standard of care is what the nurse experts testify that standard to be and ultimately what the jury believes (Sloan, 2004).

One of the first and most important cases to discuss a nurse's liability was *Darling v Charleston Community Memorial Hospital.* It involved an 18-year-old man with a fractured leg. The emergency department physician applied a cast with insufficient padding. The man's toes became swollen and discolored, and he developed decreased sensation. He complained to the nursing staff many times. Although the nurses recognized the symptoms as signs of impaired circulation, they failed to tell their supervisor that the physician did not respond to their calls or the client's needs. Gangrene developed, and the man's leg was amputated. Although the physician was held liable for incorrectly applying the cast, the nursing staff was also held liable for failing to adhere to the standards of care for monitoring and reporting the client's symptoms. Even though the nurses attempted to contact the physician, this case holds that when the physician fails to respond, the nurse must go over the physician's or health care provider's head to make sure that the client is appropriately treated. Almost every state uses this 1965 Illinois Supreme Court case as legal precedence.

The best way for nurses to keep up with the current legal issues affecting nursing practice is to maintain familiarity with standards of care and the policies and procedures of their employing agency and to read current nursing literature in their practice area (ANA, 2004).

Federal Statutory Issues in Nursing Practice

Americans With Disabilities Act

The ADA (1990) is a very broad civil rights statute. It protects the rights of disabled people. It is also the most extensive law on how employers must treat health care workers and clients infected with the human immunodeficiency virus (HIV). The Supreme Court ruled in 1998 in *Bragdon v Abbott* that even asymptomatic HIV constitutes a disability within the meaning of the ADA. This means that the ADA protects an HIV-positive individual who does not have acquired immunodeficiency syndrome (AIDS). The ADA regulations protect the privacy of infected people by giving individuals the opportunity to decide whether to disclose their disability. However, several cases have held that the health care provider has to disclose the fact that he or she has HIV. Despite these rulings, ADA protects health care workers in the workplace with disabilities, such as HIV infection. Likewise, health care workers may not discriminate against HIV-positive clients (Guido, 2006).

Emergency Medical Treatment and Active Labor Act

As a result of clients' being transferred from private hospitals to public hospitals without appropriate screening and stabilization (referred to as "patient dumping"), Congress enacted the Emergency Medical Treatment and Active Labor Act (EMTALA) (1986). This act provides that when a client comes to the emergency department or the hospital, an appropriate medical screening occurs within the hospital's capacity. If an emergency condition exists, the hospital is not to discharge or transfer the client until the condition stabilizes. Exceptions to this include if the client requests transfer or discharge in writing after receiving information on the benefits and risks or if a physician or health care provider certifies that the benefits of transfer outweigh the risks. In this example, a client transfer could occur without an EMTALA violation. The transfer always needs to be appropriate.

Mental Health Parity Act

Health insurance plans are free to eliminate coverage for certain specialties and impose limits on the amount of coverage that they will pay for certain illnesses. However, if health insurance plans provide mental health benefits, a recent federal statute regulates restrictions on mental health benefits. The Mental Health Parity Act of 1996 forbids health plans from placing lifetime or annual limits on mental health coverage that are less generous than those placed on medical or surgical benefits.

Admission of a client to a psychiatric unit occurs involuntarily or on a voluntary basis. Involuntary detention occurs when an individual files with the court within 96 hours of the client's initial detention. A judge may determine that the client is a danger to self or others; then the judge will grant the involuntary detention, and the client can be detained for 21 more days for psychiatric treatment.

Potentially suicidal clients are admitted to psychiatric units. If the client's history and medical records indicate suicidal tendencies, the client must be kept under supervision. Lawsuits result from clients' attempts at suicide within the hospital. The allegations in the lawsuits are that the health care provider failed to provide adequate supervision and failed to safeguard the facilities. Documentation of precautions against suicide is essential.

Advance Directives

There are two basic advance directives: living wills and durable powers of attorney for health care (Cady, 2005). Both living wills and durable powers of attorney for health care are based on values of informed consent, client autonomy over end-of-life decisions, truth telling, and control over the dying process. The Patient Self-Determination Act (PSDA) (1991) requires health care institutions to provide written information to clients concerning the clients' rights under state law to make decisions, including the right to refuse treatment and formulate advance directives. Under the act, the client's record must contain documentation whether the client has signed an advance directive. In order for living wills or durable powers of attorney for health care to be enforceable, the client must be legally incompetent or lack decisional capacity to make decisions regarding health care treatment. A judge makes the determination of legal competency, and the physician or health care provider and family usually make the determination of decisional capacity. Decisional capacity is the ability to make right choices for oneself as it relates to medical care. Be familiar with your institution's policies complying with the act. Likewise, check with state laws to see if a state honors an advance directive that originates in another state.

Living Wills.
Living wills represent written documents that direct treatment in accordance with a client's wishes in the event of a terminal illness or condition. With this legal document the client is able to declare which medical procedures he or she wants or does not want when terminally ill or in a persistent vegetative state. Living wills are often difficult to interpret and not clinically specific in unforeseen circumstances. Each state providing for living wills has its own requirements for executing them. If health care workers follow the directions of the living will, they should be immune from liability (Bross, 2006).

Durable Power of Attorney for Health Care.
A **Durable Power of Attorney for Health Care** (DPAHC) is a legal document that designates a person or persons of one's choosing to make health care decisions when the client is no longer able to make decisions on his or her own behalf. This agent makes health care treatment decisions based on the client's wishes (Cady, 2005).

In addition to federal statutes, the ethical doctrine of autonomy ensures the client the right to refuse medical treatment. Courts upheld the right to refuse medical treatment in the 1986 *Bouvia v Superior Court* case. This case allowed the discontinuation of the client's tube feedings at her request. The courts have also upheld the right of a legally competent client to refuse medical treatment for religious reasons. Christian Scientists refuse medical treatment based on religious beliefs, and Jehovah's Witnesses accept medical treatment but refuse blood transfusions for religious beliefs. In the absence of a truly compelling reason otherwise, clients have the right to make those choices. The U.S. Supreme Court stated in the *Cruzan v Director of Missouri Department of Health* case in 1990 that "we assume that the U.S. Constitution would grant a constitutionally protected competent person the right to refuse lifesaving hydration and nutrition." In cases involving the client's right to refuse or withdraw medical treatment, the courts balance the client's interest with the state's interest in protecting life, preserving medical ethics, preventing suicide, and protecting innocent third parties. Children are generally the innocent third parties. Although the courts will not force adults to undergo treatment refused for religious reasons, they will grant an order allowing hospitals and physicians or health care providers to treat children of Christian Scientists or Jehovah's Witnesses who have denied consent for treatment of their minor children.

When clients are legally incompetent and are unable to make health care decisions, the courts balance the state's interest with what the client would have wanted. The courts attempt to substitute their judgment as to what the client would have chosen if the client were competent. The Supreme Court held in the Cruzan case that states had the right to require "clear and convincing evidence" of a legally incompetent client's prior wishes when making determinations to discontinue life-sustaining treatment. In that case, nutrition and hydration were recognized as life-sustaining medical treatment that could be withdrawn.

In addition to client refusals of treatment, the nurse will frequently encounter the DNR order. DNR means "do not resuscitate" or "no code." The DNR order was first developed in 1976 and marks an important change in health care because it was the first order to withhold treatment instead of deliver treatment (Burns and others, 2003). A DNR order should be written, not verbal. Typically, institutions have policies directing physicians or health care providers to notify the client and family before issuing a DNR order. The physician or health care provider needs to review DNR orders routinely in case the client's condition demands a change. If a client does not have a DNR order, the health care providers need to make every effort to revive the client. Some states, such as Ohio, offer a DNR Comfort Care and DNR Comfort Care Arrest protocols. Protocols in these instances list specific actions that health care providers will take when providing CPR.

Cardiopulmonary resuscitation (CPR) is an emergency treatment provided without client consent. Health care providers perform CPR on an appropriate client unless there is a DNR order in the client's chart. New York's law, the first adopted legislation regarding DNR, is one of the most comprehensive in the United States (New York DNR Statute, 1988). The statutes assume that all clients will be resuscitated unless there is a written DNR order in the chart. Legally competent adult clients consent to a DNR order verbally or in writing after receiving the appropriate information by the physician or health care provider. Be familiar with the DNR protocols of your state.

Uniform Anatomical Gift Act

An individual who is at least 18 years of age has the right to make an organ donation (defined as a "donation of all or part of a human body to take effect upon or after death"). Donors need to make the gift in writing with their signature. In many states, adults sign the back of their driver's license, indicating consent to organ donation.

In most states, Required Request laws mandate that at the time of admission to a hospital, a qualified health care provider has to ask each client over age 18 whether the client is an organ or tissue donor. If the answer is affirmative, the health care provider obtains a copy of the document. If the answer is negative and the attending health care provider consents, the health care provider discusses the option to make or refuse an organ donation and places such documentation in the client's medical record. The health care provider who certifies death shall not be involved in the removal or transplantation of organs (see Chapter 30).

The National Organ Transplant Act of 1984 prohibits the purchase or sale of organs. The act provides civil and criminal immunity to the hospital and health care provider who performs in accordance with the act. The act also protects the donor's estate from liability for injury or damage that results from the use of the gift. Organ transplantation is extremely expensive. Clients in end-stage renal disease are eligible for Medicare coverage for a kidney transplant, but private insurance pays for other transplants. The United Network for Organ Sharing (UNOS) has a contract with the federal government and sets policies and guidelines for the procurement of organs. Most clients who require organ transplantation are on a waiting list for an organ in their geographical area. Recently, the geographical system has changed to give priority to clients who demonstrate the greatest need. Be familiar with your employing institution's policies and procedures regarding organ donation.

Health Insurance Portability and Accountability Act

The Health Insurance Portability and Accountability Act of 1996 (HIPAA) represents one of the more recent federal statutory acts affecting nursing care. This law provides rights to clients and protects employees. It protects individuals from losing their health insurance when changing jobs by providing portability. Portability allows employees to change jobs without losing coverage as a result of preexisting coverage exclusion as long as they have had 12 months of continuous group health insurance coverage (Harman, 2005).

In the Privacy Section of HIPAA, there are standards regarding accountability in the health care setting (Erickson and Millar, 2005). These rules create client rights to consent to use and disclose protected health information, to inspect and copy one's medical record, and to amend mistaken or incomplete information. It limits who is able to access a client's record. It establishes the basis for privacy and confidentiality concerns, viewed as two basic rights within the U.S. health care setting. **Privacy** is the right of clients to keep information about themselves from being disclosed. **Confidentiality** is how health care providers treat client private information once it has been disclosed to others. Client confidentiality is a sacred trust. Nurses help organizations protect clients' rights to confidentiality. Although HIPAA does not require such measures as soundproof rooms in hospitals, it does mean that nurses and all health care providers need to avoid discussing clients in public hallways and provide reasonable levels of privacy in communicating with and about clients in any manner. Message boards used in clients' hospital rooms to post daily nursing care information can no longer contain information revealing the client's medical condition. With the increased use of technology in the health care setting, such as with use of electronic health records, nurses have a challenging task to maintain client privacy and confidentiality. HIPAA violations have civil and criminal sanctions.

Restraints

The Federal Nursing Home Reform Act (1987) gave residents in certified nursing homes the right to be free of unnecessary and inappropriate restraints. The Centers for Medicare and Medicaid Services (2004) standards state that clients have the right to be free from restraints. TJC sets forth specific guidelines regarding use of restraints. TJC (2006) guidelines state that health care providers can use restraints (1) only to ensure the physical safety of the resident or other residents, (2) when less restrictive interventions are not successful, and (3) only on the written order of a physician or health care provider. Written orders include a specific episode with start and end times. Litigation arising from improper restraint use is one of the most common legal issues nurses encounter (Kleen, 2004). Nurses are negligent for failure to initiate safety procedures when the client condition necessitates it. Know when and how to use restraints correctly (Chapter 38). Liability for improper or unlawful restraint, as well as liability for client injury from unprotected falls, lies with the nurse and the health care institution. It is important to note that application of restraints in violation of state and federal regulations constitutes abuse.

State Statutory Issues in Nursing Practice

Licensure

The State Board of Nursing licenses all registered nurses in the state in which they practice. The requirements for licensure vary among states, but most states have minimum education requirements and require a licensure examination. All states use the National Council Licensure Examinations (NCLEX® examination) for registered nurse and licensed practical nurse examinations. Licensure permits persons to offer special skills to the public, but it also provides legal guidelines for protection of the public.

The State Board of Nursing suspends or revokes a license if a nurse's conduct violates provisions in the licensing statute based on administrative law rules that implement and enforce the statute. For example, nurses who perform illegal acts such as selling or taking controlled substances jeopardize their license status. Because a license is a property right, the State Board has to follow due process before revoking or suspending a license. Due process means that nurses must be notified of the charges brought against them and that the nurses have an opportunity to defend against the charges in a hearing. Hearings for suspension or revocation of a license do not occur in court. Usually a panel of professionals conducts the hearing. Some states provide administrative and judicial review of such cases after nurses have exhausted all other forms of appeal (State of Illinois, 2005).

Good Samaritan Laws

Nurses act as Good Samaritans by providing emergency assistance at an accident scene (Good Samaritan Act, 1997). All states have Good Samaritan laws enacted to encourage health care professionals to assist in emergencies (Guido, 2006). Although provisions vary among states, these laws limit liability and offer legal immunity for nurses who help at the scene of an accident. Check your own state's Good Samaritan statute, because some states (e.g., Minnesota and Vermont) require nurses to stop and help in an emergency.

Public Health Laws

Nurses need to understand public health laws, especially those employed in community health settings. State legislatures enact statutes under the health code, which describes the reporting laws for communicable diseases, school immunizations, and laws intended to promote health and reduce health risks in communities. The Centers for Disease Control and Prevention (CDC) (http://www.CDC.gov) and the Occupational Health and Safety Act (OHSA) (http://www.osha.gov) provide guidelines on a national level for safe and healthy communities and work environments. The purposes of public health laws are protection of the public's health, advocating for the rights of people, regulating health care and health care financing, and ensuring professional accountability for the care provided. Community and public health nurses have the legal responsibility to enforce the laws enacted to protect the public's health (see Chapter 3). These laws include reporting suspected abuse and neglect, such as child abuse, elder abuse, or domestic violence, reporting communicable diseases, ensuring that clients in the community have received required immunizations, and reporting of other health-related issues enacted to protect the public's health. To encourage reports of suspected cases, states provide legal immunity for the reporter if the report is made in good faith. Health care professionals who do not report suspected child abuse or neglect are sometimes liable for civil or criminal legal action.

The Uniform Determination of Death Act

Many legal issues surround the event of death, including a basic definition of the actual point at which a person is legally dead. There are essentially two standards for the determination of death. The cardiopulmonary standard requires irreversible cessation of circulatory and respiratory functions. The whole-brain standard requires irreversible cessation of all functions of the entire brain, including the brain stem. The reason for the development of different definitions is to facilitate recovery of organs for transplantation. Even though the client is legally "brain dead," the client's organs are sometimes healthy for donation to other clients. Most states have adopted the Uniform Determination of Death Act (1980). It states that health care providers can use either the cardiopulmonary definition or the whole-brain definition to determine death. Be aware of legal definitions of death because you will need to document all events that occur when the client is in your care. Nurses have a specific legal obligation to treat the deceased person's remains with dignity (see Chapter 30). Wrongful handling of a deceased person's remains cause emotional harm to the surviving family.

Physician-Assisted Suicide

Providing end-of-life care in today's world is challenging for health care professionals because people are living longer. The Oregon Death With Dignity Act (1994) was the first statute that permitted physician or health care provider–assisted suicide. The statute stated that a competent individual with a terminal disease could make an oral and written request for medication to end his or her life in a humane and dignified manner. A terminal disease is an "incurable and irreversible disease that has been medically confirmed and will, within reasonable medical judgment, produce death within 6 months." The Oregon Death With Dignity Act remains the object of several challenges in federal court (Follin, 2004). Individual autonomy is the most prominent argument for assisted death. The ANA states that the Act "violates the *Code for Nurses*" and goes against the profession's role integrity (Ersek, 2004). Be familiar with state laws pertaining to assisted suicide to avoid legal action.

Two court cases, *Compassion in Dying v Washington* (1997) and *Quill v Vacco* (1997), raise challenges to state statutes that made assisting in suicide a criminal act in Washington and New York, respectively. The lower courts both held that the criminal statutes were unconstitutional. The Supreme Court heard the cases. It held in *Washington v Glucksberg* (1997) that there is no fundamental constitutional right to assisted suicide. In making its ruling, the Supreme Court did not prevent the states from passing legislation legalizing assisted suicide. The Supreme Court also relied on the fact that there are no legal barriers to obtaining pain medication and that dying persons in Washington and New York could "obtain palliative care, even when doing so would hasten their deaths."

Another area of health care treatment that falls within the realms of assisted suicide deals with feeding tubes (Orentlicher and Callahan, 2004). Courts have hesitated to authorize withdrawals of feeding tubes unless there is very clear evidence that the client previously expressed a preference against a tube feeding.

Civil and Common Law Issues in Nursing Practice

Torts

A **tort** is a civil wrong made against a person or property. Classifications for torts include intentional, quasi-intentional, or unintentional. **Intentional torts** are willful acts that violate another's rights, such as assault, battery, and false imprisonment. Quasi-intentional torts are acts where intent is lacking but volitional action and direct causation occur, such as found with invasion of privacy and defamation of character. The third classification of tort is the unintentional tort, which includes negligence or malpractice.

Intentional Torts

Assault **Assault** is any intentional threat to bring about harmful or offensive contact. No actual contact is necessary. The law protects clients who are afraid of harmful contact. It is an assault for a nurse to threaten to give a client an injection or to threaten to restrain a client for an x-ray procedure when the client has refused consent. The key issue is the client's consent. In an assault lawsuit, if the client gives consent, the nurse is not responsible for assault.

Battery. **Battery** is any intentional touching without consent. The contact can be harmful to the client and cause an injury, or it can be merely offensive to the client's personal dignity. A battery always includes an assault, which is why the terms *assault* and *battery* are commonly combined. In the example of a nurse threatening to give a client an injection without the client's consent, if the nurse actually gives the injection, it is battery. Battery also results if the health care provider performs a procedure that exceeds the client's consent. For example, if the client gives consent for an appendectomy and the health care provider performs a tonsillectomy, battery has occurred. Once again, the key issue is the client's consent.

In some situations, consent is implied. For example, if a client gets into a wheelchair or transfers to a stretcher after receiving advice that it is time to be taken for an x-ray procedure, the client has given implied consent to the procedure. If the client learns that they will have an x-ray film of the head instead of the foot and the client refuses to have the x-ray film taken, the consent has been revoked or withdrawn.

False Imprisonment. The tort of false imprisonment occurs with unjustified restraining of a person without legal warrant. For example, this occurs when nurses restrain a client in a bounded area to keep the person from freedom.

Quasi-Intentional Torts

Invasion of Privacy. The tort of invasion of privacy protects the client's right to be free from unwanted intrusion into his or her private affairs. HIPAA Privacy Standards have raised awareness of the need for health care professionals to provide confidentiality and privacy. The four types of invasion of privacy torts are intrusion on seclusion, appropriation of name or likeness, publication of private or embarrassing facts, and publicity placing one in a false light in the public's eye (Cady, 2005).

HIPAA sets forth standards indicating that clients are entitled to confidential health care. For example, in a classic case, reporters published photographs of a female client in her hospital room without her consent. Courts upheld a claim for invasion of privacy. This case is an example of intrusion on seclusion or publication of private, embarrassing facts (*Barber v Time Magazine*, 1942).

Another form of invasion of privacy is the release of a client's medical information to an unauthorized person, such as a member of the press or the client's employer. The information that is in a client's medical record is a confidential communication. You share it with health care providers for the purpose of medical treatment only.

A client's medical record is confidential. Do not disclose the client's confidential medical information without the client's consent. For example, respect the wish not to inform the client's family of a terminal illness. Similarly, do not assume that a client's spouse or family members know all of the client's history, particularly with respect to private issues such as mental illness, medications, pregnancy, abortion, birth control, or sexually transmitted diseases.

An individual's right to privacy sometimes conflicts with the public's right to know. In one case, a television crew filmed a married couple who were participating in a hospital program. The couple had previously told no one but their immediate family that they were involved in the in vitro fertilization program and had received assurance that there would be no publicity or public exposure. After the newscast, they received phone calls and embarrassing questions. The couple filed a lawsuit. The court held that the husband and wife stated a claim for invasion of privacy and that even though the in vitro fertilization program was of public interest, the identity of the plaintiffs was a private matter (*YG v Jewish Hospital*, 1990).

Many states, through their respective public health departments, require that hospitals report certain infectious or communicable diseases. Sometimes the client is a public figure whose physical condition is newsworthy (Guido, 2006). There are also cases in which information about a scientific discovery or a major medical breakthrough is newsworthy, as with the first heart transplant case or the first artificial heart recipient. If an event falls into any of these categories, guide information through the public relations department of the institution to ensure that invasion of privacy does not occur. It is not the nurse's responsibility to decide independently the legality of disclosing information.

Defamation of Character. **Defamation of character** is the publication of false statements that result in damage to a person's reputation. The statements must be published with malice in the case of a public official or public figure. **Malice** means that the person publishing the information knows it is false and publishes it anyway or publishes it with reckless disregard as to the truth. **Slander** occurs when one verbalizes the false statement. For example, if a nurse tells people erroneously that a client has venereal disease and the disclosure affects the client's business, the nurse is liable for slander. **Libel** is the written defamation of character. Charting false entries is another example of defamation.

Unintentional Torts

Negligence.
Negligence is conduct that falls below a standard of care. The law established the standard of care for the protection of others against an unreasonably great risk of harm (Black, 2004). For example, if a driver of a car acts unreasonably in failing to stop at a stop sign, it is negligence. In general, courts define negligence in car accident cases and other negligence cases as that degree of care that an ordinarily careful and prudent person would use under the same or similar circumstances. Negligent acts such as hanging the wrong intravenous solution for a client or allowing a nursing assistant to administer a medication often will lead to disciplinary action by a state (State of Illinois, 2005).

Malpractice.
Malpractice is one type of negligence and often referred to as professional negligence. When nursing care falls below a standard of care, nursing malpractice results. To establish nursing malpractice, there are certain criteria: (1) the nurse (defendant) owed a duty to the client (plaintiff), (2) the nurse did not carry out that duty, (3) the client was injured, and (4) the nurse's failure to carry out the duty caused the injury. Even though nurses do not intend to injure clients, some clients file claims of negligence if nurses give care that does not meet the appropriate standards. Negligence sometimes involves failing to check a client's armband and then administering medication to the wrong client. Negligence also involves administering a medication to a client even though the medical record contains documentation that the client has an allergy to that medication. In general, courts define nursing negligence as the failure to use that degree of skill or learning ordinarily used under the same or similar circumstances by members of the nursing profession (Box 23-2) (Austin, 2006).

The best way for nurses to avoid negligence is to follow standards of care, give competent health care, and communicate with other health care providers. You will also avoid negligence by developing a caring rapport with the client and documenting assessments, interventions, and evaluations fully. Nurses need to know the current nursing literature in their areas of practice. Know and follow the policies and procedures of the institution where you work. Be sensitive to common sources of client injury, such as falls and medication errors. Finally, communicate with the client; explain the tests and treatment, document that you provided specific explanations to the client, and listen to the client's concerns about the treatment. You are accountable for reporting any significant changes in the client's condition to the health care provider and documenting these changes in the chart (see Chapter 26). Timely and truthful documentation is important to provide the communication necessary among the health care team members. Be certain that documentation is legible and signed (Austin, 2006).

✳ BOX 23-2 Common Negligent Acts

- Failure to assess and/or monitor, including making a nursing diagnosis
  - Failure to monitor in timely fashion
  - Failure to use proper equipment to monitor the client
  - Failure to document the monitoring
- Failure to notify the health care provider of problems
- Failure to follow orders
- Failure to follow the six rights of medication administration
- Failure to convey discharge instructions
- Failure to ensure client safety, especially those who have a history of falling, are heavily sedated, have disequilibrium problems, are frail, are mentally impaired, get up in the night, and are uncooperative
- Failure to follow policies and procedures
- Failure to properly delegate and supervise

A number of courts have stated that when a health care provider negligently alters or loses medical records relevant to a malpractice claim, the health care provider has to demonstrate why these events occurred. An institution has a duty to maintain nursing records. Statutes and accreditation regulations establish these duties. Nursing notes contain substantial evidence needed to understand the care received by a client. If records are lost or incomplete, there is a presumption that the care was negligent and therefore the cause of the client's injuries. In addition, incomplete or illegible records make the health care provider less credible or believable.

Consent

A signed consent form is required for all routine treatment, hazardous procedures such as surgery, some treatment programs such as chemotherapy, and research involving clients (TJC, 2006). A client signs general consent forms when admitted to the hospital or other health care facility. The client or a representative needs to sign separate special consent or treatment forms before the performing of specialized procedures.

State statutes provide the designation of individuals who are legally able to give consent to medical treatment (Medical Patient Rights Act, 1994). Nurses need to know the law in their own states and be familiar with the policies and procedures of their employing institution regarding consent (Box 23-3).

If a client is deaf, illiterate, or speaks a foreign language, there needs to be an official interpreter to explain the terms of consent. A family member or acquaintance who speaks a client's language should not interpret health information. Make every effort to assist the client in making an informed choice.

Informed Consent.
Informed consent is a person's agreement to allow something to happen, such as surgery or an invasive diagnostic procedure, based on a full disclosure of risks, benefits, alternatives, and consequences of refusal (Black, 2004). Informed consent creates a legal duty for the health care provider to disclose material facts in terms the client is able to understand to make an informed choice (Dalinis, 2005). The explanation also describes treatment alternatives, as well as the risks involved in all treatment options. Failure to obtain consent in situations other than emer-

BOX 23-3 Statutory Guidelines for Legal Consent for Medical Treatment

Those who consent to medical treatment are governed by state law but generally include the following:

I. Adults
A. Any competent individual 18 years of age or older for himself or herself
B. Any parent for his or her unemancipated minor
C. Any guardian for his or her ward
D. Any adult for the treatment of his or her minor brother or sister (if an emergency and parents are not present)
E. Any grandparent for a minor grandchild (if an emergency and parents are not present)

II. Minors
A. For his or her child and any child in his or her legal custody
B. For himself or herself in the following situations:
1. Lawfully married or a parent (emancipated)
2. Pregnancy (excluding abortions)
3. Venereal disease
4. Drug or substance abuse
C. Unemancipated minors may not consent to abortions without one of the following:
1. Consent of one parent
2. Self-consent being granted by court order
3. Consent specifically given by a court

gencies will possibly result in a claim of battery. Without informed consent, a client may bring a lawsuit against the health care provider for negligence.

Informed consent is part of the health care provider–client relationship. Informed consent needs to be obtained and witnessed only when the client is not under the influence of medication, such as narcotics. Because nurses do not perform surgery or direct medical procedures, in most situations, obtaining clients' informed consent does not fall within the nursing duty. The person responsible for performing the procedure has the responsibility to obtain the informed consent (Figure 23-1).

The nurse's signature witnessing the consent means that the client voluntarily gave consent, that the client's signature is authentic, and that the client appears to be competent to give consent (Ohio Nurses Foundation [ONF], 2005). When nurses provide consent forms for clients to sign, nurses must ask the clients if they understand the procedure for which they are giving consent. If clients deny understanding or you suspect they do not understand, notify the physician, health care provider, or nursing supervisor. Health care providers must inform a client refusing surgery or other medical treatment about any harmful consequences of refusal. If the client persists in refusing the treatment, this rejection needs to be written, signed, and witnessed. It is important to note that nursing students cannot be and should not be responsible for or asked to witness consent forms due to the legal nature of the document.

Parents are usually the legal guardians of pediatric clients, and therefore they are the persons who sign consent forms for treatment. If the parents are divorced, the parent with legal custody gives consent. Occasionally a parent or guardian refuses treatment for a child. In those cases, the court sometimes intervenes on the child's behalf.

In some instances, obtaining informed consent is difficult. If, for example, the client is unconscious, you must obtain consent from a person legally authorized to give consent on the client's behalf. Sometimes the client has legally designated other surrogate decision makers with this authority through special power of attorney documents or through court guardianship procedures. In emergencies, if it is impossible to obtain consent from the client or an authorized person, a health care provider may perform a procedure required to benefit the client or save a life without liability for failure to obtain consent. In such cases the law assumes that the client would wish to be treated.

Psychiatric clients must also give consent. They retain the right to refuse treatment until a court has legally determined that they are incompetent to decide for themselves.

Abortion Issues

In 1973 in the case of *Roe v Wade,* the U.S. Supreme Court ruled that there is a fundamental right to privacy, which includes a woman's decision to have an abortion. The court ruled that during the first trimester a woman could end her pregnancy without state regulation because the risk of natural mortality from abortion is less than with normal childbirth. During the second trimester, the state has an interest in protecting maternal health, and the state enforces regulations regarding the person performing the abortion and the abortion facility. By the third trimester, when the fetus becomes viable, the state's interest is to protect the fetus, so the state therefore prohibits abortion except when necessary to save the mother.

In 1989 in the case of *Webster v Reproductive Health Services* the court substantially narrowed the *Roe v Wade* case. Some states require viability tests before conducting abortions if the fetus is over 28 weeks' gestational age. Some states also require a minor's parental consent or a judicial decision that the minor is mature and can self-consent.

Nursing Students

Nursing students are liable if their actions cause harm to clients. If a student harms a client as a direct result of his or her actions or lack of action, the student, instructor, hospital or health care facility, and university or educational institution generally share the liability for the incorrect action. Nursing students should never be assigned to perform tasks for which they are unprepared, and instructors should carefully supervise them as they learn new skills. Although nursing students are not employees of the hospital, the institution has a responsibility to monitor the acts of nursing students. Nursing students are expected to perform as professional nurses would in providing safe client care. Faculty members are usually responsible for instructing and observing students, but in some situations staff nurses serving as preceptors share these responsibilities. Every nursing school should provide clear definitions of preceptor and faculty responsibility.

When students work as nursing assistants or nurse's aides when not attending classes, they should not perform tasks that do not appear in a job description for a nurse's aide or assistant. For example, even if a student has learned to administer intramuscular medications in class, the student now working as a nurse's aide may not perform this task. If a staff nurse overseeing the nursing assistant or aide knowingly assigns work without regard for the

OSF Saint Francis Medical Center - Peoria Children's Hospital of Illinois

Consent To Surgery/Procedure

FORM NO. 113-0672 (REV. 08/05) *MS*
PAGE 1 of 2

CONSENT TO SURGERY / PROCEDURE

I ______________________________ hereby authorize Dr. ______________________________

and such assistants and associates as may be selected by him/her and OSF Saint Francis Medical Center to perform the following procedure(s)/treatment(s) upon myself/the patient: ______________________________

____

Stated in Medical Terminology

____

Stated in Common Language

2. I understand that this procedure(s)/treatment(s) appears indicated by the diagnostic and/or observations performed. My physician has explained to me the following:
   A. The nature of the proposed procedure, care, treatment, services, medications, or interventions.
   B. The purpose of and need for the recommended procedure(s)/treatment(s).
   C. The potential benefits, risks, side effects, including potential problems related to recuperation.
   D. The alternatives, if any to the recommended procedure(s)/treatment(s), service, or care. I understand the explanation provided and give this consent voluntarily.
   E. The relevant risk, benefits, and side effects related to alternatives, including the possible results of not receiving care, treatment, and services.

3. I understand that the explanation I have received is not exhaustive and I acknowledge that I have received no warranties or guarantees with respect to the benefits to be realized or consequences of the aforementioned procedures(s)/treatment(s).

4. I agree to allow the performance of additional procedure(s)/treatment(s) as deemed necessary by my physician during the course of this procedure(s)/treatment(s).

5. I agree to allow the use of anesthetics/anesthesia agents by the healthcare professionals responsible for their administration and have been fully advised by them as to the nature/purpose of the planned anesthesia, the possible risks and/or complications of anesthesia and possible alternative methods. I have been fully advised of the above prior to the procedure(s)/treatment(s) and anesthesia episode.

6. I agree to imagery of the procedure(s)/treatment(s) such as for educational and performance improvement, or scientific purposes. I realize that my identity may become apparent.

Figure 23-1 Sample consent to surgery/procedure. (Courtesy OSF Saint Francis Medical Center, Peoria, Ill.)

person's ability to safely conduct the task defined in the job description, the staff nurse will also be liable. If someone requests students employed as nurse's aides to perform tasks that they are not prepared to complete safely, they need to bring this information to the supervisor's attention so that they are able to obtain the needed help.

Malpractice Insurance

Malpractice or professional liability insurance is a contract between the nurse and the insurance company. Malpractice insurance provides for a defense when a nurse is in a lawsuit involving professional negligence or medical malpractice. As part of the insurance contract, the insurance company pays for any judgment or settlement of the case and pays for the attorney's fees generated in the representation of the nurse. Nurses employed by health care institutions generally are covered by that institution's insurance and do not need to purchase any supplemental insurance unless the nurse plans to practice nursing outside of the employing institution. The employing institution's insurance, however, only covers nurses while they are working within the scope of their employment. Because nurses are professionals and it is often difficult to separate their private lives from their professional skills, nurses need to consider purchasing individual professional liability insurance, even if the employing institution has coverage. For example, a hospital policy does not cover a nurse whom neighbors and friends call upon to provide nursing care on a volunteer basis if the neighbor or friend filed suit (Sloan, 2004). Nursing students should check with their educational institution regarding the need for liability insurance.

Nurses need to consult their lawyers on what types of policies to purchase and what rights or duties, if any, exist under the policy. If both the employing institution and the nurse are sued in a professional liability case, even though the nurse has insurance with the hospital, the nurse needs to notify his or her private insurance carrier of the lawsuit. If both the hospital policy and the private policy are considered primary and the hospital loses as a result of the nurse's acts, theoretically the hospital could sue the nurse's private insurer to recover its losses. Most private insurance policies for nurses, however, are excess policies and only begin covering the nurse after all of the primary (hospital) insurance coverage has been exhausted. Because the hospital insurance coverage is generally much greater than the private insurance coverage, hospitals very rarely sue nurses' private insurers.

OSF Saint Francis Medical Center - Peoria Children's Hospital of Illinois

Consent To Surgery/Procedure

FORM NO. 113-0672 (REV. 08/05) *MS*
PAGE 2 of 2

7. I understand those involved or needing to have knowledge of my care, treatment, and services will have access to my applicable medical information. This includes equipment / supply / implant company representatives who may be present in the operating / procedure room to provide the physician with technical information related to a specific product relating to my case.

8. I understand that it is standard practice to initiate cardiopulmonary resuscitation (CPR) if need arises during the procedure(s)/treatment(s). See my wishes below:

   A. __ Initiate CPR if the need arises. I do not have a DNR *OR* I have a DNR but wish to have CPR initiated. Outpatient areas initiate CPR.

   B. __ Please follow my previously established DNR status. Maintaining my current DNR status has been reviewed with and approved by my physician.

9. I agree to allow OSF Saint Francis Medical Center to dispose of any removed tissue and/or body part.

10. I have informed the Medical Center and my attending physician that, to my knowledge, I have allergies to the following substances and drugs: _____

11. I have read this consent form in its entirety, understand its content and significance, have had all my questions answered and have no further questions.

Patient: _____ Date: _____ Time: _____
Representative: _____ Relationship: _____
Witness: _____
Physician _____

TIME OUT
To be completed prior to the procedure(s)/treatment(s) at the place where the procedure(s)/treatment(s) takes place. (Surgery and other approved departments may use their own "correct site surgery checklist")" This should be done with patient agreement unless the patient is sedated or unable to participate.

• Relevant documents and studies have been reviewed prior to the procedure that includes the following as applicable:
   • History and Physical (H&P within 24hrs for new admit. progress notes serve as update/ H&P within 30 days for AM admit or OP surgery requiring update at time of admission)
   • Imaging reports
• Site is marked with assistance from the patient, when possible. Applicable when procedure involves laterality, multiple structures (fingers, toes, lesions) or multiple levels (spine):
• The following are checked immediately prior to incision/injection/procedure:
   • Correct Patient Identity
   • Correct Side and Site
   • Agreement on the procedure to be done
   • Correct patient position
   • Correct implants, special equipment or special requirements needed are available and prepared

Staff: _____ Date: _____ Time: _____
Signature

Figure 23-1, cont'd Sample consent to surgery/procedure. (Courtesy OSF Saint Francis Medical Center, Peoria, Ill.)

Abandonment and Assignment Issues

Short Staffing. During nursing shortages or staff downsizing periods, the issue of inadequate staffing occurs (TJC, 2006). The Community Health Accreditation Program (CHAP), as well as other state and federal standards, requires institutions to have guidelines for determining the number (staffing ratios) of nurses required to give care to a specific number of clients. Legal problems occur if there are not enough nurses to provide competent care or nurses work excessive overtime (Box 23-4). One such example is in a class-action suit, *Spires v. Hospital Corporation of America,* filed on April 10, 2006. The wife claims there was poor client care related to insufficient registered nurse (RN) staffing and that the poor nurse-staffing levels led to the resultant death of her husband. This suit emphasizes the potential seriousness of short staffing and the importance of nurses' asserting employee rights.

In an attempt to address the short-staffing problem, California is the first state and so far only state to adopt legislation (California Assembly Bill 394 [AB394]) mandating a fixed nurse-to-client ratio for all areas of acute care nursing. The standards became effective January 1, 2004. Approximately 15 other states are currently addressing similar legislation. The safe staffing ratio debate is occurring throughout the country and demands close attention by all nurses (Benko, 2004).

If nurses are assigned to care for more clients than is reasonable, they need to bring this information to the attention of the nursing supervisor (Blair, 2003). If nurses have to accept assignments, they need to make written protests to nursing administrators. Although these protests do not relieve nurses of responsibility if a client suffers an injury because of inattention, it shows that the nurses were attempting to act reasonably. Whenever you make a written protest, keep a copy of this document in your own personal file. Most administrators recognize that knowledge of a potential problem shifts some of the responsibility to the institution. Do not walk out when staffing is inadequate, because this constitutes abandonment. A nurse who refuses to accept an assignment is considered insubordinate. It is important to know the institution's policies and procedures on how to handle such reports before the situation occurs (Mrayyan and Huber, 2003).

Floating. Nurses are sometimes required to "float" from the area in which they normally practice to other nursing units based on census load and client acuities. In one case a nurse in obstetrics was assigned to an emergency department. A client entered the

* BOX 23-4   EVIDENCE-BASED PRACTICE

Consequences of Working Overtime

Evidence Summary

As hospitals struggle with the nurse shortage, nurses find themselves working more hours, longer hours, and taking care of more clients. Researchers studied the work patterns of hospital staff nurses and compared the relationship between hours worked and frequency of errors. A sample of 393 unit-based hospital staff nurses who worked full-time completed logbooks that covered a 2-week period. Researchers collected information about hours and time of day worked, overtime, days off, and sleep-wake patterns. Other questions focused on errors and near errors. Results showed that nurses who worked shifts lasting 12.5 hours or more had a three-times greater likelihood of making an error. Overtime increased the odds of making at least one error, regardless of length of original shift scheduled.

Application to Nursing Practice

• The longer a nurse stays at work, especially if over 12.5 hours, the greater the likelihood he or she will make an error or near error related to client care.
• When a nurse agrees to work longer than either 40 or 50 hours per week, this increases the chance of making an error affecting client care.
• Nurses who volunteer to work overtime are subjecting themselves to making potential medical errors.
• Nursing is not a profession where one can predictably leave work at a given time.

Reference

Rogers AE and others: The working hours of hospital staff nurses and patient safety, *Health Affairs,* 23(4): 202, 2004.

emergency department and complained of chest pain. The client received an incorrect dosage of lidocaine by the obstetrical nurse and died after suffering irreversible brain damage and cardiac arrest. The nurse lost the malpractice lawsuit. Nurses who float need to inform the supervisor of any lack of experience in caring for the type of clients on the nursing unit. They also need to request and receive an orientation to the unit. Supervisors are liable if they give a staff nurse an assignment he or she cannot safely handle. In the case of *Winkelman v Beloit Memorial Hospital* (1992), the court found that the employer needed to provide the training and education to prepare nurses to work in an area outside of their normal assignment. Before accepting employment, find out the institution's policies regarding floating and have an understanding as to what is expected (Kane-Urrabazo, 2006).

Physicians' Orders. The physician is responsible for directing medical treatment. Nurses follow physicians' orders unless they believe the orders are in error or harm clients. Therefore you need to assess all orders, and if you find one to be erroneous or harmful, further clarification from the physician is necessary. If the physician or health care provider confirms an order and you still believe it is inappropriate, inform the supervising nurse or follow the established chain of command. The supervising nurse should help resolve the questionable order. A medical consultant sometimes helps clarify the appropriateness or inappropriateness of the order. A nurse carrying out an inaccurate or inappropriate order is legally responsible for any harm the client suffers.

In a malpractice lawsuit against a physician or health care provider and a hospital, one of the most frequently litigated issues is whether the nurse kept the physician or health care provider informed of the client's condition. To inform a physician or health care provider properly, you perform a competent nursing assessment of the client to determine the signs and symptoms that are significant in relation to the attending physician's or health care provider's tasks of diagnosis and treatment. Be certain to document that you notified the physician or health care provider and document his or her response, your follow-up, and the client's response.

The physician or health care provider should write all orders. The nurse is responsible for transcribing correctly written orders. If a verbal order is necessary (e.g., during an emergency), have it written and signed by the physician or health care provider as soon as possible, usually within 24 hours. The 2007 TJC National Patient Safety Goals direct the nurse to "verify the complete order or test result by having the person receiving the information record and 'read-back' the complete order or test result" (http://www.jcipatientsafety.org/). Be familiar with the institution's policy and procedures regarding verbal orders.

Risk Management

Risk management is a system of ensuring appropriate nursing care that attempts to identify potential hazards and eliminate them before harm occurs (Guido, 2006). The steps involved in risk management include identifying possible risks, analyzing them, acting to reduce the risks, and evaluating the steps taken. One tool used in risk management is the **incident report** or **occurrence report.**

Occurrence reporting provides a database for further investigation in an attempt to determine deviations from standards of care and corrective measures needed to prevent recurrence and to alert risk management to a potential claim situation. Examples of an occurrence include client or visitor falls or injury; failure to follow physician or health care provider orders; significant complaint by client, family, physician or health care provider, or other hospital department; error in technique or procedure; and malfunctioning device or product. Institutions generally have specific guidelines to direct health care providers in how to complete the occurrence report. The report is confidential and separate from the medical record. The nurse is responsible for providing information in the medical record about the occurrence. **Never document in the client's medical record that an occurrence report was completed.**

Risk management also requires good documentation. The nurse's documentation is often the evidence of care received by a client and serves as proof that the nurse acted reasonably and safely. When a lawsuit is filed, very often the nurses' notes are the first thing an attorney reviews (Austin, 2006). The nurse's assessments and the reporting of significant changes in the assessments are very important factors in defending a lawsuit. Therefore identifying the physician or health care provider contacted, the information communicated to the physician or health care provider, and the physician's or health care provider's response is essential.

For nurses in practice the underlying rationale for quality improvement and risk management programs is the highest possible quality of care. Some insurance companies, medical and nursing organizations, and TJC require the use of quality improvement and risk management procedures (TJC, 2006).

One area of potential risk is associated with the use of electronic monitoring devices. No monitor is reliable at all times, so do not completely depend on monitoring devices. Continual assessment of a client is necessary to help document the accuracy of electronic monitoring. There are also electrical hazards to the nurse and the client. Biomedical engineers are responsible for checking equipment to ensure that it is in proper working order and that a client will not receive an electrical shock.

In the operating room, sponge, needle, and instrument counts are routine surgical standards to prevent client injury and lawsuits. Physicians or health care providers rely on nurses to provide an accurate count of sponges and instruments inserted at the end of a procedure even though it is the physician or health care provider who inserts sponges and instruments into the surgical wound. Generally, when the chart records a correct sponge count and the client suffers an injury because of a retained sponge, the hospital is liable because the nurse charted a correct count when it was not correct. All nurses need to be risk managers.

Professional Involvement

Nurses need to be involved in their professional organizations and on committees that define the standards of care for nursing practice. If current laws, rules and regulations, or policies under which nurses practice do not reflect reality, nurses need to become involved as advocates to see that the scope of nursing practice is defined accurately. Be willing to represent nursing and the client's perspective in the community as well. The voice of nursing is powerful and effective when the organizing focus is the protection and welfare of the public entrusted to nurses' care (Mrayyan and Huber, 2003).

✳ Key Concepts

- Registered nurses and licensed practical nurses are licensed by the state in which they practice; licensing is based on educational requirements, the passing of an examination, and other criteria.
- The civil law system is concerned with the protection of a person's private rights, and the criminal law system deals with the rights of individuals and society as defined by legislative statutes.
- A nurse is liable for malpractice if the nurse (defendant) owed a duty to the client (plaintiff), the nurse did not carry out that duty, the client was injured, and the nurse's failure to carry out the duty caused the client's injury.
- All clients are entitled to confidential health care and freedom from unauthorized release of information.
- Under the law, practicing nurses must follow standards of care, the guidelines of professional organizations, and the written policies and procedures of employing institutions.
- Nurses who witness consents are responsible for confirming that clients have voluntarily given informed consent for any surgery or other medical procedure before the procedure is performed.
- Nurses are responsible for performing all procedures correctly and exercising professional judgment as they carry out physicians' or health care providers' orders.

- Nurses follow physicians' or health care providers' orders unless they believe the orders are in error or are harmful to clients.
- Staffing standards determine the ratio of nurses to clients, and if the nurse has to care for more clients than is reasonable, the nurse needs to make a formal protest to the nursing administration.
- Legal issues involving death include documenting all events surrounding the death and treating a deceased person with dignity.
- All nurses need to know the laws that apply to their area of practice.
- Depending on state laws, nurses are required to report possible criminal activities such as child abuse, as well as certain communicable diseases.
- Nurses are client advocates and ensure quality of care through risk management and lobbying for safe nursing practice standards.
- Nurses must file incident/occurrence reports in all situations when someone was hurt.

✳ Critical Thinking Exercises

You are working the first shift on the hematology-oncology unit and receive report on your assigned team of four clients. You have a nursing assistive personnel assigned to help you with routine care. You make quick rounds on your clients to ensure there are no immediate needs before you begin checking medications. Client No. 1 is scheduled for surgery later in the morning for a biopsy and needs the consent signed. Client No. 2 is receiving blood products for an HIV complication and needs frequent vital sign monitoring. Client No. 3 is receiving comfort care only for a terminal condition. The client is unresponsive. Family is at the bedside. You find client No. 4, an 83-year-old confused man, lying on the floor. He stated he needed to go to the restroom and no one was there to assist. You call for help to get the client back in bed, and assess for further injuries.

1. The nurse prepares the surgical consent form for client No. 1. What key points does the nurse need to ensure the client received before witnessing informed consent?

2. The son of client No. 2 calls to talk to the nurse caring for his father. The son asks questions about the reason for the blood administration. What guidelines must the nurse follow in responding to the son's questions about the father's condition? What federal statutes are involved in this scenario?

3. The family alerts the nurse that they believe client No. 3 has stopped breathing. What is the nurse's responsibility in this situation? How should the nurse best proceed in responding to this emergency?

4. One week after discharge from the hospital, the hospital received a written complaint from the family of client No. 4 about the incident related to the fall and the intent to take legal action.
   a. What must client No. 4 establish to prove negligence against the nurse?
   b. Describe those situations in which restraints may be legally applied to prevent falls.

✳ NCLEX®-Style Review Questions

1. A nurse works on a cardiac unit. She is taking care of a client who recently had coronary bypass surgery. Which of the following represent legal sources of standards of care nurses use to deliver safe health care? (Choose all that apply.)
   1. Information provided by the head nurse
   2. Policies and procedures of the employing hospital
   3. Nurse Practice Act of the state the nurse is working in
   4. Regulations identified in The Joint Commission's manual
   5. The American Nurses Association standards of nursing practice

2. A nurse is sued for failure to monitor a client appropriately. Which statements are correct about professional negligence lawsuits? (Choose all that apply.)
   1. The nurse represents the plaintiff.
   2. The defendant must prove injury, damage, or loss.
   3. The person filing the lawsuit has the burden of proof.
   4. The plaintiff must prove that a breach in the prevailing standard of care caused an injury.

3. When the nurse stops to help in an emergency at the scene of an accident, if the injured party files suit and the nurse's employing institution's insurance does not cover the nurse, the nurse would probably be covered by:
   1. The nurse's automobile insurance
   2. The nurse's homeowner's insurance
   3. The Good Samaritan laws, which grant immunity from suit if there is no gross negligence
   4. The Patient Care Partnership, which may grant immunity from suit if the injured party consents

4. Even though the nurse may obtain the client's signature on a form, obtaining informed consent is the responsibility of the:
   1. Client
   2. Physician
   3. Nursing student
   4. Supervising nurse

5. The legal definition of death that facilitates organ donation is cessation of:
   1. Pulse
   2. Respirations
   3. Functions of entire brain
   4. Circulatory and respiratory functions

6. The nurse notes that an advance directive is on the client's medical record. Which of the following statements represents the best description of guidelines a nurse would follow?
   1. A living will allows an appointed person to make health care decisions when the client is in an incapacitated state.

   2. A living will is invoked only when the client has a terminal condition or is in a persistent vegetative state.
   3. The client cannot make changes in the advance directive once admitted to the hospital.
   4. A Durable Power of Attorney for Health Care is invoked only when the client has a terminal condition or is in a persistent vegetative state.

7. A nurse notes that the health care unit keeps a listing of the client names at the front desk in easy view for health care providers to more efficiently locate the client. The nurse knows that this action would be a violation of:
   1. Mental Health Parity Act
   2. Patient Self-Determination Act
   3. Health Insurance Portability and Accountability Act
   4. Emergency Medical Treatment and Active Labor Act

8. Which of the following statements represent actions that may result in a registered nurse's receiving either disciplinary action by the nurse's State Board of Nursing or revocation of the nurse's professional license? (Choose all that apply.)
   1. Taking or selling controlled substances
   2. Assisting with physician-assisted suicide
   3. Reporting suspected abuse and neglect of children
   4. Applying physical restraints without a written physician's order

9. The Health Insurance Portability and Accountability Act of 1996 (HIPAA) provides clients basic rights pertaining to their medical records. Which statement reflects a violation of HIPAA?
   1. Discussing client conditions in the nursing report room at the change of shift
   2. Allowing nursing students to review client charts before caring for clients to whom they are assigned
   3. Posting daily nursing care information along with the medical condition of the client on a message board in the client's room
   4. Releasing client information regarding terminal illness to family when the client has given permission for information to be shared

10. The nurse must follow standards of care to avoid potential litigation and suits of negligence. Which of the following statements represents a potential nursing malpractice situation? (Choose all that apply.)
   1. Failure to make a nursing diagnosis
   2. Failure to provide discharge instructions
   3. Failure to follow the six rights of medication administration
   4. Failure to use proper medical equipment ordered for client monitoring
   5. Failure to question a health care provider about appropriateness of a client order

24 | Communication

※ OBJECTIVES

Mastery of the content in this chapter will enable the student to:

- Describe aspects of critical thinking that are important to the communication process.
- Describe the five levels of communication and their uses in nursing.
- Describe the basic elements of the communication process.
- Identify significant features and therapeutic outcomes of nurse-client helping relationships.
- List nursing focus areas within the four phases of a nurse-client helping relationship.
- Identify significant features and desired outcomes of nurse–health care team member relationships.

- Describe qualities, behaviors, and communication techniques that affect professional communication.
- Discuss effective communication techniques for clients at various developmental levels.
- Identify client health states that contribute to impaired communication.
- Discuss nursing care measures for clients with special communication needs.

※ MEDIA RESOURCES ※ KEY TERMS

 Companion CD
- NCLEX®-Style Review Questions
- Audio Glossary
- Interactive Learning Activities
- English/Spanish Glossary

evolve Website
- NCLEX®-Style Review Questions
- Audio Glossary
- English/Spanish Glossary
- Interactive Learning Activities
- WebLinks
- Audio Summaries

Active listening, p. 352
Assertiveness, p. 348
Autonomy, p. 348
Channels, p. 343
Communication, p. 340
Empathy, p. 353
Environment, p. 344
Feedback, p. 343
Interpersonal communication, p. 342
Interpersonal variables, p. 343
Intrapersonal communication, p. 342
Message, p. 343
Metacommunication, p. 346
Nonverbal communication, p. 344

Perceptions, p. 341
Perceptual biases, p. 341
Public communication, p. 342
Receiver, p. 343
Referent, p. 343
Sender, p. 343
Small-group communication, p. 342
Symbolic communication, p. 346
Sympathy, p. 356
Therapeutic communication techniques, p. 352
Transpersonal communication, p. 342
Verbal communication, p. 344

Communication and Nursing Practice

Communication is a lifelong learning process for the nurse. Nurses make the intimate journey with clients and their families from the miracle of birth to the mystery of death. It is necessary to build therapeutic communications for this journey. Nurses communicate with people under stress: clients, families, and colleagues.

Nurses function as client advocates and as members of interdisciplinary teams that sometimes have different ideas about priorities for care. In addition, nurses need to be assertive to ask the right questions and make their voices heard. Being assertive to communicate one's own needs ensures balance in a nurse's life. Without such balance, the high-stress environment contributes to burnout and diminishes the nurse's effectiveness (Balzer Riley, 2004).

Despite the complexity of technology and the multiple demands on nurses' time, it is the intimate moment of connection that makes all the difference in the quality of care and meaning for the client and the nurse. As nurses refine their communication skills and increase their confidence, they progress professionally to become experts (Balzer Riley, 2004).

Effective communication is an essential attribute of professional nursing practice (Apker and others, 2006). Competency in communication helps maintain effective relationships within the entire sphere of professional practice and helps meet legal, ethical, and clinical standards of care. Breakdown in communication is a top contributor to errors in the workplace and threatens professional credibility (The Joint Commission, 2006). The American Association of Critical-Care Nurses (2005) identified skilled communication as one of the standards for establishing and sustaining healthy work environments.

The qualities, behaviors, and therapeutic communication techniques described in this chapter characterize professionalism in helping relationships. Although the term *client* is often used, the same principles apply when communicating with any person, in any nursing situation.

Communication and Interpersonal Relationships

Caring relationships formed between the nurse and those affected by the nurse's practice are at the core of nursing (see Chapter 8). Communication is the means to establish these helping-healing relationships. All behavior communicates, and all communication influences behavior. For these reasons, communication is essential to the nurse-client relationship.

Nurses with expertise in communication express caring by the following (Watson, 1985):

- Becoming sensitive to self and others
- Promoting and accepting the expression of positive and negative feelings
- Developing helping-trust relationships
- Instilling faith and hope
- Promoting interpersonal teaching and learning
- Providing a supportive environment
- Assisting with gratification of human needs
- Allowing for spiritual expression

The nurse's ability to relate to others is important for interpersonal communication. This includes the nurse's ability to take initiative in establishing and maintaining communication, to be authentic (one's self), and to respond appropriately to the other person. Good interpersonal communication also requires a sense of mutuality, a belief that the nurse-client relationship is a partnership and that both are equal participants. Nurses honor the fact that people are very complex and ambiguous. There is often more communicated than first meets the eye, and client responses will not always be what you expect. By giving all of your attention to the client, you will be able to attend to the client's needs and aid the healing process (Tavernier, 2006).

A new perspective of human relationships suggests energy fields connect everything to each other. Although the idea of using energy for healing has recently reemerged in the West, Eastern cultures have used this method for a long time. Healers in Eastern and primitive cultures treated their clients holistically and focused on the concept of maintaining balance in vital energy to maintain health (McCaffrey and Fowler, 2003). Considering these principles, it is not surprising that nurses often perceive the strong sense of connection to others that occurs within a helping relationship. Most nurses embrace the profession's view of the holistic nature of people and have experienced synergy in human interaction. When clients and nurses work together, they accomplish much more.

Accepting that humans are energy-based beings means that nurses need to look at communication in new ways. Therapeutic communication occurs within a healing relationship between a nurse and client (Arnold and Boggs, 2003). Like any powerful therapeutic agent, the nurse's communication can result in both harm and good. Every nuance of posture, every small expression and gesture, every word chosen, every attitude held—all have the potential to hurt or heal, affecting others through the transmission of human energy. Knowing that intention and behavior directly influence human energy fields, and therefore health, gives nurses tremendous ethical responsibility to do no harm to those entrusted to their care. Respect the potential power of communication, and do not carelessly misuse communication to hurt, manipulate, or coerce others. Good communication empowers others and enables people to know themselves and make their own choices, an essential aspect of the healing process. Nurses have wonderful opportunities to bring about good things for themselves, their clients, and their colleagues through this kind of therapeutic communication.

Developing Communication Skills

Gaining expertise in communication, as in any aspect of nursing, requires both an understanding of the communication process and reflection about one's communication experiences as a nurse. Nurses who develop good critical thinking skills make the best communicators. They draw on theoretical knowledge about communication and integrate this knowledge with previously learned knowledge through personal experience. They interpret messages received from others, analyze their content, make inferences about their meaning, evaluate their effect, explain rationale for communication techniques used, and self-examine personal communication skills (Balzer Riley, 2004).

Other qualities of good critical thinking are also important to the communication process. Critical thinking attitudes offer

✳ BOX 24-1 Communication Throughout the Nursing Process

Assessment
Verbal interviewing and history taking
Visual and intuitive observation of nonverbal behavior
Visual, tactile, and auditory data gathering during physical examination
Written medial records, diagnostic tests, and literature review

Nursing Diagnosis
Intrapersonal analysis of assessment findings
Validation of health care needs and priorities via verbal discussion with client
Handwritten or computer-mediated documentation of nursing diagnosis

Planning
Interpersonal or small-group health care team planning sessions
Interpersonal collaboration with client and family to determine implementation methods
Written documentation of expected outcomes
Written or verbal referral to health care team members

Implementation
Delegation and verbal discussion with health care team
Verbal, visual, auditory, and tactile health teaching activities
Provision of support via therapeutic communication techniques
Contact with other health resources
Written documentation of client's progress in medical record

Evaluation
Acquisition of verbal and nonverbal feedback
Comparison of actual and expected outcomes
Identification of factors affecting outcomes
Modification and update of care plan
Verbal and/or written explanation of revisions of care plan to client

---

guidelines for how to approach a problem. These attitudes include being curious. Curiosity motivates the nurse to communicate and know more about a person. Clients are more likely to communicate with nurses who express an interest in them. Perseverance and creativity are also attitudes conducive to communication because they motivate the nurse to communicate and identify innovative solutions. A self-confident attitude is important because the nurse who conveys confidence and comfort while communicating more readily establishes an interpersonal helping-trust relationships. In addition, an independent attitude encourages the nurse to communicate with colleagues and share ideas about nursing interventions. Such an attitude sometimes involves risk taking because colleagues sometimes question the suggested nursing interventions. At the same time, an attitude of fairness goes a long way in the ability to listen to both sides in any discussion. An additional critical thinking attitude, integrity, allows nurses to recognize when their opinions conflict with those of the client, to review positions, and to decide how to communicate to reach mutually beneficial decisions. It is also very important for the nurse to communicate responsibly and ask for help if uncertain or uncomfortable about an aspect of client care. Furthermore, an attitude of humility is necessary to recognize and communicate the need for more information before making a decision (Paul, 1993).

Critical thinking in nursing based on established standards of nursing care and ethical standards promotes effective communication. When you consider a client's problems, it is important to apply the standards to ensure sound effective communication (Chitty, 2005).

It is challenging to understand human communication within interpersonal relationships. Each individual bases his or her **perceptions** on information received through the five senses of sight, hearing, taste, touch, and smell (Arnold and Boggs, 2003). An individual's culture and education also influence perception. Critical thinking helps the nurse overcome **perceptual biases,** or human tendencies that interfere with accurately perceiving and interpret-

ing messages from others. People often assume that others think, feel, act, react, and behave as they would in similar circumstances. They tend to distort or ignore information that goes against their expectations, preconceptions, or stereotypes (Beebe, Beebe, and Redmond, 2005). By thinking critically about personal communication habits, you will learn to control these tendencies and become more effective in interpersonal relationships.

As communication skills develop, the nurse's competence in the nursing process will also grow. You need to integrate communication skills throughout the nursing process as you collaborate with clients and health care team members to achieve goals (Box 24-1). Use your communication skills to gather, analyze, and transmit information and to accomplish the work of each step of the process. Assessment, diagnosis, planning, implementation, and evaluation all depend on effective communication among nurse, client, family, and others on the health care team. Although the nursing process is a reliable framework for client care, it will not work well unless you master the art of effective interpersonal communication.

The nature of the communication process requires you to constantly make decisions about what, when, where, why, and how to convey a message. The nurse's decision making is always contextual—the unique features of any situation influence the nature of the decisions made. For example, the explanation of the importance of following a prescribed diet to a client with a newly diagnosed medical condition will differ from the explanation to a client who has repeatedly chosen not to follow diet restrictions. Effective communication techniques are easy to learn, but their application is more difficult. Deciding which techniques best fit each unique nursing situation is challenging. Communication about specific diagnoses such as cancer or end of life and dealing with client and family emotions can be challenging, and some nurses struggle to cope with their own reactions and emotions (Sheldon, Barett, and Ellington, 2006).

Throughout this chapter, brief clinical examples guide you in the use of effective communication techniques. Situations that challenge the nurse's decision-making skills and call for careful use

---

✳ BOX 24-2   Challenging Communication Situations

- Silent, withdrawn persons who do not express any feelings or needs
- Sad, depressed persons who have slow mental and motor responses
- Angry, hostile persons who do not listen to explanations
- Uncooperative persons who resent being asked to do something
- Talkative, lonely persons who want someone with them all the time
- Demanding persons who want someone to wait on them or meet their requests
- Ranting and raving persons who blame nursing staff unfairly
- Sensory impaired persons who cannot hear or see well
- Verbally impaired persons who cannot articulate words
- Gossiping persons who violate confidentiality and cause friction
- Mentally handicapped persons who are frightened and distrustful
- Confused, disoriented persons who are bewildered and uncooperative
- Foreign-born persons who speak very little English
- Anxious, nervous persons who cannot cope with what is happening
- Grieving, crying persons who have had a major loss
- Screaming, kicking toddlers who want their mother
- Flirtatious, sexually inappropriate persons
- Loud, obscene persons causing a disturbance or violating a rule

---

of therapeutic techniques often involve the types of persons described in Box 24-2. Because the best way to acquire skill is through practice, it is useful for you to discuss and role-play these scenarios before experiencing them in the clinical setting. Consider who is involved in the situation to decide which communication will be most effective.

Levels of Communication

Nurses use different levels of communication in their professional role. The nurse's communication skills need to include techniques that reflect competence in each level.

Intrapersonal Communication

Intrapersonal communication is a powerful form of communication that occurs within an individual. This level of communication is also called self-talk, self-verbalization, and inner thought (Balzer Riley, 2004). People's thoughts strongly influence perceptions, feelings, behavior, and self-concept, and you need to be aware of the nature and content of your own thinking. Nurses and clients use intrapersonal communication to develop self-awareness and a positive self-concept that will enhance appropriate self-expression. For example, you may improve health and self-esteem through positive self-talk by replacing negative thoughts with positive assertions. Another type of intrapersonal communication, self-instruction provides a mental rehearsal for difficult tasks or situations so individuals are able to deal with them more effectively.

Interpersonal Communication

Interpersonal communication is one-to-one interaction between the nurse and another person that often occurs face to face. It is the level most frequently used in nursing situations and lies at the heart of nursing practice. It takes place within a social context and includes all the symbols and cues used to give and receive meaning. Because meaning resides in persons and not in words, messages received are sometimes different from messages intended. Nurses work with people who have different opinions, experiences, values, and belief systems, so it is important to validate meaning or mutually negotiate it between participants. For example, when teaching a client about a health concern, you use interaction to assess understanding and clarify misinterpretations. Meaningful interpersonal communication results in exchange of ideas, problem solving, expression of feelings, decision making, goal accomplishment, team building, and personal growth.

Transpersonal Communication

Transpersonal communication is interaction that occurs within a person's spiritual domain. Study of the influence of religion and spirituality has increased dramatically over the past decade, and ongoing research helps us understand the role of spirituality in health and coping (Stefanek, McDonald, and Hess, 2005). Many persons use prayer, meditation, guided reflection, religious rituals, or other means to communicate with their "higher power." Nurses who value the importance of human spirituality often use this form of communication with clients and for themselves. Nurses have a responsibility to assess client's spiritual needs and intervene to meet those needs.

Small-Group Communication

Small-group communication is interaction that occurs when a small number of persons meet together. This type of communication is usually goal directed and requires an understanding of group dynamics. When nurses work on committees, lead client support groups, form research teams, or participate in client care conferences, they use a small-group communication process. Small groups are more effective when they are a workable size, have an appropriate meeting place, suitable seating arrangements, and cohesiveness and commitment among group members (Arnold and Boggs, 2003). Group participants need to feel accepted, to feel able to communicate openly and honestly, and to actively listen to others in the group (Sully and Dallas, 2005).

Public Communication

Public communication is interaction with an audience. Nurses have opportunities to speak with groups of consumers about health-related topics, present scholarly work to colleagues at conferences, or lead classroom discussions with peers or students. Public communication requires special adaptations in eye contact, gestures, voice inflection, and use of media materials to communicate messages effectively. Effective public communication increases audience knowledge about health-related topics, health issues, and other issues important to the nursing profession.

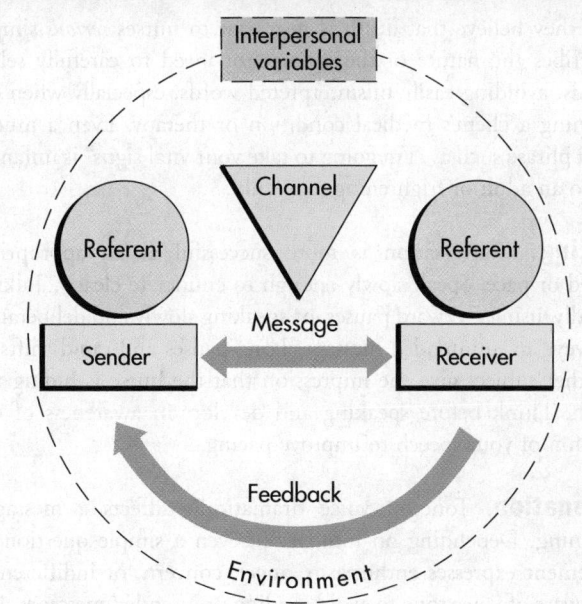

Figure 24-1 Communication as active process between sender and receiver.

Basic Elements of the Communication Process

Communication is an ongoing, dynamic, and multidimensional process. Figure 24-1 shows the basic elements of the communication process. This simple linear model represents a very complex process, but it helps identify its essential components. Nursing situations have many unique aspects that influence the nature of communication and interpersonal relationships. In the professional role, you will use critical thinking to focus on each aspect of communication so your interactions are purposeful and effective.

Referent

The **referent** motivates one person to communicate with another. In a health care setting, sights, sounds, odors, time schedules, messages, objects, emotions, sensations, perceptions, ideas, and other cues initiate communication. The nurse who knows what stimulus initiated communication is able to develop and organize messages more efficiently and better perceive meaning in another's message. A client request for help prompted by difficulty breathing brings a different nursing response than a request prompted by boredom.

Sender and Receiver

The **sender** is the person who encodes and delivers the message, and the **receiver** is the person who receives and decodes the message. The sender puts ideas or feelings into a form that is transmitted and is responsible for the accuracy of its content and emotional tone. The sender's message acts as a referent for the receiver, who is responsible for attending to, translating, and responding to the sender's message. Sender and receiver roles are fluid and change back and forth as two persons interact; sometimes sending

and receiving occurs simultaneously. The more the sender and receiver have in common and the closer the relationship, the more likely they will accurately perceive one another's meaning and respond accordingly.

Messages

The **message** is the content of the communication. It contains verbal, nonverbal, and symbolic language. Personal perceptions sometimes distort the receiver's interpretation of the message. Two nurses can provide the same information yet convey very different messages according to their personal communication styles. Two persons understand the same message differently. You send effective messages by expressing clearly, directly, and in a manner familiar to the receiver. You determine the need for clarification by watching the listener for nonverbal cues that suggest confusion or misunderstanding. Communication is difficult when participants have different levels of education and experience. "Your incision is well approximated without purulent drainage" means the same as "Your wound edges are together, and there are no signs of infection," but the latter is easier to understand. You can also send messages in writing, but be sure clients are able to read.

Channels

Channels are means of conveying and receiving messages through visual, auditory, and tactile senses. Facial expressions send visual messages, spoken words travel through auditory channels, and touch uses tactile channels. Individuals usually understand a message more clearly when the sender uses more channels to convey the message. For example, when teaching about insulin self-injection, the nurse talks about and demonstrates the technique, gives the client printed information, and encourages hands-on practice with the vial and syringe. Nurses use verbal, nonverbal, and mediated (technological) communication channels. They send and receive information in person, by informal or formal writing, over the telephone or pager, by audiotape and videotape, through fax and electronic mail, and through computer interactive and information sites.

Feedback

Feedback is the message the receiver returns. It indicates whether the receiver understood the meaning of the sender's message. Senders need to seek verbal and nonverbal feedback to ensure that good communication has occurred. To be effective, the sender and receiver need to be sensitive and open to each other's messages, clarify the messages, and modify behavior accordingly. In a social relationship, both persons assume equal responsibility for seeking openness and clarification, but the nurse assumes primary responsibility in the nurse-client relationship.

Interpersonal Variables

Interpersonal variables are factors within both the sender and receiver that influence communication. Perception is one such variable that provides a uniquely personal view of reality formed by an individual's expectations and experiences. Each person senses, interprets, and understands events differently. A nurse says, "You have been very quiet since your family left. Is there something on your mind?" Some clients will possibly perceive the nurse's question as caring and concerned; another perceives the nurse as invading privacy and is less willing to talk. Other interpersonal variables include educational and developmental levels, sociocultural backgrounds, values and beliefs, emotions, gender, physical health status, and roles and relationships. Variables associated with illness, such as pain, anxiety, and medication effects, also affect nurse-client communication (Feldman-Stewart, Brundage, and Tishelman, 2005).

Environment

The **environment** is the setting for sender-receiver interaction. For effective communication, the environment needs to meet participant needs for physical and emotional comfort and safety. Noise, temperature extremes, distractions, and lack of privacy or space create confusion, tension, and discomfort. Environmental distractions are common in health care settings and interfere with messages sent between people, so nurses need to try to control the environment as much as possible to create favorable conditions for effective communication.

Forms of Communication

Messages are conveyed verbally and nonverbally, concretely and symbolically. As people communicate, they express themselves through words, movements, voice inflection, facial expressions, and use of space. These elements work in harmony to enhance a message or conflict with one another to contradict and confuse it.

Verbal Communication

Verbal communication uses spoken or written words. Verbal language is a code that conveys specific meaning through combination of words. The most important aspects of verbal communication are presented below.

Vocabulary. Communication is unsuccessful if senders and receivers cannot translate each other's words and phrases. When a nurse cares for a client who speaks another language, an interpreter is often necessary. Even those who speak the same language use subcultural variations of certain words: *dinner* means a noon meal to one person and the last meal of the day to another. Medical jargon (technical terminology used by health care providers) sounds like a foreign language to clients unfamiliar with the health care setting. Limiting use of medical jargon to conversations with other health care team members will improve communication. Children have a more limited vocabulary than adults. They may use special words to describe bodily functions or a favorite blanket or toy. Teenagers often use words in unique ways that are unfamiliar to adults.

Denotative and Connotative Meaning. Some words have several meanings. Individuals who use a common language share the denotative meaning: *baseball* has the same meaning for everyone who speaks English, but *code* denotes cardiac arrest primarily to health care providers. The connotative meaning is the shade or interpretation of a word's meaning influenced by the thoughts, feelings, or ideas people have about the word. For example, health care providers tell a family that a loved one is in serious condition

and they believe that death is near, but to nurses *serious* simply describes the nature of the illness. You need to carefully select words, avoiding easily misinterpreted words, especially when explaining a client's medical condition or therapy. Even a much-used phrase such as "I'm going to take your vital signs" is unfamiliar to an adult or frightening to a child.

Pacing. Conversation is more successful at an appropriate speed or pace. Speak slowly enough to enunciate clearly. Talking rapidly, using awkward pauses, or speaking slowly and deliberately conveys an unintended message. Long pauses and rapid shifts to another subject give the impression that the nurse is hiding the truth. Think before speaking and develop an awareness of the rhythm of your speech to improve pacing.

Intonation. Tone of voice dramatically affects a message's meaning. Depending on intonation, even a simple question or statement expresses enthusiasm, anger, concern, or indifference. Be aware of voice tone to avoid sending unintended messages. For example, clients interpret a nurse's patronizing tone of voice as condescending, and this inhibits further communication. A client's voice tone often provides information about his or her emotional state or energy level.

Clarity and Brevity. Effective communication is simple, brief, and direct. Fewer words result in less confusion. Speaking slowly, enunciating clearly, and using examples to make explanations easier to understand improves clarity. Repeating important parts of a message also clarifies communication. Phrases such as "you know" or "OK?" at the end of every sentence detract from clarity. Use short sentences and words that express an idea simply and directly. "Where is your pain?" is much better than "I would like you to describe for me the location of your discomfort."

Timing and Relevance. Timing is critical in communication. Even though a message is clear, poor timing prevents it from being effective. For example, you do not begin routine teaching when a client is in severe pain or emotional distress. Often the best time for interaction is when a client expresses an interest in communicating. If messages are relevant or important to the situation at hand, they are more effective. When a client is facing emergency surgery, discussing the risks of smoking is less relevant than explaining presurgical procedures.

Nonverbal Communication

Nonverbal communication includes all of the five senses and everything that does not involve the spoken or written word. Researchers have estimated that approximately 7% of meaning is transmitted by words, 38% is transmitted by vocal cues, and 55% is transmitted by body cues. Hence, nonverbal communication is unconsciously motivated and more accurately indicates a person's intended meaning than the spoken words (Stuart and Laraia, 2005). When there is incongruity between verbal and nonverbal communication, the receiver usually "hears" the nonverbal message as the true message.

All kinds of nonverbal communication are important, but interpreting them is often problematic. Sociocultural background is a major influence on the meaning of nonverbal behavior. In the

United States, with its diverse cultural communities, nonverbal messages between people of different cultures are easily misinterpreted. Because the meaning attached to nonverbal behavior is so subjective, it is imperative that you check its meaning (Stuart and Laraia, 2005). Assessing nonverbal messages is an important nursing skill (Grover, 2005).

Personal Appearance. Personal appearance includes physical characteristics, facial expression, and manner of dress and grooming. These factors help communicate physical well-being, personality, social status, occupation, religion, culture, and self-concept. First impressions are largely based on appearance. Nurses learn to develop a general impression of client health and emotional status through appearance, and clients develop a general impression of the nurse's professionalism and caring in the same way.

Posture and Gait. Posture and gait (way of walking) are forms of self-expression. The way people sit, stand, and move reflect attitudes, emotions, self-concept, and health status. For example, an erect posture and a quick, purposeful gait communicate a sense of well-being and confidence. Leaning forward conveys attention. A slumped posture and slow shuffling gait indicates depression, illness, or fatigue.

Facial Expression. The face is the most expressive part of the body. Facial expressions convey emotions such as surprise, fear, anger, happiness, and sadness. Some persons have an expressionless face, or flat affect, which reveals little about what they are thinking or feeling. An inappropriate affect is a facial expression that does not match the content of a verbal message, for example, smiling when describing a sad situation. People are sometimes unaware of the messages their expressions convey. For example, a nurse frowns in concentration while doing a procedure and the client interprets this as anger or disapproval. Clients closely observe nurses. Consider the impact a nurse's facial expression has on a person who asks, "Am I going to die?" The slightest change in the eyes, lips, or facial muscles will reveal the nurse's feelings. Although it is hard to control all facial expression, try to avoid showing shock, disgust, dismay, or other distressing reactions in the client's presence.

Eye Contact. People signal readiness to communicate through eye contact. Maintaining eye contact during conversation shows respect and willingness to listen. Eye contact also allows people to closely observe one another. Lack of eye contact may indicate anxiety, defensiveness, discomfort, or lack of confidence in communicating. However, persons from some cultures consider eye contact intrusive, threatening, or harmful and minimize or avoid its use. Eye movements communicate feelings and emotions. Looking down on a person establishes authority, whereas interacting at the same eye level indicates equality in the relationship. Rising to the same eye level as an angry person helps establish autonomy.

Gestures. Gestures emphasize, punctuate, and clarify the spoken word. Gestures alone carry specific meanings, or they create messages with other communication cues. A finger pointed toward a person communicates several meanings, but when accom-

panied by a frown and stern voice, the gesture becomes an accusation or threat. Pointing to an area of pain is sometimes more accurate than describing the pain's location.

Sounds. Sounds such as sighs, moans, groans, or sobs also communicate feelings and thoughts. Combined with other nonverbal communication, sounds help send clear messages. Sounds have several interpretations: moaning conveys pleasure or suffering, and crying communicates happiness, sadness, or anger. You need to validate such nonverbal messages with the client to interpret them accurately.

Territoriality and Personal Space. Territoriality is the need to gain, maintain, and defend one's right to space. Territory is important because it provides people with a sense of identity, security, and control. Territory is sometimes separated and made visible to others, such as a fence around a yard or a bed in a hospital room. Personal space is invisible, individual, and travels with the person. During interpersonal interaction, people maintain varying distances between each other depending on their culture, the nature of their relationship, and the situation. When personal space becomes threatened, people respond defensively and communicate less effectively. Situations dictate whether the interpersonal distance between nurse and client is appropriate. Box 24-3 provides examples of nursing actions within zones of personal

---

✳ BOX 24-3 Zones of Personal Space and Touch

Zones of Personal Space
Intimate Zone (0 to 18 inches)
Holding a crying infant
Performing physical assessment
Bathing, grooming, dressing, feeding, and toileting a client
Changing a client's dressing

Personal Zone (18 inches to 4 feet)
Sitting at a client's bedside
Taking the client's nursing history
Teaching an individual client
Exchanging information at change of shift

Social Zone (4 to 12 feet)
Making rounds with a physician
Sitting at the head of a conference table
Teaching a class for clients with diabetes
Conducting a family support group

Public Zone (12 feet and greater)
Speaking at a community forum
Testifying at a legislative hearing
Lecturing to a class of students

Zones of Touch
Social Zone (permission not needed)
Hands, arms, shoulders, back

Consent Zone (permission needed)
Mouth, wrists, feet

Vulnerable Zone (special care needed)
Face, neck, front of body

Intimate Zone (great sensitivity needed)
Genitalia, rectum

space (Stuart and Laraia, 2005) and zones of touch. Nurses frequently move into clients' territory and personal space due to the nature of caregiving. You need to convey confidence, gentleness, and respect for privacy, especially when your actions require intimate contact or involve a client's vulnerable zone.

Symbolic Communication

Good communication requires awareness of **symbolic communication,** the verbal and nonverbal symbolism used by others to convey meaning. Art and music are forms of symbolic communication used by the nurse to enhance understanding and promote healing. Lane (2006) found creative expressions such as art, music, and dance have a healing effect on clients. Clients reported decreased pain and a greater sense of joy and hope.

Metacommunication

Metacommunication is a broad term that refers to all factors that influence communication. Awareness of influencing factors helps people better understand what is communicated (Arnold and Boggs, 2003). For example, the nurse observes a young client holding his body rigidly and his voice is sharp as he says, "Going to surgery is no big deal." The nurse replies, "You say having surgery doesn't bother you, but you look and sound tense. I'd like to help." Awareness of the tone of the verbal response and the nonverbal behavior results in further exploration of the client's feelings and concerns.

Professional Nursing Relationships

The nurse's application of knowledge, understanding of human behavior and communication, and commitment to ethical behavior help create professional relationships. Having a philosophy based on caring and respect for others will help the nurse be more successful in establishing relationships of this nature.

Nurse-Client Helping Relationships

Helping relationships are the foundation of clinical nursing practice. In such relationships, the nurse assumes the role of professional helper and comes to know the client as an individual who has unique health needs, human responses, and patterns of living. The relationship is therapeutic, promoting a psychological climate that facilitates positive change and growth. Therapeutic communication between the nurse and client allows the attainment of health-related goals (Arnold and Boggs, 2003). The goals of a therapeutic relationship focus on the client's achieving optimal personal growth (Stuart and Laraia, 2005). There is an explicit time frame, a goal-directed approach, and a high expectation of confidentiality. The nurse establishes, directs, and takes responsibility for the interaction, and the client's needs take priority over the nurse's needs. The nurse's nonjudgmental acceptance of the client is an important characteristic of the relationship. Acceptance conveys a willingness to hear a message or to acknowledge feelings. It does not mean you always agree with the other person or approve of the client's decisions or actions. A helping

relationship between nurse and client does not just happen—you create it with care, skill and trust.

A natural progression of four goal-directed phases characterizes the nurse-client relationship. The relationship often begins before the nurse meets the client and continues until the caregiving relationship ends (Box 24-4). Even a brief interaction uses an abbreviated version of the same preinteraction, orientation, working, and termination phases (Arnold and Boggs, 2003). For example, the student nurse gathers client information to prepare in advance for caregiving, meets the client and establishes trust, accomplishes health-related goals through use of the nursing process, and says goodbye at the end of the day.

Socializing is an important initial component of interpersonal communication. It helps people get to know one another and relax. It is easy, superficial, and not deeply personal, whereas therapeutic interactions are often more intense, difficult, and uncomfortable. A nurse often uses social conversation to lay a foundation for a closer relationship: "Hi, Mr. Simpson, I hear it's your birthday today. How old are you?" A friendly, informal, and warm communication style helps establish trust, but nurses have to get beyond social conversation to talk about issues or concerns affecting the client's health. During social conversation, some clients ask personal questions about the nurse's family, place of residence, and so forth. Students often wonder whether it is appropriate to reveal such information. The skillful nurse uses judgment about what to share and provides minimal information or deflects such questions with gentle humor and refocuses conversation back to the client.

Creating a therapeutic environment depends on your ability to communicate, to comfort, and to help clients meet their needs. Comfort is a critical value inherent in the practice of nursing. Therapeutic interactions increase feelings of personal control by helping the person feel secure, informed, and valued. Optimizing personal control facilitates emotional comfort, which minimizes physical discomfort and enhances recovery activities (Williams and Irurita, 2006) (Box 24-5).

In a therapeutic relationship, nurses often encourage clients to share personal stories. Sharing of stories is called narrative interaction. Through narrative interactions, nurses begin to understand the context of others' lives and learn what is meaningful for them from their perspective (Shattell and Hogan, 2005). For example, a nurse asked a client to tell about a time in his life when he had to make a hard decision. He related the following story:

When I was a young man, I worked on the family farm. An uncle died and left me some money. All of a sudden I could afford to go to college, but Dad didn't want me to go because he needed me there. I had to decide whether to stay or go, and it was real hard, because at first I just wanted to get away. I talked to our preacher, and he said it was up to me, to pray about it and do what my heart told me to. So I stayed. Oh, I've thought from time to time what I might have made of myself, but I never regretted it. I had a good life in farming.

From this brief story, the nurse understood that it was important to the client to put his family's needs above his personal desires and that seeking spiritual guidance was an important component of his decision making. This same information may not

✳ BOX 24-4 Phases of the Helping Relationship

Preinteraction Phase
Before meeting the client:
Review available data, including the medical and nursing history
Talk to other caregivers who have information about the client
Anticipate health concerns or issues that arise
Identify a location and setting that will foster comfortable, private interaction
Plan enough time for the initial interaction

Orientation Phase
When the nurse and client meet and get to know one another:
Set the tone for the relationship by adopting a warm, empathetic, caring manner
Recognize that the initial relationship is often superficial, uncertain, and tentative
Expect the client to test the nurse's competence and commitment
Closely observe the client, and expect to be closely observed by the client
Begin to make inferences and form judgments about client messages and behaviors
Assess the client's health status
Prioritize the client's problems, and identify the client's goals
Clarify the client's and nurse's roles
Form contracts with the client that specify who will do what
Let the client know when to expect the relationship to be terminated

Working Phase
When the nurse and client work together to solve problems and accomplish goals:
Encourage and help the client to express feelings about his or her health
Encourage and help the client with self-exploration
Provide information needed to understand and change behavior
Encourage and help the client to set goals
Take action to meet the goals set with the client
Use therapeutic communication skills to facilitate successful interactions
Use appropriate self-disclosure and confrontation

Termination Phase
During the ending of the relationship:
Remind the client that termination is near
Evaluate goal achievement with the client
Reminisce about the relationship with the client
Separate from the client by relinquishing responsibility for his or her care
Achieve a smooth transition for the client to other caregivers as needed

---

have been revealed had the nurse used a standard history form that usually only elicits short answers.

Nurse-Family Relationships

Many nursing situations, especially those in community and home care settings, require the nurse to form helping relationships with entire families. The same principles that guide one-to-one helping relationships also apply when the client is a family unit, although communication within families requires additional understanding of the complexities of family dynamics, needs, and relationships (see Chapter 10).

Nurse–Health Care Team Relationships

Nurses function in roles that require interaction with multiple health care team members. Many elements of the nurse-client helping relationship also apply to collegial relationships, which focus on establishing a healthy work environment and accomplishing the work and goals of the clinical setting (Triola, 2006). Communication in such relationships focuses on team building, facilitating group process, collaboration, consultation, delegation, supervision, leadership, and management (see Chapter 21). A variety of communication skills are necessary, including presentational speaking, persuasion, group problem solving, providing performance reviews, and writing business reports.

Within the work setting, the nurse and health care team need social and therapeutic interactions to build morale and strengthen relationships. Everyone has interpersonal needs for acceptance, inclusion, identity, privacy, power and control, and affection (Stewart and Logan, 2005). Nurses need friendship, support,

✳ BOX 24-5   EVIDENCE-BASED PRACTICE

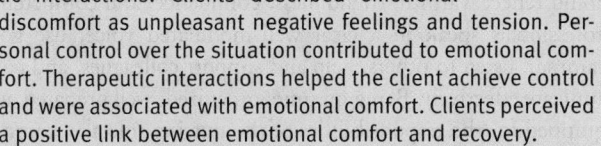

Emotional Comfort
Evidence Summary
Recently hospitalized clients described emotional comfort as a pleasant positive feeling and state of relaxation that resulted from therapeutic interactions. Clients described emotional discomfort as unpleasant negative feelings and tension. Personal control over the situation contributed to emotional comfort. Therapeutic interactions helped the client achieve control and were associated with emotional comfort. Clients perceived a positive link between emotional comfort and recovery.

Application to Nursing Practice
- Clients perceive a connection between the mind and body.
- Increased emotional comfort increases physical comfort and enhances recovery.
- Nurse-client therapeutic interactions improve the client's emotional and physical comfort.
- Using therapeutic communication to increase the client's perceived control of the situation and the environment increases comfort.

Reference
Williams AM, Irurita VF: Emotional comfort: the patient's perspective of a therapeutic context, *Int J Nurs Stud* 43(4): 405:2006.

guidance, and encouragement from one another to cope with the many stressors imposed by the nursing role and need to extend the same caring communication used with clients to build positive relationships with colleagues and co-workers.

Nurse-Community Relationships

Many nurses form relationships with community groups by participating in local organizations, volunteering for community service, or becoming politically active. Nurses in a community-based practice need to be able to establish relationships with their community to be effective change agents (see Chapter 3). Understanding the importance of community-oriented, population-focused nursing practice and developing the skills to practice it are critical in attaining a leadership role in health care regardless of the practice setting (Stanhope and Lancaster, 2004). Communication within the community occurs through channels such as neighborhood newsletters, public bulletin boards, newspapers, radio, television, and electronic information sites. Nurses use these forms of communication to share information and discuss issues important to community health.

Elements of Professional Communication

Professional appearance, demeanor, and behavior are important in establishing the nurse's trustworthiness and competence. They communicate that the nurse has assumed the professional helping role, is clinically skilled, and is focused on the client. Nothing harms nursing's professional image like an individual nurse's inappropriate appearance or behavior.

A professional is expected to be clean, neat, well groomed, conservatively dressed, and odor-free. Tattoos and piercings are not acceptable in the professional setting. Professional behavior should reflect warmth, friendliness, confidence, and competence. Professionals speak in a clear well-modulated voice, use good grammar, listen to others, help and support colleagues, and communicate effectively. Being on time, organized, well prepared, and equipped for the responsibilities of the nursing role also communicate professionalism.

Courtesy

Common courtesy is part of professional communication. To practice courtesy, say hello and goodbye to clients, knock on doors before entering, and use self-introduction. A nurse also states his or her purpose, addresses people by name, and says please and thank you to team members. When a nurse is discourteous, others perceive the nurse as rude or insensitive. It sets up barriers between nurse and client and causes friction among team members.

Use of Names

Self-introduction is important. Failure to give a name, indicate status (e.g., registered nurse or licensed practical nurse), or acknowledge the client creates uncertainty about the interaction and conveys an impersonal lack of commitment or caring. Making eye contact and smiling at others gives them recognition.

Addressing others by name conveys respect for human dignity and uniqueness. Because using last names is respectful in most cultures, nurses usually use the client's last name in the initial interaction and then use the first name if the client requests it. Ask others how they would like to be addressed, and honor their personal preferences. Using first names is appropriate for infants, young children, confused or unconscious clients, and close team members. Avoid terms of endearment such as "honey," "dear," "grandma," or "sweetheart." Avoid referring to clients by diagnosis, room number, or other attribute, which is demeaning and sends the message that the nurse does not care enough to know the person as an individual.

Trustworthiness

Trust is relying on someone without doubt or question. Being trustworthy means helping others without hesitation. To foster trust, the nurse communicates warmth and demonstrates consistency, reliability, honesty, competence, and respect. Sometimes it is not easy for a client to ask for help. Trusting another person involves risk and vulnerability, but it also fosters open, therapeutic communication and enhances the expression of feelings, thoughts, and needs. Without trust, a nurse-client relationship rarely progresses beyond social interaction and superficial care. Avoid dishonesty at all costs. Knowingly withholding key information, lying, or distorting the truth violates both legal and ethical standards of practice. Sharing personal information or gossiping about others sends the message you cannot be trusted and damages interpersonal relationships.

Autonomy and Responsibility

Autonomy is the ability to be self-directed and independent in accomplishing goals and advocating for others. Professional nurses make choices and accept responsibility for the outcomes of their actions (Townsend, 2003). The nurse takes initiative in problem solving and communicates in a manner that reflects the importance and purpose of the therapeutic conversation (Arnold and Boggs, 2003). The nurse also recognizes the client's autonomy because people who seek health care are often concerned about losing control of decisions that influence how they live.

Assertiveness

Assertive communication allows you to express feelings and ideas without judging or hurting others (Grover, 2005). **Assertiveness** conveys a sense of self-assurance while also communicating respect for the other person (Stuart and Laraia, 2005). The advantages of assertive behavior include the following (Balzer Riley, 2004):

- It is more likely you will get what you want when you ask for it.
- People respect clear, open, honest communication.
- You stand up for your own rights and experience self-respect.
- You avoid the invitation of aggression.
- You are more independent.
- You become a decision maker.
- You feel more peaceful and comfortable with yourself.

Nurses teach assertiveness skills to others as a means for promoting personal health. Assertive people express feelings and emotions confidently, spontaneously, and honestly. They make decisions and control their lives more effectively than nonassertive individuals.

They deal with criticism and manipulation by others and learn to say no, set limits, and resist intentionally imposed guilt.

Feelings of security, competence, power, optimism, and professionalism characterize assertive responses. They are good tools for dealing with criticism, change, negative conditions in personal or professional life, and conflict or stress in relationships. Assertive responses often contain "I" messages, such as "I want," "I need," "I think," or "I feel."

Communication Within the Nursing Process

In the following section, the focus of the nursing process is on providing care for clients who need special assistance with communication. However, the nursing intervention section contains examples of therapeutic communication techniques that are appropriate strategies for use in any interpersonal nursing situation.

Assessment

Assessment of a client's ability to communicate includes gathering data about the many contextual factors that influence communication. The word *context* refers to all the parts of something that help determine its meaning. A context is the situation that influences the nature of communication, interpersonal relationships, and client needs (Beebe and others, 2005). This includes the participants' internal factors and characteristics, the nature of their relationship, the situation prompting communication, the environment, and the sociocultural elements present. Box 24-6 lists the contextual factors that influence communication. Assessing these contextual factors will help you make sound decisions during the communication process.

Physical and Emotional Factors. It is especially important to assess the psychophysiological factors that influence communication. Many altered health states and human responses limit communication. Persons with hearing or visual impairments have fewer channels through which to receive messages (see Chapter 49). Facial trauma, laryngeal cancer, or endotracheal intubation often prevents movement of air past vocal cords or mobility of the tongue, resulting in inability to articulate words. An extremely breathless person needs to use oxygen to breathe rather than speak. Persons with aphasia after a stroke or in late-stage Alzheimer's disease often cannot understand or form words. Certain mental illnesses such as psychoses or depression cause clients to demonstrate jumping from one topic to another, constant verbalization of the same words or phrases, or slowed speech pattern. Persons with high anxiety are sometimes unable to perceive environmental stimuli or hear explanations. Finally, unresponsive or heavily sedated persons cannot send or respond to verbal messages.

Review of the client's medical record helps provide relevant information about the client's ability to communicate. The medical history and physical examination documents physical barriers to speech, neurological deficits, and pathophysiology affecting hearing or vision. Reviewing the client's medication record is also important. For example, opiates, antidepressants, neuroleptics, hypnotics, or sedatives may cause a client to slur words or use incomplete sentences. The nursing progress notes sometimes reveal other factors that contribute to communication difficulties, such as the absence of family members to provide more information about a confused client.

Assessment should include communicating directly with clients to provide information about their ability to attend to, interpret, and respond to stimuli. If clients have difficulty communicating, it is important to assess the effect of the problem. The client who cannot communicate effectively will often have difficulty expressing needs and responding appropriately to the environment. A client who is unable to speak is at risk for injury un-

---

✳ BOX 24-6 Contextual Factors Influencing Communication

Psychophysiological Context
The internal factors influencing communication:
Physiological status (e.g., pain, hunger, weakness, dyspnea)
Emotional status (e.g., anxiety, anger, hopelessness, euphoria)
Growth and development status (e.g., age, developmental tasks)
Unmet needs (e.g., safety/security, love/belonging)
Attitudes, values, and beliefs (e.g., meaning of illness experience)
Perceptions and personality (e.g., optimist/pessimist, introvert/ extrovert)
Self-concept and self-esteem (e.g., positive or negative)

Relational Context
The nature of the relationship between the participants:
Social, helping, or working relationship
Level of trust between participants
Level of caring expressed
Level of self-disclosure between participants
Shared history of participants
Balance of power and control

Situational Context
The reason for the communication:
Information exchange
Goal achievement
Problem resolution
Expression of feelings

Environmental Context
The physical surroundings in which communication takes place:
Privacy level
Noise level
Comfort and safety level
Distraction level

Cultural Context
The sociocultural elements that affect the interaction:
Educational level of participants
Language and self-expression patterns
Customs and expectations

less the nurse identifies an alternate communication method. If there are barriers that make it difficult to communicate directly with the client, family or friends become important sources about the client's communication patterns and abilities.

Developmental Factors. Aspects of a client's growth and development also influence nurse-client interaction. For example, an infant's self-expression is limited to crying, body movement, and facial expression, whereas older children express their needs more directly. The nurse adapts communication techniques to the special needs of infants and children. Communication with children and their parents requires special considerations. The nurse includes the parents, child, or both as sources of information about the child's health, depending on the child's age. Giving a young child toys or other distractions allows the parent to give full attention to the nurse. Children are especially responsive to nonverbal messages, and sudden movements, loud noises, or threatening gestures are frightening. Children often prefer to make the first move in interpersonal contacts and do not like adults to stare or look down at them. A child who has received little environmental stimulation is possibly behind in language development, thus making communication more challenging.

Age also influences communication. Age alone does not determine an adult's capacity for communication. However, approximately one fifth of the adults in the United States over age 70 have vision and hearing impairments (Berry, Mascia, and Steinman, 2004), and more than one million Americans have a speech disorder that prevents them from expressing themselves, such as expressive aphasia, or limits their ability to understand others, such as receptive aphasia (Goldfarb and Pietro, 2004). Even though some older adults have communication barriers, you need to communicate with them on an adult level and avoid patronizing or speaking in a condescending manner (Williams, Kemper, and Hummert, 2004). Box 24-7 highlights communication needs and barriers of older adults. Your awareness of these factors will facilitate the communication process with those older adults who do experience communication problems.

Sociocultural Factors. Culture influences thinking, feeling, behaving, and communicating. Nurses need to be aware of the typical patterns of interaction that characterize various cultures. For example, European Americans are more open and willing to discuss private family matters, whereas Hispanics, African Americans, and Asian Americans are sometimes reluctant to reveal personal or family information to strangers. Hispanics and Asian Americans value a quiet demeanor and self-restraint; to be open or argumentative reflects negatively on family honor. Native Americans also value silence and are comfortable with it.

Foreign-born persons do not always speak or understand English. Those who speak English as a second language often experience difficulty with self-expression or language comprehension. To practice cultural sensitivity in communication, understand that persons of different cultures use different degrees of eye contact, personal space, gestures, loudness of voice, pace of speech, touch, silence, and meaning of language. Make a conscious effort not to interpret messages through your cultural perspective, but consider the communication within the context of the other indi-

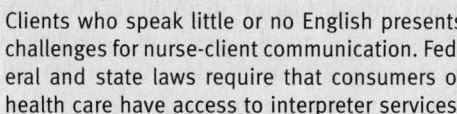
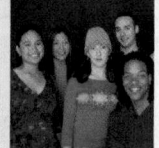

> ✴ **BOX 24-7**   **FOCUS ON OLDER ADULTS**
>
> ***Tips for Improved Communication With Older Adults Who Have Communication Needs/Barriers***
> - Get the client's attention before speaking.
> - Check for hearing aids and glasses.
> - Introduce yourself.
> - Be sure your face is visible to the client, and use facial expressions and gestures.
> - Choose a quiet, well-lit environment with minimal distractions.
> - Do not shout, it distorts sounds. Speak clearly at a moderate speed.
> - Allow time for the client to respond. Do not assume the client is being uncooperative if does not reply or takes a long time to reply.
> - Give client a chance to ask questions.
> - Do not talk to the client like a child. Use words appropriate to the client's developmental level.

> ✴ **BOX 24-8**   **CULTURAL ASPECTS OF CARE**
>
> ***Communication With Non–English-Speaking Clients***
>
> Clients who speak little or no English presents challenges for nurse-client communication. Federal and state laws require that consumers of health care have access to interpreter services, but these services are costly, so use is often limited to crucial interactions. Sometimes there is a delay in interpreter services, yet some clients require urgent care. Use of family members, children, or auxiliary personnel poses legal liabilities. Language is not the only barrier. Cultural differences also lead to misunderstanding. Developing cultural competence increases understanding.
>
> **Implications for Practice**
> - Understand your own cultural values and biases.
> - Client's culture will possibly affect willingness to share private information.
> - Determine level of fluency in English.
> - Avoid body language that can be misunderstood.
> - Speak directly to the client even if an interpreter is present.
> - Nodding or statements such as "okay" do not necessarily mean the client understands.
>
> Data from Lehna C: Interpreter services in pediatric nursing, *Pediatr Nurs* 31(4):292, 2005; and Gravely S: When your patient speaks Spanish—and you don't, *RN* 64(5):65, 2001.

vidual's background. Avoid stereotyping, patronizing, or making fun of other cultures. Language and cultural barriers are not only frustrating, but also dangerous, causing delay in care (Box 24-8). Culture also affects a client who needs to learn information or skills. To be effective, make sure client teaching is culturally sensitive (Box 24-9).

Gender. Gender is another factor influencing how we think, act, feel, and communicate. Males tend to use less verbal com-

✳ **BOX 24-9**   **CLIENT TEACHING**

Providing Culturally Congruent Client Education

Objective
- Client will demonstrate understanding of the health teaching.

Teaching Strategies
- Assess the client's understanding of the illness and health care system.
- Establish communication—use an interpreter service if needed.
- Keep instructions simple and to the point.
- Incorporate a member of the cultural community such as an elder or a health professional as a "cultural guide."
- Negotiate with the client to resolve conflicts between Western health care and the client's cultural understanding.
- For teaching in the community, work with community leaders to increase acceptance.
- Use written material, videos, or computer sites in the client's native language.

Evaluation
- Have client restate information to show understanding.
- Have client demonstrate procedures.

Modified from Cutilli CC: Do your patients understand? Providing culturally congruent patient education, *Orthop Nurs* 25(3):218, 2005.

munication but are more likely to initiate communication and address issues more directly. Males are also more likely to talk about issues. Females tend to disclose more personal information and use more active listening, responding with responses that encourage the other person to continue the conversation. Nilsson and Larsson (2005) found that male nurses generally communicate more directly and females communicate in a more roundabout manner. For example, a male nurse says to his colleague, "Help me turn Jeremy." In contrast, a female nurse says, "Jeremy needs to be turned," expecting her colleague to understand the implied request for help.

Rudan (2003) found females place more value on relationships and communicate to build connections with others, include others, and cooperate with, respond to, show interest in, and support others. Males are "all business" and limit discussion to work-related issues.

To practice gender sensitivity in communication, recognize the differences in male and female patterns to avoid misinterpretation of messages sent by someone of the opposite gender. Avoid conversations with sexual overtones, gender-denigrating jokes, and male-female stereotyping. Because of gender differences, communication is sometimes more effective when the nurse and the client are of the same gender (Arnold and Boggs, 2003).

◆ Nursing Diagnosis

Most individuals experience difficulty with some aspect of communication. Persons who are free of illness or disability sometimes lack skills in attending, listening, responding, and self-expression.

Most often, you will direct your care toward those individuals who experience more serious impairments in communication.

The primary nursing diagnostic label used to describe the client with limited or no ability to communicate verbally is *impaired verbal communication*. This is the state in which an individual experiences a decreased, delayed, or absent ability to receive, process, transmit, and use symbols (Doenges, Moorhouse, and Murr, 2005). A client will have defining characteristics such as the inability to articulate words, inappropriate verbalization, difficulty forming words, and difficulty in comprehending, which the nurse clusters together to form the diagnosis. This diagnosis is useful for a wide variety of clients with special problems and needs related to communication, such as impaired perception, reception, and articulation. Although a client's primary problem is impaired verbal communication, the associated difficulty in self-expression or altered communication patterns may also contribute to other nursing diagnoses:

- Anxiety
- Social isolation
- Ineffective coping
- Compromised family coping
- Powerlessness
- Impaired social interaction

The related (contributing) factors for a nursing diagnosis focus on the causes of the communication disorder. In the case of impaired verbal communication, these are physiological, mechanical, anatomical, psychological, cultural, or developmental in nature. Accuracy in the identification of related factors is necessary so that you select interventions that will effectively resolve the diagnostic problem. For example, you manage the diagnosis of *impaired verbal communication related to cultural difference (Hispanic heritage)* very differently than the diagnosis of *impaired verbal communication related to deafness.*

◆ Planning

Once you have identified the nature of the client's communication dysfunction, you have to consider several factors when designing the care plan. Motivation is a factor in improving communication, and clients often require encouragement to try different approaches that involve significant change. It is especially important to involve the client and family in decisions about the plan of care to determine whether suggested methods are acceptable. Make sure to meet basic comfort and safety needs before introducing new communication methods and techniques. Allow adequate time for practice. Participants need to be patient with themselves and one another in order to achieve effective communication. When the focus is on practicing communication, arrange for a quiet, private place that is free of distractions such as television or visitors. Communication aids such as a writing board for a client with a tracheostomy or a special call system for a paralyzed client enhance communication.

Goals and Outcomes. In general, effective nursing interventions will have the goal of the client experiencing a sense of trust in the nurse and health care team. Expected outcomes for the client with impaired communication are also important to identify. Outcomes are very specific and measurable and a way to determine if the broader goal is met. For example, outcomes for the client will possibly include the following:

- Client initiates conversation about diagnosis or health care problem.
- Client is able to attend to appropriate stimuli.
- Client conveys clear and understandable messages with family members and health care team.
- Client will express increased satisfaction with the communication process.

At times you will care for well clients whose difficulty in sending, receiving, and interpreting messages interferes with healthy interpersonal relationships. In this case, impaired communication will possibly be a contributing factor to other nursing diagnoses such as *impaired social interaction* or *ineffective coping*. You plan interventions to help such clients improve their communication skills. For example, you can model effective communication techniques and provide feedback regarding the client's communication. Role play helps clients rehearse situations in which they have difficulty communicating. Expected outcomes for a client in this situation possibly include demonstrating the ability to appropriately express needs, feelings, and concerns; communicating thoughts and feelings more clearly; engaging in appropriate social conversation with peers and staff; and increasing feelings of autonomy and assertiveness.

Setting of Priorities. It is essential for the nurse to always maintain an open line of communication so that the client is able to express any emergent needs or problems. This sometimes involves an intervention as simple as keeping a call light in reach for a client restricted to bed or providing communication augmentative devices (e.g., message board or Braille computer). When you plan to have lengthy interactions with a client, it is important to address physical care priorities, so that the discussion is not interrupted. Make the client comfortable by ensuring that any symptoms are under control and that any elimination needs have been met.

Continuity of Care. To ensure an effective plan of care, you will sometimes need to collaborate with other health care team members who have expertise in communication strategies. Speech therapists help clients with aphasia, interpreters are often necessary for clients who speak a foreign language, and psychiatric nurse specialists help angry or highly anxious clients to communicate more effectively.

◆Implementation

In carrying out any plan of care, nurses use communication techniques that are appropriate for the client's individual needs. Before learning how to adapt communication methods to help clients with serious communication impairments, it is necessary to learn the communication techniques that serve as the foundation for professional communication. It is also important to understand those communication techniques that create barriers to effective interaction.

Therapeutic Communication Techniques. Therapeutic communication techniques are specific responses that encourage the expression of feelings and ideas and convey acceptance and respect. Learning these techniques will help you develop awareness of the variety of nursing responses available for use in different situations. Although some of the techniques seem artificial at first, skill and comfort will increase with practice. Tremendous satisfaction will result from the development of therapeutic relationships and achievement of desired client outcomes.

Active Listening. Active listening means being attentive to what the client is saying both verbally and nonverbally. Active listening facilitates client communication. Crouch (2002) suggests it is important to remember that we have two ears and one mouth; and we should use them in that 2:1 ratio. Active listening enhances trust because the nurse communicates acceptance and respect for the client. Several nonverbal skills facilitate attentive listening. You identify them by the acronym SOLER (Townsend, 2003):

S—Sit facing the client. This posture gives the message that the nurse is there to listen and is interested in what the client is saying.

O—Observe an open posture (i.e., keep arms and legs uncrossed). This posture suggests that the nurse is "open" to what the client says. A "closed" position conveys a defensive attitude, possibly provoking a similar response in the client.

L—Lean toward the client. This posture conveys that the nurse is involved and interested in the interaction.

E—Establish and maintain intermittent eye contact. This behavior conveys the nurse's involvement in and willingness to listen to what the client is saying. Absence of eye contact or shifting of the eyes gives the message that the nurse is not interested in what the client is saying.

R—Relax. It is important to communicate a sense of being relaxed and comfortable with the client. Restlessness communicates a lack of interest and also conveys a feeling of discomfort to the client.

Sharing Observations. Nurses make observations by commenting on how the other person looks, sounds, or acts. Stating observations often helps the client communicate without the need for extensive questioning, focusing, or clarification. This technique helps start a conversation with quiet or withdrawn persons. Do not state observations that will embarrass or anger the client, such as telling someone "You look a mess!" Even if such an observation is made with humor, the client can become resentful.

Sharing observations differs from making assumptions, which means drawing unnecessary conclusions about the other person without validating them. Making assumptions puts the client in the position of having to contradict the nurse. Examples include the nurse interpreting fatigue as depression or assuming that untouched food indicates lack of interest in meeting nutritional goals. Making observations is a gentler and safer technique: "You look tired . . . ," "You seem different today . . . ," or "I see you haven't eaten anything."

Sharing Empathy. **Empathy** is the ability to understand and accept another person's reality, to accurately perceive feelings, and to communicate this understanding to the other. Balzer Riley (2004) states: "When clients or colleagues are hurting, confused, troubled, anxious, alienated, terrified, doubtful of self-worth, or uncertain as to identity, then understanding is called for" (p. 130). To express empathy, the nurse reflects understanding of the importance of what the other person communicated on a feeling level. Such empathic understanding requires the nurse to be both sensitive and imaginative, especially if the nurse has not had similar experiences. Although nurses are rarely empathetic in every situation, it is an important goal to work for, a key to unlocking concern and communicating support for others. Statements reflecting empathy are highly effective because they tell the person that the nurse heard the feeling content, as well as factual content, of the communication. Empathy statements are neutral and nonjudgmental and help establish trust in difficult situations. For example, the nurse says to an angry client who has low mobility after a stroke: "It must be very frustrating to know what you want and not be able to do it."

Sharing Hope. Nurses recognize that hope is essential for healing and learn to communicate a "sense of possibility" to others. Appropriate encouragement and positive feedback are important in fostering hope and self-confidence and for helping people achieve their potential and reach their goals. You give hope by commenting on the positive aspects of the other person's behavior, performance, or response. Sharing a vision of the future and reminding others of their resources and strengths also strengthens hope. You can reassure clients that there are many kinds of hope and that meaning and personal growth can come from illness experiences. For example, the nurse says to a client discouraged about a poor prognosis, "I believe you will find a way to face your situation, because I have seen your courage and creativity in the past."

Sharing Humor. Humor is an important but underused resource in nursing interactions. McCabe (2004) found humor improved the client's self-esteem and made the nurses seem more approachable. Laughter signifies positive events to people; it also contributes to feelings of togetherness, closeness, and friendliness. The use of humor is one indicator of mental well-being. Furthermore, humor tends to minimize the effect of negative factors and protects from difficulties. Nurses report that humor in health care does the following:

- Shows you care
- Reduces tension and helps you get on with work
- Shows you your clients' personalities with their defenses down
- Makes us equals, because we all laugh at the same things
- Makes us more likely to be accepted (Balzer Riley, 2004)

Furthermore, Balzer Riley (2004) suggests that humor works to promote positive communication in the following three ways:

- *Prevention:* Using humor when a crisis occurs in a work environment makes staff more willing to work together when tension can be great.
- *Perception:* Injecting humor into a situation changes the perception that the situation is so terrible that it cannot be handled.

- *Perspective:* Humor assists us in keeping the big picture in view and not taking ourselves too seriously.

The goal in using humor as a health care provider is to bring hope and joy to the situation and to enhance the client's well-being and the therapeutic relationship. According to Stuart and Laraia (2005), humor serves several additional functions. It helps reduce stress and tension, provides social control, permits cognitive reframing, reflects social change, and expresses emotion.

Today it is common that nurses care for clients from different cultures. When the nurse interacts with clients who do not have a full grasp of the language, it is important to realize that clients may misunderstand or misinterpret jokes and statements meant to be humorous. It is also important to recognize that when either a nurse or client tries to speak in another language, mistakes sometimes occur.

Health care professionals sometimes use a kind of dark, negative humor after difficult or traumatic situations as a way to deal with unbearable tension and stress. This coping humor has a high potential for misinterpretation as uncaring by persons not involved in the situation. For example, student nurses are sometimes offended and wonder how staff is able to laugh and joke after unsuccessful resuscitation efforts. When nurses use coping humor within earshot of clients or their loved ones, great emotional distress results.

Sharing Feelings. Emotions are subjective feelings that result from one's thought and perceptions. Feelings are not right, wrong, good, or bad, although they are pleasant or unpleasant. If individuals do not express feelings, stress and illness will worsen. You help clients express emotions by making observations, acknowledging feelings, encouraging communication, giving permission to express "negative" feelings, and modeling healthy emotional self-expression. At times, clients direct anger or frustration prompted by their illness toward the nurse. Do not take such expressions personally. Acknowledging clients' feelings communicates that you listened to and understood the emotional aspects of their illness situation.

When you care for clients, be aware of your own emotions, because feelings are difficult to hide. Students sometimes wonder whether it is helpful for the nurse to share feelings with clients. Sharing emotion makes nurses seem more human and brings people closer. It is appropriate to share feelings of caring, or even cry with others, as long as the nurse is in control of the expression of those feelings and does so in a way that does not burden the client or break confidentiality. Clients are perceptive and will sense a nurse's emotions. It is usually inappropriate to discuss negative personal emotions such as anger or sadness with clients. A social support system of colleagues is helpful, and employee assistance programs, peer group meetings, and the use of interdisciplinary teams such as social work and pastoral care provide other means for nurses to safely express feelings away from clients.

Using Touch. In today's fast-paced technical environments, nurses are required more than ever to bring the sense of caring and human connection to their clients (see Chapter 8). Touch is one of the nurse's most potent forms of communication. Nurses are privileged to experience more of this intimate form of personal contact than almost any other professional. Touch conveys many

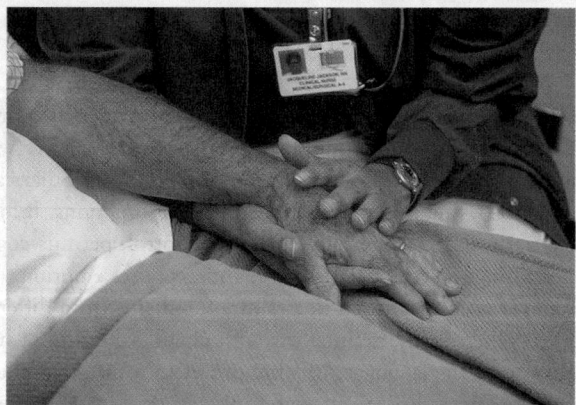

Figure 24-2 The nurse uses touch to communicate.

messages, such as affection, emotional support, encouragement, tenderness, and personal attention. Comfort touch, such as holding a hand, is especially important for vulnerable clients who are experiencing severe illness with its accompanying physical and emotional losses (Figure 24-2). In older persons, touch increases a sense of safety, increases self-confidence, and decreases anxiety (Gleeson and Timmons, 2004). Research has found that in children having a lumbar puncture, a medical procedure, a nurse's soothing nonessential touch decreased anxiety and lowered the child's distress (Vannorsdall and others, 2004).

Students may initially find giving intimate care stressful, especially when caring for clients of the opposite gender (Seed, 1995). Students learn to cope with intimate contact by changing their perception of the situation. Since much of what nurses do involves touching, you need to learn to be sensitive to others' reactions to touch and use it wisely. Touch should be as gentle or as firm as needed and delivered in a comforting, nonthreatening manner. There are times when you withhold touch; for example, highly suspicious or angry persons respond negatively or even violently to the nurse's touch.

Using Silence. It takes time and experience to become comfortable with silence. Most people have a natural tendency to fill empty spaces with words, but sometimes what those spaces really need is time for the nurse and client to observe one another, sort out feelings, think how to say things, and consider what has been communicated. Silence prompts some people to talk. Silence allows the client to think and gain insight. In general, allow the client to break the silence, particularly when the client has initiated it (Stuart and Laraia, 2005).

Silence is particularly useful when people are confronted with decisions that require much thought. For example, silence helps a client gain confidence needed to share the decision to refuse medical treatment. Silence also allows the nurse to pay particular attention to nonverbal messages such as worried expressions or loss of eye contact. Remaining silent demonstrates the nurse's patience and willingness to wait for a response when the other person is unable to reply quickly. Silence is especially therapeutic during times of profound sadness or grief.

Providing Information. Providing relevant information tells other persons what they need or want to know so they are

able to make decisions, experience less anxiety, and feel safe and secure. It is also an integral aspect of health teaching. It is usually not helpful to hide information from clients, particularly when they seek it. If a physician withholds information, the nurse needs to clarify the reason with the physician. Clients have a right to know about their health status and what is happening in their environment. Information of a distressing nature needs to be communicated with sensitivity, at a pace appropriate to what the client can absorb, and in general terms at first: "John, your heart sounds have changed from earlier today, and so has your blood pressure. I'll let your doctor know." The nurse provides information that enables others to understand what is happening and what to expect: "Mrs. Evans, John is getting an echocardiogram right now. This test uses painless sound waves to create a moving picture of his heart structures and valves and should tell us what is causing his murmur."

Clarifying. To check whether understanding is accurate, restate an unclear or ambiguous message to clarify the sender's meaning. Also, ask the other person to rephrase it, explain further, or give an example of what the person means. Without clarification, you may make invalid assumptions and miss valuable information. Despite efforts at paraphrasing, sometimes you will not understand the client's message and you need to let the client know if this is the case: "I'm not sure I understand what you mean by 'sicker than usual.' What is different now?"

Focusing. Focusing centers on key elements or concepts of a message. If conversation is vague or rambling or clients begin to repeat themselves, focusing is a useful technique. The nurse does not use focusing if it interrupts clients while discussing an important issue. Rather, the nurse uses focusing to guide the direction of conversation to important areas: "We've talked a lot about your medications, but let's look more closely at the trouble you're having in taking them on time."

Paraphrasing. Paraphrasing is restating another's message more briefly using one's own words. Through paraphrasing the nurse sends feedback that lets the client know that the nurse is actively involved in the search for understanding. Practice is required to paraphrase accurately. If the meaning of a message is changed or distorted through paraphrasing, communication becomes ineffective. For example, a client says, "I've been overweight all my life and never had any problems. I can't understand why I need to be on a diet." Paraphrasing this statement by saying, "You don't care if you're overweight or not," is incorrect. It is more accurate to say, "You're not convinced you need a diet because you've stayed healthy."

Asking Relevant Questions. Nurses ask relevant questions to seek information needed for decision making. You need to ask only one question at a time and fully explore one topic before moving to another area. During client assessment, questions follow a logical sequence and usually proceed from general to more specific. Open-ended questions allow the client to take the conversational lead and introduce pertinent information about a topic. For example, "What's your biggest problem at the moment?" Focused questions are used when information that is more specific is needed in an area: "How has your pain affected your life at home?" Allow clients to fully respond to an open-ended question before asking more focused questions. Closed-ended questions elicit a yes, no, or one-word response: "How many times a day are you taking pain medication?" Although they are helpful during assessment, they are generally less useful during therapeutic exchanges.

Asking too many questions is sometimes dehumanizing. Seeking factual information does not allow the nurse or client to establish a meaningful relationship or deal with important emotional issues. It is a way for the nurse to ignore uncomfortable areas in favor of more comfortable, neutral topics. A useful exercise is to try conversing without asking the other person a single question. By giving general leads ("tell me about it . . ."), making observations, paraphrasing, focusing, providing information, and so forth, you will discover important information that would have remained hidden if the nurse limited the communication process to questions alone.

Summarizing. Summarizing is a concise review of key aspects of an interaction. Summarizing brings a sense of satisfaction and closure to an individual conversation and is especially helpful during the termination phase of a nurse-client relationship. By reviewing a conversation, participants focus on key issues and add additional relevant information as needed. Beginning a new interaction by summarizing a previous one helps the client recall topics discussed and shows the client that the nurse has analyzed communication. Summarizing also clarifies expectations, as in this example of a nurse manager who has been working with a dissatisfied employee: "You've told me a lot of things about why you don't like this job and how unhappy you've been. We've also come up with some possible ways to make things better, and you've agreed to try some and let me know if any of them help."

Self-Disclosure. Self-disclosures are subjectively true, personal experiences about the self that are intentionally revealed to another person. This is not therapy for the nurse; rather, it shows clients that the nurse understands their experiences and their experiences are not unique. You will choose to share experiences or feelings that are similar to those of the client and emphasize both the similarities and differences. This kind of self-disclosure is indicative of the closeness of the nurse-client relationship and involves a particular kind of respect for the client. You offer it as an expression of genuineness and honesty, and it is an aspect of empathy (Stuart and Laraia, 2005). Self-disclosures needs to be relevant and appropriate and made to benefit the client rather than the nurse. Use it sparingly, so the client is the focus of the interaction: "That happened to me once, too. It was devastating, and I had to face some things about myself that I didn't like. I went for counseling, and it really helped. . . . What are your thoughts about seeing a counselor?"

Confrontation. To confront someone in a therapeutic way, you help the other person become more aware of inconsistencies in his or her feelings, attitudes, beliefs, and behaviors (Stuart and Laraia, 2005). This technique improves client self-awareness and helps the client recognize growth and deal with important issues. Use confrontation only after you have established trust, and do it gently, with sensitivity: "You say you've already decided what to do, yet you're still talking a lot about your options."

Nontherapeutic Communication Techniques. Certain communication techniques hinder or damage professional rela-

tionships. These specific techniques are referred to as nontherapeutic or blocking and will often cause recipients to activate defenses to avoid being hurt or negatively affected. Nontherapeutic techniques tend to discourage further expression of feelings and ideas and engender negative responses or behaviors in others.

Asking Personal Questions. "Why don't you and John get married?" Asking personal questions that are not relevant to the situation, simply to satisfy the nurse's curiosity, is not appropriate professional communication. Such questions are nosy, invasive, and unnecessary. If clients wish to share private information, they will. To learn more about the client's interpersonal roles and relationships, ask a question such as "How would you describe your relationship with John?"

Giving Personal Opinions. "If I were you, I'd put your mother in a nursing home." When the nurse gives a personal opinion, it takes decision making away from the client. It inhibits spontaneity, stalls problem solving, and creates doubt. Personal opinions differ from professional advice. At times, clients need suggestions and help to make choices. Suggestions you present are options to the client; he or she will make the final decision. Remember, the problem and its solution belongs to the other person and not the nurse. A much better response is, "Let's talk about what options are available for your mother's care."

Changing the Subject. "Let's not talk about your problems with the insurance company. It's time for your walk." Changing the subject when another person is trying to communicate something important is rude and shows a lack of empathy. It tends to block further communication, and the sender then withholds important messages or fails to openly express feelings. Thoughts and spontaneity are interrupted, ideas become tangled, and information provided is sometimes inadequate. In some instances, changing the subject serves as a face-saving maneuver. If this happens, reassure the client you will return to his or her concerns: "After your walk, let's talk some more about what's going on with your insurance company."

Automatic Responses. "Older adults are always confused." "Administration doesn't care about the staff." Stereotypes are generalized beliefs held about people. Making stereotyped remarks about others reflects poor nursing judgment and threatens nurse-client or team relationships. A cliché is a stereotyped comment, such as "You can't win them all," that tends to belittle the other person's feelings and minimize the importance of his or her message. These automatic phrases communicate that the nurse is not taking concerns seriously or responding thoughtfully. Another kind of automatic response is parroting, repeating what the other person has said, word for word. Parroting is easily overused and is not as effective as paraphrasing. A simple "oh?" gives the nurse time to think if the other person says something that takes one by surprise.

A nurse who is task oriented automatically makes the task or procedure the entire focus of interaction with clients, missing opportunities to communicate with them as individuals and meet their needs. Task-oriented nurses are often perceived as cold, uncaring, and unapproachable. When students first perform technical skills, it is difficult to integrate therapeutic communication due to the need to focus on the procedure. In time, you will learn to integrate communication with high-visibility tasks and accomplish several goals simultaneously.

False Reassurance. "Don't worry, everything will be all right." When a client is seriously ill or distressed, you may be tempted to offer hope to the client with statements such as "You'll be fine" or "There's nothing to worry about." When a client is reaching for understanding, false reassurance discourages open communication. Offering reassurance not supported by facts or based in reality will do more harm than good. Although the nurse is trying to be kind, it has the secondary effect of helping the nurse avoid the other person's distress, and it tends to block conversation and discourage further expression of feelings. A more facilitative nursing response is "It must be difficult not to know what the surgeon will find. What can I do to help?"

Sympathy. "I'm so sorry about your mastectomy; it must be terrible to lose a breast." **Sympathy** is concern, sorrow, or pity felt for the client generated by the nurse's personal identification with the client's needs (Grover, 2005). Sympathy is a subjective look at another person's world that prevents a clear perspective of the issues confronting that person. If a nurse overidentifies with the client, objectivity is lost and the nurse is not able to help the client work through the situation (Arnold and Boggs, 2003). Although sympathy is a compassionate response to another's situation, it is not as therapeutic as empathy. The nurse's own emotional issues sometimes prevent effective problem solving and impair good judgment. A more empathetic approach is "The loss of a breast is a major change. How do you think it will affect your life?"

Asking for Explanations. "Why are you so anxious?" Some nurses are tempted to ask the other person to explain why the person believes, feels, or has acted in a certain way. Clients frequently interpret "why" questions as accusations or think the nurse knows the reason and is simply testing them. Regardless of client perception of the nurse's motivation, "why" questions cause resentment, insecurity, and mistrust. If the nurse needs additional information, it is best to phrase a question to avoid using the word "why." "You seem upset. What's on your mind?" is more likely to help the anxious client to communicate.

Approval or Disapproval. "You shouldn't even think about assisted suicide; it's not right." Do not impose your own attitudes, values, beliefs, and moral standards on others while in the professional helping role. Other people have the right to be themselves and make their own decisions. Judgmental responses by the nurse often contain terms such as *should, ought, good, bad, right,* or *wrong.* Agreeing or disagreeing sends the subtle message you have the right to make value judgments about client decisions. Approving implies that the behavior being praised is the only acceptable one. Often the client shares a decision with the nurse, not in an effort to seek approval but to provide a means to discuss feelings. On the other hand, disapproving implies that the client needs to meet the nurse's expectations or standards. Instead, help clients explore their own beliefs and decisions. The nursing response "I'm surprised you are considering assisted suicide. Tell me more about it . . ." gives the client a chance to express ideas or feelings without fear of being judged.

Defensive Responses. "No one here would intentionally lie to you." Becoming defensive in the face of criticism implies the other person has no right to an opinion. The sender's concerns are ignored when the nurse focuses on the need for self-defense, defense of the health care team, or defense of others. When clients express criticism, listen to what they have to say. Listening does not imply agreement. To discover reasons for the client's anger or dissatisfaction, you need to listen uncritically. By avoiding defensiveness, you are able to defuse anger and uncover deeper concerns: "You believe people have been dishonest with you. It must be hard to trust anyone."

Passive or Aggressive Responses. "Things are bad, and there's nothing I can do about it." "Things are bad, and it's all your fault." Passive responses serve to avoid conflict or sidestep issues. They reflect feelings of sadness, depression, anxiety, powerlessness, and hopelessness. Aggressive responses provoke confrontation at the other person's expense. They reflect feelings of anger, frustration, resentment, and stress. Nurses who lack assertive skills also use triangulation, complaining to a third party rather than confronting the problem or expressing concerns directly to the source. This lowers team morale and draws others into the conflict situation. Assertive communication is a far more professional approach for the nurse to take.

Arguing. "How can you say you didn't sleep a wink, when I heard you snoring all night long?" Challenging or arguing against perceptions denies that they are real and valid to the other person. They imply that the other person is lying, misinformed, or uneducated. The skillful nurse gives information or presents reality in a way that avoids argument: "You feel like you didn't get any rest at all last night, even though I thought you slept well since I heard you snoring."

Adapting Communication Techniques for the Client With Special Needs.

With our aging population, there is increased incidence of clients who have difficulty communicating. One study found that 55% of Medicare recipients had some kind of communication disability (Hoffman and others, 2005). Interacting with those who have conditions that impair communication requires special thought and sensitivity. Such clients benefit greatly when the nurse adapts communication techniques to their unique circumstances or developmental level. For example, the nurse caring for a client with impaired verbal communication related to cultural differences provides a table of simple words in the client's language. The nurse and client use the table to help communicate about basic needs such as food, water, toileting, pain relief, sleep, and so forth. Research findings suggest that many of the difficulties in communicating with clients with severe communication impairment come from the lack of an understandable nurse-client communication system (Hemsley and others, 2001).

The nurse directs actions toward meeting the goals and expected outcomes identified in the plan of care, addressing both the communication impairment and its contributing factors. Box 24-10 lists many methods available to encourage, enhance, restore, or substitute for verbal communication. You need to be sure that the client is physically able to use the chosen method and that it does not cause frustration by being too complicated or difficult. A study of persons who were deaf or hard of hearing indicated one of the most important things for the nurse to do was ask the client how to best communicate with him or her (Iezzoni and others, 2004).

Because nursing care of the older adult is ideally delivered through an interdisciplinary model, the primary goal is to estab-

✳ BOX 24-10 Communicating With Clients Who Have Special Needs

Clients Who Cannot Speak Clearly (Aphasia, Dysarthria, Muteness)

Listen attentively, be patient, and do not interrupt.
Ask simple questions that require "yes" or "no" answers.
Allow time for understanding and response.
Use visual cues (e.g., words, pictures, and objects) when possible.
Allow only one person to speak at a time.
Do not shout or speak too loudly.
Encourage the client to converse.
Let client know if you have not understood him or her.
Collaborate with speech therapist as needed.
Use communication aids:
    Pad and felt-tipped pen or Magic Slate
    Communication board with commonly used words, letters, or pictures denoting basic needs
    Call bells or alarms
    Sign language
    Use of eye blinks or movement of fingers for simple responses ("yes" or "no")

Clients Who Are Cognitively Impaired

Reduce environmental distractions while conversing.
Get client's attention before speaking.
Use simple sentences, and avoid long explanations.
Ask one question at a time.
Allow time for client to respond.
Be an attentive listener.
Include family and friends in conversations, especially in subjects known to client.

Clients Who Are Hearing Impaired

Check for hearing aids and glasses.
Reduce environmental noise.
Get client's attention before speaking.
Face client with mouth visible.
Do not chew gum.
Speak at normal volume—do not shout.
Rephrase rather than repeat if misunderstood.
Provide a sign language interpreter if indicated.

Clients Who Are Visually Impaired

Check for use of glasses or contact lenses.
Identify yourself when you enter room, and notify client when you leave room.
Speak in a normal tone of voice.
Do not rely on gestures or nonverbal communication to convey messages.
Use indirect lighting, avoiding glare.
Use at least 14-point print.

Clients Who Are Unresponsive

Call client by name during interactions.
Communicate both verbally and by touch.
Speak to client as though he or she could hear.
Explain all procedures and sensations.
Provide orientation to person, place, and time.
Avoid talking about client to others in his or her presence.
Avoid saying things client should not hear.

Clients Who Do Not Speak English

Speak to client in normal tone of voice (shouting may be interpreted as anger).
Establish method for client to signal desire to communicate (call light or bell).
Provide an interpreter (translator) as needed.
Avoid using family members, especially children, as interpreters.
Develop communication board, pictures, or cards.
Translate words from native language into English list for client to make basic requests.
Have dictionary (English/Spanish and so forth) available if client can read.

---

lish a reliable communication system that all health care team members can understand easily. Effective communication involves adapting to any special needs resulting from sensory, motor, or cognitive impairments that are present. You can also encourage older adults to share life stories and reminisce about the past, which has a therapeutic effect and increases their sense of well-being. Avoid sudden shifts from subject to subject. It is helpful to include the client's family and friends and to become familiar with the client's favorite topics for conversation.

◆ Evaluation

The nurse and client determine whether the plan of care has been successful by evaluating the client communication outcomes. You evaluate nursing interventions to determine what strategies or interventions were effective and what client changes resulted because of the interventions. For example, if using a pen and paper

proves frustrating for a nonverbal client whose handwriting is shaky, you revise the care plan to include use of a picture board instead. If expected outcomes are not met or progress is not satisfactory, you will need to determine what factors influenced the outcomes, then modify the plan of care.

You evaluate the effectiveness of your own communication by videotaping practice sessions with peers or making process recordings, written records of your verbal and nonverbal interactions with clients. Process recording analysis reveals how to improve personal communication techniques to make them more effective. Box 24-11 contains a sample communication analysis of such a record. Analysis of a process recording enables the nurse to evaluate the following:

- Determine whether he or she encouraged openness and allowed the client to "tell his story," expressing both thoughts and feelings
- Identify any missed verbal or nonverbal cues or conversational themes

✳ BOX 24-11 Sample Communication Analysis

Nurse: "Good morning, Mr. Simpson."
(Smiles, approaches bed holding clipboard)
Acknowledging by name, social greeting to begin conversation

Client: "What's good about it?"
(Arms crossed over chest, frowning, direct stare)
Nonverbal signs of anger

Nurse: "You sound unhappy."
(Pulls up chair and sits at bedside)
Sharing observation, nonverbal communication of availability

Client: "You'd be unhappy, too, if nobody would answer your questions."
(Angry voice tone, challenging expression)
Further expression of feelings facilitated by nurse making accurate observation

Nurse: "This hospital has a fine staff, Mr. Simpson. I'm sure no one would intentionally keep information from you."
Feeling threatened and being defensive, a nontherapeutic technique

Client: "All right then: Why wouldn't that girl tell me what my blood sugar was?"

Nurse: "I'm not sure. If I were you, I'd forget about it and get a fresh start."
Giving advice and using cliché, which was nontherapeutic; it is better to acknowledge that client had a right to know the information

Nurse: "I'm going to test your glucose in a minute, and I'll tell you the results." (Does test) "Your blood sugar was 350."
Providing information, demonstrating trustworthiness

Client: "I'm so afraid complications will set in since my blood sugar is high."
(Stares out window)
Feels free to express deeper concerns, but they are hard to face

Nurse: "What kinds of things are you worried about?"
Open-ended question to seek information

Client: "I could lose a leg, like my mother did. Or go blind. Or have to live hooked up to a kidney machine for the rest of my life.

Nurse: "You've been thinking about all kinds of things that could go wrong, and it adds to your worry not to be told what your blood sugar is."
Summarizing to let client "hear" what he has communicated

Client: "I always think the worst."
(Shakes head in exasperation)
Expressing insight into his "inner dialogue"

Nurse: "I'll pass along to the tech that it's OK to tell you your glucose levels. And later this afternoon, I'd like us to talk more about some things you can do to help avoid these complications and set some goals for controlling your glucose."
(Stands up, keeps looking at client)
Providing information, encouraging collaboration and goal setting
Giving nonverbal cue that conversation is nearing end

Client: "OK, I'll see you later.

- Examine whether nursing responses blocked or facilitated the client's efforts to communicate
- Determine whether nursing responses were positive and supportive or superficial and judgmental
- Examine the type and number of questions that were asked
- Determine the type and number of therapeutic communication techniques used
- Discover any missed opportunities to use humor, silence, or touch

Evaluation of the communication process will help nurses gain confidence and competence in interpersonal skills. Becoming an effective communicator greatly increases the nurse's professional satisfaction and success. There is no skill more basic, no tool more powerful.

✳ Key Concepts

- Communication is a powerful therapeutic tool and an essential nursing skill that influences others and achieves positive health outcomes.
- Critical thinking facilitates communication through creative inquiry, focused self-awareness and awareness of others, purposeful analysis, and control of perceptual biases.

- Nurses consider many contexts and factors influencing communication when making decisions about what, when, where, how, why, and with whom to communicate.
- Communication is most effective when the receiver and sender accurately perceive the meaning of one another's messages.
- The sender's and receiver's physical and developmental status, perceptions, values, emotions, knowledge, sociocultural background, roles, and environment all influence message transmission.
- Effective verbal communication requires appropriate intonation, clear and concise phrasing, proper pacing of statements, and proper timing and relevance of a message.
- Effective nonverbal communication complements and strengthens the message conveyed by verbal communication.
- Nurses use intrapersonal, interpersonal, transpersonal, small-group, and public interaction to achieve positive change and health goals.
- Nurses strengthen helping relationships by establishing trust, empathy, autonomy, confidentiality, and professional competence.
- Effective communication techniques are facilitative and tend to encourage the other person to openly express ideas, feelings, or concerns.

- Ineffective communication techniques are inhibiting and tend to block the other person's willingness to openly express ideas, feelings, or concerns.
- The nurse blends social and informational interactions with therapeutic communication techniques so that others are able to explore feelings and manage health issues.
- Older adult clients with sensory, motor, or cognitive impairments require the adaptation of communication techniques to compensate for their loss of function and special needs.
- Clients with impaired verbal communication require special consideration and alterations in communication techniques to facilitate the sending, receiving, and interpreting of messages.
- Desired outcomes for clients with impaired verbal communication include increased satisfaction with interpersonal interactions, the ability to send and receive clear messages, and attending to and accurately interpreting verbal and nonverbal cues.

Critical Thinking Exercises

1. Mrs. Maria Ramirez, an American of Puerto Rican descent, is faced with the difficult decision of whether or not to continue chemotherapy in the face of a rapidly spreading malignancy. What communication techniques could the nurse use to help her at this point, and what traps must the nurse avoid in such a situation?

2. Jan, a nurse colleague, is having difficulty standing up to a health care provider who has an abrupt, intimidating communication style. She often ends up with a lot of unspoken anger, developing tension headaches and easily becoming tearful. What could the nurse do to help?

3. Mr. Hess, a client with Parkinson's disease living at an extended care facility, has a stiff, expressionless face. He sits slumped in a recliner chair all day and seems lost in his own world, rarely looking at or interacting with anyone. When he does talk, he mumbles in a soft voice and his words are difficult to understand. What kinds of things could the nurse do to establish a helping-healing relationship with Mr. Hess?

4. Jennifer Hughes, a new graduate, is very discouraged. In school she had felt a great deal of anxiety about her own performance, and even now she finds it difficult to be positive about herself or her job. What knowledge about communication could she use to help improve her situation?

5. Mrs. Esther Larson, a client who has been recently admitted to a hospice program, confides in the nurse that she feels overwhelmed with the number of things she must attend to now that she is facing the possibility of death. She says, "My thoughts are all over the place. I don't know where to start." What communication techniques, based on the critical thinking model, could the nurse use to help her at this point?

NCLEX®-Style Review Questions

1. As a nursing student, you give yourself positive messages regarding your ability to do well on a test. This is an example of what level of communication?
   1. Public
   2. Intrapersonal
   3. Interpersonal
   4. Transpersonal

2. The nurse demonstrates active listening by:
   1. Agreeing with the client
   2. Repeating everything the client says to clarify
   3. Assuming a relaxed posture and leaning toward the client
   4. Smiling and nodding continuously throughout the interview

3. During the orientation phase of the helping relationship, the nurse might do which of the following?
   1. Discuss the cards and flowers in the room
   2. Work together with the client to establish goals
   3. Review the client's history to identify possible health concerns
   4. Use therapeutic communication to manage the client's confusion

4. If the nurse is working with a client who has expressive aphasia, it would be most helpful for the nurse to:
   1. Ask open-ended questions
   2. Speak loudly and use simple sentences
   3. Allow extra time for the client to respond
   4. Encourage a family member to answer for the client

5. The statement that best explains the role of collaboration with others for the client's plan of care is which of the following?
   1. The professional nurse consults the physician for direction in establishing goals for clients.
   2. The professional nurse depends on the latest literature to complete an excellent plan of care for clients.
   3. The professional nurse works independently to plan and deliver care and does not depend on other staff for assistance.
   4. The professional nurse collaborates with colleagues and the client's family to provide combined expertise in planning care.

6. "I'm not sure I understand what you mean by 'sicker than usual.' What is different now?" The nurse is using the therapeutic technique:
   1. Focusing
   2. Clarifying
   3. Paraphrasing
   4. Providing information

7. "We've talked a lot about your medications, but let's look more closely at the trouble you're having in taking them on time." The nurse is using the therapeutic technique:
   1. Focusing
   2. Clarifying
   3. Paraphrasing
   4. Providing information

8. When working with an older adult, the nurse should remember to avoid:
   1. Touching the client
   2. Allowing the client to reminisce
   3. Shifting from subject to subject
   4. Asking the client how he or she feels

9. Which of the following nurse statements would be nontherapeutic and tend to block communication? (Choose all that apply.)
   1. "You look sad today."
   2. "Why are you so nervous?"
   3. "If I were you, I'd have the surgery."
   4. "I'm sure the test will come out fine."
   5. "Tell me what it's like to live with dizziness."

10. A nurse should consider zones of personal space and touch when caring for clients. If the nurse is taking the client's nursing history, she should:
    1. Sit next to the client
    2. Be 4 to 12 feet from the client
    3. Be 18 inches to 4 feet from the client
    4. Be 12 inches to 3 feet from the client

25 | Client Education

✳ OBJECTIVES

Mastery of the content in this chapter will enable the student to:

- Identify appropriate topics for a client's health education needs.
- Describe the similarities and differences between teaching and learning.
- Identify the role of the nurse in client education.
- Identify the purposes of client education.
- Use communication principles when providing client education.
- Describe the domains of learning.

- Identify basic learning principles.
- Differentiate factors that determine the readiness to learn from those that determine the ability to learn.
- Compare and contrast the nursing and teaching processes.
- Write learning objectives for a teaching plan.
- Establish an environment that promotes learning.
- Include patient teaching while performing routine nursing care.
- Use appropriate methods to evaluate learning.

✳ MEDIA RESOURCES ✳ KEY TERMS

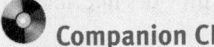 **Companion CD**
- NCLEX®-Style Review Questions
- Audio Glossary
- Interactive Learning Activities
- English/Spanish Glossary

evolve **Website**
- NCLEX®-Style Review Questions
- Audio Glossary
- English/Spanish Glossary
- Interactive Learning Activities
- Weblinks
- Audio Summaries

Affective learning, p. 365
Analogies, p. 378
Cognitive learning, p. 365
Compliance, p. 366
Functional illiteracy, p. 372
Learning, p. 362
Learning objective, p. 362

Motivation, p. 366
Psychomotor learning, p. 366
Reinforcement, p. 377
Return demonstrations, p. 378
Self-efficacy, p. 367
Teaching, p. 362

Client education is one of the most important roles for a nurse in any health care setting. Shorter hospital stays, increased demands on nurses' time, an increase in the number of chronically ill clients, and the need to give acutely ill clients meaningful information as soon as possible emphasize the importance of quality client education. As nurses try to find the best way to educate clients, the general public has become more assertive in seeking knowledge, understanding health, and finding resources available within the health care system. Nurses provide clients with information needed for self-care to ensure continuity of care from the hospital to the home (Falvo, 2004).

Clients have the right to know and to be informed about their diagnoses, prognoses, and available treatments to help them make intelligent, informed decisions about their health and lifestyle. Creating a well-designed, comprehensive teaching plan that fits a client's unique learning needs reduces health care costs, improves the quality of care, and provides information about treatment. Ultimately, this helps clients make informed decisions about their care and helps clients become healthier and more independent (Behar-Horenstein and others, 2005; Oermann and others, 2002).

Standards for Client Education

Client education has long been a standard for professional nursing practice. All state Nurse Practice Acts recognize that client teaching falls within the scope of nursing practice (Bastable, 2006). In addition, various accrediting agencies set guidelines for providing client education in health care institutions. The Joint Commission (TJC, 2006) sets standards for client and family education. These standards require nurses and the health care team to assess the client's learning needs and provide education about many topics,

including medications, nutrition, use of medical equipment, pain, and the client's plan of care. The successful accomplishment of the standards requires collaboration among health care professionals and enhances client recovery. Educational efforts need to take into consideration clients' psychosocial, spiritual, and cultural values, as well as the desire to actively participate in the educational process. It is important to document evidence of successful client education in the client's medical record. Standards such as these help to direct nurses in client education.

Purposes of Client Education

The goal of educating others about their health is to assist individuals, families, or communities in achieving optimal levels of health (Edelman and Mandle, 2006). The American Nurses Association's *Position Statement on Health Promotion and Disease Prevention* (1997) supports a focus on promoting health and preventing illness. Preventative health care is essential in reducing health care costs, as well as reducing hardships on individuals, families, and communities. Clients now know more about health and want to be involved in health maintenance. Nurses need to provide education about health and health care in places that are convenient and familiar to clients. Comprehensive client education includes three important purposes, each involving a separate phase of health care (Box 25-1).

Maintenance and Promotion of Health and Illness Prevention

The nurse is a visible, competent resource for clients who want to improve their physical and psychological well-being. In the school, home, clinic, or workplace the nurse provides information

---

✳ BOX 25-1 Topics for Health Education

Health Maintenance and Promotion and Illness Prevention
First aid
Avoidance of risk factors (e.g., smoking, alcohol, other substances)
Stress management
Growth and development
Hygiene
Immunizations
Prenatal care and normal childbearing
Nutrition
Exercise
Safety (in home and health care setting)
Screening (e.g., blood pressure, vision, cholesterol level)
Behavior modification to change risk behaviors (e.g., smoking cessation, substance abuse treatment)

Restoration of Health
Client's disease or condition
Anatomy and physiology of body system affected
Cause of disease
Origin of symptoms
Expected effects on other body systems
Prognosis
Limitations on function
Rationale for treatment and explanation of treatment methods
Medications

Intravenous therapy
Diet choices
Activity
Tests and therapies
Nursing measures
Surgical intervention
Expected duration of care
Hospital or clinic environment
Hospital or clinic staff
Long-term care
Methods for client participation in care
Limitations posed by disease or surgery

Coping With Impaired Functions
Home care
Self-help devices
Rehabilitation of remaining function
Physical therapy
Occupational therapy
Speech therapy
Prevention of complications
Knowledge of risk factors
Implications of noncompliance with therapy
Environmental alterations

and skills that allow clients to assume healthier behaviors (see Box 25-1). For example, in childbearing classes, nurses teach expectant parents about physical and psychological changes in the woman and about fetal development. After learning about normal childbearing, the mother is more likely to eat healthy foods, engage in physical exercise, and avoid substances that can harm the fetus. Promoting healthy behavior through education allows clients to assume more responsibility for their health. Greater knowledge results in better health maintenance habits. When clients become more health conscious, they are more likely to seek early diagnosis of health problems (Redman, 2007).

Restoration of Health

Injured or ill clients need information and skills to help them regain or maintain their levels of health (see Box 25-1). Clients recovering from and adapting to changes resulting from illness or injury often seek information about their conditions. For example, a woman who recently had a hysterectomy asks about her pathology reports and expected length of recovery. However, some clients who find it difficult to adapt to illness become passive and uninterested in learning. As the nurse, you learn to identify clients' willingness to learn and motivate interest in learning (Redman, 2007). The family often is a vital part of a client's return to health and usually needs to know as much as the client. If you exclude the family from a teaching plan, conflicts will possibly occur. However, do not assume that the family should be involved; assess the client-family relationship before providing education to the family.

Coping With Impaired Functions

Not all clients fully recover from illness or injury. Many have to learn to cope with permanent health alterations. New knowledge and skills are often necessary for clients to continue activities of daily living (see Box 25-1). For example, a client loses the ability to speak after surgery of the larynx and has to learn new ways of communicating. Changes in function are physical or psychosocial. In the case of serious disability, such as following a stroke or a spinal cord injury, the client's family needs to understand and accept many changes in the client's physical capabilities. The family's ability to provide support results in part from education, which begins as soon as the nurse identifies the client's needs and the family displays a willingness to help. Teach family members to help the client with health care management (e.g., giving medications through gastric tubes and doing passive range-of-motion exercises). Families of clients with alterations such as alcoholism, mental retardation, or drug dependence learn to adapt to the emotional effects of these chronic conditions and provide psychosocial support to facilitate the client's health. Comparing the desired level of health with the actual state enables you to plan effective teaching programs.

Teaching and Learning

It is impossible to separate teaching from learning. **Teaching** is an interactive process that promotes learning. It consists of a conscious, deliberate set of actions that help individuals gain new knowledge, change attitudes, adopt new behaviors, or perform new skills (Bastable, 2006; Redman, 2007). A teacher provides information that prompts the learner to engage in activities that lead to a desired change.

Learning is the purposeful acquisition of new knowledge, attitudes, behaviors, and skills (Bastable, 2003). Complex patterns are required if the client is to learn new skills, change existing attitudes, transfer learning to new situations, or solve problems (Redman, 2007). A new mother exhibits learning when she demonstrates to the nurse how to bathe her newborn. The mother shows transfer of learning when she uses the principles she learned about bathing a newborn when she bathes her older child. Generally, teaching and learning begin when a person identifies a need for knowing or acquiring an ability to do something. Teaching is most effective when it responds to the learner's needs (Redman, 2007). The teacher assesses these needs by asking questions and determining the learner's interests. Interpersonal communication is essential for successful teaching to occur (see Chapter 24).

Role of the Nurse in Teaching and Learning

Nurses have an ethical responsibility to teach their clients (Redman, 2005, 2007). In *The Patient Care Partnership,* formerly called *A Patient's Bill of Rights,* the American Hospital Association (2003) indicates that clients have the right to make informed decisions about their care. The information required to make informed decisions needs to be accurate, complete, and relevant to the client's needs.

In 2007, TJC launched its "Know Your Rights" campaign to help clients understand their rights when receiving medical care (TJC, 2007). The assumption is that clients who ask questions and are aware of their rights have a greater chance of getting the care they need when they need it. The campaign offers tips to help clients become more involved in their treatment. Clients are advised that they have a right to be informed about the care they will receive, get information about care in their preferred language, know the names of their caregivers, receive treatment for pain, receive an up-to-date list of current medications, and expect that they will be heard and treated with respect.

The nurse's responsibility is to teach the information that clients and their families need. The nurse often clarifies information provided by physicians and other health care providers and is usually the primary source of information needed for adjusting to health problems (Bastable, 2006).

Clients and their families often ask nurses for health information. For example, a client requests information about a new medication, or family members question the reason for their mother's pain. Identification of the need for teaching is easy when clients request information. However, a client's need for teaching is usually less obvious. To be an effective educator, the nurse has to do more than just pass on facts. Carefully determine what clients need to know and find the time when they are ready to learn. When nurses value and provide education, clients are better prepared to assume health care responsibilities. Evaluating the positive impact of client education on client outcomes is an important nursing issue (Bastable, 2003, 2006; Redman, 2007) (Box 25-2).

Teaching as Communication

The teaching process closely parallels the communication process (see Chapter 24). Effective teaching depends in part on effective interpersonal communication. A teacher applies each element of

BOX 25-2   **EVIDENCE-BASED PRACTICE**

The Effectiveness of Nurse-Directed Client Education

Evidence Summary

Clients living with heart failure need education about their diagnosis and related care to prevent multiple hospitalizations and promote optimal functioning. The researchers in this study wanted to know if clients who participated in a nurse-directed client education program had fewer admissions to the hospital, were more knowledgeable about self-management, and had improved quality of life and functional ability. Clients in the treatment group saw a medical physician with a subspecialty in cardiology. The cardiac clinical nurse specialists performed physical assessments and taught the clients the importance of doing and recording daily weights. They used an educational booklet outlining behaviors to successfully manage heart failure with the clients and their families. The clinical nurse specialists also provided individualized counseling and telephone follow-up between monthly clinic visits. The clients in the control group saw a cardiologist every 3 months in a cardiology clinic and received standard care. Both groups completed a quality of life survey and a walking test to measure functional status. The re-

sults of this study showed that there was no difference in functional capacity between the two groups. However, the treatment group reported greater quality of life and a positive correlation between quality of life and functional capacity.

Application to Nursing Practice
- Nurse-directed client education about lifestyle choices and exercise enhances quality of life in clients with heart failure.
- Cardiac clinical nurse specialists who collaborate with physicians successfully manage clients with heart failure in the outpatient setting.
- Improving quality of life enhances functional ability in clients with heart failure.
- Clients who receive nurse-directed client education improve their ability to manage their diet and medications.

Reference

Kutzleb J, Reiner D: The impact of nurse-directed patient education on quality of life and functional capacity in people with heart failure, *J Am Acad Nurse Pract* 18(3):116, 2006.

TABLE 25-1   Comparison of Terms Used in Teaching and Communication

COMMUNICATION	TEACHING
Referent	
Idea that initiates reason for communication	Perceived need to provide person with information; establishment of relevant learning objectives by teacher
Sender	
Person who conveys message to another	Teacher who performs activities aimed at helping other person to learn
Intrapersonal Variables (Sender)	
Knowledge, values, emotions, and sociocultural influences that affect sender's thoughts	Teacher's philosophy of education (based on learning theory); knowledge of teaching content; teaching approach; experiences in teaching; teacher's emotions and values
Message	
Information expressed or transmitted by sender	Content or information taught
Channels	
Methods used to transmit message (e.g., visual, auditory, touch)	Methods used to present content (e.g., visual and auditory materials, touch, taste, smell)
Receiver	
Person to whom message is transmitted	Learner
Intrapersonal Variables (Receiver)	
Knowledge, values, emotions, and sociocultural influences that affect receiver's thoughts	Willingness and ability to learn (e.g., physical and emotional health, education, experience, developmental level)
Feedback	
Information revealing that true meaning of message was received	Determination of whether client achieved learning objectives

the communication process while providing information to learners. Thus the teacher and learner become involved together in a teaching process that increases the learner's knowledge and skills.

The steps of the teaching process are similar to the steps of the communication process (Table 25-1). The nurse uses client requests for information or perceives a need for information because of a client's health restrictions or the recent diagnosis of an illness. The nurse then identifies specific learning objectives. A

learning objective describes what the learner will be able to do after successful instruction.

The nurse is the sender who conveys a message to the client. Many intrapersonal variables influence the nurse's style and approach. The nurse's attitudes, values, emotions, and knowledge influence the way information is delivered. Past experiences with teaching are also helpful for choosing the best way to present the necessary content.

✳ BOX 25-3   Appropriate Teaching Methods Based on Domains of Learning

Cognitive

Discussion (one-on-one or group)
- Involves nurse and one client or nurse with several clients
- Promotes active participation and focuses on topics of interest to client
- Allows peer support
- Enhances application and analysis of new information

Lecture
- Is more formal method of instruction because it is teacher controlled
- Helps learner acquire new knowledge and gain comprehension

Question-and-answer session
- Addresses client's specific concerns
- Assists client in applying knowledge

Role play, discovery
- Allows client to actively apply knowledge in controlled situation
- Promotes synthesis of information and problem solving

Independent project (computer-assisted instruction), field experience
- Allows client to assume responsibility for completing learning activities at own pace
- Promotes analysis, synthesis, and evaluation of new information and skills

Affective

Role play
- Allows expression of values, feelings, and attitudes

Discussion (group)
- Allows client to receive support from others in group
- Helps client learn from others' experiences
- Promotes responding, valuing, and organization

Discussion (one-on-one)
- Allows discussion of personal, sensitive topics of interest or concern

Psychomotor

Demonstration
- Provides presentation of procedures or skills by nurse
- Permits client to incorporate modeling of nurse's behavior
- Allows nurse to control questioning during demonstration

Practice
- Gives client opportunity to perform skills using equipment in a controlled setting
- Provides repetition

Return demonstration
- Permits client to perform skill as nurse observes
- Provides excellent source of feedback and reinforcement

Independent projects, games
- Requires teaching method that promotes adaptation and origination of psychomotor learning
- Permits learner to use new skills

The receiver in the teaching-learning process is the learner. A number of intrapersonal variables affect motivation and ability to learn. Clients are ready to learn when they express a desire to do so and are more likely to receive the message when they understand the content. Attitudes, anxiety, and values influence the ability to understand a message. The ability to learn depends on factors such as emotional and physical health, education, the stage of development, and previous knowledge.

Effective communication involves feedback. An effective teacher provides a mechanism for evaluating the success of a teaching plan and then providing positive reinforcement (Bastable, 2003; Redman, 2007). Examples of ways to evaluate teaching sessions include having a client demonstrate a newly learned skill or asking the client to describe how the correct dosage schedule for a new medication will be incorporated into a daily routine. Feedback needs to show the success of the learner in achieving objectives; that is, the learner verbalizes information or provides a return demonstration of skills learned.

Domains of Learning

Learning occurs in three domains: cognitive (understanding), affective (attitudes), and psychomotor (motor skills) (Bloom, 1956). Any topic a nurse teaches involves one or all domains or any combination of the three. Nurses often work with clients who need to learn in each domain. For example, clients diagnosed with diabetes need to learn how diabetes affects the body and how to control blood glucose levels for healthier lifestyles (cognitive domain). In addition, clients begin to accept the chronic nature of diabetes by learning

positive coping mechanisms (affective domain). Finally, many clients living with diabetes learn to test their blood glucose levels at home. This requires learning how to use a glucose meter (psychomotor domain). The characteristics of learning within each domain influence the teaching and evaluation methods used. Understanding each learning domain prepares the nurse to select proper teaching techniques and apply the basic principles of learning (Box 25-3).

Cognitive Learning

Cognitive learning includes all intellectual behaviors and requires thinking (Bastable, 2003). In the hierarchy of cognitive behaviors the simplest behavior is acquiring knowledge, whereas the most complex is evaluation. Cognitive learning includes the following:

- Knowledge: learning new facts or information and being able to recall them
- Comprehension: the ability to understand the meaning of learned material
- Application: using abstract, newly learned ideas in a concrete situation
- Analysis: breaking down information into organized parts
- Synthesis: the ability to apply knowledge and skills to produce a new whole
- Evaluation: a judgment of the worth of a body of information for a given purpose

Affective Learning

Affective learning deals with expression of feelings and acceptance of attitudes, opinions, or values. Values clarification (see Chapter 22) is an example of affective learning. The simplest behavior in the hierarchy is receiving, and the most complex is characterizing (Krathwohl and others, 1964). Affective learning includes the following:

- Receiving: being willing to attend to another person's words
- Responding: active participation through listening and reacting verbally and nonverbally
- Valuing: attaching worth to an object or behavior demonstrated by the learner's behavior
- Organizing: developing a value system by identifying and organizing values and resolving conflicts
- Characterizing: acting and responding with a consistent value system

Psychomotor Learning

Psychomotor learning involves acquiring skills that require the integration of mental and muscular activity, such as the ability to walk or to use an eating utensil (Redman, 2007). The simplest behavior in the hierarchy is perception, whereas the most complex is origination. Psychomotor learning includes the following:

- *Perception:* Being aware of objects or qualities through the use of sense organs.
- *Set:* A readiness to take a particular action. There are three sets: mental, physical, and emotional.
- *Guided response:* The performance of an act under the guidance of an instructor involving imitation of a demonstrated act.
- *Mechanism:* A higher level of behavior by which a person gains confidence and skill in performing a behavior that is more complex or involves several more steps than a guided response.
- *Complex overt response:* Smoothly and accurately performing a motor skill that requires a complex movement pattern.
- *Adaptation:* The ability to change a motor response when unexpected problems occur.
- *Origination:* Using existing psychomotor skills and abilities to perform a highly complex motor act that involves creating new movement patterns.

Basic Learning Principles

To teach effectively and efficiently, the nurse first needs to understand how people learn (Black, 2004). Motivation addresses a person's desire or willingness to learn (Redman, 2007). The client's willingness to become involved in learning influences a nurse's teaching approach. Previous knowledge, attitudes, and sociocultural factors influence motivation. The ability to learn depends on physical and cognitive attributes, developmental level, physical wellness, and intellectual thought processes. An ideal learning environment allows a person to attend to instruction.

A person's learning style affects preferences for learning. People process information in the following ways: by seeing and hearing, reflecting and acting, reasoning logically and intuitively, and analyzing and visualizing. Some people learn information gradually, whereas others learn more sporadically. Effective teaching plans include a combination of approaches that meet multiple learning styles (Felder, 2006).

Motivation to Learn

Attentional Set. An attentional set is the mental state that allows the learner to focus on and comprehend a learning activity. Before learning anything, clients need to give attention to, or concentrate on, the information to be learned. Physical discomfort, anxiety, and environmental distractions influence the ability to attend. Therefore determine the client's level of comfort before beginning a teaching plan, and ensure that the client is able to focus on the information.

As anxiety increases, the client's ability to pay attention often decreases. Anxiety is uneasiness or worry resulting from anticipating a threat or danger. When faced with change or the need to act differently, a person feels anxious. Learning requires a change in behavior and thus produces anxiety. A mild level of anxiety motivates learning. However, a high level of anxiety prevents learning from occurring. It incapacitates a person, creating an inability to focus on anything other than relieving the anxiety. Manage the client's anxiety before providing education to improve the client's comprehension and understanding of the information given (Stephenson, 2006).

Motivation. Motivation is a force that acts on or within a person (e.g., an idea, emotion, or a physical need) that causes the person to behave in a particular way (Redman, 2007). If a person does not want to learn, it is unlikely that learning will occur. Motivation sometimes results from a social, task, or physical motive.

A social motive is a need for connection, social approval, or self-esteem. People normally seek out others with whom they can compare opinions, abilities, and emotions. For example, new parents often seek validation of ideas and parenting techniques from others whom they have identified as role models in their social environment or health care workers with whom they have established a relationship.

Task mastery motives are based on needs such as achievement and competence. For example, a high school senior who has diabetes begins to test blood glucose levels and make decisions about insulin dosages in preparation for leaving home and establishing independence. The ability to successfully manage diabetes provides the motivation to master the task or skill. After a person succeeds at a task, the person is usually motivated to achieve more.

Often client motives are physical. Some clients are motivated to return to a level of physical normalcy. For example, a client with a below-the-knee amputation is motivated to learn how to walk with assistive devices. Knowledge that is necessary for survival, problem recognition, and critical decision making creates a stronger stimulus for learning than knowledge that merely promotes health (Bastable, 2006).

Know what motivates clients to learn in order to promote compliance. **Compliance** is a client's adherence to the prescribed course of therapy. Unfortunately, not all persons are interested in maintaining health. Many people will not adopt new health behaviors or change unhealthy behaviors unless they perceive a disease as a threat, they overcome barriers to changing health practices, and they see the benefits to adopting a healthy behavior. For example, some clients with lung disease continue to smoke. No therapy will have an effect unless a person believes that health is important. The nurse assesses the client's motivation to learn and what the client needs to know in order to promote compliance with the prescribed therapy.

Use of Theory to Enhance Motivation and Learning.

Health education often involves changing attitudes and values that are not easy to change by simply teaching facts. Therefore use various interventions, based on theory, when developing client education plans. Thoroughly assess the client's ideas, beliefs, and motivation in order for learning to occur.

Because of the complexity of the client education process, different theories and models are available to guide client education (Bastable, 2003; Redman, 2007). Using a theory that matches the client's needs in practice will help provide effective client education. Social learning theory provides one of the most useful approaches to client education because it explains the characteristics of the learner and guides the educator in developing effective teaching interventions that result in enhanced learning and improved motivation (Bandura, 2001; Bastable, 2003; Saarmann, Daugherty, and Riegel, 2002).

According to social learning theory, people continuously attempt to control events that affect their lives. This allows people to attain desired outcomes and avoid undesired outcomes, resulting in improved motivation. **Self-efficacy,** a concept included in social learning theory, refers to a person's perceived ability to successfully complete a task. When people believe that they are able to execute a particular behavior, they are more likely to actually perform the behavior consistently and correctly (Bandura, 1997).

Self-efficacy beliefs come from four sources: enactive mastery experiences, vicarious experiences, verbal persuasion, and physiological and affective states (Bandura, 1997). Understanding the four sources of self-efficacy allows nurses to develop interventions to help clients adopt healthy behaviors. For example, a nurse wishing to teach a child recently diagnosed with asthma to correctly use an inhaler expresses personal beliefs in the child's ability to use the inhaler (verbal persuasion). Then the nurse demonstrates how to use the inhaler (vicarious experience). Once the demonstration is complete, the child uses the inhaler (enactive mastery experience). As the child's wheezing and anxiety decrease after the correct use of the inhaler, the child experiences positive feedback, further enhancing the child's confidence to use the inhaler (physiological and affective states). Interventions such as these enhance perceived self-efficacy, which in turn improves the achievement of desired outcomes.

Self-efficacy is a concept included in many health promotion theories because it often is a strong predictor of healthy behaviors and because nurses and other health care providers can implement interventions that improve self-efficacy, which results in improved lifestyle choices (Bandura, 1997). Because of its use in theories and in research studies, many evidence-based teaching interventions include a focus on self-efficacy. When nurses implement interventions to enhance self-efficacy, their clients frequently experience positive outcomes. For example, researchers associated interventions that include self-efficacy with effective diabetes self-management (Sousa and Zauszniewski, 2005/2006; Strut and others, 2006), improved asthma management in urban Latino and African American families (Bonner and others, 2002), healthy lifestyle behaviors in rural older women (Noble Walker and others, 2006), and adoption of human immunodeficiency virus (HIV) prevention behaviors by urban African Americans (Oliva and others, 2005).

Psychosocial Adaptation to Illness. A temporary or permanent loss of health is difficult for clients to accept. Clients need to grieve, and the process of grieving gives clients time to adapt psychologically to the emotional and physical implications of illness. The stages of grieving (see Chapter 30) include a series of responses that clients experience during a loss such as illness. People experience these stages at different rates and sequences, depending on their self-concept before illness, the severity of the illness, and the changes in lifestyle that the illness creates. Effective, supportive care guides the client through the grieving process.

Readiness to learn is related to the stage of grieving (Table 25-2). Clients cannot learn when they are unwilling or unable to accept the reality of illness. However, properly timed teaching facilitates adjustment to illness or disability. Identify the client's stage of grieving on the basis of the client's behaviors. When the client enters the stage of acceptance, the stage compatible with learning, introduce a teaching plan. Continuous assessment of the client's behaviors determines the stages of grieving. Teaching continues as long as the client remains in a stage conducive to learning.

Active Participation. Learning occurs when the client is actively involved in the educational session (Edelman and Mandle, 2006). A client's involvement in learning implies an eagerness to acquire knowledge or skills. It also improves the opportunity for the client to make decisions during teaching sessions. For example, when teaching car seat safety during a parenting class, hold one teaching session in the parking lot where the participants park their cars. Encourage active participation by providing the learners with several different car seats for the participants to actually place in their cars. At the completion of this session, the parents are able to decide the types of car seats that fit in their cars and which are the easiest to use. This provides participants with the information needed to purchase the appropriate car seat.

Ability to Learn

Developmental Capability. Cognitive development influences the client's ability to learn. A nurse can be a competent teacher, but if the nurse does not consider the client's intellectual abilities, teaching will be unsuccessful. Learning, like developmental growth, is an evolving process. You need to know the client's level of knowledge and intellectual skills before beginning a teaching plan. Learning occurs more readily when new information complements existing knowledge. For example, measuring liquid or solid food portions requires the ability to perform mathematical calculations. Reading a medication label or discharge instructions requires reading and comprehension skills. Learning to regulate insulin dosages requires problem-solving skills. Following directions when performing self-care in accordance with limitations requires comprehension and application skills.

Learning in Children. The capability for learning and the type of behaviors that children are able to learn depend on the child's maturation. Without proper physiological, motor, language, and social development, many types of learning cannot take place. However, learning occurs in children of all ages. Intel-

✳ TABLE 25-2   Relationship Between Psychosocial Adaptation to Illness, Grief, and Learning

STAGE	CLIENT'S BEHAVIOR	LEARNING IMPLICATIONS FOR NURSE AND FAMILY CAREGIVER	RATIONALE
Denial or disbelief	Client avoids discussion of illness ("There's nothing wrong with me"), withdraws from others, and disregards physical restrictions. Client suppresses and distorts information that has not been presented clearly.	Provide support, empathy, and careful explanations of all procedures while they are being done. Let client know you are available for discussion. Explain situation to family or significant other if appropriate. Teach in present tense (e.g., explain current therapy).	Client is not prepared to deal with problem. Any attempt to convince or tell client about illness will result in further anger or withdrawal. Provide only information client pursues or absolutely requires.
Anger	Client blames and complains and often directs anger toward nurse or others.	Do not argue with client but listen to concerns. Teach in present tense. Reassure family/significant other of client's normalcy.	Client needs opportunity to express feelings and anger; client is still not prepared to face future.
Bargaining	Client offers to live better life in exchange for promise of better health ("If God lets me live, I promise to manage my disease better").	Continue to introduce only reality. Teach only in present tense.	Client is still unwilling to accept limitations.
Resolution	Client begins to express emotions openly, realizes that illness has created changes, and begins to ask questions.	Encourage expression of feelings. Begin to share information needed for future, and set aside formal times for discussion.	Client begins to perceive need for assistance and is ready to accept responsibility for learning.
Acceptance	Client recognizes reality of condition, actively pursues information, and strives for independence.	Focus teaching on future skills and knowledge required. Continue to teach about present occurrences. Involve family/significant other in teaching information for discharge.	Client is more easily motivated to learn. Acceptance of illness reflects willingness to deal with its implications.

✳ BOX 25-4   Teaching Methods Based on Client's Developmental Capacity

Infant
Keep routines (e.g., feeding, bathing) consistent.
Hold infant firmly while smiling and speaking softly to convey sense of trust.
Have infant touch different textures (e.g., soft fabric, hard plastic).

Toddler
Use play to teach procedure or activity (e.g., handling examination equipment, applying bandage to doll).
Offer picture books that describe story of children in hospital or clinic.
Use simple words such as *cut* instead of *laceration* to promote understanding.

Preschooler
Use role play, imitation, and play to make learning fun.
Encourage questions, and offer explanations. Use simple explanations and demonstrations.
Encourage children to learn together through pictures and short stories about how to perform hygiene.

School-Age Child
Teach psychomotor skills needed to maintain health. (Complicated skills, such as learning to use a syringe, take considerable practice.)
Offer opportunities to discuss health problems and answer questions.

Adolescent
Help adolescent learn about feelings and need for self-expression.
Use teaching as collaborative activity.
Allow adolescents to make decisions about health and health promotion (safety, sex education, substance abuse).
Use problem solving to help adolescents make choices.

Young or Middle Adult
Encourage participation in teaching plan by setting mutual goals.
Encourage independent learning.
Offer information so that adult understands effects of health problem.

Older Adult
Teach when client is alert and rested.
Involve adult in discussion or activity.
Focus on wellness and the person's strength.
Use approaches that enhance sensorially impaired client's reception of stimuli (see Chapter 49).
Keep teaching sessions short.

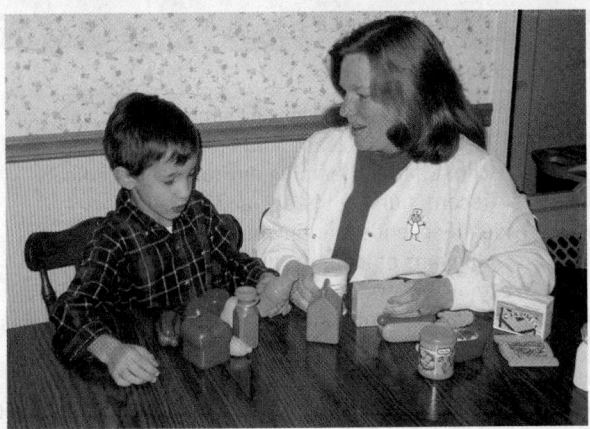

Figure 25-1 The nurse uses developmentally appropriate food models to teach healthy eating behaviors to the school-age child.

lectual growth moves from the concrete to the abstract as the child matures. Therefore information presented to children needs to be understandable, and the expected outcomes must be realistic, based on the child's developmental stage (Box 25-4). Use teaching aids that are developmentally appropriate (Figure 25-1). Learning occurs when behavior changes as a result of experience or growth (Hockenberry and Wilson, 2007).

Adult Learning. Teaching adults differs from teaching children. Adults are able to critically reflect on their current situation and sometimes need help to see their problems and change their perspectives (Redman, 2007). Because adults become independent and self-directed as they mature, they are often able to identify their own learning needs. Learning needs come from problems or tasks that result from real-life situations. Although adults tend to be self-directed learners, they often become dependent in new learning situations. The amount of information provided and the amount of time that is spent with the adult client vary depending on the client's personal situation and readiness to learn. An adult's readiness to learn is often associated with his or her developmental stage and what other events are occurring in his or her life. Resolve any needs or issues that the client perceives as extremely important so learning can occur.

Adults have a wide variety of personal and life experiences to draw on. Therefore enhance adult learning by encouraging them to use these experiences to solve problems. Furthermore, develop educational topics and goals in collaboration with the adult client. Adult clients are ultimately responsible for changing their own behavior. Assessing what the adult client currently knows, teaching what the client wants to know, and setting mutual goals will improve the outcomes of client education (Bastable, 2003).

Physical Capability. The ability to learn often depends on the client's level of physical development and overall physical health. To learn psychomotor skills, a client needs to possess a certain level of strength, coordination, and sensory acuity. For example, it is useless to teach a client to transfer from a bed to a wheelchair if the client has insufficient upper body strength. An older client with poor eyesight or the inability to grasp objects tightly cannot learn to apply an elastic bandage. Therefore do not overestimate the client's physical development or status. The following physical characteristics are necessary to learn psychomotor skills:

- Size (height and weight match the task to perform or the equipment to use [e.g., crutch walking])
- Strength (ability of the client to follow a strenuous exercise program)
- Coordination (dexterity needed for complicated motor skills, such as using utensils or changing a bandage)
- Sensory acuity (visual, auditory, tactile, gustatory, and olfactory; sensory resources needed to receive and respond to messages taught)

Any condition (e.g., pain or fatigue) that depletes a person's energy also impairs the ability to learn. For example, a client who spends a morning having rigorous diagnostic studies is unlikely to be able to learn due to fatigue. Postpone teaching when an illness becomes aggravated by complications, such as a high fever or respiratory difficulty. After working with a client, assess the client's energy level by noting the client's willingness to communicate, the amount of activity initiated, and the client's responsiveness toward questions. Temporarily stop teaching if the client needs rest. The nurse achieves greater teaching success when the client is physically able to actively participate in learning.

Learning Environment

Factors in the physical environment where teaching takes place make learning either a pleasant or a difficult experience. The ideal setting helps the client focus on the learning task. The number of persons the nurse will teach, the need for privacy, the room temperature, the room lighting, noise, the room ventilation, and the room furniture are important factors when choosing the setting. The ideal environment for learning is a room that is well lit and has good ventilation, appropriate furniture, and a comfortable temperature. A darkened room interferes with the client's ability to watch the nurse's actions, especially when demonstrating a skill or using visual aids such as posters or pamphlets. A room that is cold, hot, or stuffy will make the client too uncomfortable to focus on the information being presented.

It is also important to choose a quiet setting. A quiet setting offers privacy; infrequent interruptions are best. Provide privacy even in a busy hospital by closing cubicle curtains or taking the client to a quiet spot. Family members or significant others will often share in discussions in the home. However, clients who are reluctant to discuss the nature of the illness when others are in the room benefit from receiving education in a room separate from household activities, such as a bedroom.

Teaching a group of clients requires a room that allows everyone to be seated comfortably and within hearing distance of the teacher. Make sure the size of the room does not overwhelm the group. Arranging the group to allow participants to observe one another further enhances learning. More effective communication occurs as learners observe others' verbal and nonverbal interactions.

✳ TABLE 25-3 Comparison of the Nursing and Teaching Processes

BASIC STEPS	NURSING PROCESS	TEACHING PROCESS
Assessment	Collect data about client's physical, psychological, social, cultural, developmental, and spiritual needs from client, family, diagnostic tests, medical record, nursing history, and literature.	Gather data about client's learning needs, motivation, ability to learn, and teaching resources from client, family, learning environment, medical record, nursing history, and literature.
Nursing diagnosis	Identify appropriate nursing diagnoses based on assessment findings.	Identify client's learning needs on basis of three domains of learning.
Planning	Develop individualized care plan. Set diagnosis priorities based on client's immediate needs. Collaborate with client on care plan.	Establish learning objectives, stated in behavioral terms. Identify priorities regarding learning needs. Collaborate with client on teaching plan. Identify type of teaching method to use.
Implementation	Perform nursing care therapies. Include client as active participant in care. Involve family/significant other in care as appropriate.	Implement teaching methods. Actively involve client in learning activities. Include family/significant other participation as appropriate.
Evaluation	Identify success in meeting desired outcomes and goals of nursing care. Alter interventions as indicated when goals are not met.	Determine outcomes of teaching-learning process. Measure client's achievement of learning objectives. Reinforce information as needed.

Integrating the Nursing and Teaching Processes

A relationship exists between the nursing and teaching processes (Redman, 2007). During the assessment phase of the nursing process, the nurse determines the client's health care needs (see Unit III). At times assessment reveals a client's need for health care information. Individualize the nursing diagnoses to the client's situation, and establish the plan of care to meet desired goals and outcomes and to prescribe evidence-based nursing interventions for improving or maintaining the client's health. Evaluation determines the level of success in meeting goals of care.

While diagnosing a client's health care problems, you will often identify the need for education. When education becomes a part of the care plan, the teaching process begins. Like the nursing process, the teaching process requires assessment, in this case, analyzing the client's needs, motivation, and ability to learn. A diagnostic statement specifies the information or skills that the client requires. Develop specific learning objectives and implement the teaching plan using teaching and learning principles to ensure that the client acquires knowledge and skills. Finally, the teaching process requires an evaluation of learning based on learning objectives.

The nursing and teaching processes are not the same. The nursing process requires assessment of all sources of data to determine a client's total health care needs. The teaching process focuses on the client's learning needs and willingness and capability to learn. Table 25-3 compares the teaching and nursing processes.

◆ Assessment

To be successful in teaching a client, you need to assess all factors influencing relevant content, the client's ability to learn, and the resources available for instruction. Learning needs, identified by both you and the client, determine the choice of teaching content. An effective assessment provides the basis for individualized client

✳ BOX 25-5 NURSING ASSESSMENT QUESTIONS

Ask Clients
- What do you want to know?
- What do you know about your illness and your treatment plan?
- How does (or will) your illness affect your current lifestyle?
- What barriers currently exist that are preventing you from managing your illness the way you would like to manage it?
- What cultural or spiritual beliefs do you have regarding your illness and the prescribed treatment?
- What experiences have you had in the past that are similar to what you are experiencing now?
- Together we can choose the best way for you to learn about your disease. How can I best help you?
- What role do you believe your health care providers should take in helping you manage your illness or maintain health?
- When you learn new information, do you prefer to have the information given to you in pictures or written down in words?
- When you give someone directions to your house, do you tell the person how to get there, write out the instructions or draw a map?
- How involved do you want your family to be in the management of your illness?

Ask Family Members
- When are you available to help, and how do you plan to help your loved one?
- Your spouse needs some help. How do you feel about learning how to assist him (her)?

teaching (Wingard, 2005). Ask specific questions to assess a client's unique learning needs (Box 25-5).

Expectations of Learning. Sometimes nurses use formal educational assessment tools to determine their clients' perceived learning needs. Other times nurses simply identify their clients' expectations during routine assessments. Clients identify their own learning needs based on the implications of living with their illness. To meet these learning needs, assess what clients view as important information to know. When a client feels a need to know something, the client is likely to be receptive to information presented. For example, many parents need to know how to take care of their child after the arrival of a new baby. Therefore new parents are often very receptive to information about baby care (e.g., how to feed the baby and how to make sure the baby gets enough sleep).

Learning Needs. Determine information that is critical for the client to learn. Learning needs change depending on the client's current health status. Because a client's health status is dynamic, assessment is an ongoing activity. Assess the following:

- Information or skills needed by the client to perform self-care and to understand the implications of a health problem. Health care team members anticipate learning needs related to specific health problems. For example, the nurse teaches a boy who has just entered high school to perform testicular self-examination.
- Client's experiences that influence the need to learn.
- Information that family members or significant others require to support the client's needs. The amount of information needed depends on the extent of the family's role in helping the client.

Motivation to Learn. Ask questions that identify and define the client's motivation. These questions help to determine if the client is prepared and willing to learn. Assess the following motivational factors in clients:

- Behavior (e.g., attention span, tendency to ask questions, memory, and ability to concentrate during the teaching session).
- Health beliefs and sociocultural background. Sociocultural norms, values, and traditions all influence a client's beliefs and values about health and various therapies, as well as communication patterns and perceptions of time (see Chapter 9 and Box 25-6).
- Perception of the severity and susceptibility of a health problem and the benefits and barriers to treatment.
- Perceived ability to perform health behaviors.
- Desire to learn.
- Attitudes about health care providers (e.g., role of client and nurse in making decisions).
- Learning style preference. Clients who learn better by seeing and hearing benefit from watching a videotape. Clients who learn best by reasoning logically and intuitively learn better if presented with a case study that requires careful analysis and discussion with others to arrive at conclusions (Black, 2004).

Ability to Learn. Determine the client's physical and cognitive ability to learn. Health care providers often underestimate the client's cognitive deficits. Many factors impair the ability to learn, including fatigue, body temperature, electrolyte levels, oxygenation status, and blood glucose level. In any health care setting, several of these factors often influence a client at the same time. Assess the following factors related to the ability to learn:

- Physical strength, endurance, movement, dexterity, and coordination. Determine the extent to which the client can perform skills. For example, have the client manipulate equipment that will be used in self-care at home.

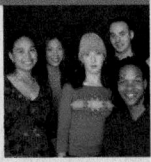

※ BOX 25-6   CULTURAL ASPECTS OF CARE

Client Education

Client education needs to be culturally sensitive in order for learning to occur. Assessing clients' preferred learning approaches and adapting education to meet clients' needs facilitates the attainment of educational outcomes. Sociocultural norms, values, and traditions often determine the importance of different health education topics and the preference of one learning approach over another. Educational efforts are especially challenging when clients and educators do not speak the same language or when written materials are not culturally sensitive and are written above the clients' reading abilities.

Implications for Practice

- Sociocultural background influences a client's desire to learn, as well as what information the client perceives as important to learn.
- Carefully assessing a client's preference for educational delivery method is vital to ensure successful learning.
- Nurses need to have a wide variety of culturally sensitive educational resources available to them to meet the needs of diverse populations.
- When the client and nurse do not speak the same language, accurate translators are necessary.

Data from Jack L and others: Understanding the environmental issues in diabetes self management education research: a re-examination of 8 studies in community-based settings, *Ann Intern Med* 140(11):964, 2004; Steven D and others: Knowledge, attitudes, beliefs and practices regarding breast and cervical cancer screening in selected ethnocultural groups in northwestern Ontario, *Oncol Nurs Forum* 31(2):305, 2004; and Wilson FL and others: Literacy, readability and cultural barriers: critical factors to consider when educating older African Americans about anticoagulation therapy, *J Clin Nurs* 12(2):275, 2003.

- Sensory deficits (see Chapter 49) that affect the client's ability to understand or follow instruction.
- Client's reading level. This is often difficult to assess because a functionally illiterate client is often able to conceal it by using excuses such as not having the time or not being able to see. One way to assess a client's reading level and level of understanding is to ask the client to read instructions from an educational handout and then explain their meaning (see the discussion of health literacy on p. 372).
- Client's developmental level. This influences the selection of teaching approaches (see Box 25-4).
- Client's cognitive function, including memory, knowledge, association, and judgment.
- Pain, fatigue, anxiety, or other physical symptoms that interfere with the ability to maintain attention and participate. In acute care settings a client's physical condition can easily prevent a client from learning.

Teaching Environment. The environment for a teaching session needs to be conducive to learning. Assess the following environmental factors:

- Distractions or persistent noise. A quiet area is essential for effective learning.

- Comfort of the room, including ventilation, temperature, lighting, and furniture.
- Room facilities and available equipment.

Resources for Learning. A client frequently requires the support of family members or significant others. In this case, assess the readiness and ability of family and friends to learn the information necessary for the care of the client. Also review resources within the home environment. Assessment of resources includes a review of any teaching tools available. Assess the following:

- Client's willingness to have family members and significant others involved in the teaching plan and to provide health care. Information about the client's health care is confidential unless the client chooses to share it. Sometimes it is difficult for the client to accept the help of family members, especially when bodily functions are involved.
- Family members' perceptions and understanding of the client's illness and its implications. Family members' perceptions should match those of the client; otherwise, conflicts will occur in the teaching plan.
- Family's or significant other's willingness and ability to participate in care. If the client chooses to share information about his or her health status with family members, the family members need to be responsible, willing, or physically and cognitively able to assist in care activities, such as bathing or administering medications. Not all family members meet these requirements.
- Resources. These include financial or material resources, such as having the ability to obtain health care equipment.
- Teaching tools, including brochures, audiovisual materials, or posters. Printed material needs to present current information that is written clearly and logically and that matches the client's reading level.

Health Literacy and Learning Disabilities. Current research shows that health literacy is a strong predictor of health status (Speros, 2005). Therefore assess clients' health literacy before providing instruction. **Functional illiteracy,** the inability to read above a fifth-grade level, is a major problem in America today. The National Assessment of Adult Literacy Survey (NAALS), conducted in 2003 by the National Center for Education Statistics assessed the extent of literacy skills in Americans over the age of 16 (Kutner and others, 2006). Results from the NAALS reflected that over 75 million American adults had basic or below basic levels of health literacy. Approximately 14% of adults could not understand a basic client education pamphlet, and 36% could not perform moderately difficult tasks (e.g., reading a childhood vaccination chart or determining possible medication interactions from a prescription label). Older adults, men, people who did not speak English before entering school, people living below poverty level, and people without a high school education tended to have lower health literacy scores. White and Asian/Pacific Islander adults had higher literacy levels than African American, Native American/Alaska Native, and multiracial adults. Furthermore, Hispanic adults had the lowest levels of health literacy.

To compound the problem, the readability of printed health education material ranges from elementary school level to college level. Currently, printed educational materials are often above the client's reading level (Cutilli, 2005; Dreger and Trembeck, 2002; Wilson and others, 2003). Unfortunately, health care professionals do not always address the gap between the client's reading level and the readability of educational materials (Minerd, 2006; Wilson and others, 2003). This results in unsafe care. To ensure client safety, all health care providers need to ensure that information is presented clearly and in a culturally sensitive manner (TJC, 2007).

Although assessing health literacy is challenging, all health care providers need to identify problems with health literacy and provide appropriate education to people who have special health literacy needs to ensure safe care (TJC, 2007). Research shows that many Americans read and understand information that is 3 to 5 years below their last year of formal education. In addition, most people will say that they are good readers, even if they cannot read (Cutilli, 2005). Nurses use a variety of screening tools to test literacy. The Wide Range Achievement Test (WRAT 3) evaluates reading, spelling, and arithmetic skills for clients from 5 to 74 years of age. The Rapid Estimate of Adult Literacy in Medicine (REALM) uses pronunciation of health care terms to determine approximate reading level (Figure 25-2). The Cloze test, a test of reading comprehension, asks clients to fill in the blanks that are in a written paragraph. Nurses need to assess the client's ability to understand mathematical calculations in addition to reading skills. If these tests are not available or not appropriate, nurses can assess their clients' literacy skills by having clients read a written client education handout and then describe in their own words what the information means to them.

In addition to illiteracy, nurses need to assess their clients for learning disabilities that impair the ability to learn. For example, many self-care behaviors require an understanding of math, including computation and fractions. If a client's learning disability impairs the ability to effectively use math skills, teaching will be challenging, especially when trying to teach clients about complex medication dosages and frequencies. Another learning disability that affects the client's ability to learn includes attention-deficit/hyperactivity disorder (ADHD). Clients with ADHD frequently have difficulty recalling information and staying focused during educational sessions in addition to having a low threshold of frustration.

◆Nursing Diagnosis

After assessing information related to the client's ability and need to learn, interpret data and cluster defining characteristics to form diagnoses that reflect the client's specific learning needs (Box 25-7). This ensures that teaching will be goal directed and individualized. If a client has several learning needs, the nursing diagnoses guide priority setting. When the nursing diagnosis is *deficient knowledge,* the diagnostic statement describes the specific type of learning need and its cause; for example, *deficient knowledge regarding psychomotor learning related to inexperience with medication self-administration.* Classifying diagnoses by the three learning domains helps the nurse focus specifically on subject matter and teaching methods. Clients often require education to support resolution of their various health problems.

List 1		List 2		List 3	
fat	___	fatigue	___	allergic	___
flu	___	pelvic	___	menstrual	___
pill	___	jaundice	___	testicle	___
dose	___	infection	___	colitis	___
eye	___	exercise	___	emergency	___
stress	___	behavior	___	medication	___
smear	___	prescription	___	occupation	___
nerves	___	notify	___	sexually	___
germs	___	gallbladder	___	alcoholism	___
meals	___	calories	___	irritation	___
disease	___	depression	___	constipation	___
cancer	___	miscarriage	___	gonorrhea	___
caffeine	___	pregnancy	___	inflammatory	___
attack	___	arthritis	___	diabetes	___
kidney	___	nutrition	___	hepatitis	___
hormones	___	menopause	___	antibiotics	___
herpes	___	appendix	___	diagnosis	___
seizure	___	abnormal	___	potassium	___
bowel	___	syphilis	___	anemia	___
asthma	___	hemorrhoids	___	obesity	___
rectal	___	nausea	___	osteoporosis	___
incest	___	directed	___	impetigo	___

Score

List 1 _____
List 2 _____
List 3 _____

Raw Score _____

A

Directions:

1. Give the patient a laminated copy of the REALM and ask the patient to read the words in each list. Use an unlaminated copy of the REALM on a clipboard to score the test. Hold the clipboard so that the patient is not distracted by the scoring.
2. Give the patient the following instructions:
   "I want to hear you read as many words as you can from this list. Begin with the first word on List 1 and read aloud. When you come to a word you cannot read, do the best you can or say 'blank' and go on to the next word."
3. If a patient takes more than 5 seconds on a word, say "blank" and point to the next word, if necessary to move the patient along. If the patient begins to miss every word, have him or her pronounce only known words.
4. Count as an error any word not attempted or mispronounced. Score by making a (+) after each correct word, a check (√) after each mispronounced words, and a minus (−) after words not attempted. Count as correct any self-corrected words. Count the number of correct words and this is the total score.

Scoring:

Raw Score	Grade Range
0–18	3rd grade and below
	Will not be able to read most low literacy materials; will need repeated oral instructions, materials composed primarily of illustrations, or audio or video tapes.
19–44	4th to 6th grade
	Will need low literacy materials; may not be able to read prescription labels.
45–60	7th to 8th grade
	Will struggle with most patient education materials; will not be offended by low literacy materials.
61–66	High school
	Will be able to read most patient education materials.

Figure 25-2 A, The Rapid Estimate of Adult Literacy in Medicine (REALM). (**A,** Permission from Terry Davis, PhD, Louisiana State University.)

Continued

Cloze Test

When one is injured it is possible that a bone has been broken. Bones can break in _____ places in the body. A _____ bone can be as _____ as a little crack or _____ or as large as a _____ broken in many places (_____). The first step in _____ fixing of a bone is _____ have the broken part _____. The next step is to _____ the bone put in the _____ position for it to _____. This may be as _____ as not using the bone _____ (not running on your _____) or as complex as _____ metal plates screwed into the _____ to keep it in _____. Many other ways the _____ can be put into a _____ position include ace wraps, _____, boots, and casts.

List of words:
splints, healing, bone, place, bone, having, foot, hard, simple, heal, best, have, identified, to, the, shattered, bone, chip, small, broken, many

B

Figure 25-2, cont'd **B,** Cloze test for reading comprehension.

BOX 25-7   NURSING DIAGNOSTIC PROCESS

Deficient Knowledge (Psychomotor) Regarding Use of Crutches Related to Lack of Experience

Assessment Activities	Defining Characteristics
Have client describe how to walk with crutches.	Client states that he or she has not received information about use of crutches Asks questions about how to use crutches
Have client demonstrate three-point crutch walking on level surfaces and up stairs.	Uses crutches inappropriately Cannot go up or down stairs on crutches

Examples of additional nursing diagnoses that indicate a need for education include the following:

- Ineffective health maintenance
- Health-seeking behaviors
- Impaired home maintenance
- Ineffective therapeutic regimen management
- Ineffective community therapeutic regimen management
- Ineffective family therapeutic regimen management
- Noncompliance

When the nurse can manage or eliminate health care problems through education, the related factor of the diagnostic statement is *deficient knowledge.* For example, an older adult client is having difficulty managing a medication regimen because of the number of medications that she has to take at different times of the day. In this case educating the client about the medications will improve the client's ability to schedule and take the medications as directed. When the nurse identifies conditions that cause barriers to effective learning (e.g., nursing diagnosis of *acute pain* or *activity intolerance*), teaching is inappropriate. In these cases delay teaching until the nursing diagnosis is resolved or the health problem is controlled.

◆ Planning

After determining the nursing diagnoses that identify a client's learning needs, develop a teaching plan, determine goals and expected outcomes, and involve the client in selecting learning ex-

periences (see care plan). Expected outcomes (or learning objectives) guide the choice of teaching strategies and approaches with a client. Client participation ensures a more relevant, meaningful plan.

Goals and Outcomes. Goals of client education indicate that the client better understands information provided and is able to attain health or better manage illness. Include the client if possible when establishing learning goals and outcomes, and serve as a resource in setting the minimum criteria for success. Outcomes often describe a behavior that identifies the client's ability to do something upon completion of teaching, such as *will empty* colostomy bag, or *will administer* an injection. When developing outcomes, conditions or time frames need to be realistic and meet the client's needs (e.g., "will identify the side effects of aspirin by discharge"). Consider conditions under which the client or family will typically perform the behavior (e.g., "will walk from bedroom to bathroom using crutches").

In some health care settings, nurses develop written teaching plans. The teaching plan includes topics for instruction, resources (e.g., equipment, teaching booklets, and referrals to special educational programs), recommendations for involving family, and objectives of the teaching plan. Some plans are very detailed, whereas others are in outline form. Nurses use the plan to provide continuity of instruction. The more specific the plan, the easier it is to follow.

The setting influences the complexity of any teaching plan. In an acute care setting, plans are concise and focused on the primary learning needs of the client because there is limited time for teaching. Home care and outpatient clinic teaching plans are usually more comprehensive in scope because nurses often have more time to instruct clients and clients are often less anxious in outpatient settings.

Setting Priorities. Include the client when determining priorities for client education. Base priorities on the client's immediate needs, nursing diagnoses, and the goals and outcomes established for the client. Priorities also depend on what the client perceives to be most important, the client's anxiety level, and the amount of time available to teach. A client's learning needs are set in order of priority to conserve the time and energy of the client and nurse. For example, a client recently diagnosed with coronary artery disease has deficient knowledge related to the illness and its implications. The client benefits most by first learning about the

NURSING CARE PLAN

Deficient Knowledge: Surgical Procedure

Assessment

Connie, a nurse in a surgeon's office, is preparing Mr. Holland for a colon resection, which is scheduled in 1 week. Mr. Holland is 75 years old and has recently been diagnosed with colorectal cancer.

Connie's assessment focuses on Mr. Holland's readiness to learn and factors that affect his ability to understand the procedure and related postoperative care.

Assessment Activities*

Assess Mr. Holland's readiness to learn, and ask what the surgeon has already told him about the surgery.

Ask Mr. Holland to explain postoperative care, including performing a return demonstration of deep breathing and coughing.

Findings/Defining Characteristics

Mr. Holland responds, **"I can't remember what the doctor told me** at my last appointment. But, **I need to know how to take care of myself.** My surgery is scheduled for next week."
Mr. Holland is **unable to describe postoperative care or provide a return demonstration of deep breathing and coughing.**

*Defining characteristics are shown in bold type.

Nursing Diagnosis: Deficient knowledge: surgical procedure related to lack of recall and exposure to information.

Planning

Goal

Mr. Holland will describe preoperative and postoperative care activities before surgery.

Mr. Holland will participate in postoperative care during hospitalization.

Expected Outcomes (NOC)†

Knowledge: Treatment Procedure

Mr. Holland will verbalize understanding of surgical procedure and postoperative monitoring and activity planned on the day of surgery.
Mr. Holland will demonstrate deep breathing and coughing and will advance his level of activity after his surgery.

†Outcome classification labels from Moorhead S and others: *Nursing outcomes classification (NOC)*, ed 4, St. Louis, 2008, Mosby.

Interventions (NIC)‡

Learning Readiness Enhancement
Determine readiness to learn and information Mr. Holland thinks is important to know.

Learning Facilitation
Offer Mr. Holland multiple teaching modalities (e.g., brochure and audiotape describing preoperative and postoperative care).
Explain postoperative care, demonstrating deep breathing and coughing, and having Mr. Holland perform return demonstration.

Rationale

The adult client's learning is enhanced when the client is ready to learn and when the client perceives the information as important (Bastable, 2003).

Providing clients with educational methods that use multiple senses is effective in educating older adults. Older adults prefer written handouts in large fonts (Wendell and others, 2003).
Improving self-efficacy by using role-modeling and having the client perform behaviors enhances the successful adoption of healthy behaviors (Bandura, 1997).

‡Intervention classification labels from Bulechek GM, Butcher HK, and Dochterman JM: *Nursing interventions classification (NIC)*, ed 5, St. Louis, 2008, Mosby.

Evaluation

Nursing Actions	Client Response/Finding	Achievement of Outcome
Ask Mr. Holland to describe what will happen before and after surgery.	Mr. Holland is able to state understanding of preoperative and postoperative care activities.	Mr. Holland's anxiety level has decreased, and he reports he is ready for surgery.
Observe client as he demonstrates deep breathing and coughing and advances his activity postoperatively.	Mr. Holland is able to deep breathe and cough postoperatively, but he is hesitant to advance his activity level after surgery.	Client has not totally achieved outcome of advancing activity postoperatively. Manage barriers inhibiting attainment of this outcome (e.g., pain), and continue to encourage and educate client.

correct way to take nitroglycerin and how long to wait before calling for help when chest pain occurs. Once these needs related to basic survival are met, then other topics, such as exercise and nutritional changes, are discussed.

Timing. When is the right time to teach? Before a client enters a hospital? When a client first enters a clinic? At dis-

charge? At home? Each is appropriate because clients continue to have learning needs and opportunities as long as they stay in the health care system. Plan teaching activities for a time when the client is most attentive, receptive, and alert, and organize the client's activities to provide time for rest and teaching-learning interactions.

Timing is sometimes difficult because the emphasis is often on a client's early discharge from a hospital. For example, it takes several days after surgery for a client to be alert and comfortable enough to learn. By the time the client feels ready to learn, sometimes discharge is already scheduled. Therefore, to improve client outcomes, anticipate educational needs of clients before they occur.

Although prolonged sessions cause concentration and attentiveness to decrease, make sure teaching sessions are not too brief. The client needs time to comprehend the information and to give feedback. Frequent sessions lasting 20 minutes are easier to tolerate and retain interest in the material. However, factors such as shorter hospital stays and lack of insurance reimbursement for outpatient education sessions often necessitate longer teaching sessions.

The frequency of sessions depends on the learner's abilities and the complexity of the material. For example, a child newly diagnosed with diabetes will require more visits to an outpatient center than the older adult client who has had diabetes for 15 years and who lives in a nursing home. Make sure intervals between teaching sessions are not so long that the client forgets information. Home care nurses frequently reinforce learning during home visits when clients are discharged from the hospital.

Organizing Teaching Material. An effective teacher carefully considers the order of information to present. An outline of content helps organize information into a logical sequence. Material needs to progress from simple to complex ideas because a person must learn the simple facts and concepts before learning how to make associations or complex interpretations of ideas. For example, to teach a woman how to feed her husband who has a gastric tube, the nurse first teaches the wife how to measure the tube feeding and how to manipulate the equipment. Once the wife has accomplished this, the process of administering the feeding occurs.

Begin any instruction with essential content because clients are more likely to remember information that the nurse teaches early in the teaching session. For example, immediately after surgical removal of a malignant breast tumor, the client has many learning needs. Start with essential information such as how to monitor the incision site for signs of infection and how to deal with the emotional aspects of a cancer diagnosis, and then complete the teaching session with informative but less critical content including the warning signs of cancer. Repetition reinforces learning. A concise summary of key topics helps the learner remember the most important information (Bastable, 2003).

Collaborative Care. During planning, choose appropriate teaching methods, encourage the client to offer suggestions, and make referrals to other health care professionals (e.g., dietitians and physical, speech, or occupational therapists) when appropriate. The nurse is the primary member of the health care team responsible for ensuring that all client educational needs are met. However, sometimes client needs are highly complex. In these cases the nurse identifies appropriate health education resources within the health care system or the community during planning. Examples of resources for client education include diabetes education clinics, cardiac rehabilitation programs, prenatal classes, and support groups. When clients receive education and support from these types of resources, the nurse is responsible for obtaining a referral if necessary, encouraging clients to attend these resources,

and reinforcing information taught. Resources that specialize in a particular health need are integral to successful client education.

Implementation

The implementation of client education depends on your ability to critically analyze assessment data when identifying learning needs and developing the teaching plan (see care plan). Carefully evaluate the learning objectives, and determine which teaching and learning principles will most effectively and efficiently assist the client in meeting expected goals and outcomes. Implementation involves believing that each interaction with a client is an opportunity to teach. Use evidence-based interventions to create an effective learning environment.

Maintaining Learning Attention and Participation. Active participation is key to learning. Persons learn better when more than one of the body's senses are stimulated. Audiovisual aids and role play are good teaching strategies. By actively experiencing a learning event, the person will be more likely to retain knowledge. A teacher's actions also increase learner attention and interest. When conducting a discussion with a learner, the teacher stays active by changing the tone and intensity of his or her voice, making eye contact, and using gestures that accentuate key points of discussion. An effective teacher often uses as much energy as the learner, talking and moving among a group rather than remaining stationary behind a lectern or table. A learner remains interested in a teacher who is actively enthusiastic about the subject under discussion.

Building on Existing Knowledge. A client learns best on the basis of preexisting cognitive abilities and knowledge. Thus a teacher is more effective by presenting information that builds on a learner's existing knowledge. A client quickly loses interest if a nurse begins with familiar information. For example, a client who has lived with multiple sclerosis for several years is beginning a new medication that is given subcutaneously. Before teaching the client how to prepare the medication and give the injection, the nurse asks the client about previous experience with injections. On assessment the nurse learns that the client's father had diabetes and that the client administered the insulin injections. The nurse individualizes the teaching plan by building on the client's previous knowledge and experience with insulin injections.

Teaching Approaches. A nurse's approach in teaching is different from teaching methods. Some situations require a teacher to be directive. Others require a nondirective approach. An effective teacher concentrates on the task and uses teaching approaches according to the learner's needs. A learner's needs and motives frequently change over time. Thus the effective teacher is always aware of the need to modify teaching approaches.

Telling. Use the telling approach when teaching limited information (e.g., preparing a client for an emergent diagnostic procedure). If a client is highly anxious but it is vital for information to be given, telling is effective. When using telling, the nurse outlines the task the client will perform and gives explicit instructions. There is no opportunity for feedback with this method.

Participating. In the participating approach the nurse and client set objectives and become involved in the learning process together. The client helps decide content, and the nurse guides and counsels the client with pertinent information. In this method there is opportunity for discussion, feedback, mutual goal setting, and revision of the teaching plan. For example, a parent caring for a child with leukemia learns how to care for the child at home and how to recognize problems that need to be reported immediately. The parent and the nurse collaborate on developing an appropriate teaching plan. After each teaching session is completed, the parent and nurse review the objectives together, determine if the objectives were met, and plan what will be covered in the next session.

Entrusting. The entrusting approach provides the client the opportunity to manage self-care. The client accepts responsibilities and performs tasks correctly and consistently. The nurse observes the client's progress and remains available to assist without introducing more new information. For example, a client has been managing diabetes well for 10 years. Because of the development of a complication of diabetes, the client now has to walk instead of jog during exercise. The client understands how to adjust insulin when exercising to prevent hypoglycemia. The nurse instructs the client about the newly prescribed exercise therapy and allows the client to adjust insulin dosages independently.

Reinforcing. Reinforcement requires using a stimulus that increases the probability for a response. A learner who receives reinforcement before or after a desired learning behavior is likely to repeat the behavior. Feedback is a common form of reinforcement. Reinforcers are positive or negative. Positive reinforcement, such as a smile or spoken approval, produces desired responses. Although negative reinforcement, such as frowning or criticizing, will decrease an undesired response, people usually respond better to positive reinforcement (Bastable, 2003). The effects of negative reinforcement are less predictable and often undesirable.

Three types of reinforcers are social, material, and activity. When a nurse works with a client, most reinforcers are social ones (e.g., smiles, compliments, or words of encouragement), which are used to acknowledge a learned behavior. Examples of material reinforcers are food, toys, and music. These work best with young children. Activity reinforcers rely on the principle that a person is motivated to engage in an activity if he or she will have the opportunity to engage in more desirable activity after completion of the task. For example, a client will more likely go to a mental health counseling session if he or she is given the chance to go outside for a walk with the nurse afterward.

Choosing an appropriate reinforcer involves giving careful thought and attention to individual preferences. Observing behavior often helps reveal the best reinforcer to use. Do not use reinforcers as threats. Reinforcers are not always effective with every client. A young child responds more to social reinforcers than do older children or adults. In adults, reinforcement is more effective when the client establishes a therapeutic relationship with the nurse.

Incorporating Teaching With Nursing Care.

Many nurses find they are able to teach more effectively while delivering nursing care. This becomes easier as nurses gain confidence

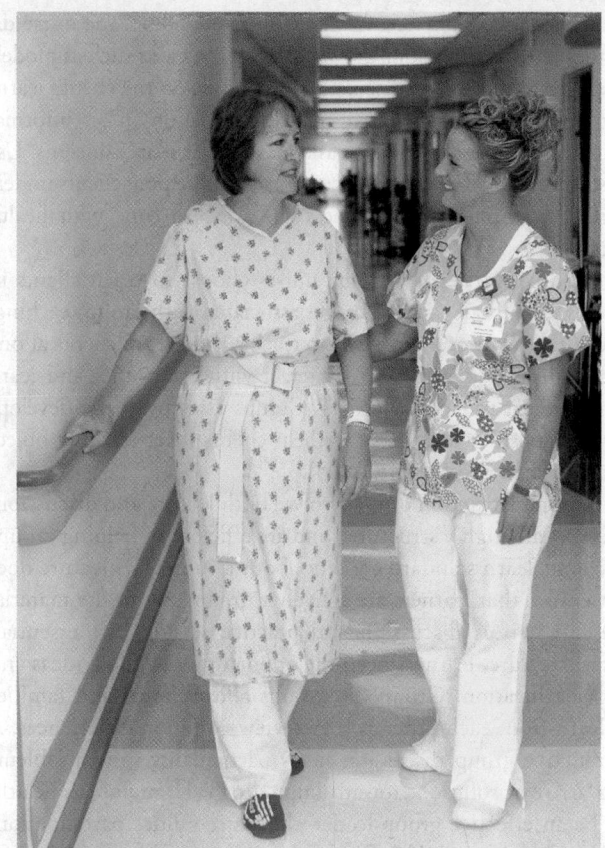

Figure 25-3 Teaching postoperative care while walking with the client uses time efficiently.

in their own clinical skills. For example, while hanging blood, the nurse explains why the blood is necessary and the symptoms indicated with transfusion reactions that need to be reported immediately. Another example is the nurse who explains a medication's side effects while administering the medication. An informal, unstructured style relies on the positive therapeutic relationship between nurse and client, which fosters spontaneity in the teaching-learning process. Teaching during routine care is efficient and cost-effective (Figure 25-3).

Instructional Methods. Choose instructional methods to meet the client's learning needs, the time available for teaching, the setting, the resources available, and the nurse's own comfort level with teaching. Skilled teachers are flexible in altering teaching methods according to the learner's responses. An experienced teacher uses a variety of techniques and teaching aids. Do not expect to be an expert educator when first entering nursing practice. Learning to become an effective educator takes time and practice.

When first starting to teach clients, it helps to remember that clients perceive the nurse as an expert. However, this does not mean that clients expect the nurse to have all of the answers. It simply means that clients expect that the nurse will keep them appropriately informed. Effective nurses keep the teaching plan simple and focused on clients' needs.

One-on-One Discussion. Perhaps the most common method of instruction is one-on-one discussion. When teaching a client at the bedside, in a physician's office, or in the home, the nurse directly shares information. Use various teaching aids such as models or diagrams during the discussion, depending on the client's learning needs. The nurse usually gives information in an informal manner, allowing the client to ask questions or share concerns. Use unstructured and informal discussions when helping clients understand the implications of illness and ways to cope with health stressors.

Group Instruction. Some nurses choose to teach clients in groups because of the advantages associated with group teaching. Groups are an economical way to teach a number of clients at one time, and clients are able to interact with each other and learn from the experiences of others. Groups also foster the development of positive attitudes that help clients meet learning objectives (Kuiken and Seiffert, 2005).

Group instruction often involves both lecture and discussion. Lectures are highly structured and are efficient in helping groups of clients learn standard content about a subject. A lecture does not ensure that learners are actively thinking about the material presented; thus discussion and practice sessions are essential. After a lecture, learners need the opportunity to share ideas and seek clarification. Group discussions allow clients and families to learn from each other as they review common experiences. A productive group discussion helps participants solve problems and arrive at solutions toward improving each member's health. To be an effective group leader, the nurse guides participation. Acknowledging a look of interest, asking questions, and summarizing key points foster group involvement. However, not all clients benefit from group discussions, and sometimes the physical or emotional level of wellness makes participation difficult or impossible.

Preparatory Instruction. Clients frequently face unfamiliar tests or procedures that create significant anxiety. Providing information about procedures often decreases anxiety because clients have a better idea of what to expect during the procedure, which helps to give them a sense of control. The known is less threatening than the unknown. Use the following guidelines for giving preparatory explanations:

- Describe physical sensations during the procedure. For example, when drawing a blood specimen, explain that the client will feel a sticking sensation as the needle punctures the skin.
- Describe the cause of the sensation, preventing misinterpretation of the experience. For example, explain that a needle stick burns because the alcohol used to clean the skin enters the puncture site.
- Prepare clients only for aspects of the experience that others have commonly noticed. For example, explain that it is normal for a tight tourniquet to cause a person's hand to tingle and feel numb.

Demonstrations. Use demonstrations when teaching psychomotor skills such as preparation of a syringe, bathing an infant, crutch walking, or taking a pulse. Demonstrations are most effective when learners first observe the teacher and then during a **return demonstration** have the chance to practice the skill. Combine a demonstration with discussion to clarify concepts and feelings. An effective demonstration requires advanced planning:

1. Be sure the learner can easily see each step of the demonstration. Position the learner to provide a clear view of the skill being performed.
2. Assemble and organize equipment. Be sure that all equipment works.
3. Perform each step slowly and accurately in sequence while analyzing the knowledge and skills involved, and allow the client to handle equipment
4. Review the rationale and steps of the procedure.
5. Encourage the client to ask questions so that he or she will understand each step.
6. Judge proper speed and timing of the demonstration, based on the client's cognitive abilities and anxiety level.
7. Have the client perform a return demonstration under the same conditions that will be experienced at home or in the place where the skill is to be performed to demonstrate mastery of the skill. For example, when a client needs to learn to walk with crutches, the nurse simulates the home environment. If the client's home has stairs, the client practices going up and down a staircase in the hospital.

Analogies. Learning occurs when a teacher translates complex language or ideas into words or concepts that the client understands. **Analogies** supplement verbal instruction with familiar images that make complex information more real and understandable. For example, when explaining arterial blood pressure, the nurse uses an analogy of the flow of water through a hose. Following these general principles when using analogies:

- Be familiar with the concept.
- Know the client's background, experience, and culture.
- Keep the analogy simple and clear.

Role Play. During role play, people are asked to play themselves or someone else. Clients learn required skills and feel more confident in being able to perform them independently. The technique involves rehearsing a desired behavior. For example, a nurse who is teaching a parent how to respond to a child's behavior pretends to be a child who is having a temper tantrum. The parent responds to the nurse who is pretending to be the child. Afterward, the nurse evaluates the parent's response and determines whether an alternative approach would have been more appropriate.

Simulation. Simulation is a useful technique for teaching clients problem solving, application, and independent thinking. During individual or group discussion a nurse poses a pertinent problem or situation for clients to solve. For example, clients with heart disease plan a meal that is low in cholesterol and fat. The clients in the group decide which foods are appropriate. The nurse asks the group members to present their diet, providing an opportunity to identify mistakes and reinforce correct information.

Illiteracy and Other Disabilities.

It is important to use words a client is able to understand. Medical jargon is confusing. Implications of illiteracy and learning disabilities include an impaired ability to analyze instructions or synthesize information. Also, many of these clients have not acquired the problem-solving skills of drawing conclusions and inferences from experience, and

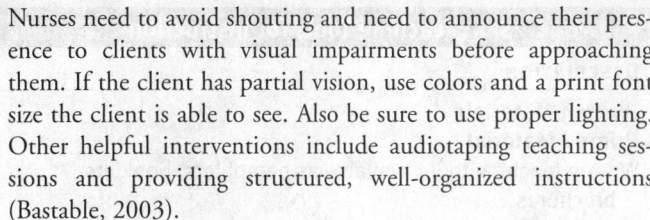

✳ BOX 25-8   **CLIENT TEACHING**

*Illiterate Client or the Client
With a Learning Disability*

Objectives
- Client will understand information presented.
- Client will perform desired behaviors accurately.

Teaching Strategies
- Establish trust with the client before beginning the teaching-learning session.
- Use simple terminology to enhance the client's understanding.
- Avoid medical jargon. If necessary, explain medical terms using basic one- or two-syllable words.
- Keep teaching sessions short and to the point, and minimize distractions.
- Include the most important information at the beginning of the session.
- Relate practical information to personal experiences or real-life situations.
- Use visual cues and simple analogies when appropriate.
- Frequently ask the client for feedback to determine if the client comprehends information.
- Ask for return demonstrations (provides opportunity to clarify instructions and time to review procedures).
- Provide teaching materials that reflect the reading level of the client, with attention given to short words and sentences, large type, and simple format (generally, information written on a fifth-grade reading level is recommended for adult learners).
- Reinforce the most important information at the end of the session.
- Schedule teaching sessions at frequent intervals.
- Model appropriate behavior, and use role play to help client learn how to ask questions and ask for help effectively.

Evaluation
- Ask the client to verbalize understanding of information taught.
- Observe and evaluate the client's ability to perform desired behaviors.

Data from Bastable S: *Nurse as educator: principles of teaching and learning for nursing practice*, Sudbury, Mass, 2003, Jones & Bartlett; Mika VS and others: The ABCs of health literacy, *Fam Community Health* 28(4):351, 2005; Osborne H: *Health literacy from A to Z: practical ways to communicate your health message*, Boston, 2005, Jones & Bartlett.

they will not ask questions to obtain or clarify information that has been presented. Box 25-8 summarizes nursing interventions nurses use when caring for clients who are illiterate or who have learning disabilities.

Some clients have sensory deficits that affect how the nurse presents information (see Chapter 49). For example, some clients who have hearing impairments require a sign language interpreter. Not all people who are deaf read lips. Therefore it is very important to provide clear written materials. Written materials for the deaf population need to match the clients' reading level. Visual impairments also impact the teaching strategy used by the nurse. Many people who are blind have acute listening skills.

Nurses need to avoid shouting and need to announce their presence to clients with visual impairments before approaching them. If the client has partial vision, use colors and a print font size the client is able to see. Also be sure to use proper lighting. Other helpful interventions include audiotaping teaching sessions and providing structured, well-organized instructions (Bastable, 2003).

Cultural Diversity. You need to have knowledge of the client's cultural background and beliefs, as well as the client's ability to understand instructions developed outside of his or her native language (see Chapter 9). The cultural diversity of clients poses a great challenge when you are trying to provide culturally sensitive care. When educating clients of different ethnic groups, be aware of the distinctive aspects of each culture, being careful not to stereotype clients. Collaborate with other nurses and educators to assist in dealing with cultural diversity and ask the people in the cultural group to help by sharing values and beliefs. Ethnic nurses are excellent resources who are able to provide input through their experiences to improve the care provided to members of their own community (Bastable, 2003). When clients cannot understand English, use trained and certified health care interpreters to provide health care information (Cutilli, 2006; TJC, 2007).

In addition, be aware of intergenerational conflict of values. This occurs when immigrant parents uphold their traditional values and their children, who are exposed to American values in social encounters, develop beliefs similar to those of their American peers. Consider this conflict in values when providing information to families or groups that have members from different generations. To enhance client education in culturally diverse populations, know when and how to provide education while respecting cultural values. Modify teaching regarding interventions or desired behaviors to accommodate for cultural differences. Effective educational strategies often require the nurse to use different patterns of communication (Cutilli, 2006; TJC, 2007).

Using Teaching Tools. Many teaching tools are available for client education. Selection of the right tool depends on the instructional method chosen, the client's learning needs, and the client's ability to learn (Table 25-4). For example, a printed pamphlet is not the best tool to use for a client with poor reading comprehension, but an audiotape is the best choice for a client with visual impairment.

Special Needs of Children and Older Adults. Children, adults, and older adults learn differently. The nurse adapts teaching strategies to each learner. Children pass through several developmental stages (see Unit II). In each developmental stage, children acquire new cognitive and psychomotor abilities that respond to different types of teaching methods (Figure 25-4). Incorporate parental input in planning health education for children.

Older adults experience numerous physical and psychological changes as they age (see Chapter 14). These changes not only increase the educational needs of older adults, they also create bar-

✳ **TABLE 25-4** **Teaching Tools for Instruction**

Description	Learning Implications
Written Materials	
Printed Material	
Written teaching tools available as pamphlets, booklets, brochures	Material needs to be easy to read. Information must be accurate and current. Method is ideal for understanding complex concepts and relationships.
Programmed Instruction	
Written sequential presentation of learning steps requiring that learners answer questions and that teachers tell them whether they are right or wrong	Instruction is primarily verbal, but teacher sometimes uses pictures or diagrams. Method requires active learning, giving immediate feedback, correcting wrong answers, and reinforcing right answers. Learner works at own pace.
Computer Instruction	
Use of programmed instruction format in which computers store response patterns for learners and select further lessons on basis of these patterns (programs can be individualized)	Method requires reading comprehension, psychomotor skills, and familiarity with computer.
Nonprint Materials	
Diagrams	
Illustrations that show interrelationships by means of lines and symbols	Method demonstrates key ideas, summarizes, and clarifies key concept.
Graphs (Bar, Circle, or Line)	
Visual presentations of numerical data	Graphs help learner to grasp information quickly about single concept.
Charts	
Highly condensed visual summary of ideas and facts that highlights series of ideas, steps, or events	Charts demonstrate relationship of several ideas or concepts. Method helps learners know what to do.
Pictures	
Photographs or drawings used to teach concepts in which the third dimension of shape and space is not important	Photographs are more desirable than diagrams because they more accurately portray the details of the real item.
Physical Objects	
Use of actual equipment, objects, or models to teach concepts or skills	Models are useful when real objects are too small, large, or complicated or are unavailable. Allows learners to manipulate objects that they will use later in skill.
Other Audiovisual Materials	
Slides, audiotapes, television, and videotapes used with printed material or discussion	Materials are useful for clients with reading comprehension problems and visual deficits.

riers to learning unless adjustments are made in nursing interventions. Sensory changes such as visual and hearing changes require adaptation of teaching methods to enhance functioning. Older adults learn and remember effectively if the nurse paces the learning properly and if the material is relevant to the learner's needs and abilities. Although many older adults have slower cognitive function and reduced short-term memory, nurses facilitate learning in several ways to support behaviors that maximize the individual's capacity for self-care (Box 25-9).

Establish short-term goals when teaching older clients. Include family members who assume care for the client. However, be sensitive to the client's desire for assistance, because offering unwanted support often results in negative outcomes and perceptions of nagging and interference. Furthermore, not all relation-

ships between older adults and other family members are therapeutic. Because of the high incidence of abuse and neglect of older adults, assess family dynamics before including family members in educational sessions.

Evaluation

Client education is not complete until the nurse evaluates outcomes of the teaching-learning process (see care plan). The nurse determines whether clients have learned the material. Evaluation reinforces correct behavior, helps learners realize how to change incorrect behavior, and helps the teacher determine adequacy of teaching (Redman, 2007).

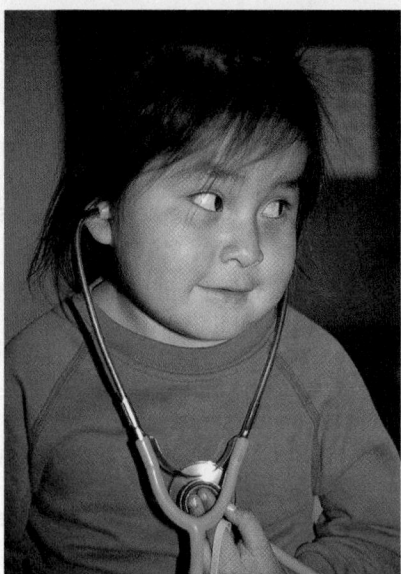

Figure 25-4 The preschool child learns not to be afraid of medical equipment by being allowed to handle the stethoscope and imitating its use.

The nurse is legally responsible for providing accurate, timely client information that promotes continuity of care; therefore it is essential to document the outcomes of teaching. Documentation of client teaching also supports quality improvement efforts, meets TJC standards, and promotes third-party reimbursement. Many institutions have special forms that allow easy documentation. Teaching flow sheets and written plans of care (e.g., care maps) are excellent records that document the plan, implementation, and evaluation of learning.

The nurse evaluates success by observing the client's performance of each expected behavior. Success depends on the client's ability to meet the established outcome and goals. The nurse carefully phrases questions to ensure that the learner understands them and that objectives are truly measured. Questions to ask when evaluating client education include the following:

- Were the client's goals or outcomes realistic and observable?
- Did the client value the information provided?
- Was the client willing to change an existing or adopt a new behavior?
- What barriers prevented learning or change in behaviors?
- Is the client able to perform the behavior or skill in the natural setting (e.g., home)?
- How well is the client able to answer questions about topic?
- If the client is completing a log, how well does the log match what was taught?
- Does the client continue to have problems understanding the information or performing a skill? If so, how can the nurse change the interventions to enhance knowledge or skill performance?

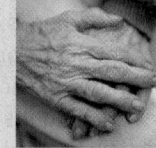

✳ BOX 25-9   FOCUS ON OLDER ADULTS

Providing Client Education

Nurses facilitate learning by using the following interventions when providing client education to older adults:

- Begin and end each teaching session with the most important information.
- Present information slowly.
- Speak in a low tone of voice (lower tones are easier to hear than higher tones).
- Allow enough time for understanding of the material.
- Emphasize concrete material that applies to current situations.
- Present only crucial information to avoid overwhelming the learner.
- Provide specific information in frequent, small amounts.
- Repeat important information.
- Relate new material to previous life experiences.
- Build on existing knowledge.
- Allow clients to progress at their own pace (older adults are more cautious, so it may take longer to adopt a behavior change).
- Use group experiences if appropriate to enhance problem solving.
- If using written material, assess the client's ability to read and use information that is printed in a large type size and in a color that contrasts highly with the background (e.g., black 14-point print on buff-colored paper). Avoid blues and greens because they are more difficult to see.

Data from Edelman CL, Mandle CL: *Health promotion throughout the lifespan*, ed 6, St. Louis, 2006, Mosby; and Mauk KL: Reaching and teaching older adults, *Nursing* 36(2):17, 2006.

✳ Key Concepts

- The nurse ensures that clients, families, and communities receive information needed to promote, restore, and maintain optimal health.
- Teaching is most effective when it is responsive to the learner's needs.
- Teaching is a form of interpersonal communication, with the teacher and learner actively involved in a process that increases the learner's knowledge and skills.
- The ability to learn depends on a person's physical and cognitive attributes.
- The ability to attend to the learning process depends on physical comfort and anxiety levels and the presence of environmental distraction.
- A person's health beliefs influence the willingness to gain knowledge and skills necessary to maintain health.
- Use of a theory (e.g., social learning theory) or theoretical concepts (e.g., self-efficacy) enhance learning.
- Time teaching so it occurs when the client is ready to learn.
- Clients of different age-groups require different teaching strategies as a result of developmental capabilities.
- Involve the client actively in all aspects of the teaching plan.
- Nurses use learning objectives to set priorities for learning.

- A combination of teaching methods improves the learner's attentiveness and involvement.
- A teacher is more effective when presenting information that builds on a learner's existing knowledge.
- Effective teachers use positive reinforcement.
- Older adults learn most effectively when information is slowly paced and presented in small amounts.
- Evaluate a client's learning by observing performance of expected learning behaviors under desired conditions.
- Effective documentation describes the entire process of client education, promotes continuity of care, and demonstrates that educational standards have been met.

Critical Thinking Exercises

1. As Connie provides Mr. Holland with an educational client teaching brochure about surgery, Connie asks Mr. Holland to verbalize what he read in his own words. However, Mr. Holland has trouble describing what he read, and he misunderstood much of the information included in the brochure. What does this assessment data suggest about Mr. Holland's health literacy? What special considerations does Connie need to implement based on this assessment data?

2. The surgeon comes to see Mr. Holland after surgery. Connie is in the hospital room at this time. The surgeon tells Mr. Holland that his cancer is aggressive and that he will probably need to have chemotherapy once the incision is healed. The surgeon leaves the room. Connie turns to Mr. Holland. He states, "I am sure the doctor is wrong. After all, he's a surgeon, not an oncologist." Which stage of grieving is Mr. Holland experiencing? What approach should Connie take in planning education for him?

3. Mr. Holland has been discharged. In planning discharge teaching, Connie reviews the medications Mr. Holland will be taking at home. She notices that his physician has prescribed three new medications for home. When Connie asks Mr. Holland what he understands about these medications, Mr. Holland states, "I have never heard of these medications before." What is the priority nursing diagnosis at this time?

4. Mrs. Holland enters the room while Connie is going over discharge instructions with Mr. Holland. What does Connie need to do before proceeding with her teaching?

NCLEX®-Style Review Questions

1. A client needs to learn to use a walker. Acquisition of this skill will require learning in the:
   1. Affective domain
   2. Cognitive domain
   3. Attentional domain
   4. Psychomotor domain

2. The nurse plans to teach a client about the importance of exercise:
   1. When there are visitors in the room
   2. When the client's pain medications are working
   3. Just before lunch, when the client is most awake and alert
   4. When the client is talking about current stressors in his or her life

3. A client newly diagnosed with cervical cancer is going home. The client is avoiding discussion of her illness and postoperative orders. In teaching the client about discharge instructions, the nurse:
   1. Teaches the client's spouse
   2. Provides only the information the client needs to go home
   3. Focuses on knowledge the client will need in a few weeks
   4. Convinces the client that learning about her health is necessary

4. The school nurse is about to teach a freshman-level health class about nutrition. To achieve the best learning outcomes, the nurse:
   1. Provides information using a lecture
   2. Uses simple words to promote understanding
   3. Develops topics for discussion that require problem solving
   4. Completes an extensive literature search focusing on eating disorders

5. A nurse is going to teach a client how to perform a breast self-examination. The behavioral objective that best measures the client's ability to perform the examination is:
   1. The client will verbalize the steps involved in breast self-examination within 1 week
   2. The nurse will explain the importance of performing breast self-examination once a month
   3. The client will perform breast self-examination correctly on herself before the end of the teaching session
   4. The nurse will demonstrate breast self-examination on a breast model provided by the American Cancer Society

6. A client who is having chest pain is going for an emergency cardiac catheterization. The most appropriate teaching approach in this situation is the:
   1. Telling approach
   2. Selling approach
   3. Entrusting approach
   4. Participating approach

7. The nurse is teaching a parenting class to a group of pregnant adolescents and has given the adolescents baby dolls to bathe and talk to. This is an example of:
   1. Role play
   2. Discovery
   3. An analogy
   4. A demonstration

8. An older adult is being started on a new antihypertensive medication. In teaching the client about the medication, the nurse:
   1. Speaks loudly
   2. Presents the information once
   3. Expects the client to understand the information quickly
   4. Allows the client time to express himself or herself and ask questions

9. A client needs to learn how to administer a subcutaneous injection. The nurse knows the client is ready to learn when the client:
   1. Has walked 400 feet
   2. Expresses the importance of learning the skill
   3. Can see and understand the markings on the syringe
   4. Has the dexterity needed to prepare and inject the medication

10. A client who is hospitalized has just been diagnosed with diabetes. He is going to need to learn how to give himself injections. The best teaching method would be:
    1. Simulation
    2. Demonstration
    3. Group instruction
    4. One-on-one discussion

26 | Documentation and Informatics

※ OBJECTIVES

Mastery of content in this chapter will enable the student to:

- Describe multidisciplinary communication within the health care team.
- Identify purposes of a health care record.
- Discuss legal guidelines for documentation.
- Identify ways to maintain confidentiality of records and reports.
- Describe five quality guidelines for documentation and reporting.
- Discuss the relationship between documentation and health care financial reimbursement.
- Describe the different methods used in record keeping.

- Discuss the advantages of standardized documentation forms.
- Identify elements to include when documenting a client's discharge plan.
- Identify the important aspects of home care and long-term care documentation.
- Describe the purpose and content of a change-of-shift report.
- Explain how to verify telephone orders.
- Discuss the relationship between informatics and quality health care.
- Identify ways to reduce data entry errors.

※ MEDIA RESOURCES   ※ KEY TERMS

 Companion CD
- NCLEX®-Style Review Questions
- Audio Glossary
- Interactive Learning Activities
- English/Spanish Glossary

 Website
- NCLEX®-Style Review Questions
- Audio Glossary
- English/Spanish Glossary
- Interactive Learning Activities
- Weblinks
- Audio Summaries

Accreditation, p. 385
Acuity records, p. 397
Case management, p. 393
Change-of-shift report, p. 399
Charting by exception (CBE), p. 392
Computerized physician order entry (CPOE), p. 407
Consultations, p. 386
Critical pathways, p. 393
DAR, p. 391
Diagnosis-related group (DRG), p. 385
Documentation, p. 385
Flow sheets, p. 394
Focus charting, p. 391
Incident (occurrence) reports, p. 403

Information technology, p. 404
Kardex, p. 397
Menu, p. 405
Nursing informatics, p. 404
Password, p. 406
PIE, p. 391
Problem-oriented medical record (POMR), p. 390
Record, p. 386
Referrals, p. 386
Reports, p. 386
Residents, p. 399
SOAP, p. 391
SOAPIE, p. 391
Source record, p. 391
Standardized care plans, p. 397
Transfer reports, p. 403
Variances, p. 393

Documentation is anything written or printed you rely on as record or proof for authorized persons. Documentation within a client's medical record is a vital aspect of nursing practice. Nursing documentation must be accurate, comprehensive, and flexible enough to retrieve critical data, maintain continuity of care, track client outcomes, and reflect current standards of nursing practice. Information in the client record provides a detailed account of the level of quality of care delivered to clients. Effective documentation ensures continuity of care, saves time, and minimizes the risk of errors (Yocum, 2002). Today's health care environment creates many challenges for accurately documenting and recording care provided to clients.

Accreditation agencies such as The Joint Commission (TJC) specify guidelines for documentation. Under the prospective payment system, Medicare reimburses hospitals a set dollar amount for each **diagnosis-related group (DRG)** (Box 26-1). Everything that is done for a client must be documented in the medical record for the health care institution to recover its costs.

As a member of the health care team, you will need to communicate information about clients accurately and in a timely, effective manner. The quality of client care depends on caregivers' ability to communicate with one another. All health care providers require the same information about clients so that they can plan an organized, comprehensive care plan. When a care plan is not communicated to all members of the health care team, care becomes fragmented, repetition of tasks occurs, and there are often delays or omissions in therapy. Data recorded, reported, or communicated to other health care professionals are confidential and must be protected.

The health care environment creates many challenges for accurately documenting and reporting the care delivered to clients. The quality of care, the standards of regulatory agencies and nursing practice, the reimbursement structure in the health care system, and legal guidelines make documentation and reporting an extremely important responsibility of a nurse. Whether the transfer of client information occurs through verbal reports, written documents, or electronic transfer, you need to follow basic principles to maintain confidentiality of information.

Confidentiality

Nurses are legally and ethically obligated to keep information about clients confidential. Nurses may not discuss a client's examination, observation, conversation, or treatment with other clients or staff not involved in the client's care. Only staff directly involved in a specific client's care have legitimate access to the records. Clients frequently request copies of their medical records, and they have the right to read those records. Each institution has policies to control the manner for sharing records. In most situations, clients are required to give written permission for release of medical information.

Nurses are responsible for protecting the client's records from all unauthorized readers. When nurses and other health care professionals have a legitimate reason to use records for data gathering, research, or continuing education, they obtain appropriate authorization according to agency policy. Nursing students and faculty may be required to present identification indicating access to the record is authorized. The health care agency stores the records.

Legislation to protect client privacy for health information, the Health Insurance Portability and Accountability Act (HIPAA), became a final rule in April 2001 and took effect in April 2003. This legislation governs all areas of information management. Health care providers (e.g., hospitals, clinics, physicians' or other health care providers' offices, and pharmacies) are required to provide clients with greater control over personal health care information. Previously the rule required written consent for disclosure of all client information. Under new regulations, in order to eliminate barriers that could delay access to care, providers are required only to notify clients of their privacy policy and make a reasonable effort to get written acknowledgment of this notification (Frank-Stromborg and Gauschow, 2002).

HIPAA requires that disclosure or requests regarding health information are limited to the minimum necessary. This includes only the specific information required for a particular purpose. For example, if you need a client's home telephone number to reschedule an appointment, access to the medical records will be limited solely to telephone information. According to the U.S. Department of Health and Human Services (USDHHS) (2001), clients have significant rights to understand and control the use of their health information.

- **Client education on privacy protections:** Providers and health plans give clients a clear written explanation of how the covered entity may use and disclose their health information.
- **Ensuring clients' access to their medical records:** Clients are able to see and get copies of their records and request amendments.
- **Receiving client consent before information is released:** Health care providers who see clients need to obtain client consent before sharing their information for treatment, payment, and health care operations. In addition, providers must obtain separate client authorization for disclosure of drug and alcohol treatment, mental health, and human immunodeficiency virus (HIV) information, as well as for health care purposes. Clients have the right to request restrictions on the uses and disclosures of their information.
- **Providing recourse if privacy protections are violated:** People have the right to file a formal complaint with a covered provider or health plan, or with the USDHHS, about violations of the provisions of this rule or the policies and procedures of the covered entity.

✳ **BOX 26-1 Diagnosis-Related Groups**

- A diagnosis-related group (DRG) is a series of decision trees designed to cluster groups of clients together by diagnosis, surgical procedures, complications, comorbidities (preexisting illness), and age.
- A hospital is reimbursed a fixed amount based on the hospital's specific rate of reimbursement.
- Each client with a particular diagnosis is reimbursed the same regardless of length of stay or cost of treatment.
- An assigned DRG may change on the basis of documentation.

Standards

Current TJC standards require that all clients who are admitted to a health care institution have an assessment of physical, psychosocial, environmental, self-care, client education, and discharge planning needs (TJC, 2007). TJC requires documentation within the context of the nursing process, as well as evidence of client and family teaching and discharge planning.

TJC also stresses the importance of evaluating client outcomes, including the client's response to treatments, teaching, or preventive care. If more than one discipline regularly cares for a client, TJC also expects a multidisciplinary care plan. For example, TJC standards recently incorporated a collaborative and interdisciplinary approach to pain management. This includes individualized pain control strategies involving frequent reassessment of pain, use of both pharmacological and nonpharmacological strategies, and a formalized approach to the implementation and evaluation of pain management (see Chapter 43).

The nursing service department of each health care agency selects a method for documenting client care. The method reflects the philosophy of the nursing department and incorporates the standards of care. For example, if a nursing department's standards of practice use nursing diagnosis or a framework such as Gordon's functional health patterns (Gordon, 2002), the documentation system uses nursing diagnoses and health patterns in care plans and other forms. Because the nursing process shapes a nurse's approach and direction of care, effective documentation reflects the nursing process.

Federal and state regulations, state statues, standards of care, and accrediting agencies set nursing documentation standards. The American Nurses Association's (ANA's) standard of nursing documentation states that "documentation must be systematic, continuous, accessible, communicated, recorded and readily available to all members of the health care team." It is expected that all nurses will maintain the client's record in accordance with the standard of care and the institution's policy and practice.

Multidisciplinary Communication Within the Health Care Team

Client care requires effective communication among members of the health care team. Effective communication takes place along two approaches. A client's **record** or chart is a confidential, permanent legal documentation of information relevant to a client's health care. Record information about the client's health care after each client contact. The record is a continuing account of the client's health care status and is available to all members of the health care team. All records basically contain the following information:

- Client identification and demographic data
- Informed consent for treatment and procedures
- Admission nursing history
- Nursing diagnoses or problems and nursing or multidisciplinary care plan

- Record of nursing care treatment and evaluation
- Medical history
- Medical diagnosis
- Therapeutic orders
- Medical and health discipline's progress notes
- Reports of physical examinations
- Reports of diagnostic studies
- Client education
- Summary of operative procedures
- Discharge plan and summary

Reports are oral, written, or audiotaped exchanges of information between caregivers. Common reports given by nurses include change-of-shift reports, telephone reports, transfer reports, and incident reports. A physician calls a nursing unit to receive a verbal report on a client's condition. The laboratory submits a written report providing the results of diagnostic tests. Nurses submit incident reports on a record that is not part of the client medical record (see Chapter 23).

Team members communicate information through discussions or conferences. For example, a discharge planning conference often involves members of all disciplines (e.g., nursing, social work, dietary, medicine, and physical therapy), who meet to discuss the client's progress toward established discharge goals. **Consultations** are another form of discussion whereby one professional caregiver gives formal advice about the care of a client to another caregiver. For example, a nurse caring for a client with a chronic wound consults with a wound care specialist. Nurses document **referrals** (an arrangement for services by another care provider), consultations, and conferences in a client's permanent record so that all caregivers can plan care accordingly.

Purposes of Records

A record is a valuable source of data for all members of the health care team. Its purposes include communication, legal documentation, financial billing, education, research, and auditing-monitoring.

Communication

The record is a means by which health care team members communicate client needs and progress, individual therapies, content of conferences, client education, and discharge planning. The plan of care needs to be clear to anyone reading the chart (see Unit III). The record should be the most current and accurate continuous source of information about a client's health care status.

Always communicate the manner in which you conduct the nursing process with a client in the record. The admitting nursing history and physical assessment is comprehensive and provides a baseline of the client's health status on admission to the facility. These data usually contain biographical data (e.g., age and marital status), method of admission, reason for admission, a brief past medical-surgical history (e.g., previous surgeries or illnesses), allergies, current medication (prescribed and over-the-counter), the client's perceptions about illness or hospitalization, and a review of health risk factors (see Chapter 16). A physical assessment of all body systems is either documented in the nursing history or on a separate form (see Chapter 33).

The medical progress notes should complement nursing process information. The notes detail the physician's findings at the time of assessment. While caring for any client, first refer to the medical record for relevant assessment findings. You are then able to enter a client's room, anticipate the status of the client, and then conduct your own individualized client assessment.

The record provides data that you use to identify and support nursing diagnoses, establish expected outcomes of care, plan interventions, and evaluate the care according to clients' responses to the care provided. Information from the record adds to your observations and assessment. It is unnecessary to collect information that is already available. If there is reason to believe that the information is inaccurate, verify the information and make appropriate notations in the client's record.

Legal Documentation

Accurate documentation is one of the best defenses for legal claims associated with nursing care (see Chapter 23). To limit nursing liability, nursing documentation must clearly indicate that individualized, goal-directed nursing care was provided to a client based on the nursing assessment. The record needs to describe exactly what happened to a client. This is best achieved when you chart immediately after providing care. Even though nursing care may have been excellent, in a court of law "care not documented is care not provided." Nurses need to indicate all assessments, interventions, client responses, instructions, and referrals in the medical record. Complete all documentation on appropriate forms, and be sure client identifying information (client's name and identification number) is on every page of documentation.

The Nurses Service Organization (medical malpractice, professional liability, and risk management company) (2006) has identified common charting mistakes that can result in malpractice: (1) failing to record pertinent health or drug information; (2) failing to record nursing actions; (3) failing to record that medications have been given; (4) failing to record drug reactions or changes in client's condition; (5) writing illegible or incomplete records; and (6) failing to document a discontinued medication. Table 26-1 provides guidelines for legally sound documentation.

Financial Billing

DRGs have become the basis for establishing reimbursement for client care. DRGs are a prospective payment system. Hospitals are reimbursed a preestablished dollar amount by Medicare for each DRG. Detailed recording establishes codable diagnoses for determining a DRG. Your documentation can help clarify the type of treatment a client receives and help support the reimbursement to the health care agency.

A medical record audit reviews financial charges used in the client's care. Private insurance carriers and auditors from federal agencies review records to determine the reimbursement that a client or a health care agency receives. Accurate documentation of supplies and equipment used assists in accurate and timely reimbursement.

Education

A client's record contains a variety of information, including diagnoses, signs and symptoms of disease, successful and unsuccessful therapies, diagnostic findings, and client behaviors. One way to learn the nature of an illness and the individual client's response to it is to read the client care record. No two clients have identical records, but patterns of information can be identified in records of clients who have similar health problems. With this information, students identify patterns for various health problems and learn to anticipate the type of care required for a client.

Research

Statistical data on the frequency of clinical disorders, complications, use of specific medical and nursing therapies, recovery from illness, and deaths can be gathered from client records. For example, as a part of a quality improvement program (see Chapter 5) for clients receiving intravenous therapy, a nurse manager reviews clients' records to investigate the incidence of infection in clients with a specific type of intravenous catheter. The record review indicates that the infection rate is increased, and the nurse manager and staff nurses design a new specific method for intravenous catheter care. Once this new intervention is implemented, the manager again reviews clients' records to determine if the infection rate decreases.

A nurse may use clients' records during a clinical research study to investigate a new nursing intervention. For example, a nurse wants to compare a new method of pain control with a standard pain protocol using two groups of clients. The records provide data on the two types of interventions: the new method and the standard pain control. The nurse researcher collects data from the records that describe the type and dose of analgesic medications used, objective assessment data, and clients' subjective reports of pain relief. The researcher then compares the findings to determine if the new method was more effective than the standard pain control protocol.

Auditing-Monitoring

TJC (2007) requires hospitals to establish quality improvement programs for conducting objective, ongoing reviews of client care. TJC has standards for the information located in the client's record, including indications that a plan of care is developed with the client as a participant and that discharge planning and client education have occurred. TJC asks institutions to establish standards for quality care. Nurses monitor or review records throughout the year to determine the degree to which quality improvement standards are met (see Chapter 5). Nurses share deficiencies identified during monitoring with all members of the nursing staff to make corrections in policy or practice. Quality improvement programs keep nurses informed of standards of nursing practice to maintain excellence in nursing care.

Guidelines for Quality Documentation and Reporting

High-quality documentation and reporting are necessary to enhance efficient, individualized client care. Quality documentation and reporting have five important characteristics: they are factual, accurate, complete, current, and organized.

✳ TABLE 26-1 Legal Guidelines for Recording

GUIDELINES	RATIONALE	CORRECT ACTION
Do not erase, apply correction fluid, or scratch out errors made while recording.	Charting becomes illegible: it may appear as if you were attempting to hide information or deface record.	Draw single line through error, write word *error* above it, and sign your name or initials and date it. Then record note correctly.
Do not write retaliatory or critical comments about client or care by other health care professionals. Do not write personal opinions.	Statements can be used as evidence for nonprofessional behavior or poor quality of care.	Enter only objective and factual observations of client's behavior; quote all client comments.
Correct all errors promptly.	Errors in recording can lead to errors in treatment or may imply an attempt to mislead or hide evidence.	Avoid rushing to complete charting; be sure information is accurate and complete.
Record all facts.	Record must be accurate, factual, and objective.	Be certain entry is factual and thorough. A person reading the documentation should be able to determine the client was adequately cared for.
Do not leave blank spaces in nurses' notes.	Another person can add incorrect information in space.	Chart consecutively, line by line; if space is left, draw line horizontally through it and sign your name at end.
Record all entries legibly and in black ink. Do not use felt tip pens or erasable ink.	Illegible entries can be misinterpreted, causing errors and lawsuits; felt tip pen ink will smudge or run when wet and may destroy documentation; erasures are not permitted in client charting; black ink is more legible when records are photocopied or transferred to microfilm.	Never erase entries or use correction fluid, and never use pencil.
If order is questioned, record that clarification was sought.	If you perform order known to be incorrect, you are just as liable for prosecution as the physician is.	Do not record "physician made error." Instead, chart that "Dr. Smith was called to clarify order for analgesic." Include the date and time of phone call, whom you spoke with, and the outcome.
Chart only for yourself.	You are accountable for information you enter into chart.	Never chart for someone else (exception: if caregiver has left unit for day and calls with information that needs to be documented, include the date and time of entry and reference the specific date and time you are referring to, name of the source of information in the entry, and include that the information was provided via telephone).
Avoid using generalized, empty phrases such as "status unchanged" or "had good day."	This type of documentation is subjective and does not reflect client assessment.	Use complete, concise descriptions of care so that documentation is objective and factual.
Begin each entry with date and time, and end with your signature and title.	This guideline ensures that correct sequence of events is recorded; signature documents who is accountable for care delivered.	Do not wait until end of shift to record important changes that occurred several hours earlier; be sure to sign each entry (for example, Mary Marcus, RN).
For computer documentation keep your password to yourself.	This maintains security and confidentiality.	Once logged into the computer, do not leave the computer screen unattended. Make sure the computer screen is not accessible for public viewing.

Factual

A factual record contains descriptive, objective information about what a nurse sees, hears, feels, and smells. An objective description is the result of direct observation and measurement. For example, "B/P 80/50, client diaphoretic, heart rate 102 and regular." The use of inferences (e.g., "client appears to be in shock") without supporting factual data is not acceptable because it can be misunderstood.

The use of vague terms, such as *appears, seems,* or *apparently,* is not acceptable because these words suggest that you are stating an opinion. For example, the description "the client seems anxious" does not accurately communicate facts and does not inform another caregiver of the details regarding the behaviors exhibited by the client that led to the use of the word *anxious*. The phrase *seems anxious* is a conclusion without supported facts. Objective documentation includes the observations of the client's behaviors. For example, objective signs of anxiety include increased pulse rate, increased respiration, and increased restlessness.

When recording subjective data, document the client's exact words within quotation marks whenever possible. For example, when a client exhibits anxiety you record, "Client states, 'I feel very nervous.'"

Accurate

The use of exact measurements establishes accuracy. For example, a description such as "Intake, 360 mL of water" is more accurate than "Client drank an adequate amount of fluid." These measurements can later determine whether a client's condition has changed. Charting that an abdominal wound is "5 cm in length without redness, drainage, or edema" is more descriptive than "large wound healing well."

Documentation of concise data is clear and easy to understand. It is essential to avoid the use of unnecessary words and irrelevant detail. For example, the fact that the client is watching TV is only necessary when this activity is significant to the client's status and plan of care.

Use of an institution's accepted abbreviations, symbols, and system of measures (e.g., metric) ensures that all staff members use the same language in their reports and records. Always use abbreviations carefully to avoid misinterpretation. To minimize errors, abbreviations are spelled in their entirety when abbreviations become confusing. In the interest of client safety, TJC requires that health care institutions develop a list of standard abbreviations, symbols, and acronyms to be used by all members of the health care team when documenting or communicating client care and treatment. Approved abbreviations and acronyms will vary depending on the type of facility (i.e., long-term care versus acute care facility). Each member of the health care team is responsible for knowing and using the appropriate documentation for their institution.

TJC's "do not use" list of abbreviations (see Chapter 35) is intended to be used by all health care providers to promote client safety. These abbreviations were often confused with other words or symbols. TJC is looking at additional abbreviations to add to this list in the future.

Correct spelling demonstrates a level of competency and attention to detail. Many terms can easily be misinterpreted (e.g., *dysphagia* or *dysphasia* and *dram* or *gram*). Some spelling errors can also result in serious treatment errors; for example, the names of certain medications such as digitoxin and digoxin or morphine and Numorphan are similar. Transcribe such terms carefully to ensure that the client receives the correct medication.

TJC standards (2007) require that "all entries in medical records are dated and a method is established to identify the authors of entries." Therefore each entry in a client's record ends with the caregiver's full name or initials and status, such as "Julie Smith, RN." Each time initials are used, the full name and status must previously appear on the same page so the individual entering initials can be readily identified. A nursing student enters full name, student nurse abbreviation (e.g., SN or NS), and educa-tional institution, such as "David Jones, SN (student nurse), CMTC (Central Maine Technical College)."

Records need to reflect accountability during the time frame of the entry. This is accomplished when nurses chart only their own observations and actions. The signature holds that nurse accountable for information recorded. If information was inadvertently omitted from the record, it is acceptable for nurses to ask colleagues to chart information after they leave work. The entry needs to clearly show what was done and by whom (e.g., "At 11 AM Sam Turner, RN, called and reported that at 8 AM morphine sulfate 15 mg IM was administered to client for abdominal pain").

Complete

The information within a recorded entry or a report needs to be complete, containing appropriate and essential information. Criteria for thorough communication exist for certain health problems or nursing activities (Table 26-2). Your written entries in the client's medical record describe the nursing care you administer and the client's response. An example of a thorough nurse's note follows:

1915 Client verbalizes sharp, throbbing pain localized along lateral side of right ankle, beginning approximately 15 minutes ago after twisting his foot on the stairs. Client rates pain as 8 on a scale of 0-10. Pain increased with movement, slightly relieved with elevation. Pedal pulses equal bilaterally. Right ankle circumference 1 cm larger than left. Capillary refill less than 3 seconds bilaterally, right foot warm to touch and pale pink; skin intact on right foot; responds to tactile stimulation on right foot. Ice applied. Percocet 2 tabs (PO) given for pain. Client states pain somewhat relieved with ice, rates pain as 6 on a scale of 0-10. Dr. M. Smith notified. Lee Turno, RN.

Current

Timely entries are essential in the client's ongoing care (TJC, 2007). To increase accuracy and decrease unnecessary duplication, many health care agencies keep records near the client's bedside to facilitate immediate documentation of information as it is collected from a client. Flow sheets offer a means to enter current information quickly. Portable electronic work stations or secure wall cabinets help to ensure client confidentiality is maintained. Nurses often keep notes on a worksheet when caring for several clients, making notes as the care occurs to ensure that entries recorded later in the record are accurate. Activities or findings to communicate at the time of occurrence include the following:

- Vital signs
- Administration of medications and treatments
- Preparation for diagnostic tests or surgery
- Change in client's status and who was notified, (e.g., physician, manager, client's family)
- Admission, transfer, discharge, or death of a client
- Treatment for a sudden change in client's status
- Client's response to treatment or intervention

Most health care agencies use military time, a 24-hour system that avoids misinterpretation of AM and PM times (Figure 26-1). Instead of two 12-hour cycles in standard time, the military clock is one 24-hour time cycle. The military clock ends with midnight at

✳ TABLE 26-2 Examples of Criteria for Reporting and Recording

TOPIC	CRITERIA TO REPORT OR RECORD
Assessment	
Subjective data	Client's description of episode in quotation marks; for example, "I feel like I have an elephant sitting on my chest, and I can't catch my breath." Onset, location, description of condition (severity, duration, frequency, precipitating, aggravating and relieving factors); for example, "The pain in my left knee started last week after I knelt on the ground. Every time I bend my knee I have a shooting pain on the inside of my knee."
Client behavior (e.g., anxiety, confusion, hostility)	Onset, behaviors exhibited, precipitating factors, client's verbal behavior; for example, "Client observed pacing in her room, avoiding eye contact with nurse and repeatedly stating 'I have to go home now.'"
Objective data (e.g., rash, tenderness, breath sounds)	Onset, location, description of condition (see above); for example, "1100: 2-cm raised pale red area noted on back of left hand."
Nursing Interventions and Evaluation	
Treatments (e.g., enema, bath, dressing change)	Time administered, equipment used (if appropriate), client's response (objective and subjective changes) compared to previous treatment; for example, "Client denied incisional pain during abdominal dressing change" or "Client ambulated 300 feet in hallway without assistance. Denied incisional pain during or after ambulation."
Medication administration	Immediately after administration, document: time medication given, preliminary assessment (e.g., pain level, vital signs), client response or effect of medication; for example, "1500 Client reports a 'throbbing headache all over her head.' Rates pain at 6 (scale 0-10). Tylenol 650 mg given PO 1530: Client reports pain level 2 (scale 0-10) and states 'the throbbing has stopped.'"
Client teaching	Information presented, method of instruction (e.g., discussion, demonstration, videotape, booklet), and client response, including questions and evidence of understanding such as return demonstration or change in behavior.
Discharge planning	Measurable client goals or expected outcomes, progress toward goals, need for referrals.

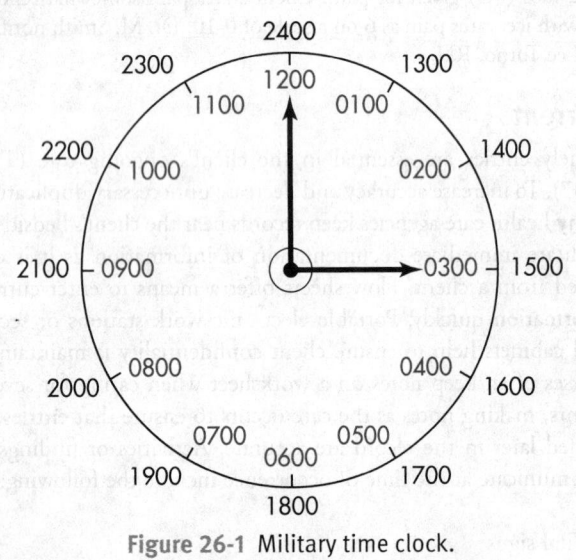

Figure 26-1 Military time clock.

2400 and begins at 1 minute after midnight as 0001. For example, 10:22 AM is 1022 military time; 1:00 PM is 1300 military time.

Organized

As a nurse, you want to communicate information in a logical order. For example, an organized note describes the client's pain, your assessment and interventions, and the client's response. To write notes about complex situations in an organized fashion think about the situation and make notes of what to include be-

fore beginning to write in the permanent legal record. Applying critical thinking skills and the nursing process gives logic and order to nursing documentation.

Methods of Recording

There are several documentation systems for recording client data. Each nursing service selects a documentation system that reflects the philosophy of the department. The same documentation system is used throughout a specific agency and may be used throughout a health care system as well.

Narrative Documentation

Narrative documentation is the traditional method for recording nursing care. It is simply the use of a storylike format to document information specific to client conditions and nursing care. Narrative charting, however, has many disadvantages, including the tendency to have repetitious information, to be time consuming, and to require the reader to sort through much information to locate desired data. There are several formats for recording health care information.

Problem-Oriented Medical Record

The **problem-oriented medical record** (POMR) is a method of documentation that emphasizes the client's problems. Data are organized by problem or diagnosis. Ideally each member of the health care team contributes to a single list of identified client problems. This approach coordinates a common plan of care. The

POMR has the following major sections: database, problem list, care plan, and progress notes.

Database. The database section contains all available assessment information pertaining to the client (e.g., history and physical examination, the nurse's admission history and ongoing assessment, the dietitian's assessment, laboratory reports, and radiological test results). The database is the foundation for identifying client problems and planning care. As new data become available, you revise the database. It accompanies clients through successive hospitalizations or clinic visits.

Problem List. After analyzing data, health care team members identify problems and make a single problem list. The problem list includes the client's physiological, psychological, social, cultural, spiritual, developmental, and environmental needs. Team members list the problems in chronological order and file the list in the front of the client's record to serve as an organizing guide for the client's care. Add new problems as you identify them. When a problem is resolved, record the date and highlight it or draw a line through the problem and its number.

Nursing Care Plan. Disciplines involved in the client's care develop a care plan for each problem (see Chapter 18). Nurses document the plan of care in a variety of formats. Generally these plans of care include nursing diagnoses, expected outcomes, and interventions.

Progress Notes. Health care team members monitor and record the progress of a client's problems (Box 26-2). Progress notes come in various formats or structured notes. One method is SOAP charting. The acronym **SOAP** stands for: S—subjective data (verbalizations of the client), O—objective data (that which is measured and observed), A—assessment (diagnosis based on the data), P—plan (what the caregiver plans to do). An I and E are sometimes added (i.e., **SOAPIE**) in some institutions. The I stands for intervention, and the E represents evaluation. The logic for SOAPIE notes is similar to that of the nursing process. Collect data about the client's problems, draw conclusions, and develop a plan of care. The nurse numbers each SOAP note and titles it according to the problem on the list.

A second progress note method is the **PIE** format. It is similar to SOAP charting in its problem-oriented nature. However, it differs from the SOAP method in that PIE charting has a nursing origin, whereas SOAP originated from medical records. The format simplifies documentation by unifying the care plan and progress notes. PIE differs from SOAP notes because the narrative does not include assessment information. A nurse's daily assessment data appear on flow sheets, preventing duplication of data. The narrative note includes P—problem, I—intervention, and E—evaluation. The PIE notes are numbered or labeled according to the client's problems. Resolved problems are dropped from daily documentation after the nurse's review. Continuing problems are documented daily.

A third narrative format is **focus charting.** It involves use of **DAR** notes, which include D—data (both subjective and objective), A—action or nursing intervention, and R—response of the client (i.e., evaluation of effectiveness). One distinction of focus

---

> ### ✳ BOX 26-2   Examples of Progress Notes Written in Different Formats
>
> **SOAP (Subjective—Objective—Assessment—Plan)**
> 1/19/06 Deficient knowledge related to inexperience regarding surgery
> 4:30 PM
> **S**— "I'm worried about what it will be like after surgery."
> **O**— Client asking frequent questions about surgery. Has had no previous experience with surgery. Wife present, acts as a support person.
> **A**— Deficient knowledge regarding surgery related to inexperience. Client also expressing anxiety.
> **P**— Explain routine preoperative preparation. Demonstrate and explain rationale for turning, coughing, and deep breathing (TCDB) exercises. Provide explanation and teaching booklet on postoperative nursing care. Sue Lazarus, RN
>
> **PIE (Problem—Intervention—Evaluation)**
> **P**— Deficient knowledge regarding surgery related to inexperience.
> **I**— Explained to client normal preoperative preparations for surgery. Demonstrated TCDB exercises. Provided booklet to client on postoperative nursing care.
> **E**— Client demonstrates TCBD exercises correctly. Needs review of postoperative nursing care. Sue Lazarus, RN
>
> **Focus Charting (Data—Action—Response)**
> **D**— Client stated, "I'm worried about what it will be like after surgery." Client asking frequent questions about surgery. Has had no previous experience with surgery. Wife present, acts as a support person.
> **A**— Explained to client normal preoperative preparations for surgery. Demonstrated TCDB exercises. Provided booklet to client on postoperative nursing care.
> **R**— Client demonstrates TCDB exercises correctly. Needs review of postoperative nursing care. Client states "I feel better knowing a little bit of what to expect." Sue Lazarus, RN

---

charting is its movement away from charting only problems, which has a negative connotation. Instead a DAR note addresses client concerns: a sign or symptom, a condition, a nursing diagnosis, a behavior, a significant event, or a change in a client's condition. Documentation is written in accordance with the nursing process. Nurses broaden their thinking to include any client concerns, not just problem areas. This method encourages critical thinking.. The benefits to focus charting is that it incorporates all aspects of the nursing process, highlights the client's concerns, and can be integrated into any clinical setting (*Mosby's Surefire Documentation,* 2006).

Source Records

In a **source record** the client's chart has a separate section for each discipline (e.g., nursing, medicine, social work, or respiratory therapy) to record data. One advantage of a source record is that caregivers can easily locate the proper section of the record in which to make entries. Table 26-3 lists the components of a source record.

A disadvantage of the source record is that details about a specific problem are distributed throughout the record. For example, the nurse describes the character of abdominal pain and use of relaxation therapy and analgesic medication in the nurses' notes.

✳ TABLE 26-3 Organization of Traditional Source Record

SECTIONS	CONTENTS
Admission sheet	Specific demographic data about client: legal name, identification number, gender, age, birth date, marital status, occupation and employer, health insurance, nearest relative to notify in an emergency, religious preference, name of attending physician, date and time of admission
Physician's order sheet	Record of physician's or other health care provider's orders for treatment and medications, with date, time, and signature
Nurse's admission assessment	Summary of nursing history and physical examination
Graphic sheet and flow sheet	Record of repeated observations and measurements such as vital signs, daily weights, and intake and output
Medical history and examination	Results of initial examination performed by physician, including findings, family history, confirmed diagnoses, and medical plan of care
Nurses' notes	Narrative record of nursing process: assessment, nursing diagnosis, planning, implementation, and evaluation of care
Medication records	Accurate documentation of all medications administered to client: date, time, dose, route, and nurse's signature
Physician's progress notes	Ongoing record of client's progress and response to medical therapy and review of disease process
Health care disciplines' records	Entries made into record by all health-related disciplines: radiology, social work, and laboratories
Discharge summary	Summary of client's condition, progress, prognosis, rehabilitation, and teaching needs at time of dismissal from hospital or health care agency

✳ BOX 26-3 Sample Narrative Note

8/6/04 1100

Client states, "I'm having a hard time catching my breath." Respirations, labored at 32/min; P, 120; BP, 112/70, Pulse ox 90% on room air. Skin color pale, skin warm and dry, lips and nail beds cyanotic. Client alert and oriented ×3. Client using intercostal muscles during inhalation. Breath sounds auscultated, crackles and wheezes over both lower lobes. Chest excursion equal bilaterally. Elevated head of bed to high-Fowler's position. Obtained arterial blood gas analysis at 1045 and O_2 started at 2 L/min per mask as ordered. Remained at bedside to calm client. Pat Haske, RN

1130 Results of ABGs reported to Dr Stein are pH, 7.34; PCO_2, 44 mm Hg; PO_2, 80 mm Hg. Client states "it is easier to breathe now." R, 24/min; P, 96; BP, 110/72. Pulse ox 97% on 2 L O_2, lips pale pink; capillary refill greater than 3 seconds. Crackles and wheezing still apparent. Client remains in high-Fowler's position. Pat Haske, RN

The physician's notes describe the progress of the client's bowel obstruction and the plan for surgery in a separate section of the record. The results of x-ray examinations that show the location of the bowel obstruction are in the test results section of the record. The method by which source records are organized does not show how information from the disciplines is related or how care is coordinated to meet all of the client's needs.

The notes section is where nurses enter a narrative description of nursing care and the client's response (Box 26-3). It is also a section for documenting care that a physician or other health care provider administers in the nurse's presence. The nurse also records key diagnostic test results from other sections of the record in the notes if they are of major importance in the care of the client.

Charting by Exception

Charting by exception (CBE) focuses on documenting deviations from the established norm or abnormal findings. This approach reduces documentation time and highlights trends or changes in the client's condition (*Mosby's Surefire Documentation,* 2006). It is a shorthand method for documenting normal findings and routine care based on clearly defined standards of practice and predetermined criteria for nursing assessments and interventions. Clearly defined standards of practice that specify nurses' responsibilities to clients provide the framework for routine care of all clients. With standards integrated into documentation forms, such as predefined normal assessment findings or predetermined interventions, a nurse need only document significant findings or exceptions to the predefined norms. In other words, the nurse writes a progress note only when the standardized statement on the form is not met. Assessments are standardized on forms so that all caregivers evaluate and document findings consistently (Figure 26-2).

Because standard assessments are in the chart, client data are already present on the permanent record, so nurses do not have to keep temporary notes for later transcription and caregivers have easy access to current data. The assumption with charting by exception is that all standards are met unless otherwise documented. When nurses see entries in the chart, they know that something out of the ordinary has been observed or has occurred. For that reason when changes in a client's condition have developed, it is easy to track them. When clients' conditions change, thorough and precise descriptions of what happens to clients and the actions taken are essential.

Charting by exception can pose legal risks if nurses are not disciplined in documenting exceptions. The charting method fails to provide a thorough picture of a client's developing condition and does not reflect communication among members of the health care team. If nurses rely too heavily on charting standard categories and do not enter exception notes, a clear picture of the client's situation will not be available.

Case Management Plan and Critical Pathways

The **case management** model of delivering care (see Chapter 2) incorporates a multidisciplinary approach to documenting client care. In many organizations the standardized plan of care is summarized into critical pathways for a specific disease or condition. The **critical pathways** are multidisciplinary care plans that include client problems, key interventions, and expected outcomes within an established time frame (Figure 26-3). A computerized charting system allows for integration of the chart by many disciplines. The nurse and other team members use the same critical pathway to monitor the client's progress during each shift or in the case of home care, every visit. With the computerized record available at every computer terminal, each care provider can access it at any time.

Critical pathways eliminate nurses' notes, flow sheets, and nursing care plans because the pathway document integrates all relevant information. Unexpected outcomes, unmet goals, and interventions not specified within the critical pathway time frame are called **variances.** A variance occurs when the activities on the critical pathway are not completed as predicted or the client does not meet the expected outcomes. An example of a variance is when a client develops pulmonary complications after surgery requiring oxygen therapy and monitoring with pulse oximetry. A positive variance occurs when a client progresses more rapidly than expected (e.g., use of a Foley catheter may be discontinued a

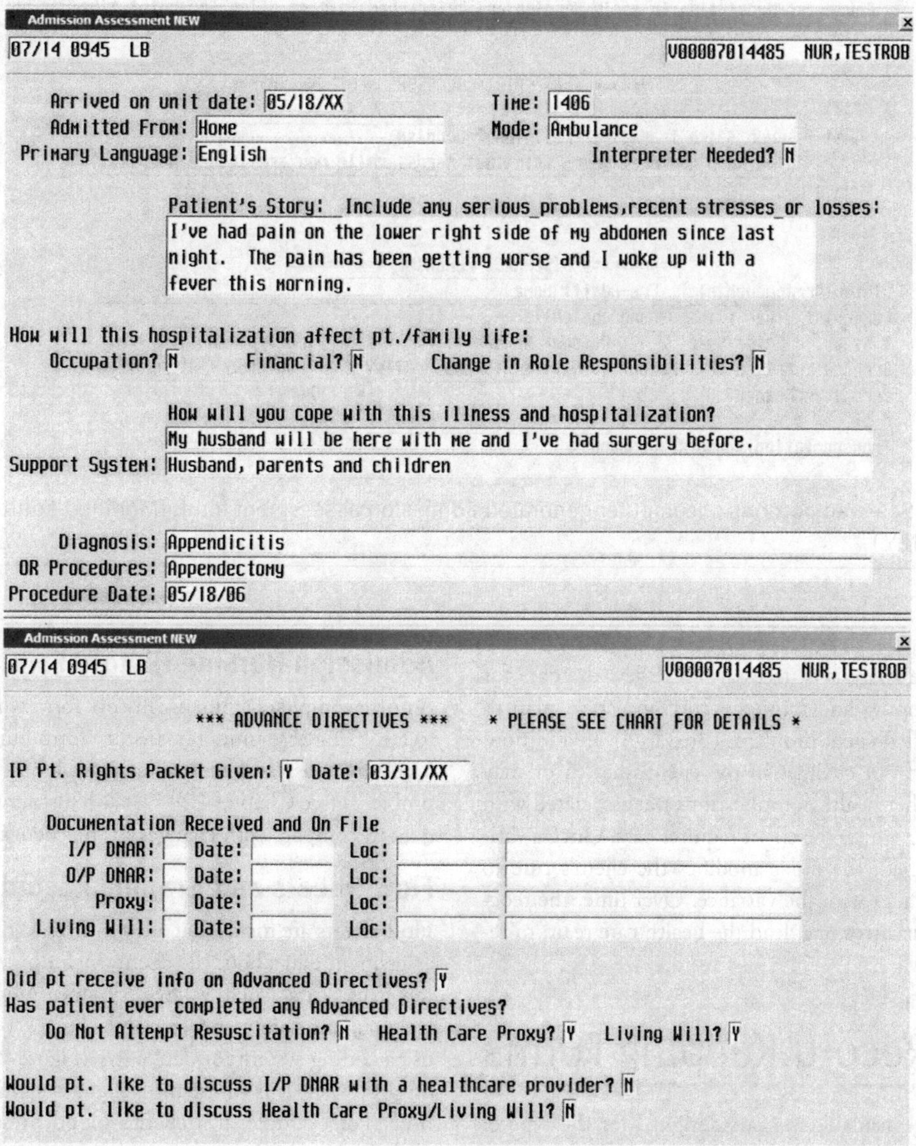
Admission Assessment NEW

07/14 0945 LB   V00007014485 NUR,TESTROB

Arrived on unit date: 05/18/XX   Time: 1406
Admitted From: Home   Mode: Ambulance
Primary Language: English   Interpreter Needed? N

Patient's Story: Include any serious_problems,recent stresses_or losses:
I've had pain on the lower right side of my abdomen since last night. The pain has been getting worse and I woke up with a fever this morning.

How will this hospitalization affect pt./family life:
Occupation? N   Financial? N   Change in Role Responsibilities? N

How will you cope with this illness and hospitalization?
My husband will be here with me and I've had surgery before.
Support System: Husband, parents and children

Diagnosis: Appendicitis
OR Procedures: Appendectomy
Procedure Date: 05/18/06

Admission Assessment NEW

07/14 0945 LB   V00007014485 NUR,TESTROB

*** ADVANCE DIRECTIVES ***   * PLEASE SEE CHART FOR DETAILS *

IP Pt. Rights Packet Given: Y Date: 03/31/XX

Documentation Received and On File
I/P DNAR: Date: Loc:
O/P DNAR: Date: Loc:
Proxy: Date: Loc:
Living Will: Date: Loc:

Did pt receive info on Advanced Directives? Y
Has patient ever completed any Advanced Directives?
Do Not Attempt Resuscitation? N   Health Care Proxy? Y   Living Will? Y

Would pt. like to discuss I/P DNAR with a healthcare provider? N
Would pt. like to discuss Health Care Proxy/Living Will? N

Figure 26-2 Selected portions of computer-generated admission assessment form. (Modified Courtesy Bassett Healthcare, Cooperstown, N.Y.)

Continued

```
                        Fall Risk Assessment-
Fall History:
               Recent fall? N : 0
     Fall during this admission? N : 0    Date: [        ]

Mentation:                                Elimination:
       Comatose/unresponsive ? N : [  ]              Incontinent? N : 0
        Confused at all times? N : 0     Needs assistance w/toileting? N : 0
           Periodic confusion? N : 0   Independent but frequency/diarrhea? N : 0
          Alert and oriented x 3? N : Y              Independent? N : Y
Mobility:
     Unable to amb./transfer (bedrest only)? N : [  ]
Unsteady gait & amb/trans w/assist/devices? N : 0
           Unsteady gait w/o assistance? N : 0
     Amb. independently -No gait disturbance? N : Y
Medication:
Ordered/receiving any anticonvulsants, tranquilizers, psychotropics, or hypnotics? N : 0
           * 3 or greater = HIGH FALL RISK              Total: 0
    +------------------------------------------+
    | Options                              [x] |    Fall Protocol? N
    +------------------------------------------+    Green Wrist Band On? N
         <Prev>  <Return>  <Exit>          |

         ========== CULTURAL ASSESSMENT ==========
       Do you have any cultural needs that will help us care for you? Y
Comments: Meditation in early morning and before bed, please allow for quiet time.


         =========== SPIRITUAL ASSESSMENT ============

  What is your faith tradition (religion)? buddism
       May we help you meet your  spiritual needs, while you are in the hospital? N
Comments: [                                                         ]


         ========== DISCHARGE PLANNING ==========
Living Arrangements:    Pre-Admit: Home
Comments: Lives with husband and children
# Steps to Enter Home: 3    Outdoor Handrail? N    # of Floors at Home: 2
Bedroom Location: 2    Number of Stairs: 13  Handrails? N    Bathroom(s) Location: [  ]
Caregiver Needed? N    Name: [              ]  *  Phone: [          ]  *

Transportation/Vendor: [Husband            ]
```

Figure 26-2, cont'd Selected portions of computer-generated admission assessment form. (Modified Courtesy Bassett Healthcare, Cooperstown, N.Y.)

day early). A variance analysis is necessary to review the data for trends and for developing and implementing an action plan to respond to the identified client problems (Box 26-4). In addition, variances may result from changes in the client's health or may occur as a result of other health complications not associated with the primary reason for which the client requires care. Once a variance has been identified, the nurse modifies the client's care to meet the needs associated with the variance. Over time, the reoccurrence of similar variances may lead the health care team to revise a critical pathway.

Common Record-Keeping Forms

A variety of forms are available that are designed for the type of information nurses routinely document. The categories within a form are usually derived from institutional standards of practice or guidelines established by accrediting agencies.

Admission Nursing History Forms

A nurse completes a nursing history form when a client is admitted to a nursing care unit. The history form guides the nurse through a complete assessment to identify relevant nursing diagnoses or problems (see Chapter 16). Data on history forms provide baseline data to compare with changes in the client's condition.

Flow Sheets and Graphic Records

Flow sheets are forms that allow nurses to quickly and easily enter assessment data about the client, including vital signs and routine repetitive care, such as hygiene measures, ambulation, meals, weights, and safety and restraint checks (Box 26-5). Flow sheets use a coding system for data entry (Figure 26-4). If an occurrence on a flow sheet is unusual or changes significantly, enter a focus note. For example, if a client's blood pressure becomes dangerously high, complete a focus assessment and record this, as well as action taken, in the progress notes. Flow sheets provide a quick, easy reference for the health care team members in assessing a

Text continued on page 397

Norman Regional Hospital CareMap®
Community Acquired Pneumonia

Check (✓) Precautions

	Falls	Skin	DNR
	☐	☐	☐

Page 1

Admitting Physician:	Primary Care Physician:	Consulting Physician(s):	Expected LOS	M&R LOS

Allergy/Reaction

Secondary Diagnosis

Prob	Patient Problem	Expected Outcome (Responsible Discipline)	Outcome	Date	Signature
#1 ★	Infection	Blood cultures obtained prior to start of antibiotics? (RN)	☐YES ☐NO		
#2	Activity Tolerance	Patient is at or above baseline activity (endurance) level? (RN)	☐YES ☐NO		
#3	Knowledge Deficit	Patient able to verbalize understanding of pneumonia signs and symptoms? (RN)	☐YES ☐NO		
#4 ★	Timeliness of Antibiotic Administration	First dose of antibiotic administered within 2 hours of order? (RN, RPh)	☐YES ☐NO		
#5 ★	Discharge Preparation	Patient switched from IV to oral antibiotic within 48 hrs after delivery of 1st dose? (RN, RPh)	☐YES ☐NO		

★ = Key Exception
__ = Documentaion Required

Copyright©2000 Norman Regional Hospital

Statement of Intent:
The CareMap® serves as an optional guideline for patient care and is subject to alteration based on the individual needs of the patient.
(CareMap® used with permission of the Center for Case Management.)

Authors: **Rosalie Lavon, M.D., Jerry Leu, M.D., John McCarter, M.D., Tom Merrill, M.D., Bruce Naylor, M.D., J. Kin Pirtle, M.D., Joe Riddle, M.D., Christian Sieck, M.D., Jackie Evans, Linda Fielder, Vicki Johnson, Wanda Maddox, Yvette Morrison, Wanda Morrow, Joyce Nolen, Barbara Poe, Michelle Rausch, Darin Smith, Brenda Wilson**

Date: 7/00	Form# CMAP 114	Revised:

Patient Sticker

Figure 26-3 Example of a critical pathway for pneumonia. (From Norman Regional Hospital CareMap®, Community Acquired Pneumonia. Copyright 2000, Norman Regional Hospital. Used with the permission of Norman Regional Hospital, Norman, Okla.)

Continued

PATIENT STICKER	Time Admitted: _____	Day #1 (ER/Floor) Date _____	Day #2 Date _____
Page 2			
Additional Daily Treatments/Other			
	Assessments/Monitoring	VS qshift (and Temp q4h if T>99.5) Nursing Assessment qshift Weight I&O Pain Assessment	VS qshift (and Temp q4h if T>99.5) Nursing Assessment qshift I&O Pain Assessment
Isolation Precautions	**Consults**	Respiratory Therapy Assess need for Social Work Consult	
Special Procedures/Surgeries:	**Procedures/Tests**	CBC with diff, Basic Metabolic Panel, UA, Sputum gram stain + C&S Stat (induce if necessary), Blood cultures x2 (15 minutes apart), CXR (PA & Lateral)	CBC with diff
	Treatments	Oxygen Therapy per protocol C&DB q2hr Suction prn Albuterol AN treatments/MDI per RT/RN if ordered Incentive Spirometry q2hr WA @ bedside if ordered	Continue oxygen therapy per protocol, evaluate for discontinuation of O2 RT to convert to MDI prn Incentive Spirometry q2hr WA @ bedside if ordered
Additional Daily Lab: Order for CareMap entered into computer: initial (RN/US) _____	**Medications/IV**	Initial Antibiotic STAT (to be administered within one hour of order) IV Fluids	Cont Abx–consider oral switch Evaluate and change to HL or DC IV if applicable
	Nutrition	Diet as tolerated Encourage oral fluids if appropriate	Diet as tolerated Encourage oral fluids if appropriate Goal: 3-4 glasses H$_2$O if not fluid restricted
Other Pertinent Information:	**Activity/Safety**	Activity as tolerated (Encourage up in chair for meals) Fall prevention program initiated if appropriate	Activity as tolerated (Encourage up in chair for meals) Goal: Ambulate 25-50ft x 2
	Patient/Family Education	Assess knowledge level concerning disease process and medication Teach use of MDI if applicable	Reasses patient's ability to use MDI Reinforce med education, activity and follow-up
Family Spokesperson:	**Discharge Planning**	RN/SW initiates discharge planning	Interview patient/family re: discharge planning
Emergency Phone #:	**Psychosocial/Emotional/ Spiritual**	Explain procedures Encourage verbalization of feelings	Notify Chaplain to visit if requested
_____	**CMAP # 114**		

Norman Regional Hospital CareMap®
Community Acquired Pneumonia
CareMap® Summary

Copyright©2000 Norman Regional Hospital

Figure 26-3, cont'd Example of a critical pathway for pneumonia. (From Norman Regional Hospital CareMap®, Community Acquired Pneumonia. Copyright 2000, Norman Regional Hospital. Used with the permission of Norman Regional Hospital, Norman, Okla.)

> ✳ **BOX 26-4 Example of Variance Documentation**
>
> A 56-year-old client is on a surgical unit 1 day after cholecystectomy. He is beginning to have an elevated temperature, his breath sounds are decreased bilaterally in the bases of both lobes of the lungs, and he is slightly confused. Ordinarily, 1 day after surgery the client should be afebrile with lungs clear. The following is an example of the variance documentation for this client.
>
> 9/23/05 1000
>
> Breath sounds diminished bilaterally at the bases. T, 100.4; P, 92; R, 28/min; oxygen sat, 84%. Daughter states he is "confused" and did not recognize her when she arrived a few minutes ago. Oxygen started at 2 L per standing orders. Will monitor pulse oximetry and vital signs every 15 minutes. Physician notified of change in status. Daughter at bedside.
> (signature)

> ✳ **BOX 26-5 Benefits of Using a Flow Sheet**
>
> - Information is accessible to all members of the health care team.
> - Decreases time spent on writing a narrative note.
> - Information is current.
> - Decreases errors resulting from transfer of information.
> - Team members can quickly see trends over time.

client's status. Critical care and acute care units commonly use flow sheets for all types of physiological data.

Client Care Summary or Kardex

Many hospitals now have computerized systems that provide basic, summative information in the form of a client care summary. This is printed out for each client during each shift. Nurses continually update the summary, which provides a current detailed list of orders, treatment, and diagnostic testing. In some settings a **Kardex,** a portable "flip-over" file or notebook, is kept at the nurses' station. Most Kardex forms have an activity and treatment section and a nursing care plan section that organize information for quick reference as nurses give change-of-shift reports or make walking rounds. An updated Kardex eliminates the need for repeated referral to the chart for routine information throughout the day. In many institutions nurses make Kardex entries in pencil because of the need for frequent revisions as the client's needs change. In settings in which the Kardex is a permanent part of the client's record, nurses make entries in ink. The client care summary or Kardex includes the following information:

- Basic demographic data (e.g., age, religion)
- HIPAA code word
- Physician's or health care provider's name
- Primary medical diagnosis
- Medical and surgical history
- Current treatment orders from health care provider to be carried out by the nurse (e.g., dressing changes, ambulation, glucose monitoring)
- Nursing care plan
- Nursing orders (e.g., education sessions, symptom relief measures, counseling)
- Scheduled tests and procedures
- Safety precautions to be used in the client's care
- Factors related to activities of daily living
- Nearest relative/guardian or person to contact in an emergency
- Emergency code status
- Allergies

Acuity Records

Acuity records offer a way to determine the hours of care and staff required for a given group of clients. A client's acuity level is based on the type and number of nursing interventions (e.g., intravenous [IV] therapy, wound care, or ambulation assistance) required over a 24-hour period. The acuity level rates clients in comparison with one another. For example, an acuity system might rate bathing clients from 1 to 5 (1 is totally dependent, and 5 is independent). A client returning from surgery requiring frequent monitoring and extensive care may be listed with an acuity level of 1, compared with another client awaiting discharge after a successful recovery from surgery who has an acuity level of 5. Accurate acuity ratings justify overtime and the number and qualifications of staff needed to safely care for clients. The client-to-staff ratios established for a unit depend on a composite gathering of 24-hour acuity data for each client receiving care.

Standardized Care Plans

Many institutions have made documentation easier for nurses with **standardized care plans.** The plans, based on the institution's standards of nursing practice, are preprinted, established guidelines that are used to care for clients who have similar health problems. After completing a nursing assessment, the staff nurse identifies the standard care plans that are appropriate for the client and places the plans in the client's medical record. The nurse modifies standardized plans in ink to individualize the therapies. Most standardized care plans also allow the nurse to write in specific goals or desired outcomes of care and the dates by which these outcomes should be achieved.

One advantage of standardized care plans is establishment of clinically sound standards of care for similar groups of clients. These standards are useful when conducting quality improvement audits. Another advantage is education. Nurses learn to recognize the accepted requirements of care for clients. The standardized care plans can also improve continuity of care among professional nurses.

The use of standardized care plans is controversial. The major disadvantage is the risk that the standardized plans inhibit nurses' identification of unique, individualized therapies for clients. When standardized care plans are used in a health care facility, the nurse remains responsible for an individualized approach to care. Standardized care plans cannot replace the nurse's professional judgment and decision making. In addition, care plans need to be updated on a regular basis to ensure that content is current and appropriate.

Discharge Summary Forms

It is important to prepare clients for an effective, timely discharge from a health care institution. A prospective payment system based on DRGs encourages health care institutions to be more efficient and to discharge clients as soon as possible. The earlier a client is discharged, the more likely it is that a hospital will be fully reimbursed. However, it is important to ensure that a client's

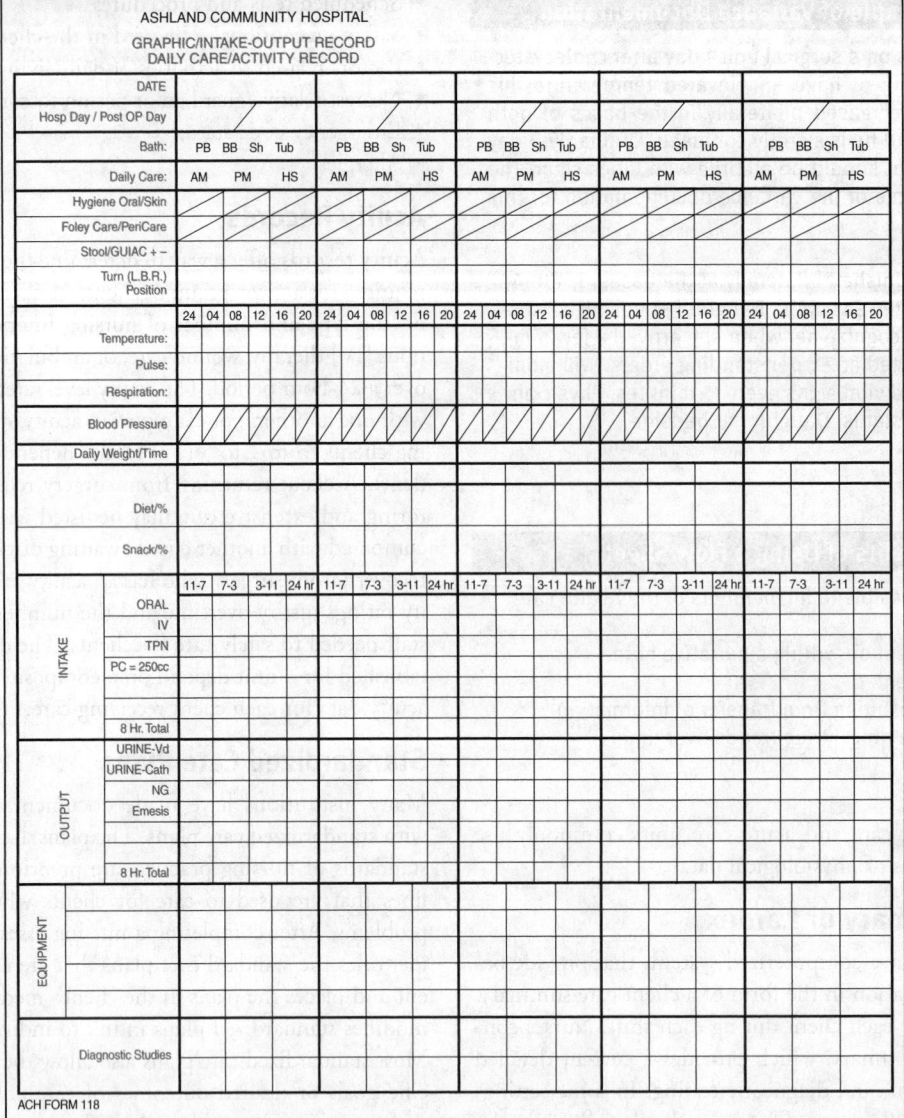

Figure 26-4 Nursing assessment flow sheet. (Courtesy Ashland Community Hospital, Ashland, Ore.)

BOX 26-6   Discharge Summary Information

- Use clear, concise descriptions in client's own language.
- Provide step-by-step description of how to perform a procedure (e.g., home medication administration). Reinforce explanation with printed instructions.
- Identify precautions to follow when performing self-care or administering medications.
- Review signs and symptoms of complications that should be reported to a physician or other health care provider.
- List names and phone numbers of health care providers and community resources that the client can contact.
- Identify any unresolved problem, including plans for follow-up and continuous treatment.
- List actual time of discharge, mode of transportation, and who accompanied the client.

discharge results in desirable outcomes. Multidisciplinary discharge planning ensures that a client leaves the hospital in a timely manner with the necessary resources (Box 26-6).

Ideally discharge planning begins at admission. Nurses revise the plan of care as the client's condition changes. There needs to be evidence of the involvement of the client and family members in the discharge planning process so that the client and family have the necessary information and resources to return home. TJC (2007) has standards for client education necessary for effective discharge planning:

- Instruction in potential food-drug interactions, nutrition intervention, and modified diets
- Rehabilitation techniques to support adaptation to and/or functional independence in the environment
- Access to available community resources
- Under what circumstances clients should obtain further treatment or follow-up care
- Methods of obtaining follow-up care

- The client's and family's responsibilities in the client's care
- Medication instructions, including when to take each medication and why, the dose, the route, precautions, and possible adverse reactions, and when and how to get prescriptions refilled.

In addition to TJC standards, a common standard in nursing practice is to educate clients about the nature of their disease process, its likely progress, and the signs and symptoms of complications. When a client is discharged from inpatient care, various members of the health care team prepare a discharge summary. The summary goes to the client or family or to the home care, rehabilitation, or long-term care agency (TJC, 2006-2007). Discharge summary forms (Figure 26-5) make the summary concise and instructive. A summary form emphasizes previous learning by the client and family and the care that should be continued in any restorative care setting. When given directly to clients, the form may be attached to pamphlets or teaching brochures.

Home Care Documentation

The home care business continues to grow with shorter hospitalizations and larger numbers of older adults requiring home care services. Medicare has specific guidelines for establishing eligibility for home care reimbursement. Documentation in the home care system has different implications than in other areas of nursing. One primary difference is that the client and family witness the majority of care rather than the nurse. Nurses must have astute assessment skills to gather the needed information about changes in the client's health care status. In addition, documentation systems need to provide the entire health care team with the necessary information to be able to work together effectively (Box 26-7). The documentation is both the quality control and the justification for reimbursement from Medicare, Medicaid, or private insurance companies. Nurses need to document all their services for payment (e.g., direct skilled care, client instructions, skilled observation, and evaluation visits) (TJC, 2006-2007).

Some parts of the record are needed in the home with the client; other information is needed in an office setting. Thus duplication of documentation is necessary, or agency policies are needed regarding what forms nurses need to leave at their office versus what forms need to be taken into the homes. Computerized client records are evolving to address these different needs. With the use of modems and laptop computers it is becoming possible for the records to be available in multiple locations, which allows greater access to information about the multidisciplinary needs that are often present in home care.

Long-Term Health Care Documentation

An increasing number of older adults require care in long-term health care facilities. Because many individuals will live in this setting for the rest of their lives, they are referred to as **residents** rather than clients. In long-term care, governmental agencies are instrumental in determining the standards and policies for documentation. The Omnibus Budget Reconciliation Act of 1987 includes extremely significant Medicare and Medicaid legislation for long-term care documentation. Each resident is viewed holistically by using the Resident Assessment Instrument (RAI). A registered nurse who has clinical competence, observational skills, and assessment expertise gathers the RAI. The goal is a system of clinical documentation that improves care for residents and increases reimbursement for that care (Boroughs, 1999).

In addition, the department of health in each state governs the frequency of written nursing records of the residents in long-term care facilities. Because residents are often stable, daily documentation is done using flow sheets. Assessments done several times a day in the acute care setting may be required only weekly or monthly in the long-term care setting.

Long-term care agencies also may have skilled care units where clients require increased levels of care in response to mandates for shorter hospital stays. Multidisciplinary communication among such health care providers as nurses, social workers, recreational therapists, and dietitians is essential in these settings as well. The fiscal support for long-term care residents hinges on the justification of nursing care as demonstrated in documentation of the services rendered.

Reporting

Nurses communicate information about clients so that all team members can make appropriate decisions about their care. It is important that any form of verbal report be timely, accurate, and relevant. Nurses make four types of reports, including change-of-shift reports, telephone reports, transfer reports, and incident reports.

Change-of-Shift Reports

At the end of each shift nurses report information about their assigned clients to the nurses working on the next shift. The report provides continuity of care among nurses who are caring for a client. For example, if one nurse finds a certain pain-relief measure effective for a client, it is important that the information be relayed to the next nurse caring for the client so that pain-control interventions can be continued.

Nurses give a **change-of-shift report** orally in person, by audiotape recording, or during "walking-planning" rounds at each client's bedside. Oral reports are given in conference rooms, with staff members from both shifts participating. An advantage of oral reports is that they allow staff members to ask questions or clarify explanations. When nurses make rounds, the client and family members also have the opportunity to participate in any decisions. The nurses can see the client together to perform needed assessments, evaluate progress, and discuss the interventions best suited to the client's needs. An audiotape report is given by the nurse who has completed care for the client and is left for the nurse on the next shift to review. Taped reports improve efficiency by taping report before the end of the shift when time is available and by avoiding social conversations between peers. It is essential to schedule an opportunity for the oncoming nurses to ask questions for clarification after listening to the taped report.

Text continued on page 402

The Kingston Hospital

Interdisciplinary Discharge Instructions
(Physician to complete items 1-5)

Date:_____   Time:_____

Addressograph

Discharge to:
- ❏ Skilled Nursing   ❏ Home
- ❏ Acute Rehab   ❏ Home with home health   ❏ Adult home

1. Diet
- ❏ No restrictions ❏ Low cholesterol   ❏ Fluid restrictions_____ oz/day ❏ Cardiac   ❏ Diabetic
- ❏ Low sodium_____ gm/day ❏ Potassium supplement ❏ Special (copy given to patient): _____

2. Activity (check all that apply)
- ❏ Resume normal activities as tolerated   ❏ May walk ____feet   ❏ Limit lifting to _____lbs
- ❏ Resume sexual activity in____days   ❏ May not drive for:_____ days ❏ Limit pushing, pulling, straining
- ❏ May not shower for:_____ days   ❏ May climb _____ stairs_____ times per day
- May walk with: ❏ crutches ❏ walker ❏ wheelchair ❏ bed rest ❏ Other: _____

3. Medications   IMPORTANT: Remember to check expiration dates on all medications and discard if outdated

CONSIDER FOR CARDIAC PATIENT				
*ASPIRIN	*ACE INHIBITOR	*BETA BLOCKER	*STATIN THERAPY	
Medication and Dose	Purpose	Time to be taken	Comments/ Special Instructions (with food, etc.)	Med Info Given to Pt (RN to initial each-N/A if no sheet to provide)
1				
2				
3				
4				
5				
6				
7				
8				
9				
10				
11				
12				
13				
14				

Take no medications other than those listed. If you have any questions concerning your medications call your primary physician.
- ❏ Patient / support person understands medication instructions _____ (initial)
- ❏ Patient / support person understands importance of getting medications filled. ❏ Prescription changes have been made on this admission

4. Follow up Appointment
- ❏ Call Dr._____ at phone #:_____ to schedule follow up appointment.
- ❏ Call Dr._____ at phone #:_____ to schedule follow up appointment.
- ❏ Follow up appointment scheduled with Dr._____ on_____ at _____am/pm.

5. Wound care
- ❏ Keep wound clean/dry ❏ N/A ❏ Other:_____

Physician Signature_____   Date_____

Page 1 of 2

Revised 6/22/2006

Figure 26-5 Interdisciplinary discharge summary form. (Courtesy Kingston Hospital, Kingston, NY.)

The Kingston Hospital
Interdisciplinary Discharge Instructions

Check **all** areas that apply

6. <u>Nursing</u> *(Be sure patient medications are returned to patient upon discharge, as appropriate)*
   - ❏ Diagnosis specific discharge instructions given to patient (specify dx):_____
   - ❏ **CHF patients**: Weigh yourself every morning at the same time after you empty your bladder. Use the same scale and wear the same amount of clothes. Keep a daily log of your weight and bring it to your doctor appointment. Call your doctor if you have weight gain of 2-4 lbs. over 1-3 days. CHF Booklet given to patient/family.
   - ❏ **AMI patients**: MI booklet provided to patient/family.
   - ❏ **Pneumonia patients**: Tips on Pneumonia Care booklet provided to patient/family.
   - ❏ **Medical Oncology** (Discharge instructions given to patients/family)
7. <u>Smoking</u>   ❏ Patient does not smoke
   - ❏ Patient currently smokes or has quit in the past 12 months.   ❏ If YES, smoking cessation advice/counseling provided to patient
8. <u>Case Management</u>
   - ❏ No needs identified
   - ❏ Case Manager_____
   - ❏ Home health (agency):_____
        - phone:_____
        - ❏ RN ❏ OT ❏ PT ❏ Other:_____
   - ❏ Equipment: ❏ Cane ❏ Commode ❏ Walker ❏ Wheelchair ❏ Hospital bed ❏ Lifeline
   - ❏ Other:_____
        - ❏ Equipment delivered to hospital (specify)_____ To home (specify):_____
        - ❏ You will be contacted by (agency):_____
        - phone:_____
   - ❏ Respiratory services (specify): ❏ Oxygen   ❏ Nebulizers   ❏Other_____
        - ❏ You will be contacted by (agency):_____
        - phone:_____
   Other:_____

Additional Notes (for all disciplines):
_____
_____
_____
_____
_____
_____
_____

<u>**If you have any questions after discharge from the hospital, please call your physician.**</u>

I have received a copy of these discharge instructions and they have been explained to me. I understand that these instructions are necessary for my continuing medical care after I leave the hospital. Also, I give the hospital permission to release my patient information to referral agencies, as necessary to provide proper service, equipment and treatment.

_____
Patient/representative Signature
Date_____

_____
Nurse Signature
Time_____

Page 2 of 2

Revised 6/22/2006

Figure 26-5, cont'd Interdisciplinary discharge summary form. (Courtesy Kingston Hospital, Kingston, NY.)

✳ BOX 26-7 **Home Care Forms for Documentation**

The usual forms used to document home care include the following:

- Client assessment
- Referral source information/intake form
- Discipline-specific care plans
- Physician's plan of treatment
- Medication sheet
- Clinical progress notes
- Miscellaneous (conference notes, verbal order forms, telephone calls)
- Discharge summary
- Reports to third-party payers

Modified from Iyer PW, Camp NH: *Nursing documentation: a nursing process approach*, St. Louis, 1999, Mosby.

Because nurses have many responsibilities, it is important to a conduct a change-of-shift report quickly and efficiently (Table 26-4). An effective report describes each client's health status and lets staff on the next shift know what care the clients will require. A change-of-shift report should *not* simply be the reading of documented information. Instead, nurses review significant information about clients (e.g., the condition of wounds or episodes of chest pain) to provide a baseline for comparison during the next shift. Data about clients need to be objective, current, and concise.

An organized report follows a logical sequence. To prepare for a report, gather information from work sheets, the client's records, and the client's care plan. A systematic approach such as using the nursing process can provide staff with critical information that is needed to continue care. The following is an example of a change-of-shift report:

Background information: *Cy Tolan in bed 4, a 32-year-old client of Dr. Lang, is scheduled for a colon resection this morning. He has had ulcerative colitis for 2 years with recent bouts of frank bleeding in stools. He was admitted last night with slight abdominal discomfort. This is his first experience with surgery. He knows he may require a colostomy. He has been NPO since midnight.*

Assessment: *Mr. Tolan expressed difficulty falling asleep last night. He had several questions about surgery. Early in the night he called for assistance several times.*

Nursing diagnosis: *His chief concerns are anxiety related to inexperience with surgery and risk for body image disturbance.*

Teaching plan: *He asks appropriate questions about surgery. Staff on evenings explained postoperative routines. I reinforced information with him early in the night. He stated that he feels less anxious now that he knows more what to expect.*

Treatments: *A cleansing enema was administered until clear at 2100; no blood was noted in the return. He complained of some abdominal cramping immediately afterward, and that subsided within an hour. He received Restoril 15 mg PO at 2100, and I gave him a back rub. When he awakened at 0630, he stated he slept OK.*

Family information: *His wife remained with him last evening until the end of visiting hours. She has returned and is in the room this morning.*

Discharge plan: *Mr. Tolan is a very active person at home. He participates in strenuous sports such as tennis, basketball, and swimming, and for this reason Mrs. Tolan is concerned about how he might react to a colostomy. I suggest making a referral to the enterostomal therapist early, if the colostomy is performed.*

Priority needs: *Right now, Mr. Tolan is relaxing in his room. The operative permit has been signed. All preoperative procedures have been completed except for his preop medications, due on call to the operating room.*

A professional demeanor is essential when you give a report about clients or family members. It is often necessary to describe the interactions among clients, nurses, and family members in behavioral terms. Avoid using judgmental language such as *uncooperative, difficult,* or *bad* when describing such behaviors. In many settings nursing assistive personnel participate in the change-of-shift report. Nursing assistive personnel are part of the team and can contribute more when they also know a client's condition and the nursing team's priorities in care. The registered professional nurse (RN) uses the report to emphasize to nursing assistive personnel the tasks to be done.

Telephone Reports

Nurses inform physicians or other health care providers of changes in a client's condition and communicate information to nurses on other units about client transfer. The laboratory staff or a radiologist may report results of diagnostic tests. Persons involved with a telephone report also must provide clear, accurate, and concise information. In many cases information in a telephone report is documented when significant events or changes in a client's condition have occurred. To document a phone call, the nurse includes when the call was made, who made it (if other than the writer of the information), who was called, to whom information was given, what information was given, and what information was received, for example, "At 1022 called Dr. Morgan's office; S. Thomas, RN, will inform Dr. Morgan that Mr. Rush's STAT potassium level drawn at 0800 was 3.2. C. Towns, RN."

Telephone or Verbal Orders

A telephone order (TO) involves a physician's or health care provider's stating a prescribed therapy over the phone to a registered nurse. A verbal order (VO) may be accepted when there is no opportunity for a physician or health care provider to write the order, as in emergency situations. TJC's 2007 National Patient Safety Goals requires nurses to verify verbal or telephone orders by having the person receiving the information record or read back the complete order (www.jointcommission.org). The registered nurse is responsible for writing the order on the physician's or other health care provider's order sheet in the client's permanent record and signs it. An example follows: "1/16/2004: 1920 acetaminophen 650 mg PO, 1 tab now and q4h prn. TO. Dr. Reiss/Carol Towns, RN." The physician or other health care provider later verifies the telephone order legally by signing it within a set time period (e.g., 24 hours). Physicians and other health care providers frequently give telephone orders at night or during an emergency; telephone orders need to be used only when absolutely necessary. In some situations it may be prudent to have a second person listen to telephone orders. Check agency policy. Box 26-8 provides some guidelines to prevent errors in receiving telephone and verbal orders.

✳ **TABLE 26-4 Comparison of Do's and Don'ts of Change-of-Shift Report**

Do's	Don'ts
Provide only essential background information about client (i.e., name, gender, medical diagnosis, and history).	Don't review all routine care procedures or tasks (e.g., bathing, scheduled changes).
Identify client's nursing diagnoses or health care problems and their related causes.	Don't review all biographical information already available in written form.
Describe objective measurements or observations about client's condition and response to health problem: emphasize recent changes.	Don't use critical comments about client's behavior, such as "Mrs. Wills is so demanding."
Share significant information about family members as it relates to client's problems.	Don't make assumptions about relationships between family members.
Continuously review ongoing discharge plan (e.g., need for resources, client's level of preparation to go home).	Don't engage in idle gossip.
Relay significant changes to staff in the way therapies are to be given (e.g., different position for pain relief, new medication).	Don't describe basic steps of a procedure.
Describe instructions given in teaching plan and client's response.	Don't explain detailed content unless staff members ask for clarification.
Evaluate results of nursing or medical care measures (e.g., effect of back rub or analgesic administration).	Don't simply describe results as "good" or "poor." Be specific.
Be clear about priorities to which oncoming staff must attend.	Don't force oncoming staff to guess what to do first.

✳ **BOX 26-8 Guidelines for Telephone Orders and Verbal Orders**

- Clearly determine the client's name, room number, and diagnosis.
- Repeat any prescribed orders back to the physician or health care provider.
- Use clarification questions to avoid misunderstandings.
- Write TO (telephone order) or VO (verbal order), including date and time, name of client, the complete order; and sign the name of the physician or health care provider and nurse.
- Follow agency policies; some institutions require telephone (and verbal) orders to be reviewed and signed by two nurses.
- The physician or health care provider must cosign the order within the time frame required by the institution (usually 24 hours).

Transfer Reports

Clients often transfer from one unit to another to receive different levels of care. For example, clients transfer from an intensive care unit or the recovery room to general nursing units when the client no longer requires such intense monitoring. To promote continuity of care, you may give **transfer reports** by phone or in person. When giving a transfer report, include the following information:

1. Client's name, age, primary physician or health care provider, and medical diagnosis
2. Summary of progress up to the time of transfer
3. Current health status (physical and psychosocial)
4. Allergies
5. Emergency code status
6. Family support
7. Current nursing diagnoses or problem and care plan
8. Any critical assessments or interventions to be completed shortly after transfer (helps receiving nurse to establish priorities of care)
9. Need for any special equipment, such as isolation equipment, suction equipment, or traction

After completion of the transfer report, the receiving nurse needs an opportunity to ask questions about the client's status. In some cases written documentation must include a record of information reported.

Incident or Occurrence Reports

An incident is any event that is not consistent with the routine operation of a health care unit or routine care of a client. Examples of incidents include client falls, needle-stick injuries, a visitor having symptoms of illness, medication administration errors, accidental omission of ordered therapies, and circumstances that led to injury or a risk for client injury. Analysis of incident reports helps with the identification of trends in systems and unit operations that provide justification for changes in policies and procedures or for in-service seminars. **Incident (or occurrence) reports** are an important part of a unit's quality improvement program (see Chapter 5).

Nursing Informatics

All nurses deal with data, information, and knowledge (Hebda and others, 2005). As explained in the previous section on documentation, it is important that nurses know how to record and report data and information and to critically think and apply knowledge to use information for client care. Data include numbers, characters, or facts that are collected according to a perceived need for analysis and possible action. An example is a nurse's observation of a wound's edges, color of drainage, and measurement of the wound's length. Information is data that has been interpreted (Hebda and others, 2005). When the nurse examines the data describing the condition of the wound over time, a pattern develops showing that the wound is not healing (information). Knowledge is the synthesis of information derived from several sources to produce a single concept (Hebda and others, 2005). Based on evidence available in the scientific literature, the nurse applies knowledge of wound care principles and intervenes to manage the client's wound.

It is a challenge in health care settings to easily access data and information about clients. This is especially the case when information is recorded manually on printed forms. For example, a nurse working in risk management who is interested in investigating client falls has to review page by page the records of clients who have fallen to identify the common factors contributing to falls. Remember, three important purposes of medical records are communication, education, and research. When a health care organization relies on handwritten client records, locating, summarizing, and comparing information is slow and difficult. Thus it becomes even more difficult to access information in a timely manner to provide or improve client care. It also becomes difficult to locate data sources for research purposes. Furthermore, when data about clients must be compared manually, it is more difficult to see the trends that help educate staff about client care. The Institute of Medicine (2001) recognized that the only way to use data and information to improve care delivery, as well as quality improvement, research, and education, is through information technology.

Information technology (IT) refers to the management and processing of information, generally with the assistance of computers (Hebda and others, 2005). Advances in technology allow health care agencies to move from paper-based medical records to computer-based records. More and more health care agencies are adopting computerized information systems to support and enhance health care delivery.

A health care information system (HIS) is a group of systems used within a health care enterprise that support and enhance health care (Hebda and others, 2005). A HIS consists of two majors types of information systems: clinical information systems (CIS) and administrative information systems. Together, the two systems operate to make the entry and communication of data and information more efficient. You will find that any single health care agency will use one or several of the CIS and administrative information systems. For example, a small community hospital uses a nursing information system (NIS), an order entry system, and laboratory, radiology, and pharmacy systems to coordinate their core client care services. A nurse working in such a hospital documents nursing care on a computer, locates and reviews laboratory test results, orders sterile supplies, and enters health care provider orders for x-ray films and clients' medications.

Many hospitals now use nursing information systems to support the documentation of nursing process activities and offer resources for managing nursing care delivery (Figure 26-6). A reliable NIS is the product of nursing informatics. **Nursing informatics** is defined by the American Nurses Association (2001) as a specialty that integrates nursing science, computer science, and information science to manage and communicate data, information, and knowledge in nursing practice. Nursing informatics facilitates the integration of data, information, and knowledge to support clients, nurses, and other providers in decision making in all roles and settings. The application of nursing informatics results in an efficient and effective nursing information system. An expertly designed clinical information system based on nursing informatics integrates and supports clinical judgments with up-to-date evidence-based practice (Healthcare Information and Management Systems Society [HIMSS] NI Awareness Task Force, 2007). An effective nursing information system meets two goals. First, it supports the way that nurses function and work by providing nurses the flexibility to use the system to view data and

collect information, provide client care, and document the client's condition and care provided. Secondly, it supports and enhances nursing practice through improved access to information and clinical decision-making tools (Hebda and others, 2005).

In the fast-paced world of nursing, nursing informatics plays an important role in helping nurses make decisions more rapidly and more accurately. Examples of this include streamlining documentation, integrating safety measures online, and participating in new, innovative technologies such as medication safety distribution systems, telemedicine, privacy protection programs, and wireless applications (Bailey, 2006). Nursing informatics has revolutionized how health care providers locate or mine client data to look for trends and patterns between client outcomes and care provided by nurses. New technologies also allow nurses to study the impact of systems on error reduction and client safety. Through the application of nursing informatics, practical applications of technology enhance bedside care and education.

Numerous groups, including the ANA (2001) and the PEW Health Professions Commission (1998), have recommended that all nurses acquire a minimal level of awareness and competence in informatics and use of information technology. Competence in informatics is not the same as computer competency. To become competent in informatics you must be able to use evolving methods of discovering, retrieving, and using information in your practice (Hebda, 2005). This means that you learn to recognize when information is needed and have the skills to find, evaluate, and use needed information effectively. The evidence-based practice chapter in this text describes a model to acquire, critique, and apply scientific evidence from literature databases (see Chapter 5). As a nurse, you must also know how to use clinical databases within your institution and apply the information so that you can deliver high-quality, appropriate client care.

Nursing Information Systems

A good information system, which incorporates principles of nursing informatics, supports the work you do. As a nurse, you want to be able to easily access a computer program, review the client's medical history and physician or other health care provider orders, and then go to the client's bedside to conduct a comprehensive assessment. Once you have completed the assessment, you enter data into the computer terminal at the client's bedside and develop a plan of care from the information gathered. This allows you to quickly share the plan of care with the client. Periodically, you will return to the computer to check on laboratory test results and document the therapies you administer. The computer screens and optional pop-up windows make it easy to locate information, enter and compare data, and make changes.

Nursing information systems basically have two designs. The nursing process design is the most traditional. It organizes documentation within well-established formats, such as admission and postoperative assessments, problem lists, care plans, discharge planning instructions, and intervention lists or notes. In the more advanced systems, standardized nursing languages such as the NANDA International nursing diagnoses, the Nursing Interventions Classification (NIC), and the Nursing Outcomes Classification (NOC) are incorporated into the software programs. For example, the documentation of nursing admis-

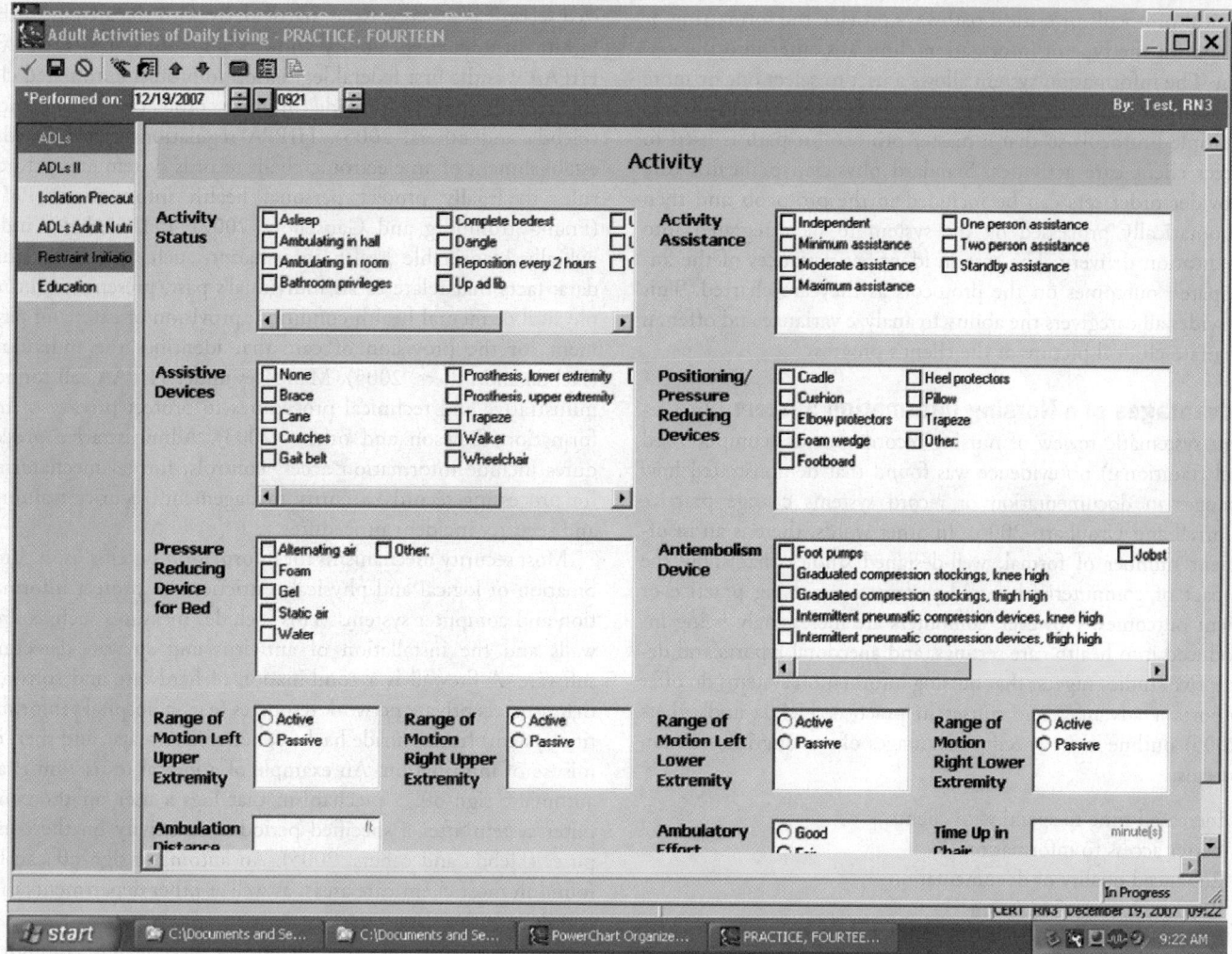

Figure 26-6 Example of a screen for nursing assessment of activity, part of a clinical information system program.

sion assessment findings relies on a menu-driven approach. A **menu** lists related commands that the nurse selects from the computer screen to complete the client assessment. The commands direct the nurse through the various assessment categories, such as a client's medication history, nutritional status, psychosocial history, and review of systems. After a nurse enters assessment data into a computer, a program will offer menu lists for the selection of nursing diagnoses and interventions, allowing the nurse to individualize a client's care plan. Another example is a program for discharge instructions. After a nurse enters the necessary information for a client's discharge instructions, follow-up appointments, and medication information, the system generates printed copies of the instructions for nurses to review and give to clients on discharge. A copy is stored in the client's record and is available for home care staff, as well as the client's health care provider.

The nursing process design also includes formats for the following:

- Generation of a nursing work list that indicates routine scheduled activities related to the care of each client

- Documentation of routine aspects of client care, such as hygiene, positioning, fluid intake and output, wound care measures, and blood glucose measurements
- Progress note entries using narrative notes, charting by exception, and flow sheet charting
- Documentation of medication administration (see Chapter 35)

One of the challenges of computerized documentation is inclusion of the nursing process (Ammenwerth and others, 2001). Successful implementation of computer-based nursing process documentation requires a high acceptance of the nursing process, careful preparation of predefined care plans, organizational preparation, and inclusion of future users, including bedside nurses, in the development process. It is also essential to have sufficient technical equipment with integration into the hospital information system.

The second design model for a nursing information system is the protocol or critical pathway design (Hebda and others, 2005). This designs offers a multidisciplinary format to managing information. All health care providers use a protocol system to document the care they provide clients. Evidence-based clinical protocols or critical pathways provide the formatting or design for the type of information clinicians enter into the system. The information system allows a user to select one or more appropriate protocols for a client. An advanced system merges multiple protocols so that a master protocol or path is used to direct client care activities. Standard physician or health care provider order sets can be included in the protocols and then automatically processed by the system to be integrated into medication delivery. The system identifies variances of the anticipated outcomes on the protocols as they are charted. This provides all caregivers the ability to analyze variance and offer an accurate clinical picture of the client's progress.

Advantages of a Nursing Information System.
In a recent systematic review of nursing record systems (computerized and traditional) no evidence was found that demonstrated how changes in documentation or record systems change practice (Currell and Urquhart, 2006). In other words, there is an insufficient number of formal, well-designed studies that show the impact of computerized record systems on nursing practice or client outcomes. However, computers are increasingly being introduced into health care settings, and anecdotal reports and descriptive studies suggest that nursing information systems do offer important advantages to nurses in practice. Hebda and others (2005) outline some specific advantages of nursing information systems:

- Increased time to spend with clients
- Better access to information
- Enhanced quality of documentation
- Reduced errors of omission
- Reduced hospital costs
- Increased nurse job satisfaction
- Compliance with TJC and other accrediting agencies
- Development of a common clinical database

The transition to computerized documentation presents both opportunities and challenges to nurses and nurse managers. A barrier to the successful implementation of a clinical information system is the reluctance on the part of some nurses and other clinical staff to accept technological advances. Often clinicians fail to understand how technology can improve the way they deliver care and enhance clinical decision processes. The successful implementation of a nursing information system requires preparation, involvement, and commitment of the entire nursing staff. The transition from paper to computer presents challenges for nursing staff. There are available tools for transforming existing documents into interactive interdisciplinary computerized forms (Wenzel, 2002). Research shows that during the transition when charting must be done on both paper and the computer, the amount of time spent on documentation is not excessive (Korst, 2003).

Security Mechanisms.
Computerized documentation has legal risks. Any given person could theoretically access a computer station within a health care agency and gain information on almost any client. Protection of information and computer systems is a top priority. Confidentiality of access to computerized records is a major issue, particularly with the advent of the Health Insurance Portability and Accountability Act (HIPAA). HIPAA was the first federal legislation to protect automated client records and to provide uniform protection nationwide (Hebda and others, 2005). HIPPA regulations called for the establishment of an electronic client records system and privacy rules to legally protect personal health information (PHI) (Frank-Stromborg and Ganschow, 2002). PHI includes individually identifiable health information such as demographic data; facts that relate to an individual's past, present, or future physical or mental health condition; provision of care; and payment for the provision of care that identifies the individual (Hebda and others, 2005). Mandates under HIPAA call for administrative and technical procedures to protect privacy of information (Lawson and others, 2003). Administrative procedures include information access controls, formal mechanisms for processing records, security management, security training, and security incident procedures.

Most security mechanisms for information systems use a combination of logical and physical restrictions to protect information and computer systems. This includes measures such as firewalls and the installation of antivirus and spyware-detection software. A firewall is a combination of hardware and software that protects private network resources (e.g., a hospital's information system) from outside hackers, network damage, and theft or misuse of information. An example of a logical restriction is an automatic sign-off, a mechanism that logs a user off the computer system after a specified period of inactivity on the computer (Hebda and others, 2005). An automatic sign-off can be found in most client care areas, as well as other departments that handle sensitive data.

Physical security measures include the placement of computers or file servers in restricted areas. This form of security may have limited benefit, especially if an organization uses mobile wireless devices such as notebooks, tablet personal computers (PCs), and personal digital assistants (PDAs). These devices can easily be misplaced or lost, falling into the wrong hands. An organization may use motion detectors or alarms with these devices to help prevent theft.

A familiar and inexpensive technology for authenticating access to automated records is the use of access codes and passwords (Fratto, 2002). A **password** is a collection of alphanumeric characters that a user types into the computer before accessing a program. A user is usually required to enter a password after the entry and acceptance of an access code or user name. A password does not appear on the computer screen when it is typed, nor should it be known to anyone but the user and information systems (IS) administrators (Hebda and others, 2005). Strong passwords use combinations of letters, numbers, and symbols that are not easily guessed. When using a health care agency computer system, it is essential that you not share your computer password, under any circumstances, with anyone. A good system requires frequent and random changes in personal passwords to prevent unauthorized persons from tampering with records. In addition, most staff have access only to clients in their work area. Select staff (e.g., administrators or risk managers) may be given authority to access all client records.

Handling and Disposal of Information.

After reading the first section of this chapter, it is clear how important it is to keep medical records confidential. However, it is equally important to safeguard the information that is printed from the record or extracted for report purposes. For example, a nurse prints a copy of a nursing activities work list to use as a day planner while administering care to clients. The nurse refers to information on the list and writes handwritten notes to later enter into the computer. Information on the list is considered to be PHI and must be kept confidential and not left out for view by unauthorized persons. The nurse destroys anything that is printed when the printed information is no longer needed.

The printing and faxing of information from a client's record is a primary source for the unauthorized release of information. All papers containing PHI (e.g., Social Security number, date of birth or age, client's name or address) must be destroyed. Most agencies have shredders or locked receptacles for shredding and later incineration. Nurses also work in settings where they are responsible for erasing computer files from the hard drive containing calendars, surgery or diagnostic procedure schedules, or other daily records that contain PHI (Hebda and others, 2005). Be sure you know the disposal policies for records in the institution where you work.

An institution needs to have sound policies for the use of fax machines, specifically what types of information can be sent and to which departments. Information that you send by fax should not exceed that requested or required for immediate clinical needs. The following are some steps to take to enhance fax security (Hebda and others, 2005):

- Confirm that fax numbers are correct before sending, to be sure you direct information properly.
- Use a cover sheet, especially if a fax machine serves a number of different users.
- Authenticate at both ends of the transmission before data transmission to verify the source and destination are correct.
- Use programmed speed-dial keys to eliminate the chance of a dialing error and misdirected information.
- Place fax machines in a secure area.
- Limit machine access to designated individuals.
- Log fax transmissions. This feature is often available electronically on the machine.

Clinical Information Systems

Any clinician, including nurses, physicians, pharmacists, social workers, and therapists, will use programs available on a CIS. These programs include monitoring systems, order entry systems, and laboratory, radiology, and pharmacy systems. A monitoring system includes devices that automatically monitor and record biometric measurements (e.g., vital signs, oxygen saturation, cardiac index, and stroke volume) in critical care and specialty areas. The devices electronically send measurements direct to the nursing documentation system.

Order entry systems allow nurses to order supplies and services from another department. An example is the ability to order sterile supplies from the central supply processing department. This eliminates written order forms and expedites the delivery of needed supplies to a nursing unit. The **computerized physician order entry (CPOE)** is one type of order entry system gaining popularity in the larger medical centers across the country. CPOE is a process by which the physician or an advanced practice nurse directly enters orders for client care into the hospital information system. In advanced systems, CPOE has built-in reminders and alerts that help the client's health care provider to select the most appropriate medication or diagnostic test. There are major initiatives from the Institute of Medicine to improve the quality of care and reduce medication errors. Many believe CPOE is the answer. CPOE allows direct entry of orders to eliminate issues related to illegible handwriting and transcription errors. In addition, a CPOE system speeds the implementation of ordered diagnostic tests and treatments, which improves staff productivity and saves money (Dorenfest, 2003). A unit secretary no longer has to transcribe a written order onto a nursing order form. Orders made through CPOE are integrated within the record and sent to the appropriate departments (e.g., pharmacy and radiology). The implementation of CPOE is slowed by such factors as difficult system sign-on procedures, limited system access or response time, lack of funding, inadequate access to clinical data to support the expert decision-making features, and the perception by physicians that CPOE offers them few benefits (Hebda and others, 2005).

The Electronic Health Record

As a result of government, professional organization, and accrediting body initiatives, the management of health care information is a major national issue. The traditional paper medical record no longer meets the needs of today's health care industry. A paper record is episode-oriented, with a separate record for each client visit to a health care agency (Hebda, 2005). Key information, such as client allergies, current medications, and complications from treatment may be lost from one episode of care (e.g., hospitalization or clinic visit) to the next, jeopardizing a client's safety. The electronic health record (EHR) is a longitudinal electronic record of client health information generated by one or more encounters in any care delivery setting (HIMSS, 2007). The EHR provides access to a client's health record information at the time and place that clinicians need it. A unique feature of an EHR is its ability to integrate all pertinent client information into one record, regardless of the number of times a client enters a health care system. An EHR also includes results of diagnostic studies that may include images and sound, as well as decision-support software programs. Because an unlimited number of client records can be potentially stored within an EHR system, health care providers can access clinical data to identify quality issues, link interventions with positive outcomes, and make evidence-based decisions.

The Healthcare Information and Management Systems Society (HIMSS) (2003) has developed a definitional model for an EHR. The model outlines the definitions, attributes, and requirements for assessing the extent to which an organization is using an EHR. Attributes of an EHR include the following:

- Provides secure, reliable, real-time access to client health record information where and when it is needed to support care

- Captures and manages episodic and longitudinal EHR information
- Functions as clinicians' primary information resource during the provision of client care
- Assists with the work of planning and delivering evidence-based care to individuals and groups of clients
- Captures data used for continuous quality improvement, utilization review, risk management, resource planning, and performance management
- Captures the client health-related information needed for medical records and reimbursement
- Provides longitudinal, appropriately masked information to support clinical research, public health reporting, and population health initiatives
- Supports clinical trials and evidence-based research

Those who support the development of an EHR believe that it will improve client and clinician satisfaction because it will improve continuity of health care from one episode of illness to another. A clinician can access relevant and timely information about a client so as to focus on the priority problems of care and to make timely well-informed clinical decisions. An EHR is a powerful tool because of the decision-support resources it contains. For example, in a hospital setting an EHR gathers data and performs checking to support regulatory and accreditation requirements. It also includes tools to guide and critique medication administration—right client, right drug, right route, right dose, right time, and right documentation. An EHR also contains basic decision-support tools such as physician order sets, interdisciplinary treatment plans, and rules based on documentation templates. The evidence that is derived from the clinical information in an EHR provides an excellent foundation for an organization to identify clinical problem areas and to initiate clinical research trials.

The ultimate development of an EHR for clients will affect the entire health care community. Currently the American Medical Association, American Nurses Association, the HIMSS, and the American Medical Informatics Association are just some of the organizations charged with the task of facilitating rapid input to support the adoption of EHR standards (Hebda and others, 2005). All disciplines and health care organizations will benefit. The key advantages for nursing include providing a means to easily compare data from different health care encounters, maintaining an ongoing record of a client's education and learning in all health care encounters, offering better quality and easily accessible data for research, automating critical and clinical pathways of care, and comparing ongoing clinical data about a client with original baseline information.

Key Concepts

- The medical record is a legal document and requires information describing the care that is delivered to a client.
- All information pertaining to a client's health care management that is gathered by examination, observation, conversation, or treatment is confidential.
- Multidisciplinary communication is essential within the health care team.

- Accurate record keeping requires an objective interpretation of data with precise measurements, correct spelling, and proper use of abbreviations.
- A nurse's signature on an entry in a record designates accountability for the contents of that entry.
- Any change in a client's condition warrants immediate documentation to keep a record accurate.
- The medical record is a financial record that serves as the basis for reimbursement.
- Problem-oriented medical records are organized by the client's health care problems.
- The intent of SOAP, SOAPIE, PIE, or DAR charting formats is to organize entries in the progress notes according to the nursing process.
- Medicare guidelines for establishing a client's home care cost reimbursement is the basis for documentation by home care nurses.
- Long-term care documentation is multidisciplinary and closely linked with fiscal requirements of outside agencies.
- Computerized information systems provide information about clients in an organized and easily accessible fashion.
- The major purpose of the change-of-shift report is to maintain continuity of care.
- Rounds allow nurses to perform needed assessments, evaluate clients' progress, and determine the best interventions for a client's needs.
- Always verify client care information communicated by telephone.
- A hospital information system (HIS) consists of two major types of information systems: clinical information systems (CIS) and administrative information systems.
- Nursing informatics facilitates the integration of data, information, and knowledge to support clients, nurses, and other providers in decision making in all roles and settings.
- Protection of the confidentiality of clients' health information and the security of computer systems should be a top priority.

Critical Thinking Exercises

1. Joseph Page is an 80-year-old man admitted with a diagnosis of possible pneumonia. He complains of general malaise and a frequent productive cough, worse at night. Vital signs are as follows: blood pressure, 150/90 mm Hg; pulse rate, 92 beats per minute; respirations, 22 breaths per minute; and temperature, 38.5° C (101.3° F). During your initial assessment he coughs violently for 40 to 45 seconds without expectorating. His lungs have wheezes and rhonchi in both bases and are otherwise clear. He states, "It hurts in my chest when I cough." Differentiate between objective and subjective data in this case example.

2. The nurse positions Mr. Page in a semi-Fowler's position, encourages increased fluid intake, and gives Tylenol 650 mg by mouth (PO) as ordered for fever. One hour later the client is resting in bed. Vital signs are as follows: blood pressure, 130/86 mm Hg; pulse rate, 86 beats per minute; respirations, 22 breaths per minute; and temperature, 37.7° C (99.8° F). He states he has been unable to

sleep. His fluid intake has been 200 mL of water. Use the given information to write a nurse's progress note using the PIE format.

3. At the end of your shift you have identified *deficient fluid volume* as a nursing diagnosis for Mr. Page. The client entered the hospital by way of the emergency department 8 hours ago. He was accompanied at that time by his family. Since his admission he has had fluid intake of about 600 mL, and his urine output was 300 mL of dark concentrated urine. His temperature is back up to 38.3° C (101° F), his mucous membranes are dry, and he states he feels very weak. Describe what should be included in the change-of-shift report.

4. Several days later, following treatment with intravenous antibiotics, Mr. Page is feeling much better and preparations are being made for discharge. He is to take Keflex 500 mg every 6 hours for the next 10 days, continue to drink extra fluids, and get extra rest. He lives alone. Although he is generally cooperative, he does not like drinking water or taking pills. He is to make an appointment with his physician for 1 week from today and should call the physician if he develops symptoms of recurrence. Write a discharge summary that is concise and instructive.

✳ NCLEX®-Style Review Questions

1. A manager is reviewing the nurses' notes in a client's medical record. She finds the following entry, "Client is difficult to care for, refuses suggestion for improving appetite." Which of the following directions should the manager give to the staff nurse who entered the note?
   1. Avoid rushing when charting an entry
   2. Use correction fluid to remove the entry.
   3. Draw a single line through the statement and initial it.
   4. Enter only objective and factual information about the client.

2. A client tells the nurse, "I have stomach cramps and feel nauseous." This is an example of what type of data?
   1. Objective
   2. Historical
   3. Subjective
   4. Assessment

3. As you enter the client's room, you notice he is anxious to say something. He quickly states, "I do not know what is going on; I cannot get an explanation from my doctor about the results of my test. I want something done about this." Which of the following is most appropriate documentation of the client's emotional status?
   1. The client has a defiant attitude.
   2. The client appears to be upset with his physician.
   3. The client is demanding and complains frequently.
   4. The client stated "he felt frustrated by the lack of information he has received regarding his diagnostic tests."

4. A primary benefit of HIPAA regulations is to:
   1. Allow access of the medical record to all hospital staff
   2. Limit what information must be documented in the client's record
   3. Provide clients with greater control over personal health care information
   4. Enable health care institutions to release any client-related information with a general client authorization

5. Clients frequently request copies of their medical records. The nurse understands:
   1. Only the families may read the records
   2. They have the right to read those records
   3. They are not allowed to read those records
   4. Only the health care workers have access to the records

6. Accurate entries are an important characteristic of good documentation. Which of the following charting entries is most accurate in the way it is written?
   1. Client up, out of bed, walked down hallway with assistance, tolerated well.
   2. Client up, out of bed, walked 50 feet and back down hallway, tolerated well.
   3. Client up, out of bed, walked 50 feet and back down hallway with assistance from nurse.
   4. Client up, out of bed, walked 50 feet and back down hallway with assistance from nurse, HR 88 and regular before exercise, 94 and regular following exercise.

7. Match the correct entry with the appropriate SOAP category.
   S
   O
   A
   P
   Repositioned client on right side. Encouraged client to use PCA device.
   The pain increases every time I try to turn on my left side.
   Acute pain related to tissue injury from surgical incision.
   Left lower abdominal surgical incision, 3 inches in length, closed, sutures intact, no drainage. Pain noted on mild palpation.

8. On the nursing unit at Stevens Health Center a nurse is able to access a client's medical record and review the education that nurses provided the client during an initial hospitalization and three subsequent clinic visits. This type of record system is an example of:
   1. Information technology
   2. Electronic health record
   3. Personal health information
   4. Administrative information system

27 | Self-Concept

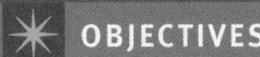

OBJECTIVES

Mastery of content in this chapter will enable the student to:

- Discuss factors that influence the following components of self-concept: identity, body image, and role performance.
- Identify stressors that affect self-concept and self-esteem.
- Describe the components of self-concept as related to psychosocial and cognitive developmental stages.
- Explore ways in which the nurse's self-concept and nursing actions affect the client's self-concept and self-esteem.

- Discuss evidence-based practice applicable for identity confusion, disturbed body image, low self-esteem, and role conflict.
- Examine cultural considerations that affect self-concept.
- Apply the nursing process to promote a client's self-concept.

MEDIA RESOURCES   KEY TERMS

 Companion CD
- NCLEX®-Style Review Questions
- Audio Glossary
- Interactive Learning Activities
- English/Spanish Glossary

Body image, p. 413
Identity, p. 412
Identity confusion, p. 415
Role ambiguity, p. 415
Role conflict, p. 415
Role overload, p. 416

Role performance, p. 414
Role strain, p. 416
Self-concept, p. 411
Self-esteem, p. 414
Sick role, p. 415

evolve Website
- NCLEX®-Style Review Questions
- Audio Glossary
- English/Spanish Glossary
- Interactive Learning Activities
- Weblinks
- Audio Summaries

Self-concept is an individual's conceptualization of himself or herself. It is a subjective sense of self and a complex mixture of unconscious and conscious thoughts, attitudes, and perceptions. Self-concept directly affects one's self-esteem, or how one feels about himself or herself. Although these two terms are often used interchangeably, nurses need to differentiate the two so they will correctly and completely assess clients and develop an individualized plan of care based on the client's needs.

Nurses care for clients who face a variety of health problems that threaten their self-concept and self-esteem. The loss of bodily function, a decline in activity tolerance, and difficulty in managing a chronic illness are examples of situations that change a client's self-concept. Nurses need to help clients adjust to alterations in self-concept and support components of self-concept to promote successful coping.

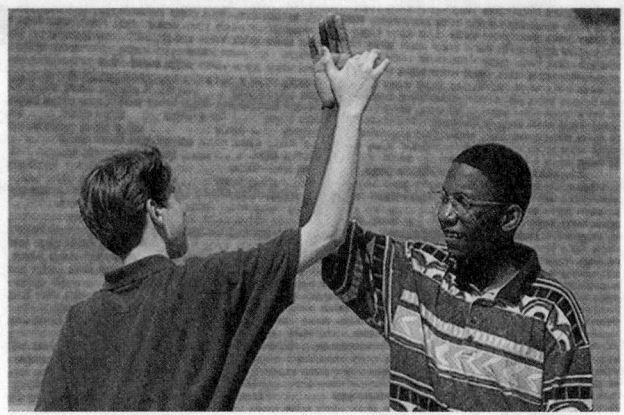

Figure 27-1 Adolescents' participating in group activities can foster self-esteem. (From Birchenall J, Streight E: *Mosby's textbook for the home care aide,* ed 2, St. Louis, 2003, Mosby.)

Scientific Knowledge Base

Development and maintenance of self-concept and self-esteem begin at a young age and continue across the life span. There is a tendency for males to report higher self-esteem than females (Birndorf and others, 2005). However, the exact amount of this gender difference and the way it varies across the life span remain unclear. Parents and other primary caregivers influence the development of a child's self-concept and self-esteem. In addition, individuals learn and internalize cultural influences on self-concept and self-esteem in childhood and adolescence. There is a significant amount of emphasis on fostering a school-age child's self-concept. In general, young children tend to rate themselves higher than they rate other children, suggesting that their view of themselves is positively inflated. Adolescence is a particularly critical time when many variables affect self-concept and self-esteem (Figure 27-1). The adolescent experience appears to adversely affect self-esteem, more strongly for girls than for boys. For example, some adolescent girls are more sensitive about their appearance and how others view them. Thus it is important to assess changes in self-esteem between early, middle, and late adolescence because changes in self-concept occur over time.

Job satisfaction and job performance in adulthood are also linked to self-esteem. Sometimes when individuals lose a job, their sense of self diminishes, they lose motivation to be socially active, or they even become depressed. They lose their job identity, and as a result, this alters their self-perceptions. The establishment of a sense of self that is stable and that transcends relationships and situations is a developmental goal of adulthood.

Evidence suggests that sense of self is often negatively affected in older adulthood because of the intensity of emotional and physical changes associated with aging (Robins and others, 2002). For example, when the older adult loses a partner or has a change in health, sometimes there is a change in social interaction or even personal hygiene care.

Researchers have also found ethnic and cultural differences in self-concept and self-esteem across the life span (Twenge and Crocker, 2002). For boys, family income above the federal poverty level, positive family communication, and involvement in a religious community are associated with high self-esteem; for girls, being of African American or Hispanic race/ethnicity, positive family communication, and feeling safe are predictive of higher self-esteem (Birndorf and others, 2005). Sensitivity to factors that affect self-concept and self-esteem in diverse cultures is essential to ensure an individualized approach to health care.

How individuals view themselves and their perception of their health are closely related. A client's belief in personal health often enhances his or her self-concept. Statements such as "I can get through anything" or "I've never been sick a day in my life" indicate that a person's thoughts about personal health are positive. Illness, hospitalization, and surgery also affect self-concept. Chronic illness often affects the ability to provide financial support, which then affects an individual's self-esteem and perceived roles within the family. Negative perceptions regarding health status are reflected in such statements as "It's not worth it anymore" or "I'm a burden to my family." Further, chronic illness affects identity and body image as reflected by verbalizations such as "I'll never get any better" or "I can't stand to look at myself any more."

What individuals think and how they feel about themselves affects the way in which they care for themselves physically and emotionally, as well as the way in which they care for others. Further, how a person behaves is generally consistent with both self-concept and self-esteem. Individuals who have poor self-concepts often do not feel in control of situations and do not feel worthy of care, which influences decisions regarding health care. Knowledge of variables that affect self-concept and self-esteem is critical to provide effective treatment.

Nursing Knowledge Base

In providing evidence-based practice to clients, incorporate professional nursing knowledge developed from the humanities and sciences, nursing research, and clinical practice. A broad knowledge base allows nurses to have a holistic view of clients, thus promoting quality client care that will best meet the self-concept needs of each client and family.

✳ BOX 27-1   Self-Concept: Developmental Tasks

Trust Versus Mistrust (Birth to 1 Year)
Develops trust following consistency in caregiving and nurturing interactions
Distinguishes self from environment

Autonomy Versus Shame and Doubt (1 to 3 Years)
Begins to communicate likes and dislikes
Increasingly independent in thoughts and actions
Appreciates body appearance and function (including dressing, feeding, talking, and walking)

Initiative Versus Guilt (3 to 6 Years)
Identifies with a gender
Enhances self-awareness
Increases language skills, including identification of feelings

Industry Versus Inferiority (6 to 12 Years)
Incorporates feedback from peers and teachers
Increases self-esteem with new skill mastery (e.g., reading, math, sports, music)
Aware of strengths and limitations

Identity Versus Role Confusion (12 to 20 Years)
Accepts body changes/maturation
Examines attitudes, values, and beliefs; establishes goals for the future
Feels positive about expanded sense of self

Intimacy Versus Isolation (Mid-20s to Mid-40s)
Has stable, positive feelings about self
Experiences successful role transitions and increased responsibilities

Generativity Versus Self-Absorption (Mid-40s to Mid-60s)
Able to accept changes in appearance and physical endurance
Reassesses life goals
Shows contentment with aging

Ego Integrity Versus Despair (Late 60s to Death)
Feels positive about life and its meaning
Interested in providing a legacy for the next generation

Development of Self-Concept

The development of self-concept is a complex lifelong process that involves many factors. Erikson's psychosocial theory of development (1963) remains helpful in understanding key tasks that individuals face at various stages of development. Each stage builds on the tasks of the previous stage. Successful mastery of each stage leads to a solid sense of self (Box 27-1).

A nurse learns to recognize an individual's failure in achieving an age-appropriate developmental stage or an individual's regression to an earlier stage in a period of crisis. This understanding allows a nurse to individualize care and determine appropriate nursing interventions. Self-concept is always changing and is based on the following:

- Sense of competency
- Perceived reactions of others to one's body
- Ongoing perceptions and interpretations of the thoughts and feelings of others
- Personal and professional relationships
- Academic and employment-related identity

- Personality characteristics that affect self-expectations
- Perceptions of events that have an impact on the self
- Mastery of prior and new experiences
- Ethnic, racial, and spiritual identity

Self-esteem is usually highest in childhood, drops during adolescence, rises gradually throughout adulthood, and declines again in old age (Robins and others, 2002). Although variability exists, in general this pattern holds true across gender, socioeconomic status, and ethnicity. Children often report high self-esteem because their sense of self is inflated by a variety of extremely positive sources, and the subsequent decline is sometimes associated with a shift to more realistic information about the self.

> **SAFETY ALERT** For some adolescents, a decline in self-esteem results in increased risk-taking behavior. This is demonstrated in unsafe behaviors such as premature sexual activity, unprotected sex, risky driving, or substance abuse. In addition, low self-esteem and stressful life events significantly predict suicidal ideations in older adolescents (Wilburn and Smith, 2005). Nurses in all health care settings need to initiate suicide screening for early detection for suicide risk and implement nursing interventions directed toward suicide prevention (Folse and others, 2006).

Erikson's emphasis on the generativity stage (1963) (see Chapter 11) explains the rise in self-esteem and self-concept in adulthood. The individual focuses on being increasingly productive and creative at work, while at the same time promoting and guiding the next generation. Other than childhood, the mid-60s seem to represent the highest level of self-esteem across the life span. Researchers have reported a sharp decline in self-esteem around age 70 (Robins and others, 2002). Based on Erikson's stages of development, a decline in self-concept at this advanced age reflects a diminished need for self-promotion and a shift in self-concept to a more modest and balanced view of the self. Identification of specific nursing interventions to address the unique needs of clients at various life stages is essential.

Components and Interrelated Terms of Self-Concept

A positive self-concept gives a sense of meaning, wholeness, and consistency to a person. A healthy self-concept has a high degree of stability and generates positive feelings toward the self. The components of self-concept frequently considered by nurses are identity, body image, and role performance. Self-esteem is a closely related concept. Self-esteem comes from self-concept, and self-esteem influences self-concept.

Identity. Identity involves the internal sense of individuality, wholeness, and consistency of a person over time and in different situations. Identity implies being distinct and separate from others. Being "oneself" or living an authentic life is the basis of true identity. Children learn culturally accepted values, behaviors, and roles through identification and modeling. They often gain an identity from self-observations and from what individuals tell them. An individual first identifies with parenting figures and later with other role models such as teachers or peers. To form an identity, the child must be able to bring together learned behaviors and expectations into a coherent, consistent, and unique whole (Erikson, 1963).

✳ BOX 27-2   CULTURAL ASPECTS OF CARE

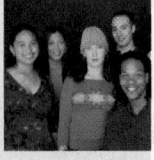

Racial and cultural identity are important components of a person's self-concept. Early in growth and development, an individual develops this identity within the context of family. As the individual grows, the cultural aspects of his or her self-concept are reinforced through social, family, or cultural experiences. In addition, a person's self-concept is strengthened or questioned through political, social, or cultural influences experienced in the school and workplace environments. Positive or negative cultural role modeling or past experiences influence self-concept.

Implications for Practice

- Develop an open, nonrestrictive attitude for assessing and encouraging cultural practices to improve clients' self-concept.
- Ask clients what they think is important to help them feel better or gain a stronger sense of self.
- Encourage cultural identity by individualizing self-care practices and offering treatment choices to meet clients' self-concept needs.
- Facilitate culturally sensitive health promotion activities that address at-risk behaviors identified through evidence-based practice (e.g., sexual risk behaviors, weight and shape issues).

Data from Birndorf S and others: High self-esteem among adolescents: longitudinal trends, sex differences, and protective factors, *J Adolesc Health* 37:194, 2005; Robins RW and others: Global self-esteem across the life span, *Psychol Aging* 17(3):423, 2002; Ruiz SY and others: Predictors of self-esteem for Mexican American and European American youths: a reexamination of the influence of parenting, *J Fam Psychol* 16(1):70, 2002; Sterk CE and others: Self-esteem and at risk women: determinants and relevance to sexual and HIV-related risk behaviors, *Women Health* 40(4):75, 2004; and Twenge JM, Crocker J: Race and self-esteem: meta-analyses comparing whites, blacks, Hispanics, Asians, and American Indians, *Psychol Bull* 128(3):371, 2002.

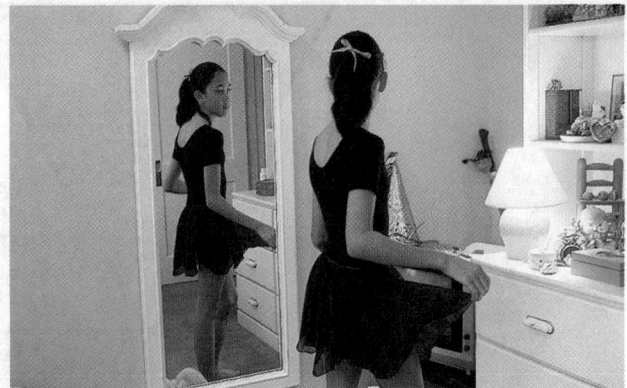

Figure 27-2 An individual's appearance influences self-concept. (From Sorrentino SA: *Mosby's textbook for nursing assistants,* ed 6, St. Louis, 2004, Mosby.)

The achievement of identity is necessary for intimate relationships because individuals express identity in relationships with others (Stuart and Laraia, 2005). Sexuality is a part of identity. Gender identity is a person's private view of maleness or femaleness; gender role is the masculine or feminine behavior exhibited. This image and its meaning depend on culturally determined values (see Chapter 28).

Cultural differences in identity exist (Box 27-2). Racial or cultural identity develops from identification and socialization within an established group, as well as through the experience of integrating the response of individuals outside the cultural or racial group into one's self-concept. Differences in ethnic identity (e.g., Mexican American or Cuban American) exist through identification with traditions, customs, and rituals within one's race/ethnic group (e.g., Hispanic/Latino). In general, the more a person identifies with social groups, the greater the person's self-esteem. In addition, when racial identity is central to self-concept and is positive, self-esteem tends to be high (Twenge and Crocker, 2002). An individual who experiences discrimination, prejudice, or environmental stressors such as low income or high-crime neighborhoods, often conceptualizes himself or herself differently than an individual who has had different living conditions (Ruiz and others, 2002). The influence of race/ethnicity on self-esteem

is evident within families of adolescents: African American and Hispanic/Latino fathers report higher perceptions of physical appearance and global self-worth than white fathers, and African American mothers describe more athletic competence than white or Hispanic/Latina mothers (Phares and others, 2005).

Body Image. **Body image** involves attitudes related to the body, including physical appearance, structure, or function. Feelings about body image include those related to sexuality, femininity and masculinity, youthfulness, health, and strength. These mental images are not always consistent with a person's actual physical structure or appearance. Some body image distortions have deep psychological origins, such as the eating disorder anorexia nervosa. Other alterations occur as a result of situational events such as the loss or change in a body part. Nurses need to be aware that the majority of men and women experience some degree of dissatisfaction with their bodies, which affects body image and overall self-concept. Individuals often exaggerate disturbances in body image when a change in health status occurs. The way others view a person's body and the feedback offered is also influential. For example, a controlling, violent husband tells his wife that she is ugly and that no one else would want her. Over the years of marriage, she incorporates this devaluation into her self-concept.

Cognitive growth and physical development also affect body image. Normal developmental changes such as puberty and aging have a more apparent effect on body image than on other aspects of self-concept. Hormonal changes during adolescence and menopause influence body image. The development of secondary sex characteristics and changes in body fat distribution have a tremendous impact on the self-concept of an adolescent. Changes associated with aging (i.e., wrinkles; graying hair; and decrease in visual acuity, hearing, and mobility) also affect body image in an older adult.

Cultural and societal attitudes and values also influence body image. Culture and society dictate the accepted norms of body image and influence one's attitudes (Figure 27-2). Racial and ethnic background plays an integral role in body satisfaction in adolescent girls as reflected in the higher incidence of body satisfaction among African American girls compared to white girls (Kelly and others, 2005). Further, African American girls de-

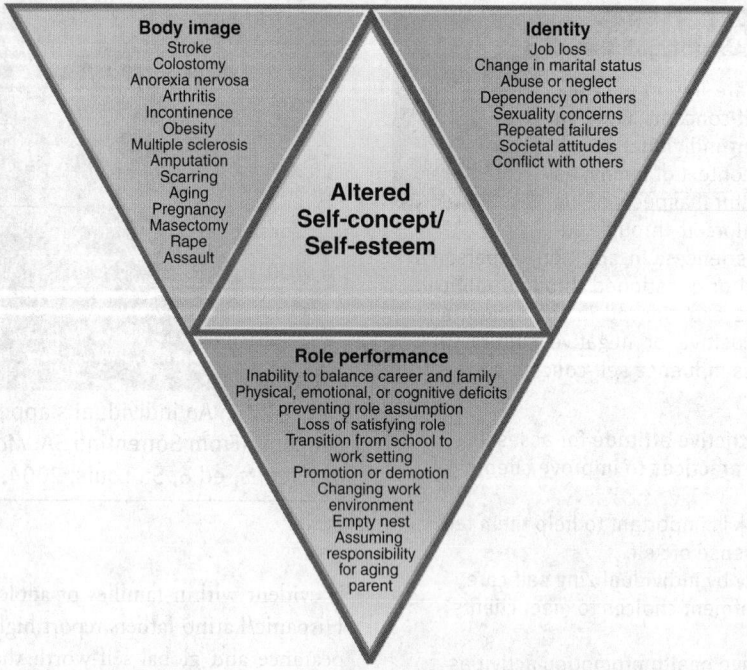

Figure 27-3 Common stressors that influence self-concept.

scribed more favorable views about physical appearance, reported less social pressure for thinness, and less tendency to base self-esteem on body image than did white girls (White and others, 2003). Values such as ideal body weight and shape, as well as attitudes toward piercing and tattoos, are culturally based. American society emphasizes youth, beauty, and wholeness. Western cultures have been socialized to dread the normal aging process, whereas Eastern cultures view aging very positively and respect older adults. Body image issues are often associated with impaired self-concept and self-esteem.

Role Performance. Role performance is the way in which individuals perceive their ability to carry out significant roles. This includes roles such as parent, supervisor, or close friend. Roles that individuals follow in given situations involve socialization to expectations or standards of behavior. The patterns are stable and change only minimally during adulthood. Individuals develop and maintain behaviors that society approves through the following processes:

- *Reinforcement-extinction:* Certain behaviors become common or are avoided, depending on whether they are approved and reinforced or discouraged and punished.
- *Inhibition:* An individual learns to refrain from behaviors, even when tempted to engage in them.
- *Substitution:* An individual replaces one behavior with another, which provides the same personal gratification.
- *Imitation:* An individual acquires knowledge, skills, or behaviors from members of the social or cultural group.
- *Identification:* An individual internalizes the beliefs, behavior, and values of role models into a personal, unique expression of self.

Ideal societal role behaviors are often hard to achieve in real life. Individuals have multiple roles and personal needs that some-

times conflict. Successful adults learn to distinguish between ideal role expectations and realistic possibilities. To function effectively in multiple roles, a person must know the expected behavior and values, desire to conform to them, and be able to meet the role requirements. Fulfillment of role expectations leads to an enhanced sense of self. Difficulty or failure in meeting role expectations leads to deficits and often contributes to decreased self-esteem or altered self-concept.

Self-Esteem. Self-esteem is an individual's overall feeling of self-worth or the emotional appraisal of self-concept. It is the most fundamental self-evaluation because it represents the overall judgment of personal worth or value. Self-esteem is positive when one feels capable, worthwhile, and competent (Rosenberg, 1965). A child's self-esteem is related to the child's evaluation of his or her effectiveness at school, within the family, and in social settings. The evaluation of others also is likely to have a profound influence on the child's self-esteem.

Considering the relationship between a person's actual self-concept and his or her ideal self enhances understanding self-esteem. The ideal self consists of the aspirations, goals, values, and standards of behavior that a person considers ideal and strives to attain. In general, a person whose self-concept comes close to matching the ideal self has high self-esteem, whereas a person whose self-concept varies widely from the ideal self suffers from low self-esteem. Once established, basic feelings about the self tend to be constant, even though a situational crisis temporarily affects self-esteem.

Stressors Affecting Self-Concept

A self-concept stressor is any real or perceived change that threatens identity, body image, or role performance (Figure 27-3). The individual's perception of the stressor is the most important factor in determining his or her response. The ability to reestablish balance following a stressor is related to numerous factors, including the number of stressors, duration of the stressor, and health status (see Chapter 31). Stressors challenge a person's adaptive capacities. Changes that occur in physical, spiritual, emotional, sexual, familial, and sociocultural health affect self-concept. Being able to adapt to stressors is likely to lead to a positive sense of self, whereas failure to adapt often leads to a negative self-concept.

Any change in health is a stressor that potentially affects self-concept. A physical change in the body sometimes leads to an altered body image affecting identity and self-esteem. Chronic illnesses often alter role performance, which change an individual's identity and self-esteem. Further, an essential process in the adjustment to loss is the development of a new self-concept. A loss of a partner will possibly lead to a loss of identity and a lower self-esteem (Van Baarsen, 2002). Unlike the loss in self-esteem shown in vulnerable older adults, the resiliency demonstrated in some older adults reflects sophisticated cognitive strategies to manage losses (Collins and Smyer, 2005).

The stressors created as a result of a crisis also affect a person's health. If the resulting identity confusion, disturbed body image, low self-esteem, or role conflict is not relieved, illness will possibly result. For example, the diagnosis of cancer places additional demands on a person's established living pattern. It changes the person's appraisal of and satisfaction with the current level of physical, emotional, and social functioning. In this case, assess self-esteem, effectiveness of coping strategies, and social support. During self-concept crises, supportive and educative resources are valuable in helping a person learn new ways of coping with and responding to the stressful event or situation to maintain or enhance self-concept.

Identity Stressors. Stressors affect an individual's identity throughout life, but individuals are particularly vulnerable during adolescence. Adolescents are trying to adjust to the physical, emotional, and mental changes of increasing maturity, which result in insecurity and anxiety. It is also a time when the adolescent is developing psychosocial competence, including coping strategies (see Chapter 31).

An adult generally has a more stable identity and thus a more firmly developed self-concept. Cultural and social stressors, rather than personal stressors, have more impact on an adult's identity. For example, an adult has to balance career and family or make choices regarding honoring religious traditions from one's family of origin. **Identity confusion** results when people do not maintain a clear, consistent, and continuous consciousness of personal identity. It occurs at any stage of life if a person is unable to adapt to identity stressors.

Body Image Stressors. Changes in the appearance, structure, or function of a body part requires an adjustment in body image. An individual's perception of the change and the relative importance placed on body image will affect the significance of a loss of function or change in appearance. For example, if a woman's body image incorporates reproductive organs as the ideal, a hysterectomy needed because of a diagnosis of uterine cancer is a significant alteration and will possibly result in a perceived loss of femininity or wholeness. Changes in the appearance of the body, such as an amputation, facial disfigurement, or scars from burns,

are obvious stressors affecting body image. Mastectomy and colostomy are surgical procedures that alter the appearance and function of the body, yet the changes are not apparent to others when the individual is dressed. Although potentially undetected by others, these bodily changes have a significant impact on the individual. Even some elective changes such as breast augmentation or reduction affect body image. Chronic illnesses such as heart and renal disease affect body image because the body no longer functions at an optimal level. In addition, the effects of pregnancy, significant weight gain or loss, pharmacological management of illness, or radiation therapy change body image. Negative body image often leads to adverse health outcomes.

Society's response to physical changes in an individual often depends on the conditions surrounding the alteration. Overall, positive social changes with regard to how the public responds to illness and altered body image have occurred. The media frequently present positive stories about persons adjusting in a healthy manner following serious disabilities (e.g., Christopher Reeve's spinal cord injury) or adapting to a debilitating illness (e.g., Michael J. Fox's Parkinson's disease). These stories change public perception of what constitutes a disability and certainly have provided positive role models for individuals undergoing self-concept stressors, as well as for their families, friends, and society as a whole. In view of the growing epidemic of obesity in Western cultures, parents and health care providers need to address weight management issues without causing further injury to body image. Providing a social environment that focuses on health and fitness, rather than on weight control, will possibly increase adolescent girls' satisfaction with their bodies (Kelly and others, 2005).

Role Performance Stressors. Throughout life a person undergoes numerous role changes. Situational transitions occur when parents, spouses, children, or close friends die or people move, marry, divorce, or change jobs. It is important to recognize that a shift along the continuum from illness to wellness is as stressful as a shift from wellness to illness. Any of these transitions may lead to role conflict, role ambiguity, role strain, or role overload.

Role conflict results when a person has to simultaneously assume two or more roles that are inconsistent, contradictory, or mutually exclusive. For example, when a middle-age woman with teenage children assumes responsibility for the care of her older parents, conflicts occur in relation to being both a parent to her children and the child of her parents. Negotiating a balance of time and energy between her children and parents create role conflicts. The perceived importance of each conflicting role influences the degree of conflict experienced. The **sick role** involves the expectations of others and society regarding how an individual behaves when sick. Role conflict occurs when general societal expectations (take care of yourself, and you will get better) and the expectations of co-workers (need to get the job done) collide. The conflict of taking care of oneself while getting everything done is often a major challenge.

Role ambiguity involves unclear role expectations, which makes people unsure about what to do or how to do it, creating stress and confusion. Role ambiguity is common in the adolescent years. Parents, peers, and the media pressure adolescents to assume adultlike roles, yet many lack the resources to move beyond the role of a dependent child. Role ambiguity is also common in employment situations. In complex, rapidly changing, or highly specialized organizations, employees often become unsure about job expectations.

Role strain combines role conflict and role ambiguity. Some express role strain as a feeling of frustration when a person feels inadequate or unsuited to a role (Stuart and Laraia, 2005), such as providing care to a family member with Alzheimer's disease.

Role overload involves having more roles or responsibilities within a role than are manageable. This is common in an individual who unsuccessfully attempts to meet the demands of work and family while carving out some personal time. Often during periods of illness or change, those involved either as the one who is ill or as a significant other find themselves in role overload.

Self-Esteem Stressors. Individuals with high self-esteem are generally more resilient and are better able to cope with demands and stressors than those with low self-esteem. Low self-worth contributes to feeling unfulfilled and disconnected to others and sometimes results in depression and unremitting uneasiness or anxiety. Illness, surgery, or accidents that change life patterns also influence feelings of self-worth. Chronic illnesses such as diabetes, arthritis, and cardiac dysfunction require changes in accepted and long-assumed behavioral patterns. The more the chronic illness interferes with the ability to engage in activities contributing to feelings of worth or success, the more it affects self-esteem.

Self-esteem stressors vary with developmental stages. Perceived inability to meet parental expectations, harsh criticism, inconsistent discipline, and unresolved sibling rivalry reduce the level of self-worth of children. Low self-esteem and stressful life events in college-age adolescents are potential predictors for suicidal thoughts and behavior (Wilburn and Smith, 2005). A developmental milestone, such as pregnancy, introduces unique self-concept stressors and has significant health care implications. Recent findings suggest that for some economically disadvantaged African American adolescents, safe sex behaviors are not always valued and pregnancy is an affirmation of ethnic identity (Salazar and others, 2005). Low self-esteem during adolescence also has significant real world consequences in adulthood, including poor health, criminal behavior, and limited economic prospects compared to adolescents with high self-esteem (Trzesniewski and others, 2006). The link between sexual and human immunodeficiency virus (HIV)–related risk behaviors in African American women suggests that self-esteem and health behaviors are intertwined (Sterk and others, 2004). Stressors affecting the self-esteem of an adult include failure in work and unsuccessful relationships. Self-concept stressors in older adults include health problems, declining socioeconomic status, spousal loss or bereavement, loss of social support, and decline in achievement experiences following retirement (Box 27-3).

Family Effect on Self-Concept Development

The family plays a key role in creating and maintaining the self-concepts of its members. Children develop a basic sense of who they are from their family caregivers. A child also gains accepted norms for thinking, feeling, and behaving from family mem-

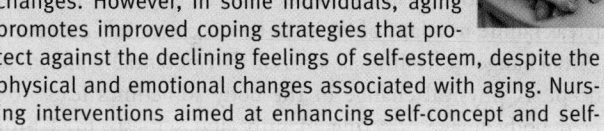

✳ BOX 27-3 **FOCUS ON OLDER ADULTS**

Enhancing Self-Concept
Self-concept is sometimes negatively affected in older adulthood because of a number of life changes. However, in some individuals, aging promotes improved coping strategies that protect against the declining feelings of self-esteem, despite the physical and emotional changes associated with aging. Nursing interventions aimed at enhancing self-concept and self-esteem in older adults is essential.

Implications for Practice
- Clarify what the life changes mean and the effect on self-concept. Discuss health problems, declining socioeconomic status, spousal loss or bereavement, and loss of social support following retirement.
- Be alert to preoccupation with physical complaints. Assess complaints thoroughly and if no physical explanation exists, encourage older adult to verbalize needs (fear, insecurity, loneliness) in a nonphysical way.
- Identify positive and negative coping mechanisms. Support effective strategies.
- Encourage the use of storytelling and review of old photographs.
- Communicate that the older adult is worthwhile by actively listening to and accepting the person's feelings, being respectful, and praising healthy behaviors.
- Allow additional time to complete tasks. Reinforce the older adult's efforts at independence.

Data from Collins A, Smyer MA: The resilience of self-esteem in late adulthood: *J Aging Health* 17(4):471, 2005; Ebersole P and others: *Gerontological nursing and healthy aging*, ed 2, St. Louis, 2005, Mosby; and Robins RW and others: Global self-esteem across the life span, *Psychol Aging* 17(3):423, 2002.

bers. Sometimes well-meaning parents cultivate negative self-concepts in children. Some literature suggests that parents are the most important influences on a child's development, yet variations in approach depend on the culture. Specifically, a relationship exists between parents who respond in a firm, consistent, and warm manner and a child's positive self-esteem and school achievement (Ruiz and others, 2002). High parental support and parental monitoring are related to greater self-esteem and lower risk behaviors (Parker and Benson, 2004). Parents who are harsh, inconsistent, or have low self-esteem themselves often behave in ways that foster negative self-concepts in their children. Positive communication and social support fosters self-esteem and well-being in adolescence (Birndorf and others, 2005). To reverse a client's negative self-concept, first assess the family's style of relating (see Chapter 10). Family and cultural factors sometimes influence negative health practices, such as cigarette smoking (Box 27-4). Self-concept change demands an evidence-based practice approach, supported by the entire health care team.

The Nurse's Effect on the Client's Self-Concept

A nurse's acceptance of a client with an altered self-concept helps promote positive change. When a client's physical appearance has changed, it is likely that both the client and the family will look

BOX 27-4 EVIDENCE-BASED PRACTICE

Self-Concept and Risk of Smoking

Evidence Summary

Cigarette smoking by young women is a growing health concern. The decision to smoke is perhaps reflective of self-concept issues and is possibly influenced by culture. Awareness of risk factors is essential for implementation of preventative health care in a variety of nursing settings.

The purpose of this 10-year study was to identify early predictors of daily smoking in young women. This study of 1,213 black and 1,166 white girls revealed that white girls were at higher risk of becoming daily smokers than black girls. Early predictors of daily smoking included parental education, single-family home, drinking alcohol at ages 11 to 12, higher drive for thinness at ages 11 to 12, lower behavioral conduct at ages 11 to 12, and a perceived increase in stress from ages 10 to 11 to ages 12 to 13.

Application to Nursing Practice

- Body weight concerns, as well as family, social environment, and behavioral factors, are important issues to address with preadolescents.
- Nurses need to implement effective, healthy, and realistic weight management methods for young adolescent girls; techniques include promoting fun, family-oriented physical activity and the elimination of dieting.
- A priority nursing action is the assessment of child and adolescent coping strategies; appropriate techniques, including effective communication, conflict resolution, and stress management, must be taught to children.
- Identification of risk factors for early drug and alcohol use, including genetic predisposition and family environment, needs to be a priority for health care providers.

Reference

Voorhees CC and others: Early predictors of daily smoking. in young women: the National Heart, Lung, and Blood Institute growth and health study, *Prev Med* 34:616, 2002.

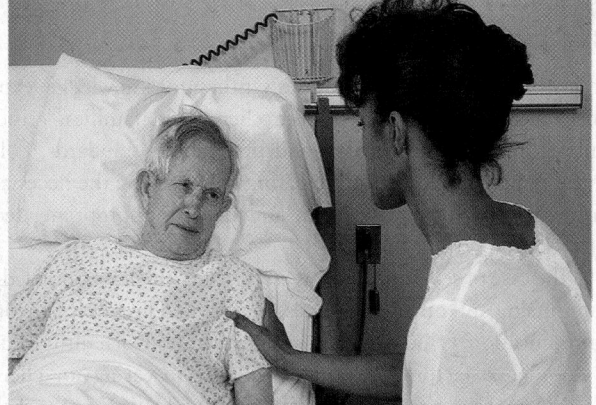

Figure 27-4 Nurses can use touch and eye contact to enhance a client's self-esteem.

to nurses and observe their verbal and nonverbal responses and reactions to the changed appearance. Nurses need to remain aware of their own feelings, ideas, values, expectations, and judgments. Self-awareness is critical in understanding and accepting others. Nurses need to assess and clarify the following self-concept issues about themselves:

- Thoughts and feelings about lifestyle, health, and illness
- Awareness of how own nonverbal communication affects clients and families
- Personal values and expectations and how these affect clients
- Ability to convey a nonjudgmental attitude toward clients
- Preconceived attitudes toward cultural differences in self-concept and self-esteem

Some clients with a change in body appearance or function are extremely sensitive to the verbal and nonverbal responses of the health care team. A positive and matter-of-fact approach to care provides a model for the client and family to follow. Nurses have a significant effect on clients by conveying genuine interest and acceptance. Recognizing and including self-concept issues in the planning and delivery of care positively influence client outcomes. Building a trusting nurse-client relationship and appropriately involving the client and family in decision making will enhance self-concept. Nurses individualize their approach by highlighting a client's unique needs or by incorporating alternative health care practices or methods of spiritual expression in the plan of care.

Nurses also have a significant impact on their client's body image. For example, the body image of a woman who has had a mastectomy is influenced in a positive way by showing acceptance of the mastectomy scar. On the other hand, a nurse who has a shocked or disgusted facial expression will contribute to the woman developing a negative body image. Clients closely watch the reactions of others to their wounds and scars, and it is very important for the nurse to monitor responses toward the client. Statements such as "This wound is healing nicely" or "This tissue looks healthy" are very affirming for the body image of the client. Nonverbal behaviors help to convey the level of caring that exists for a client and affect self-esteem (Figure 27-4). Anticipate personal reactions, acknowledge them, and focus on the client instead of the unpleasant task or situation. Nurses who put themselves in the client's position, will incorporate measures to ease embarrassment, frustration, anger, and denial.

Preventative measures, early identification, and appropriate treatment minimize the intensity of self-esteem stressors and the potential effects for the client and family. Learn to design specific self-concept interventions to fit a client's profile of risk factors. It is essential to assess the client's perception of a problem and to work collaboratively to resolve self-concept issues. For example, self-esteem and HIV high-risk behavior practices were linked in a study of predominantly urban African American women (Sterk and others, 2004). Researchers predicted self-esteem levels in these "at-risk" women by race, religion, childhood experiences with emotional neglect, the number of money-related problems experienced, and the number of drug-related problems. Thus, a different set of interventions for this group of clients to incorporate self-esteem building components and improve health outcomes is necessary.

Critical Thinking

Successful critical thinking requires synthesis of knowledge, experience, information gathered from clients and families, critical thinking attitudes, and ethical and professional standards. Solid clinical judgment requires anticipating and securing the necessary information, analyzing the data, and making appropriate decisions regarding client care.

In the case of self-concept, it is essential to integrate knowledge from nursing and other disciplines, including self-concept theory, communication principles, and a consideration of cultural and developmental factors. Previous experience in caring for clients with self-concept alterations assists in individualizing care. Self-concept profoundly influences a person's response to illness. A critical thinking approach to care is essential. The nursing process is continuous until the client's self-concept is improved, restored, or maintained.

Self-Concept and the Nursing Process

◆ Assessment

In assessing self-concept and self-esteem, first focus on each component of self-concept (identity, body image, and role performance). Assessment needs to include behaviors suggestive of an altered self-concept or self-esteem (Box 27-5), actual and potential self-concept stressors (see Figure 27-3), and coping patterns. Gathering comprehensive assessment data requires the critical synthesis of information from multiple sources (Figure 27-5). In addition to direct questioning (Box 27-6), nurses gather much of the data regarding self-concept through observation of the client's nonverbal behavior and by paying attention to the content of the client's conversation. Take note of the manner in which clients talk about the people in their lives, because this will provide clues to both stressful and supportive relationships, as well as to key roles the client assumes. Using knowledge of developmental stages to determine what areas are likely to be important to the client, inquire about these aspects of the person's life. For example, ask a 70-year-old client about his life and what has been important to him. The individual's conversation will likely provide data relating to role performance, identity, self-esteem, stressors, and coping patterns.

Coping Behaviors. The nursing assessment also includes consideration of previous coping behaviors; the nature, number, and intensity of the stressors; and the client's internal and external resources. Knowledge of how a client has dealt with stressors in the past provides insight into the client's style of coping. Clients do not address all issues in the same ways, but they often use a familiar coping pattern for newly encountered stressors. Identify previous coping strategies to determine whether these patterns have contributed to healthy functioning or created more problems. For example, the use of drugs or alcohol during times of stress often creates additional stressors (see Chapter 31).

✳ BOX 27-5 Behaviors Suggestive of Altered Self-Concept

- Avoidance of eye contact
- Slumped posture
- Unkempt appearance
- Overly apologetic
- Hesitant speech
- Overly critical or angry
- Frequent or inappropriate crying
- Negative self-evaluation
- Excessively dependent
- Hesitant to express views or opinions
- Lack of interest in what is happening
- Passive attitude
- Difficulty in making decisions

✳ BOX 27-6 NURSING ASSESSMENT QUESTIONS

Nature of the Problem
- How would you describe yourself?
- What aspects of your appearance do you like?
- Tell me about the things you do that make you feel good about yourself.
- Tell me about your primary roles. How effective are you at carrying out each of these roles?

Onset and Duration
- When did you start to think or feel differently about yourself?
- How long have you struggled with _____ (specify identity, body image, role performance, or self-esteem)?
- Can you remember a time when you felt good about yourself?

Effect on Client
- Tell me how your self-concept affects your ability to take care of yourself.
- What impact does your self-esteem have on relationships?
- How does your self-esteem affect other areas of your life?

Significant Others. Exploring resources and strengths, such as availability of significant others or prior use of community resources, is important in formulating a realistic and effective plan of care. Valuable information comes from conversations with family and significant others. Significant others sometimes have insights into the person's way of dealing with stressors. They also have knowledge about what is important to the person's self-concept. The way in which a significant other talks about the client and the significant other's nonverbal behaviors provide information about what kind of support is available for the client.

Client Expectations. Another important factor in assessing self-concept is the person's expectations. Asking the client how interventions will make a difference provides useful information regarding the client's expectations. It is also an opportunity to discuss the client's goals. For example, a nurse working with a client who is experiencing anxiety related to an upcoming diagnostic study asks the client about his expectations of the relaxation exer-

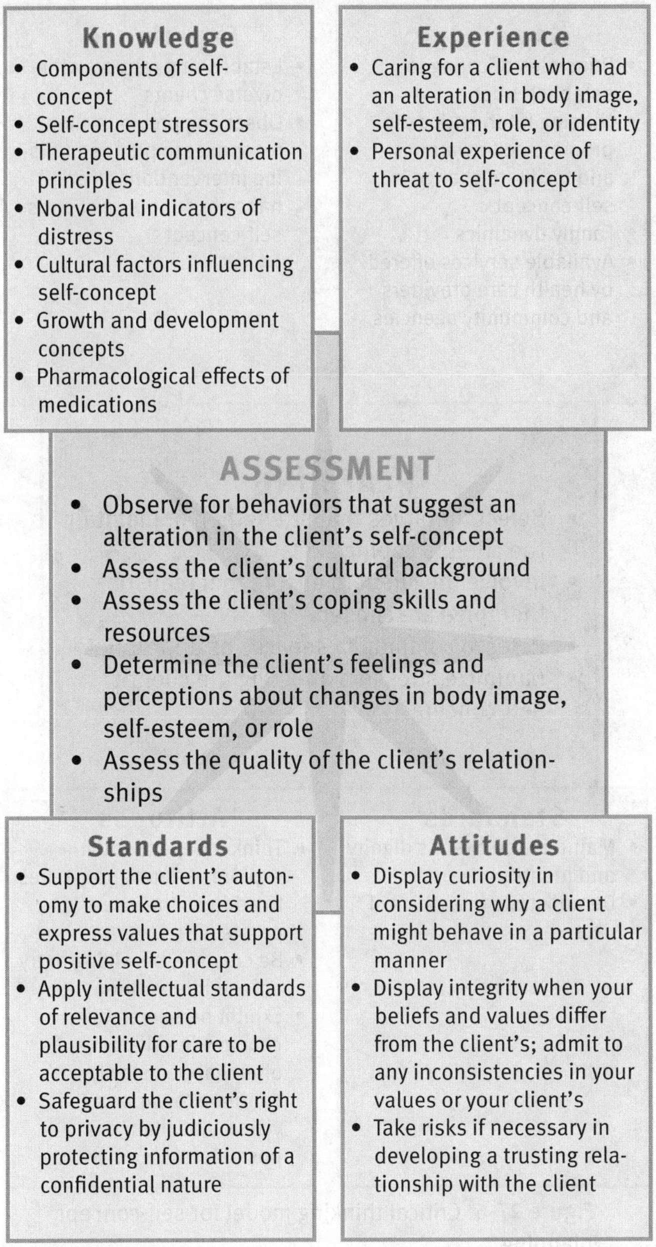

Knowledge

- Components of self-concept
- Self-concept stressors
- Therapeutic communication principles
- Nonverbal indicators of distress
- Cultural factors influencing self-concept
- Growth and development concepts
- Pharmacological effects of medications

Experience

- Caring for a client who had an alteration in body image, self-esteem, role, or identity
- Personal experience of threat to self-concept

ASSESSMENT

- Observe for behaviors that suggest an alteration in the client's self-concept
- Assess the client's cultural background
- Assess the client's coping skills and resources
- Determine the client's feelings and perceptions about changes in body image, self-esteem, or role
- Assess the quality of the client's relationships

Standards

- Support the client's autonomy to make choices and express values that support positive self-concept
- Apply intellectual standards of relevance and plausibility for care to be acceptable to the client
- Safeguard the client's right to privacy by judiciously protecting information of a confidential nature

Attitudes

- Display curiosity in considering why a client might behave in a particular manner
- Display integrity when your beliefs and values differ from the client's; admit to any inconsistencies in your values or your client's
- Take risks if necessary in developing a trusting relationship with the client

Figure 27-5 Critical thinking model for self-concept assessment.

cise that they have been practicing together. The client's response gives the nurse valuable information about the client's beliefs and attitudes regarding the efficacy of the interventions, as well as the potential need to modify the nursing approach.

◆Nursing Diagnosis

Carefully consider the assessment data to identify a client's actual or potential problem areas. Rely on knowledge and experience, apply appropriate professional standards, and look for clusters of defining characteristics that indicate a nursing diagnosis. Although there are four nursing diagnostic labels for altered self-

✳ BOX 27-7   NURSING DIAGNOSTIC PROCESS

Situational Low Self-Esteem

Assessment Activities	Defining Characteristics
Ask client to explain thoughts and feeling about self.	Client is tearful and reports negative thoughts about self. Client reports not wanting to have any visitors.
Observe client's behavior, and ask family if client is experiencing emotional or behavior changes.	Spouse describes withdrawal and avoidance of intimacy. Spouse states wife is unable to make decisions.
Determine if client has had issues with self-esteem in the past and her plans to improve her self-esteem.	Client denies any self-esteem issues since adolescence. She describes a willingness to bring her husband to a counselor to discuss ways he can support her return to high self-esteem.

concept, the following list (NANDA International, 2007) also provides examples of self-concept–related nursing diagnoses:

- Disturbed body image
- Caregiver role strain
- Disturbed personal identity
- Ineffective role performance
- Readiness for enhanced self-concept
- Chronic low self-esteem
- Situational low self-esteem
- Risk for situational low self-esteem

Making nursing diagnoses about self-concept is complex. Often, isolated data are defining characteristics for more than one nursing diagnosis (Box 27-7). For example, a client expresses feelings of uncertainty and inadequacy. These are defining characteristics for both *anxiety* and *situational low self-esteem*. Realizing that the client is demonstrating defining characteristics of more than one nursing diagnosis guides the nurse to gather specific data to validate and differentiate the underlying problem. To further assess the possibility of *anxiety* as the nursing diagnosis, consider whether the person has any of the following defining characteristics: Is the person experiencing increased muscle tension, shakiness, a sense of being "rattled," or restlessness? These symptoms suggest *anxiety* as the more appropriate diagnosis. On the other hand, if the person expresses a predominantly negative self-appraisal, including inability to handle situations or events and difficulty making decisions, these characteristics suggest that *situational low self-esteem* is more appropriate. To further aid in differentiating between the two demonstrated diagnoses, information regarding recent events in the person's life and how the person has viewed himself or herself in the past provide insight into the most appropriate nursing diagnosis. As the nurse gathers additional data, usually the priority nursing diagnosis becomes evident.

To validate critical thinking regarding a nursing diagnosis, share observations with the client and allow the client to verify perceptions. This approach often results in the client's providing additional data, which further clarifies the situation. For example, "I noticed that you jumped when I touched your arm. Are you feeling uneasy today?" allows the client to verify whether he or she is in fact anxious and describe his or her concerns.

◆ Planning

During planning, synthesize knowledge, experience, critical thinking attitudes, and standards (Figure 27-6). Critical thinking ensures that the client's plan of care integrates information known about the individual, as well as key critical thinking elements (see Care Plan). Professional standards are especially important to consider when developing a plan of care. These standards often establish ethical or evidence-based practice guidelines for selecting effective nursing interventions.

Another method to assist in planning care is a concept map. An illustrative concept map (Figure 27-7) shows the relationship of a medical diagnosis, postoperative reconstruction of severe facial scars, with four nursing diagnoses. The concept map shows how the nursing diagnoses are interrelated. It also assists in showing the interrelationships between nursing interventions. A single intervention can be effective for more than one diagnosis.

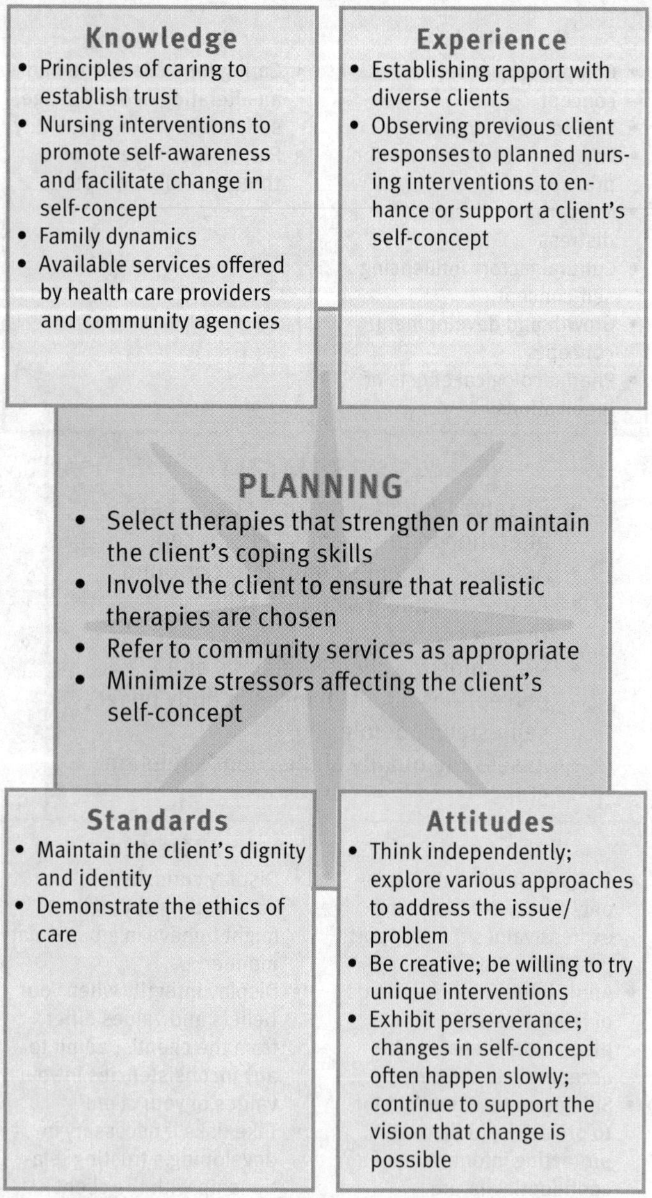

Goals and Outcomes. Develop an individualized plan of care for each nursing diagnosis. Work collaboratively with the client to set realistic expectations for care. Make sure goals are individualized and realistic with measurable outcomes. In establishing goals, consult with the client about whether the goals are achievable. Consultation with significant others, mental health clinicians, and community resources will result in a more comprehensive and workable plan. Once the goal is formulated, consider how the data that illustrated the problem would change if the problem were diminished. The outcome criteria should reflect these changes. For example, a client is diagnosed with *situational low self-esteem related to a recent job layoff*. Establish a goal: "Client's self-esteem and self-concept will begin to improve in 1 week." Examples of expected outcomes directed toward that goal include the following:

- The client will discuss a minimum of three areas of her life where she is functioning well.
- The client will be able to voice the recognition that losing her job is not reflective of her worth as a person.
- The client will attend a support group for out-of-work professionals.

Setting Priorities. The care plan presents the goals, expected outcomes, and interventions for a client with an alteration in self-concept. Interventions help the client adapt to the stressors that led to the self-concept disturbance and support and reinforce the development of coping methods. Often a client perceives a situation as overwhelming and feels hopeless about returning to the level of previous functioning. The client often needs time to adapt to physical changes but can work toward progressive improvement in self-concept and self-esteem.

Establishing priorities includes using therapeutic communication to address self-concept issues, which ensures that the client's

Knowledge
- Principles of caring to establish trust
- Nursing interventions to promote self-awareness and facilitate change in self-concept
- Family dynamics
- Available services offered by health care providers and community agencies

Experience
- Establishing rapport with diverse clients
- Observing previous client responses to planned nursing interventions to enhance or support a client's self-concept

PLANNING
- Select therapies that strengthen or maintain the client's coping skills
- Involve the client to ensure that realistic therapies are chosen
- Refer to community services as appropriate
- Minimize stressors affecting the client's self-concept

Standards
- Maintain the client's dignity and identity
- Demonstrate the ethics of care

Attitudes
- Think independently; explore various approaches to address the issue/problem
- Be creative; be willing to try unique interventions
- Exhibit perserverance; changes in self-concept often happen slowly; continue to support the vision that change is possible

Figure 27-6 Critical thinking model for self-concept planning.

ability to address physical needs is maximized. Look for strengths in both the individual and the family, and provide resources and education to turn limitations into strengths. Client teaching creates understanding of the normalcy of certain situations (e.g., nature of a chronic disease, change in relationships, or effect of a loss). Often, once clients understand their situations, their sense of hopelessness and helplessness is lessened.

Collaborative Care. The perceptions of significant others are important to incorporate into the plan of care. Individuals who have experienced deficits in self-concept before the current episode of treatment have often established a system of support including mental health clinicians, clergy, and other community resources. Before including the family, consider the client's desires for their involvement and cultural norms regarding who most frequently

NURSING CARE PLAN
Situational Low Self-Esteem

Assessment

Mrs. Johnson, a 45-year-old married woman who had a unilateral radical mastectomy due to malignant breast cancer, has been assigned to Susan Carr, nursing student. Susan completed Mrs. Johnson's physical assessment. Mrs. Johnson has been adequately medicated for pain. Ms. Carr sits down to discuss how the mastectomy has affected Mrs. Johnson's self-concept and self-esteem.

Assessment Activities

Assess identity concerns (e.g., sexual role, femininity). Ask how the loss of a breast has affected her sense of self.

Observe Mrs. Johnson's mood and affect and her nonverbal communication and interactions with others.

Determine Mrs. Johnson's interest and involvement in self-care activities.

Offer opportunities to participate in treatment and provide supportive-educative nursing care.

Findings/Defining Characteristics*

Mrs. Johnson **looks away, shakes her head**, and states, **"I feel like less of a woman**. My husband says I'm still sexy, but I don't believe him."

Mrs. Johnson demonstrates **intermittent eye contact, frequent crying when alone, pulling hospital gown tightly across chest**, and **superficial conversations** with family members.

Mrs. Johnson **refuses to bathe, comb hair, and apply typical makeup and avoids looking in a mirror.** She **eats less** than 50% of meals.

Mrs. Johnson avoids looking at or touching her chest and **does not ask questions** about her condition.

****Defining characteristics** are shown in bold type.

Nursing Diagnosis: Situational low self-esteem related to negative view of self as less than whole following mastectomy and uncertainty of future identity and roles.

Planning

Goal

Mrs. Johnson's self-concept will improve, including a more positive self-esteem and ability to achieve role performance before discharge.

Expected Outcomes (NOC)†

Self-Esteem

Mrs. Johnson will verbalize feelings of self-acceptance and self-worth within 4 days.

Mrs. Johnson will demonstrate maintenance of basic grooming and hygiene needs within 2 days.

Role Performance

Mrs. Johnson will describe role changes associated with mastectomy and will verbalize commitment to accessing community resources by day of discharge.

†Outcome classification labels from Moorhead S and others: *Nursing outcomes classification (NOC)*, ed 4, St. Louis, 2008, Mosby.

Interventions (NIC)‡

Self-Esteem Enhancement

- Facilitate an environment and activities that will increase self-esteem.

- Monitor Mrs. Johnson's statements of self-worth.

- Encourage increased responsibility for self and assist client with accepting dependence on others, as appropriate.

Role Enhancement

- Assist Mrs. Johnson with identifying specific role changes brought on by mastectomy.

Rationale

A therapeutic nurse-client relationship promotes positive client outcome, including the client's assuming responsibility for her own care (Stuart and Laraia, 2005).

The nurse must assess thoughts and feelings, including depression, to ensure the client's safety and make appropriate referrals (Folse and others, 2006).

Promoting self-care enhances self-concept, including improving role performance (Stuart and Laraia, 2005).

Only after the problem is accurately defined can alternative choices be proposed (Stuart and Laraia, 2005).

‡Intervention classification labels from Bulechek GM, Butcher HK, and Dochterman JM: *Nursing interventions classification (NIC)*, ed 5, St. Louis, 2008, Mosby.

Continued

NURSING CARE PLAN
===

NURSING CARE PLAN

Situational Low Self-Esteem—cont'd

Evaluation

Nursing Actions	Client Response/Finding	Achievement of Outcome
Ask Mrs. Johnson how effective she feels in her ability to identify and express feelings verbally and nonverbally.	Mrs. Johnson reports, "I've been able to talk with my husband, even about my concerns that he won't find me attractive anymore."	Improved verbal and nonverbal communication noted.
Monitor changes in Mrs. Johnson's statements about herself.	Mrs. Johnson is making fewer negative comments and is evaluating body image more realistically but remains dissatisfied with appearance.	Small improvement in self-esteem; body image more realistic, but remains negative. Discusses body image with husband and nursing student.
Observe Mrs. Johnson's participation in self-care related to mastectomy.	Mrs. Johnson assumed responsibility for basic hygiene; has used a mirror to examine mastectomy scar.	Meeting self-care needs.
Ask Mrs. Johnson to identify resources outside the hospital.	Mrs. Johnson has expressed interest in attending local breast cancer survivors' support group	Scheduled to attend mastectomy support group 2 days after scheduled discharge.

CONCEPT MAP

Nursing diagnosis: Disturbed body image
- Does not touch her face
- Unable to look in mirror
- Avoids new social interactions
- Fears losing husband if surgeries "don't work"

Interventions
- Assist to develop a realistic perception of her body image
- Tell client that her feelings are similar to feelings of other people in the same situation
- Show acceptance of facial scars when providing care

Nursing diagnosis: Acute pain
- Rates postoperative facial pain as 9 on 0 to 10 scale
- States "no relief from pain" with PCA
- Poor sleeping patterns
- Lack of appetite
- Decreased nutritional intake

Interventions
- Ask client to describe past methods used to control pain
- Explore the need for opioid and nonnarcotic analgesics
- Discuss client's fears of undertreated pain and addiction

Client's chief medical diagnosis: Postoperative reconstruction of severe facial scars
Priority assessments: Self-esteem, effects of scars on body image, pain level, and feelings of fear and anxiety

Nursing diagnosis: Situational low self-esteem
- States she is unable to "cope"
- Difficulty making decisions
- Feelings of uselessness

Interventions
- Assess client for signs and symptoms of depression and potential for suicide
- Actively listen to and demonstrate respect for client
- Ask client to identify personal strengths and talents

Nursing diagnosis: Fear
- Decreased self-confidence
- Reports being unable to solve personal problems
- Panics when people ask about the accident
- Daily fatigue
- Worries that surgeries "won't work"

Interventions
- Help client distinguish between real and imagined threats
- Encourage client to write about fears in a journal
- Explore feelings that contribute to fear

——— Link between medical diagnosis and nursing diagnosis   - - - - Link between nursing diagnoses

Figure 27-7 Concept map for client who is postoperative for reconstruction of severe facial scars.

makes decisions in the family. Clients who are experiencing threats to or alterations in self-concept often benefit from collaboration with mental health and community resources to promote increased awareness. Additional resources include physical therapy, occupational therapy, behavioral health, social services, and pastoral care. Knowledge of available resources allows appropriate referrals.

◆Implementation

As with all the steps of the nursing process, a therapeutic nurse-client relationship is central to the implementation phase. The nurse develops the goals and outcome criteria, then considers nursing interventions for promoting a healthy self-concept and helping the client move toward the goals. To develop effective nursing interventions, consider the nursing diagnosis and individualize interventions that address the diagnosis. Collaborating with members of the health care team will maximize the comprehensiveness of the approach to self-concept issues. Regardless of the health care setting, it is important to work with clients and their families or significant others to promote a healthy self-concept. For example, select nursing interventions that help clients regain or restore the elements that contribute to a strong and secure sense of self. The approaches chosen will vary according to the level of care required.

Health Promotion. Work with clients to help them develop healthy lifestyle behaviors that contribute to a positive self-concept. Measures that support adaptation to stress, such as proper nutrition, regular exercise within the client's capabilities, adequate sleep and rest, and stress-reducing practices contribute to a healthy self-concept. Nurses are in a unique position to identify lifestyle practices that put a person's self-concept at risk or are suggestive of altered self-concepts. For example, a young teacher visits a clinic, with complaints of being unable to sleep and experiencing anxiety attacks. In gathering the nursing history, lifestyle practices such as too little rest, a large number of life changes occurring simultaneously, and excessive use of alcohol emerge. These data, when taken together, are suggestive of actual or potential self-concept disturbances. Determine how the client views the various lifestyle elements to facilitate the client's insight into behaviors and to make referrals or provide needed health teaching.

Acute Care. In the acute care setting, some clients experience potential threats to their self-concept because of the nature of the treatment and diagnostic procedures. Threats to a person's self-concept often result in anxiety and/or fear. Numerous stressors, including unknown diagnoses, the need to modify lifestyle, and change in functioning, are often present, and the nurse needs to address them. In the acute care setting there is often more than one stressor, thus increasing the overall stress level for the client and family.

Nurses in the acute care setting also encounter clients who face the need to adapt to an altered body image as a result of surgery or other physical change. Because addressing these needs is difficult to do while in an acute care setting, appropriate follow-up and referrals, including home care, are essential. Remain sensitive to the client's level of acceptance of the change. Forcing confrontation with the change before the client is ready will likely delay the person's acceptance. Signs that a person is receptive to such a

---

✳ BOX 27-8   **CLIENT TEACHING**

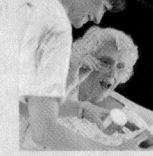

Alterations in Self-Concept

Objective
- Situational low self-esteem will be reduced in the home care setting.

Teaching Strategies
- Encourage opportunities for client to care for self.
- Elicit client's perceptions of strengths and weaknesses.
- Express verbally and behaviorally that client is responsible for behavior.
- Identify relevant stressors with client, and ask for appraisal of them.
- Explore client's adaptive and maladaptive coping responses to problems.
- Collaboratively identify alternative solutions; encourage alternatives not previously tried.
- Continue to reinforce strengths and successes.

Evaluation
- Confirm perception of and actual use of improved communication skills.
- Observe level of participation in decisions that affect care.
- Observe the client's establishment of a simple routine.
- Observe client taking necessary action to change maladaptive coping responses and maintaining adaptive ones.
- Confirm with client and family how to apply new coping resources to continued change.

Modified from Stuart GW, Laraia MT: *Principles and practice of psychiatric nursing,* ed 8, St. Louis, 2005, Mosby.

---

visit include asking questions related to how to manage a particular aspect of what has happened or looking at the changed area. As the client expresses readiness to integrate the body change into his or her self-concept, let the client know about groups that are available and make the initial contact.

Restorative and Continuing Care. Often, in a home care environment a nurse has more of an opportunity to work with a client to obtain the goal of attaining a more positive self-concept. Interventions designed to help a client reach the goal of adapting to changes in self-concept or attaining a positive self-concept are based on the premise that the client first develops insight and self-awareness concerning problems and stressors and then acts to solve the problems and cope with the stressors. Incorporate this approach into client teaching for alterations in self-concept, including situational low self-esteem, which sometimes present in the home care setting (Box 27-8).

Increase the client's self-awareness by allowing the client to openly explore thoughts and feelings. A priority nursing intervention is the expert use of communication skills to clarify the expectations of the client and family. Open exploration makes the situation less threatening for the client and encourages behaviors that expand self-awareness. Accept the client's thoughts and feelings, help the client to clarify interactions with others, and be empathic. Support self-expression, and stress the client's self-responsibility.

Help the client to define problems clearly and to identify positive and negative coping mechanisms. Work closely with the client to analyze adaptive and maladaptive responses, contrast different

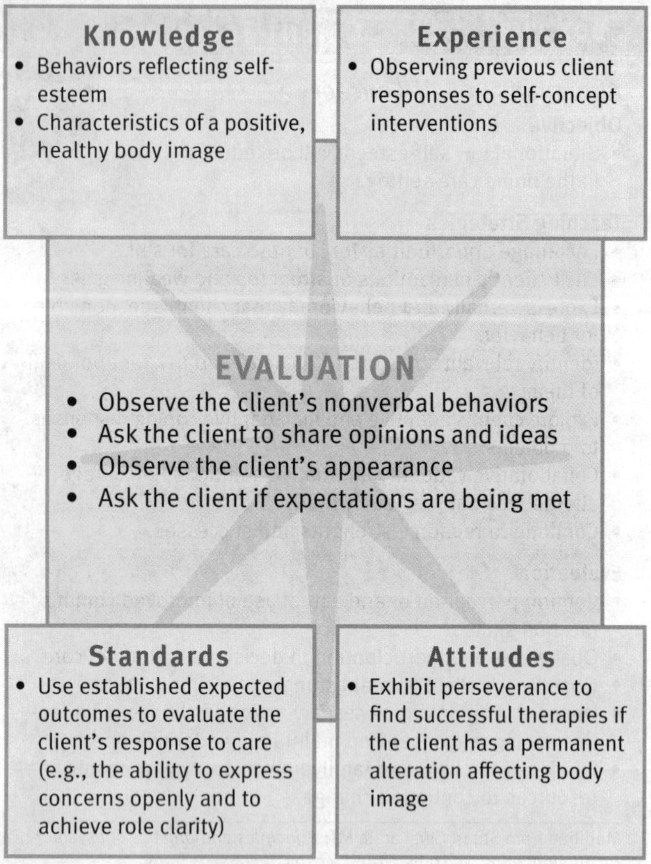

Figure 27-8 Critical thinking model for self-concept evaluation.

Knowledge
- Behaviors reflecting self-esteem
- Characteristics of a positive, healthy body image

Experience
- Observing previous client responses to self-concept interventions

EVALUATION
- Observe the client's nonverbal behaviors
- Ask the client to share opinions and ideas
- Observe the client's appearance
- Ask the client if expectations are being met

Standards
- Use established expected outcomes to evaluate the client's response to care (e.g., the ability to express concerns openly and to achieve role clarity)

Attitudes
- Exhibit perseverance to find successful therapies if the client has a permanent alteration affecting body image

alternatives, devise a plan, and discuss outcomes. Collaborate with the client to identify alternative solutions and develop realistic goals to facilitate real change and encourage further goal-setting behaviors. Design opportunities that result in success, reinforce the client's skills and strengths, and help the client find needed assistance. Encourage the client to commit to decisions and actions to achieve goals by teaching the client to move away from ineffective coping mechanisms and develop successful coping strategies. Supporting attempts that are helpful is essential, because with each success the client is able to make another attempt.

◆ Evaluation

Use critical thinking to evaluate the client's success in meeting each goal and the established expected outcomes (Figure 27-8). Frequent evaluation of client progress is necessary. Apply knowledge of behaviors and characteristics of a healthy self-concept when reviewing the actual behaviors clients display. This determines whether outcomes have been met.

Expected outcomes for a client with a self-concept disturbance include nonverbal behaviors indicating a positive self-concept, statements of self-acceptance, and acceptance of change in appearance or function. Key indicators of a client's self-concept are nonverbal behaviors. For example, a client who has had difficulty making eye contact demonstrates a more positive self-concept by

making more frequent eye contact during conversation. Social interaction, adequate self-care, acceptance of the use of prosthetic devices, and statements indicating understanding of teaching all indicate progress. A positive attitude toward rehabilitation and increased movement toward independence facilitate a return to preexisting roles at work or at home. Patterns of interacting also reflect changes in self-concept. For example, a client who has been hesitant to express personal views more readily offers opinions and ideas as self-esteem increases.

The goals of care sometimes become unrealistic or inappropriate as the client's condition changes. Revise the plan if needed, reflecting on successful experiences with other clients. Client adaptation to major changes takes a year or longer, but the fact that this period is long does not suggest problems with adaptation. Look for signs that the client has reduced some stressors and that some behaviors have become more adaptive. If initial outcomes regarding self-concept are not met, the nurse often asks, "Tell me what you will do if you are not able to return to work," or "Describe whom you will contact if you are not feeling any better about yourself in 2 weeks." Changes in self-concept take time. Although change is often slow, care of the client with a self-concept disturbance is rewarding.

✳ Key Concepts

- Self-concept is an integrated set of conscious and unconscious attitudes and perceptions about the self.
- Components of self-concept are identity, body image, and role performance.
- Each developmental stage involves factors that are important to the development of a healthy, positive self-concept.
- Identity is particularly vulnerable during adolescence.
- Body image is the mental picture of one's body and is not necessarily consistent with a person's actual body structure or appearance.
- Body image stressors include changes in physical appearance, structure, or functioning caused by normal developmental changes or illness.
- Self-esteem stressors include developmental and relationship changes, illness, surgery, accidents, and the responses of other individuals to changes resulting from these events.
- Role stressors, including role conflict, role ambiguity, and role strain, originate in unclear or conflicting role expectations; the effects of illness often aggravate this.
- The nurse's self-concept and nursing actions have an effect on a client's self-concept.
- Planning and implementing nursing interventions for self-concept disturbance involve expanding the client's self-awareness, encouraging self-exploration, aiding in self-evaluation, helping formulate goals in regard to adaptation, and assisting the client in achieving those goals.

✳ Critical Thinking Exercises

1. On the second postoperative day you enter the room and find Mrs. Johnson crying. She states she has just gotten off the phone with her 23-year-old daughter and has agreed to care for her daughter's 3-month-old daughter while the daughter returns to work. You were informed in

shift report that Mrs. Johnson had a restless night and has not taken pain medication since 2030. You assess she is in moderate pain, which you immediately treat with morphine. Within 40 minutes, Mrs. Johnson reports the morphine has decreased her pain rating from a 6 to a 3 on a scale of 0 to 10 but has left her somewhat drowsy. Mrs. Johnson has shared with you some of her concerns about whether or not she can actually provide child care for her granddaughter but states, "Maybe it will make me feel worthwhile and will take my mind off of how disgusting I look." She continues, "I just want to be normal again." How would you address her comment regarding "being normal again" and her lack of understanding of her physical condition, including pain management, increased fatigue, and limitations regarding lifting?

2. As a part of your home care experience, you are assigned to visit Mrs. Johnson who, in addition to caring for her infant granddaughter, is also caring for her mother, who is increasingly agitated and aggressive secondary to Alzheimer's disease. When you go to the home, you find Mrs. Johnson tearful. She says, "I can't do this anymore. She doesn't like anything I cook. She calls me two or three times during the night to sit with her; sometimes she doesn't even recognize me. The baby is constantly crying; I think she senses my stress. I feel so overwhelmed." What additional assessment data would be important to gather? What priority nursing diagnosis could be made for Mrs. Johnson?

✳ NCLEX®-Style Review Questions

1. Following a bilateral mastectomy, a 50-year-old client refuses to eat, discourages visitors, and pays little attention to her appearance. One morning the nurse enters the room to see the client with her hair combed and makeup applied. Which of the following is the best response from the nurse?
   1. "What's the special occasion?"
   2. "You must be feeling better today."
   3. "This is the first time I have seen you look this good."
   4. "I see you have combed your hair and put on makeup."

2. When developing an appropriate outcome for a 15-year-old girl, the nurse considers that a primary developmental task of adolescence is to:
   1. Form a sense of identity
   2. Create intimate relationships
   3. Separate from parents and live independently
   4. Achieve positive self-esteem through experimentation

3. Several staff members complain about a client's constant questions, such as "Should I have a cup of coffee or a cup of tea?" and "Should I take a shower now or wait until later?" Which interpretation of the client's behavior will help the nurses provide optimal care?
   1. Asking questions is attention-seeking behavior.
   2. Inability to make decisions reflects a self-concept issue.
   3. Dependence on staff needs to be stopped immediately.
   4. Indecisiveness is aimed at testing how the staff reacts.

4. A depressed client is crying and verbalizes feelings of low self-esteem and self-worth such as "I'm such a failure . . . I can't do anything right." The best nursing response would be to:
   1. Remain with the client until the client stops crying
   2. Tell the client that is not true and that every person has a purpose in life
   3. Review recent behaviors or accomplishments that demonstrate skill ability
   4. Reassure the client you know how he is feeling and that things will get better

5. When an individual internalizes the beliefs, behavior, and values of role models into a personal, unique expression of self, the nurse would document this as:
   1. Inhibition
   2. Substitution
   3. Identification
   4. Reinforcement-extinction

6. When caring for an 87-year-old client, the nurse needs to understand which of the following most directly influences the client's self-concept:
   1. Attitude and behaviors of relatives providing care
   2. Caring behaviors of the nurse and health care team
   3. Level of education, economic status, and living conditions
   4. Adjustment to role change, loss of loved ones, and physical energy

7. An appropriate nursing diagnosis for an individual who experiences confusion in the mental picture of his physical self is:
   1. Acute confusion
   2. Disturbed body image
   3. Chronic low self-esteem
   4. Situational low self-esteem

8. The nurse asks the client, "How do you feel about yourself?" The nurse is assessing the client's:
   1. Identify
   2. Self-esteem
   3. Body image
   4. Role performance

9. The nurse can increase a client's self-awareness by which of the following? (Choose all that apply.)
   1. Helping the client to define her problems clearly
   2. Allowing the client to openly explore thoughts and feelings
   3. Reframing the client's thoughts and feelings in a more positive way
   4. Having the client identify her positive and negative coping mechanisms

28 | Sexuality

OBJECTIVES

Mastery of content in this chapter will enable the student to:

- Identify personal attitudes, beliefs, and biases related to sexuality.
- Discuss the nurse's role in maintaining or enhancing a client's sexual health.
- Describe key concepts of sexual development across the life span.
- Identify causes of sexual dysfunction.
- Assess a client's sexuality.
- Formulate appropriate nursing diagnoses for clients with alterations in sexuality.

- Identify client risk factors in the area of sexual health.
- Identify and describe nursing interventions to promote sexual health.
- Evaluate client outcomes related to sexual health needs.
- Identify other health care providers and community resources available to help clients resolve sexual concerns that are outside the nurse's level of expertise.
- Use critical thinking skills when helping clients meet their sexual needs.

 MEDIA RESOURCES   KEY TERMS

 Companion CD
- NCLEX®-Style Review Questions
- Audio Glossary
- Interactive Learning Activities
- English/Spanish Glossary

***evolve* Website**
- NCLEX®-Style Review Questions
- Audio Glossary
- English/Spanish Glossary
- Interactive Learning Activities
- Weblinks
- Audio Summaries

Bisexual, p. 428
Climacteric, p. 438
Condom, p. 429
Contraception, p. 427
Diaphragm, p. 429
Dyspareunia, p. 428
Gay, p. 430
Gender identity, p. 427
Gender roles, p. 427
Heterosexual, p. 428
Homosexual, p. 428
Infertility, p. 430
Intercourse, p. 427

Lesbian, p. 428
Perimenopausal, p. 428
Sexual dysfunction, p. 432
Sexual health, p. 427
Sexual orientation, p. 427
Sexuality, p. 427
Sexually transmitted diseases (STDs), p. 427
Sterilization, p. 429
Tubal ligation, p. 429
Vaginismus, p. 432
Vasectomy, p. 429

Sexuality is part of a person's personality and is important for overall health. Even though openness to sexual topics and discussion has increased over the years, many adults lack knowledge regarding **sexuality** and are reluctant to raise questions related to sexuality. For example, clients who have had a myocardial infarction (MI) frequently have concerns about resuming sexual **intercourse** and experience anxiety about the effects new medications will have on sexual functioning. Although these clients are often hesitant to bring up their concerns, they will often share their feelings when the nurse addresses sexuality in a relaxed, matter-of-fact manner. In order to feel comfortable addressing sexuality, nurses need to have an adequate knowledge base regarding sexual functioning and sexual issues; well-developed communication skills; knowledge of areas to assess in regard to sexuality; personal comfort in discussing sexuality; and a caring, sensitive attitude. It is also critical to recognize that there are many values and issues surrounding sexuality. Religious teachings, cultural influences on **gender roles**, beliefs about **sexual orientation**, and social and environmental climates influence the values systems for both clients and health care providers.

Sexuality is more than genital physical activity. It includes a sense of femaleness and maleness as well as biological, sociological, psychological, spiritual, and cultural dimensions of each person's being (Andrews, 2005). In addition, values, attitudes, behaviors, relationships with others, and the need to establish emotional closeness with others influence sexuality. According to the World Health Organization (2004), **sexual health** is "a state of physical, emotional, mental and social well-being in relation to sexuality; it is not merely the absence of disease, dysfunction or infirmity." People who are sexually healthy have a positive and respectful approach to sexuality and sexual relationships. They also have a potential for having pleasurable and safe sexual experiences that are free from coercion, discrimination, and violence.

Scientific Knowledge Base

Nurses help clients achieve sexual health by having a sound scientific knowledge base regarding sexuality. A basic understanding of sexual development, sexual orientation, **contraception**, abortion, and **sexually transmitted diseases (STDs)** is necessary.

Sexual Development

Sexuality changes as a person grows and develops (King, 2005). Each stage of development brings changes in sexual functioning and the role of sexuality in relationships.

Infancy and Early Childhood.
From birth on, children are treated differently according to their gender (Andrews, 2005). The first 3 years of life are crucial in the development of **gender identity** (DeLemaster and Friedrich, 2002). The child identifies with the parent of the same sex and develops a complementary relationship with the parent of the opposite sex. Children become aware of differences between the sexes, begin to perceive that they are either male or female, and interpret the behaviors of others as behavior appropriate for a female or a male.

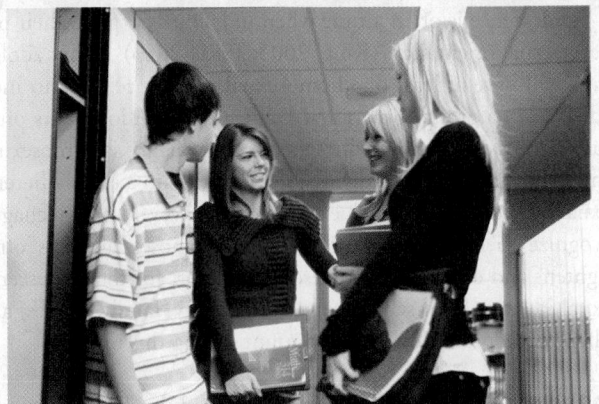

Figure 28-1 Adolescents function within a powerful network of peers as they explore their sexual identity. (Copyright 2007 Jupiter Images Corporation.)

School-Age Years.
During the school years, parents, teachers, and peer groups serve as role models and teachers about how men and women act and relate with each other. School-age children generally have questions regarding the physical and emotional aspects of sex. They need accurate information from home and school about changes in their bodies and emotions during this period and what to expect as they move into puberty (Edleman and Mandle, 2006). Knowledge about normal emotional and physical changes associated with puberty will decrease anxiety as these changes begin to happen. Menstruation or nocturnal emission is sometimes frightening for uninformed children, and some view them as evidence of a dreadful disease.

Puberty/Adolescence.
The emotional changes during puberty and adolescence are as dramatic as the physical ones. The adolescent functions within a powerful peer group, with the almost constant anxiety of "Am I normal?" and "Will I be accepted?" (Figure 28-1). Adolescents face many decisions and need accurate information on topics such as body changes, sexual activity, emotional responses within intimate sexual relationships, STDs, contraception, and pregnancy.

In the United States approximately 47% of high school students report that they have had sexual intercourse at least one time (Centers for Disease Control and Prevention [CDC], 2006c). One reason why adolescents are sexually active is because many believe that sexual intercourse helps them achieve goals of intimacy, social status, and pleasure (Ott and others, 2006). A substantial number of sexually active teenagers do not protect themselves from pregnancy or STDs. The dynamics of sexual risk taking are not fully understood, but numerous studies have found correlations between drug/alcohol use, sexual abuse, and unsafe sex (Morrison-Beedy and others, 2005; Price, 2003). Adolescents tend to think they are invincible and believe that unwanted pregnancy, STDs, and other negative outcomes of sexual behavior are not likely to happen to them (Metcalfe, 2004). Parents need to understand the importance of providing factual information, sharing their values, and promoting sound decision-making skills. They need to know that even with the best guidance and information, adolescents will make their own decisions and need to be held accountable for those decisions.

Adolescence is often a time when individuals explore their primary sexual orientation (King, 2005; Price, 2003). Many adolescents will have at least one **homosexual** experience with an individual or in a group (Stuart and Laraia, 2005). Adolescents often fear that this experience defines their total sexuality as homosexual. This is not true. Many individuals continue with a strictly **heterosexual** orientation after such experiences. However, some teenagers recognize their preference as distinctly homosexual. This often frightens and confuses an adolescent. Support for the adolescent's sexual identity from school counselors, clergy, family, nurses, and other health professionals is important during this time.

Young Adulthood. Although young adults have physically matured, they continue to explore and mature emotionally in relationships. Intimacy and sexuality are issues for all young adults whether they are in a sexual relationship, choose to abstain from sex, remain single by choice, are homosexual, or are widowed. People are sexually healthy in numerous ways. Sexual activity is often defined as a basic need, and healthy sexual desire is channeled into forms of intimacy throughout a lifetime.

As sexually active adults develop intimate relationships, they learn techniques of stimulation that are satisfying to both themselves and their sexual partners. Some adults need permission or affirmation that alternative ways of sexual expression other than penile-vaginal intercourse are normal. Other individuals require significant education or therapy to achieve mutually satisfying sexual relationships. Young adults, especially those with a lower socioeconomic status, are at a high risk for developing STDs.

Middle Adulthood. Changes in physical appearance in middle adulthood sometimes lead to concerns about sexual attractiveness. In addition, actual physical changes related to aging affect sexual functioning. Decreasing levels of estrogen in the **perimenopausal** woman lead to diminished vaginal lubrication and decreased vaginal elasticity. Both of these changes often lead to **dyspareunia**, or the occurrence of pain during intercourse. Decreasing levels of estrogen also result in a decreased desire for sexual activity. As men age, they are likely to experience changes such as an increase in the postejaculatory refractory period and delayed ejaculation. Anticipatory guidance regarding these normal changes, using vaginal lubrication, and creating time for caressing and tenderness ease concerns regarding sexual functioning. Some aging adults also need to adjust to the impact of chronic illness, medications, aches, pains, and other health concerns on sexuality.

Later in the adult years, some individuals have to adjust to the social and emotional changes associated with children moving away from home. This results in either a time of renewed intimacy between partners or a time when formerly intimate partners realize that they no longer care for each other or have common interests. In either case, children leaving home usually creates a change in intimate relationships.

Older Adulthood. Studies of sexuality in older adults are limited and inconsistent in their findings. Many studies suggest that older adults retain an interest in sexual function and are sexually active (Nusbaum and others, 2005). Other studies conclude that there is a decline of sexual interest and behavior among older adults (Box 28-1). Factors that determine sexual activity in older adults

---

BOX 28-1   FOCUS ON OLDER ADULTS

Sexuality in Older Adults

- Sexuality and continued interest in sex throughout late life generally reflects life patterns (Meiner and Lueckenotte, 2006).
- Pathological problems with the aging sexual response are often related to illnesses and medications. For example, impotence is often due to the use of tranquilizers, antidepressants, antihypertensives, or phenothiazines. Removal of causative agent generally results in resolution of the problem (Meiner and Lueckenotte, 2006).
- Older men are often reluctant to discuss sexual problems with health care providers (Nusbaum and others, 2005).
- Older adults who live in assisted living or extended care facilities lose their privacy and experience a decline in physical and cognitive abilities that affects their sexual expression (Nusbaum and others, 2005).
- Some older adults fear that sexual activity will be harmful (Steinke, 2005).
- Many older adults are unfamiliar with the use of condoms and other health promotion activities (e.g., having protected sex with a limited number of sexual partners) related to prevention of sexually transmitted diseases (Nusbaum and others, 2005).

---

include present health status, past and present life satisfaction, and the status of marital or intimate relationships. For example, many older women are widowed or divorced and lack available sexual partners, which accounts for their decline in sexual activity. Nurses working with older adults need to be aware of the sexuality of their clients, assess interest and functioning, and plan accordingly (Meiner and Lueckenotte, 2006). It is essential to maintain a nonjudgmental attitude and convey that sexual activity is normal in later years. Emphasize that sexual activity is not essential to maintaining quality of life, especially when clients have decided not to remain sexually active (Nusbaum and others, 2005).

Nurses need to understand the normal sexual changes that occur as people age to be effective in promoting sexual health (Meiner and Lueckenotte, 2006; Nusbaum and others, 2005). The excitement phase prolongs in both men and women and it usually takes longer for them to reach orgasm. The refractory time following orgasm is also longer. Both genders experience a reduced availability of sex hormones. Men often have erections that are less firm and shorter acting. Women usually do not have difficulty maintaining sexual function unless they have a medical condition that impairs their sexual activity. Typically the infrequency of sex in older women is related to the age, health, and sexual function of their partner. Women continue to experience changes related to menopause, and those with problems related to urinary incontinence often experience embarrassment during intercourse. Couples who experience physically disabling conditions often need information about which positions are more comfortable when having sexual intercourse.

Sexual Orientation

Sexual orientation describes the predominant gender preference of a person's sexual attraction over time. Many stereotypical myths remain about people who are homosexual, **lesbian**, or **bisexual**.

Current evidence indicates that they experience decreased access to health care and do not readily seek preventive care (Heck and others, 2006). Nonjudgmental nurses who have a solid knowledge base help to discourage these myths and provide nursing care that includes attention to the person's sexual orientation.

Contraception

Numerous contraceptive options are available to sexually active couples today. They provide varying levels of protection against unwanted pregnancies. Some methods do not require a prescription, whereas others require a prescription or some other type of intervention from a health care provider. Methods that are effective for contraception do not always reduce the risk of STDs. For example, the pill and intrauterine device (IUD) are effective as birth control but not for protection from STDs. Effectiveness varies with each contraceptive method and the consistency of use. Unplanned pregnancies occur because contraceptives are not used, are used inconsistently, or are used improperly (Running and Berndt, 2003).

Nonprescription Contraceptive Methods. Nonprescription methods for contraception include abstinence, barrier methods, and timing of intercourse in regard to the menstrual cycle. Although abstinence from sexual intercourse is 100% effective, it is often difficult for both men and women to use consistently. Any act of unprotected intercourse potentially results in pregnancy and exposure to STDs.

Barrier methods include over-the-counter spermicidal products and condoms. Spermicidal products (e.g., creams, jellies, foams, and sponges) are put into the vagina before intercourse to create a spermicidal barrier between the uterus and ejaculated sperm. A **condom** is a thin rubber sheath that fits over the penis to prevent entrance of sperm into the vagina. Vaginal spermicides and condoms are most effective when instructions are carefully followed; their combined use is more effective in preventing pregnancy than the use of either one alone (Running and Berndt, 2003).

Nonprescription methods of contraception based on the physiological changes of the menstrual cycle include the rhythm, basal body temperature, cervical mucus, and fertility awareness methods. Couples who use these methods need to understand the reproductive cycle of the woman's body and the subtle signs and signals her body gives during the cycle. To prevent pregnancy, couples abstain from sexual intercourse during designated fertile periods.

Methods That Require a Health Care Provider's Intervention. Contraceptive methods that require the intervention of a health care provider include hormonal contraception, IUDs, the **diaphragm**, the cervical cap, and **sterilization**. Hormonal contraception is available in several forms: oral contraceptive pills, vaginal contraceptive rings, intramuscular injection, subdermal implant, transdermal skin patches, and IUDs. Hormonal contraception alters the hormonal environment to prevent ovulation and thicken cervical mucus.

An IUD is a plastic device inserted by a health care provider into the uterus through the cervical opening. IUDs vary in shape and some contain copper or progesterone. The IUD makes the lining of the uterus less favorable for the implantation of a fertilized ovum.

The diaphragm is a round, rubber dome that has a flexible spring around the edge. It must be used with a contraceptive cream or jelly and is inserted in the vagina so that it provides a contraceptive barrier over the cervical opening. The woman needs to be refitted after a significant change in weight (10 lb gain or loss) or pregnancy. The cervical cap functions like the diaphragm; however, it covers only the cervix. It may be left in place longer, and some perceive it as more comfortable than the diaphragm.

Sterilization is the most effective contraception method other than abstinence. Female sterilization, or **tubal ligation**, involves cutting, tying, or otherwise ligating the fallopian tubes. In male sterilization, or **vasectomy,** the vas deferens, which carries the sperm away from the testicles, is cut and tied. Both a tubal ligation and a vasectomy are considered permanent surgical procedures.

Sexually Transmitted Diseases

The incidence of STDs continues to increase. About 15 million people in the United States are diagnosed with an STD each year; almost 4 million of them are adolescents (U.S. Department of Health and Human Services [USDHHS], 2000). The prevalence of STDs is a major health concern for several reasons. African American and Hispanic populations are diagnosed with STDs more frequently than whites, and women have more complications associated with STDs than men. In addition, social factors such as poverty, low literacy, discrimination, use of illegal drugs (e.g., crack cocaine, methamphetamine), incarceration, sexual abuse, and racial segregation contribute to racial disparities in rates of STDs (Adimora and Schoenbach, 2005; Whyte, 2006). Treatment of STDs in America costs about $17 billion annually (USDHHS, 2000). Commonly diagnosed STDs include syphilis, gonorrhea, chlamydia, trichomoniasis, and infection with the human papillomavirus (HPV) and herpes simplex virus (HSV) type II (genital warts and genital herpes, respectively).

As the name implies, STDs are transmitted from infected individuals to partners during intimate sexual contact. The site of transmission is usually genital, but sometimes it is oral-genital or anal-genital. People most likely to be infected share one key characteristic: unprotected sex with multiple partners. Gonorrhea, chlamydia, syphilis, and pelvic inflammatory disease (PID) are caused by bacteria and are usually curable with antibiotics. All clients need to understand that antibiotics need to be taken for the full course of treatment. An emerging concern, however, is that some of these bacterial infections (e.g., gonorrhea and syphilis) are now developing antibiotic-resistant strains. Two diseases—genital herpes and genital warts—are caused by viruses and cannot be cured.

A major problem in dealing with STDs is finding and treating the people who have them. Some people do not know that they are infected because symptoms are sometimes absent or go unnoticed. However, common symptoms of an STD include discharge from the vagina, penis, or anus; pain during sex or when urinating; blisters or sores in the genital area; and fever (King, 2005). Because sexual behavior often includes the whole body rather than just the genitalia, many parts of the body are potential sites for an STD. The ears, mouth, throat, tongue, nose, and eyelids are sometimes used for sexual pleasure. The perineum, anus, and rectum are also frequently included in sexual activity. Furthermore, any contact with another person's body fluids around the head or an open lesion on the skin, anus, or genitalia can transmit an STD.

Sometimes people do not seek treatment because they are embarrassed to discuss sexual symptoms or concerns. They are also often hesitant to talk about their sexual behavior if they believe that it is not "normal." Any sexual behavior that embarrasses the client often hinders the detection of an STD.

Develop communication skills and a nonjudgmental attitude to provide effective care for those diagnosed with STDs. Detect valuable clues about an STD by establishing trust and talking with clients and asking questions in a caring manner. Assess attitudes toward sexuality, and adjust the intervention to make it acceptable to the client's sexual value system.

Human Immunodeficiency Virus Infection. Human immunodeficiency virus (HIV) infection is sometimes spread through sexual contact. Although HIV is present in the majority of body fluids, it is a blood-borne pathogen. Transmission occurs when there is an exchange of body fluid. Primary routes of transmission include contaminated intravenous (IV) needles, anal intercourse, vaginal intercourse, oral-genital sex, and transfusion of blood and blood products. Populations that are at risk for HIV include gay men, IV drug users, individuals with hemophilia, and heterosexual persons who have unprotected sex with multiple partners.

The natural history of HIV is made up of three stages. The primary infection stage lasts for about a month after contracting the virus. During this time, the person often experiences flulike symptoms. Then the person enters the clinical latency phase; at this time the person has no symptoms of infection. HIV antibodies appear in the blood about 6 weeks to 3 months following infection. If left untreated, people who are infected with HIV will live about 10 years. The last stage, acquired immunodeficiency syndrome (AIDS), happens when the person begins to show symptoms of the disease. AIDS is a serious, debilitating, and eventually fatal disease. Highly active antiretroviral therapy (HAART) has greatly increased the survival time of persons who live with HIV/AIDS (Stanhope and Lancaster, 2004).

Human Papillomavirus Infection. HPV infection, or genital warts, is spread through direct contact with warts, semen, and other body fluids from others who have HPV. The textured warts often have a cauliflower appearance and are most common on the penis and scrotum in men and on the vagina and cervix in women. About 16% of women have genital HPV. HPV is a serious health concern, especially for women. Researchers estimate that 80% to 90% of cervical cancer cases are linked to HPV infection (Stanhope and Lancaster, 2004).

Chlamydia. An infection of the bacteria *Chlamydia trachomatis* causes chlamydia. It is the most commonly reported bacterial STD in the United States, affecting about 2.8 million Americans each year (CDC, 2006a). Chlamydia infects the genitourinary tract and rectum in adults, and it causes conjunctivitis and pneumonia in newborn babies. Transmission occurs when the person comes in contact with fluids from infected sites (e.g., cervix or urethra). It is a major health issue because if it is not treated, it causes PID, ectopic pregnancy, **infertility**, and neonatal complications. The risk of infection is higher in people who are less than 25 years old and who do not consistently use barrier contraceptives. It is also common in people who have multiple sex partners and who are infected with other STDs (Stanhope and Lancaster, 2004). Chlamydia is considered a "silent" disease because about three quarters of women and half of men do not have symptoms (CDC, 2006a). Symptoms in women include dysuria, urinary frequency, and purulent vaginal discharge. In men, it usually infects the urethra and causes nongonococcal urethritis (NGU). Dysuria and urethral discharge are common symptoms of NGU (Stanhope and Lancaster, 2004).

Nursing Knowledge Base

Use critical thinking skills and basic nursing knowledge when addressing clients' sexual health needs. Draw from the following areas of nursing knowledge: sociocultural dimensions of sexuality, decisional issues, and alterations in sexual health.

Sociocultural Dimensions of Sexuality

Cultural rules and norms regarding acceptable behavior within the culture influence sexuality. People assign different meanings to sexuality based on their culture, gender, education, socioeconomic status, and religion (McCarthy and Bodnar, 2005). Society plays a powerful role in shaping sexual values and attitudes and in supporting specific expression of sexuality in its members.

Each cultural and social group has its own set of rules and norms that guide sexual behavior, sexual health, and the willingness to discuss this private part of life. For example, cultural norms influence how people find partners, whom they choose as partners, how they relate to one another, how often they have sex, and what they do when they have sex. Personal beliefs enable certain practices and prohibit others (Box 28-2). For example, the teachings of the Roman Catholic Church prohibit the use of artificial contraception.

Impact of Pregnancy and Menstruation on Sexuality.

Sexual interest and activity of women and their partners varies during pregnancy and menstruation. Some cultures encourage sexual intercourse or male-female contact during menstruation and pregnancy, but other cultures strictly forbid it. For example, in the Hindu culture a woman avoids worship, cooking, and other members of the family during menstruation. Research has found no physiological contraindication to intercourse during menstruation or during most pregnancies. Female sexual interest tends to fluctuate during pregnancy, with increased interest during the second trimester and often decreased interest during the first and third trimesters. There is often a decrease in libido during the first trimester because of nausea, fatigue, and breast tenderness. During the second trimester, there is an increased blood flow to the pelvic area to supply the placenta, resulting in increased sexual enjoyment and libido. During the third trimester the increased abdominal size often makes finding a comfortable position difficult (Murray and McKinney, 2006).

✳ BOX 28-2   CULTURAL ASPECTS OF CARE

Latinos and HIV/AIDS Risk Factors

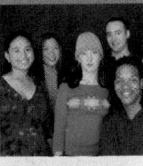

Latino men and women (Latinas) have a higher incidence of HIV/AIDS than non-Hispanic white men and women. Sociocultural factors such as lack of knowledge, limited communication between parents and children about use of contraceptives, and limited exposure to sex education in school contribute to this discrepancy. Low health literacy is sometimes a factor. Latino men are not as comfortable in using condoms, and Latinas are less likely to seek HIV/AIDS testing. Traditional Latino culture supports beliefs in abstinence until marriage, and many believe that teaching children about sex promotes sexual activity. Parents also are not comfortable teaching their children, especially their daughters, about sex.

Implications for Practice

- Whenever possible, first establish a strong therapeutic relationship with the client and family before discussing sexual health.
- Design culturally sensitive and specific nursing interventions for Latinas, potential male partners, and parents.
- Include information about sex education, assertive communication, power in relationships, and negotiation skills.
- Encourage community resources such as churches and schools to improve sex education in Latino communities.
- Continuously assess the client's level of emotional, social, and psychological comfort with sexual health issues.

Data from Zambrana RE and others: Latinas and HIV/AIDS risk factors: implications for harm reduction strategies, *Am J Public Health* 94(7):1152, 2004.

Discussing Sexual Issues. Sexuality is a significant part of each person's being, yet sexual assessment and interventions are not always included in health care. The area of sexuality is often emotionally charged for nurses and clients. Sometimes nurses avoid discussing sexual issues with clients because they lack information or have different values than their clients. Nurses who have difficulty discussing topics related to sexuality need to explore their discomfort and develop a plan to address it. If you are uncomfortable with topics related to sexuality, the client is unlikely to share sexual concerns with you.

Decisional Issues

Individuals make many decisions about their sexuality. Some nurses help clients make decisions about contraception and abortion.

Contraception. Decisions clients make regarding contraception have far-reaching effects on their lives. Pregnancy, whether planned or unplanned, significantly affects the life of the mother and father and often affects their support network. Effects are physical, interpersonal, social, financial, and societal. The choice to use contraception is multifaceted and is not completely understood. Factors that affect the effectiveness of contraception include the method of contraception, the couple's understanding of the contraceptive method, the consistency of use, and the compliance with the requirements of the chosen method. Personal char-

acteristics that positively influence contraceptive use include motivation to avoid unplanned pregnancy, ability to plan, comfort with sexuality, and previous contraceptive use (Running and Berndt, 2003). Some cultural and religious backgrounds permit certain contraceptive practices and prohibit others.

Abortion. Half of all pregnancies in the United States are unplanned; the majority of unplanned pregnancies occur in teenagers, women over 40 years of age and low-income African American women. Almost half of unintended pregnancies end in abortion (USDHHS, 2000). Abortions have been performed since ancient times. The safety and availability of abortions in the United States improved after the 1973 Supreme Court decision *Roe v Wade*, which established the right of every woman to have an abortion. Abortions are safer and less costly when performed in the early weeks of pregnancy.

Abortion is a hotly debated issue. Women and their partners who face an unwanted pregnancy often consider abortion. If caring for a client contemplating abortion, provide an environment in which the client is able to discuss the issue of abortion openly, allowing exploration of various options with an unwanted pregnancy. Discuss religious, social, and personal issues in a nonjudgmental manner with clients. Reasons for choosing an abortion vary and include terminating an unwanted pregnancy or aborting a fetus known to have birth defects. When a woman chooses abortion as a way of dealing with an unwanted pregnancy, the woman, and often her partner, experience a sense of loss, grief, and/or guilt.

Be aware of personal values related to abortion. Nurses are entitled to their personal views and should not be forced to participate in counseling or procedures contrary to beliefs and values. It is essential to choose specialties or places of employment where personal values are not compromised and the care of a client in need of health care is not jeopardized.

STD Prevention. "Safe sex" is a term that describes responsible sexual behavior aimed at preventing the spread of STDs, including HIV/AIDS. Responsible sexual behavior includes knowing one's sexual partner, being able to openly discuss sexual and drug-use history with the partner, not allowing drugs or alcohol to influence decision making, and using protective devices.

Alterations in Sexual Health

Infertility. Infertility is the inability to conceive after 1 year of unprotected intercourse. A couple who wants to conceive and cannot has special needs. Some experience a sense of failure and feel that their bodies are defective. Sometimes the desire to become pregnant grows until it permeates most waking moments. Some individuals become preoccupied with creating just the right circumstances for conception. With advances in reproductive technology, infertile couples face many choices that involve religious and ethical values and financial limitations.

Choices for the infertile couple include pursuit of adoption, medical assistance with fertilization, or adapting to the probability of remaining childless. Organizations such as RESOLVE, a national support group for couples with infertility, or international adoption groups provide couples with support and offer referral sources.

Sexual Abuse. Sexual abuse is a widespread health problem. Abuse crosses all gender, socioeconomic, age, and ethnic groups. Most often abuse is at the hands of a former intimate partner or family member. Sexual abuse has far-ranging effects on physical and psychological functioning (Edelman and Mandle, 2006).

Sometimes sexual abuse begins, continues, or even intensifies during pregnancy. Cues that raise a question of possible sexual abuse include extreme jealousy and refusal to leave a woman's presence. The overall appearance is sometimes that of a very concerned and caring husband or boyfriend when the underlying reason for this behavior is very different.

When you recognize abuse, mobilize support for the victim and the family. All family members usually require therapy to promote healthy interactions and relationships. Rape victims often need to work through the crisis before feeling comfortable with intimate expressions of affection. The partner needs to know how to help and support the victim. Children who have been sexually molested need to understand that they are not at fault for the incident. The parents need to understand that their response is critical to how the child reacts and adapts. Nurses are in an ideal position to assess occurrences of sexual violence, to help clients confronting these stressors, and to educate individuals regarding community services.

Personal and Emotional Conflicts. Ideally, sex is a natural, spontaneous act that passes easily through a number of recognizable physiological stages and ends in one or more orgasms. In reality, this sequence of events is more the exception than the rule. Nurses meet clients who have problems with one or more of the stages of sexual activity, including the feeling of wanting sex, the physiological processes and emotions of having sex, and the feelings experienced after sex. For example, some women and men who are taking antidepressants report that their ability to reach orgasm is negatively affected.

Sexual Dysfunction. Sexual dysfunction, the absence of complete sexual functioning, is common. The incidence of sexual dysfunction in the general population is estimated as high as 52% in men and 63% in women (Nusbaum and Hamilton, 2002). Sexual dysfunction is more prevalent in men and women with poor emotional and physical health (Box 28-3). Sometimes the exact cause cannot be determined.

Erectile dysfunction (ED) affects about 30 million men in the United States and is often unreported (Running and Berndt, 2003). ED occurs more frequently in older men, but it occurs in younger men as well. Risk factors are similar to those for heart disease (e.g., diabetes mellitus, hyperlipidemia, hypertension, hypothyroidism, chronic renal failure, smoking, obesity, alcohol abuse, and lack of exercise). The etiology of ED is often multifactorial. Neurogenic problems, medications, or endocrine or psychogenic factors can cause ED. An age-related decrease in testosterone often results in decreased tone of the erectile tissues.

Sexual dysfunction in women is commonly caused by vaginismus or orgasmic dysfunction. **Vaginismus** is a spastic contraction or tightening of the vagina during or before penetration for intercourse. Orgasmic dysfunction is the inability to achieve orgasm or

---

✱ BOX 28-3 Illnesses and Medications That Affect Sexual Functioning of Men and Women

Illnesses
Diabetes mellitus
Cancer (e.g., prostate, breast, colon, ovarian, testicular, rectal)
Neuropathy
Spina bifida
Spinal cord injury
Unstable angina
Uncontrolled hypertension
Chronic obstructive pulmonary disease
Human immunodeficiency virus (HIV) infection
Substance abuse
Depression

Medications
Antihypertensives
Antipsychotics
Antidepressants
Anxiolytics
Diuretics
Oncologic agents
Recreational or illicit drugs

Data from Burt J and others: Radical prostatectomy: men's experiences and postoperative needs, *J Clin Nurs* 14(7):883, 2005; Nusbaum MRH and others: Chronic illness and sexual functioning, *Am Fam Physician* 67(2):347, 2003; and Townley Bakewell R, Volker DL: Sexual dysfunction related to the treatment of young women with breast cancer *Clin J Oncol Nurs* 9(6):697, 2005.

---

difficulty attaining orgasm in certain situations. Physical causes include infection, diabetes, neurological disease, drug or alcohol use, and aging changes. Unresolved anger, fear of pregnancy, fatigue, anxiety, stress, and depression sometimes cause a lack of desire and loss of interest in being sexually active.

Critical Thinking

Successful critical thinking requires synthesis of knowledge, experience, information gathered from clients, critical thinking attitudes, and intellectual and professional standards. Nurses use clinical judgment to anticipate information needs, analyze assessment data, and make appropriate decisions regarding client care. Figure 28-2 shows how to use elements of critical thinking and client assessment data to develop appropriate nursing diagnoses.

In the case of sexuality, integrate knowledge from nursing and other disciplines. Have a good understanding of safe sex practices and the risks and behaviors associated with sexual problems to anticipate how to assess a client and then how to interpret findings. Use previous experiences to provide care for clients with sexual issues in a more reflective and helpful way. Clients will have different customs and values from those of the nurse. Professional standards require respect for each client as an individual. Critical thinking attitudes such as integrity require you to recognize when personal opinions and values are in conflict with those of the client and to consider how to proceed in a way that is mutually beneficial.

Sexuality and the Nursing Process

A person's sexuality has physical, psychological, social, and cultural elements. Assess all relevant elements to determine a client's sexual well-being. Many nurses find that they are uncomfortable talking about sexuality with clients. To increase comfort in discussing sexuality, build a sound knowledge base and be willing to explore personal issues regarding sexuality. The nursing role in addressing sexual concerns ranges from ongoing assessment to providing information, counseling, and referral. Keep in mind that nurses are not expected to have answers to all of the sexual issues and concerns identified.

◆Assessment

Factors Affecting Sexuality. In gathering a sexual history, consider physical, functional, relationship, lifestyle, developmental, and self-esteem factors that influence sexual functioning. Sexual desire varies among individuals; some people want and enjoy sex every day, whereas others want sex only once a month, and still others have no sexual desire and are quite comfortable with that fact. Sexual desire becomes an issue if the person wants to feel sexual desire more often, if the person believes it is necessary to measure up to some cultural norm, or if there is a discrepancy between the sexual desires of the partners in a relationship.

Ask clients to describe factors that typically influence their sexual desire. Knowing the clients' medical history and probing for information is helpful. For example, minor illness, medications, and fatigue often decrease sexual desire. Lifestyle factors, such as the use or abuse of alcohol, lack of sleep, lack of time, or the demands of caring for a new baby are other influencing factors. Working parents, for example, sometimes feel so overburdened that they perceive sexual advances from a partner as an additional demand on them. Confirm factors that potentially affect sexual desire, and determine the extent to which sexual function is impaired with the client.

Self-concept issues (see Chapter 27), including identity, body image, role performance, and self-esteem, affect a client's sexuality. Consider how these factors relate to the client's condition. For example, poor body image associated with chronic disease magnifies feelings of rejection. This often results in diminished or absent sexual desire. Problems with a person's self-esteem frequently lead to conflicts involving sexuality. Clients who experience negative feelings often suppress sexual feelings when they have not developed a healthy sense of a sexual self. Low sexual self-esteem negatively affects a person's self-concept.

Issues in a relationship often affect sexual desire. After the initial glow of a new relationship has faded, some couples find that they have major differences in their values or lifestyles. Ask couples to describe how close they feel to each other and how often they interact on an intimate level. Assess communication patterns between sexual partners to determine sexual satisfaction within a relationship.

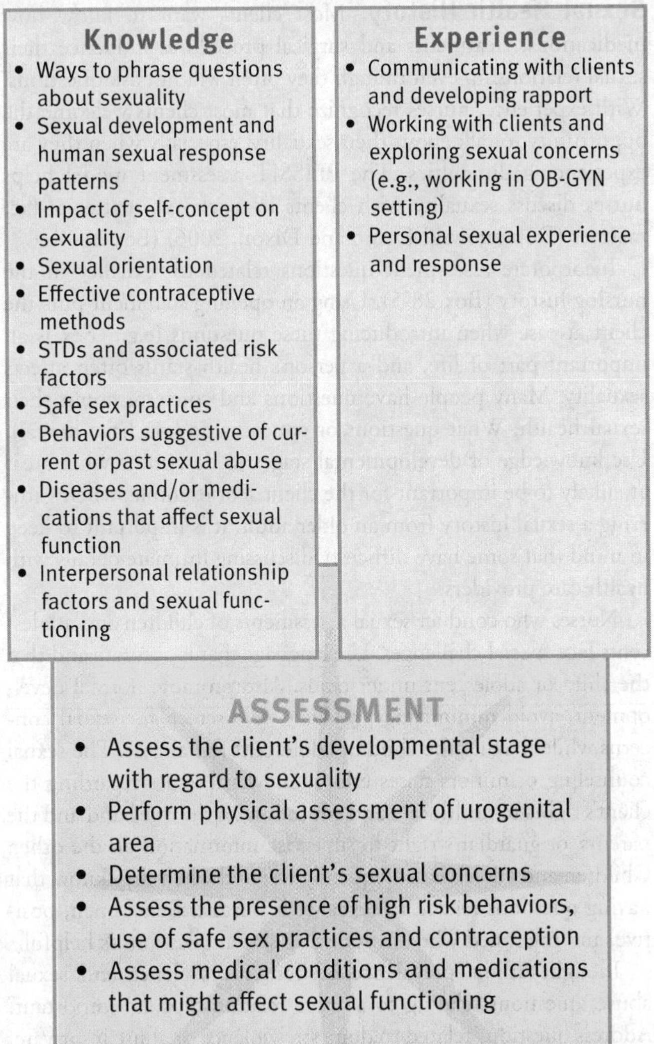

Knowledge
- Ways to phrase questions about sexuality
- Sexual development and human sexual response patterns
- Impact of self-concept on sexuality
- Sexual orientation
- Effective contraceptive methods
- STDs and associated risk factors
- Safe sex practices
- Behaviors suggestive of current or past sexual abuse
- Diseases and/or medications that affect sexual function
- Interpersonal relationship factors and sexual functioning

Experience
- Communicating with clients and developing rapport
- Working with clients and exploring sexual concerns (e.g., working in OB-GYN setting)
- Personal sexual experience and response

ASSESSMENT
- Assess the client's developmental stage with regard to sexuality
- Perform physical assessment of urogenital area
- Determine the client's sexual concerns
- Assess the presence of high risk behaviors, use of safe sex practices and contraception
- Assess medical conditions and medications that might affect sexual functioning

Standards
- Apply intellectual standards of relevance and plausibility for care to be acceptable to the client
- Safeguard the client's right to privacy by judiciously protecting information of a confidential nature
- Apply ethic of care

Attitudes
- Display curiosity; consider why a client might behave or respond in a particular manner
- Display integrity; your beliefs and values differ from client's; admit to any inconsistencies in your values and in the client's
- Take risks if necessary to explore both personal sexual issues and concerns and those of the client

Figure 28-2 Critical thinking model for sexuality assessment.

Sexual Health History. Most clients want to know how medications, treatments and surgical procedures influence their sexual relationship even though they often will not ask questions. With experience, nurses recognize that most clients welcome the opportunity to talk about their sexuality, especially when they are experiencing difficulties. The PLISSIT assessment model helps nurses discuss sexuality with clients in a relaxed, matter-of-fact manner (Dobranowski-Dixon and Dixon, 2006) (Box 28-4).

Incorporate assessment questions related to sexuality in the nursing history (Box 28-5). Using an opening statement puts the client at ease when introducing these questions (e.g., "Sex is an important part of life, and a person's health status often affects sexuality. Many people have questions and concerns about their sexual health. What questions or concerns do you have now?"). Use knowledge of developmental stages to determine what areas are likely to be important for the client. For example, when gathering a sexual history from an older adult, it is important to keep in mind that some have difficulty discussing intimate details with health care providers.

Nurses who conduct sexual assessments of children and adolescents face special challenges. Use language that is accurate and that the child or adolescent understands. Also promote normal development, avoid minimizing problems, and screen for sexual concerns while making the child or adolescent feel at ease. The sexual counseling of minors raises ethical and legal issues regarding the client's rights to health care and education on the one hand and the parents' or guardian's right to supervise information on the other. Children and adolescents frequently respond when they know that having questions related to sexuality is normal. Being open, positive, and interested when introducing sexual questions is helpful.

In light of the prevalence of domestic violence and sexual abuse, questions relating to abusive relationships are important. Address questions related to domestic violence or abuse in private. Recognizing both subjective and objective signs and symptoms of abuse in children and adults will aid in identification of this too-common problem (Table 28-1).

Some individuals are too embarrassed or do not know how to ask sexual questions directly. Look for clues that a person has questions. For example, a client expresses concern about how his or her partner will respond now or makes a sexual comment or joke. Observing for and listening to concerns about sexuality takes practice. With experience a nurse develops skill in clarifying and paraphrasing to help individuals express sexual concerns. By including sexuality in the nursing history, the nurse acknowledges that sexuality is an important component of health and creates an opportunity for the person to discuss sexual concerns.

Sexual Dysfunction. Many illnesses, injuries, medications and aging changes have a negative effect on sexual health. Sexual dysfunction is either temporary or permanent. Apply knowledge about conditions that frequently cause sexual dysfunction while assessing a client's risks (see Box 28-3). Awareness of the possible effects of physical problems, altered self-concept, medications, and the factors addressed thus far on sexual functioning will assist in conducting a thorough assessment. Some clients bring up the topic of sexual dysfunction. Other times issues become evident as the client answers other nursing history questions.

BOX 28-4   PLISSIT Assessment of Sexuality

Permission to discuss sexuality issues
Limited **I**nformation related to sexual health problems being experienced
Specific **S**uggestions—only when the nurse is clear about the problem
Intensive **T**herapy—referral to professional with advanced training if necessary

Modified from Annon JS: The PLISSIT model: a proposed conceptual scheme for the behavioral treatment of sexual problems, *J Sex Educ Ther* 2(2):1, 1976.

BOX 28-5   NURSING ASSESSMENT QUESTIONS

- Are you sexually active?
- How do you feel about the sexual aspects of your life?
- Have you noticed any changes in the way you feel about yourself?
- How has your illness, medication, or surgery affected your sex life?
- It is not unusual for people with your condition to be experiencing some sexual changes. Have you noticed any changes, or do you have any concerns?
- Are you in a relationship in which someone is hurting you?
- Has anyone ever forced you to have sex you did not wish to participate in?
- How many sexual partners do you have (or have you ever had)?
- Tell me what you know about safe sexual practices, use of contraceptives, or prevention of STDs.

Physical Assessment. The physical examination is important in evaluating the cause of sexual concerns or problems and usually provides the best opportunity to teach an individual about sexuality. In examining a woman's breasts and the external and internal genitalia, a nurse has the opportunity to assess the woman's reaction, answer questions, and provide information about the examination of anatomical and physiological structures. For example, a nurse teaches a woman how to perform a breast self-examination during physical assessment (see Chapter 33). During physical assessment of the genitalia, teach men how to perform testicular self-examination (see Chapter 33). Knowledge of normal scrotal anatomical structures helps men detect signs of testicular cancer. Instruct both men and women on signs and symptoms of STDs during the examination when clients' histories suggest risks for STDs.

Client Expectations. As in the case of any client assessment, it is important to understand the client's expectations regarding care. Questions such as "What would you like to have happen in regard to your sexual health problems?" and "What initial steps might you take?" help the client identify desired outcomes. It is important to set aside personal views and not assume the client's expectations.

✳ TABLE 28-1 Signs and Symptoms That Indicate Possible Current Sexual Abuse or a History of Sexual Abuse

TYPES OF FINDINGS	SYMPTOMS OFTEN FOUND IN CHILDREN	SYMPTOMS OFTEN FOUND IN ADULTS
Injuries and/or physical signs	• Bruises, bleeding, soreness, or irritation of external genitalia, anus, mouth, or throat • Sexually transmitted infections • Recurrent urinary tract infections • Unintended pregnancy • Chronic pain • Difficulty walking or sitting • Unusual odor in genital area • Penile discharge • Torn, stained, or bloody underclothing	• Welts, bruising, swelling, scars, burns, or lacerations on arms, legs, breasts, or abdomen • Wounds that do not match the client's "story" • Multiple bruises in various stages of healing • Vaginal or rectal bleeding • Fractures of face, nose, ribs or arms • Trauma to labia, vagina, cervix, or anus • Vomiting or abdominal tenderness
Behavior, nonverbal and/or vague somatic complaints	• Physical aggression • Sexual acting out • Excessive masturbation • Expressions of low self-esteem • Poor school performance • Poor peer relationships • Sleep disturbances • Social withdrawal and excessive daydreaming • Running away from home • Substance abuse or suicide attempts	• Facial grimacing • Absence of facial response or flat affect • Anxiety • Depression • Panic attacks • Difficulty sleeping • Anorexia • Slow, unsteady gait

Data from Hockenberry MJ, Wilson D: *Wong's nursing care of infants and children*, ed 8, St. Louis, 2007, Elsevier; Stuart GW, Laraia MT: *Principles and practice of psychiatric nursing*, ed 8, St. Louis, 2005, Mosby; and Murray SS, McKinney ES: *Foundations of maternal-newborn nursing*, ed 4, St. Louis, 2006, Saunders.

◆ Nursing Diagnosis

After completing an assessment and applying critical thought to the diagnostic process, select diagnoses applicable to the client's needs. Possible nursing diagnoses related to sexual functioning are listed below:

- Anxiety
- Ineffective coping
- Interrupted family processes
- Deficient knowledge (contraception/STDs)
- Sexual dysfunction
- Ineffective sexuality pattern
- Social isolation
- Risk for other-directed violence
- Risk for self-directed violence

Assessment data that signal a nursing diagnosis related to sexuality often include history of surgery of reproductive organs, changes in appearance or body image, a history of or current physical or sexual abuse, chronic illness, or developmental milestones such as puberty or menopause. To make a nursing diagnosis related to sexual dysfunction, assess anatomical, physiological, sociocultural, ethical, and situational issues thoroughly.

As with making any nursing diagnosis, clarify that the defining characteristics exist and that the client perceives a problem or difficulty with regard to sexuality. Determining the etiological or contributing factors helps the nurse plan effectively and select appropriate nursing interventions. For example, the nursing interventions appropriate for the nursing diagnosis of *sexual dysfunction* are different for different etiological factors. *Sexual dysfunction related to misinformation about the risk of sexually transmitted diseases* requires counseling and education on how to maintain safe sexual practices. In contrast, clients who experience *sexual dysfunction related to physical abuse* need counseling and referral to community resources (e.g., crisis services and physical abuse support group).

◆ Planning

Goals and Outcomes. Synthesize information from multiple resources to develop an individualized plan of care (Figure 28-3). Critical thinking ensures that the client's plan of care integrates all that a nurse knows about the individual, as well as critical thinking elements as they pertain to sexuality. Professional standards are especially important to consider when developing a plan of care. Maintaining a client's dignity and identity is a significant consideration. For example, to convey respect for the client's gender preferences, include a lesbian or gay partner in the plan to the degree that the client wishes.

Develop an individualized plan of care for each nursing diagnosis (see Care Plan). Set realistic goals and measurable outcomes with the client. Goals and outcomes need to be individualized and realistic. For example, a client who has dyspareunia has a nursing diagnosis of *sexual dysfunction related to decreased sexual desire*. The nurse and client develop a goal to report decreased anxiety and greater satisfaction with sexual activity within 1 month. Expected outcomes include that the client will do the following:

- Consistently use a water-soluble lubricant before sexual intercourse within 1 week
- Discuss stressors that contribute to sexual dysfunction with partner within 2 weeks

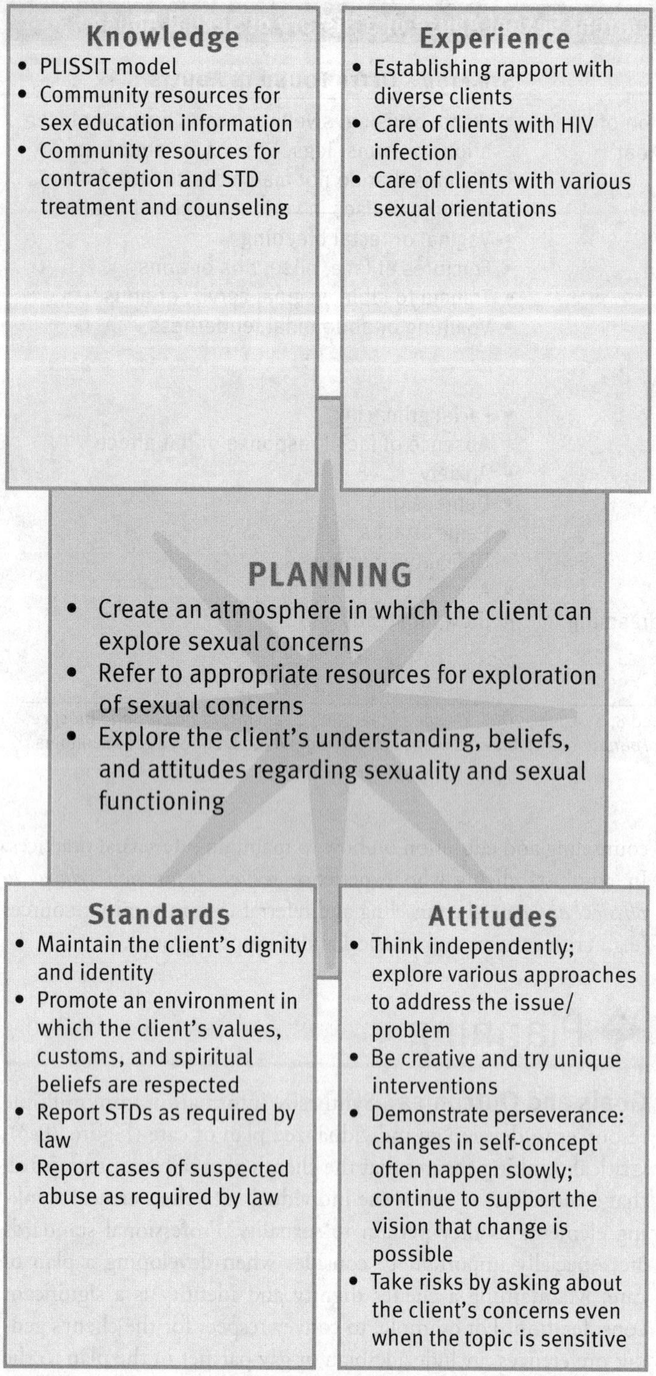

Knowledge

- PLISSIT model
- Community resources for sex education information
- Community resources for contraception and STD treatment and counseling

Experience

- Establishing rapport with diverse clients
- Care of clients with HIV infection
- Care of clients with various sexual orientations

PLANNING

- Create an atmosphere in which the client can explore sexual concerns
- Refer to appropriate resources for exploration of sexual concerns
- Explore the client's understanding, beliefs, and attitudes regarding sexuality and sexual functioning

Standards

- Maintain the client's dignity and identity
- Promote an environment in which the client's values, customs, and spiritual beliefs are respected
- Report STDs as required by law
- Report cases of suspected abuse as required by law

Attitudes

- Think independently; explore various approaches to address the issue/problem
- Be creative and try unique interventions
- Demonstrate perseverance: changes in self-concept often happen slowly; continue to support the vision that change is possible
- Take risks by asking about the client's concerns even when the topic is sensitive

Figure 28-3 Critical thinking model for sexuality planning.

- Identify alternative, satisfying, and acceptable sexual practices for self and partner within 4 weeks

A concept map is another method that is useful in organizing client care (Figure 28-4). This concept map shows the relationship of a medical diagnosis (decreased libido and depression) with the four nursing diagnoses identified from the client assessment data. The map also shows the links and relationship with the nursing diagnosis and interventions appropriate for each diagnosis. For example, ineffective coping affects and contributes to social isolation, and as long as the client has ineffective coping, the social isolation continues or perhaps worsens.

Setting Priorities. The care plan shows the goals, expected outcomes, and interventions for a client experiencing sexual dysfunction. Nursing interventions for clients with sexual concerns focus on supporting the client's need for intimacy and sexual activity. Clients often feel overwhelmed and hopeless about returning to the level of previous sexual functioning. Clients usually need time to adapt to physical and psychosocial changes that affect their sexuality and sexual health.

The priority in addressing needs related to sexuality includes establishing a therapeutic relationship in order for the client to feel comfortable in discussing issues related to sexuality. Look for strengths in both the client and the family while providing education and access to resources to turn limitations into strengths. Client teaching communicates the normalcy of feelings following certain situations (e.g., the diagnosis of a chronic illness or the loss of a body part). The nurse determines the client's needs and plans accordingly.

The client's current problems and needs help the nurse determine the priorities related to the client's sexual health. Priorities for sexual health often include resuming sexual activities. For example, if the client is recovering from a mastectomy and is having problems resuming an intimate relationship with her spouse because of problems related to body image, the nurse helps the client adapt to and cope with the changes in her body image associated with the mastectomy. Once the client's issues related to body image are resolved, she is able to restore intimacy with her spouse and then address her sexual health needs.

Collaborative Care. Planning in the area of sexuality often includes collaboration with other health care providers as well as referrals to community resources (Box 28-6). Nurses generally raise awareness of sexual issues, assist in clarifying concerns, and/or provide information. Nurses who have specialized education in sexual functioning and counseling provide more intensive sex therapy. It is necessary for nurses to understand the limits of their own knowledge base and include other health care providers such as sex therapists, clinical psychologists, and social workers appropriately in order to meet their clients' needs for sexual health. For example, conflicts in marriage usually require intensive treatment with a mental health professional or certified sex therapist. For the woman who is currently in an abusive relationship, the nurse collaborates with special women's shelters that provide counseling and serve as a safe place for the woman while further plans are made.

◆ Implementation

As a nurse, promote sexual health as a component of overall wellness by identifying clients at increased risk (Box 28-7), by providing appropriate information, by helping individuals gain insight into their problems, and by exploring methods to deal with them effectively.

Health Promotion. Helping clients maintain or gain sexual health involves consideration of factors that influence sexual satisfaction. Educate clients about sexual health, including measures for contraception, safe sex practices, and prevention of STDs.

NURSING CARE PLAN
Sexual Dysfunction

Assessment

Mr. Clements is a 65-year-old African American client who had an uncomplicated myocardial infarction (MI) 3 days ago. He is stable and experienced no complications following his MI. He currently is on a cardiac telemetry nursing unit. According to Mr. Clements' medical record, he last visited his advanced practice nurse in the office 2 months ago and was diagnosed with hypertension. He was given a prescription for propranolol (Inderal). Mr. Clements is married and lives with his wife.

His blood pressure today is 122/82 mm Hg. Mr. Clements reports that he has been taking his medication regularly. The nurse knows that clients who have had MIs and who are on antihypertensive medications often experience sexual problems. When assessed by the nurse, Mrs. Clements expresses that she is still interested in having a sexual relationship with her spouse.

Assessment Activities

Ask Mr. Clements if his interest in sex has changed since he started taking propranolol.

Ask Mr. Clements to compare his sexual relationship with his wife before and after taking propranolol.

Ask Mr. Clements if he has noticed any changes in his erect penis.

Ask Mr. Clements what concerns or fears he has about resuming his sexual relationship with his wife now that he has had a myocardial infarction.

Findings/Defining Characteristics*

He responds that he has been **less interested in having sexual intercourse with his wife** since he started taking propranolol.

He states they used to have intercourse 1 to 3 times per week and since he started taking propranolol **they rarely have intercourse.**

He states he **sometimes has trouble having an erection.**

He states that **he is afraid that after discharge he will have chest pain or another heart attack if he has sexual intercourse** with his wife.

*__Defining characteristics__ are shown in bold type.

Nursing Diagnosis: Sexual dysfunction related to altered body function (side effects of propranolol) and lack of knowledge.

Planning

Goal

Client will express satisfaction with sexual relationship with wife within 1 month.

Expected Outcomes (NOC)†
Sexual Functioning

Client will express renewed sexual interest within 2 weeks.

Client will sustain arousal through orgasm within 3 weeks.

†Outcome classification labels from Moorhead S and others: *Nursing outcomes classification (NOC)*, ed 4, St. Louis, 2008, Mosby.

Interventions (NIC)‡

Sexual Counseling

Establish trust and respect with Mr. Clements. Offer privacy during conversations.

Discuss possible effects of MI and propranolol on sexual functioning and that it is safe to resume sexual intercourse 10 days to 3 weeks following an uncomplicated MI (Steinke, 2005).

Include Mrs. Clements in discussions about sexual issues as frequently as possible and when appropriate.

Anxiety Reduction

Encourage Mr. Clements to express fears about resuming sexual activity, and assure him that others who have had MIs experience similar fears.

Rationale

Expresses sense of caring, increasing likelihood of client's ability to express concerns fully (Steinke, 2005).

Enhances understanding about reasons for sexual difficulties and provides safe guidelines for resumption of sexual intercourse following MI (Crumlish, 2004).

Including family members in the plan of care helps clients cope better with problems associated with MIs (Kristofferzon and others, 2005).

Knowing that feelings and fears are normal helps decrease anxiety and encourages return of sexual activity (Steinke, 2005).

‡Intervention classification labels from Bulechek GM, Butcher HK, and Dochterman JM: *Nursing interventions classification (NIC)*, ed 5, St. Louis, 2008, Mosby.

Evaluation

Nursing Actions	Client Response/Finding	Achievement of Outcome
Ask Mr. Clements if he and his wife are satisfied with their sexual relationship during return office visit.	Mr. Clements reports that his interest in sex is back to normal, and he is able to have an erection.	Mr. Clements reports sexual interest and function; he and his wife are satisfied with their relationship.

Regular breast self-examinations, mammograms, and Papanicolaou (Pap) smears are important sexual health measures for women, whereas testicular self-examinations are important for men. Offer the vaccine for HPV to girls who are between 11 and 12 years of age. The vaccine is safe for girls as young as 9 years old and is recommended for females age 13 to 26 if they have not already completed the three required injections. Current evidence shows that the vaccine is effective for at least 5 years (CDC, 2006b).

Exploring an individual's values, discussing levels of satisfaction, and providing sex education require therapeutic communica-

CONCEPT MAP

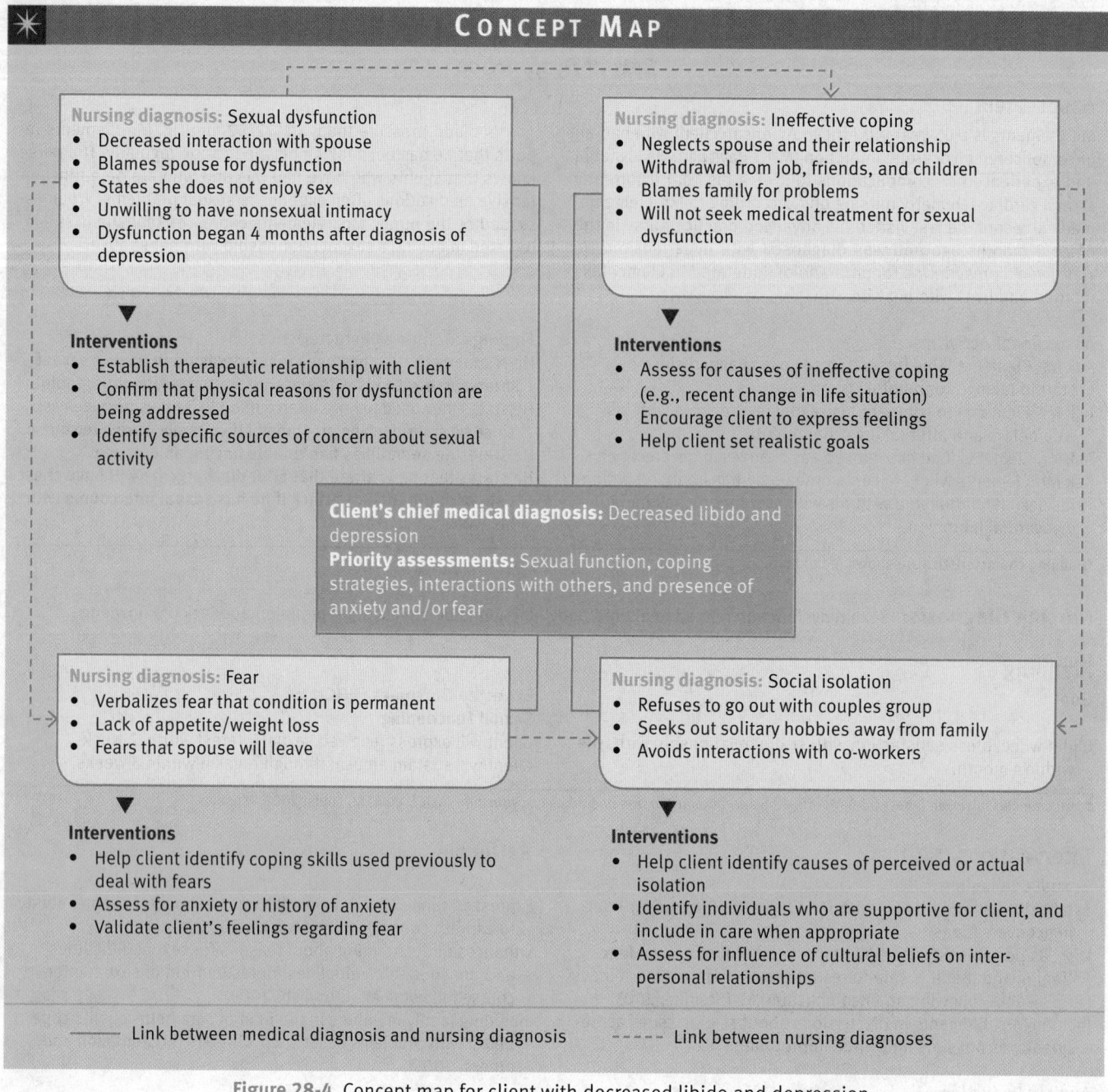

Nursing diagnosis: Sexual dysfunction
- Decreased interaction with spouse
- Blames spouse for dysfunction
- States she does not enjoy sex
- Unwilling to have nonsexual intimacy
- Dysfunction began 4 months after diagnosis of depression

Interventions
- Establish therapeutic relationship with client
- Confirm that physical reasons for dysfunction are being addressed
- Identify specific sources of concern about sexual activity

Nursing diagnosis: Ineffective coping
- Neglects spouse and their relationship
- Withdrawal from job, friends, and children
- Blames family for problems
- Will not seek medical treatment for sexual dysfunction

Interventions
- Assess for causes of ineffective coping (e.g., recent change in life situation)
- Encourage client to express feelings
- Help client set realistic goals

Client's chief medical diagnosis: Decreased libido and depression
Priority assessments: Sexual function, coping strategies, interactions with others, and presence of anxiety and/or fear

Nursing diagnosis: Fear
- Verbalizes fear that condition is permanent
- Lack of appetite/weight loss
- Fears that spouse will leave

Interventions
- Help client identify coping skills used previously to deal with fears
- Assess for anxiety or history of anxiety
- Validate client's feelings regarding fear

Nursing diagnosis: Social isolation
- Refuses to go out with couples group
- Seeks out solitary hobbies away from family
- Avoids interactions with co-workers

Interventions
- Help client identify causes of perceived or actual isolation
- Identify individuals who are supportive for client, and include in care when appropriate
- Assess for influence of cultural beliefs on interpersonal relationships

——— Link between medical diagnosis and nursing diagnosis   - - - - - Link between nursing diagnoses

Figure 28-4 Concept map for client with decreased libido and depression.

---

tion skills. Structure the environment and timing to provide privacy, comfort, and uninterrupted time (Steinke, 2005). For example, when discussing methods of contraception with a woman, provide education in a private area rather than discussing this in the examination room when the client is only partially clothed.

Topics of education vary and often are related to the client's developmental level. For example, a nurse talks to school-age children regarding the appearance of breast buds or pubic hair. When discussing sexual health with clients of childbearing age, always consider the client's cultural and religious beliefs regarding contraception. The discussion includes the desire for children, usual sexual practices, and acceptable methods of contraception.

Nurses review all methods of contraception to allow clients to make informed decisions.

Major developmental crises (e.g., puberty, **climacteric**, or menopause) prompt education about sexuality. Situational crises such as a life change with pregnancy, illness, extreme financial stress, placement of a spouse in a nursing home, or loss and grief affect sexuality. Effects often last for days, months, or years and are often minimized when the individual is prepared for possible changes in sexual functioning.

Demonstrate recognition, acceptance, and respect for an older adult's sexuality by displaying a willingness to openly discuss sex and sexuality-related concerns. Strategies that enhance sexual

✳ BOX 28-6 Examples of Community Resources Relating to Sexuality

- Planned Parenthood
- Health department (often for both family planning and sexually transmitted diseases)
- Groups that provide education/services for those with particular conditions include the following:
  - American Diabetes Association
  - American Heart Association
  - Muscular Dystrophy Association
  - Muscular Sclerosis Society
- Sexual abuse support groups and hot lines
- Women's shelters (for those who have been physically and/or sexually abused)
- Resolve Inc national office, http://www.resolve.org
- North America Menopause Society, http://www.menopause.org

✳ BOX 28-7 EVIDENCE-BASED PRACTICE

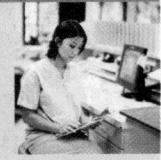

The Effects of Prostate Cancer on Survivors and Their Partners

Evidence Summary

This longitudinal study described health-related quality of life (QOL) and the symptoms caused by prostate cancer treatment of 137 men who received a variety of different treatments for early-stage prostate cancer over 5½ years. The researchers also investigated health-related QOL, health status, and marital satisfaction in 102 of the men's partners. Participants completed several surveys that measured quality of life, medical outcomes, symptoms related to the treatment of prostate cancer, and quality of the marriage. The average age of the men in the study was about 70 years, whereas the average age of the women was 66 years. QOL diminished in all men, and men who received "watchful waiting" or no treatment reported poorer health status and more urinary and sexual symptoms over time. Overall, the men stated sexual issues caused more distress than any other effects of the treatment of prostate cancer. Few men were satisfied with their sexual functioning, and almost 60% were bothered by the lack of sexual relations. Although the wives' QOL, marital satisfaction, and health status were similar to their partners early in the study, the associations did not continue 5½ years after treatment.

Application to Nursing Practice

- Men who have prostate cancer, especially those who opt for watchful waiting, are at risk for a wide variety of health issues, including problems with sexual function.
- Men continue to have concerns about sexual issues as they age; however, few seek treatment for erectile dysfunction.
- Assess men and their partners for the effects of prostate cancer treatment on sexuality and intimacy.
- Provide education to men and their partners about the potential consequences of prostate cancer, available treatment options for erectile dysfunction, and alternative methods to achieve sexual satisfaction.
- Focusing on communication, intimacy, and educational needs is essential in helping men and their partners overcome the challenges related to prostate cancer.

Reference

Galbraith ME and others: Prostate cancer survivors' and partners' self-reports of health-related quality of life, treatment symptoms, and marital satisfaction 2.5-5.5 years after treatment, *Oncol Nurs Forum* 32(2):E30, 2005.

---

functioning include the following (Meiner and Lueckenotte, 2006; Nusbaum and others, 2005):

- Avoid alcohol and tobacco.
- Eat well-balanced meals.
- Plan sexual activity for times when the couple feels rested.
- Take pain medication if needed before sexual intercourse.
- Use pillows and alternate positioning to enhance comfort.
- Encourage touch, kissing, hugging, and other tactile stimulation.
- Communicate concerns and fears with partner and health care provider.

Individuals who have more than one sex partner or whose partner has other sexual experiences need to learn about safe sex practices. Provide information about STD symptoms and transmission, use of condoms and risky sexual activities (e.g., trauma from penile-anal sex). To prevent HIV infection, teach clients to avoid having multiple sexual partners and use condoms to reduce the risk of HIV/AIDS. Role play is a useful educational tool in helping a person learn to say no or negotiate with a partner to use a condom (Box 28-8). Also teach clients to avoid the use of IV drugs. If people do use IV drugs, tell them to avoid sharing needles with others and to always use new needles. Safe sex considers clients' physical and emotional health.

Encourage clients to have regular health examinations to maintain sexual health. Often asymptomatic STDs (e.g., chlamydia or gonorrhea) are diagnosed during a physical examination with appropriate laboratory work. Annual health examinations provide an opportunity to discuss contraception and safe sex practices. However, some people do not routinely seek annual health examinations. Barriers to annual health screenings include cultural beliefs, low socioeconomic status, and low health literacy (Juon and others, 2003; Shah and others, 2006). For example, women who are Muslim do not frequently have breast examinations, mammograms, and cervical cancer screening because of religious and cultural beliefs of modesty (Matin and LeBaron, 2004). African American men often do not seek prostate cancer screening (Plowden, 2006). Develop a therapeutic relationship with clients, and provide culturally appropriate education that is written at an appropriate reading level (see Chapter 25). Encourage clients to find health care providers that they can trust, and help clients who are uninsured or underinsured to locate resources that will help them pay for important sexual health screenings (Amy and others, 2006; Farmer and others, 2007).

Acute Care. Illness and surgery create situational stressors that often affect a person's sexuality. During periods of illness, individuals experience major physical changes, the effects of drugs or treatments, the emotional stress of a prognosis, concern about future functioning, and separation from significant others. Never assume that sexual functioning is not a concern merely because of an individual's age or severity of prognosis. After identifying concerns, address them in the context of the individual's value system.

✳ BOX 28-8   **CLIENT TEACHING**

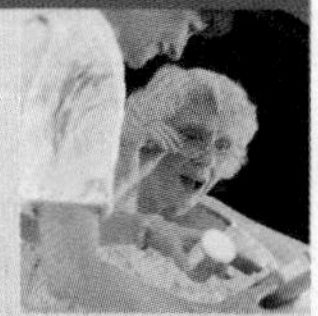

Using a Condom Correctly

Objective
- Client will verbalize correct use of a condom

Teaching Strategies
- Develop a trusting relationship with the client.
- Explain to always use a latex or rubber condom when having vaginal, oral, or anal sex and to store condoms in a cool, dry place away from sunlight.
- Encourage to read the label on the condom package to check the expiration date and ensure that the condom protects against STDs.
- Instruct the client to never reuse a condom or never use a damaged condom.
- Explain how to correctly apply the condom (e.g., put it on as soon as the penis is hard and before vaginal, anal, or oral contact; gently squeeze any air out from the tip of the condom, leaving space for semen; unroll the condom to the base of the penis).
- Teach client to pull out right after coming and hold onto the condom when pulling out.
- Instruct the client to only use water-based lubricants (e.g., K-Y Jelly or WET) to prevent the condom from breaking; do not use petroleum jelly, massage oils, body lotions, or cooking oil.

Evaluation
- Ask client to describe where condoms are stored.
- Ask client questions that verify understanding of instruction (e.g., What would you do if you noticed that a condom you just opened had an open slit in it?).

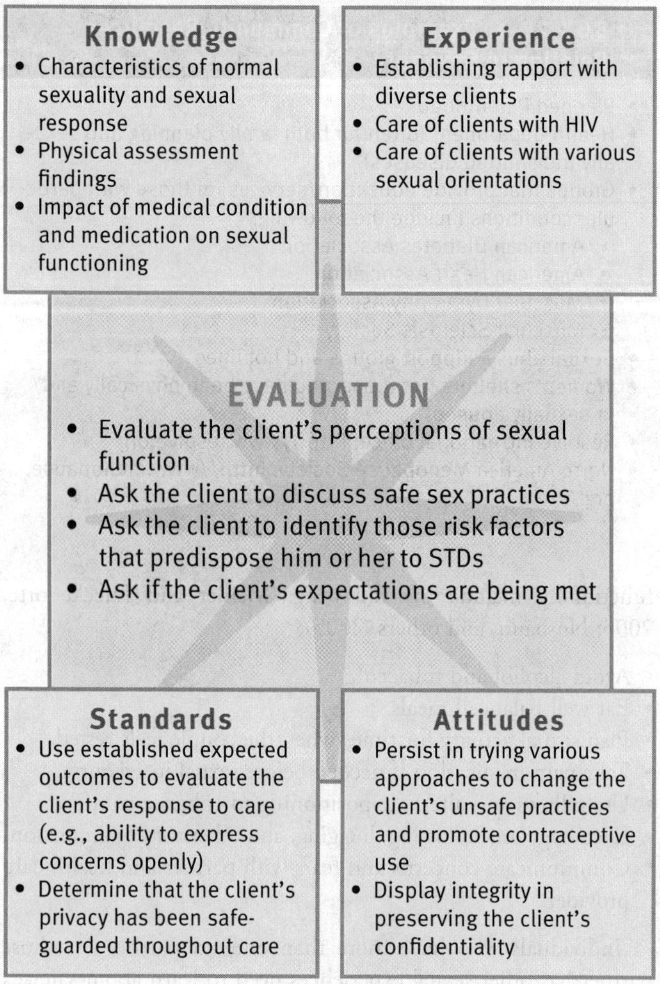

Knowledge
- Characteristics of normal sexuality and sexual response
- Physical assessment findings
- Impact of medical condition and medication on sexual functioning

Experience
- Establishing rapport with diverse clients
- Care of clients with HIV
- Care of clients with various sexual orientations

EVALUATION
- Evaluate the client's perceptions of sexual function
- Ask the client to discuss safe sex practices
- Ask the client to identify those risk factors that predispose him or her to STDs
- Ask if the client's expectations are being met

Standards
- Use established expected outcomes to evaluate the client's response to care (e.g., ability to express concerns openly)
- Determine that the client's privacy has been safeguarded throughout care

Attitudes
- Persist in trying various approaches to change the client's unsafe practices and promote contraceptive use
- Display integrity in preserving the client's confidentiality

Figure 28-5 Critical thinking model for sexuality evaluation.

When a client identifies sexual concerns, initiate discussion and education appropriately. Nurses often provide the following suggestions: planning sexual activity when the client is rested, experimenting with positions that are more comfortable, encouraging partners to give each other more time and encouraging the use of foreplay to achieve arousal. Help clients to anticipate how their illness or disease will change over time and the adjustments that will be necessary to achieve sexual fulfillment.

Restorative and Continuing Care. Frequently nurses establish relationships with couples that encourage honest and open discussions about sexual health during restorative or continuing care. Address needs by taking a sexual health history and implementing a basic model such as PLISSIT to provide options for clients (see Box 28-4). Assessment and management of sexual concerns is important when promoting sexual intimacy and providing closeness and closure between partners at the end of life (Stausmire, 2004).

In the home environment it is important to provide information on how an illness will limit sexual activity and give ideas for adapting or facilitating sexual activity. Interventions range from giving permission for a partner to lie in bed and hold a client to coordinating nursing care and medications to provide opportunity for privacy and intimacy. Often, nurses help individuals create an environment that is comfortable for sexual activity in the home. This sometimes involves making recommendations for

ways to arrange the bedroom to accommodate physical limitations. For example, some individuals who are in a wheelchair prefer being able to move the chair close to the side of the bed at an angle that allows for more ease in touching and caressing. Suggestions regarding how to accommodate barriers such as Foley catheters or drainage tubes contribute to sexual activity.

In the long-term care setting, facilities need to make proper arrangements for privacy during residents' sexual experiences (Meiner and Lueckenotte, 2006). The ideal situation is to set up a pleasant room that is used for a variety of activities that the resident is able to reserve for private visits with a spouse or partner. If this is not possible, make arrangements for the roommate of a client to be somewhere else to allow a couple time alone. Never leave clients alone in a situation in which they will injure themselves.

◆ Evaluation

Evaluate client responses to nursing interventions to determine if goals and outcome criteria have been met (Figure 28-5). Critical thinking ensures that the nurse applies what is known about sexuality and the client's unique situation.

Have follow-up discussions with the client or partner to determine whether goals and outcomes have been achieved. Sexuality is felt more than observed, and sexual expression requires an intimacy that is not amenable to observation. Therefore ask clients questions about risk factors, sexual concerns, and their level of satisfaction. Nurses also observe behavioral cues, such as eye contact, posture, and extraneous hand movements, that indicate comfort or suggest continued anxiety or concern as topics are addressed. Anticipate the need to modify expectations with the individual and partner when evaluating outcomes. Sometimes a nurse will need to establish more appropriate time frames in which to achieve the target goals. Ask clients to define what is acceptable and satisfying while considering the partner's level of sexual satisfaction.

When outcomes are not met, begin to ask questions to determine appropriate changes in interventions. Examples of questions include the following:

- What other questions do you have about your sexual health?
- Did you experience less pain during sexual intercourse after taking your pain medication?
- What positions did you find most comfortable when you had sexual intercourse? What positions were most awkward?
- What barriers are preventing you from discussing your feelings and fears with your partner?

Key Concepts

- Sexuality is related to all dimensions of health; therefore nurses address sexual concerns or problems while providing routine nursing care.
- Sexuality is a part of each individual's identity and includes biological sex, gender identity, gender role, and sexual partner preference.
- Attitudes toward sexuality vary widely. Religious beliefs, society's values, the media, the family, and other factors all influence sexuality.
- Nurses' attitudes toward sexuality vary and often differ from those of clients; be sensitive to clients' sexual preferences and needs.
- Sexual development begins in infancy and involves some level of sexual behavior or growth in all developmental stages.
- The physiological sexual response changes with aging, but aging does not lead to diminished sexuality.
- Sexual health contributes to an individual's sense of self-worth and positive interpersonal relationships.
- Sexual dysfunctions result from varied and complex etiologies.
- Interventions for sexual dysfunctions depend on the condition and the client; interventions often include giving information, teaching specific exercises, improving communication between partners, and referral to a knowledgeable professional.
- Sexual biases, comfort with touching genitalia, desire for future fertility, financial status, ability to plan sexual contact, and ability to communicate with the sex partner all affect the choice and use of effective contraceptive methods.
- Include a brief review of sexuality whenever assessing a client's level of wellness.
- Most nursing interventions that enhance sexual health require providing education.
- Evaluate outcomes of care by talking with clients regarding satisfaction with sexual functioning and through observations of nonverbal behaviors that suggest anxiety. Include the partner when appropriate.

Critical Thinking Exercises

1. Mr. Clements returns to see the advanced practice nurse (APN) in his cardiologist's office for a routine visit. During the visit the APN plans to assess Mr. Clements' sexuality. What can the APN do to help Mr. Clements feel comfortable in discussing his sexuality? Develop an opening statement that would be effective in decreasing Mr. Clements' anxiety about discussing this private aspect of his life.

2. During the office visit, Mr. and Mrs. Clements state that although they are able to engage in sexual intercourse, it is taking both of them longer to reach orgasm. Explain why they are experiencing this change, and describe at least three strategies they could use to enhance their sexual functioning.

NCLEX®-Style Review Questions

1. The nurse is providing education to a new mother about her infant son's sexual development. The nurse knows the mother understands the teaching about the baby's development at this time when the mother states:
   1. "As soon as he begins to talk, my son will have a lot of questions about sex."
   2. "My son is beginning to be able to tell the difference between men and women."
   3. "The relationship my son has with peers of the same sex will influence his sexual identity."
   4. "My son is in a self-centered, egocentric stage that will help him determine appropriate sexual behavior."

2. A 25-year-old client is in the emergency department and states she is having problems with a cough and fever for the past 3 days. While performing a physical assessment, the nurse finds several bruises that are in various stages of healing. The nurse suspects that the client may be a victim of sexual abuse. Which of the following is the nurse's first action?
   1. Refer the client to a sexual counselor.
   2. Tell the client about the safe house for women.
   3. Ask the client to describe how she got the bruises.
   4. Report the abuse immediately to the proper authorities.

3. A 17-year-old male client states that he has been dating the same girlfriend for the past 6 months and that he is currently sexually active. Which of the following state-

ments made by the client indicates that he needs further education about contraceptive methods and the prevention of STDs?
1. "If we do not use contraceptives the right way, we could get pregnant or get an STD."
2. "If my girlfriend has an IUD, she probably will not get pregnant, but we both might still get an STD."
3. "Since my girlfriend is taking a birth control pill, we do not have to worry about getting pregnant or getting an STD."
4. "Using a condom with spermicide will keep my girlfriend from getting pregnant and will keep us both from getting an STD."

4. Which of the following clients are highest at risk for developing HPV?
1. An overweight 8-year-old boy
2. A sexually active 15-year-old girl
3. A 42-year-old divorced woman with hypertension
4. A 28-year-old married man who has type 2 diabetes

5. A 26-year-old married woman recently discovered she is pregnant and is at her first prenatal visit. While assessing the client, the woman's health nurse practitioner discovers that the client has purulent vaginal discharge. The client states, "It burns when I urinate, and I seem to have to go to the bathroom frequently." Based on these symptoms, the nurse practitioner determines that the client:
1. Should be tested for HIV
2. May have an STD such as chlamydia
3. Is experiencing normal signs of pregnancy
4. Needs education on proper perineal hygiene

6. A new graduate nurse has started working in a rehabilitation center that specializes in the care of clients with spinal cord injuries (SCIs). The new graduate knows that sexual issues are common among clients with SCIs. Which of the following actions would enhance the nurse's comfort in discussing sexual issues with the clients? (Choose all that apply)
1. Clarify personal values related to sexuality.
2. Role play discussion of sexual concerns with another nurse.
3. Attend a conference to enhance knowledge about sexuality.
4. Avoid discussing sexual concerns until after completing new nurse orientation.

7. A couple has six children. The wife states, "We just really do not want to have any more children. Six is enough." The husband is thinking about having a vasectomy. Which of the following statements made by the husband reflects that he understands the procedure?
1. "The diaphragm works better than a vasectomy."
2. "Vasectomies are usually less effective than birth control pills."
3. "A vasectomy is not considered permanent because it is easy to reverse."
4. "I should only have a vasectomy if we are certain we do not want any other children."

8. Which of the following male clients is least at risk for experiencing sexual dysfunction?
1. A 50-year-old who is taking one aspirin a day
2. A 20-year-old who was born with spina bifida
3. A 63-year-old who has had diabetes mellitus for 10 years
4. A 72-year-old who receives hemodialysis 3 times a week for his chronic renal failure

9. When the nurse is gathering a sexual history from an older adult, the nurse must keep in mind:
1. Older men lose fertility
2. Older adults may not reveal intimate details
3. Older men and women have sexual dysfunction
4. Older adults do not usually participate in sexual activity

10. A useful framework for the nurse in guiding planning and setting priorities regarding sexual activity for a client is the:
1. PLISSIT model
2. NIC and NOC guidelines
3. NANDA International guidelines
4. The nurse's own theory of sexual behavior

29 | Spiritual Health

⁕ OBJECTIVES

Mastery of content in this chapter will enable the student to:

- Discuss the influence of spiritual practices on the health status of clients.
- Describe the relationship between faith, hope, and spiritual well-being.
- Compare and contrast the concepts of religion and spirituality.
- Perform an assessment of a client's spirituality.

- Explain the importance of establishing a caring relationship with clients to gain spiritual insight.
- Discuss nursing interventions designed to promote spiritual health.
- Establish presence with clients.
- Evaluate how clients attain spiritual health.

⁕ MEDIA RESOURCES   ⁕ KEY TERMS

 Companion CD

- NCLEX®-Style Review Questions
- Audio Glossary
- Interactive Learning Activities
- English/Spanish Glossary

 Website

- NCLEX®-Style Review Questions
- Audio Glossary
- English/Spanish Glossary
- Interactive Learning Activities
- Weblinks
- Audio Summaries

Agnostic, p. 445
Atheist, p. 445
Connectedness, p. 445
Faith, p. 446
Holistic, p. 456

Hope, p. 446
Self-transcendence, p. 444
Spiritual distress, p. 445
Spirituality, p. 444
Spiritual well-being, p. 445

The word *spirituality* derives from the Latin word *spiritus,* which refers to breath or wind. The spirit gives life to a person. It signifies whatever is at the center of all aspects of a person's life (McEwan, 2005). Florence Nightingale believed that spirituality was a force that provided energy needed to promote a healthy hospital environment and that caring for a person's spiritual needs was just as essential as caring for a person's physical needs (Delgado, 2005; Kelly, 2004). Today, **spirituality** is often defined as an awareness of one's inner self and a sense of connection to a higher being, nature, or to some purpose greater than oneself (Mauk and Schmidt, 2004). A person's health depends on a balance of physical, psychological, sociological, cultural, developmental, and spiritual factors. Spirituality is an important factor that helps individuals achieve the balance needed to maintain health and well-being and to cope with illness. Research shows that spirituality positively affects and enhances health, quality of life, health promotion behaviors, and disease prevention activities (Aaron and others, 2003; Figueroa and others, 2006; Gibson and Hendricks, 2006; Grey and others, 2004; Grimsley, 2006).

Too often, nurses and other health care providers fail to recognize the spiritual dimension of their clients, because spirituality is not scientific enough, it has many definitions, and it is difficult to measure (Delgado, 2005; Gray, 2006). In addition, some nurses and health care providers do not believe in God or an ultimate being (Friedemann and others, 2002), some are not comfortable with discussing the topic, and others claim they do not have time to address spiritual needs. The concepts of spirituality and religion are often interchanged, but spirituality is a much broader and more unifying concept than religion (Hollins, 2005).

The human spirit is powerful, and spirituality has different meanings for different people. Therefore nurses need an awareness of their own spirituality in order to provide appropriate and relevant spiritual care to others. Nurses need to care for the whole person and accept the client's beliefs and experiences when providing spiritual care (Bash, 2004). Being able to determine the importance spirituality holds for clients depends on a nurse's ability to develop a caring relationship (see Chapter 8). Nursing care involves helping clients use their spiritual resources as they identify and explore what is meaningful in their lives and find ways to cope with the impact of illness and the ongoing stressors of life (Krebs, 2003).

Scientific Knowledge Base

Health care research shows the association between spirituality and health. There are beneficial health outcomes when an individual is able to engage his or her beliefs in a higher power and sense a source of strength or support. For example, Spurlock (2005) found that caregivers who reported higher levels of spiritual well-being experienced less caregiver burden when providing care to family members diagnosed with Alzheimer's disease at home. Holstad and others (2006) found that clients diagnosed with human immunodeficiency virus/ acquired immunodeficiency syndrome (HIV/AIDS) who found meaning and hope in their lives were more likely to follow their prescribed antiretroviral therapy. Many people use prayer as a method of coping because it is effective in minimizing physical stressors. Attending church and

praying often positively impacts health and the decision to participate in health promotion practices (Aaron and others, 2003; Banks-Wallace and Parks, 2004). The increased interest in studying the relationship between spirituality and health has greatly contributed to nursing science (Gray, 2006; Smith, 2006).

The relationship between spirituality and healing is not completely understood. However, it is the individual's intrinsic spirit that seems to be an important factor in healing. Healing often takes place because of believing. Current evidence shows a link between mind, body, and spirit. An individual's beliefs and expectations often have effects on the person's physical and psychological well-being (Smith, 2006). Many of these effects are tied to hormonal and neurological function. For example, relaxation exercises and guided imagery improve immune function (Lindberg, 2005) and reduce perceptions of pain and anxiety (Antall and Kresevic, 2004). Laughter raises pain thresholds, boosts the immune system, reduces stress hormones, relieves tension, and elevates mood (Bennet and Lengacher, 2006; Hoare, 2004; Hsieh and others, 2005; MacDonald, 2004). In one study, researchers found that adults who believed they were both religious and spiritual and who participated in religious activities reported better physical health, less depression, and better social support (Koenig and others, 2004). A person's inner beliefs and convictions are powerful resources for healing. Nurses who support the spirituality of clients and their families are successful in helping clients achieve desirable health outcomes.

Nursing Knowledge Base

Current Concepts in Spiritual Health

A variety of concepts describe spiritual health. To provide meaningful and supportive spiritual care, it is important for nurses to understand the concepts of spirituality, spiritual well-being, faith, religion, and hope. Each concept offers direction in understanding the views individuals have of life and its value.

Spirituality. Spirituality is a complex concept that is unique to each individual, and is dependent upon a person's culture, development, life experiences, beliefs, and ideas about life (Mauk and Schmidt, 2004). Furthermore, spirituality is an inherent human characteristic. Therefore spirituality exists in all people regardless of their religious beliefs (Delgado, 2005). An individual's spirituality enables the person to love, have faith and hope, seek meaning in life, and to nurture relationships with others. There are two important characteristics of spirituality agreed upon by most authors: (1) it is a unifying theme in people's lives, and (2) it is a state of being. Current definitions of spirituality include eight distinct but overlapping constructs (Figure 29-1).

Spirituality gives individuals the *energy* needed to discover themselves, to cope with difficult situations, and to maintain health. Energy generated by spirituality helps clients feel well and guides choices made throughout life (Chiu and others, 2004). **Self-transcendence** is the belief that there is a force outside of and greater than the person. This force goes beyond space and time. Individuals usually see this force as positive, and it allows people to have new experiences and develop new perspectives that are beyond ordinary physical boundaries. Examples of transcendent

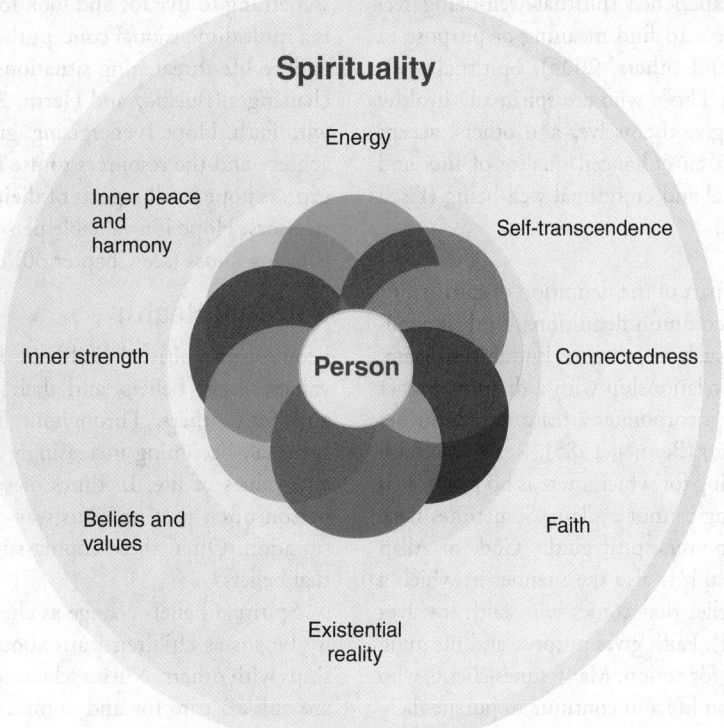

Figure 29-1 The concept of spirituality has eight distinct but overlapping constructs. (Modified from Villagomeza LR: Mending broken hearts: the role of spirituality in cardiac illness: a research synthesis, 1991-2004, *Holist Nurs Pract* 20[4]:169, 2006.)

moments include the feeling of awe when holding a new baby or looking at a beautiful sunset (Davis, 2003; Delgado, 2005; Hollins, 2005). Spirituality offers a sense of **connectedness** intrapersonally (connected within oneself), interpersonally (connected with others and the environment), and transpersonally (connected with the unseen, God, or a higher power) (Miner-Williams, 2006). Through connectedness, clients are able to move beyond the stressors of everyday life and find comfort, faith, hope, peace, and empowerment (Chiu and others, 2004; Delgado, 2005; Tanyi, 2002; Villagomeza, 2005). *Faith* allows people to have firm beliefs despite lack of physical evidence. It enables people to believe in and establish transpersonal connections. Although many people associate faith with religious beliefs, faith exists without religious beliefs (Villagomeza, 2005).

Spirituality includes an *existential reality* that provides unique and subjective experiences for all people. This personal lifelong journey allows people to discover and develop a sense of life's meaning and purpose. The search for purpose is often connected to vocation or a calling in life (Delgado, 2005). Existential reality helps people deal with the unknown and allows people to love, comfort, and forgive others (Chiu and others, 2004). *Beliefs and values* provide the foundation for truth. Values allow people to determine what is important to them and help people appreciate the beauty and worth of thoughts, objects, and behaviors (Hollins, 2005; Villagomeza, 2005). Spirituality gives people the ability to find a dynamic and creative sense of *inner strength* that is often used when making difficult decisions (Banks-Wallace and Parks, 2004). Inner strength is a source of energy that instills hope, provides motivation, and promotes a positive outlook on

life (Chiu and others, 2004; Villagomeza, 2005). *Inner peace and harmony* fosters calm, positive, and peaceful feelings despite life experiences of chaos, fear, and uncertainty. These feelings help people feel comforted even in times of great distress (Banks-Wallace and Parks, 2004; Villagomeza, 2005).

There are individuals who either do not believe in the existence of God (**atheist**) or who believe that there is no known ultimate reality (**agnostic**). This does not mean that spirituality is not an important concept for the atheist or agnostic (Taylor, 2002). Atheists search for meaning in life through their work and their relationships with others. Agnostics discover meaning in what they do or how they live because they find no ultimate meaning for the way things are. They believe that people bring meaning to what they do.

Spirituality is an integrating theme. A person's concept of spirituality begins in childhood and continues to grow throughout adulthood (Narayanasamy and others, 2004; Smith and McSherry, 2004). Spirituality represents the totality of one's being, serving as the overriding perspective that unifies the various aspects of an individual. Spirituality spreads through the physiological, psychological, and sociocultural dimensions of a person's life, whether or not the person acknowledges or develops it.

Spiritual Well-Being. The concept of **spiritual well-being** is often described as having two dimensions. The vertical dimension supports the transcendent relationship between a person and God or some other higher power. The horizontal dimension describes positive relationships and connections people have with others (Gray, 2006; Smith, 2006). Spiritual well-being has a positive effect on health. Those who experience spiritual well-being feel connected to others and are able to find meaning or purpose in their lives (Hammermeister and others, 2005). Spiritual well-being leads to spiritual health. Those who are spiritually healthy experience joy, are able to forgive themselves and others, accept hardship and mortality, report an enhanced quality of life, and have a positive sense of physical and emotional well-being (Fisch and others, 2003; Tanyi, 2002).

Faith. In addition to being a part of the definition of spirituality, the concept of **faith** has other common definitions. Faith is a cultural or institutional religion, such as Judaism, Buddhism, Islam, or Christianity. Faith is also a relationship with a divinity, higher power, authority, or spirit that incorporates a reasoning faith (belief) and a trusting faith (action) (Benner, 1985). Reasoning faith provides confidence in something for which there is no proof. It is an acceptance of what reasoning cannot explain. Sometimes faith involves a belief in a higher power, spirit guide, God, or Allah (Mauk and Schmidt, 2004). Faith is also the manner in which a person chooses to live. The belief that comes with faith involves self-transcendence (Perry, 2004). Faith gives purpose and meaning to an individual's life, allowing for action. Many times clients who are ill have a positive outlook on life and continue to pursue daily activities rather than resign themselves to the disease's symptoms. Their faith often becomes stronger because they view their illness as an opportunity for personal growth.

Religion. Religion is associated with the "state of doing," or a specific system of practices associated with a particular denomination, sect, or form of worship. Religion refers to the system of organized beliefs and worship that a person practices to outwardly express spirituality (Tanyi, 2002). Many people practice a faith or belief in the doctrines and expressions of a specific religion or sect, such as the Lutheran church or Orthodox Judaism. People from different religions view spirituality differently (McSherry and others, 2004). For example, a Buddhist believes in Four Noble Truths: life is suffering; suffering is caused by clinging; suffering can be eliminated by eliminating clinging; and to eliminate clinging and suffering, one follows an eightfold path. The path includes right understanding, intention, speech, action, livelihood, effort, mindfulness, and concentration. This path promotes wisdom, moral behavior, and meditation (Mauk and Schmidt, 2004). A Buddhist turns inward, valuing self-control, whereas a Christian looks to the love of God to provide enlightenment and direction in life.

When providing spiritual care to clients it is important to understand the differences between religion and spirituality. Many people tend to use the terms *spirituality* and *religion* interchangeably. Although closely associated, these terms are not synonymous. Religious practices encompass spirituality, but spirituality does not need to include religious practice. Religious care is helping clients maintain their faithfulness to their belief systems and worship practices. Spiritual care helps people identify meaning and purpose in life, look beyond the present, and maintain personal relationships as well as a relationship with a higher being or life force.

Hope. Spirituality and faith bring **hope** (Buckley and Herth, 2004; Chiu and others, 2004). When a person has the attitude of something to live for and look forward to, hope is present. Hope is a multidimensional concept that provides comfort while people endure life-threatening situations, hardships, and other personal challenges (Buckley and Herth, 2004). Hope is closely associated with faith. Hope is energizing, giving individuals a motivation to achieve and the resources to use toward that achievement. People express hope in all aspects of their lives to help them deal with life stressors. Hope is a valuable personal resource whenever someone is facing a loss (see Chapter 30) or a difficult challenge.

Spiritual Health

People gain spiritual health by finding a balance between their values, goals, beliefs, and their relationships within themselves and with others. Throughout life a person often grows more spiritual, becoming increasingly aware of the meaning, purpose, and values of life. In times of stress, illness, loss, or recovery, a person often uses previous ways of responding or adjusting to a situation. Often these coping styles lie within the person's spiritual beliefs.

Spiritual beliefs change as clients grow and develop. Spirituality begins as children learn about themselves and their relationships with others. Nurses who understand a child's spiritual beliefs are able to care for and comfort the child (McEvoy, 2003). As children mature into adulthood, they experience spiritual growth by entering into lifelong relationships. An ability to care meaningfully for others and self is evidence of a healthy spirituality.

Beliefs among older people vary based on many factors, such as gender, past experience, religion, economic status, and ethnic background. Healthy spirituality in older adults is one that gives peace and acceptance of the self. It is often based on a lifelong relationship with a supreme being. Illness and loss sometimes threaten and challenge the spiritual developmental process. Older adults often express their spirituality by turning to important relationships and giving of themselves to others (Edelman and Mandle, 2006; Young and Koopsen, 2005).

Spiritual Problems

When illness, loss, grief, or a major life change occur, people either use spiritual resources to help them cope or spiritual needs and concerns develop. **Spiritual distress** is the "impaired ability to experience and integrate meaning and purpose in life through connectedness with self, others, art, music, literature, nature, and/or a power greater than oneself" (NANDA International, 2007). A catastrophic illness, for example, can upset a person's spiritual well-being sufficiently to cause doubt and loss of faith. Spiritual distress often causes the person to feel alone or even abandoned. Individuals often question their spiritual values, raising questions about their way of life, purpose for living, and source of meaning. Spiritual distress also occurs when there is conflict between a person's beliefs and prescribed health regimens or the inability to practice usual rituals.

Acute Illness. Sudden, unexpected illness that poses both an immediate and a long-term threat to a client's life, health, and/or well-being frequently creates significant spiritual distress. For example, both the 50-year-old client who has a heart attack and the 20-year-old client who is in a motor vehicle accident face crises that threaten their spiritual health. The illness or injury creates an unanticipated scramble to integrate and cope with new realities (e.g., disability). People often look for ways to remain faithful to their beliefs and value systems. Some pray, attend religious services more often, or spend time reflecting on the positive aspects of their lives. Often conflicts develop around a person's beliefs and the meaning of life. Anger is common, and clients sometimes express it against God, their families, themselves, or the nurse. The strength of a client's spirituality influences how he or she copes with sudden illness and how quickly he or she moves to recovery. Nurses use knowledge of a person's spiritual well-being and implement spiritual interventions to maximize inner peace and healing (Grant, 2004).

Chronic Illness. Many chronic illnesses threaten the person's independence, causing fear, anxiety, and spiritual distress. Dependence on others for routine self-care needs often creates feelings of powerlessness. Powerlessness and the loss of a sense of purpose in life impairs the ability to cope with alterations in functioning. Spirituality significantly helps clients and their caregivers adapt to the changes that result from chronic illness (Box 29-1). Successful adaptation often provides spiritual growth. Clients who have a sense of spiritual well-being, who feel connected with a higher power and others, and who are able to find meaning and purpose in life are better able to cope with their chronic illness, which helps them achieve their potential and experience enhanced quality of life (Adegbola, 2006; Narayanasamy, 2004).

Terminal Illness. Terminal illness commonly causes fears of physical pain, isolation, the unknown, and dying. Terminal illness creates an uncertainty about what death means and thus makes clients susceptible to spiritual distress. However, some clients have a spiritual sense of peace that enables them to face death without fear. Spirituality helps these clients find peace in themselves and their death. Individuals experiencing a terminal illness will often find themselves reviewing their life and questioning its meaning. Common questions they ask include "Why is this happening to me?" or "What have I done?" Terminal illness often affects family and friends just as much as the client. Terminal illness causes members of the family to ask important questions about its meaning and how it will affect their relationship with the client (see Chapter 30).

In addition to managing clients' physical and psychosocial symptoms experienced at the end of life, empower them to have a greater sense of control over their disease regardless of whether the client receives care in a hospital or at home. Providing holistic care is essential because dying is a part of life that encompasses the client's physical, social, psychological, and spiritual health (Peters and Sellick, 2006).

Near-Death Experience. Some nurses will care for clients who have had a near-death experience (NDE). An NDE is a psychological phenomenon of people who either have been close to clinical death or have recovered after being declared dead. It is not associated with a mental disorder. Persons who experience an NDE often tell the same story of feeling themselves rising above their bodies and watching caregivers initiate lifesaving measures. Most individuals describe passing through a tunnel to a bright light, encountering people who had preceded them in death, and

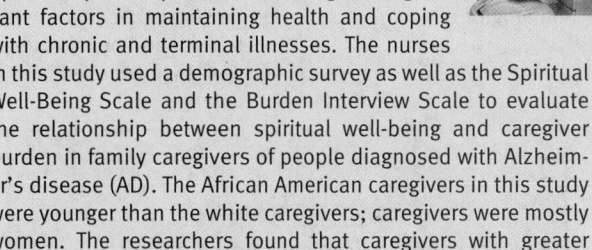

BOX 29-1   EVIDENCE-BASED PRACTICE

Alzheimer's Disease, Spiritual Well-Being, and Caregiver Burden

Evidence Summary
Spirituality and spiritual well-being are significant factors in maintaining health and coping with chronic and terminal illnesses. The nurses in this study used a demographic survey as well as the Spiritual Well-Being Scale and the Burden Interview Scale to evaluate the relationship between spiritual well-being and caregiver burden in family caregivers of people diagnosed with Alzheimer's disease (AD). The African American caregivers in this study were younger than the white caregivers; caregivers were mostly women. The researchers found that caregivers with greater spiritual well-being experienced less caregiver burden. They also found that African American caregivers reported a higher level of spiritual well-being than white caregivers.

Application to Nursing Practice
- Use assessment data about the spirituality and spiritual behaviors or practices from caregivers of family members with AD to identify areas of strength and support.
- Encourage caregivers to participate in spiritual behaviors or practices (e.g., prayer, attending religious services) to enhance spiritual well-being when appropriate.
- It is essential to consider cultural differences and explore personal preferences when determining nursing interventions to enhance spiritual well-being.
- Inform caregivers of spiritual resources available in the community (e.g., parish nurses, community- or faith-based support groups, clergy, social services).

Reference
Spurlock WR: Spiritual well-being and caregiver burden in Alzheimer's caregivers, *Geriatr Nurs* 26(3):154, 2005.

feeling an inner tranquility and peace. Instead of moving toward the light, they learn it is not time for them to die, and they return to life (James, 2004).

Clients who have an NDE are often reluctant to discuss it, thinking family or caregivers will not understand. However, individuals experiencing an NDE who discuss it with family or caregivers find acceptance and meaning from this powerful experience. They are often no longer afraid of death. After a client has survived an NDE, it is important to remain open and give the client a chance to explore what happened. Provide support if the client decides to share the experience with significant others (James, 2004).

Critical Thinking

The helping role is important in nursing practice (Benner, 1984). Clients look to nurses for help that is different than the help they seek from other health care professionals. Expert nurses acquire the ability to anticipate personal issues affecting clients and their spiritual well-being. Critical thinking knowledge and skills help nurses enhance clients' spiritual well-being and health. While using the nursing process, apply knowledge, experience, attitudes, and standards in providing appropriate spiritual care (Figure 29-2).

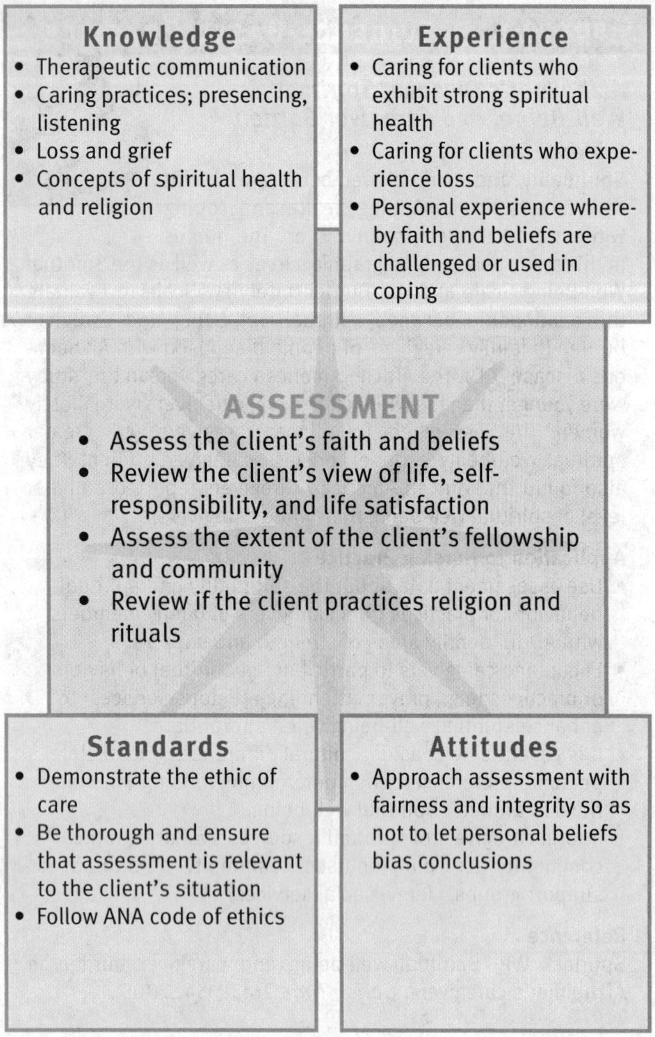

Knowledge

- Therapeutic communication
- Caring practices; presencing, listening
- Loss and grief
- Concepts of spiritual health and religion

Experience

- Caring for clients who exhibit strong spiritual health
- Caring for clients who experience loss
- Personal experience whereby faith and beliefs are challenged or used in coping

ASSESSMENT

- Assess the client's faith and beliefs
- Review the client's view of life, self-responsibility, and life satisfaction
- Assess the extent of the client's fellowship and community
- Review if the client practices religion and rituals

Standards

- Demonstrate the ethic of care
- Be thorough and ensure that assessment is relevant to the client's situation
- Follow ANA code of ethics

Attitudes

- Approach assessment with fairness and integrity so as not to let personal beliefs bias conclusions

Figure 29-2 Critical thinking model for spiritual health assessment.

Nurses who are comfortable with their own spirituality often are more likely to care for their clients' spiritual needs (Miner-Williams, 2006). Nurses who foster their own personal, emotional, and spiritual health become resources for their clients and use their own spirituality as a tool when caring for themselves and their clients (Gray, 2006; Jackson, 2004).

Taking a faith history reveals client's beliefs about life, health, and a supreme being. Knowing the client's cultural preferences provides additional insight into the client's spiritual practices. Applying knowledge of spiritual concepts, principles of caring (see Chapter 8), and therapeutic communication skills (see Chapter 24) helps nurses readily recognize and understand their clients' spiritual needs. Convey caring and openness to successfully promote honest discussion about clients' spiritual beliefs.

A sound understanding of ethics and values (Chapter 22) is essential when providing spiritual care. A person's values or beliefs about the worth of a given idea, attitude, or custom are linked to the individual's spiritual well-being. Application of ethical principles ensures respect for a client's spiritual and religious convictions.

Personal experience in caring for clients in spiritual distress is valuable when helping clients select coping options. Nurses need to determine if their own spirituality is beneficial in assisting clients. Nurses who sense a personal faith and hope regarding life are usually better able to help their clients (Jackson, 2004). Previous personal and professional experiences with dying clients, clients with chronic disease, or clients who have experienced significant losses provide lessons in how to help clients face difficult challenges and how to offer support to family and friends (Wright, 2005).

Because each person has a unique spirituality, nurses need to know their own beliefs so they are able care for each client without bias. Use critical thinking when assessing each client's reaction to illness and loss and when determining if spiritual intervention is necessary. Humility is essential, especially when caring for clients from diverse cultural and/or religious backgrounds. Recognize personal limitations in knowledge about clients' spiritual beliefs and religious practices. Effective nurses show genuine concern as they assess their clients' beliefs and determine how spirituality influences their clients' health (Mazanec and Tyler, 2004). Nurses demonstrate integrity by refraining from voicing their own opinions about religion or spirituality when their beliefs conflict with their clients' beliefs.

The application of intellectual standards helps the nurse make accurate clinical decisions and helps clients find meaningful and logical ways to acquire spiritual healing. Critical thinking ensures that nurses obtain significant and relevant information when making decisions about their clients' spiritual needs. The nature of a person's spirituality is complex and highly individualized. Therefore avoid making assumptions about the client's religion and beliefs. Significance and relevance are standards of critical thinking that ensure nurses explore the issues that are most meaningful to clients and most likely to affect spiritual well-being.

In setting standards for quality health care, The Joint Commission requires health care organizations to acknowledge clients' rights to spiritual care and provide for clients' spiritual needs through pastoral care or others who are certified, ordained, or lay individuals (LaPierre, 2003). The Joint Commission requires nurses to assess their clients' denomination, beliefs, and spiritual practices (Mauk and Schmidt, 2004).

The Code of Ethics for Nurses (ANA, 2001) requires nurses to practice nursing with compassion by accepting the dignity and worth of each client despite socioeconomic status, personal characteristics, or type of health problem. It is essential to promote an environment that respects clients' values, customs, and spiritual beliefs. Routinely implementing nursing interventions such as prayer or meditation is coercive and/or unethical. Therefore determine which interventions are compatible with the client's beliefs and values before selecting nursing interventions. An ethic of caring (see Chapter 22) provides a framework for decision making and places the nurse as the client's advocate.

Nursing Process

The core of nursing includes a commitment to caring and respect for an individual's uniqueness. In the case of spirituality, it is even more important to respect each client's personal beliefs. People experience the world and find meaning in that experience in different ways. Application of the nursing process from the perspective of a client's spiritual needs is not simple. It goes beyond assessing a client's religious practices. Understanding a client's spirituality and then appropriately identifying the level of support and resources needed requires a compassionate perspective. Remove any personal biases or misconceptions from client assessments, and be willing to share and discover another person's meaning and purpose in life, illness, and health. Learn to look beyond a personal view when establishing relationships with clients. Identifying common values and respecting unique commitments and values requires quiet conversations, effective listening, and communication through presence and touch (Smith and McSherry, 2004; Villagomeza, 2005).

Love, trust, hope, forgiveness, meaning, and community are universal spiritual needs. Learning to share these needs helps the nurse find a way to give clients spiritual care and support. Recognize that a client does not have to have a spiritual problem. Clients bring certain spiritual resources that help them assume healthier lives, recover from illness, or face impending death. Supporting and recognizing the positive side of a client's spiritually goes a long way toward delivering effective, individualized nursing care.

◆ Assessment

Because spirituality is deeply subjective, it means different things to different people (McSherry and Ross, 2002). The ability to gain a reliable picture of clients' spirituality is limited when nurses have limited contact with their clients or when they fail to build therapeutic relationships with their clients. Once the nurse establishes a trusting relationship with a client and they reach a point of learning together, spiritual caring occurs (Taylor, 2003). Focus nursing assessment on aspects of spirituality that life experiences and events will most likely influence. Conducting an assessment is therapeutic because it expresses a level of caring and support.

Spiritual assessment is a fundamental part of the nursing assessment. Because nurses often have limited time to spend with their clients, it is often difficult to obtain an in-depth spiritual assessment. A key to success is to conduct an ongoing assessment over the course of the client's stay in the health care setting. Establish trust and rapport, and make the opportunity to conduct meaningful discussions with clients a priority. Assess a client's spiritual health in several different ways. One way is to ask direct questions (Box 29-2). This approach requires you to feel comfortable asking others about their spirituality.

Many spiritual assessment tools are available to help nurses clarify values and assess spirituality (Elkins and Cavendish, 2004). The B-E-L-I-E-F assessment tool helps pediatric nurses evaluate the child and family's spiritual and religious needs (McEvoy, 2003). The acronym stands for the following:

B—Belief system
E—Ethics or values
L—Lifestyle
I—Involvement in a spiritual community
E—Education
F—Future events

> ## ✴ BOX 29-2 NURSING ASSESSMENT QUESTIONS
>
> ### Spirituality and Spiritual Health
> - What gives you energy during difficult times?
> - What aspects of your spirituality have been most helpful to you?
> - What aspects of your spirituality would you like to discuss?
>
> ### Faith, Belief, Fellowship, and Community
> - To what or whom do you look as a source of strength, hope, or faith in times of difficulty?
> - How does your faith help you cope?
> - Do you use prayer?
> - What can I do to support your religious beliefs or faith commitment?
> - What gives your life meaning?
>
> ### Life and Self-Responsibility
> - How do you feel about the changes this illness has caused?
> - How do these changes affect what you now need to do?
>
> ### Life Satisfaction
> - How happy or satisfied are you with your life?
> - What accomplishments help you feel satisfied with your life?
>
> ### Connectedness
> - What feelings do you have after you pray?
> - Who do you feel is the most important person to you?
>
> ### Vocation
> - How has your illness affected the way you live your life spiritually, at home, or where you work?
> - In what way has your illness affected your ability to express what is important in life to you?

The Spiritual Well-Being Scale (SWB) has 20 items that assess the individual's view of life and relationship with a higher power (Gray, 2006). The Spiritual Perspective Scale (SPS) is a 10-item tool that was developed by a nurse. It measures connectedness to a higher power, others, and self (Gray, 2006). The JAREL spiritual well-being scale also provides nurses and other health care professionals with a simple tool for assessing a client's spiritual well-being (Hungelmann and others, 1996). Items on the tool are made up of three key dimensions: faith/belief, life/self-responsibility, and life-satisfaction/self-actualization.

Effective spiritual assessment tools like B-E-L-I-E-F and the SWB scale are easy to use and help nurses remember important areas to assess. Responses to assessment tools often indicate areas that need further investigation. For example, if after using an assessment tool, a nurse finds that a client has difficulty accepting change, the nurse will need to spend time understanding how the client is accepting and managing the new illness. Whether a nurse uses an assessment tool or directs an assessment with questions that are based on principles of spirituality, it is important not to impose personal value systems on the client. This is particularly true when the client's values and beliefs are similar to those of the nurse, because it then becomes very easy to make false assumptions. When nurses understand the overall approach to spiritual assessment, they are able to enter into thoughtful discussions with their clients, gain a greater awareness of the personal resources clients bring to a situation, and incorporate the resources into an effective plan of care.

Faith/Belief. Assess the source of authority and guidance that clients use in life to choose and act on their beliefs. Determine if the client has a religious source of guidance that conflicts with medical treatment plans. This seriously affects the options nurses and other health care providers are able to offer clients. For example, if a client is a Jehovah's Witness, blood products are not an acceptable form of treatment. Christian Scientists often refuse any medical intervention, believing that their faith will heal them. It is also important to understand a client's philosophy of life. Assessment data reveal the basis of the client's belief system regarding meaning and purpose in life and the client's spiritual focus. This information often reflects the impact that illness, loss, or disability has on the person's life. There is considerable religious diversity in the United States. A client's religious faith and practices, views about health, and the response to illness often influence how nurses provide support (Table 29-1).

Life and Self-Responsibility. Spiritual well-being includes life and self-responsibility. Individuals who accept change in life, make decisions about their lives, and are able to forgive others in times of difficulty have a higher level of spiritual well-being. During illness clients often are unable to accept limitations or do not know how to regain a functional and meaningful life. Their sense of helplessness reflects spiritual distress. However, clients often use their spiritual well-being as a resource as they adapt to changes and seek solutions to deal with limitations. Assess the extent to which a client understands the limitations or threats posed by an illness and the manner in which the client chooses to adjust to them.

Connectedness. People who are connected to themselves, others, nature, and God or another supreme being cope with the stress brought on by crisis and chronic illness (Narayanasamy, 2004). Clients remain connected with God by praying (Figure 29-3). Prayer is personal communication with one's god. It provides a sense of hope, strength, and security, and it is a part of faith (Cavendish and others, 2006). Help clients become or remain connected by respecting each client's unique sense of spirituality. Assess whether the client loses the ability to express a sense of relatedness to something greater than the self.

Life Satisfaction. Spiritual well-being is tied to a person's satisfaction with life and what he or she has accomplished (Krebs, 2003). Assessing satisfaction with life often provides insight to

appropriate nursing care. When people are satisfied with life, more energy is available to deal with new difficulties and to resolve problems.

Culture. Spirituality is a personal experience within a cultural context (Pincharoen and Congdon, 2003). It is important to know a client's culture of origin and to assess a client's values. It is common in many cultures for individuals to feel that they have led a worthwhile and purposeful life. Remaining connected with their cultural heritage often helps clients define their place in the world and to express their spirituality. Asking clients about their faith and belief systems is a good beginning for understanding the relationship between culture and spirituality (Box 29-3).

Fellowship and Community. Fellowship is a type of relationship an individual has with other persons (e.g., family, close friends, fellow members of a church, or neighbors). Explore the extent and nature of the client's support networks. It is unwise to assume that a given network offers the kind of support a client desires. For example, calling the client's clergy to request a visit is inappropriate if the client finds little fellowship with that individual.

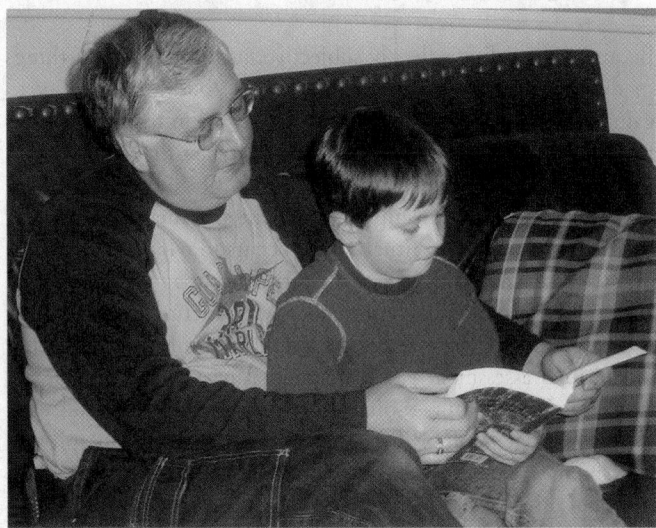

Figure 29-3 Praying together enhances the connectedness between parents and their children.

✳ TABLE 29-1 Religious Beliefs About Health			
RELIGIOUS OR CULTURAL GROUP	**HEALTH CARE BELIEFS**	**RESPONSE TO ILLNESS**	**IMPLICATIONS FOR HEALTH AND NURSING**
Hinduism	Accepts modern medical science.	Past sins cause illness. Prolonging life is discouraged.	Allow time for prayer and purity rituals. Allow use of amulets, rituals, and symbols.
Sikhism	Accepts modern medical science.	Females to be examined by females. Removing undergarments causes great distress.	Provide time for devotional prayer. Allow use of religious symbols.

✳ **TABLE 29-1 Religious Beliefs About Health, cont'd**

RELIGIOUS OR CULTURAL GROUP	HEALTH CARE BELIEFS	RESPONSE TO ILLNESS	IMPLICATIONS FOR HEALTH AND NURSING
Buddhism	Accepts modern medical science.	Sometimes refuses treatment on Holy Days. Nonhuman spirits invading the body cause illness. Sometimes wants a Buddhist priest. Usually accepts death as last stage of life and usually permits withdrawal of life support. Does not practice euthanasia. Often will not take time off from work or family responsibilities when sick.	Health is an important part of life. Maintain good health by caring for self and others. Does not always accept medications because of belief that chemical substances in the body are harmful.
Islam	Must be able to practice the Five Pillars of Islam. Sometimes has a fatalistic view of health.	Uses faith healing. Family members are a comfort. Group prayer is strengthening. Often permits withdrawal of life support. Does not practice euthanasia. Believes time of death is predetermined and cannot be changed. Maintains a sense of hope and often avoids discussions of death.	Women prefer female health care providers. During month of Ramadan, women cannot eat until after the sun goes down. Health and spirituality are connected. Family and friends visit during time of illness. Usually does not consider organ transplantation or donation and postmortem examinations.
Judaism	Believes in the sanctity of life. God and medicine have a balance. Observance of the Sabbath is important. Some refuse treatments on the Sabbath.	Visiting the sick is an obligation. Obligation to seek care, exercise, sleep, eat well, and avoid drug and alcohol abuse. Euthanasia is forbidden. Discourages life support.	Believes it is important to stay healthy. Expects nurse to provide competent health care. Allow clients to express their feelings. Allow family to stay with dying client.
Christianity	Accepts modern medical science. Many follow complementary or alternative medicine (see Chapter 36).	Uses prayer, faith healing. Appreciates visits from clergy. Some will use laying on of hands. Holy Communion is sometimes practiced. Anointing of the Sick given when client is ill or near death (Catholic).	Is usually in favor of organ donation. Health is important to maintain. Allow time for clients to pray by themselves, with family or friends.
Navajos	Concepts of health have a fundamental place in their concept of humans and their place in the universe.	Blessingway is a practice that attempts to remove ill health by means of stories, songs, rituals, prayers, symbols, and sand paintings.	Prefer holistic approach to health care. Often are not on time for appointments. Promote physical, mental, spiritual, and social health of persons, families, and communities. Allow family members to visit. Provide teaching about wellness, not disease prevention, when possible.
Appalachians	External locus of control. Nature controls life and health. Accept folk healers. Good Christian members of community are called as servants to minister to disabled.	Dislike hospitals. Tend to not follow medical regimens but expect to be helped directly when seeking episodic treatment.	Become anxious in unfamiliar settings. Encourage communication with family and friends when ill.

✳ **BOX 29-3**   **CULTURAL ASPECTS OF CARE**

Spirituality Affected by Culture

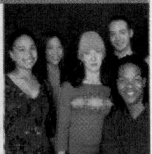

Spirituality and spiritual health vary among cultures. Therefore nurses need to assess how their clients' culture affects spirituality. Spiritual aspects of life are frequently important to Latinos. *Personalismo* is a cultural value that indicates warmth, closeness, and empathy in relationships with other people and a universal being. *Familismo*, another Latino cultural value, indicates commitment and loyalty to immediate and extended family. For Thai older adults finding harmony through a healthy mind and body is critical to maintaining health. For African Americans, spirituality is associated with guidance, coping, strength, and peace. Spirituality is often a catalyst for recovery, and community- and faith-based programs are effective in promoting health. Although people who practice Tibetan Buddhism believe that suffering is a part of life, they try to avoid suffering when possible. At the end of life, they prepare for "a good death," which requires quiet time for meditation and prayer.

Implications for Practice

- Explore the spirituality of clients from different cultures by assessing the meaning of health and how clients achieve balance, stability, peace, or comfort in their lives.
- Offer a universal and holistic approach to assessing clients' needs by demonstrating caring and using therapeutic communication techniques.
- Promote an environment during assessment that respects human rights, values, customs, and spiritual beliefs.
- Include appropriate pastoral care professionals in the assessment process.
- Avoid use of language that alienates or discriminates between different religions.

Data from Boyd AS, Wilmoth MC: An innovative community-based intervention for African American women with breast cancer: the witness project ®, *Health Soc Work* 31(1):77, 2006; Campesino M, Schwartz GE: Spirituality among Latinas/os: implications of culture in conceptualization and measurement, *ANS Adv Nurs Sci* 29(1):69, 2006; Newlin K and others: African-American spirituality: a concept analysis, *ANS Adv Nurs Sci* 25(2):57, 2002; Perdue B and others: Assessing spirituality in mentally ill African Americans, *ABNF J* 17(2):78, 2006; and Smith-Stoner M: End-of-life needs of patients who practice Tibetan Buddhism, *J Hosp Palliat Nurs* 7(4):228, 2005.

Ritual and Practice. Assessing the use of rituals and practices helps nurses understand a client's spirituality. Rituals include participation in worship, prayer, sacraments (e.g., baptism or communion), fasting, singing, meditating, scripture reading, and making offerings or sacrifices. Different religions have different rituals for life events. For example, Buddhists practice baptism later in life and find burial or cremation acceptable at death. Muslims wash the body of a dead family member and wrap it in white cloth with the head turned toward the right shoulder. Orthodox and Conservative Jews circumcise their newborn sons 8 days after birth. Determine whether illness or hospitalization has interrupted a client's usual rituals or practices. A ritual often provides the client with structure and support during difficult times. If rituals are important to the client, use them as part of nursing intervention.

Vocation. Individuals express their spirituality on a daily basis in life routines, work, play, and relationships. Spirituality is often a part of a person's identity and vocation in life (Skalla and McCoy, 2006). Determine if illness or hospitalization alters the ability to express some aspect of spirituality as it relates to the person's work or daily activities. Expression of spirituality is highly individual and includes showing an appreciation for life in the variety of things people do, living in the moment and not worrying about tomorrow, appreciating nature, expressing love towards others, and being productive (McSherry and others, 2004). When illness or loss prevents clients from expressing their spirituality, understand the psychological, social, and spiritual implications, and provide appropriate guidance and support.

◆Nursing Diagnosis

A spiritual assessment allows a nurse to learn a great deal about the client and the extent that spirituality plays in the client's life. Exploring the client's spirituality sometimes reveals responses to health problems that require nursing intervention or the existence of a strong set of resources that allow the client to cope effectively. Analyze data to find patterns of defining characteristics, and select appropriate nursing diagnoses (Box 29-4). In identifying diagnoses, recognize the significance that spirituality has for all types of health problems. Be sure each diagnosis has an accurate related factor to guide the selection of individualized, purposeful, and goal-directed interventions. Potential nursing diagnoses for spiritual health include the following:

- Anxiety
- Ineffective coping
- Fear
- Complicated grieving
- Hopelessness
- Powerlessness
- Readiness for enhanced spiritual well-being
- Spiritual distress
- Risk for spiritual distress

Three nursing diagnoses accepted by NANDA International (2007) pertain specifically to spirituality. *Readiness for enhanced spiritual well-being* is based on defining characteristics that show a person's ability to experience and integrate meaning and purpose in life through connectedness with self and others. A client with this nursing diagnosis has potential resources to draw on when faced with illness or a threat to well-being. If the client does not know how to engage personal resources to cope with health problems, offer support in exploring options.

The nursing diagnosis of *spiritual distress* and *risk for spiritual distress* create different clinical pictures. Defining characteristics from a nurse's assessment reveal patterns that reflect a person's actual or potential dispiritedness (e.g., expressing lack of hope, meaning, or purpose in life; anger toward God; or verbalizing conflicts about personal beliefs). Clients likely to be at risk for spiritual distress include those who have poor relationships, have experienced a recent loss, or are suffering some form of mental or physical illness.

✷ BOX 29-4 ✷ NURSING DIAGNOSTIC PROCESS

Readiness for Enhanced Spiritual Well-Being

Assessment Activities	Defining Characteristics
Ask client to describe personal source of faith and hope.	Client expresses an inner strength and source of guidance.
Have client describe level of satisfaction with life.	Life has purpose and meaning, provides community service as a volunteer.
Determine who provides the greatest source of strength and support to the client during times of difficulty.	Person pursues interactions with friends and family.

Accurate selection of diagnoses requires critical thinking. The nurse reviews concrete data (e.g., religious rituals and sources of fellowship), an assessment of previous client experiences, the nurse's own spirituality, and the appraisal of the client's spiritual well-being. Validate and clarify defining characteristics with the client before making a diagnosis and plan of care. Commonly clients have multiple nursing diagnoses.

◆ Planning

During the planning step of the nursing process, develop a plan of care for each of the client's nursing diagnoses. Critical thinking at this step is important because you will reflect on previous experiences and apply knowledge and critical thinking attitudes and standards in selecting the most appropriate nursing interventions (Figure 29-4). Prior experience in selecting interventions that support clients' spiritual well-being is valuable when considering the best options for clients with similar types of situations or problems. Integrate knowledge gathered from assessment and knowledge relating to resources and therapies available for spiritual care to develop an individualized plan of care (see Care Plan). Match the client's needs with evidence-based interventions that are supported and recommended in the clinical and research literature. Use a concept map (Figure 29-5) to organize client care and to show how the client's medical diagnosis, assessment data, and nursing diagnoses are interrelated.

Confidence becomes an important critical thinking attitude when building a caring relationship with the client. Confidence builds trust, enabling the nurse and client to enter into a healing relationship together. Attempting to meet or support clients' spiritual needs is not simple, and frequently nurses will need additional resources. For example, sometimes a nurse's skills in helping clients interpret and understand the meaning of illness and loss are limited. Because spiritual care is so personal, standards of autonomy and self-determination are critical in supporting the client's decisions about the plan of care.

Goals and Outcomes. A spiritual care plan includes realistic and individualized goals along with relevant outcomes. It is impor-

Knowledge
- Caring practices in the individualization of an approach with a client
- Available services offered by health care providers and community agencies
- Nursing interventions that instill hope and provide spiritual support

Experience
- Previous client responses to nursing interventions designed to support the client's spiritual well-being

PLANNING
- Collaborate with the client and family on choice of interventions
- Consult with pastoral care or other clergy or spiritual leaders as appropriate
- Incorporate spiritual rituals and observances

Standards
- Support the client's autonomy to make choices
- Promote self-determination

Attitudes
- Exhibit confidence in your skills and knowledge to develop a trusting relationship with the client

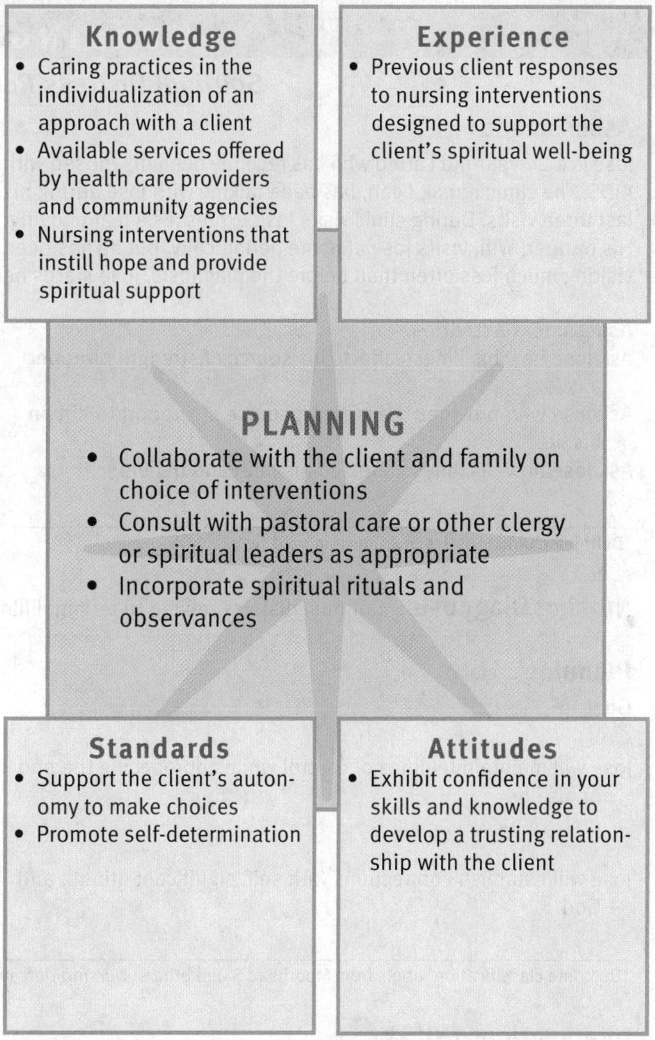

Figure 29-4 Critical thinking model for spiritual health planning.

tant for both nurse and client to collaborate closely in setting goals and choosing related interventions. Setting realistic goals requires the nurse to know the client well. When spiritual care requires helping clients adjust to loss or stressful life situations, goals are long-term. However, short-term outcomes, such as renewing participation in religious practices, help the client progressively reach a more spiritually healthy situation. In establishing a plan of care, an example of a goal and associated outcomes follows:

The client will improve personal harmony and connections with members of his or her support system.

- The client will express an acceptance of his or her illness.
- The client reports the ability to rely on family members for support.
- The client initiates social interactions with family and friends.

Setting Priorities. Spiritual care is very personalized. The nurse's relationship with the client allows the nurse to understand the client's priorities. When establishing a mutually agreed-upon plan with the client, he or she will be able to identify what is most

Spiritual Distress Related to Terminal Illness

Assessment

Jose is a 24-year-old Latino who has recently been diagnosed with AIDS. The clinic nurse, Leah, has been talking with Jose during his last three visits. During clinic visits Jose expresses a fear of dying. His partner, Will, visits Jose at home periodically, but he has been visiting much less often than before the diagnosis. Jose states he "used to go to a Catholic church" when he was younger and explains that he currently has a poor relationship with his mother and his brother. His physician recently told Jose that he is in the end stage of his illness and suggested that he consider hospice care. Leah now talks with Jose in a private conference area.

Assessment Activities	Findings/Defining Characteristics*
Ask Jose how his illness affects his source of strength or hope. Ask Jose who provides the greatest source of support to him in his life. Ask Jose how his illness affected his faith and beliefs.	Jose responds, "**How can God do this to me**? There are moments when I just **feel so angry**. What is going to happen to me?" He begins to cry and admits, "**I feel so alone. Will has not been there** when I need him." Jose responds, "My church does not accept homosexuality, so **I don't feel like I fit in** there. I have always had a faith in God."

*__Defining characteristics__ are shown in bold type.

Nursing Diagnosis: Spiritual distress related to terminal illness.

Planning

Goal	Expected Outcomes (NOC)†
	Dignified Life Closure
Jose will maintain feelings of control while approaching the end of his life.	Jose will share feelings about dying in 1 week. Jose will initiate contact and begin to heal relationships with his family within 3 weeks.
	Spiritual Health
Jose will establish connections with self, significant others, and God.	Jose will visit with Will in the next 2 weeks to share his thoughts, feelings, and beliefs. Jose will identify and participate in spiritual activites in 1 month.

†Outcome classification labels from Moorhead S and others: *Nursing outcomes classification (NOC)*, ed 4, St. Louis, 2008, Mosby.

Interventions (NIC)‡	Rationale
Spiritual Growth Facilitation Ask Jose to identify activities that will help heal his body, mind, and spirit. Encourage Jose to pray; offer to pray with him.	Spirituality helps men who are HIV positive cope with their illness and enhances quality of life (Grimsley, 2006). People who are Latino sometimes pray more frequently than they attend church; prayer often provides spiritual strength (Campesino and Schwartz, 2006).
Spiritual Support Use therapeutic communication to establish trust and a caring presence. Encourage Jose to renew his relationships with Will, his mother, and his brother. Teach Jose methods of relaxation, meditation, and guided imagery.	Providing spiritual care requires caring, compassion, and respect (Cavendish and others, 2006). The Latino cultural values of *personalismo* and *simpático* (close, personal relationships with others) enhance connection with God (Campesino and Schwartz, 2006). Relaxation methods such as controlled breathing and yoga often help clients with HIV enhance their self-awareness and manage personal issues related to their illness more positively (Brazier and others, 2006).

‡Intervention classification labels from Bulechek GM, Butcher HK, and Dochterman JM: *Nursing interventions classification (NIC)*, ed 5, St. Louis, 2008, Mosby.

NURSING CARE PLAN

Spiritual Distress Related to Terminal Illness—cont'd

Evaluation

Nursing Actions	Client Response/Finding	Achievement of Outcome
Ask Jose how he currently feels about having end-stage AIDS.	"I am not quite as frightened as I was a few weeks ago."	Jose reports an improved outlook. Will probably continue to have fears about dying.
Ask Jose about his relationships with Will, his mother, and his brother.	"It meant a great deal to tell Will and my family how I feel. They did not know how to help me. We now talk on the phone almost every day."	Successfully increased connection with significant others.
Ask Jose which spiritual activities he finds helpful.	"I have been praying and have been using the breathing techniques you taught me every day. They have helped me feel better about myself and my situation. I don't seem to feel so angry anymore."	Prayer and relaxation activities have enhanced positive feelings about self and have reduced feelings of anger.

CONCEPT MAP

Nursing diagnosis: Spiritual distress
- Expresses anger in having cancer and in having to deal with an ostomy
- States "Why has God done this to me?"
- No longer attending spiritual services at church

Interventions
- Establish therapeutic relationship by being physically present and actively listening to client
- Help the client find a reason for living
- Encourage use of humor, as appropriate, to enhance spiritual well-being

Nursing diagnosis: Ineffective coping
- Calls in sick at work without reason
- Becomes angry with friends who offer support
- Reports inability to sleep
- Avoids social contact

Interventions
- Assess for risk of client harming self or others
- Encourage client to walk for 15 to 20 minutes a day
- Refer client for counseling as needed
- Recommend good sleep hygiene habits

Client's chief medical diagnosis: Colon resection with formation of permanent transverse colostomy, depression 1 month postoperatively
Priority assessments: Coping strategies, acceptance of diagnosis of cancer and ostomy, and effect of diagnosis on spirituality

Nursing diagnosis: Disturbed body image
- Verbalizes "I can barely look at myself in the mirror"
- Ostomy is incontinent form; requires routine changing of ostomy bag
- Avoids social activities

Interventions
- Assess stage of grieving and acceptance of colostomy, including effect of colostomy on sexuality
- Help client develop a realistic perception of body image
- Focus on remaining abilities by having client make a list of current strengths, gifts, and talents

——— Link between medical diagnosis and nursing diagnosis   - - - - Link between nursing diagnoses

Figure 29-5 Concept map for client with colon resection with formation of permanent transverse colostomy and depression 1 month postoperatively.

important. Spiritual priorities do not need to be sacrificed for physical care priorities. For example, when a client is in acute distress, focus care to provide the client a sense of control. When a client is terminally ill, spiritual care is possibly the most important nursing intervention.

Collaborative Care.
If the client participates in a formal religion, involve members of the clergy or members of the church, temple, mosque, or synagogue in the plan of care. In a hospital setting the pastoral care department is a valuable resource. These professionals provide insight about how and when to best support clients and their families. In addition, significant others, such as spouses, siblings, parents, and friends, need to be involved in the client's care, as appropriate. This means that the nurse learns from the assessment what individuals or groups have formed a relationship with the client. These individuals sometimes become involved in all levels of the nurse's plan. They often assist in giving physical care, providing emotional comfort, and sharing spiritual support.

Implementation

Establish a caring relationship with a client to discover the client's meaning of illness or loss and the effect it has on the meaning and purpose of life. Achieving this level of understanding with a client enables the nurse to deliver care in a sensitive, creative, and appropriate manner.

Health Promotion.
Spiritual care needs to be a central theme in promoting an individual's overall well-being (Grant, 2004). Spirituality is one personal resource that affects the balance between health and illness. In settings where health promotion activities occur, clients are often in need of information, counseling, and guidance to make the necessary choices to remain healthy.

Establishing Presence. Nurses contribute to a sense of well-being and provide hope for recovery when they spend time with their clients (Krebs, 2003). Behaviors that establish the nurse's presence include giving attention, answering questions, listening, and having a positive and encouraging (but realistic) attitude. Establishing presence is part of the art of nursing. It is not simply being in the same room with a client while performing procedures or sharing technical information with a client. Presence involves "being with" a client versus "doing for" a client (Benner, 1984). Presence involves offering a closeness with the client, physically, psychologically, and spiritually (see Chapter 8).

When health promotion is the focus of care, the nurse's presence becomes important in giving clients the confidence needed to remain healthy. Demonstrate a caring presence by listening to clients' concerns and willingly involving family in discussions about the clients' health. Show self-confidence when providing health instruction, and support clients as they make decisions about their health. The client who seeks health care is often fearful of experiencing an illness that threatens loss of control and looks for someone to offer competent direction. Encouraging words of support and a calm, decisive approach establish a presence that builds trust and well-being.

Supporting a Healing Relationship.
Learn to look beyond isolated client problems and recognize the broader picture of a client's holistic needs. For example, do not just look at a client's back pain as a problem to solve with quick remedies, but rather look at how the pain influences the client's ability to function and achieve goals established in life. A **holistic** view enables the nurse to establish a helping role and a healing relationship. Three factors are evident when a healing relationship develops between nurse and client:

1. Mobilizing hope for the nurse, as well as for the client
2. Finding an interpretation or understanding of the illness, pain, anxiety, or other stressful emotion that is acceptable to the client
3. Assisting the client in using social, emotional, and spiritual resources (Benner, 1984)

Mobilizing the client's hope is central to a healing relationship. Hope motivates people with strategies to face challenges in life (Lohne and Severinsson, 2004). Help clients find things to hope for. For example, a client newly diagnosed with diabetes wants to learn how to manage the disease to continue a productive and satisfying way of life. An adult daughter who has decided to become caregiver to her older adult parent hopes to be able to protect the parent from injury or worsening disability. Hope helps a client work toward recovery. To help clients achieve hope, work together to find an explanation of the situation that is acceptable to both the nurse and the client. Help the client realistically exercise hope by supporting a client's positive attitude toward life or a desire to be informed and to make decisions.

To further support a healing relationship, remain aware of the client's spiritual resources and needs. It is always important for a client to be able to express and exercise his or her beliefs and to find spiritual comfort. When life stressors or illness create confusion or uncertainty, recognize the possible effect on a client's well-being. How does the nurse use and strengthen spiritual resources? Begin by encouraging a client to discuss the effect illness has had on personal beliefs and faith, thus giving the chance to clarify any misconceptions or inaccuracies in information. Having a clear sense of what illness will be like for an individual helps the person to apply all resources toward recovery.

Acute Care.
Within acute care settings, clients experience multiple stressors that threaten their sense of control. Ongoing assessment of spiritual needs is essential because the client's needs often change rapidly (Smith, 2006). Support and enhancement of a client's spiritual well-being is a challenge when the focus of health care seems to be one of treatment and cure rather than care (McEwen, 2005). To overcome these challenges, display a soothing presence and supportive touch when providing nursing care. The artful use of hands, encouraging words of support, promotion of connectedness, and a calm and decisive approach establishes a presence that builds trust.

Support Systems. Use of support systems is important in any health care setting. Support systems provide clients with the greatest sense of well-being during hospitalization and serve as a human link connecting the client, the nurse, and the client's lifestyle before an illness. Part of the client's caregiving environment is the regular presence of supportive family and friends. Provide

✳ TABLE 29-2 Religious Dietary Regulations Affecting Health Care

RELIGION	DIETARY PRACTICES
Hinduism	Some sects are vegetarians. The belief is not to kill *any* living creature.
Buddhism	Some are vegetarians and will not use alcohol. Many will fast on Holy Days.
Islam	Prohibits consumption of pork and alcohol. Fasts during the month of Ramadan.
Judaism	Some observe the kosher dietary restrictions (e.g., avoid pork and shellfish, do not prepare and eat milk and meat at the same time).
Christianity	Some Baptists, Evangelicals, and Pentecostals discourage the use of alcohol and caffeine.
	Roman Catholics fast on Ash Wednesday, Good Friday, and 1 hour before receiving Communion; do not eat meat on Fridays during Lent.
Jehovah's Witnesses	Members avoid food prepared with or containing blood.
Mormonism	Members abstain from alcohol and caffeine.
Russian Orthodox Church	Followers observe fast days as well as a "no meat" rule on Wednesdays and Fridays. During Lent all animal products, including dairy products and butter, are forbidden.
Native Americans	Individual tribal beliefs influence food practices.

privacy during visits, and plan care with the client and the client's support network to promote the interpersonal bonding that is needed for recovery. The support system is a source of faith and hope, and it often is an important resource in conducting meaningful religious rituals.

When clients depend on family and friends for support, encourage them to visit the client regularly. Encourage family to be themselves during visits to facilitate spiritual comfort. Help family members feel comfortable in the health care setting, and use their support and presence to promote the client's healing. Including family members in prayer, for example, is a thoughtful gesture if it is appropriate to the client's religion and if family members are comfortable participating. Encouraging the family to bring meaningful religious symbols to the client's bedside offers significant spiritual support.

Other important resources to clients are spiritual advisors and members of the clergy. Many hospitals have pastoral care departments. Pastoral care professionals have expertise in understanding how an illness influences a person's beliefs and how the beliefs of the person influence illness and recovery. Ask if clients desire to have a member of the clergy visit during their hospitalization. When requested by clients or families, keep clergy informed of any physical, psychosocial, or spiritual concerns affecting the client. Show respect for clients' spiritual values and needs by willingly cooperating with others giving spiritual care and by facilitating the administration of sacraments, rites, and rituals.

Diet Therapies. Food and nutrition are important aspects of client care and often an important component of some religious observances (Table 29-2). Food and the rituals surrounding the preparation and serving of food are sometimes important to a person's spirituality. Consult with the dietitian to integrate the client's dietary preferences into daily care. In the event that a hospital or other health care agency cannot prepare food in the preferred way, ask the family to bring meals that fit into dietary restrictions posed by the client's condition.

Supporting Rituals. Nurses provide spiritual care by supporting clients' participation in spiritual rituals and activities. Plan care to allow time for religious readings, spiritual visitations, or attendance at religious services. Allow family members to plan a prayer session or an organized reading of scriptures on a regular basis. Make arrangements with pastoral care staff for the client

and family to participate in religious practices (e.g., receiving sacraments). Clergy often visit people who are unable to attend religious services. Taped meditations, classical or religious music, and televised religious services provide other effective options. The nurse respects icons, medals, prayer rugs, or crosses that clients bring to a health setting and ensure they are not accidentally lost, damaged, or misplaced. Supporting spiritual rituals is especially important for older adults (Box 29-5).

Restorative and Continuing Care. For clients who are recovering from a long-term illness or disability or who suffer chronic or terminal disease, spiritual care becomes especially important. Many of the nursing interventions applicable in health promotion and acute care apply to this level of health care as well.

Prayer. Prayer offers an opportunity to renew personal faith and belief in a higher being in a specific, focused way that is either highly ritualized and formal or quite spontaneous and informal. Prayer is an effective coping resource for physical as well as psychological symptoms (Wright, 2005). Clients pray in private or pursue opportunities for group prayer with family, friends, or clergy. Nurses are supportive of prayer by giving clients privacy, by suggesting prayer when they know clients use it as a coping resource, and by participating in prayer with clients (Cavendish and others, 2006). If prayer is not suitable for a client, alternatives include listening to music or reading a book, poetry, or other inspirational texts selected by the client.

Meditation. Meditation effectively creates a relaxation response that reduces daily stress. Meditation reduces blood pressure, slows the aging process, reduces pain, and enhances the function of the immune system (Lindberg, 2005). Nurses often use guided imagery to help clients learn meditation (see Chapter 36). When clients use meditation in conjunction with their spiritual beliefs, they often report an increased spirituality that they commonly describe as experiencing the presence of a power, force, or energy, or what was perceived as God (Box 29-6).

Supporting Grief Work. Clients who experience terminal illness or who have suffered permanent loss in body function because of a disabling disease or injury require the nurse's support in grieving over and coping with their loss (see Chapter 30). The nurse's ability to enter into a therapeutic and spiritual relationship with the client will support a client during times of grief.

✳ BOX 29-5   FOCUS ON OLDER ADULTS

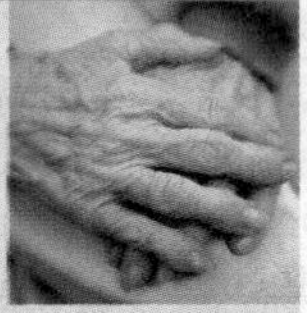

Spirituality and Spiritual Health

- There is an association between an older adult's spirituality and ability to adjust or cope with illness (Ebersole and others, 2004).
- Religious activities and spiritual experiences are very common among older adults. Those who experience spiritual well-being have strong social support, better emotional health, and to some extent, improved physical health (Koenig and others, 2004).
- Respecting privacy and dignity is an essential part of nursing care, especially when meeting spiritual needs of the older adult (Narayanasamy and others, 2004).
- Older adults use a variety of strategies such as spiritual rituals, exercise, and complementary medicine to cope with pain and chronic illness. Including religious activities and meditation positively enhance coping and feelings of peace (Barry and others, 2004; Lindberg, 2005).
- Feelings of connectedness are important for the older adult. Enhance connectedness by helping older clients find meaning and purpose in life, listening actively to concerns, and being present (Narayanasamy and others, 2004).
- Beliefs in the afterlife increase as adults grow older. Make visits from clergy, social workers, lawyers, and financial advisors available so clients feel as though they have completed all unfinished business. Leaving a legacy to loved ones prepares the older adult to leave the world with a sense of meaning (Ebersole and others, 2004). Legacies include oral histories, works of art, publications, photographs, or other objects of significance.
- Older adult caregivers, such as those caring for another with Alzheimer's dementia, often use their spirituality and spiritual behaviors or practices to help them deal with crisis and conflict (Spurlock, 2005).

✳ BOX 29-6   CLIENT TEACHING

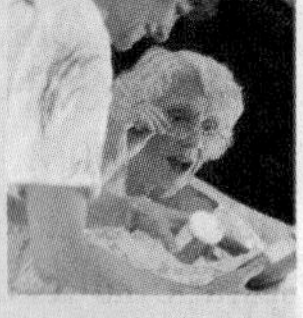

Meditation Techniques

Objective
- The client will verbalize feelings of relaxation and self-transcendence after meditation.

Teaching Strategies
- Provide client a brief description of information that will be provided, as well as a printed teaching guide that describes how to meditate.
- Help client identify a quiet room in the home that has minimal interruptions.
- Explain that peaceful music or the quiet whirring of a fan will block out distractions.
- Teach steps of meditation—sit in a comfortable position with the back straight; breathe slowly; and focus on a sound, prayer, or image.
- Encourage to meditate for 10 to 20 minutes twice a day.
- Answer questions, and reinforce information as needed.

Evaluation
- Have the client describe feelings following meditation.

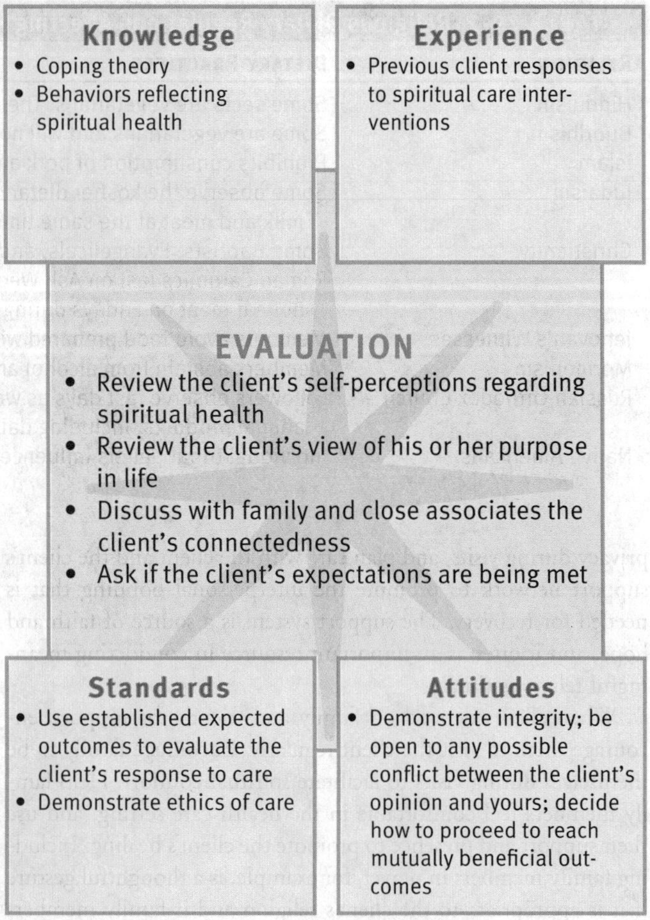

Knowledge
- Coping theory
- Behaviors reflecting spiritual health

Experience
- Previous client responses to spiritual care interventions

EVALUATION
- Review the client's self-perceptions regarding spiritual health
- Review the client's view of his or her purpose in life
- Discuss with family and close associates the client's connectedness
- Ask if the client's expectations are being met

Standards
- Use established expected outcomes to evaluate the client's response to care
- Demonstrate ethics of care

Attitudes
- Demonstrate integrity; be open to any possible conflict between the client's opinion and yours; decide how to proceed to reach mutually beneficial outcomes

Figure 29-6 Critical thinking model for spiritual health evaluation.

◆ Evaluation

The evaluation of a client's spiritual care requires the nurse to think critically in determining if efforts at restoring or maintaining the client's spiritual health were successful (Figure 29-6). Outcomes established during the planning phase serve as the standards to evaluate the client's progress. In addition, the nurse evaluates any ethical concerns that arise in the course of the client's spiritual care and support. Apply critical thinking attitudes to ensure sound nursing judgments.

Attainment of spiritual health is a lifelong goal. In evaluating outcomes, compare the client's level of spiritual health with the behaviors and perceptions noted in the nursing assessment. Evaluation data related to spiritual health is usually subjective. For example, if the nurse's assessment finds the client losing hope, the follow-up evaluation involves asking the client if feelings of hope have been restored. Include family and friends when gathering evaluative information. Successful outcomes reveal the client developing an increased or restored sense of connectedness with family; maintaining, renewing, or reforming a sense of purpose in life and, for some, a confidence and trust in a supreme being or power. When outcomes are not met, ask questions to determine appropriate continuing care. Examples of questions to ask include the following:

- Do you feel the need to forgive someone or to be forgiven by someone?
- What spiritual activities, such as prayer or meditation, were helpful in the past?
- Would you like for me to ask a friend, family member, or someone from pastoral care to come talk with you?
- What can I do to help you feel more at peace?
- Sometimes people need to give themselves permission to feel hope when they experience difficult events. What can you do to allow yourself to feel hope again?

✳ Key Concepts

- Attending to a client's spirituality ensures a holistic focus to nursing practice.
- Beneficial health outcomes occur when individuals are able to exercise their spiritual beliefs.
- Frequently spirituality and religion are interchanged, but spirituality is a much broader and more unifying concept than religion.
- Spirituality is highly personal and unique to each individual.
- Faith and hope are closely linked to a person's spiritual well-being, providing an inner strength for dealing with illness and disability.
- When clients experience acute or chronic illness or a terminal disease, spiritual resources either help a person move to recovery or spiritual distress develops.
- Common religious rituals include private worship, prayer, singing, use of a rosary, and scripture reading.
- A spiritual assessment is most successful when the nurse applies knowledge that is relevant to therapeutic communication, principles of loss and grief, and knowledge of caring practices.
- The personal nature of spirituality requires open communication and the establishment of trust between nurse and client.
- Nurses need to determine if a client's religious beliefs conflict with medical treatment.
- An important part of spiritual assessment is learning who makes up the client's community of faith (e.g., friends, family, religious leaders).
- A hospital's pastoral care department is a valuable resource to use in planning a client's spiritual care.
- Establishing presence involves giving attention, answering questions, having an encouraging attitude and expressing a sense of trust.
- Connectedness and fellowship with other persons are a source of hope for a client.
- Part of a client's caregiving environment is the regular presence of family, friends, and spiritual advisors.
- Prayer is an effective coping resource for physical and psychological symptoms.
- When evaluating spiritual care, successful outcomes reveal the client developing an increased or restored sense of connectedness with family and maintaining, renewing, or reforming a sense of purpose in life.

✳ Critical Thinking Exercises

1. Jose continues to regularly visit the HIV/AIDS clinic. The nurse wants to incorporate a spiritual assessment with the physical assessment. During the assessment the nurse asks Jose if he has any questions. Jose asks the nurse about a Buddhist ritual he heard about from a friend of his. The nurse has not heard about that ritual before. The nurse states, "I am not sure what you are asking about. After we are done here, I will try to find some information for you."

   In this interaction, the nurse is exhibiting the attitude for critical thinking known as _____.

2. Jose's mother comes with Jose to a clinic visit. During the visit the nurse asks Jose's mother, "What spiritual activities do you participate in?" Jose's mother responds that she goes to daily mass, listens to religious music, and spends time praying while she sits in her garden. When asked if there is anything the nurse can do for Jose's mother, she responds that she would like to meet with a priest while she is visiting Jose. She then states, "My biggest concern is remaining strong for Jose. It is so hard to watch your child die."
   a. What nursing diagnosis is appropriate for Jose's mother at this time?
   b. Provide an appropriate outcome with two nursing interventions and rationale.

3. Jose is too ill to come to the clinic. He now is being seen every other day by the hospice team. Jose's family and his partner, Will, are at his side. Describe two nursing interventions the hospice nurse could implement to enhance the family's connectedness.

✳ NCLEX®-Style Review Questions

1. An emergency department nurse is caring for a client who was severely injured in a car accident. The client's family is in the waiting room. They are crying softly. The nurse sits down next to the family, takes the mother's hand, and says, "I can only imagine how you are feeling. What can I do to help you feel more at peace right now?" In this example, the nurse is demonstrating:
   1. Prayer
   2. Presence
   3. Coaching
   4. Instilling hope

2. A client states that he does not believe in the existence of God. This client most likely is an:
   1. Agenic
   2. Atheist
   3. Agnostic
   4. Anarchist

3. As the nurse cares for a client in an outpatient clinic, the client states that he recently lost his position as a volunteer coordinator at a local community center. He expresses that he is angry with his former boss and with

God. The nurse knows the priority at this time is to assess the client's spirituality in relation to his:
1. Vocation
2. Life satisfaction
3. Fellowship and community
4. Connectedness with his family and co-workers

4. A client who is hospitalized with congestive heart failure states that she sees her illness as an opportunity and a challenge. Despite her illness, she is still able to see that life is worth living. This is an example of:
1. Hope
2. Faith
3. Values
4. Connectedness

5. Which of the following statements made by an older adult woman whose husband recently died most indicates the need for follow-up by the nurse?
1. "I cry almost every day."
2. "I have been unable to talk with my children lately."
3. "My friends think that I need to go to a grief support group."
4. "I believe that some day I will meet my husband in heaven."

6. Which of the following nursing interventions support a healing relationship with a client? (Choose all that apply):
1. Praying with the client
2. Giving pain medications
3. Telling a client that it is time to take a bath
4. Making the client's bed following hospital protocol
5. Helping a client see positive aspects related to a chronic illness

7. A client expresses the desire to learn how to meditate. What does the nurse need to do first?
1. Answer the client's questions
2. Help the client get into a comfortable position
3. Select a teaching environment that is free from distractions
4. Encourage the client to meditate for 10 to 20 minutes 2 times a day

8. An older adult is receiving hospice care. What nursing interventions will help the client cope with feelings related to death and dying? (Choose all that apply.)
1. Teaching the client how to use guided imagery
2. Encouraging the family to visit the client frequently
3. Taking the client's vital signs every time the nurse visits
4. Teaching the client how to manage pain and how to take pain medications
5. Helping the client put significant photographs in a scrapbook for the family

30 | The Experience of Loss, Death, and Grief

✳ OBJECTIVES

Mastery of content in this chapter will enable the student to:

- Identify the nurse's role in assisting clients experiencing loss, grief, or death.
- Describe the types of loss experienced throughout life.
- Discuss grief theories.
- Identify types of grief.
- Describe characteristics of a person experiencing grief.
- Discuss variables that influence a person's response to grief.
- Develop a nursing care plan for a client and family experiencing loss and grief.

- Identify ways to involve family members in palliative care.
- Discuss the criteria for hospice care.
- Describe care of the body after death.
- Discuss the nurse's own grief experience when caring for dying clients.
- Identify methods for nurse self-care in grief and loss.

✳ MEDIA RESOURCES   ✳ KEY TERMS

Companion CD
- NCLEX®-Style Review Questions
- Audio Glossary
- Interactive Learning Activities
- English/Spanish Glossary

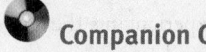 **Website**
- NCLEX®-Style Review Questions
- Audio Glossary
- English/Spanish Glossary
- Interactive Learning Activities
- Weblinks
- Audio Summaries

Acceptance, p. 464
Actual loss, p. 462
Anger, p. 464
Anticipatory grief, p. 463
Autopsy, p. 479
Bargaining, p. 464
Bereavement, p. 463
Complicated (or dysfunctional) grief, p. 463
Denial, p. 464
Depression, p. 464
Disenfranchised grief, p. 463
Disorganization and despair, p. 464
Grief, p. 463
Hope, p. 467

Hospice, p. 478
Maturational loss, p. 462
Mourning, p. 463
Necessary loss, p. 462
Normal (uncomplicated) grief, p. 463
Numbing, p. 464
Organ and tissue donation, p. 479
Palliative care, p. 471
Perceived loss, p. 462
Postmortem care, p. 480
Reorganization, p. 464
Situational loss, p. 462
Spiritual integration, p. 467
Yearning and searching, p. 464

Every person who experiences illness or injury will likely also experience loss or grief. A client may grieve the loss of multiple things: the loss of body parts or function, self-esteem, confidence, or income. Illness can change or threaten a person's identity, and at some time everyone will die. Nurses have a primary duty to prevent illness and injury and help clients return to health. They also play an important role in helping clients and families cope with things that cannot be changed and facilitate a peaceful death.

Several barriers exist in the delivery of expert care at the end of life. Before the development of medical technology, death occurred at home, in a familiar, nontechnical setting with family and friends caring for the dying. Now, death most often takes place in institutions offering technical, efficient interventions designed to prolong life and avoid death. Strangers, often unfamiliar with client and family values and wishes, care for the dying. Health care professionals sometimes resist feeling the uncomfortable emotions associated with grief and death and view death as a personal and professional failure. Talking openly about death is discouraged in American society, our everyday lives, our language, and even our thinking (Matzo and Sherman, 2006). Terminal illness reminds friends and family members of their own mortality, which may cause them, often unconsciously, to withdraw from the dying person. Nurses grieve themselves when they witness the suffering of others (Sherman, 2004).

Despite the barriers to providing end-of-life care, nurses have a long and proud history of assuming primary responsibility for the direct care of the grieving and dying (Blum, 2006). Clients and families need expert nursing care through grief and death, perhaps more than at any other time. Providing care for clients at the end of life requires knowledge and caring to bring comfort, even when the hope for cure or continued life is not possible (Virani and Sofer, 2003).

Scientific Knowledge Base

Loss

From birth to death we form attachments and suffer losses. We develop independence from the adults who raise us, start and leave school, change friends, begin careers, and form new relationships. The values learned in one's family, religious community, society, and culture shape what a person regards as loss and how to grieve (Hooyman and Kramer, 2006). People experience loss when another person, possession, body part, familiar environment, or sense of self changes or is no longer present (Table 30-1).

Life changes are natural and often positive. As we move forward in life, we learn that change always involves **necessary losses,** which are a part of life. We learn to expect that most of our necessary losses are eventually replaced by something different or better. Some losses, however, cause us to undergo permanent changes in our lives and threaten our sense of belonging and security. The death of a loved one, divorce, or loss of independence changes life forever and often significantly disrupts a person's physical, psychological, and spiritual health. **Maturational losses** are a form of necessary loss and include all normally expected life changes across the life span. A mother feels loss when her child leaves home for the first day of school. A grade school child does not want to lose her favorite teacher and classroom. Maturational losses associated with normal life transitions help people develop coping skills to use when experiencing unplanned, unwanted, or unexpected loss.

Some losses seem unnecessary and are not part of expected maturation experiences. Sudden, unpredictable external events bring about **situational loss.** An automobile accident, for example, might involve an injury with physical changes that makes it impossible for a person to return to work or school, leading to loss of function, income, life goals, or self-esteem.

Losses may be actual or perceived. An **actual loss** occurs when a person can no longer feel, hear, or know a person or object. Examples include the loss of a body part, death of a family member, or loss of a job. Lost valued objects include those that wear out or are misplaced, stolen, or ruined by disaster. A child may grieve the loss of a favorite toy washed away in a flood. **Perceived losses** are uniquely defined by the person experiencing the loss and are less obvious to other people. Some people perceive rejection by a friend, for example, or sense a loss of confidence or status in a group. How an individual interprets the meaning of the perceived loss affects the intensity of grief response. Perceived losses are easy to overlook because they are so internally and individually experienced, although they are grieved in the same way as an actual loss.

Each person responds to loss differently. The type of loss and the person's perception of it influence the depth and duration of

---

✳ TABLE 30-1 Types of Loss

DEFINITION	IMPLICATIONS OF LOSS
Loss of possessions or objects (e.g., theft, deterioration, misplacement, or destruction)	Extent of grieving depends on object's value, sentiment attached to it, or its usefulness.
Loss of known environment (e.g., leaving home, hospitalization, new job, moving out of a rehabilitation unit)	Loss occurs through maturational or situational events or by injury/ illness. Loneliness in an unfamiliar setting threatens self-esteem, hopefulness, or belonging.
Loss of a significant other (e.g., divorce, loss of friend, trusted caregiver, or pet)	Close friends, family members, and pets fulfill psychological, safety, love, belonging, and self-esteem needs.
Loss of an aspect of self (e.g., body part, job, psychological or physiological function)	Illness, injury, or developmental changes result in loss of a valued aspect of self, altering personal identity and self-concept.
Loss of life (e.g., death of family member, friend, co-worker, or one's own death)	Loss of life grieves those left behind. Dying persons also feel sadness or fear pain, loss of control, and dependency on others.

the grief response. For some individuals, the loss of an object (e.g., home or treasured, inherited gift) generates the same level of distress as the loss of a person, depending on the value the person places on the object. Chronic illnesses, disabilities, and hospitalization produce multiple losses. When entering an institution for care, clients lose access to familiar people and environments, privacy, and control over body functions and daily routines. A chronic illness or disability adds financial hardships for most people and often brings about changes in lifestyle and dependence on others. Even brief illnesses or hospitalizations cause temporary shifts in family role functioning and daily activities and change relationships.

Death is the ultimate loss. Although part of the continuum of life and a part of being human, death represents the unknown and generates anxiety, fear, and uncertainty for many people. Death permanently separates people physically from important persons in their lives and causes fear, sadness, and regret for the dying person, family members, friends, and caregivers (Craib, 2003). A person's culture, spirituality, personal beliefs and values, previous experiences with death, and degree of social support influence the way he or she approaches death.

Grief

Grief is the emotional response to a loss, manifested in ways unique to an individual, based on personal experiences, cultural expectations, and spiritual beliefs (Hooyman and Kramer, 2006) (see Chapters 9 and 29). Coping with grief involves a period of **mourning,** the outward, social expressions of grief and the behavior associated with loss. Mourning rituals are culturally influenced and as such are learned behaviors. For example, the Jewish mourning ritual of *shiva* incorporates the community's helping behaviors toward those experiencing death, sets expectations for survivor behavior, and sustains the community with tradition and rituals (Clements and others, 2003). The term **bereavement** captures both grief and mourning and includes the emotional responses and outward behaviors of a person experiencing loss (End-of-Life Nursing Education Consortium [ELNEC], 2003).

The Continuum of Grief. It is important to differentiate the expression of grief as a normal, healthy response to loss, which requires support and public acknowledgment, from grief as a response with greater distress and personal disruption, which requires more intensive intervention. Recognizing that there are different types of grief can help nurses plan and implement appropriate care.

Normal Grief. When people are grieving, it means that they are in the process of coping with the death of a loved one. **Normal (uncomplicated) grief** is the most common reaction to death. Though manner of death (violent, unexpected, traumatic) does pose greater risk to survivors, it does not always determine how an individual will grieve. Coping styles, such as hardiness, and resilience and a personal sense of control, as well as the ability to make sense of the loss, and to find benefit in the loss are factors that have been found to be helpful (Holland and others, 2006; Ong and others, 2006; Onrus and others, 2006; Matthews, 2007). Normal grief is a complex response with emotional, cognitive, social, physical, behavioral, and spiritual concepts.

A recent study found that feelings of acceptance, disbelief, yearning, anger, and depression were displayed in normal bereavement grief (Maciejewski and others, 2007). The research identified patterns in how these feelings changed over the 2 years of the study. Yearning, which is a longing or searching for the deceased person, was the most common negative feeling, peaking around 2 months after the loss. Acceptance was the strongest initial response and grew increasingly stronger over time. Negative emotions (anger and depression) peaked around 4 months and were in decline by 6 months.

Complicated Grief. For a minority of people, normal grief adjustment does not occur. In **complicated (dysfunctional) grief** the grieving person has a prolonged or significantly difficult time moving forward after a loss. Following the loss of a loved one, those with complicated grief experience a chronic and disruptive yearning for the deceased and are likely to have trouble accepting the death and trusting others, feel excessively bitter, or are uneasy about the future. They may also feel emotionally numb. Complicated grief occurs more often in situations of conflicted relationships with the deceased, prior or multiple losses or stressors, mental health issues, or lack of social support. Loss associated with homicide, suicide, sudden accidents, or the loss of a child have the potential to become complicated. Symptoms and disturbances of complicated grief last at least 6 months after a loss, and they interrupt every dimension of the person's life.

Anticipatory Grief. A person experiences **anticipatory grief,** the unconscious process of disengaging or "letting go" before the actual loss or death occurs, especially in situations of prolonged or predicted loss (Corless, 2006). When grief extends over a long period of time, people absorb loss more gradually and begin to prepare for its inevitability. They experience their more intense responses to grief (e.g., shock, denial, and tearfulness) before the actual death occurs and often feel relief when it finally happens. The idea that people actually grieve in anticipation (rather than following a loss) is hotly debated by researchers. Another way to think about anticipatory grief is that it is a form of forewarning or cushion to give families time to prepare for death or to complete the tasks related to the impending death. However, this idea may not apply in every situation. Saldiner and Cain (2004) found that the stress and strain of a terminal illness, including ruptures in spousal intimacy, separation anxiety, security threats, and the traumatic helplessness of watching a loved one die, outweigh the supposed benefits of anticipatory grieving. Although forewarning may be a buffer for some, it may increase stress for others, posing a sort of emotional roller coaster of highs and lows.

Disenfranchised Grief. People experience **disenfranchised grief,** also known as marginal or unsupported grief, when their relationship to the deceased person is not socially sanctioned, cannot be openly acknowledged or publicly shared, or seems of lesser significance (Hooyman and Kramer, 2006). Examples include the death of a very old person, an ex-spouse, a gay partner, or even a loved pet.

Theories of Grief and Mourning

Knowledge of grief theories and "normal" responses to loss and bereavement aids the nurse's understanding of these complex experiences. Grief theorists consistently acknowledge the individuality of grief responses. Do not assume that people who vary from

TABLE 30-2   Theories of Loss, Grief, and Mourning

FIVE STAGES OF DYING (KÜBLER-ROSS)	ATTACHMENT THEORY (BOWLBY)	TASKS OF MOURNING (WORDEN)	THE R PROCESS MODEL (RANDO)
Denial	Numbing	Accepting the reality of loss	Recognize and accept the reality of the loss
Anger	Yearning and searching	Working through the pain of grief	React to, experience, and express the pain of separation
Bargaining	Disorganization and despair	Adjusting to the environment without the deceased	Reminisce
Depression	Reorganization	Emotionally relocating the deceased and moving on with life	Relinquish old attachments
Acceptance			Readjust and Reinvest

normal grief responses are abnormal. Although most grief theories describe how people cope with death, they can also be used to understand responses to other significant losses. A review of some classic grief theories follows (Table 30-2).

Stages of Dying. Kübler-Ross' classic behavioral theory (1969) describes five stages of dying. Although the stages are listed in an order, grieving people do not experience them in any particular order or for any length of time and often move back and forth between the stages. In the **denial** stage, a person acts as though nothing has happened and refuses to accept the fact of the loss. The person shows no understanding of what has occurred. When experiencing the **anger** stage of adjustment to loss, a person expresses resistance and sometimes feels intense anger at God, other people, or the situation. **Bargaining** cushions and postpones awareness of the loss by trying to prevent it from happening. Grieving or dying people make promises to self, God, or loved ones that they will live or believe differently if they can be spared the dreaded outcome. When a person realizes the full impact of the loss, **depression** occurs. Some individuals feel overwhelmingly sad, hopeless, and lonely. Resigned to the bad outcome, they sometimes withdraw from relationships and life. In **acceptance,** the person incorporates the loss into life and finds ways to move forward.

Stage and phase theories such as Kübler-Ross' have been criticized for a lack of empirical evidence, inattention to cultural difference and the assumption that there is an end-point in grieving (Rothaups and Becker, 2007). A recent study validated that the stage-like emotions of acceptance, disbelief, yearning, anger, and depression are present following natural death in normal grief, although no in the expected order predicted by stage theory (Maciejewski and others, 2007). Nevertheless, stage theory should never be considered as a prescription for grief or an indication that anyone can assert control over the dying process. That grief has a time course is another area of contention. Widows reported that they continued to think about deceased spouses once or twice a month and had a conversation about the spouse on average of once a month even when the loss occurred as much as 20 years earlier (Carnelly and others, 2006).

Attachment Theory. Bowlby's attachment theory (1980) describes the experience of mourning. Attachment, an instinctive behavior, leads to the development of affectional bonds between children and their primary caregivers. Relational bonds are present and active throughout the life cycle, and individuals later generalize them to persons in other relationships. Attachment

behavior ensures survival because it keeps people close to those who offer love, protection, and support.

Bowlby describes four phases of mourning. As with other staged grief theories, a person can move back and forth between any two of the phases in response to loss. **Numbing,** the shortest phase of mourning, may last from a few hours to a week or more. The grieving person describes this phase as feeling "stunned" or "unreal." Numbing protects the person from the full impact of the loss. Emotional outbursts of tearful sobbing and acute distress characterize the second bereavement phase, **yearning and searching.** Common physical symptoms in this phase include tightness in the chest and throat, shortness of breath, a feeling of lethargy, insomnia, and loss of appetite. A person also experiences an inner, intense yearning for the lost person or object. This phase lasts for months or considerably longer. During the phase of **disorganization and despair** a person endlessly examines how and why the loss occurred or expresses anger at anyone who seems responsible for the loss. The grieving person retells the loss story again and again. Gradually the person realizes the loss is permanent. With **reorganization,** which usually takes a year or more, the person begins to accept change, assume unfamiliar roles, acquire new skills, and build new relationships. Persons who are reorganizing begin to untie themselves from their lost relationship without feeling that they are lessening its importance.

Grief Tasks Model. Worden (1982) proposes four tasks of mourning and suggests that mourning persons actively engage in behaviors to help themselves and respond to outside interventions. Working through the grief tasks typically requires a minimum of a full year, although the time varies from person to person.

- *Task I: Accept the reality of the loss.* Even when a death is expected, survivors register some disbelief and surprise that the event has really happened. Task I involves the process of accepting that the person or object is gone and will not return.
- *Task II: Work through the pain of grief.* Even though people respond to loss differently, it is impossible to experience a significant loss without some emotional pain. People react with sadness, loneliness, despair, or regret and will work through painful feelings using the coping mechanisms most familiar and comfortable to them.
- *Task III: Adjust to the environment in which the deceased is missing.* A person does not realize the full impact of a loss for at least 3 months. Family members or friends pay less attention to the bereaved person at about the same time, just as the fi-

nality of the loss becomes real. People completing this task begin to take on roles formerly filled by the deceased, including some jobs they do not want.

- *Task IV: Emotionally relocate the deceased and move on with life.* The deceased person is not forgotten, but rather takes a different and less prominent place in the survivor's emotional life. People often fear that in making new attachments they will forget their loved one or seem disloyal, making this a potentially difficult task to complete. Realizing that it is possible to love other people without betraying the deceased, the person moves forward.

Dual Process Model. Although phase and task-oriented grief theories provide useful guiding principles, many theorists note that the grief process does not unfold in predictable, sequential stages. Newer theories account for gender and cultural variations and point out the limitations of focusing mainly on internal, emotional responses to grief. The dual process model of coping with bereavement, for example, describes the everyday life experiences of grief as moving back and forth between loss-oriented and restoration-oriented processes (Hooyman and Kramer, 2006; Stroebe and Schut, 1999). Loss-oriented behaviors include grief work, dwelling on the loss, breaking connections to the deceased, and resisting activities to get past the grief. Restoration-oriented activities, such as attending to life changes, finding new roles or relationships, coping with finances, and participating in distractions, provide balance to the loss-oriented state. The extent to which an individual engages in loss- or restoration-oriented processes depends on factors such as personality, coping styles, or cultural practices.

Nursing Knowledge Base

Nurses develop plans of care to help clients and family members undergoing loss, grief, or death experiences. Based on nursing research, practice evidence, nursing experience, and client and family preferences, nurses implement plans of care in acute care, nursing home, hospice, home care, and community settings. Recent developments in nursing education support the effort to improve end-of-life care with changes occurring at every level of practice (Virani and Sofer, 2003). The End-of-Life Nursing Consortium (ELNEC), funded by the Robert Wood Johnson Foundation, provides nurses with basic and advanced curricula to care for clients and families experiencing loss, grief, death, and bereavement (ELNEC, 2003; Matzo and others, 2003). Professional nursing organizations such as the American Nurses Association, the American Society of Pain Management Nurses, and the Hospice and Palliative Care Nurses Association have developed evidence-based practice guidelines for managing clinical and ethical issues at the end of life.

Factors Influencing Loss and Grief

Multiple variables influence the way a person perceives and responds to loss. Those variables include developmental factors, personal relationships, the nature of the loss, coping strategies, socioeconomic status, and cultural and spiritual influences and beliefs.

✱ BOX 30-1 **FOCUS ON OLDER ADULTS**

Grief Expression and Interventions in Older Adults

- There is little evidence that grief experiences differ due to age alone. Responses to loss are more likely related to the nature of the specific loss experience.
- Increased age increases the likelihood that older adults have faced multiple losses—loved ones, friends, valued objects, outliving a child, or declining health. Older adults residing in communal living situations experience many losses as friends die.
- Some older adults are at risk for complicated grieving due to multiple losses, potential for cognitive impairment, or decreased physical resources. The risks include depression, loneliness, and accompanying functional decline.
- Physical decline due to chronic illness sometimes leads to grief over lost health, function, and roles.
- Older adults benefit from the same therapeutic techniques as persons in other age-groups. Evidence indicates that positive reappraisal (cognitive restructuring) helps older adults adapt to significant losses.
- Relieving depression and maintaining physical function are therapeutic goals for grieving older adults.

Data from Talerico K: Aging matters: addressing issues related to geropsychiatry and the well-being of older adults, *J Psychosoc Nurs* 41(7):12, 2006.

Human Development. Client age and stage of development affect the grief response. For example, toddlers cannot understand loss or death but often feel anxiety over the loss of objects and separation from parents. They sometimes express the sense of absence they feel with changes in eating and sleeping patterns, fussiness, or bowel and bladder disturbances. School-age children understand the concepts of permanence and irreversibility but do not always understand the causes of a loss. Some have intense periods of emotional expression. Young adults undergo many necessary, developmental losses related to their evolving futures. They leave home, begin school or a work life, or form significant relationships. Illness or death disrupts one's future and the necessary young adult task of establishing an autonomous sense of self. Midlife adults also experience major life transitions such as caring for aging parents, dealing with changes in marital status, and adapting to new family roles (Hooyman and Kramer, 2006). For older adults the aging process leads to some necessary and developmental losses. Some experience age discrimination, especially when they become dependent or are near death. Older adults also show resilience after a loss as a result of their prior experiences (Box 30-1).

Personal Relationships. When loss involves another person, the quality and meaning of the lost relationship influences the grief response. When a relationship between two people has been very close and well connected, understandably the survivor finds it difficult to go on. Grief resolution may be hampered by regret and a sense of unfinished business when people are closely related but did not have a good relationship at the time of death. Social support and the ability to accept help from others are critical variables in recovery from loss and grief. When clients do not receive supportive understanding and compassion from others, grief becomes complicated or prolonged (Hooyman and Kramer, 2006).

Nature of the Loss. Exploring the meaning a loss has for a client helps the nurse better understand the impact of the loss on the client's behavior, health, and well-being (Corless, 2006). Highly visible losses generally stimulate a helping response from others. For example, the loss of one's home from a tornado often brings community and governmental support. A more private loss, such as a miscarriage, brings less support from others. The stressors in a sudden and unexpected death pose different challenges than those in a debilitating chronic illness. In the first case, the survivors do not have time to let go. In chronic illness, survivors have memories of prolonged suffering, pain, and loss of function. Death by violence or suicide or multiple losses by their very nature complicate the grieving process in unique ways (Stroebe and Schut, 2006).

Coping Strategies. Life experiences shape the coping strategies a person uses to deal with the stress of loss. Clients rely first on their familiar coping strategies when under the stress of a loss. When a person's usual coping strategies do not work, he or she needs new ones. Emotional disclosure (venting, or talking about one's feelings) has been viewed as an important way to cope with loss. In the past, emphasis would have been on helping people express anger or other negative feelings associated with loss. Recent research, however, shows that focusing on positive emotions and optimistic feelings might be an even more important indication of successful coping in bereavement (Ong and others, 2004). Negative themes that are present when people talk about grief may also be predictive of more distressful reactions (Maciejewski, 2007; Maercker and others, 1998). Emotional disclosure is often accomplished by having people write about their feelings. Research studies exploring the benefits of written disclosure have found that this technique was worthwhile, particularly because mourners perceive it as a pleasant activity—it requires little time and it is virtually cost-free (Frattaroli, 2006).

Socioeconomic Status. Socioeconomic status influences a person's ability to access support and resources for coping with loss and physical responses to stress (Cohen, Doyle, and Baum, 2006). When people lack financial, educational, or occupational resources, the burdens of loss multiply. For example, a client with limited finances is not able to replace a car demolished in an accident and pay for the associated medical expenses.

Culture and Ethnicity. A person's culture and other social structures (e.g., family or religious affiliation) influence the interpretations of loss, establish acceptable expressions of grief, and provide stability and structure in the midst of chaos and loss (Box 30-2). Expressions of grief in one culture may not make sense to persons from a different culture (see Chapter 9). Try to understand and appreciate each client's cultural values related to loss, death, and grieving.

Grief theories commonly used to understand loss and death have cultural limitations. For example, some theorists describe

---

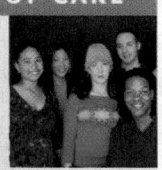

✳ BOX 30-2   CULTURAL ASPECTS OF CARE

Importance of Culture in Death Rituals, Mourning Practices, and Grief

Every culture has death rituals, mourning practices, and expected grief behaviors that offer structure, guidance, and comfort to the survivors of a death. These practices vary widely across the world. The importance of honoring cultural variations is essential if nurses are to obtain positive outcomes in cross-cultural situations and in multicultural health care settings. Cultural differences in end-of-life care become evident in the areas of language, family relationships and involvement, religious beliefs, ethical issues, expressions of pain and suffering, and care of the body after death (Kemp, 2005). Great variation in individual practices within a culture exist, with some people following traditional beliefs more strictly than others. A brief description of some common traditional understandings of death in different cultural groups follows:

- Hispanic cultures: Extended family cares for ill, sharing information and decisions. They often use special objects, such as amulets or rosary beads, and prayer. In traditional Hispanic families, respect, especially for elders, is a cherished value. Grief is expressed openly. Religious and spiritual rituals (dominantly Catholic) are essential at the end of life (Clements and others, 2003).
- African Americans have a number of differing religious and secular ceremonies. Family unit is important in grief, including the church family. Death is not the end of life, but passing on to another life. Loss of a loved one is temporary, and all will be united in heaven (Holloway, 2002).
- Native Americans encompass diverse tribal groups with differing practices, traditions, and ceremonies. General approaches to death envision the land of the dead as a parallel world, where the spirits of the dead affect the lives of those still living. Navajos use songs, chants, prayers, and sand paintings as rituals.

Implications for Practice

- Cultural beliefs influence who makes up a client's support network and the acceptable, expected forms of giving and receiving care at the end of life.
- Assess each client and family for culturally meaningful practices for end-of-life care. Ask which general, traditional understandings are important to them.
- Nurses have a cultural orientation to death and loss that sometimes differs from the client's. Honoring client and family cultural values characterizes expert end-of-life care.
- Care provided at the end of life within the client and family's cultural context draws on the resources of their entire lives.

---

grief as a process of "work" or "tasks" that occur in stages or on projected timelines. North Americans, who respond to problems by "working at" them, may better understand work, task, and process grief concepts than cultural groups not defined by work achievement. Some cultural groups may experience grief, instead, as a communal expression or state of being (Wortman and Silver, 1989). Many people in Western European and American cultures hold back their public displays of emotion. In other cultures, behaviors such as public wailing and physical demonstrations of grief, including survivor body mutilation, show respect for the dead. Core American cultural values of individualism and self-determination stand in contrast with communal, family, or tribal ways of life. These differences influence processes such as obtaining informed consent or making life support decisions (Kemp, 2005).

Spiritual and Religious Beliefs. The care of seriously ill clients usually involves medical interventions to restore or maintain health. A second set of practices, transformative strategies, acknowledge life's limits and help dying people find meaning in suffering so that they are able to transcend, or go beyond, their personal existence. Transformative practices are associated with healing, spiritual or religious communities and beliefs (Myers, 2003). Spiritual resources include faith in a higher power, communities of support, friends, a sense of hope and meaning in life, and religious practices. Client and family members' spirituality affects their ability to cope with loss. Individuals who have a strong interconnectedness with a higher power show resilience and ability to experience healing in loss (Matheis, Tulsky, and Matheis, 2006). **Spiritual integration** occurs when an individual comes to terms with his or her life and puts life's pieces together in a way consistent with one's entire life. Near the end of life, integration helps a person attend to broken relationships or unfinished business (O'Gorman, 2002).

Hope. Hope, a multidimensional component of spirituality, energizes and provides comfort to individuals experiencing personal challenges. Hopefulness gives a person the ability to see life as enduring or as having meaning or purpose. As a future-shaping, motivating force, hope helps clients maintain anticipation of a continued good, an improvement in their circumstances, or a lessening of something unpleasant. With hope, a client moves from feelings of weakness and vulnerability to living as fully as possible (Arnaert, Filteau, and Sourial, 2006).

Maintaining a sense of hope depends, in part, on a person having strong relationships and emotional connectedness to others. Nurses and other health care professionals help provide the sense of belonging, which is so essential to hope. On the other hand, the experience of spiritual distress often arises from a client's inability to feel hopeful or foresee any favorable outcomes. Spirituality and hope play a vital role in a client's adjustment to loss and death (see Chapter 29).

Critical Thinking

To provide appropriate and responsive care for the grieving client and family, use critical thinking skills to synthesize scientific knowledge from nursing and nonnursing disciplines, professional standards, evidence-based practice, client-specific assessments, previous caregiving experiences, and self-knowledge. Critical thinking informs all steps of the nursing process (see Chapter 15).

During the assessment phase, use critical thinking to gather and analyze the data that leads to the selection of appropriate nursing diagnoses (Figure 30-1). To understand a client's subjective experiences of loss, form assessment questions based on your knowledge of grief theory, but then listen carefully to the client's

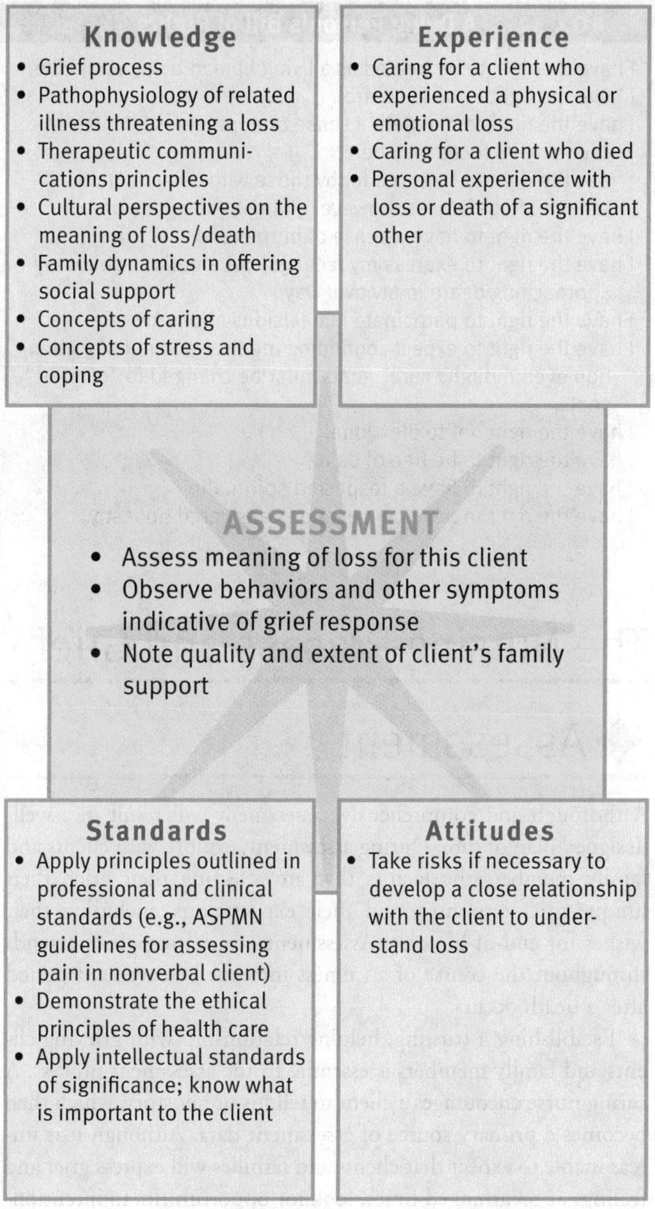

Figure 30-1 Critical thinking model for loss, death, and grieving assessment.

perceptions. A culturally competent nurse uses culture-specific descriptions of grief to explore the meaning of loss with a client.

Knowing the theoretical stages of grief will enable you to better understand a client's emotions and behaviors. During implementation of care some clients ignore, lash out, plead with, or withdraw from caregivers and other people as part of a normal response to loss. Instead of "taking things personally," a critically thinking nurse integrates theory, prior experience, appreciation of subjective experiences, and self-knowledge to respond to the client's emotions with patience and understanding. In designing plans of care, use professional standards, including the Nursing Code of Ethics (see Chapter 22), the dying person's bill of rights (Box 30-3), and clinical standards, such as the American Society of Pain Management Nurses' guidelines for pain assessment in the nonverbal client (Herr, Bjoro, and Decker 2006).

✳ BOX 30-3 A Dying Person's Bill of Rights

I have the right to be treated as a living human being until I die.

I have the right to be in control.

I have the right to maintain a sense of hopefulness, however changing its focus may be.

I have the right to be cared for by those who can maintain a sense of hopefulness, however changing this may be.

I have the right to have a sense of purpose.

I have the right to express my feelings and emotions about my approaching death in my own way.

I have the right to participate in decisions about my care.

I have the right to expect continuing medical and nursing attention even though "cure" goals must be changed to "comfort" goals.

I have the right not to die alone.

I have the right to be free of pain.

I have the right to have a respected spirituality.

I have the right to have my questions answered honestly.

I have the right not to be deceived.

I have the right to have help from and for my family in accepting my death.

I have the right to die in peace and dignity.

I have the right to retain my individuality and not be judged for my decisions that may be contrary to beliefs of others.

I have the right to discuss and enlarge my religious and/or spiritual experiences, whatever these may mean to others.

I have a right to expect that the sanctity of the human body will be respected after death.

I have the right to be cared for by caring, sensitive, knowledgeable people who will try to understand my needs and will be able to gain some satisfaction in helping me face my death.

Modified from Barbus AJ: The dying person's bill of rights, *Am J Nurs* 75:99, 1975; and *Dying person's bill of rights*, 2004, http://learningplaceonline.com/stages/together/dying-rights.htm.

The Nursing Process and Grief

 ## Assessment

A thorough and comprehensive assessment will result in a well-designed plan of care. During assessment, explore with clients and family members the factors that are affecting their grief, their unique grief responses, and their expectations, including their wishes for end-of-life care. Assessment of grief responses extends throughout the course of an illness into the bereavement period after a death occurs.

Establishing a trusting, helping relationship with grieving clients and family members is essential to the assessment process. A caring nurse encourages a client to tell his or her story, which then becomes a primary source of assessment data. Although it is unreasonable to expect that clients and families will express grief and feelings at prearranged times, look for opportunities to intentionally invite clients to share their experiences if they so wish. Be aware that attitudes about self-disclosure, sharing emotions, or talking about illness, fears, and death are shaped by an individual's personality, coping style, and culture. Research has not always supported the belief that "talking about things" facilitates healing and a quicker recovery from loss (Stroebe, Schut, and Stroebe, 2005).

Speak to clients and family members using honest and open communication. Keep an open mind, listen carefully, and observe the client's verbal and nonverbal responses. Facial expressions, voice tones, and avoided topics often say more than words. Anticipate common grief responses, but allow clients to describe their experiences in their own words. Open-ended questions such as, "Tell me how you feel about your cancer diagnosis" or "You seem sad today. Can you tell me more?" may open the door to a client-centered discussion. Many people find it difficult to talk about loss, fears, death, or grief. The use of pauses, gentle questioning, and silence honors the client's privacy and readiness to talk (Green, 2006). As you gather assessment data, summarize and validate your impressions with the client or family member.

Information from other members of the health care team, physicians, social workers, and spiritual care providers also contributes to your assessment data.

Interview clients and families separately in a private, quiet setting. A client or family member sometimes has important concerns that they are not comfortable expressing in the other's presence. At other times a client will want to have family members present so that everyone hears the same thing and has an opportunity to add to the conversation. Ask clients and family members about their preferences.

Factors That Affect Grief. Conversations about the meaning of a loss to the client may lead to other important areas of assessment, including the client's coping style, the nature of family relationships, personal goals, cultural and spiritual beliefs, sources of hope, and the availability of support systems (Box 30-4). Use skills appropriate for assessing the client's culture, family, self-concept, or spiritual beliefs (see Chapters 9, 10, 27, and 29) to acquire a deeper understanding of the client's loss.

Knowing the theoretical descriptions of grief stages, phases, types, and tasks guides your critical thinking and assessment skills. A single behavior can occur in all types of grief. If a grieving client describes loneliness and difficulty falling asleep, consider all factors surrounding the loss in context. What was the loss? When did the loss occur? What was the meaning of the loss to the client? The client may be having a normal grief reaction, but if you learn that the loss occurred 2 years ago, it is more likely the client has a complicated, chronic grief response. Most importantly, focus assessment on how a client is currently reacting to loss or grief, not on how you believe the client should be reacting.

Grief Reactions. Use psychological and physical assessment skills to assess a client's unique grief responses. Most grieving people show some common outward signs and symptoms (Box 30-5). Analyze the assessment data, and identify possible related causes for your findings. For example, after a significant loss a client has a sad affect, withdrawn behaviors, headaches, upset stomach, and decreased ability to concentrate. You associate these

✳ BOX 30-4   NURSING ASSESSMENT QUESTIONS

Nature of Relationships
- How long have you known your friend?
- What role did your mother/father play in your family?
- How have family relationships changed as a result of your loss?

Social Support Systems
- Who is present? Absent? Supportive? Nonsupportive?
- What do family/friends do that is most meaningful?
- Are family/friends available when needed? Who do you wish was here?

Nature of the Loss
- What helps you grieve? What interferes with grieving?
- How have you handled loss in the past?
- What does this loss mean to you?

Cultural and Spiritual Beliefs
- What is your belief about death? Meaning of life?
- What rituals are important to you at the time of death?
- How do members of your culture or religious group view this loss?

Loss of Personal Life Goals
- What are your life goals at this time?
- How have your goals changed since your diagnosis?
- Have you made plans for returning to work after treatment?

Family Grief Responses
- How has your family dealt with problems in the past?
- What are your family's strengths?
- What role do you assume in your family during stressful situations?

Survivor Risk Factors
- Tell me how you are feeling.
- What are you doing to take care of yourself now?

Hope
- What do you hope your treatment will accomplish?
- What helps you remain hopeful? What causes you to lose hope?

✳ BOX 30-5   Symptoms of Normal Grief

Feelings
Sorrow
Fear
Anger
Guilt or self-reproach
Anxiety
Loneliness
Fatigue
Helplessness/ hopelessness
Yearning
Relief

Cognitions (Thought Patterns)
Disbelief
Confusion or memory problems
Problems with decision making
Inability to concentrate
Feeling the presence of the deceased

Physical Sensations
Headaches
Nausea and appetite disturbances
Tightness in the chest and throat
Insomnia
Oversensitivity to noise
Sense of depersonalization ("Nothing seems real")
Feeling short of breath, choking sensation
Muscle weakness
Lack of energy
Dry mouth

Behaviors
Crying and frequent sighing
Distancing from people
Absentmindedness
Dreams of the deceased
Keeping the deceased's room intact
Loss of interest in regular life events
Wearing objects that belonged to the deceased

symptoms with several potential causes, including anxiety, gastrointestinal disturbances, medication side effects, or impaired memory. Careful analysis of the symptoms in context will lead you to an accurate nursing diagnosis. Ask: How are the symptoms related to one another when they occur? When did the symptoms begin? Were they present before the loss? To what does the client attribute the symptoms?

Loss takes place in a social context, so family assessment is a vital part of your data gathering. If a father of a young family is dying, he will not be able to fulfill certain roles, causing a change in family structure. When a person develops a disability, the client and family members realign their roles and responsibilities to meet new demands. Family members also experience a variety of physical and psychological symptoms. Assess the family's response to loss, and recognize that they are sometimes dealing with their grief at a different pace than the client (Kristjanson and Aoun, 2004).

Client Expectations. In situations as personally and culturally experienced as grief and loss, explore the client's and family's

expectations for nursing care. Client perceptions and expectations influence how to prioritize nursing diagnoses. Assess the client's expectations by asking a question such as, "What is the most important thing I can do for you right now?"

Encourage family members also to share their goals with the health care team and their perceptions of the nurse's role. Their input into the assessment process may help clarify misunderstandings or identify overlooked or hidden information. Assess client and family understanding of treatment options, and provide appropriate information and teaching so that an individualized, mutually developed care plan can be implemented.

End-of-Life Decisions. Clients with advanced chronic illness and their families will all eventually face end-of-life care decisions. Most deaths are now "negotiated" among clients, family members, and the health care team, making it imperative that end-of-life care preferences are discussed in a timely manner. Highly stressed clients and family members often rely on the nurse and other members of the health care team to initiate discussions regarding end-of-life care and to pose options that fam-

✳ BOX 30-6   NURSING DIAGNOSTIC PROCESS

Hopelessness Related to Diagnosis of Terminal Illness

Assessment Activities	Defining Characteristics
Ask client to discuss future goals and plans.	Client sighs and says, "I have no future."
Observe client's nonverbal behavior.	Client avoids eye contact, has a flat affect, covers head with blanket.
Observe client responses to care options.	Client shrugs and says, "What does it matter?"
Assess activity level.	Client refuses to eat, sleeps all the time, keeps lights out.
Observe client interactions with family or friends.	Shows lack of interest in others. Communicates only when spoken to.

ily members do not know are available (Doka, 2005; Scanlon, 2003). Nurses provide essential advocacy roles for clients and family members making decisions at the end of life (McSteen and Peden-McAlpine, 2006).

✦ Nursing Diagnosis

Use critical thinking to cluster assessment data cues, identify defining characteristics, draw conclusions regarding the client's actual or potential needs or resources, and identify nursing diagnoses applicable to the client's situation (Box 30-6). Some nursing diagnoses relevant for clients experiencing grief, loss, or death include the following:

- Death anxiety
- Caregiver role strain
- Compromised family coping
- Readiness for enhanced comfort
- Disturbed personal identity
- Ineffective denial
- Fear
- Grieving
- Complicated grieving
- Risk for complicated grieving
- Hopelessness
- Risk for loneliness
- Spiritual distress
- Readiness for enhanced spiritual well-being

You cannot make accurate nursing diagnosis on the basis of just one or two defining characteristics. Carefully review the data to consider if more than one diagnosis may apply. For example, a dying client who cries often, has angry outbursts, and reports nightmares could be giving evidence of several possible nursing diagnoses: *pain (acute or chronic), ineffective coping, grieving,* or

spiritual distress. Examine the available data, validate assumptions with the client, and look for other validating behaviors and symptoms before making a diagnosis.

As part of the diagnostic process, identify the appropriate "related to" factor for each diagnosis. Clarification of the related factors will ensure that you select appropriate interventions. For example, a nursing diagnosis of *risk for complicated grieving related to the permanent loss of mobility* requires completely different interventions than a diagnosis of *risk for complicated grieving related to infertility after an ectopic pregnancy.*

When identifying nursing diagnoses related to the client's grief or loss, you will sometimes identify other related diagnoses. Clients experiencing grief or impending death may have nursing diagnoses such as *disturbed body image* or *impaired physical mobility.* A client entering the phase of active dying will often have diagnoses related to physical changes, including *impaired urinary elimination, bowel incontinence, acute pain, nausea, disturbed sensory perception,* and *ineffective breathing pattern.*

✦ Planning

Nurses provide holistic physical, emotional, social, and spiritual care to the client experiencing grief, death, or loss. Figure 30-2 illustrates the interrelatedness of critical thinking factors during the planning phase of the nursing process. The use of critical thinking ensures a well-designed care plan that supports a client's self-esteem and autonomy by including him or her in the planning process. A care plan for the dying client focuses on comfort, preserving dignity and quality of life, and providing family members with emotional, social, and spiritual support (see Care Plan, p. 472).

Goals and Outcomes. During planning, establish realistic goals and expected outcomes based on the nursing diagnoses. Consider the client's own resources, such as physical energy and activity tolerance, family support, and coping style. A nursing diagnosis of *powerlessness related to planned cancer therapy* with a goal of "Client will be able to discuss expected course of disease" is realistic for a client who frequently asks for clarification about the treatment plan and participates in educational discussions. In contrast, an expected outcome of "Client will identify effective coping skills" is appropriate for a client with the same nursing diagnosis who is experiencing depression from feeling powerless about having cancer treatment.

The goals of care for a client experiencing loss are either short or long term, depending on the nature of the loss and the client's grief. Some nursing care goals for clients facing loss or death include accommodating grief, accepting the reality of a loss, or maintaining meaningful relationships. A possible goal for a young woman with breast cancer is "Maintain a sense of control," with the following potential expected outcomes:

- Client will participate in treatment decisions.
- Client will be able to continue parental responsibilities in care of toddler.
- Client will communicate treatment side effects or concerns to the health care team.

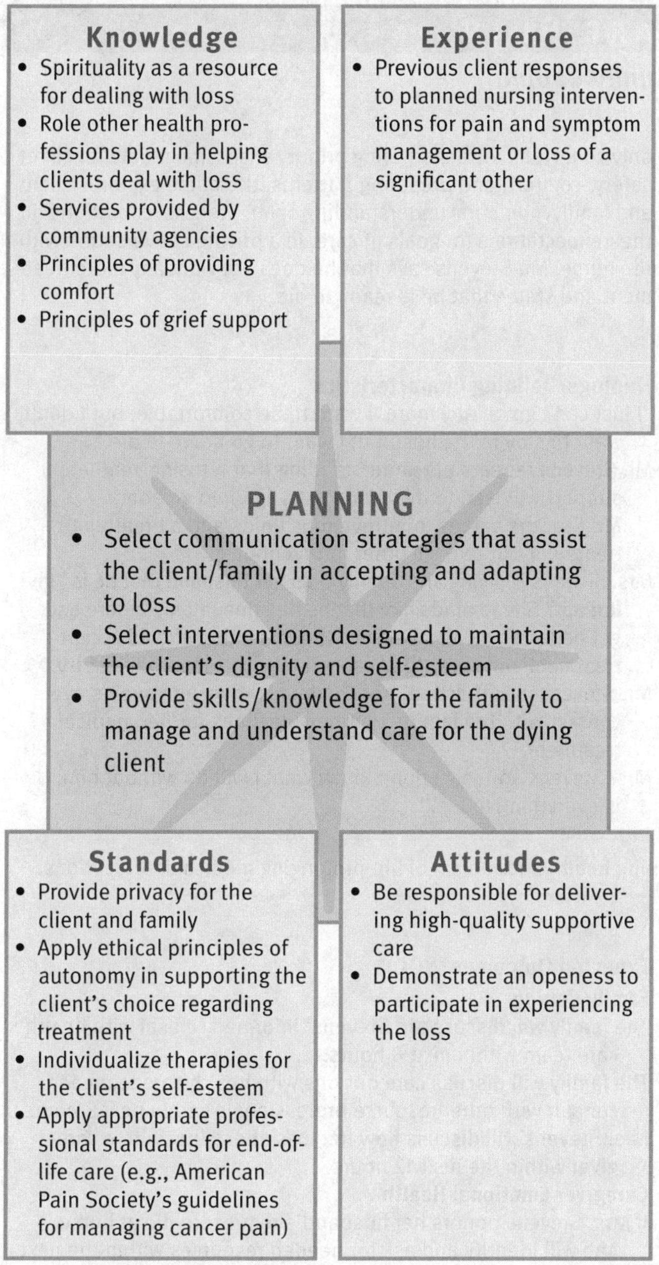

Knowledge
- Spirituality as a resource for dealing with loss
- Role other health professions play in helping clients deal with loss
- Services provided by community agencies
- Principles of providing comfort
- Principles of grief support

Experience
- Previous client responses to planned nursing interventions for pain and symptom management or loss of a significant other

PLANNING
- Select communication strategies that assist the client/family in accepting and adapting to loss
- Select interventions designed to maintain the client's dignity and self-esteem
- Provide skills/knowledge for the family to manage and understand care for the dying client

Standards
- Provide privacy for the client and family
- Apply ethical principles of autonomy in supporting the client's choice regarding treatment
- Individualize therapies for the client's self-esteem
- Apply appropriate professional standards for end-of-life care (e.g., American Pain Society's guidelines for managing cancer pain)

Attitudes
- Be responsible for delivering high-quality supportive care
- Demonstrate an openess to participate in experiencing the loss

Figure 30-2 Critical thinking model for loss, death, and grieving planning.

Setting Priorities. Encourage clients and family members to share their priorities for care at the end of life. Dying clients or those with advanced chronic illness are more likely to want their comfort, social, or spiritual needs met rather than pursuing medical cures. Give priority to a client's most urgent physical or psychological needs, while also considering the client's expectations and priorities. If a terminally ill client's goals include pain control and promoting self-esteem, pain control will take priority when the client experiences acute physical discomfort. When comfort needs have been met, other issues important to the client and family can be addressed. When it is realistic for the client to remain independent, strategies that foster the client's sense of

autonomy and ability to function independently take priority (Chochinov, 2002). Because a client's condition at the end of life often changes quickly, maintain an ongoing assessment to revise the plan of care according to client needs and preferences.

When a client has multiple nursing diagnoses, it is not possible to address them all simultaneously. Figure 30-3 illustrates a concept map developed for a client with a medical diagnosis of depression following the death of his wife 6 months ago. As a result of the client's depression, he experiences other health problems, identified in the nursing diagnoses *risk for complicated grieving, insomnia,* and *imbalanced nutrition: less than body requirements.* In such a situation, determine which of the three diagnoses should take priority. The continuing grief experienced by the client is possibly the first focus. Until the client is able to accept his wife's absence and begin to adjust psychologically, changes in his physical responses to loss will be difficult to achieve.

Collaborative Care. As described above, grief, loss, and death affect people physically, emotionally, spiritually, and culturally. No one professional group is able to address all of these dimensions alone. A team composed of nurses, physicians, social workers, spiritual care providers, nutritionists, pharmacists, physical and occupational therapists, clients, and family members works together to provide grief, palliative, and hospice care. Massage or music/art therapists who provide alternative therapies are sometimes part of the team (see Chapter 36). As a client's care needs change, team members take a more or less active role, depending on the client's shifting priorities. Team members communicate with each other on a regular basis to ensure coordination and effectiveness of care.

◆Implementation

Health Promotion. Health promotion in serious chronic illness or death focuses on facilitating successful coping and optimizing physical, emotional, and spiritual health. Many people continue to look for and find meaning even in difficult life circumstances. They often find personal growth and spiritual insights unlike anything they have ever experienced and need family and nurse support as they learn to live with loss, make health care decisions, and adjust to disappointments, frustration, and anxieties along the way (Wayman and Gaydos, 2005).

Palliative Care. Interventions for people who face chronic life-threatening illnesses or who are at the end of life have a palliative focus. **Palliative care** is the prevention, relief, reduction, or soothing of symptoms of disease or disorders throughout the entire course of an illness, including care of the dying and bereavement follow-up for the family (Ferrell and Coyle, 2006). The primary goal of palliative care is to help clients and families achieve the best possible quality of life. Although palliative care is especially important in advanced or chronic illness, it is appropriate for clients of any age, any diagnosis, at any time, or in any setting.

Clients who have complex, serious illnesses often benefit from palliative care throughout the course of their illness, even while seeking treatment for their disease. As the goals of care change and

NURSING CARE PLAN
Compromised Family Coping

Assessment

A 79-year-old client, Mr. Stevens, is admitted to the hospital for acute shortness of breath, increased sputum production, fever, fatigue, and decreased appetite. He has lived with advanced, end-stage lung disease for 10 years and has increasingly lost functional abilities. He will possibly require the assistance of a ventilator within the next day or two. Mrs. Stevens, who cares for her husband at home, has come with him to the hospital with their only son, Frank. After gathering priority assessment data for client safety, comfort, and breathing patterns, the nurse explores client and family members' understanding of Mr. Stevens' condition and their expectations for goals of care. In a private conversation with the nurse, Mr. Stevens says that he does not want any more treatment and states that he is ready to die.

Assessment Activities

Ask open-ended questions regarding goals of care. "Tell me, Mr. Stevens, what you hope for right now."

Observe Mr. Stevens' behaviors and communication with other health care team members.

Note conversations between Mr. and Mrs. Stevens and their son, Frank.

Observe Mr. Stevens' interactions with others.

Assess meaning of treatment refusal to Mrs. Stevens.

Findings/Defining Characteristics

"I just can't go on any more. I want to be comfortable, but I don't want to stay in the hospital. I want to go home to die."

Mr. Stevens repeats his understanding that refusing ventilatory support will lead to death. He asks again to go home.
Mr. Stevens agrees to intravenous fluids and a breathing treatment but refuses other interventions.

Mrs. Stevens is crying and angrily **tells her husband that he is "giving up."** She reminds him that he had pneumonia before and got better. Frank also **believes that his father should accept treatment** and says, **"Dad can get over this if he will just try."**

Mr. Stevens is **withdrawn, noncommunicative, and avoids eye contact with his family.** He firmly declines further medical treatment.

Mrs. Stevens states, "I don't know what I will do without him. He is everything to me."

Nursing Diagnosis: Compromised family coping related to declining health and refusal of life-prolonging medical interventions.

Planning

Goal

Identify and support Mr. Stevens' care priorities and preferences.

The Stevens family will agree on care goals.

Mrs. Stevens will demonstrate effective expression of grief within next 12 hours.

The family will arrange for Mr. Stevens' caregiving needs.

Expected Outcomes (NOC)*

Family Coping

The family will discuss Mr. Stevens' informed refusal with health care team within next 8 hours.

The family will discuss care options with health care team and consult with other resource professionals within next 8 hours.

Mrs. Stevens will discuss how her loss affects her with a caregiver within the next 12 hours.

Caregiver Emotional Health

If Mrs. Stevens honors her husband's request to die at home, she will identify and ask for needed resources within the next 36 hours.

---

†Outcome classification labels from Moorhead S and others: *Nursing outcomes classification (NOC),* ed 4, St. Louis, 2008, Mosby.

Interventions (NIC)†

Presence

Provide active listening and emotional support to Mr. Stevens and his family. Display interest in Mrs. Stevens' situation, and accept her coping behaviors.

Establish trust and positive regard with understanding and empathy. Create an environment of emotional safety and privacy.

Rationale

Recognize denial (Kübler-Ross' theory) as an anticipated grief phase to help client's family cope with his treatment refusal.

A privacy setting encourages greater freedom of expression to work through feelings (Green, 2006). Fear of losing self-control in front of others will not promote honest expression of feelings.

NURSING CARE PLAN

Compromised Family Coping—cont'd

Interventions (NIC)†

Grief Work Facilitation

Offer Mrs. Stevens encouragement to explore and verbalize feelings of grief and identify new coping strategies.

Identify personal coping strategies used in the past. Evaluate effectiveness, and promote when appropriate.

Determine Mrs. Stevens' willingness to accept available resources such as hospice, home care, and social services. Initiate as appropriate.

Rationale

Encouragement focuses on current needs and minimizes compromised coping behaviors by facilitating new problem-solving skills (Briggs and Colvin, 2002).

Under stress, people first use their most comfortable coping strategies (Kristjanson and Aoun, 2004). Effective handling of end-of-life decisions facilitates a healthy grief response (Doka, 2005).

Professionals use their expertise to facilitate the grieving process. Trust in relationships already formed will speed the therapeutic communication process (Scanlon, 2003).

†Interventions classification labels from Bulechek GM, Butcher HK, and Dochterman JM: *Nursing interventions classification (NIC)*, ed 5, St. Louis, 2008, Mosby.

Evaluation

Nursing Actions	Client Response/Finding	Achievement of Outcome
Validate Mrs. Stevens' experience: "It must be difficult to face such a big change in your life."	Mrs. Stevens responds, "I don't understand why he wants to leave me, but I can't make him go on a ventilator."	Shows beginning acceptance of client's wishes to not seek invasive medical interventions.
Use open-ended question: "Tell me how you are feeling now."	Mrs. Stevens explains, "I'm so confused. I don't know what to do next. I wish he hadn't gotten so sick."	Able to express normal grieving behaviors.
Observe Mrs. Stevens planning activities and behavior with family.	Mrs. Stevens discusses with Frank what they will do to get Mr. Stevens home for hospice care.	Indicates ability to make plans for a change of care location. Son supports revised plans.

cure for illnesses becomes less likely, the focus shifts to more palliative care strategies. Hospice care is a final phase of palliative care, designed for clients who no longer benefit from medical treatments, who will likely not live more than 6 months, or who are actively dying (Figure 30-4). Palliative care interventions are not just for hospice or end-of-life care. Making this distinction is important, because some clients, family members, or health care professionals refuse helpful palliative care interventions, believing that palliative care is only for the dying (Douglass, Maxwell, and Whitecar, 2004). The World Health Organization (2003) defines the primary obligations of the collaborative team offering palliative care:

- Affirm life, and regard dying as a normal process.
- Neither hasten nor postpone death.
- Provide relief from pain and other distressing symptoms.
- Integrate psychological and spiritual aspects of client care.
- Offer a support system to help clients live as actively as possible until death.
- Offer a support system to help families cope during the client's illness and their own bereavement.
- Enhance the quality of life.

Members of a collaborative, interdisciplinary health care team, together with clients and family members, determine the goals of care and select appropriate interventions. The nurse provides psychosocial care and expert symptom management, promotes client dignity and self-esteem, maintains a comfortable and peaceful environment, provides spiritual comfort and hope, protects against abandonment or isolation, offers family support, assists with ethical decision making, and facilitates mourning.

Use Therapeutic Communication. Establishing a caring, trusting relationship with the client and family through the use of therapeutic communication forms the basis for palliative care interventions (Mok and Chiu, 2004). Normal grief responses of sadness, numbing, denial, or anger make talking about these situations especially difficult. A grieving client may experience anger, for example, and become hostile with family members or caregivers. Some clients become demanding and accusing. Remain supportive by letting clients and family members know that feelings such as anger are normal by saying, for example, "You are understandably upset right now. I just want you to know I am here to talk with you if you want." Invite clients to reveal the emotions and concerns of greatest importance to them, and acknowledge their feelings and concerns in a nonjudgmental manner.

If a client chooses not to share feelings or concerns, express a willingness to be available at any time. Some clients will not discuss emotions for personal or cultural reasons, and other clients hesitate to express their emotions for fear that others will abandon them (Buckley and Herth, 2004). If you are reassuring and respectful of the client's privacy, a therapeutic relationship will likely develop. Sometimes clients need to begin resolving their grief privately before they will discuss their loss with others, especially strangers.

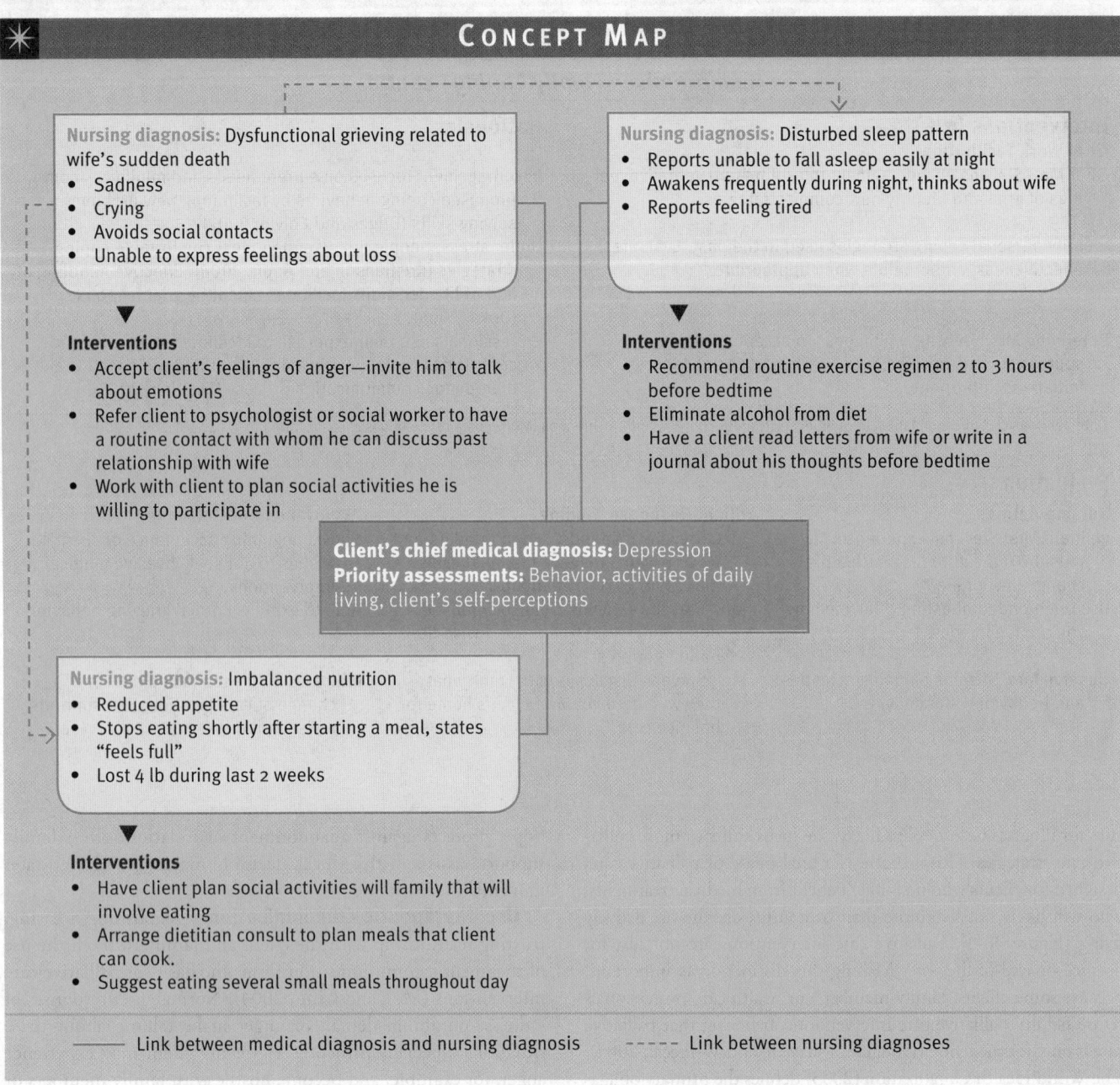

CONCEPT MAP

Nursing diagnosis: Dysfunctional grieving related to wife's sudden death
- Sadness
- Crying
- Avoids social contacts
- Unable to express feelings about loss

Interventions
- Accept client's feelings of anger—invite him to talk about emotions
- Refer client to psychologist or social worker to have a routine contact with whom he can discuss past relationship with wife
- Work with client to plan social activities he is willing to participate in

Nursing diagnosis: Disturbed sleep pattern
- Reports unable to fall asleep easily at night
- Awakens frequently during night, thinks about wife
- Reports feeling tired

Interventions
- Recommend routine exercise regimen 2 to 3 hours before bedtime
- Eliminate alcohol from diet
- Have a client read letters from wife or write in a journal about his thoughts before bedtime

Client's chief medical diagnosis: Depression
Priority assessments: Behavior, activities of daily living, client's self-perceptions

Nursing diagnosis: Imbalanced nutrition
- Reduced appetite
- Stops eating shortly after starting a meal, states "feels full"
- Lost 4 lb during last 2 weeks

Interventions
- Have client plan social activities will family that will involve eating
- Arrange dietitian consult to plan meals that client can cook.
- Suggest eating several small meals throughout day

——— Link between medical diagnosis and nursing diagnosis   - - - - Link between nursing diagnoses

Figure 30-3 Concept map for a client with depression following death of spouse.

Avoid communication barriers such as denying the client's grief, providing false reassurance, or avoiding discussion of sensitive issues (see Chapter 24). When you sense that a client wants to talk about something, make time right then, if at all possible. This is very challenging if you have limited experience with dying clients or are in a busy acute care setting. Above all, remember that a client's emotions are not something you can "fix." Instead, view emotional expression as a necessary part of the client's adjustment to significant life changes and development of effective coping skills. Help family members access other professional resources. Spiritual care providers, for example, help clients and family members discuss difficult issues related to personal meanings and values, death, and loss (Figure 30-5).

Provide Psychosocial Care. Clients at the end of life experience a range of psychological symptoms, including anxiety, de-

pression, altered body image, denial, powerlessness, uncertainty, and isolation (Carroll-Johnson, Gorman, and Bush, 2006). Clients and families face "hard work" when facing death and dying, including managing their symptoms, creating a support system, feeling safe, and finding meaning in their circumstances (Coyle, 2006).

Clients experience anguish from not knowing or being unaware of aspects of their health status or treatment. Worry or fear is common in many clients and often heightens their perception of discomfort. Provide information that helps clients understand their condition, the course of their disease, the benefits and burdens of treatment options, and their values and goals to preserve the autonomy of clients who are plagued by not knowing what the future holds or are uncertain about the goals of care (Weiner and Roth, 2006).

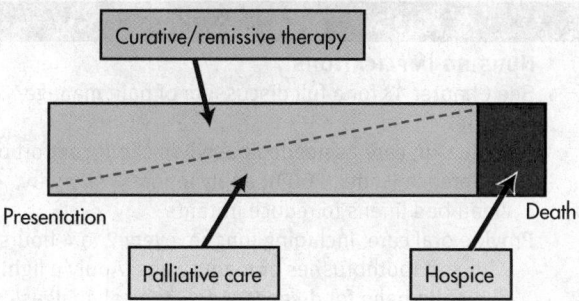

Figure 30-4 Palliative care. (From Emanuel L, VonGunten C, Ferris F: *The education in palliative and end of life care [EPEC] curriculum: The EPEC Project,* Chicago, 2003, Northwestern University.)

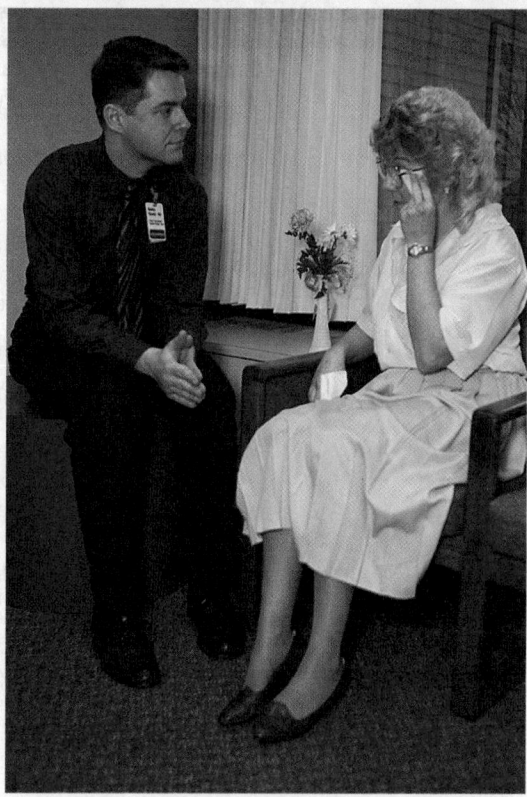

Figure 30-5 Nurses assist family members in finding resources to help with grief.

Manage Symptoms. Managing the multiple symptoms commonly experienced by chronically ill or dying clients remains a primary goal of palliative care nursing. Symptom distress, discomfort, or anguish often complicate a client's dying experience. Despite the availability of good treatment options for pain, many clients suffer with avoidable pain at the end of life. Take responsibility for maintaining an ongoing assessment, reassessing pain and medication side effects, developing pain management expertise, and advocating for change if the client does not get relief from the prescribed regimen. Excellent evidence-based pain management protocols have been developed (Paice and Fine, 2006) (see Chapter 43). Seriously debilitated or dying clients often lose their ability to communicate or to self-advocate, making it essential for you to learn how to assess pain in the nonverbal client (Herr and others, 2006). As renal and liver function decline in the dying client, metabolism and rate of drug clearance diminish, indicating the potential need for decreased dosages at the end of life to avoid toxicities. Also be aware that advancing disease pathology, anxiety, or delirium often call for higher doses or different drug therapies.

Remain alert to the potential side effects of opioid administration: constipation, nausea, sedation, respiratory depression, or myoclonus. Family members often worry about potential addiction to opioid medications. Not only is the incidence of true addiction very low, but the client's need for pain relief at the end of life takes priority (see Chapter 43). Consider nonpharmacological interventions to increase client comfort and manage pain. Family members are often able to provide these interventions, increasing their sense of positive contribution. Table 30-3 outlines nursing interventions to address other comfort needs and common symptoms.

Promote Dignity and Self-Esteem. A sense of dignity includes a person's positive self-regard, an ability to invest in and gain strength from one's own meaning in life, feeling valued by others, and how one is treated by caregivers. Nurses promote a client's self-esteem and dignity by respecting him or her as a whole person with feelings, accomplishments, and passions independent of the illness experience (Chochinov, 2002). Giving importance to the things that a client cares about validates the person, at the same time strengthening communication among the client, family members, and the nurse. Spending time with clients as they share their life experiences, particularly what has been meaningful, helps you know the client better and facilitates the develop-

ment of individualized interventions. Show respect for older clients by calling them by surnames and titles and by obtaining their permission to include others in private conversations.

Attending to the client's physical appearance promotes dignity and self-esteem. Cleanliness, absence of body odors, and attractive clothing give clients a sense of worth. When caring for a client's bodily functions, show patience and respect, especially after the client becomes dependent. Allow clients to make decisions, such as how and when to administer personal hygiene, diet preferences, and timing of nursing interventions. Keep the client and family members informed about daily activities, tests, or therapies, their purpose, and anticipated effects. Provide privacy during nursing care procedures, and be sensitive to when the client and family need time alone together.

Maintain a Comfortable and Peaceful Environment. A comfortable, clean, pleasant environment helps clients relax, promotes good sleep patterns, and minimizes symptom severity. Keep a client comfortable through frequent repositioning, making sure bed linens are dry, and controlling extraneous environmental noise and odors. Pictures, cherished objects, and cards or letters from family members and friends create a familiar and comforting environment for the dying client in an institutional setting. Offer the client back, foot, or hand massage (Kolcaba and others, 2004). Using client-preferred music in the background, provide guided imagery exercises.

Promote Spiritual Comfort and Hope. Help clients make connections to their spiritual practice or cultural community. Clients are comforted when they have assurance that some aspect

✳ TABLE 30-3 Promoting Comfort in the Terminally Ill Client

SYMPTOMS	CHARACTERISTICS OR CAUSES	NURSING IMPLICATIONS
Pain	Multiple causes, depending on client diagnosis.	See Chapter 43 for a full discussion of pain management.
Skin and mucous membrane discomfort	Any source of skin irritation increases discomfort.	Provide skin care as needed based on client comfort or preference (Lentz, 2003); apply lotion to skin; dry, clean bed linens to reduce irritants.
	Mouth breathing or dehydration leads to dry mucous membranes; tongue and lips become dry or chapped.	Provide oral care, including tongue, every 2 to 4 hours with soft toothbrushes or foam swabs. Apply a light film of lip balm for dryness. Apply topical analgesics to oral lesions (Dahlin, 2004).
	Blinking reflexes diminish near death, causing drying of cornea.	Optical lubricants or artificial tears reduce corneal drying. Eye care with warm water removes crusts from eyelid margins.
Fatigue	Metabolic demands, decreased oral intake and heart function, stress, disease states cause weakness and fatigue.	Balance activity and rest periods according to client's priorities and preferred time of day. Conserve client energy by modifying environment (Whitecar, Maxwell, and Douglass, 2004).
Anxiety	Physical, social or spiritual distress causes anxiety; causes may be situational or event specific.	Address underlying cause; provide calm, supportive environment, active listening; benzodiazepines used for acute anxiety (Whitecar and others, 2004).
Nausea	Medications, pain, or decreased intestinal blood flow with impending death.	Administer antiemetics or promotility agents; discontinue medications or foods that incite nausea; provide oral care at least every 2 to 4 hours; offer clear liquid diet and ice chips; avoid liquids that increase stomach acidity (Ferrell and Coyle, 2006).
Constipation	Opioids, medications, and immobility slow peristalsis.	Use a stimulant laxative with opioids. Make dietary alterations as preferred or tolerated; increase fluid intake if tolerated (Matzo and Sherman, 2006).
	Lack of bulk in diet or reduced fluid intake contributes to constipation.	
Diarrhea	Disease processes, treatment or medications, gastrointestinal (GI) infections.	Assess for fecal impaction. Confer with health care provider to change medication if cause.
		Protect skin with moisture barrier.
Urinary incontinence	Progressive disease and decreased level of consciousness.	Protect skin from irritation or breakdown by maintaining dry linens and clothing. Use indwelling urinary catheter or condom catheters for comfort or skin problems.
Altered nutrition	Medications, depression, decreased activity, decreased blood flow to the GI tract; nausea produces anorexia.	Offer smaller portions of client-preferred foods. Treat underlying cause of anorexia. Do not force food on actively dying client (Pitorak, 2003).
Dehydration	Client is less willing or able to maintain oral fluid intake; fever.	Reduce discomfort from dehydration; give mouth care at least every 2 to 4 hours; offer ice chips or moist cloth to lips. Keep lips and tongue moist.
Ineffective breathing patterns (e.g., dyspnea, shortness of breath)	Anxiety, fever, pain, increased oxygen demand.	Treat or control underlying cause.
	Disease processes or anemia, which reduces oxygen-carrying capacity.	Position for comfort and maximal respiratory excursion, provide supplemental oxygen if comforting; reduce anxiety or fever; provide effective pain management. Use fan for air movement, stimulating trigeminal nerve in cheek, which decreases dyspneic sensation (Pitorak, 2003).
		Administer anxiolytics, bronchodilators, inhaled steroids, or opioids to suppress cough and ease breathing and apprehension (Matzo and Sherman, 2006).

of their lives will transcend death. Draw on the resources of spiritual care providers in an institutional setting, or collaborate with the client's own spiritual leader and community. Making an audiotape or videotape for the family, writing letters, or keeping a journal assures clients that something of their essence will survive past their death.

The spiritual concept of hope takes on special significance near the end of life. Nursing strategies that promote hope are often quite simple: demonstrating patience, treating the client's family well, and being friendly. Clients perceive the love of family and friends, faith, goal setting, positive relationships with professional caregivers, humor, and uplifting memories as hope promoting.

Circumstances that hinder the preservation of hope include abandonment or isolation, uncontrolled symptoms, or being devalued as a person (Buckley and Herth, 2004).

Dying clients and their families hope for different things over the course of their experience with illness and death. Some hope to live for an anniversary, to sit outdoors for a meal, to see an important person one last time, to gain pain relief, or to have a peaceful death. Listen for shifts in what clients hope for and find ways to help them meet their desired goals.

Protect Against Abandonment and Isolation. Many terminally ill clients fear dying alone. Clients feel more hopeful when others are near to help them. Alone, they can become fearful and feel hopeless. Nurses in an institutional setting need to answer call lights promptly and check on clients often to reassure them that someone is close at hand (Stanley, 2002). Consider carefully whether or not to place a dying client in a private room. If family members plan to stay with the client at all times, or if you have assessed high privacy needs for the client and family, a private room will be best. Many clients, on the other hand, appreciate being able to stay involved and interact with others, which is possible when sharing a room.

Family members who have a difficult time accepting the client's impending death might cope by making fewer visits. When they do visit, inform them of the client's status and share meaningful insights or encounters you have had with the client. Find simple and appropriate care activities for the family to perform, such as offering food, cooling the client's face, combing hair, or filling out a menu. Nighttime can be particularly lonely. Suggest that a family member stay through the night, if possible. Make exceptions to institutional visiting policies, allowing family members to remain with dying clients at any time. Family members regard open access or closeness to their loved one as an indicator of good care through the grieving process (Harstäde and Andershed, 2004). Record contact information for family members so you can reach them at any time.

Support the Grieving Family. Family members of clients receiving palliative care are affected by the challenges of caregiving and grief. They often report being unable to get the information they need in terms they can understand. Lack of information is the major reported concern of family members of dying clients (Kristjanson and Aoun, 2004). They need the nurse's support, guidance, and education as they care for their loved one (Box 30-7). When the client chooses to die at home, family members provide direct care, which is often emotionally stressful and physically exhausting.

In the home setting, fatigued family caregivers benefit from respite care. During respite care, the client temporarily receives care from others so that family members are able to get away to rest and relax. Hospice program benefits include some days of respite care. Inform family members of home care, hospice, and community service options so that they access the best resources for their situation. In some cases, families need assistance and support in making the very difficult decision about nursing home placement (Holmberg, 2006).

Educate the family on the symptoms the client will likely experience and the implications for care. It is common for clients in the last days of life to have decreased appetite or feel nauseated by food. Illness, decreased activity, treatments, and fatigue decrease a client's caloric needs and intake. Family members, distressed with

---

★ BOX 30-7   **CLIENT TEACHING**

Preparing the Dying Client's Family
Objectives
- Family will provide physical care for the dying client in the home.
- Family will provide psychological support to the dying client in the home.

Teaching Strategies
- Discuss feeding techniques and food choices that facilitate chewing and swallowing.
- Demonstrate hygiene measures (bathing, skin and oral care), with return demonstration.
- Demonstrate safe transfer techniques to bed, chair, toilet, with return demonstration.
- Discuss need to balance activity and rest, adjusting to client preference.
- Discuss recognition of changes in client comfort status (e.g. pain, constipation, thirst).
- Discuss common emotional responses to impending death and how to encourage client expression of feelings and/or concerns.
- Discuss client's needs for presence of particular people, company, or for solitude.
- Discuss changes in client condition that signal impending death, such as irregular breathing patterns, noisy respirations, decreased level of consciousness, skin changes of the lower extremities, cold hands and feet, weak pulse, decreased urine output, diminished swallow.
- Inform family members about who to call for questions, emergencies, and at time of death.

Evaluation
- Family members will successfully demonstrate physical care techniques (e.g., turning, feeding, oral care).
- Ask how family members vary their care in response to changing client needs or symptoms.
- Have family members describe the physical changes that occur with impending death.
- Ask family members about their ability to give care and emotional support to the client.

---

the decline, often believe they should encourage or force the client to eat. Forcing food or fluids will stress the client's failing gastrointestinal and cardiovascular systems, potentially creating increased discomfort (Ersek, 2003). When family members understand the burdens that eating causes the dying person, they shift their focus to other helping activities.

Family members often seek out personal time with the nurse to share their concerns, ask about treatment options, validate perceived changes in the client's status, explore the possible meaning of client behaviors, or suggest ideas for care. Whenever possible, communicate news of a client's declining condition or impending death when family members are together so they can provide support for one another. Give the news in privacy, and stay with the family as long as needed or desired.

With the death of the client, grieving family members benefit from the many resources of the health care team. For example, spiritual care providers offer comfort and support for grieving families during and after a death (see Figure 30-5). After a death, assist the family with decision making such as notification of a funeral home, transportation of family members, and collection of the client's belongings. Nurses are a primary source of family support in hospice or home care. Remember that because of differing responses to grief, some family members prefer to be alone at the time of a death, whereas others want to be surrounded by a support community. When uncertain about what a family member prefers for support, pose simple questions and offer suggestions for assistance.

Assist With End-of-Life Decision Making. Clients and family members often face complex treatment decisions with limited knowledge, no prior experiences with death, and at times, unresolved feelings of fear or guilt. They need time and careful explanations by nurses and other health care providers to make decisions. Preferences for end-of-life care rank among the most important discussions a nurse can have with a client and family (Scanlon, 2003).

Clients and family members face a wide range of difficult questions. What medical interventions would the client want to use? Should life-extending treatments be stopped if there appears to be little chance of recovery? Should artificial nutrition and hydration be provided when a client is near death and is no longer able to eat? (Amella, Lawrence, and Gresle, 2005). Nurses caring for terminally ill older adult clients face ethical issues specific to this group of clients (Enes and de Vries, 2004). Difficult ethical decisions at the end of life complicate a survivor's grief, create family divisions, or increase family uncertainty at the time of death (see Chapter 22). When ethical decisions are handled well, survivors achieve a sense of control and experience a meaningful conclusion to their loved one's death (Doka, 2005). Family members whose loved ones have advance directives in place when decisions have to be made experience less stress than those families who cannot consult an advance directive (Davis and others, 2005).

Conversations regarding chronic illness or end-of-life decisions are of major consequence to the client, and he or she needs to be included (Derby and O'Mahony, 2006). Suggest to clients that they clearly communicate their wishes for end-of-life care so that family members are able to act as faithful surrogates when the client can no longer speak for him or herself (see Chapter 23). Several sample documents exist for guiding family discussions for end-of-life care preferences. The publication *Five Wishes* recommends that clients consider five things: who you want to make your health care decisions if you are unable to do so; what medical treatment you do or do not want; how comfortable do you wish to be; how you want to be treated by others; and what you want your loved ones to know (Aging With Dignity, 2005). If you feel uncomfortable in assessing a client's wishes, ask a health care provider experienced in discussing end-of-life issues to assist you. Communicate what you know about client preferences during change-of-shift reports, at health care team conferences, in written care plans, and through ongoing consultation (see Chapter 26).

Facilitate Mourning. Nurses who work with grieving family members often provide bereavement care after the client's death. These guidelines assist persons who care for people in grief (Clements, 2003):

- Help the survivor accept that the loss is real. Discuss how the loss or illness occurred or was discovered, when, under what circumstances, who told them about it, and other factual topics to reinforce the reality of the event and to put it in perspective.

- Support efforts to adjust to the loss. Use a problem-solving approach. Have survivors make a list of their concerns or needs, help them prioritize, and then lead them step-by-step through a discussion of how to proceed. Encourage survivors to ask for help.

- Encourage establishment of new relationships. Reassure people that new relationships do not mean that they are replacing the person who has died. Encourage involvement in non-threatening group social activities (e.g., volunteer activities or church events).

- Allow time to grieve. "Anniversary reactions," renewed grief around the time of the loss in subsequent years, are common. A return to sadness or the pain of grief is often worrisome. Openly acknowledge the loss, give reassurance that the reaction is normal, and encourage the survivor to reminisce.

- Interpret "normal" behavior. Being distractible, having difficulty sleeping or eating, and thinking they have heard the deceased's voice are common behaviors following loss. These symptoms do not mean an individual has an emotional problem or is becoming ill. Reinforce that these behaviors are normal and will resolve over time.

- Provide continuing support. Survivors need the support of a nurse with whom they have bonded for a time following a loss, especially in home care or hospice nursing. The nurse has become an important "actor" in the drama of the deceased's life and death and has helped them through some very intimate and memorable times. Attachment for a while after the death is appropriate and healing for both the survivor and the nurse.

- Be alert for signs of ineffective, potentially harmful coping mechanisms, such as alcohol and substance abuse or excessive use of over-the-counter analgesics or sleep aids.

Hospice Care. **Hospice** care is a philosophy and a model for the care of terminally ill clients and their families. Hospice is not a place, but rather a client- and family-centered approach to care. It gives priority to managing the client's pain and other symptoms, comfort, quality of life, and attention to physical, psychological, social, and spiritual needs and resources. Research shows the effectiveness of hospice care in meeting those goals (Box 30-8). Clients accepted into a hospice program usually have less than 6 months to live. Hospice services are available in home, hospital, extended care, or nursing home settings. Hospice care focuses on the following:

- Client and family as the unit of care
- Coordinated home care with access to available inpatient and nursing home beds
- Control of symptoms (physical, sociological, psychological, and spiritual)
- Physician-directed services
- Provision of an interdisciplinary care team of physicians, nurses, spiritual advisers, social worker, and counselors
- Medical and nursing services available at all times
- Bereavement follow-up after a client's death
- Use of trained volunteers for frequent visitation and respite support
- Acceptance into the program based on need rather than the ability to pay (Hospice Foundation of America, 2004).

✷ BOX 30-8   **EVIDENCE-BASED PRACTICE**

Improving End-of-Life Pain Management in Nursing Homes With Use of Hospice

Evidence Summary

Study findings indicate that the daily pain management for dying nursing home clients enrolled in hospice is better than for dying residents not receiving hospice care. Hospice residents are twice as likely than nonhospice residents to get daily, regular treatment for pain at the end of life. Of the residents in hospice care, 51% receive daily pain treatment compared to 33% of nonhospice residents. The type of pain medication used to manage pain in hospice residents is more consistent with recommended prescribing practices for pain at the end of life. Nonhospice residents frequently receive acetaminophen (Tylenol), whereas hospice residents usually receive morphine derivatives. Study results also demonstrate that while residents enrolled in hospice receive better pain management at the end of life, undertreatment of pain in dying nursing home residents for both hospice and nonhospice groups remains a significant problem.

Application to Nursing Practice

- Pain management practices for dying nursing home residents are better for residents enrolled in hospice programs.
- Become familiar with hospice services to better inform clients and families about the availability of hospice in nursing homes.
- Daily pain management in dying nursing home residents remains suboptimal for both hospice and nonhospice clients, underscoring the need for continued professional end-of-life and pain management education.
- Advocate for better pain management practices for nursing home residents at the end of life.

Reference

Miller S and others: Does receipt of hospice care in nursing homes improve the management of pain at the end-of-life? *J Am Geriatr Soc* 50(3):507, 2002.

Many clients prefer to die at home in a familiar setting, whereas others fear burdening their families or prefer to die in a hospital or nursing home. It is important that the hospice team knows the client's preference. When family issues complicate the options, hospice caregivers try to support the client's wishes but also consider what is best for everyone. Sometimes the complexity or severity of clients' symptoms prevent them from being cared for at home, despite the willingness of family and friends to provide care.

Nurses providing hospice care involve the dying client and family members as active participants in all aspects of care and prioritize care according to their wishes. Client care goals are mutually set, and all participants fully understand the client's care preferences and try to honor them. Hospice services provide for bereavement visits made by the staff after the death of the client to help the family move through the grieving process.

To be eligible for home hospice services a client must have a family caregiver to provide daily basic care. Home care aides offer help with hygienic needs, and a nurse is available to coordinate and manage symptom relief. Hospice team members offer 24-hour accessibility and coordinate care between the home and in-

patient setting. A client receiving home hospice care may enter the hospital for stabilization of symptoms or for caregiver respite. As a client's death comes closer, the hospice team provides intensive support to the client and family (Hospice Foundation of America, 2004).

Care After Death. Federal and state laws require that institutions develop policies and procedures for certain events that occur after death: requesting organ or tissue donation, autopsy, certifying and documenting the occurrence of a death, and providing safe and appropriate postmortem care. In accord with federal law, a specially trained professional (e.g., transplant coordinator or social worker) makes requests for **organ and tissue donation** at the time of every death. The person requesting organ or tissue donation provides information about who can legally give consent, which organs or tissues can be donated, associated costs, and how donation will affect burial or cremation.

Nurses provide support and reinforce explanations to grieving family members, who often need clarification of what they were told during the request process. In extremely stressful circumstances created by the loss of a loved one, grieving survivors usually cannot remember all they were told. Also, understanding the physiology of organ donation is often difficult for family members. Even though the client with brain death has been declared legally dead, he or she remains on life support to provide the vital organs with blood and oxygen before transplant. The appearance of a live-looking body confuses the family, and they need help to understand that the life support is only preserving the vital organs. Nonvital tissues such as corneas, skin, long bones, and middle ear bones are taken at the time of death without artificially maintaining vital functions. If the deceased has not left behind instructions of preference for organ and tissue donation, the family may give consent at the time of death. Review your state organ retrieval laws and institutional policy and procedure regarding the formal consent process. Be aware that the laws governing who to approach for organ donation may not be acceptable in other cultures.

Family members give consent for an **autopsy**, the surgical dissection of a body after death to determine the exact cause and circumstances of death or discover the pathway of a disease (see Chapter 23). In most cases a coroner or medical examiner determines the need to perform an autopsy. Law sometimes requires that an autopsy be performed when death is due to foul play, homicide, suicide, or accidental causes such as motor vehicle crashes, falls, the ingestion of drugs, or deaths within 24 hours of hospital admission. Unattended deaths or those that occur in the workplace or during incarceration also usually require an autopsy (American Medical Association, 2004).

Usually the physician or other designated health care provider will ask for autopsy permission, but the nurse might answer questions and support the family's choices. Inform family members that an autopsy does not deform the body and that all organs are replaced in the body. Family members are often comforted to know that others may be helped by either the gift of organ and tissue donation or through autopsy. Respect and honor family wishes and final decisions.

Documentation of a death provides a legal record of the event. Follow agency policies and procedures carefully to provide an accurate and reliable medical record of all assessments and activities

---

✳ BOX 30-9 Documentation of End-of-Life Care

- Time and date of death and all actions taken to respond to the impending death
- Name of health care provider certifying the death
- Persons notified of the death (e.g., health care providers, family members, organ request team, morgue, funeral home, spiritual care providers) and who comes to the setting at time of death
- Request for organ or tissue donation made and by whom
- Special preparations of the body (e.g., desired or required religious/cultural rituals)
- Medical tubes, devices, or lines left in or on the body
- Personal articles left on and secured to the body
- Personal items given to the family with description, date, time, to whom given
- Location of body identification tags
- Time of body transfer and destination
- Any other relevant information or family requests that help clarify special circumstances

---

surrounding a death. Some medical forms, such as a request for autopsy, must be signed by a physician or coroner, but the registered nurse gathers and records much of the remaining information surrounding a death. A licensed professional or his or her designee witnesses the signing of forms (e.g., release of body or personal belongings forms). Nursing documentation becomes relevant in risk management or legal investigations into a death, underscoring the importance of accurate, legal reporting. Documentation also validates success in meeting client goals or provides justification for changes in treatment or expected outcomes. Box 30-9 lists important documentation elements for end-of-life care.

Family members deserve and expect a clear description of what happened to their loved one, especially in cases of sudden, unusual, or unexpected circumstances. Give only factual information in a nonjudgmental, objective manner, and avoid sharing your opinions. State law and agency policy govern the sharing of the written medical record information, which usually involves a written request. Follow legal guidelines for documentation and the sharing of medical records (see Chapter 23).

When a client dies in an institutional or home care setting, nurses provide or delegate **postmortem care**, the care of a body after death. Above all, a human body deserves the same respect and dignity as a living person and needs to be prepared in a manner consistent with the client's cultural and religious beliefs. Death produces physical changes in the body quite quickly, so you should perform postmortem care as soon as possible to prevent discoloration, tissue damage, or deformities.

Maintaining the integrity of rituals and mourning practices gives families a sense of fulfilled obligations and promotes acceptance of the client's death (Box 30-10). The ability of families to mourn in a manner consistent with cultural values helps survivors experience some predictability and control in an otherwise uncertain and confusing time (see Chapter 9). Some cultures consider "family" as more than a nuclear biological unit. Health care providers need to understand the makeup of a family network and know which individuals to involve in end-of-life decisions.

The nurse coordinates client and family care during and after a death. Become familiar with applicable policies and procedures for postmortem care, because they may vary among settings or institutions. The procedural guideline (Box 30-11) outlines standard activities for care of the body after death.

◆ Evaluation

Effective evaluation strategies enable the nurse to determine if outcomes were met to support the goals of care. Even when a client is not seeking care specifically related to a loss, be on the alert for signs and symptoms of grief. These signs and symptoms provide the criteria for evaluating whether a client is coping with a loss and how he or she is moving through the grief process. Critical thinking ensures that the evaluation process accurately reflects the client's situation and desired outcomes (Figure 30-6).

Refer back to the goals and expected outcomes established during the planning phase to determine the effectiveness of nursing interventions. You evaluate the client's progress by comparing actual client behaviors with expected outcomes to determine whether or not to revise the care plan. For example, if the goal is to have the client communicate a sense of hope to family members, evaluate the verbal and nonverbal communication and behaviors for cues related to expressions of hope. The client's responses will determine if the existing plan of care is effective or if different strategies are necessary. Continue to evaluate the client's progress, the effectiveness of the interventions, and client and family interactions.

The success of the evaluation process depends partially on the bond you have formed with the client. Unless the client trusts you, the sharing of personal expectations or desires is not likely to occur. The following questions will help you validate achievement of client goals and expectations:

- What is the most important thing I can do for you at this time?
- Are your needs being attended to in a timely manner?
- Are you getting the care you have hoped for?
- Would you like me to assist you in a different way?
- Do you have a specific request that I have not been able to meet?

Include family members in the evaluation process. The short- and long-term outcomes that signal a family's recovery from a loss will guide your evaluation. Short-term outcomes indicating effectiveness of grief interventions include talking about the loss without feeling overwhelmed, improved energy level, normalized sleep and dietary patterns, reorganization of life patterns, improved ability to make decisions, and finding it easier to be around other people. Long-term achievements include the return of a sense of humor and normal life patterns, renewed or new personal relationships, and decrease of inner pain (Clements, 2003).

Care for the Grieving Nurse

When caring for dying clients and families, nurses, too, experience grief and loss. Hospice nurses often lose many clients, some of whom they have cared for over long periods of time. Before

---

✴ BOX 30-10   Cultural Considerations in Care of the Body After Death

African Americans: Prefer having a member of the health care team clean and prepare the deceased's body. Relatively short mourning period with a memorial service and a public viewing of the body or a wake before burial. Organ donation and autopsy allowable. African Americans of Christian faith have no prescribed body preparation.

Chinese Americans: Family usually stays with deceased for up to 8 hours after death. Chinese oldest son or daughter bathes the body under direction from older relative or temple priest. Often believe the body should remain intact, so organ donation and autopsy are uncommon.

Hispanic or Latino culture: Central focus is on extended family at time of death. Family members may help with care of the body and are likely to want time with the body. Organ donation and autopsy are not common, but they are not prohibited.

Native Americans: Care of the body in the large Navajo tribe includes cleansing the body, painting the deceased's face, dressing in clothing, and attaching an eagle feather to symbolize a return home. Mourners also have ritual cleansing of their bodies. Burial sites are on the deceased's homeland.

Islamic cultures: Deceased's body is ritualistically washed, wrapped, cried over, prayed for, and buried. Non-Muslims should not touch body. Islamic law forbids cremation, because the body continues after death. At time of death deceased faces Mecca. Modesty is important, so use same-sex caregivers when possible. Autopsies are not allowed; organ donation is sometimes allowed.

Asian cultures, Buddhist faith: Recommend not touching body after death to give deceased smoother transition to the afterlife. Individuals usually minimize emotional expressions and maintain a peaceful, compassionate atmosphere. Persons often say prayers while touching and standing at the deceased's head.

Jewish cultures: In orthodox Judaism, there should be no preparation of the body until it is known whether members from the Jewish Burial Society are coming to the facility. A family member may stay with the body until burial. Usually the burial occurs within 24 hours, but not on the Sabbath. Families participate in a mourning period during which grief is expressed openly and in keeping with ritual. In some, but not all types of Judaism, cremation, autopsy, and embalming are avoided.

Data from Clements P and others: Cultural perspectives of death, grief, and bereavement, *J Psychosoc Nurs Ment Health Serv* 41(7):18, 2003; Kemp C, Bhungalia S: Culture and the end-of-life: a review of major world religions, *J Hosp Palliat Nurs* 4(4):235, 2002; Kemp C, Chang B: Culture and the end-of-life: Chinese, *J Hosp Palliat Nurs* 4(3):173, 2002.

✴ BOX 30-11   PROCEDURAL GUIDELINES

Care of the Body After Death

Delegation: You can delegate care of the body after death to nursing assistive personnel except for organ/tissue donation and autopsy requests.

Equipment: Bath towels, washcloths, washbasin, scissors, shroud kit with name tags, bed linen, documentation forms.

1. A physician or other designated health care provider certifies the death and documents the time of death and actions taken.
2. A physician or designated health care provider requests an autopsy. An autopsy is sometimes required for deaths that occur under certain circumstances.
3. Validate the status of request for organ or tissue donation. Given the complex and sensitive nature of such requests, only specially trained personnel make the requests. Maintain sensitivity to personal, religious, and cultural beliefs in this process.
4. Provide sensitive and dignified nursing care to the client and the family.
   a. Note if you need to collect any specimens.
   b. Ask if the family wishes to participate in the preparation of the body. If not, offer to make arrangements for supportive company for the family (client/family religious leader, spiritual care personnel, or bereavement specialist) during body preparation.
   c. Ask about family requests for body preparation, such as the wearing of special clothing or religious artifacts. Be aware that personal, religious, or cultural practices determine whether or not to shave male facial hair. Get permission before shaving a beard.
   d. Remove all equipment, tubes, and indwelling lines. Note that autopsy or organ donation often pose exceptions to removal, so consult agency policy in these situations.
   e. Cleanse the body thoroughly, maintaining safety standards for body fluids and contamination when indicated. Comb client's hair, or apply personal hairpieces.
   f. Cover body with a clean sheet, place head on a pillow, and leave arms outside covers, if possible. Close eyes by gently holding them shut; leave dentures in the mouth to maintain facial shape; cover any signs of body trauma or packings.
   g. Prepare and clean the environment, deodorize room if needed, and lower the lights.
   h. Offer family members the option to view the body, and ask if they would like you or other support persons to accompany them. Honor and respect individual choices.
   i. Encourage grievers to say good-bye in their own way: words, touch, singing, religious rituals, or prayers.
   j. Provide privacy and an unrushed atmosphere. Assess family members' need or desire for your presence at this time. If you leave, tell them how to reach you.
   k. Determine which personal belongings stay with the body (e.g., wedding or religious symbol), and give other personal items to family members. Document time, date, description of the items taken, and who received them. Save any items that are accidentally left behind, and contact family for further instructions.
   l. Apply identifying name tags to the body, and shroud according to agency policy before transporting the body. Follow safety procedures for body fluid precautions or contamination concerns.
   m. Complete documentation in the nursing notes (see Box 30-9).
   n. Maintain privacy and dignity when transporting the body to another location; cover the body or stretcher with a clean sheet.

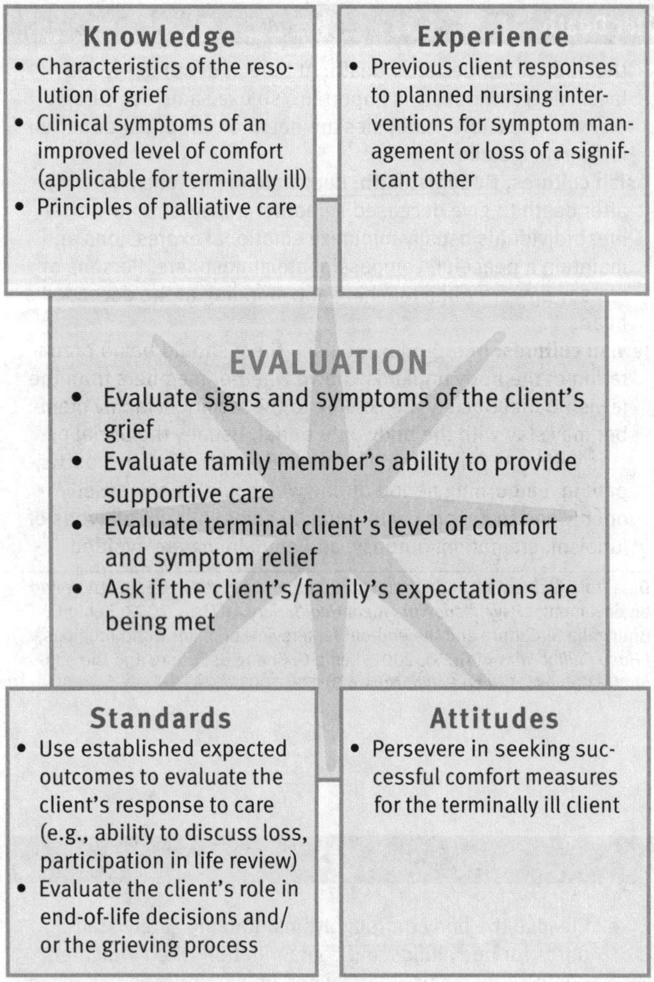

Knowledge
- Characteristics of the resolution of grief
- Clinical symptoms of an improved level of comfort (applicable for terminally ill)
- Principles of palliative care

Experience
- Previous client responses to planned nursing interventions for symptom management or loss of a significant other

EVALUATION
- Evaluate signs and symptoms of the client's grief
- Evaluate family member's ability to provide supportive care
- Evaluate terminal client's level of comfort and symptom relief
- Ask if the client's/family's expectations are being met

Standards
- Use established expected outcomes to evaluate the client's response to care (e.g., ability to discuss loss, participation in life review)
- Evaluate the client's role in end-of-life decisions and/or the grieving process

Attitudes
- Persevere in seeking successful comfort measures for the terminally ill client

Figure 30-6 Critical thinking model for loss, death, and grieving evaluation.

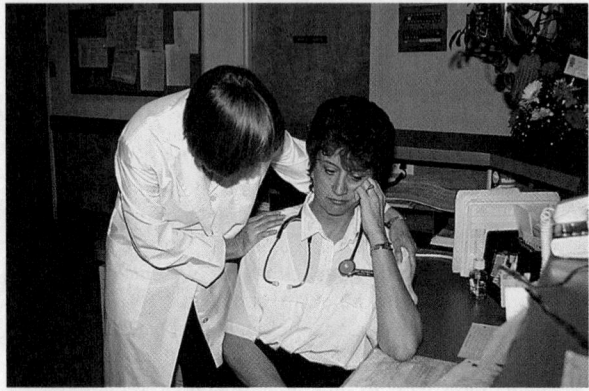

Figure 30-7 Nurses benefit from support of colleagues during their time of loss.

they recover from one loss, they are introduced to another difficult human story. Nurses in acute care settings often witness prolonged, concentrated suffering on a daily basis, leading to feelings of frustration, anger, guilt, sadness, or anxiety. Nursing students report feeling initially hesitant and uncomfortable with their first encounters with a dying client and identify feelings of sadness, anxiety, and discomfort (Allchin, 2006).

Self-reflection, an element of critical thinking, leads you to ask if your sadness is related to caring for the client or to unresolved past personal experiences. Talking with friends, a spiritual care provider, or a close professional colleague helps you begin to recognize your own grief and reflect on the meaning of caring for dying clients (Figure 30-7). Creative strategies help you cope with the loss of a person to whom you have become attached. You can gain some closure by attending a mortuary viewing or a funeral or writing a sympathy letter to the family. Develop support systems that allow time away from caregiving and focus on pleasant, nonstressful activities. Stress management techniques (see Chapter 31) help to restore your energy and continued enjoyment in caring for clients. In some instances, nurses choose to work temporarily in settings where grief and death occur less frequently.

Care for your physical health by eating well, exercising, engaging in relaxing activities, and by getting enough sleep. To promote emotional health, participate in calming activities such as meditation, walking, or listening to music. As noted above, developing awareness of your feelings and their source is the first step to effective emotional self-care. Given the relentless demands of caregiving, set limits on the how much you do and spend time enjoying your favorite activities. Pay attention to the people and activities that provide nurture. Learn to ask for help and accept it when someone offers (Sherman, 2004).

As difficult as caregiving in situations of loss and death is, nurses who work primarily in palliative care or hospice report that they experience personal growth, a sense of being able to "let go," and satisfaction with life. Caring for seriously ill and dying people gives nurses an opportunity to see the meaning and importance of their work. They look for joy and beauty in their own lives and become more open to others (Mok and Chiu, 2004). The same nursing students who experience discomfort in their first experiences with death also note that they reflect on those experiences well beyond their clinical time and were able to identify personal and professional benefits to their experience (Allchin, 2006). Although the possibilities of compassion fatigue exist for nurses, those who practice self-care experience professional and personal growth and find much meaning in their work.

✳ Key Concepts

- When caring for clients who have experienced a loss, facilitate the grief process by assisting survivors in feeling the loss, expressing the loss, and moving through their grief.
- Loss comes in many forms, based on the values and priorities learned within a person's sphere of influence—family, friends, religion, society, and culture.
- The type of loss and the perception of the loss influence how a person experiences grief.
- Death is difficult for the dying person, as well as for the person's family, friends, and caregivers.
- Survivors move back and forth through a series of stages and/or tasks many times, possibly extending over a long period of time.
- Theorists described stages of the grieving process and a series of tasks for survivors to successfully complete their bereavement and adapt to life with a loss.

- Knowledge of the types of grief helps the nurse identify appropriate interventions.
- A person's development, coping strategies, socioeconomic status, personal relationships, nature of loss, and cultural and spiritual beliefs influence the way he or she perceives and responds to grief.
- Nursing interventions involve reinforcement of clients' successful coping mechanisms and introduction of new coping approaches when needed.
- Do not assume how or if clients experience grief or that a particular behavior indicates grief. Allow clients to share the experience in their own way.
- Assess the terminally ill client and family wishes for end-of-life care, including the preferred place for death, desired level of intervention, and expectations for pain and symptom management.
- Establish a caring presence, and use effective communication strategies to encourage clients to share to the degree they are comfortable.
- Palliative care allows clients to make more informed choices, achieve better alleviation of symptoms, and experience a higher quality of life through an illness or death experience.
- Hospice is not a place, but rather a philosophy of family-centered, whole person care at the end of life.
- Practice self-care, ask for and accept help, and reflect on the meaning of nursing experiences of caring for the dying client and family.

✳ Critical Thinking Exercises

1. Mr. Stevens agrees to receive antibiotic therapy, intravenous fluids, and breathing treatments for his newly diagnosed pneumonia. He has recovered enough to return home and receive hospice care. Mr. Stevens' son does not understand hospice care and wants the nurse to tell him what to expect. What major points would the nurse include in a conversation with the client and family before discharge related to hospice philosophy, services, and impact on the family?

2. Mr. Stevens' family members express concern about their ability to provide care for Mr. Stevens. What would you include in a family teaching plan?

✳ NCLEX®-Style Review Questions

1. Regarding the request for organ and tissue donation at the time of death, the nurse should be aware that:
   1. Specially educated personnel make requests
   2. Requests are usually made by the nurse caring for the client at the time of death
   3. Only clients who have given prior instruction regarding donation can become donors
   4. Professionals should be very selective in whom they ask for organ and tissue donation

2. The nurse notes that a woman recently beginning cancer treatment appears quiet and withdrawn, states she does not believe the treatments will make any difference, does not ask about her progress, and has missed two chemo-

therapy sessions. Based on the above assessment data, the nurse would gather more information to consider making which of the following nursing diagnoses?
   1. Anxiety
   2. Powerlessness
   3. Spiritual distress
   4. Anticipatory grieving
   5. 1 and 2
   6. 1, 3, and 4

3. A home care nurse is asked by a family member what he should do if the client's serious chronic illness continues to worsen even with increased medical interventions. The nurse recognizes that the family member is posing a question about goals of care at the end of life. The nurse should:
   1. Encourage the family to think more positively about the client's new therapy
   2. Avoid the discussion because it has to do with medical, not nursing, diagnoses
   3. Initiate a discussion about advance directives with the client, family, and health care team
   4. Begin the discussion by asking the family member what he believes the goals should be

4. The nurse suggests that a client receive a palliative care consultation for symptom management related to anxiety and increasing pain. A family member asks the nurse if this means the client is dying and is now "in hospice." The nurse explains that:
   1. Hospice (end-of-life care) and palliative care are the same thing
   2. Palliative care is for any client, any time, any disease, in any setting
   3. Palliative care interventions relieve the symptoms of illness and treatment
   4. Palliative care strategies are primarily designed to treat the client's illness
   5. 1 and 3
   6. 1 and 4

5. A young man is diagnosed with a serious, life-changing illness. His conversations during his first 2 days of hospitalization are abrupt, superficial, and unrelated to his illness. Regarding the use of therapeutic communication, the nurse knows that:
   1. Younger clients are usually less talkative about their diagnoses
   2. All clients benefit by talking about their loss feelings with another person
   3. The nurse should avoid discussing illness-related topics with quiet clients
   4. The nurse should remain alert for signals the client wants to discuss his illness
   5. 2 and 4
   6. 1, 2, and 4

6. A woman experiences the loss of a very early term pregnancy. Her friends do not mention the loss, and someone suggests to her that she can "always try again." The

woman feels confusion over her sadness and stops talking about it with others. The type of grief the woman may be experiencing is:
1. Delayed
2. Anticipated
3. Exaggerated
4. Disenfranchised

7. A nurse has the responsibility of managing a deceased client's postmortem care. Arrange the steps for postmortem care in the proper order.
1. Bathe the deceased's body.
2. Collect any needed specimens.
3. Remove all drains and indwelling tubes.
4. Position the body for family visit/viewing.
5. Speak to the family members about their possible participation.
6. Confirm that request for organ/tissue donation and/or autopsy has been made.
7. Notify a support person (e.g., spiritual care provider, bereavement specialist) for the family.
8. Accurately tag the body, indicating deceased's identity and safety issues regarding infection control.

8. A family member of a recently deceased client talks casually with the nurse at the time of the client's death and expresses relief that she will not have to visit at the hospital anymore. What theoretical description of grief may apply to this family member?
1. Denial
2. Anticipatory grief
3. Dysfunctional grief
4. Yearning and searching

9. A self-care goal for the nurse who cares for dying and grieving clients might be:
1. Learn not to take the loss so seriously
2. Limit involvement with clients who are grieving
3. Maintain life balance, and reflect on the meaning of one's work
4. Admit that you are not well suited to care for grieving clients and families

10. During postmortem care the nurse should give priority to:
1. Locating the client's clothing
2. Providing culturally and religiously sensitive care in body preparation
3. Transporting the body to the morgue as soon as possible to prevent body decomposition
4. Providing all postmortem care to protecting the deceased's family from having to see the body

31 | Stress and Coping

Mastery of content in this chapter will enable the student to:

- Describe the three stages of the general adaptation syndrome.
- Differentiate acute stress disorder and posttraumatic stress disorder.
- Discuss the integration of stress theory with nursing theories.
- Describe stress management techniques beneficial for coping with stress.

- Discuss the process of crisis intervention.
- Develop a care plan for clients experiencing stress.
- Discuss how stress in the workplace affects the nurse.

✳ MEDIA RESOURCES   ✳ KEY TERMS

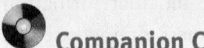 **Companion CD**
- NCLEX®-Style Review Questions
- Audio Glossary
- Interactive Learning Activities
- English/Spanish Glossary

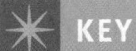 **Website**
- NCLEX®-Style Review Questions
- Audio Glossary
- English/Spanish Glossary
- Interactive Learning Activities
- Weblinks
- Audio Summaries

Acute stress disorder (ASD), p. 489
Alarm reaction, p. 487
Appraisal, p. 486
Burnout, p. 497
Coping, p. 488
Crisis, p. 486
Crisis intervention, p. 499
Developmental crises, p. 489
Distress, p. 489
Ego-defense mechanisms, p. 488
Endorphins, p. 486
Eustress, p. 489

Exhaustion stage, p. 487
Fight-or-flight response, p. 486
Flashback, p. 489
General adaptation syndrome (GAS), p. 486
Posttraumatic stress disorder (PTSD), p. 489
Primary appraisal, p. 488
Resistance stage, p. 487
Secondary appraisal, p. 488
Situational crises, p. 489
Stress, p. 486
Stressors, p. 486
Trauma, p. 486

Health care professionals need to know about stress so they are able to recognize it in clients and families and intervene effectively. In addition, health care professionals need to know how stressful events that occur in the course of clinical practice affect them. It is important to recognize the signs and symptoms of stress and understand stress management techniques to aid personal coping, as well as to design stress management interventions for clients and their families.

People use the term **stress** in many ways. First, stress is an experience a person is exposed to, through a stimulus or stressor. **Stressors** are disruptive forces operating within or on any system (Neuman and Fawcett, 2002). Stress is also the appraisal, or perception, of a stressor. **Appraisal** is how people interpret the impact of the stressor on themselves, of what is happening, and what they are able to do about it (Lazarus, 2007). Finally, stress is a general term that links environmental demands and the person's perception of those demands as challenging, threatening, or damaging (Varcarolis, Carson, and Shoemaker, 2006). Stress in this context refers to the consequences of the stressor, as well as to the person's appraisal of the stressor.

People experience stress as a consequence of daily life events and experiences. Stress is helpful by stimulating thinking processes and helping people stay alert to their environment. Furthermore, stress results in personal growth and facilitate development (Aguilera, 1998). How people react to stress depends on how they view and evaluate the impact of the stressor, its effect on their situation and support at the time of the stress, and their usual coping mechanisms. When stress overwhelms a person's existing coping mechanisms, disequilibrium occurs, and a **crisis** results (Aguilera, 1998). If symptoms of stress persist beyond the duration of the stressor, a person has experienced a **trauma** (Hyer and Sohnle, 2001).

Scientific Knowledge Base

Over 60 years ago Walter Cannon proposed the **fight-or-flight response** to stress, which is arousal of the sympathetic nervous system (Aldwin and Werner, 2007). This reaction prepares a person for action by increasing heart rate; diverting blood from the intestines to the brain and striated muscles; and increasing blood pressure, respiratory rate, and blood glucose levels (Figure 31-1).

Neurophysiological responses to stress function through negative feedback. The process of negative feedback senses an abnormal state, such as lowered body temperature, and makes an adaptive response, such as initiating shivering to generate body heat. Three structures, the medulla oblongata, the reticular formation, and the pituitary gland, control the body's response to a stressor.

Medulla Oblongata

The medulla oblongata controls heart rate, blood pressure, and respiration. Impulses traveling to and from the medulla oblongata increase or decrease these vital functions. For example, sympathetic or parasympathetic nervous system impulses traveling from the medulla oblongata to the heart control regulation of the heartbeat. The heart rate increases in response to impulses from sympathetic fibers and decreases with impulses from parasympathetic fibers.

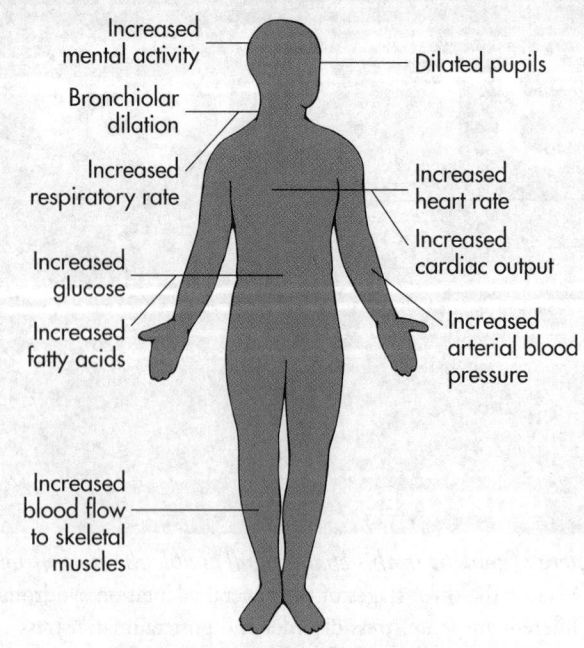

Figure 31-1 Fight-or-flight response.

Reticular Formation

The reticular formation, a small cluster of neurons in the brain stem and spinal cord, continuously monitors the physiological status of the body through connections with sensory and motor tracts. For example, certain cells within the reticular formation cause a sleeping person to regain consciousness or increase the level of consciousness when a need arises.

Pituitary Gland

The pituitary gland, a small gland attached to the hypothalamus, produces hormones necessary for adaptation to stress, such as adrenocorticotropic hormone (ACTH), which in turn produces cortisol. In addition, the pituitary gland regulates the secretion of thyroid, gonadal, and parathyroid hormones. A feedback mechanism continuously monitors hormone levels in the blood and regulates hormone secretion. When hormone levels drop, the pituitary gland receives a message to increase hormone secretion. When hormone levels rise, the pituitary gland decreases hormone production.

General Adaptation Syndrome

From the 1930s to the 1950s, Hans Selye enlarged on Cannon's fight-or-flight hypothesis to describe the **general adaptation syndrome (GAS)**, a three-stage reaction to stress (Page and Lindsey, 2003). The GAS describes how the body responds to stressors through the alarm reaction, the resistance stage, and the exhaustion stage. The GAS is triggered either directly by a physical event or indirectly by a psychological event (Lazarus, 1999).

The GAS involves several body systems, especially the autonomic nervous system and the endocrine system, and responds immediately to stress (Figure 31-2). When the body encounters a physical demand, such as an injury, the pituitary gland initiates the GAS. The pituitary gland communicates with the hypothalamus, which secretes **endorphins**. Endorphins, hormones that act on the

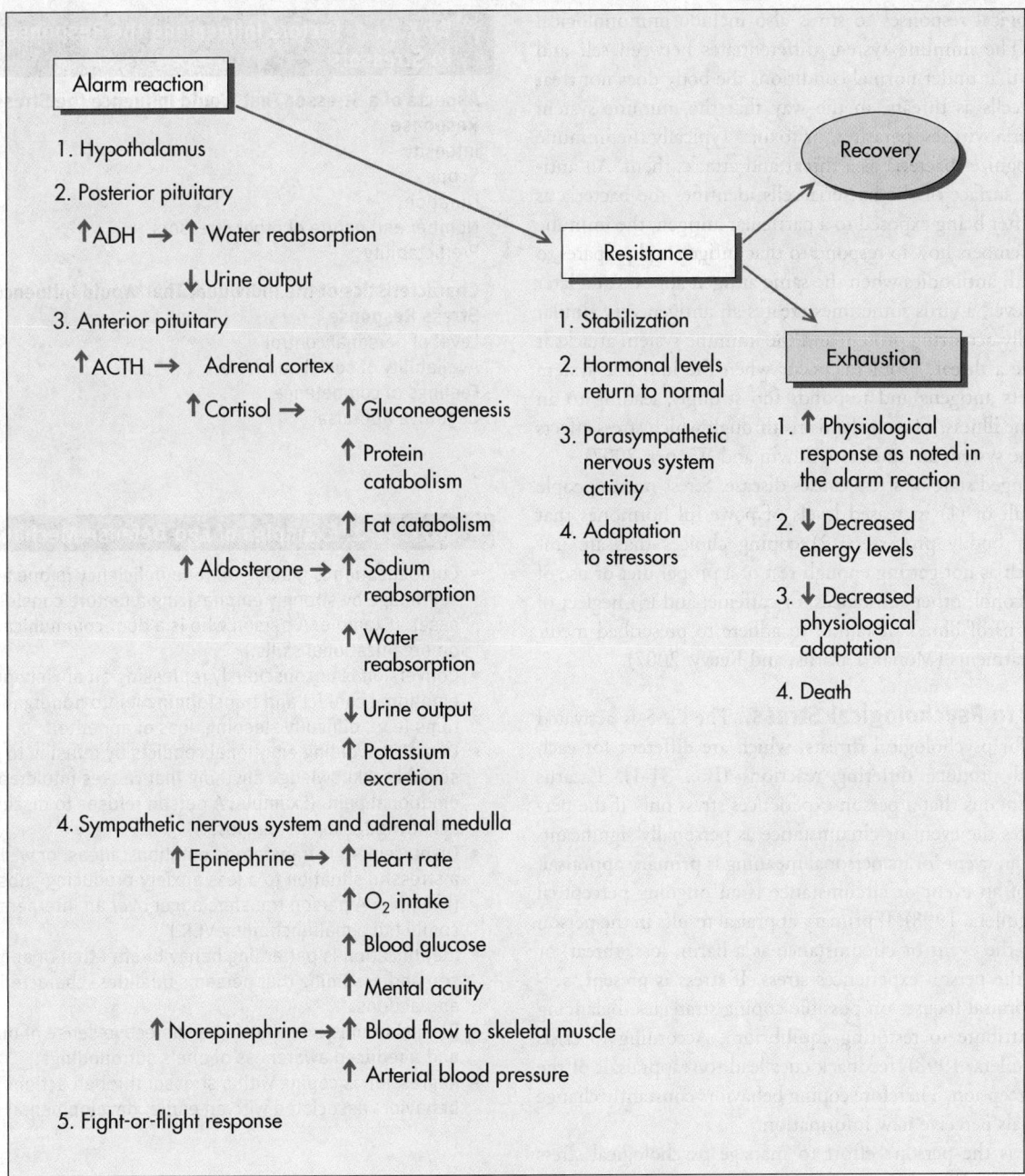

Figure 31-2 General adaptation syndrome (GAS).

mind like morphine and opiates, produce a sense of well-being and reduce pain (Lazarus, 1999). In this way the GAS defends against stress both by activating the neuroendocrine system and by providing endorphins that decrease awareness of the pain.

During the **alarm reaction** rising hormone levels result in increased blood volume, blood glucose levels, epinephrine and norepinephrine amounts, heart rate, blood flow to muscles, oxygen intake, and mental alertness (Page and Lindsey, 2003). In addition, the pupils of the eyes dilate to produce a greater visual field. This change in body systems prepares an individual for fight or flight and lasts from 1 minute to many hours. If the stressor poses an extreme threat to life or remains for a long time, the person progresses to the second stage, resistance.

During the **resistance stage** the body stabilizes and responds in an opposite manner to the alarm reaction. Hormone levels, heart rate, blood pressure, and cardiac output return to normal, and the body repairs any damage that has occurred. However, if the stressor remains, and the body does not adapt, the person enters the third stage, exhaustion.

The **exhaustion stage** occurs when the body is no longer able to resist the effects of the stressor and when the body has depleted the energy necessary to maintain adaptation. The physiological response has intensified, but with a compromised energy level, the person's adaptation to the stressor diminishes. The body cannot defend itself against the impact of the event, physiological regulation diminishes, and, if the stress continues, death results.

Physiological responses to stress also include immunological responses. The immune system differentiates between self and nonself, so that under normal conditions the body does not treat one's own cells as threats, in the way that the immune system treats bacteria, viruses, parasites, or toxins. Typically the immune system recognizes bacteria as a threat and attacks them. An antigen on the surface of the bacteria cells identifies the bacteria as invaders. After being exposed to a particular antigen, the immune system remembers how to respond to that antigen and prepares to respond with antibodies when the same antigen appears at a later time. However, a virus sometimes creates an antigen very similar to a naturally occurring protein and the immune system attacks it as if it were a threat. Problems occur when the immune system misinterprets antigens and responds too strongly, leading to an autoimmune illness. The mechanisms through which stress affects the immune system are unclear (Aldwin and Werner, 2007).

A prolonged state of stress causes disease. Stress makes people ill as a result of (1) increased levels of powerful hormones that change our bodily processes; (2) coping choices that are unhealthy, such as not getting enough rest or a proper diet or use of tobacco, alcohol, other substances, or caffeine; and (3) neglect of warning signs of illness or failure to adhere to prescribed medicines or treatments (Monat, Lazarus, and Reevy, 2007).

Reaction to Psychological Stress.

The GAS is activated indirectly for psychological threats, which are different for each person and produce differing reactions (Box 31-1). Lazarus (1999) maintains that a person experiences stress only if the person evaluates the event or circumstance as personally significant. Evaluating an event for its personal meaning is **primary appraisal**. Appraisal of an event or circumstance is an ongoing perceptual process (Aguilera, 1998). If primary appraisal results in the person identifying the event or circumstance as a harm, loss, threat, or challenge, the person experiences stress. If stress is present, **secondary appraisal** focuses on possible coping strategies. Balancing factors contribute to restoring equilibrium. According to crisis theory (Aguilera, 1998), feedback cues lead to reappraisals of the original perception. Therefore coping behaviors constantly change as individuals perceive new information.

Coping is the person's effort to manage psychological stress (Lazarus, 2007). Effectiveness of coping strategies depends on the individual's needs. A person's age and cultural background influence these needs. For this reason no single coping strategy works for everyone or for every stress. The same person may cope differently from one time to another. In stressful situations most people use a combination of problem-focused coping and emotion-focused coping strategies. In other words, when under stress, a person obtains information and takes action to change the situation, as well as regulating emotions tied to the stress. In some cases a person avoids thinking about the situation or changes the way he or she thinks about it, without changing the actual situation itself (Lazarus, 2007).

Lazarus (2007) suggests that not only does the type of stress make a difference, but that people's goals, their beliefs about themselves and the world, and personal resources determine how they cope with stress. Resources include intelligence, money, social skills, supportive family and friends, physical at-

---

BOX 31-1   Factors Influencing the Response to Stressors

Aspects of a Stressor That Would Influence the Stress Response
Intensity
Scope
Duration
Number and nature of other stressors
Predictability

Characteristics of the Individual That Would Influence the Stress Response
Level of personal control
Availability of social supports
Feelings of competence
Cognitive appraisal

BOX 31-2   Examples of Ego-Defense Mechanisms

- Compensation is making up for a deficiency in one aspect of self-image by strongly emphasizing a feature considered an asset. (Example: A person who is a poor communicator relies on organizational skills.)
- Conversion is unconsciously repressing an anxiety-producing emotional conflict and transforming it into nonorganic symptoms (e.g., difficulty sleeping, loss of appetite).
- Denial is avoiding emotional conflicts by refusing to consciously acknowledge anything that causes intolerable emotional pain. (Example: A person refuses to discuss or acknowledge a personal loss.)
- Displacement is transferring emotions, ideas, or wishes from a stressful situation to a less anxiety-producing substitute. (Example: A person transfers anger over an interpersonal conflict to a malfunctioning VCR.)
- Identification is patterning behavior after that of another person and assuming that person's qualities, characteristics, and actions.
- Dissociation is experiencing a subjective sense of numbing and a reduced awareness of one's surroundings.
- Regression is coping with a stressor through actions and behaviors associated with an earlier developmental period.

---

tractiveness, health and energy, and ways of thinking, such as optimism (Lazarus, 2007).

Coping mechanisms include psychological adaptive behaviors. Such behaviors are often task oriented, involving the use of direct problem-solving techniques to cope with the threats. They are also **ego-defense mechanisms,** the purpose of which is to regulate emotional distress and thus give a person protection from anxiety and stress. Ego-defense mechanisms help a person cope with stress indirectly.

Ego-defense mechanisms, first described by Sigmund Freud, offer psychological protection from a stressful event. Everyone uses them unconsciously to protect against feelings of worthlessness and anxiety. Occasionally a defense mechanism becomes distorted and no longer assists the person in adapting to a stressor. Generally, however, people find them very helpful in coping and use them spontaneously (Box 31-2). Frequently, short-term stressors activate ego-defense mechanisms. These usually do not result in psychiatric disorders.

Types of Stress

Selye identified two types of stress: **distress,** or damaging stress, and **eustress,** stress that protects health. Eustress is motivating energy, such as happiness, hopefulness, and purposeful movement (Varcarolis and others, 2006). However, the idea of healthy stress is controversial because it is difficult to tell whether a person has benefited from stress or is coping by denying the stress in some way (Aldwin and Werner, 2007). Stress includes work stress, family stress, chronic stress, acute stress, daily hassles, trauma, and crisis. One person looks at a stimulus and sees it as a challenge, leading to mastery and growth. Another sees the same stimulus as a threat, leading to stagnation and loss. Lazarus suggests a spillover of stresses between work and home. The individual with family responsibilities and a full-time job outside the home possibly experiences chronic stress. Chronic stress occurs in stable conditions and from stressful roles. Living with a long-term illness produces chronic stress. Conversely, time-limited events that threaten a person for a relatively brief period provoke acute stress. Recurrent daily hassles, such as commuting to work, maintaining a house, dealing with difficult people, and managing money will further complicate chronic or acute stress.

When a trauma occurs, its effects will sometimes last well after the traumatizing event ends (Hyer and Sohnle, 2001). **Posttraumatic stress disorder (PTSD)** begins with an **acute stress disorder (ASD)** (Hyer and Sohnle, 2001). An acute stress disorder begins with the person experiencing, witnessing, or being confronted with a traumatic event and responding with intense fear, helplessness, or horror (American Psychiatric Association [APA], 2000). Other criteria of the acute stress disorder consist of the person displaying at least three acute dissociative symptoms, having at least one reexperiencing symptom, displaying marked avoidance of stimuli that arouse memories of the trauma, showing marked hyperarousal, and having these symptoms between 2 days and 4 weeks after the trauma (Hyer and Sohnle, 2001). Some examples of traumatic events that lead to ASD include motor vehicle crashes, natural disasters, violent personal assault, and military combat. Symptoms of PTSD sometimes have a delayed onset longer than 4 weeks and persist longer than 1 month (APA, 2000). Some people with PTSD experience **flashbacks,** or recurrent and intrusive recollections of the event. Traumatic events that lead to PTSD include the same events that lead to ASD.

Conversely, research has shown that trauma sometimes has positive effects. Benefits enable the person to improve in coping skills and self-knowledge, social ties, and changes in values and perspectives (Hyer and Sohnle, 2001).

A crisis implies that a person is facing a turning point in life. This means that previous ways of coping are not effective and the person must change. Gerald Caplan, in 1964, first described crisis intervention. Caplan distinguished two types of crises, those associated with changing developmental levels, or **developmental crises,** and **situational crises.** A new developmental stage, such as marriage, birth of a child, or retirement, requires new coping styles. Developmental crises occur as a person moves through life's

stages. A situational crisis, on the other hand, can be provoked by an external source such as a job change, a motor vehicle crash, a death, or severe illness (Varcarolis and others, 2006).

The view of the person experiencing a crisis provides the frame of reference for the crisis. Aguilera's crisis theory (1998) maintains that the vital question for a person in crisis is, "What does this mean to you; how is it going to affect your life?" What causes extreme stress for one person is not always stressful to another. The perception of the event, the situational supports, and the coping mechanisms all influence return of equilibrium or homeostasis. A person either advances or regresses as a result of a crisis, depending upon how the person manages the crisis (Lazarus, 2007).

Nursing Knowledge Base

Nurses have proposed theories related to stress and coping. Because stress plays a central role in vulnerability to disease, symptoms of stress often require nursing intervention.

Nursing Theory and the Role of Stress

Neuman Systems Model is based on the concepts of stress and reaction to stress. This nursing theory views nursing as being responsible for developing interventions to prevent or reduce stressors on the client or to make them more bearable for the client (Neuman and Fawcett, 2002). Because Neuman Systems Model is a systems model, you apply it to understand the client's individual, family's, and community's responses to stressors. All systems experience multiple stressors, each of which has a differing potential to disturb the person's, family's, or community's balance. Examples of stress include intrapersonal stressors, such as an illness or injury; interpersonal stressors, such as an argument or misunderstanding between two people; or extrapersonal stressors, such as financial concerns. Every person develops a set of responses to stress that constitute the "normal line of defense" (Neuman and Fawcett, 2002). This line of defense helps to maintain health and wellness. However, when "physiological, psychological, sociocultural, developmental, or spiritual influences" are unable to buffer stress, the normal line of defense is broken, and disease can result.

Neuman Systems Model (2002) stresses the importance of accuracy in assessment and interventions that promote optimal wellness using primary, secondary, and tertiary prevention strategies. According to Neuman's theory, the goal of primary prevention is to promote client wellness by stress prevention and reduction of risk factors. Secondary prevention occurs after symptoms appear. The nurse determines the meaning of the illness and stress to the client and the client's needs and resources for meeting them. Tertiary prevention begins when the client system becomes more stable and recovers. At the tertiary level of prevention the nurse supports rehabilitation processes involved in healing, moving the client back to wellness and the primary level of disease prevention. Neuman Systems Model of nursing views the person, family, or community as constantly changing in response to the environment and stressors.

Pender's health promotion model proposes that health promotion means increasing the level of well-being of an individual or

---

Reducing Stress for Family Members by Involving Them in Caregiving

Evidence Summary

Family caregivers of clients in residential long-term care experience stress even though the client is no longer living at home. The decision to institutionalize their family member and the aftermath of that decision causes emotional distress and is a threat to the family member's psychological well-being. This study examined the effect of family members assisting with the personal care and activities of daily living (ADLs) of institutionalized clients with Alzheimer's disease as a strategy to reduce the stress. The sample included 185 clients with an average age of 76 years. The average age of the caregivers was 61 years. The average caregiver spent 8 hours per week visiting their relative. Researchers found that the more frequent the visits, the less emotional and physical fatigue the family member felt. The researchers suggested that when the nursing home staff carried out physically draining tasks such as toileting and bathing, family caregivers were able to provide more emotionally fulfilling aspects such as socializing and sharing meals. Furthermore, visiting provided the opportunity for family members to monitor the care given by the nursing home staff, thus reducing the caregiver's stress. In addition, when their role shifted from primary caregiver to advocate for the client, the family members felt empowered. Previous studies showed that institutionalized residents have a better

quality of life when family members are involved. This study shows that the emotional well-being of the involved family members improved and the stress level was reduced.

Application to Nursing Practice

- Have a welcoming attitude toward family members who have been providing care at home. Listen to their suggestions about care.
- Communicate with family caregivers of clients in residential long-term care about the client's daily care, in addition to the required care plan conferences.
- Provide opportunities for family members to share meals with clients.
- Encourage family members to assist with personal care such as feeding, combing hair, selecting clothes, and straightening the client's room when the family member expresses an interest.
- Recognize when family members are able to carry out activities that preserve the identity of the institutionalized relative and maintain the family member–resident relationship, such as displaying family pictures and celebrating family events.

Reference

Gaugler JE and others: Family involvement in nursing homes: effects on stress and well-being, *Aging Ment Health* 8(1):65, 2004.

---

group (Pender, Murdaugh, and Parsons, 2006). Conversely, primary, secondary, and tertiary prevention (health protection) focus on avoiding negative events. Pender considers stress reduction strategies important to reduce threats to well-being, to help people fulfill their potential, and to shape and maintain health behaviors. To change behavior, the client must initiate the change and behave differently in interactions. People want to live in ways that enable them to be as healthy as possible and to be capable of assessing their own abilities and assets. Based on these assumptions of the capability and desire of people to be healthy, Pender suggests strategies for prevention and health promotion related to stress management.

Situational, Maturational, and Sociocultural Factors

Potential stressors and coping mechanisms vary across the life span. Adolescence, adulthood, and old age bring different stressors. The appraisal of stressors, the amount and type of social support, and coping strategies all balance when assessing stress, and all depend on previous life experiences (Aguilera, 1998). Furthermore, situational and social stressors place people who are vulnerable at higher risk for prolonged stress.

Situational Factors.

Situational stress arises from job changes, either one's own or that of a family member, and relocation. Stressful job changes include promotions, transfers, downsizing, restructuring, changes in supervisors, and additional responsibilities. Adjusting to chronic illness leads to situational stress. Common diseases, such as obesity, hypertension, diabetes, depression, asthma, and coronary artery disease, provoke stress. Uncertainty associated with treatment and illness triggers stress in clients of all ages. Stress related to paying for treatment and limited access to

providers cannot be overlooked. Although being a family caregiver for someone with a chronic illness such as Alzheimer's disease is associated with stress, the actions of competent health care providers can often minimize the stress for caregivers (Gaugler and others, 2004) (Box 31-3).

Maturational Factors.

Stressors vary with life stage. Children identify stressors related to their physical appearance, their families, their friends, and school (Chen and others, 2005). Preadolescents experience stress related to self-esteem issues, changing family structure due to divorce or death of a parent, or hospitalizations. As adolescents search for their identity with peer groups and separate from their families, they experience stress. In addition, they face questions about using mind-altering substances, sexuality, jobs, school, and career choices that cause stress. Stress for adults center around major changes in life circumstances (Aguilera, 1998). These include the many milestones of beginning a family and a career, losing parents, seeing children leave home, and accepting physical aging. In old age, stressors include the loss of autonomy and mastery due to general frailty or health problems that limit stamina and strength (Box 31-4).

Sociocultural Factors.

Environmental and social stressors lead to developmental problems. Potential stressors that affect any age-group, but that are especially stressful for young people, include prolonged poverty and physical handicap. Children become vulnerable when they lose parents and caregivers through divorce, imprisonment, or death or when parents have mental illness or substance abuse disorders. Furthermore, living under conditions of continuing violence, disintegrated neighborhoods, or homelessness damage people of any age, but especially young people (Pender and others, 2006) (Box 31-5).

BOX 31-4   FOCUS ON OLDER ADULTS

Understanding Differences in Stress Among Older Adults

- There are very few age-related differences in coping strategies, and older adults are just as effective at coping as younger adults (Varcarolis and others, 2006).
- Older adults with depression and anxiety are less likely than young adults to be accurately diagnosed (Varcarolis and others, 2006).
- Life experiences and perspectives of older adults make most problems seem insignificant, and many older adults have acquired appropriate stress management techniques.
- The timing of stress-inducing events significantly influences older adults' ability to cope. The fact that older adults have several stressful events (e.g., loss of a spouse and new medical diagnosis) occur with a short period of time often results in negative effects on coping ability.
- Anxiety disorders are the most prevalent disorders in later life and are continuations of life-long illnesses (Hyer and Sohnle, 2001).

Critical Thinking

When caring for a client experiencing stress, use critical thinking skills to understand the client's stressor and the stress response. Integrate knowledge from nursing and other disciplines, previous experiences, and information gathered from clients to understand stress and its impact on the client and family.

Know the neurophysiological changes that occur in the client experiencing the alarm reaction, resistance stage, and exhaustion stage of the general adaptation syndrome. In addition, know communication principles that contribute to assessing client's behaviors (see Chapter 24). Give utmost attention to determining the client's perception of the situation and the ability of the client to cope with the stress. If the client's usual coping skills have not helped or the client's support systems have failed, use crisis intervention counseling.

Experience teaches you to understand the client's unique perspective and to view every person as an individual, recognizing that no two people are exactly alike. Experience with clients will also help you to recognize responses to stress. In addition, your own personal experiences with stress and coping will increase your ability to empathize with a client temporarily immobilized by stress.

Be confident in the belief that you can effectively manage stress, if necessary, and so can the client. Clients who feel overwhelmed and perceive events as being beyond their capacity to cope will rely on you as an expert. Clients will respect your advice and counsel and gain confidence from your belief in the client's ability to move past the stressful event or illness. Clients overwhelmed by life events are often unable, at least initially, to act on their own behalf and require either direct intervention or guidance. Integrity is an essential attitude through which you respect the client's perception of the stressor. Make the effort to have the client explain his or her unique viewpoint and situation.

The Standards of Care for Psychiatric Mental Health Nursing Practice (ANA, 2000) are useful to guide an accurate assessment

BOX 31-5   CULTURAL ASPECTS OF CARE

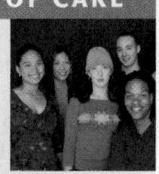

Cultural Variations in Stress Appraisal and Coping Strategies

A client's culture defines what is stressful to the person and ways of coping with stress (Aldwin, 2000). Cultural context shapes the types of environmental stimuli that produce stress. For example, diverse cultures address developmental transitions and life's turning points differently. How a person leaves the parental home, experiences health crises or chronic illness, cares for the family or becomes disabled or dependent are all culturally bound. Furthermore, how a person appraises stress is also dependent upon the person's culture. What is perceived as a stressor in one culture might be viewed as a minor problem in another culture. A person's response to the stress of pain is an example of a culture-based response to stress, whether a person maintains personal control or becomes emotionally expressive. Coping strategies are also influenced by one's cultural background. According to Aldwin, cultures vary in their emotion-focused and problem-focused coping strategies. Related to emotion-focused coping, some cultures stress that emotions should be controlled whereas others believe in expressing emotions. Problem-focused coping refers to controlling or managing stress. Different cultures control stress in different ways. Finally, cultures provide different institutions for coping with stress. These include the legal system for conflict resolution, advice givers or support groups, and rituals.

Implications for Practice

- Realize that stressors and coping styles vary with different cultures.
- Use introspection to examine one's own perceptions of stress and coping in a cultural context.
- Assess the influence of culture on a client's appraisal of stress.
- Determine the institutions within a client's culture that facilitate coping.

Aldwin CM and Werner EE: Stress, coping and development: an integrative perspective, ed 2, New York, 2007, Guilford Press.

of a client's stress, coping mechanisms, and support system before intervening. Use linguistic and culturally effective communication skills to clearly and precisely understand a client's perception of the stress. Focus on factors relevant to the client's well-being. In addition, the client will expect you to exhibit confidence and integrity if the client feels temporarily vulnerable. Be especially aware of the ethical responsibility in caring for someone who has diminished autonomy due to stress.

Nursing Process

◆ Assessment

Assessment of a client's stress level and coping resources requires that you first establish a trusting nurse-client relationship because you will be asking the client to share personal and sensitive information. Learn from the client both by asking questions and by making

Knowledge
- Basic stress response
- Factors influencing stress
- Physiological, emotional, and behavioral risks associated with a stressor
- Basic defense mechanisms
- Cultural influences
- Communication principles

Experience
- Caring for clients whose illness, lifestyle, family interactions, and personal/professional demands resulted in stress
- Personal experience in dealing with stressful situations

ASSESSMENT
- Identify actual or potential stressors
- Identify client's appraisal of stressor
- Obtain data regarding the client's previous experience with stress
- Determine the impact of illness on the client's lifestyle

Standards
- Apply intellectual standards of completeness, relevance, precision, and accuracy when assessing the client's stress response
- Apply ANA Standards of Care for Psychiatric Mental Health Nursing Practice by using linguistic and culturally effective communication skills and comprehensive assessment

Attitudes
- Exhibit confidence that stress can be managed
- Approach assessment with fairness and integrity to collect data in an unbiased manner and convey that client information remains confidential

Figure 31-3 Critical thinking model for stress and coping assessment.

observations of nonverbal behavior and the client's environment. Synthesize the information and adopt a critical thinking attitude while observing and analyzing your client's behavior (Figure 31-3). Often the client has difficulty expressing exactly what is most bothersome about the situation until there is an opportunity to discuss it with someone who has time to listen.

Stress occurs in a family or a community, as well as to an individual. Stress in a family is sometimes from a critically ill family member, the sudden loss of a job, a move, or becoming homeless. An example of stress in a community is a natural disaster such as a major flood or the sudden, unexpected death of a beloved teacher or teenager. Individuals experience stress and difficulty in coping, while others are also experiencing the stress in their own ways.

Subjective Findings. When assessing a client's level of stress and coping resources, create a nonthreatening physical environ-

---

BOX 31-6 NURSING ASSESSMENT QUESTIONS

Perception of Stressor
- What is bothering you most right now?
- What do you think about when you are lying awake?

Maladaptive Coping Used
- Do you live alone or with others?
- Who helps you?
- Have you started drinking or smoking?
- Has your caffiene intake increased?

Adherence to Healthy Practices
- Do you have high blood pressure?
- Have you noticed an increase or decrease in weight?
- Are you taking your prescribed medications?
- Have you increased any medications?

ment, without a desk as a barrier, for the interaction (Varcarolis and others, 2006). Assume the same height as the client, arranging the interview environment so that you can maintain or avoid eye contact comfortably. You accomplish this by placing chairs at a 90-degree angle or side by side to reduce the intensity of the interaction (Varcarolis and others, 2006). Gather information about the health status of the client from the client's perspective, and begin the process of developing a trusting relationship with the client. Use the interview to determine the client's view of the stress, coping resources, any possible maladaptive coping, and adherence to prescribed medical recommendations, such as medication or diet (Monat and Lazarus, 1991) (Box 31-6). If the client is using denial as a coping mechanism, be alert to whether the person is overlooking necessary information. As in all interactions with the client, respect the confidentiality and sensitivity of the information shared.

Objective Findings. Obtain objective findings related to stress and coping through observation of the appearance and nonverbal behavior of the client. Observe the client's grooming and hygiene, gait, characteristics of the handshake, actions while sitting, quality of speech, eye contact, and the attitude of the client during the interview. Before the interview begins or at the end of the interview, depending upon the anxiety level of the client, obtain basic vital signs to assess for physiological signs of stress such as elevated blood pressure, heart rate, or respiratory rate.

SAFETY ALERT Medical conditions such as hypoxia and thyroid dysfunction that are common in older adults initially present symptoms that mimic the consequences of stress and anxiety. For this reason, a thorough physical assessment of an older adult appearing stressed or anxious is necessary to rule out potentially serious medical disorders. In addition, it is critical to differentiate signs of stress and crisis in older adults from dementia and from acute confusion, a condition that is life threatening.

Client Expectations. A central point relating to stress is the importance of an understanding of the meaning of the precipitating event to the client and the ways in which stress is affecting the client's life. Allow time for the client to express priorities for

✳ **BOX 31-7** **NURSING DIAGNOSTIC PROCESS**

Ineffective Coping

Assessment Activities	Defining Characteristics
Ask client about change in sleeping patterns.	Sleep disturbance; difficulty falling asleep at night; sighing
Ask client to complete a sleep diary for 2 weeks.	Excessive sleeping
Observe client's behavior and response to questions during assessment.	Fatigue Inability to concentrate Inaccurate response to questions Inappropriate laugh or crying
Observe client's appearance.	Poor grooming Self-harm
Ask client about changes in eating patterns.	Weight gain or loss Lack of interest in food

coping with stress. For example, in the case of a woman who has just been told that a breast mass was identified on a routine mammogram, it is important to know what the client wants and needs most from the nurse. Although some persons in this situation identify their need for information about biopsy or mastectomy as their personal priority, other women need guidance and support in discussing how to share the news with family members. In some cases, when there is nothing that will change or improve the situation, allowing the client to use denial as a coping mechanism is helpful. Gaining an understanding of client expectations does not mean excluding certain types of care that are important simply because a client does not identify them as needs. However, by inquiring about client expectations and priorities, you will be better able to ensure that you address *all* the client's needs in some way.

◆ Nursing Diagnosis

A review of assessment data leads the nurse to cluster data that indicate a potential or actual stressor and the client's response. Clustering data, along with the application of the nurse's knowledge and experiences with clients in stress, leads to individualized nursing diagnoses (Box 31-7).

Nursing diagnoses for people experiencing stress generally focus on coping. Specifically, major defining characteristics of *ineffective coping* include verbalization of an inability to cope and an inability to ask for help. Identify defining characteristics when asking the client what is of most concern at the time of the interview and, importantly, then allowing the client sufficient time to answer. Observe for nonverbal signs of anxiety, fear, anger, irritability, and tension in a client who is experiencing ineffective coping. Other defining characteristics include the presence of life stress, an inability to meet role expectations and basic needs, alteration in societal participation, self-destructive behavior, change in usual communication patterns, high rate of accidents, excessive food intake, drinking, smoking, and sleep disturbances. Stress often results in multiple nursing diagnoses.

Examples of these diagnoses include but are not limited to the following:

- Anxiety
- Caregiver role strain
- Ineffective coping
- Fear
- Risk for post-trauma syndrome
- Insomnia
- Self-esteem disturbance

Crisis differs from stress in the degree of severity, although there are many similarities between stress and crisis. A client who perceives a situation as stressful, who is unable to cope in any ways that have worked before, and who has insufficient supports is experiencing a crisis. A crisis is devastating and requires use of all resources available (Aguilera, 1998). Unlike stress, which ends when the stressor is gone, the effects of a trauma last for years (Hyer and Sohnle, 2001).

◆ Planning

Goals and Outcomes. Desirable outcomes for persons experiencing stress may include effective coping, family coping, caregiver emotional health, and psychosocial adjustment: life change. The nurse may select interventions for stress and improved coping such as coping enhancement and crisis intervention. In addition, the nurse selects individualized interventions after considering the nursing diagnosis, the resources available to the client, and the goals identified by the client and nurse (Figure 31-4).

Nursing interventions are designed within the framework of primary, secondary, and tertiary prevention. At the primary level of prevention, you direct nursing activities to identifying individuals and populations who are possibly at risk for stress. Nursing interventions at the secondary level include actions directed at symptoms, such as protecting the client from self-harm. Tertiary-level interventions have the purpose of assisting the client in readapting and will possibly include relaxation training and time management training. According to Pender's health promotion model (Pender and others, 2006), the nurse and the client assess the level and source of the existing stress and determine the appropriate points for intervention to reduce the stress (see Care Plan).

Another method of planning care is through the use of a concept map (Figure 31-5). This concept map identifies multiple nursing diagnoses from the assessment database and shows how they are related. In this example, the nursing diagnoses are linked to the client's diagnosis of caregiver role strain. In addition, the concept map shows the relationships with the nursing diagnoses *chronic low self-esteem, ineffective coping, anxiety,* and *imbalanced nutrition: less than body requirements* (Ackley and Ladwig, 2006). Use of a concept map requires critical thinking skills to organize client data and assists in planning for client-centered care.

Just as the nursing assessment of the client's stress and coping depends on the client's perception of the problem and coping resources, the interventions focus on a partnership with the client and support system, usually the family. In the case of a family or

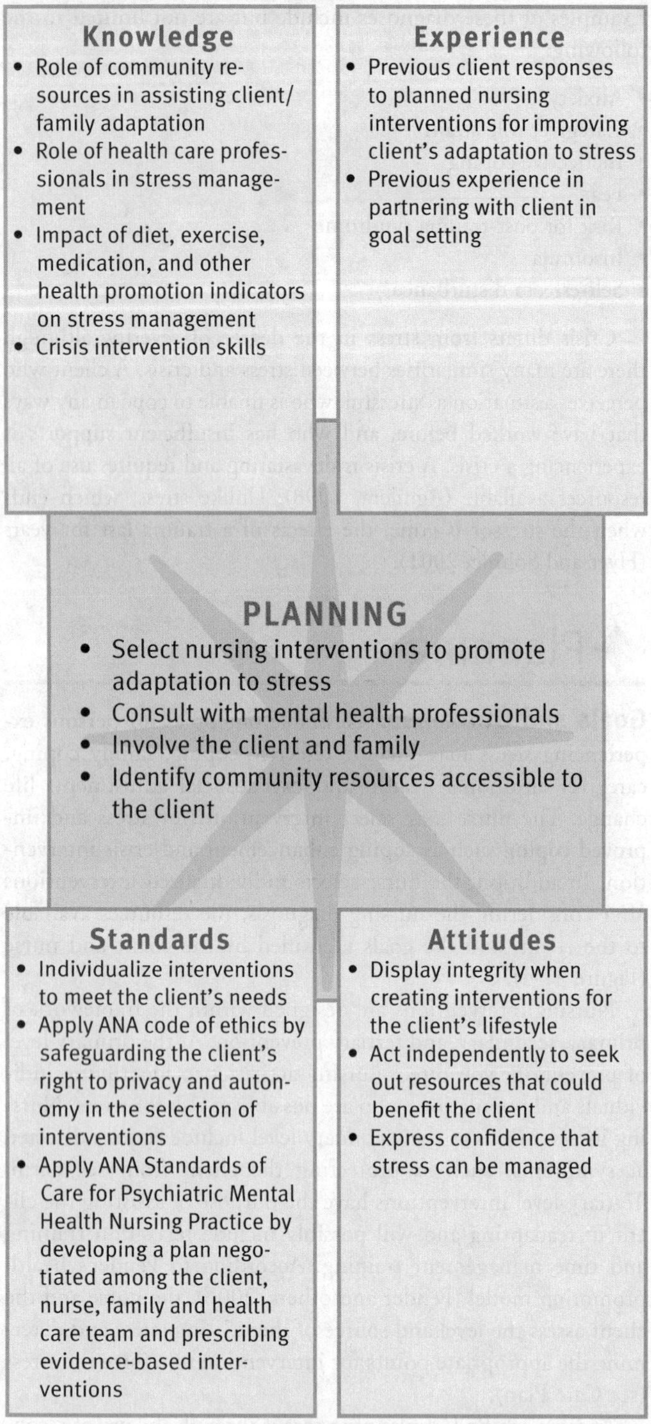

Knowledge
- Role of community resources in assisting client/family adaptation
- Role of health care professionals in stress management
- Impact of diet, exercise, medication, and other health promotion indicators on stress management
- Crisis intervention skills

Experience
- Previous client responses to planned nursing interventions for improving client's adaptation to stress
- Previous experience in partnering with client in goal setting

PLANNING
- Select nursing interventions to promote adaptation to stress
- Consult with mental health professionals
- Involve the client and family
- Identify community resources accessible to the client

Standards
- Individualize interventions to meet the client's needs
- Apply ANA code of ethics by safeguarding the client's right to privacy and autonomy in the selection of interventions
- Apply ANA Standards of Care for Psychiatric Mental Health Nursing Practice by developing a plan negotiated among the client, nurse, family and health care team and prescribing evidence-based interventions

Attitudes
- Display integrity when creating interventions for the client's lifestyle
- Act independently to seek out resources that could benefit the client
- Express confidence that stress can be managed

Figure 31-4 Critical thinking model for stress and coping planning.

community stressor and impaired family or community coping, the view of the situation and resources would be broader.

Setting Priorities. Prioritizing needs has special meaning for a person experiencing stress or crisis (see care plan). The first question to ask is, "What is happening in your life that you needed to come today?" or "What happened in your life that is *different?*" This requires some focusing by the client. Next, assess the client's

perception of the event, available situational supports, and what the person usually does when there is a problem the client cannot solve (Aguilera, 1998). As in all areas of nursing, safety of the client and others in the client's environment is the first priority.

SAFETY ALERT Determine if the person is suicidal or homicidal by asking directly. For example, ask, "Are you thinking of killing yourself or someone else?" If so, determine in a caring and concerned manner if the person has a plan and determine how lethal the means are. If suicide or homicide is not an issue, examine other potential threats to the safety of vulnerable people who are under the care of the client. Provide for their temporary care or supervision if necessary. Determine the degree of disruption in the person's life with work, school, home, and family. When you have completed immediate assessment and ensured safety, begin the problem-solving process (Aguilera, 1998).

Collaborative Care. Collaborate with occupational therapists, dietitians, pastoral care professionals, and health care professionals from other clinical specialties depending upon the client's situation. The scope of your nursing practice cannot meet all of the client's needs. Clients experiencing stress from medical conditions or psychiatric disorders will present needs that will make it necessary for you to consult with advanced practice mental health nurses, psychiatrists, psychologists, or psychiatric social workers. Such a multidisciplinary approach addresses the holistic needs of the client. In this role the nurse recognizes the need for collaboration and consultation, informs the client about potential resources, and makes arrangements for interventions, such as consultations, group sessions, or therapy as needed. A hospital social worker shares ideas for available resources both within the hospital and in the community. A home care nurse knows community services, groups, and appropriate contacts.

In addition to maximizing use of available resources for the client, collaborative care benefits the nurse as well. While working with clients experiencing stress, you will gain a broad understanding of the multitude of health care disciplines. Work becomes more satisfying for the nurse. Contacts with other members of the multidisciplinary team and the community provide a feeling of contributing to the teamwork of providing holistic care.

◆Implementation

Health Promotion. Three primary modes of intervention for stress are to decrease stress-producing situations, increase resistance to stress, and learn skills that reduce physiological response to stress (Pender and others, 2006) (Box 31-8). The nurse is in a position to educate clients and families about the importance of health promotion.

Regular Exercise. A regular exercise program improves muscle tone and posture, controls weight, reduces tension, and promotes relaxation. In addition, exercise reduces the risk of cardiovascular disease and improves cardiopulmonary functioning. Clients who have a history of a chronic illness, who are at risk for developing an illness, or who are older than 35 years of age need to begin a physical exercise program only after discussing the plan with a health care provider. In general, for a fitness program to have positive physical effects, a person needs to exercise daily for an hour (Figure 31-6).

NURSING CARE PLAN
Caregiver Role Strain

Assessment

When Janet Rich first goes to Carl's house, she finds the home in slight disarray. Carl has been providing Evelyn's care. The lawn is overgrown, there are dirty dishes in the sink, and an empty can of soup is sitting on the kitchen counter. Carl, 80, is standing in the living room folding clothes from a laundry basket, and Evelyn, Carl's wife, is watching TV. Evelyn, 81, was recently diagnosed with Alzheimer's dementia. Her health care provider has concerns about Evelyn's nutrition.

Assessment Activities	Findings/Defining Characteristics*
Ask Carl about his recent stressors and coping strategies.	He continues to fold clothes during the visit, stating, **"There's so much to do that I don't even know where to begin."** Carl describes **awakening 3 to 4 times per night** to find Evelyn wandering about. He states that he has **no outside activities,** and his children live in other states.
Observe Carl's grooming and hygiene.	Carl is **unshaven and appears disheveled.**
Ask Carl about his sleep and nutrition patterns.	Carl states that he has **lost 20 pounds in the past 6 months** and that his **appetite has been poor.**
Assess Carl's mood and affect by asking how he is feeling.	Carl states, **"I feel very tired. Everything feels overwhelming."**
Assess Carl's suicide potential.	Carl denies being suicidal.
Assess health status and health care status.	Carl **has not seen a health care provider for his own health in over a year.**

*Defining characteristics are shown in bold type.

Nursing Diagnosis: Caregiver role strain related to recent diagnosis of wife's Alzheimer's dementia.

Planning

Goal	Expected Outcomes (NOC)†
	Caregiver Physical Health
Carl will appear rested in 1 month.	Carl will verbalize approaches used to involve others in Evelyn's caregiving activities within 2 weeks.
Carl will maintain a stable weight over next 4 weeks.	Carl will reestablish normal eating pattern within 1 week.
	Caregiver Lifestyle Disruption
Carl will state that he has resumed one outside activity within 1 month.	Carl will report a balanced routine that incorporates time for own rest or relaxation within 1 week.

†Outcome classification labels from Moorhead S and others: *Nursing outcomes classification (NOC),* ed 4, St. Louis, 2008, Mosby.

Interventions (NIC)‡

Caregiver Support
- Assist Carl in establishing a consistent care routine.
- Discuss ways that Carl agrees will simplify care routine such as hiring a teenage neighbor to mow the lawn, buying frozen meals, having groceries delivered, having a cleaning service twice a month.
- Identify sources of respite care by encouraging Carl to identify available friends who assist with caregiving.

- Explore community resources such as home care, adult day care, and Meals on Wheels with Carl.
- Teach Carl stress management techniques.
- Set up monthly health checks for Carl that including vital sign and weight checks.

Rationale

Routines help simplify tasks and make them more time efficient.
Caregivers experience stress outside of their caregiving roles. Frequently, providing ways to assist the caregiver with home maintenance, meal planning, and shopping assists caregivers with stress management (Aldwin and Werner, 2007).
Successful caregiving cannot normally occur with only one caregiver. Caregiver is often hesitant to ask for help because of past family conflict (Gulanick and others, 2003).
Social support reduces caregiver stress.

Long-term stress causes physical illness.
Teaching the caregiver health maintenance strategies will sustain his own health.

‡Intervention classification labels from Bulechek GM, Butcher HK, and Dochterman JM: *Nursing interventions classification (NIC),* ed 5, St. Louis, 2008, Mosby.

Continued

NURSING CARE PLAN

Caregiver Role Strain—cont'd

Evaluation

Nursing Actions	Client Response/Finding	Achievement of Outcome
Observe for signs of fatigue.	Carl states he feels more rested and less depressed.	Carl sleeps for 6 hours at night and takes a 30-minute nap in the afternoon.
Ask Carl what other modifications he can make in his routine.	Carl buys frozen meals to use when he is busy with other caregiving.	Carl has reduced his personal expectation that he must cook every meal himself.
Ask Carl how community support is reducing his stress.	Meals on Wheels delivers lunch 5 days per week.	Carl is mobilizing community resources.
Ask Carl to compare past and present energy levels.	A neighbor mows the lawn for Carl.	Carl has improved the balance in his life.
Weigh Carl regularly.	Carl reports 5 pound weight gain in 1 month.	Carl has resumed a normal eating pattern.

CONCEPT MAP

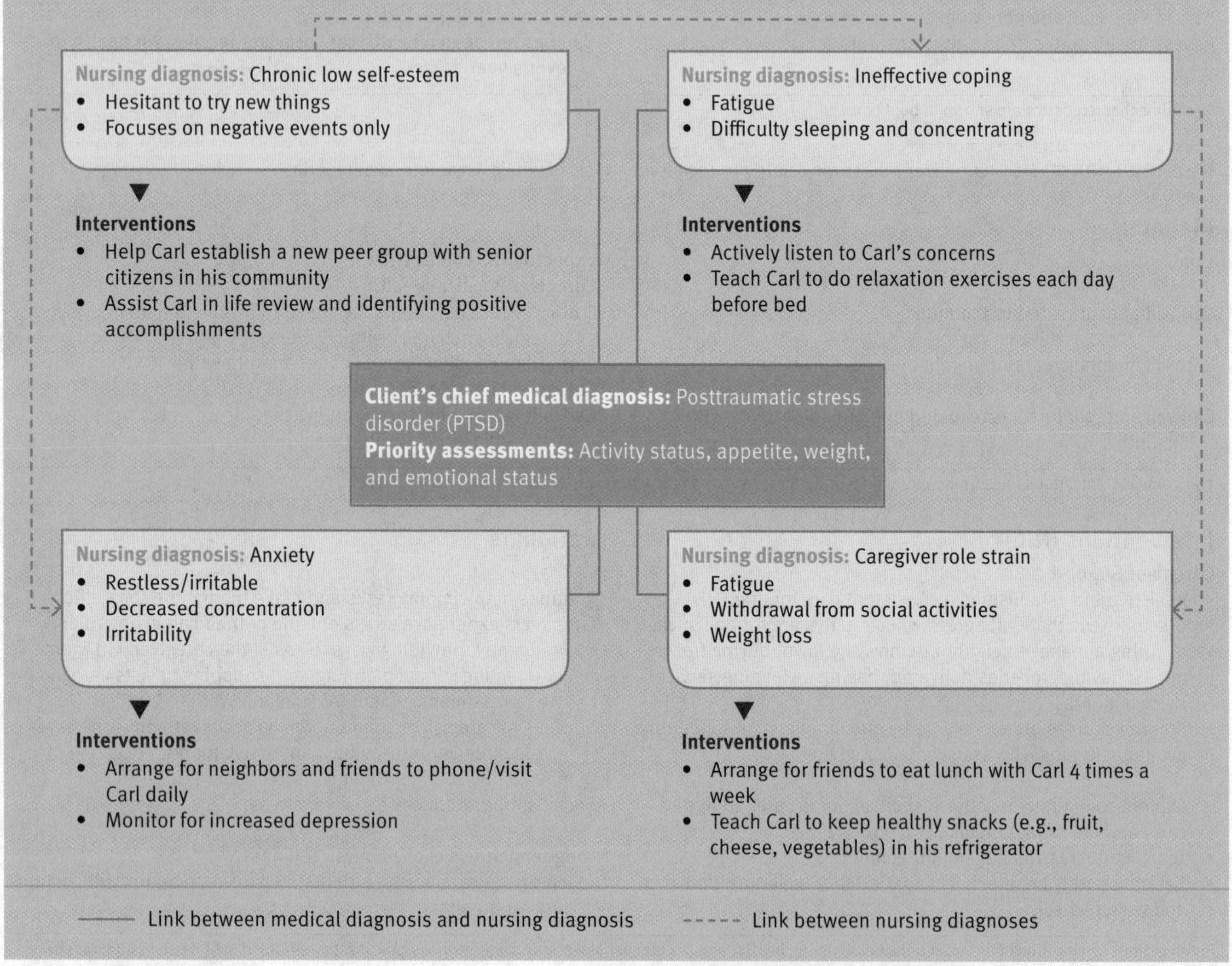

Nursing diagnosis: Chronic low self-esteem
- Hesitant to try new things
- Focuses on negative events only

Interventions
- Help Carl establish a new peer group with senior citizens in his community
- Assist Carl in life review and identifying positive accomplishments

Nursing diagnosis: Ineffective coping
- Fatigue
- Difficulty sleeping and concentrating

Interventions
- Actively listen to Carl's concerns
- Teach Carl to do relaxation exercises each day before bed

Client's chief medical diagnosis: Posttraumatic stress disorder (PTSD)
Priority assessments: Activity status, appetite, weight, and emotional status

Nursing diagnosis: Anxiety
- Restless/irritable
- Decreased concentration
- Irritability

Interventions
- Arrange for neighbors and friends to phone/visit Carl daily
- Monitor for increased depression

Nursing diagnosis: Caregiver role strain
- Fatigue
- Withdrawal from social activities
- Weight loss

Interventions
- Arrange for friends to eat lunch with Carl 4 times a week
- Teach Carl to keep healthy snacks (e.g., fruit, cheese, vegetables) in his refrigerator

——— Link between medical diagnosis and nursing diagnosis   - - - - - Link between nursing diagnoses

Figure 31-5 Concept map for Carl with caregiver role strain.

BOX 31-8   **CLIENT TEACHING**

Stress Management

Objective

- Client will report using strategies to relieve chronic stress.

Teaching Strategies

- Go to sleep 30 to 60 minutes earlier each night for a few weeks. However, sleeping later in the morning is not helpful because it disturbs body rhythms.
- Exercise for at least 30 minutes every day.
- Lower or stop caffeine intake as found in coffee, tea, and soda.
- Listen to music that you enjoy.
- Consider whether or not having a pet would reduce stress by providing social support.
- Have a massage.
- Keep a journal of your thoughts and feelings.
- Replace time-consuming activities that are not necessary with activities that are pleasurable or interesting.
- Look for the humor in a stressful situation.
- Use meditation, guided imagery, or yoga for deep relaxation.

Evaluation

- Observe client for signs of stress.
- Ask client to keep a record of hours of sleep.
- Ask client to list participation in activities that are soothing or enjoyable.

Data from Varcarolis EM, Carson VB, Shoemaker NC: *Foundations of psychiatric mental health nursing: a clinical approach,* ed 5, St. Louis, Saunders Elsevier, 2006.

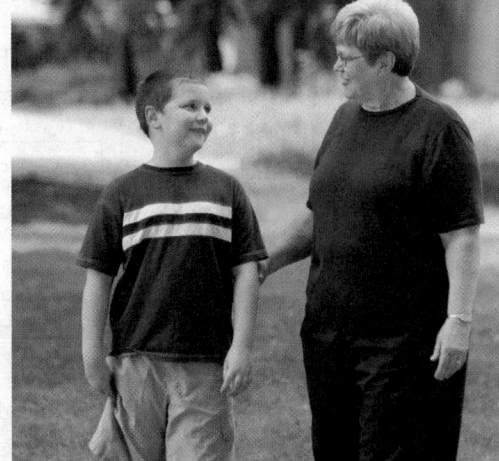

Figure 31-6 Regular exercise assists in coping with stress.

Support Systems. A support system of family, friends, and colleagues who will listen, offer advice, and provide emotional support benefits a client experiencing stress. There are many support groups available to individuals, such as those sponsored by the American Heart Association, the American Cancer Society, local hospitals and churches, and mental health organizations.

Time Management. Time management techniques include developing lists of prioritized tasks. For example, list those tasks that require immediate attention, those that are important and can be delayed, and those tasks that are routine and can be accomplished when time becomes available. In many cases setting priorities helps individuals identify tasks that are not necessary or perhaps tasks to delegate to someone else.

Guided Imagery and Visualization. Guided imagery is based on the belief that a person significantly reduces stress with imagination. Guided imagery is a relaxed state in which a person actively uses imagination in a way that allows visualization of a soothing, peaceful setting. Typically the image created or suggested uses many sensory words to engage the mind and offer distraction and relaxation.

Progressive Muscle Relaxation. In the presence of anxiety-provoking thoughts and events, a common physiological symptom is muscle tension. You diminish physiological tension through a systematic approach to releasing tension in major muscle groups. Typically an individual achieves a relaxed state through deep chest breathing. Once the client is breathing deeply, you direct the client to alternately tighten and relax muscles in specific groupings.

Assertiveness Training. Assertiveness comprises skills for helping individuals communicate effectively regarding their needs and desires. The ability to resolve conflict with others through assertiveness training is important for reducing stress. Teaching assertiveness in a group setting increases the benefits of the experience.

Journal Writing. For many people, keeping a private, personal journal provides a therapeutic outlet for stress, and it is well within the realm of nursing to suggest journal keeping to clients experiencing difficult situations. In a private journal, clients are able to express a full range of emotion and vent their honest feelings without hurting anyone's feelings and without concern for how they appear to others.

Stress Management in the Workplace. Rapid changes in health care technology, diversity in the workforce, organizational restructuring, and changing work systems place stress on nurses. **Burnout** occurs as a result of chronic stress. Burnout is "a syndrome of emotional exhaustion, depersonalization of others, and perceptions of reduced personal accomplishment, resulting from intense involvement with people in a care-giving environment" (Aguilera, 1998).

If you recognize feelings of burnout, you can make changes in your behavior to cope with workplace stress. An important step is identifying the limits and scope of your responsibilities at work (Aguilera, 1998). Recognizing the areas over which you have control and can change and those that you do not have responsibility for is a vital insight. Making a clear separation between work and home life is crucial as well. Strengthening friendships outside of the workplace, arranging for temporary social isolation for personal "recharging" of emotional energy, and spending off-duty hours in interesting activities all help reduce burnout.

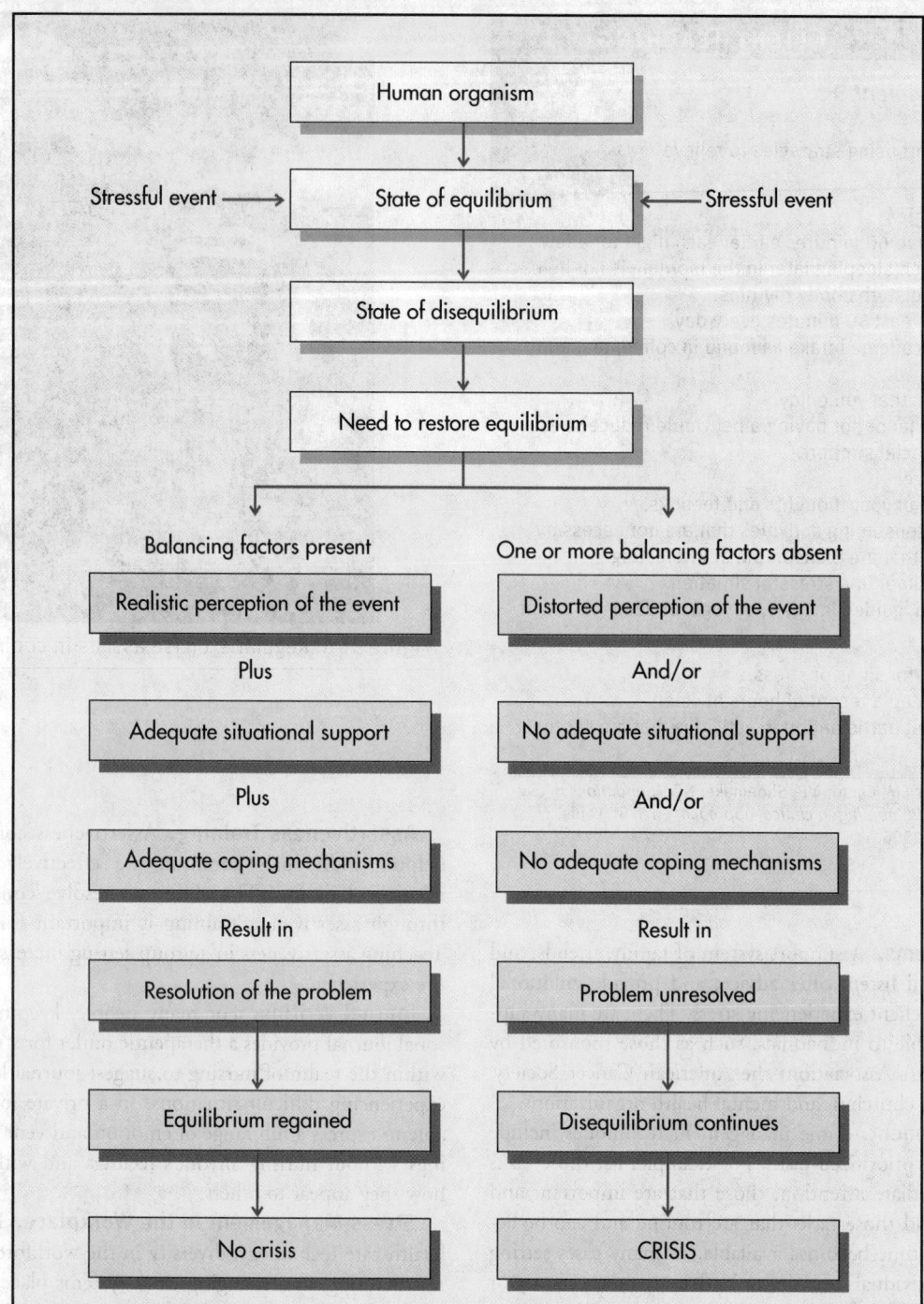

Figure 31-7 Crisis intervention model. (Redrawn from Aguilera DC: *Crisis intervention: theory and methodology,* ed 8, St. Louis, 1998, Mosby.)

Acute Care
Crisis Intervention. When stress overwhelms a person's usual coping mechanisms and demands mobilization of all available resources, it becomes a crisis (Aguilera, 1998). A crisis creates a turning point in a person's life because it changes the direction of a person's life in some way. According to Aguilera (1998), the precipitating event usually occurs from 1 to 2 weeks before the individual seeks help, but sometimes it has occurred within the

past 24 hours. Generally a person resolves the crisis in some way within approximately 6 weeks. Crisis intervention aims to return the person to a precrisis level of functioning and to promote growth (Figure 31-7).

Because an individual's or family's usual coping strategies are ineffective in managing the stress of the precipitating event, the use of new coping mechanisms is necessary. This experience, which forces the use of unfamiliar strategies, results either in a heightened awareness of previously unrecognized strengths and resources or in deterioration in functioning. Thus a crisis is often referred to as a situation of both danger and opportunity. Some persons or families will emerge from a crisis state functioning more effectively, whereas others find themselves weakened, and still others completely dysfunctional.

Crisis intervention is a specific type of brief psychotherapy with prescribed steps (Aguilera, 1998). Crisis intervention is more directive than traditional psychotherapy or counseling, and any member of the health care team who has been trained in its techniques can use it. The basic approach is problem solving and focuses only on the problem presented by the crisis.

When using a crisis intervention approach, the nurse helps the client make the mental connection between the stressful event and the client's reaction to it. This is crucial because the person is sometimes unable to see the whole situation clearly. The nurse also helps the person become aware of present feelings, such as anger, grief, or guilt, to help the individual reduce feelings of tension. In addition, the nurse helps the client explore coping mechanisms, perhaps identifying new methods of coping. Finally, the nurse needs to help increase the scope of the person's social contacts if the person had been internally focused and isolated (Aguilera, 1998).

Restorative and Continuing Care. A person under stress recovers when the stress is removed or coping strategies are successful; however, a person who has experienced a crisis has changed, and the effects often last for years or for the rest of the person's life. The final stage of adapting to a crisis is acknowledgment of the long-term implications of the crisis. If a person has successfully coped with a crisis and its consequences, he or she becomes a more mature and healthy person. When a person has recovered from a stressful situation, the time is right for introducing stress management skills to reduce the number and intensity of stressful situations in the future.

◆ Evaluation

A client recovering from acute stress often spontaneously reports feeling better when the stressor is gone. The recovery from chronic stress occurs more gradually as the client emerges from the strain. In either situation, reassess the client for the presence of new or recurring stress-related symptoms (Figure 31-8). Observe client behaviors, and talk with the client and family, if appropriate. Ask the client about sleep patterns, appetite, and ability to concentrate. Ask about coping strategies that the client uses effectively. Ask the client to compare his or her current feelings and behaviors with feelings and behaviors 6 months ago. If desired outcomes have been met, the client will report feeling better now than 6 months ago.

Remember that coping with stress takes time. Maintain ongoing communication with clients regarding their coping. Clients under severe stress, or trauma, often experience feelings of powerlessness, vulnerability, and loss of control. The nurse addresses these feelings by actively involving clients and families in the process of problem identification (assessment), prioritizing, and

Knowledge
- Characteristics of adaptive behaviors
- Characteristics of continuing stress response
- Differentiation of stress and trauma

Experience
- Previous client responses to planned nursing interventions

EVALUATION
- Reassess the client for the presence of new or recurring stress-related problems or symptoms
- Determine if change in care promoted the client's adaptation to stress
- Ask if the client's expectations are being met

Standards
- Use established expected outcomes to evaluate the client's response to care (e.g., return to normal sleep pattern)
- Apply the intellectual standard of relevance; be sure the client achieves goals relevant to his or her needs

Attitudes
- Demonstrate perseverance in redesigning interventions to promote the client's adaptation to stress
- Display integrity in accurately evaluating nursing interventions

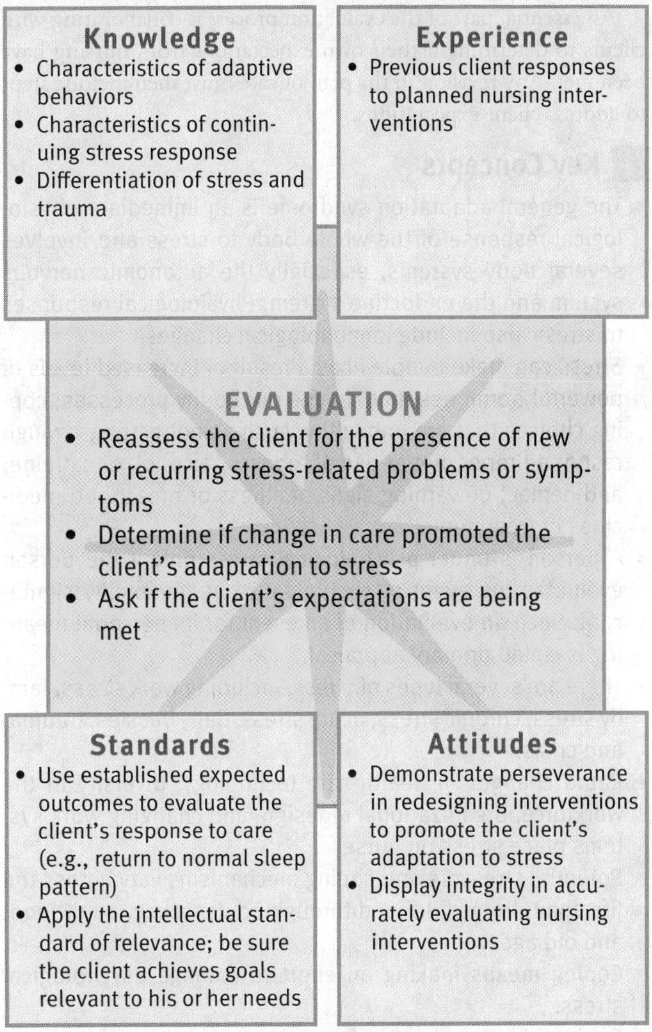

Figure 31-8 Critical thinking model for stress and coping evaluation.

goal setting and evaluation. Involving clients in these processes gives them an opportunity to direct their energy in a positive way and moves them toward taking greater responsibility for health maintenance and promotion.

Engaging the client as a partner in health care sets the stage for open communication. In such an environment the client will feel more freedom to give important feedback about interventions that are successful and will help the nurse better understand why some interventions fail to meet the established goals. If the client reports continued acute stress, assess for safety by asking about whether or not there have been any recent accidents at home, in the car, or at work. Ask about coping strategies to determine if the client is using unsafe, maladaptive strategies. If the client reports continued chronic stress, ask about the client's perception of the stressor and coping behaviors used. Discuss the stressor with the client to determine if the stressor needs to be redefined. If contact with a client must end before you have achieved the resolution of goals, it is important to refer clients to appropriate resources so that progress is not delayed or interrupted.

An essential part of the evaluation process is collaborating with clients to determine if their own expectations from nursing have been met. Any revision in the plan of care must then include steps to address client expectations.

✳ Key Concepts

- The general adaptation syndrome is an immediate physiological response of the whole body to stress and involves several body systems, especially the autonomic nervous system and the endocrine system. Physiological responses to stress also include immunological changes.
- Stress can make people ill as a result of increased levels of powerful hormones that change our bodily processes; coping choices that are unhealthy, such as not getting enough rest or a proper diet or use of tobacco, alcohol, or caffeine; and neglect of warning signs of illness or prescribed medicines or treatments.
- A person is under psychological stress only if the person evaluates the event or circumstance as personally significant. Such an evaluation of an event for its personal meaning is called primary appraisal.
- There are several types of stress, including work stress, family stress, chronic stress, acute stress, daily hassles, trauma, and crisis.
- Rapid changes in health care technology, diversity in the workforce, organizational redesign, and changing work systems place stress on nurses.
- Potential stressors and coping mechanisms vary across the life span, from childhood through adolescence, adulthood, and old age.
- Coping means making an effort to manage psychological stress.
- Coping is a process that is constantly changing to manage demands on a person's resources.
- Three primary modes for stress intervention are to decrease stress-producing situations, increase resistance to stress, and learn skills that reduce physiological response to stress.
- A client whose stress is so severe that the person is unable to cope in any ways that have worked before is experiencing a crisis.
- A crisis is a turning point in life and is either developmental or situational.
- Generally a crisis is resolved in some way within approximately 6 weeks. Crisis intervention aims to return the person to a precrisis level of functioning and to promote growth.

✳ Critical Thinking Exercises

1. You are making a home visit to see 80-year-old Carl and 81-year-old Evelyn because Evelyn has Alzheimer's dementia and her health care provider is concerned about her nutrition. He also wants to know if she is taking her medications. Carl has been providing Evelyn's care, and he is also worried about his own health. Discuss the various stressors that will need to be considered when assessing their situation.

2. Carl reports dizziness, but you do not identify any physical findings, based on your thorough assessment, that would account for this. As you talk with Carl, he tells you that his life is very stressful and he is barely coping. He is the sole caregiver for his wife, Evelyn, who has dementia. He is worried about what might happen to her if his health failed. He has not been able to play golf with his friends or go to church in months. His only social activity is a trip to the grocery store while his neighbor stays with Evelyn. He is worried that they will spend all their life savings if she needs to go to a nursing home, and he loses his patience with her. Develop nursing diagnoses related to this situation.

3. Carl is admitted to the hospital with a fractured hip sustained from a fall when he got up during the night to check on his wife, Evelyn, who was wandering in the house. Before his injury he cared for Evelyn, who suffers from advancing Alzheimer's disease. While he is hospitalized, Evelyn is staying with a niece who lives 100 miles away, but this cannot be a permanent situation because their niece is also in frail health. Carl and Evelyn's children live across the country and are very involved in their careers. He is concerned about who will care for them. What approach would be the best to take in establishing goals for treatment?

✳ NCLEX®-Style Review Questions

1. The vital functions necessary for survival, which include heart rate, blood pressure, and respiration, are controlled by the:
   1. Adrenal gland
   2. Pituitary gland
   3. Medulla oblongata
   4. Reticular formation

2. While assessing a person for effects of the general adaptation syndrome, the nurse should be aware that:
   1. Heart rate increases in the resistance state
   2. Blood volume increases in the exhaustion stage
   3. Vital signs return to normal in the exhaustion stage
   4. Blood glucose level increases during the alarm reaction stage

3. A client avoids emotional conflict by refusing to consciously acknowledge anything that might cause intolerable emotional pain. The client is using the defense mechanism:
   1. Denial
   2. Conversion
   3. Dissociation
   4. Displacement

4. When doing an assessment of a young woman who was in an automobile accident 6 months before, the nurse learns that the woman has vivid images of the crash whenever she hears a loud, sudden noise. The nurse recognizes this as:
   1. Acute anxiety
   2. Social phobia

3. Posttraumatic stress disorder
4. Borderline personality disorder

5. A man is adjusting to chronic illness; this is an example of:
   1. A situational factor
   2. A maturational factor
   3. A sociocultural factor
   4. A developmental factor

6. A child who has been in a house fire comes to the emergency department with her parents. The child and parents are upset and tearful. During the nurse's first assessment for stress she should say:
   1. "Tell me whom I can call to help you."
   2. "Tell me what bothers you the most about this experience."
   3. "I will contact someone who can help get you temporary housing."
   4. "I will sit with you until other family members can come help you get settled."

7. The nurse is evaluating the coping success of a client experiencing stress from being newly diagnosed with multiple sclerosis and psychomotor impairment. The nurse realizes that the client is coping successfully when the client says:
   1. "I am going to learn to drive a car so I can be more independent."
   2. "My sister says she feels better when she goes shopping, so I will go shopping."
   3. "I have always felt better when I go for a long walk. I will do that when I get home."
   4. "I am going to attend a support group to learn more about multiple sclerosis and what I will be able to do."

8. A client newly diagnosed with type 2 diabetes exhibits denial when she says, "My blood sugar was just a little high. I don't have diabetes." The nurse responds:
   1. "Let's talk about something cheerful."
   2. "Do other members of your family have diabetes?"
   3. "I can tell that you feel stressed to learn that you have diabetes."
   4. With silence; the nurse understands the denial is a defense mechanism that assists in coping with a shock.

9. A staff nurse is talking with her nursing supervisor about the stress she feels on the job. The supervising nurse recognizes that:
   1. Nurses who feel stress usually pass the stress along to their clients
   2. A nurse who feels stress is ineffective as a nurse and should not be working
   3. Nurses who talk about feeling stress are unprofessional and should calm down
   4. Nurses frequently experience stress with the rapid changes in health care technology and organizational restructuring

10. Generally a person's crisis is resolved in some way within approximately:
    1. 2 weeks
    2. 6 weeks
    3. 1 month
    4. 6 months

32 | Vital Signs

✳ OBJECTIVES

Mastery of content in this chapter will enable the student to:

- Explain the principles and mechanisms of thermoregulation.
- Describe nursing measures that promote heat loss and heat conservation.
- Discuss physiological changes associated with fever.
- Accurately assess tympanic, oral, rectal, and axillary temperatures.
- Accurately assess pulse, respirations, oxygen saturation, and blood pressure.
- Explain the physiology of normal regulation of blood pressure, pulse, oxygen saturation, and respirations.
- Describe factors that cause variations in body temperature, pulse, oxygen saturation, respirations, and blood pressure.

- Describe cultural and ethnic variations with blood pressure assessment.
- Identify ranges of acceptable vital sign values for an infant, a child, and an adult.
- Explain variations in technique used to assess an infant's, a child's, and an adult's vital signs.
- Describe the benefits and precautions involving self-measurement of blood pressure.
- Identify when to take vital signs.
- Accurately record and report vital sign measurements.
- Appropriately delegate vital sign measurement.

✳ MEDIA RESOURCES   ✳ KEY TERMS

 Companion CD
- NCLEX®-Style Review Questions
- Audio Glossary
- Interactive Learning Activities
- English/Spanish Glossary

 Website
- NCLEX®-Style Review Questions
- Audio Glossary
- English/Spanish Glossary
- Interactive Learning Activities
- Weblinks
- Audio Summaries
- Video Clips
- Nursing Skills Online

Afebrile, p. 507
Antipyretics, p. 518
Auscultatory gap, p. 545
Basal metabolic rate (BMR), p. 504
Blood pressure, p. 536
Bradycardia, p. 527
Cardiac output, p. 520
Celsius, p. 509
Conduction, p. 505
Convection, p. 505
Core temperature, p. 504
Diaphoresis, p. 505
Diastolic pressure, p. 536
Diffusion, p. 528
Dysrhythmia, p. 527
Eupnea, p. 529
Evaporation, p. 505
Fahrenheit, p. 509

Febrile, p. 507
Fever, p. 507
Fever of unknown origin (FUO), p. 507
Frostbite, p. 508
Heat exhaustion, p. 508
Heatstroke, p. 508
Hematocrit, p. 536
Hypertension, p. 537
Hyperthermia, p.507
Hypotension, p. 538
Hypothalamus, p. 504
Hypothermia, p. 508
Hypoxemia, p. 528
Malignant hyperthermia, p. 507
Nonshivering thermogenesis, p. 505

Orthostatic hypotension, p. 538
Perfusion, p. 528
Postural hypotension, p. 538
Pulse deficit, p. 527
Pulse pressure, p. 536
Pyrexia, p. 507
Pyrogens, p. 507
Radial pulse, p. 521
Radiation, p. 505
Shivering, p. 505
Sphygmomanometer, p. 543
Systolic pressure, p. 536
Tachycardia, p. 527
Thermoregulation, p. 504
Ventilation, p. 528
Vital signs, p. 503

The most frequent measurements obtained by health care providers are those of temperature, pulse, blood pressure (BP), respiratory rate, and oxygen saturation. As indicators of health status, these measures indicate the effectiveness of circulatory, respiratory, neural, and endocrine body functions. Because of their importance they are referred to as **vital signs.** Pain, a subjective symptom, is also a vital sign that is frequently measured along with vital signs (see Chapter 43). Measurement of vital signs provides data to determine a client's usual state of health (baseline data). Many factors, such as the temperature of the environment, the client's physical exertion, and the effects of illness, cause vital signs to change, sometimes outside an acceptable range. A change in vital signs indicates a change in physiological function. Assessment of vital signs provides data to identify nursing diagnoses, to implement planned interventions, and to evaluate outcomes of care. An alteration in vital signs signals the need for medical or nursing intervention.

Vital signs are a quick and efficient way of monitoring a client's condition or identifying problems and evaluating the client's response to intervention. When you learn the physiological variables influencing vital signs and recognize the relationship of vital sign changes to other physical assessment findings, you can make precise determinations of the client's health problems. You use the basic techniques of inspection, palpation, and auscultation to obtain vital signs. These skills are simple, but do not take them for granted. Careful measurement techniques ensure accurate findings. Vital signs and other physiological measurements are the basis for clinical problem solving.

Guidelines for Measuring Vital Signs

Vital signs are a part of the assessment database (Box 32-1). You include vital signs in a complete physical assessment (see Chapter 33), or obtain them individually to assess a client's condition. Establishing a database of vital signs during a routine physical examination serves as a baseline for future assessments. The client's needs and condition determine when, where, how, and by whom vital signs are measured. You need to be able to measure vital signs correctly or appropriately delegate the measurement of vital signs. When obtaining vital signs, you need to understand and interpret the values, communicate findings appropriately, and begin interventions as needed. Use the following guidelines to incorporate vital sign measurements into nursing practice:

- The nurse caring for the client is responsible for vital sign measurement. You may delegate measurement of selected vital signs (i.e., in stable clients). However, you need to analyze the vital signs to interpret their significance and make decisions about interventions.
- Make sure equipment is functional and appropriate for the size and the age of the client. Equipment used to measure vital signs (e.g., a thermometer) needs to work properly to ensure accurate findings.

✳ BOX 32-1 Vital Signs: Acceptable Ranges for Adults

Temperature Range: 36° to 38° C (96.8° to 100.4° F)
Average oral/tympanic: 37° C (98.6° F)
Average rectal: 37.5° C (99.5° F)
Average axillary: 36.5° C (97.7° F)

Pulse
60 to 100 beats per minute

Respirations
12 to 20 breaths per minute

Blood Pressure
Average: <120/80
Pulse pressure: 30 to 50 mm Hg

- Select equipment based on the client's condition and characteristics (e.g., do not use an adult-size blood pressure cuff for a child).
- Know the client's usual range of vital signs. A client's usual values often differ from the acceptable range for that age or physical state. The client's usual values serve as a baseline for comparison with later findings. Thus you are able to detect a change in condition over time.
- Learn the client's medical history, therapies, and prescribed medications. Some illnesses or treatments cause predictable vital sign changes. Some medications affect one or more of the vital signs.
- Control or minimize environmental factors that affect vital signs. For example, assessing the client's temperature in a warm, humid room may yield a value that is not a true indicator of the client's condition.
- Use an organized, systematic approach when taking vital signs. Each procedure requires a step-by-step approach to ensure accuracy.
- Based on the client's condition, collaborate with health care providers to decide the frequency of vital sign assessment. In the hospital, the health care provider will order a minimum frequency of vital sign measurements for each client. Following surgery or treatment intervention, you measure vital signs more frequently to detect complications. In a clinic or outpatient setting, you take vital signs before the health care provider examines the client and after any invasive procedures. As a client's physical condition worsens, it is often necessary to monitor vital signs as often as every 5 to 10 minutes. The nurse is responsible for judging whether more frequent assessments are necessary (Box 32-2).
- Use vital sign measurements to determine indications for medication administration. For example, you give certain cardiac drugs only within a range of pulse or blood pressure values. Administer antipyretics when temperature is elevated outside of the acceptable range for the client. Do not administer these drugs if the vital sign assessment indicates the measurements are within the specified acceptable range.
- Analyze the results of vital sign measurement. Vital signs are not interpreted in isolation. You need to also know related physical signs or symptoms and be aware of the client's ongoing health status.

✳ **BOX 32-2 When to Measure Vital Signs**

- On admission to a health care facility
- When assessing the client during home care visits
- In a hospital on a routine schedule according to the health care provider's order or the hospital's standards of practice
- Before and after a surgical procedure or invasive diagnostic procedure
- Before, during, and after a transfusion of blood products
- Before, during, and after the administration of medication or therapies that affect cardiovascular, respiratory, or temperature-control functions
- When the client's general physical condition changes (e.g., loss of consciousness or increased intensity of pain)
- Before and after nursing interventions influencing a vital sign (e.g., before a client previously on bed rest ambulates or before a client performs range-of-motion exercises)
- When the client reports nonspecific symptoms of physical distress (e.g., feeling "funny" or "different")

- Verify and communicate significant changes in vital signs. Document vital signs, and communicate information to the client's caregivers. Baseline measurements allow a nurse to identify changes in vital signs. When vital signs appear abnormal, it helps to have another nurse or health care provider repeat the measurement. Inform the health care provider or nurse in charge of abnormal vital signs.
- Develop a teaching plan to instruct the client or caregiver in vital sign assessment and the significance of findings.

Body Temperature

Physiology

The body temperature is the difference between the amount of heat produced by body processes and the amount of heat lost to the external environment.

$$\text{Heat produced} - \text{Heat lost} = \text{Body temperature}$$

Despite extremes in environmental conditions and physical activity, temperature-control mechanisms of human beings keep the body's **core temperature** (temperature of the deep tissues) relatively constant (Figure 32-1). However, surface temperature varies depending on blood flow to the skin and the amount of heat lost to the external environment. Because of these surface temperature changes, the acceptable temperature of human beings ranges from 36° to 38° C (96.8° to 100.4° F). The body's tissues and cells function best within the relatively narrow temperature range.

The site of temperature measurement (oral, rectal, axillary, tympanic membrane, temporal artery, esophageal, pulmonary artery, or even urinary bladder) is one factor that determines the client's temperature. For healthy young adults the average oral temperature is 37° C (98.6° F). In clinical practice, you will learn the temperature range of individual clients. No single temperature is normal for all people.

The measurement of body temperature aims to obtain a representative average temperature of core body tissues. Sites reflecting core temperatures are more reliable indicators of body temperature than sites reflecting surface temperatures (Box 32-3). In addition, the temperature value obtained often differs depending on the measurement site.

Regulation. Physiological and behavioral mechanisms regulate the balance between heat lost and heat produced, or **thermoregulation.** For the body temperature to stay constant and within an acceptable range, body mechanisms must maintain the relationship between heat production and heat loss. This relationship is regulated by neurological and cardiovascular mechanisms. Apply knowledge of temperature-control mechanisms to promote temperature regulation.

Neural and Vascular Control. The **hypothalamus,** located between the cerebral hemispheres, controls body temperature the same way a thermostat works in the home. A comfortable temperature is the "set point" at which a heating system operates. In the home a fall in environmental temperature activates the furnace, whereas a rise in temperature shuts the system down.

The hypothalamus senses minor changes in body temperature. The anterior hypothalamus controls heat loss, and the posterior hypothalamus controls heat production. When nerve cells in the anterior hypothalamus become heated beyond the set point, impulses are sent out to reduce body temperature. Mechanisms of heat loss include sweating, vasodilation (widening) of blood vessels, and inhibition of heat production. The body redistributes blood to surface vessels to promote heat loss.

If the posterior hypothalamus senses the body's temperature is lower than the set point, the body initiates heat conservation mechanisms. Vasoconstriction (narrowing) of blood vessels reduces blood flow to the skin and extremities. Compensatory heat production is stimulated through voluntary muscle contraction and muscle shivering. When vasoconstriction is ineffective in preventing additional heat loss, shivering begins. Disease or trauma to the hypothalamus or to the spinal cord, which carries hypothalamic messages, causes serious alterations in temperature control.

Heat Production. Thermoregulation depends on the normal function of heat production processes. Heat produced by the body is a by-product of metabolism, which is the chemical reaction in all body cells. Food is the primary fuel source for metabolism. Activities requiring additional chemical reactions increase the metabolic rate. As metabolism increases, additional heat is produced. When metabolism decreases, less heat is produced. Heat production occurs during rest, voluntary movements, involuntary shivering, and nonshivering thermogenesis.

- Basal metabolism accounts for the heat produced by the body at absolute rest. The average **basal metabolic rate (BMR)** depends on the body surface area. Thyroid hormones also affect the BMR. By promoting the breakdown of body glucose and fat, thyroid hormones increase the rate of chemical reactions in almost all cells of the body. When large amounts of thyroid hormones are secreted, the BMR can increase 100% above normal. Absence of thyroid hormones cut the BMR in half, causing a decrease in heat production. The male sex hormone testosterone increases BMR. Men have a higher BMR than women.
- Voluntary movements such as muscular activity during exercise require additional energy. The metabolic rate increases

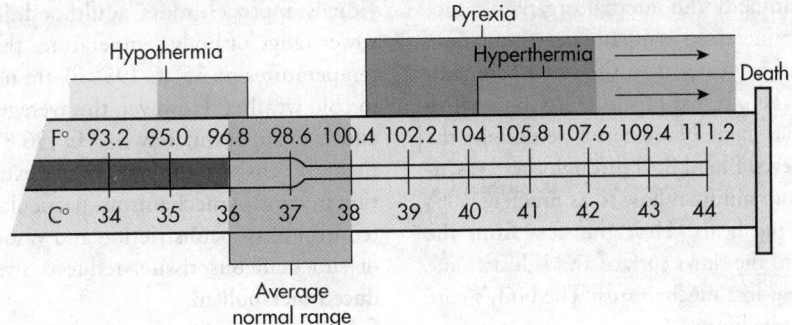

Figure 32-1 Ranges of normal temperature values and physiological consequences of abnormal body temperature.

✳ BOX 32-3 Core and Surface Temperature Measurement Sites

Core Temperature	Surface Temperature
Rectum	Skin
Tympanic membrane	Oral
Temporal artery	Axillae
Esophagus	
Pulmonary artery	
Urinary bladder	

during activity, sometimes causing heat production to increase up to 50 times normal.

- **Shivering** is an involuntary body response to temperature differences in the body. The skeletal muscle movement during shivering requires significant energy. Shivering sometimes increases heat production 4 to 5 times greater than normal. The heat that is produced assists in equalizing the body temperature, and the shivering ceases. In vulnerable clients shivering seriously drains energy sources, resulting in further physiological deterioration.
- **Nonshivering thermogenesis** occurs primarily in neonates. Because neonates cannot shiver, a limited amount of vascular brown tissue, present at birth, is metabolized for heat production.

Heat Loss. Heat loss and heat production occur simultaneously. The skin's structure and exposure to the environment result in constant, normal heat loss through radiation, conduction, convection, and evaporation.

Radiation is the transfer of heat from the surface of one object to the surface of another without direct contact between the two. Up to 85% of the human body's surface area radiates heat to the environment. Peripheral vasodilation increases blood flow from the internal organs to the skin to increase radiant heat loss. Peripheral vasoconstriction minimizes radiant heat loss. Radiation increases as the temperature difference between the objects increases. However, if the environment is warmer than the skin, the body absorbs heat through radiation.

The client's position enhances radiation heat loss (e.g., standing exposes a greater radiating surface area and lying in a fetal position minimizes heat radiation). Help promote heat loss through radiation by removing clothing or blankets. Covering the body with dark, closely woven clothing decreases the amount of heat lost from radiation.

Conduction is the transfer of heat from one object to another with direct contact. Solids, liquids, and gases conduct heat through contact. When the warm skin touches a cooler object, heat is lost. Conduction normally accounts for a small amount of heat loss. Applying an ice pack or bathing a client with a cool cloth increases conductive heat loss. Applying several layers of clothing reduces conductive loss. The body gains heat by conduction when it makes contact with materials warmer than skin temperature (e.g., application of an aquathermia pad).

Convection is the transfer of heat away by air movement. A fan promotes heat loss through convection. Convective heat loss increases when moistened skin comes into contact with slightly moving air.

Evaporation is the transfer of heat energy when a liquid is changed to a gas. The body continuously loses heat by evaporation. About 600 to 900 mL a day evaporates from the skin and lungs, resulting in water and heat loss. By regulating perspiration or sweating, the body promotes additional evaporative heat loss. When body temperature rises, the anterior hypothalamus signals the sweat glands to release sweat through tiny ducts on the skin's surface. Sweat evaporates, resulting in heat loss. During exercise and emotional or mental stress, sweating is one way to lose excessive heat produced by the increased metabolic rate. **Diaphoresis** is visible perspiration primarily occurring on the forehead and upper thorax, though you can see it in other places on the body. Excessive evaporation causes skin scaling and itching, as well as drying of the nares and pharynx. A lowered body temperature inhibits sweat gland secretion. People who have a congenital absence of sweat glands or a serious skin disease that impairs sweating are unable to tolerate warm temperatures because they cannot cool themselves adequately.

Skin in Temperature Regulation. The skin regulates temperature through insulation of the body, vasoconstriction (which affects the amount of blood flow and heat loss to the skin), and temperature sensation. The skin, subcutaneous tissue, and fat keep heat inside the body. Persons with more body fat have more natural insulation than do slim and muscular people.

The way the skin controls body temperature is similar to the way an automobile radiator controls engine temperature. The engine of an automobile generates a great deal of heat. Water is pumped through the engine's system to collect the heat and carry it to the radiator, where a fan transfers the heat from the water to the outside air. In the human body the internal organs produce heat, and during exercise or increased sympathetic stimulation, the amount of heat produced is greater than the usual core temperature. Blood flows from the internal organs, carrying heat to the body surface. The skin has many blood vessels, especially the areas of the hands, feet, and ears. Blood flow through these vascular areas of the skin varies from minimal flow to as much as 30% of the blood ejected from the heart. Heat transfers from the blood, through vessel walls, to the skin's surface and is lost to the environment through the heat-loss mechanisms. The body's core temperature remains within safe limits.

The degree of vasoconstriction determines the amount of blood flow and heat loss to the skin. If the core temperature is too high, the hypothalamus inhibits vasoconstriction. As a result, blood vessels dilate, and more blood reaches the skin's surface. On a hot, humid day the blood vessels in the hands are dilated and easily visible. In contrast, if the core temperature becomes too low, the hypothalamus initiates vasoconstriction and blood flow to the skin lessens. Thus body heat is conserved.

Behavioral Control. Healthy individuals are able to maintain comfortable body temperature when exposed to temperature extremes. The ability of a person to control body temperature depends on (1) the degree of temperature extreme, (2) the person's ability to sense feeling comfortable or uncomfortable, (3) thought processes or emotions, and (4) the person's mobility or ability to remove or add clothes. Individuals are unable to control body temperature if any of these abilities are lost. For example, infants are able to sense uncomfortable warm conditions but need assistance in changing their environment. Older adults sometimes need help in detecting cold environments and minimizing heat loss. Illness, a decreased level of consciousness, or impaired thought processes result in an inability to recognize the need to change behavior for temperature control. When temperatures become extremely hot or cold, health-promoting behaviors, such as removing or adding clothing, have a limited effect on controlling temperature. Assess for factors that place clients at high risk for ineffective thermoregulation.

Factors Affecting Body Temperature

Many factors affect body temperature. Changes in body temperature within an acceptable range occur when physiological or behavioral mechanisms alter the relationship between heat production and heat loss. Be aware of these factors when assessing temperature variations and evaluating deviations from normal.

Age. At birth the newborn leaves a warm, relatively constant environment and enters one in which temperatures fluctuate widely. Temperature-control mechanisms are immature. An infant's temperature responds drastically to changes in the environment. Take extra care to protect the newborn from environmental temperatures. Clothing needs to be adequate, and the infant's exposure to temperature extremes avoided. A newborn loses up to 30% of body heat through the head and therefore needs to wear a cap to prevent heat loss. When protected from environmental extremes, the newborn's body temperature is usually within 35.5° to 37.5° C (95.9° to 99.5° F).

Temperature regulation is unstable until children reach puberty. The normal temperature range gradually drops as individuals approach older adulthood. The older adult has a narrower range of body temperatures than the younger adult. Oral temperatures of 35° C (95° F) are not unusual for older adults in cold weather. However, the average body temperature of older adults is approximately 36° C (96.8° F). Older adults are particularly sensitive to temperature extremes because of deterioration in control mechanisms, particularly poor vasomotor control (control of vasoconstriction and vasodilation), reduced amounts of subcutaneous tissue, reduced sweat gland activity, and reduced metabolism.

Exercise. Muscle activity requires an increased blood supply and an increased carbohydrate and fat breakdown. Any form of exercise increases metabolism and will increase heat production and thus body temperature. Prolonged strenuous exercise, such as long distance running, temporarily raises body temperatures up to 41° C (105.8° F).

Hormone Level. Women generally experience greater fluctuations in body temperature than men. Hormonal variations during the menstrual cycle cause body temperature fluctuations. Progesterone levels rise and fall cyclically during the menstrual cycle. When progesterone levels are low, the body temperature is a few tenths of a degree below the baseline level. The lower temperature persists until ovulation occurs. During ovulation, greater amounts of progesterone enter the circulatory system and raise the body temperature to previous baseline levels or higher. These temperature variations help to predict a woman's most fertile time to achieve pregnancy.

Body temperature changes also occur in women during menopause (cessation of menstruation). Women who have stopped menstruating often experience periods of intense body heat and sweating lasting from 30 seconds to 5 minutes. During these periods there are often intermittent increases in skin temperature of up to 4° C (7.2° F), referred to as hot flashes. This is due to the instability of the vasomotor controls for vasodilation and vasoconstriction.

Circadian Rhythm. Body temperature normally changes 0.5° to 1° C (0.9° to 1.8° F) during a 24-hour period. However, temperature is one of the most stable rhythms in humans. The temperature is usually lowest between 1:00 and 4:00 AM (Figure 32-2). During the day, body temperature rises steadily, until a maximum temperature value at about 6:00 PM, and then declines to early morning levels. Temperature patterns are not automatically reversed in people who work at night and sleep during the day. It takes 1 to 3 weeks for the cycle to reverse. In general, the circadian temperature rhythm does not change with age.

Stress. Physical and emotional stress increase body temperature through hormonal and neural stimulation. These physiological changes increase metabolism, which increases heat production. The client who is anxious about entering a hospital or a health care provider's office often has a higher normal temperature (see Chapter 31).

Environment. Environment influences body temperature. When placed in a warm room a client may be unable to regulate

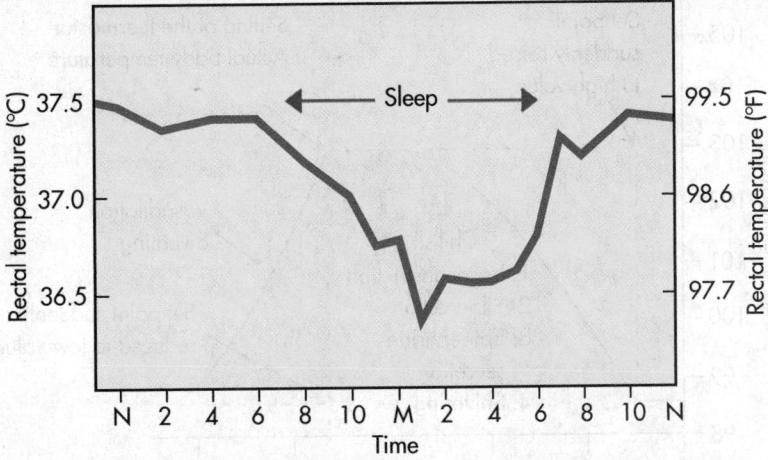

Figure 32-2 Temperature cycle for 24 hours.

body temperature by heat-loss mechanisms, and the body temperature may elevate. If the client was outside in the cold without warm clothing, body temperature may be low due to extensive radiant and conductive heat loss. Environmental temperatures affect infants and older adults more often because their temperature-regulating mechanisms are less efficient.

Temperature Alterations. Changes in body temperature outside the usual range affect the hypothalamic set point. These changes are related to excess heat production, excessive heat loss, minimal heat production, minimal heat loss, or any combination of these alterations. The nature of the change affects the type of clinical problems a client experiences.

Fever. Pyrexia, or **fever**, occurs because heat-loss mechanisms are unable to keep pace with excess heat production, resulting in an abnormal rise in body temperature. A fever is usually not harmful if it stays below 39° C (102.2° F), and a single temperature reading does not always indicate a fever. In addition to physical signs and symptoms of infection, a fever determination is based on several temperature readings at different times of the day compared with the usual value for that person at that time.

A true fever results from an alteration in the hypothalamic set point. **Pyrogens**, such as bacteria and viruses, elevate body temperature. Pyrogens act as antigens, triggering immune system responses. The hypothalamus reacts to raise the set point, and the body responds by producing and conserving heat. Several hours pass before the body temperature reaches the new set point. During this period the person experiences chills, shivers, and feels cold, even though the body temperature is rising (Figure 32-3). The chill phase resolves when the new set point, a higher temperature, is achieved. During the next phase, the plateau, the chills subside and the person feels warm and dry. If the new set point is "overshot," or the pyrogens are removed (e.g., destruction of bacteria by antibiotics), the third phase of a **febrile** episode occurs. The hypothalamus set point drops, initiating heat loss responses. The skin becomes warm and flushed because of vasodilation. Diaphoresis assists in evaporative heat loss. When the fever "breaks," the client becomes **afebrile.**

Fever is an important defense mechanism. Mild temperature elevations up to 39° C (102.2° F) enhance the body's immune system. During a febrile episode, white blood cell production is stimulated. Increased temperature reduces the concentration of iron in the blood plasma, suppressing the growth of bacteria. Fever also fights viral infections by stimulating interferon, the body's natural virus-fighting substance.

Fevers and fever patterns serve a diagnostic purpose. Fever patterns differ depending on the causative pyrogen (Box 32-4). The increase or decrease in pyrogen activity results in fever spikes and declines at different times of the day. The duration and degree of fever depend on the pyrogen's strength and the ability of the individual to respond. The term **fever of unknown origin** (FUO) refers to a fever whose etiology (cause) cannot be determined.

During a fever, cellular metabolism increases and oxygen consumption rises. The body's metabolism increases 10% for every degree Celsius of temperature elevation (Henker and Carlson, 2007). Heart and respiratory rates increase to meet the metabolic needs of the body for nutrients. The increased metabolism uses energy that produces additional heat. If the client has a cardiac or respiratory problem, the stress of a fever is great. A prolonged fever weakens a client by exhausting energy stores. Increased metabolism requires additional oxygen. If the body cannot meet the demand for additional oxygen, cellular hypoxia (inadequate oxygen) occurs. Myocardial hypoxia produces angina (chest pain). Cerebral hypoxia produces confusion. Interventions during a fever include oxygen therapy. When water loss through increased respiration and diaphoresis is excessive, the client is at risk for fluid volume deficit. Dehydration is a serious problem for older adults and children with low body weight. Maintaining optimum fluid volume status is an important nursing action (see Chapter 41).

Hyperthermia. An elevated body temperature related to the body's inability to promote heat loss or reduce heat production is **hyperthermia.** Whereas fever is an upward shift in the set point, hyperthermia results from an overload of the body's thermoregulatory mechanisms. Any disease or trauma to the hypothalamus impairs heat-loss mechanisms. **Malignant hyperthermia** is a hereditary condition of uncontrolled heat production, occurring when susceptible persons receive certain anesthetic drugs.

Heatstroke. Heat depresses hypothalamic function. Prolonged exposure to the sun or high environmental temperatures

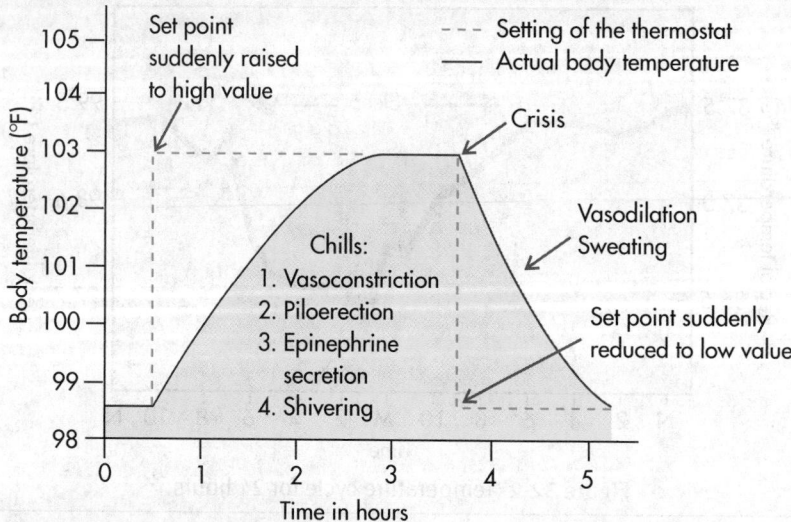

Figure 32-3 Effect of changing the set point of the hypothalamic temperature control during a fever. (Modified from Guyton AC, Hall JE: *Textbook of medical physiology,* ed 10, Philadelphia, 2000, WB Saunders.)

BOX 32-4 Patterns of Fever

Sustained: A constant body temperature continuously above 38° C (100.4° F) that has little fluctuation.

Intermittent: Fever spikes interspersed with usual temperature levels. Temperature returns to acceptable value at least once in 24 hours.

Remittent: Fever spikes and falls without a return to normal temperature levels.

Relapsing: Periods of febrile episodes and periods with acceptable temperature values. Febrile episodes and periods of normothermia are often longer than 24 hours.

TABLE 32-1 Classification of Hypothermia

	C	F
Mild	34°-36°	93.2°-96.8°
Moderate	30°-34°	86.0°-93.2°
Severe	<30°	<86.0°

---

overwhelm the body's heat-loss mechanisms. These conditions cause **heatstroke,** a dangerous heat emergency with a high mortality rate. Clients at risk include those who are very young or very old and those who have cardiovascular disease, hypothyroidism, diabetes, or alcoholism. Also at risk are those who take medications that decrease the body's ability to lose heat (e.g., phenothiazines, anticholinergics, diuretics, amphetamines, and beta-adrenergic receptor antagonists) and those who exercise or work strenuously (e.g., athletes, construction workers, and farmers).

Signs and symptoms of heatstroke include giddiness, confusion, delirium, excess thirst, nausea, muscle cramps, visual disturbances, and even incontinence. Vital signs reveal a body temperature sometimes as high as 45° C (113° F) with an increase in heart rate and lowering of blood pressure. The most important sign of heatstroke is hot, dry skin. Victims of heatstroke do not sweat because of severe electrolyte loss and hypothalamic malfunction. If the condition progresses, the client with heatstroke becomes unconscious with fixed, nonreactive pupils. Permanent neurological damage occurs unless cooling measures are rapidly started.

Heat Exhaustion. Heat exhaustion occurs when profuse diaphoresis results in excess water and electrolyte loss. Caused by environmental heat exposure, the client exhibits signs and symp-

toms of fluid volume deficit (see Chapter 41). First aid includes transporting the client to a cooler environment and restoring fluid and electrolyte balance.

Hypothermia. Heat loss during prolonged exposure to cold overwhelms the body's ability to produce heat, causing hypothermia. **Hypothermia** is classified by core temperature measurements (Table 32-1). It is sometimes unintentional, such as falling through the ice of a frozen lake. Occasionally, hypothermia is intentionally induced during surgical procedures to reduce metabolic demand and the body's need for oxygen.

Accidental hypothermia usually develops gradually and usually goes unnoticed for several hours. When skin temperature drops to 35° C (95° F), the client suffers uncontrolled shivering, loss of memory, depression, and poor judgment. As the body temperature falls below 34.4° C (94° F), heart rate, respiratory rate, and blood pressure fall. The skin becomes cyanotic. If hypothermia progresses, a client experiences cardiac dysrhythmias, loss of consciousness, and unresponsiveness to painful stimuli. In cases of severe hypothermia a person demonstrates clinical signs similar to death (e.g., lack of response to stimuli and extremely slow respirations and pulse). When you suspect hypothermia, assessment of core temperature is critical. A special low-reading thermometer is required because standard devices do not register below 35° C (95° F).

Frostbite occurs when the body is exposed to subnormal temperatures. Ice crystals form inside the cell, and permanent circulatory and tissue damage occurs. Areas particularly susceptible to frostbite are the earlobes, tip of the nose, and fingers and toes. The injured area becomes white, waxy, and firm to the touch. The client loses sensation in the affected area. Interventions include gradual warming measures, analgesia, and protection of the injured tissue.

Nursing Process and Thermoregulation

Knowledge of the physiology of body temperature regulation is essential to assess and evaluate the client's response to temperature alterations and to intervene safely. You can implement independent measures to increase or minimize heat loss, to promote heat conservation, and to increase comfort. These measures complement the effects of medically ordered therapies during illness. You can also teach many measures to family members, parents of children, or other caregivers.

◆Assessment

Sites. There are several sites for measuring core and surface body temperature. Intensive care units use the core temperatures of the pulmonary artery, esophagus, and urinary bladder. These measurements require the use of continuous invasive devices placed in body cavities or organs and continually display readings on an electronic monitor.

Obtain intermittent temperature measurements from the routinely used sites of the mouth, rectum, tympanic membrane, temporal artery, and axilla. You can also apply noninvasive chemically prepared thermometer patches to the skin. Oral, rectal, axillary, and skin temperature sites rely on effective blood circulation at the measurement site. The heat of the blood is conducted to the thermometer probe. Tympanic temperature relies on the radiation of body heat to an infrared sensor. Because the tympanic membrane shares the same arterial blood supply as the hypothalamus, the tympanic temperature is a core temperature. Temporal artery measurements detect the temperature of cutaneous blood flow.

To ensure accurate temperature readings, measure each site correctly (Skill 32-1). The temperature obtained varies, depending on the site used, but it is usually between 36.0° C (96.8° F) and 38.0° C (100.4° F). Rectal temperatures are usually 0.5° C (0.9° F) higher than oral temperatures, and axillary temperatures are usually 0.5° C (0.9° F) lower than oral temperatures. Each of the common temperature measurement sites has advantages and disadvantages (Box 32-5). Choose the safest and most accurate site for the client. When possible, use the same site when repeated measurements are necessary.

Thermometers. Two types of thermometers are available for measuring body temperature: electronic and disposable. A third type, the mercury-in-glass thermometer, was once the standard device found in the clinical setting. However, most municipalities have prohibited the sale or use of mercury-containing medical devices because of the potential hazards.

Each device measures temperature using the **Celsius** or **Fahrenheit** scale. Electronic thermometers convert the temperature scales by activating a switch. When it is necessary to convert temperature readings, use the following formulas:

1. To convert Fahrenheit to Celsius, subtract 32 from the Fahrenheit reading and multiply the result by 5/9.

$$C = (F - 32°) \times 5/9$$
Example: $40° C = (104° F - 32° F) \times 5/9$

2. To convert Celsius to Fahrenheit, multiply the Celsius reading by 9/5 and add 32 to the product.

$$F = (9/5 \times C) + 32°$$
Example: $104° F = (9/5 \times 40° C) + 32°$

Electronic Thermometer. The electronic thermometer consists of a rechargeable battery-powered display unit, a thin wire cord, and a temperature-processing probe covered by a disposable probe cover (Figure 32-4). Separate unbreakable probes are available for oral and rectal use. You can also use the oral probe for axillary temperature measurement. Electronic thermometers provide two modes of operation: a 4-second predictive temperature and a 3-minute standard temperature. In day-to-day clinical situations, most nurses use the 4-second predictive mode. A sound signals and a reading appears on the display unit when the peak temperature reading has been measured.

Another form of electronic thermometer is used exclusively for tympanic temperature. An otoscope-like speculum with an infrared sensor tip detects heat radiated from the tympanic membrane. Within seconds of placement in the auditory canal, a sound signals and a reading appears on the display unit when the peak temperature reading has been measured.

A newer type of electronic thermometer measures the temperature of the superficial temporal artery. A handheld scanner with an infrared sensor tip detects the temperature of cutaneous blood flow by sweeping the sensor across the forehead and just behind the ear (Figure 32-5). After scanning is complete, a reading appears on the display unit. Temporal artery temperature is a reliable noninvasive measure of core temperature (Sidberry and others, 2002) (Box 32-6).

The greatest advantages of electronic thermometers are that their readings appear within seconds and they are easy to read. The plastic sheath is unbreakable and ideal for children. Their expense is a major disadvantage. Maintaining cleanliness of the probes is an important consideration. If not properly cleaned between clients, gastrointestinal contamination of the rectal probe will cause disease transmission. Wipe the thermometer daily with alcohol, and wipe the thermometer probe with an alcohol swab after each client. Pay particular attention to the probe hub, which has ridges, where the probe cover is secured to the probe.

Chemical Dot Thermometers. Single-use or reusable chemical dot thermometers (Figure 32-6) are thin strips of plastic with a temperature sensor at one end. The sensor consists of a matrix of chemically impregnated dots that change color at different temperatures. In the Celsius version there are 50 dots, each representing a temperature increment of 0.1° C, over a range of 35.5° C to 40.4° C. The Fahrenheit version has 45 dots with increments of 0.2° F and a range of 96.0° F to 104.8° F. Chemical dots on the thermometer change color to reflect temperature reading, usually within 60 seconds. Most are for single use.

Text continued on p. 516

✳ **SKILL 32-1**   **MEASURING BODY TEMPERATURE**   Video

Delegation Considerations

The skill of temperature measurement can be delegated. The nurse is responsible for assessing changes in body temperature. The nurse instructs nursing assistive personnel to:

- Select appropriate route and device to measure temperature.
- Take appropriate precautions when properly positioning the client for rectal temperature measurement.
- Consider specific client-related factors that falsely raise or lower temperature.
- Obtain temperature measurement at ordered frequency.

- Be aware of the usual values for client.
- Report abnormalities to the nurse for further assessment.

Equipment

- Appropriate thermometer
- Soft tissue or wipe
- Lubricant (for rectal measurements only)
- Pen, pencil, vital sign flow sheet or record form
- Clean gloves, plastic thermometer sleeve or disposable probe cover
- Towel

STEPS

1. Assess for signs and symptoms of temperature alterations and for factors that influence body temperature.
2. Determine any previous activity that interferes with accuracy of temperature measurement. When taking oral temperature, wait 20 to 30 minutes before measuring temperature if client has smoked or ingested hot or cold liquids or foods.
3. Determine appropriate temperature site and device for client.

4. Explain route by which temperature will be taken and importance of maintaining proper position until reading is complete.
5. Perform hand hygiene.
6. Assist client in assuming comfortable position that provides easy access to temperature measurement site.
7. Obtain temperature reading.
   A. **Oral temperature measurement with electronic thermometer**
      (1) Apply clean gloves (optional).

      (2) Remove thermometer pack from charging unit. Attach oral thermometer probe stem (blue tip) to thermometer unit. Grasp top of probe stem, being careful not to apply pressure on the ejection button.
      (3) Slide disposable plastic probe cover over thermometer probe stem until cover locks in place (see illustration).

RATIONALE

Physical signs and symptoms indicate abnormal temperature. Enables you to accurately assess the nature of variations.
Smoking, mouth breathing, and oral intake causes false oral temperature readings (Henker and Carlson, 2007).

Chosen based on advantages and disadvantages of each site (see Box 32-5). Use disposable single-use thermometer for client on isolation precautions.
Clients are often curious about such measurements and need to be cautioned against prematurely removing thermometer to read results.
Reduces transmission of microorganisms.
Ensures comfort and accuracy of temperature reading.

Use of oral probe cover, which you can remove without physical contact, minimizes need to wear gloves.
Charging provides battery power. Ejection button releases plastic probe cover from probe stem.

Soft plastic cover will not break in client's mouth and prevents transmission of microorganisms between clients.

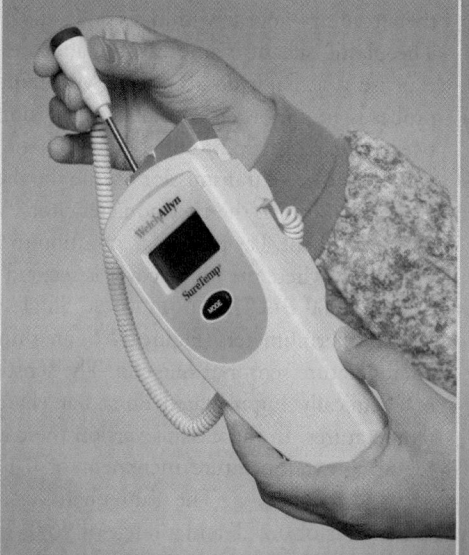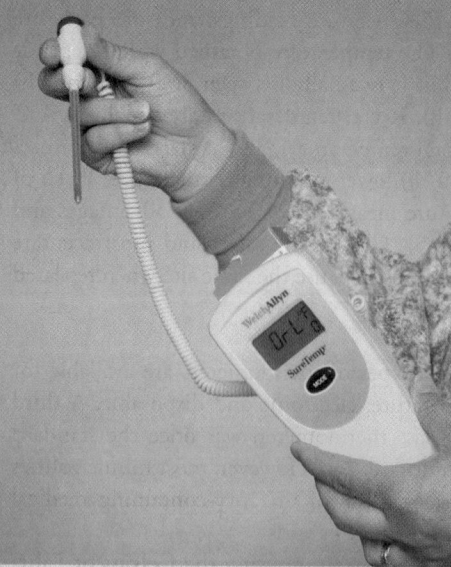

STEP 7A(3) Disposable plastic cover is placed over the probe.

STEPS	RATIONALE
(4) Ask client to open mouth; then gently place thermometer probe under tongue in posterior sublingual pocket lateral to center of lower jaw (see illustration).	Heat from superficial blood vessels in sublingual pocket produces temperature reading. With electronic thermometer, temperatures in right and left posterior sublingual pocket are significantly higher than in area under front of tongue.
(5) Ask client to hold thermometer probe with lips closed.	Maintains proper position of thermometer during recording.
(6) Leave thermometer probe in place until audible signal indicates completion and temperate reading appears on digital display; remove thermometer probe from under client's tongue.	Probe needs to stay in place until signal occurs to ensure accurate reading.
(7) Push ejection button on thermometer probe stem to discard plastic probe cover into appropriate receptacle.	Reduces transmission of microorganisms.
(8) Return thermometer probe stem to storage position of recording unit.	Storage position protects probe stem. Returning probe stem automatically causes digital reading to disappear.
(9) If gloves worn, remove and dispose in appropriate receptacle. Perform hand hygiene.	Reduces transmission of microorganisms.
(10) Return thermometer to charger.	Maintains battery charge.

B. Rectal temperature measurement with electronic thermometer

(1) Draw curtain around bed, and/or close room door. Assist client to Sims' position with upper leg flexed. Move aside bed linen to expose only anal area. Keep client's upper body and lower extremities covered with sheet or blanket.	Maintains client's privacy, minimizes embarrassment, and promotes comfort. Exposes anal area for correct thermometer placement.
(2) Apply clean gloves.	Maintains standard precautions when exposed to items soiled with body fluids (e.g., feces).
(3) Remove thermometer pack from charging unit. Attach rectal probe stem (red tip) to thermometer unit. Grasp top of probe stem, being careful not to apply pressure on the ejection button.	Charging provides battery power. Ejection button releases plastic cover from probe stem.
(4) Slide disposable plastic probe cover over thermometer probe stem until cover locks in place.	Soft plastic probe cover prevents transmission of microorganisms between clients.
(5) Squeeze liberal portion of lubricant on tissue. Dip probe cover's end into lubricant, covering 2.5 to 3.5 cm (1 to 1½ inches) for adult.	Lubrication minimizes trauma to rectal mucosa during insertion. Tissue avoids contamination of remaining lubricant in container.
(6) With nondominant hand, separate client's buttocks to expose anus. Ask client to breathe slowly and relax.	Fully exposes anus for thermometer insertion. Relaxes anal sphincter for easier thermometer insertion.

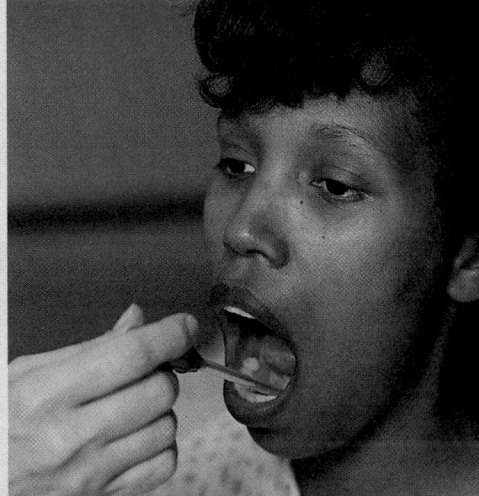

STEP 7A(4) Probe under tongue in posterior sublingual pocket.

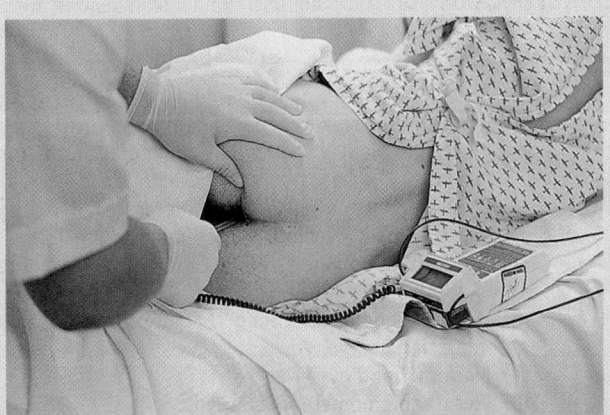

STEP 7B(8) Probe position in anus.

Continued

✳ **SKILL 32-1** | **MEASURING BODY TEMPERATURE—CONT'D**

STEPS	RATIONALE
(7) Gently insert thermometer probe into anus in direction of umbilicus 2.5 to 3.5 cm (1 to 1½ inches) for adult. Do not force thermometer.	Ensures adequate exposure against blood vessels in rectal wall.

Critical Decision Point: If you cannot adequately insert thermometer into rectum, remove thermometer and consider alternative method for obtaining temperature.

STEPS	RATIONALE
(8) Once positioned, hold thermometer probe in place (see illustration) until audible signal indicates completion and client's temperature appears on digital display; remove thermometer probe from anus.	Probe needs to stay in place until signal occurs to ensure accurate reading.
(9) Push ejection button on thermometer stem to discard plastic probe cover into an appropriate receptacle. Wipe probe stem with alcohol swab, paying particular attention to ridges where probe stem cover connects to probe.	Reduces transmission of microorganisms.
(10) Return thermometer probe stem to storage position of recording unit.	Protects probe stem from damage. Returning probe stem automatically causes digital reading to disappear.
(11) Wipe client's anal area with soft tissue to remove lubricant or feces, and discard tissue. Assist client in assuming a comfortable position.	Provides for comfort and hygiene.
(12) Remove and dispose of gloves in appropriate receptacle. Perform hand hygiene.	Reduces transmission of microorganisms.
(13) Return thermometer to charger. Verify that charger and probes are wiped with alcohol daily.	Maintains battery charge of thermometer unit. Reduces transmission of microorganisms.

C. Axillary temperature measurement with electronic thermometer

STEPS	RATIONALE
(1) Draw curtain around bed and/or close door. Assist client to a supine or sitting position. Move clothing or gown away from shoulder and arm.	Maintains client's privacy, minimizes embarrassment. Position provides easy access to axilla. Exposes axilla for correct thermometer probe placement.
(2) Remove thermometer pack from charging unit. Be sure oral probe stem (blue tip) is attached to thermometer unit. Grasp top of thermometer probe stem, being careful not to apply pressure on the ejection button.	Charging provides battery power. Ejection button releases plastic cover from probe.
(3) Slide disposable plastic probe cover over thermometer stem until cover locks in place.	Soft plastic probe cover prevents transmission of microorganisms between clients.
(4) Raise client's arm away from torso; inspect for skin lesion and excessive perspiration. Insert thermometer probe into center of axilla, lower arm over probe, and place arm across client's chest (see illustration).	Maintains proper position of probe against blood vessels in axilla.

Critical Decision Point: Do not use axilla if skin lesions are present because lesions alter local temperature and areas are painful to touch.

STEPS	RATIONALE
(5) Once positioned, hold thermometer probe in place until audible signal occurs and temperature appears on digital display. Remove thermometer probe from axilla.	Thermometer probe needs to stay in place until signal occurs to ensure accurate reading.
(6) Push ejection button on thermometer stem to discard plastic probe cover into appropriate receptacle.	Reduces transmission of microorganisms.
(7) Return thermometer stem to storage position of recording unit.	Storage position protects stem. Returning probe automatically causes digital reading to disappear.
(8) Assist client in assuming a comfortable position, replacing linen or gown.	Restores comfort and promotes privacy.
(9) Perform hand hygiene.	Reduces transmission of microorganisms.
(10) Return thermometer to charger.	Maintains battery charge.

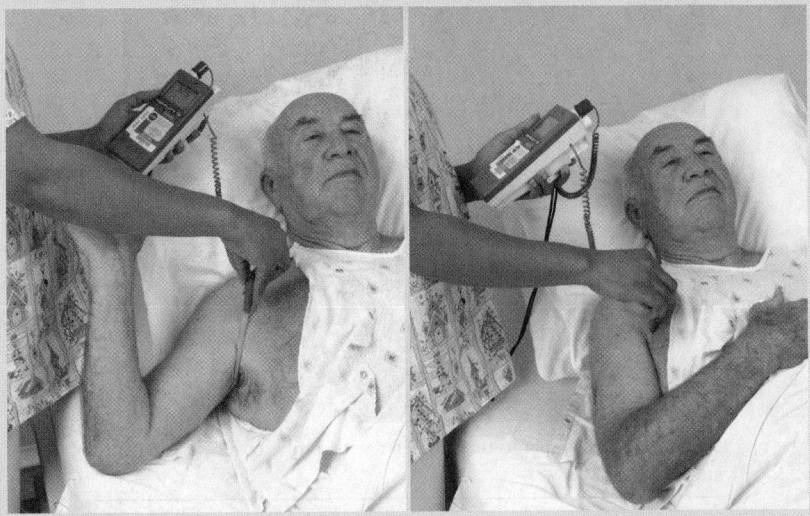

STEP 7C(4) Thermometer tip in axilla.

STEPS	RATIONALE
D. Tympanic membrane temperature with electronic thermometer	
(1) Assist client in assuming comfortable position with head turned toward side, away from nurse. If client has been lying on one side, use upper ear. Right-handed persons need to obtain temperature from client's right ear. Left-handed people need to obtain temperature from client's left ear.	Ensures comfort and exposes auditory canal for accurate temperature measurement. Heat trapped in lower ear will cause false high temperature readings. The less acute the angle of approach, the better the probe seal.
(2) Note if there is obvious earwax in the client's ear canal.	To ensure clear optical pathway, make sure earwax is not blocking the lens cover of speculum. Switch to other ear or select alternative measurement site if needed.
(3) Remove thermometer handheld unit from charging base, being careful not to apply pressure to the ejection button.	Base provides battery power. Removal of handheld unit from base prepares it to measure temperature. Ejection button releases plastic probe cover from thermometer tip.
(4) Slide clean disposable speculum cover over otoscope-like lens tip until it locks into place, being careful not to touch lens cover.	Lens cover must be unimpeded by dust, fingerprints, or earwax to ensure clear optical pathway.
(5) If holding handheld unit with right hand, obtain temperature from client's right ear; left-handed persons obtain temperature from client's left ear.	The less acute angle of approach, the better the probe will seal inside the auditory canal.
(6) Insert speculum into ear canal following manufacturer's instructions for tympanic probe positioning:	The ear tug straightens the external auditory canal, allowing maximum exposure of the tympanic membrane (Hockenberry and others, 2007).
a. Pull ear pinna backward, up, and out for an adult. For children 3 years and younger, pull the pinna down and back. For children older than 3 years, pull the pinna up and back (Hockenberry and Wilson, 2007).	Correct positioning of the speculum tip with respect to ear canal ensures accurate readings.
b. Move thermometer in a figure-eight pattern.	Some manufacturers recommend movement of the speculum tip in a figure-eight pattern, which allows the sensor to detect maximum tympanic membrane heat radiation.
c. Fit speculum tip snugly into canal, and do not move (see illustration), pointing speculum tip toward nose.	Gentle pressure seals ear canal from ambient temperature, which alters readings as much as 2.8° C (5° F). Operator error will lead to false low temperatures.

Continued

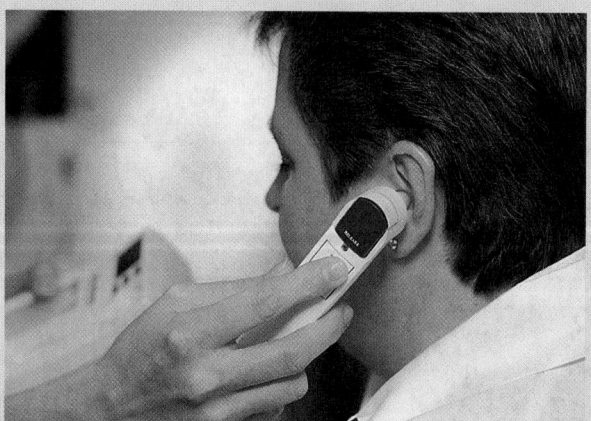

STEP 7D(6)c Tympanic thermometer with probe cover inserted into auditory canal.

STEPS	RATIONALE
(7) Once positioned, press scan button on handheld unit. Leave speculum in place until audible signal indicates completion and client's temperature appears on digital display.	Pressing scan button causes detection of infrared energy. Speculum needs to stay in place until signal occurs to ensure accurate reading.
(8) Carefully remove speculum from auditory meatus.	Prevents rubbing of sensitive outer ear lining.
(9) Push ejection button on handheld unit to discard speculum cover into appropriate receptacle.	Reduces transmission of microorganisms. Automatically causes digital reading to disappear.
(10) If temperature is abnormal or a second reading is necessary, replace speculum cover and wait 2 to 3 minutes before repeating the measurement in the same ear. Repeat measurement in other ear, or try an alternative temperature site or instrument.	Lens cover needs to be free of cerumen to maintain optical path. Time allows ear canal to regain usual temperature.
(11) Return handheld unit to charging base.	Protects sensor tip from damage.
(12) Assist client in assuming a comfortable position.	Restores comfort and sense of well-being.
(13) Perform hand hygiene.	Reduces transmission of microorganisms.
8. Discuss findings with client as needed.	Promotes participation in care and understanding of health status.
9. If temperature is assessed for the first time, establish temperature as baseline if it is within normal range.	Used to compare future temperature measurements.
10. Compare temperature reading with client's previous baseline and acceptable temperature range for client's age-group.	Body temperature fluctuates within narrow range; comparison reveals presence of abnormality. Improper placement or movement of thermometer causes inaccuracies. Second measurement confirms initial findings of abnormal body temperature.

Unexpected Outcomes and Related Interventions

- Temperature 1° C above usual range
  - Assess possible sites (e.g., central line catheter, wounds) for localized infection and for related data suggesting a systemic infection.
  - Follow interventions listed in Box 32-10, p. 520.
- Persistent fever
  - Notify health care provider, and administer antipyretic and antibiotics as ordered.
- Temperature 1° C below usual range
  - Remove any drafts, wet clothing, or linen.
  - Apply extra blankets, and unless contraindicated offer warm liquids.

Recording and Reporting

- Record temperature in nurses' notes or vital sign flow sheet. Document measurement of temperature after administration of specific therapies in narrative form in nurses' notes.
- Report abnormal findings to nurse in charge or health care provider.

Home Care Considerations

- Assess temperature and ventilation of client's environment to determine existence of any environmental condition that will influence outcome of client's temperature.
- In the home, clients often continue to use mercury-in-glass thermometers (see Box 32-7, p. 517). Assess safe storage of mercury-in-glass thermometers to protect from breakage and mercury spills. Educate client and caregiver about mercury hazards.

✳ BOX 32-5 Advantages and Disadvantages of Select Temperature Measurement Sites

Site Advantages	**Site Limitations**
Oral	
Easily accessible—requires no position change.	Causes delay in measurement if client recently ingested hot/cold fluids or foods, smoked, or is receiving oxygen by mask/cannula
Comfortable for client	Not for clients who had oral surgery, trauma, history of epilepsy, or shaking chills
Provides accurate surface temperature reading	
Reflects rapid change in core temperature	Not for infants, small children, or confused, unconscious, or unco-operative clients
Reliable route to measure temperature in intubated clients	Risk of body fluid exposure

Tympanic Membrane

Easily accessible site	More variability of measurement than with other core temperature devices
Minimal client repositioning required	Requires removal of hearing aids before measurement
Obtained without disturbing, waking, or repositioning clients	Requires disposable sensor cover with only one size available
Used for clients with tachypnea without affecting breathing	Otitis media and cerumen impaction distorts readings
Provides accurate core reading because eardrum close to hypothalamus; sensitive to core temperature changes	Do not use in clients who had surgery of the ear or tympanic membrane
Very rapid measurement (2 to 5 seconds)	Does not accurately measure core temperature changes during and after exercise
Unaffected by oral intake of food or fluids or smoking	Does not obtain continuous measurement
Used in newborns to reduce infant handling and heat loss	Affected by ambient temperature devices such as incubators, radiant warmers, and facial fans
	When used in neonates, infants, and children under 3 years old, use care to position device correctly because the anatomy of ear canal makes it difficult to position (Holtzclaw, 2003)
	Inaccuracies reported due to incorrect positioning of handheld unit (Maxton, Justin, and Gilles, 2004)

Rectal

Argued to be more reliable when oral temperature cannot be obtained	Lags behind core temperature during rapid temperature changes (Maxton and others, 2004)
	Not for clients with diarrhea, clients who had rectal surgery, rectal disorders, or bleeding tendencies
	Requires positioning and is often source of client embarrassment and anxiety
	Risk of body fluid exposure
	Requires lubrication
	Not for routine vital signs in newborns
	Impacted stool influences readings (Maxton and others, 2004)

Axilla

Safe and inexpensive	Long measurement time
Used with newborns and unconscious clients	Requires continuous positioning by nurse
	Measurement lags behind core temperature during rapid temperature changes
	Not recommended to detect fever in infants and young children
	Requires exposure of thorax, which results in temperature loss, especially in newborns
	Affected by exposure to the environment, including time to place thermometer (Maxton and others, 2004)

Skin

Inexpensive	Measurement lags behind other sites during temperature changes, especially during hyperthermia
Provides continuous reading	Adhesion impaired by diaphoresis or sweat
Safe and noninvasive	Reading affected by environmental temperature
Used for neonates	Cannot be use for clients with allergy to adhesive

Continued

⁎ BOX 32-5 **Advantages and Disadvantages of Select Temperature Measurement Sites—cont'd**

Site Advantages
Temporal Artery
Easy to access without position change
Very rapid measurement
No risk of injury to client or nurse
Eliminates need to disrobe or be unbundled
Comfortable for client
Used in premature infants, newborns, and children (Sidberry and others, 2002)
Reflects rapid change in core temperature
Sensor cover not required

Site Limitations

Inaccurate with head covering or hair on forehead
Affected by skin moisture such as diaphoresis or sweating
Cannot use if continuous measurement is required

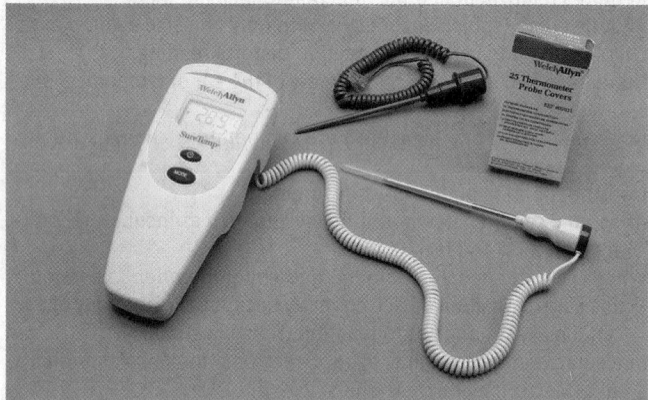

Figure 32-4 Electronic thermometer. Blue probe is for oral or axillary use. Red probe is for rectal use.

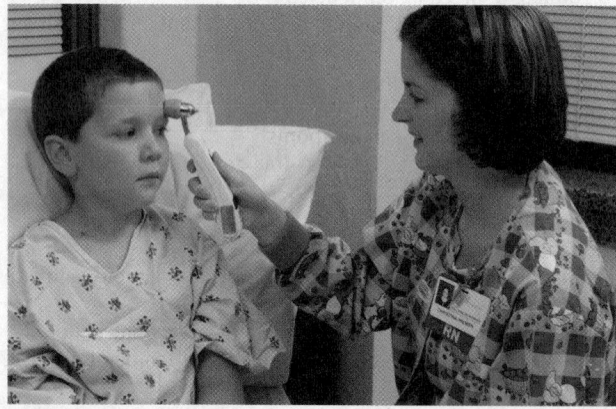

Figure 32-5 Temporal artery thermometer scanning the child's forehead.

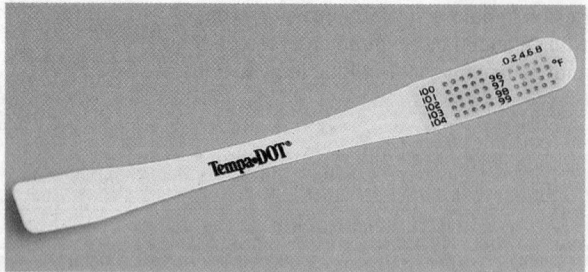

Figure 32-6 Disposable, single-use thermometer strip.

⁎ BOX 32-6 **PROCEDURAL GUIDELINES**

Measurement of Temporal Artery Temperature
Delegation Considerations: The skill of measurement of temporal artery temperature can be delegated. It is the nurse's responsibility to assess the significance of the findings. Instruct nursing assistive personnel about:

• Frequency of temperature measurement
• Factors that falsely raise or lower temperature readings
• Reporting abnormalities to the nurse for further assessment

Equipment: Temporal artery thermometer, alcohol wipes or probe cover (optional).

1. Perform hand hygiene.
2. Ensure that forehead is dry; wipe with towel if needed.
3. Place probe flush on client's forehead to avoid measuring ambient temperature.
4. Press the red scan button with your thumb. Continuous scanning for the highest temperature will occur until you release the scan button.
5. Slowly slide thermometer straight across forehead while keeping probe flush on skin.
6. Keeping the scan button pressed, lift probe from forehead and touch probe to neck just behind earlobe (the area where perfume is typically applied).
7. While scanning, a clicking sound occurs and stops when peak temperature is reached.
8. Release the scan button; read and record temperature. The reading remains on for 15 seconds after you release the button.
9. Clean probe with alcohol wipe, or remove and dispose of probe cover if used.

In one reusable brand for a single client the chemical dots return to the original color within a few seconds. Chemical dot thermometers are usually for oral temperatures. You also use them at axillary or rectal sites, covered by a plastic sheath at the latter site, with a placement time of 3 minutes. Chemical dot thermometers are useful for screening temperatures, especially in infants and young children. Research has also demonstrated the ability of oral chemical dot thermometers to screen temperatures in orally intubated critical care clients (Potter and others, 2003). Because chemical dot thermometers often underestimate oral temperature by 0.4° C or more, use electronic thermometers to confirm measurements made with a chemical dot thermometer when treatment decisions are involved (Potter and others, 2003). They

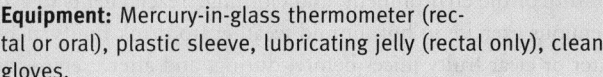

BOX 32-7 CLIENT TEACHING

Use of a Mercury-in-Glass Thermometer by Caregivers in the Home

Objective: Client and family member will correctly perform temperature measurement.

Equipment: Mercury-in-glass thermometer (rectal or oral), plastic sleeve, lubricating jelly (rectal only), clean gloves.

Teaching Strategies

Explain to the client the following steps for oral temperature:

1. Wash hands.
2. Hold end (tip will be blue) of glass thermometer with fingertips to reduce contamination of bulb.
3. Read mercury level while gently rotating thermometer at eye level. If mercury is above desired level, grasp tip of thermometer securely, stand away from solid objects, and sharply flick wrist downward. Briskly shaking lowers mercury level in glass tube. Continue shaking until reading is below 35.5° C (96° F). Make sure thermometer reading is below client's actual temperature before use.
4. Place thermometer into oral sublingual pocket using technique appropriate to oral site (see Skill 32-1, p. 510).
5. Leave thermometer in place 3 minutes.
6. Remove the thermometer. Carefully discard the plastic sleeve. Wipe off secretions with clean tissue, moving toward the bulb.
7. With thermometer at eye level, read findings, store thermometer in storage container. Perform hand washing.

Evaluation

- Observe client perform temperature measurement.
- Have client explain how to measure temperature.

BOX 32-8 Steps to Take in the Event of a Mercury Spill

1. **DO NOT** touch spilled mercury droplets. If skin contact occurs, immediately flush area with water for 15 minutes.
2. If possible, remove client from immediate contaminated area; shut door of contaminated area; turn off ventilation system to enclosed area.
3. Using rubber gloves, remove any clothing, linen, or shoes that have been contaminated with mercury and place in plastic trash bag. Contaminated clothing, including shoes, can spread mercury.
4. Using rubber gloves, wipe off visible mercury beads with moistened paper towels and put into plastic trash bag.
5. Notify agency's environmental services department, or obtain a mercury spill kit if available.
6. Follow procedures for mercury removal as directed by material safety data sheet (MSDS) and agency policy. Remove spills using special absorbent materials. Seal everything contaminated with mercury in a plastic bag and discard.
7. After affected area is clean, keep area well ventilated to the outside for at least 24 hours.
8. Complete occurrence report as directed by institution procedure.

Data from Environmental Protection Agency: *What should I do if I have a mercury spill?* Updated May 21, 2007, http://www.epa.gov/epaoswer/hazwaste/mercury/spills.htm, accessed June 23, 2007.

---

are useful when caring for clients on protective isolation to avoid the need to take electronic instruments into client rooms (see Chapter 34).

Another form of disposable thermometer is a temperature-sensitive patch or tape. Applied to the forehead or abdomen, chemical sensitive areas of the patch change color at different temperatures.

Glass Thermometers. The mercury-in-glass thermometer is a glass tube sealed at one end, with a mercury-filled bulb at the other. Exposure of the bulb to heat causes the mercury to expand and rise in the enclosed tube. The length of the thermometer has either Fahrenheit or Celsius calibrations. Obtaining a temperature with a mercury-in-glass thermometer requires careful preparation of the device (Box 32-7). In addition to proper positioning of the thermometer using the oral, rectal, or axillary site, you need to maintain the position for the appropriate length of time to obtain an accurate reading. In addition to the time delay, the mercury-in-glass device is easily breakable and when broken, releases hazardous mercury. If a thermometer is broken or if you suspect a mercury spill, take immediate action (Box 32-8). Although health care agencies no longer use glass thermometers, some clients have mercury-in-glass thermometers in their homes. It is important to teach clients and their families how to use the thermometer correctly and what to do if a mercury-in-glass thermometer breaks.

✦ Nursing Diagnosis

After concluding your assessment, cluster defining characteristics to form a nursing diagnosis (Box 32-9). For example, an increase in body temperature, flushed skin, skin warm to touch, and tachycardia indicate the diagnosis *hyperthermia*. State the nursing diagnosis as either an at-risk or actual temperature alteration. If the client possesses risk factors for temperature alterations, you implement actions to minimize or eliminate the risk factors. Examples of nursing diagnoses for clients with body temperature alterations include the following:

- Risk for imbalanced body temperature
- Hyperthermia
- Hypothermia
- Ineffective thermoregulation

Once you determine a diagnosis, accurately select the related factor or etiology. The related factor allows you to select appropriate nursing interventions. In the example of hyperthermia, a related factor of vigorous activity will result in much different interventions than a related factor of decreased ability to perspire.

✦ Planning

During planning, integrate the knowledge gathered from assessment and the client history to develop an individualized plan of care (see Care Plan). Match the client's needs with those interventions that are supported and recommended in the clinical research literature.

❋ **BOX 32-9** **NURSING DIAGNOSTIC PROCESS**

Ineffective Thermoregulation Related to Aging and Inability to Adapt to Environmental Temperature

Assessment Activities	Defining Characteristics
Obtain vital signs, including temperature, pulse (see Skill 32-2, p. 522), respirations (see Skill 32-3, p. 530), SpO$_2$ (see Skill 32-4, p. 534).	Increased body temperature above usual range Tachycardia Tachypnea Hypoxemia
Palpate skin.	Warm, dry skin
Observe client's appearance and behavior while talking and resting.	Restlessness Confusion Flushed appearance
Review medical history.	Found in unventilated apartment during heat wave; 85 years old with history of dementia

Goals and Outcomes. The plan of care for a client with alteration in temperature includes realistic and individualized goals along with relevant outcomes. This requires collaboration with the client and family in setting goals and outcomes and selecting nursing interventions. Establish expected outcomes to gauge progress toward returning the body temperature to an acceptable range. In cases where the temperature alteration requires helping clients modify their environment, goals may be long term (e.g., obtaining appropriate clothing to wear in cold weather). Short-term goals, such as regaining normal range of body temperature, improve client health. In the example of a client who has an elevated fever and has had excessive diaphoresis, the goal of care is attaining fluid and electrolyte balance. The outcome is that client intake and output will be equal for the next 24 hours.

Setting Priorities. Set priorities of care with regard to the extent the temperature alteration affects a client. The severity of a temperature alteration and its effects, together with the client's general health status, will influence your priorities in the care of a client. Safety is a top priority. Often, other medical problems complicate the care plan. For instance, body temperature imbalance affects the body's requirements for fluids. Clients with heart problems often have difficulty tolerating required fluid replacement therapy.

Collaborative Care. Clients at risk for imbalanced body temperature require an individualized care plan directed at maintaining normothermia and reducing risk factors. For example, it is important to establish the outcome that the client can explain appropriate actions to take during a heat wave. Teach the client and caregiver the importance of thermoregulation and actions to take during excessive environmental heat. Education is particularly important for parents, who need to know how to take action at home when an infant or child develops a temperature imbalance.

◆ Implementation

Health Promotion. By maintaining balance between heat production and heat loss you promote the health of clients at risk for imbalanced body temperature. Consider client activity, temperature of the environment, and clothing. Teach clients to avoid strenuous exercise in hot, humid weather; to drink fluids such as water or clear fruity juices before, during, and after exercise; and to wear light, loose-fitting, light-colored clothes. Also teach clients to avoid exercising in areas with poor ventilation, to wear a protective covering over the head when outdoors, and to expose themselves to hot climates gradually.

Prevention is the key for clients at risk for hypothermia. Prevention involves educating clients, family members, and friends. Clients at risk include the very young and the very old and persons debilitated by trauma, stroke, diabetes, drug or alcohol intoxication, sepsis, and Raynaud's disease. Mentally ill or handicapped clients sometimes fall victim to hypothermia because they are unaware of the dangers of cold conditions. Persons without adequate home heating, shelter, diet, or clothing are also at risk. Fatigue, skin color (African Americans are more susceptible), malnutrition, and hypoxemia also contribute to the risk of frostbite.

Acute Care

Fever. When an elevated body temperature develops, initiate interventions to treat fever. The objective of therapy is to increase heat loss, reduce heat production, and prevent complications.

The choice of interventions depends on the cause, any adverse effects, and the strength, intensity, and duration of the temperature elevation. Nurses are essential in assessing and implementing temperature-reducing strategies (Box 32-10). The health care provider attempts to determine the cause of the elevated temperature by isolating the causative pyrogen. Sometimes it is necessary to obtain culture specimens for laboratory analysis such as urine, blood, sputum, and wound sites (see Chapter 34). Some antibiotic medications are ordered to be given after the cultures have been obtained. Administering antibiotics destroys pyrogenic bacteria and eliminates the body's stimulus for the elevated temperature.

Most fevers in children are of a viral origin, last only briefly, and have limited effects. However, children still have immature temperature-control mechanisms and temperatures can rise rapidly. Dehydration and febrile seizures occur during rising temperatures of children between 6 months and 3 years of age. Febrile seizures are unusual in children more than 5 years of age. The extent of the temperature, often exceeding 38.8° C (101.8° F), seems to be a more important factor than the rapidity of the temperature increase. Children are at particular risk for fluid volume deficit because they can quickly lose large amounts of fluids in proportion to their body weight. It is important to maintain accurate intake and output records and encourage fluids.

Sometimes a fever is a hypersensitivity response to a drug. Drug fevers are often accompanied by other allergy symptoms such as rash or pruritus (itching). Treatment involves withdrawing the medication.

Antipyretics are drugs that reduce fever. Nonsteroidal drugs such as acetaminophen, salicylates, indomethacin, and ketorolac

NURSING CARE PLAN
Elevated Body Temperature

Assessment
Mr. Coburn is a 56-year-old school teacher who arrives at the outpatient clinic with the complaint of malaise. His medical history includes a past urinary tract infection. Several of his students have been out of school lately with colds. He has been feeling poorly for the past 3 days.

Assessment Activities	Findings/Defining Characteristics*
Palpate skin.	Mr. Coburn's skin is **warm and dry** to touch.
Observe client's behavior while talking and resting.	Mr. Coburn appears to have labored breathing. His face is **flushed**.
Obtain vital signs.	Blood pressure right arm 116/62 mm Hg, left arm 114/64 mm Hg; right radial pulse **128 beats per minute**, regular and bounding; respiratory rate **26 breaths per minute**; SpO₂ 98% on room air; oral temperature **39.2° C** (102.6° F).
Review medical history.	He admits to smoking one pack of cigarettes per day and recently began expectorating **yellow-green sputum**. He has been **tired** for the past 3 days and upon rising in the morning has been dizzy.

*Defining characteristics are shown in bold type.

Nursing Diagnosis: Hyperthermia related to infectious process.

Planning

Goals	Expected Outcomes†
	Thermoregulation
Client will regain normal range of body temperature within next 24 hours.	Body temperature will decline at least 1° C (1.8° F) within next 8 hours.
Client will attain sense of comfort and rest within next 48 hours.	Client will verbalize increased satisfaction with rest and sleep pattern.
	Client will report increase in energy level within next 3 days.
Fluid and electrolyte balance will be maintained during next 3 days.	Intake will equal output within next 24 hours.
	No evidence of postural hypotension during ambulation.

†Outcome classification labels from Moorhead S and others: *Nursing outcomes classification (NOC)*, ed 4, St. Louis, 2008, Mosby.

Interventions‡	Rationale
Fever Treatment	
• Instruct client to reduce external coverings and keep clothing and bed linen dry.	Promotes heat loss through conduction and convection.
• Instruct client to monitor temperature at home and administer acetaminophen every 4 hours as ordered for temperature over 39° C (102.2° F).	Antipyretics reduce set point.
• Instruct client to limit physical activity and increase frequency of rest periods over next 2 days.	Activity and stress increase metabolic rate, contributing to heat production.
• Instruct client to increase oral fluids of choice.	Fluids lost through insensible water loss require replacement.

‡Intervention classification labels from Bulechek GM, Butcher HK, and Dochterman JM: *Nursing interventions classification (NIC)*, ed 5, St. Louis, 2008, Mosby.

Evaluation

Nursing Actions	Client Response/Finding	Achievement of Outcome
Obtain body temperature measurement.	Body temperature 37.8° C.	Body temperature within normal limits.
Obtain orthostatic blood pressure measurements.	Blood pressure measurements lying, sitting, and standing are within 5 mm Hg of each other.	No evidence of postural hypotension.
Ask Mr. Coburn if he has had any episodes of dizziness.	Mr. Coburn denies dizziness.	
Ask Mr. Coburn if his energy level has changed since the last visit.	He responds, "I am sleeping much better and have returned to work with a lot more energy."	Improved rest and sleep pattern and increased energy level.

✳ BOX 32-10 Nursing Interventions for Clients With a Fever

Interventions (Unless Contraindicated)

- Obtain blood cultures if ordered. Blood specimens are obtained to coincide with temperature spikes when the antigen-producing organism is most prevalent.
- Minimize heat production: reduce the frequency of activities that increase oxygen demand, such as excessive turning and ambulation; allow rest periods; limit physical activity.
- Maximize heat loss: reduce external covering on client's body without causing shivering; keep clothing and bed linen dry.
- Satisfy requirements for increased metabolic rate: provide supplemental oxygen therapy as ordered to improve oxygen delivery to body cells; provide measures to stimulate appetite, and offer well-balanced meals; provide fluids (at least 3 L/day for a client with normal cardiac and renal function) to replace fluids lost through insensible water loss and sweating.
- Promote client comfort: encourage oral hygiene because oral mucous membranes dry easily from dehydration; control temperature of the environment without inducing shivering; apply damp cloth to client forehead.
- Identify onset and duration of febrile episode phases: examine previous temperature measurements for trends.
- Initiate health teaching as indicated.
- Control environmental temperature to 21° to 27° C (70° to 80° F).

reduce fever by increasing heat loss. Corticosteroids reduce heat production by interfering with the immune system and mask signs of infection. Corticosteroids are not used to treat a fever. However, corticosteroids can suppress a client's fever in response to a pyrogen.

Nonpharmacological therapy for fever uses methods that increase heat loss by evaporation, conduction, convection, or radiation. Tepid sponge baths, bathing with alcohol water solutions, applying ice packs to axillae and groin areas, and cooling fans were previously used to reduce fever; however, avoid these therapies because they lead to shivering. There is no advantage of these methods over antipyretic medications.

Blankets cooled by circulating water delivered by motorized units increase conductive heat loss. Follow the manufacturer's instructions for applying these hypothermia blankets because of the risk for skin breakdown and "freeze burns." Placing a bath blanket between the client and the hypothermia blanket and wrapping distal extremities (fingers, toes, and genitalia) reduces the risk of injury to the skin and tissue from hypothermia therapy.

Make sure nursing measures to enhance body cooling do not stimulate shivering. Shivering is counterproductive and increases energy expenditure up to 400%. Wrapping the client's extremities reduces the incidence and intensity of shivering. Medications, such as meperidine or butorphanol reduce shivering.

Heatstroke. Heatstroke is an emergency situation. First aid treatment for heatstroke includes moving the client to a cooler environment, removing excess body clothing, placing cool wet towels over the skin, and using oscillating fans to increase convective heat loss. Emergency medical treatment includes intravenous (IV) fluids, irrigating the stomach and lower bowel with cool solutions, and hypothermia blankets.

Hypothermia. The priority treatment for hypothermia is to prevent a further decrease in body temperature. Removing wet clothes, replacing them with dry ones, and wrapping the client in blankets are key nursing interventions. In emergencies away from a health care setting, have the client lie under blankets next to a warm person. A conscious client benefits from drinking hot liquids such as soup, while avoiding alcohol and caffeinated fluids. It is also helpful to keep the head covered, place the client near a fire or in a warm room, or place heating pads next to areas of the body (head and neck) that lose heat the quickest.

Restorative and Continuing Care. Educate the client with a fever about the importance of taking and continuing any antibiotics as directed until the course of treatment is completed. Children and older adults are at risk for fluid volume deficit because they can quickly lose large amounts of fluids in proportion to their body weight. Identifying preferred fluids and encouraging oral fluid intake is an important ongoing nursing intervention.

◆ Evaluation

Evaluate all nursing interventions by comparing the client's actual response to the expected outcomes of the care plan. Determine whether goals of care were met or if a revision to the plan is necessary. After any intervention measure the client's temperature to evaluate for change. In addition, use other evaluative measures such as palpation of the skin and assessment of pulse and respirations. If therapies are effective, body temperature will return to an acceptable range, other vital signs will stabilize, and the client will report a sense of comfort.

Pulse

The pulse is the palpable bounding of blood flow noted at various points on the body. Blood flows through the body in a continuous circuit. The pulse is an indicator of circulatory status.

Physiology and Regulation

Electrical impulses originating from the sinoatrial (SA) node travel through heart muscle to stimulate cardiac contraction. Approximately 60 to 70 mL of blood enters the aorta with each ventricular contraction (stroke volume). With each stroke volume ejection, the walls of the aorta distend, creating a pulse wave that travels rapidly toward the distal ends of the arteries. The pulse wave moves 15 times faster through the aorta and 100 times faster through the small arteries than the ejected volume of blood. When a pulse wave reaches a peripheral artery, you can feel it by palpating the artery lightly against underlying bone or muscle. The pulse is the palpable bounding of the blood flow in the peripheral artery. The number of pulsing sensations occurring in 1 minute is the pulse rate.

The volume of blood pumped by the heart during 1 minute is the **cardiac output**, the product of heart rate (HR) and the ventricle's stroke volume (SV). In an adult the heart normally pumps

✳ TABLE 32-2 Pulse Sites

SITE	LOCATION	ASSESSMENT CRITERIA
Temporal	Over temporal bone of head, above and lateral to eye	Easily accessible site used to assess pulse in children
Carotid	Along medial edge of sternocleidomastoid muscle in neck	Easily accessible site used during physiological shock or cardiac arrest when other sites are not palpable
Apical	Fourth to fifth intercostal space at left midclavicular line	Site used to auscultate for apical pulse
Brachial	Groove between biceps and triceps muscles at antecubital fossa	Site used to assess status of circulation to lower arm Site used to auscultate blood pressure
Radial	Radial or thumb side of forearm at wrist	Common site used to assess character of pulse peripherally and assess status of circulation to hand
Ulnar	Ulnar side of forearm at wrist	Site used to assess status of circulation to hand; also used to perform an Allen's test
Femoral	Below inguinal ligament, midway between symphysis pubis and anterior superior iliac spine	Site used to assess character of pulse during physiological shock or cardiac arrest when other pulses are not palpable; used to assess status of circulation to leg
Popliteal	Behind knee in popliteal fossa	Site used to assess status of circulation to lower leg
Posterior tibial	Inner side of ankle, below medial malleolus	Site used to assess status of circulation to foot
Dorsalis pedis	Along top of foot, between extension tendons of great and first toe	Site used to assess status of circulation to foot

5000 ml of blood per minute. A change in heart rate or stroke volume does not always change the heart's output or the amount of blood in the arteries. For example, if a person's heart rate is 70 beats per minute and the stroke volume is 70 mL, the cardiac output is 4900 mL per minute (70 beats per minute times 70 mL per beat). If the heart rate drops to 60 beats per minute and the stroke volume rises to 85 mL per beat, then the cardiac output increases to 5100 mL or 5.1 L per minute (60 beats per minute times 85 mL per beat).

Mechanical, neural, and chemical factors regulate the strength of ventricular contraction and its stroke volume. But when mechanical, neural, or chemical factors are unable to alter stroke volume, a change in heart rate will result in a change in cardiac output, which affects blood pressure. As heart rate increases, there is less time for the heart to fill. As heart rate increases without a change in stroke volume, blood pressure will decrease. As the heart rate slows, filling time is increased and blood pressure increases. The inability of blood pressure to respond to increases or decreases in heart rate indicates a possible health problem. Report this to the health care provider.

An abnormally slow, rapid, or irregular pulse alters cardiac output. Assess the heart's ability to meet the demands of the body's tissue for nutrients by palpating a peripheral pulse or by using a stethoscope to listen to heart sounds (apical rate).

Assessment of Pulse

You can assess any artery for pulse rate, but you will typically use the radial or carotid arteries because they are easy to palpate. When a client's condition suddenly worsens, the carotid site is recommended for quickly finding a pulse. The heart continues delivering blood through the carotid artery to the brain as long as possible. When cardiac output declines significantly, peripheral pulses weaken and are difficult to palpate.

The radial and apical locations are the most common sites for pulse rate assessment. Use the **radial pulse** to teach clients to learn how to monitor their own heart rates (e.g., athletes, persons taking heart medications, and clients starting a prescribed exercise regimen). If the radial pulse is abnormal or intermittent resulting from dysrhythmias, or if it is inaccessible because of a dressing or cast, assess the apical pulse. When a client takes medication that affects the heart rate, the apical pulse provides a more accurate assessment of heart function. The brachial or apical pulse is the best site for assessing an infant's or young child's pulse because other peripheral pulses are deep and difficult to palpate accurately.

Assessment of other peripheral pulse sites such as the brachial or femoral artery is unnecessary when routinely obtaining vital signs. You assess other peripheral pulses when conducting a complete physical, when surgery or treatment has impaired blood flow to a body part, or when there are clinical indications of impaired peripheral blood flow (see Chapter 33). Table 32-2 summarizes pulse sites and criteria for measurement. Skill 32-2 outlines pulse rate assessment.

Use of a Stethoscope. Assessing the apical rate requires a stethoscope. The five major parts of the stethoscope are the earpieces, binaurals, tubing, bell chestpiece, and diaphragm chestpiece (Figure 32-7).

The plastic or rubber earpieces should fit snugly and comfortably in your ears. The binaurals should be angled and strong enough so the earpieces stay firmly in the ears without causing discomfort. To ensure the best reception of sound, the earpieces follow the contour of the ear canal pointing toward the face when the stethoscope is in place.

The polyvinyl tubing is flexible and 30 to 40 cm (12 to 18 inches) in length. Longer tubing decreases the transmission of sound waves. Thick-walled and moderately rigid tubing eliminates

Text continued on p. 526

Delegation Considerations

The skill of pulse measurement can be delegated. The nurse is responsible for assessing the impact of changes in the pulse. The nurse instructs nursing assistive personnel to:

- Consider specific factors related to client history, usual values, or risk for irregular pulse.
- Obtain appropriate pulse measurements and position for se-lect client.
- Report specific abnormalities to the nurse for further assessment.

Equipment

- Stethoscope (apical pulse only)
- Wristwatch with second hand or digital display
- Pen, pencil, vital sign flow sheet, or record form
- Alcohol swab

STEPS	RATIONALE
1. Determine need to assess radial or apical pulse:	Nurse uses clinical judgment to determine need for assessment.
a. Assess for any risk factors for pulse alterations.	Certain conditions place clients at risk for pulse alterations. Heart disease, cardiac dysrhythmias, onset of sudden chest pain, or acute pain from any site affects the pulse. Invasive cardiovas-cular diagnostic tests, surgery, sudden infusion of large volume of IV fluid, internal or external hemorrhage, and administration of medications that alter heart function also affect the pulse.
b. Assess for signs and symptoms of altered stroke volume and cardiac output, such as dyspnea, fatigue, chest pain, orthopnea, syncope, palpitations (person's un-pleasant awareness of heartbeat), jugular venous disten-tion, edema of dependent body parts, cyanosis, or pallor of skin.	Physical signs and symptoms indicate alteration in cardiac function.
c. Assess for signs and symptoms of peripheral vascular disease such as pale, cool extremities; thin, shiny skin with decreased hair growth; thickened nails.	Physical signs and symptoms indicate alteration in local arterial blood flow.
2. Assess for factors that influence pulse rate and rhythm: age, exercise, position changes, fluid balance, medications, tem-perature, and sympathetic stimulation.	Allows for accurate assessment of presence and significance of pulse alterations. Acceptable range of pulse rate changes with age (see Table 32-3).
3. Determine previous baseline apical rate (if available) from client's record. Otherwise note baseline radial rate.	Allows for accurate assessment of change in condition. Provides comparison with future apical pulse measurements.
4. Explain that you will assess pulse or heart rate. Encourage client to relax and not speak. If client was active, wait 5 to 10 minutes before assessing pulse.	Activity and anxiety elevate heart rate. Client's voice interferes with your ability to hear sound when assessing apical rate. Obtaining pulse rates at rest allows for objective comparison of values.
5. Perform hand hygiene.	Reduces transmission of microorganisms.
6. If necessary, draw curtain around bed and/or close door.	Maintains privacy.
7. Obtain pulse measurement.	
A. Radial pulse	
(1) Assist client in assuming a supine or sitting position.	Provides easy access to pulse sites.
(2) If supine, place client's forearm straight alongside body or across lower chest or upper abdomen with wrist extended straight (see illustration). If sitting, bend client's elbow 90 degrees and support lower arm on chair or on your arm.	Relaxed position of lower arm and slight flexion of wrist promotes exposure of artery to palpation without restriction.

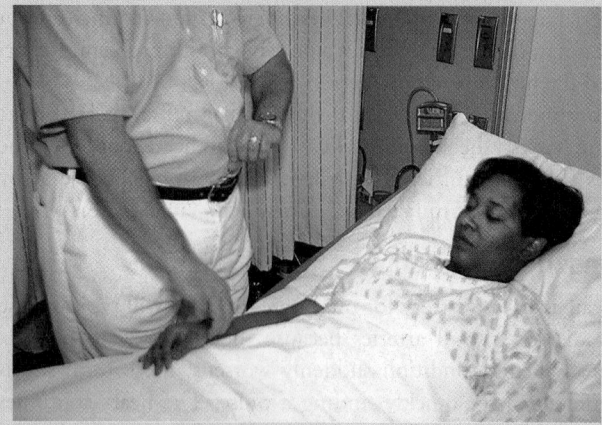

STEP 7A(2) Pulse check with client's forearm at side with wrist extended.

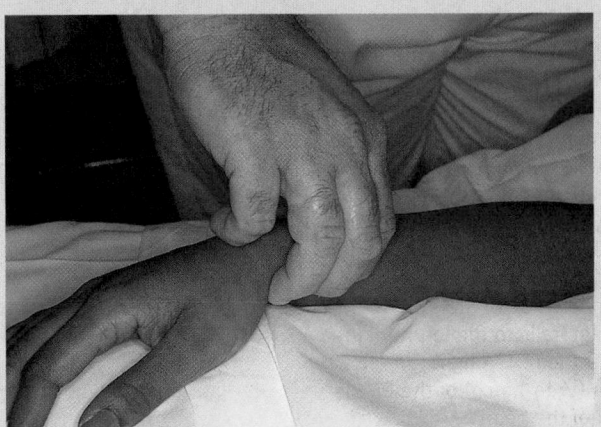

STEP 7A(3) Hand placement for pulse checks.

STEPS

(3) Place tips of first two or middle three fingers of hand over groove along radial or thumb side of client's inner wrist. Slightly extend the wrist with palm down until you note the strongest pulse (see illustration).

(4) Lightly compress against radius, obliterate pulse initially, and then relax pressure so pulse becomes easily palpable.

(5) Determine strength of pulse. Note whether thrust of vessel against fingertips is strong, bounding (4+), full, easy to palpate (3+), normal, easy to palpate (2+), diminished, difficult to palpate weak and thready (1+), or absent (0).

(6) After feeling a regular pulse, look at watch's second hand and begin to count rate: count the first beat after the second hand hits the number on the dial, count as one, then two, and so on.

(7) If pulse is regular, count rate for 30 seconds and multiply total by 2.

(8) If pulse is irregular, count rate for 1 minute (60 seconds). Assess frequency and pattern of irregularity. Compare radial pulses bilaterally.

RATIONALE

Fingertips are most sensitive parts of hand to palpate arterial pulsation. Your thumb has a pulsation that interferes with accuracy.

Pulse is more accurately assessed with moderate pressure. Too much pressure occludes pulse and impairs blood flow.

Strength reflects volume of blood ejected against arterial wall with each heart contraction. Accurate description of strength improves communication among nurses and other health care providers.

Determine rate only after knowing that you can palpate pulse. Timing begins with zero. Count of one is first beat palpated after timing begins.

A 30-second count is accurate for rapid, slow, or regular pulse rates.

Inefficient contraction of heart fails to transmit pulse wave, interfering with cardiac output, resulting in irregular pulse. Longer time ensures accurate count (Evans and others, 2004).

Critical Decision Point: If pulse is irregular, do an apical/radial pulse assessment to detect a pulse deficit. Count apical pulse while a colleague counts radial pulse. Begin apical pulse count out loud to simultaneously assess pulses. If pulse count differs by more than 2, a pulse deficit exists, which sometimes indicates alterations in cardiac output.

B. **Apical pulse**

(1) Perform hand hygiene, and clean earpieces and diaphragm of stethoscope with alcohol swab.

(2) Draw curtain around bed, and/or close room door.

(3) Assist client to supine or sitting position. Move aside bed linen and gown to expose sternum and left side of chest.

Reduces transmission of microorganisms.

Maintains privacy.
Exposes portion of chest wall for selection of auscultatory site.

Continued

✳ **SKILL 32-2** ASSESSING THE RADIAL AND APICAL PULSES—CONT'D

STEPS

(4) Locate anatomical landmarks to identify the point of maximal impulse (PMI), also called the apical impulse (see illustrations A-D). Heart is located behind and to left of sternum with base at top and apex at bottom. Find angle of Louis just below suprasternal notch between sternal body and manubrium; feels like a bony prominence (illustration A). Slip fingers down each side of angle to find second intercostal space (ICS) (illustration B). Carefully move fingers down left side of sternum to fifth ICS (illustration C) and laterally to the left midclavicular line (MCL) (illustration D). A light tap felt within an area 1 to 2 cm (½ to 1 inch) of the PMI is reflected from the apex of the heart.

(5) Place diaphragm of stethoscope in palm of hand for 5 to 10 seconds.

RATIONALE

Use of anatomical landmarks allows correct placement of stethoscope over apex of heart, enhancing ability to hear heart sounds clearly. If unable to palpate the PMI, reposition client on left side. In the presence of serious heart disease, the PMI is located to the left of the MCL or at the sixth ICS.

Warming of metal or plastic diaphragm prevents client from being startled and promotes comfort.

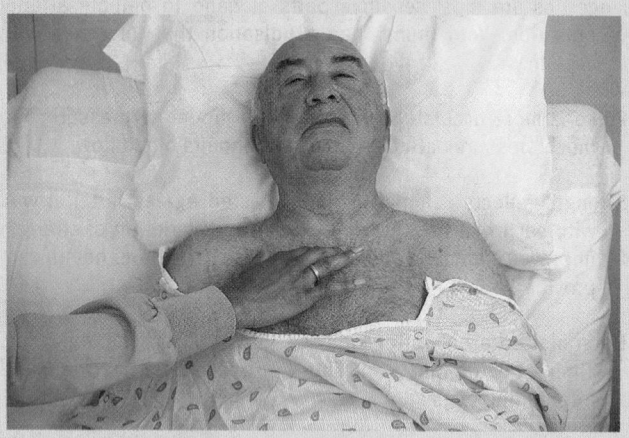

STEP 7B(4) A, Locating the angle of Louis.

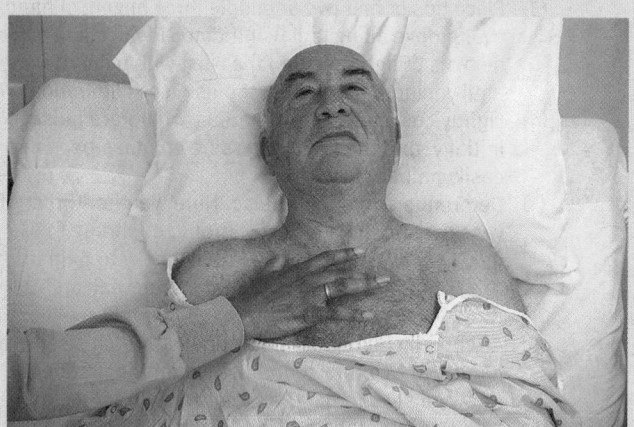

STEP 7B(4) B, Locating the second intercostal space (ICS).

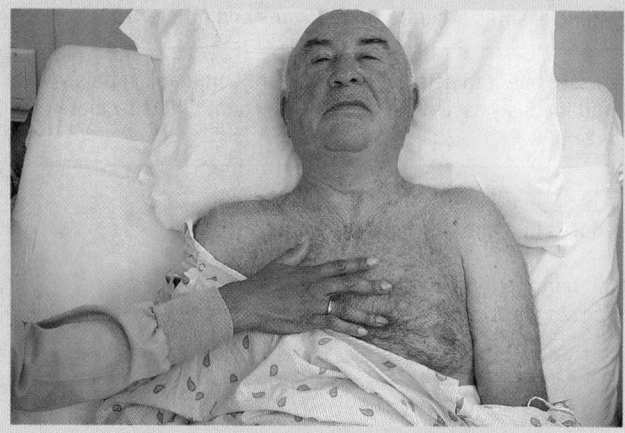

STEP 7B(4) C, Locating the fifth ICS.

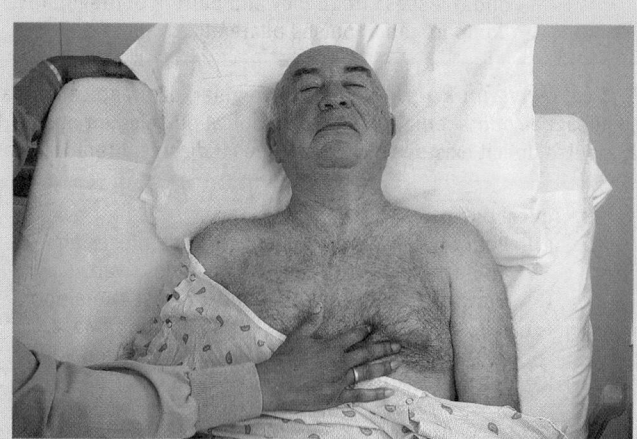

STEP 4B(4) D, Identifying the midclavicular line (MCL).

✳ **SKILL 32-2** **ASSESSING THE RADIAL AND APICAL PULSES—CONT'D**

STEPS

(6) Place diaphragm of stethoscope over PMI at the fifth ICS, at left MCL, and auscultate for normal S_1 and S_2 heart sounds (heard as "lub-dub") (see illustrations).

(7) When S_1 and S_2 are heard with regularity, use watch's second hand and begin to count rate: when sweep hand hits number 12 on dial, start counting with zero, then one, two, and so on.

(8) If apical rate is regular, count for 30 seconds and multiply by 2.

RATIONALE

Allow stethoscope tubing to extend straight without kinks that would distort sound transmission. Normal sounds S_1 and S_2 are high pitched and best heard with the diaphragm.

Determine apical rate accurately only after you are able to auscultate sounds clearly. Timing begins with zero. Count of one is first sound auscultated after timing begins.

Regular rate is accurate when measured for 30 seconds.

Critical Decision Point: If heart rate is irregular or client is receiving cardiovascular medication, count for 1 minute (60 seconds). Irregular rate is more accurately assessed when measured over a longer interval (Evans and others, 2004).

---

(9) Note if heart rate is irregular, and describe pattern or irregularity (S_1 and S_2 occurring early or later after previous sequence of sounds; for example, every third or every fourth beat is skipped).

(10) Replace client's gown and bed linen; assist client in returning to comfortable position.

(11) Perform hand hygiene.

(12) Clean earpieces and diaphragm of stethoscope with alcohol swab as needed (optional).

8. Perform hand hygiene.

9. Discuss findings with client as needed.

10. Compare readings with previous baseline and/or acceptable range of heart rate for client's age (see Table 32-3).

11. Compare peripheral pulse rate with apical rate, and note discrepancy.

12. Compare radial pulse equality, and note discrepancy.

13. Correlate pulse rate with data obtained from blood pressure and related signs and symptoms (palpitations, dizziness).

Regular occurrence of dysrhythmia within 1 minute indicates inefficient contraction of heart and alteration in cardiac output.

Restores comfort and promotes sense of well-being.

Reduces transmission of microorganisms.

Controls transmission of microorganisms when providers share stethoscopes.

Reduces transmission of microorganisms.

Promotes participation in care and understanding of health status.

Evaluates for change in condition and alterations.

Differences between measurements indicate pulse deficit and warn of cardiovascular compromise. Abnormalities often require therapy.

Differences between radial arteries indicate compromised peripheral vascular system.

Pulse rate and blood pressure are interrelated.

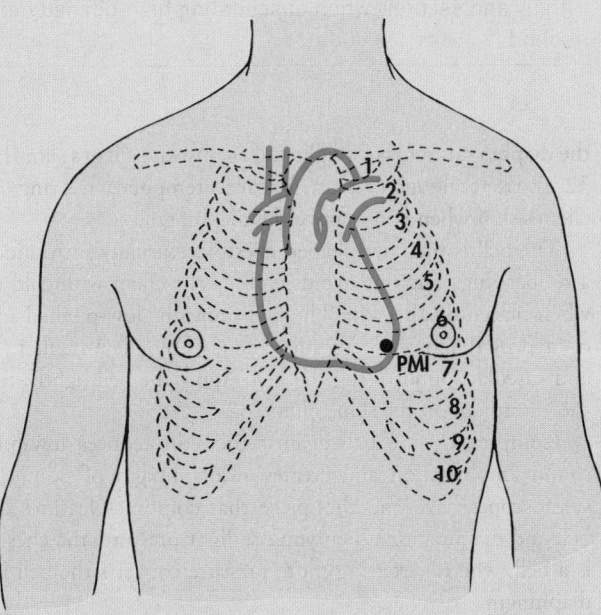

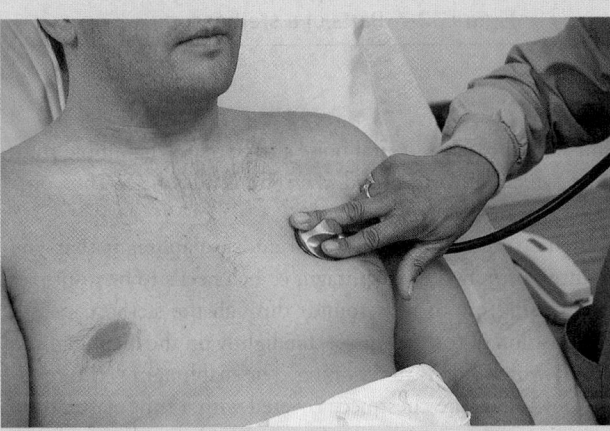

A **B**

STEP 7B(6) **A,** Location of point of maximal impulse (PMI) in adult. **B,** Stethoscope over PMI.

Continued

✳ **SKILL 32-2**   **ASSESSING THE RADIAL AND APICAL PULSES—CONT'D**

Unexpected Outcomes and Related Interventions

- Radial pulse is weak and thready.
  - Assess both radial pulses, and compare findings. Local obstruction to one extremity (e.g., clot, edema) decreases peripheral blood flow.
  - Perform complete assessment of all pulses (see Chapter 33).
  - Observe for symptoms associated with decreased tissue perfusion, including pallor and cool skin temperature of tissue distal to the weak pulse.
  - Measure apical and radial pulse simultaneously to determine presence of pulse deficit.
- Apical pulse is greater than 100 beats per minute (tachycardia).
  - Identify related data, including fever, anxiety, pain, recent exercise, hypotension, decreased oxygenation, or dehydration.
  - Observe for signs and symptoms of inadequate cardiac output, including fatigue, chest pain, orthopnea, cyanosis, and dizziness.

- Apical pulse is less than 60 beats per minute (bradycardia).
  - Observe for factors that alter heart rate such as digoxin and antidysrhythmics: it is sometimes necessary to withhold prescribed medications until the health care provider is able to evaluate the need to adjust dosage.
  - Observe for signs and symptoms of inadequate cardiac output, including fatigue, chest pain, orthopnea, cyanosis, dizziness.

Recording and Reporting

- Record pulse rate with assessment site in nurses' notes or vital signs flow sheet. Document pulse rate after administration of specific therapies in narrative form in nurses' notes.
- Report abnormal findings to nurse in charge or health care provider.

Home Care Considerations

- Assess home environment to determine room that will afford quiet environment for auscultating apical rate.

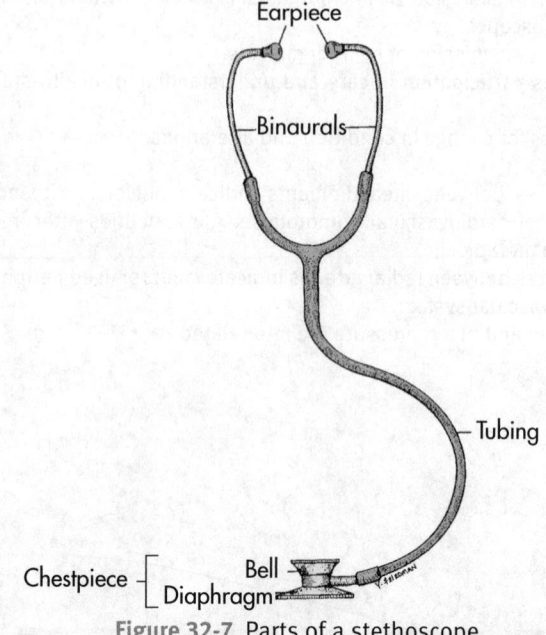

Figure 32-7 Parts of a stethoscope.

- Earpiece
- Binaurals
- Tubing
- Chestpiece [Bell / Diaphragm]

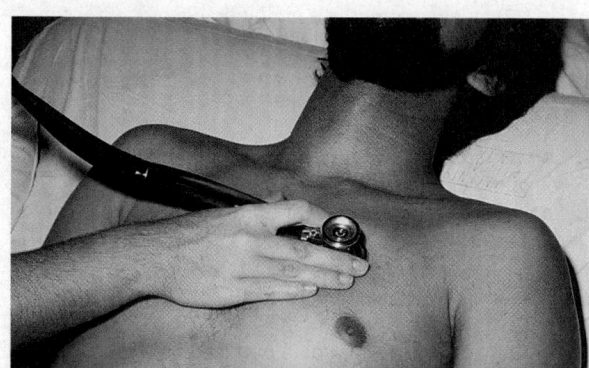

Figure 32-8 Positioning the diaphragm of the stethoscope firmly and securely when auscultating high-pitched heart sounds.

transmission of environmental noise and prevents the tubing from kinking, which distorts sound wave transmission. Stethoscopes have single or dual tubes.

The chestpiece consists of a bell and a diaphragm that you rotate into position. The diaphragm or bell needs to be in proper position during use to hear sounds through the stethoscope. To test the position of the chestpiece, tap lightly on the diaphragm to determine which side is functioning. The diaphragm is the circular, flat portion of the chestpiece covered with a thin plastic disk. It transmits high-pitched sounds created by the high-velocity movement of air and blood. Auscultate bowel, lung, and heart sounds using the diaphragm. Always place the stethoscope directly on the skin, because clothing obscures the sound. Position

the diaphragm to make a tight seal against the client's skin (Figure 32-8). Exert enough pressure to leave a temporary red ring on the client's skin when you remove the diaphragm.

The bell is the bowl-shaped chestpiece usually surrounded by a rubber ring. The ring avoids chilling the client with cold metal when placed on the skin. The bell transmits low-pitched sounds created by the low-velocity movement of blood. Auscultate heart and vascular sounds using the bell. Apply the bell lightly, resting the chestpiece on the skin (Figure 32-9).

Compressing the bell against the skin reduces low-pitched sound amplification and creates a "diaphragm of skin." Some stethoscopes have one chestpiece that combines features of the bell and diaphragm. When you use light pressure, the chestpiece is a bell, whereas exerting more pressure converts the bell into a diaphragm.

The stethoscope is a delicate instrument and requires proper care for optimal function. Remove the earpieces regularly, and clean them of cerumen (earwax). Clean the bell and diaphragm of dust, lint, and body oils. Clean the tubing with mild soap and water.

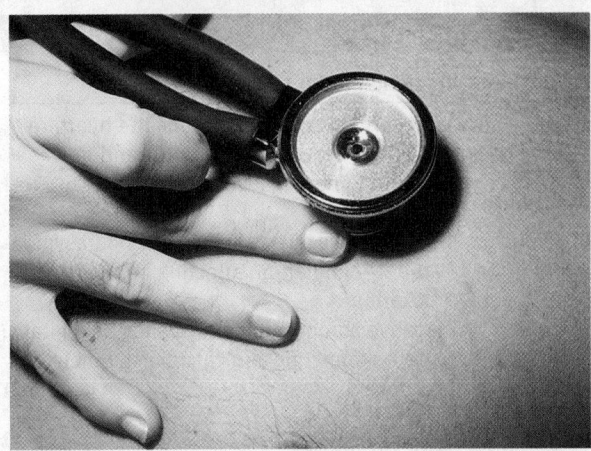

Figure 32-9 Positioning the bell of the stethoscope lightly on the skin to hear low-pitched heart sounds.

✳ TABLE 32-3 Acceptable Ranges of Heart Rates

AGE	HEART RATE (BEATS PER MINUTE)
Infant	120-160
Toddler	90-140
Preschooler	80-110
School-age child	75-100
Adolescent	60-90
Adult	60-100

Character of the Pulse

Assessment of the radial pulse includes measurement of the rate, rhythm, strength, and equality. When auscultating an apical pulse, assess rate and rhythm only.

Rate. Before measuring a pulse, review the client's baseline rate for comparison (Table 32-3). Some practitioners prefer to make baseline measurements of the pulse rate as the client assumes a sitting, standing, and lying position. Postural changes affect the pulse rate because of alterations in blood volume and sympathetic activity. The heart rate temporarily increases when a person changes from a lying to a sitting or standing position.

When assessing the pulse, consider the variety of factors influencing the pulse rate (Table 32-4). A single factor or a combination of these factors often causes significant changes. If you detect an abnormal rate while palpating a peripheral pulse, the next step is to assess the apical rate. The apical rate requires auscultation of heart sounds, which provides a more accurate assessment of cardiac contraction.

Assess the apical rate by listening for heart sounds (see Chapter 33). Try to identify the first and second heart sounds (S_1 and S_2). At normal slow rates, S_1 is low pitched and dull, sounding like a "lub." S_2 is higher pitched and shorter, creating the sound "dub." Count each set of "lub-dub" as one heartbeat. Using the diaphragm or bell of the stethoscope, count the number of lub-dubs occurring in 1 minute.

Peripheral and apical pulse rate assessment often reveals variations in heart rate. Two common abnormalities in pulse rate are tachycardia and bradycardia. **Tachycardia** is an abnormally elevated heart rate, above 100 beats per minute in adults. **Bradycardia** is a slow rate, below 60 beats per minute in adults.

An inefficient contraction of the heart that fails to transmit a pulse wave to the peripheral pulse site creates a **pulse deficit**. To assess a pulse deficit you and a colleague assess radial and apical rates simultaneously and then compare rates. The difference between the apical and radial pulse rates is the pulse deficit. For example, an apical rate of 92 with a radial rate of 78 leaves a pulse deficit of 14 beats. Pulse deficits are often associated with abnormal rhythms.

Rhythm. Normally a regular interval occurs between each pulse or heartbeat. An interval interrupted by an early or late beat or a missed beat indicates an abnormal rhythm or **dysrhythmia.** A dysrhythmia threatens the heart's ability to provide adequate cardiac output, particularly if it occurs repetitively. Identify a dysrhythmia by palpating an interruption in successive pulse waves or auscultating an interruption between heart sounds. If a dysrhythmia is present, assess the regularity of its occurrence and auscultate the apical rate (see Chapter 33). Dysrhythmias are described as regularly irregular or irregularly irregular.

To document a dysrhythmia, the health care provider will often order an electrocardiogram, Holter monitor, or telemetry. An electrocardiogram records the electrical activity of the heart for a 12-second interval. This test requires placement of electrodes across the client's chest followed by recording of the heart rhythm. The Holter monitor records 24 hours of electrical activity in a small tape recorder that the client wears. Access to the information recorded is not available until after the 24 hours have passed and the data are reviewed. Cardiac telemetry provides continuous monitoring of the heart's electrical activity transmitted to a stationary monitor. Telemetry permits continuous observation of heart rhythm during all of the client's daily activities and thus allows for immediate treatment if the rhythm becomes erratic or unstable.

Children often have a sinus dysrhythmia, which is an irregular heartbeat that speeds up with inspiration and slows down with expiration. This is a normal finding that you can verify by having the child hold his or her breath; the heart rate usually becomes regular.

Strength. The strength or amplitude of a pulse reflects the volume of blood ejected against the arterial wall with each heart contraction and the condition of the arterial vascular system leading to the pulse site. Normally the pulse strength remains the same with each heartbeat. Document the pulse strength as strong, weak, thready, or bounding. Assessment of pulse strength is included in the assessment of the vascular system (see Chapter 33).

Equality. Assess radial pulses on both sides of the peripheral vascular system, comparing the characteristics of each. A pulse in one extremity is sometimes unequal in strength or absent in many disease states (e.g., thrombus [clot] formation, aberrant blood vessels, cervical rib syndrome, or aortic dissection). Assess all symmetrical pulses simultaneously except for the carotid pulse. Never

✳ TABLE 32-4 Factors Influencing Pulse Rate

FACTOR	INCREASES PULSE RATE	DECREASES PULSE RATE
Exercise	Short-term exercise.	Long-term exercise conditions the heart, resulting in lower resting pulse and quicker return to resting level after exercise.
Temperature	Fever and heat.	Hypothermia.
Emotions	Acute pain and anxiety increase sympathetic stimulation, affecting heart rate. The effect of chronic pain on heart rate varies.	Unrelieved severe pain increases parasympathetic stimulation, affecting heart rate; relaxation.
Drugs	Positive chronotropic drugs such as epinephrine.	Negative chronotropic drugs such as digitalis; beta-adrenergic and calcium channel blockers.
Hemorrhage	Loss of blood increases sympathetic stimulation.	
Postural changes	Standing or sitting.	Lying down.
Pulmonary conditions	Diseases causing poor oxygenation such as asthma, chronic obstructive pulmonary disease (COPD).	

measure the carotid pulses simultaneously because excessive pressure occludes blood supply to the brain.

Nursing Process and Pulse Determination

Pulse assessment determines the general state of cardiovascular health and the body's response to other system imbalances. Tachycardia, bradycardia, and dysrhythmias are defining characteristics of many nursing diagnoses, including the following:

- Activity intolerance
- Anxiety
- Decreased cardiac output
- Fear
- Deficient/excess fluid volume
- Impaired gas exchange
- Hyperthermia
- Hypothermia
- Acute pain
- Ineffective tissue perfusion

The nursing care plan includes interventions based on the nursing diagnosis identified and the related factors. For example, the defining characteristics of an abnormal heart rate, exertional dyspnea, and a client's verbal report of fatigue lead to a diagnosis of *activity intolerance*. When the related factor is "inactivity following a prolonged illness," interventions will focus on increasing the client's daily exercise routine. Once the plan is implemented, evaluate client outcomes by assessing the client's pulse.

Respiration

Human survival depends on the ability of oxygen (O_2) to reach body cells and for carbon dioxide (CO_2) to be removed from the cells. Respiration is the mechanism the body uses to exchange gases between the atmosphere and the blood and the blood and the cells. Respiration involves **ventilation** (the movement of gases in and out of the lungs), **diffusion** (the movement of oxygen and

carbon dioxide between the alveoli and the red blood cells), and **perfusion** (the distribution of red blood cells to and from the pulmonary capillaries). Analyzing respiratory efficiency requires integrating assessment data from all three processes. Assess ventilation by determining respiratory rate, respiratory depth, and respiratory rhythm. Assess diffusion and perfusion by determining oxygen saturation.

Physiological Control

Breathing is generally a passive process. Normally a person thinks little about it. The respiratory center in the brain stem regulates the involuntary control of respirations. Adults normally breathe in a smooth, uninterrupted pattern, 12 to 20 times a minute.

The body regulates ventilation using levels of CO_2, O_2, and hydrogen ion concentration (pH) in the arterial blood. The most important factor in the control of ventilation is the level of CO_2 in the arterial blood. An elevation in the CO_2 level causes the respiratory control system in the brain to increase the rate and depth of breathing. The increased ventilatory effort removes excess CO_2 (hypercarbia) by increasing exhalation. However, clients with chronic lung disease have ongoing hypercarbia. For these clients chemoreceptors in the carotid artery and aorta become sensitive to **hypoxemia**, or low levels of arterial O_2. If arterial oxygen levels fall, these receptors signal the brain to increase the rate and depth of ventilation. Hypoxemia helps to control ventilation in clients with chronic lung disease. Because low levels of arterial O_2 provide the stimulus that allows the client to breathe, administration of high oxygen levels will be fatal for clients with chronic lung disease.

Mechanics of Breathing

Although breathing is normally passive, muscular work is involved in moving the lungs and chest wall. Inspiration is an active process. During inspiration the respiratory center sends impulses along the phrenic nerve, causing the diaphragm to contract. Abdominal organs move downward and forward, increasing the length of the chest cavity to move air into the lungs. The diaphragm moves approximately 1 cm ($\frac{4}{10}$ inch), and the ribs retract upward from the body's midline approximately 1.2 to 2.5 cm

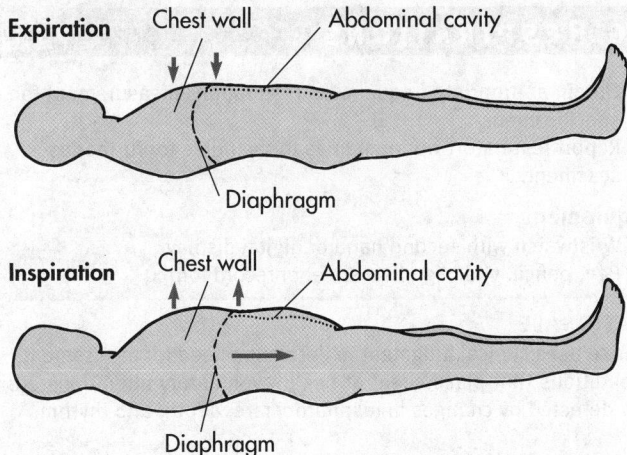

Figure 32-10 Illustration of diaphragmatic and chest wall movement during inspiration and expiration.

(½ to 1 inch). During a normal, relaxed breath, a person inhales 500 ml of air. This amount is referred to as the tidal volume. During expiration the diaphragm relaxes, and the abdominal organs return to their original positions. The lung and chest wall return to a relaxed position (Figure 32-10). Expiration is a passive process. Sighing interrupts the normal rate and depth of ventilation, **eupnea**. The sigh, a prolonged deeper breath, is a protective physiological mechanism for expanding small airways and alveoli not ventilated during a normal breath.

The accurate assessment of respirations depends on the recognition of normal thoracic and abdominal movements. During quiet breathing the chest wall gently rises and falls. Contraction of the intercostal muscles between the ribs or contraction of the muscles in the neck and shoulders, the accessory muscles of breathing, is not visible. During normal quiet breathing, diaphragmatic movement causes the abdominal cavity to rise and fall slowly.

Assessment of Ventilation

Respirations are the easiest of all vital signs to assess, but they are often the most haphazardly measured. Do not estimate respirations. Accurate measurement requires observation and palpation of chest wall movement.

A sudden change in the character of respirations is important. Because respiration is tied to the function of numerous body systems, consider all variables when changes occur (Box 32-11). For example, a drop in respirations occurring in a client after head trauma often signifies injury to the brain stem. Abdominal trauma injures the phrenic nerve, which is responsible for diaphragmatic contraction.

Do not let a client know that you are assessing respirations. A client aware of the assessment can alter the rate and depth of breathing. Assess respirations immediately after measuring pulse rate, with your hand still on the client's wrist as it rests over the chest or abdomen. When assessing a client's respirations, keep in mind the client's usual ventilatory rate and pattern, the influence any disease or illness has on respiratory function, the relationship between respiratory and cardiovascular function, and the influence of therapies on respirations. The objective measurements of

respiratory status include the rate and depth of breathing and the rhythm of ventilatory movements (Skill 32-3).

Respiratory Rate. Observe a full inspiration and expiration when counting ventilation or respiration rate. The respiratory rate varies with age (Table 32-5). The usual range of respiratory rate declines throughout life.

BOX 32-11 Factors Influencing Character of Respirations

Exercise
Exercise increases rate and depth to meet the body's need for additional oxygen and to rid the body of CO_2.

Acute Pain
Pain alters rate and rhythm of respirations; breathing becomes shallow.
Client inhibits or splints chest wall movement when pain is in area of chest or abdomen.

Anxiety
Anxiety increases respiration rate and depth as a result of sympathetic stimulation.

Smoking
Chronic smoking changes pulmonary airways, resulting in increased rate of respirations at rest when not smoking.

Body Position
A straight, erect posture promotes full chest expansion.
A stooped or slumped position impairs ventilatory movement.
Lying flat prevents full chest expansion.

Medications
Opioid analgesics, general anesthetics, and sedative hypnotics depress rate and depth.
Amphetamines and cocaine sometimes increase rate and depth.
Bronchodilators slow rate by causing airway dilation.

Neurological Injury
Injury to the brain stem impairs the respiratory center and inhibits respiratory rate and rhythm.

Hemoglobin Function
Decreased hemoglobin levels (anemia) reduce oxygen-carrying capacity of the blood, which increases respiratory rate.
Increased altitude lowers the amount of saturated hemoglobin, which increases respiratory rate and depth.
Abnormal blood cell function (e.g., sickle cell disease) reduces ability of hemoglobin to carry oxygen, which increases respiratory rate and depth.

TABLE 32-5 Acceptable Ranges of Respiratory Rate

AGE	RATE (BREATHS PER MINUTE)
Newborn	30-60
Infant (6 months)	30-50
Toddler (2 years)	25-32
Child	20-30
Adolescent	16-19
Adult	12-20

✳ **SKILL 32-3**   ASSESSING RESPIRATIONS   `Video`

Delegation Considerations

The skill of respiration measurement can be delegated. The nurse is responsible for assessing the impact of changes in respiratory rate, rhythm, and depth. The nurse instructs nursing assistive personnel to:

- Consider specific factors related to client history that increase risk for abnormal respirations.

- Obtain appropriate frequency of respirations measurement for specific client.
- Report respiratory abnormalities to the nurse for further assessment.

Equipment

- Wristwatch with second hand or digital display
- Pen, pencil, vital sign flow sheet or record form

STEPS	RATIONALE
1. Determine need to assess client's respirations:	Nurse uses clinical judgment to determine need for assessment. Conditions that place client at risk for ventilatory alterations are detected by changes in respiratory rate, depth, and rhythm.
a. Identify risk factors for respiratory alterations including: fever, pain, anxiety, diseases of chest wall or muscles, constrictive chest or abdominal dressings, gastric distention, chronic pulmonary disease (emphysema, bronchitis, asthma), traumatic injury to chest wall with or without collapse of underlying lung tissue, presence of a chest tube, respiratory infection (pneumonia, acute bronchitis), pulmonary edema and emboli, head injury with damage to brain stem, and anemia.	
b. Assess for signs and symptoms of respiratory alterations such as bluish or cyanotic appearance of nail beds, lips, mucous membranes, and skin; restlessness, irritability, confusion, reduced level of consciousness; pain during inspiration; labored or difficult breathing; adventitious breath sounds (see Chapter 33), inability to breathe spontaneously; thick, frothy, blood-tinged, or copious sputum produced on coughing.	Physical signs and symptoms indicate alterations in respiratory status related to ventilation.
2. Assess pertinent laboratory values:	
A. **Arterial blood gases (ABGs):** Normal ABGs (values vary slightly among institutions): pH: 7.35-7.45 $PaCO_2$: 35-45 mm Hg PaO_2: 80-100 mm Hg SaO_2: 95%-100%	Arterial blood gases measure arterial blood pH, partial pressure of O_2 and CO_2, and arterial O_2 saturation, which reflects client's oxygenation status.
B. **Pulse oximetry (SpO_2):** Acceptable SpO_2 ranges from 90% to 100%; however, a range from 85% to 89% is acceptable for certain chronic disease conditions; less than 85% is abnormal (see Skill 32-4).	Although 95% is considered normal, clients with sleep disorders may have an acceptable value of 90%. Changes in respiratory rate, depth, and rhythm often accompany changes in SpO_2 less than 85%.
C. **Complete blood count (CBC):** Normal CBC for adults (values vary among institutions): *Hemoglobin:* 14 to 18 g/100 mL, males; 12 to 16 g/100 mL, females *Hematocrit:* 42% to 52%, males; 37% to 47%, females *Red blood cell count:* 4.7 to 6.1 million/mm³, males; 4.2 to 5.4 million/mm³, females	Complete blood count measures red blood cell count, volume of red blood cells, and concentration of hemoglobin, which reflects client's capacity to carry O_2.
3. Determine previous baseline respiratory rate (if available) from client's record.	Allows nurse to assess for change in condition. Provides comparison with future respiratory measurements.
4. Perform hand hygiene. Draw curtain around bed, and/or close door.	Prevents transmission of microorganisms. Maintains privacy.

Critical Decision Point: Assess clients with difficulty breathing (dyspnea), such as those with congestive heart failure or abdominal ascites or in late stages of pregnancy, in the position of greatest comfort. Repositioning sometimes increases the work of breathing, which will increase respiratory rate.

---

5. Be sure client is in comfortable position, preferably sitting or lying with the head of the bed elevated 45 to 60 degrees. Be sure client's chest is visible. If necessary, move bed linen or gown.	Sitting erect promotes full ventilatory movement. Ensures clear view of chest wall and abdominal movements.

SKILL 32-3   ASSESSING RESPIRATIONS—CONT'D

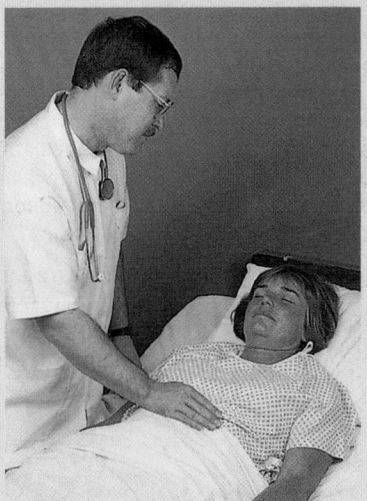

STEP 6 Nurse's hand over client's abdomen to check respiration.

STEPS	RATIONALE
6. Place client's arm in relaxed position across the abdomen or lower chest, or place nurse's hand directly over client's upper abdomen (see illustration).	A similar position used during pulse assessment allows respiratory rate assessment to be inconspicuous. Client's hand or your hand rises and falls during respiratory cycle.
7. Observe complete respiratory cycle (one inspiration and one expiration).	Rate is accurately determined only after you have observed a respiratory cycle.
8. After cycle is observed, look at watch's second hand and begin to count rate: when sweep hand hits number on dial, begin time frame, counting one with first full respiratory cycle.	Timing begins with count of one. Respirations occur more slowly than pulse; thus timing does not begin with zero.
9. If rhythm is regular, count number of respirations in 30 seconds and multiply by 2. If rhythm is irregular, less than 12, or greater than 20, count for 1 full minute.	Respiratory rate is equivalent to number of respirations per minute. Suspected irregularities require assessment for at least 1 minute.
10. Note depth of respirations. Subjectively assess by observing degree of chest wall movement while counting rate. Objectively assess depth by palpating chest wall excursion or auscultating the posterior thorax after rate has been counted (see Chapter 33). Describe depth as shallow, normal, or deep.	Character of ventilatory movement reveals specific disease states that restrict volume of air from moving into and out of the lungs.
11. Note rhythm of ventilatory cycle. Normal breathing is regular and uninterrupted. Do not confuse sighing with abnormal rhythm.	Character of ventilations reveals specific types of alterations. Periodically people unconsciously take single deep breaths or sighs to expand small airways prone to collapse.

Critical Decision Point: Any irregular respiratory pattern or periods of apnea (the cessation of respiration for several seconds) are symptoms of underlying disease in the adult and need to be reported to the health care provider or nurse in charge. Further assessment (see Chapter 33) and immediate intervention are often necessary. An irregular respiratory rate and short apneic spells are normal for newborns.

12. Replace bed linen and client's gown.	Restores comfort and promotes sense of well-being.
13. Perform hand hygiene.	Reduces transmission of microorganisms.
14. Discuss findings with client as needed.	Promotes participation in care and understanding of health status.
15. If assessing respirations for the first time, establish rate, rhythm, and depth as baseline if within normal range.	Used to compare future respiratory assessment.
16. Compare respirations with client's previous baseline and normal rate, rhythm, and depth.	Allows nurse to assess for changes in client's condition and for presence of respiratory alterations.

Continued

✳ **SKILL 32-3**   **ASSESSING RESPIRATIONS—CONT'D**

Unexpected Outcomes and Related Interventions

- Client has respiratory rate less than 12 (bradypnea) or above 20 (tachypnea) breaths per minute. Breathing pattern is irregular. Depth of respirations increase or decrease: client complains of feeling short of breath.
  - Observe for related factors, including obstructed airway, abnormal breath sounds, productive cough, restlessness, irritability, anxiety, confusion.
  - Assist client to supported sitting position (semi- or high-Fowler's) unless contraindicated, which improves ventilation.
  - Provide oxygen as ordered.
  - Assess for environmental factors that influence client's respiratory rate such as secondhand smoke, poor ventilation, or gas fumes.

Recording and Reporting

- Record respiratory rate and character in nurses' notes or vital sign flow sheet. Indicate type and amount of oxygen therapy if used by client during assessment. Document respiratory assessment after administration of specific therapies in narrative form in nurses' notes.
- Report abnormal findings to nurse in charge or health care provider.

Home Care Considerations

- Assess for environmental factors in the home that influence client's respiratory rate such as secondhand smoke, poor ventilation, or gas fumes.

✳ **TABLE 32-6 Alterations in Breathing Pattern**

ALTERATION	DESCRIPTION
Bradypnea	Rate of breathing is regular but abnormally slow (less than 12 breaths per minute).
Tachypnea	Rate of breathing is regular but abnormally rapid (greater than 20 breaths per minute).
Hyperpnea	Respirations are labored, increased in depth, and increased in rate (greater than 20 breaths per minute). Occurs normally during exercise.
Apnea	Respirations cease for several seconds. Persistent cessation results in respiratory arrest.
Hyperventilation	Rate and depth of respirations increase. Hypocarbia sometimes occurs.
Hypoventilation	Respiratory rate is abnormally low, and depth of ventilation is depressed. Hypercarbia sometimes occurs.
Cheyne-Stokes respiration	Respiratory rate and depth are irregular, characterized by alternating periods of apnea and hyperventilation. Respiratory cycle begins with slow, shallow breaths that gradually increase to abnormal rate and depth. The pattern reverses, breathing slows and becomes shallow, climaxing in apnea before respiration resumes.
Kussmaul's respiration	Respirations are abnormally deep, regular, and increased in rate.
Biot's respiration	Respirations are abnormally shallow for two to three breaths followed by irregular period of apnea.

The apnea monitor is a device that aids respiratory rate assessment. This device uses leads attached to the client's chest wall that sense movement. The absence of chest wall movement triggers the apnea alarm. Apnea monitoring is used frequently with infants in the hospital and at home to observe clients at risk for prolonged apneic events.

Ventilatory Depth. Assess the depth of respirations by observing the degree of excursion or movement in the chest wall. Describe ventilatory movements as deep, normal, or shallow. A deep respiration involves a full expansion of the lungs with full exhalation. Respirations are shallow when only a small quantity of air passes through the lungs and ventilatory movement is difficult to see. Use more objective techniques if you observe that chest excursion is unusually shallow (see Chapter 33). Table 32-6 summarizes types of breathing patterns.

Ventilatory Rhythm. Determine breathing pattern by observing the chest or the abdomen. Diaphragmatic breathing results from the contraction and relaxation of the diaphragm, and

you observe it best by watching abdominal movements. Healthy men and children usually demonstrate diaphragmatic breathing. Women tend to use thoracic muscles to breathe, assessed by observing movements in the upper chest. Labored respirations usually involve the accessory muscles of respiration visible in the neck. When something such as a foreign body interferes with the movement of air in and out of the lungs, the intercostal spaces retract during inspiration. A longer expiration phase is evident when the outward flow of air is obstructed (e.g., asthma).

With normal breathing a regular interval occurs after each respiratory cycle. Infants tend to breathe less regularly. The young child often breathes slowly for a few seconds and then suddenly breathes more rapidly. While assessing respirations, estimate the time interval after each respiratory cycle. Respiration is regular or irregular in rhythm.

Assessment of Diffusion and Perfusion

Evaluate the respiratory processes of diffusion and perfusion by measuring the oxygen saturation of the blood. Blood flow through the pulmonary capillaries provides red blood cells for oxygen attachment. After oxygen diffuses from the alveoli into the pulmonary blood, most of the oxygen attaches to hemoglobin molecules in red blood cells. Red blood cells carry the oxygenated hemoglobin molecules through the left side of the heart and out to the peripheral capillaries, where the oxygen detaches, depending on the needs of the tissues.

The percent of hemoglobin that is bound with oxygen in the arteries is the percent of saturation of hemoglobin (or SaO_2). It is usually between 95% and 100%. SaO_2 is affected by factors that interfere with ventilation, perfusion, or diffusion (see Chapter 40). The saturation of venous blood (SvO_2) is lower because the tissues have removed some of the oxygen from the hemoglobin molecules. Factors that interfere with or increases tissue oxygen demand affect the usual value for SvO_2, which is 70%.

Measurement of Arterial Oxygen Saturation.
A pulse oximeter permits the indirect measurement of oxygen saturation (Skill 32-4). The pulse oximeter is a probe with a light-emitting diode (LED) and photodetector connected by cable to an oximeter (Figure 32-11). The LED emits light wavelengths that the oxygenated and deoxygenated hemoglobin molecules absorb differently. The photodetector detects the amount of oxygen bound to hemoglobin molecules, and the oximeter calculates the pulse saturation (SpO_2). SpO_2 is a reliable estimate of SaO_2 when the SaO_2 is over 70%. Values obtained with pulse oximetry are less accurate at saturations less than 70% (Grap, 2002).

The photodetector is in the oximeter probe. Selecting the appropriate probe is important to reduce measurement error. Digit probes are spring loaded and conform to various sizes. Earlobe probes have greater accuracy at lower saturations and are least affected by peripheral vasoconstriction (Grap, 2002). You can apply disposable sensor pads to a variety of sites, even the bridge of an adult's nose or the sole of an infant's foot. Factors that affect light transmission or peripheral arterial pulsations affect the ability of the photodetector to measure SpO_2 (Box 32-12). An awareness of these factors allows accurate interpretation of abnormal SpO_2 measurements.

Nursing Process and Respiratory Vital Signs

Vital sign measurement of respiratory rate, pattern, and depth, along with SpO_2 assesses ventilation, diffusion, and perfusion. You also conduct other assessments to measure respiratory status (see Chapter 33). Each measurement provides clues in determining the nature of a client's problem. Respiratory assessment data are defining characteristics of many nursing diagnoses, including the following:

- Activity intolerance
- Ineffective airway clearance
- Anxiety
- Ineffective breathing pattern
- Impaired gas exchange
- Acute pain
- Ineffective tissue perfusion
- Dysfunctional ventilatory weaning response

The nursing care plan includes interventions based on the nursing diagnosis identified and the related factors. For example,

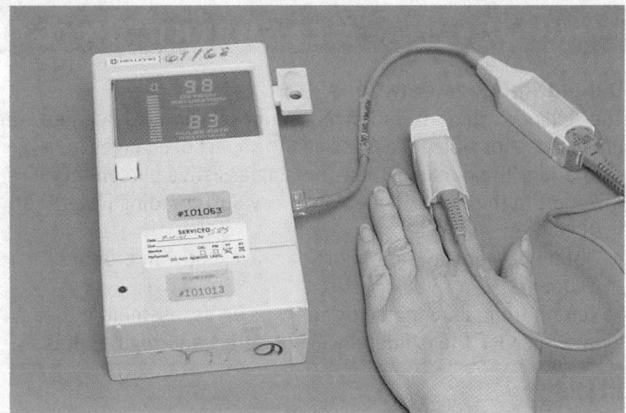

Figure 32-11 Portable pulse oximeter with digit probe.

✳ BOX 32-12   Factors Affecting Determination of Pulse Oxygen Saturation (SpO_2)

Interference With Light Transmission

Outside light sources interfere with the oximeter's ability to process reflected light.

Carbon monoxide (caused by smoke inhalation or poisoning) artificially elevates SpO_2 by absorbing light similar to oxygen.

Client motion interferes with the oximeter's ability to process reflected light.

Jaundice interferes with the oximeter's ability to process reflected light.

Intravascular dyes (methylene blue) absorb light similar to deoxyhemoglobin and artificially lower saturation.

Nail polish, artificial nails, or metal studs in nails can interfere with light absorption and the ability of the oximeter to process reflected light.

Dark skin pigment sometimes results in signal loss or overestimation of saturation.

Interference With Arterial Pulsations

Peripheral vascular disease (atherosclerosis) reduces pulse volume.

Hypothermia at assessment site decreases peripheral blood flow.

Pharmacological vasoconstrictors (e.g., epinephrine) decrease peripheral pulse volume.

Low cardiac output and hypotension decrease blood flow to peripheral arteries.

Peripheral edema obscures arterial pulsation.

Tight probe will record venous pulsations in the finger that compete with arterial pulsations.

---

the defining characteristics of tachypnea, changes in depth of respirations, use of accessory muscles, cyanosis, and a decline in SpO_2, lead to a diagnosis of *impaired gas exchange*. Related factors could include an infectious process or a history of chronic obstructive lung disease with a 30 pack-year history of smoking. Interventions will be based on the related factor. For example, evaluate client outcomes by assessing the respiratory rate, ventilatory depth, rhythm, and SpO_2 following each intervention.

Text continued on p. 536

✳ **SKILL 32-4**   **MEASURING OXYGEN SATURATION (PULSE OXIMETRY)**

Delegation Considerations

The skill of oxygen saturation measurement can be delegated. The nurse is responsible for assessing the impact of changes in oxygen saturation. The nurse instructs nursing assistive personnel to:

- Report to the nurse immediately any SpO_2 reading lower than 90%.
- Obtain oxygen saturation for specific client with ordered frequency.
- Refrain from using pulse oximetry as an assessment of heart rate because the oximeter will not detect an irregular pulse.

Equipment

- Oximeter
- Oximeter probe appropriate for client and recommended by manufacturer
- Acetone or nail polish remover if needed
- Pen, pencil, vital sign flow sheet, or record form

STEPS	RATIONALE
1. Determine need to measure client's oxygen saturation:	Clinical judgment determines need for assessment.
a. Identify risk factors of decreased oxygen saturation, including: acute or chronic compromised respiratory function, recovery from general anesthesia or conscious sedation, or traumatic injury to chest wall with or without collapse of underlying lung tissue, ventilator dependence, changes in supplemental oxygen therapy (Grap, 2002).	Certain conditions place clients at risk for decreased oxygen saturation.
b. Assess for signs and symptoms of alterations in oxygen saturation such as altered respiratory rate, depth, or rhythm; adventitious breath sounds (see Chapter 33); cyanotic appearance of nail beds, lips, mucous membranes, and skin; restlessness, irritability, confusion; reduced level of consciousness; labored or difficult breathing.	Physical signs and symptoms often indicate abnormal oxygen saturation.
2. Assess for factors that normally influence measurement of SpO_2 (see Box 32-12) in addition to oxygen therapy, hemoglobin level, body temperature, and medications such as bronchodilators.	Allows nurse to accurately assess oxygen saturation variations.
3. Review client's medical record for order or consult agency policy or procedure manual for standard of care.	Medical order is sometimes required to assess oxygen saturation.
4. Determine most appropriate client-specific site (e.g., finger, earlobe) for sensor probe placement by measuring capillary refill (see Chapter 33). If capillary refill is greater than 3 seconds, select alternate site.	Sensor requires pulsating vascular bed to identify hemoglobin molecules that absorb emitted light. Changes in SpO_2 are reflected in the circulation of finger capillary bed within 30 seconds and the capillary bed of ear lobe within 5-10 seconds. Moisture prevents the sensor from detecting SpO_2 levels. Artificial nails and certain nail polish colors will alter readings (Grap, 2002). Motion artifact is the most common cause of inaccurate readings.
a. Site needs to have adequate local circulation and be free of moisture.	
b. Place probe on finger free of polish or artificial nail.	
c. If tremors are present, use earlobe as site.	
d. If client is obese, clip-on probe may not fit properly; obtain a single-use (tape-on) probe.	
5. Determine previous baseline SpO_2 (if available) from client's record.	Baseline information provides basis for comparison and assists in assessment of current status and evaluation of interventions.
6. Explain purpose of procedure to client and how you will measure oxygen saturation. Instruct client to breathe normally.	Promotes client cooperation and increases compliance. Prevents large fluctuations in minute ventilation and possible error in SpO_2 readings.
7. Perform hand hygiene.	Reduces transmission of microorganisms.
8. Position client comfortably. When using finger as monitoring site, support lower arm.	Ensures probe positioning and decreases motion artifact that interferes with SpO_2 determination.
9. Instruct client to breathe normally.	Prevents large fluctuations in respiratory rate and depth and possible changes in SpO_2.
10. When using finger as monitoring site, remove any fingernail polish with acetone.	Ensures accurate readings. Opaque coatings decrease light transmission; nail polish containing blue pigment absorbs light emissions and falsely alters saturation (Grap, 2002).
11. Attach sensor probe to monitoring site. Instruct client that clip-on probe feels like a clothespin on the finger but will not hurt.	Pressure of sensor probe's spring tension on a peripheral digit or earlobe is unexpected.

✳ SKILL 32-4   MEASURING OXYGEN SATURATION (PULSE OXIMETRY)—CONT'D

STEPS	RATIONALE

Critical Decision Point: Do not attach probe to finger, ear, or bridge of nose if area is edematous or skin integrity is compromised. Do not attach probe to fingers that are hypothermic. Select ear or bridge of nose if adult client has history of peripheral vascular disease. Do not use earlobe and bridge of nose sensors for infants and toddlers because of skin fragility. Do not use disposable adhesive probes if client has latex allergy. Do not place sensor on same extremity as electronic blood pressure cuff because blood flow to finger will be temporarily interrupted when cuff inflates and causes inaccurate readings that trigger alarms.

STEPS	RATIONALE
12. Once sensor is in place, turn on oximeter by activating power. Observe pulse waveform/intensity display and audible beep. Correlate oximeter pulse rate with client's radial pulse. Differences require reevaluation of oximeter probe placement and may require reassessment of pulse rates.	Pulse waveform/intensity display enables detection of valid pulse or presence of interfering signal. Pitch of audible beep is proportional to SpO_2 value. Double-checking pulse rate ensures oximeter accuracy. Oximeter pulse rate, client's radial pulse, and apical pulse rate should be the same. Any difference requires reevaluation of oximeter sensor probe placement and reassessment of pulse rates.
13. Leave probe in place until oximeter readout reaches constant value and pulse display reaches full strength during each cardiac cycle. Inform client that oximeter will alarm if the probe falls off or if client moves the probe. Read SpO_2 on digital display.	Reading takes 10 to 30 seconds, depending on site selected.
14. If continuous SpO_2 monitoring is necessary, verify SpO_2 alarm limits and alarm volume, which are preset by the manufacturer at a low of 85% and a high of 100%. You determine limits for SpO_2 and pulse rate alarms based on each client's condition. Verify that alarms are on. Assess skin integrity every 2 hours under sensor probe. Relocate sensor probe at least every 24 hours or more frequently if skin integrity is altered or tissue perfusion compromised.	Alarms are set at appropriate limits and volumes to avoid frightening clients and visitors. Sensor probe tension or sensitivity to disposable sensor probe adhesive causes skin irritation and leads to disruption of skin integrity.
15. Assist client in returning to comfortable position.	Restores comfort and promotes sense of well-being.
16. Perform hand hygiene.	Reduces transmission of microorganisms.
17. Discuss findings with client as needed.	Promotes participation in care and understanding of health status.
18. If planning intermittent or spot-checking SpO_2 measurements, remove probe and turn oximeter power off. Store probe in appropriate location.	Batteries will run out if oximeter is left on. Sensor probes are expensive and vulnerable to damage.
19. Compare SpO_2 readings with client baseline and acceptable values.	Comparison reveals presence of abnormality.
20. Correlate SpO_2 with SaO_2 obtained from arterial blood gas measurements (see Chapter 41) if available.	Documents reliability of noninvasive assessment.
21. Correlate SpO_2 reading with data obtained from respiratory rate, depth, and rhythm assessment (see Skill 32-3, p. 530).	Measurements assessing ventilation, perfusion, and diffusion are interrelated.

Unexpected Outcomes and Related Interventions

- SpO_2 is less than 90%.
  - Verify that oximeter probe is intact and that outside light transmission does not influence measurement.
  - Observe for signs and symptoms of decreased oxygenation: anxiety, restlessness, tachycardia, cyanosis.
  - Verify that supplemental oxygen delivery system is delivered as ordered and is functioning properly.
  - Observe for and minimize factors that decrease SpO_2 such as lung secretions, increased activity, and hyperthermia.
  - Assist client to a position that maximizes ventilatory effort; for example, place an obese client in a high-Fowler's position.
- Pulse rate indicated on the oximeter is less than client's radial or apical pulse.
  - Reposition sensor probe to an alternative site with increased blood flow.
  - Assess client for signs of altered cardiac output (e.g., decreased blood pressure, cool skin, confusion).

Recording and Reporting

- Record SpO_2 value on nurses' notes or vital sign flow sheet, indicating type and amount of oxygen therapy used by client during assessment. Also record any signs and symptoms of oxygen desaturation in narrative form in nurses' notes. Report abnormal findings to nurse in charge or health care provider
- Document oxygen saturation after administration of specific therapies in narrative form in nurses' notes.
- Record in nurses' notes client's use of continuous or intermittent pulse oximetry. Documents use of equipment for third-party payers.

Home Care Considerations

- Pulse oximetry is used in home care to noninvasively monitor oxygen therapy or changes in oxygen therapy.
- Instruct caregivers to examine oximeter site before applying sensor.
- Instruct caregivers on procedure to implement when oxygen saturation is not within acceptable values.

Blood Pressure

Blood pressure is the force exerted on the walls of an artery by the pulsing blood under pressure from the heart. Blood flows throughout the circulatory system because of pressure changes. It moves from an area of high pressure to an area of low pressure. Systemic or arterial blood pressure, the blood pressure in the system of arteries in the body, is a good indicator of cardiovascular health. The heart's contraction forces blood under high pressure into the aorta. The peak of maximum pressure when ejection occurs is the **systolic pressure.** When the ventricles relax, the blood remaining in the arteries exerts a minimum or **diastolic pressure.** Diastolic pressure is the minimal pressure exerted against the arterial walls at all times.

The standard unit for measuring blood pressure is millimeters of mercury (mm Hg). The measurement indicates the height to which the blood pressure raises a column of mercury. Record blood pressure with the systolic reading before the diastolic (e.g., 120/80). The difference between systolic and diastolic pressure is the **pulse pressure.** For a blood pressure of 120/80, the pulse pressure is 40.

Physiology of Arterial Blood Pressure

Blood pressure reflects the interrelationships of cardiac output, peripheral vascular resistance, blood volume, blood viscosity, and artery elasticity. Your knowledge of these hemodynamic variables helps in the assessment of blood pressure alterations.

Cardiac Output.
The blood pressure depends on the cardiac output. When volume increases in an enclosed space, such as a blood vessel, the pressure in that space rises. Thus, as cardiac output increases, more blood is pumped against arterial walls, causing the blood pressure to rise. Cardiac output increases as a result of an increase in heart rate, greater heart muscle contractility, or an increase in blood volume. Changes in heart rate occur faster than changes in heart muscle contractility or blood volume. A rapid or significant increase in heart rate decreases the heart's filling time. As a result, there is a decrease in blood pressure.

Peripheral Resistance.
The blood pressure depends on peripheral vascular resistance. Blood circulates through a network of arteries, arterioles, capillaries, venules, and veins. Arteries and arterioles are surrounded by smooth muscle that contracts or relaxes to change the size of the lumen. The size of arteries and arterioles changes to adjust blood flow to the needs of local tissues. For example, when a major organ needs more blood, the peripheral arteries constrict, decreasing their supply of blood. More blood becomes available to the major organ because of the resistance change in the periphery. Normally, arteries and arterioles remain partially constricted to maintain a constant flow of blood. Peripheral vascular resistance is the resistance to blood flow determined by the tone of vascular musculature and diameter of blood vessels. The smaller the lumen of a vessel, the greater peripheral vascular resistance to blood flow. As resistance rises, arterial blood pressure rises. As vessels dilate and resistance falls, blood pressure drops.

Blood Volume.
The volume of blood circulating within the vascular system affects blood pressure. Most adults have a circulating blood volume of 5000 mL. Normally the blood volume remains constant. However, if volume increases, this exerts more pressure against arterial walls. For example, the rapid, uncontrolled infusion of intravenous fluids elevates blood pressure. When circulating blood volume falls, as in the case of hemorrhage or dehydration, blood pressure falls.

Viscosity.
The thickness or viscosity of blood affects the ease with which blood flows through small vessels. The **hematocrit,** or percentage of red blood cells in the blood, determines blood viscosity. When the hematocrit rises and blood flow slows, arterial blood pressure increases. The heart contracts more forcefully to move the viscous blood through the circulatory system.

Elasticity.
Normally the walls of an artery are elastic and easily distensible. As pressure within the arteries increases, the diameter of vessel walls increases to accommodate the pressure change. Arterial distensibility prevents wide fluctuations in blood pressure. However, in certain diseases, such as arteriosclerosis, the vessel walls lose their elasticity and are replaced by fibrous tissue that cannot stretch well. With reduced elasticity there is greater resistance to blood flow. As a result, when the left ventricle ejects its stroke volume, the vessels no longer yield to pressure. Instead, a given volume of blood is forced through the rigid arterial walls, and the systemic pressure rises. Systolic pressure is more significantly elevated than diastolic pressure as a result of reduced arterial elasticity.

Each hemodynamic factor significantly affects the others. For example, as arterial elasticity declines, peripheral vascular resistance increases. The complex control of the cardiovascular system normally prevents any single factor from permanently changing the blood pressure. For example, if the blood volume falls, the body compensates with an increased vascular resistance.

Factors Influencing Blood Pressure

Blood pressure is not constant. Many factors continually influence blood pressure. One measurement cannot adequately reflect a client's usual blood pressure. Even under the best conditions, blood pressure changes from heartbeat to heartbeat. Blood pressure trends, not individual measurements, guide nursing interventions. Understanding these factors ensures a more accurate interpretation of blood pressure readings.

Age.
Normal blood pressure levels vary throughout life (Table 32-7). Blood pressure increases during childhood. Evaluate the level of a child or adolescent's blood pressure with respect to body size and age. An infant's blood pressure ranges from 65-115/42-80 mm Hg. The normal blood pressure for a 7-year-old is 87-117/48-64 mm Hg. Larger children (heavier and/or taller) have higher blood pressures than smaller children of the same age. During adolescence, blood pressure continues to vary according to body size.

An adult's blood pressure tends to rise with advancing age. The optimal blood pressure for a healthy, middle-age adult is less than 120/80 mm Hg. Values of 120-139/80-89 mm Hg are considered prehypertension (National High Blood Pressure Education Program

TABLE 32-7 Average Optimal Blood Pressure for Age

AGE	BLOOD PRESSURE (mm Hg)
Newborn (3000 g [6.6 lb])	40 (mean)
1 month	85/54
1 year	95/65
6 years*	105/65
10-13 years*	110/65
14-17 years*	120/75
>18	<120/80

From National High Blood Pressure Education Program (NHBPEP); National Heart, Lung, and Blood Institute; National Institutes of Health: The seventh report of the Joint National Committee on Detection, Evaluation, and Treatment of High Blood Pressure, *JAMA* 289(19):2560, 2003.

*In children and adolescents, hypertension is defined as BP that is, on repeated measurement, at the 95th percentile or greater adjusted for age, height, and gender (NHBPEP, 2003).

TABLE 32-8 Classification of Blood Pressure for Adults Ages 18 and Older

CATEGORY	SYSTOLIC (mm Hg)*		DIASTOLIC (mm Hg)*
Normal	<120		<80
Prehypertension†	120-139	or	80-89
Stage 1 hypertension	140-159	or	90-99
Stage 2 hypertension	≥160	or	≥100

Data from National High Blood Pressure Education Program (NHBPEP); National Heart, Lung, and Blood Institute; National Institutes of Health: The seventh report of the Joint National Committee on Detection, Evaluation, and Treatment of High Blood Pressure, *JAMA* 289(19):2560, 2003.

*Treatment based on highest category.

†Based on average of two or more readings.

[NHBPEP], 2003) (Table 32-8). Older adults often have a rise in systolic pressure related to decreased vessel elasticity; however, blood pressure greater than 140/90—is defined as hypertension and increases an older adult's risk for hypertension-related illness.

Stress. Anxiety, fear, pain, and emotional stress result in sympathetic stimulation, which increases heart rate, cardiac output, and vascular resistance. The effects of sympathetic stimulation increase blood pressure. Anxiety raises BP as much as 30 mm Hg.

Ethnicity. The incidence of hypertension (high blood pressure) is higher in African Americans than in European Americans. African Americans tend to develop more severe hypertension at an earlier age and have twice the risk for complications such as stroke and heart attack. Genetic and environmental factors are often contributing factors. Hypertension-related deaths are also higher among African Americans.

Gender. There is no clinically significant difference in blood pressure levels between boys and girls. After puberty, males tend to have higher blood pressure readings. After menopause, women tend to have higher levels of blood pressure than men of similar age.

Daily Variation. Blood pressure varies throughout the day with lower blood pressure during sleep between midnight and 3:00 AM (Jones and others, 2006). Between 3:00 AM and 6:00 AM there is a slow and steady rise in blood pressure. When a client awakens, there is an early morning blood pressure surge (Redon, 2004). Blood pressure is highest during the day between 10:00 AM and 6 PM (Redon, 2004). No two persons have the same pattern or degree of variation. Students may find it interesting to have their blood pressure checked by a friend at intervals over 24 hours.

Medications. Some medications directly or indirectly affect blood pressure. Before blood pressure assessment, ask whether the client is receiving antihypertensive or other cardiac medications, which lower blood pressure (Table 32-9). Another class of medications affecting blood pressure is opioid analgesics, which can lower blood pressure. Vasoconstrictors and an excess volume of intravenous fluids increase blood pressure.

Activity and Weight. A period of exercise can reduce blood pressure for several hours afterwards. Older adults often experience a 5- to 10-mm fall in blood pressure about 1 hour after eating. Increase in oxygen demand by the body during activity increases BP. Inadequate exercise frequently contributes to weight gain, and obesity is a factor in the development of hypertension (Thomas and others, 2002).

Smoking. Smoking results in vasoconstriction, a narrowing of blood vessels. BP rises when a person smokes and returns to baseline in about 15 minutes after stopping smoking (NHBPEP, 2003).

Hypertension

The most common alteration in blood pressure is **hypertension.** Hypertension is often asymptomatic. Prehypertension is diagnosed in adults when an average of two or more diastolic readings on at least two subsequent visits is between 80 and 89 mm Hg or when the average of multiple systolic blood pressures on two or more subsequent visits is between 120 and 139 mm Hg. Diastolic readings greater than 90 mm Hg and systolic readings greater than 140 mm Hg (NHBPEP, 2003) define hypertension. Categories of hypertension have been developed (see Table 32-8) and determine medical intervention. One elevated blood pressure measurement does not qualify as a diagnosis of hypertension. However, if a high reading during the first blood pressure measurement (e.g., 150/90 mm Hg) is obtained, the client is encouraged to return for another checkup within 2 months.

Hypertension is associated with the thickening and loss of elasticity in the arterial walls. Peripheral vascular resistance increases within thick and inelastic vessels. The heart continually pumps against greater resistance. As a result, blood flow to vital organs such as the heart, brain, and kidney decreases.

Persons with a family history of hypertension are at significant risk. Modifiable risk factors include obesity, cigarette smoking, heavy alcohol consumption, and high sodium (salt) intake. Sedentary lifestyle and continued exposure to stress are also linked to

✴ **TABLE 32-9** Antihypertensive Medications

MEDICATION TYPE	NAMES	ACTION
Diuretics	Furosemide (Lasix), spironolactone (Aldactone), metolazone, polythiazide, benzthiazide	Lower blood pressure by reducing reabsorption of sodium and water by the kidneys, thus lowering circulating fluid volume
Beta-adrenergic blockers	Atenolol (Tenormin), nadolol (Corgard), timolol maleate (Blocadren), propranolol (Inderal)	Combine with beta-adrenergic receptors in the heart, arteries, and arterioles to block response to sympathetic nerve impulses; reduce heart rate and thus cardiac output
Vasodilators	Hydralazine hydrochloride (Apresoline), minoxidil (Loniten)	Act on arteriolar smooth muscle to cause relaxation and reduce peripheral vascular resistance
Calcium channel blockers	Diltiazem (Cardizem, Dilacor XR), verapamil hydrochloride (Calan SR), nifedipine (Procardia), nicardipine (Cardene)	Reduce peripheral vascular resistance by systemic vasodilation
Angiotensin-converting enzyme (ACE) inhibitors	Captopril (Capoten), enalapril (Vasotec), lisinopril (Prinivil, Zestril), benazepril (Lotensin)	Lower blood pressure by blocking the conversion of angiotensin I to angiotensin II, preventing vasoconstriction; reduce aldosterone production and fluid retention, lowering circulating fluid volume
Angiotensin-II receptor blockers (ARBs)	Losartan (Cozaar), olmesartan (Benicar)	Lowers the blood pressure by blocking the binding of angiotensin II, which prevents vasoconstriction

hypertension. The incidence of hypertension is greater in diabetic clients, older adults, and African Americans. It is a major factor underlying deaths from strokes and is a contributing factor to myocardial infarctions (heart attacks). When clients are diagnosed with hypertension, educate them about blood pressure values; long-term follow-up care and therapy; the usual lack of symptoms (the fact that it may not be "felt"); therapy's ability to control, but not cure, hypertension; and a consistently followed treatment plan that ensures a relatively normal lifestyle (NHBPEP, 2003).

Hypotension

Hypotension is present when the systolic blood pressure falls to 90 mm Hg or below. Although some adults have a low blood pressure normally, for the majority of people, low blood pressure is an abnormal finding associated with illness.

Hypotension occurs because of the dilation of the arteries in the vascular bed, the loss of a substantial amount of blood volume (e.g., hemorrhage), or the failure of the heart muscle to pump adequately (e.g., myocardial infarction). Hypotension associated with pallor, skin mottling, clamminess, confusion, increased heart rate, or decreased urine output is life threatening and is reported to a health care provider immediately.

Orthostatic hypotension, also referred to as **postural hypotension**, occurs when a normotensive person develops symptoms and low blood pressure when rising to an upright position. When a healthy individual changes from a lying, to sitting, to standing position, the peripheral blood vessels in the legs constrict. Constriction of the lower extremity vessels when standing prevents the pooling of blood in the legs due to gravity. Thus an individual normally does not feel any symptoms when standing. In contrast, when clients have a decreased blood volume, their blood vessels are already constricted. When a volume-depleted client stands, there is a significant drop in blood pressure with an increase in heart rate to compensate for

the drop in cardiac output. Clients who are dehydrated, anemic, or have experienced prolonged bed rest or recent blood loss are at risk for orthostatic hypotension. Some medications cause orthostatic hypotension if misused, especially in older adults or young clients. Always measure blood pressure before administering such medications.

Assess for orthostatic hypotension during vital sign measurements by obtaining blood pressure and pulse with the client supine, sitting, and standing. Obtain blood pressure readings 1 to 3 minutes after the client changes position. In most cases, orthostatic hypotension is detected within a minute of standing. If orthostatic hypotension occurs, assist the client to a lying position and notify the health care provider or nurse in charge. While obtaining orthostatic measurements, observe for other symptoms of hypotension such as fainting, weakness, or light-headedness. When recording orthostatic blood pressure measurements, record the client's position in addition to the blood pressure measurement; for example: 140/80 mm Hg supine, 132/72 mm Hg sitting, 108/60 mm Hg standing. Because the skill of orthostatic measurements requires critical thinking and ongoing nursing judgment, do not delegate this procedure.

Measurement of Blood Pressure

Arterial blood pressure measurements are obtained either directly (invasively) or indirectly (noninvasively). The direct method requires the insertion of a thin catheter into an artery. Tubing connects the catheter with electronic hemodynamic monitoring equipment. The monitor displays a constant arterial pressure waveform and reading. Because of the risk of sudden blood loss from an artery, invasive blood pressure monitoring is used only in intensive care settings. The common indirect method requires a sphygmomanometer and stethoscope. Auscultation or palpation with auscultation is the most widely used technique (Skill 32-5).

Text continued on p. 543

Delegation Considerations

The skill of blood pressure measurement can be delegated. The nurse is responsible for assessing the impact of changes in blood pressure. The nurse instructs nursing assistive personnel to:
- Select appropriate limb for blood pressure measurement.
- Select appropriate-size blood pressure cuff for designated limb.
- Consider specific client-related factors that influence blood pressure and risk of orthostatic hypotension.
- Obtain blood pressure measurement for select client with ordered frequency.
- Report abnormalities to the nurse for further assessment.

Equipment
- Aneroid sphygmomanometer
- Cloth or disposable vinyl pressure cuff of appropriate size for client's extremity
- Stethoscope
- Alcohol swab
- Pen, pencil, vital sign flow sheet or record form

STEPS

1. Determine need to assess client's BP:
   a. Identify risk factors, including: history of cardiovascular disease, renal disease, diabetes, circulatory shock (hypovolemic, septic, cardiogenic, or neurogenic), acute or chronic pain, rapid intravenous infusion of fluids or blood products, increased intracranial pressure, postoperative conditions, toxemia of pregnancy.
   b. Observe for signs and symptoms of BP alterations:
      (1) High BP (hypertension): headache (usually occipital), flushing of face, nosebleed, and fatigue in older adults.
      (2) Low BP (hypotension): dizziness, mental confusion; restlessness; pale, dusky, or cyanotic skin and mucous membranes; cool, mottled skin over extremities.
2. Determine best site for BP assessment. Avoid applying cuff to extremity when intravenous fluids are infusing; an arteriovenous shunt or fistula is present; breast or axillary surgery has been performed on that side; extremity has been traumatized, diseased, or requires a cast or bulky bandage. Use the lower extremities when the brachial arteries are inaccessible.
3. Determine previous baseline BP (if available) from client's record.
4. Encourage client to avoid caffeine and smoking before BP assessment.
5. Explain to client that you will assess BP. Have client rest at least 5 minutes before measuring client BP sitting or lying down; wait 1 minute if client standing. When possible, have client sit in a chair (NHBPEP, 2003). Ask client not to speak while measuring BP.
6. Select appropriate cuff size.
7. Perform hand hygiene.
8. Have client assume sitting or lying position. Be sure room is warm, quiet, and relaxing.
9. With client sitting or lying, position client's forearm at heart level, position thigh flat (provide support as needed). For arm, turn palm up (see illustration); for thigh, position with knee slightly flexed. If sitting, instruct client to keep feet flat on floor without crossing legs.
10. Expose extremity (arm or leg) fully by removing constricting clothing.

RATIONALE

Nurse uses clinical judgment to determine need for assessment. Certain conditions place clients at risk for BP alteration.

Physical signs and symptoms often indicate alterations in BP. High BP is often asymptomatic until pressure is very high.

Inappropriate site selection results in poor amplification of sounds, causing inaccurate readings. Application of pressure from inflated bladder temporarily restricts blood flow and further compromises circulation in extremity that already has impaired blood flow.

Allows nurse to assess for change in condition. Provides comparison with future BP measurements.
Caffeine or nicotine causes false BP elevations. Smoking immediately increases BP and lasts up to 15 minutes, caffeine increases BP up to 3 hours.
Allows client to relax and helps to avoid falsely elevated readings. When assessed at rest, blood pressure readings taken at different times are comparable (NHBPEP, 2003). Talking to a client when assessing the BP will increase readings 10% to 40% (Thomas and others, 2002).
Improper cuff size results in inaccurate readings (see Table 32-10). If cuff is too small, it tends to come loose when being inflated or results in false high readings. If the cuff is too large, you may obtain false low readings.
Reduces transmission of microorganisms.
Maintains client's comfort during measurement. The client's perceptions that the physical or interpersonal environment is stressful affect the BP measurement.
If extremity is unsupported, client will perform isometric exercise that increases diastolic blood pressure. Leg crossing falsely elevates BP.

Ensures proper cuff application.

Continued

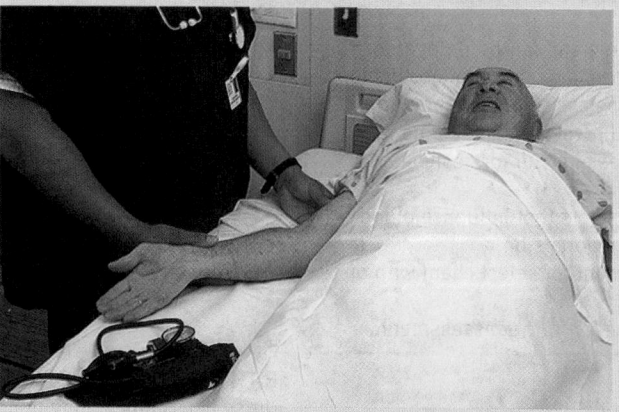

STEP 9 Client's forearm supported in bed.

A

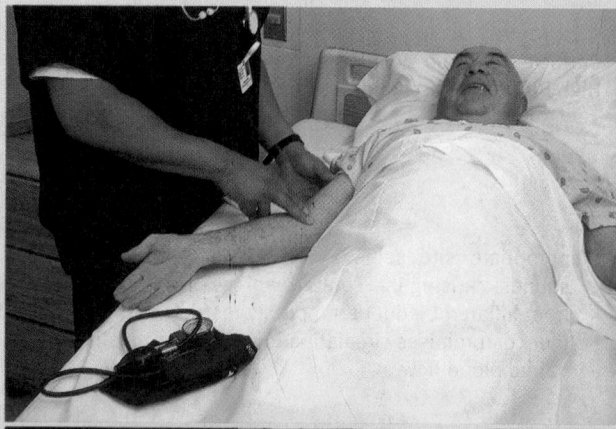

B

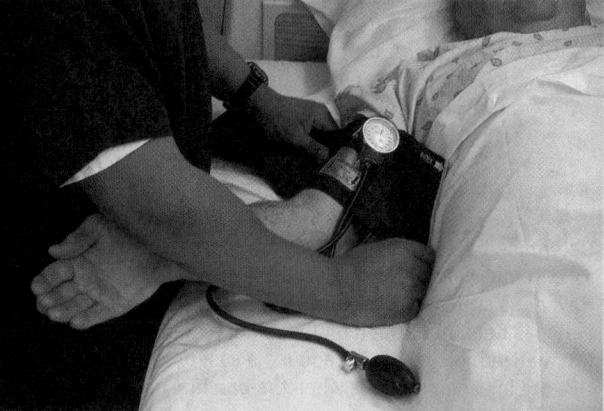

C

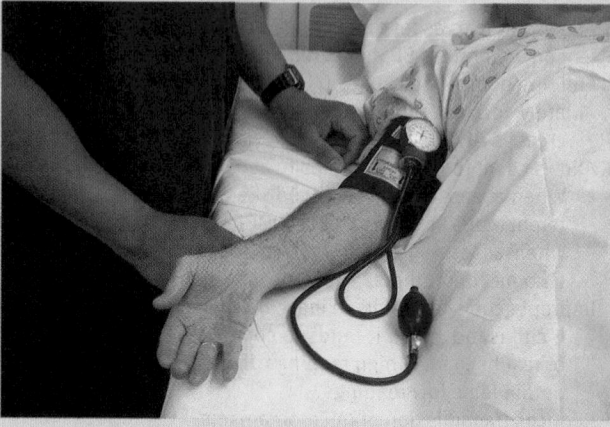

STEP 11 **A,** Nurse palpating client's brachial artery. **B,** Center bladder cuff above artery. **C,** Blood pressure cuff wrapped around upper arm.

STEPS

11. Palpate brachial artery (arm) (see illustration) or popliteal artery (leg). With cuff fully deflated, apply bladder of cuff above artery by centering arrows marked on cuff over artery. If there are no center arrows on cuff, estimate the center of the bladder and place this center over artery. Position cuff 2.5 cm (1 inch) above site of pulsation (antecubital or popliteal space). Wrap cuff evenly and snugly around extremity (see illustrations).

RATIONALE

Inflating bladder directly over artery ensures proper pressure is applied during inflation. Loose-fitting cuff causes false high readings.

✳ **SKILL 32-5**   **MEASURING BLOOD PRESSURE—CONT'D**

STEPS

12. Position aneroid needle no farther that 1 m (approximately 1 yard) away.
13. Measure blood pressure.
    A. Two-Step Method
    (1) Relocate brachial pulse. Palpate the artery distal to the cuff with fingertips of nondominant hand while inflating cuff rapidly to pressure 30 mm Hg above point at which pulse disappears. Slowly deflate cuff and note point when pulse reappears. Deflate cuff fully and wait 30 seconds.
    (2) Place stethoscope earpieces in ears, and be sure sounds are clear, not muffled.
    (3) Relocate brachial or popliteal artery, and place bell or diaphragm chestpiece of stethoscope over it. Do not allow chestpiece to touch cuff or clothing (see illustration).
    (4) Close valve of pressure bulb clockwise until tight.
    (5) Quickly inflate cuff to 30 mm Hg above palpated systolic pressure (client's estimated systolic pressure) (see illustration).
    (6) Slowly release pressure bulb valve, and allow needle of manometer gauge to fall at rate of 2 to 3 mm Hg/sec. Make sure there are no extraneous sounds.
    (7) Note point on manometer when you hear the first clear sound. The sound will slowly increase in intensity.
    (8) Continue to deflate cuff, noting point at which muffled or dampened sound appears.
    (9) Continue to deflate cuff gradually, noting point at which sound disappears in adults. Listen for 10 to 20 mm Hg after the last sound, and then allow remaining air to escape quickly.

    B. One-Step Method
    (1) Place stethoscope earpieces in ears, and be sure sounds are clear, not muffled.
    (2) Relocate brachial or popliteal artery, and place bell or diaphragm chestpiece of stethoscope over it. Do not allow chestpiece to touch cuff or clothing.
    (3) Close valve of pressure bulb clockwise until tight. Quickly inflate cuff to 30 mm Hg above palpated systolic pressure.
    (4) Slowly release pressure bulb valve and allow needle of manometer gauge to fall at rate of 2 to 3 mm Hg/sec.

RATIONALE

Obtain correct readings by looking at the aneroid needle.

Estimating prevents false low readings. Determine maximal inflation point for accurate reading by palpation. If unable to palpate artery because of weakened pulse, use an ultrasonic stethoscope (see Chapter 33). Completely deflating cuff prevents venous congestion and false high readings.

Each earpiece follows angle of ear canal to facilitate hearing.

Proper stethoscope placement ensures the best sound reception. Stethoscope improperly positioned causes muffled sounds that often result in false low systolic and false high diastolic readings.
Tightening of valve prevents air leak during inflation.
Rapid inflation ensures accurate measurement of systolic pressure.

Too rapid or slow a decline in pressure causes inaccurate readings. Noise interferes with precise determination of Korotkoff phases.
First Korotkoff reflects systolic blood pressure.

Fourth Korotkoff sound involves distinct muffling of sounds and is an indicator of diastolic pressure in children (NHBPEP, 2003).
Beginning of the fifth Korotkoff sound is an indicator of diastolic pressure in adults (NHBPEP, 2003).
Continuous cuff inflation causes arterial occlusion, resulting in numbness and tingling of client's arm.

Each earpiece follows angle of ear canal to facilitate hearing.

Proper stethoscope placement ensures optimal sound reception. Stethoscope improperly positioned causes muffled sounds that results in false low systolic and false high diastolic readings.
Tightening of valve prevents air leak during inflation. Inflation above systolic level ensures accurate measurement of systolic blood pressure.
Too rapid or slow a decline in pressure causes inaccurate readings.

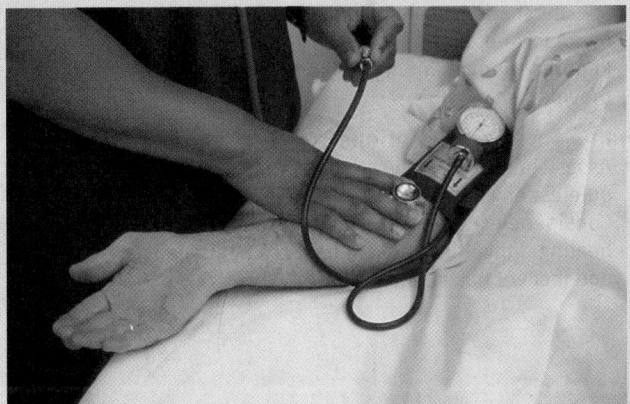

STEP 13A(3) Stethoscope over brachial artery to measure blood pressure (BP).

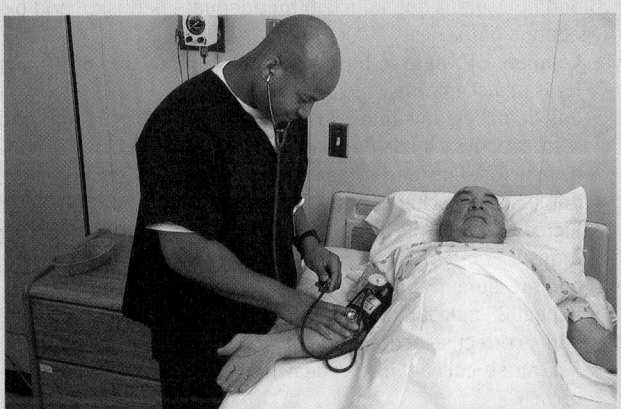

STEP 13A(5) Inflating BP cuff.

Continued

✷ SKILL 32-5   MEASURING BLOOD PRESSURE—CONT'D

STEPS

    (5) Note point on manometer when you hear the first clear sound. The sound will slowly increase in intensity.

    (6) Continue to deflate cuff, noting point at which muffled or dampened sound appears.

    (7) While gradually deflating cuff, note point at which sound disappears in adults. Listen for 10 to 20 mm Hg after the last sound, and then allow remaining air to escape quickly.

14. The Joint National Commission (NHBPEP, 2003) recommends the average of two sets of BP measurement, 2 minutes apart. Use the second set of BP measurements as the baseline. If readings are different by more than 5 mm Hg, additional readings are necessary.

15. Remove cuff from extremity unless you need to repeat measurement. If this is the first assessment of client, repeat blood pressure assessment on other extremity.

16. Assist client in returning to comfortable position, and cover upper arm if previously clothed.

17. Discuss findings with client as needed.

18. Perform hand hygiene.

19. Compare reading with previous baseline and/or acceptable value of blood pressure for client's age.

RATIONALE

First Korotkoff sound reflects systolic pressure.

Fourth Korotkoff sound involves distinct muffling of sounds and indicates the diastolic pressure in children (NNBPEP, 2003).

Beginning of the fifth Korotkoff sound indicates the diastolic pressure in adults (NHBPEP, 2003). Continuous cuff inflation causes arterial occlusion, resulting in numbness and tingling of client's arm.

Two sets of BP measurements help to prevent false positives based on a client's sympathetic response (alert reaction). Averaging minimizes the effect of anxiety, which often causes a first reading to be higher than subsequent measurements (NHBPEP, 2003).

Comparison of BP in both extremities detects circulation problems. (Normal difference of 5 to 10 mm Hg exists between extremities.)

Restores comfort and promotes sense of well-being.

Promotes participation in care and understanding of health status.

Reduces transmission of microorganisms.

Evaluates for change in condition and alterations.

Critical Decision Point: In some situations (e.g., critically ill clients or clients with peripheral vascular diseases) it is often necessary to compare blood pressure readings in both arms and/or legs. If using upper extremities, use the arm with the higher pressure for subsequent assessments unless contraindicated.

---

20. Correlate blood pressure with data obtained from pulse assessment and related cardiovascular signs and symptoms.

Blood pressure and heart rate are interrelated.

Unexpected Outcomes and Related Interventions

- Unable to obtain BP reading
  - Determine that no immediate crisis is present by obtaining pulse and respiratory rate.
  - Assess for signs of decreased cardiac output; if present, notify nurse in charge or health care provider immediately.
  - Use alternative sites or procedures to obtain BP: auscultate BP in lower extremity, use a Doppler ultrasonic instrument, implement palpation method to obtain systolic blood pressure.
  - Repeat BP measurement with sphygmomanometer. Electronic BP devices are less accurate in low blood flow conditions.
- Blood pressure is not sufficient for adequate perfusion and oxygenation of tissues.
  - Compare BP value to baseline. A systolic reading of 90 mm Hg is an acceptable value for some clients.
  - Position client in supine position to enhance circulation and restrict activity if it is decreasing BP.
  - Assess for signs and symptoms of decreased CO; if present, notify nurse in charge or health care provider.
  - Increase rate of IV infusion, or administer vasoconstricting drugs if ordered.
- Blood pressure is above acceptable range.
  - Repeat BP measurement in other arm, and compare findings. Verify correct selection and placement of cuff.
  - Ask nurse colleague to repeat measurement in 1 to 2 minutes.

- Observe for related symptoms, though symptoms are sometimes not apparent until blood pressure is extremely elevated.
- Report elevated BP to nurse in charge or health care provider to initiate appropriate evaluation and treatment.
- Administer antihypertensive medications as ordered.

Recording and Reporting

- Inform client of value and need for periodic reassessment of blood pressure.
- Record blood pressure in nurses' notes or vital sign flow sheet. Measurement of blood pressure after administration of specific therapies needs to be documented in narrative form in nurses' notes.
- Report abnormal findings to nurse in charge or health care provider.

Home Care Considerations

- Assess home noise level to determine room that will provide quietest environment for assessing BP.
- Consider electronic blood pressure cuff for home if client has hearing difficulties, if client has sufficient financial resources, and if client has adequate dexterity.

Blood Pressure Equipment. Before assessing blood pressure, make sure you are comfortable using a sphygmomanometer and stethoscope. A **sphygmomanometer** includes a pressure manometer, an occlusive cloth or vinyl cuff that encloses an inflatable rubber bladder, and a pressure bulb with a release valve that inflates the bladder. The two types of manometers are the aneroid and the mercury (Figure 32-12). Aneroid manometers have the advantages of being safe, lightweight, portable, and compact. The aneroid manometer has a glass-enclosed circular gauge containing a needle that registers millimeter calibrations. Before using the aneroid model, make sure that the needle points to zero and that the manometer is correctly calibrated. Aneroid sphygmomanometers require biomedical calibration every 6 months to verify their accuracy (Jones and others, 2003).

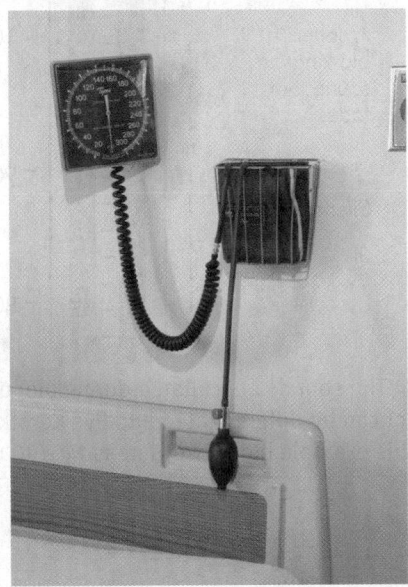

Figure 32-12 Wall-mounted aneroid sphygmomanometer.

Mercury manometers, once the gold standard, are less common because they contain mercury, a hazardous substance. Many cities have prohibited the sale or use of devices containing mercury. However, some facilities or nursing units still have mercury manometers. Pressure created by the inflation of the compression cuff moves the column of mercury upward against the force of gravity. Millimeter calibrations mark the height of the mercury column. To ensure accurate readings, the mercury column needs to fall freely as pressure is released and is always at zero when the cuff is deflated.

Cloth or disposable vinyl compression cuffs contain an inflatable bladder and come in different sizes. The size selected is proportional to the circumference of the limb being assessed (Figure 32-13). Ideally, the width of the cuff is 40% of the circumference (or 20% wider than the diameter) of the midpoint of the limb on which the cuff is used to measure blood pressure. The bladder, enclosed by the cuff, encircles at least 80% of the upper arm of an adult and the entire arm of a child (NHBPEP, 2003). Place the lower edge of the cuff above the antecubital fossa, allowing room for positioning the stethoscope bell or diaphragm. Many adults require a large adult cuff. Using the forearm when a larger cuff is not readily available is not recommended (Box 32-13). An improperly fitting cuff causes inaccurate BP measurements (see Table 32-10).

The release valve of the aneroid and mercury sphygmomanometers needs to be clean and freely movable in either direction. The value, when closed, holds the pressure constant. A sticky valve makes pressure cuff deflation hard to regulate.

Auscultation. The best environment for blood pressure measurement by auscultation is a quiet room at a comfortable temperature. Although the client may lie or stand, sitting is the preferred position. In most cases blood pressure readings obtained with the client in the supine, sitting, and standing positions are similar.

The client's position during routine blood pressure determination needs to be the same during each measurement to permit a

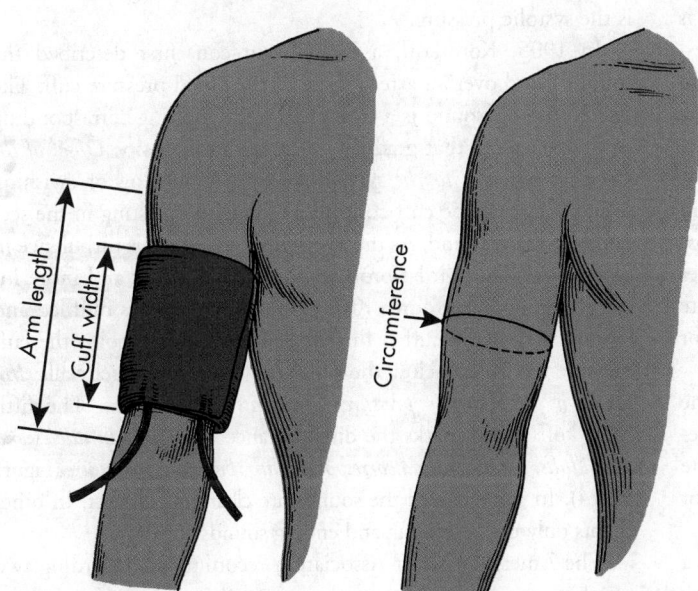

Figure 32-13 Guidelines for proper blood pressure cuff size. Cuff width 20% more than upper arm diameter, or 40% of circumference and two thirds of arm length.

✳ **BOX 32-13**   **EVIDENCE-BASED PRACTICE**

Forearm Versus Upper Arm Blood Pressure Measurements

Evidence Summary

Blood pressure measurement is an important factor when determining the diagnosis of hypertension and evaluating therapies. Because hypertension leads to serious complications, eliminating errors in measuring blood pressure is important. When the upper arm is not accessible or when the blood pressure (BP) cuff does not fit the client's upper arm, the forearm has been used for BP measurement. In this research study BP measurements taken on the forearm and the upper arm were compared when clients were supine and when the head of the bed was elevated at 45 degrees. The researchers wanted to know if placement of the BP cuff affected systolic and diastolic BP. Two hundred twenty-one medical surgical inpatients had their BP measured at both arm locations in the supine and head-elevated positions. Researchers selected cuff size based on forearm and upper arm circumference. Results indicated a significant difference between upper arm and forearm blood pressures in both positions. Both systolic and diastolic blood pressure differed as much as 33 mm Hg.

Application to Nursing Practice

- A consistent approach to the placement of upper extremity blood pressure cuff allows accurate assessment of change in condition.
- Appropriate cuff size is essential for accurate measurement.
- You cannot substitute forearm BP measurements for upper arm blood pressure measurements.

Reference

Schell K and others: Clinical comparison of automatic noninvasive measurements of blood pressure in the forearm and upper arm with the client supine or with the head of the bed raised 45 degrees: a follow-up study, *Am J Crit Care* 15(2):196, 2006.

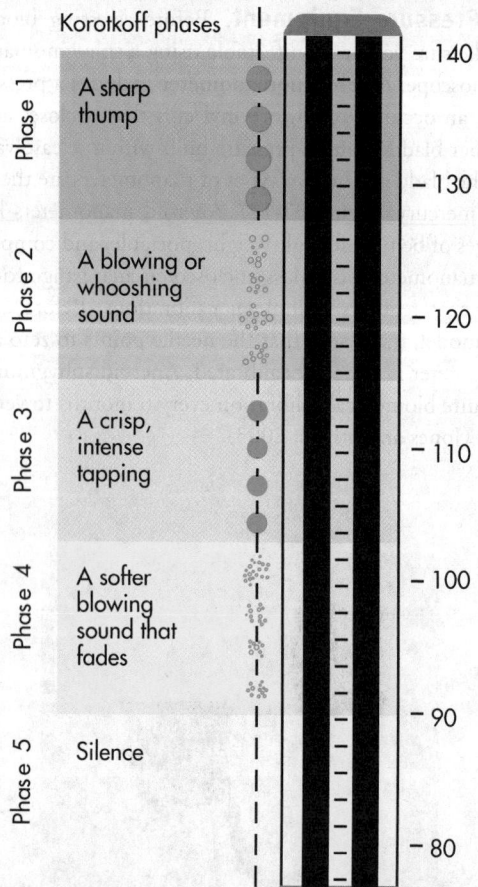

Figure 32-14 The sounds auscultated during blood pressure measurement can be differentiated into five Korotkoff phases. In this example blood pressure is 140/90 mm Hg.

meaningful comparison of values. Before obtaining the client's blood pressure, attempt to control factors responsible for artificially high readings, such as pain, anxiety, or exertion. The client's perception that the physical or interpersonal environment is stressful will affect the blood pressure measurement. Blood pressure measurements taken at the client's place of employment or in a health care provider's office are higher than those taken at the client's home.

During the initial assessment obtain and record the blood pressure in both arms. Normally there is a difference of 5 to 10 mm Hg between the arms (Lane and others, 2002). In subsequent assessments measure the blood pressure in the arm with the higher pressure. Pressure differences greater than 10 mm Hg indicate vascular problems and are reported to the health care provider or nurse in charge.

Ask the client to state his or her usual blood pressure. If the client does not know, inform the client after measuring and recording the blood pressure. This is a good opportunity to educate a client about optimal values of blood pressure, the risk factors for developing hypertension, and dangers of hypertension.

Indirect measurement of arterial blood pressure works on a basic principle of pressure. Blood flows freely through an artery until an inflated cuff applies pressure to tissues and causes the artery to collapse. After releasing the cuff pressure, the point at which blood flow returns and sound appears through auscultation is the systolic pressure.

In 1905, Korotkoff, a Russian surgeon, first described the sounds heard over an artery distal to the blood pressure cuff. The first Korotkoff sound is a clear rhythmical tapping corresponding to the pulse rate that gradually increases in intensity. *Onset of the sound corresponds to the systolic pressure.* A blowing or swishing sound occurs as the cuff continues to deflate, resulting in the second Korotkoff sound. As the artery distends, there is turbulence in blood flow. The third Korotkoff sound is a crisper and more intense tapping. The fourth Korotkoff sound becomes muffled and low pitched as the cuff is further deflated. At this point the cuff pressure has fallen below the pressure within the vessel walls; *this sound is the diastolic pressure in infants and children.* The fifth Korotkoff sound marks the disappearance of sound. *In adolescents and adults, the fifth sound corresponds with the diastolic pressure* (Figure 32-14). In some clients the sounds are clear and distinct. In other clients only the beginning and ending sounds are clear.

The American Heart Association recommends recording two numbers for a blood pressure measurement: the point on the

TABLE 32-10 Common Errors in Blood Pressure Assessment

ERROR	EFFECT
Bladder or cuff too wide	False low reading
Bladder or cuff too narrow or too short	False high reading
Cuff wrapped too loosely or unevenly	False high reading
Deflating cuff too slowly	False high diastolic reading
Deflating cuff too quickly	False low systolic and false high diastolic reading
Arm below heart level	False high reading
Arm above heart level	False low reading
Arm not supported	False high reading
Stethoscope that fits poorly or impairment of the examiner's hearing, causing sounds to be muffled	False low systolic and false high diastolic reading
Stethoscope applied too firmly against antecubital fossa	False low diastolic reading
Inflating too slowly	False high diastolic reading
Repeating assessments too quickly	False high systolic reading
Inadequate inflation level	False low systolic reading
Multiple examiners using different Korotkoff sounds for diastolic readings	False high systolic and false low diastolic reading

BOX 32-14 PROCEDURAL GUIDELINES

Palpating the Systolic Blood Pressure

Delegation Considerations: The skill of palpation of blood pressure may not be delegated.

Equipment: Sphygmomanometer.

1. Perform hand hygiene.
2. Apply blood pressure (BP) cuff to the extremity selected for measurement.
3. Continually palpate the pulse of the brachial, radial, or popliteal artery with fingertips of one hand.
4. Inflate BP cuff 30 mm Hg above the point at which you no longer can palpate the pulse.
5. Slowly release valve and deflate cuff, allowing manometer needle mercury to fall 2 mm Hg per second.
6. Note point on manometer when pulse is again palpable; this is the systolic blood pressure.
7. Deflate cuff rapidly and completely. Remove cuff from client extremity unless you need to repeat the measurement.
8. Perform hand hygiene. Record pressure as systolic/−, palpated (e.g., BP 108/−, palpated).

manometer when you hear the first sound for systolic and the point on the manometer when you hear the fifth sound for diastolic (NHBPEP, 2003). Some institutions recommend recording the point when you hear the fourth sound as well, especially for clients with hypertension. Divide the numbers by slashed lines (e.g., 120/80 or 120/100/80). Note the arm used to measure the blood pressure (e.g., right arm [RA] 130/70), and the client's position (e.g., sitting).

Blood pressure assessment results in many medical decisions and nursing interventions. Obtaining an accurate blood pressure measurement is essential. There are several sources for error. Table 32-10 summarizes common mistakes in measurement. When you are unsure of a reading, have a colleague reassess the blood pressure.

Assessment in Children.
All children 3 years of age through adolescence need to have blood pressure checked at least yearly. Blood pressure in children changes with growth and development. Help parents to understand the importance of this routine screening to detect children who are at risk for hypertension. The measurement of blood pressure in infants and children is difficult for several reasons:

- Different arm size requires careful and appropriate cuff size selection. Do not choose a cuff based on the name of the cuff. An "infant" cuff is often too small for some infants.
- Readings are difficult to obtain in restless or anxious infants and children. Allow at least 15 minutes for children to recover from recent activities and become less apprehensive. Preparing

the child for the blood pressure cuff's unusual sensation increases cooperation. Most children will understand the analogy of a "tight hug on your arm."
- Placing the stethoscope too firmly on the antecubital fossa causes errors in auscultation.
- Korotkoff sounds are difficult to hear in children because of low frequency and amplitude. A pediatric stethoscope bell is often helpful.

Ultrasonic Stethoscope.
When you are unable to auscultate sounds because of a weakened arterial pulse, you can use an ultrasonic stethoscope (see Chapter 33). This stethoscope allows you to hear low-frequency systolic sounds. You will frequently use this device when measuring the blood pressure of infants, children, and low blood pressure in adults.

Palpation.
Indirect measurement of blood pressure by palpation is useful for clients whose arterial pulsations are too weak to create Korotkoff sounds. Severe blood loss and decreased heart contractility are examples of conditions that result in blood pressures too low to auscultate accurately. In these cases, you can assess the systolic blood pressure by palpation. The diastolic blood pressure is difficult to determine by palpation (Box 32-14). When using the palpation technique, record the systolic value and how you measured it (e.g., RA 90/−, palpated, supine).

You can use the palpation technique along with auscultation. In some hypertensive clients the sounds usually heard over the brachial artery when the cuff pressure is high disappear as pressure is reduced and then reappear at a lower level. This temporary disappearance of sound is the **auscultatory gap**. It typically occurs between the first and second Korotkoff sounds. The gap in sound covers a range of 40 mm Hg and thus causes an underestimation of systolic pressure or overestimation of diastolic pressure. The examiner needs to be certain to inflate the cuff high enough to hear the true systolic pressure before the auscultatory gap. Palpation of

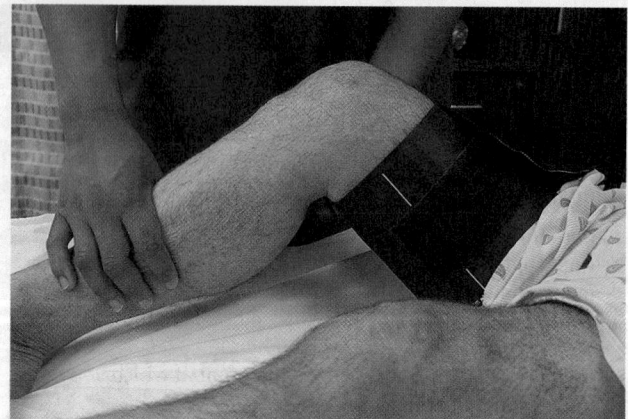

Figure 32-15 Lower extremity blood pressure cuff positioned above popliteal artery at midthigh with knee flexed.

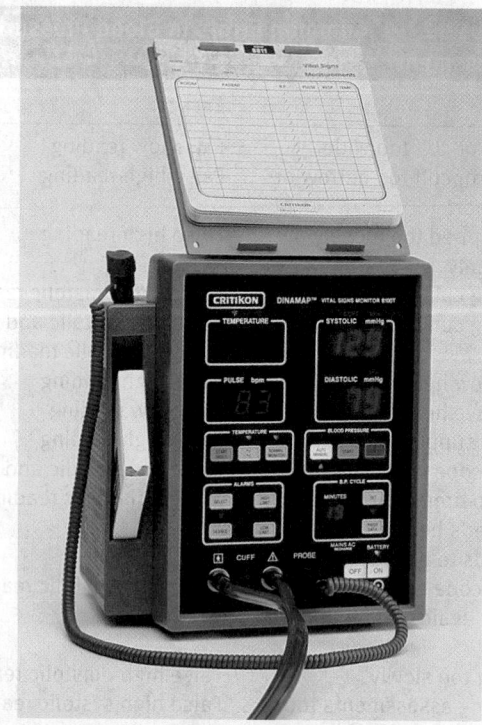

Figure 32-16 Automatic blood pressure monitor. (Dinamap Vital Signs Monitor is a trademark of Critikon, Inc. Photo courtesy Critikon, Inc, Tampa, Fla.)

the radial artery helps to determine how high to inflate the cuff. The examiner inflates the cuff 30 mm Hg above the pressure at which the radial pulse was palpated. Record the range of pressures in which the auscultatory gap occurs (e.g., BP RA 180/94 mm Hg with an auscultatory gap from 180 to 160 mm Hg, sitting).

Lower Extremity Blood Pressure. Dressings, casts, intravenous catheters, or arteriovenous fistulas or shunts make the upper extremities inaccessible for blood pressure measurement. You then need to obtain the blood pressure in a lower extremity. Comparing upper extremity blood pressure with that in the legs is also necessary for clients with certain cardiac and BP abnormalities. The popliteal artery, palpable behind the knee in the popliteal space, is the site for auscultation. The cuff needs to be wide and long enough to allow for the larger girth of the thigh. Placing the client in a prone position is best. If such a position is impossible, ask the client to flex the knee slightly for easier access to the artery. Position the cuff 2.5 cm (1 inch) above the popliteal artery with the bladder over the posterior aspect of the midthigh (Figure 32-15). The procedure is identical to brachial artery auscultation. Systolic pressure in the legs is usually higher by 10 to 40 mm Hg than in the brachial artery, but the diastolic pressure is the same.

Electronic Blood Pressure Devices. Many different styles of electronic BP machines are available to determine BP automatically (Figure 32-16). Electronic BP machines rely on an electronic sensor to detect the vibrations caused by the rush of blood through an artery. When the cuff deflates, one style of BP machine determines the initial burst of oscillations and translates the information in a systolic pressure reading. The machine makes the diastolic measurement when the oscillations are lowest, just before they stop. Use electronic devices when frequent blood pressure assessment is necessary, such as in the critically ill or potentially unstable client, during or after invasive procedures, or when therapies require frequent monitoring (e.g., intravenous heart and blood pressure medications) (Box 32-15). However, some client conditions are not appropriate for automatic blood pressure devices (Box 32-16).

The advantages of automatic devices are the ease of use and efficiency when repeated or when frequent measurements are indicated. The ability to use a stethoscope is not necessary. However, automatic devices are more sensitive to outside interference and are susceptible to error. Most electronic blood pressure devices are unable to process sounds or vibrations of low blood pressure. The range of device sophistication also makes blood pressure measurement comparisons difficult. The use of automatic blood pressure devices permits assessment of blood pressure during interpersonal interactions. However, avoid speaking to the client for at least a minute before initiating a blood pressure recording. Talking to a client while assessing the blood pressure will increase readings 10% to 40% (Pickering, 2001).

Self-Measurement of Blood Pressure. Improved technology in electronic monitoring devices allows individuals to measure their own blood pressures in their home. The portable home devices include the aneroid sphygmomanometer and electronic digital readout devices that do not require use of a stethoscope. The electronic devices inflate and deflate cuffs with the push of a button. The electronic devices are easier to manipulate but require frequent recalibration, more than once a year. Because of their sensitivity, improper cuff placement or movement of the arm causes electronic devices to give incorrect readings.

Stationary automatic blood pressure devices are often found in public places such as grocery stores, fitness clubs, airports, or work sites. Users simply rest their arms within the machine's inflatable cuff, which contains a pressure sensor. The cuff fits over clothing.

✳ BOX 32-15   PROCEDURAL GUIDELINES

Electronic Blood Pressure Measurement

Delegation Considerations: The skill of obtaining an electronic blood pressure measurement can be delegated unless the client is considered unstable or needs to be closely monitored for evaluating response to medications. The nurse is responsible for assessing the impact of changes in blood pressure. The nurse instructs nursing assistive personnel to:

- Select appropriate limb for blood pressure measurement.
- Select appropriate-size blood pressure cuff for designated limb.
- Select blood pressure cuff recommended by manufacturer.
- Obtain blood pressure measurement for select client with ordered frequency.
- Report abnormalities to the nurse for further assessment.

Equipment: Electronic BP machine, BP cuff of appropriate size as recommended by manufacturer.

1. Determine appropriateness of using electronic BP measurement. Clients with irregular heart rates, peripheral vascular disease, seizures, tremors, and shivering are not candidates for this device.
2. Determine best site for cuff placement (see Skill 32-5, Step 2).
3. Assist client to comfortable position, either lying or sitting. Plug in device, and place device near client, ensuring that the connector hose, between cuff and machine, will reach.
4. Locate on/off switch, and turn machine on to enable device to self-test computer systems.
5. Select appropriate cuff size for client extremity (see Table 32-10) and appropriate cuff for machine. Electronic BP cuff and machine are matched by the manufacturer and are not interchangeable.
6. Expose extremity for measurement by removing restrictive clothing to ensure proper cuff application. Do not place BP cuff over clothing.
7. Prepare BP cuff by manually squeezing all the air out of the cuff and connecting cuff to connector hose.
8. Wrap flattened cuff snugly around extremity, verifying that only one finger fits between cuff and client's skin. Make sure the "artery" arrow marked on the outside of the cuff is correctly placed (see illustration for Skill 32-5, Step 11).
9. Verify that connector hose between cuff and machine is not kinked. Kinking prevents proper inflation and deflation of cuff.

10. Following manufacturer's directions, set the frequency control of automatic or manual, then press the start button. The first BP measurement will pump the cuff to a pressure of about 180 mm Hg. After this pressure is reached, the machine begins a deflation sequence that determines the BP. The first reading determines the peak pressure inflation for additional measurements.

Critical Decision Point: If unable to obtain BP with electronic device, verify machine connections (e.g., plugged into working electrical outlet, hose-cuff connections tight, machine on, correct cuff). Repeat electronic BP; if unable to obtain, use auscultatory technique (see Skill 32-5).

11. When deflation is complete, digital display will provide most recent values and flash time in minutes that has elapsed since measurement occurred.
12. Set frequency of BP measurements, upper and lower alarm limits for systolic, diastolic, and mean BP readings. Intervals between BP measurements are set from 1 to 90 minutes. Determine measurement frequency and alarm limits based on client's acceptable range of blood pressure, nursing judgment, and health care provider order.
13. Obtain additional readings at any time by pressing the start button. (Sometimes you will need these for unstable clients.) Pressing the cancel button immediately deflates the cuff.
14. If frequent BP determinations are necessary, leave the cuff in place. Remove cuff at least every 2 hours to assess underlying skin integrity, and if possible, alternate BP sites. Clients with abnormal bleeding tendencies are at risk for microvascular rupture from repeated inflations. When the client no longer requires the electronic BP machine, clean BP cuff according to facility policy to reduce transmission of microorganisms.
15. Compare electronic BP readings with auscultatory BP to verify accuracy of the electronic BP device.
16. Record BP and site assessed on vital sign flow sheet or in nurses' notes (per agency policy). Record any signs of BP alterations in nurses' notes. Report abnormal findings to nurse in charge or health care provider.

A visual display tells users their blood pressure within 60 to 90 seconds. The reliability of the stationary machines is limited. Blood pressure values vary by 5 to 10 mm Hg or more (for both systolic and diastolic values) compared with pressures taken with a manual sphygmomanometer.

Self-measurement of blood pressure has several benefits. Sometimes elevated blood pressure is detected in persons previously unaware of a problem. Persons with prehypertension provide information about the pattern of blood pressure values to their health care provider. Clients with hypertension benefit from participating actively in their treatment through self-monitoring, which helps compliance with treatment. The disadvantages of self-measurement include improper use of the device and risk of

✳ BOX 32-16   Client Conditions Not Appropriate for Electronic Blood Pressure Measurement

- Irregular heart rate
- Peripheral vascular obstruction (e.g., clots, narrowed vessels)
- Shivering
- Seizures
- Excessive tremors
- Inability to cooperate
- Blood pressure less than 90 mm Hg systolic

Health Promotion

Temperature

- Identify client's ability to initiate preventive health measures and recognize alteration in body temperature. Educate client and caregiver about measures to prevent body temperature alterations.
- Teach clients risk factors for hypothermia and frostbite: fatigue; malnutrition; hypoxemia; cold, wet clothing; alcohol intoxication.
- Teach clients risk factors for heat stroke: strenuous exercise in hot, humid weather; tight-fitting clothing in hot environments; exercising in poorly ventilated areas; sudden exposures to hot climates; poor fluid intake before, during, and after exercise.
- Teach clients the importance of taking and continuing antibiotics as directed until course of treatment is completed.

Pulse Rate

- Clients taking certain prescribed cardiac medications need to learn to assess their own pulse rates to detect side effects of medications.
- Clients undergoing cardiac rehabilitation need to learn to assess their own pulse rates to determine their response to exercise.

Blood Pressure

- Teach client risk factors for hypertension. Persons with family history of hypertension are at significant risk. Obesity, cigarette smoking, heavy alcohol consumption, high blood cholesterol and triglyceride levels, and continued exposure to stress are risk factors linked to hypertension.

- Clients with hypertension need to learn about their blood pressure (BP) values, long-term follow-up care and therapy, the usual lack of symptoms, therapy's ability to control but not cure, and benefits of a consistently followed treatment plan.
- Instruct clients in the importance of appropriate-size blood pressure cuff for home use.
- Instruct client or primary caregiver to take BP at same time each day and after client has had a brief rest. Take BP sitting or lying down; use same position and arm each time pressure is taken.
- Instruct client or primary caregiver that if it is difficult to hear the pressure, the cuff is probably too loose, not big enough, or too narrow; the stethoscope is not over arterial pulse; the cuff deflated too quickly or too slowly; or the cuff was not inflated enough for systolic readings.

Respirations

- Clients who demonstrate decreased ventilation will benefit from learning deep breathing and coughing exercises (see Chapter 50).
- Instruct caregiver to contact home care nurse or health care provider if unusual fluctuations in respiratory rate occur.
- Teach client signs and symptoms of hypoxemia: headache, somnolence, confusion, dusky color, shortness of breath, dyspnea.
- Teach client effect of high-risk behaviors such as cigarette smoking on oxygen saturation.

inaccurate readings. Some clients are needlessly alarmed with one elevated reading. Some clients with hypertension become overly conscious of their blood pressure and make inappropriate self-adjustment of medications.

Consumers can learn to use self-measurement devices if they have the information needed to perform the procedure correctly and if they know when to seek medical attention. Advise clients of possible inaccuracies in the blood pressure devices, help clients understand the meaning and implications of readings, and teach them proper measurement techniques.

Nursing Process and Blood Pressure Determination

The assessment of blood pressure along with pulse assessment evaluates the general state of cardiovascular health and responses to other system imbalances. Hypotension, hypertension, orthostatic hypotension, and narrow or wide pulse pressures are defining characteristics of certain nursing diagnoses, including the following:

- Activity intolerance
- Anxiety
- Decreased cardiac output
- Deficient/excess fluid volume
- Risk for injury
- Acute pain
- Ineffective tissue perfusion

The nursing care plan includes interventions based on the nursing diagnosis identified and the related factors. For example, the defining characteristics of hypotension, dizziness, pulse deficit, and dysrhythmia lead to a diagnosis of *decreased cardiac output*. Related factors might include poor oral intake, excessive heat exposure, and a history of valvular heart disease. The related factor guides the choice of nursing interventions. Evaluate client outcomes by assessing the blood pressure following each intervention.

Health Promotion and Vital Signs

The emphasis on health promotion and health maintenance, as well as early discharge from hospital settings, has resulted in an increase in the need for clients and their families to monitor vital signs in the home. Teaching considerations affect all vital sign measurements, and you need to incorporate them within the client's plan of care (Box 32-17).

When considering how to teach clients and their families about vital sign measurements and their importance and significance, the client's age is an important factor. With an increase in the older adult population there is a greater need for caregivers to be aware of changes that are unique to older adults. Box 32-18 identifies some of these variations unique to the older adult.

Vital Signs

Temperature

- The temperature of older adults is at the lower end of the normal temperature range, 36° to 36.8° C (96.8° to 98.3° F) orally and 36.6° to 37.2° C (98° to 99° F) rectally. Therefore temperatures considered within normal range sometimes reflect a fever in an older adult.
- Older adults are very sensitive to slight changes in environmental temperature because their thermoregulatory systems are not as efficient (Ebersole and others, 2004).
- A decrease in sweat gland reactivity in the older adult results in a higher threshold for sweating at high temperatures, which leads to hyperthermia and heatstroke.
- Be especially attentive to subtle temperature changes and other manifestations of fever in this population, such as tachypnea, anorexia, falls, delirium, and overall functional decline.
- With aging, loss of subcutaneous fat reduces the insulating capacity of the skin; older men are especially high risk for hypothermia.

Pulse Rate

- If it is difficult to palpate the pulse of an older adult or obese client, a Doppler device will provide a more accurate reading.
- The older adult has a decreased heart rate at rest (Ebersole and others, 2004).
- It takes longer for the heart rate to rise in the older adult to meet sudden increased demands that result from stress, illness, or excitement. Once elevated, the pulse rate of an older adult takes longer to return to normal resting rate (Ebersole and others, 2004).
- When assessing the apical rate of an older woman, the breast tissue is gently lifted and the stethoscope placed at the fifth intercostal space (ICS) or the lower edge of the breast.
- Heart sounds are sometimes muffled or difficult to hear in older adults because of an increase in air space in the lungs.

Blood Pressure

- The normal range for blood pressure (BP) is the same for older adults and younger people (NHBPEP, 2003).
- Older adults often have decreased upper arm mass, which requires special attention to selection of BP cuff size.
- Older adults sometimes have an increase in systolic pressure related to decreased vessel elasticity while the diastolic pressure remains the same, resulting in a wider pulse pressure.
- Instruct older adults to change position slowly and wait after each change to avoid postural hypotension and prevent injuries.

Respirations

- Aging causes ossification of costal cartilage and downward slant of ribs, resulting in a more rigid rib cage, which reduces chest wall expansion. Kyphosis and scoliosis that occur in older adults also restrict chest expansion and decrease tidal volume.
- Older adults depend more on accessory abdominal muscles during respiration than on weaker thoracic muscles.
- The respiratory system matures by the time a person reaches 20 years of age and begins to decline in healthy people after the age of 25. Despite this decline, older adults are able to breathe effortlessly as long as they are healthy. However, sudden events that require an increased demand for oxygen (e.g., exercise, stress, illness) create shortness of breath in the older adult (Ebersole and others, 2004).
- Identifying an acceptable pulse oximeter probe site is difficult with older adults because of the likelihood of peripheral vascular disease, decreased cardiac output, cold-induced vasoconstriction, and anemia.

Recording Vital Signs

Special graphic flow sheets exist for recording vital signs (see Chapter 26). Identify the institution's procedure for documenting on the graphic or vital sign flow sheet. In addition to the actual vital sign values, record in the nurses' notes any accompanying or precipitating symptoms such as chest pain and dizziness with abnormal blood pressure, shortness of breath with abnormal respirations, cyanosis with hypoxemia, or flushing and diaphoresis with elevated temperature. Document any interventions initiated as a result of vital sign measurement, such as administration of oxygen therapy or an antihypertensive medication.

Clients being managed on critical paths or CareMaps often have vital sign values listed as outcomes. If a vital sign value is above or below the anticipated outcomes, write a variance note to explain the nature of the variance and the nursing course of action. For example, a CareMap for a client who has undergone a thoracotomy often has an outcome during the postoperative period of "afebrile." If the client has a fever, the nurse's variance note addresses possible sources of fever (e.g., retained pulmonary secretions) and nursing interventions (e.g., increased suctioning, postural drainage, or hydration).

✳ Key Concepts

- Vital sign measurement includes the physiological measurement of temperature, pulse, blood pressure, respirations, and oxygen saturation.
- Nurses measure vital signs as part of a complete physical examination or in a review of a client's condition.
- Nurses assess vital sign changes with other physical assessment findings, using clinical judgment to determine measurement frequency.
- Knowledge of the factors influencing vital signs assists in determining and evaluating abnormal values.
- Vital signs provide a basis for evaluating response to nursing interventions.
- Measure vital signs when the client is inactive and the environment is controlled for comfort.
- Nurses assist clients in maintaining body temperature by initiating interventions that promote heat loss, production, or conservation.
- A fever is one of the body's normal defense mechanisms.
- Measurement of temperature using the temporal artery is the least invasive, most accurate method of obtaining core temperature.

- Respiratory assessment includes determining the effectiveness of ventilation, perfusion, and diffusion.
- Assessment of respiration involves observing ventilatory movements through the respiratory cycle.
- Variables affecting ventilation, perfusion, and diffusion influence oxygen saturation.
- To assess cardiac function, it is easy to measure pulse rate and rhythm using the radial or apical pulses.
- Hypertension is diagnosed only after an average of readings made during two or more subsequent visits reveals an elevated blood pressure.
- Selecting and applying the blood pressure measurement cuff improperly will result in errors in blood pressure measurement.
- Changes in one vital sign often influence characteristics of the other vital signs.

✳ Critical Thinking Exercises

Mr. Coburn, the 56-year-old schoolteacher who was seen earlier in the week for hyperthermia, arrives at the walk-in health center complaining of feeling dizzy and nauseated. You immediately note that he appears to be having some difficulty catching his breath during coughing spells.

1. List in priority order the vital signs to be measured for Mr. Coburn.
2. Which of the vital signs do you delegate to the nursing assistant?

The electronic blood pressure machine alarm is sounding. You note that it is flashing "72 systolic" with no diastolic reading.

3. What actions do you take?

Mr. Coburn's blood pressure according to the BP machine is 82/38 mm Hg. His radial pulse is 1+, slightly irregular, and 112 beats per minute.

4. What actions do you take?

You have difficulty auscultating Mr. Coburn's blood pressure in his left upper arm.

5. List three actions that you could take to obtain Mr. Coburn's blood pressure.

✳ NCLEX®-Style Review Questions

A 52-year-old woman is admitted with dyspnea and discomfort in her left chest with deep breaths. She has smoked for 35 years and recently lost over 10 pounds.

1. Which vital sign should not be delegated to a nursing assistant?
   1. Temperature
   2. Radial pulse
   3. Respiratory rate
   4. Oxygen saturation

2. Place the vital signs in order of priority for your nursing interventions.
   1. SpO_2 = 89%
   2. BP = 160/86 mm Hg
   3. Temperature = 37.3° C, tympanic
   4. Heart (HR) = 72 beats per minute
   5. Respiratory rate (RR) = 28 breaths per minute

An 82-year-old widower is admitted via ambulance to the emergency department with complaints of shortness of breath, anorexia, and malaise. He recently visited his health care provider and was begun on an antibiotic for pneumonia. The client indicates that he also takes a diuretic and a beta-adrenergic blocker, which helps his "high blood."

3. What vitals signs do you delegate to the nursing assistant?
   1. BP, HR, SpO_2
   2. HR, RR, SpO_2
   3. BP, RR, temperature
   4. Temperature, SpO_2, RR

4. The client requests to get out of bed to go to the bathroom. He has orders for "up ad lib." What action do you take?
   1. Obtain orthostatic BP measurements.
   2. Tell him it is not a good idea, and provide a urinal.
   3. Ask the nursing assistant to assist him to the bathroom.
   4. Give him some slippers, and tell him where the bathroom is located.

5. The client has a temperature of 38.2° C via the temporal artery. What additional information do you need to plan your interventions? (Choose all that apply.)
   1. Heart rate
   2. Skin turgor
   3. Smoking history
   4. Allergies to antibiotics
   5. Recent bowel movement
   6. Blood pressure in right arm
   7. Client's normal temperature
   8. Blood pressure in distal extremity

Ms. Kilty is a 55-year-old widowed client who was in a motor vehicle accident and is admitted to your surgical unit after repair of fractured left arm and left leg. She also has a laceration on her forehead. An IV is infusing in the right antecubital fossa, and pneumatic compression stockings are on the right lower leg. She is receiving oxygen via a simple face mask.

6. Which vital sign measurements do you delegate to the nursing assistant?

7. What site should you instruct the nursing assistant to use for obtaining Ms. Kilty's temperature? Provide your rationale for selecting this site.

8. The nursing assistant informs you that the electronic blood pressure machine that is taking Ms. Kilty's blood pressure on her right arm is reading 210/100 mm Hg. You are aware that the client's preoperative blood pressure was 138/84 mm Hg. Select the appropriate nursing interventions, and place them in order of priority. If you do not select an intervention, provide a rationale.

1. Obtain a complete set of vital signs.
2. Notify the physician or nurse in charge.
3. Administer antihypertensive medication as ordered.
4. Assess the client for pain, and medicate as ordered.
5. Obtain the client's blood pressure using the right lower extremity.
6. Verify the client's right arm blood pressure yourself using auscultation.
7. Ask the nursing assistant to try a different electronic blood pressure machine.
8. Ask the nursing assistant to take another reading with the electronic blood pressure machine in 15 minutes.

9. Mr. Achilles has been transferred to your unit from the respiratory intensive care unit, where he has been for the past 2 weeks recovering from pneumonia. He is receiving oxygen via 4 L nasal cannula. His respiratory rate is 26 breaths per minute, and his oxygen saturation is 92%. In planning his care, what information would be most helpful in determining your priority nursing interventions?

1. Activity order
2. Medication list
3. Baseline vital signs
4. Client's perception of dyspnea

10. You assess Mrs. Morgan's vital signs during her routine yearly physical. She tells you she has noted that her heart feels like it is "racing," usually in the later morning, early afternoon, or just before she goes to bed. Her radial pulse rate is 68 beats per minute and regular; her blood pressure is 134/82 mm Hg. How would the following information be helpful in evaluating Mrs. Morgan's racing heart?

1. Dietary habits
2. Medication list
3. Exercise regimen
4. Age, weight, and height

33 | Health Assessment and Physical Examination

✳ OBJECTIVES

Mastery of content in this chapter will enable the student to:

- Discuss the purposes of physical assessment.
- Demonstrate the techniques used with each physical assessment skill.
- Discuss how cultural diversity influences health assessment.
- List techniques used to prepare a client physically and psychologically before and during an examination.
- Describe interview techniques used to enhance communication during history taking.
- Make environmental preparations before an examination.
- Identify data to collect from the nursing history before an examination.
- Discuss normal physical findings in a young, middle-age, and older adult.
- Discuss ways to incorporate health promotion and health teaching into the examination.
- Use physical assessment skills during routine nursing care.
- Describe physical measurements made in assessing each body system.
- Identify self-screening examinations commonly performed by clients.
- Identify preventive screenings and the appropriate age(s) for each screening to occur.

✳ MEDIA RESOURCES   ✳ KEY TERMS

Companion CD
- NCLEX®-Style Review Questions
- Audio Glossary
- Interactive Learning Activities
- English/Spanish Glossary

evolve **Website**
- NCLEX®-Style Review Questions
- Audio Glossary
- English/Spanish Glossary
- Interactive Learning Activities
- Weblinks
- Audio Summaries

Acromegaly, p. 575
Adventitious sounds, p. 597
Alopecia, p. 570
Aneurysm, p. 618
Aphasia, p. 633
Apical impulse, p. 598
Arcus senilis, p. 579
Atherosclerosis, p. 603
Atrophied, p. 631
Basal cell carcinoma, p. 569
Benign (fibrocystic) breast disease, p. 614
Borborygmi, p. 617
Bronchophony, p. 597
Bruit, p. 603
Capillary refill, p. 608
Caries, p. 587
Cerumen, p. 582
Chancre, p. 620
Cherry angiomas, p. 569
Cholecystitis, p. 618
Cirrhosis, p. 574
Clubbing, p. 608
Conjunctivitis, p. 579
Cyanosis, p. 566
Dermatitis, p. 568
Distention, p. 616
Dysrhythmia, p. 600
Ectropion, p. 579
Eczema, p. 568

Edema, p. 569
Entropion, p. 579
Erythema, p. 567
Excoriation, p. 585
Exophthalmos, p. 579
Exostosis, p. 588
Goniometer, p. 626
Hemorrhoids, p. 624
Hepatitis B virus, p. 615
Hernias, p. 616
Hirsutism, p. 570
Hydrocephalus, p. 575
Hypertonicity, p. 627
Hypotonicity, p. 627
Indurated, p. 569
Integument, p. 566
Jaundice, p. 567
Kyphosis, p. 625
Leukoplakia, p. 587
Lordosis, p. 625
Melanoma, p. 566
Metastasize, p. 612
Murmurs, p. 600
Nystagmus, p. 578
Occlusion, p. 602
Ophthalmoscope, p. 580
Orthopnea, p. 594
Osteoporosis, p. 625
Otoscope, p. 582
Ototoxicity, p. 583

Palpation, p. 554
Pancreatitis, p. 618
Papanicolaou (Pap) test, p. 620
Paralytic ileus, p. 617
Peristalsis, p. 617
Peritonitis, p. 617
PERRLA, p. 580
Petechiae, p. 569
Phlebitis, p. 609
Pigmentation, p. 567
Point of maximal impulse (PMI), p. 598
Polyps, p. 585
Ptosis, p. 579
Pulse deficit, p. 600
Scoliosis, p. 625
Senile keratosis, p. 569
Squamous cell carcinoma, p. 569
Stenosis, p. 602
Striae, p. 616
Syncope, p. 602
Tactile fremitus, p. 594
Thrill, p. 601
Turgor, p. 569
Varicosities, p. 588
Ventricular gallop, p. 600
Vocal fremitus, p. 594
Whispered pectoriloquy, p. 597

A nurse is sometimes the first person to detect changes in a client's condition, regardless of the setting. For this reason, the ability to critically think and interpret the meaning of a client's behavior and presenting physiological changes is very important. The skills of physical assessment and examination provide powerful tools to detect subtle, as well as obvious, changes in a client's health. Physical assessment enables the nurse to assess patterns reflecting health problems and to evaluate the client's progress following therapy.

While working in various settings, nurses seek information about clients' health status. The nurse conducts health assessments at health fairs, at screening clinics, in physicians' offices, in acute care agencies, and in the client's home. Health screenings focus on a specific physical problem. For example, blood pressure screenings detect the risk for high blood pressure. If screening determines that a client has a risk for disease, the nurse refers the client for a more complete physical examination.

A complete health assessment involves a nursing history (see Chapter 16) and a behavioral and physical examination. The health history involves a lengthy client interview to gather subjective data about the client's condition. A physical examination is a head-to-toe review of each body system that offers objective information about the client. This allows the nurse to make clinical judgments. The client's condition and response affect the extent of the examination. The accuracy of the physical assessment will influence the choice of therapies a client receives and the evaluation of the response to those therapies. Continuity in health care improves when the nurse makes ongoing, objective, and comprehensive assessment.

Purposes of Physical Examination

An examination is designed for the client's needs. In an acutely ill client the nurse assesses only the involved body system(s). When a client is having an asthmatic attack, the nurse initially assesses the pulmonary and cardiac systems. Then a more comprehensive examination about the client's total health status is completed when the client feels more at ease. You perform a complete physical examination for routine screening to promote wellness behaviors and preventive health care measures; to determine eligibility for health insurance, military service, or a new job; and to admit to a hospital or long-term care facility. Use physical examination to do the following:

- Gather baseline data about the client's health status
- Supplement, confirm, or refute data obtained in the history
- Confirm and identify nursing diagnoses
- Make clinical judgments about a client's changing health status and management
- Evaluate the outcomes of care

Gathering a Health History

The main objective of interacting with clients is to find out what their concerns are and to help them find solutions. Pay close attention to a client's concerns. Direct the interview and examination so that you can create a clear picture of the client's condition. Collection of a health history and a physical examination require patience and a dedication to thoroughness and detail. Conducting a successful interview and physical examination is based on several principles (see Chapter 16). The interview allows for formation of a partnership with the client. Orient the interview to the client, not to a disease. Make sure you know your own idiosyncrasies (e.g., wanting to be liked, fear of harming the client, or catching a disease) so you are able to prevent these feelings from harming the relationship with the client.

Developing Nursing Diagnoses and a Care Plan

Gather information about the client's health from the health history. A subsequent physical assessment can reveal information that refutes, confirms, or supplements the history. Think critically about the information the client provides, apply knowledge from previous clinical care, and methodically conduct the examination to create a clear picture of the client's status. For example, if a client complains of back pain, ask the client several questions to clarify the nature of the pain. During the examination, look carefully for the source of the pain (e.g., discomfort when changing position or a bruise across the client's back) to rule out a variety of potential ailments.

One assessment finding does not conclusively reveal the nature of an abnormality. A complete assessment is necessary to form a definitive nursing diagnosis. Learn to group significant findings into clusters of data that reveal actual or "risk for" nursing diagnoses (see Chapter 17). In addition, each abnormal finding provides direction to gather additional information. Gather information during the initial physical assessment to provide a baseline of the client's functional abilities. The baseline is not necessarily the normal range of physical findings but rather the pattern of findings identified when the client was first assessed. Use this baseline as a comparison for future assessment findings. Determine whether the client's condition is changing during subsequent assessments.

The accuracy of the database allows for the development of an individualized nursing diagnosis (Table 33-1). Physical assessment findings determine the etiology of the diagnosis so that the selection of interventions is appropriate for the care plan. Physical assessment is ongoing, and thus the care plan changes with the client's condition. Monitor the client's progress and responses to therapies to review existing diagnoses and identify new problems.

Managing Client Problems

When caring for clients, the nurse assesses and performs a variety of interventions. Yet the nurse's success in giving care depends on the ability to recognize change in status and to modify interventions so that clients gain the most desirable outcomes. Physical assessment skills allow nurses to judge the status of clients' health and direct the management of care. For example, the nurse inspects the skin during a routine bath and finds it excessively dry. The nurse does not use soap and applies body lotion to the skin. The nurse revises the written care plan so that other nurses know the type of skin care to provide and instructs the client about skin care. Performing the mechanics of physical assessment is relatively simple. The more difficult challenge lies in using findings to make decisions.

✳ **TABLE 33-1 Development of Individualized Nursing Diagnoses**

ASSESSMENT METHOD	FINDINGS	PATTERNS	NURSING DIAGNOSIS
Inspection of skin	Skin along sacral area is intact. There is 3-cm area of redness around coccyx; skin blanches on palpation. There are no skin lesions.	There is pressure area around coccyx.	Risk for impaired skin integrity.
Palpation of skin	Skin is moist from diaphoresis. There is tenderness to palpation around sacral area. There is elastic skin turgor.	Skin moisture promotes maceration.	
Historical data	Client suffered fractured left leg. Client's mobility is reduced as a result of left leg traction.		

Evaluating Nursing Care

Nurses demonstrate accountability for their nursing care through evaluating the results of nursing interventions. Physical assessment skills enhance the evaluation of nursing measures through monitoring physiological and behavioral outcomes of care. You use the same physical assessment skills to assess a condition (e.g., palpation of the client's pulse) and evaluate a client's response to care (e.g., an evaluation of a client's tolerance to an exercise plan).

Nurses make accurate, detailed, objective measurements through physical assessment. These measurements determine whether the expected outcomes of care are met.

Cultural Sensitivity

Respect the cultural differences of the clients when completing an examination (see Chapter 9). It is important to remember that cultural differences influence a client's behavior. Consider the client's health beliefs, use of alternative therapies, nutritional habits, relationships with family, and comfort with your physical closeness during the examination and history.

Be culturally aware, and avoid stereotyping on the basis of gender or race. There is a difference between cultural characteristics and physical characteristics. Learn to recognize common disorders of those ethnic populations within the community. For example, Navajo Indians often have ear anomalies, Polynesians often suffer clubfoot, and many African Americans experience sickle cell disease. Similarly, it is important to know variations in physical characteristics, such as in the skin and musculoskeletal system, that are related to racial variables. Recognition of cultural diversity helps to respect a client's uniqueness and to provide care of a higher quality (see Chapter 9). Recognition and respect of cultural diversity leads to greater client satisfaction and improved clinical outcomes (Galanti, 2004).

Integration of Physical Assessment With Nursing Care

Learn to integrate an examination during routine client care. For example, assess the condition of the skin during a bed bath, or observe a client's gait, range of motion (ROM), and balance as the client ambulates. Assisting with activities of daily living offers an additional opportunity to obtain assessment data. This practice makes more efficient use of time.

Skills of Physical Assessment

A comprehensive physical examination involves the use of five skills: inspection, palpation, percussion, auscultation, and olfaction.

Inspection

Inspection is the use of vision and hearing to distinguish normal from abnormal findings. It is important to know what to consider normal for clients of different age-groups. You will need experience to recognize normal variations among clients. Inspection is a simple technique, and the quality of an inspection depends on the nurse's willingness to spend time doing a thorough job. To inspect body parts accurately, follow these principles:

- Make sure adequate lighting is available.
- Position and expose body parts so all surfaces can be viewed.
- Inspect each area for size, shape, color, symmetry, position, and abnormalities.
- When possible, compare each area inspected with the same area on the opposite side of the body.
- Use additional light (e.g., a penlight) to inspect body cavities.
- Do not hurry inspection. Pay attention to detail.

After inspection of a body part, findings sometimes indicate the need for further examination. Use palpation with or after visual inspection.

Palpation

Palpation involves the use of the hands to touch body parts to make sensitive assessments. Use palpation to examine all accessible parts of the body. For example, palpate the skin for temperature, moisture, texture, turgor, tenderness, and thickness. Palpate the abdomen for tenderness, distention, or masses. Use different parts of the hand to detect characteristics such as texture, temperature, and perception of movement (Table 33-2).

Before palpation, help the client relax and be comfortable because muscle tension during palpation impairs effective assessment. To promote relaxation, have the client take slow, deep breaths and place the arms along the side of the body. *Palpate tender areas last.* Be sure to ask the client to point out the more sensitive areas, and note any nonverbal signs of discomfort.

✳ **TABLE 33-2 Examples of Characteristics Measured by Palpation**

Area Examined	Criteria Measured	Portion of Hand to Use
Skin	Temperature	Dorsum of hand/fingers
	Moisture	Palmar surface
	Texture	
	Turgor and elasticity	Grasping with fingertips
	Tenderness	
	Thickness	Palmar surface
Organs (e.g., liver and intestine)	Size	Entire palmar surface of hand or palmar surface of fingers
	Shape	
	Tenderness	
	Absence of masses	
Glands (e.g., thyroid and lymph)	Swelling	Pads of fingers
	Symmetry and mobility	
Blood vessels (e.g., carotid or femoral artery)	Pulse amplitude	Palmar surface/pads of fingertips
	Elasticity	
	Rate	
	Rhythm	
Thorax	Excursion	Palmar surface
	Tenderness	Finger pads/palmar surface of fingers
	Fremitus	Palmar or ulnar surface of entire hand

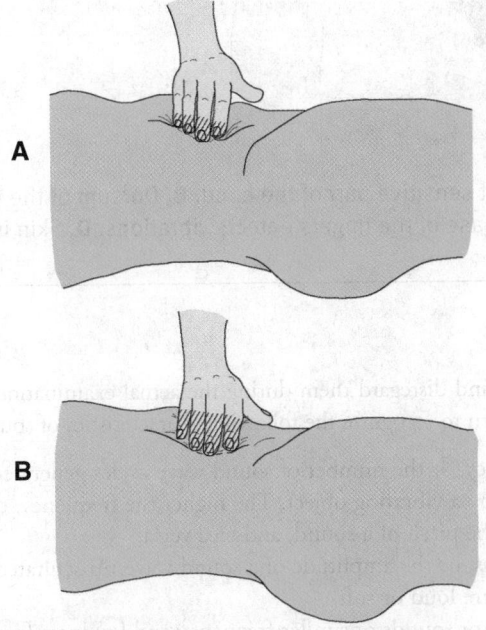

Figure 33-1 A, During light palpation, gentle pressure against underlying skin and tissues can detect areas of irregularity and tenderness. **B,** During deep palpation, depress the tissue to assess the condition of underlying organs.

You need warm hands, short fingernails, and a gentle approach for this technique. Perform palpation slowly, gently, and deliberately. Light palpation of structures such as the abdomen determines areas of tenderness (Figure 33-1, *A*). Place the hand on the part you will examine, and depress about 1 cm (½ inch). Examine tender areas further for potentially serious abnormalities. Light, intermittent pressure is best when palpating; heavy, prolonged pressure causes a loss of sensitivity in the hand.

After light palpation, use deeper palpation to examine the condition of organs, such as those in the abdomen (Figure 33-1, *B*).

Depress the area you are examining approximately 4 cm (2 inches) (Seidel and others, 2006). Caution is the rule. To avoid injuring a client, do not attempt deep palpation without clinical supervision. Apply deep palpation with one hand or both hands (bimanually). When using bimanual palpation, relax one hand (sensing hand), and place it lightly over the client's skin. Use the other hand (active hand) to apply pressure to the sensing hand. The lower hand does not exert pressure directly and thus remains sensitive to detect organ characteristics.

Use the most sensitive parts of the hand, the palmar surface of the fingers and finger pads, to determine position, texture, size, consistency, masses, fluid, and crepitus (Figure 33-2, *A*). Measure temperature using the dorsal surface or back of the hand (Figure 33-2, *B*). The palmar surface of the hand and finger (Figure 33-2, *C*) is more sensitive to vibration. Measure position, consistency, and turgor by lightly grasping the body part with the fingertips (Figure 33-2, *D*).

Do not palpate without considering the client's condition. For example, if the client has a fractured rib, use extra care to locate the painful area. Do not palpate a vital artery with pressure that obstructs blood flow. Also consider the body area being palpated, as well as the reason for using palpation.

Percussion

Percussion involves tapping the body with the fingertips to produce a vibration that travels through body tissues. The character of the sound determines the location, size, and density of underlying structures to verify abnormalities assessed by palpation and auscultation. This vibration is transmitted through body tissues, and the character of the sound heard depends on the density of the underlying tissue. By knowing the way various densities influence sound, you locate organs or masses, map their boundaries, and determine their size. An abnormal sound suggests a mass or substance such as air or fluid within an organ or body cavity. The skill of percussion requires dexterity and is usually for advanced practitioners.

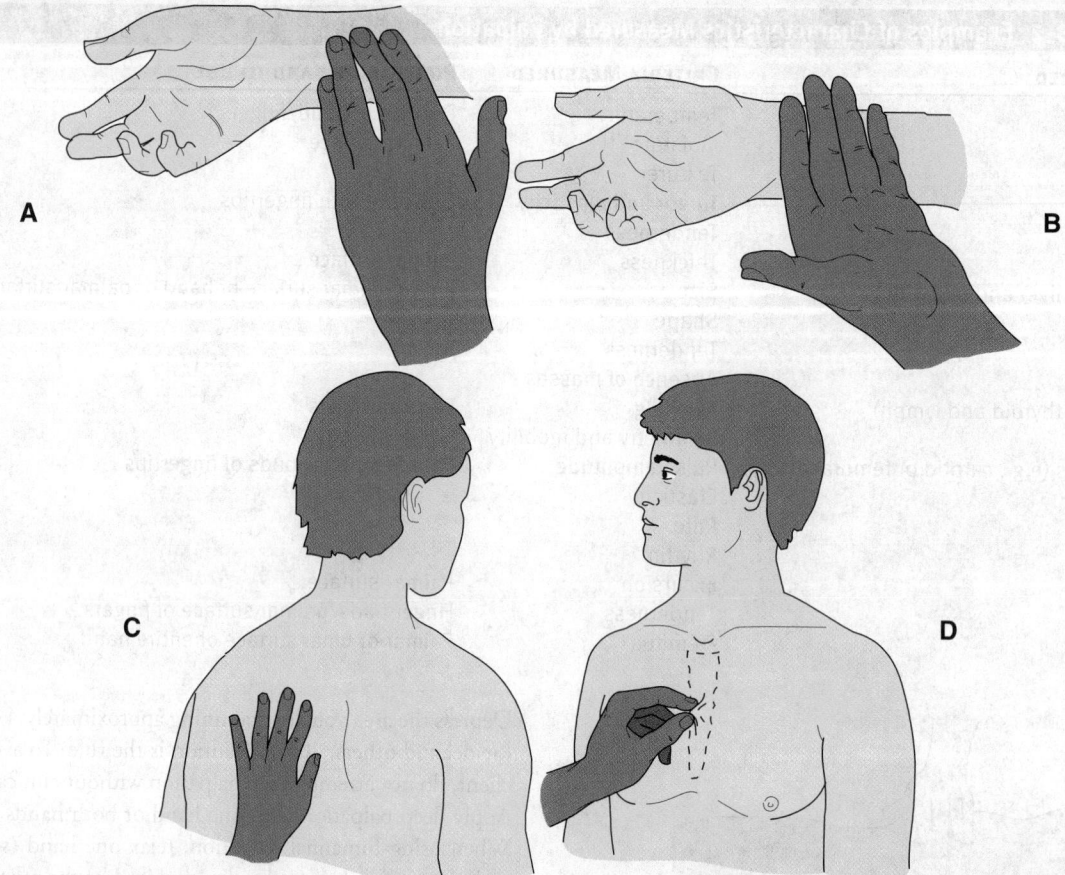

Figure 33-2 A, Radial pulse is detected with the pads of fingertips, the most sensitive part of the hand. **B,** Dorsum of the hand detects temperature variations in skin. **C,** The bony part of the palm at the base of the fingers detects vibrations. **D,** Skin is grasped with the fingertips to assess turgor.

Auscultation

Auscultation involves listening to sounds the body makes to detect variations from normal. You are able to hear some sounds without assistance but will need a stethoscope for most sounds.

First learn the normal sounds created by the cardiovascular, respiratory, and gastrointestinal (GI) systems, such as the passage of blood through an artery. Recognize abnormal sounds after learning normal variations. Becoming more proficient in auscultation occurs by knowing the types of sounds each body structure makes and the location in which you hear the sounds best. Also, learn which areas do not normally emit sounds.

To auscultate correctly, the nurse needs to hear well, have a good stethoscope, and know how to use it properly. For those with a hearing disorder, use a stethoscope with greater sound amplification. Always place the stethoscope on skin, because clothing obscures sound. Chapter 32 describes the parts of the stethoscope and its general use. The bell is best for low-pitched sounds, such as vascular and certain heart sounds, and the diaphragm is best for high-pitched sounds, such as bowel and lung sounds.

Be familiar with the stethoscope before attempting to use it. Practice using the stethoscope. Extraneous sounds created by movement of the tubing or chestpiece interfere with auscultation of body organ sounds. By deliberately producing these sounds, learn to

recognize and disregard them during the actual examination (Box 33-1). Learn to recognize the following characteristics of sounds:

- Frequency, or the number of sound wave cycles generated per second by a vibrating object. The higher the frequency, the higher the pitch of a sound, and vice versa.
- Loudness, or the amplitude of a sound wave. Auscultated sounds are loud or soft.
- Quality, or sounds of similar frequency and loudness from different sources. Terms such as *blowing* or *gurgling* describe the quality of sound.
- Duration, or the length of time that sound vibrations last. The duration of sound is short, medium, or long. Layers of soft tissue dampen the duration of sounds from deep internal organs.

Auscultation requires concentration and practice. Always consider the part of the body auscultated and the cause of the sound. For example, closure of the mitral valve causes the first heart sound. Learn where you hear the sounds best. You typically hear the first heart sound best when auscultated at the left fifth intercostal space along the midclavicular line. It is also important to learn the characteristics of normal sounds. The first heart sound has the quality of a loud "lub," whereas the second sound is a

---

✳ BOX 33-1 Exercises to Increase Familiarity With the Stethoscope

- Ensure that the earpiece follows the contour of the ear canals. Learn what fit is best for you by comparing amplification of sounds with the earpieces in both directions.
- Place the earpieces in your ears with the tips of the earpieces turned toward the face. *Lightly* blow into the diaphragm. Again place the earpieces in your ears, this time with the ends turned toward the back of the head. *Lightly* blow into the diaphragm. You will find that you hear clearer sounds with the earpiece turned toward the face. After you have learned the right fit for the loudest amplification, wear the stethoscope the same way each time.
- Put on the stethoscope, and *lightly* blow into the diaphragm. If the sound is barely audible, *lightly* blow into the bell. Sound is carried through only one part of the chestpiece at a time. If the sound is greatly amplified through the diaphragm, the diaphragm is in position for use. If the sound is barely audible through the diaphragm, the bell is in position for use. Rotation of the diaphragm and bell places the chestpiece in the desired position. Leave the diaphragm in position for the next exercise.
- Place the diaphragm over the anterior part of your chest. Ask a friend to speak in a normal conversational tone. Environmental noise seriously detracts from hearing the noise created by body organs. When using a stethoscope, the client and the examiner need to remain quiet.
- Put the stethoscope on, and gently tap the tubing. It is often difficult to avoid stretching or moving the stethoscope's tubing. The examiner is in a position so that the tubing hangs free. Moving or touching the tubing creates extraneous sounds.
- *Care of the stethoscope:* Remove earpieces regularly and clean; remove cerumen (earwax). Keep the bell and diaphragm free of dust, lint, and body oils. Keep the tubing away from nurse's body oils. Avoid draping the stethoscope around the neck next to the skin. To clean, wipe the entire stethoscope (diaphragm, tubing, etc.) with alcohol or soapy water. Be sure to dry all parts thoroughly. Follow the manufacturer's recommendations.
- *Infection Control:* Harmful bacteria, even antibiotic-resistant microorganisms, can be transferred from client to client when using portable equipment such as stethoscopes (Truscott, 2005). Cleanse the stethoscope (diaphragm/bell) with a disinfectant *before* reuse on another client. Using a disinfectant such as isopropyl alcohol (with or without chlorhexidine), benzalkonium, or sodium hypochlorite are effective in reducing the number of bacterial colonies (Guinto and others, 2002). Earpieces of stethoscopes are sources of transferable bacteria. When you inadvertently touch your ears and care for the client potential pathogens could contaminate the earpieces. Using hand hygiene, before and after client contact, decreases the risk of transmitting microorganisms from your ear to your client (Guinto and others, 2002). Follow institution infection control guidelines, especially contact precautions, to decrease this risk.

✳ TABLE 33-3 Assessment of Characteristic Odors

Odor	Site or Source	Potential Causes
Alcohol	Oral cavity	Ingestion of alcohol, diabetes
Ammonia	Urine	Urinary tract infection, renal failure
Body odor	Skin, particularly in areas where body parts rub together (e.g., underarms and under breasts)	Poor hygiene, excess perspiration (hyperhidrosis), foul-smelling perspiration (bromhidrosis)
	Wound site	Wound abscess
	Vomitus	Abdominal irritation, contaminated food
Feces	Vomitus/oral cavity (fecal odor)	Bowel obstruction
	Rectal area	Fecal incontinence
Foul-smelling stools in infant	Stool	Malabsorption syndrome
Halitosis	Oral cavity	Poor dental and oral hygiene, gum disease
Sweet, fruity ketones	Oral cavity	Diabetic acidosis
Stale urine	Skin	Uremic acidosis
Sweet, heavy, thick odor	Draining wound	*Pseudomonas* (bacterial) infection
Musty odor	Casted body part	Infection inside cast
Fetid, sweet odor	Tracheostomy or mucus secretions	Infection of bronchial tree (*Pseudomonas* bacteria)

"dub." After understanding the cause and character of normal auscultated sounds, it becomes easier to recognize abnormal sounds and their origins.

Olfaction

While assessing a client, become familiar with the nature and source of body odors (Table 33-3). Olfaction helps to detect abnormalities that you cannot recognize by any other means. For example, if a client's cast has a sweet, heavy, thick odor, this indicates an underlying infection. Findings from olfaction and other assessment skills allow detection of serious abnormalities.

Preparation for Examination

Proper preparation of the environment, equipment, and client ensures a smooth physical examination with few interruptions. A disorganized approach when preparing for a physical examination will cause errors and incomplete findings.

Infection Control

During an examination some clients will present with open skin lesions or weeping wounds. Use standard precautions throughout the examination (see Chapter 34) as appropriate. It is necessary to wear gloves during palpation and percussion to reduce contact with microorganisms. If a client has excessive drainage or risk of spray from a wound, wear a gown and other personal protective equipment as needed. Follow agency hand hygiene policies before initiating and after completing a physical assessment.

Environment

A physical examination requires privacy. A well-equipped examination room is preferable, but often the examination occurs in the client's room. In the home, you will often perform an examination in the client's bedroom.

Any examination room needs to be well equipped for all necessary procedures. Adequate lighting is necessary for proper illumination of body parts. Ideally an examination room is soundproof, so clients feel comfortable discussing their conditions. Be sure to eliminate sources of noise, take precautions to prevent interruptions from others, and make sure the room is warm enough to maintain comfort.

Sometimes it is difficult to perform a complete examination when clients are in beds or on stretchers. Special examination tables make clients easily accessible and help them assume special positions. Carefully assist clients so that they do not fall while getting on and off the table. Do not leave a confused, combative, or uncooperative client unsupervised on an examination table.

Examination tables are often hard and uncomfortable. When the client lies supine, raise the head of the table about 30 degrees. Also give the client a small pillow to use. When examining a client in bed, raise the bed to reach the client's body parts more easily.

Equipment

Perform hand hygiene thoroughly before equipment preparation and the examination. Set up equipment so it is readily available and arranged in order for easy use (Figure 33-3). Keep equipment as warm as appropriate. Rub the diaphragm of the stethoscope briskly between the hands before applying it to the skin. Run warm water over the vaginal speculum just before using. Check all equipment to ensure that it functions properly. The ophthalmoscope and otoscope require good batteries and light bulbs. Box 33-2 lists typical physical assessment equipment.

Physical Preparation of the Client

The client's physical comfort is vital for a successful examination. Before starting, ask if the client needs to use the restroom. An empty bladder and bowel facilitate examination of the abdomen, genitalia, and rectum. Collection of urine or fecal specimens occurs at this time if needed. Be sure to explain the proper method for collecting specimens, and make sure to label each specimen properly.

Physical preparation involves being sure the client is dressed and draped properly. The client in the hospital will likely be wearing only a simple gown. An outpatient will have to undress and wear a light cover gown. If the examination is limited to certain body systems, it is not always necessary for the client to undress completely. Provide the client privacy and plenty of time during undressing. Walking into the room as the client undresses causes embarrassment. Drapes and gowns are made of linen or disposable paper. After clients have undressed and put on a gown, they

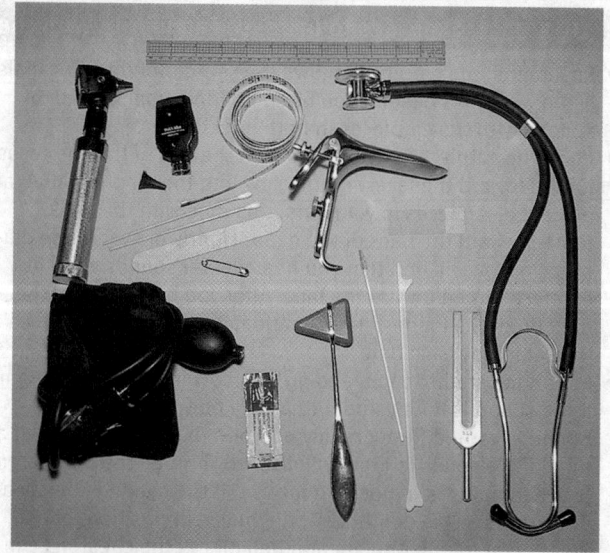

Figure 33-3 Equipment used during a physical examination.

✳ BOX 33-2 Equipment and Supplies for Physical Assessment

- Cervical brush or broom devices (if needed)
- Cotton applicators
- Disposable pad/paper towels
- Drapes
- Eye chart (e.g., Snellen chart)
- Flashlight and spotlight
- Forms (e.g., physical, laboratory)
- Gloves (sterile and clean)
- Gown for client
- Ophthalmoscope
- Otoscope
- Papanicolaou (Pap) liquid prep (if needed)
- Percussion (reflex) hammer
- Pulse oximeter
- Ruler
- Scale with height measurement rod
- Specimen containers, slides, wooden or plastic spatula, and cytologic fixative (if needed)
- Sphygmomanometer and cuff
- Sterile swabs
- Stethoscope
- Tape measure
- Thermometer
- Tissues
- Tongue depressors
- Tuning fork
- Vaginal speculum (if needed)
- Water-soluble lubricant
- Wristwatch with second hand or digital display

sit or lie down on the examination table with the drape over the lap or lower trunk. Make sure the client stays warm by eliminating drafts, controlling room temperature, and providing warm blankets. Routinely ask if the client is comfortable.

Positioning. During the examination ask the client to assume proper positions so that body parts are accessible and the client stays comfortable. Table 33-4 lists the preferred positions for each part of the examination and contains figures illustrating these positions. Clients' abilities to assume positions will depend on their physical strength, mobility, ease of breathing, age, and degree of wellness. Explain the positions, and assist clients in assuming them. Adjust the drapes so that the area examined is accessible, making sure not to unnecessarily expose a body part. A client may assume more than one position. To decrease the number of times the client changes positions, organize the examination so that you

✳ TABLE 33-4 Positions for Examination

POSITION	AREAS ASSESSED	RATIONALE	LIMITATIONS
Sitting	Head and neck, back, posterior thorax and lungs, anterior thorax and lungs, breasts, axillae, heart, vital signs, and upper extremities	Sitting upright provides full expansion of lungs and provides better visualization of symmetry of upper body parts.	Physically weakened client is sometimes unable to sit. Use supine position with head of bed elevated instead.
Supine	Head and neck, anterior thorax and lungs, breasts, axillae, heart, abdomen, extremities, pulses	This is most normally relaxed position. It provides easy access to pulse sites.	If client becomes short of breath easily, raise the head of bed.
Dorsal recumbent	Head and neck, anterior thorax and lungs, breasts, axillae, heart, abdomen	Position is for abdominal assessment because it promotes relaxation of abdominal muscles.	Clients with painful disorders are more comfortable with knees flexed.
Lithotomy*	Female genitalia and genital tract	This position provides maximal exposure of genitalia and facilitates insertion of vaginal speculum.	Lithotomy position is embarrassing and uncomfortable, so examiner minimizes time that client spends in it. Keep client well draped.
Sims'	Rectum and vagina	Flexion of hip and knee improves exposure of rectal area.	Joint deformities hinder client's ability to bend hip and knee.
Prone	Musculoskeletal system	This position is only for assessing extension of hip joint, skin, buttocks.	Clients with respiratory difficulties do not tolerate this position well.
Lateral recumbent	Heart	This position aids in detecting murmurs.	Clients with respiratory difficulties do not tolerate this position well.
Knee-chest*	Rectum	This position provides maximal exposure of rectal area.	This position is embarrassing and uncomfortable.

*Some clients with arthritis or other joint deformities are unable to assume this position.

perform all techniques requiring a sitting position first, then perform those that require a supine position next, and so forth. Be sure to use extra care when positioning older adults, because they are more prone to having disabilities and limitation.

Psychological Preparation of the Client

Many clients find an examination stressful or tiring, or they experience anxiety about possible findings. A thorough explanation of the purpose and steps of each assessment lets clients know what to expect and what to do so that they can cooperate. Keep explanations simple and in understandable terms. Help clients to feel free to ask questions and mention any discomfort. As you examine each body system, give a more detailed explanation. Convey an open, professional approach while remaining relaxed. A still, formal demeanor will inhibit the client's ability to communicate, but a style that is too casual will fail to assure the client (Seidel and others, 2006).

When the client and nurse are of opposite gender, it helps to have a third person of the client's gender in the room. The presence of a third person assures the client that the examiner will behave ethically. This person is also a witness to the examiner's conduct and the client's.

During the examination watch the client's emotional responses. Observe whether the client's facial expression shows fear or concern and if body movements show anxiety. Remain calm, and explain each step clearly. It is sometimes necessary to stop the examination and ask how the client feels. Do not force the client to continue. Postponing the examination is advantageous because the findings may be more accurate when the client can cooperate and relax. If the client's fears result from misconceptions, clarify the purpose of the examination and how you will perform it.

Assessment of Age-Groups

It is necessary to use different interview styles and approaches to physical examination for clients of different age-groups. When assessing children, be sensitive and anticipate the child's reaction to the examination as a strange and unfamiliar experience. Routine pediatric examinations focus on health promotion and illness prevention particularly for the care of well children who receive competent parenting and have no serious health problems (Hockenberry and Wilson, 2007). This examination focuses on growth and development, sensory screening, dental examination, and behavioral assessment. Children who are chronically ill or disabled, foster children, foreign-born, or adopted sometimes require additional examination visits. When examining children, the following tips assist in data collection:

- Gather all or part of the histories on infants and children from parents or guardians.
- Perform the examination in a nonthreatening area; provide time for play to become acquainted.
- Because parents sometimes think the examiner is testing them, offer support during the examination and do not pass judgment.
- Call children by their first name, and address the parents as "Mr., Mrs., or Ms." rather than by their first names.
- Use open-ended questions to allow parents to share more information and describe more of the children's problems.

This also allows observation of parent-child interactions. Interview older children, who often provide details about their health history and severity of symptoms.

- Treat adolescents as adults and individuals because they tend to respond best when treated as such.
- Remember that adolescents have the right to confidentiality. After talking with parents about historical information, speak alone with adolescents.

A comprehensive health assessment and examination of older adults includes physical data, developmental stage, family relationships, group involvement, and religious and occupational pursuits, as well as a review of the client's cognitive, affective, and social level (Ebersole and others, 2004; Meiner and Lueckenotte, 2006). An important aspect is to assess basic activities of daily living as well as complex instrumental activities of daily living.

Throughout the examination, recognize that with advancing age the body does not respond vigorously to injury or disease. Therefore older persons do not always exhibit the expected signs and symptoms (Meiner and Lueckenotte, 2006). Characteristically, older adults present more blunted or atypical signs and symptoms. Principles to follow during examination of an older adult include the following:

- Do not stereotype aging clients. Most are able to adapt to change and to learn about their health. Similarly, most are reliable historians.
- Recognize that sensory or physical limitations affect how quickly you are able to interview older adults and conduct examinations. Plan for more than one examination session. Sometimes it helps to give clients an initial health questionnaire before they come to a clinic or office (Ebersole and others, 2004; Meiner and Lueckenotte, 2006).
- Perform the examination with adequate space; this is especially important for clients with mobility aids such as a cane or walker.
- During the examination use patience, allow for pauses, and observe for details. Recognize normalities of later life.
- Certain types of health information are stressful for older clients to give. Some view illness as a threat to independence and a step toward institutionalization.
- Perform the examination near bathroom facilities if the client has an urgent need to eliminate.
- Be alert to signs of increasing fatigue, such as sighing, grimacing, irritability, leaning against objects for support, and drooping of the head and shoulders.

Organization of the Examination

The physical examination is made up of individual assessments for each body system. Clients with specific symptoms or needs require only portions of an examination. A client who comes to a clinic with symptoms of a severe chest cold will not routinely require a neurological assessment. A client entering the emergency department with an acute illness requires assessment of the body

✳ TABLE 33-5 Recommended Preventive Screenings

DISEASE/CONDITION	AGE-GROUP	SCREENING MEASURES
Breast cancer*	Ages 20 to 39	Monthly breast self-examination (BSE). Clinical breast examination by health care professional every 3 years.
	Ages 40 and up	Monthly BSE. Annual clinical breast examination by health care professional. Yearly mammograms. Women at increased risk need to speak to health care provider regarding screening options.
Colon/rectal cancer*	Ages 50 and up	Men and women need to have one of the following: fecal occult blood test (FOBT) or fecal immunochemical test (FIT) yearly; or flexible sigmoidoscopy (FSIG) every 5 years; the combination of FOBT or FIT yearly and a flexible sigmoidoscopy every 5 years is preferred over either of these options above; or double-contrast barium enema every 5 years; or colonoscopy every 10 years. They also need a digital rectal examination at the same time as above. Earlier screening is necessary if risk factors exist.
Ear disorders	All ages Over age 65	Periodic hearing checks as needed. Regular hearing checks.
Eye disorders	Age 40 and under Ages 40 to 64 Age 65 and up	Complete eye examination every 3 to 5 years (more if positive history). Complete eye examination every 2 years. Complete eye examination every year.
Heart/vascular disorders	Men age 45 to 65 Women age 45 to 65	Regular measurement of total blood cholesterol levels, lipids, and triglycerides; blood pressure screenings. If client has risk factors for coronary artery disease (CAD), blood pressure screening needs to begin at age 20-35 for men, 20-45 for women.
Obesity	All ages	Periodic height and weight measurements.
Oral cavity/pharyngeal disorders/cancer	All ages (children, adults, older adults)	Regular dental examinations every 6 months.
Ovarian cancer*	Age 18 and up or on becoming sexually active	Annual pelvic examinations by health care provider. This screening occasionally detects ovarian cancer in its advanced stage. Those at high risk need to have a thorough pelvic examination, a transvaginal ultrasound, and a blood test (tumor marker CA 125).
Prostate cancer*	Ages 50 and up	Men who have at least a 10-year life expectancy need to have a digital rectal examination (DRE) and prostate-specific antigen (PSA) blood test annually. Men at high risk require earlier screening.
Skin cancer*	All ages Ages 20 to 40 Over 40	Regular skin self-examination. See specialist every 3 years. Annual skin checkups with biopsy of suspicious lesions.
Testicular cancer*	Age 15 and up	Monthly testicular self-examination (TSE).
Uterine cancer*	Screening begins 3 years after having vaginal intercourse, but not later than age 21	Annual pelvic examination by health care provider plus an annual Papanicolaou (Pap) test.
Cervical cancer	Screening begins 3 years after vaginal intercourse, but not later than 21 years of age	Annual pelvic examination by health care provider, plus an annual Pap test. At age 30 or after, those who have had three normal tests consecutively may be screened every 2 to 3 years. If client has risk factors, screening needs to occur more frequently. Contact health care provider.
Endometrial cancer	Same as above	Endometrial biopsy at age 35 for high-risk clients (those with or at risk for hereditary nonpolyposis colon cancer [HNPCC]). At menopause women at average and high risk need to be informed about signs and symptoms to report.

*Data from American Cancer Society: *Cancer facts and figures 2006*, Atlanta, 2006, The Society.

Website for further information on preventative screenings: *Guide to clinical preventive services*, AHRQ Publication No. 05-0570, Rockville, Md, 2005, Agency for Healthcare Research and Quality, http://www.ahrp.gov/clinic/pocketgd.htm.

systems most at risk for being abnormal. When a client is admitted to the hospital, a complete examination is performed. A client who is receiving a routine health promotion examination undergoes specific preventive screenings, depending on the client's age or health risk (Table 33-5). Clients with specific symptoms or needs often require only portions of an examination. Use judgment to ensure that an examination is relevant and includes the correct observations.

The performance of a complete health assessment follows the format of the nursing history (see Chapter 16). Obtain information from the history to focus attention on specific parts of the examination. Findings from the history generally reveal a pattern of related signs and symptoms. The physical examination supplements information from the history to confirm or refute the data.

Be systematic and well organized about the examination so you do not miss important assessments. A head-to-toe approach includes all body systems and helps to anticipate each step. In an adult begin by assessing the head and neck, progressing methodically down the body to incorporate all body systems. The following tips help keep an examination well organized:

- Compare both sides of the body for symmetry. A degree of asymmetry is normal (e.g., the biceps muscles in the dominant arm are sometimes more developed than the same muscles in the nondominant arm).
- If a client is seriously ill, first assess the systems of the body more at risk for being abnormal. For example, a client with chest pain first undergoes a cardiovascular assessment.
- If a client becomes fatigued, offer rest periods between assessments.
- Perform painful procedures near the end of the examination.
- Record assessments in specific terms on a physical assessment form or in the nurses' notes.
- Use common and accepted medical abbreviations to keep notes brief and concise.
- Record quick notes during the examination to avoid keeping the client waiting. Complete any observations at the end of the examination.
- A physical assessment form allows you to record information in the same sequence as you gather it.

General Survey

Assessment begins when first meeting the client. Determine the client's reason for seeking health care. Initial data from the general survey begins with a review of the client's primary health problems. Make mental notes of the client's behavior and appearance. Begin the examination with a general survey. The survey provides information about characteristics of an illness, a client's hygiene and body image, emotional state, recent changes in weight, and developmental status. If there are abnormalities or problems, closely assess the affected body system later.

General Appearance and Behavior

Assess appearance and behavior while preparing the client for the examination. The review of general appearance and behavior includes the following:

- *Gender and race:* A person's gender affects the type of examination performed and the manner in which you make assessments. Different physical features are related to gender and race. Certain illnesses are more likely to affect a specific gender or race; for example, the incidence of skin cancer is more common in whites than in African Americans, prostate cancer is higher in African American men than in white men, and

cancer of the bladder is four times higher in men than women (American Cancer Society [ACS], 2006).
- *Age:* Age influences normal physical characteristics and a person's ability to participate in some parts of the examination.
- *Signs of distress:* There are sometimes obvious signs or symptoms indicating pain (grimacing, splinting painful area), or difficulty in breathing (shortness of breath, sternal retractions), or anxiety. These signs establish priorities regarding what to examine first.
- *Body type:* Observe if a client appears trim and muscular, obese, or excessively thin. Body type reflects the level of health, age, and lifestyle.
- *Posture:* Normal standing posture is an upright stance with parallel alignment of the hips and shoulders. Normal sitting posture involves some degree of rounding of the shoulders. Observe whether the client has a slumped, erect, or bent posture. Posture often reflects mood or pain. Many older adults assume a stooped, forward-bent posture, with the hips and knees somewhat flexed and the arms bent at the elbows, raising the level of the arms.
- *Gait:* Observe the client walking into the room or at the bedside (if the client is ambulatory). Note whether movements are coordinated or uncoordinated. A person normally walks with the arms swinging freely at the sides, with the head and face leading the body.
- *Body movements:* Observe whether movements are purposeful, and note if there are any tremors involving the extremities. Determine if any body parts are immobile.
- *Hygiene and grooming:* Note the client's level of cleanliness by observing the appearance of the hair, skin, and fingernails. Note if the client's clothes are clean. Grooming depends on the activities being performed just before the examination, as well as the client's occupation. Also note the amount and type of cosmetics used.
- *Dress:* Culture, lifestyle, socioeconomic level, and personal preference affect the type of clothes worn. Note if the type of clothing worn is appropriate for the temperature and weather conditions. Depressed or mentally ill persons are often unable to choose proper clothing. An older adult tends to wear extra clothing because of the sensitivity to cold.
- *Body odor:* An unpleasant body odor often results from physical exercise, poor hygiene, or certain disease states.
- *Affect and mood:* Affect is a person's feelings as they appear to others. Clients express mood or emotional state verbally and nonverbally. Note if verbal expressions match nonverbal behavior. Observe if mood is appropriate for the situation. Observe facial expressions while asking questions.
- *Speech:* Normal speech is understandable and moderately paced. It shows an association with the person's thoughts. Note if the client talks rapidly or slowly. Emotions or neurological impairment sometimes cause an abnormal pace. Observe whether the client speaks in a normal tone with clear inflection of words.
- *Client abuse:* Abuse of children, women, and older adults is a growing health problem. Obvious physical injury or neglect are signs of possible abuse (e.g., evidence of malnutrition or presence of bruising on the extremities or trunk). Assess for the client's fear of the spouse or partner, caregiver, parent, or

---

✳ BOX 33-3 Clinical Indicators of Abuse

Physical Findings

Child Sexual Abuse

Vaginal or penile discharge
Blood on underclothing
Pain, itching, or unusual odor in genital area
Genital injuries
Difficulty sitting or walking
Pain while urinating; recurrent urinary tract infections
Foreign bodies in rectum, urethra, or vagina
Sexually transmitted diseases
Pregnancy in young adolescent

Domestic Abuse

Injuries and trauma are inconsistent with reported cause
Multiple injuries involving head, face, neck, breasts, abdomen, and genitalia (black eyes, orbital fractures, broken nose, fractured skull, lip lacerations, broken teeth, strangulation marks)
X-ray films show old and new fractures in different stages of healing
Abrasions, lacerations, bruises/welts
Burns
Human bites

Older Adult Abuse

Injuries and trauma are inconsistent with reported cause (cigarette burn, scratch, bruise, or bite)
Hematomas
Bruises at various stages of resolution
Bruises, chafing, excoriation on wrist or legs (restraints)
Burns
Fractures inconsistent with cause described
Dried blood

Behavioral Findings

Problem in sleeping or eating
Fear of certain people or places
Play activities recreate the abuse situation
Regressed behavior
Sexual acting out
Knowledge of explicit sexual matters
Preoccupation with others' or own genitals
Profound and rapid personality changes
Rapidly declining school performance
Poor relationship with peers

Attempted suicide
Eating or sleeping disorders
Anxiety
Panic attacks
Pattern of substance abuse (follows physical abuse)
Low self-esteem
Depression
Sense of helplessness
Guilt
Increased forgetfulness
Stress-related complaints (headache, anxiety)

Dependent on caregiver
Physically and/or cognitively impaired
Combative
Wandering
Verbally aggressive
Minimal social support
Prolonged interval between injury and medical treatment

Data from Kovach K: Intimate partner violence, *RN* 67(8):38, 2004; Quinn MJ: Undue influence and elder abuse: recognition and intervention strategies, *Geriatr Nurs* 23(1):11, 2002; Fulmer T: Elder abuse and neglect assessment, *J Gerontol Nurs* 29(1):8; and Hockenberry MJ, Wilson P: *Wong's nursing care of infants and children*, ed 8, St. Louis, 2007, Mosby.

---

adult child. Note if the partner or caregiver has a history of violence, alcoholism, or drug abuse. Is the person unemployed, ill, or frustrated in caring for the client? Most states mandate a report to a social service center if you suspect abuse or neglect (Box 33-3). When you suspect abuse, interview the client in private. It is difficult to detect abuse, because victims often will not complain or report that they are in an abusive situation (Kovach, 2004). Clients are more likely to reveal any problems when the suspected abuser is absent from the room (Kovach, 2004).

SAFETY ALERT The risk for further abuse is high once the victim has reported the abuse or tries to leave the abusive situation. Provide counseling options for these individuals.

- *Substance abuse:* Substance abuse affects all socioeconomic groups. A single visit to a clinic does not always reveal the problem. Several visits often reveal behaviors that you can confirm with a well-focused history and physical examination. Approach the client in a caring and nonjudgmental way, because issues of substance abuse involve both emotional and lifestyle issues. Box 33-4 lists clients to suspect for substance

abuse. When you suspect substance abuse, ask the following CAGE questions (CAGE is an acronym for the following):

- Have you ever felt the need to **Cut down** on your drinking or drug use?
- Have people **Annoyed** you by criticizing your drinking or drug use?
- Have you ever felt bad or **Guilty** about your drinking or drug use?
- Have you ever used or had a drink first thing in the morning as an **Eye-opener** to steady your nerves or feel normal?

If two or more of the CAGE questions are positive, strongly suspect substance abuse and consider how to motivate the client to seek treatment (Stuart and Laraia, 2005; Widlitz and Marin, 2002).

Vital Signs

Assessment of vital signs (see Chapter 32) is the first part of the physical examination. Positioning or moving the client during the examination interferes with obtaining accurate values. You can also measure specific vital signs during assessment of individual body systems.

✳ **BOX 33-4** **Red Flags for Suspicion of Substance Abuse**

- Clients who frequently miss appointments
- Clients who frequently request written excuses for absence from work
- Clients who have chief complaints of insomnia, "bad nerves," or pain that does not fit a particular pattern
- Clients who often report lost prescriptions (e.g., tranquilizers or pain medications) or ask for frequent refills
- Clients who make frequent emergency department visits
- Clients who have a history of changing health care providers or who bring in medication bottles prescribed by several different providers
- Clients with a history of gastrointestinal bleeds, peptic ulcers, pancreatitis, cellulitis, or frequent pulmonary infections
- Clients with frequent sexually transmitted diseases (STDs), complicated pregnancies, multiple abortions, or sexual dysfunction
- Clients who complain of chest pains or palpitations or who have a history of admissions to rule out myocardial infarctions
- Clients who give histories of activities that place them at risk for human immunodeficiency virus (HIV) infections (multiple partners, multiple rapes)
- Clients with a family history of addiction; history of childhood sexual, physical, or emotional abuse; or social and financial or marital problems

Data from American Psychiatric Association: *Diagnostic and statistical manual of mental disorders*, ed 4, text revision, Washington, DC, 2000, The Association; Graham A and others: *Principles of addiction medicine*, ed 3, Chevy Chase, Md, 2003, American Society of Addiction Medicine, Inc.; and Widlitz M, Marin D: Substance abuse in older adults: an overview, *Geriatrics* 57(12):29, 2002.

✳ **BOX 33-5** **Dietary History for Older Adults**

- Does the older adult need or have help in shopping for or preparing meals?
- Is income adequate for food purchasing? Food stamps or public assistance required?
- Does the client ever skip meals?
- Are the five primary food groups from the food guide pyramid represented in the daily diet (bread, cereal, rice, and pasta group, 6 ounces daily; fruit group, 2 cups daily; vegetable group, 2½ cups daily; meat, poultry, fish, dry beans, eggs, and nut group, 5½ ounces; and milk, yogurt, and cheese group, 3 cups daily) (see Chapter 44) (U.S. Department of Agriculture, 2005)? (Based on a 2000-calorie/day diet.)
- Does the older adult take nutritional supplements, such as multivitamins?
- Does the older adult take any medication affecting appetite or absorption of nutrients?
- Does the older adult have any religious or cultural beliefs and practices that influence diet?
- Does the older adult have a special diet, food intolerances, or allergies? Does the client's diet contain an unusual amount of alcohol, sweets, or fried food?
- Does the older adult have problems with chewing, swallowing, or salivation?
- Does the older adult have gastrointestinal problems that interfere with food intake?

Data from Meiner SE, Lueckenotte A: *Gerontologic nursing*, ed 3, St. Louis, 2006, Mosby; Moore MC: *Pocket guide to nutritional assessment and care*, ed 5, St. Louis, 2005, Mosby; and U.S. Department of Agriculture, Center for Nutrition Policy and Promotion, 2005, http://www.mypyramid.gov.

Height and Weight

Height and weight reflect a person's general level of health. Weight is a routine measure during health screenings and visits to physicians' offices or clinics. Both measures are routine when clients are admitted to a health care setting. Health care providers measure an infant or child's height and weight to assess growth and development. In older adults, height and weight coupled with a nutritional assessment determine the cause of and treatment for chronic disease or help to identify the older adult who has difficulty with feeding and other functional activities (Box 33-5). Be sure to look for overall trends in height and weight changes.

A client's weight will normally vary daily because of fluid loss or retention. A downward trend in a frail older adult indicates serious reduction in nutritional reserves. Assessments screen for abnormal weight changes. The nursing history helps to focus on possible causes for a change in weight (Table 33-6). First ask the client his or her current height and weight. Also assess weight gains or losses. Standardized tables help reveal the normal expected weight for a client at a given height (Table 33-7). A weight gain of 5 pounds (2.3 kg) in a day indicates fluid retention problems. If the client has lost more than 5% of body weight in a month or 10% in 6 months, the loss is significant.

You need to weigh clients at the same time of day, on the same scale, and in the same clothes to allow an objective comparison of subsequent weights. Accuracy of weight measurement is impor-

tant because health care providers will base medical and nursing decisions (e.g., drug dosage determinations, lifting, and positioning) on changes. Clients capable of bearing their own weight use a standing scale. Calibrate a standard platform scale by moving the large and small weights to zero. Make the balance beam level and steady by adjusting the calibrating knob. The client stands on the scale platform and remains still. Move the largest weight to the 50-pound or 22.5-kg increment under the client's weight. Then adjust the smaller weight to balance the scale at the nearest ¼ pound or 0.1 kg (Seidel and others, 2006). Electronic scales automatically display the weight within seconds. Electronic scales are automatically calibrated each time they are used.

Stretcher and chair scales are available for clients unable to bear weight. After you transfer the client to the scale, a hydraulic device lifts the client above the bed and measures the weight on a balance beam or digital display. Use caution when transferring clients to and from the scales.

Always weigh infants in baskets or on platform scales. Remove the infant's clothing, and weigh the infant in dry, disposable diapers. Adjust the measurement later for the weight of the diaper, ensuring an accurate reading. Keep the room warm to prevent chills. A light cloth or paper placed on the scale's surface prevents cross infection from urine or feces. When placing infants in baskets or on platforms, hold a hand lightly above to prevent accidental falls. You measure weight in ounces and grams.

TABLE 33-6 Nursing History for Weight Assessment

Assessment Category	Rationale
Ask about total weight lost or gained; compare with usual weight; note time period for loss (e.g., gradual, sudden, desired, or undesired).	Determines severity of problem and reveals if weight change is related to disease process, change in eating pattern, or pregnancy.
If weight loss desired, ask about eating habits, diet plan followed, food preparation, calorie intake, appetite, exercise pattern, support group participation, weight goal.	Helps to determine appropriateness of diet plan followed.
If weight loss undesired, ask about anorexia, vomiting, diarrhea, thirst, frequent urination, and change in lifestyle, activity, and stress levels.	Focuses on problems that cause weight loss (e.g., gastrointestinal problems).
Assess if client has noted changes in social aspects of eating: more meals in restaurants, rushing to eat meals, stress at work, or skipping meals.	Lifestyle changes sometimes contribute to weight changes.
Assess if client takes chemotherapy, diuretics, insulin, fluoxetine, prescription and nonprescription appetite suppressants, laxatives, oral hypoglycemics, and herbal supplements (weight loss); steroids, oral contraceptives, antidepressants, insulin (weight gain).	Weight gain or loss is a side effect of these medications.
Assess for preoccupation with body weight or body shape such as fasting, never feeling thin enough, unusually strict caloric intake or restrictions, laxative abuse, induced vomiting, amenorrhea, excessive exercise, alcohol intake.	Indicates an eating disorder.

TABLE 33-7 Height and Weight Table: Weights for Persons 25 to 59 Years According to Build*

Men					Women				
Height		Small Frame	Medium Frame	Large Frame	Height†		Small Frame	Medium Frame	Large Frame
Feet	Inches				Feet	Inches			
5	2	128-134	131-141	138-150	4	10	102-111	109-121	118-131
5	3	130-136	133-143	140-153	4	11	102-111	111-123	120-134
5	4	132-138	135-145	142-156	5	0	103-113	113-126	122-137
5	5	134-140	137-148	144-160	5	1	104-115	115-129	125-140
5	6	136-142	139-151	146-164	5	2	106-118	118-132	128-143
5	7	138-145	142-154	149-168	5	3	108-121	121-135	131-147
5	8	140-148	145-157	152-172	5	4	111-124	124-138	134-151
5	9	142-151	148-160	155-176	5	5	114-127	127-141	137-155
5	10	144-154	151-163	158-180	5	6	117-130	130-144	140-159
5	11	146-157	154-166	161-184	5	7	120-133	133-147	143-163
6	0	149-160	157-170	164-188	5	8	123-136	136-150	146-167
6	1	152-164	160-174	168-192	5	9	126-139	139-153	149-170
6	2	155-168	164-178	172-197	5	10	129-142	142-156	152-173
6	3	158-172	167-182	176-207	5	11	132-145	145-159	155-176
6	4	162-176	171-187	181-207	6	0	138-151	148-162	158-179

Courtesy Metropolitan Life Insurance Company: *Statistical bulletin*, New York, 2000, Metropolitan.
*Indoor clothing weighing 5 pounds for men and 3 pounds for women.
†Shoes with 1-inch heels.

To measure the height of weight-bearing clients, have them remove their shoes. Place a paper towel on the scale platform or floor so the client's feet remain clean. A measuring stick or tape is attached vertically to the weight scales or wall. Have the client stand erect. The platform scale has a metal rod attached to the back of the scale; this swings out and over the crown of the head. You can also place a measuring stick or flat book on the head when a scale is unavailable. With the rod or stick placed level horizontally at a 90-degree angle to the measuring stick, measure the client's height in inches or centimeters.

Remove the shoes of a non–weight-bearing client, and position the client (such as an infant) supine on a firm surface. Portable devices are available that provide a reliable means to measure height. Place the infant on the device, having the parent hold the

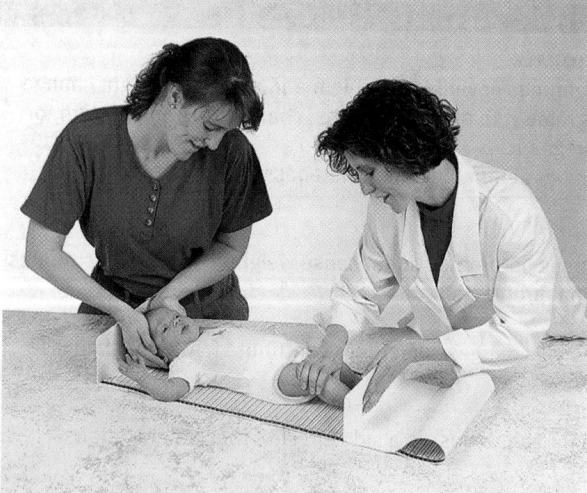

Figure 33-4 Measurement of infant length. (From Seidel HM and others: *Mosby's guide to physical examination,* ed 6, St. Louis, 2006, Mosby.)

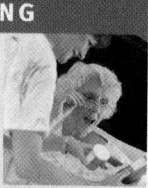

BOX 33-6   CLIENT TEACHING

Skin Assessment
Objectives
- Client will perform a monthly self-examination of the skin.
- Client will identify factors that increase the risk of skin cancer.
- Client will follow hygiene practices aimed at maintaining skin integrity.

Teaching Strategies
- Instruct client to conduct a complete monthly self-examination of the skin, noting moles, blemishes, and birthmarks. Tell client to inspect all skin surfaces. Cancerous melanomas start as small, molelike growths that increase in size, change color, become ulcerated, and bleed (see Box 33-8, p. 571).
- Tell client to report to a physician or health care provider any change in skin lesions or a sore that does not heal.
- Instruct client to report any lesion that bleeds or fails to heal to a physician. Especially instruct older adults, who tend to have delayed wound healing.
- To treat excessively dry skin, tell client to avoid hot water, harsh soaps, and drying agents such as rubbing alcohol. Use a superfatted (Dove) soap, and pat rather than rub the skin after bathing.
- Apply moisturizers (mineral oil) to the skin regularly to reduce itching and drying, and wear cotton clothing (Hardy, 1996).

Evaluation
- Observe client perform skin assessment.
- Have client describe signs of skin cancer and measures to take to prevent skin cancer.
- Ask client to describe methods for keeping the skin lubricated and supple.

infant's head against the headboard. With the infant's legs straight at the knees, place the footboard against the bottom of the infant's feet (Figure 33-4). Record the infant's length to the nearest 0.5 cm or ¼ inch.

Skin, Hair, and Nails

The **integument** consist of the skin, hair, scalp, and nails. First inspect all skin surfaces, or assess the skin gradually while examining other body systems. Use the skills of inspection, palpation, and olfaction to assess the integument's function and integrity.

Skin

Assessment of the skin reveals changes in oxygenation, circulation, nutrition, local tissue damage, and hydration. In a hospital setting the majority of clients are older adults, debilitated clients, or young but seriously ill clients. There are significant risks for skin lesions resulting from trauma to the skin during administration of care, from exposure to pressure during immobilization, or from reaction to various medications used in treatment. Clients at high risk are the neurologically impaired; chronically ill; and orthopedic clients. Others at risk are clients with diminished mental status, poor tissue oxygenation, low cardiac output, or inadequate nutrition. In nursing homes and extended care facilities, clients are often at risk for many of the same problems, depending on their level of mobility and the presence of chronic illness. Routinely assess the skin to look for primary or initial lesions that develop. Without proper care, primary lesions can deteriorate to become secondary lesions that require more extensive nursing care. The development of a pressure ulcer, for example, will lengthen a hospital stay unless you prevent or discover it early and treat it properly (see Chapter 48).

There will be approximately 59,940 new cases of **melanoma,** an aggressive form of skin cancer, diagnosed in 2007 (ACS, 2007). In addition, health care providers will see more than one million new cases of the highly curable basal cell and squamous cell cancers (ACS, 2007). Cutaneous malignancies are the most common neoplasms seen in clients. Incorporate performing a thorough skin assessment on all clients with educating them about self-examination (Box 33-6).

The condition of the client's skin reveals the need for nursing intervention. Use assessment findings to determine the type of hygiene measures required to maintain integrity of the integument (see Chapter 39). Adequate nutrition and hydration become goals of therapy if you identify an alteration in the integument's status (see Chapter 44).

You need adequate lighting to accurately observe a client's skin. The recommended choice is natural or halogen lighting. For detecting skin changes in the dark-skinned client, sunlight is the best choice (Talbot and Curtis, 1996). Room temperature also affects skin assessment. A room that is too warm causes superficial vasodilation, resulting in an increased redness of the skin. A cool environment causes the sensitive client to develop **cyanosis** around the lips and nail beds (Talbot and Curtis, 1996).

Use disposable gloves for palpation if open, moist, or draining lesions are present. Although you inspect each part of the body during an examination, it is helpful to make a brief but careful overall visual sweep of the entire body. This provides a good idea of the distribution and extent of any lesions, as well as the overall symmetry of skin color. Because you need to inspect all skin sur-

✳ TABLE 33-8 Nursing History for Skin Assessment

ASSESSMENT CATEGORY	RATIONALE
Ask client about history of changes in the skin: dryness, pruritus, sores, rashes, lumps, color, texture, odor, lesion that does not heal.	Client is best source to recognize change. Usually skin cancer is first noticed as a localized change in skin color.
Consider if the client has the following history: fair, freckled, ruddy complexion; light-colored hair or eyes; tendency to burn easily.	Characteristics are risk factors for skin cancer.
Determine whether client works or spends excessive time outside. If so, ask whether client wears sunscreen and the level of protection.	Exposed areas such as face and arms will be more pigmented than rest of body. The American Cancer Society (2000) recommends use of sunscreen.
Determine whether client has noted lesions, rashes, or bruises.	Most skin changes do not develop suddenly. Change in character of lesion possibly indicates cancer. Bruising indicates trauma or bleeding disorder.
Question client about frequency of bathing and type of soap used.	Excessive bathing and use of harsh soaps cause dry skin.
Ask if client has had recent trauma to skin.	Some injuries cause bruising and changes in skin texture.
Determine whether client has history of allergies.	Skin rashes commonly occur from allergies.
Ask if client uses topical medications or home remedies on skin.	Incorrect use of topical agents causes inflammation or irritation.
Ask if client goes to tanning parlors, uses sun lamps, or takes tanning pills.	Overexposure of skin to these irritants will possibly cause skin cancer.
Ask if client has family history of serious skin disorders such as skin cancer or psoriasis.	Family history will possibly reveal information about client's condition.
Determine if client works with creosote, coal, tar, petroleum products, arsenic compounds, or radium.	Exposure to these agents creates risk for skin cancer.

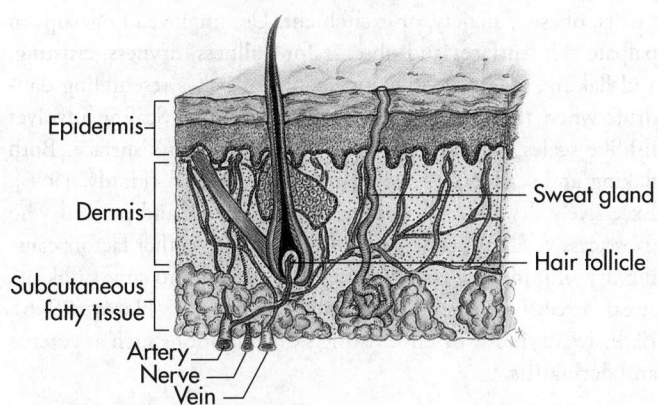

Figure 33-5 A cross section of the skin reveals three layers: epidermis, dermis, and subcutaneous fatty tissues.

faces, the client will assume several positions. Table 33-8 outlines the nursing history for skin assessment. If you notice abnormalities during an examination, palpate the involved areas. Skin odors are usually apparent in the folds of the skin, such as the axillae or under the female client's breasts. Figure 33-5 illustrates a normal cross section of the skin.

Color. Skin color varies from body part to body part and from person to person. Despite individual variations, skin color is usually uniform over the body. Table 33-9 lists common variations. Normal skin pigmentation ranges in tone from ivory or light pink to ruddy pink in light skin and from light to deep brown or olive in dark skin. In older adults, **pigmentation** increases unevenly, causing discolored skin. While inspecting the skin, be aware that cosmetics or tanning agents sometimes mask color.

The assessment of color first involves areas of the skin not exposed to the sun, such as the palms of the hands. Note if the skin is unusually pale or dark. Areas exposed to the sun, such as the face and arms, will be darker. It is more difficult to note changes such as pallor or cyanosis in clients with dark skin. Usually you see color hues best in the palms, soles of the feet, lips, tongue, and nail beds. Areas of increased color (hyperpigmentation) and decreased color (hypopigmentation) are common. Skin creases and folds are darker than the rest of the body in the dark-skinned client.

Inspect sites where you are able to identify abnormalities more easily. For example, you can see pallor more easily in the face, buccal (mouth) mucosa, conjunctiva, and nail beds. Observe for **cyanosis** (bluish discoloration) in the lips, nail beds, palpebral conjunctivae, and palms. In recognizing pallor in the dark-skinned client, observe that normal brown skin appears to be yellow-brown and normal black skin appears to be ashen gray. Also assess the lips, nail beds, and mucous membranes for generalized pallor; if pallor is present, the mucous membranes will be ashen gray. Assessment of cyanosis in the dark-skinned client requires observation of areas where pigmentation occurs the least (conjunctiva, sclera, buccal mucosa, tongue, lips, nail beds, and palms and soles). In addition, verify these findings with clinical manifestations (Talbot and Curtis, 1996).

The best site to inspect for **jaundice** (yellow-orange discoloration) is the client's sclera. You can see normal reactive hyperemia, or redness, most often in regions exposed to pressure such as the sacrum, heels, and greater trochanter. Inspect for any patches or areas of skin color variation. Localized skin changes, such as pallor or **erythema** (red discoloration), indicate circulatory changes. For example, an area of erythema is due to localized vasodilation resulting from a sunburn, inflammation, or fever. It is difficult to observe erythema in the dark-skinned client, so palpate the area

✳ **TABLE 33-9** Skin Color Variations

COLOR	CONDITION	CAUSES	ASSESSMENT LOCATIONS
Bluish (cyanosis)	Increased amount of deoxy-genated hemoglobin (associated with hypoxia)	Heart or lung disease, cold environment	Nail beds, lips, mouth, skin (severe cases)
Pallor (decrease in color)	Reduced amount of oxyhemoglobin	Anemia	Face, conjunctivae, nail beds, palms of hands
	Reduced visibility of oxyhemoglobin resulting from decreased blood flow	Shock	Skin, nail beds, conjunctivae, lips
Loss of pigmentation	Vitiligo	Congenital or autoimmune condition causing lack of pigment	Patchy areas on skin over face, hands, arms
Yellow-orange (jaundice)	Increased deposit of bilirubin in tissues	Liver disease, destruction of red blood cells	Sclera, mucous membranes, skin
Red (erythema)	Increased visibility of oxyhemoglobin caused by dilation or increased blood flow	Fever, direct trauma, blushing, alcohol intake	Face, area of trauma, sacrum, shoulders, other common sites for pressure ulcers
Tan-brown	Increased amount of melanin	Suntan, pregnancy	Areas exposed to sun: face, arms, areolae, nipples

✳ **TABLE 33-10** Physical Findings of the Skin Indicative of Substance Abuse

BODY SYSTEM	COMMONLY ASSOCIATED DRUG
Diaphoresis	Sedative hypnotic (including alcohol)
Spider angiomas	Alcohol, stimulants
Burns (especially fingers)	Alcohol
Needle marks	Opioids
Contusion, abrasions, cuts, scars	Alcohol, other sedative hypnotics
"Homemade" tattoos	Cocaine, intravenous (IV) opioids (prevents detection of injection sites)
Increased vascularity of face	Alcohol
Red, dry skin	Phencyclidine (PCP)

Data from Friedman L and others: *Source book of substance abuse and addiction*, Baltimore, 1996, Williams & Wilkins; McKenry L and others: *Mosby's pharmacology in nursing*, ed 22, St. Louis, 2006, Mosby; and Smith DE, Seymour RB: *Clinician's guide to substance abuse*, New York, 2001, McGraw-Hill.

for heat and warmth to note the presence of skin inflammation (Talbot and Curtis, 1996). An area of an extremity that appears unusually pale results from arterial occlusion or edema. Be sure to ask if the client has noticed any changes in skin coloring.

There is also a pattern of findings associated with clients who are chemically dependent or are intravenous (IV) drug abusers (Table 33-10). It is sometimes difficult to recognize signs and symptoms after one examination. A client who takes repeated IV injections has edematous, reddened, and warm areas along the arms and legs. This pattern suggests recent injections. Evidence of old injection sites appears as hyperpigmented and shiny or scarred areas.

Moisture. The hydration of skin and mucous membranes helps to reveal body fluid imbalances, changes in the skin's environment, and regulation of body temperature. Moisture refers to wetness and oiliness. The skin is normally smooth and dry. Skin folds such as the axillae are normally moist. Minimal perspiration or oiliness is often present (Seidel and others, 2006). Increased perspiration is sometimes associated with activity, warm environments, obesity, anxiety, or excitement. Use ungloved fingertips to palpate skin surfaces and observe for dullness, dryness, crusting, and flaking. Flaking is the appearance of flakes resembling dandruff when the skin surface is lightly rubbed. Scaling involves fishlike scales that are easily rubbed off the skin's surface. Both flaking and scaling indicate abnormally dry skin (Hardy, 1996). Excessively dry skin is common in older adults and persons who use excessive amounts of soap during bathing. Other factors causing dry skin include lack of humidity, exposure to sun, smoking, stress, excessive perspiration, and dehydration (Hardy, 1996). Excessive dryness worsens existing skin conditions such as **eczema** and **dermatitis.**

Temperature. The temperature of the skin depends on the amount of blood circulating through the dermis. Increased or decreased skin temperature indicates an increase or decrease in blood flow. An increase in skin temperature often accompanies localized erythema or redness of the skin. A reduction in skin temperature reflects a decrease in blood flow. It is important to remember that if an examination room is cold, this will affect the client's skin temperature and color.

Accurately assess temperature by palpating the skin with the dorsum or back of the hand. Compare symmetrical body parts. Normally the skin temperature is warm. Sometimes skin temperature is the same throughout the body, and other times it varies in one area. Always assess skin temperature for clients at risk of having impaired circulation, such as after a cast application or vascular surgery. You can identify a stage I pressure ulcer early by noting warmth and erythema on an area of the skin (see Chapter 48).

Texture. The character of the skin's surface and the feel of deeper portions are its texture. Determine whether the client's

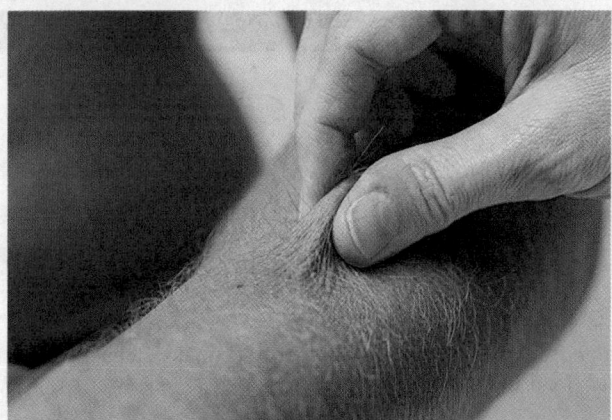

Figure 33-6 Assessment for skin turgor. (From Seidel HM and others: *Mosby's guide to physical examination,* ed 6, St. Louis, 2006, Mosby.)

skin is smooth or rough, thin or thick, tight or supple, and **indurated** (hardened) or soft by stroking it lightly with the fingertips. The texture of the skin is normally smooth, soft, even, and flexible in children and adults. However, the texture is usually not uniform throughout. The palms of the hand and soles of the feet tend to be thicker. In older adults the skin becomes wrinkled and leathery because of a decrease in collagen, subcutaneous fat, and sweat glands.

Localized changes result from trauma, surgical wounds, or lesions. When finding irregularities in texture such as scars or induration, ask the client if a recent injury to the skin has occurred. Deeper palpation sometimes reveals irregularities such as tenderness or localized areas of induration commonly caused by repeated injections.

Turgor. **Turgor** is the skin's elasticity. Edema or dehydration diminish turgor. Normally the skin loses its elasticity with age. To assess the skin turgor, grasp a fold of skin on the back of the forearm or sternal area with the fingertips and release (Figure 33-6). Normally the skin lifts easily and snaps back immediately to its resting position. The back of the hand is not the best place to test for turgor, because the skin is normally loose and thin (Seidel and others, 2006). The skin stays pinched when turgor is poor. Note the ease with which the skin moves and the speed at which it returns to place. Failure of the skin to reassume its normal contour or shape indicates dehydration. The client with poor skin turgor does not have a resilience to the normal wear and tear on the skin. The skin tends to stay pinched or tented when turgor is poor. A decrease in turgor predisposes the client to skin breakdown.

Vascularity. The circulation of the skin affects color in localized areas and the appearance of superficial blood vessels. With aging, capillaries become fragile. Localized pressure areas, found after a client has remained in one position, appear reddened, pink, or pale (see Chapter 48). **Petechiae** are pinpoint-sized, red or purple spots on the skin caused by small hemorrhages in the skin layers. Petechiae do not blanch, but may indicate serious blood-clotting disorders, drug reactions, or liver disease.

Edema. Areas of the skin become swollen or edematous from a buildup of fluid in the tissues. Direct trauma and impairment of venous return are two common causes of **edema.** Inspect edematous areas for location, color, and shape. The formation of edema separates the skin's surface from the pigmented and vascular layers, masking skin color. Edematous skin also appears stretched and shiny. Palpate edematous areas to determine mobility, consistency, and tenderness. When pressure from the examiner's fingers leaves an indentation in the edematous area, it is called pitting edema. To assess the degree of pitting edema, press the edematous area firmly with the thumb for several seconds and release. The depth of pitting, recorded in millimeters, determines the degree of edema (Seidel and others, 2006). For example, 1+ edema equals a 2-mm depth, 2+ edema equals a 4-mm depth, 3+ equals 6-mm, and 4+ equals 8-mm (see Figure 33-58, p. 609).

Lesions. The skin is normally free of lesions, except for common freckles or age-related changes such as skin tags, **senile keratosis** (thickening of skin), **cherry angiomas** (ruby red papules), and atrophic warts. Lesions are primary (occurring as initial spontaneous manifestations of a pathological process), such as an insect bite, or secondary (resulting from later formation or trauma to a primary lesion), such as a pressure ulcer. When you detect a lesion, inspect it for color, location, texture, size, shape, type, grouping (clustered or linear), and distribution (localized or generalized). Observe any exudate for color, odor, amount, and consistency. Measure the size of the lesion by using a small, clear, flexible ruler divided in centimeters. Comparing a lesion with a household measure, such as a coin or eraser, is not reliable (Seidel and others, 2006). Measure lesions in height, width, and depth.

Palpation determines the lesion's mobility, contour (flat, raised, or depressed), and consistency (soft or indurated). Certain types of lesions present a characteristic pattern. For example, a tumor is usually an elevated, solid lesion larger than 2 cm. Primary lesions, such as macules and nodules, come from some stimulus to the skin (Box 33-7). Secondary lesions, such as ulcers, occur as alterations in primary lesions. After you identify a lesion, closely inspect it in good lighting. Palpate gently, covering the entire area of the lesion. If the lesion is moist or draining fluid, wear gloves during palpation.

Note if the client complains of tenderness during palpation. Cancerous lesions frequently undergo changes in color and size (Box 33-8). **Basal cell carcinoma** is most common in sun-exposed areas and frequently occurs in a background of sun-damaged skin; it almost never spreads to other parts of the body. **Squamous cell carcinoma** is more serious than basal cell and develops on the outer layers of sun-exposed skin; these cells may travel to lymph nodes and throughout the body. Report abnormal lesions to the health care provider for further examination.

SAFETY ALERT Individuals exposed to the sun through sunbathing or artificial means increase their risk for development of skin cancer. Provide appropriate teaching to inform clients of ways to decrease their risk (see Boxes 33-6, p. 566, and 33-8, p. 571).

Hair and Scalp

The following types of hair cover the body: terminal hair (long, coarse, thick hair easily visible on the scalp, axillae, pubic areas, and in the beard in men) and vellus hair (small, soft, tiny hairs

✳ BOX 33-7 Types of Primary Skin Lesions

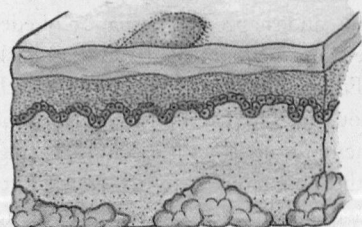

Macule: Flat, nonpalpable change in skin color, smaller than 1 cm (e.g., freckle, petechia)

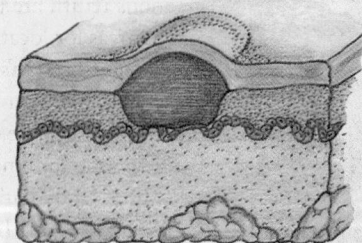

Papule: Palpable, circumscribed, solid elevation in skin, smaller than 1 cm (e.g., elevated nevus)

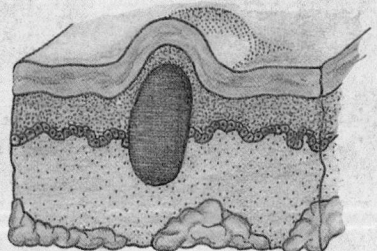

Nodule: Elevated solid mass, deeper and firmer than papule, 1-2 cm (e.g., wart)

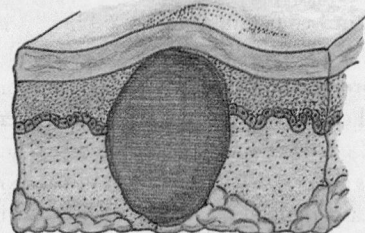

Tumor: Solid mass that extends deep through subcutaneous tissue, larger than 1-2 cm (e.g., epithelioma)

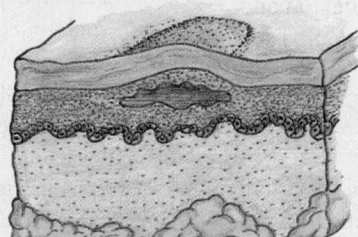

Wheal: Irregularly shaped, elevated area or superficial localized edema; varies in size (e.g., hive, mosquito bite)

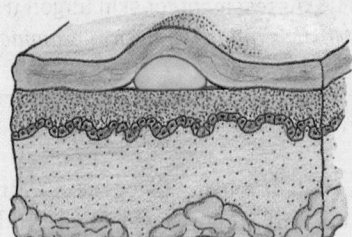

Vesicle: Circumscribed elevation of skin filled with serous fluid, smaller than 1 cm (e.g., herpes simplex, chickenpox)

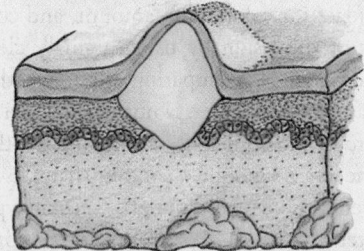

Pustule: Circumscribed elevation of skin similar to vesicle but filled with pus; varies in size (e.g., acne, staphylococcal infection)

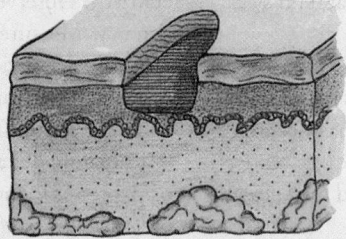

Ulcer: Deep loss of skin surface that extends to dermis and frequently bleeds and scars; varies in size (e.g., venous stasis ulcer)

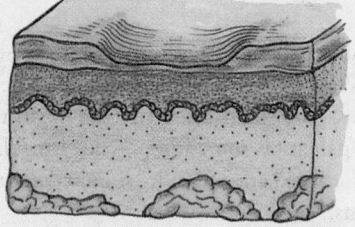

Atrophy: Thinning of skin with loss of normal skin furrow, with skin appearing shiny and translucent; varies in size (e.g., arterial insufficiency)

covering the whole body except for the palms and soles). Inspecting the condition and distribution of hair and the integrity of the scalp requires good lighting. Assessment of the hair occurs during all portions of the examination.

Inspection. During inspection explain that it is necessary to separate parts of the hair to detect abnormalities. If lesions or lice are probable, wear clean gloves to avoid infection. Table 33-11 describes the nursing history for assessment of the hair and scalp.

First inspect the color, distribution, quantity, thickness, texture, and lubrication of body hair. Scalp hair is coarse or fine; curly or straight; and should be shiny, smooth, and pliant. While separating sections of scalp hair, observe characteristics of color and coarseness. Color varies from very light blond to black to gray and sometimes shows alterations from rinses or dyes. In older adults the hair becomes dull gray, white, or yellow. The hair also thins over the scalp, axillae, and pubic areas. Older men often lose

facial hair, whereas some older women develop hair on the chin and upper lip.

Be aware of the normal distribution of hair growth in a man and a woman. At puberty a change in the amount and distribution of hair growth occurs. Some clients with hormone disorders experience an unusual distribution and growth. A woman with **hirsutism** has hair growth on the upper lip, chin, and cheeks, with vellus hair becoming coarser over the body. For some, a change in hair growth negatively affects body image and emotional well-being.

Some changes occur in the thickness, texture, and lubrication of scalp hair. Disturbances such as a febrile illness or scalp disease sometimes result in hair loss. Conditions such as thyroid disease alter the condition of the hair, making it fine and brittle. Hair loss **(alopecia)** or thinning of the hair is usually related to genetic tendencies and endocrine disorders such as diabetes, thyroiditis, and even menopause. Poor nutrition causes stringy, dull, dry, and thin hair. The oil of sebaceous glands lubricates the hair. Exces-

✳ BOX 33-8 Skin Malignancies

Basal Cell Carcinoma
0.5- to 1.0-cm crusted lesion that is flat or raised and has a rolled, somewhat scaly border.
Frequently there are underlying, widely dilated blood vessels that appear
  within the lesion.

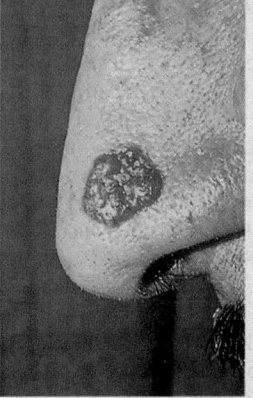

Squamous Cell Carcinoma
Occurs more often on mucosal surfaces and nonexposed areas of skin,
  compared with basal cell.
0.5- to 1.5-cm scaly lesion is sometimes ulcerated or crusted. Appears
  frequently and grows more rapidly than basal cell.

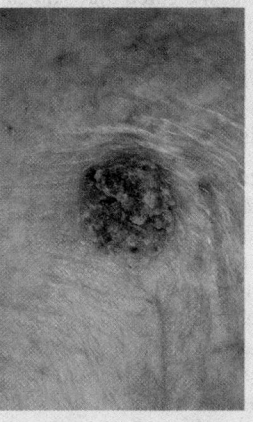

Melanoma
0.5- to 1.0-cm brown, flat lesion that appears on sun-exposed or nonexposed skin. Variegated pigmentation, irregular borders, and indistinct
  margins.
Ulceration, recent growth, or recent changes in long-standing mole are
  ominous signs.

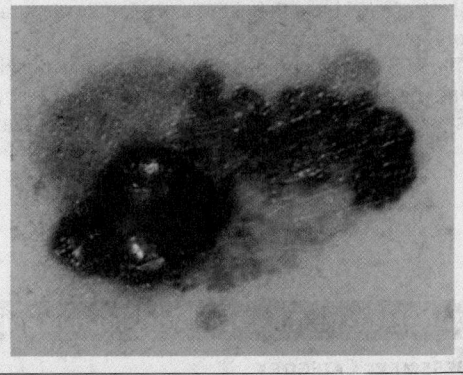

Illustrations from Belcher AE: *Cancer nursing*, St. Louis, 1992, Mosby; Habif TP: *Clinical dermatology: a color guide to diagnosis and therapy*, ed 3, St. Louis, 1996, Mosby; and Zitelli B, Davis H: *Atlas of pediatric physical diagnosis*, ed 2, St. Louis, 1991, Mosby.

sively oily hair is associated with androgen hormone stimulation. Dry, brittle hair occurs with aging and with excessive use of chemical agents.

The amount of hair covering the extremities is sometimes reduced as a result of aging. Arterial insufficiency is most common over the lower extremities. In women, do not confuse a loss of hair with shaven legs.

Inspect the scalp for lesions, which are not easy to notice in thick hair. The scalp is normally smooth and inelastic, with even coloration. By carefully separating strands of hair, thoroughly examine the scalp for lesions. Note the characteristics of any scalp

lesion. If you find lumps or bruises, ask if the client has experienced recent head trauma. Moles on the scalp are common. Warn the client that combing or brushing sometimes causes a mole to bleed. Dandruff or psoriasis frequently causes scaliness or dryness of the scalp.

Careful inspection of hair follicles on the scalp and pubic areas will possibly reveal lice or other parasites. The three types of lice are *Pediculus humanus capitis* (head lice), *Pediculus humanus corporis* (body lice), and *Pediculus pubis* (crab lice). Head and crab lice attach their eggs to hair. The tiny eggs look like oval particles of dandruff. The lice themselves are difficult to see. Head and body

* BOX 33-9 **EVIDENCE-BASED PRACTICE**

Skin Cancer Prevention

Research Summary

What is cancer? More specifically, what is skin cancer? Cancer by definition is an "uncontrolled growth and spread of abnormal cells" (ACS, 2006). Therefore skin cancer is characterized by abnormal skin cells, which can spread and invade other tissues. More importantly, what can we do about skin cancer? As nurses, it becomes our responsibility to assess for and educate our clients about all types of skin cancers, especially for the most serious form called melanoma. There are several risk factors for melanoma: major factors are positive family history of melanoma, a prior melanoma, and multiple or unusual moles. Other factors include fair complexion/skin that is sensitive to the sun; excessive exposure to the sun (especially before age 18), and the use of tanning beds/booths.

Research has indicated that skin cancer, when detected early and treated properly, is highly curable. Overall survival rates for melanoma at the 5-year mark are 92%, with 98% for localized melanoma; when it is grouped in regional and distant stages, the survival rates dramatically decrease (ACS, 2006). Therefore early intervention is of utmost importance.

Application to Nursing Practice

The results from the research studies have made it a nursing responsibility to screen and intervene for our clients' best interest. It is a necessity that we promote self-screening for all clients and their family members. We must also educate the general public.

- Instruct clients to conduct a complete monthly self-examination of the skin and scalp, noting moles, blemishes, and birthmarks.
- Perform the examination after a bath or shower, including a head-to-toe check.
- Use a well-lit room and mirrors to examine all skin surfaces. If necessary, have the client ask a family member/significant other to aid in the investigation.
- The ACS (2006) outlines the warning signs of skin cancer using the ABCD mnemonic: A is for Asymmetry—look for uneven shape; B is for Border irregularity—look for edges that are blurred, notched, or ragged; C is for Color—pigmentation is not uniform; blue, black, brown variegated and areas of pink, white, gray, blue, or red are abnormal (Hayes, 2003); and D is for Diameter, greater than the size of a typical pencil eraser.
- Teach your clients to contact their health care provider if a skin lesion or mole starts to bleed or ooze or feels different (swollen, hard, lumpy, itchy, or tender to the touch). Especially instruct older adults, who tend to have delayed wound healing.
- Inform your clients of ways to prevent skin cancer by avoiding overexposure to the sun:
  - Wear wide-brimmed hats and long sleeves.
  - Apply broad-spectrum sunscreens with SPF of 15 or greater to protect against ultraviolet B (UVB) and ultraviolet A (UVA) rays approximately 15 minutes before going into the sun and after swimming or perspiring.
  - Avoid tanning under the direct sun at midday (10 AM to 4 PM).
  - Do not use indoor sunlamps, tanning parlors, or tanning pills.
- Inform clients who are on medications that make the skin more sensitive to the sun (e.g., oral contraceptives, antibiotics, antiinflammatories, antihypertensives, immunosuppressives) to take extra precautions when spending time in the sun.
- Inform clients to protect their children from the sun. Severe sunburns in childhood greatly increase melanoma risk later in life (ACS, 2006).
- These interventions will provide the client with self-screening measures to detect, prevent, and seek early treatment for skin cancer.

Data from American Cancer Society: *Cancer facts and figures 2006*, Atlanta, 2006, The Society; and Hayes JL: Are you assessing for melanoma? *RN* 66(2):36, 2003.

ACS, American Cancer Society.

TABLE 33-11 Nursing History for Hair and Scalp Assessment

ASSESSMENT CATEGORY	RATIONALE
Ask client if he or she is wearing a wig or hairpiece, and ask him or her to remove it.	Wigs or hairpieces interfere with inspection of hair and scalp. (Client sometimes requests to omit this part of examination.)
Determine if client has noted change in growth or loss of hair; change in texture or color.	Change often occurs slowly over time.
Identify type of hair care products used for grooming.	Excessive use of chemical agents and burning of hair causes drying and brittleness.
Determine if client has recently had chemotherapy (drugs that cause hair loss) or taken a vasodilator (minoxidil) for hair growth.	Chemotherapeutic agents kill cells that rapidly multiply, such as tumor cells and normal hair cells. Minoxidil causes excessive hair growth.
Has client noted changes in diet or appetite?	Nutrition influences condition of hair.

✳ **BOX 33-10** ㅤㅤㅤㅤㅤㅤㅤㅤㅤㅤㅤㅤ **CLIENT TEACHING**

Hair and Scalp Assessment

Objective
- Client will perform proper hygiene practices for care of the hair and scalp.

Teaching Strategies
- Instruct client about basic hygiene practices for care of the hair and scalp (see Chapter 39).
- Instruct clients who have head lice to shampoo thoroughly with pediculicide (shampoo available at drugstores) in cold water, comb thoroughly with a fine-tooth comb (following product directions), and discard comb. Caution against use of products containing lindane, a toxic ingredient known to cause adverse reactions. Repeat shampoo treatment 12 to 24 hours later.
- After combing, remove any detectable nits or nit cases with tweezers or between the fingernails. A dilute solution of vinegar and water helps loosen nits.
- Instruct clients and parents about ways to reduce transmission of lice:
  - Do not share personal care items with others.
  - Vacuum all rugs, car seats, pillows, furniture, and flooring thoroughly, and discard vacuum bag.
- Seal nonwashable items in plastic bags for 14 days if unable to dry-clean or vacuum.
- Use thorough hand hygiene practices.
- Launder all clothing, linen, and bedding in hot soap and water, and dry in a hot dryer for at least 20 minutes. Dry-clean nonwashable items.
- Do not use insecticide.
- Instruct client to notify his or her partner if lice were sexually transmitted.
- Avoid physical contact with infested individuals and their belongings, especially clothing and bedding.
- Soak combs, brushes, and hair accessories in lice-killing products for 1 hour or in boiling water for 10 minutes.

Evaluation
- Have client describe methods used to care for the hair and scalp.
- Have client explain the steps to take to reduce lice transmission in the home.

Data from Chin J, editor: *Control of communicable diseases manual*, Washington, DC, 2000, American Public Health Association; and National Pediculosis Association: *Child care provider's guide to controlling head lice*, http://www.headlice.org.

✳ **TABLE 33-12 Nursing History for Nail Assessment**

ASSESSMENT CATEGORY	RATIONALE
Ask if client has experienced recent trauma or changes in nails (splitting, breaking, discoloration, thickening).	Trauma changes shape and growth of nail. Systemic conditions cause changes in color, growth, and shape.
Has the client had other symptoms of pain, swelling, presence of systemic disease with fever, or psychological or physical stress?	Alterations sometimes occur slowly over time.
Question client's nail care practices. Determine if client has acrylic nails or silk wraps.	Helps to indicate if change in nails is due to local or systemic problem. Acrylic nails and silk wraps are areas for fungal growth. Chemical agents cause drying of nails. Improper care damages nails and cuticles.
Determine if client has risks for nail or foot problems (e.g., diabetes, peripheral vascular disease, older adulthood, obesity).	Vascular changes associated with diabetes and peripheral vascular disease reduce blood flow to peripheral tissues; foot lesions and thickened nails are common. Some older adults have trouble performing foot and nail care because of poor vision, incoordination, or inability to bend over. Obese clients have difficulty bending over.

lice are very small with grayish white bodies. Crab lice have red legs. Observe for bites or pustular eruptions in the hair follicles and in areas where skin surfaces meet, such as behind the ears and in the groin. The discovery of lice requires immediate treatment (Box 33-10).

Nails

The condition of the nails reflects general health, state of nutrition, a person's occupation, and level of self-care. Nail biting can reveal a person's psychological state. Before assessing the nails, gather a brief history (Table 33-12). The most visible portion of the nails is the nail plate, the transparent layer of epithelial cells

covering the nail bed (Figure 33-7). The vascularity of the nail bed creates the nail's underlying color. The semilunar, whitish area at the base of the nail bed is called the lunula, from which the nail plate develops.

Inspection and Palpation. Inspect the nail bed for color, cleanliness, and length; the thickness and shape of the nail, the texture of the nail; the angle between the nail and the nail bed; and the condition of the lateral and proximal nail folds around the nail. Also palpate the nail base. When inspecting the nails, you will obtain a quick sense about the client's hygiene practices. The nails are normally transparent, smooth, well rounded, and con-

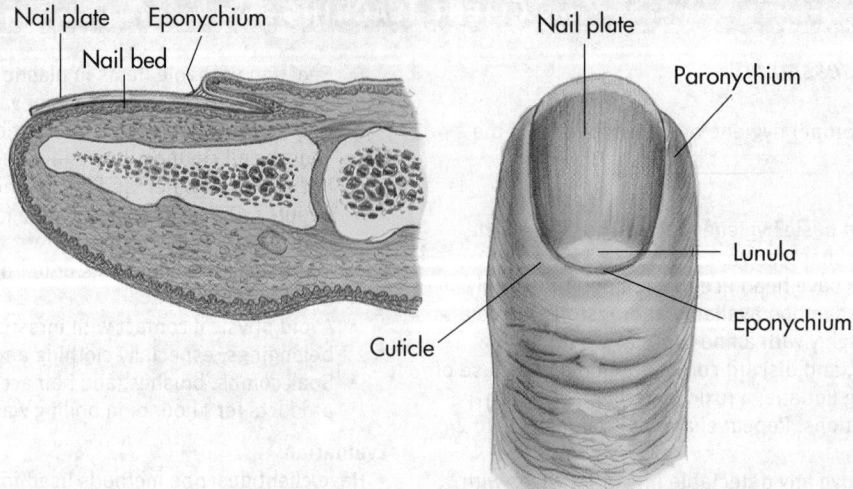

Figure 33-7 Components of the nail unit. (Redrawn from Thompson JM and others: *Mosby's clinical nursing,* ed 5, St. Louis, 2001, Mosby.)

vex, with a nail bed angle of about 160 degrees. The surrounding cuticles are smooth, intact, and without inflammation. If the nails are ragged, dirty, and poorly kept, this is a good indication that either the client practices infrequent nail care or is physically unable to perform care. However, consider the client's profession, because some individuals have dirty nails as part of their employment (e.g., mechanics, coal miners, and farmers) despite excellent nail care. Jagged, bitten, or broken nail edges or cuticles predispose a client to localized infection. Report any abnormalities such as erythema or swelling.

SAFETY ALERT Clients with impaired circulation are at greater risk for localized infection. It is important to observe the condition of hand and foot nails and nail beds to identify risks for and early signs of infection.

In whites, nail beds are pink with translucent white tips. In dark-skinned clients, nail beds are darkly pigmented with a blue or reddish hue. A brown or black pigmentation is normal with longitudinal streaks (Figure 33-8). Trauma, **cirrhosis**, diabetes mellitus, and hypertension cause splinter hemorrhages. Vitamin, protein, and electrolyte changes cause various lines or bands to form on the nail beds.

Nails normally grow at a constant rate, but direct injury or generalized disease impairs growth. With aging, the nails of the fingers and toes become harder and thicker. Longitudinal striations develop, and the rate of nail growth slows. Nails become more brittle, dull, and opaque and turn yellow in older adults because of insufficient calcium. Also with age, the cuticle becomes less thick and wide.

Inspection of the angle between the nail and nail bed normally reveals an angle of 160 degrees (Box 33-11). A larger angle and softening of the nail bed indicates chronic oxygenation problems. Palpate the nail base to determine firmness and the condition of circulation. The nail base is normally firm.

To palpate, gently grasp the client's finger and observe the color of the nail bed. Next, apply gentle, firm, quick pressure with

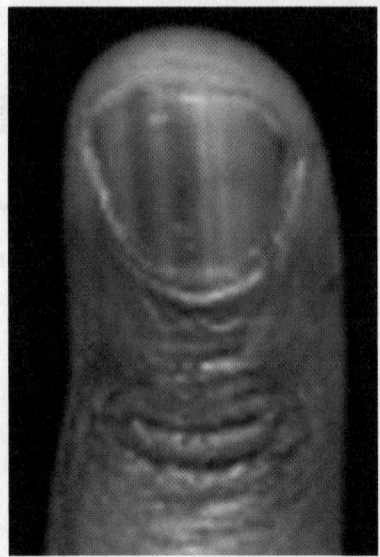

Figure 33-8 Pigmented bands in nail of client with dark skin. (From Seidel HM and others: *Mosby's guide to physical examination,* ed 6, St. Louis, 2006, Mosby.)

the thumb to the nail bed and release and observe capillary refill. As you apply pressure, the nail bed will appear white or blanched; however, the pink color should return immediately on release of pressure. Capillary refill is measured in seconds; less than 2 seconds is brisk, while greater than 4 seconds is sluggish. Failure of the pinkness to return promptly indicates circulatory insufficiency. An ongoing bluish or purplish cast to the nail bed occurs with cyanosis. A white cast or pallor results from anemia.

Calluses and corns are commonly found on the toes or fingers. A callus is flat and painless resulting from a thickening of the epidermis. Friction and pressure from shoes causes corns, usually over bony prominences. During the examination instruct the client in proper nail care (Box 33-12).

✳ BOX 33-11 Abnormalities of the Nail Bed

Normal nail: Approximately 160-degree angle between nail plate and nail

Clubbing: Change in angle between nail and nail base (eventually larger than 180 degrees); nail bed softening, with nail flattening; often, enlargement of fingertips
Causes: Chronic lack of oxygen: heart or pulmonary disease

Beau's lines: Transverse depressions in nails indicating temporary disturbance of nail growth (Nail grows out over several months.)
Causes: Systemic illness such as severe infection; nail injury
Koilonychia (spoon nail): Concave curves
Causes: Iron deficiency anemia, syphilis, use of strong detergents
Splinter hemorrhages: Red or brown linear streaks in nail bed
Causes: Minor trauma, subacute bacterial endocarditis, trichinosis
Paronychia: Inflammation of skin at base of nail
Causes: Local infection, trauma

✳ BOX 33-12 CLIENT TEACHING

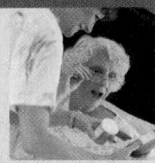

Nail Assessment
Objective
- Client properly cares for fingernails, feet, and toenails.

Teaching Strategies
- Instruct client to cut nails only after soaking them about 10 minutes in warm water. (Exception: Diabetic clients are warned against soaking nails because this dries the hands and feet out; dry skin leads to infection.)
- Caution client against over-the-counter preparations to treat corns, calluses, or ingrown toenails.
- Tell the client to cut nails straight across and even with the tops of the fingers or toes. If client has diabetes, tell client to file rather than cut the nails (see Chapter 39).
- Instruct client to shape nails with a file or emery board.
- If client is diabetic:
  - Wash feet daily in warm water, and carefully dry them, especially between the toes. Inspect feet each day in good lighting, looking for dry places and cracks in the skin. Soften dry feet by applying a cream or lotion such as Nivea, Eucerin, or Alpha Keri.
  - Do not put lotion between the toes; moisture between the toes allows microorganisms to grow, leading to infections.
  - Caution client against using sharp objects to poke or dig under the toenail or around the cuticle.
  - Have client see a podiatrist for treatment of ingrown toenails and nails that are thick or tend to split.

Evaluation
- Inspect nails during the next home visit.
- Have client explain steps to take to avoid injury.

Head and Neck

An examination of the head and neck includes assessment of the head, eyes, ears, nose, mouth, pharynx, and neck (lymph nodes, carotid arteries, thyroid gland, and trachea). During assessment of peripheral arteries also assess the carotid arteries. Assessment of the head and neck uses inspection, palpation, and auscultation, with inspection and palpation often used simultaneously.

Head

Inspection and Palpation. The nursing history screens for intracranial injury and local or congenital deformities (Table 33-13). Inspect the client's head, noting the position, size, shape, and contour. The head is normally held upright and midline to the trunk. Holding the head tilted to one side is perhaps an indication of unilateral hearing or visual loss. A horizontal jerking or bobbing indicates a tremor.

Note the client's facial features, looking at the eyelids, eyebrows, nasolabial folds, and mouth for shape and symmetry. It is normal for slight asymmetry to exist. If there is facial asymmetry, note if all features on one side of the face are affected or if only a portion of the face is involved. Various neurological disorders (e.g., facial nerve paralysis) affect different nerves that innervate muscles of the face.

Examine the size, shape, and contour of the skull. The skull is generally round with prominences in the frontal area anteriorly and the occipital area posteriorly. Trauma typically causes local skull deformities. In infants, a large head results from congenital anomaly or the buildup of cerebrospinal fluid in the ventricles (**hydrocephalus**). Some adults have enlarged jaws and facial bones resulting from **acromegaly,** a disorder caused by excessive secretion of growth hormone. Palpate the skull for nodules or masses. Gently rotate the fingertips down the midline of the scalp and then along the sides of the head to identify abnormalities. Then palpate the temporomandibular joint (TMJ) space bilaterally. Place the fingertips just anterior to the tragus of each ear. The fingertips should slip into the joint space as the client's mouth opens, to gently palpate the joint spaces. Normally the movements should be smooth, although it is not unusual to hear or feel a clicking or snapping in the TMJ (Seidel and others, 2006).

⋇ TABLE 33-13 Nursing History for Head Assessment

ASSESSMENT CATEGORY	RATIONALE
Determine if client experienced recent head trauma. If so, assess state of consciousness after injury (immediately on return and 5 minutes later), duration of unconsciousness, and predisposing factors (e.g., seizure, poor vision, blackout).	Trauma is major cause for lumps, bumps, cuts, bruises, or deformities of scalp or skull. Loss of consciousness following head injury indicates possible brain injury.
Ask if client has history of headache; note onset, duration, character, pattern, and associated symptoms.	Character of headache helps to reveal causative factors such as sinus infection, migraine, or neurological disorders.
Determine length of time client has experienced neurological symptoms.	Duration of signs or symptoms reveal severity of problem.
Review client's occupational history for use of safety helmets.	Nature of some occupations creates a risk for head injury.
Ask if client participates in contact sports, cycling, rollerblading, or skateboarding.	These activities require use of safety helmets.

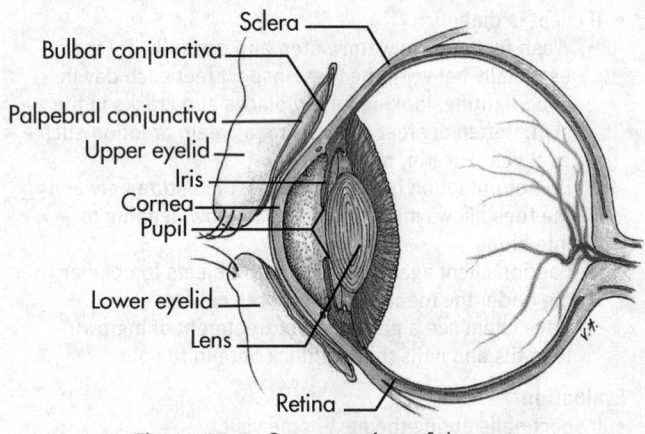

Figure 33-9 Cross section of the eye.

Eyes

Examination of the eyes includes assessment of visual acuity, visual fields, extraocular movements, and external and internal eye structures. Figure 33-9 shows a cross section of the eye. The assessment detects visual alterations and determines the level of assistance that clients require when ambulating or performing self-care activities. Some clients with visual problems also need special aids for reading educational materials or instructions (e.g., medication labels). Table 33-14 reviews the nursing history for an eye examination. Box 33-13 describes common types of visual problems.

Visual Acuity. The assessment of visual acuity, the ability to see small details, tests central vision. The easiest way to assess near vision is to ask clients to read printed material under adequate lighting. If clients wear glasses, make sure they wear them during assessment. Determine the language the client speaks and reading ability. Asking clients to read aloud will help determine literacy. If the client has difficulty reading, move to the next step.

Assessment of distant vision requires using a Snellen chart (paper chart or projection screen). The chart is well lighted. Test vision without corrective lenses first. Have the client sit or stand 20 feet (6.1 m) away from the chart and try to read all of the letters beginning at any line with both eyes open. Then have the client read the line with each eye separately (client covers the op-

posite eye with an index card or eye cover). The client avoids applying pressure to the eye. Note the smallest line in which the client is able to read all of the letters correctly, and record the visual acuity for that line. Repeat the test with the client wearing corrective lenses. Complete the test rapidly enough so that the client does not memorize the chart (Seidel and others, 2006).

If a client is unable to read, use an *E* chart or one with pictures of familiar objects. Instead of reading letters, clients tell which direction each *E* is pointing or the name of the object. Record the visual acuity score for each eye and for both eyes.

The Snellen chart has standardized numbers at the end of each line of the chart. The numerator is the number 20, or the distance the client stands from the chart. The denominator is the distance from which the normal eye is able to read the chart. Normal vision is 20/20. The larger the denominator, the poorer the client's visual acuity. For example, a value of 20/40 means that the client, standing 20 feet away, can read a line that a person with normal vision can read from 40 feet away. Record visual acuity as *sc* (without correction) or *cc* (with correction), depending on whether or not the client wears glasses or contact lenses.

If clients cannot read even the largest letters or figures of a Snellen chart, test their ability to count upraised fingers or distinguish light. Hold a hand 30 cm (1 foot) from the client's face, and have the client count the upraised fingers. To check light perception, shine a penlight into the eye and then turn the light off. If the client notes when the light is turned on or off, light perception is intact.

You assess near vision by asking the client to read a handheld card containing a vision screening chart. Instruct the client to hold the card a comfortable distance (5 to 6 cm, or about 12½ to 14 inches) from the eyes and read the smallest line possible. This portion of the examination is a good time to discuss the need for routine eye examinations (see Box 33-14, p. 578).

Extraocular Movements. Six small muscles guide the movement of each eye. Both eyes move parallel to each other in each of the six directions of gaze (Figure 33-10). To assess extraocular movements have the client sit or stand 60 cm (2 feet) away, facing you. Hold a finger at a comfortable distance (15 to 30 cm, or 6 to 12 inches) from the client's eyes. Have the client maintain his or her head in a fixed position facing forward and follow the movement of the finger with the eyes only. Have the client look to the right, to the left, and diagonally up and down to the left

✳ TABLE 33-14   Nursing History for Eye Assessment

ASSESSMENT CATEGORY	RATIONALE
Determine if client has history of eye disease, (e.g., glaucoma, retinopathy, cataracts), eye trauma, diabetes, hypertension, or eye surgery.	Some diseases or trauma cause risk for partial or complete visual loss. Client may have had surgery for a visual disorder.
Determine problems that prompted client to seek health care. Ask client about eye pain, photophobia (sensitivity to light), burning or itching, excess tearing or crusting, diplopia (double vision) or blurred vision, awareness of a "film" or "curtain" over field of vision, floaters (small, black spots that seem to float across field of vision), flashing lights, or halos around lights.	Common symptoms of eye disease indicate need for health care provider.
Determine whether there is family history of eye disorders or diseases.	Certain eye problems such as glaucoma or retinitis pigmentosa are inherited.
Review client's occupational history and recreational hobbies; are safety glasses worn?	Performance of close, intricate work causes eye fatigue. Working with computers causes eye strain. Certain occupational tasks (e.g., working with chemicals) and recreational activities (e.g., fencing, motorcycle riding) place persons at risk for eye injury unless clients take precautions.
Ask client if he or she wears glasses or contacts and if so, how often.	Clients need to wear glasses or contacts during certain portions of examination for accurate assessment.
Determine when client last visited ophthalmologist or optometrist.	Date of last eye examination reveals level of preventive care client takes.
Assess medications client is taking, including eye drops or ointment.	Determines need to assess client's knowledge of medications. Certain medications cause visual symptoms.

✳ BOX 33-13   Common Eye and Visual Problems

Hyperopia
Hyperopia is farsightedness, a refractive error in which rays of light enter the eye and focus behind the retina. Persons are able to clearly see distant objects but not close objects.

Myopia
Myopia is nearsightedness, a refractive error in which rays of light enter the eye and focus in front of the retina. Persons are able to clearly see close objects but not distant objects.

Presbyopia
Presbyopia is impaired near vision in middle-age and older adults, caused by loss of elasticity of the lens and associated with the aging process.

Retinopathy
Retinopathy is a noninflammatory eye disorder resulting from changes in retinal blood vessels. It is a leading cause of blindness.

Strabismus
Strabismus is a (congenital) condition in which both eyes do not focus on an object simultaneously; these eyes appear crossed. Impairment of the extraocular muscles or their nerve supply cause strabismus.

Cataracts
A cataract is an increased opacity of the lens, which blocks light rays from entering the eye. Cataracts sometimes develop slowly and progressively after age 35 or suddenly after trauma. Cataracts are one of the most common eye disorders. Most older adults (65 year old and up) have some evidence of visual impairment from cataracts.

Glaucoma
Glaucoma is intraocular structural damage resulting from elevated intraocular pressure. Obstruction of the outflow of aqueous humor causes this. Without treatment the disorder will lead to blindness.

Macular Degeneration
Macular degeneration is blurred central vision often occurring suddenly, caused by a progressive degeneration of the center of the retina. It is the most common visual impairment of individuals over age 50 and the most common cause of blindness in older adults. There is no cure.

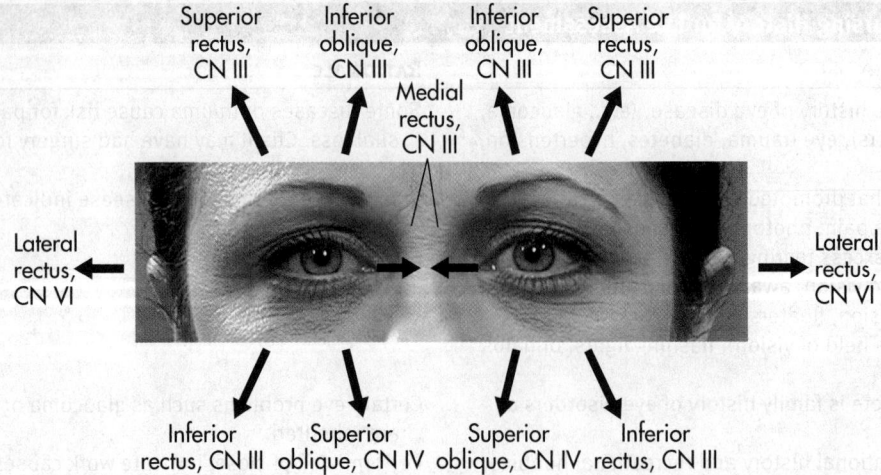

Figure 33-10 Six directions of gaze. Direct the client to follow finger movement through each gaze. (From Seidel HM and others: *Mosby's guide to physical examination,* ed 6, St. Louis, 2006, Mosby.)

✳ **BOX 33-14**   CLIENT TEACHING

Eye Assessment
Objectives
- Client follows recommendations for regular eye examinations.
- Client recognizes warning signs and symptoms of eye disease.
- Client takes appropriate safety precautions for visual deficits.

Teaching Strategies
- Tell client that persons under age 40 need to have a complete eye examination every 3 to 5 years (or more often if family histories reveal risks such as diabetes or hypertension).
- Tell client that persons over age 40 need to have eye examinations every 2 years to screen for conditions that may develop without awareness (e.g., glaucoma).
- Tell client that persons over age 65 should have yearly eye examinations.
- Describe the typical symptoms of eye disease (see Table 33-14).

- Instruct older adult to take the following precautions because of normal visual changes: avoid or use caution while driving at night, increase lighting in the home to reduce risk of falls, and paint the first and last steps of a staircase and the edge of each step in between a bright color to aid depth perception.

Evaluation
- Ask client or family member to report on client's most recent visit to an ophthalmologist.
- Have client describe when to have an eye examination.
- Ask client to describe common symptoms of eye disease.
- Observe the home environment of a client with visual deficits.

Guide to clinical preventive services, AHRQ Publication No. 05-0570, Rockville, MD, 2005. Agency for Healthcare Research and Quality, http://www.ahrp.gov/clinic/pocketgd.htm.

---

and right. The finger moves smoothly and slowly within the normal field of vision.

As the client gazes in each direction, observe for parallel eye movement, the position of the upper eyelid in relation to the iris, and the presence of abnormal movements. As the eyes move through each direction of gaze, the upper eyelid covers the iris only slightly. You assess **nystagmus,** an involuntary, rhythmical oscillation of the eyes, by periodically stopping movement of the finger. You initiate nystagmus in clients with normal eye movements by having them gaze to the far left or right. Disturbances in eye movement reflect local injury to eye muscles and supporting structures or a disorder of the cranial nerves innervating the muscles.

Visual Fields. As a person looks straight ahead, he or she is normally able to see all objects in the periphery. To assess visual fields, have the client stand or sit 60 cm (2 feet) away, facing you at eye level. The client gently closes or covers one eye (e.g., the

left) and looks at your eye directly opposite. Close the opposite eye (in this case the right) so that the field of vision is superimposed on that of the client. Move a finger equidistant from you and the client outside the field of vision, then slowly bring it back into the visual field. Ask the client to tell when he or she is able to see the finger. If you see the finger before the client does, a portion of the client's visual field is reduced. To test temporal field vision, the object should be slightly behind the client. (NOTE: The nurse can see the finger.) Repeat the procedure for each field of vision for the other eye.

SAFETY ALERT Some clients with visual field problems are at risk for injury because they cannot see all of the objects in front of them. Older adults commonly have loss of peripheral vision caused by changes in the lens.

External Eye Structures. To inspect external eye structures, stand directly in front of the client at eye level and ask the client to look at your face.

Position and Alignment. Assess the position of the eyes in relation to one another. Normally they are parallel to each other. Bulging eyes (**exophthalmos**) usually indicate hyperthyroidism. The crossing of eyes (strabismus) results from neuromuscular injury or inherited abnormalities. Tumors or inflammation of the orbit often cause abnormal eye protrusion.

For the remainder of the eye examination, have the client remove contact lenses.

Eyebrows. Inspect the eyebrows for size, extension, texture of hair, alignment, and movement. Normally, the eyebrows are symmetrical. Coarseness of hair and failure to extend beyond the temporal canthus possibly reveals hypothyroidism. If the brows are thinned, this is possibly a result of waxing or plucking. Aging causes loss of the lateral third of the eyebrows. Have the client raise and lower the eyebrows. The brows normally raise and lower symmetrically. An inability to move the eyebrows indicates a facial nerve paralysis (cranial nerve VII).

Eyelids. Inspect the eyelids for position, color, condition of the surface, condition and direction of the eyelashes, and the client's ability to open, close, and blink. When the eyes are open in a normal position, the lids do not cover the pupil and you cannot see the sclera above the iris. The lids are also close to the eyeball. An abnormal drooping of the lid over the pupil is called **ptosis** (pronounced "toe-sis"), caused by edema or impairment of the third cranial nerve. In the older adult, ptosis results from a loss of elasticity that accompanies aging. Observe for defects in the position of the lid margins. An older adult frequently has lid margins that turn out (**ectropion**) or in (**entropion**). An entropion sometimes leads to the lashes of the lid irritating the conjunctiva and cornea, increasing the risk of infection. The eyelashes are normally distributed evenly and curved outward away from the eye. An erythematous or yellow lump (hordeolum or sty) on the follicle of an eyelash indicates an acute suppurative inflammation.

To inspect the surface of the upper lids, ask the client to close his or her eyes. Then raise both eyebrows gently with the thumb and index finger to stretch the skin. The lids are normally smooth and the same color as the skin. Redness indicates inflammation or infection. Lid edema is sometimes due to allergies or to heart or kidney failure. Edema of the eyelids prevents them from closing. Inspect lesions for typical characteristics and discomfort or drainage. Wear clean gloves if drainage is present.

The lids normally close symmetrically. Failure of the lids to close exposes the cornea to drying. This condition is common in unconscious clients or in those with facial nerve paralysis Ask the client to open the eyes for inspection of the lower lids. You assess the same characteristics noted for the upper lids. Normally a client blinks involuntarily and bilaterally up to 20 times a minute. The blink reflex lubricates the cornea. Report absent or infrequent, rapid, or monocular (one-eyed) blinking.

Lacrimal Apparatus. The lacrimal gland (Figure 33-11), located in the upper outer wall of the anterior part of the orbit, is responsible for tear production. Tears flow from the gland across the eye's surface to the lacrimal duct, which is in the nasal corner or inner canthus of the eye. The lacrimal gland is sometimes the site of tumors or infections. Inspect this area for edema and redness. Palpate the gland gently to detect tenderness. Normally you cannot feel the gland.

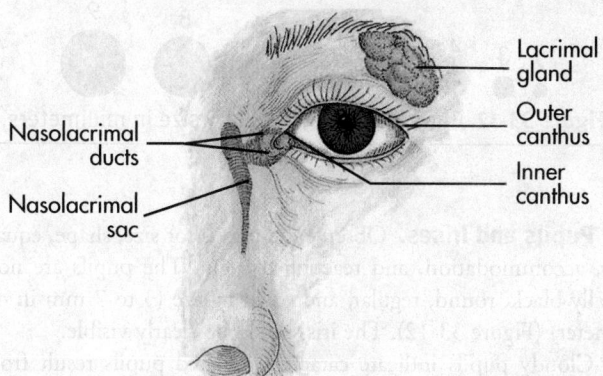

Figure 33-11 The lacrimal apparatus secretes and drains tears, which moisten and lubricate eye structures.

The nasolacrimal duct sometimes becomes obstructed, blocking the flow of tears. Observe for evidence of edema in the inner canthus. Gentle palpation of the duct at the lower eyelid just inside the lower orbital rim causes a regurgitation of tears.

Conjunctivae and Sclerae. The bulbar conjunctiva covers the exposed surface of the eyeball up to the outer edge of the cornea. Observe the sclera under the bulbar conjunctiva, it normally has the color of white porcelain in whites and light yellow in dark-skinned clients. Sclerae become pigmented and appear either yellow or green if liver disease is present.

Take care when inspecting the conjunctivae. For adequate exposure of the bulbar conjunctiva, retract the eyelids without placing pressure directly on the eyeball. Gently retract both lids, with the thumb and index finger pressed against the lower and upper bony orbits. Ask the client to look up, down, and from side to side. Many clients begin to blink, making the examination difficult. Inspect for color, texture, and the presence of edema or lesions. Normally the conjunctivae are free of erythema. The presence of redness indicates an allergic or infectious **conjunctivitis.** Bright red blood in a localized area surrounded by normal-appearing conjunctiva usually indicates subconjunctival hemorrhage. Conjunctivitis is a highly contagious infection. It is easy to spread the crusty drainage that collects on eyelid margins from one eye to the other. Wear clean gloves during the examination. Performing proper hand hygiene is necessary before and after the examination.

Corneas. The cornea is the transparent, colorless portion of the eye covering the pupil and iris. From a side view, it looks like the crystal of a wristwatch. While the client looks straight ahead, inspect the cornea for clarity and texture while shining a penlight obliquely across the cornea's entire surface. The cornea is normally shiny, transparent, and smooth. In older adults the cornea loses its luster. Any irregularity in the surface indicates an abrasion or tear that requires further examination by a health care provider. Both conditions are very painful. Note the color and details of the underlying iris. In an older adult the iris becomes faded. A thin white ring along the margin of the iris, called an **arcus senilis,** is common with aging but is abnormal in anyone under age 40. To test for the corneal blink reflex, see the cranial nerve test section of this chapter.

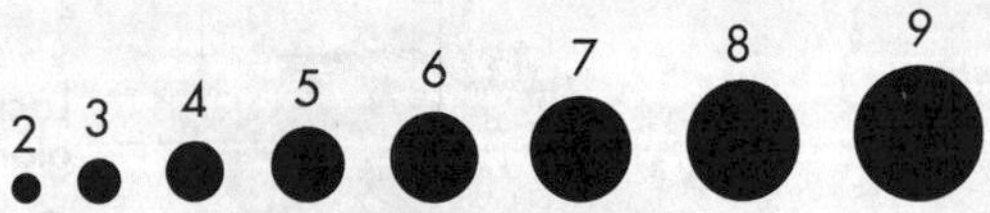

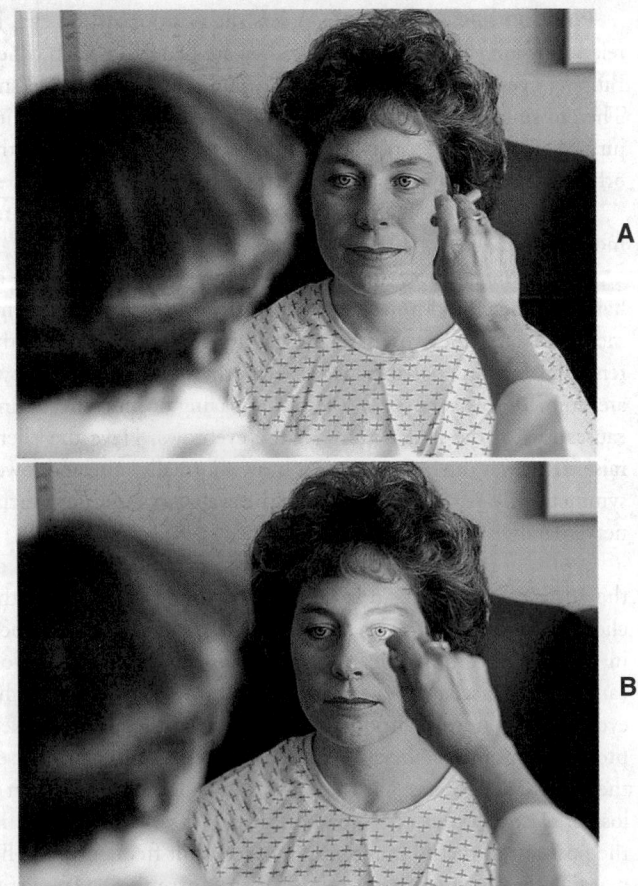

Figure 33-12 Chart depicting pupillary size in millimeters.

Pupils and Irises. Observe the pupils for size, shape, equality, accommodation, and reaction to light. The pupils are normally black, round, regular, and equal in size (3 to 7 mm in diameter) (Figure 33-12). The iris should be clearly visible.

Cloudy pupils indicate cataracts. Dilated pupils result from glaucoma, trauma, neurological disorders, eye medications (e.g., atropine), or withdrawal from opioids. Inflammation of the iris or use of drugs (e.g., pilocarpine, morphine, or cocaine) causes constricted pupils. Pinpoint pupils are a common sign of opioid intoxication. When shinning a beam of light through the pupil and onto the retina, this stimulates the third cranial nerve and causes the muscles of the iris to constrict. Any abnormality along the nerve pathways from the retina to the iris alters the ability of the pupils to react to light. Changes in intracranial pressure, lesions along the nerve pathways, locally applied ophthalmic medications, and direct trauma to the eye alter pupillary reaction.

Test pupillary reflexes (to light and accommodation) in a dimly lit room. While the client looks straight ahead, bring a penlight from the side of the client's face, directing the light onto the pupil (Figure 33-13). If the client looks at the light, there will be a false reaction to accommodation. A directly illuminated pupil constricts, and the opposite pupil constricts consensually. Observe the quickness and equality of the reflex. Repeat the examination for the opposite eye.

To test for accommodation, ask the client to gaze at a distant object (the far wall) and then at a test object (finger or pencil) held approximately 10 cm (4 inches) from the bridge of the client's nose. The pupils normally converge and accommodate by constricting when looking at close objects. The pupillary responses are equal. Testing for accommodation is only important if the client has a defect in the pupillary response to light (Seidel and others, 2006). If assessment of pupillary reaction is normal in all tests, record the abbreviation **PERRLA** (pupils equal, round, reactive to light, and accommodation).

Internal Eye Structures. The examination of the internal eye structures through the use of an ophthalmoscope is beyond the scope of new graduate nurses' practice. Advanced nurse practitioners use the **ophthalmoscope** to inspect the fundus (Figure 33-14), which includes the retina, choroid, optic nerve disc, macula, fovea centralis, and retinal vessels. Clients in greatest need of an examination are those with diabetes, hypertension, and intracranial disorders.

Ears

The ear assessment determines the integrity of ear structures and hearing acuity. The three parts of the ear are the external, middle, and inner ear (Figure 33-15). Inspect and palpate external ear structures, inspect middle ear structures with an otoscope, and test the inner ear by measuring the client's hearing acuity. External ear structures consist of the auricle, outer ear canal, and tympanic

Figure 33-13 A, To check pupillary reflexes, the nurse first holds the penlight to the side of the client's face. **B,** Illumination of the pupil causes pupillary constriction.

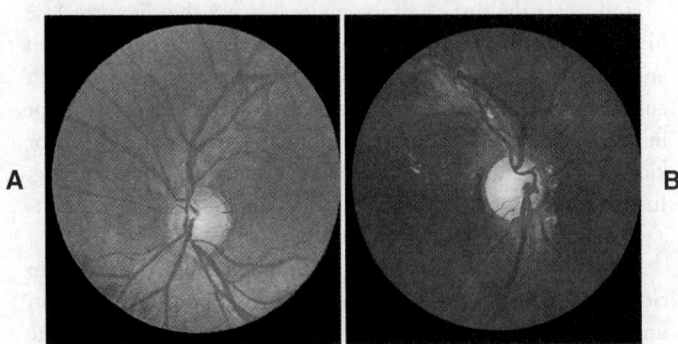

Figure 33-14 Fundus of, **A,** white client and, **B,** African American client. (Courtesy MEDCOM, Cypress, Calif.)

membrane (eardrum). The ear canal is normally curved and approximately 2.5 cm (1 inch) long in an adult. It is lined with skin containing fine hairs, nerve endings, and glands secreting cerumen. The middle ear is an air-filled cavity containing the three bony ossicles (malleus, incus, and stapes). The eustachian tube connects the middle ear to the nasopharynx. Pressure between the outer atmosphere and the middle ear is stabilized through the eustachian tube.

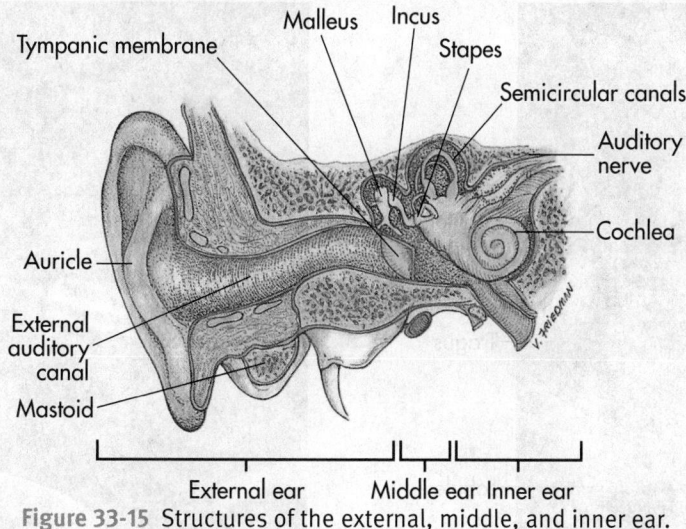

Figure 33-15 Structures of the external, middle, and inner ear.

✳ TABLE 33-15 Nursing History for Ear Assessment

ASSESSMENT CATEGORY	RATIONALE
Ask if client has experienced ear pain, itching, discharge, vertigo, tinnitus (ringing in ears), or change in hearing.	These signs and symptoms indicate infection or hearing loss.
Assess risks for hearing problem.	Risk factors predispose client to permanent hearing loss.
Infants/children: Hypoxia at birth, meningitis, birth weight less than 1500 g, family history of hearing loss, congenital anomalies of skull or face, nonbacterial intrauterine infections (rubella, herpes), maternal drug use, excessively high bilirubin, head trauma	It is difficult to assess infant's hearing status with examination only.
Adults: Exposure to industrial or recreational noise, genetic disease (Meniere's disease), neurodegenerative disorder	
Determine client's exposure to loud noises at work and availability of protective devices.	Prolonged noise exposure causes temporary or permanent hearing loss.
Note behaviors indicative of hearing loss, such as failure to respond when spoken to, requests to repeat comments, leaning forward to hear, and child's inattentiveness or use of monotonous voice tone.	Persons with hearing loss cope with sensory deficit through a variety of behavioral cues.
Assess if client takes large doses of aspirin or other ototoxic drugs (e.g., aminoglycosides, furosemide, streptomycin, cisplatin, ethacrynic acid).	Medications have side effects of hearing loss.
Determine whether client uses hearing aid.	Determination allows nurse to assess ability to care for device and allows nurse to adjust voice tone to communicate.
If client had recent hearing problem, note onset, contributing factors, affected ear, and effect on activities of daily living.	Helps determine nature and severity of hearing problem.
Determine whether client has repeated history of cerumen buildup in ear.	Cerumen impaction is common cause for conduction deafness.

The inner ear contains the cochlea, vestibule, and semicircular canals. Assessing the ears determines the integrity of ear structures and the condition of hearing. Nursing history data (Table 33-15) aid in identifying risks for hearing disorders.

Understanding the mechanisms for sound transmission helps identify the nature of hearing disorders. Sound travels through the ear by air and bone conduction; the following explains the steps of hearing:

1. Sound waves in the air enter the external ear, passing through the outer ear canal.

2. The sound waves reach the tympanic membrane, causing it to vibrate.

3. Vibrations are transmitted through the middle ear by the bony ossicular chain to the oval window at the opening of the inner ear.

4. The cochlea receives the sound vibration.

5. Nerve impulses from the cochlea travel to the auditory (eighth cranial) nerve and to the cerebral cortex.

Disorders of the ear result from several types of problems, including mechanical dysfunction (blockage by earwax or foreign

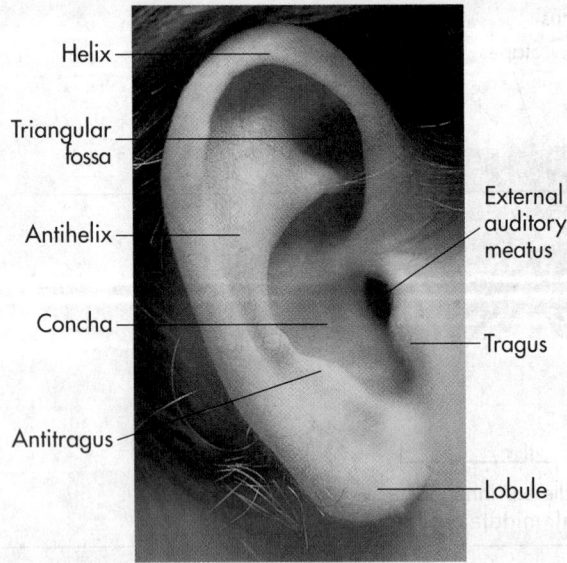

Figure 33-16 Anatomical structures of the auricle. (From Seidel HM and others: *Mosby's guide to physical examination,* ed 6, St. Louis, 2006, Mosby.)

Helix
Triangular fossa
Antihelix
Concha
Antitragus
External auditory meatus
Tragus
Lobule

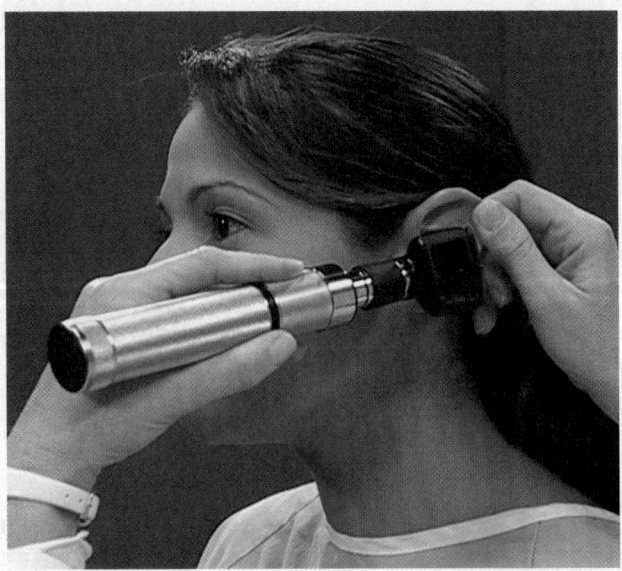

Figure 33-17 Otoscopic examination. (From Seidel HM and others: *Mosby's guide to physical examination,* ed 6, St. Louis, 2006, Mosby.)

body), trauma (foreign bodies or noise exposure), neurological disorders (auditory nerve damage), acute illnesses (viral infection), and toxic effects of medications.

Auricles. With the client sitting comfortably, inspect the auricle's size, shape, symmetry, landmarks, position, and color (Figure 33-16). The auricles are normally of equal size and level with each other. The upper point of attachment is in a straight line with the lateral canthus, or corner of the eye. The position of the auricle is almost vertical. Ears that are low set or at an unusual angle are a sign of chromosome abnormality (e.g., Down syndrome). Ear color is usually the same as that of the face, without moles, cysts, deformities, or nodules. Redness is a sign of inflammation or fever. Extreme pallor indicates frostbite.

Palpate the auricles for texture, tenderness, and skin lesions. Auricles are normally smooth, and without lesions. If the client complains of pain, gently pull the auricle, press on the tragus, and palpate behind the ear over the mastoid process. If palpating the external ear increases the pain, an external ear infection is likely. If palpation of the auricle and tragus does not influence the pain, the client possibly has a middle ear infection. Tenderness in the mastoid area indicates mastoiditis.

Inspect the opening of the ear canal for size and presence of discharge. If discharge is present, wear clean gloves during the examination. A swollen or occluded meatus is not normal. A yellow, waxy substance called **cerumen** is common. Yellow or green, foul-smelling discharge indicates infection or a foreign body.

Ear Canals and Eardrums. Observe the deeper structures of the external and middle ear with the use of an **otoscope.** A special ear speculum attaches to the handle of the ophthalmoscope. For best visualization select the largest speculum that fits comfortably in the client's ear. Before inserting the speculum, check for foreign bodies in the opening of the auditory canal.

Make sure the client avoids moving the head during the examination to avoid damage to the canal and tympanic membrane. You often need to restrain infants and young children. Lay infants supine with their heads turned to one side and their arms held securely at their sides. Have young children sit on their parents' laps with their legs held between the parents' knees.

Turn on the otoscope by rotating the dial at the top of the handle. To insert the speculum properly, ask the client to tip the head slightly toward the opposite shoulder. Hold the handle of the otoscope in the space between the thumb and index finger, supported on the middle finger. This leaves the ulnar side of the hand to rest against the client's head, stabilizing the otoscope as you insert it into the canal (Seidel and others, 2006). There are two types of grips for the otoscope. In one, hold the handle along the client's face with the fingers against the face or neck. In the other grip, lightly brace the inverted otoscope against the side of the client's head or cheek. This grip, used with children, prevents accidental movement of the otoscope deeper into the ear canal. Insert the scope while pulling the auricle upward and backward in the adult and older child (Figure 33-17). This maneuver straightens the ear canal. In infants pull the auricle down and back.

Insert the speculum slightly down and forward 1 to 1.5 cm (½ inch) into the ear canal. Take care not to scrape the sensitive lining of the ear canal, which is painful. The ear canal normally has little cerumen and is uniformly pink with tiny hairs in the outer third of the canal. Observe for color, discharge, scaling, lesions, foreign bodies, and cerumen. Normally cerumen is dry (light brown to gray and flaky) or moist (dark yellow or brown) and sticky. Dry cerumen occurs in Asians and Native Americans about 85% of the time (Seidel and others, 2006). A reddened canal with discharge is a sign of inflammation or infection. In other adults, accumulated cerumen is a common problem. Buildup of cerumen creates a mild hearing loss. During the ex-

✳ BOX 33-15   **CLIENT TEACHING**

Ear Assessment

Objectives
- Client uses proper technique for cleansing the ears.
- Client follows preventive guidelines for screening of hearing loss.
- Client with hearing loss communicates effectively.

Teaching Strategies
- Instruct client in the proper way to clean the outer ear (see Chapter 39), avoiding use of cotton-tipped applicators and sharp objects such as hairpins, which cause impaction of cerumen deep in the ear canal or cause trauma.
- Tell client to avoid inserting pointed objects into the ear canal.
- Encourage clients over age 65 to have regular hearing checks. Explain that a reduction in hearing is a normal part of aging (see Chapter 49).
- Instruct family members of clients with hearing losses to avoid shouting and instead speak in low tones, and to be sure the client is able to see the speaker's face.

Evaluation
- Ask client to explain the proper technique for cleansing the ears.
- In a follow-up visit, question client about frequency of hearing checks.
- Observe client with hearing loss interacting with family members.

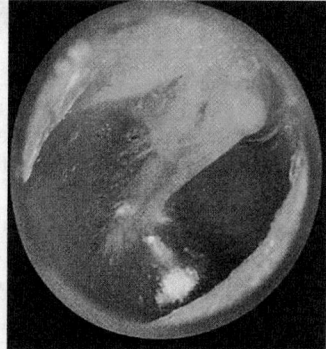

Figure 33-18   Normal right tympanic membrane. (Courtesy Dr. Richard A. Buckingham, Abraham Lincoln School of Medicine, University of Illinois, Chicago.)

amination ask about methods that the client uses to clean the ear canal (Box 33-15).

The light from the otoscope allows visualization of the tympanic membrane. Know the common anatomical landmarks and their appearances (Figure 33-18). Gently move the otoscope so that you are able to see the entire tympanic membrane and its periphery. Because the tympanic membrane is angled away from the ear canal, the light from the otoscope appears as a cone shape rather than a circle. A ring of fibrous cartilage surrounds the oval membrane. The umbo is near the center of the membrane, behind which is the attachment of the malleus. The underlying short process of the malleus creates a knoblike structure at the top of the drum. Check carefully to make sure that there are no tears or breaks in the membrane. The normal tympanic membrane is translucent, shiny, and pearly gray. It is free from tears or breaks. A pink or red bulging membrane indicates inflammation. A white color reveals pus behind it. The membrane is taut, except for the small triangular pars flaccida near the top. If cerumen is blocking the tympanic membrane, warm water irrigation will safely remove the wax.

Hearing Acuity.   A client with a hearing loss often fails to respond to conversation. The three types of hearing loss are conduction, sensorineural, and mixed. A conduction loss interrupts sound waves as they travel from the outer ear to the cochlea of the inner ear because the sound waves are not transmitted through the outer and middle ear structures. Examples of causes of a conduction loss are swelling of the auditory canal or tears in the

tympanic membrane. A sensorineural loss involves the inner ear, auditory nerve, or hearing center of the brain. Sound is conducted through the outer and middle ear structures, but the continued transmission of sound becomes interrupted at some point beyond the bony ossicles. A mixed loss involves a combination of conduction and sensorineural loss.

SAFETY ALERT   Clients working or living around loud noises are at risk for hearing loss. In addition, adolescents are at risk for premature hearing loss from continued exposure to loud music in their car or home or at concert events. The use of IPODs and MP3 players also increase the risk for hearing loss in all clients.

Older adults experience an inability to hear high-frequency sounds and consonants (e.g., *S, Z, T,* and *G*). Deterioration of the cochlea and thickening of the tympanic membrane cause older adults to gradually lose hearing acuity. They are especially at risk for hearing loss due to **ototoxicity** (injury to auditory nerve) resulting from high maintenance doses of antibiotics (e.g., aminoglycosides).

To conduct a hearing assessment, have the client remove any hearing aid if worn. Note the client's response to questions. Normally the client responds without excessive requests to have the questions repeated. If you suspect hearing loss, check the client's response to the whispered voice. Test one ear at a time while the client occludes the other ear with a finger. Ask the client to gently move the finger up and down during the test. While standing 30 to 60 cm (1 to 2 feet) from the testing ear, cover the mouth so that the client is unable to read lips. After exhaling fully, whisper softly toward the unoccluded ear, reciting random numbers with equally accented syllables, such as *nine-four-ten.* If necessary, gradually increase voice intensity until the client correctly repeats the numbers. Then test the other ear for comparison. Seidel and others (2006) report that clients normally hear numbers clearly when whispered, responding correctly at least 50% of the time.

If a hearing loss is present, there are tests that you perform using a tuning fork or audiometry. A tuning fork of 256 to 512 hertz (Hz) is most commonly used. The tuning fork allows for comparison of hearing by bone conduction with that of air conduction. Hold the base of the tuning fork with one hand without touching the tines. Tap the fork lightly against the palm of the other hand to set the fork in vibration (Table 33-16).

✳ TABLE 33-16 Tuning Fork Tests

TESTS AND STEPS	RATIONALE
Weber's Test (Lateralization of Sound) Hold fork at its base and tap it lightly against heel of palm. Place base of vibrating fork on midline vertex of client's head or middle of forehead (see illustration *A*). Ask client if he or she hears the sound equally in both ears or better in one ear.	Client with normal hearing hears sound equally in both ears. In conduction deafness, sound is heard best in impaired ear. In unilateral sensorineural hearing loss, sound is identified only in normal ear.
Rinne Test (Comparison of Air and Bone Conduction) Place stem of vibrating tuning fork against client's mastoid process (see illustration *B*). Begin counting the interval with your watch. Ask client to tell you when he or she no longer hears the sound; note number of seconds. Quickly place still-vibrating tines 1 to 2 cm (½ to 1 inch) from ear canal, and ask client to tell you when he or she no longer hears the sound (see illustration *C*). Continue counting time the sound is heard by air conduction. Compare number of seconds the sound is heard by bone conduction versus air conduction.	Client should hear air-conducted sound twice as long as bone-conducted sound (2:1 ratio). For example; if client hears bone-conducted sound for 10 seconds, he or she should hear air-conducted sound for an additional 10 seconds. In conduction deafness, client can no longer hear bone-conducted sound. In sensorineural loss, sound is reduced and heard longer through air but less than 2:1 ratio.

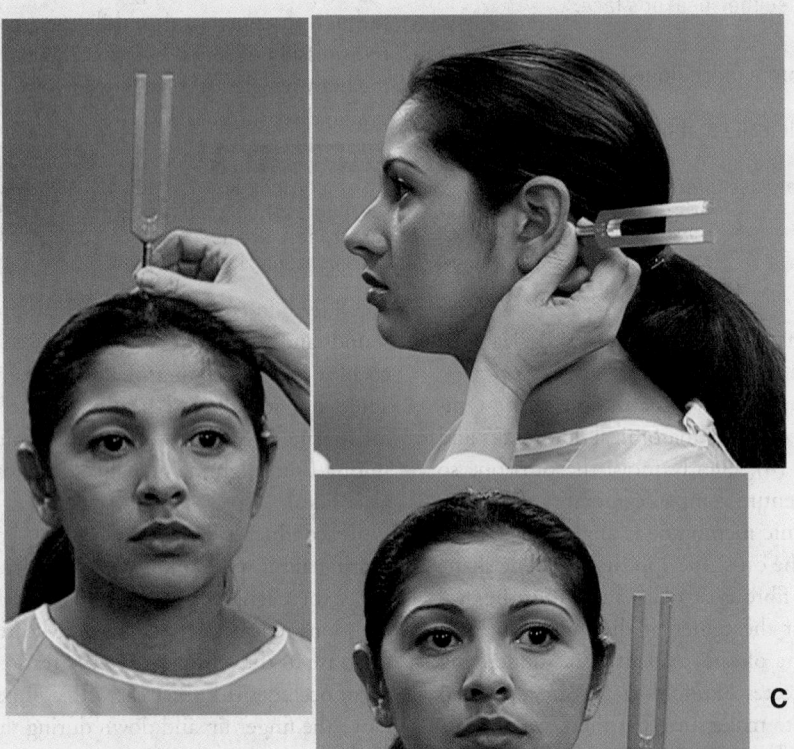

Illustrations from Seidel HM and others: *Mosby's guide to physical examination*, ed 6, St. Louis, 2006, Mosby.

✳ TABLE 33-17 Nursing History for Nose and Sinus Assessment

ASSESSMENT CATEGORY	RATIONALE
Ask if client has had trauma to nose.	Trauma causes septal deviation and asymmetry of external nose.
Ask if client has history of allergies, nasal discharge, epistaxis (nosebleeds), or postnasal drip.	History is useful in determining source or nature of nasal and sinus drainage.
If there is history of nasal discharge, assess color, amount, odor, duration, and associated symptoms (e.g., sneezing, nasal congestion, obstruction, or mouth breathing).	Aids in ruling out presence of infection, allergy, or drug use.
Assess for history of nosebleed, including site, frequency, amount of bleeding, treatment, and difficulty stopping bleeding.	Characteristics sometimes reveal trauma, medication use, or excessive dryness as causative factors.
Ask if client uses nasal spray or drops, including amount, frequency, and duration of use.	Overuse of over-the-counter nasal preparations causes physical change in mucosa.
Ask if client snores at night or has difficulty breathing.	Difficulty with breathing or snoring indicates septal deviation or obstruction.

Nose and Sinuses

Assess the integrity of the nose and sinuses by using inspection and palpation. The client sits during the examination. A penlight allows for gross examination of each naris. A more detailed examination requires use of a nasal speculum to inspect the deeper nasal turbinates. Do not use a speculum unless a qualified practitioner is present. Table 33-17 lists components of the nursing history.

Nose. When inspecting the external nose, observe for shape, size, skin, color, and the presence of deformity or inflammation. The nose is normally smooth and symmetric with the same color as the face. Recent trauma sometimes causes edema and discoloration. If swelling or deformities exist, gently palpate the ridge and soft tissue of the nose by placing one finger on each side of the nasal arch and gently moving the fingers from the nasal bridge to the tip. Note any tenderness, masses, or underlying deviations. Nasal structures are usually firm and stable.

Air normally passes freely through the nose when a person breathes. To assess patency of the nares, place a finger on the side of the client's nose and occlude one naris. Ask the client to breathe with the mouth closed. Repeat the procedure for the other naris.

While illuminating the anterior nares, inspect the mucosa for color, lesions, discharge, swelling, and evidence of bleeding. If discharge is present, apply gloves. Normal mucosa is pink and moist without lesions. Pale mucosa with clear discharge indicates allergy. A mucoid discharge indicates rhinitis. A sinus infection results in yellowish or greenish discharge. Habitual use of intranasal cocaine and opioids cause puffiness and increased vascularity of the nasal mucosa. For the client with a nasogastric tube, routinely check for local skin breakdown (**excoriation**) of the naris, characterized by redness and skin sloughing.

To view the septum and turbinates, have the client tip the head back slightly to provide a clear view. Illuminate the septum and observe for alignment, perforation, or bleeding. Normally the septum is close to the midline, and thicker anteriorly than posteriorly. The turbinates are covered with mucous membranes that warm and moisten inspired air. Normal mucosa is pink and

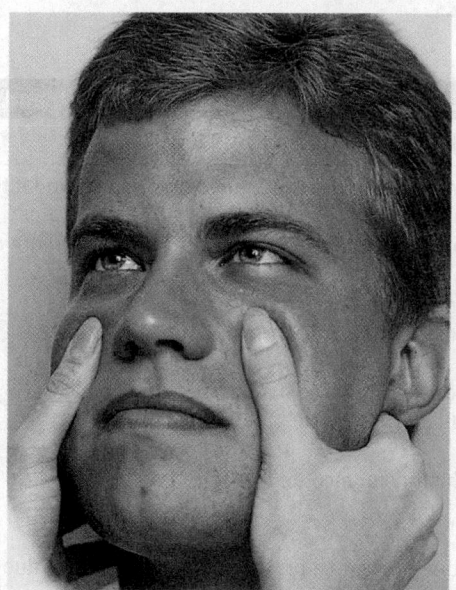

Figure 33-19 Palpation of maxillary sinuses.

moist, without lesions. A deviated septum obstructs breathing and interferes with passage of a nasogastric tube. Perforation of the septum often occurs after repeated use of intranasal cocaine. Note any **polyps** (tumorlike growths) or purulent drainage.

Sinuses. Examination of the sinuses involves palpation. In cases of allergies or infection, the interior of the sinuses become inflamed and swollen. The most effective way to assess for tenderness is by externally palpating the frontal and maxillary facial areas (Figure 33-19). Palpate the frontal sinus by exerting pressure with the thumb up and under the client's eyebrow. Gentle, upward pressure elicits tenderness easily if sinus irritation is present. Do not apply pressure to the eyes. If tenderness of sinuses is present, the sinuses may be transilluminated. This procedure, however, requires advanced experience. Box 33-16 describes teaching guidelines during nose and sinus assessment.

BOX 33-16   CLIENT TEACHING

Nose and Sinus Assessment

Objectives
- Client will safely use over-the-counter nasal sprays.
- Parents will take proper measures to stop a child's nosebleed.
- Older adult will take safety precautions with loss of olfaction.

Teaching Strategies
- Caution client against overuse of over-the-counter nasal sprays, which leads to "rebound" effect, causing excess nasal congestion.
- Instruct parents in care of a child with nosebleeds: have child sit up and lean forward to avoid aspiration of blood, apply pressure to the anterior nose with the thumb and forefinger as the child breathes through the mouth, and apply ice or a cold cloth to the bridge of the nose if pressure fails to stop bleeding.

- Instruct older adults to install smoke detectors on each floor of their home.
- Instruct older adults to always check dated labels on food to ensure against spoilage.

Evaluation
- Have client explain proper use of over-the-counter nasal sprays.
- Have parents demonstrate and describe technique for stopping a nosebleed.
- Inspect client's home during visit, and look for smoke detectors. Ask to check some food items in the refrigerator.

TABLE 33-18   Nursing History for Mouth and Pharyngeal Assessment

ASSESSMENT CATEGORY	RATIONALE
Determine if client wears dentures or retainers and if they are comfortable.	Client needs to remove dentures to visualize and palpate gums. Ill-fitting dentures chronically irritate mucosa and gums.
Determine if client has had recent change in appetite or weight.	Symptoms result from painful mouth conditions or poor hygiene.
Determine if client uses tobacco products:	
• Smoking of cigarette, cigar, or pipe	Smoking of these products increases risk for lung, oral cavity, larynx, and esophageal cancers (American Cancer Society [ACS], 2006).
• Smokeless tobacco: use of chewing tobacco and snuff	Smokeless tobacco causes various cancers and noncancerous oral disorders. Long-term snuff users have increased risk for cancer of the gums and cheeks (ACS, 2006).
Review history for alcohol consumption.	Excessive alcohol consumption appears to have greater risk for oral cavity and pharynx cancer. Effects of alcohol are independent of tobacco use.
Assess dental hygiene practices, including use of fluoride toothpaste, frequency of brushing and flossing, and frequency of dental visits.	Assessment reveals client's need for education and/or financial support. Periodontal disease has a higher prevalence in older adults who have history of high plaque buildup, use tobacco, and visit the dentist infrequently.
Ask if client has pain from chewing or eating. If so, ask if mouth lesions are present, including duration and associated symptoms.	Pain is often associated with broken tooth, tooth grinding, or temporomandibular joint problems. Extra care is needed during oral hygiene administration.

Mouth and Pharynx

Assess the mouth and pharynx to detect signs of overall health, determine oral hygiene needs, and develop therapies for clients with dehydration, restricted intake, oral trauma, or oral airway obstruction. To assess the oral cavity, use a penlight and tongue depressor or a single gauze square. Wear clean gloves during the examination. Have the client sit or lie down during the examination. Assess the oral cavity also while administering oral hygiene (see Chapter 39). Table 33-18 describes the nursing history for assessment of the mouth and pharynx.

Lips. Inspect the lips for color, texture, hydration, contour, and lesions. With the client's mouth closed, view the lips from end to end. Normally they are pink, moist, symmetrical, and smooth (Figure 33-20). Lip color in the dark-skinned client varies from pink to plum. Have female clients remove their lipstick before the examination. Anemia causes pallor of the lips, with cyanosis caused by respiratory or cardiovascular problems. Cherry-colored lips indicate carbon monoxide poisoning. Any lesions such as nodules or ulcerations are related to infection, irritation, or skin cancer.

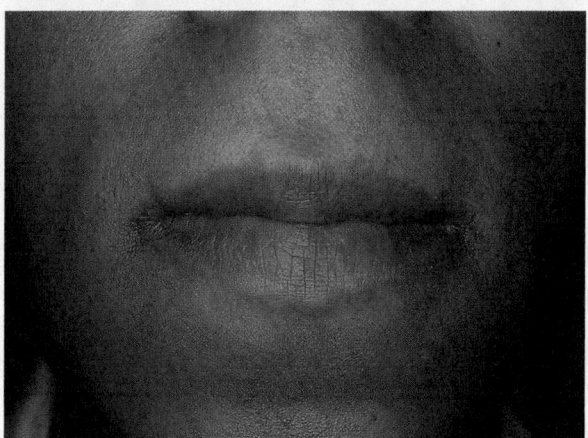

Figure 33-20 The lips are normally pink, symmetrical, smooth, and moist.

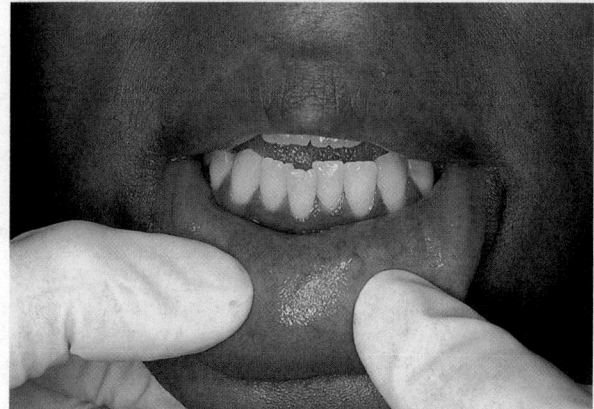

Figure 33-21 Inspection of inner oral mucosa of the lower lip.

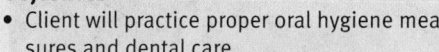
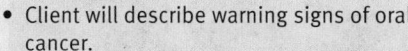

BOX 33-17   **CLIENT TEACHING**

Mouth and Pharyngeal Assessment

Objectives
- Client will practice proper oral hygiene measures and dental care.
- Client will describe warning signs of oral cancer.
- Older adult will maintain normal solid food intake.

Teaching Strategies
- Discuss proper techniques for oral hygiene, including brushing and flossing (see Chapter 39).
- Explain the early warning signs of oral cavity and pharynx cancer, including a sore that bleeds easily and does not heal, a lump or thickening, and a red or white patch on the mucosa that persists. Difficulty chewing, swallowing, or moving the tongue or jaw are late symptoms (American Cancer Society, 2006).
- Encourage regular dental examination every 6 months for children, adults, and older adults.
- Identify older clients who have difficulty in chewing and changes in the teeth. Teach clients to eat soft foods and cut food into small pieces.

Evaluation
- Ask client to demonstrate brushing.
- Have client identify when to have regular dental checkups.
- Have client identify the warning signs of oral cavity and pharynx cancer.
- Ask older adult to keep a diet record for 3 days.

Buccal Mucosa, Gums, and Teeth. Ask the client to clench the teeth and smile to observe teeth occlusion. The upper molars normally rest directly on the lower molars, and the upper incisors slightly override the lower incisors. A symmetrical smile reveals normal facial nerve function.

Inspect the teeth to determine the quality of dental hygiene (Box 33-17). Note the position and alignment of the teeth. To examine the posterior surface of the teeth, have the client open

the mouth with the lips relaxed. Use a tongue depressor to retract the lips and cheeks, especially when viewing the molars. Note the color of teeth and presence of dental **caries** (cavities), tartar, and extraction sites. Normal, healthy teeth are smooth, white, and shiny. A chalky white discoloration of the enamel is an early indication of caries formation. Brown or black discolorations indicate the formation of caries. A stained yellow color is from tobacco use, whereas coffee, tea, and colas cause a brown stain. In the older adult, loose or missing teeth are common because bone resorption increases. An older adult's teeth often feel rough when tooth enamel calcifies. Yellow or darkened teeth are also common in the older adult because of the general wear and tear that exposes the darker, underlying dentin.

To view the mucosa and gums, ask the client to first remove any dental appliance. View the inner oral mucosa by having the client open and relax the mouth slightly and then gently retract the client's lower lip away from the teeth (Figure 33-21). Repeat this process for the upper lip. Inspect the mucosa for color, hydration, texture, and lesions such as ulcers, abrasions, or cysts. Normally the mucosa is a glistening pink, smooth, and moist. Some common small, yellow-white raised lesions on the buccal mucosa and lips are Fordyce spots, or ectopic sebaceous glands (Seidel and others, 2006). If lesions are present, palpate them gently with a gloved hand for tenderness, size, and consistency.

To inspect the buccal mucosa, ask the client to open the mouth and then gently retract the cheeks with a tongue depressor or gloved finger covered with gauze (Figure 33-22). View the surface of the mucosa from right to left and top to bottom. A penlight illuminates the most posterior portion of the mucosa. Normal mucosa is glistening, pink, soft, moist, and smooth. Varying shades of hyperpigmentation are normal in 10% of whites after age 50 and up to 90% of African Americans by the same age. For clients with normal pigmentation, the buccal mucosa is a good site to inspect for jaundice and pallor. In older adults the mucosa is normally dry because of reduced salivation. Thick white patches (**leukoplakia**) are often a precancerous lesion seen in heavy smokers and alcoholics. Palpate for any buccal lesions by placing the index finger within the buccal cavity and the thumb on the outer surface of the cheek.

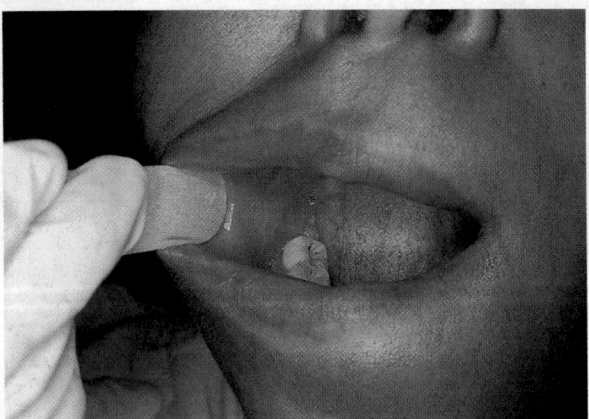

Figure 33-22 Retraction of the buccal mucosa allows for clear visualization.

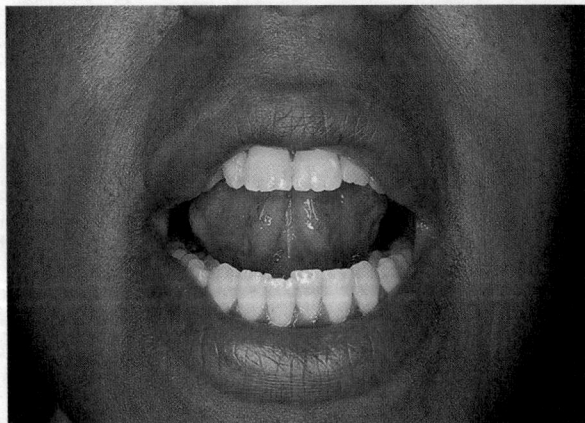

Figure 33-23 The undersurface of the tongue is highly vascular.

> **SAFETY ALERT** Clients who smoke cigarettes, cigars, or pipes and those who use smokeless tobacco have an increased risk of oral, laryngeal, and esophageal cancer. These individuals have leukoplakia or other lesions anywhere in their oral cavity (e.g., lips, gums, or tongue) at an early age.

Inspect the gums (gingivae) for color, edema, retraction, bleeding, and lesions while retracting the cheeks. Healthy gums are pink, smooth, and moist and tightly fit around each tooth. Dark-skinned clients often have patchy pigmentation. In older adults the gums are usually pale. Using clean gloves, palpate the gums to assess for lesions, thickening, or masses. Normally there is no tenderness. Spongy gums that bleed easily indicate periodontal disease and vitamin C deficiency. If the client has loose or mobile teeth, swollen gums, or pockets containing debris at the tooth margins, suspect periodontal disease or gingivitis.

Tongue and Floor of Mouth. Carefully inspect the tongue on all sides, as well as the floor of the mouth. Have the client relax the mouth and stick the tongue out halfway. Note any deviation, tremor, or limitation in movement. This tests hypoglossal nerve function. If the client protrudes the tongue too far, this will elicit the gag reflex. When the tongue protrudes, it lies midline. To test for tongue mobility, ask the client to raise the tongue up and move it from side to side. The tongue should move freely.

Using a penlight for illumination, examine the tongue for color, size, position, texture, and coatings or lesions. A normal tongue is medium or dull red in color, moist, slightly rough on the top surface, and smooth along the lateral margins. The undersurface of the tongue and the floor of the mouth are highly vascular (Figure 33-23). Take extra care to inspect this area, a common site for oral cancer lesions. The client lifts the tongue by placing its tip on the palate behind the upper incisors. Inspect for color, swelling, and lesions such as nodules or cysts. The ventral surface of the tongue is pink and smooth, with large veins between the frenulum folds. To palpate the tongue, explain the procedure and ask the client to protrude the tongue. Grasp the tip with a gauze square and gently pulls it to one side. With a gloved hand, palpate the full length of the tongue and the base for any areas of hardening or ulceration. **Varicosities** (swollen, tortuous veins) are common in the older adult and rarely cause problems.

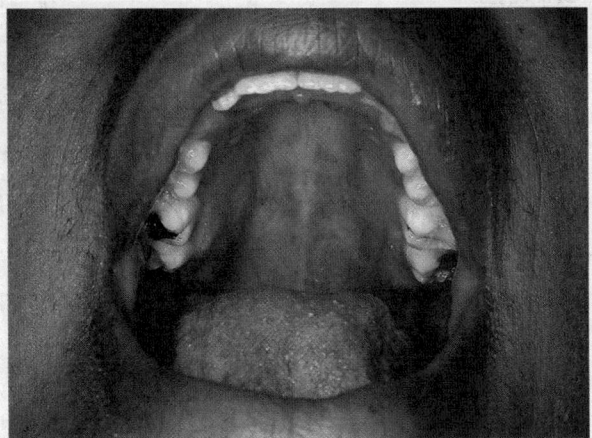

Figure 33-24 The hard palate is located anteriorly in the roof of the mouth.

Palate. Have the client extend the head backward, holding the mouth open to inspect the hard and soft palates. The hard palate, or roof of the mouth, is located anteriorly. The whitish hard palate is dome shaped. The soft palate extends posteriorly toward the pharynx. It is normally light pink and smooth. Observe the palates for color, shape, texture, and extra bony prominences or defects (Figure 33-24). A bony growth, or **exostosis**, between the two palates is common.

Pharynx. Perform an examination of pharyngeal structures to rule out infection, inflammation, or lesions. Have the client tip the head back slightly, open the mouth wide, and say "Ah" while you place the tip of a tongue depressor on the middle third of the tongue. Take care not to press the lower lip against the teeth. By placing the tongue depressor too far anteriorly, the posterior part of the tongue mounds up, obstructing the view. Placing the tongue depressor on the posterior tongue elicits the gag reflex.

With a penlight, first inspect the uvula and soft palate (Figure 33-25). Both structures, which are innervated by the tenth cranial (vagus) nerve, should rise centrally as the client says "Ah." Examine the anterior and posterior pillars, soft palate, and uvula. View

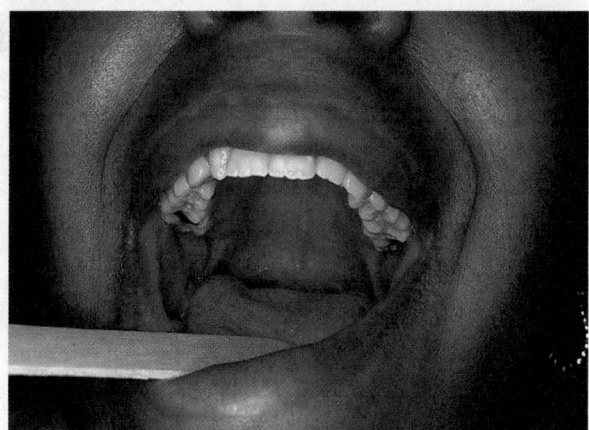

Figure 33-25 A penlight and tongue depressor allow the visualization of the uvula and posterior soft palate.

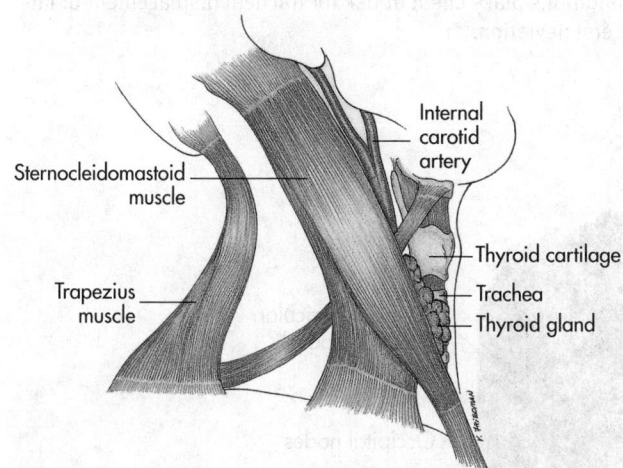

Figure 33-26 Anatomical position of the major neck structures. Note the triangles formed by the sternocleidomastoid muscle, lower jaw, and anterior neck anteriorly and by the sternocleidomastoid muscle, trapezius muscle, and lower neck posteriorly.

the tonsils in the cavities between the anterior and posterior pillars and note the presence or absence of tissue. The posterior pharynx is behind the pillars. Normally pharyngeal tissues are pink and smooth and well hydrated. Small irregular spots of lymphatic tissue and small blood vessels are normal. Note edema, petechiae (small hemorrhages), lesions, or exudate. Clients with chronic sinus problems frequently exhibit a clear exudate that drains along the wall of the posterior pharynx. Yellow or green exudate indicates infection. A client with a typical sore throat has a red and edematous uvula and tonsillar pillars with possible presence of yellow exudate.

Neck

Assessment of the neck includes assessing the neck muscles, lymph nodes of the head and neck, carotid arteries, jugular veins, thyroid gland, and trachea (Figure 33-26). Postpone the examination of the jugular veins and carotid arteries until the vascular

system assessment. Inspect and palpate the neck to determine the integrity of the neck structures and to examine the lymphatic system. Examine the lymphatic system region by region during the assessment of other body systems (head and neck, breast, genitalia, and extremities). An abnormality of superficial lymph nodes sometimes reveals the presence of an infection or malignancy. Examination of the thyroid gland and trachea also aids in ruling out malignancies. Perform this examination with the client sitting. The sternocleidomastoid and trapezius muscles outline the areas of the neck, dividing each side of the neck into two triangles. The anterior triangle contains the trachea, thyroid gland, carotid artery, and anterior cervical lymph nodes. The posterior triangle contains the posterior lymph nodes. Table 33-19 reviews the nursing history for the head and neck examination.

Neck Muscles. First inspect the neck in the usual anatomical position, with slight hyperextension. Observe for symmetry of the neck muscles. Ask the client to flex the neck with the chin to the chest, hyperextend the neck backward, and move the head laterally to each side and then sideways with the ear moving toward the shoulder. This tests the sternocleidomastoid and trapezius muscles. The neck normally moves without discomfort. Perform other tests for muscle strength and function during assessment of the musculoskeletal system.

Lymph Nodes. An extensive system of lymph nodes collects lymph from the head, ears, nose, cheeks, and lips (Figure 33-27). The immune system protects the body from foreign antigens, removes damaged cells from the circulation, and provides a partial barrier to growth of malignant cells within the body. Assessing the lymph nodes requires competence when caring for clients with suspected immunoincompetence, which is often linked to allergies, human immunodeficiency virus (HIV) infection, autoimmune disease (e.g., lupus erythematosus), or serious infection.

With the client's chin raised and head tilted slightly, first inspect the area where lymph nodes are distributed and compare both sides. This position stretches the skin slightly over any possible enlarged nodes. Inspect visible nodes for edema, erythema, or red streaks. Nodes are not normally visible.

Use a methodical approach to palpate the lymph nodes to avoid overlooking any single node or chain. The client relaxes with the neck flexed slightly forward. Inspect and palpate both sides of the neck for comparison. During palpation either face or stand to the side of the client for easy access to all nodes. Using the pads of the middle three fingers of each hand, gently palpate in a rotary motion over the nodes (Figure 33-28). Check each node methodically in the following sequence: occipital nodes at the base of the skull, postauricular nodes over the mastoid, preauricular nodes just in front of the ear, retropharyngeal nodes at the angle of the mandible, submandibular nodes, and submental nodes in the midline behind the mandibular tip. Try to detect enlargement and note the location, size, shape, surface characteristics, consistency, mobility, tenderness, and warmth of the nodes. If the skin is mobile, move the skin over the area of the nodes. It is important to press underlying tissue in each area and not simply move the fingers over the skin. However, if you apply excessive pressure, you will miss small nodes and destroy palpable nodes.

※ **TABLE 33-19** Nursing History for Neck Assessment

ASSESSMENT CATEGORY	RATIONALE
Assess for history of recent cold or infection or enlarged lymph nodes, exposure to radiation or toxic chemicals.	Colds or infections cause temporary or permanent lymph node enlargement. Lymph nodes are also enlarged in various diseases such as cancer.
If there is an enlarged lymph node, consider reviewing history of intravenous drug use, hemophilia, sexual contact with persons infected with human immunodeficiency virus (HIV), history of blood transfusion, multiple and indiscriminate sexual contacts, or male with homosexual or bisexual activities.	These are risk factors for HIV infection.
Ask if client has had history of neck pain with restriction in movement.	Indicates muscle strain, head injury, local nerve injury, or enlarged or swollen lymph node.
Ask if client has had change in temperature preference (more or less clothing); swelling in neck; change in texture of hair, skin, or nails; or change in emotional stability.	Symptoms indicative of thyroid disease.
Ask if client has history of hypothyroidism or hyperthyroidism or takes thyroid medication or has a family history of thyroid disease.	Disease or medications influence tissue growth of gland.
Review medical history of pneumothorax (collapsed lung) or bronchial tumor.	Conditions place client at risk for tracheal displacement or lateral deviation.

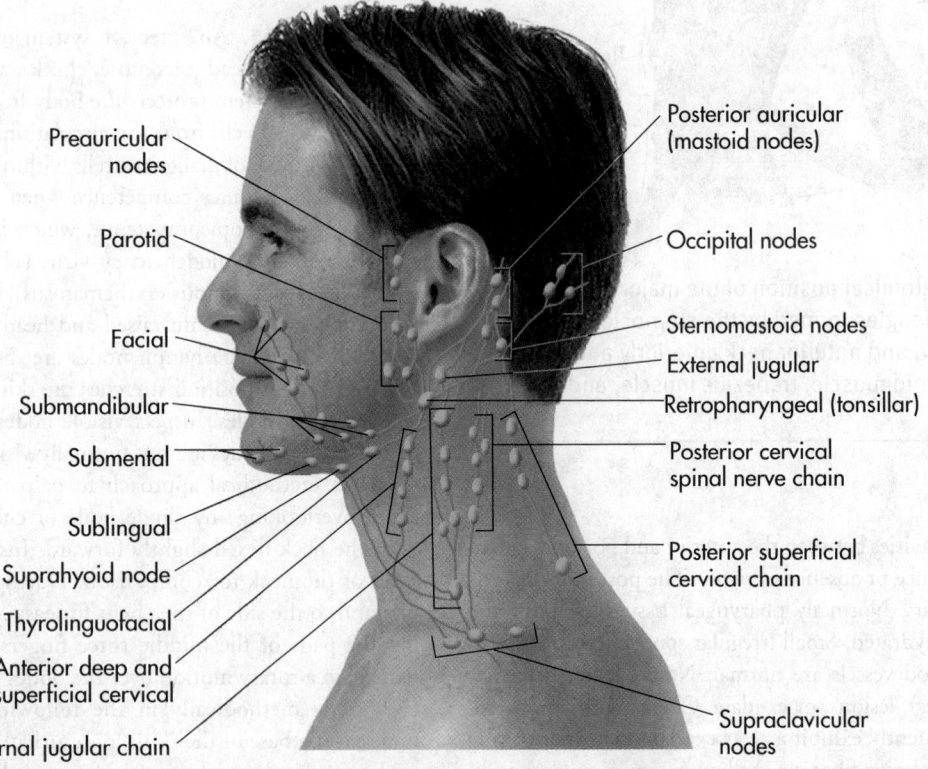

Figure 33-27 Palpable lymph nodes in the head and neck. (From Seidel HM and others: *Mosby's guide to physical examination,* ed 6, St. Louis, 2006, Mosby.)

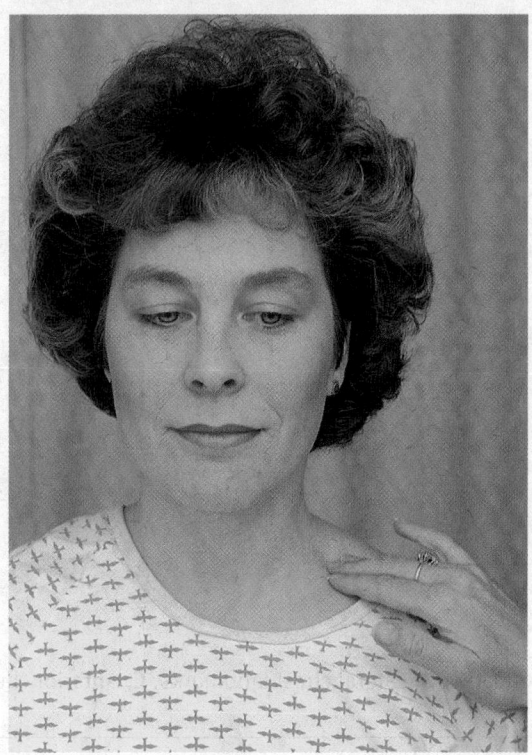

Figure 33-28 Supraclavicular lymph node palpation.

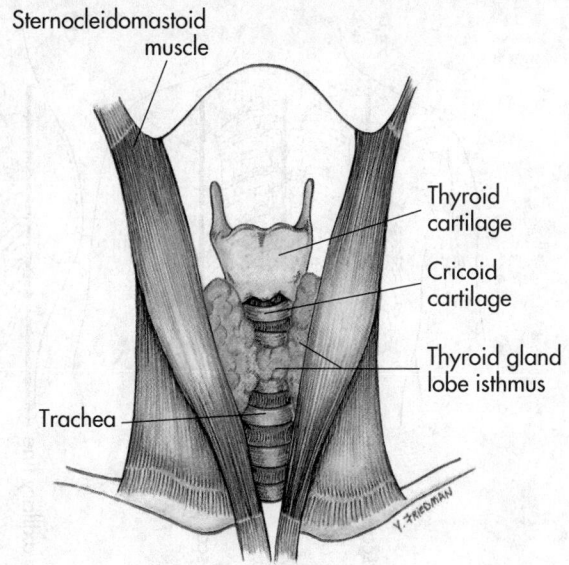

Figure 33-29 Anatomical position of the thyroid gland.

Sternocleidomastoid muscle

Thyroid cartilage

Cricoid cartilage

Thyroid gland lobe isthmus

Trachea

To palpate supraclavicular nodes, ask the client to bend the head forward and relax the shoulders. Palpate these nodes by hooking the index and third finger over the clavicle, lateral to the sternocleidomastoid muscle. Palpate the deep cervical nodes only with the fingers hooked around the sternocleidomastoid muscle.

Normally lymph nodes are not easily palpable. However, small, mobile, nontender nodes are common. Lymph nodes that are large, fixed, inflamed, or tender indicate a problem such as local infection, systemic disease, or neoplasm (Seidel and others, 2006) (Box 33-18). When you find enlarged nodes, explore the adjacent areas and regions drained by the nodes. Tenderness almost always indicates inflammation. A problem involving a lymph node of the head and neck means an abnormality in the mouth, throat, abdomen, breasts, thorax, or arms. These are the areas drained by the head and neck nodes.

Thyroid Gland. The thyroid gland lies in the anterior lower neck, in front of and to both sides of the trachea. The gland is fixed to the trachea with the isthmus overlying the trachea and connecting the two irregular, cone-shaped lobes (Figure 33-29). Inspect the lower neck overlying the thyroid gland for obvious masses, symmetry, and any subtle fullness at the base of the neck. Ask the client to hyperextend the neck, which helps tighten the skin for better visualization. Offer the client a glass of water, and, while observing the neck, have the client swallow. This maneuver helps to visualize an abnormally enlarged thyroid. Normally you cannot visualize the thyroid.

More experienced nurses examine the thyroid by palpating for more subtle masses; this technique will not be discussed here.

✴ **BOX 33-18**   **CLIENT TEACHING**

Neck Assessment
Objective
• Client takes proper preventive action if he or she notices a mass in the neck.

Teaching Strategies
• Stress importance of regular compliance with medication schedule to clients with thyroid disease.
• Instruct client about the lymph nodes and how infection commonly causes node tenderness.
• Instruct client to call a health care provider when he or she notices an enlarged lump or mass in the neck.
• Teach client risk factors for HIV infection and other sexually transmitted diseases.

Evaluation
• Have client explain when to notify a physician about a neck mass.

HIV, Human immunodeficiency virus.

Carotid Artery and Jugular Vein. This portion of the examination is described under examination of the vascular system (see later section).

Trachea. The trachea is a part of the upper respiratory system that you directly palpate. It is normally located in the midline above the suprasternal notch. Masses in the neck or mediastinum and pulmonary abnormalities cause displacement laterally. Have the client sit or lie down during palpation. Determine the position of the trachea by palpating at the suprasternal notch, slipping the thumb and index fingers to each side. Note if the finger and thumb shift laterally. Do not apply forceful pressure because this elicits coughing.

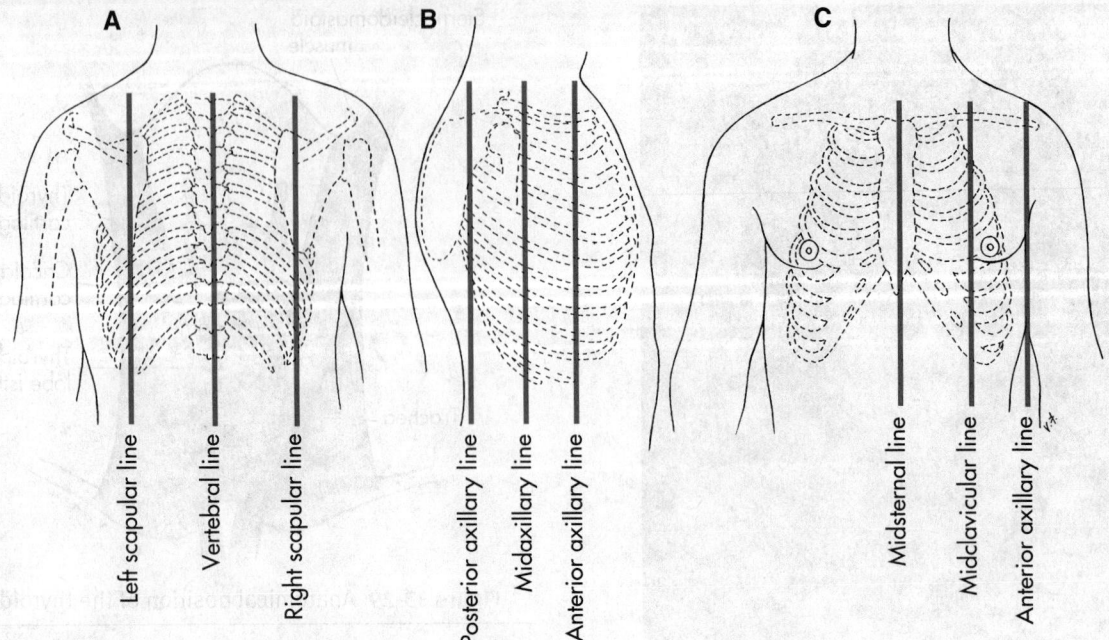

Figure 33-30 Anatomical chest wall landmarks. **A,** Posterior chest landmarks. **B,** Lateral chest landmarks. **C,** Anterior chest landmarks.

Thorax and Lungs

Accurate physical assessment of the thorax and lungs requires review of the ventilatory and respiratory functions of the lungs. If disease is affecting the lungs, this will affect other body systems as well. For example, reduced oxygenation causes changes in mental alertness because of the brain's sensitivity to lowered oxygen levels. You will use data from all body systems to determine the nature of pulmonary alterations.

Before assessing the thorax and lungs, be familiar with the landmarks of the chest (Figure 33-30). These landmarks help you identify findings and use assessment skills correctly. The client's nipples, angle of Louis, suprasternal notch, costal angle, clavicles, and vertebrae are key landmarks that provide a series of imaginary lines for sign identification. Keep a mental image of the location of the lobes of the lung and the position of each rib (Figure 33-31). The proper orientation to anatomical structures ensures a thorough assessment of the anterior, lateral, and posterior thorax.

Locating the position of each rib is critical to visualizing the lobe of the lung being assessed. To begin, locate the angle of Louis at the manubriosternal junction. The angle is a visible and palpable angulation of the sternum and is the point at which the second rib articulates with the sternum. Count the ribs and intercostal spaces (between the ribs) from this point. The number of each intercostal space corresponds with that of the rib just above it. The spinous process of the third thoracic vertebra and the fourth, fifth, and sixth ribs help to locate the lung's lobes laterally. The lower lobes project laterally and anteriorly (Figure 33-32). Posteriorly the tip or inferior margin of the scapula lies approxi-

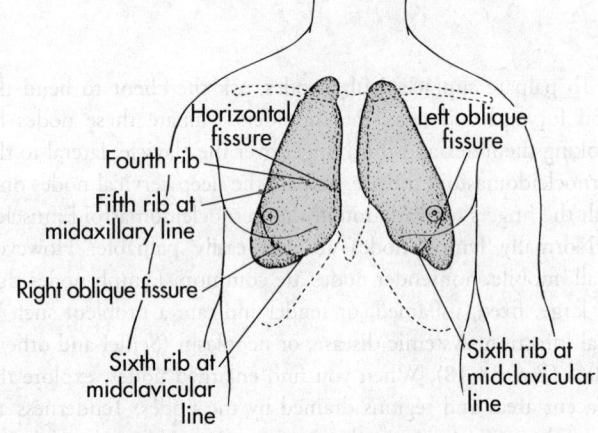

Figure 33-31 Anterior position of lung lobes in relation to anatomical landmarks.

mately at the level of the seventh rib (Figure 33-33). After identifying the seventh rib, count upward to locate the third thoracic vertebra, and align it with the inner borders of the scapula to locate the posterior lobes.

The examination requires the client to be undressed to the waist, with good lighting. Assess clients at risk for pulmonary problems, such as the client confined to bed rest or the client with chest pain who cannot fully expand the lungs. The examination begins with the client sitting for assessment of the posterior and lateral chest. Have the client sit or lie down for assessment of the anterior chest. Table 33-20 reviews the nursing history for lung examination.

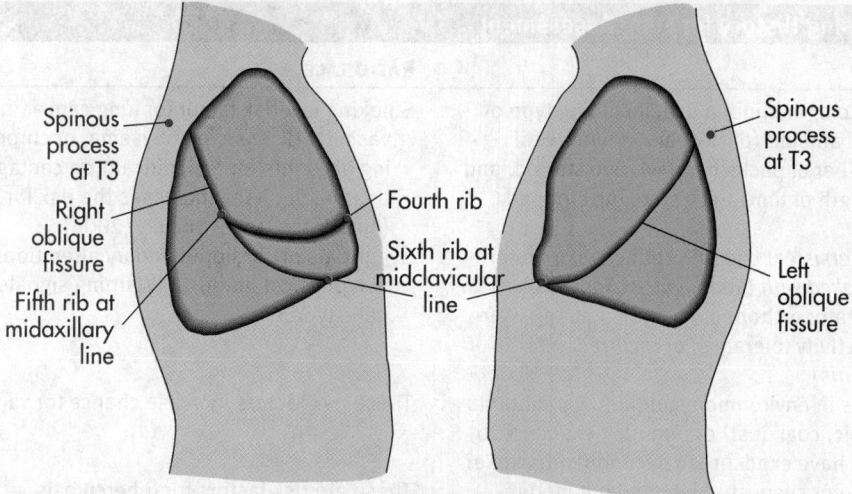

Figure 33-32 Lateral position of lung lobes in relation to anatomical landmarks.

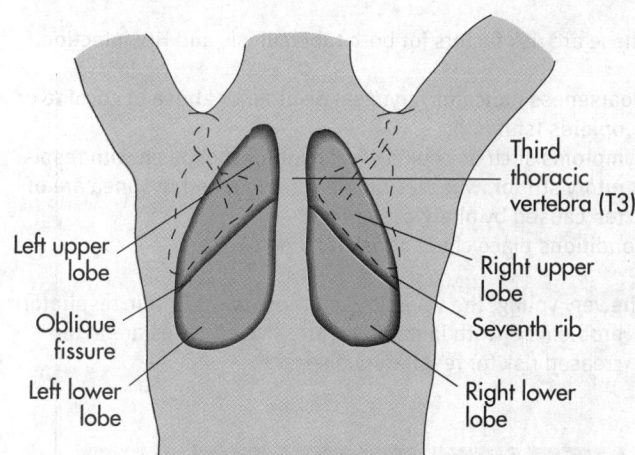

Figure 33-33 Posterior position of lung lobes in relation to anatomical landmarks.

Posterior Thorax

Begin examination of the posterior thorax by observing for any signs or symptoms in other body systems that indicate pulmonary problems. Reduced mental alertness, nasal flaring, somnolence, and cyanosis are examples of signs assessed that indicate oxygenation problems. Inspect the posterior thorax by observing the shape and symmetry of the chest from the client's back and front. Note the anteroposterior diameter. Body shape or posture significantly impairs ventilatory movement. Normally the chest contour is symmetrical, with the anteroposterior diameter one third to one half of the transverse, or side-to-side, diameter. A barrel-shaped chest (anteroposterior diameter equals transverse diameter) characterizes aging and chronic lung disease. Infants have an almost round shape. Congenital and postural alterations cause abnormal contours. Some clients lean over a table or splint the side of the chest because of a breathing problem. Splinting or holding the

chest wall because of pain causes a client to bend toward the side affected. Such a posture impairs ventilatory movement.

Standing at a midline position behind the client, look for deformities, position of the spine, slope of the ribs, retraction of the intercostal spaces during inspiration, and bulging of the intercostal spaces during expiration. The scapulae are normally symmetrical and closely attached to the thoracic wall. The normal spine is straight without lateral deviation. Posteriorly, the ribs tend to slope across and down. The ribs and intercostal spaces are easier to see in a thin person. Normally no bulging or active movement occurs within the intercostal spaces during breathing. Bulging indicates that the client is using great effort to breathe.

Also assess the rate and rhythm of breathing (see Chapter 32). Observe the thorax as a whole. The thorax normally expands and relaxes regularly with equality of movement bilaterally. In healthy adults the normal respiratory rates vary from 12 to 20 respirations per minute.

Palpation of the posterior thorax assesses further characteristics. Palpate the thoracic muscles and skeleton for lumps, masses, pulsations, and unusual movement. If you note pain or tenderness, avoid deep palpation. Fractured rib fragments could be displaced against vital organs. Normally the chest wall is not tender. If you find a suspicious mass or swollen area, lightly palpate it for size, shape, and the typical qualities of a lesion.

To measure chest excursion or depth of breathing, stand behind the client and place the thumbs along the spinal processes at the tenth rib, with the palms lightly contacting the posterolateral surfaces. Place thumbs 5 cm (2 inches) apart, pointing toward the spine and fingers pointing laterally (Figure 33-34, *A*). Press the hands toward the spine so that a small skin fold appears between the thumbs. Do not slide the hands over the skin. Instruct the client to take a deep breath after exhaling. Note movement of the thumbs (Figure 33-34, *B*). Chest excursion is symmetrical, separating the thumbs 3 to 5 cm (1¼ to 2 inches). Reduced chest excursions may be caused by pain, postural deformity, or fatigue. In older adults, chest movement normally declines because of costal cartilage calcification and respiratory muscle atrophy.

✳ **TABLE 33-20** Nursing History for Lung Assessment

ASSESSMENT CATEGORY	RATIONALE
Assess history of tobacco or marijuana use, including type of tobacco, duration and amount (pack-years = number of years smoking × number of packs per day), age started, and efforts to quit and length of time since smoking stopped.	Smoking is a risk factor for lung cancer, heart disease, cerebrovascular disease, emphysema, or chronic bronchitis. Smoking accounts for a significant percentage of all cancer deaths. Smoking increases the risk for 15 types of cancer (American Cancer Society, 2006).
Ask if client has had a *persistent cough* (productive or nonproductive), *sputum streaked with blood, voice change, chest pain,* shortness of breath, **orthopnea,** dyspnea during exertion or at rest, poor activity tolerance, or *recurrent attacks of pneumonia or bronchitis.*	Symptoms of cardiopulmonary alterations help localize objective physical findings. (Warning signals for lung cancer are in italic type.)
Determine if client works in environment containing pollutants (e.g., asbestos, arsenic, coal dust) or requiring exposure to radiation. Does client have exposure to secondhand smoke?	These risk factors increase chance for various lung diseases.
Review history for known or suspected human immunodeficiency virus (HIV) infection, substance abuse, low income, or being a resident or employee of nursing home or shelter, homeless, recent prison inmate, family member of tuberculosis (TB) client, or immigrant to the United States from a country where TB is prevalent (Frakes and Evans, 2004).	These are risk factors for tuberculosis.
Ask if client has history of persistent cough, hemoptysis, unexplained weight loss, fatigue, night sweats, or fever.	These are risk factors for both tuberculosis and HIV infection.
Does client have history of chronic hoarseness?	Hoarseness indicates laryngeal disorder or abuse of cocaine or opioids (sniffing).
Assess history of allergies to pollens, dust, or other airborne irritants and to foods, drugs, or chemical substances.	Symptoms such as choking feeling, bronchospasm with respiratory stridor, wheezes on auscultation, and dyspnea are often caused by allergic response.
Review family history for cancer, tuberculosis, allergies, or chronic obstructive pulmonary disease.	Conditions place client at risk for lung disease.
Ask if client has had a pneumonia or influenza vaccine and a TB test; if not, educate client on need to do so.	The very young, the very old, and those with chronic respiratory problems or with immunosuppressive diseases are at increased risk for respiratory disease.

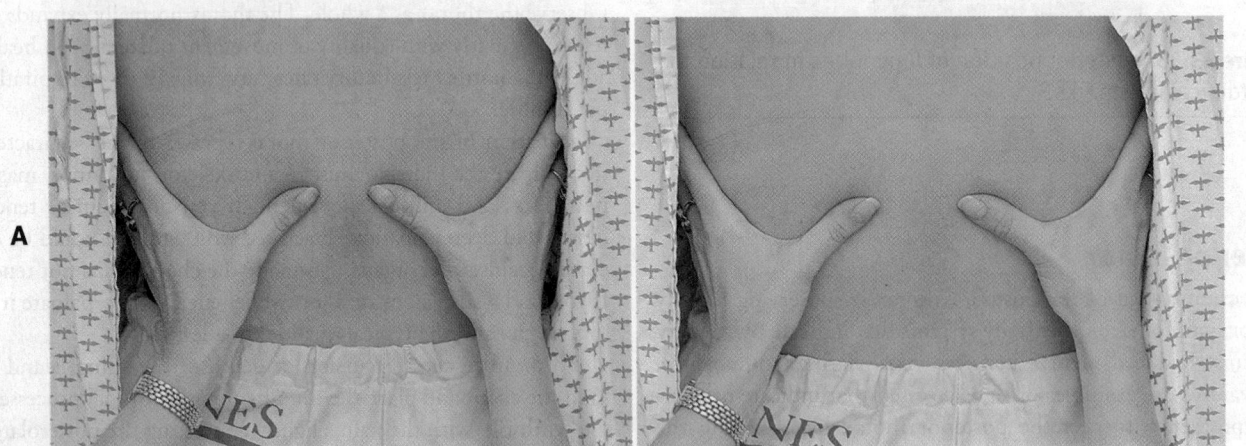

A   **B**

Figure 33-34 A, Hand position for palpation of posterior thorax excursion. **B,** As client inhales, movement of chest excursion separates the thumbs.

During speech the sound created by the vocal cords is transmitted through the lung to the chest wall. The sound waves create vibrations that you palpate externally. These vibrations are called **vocal** or **tactile fremitus.** The accumulation of mucus, the collapse of lung tissue, or the presence of lung lesions block the vibrations from reaching the chest wall.

To palpate for tactile fremitus, place the palmar surfaces of the fingers or the ulnar part of the hand over symmetrical intercostal spaces, beginning at the lung apex (Figure 33-35, *A*), using a firm, light touch. Ask the client to say "ninety-nine" or "one-one-one." Palpate both sides simultaneously and symmetrically (from top to bottom) for comparison, or use one hand, quickly alternating

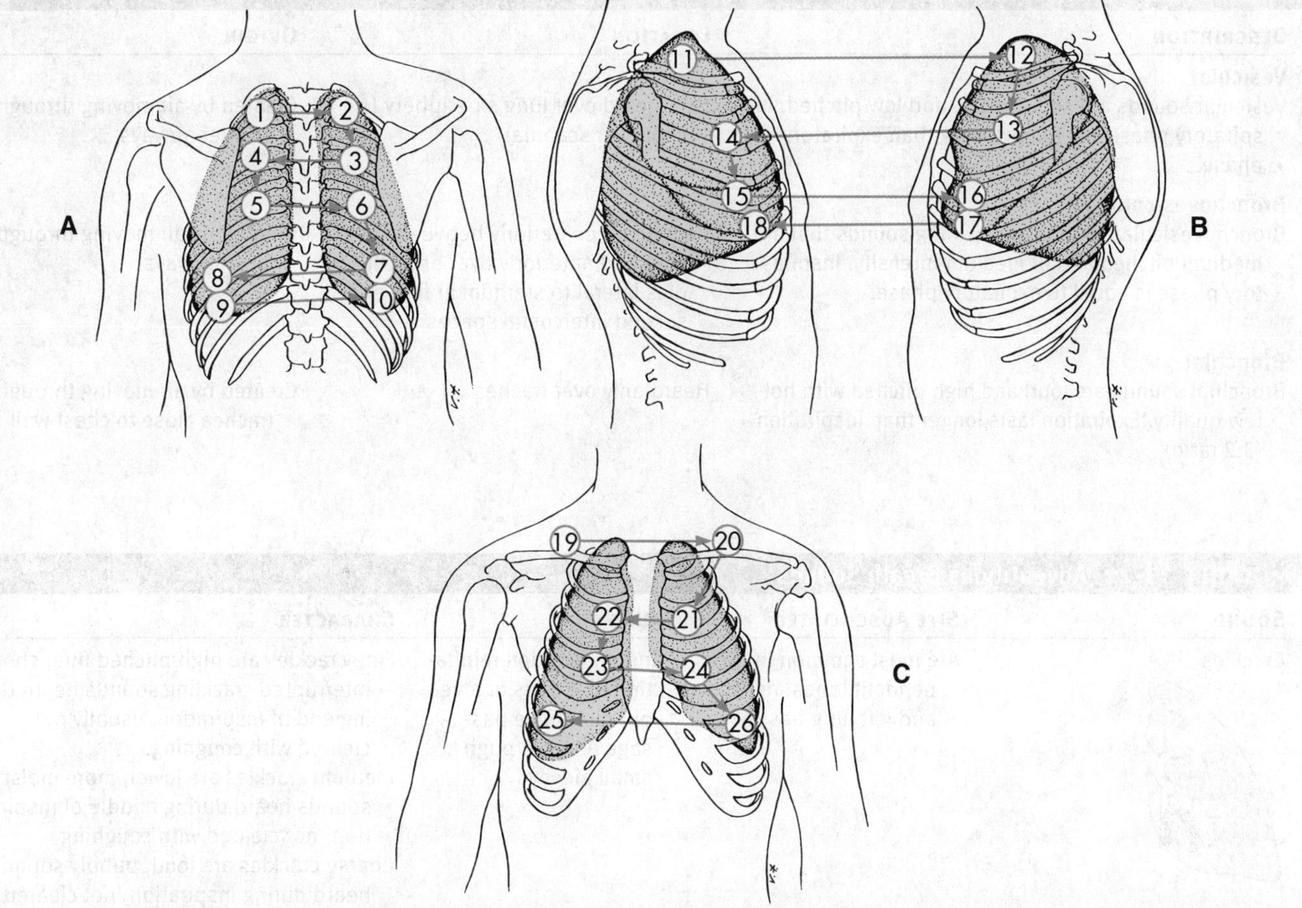

A

B

C

Figure 33-35 **A** to **C,** A systematic pattern (posterior-lateral-anterior) is followed when palpating and auscultating the thorax.

between the two sides (Seidel and others, 2006). Normally a faint vibration is present as the client speaks. If fremitus is faint, ask the client to speak in a louder or lower tone of voice. Normally fremitus is symmetrical. Vibrations are strongest at the top, near the level of the tracheal bifurcation. You assess strong vibrations through the chest wall in a crying infant.

Auscultation assesses the movement of air through the tracheobronchial tree and detects mucus or obstructed airways. Normally air flows through the airways in an unobstructed pattern. Recognizing the sounds created by normal airflow allows the nurse to detect sounds caused by airway obstruction.

Place the diaphragm of the stethoscope firmly on the skin, over the posterior chest wall between the ribs (Figure 33-36). The client folds the arms in front of the chest and keeps the head bent forward while taking slow, deep breaths with the mouth slightly open. Listen to an entire inspiration and expiration at each position of the stethoscope. If sounds are faint, as in the obese client, ask the client to breathe harder and faster temporarily. Breath sounds are much louder in children because of their thin chest walls. In children the bell works best because of a child's small chest. Use a systematic pattern comparing lung sounds in one region on one side of the body with sounds in the same region on the opposite side. It is impossible to remember the quality of all sounds noted on one side of the body

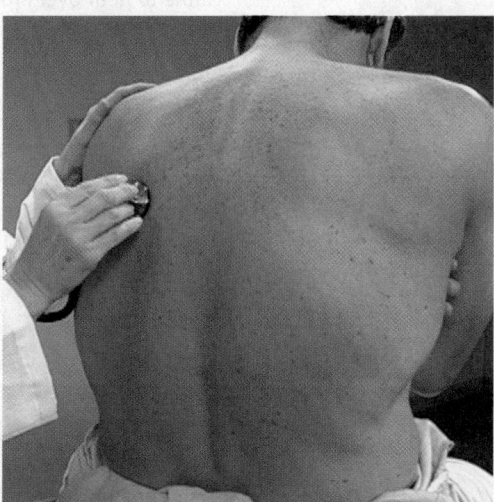

Figure 33-36 Use the diaphragm of the stethoscope to auscultate breath sounds. (From Seidel HM and others: *Mosby's guide to physical examination,* ed 6, St. Louis, 2006, Mosby.)

✳ TABLE 33-21 Normal Breath Sounds

DESCRIPTION	LOCATION	ORIGIN
Vesicular Vesicular sounds are soft, breezy, and low pitched. Inspiratory phase is 3 times longer than expiratory phase.	Best heard over lung's periphery (except over scapula)	Created by air moving through smaller airways
Bronchovesicular Bronchovesicular sounds are blowing sounds that are medium pitched and of medium intensity. Inspiratory phase is equal to expiratory phase.	Best heard posteriorly between scapulae and anteriorly over bronchioles lateral to sternum at first and second intercostal spaces	Created by air moving through large airways
Bronchial Bronchial sounds are loud and high pitched with hollow quality. Expiration lasts longer than inspiration (3:2 ratio).	Heard only over trachea	Created by air moving through trachea close to chest wall

✳ TABLE 33-22 Adventitious Breath Sounds

SOUND	SITE AUSCULTATED	CAUSE	CHARACTER
Crackles	Are most common in dependent lobes: right and left lung bases	Random, sudden reinflation of groups of alveoli; disruptive passage of air through small airways	Fine crackles are high-pitched fine, short, interrupted crackling sounds heard during end of inspiration, usually not cleared with coughing. Medium crackles are lower, more moist sounds heard during middle of inspiration; not cleared with coughing. Coarse crackles are loud, bubbly sounds heard during inspiration; not cleared with coughing.
Rhonchi (sonorous wheeze)	Are primarily heard over trachea and bronchi; if loud enough, you are able to hear over most lung fields	Muscular spasm, fluid, or mucus in larger airways, new growth or external pressure causing turbulence	Loud, low-pitched, rumbling coarse sounds heard either during inspiration or expiration; sometimes cleared by coughing.
Wheezes (sibilant wheeze)	Heard over all lung fields	High-velocity airflow through severely narrowed or obstructed airway	High-pitched, continuous musical sounds like a squeak heard continuously during inspiration or expiration; usually louder on expiration.
Pleural friction rub	Heard over anterior lateral lung field (if client is sitting upright)	Inflamed pleura, parietal pleura rubbing against visceral pleura	Has dry, rubbing, or grating quality heard during inspiration or expiration; does not clear with coughing; heard loudest over lower lateral anterior surface.

Data from Seidel HM and others: *Mosby's guide to physical examination*, ed 6, St. Louis, 2006, Mosby.

and then compare them with sounds on the other side (see Figure 33-35, *A*).

Auscultate for normal breath sounds and abnormal or **adventitious sounds.** Normal breath sounds differ in character, depending on the area you are auscultating. You normally hear bronchovesicular and vesicular sounds over the posterior thorax (Table 33-21).

Abnormal sounds result from air passing through moisture, mucus, or narrowed airways. They also result from alveoli suddenly reinflating or from an inflammation between the pleural linings of the lung. Adventitious sounds often occur superimposed over normal sounds. The four types of adventitious sounds are crackles, rhonchi, wheezes, and pleural friction rub. A specific entity causes each sound, and each has typical auditory features (Table 33-22). During auscultation note the location and characteristics of the sounds, and listen for the absence of breath sounds (found in clients with collapsed or surgically removed lobes).

If there are abnormalities in tactile fremitus or auscultation, perform the vocal resonance tests (spoken and whispered voice sounds). Place the stethoscope over the same locations used to assess breath sounds, have the client say "ninety-nine" in a normal voice tone. Normally the sound is muffled. If fluid is compressing the lung, the vibrations from the client's voice are transmitted to the chest wall and the sound becomes clear (**bronchophony**). Then ask the client to whisper "ninety-nine." The whispered voice is usually faint and indistinct. Certain lung abnormalities cause the whispered voice to become clear and distinct (**whispered pectoriloquy**).

Lateral Thorax

Extend the assessment of the posterior thorax to the lateral sides of the chest. The client sits during examination of the lateral chest. Have the client raise the arms, to improve access to lateral thoracic structures. Use inspection, palpation, and auscultation skills to examine the lateral thorax (see Figure 33-35, *B*). Do not assess excursion laterally. Normally, the breath sounds you hear are vesicular.

Anterior Thorax

Inspect the anterior thorax for the same features as the posterior thorax. The client sits or lies down with the head elevated (Box 33-19). Observe the accessory muscles of breathing: sternocleidomastoid, trapezius, and abdominal muscles. The accessory muscles move little with normal passive breathing. When a client requires effort to breathe as a result of strenuous exercise or disease (e.g., chronic obstructive pulmonary disease), the accessory muscles and abdominal muscles contract. Some clients produce a grunting sound.

Observe the width of the costal angle. It is usually larger than 90 degrees between the two costal margins. Observe the breathing pattern. Normal breathing is quiet and barely audible near the open mouth. You most often assess respiratory rate and rhythm anteriorly (see Chapter 32). The male client's respirations are usually diaphragmatic, whereas a female's are more costal. Accurate assessment occurs as a client breathes passively.

Palpate the anterior thoracic muscles and skeleton for lumps, masses, tenderness, or unusual movement. The sternum and xiphoid are relatively inflexible. Place the thumbs parallel approxi-

BOX 33-19 CLIENT TEACHING

Lung Assessment

Objectives
- Client describes warning signs of lung disease.
- Older adult receives influenza and pneumonia vaccines as appropriate.
- Client with chronic obstructive pulmonary disease (COPD) clears airways more effectively and reports less shortness of breath.

Teaching Strategies
- Explain risk factors for chronic lung disease and lung cancer, including cigarette smoking, history of smoking for over 20 years, exposure to environmental pollution, and radiation exposure from occupational, medical, and environmental sources. Exposure to radon and asbestos also increases risk especially for cigarette smokers. Other risk factors include certain metals (arsenic, cadmium, chromium), some organic chemicals, and tuberculosis. Exposure to secondhand cigarette smoke increases risk for nonsmokers (American Cancer Society, 2006).
- Share brochures on lung cancer from American Cancer Society with client and family.
- Discuss warning signs of lung cancer, such as a persistent cough, sputum streaked with blood, chest pains, and recurrent attacks of pneumonia or bronchitis.
- Counsel older adult on benefits from receiving influenza and pneumonia vaccinations because of a greater susceptibility to respiratory infection.
- Instruct client with COPD in coughing and pursed-lip breathing exercises.
- Refer persons at risk for tuberculosis who visit clinics or health care centers for skin testing.

Evaluation
- Have client describe risk factors for lung disease and cancer.
- Ask client to identify any known risks for cancer.
- Ask client to name warning signs for cancer.
- In a follow-up visit, review client's immunization record.
- Observe client performing breathing exercises and coughing.

mately along the costal margin 6 cm (2½ inches) apart with the palms touching the anterolateral chest. Push the thumbs toward the midline to create a skin fold. As the client inhales deeply, the thumbs normally separate approximately 3 to 5 cm (1¼ to 2 inches), with each side expanding equally.

Assess tactile fremitus over the anterior chest wall. Anterior findings differ from posterior findings because of the heart and female breast tissue. You feel fremitus next to the sternum at the second intercostal space, at the level of the bronchial bifurcation. It decreases over the heart, lower thorax, and breast tissue.

Auscultation of the anterior thorax follows a systematic pattern (see Figure 33-35, *C*). Have the client sit, if possible, to maximize chest expansion. Give special attention to the lower lobes, where mucus secretions commonly gather. Listen for bronchovesicular and vesicular sounds above and below the clavicles and along the lung periphery. Auscultate also for bronchial sounds, which are loud, high pitched, and hollow sounding, with expiration lasting longer than inspiration (3:2 ratio). You normally hear this sound over the trachea.

TABLE 33-23 Nursing History for Heart Assessment

ASSESSMENT CATEGORY	RATIONALE
Determine history of smoking, alcohol intake, caffeine intake, use of prescriptive and recreational drugs, exercise habits, and dietary patterns and intake (including fat and sodium intake).	Smoking, alcohol ingestion, cocaine use, lack of regular exercise, and intake of foods high in carbohydrates, fats, and cholesterol are risk factors for cardiovascular disease. Caffeine can cause heart dysrhythmias.
Determine if client is taking medications for cardiovascular function (e.g., antidysrhythmias, antihypertensives) and if client knows their purpose, dosage, and side effects.	Knowledge allows nurse to assess compliance with drug therapies. Medications sometimes affect vital sign values.
Assess for chest pain or discomfort, palpitations, excess fatigue, cough, dyspnea, leg pain or cramps, edema of feet, cyanosis, fainting, and orthopnea. Ask if symptoms occur at rest or during exercise.	These are key symptoms of heart disease. Cardiovascular function is sometimes adequate during rest but not during exercise.
If client reports chest pain, determine if it is cardiac in nature. Anginal pain is usually a deep pressure or ache that is substernal and diffuse, radiating to one or both arms, neck, or jaw.	Determines nature of pain and need to initiate care immediately.
Determine whether client has a stressful lifestyle. What physical demands or emotional stress exists?	Repeated exposure to stress increases risk for heart disease.
Assess family history for heart disease, diabetes, high cholesterol levels, hypertension, stroke, or rheumatic heart disease.	Factors increase risk for heart disease.
Ask client about history of heart trouble (e.g., congestive heart failure, congenital heart disease, coronary artery disease, dysrhythmias, murmurs).	Knowledge reveals client's level of understanding of condition. Preexisting condition influences examination techniques used, as well as findings to expect.
Determine whether client has preexisting diabetes, lung disease, obesity, or hypertension.	These disorders alter heart function.

Use a systematic pattern when comparing the right and left sides (see Figure 33-36). Initially you may want to auscultate all of the left side and then return to the right side. This is incorrect. You need to compare lung sounds in one region on one side of the body with sounds in the same region on the opposite of the body.

Heart

Compare the assessment of heart function with findings from the vascular assessment (see later section). Alterations in either system sometimes manifest as changes in the other. Some clients with signs or symptoms of heart (cardiac) problems have a life-threatening condition requiring immediate attention. In this case, act quickly and conduct only the portions of the examination that are absolutely necessary. When a client is more stable, conduct a more thorough assessment. The nursing history (Table 33-23) provides data to help interpret physical findings.

Assess cardiac function through the anterior thorax. Form a mental image of the heart's exact location (Figure 33-37). In the adult, the heart is located in the center of the chest (precordium), behind and to the left of the sternum, with a small section of the right atrium extending to the right of the sternum. The base of the heart is the upper portion, and the apex is the bottom tip. The surface of the right ventricle composes most of the heart's anterior surface. A section of the left ventricle shapes the left anterior side of the apex. The apex actually touches the anterior chest wall at approximately the fourth to fifth intercostal space just medial to the left midclavicular line. This is the **apical impulse** or **point of maximal impulse (PMI)**.

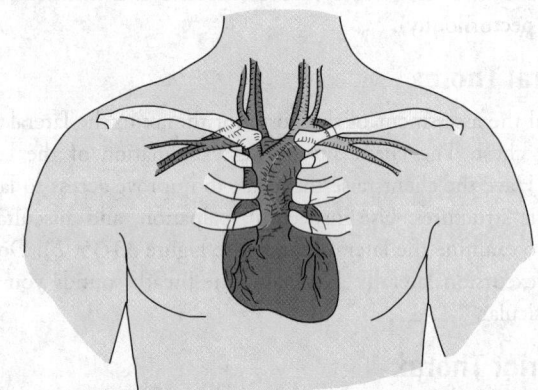

Figure 33-37 Anatomical position of the heart.

An infant's heart is positioned more horizontally. The apex of the heart is at the third or fourth intercostal space, just to the left of the midclavicular line. By the age of 7, a child's PMI is in the same location as the adult's. In tall, slender persons the heart hangs more vertically and is positioned more centrally. With increased stockiness and shortness, the heart tends to lie more to the left and horizontally (Seidel and others, 2006).

To assess heart function, a clear understanding of the cardiac cycle and associated physiological events is of utmost importance (Figure 33-38). The heart normally pumps blood through its four chambers in a methodical, even sequence. Events on the left side occur just before those on the right. As blood flows through each chamber, the valves open and close, the pressures within chambers rise and fall, and the chambers contract. Each event creates a

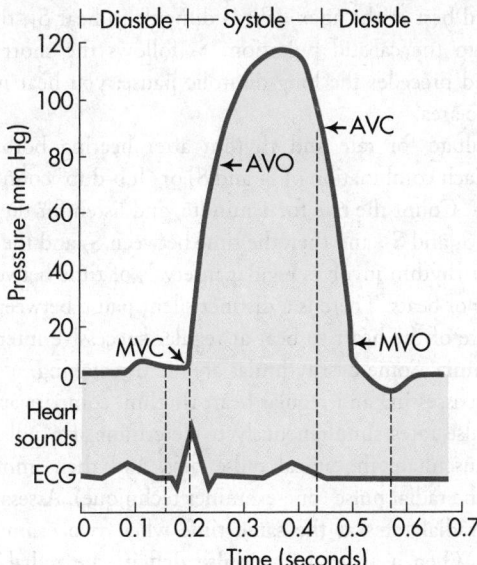

Figure 33-38 Cardiac cycle. *MVC,* Mitral valve closes; *AVO,* aortic valve opens; *AVC,* aortic valve closes; *MVO,* mitral valve opens.

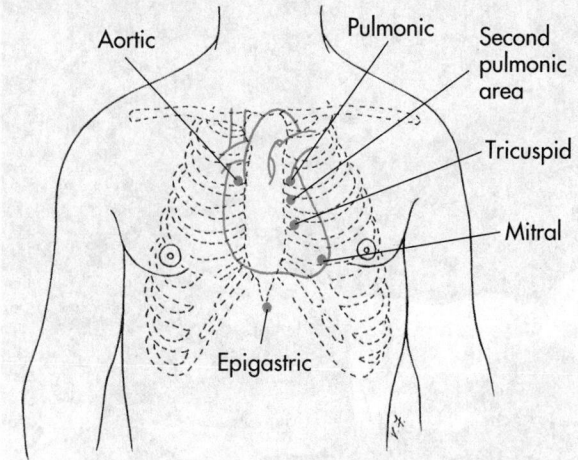

Figure 33-39 Anatomical sites for assessment of cardiac function.

physiological sign. Both sides of the heart function in a coordinated fashion.

There are two phases to the cardiac cycle: systole and diastole. During systole the ventricles contract and eject blood from the left ventricle into the aorta and from the right ventricle into the pulmonary artery. During diastole the ventricles relax and the atria contract to move blood into the ventricles and fill the coronary arteries.

Heart sounds occur in relation to physiological events in the cardiac cycle. As systole begins, ventricular pressure rises and closes the mitral and tricuspid valves. Valve closure causes the first heart sound (S_1), often described as "lub." The ventricles then contract, and blood flows through the aorta and pulmonary circulation. After the ventricles empty, ventricular pressure falls below that in the aorta and pulmonary artery. This allows the aortic and pulmonic valves to close, causing the second heart sound (S_2), described as "dub." As ventricular pressure continues to fall, it drops below that of the atria. The mitral and tricuspid valves reopen to allow ventricular filling. Rapid ventricular filling creates a third heart sound (S_3), heard more often in children and young adults. An S_3 is also an abnormality in adults over 30 years of age. A fourth heart sound (S_4) occurs when the atria contract to enhance ventricular filling. You will hear an S_4 in healthy older adults, children, and athletes, but it is not normal in adults. Because S_4 also indicates an abnormal condition, report it to a health care provider.

Inspection and Palpation

Before the examination, ensure that the client is relaxed and comfortable. Explain the procedure to relieve the client's anxiety. An anxious or uncomfortable client will have mild tachycardia, which will lead to inaccurate findings.

Use the skills of inspection and palpation simultaneously. The examination begins with the client in the supine position or with the upper body elevated 45 degrees because clients with heart disease frequently suffer shortness of breath while lying flat. Stand at the client's right side. Do not let the client talk, especially when auscultating heart sounds. Good lighting in the room is essential.

Direct your attention to the anatomical sites best suited for assessment of cardiac function. During inspection and palpation look for visible pulsations and exaggerated lifts, and palpate for the apical impulse and any source of vibrations (thrills). Follow an orderly sequence beginning with assessment of the base of the heart and moving toward the apex. First inspect the angle of Louis, which lies between the sternal body and manubrium, and feel the ridge in the sternum approximately 5 cm (2 inches) below the sternal notch. Slip the fingers along the angle on each side of the sternum to feel adjacent ribs. The intercostal spaces are just below each rib. The second intercostal space allows identification of each of the six anatomical landmarks (Figure 33-39). The second intercostal space on the right is the aortic area, and the left second intercostal space is the pulmonic area. You will need deeper palpation to feel the spaces in obese or heavily muscled clients. After locating the pulmonic area, move the fingers down the client's left sternal border to the third intercostal space, called the second pulmonic area. The tricuspid area is located at the fourth or fifth intercostal space along the sternum. To find the apical or mitral area, locate the fifth intercostal space just to the left of the sternum and move the fingers laterally, to the left midclavicular line. Locate the apical area with the palm of the hand or the fingertips. Normally you feel the apical impulse as a light tap in an area 1 to 2 cm (½ to ¾ inch) in diameter at the apex (Figure 33-40). Another landmark is the epigastric area at the tip of the sternum. You typically use it to palpate for aortic abnormalities.

Locate the six anatomical landmarks of the heart, and inspect and palpate each area. Look for the appearance of pulsations, viewing each area over the chest at an angle to the side. Normally you will not see any pulsations, except perhaps at the PMI in thin clients or at the epigastric area as a result of abdominal aorta pulsation. Use the proximal halves of the four fingers together, and then alternate this with the ball of the hand to palpate for pulsa-

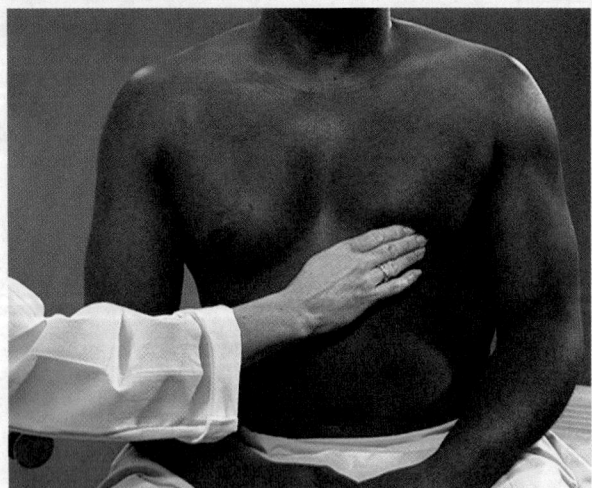

Figure 33-40 Palpation of apical pulse. (From Seidel HM and others: *Mosby's guide to physical examination,* ed 6, St. Louis, 2006, Mosby.)

tions. Touch the areas gently to allow movements to lift the hand. Normally you will not feel any pulsations or vibrations in the second, third, or fourth intercostal spaces. Loud murmurs cause a vibration. Time palpated pulsations or vibrations and their occurrence in relation to systole or diastole by auscultating heart sounds simultaneously.

You should feel the apical impulse or PMI easily. If you do not find it, have the client roll onto the left side, moving the heart closer to the chest wall. Estimate the size of the heart by noting the diameter of the PMI and its position relative to the midclavicular line. In cases of serious heart disease, the cardiac muscle enlarges, with the PMI found to the left of the midclavicular line. The PMI is sometimes difficult to find in the older adult because the chest deepens in its anteroposterior diameters. It is also difficult to find in muscular or overweight clients. You usually find an infant's PMI near the third or fourth intercostal space. It is easy to palpate because of the child's thin chest wall.

Auscultation

Auscultation of the heart detects normal heart sounds, extra heart sounds, and murmurs. Concentrate on detecting low-intensity sounds created by valve closures. To begin auscultation, eliminate all sources of room noise and explain the procedure to reduce the client's anxiety. Follow a systematic pattern beginning at the aortic area and inching the stethoscope across each of the anatomical sites (see Figure 33-41*A*). Listen for the complete cycle ("lub-dub") of heart sounds clearly at each location. Then repeat the sequence using the bell of the stethoscope. Sometimes the client will assume three different positions during the examination (Figure 33-41): sitting up and leaning forward (good for all areas and to hear high-pitched murmurs), supine (good for all areas), and left lateral recumbent (good for all areas; best position to hear low-pitched sounds in diastole).

Learn to identify the first (S_1) and second (S_2) heart sounds. At normal rates, S_1 occurs after the long diastolic pause and preceding the short systolic pause. S_1 is high pitched, dull in quality,

and heard best at the apex. If it is difficult to hear S_1, time it in relation to the carotid pulsation. S_2 follows the short systolic pause and precedes the long diastolic pause; you hear it best at the aortic area.

Auscultate for rate and rhythm after hearing both sounds clearly. Each combination of S_1 and S_2 or "lub-dub" counts as one heartbeat. Count the rate for 1 minute, and listen for the interval between S_1 and S_2, and then the time between S_2 and the next S_1. A regular rhythm involves regular intervals of time between each sequence of beats. There is a distinct silent pause between S_1 and S_2. Failure of the heart to beat at regular successive intervals is a **dysrhythmia.** Some dysrhythmias are life threatening.

When assessing an irregular heart rhythm, compare apical and radial pulse rates simultaneously to determine if a pulse deficit exists. Auscultate the apical pulse first, and then immediately palpate the radial pulse (one-examiner technique). Assess the apical and radial rates at the same time when two examiners are present. When a client has a **pulse deficit,** the radial pulse is slower than the apical pulse because ineffective contractions fail to send pulse waves to the periphery. Report a difference in pulse rates to the health care provider immediately.

Assess for extra heart sounds at each auscultatory site. Use the bell of the stethoscope, and listen for low-pitched extra heart sounds such as S_3 and S_4 gallops, clicks, and rubs. Auscultate over all anatomical areas. S_3, or a **ventricular gallop,** occurs just after S_2 at the end of ventricular diastole. This is due to a premature rush of blood into a ventricle that is stiff or dilated as a result of heart failure and hypertension. The combination of S_1, S_2, and S_3 sounds like "Ken-tuck´-y."

S_4, or an **atrial gallop,** occurs just before S_1 or ventricular systole. The sound of an S_4 is similar to that of "Ten´-es- see." Physiologically it is due to an atrial contraction pushing against a ventricle that is not accepting blood because of heart failure or other alterations. You hear extra heart sounds more easily with the client lying on the left side and the stethoscope at the apical site.

The final portion of the examination includes assessment for heart murmurs. **Murmurs** are sustained swishing or blowing sounds heard at the beginning, middle, or end of the systolic or diastolic phase. They are due to increased blood flow through a normal valve, forward flow through a stenotic valve or into a dilated vessel or heart chamber, or backward flow through a valve that fails to close. A murmur is asymptomatic or a sign of heart disease (Box 33-20). Murmurs are common in children. Keep the following factors in mind when auscultating to detect murmurs:

- When you detect a murmur, auscultate the mitral, tricuspid, aortic, and pulmonic valve areas for placement in the cardiac cycle (timing), the place it is heard best (location), radiation, loudness, pitch, and quality.
- If a murmur occurs between S_1 and S_2, it is a systolic murmur. If it occurs between S_2 and the next S_1, it is a diastolic murmur.
- The location of a murmur is not necessarily directly over the valves. With experience, you will learn where each type of murmur is best heard. For example, you hear mitral murmurs best at the apex of the heart.
- To assess for radiation, listen over areas besides where it is heard best. You also hear murmurs over the neck or back.

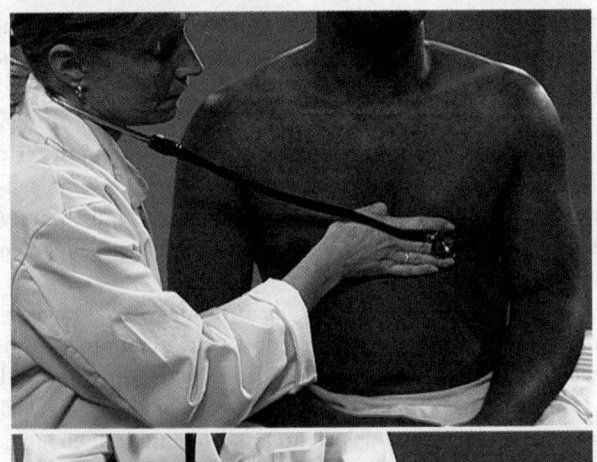
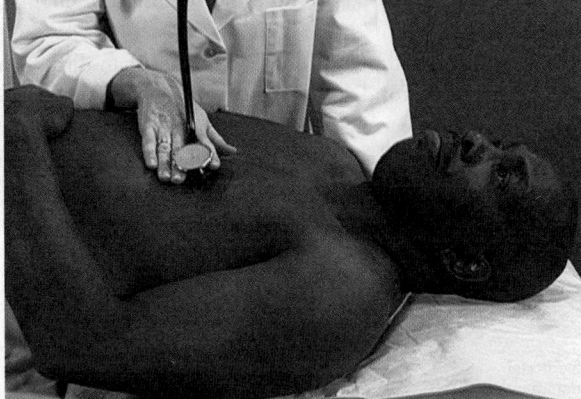
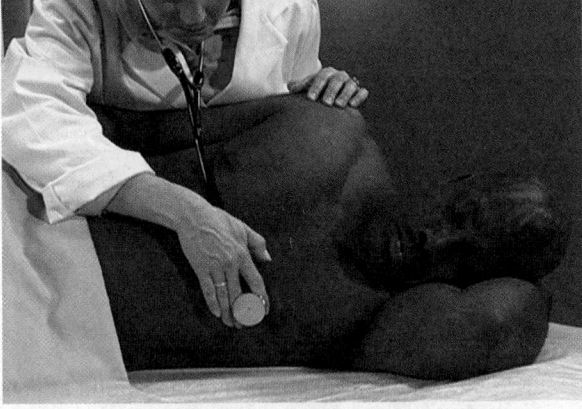

Figure 33-41 Sequence of client positions for heart auscultation. **A,** Sitting, **B,** Supine, **C,** Left lateral recumbent. (From Seidel HM and others: *Mosby's guide to physical examination,* ed 6, St. Louis, 2006, Mosby.)

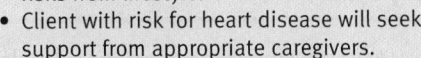
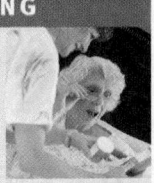

BOX 33-20   CLIENT TEACHING

Heart Assessment

Objectives
- Client describes risk factors for heart disease and takes appropriate steps to eliminate risks from lifestyle.
- Client with risk for heart disease will seek support from appropriate caregivers.

Teaching Strategies
- Explain risk factors for heart disease, including high dietary intake of saturated fat or cholesterol, lack of regular aerobic exercise, smoking, excess weight, stressful lifestyle, hypertension, and family history of heart disease.
- Refer client (if appropriate) to resources available for controlling or reducing risks (e.g., nutritional counseling, exercise class, stress reduction programs).
- Explain that research shows clinical benefit from reducing dietary intake of cholesterol and saturated fats. Tell client that about 70% to 75% of saturated fatty acids come from meats, poultry, fish, and dairy products. The American Heart Association recommends a diet that includes an intake of total fat less than 35% of calories, saturated fatty acids less than 10% of calories, and cholesterol less than 300 mg/100 mL (Moore, 2005).
- Encourage client to have regular measurement of total blood cholesterol levels and triglycerides. Desirable levels are less than 200 mg/100 mL. You need more than one cholesterol measurement to assess the blood cholesterol level accurately. Low-density lipoprotein (LDL) cholesterol is the major component of atherosclerotic plaques. Separate measurement of LDL cholesterol is wise in a client with high total blood cholesterol levels. In an individual with no other risk factors, an LDL cholesterol level of 160 mg/100 mL or higher is high risk (Moore, 2005).
- Encourage client to discuss with health care provider the need for periodic C-reactive protein (CRP) testing. CRP levels assess a client's cardiovascular disease risk.
- Advise client to avoid cigarette smoke because nicotine causes vasoconstriction.
- Advise client to quit smoking because this lowers the risk for coronary heart disease and coronary vascular disease (American Cancer Society, 2006).
- Clients who are at risk benefit from taking a daily low dose of aspirin. Consult health care provider before starting therapy.

Evaluation
- Ask client to identify risk factors for heart disease.
- Have client develop a meal plan low in saturated fat and cholesterol.
- Check client's cholesterol level during follow-up appointments at the clinic or physician's office.

- Intensity or loudness is related to the rate of blood flow through the heart or the amount of blood regurgitated. In serious murmurs feel for a thrust or intermittent palpable sensation at the auscultation site. A **thrill** is a continuous palpable sensation like the purring of a cat. You record intensity in the following grades (Seidel and others, 2006):

Grade 1	Barely audible in a quiet room
Grade 2	Clearly audible but quiet
Grade 3	Moderately loud
Grade 4	Loud, with associated thrill
Grade 5	Very loud, thrill easily palpable
Grade 6	Louder, may be heard without stethoscope, thrill palpable and visible

- A murmur is low, medium, or high in pitch, depending on the velocity of blood flow through the valves. You hear a low-pitched murmur best with the bell of the stethoscope. If you hear it best with the diaphragm, the murmur is high pitched.

The quality of a murmur refers to its characteristic pattern and sound. A crescendo murmur starts softly and builds in loudness. A decrescendo murmur starts loudly and then becomes less intense.

Vascular System

Examination of the vascular system includes measuring the blood pressure (see Chapter 32) and assessing the integrity of the peripheral vascular system. Table 33-24 reviews the nursing history data collected before the examination. Use the skills of inspection, palpation, and auscultation. Perform portions of the vascular examination during other body systems assessments. For example, check the carotid pulse after palpating the cervical lymph nodes. Note signs and symptoms of arterial and venous insufficiency when assessing the skin.

Blood Pressure

When auscultating blood pressure, know that readings between the arms vary by as much as 10 mm Hg and tend to be higher in the right arm (Seidel and others, 2006). Always record the higher reading. Systolic readings that differ by 15 mm Hg or more suggest atherosclerosis or disease of the aorta.

Carotid Arteries

When the left ventricle pumps blood into the aorta, the arterial system transmits pressure waves. The carotid arteries reflect heart function better than peripheral arteries because their pressure correlates with that of the aorta. The carotid artery supplies oxygenated blood to the head and neck (Figure 33-42). The overlying sternocleidomastoid muscle protects it.

To examine the carotid arteries, have the client sit or lie supine with the head of the bed elevated 30 degrees. Examine one carotid artery at a time. If both arteries are simultaneously occluded during palpation, the client will lose consciousness as a result of inadequate circulation to the brain. Do not palpate or massage the carotid arteries vigorously because the carotid sinus is located at the bifurcation of the common carotid arteries in the upper third of the neck. This sinus sends impulses along the vagus nerve. Its stimulation causes a reflex drop in heart rate and blood pressure, which causes **syncope** or circulatory arrest. This is a particular problem for older adults.

Begin inspection of the neck for obvious pulsation of the artery. Have the client turn the head slightly away from the artery being examined. Sometimes the wave of the pulse is visible. The carotid is the only site for assessing the quality of a pulse wave. An absent pulse wave indicates arterial **occlusion** (blockage) or **stenosis** (narrowing).

To palpate the pulse, ask the client to look straight ahead or turn the head slightly toward the side you are examining. Turning relaxes the sternocleidomastoid muscle. Slide the tips of the index and middle fingers around the medial edge of the sternocleidomastoid muscle. Gently palpate to avoid occlusion of circulation (Figure 33-43).

The normal carotid pulse is localized rather than diffuse. As a strong pulse, the carotid has a thrusting quality. As the client breathes, no change occurs. Rotation of the neck or a shift from a sitting to a supine position does not change the carotid artery's

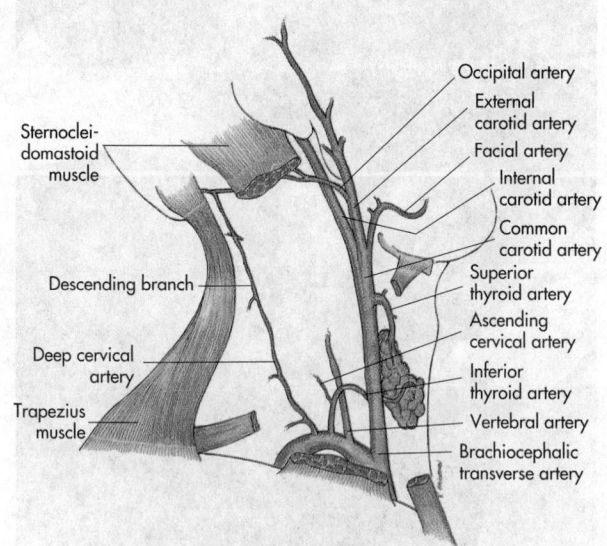

Figure 33-42 Anatomical position of the carotid artery.

✳ TABLE 33-24 Nursing History for Vascular Assessment	
ASSESSMENT CATEGORY	**RATIONALE**
Determine if client experiences leg cramps, numbness or tingling in extremities, sensation of cold hands or feet, pain in legs, or swelling or cyanosis of feet, ankles, or hand.	These signs and symptoms indicate vascular disease.
If client experiences leg pain or cramping in lower extremities, ask if walking or standing for long periods or during sleep aggravate or relieve it.	Relationship of symptoms to exercise will clarify whether problem is vascular or musculoskeletal. Pain caused by vascular condition tends to increase with activity. Musculoskeletal pain is not usually relieved when exercise ends.
Ask clients if they wear tight-fitting garters or hosiery and sit or lie in bed with legs crossed.	Tight hosiery around lower extremities and crossing legs can impair venous return.
Reconsider previous heart risk factors (e.g., smoking, exercise, nutritional problems).	These predispose client to vascular disease.
Assess medical history for heart disease, hypertension, phlebitis, diabetes, or varicose veins.	Circulatory and vascular disorders influence findings gathered during examination.

quality. Both carotid arteries are normally equal in pulse rate, rhythm, and strength and are equally elastic. Diminished or unequal carotid pulsations indicate **atherosclerosis** or other forms of arterial disease.

The carotid is the most commonly auscultated pulse. Auscultation is especially important for middle-age or older adults or clients suspected of having cerebrovascular disease. When the lumen of a blood vessel is narrowed, this disturbs blood flow. As blood passes through the narrowed section, this creates turbulence, causing a blowing or swishing sound. The blowing sound is called a **bruit** (pronounced "brew-ee") (Figure 33-44).

Place the bell of the stethoscope over the carotid artery at the lateral end of the clavicle and the posterior margin of the sternocleidomastoid muscle. Have the client turn the head slightly away from the side being examined (Figure 33-45). Ask the client to hold the breath for a moment so that breath sounds do not obscure a bruit. Normally you do not hear any sounds during carotid auscultation. Palpate the artery lightly for a thrill (palpable bruit) if you hear a bruit.

Jugular Veins

The most accessible veins for examination are the internal and external jugular veins in the neck. Both veins drain bilaterally from the head and neck into the superior vena cava. The external jugular vein lies superficially and is just above the clavicle. The internal jugular vein lies deeper, along the carotid artery.

It is best to examine the right internal jugular vein because it follows a more direct anatomical path to the right atrium of the heart. The column of blood inside the internal jugular vein serves as a manometer, reflecting pressure in the right atrium. The higher the column, the greater the venous pressure. Raised venous pressure reflects right-sided heart failure.

Normally when a client lies in the supine position, the external jugular vein distends and becomes easily visible. In contrast, the jugular veins normally flatten when the client is in a sitting or standing position. Some clients with heart disease, however, have distended jugular veins when sitting.

To measure venous pressure inspect the jugular veins. Blood volume, the capacity of the right atrium to receive blood and send it to the right ventricle, and the ability of the right ventricle to contract and force blood into the pulmonary artery all influence venous pressure. Any factor resulting in greater blood volume

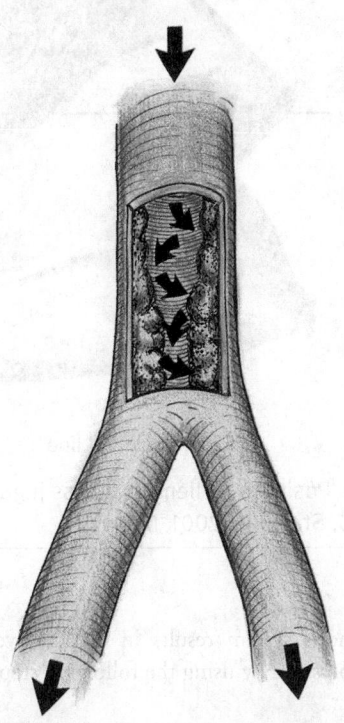

Figure 33-44 Occlusion or narrowing of the carotid artery disrupts normal blood flow. The resultant turbulence creates a sound (bruit) that is auscultated.

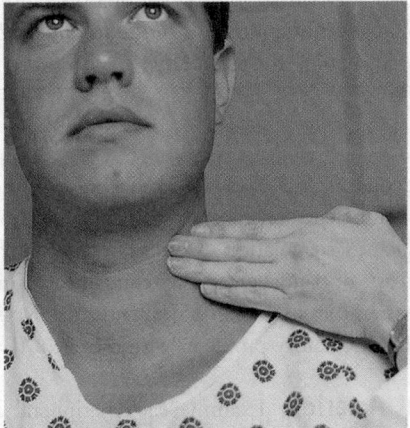

Figure 33-43 Palpation of internal carotid artery along the margin of the sternocleidomastoid muscle.

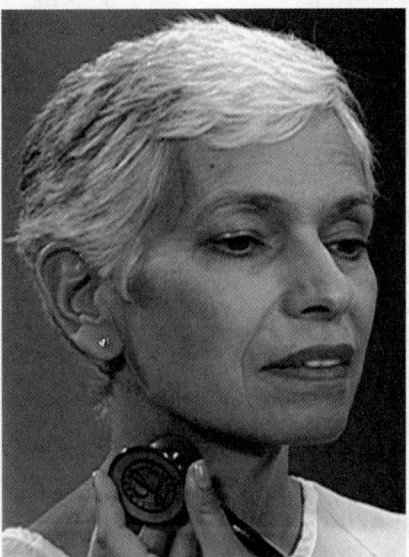

Figure 33-45 Auscultation for carotid artery bruit. (From Seidel HM and others: *Mosby's guide to physical examination,* ed 6, St. Louis 2006, Mosby.)

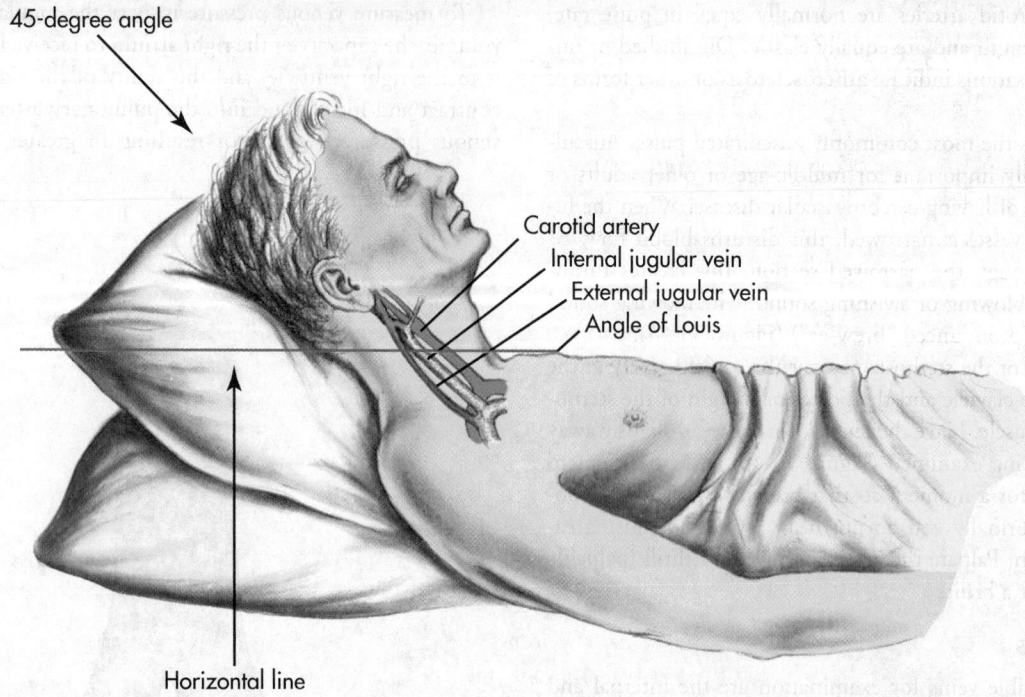

Figure 33-46 Position of client to assess jugular vein distention. (From Thompson JM and others: *Mosby's manual of clinical nursing,* ed 5, St. Louis, 2001, Mosby.)

within the venous system results in elevated venous pressure. Assess venous pressure by using the following steps:

1. Ask the client to lie supine with the head elevated 30 to 45 degrees (semi-Fowler's position).
2. Expose the neck and upper thorax. Use a pillow to align the head. Avoid neck hyperextension or flexion to ensure that the vein is not stretched or kinked (Figure 33-46).
3. Usually pulsations are not evident with the client sitting up. As the client slowly leans back into a supine position, the level of venous pulsations begins to rise above the level of the manubrium as much as 1 or 2 cm as the client reaches a 45-degree angle. Measure venous pressure by measuring the vertical distance between the angle of Louis and the highest level of the visible point of the internal jugular vein pulsation.
4. Use two rulers. Line up the bottom edge of a regular ruler with the top of the area of pulsation in the jugular vein. Then take a centimeter ruler and align it perpendicular to the first ruler at the level of the sternal angle. Measure in centimeters the distance between the second ruler and the sternal angle (Figure 33-47).
5. Repeat the same measurement on the other side. Bilateral pressures higher than 2.5 cm (1 inch) are considered elevated and are a sign of right-sided heart failure. One-sided pressure elevation is due to obstruction.

Peripheral Arteries and Veins

To examine the peripheral vascular system, first assess the adequacy of blood flow to the extremities by measuring arterial pulses and inspecting the condition of the skin and nails. Next assess the integ-

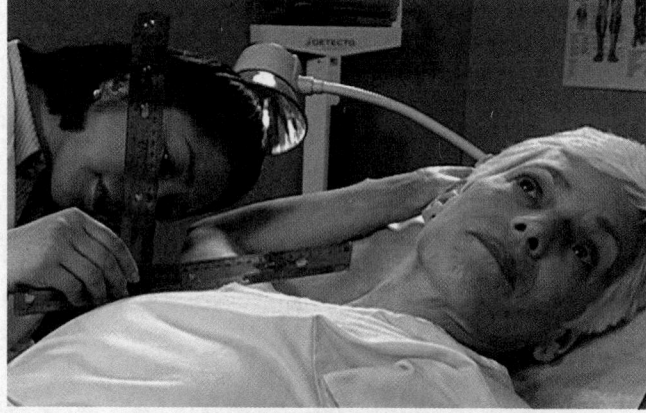

Figure 33-47 Measuring jugular venous pressure. (From Seidel HM and others: *Mosby's guide to physical examination,* ed 6, St. Louis, 2006, Mosby.)

rity of the venous system. Assess the arterial pulses in the extremities to determine sufficiency of the entire arterial circulation.

Factors such as coagulation disorders, local trauma or surgery, constricting casts or bandages, and systemic diseases impair circulation to the extremities (Table 33-25). Discuss risk factors and ways to monitor for circulatory problems with the client (Box 33-21).

Peripheral Arteries. Examine each peripheral artery using the distal pads of the second and third fingers. The thumb helps anchor the brachial and femoral artery. Apply firm pressure but avoid occluding a pulse. When a pulse is difficult to find, it helps

✳ TABLE 33-25 Indicators for Assessing Local Blood Flow

INDICATOR	RATIONALE
Systemic diseases (e.g., arteriosclerosis, atherosclerosis, diabetes)	Diseases result in changes in integrity of walls of arteries and smaller blood vessels.
Coagulation disorders (e.g., thrombosis, embolus)	Blood clot causes mechanical obstruction to blood flow.
Local trauma or surgery (e.g., contusion, fracture, vascular surgery)	Direct manipulation of vessels or localized edema impairs blood flow.
Application of constricting devices (e.g., casts, dressings, elastic bandages, restraints)	Constriction causes tourniquet effect, impairing blood flow to areas below site of constriction.

✳ BOX 33-21   CLIENT TEACHING

Vascular Assessment

Objectives

- Client will know normal blood pressure range for age and compare it with own blood pressure readings to identify normalcy of blood pressure.
- Client with vascular insufficiency will avoid activities that worsen circulatory status.

Teaching Strategies

- Tell client the blood pressure reading. Explain the normal reading for the client's age. Discuss implications of abnormalities.
- Instruct client with risk or evidence of vascular insufficiency in the lower extremities to avoid tight clothing over the lower body or legs, to avoid sitting or standing for long periods, to walk regularly, and to elevate feet when sitting.
- Advise client to avoid cigarette smoking because nicotine causes vasoconstriction.
- Identify client with hypertension who sometimes benefit from regular monitoring of blood pressure (daily, weekly, or monthly). Teach client how to use home monitoring kits (see Chapter 32).

Evaluation

- Ask client to identify if blood pressure reading is within normal limits for age.
- Have client with vascular insufficiency describe precautions to take to avoid further circulatory deficiency.
- Have client demonstrate self-monitoring of blood pressure.

to vary pressure and feel all around the pulse site. Be sure not to palpate your own pulse.

Routine vital signs usually include assessment of the rate and rhythm of the radial artery because it is easily accessible. Count the pulse for either 30 seconds or a full minute, depending on the character of the pulse. Always count an irregular pulse for 60 seconds. With palpation, normally feel the pulse wave at regular intervals. When an interval is interrupted by an early, late, or missed beat, the pulse rhythm is irregular. In emergencies health care providers usually assess the carotid artery because it is accessible and most useful in evaluating heart activity. To check local circulatory status of tissues, palpate the peripheral arteries long enough to note that a pulse is present.

Assess each peripheral artery for elasticity of the vessel wall, strength, and equality. The arterial wall is normally elastic, mak-

ing it easily palpable. After depressing the artery, it will spring back to shape when releasing the pressure. An abnormal artery is hard, inelastic, or calcified.

The strength of a pulse is a measurement of the force at which blood is ejected against the arterial wall. Some examiners use a scale rating from 0 to 4+ for the strength of a pulse (Seidel and others, 2006):

0	Absent, not palpable
1+	Pulse diminished, barely palpable
2+	Expected/normal
3+	Full pulse, increased
4+	Bounding pulse

Measure all peripheral pulses for equality and symmetry. Compare the left radial pulse with that of the right, and so on. Lack of symmetry indicates impaired circulation such as a localized obstruction or an abnormally positioned artery.

In the upper extremities the brachial artery channels blood to the radial and ulnar arteries of the forearm and hand. If circulation in this artery becomes blocked, the hands will not receive adequate blood flow. If circulation in the radial or ulnar arteries becomes impaired, the hand will still receive adequate perfusion. An interconnection between the radial and ulnar arteries guards against arterial occlusion (Figure 33-48).

To locate pulses in the arm have the client sit or lie down. Find the radial pulse along the radial side of the forearm at the wrist. Thin individuals have a groove lateral to the flexor tendon of the wrist. Feel the radial pulse with light palpation in the groove (Figure 33-49). The ulnar pulse is on the opposite side of the wrist and feels less prominent (Figure 33-50). Palpate the ulnar pulse only when evaluating arterial insufficiency to the hand.

To palpate the brachial pulse, find the groove between the biceps and triceps muscle above the elbow at the antecubital fossa (Figure 33-51). The artery runs along the medial side of the extended arm. Palpate the artery with the fingertips of the first three fingers in the muscle groove.

The femoral artery is the primary artery in the leg, delivering blood to the popliteal, posterior tibial, and dorsalis pedis arteries (Figure 33-52). An interconnection between the posterior tibial and dorsalis pedis arteries guards against local arterial occlusion.

Find the femoral pulse with the client lying down with the inguinal area exposed (Figure 33-53). The femoral artery runs below the inguinal ligament, midway between the symphysis pubis and the anterosuperior iliac spine. Sometimes you will use deep palpation to feel the pulse. Bimanual palpation is effective in

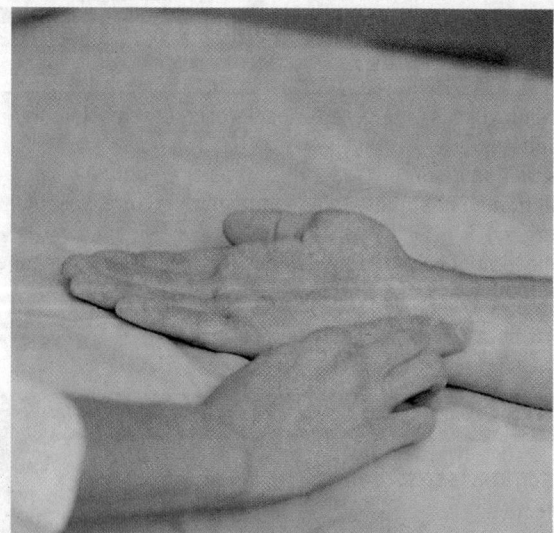

Figure 33-50 Palpation of ulnar pulse.

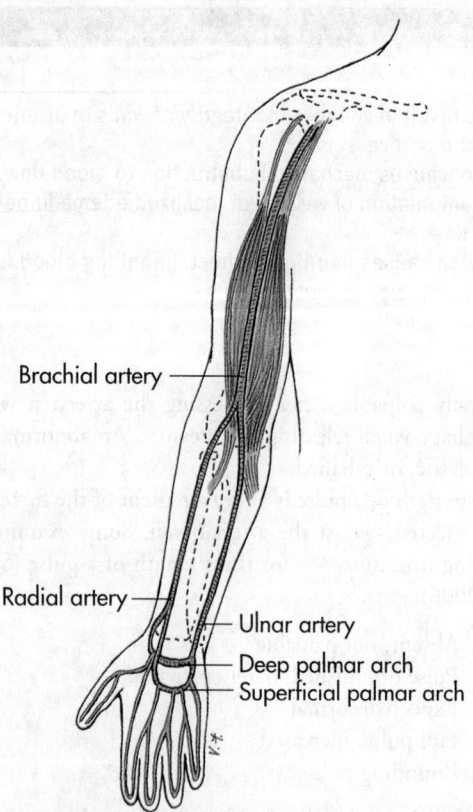

Figure 33-48 Anatomical positions of brachial, radial, and ulnar arteries.

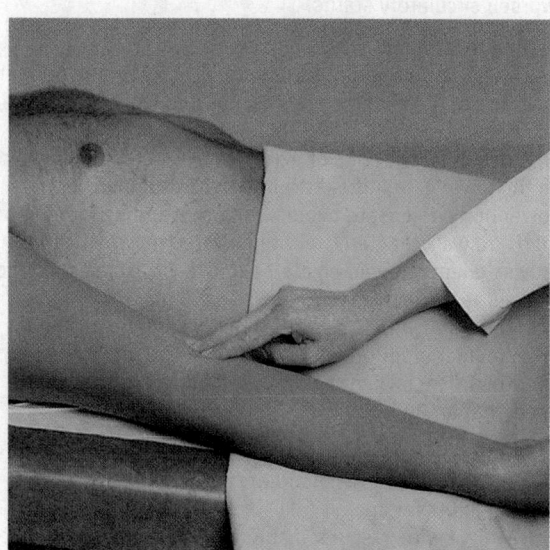

Figure 33-51 Palpation of brachial pulse.

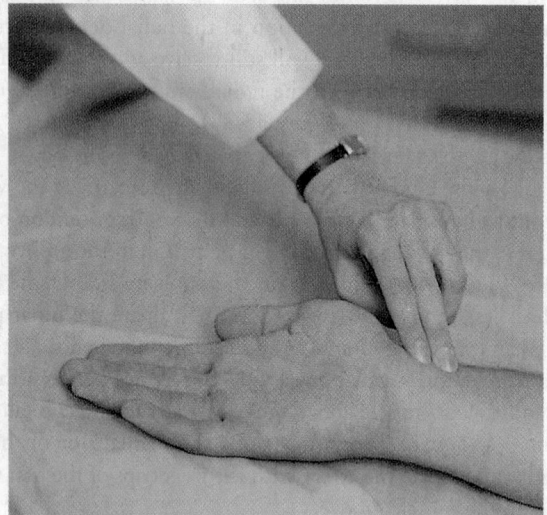

Figure 33-49 Palpation of radial pulse.

obese clients. Place the fingertips of both hands on opposite sides of the pulse site. Feel a pulsatile sensation when the arterial pulsation pushes the fingertips apart.

The popliteal pulse runs behind the knee. Have the client slightly flex the knee, with the foot resting on the examination table, or assume a prone position with the knee slightly flexed (Figure 33-54). Instruct the client to keep leg muscles relaxed. Palpate with the fingers of both hands deeply into the popliteal fossa, just lateral to the midline. The popliteal pulse is difficult to locate.

With the client's foot relaxed, locate the dorsalis pedis pulse. The artery runs along the top of the foot in line with the groove between the extensor tendons of the great toe and first toe (Figure 33-55). To find the pulse, place the fingertips between the first and second toes and slowly move up the dorsum of the foot. This pulse is sometimes congenitally absent.

Find the posterior tibial pulse on the inner side of each ankle (Figure 33-56). Place the fingers behind and below the medial malleolus (ankle bone). With the foot relaxed and slightly extended, palpate the artery.

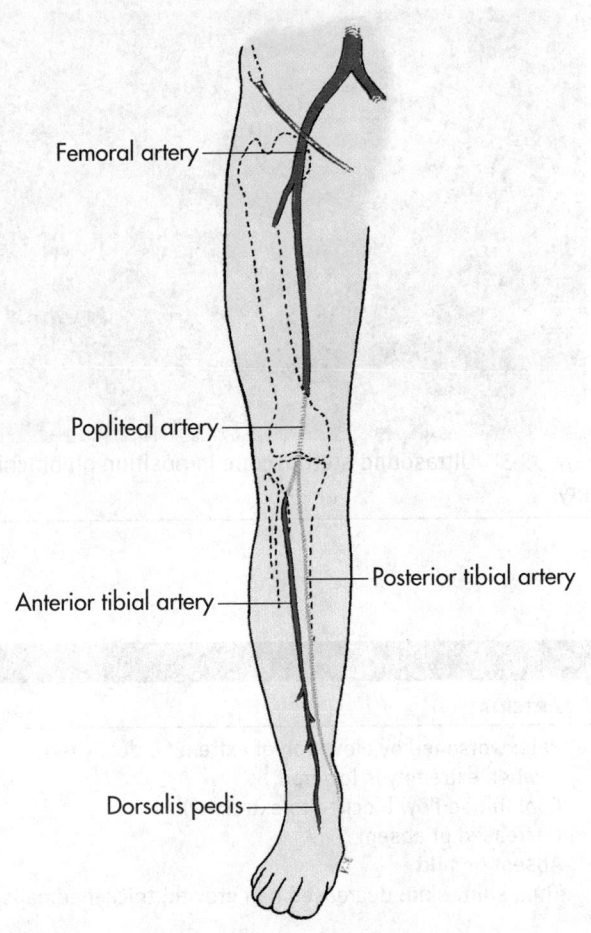

Figure 33-52 Anatomical position of femoral, popliteal, dorsalis pedis, and posterior tibial arteries.

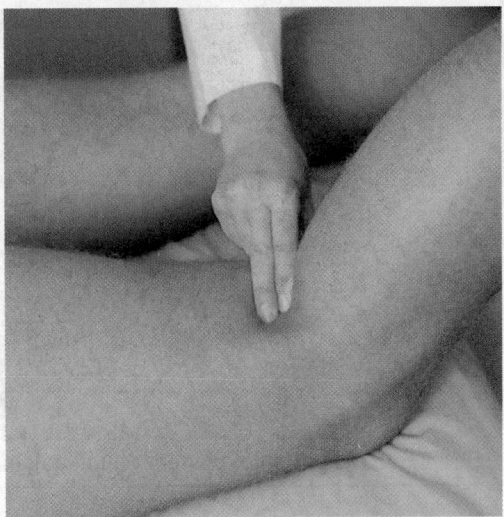

Figure 33-54 Palpation of popliteal pulse.

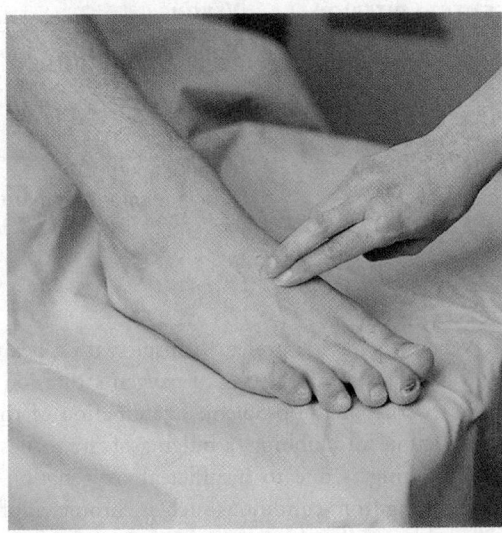

Figure 33-55 Palpation of dorsalis pedis pulse.

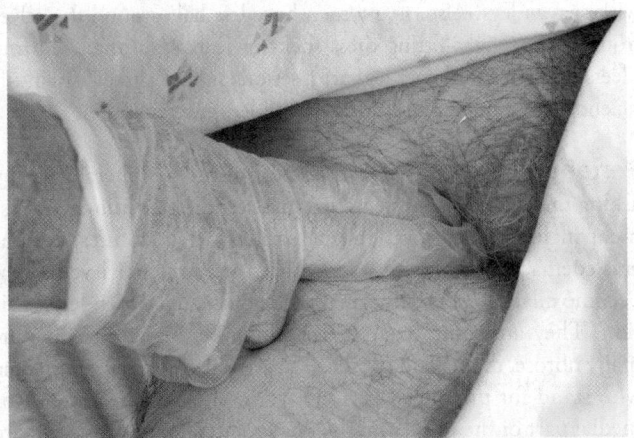

Figure 33-53 Palpation of femoral pulse.

Ultrasound Stethoscopes. If a pulse is difficult to palpate, an ultrasound (Doppler) stethoscope is a useful tool that amplifies the sounds of a pulse wave. Factors that weaken a pulse or make palpation difficult include obesity, reduction in the heart's stroke volume, diminished blood volume, or arterial obstruction. Apply a thin layer of transmission gel to the client's skin at the pulse site

or directly onto the transducer tip of the probe. Turn on the volume control, and place the tip of the transducer at a 45- to 90-degree angle on the skin (Figure 33-57). Move the transducer until you hear a pulsating "whooshing" sound that indicates arterial blood flow is present.

Tissue Perfusion. The condition of the skin, mucosa, and nail beds offers useful data about the status of circulatory blood flow. Examine the face and upper extremities, looking at the color of the skin, mucosa, and nail beds. The presence of cyanosis requires special attention. Heart disease sometimes causes central cyanosis, which indicates poor arterial oxygenation. Some characteristics of this are a bluish discoloration of the lips, mouth, and conjunctivae. Blue lips, earlobes, and nail beds are signs of peripheral cyanosis, which indicates peripheral vasocon-

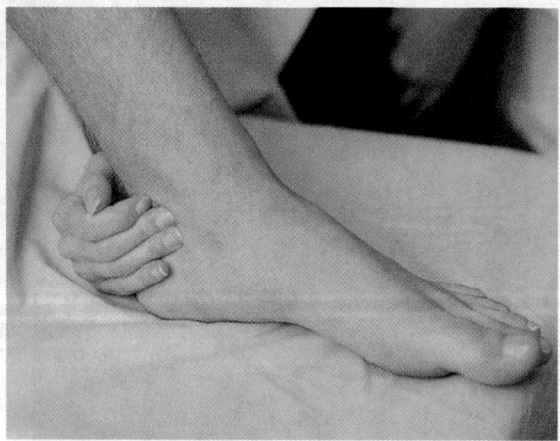

Figure 33-56 Palpation of posterior tibial pulse.

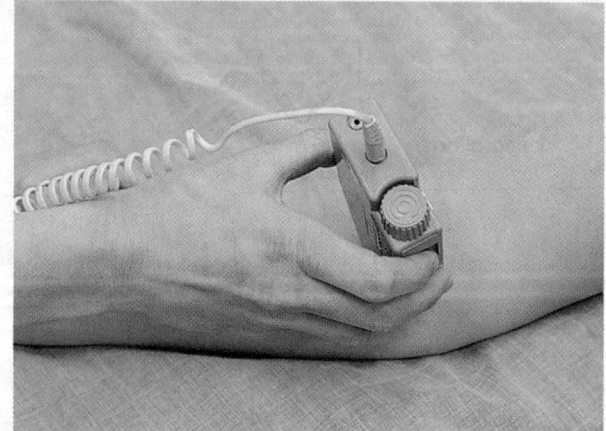

Figure 33-57 Ultrasound stethoscope in position on brachial artery.

TABLE 33-26 Signs of Venous and Arterial Insufficiency

ASSESSMENT CRITERION	VENOUS	ARTERIAL
Color	Normal or cyanotic	Pale; worsened by elevation of extremity; dusky red when extremity is lowered
Temperature	Normal	Cool (blood flow blocked to extremity)
Pulse	Normal	Decreased or absent
Edema	Often marked	Absent or mild
Skin changes	Brown pigmentation around ankles	Thin, shiny skin; decreased hair growth; thickened nails

striction. When cyanosis is present, consult with a health care provider to have laboratory testing of oxygen saturation to determine the severity of the problem. Examination of the nails involves inspection for clubbing, a bulging of the tissues at the nail base. **Clubbing** is due to insufficient oxygenation at the periphery resulting from conditions such as chronic emphysema and congenital heart disease.

Inspect the lower extremities for changes in color, temperature, and condition of the skin indicating either arterial or venous alterations (Table 33-26). This is a good time to ask the client about any history of pain in the legs. If an arterial occlusion is present, the client has signs resulting from an absence of blood flow. Pain will be distal to the occlusion. The *P*'s—pain, pallor, pulselessness, paresthesias, and paralysis—characterize an occlusion. Venous congestion causes tissue changes indicating an inadequate circulatory flow back to the heart.

During examination of the lower extremities, also inspect skin and nail texture; hair distribution on the lower legs, feet, and toes; the venous pattern; and scars, pigmentation, or ulcers. Palpate the legs and feet for color and temperature. Also assess **capillary refill**. Measure capillary refill by blanching the nail bed with a substantial pressure for several seconds. Release the pressure, and observe the time elapsed before the nail regains its full color. An acceptable capillary refill time is less than 2 seconds (Seidel and others, 2006).

The absence of hair growth over the legs indicates circulatory insufficiency. Remember, do not confuse absence of hair on the legs with shaven legs. Also, many men have less hair around the calves from wearing tight-fitting dress socks or jeans. Chronic recurring ulcers of the feet or lower legs are a serious sign of circulatory insufficiency and require a health care provider's intervention.

Peripheral Veins. Assess the status of the peripheral veins by asking the client to assume sitting and standing positions. Assessment includes inspection and palpation for varicosities, peripheral edema, and phlebitis. Varicosities are superficial veins that become dilated, especially when the legs are in a dependent position. They are common in older adults because the veins normally fibrose, dilate, and stretch. They are also common in people who stand for prolonged periods. Varicosities in the anterior or medial part of the thigh and the posterolateral part of the calf are abnormal.

Dependent edema around the area of the feet and ankles is a sign of venous insufficiency or right-sided heart failure. Dependent edema is common in older adults and persons who spend a lot of time standing (e.g., waitresses, security guards, and nurses). To assess for pitting edema, use the index finger to press firmly for several seconds and then release over the medial malleolus or the shins. A depression left in the skin indicates edema. Grading 1+ through 4+ characterizes the severity of the edema (Figure 33-58).

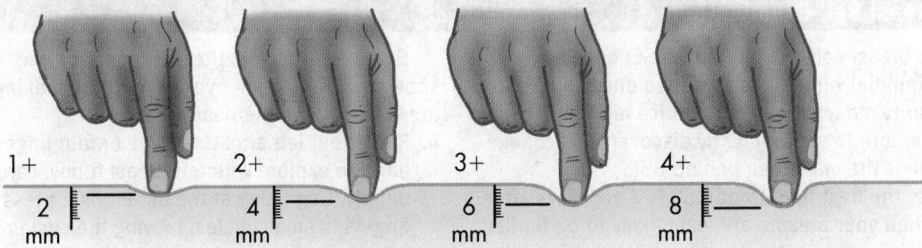

Figure 33-58 Assessing for pitting edema. (From Seidel HM and others: *Mosby's guide to physical examination,* ed 6, St. Louis, 2006, Mosby.)

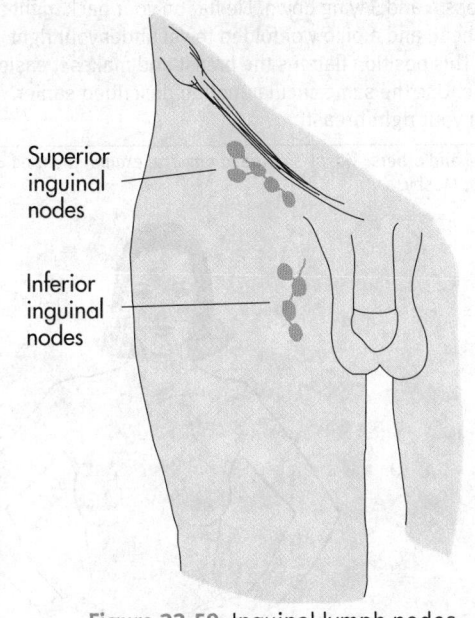

Figure 33-59 Inguinal lymph nodes.

Lymphatic System

Assess the lymphatic drainage of the lower extremities during examination of the vascular system or during the female or male genital examination. Superficial and deep nodes drain the legs, but only two groups of superficial nodes are palpable. With the client supine, palpate the area of the superficial inguinal nodes in the groin area (Figure 33-59). Then move the fingertips toward the inner thigh, feeling for any inferior nodes. Use a firm but gentle pressure when palpating over each lymphatic chain. Multiple nodes are not normally palpable, although a few soft, nontender nodes are not unusual. Enlarged, hardened, tender nodes reveal potential sites of infection or metastatic disease.

Breasts

It is important to examine the breasts of female and male clients. Males have a small amount of glandular tissue, a potential site for the growth of cancer cells, in the breast. In contrast, the majority of the female breast is glandular tissue.

Female Breasts

Researchers predicted that new cases of invasive breast cancer will affect 178,480 women in the United States in 2007 (ACS, 2007). The disease is second to lung cancer as the leading cause of death in women with cancer. Early detection is the key to cure. A major responsibility for you is to teach clients health behaviors such as breast self-examination (BSE) (Box 33-22).

If the client already performs self-examination, assess the method she uses and times she does the examination in relation to her menstrual cycle. The best time for a BSE is the fourth through seventh day of the menstrual cycle or right after the menstrual cycle ends, when the breast is no longer swollen or tender from hormone elevations. If the woman is postmenopausal, advise her to check her breasts on the same day each month. The pregnant woman should also check her breasts on a monthly basis.

Older women require special attention when reviewing the need for regular BSE. Fixed incomes limit many older women, and thus they fail to pursue regular clinical breast examination and mammography. Unfortunately, many older women ignore changes in their breasts, assuming that they are a part of aging. In addition, physiological factors affect the ease with which older women perform a BSE. Musculoskeletal limitations, diminished

Phlebitis is an inflammation of a vein that occurs commonly after trauma to the vessel wall, infection, immobilization, and prolonged insertion of IV catheters (see Chapter 41). Phlebitis promotes clot formation, a potentially dangerous situation because a clot within a deep vein of the leg can become dislodged and travel through the heart, causing a pulmonary embolus. To assess for phlebitis, inspect the calves for localized redness, tenderness, and swelling over vein sites. Gentle palpation of calf muscles reveals warmth, tenderness, and firmness of the muscle. Unilateral edema of the affected leg is one of the most reliable findings of phlebitis (Day, 2003). Determine if dorsiflexion of the foot (Homans' sign) causes pain in the calf. However, Homans' sign is not always a reliable indicator of phlebitis and is present in other conditions (Crowther and McCourt, 2004; Day, 2003). Performing the Homans' sign test is contraindicated in clients with deep vein thrombosis. If a clot is present, it may become dislodged from its original site during this test, resulting in a pulmonary embolism.

✳ BOX 33-22   Breast Self-Examination

You need to perform breast self-examination (BSE) once a month so that you become familiar with the usual appearance and feel of your breasts. Familiarity makes it easier to notice any changes in the breast from one month to another. Early discovery of a change from what is baseline is the main idea behind BSE.

If you menstruate, the best time to do BSE is 2 or 3 days after your period ends, when your breasts are least likely to be tender or swollen. If you no longer menstruate, pick a day, such as the first day of the month, to remind yourself it is time to do BSE.

Here is how to do BSE:

1. Stand before a mirror. Inspect both breasts for anything unusual, such as any discharge from the nipples, puckering, dimpling, or scaling of the skin.

The next two steps are designed to emphasize any change in the shape or contour of your breasts. As you do them, you will feel your chest muscles tighten.

2. Watching closely in the mirror, clasp hands behind your head and swing elbows forward.

3. Next, press hands firmly on hips and bow slightly toward your mirror as you pull your shoulders and elbows forward.

Some women do the next part of the examination in the shower. Fingers glide over soapy skin, making it easy to appreciate the texture underneath.

4. Raise your left arm. Use three or four fingers of your right hand to explore your left breast firmly, carefully, and thoroughly. Beginning at the outer edge, press the flat part of your fingers in small circles, moving the circles slowly around the breast. Gradually work toward the nipple. Be sure to cover the entire breast. Pay special attention to the area between the breast and the armpit, including the armpit itself. Feel for any unusual lump or mass under the skin.

5. Gently squeeze the nipple and look for discharge. Repeat the exam on your right breast.

6. Repeat steps 4 and 5 lying down. Lie flat on your back, right arm over your head and a pillow or folded towel under your right shoulder. This position flattens the breast and makes it easier to examine. Use the same circular motion described earlier.

7. Repeat on your right breast.

From Seidel HM and others: *Mosby's guide to physical examination*, ed 6, St. Louis, 2006, Mosby.

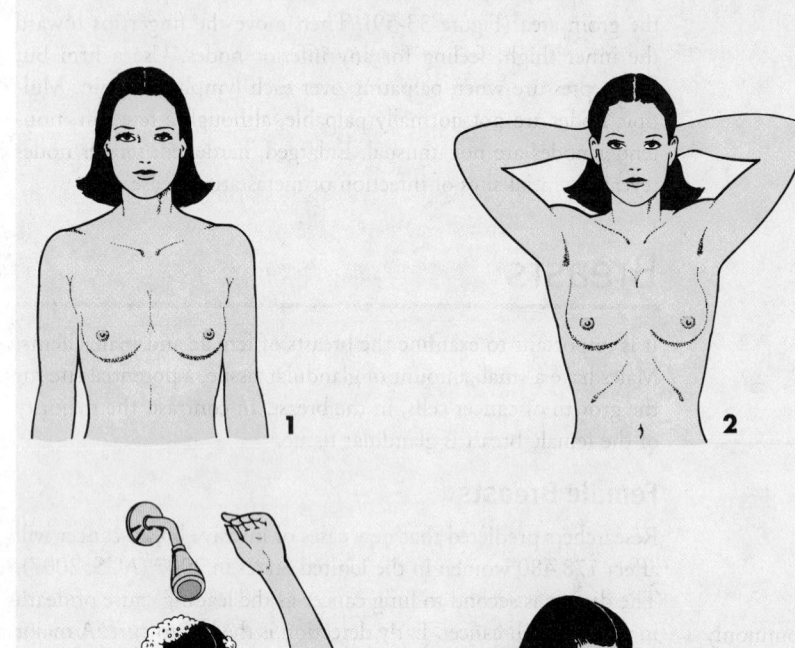

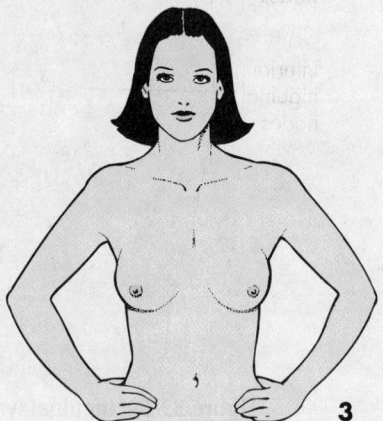

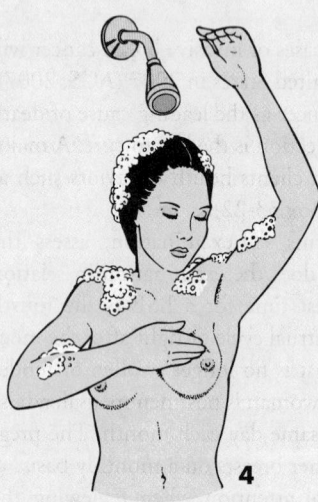

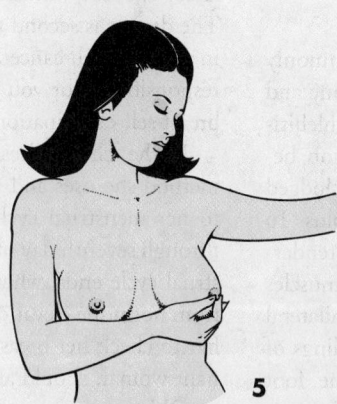

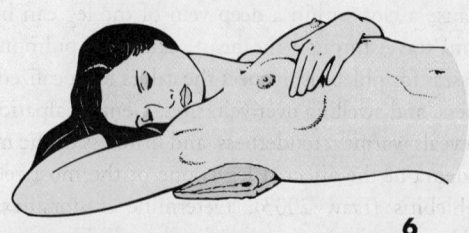

✳ TABLE 33-27 Nursing History for Breast Assessment

ASSESSMENT CATEGORY	RATIONALE
Determine if woman is over age 40; has a personal or family history of breast cancer, early-onset menarche (before age 13), or late-age menopause (after age 50); never had children or gave birth to first child after age 30; or has recent used of oral contraceptives.	These are risk factors for breast cancer (American Cancer Society [ACS], 2006).
Ask if client (both sexes) has noticed lump, thickening, pain, or tenderness of breast; discharge, distortion, retraction, or scaling of the nipple; or change in size of breast.	Potential signs and symptoms of breast cancer allow nurse to focus on specific areas of breast during assessment.
Determine client's use of medications (oral contraceptives, digitalis, diuretics, steroids, or estrogen). Determine client's caffeine intake.	Some medications cause nipple discharge. Hormones and caffeine cause fibrocystic changes in breast.
Determine client's level of activity, alcoholic intake, and weight.	Breast cancer incidence rates correlate with being overweight or obese (postmenopausal), physical inactivity, and consumption of one or more alcoholic beverages per day (ACS, 2006; Moore, 2005).
Ask if client performs monthly breast self-examination (BSE). If so, determine time of month she performs examination in relation to menstrual cycle. Have client describe or demonstrate method used.	Nurse's role is to educate client about breast cancer and techniques for BSE.
If client reports a breast mass, ask about length of time since client first noticed the lump. Does lump come and go, or is it always present? Have there been changes in the lump (e.g., size, relationship to menses), and are there associated symptoms?	Helps to determine nature of mass, (e.g., breast cancer versus fibrocystic disease).

peripheral sensation, reduced eyesight, and changes in joint range of motion limit palpation and inspection abilities. Find resources for older women, including free screening programs. Teach family members to perform the client's examination.

The American Cancer Society (ACS, 2006) recommends the following guidelines for the early detection of breast cancer:

- BSE monthly is an option for women in their 20s.
- Women 20 years of age and older need to report any breast changes to a health care provider immediately.
- Women need a clinical breast examination by a health care provider every 3 years from ages 20 to 40, and yearly for women over age 40.
- Women with a family history of breast cancer need a yearly examination by a health care provider.
- Asymptomatic women need a screening mammogram by age 40; women age 40 and over need to have a mammogram annually.
- For women at increased risk, the ACS recommends talking with the health care provider for screening options and additional testing.

The client's history (Table 33-27) reveals normal developmental changes, as well as signs of breast disease. Because of its glandular structure, the breast undergoes changes during a woman's life. Knowing these changes (Box 33-23) allows complete and accurate assessment. Encourage both men and women to observe their breasts for changes.

Inspection. Have the client remove the top gown or drape to allow simultaneous visualization of both breasts. Have the client stand or sit with her arms hanging loosely at her sides. If possible, place a mirror in front of the client during inspection so she sees what to look for when performing a BSE. To recognize abnormalities, the client needs to be familiar with the normal appearance of her breasts. Describe observations or findings in relation to imaginary lines that divide the breast into four quadrants and a tail. The lines cross at the center of the nipple. Each tail extends outward from the upper outer quadrant (Figure 33-60).

Inspect the breasts for size and symmetry. Normally the breasts extend from the third to the sixth ribs, with the nipple at the level of the fourth intercostal space. It is common for one breast to be smaller. However, inflammation or a mass causes a difference in size. As the woman becomes older, the ligaments supporting the breast tissue weaken, causing the breasts to sag and the nipples to lower.

Observe the contour or shape of the breasts, and note masses, flattening, retraction, or dimpling. Breasts vary in shape from convex to pendulous or conical. Retraction or dimpling results from invasion of underlying ligaments by tumors. The ligaments fibrose and pull the overlying skin inward toward the tumor. Edema also changes the contour of the breasts. To bring out retraction or changes in the shape of breasts, ask the client to assume three positions: raise arms above the head, press hands against the hips, and extend arms straight ahead while sitting and leaning forward. Each maneuver causes a contraction of the pectoral muscles, which will accentuate the presence of any retraction.

Carefully inspect the skin for color; venous pattern; and the presence of lesions, edema, or inflammation. Lift each breast when necessary to observe lower and lateral aspects for color and texture changes. The breasts are the color of neighboring skin, and

✳ BOX 33-23 Normal Changes in the Breast During a Woman's Life Span

Puberty (8 to 20 Years)
Breasts mature in five stages. One breast may grow more rapidly than the other. The ages at which changes occur and rate of developmental progression vary.

Stage 1 (Preadolescent)
This stage involves elevation of the nipple only.

Stage 2
The breast and nipple elevate as a small mound, and the areolar diameters enlarge.

Stage 3
There is further enlargement and elevation of the breast and areola, with no separation of contour.

Stage 4
The areola and nipple project into the secondary mound above the level of the breast (does not occur in all girls).

Stage 5 (Mature Breast)
Only the nipple projects, and the areola recedes (varies in some women).

Young Adulthood (20 to 30 Years)
Breasts reach full (nonpregnant) size. Shape is generally symmetrical. Breasts are sometimes unequal in size.

Pregnancy
Breast size gradually enlarges to 2 to 3 times the previous size. Nipples enlarge and become erect. Areolae darken, and diameters increase. Superficial veins become prominent. The nipples expel a yellowish fluid (colostrum).

Menopause
Breasts shrink. Tissue becomes softer, sometimes flabby.

Older Adulthood
Breasts become elongated, pendulous, and flaccid as a result of glandular tissue atrophy. The skin of the breasts tends to wrinkle, appearing loose and flabby.
 Nipples become smaller and flatter and lose erectile ability. Nipples sometimes invert because of shrinkage and fibrotic changes.

Data from Hockenberry MJ, Wilson D: *Wong's nursing care of infants and children,* ed 8, St. Louis, 2007, Mosby; Seidel HM and others: *Mosby's guide to physical examination,* ed 6, St. Louis, 2006, Mosby; and Ebersole P and others: *Toward healthy aging,* ed 6, St. Louis, 2004, Mosby.

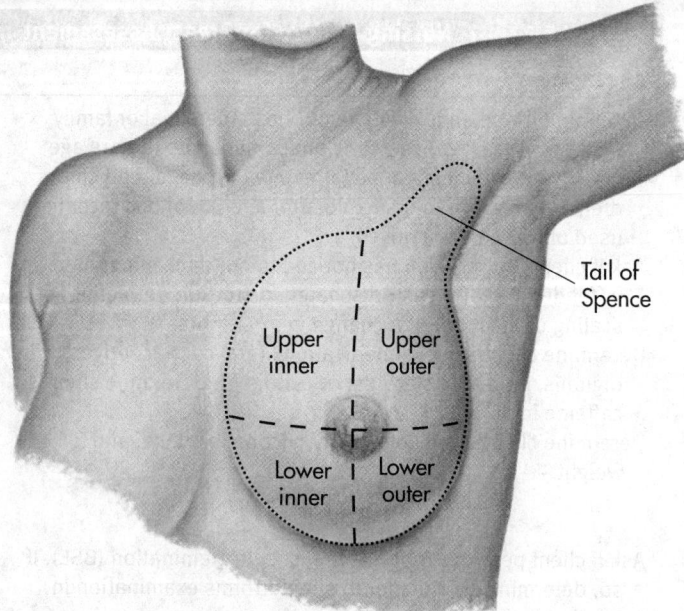

Figure 33-60 Quadrants of the left breast and axillary tail of Spence. (From Seidel HM and others: *Mosby's guide to physical examination,* ed 6, St. Louis, 2006, Mosby.)

venous patterns are the same bilaterally. Venous patterns are easily visible in thin or pregnant women. Women with large breasts often have redness and excoriation of the undersurfaces caused by rubbing of skin surfaces.

Inspect the nipple and areola for size, color, shape, discharge, and the direction the nipples point. The normal areolae are round or oval and nearly equal bilaterally. Color ranges from pink to brown. In light-skinned women the areola turns brown during pregnancy and remains dark. In dark-skinned women the areola is brown before pregnancy (Seidel and others, 2006). Normally the nipples point in symmetrical directions, are everted, and have no drainage. If the nipples are inverted, ask if this has been a lifetime history. A recent inversion or inward turning of the nipple indicates an underlying growth. Rashes or ulcerations are not

normal on the breast or nipples. Note any bleeding or discharge from the nipple. Clear yellow discharge 2 days after childbirth is common. While inspecting the breasts, explain the characteristics you see. Teach the client the significance of abnormal signs or symptoms.

Palpation. Palpation assesses the condition of underlying breast tissue and lymph nodes. Breast tissue consists of glandular tissue, fibrous supportive ligaments, and fat. Glandular tissue is organized into lobes that end in ducts that open onto the nipple's surface. The largest portion of glandular tissue is in the upper outer quadrant and tail of each breast. Suspensory ligaments connect to skin and fascia underlying the breast to support the breast and maintain its upright position. Fatty tissue is located superficially and to the sides of the breast.

A large portion of lymph from the breasts drains into axillary lymph nodes. If cancerous lesions **metastasize** (spread), the nodes commonly become involved. Study the location of supraclavicular, infraclavicular, and axillary nodes (Figure 33-61). The axillary nodes drain lymph from the chest wall, breasts, arms, and hands. A tumor of one breast sometimes involves nodes on the opposite side, as well as those on the same side.

To palpate the lymph nodes have the client sit with the her arms at her sides and muscles relaxed. While facing the client and standing on the side you are examining, support the client's arm in a flexed position and abduct the arm from the chest wall. Place the free hand against the client's chest wall and high in the axillary hollow. With the fingertips press gently down over the surface of the ribs and muscles. Palpate the axillary nodes with the fingertips gently rolling soft tissue (Figure 33-62). Palpate four areas of the axilla: at the edge of the pectoralis major muscle along the anterior axillary line, the chest wall in the midaxillary area, the upper part

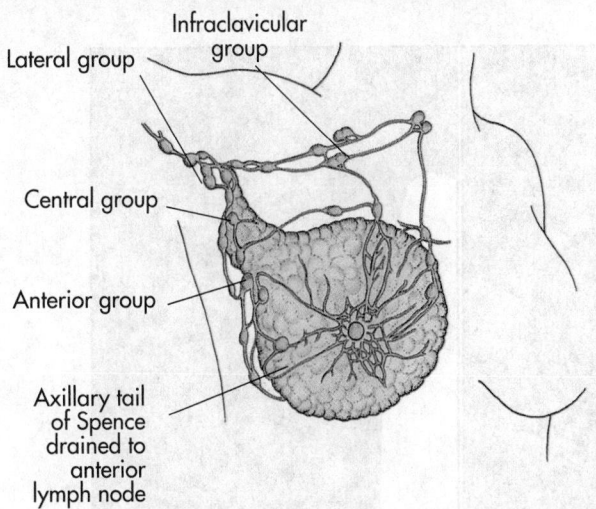

Figure 33-61 Anatomical position of axillary and clavicular lymph nodes.

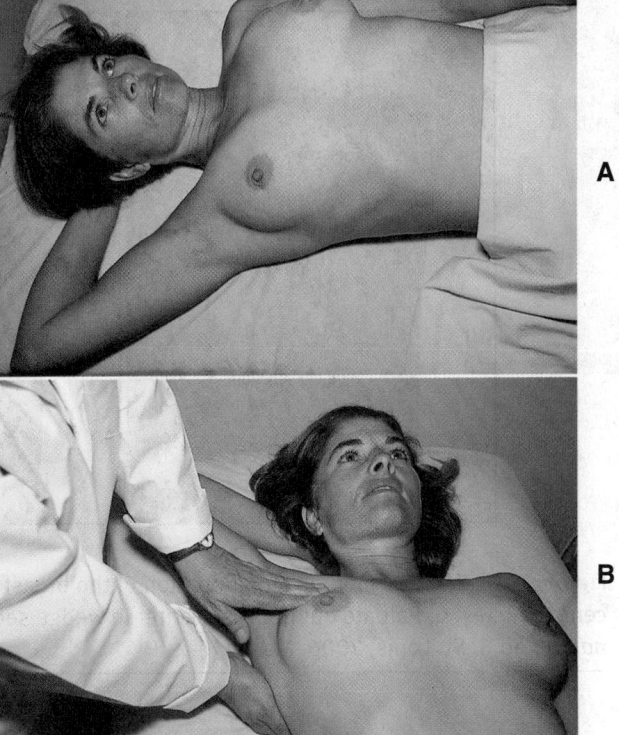

Figure 33-63 **A,** The client lies flat with arm abducted and hand under head to help flatten breast tissue evenly over the chest wall. **B,** Each breast is palpated in a systematic fashion.

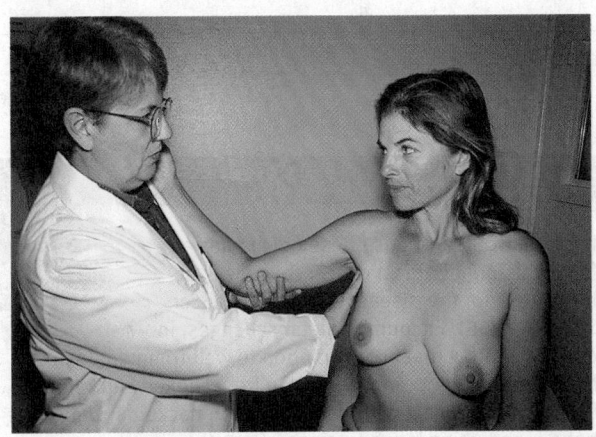

Figure 33-62 Support the client's arm, and palpate axillary lymph nodes.

of the humerus, and the anterior edge of the latissimus dorsi muscle along the posterior axillary line.

Normally lymph nodes are not palpable. Carefully assess each area, and note their number, consistency, mobility, and size. One or two small, soft, nontender palpable nodes are normal. A palpable node feels like a small mass that is hard, tender, and immobile. Also palpate along the upper and lower clavicular ridges. Reverse the procedure for the client's other side.

It is sometimes difficult for the client to learn to palpate for lymph nodes. Lying down with the arm abducted makes the area more accessible. Instruct the client to use her left hand for the right axillary and clavicular areas. Take the client's fingertips and move them in the proper fashion. Then have the client use her right hand to palpate for nodes on the left side.

With the client lying supine and one arm behind the head (alternating with each breast) palpate client's breast tissue. The supine position allows the breast tissue to flatten evenly against the chest wall. The client raises her hand and places it behind the

neck to further stretch and position breast tissue evenly (Figure 33-63, *A*). Place a small pillow or towel under the client's shoulder blade to further position breast tissue.

The consistency of normal breast tissue varies widely. The breasts of a young client are firm and elastic. In an older client the tissue sometimes feels stringy and nodular. The client's familiarity with the texture of her own breasts is very important. Client's gain familiarity through monthly BSE (Box 33-24).

If the client complains of a mass, examine the opposite breast to ensure an objective comparison of normal and abnormal tissue. Use the pads of the first three fingers to compress breast tissue gently against the chest wall, noting tissue consistency (Figure 33-63, *B*). Perform palpation systematically in one of three ways: (1) clockwise or counterclockwise, forming small circles with the fingers along each quadrant and the tail; (2) using a vertical technique with the fingers moving up and down each quadrant; or (3) palpating from the center of the breast in a radial fashion, returning to the areola to begin each spoke (Figure 33-64). Whatever approach you use, be sure to cover the entire breast and tail, directing attention to any areas of tenderness.

When palpating large, pendulous breasts, use a bimanual technique. Support the inferior portion of the breast in one hand while using the other hand to palpate breast tissue against the supporting hand.

During palpation note the consistency of breast tissue. It normally feels dense, firm, and elastic. With menopause, breast tissue

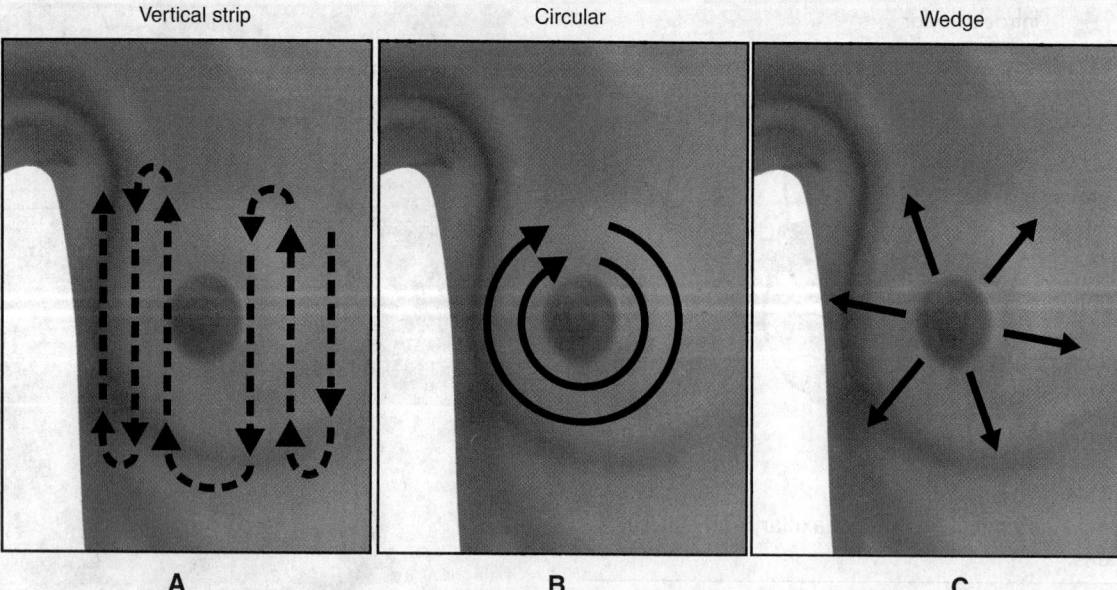

Vertical strip · Circular · Wedge

A **B** **C**

Figure 33-64 Various methods for palpation of the breast. **A,** Palpate from top to bottom in vertical strips. **B,** Palpate in concentric circles. **C,** Palpate out from the center in wedge sections. (From Seidel HM and others: *Mosby's guide to physical examination,* ed 6, St. Louis, 2006, Mosby.)

✴ BOX 33-24 **CLIENT TEACHING**

Female Breast Assessment
Objectives
- Client will perform breast self-examination (BSE) (see Box 33-22, p. 610).
- Client will have screening mammography performed at recommended intervals, beginning at age 40.
- Client will identify signs and symptoms of breast cancer.
- Client will identify signs and symptoms of benign (fibrocystic) breast disease.
- Client will follow a low-fat diet.

Teaching Strategies
- Have client perform return demonstration of BSE, and offer the opportunity to ask questions.
- Explain recommended frequency of mammography and assessment by a health care provider.
- Discuss signs and symptoms of breast cancer.
- Discuss signs and symptoms of benign (fibrocystic) breast disease.

- Inform a woman who is obese or who has a family history of breast cancer that she is at higher risk for the disease (American Cancer Society, 2006). Encourage dietary changes, including limiting meat consumption to well-trimmed, lean beef, pork, or lamb; removing skin from cooked chicken before eating it; selecting tuna and salmon packed in water and not oil; and using low-fat dairy products.
- Encourage client to reduce intake of caffeine and theophyllines. Although this approach is controversial, it will possibly reduce symptoms of benign (fibrocystic) breast disease.

Evaluation
- Have client demonstrate BSE.
- During follow-up visit, determine whether client has had mammography performed.
- Ask client to explain frequency of mammography.
- Have client describe signs and symptoms of breast cancer compared with benign (fibrocystic) breast disease.

---

shrinks and becomes softer. The lobular feel of glandular tissue is normal. The lower edge of each breast sometimes feels firm and hard. This is the normal inframammary ridge and not a tumor. It helps to move the client's hand so that she can feel normal tissue variations. Palpate abnormal masses to determine location in relation to quadrants, diameter in centimeters, shape (e.g., round or discoid), consistency (soft, firm, or hard), tenderness, mobility, and discreteness (clear or unclear boundaries).

Cancerous lesions are hard, fixed, nontender, irregular in shape, and usually unilateral. A common benign condition of the breast is **benign (fibrocystic) breast disease.** Bilateral lumpy, painful breasts and sometimes nipple discharge characterize this condition. Symptoms are more apparent during the menstrual period. When palpated, the cysts (lumps) are soft, well differentiated, and movable. Deep cysts feel hard.

Give special attention palpating the nipple and areola. Palpate the entire surface gently. Use the thumb and index finger to compress the nipple, and note any discharge. During the examination of the nipple and areola, the nipple sometimes becomes erect with wrinkling of the areola. These changes are normal.

✳ TABLE 33-28 Nursing History for Abdominal Assessment

ASSESSMENT CATEGORY	RATIONALE
If client has abdominal or low back pain, assess character of pain in detail (location, onset, frequency, precipitating factors, aggravating factors, type of pain, severity, course).	Pattern of characteristics of pain helps determine its source.
Carefully observe client's movement and position, including lying still with knees drawn up, moving restlessly to find comfortable position, and lying on one side or sitting with knees drawn to chest.	Positions assumed by client reveals nature and source of pain, including peritonitis, renal stone, and pancreatitis.
Assess normal bowel habits and stool character; ask if client uses laxatives.	Data compared with physical findings help identify cause and nature of elimination problems.
Determine if client has had abdominal surgery, trauma, or diagnostic tests of gastrointestinal (GI) tract.	Surgical or traumatic alterations of abdominal organs cause changes in expected findings (e.g., position of underlying organs). Diagnostic tests change character of stool.
Assess if client has had recent weight changes or intolerance to diet (e.g., nausea, vomiting, cramping, especially in last 24 hours).	Data possibly indicate alterations in upper GI tract (stomach or gallbladder) or lower colon.
Assess for difficulty in swallowing, belching, flatulence (gas), bloody emesis (hematemesis), black or tarry stools (melena), heartburn, diarrhea, or constipation.	These characteristic signs and symptoms indicate gastrointestinal alterations.
Ask if client takes antiinflammatory medication (e.g., aspirin, ibuprofen, steroids) or antibiotics.	Pharmacological agents cause GI upset or bleeding.
Ask client to locate tender areas before examination begins.	Assess painful areas last to minimize discomfort and anxiety.
Inquire about family history of cancer, kidney disease, alcoholism, hypertension, or heart disease.	Data possibly reveal risk for alterations identifiable during examination.
Determine if female client is pregnant; note last menstrual period.	Pregnancy causes changes in abdominal shape and contour.
Assess client's usual intake of alcohol.	Chronic alcohol ingestion causes gastrointestinal and liver problems.
Review client's history for the following: health care occupation, hemodialysis, intravenous drug user, household or sexual contact with hepatitis B virus (HBV) carrier, heterosexual person with more than one sex partner in previous 6 months, sexually active homosexual or bisexual male, international traveler in area of high HBV infection rate.	Risk factors for HBV exposure.

After completing the examination, have the client demonstrate self-palpation. Observe the client's technique, and emphasize the importance of a systematic approach. Urge the client to see her health care provider if she discovers an abnormal mass during routine monthly self-examination. She also needs to know all of the signs and symptoms of breast cancer.

Male Breasts

Examination of the male breast is relatively easy. Inspect the nipple and areola for nodules, edema, and ulceration. An enlarged male breast results from obesity or glandular enlargement. Breast enlargement in young males results from steroid use. Fatty tissue feels soft, whereas glandular tissue is firm. Use the same techniques to palpate for masses used in examination of the female breast. Because breast cancer in men is relatively rare, routine self-examinations are unnecessary.

SAFETY ALERT Men, especially men who have a first-degree relative (e.g., mother or sister) with breast cancer, are at risk for breast cancer and need to palpate their breasts at regular intervals. In discussion with their health care provider these men may also be scheduled for routine mammograms.

Abdomen

The abdominal examination is complex because of the number of organs located within and near the abdominal cavity. A thorough nursing history (Table 33-28) helps interpret physical signs. The examination includes an assessment of structures of the lower GI tract in addition to the liver, stomach, uterus, ovaries, kidneys, and bladder. Abdominal pain is one of the most common symptoms that clients report when seeking medical care. An accurate assessment requires matching client history data with a careful assessment of the location of physical symptoms.

Assess the organs anteriorly and posteriorly. A system of landmarks help map out the abdominal region. The xiphoid process (tip of the sternum) is the upper boundary of the anterior abdominal region. The symphysis pubis marks the lower boundary. Divide the abdomen into four imaginary quadrants (Figure 33-65, *A*), and refer to assessment findings and record them in relation to each quadrant. Posteriorly, the lower ribs and heavy back muscles protect the kidneys, which are located from the T12 to L3 vertebrae (Figure 33-65, *B*). The costovertebral angle formed by the last rib and vertebral column is a landmark used during kidney palpation.

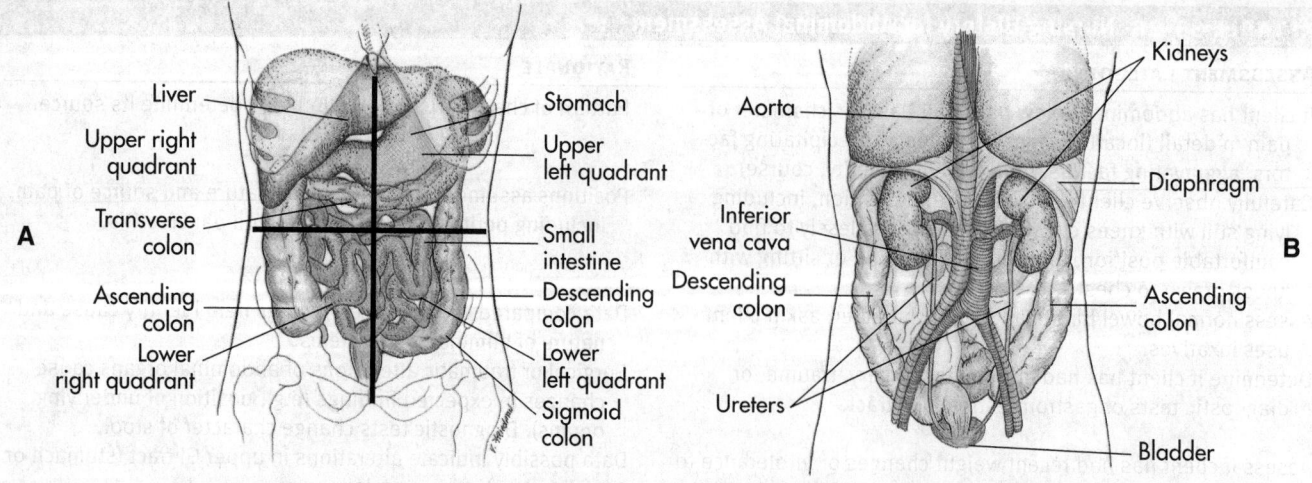

Figure 33-65 A, Anterior view of abdomen divided by quadrants. **B,** Posterior view of abdominal section.

During the abdominal examination the client needs to relax. A tightening of abdominal muscles hinders palpation. Ask the client to void before beginning. Be sure the room is warm, and drape upper chest and legs. The client lies supine or in a dorsal recumbent position with the arms at the sides and knees slightly bent. Place small pillows beneath the knees. If the client places the arms under the head, the abdominal muscles tighten. Proceed calmly and slowly, being sure that there is adequate lighting. Expose the abdomen from just above the xiphoid process down to the symphysis pubis. Warm hands and stethoscope further promote relaxation. Ask the client to report pain and point out tender areas. Assess tender areas last.

The order of an abdominal examination differs slightly from previous assessments. Begin with inspection and follow with auscultation. By using auscultation before palpation there is less chance of altering the frequency and character of bowel sounds. Be sure to have a tape measure and marking pen available during the examination.

Inspection

Make it a habit to observe the client during routine care activities. Note the client's posture and look for evidence of abdominal splinting: lying with the knees drawn up or moving restlessly in bed. A client free from abdominal pain will not guard or splint the abdomen. To inspect the abdomen for abnormal movement or shadows, stand on the client's right side and inspect from above the abdomen. By sitting down to look across the abdomen, assess abdominal contour. Direct the examination light over the abdomen.

Skin. Inspect the skin over the abdomen for color, scars, venous patterns, lesions, and **striae** (stretch marks). The skin is subject to the same color variations as the rest of the body. Venous patterns are normally faint, except in thin clients. Striae result from stretching of tissue by obesity or pregnancy. Artificial openings indicate drainage sites resulting from surgery (see Chapter 50) or an ostomy (see Chapters 45 and 46). Scars reveal evidence of past trauma or surgery that has created permanent changes in underlying organ anatomy. Bruising indicates accidental injury, physical abuse, or a

type of bleeding disorder. Ask if the client self-administers injections (e.g., low-molecular-weight heparin or insulin). Unexpected findings include generalized color changes such as jaundice or cyanosis. A glistening, taut (tight) appearance indicates ascites.

Umbilicus. Note the position; shape; color; and signs of inflammation, discharge, or protruding masses. A normal umbilicus is flat or concave with the color the same as that of the surrounding skin. Underlying masses cause displacement of the umbilicus. An everted (pouched-out) umbilicus usually indicates distention. **Hernias** (protrusion of abdominal organs through the muscle wall) cause upward protrusion of the umbilicus. Normally the umbilical area does not emit discharge.

Contour and Symmetry. Inspect for contour, symmetry, and surface motion of the abdomen, noting any masses, bulging, or distention. A flat abdomen forms a horizontal plane from the xiphoid process to the symphysis pubis. A round abdomen protrudes in a convex sphere from the horizontal plane. A concave abdomen appears to sink into the muscular wall. Each of these findings is normal if the abdomen's shape is symmetrical. In older adults there is often an overall increased distribution of adipose tissue. The presence of masses on only one side, or asymmetry, possibly indicates an underlying pathological condition.

Intestinal gas, a tumor, or fluid in the abdominal cavity causes **distention** (swelling). When distention is generalized, the entire abdomen protrudes. The skin often appears taut, as if it were stretched over the abdomen. When gas causes distention, the flanks do not bulge. However, if fluid is the source of the problem, the flanks bulge. Ask the client to roll onto one side. A protuberance forms on the dependent side if fluid is the cause of the distention. Ask the client if the abdomen feels unusually tight. Be careful not to confuse distention with obesity. In obesity the abdomen is large, rolls of adipose tissue are often present along the flanks, and the client does not complain of tightness in the abdomen. If abdominal distention is expected, measure the abdomen by placing a tape measure around the abdomen at the level of the umbilicus. Consecutive measurements will show any increase or decrease in distention. Use a marking pen to indicate the location of tape measure.

Enlarged Organs or Masses. Observe the contour of the abdomen while asking the client to take a deep breath and hold it. Normally, the contour remains smooth and symmetrical. This maneuver forces the diaphragm downward and reduces the size of the abdominal cavity. Any enlarged organs in the upper abdominal cavity (e.g., liver or spleen) will descend below the rib cage to cause a bulge. Perform a closer examination with palpation.

To evaluate the abdominal musculature, have the client raise the head. This position causes superficial abdominal wall masses, hernias, and muscle separations to become more apparent.

Movement or Pulsations. Inspect for movement. Normally men breathe abdominally and women breathe more costally. A client with severe pain has diminished respiratory movement and tightens the abdominal muscles to guard against the pain. Closely inspect for peristaltic movement and aortic pulsation by looking across the abdomen from the side. These movements are visible in thin clients; otherwise no movement is present.

Auscultation

Auscultate before palpation during the abdominal assessment because manipulation of the abdomen alters the frequency and intensity of bowel sounds. Ask the client not to talk. Clients with GI tubes connected to suction need them temporarily turned off before beginning the examination.

Bowel Motility. **Peristalsis**, or the movement of contents through the intestines, is a normal function of the small and large intestine. Bowel sounds are the audible passage of air and fluid that peristalsis creates. Place the warmed diaphragm of the stethoscope lightly over each of the four quadrants. Normally air and fluid move through the intestines, creating soft gurgling or clicking sounds that occur irregularly 5 to 35 times per minute (Seidel and others, 2006). Sounds usually last ½ second to several seconds. It normally takes 5 to 20 seconds to hear a bowel sound. However, it takes 5 minutes of continuous listening before determining that bowel sounds are absent (Seidel and others, 2006). Auscultate all four quadrants to be sure that you do not miss any sounds. The best time to auscultate is between meals. Sounds are generally described as normal, audible, absent, hyperactive, or hypoactive. Absent sounds indicate a lack of peristalsis, possibly due to late-stage bowel obstruction, **paralytic ileus**, or **peritonitis**. Normally, absent or hypoactive bowel sounds occur postoperatively following general anesthesia. Hyperactive sounds are loud, "growling" sounds called **borborygmi**, which indicate increased gastrointestinal motility. Inflammation of the bowel, anxiety, diarrhea, bleeding, excessive ingestion of laxatives, and reaction of the intestines to certain foods cause increased motility (Box 33-25).

Vascular Sounds. Bruits indicate narrowing of the major blood vessels and disruption of blood flow. The presence of bruits in the abdominal area will possibly reveal aneurysms or stenotic vessels. Use the bell of the stethoscope to auscultate in the epigastric region and each of the four quadrants. Normally there are no vascular sounds over the aorta (midline through the abdomen) or femoral arteries (lower quadrants). Renal artery bruits are heard by placing the stethoscope over each upper quadrant anteriorly or

---

BOX 33-25 CLIENT TEACHING

Abdominal Assessment

Objectives
- Client will maintain normal bowel elimination.
- Client will achieve pain relief.
- Clients at high risk for hepatitis B virus (HBV) will receive immunization.
- Client will identify signs and symptoms of colon cancer.

Teaching Strategies
- Explain factors that promote normal bowel elimination, such as diet, regular exercise, limited use of over-the-counter drugs causing constipation, establishment of regular elimination schedule, and a good fluid intake (see Chapter 46). Stress importance for older adults.
- Caution clients about dangers of excessive use of laxatives or enemas.
- Instruct client to have acute abdominal pain evaluated by a health care provider.
- If client has chronic pain, explain measures used for pain relief (e.g., relaxation exercises, positioning) (see Chapter 43).
- If client is a health care worker or has contact with blood or fluids of affected person, encourage client to receive the series of three HBV vaccine doses.
- Instruct client about warning signs of colon cancer, including rectal bleeding, cramping pain in lower abdomen, black or tarry stools, blood in stool, and a change in bowel habits (constipation or diarrhea).

Evaluation
- Reassess client's bowel elimination pattern and stool character after therapies begin.
- Observe client using pain-relief measures and reassess character of pain.
- During follow-up clinic or office visit, check client's compliance with HBV vaccine schedule.
- Ask client to state signs and symptoms of colon cancer.

---

over the costovertebral angle posteriorly. Report a bruit immediately to a health care provider.

Kidney Tenderness. With the client sitting or standing erect, use direct or indirect percussion to assess for kidney inflammation. With the ulnar surface of the partially closed fist, percuss posteriorly the costovertebral angle at the scapular line. If the kidneys are inflamed, the client feels tenderness during percussion.

Palpation

Palpation primarily detects areas of abdominal tenderness, distention, or masses. As skill base increases, learn to palpate for specific organs. Use light and deep palpation.

Use light palpation over each abdominal quadrant. Initially avoid areas previously identified as problem spots. Lay the palm of the hand with fingers extended and approximated lightly on the abdomen. Explain the maneuver to the client, and then with the palmar surface of the fingers depress approximately 1.3 cm (½ inch) in a gentle dipping motion (Figure 33-66). Avoid quick jabs, and use smooth, coordinated movements. For ticklish cli-

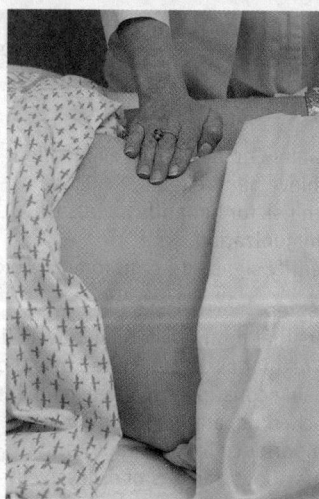

Figure 33-66 Light palpation of abdomen.

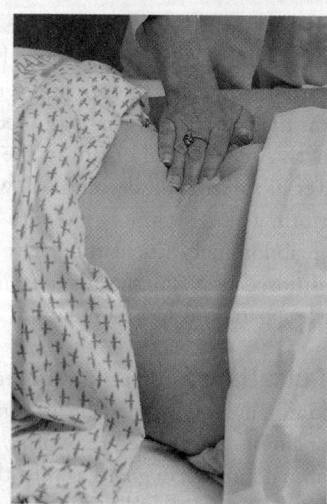

Figure 33-67 Deep palpation of abdomen.

ents, first place the client's hand on the abdomen with your hand on the client's; continue this until the client tolerates palpation.

Use a systematic palpation approach for each quadrant and assess for muscular resistance, distention, tenderness, and superficial organs or masses. Observe the client's face for signs of discomfort. The abdomen is normally smooth with consistent softness and nontender without masses. The older adult often lacks abdominal tone. Guarding or muscle tenseness sometimes occurs while palpating a sensitive area. If tightening remains after the client relaxes, peritonitis, acute **cholecystitis**, or appendicitis is sometimes the cause. It is easy to detect a distended bladder with light palpation. Normally the bladder lies below the umbilicus and above the symphysis pubis. Routinely check for a distended bladder if a client has been unable to void (e.g., because of anesthesia or sedation), has been incontinent, or if an indwelling urinary catheter is not draining well.

With practice and experience perform deep palpation to delineate abdominal organs and to detect less obvious masses. You will need short fingernails. It is important for the client to be relaxed while the hands depress approximately 2.5 to 7.5 cm (1 to 3 inches) into the abdomen (Figure 33-67). Never use deep palpation over a surgical incision or over extremely tender organs. It is also unwise to use palpation on abnormal masses. Deep pressure causes tenderness in the healthy client over the cecum, sigmoid colon, aorta, and the midline near the xiphoid process (Seidel and others, 2006).

Survey each quadrant systematically. Palpate masses for size, location, shape, consistency, tenderness, pulsation, and mobility. Test for rebound tenderness by pressing a hand slowly and deeply into the involved area and then letting go quickly. The test is positive if the client feels pain with the release of the hand. Rebound tenderness occurs in clients with peritoneal irritation such as occurs in appendicitis; **pancreatitis;** or any peritoneal injury causing bile, blood, or enzymes to enter the peritoneal cavity.

Aortic Pulsation. To assess aortic pulsation, palpate with the thumb and forefinger of one hand deeply into the upper abdomen, just left of the midline. Normally a pulsation is transmitted

forward. If there is enlargement of the aorta from an **aneurysm** (localized dilation of a vessel wall), the pulsation expands laterally. Do not palpate a pulsating abdominal mass. In obese clients it is often necessary to palpate with both hands, one on each side of the aorta.

> **SAFETY ALERT** When enlargement from an aneurysm is present, only lightly palpate this area. In addition, only someone with advanced education and experience should perform palpation of this area.

Female Genitalia and Reproductive Tract

Examination of the female genitalia is embarrassing to the client unless you use a calm, relaxed approach. The gynecological examination is one of the most difficult experiences for adolescents. Cultural background further adds to apprehension. For example, female Mexican Americans have a strong social value that women do not expose their bodies to men or even to other women. Similarly, Chinese Americans believe the examination of genitalia is offensive. Provide a thorough explanation as to the reason for the procedures used in the examination. The lithotomy position assumed during the examination is an added source of embarrassment. You achieve comfort through correct positioning and draping. Be sure to explain each portion of the examination in advance so that clients will anticipate necessary actions. Adolescents sometimes choose to have parents present in the examination room.

Sometimes a client requires a complete examination of the female reproductive organs, including assessment of the external genitalia and performing a vaginal examination. The nurse will examine external genitalia while performing routing hygiene measures or preparing to insert a urinary catheter. An internal examination is part of each woman's preventive health care because ovarian cancer causes more deaths than any other cancer of the female reproductive system (ACS, 2006, 2007).

Adolescents and young adults are examined because of the growing incidence of sexually transmitted diseases (STDs). The

※ **TABLE 33-29 Nursing History for Female Genitalia and Reproductive Tract Assessment**

Assessment Category	Rationale
Determine if client has had previous illness or surgery involving reproductive organs, including sexually transmitted diseases (STDs).	Illness or surgery influences appearance and position of organs being examined.
Determine if client has received human papillomavirus (HPV) vaccine.	HPV vaccine is recommended for females (ages 9-26) to prevent cervical cancer (American Cancer Society [ACS], 2007). HPV increases client's risk for development of cervical cancer.
Review menstrual history, including age at menarche, frequency and duration of menstrual cycle, character of flow (e.g., amount, presence of clots), presence of dysmenorrhea (painful menstruation), pelvic pain, dates of last two menstrual periods, and premenstrual symptoms.	This information helps to reveal level of reproductive health, including normalcy of menstrual cycle.
Ask client to describe obstetrical history, including each pregnancy and history of abortions or miscarriages.	Observed physical findings will vary, depending on woman's history of pregnancy.
Ask client to describe current and past contraceptive practices and problems encountered. Determine whether client uses safe sex practices. Discuss risk of STDs and HIV infection.	Use of certain types of contraceptives influence reproductive health (e.g., sensitivity reaction to spermicidal jelly).
Sexual history reveals risk for and understanding of STDs.	
Assess if client has signs and symptoms of vaginal discharge, painful or swollen perianal tissues, or genital lesions.	These signs and symptoms may indicate STD or other pathologic condition.
Determine if client has symptoms or history of genitourinary problems, including burning during urination, frequency, urgency, nocturia, hematuria, incontinence, or stress incontinence (see Chapter 45).	Urinary problems are associated with gynecological disorders, including STDs.
Ask if client has had signs of bleeding outside of normal menstrual period or after menopause or has had unusual vaginal discharge.	These are warning signs for cervical and endometrial cancer or vaginal infection.
Determine if client has history of HPV (condyloma acuminatum, herpes simplex, or cervical dysplasia); has multiple sex partners; smokes cigarettes; has had multiple pregnancies; or was young at first intercourse.	These are risk factors for cervical cancer (ACS, 2007). Vaccines are available for HPV for females 9-26 years of age.
Determine if client is older than 40, obese, and has history of ovarian dysfunction, breast or endometrial cancer, irradiation of pelvic organs, or endometriosis; has family history of ovarian, breast, or colon cancer; has history of infertility or nulliparity; or use of estrogen (alone) hormone replacement therapy.	These are risk factors for ovarian cancer (ACS, 2007).
Determine if client is postmenopausal, obese, or infertile; had early menarche; had late menopause; has history of hypertension, diabetes, gallbladder disease, or polycystic ovary disease; has family history of endometrial, breast, or colon cancer; or has a history of estrogen-related exposure (estrogen replacement therapy, tamoxifen use).	These are risk factors for endometrial cancer (ACS, 2007).

average age of menarche among young girls has declined, and the majority of male and female teenagers are sexually active by age 19 (Hockenberry and Wilson, 2007). It is important to assess the client's level of anxiety as you obtain the nursing history (Table 33-29). Rectal and anal assessment are combined with this examination because the client assumes a lithotomy or dorsal recumbent position.

Preparation of the Client

As a beginning nurse, your responsibility will be assisting the client's health care provider with the examination. For a complete examination, you will need the following special equipment: examination table with stirrups, vaginal speculum of correct size, adjustable light source, sink, clean disposable gloves, sterile cotton swabs, glass slides, plastic or wooden spatula, cervical brush or broom device, cytologic fixative, and culture plates or media (Seidel and others, 2006).

Make sure the equipment is ready before the examination begins. Ask the client to empty her bladder so that the uterus and ovaries are readily palpable. Often it is necessary to collect a urine specimen. Assist the client to the lithotomy position, in bed or on an examination table for the external genitalia assessment. Assist the client into stirrups for a speculum examination. Have the woman stabilize each foot in a stirrup and then have her slide the buttocks down to the edge of the examining table. Place a hand at the edge of the table and instruct the client to move until touching the hand. The client's arms should be at her sides or folded across the chest to prevent tightening of abdominal muscles.

Some women suffering from pain or deformity of the joints are unable to assume a lithotomy position. In this situation it is necessary to have the client abduct only one leg or to have another assist in separating the client's thighs. Also, use the side-lying position with the client on the left side with the right thigh and knee drawn up to her chest.

Give a square drape or sheet to the client. She holds one corner over her sternum, the adjacent corners fall over each knee, and the fourth corner covers the perineum. After the examination begins, lift the drape over the perineum. The male examiner always needs to have a female attendant present during the examination. A female examiner may prefer to work alone but should have a female attendant if the client is particularly anxious or emotionally unstable.

External Genitalia

Make sure the perineal area is well illuminated. Apply clean gloves on both hands to prevent contact with infectious organisms. The perineum is extremely sensitive and tender; do not touch the area suddenly without warning the client. It is best to touch the neighboring thigh first before advancing to the perineum.

While sitting at the end of the examination table or bed, inspect the quantity and distribution of hair growth. Preadolescents have no pubic hair. During adolescence, hair grows along the labia, becoming darker, coarser, and curlier. In an adult, hair grows in a triangle over the female perineum and along the medial surfaces of the thighs. Hair is normally free of nits and lice. The underlying skin is free of inflammation, irritation, or lesions.

Inspect surface characteristics of the labia majora. The skin of the perineum is smooth, clean, and slightly darker than other skin. The mucous membranes appear dark pink and moist. The labia majora are gaping or closed and appear dry or moist. They are usually symmetrical. After childbirth the labia majora separate, causing the labia minora to become more prominent. When a woman reaches menopause, the labia majora become thinned. With advancing age, they become atrophied. The labia majora are normally without inflammation, edema, lesions, or lacerations.

To inspect the remaining external structures, use your nondominant hand and gently place the thumb and index finger inside the labia minora and retract the tissues outwardly (Figure 33-68). Be sure to have a firm hold to avoid repeated retraction against the sensitive tissues. Use the other hand to palpate the labia minora between the thumb and second finger. On inspection, the labia minora are normally thinner than the labia majora, and one side is sometimes larger. The tissue feels soft on palpation and without tenderness. The size of the clitoris is variable, but it normally does not exceed 2 cm in length and 0.5 cm in width. Look for atrophy, inflammation, or adhesions. If inflamed, the clitoris will be a bright cherry red. In young women it is a common site for syphilitic lesions, or **chancres,** which appear as small open ulcers that drain serous material. Some older women have malignant changes that result in dry, scaly, nodular lesions.

Inspect the urethral orifice carefully for color and position. It is normally intact without inflammation. The urethral meatus is anterior to the vaginal orifice and is pink. It appears as a small slit or pinhole opening just above the vaginal canal. Note any discharge, polyps, or fistulas.

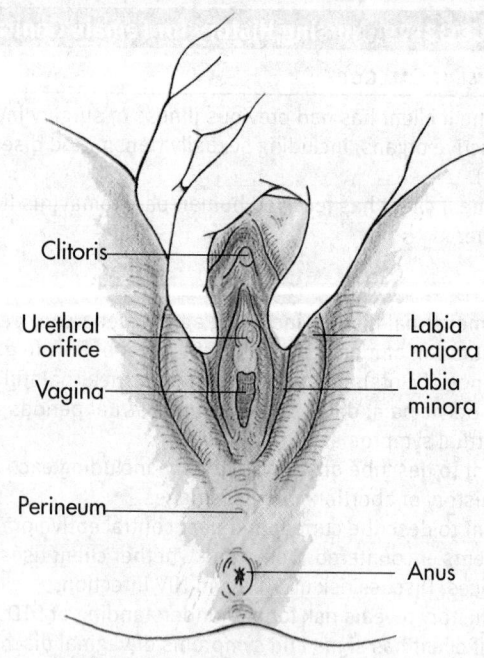

Figure 33-68 Female external genitalia.

Inspect the vaginal orifice (introitus), for inflammation, edema, discoloration, discharge, and lesions. Normally the introitus is a thin, vertical slit or a large orifice. The tissue is moist. While inspecting the vaginal orifice, note the condition of the hymen, which is just inside the introitus. In the virgin the hymen restricts the opening of the vagina. Only remnants of the hymen remain after sexual intercourse.

Inspect the anus, looking for lesions and hemorrhoids (see rectal examination). After completion of the external examination, dispose of examination gloves and offer the client perineal hygiene.

Clients who are at risk for contracting an STD need to learn to perform a genital self-examination (GSE) (Box 33-26). The purpose of the examination is to detect any signs or symptoms of an STD. Many persons do not know they have an STD (e.g., chlamydia), and some STDs (e.g., syphilis) remain undetected for years.

Speculum Examination of Internal Genitalia

An examination of the internal genitalia requires much skill and practice. Advanced nurse practitioners and primary care providers will perform this examination. Beginning students will more than likely only observe the procedure or assist the examiner by helping the client with positioning, handing off specimen supplies, and comforting the client.

The examination involves use of a plastic or metal speculum, consisting of two blades and an adjustment device. The examiner inserts the speculum into the vagina to assess the internal genitalia for cancerous lesions and other abnormalities. During the examination, the examiner will collect a specimen for a **Papanicolaou (Pap) test** for cervical and vaginal cancer. This examination will not be discussed here.

✴ **BOX 33-26** CLIENT TEACHING

Female Genitalia and Reproductive Tract Assessment

Objectives

- Client will pursue routine gynecological examinations based on her level of risk for cervical cancer and other gynecological pathology.
- Client with a sexually transmitted disease (STD) will follow safe sex practices.
- Client will use measures to prevent acquisition and transmission of STDs.

Teaching Strategies

- Instruct client about purpose and recommended frequency of Papanicolaou (Pap) smears and gynecological examinations. Explain that the Pap smear is relatively painless and needed annually with a pelvic examination for women who are sexually active or who are over the age of 21. Clients are screened more often if certain risk factors exist such as a weak immune system, multiple sex partners, smoking, and a history of infections (e.g., human papillomavirus [HPV]).
- Counsel client with an STD about diagnosis and treatment.
- Instruct in genital self-examination (GSE): Using a mirror, position self in order to examine the area covered by the pubic hair. Spread the hair apart, looking for bumps, sores, or blisters. Also, look for any warts, which appear as small, bumpy spots and that enlarge to fleshy, cauliflower-like lesions. Next, spread the outer vaginal lips apart and look at the clitoris for bumps, blisters, sores, or warts. Also look at both sides of the inner vaginal lips. Inspect the area around the urinary and vaginal opening for bumps, blisters, sores, or warts.
- Explain warning signs of STDs: pain or burning on urination, pain during sex, pain in pelvic area, bleeding between menstruation, itchy rash around vagina, and abnormal vaginal discharge.
- Teach measures to prevent STDs: male partner's use of condoms, restricting number of sexual partners, avoiding sex with persons who have several other partners, and perineal hygiene measures.
- Tell clients with an STD to inform sexual partners of the need for an examination.
- Reinforce the importance of performing perineal hygiene (as appropriate).

Evaluation

- Ask client to explain when she should routinely have a gynecological examination and Pap test.
- Have client describe ways to prevent transmission of STDs.
- For client with an STD, determine during follow-up visit if client has followed safe sexual practices (use nonthreatening inquiry).

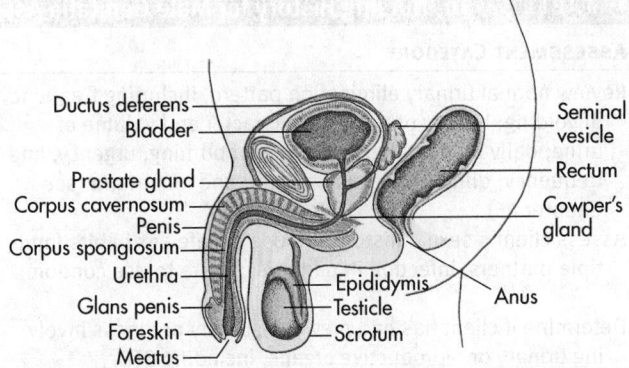

Figure 33-69 External and internal male sex organs.

(Labels: Ductus deferens, Bladder, Prostate gland, Corpus cavernosum, Penis, Corpus spongiosum, Urethra, Glans penis, Foreskin, Meatus, Seminal vesicle, Rectum, Cowper's gland, Epididymis, Testicle, Anus, Scrotum)

✴ **BOX 33-27** CLIENT TEACHING

Male Genitalia Assessment

Objectives

- Client will describe methods to prevent transmission of sexually transmitted diseases (STDs).
- Client will perform genital self-examination.
- Client with an STD will follow safe sex practices.

Teaching Strategies

- Counsel client with an STD about diagnosis and treatment.
- Explain warning signs of STDs: pain on urination and during sex, abnormal penile discharge (different from usual), swollen lymph nodes, or rash or ulcer on skin or genitalia.
- Teach measures to prevent STDs: use of condoms, avoiding sex with infected partner, restricting number of sexual partners, avoiding sex with persons who have multiple partners, and using regular perineal hygiene.
- Tell clients with an STD to inform their sexual partners of the need to have an examination.
- Instruct client to seek treatment as soon as possible if partner becomes infected with an STD.
- Instruct client in how to perform genital self-examination (see Box 33-28).

Evaluation

- Ask client to describe methods for preventing and treating STDs.
- During a follow-up visit, determine whether client with an STD has used safe sex practices.

Male Genitalia

An examination of the male genitalia assesses the integrity of the external genitalia (Figure 33-69) inguinal ring, and canal. Because the incidence of STDs in adolescents and young adults is high, an assessment of the genitalia needs to be a routine part of any health maintenance examination for this age-group (Box 33-27). The examination begins by having the client void. Make sure the examination room is warm. Have the client lie supine with the chest, abdomen, and lower legs draped or stand during the examination. Apply clean gloves.

Use a calm, gentle approach to lessen the client's anxiety. The position and exposure of the body during the examination is embarrassing for some. To minimize the client's anxiety, it often helps to offer explanations of the steps of examination so the cli-

✳ TABLE 33-30 Nursing History for Male Genitalia Assessment

ASSESSMENT CATEGORY	RATIONALE
Review normal urinary elimination pattern, including frequency of voiding; history of nocturia; character and volume of urine; daily fluid intake; symptoms of burning, urgency, and frequency; difficulty starting stream; and hematuria (see Chapter 45).	Urinary problems are directly associated with genitourinary problems because of anatomical structure of men's reproductive and urinary systems.
Assess client's sexual history and use of safe sex habits (multiple partners, infection in partners, failure to use condom).	Sexual history reveals risk for and understanding of sexually transmitted diseases (STDs) and human immunodeficiency virus (HIV).
Determine if client has had previous surgery or illness involving urinary or reproductive organs, including STD.	Alterations resulting from disease or surgery are sometimes responsible for symptoms or changes in organ structure or function.
Ask if client has noted penile pain or swelling, genital lesions, or urethral discharge.	These signs and symptoms may indicate STD.
Determine if client has noticed heaviness or painless enlargement of testis or irregular lumps.	These signs and symptoms are early warning signs for testicular cancer.
If client reports an enlargement in inguinal area, assess if it is intermittent or constant, associated with straining or lifting, and painful, and whether pain is affected by coughing, lifting, or straining at stool.	Signs and symptoms reflect potential inguinal hernia.
Ask if client has difficulty achieving erection or ejaculation; also review whether client is taking diuretics, sedatives, antihypertensives, or tranquilizers.	These medications influence sexual performance.

ent anticipates all actions. Manipulate the genitalia gently to avoid causing erection or discomfort. Obtain a thorough history (Table 33-30) before the examination, ensuring that the assessment is complete.

Sexual Maturity

First, note the sexual maturity of the client by observing the size and shape of the penis and testes; the size, color, and texture of the scrotal skin; and the character and distribution of pubic hair. The testes first increase in size in preadolescence. During this time there is no pubic hair. By the end of puberty, the testes and penis enlarge to adult size and shape and scrotal skin darkens and becomes wrinkled. With puberty, hair is coarse and abundant in the pubic area. The penis has no hair, and the scrotum has very little hair (Figure 33-70). Also inspect the skin covering the genitalia for lice, rashes, excoriations, or lesions. Normally the skin is clear, without lesions.

Penis

To inspect penile surfaces thoroughly, manipulate the genitalia or have the client assist. Inspect the shaft, corona, prepuce (foreskin), glans, and urethral meatus. The dorsal vein is apparent on inspection. In uncircumcised males retract the foreskin to reveal the glans and urethral meatus. The foreskin usually retracts easily. A small amount of white, thick smegma sometimes collects under this foreskin. Obtain a culture if abnormal discharge is present. The urethral meatus is slitlike and is positioned on the ventral surface just millimeters from the tip of the glans. In some congenital conditions the meatus is displaced along the penile shaft. The area between the foreskin and glans is a common site for venereal lesions. Gently compress the glans between thumb and

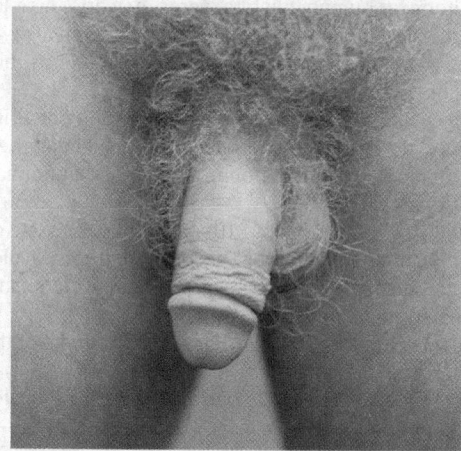

Figure 33-70 Normal male genitalia (circumcised). (From Seidel HM and others: *Mosby's guide to physical examination*, ed 6, St. Louis, 2006, Mosby.)

index finger, this opens the urethral meatus for inspection of lesions, edema, and inflammation. Normally the opening is glistening and pink without discharge. Palpate any lesion gently to note tenderness, size, consistency, and shape. When inspection and palpation of the glans is complete, pull the foreskin down to its original position.

Continue by inspecting the entire shaft of the penis, including the undersurface, looking for lesions, scars, or edema. Palpate the shaft between the thumb and first two fingers to detect localized areas of hardness or tenderness. A client who has lain in bed for a

✳ BOX 33-28 Male Genital Self-Examination

All men 15 years and older need to perform this examination monthly using the following steps.

Genital Examination

Perform the examination after a warm bath or shower when the scrotal skin is less thick.

Stand naked in front of a mirror, and hold the penis in your hand and examine the head. Pull back the foreskin if uncircumcised to expose the glans.

Inspect and palpate the entire head of the penis in a clockwise motion, looking carefully for any bumps, sores, or blisters (bumps and blisters may be light colored or red, resemble pimples).

Look also for any genital warts (see illustration).

Look at the opening (urethral meatus) at the end of the penis for discharge.

Look along the entire shaft of the penis for the same signs.

Be sure to separate pubic hair at the base of the penis and carefully examine the skin underneath.

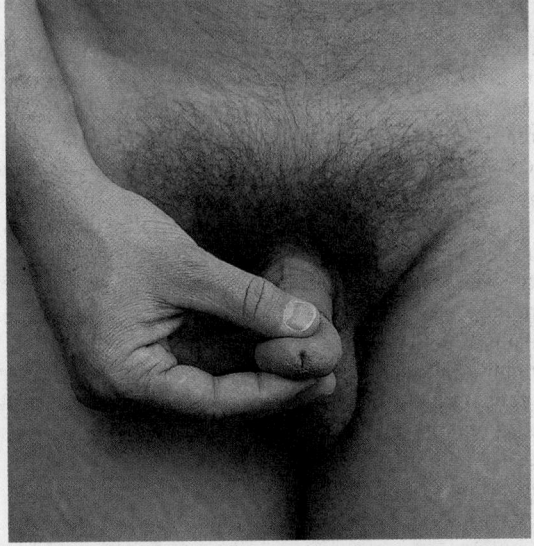

Testicular Self-Examination

Look for swelling or lumps in the skin of the scrotum while looking in the mirror.

Use both hands, placing the index and middle fingers under the testicles and the thumb on top (see illustration).

Gently roll the testicle, feeling for lumps, swelling, soreness, or a change in consistency (hardening).

Find the epididymis (a cordlike structure on the top and back of the testicle; it is not a lump).

Feel for small, pea-size lumps on the front and side of the testicle. The lumps are usually painless and are abnormal.

Call your health care provider for abnormal findings.

Illustrations from Seidel HM and others: *Mosby's guide to physical examination,* ed 6, St. Louis, 2006, Mosby.

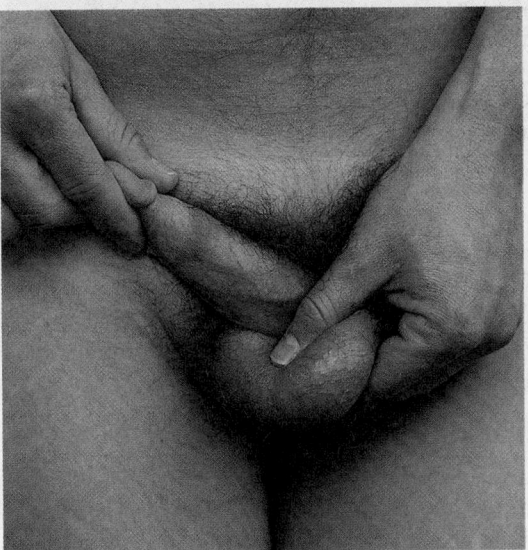

prolonged time sometimes develops dependent edema in the penis shaft.

It is important for any male client to learn to perform a genital self-examination to detect signs or symptoms of STDs. Many people who have an STD do not know it. Self-examination is a routine part of self-care (Box 33-28).

Scrotum

Be particularly cautious while inspecting and palpating the scrotum because the structures lying within the scrotal sac are very sensitive. The scrotum is divided internally into two halves. Each half contains a testicle, epididymis, and the vas deferens, which travels upward into the inguinal ring. Normally the left testicle is lower than the right. Inspect the scrotum's size, shape, and symmetry while observing for lesions or edema. Gently lift the scrotum to view the posterior surface. The scrotal skin is usually loose, and the surface is coarse. The scrotal skin is more deeply pig-

mented than body skin. Tightening or loss or wrinkling reveal edema. The size of the scrotum normally changes with temperature variations because the dartos muscle contracts in cold and relaxes in warm temperatures. Lumps in the scrotal skin are commonly sebaceous cysts.

Testicular cancer is a solid tumor common in young men ages 18 to 34 years. Early detection is critical. Explain testicular self-examination (see Box 33-29) while examining the client. The testes are normally sensitive but not tender. The underlying testicles are normally ovoid and approximately 2 to 4 cm (⅘ to 1⅗ inches) in size. Gently palpate the testicles and epididymis between the thumb and first two fingers. The testes feel smooth, rubbery, and free of nodules. The epididymis is resilient. Note the size, shape, and consistency of the organs. The most common symptoms of testicular cancer are a painless enlargement of one testis and the appearance of a palpable, small, hard lump, about the size of a pea, on the front or side of the testicle. In the older

✳ **TABLE 33-31 Nursing History for Rectal and Anal Assessment**

ASSESSMENT CATEGORY	RATIONALE
Determine whether client has experienced bleeding from rectum, black or tarry stools (melena), rectal pain, or change in bowel habits (constipation or diarrhea).	These are warning signs of colorectal cancer* or other gastrointestinal alterations.
Determine whether client has personal or strong family history of colorectal cancer, polyps, or chronic inflammatory bowel disease. Ask if client is over age 40.	These are risk factors for colorectal cancer.*
Assess dietary habits, including high fat intake, diet high in processed or red meats, or deficient fiber content (inadequate fruits and vegetables).	Bowel cancer is often linked to dietary intake of fat or insufficient fiber intake.*
Determine if client is obese, physically inactive, smokes, or consumes alcohol.	Risk factors for colorectal cancer.
Determine whether client has undergone screening for colorectal cancer (digital examination, fecal occult blood test, flexible sigmoidoscopy, and colonoscopy).	Undergoing this screening reflects understanding and compliance with preventive health care measures.
Assess medication history for use of laxatives or cathartic medications.	Repeated use causes diarrhea and eventual loss of intestinal muscle tone.
Assess for use of codeine or iron preparations.	Codeine causes constipation. Iron turns the color of feces black and tarry.
Ask male client if he has experienced weak or interrupted urine flow, inability to urinate, difficulty in starting or stopping urine flow, polyuria, nocturia, hematuria, or dysuria. Does client have continuing pain in lower back, pelvis, or upper thighs?	These are warning signs of prostatic cancer.* Symptoms also suggest infection or prostate enlargement.

*Data from American Cancer Society: *Cancer facts and figures 2006*, Atlanta, 2006, The Society.

adult the testicles decrease in size and are less firm during palpation. Continue to palpate the vas deferens separately as it forms the spermatic cord toward the inguinal ring, noting nodules or swelling. It normally feels smooth and discrete.

Inguinal Ring and Canal

The external inguinal ring provides the opening for the spermatic cord to pass into the inguinal canal. The canal forms a passage through the abdominal wall, a potential site for hernia formation. A hernia is a protrusion of a portion of intestine through the inguinal wall or canal. Sometimes an intestinal loop enters the scrotum. Have the client stand during this portion of the examination.

During inspection, ask the client to strain or bear down. The maneuver will help to make a hernia more visible. Look for obvious bulging in the inguinal area.

Complete the examination by palpating for inguinal lymph nodes. Normally, small, nontender, mobile horizontal nodes are palpable. Any abnormality indicates local or systemic infection or malignant disease.

Rectum and Anus

A good time to perform the rectal examination is after the genital examination. Usually you do not perform the examination in young children or adolescents. The examination detects colorectal cancer in its early stages. In men, the rectal examination also detects prostatic tumors. Collect a thorough history (Table 33-31) to detect the client's risk for bowel or rectal disease or prostatic disease.

The rectal examination is uncomfortable, so explaining all steps helps the client relax. Use a calm, slow-paced, gentle approach during the examination. Female clients remain in the dorsal recumbent position following genitalia examination or they assume a side-lying (Sims') position. The best way to examine men is to have the client stand and bend over forward with hips flexed and upper body resting across the examination table. Examine a nonambulatory client in Sims' position. Use disposable gloves.

Inspection

Using the nondominant hand, gently retract the buttocks to view the perianal and sacrococcygeal areas. Perianal skin is smooth and more pigmented and coarser than skin over the buttocks. Inspect anal tissue for skin characteristics, lesions, external **hemorrhoids** (dilated veins that appear as reddened protrusions), ulcers, fissures and fistulas, inflammation, rashes, or excoriation. Anal tissues are moist and hairless and the voluntary external muscle sphincter holds the anus closed. Next, ask the client to bear down as though having a bowel movement. Any internal hemorrhoids or fissures will appear at this time. Use clock reference (e.g., 3 o'clock or 8 o'clock) to describe location of findings. Normally there is no protrusion of tissue.

Digital Palpation

Examine the anal canal and sphincters with digital palpation, and in male clients, palpate the prostate gland to rule out enlargement (Box 33-29). Usually advanced practitioners perform this portion of the examination. This technique will not be discussed here.

✴ **BOX 33-29** **CLIENT TEACHING**

Rectal and Anal Assessment

Objectives
- Client will have a regular digital examination performed appropriate to age.
- Client will be able to identify symptoms of colorectal and prostatic cancer.
- Client will follow a nutritiously sound diet.

Teaching Strategies
- Discuss the American Cancer Society's (ACS's) guidelines (2006) for early detection of colorectal cancer with one of the following examination schedules beginning at age 50:
  - Digital rectal examination yearly
  - Fecal occult blood test (FOBT) yearly
  - Flexible sigmoidoscopy (FSIG): visual inspection of the rectum and lower colon with a hollow, lighted tube, performed by a physician every 5 years
  - Annual FOBT and FSIG every 5 years (preferred)
  - Double-contrast barium enema every 5 years
  - Colonoscopy every 10 years
  - Individuals at increased risk should discuss options with their health care provider.
- Discuss warning signs of colorectal cancer (see Table 33-6).
- Discuss dietary planning and healthy lifestyle choices to maintain or improve colon health.
- Warn client against problems caused by overuse of laxatives, cathartic medications, codeine, or enemas.
- Discuss with male client the ACS's guidelines (2006) for early detection of prostatic cancer:
  - Digital rectal examination performed annually after age 50
  - Annual prostate-specific antigen (PSA) blood test for men age 50 and over
  - Prostate ultrasound testing if results of either digital rectal examination or PSA test are suspicious
  - African American men or those with a first-degree relative diagnosed with prostate cancer need to begin testing at age 45
- Discuss the warning signs of prostatic cancer.

Evaluation
- During follow-up visits, determine whether client has had a rectal examination performed.
- Have client explain warning signs of colorectal and prostatic cancer.
- Ask client to describe appropriate lifestyle and food choices for healthy colon.

Musculoskeletal System

You conduct the musculoskeletal assessment as a separate examination or integrate it with other portions of the total physical examination. Assess this system while performing other nursing care measures such as bathing or positioning. The assessment of musculoskeletal function focuses on determining range of joint motion, muscle strength and tone, and joint and muscle condition. The assessment of musculoskeletal integrity is especially important when the client reports pain or loss of function in a joint or muscle. Frequently, muscular disorders are the result of neurological disease. For this reason, health care providers often conduct a neurological assessment simultaneously.

While examining the client's musculoskeletal function, visualize the anatomy of bone and muscle placement and joint structure (see Chapter 47). Joints vary in their degree of mobility. Some, as in the knee, are freely movable. The spinal vertebrae are examples of slightly movable joints.

For a complete examination expose the muscles and joints so they are free to move. Have the client assume a sitting, supine, prone, or standing position while assessing certain muscle groups. Table 33-32 lists the information gathered in the nursing history.

General Inspection

Observe the client's gait when entering the examination room. When a client is unaware of the nature of the observation, gait is more natural. Later a more formal test has the client walk in a straight line away and then return to point of origin. Note how the client walks, sits, and rises from a sitting position. Normally clients walk with the arms swinging freely at the sides and the head leading the body. Older adults often walk with smaller steps and a wider base of support. Note foot dragging, limping, shuffling, and the position of the trunk in relation to the legs.

Observe the client from the side in a standing position. The normal standing posture is upright with parallel alignment of the hips and shoulders (Figure 33-71). There is an even contour of the shoulders, level scapulae and iliac crests, alignment of the head over the gluteal folds, and symmetry of extremities. Looking sideways at the client, note the normal cervical, thoracic, and lumbar curves. Holding the head erect is normal. As the client sits, some degree of rounding of the shoulders is normal. Older adults tend to assume a stooped, forward-bent posture with the hips and knees somewhat flexed and arms bent at the elbows, raising the level of the arms.

Common postural abnormalities include lordosis, kyphosis, and scoliosis (Figure 33-72). **Kyphosis,** or hunchback, is an exaggeration of the posterior curvature of the thoracic spine. This postural abnormality is common in the older adult. **Lordosis,** or swayback, is an increased lumbar curvature. A lateral spinal curvature is called **scoliosis.** Loss of height is frequently the first clinical sign of osteoporosis, in which height loss occurs in the trunk as a result of vertebral fracture and collapse. **Osteoporosis** is a metabolic bone disease that causes a decrease in quality and quantity of bone. Lewis (2003) reports that osteoporosis affects 28 million Americans, the majority of which are women. This disease now affects 2 million men, and it will affect another 3 million men (Lewis, 2003). Osteoporosis not only affects adults, it strikes any age-group, including children (Holcomb, 2005). Although a small amount of height loss is to be expected with aging, if the amount of loss is great, osteoporosis is likely (Box 33-30, p. 628). As men and women age, they are more likely to have osteoporotic fractures of the forearm/wrists, hips, and vertebrae (Holcomb, 2005).

During general inspection look at the extremities for overall size, gross deformity, bony enlargement, alignment, and symmetry. Normally there is bilateral symmetry in length, circumference, alignment, and position and in the number of skin folds (Seidel and others, 2006). A general review pinpoints areas requiring specialized assessment.

✳ TABLE 33-32 Nursing History for Musculoskeletal Assessment

ASSESSMENT CATEGORY	RATIONALE
Determine if client is involved in competitive sports (particularly involving collision and contact), fails to warm up adequately, is in poor physical condition, or had had a rapid growth spurt (adolescents).	These are risk factors for sports injury.
Review client history for use of alcohol and/or caffeine; cigarette smoking; constant dieting; calcium intake less than 500 mg daily; thin and light body frame; nulliparous status; menopause before age 45; estrogen deficiency; postmenopause status; family history of osteoporosis; white, Asian, Native American, or northern European ancestry; advanced age; history of fractures/falls; inadequate calcium intake and vitamin D; sedentary lifestyle; chronic diseases (Cushing's hyperthyroidism and hypothyroidism, malabsorption/malnutrition disorders, neoplasm); long-term use of corticosteroids, methotrexate, phenytoin, aluminum-containing antacids; lack of weight-bearing exercise; lack of exposure to sunlight (Holcomb, 2005).	These are risk factors for osteoporosis.
Ask client to describe history of problems in bone, muscle, or joint function (e.g., recent fall, trauma, lifting of heavy objects, history of bone or joint disease with sudden or gradual onset, location of alteration).	History assists in assessing nature of musculoskeletal problem.
Assess nature and extent of pain, including location, duration, severity, predisposing and aggravating factors, relieving factors, and type.	Pain frequently accompanies alterations in bone, joints, or muscle. This has implications for not only comfort, but also ability to perform activities of daily living.
Assess client's normal activity pattern, including type of exercise routinely performed.	Provides baseline in assessment. Sedentary lifestyle and lack of appropriate exercise increases bone loss and risk of fractures.
Determine how alteration influences ability to perform activities of daily living (e.g., bathing, feeding, dressing, toileting, ambulating) and social functions (e.g., household chores, work, recreation, sexual activities).	The extent to which client is able to perform self-care will determine the level of nursing care. Type and degree of restriction in continuing social activities influence topics for client education and ability of nurse to identify alternative ways to maintain function.
Assess height loss of woman over age 50 by subtracting current height from recall of maximum adult height.	Measurement is useful screening tool to predict osteoporosis.

Palpation

Apply gentle palpation to all bones, joints, and surrounding muscles during a complete examination. In the case of a focused assessment, only examine the involved area. Note any heat, tenderness, edema, or resistance to pressure. The client should not feel any discomfort when you palpate. Muscles should be firm.

Range of Joint Motion

The examination includes comparison of both active and passive ROM. Ask the client to put each major joint through active and passive full ROM (see Chapter 47). Learn the correct terminology for the movements that the joints are capable of making (Table 33-33, p. 629), and instruct the client in how to move through each range of motion. Demonstrate range of motion to the client when possible. To assess ROM passively, ask the client to relax and then passively move the extremities through their range of motion. Compare the same body parts for equality in movement. Figure 33-73 shows an example of range-of-motion positions for the hand and wrist. Do not force a joint into a painful position. Know the normal range of each joint and the extent to which you can move the client's joints. Range of motion is equal between contra-

lateral joints. Ideally, assess the client's normal range to determine a baseline for assessing later change.

A **goniometer**, frequently used by physical and occupational therapists, measures the precise degree of motion in a particular joint and is mainly for clients who have a suspected reduction in joint movement. The instrument has two flexible arms with a 180-degree protractor in the center. Position the center of the protractor at the center of the joint you are measuring (Figure 33-74, p. 630). The arms extend along the body parts on each side of the protractor. You take a measurement of the joint angle before moving the joint. After taking the joint through a full range of motion, measure the angle again to determine the degree of movement. Compare the reading with the normal degree of joint movement.

Joints are typically free from stiffness, instability, swelling, or inflammation. There should be no discomfort when applying pressure to bones and joints. In older adults, joints often become swollen and stiff with reduced range of motion resulting from cartilage erosion and fibrosis of synovial membranes (see Chapter 47). If a joint appears swollen and inflamed, palpate it for warmth.

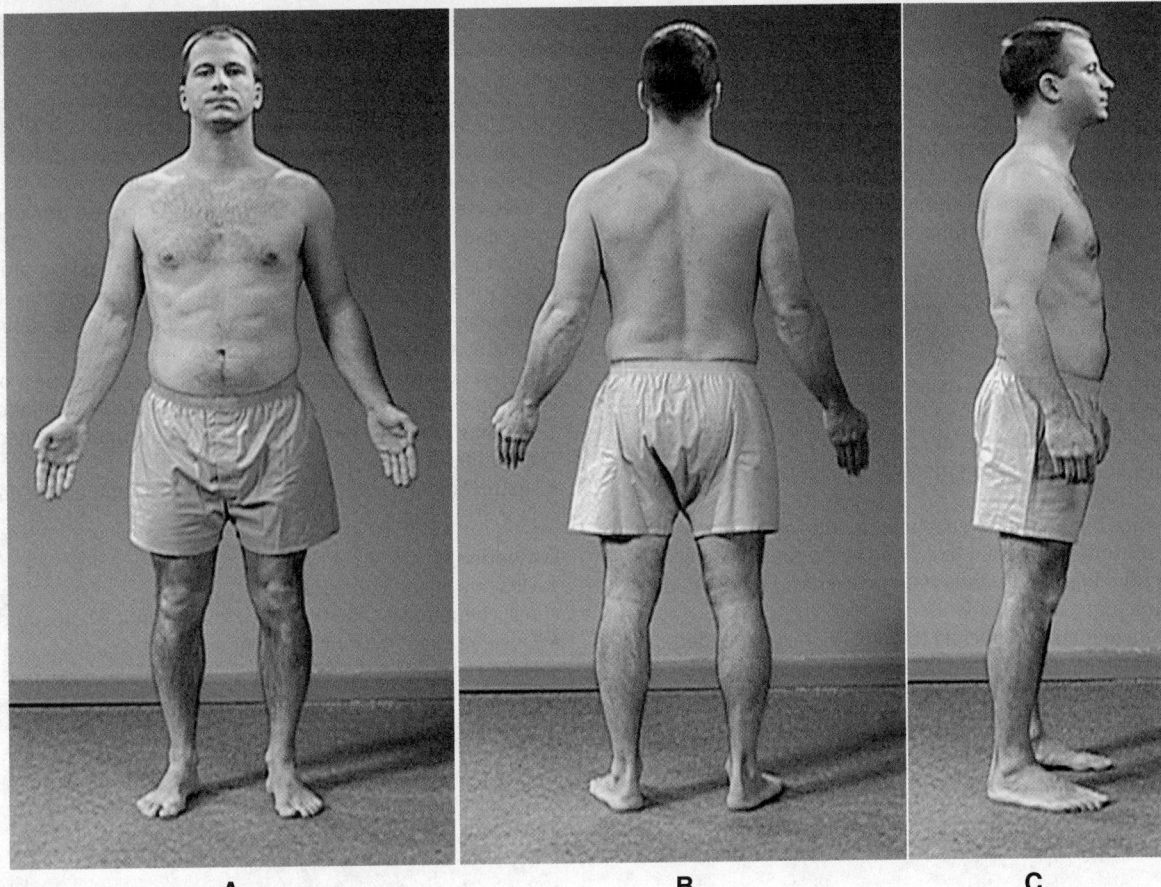

A   **B**   **C**

Figure 33-71 Inspection of overall body posture. **A,** Anterior view. **B,** Posterior view. **C,** Lateral view. (From Seidel HM and others: *Mosby's guide to physical examination,* ed 6, St. Louis, 2006, Mosby.)

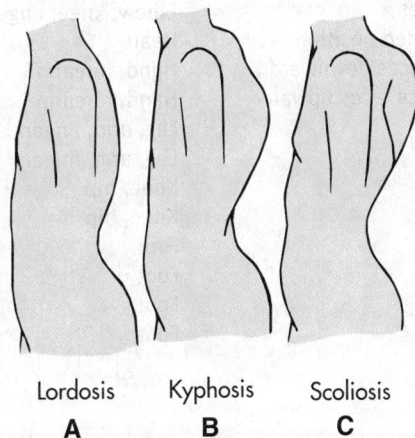

Lordosis   Kyphosis   Scoliosis
A   **B**   **C**

Figure 33-72 Common postural abnormalities. **A,** Lordosis. **B,** Kyphosis. **C,** Scoliosis.

Muscle Tone and Strength

Assess muscle strength and tone during ROM measurement. Integrate these findings with those from the neurological assessment. Note muscle tone, the slight muscular resistance felt as you move the relaxed extremity passively through its range of motion.

Ask the client to allow an extremity to relax or hang limp. This is often difficult, particularly if the client feels pain in the extremity. Support the extremity, and grasp each limb, moving it through the normal ROM (Figure 33-75, p. 630). Normal tone causes a mild, even resistance to movement through the entire range.

If a muscle has increased tone, or **hypertonicity,** you will meet considerable resistance with any sudden passive movement of a joint. Continued movement eventually causes the muscle to relax. A muscle that has little tone (**hypotonicity**) feels flabby. The involved extremity hangs loosely in a position determined by gravity.

For assessment of muscle strength, the client assumes a stable position. The client performs maneuvers demonstrating strength of major muscle groups (Table 33-34, p. 630). Compare symmetrical muscle pairs for strength based on a grading scale of 0 to 5 (Table 33-35, p. 630). The arm on the dominant side is normally stronger than the arm on the nondominant side. In the older adult a loss of muscle mass causes bilateral weakness, but muscle strength remains greater in the dominant arm or leg.

Examine each muscle group. Ask the client to first flex the muscle you are examining and then to resist when you apply an opposing force against that flexion. It is important to not allow the client to move the joint. Gradually increase pressure to a muscle group (e.g., elbow extension). Have the client resist the

✱ BOX 33-30   CLIENT TEACHING

Musculoskeletal Assessment

Objectives
- Client will follow measures to prevent or minimize osteoporosis.
- Client will assume proper body posture.
- Client will be able to perform self-care measures.

Teaching Strategies
- Instruct client in correct postural alignment. Consult with physical therapist to provide client with exercises for improving posture.
- Recommend women age 65 and older for routine screening for osteoporosis (U.S. Preventative Services Task Force, 2003). Recommend men for screening as well; they are equally at risk for development of osteoporosis as they age (Lewis, 2003).
- To reduce bone demineralization, instruct older adults in a proper exercise program (e.g., weight-bearing, muscle-strengthening and balance-training exercise) to be followed 3 or more times a week.
- Encourage intake of calcium to meet the recommended daily allowance. Increased vitamin D will aid calcium absorption.
- Recommendation for calcium supplements for adults over age 25 is 1000 to 1500 mg/day. Instruct client to take no more than 600 mg of calcium at one time.

- Explain to clients with low back pain that they will benefit from modification of worker risk factors (e.g., lifting heavy weights, use of protective equipment), regular aerobic exercise, exercises that strengthen the back and increase trunk flexibility, and learning how to lift properly.
- Instruct older adults and those with osteoporosis in proper body mechanics and range-of-motion and moderate weight-bearing exercises (e.g., swimming and walking) to minimize trauma and subsequent fracture of bones.
- Instruct client in use of assistive devices (e.g., zippers on clothing instead of buttons; elevation of chairs to minimize bending of knees and hips) when client is unable to perform activities of daily living.
- Instruct older clients to pace activities to compensate for loss in muscle strength.

Evaluation
- Observe client's posture.
- Ask client to describe therapies for preventing osteoporosis.
- Observe client perform range-of-motion exercises.
- Have client keep log of regular weight-training exercises.
- Ask client or family members to describe client's use of self-care aids.

✱ TABLE 33-33 Terminology for Normal Range-of-Motion Positions

TERM	RANGE OF MOTION	EXAMPLES OF JOINTS
Flexion	Movement decreasing angle between two adjoining bones; bending of limb	Elbow, fingers, knee
Extension	Movement increasing angle between two adjoining bones	Elbow, knee, fingers
Hyperextension	Movement of body part beyond its normal resting extended position	Head
Pronation	Movement of body part so that front or ventral surface faces downward	Hand, forearm
Supination	Movement of body part so that the front or ventral surface faces upward	Hand, forearm
Abduction	Movement of extremity away from midline of body	Leg, arm, fingers
Adduction	Movement of extremity toward midline of body	Leg, arm, fingers
Internal rotation	Rotation of joint inward	Knee, hip
External rotation	Rotation of joint outward	Knee, hip
Eversion	Turning of body part away from midline	Foot
Inversion	Turning of body part toward midline	Foot
Dorsiflexion	Flexion of toes and foot upward	Foot
Plantar flexion	Bending of toes and foot downward	Foot

pressure applied by attempting to move against resistance (e.g., elbow flexion). The client resists until instructed to stop. Vary the amount of pressure applied, then observe the joint move. If you identify a weakness, compare the size of the muscle with its opposite counterpart by measuring the circumference of the muscle body with a tape measure. A muscle that has **atrophied** (reduced in size) feels soft and boggy when palpated.

Neurological System

The neurological system is responsible for many functions, including initiation and coordination of movement, reception and perception of sensory stimuli, organization of thought processes, control of speech, and storage of memory. A close integration exists between the neurological system and all other body systems. For example, urine production relies in part on the adequacy of blood flow to the kidneys, and the size of arterioles supplying the kidneys is under neural control.

An assessment of neurological function alone is quite time consuming. For efficiency, integrate neurological measurements with other parts of the physical examination. For example, test cranial nerve function during the survey of the head and neck. Observe mental and emotional status during the initial interview.

Consider many variables when deciding the extent of the examination. A client's level of consciousness influences the ability to follow directions. General physical status influences tolerance

to assessment. The client's chief complaint also helps determine the need for a thorough neurological assessment. If the client complains of headache or a recent loss of function in an extremity, the client will need a complete neurological review. Table 33-36 reviews the data collected in the nursing history. For a complete examination, you will need the following special equipment:

- Reading material
- Vials containing aromatic substances (e.g., vanilla extract and coffee)
- Opposite tip of cotton swab or tongue blade broken in half
- Snellen eye chart
- Penlight
- Vials containing sugar or salt
- Tongue blade
- Two test tubes, one filled with hot water and the other with cold water
- Cotton balls or cotton-tipped applicators
- Tuning fork
- Reflex hammer

Mental and Emotional Status

You learn a great deal about mental capacities and emotional state by simply interacting with the client. Ask questions during an examination to gather data and observe the appropriateness of emotions and thoughts. There are special assessment tools designed to assess a client's mental status. The Mental Status Questionnaire

TABLE 33-36 Nursing History for Neurological Assessment

ASSESSMENT CATEGORY	RATIONALE
Determine client use of analgesics, alcohol, sedatives, hypnotics, antipsychotics, antidepressants, nervous system stimulants, or recreational drugs.	These medications alter level of consciousness or cause behavioral changes. Abuse sometimes causes tremors, ataxia, and changes in peripheral nerve function.
Determine if client has recent history of seizures/convulsions: clarify sequence of events (aura, fall to ground, motor activity, loss of consciousness); character of any symptoms; and relationship of seizure to time of day, fatigue, or emotional stress.	Seizure activity often originates from central nervous system alteration. Characteristics of seizure help determine its origin.
Screen client for symptoms of headache, tremors, dizziness, vertigo, numbness or tingling of body part, visual changes, weakness, pain, or changes in speech. Presence of any symptom requires more detailed review (onset, severity, precipitating factors or sequence of events).	These symptoms frequently originate from alterations in central nervous system or peripheral nervous system function. Identification of specific patterns aids in diagnosis of pathological condition.
Discuss with client's family any recent changes in client's behavior (e.g., increased irritability, mood swings, memory loss, change in energy level).	Behavioral changes sometimes result from intracranial pathological states.
Assess client for history of change in vision, hearing, smell, taste, or touch.	Major sensory nerves originate from brain stem. These symptoms help to localize nature of problem.
If an older client displays sudden acute confusion (delirium), review history for drug toxicity (anticholinergics, diuretics, digoxin, cimetidine, sedatives, antihypertensives, antiarrhythmics), serious infections, metabolic disturbances, heart failure, and severe anemia.	This is one of the most common mental disorders in older persons. Condition is always potentially reversible (see Box 33-32).
Review past history for head or spinal cord injury, meningitis, congenital anomalies, neurological disease, or psychiatric counseling.	Factors cause neurological symptoms or behavioral changes to develop, focusing assessment on possible cause.

※ **BOX 33-31 MMSE Sample Questions**

- Orientation to time
  "What is the date?"
- Registration
  "Listen carefully. I am going to say three words. You say them back after I stop.
  Ready? Here they are . . .
  HOUSE (pause), CAR (pause), LAKE (pause). Now repeat those words back to me."
  [Repeat up to five times, but score only the first trial.]
- Naming
  "What is this?" [Point to a pencil or pen.]
- Reading
  "Please read this and do what it says." [Show examinee the words on the stimulus form.]
  CLOSE YOUR EYES

Reproduced by special permission of the Publisher, Psychological Assessment Resources, Inc., 16204 North Florida Avenue, Lutz, Florida 33549, from Mini-Mental State Examination, by Marshal Folstein and Susan Folstein, Copyright 1975, 1998, 2001 by Mini Mental, LLC, Inc. Published 2001 by Psychological Assessment Resources, Inc. Further reproduction is prohibited without permission of PAR, Inc. The MMSE can be purchased from PAR, Inc. by calling (800) 331-8378 or (813) 968-3003.

※ **BOX 33-32 Clinical Criteria for Delirium**

- *Definition:* An acute disturbance of consciousness that is accompanied by a change in cognition. It is not due to a preexisting or evolving dementia. Delirium develops over a short period of time, usually hours to days, and tends to fluctuate during the course of the day. It is usually a direct physiological consequence of a general medical condition. It is most common in older adults, but occurs occasionally in younger clients.
- There is reduced clarity of awareness of the environment.
- Ability to focus, sustain, or shift attention is impaired (questions must be repeated).
- Irrelevant stimuli easily distract the person.
- There is an accompanying change in cognition (memory impairment, disorientation, or language disturbance).
- Commonly affects recent memory.
- Disorientation usually occurs, with client disoriented to time, place, or person.
- Language disturbance involves impaired ability to name objects or ability to write; speech is sometimes rambling.
- Perceptual disturbances include misinterpretations, delusions, or visual and auditory hallucinations. Neurologic signs include tremor, unsteady gait, asterixis, or myoclonus.

Modified from American Psychiatric Association: *Diagnostic and statistical manual of mental disorders,* ed 4, text revision, Washington, DC, 2000, The Association; Stuart G, Laraia M: *Principles and practice of psychiatric nursing,* ed 8, St. Louis, 2005, Mosby; and Gray-Vickrey, P: What's behind acute delirium, *Nursing made incredibly easy* 3(1):20, 2005.

(MSQ) developed by Kahn and others (1960) is a 10-item instrument and a widely used tool. The Mini-Mental State Examination (MMSE) is another instrument developed by Folstein, Folstein, and McHugh (1975) that measures orientation and cognitive function. The sample questions in Box 33-31 offer examples of questions found on the MMSE. A maximum score on the MMSE is 30. Clients with scores of 21 or less generally reveal cognitive impairment requiring further evaluation.

To ensure an objective assessment, consider the client's cultural and educational background, values, beliefs, and previous experiences. Such factors influence response to questions. An alteration in mental or emotional status reflects a disturbance in cerebral functioning. The cerebral cortex controls and integrates intellectual and emotional functioning. Primary brain disorders, medication, and metabolic changes are examples of factors that change cerebral function.

Delirium is a common mental disorder among older adults. It is an acute mental disorder characterized by confusion, disorientation, and restlessness. The acute condition is often misdiagnosed as a form of dementia, a more progressive, organic mental disorder such as Alzheimer's disease. Thus many health care providers miss the underlying cause of the condition. When it occurs, many think it is common older adult behavior. Delirium is often overlooked in older adults because of a failure to adequately assess mental status. Fortunately, the condition often reverses when it is correctly assessed and the underlying cause is treated (central nervous system [CNS], metabolic, and cardiopulmonary disorders; systemic illnesses; and sensory deprivation or overload) (Stuart and Laraia, 2005). Frequently clients who develop delirium are labeled with sundown syndrome because the delirium frequently worsens at night. Many practitioners mistake this as being common with old age. Be aware that delirium has occurred in children having surgery (20%) and hospitalized children (8%)

(Gray-Vickrey, 2005). Obtain a good history of the client's behavior before delirium develops so as to recognize the condition early. Family members are usually a good resource. Box 33-32 summarizes clinical criteria for delirium.

Level of Consciousness. A person's level of consciousness exists along a continuum from full awakening, alertness, and cooperation to unresponsiveness to any form of external stimuli. Talk with the client, asking questions about events involving the client or concerns about any health problems. A fully conscious client responds to questions quickly and expresses ideas logically. With a lowering of the client's consciousness, use the Glasgow Coma Scale (GCS) for an objective measurement of consciousness on a numerical scale (Table 33-37). The client needs to be as alert as possible before testing. Use caution when using the scale if a client has sensory losses (e.g., vision or hearing). The GCS allows evaluation of a client's neurological status over time. The higher the score, the better the client's neurological function. Ask short, simple questions such as "What is your name?" "Where are you?" and "What day is this?" Also ask the client to follow simple commands, such as "Move your toes."

If a client is not conscious enough to follow commands, try to elicit the pain response. Apply firm pressure with the thumb over the root of the client's fingernail. The normal response to the painful stimuli is withdrawal of the body part from the stimulus. A client with serious neurological impairment exhibits abnormal posturing in response to pain. A flaccid response indicates the absence of muscle tone in the extremities and severe injury to brain tissue.

TABLE 33-37 Glasgow Coma Scale

ACTION	RESPONSE	SCORE
Eyes open	Spontaneously	4
	To speech	3
	To pain	2
	None	1
Best verbal response	Oriented	5
	Confused	4
	Inappropriate words	3
	Incomprehensible sounds	2
	None	1
Best motor response	Obeys commands	6
	Localized pain	5
	Flexion withdrawal	4
	Abnormal flexion	3
	Abnormal extension	2
	Flaccid	1
	TOTAL SCORE	15

Behavior and Appearance. Behavior, moods, hygiene, grooming, and choice of dress reveal pertinent information about mental status. Remain perceptive of the client's mannerisms and actions during the entire physical assessment. Note nonverbal and verbal behaviors. Does the client respond appropriately to directions? Does the client's mood vary with no apparent cause? Does the client show concern about appearance? Is the client's hair clean and neatly groomed, and are the nails trim and clean? The client should behave in a manner expressing concern and interest in the examination. The client should make eye contact with the nurse and express appropriate feelings that correspond to the situation. Normally the client will show some degree of personal hygiene.

Choice and fit of clothing reflect socioeconomic background or personal taste rather than deficiency in self-concept or self-care. Avoid being judgmental, and focus assessment on the appropriateness of clothing for the weather. Older adults sometimes neglect their appearance because of a lack of energy, finances, or reduced vision.

Language. Normal cerebral function allows a person to understand spoken or written words and to express the self through written words or gestures. Assess the client's voice inflection, tone, and manner of speech. Normally the client's voice has inflections, is clear and strong, and increases in volume appropriately. Speech is fluent. When communication is clearly ineffective (e.g., omission or addition of letters and words, misuse of words, or hesitations), assess for **aphasia**. Injury to the cerebral cortex results in aphasia.

The two types of aphasia are sensory (or receptive) and motor (or expressive). With receptive aphasia a person cannot understand written or verbal speech. With expressive aphasia a person understands written and verbal speech but cannot write or speak appropriately when attempting to communicate. A client sometimes suffers a combination of receptive and expressive aphasia.

Assess language capabilities when it is clear that ineffective communication with the client exists. Some simple assessment techniques include the following:

- Point to a familiar object, and ask the client to name it.
- Ask the client to respond to simple verbal and written commands, such as "Stand up" or "Sit down"
- Ask the client to read simple sentences out loud.

Normally a client names objects correctly, follows commands, and reads sentences correctly.

Intellectual Function

Intellectual function includes memory (recent, immediate, and past), knowledge, abstract thinking, association, and judgment. Testing each aspect of function involves a specific technique. However, because cultural and educational background influences the ability to respond to test questions, do not ask questions related to concepts or ideas with which the client is unfamiliar.

Memory. Assess immediate recall and recent and remote memory. Clients demonstrate immediate recall by repeating a series of numbers (e.g., *7, 4, 1*) in the order they are presented or in reverse order. Clients normally recall a series of five to eight digits forward and four to six digits backward.

First ask to test the client's memory. Then state clearly and slowly the name of three unrelated objects. After mentioning all three, ask the client to repeat each. Continue until the client is successful. Then, later in the assessment, ask the client to repeat the three words again. The client should be able to identify the three words. Another test for recent memory involves asking the client to recall events occurring during the same day (e.g., what was eaten for breakfast). Validate information with a family member.

To assess past memory, ask the client to recall the maiden name of the client's mother, a birthday, or a special date in history. It is best to ask open-ended questions rather than simple yes/no questions. A client usually has immediate recall of such information. With older adults do not interpret a hearing loss as confusion. Good communication techniques are essential throughout the examination to ensure that the client clearly understands all directions and testing.

Knowledge. Assess knowledge by asking how much the client knows about his or her illness or the reason for seeking health care. By assessing a client's knowledge, a client's ability to learn or understand can be determined. If there is an opportunity to teach, test the client's mental status by asking for feedback during a follow-up visit.

Abstract Thinking. Interpreting abstract ideas or concepts reflects the capacity for abstract thinking. For an individual to explain common phrases such as "A stitch in time saves nine" or "Don't count your chickens before they're hatched" requires a higher level of intellectual function. Note whether the client's explanations are relevant and concrete. The client with altered mental status will probably interpret the phrase literally or merely rephrase the words.

Association. Another higher level of intellectual functioning involves finding similarities or associations between concepts: a dog is to a beagle as a cat is to a Siamese. Name related concepts, and ask the client to identify their associations. Questions are appropriate to the client's level of intelligence. Using simple concepts is sufficient.

Judgment. Judgment requires a comparison and evaluation of facts and ideas to understand their relationships and to form appropriate conclusions. Attempt to measure the client's ability to make logical decisions with questions such as "Why did you seek health care?" or "What would you do if you became ill at home?" Normally a client makes logical decisions.

Cranial Nerve Function

To assess cranial nerve function, you may test all 12 cranial nerves or a single nerve or related group of nerves. A dysfunction in one nerve reflects an alteration at some point along the distribution of the cranial nerve. Measurements used to assess the integrity of organs within the head and neck also assess cranial nerve func-

tion. A complete assessment involves testing the 12 cranial nerves in order of their numbers. To remember the order of the nerves, use this simple phrase, "On old Olympus' towering tops, a Finn and German viewed some hops." The first letter of each word in the phrase is the same as the first letter of the names of the cranial nerves listed in order (Table 33-38).

Sensory Function

The sensory pathways of the central nervous system conduct sensations of pain, temperature, position, vibration, and crude and finely localized touch. Different nerve pathways relay the sensations. Most clients require only a quick screening of sensory function unless there are symptoms of reduced sensation, motor impairment, or paralysis.

> **SAFETY ALERT** The risk of skin breakdown is greater in a client with impaired sensation. When assessing decreased sensation, complete a skin and tissue assessment of the area affected by the sensory loss. In addition, teach the client to avoid pressure, thermal, and/or chemical trauma to the area.

✳ **TABLE 33-38 Cranial Nerve Function and Assessment**

Number	Name	Type	Function	Method
I	Olfactory	Sensory	Sense of smell	Ask client to identify different nonirritating aromas such as coffee and vanilla.
II	Optic	Sensory	Visual acuity	Use Snellen chart, or ask client to read printed material while wearing glasses.
III	Oculomotor	Motor	Extraocular eye movement	Assess directions of gaze.
IV	Trochlear	Motor	Pupil constriction and dilation	Measure pupillary reaction to light reflex and accommodation.
			Upward and downward movement of eyeball	Assess directions of gaze.
V	Trigeminal	Sensory and motor	Sensory nerve to skin of face	Lightly touch cornea with wisp of cotton. Assess corneal reflex. Measure sensation of light pain and touch across skin of face.
			Motor nerve to muscles of jaw	Palpate temples as client clenches teeth.
VI	Abducens	Motor	Lateral movement of eyeballs	Assess directions of gaze.
VII	Facial	Sensory and motor	Facial expression	As client smiles, frowns, puffs out cheeks, and raises and lowers eyebrows, look for asymmetry.
			Taste	Have client identify salty or sweet taste on front of tongue.
VIII	Auditory	Sensory	Hearing	Assess ability to hear spoken word.
IX	Glossopharyngeal	Sensory and motor	Taste	Ask client to identify sour or sweet taste on back of tongue.
			Ability to swallow	Use tongue blade to elicit gag reflex.
X	Vagus	Sensory and motor	Sensation of pharynx	Ask client to say "ah." Observe movement of palate and pharynx.
			Movement of vocal cords	Assess speech for hoarseness.
XI	Spinal accessory	Motor	Movement of head and shoulders	Ask client to shrug shoulders and turn head against passive resistance.
XII	Hypoglossal	Motor	Position of tongue	Ask client to stick out tongue to midline and move it from side to side.

Normally a client has sensory responses to all stimuli that are tested. A client feels sensations equally on both sides of the body in all areas. Assess the major sensory nerves by knowing the sensory dermatome zones (Figure 33-76). Some areas of the skin are innervated by specific dorsal root cutaneous nerves. For example, if assessment reveals reduced sensation when checking for light touch along an area of the skin (e.g., the lower neck), this determines, in general, where a neurological lesion exists (e.g., fourth cervical spinal cord segment).

Perform all sensory testing with the client's eyes closed so that the client is unable to see when or where a stimulus strikes the skin (Table 33-39). Then apply stimuli in a random, unpredictable order to maintain the client's attention and prevent detection of a predictable pattern. Ask the client to describe when, what, and where he or she feels each stimulus. Compare symmetrical areas of the body while applying stimuli to the client's arms, trunk, and legs.

Motor Function

An assessment of motor function includes measurements made during the musculoskeletal examination. In addition, you assess cerebellar function. The cerebellum coordinates muscular activity, maintains balance and equilibrium, and controls posture.

Coordination. To avoid confusion, demonstrate each maneuver and then have the client repeat it, observing for smoothness and balance in the client's movements (Box 33-33). In older adults normally slow reaction time causes movements to be less rhythmical.

To assess fine motor function, have the client extend the arms out to the sides and touch each forefinger alternately to the nose (first with eyes open, then with eyes closed). Normally the client alternately touches the nose smoothly. Performing rapid, rhythmical, alternating movements demonstrates coordination in the

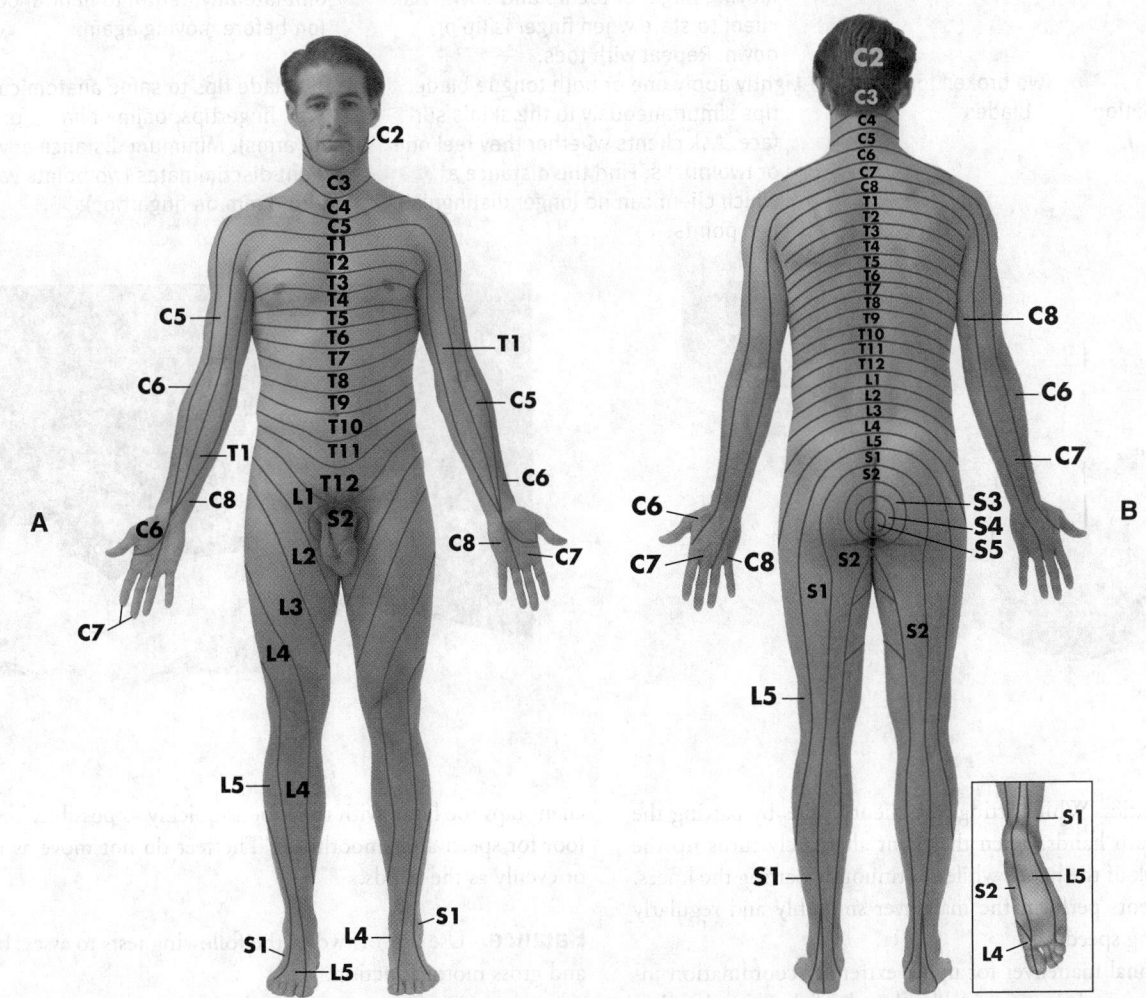

Figure 33-76 Dermatomes of the body, the body surface areas innervated by particular spinal nerves; C1 usually has no cutaneous distribution. **A,** Anterior view. (From Seidel HM and others: *Mosby's guide to physical examination,* ed 6, St. Louis, 2006, Mosby.) **B,** Posterior view. It appears that there is a distinct separation of surface area controlled by each dermatome, but there is almost always overlap between spinal nerves. (From Seidel HM and others: *Mosby's guide to physical examination,* ed 6, St. Louis, 2006, Mosby.)

TABLE 33-39 Assessment of Sensory Nerve Function

FUNCTION	EQUIPMENT	METHOD	PRECAUTIONS
Pain	Broken tongue blade or wooden end of cotton applicator	Ask clients to voice when they feel dull or sharp sensation. Alternately apply sharp and blunt ends of tongue blade to skin's surface. Note areas of numbness or increased sensitivity.	Remember that areas where skin is thick, such as heel or sole of foot, are less sensitive to pain.
Temperature	Two test tubes, one filled with hot water and other with cold	Touch skin with tube. Ask client to identify hot or cold sensation.	Omit test if pain sensation is normal.
Light touch	Cotton ball or cotton-tip applicator	Apply light wisp of cotton to different points along skin's surface. Ask clients to voice when they feel a sensation.	Apply at areas where skin is thin or more sensitive (e.g., face, neck, inner aspect of arms, top of feet and hands).
Vibration	Tuning fork	Apply stem of vibrating fork to distal interphalangeal joint of fingers and interphalangeal joint of great toe, elbow, and wrist. Have clients voice when and where they feel vibration.	Be sure client feels vibration and not merely pressure.
Position		Grasp finger or toe, holding it by its sides with thumb and index finger. Alternate moving finger or toe up and down. Ask client to state when finger is up or down. Repeat with toes.	Avoid rubbing adjacent appendages as you move finger or toe. Do not move joint laterally; return to neutral position before moving again.
Two-point discrimination	Two broken tongue blades	Lightly apply one or both tongue blade tips simultaneously to the skin's surface. Ask clients whether they feel one or two pricks. Find the distance at which client can no longer distinguish two points.	Apply blade tips to same anatomical site (e.g., fingertips, palm of hand, or upper arms). Minimum distance at which client discriminates two points varies (2 to 8 mm on fingertips).

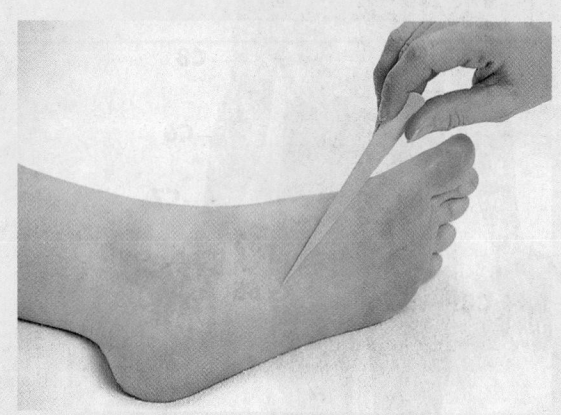
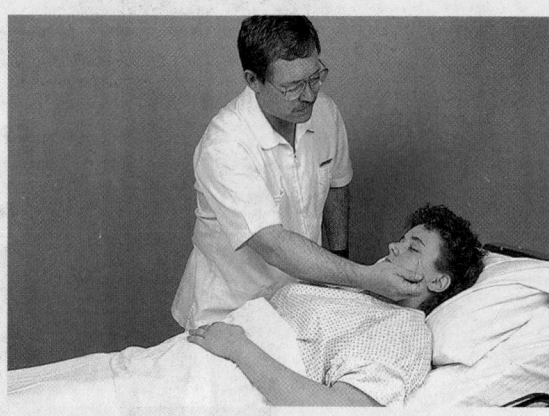

upper extremities. While sitting, the client begins by patting the knees with both hands. Then the client alternately turns up the palm and back of the hands while continuously patting the knees. Normally clients perform the maneuver smoothly and regularly with increasing speed.

An additional maneuver for upper extremity coordination involves touching each finger with the thumb of the same hand in rapid sequence. The client moves from the index finger to the little finger and back, with one hand tested at a time. The client's dominant hand is slightly less awkward when performing this movement. Movement is smooth and in succession.

Test lower extremity coordination with the client lying supine, legs extended. Place a hand at the ball of the client's foot. The client taps the hand with the foot as quickly as possible. Test each foot for speed and smoothness. The feet do not move as rapidly or evenly as the hands.

Balance. Use one or two of the following tests to assess balance and gross motor function:

• Have the client perform a Romberg's test by standing with feet together, arms at the sides, both with eyes open and eyes closed. Protect the client's safety by standing at the side, observe for swaying. Expect slight swaying of the body in the Romberg's test. A loss of balance (positive Romberg) causes a client to fall to the side. Normally the client does not break the stance.

✳ BOX 33-33   CLIENT TEACHING

Neurological Assessment

Objectives
- Client's family will understand relationship of client's behavioral and mental changes to physical status.
- Client with sensory or motor impairment will select safety measures for self-care.
- Older adult will routinely inspect skin for injuries.

Teaching Strategies
- Explain to family or friends the implications of any behavioral or mental impairment shown by client.
- If client has sensory or motor impairments, explain measures to ensure safety (e.g., use of ambulation aids or safety bars in bathrooms or stairways).
- Teach older adult to plan enough time to complete tasks because reaction time is slow.
- Teach older adult to observe skin surfaces for areas of trauma, because perception of pain is reduced.

Evaluation
- Ask family to discuss client behaviors that result from neurological impairments.
- Have client explain safety measures used to avoid injury from sensory and motor limitations.
- Have older client explain reason for inspecting skin surface routinely.

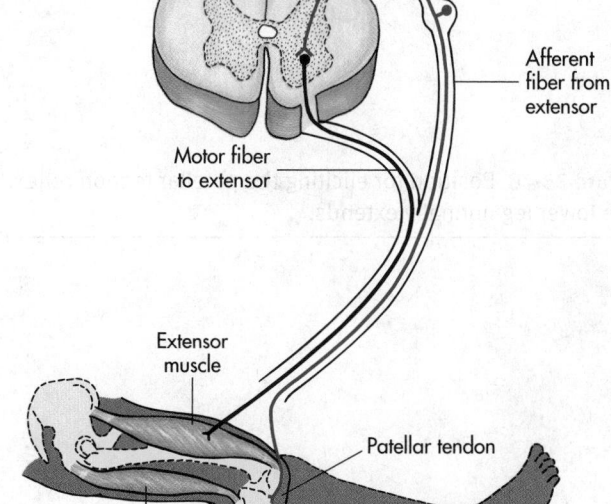

Figure 33-77 Pathway of the reflex arc.

- Have the client close the eyes, with arms held straight at the sides, and stand on one foot and then the other. Normally clients are able to maintain balance for 5 seconds with slight swaying.
- Ask the client to walk a straight line by placing the heel of one foot directly in front of the toes of the other foot.

SAFETY ALERT When examining the older adult client's gait, be aware of the risk for falls. Some older adult clients need assistance with this portion of the examination.

Reflexes

Eliciting reflex reactions provides data about the integrity of sensory and motor pathways of the reflex arc and specific spinal cord segments. Assessment of reflexes does not determine higher neural center functioning. Figure 33-77 traces the pathway of the reflex arc. Each muscle contains a small sensory unit called a muscle spindle, which controls muscle tone and detects changes in the length of muscle fibers. Tapping a tendon with a reflex hammer stretches the muscle and tendon, lengthening the spindle. The spindle sends nerve impulses along afferent nerve pathways to the dorsal horn of the spinal cord segment. Within milliseconds the impulses reach the spinal cord and synapse to travel to the efferent motor neuron in the spinal cord. A motor nerve sends the impulses back to the muscle, causing the reflex response.

The two categories of normal reflexes are deep tendon reflexes, elicited by mildly stretching a muscle and tapping a tendon, and cutaneous reflexes, elicited by stimulating the skin superficially. Grade reflexes as follows (Seidel and others, 2006):

0	No response
1+	Sluggish or diminished
2+	Active or expected response
3+	More brisk than expected, slightly hyperactive
4+	Brisk and hyperactive with intermittent or transient clonus

When assessing reflexes have the client relax as much as possible to avoid voluntary movement or tensing of muscles. Position the limbs to slightly stretch the muscle being tested. Hold the reflex hammer loosely between the thumb and fingers so that it is able to swing freely and tap the tendon briskly (Figure 33-78). Compare the responses on corresponding sides. Normally the older adult presents with diminished reflexes. Reflexes are hyperactive in clients with alcohol, cocaine, or opioid intoxication (Caulker-Burnett, 1994). Stick figures are sometimes used to record reflexes. Table 33-40 summarizes common deep tendon and cutaneous reflexes.

After the Examination

Record findings from the physical assessment during the examination or at the end. Special forms are available to record data. Review all findings before assisting the client with dressing, in case

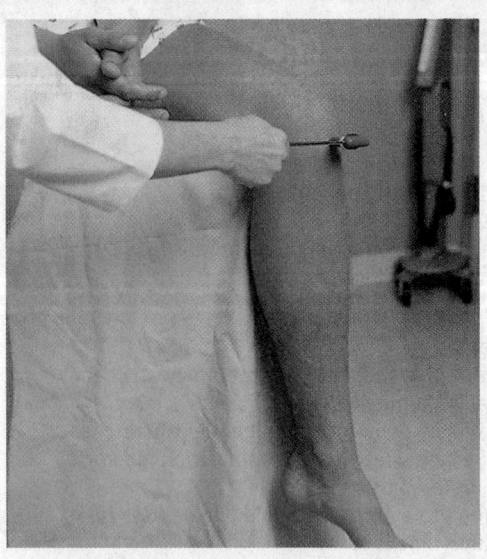

Figure 33-78 Position for eliciting the patellar tendon reflex. The lower leg normally extends.

✳ TABLE 33-40	Assessment of Common Reflexes	
TYPE	**PROCEDURE**	**NORMAL REFLEX**
Deep Tendon Reflexes		
Biceps	Flex client's arm up to 45 degrees at elbow with palms down. Place your thumb in antecubital fossa at base of biceps tendon and your fingers over biceps muscle. Strike triceps tendon with reflex hammer.	Flexion of arm at elbow
Triceps	Flex client's arm at elbow, holding arm across chest, or hold upper arm horizontally and allow lower arm to go limp. Strike triceps tendon just above elbow.	Extension at elbow
Patellar	Have client sit with legs hanging freely over side of table or chair, or have client lie supine and support knee in a flexed 90-degree position. Briskly tap patellar tendon just below patella.	Extension of lower leg
Achilles	Have client assume same position as for patellar reflex. Slightly dorsiflex client's ankle by grasping toes in palm of your hand. Strike Achilles tendon just above heel at ankle malleolus.	Plantar flexion of foot
Cutaneous Reflexes		
Plantar	Have client lie supine with legs straight and feet relaxed. Take handle end of reflex hammer and stroke lateral aspect of sole from heel to ball of foot, curving across ball of foot toward big toe.	Plantar flexion of all toes
Gluteal	Have client assume side-lying position. Spread buttocks apart and lightly stimulate perineal area with cotton applicator.	Contraction of anal sphincter
Abdominal	Have client stand or lie supine. Stroke abdominal skin with base of cotton applicator over lateral borders of rectus abdominis muscle toward midline. Repeat test in each abdominal quadrant.	Contraction of rectus abdominis muscle with pulling of umbilicus toward stimulated side

of a need to recheck any information or gather additional data. Integrate physical assessment findings into the plan of care.

After completing the assessment, give the client time to dress. The hospitalized client sometimes needs help with hygiene and returning to bed. When the client is comfortable, it helps to share a summary of the assessment findings. If the findings have revealed serious abnormalities, such as a mass or highly irregular heart rate, consult the client's health care provider before revealing any findings. It is the health care provider's responsibility to make definitive medical diagnoses. Explain the type of abnormality found and the need for the health care provider to conduct an additional examination.

Delegate the cleaning of the examination area to support staff if needed. Use infection-control practices in removing materials or instruments soiled with potentially infectious wastes. If the client's bedside was the examination site, clear away soiled items from the bedside table, and make sure that the bed linen is dry and clean. The client will appreciate a clean gown and the opportunity to wash the face and hands. Afterward, be sure to perform hand hygiene.

Be sure to record a complete assessment. If you delayed entering any items into the assessment form, record them at this time to avoid forgetting any important information. If you made entries periodically during the examination, review them for accuracy and thoroughness. Communicate significant findings to appropriate medical and nursing personnel, either verbally or in the client's written care plan.

The client often needs a number of ancillary examinations, such as x-ray examinations, laboratory tests, or ultrasonography, after a physical examination. The tests provide additional screening information to rule out the presence of abnormalities and help in the diagnosis of specific abnormalities found during the examination. Explain the purpose of these tests and the sensations that the client will experience.

✳ Key Concepts

- Baseline assessment findings reflect the client's functional abilities and serve as the basis for comparison with subsequent assessment findings.
- Physical assessment of a child or infant requires the application of the principles of growth and development.
- Recognize that the normal process of aging affects physical findings collected from an older adult.
- Integrate client teaching throughout the examination to help clients learn about health promotion and disease prevention.
- Inspection requires good lighting, full exposure of the body part, and a careful comparison of the part with its counterpart on the opposite side of the body.
- Palpation involves the use of parts of the hand to detect different types of physical characteristics.
- Use auscultation to assess the character of sounds created in various body organs.
- Perform a physical examination only after proper preparation of the environment and equipment and after preparing the client physically and psychologically.
- Throughout the examination keep the client warm, comfortable, and informed of each step of the process.
- A competent examiner is systematic while combining assessment of different body systems simultaneously.
- Information from the history helps to focus on body systems likely to be affected.
- When assessing a seriously ill client, concentrate on the body systems most likely to be affected.
- Creating a mental image of internal organs in relation to external anatomical landmarks enhances accuracy in assessing the thorax, heart, and abdomen.
- When assessing heart sounds, imagine events occurring during the cardiac cycle.
- Never palpate the carotid arteries simultaneously.
- When examining a woman's breasts, explain the techniques for breast self-examination.

- The abdominal assessment differs from other portions of the examination in that auscultation follows inspection.
- During assessment of the genitalia, explain the technique for genital self-examination.
- Conduct an assessment of musculoskeletal function when observing the client ambulate or participate in other active movements.
- Assess mental and emotional status by interacting with the client throughout the examination.
- At the end of the examination provide for the client's comfort, and then document a detailed summary of physical assessment findings.

✳ Critical Thinking Exercises

You are caring for Mrs. Brown, a 75-year-old retired schoolteacher who underwent repair of right fractured femur attributed to osteoporosis. This is her first postoperative day on your clinical unit. The night nurse reported that the client had an "uneventful" night. She has an intravenous line (IV) for fluids and medication, a right hip dressing, a Jackson-Pratt drain, a Foley (urethral) catheter to gravity and is on bed rest.

1. What body systems would you assess for this client?
   A. Describe the key elements in these assessments.

2. Upon entrance to the room, you observe that Mrs. Brown appears agitated and confused. How do you further evaluate her mental status? What condition may these symptoms indicate?

3. After you reorient Mrs. Brown, she allows you to continue with your assessment. Upon auscultation of her posterior lung field bases, you hear a crackling noise upon inspiration. What is this sound, and what does it indicate?

4. You next assess her cardiac status. Her apical heart rate is 72 beats per minute, rhythm regular. You interpret this finding as:
   a. Abnormal
   b. Bradycardia
   c. Normal
   d. Tachycardia

5. You are performing neurovascular checks of the lower extremities. Describe how you would evaluate for capillary refill.

✳ NCLEX®-Style Review Questions

1. The nurse conducts a general survey on an adult client, which includes:
   1. Appearance and behavior
   2. Measurement of vital signs
   3. Observing specific body systems
   4. Conducting a detailed health history

2. To correctly palpate the client's skin for temperature, the nurse uses the:
   1. Base of the hands
   2. Fingertips of the hands.
   3. Dorsal surface of the hands.
   4. Palmar surface of the hands.

3. To assess a client's superficial lymph nodes, the nurse:
   1. Deeply palpates using the entire hand
   2. Lightly palpates using a bimanual technique
   3. Deeply palpates using a bimanual technique
   4. Gently palpates using the pads of the index and middle fingers

4. The nurse is teaching the client to inspect all skin surfaces and to report pigmented skin lesions that:
   1. Are symmetrical
   2. Are uniform in color
   3. Have irregular borders
   4. Are less than 6 mm in diameter

5. To auscultate the client's lung fields, the nurse uses a systematic pattern comparing:
   1. Top to bottom
   2. Anterior to posterior
   3. Side to side
   4. Interspace to interspace

6. The client's respiratory assessment reveals a loud, low-pitched, rumbling coarse sound heard during inspiration and expiration. The nurse interprets these sounds as:
   1. Crackles
   2. Normal
   3. Rhonchi
   4. Wheezes

7. While auscultating heart sounds, the nurse documents that S_2 is best heard at the base. This sound (S_2) correlates with closure of the:
   1. Aortic and mitral valves
   2. Mitral and tricuspid valves
   3. Aortic and pulmonic valves
   4. Tricuspid and pulmonic valves

8. To assess the client's dorsalis pedis pulse, the nurse palpates:
   1. Behind the knee
   2. Over the lateral malleolus
   3. In the groove behind the medial malleolus
   4. Lateral to the extensor tendon of the great toe

9. To spread breast tissue evenly over the chest wall during an examination, the nurse asks the client to lie supine with:
   1. Both arms overhead with palms upward
   2. Hands clasped just above the umbilicus
   3. The dominant arm straight along side the body
   4. The ipsilateral arm overhead with a small pillow under the shoulder

10. Place in order the assessment techniques employed during an abdominal examination.
    1. Palpation
    2. Inspection
    3. Percussion
    4. Auscultation

11. The nurse is teaching a client how to perform a testicular self-examination. The nurse informs the client:
    1. "The testes are normally round, movable, and have a lumpy consistency."
    2. "Contact your health care provider if you feel a painless pea-size nodule."
    3. "The best time to do a testicular self-examination is before your bath or shower."
    4. "Perform a testicular self-examination weekly to detect signs of testicular cancer."

12. The client is being assessed for range of joint movement. You ask the client to move the arm toward the body, evaluating the movement of:
    1. Flexion
    2. Extension
    3. Abduction
    4. Adduction

13. The nurse asks the client to interpret the saying "Don't count your chickens before they're hatched." The client's response reveals:
    1. Judgment
    2. Knowledge
    3. Association
    4. Abstract reasoning

14. The nurse asks the client to shrug the shoulders and turn the head side to side against the resistance of the examiner's hand; these actions evaluate cranial nerve number:
    1. VII—facial
    2. V—trigeminal
    3. XII—hypoglossal
    4. XI—spinal accessory

34 | Infection Prevention and Control

OBJECTIVES

Mastery of content in this chapter will enable the student to:
- Explain the relationship between the chain of infection and transmission of infection.
- Give an example for preventing infection for each element of the infection chain.
- Identify the body's normal defenses against infection.
- Discuss the events in the inflammatory response.
- Identify clients most at risk for infection.
- Describe the signs/symptoms of a localized infection and those of a systemic infection.
- Explain conditions that promote the transmission of health care–associated infection.
- Explain the difference between medical and surgical asepsis.
- Explain the rationale for standard precautions.
- Perform proper procedures for hand hygiene.
- Explain how infection control measures may differ in the home versus the hospital.
- Properly don a surgical mask, sterile gown, and sterile gloves.
- Explain procedures for each isolation category.
- Understand the definition of occupational exposure.
- Explain the postexposure process.

MEDIA RESOURCES

 Companion CD
- NCLEX®-Style Review Questions
- Audio Glossary
- Interactive Learning Activities
- English/Spanish Glossary

 Website
- NCLEX®-Style Review Questions
- Audio Glossary
- English/Spanish Glossary
- Interactive Learning Activities
- Weblinks
- Audio Summaries
- Video Clips
- Nursing Skills Online

KEY TERMS

Aerobic, p. 643
Anaerobic, p. 643
Asepsis, p. 654
Asymptomatic, p. 642
Bactericidal, p. 644
Bacteriostasis, p. 644
Broad-spectrum antibiotics, p. 646
Carriers, p. 643
Colonization, p. 642
Communicable disease, p. 642
Contaminated, p. 644
Cough etiquette, p. 661
Disinfection, p. 658
Dose, p. 643
Edema, p. 647
Endogenous infection, p. 648
Epidemiology, p. 668
Exogenous infection, p. 648

Exudates, p. 647
Granulation tissue, p. 648
Hand hygiene, p. 655
Hand washing, p. 655
Health care–acquired infections, p. 648
Health care–associated infections, p. 648
Host resistance, p. 643
Iatrogenic infections, p. 648
Immunocompromised, p. 643
Infectious, p. 642
Inflammatory response, p. 646
Invasive, p. 642
Leukocytosis, p. 648
Localized, p. 645
Medical asepsis, p. 655
Microorganisms, p. 642
Necrotic, p. 646

Normal flora, p. 646
Nosocomial infections, p. 648
Pathogen, p. 642
Pathogenicity, p. 645
Phagocytosis, p. 648
Purulent, p. 648
Sanguineous, p. 648
Serous, p. 648
Standard precautions, p. 655
Sterile field, p. 671
Sterilization, p. 659
Suprainfection, p. 646
Surgical asepsis, p. 668
Susceptibility, p. 645
Suppurative, p. 651
Symptomatic, p. 642
Systemic, p. 645
Vector, p. 644
Virulence, p. 643

The incident rate of clients developing infections as the direct result of hospital stay and hospital procedures is increasing. Several states have passed legislation requiring hospitals to report their infection rates and specific type of infections. This reporting permits clients to see infection rates for facilities and select their point of care. The Joint Commission (TJC) (2007) is viewing this as a client safety issue. Infection prevention and control are essential for creating a safe health care environment for clients and staff. As a nurse, you play a primary role in infection prevention and control in all health care settings. Clients in all health care settings are at risk for acquiring infections because of lower resistance to infectious **microorganisms,** increased exposure to numbers and types of disease-causing microorganisms, and **invasive** procedures. Staff are at risk for exposure to infections as the result of contact with client blood, body fluids, and contaminated equipment and surfaces. In acute care or ambulatory care facilities, clients can be exposed to pathogens, some of which may be resistant to most antibiotics. By practicing basic infection prevention and control techniques, you can avoid spreading microorganisms to clients and sustaining an exposure when providing direct care.

In all settings, clients and their families need to be able to recognize sources of infections and institute protective measures. Client teaching needs to include basic information on infection, the various modes of transmission, and methods of prevention appropriate to their care needs.

Health care workers protect themselves from contact with infectious material, sharps injury and/or exposure to a communicable disease by using knowledge of the infectious process and appropriate personal protective equipment (PPE). Diseases such as hepatitis B and C, human immunodeficiency virus (HIV) infection, acquired immunodeficiency syndrome (AIDS), tuberculosis (TB), and multidrug-resistant organisms require a greater emphasis on infection prevention and control techniques.

Nature of Infection

Infection is the entry and multiplication of an organism (infectious agent) in a host. If an infectious agent (**pathogen**) is merely present in a host, it does not mean that infection will occur. If a microorganism is present or invades a host, grows and/or multiplies but does not cause infection, this is referred to as **colonization.** Infections are infectious or communicable. An **infectious** disease may not pose a risk for transmission. Illness such as viral meningitis or pneumonia are infectious. The illness, although possibly serious for the client, does not pose a risk to others, including caregivers.

If the infectious disease can be transmitted directly from one person to another, it is termed a **communicable disease.** If the pathogens multiply and cause clinical signs and symptoms, the infection is **symptomatic.** If clinical signs and symptoms are not present, the illness is termed **asymptomatic.** Hepatitis C is a communicable disease that can be asymptomatic. It is most efficiently transmitted through the direct passage of blood into the skin from a percutaneous exposure even if the source client is asymptomatic (Centers for Disease Control and Prevention [CDC], 2001).

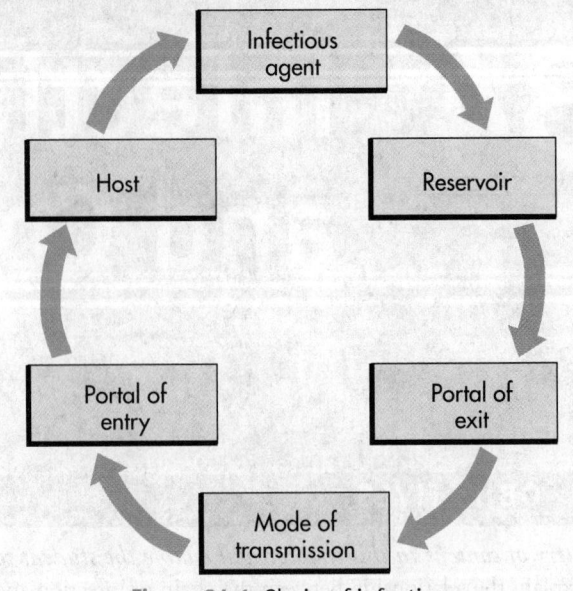

Figure 34-1 Chain of infection.

Chain of Infection

The presence of a pathogen does not mean that an infection will occur. Infection occurs in a cycle that depends on the presence of all of the following elements:

- An infectious agent or pathogen
- A reservoir or source for pathogen growth
- A portal of exit from the reservoir
- A mode of transmission
- A portal of entry to a host
- A susceptible host

Infection can develop if this chain remains uninterrupted (Figure 34-1). It is imperative that nurses follow infection prevention and control practices to break the chain so that infection will not develop.

Infectious Agent. Microorganisms include bacteria, viruses, fungi, and protozoa (Table 34-1). Microorganisms on the skin are either resident or transient flora. Resident organisms (normal flora) are permanent residents of the skin, where they survive and multiply without causing illness. It fact, they serve as a major part of the body's protection. Resident flora on the skin covers the entire exterior of the body and protects against pathogens. It is important to retain and maintain resident flora (CDC, 2002b).

Transient microorganisms attach to the skin when a person has contact with another person or object during normal activities. For example, when a nurse touches a bedpan or a contaminated dressing, transient bacteria adhere to the nurse's skin. The organisms attach loosely to the skin in dirt and grease or under fingernails. These organisms may be readily transmitted unless removed using hand hygiene (Larson, 2005). If hands are visibly soiled with proteinaceous material, soap and water is the preferred prac-

✳ **TABLE 34-1 Common Pathogens and Some Infections or Diseases They Produce**

Organism	Major Reservoir(s)	Major Infections/Diseases
Bacteria		
Escherichia coli	Colon	Gastroenteritis, urinary tract infection
Staphylococcus aureus	Skin, hair, anterior nares, mouth	Wound infection, pneumonia, food poisoning, cellulitis
Streptococcus (beta-hemolytic group A) organisms	Oropharynx, skin, perianal area	"Strep throat," rheumatic fever, scarlet fever, impetigo, wound infection
Streptococcus (beta-hemolytic group B) organisms	Adult genitalia	Urinary tract infection, wound infection, postpartum sepsis, neonatal sepsis
Mycobacterium tuberculosis	Droplet nuclei from lungs, larynx	Tuberculosis
Neisseria gonorrhoeae	Genitourinary tract, rectum, mouth	Gonorrhea, pelvic inflammatory disease, infectious arthritis, conjunctivitis
Rickettsia rickettsii	Wood tick	Rocky Mountain spotted fever
Staphylococcus epidermidis	Skin	Wound infection, bacteremia
Viruses		
Hepatitis A virus	Feces	Hepatitis A
Hepatitis B virus	Blood and certain body fluids, sexual contact	Hepatitis B
Hepatitis C virus	Blood, certain body fluids, sexual contact	Hepatitis C
Herpes simplex virus (type 1)	Lesions of mouth or skin, saliva, genitalia	Cold sores, aseptic meningitis, sexually transmitted disease, herpetic whitlow
Human immunodeficiency virus (HIV)	Blood, semen, vaginal secretions via sexual contact	Acquired immunodeficiency syndrome (AIDS)
Fungi		
Aspergillus organisms	Soil, dust, mouth, skin, colon, genital tract	Aspergillosis, pneumonia, sepsis
Candida albicans	Mouth, skin, colon, genital tract	Candidiasis, pneumonia, sepsis
Protozoa		
Plasmodium falciparum	Blood	Malaria

Modified from Ritter H: Clinical microbiology. In Carrico R, editor: *APIC text of infection control and epidemiology,* Washington, DC, 2005, Association for Professionals in Infection Control and Epidemiology.

tice. If hands are not visibly soiled, use of an alcohol-based hand product or hand washing with soap and water is acceptable for disinfecting hands of health care workers (CDC, 2002).

The potential for microorganisms or parasites to cause disease depends on the following factors:

- Sufficient number of organisms (**dose**)
- **Virulence,** or ability to survive in the host or outside the body
- Ability to enter and survive in the host
- Susceptibility of the host (**host resistance**)

Resident skin microorganisms are not virulent. However, they can cause serious infection when surgery or other invasive procedures allow them to enter deep tissues or when a client is severely **immunocompromised** (has an impaired immune system).

Reservoir. A reservoir is a place where a pathogen can survive but may or may not multiply. For example, hepatitis A virus survives in shellfish but does not multiply; *Pseudomonas* organisms may survive and multiply in nebulizer reservoirs used in the care of clients with respiratory problems. The most common reservoir is the human body. A variety of microorganisms live on the skin and within the body cavities, fluids, and discharges. The presence of microorganisms does not always cause a person to become ill. **Carriers** are persons who show no symptoms of illness but who

have pathogens on or in their bodies that can be transferred to others. For example, a person can be a carrier of hepatitis B virus without having signs or symptoms of infection. These persons transmit the disease to others through their blood or through sexual contact. Animals, food, water, insects, and inanimate objects can also be reservoirs for infectious organisms. *Clostridium botulinum* toxin, which causes botulism, survives in improperly processed foods (e.g., home-canned green beans and infant formulas). The bacterium *Legionella pneumophila,* which causes legionnaires' disease, survives in contaminated water and water systems. To thrive, organisms require a proper environment, including appropriate food, oxygen, water, temperature, pH, and light.

Food. Microorganisms require nourishment. Some, such as *Clostridium perfringens,* the microbe that causes gas gangrene, thrive on organic matter. Others, such as *Escherichia coli,* consume undigested foodstuff in the bowel. Carbon dioxide and inorganic material such as soil provide nourishment for other organisms.

Oxygen. **Aerobic** bacteria require oxygen for survival and for multiplication sufficient to cause disease. Aerobic organisms cause more infections in humans, when compared with **anaerobic** organisms. Examples of aerobic organisms are *Staphylococcus aureus* and strains of *Streptococcus* organisms. Anaerobic bacteria thrive where little or no free oxygen is available. Infections deep within the pleural cavity, in a joint, or in a deep sinus tract are typically caused by anaerobes. Bacteria that cause tetanus, gas gangrene, and botulism are anaerobes. An example of an anaerobic organism is *Clostridium difficile,* an organism that causes antibiotic-induced diarrhea.

Water. Most organisms require water or moisture for survival. For example, a frequent place for microorganisms is the moist drainage from a surgical wound. Some bacteria assume a form, called a spore, that is resistant to drying. Spore-forming bacteria include organisms such as those that cause anthrax, botulism, and tetanus. These can live without water.

Temperature. Microorganisms can live only in certain temperature ranges. Each species of bacteria has a specific temperature at which it grows best. The ideal temperature for most human pathogens is 20° to 43° C (68° to 109° F). For example, *Legionella pneumophila* grows best in water at 77° to 108° F (Ritter, 2005). However, some can survive temperature extremes that would be fatal to humans. Cold temperatures tend to prevent growth and reproduction of bacteria (**bacteriostasis**). A temperature or chemical that destroys bacteria is **bactericidal**.

pH. The acidity of an environment determines the viability of microorganisms. Most microorganisms prefer an environment within a pH range of 5 to 7. Bacteria in particular thrive in urine with an alkaline pH. Most organisms cannot survive the acid environment of the stomach. Acid-reducing medications (e.g., antacids and H_2 blockers) may cause an overgrowth of gastrointestinal organisms, which can contribute to health care–associated pneumonia in a client receiving these medications (CDC, 2005b).

Light. Microorganisms thrive in dark environments such as those under dressings and within body cavities.

Portal of Exit.

After microorganisms find a site to grow and multiply, they must find a portal of exit if they are to enter another host and cause disease. Portals of exit include sites such as blood, skin and mucous membranes, respiratory tract, genitourinary tract, gastrointestinal tract, and transplacental (mother to fetus).

Skin and Mucous Membranes. The skin may be considered a portal of exit because any break in the integrity of the skin and mucous membranes may allow pathogens to exit the body. This may be exhibited by the creation of purulent drainage. For example, *S. aureus* causes a characteristic yellow, creamy drainage, and infection with *Pseudomonas aeruginosa* causes a greenish, creamy drainage. The presence of purulent drainage is a potential portal of exit.

Respiratory Tract. Pathogens that infect the respiratory tract, such as *Mycobacterium tuberculosis* or influenza virus, can be released from the body when an infected person sneezes or coughs. The act of coughing or sneezing allows for organisms to exit the respiratory tract. In clients with artificial airways such as tracheostomy or endotracheal tubes, organisms easily exit the respiratory tract through these devices when the device is manipulated or suctioned (see Chapter 40).

Urinary Tract. Normally urine is sterile. However, when a client has a urinary tract infection (UTI), microorganisms exit during urination or through urinary diversions such as ileostomies and suprapubic drains (see Chapter 45).

Gastrointestinal Tract. The mouth is one of the most bacterially contaminated sites of the human body, but most of the organisms are normal flora. Organisms that are normal flora in one person can be pathogens in another. Organisms, for example, exit when a person expectorates saliva. Kissing can also provide a means of exit. For example, *Neisseria,* the organism responsible for meningitis in young adults, is normal flora in the mouth and is transmitted to another person via kissing. In addition, gastrointestinal portals of exit include bowel elimination, drainage of bile via surgical wounds, or drainage tubes.

Reproductive Tract. Organisms such as *Neisseria gonorrhoeae* and HIV may exit through a man's urethral meatus or a woman's vaginal canal during sexual contact. HIV is present in much higher numbers in semen than in female vaginal secretions.

Blood. The blood is normally a sterile body fluid, but in the case of communicable diseases such as hepatitis B or C or HIV it becomes a reservoir for pathogens. Caregivers may become exposed during activities such as blood drawing, starting an intravenous (IV) line, or giving an injection unless standard precautions are taken and needle-safe devices are used. A blood-borne pathogen exposure involves being stuck with a sharp **contaminated** with infected blood.

Modes of Transmission.

Each disease has a specific mode of transmission. For example, some types of encephalitis are transmitted by infected mosquitoes. The mosquito serves as a **vector**, transmitting the virus when it bites the host. Table 34-2 summarizes the most common modes of transmission. However, some microorganisms may be transmitted by more than one route. For example, varicella zoster (chickenpox) may be spread by the airborne route in droplet nuclei or by direct contact.

The major route of transmission for pathogens identified in the health care setting is the unwashed hands of the health care worker (CDC, 2002b; Cipriano, 2007). Equipment used within the environment (e.g., a stethoscope, blood pressure cuff, bedside commode, or shower chair) can become a source for the transmission of pathogens. All hospital personnel providing direct care (e.g., nurses, physical therapists, and physicians) and persons performing diagnostic and support services (e.g., laboratory technicians, respiratory therapists, and dietary workers) must follow infection prevention and control practices to minimize the spread of infection. Each group follows procedures for handling and cleaning equipment and supplies used by a client. For example, respiratory therapists perform hand hygiene before working with each client and dispose of or clean contaminated therapy equipment according to established infection prevention and control procedures. Medical devices and the performance of diagnostic procedures provide a mode of entry for pathogens. For example, starting a line for IV infusion introduces bacteria if the skin is not properly cleansed. Invasive procedures such as cystoscopy (visualization of the bladder) also increase the risk of introducing infection. Because so many factors promote the spread of infection to a client, all health care workers must be diligent in using infection prevention and control practices, such as proper hand hygiene and ensuring that shared equipment is adequately cleaned, disinfected, and/or sterilized before it is used again.

Portal of Entry.

Organisms enter the body through the same routes they use for exiting. For example, when a needle pierces a client's skin, organisms enter the body if a proper skin preparation

✳ TABLE 34-2   Modes of Transmission

ROUTES AND MEANS	EXAMPLES OF ORGANISMS
Contact	
DIRECT	
Person-to-person (fecal, oral)	
Physical contact between source and susceptible host (e.g., touching client feces and then touching your inner mouth or consuming contaminated food)	Hepatitis A virus, *Shigella, Staphylococcus*
INDIRECT	
Personal contact of susceptible host with contaminated inanimate object (e.g., needles or sharp objects, dressings, environment)	Hepatitis B virus, hepatitis C virus, human immunodeficiency virus (HIV), *Staphylococcus,* respiratory syncytial virus (RSV), *Pseudomonas,* methicillin-resistant *Staphylococcus aureus* (MRSA)
DROPLET	
Large particles that travel up to 3 feet and come in contact with susceptible host (e.g., coughing, sneezing, or talking)	Influenza virus, rubella virus, bacterial meningitis
Airborne	
Droplet nuclei, or residue or evaporated droplets suspended in air (e.g., coughing, sneezing) or carried on dust particles	*Mycobacterium tuberculosis* (tuberculosis), varicella zoster virus (chickenpox), *Aspergillus,* measles virus
Vehicles	
Contaminated items	*Vibrio cholerae,* MRSA
Water	*Pseudomonas, Legionella*
Drugs, solutions	*Pseudomonas*
Blood	Hepatitis B virus, hepatitis C virus, HIV, syphilis
Food (improperly handled, stored, or cooked; fresh or thawed meats)	*Salmonella, Escherichia coli, Clostridium botulinum*
Vector	
External mechanical transfer (flies)	*V. cholerae*
Internal transmission such as parasitic conditions between **vector** and host, such as:	
Mosquito	*Plasmodium falciparum* (malaria), West Nile virus
Louse	*Rickettsia typhi*
Flea	*Yersinia pestis* (plague)
Tick	*Borrelia burgdorferi* (Lyme disease)

is not performed. Any obstruction to the flow of urine from a urinary catheter allows organisms to migrate up the urethra. Factors that reduce the body's defenses enhance the chances of pathogens entering the body.

Susceptible Host. Whether a person acquires an infection depends on susceptibility to an infectious agent. **Susceptibility** depends on the individual degree of resistance to a pathogen (immune response). Although everyone is constantly in contact with large numbers of microorganisms, an infection does not develop until an individual becomes susceptible to the strength and numbers of microorganisms (dose) capable of producing infection. The more virulent an organism, the greater the dose, the more likely a person will develop an infection. Some of the factors that influence a person's susceptibility (resistance) include age, nutritional status, presence of chronic disease, trauma, and smoking. Organisms with resistance to key antibiotics are becoming more common in all health care settings, but especially acute care. This is associated with the frequent and sometimes inappropriate use of antibiotics over the years in all settings (i.e., acute care, ambulatory care, clinics, and long-term care).

The Infectious Process

By understanding the chain of infection, you are vital in preventing infections. When the client acquires an infection, observe for signs and symptoms of infection and take appropriate actions to prevent its spread. Infections follow a progressive course (Box 34-1). The severity of the client's illness depends on the extent of the infection, the **pathogenicity** of the microorganisms, dose of the organism, and the susceptibility of the host.

If an infection is **localized** (e.g., a wound infection), the client usually experiences localized symptoms, such as pain and tenderness and redness at the wound site. Use standard precautions, appropriate PPE, and hand hygiene when assessing the wound. The use of these precautions and hand hygiene will block the spread of infection to other sites or clients. An infection that affects the entire body instead of just a single organ or part is **systemic** and can become fatal if undetected and untreated.

The course of an infection influences the level of nursing care provided. The nurse is responsible for properly administering antibiotics, monitoring the response to drug therapy (see Chap-

---

✳ BOX 34-1 Course of Infection by Stage

Incubation Period
Interval between entrance of pathogen into body and appearance of first symptoms (e.g., chickenpox, 10 to 21 days post exposure; common cold, 1 to 2 days; influenza, 1 to 5 days; mumps, 12 to 26 days).

Prodromal Stage
Interval from onset of nonspecific signs and symptoms (malaise, low-grade fever, fatigue) to more specific symptoms. (During this time, microorganisms grow and multiply, and client may be capable of spreading disease to others.) For example, herpes simplex begins with itching and tingling at the site before the lesion appears.

Illness Stage
Interval when client manifests signs and symptoms specific to type of infection. (For example, strep throat is manifested by sore throat, pain, and swelling; mumps is manifested by high fever, parotid and salivary gland swelling.)

Convalescence
Interval when acute symptoms of infection disappear. (Length of recovery depends on severity of infection and client's host resistance; recovery may take several days to months.)

---

ter 35), and using proper hand hygiene and standard precautions. Supportive therapy includes providing adequate nutrition and rest to bolster defenses against the infectious process. The course of care for the client may have additional effects on body systems affected by the infection.

The nurse plays a vital role in the control of infection whether infection is localized or systemic. For example, if the nurse uses improper hand hygiene and skin preparation technique, the organism causing wound infection can be transferred to that same client's IV site. Infection from one client's wound infection can transfer to another clients' tracheostomy site. Nurses who have breaks in their own skin are at risk for infections from blood or tissues if proper infection prevention and control practices, such as gloves and proper hand hygiene, are not used. However, if the nurse has an open area too large to be covered with a dressing, the nurse should not perform client care procedures (CDC, 2002b; Occupational Safety and Health Administration [OSHA], 2001).

Defenses Against Infection

The body has normal defenses, which protect against infection. Normal body flora that reside inside and outside of the body protect a person against pathogens. Intact skin protects from pathogens, and linings of the nasal passageways act to prevent organisms from entering the lungs. Each organ system has defense mechanisms that work to prevent exposure to infection. The **inflammatory response** is a protective reaction that serves to neutralize pathogens and repair body cells. Normal flora, body system defenses, and inflammation are all nonspecific defenses that protect against microorganisms regardless of prior exposure. The immune system is composed of separate cells that help the body resist disease. Certain responses of the immune system are nonspecific, whereas others are specific defenses against specific pathogens. If any of the body's defenses fail, an infection can occur. This infection may lead to a serious health problem.

Normal Flora. The body normally contains microorganisms that reside on the surface and deep layers of skin, in the saliva and oral mucosa, and in the gastrointestinal and genitourinary tracts. A person normally excretes trillions of microbes daily through the intestines. **Normal flora** do not usually cause disease when residing in their usual area of the body but instead participate in maintaining health.

Normal flora of the large intestine exist in large numbers without causing illness. Normal flora also secrete antibacterial substances within the intestine's walls. The skin's normal flora exert a protective, bactericidal action that kills organisms landing on the skin. The mouth and pharynx are also protected by flora that impair growth of invading microbes. Normal flora maintain a sensitive balance with other microorganisms to prevent infection. Any factor that disrupts this balance places a person at increased risk for acquiring a disease. For example, the use of **broad-spectrum antibiotics** for the treatment of infection can lead to **suprainfection**. A suprainfection develops when broad-spectrum antibiotics eliminate a wide range of normal flora organisms, not just those causing infection. When normal bacterial flora are eliminated, the body's defenses are reduced, which allows for disease-producing microorganisms to multiply, causing illness.

Body System Defenses. A number of the body's organ systems have unique defenses against infection (Table 34-3). The skin, respiratory tract, and gastrointestinal tract are easily accessible to microorganisms. Pathogenic organisms can adhere to the skin's surface, be inhaled into the lungs, or be ingested with food. Each organ system has defense mechanisms physiologically suited to its specific structure and function. For example, the lungs cannot completely control the entrance of microorganisms. However, the airways are lined with moist mucous membranes and with hairlike projections, or cilia, that rhythmically beat to move mucus or cellular debris up to the pharynx to be expelled.

Inflammation. The body's cellular response to injury, infection, or irritation is termed inflammation. Inflammation is a protective vascular reaction that delivers fluid, blood products, and nutrients to an area of injury. The process neutralizes and eliminates pathogens or dead (**necrotic**) tissues and establishes a means of repairing body cells and tissues. Signs of localized inflammation may include swelling, redness, heat, pain or tenderness, and loss of function in the affected body part. When inflammation becomes systemic, other signs and symptoms develop, including fever, leukocytosis, malaise, anorexia, nausea, vomiting, lymph node enlargement, or organ failure.

The inflammatory response may be triggered by physical agents, chemical agents, or microorganisms. Mechanical trauma, temperature extremes, and radiation are examples of physical agents. Chemical agents include external and internal irritants such as harsh poisons or gastric acid. Microorganisms may also trigger this response.

TABLE 34-3 Normal Defense Mechanisms Against Infection

DEFENSE MECHANISMS	ACTION	FACTORS THAT MAY ALTER DEFENSE MECHANISMS
Skin		
Intact multilayered surface (body's first line of defense against infection)	Provides barrier to microorganisms and antibacterial activity	Cuts, abrasions, puncture wounds, areas of maceration
Shedding of outer layer of skin cells	Removes organisms that adhere to skin's outer layers	Failure to bathe regularly, improper hand-washing technique
Sebum	Contains fatty acid that kills some bacteria	Excessive bathing
Mouth		
Intact multilayered mucosa	Provides mechanical barrier to microorganisms	Lacerations, trauma, extracted teeth
Saliva	Washes away particles containing microorganisms	Poor oral hygiene, dehydration
	Contains microbial inhibitors (e.g., lysozyme)	
Eye		
Tearing and blinking	Provides mechanisms to reduce entry (blinking) or to assist in washing away (tearing) particles containing pathogens, thus reducing dose of organisms	Injury, exposure—splash/splatter of blood or other potentially infectious material into the eye
Respiratory Tract		
Cilia lining upper airway, coated by mucus	Trap inhaled microbes and sweep them outward in mucus to be expectorated or swallowed	Smoking, high concentration of oxygen and carbon dioxide, decreased humidity, cold air
Macrophages	Engulf and destroy microorganisms that reach lung's alveoli	Smoking
Urinary Tract		
Flushing action of urine flow	Washes away microorganisms on lining of bladder and urethra	Obstruction to normal flow by urinary catheter placement, obstruction from growth or tumor, delayed micturition
Intact multilayered epithelium	Provides barrier to microorganisms	Introduction of urinary catheter, continual movement of catheter in urethra
Gastrointestinal Tract		
Acidity of gastric secretions	Prevents retention of bacterial contents	Administration of antacids
Rapid peristalsis in small intestine		Delayed motility resulting from impaction of fecal contents in large bowel or mechanical obstruction by masses
Vagina		
At puberty, normal flora causing vaginal secretions to achieve low pH	Inhibit growth of many microorganisms	Antibiotics and oral contraceptives disrupting normal flora

After tissues are injured, a series of well-coordinated events occurs. The inflammatory response includes the following:

1. Vascular and cellular responses
2. Formation of inflammatory **exudates** (fluid and cells that are discharged from cells or blood vessels, e.g., pus or serum)
3. Tissue repair

Vascular and Cellular Responses. Acute inflammation is an immediate response to cellular injury. When this occurs, rapid vasodilatation occurs, which allows more blood near the location of the injury. The increase in local blood flow causes the redness at the site of inflammation. The localized warmth at the site is also the result of a greater volume of blood. Local vasodilatation delivers blood and white blood cells (WBCs) to injured tissues. Serum proteins play a major role in inflammation. These include kinins, vasoactive amines, prostaglandins, and certain complement components. These serve to increase vasodilatation. Neutrophils present at the site of infection serve as the first line of defense from microorganisms. If this does not occur, then chronic inflammation will result.

Injury causes tissue damage and possibly necrosis, and as a result the body releases chemical mediators that increase the permeability of small blood vessels. As a result, fluid, protein, and cells enter interstitial spaces. The accumulation of fluid appears as localized swelling (**edema**). Another sign of inflammation is pain. The swelling of inflamed tissues increases pressure on nerve endings, causing pain. As a result of physiological changes occurring with inflammation, the involved body part may undergo a temporary loss of function. For example, a localized infection of the hand causes the fingers to become swollen, painful, and discolored. Joints may become stiff as a result of swelling, but function of the fingers returns when inflammation subsides.

The cellular response of inflammation involves WBCs arriving at the site. WBCs pass through blood vessels and into the tissues. **Phagocytosis** is a process that involves the destruction and absorption of bacteria. Through the process of phagocytosis, specialized WBCs, called neutrophils and monocytes, ingest and destroy microorganisms or other small particles. If inflammation becomes systemic, other signs and symptoms develop. **Leukocytosis,** or an increase in the number of circulating WBCs, is the body's response to WBCs leaving blood vessels. A serum WBC count is normally 5000 to 10,000/mm^3 but may rise to 15,000 to 20,000/mm^3 and higher during inflammation. Fever is caused by phagocytic release of pyrogens from bacterial cells that cause a rise in the hypothalamic set point (see Chapter 32).

Inflammatory Exudate. Accumulation of fluid and dead tissue cells and WBCs forms an exudate at the site of inflammation. Exudate may be **serous** (clear, like plasma), **sanguineous** (containing red blood cells), or **purulent** (containing WBCs and bacteria). Usually the exudate is cleared away through lymphatic drainage. Platelets and plasma proteins such as fibrinogen form a meshlike matrix at the site of inflammation to prevent its spread.

Tissue Repair. When there is injury to tissue cells, healing involves the defensive, reconstructive, and maturative stages (see Chapter 48). Damaged cells are eventually replaced with healthy new cells. The new cells undergo a gradual maturation until they take on the same structural characteristics and appearance as the previous cells. If inflammation is chronic, tissue defects may fill with fragile **granulation tissue.** Granulation tissue is not as strong as tissue collagen and assumes the form of scar tissue.

Health Care–Associated Infections

Clients in health care settings may have an increased risk of acquiring infections. **Health care–associated infections (HAIs),** formerly called **nosocomial** or **health care–acquired infections,** result from delivery of health services in a health care facility. They can occur as the result of invasive procedures, antibiotic administration, the presence of multidrug-resistant organisms, and breaks in infection prevention and control activities.

Iatrogenic infections are a type of HAI from a diagnostic or therapeutic procedure. For example, following a gastrointestinal endoscopy the client developed a *P. aeruginosa* infection. Use critical thinking when practicing aseptic techniques and following basic infection prevention and control policies and procedures to reduce the incidence of HAIs. Always consider the client's risks for infection, and anticipate how the approach to care may increase or decrease the risk.

Health care–associated infections are exogenous or endogenous. An exogenous organism is one that is present outside the client. For example, a postoperative infection is an **exogenous infection.** Endogenous organisms are part of normal flora or virulent organisms residing that could cause infection. An **endogenous infection** can occur when part of the client's flora becomes

altered and an overgrowth results. For example, a client is placed on several antibiotics in the hospital setting and develops *C. difficile* infection as a result.

The number of health care employees having direct contact with a client, the type and number of invasive procedures, the therapy received, and the length of hospitalization influence the risk of infection. Major sites for HAIs include surgical or traumatic wounds, urinary and respiratory tracts, and the bloodstream (Box 34-2).

Health care–associated infections significantly increase costs of health care. Older adults have increased susceptibility to these infections because of their affinity to chronic disease and the aging process itself (Box 34-3). Extended stays in health care institutions, increased disability, increased costs of antibiotics, and prolonged recovery times add to the expenses of the client, as well as the expenses of the health care institution and funding bodies (e.g., Medicare). Often costs for HAIs are not reimbursed; as a result, prevention has a beneficial financial impact and is an important part of managed care. TJC has listed several national safety goals focusing

---

BOX 34-2 Sites for and Causes of Health Care–Associated Infections

Improperly performing hand hygiene increases client risk for all types of health care–associated infections.

Urinary Tract
Unsterile insertion of urinary catheter
Improper positioning of the drainage tubing
Open drainage system
Catheter and tube becoming disconnected
Drainage bag port touching contaminated surface
Improper specimen collection technique
Obstruction or interference with urinary drainage
Urine in catheter or drainage tube being allowed to reenter bladder (reflux)
Repeated catheter irrigations

Surgical or Traumatic Wounds
Improper skin preparation before surgery (i.e., shaving verses clipping hair; not performing a preoperative bath or shower)
Failure to cleanse skin surface properly
Failure to use aseptic technique during dressing changes
Use of contaminated antiseptic solutions

Respiratory Tract
Contaminated respiratory therapy equipment
Failure to use aseptic technique while suctioning airway
Improper disposal of secretions

Bloodstream
Contamination of intravenous (IV) fluids by tubing
Insertion of drug additives to IV fluid
Addition of connecting tube or stopcocks to IV system
Improper care of needle insertion site
Contaminated needles or catheters
Failure to change IV access site when inflammation first appears
Improper technique during administration of multiple blood products
Improper care of peritoneal or hemodialysis shunts
Improperly accessing an IV port

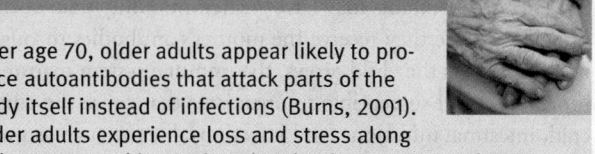

✳ BOX 34-3   FOCUS ON OLDER ADULTS

Risks for Infection

- An age-related decline in immune system function, termed immune senescence, increases the body's susceptibility to infection and slows overall immune response (Lesser and others, 2006).
- Older adults are less capable of producing lymphocytes to combat challenges to the immune system. When antibodies are produced, the duration of their response is shorter and fewer cells are produced (Burns, 2001).
- Risks associated with the development of health care–associated infections in older clients include poor nutrition, unintentional weight loss, and low serum albumin levels (Meiner and Lueckenotte, 2006).

- After age 70, older adults appear likely to produce autoantibodies that attack parts of the body itself instead of infections (Burns, 2001).
- Older adults experience loss and stress along with suppressed immunity related to bereavement, depression, and poor social support (Burns, 2001).

✳ TABLE 34-4   Assessing the Risk of Infection in Adults

COMPONENT	CAUSES	OUTCOME
Age	COPD, heart disease, diabetes	Pneumonia, skin breakdown, venous stasis ulcers
Lifestyle—high-risk behaviors	Exposure to communicable/infectious diseases Use of IV drugs Use of other drugs/substances	STDs, HIV, HBV, HCV, opportunistic infections, viral infections, yeast infections, liver failure
Occupation	Miner, unemployed, homeless	Black lung disease, pneumonia, TB, poor nutritional intake, lack of access to medical care, stress
Diagnostic procedures	Invasive radiology, transplant	Multiple IV lines, immunosuppressive drugs
Heredity	Sickle cell disease, diabetes	Anemia, delayed healing
Travel history	West Nile virus, SARS, avian flu, *Hantavirus*	Meningitis, acute respiratory distress
Trauma	Fractures, internal bleeding	Sepsis, secondary infection
Nutrition	Obesity, anorexia	Impaired immune response

Modified from Tweeten SM: General principles of epidemiology. In Carrico R, editor: *APIC text of infection control and epidemiology,* Washington, DC, 2005, Association for Professionals in Infection Control and Epidemiology.

COPD, Chronic obstructive pulmonary disease; *HBV,* hepatitis B virus; *HCV,* hepatitis C virus; *HIV,* human immunodeficiency virus; *IV,* intravenous; *SARS,* severe acute respiratory syndrome; *STDs,* sexually transmitted diseases; *TB,* tuberculosis.

on the care of older adults, for example, ensuring that older adults receive influenza and pneumonia vaccine or preventing health care–associated pressure ulcers (TJC, 2007).

The Nursing Process in Infection Control

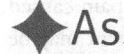Assessment

Assess the client's defense mechanisms, susceptibility, and knowledge of how infections are transmitted (Table 34-4). Conduct a review of disease and travel history with the client and family to reveal an exposure to a communicable disease. Immunization and vaccination history is also very useful. Conduct a thorough review of the client's clinical condition to identify signs and symptoms of actual infection or a risk for infection. An analysis of laboratory findings provides information about a client's defense against infection. By knowing the factors that increase susceptibility or risk

for infection and recognizing early signs and symptoms, you are able to plan appropriate interventions.

Status of Defense Mechanisms. Review physical assessment findings and the client's medical condition to determine the status of normal defense mechanisms against infection. For example, any break in the skin, such as an ulcer on the foot of a client who has diabetes, is a potential site for infection. Similarly, a client who smokes is at greater risk for acquiring a respiratory tract infection after general surgery because respiratory cilia are less likely to propel retained mucus from the client's airways. Any reduction in the body's primary or secondary defenses against infection places a client at increased risk.

Client Susceptibility. Many factors influence susceptibility to infection. Gather information about each factor through the client's and family's history.

Age. Throughout life, susceptibility to infection changes. For example, an infant has immature defenses against infection. Born with only the antibodies provided by the mother, the infant's immune system is incapable of producing the necessary immunoglobulins and WBCs to adequately fight some infections. However, breast-fed infants may have greater immunity than bottle-fed infants, because they receive the mother's antibodies through the breast milk. As the child grows, the immune system matures, but the child is still susceptible to organisms that cause the common cold, intestinal infections, and infectious diseases such as mumps, measles, and chickenpox if not vaccinated.

The young or middle-age adult has refined defenses against infection. Normal flora, body system defenses, inflammation, and the immune response provide protection against invading microorganisms. Viruses are the most common cause of communicable illness in young or middle-age adults. Since 2000, there has been a major effort to vaccinate all children against all diseases for which vaccine is available. The result is a significant decline in the number of cases occurring. For example, hepatitis B infection in children and adolescents has decreased by 89% (CDC, 2005b).

Defenses against infection change with aging (Lesser, Paiusi, and Leips, 2006). The immune response, particularly cell-mediated immunity, declines. Older adults also undergo alterations in the structure and function of the skin, urinary tract, and lungs. For example, the skin loses its turgor, and the epithelium thins. As a result, it is easier to tear or abrade the skin, and this increases the potential for invasion by pathogens.

Nutritional Status. When protein intake is inadequate as a result of poor diet or debilitating disease, the rate of protein breakdown exceeds that of tissue synthesis (see Chapter 44). A reduction in the intake of protein and other nutrients such as carbohydrates and fats reduces the body's defenses against infection and impairs wound healing (see Chapter 48).

Clients with illnesses or problems that increase protein requirements are at further risk. These problems include traumatic injury, extensive burns, and conditions causing fever. Clients who have had surgery also require increased protein.

The nurse assesses clients' dietary intakes and abilities to tolerate solid foods. Clients who have difficulty with swallowing, who experience alterations in digestion, or who are too confused or weak to feed themselves are at risk for inadequate dietary intake. Obese clients will benefit from dietary assessment. Confer with a dietitian to assist in calculating the calorie count of foods ingested.

Stress. The body responds to emotional or physical stress by the general adaptation syndrome (see Chapter 31). During the alarm stage the basal metabolic rate increases as the body uses energy stores. Adrenocorticotropic hormone (ACTH) acts to increase serum glucose levels and decrease unnecessary antiinflammatory responses through the release of cortisone. If stress continues or becomes intense, elevated cortisone levels result in decreased resistance to infection. Continued stress leads to exhaustion, in which energy stores are depleted and the body has no resistance to invading organisms. The same conditions that increase nutritional requirements, such as surgery or trauma, also increase physiological stress. For example, meningitis is a seasonal disease commonly occurring in high schools and colleges around examination time. Students are under stress, not eating properly, and not getting enough sleep. Their resistance is lowered, and they are more prone to illness.

Disease Process. Clients with diseases of the immune system are at particular risk for infection. Leukemia, AIDS, lymphoma, and aplastic anemia are conditions that compromise a host by weakening defenses against infectious organisms. For example, clients with leukemia are unable to produce enough WBCs to ward off infection. Clients with HIV are often unable to ward off simple infections and are prone to opportunistic infections.

Clients with chronic diseases such as diabetes mellitus and multiple sclerosis are also more susceptible to infection because of general debilitation and nutritional impairment. Diseases that impair body system defenses, such as emphysema and bronchitis (which impair ciliary action and thicken mucus), cancer (which alters the immune response), and peripheral vascular disease (which reduces blood flow to injured tissues), increase susceptibility to infection. Clients with burns have a very high susceptibility to infection because of the damage to skin surfaces. The greater the depth and extent of the burns, the higher the risk for infection.

Medical Therapy. Some drugs and medical therapies compromise immunity to infection. The nurse assesses the client's history to determine whether the client takes medications at home that increase infection susceptibility. The medication assessment includes any over-the-counter medications and herbal medications. A review of therapies received within the health care setting further reveals risks. Adrenal corticosteroids, prescribed for several conditions, are antiinflammatory drugs that cause protein breakdown and impair the inflammatory response against bacteria and other pathogens. Cytotoxic or antineoplastic drugs attack cancer cells but cause side effects of bone marrow depression and normal cell toxicity. With bone marrow depression the body is unable to produce lymphocytes and sufficient WBCs. When normal cells become altered by antineoplastic agents, cellular defenses against infection fail. Cyclosporine and other immunosuppressant drugs, which decrease the body's immune response, are commonly taken by clients who receive organ transplants. The immunosuppressants prevent organ and tissue rejection, but they also increase susceptibility to infection.

Clinical Appearance. The signs and symptoms of infection may be local or systemic. Localized infections are most common in areas of skin or mucous membrane breakdown, such as surgical and traumatic wounds, pressure ulcers, oral lesions, and abscesses.

To assess an area for localized infection, first inspect the area for redness and swelling caused by inflammation. Because there may be drainage from open lesions or wounds, wear clean gloves. Infected drainage may be yellow, green, or brown, depending on the pathogen. For example, green nasal secretions may indicate a sinus infection. Ask the client about pain or tenderness around the site. Some clients may complain of tightness and pain caused by edema. If the infected area is large enough, movement may be restricted. Gentle palpation of an infected area usually results in some degree of tenderness. In addition to gloves, wear a surgical mask to prevent additional contamination of the wound. Wear protective eyewear when there is a risk for splash or spray with blood or body fluids.

Systemic infections cause more generalized symptoms than local infection. They usually result in fever, fatigue, nausea/vomiting, and malaise. Lymph nodes that drain the area of infection often become enlarged, swollen, and tender during palpation. For example, an abscess in the peritoneal cavity may cause enlargement of lymph nodes in the groin. An infection of the upper respiratory tract may cause cervical lymph node enlargement. If an infection is serious and widespread, all major lymph nodes may enlarge.

Systemic infections can develop after treatment for localized infection has failed. Be alert for changes in the client's level of activity and responsiveness. As systemic infections develop, an elevation in body temperature can lead to episodes of increased heart and respiratory rates and low blood pressure. Involvement of major body systems produces specific symptoms. For example, a pulmonary infection may result in a productive cough with purulent sputum. A urinary tract infection may result in cloudy, foul-smelling urine.

An infection does not always present with typical signs and symptoms in all clients. It is not unusual to find that older adults have an advanced infection before it is identified. This is because due to age there is a reduced inflammatory and immune response. Older adults have increased fatigue and diminished pain sensitivity. A reduced or absent fever response can occur from chronic use of aspirin or nonsteroidal antiinflammatory drugs. Atypical symptoms such as confusion, incontinence, or agitation may be the only symptoms of an infectious illness (Gantz, 2005). For example, as many as 20% of older adults with pneumonia do not have the typical signs and symptoms of fever, shaking, chills, and rusty productive sputum. The only symptoms are often an increased, unexplained heart rate, confusion, or generalized fatigue. A pneumonia vaccine is available and recommended for all persons with respiratory problems and those over 65 years of age. This will greatly assist in the decline of pneumonia in the older adult population.

Laboratory Data. A review of laboratory test results may reveal infection (Table 34-5). Laboratory values, however, are not enough to detect infection. You need to assess other clinical signs. Factors other than infection may alter test values. For example, trauma and physical stress can cause an elevation in the number of neutrophils. A culture result may show growth of an organism in the absence of infection. It is also important to note that laboratory values may vary from laboratory to laboratory. Be sure to know the standard range of laboratory values for the laboratory in your facility.

Clients With Infection. Some clients with infection have a variety of problems. It is important to ask specific questions to assesses the client's and family's needs related to disease status (Box 34-4). These needs are physical, psychological, social, or economic. For example, a client with a chronic disease such as HIV/AIDS may experience serious psychological problems as a result of self-imposed isolation or rejection by family and friends. Clients or their families may not be able to afford the cost of medical

---

✴ BOX 34-4 NURSING ASSESSMENT QUESTIONS

Risk Factors
- Do you have any recent cuts or lacerations?
- Have you been diagnosed with any chronic illnesses?
- Have you had any recent diagnostic testing, such as cystoscopy, performed?

Possible Existing Infections
- Do you have or feel like you have a fever?
- Do you have any pain/burning during urination?

Medication History
- Are you taking any medication that could affect your immune system (e.g., cancer chemotherapy, rheumatoid arthritis medications, steroids)?
- Are you taking any antiviral medications?

Stressors
- Is there any major lifestyle change occurring, such as the loss of employment or place of residence, divorce, or disability?

✴ TABLE 34-5 Laboratory Tests to Screen for Infection

LABORATORY VALUE	NORMAL (ADULT) VALUES	INDICATION OF INFECTION
WBC count	5000-10,000/mm^3	Increased in acute infection, decreased in certain viral or overwhelming infections
Erythrocyte sedimentation rate	Up to 15 mm/hr for men and 20 mm/hr for women	Elevated in presence of inflammatory process
Iron level	60-90 g/100 mL	Decreased in chronic infection
Cultures of urine and blood	Normally sterile, without microorganism growth	Presence of infectious microorganism growth
Cultures and Gram stain of wound, sputum, and throat	No WBCs on Gram stain, possible normal flora	Presence of infectious microorganism growth and WBCs on Gram stain
Differential Count (Percentage of Each Type of WBC)		
Neutrophils	55%-70%	Increased in acute **suppurative** (pus-forming) infection, decreased in overwhelming bacterial infection (older adult)
Lymphocytes	20%-40%	Increased in chronic bacterial and viral infection, decreased in sepsis
Monocytes	5%-10%	Increased in protozoan, rickettsial, and tuberculosis infections
Eosinophils	1%-4%	Increased in parasitic infection
Basophils	0.5%-1.5%	Normal during infection

WBC, White blood cell.

✴ BOX 34-5   NURSING DIAGNOSTIC PROCESS

Risk for Infection Related to Impaired Immunity

Assessment Activities	Defining Characteristics
Check results of laboratory tests.	WBC count ≤5000/mm³
Review current medications.	Client receiving azathioprine (Imuran), an immunosuppressant
Identify potential sites of infection.	IV catheter in right forearm, in place for 3 days Foley catheter draining cloudy amber-colored urine

WBC, White blood cell; *IV*, intravenous.

---

care. Using a case management approach, the nurse determines the client's and family's ability to adjust to the disease and identifies available resources needed for managing health care challenges, such as referrals to area group meetings that may assist a client with acceptance of the illness or referral to local agency resources for assistance with prescription drug expenses.

✦ Nursing Diagnosis

During assessment gather objective data, such as an open incision or a reduced caloric intake, and subjective data, such as a client's complaint of tenderness over a surgical wound site. Then review the data carefully, looking for clusters of characteristics or risk factors that create a pattern. This pattern may suggest a specific nursing diagnosis (Box 34-5). The following are examples of nursing diagnoses:

• Risk for infection
• Imbalanced nutrition: less than body requirements
• Impaired oral mucous membrane
• Risk for impaired skin integrity
• Social isolation
• Impaired tissue integrity

It is necessary to validate data, such as inspecting the integrity of a wound more carefully, and to review laboratory findings as needed. Success in planning appropriate nursing interventions depends on the accuracy of the diagnosis and the ability to meet the client's needs. For example, minimizing the *risk for infection related to broken skin* requires proper hygiene measures, wound care, and use of standard precautions. Minimizing the *risk for infection related to malnutrition* requires good nutritional support and fluid balance.

✦ Planning

Goals and Outcomes. The client's care plan is based on each nursing diagnosis and related factor (see Care Plan). Develop a plan that sets realistic outcomes so that interventions are purposeful and directed. When you care for a client with the nursing di-

agnosis of *risk for infection related to broken skin,* implement skin and wound care measures to promote healing. The expected outcomes of "reduction in wound size by 1 cm" and "absence of drainage" set targets for measuring the client's improvement. Common goals of care applicable to clients with infection often include the following:

• Preventing exposure to infectious organisms
• Controlling or reducing the extent of infection
• Maintaining resistance to infection
• Verbalizing understanding of infection prevention and control techniques (e.g., hand hygiene)

Setting Priorities. Establish priorities for each goal of care. For example, your client developed an open wound, suffers a debilitating disease such as cancer, and is unable to tolerate solid foods. The priority of administering therapies to promote wound healing overrides the goal of educating the client to assume self-care therapies at home. When the client's condition improves, the priorities will change, and client education becomes an essential intervention.

Collaborative Care. The development of a care plan includes prevention and infection control practices from multiple disciplines. Select interventions in collaboration with the client, the family, and others on the health care team such as the dietitian or respiratory therapist. In addition, the infection prevention and control professional (IPCP) or home care nurses collaborate in the client's care. When care continues into the client's home, the home care nurse plans to ensure that the home environment supports good infection prevention and control practices. For example, if a client does not have running water yet requires wound care, even simple hand hygiene with soap and water is difficult to achieve. The nurse will need to bring a waterless alcohol product during visits to ensure adequate hand hygiene. Use bottled water if hands are visibly soiled. Instruct the client to use hand hygiene with either bottled water and soap or alcohol-based hand products.

✦ Implementation

By identifying and assessing a client's risk factors and implementing appropriate measures, the nurse reduces the risk of infection.

Health Promotion. Use your critical thinking skills to prevent an infection from developing or spreading. Implement procedures to minimize the numbers and kinds of organisms that could be possibly transmitted. Eliminating reservoirs of infection, controlling portals of exit and entry, and avoiding actions that transmit microorganisms prevent bacteria from finding a new site in which to grow. Proper use of sterile supplies, barrier precautions, standard precautions, transmission-based precautions, and proper hand hygiene are examples of methods to control the spread of microorganisms. A final preventive measure is to strengthen a potential host's defenses against infection. Nutritional support, rest, maintenance of physiological protective mechanisms, and

NURSING CARE PLAN

Risk for Infection

Assessment

Mr. Huntly is a 32-year-old married father of two admitted to the medical nursing unit 5 days ago with a diagnosis of HIV infection. He received his first doses of antiretroviral drugs. Before his admission he lost interest in food and noticed that his intake decreased. His children are school aged and attend public school.

Both children have stayed home from school twice in the last 2 months for colds and sore throats. Sara Jones is the nursing student caring for Mr. Huntly. She begins her shift of care by conducting a focused assessment.

Assessment Activities

Review client's chart for laboratory data reflecting immune function (e.g., WBC count; CD4 count; viral load).

Ask client to describe appetite and review food intake for last 24 hours.

Weigh client. Measure height.
Palpate client's cervical and clavicular lymph nodes.
Assess client's complete medication history.

Findings/Defining Characteristics

The number of **CD4 cells is low.**

Client reports a **decreased interest in eating** for a couple of weeks. He **lost** approximately **8 pounds in 3 weeks.** His food intake yesterday consisted of a small cup of applesauce, one-half bowl of soup, some crackers, and two glasses of juice.

His current weight is 155 pounds; height is 5 feet 10 inches.
Lymph nodes are enlarged and pain free.
Client receiving **multiagent chemotherapy.**

Nursing Diagnosis: Risk for infection related to immunosuppression and reduced food intake.

Planning

Goal

Client will remain free of infection.

Client describes risks for infection in 2 weeks.

Expected Outcomes (NOC)*

Immune Status
Client will remain afebrile.
Client will have no signs or symptoms of local infection (e.g., remains free of cough, cloudy or foul-smelling urine, oral lesions).

Knowledge: Infection Management
Client will identify routines to follow in the home that reduce risk for infection.
Client will identify signs and symptoms to report to health care provider indicating infection.

---

†Outcome classification labels from Moorhead S and others: *Nursing outcomes classification (NOC),* ed 4, St. Louis, 2008, Mosby.

Interventions†

Infection Protection

- Monitor client's body temperature routinely, inspect oral cavity for lesions, inspect urine for odor, inspect IV access site for drainage, and observe client for evidence of cough.
- Consult with dietitian in providing a high-calorie, high-protein, low-bacteria diet. Minimize intake of salads, raw fruits and vegetables and undercooked meat, pepper, and paprika. Offer small frequent meals.

Infection Control

- Teach client and family how to perform hand hygiene correctly.

- Instruct client to report the following to his caregiver: temperature greater than 100° F (38° C), persistent cough with or without sputum, urine that is cloudy or foul smelling, or burning on urination.

Rationale

Interventions help prevent and ensure early detection of infection in a client at risk (Fauerbach, 2005).

Maintaining calorie and protein intake will prevent weight loss. Foods high in fat should be avoided. Excessive amounts of omega fatty acids are immunosuppressive (Gantz, 2005).

Client can easily come in contact with organisms in the environment that can cause infection. Rigorous hand hygiene reduces bacterial counts on the hands (Larson, 2005).
Signs and symptoms are indicative of local or systemic infection.

---

†Intervention classification labels from Bulechek GM, Butcher HK, and Dochterman JM: *Nursing interventions classification (NIC),* ed 5, St. Louis, 2008, Mosby.

Continued

NURSING CARE PLAN

Risk for Infection—cont'd

Interventions†

Infection—cont'd

- Teach client and family the following:
  - Avoid crowds and large gatherings of people.
  - Do not share personal toilet items (toothbrush, washcloth, deodorant stick) with family.
  - Take temperature twice daily.
  - Do not drink water that has been standing for longer than 15 minutes.
  - Do not reuse cups or glasses without washing; whenever possible, use the dishwasher.
  - Use of condoms during intercourse. Do not pass or receive body fluids, particularly blood, semen, or vaginal secretions.

Rationale

These measures are designed to prevent infection in those clients with impaired immune function (Gantz, 2005).

†Intervention classification labels from Bulechek GM, Butcher HK, and Dochterman JM: *Nursing interventions classification (NIC)*, ed 5, St. Louis, 2008, Mosby.

Evaluation

Nursing Actions	Client Response/Finding	Achievement of Outcome
Compare client's body temperature and other physical findings with baseline data.	Client remains afebrile and denies having cough or burning on urination. No sign of oral lesions	Client has no active infection at this time.
Ask client to describe signs and symptoms to report to health care provider.	Client able to identify temperature range to report. Was able to describe cough. Unable to identify signs of urinary infection or local discharge.	Client has partial understanding of signs and symptoms to report. Will require additional instruction. Offer information sheet.
Ask client to explain the measures to take at home to reduce exposure to infectious agents.	Client able to discuss need to avoid sharing personal hygiene articles and to wash fresh produce. Asked for a listing of other precautions and requested that his wife be included in discussion.	Client has partial understanding of restrictions. Will obtain printed guidelines and include wife in discussion this evening.

recommended immunizations protect a client. For example, annual vaccination to protect against influenza is an important element of risk reduction.

Having an infection prevention and control conscience helps you apply principles of medical-surgical asepsis. When a client develops an infection, implement techniques and procedures to reduce the opportunity for health care personnel and other clients to be exposed to the infection. Clients with communicable diseases may require specific isolation precautions to break the chain of infection.

Acute Care. Treatment of an infectious process includes eliminating the infectious organisms and supporting the client's defenses. To identify the causative organism, the nurse collects specimens of body fluids such as sputum or drainage from infected body sites for cultures. When the disease process or causative organism is identified, the health care provider prescribes the most effective treatment.

Systemic infections require measures to prevent complications of fever (see Chapter 32). Maintaining intake of fluids prevents dehydration resulting from diaphoresis. The client's increased metabolic rate requires an adequate nutritional intake. Rest preserves energy for the healing process.

Localized infections often require measures to assist removal of debris to promote healing. The nurse applies principles of wound care to remove infected drainage from wound sites and support the integrity of healing wounds. When changing a dressing, wear a mask and goggles or a mask with a face shield if splashing or spraying with blood or body fluids is anticipated. Apply gloves to reduce the transmission of microorganisms into the wound (CDC, 2007). Apply special dressings to facilitate removal of drainage and promote healing of wound margins. Sometimes drainage tubes are inserted to remove infected drainage from body cavities. Use medical and surgical aseptic techniques to manage wounds and ensure correct handling of all drainage or body fluids (see Chapter 48).

During the course of infection the nurse supports the client's body defense mechanisms. For example, if a client has diarrhea, the nurse needs to maintain skin integrity to prevent breakdown and the entrance of additional microorganisms. Other routine hygiene measures such as cleansing the oral cavity and bathing protect the skin and mucous membranes from invasion and overgrowth of organisms.

Asepsis. Base efforts to minimize the onset and spread of infection on the principles of aseptic technique. **Asepsis** is the absence of pathogenic (disease-producing) microorganisms. Aseptic technique refers to practices/procedures that assist in reducing the risk for infection. The two types of aseptic technique are medical and surgical asepsis.

Medical asepsis, or clean technique, includes procedures used to reduce the number of organisms present and prevent the transfer of organisms. Hand hygiene, using clean gloves to prevent the transfer of organisms from one client to another or to prevent direct contact with client blood or body fluids, and cleaning the environment routinely are examples of medical asepsis. Principles of medical asepsis are also commonly followed in the home; hand hygiene with soap and water before preparing food is an example.

After an object becomes unsterile or unclean, it is considered contaminated. In medical asepsis an area or object is considered contaminated if it contains or is suspected of containing pathogens. For example, a used bedpan, the over-bed table, and a used dressing are considered to be contaminated items.

The nurse follows certain principles and procedures, including **standard precautions,** to prevent and control infection and its spread. During daily routine care the nurse uses basic medical aseptic techniques to break the infection chain. For example, use gloves and a mask during a dressing change to break the mode of entry for pathogens. Eyewear is indicated whenever there is the possibility for splash or splatter. The term *standard precautions* applies to all blood and body fluids except sweat even if blood is not present. Standard precautions apply to contact with blood, body fluid, nonintact skin, and mucous membranes from all clients. These precautions protect the client and provide protection of the health care staff as directed by the Occupational Safety and Health Administration (OSHA) (2001).

A major component of client and worker protection is hand hygiene (Skill 34-1). **Hand hygiene** includes using an instant alcohol hand antiseptic before and after providing client care, hand washing with soap and water when hands are visibly soiled, and performing a surgical scrub. **Hand washing** is the act of washing hands with soap and water, followed by rinsing under a stream of water for 15 seconds (CDC, 2002b). The friction used removes soil and transient organisms from the hands.

Contaminated hands of health care workers are a primary source of infection transmission in the health care settings For example, you are performing a dressing change, and the client's roommate asks for assistance with a blocked IV line. If you fail to **perform** hand hygiene before handling the IV line, organisms from the client's wound could be transferred to the roommate's IV site. TJC has identified compliance with proper hand hygiene as a National Patient Safety Goal (TJC, 2007).

The use of alcohol-based hand rubs is recommended by the Centers for Disease Control and Prevention (CDC) (2002b) to improve hand hygiene practices, protect health care worker's hands, and reduce transmission of pathogens to clients and personnel in health care settings. Alcohols have excellent germicidal activity and are as effective than either soap and water.

The CDC (2002b) recommends the following:

1. Wash hands with a non-antimicrobial soap or antimicrobial soap and water when hands are visibly soiled.

2. If hands are not visibly soiled, use an alcohol-based waterless antiseptic agent for routinely decontaminating hands in all other clinical situations:
   a. After contact with a client's intact skin (as in taking a pulse or blood pressure or lifting a client)
   b. Before eating
   c. After contact with body fluids or excretions, mucous membranes, nonintact skin, or wound dressings as long as hands are not visibly soiled
   d. When moving from a contaminated body site to a clean body site during client care
   e. After contact with inanimate objects (including medical equipment) in the immediate area of the client
   f. Before caring for clients with severe neutropenia or other forms of severe immune suppression
   g. Before inserting indwelling urinary catheters or other invasive devices
   h. After removing gloves

Instruct clients and visitors about the proper technique and times for hand hygiene. Teaching hand hygiene is particularly important if health care is to continue at home. Clients need to wash their hands before eating or handling food; after handling contaminated equipment, linen, or organic material; and after elimination. Encourage visitors to wash their hands before eating or handling food, after coming in contact with infected clients, and after handling contaminated equipment, client furniture, or organic material.

You are responsible for providing the client with a safe environment. The effectiveness of infection control practices depends on your conscientiousness and consistency in using effective aseptic technique. It is human nature to forget key procedural steps or, when hurried, to take shortcuts that break aseptic procedures. However, failure to comply with basic procedures places the client at risk for an infection that can seriously impair recovery or lead to death.

Cleaning, Disinfection, and Sterilization. Proper cleansing, disinfection, and sterilization of contaminated objects significantly reduce and often eliminate microorganisms. In health care facilities, a sterile processing department is responsible for the disinfection and sterilizing of reusable supplies and equipment. However, in the home care setting, sometimes the nurse has to perform these functions. Many principles of cleaning and disinfection also apply to the home.

Cleaning. Cleaning is the removal of all soil (e.g., organic and inorganic material) from objects and surfaces (Rutala and Weber, 2005). Generally cleaning involves use of water and mechanical action with detergents or enzymatic products. Detergents should have natural pH. When an object comes in contact with an infectious or potentially infectious material, the object is contaminated. If the object is disposable, it is discarded. Clean reusable objects must be cleaned thoroughly before reuse and then either disinfected or sterilized according to the manufacturer's recommendations. Failure to follow the manufacturer's recommendations transfers liability from the manufacturer to the health care facility or agency if an infection results from improper processing.

✱ **SKILL 34-1**   **HAND HYGIENE**   Video

Delegation Considerations
The skills of hand hygiene is performed by all caregivers. Instruct all caregivers to use proper hand hygiene.

Equipment
- Antiseptic hand rub
  - Alcohol-based waterless hand products containing emollient
- Hand washing
  - Easy-to-reach sink with warm running water
  - Antimicrobial or non-antimicrobial soap
  - Paper towels or air dryer
  - Clean orangewood stick (optional)

STEPS	RATIONALE
1. Inspect surface of hands for breaks or cuts in skin or cuticles. Cover any skin lesions with a dressing before providing care. If lesions are too large to cover, you may be restricted from direct client care (CDC, 2002b).	Open cuts or wounds can harbor high concentrations of microorganisms. Health care facility or agency policy often prevents nurses from caring for high-risk clients if open lesions are present on hands.
2. Inspect hands for visible soiling.	If hands are visibly soiled, use soap and water until soil is removed.
3. Inspect condition of nails. Natural tips should be ¼ inch from fingertip and smooth. DO NOT WEAR artificial nails or extensions.	Subungual areas of hand harbor high concentrations of bacteria. Long nails and chipped or old polish increase the number of bacteria residing on hands. Artificial applications increase microbial load on hands (CDC, 2002b) (Box 34-6).
4. Push wristwatch and long uniform sleeves above wrists. Avoid wearing rings; however, there is not definitive evidence that rings increase microbial load on the hands (CDC, 2002b).	Provides complete access to fingers, hands, and wrists. Some studies do show that the skin underneath rings is more heavily colonized. Gram-negative bacilli and *Staphylococcus aureus* are more common under rings (Boyce and Pitter, 2001).
5. Antiseptic hand rub	
a. Apply an ample amount of product to palm of one hand (see illustration).	Enough product is needed to thoroughly cover the hands.
b. Rub hands together, covering all surfaces of hands and fingers with antiseptic (see illustration).	Covering all aspects of the hands will kill bacteria that can be transmitted to the client.
c. Rub hands together for several seconds until alcohol is dry. Allow hands to dry before applying gloves.	Drying ensures full antiseptic effect.
6. Hand washing using antiseptic soap	
a. Stand in front of sink, keeping hands and uniform away from sink surface. (If hands touch sink during hand washing, repeat.)	Inside of sink is a contaminated area. Reaching over sink increases risk of touching edge, which is contaminated.
b. Turn on water. Turn faucet on or push knee pedals laterally or press pedals with foot to regulate flow and temperature (see illustration).	Knee pads within the operating room and treatment areas are preferred to prevent hand contact with faucet. Faucet handles are likely to be contaminated with organic debris and microorganisms (Griffith and others, 2003).
c. Avoid splashing water against uniform.	Microorganisms travel and grow in moisture.
d. Regulate flow of water so that temperature is warm.	Warm water removes less of the protective oils than hot water.
e. Wet hands and wrists thoroughly under running water. Keep hands and forearms lower than elbows during washing.	Hands are the most contaminated parts to be washed. Water flows from least to most contaminated area, rinsing microorganisms into the sink.

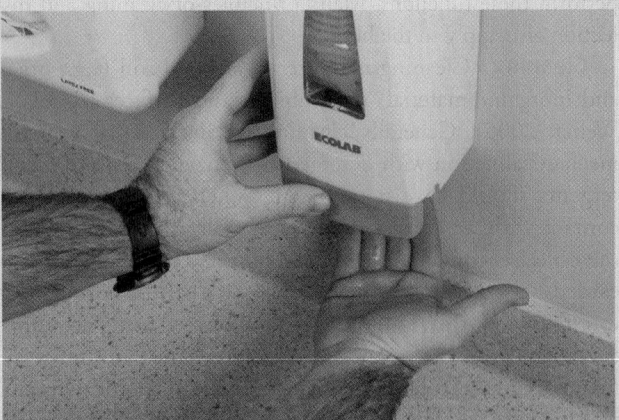

STEP 5a Apply waterless antiseptic to hands.

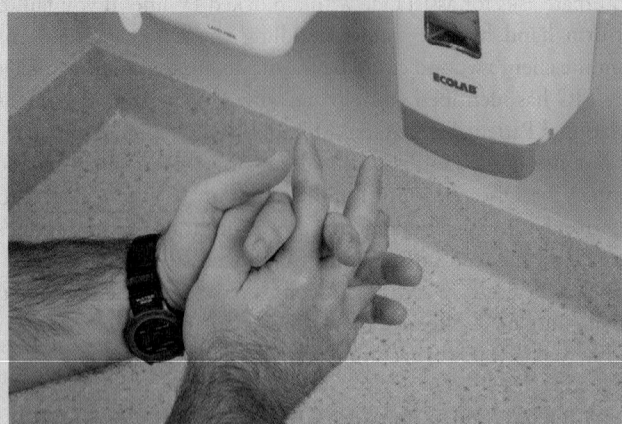

STEP 5b Rub hands thoroughly.

STEPS

f. Apply 3 to 5 mL of antiseptic soap, and rub hands together vigorously, lathering thoroughly (see illustration). Soap granules and leaflet preparations may be used.

RATIONALE

Ensures that all surface areas of the hands and fingers are cleansed.

Critical Decision Point: The decision whether to use a non-antimicrobial soap, antimicrobial soap, or alcohol-based hand antiseptic is not dependent on the procedure and the client's immune status. However, acute care hospitals usually have only antiseptic soap.

---

g. Wash hands using plenty of lather and friction for at least 15 seconds. Interlace fingers, and rub palms and back of hands with circular motion at least 5 times each. Keep fingertips down to facilitate removal of microorganisms.

h. Areas under fingernails are often soiled. Clean them with fingernails of other hand and additional soap with an orangewood stick (optional).

Soap cleanses by emulsifying fat and oil and lowering surface tension. Friction and rubbing mechanically loosen and remove dirt and transient bacteria. Interlacing fingers and thumbs ensures that all surfaces are cleansed. Adequate time is needed to expose skin surfaces to antimicrobial agent

Areas under nails are often highly contaminated, which will increase the risk of infection for the nurse or the client.

Critical Decision Point: Do not tear or cut skin under or around nail.

---

i. Rinse hands and wrists thoroughly, keeping hands down and elbows up (see illustration).

Rinsing mechanically washes away dirt and microorganisms.

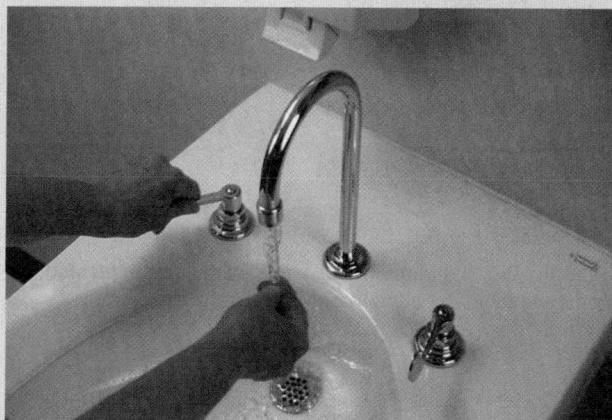
STEP 6b Turning on water.

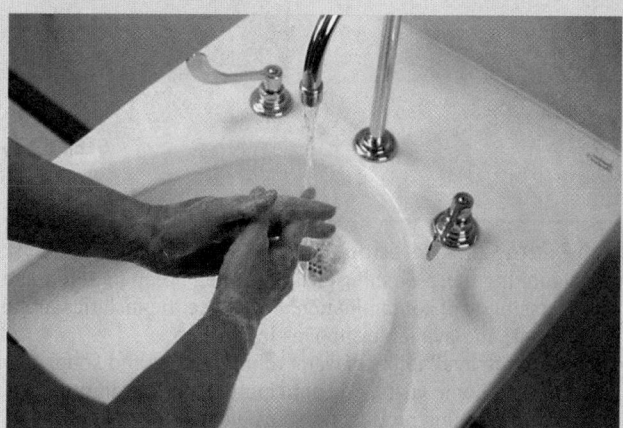
STEP 6f Lathering hands thoroughly.

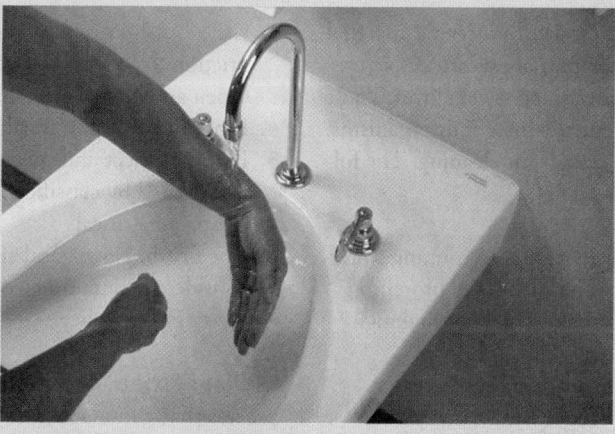
STEP 6i Rinsing hands.

Continued

STEPS	RATIONALE
j. Dry hands thoroughly from fingers to wrists and forearms with paper towel, single-use cloth, or warm air dryer.	Drying from cleanest (fingertips) to least clean (forearms) area avoids contamination. Drying hands prevents chapping and roughened skin.

Critical Decision Point: Paper towels should dispense cleanly without hand or paper towel contact with other surfaces. Reaching into the dispenser cabinet and touching the paper slot increases the risk of contamination (Harrison and others, 2003).

k. If used, discard paper towel in proper receptacle.	Prevents transfer of microorganisms.
l. Turn off water with foot or knee pedals. To turn off hand faucet, use clean, dry paper towel; avoid touching handles with hands (see illustration).	Wet towel and hands allow transfer of pathogens from faucet to hands. Faucet handles are contaminated (Griffiths and others, 2003).

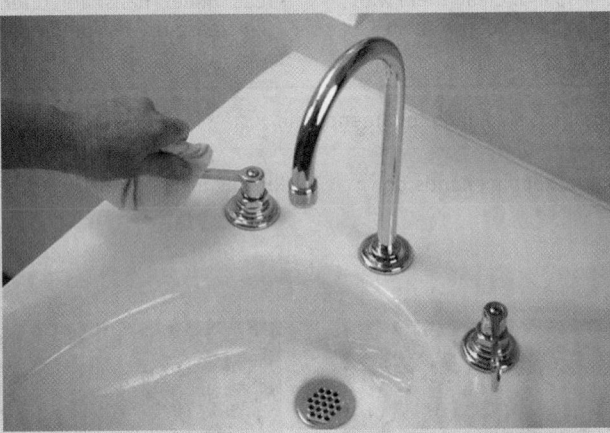

STEP 6l Turning off faucet.

Home Care Considerations

- Evaluate the hand-washing facilities in the home to determine the possibility of contamination, how close the facilities are to the client, and available supplies in the area.
- Evaluate the availability of warm running water and soap when conducting home visits, and anticipate the need for alternative hand-washing products such as alcohol-based hand rubs and/or detergent-containing towels.
- Instruct the client and primary caregiver in proper techniques and situations for hand washing.

When cleaning equipment that is soiled by organic material such as blood, fecal matter, mucus, or pus, apply protective eyewear (or a face shield) and utility (dishwashing style) gloves. These barriers provide protection from potentially infectious organisms. A brush and detergent or soap are necessary for cleaning. The following steps ensure that an object is clean:

1. Rinse contaminated object or article with cold running water to remove organic material. Hot water causes the protein in organic material to coagulate and stick to objects, making removal difficult.
2. After rinsing, wash the object with soap and warm water. Soap or detergent reduces the surface tension of water and emulsifies dirt or remaining material. Rinse the object thoroughly.
3. Use a brush to remove dirt or material in grooves or seams. Friction dislodges contaminated material for easy removal. Open any hinged items for cleaning.
4. Rinse the object in warm water.
5. Dry the object and prepare it for disinfection or sterilization if indicated by classification of the item—critical, semicritical, or noncritical.
6. The brush, gloves, and sink used to clean the equipment are considered contaminated and should be cleaned and dried according to policy.

Disinfection and Sterilization. **Disinfection** describes a process that eliminates many or all microorganisms, with the exception of bacterial spores, from inanimate objects (Rutala and Weber, 2005). There are two types of disinfection: the disinfection

✴ BOX 34-6 ・ EVIDENCE-BASED PRACTICE

Pathogens and Artificial Fingernails

Evidence Summary

Female health care workers (HCWs) frequently have artificial or manicured nails. Researchers posed the question as to whether bacteria reside in higher than normal numbers on artificial nail material.

In three separate studies the identity and quantity of microbial flora from HCWs wearing artificial nails were compared with those from HCWs with normal nails. In both studies, nail surfaces were swabbed and subungual (area under nails) debris was collected to obtain material for culture. In the first study, 12 HCWs who did not normally wear artificial nails wore polished artificial nails on their nondominant hand for 15 days. Identity and quantity of microflora were compared between the artificial nails and the polished normal nails of the other hand. Potential pathogens were isolated from more samples obtained from artificial nails than normal nails. Colonization of artificial nails increased over time. More organisms were found on the surface of artificial nails than normal nails.

In the second study the flora of the nails of 30 HCWs who wore permanent acrylic artificial nails were compared with that of HCWs who do not wear artificial nails. HCWs wearing artificial nails were more likely to have a pathogen isolated than the other group.

In this study, artificial nails were more likely to harbor pathogens, especially gram-negative bacilli and yeasts, than normal nails. The longer artificial nails were worn, the more likely that a pathogen was isolated.

The third study examined an outbreak of *Pseudomonas aeruginosa* in a neonatal intensive care unit. This outbreak was attributed to two nurses. One nurse had long artificial nails, and another nurse had long natural nails. Both nurses carried on their hands the implicated strain of *P. aeruginosa*. The investigation found that the neonates were more likely to have been cared for by the two nurses during the exposure period. This indicated that the artificial and long natural nails may have contributed to causing this outbreak.

Evidence-Based Practice

- Nurses should not wear artificial nails or extenders when performing client care (CDC, 2002).
- Natural nails should be kept well manicured at ¼ inch long and free of nail gels and acrylic products.

Reference

Boyce JM, Pittet D: HICPAC/SHEA/APIC/IDSA Hand Hygiene Task Force and the CDC Healthcare Control Practices Advisory Committee draft guidelines for hand hygiene in healthcare settings, 2001.

---

of surfaces and high-level disinfection, which is required for some client care items such as endoscopes and bronchoscopes. You accomplish disinfection using a chemical disinfectant or wet pasteurization (used for respiratory therapy equipment). Examples of disinfectants are alcohols, chlorines, glutaraldehydes, hydrogen peroxide, and phenols. Glutaraldehydes are caustic and toxic to tissues and have been shown to pose a potential health risk. **Sterilization** is the complete elimination or destruction of all microorganisms, including spores. Steam under pressure, ethylene oxide (ETO) gas, hydrogen peroxide plasma, and chemicals are the most common sterilizing agents. ETO poses a potential health risk to staff processing with this agent, and exposure must be monitored.

The decision to clean, or clean and disinfect or sterilize, depends on the intended use of the item. There are three categories of device classification (Box 34-7). Be familiar with the health care facility or agency policy and procedures for cleaning, handling, and delivering care items for eventual disinfection and sterilization. Workers in the central processing area who are specially trained in disinfection and sterilization should perform most of the procedures. The following factors influence the efficacy of the disinfecting or sterilizing method:

- *Concentration of solution and duration of contact.* A weakened concentration or shortened exposure time lessens its effectiveness.
- *Type and number of pathogens.* The greater the number of pathogens on an object, the longer the required disinfecting time.
- *Surface areas to treat.* All dirty surfaces and areas must be fully exposed to disinfecting and sterilizing agents. The type of surface is an important factor. Is the surface porous or nonporous?
- *Temperature of the environment.* Disinfectants tend to work best at room temperature.

✴ BOX 34-7 ・ Categories for Sterilization, Disinfection, and Cleaning

Critical Items

Items that enter sterile tissue or the vascular system present a high risk of infection if the items are contaminated with microorganisms, especially bacterial spores. *Critical items* must be *sterile*. Some of these items include:

- Surgical instruments
- Cardiac or intravascular catheters
- Urinary catheters
- Implants

Semicritical Items

Items that come in contact with mucous membranes or nonintact skin also present a risk. These objects must be free of all microorganisms (except bacterial spores). *Semicritical items* must be *high-level disinfected (HLD)* or *sterilized*. Some of these items include:

- Respiratory and anesthesia equipment
- Endoscopes
- Endotracheal tubes
- Gastrointestinal endoscopes
- Diaphragm fitting rings

After rinsing, dry items and store in a manner to protect from damage and contamination.

Noncritical Items

Items that come in contact with intact skin but not mucous membranes must be clean. *Noncritical items* must be *disinfected*. Some of these items include:

- Bedpans
- Blood pressure cuffs
- Bed rails
- Linens
- Stethoscopes
- Bedside trays and client furniture
- Food utensils

TABLE 34-6 Examples of Disinfection and Sterilization Processes

CHARACTERISTICS	EXAMPLES OF USE
Moist Heat Steam is moist heat under pressure. When exposed to high pressure, water vapor can attain temperature above boiling point to kill pathogens and spores.	Autoclave sterilizes heat-tolerant surgical instruments and semicritical client care items.
Chemical Sterilants—High-Level Disinfection (HLD) A number of chemical disinfectants are used in health care. These include alcohols, chlorines, formaldehyde, glutaraldehyde, hydrogen peroxide, iodophors, phenolics, and quaternary ammonium compounds. Each product performs in a unique manner and is used for a specific purpose.	Chemicals disinfect heat-sensitive instruments and equipment, such as endoscopes, respiratory therapy equipment.
Ethylene Oxide (ETO) Gas This gas destroys spores and microorganisms by altering cells' metabolic processes. Fumes are released within an autoclave-like chamber. Ethylene oxide gas is toxic to humans, and aeration time varies with products.	This gas sterilizes most medical materials.
Boiling Water Boiling is least expensive for use in home. Bacterial spores and some viruses resist boiling. It is not used in health care facilities.	Items in home care.

BOX 34-8 Infection Prevention and Control to Reduce Reservoirs of Infection

Bathing
Use soap and water to remove drainage, dried secretions, or excess perspiration.

Dressing Changes
Change dressings that become wet and/or soiled (see Chapter 48).

Contaminated Articles
Place tissues, soiled dressings, or soiled linen in fluid-resistant bags for proper disposal.

Contaminated Sharps
Place all needles, safety needles, and needleless systems into puncture-proof containers, which should be located at the site of use. Federal law requires the use of needle-safe technology. Blood tube holders are single use only (OSHA: Needlestick Safety Prevention Act of 2000, 2001).

Bedside Unit
Keep table surfaces clean and dry.

Bottled Solutions
Do not leave bottled solutions open.
Keep solutions tightly capped.
Date bottles when opened, and discard in 24 hours.

Surgical Wounds
Keep drainage tubes and collection bags patent to prevent accumulation of serous fluid under the skin surface.

Drainage Bottles and Bags
Wear gloves and protective eyewear if splashing or spraying with contaminated blood or body fluids is anticipated.
Empty and dispose of drainage suction bottles according to facility policy.
Empty all drainage systems on each shift unless otherwise ordered by a physician.
Never raise a drainage system (e.g., urinary drainage bag) above the level of the site being drained unless it is clamped off.

OSHA, Occupational Safety and Health Administration.

• *Presence of soap.* Soap cause certain disinfectants to be ineffective. Thorough rinsing of an object is necessary before disinfecting.
• *Presence of organic materials.* Disinfectants become inactivated unless blood, saliva, pus, or body excretions are washed off.

Table 34-6 lists processes for disinfection and sterilization and their characteristics. It should be noted that some delicate instruments requiring sterilization cannot tolerate steam and must be processed using gas or plasma.

Infection Prevention and Control—Client Safety. Effective prevention and control of infection requires you to remain aware of the modes of transmission and ways to control them (Box 34-8). In the hospital, home, or extended care facility a client should have a personal set of care items. Sharing bedpans, urinals, bath basins, and eating utensils can easily lead to cross infection. In facilities where health care–associated diarrhea occurs, electronic thermometers are not recommended for rectal temperatures. Do not use the same electronic thermometer for clients on contact isolation.

Always be careful when handling exudate, such as urine, feces, emesis, and blood. Contaminated fluids can easily splash while being discarded in toilets or hoppers. These containers need to be emptied at water level to reduce the risk of splash or splatter, and gloves and protective eyewear are worn. The nurse appropriately disposes of disposable soiled items in trash bags. Items contaminated with large amounts of blood are to be disposed of in biohazard bags. Check the location of the biohazard bags because their location may vary depending on the health care facility. Handle laboratory specimens from all clients as if they were infectious and place them in designated biohazard containers or bags for transport or disposal.

Even though there is no science to show that medical waste poses a health risk, the nurse must also be aware of the state regulations for the handling and disposal of medical (infectious) waste. The updated version of OSHA's regulations address the handling and disposal of blood and body fluids that potentially pose a risk for the transmission of blood-borne pathogens. These regulations defer to the state laws and regulations (OSHA, 1991).

To control organisms exiting via the respiratory tract, cover your mouth or nose when coughing or sneezing. The nurse should also teach clients respiratory hygiene or **cough etiquette** (see Table 34-7). Cough etiquette has become more important due to concerns for transmission of respiratory infections such as *M. tuberculosis* and influenza (CDC, 2007). The elements of a respiratory hygiene or cough etiquette include (1) education of health care facility staff, clients' families, and visitors; (2) posters and written material for health care facility or agency staff, clients, families, and visitors; (3) education on how to cover your nose/mouth when you cough, using a tissue, and the prompt disposal of the contaminated tissue; (4) placing a surgical mask on the client if it will not compromise respiratory function or is applicable, which may not be feasible in pediatric populations; (5) hand hygiene after contact with contaminated respiratory secretions; and (6) spatial separation greater than 3 feet away from persons with respiratory infections (CDC, 2007).

A nurse who has an upper respiratory tract infection should be placed on work restriction. Working when ill poses an additional risk to clients and co-workers. OSHA is enforcing the CDC guidelines for work restriction published in 1998. Work restriction for non–work-related illness requires the use of sick time. Work-related illness or exposures are covered by workers' compensation. Employee health and infection control services may become responsible to ensure compliance with these guidelines.

To prevent transmission of microorganisms through indirect contact, soiled items and equipment must be kept from touching your clothing. A common error is to carry dirty linen in the arms against the uniform. Use fluid-resistant linen bags, or carry soiled linen with hands held out from the body. Laundry hampers should be covered and emptied before becoming overloaded.

Many measures that control the exit of microorganisms likewise control the entrance of pathogens. Maintaining the integrity of skin and mucous membranes reduces the chances of microorganisms reaching a host. Keep the client's skin well lubricated by using lotion as appropriate. Immobilized and debilitated clients are particularly susceptible to skin breakdown. Do not position clients on tubes or objects that might cause breaks in the skin. Dry, wrinkle-free linen also reduces the chances of skin breakdown. It is important to turn and position clients before their skin becomes reddened. Frequent oral hygiene prevents drying of mucous membranes. A water-soluble ointment keeps the client's lips well lubricated.

After elimination, a woman should clean the rectum and perineum by wiping from the urinary meatus toward the rectum. Cleansing in a direction from the least to the most contaminated area helps reduce genitourinary infections. Meticulous and frequent perineal care is especially important in older adult women who wear disposable incontinent pads

Another cause for entrance of microorganisms into a host is improper handling and management of urinary catheters and drainage sets (see Chapter 45). The point of connection between a catheter and drainage tube should remain closed and intact. As long as such systems are closed, their contents are considered sterile. Outflow spigots on drainage bags should also remain

closed to prevent entrance of bacteria. Minimize movement of the catheter at the urethra by stabilizing the catheter with tape to reduce chances of microorganisms ascending the urethra into the bladder. Do not share urine-measuring containers between clients. Performing hand hygiene is an important intervention when caring for urinary drainage systems.

Sometimes you will care for clients with closed drainage systems that collect wound drainage, bile, or other body fluids. Make sure the site from which a drainage tube exits remains clear of excess moisture or accumulated drainage. All tubing should remain connected throughout use. You only open drainage receptacles when it is necessary to discard or measure the volume of drainage.

As a nurse, you will at times obtain specimens from drainage tubes or IV tubing ports. Disinfect tubes and ports by wiping the surface outward with alcohol or a chlorhexidine solution before entering the system. Temporarily placing squares of sterile gauze around the ends of an open drainage tube, such as a urinary catheter, adds further protection against bacteria. However, keeping drainage tubes closed and secure is the best practice.

A final method for reducing the entry of microorganisms is the technique for wound cleansing. The surgical wound is considered to be sterile. To prevent entry of microorganisms into the wound, always clean outward from a wound site. When applying an antiseptic or cleaning with soap and water, wipe around the wound edge first and then clean outward away from the wound (see Chapter 48). Use clean gauze for each revolution around the wound's circumference. A client's resistance to infection improves as the nurse protects normal body defenses against infection. The nurse intervenes to maintain the body's normal reparative processes (Box 34-9). Nurses also protect themselves and others through the use of isolation precautions.

The risk of transmitting HAIs or infectious disease among clients is high especially with an organism such as methicillin-resistant *S. aureus* (MRSA). When a client has a suspected or known infection, health care workers become alerted and follow infection prevention and control practices. However, in some cases, health care workers are not always aware that clients have an infection. Body substances such as feces, saliva, mucus, and wound drainage always contain potentially infectious organisms.

Isolation and Isolation Precautions. Isolation is the separation and restriction of movement of ill persons with contagious diseases. Health care facilities are required to have the capability of isolating clients. For example, facilities are required to have special negative-pressure rooms for clients suspected of or diagnosed with active pulmonary TB. However, not all communicable diseases require the placement of a client in a special private room (OSHA, 1996). You can conduct many isolation practices in standard rooms using barrier precautions.

Barrier precautions includes the appropriate use of gowns, gloves, masks, eyewear, and other protective devices or clothing. The choice of barriers depends on the task being performed. Barrier protection, using gloves for example, is for use with all clients because every client has the potential to transmit infection via blood and body fluids, and the risk for infection transmission is unknown. Because of the increased attention to the prevention of blood-borne pathogens and tuberculosis, the CDC and OSHA have stressed the

✳ BOX 34-9   Infection Prevention and Control: Protecting the Susceptible Host

Protecting Normal Defense Mechanisms

Regular bathing removes transient microorganisms from the skin's surface. Lubrication helps keep the skin hydrated and intact.

Regular oral hygiene. Saliva contains enzymes that promote digestion and has a bactericidal action to maintain control of bacteria. Flossing removes tartar and plaque that cause germ infection.

Maintenance of adequate fluid intake promotes normal urine formation and a resultant outflow of urine to flush the bladder and urethral lining of microorganisms.

For physically dependent or immobilized clients, encourage routine coughing and deep breathing to keep lower airways clear of mucus.

The nurse encourages proper immunization of children or adult clients who become exposed to certain infectious microorganisms. Children are vaccinated for measles, mumps, rubella, chickenpox, diphtheria, and other vaccine-preventable diseases. Adults should receive one booster of tetanus-diphtheria-acellular pertussis (Tdap), annual flu vaccine, and others as recommended by the CDC. Older adults should receive pneumococcal vaccine and annual influenza vaccine.

Maintaining Healing Processes

Promote intake of adequate fluids and a well-balanced diet containing essential proteins, vitamins, carbohydrates, and fats. The nurse also uses measures to increase the client's appetite.

Promote a client's comfort and sleep so that energy stores are replaced daily.

Assist the client in learning techniques to reduce stress.

---

importance of using barrier protection (OSHA, 2001). The CDC issued new isolation guidelines in 2007 that build on the two-tiered approach established in the 1996 guidelines.

The first and most important tier is standard precautions. The second tier addresses isolation precautions, which are based on the mode of transmission of the disease (Table 34-7). Isolation precautions are termed airborne, droplet, contact, and a new category, protective environment. The precautions are for clients with highly transmissible pathogens. The new category, protective environment, is designed for clients who have undergone transplants and gene therapy (CDC, 2007).

Contact transmission—Is divided into two subcategories, direct and indirect. Direct contact transmission is applied to the care and handling of contaminated body fluids. An example includes blood or other bloody body fluids from an infected client that enters the health care worker's body through direct contact with compromised skin or mucous membranes. Indirect contact transmission involves the transfer of an infectious agent through a contaminated intermediate object such as contaminated instruments or hands of health care workers. The health care worker may transmit microorganisms from one client site to another if hand hygiene is not performed between clients (CDC, 2007).

Droplet Precautions—Focus on diseases that are transmitted by large droplets that are expelled into the air 3 to 6 feet. Droplet precautions require the wearing of a surgical mask when within 3 feet of the client, proper hand hygiene, and some dedicated-care equipment. An example would be a client with influenza.

Airborne precautions—Focus on diseases that are transmitted by smaller droplets that remain in the air for long periods of time. This requires a specially equipped room with a negative air flow. The air exchanges in the room are set at a lower rate and are exhausted directly to the outside. Air is not returned to the inside ventilation system and is filtered though a high-efficiency particulate air (HEPA) filter.

Protective environment—Focuses on a very limited client population. This form of isolation requires a specialized room with positive airflow. The airflow rate is set at greater than 12 air exchanges per hour, and all air is filtered through a HEPA filter. Clients are not allowed to have dried and fresh flowers and potted plants in these rooms (CDC, 2007).

When using the CDC's isolation guidelines also refer to additional CDC documents to prevent health care–associated aspergillosis and legionnaires' disease in immunocompromised clients and the spread of multidrug-resistant organisms (CDC, 1995, 2002a, 2006b).

Regardless of the type of isolation system, follow the following basic principles:

- Use thorough hand hygiene before entering and leaving the room of a client in isolation.
- Dispose of contaminated supplies and equipment in a manner that prevents spread of microorganisms to other persons as indicated by the mode of transmission of the organism.
- Apply knowledge of a disease process and the mode of infection transmission when using protective barriers.
- Protect all persons who might be exposed during transport of a client outside the isolation room.

Psychological Implications of Isolation. When a client requires isolation in a private room, a sense of loneliness may develop because normal social relationships become disrupted. This situation can be psychologically harmful, especially for children.

As a result of the infectious process, clients' body images are altered. Some feel unclean, rejected, lonely, or guilty. Infection prevention and control practices further intensify these beliefs of difference or undesirability. Isolation in a private room limits sensory contact. Unless the nurse acts to minimize feelings of psychological and physical isolation, clients' emotional states can interfere with recovery. Another factor to consider is your attitude and body language when caring for clients in isolation. If you are uncomfortable, the client will sense this, and this will further impair the client's emotional status.

Before you institute isolation measures, the client and family need to understand the nature of the disease or condition, the purposes of isolation, and steps for carrying out specific precautions. If they are able to participate in maintaining infection prevention and control practices, the chances of reducing the spread of infection increase. Teach the client and family to perform hand

✳ TABLE 34-7 Centers for Disease Control and Prevention Isolation Guidelines

Standard Precautions—Tier 1

Standard precautions apply to all blood, all body fluids **(except sweat),** nonintact skin, and mucous membranes.

Perform hand hygiene between client contact; after contact with blood, body fluids, secretions, and excretions and after contact with equipment or articles contaminated by them; and immediately after gloves are removed.

Wear gloves when touching blood, body fluids, secretions, excretions (except sweat) nonintact skin, mucous membranes, or contaminated items or surfaces. Gloves should be removed and hand hygiene performed between client care encounters.

Wear masks, eye protection, or face shields if client care activities generate actual or risk of splashes or sprays of blood or body fluids.

Wear gowns if soiling of clothing is likely from blood and/or body fluids. Perform hand hygiene after gown removal.

Client care equipment is properly cleaned and disinfected. Single-use items are discarded (see health care facility or agency policy).

Place contaminated linen in leakproof bags and handle so as to prevent skin and mucous membrane exposure.

Discard all contaminated sharp instruments and needles in a puncture-resistant container. Health care facilities must make available needleless devices. Any needle should be disposed of uncapped, or a mechanical safety device is activated for recapping.

A private room is unnecessary unless the client's hygiene is unacceptable. Check with an infection prevention and control professional.

Respiratory hygiene/cough etiquette. Have clients cover the nose/mouth when coughing or sneezing; use tissues to contain respiratory secretions and dispose in nearest waste container; perform hand hygiene after contacting respiratory secretions and contaminated objects; contain respiratory secretions with procedure or surgical masks; sit at least 3 feet away from others if coughing.

Transmission Categories (Tier Two)

CATEGORY	DISEASE	BARRIER PROTECTION
Airborne precautions	Droplet nuclei smaller than 5 mcg; measles; chickenpox (varicella); disseminated varicella zoster; pulmonary or laryngeal TB	Private room, negative-pressure airflow of at least 6-12 air exchanges per hour via HEPA filtration; mask or respiratory protection device
Droplet precautions	Droplets larger than 5 mcg; being within 3 feet of the client; diphtheria (pharyngeal); rubella; streptococcal pharyngitis, pneumonia, or scarlet fever in infants and young children; pertussis; mumps; mycoplasmal pneumonia; meningococcal pneumonia or sepsis; pneumonic plague	Private room or cohort clients; refer to the facility policy for cohorting clients Mask or respirator is required; refer to facility policy
Contact precautions	Direct client or environmental contact; colonization or infection with multidrug-resistant organism (MDRO) such as VRE and MRSA, *Clostridium difficile,* or respiratory syncytial virus (RSV); draining wounds where secretions are not contained; scabies	Private room or cohort clients; refer to the facility policy for cohorting clients; gloves, gowns
Protective environment	Allogeneic hematopoietic stem cell transplants	Private room, positive-pressure room with 12 or more air exchanges per hour, HEPA filtration for incoming air, respirator mask, gloves, and gowns

TB, Tuberculosis; *HEPA,* high-efficiency particulate air; *VRE,* vancomycin-resistant enterococci; *MRSA,* methicillin-resistant *Staphylococcus aureus.*

hygiene and use barrier protection if appropriate. Demonstrate each procedure, and give the client and family an opportunity for practice. It is also important to explain how infectious organisms are transmitted so that the client and family understand the difference between contaminated and clean objects.

Take measures to improve the client's sensory stimulation during isolation. Make sure the room environment is clean and pleasant. Open drapes or shades, and remove excess supplies and equipment. Listen to the client's concerns or interests. If the nurse rushes through care or shows a lack of interest, the client will feel rejected and even more isolated. Mealtime is a particularly good opportunity for conversation. Providing comfort measures such as repositioning, a back massage, or a warm sponge bath increases physical stimulation. Depending on the client's condition, encourage the client to walk around the room or sit up in a chair. Recreational activities such as board games or cards are an option to keep the client mentally stimulated.

Explain to the family the client's risk for depression or loneliness. Encourage visiting family members to avoid expressions or actions that convey revulsion or disgust related to infection prevention and control practices. Discuss ways to provide meaningful stimulation.

The Isolation Environment. Private rooms used for isolation sometimes provide negative-pressure airflow to prevent infectious particles from flowing out of the room to other rooms and the air handling system. There are also special rooms with positive-pressure airflow that are used for highly susceptible immunocompromised clients such as recipients of transplanted organs. On the door or wall outside the room the nurse posts a card listing precautions for the isolation category according to health care facility policy. The card is a handy reference for health care personnel and visitors and alerts anyone who might enter the room accidentally that special precautions must be followed.

The isolation room or an adjoining anteroom needs to contain hand hygiene and personal protective equipment supplies. Soap

✳ **BOX 34-10** **PROCEDURAL GUIDELINES**

Caring for a Client on Isolation Precautions

Delegation Considerations: The skill of caring for a client on isolation precautions can be delegated. However, it is the nurse who assesses the client's status and isolation indications. Instruct nursing assistive personnel about special precautions regarding individual client needs, such as transportation to diagnostic tests.

Equipment: Barrier protection determined by type of isolation—gowns, protective eyewear, or face shield may be needed; supplies depend on procedures performed in room; sharps container; disposable blood pressure (BP) cuff

1. Assess isolation indications (e.g., client's medical history for exposure, laboratory tests, wound drainage).
2. Review agency policies and precautions necessary for the specific isolation system, and consider care measures you will perform while in client's room.
3. Review nurses' notes or speak with colleagues regarding client's emotional state and adjustment to isolation.
4. Perform hand hygiene, and prepare all equipment you will need to take into client's room. In some cases, equipment may remain in the room (stethoscope or BP cuff). Decide which isolation equipment is necessary before entering the client's room. For example, decide if you will need a gown and gloves for a client in contact precautions or if you will need a special respirator mask for a client on airborne precautions.
5. Prepare for entrance into isolation room:
   a. Apply cover gown, being sure it covers all outer garments. Pull sleeves down to wrist. Tie securely at neck and waist (see illustration).
   b. Apply either surgical mask or respirator around mouth and nose. (Type will depend on type of precautions and facility policy.) The nurse must have a medical evaluation and be fit tested before using a respirator (OSHA, 1996).
   c. If needed, apply eyewear or goggles snugly around face and eyes. If prescription glasses are worn, side shield may be used.
   d. Apply clean gloves. (NOTE: Wear unpowdered, latex-free gloves.) Wear gloves within gown, bring glove cuffs over edge of gown sleeves.
6. Enter client's room. Arrange supplies and equipment. (If equipment will be removed from room for reuse, place on clean paper towel.)
7. Explain purpose of isolation and necessary precautions to client and family. Offer opportunity to ask questions. Assess for evidence of emotional problems that can occur from isolation.
8. Assess vital signs.
   a. If client is infected or colonized with a resistant organism (e.g., vancomycin-resistant enterococcus [VRE], methicillin-resistant *Staphylococcus aureus* [MRSA]), equipment remains in room. This includes the stethoscope and blood pressure cuff.
   b. If stethoscope is to be reused, clean diaphragm or bell with alcohol. Set aside on clean surface.
   c. Use individual electronic or disposable thermometer.

Critical Decision Point: If disposable thermometer indicates a fever, assess for other signs/symptoms. Confirm fever using an electronic thermometer (Potter, 2003).

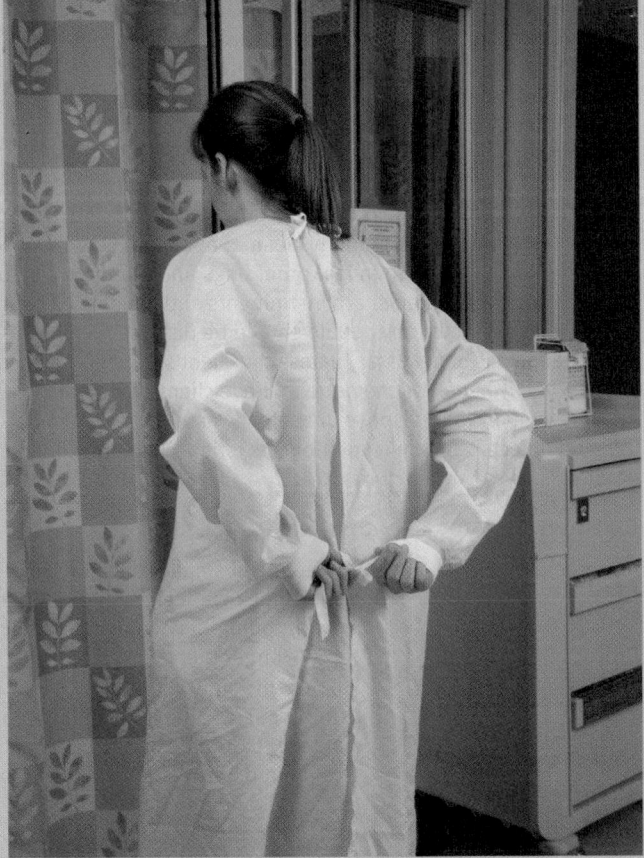

STEP 5a Tying gown at waist.

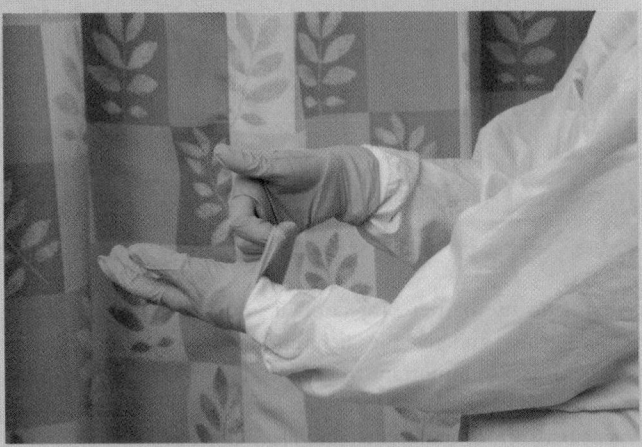

STEP 5d Applying gloves over gown sleeves.

9. Administer medications (see Chapter 35).
   a. Give oral medication in wrapper or cup.
   b. Dispose of wrapper or cup in plastic-lined receptacle.
   c. Administer injection.
   d. Discard safety needle and syringe or needle into the sharps container.
   e. If you are not wearing gloves and hands come into contact with contaminated article or body fluids, perform hand hygiene as soon as possible.

✴ **BOX 34-10**   **PROCEDURAL GUIDELINES—CONT'D**

Caring for a Client on Isolation Precautions—cont'd

10. Administer hygiene, encouraging the client to discuss questions or concerns about isolation. Use informal teaching at this time.
    a. Avoid allowing gown to become wet. Carry washbasin out away from gown; avoid leaning against any wet surface.
    b. Remove linen from bed; avoid contact with gown. Place in leakproof linen bag.
    c. Change gloves, and perform hand hygiene if hands become excessively soiled and further care is necessary.
11. Collect specimens.
    a. Place specimen containers on clean paper towel in client's bathroom. Follow procedure for collecting specimen of body fluids.
    b. Transfer specimen to container without soiling outside of container. Place container in plastic bag, and place label on outside of bag or as per facility policy. Perform hand hygiene, and reglove if additional procedures are needed.
12. Dispose of linen and trash bags as they become full.
    a. Use sturdy, moisture-resistant single bags to contain soiled articles. Use double bag if outside of bag is contaminated.
    b. Tie bags securely at top in knot (see illustration).
13. Remove all reusable equipment. Clean any contaminated surfaces (see health care facility or agency policy).
14. Resupply room as needed. Have a staff member outside the isolation room hand you new supplies.
15. Explain to client when you plan to return to room. Ask whether client requires any personal care items, books, or magazines.
16. Leave isolation room. The order for removing PPE depends on what was needed for the type of isolation. The sequence listed is based on full PPE being required.
    a. Remove gloves. Remove one glove by grasping cuff and pulling glove inside out over hand. Discard glove. With ungloved hand, tuck finger inside cuff of remaining glove and pull it off, inside out (see illustration).
    b. Remove eyewear/face shield or goggles.
    c. Untie waist and neck strings of gown. Allow gown to fall from shoulders. Remove hands from sleeves without touching outside of gown. Hold gown inside at shoulder seams, and fold inside out. Discard in laundry bag if fabric or in trash can if gown is disposable.
    d. Remove mask: If mask loops over your ears, remove from ears and pull away from face. For a tie-on mask, untie *top* mask strings, hold strings, and then untie bottom strings, pull mask away from face, and drop it into trash receptacle. Do not touch outer surface of mask.
    e. Perform hand hygiene.
    f. Leave room, and close door, if necessary. (Make sure door is closed if client is on airborne precautions.)
    g. Dispose of all contaminated supplies and equipment in a manner that prevents spread of microorganisms to other persons (see health care facility or agency policy).

OSHA, Occupational Safety and Health Administration; *PPE,* personal protective equipment.

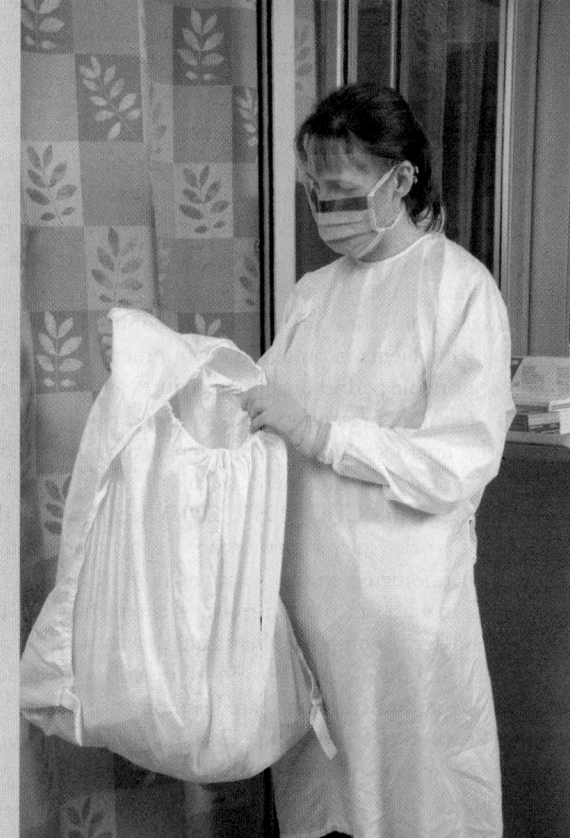

STEP 12b Tie trash bag securely.

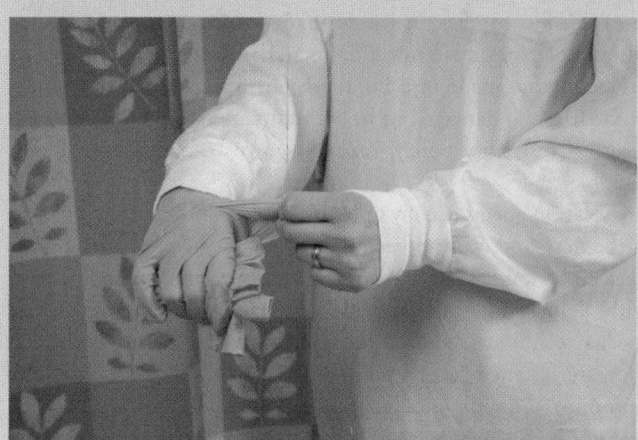

STEP 16a Removing glove.

and antiseptic (antimicrobial) solutions need to be available. Personnel and visitors perform hand hygiene before approaching the client's bedside and again before leaving the room. If toilet facilities are unavailable, there are special procedures for handling portable commodes, bedpans, or urinals.

All client care rooms, including those used for isolation, contain an impervious bag for soiled or contaminated linen, as well as a trash container with plastic liners. Impervious receptacles prevent transmission of microorganisms by preventing leaking and soiling of the outside surface. A disposable rigid container needs to be available in the room to discard used sharps such as safety needles and syringes.

Remain aware of infection prevention and control techniques while working with clients in protected environments. The nurse should feel comfortable performing all procedures and yet remain conscious of infection prevention and control principles. Depending on the microorganism and the mode of transmission, evaluate what articles or equipment to take into an isolation room. For example, the CDC (1995, 2007) recommends the dedicated use of articles such as stethoscopes, sphygmomanometers, or rectal thermometers in the isolation room of a client infected or colonized with vancomycin-resistant enterococci (VRE). Do not use these devices on other clients unless they are first adequately cleaned and disinfected. Box 34-10 describes the procedures commonly performed when shared equipment is used.

Personal Protective Equipment. Personal protective equipment (gowns, masks or respirators, protective eyewear, and gloves) should be readily available for personnel performing client care. The equipment to be used is task based.

Gowns. The primary reason for gowning is to prevent soiling clothes during contact with the client. Gowns or cover-ups protect health care personnel and visitors from coming in contact with infected material and blood or body fluid. Gowns are often required for contact precautions, depending on the expected amount of exposure to infectious material. Gowns used for barrier protection are made of a fluid-resistant material. Change gowns immediately if damaged or heavily contaminated. Depending on health care facility policy, isolation gowns can be disposable or reusable.

Isolation gowns usually open at the back and have ties or snaps at the neck and waist to keep the gown closed and secure. Gowns need to be long enough to cover all outer garments. Long sleeves with tight-fitting cuffs provide added protection. There is no special technique required for applying clean gowns as long as they are fastened securely. However, carefully remove gowns to minimize contamination of the hands and uniform, and then discard them after removal.

Respiratory Protection. Wear full-face protection (with eyes, nose, and mouth covered) when you anticipate splashing or spraying of blood or body fluid into the face. Also wear masks when working with a client placed on airborne or droplet precautions. If the client is on airborne precautions for TB, then apply an OSHA-approved respirator-style mask. The mask protects the nurse from inhaling microorganisms from a client's respiratory tract and prevents transmission of pathogens from the nurse's respiratory tract to the client. The surgical mask protects a wearer from inhaling large-particle aerosols that travel short distances (3 feet) and small-particle droplet nuclei that remain suspended in the air and travel

---

✳ BOX 34-11 **PROCEDURAL GUIDELINES**

Applying a Surgical Type of Mask

1. Find top edge of mask (some have a thin metal strip along edge). Pliable metal fits snugly against bridge of nose. Others offer an occlusive fit that does not require an adjustment.
2. Hold mask by top two strings or loops. Tie two top ties at top of back of head (see illustration), with ties above ears. (*Alternative:* Slip loops over each ear.)
3. Tie two lower ties snugly around neck with mask well under chin (see illustration).
4. Gently pinch upper metal band around bridge of nose.

NOTE: Change mask if wet, moist, or contaminated.

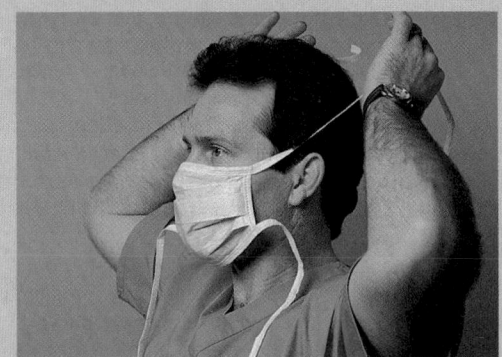

STEP 2

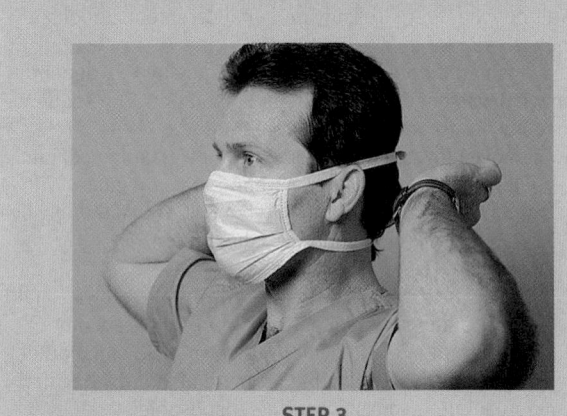

STEP 3

---

longer distances. When caring for clients on droplet precautions apply a surgical mask when entering the isolation room.

At times a client who is susceptible to infection wears a mask to prevent inhalation of pathogens. Clients on droplet or airborne precautions who are transported outside of their rooms need to wear a surgical mask to protect other clients and personnel. Masks prevent transmission of infection by direct contact with mucous membranes (CDC, 2005a). A mask discourages the wearer from touching the eyes, nose, or mouth (Box 34-11).

A properly applied mask fits snugly over the mouth and nose so that pathogens and body fluids cannot enter or escape through the sides. If a person wears glasses, the top edge of the mask fits below the glasses so that they will not cloud over as the person exhales. Keep talking to a minimum while wearing a mask to reduce respiratory airflow. A mask that has become moist does not

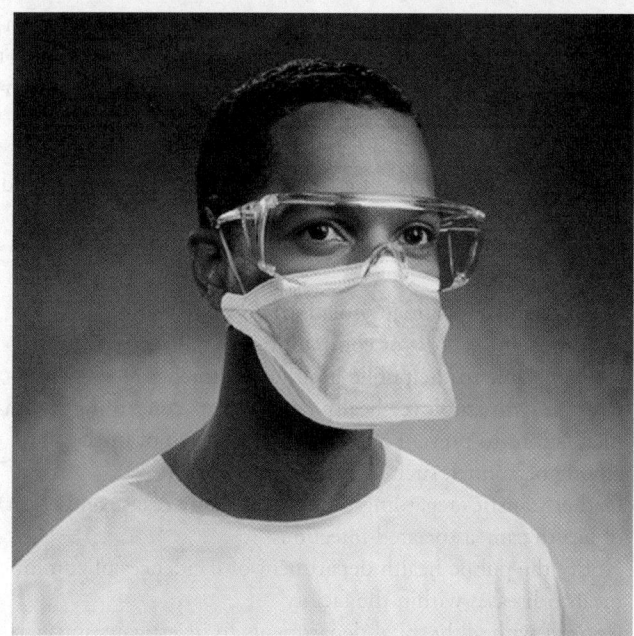

Figure 34-2 N95 respirator mask with protective eyewear. (Courtesy Kimberly-Clark Health Care, Roswell, Ga.)

provide a barrier to microorganisms and is ineffective. You will need to discard it. Never reuse a disposable mask. Warn clients and family members that a mask can cause a sensation of smothering. If family members become uncomfortable, they should leave the room and discard the mask.

Specially fitted respiratory protective devices (N95 respirator masks) are required when caring for a client with known or suspected TB (Figure 34-2) (CDC, 2005a). The mask must have a higher filtration rating than the regular surgical mask and be fitted snugly to prevent leakage around the sides. Be aware of health care facility policy regarding the type of respiratory protective device required. Special fit testing is required to establish the size and ability of the nurse to wears this type of mask (OSHA, 1995).

Eye Protection. Use either special glasses or goggles when performing procedures that generate splash or splatter. Examples of such procedures include irrigation of a large abdominal wound or insertion of an arterial catheter in which the nurse assists a health care provider. A nurse who wears prescription glasses will use removable reusable or disposable side shields over prescription glasses (OSHA, 2001). Eyewear is available in the form of plastic glasses or goggles. The eyewear needs to fit snugly around the face so that fluids cannot enter between the face and the glasses.

Gloves. Gloves help to prevent the transmission of pathogens by direct and indirect contact. The CDC notes that you should wear clean gloves when touching blood, body fluid, secretions, excretions, (except sweat), moist mucous membranes, nonintact skin, and contaminated items or surfaces. Change gloves between tasks and procedures on the same client after contact with material that contains a high concentration of microorganisms. Remove gloves promptly after use, before touching noncontaminated items and environmental surfaces, and before going to another client. Perform hand hygiene immediately to avoid transfer of microorganisms to other clients or environments. Because of allergy or sensitivity to latex gloves, facilities provide

nonlatex gloves. This is to reduce the incidence of health care providers developing latex allergy or sensitivity. Most facilities are working to become latex free to protect health care providers and clients.

When full PPE is necessary, first perform hand hygiene, then apply a gown, apply mask and eyewear or goggles (as needed), and end with applying gloves. Clean gloves are easy to apply and will fit either hand. The glove cuffs should be pulled up over the wrists or over the cuffs of the gown. If you notice a break or tear in a glove while providing care, change gloves. If the nurse does not plan to have more contact with the client, reapplying gloves is unnecessary. Perform hand hygiene when gloves are removed.

Instruct family members visiting clients on isolation precautions in how to apply gloves properly. Demonstrate application of gloves to family members and explain the reason for the use of gloves. Emphasize the importance of performing hand hygiene after removing gloves.

Specimen Collection. Many laboratory studies are often necessary when a client is suspected of having an infectious or communicable disease (Box 34-12). You will collect body fluids and secretions suspected of containing infectious organisms for culture and sensitivity tests. Place the specimen in a medium that promotes growth of organisms. After the specimen is sent to the laboratory, the laboratory technologist then identifies the microorganisms growing in the culture. Additional test results indicate antibiotics to which the organisms are resistant or sensitive. Sensitivity reports determine the antibiotics used in treatment.

The nurse obtains all culture specimens using clean gloves and sterile equipment. Collecting fresh material from the site of infection, such as wound drainage, ensures that neighboring microbes do not contaminate the specimen. Seal all specimen containers tightly to prevent spillage and contamination of the outside of the container.

Bagging Trash or Linen. Nurses use special bagging procedures for removing contaminated items from the client's environment. Bagging contaminated items prevents accidental exposure of personnel and prevents contamination of the surrounding environment.

The CDC recommends a single bag for discarding items if the bag is impervious and sturdy and if you are able to place the article in the bag without contaminating the outside of the bag. You need to place soiled linen in an impervious laundry bag in the client's room (OSHA, 2001).

The CDC recommends double bagging if it is impossible to prevent contamination of the bag's outer surface. Double bagging is not otherwise recommended. Studies have shown that this procedure is not necessary to prevent and control infection (CDC, 2007). Use of one standard-size linen bag that is not overfilled, that is tied securely, and that is intact is adequate to prevent infection transmission. Check the color code of bag that your facility uses for bagging these items.

Transporting Clients. Before transferring clients to wheelchairs or stretchers, the nurse gives them clean gowns to serve as robes. Clients infected with organisms transmitted by the airborne route normally leave their rooms only for essential purposes, such as diagnostic procedures or surgery. These clients must also wear surgical masks. Personnel transporting these clients should also wear barrier protection as needed.

✳ BOX 34-12 Specimen Collection Techniques*

Ensure that all specimen containers used have the biohazard symbol on the outside.

Wound Specimen
Clean site with sterile water or saline before wound specimen collection (see Chapter 48). Apply gloves and use cotton-tipped swab or syringe to collect as much drainage as possible. Have clean test tube or culture tube on clean paper towel. After swabbing center of wound site, grasp collection tube with a paper towel. Carefully insert swab without touching outside of tube. After securing tube's top, transfer tube into biohazard bag for transport and perform hand hygiene.

Blood Specimen (This procedure is usually performed by the laboratory technician.)
Wearing gloves, use a needle-safe syringe and culture media bottles to collect up to 10 mL of blood per culture bottle (check health care facility or agency policy). After prepping, perform venipuncture at two different sites to decrease likelihood of both specimens being contaminated with skin flora. Place blood culture bottles on a clean paper towel on bedside table or other surface; swab off bottle tops with alcohol. Inject appropriate amount of blood into each bottle. Transfer specimen into clean, labeled biohazard bag for transport. Remove gloves and perform hand hygiene.

Stool Specimen
Wearing gloves, use clean cup with seal top (need not be sterile) and tongue blade to collect small amount of stool, approximately 2 to 3 cm. Place cup on clean paper towel in client's bathroom. Using tongue blade, collect needed amount of feces from client's bedpan. Transfer feces to cup without touching cup's outside surface. Dispose of tongue blade, and place seal on cup. Transfer specimen into clean biohazard bag for transport. Remove gloves and perform hand hygiene.

Urine Specimen
Apply gloves and use sterile cup to collect 1 to 5 mL of urine. Place cup or tube on clean towel in client's bathroom. If client has a urinary catheter, use a needleless safety syringe to collect specimen from the sampling port on the catheter (see manufacturer's instructions). Have client follow procedure to obtain a clean voided specimen (see Chapter 45) if not catheterized. Secure top of transfer container, label for transport, and place in a biohazard bag. Remove gloves and perform hand hygiene.

From Pagana KD, Pagana TJ: *Mosby's diagnostic and laboratory test reference,* ed 7, St. Louis, 2005, Mosby.

*Health care facility or agency policies may differ on type of containers and amount of specimen material required.

Notify personnel in diagnostic or procedural areas or the operating room of the type of isolation precautions the client requires. Some clients being transported drain body fluids onto a stretcher or wheelchair. Use an extra layer of sheets to cover the stretcher or seat of the wheelchair. When this occurs, be sure to clean the equipment after client use and before another client uses the shared equipment.

Role of the Infection Control Professional. An infection prevention and control professional is a valuable resource for assisting nurses in controlling health care–associated infections. These professionals are specially trained in infection prevention

and control. They are responsible for advising health care personnel regarding infection prevention and control practices and for monitoring infections within the hospital. An infection prevention and control professional may do the following:

- Provide staff and client education on infection prevention and control
- Develop and review infection prevention and control policies and procedures
- Recommend appropriate isolation procedures
- Screen client records for community-acquired infections that are reportable to the public health department
- Consult with employee health departments concerning recommendations to prevent and control the spread of infection among personnel, such as TB testing
- Gather statistics regarding the **epidemiology** (cause and effect) of health care–associated infections
- Notify the public health department of incidences of communicable diseases within the facility
- Consult with all hospital departments to investigate unusual events or clusters of infection
- Monitor antibiotic-resistant organisms in the institution

Infection Prevention and Control for Hospital Personnel. Health care workers are continually at risk for exposure to infectious microorganisms. OSHA (2001) publishes rules and regulations to protect employees from blood-borne pathogens in the workplace. The OSHA regulations and CDC guidelines are incorporated into the policies and procedures of health care institutions and are part of regularly scheduled staff education programs.

Client Education. Often clients must learn to use infection prevention and control practices at home (Box 34-13). Preventive technique becomes almost second nature to the nurse who practices it daily. However, the client is less aware of factors that promote the spread of infection or ways to prevent its transmission. The home environment does not always lend itself to infection prevention and control. Often you will help a client adapt according to the resources available to maintain hygienic techniques. Generally clients in a home care setting have a decreased risk of infection because of decreased exposure to resistant organisms such as those found in a health care facility and because of fewer invasive procedures. However, it is important to educate clients about infection prevention and control techniques.

Surgical Asepsis. Surgical asepsis or sterile technique prevents contamination of an open wound, serves to isolate the operative area from the unsterile environment, and maintains a sterile field for surgery. Surgical asepsis includes procedures used to eliminate all microorganisms, including pathogens and spores, from an object or area. In surgical asepsis an area or object is considered contaminated if touched by any object that is not sterile. For example, a tear in a surgical glove exposes the outside of the glove to the skin surface, thus contaminating it. The nurse working with a sterile field or with sterile equipment needs to understand that the slightest break in technique results in contamination. Use surgical asepsis in the following situations:

✷ **BOX 34-13** **CLIENT TEACHING**

Infection Prevention and Control

Objective
- Client will assume self-care using proper infection prevention and control techniques.

Teaching Strategies
- Instruct client about cleaning equipment using soap and water and disinfecting with an appropriate disinfectant, such as diluted bleach.
- Demonstrate proper hand hygiene, explaining that the client should perform before and after all treatments and when infected body fluids are contacted.
- Instruct client in the signs and symptoms of wound infection and when to notify the health care provider.
- For clients who receive tube feedings at home, explain the importance of preparing enough formula for only 8 hours (commercially prepared) or 4 hours (home prepared). Tell client that contaminated enteral feeding sometimes causes infections. Rinse feeding bag and tubing with mild soap and water daily and dry.
- Instruct client to place contaminated dressings and other disposable items containing infectious body fluids in impervious plastic or brown paper bags. Place needles in metal or hard plastic containers such as coffee cans or laundry detergent bottles, and tape the openings shut. **Some states have specific requirements for sharps disposal. Check local regulations.**
- Clean noticeably soiled linen separate from other laundry. Wash in warm water with detergent. There are no special recommendations for setting dryer temperature (CDC, 2007).

Evaluation
- Ask client or family member to describe techniques used to reduce transmission of infection.
- Have client demonstrate select techniques.
- Ask client to explain the risks for infection based on the condition.

CDC, Centers for Disease Control and Prevention.

- During procedures that require intentional perforation of the client's skin, such as insertion of IV catheters or central lines
- When the skin's integrity is broken as a result of trauma, surgical incision, or burns
- During procedures that involve insertion of catheters or surgical instruments into sterile body cavities, such as insertion of a urinary catheter

Although surgical asepsis is common in the operating room, labor and delivery area, and major diagnostic areas, you will also use surgical aseptic techniques at the client's bedside. This includes, for example, inserting IV or urinary catheters, suctioning the tracheobronchial airway, and reapplying sterile dressings. A nurse in an operating room follows a series of steps to maintain sterile technique, including applying a mask, protective eyewear, and a cap; performing a surgical hand scrub; and applying a sterile gown and gloves. In contrast, a nurse performing a dressing change at a client's bedside only performs hand hygiene and applies sterile gloves.

Client Preparation. Because surgical asepsis requires exact techniques, you need to have the client's cooperation. Certain clients fear moving or touching objects during a sterile procedure, whereas others try to assist. Explain how you will perform a procedure and what the client can do to avoid contaminating sterile items, including the following:

- Avoid sudden movements of body parts covered by sterile drapes
- Refrain from touching sterile supplies, drapes, or the nurse's gloves and gown
- Avoid coughing, sneezing, or talking over a sterile area

Certain sterile procedures last an extended time. The nurse assesses the client's needs and anticipates factors that may disrupt a procedure. If a client is in pain, you need to administer analgesics no more than half an hour before a sterile procedure begins. Ask the client if he or she needs to use the bathroom or a bedpan. Often clients have to assume relatively uncomfortable positions during sterile procedures. The nurse helps the client to assume the most comfortable position possible. Finally, the client's condition sometimes results in actions or events that contaminate a sterile field. For example, a client with a respiratory infection transmits organisms by coughing or talking. Anticipate such a problem and place a surgical mask on the client before the procedure begins.

Principles of Surgical Asepsis. When beginning a surgically aseptic procedure, the nurse follows certain principles to ensure maintenance of asepsis. Failure to follow these principles places clients at risk for infection. The following principles are important:

1. *A sterile object remains sterile only when touched by another sterile object.* This principle guides the nurse in placement of sterile objects and how to handle them.
   a. Sterile touching sterile remains sterile; for example, sterile gloves or sterile forceps are used to handle objects on a sterile field.
   b. Sterile touching clean becomes contaminated; for example, if the tip of a syringe or other sterile object touches the surface of a clean disposable glove, the object is contaminated.
   c. Sterile touching contaminated becomes contaminated; for example, when the nurse touches a sterile object with an ungloved hand, the object is contaminated.
   d. Sterile state is questionable, for example, when you find a tear or break in the covering of a sterile object. Discard it regardless of whether the object itself appears untouched.
2. *Only sterile objects may be placed on a sterile field.* All items are properly sterilized before use. Sterile objects are kept in clean, dry storage areas. The package or container holding a sterile object must be intact and dry. A package that is torn, punctured, wet, or open is considered unsterile.
3. *A sterile object or field out of the range of vision or an object held below a person's waist is contaminated.* Nurses never turn their backs on a sterile field or a sterile tray or leave it unattended. Contamination can occur accidentally by a dangling piece of clothing, falling hair, or an unknowing client touching a sterile object. Any object held below waist level is considered contaminated because it cannot be viewed at all times. Keep sterile objects in front with the hands as close together as possible.
4. *A sterile object or field becomes contaminated by prolonged exposure to air.* Avoid activities that may create air currents, such

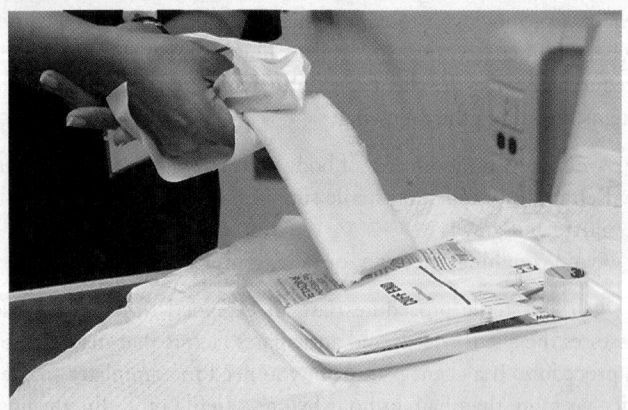

Figure 34-3 Placing sterile item on sterile field.

as excessive movements or rearranging linen after a sterile object or field becomes exposed. When you are opening sterile packages, it is important to minimize the number of people walking into the area. Microorganisms also travel by droplet through the air. No one should talk, laugh, sneeze, or cough over a sterile field or when gathering and using sterile equipment. When opening sterile packages, the nurse holds the item or piece of equipment as close as possible to the sterile field without touching the sterile surface.

5. *When a sterile surface comes in contact with a wet, contaminated surface, the sterile object or field becomes contaminated by capillary action.* If moisture leaks through a sterile package's protective covering, microorganisms travel to the sterile object. When stored sterile packages become wet, discard the objects immediately or send the equipment for resterilization. When working with a sterile field or tray, you may have to pour sterile solutions. Any spill is a source of contamination unless on a sterile surface that moisture cannot penetrate. Urinary catheterization trays contain sterile supplies that rest in a sterile, plastic container. In contrast, if a nurse places a piece of sterile gauze in its wrapper on a client's bedside table and the table surface is wet, the gauze is considered contaminated.

6. *Fluid flows in the direction of gravity.* A sterile object becomes contaminated if gravity causes a contaminated liquid to flow over the object's surface. To avoid contamination during a surgical hand scrub, hold your hands above your elbows. This allows water to flow downward without contaminating the nurse's hands and fingers. The principle of water flow by gravity is also the reason for drying from fingers to elbows, with hands held up, after the scrub.

7. *The edges of a sterile field or container are considered to be contaminated.* Frequently you will place sterile objects on a sterile towel, drape, or tray (Figure 34-3). Because the edge of the drape touches an unsterile surface, such as a table or bed linen, a 2.5-cm (1-inch) border around the drape is considered contaminated. Objects placed on the sterile field must be inside this border. The edges of sterile containers become exposed to air after they are open and are thus contaminated. After you remove a sterile needle from its protective cap or after you remove forceps from a container, the objects must not touch the container's edge.

Performing Sterile Procedures. Assemble all of the equipment that will be needed before a procedure. Have a few extra supplies available in case objects accidentally become contaminated. The nurse should not leave the sterile area. Before the sterile procedure, each step should be explained so that the client can cooperate fully. If an object becomes contaminated during the procedure, do not hesitate to discard it immediately.

Donning and Removing Caps, Masks, and Eyewear. For sterile procedures on a general nursing unit, wear a surgical mask and eyewear without a cap. Eyewear is worn as a part of standard precautions if there is a risk of fluid or blood splashing into the nurse's eyes. For sterile surgical procedures, the nurse first applies a clean cap that covers all of the hair and then the surgical mask and eyewear. A mask should fit snugly around the face and nose. After wearing a mask for several hours, the area over the mouth and nose often becomes moist. Because moisture promotes the growth of microorganisms, change the mask if it becomes moist.

Protective glasses or goggles should fit snugly around the forehead and face to fully protect the eyes. Wear eyewear only for procedures that create the risk of body fluids splashing into the eyes. Remove PPE in the following order: gloves, face shield or goggles, gown, and then mask or respirator (CDC, 2005b). After removing all PPE, perform hand hygiene.

Opening Sterile Packages. Sterile items such as syringes, gauze dressings, or catheters are packaged in paper or plastic containers and are impervious to microorganisms as long as they are dry and intact. Some institutions wrap reusable supplies in a double thickness of paper, linen, or muslin. These packages are permeable to steam and thus allow for steam autoclaving. Sterile items are kept in clean, enclosed storage cabinets and are separated from dirty equipment.

Sterile supplies have chemical tapes indicating that a sterilization process has taken place. The tapes change color during the sterilization process. Failure of the tapes to change color means that the item is not sterile. Never use a sterile item if the packaging is outdated, open, or soiled. Health care facilities apply the date processed and a lot number to the item after processing ("event-related expiration"), or they may apply an expiration date ("date-related expiration") to the item. With either system it is important for the nurse to check the packaging of the item before use.

Before opening a sterile item, perform hand hygiene. Inspect the supplies for package integrity and sterility, and assemble the supplies in the work area, such as the bedside table or treatment room, before opening packages. A bedside table or countertop provides a large, clean working area for opening items. The work area should be above waist level. Do not open sterile supplies in a confined space where contamination might occur.

Opening a Sterile Item on a Flat Surface. You must open sterile packages without contaminating the contents. Commercially packaged items are usually designed so that the nurse only has to tear away or separate the paper or plastic cover. Hold the item in one hand while pulling the wrapper away with the other (Figure 34-4). Take care to keep the inner contents sterile before use. When opening items processed by the facility and packed in paper or linen, use the following steps:

1. Place the item flat in the center of the work surface.
2. Remove the sterilization tape or seal.

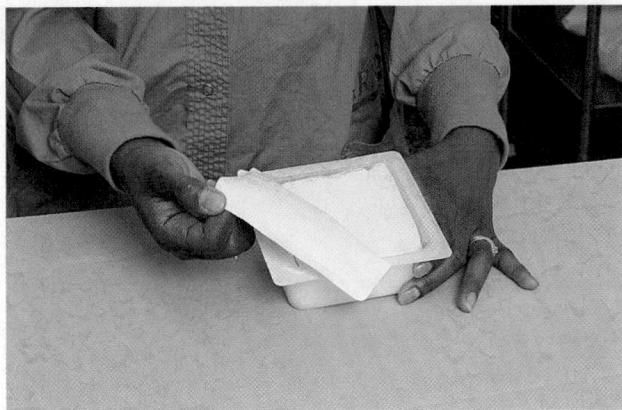

Figure 34-4 Nurse opens sterile package on work area above waist level.

3. Grasp the outer surface of the tip of the outermost flap.
4. Open the outer flap away from the body, keeping the arm outstretched and away from the sterile field (Figure 34-5, *A*).
5. Grasp the outside surface of the first side flap.
6. Open the side flap, allowing it to lie flat on the table surface. Keep the arm to the side and not over the sterile surface (Figure 34-5, *B*). Do not allow the flaps to spring back over the sterile contents.
7. Grasp the outside surface of the second side flap and allow it to lie flat on the table surface (Figure 34-5, *C*).
8. Grasp the outside surface of the last and innermost flap.
9. Stand away from the sterile package and pull the flap back, allowing it to fall flat on the surface (Figure 34-5, *D*).
10. Use the inner surface of the package (except for the 1-inch border around the edges) as a sterile field to add additional sterile items. Grasp the 1-inch border to maneuver the field on the table surface.

If you will not be using the sterile supplies immediately, close the sterile package. In this case the nurse should touch only the wrapper's outside surface. To close the package, the order of unwrapping is reversed, and the nurse does not touch the inside contents or reach over the field.

Opening a Sterile Item While Holding It. To open a small sterile item, hold the package in the nondominant hand while opening the top flap and pulling it away from the nurse. Using the dominant hand, the nurse carefully opens the sides and innermost flap away from the enclosed sterile item in the same order previously mentioned. You open the item in a hand so that you can pass the item to a person wearing sterile gloves or transfer to a sterile field.

Preparing a Sterile Field. When performing sterile procedures, the nurse needs a sterile work area that provides room for handling and placing of sterile items. A **sterile field** is an area free of microorganisms and prepared to receive sterile items. You prepare the field by using the inner surface of a sterile wrapper as the work surface or by using a sterile drape or dressing tray. After creating the surface for the field (Skill 34-2), the nurse adds sterile items by placing them directly on the field or by transferring them with a sterile forceps. Discard an object that comes in contact with the 1-inch border

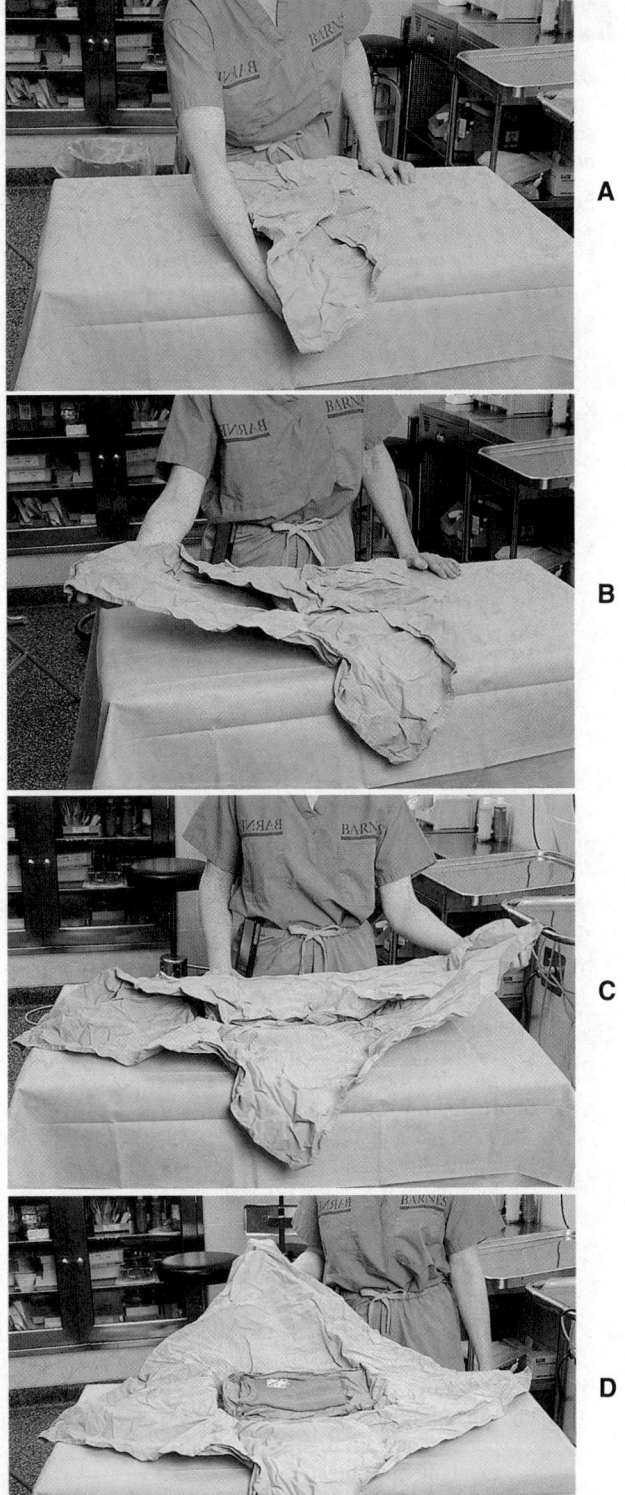

Figure 34-5 Opening sterile packaged items on a flat surface.
A, The nurse opens the top flap away from the body.
B, The nurse's arm is kept out away from the sterile field while opening a side flap. **C,** The second side flap is opened.
D, The back flap is opened.

✳ **SKILL 34-2**   **PREPARATION OF STERILE FIELD**

Delegation Considerations

The skill of preparation of a sterile field cannot be delegated. A surgical technician may prepare a sterile field as indicated by health care facility policy.

Equipment

- Sterile gloves
- Sterile drape or kit that is used as a sterile field

- Sterile gown (see health care facility policy)
- Disposable cap, mask, and/or eyewear (see health care facility policy)
- Sterile equipment and solutions specific to the procedure
- Waist-high table or surface
- Protective eyewear

STEPS	RATIONALE
1. Apply personal protective equipment as needed (consult agency policy)	
2. Select clean work surface above waist level.	Sterile object held below waist is contaminated.
3. Assemble necessary equipment, and check dates or labels on supplies for sterility of equipment.	Preparation of equipment in advance prevents break in technique. Equipment stored beyond expiration date is considered unsterile.
4. Perform hand hygiene.	Reduces transmission of microorganisms.
5. Prepare sterile field.	
a. **Sterile commercial kit or tray containing sterile items**	
(1) Place sterile kit or pack containing sterile items on work surface.	Ensures sterility of packaged drape.
(2) Open outside cover, and remove kit from dust cover. Place on work surface.	Inner kit remains sterile.
(3) Grasp outer edge of tip of outermost flap.	Outer surface of package is considered unsterile. There is a 2.5-cm (1-inch) border around any sterile drape or wrap that is considered unsterile.
(4) Open outermost flap away from body, keeping arm outstretched and away from the sterile field.	Reaching over sterile field contaminates it.
(5) Grasp outer edge of first side of flap.	Outer border is considered unsterile.
(6) Open side flap, pulling to side and allowing it to lie flat on table surface. Keep arm to the side, and do not extend it over the sterile surface.	Drape or flap should lie flat so it will not accidentally rise up and contaminate inner surface or the sterile items placed on its surface.
(7) Grasp outer edge of second side flap. Repeat for opening second side of package.	
(8) Grasp outer edge of last and innermost flap.	
(9) Stand away from sterile package, and pull flap back, allowing it to fall flat on work surface.	Reaching over sterile filed contaminates it.
b. **Sterile linen-wrapped package**	
(1) Place package on work surface.	
(2) Remove tape and seal, and unwrap both layers, following steps 5a(1) to (9) as with sterile kit.	
(3) Use opened package wrapper as a sterile field.	Inner surface of wrapper is considered sterile.
c. **Sterile drape**	
(1) Place pack containing the sterile drape on work surface.	Ensures sterility of packaged drape.
(2) Apply sterile gloves.	
(NOTE: This is an option depending on health care facility policy. You may touch outer 1-inch border of drape without wearing gloves.)	
(3) Grasp folded top edge of drape with fingertips of one hand. Gently lift drape up from its wrapper without touching any object.	If sterile object touches any nonsterile object, it becomes contaminated.
(4) Allow drape to unfold, keeping it above waist and the work surface and away from the body. (Carefully discard outer wrapper with other hand.)	Object held below person's waist or above chest is contaminated.
(5) With other hand, grasp the adjacent corner of drape. Hold drape straight over work surface (see illustration).	Drape can now be properly placed with two hands.
(6) Holding drape, first position the bottom half over top half of the intended work surface (see illustration).	Prevents nurse from reaching over sterile filed.
(7) Allow top half of drape to be placed over bottom half of work surface (see illustration).	A flat sterile surface is now available for placement of sterile items.

✳ **SKILL 34-2**   **PREPARATION OF STERILE FIELD—CONT'D**

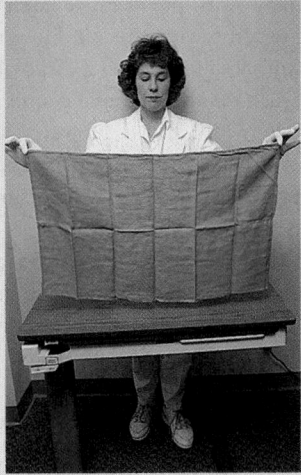

STEP 5c(5) Hold drape straight up and away from body.

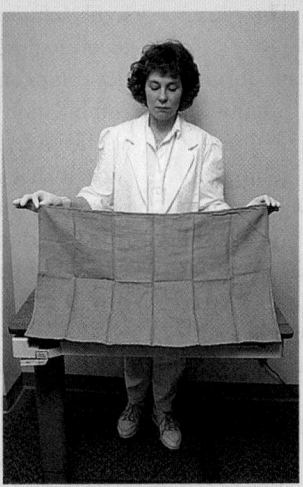

STEP 5c(6) Lay bottom half over work surface.

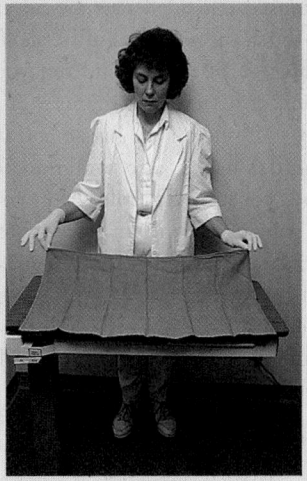

STEP 5c(7) Place top half of drape over work surface.

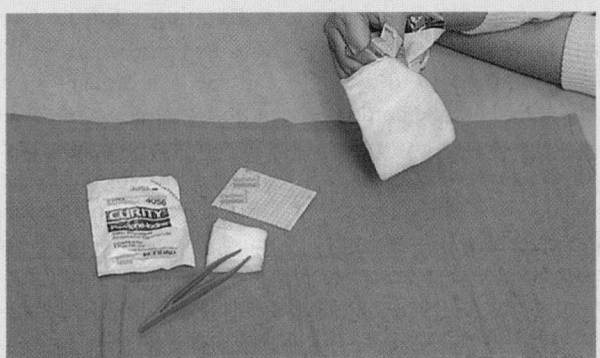

STEP 6c Adding item to sterile field.

STEPS	RATIONALE
6. Adding sterile items	
a. Open sterile item (following package directions) while holding outside wrapper in nondominant hand.	Frees dominant hand for unwrapping outer wrapper.
b. Carefully peel wrapper onto nondominant hand.	Item remains sterile. Inner surface of wrapper covers hand, making it sterile.
c. Being sure wrapper does not fall down on sterile field, place item onto field at angle. Do not hold arm over sterile field (see illustration).	Prevents reaching over field and contaminating its surface.
d. Dispose of outer wrapper.	Prevents accidental contamination of sterile field.
7. Perform procedure using sterile technique.	Prevents transmission of infection to client.

Recording and Reporting

- It is not necessary to record or report this procedure.

Sometimes you may wear sterile gloves while preparing items in the field. If you do this, you can touch the entire drape, but sterile items must be handed over by an assistant. The nurse's gloves cannot touch the wrappers of sterile items.

Pouring Sterile Solutions. Often you will have to pour sterile solutions into sterile containers. A bottle containing a sterile solution is sterile on the inside and contaminated on the outside; the bottle's neck is also contaminated, but the inside of the bottle cap is considered sterile. After you remove the cap or lid, you hold it in your hand or place it sterile side (inside) up on a clean surface. This means that you are able to see the inside of the lid as it rests on the table surface. Never rest a bottle cap or lid on a sterile surface, even though the inside of the cap is sterile. The outer edge of the cap is unsterile and will contaminate the surface. Placing a sterile cap down on an unsterile surface increases the chances of the inside of the cap becoming contaminated.

Hold the bottle with its label in the palm of the hand to prevent the possibility of the solution wetting and fading the label. Before pouring the solution into the container, the nurse pours a small amount (1 to 2 mL) into a disposable cap or plastic-lined waste receptacle. The discarded solution cleans the lip of the bottle. Keep the edge of the bottle away from the edge or inside of the receiving container. Pour the solution slowly to avoid splashing the underlying drape or field. Never hold the bottle so high above the container that even slow pouring will cause splashing. Hold the bottle outside the edge of the sterile field.

Surgical Scrub. Clients undergoing operative procedures are at an increased risk for infection. Nurses working in operating rooms perform surgical hand antisepsis (Skill 34-3) to decrease and suppress the growth of skin microorganisms in case of glove tears (Association of Perioperative Nurses [AORN], 2005). For maximum elimination of bacteria, remove all jewelry and keep the nails clean and short. Do not wear artificial nails because they often hold a greater number of bacteria (AORN 2005; CDC, 2002b). Nurses who have active skin infections, open lesions or cuts, or respiratory infections should be excluded from the surgical team.

During surgical hand antisepsis the nurse scrubs from fingertips to elbows with an antiseptic soap before each operation. The optimum duration of the surgical hand scrub is unclear, although research indicates that it may be dependent on the type of antimicrobial product (CDC, 2002b). The traditional scrub time in the United States for both the initial and the subsequent scrub has been 5 minutes. Follow the manufacturer's recommendation for scrub solutions. For many years, preoperative hand washing protocols required nurses to scrub with a brush. However, this practice can damage the skin. Scrubbing with a disposable sponge or combination sponge-brush reduces bacterial counts on the hands as effectively as scrubbing with a brush. However, several studies suggest that neither a brush nor a sponge is necessary to reduce bacterial counts on the hands, especially when using an alcohol-based product (CDC, 2002b).

Applying Sterile Gloves. Sterile gloves are an additional barrier to bacterial transfer. There are two gloving methods: open and closed. Nurses who work on general nursing units use open gloving before procedures such as dressing changes or urinary catheter insertions. The closed gloving method, which you perform after applying sterile gowns, is practiced in operating rooms and special treatment areas. Skills 34-4, p. 678, and 34-5, p. 681 review the steps of each sterile gloving technique. Make sure to select the proper glove size; the glove should not stretch so tightly that it can easily tear, yet it should be tight enough that you can pick up objects easily.

Donning a Sterile Gown. Nurses wear sterile gowns when assisting at the sterile field in the operating room, delivery room, and special treatment areas. Wearing a sterile gown allows the nurse to handle sterile objects and also be comfortable with less risk of contamination. The circulating nurse does not generally wear a sterile gown. The sterile gown acts as a barrier to decrease shedding of microorganisms from skin surfaces into the air and thus prevents wound contamination. Nurses caring for clients with large open wounds or assisting physicians during major invasive procedures (e.g., inserting an arterial catheter) will also wear sterile gowns.

The nurse does not apply a sterile gown until after applying a mask and surgical cap and performing surgical hand washing. The nurse picks up the gown from a sterile pack, or an assistant hands the gown to the nurse. Only a certain portion of the gown—the area from the anterior waist to, but not including, the collar and the anterior surface of the sleeves—is considered sterile. The back of the gown, the area under the arms, the collar, the area below the waist, and the underside of the sleeves are not sterile because the nurse cannot keep these areas in constant view and ensure their sterility. Skill 34-4 reviews the steps for applying a sterile gown.

Text continued on p. 682

✳ SKILL 34-3   SURGICAL HAND ASEPSIS

Delegation Considerations
The skill of surgical hand asepsis can be delegated to properly trained surgical technicians (know State's Nurse Practice Act).

Equipment
- Deep sink with foot or knee controls for dispensing water and soap (faucets should be high enough for hands and forearms to fit comfortably)

- Antimicrobial agent approved by the health care facility
- Surgical scrub sponge with plastic nail pick
- Paper face mask, cap or hood, surgical shoe covers
- Sterile towel
- Sterile pack containing sterile gown
- Protective eyewear (glasses or goggles)

STEPS	RATIONALE
1. Consult manufacturer's policy regarding required length of time and antiseptic to use for hand antisepsis.	Guidelines vary regarding ideal time needed and antiseptic to use for surgical scrub.
2. Remove bracelets, rings, and watches.	Jewelry may harbor or protect microorganisms from removal. Allergic skin reactions may occur as a result of scrub agent or glove powder accumulating under jewelry.
3. Be sure fingernails are short, clean, and healthy. Artificial nails should be removed. Natural nails should be less than ¼ inch long.	Long nails and chipped or old polish increase number of bacteria residing on nails. Long fingernails can puncture gloves, causing contamination. Artificial nails are known to harbor gram-negative microorganisms and fungus (AORN, 2005; AORN, 2007; CDC, 2002b).

Critical Decision Point: Remove nail polish if chipped or worn longer than 4 days because it may harbor microorganisms (AORN, 2005).

4. Inspect condition of cuticles, hands, and forearms for abrasions, cuts, or open lesions.	These conditions increase likelihood of more microorganisms residing on skin surfaces. Broken skin permits microorganisms to enter layers of the skin providing deeper microbial breeding grounds (AORN, 2005).
5. Apply surgical shoe covers, cap or hood, face mask, and protective eyewear.	Mask prevents escape into air of microorganisms that can contaminate hands. Other protective wear prevents exposure to blood and body fluid splashes during the procedure.
6. Turn on water using knee or foot controls, and adjust to comfortable temperature.	Knee or foot controls prevent contamination of hands after scrub.
7. Prescrub wash/rinse: Wet hands and arms under running lukewarm water, and lather with detergent to 5 cm (2 inches) above elbows. (Hands need to be above elbows at all times.)	Water runs by gravity from fingertips to elbows. Hands become cleanest part of upper extremity. Keeping hands elevated allows water to flow from least to most contaminated areas. Washing a wide area reduces risk of contaminating overlying gown that the nurse later applies.
8. Rinse hands and arms thoroughly under running water. **Remember to keep hands above elbows.**	Rinsing removes transient bacteria from fingers, hands, and forearms.
9. Under running water, clean under nails of both hands with nail pick. Discard after use (see illustration).	Removes dirt and organic material that harbor large numbers of microorganisms.

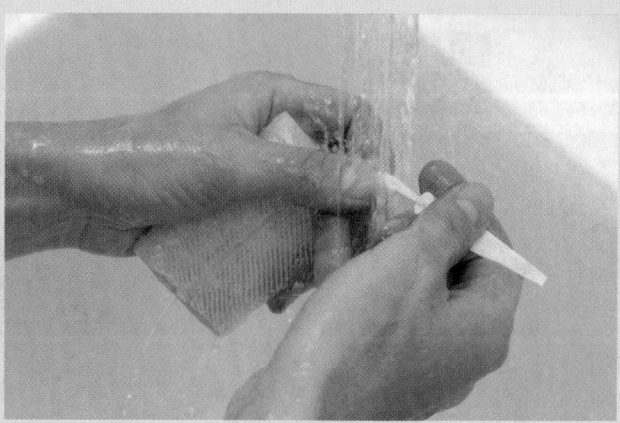

STEP 9 Cleaning under fingernails.

Continued

✳ **SKILL 34-3** **SURGICAL HAND ASEPSIS—CONT'D**

STEPS

10. Surgical hand scrub (with brush).
    a. Wet clean sponge, and apply antimicrobial agent. Visualize each finger, hand, and arm as having four sides. Wash all four sides effectively. Scrub the nails of one hand with 15 strokes. Scrub the palm, each side of thumb and fingers, and posterior side of hand with 10 strokes each (see illustration).

    b. Divide the arm mentally into thirds: scrub each third 10 times (AORN, 2005) (see illustration). Some health care facility policies require scrub by time rather than 10 strokes. Rinse brush, and repeat the sequence for the other arm. A two-brush method may be substituted (check health care facility policy).

    c. Discard brush. Flex arms, and rinse from fingertips to elbows in one continuous motion, allowing water to run off at elbow (see illustration).

    d. Turn off water with foot or knee control, with hands elevated in front of and away from body. Enter operating room suite by backing into room.

    e. Approach sterile setup; grasp sterile towel, taking care not to drip water onto the sterile setup.

    f. Bending slightly at waist, keeping hands and arms above the waist and outstretched, grasp one end of the sterile towel and dry one hand moving from fingers to elbow in a rotating motion (see illustration).

RATIONALE

Friction loosens resident bacteria that adhere to skin surfaces. Ensures coverage of all surfaces. Scrubbing is performed from cleanest area (hands) to marginal area (upper arms).

Eliminates transient microorganisms and reduces resident hand flora.

Hands remain the cleanest part of upper extremities.

Keeps hands free of microorganisms.

Water contaminates sterile setup.

Avoids sterile towel from contacting unsterile scrub attire and transferring contamination to hands. Dry skin from cleanest (hands) to least clean (elbows).

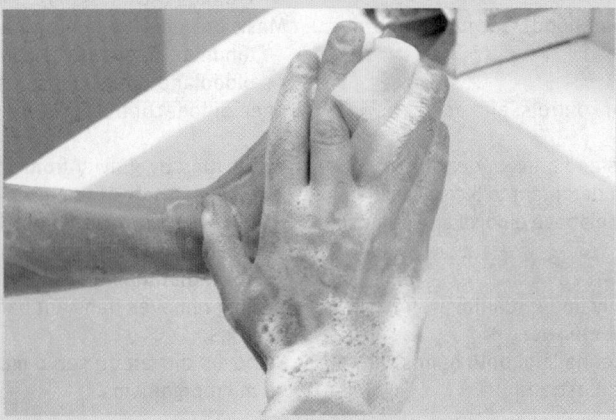

STEP 10a Scrubbing side of fingers.

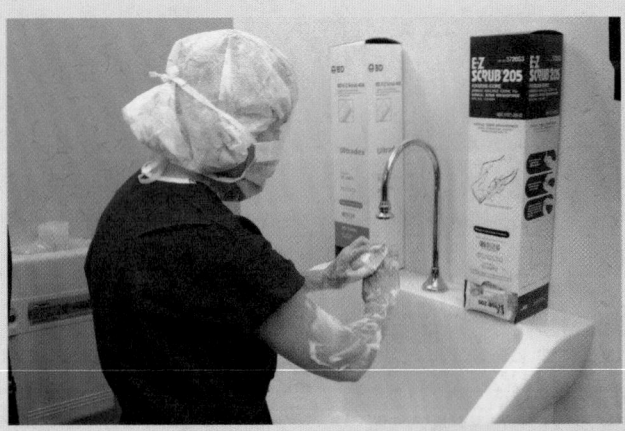

STEP 10b Scrubbing forearms.

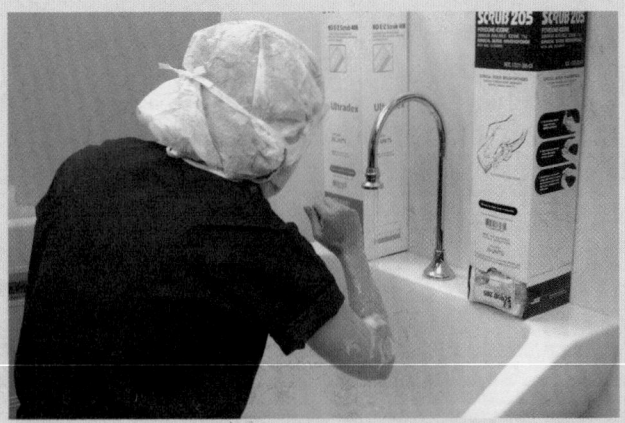

STEP 10c Rinsing arms.

✳ **SKILL 34-3**   **SURGICAL HAND ASEPSIS—CONT'D**

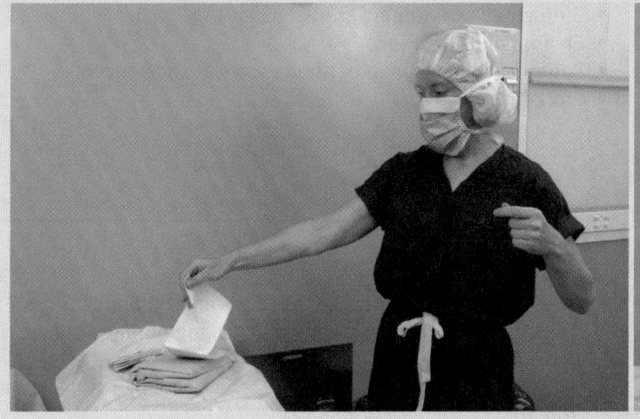
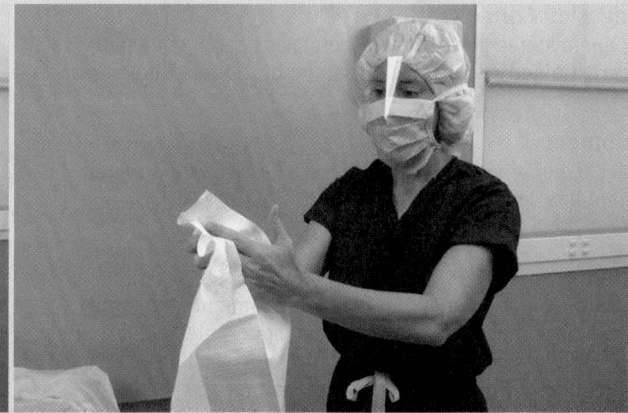

STEP 10f A, Grasping sterile towel. **B,** Drying sequence.

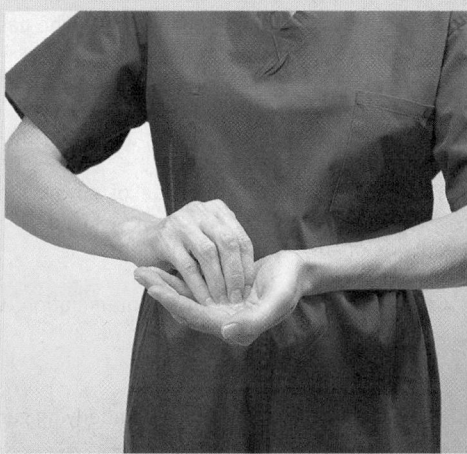
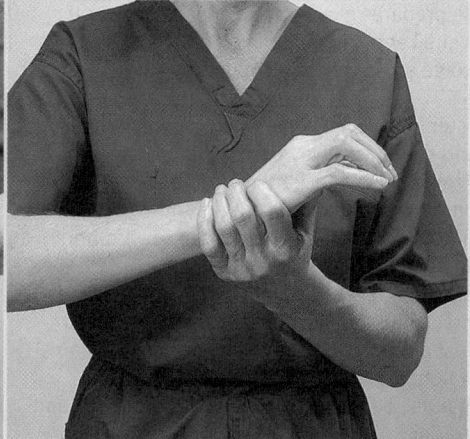

STEP 11b Application of an antimicrobial agent for brushless hand scrub. Nurse using 3M Avagard. (Photo courtesy of 3M Health Care.)

STEPS	RATIONALE
g. Repeat drying method for other hand by carefully reversing towel or using a new sterile towel.	Prevents accidental contamination.
h. Drop town into linen hamper or into circulating nurse's hand.	Prevents accidental contamination.
11. *Optional:* Brushless antiseptic hand rub	
a. After prescrub wash, dry hands and forearms thoroughly with a paper towel.	Promotes reduction in microorganisms on all surfaces of hands and arms.
b. Dispense 2 mL of antimicrobial agent hand preparation into the palm of one hand. Dip the fingertips of the opposite hand into the hand preparation and work it under the nails. Spread the remaining hand prep over the hand and up to just above the elbow, covering all surfaces (see illustration).	
c. Using another 2 mL of hand preparation, repeat with other hand.	
d. Dispense another 2 mL of hand preparation into either hand, and reapply to all aspects of both hands up to the wrist. Allow to dry before donning gloves.	
12. Proceed with sterile gowning (see Skill 34-4).	

Recording and Reporting
- It is not necessary to record or report this procedure.
- Report any dermatitis to employee health or infection control per agency policy.

✳ SKILL 34-4   APPLYING A STERILE GOWN AND PERFORMING CLOSED GLOVING

Delegation Considerations

Applying a sterile gown and closed gloving can be delegated to a properly trained surgical technician (know State's Nurse Practice Act).

Equipment

- Package of proper-size sterile gloves (latex free if nurse or client has sensitivity or allergy)

- Sterile pack containing sterile gown
- Clean, flat, dry surface
- Paper face masks, cap or hood, surgical shoe covers
- Protective eyewear/face shield

STEPS	RATIONALE
Gowning	
1. Before entering operating room or treatment area, apply cap, face mask, and eyewear. Foot covers are also required in operating room.	Prevents hair and air droplet nuclei from contaminating sterile work areas. Eyewear protects mucous membranes of eye. Foot covers are paper or cloth and fit over work shoes.
2. Perform thorough surgical hand wash (see Skill 34-3).	Removes transient and resident bacteria from fingers, hands, and forearms.
3. Circulating nurse assists by opening sterile pack containing sterile gown (folded inside out).	Gown's outer surface remains sterile.
4. Circulating nurse prepares glove package by peeling outer wrapper open while keeping inner contents sterile. Places inner glove package on sterile field created by sterile outer wrapper.	Keeps gloves sterile and allows nurse who has scrubbed to handle sterile items.
5. Reach down to sterile gown package; lift folded gown directly upward and step back away from table.	Provides wide margin of safety, avoiding contamination of gown.
6. Holding folded gown, locate neckband. With both hands, grasp inside front of gown just below neckband.	Clean hands can touch inside of gown without contaminating outer surface.
7. Allow gown to unfold, keeping inside of gown toward body. Do not touch outside of gown with bare hands.	Outside of gown will be sterile surface.
8. With hands at shoulder level, slip both arms into armholes simultaneously (see illustration). Ask circulating nurse to bring gown over shoulders by reaching inside to arm seams and pulling gown on, leaving sleeves covering hands.	Careful application prevents contamination. Gown covers hands to prepare for closed gloving.
9. Have circulating nurse securely tie back of gown at neck and waist (see illustration). (If gown is a wraparound style, do not touch sterile flap to cover gown until you are gloved.)	Gown must completely enclose underlying garments.
10. Closed gloving	
a. With hands covered by gown sleeves, open inner sterile glove package (see illustration).	Hands remain clean. Sterile gown cuff will touch sterile glove surface.
b. With dominant hand inside gown cuff, pick up glove for nondominant hand by grasping folded cuff.	Sterile gown touches sterile glove.

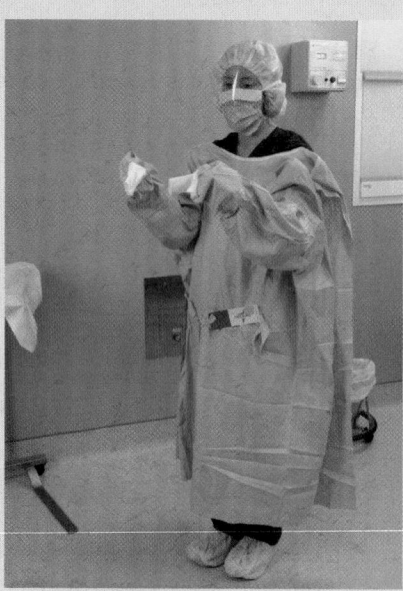

STEP 8 Placing arms in sleeves.

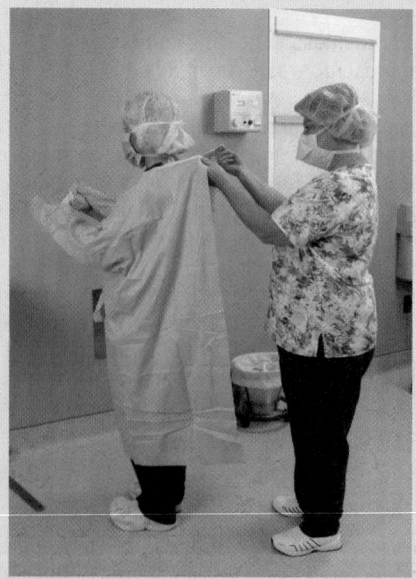

STEP 9 Circulating nurse ties scrub gown.

✳ **SKILL 34-4**

APPLYING A STERILE GOWN AND PERFORMING CLOSED GLOVING—CONT'D

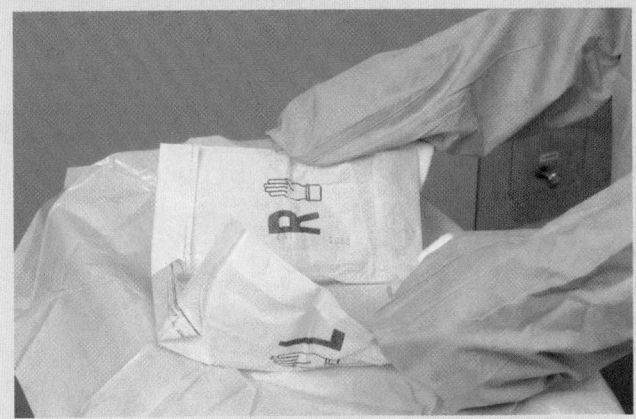

STEP 10a Scrub nurse opens glove package.

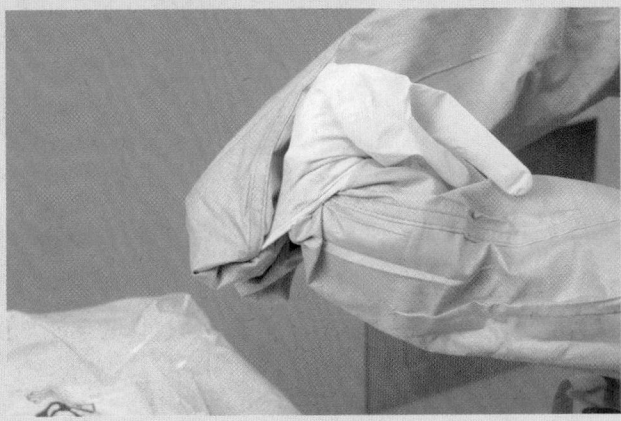

STEP 10d Glove applied to left hand as right hand remains inside cuff.

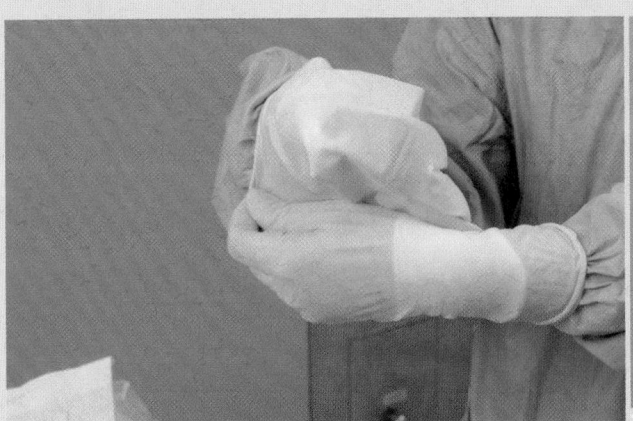

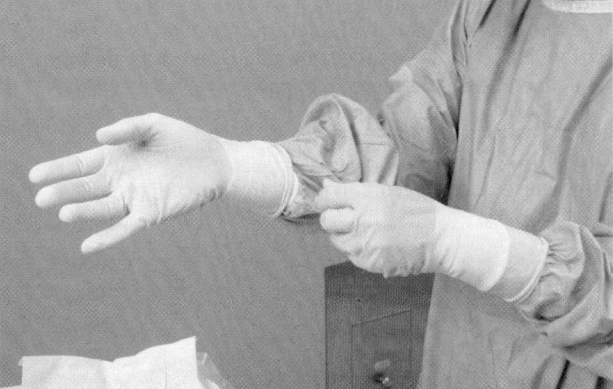

STEP 10f Second glove applied.

STEPS	RATIONALE
c. Extend nondominant forearm with palm up and place palm of glove against palm of nondominant hand. Glove fingers will point toward elbow.	Positions glove for application over cuffed hand, keeping glove sterile.
d. Grasp back of glove cuff with covered dominant hand, and turn glove cuff over end of nondominant hand and gown cuff (see illustration).	Seal created by glove cuff over gown prevents exit of microorganisms over operative sterile field.
e. Grasp top of glove and underlying gown sleeve with covered dominant hand. Carefully extend fingers into glove, being sure glove's cuff covers gown's cuff.	
f. Glove dominant hand in same manner, reversing hands (see illustration). Use gloved nondominant hand to pull on glove. Keep hand inside sleeve (see illustration).	Sterile touches sterile.
g. Be sure fingers are fully extended into both gloves.	
11. For wraparound sterile gowns: take gloved hand and release fastener or ties in front of gown.	Ensures that nurse has full dexterity while using gloved hand. Front of gown is sterile.

Continued

✳ **SKILL 34-4**

APPLYING A STERILE GOWN AND
PERFORMING CLOSED GLOVING—CONT'D

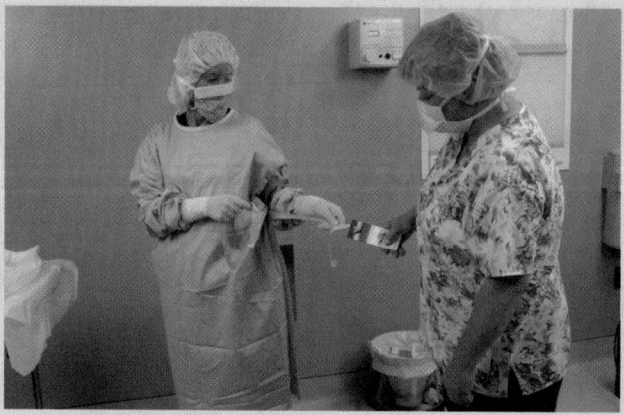

STEP 12 Handing tie to sterile team member.

STEPS	**RATIONALE**
12. Hand tie to sterile team member who stands still (see illustration). Allowing margin of safety, turn around to the left, covering back with extended gown flap. Take back tie from team member, and secure tie to gown.	Contact with team member could contaminate gown and gloves. Gown must enclose undergarments.

Recording and Reporting
• It is not necessary to record or report this procedure.

Delegation Considerations
The skill of open gloving can be delegated when personnel are trained to perform a sterile procedure.

Equipment
- Sterile gloves (proper size)

STEPS	RATIONALE
1. Perform thorough hand hygiene.	Removes bacteria from skin surfaces and reduces transmission of infection.
2. Remove outer glove package wrapper by carefully separating and peeling apart sides.	Prevents inner glove package from accidentally opening and touching contaminated objects.
3. Grasp inner package, and lay it on clean, flat surface just above waist level. Open package, keeping gloves on wrapper's inside surface (see illustration).	Sterile object held below waist is contaminated. Inner surface of glove package is sterile.
4. If gloves are not prepowdered, take packet of powder and apply lightly to hands over sink or wastebasket.	Powder allows gloves to slip on easily. (Some staff members do not use powder for fear of promoting growth of microorganisms.)
5. Identify right and left glove. Each glove has cuff approximately 5 cm (2 inches) wide. Glove dominant hand first.	Proper identification of gloves prevents contamination by improper fit. Gloving of dominant hand first improves dexterity.
6. With thumb and first two fingers of nondominant hand, grasp edge of cuff of glove for dominant hand. Touch only glove's inside surface.	Inner edge of cuff will lie against skin and thus is not sterile.
7. Carefully pull glove over dominant hand, leaving cuff and being sure cuff does not roll up wrist. Be sure thumb and fingers are in proper spaces (see illustration).	If glove's outer surface touches hand or wrist, then it is contaminated.
8. With gloved dominant hand, slip fingers underneath second glove's cuff (see illustration).	Cuff protects gloved fingers. Sterile touching sterile prevents glove contamination.
9. Carefully pull second glove over nondominant hand. Do not allow fingers and thumb of gloved dominant hand to touch any part of exposed nondominant hand. Keep thumb of dominant hand abducted back (see illustration).	Contact of gloved hand with exposed hand results in contamination.

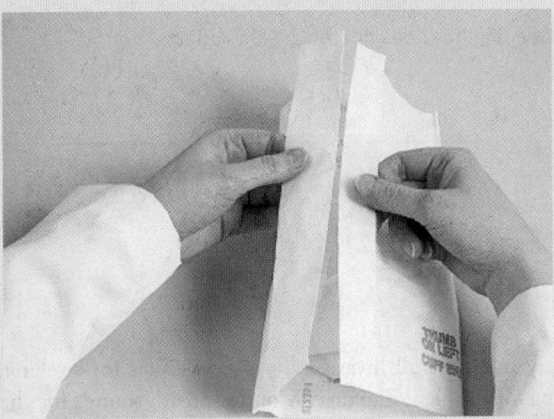

STEP 3 Opening package.

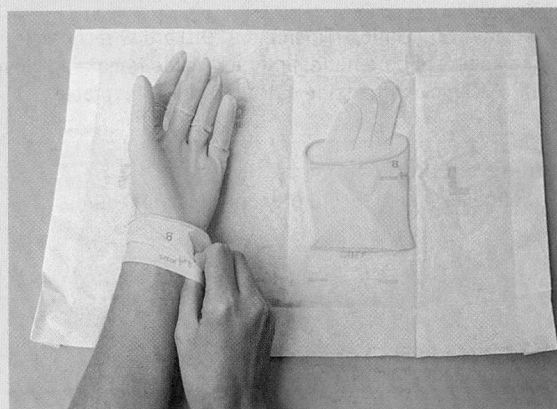

STEP 7 Pulling glove over dominant hand.

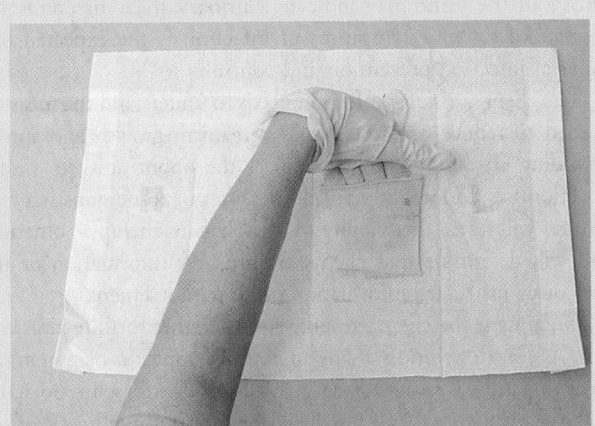

STEP 8 Slipping fingers underneath second glove's cuff.

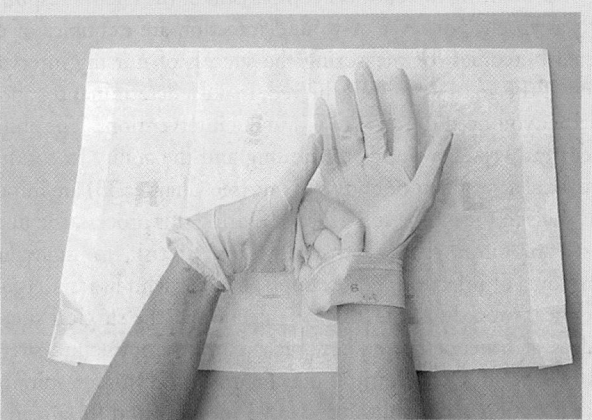

STEP 9 Pulling second glove over nondominant hand.

Continued

✳ **SKILL 34-5**   OPEN GLOVING—CONT'D

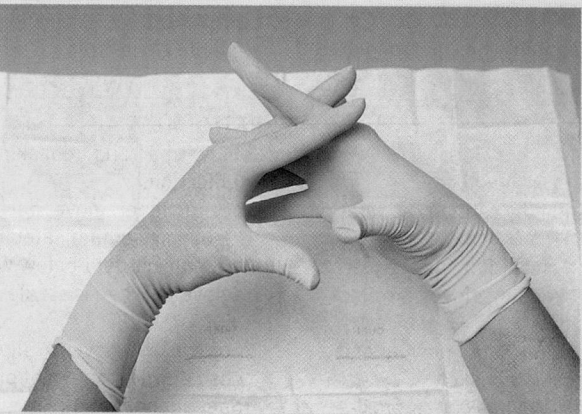

STEP 10 Hands interlocked.

STEPS	RATIONALE
10. After second glove is on, interlock hands. The cuffs usually fall down after application. Be sure to touch only sterile sides (see illustration).	Ensures smooth fit over fingers.

Glove Disposal

11. Grasp outside of one cuff with other gloved hand; avoid touching wrist. Pull half way down palm of hand. Take thumb of half-ungloved hand, and place under cuff of the other glove	Minimizes contamination of underlying skin.
12. Pull glove off, turning it inside out. Discard in receptacle.	
13. Take fingers of bare hand, and tuck inside remaining glove cuff. Peel glove off, inside out. Discard in receptacle.	Outside of glove does not touch skin surface.

Recording and Reporting

• It is not necessary to record or report this procedure.

◆Evaluation

Measure the success of infection prevention and control techniques by determining whether you achieved the goals for reducing or preventing infection. A comparison of the client's response, such as absence of fever or wound infection are examples of expected outcomes for measuring the success of nursing interventions. If the goals were not achieved, make a determination about whether you need to revise or eliminate interventions. The ability to correctly assess wounds for healing and the ability to conduct a physical assessment of body systems (see Chapter 33) are important skills in the evaluation process. During this process, the nurse closely monitors clients, especially those at risk, for signs and symptoms of infection. For example, a client who has undergone a surgical procedure is at risk for infection at the surgical site, as well as at other invasive sites, such as the venipuncture site or central line sites. In addition, the client is at risk for a respiratory tract infection as a result of decreased mobility and for a urinary tract infection if an indwelling catheter is present. The nurse closely monitors all invasive and surgical sites for swelling, erythema, or purulent drainage. Monitor breath sounds for changes, and observe sputum character for change in color or consistency. Review laboratory test results for leukocytes. For example, leukocytosis in the urine may indicate a urinary tract infection. The absence of signs or symptoms of infection is the expected outcome of infection prevention and control.

The client at risk for infection needs to understand the measures needed to reduce or prevent microorganism growth and spread. Providing clients or family members the opportunity to discuss infection prevention and control measures or to demonstrate procedures will reveal their ability to comply with therapy. Sometimes you will determine that clients require new information or that previously instructed information needs reinforcement.

Document the client's response to therapies for infection control. A clear description of any signs and symptoms of systemic or local infection is necessary to give all nurses a baseline for comparative evaluation. You also need to report the efficacy of any intervention in reducing infection.

✳ **BOX 34-14   Hepatitis B Vaccination and Follow-Up After Exposure**

1. Health care employers shall make available the hepatitis B vaccine and vaccination series to all employees who may have occupational exposures. If an employee declines the vaccine, the employee must sign a declination form. Evaluation and follow-up care will be available to all employees who have been exposed.
2. Hepatitis B vaccinations will be made available to employees within 10 working days of assignment. This means before starting to provide client care and after receiving education and training on the vaccine.
3. A blood test (titer) is offered in some facilities 1-2 months after completing the 3 dose vaccine series (check the health care facility or agency policy).
4. Vaccine is offered at no cost to employees. Vaccine does not require any boosters.
5. After exposure, no treatment is needed if there is a positive blood titer on file. If no positive titer is on file, the CDC guidelines must be followed.

Exposure to Hepatitis C (HCV)
1. If the source client is positive for HCV, the employee will receive a baseline test.
2. At 4 weeks after exposure, the employee should be offered a HCV-RNA test to determine if the employee contracted HCV.
3. If positive, the employee is started on treatment.
4. There is no prophylactic treatment for HCV after exposure.
5. Early treatment for infection can prevent chronic infection.

Exposure to HIV
1. If the client is positive for HIV infection, a viral load study should be performed to determine the amount of virus present in the blood.
2. If the exposure meets the CDC criteria for HIV prophylactic treatment (PEP), it should be started as soon as possible, preferably within 24 hours after the exposure (CDC, 2005b).

All medical evaluations and procedures, including the vaccine and vaccination series and evaluation after exposure (prophylaxis), are made available at no cost to at-risk employees.

A confidential written medical evaluation will be available to employees with exposure incidents.

From Occupational Safety and Health Administration: Occupational Safety and Health Act of 2001, 2001, 2005, *http://www.cdc.gov.*

Exposure Issues. Clients and health care personnel, which includes housekeepers and maintenance personnel, are at risk for acquiring infections from accidental needle sticks. After administering an injection or inserting an IV catheter, place the used needle safety device in a puncture-resistant box (see Chapter 35). Sharps boxes must be at the site of use; this is an OSHA requirement. With the passage of the Needlestick Safety and Prevention Act in 2000, the incidence rate of sharps injuries decreased by 50% (Jagger, 2003). All sharps must now be either needle safe or needleless. In the past a stray needle lying in bed linen or carelessly thrown into a wastebasket served as a prime source for exposure to blood-borne pathogens. Hepatitis B and hepatitis C are the infections most commonly transmitted by contaminated needles (Box 34-14). Report any contaminated needle stick immediately. Additional criteria for exposure reporting includes

blood or other potentially infectious materials (OPIM) in direct contact with an open area of the skin, blood or OPIM that is splashed into the nurse's eye, mouth or up the nose, and cuts with a sharp object that is covered with blood or OPIM. Follow-up for risk for acquiring infection will begin with source client testing, Access to testing the client (source) is stated in the testing law for each state. Some states have deemed consent, which means the state has granted the clients consent to be tested. Other states require that the client consent to testing for the presence of blood-borne pathogens. Nurses should know the testing laws in the state where they are employed. Health care facilities, agencies, and workers' compensation require the exposed employee to complete an injury report and seek appropriate treatment if needed. The need for treatment is linked to the results of the testing of the client. The client should be tested for HIV, hepatitis B virus (HBV) and hepatitis C virus (HCV). If positive for HIV or HCV, then testing for syphilis may be indicated because of the incidence of coinfection (CDC, 2005b) It is required that an exposed employee be given the client's testing results. This is **not** a violation of the Health Insurance Portability and Accountability Act (HIPAA) of 1996. Both the CDC and OSHA state that this information must be given to the exposed health care worker.

Testing the exposed employee at the time of the exposure is not needed immediately unless required by the state testing law. Testing of the exposed employee is dependent on the results of the testing of the client. If the client tests positive for a blood-borne pathogen, then testing and treatment will be started for the employee.

Exposures also occur involving non–blood-borne pathogens. Airborne and droplet diseases also pose a risk to the nonimmune nurse. The CDC has published a list of recommended immunizations and vaccinations for health care workers, and OSHA is enforcing them. The recommended vaccinations and immunizations include hepatitis B vaccine; TB testing; annual influenza vaccine; measles, mumps, rubella (MMR); chickenpox vaccine; and tetanus, diphtheria, and pertussis. Employee health should review your health history and offer appropriate prevention. Declination forms are needed if these are declined (OSHA, 2001).

✳ **Key Concepts**
- Hand hygiene is the most important technique to use in preventing and controlling transmission of infection.
- The potential for microorganisms to cause disease depends on the number of organisms, virulence, ability to enter and survive in a host, and susceptibility of the host.
- Normal body flora help to resist infection by releasing antibacterial substances and inhibiting multiplication of pathogenic microorganisms.
- The signs of local inflammation and infection are identical.
- An infection can develop as long as the six elements composing the infection chain are uninterrupted.
- Microorganisms are transmitted by direct and indirect contact, by airborne spread, and by vectors and contaminated articles.
- Increasing age, poor nutrition, stress, inherited conditions, chronic disease, and treatments or conditions that compromise the immune response increase susceptibility to infection.

- The major sites for health care–associated infections include the urinary and respiratory tracts, bloodstream, and surgical or traumatic wounds.
- The Centers for Disease Control and Prevention now recommend use of alcohol-based waterless antiseptics as an alternative to hand washing.
- Invasive procedures, medical therapies, long hospitalization, and contact with health care personnel increase a hospitalized client's risk for acquiring a health care–associated infection.
- Isolation practices may prevent personnel and clients from acquiring infections and may prevent transmission of microorganisms to other persons.
- Standard precautions use generic barrier techniques when caring for all clients.
- Proper cleansing requires mechanical removal of all soil from an object or area.
- A client in isolation is subject to sensory deprivation because of the restricted environment.
- An infection prevention and control professional monitors the incidence of infection within an institution and provides educational and consultative services to maintain infection prevention and control.
- Surgical asepsis requires more stringent techniques than medical asepsis and is directed at eliminating microorganisms.
- If the skin is broken, or if an invasive procedure into a body cavity normally free of microorganisms is performed, follow surgical aseptic practices.

✳ Critical Thinking Exercises

1. Mrs. Jaycock had an indwelling urethral catheter for 1 week. The catheter has now been out for 24 hours. She complains of frequency and pain on urination. Mrs. Jaycock suggests reinsertion of the catheter because of the need to get up frequently. What can frequency or pain on urination be an indication of? Should the catheter be reinserted? Why or why not? Describe at least one appropriate assessment measure and independent nursing action for Mrs. Jaycock.

2. You are caring for Mr. Huang, who has a large, open, and draining abdominal wound. You notice another health care worker changing Mr. Huang's dressing without wearing gloves or using sterile supplies or sterile technique. When you question the health care worker regarding his or her practice, this person says, "Don't worry, the wound is already infected, and the antibiotics and draining will take care of any contaminants." How would you respond to this comment? What would your next steps be in following up on this incident?

3. Mrs. Niles is 83 years of age and lives alone. She has difficulty walking and relies on a church volunteer group to deliver lunches during the week. Her fixed income limits her ability to buy food. Last week, Mrs. Niles's 79-year-old

sister died. The two sisters had been very close. As a home care nurse, explain the factors that might increase Mrs. Niles's risk for infection.

4. Mr. Vargas is admitted to the facility with a history of recent weight loss, a cough that has persisted for 2 months, and hemoptysis. His chest x-ray film shows a cavitary lesion in one lung, and his physician suspects tuberculosis. What type of isolation precautions would you use for Mr. Vargas? What protection would you use to provide care? What education would you provide for the client and his family?

✳ NCLEX®-Style Review Questions

1. If the infectious disease can be transmitted directly from one person to another, it is a:
   1. Susceptible host
   2. Communicable disease
   3. Portal of entry to a host
   4. Portal of exit from the reservoir

2. Infectious diseases such as hepatitis B or C become a reservoir for pathogens in:
   1. Blood
   2. The urinary tract
   3. The respiratory tract
   4. The reproductive tract

3. The interval when a client manifests signs and symptoms specific to a type of infection is the:
   1. Illness stage
   2. Convalescence
   3. Prodromal stage
   4. Incubation period

4. The most *effective* way to break the chain of infection is by:
   1. Hand hygiene
   2. Wearing gloves
   3. Placing clients in isolation
   4. Providing private rooms for clients

5. After coming in contact with infected clients, and after handling contaminated equipment or organic material, visitors are encouraged to:
   1. Wear gloves before eating or handling food
   2. Use a private room to talk with family members
   3. Leave the facility to prevent contamination of others
   4. Perform hand hygiene before eating or handling food

6. A client is isolated for pulmonary tuberculosis. The nurse notes the client seems to be angry, but he knows this is a normal response to isolation. The best intervention is to:
   1. Provide a dark, quiet room to calm the client
   2. Reduce the level of precautions to keep the client from becoming angry
   3. Explain the reasons for isolation procedures and provide meaningful stimulation
   4. Limit family and other caregiver visits to reduce the risk of spreading the infection

7. A gown should be worn when:
   1. The client's hygiene is poor
   2. The nurse is assisting with medication administration
   3. The client has acquired immunodeficiency syndrome (AIDS) or hepatitis
   4. Blood or body fluids may get on the nurse's clothing from a task the nurse plans to perform

8. The nurse has redressed a client's wound and now plans to administer a medication to the client. It is important to:
   1. Leave the gloves on to administer the medication
   2. Remove gloves and perform hand hygiene before leaving the room
   3. Remove gloves and perform hand hygiene before administering the medication
   4. Leave the medication on the bedside table to avoid having to remove gloves before leaving the client's room

9. When a nurse is performing surgical hand asepsis, the nurse must keep hands:
   1. Below elbows
   2. Above elbows
   3. At a 45-degree angle
   4. In a comfortable position

10. To sterilize surgical instruments, parenteral solutions, and surgical dressings:
    1. An autoclave is used
    2. Soap and water is used
    3. Ethylene oxide gas is used
    4. Chemicals are used for disinfection

35 | Medication Administration

✳ OBJECTIVES

Mastery of content in this chapter will enable the student to:

- Examine the nurse's role and responsibilities in medication administration.
- Describe the physiological mechanisms of medication action, including absorption, distribution, metabolism, and excretion of medications.
- Differentiate among different types of medication actions.
- Discuss developmental factors that influence pharmacokinetics.
- Discuss factors that influence medication actions.
- Discuss methods used to educate a client about prescribed medications.
- Compare and contrast the roles of the prescriber, pharmacist, and nurse in medication administration.

- Implement nursing actions to prevent medication errors.
- Describe factors to consider when choosing routes of medication administration.
- Calculate prescribed medication doses correctly.
- Discuss factors to include in assessing a client's needs for and response to medication therapy.
- Apply the six rights of medication administration in clinical settings.
- Correctly prepare and administer subcutaneous, intramuscular, and intradermal injections; intravenous medications; oral and topical skin preparations; eye, ear, and nose drops; vaginal instillations; rectal suppositories; and inhalers.

✳ MEDIA RESOURCES   ✳ KEY TERMS

 Companion CD

- NCLEX®-Style Review Questions
- Audio Glossary
- Interactive Learning Activities
- English/Spanish Glossary

 Website

- NCLEX®-Style Review Questions
- Audio Glossary
- English/Spanish Glossary
- Interactive Learning Activities
- Weblinks
- Audio Summaries
- Video Clips
- Nursing Skills Online

Absorption, p. 689
Adverse effects, p. 691
Anaphylactic reactions, p. 691
Biotransformation, p. 690
Buccal, p. 693
Concentration, p. 692
Detoxify, p. 690
Idiosyncratic reaction, p. 691
Infusions, p. 692
Inhalation, p. 695
Injection, p. 689
Instillation, p. 695
Intraarticular, p. 695
Intracardiac, p. 695
Intradermal (ID), p. 693
Intramuscular (IM), p. 693
Intraocular, p. 695
Intravenous (IV), p. 693
Irrigations, p. 696
Medication allergy, p. 691
Medication error, p. 698
Medication interaction, p. 692
Medication reconciliation,
  p. 705

Metered-dose inhalers (MDIs),
  p. 729
Metric system, p. 695
Narcotics, p. 688
Nurse Practice Acts, p. 688
Ophthalmic, p. 723
Parenteral administration,
  p. 693
Peak, p. 692
Pharmacokinetics, p. 689
Polypharmacy, p. 715
Prescriptions, p. 699
Serum half-life, p. 692
Side effects, p. 691
Solution, p. 696
Subcutaneous (Sub-Q), p. 693
Sublingual, p. 693
Synergistic effect, p. 692
Therapeutic effects, p. 691
Toxic effects, p. 691
Transdermal disk, p. 695
Verbal order, p. 699
Z-track method, p. 753

Clients with acute or chronic health alterations restore or maintain their health using a variety of strategies. A medication is a substance used in the diagnosis, treatment, cure, relief, or prevention of health alterations. Medications are the primary treatment clients associate with restoration of health. No matter where clients receive their health care—hospitals, clinics, or home—the nurse plays an essential role in medication preparation and administration, medication teaching, and evaluating clients' responses to medications.

In both acute care and restorative care settings, nurses spend a great deal of time administering medications to clients and ensure that clients or their families are adequately prepared to administer their medications when they are discharged. When clients cannot administer their own medications at home, family members or home care personnel are often responsible for doing so. In every health care setting, the nurse is responsible for evaluating the effects of medications on the client's health status, teaching clients about their medications and their side effects, ensuring adherence with the medication regimen, and evaluating the client's ability to self-administer medications. In some cases, nurses direct teaching and evaluation toward a family member who helps with medication administration.

Scientific Knowledge Base

Medications are most frequently used to manage diseases. Because medication administration and evaluation are essential to nursing practice, nurses need to have knowledge about the actions and effects of the medications their clients take. Administering medications safely requires an understanding of legal aspects of health care, pharmacology, pharmacokinetics (the study of drug concentrations), the life sciences, human anatomy, and mathematics.

Medication Legislation and Standards

Federal Regulations. The role of the U.S. government in regulation of the pharmaceutical industry is to protect the health of the people by ensuring that medications are safe and effective. The first American law to regulate medications was the Pure Food and Drug Act. This law simply requires all medications to be free of impure products. Subsequent legislation (Table 35-1) has set standards related to safety, potency, and efficacy. Enforcement of medication laws currently rests with the Food and Drug Administration (FDA), which ensures that all medications on the market undergo vigorous testing before they are sold to the public. Fed-

---

✳ **TABLE 35-1 Federal Medication Laws in the United States**

DATE	TITLE OF LAW	PROVISIONS
1906	Pure Food and Drug Act	Designated official standards for medications (USP and the National Formulary); specified standards for medication labeling especially those that were habit forming; also established the Food and Drug Administration (FDA)
1912	Sherley Amendment	Enabled the FDA to have oversight over manufacturer claims about medication efficacy and therapeutic effects
1914	Harrison Narcotic Act	Legally classified medications believed to be habit forming as narcotics; regulated importation, manufacture, sale, and use of narcotic substances
1938	Federal Food, Drug, and Cosmetic Act	Added the Homeopathic Pharmacopeia of the United States as a third medication standard; required that medication preparation be approved as safe by the FDA before marketing; further outlined criteria for medication labeling
1945	Penicillin Amendment	Required FDA testing and certification of safety and effectiveness of all penicillin products (later amendments extended this to all antibiotics); abolished in 1983 as such control was no longer needed
1951	Durham-Humphrey Amendment	Distinguished between prescription and nonprescription medications; according to the FDA, required prescription by a physician for drugs that could not be used safely without medical supervision; up until that time, all medications could be purchased over-the-counter
1962	Kefauver-Harris Amendment	Authorized FDA to supervise medication production to ensure safety and efficacy and to establish official medication names; specified greater controls on investigational medications; required that manufacturers prove their drug was effective before marketing them; this amendment occurred as a result of the drug Thalidomide and its devastating effects to newborns
1970	Comprehensive Drug Abuse Prevention and Control Act (Controlled Substances Act)	Set strict controls on manufacture and distribution of controlled medication (possession of controlled substances unlawful without prescription); established government programs to promote prevention and treatment of medication dependence; categorized drugs on basis of addiction potential
1978	Drug Regulation Reform Act	Shortened the drug investigation process to release drugs sooner to the public
1997	Food and Drug Administration and Modernization Act	Allowed new drugs and medical devices to be approved in a more efficient manner, while ensuring product safety; allowed pharmacy compounding of drugs; allowed manufacturers to market "off-label" use of drugs to health care providers

USP, United States Pharmacopeia.

eral medication law extended and refined controls on medication sales and distribution; medication testing, naming, and labeling; and the regulation of controlled substances. Official publications, such as the *United States Pharmacopeia* (USP) and the *National Formulary,* set standards for medication strength, quality, purity, packaging, safety, labeling, and dose form. In 1993 the FDA instituted the MedWatch program. This voluntary program encourages nurses and other health care professionals to report when a medication, product, or medical event causes serious harm to a client by completing the MedWatch form. The form is available on the MedWatch website (U.S. Food and Drug Administration [USFDA], 2007).

State and Local Regulation of Medication.
State and local medication laws must conform to federal legislation. States often have additional controls, including control of substances not regulated by the federal government. Local governmental bodies regulate the use of alcohol and tobacco.

Health Care Institutions and Medication Laws.
Health care institutions establish individual policies to meet federal, state, and local regulations. The size of the institution, the types of services it provides, and the types of professional personnel it employs influence these policies. Institutional policies are often more restrictive than governmental controls. An institution is concerned primarily with preventing poor health outcomes resulting from medication use. For example, a common institutional policy is the automatic discontinuation of narcotics after a set number of days. Although a prescriber can reorder the narcotic, this policy helps to control unnecessarily prolonged medication therapy and requires the prescriber to review the need for this class of medication on a regular basis.

Medication Regulations and Nursing Practice.
State **Nurse Practice Acts (NPAs)** have the most influence over nursing practice by defining the scope of a nurse's professional functions and responsibilities. Most NPAs are purposefully broad so the professional responsibilities of the nurse are not limited. Health care agencies often interpret specific actions allowed under the acts, but they are not able to modify, expand, or restrict the act's intent. The primary intent of NPAs is to protect the public from unskilled, undereducated, and unlicensed personnel.

The nurse is responsible for following legal provisions when administering controlled substances or **narcotics,** which are carefully controlled through federal and state guidelines. Violations of the Controlled Substances Act are punishable by fines, imprisonment, and loss of nurse licensure. Hospitals and other health care institutions have policies for the proper storage and distribution of narcotics (Box 35-1).

Pharmacological Concepts

Drug Names.
Some medications have as many as three different names. A medication's chemical name provides an exact description of the medication's composition and molecular structure. Nurses rarely use chemical names in clinical practice. An example of a chemical name is *N*-acetyl-para-aminophenol, which is commonly known as Tylenol. The manufacturer who first develops the medication gives the generic or nonproprietary name, with United

---

✳ BOX 35-1 Guidelines for Safe Narcotic Administration and Control

- Store all narcotics in a locked, secure cabinet or container. (Computerized, locked cabinets are preferred.)
- Narcotics are frequently counted. Usually counts are made on a continuous basis with the opening of narcotic drawers and/or at shift change.
- Report discrepancies in narcotic counts immediately.
- Use a special inventory record each time a narcotic is dispensed. Records are often kept electronically and provide an accurate ongoing count of narcotics used and remaining as well as information about narcotics that are wasted.
- Use the record to document the client's name, date, time of medication administration, name of medication, dose, and signature of nurse dispensing the medication.
- If a nurse gives only part of a premeasured dose of a controlled substance, a second nurse witnesses disposal of the unused portion. If paper records are kept, both nurses sign their names on the form. Computerized systems record the nurses' names electronically. Do not place wasted portions in the sharps containers. Instead, flush wasted portions of tablets down the toilet and wash liquids down the sink.

States Adopted Names (USAN) Council approval. Acetaminophen is an example of a generic name. It is the generic name for Tylenol. The generic name becomes the official name listed in official publications such as the USP. The trade name, brand name, or proprietary name is the name under which a manufacturer markets a medication. The trade name has the symbol ™ at the upper right of the name, indicating that the manufacturer has trademarked the medication's name (e.g., Panadol™, Tempra™, and St. Joseph Aspirin-Free Fever Reducer for Children™).

Manufacturers choose trade names that are easy to pronounce, spell, and remember. Many companies produce the same medication, so similarities in trade names are often confusing. Therefore nurses need to be careful to obtain the exact name and spelling for each medication administered to clients. Because the similarities in drug names is a common cause of medical errors, The Joint Commission (TJC) (2007) publishes on their website (http://www.jointcommission.org) a look-alike/sound-alike drug list and recommendations for nurses, prescribers, other health care providers and health care organizations to prevent mixing these medications.

Classification.
Medication classification indicates the effect of the medication on a body system, the symptoms the medication relieves, or the medication's desired effect. Usually each class contains more than one medication that is used for the same type of health problem. For example, clients who have type 2 diabetes often take oral medications to control their blood glucose levels. *Sulfonyl-ureas* is one classification of medications often used by these clients. There are at least seven different medications in the sulfonylurea classification (McKenry and others, 2006). Some medications are part of more than one class. For example, aspirin is an analgesic, an antipyretic, and an antiinflammatory medication.

Medication Forms.
Medications are available in a variety of forms, or preparations (Figure 35-1). The form of the medication

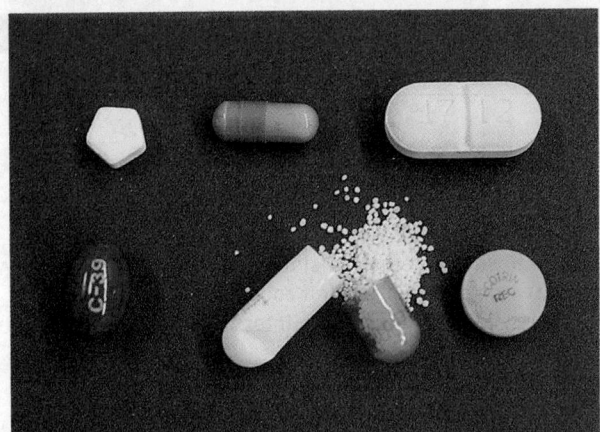

Figure 35-1 Forms of oral medications. *Top row:* Uniquely shaped tablet, capsule, scored tablet. *Bottom row:* Gelatin-coated liquid, extended-release capsule, enteric-coated tablet.

determines its route of administration. The composition of a medication enhances its absorption and metabolism. Many medications come in several forms such as tablets, capsules, elixirs, and suppositories. When administering a medication, be certain to use the proper form (Table 35-2).

Pharmacokinetics as the Basis of Medication Actions

For medications to be therapeutic they must be taken into a client's body; be absorbed and distributed to cells, tissues, or a specific organ; and alter physiological functions. **Pharmacokinetics** is the study of how medications enter the body, reach their site of action, metabolize, and exit the body. Use knowledge of pharmacokinetics when timing medication administration, selecting the route of administration, considering the client's risk for alterations in medication action, and evaluating the client's response.

Absorption. **Absorption** refers to passage of medication molecules into the blood from the site of medication administration. Factors that influence medication absorption are the route of administration, ability of the medication to dissolve, blood flow to the site of administration, body surface area, and lipid solubility of medication.

Route of Administration. Each route of medication administration has a different rate of absorption. When applying medications on the skin, absorption is slow due to the physical makeup of the skin. Medications placed on the mucous membranes and respiratory airways are quickly absorbed because these tissues contain many blood vessels. Because orally administered medications pass through the gastrointestinal (GI) tract, the overall rate of absorption is usually slow. Intravenous (IV) **injection** produces the most rapid absorption because medications are immediately available when they enter the systemic circulation.

Ability of the Medication to Dissolve. The ability of an oral medication to dissolve depends largely on its form or preparation. The body absorbs solutions and suspensions already in a liquid state more readily than tablets or capsules. Acidic medica-

tions pass through the gastric mucosa rapidly. Medications that are basic are not absorbed before reaching the small intestine.

Blood Flow to the Site of Administration. When the site of administration contains a rich blood supply, the body absorbs medications more rapidly. As blood comes in contact with the site of administration, the medication is absorbed. Therefore areas that have more blood supply will experience enhanced absorption, facilitating the passage of the medication into the blood.

Body Surface Area. When a medication comes in contact with a large surface area, the medication is absorbed at a faster rate. This helps explain why the majority of medications are absorbed in the small intestine rather than the stomach.

Lipid Solubility of a Medication. Because the cell membrane has a lipid layer, highly lipid-soluble medications easily cross the cell membrane and are absorbed quickly. Another factor that often affects absorption of medication is whether or not food is in the stomach. Some oral medications are absorbed more easily when administered between meals because food changes the structure of a medication and sometimes impairs its absorption. Some medications when administered together interfere with each other so as to impair the absorption of one or both.

Safe medication administration requires knowledge of factors that alter or impair absorption of prescribed medications. This information is based on an understanding of medication pharmacokinetics, the nursing history, the physical examination, and knowledge gained through daily interactions with clients. Use this knowledge to ensure that you administer all prescribed medications at the correct time. Because some medications interact with food, it is often appropriate to administer medications before meals or after meals, with meals, or on an empty stomach. Some medications interact with each other. If this occurs, ensure that they are not given at the same time. Consult and collaborate with the client's prescribers to ensure that the client achieves the therapeutic effect of all medications. Before administering any medication, check pharmacology books, drug references, or package inserts, or consult with pharmacists to identify medication-medication interactions or medication-food interactions.

Distribution. After a medication is absorbed, it is distributed within the body to tissues and organs and ultimately to its specific site of action. The rate and extent of distribution depend on the physical and chemical properties of medications and the physiology of the person taking the medication.

Circulation. Once a medication enters the bloodstream, it is carried throughout the tissues and organs. How fast it reaches the site depends on the vascularity of the various tissues and organs. Conditions that limit blood flow or blood perfusion inhibit the distribution of a medication. For example, clients with congestive heart failure have impaired circulation, which impairs medication delivery to the intended site of action. Therefore the efficacy of medications in these clients is delayed or altered.

Membrane Permeability. To be distributed to an organ, a medication has to pass through all of the organ's tissues and biological membranes. Some membranes serve as barriers to the passage of medications. For example, the blood-brain barrier allows only fat-soluble medications to pass into the brain and cerebral spinal fluid. Therefore central nervous system infections often require treatment with antibiotics injected directly into the sub-

✳ TABLE 35-2 Forms of Medication

FORM	DESCRIPTION
Medication Forms Commonly Prepared for Administration by Oral Route	
Solid Forms	
Caplet	Shaped like capsule and coated for ease of swallowing
Capsule	Medication encased in a gelatin shell
Tablet	Powdered medication compressed into hard disk or cylinder; in addition to primary medication, contains binders (adhesive to allow powder to stick together), disintegrators (to promote tablet dissolution), lubricants (for ease of manufacturing), and fillers (for convenient tablet size)
Enteric-coated tablet	Coated tablet that does not dissolve in stomach; coatings dissolve in intestine, where medication is absorbed
Pill	Contains one or more medications, shaped into globules, ovoids, or oblong shapes; rarely used because have been replaced by tablets
Liquid Forms	
Elixir	Clear fluid containing water and/or alcohol; often sweetened
Extract	Syrup or dried form of pharmacologically active medication, usually made by evaporating solution
Aqueous solution	Substance dissolved in water and syrups
Aqueous suspension	Finely divided drug particles dispersed in liquid medium; when suspension is left standing, particles settle to bottom of container
Syrup	Medication dissolved in a concentrated sugar solution
Tincture	Alcohol extract from plant or vegetable
Other Oral Forms and Terms Associated With Oral Preparations	
Troche (lozenge)	Flat, round tablets that dissolve in mouth to release medication; not meant for ingestion
Aerosol	Aqueous medication sprayed and absorbed in mouth and upper airway; not meant for ingestion
Sustained release	Tablet or capsule that contains small particles of a medication coated with material that requires a varying amount of time to dissolve
Medication Forms Commonly Prepared for Administration by Topical Route	
Ointment (salve or cream)	Semisolid, externally applied preparation, usually containing one or more medications
Liniment	Usually contains alcohol, oil, or soapy emollient applied to skin
Lotion	Liquid suspension that usually protects, cools, or cleanses skin
Paste	Thick ointment; absorbed through skin more slowly than ointment; often used for skin protection
Transdermal disk or patch	Medicated disk or patch absorbed through skin slowly over long period of time (e.g., 24 hours, 1 week)
Medication Forms Commonly Prepared for Administration by Parenteral Route	
Solution	Sterile preparation that contains water with one or more dissolved compounds
Powder	Sterile particles of medication that are dissolved in a sterile liquid (e.g., water, normal saline) before administration
Medication Forms Commonly Prepared for Instillation Into Body Cavities	
Solution	Substance dissolved in water or other liquid
Intraocular disk	Small, flexible oval (similar to contact lens) consisting of two soft, outer layers and a middle layer containing medication; slowly releases medication when moistened by ocular fluid
Suppository	Solid dosage form mixed with gelatin and shaped in form of pellet for insertion into body cavity (rectum or vagina); melts when it reaches body temperature, releasing medication for absorption

arachnoid space in the spinal cord. Some older clients experience adverse effects (e.g., confusion) as a result of the change in the permeability of the blood-brain barrier, with easier passage of fat-soluble medications. The placental membrane also has a nonselective barrier to medications. Fat-soluble and non–fat-soluble agents often cross the placenta and produce fetal deformities, respiratory depression, and, with narcotic abuse, withdrawal symptoms.

Protein Binding. The degree to which medications bind to serum proteins such as albumin affects medication distribution. Most medications bind to albumin to some extent. Medications bound to albumin cannot exert pharmacological activity. The unbound or "free" medication is the active form of the medication. Older adults have a decrease in albumin in the bloodstream,

probably caused by a change in liver function. The same is true for clients with liver disease or malnutrition. Because of the potential for more medication being unbound, some older adults are at risk for an increase in medication activity or toxicity or both.

Metabolism. After a medication reaches its site of action, it becomes metabolized into a less active or inactive form that is easier to excrete. **Biotransformation** occurs under the influence of enzymes that **detoxify**, degrade (break down), and remove biologically active chemicals. Most biotransformation occurs within the liver, although the lungs, kidneys, blood, and intestines also metabolize medications. The liver is especially important because its specialized structure oxidizes and transforms many toxic substances. The liver degrades many harmful chemicals before they become distributed to the tissues. If a decrease in liver function occurs, such as with aging or liver disease, a medication is usually eliminated more slowly, resulting in an accumulation of the medication. Clients are at risk for medication toxicity if their organs that metabolize medications are not functioning correctly. For example, a small sedative dose of a barbiturate causes a client with liver disease to lapse into a coma.

Excretion. After medications are metabolized, they exit the body through the kidneys, liver, bowel, lungs, and exocrine glands. The chemical makeup of a medication determines the organ of excretion. Gaseous and volatile compounds, such as nitrous oxide and alcohol, exit through the lungs. Deep breathing and coughing (see Chapter 40) help the postoperative client eliminate anesthetic gases more rapidly. The exocrine glands excrete lipid-soluble medications. When medications exit through sweat glands, the skin often becomes irritated. The nurse assists the client in good hygiene practices (see Chapter 39) to promote cleanliness and skin integrity. If a medication is excreted through the mammary glands, there is a risk that a nursing infant will ingest the chemicals. Check the safety of any medication used in breast-feeding women.

The GI tract is another route for medication excretion. Many medications enter the hepatic circulation to be broken down by the liver and excreted into the bile. After chemicals enter the intestines through the biliary tract, the intestines reabsorb them. Factors that increase peristalsis (e.g., laxatives and enemas) accelerate medication excretion through the feces, whereas factors that slow peristalsis (e.g., inactivity and improper diet) often prolong a medication's effects.

The kidneys are the main organs for medication excretion. Some medications escape extensive metabolism and exit unchanged in the urine. Other medications undergo biotransformation in the liver before the kidneys excrete them. If renal function declines, a client is at risk for medication toxicity. If the kidney cannot adequately excrete a medication, it is often necessary to reduce the dose. Maintenance of an adequate fluid intake (50 mL/kg/day) promotes proper elimination of medications for the average adult.

Types of Medication Action

Medications vary considerably in the way they act and their types of action. Clients do not always respond in the same way to each successive dose of a medication. Sometimes the same medication causes very different responses in different clients. Therefore it is essential to understand all the effects that medications have on clients.

Therapeutic Effects. The **therapeutic effect** is the expected or predictable physiological response a medication causes. Each medication has a desired therapeutic effect. For example, nitroglycerin reduces cardiac workload and increases myocardial oxygen supply. Some medications have more than one therapeutic effect. For example, prednisone, a steroid, is used to decrease swelling, inhibit inflammation, reduce allergic responses, and prevent rejection of transplanted organs. Knowing the desired therapeutic effect for each medication allows the nurse to provide client education and to accurately evaluate the medication's desired effect.

Side Effects/Adverse Effects. **Side effects** are predictable and often unavoidable secondary effects produced at a usual therapeutic dose. Side effects are either harmless or cause injury. For example, some antihypertensive medications cause impotence in men. If the side effects are serious enough to negate the beneficial effects of a medication's therapeutic action, the prescriber will discontinue the medication. Clients often stop taking medications because of side effects. **Adverse effects** are unintended, undesirable, and often unpredictable severe responses to medication. Every medication has a potential to harm a client. For example, a client becomes comatose after ingesting a drug. Unfortunately, adverse effects are sometimes immediate, but often take weeks or months to develop. Early recognition is key. When adverse responses to medications occur, the prescriber discontinues the medication immediately. Health care providers report adverse effects to the FDA using the MedWatch program (USFDA, 2007).

Toxic Effects. **Toxic effects** develop after prolonged intake of a medication or when a medication accumulates in the blood because of impaired metabolism or excretion. Excess amounts of a medication within the body sometimes have lethal effects, depending on the medication's action. For example, toxic levels of morphine, an opioid, cause severe respiratory depression and death. Antidotes are available to treat specific types of medication toxicity. For example, Narcan reverses the effects of opioid toxicity.

Idiosyncratic Reactions. Medications sometimes cause unpredictable effects such as an **idiosyncratic reaction** in which a client overreacts or underreacts to a medication or has a reaction different from normal. For example, a child receiving an antihistamine (Benadryl) becomes extremely agitated or excited instead of drowsy. It is not always possible to predict if a client will have an idiosyncratic response to a medication.

Allergic Reactions. Allergic reactions also are unpredictable responses to a medication. Some clients become immunologically sensitized to the initial dose of a medication. With repeated administration, the client develops an allergic response to the medication, its chemical preservatives, or a metabolite. The medication or chemical acts as an antigen, triggering the release of the body's antibodies. A client's **medication allergy** symptoms vary, depending on the individual and the medication (Table 35-3). Among the different classes of medications, antibiotics cause a high incidence of allergic reactions. Severe or **anaphylactic reactions,** which are life threatening, are characterized by sudden constriction of bronchiolar muscles, edema of the pharynx and larynx, and severe wheezing and shortness of breath. Immediate medical attention is required to treat anaphylactic reactions.

A client with a known history of an allergy to a medication needs to avoid exposure to that medication in the future and needs to wear an identification bracelet or medal (Figure 35-2), which alerts nurses and physicians to the allergy if the client is unconscious when receiving medical care.

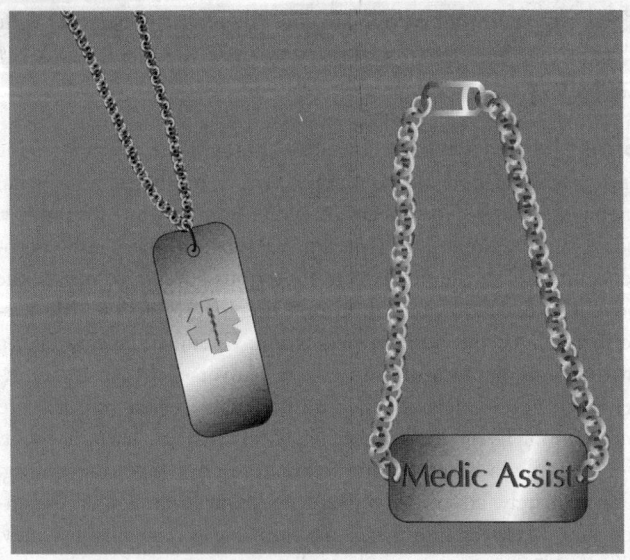

Figure 35-2 Identification bracelet and medal.

TABLE 35-3	**Mild Allergic Reactions**
SYMPTOM	**DESCRIPTION**
Urticaria	Raised, irregularly shaped skin eruptions with varying sizes and shapes; eruptions have reddened margins and pale centers
Rash	Small, raised vesicles that are usually reddened; often distributed over entire body
Pruritus	Itching of skin; accompanies most rashes
Rhinitis	Inflammation of mucous membranes lining nose; causes swelling and clear, watery discharge

Medication Interactions

When one medication modifies the action of another medication, a **medication interaction** occurs. Medication interactions are common in individuals taking several medications. Some medications increase or diminish the action of other medications and may alter the way another medication is absorbed, metabolized, or eliminated from the body. When two medications have a **synergistic effect,** the combined effect of the two medications is greater than the effect of the medications when given separately. For example, alcohol is a central nervous system depressant that has a synergistic effect on antihistamines, antidepressants, barbiturates, and narcotic analgesics. Sometimes a medication interaction is desired. Prescribers often combine medications to create an interaction that will have a beneficial effect. For example, a client with high blood pressure takes several medications such as diuretics and vasodilators that act together to control the blood pressure when one medication is not effective on its own.

Medication Dose Responses

After administration, a medication undergoes absorption, distribution, metabolism, and excretion. Except when administered intravenously, medications take time to enter the bloodstream.

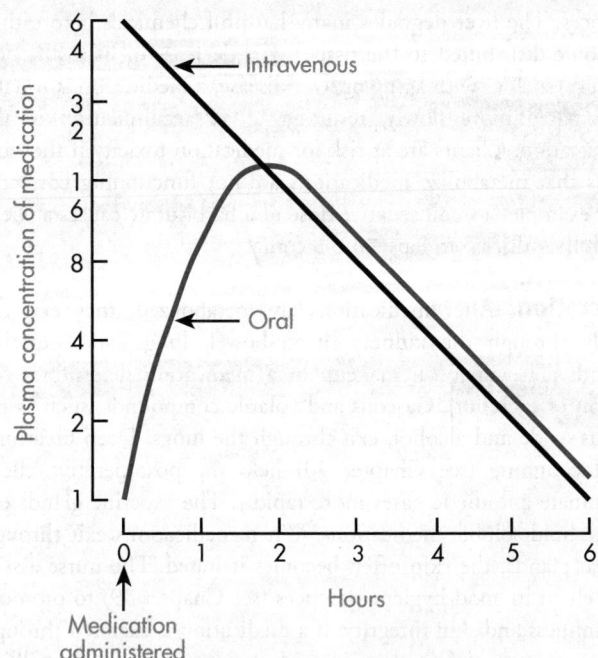

Figure 35-3 Curve showing therapeutic blood levels. (From Clark JF, Queener SF, Karb VB: *Pharmacological basis of nursing practice,* ed 6, St. Louis, 1998, Mosby.).

The quantity and distribution of a medication in different body compartments change constantly. When a medication is prescribed, the goal is a constant blood level within a safe therapeutic range. Repeated doses are required to achieve a constant therapeutic **concentration** of a medication because a portion of a medication is always being excreted. The highest serum concentration (**peak** concentration) of the medication usually occurs just before the body absorbs the last of the medication (McKenry and others, 2006). After peaking, the serum medication concentration falls progressively. With intravenous **infusions,** the peak concentration occurs quickly, but the serum level also begins to fall immediately (Figure 35-3). The point at which the lowest amount of drug is in the serum is called the trough concentration. Some medication doses (e.g., vancomycin) are based on peak and trough serum levels. The trough level is generally drawn 30 minutes before administering the drug, and the peak level is drawn whenever the drug is expected to reach its peak concentration. The time it takes for a drug to reach its peak concentration varies depending on the medication's pharmacokinetics.

All medications have a **serum half-life,** which is the time it takes for excretion processes to lower the serum medication concentration by half. To maintain a therapeutic plateau, the client needs to receive regular fixed doses. For example, current evidence shows that pain medications are most effective when they are given around-the-clock rather than when the client intermittently complains of pain because the body maintains an almost constant level of pain medication. After an initial medication dose, the client receives each successive dose when the previous dose reaches its half-life.

The client and nurse need to follow regular dosage schedules and adhere to prescribed doses and dosage intervals (Table 35-4).

✴ TABLE 35-4 Common Dosage Administration Schedules

DOSAGE SCHEDULE	ABBREVIATION
Before meals	AC, ac
As desired	ad lib
Twice a day	Do not abbreviate
Hour	h, hr
At bedtime	"nightly" or "at bedtime"
After meals	PC, pc
Whenever there is a need	prn
Every morning, every am	qAM
Every day	daily
Every hour	qh
Every 2 hours	q2h
Every 4 hours	q4h
Every 6 hours	q6h
Every 8 hours	q8h
4 times a day	Do not abbreviate
Give immediately	STAT, stat
3 times a day	Do not abbreviate

✴ TABLE 35-5 Terms Associated With Medication Actions

TERM	MEANING
Onset	Time it takes after a medication is administered for it to produce a response
Peak	Time it takes for a medication to reach its highest effective concentration
Trough	Minimum blood serum concentration of medication reached just before the next scheduled dose
Duration	Time during which the medication is present in concentration great enough to produce a response
Plateau	Blood serum concentration of a medication reached and maintained after repeated fixed doses

Some agencies set schedules for medication administration. However, nurses are able to alter this schedule based on knowledge about a medication. For example, at some agencies, medications that are to be taken once a day are given at 9:00 AM. However, if a medication works best when given before bedtime, the nurse administers the medication before the client goes to sleep.

When teaching clients about dosage schedules, use language that is familiar to the client. For example, when teaching a client about medication dosing twice a day, instruct the client to take a medication in the morning and again in the evening. Use knowledge about the time intervals of medications to anticipate a medication's effect and educate the client about when to expect a response. Table 35-5 defines common terms associated with medication actions.

Routes of Administration

The route prescribed for administering a medication depends on the medication's properties and desired effect and on the client's physical and mental condition (Table 35-6). Work with the pre-

scriber in determining the best route for a client's medication, as in the following hypothetical situation:

Mr. Koop has progressively worsened physically. His temperature is 39.2° C. He complains of nausea and is unable to tolerate oral fluids. The nurse checks Mr. Koop's order, which reads, "Acetaminophen 650 mg orally for temperature above 38.5° C." On the basis of the assessment, the nurse believes that because Mr. Koops is nauseated, he will not be able to tolerate an oral dose of acetaminophen. By consulting the physician, the nurse acquires an order for a rectal suppository instead. A rectal suppository enables the nurse to administer the appropriate medication without increasing the client's symptoms of nausea.

Oral Routes. The oral route is the easiest and the most commonly used. Medications are given by mouth and swallowed with fluid. Oral medications have a slower onset of action and a more prolonged effect than parenteral medications. Clients generally prefer the oral route.

Sublingual Administration. Some medications are readily absorbed after being placed under the tongue to dissolve (Figure 35-4). A medication given by the **sublingual** route should not be swallowed because the medication will not have the desired effect. Nurses often give nitroglycerin by the sublingual route. Tell the client not to drink anything until the medication is completely dissolved.

Buccal Administration. Administration of a medication by the **buccal** route involves placing the solid medication in the mouth and against the mucous membranes of the cheek until the medication dissolves (Figure 35-5). Teach clients to alternate cheeks with each subsequent dose to avoid mucosal irritation. Warn clients not to chew or swallow the medication or to take any liquids with it. A buccal medication acts locally on the mucosa or systemically as it is swallowed in a person's saliva.

Parenteral Routes. **Parenteral administration** involves injecting a medication into body tissues. The following are the four major sites of injection:

1. **Intradermal (ID):** Injection into the dermis just under the epidermis
2. **Subcutaneous (Sub-Q):** Injection into tissues just below the dermis of the skin
3. **Intramuscular (IM):** Injection into a muscle
4. **Intravenous (IV):** Injection into a vein

Some medications are administered into body cavities other than the four types listed above. These routes of medication administration include epidural, intrathecal, intraosseous, intraperitoneal, intrapleural, and intraarterial. Nurses often are not responsible for the administration of medications through these advanced techniques. Whether or not the nurse actually administers the medication, the nurse remains responsible for monitoring the integrity of the medication delivery system, understanding the therapeutic value of the medication, and evaluating the client's response to the therapy.

Epidural. Epidural medications are administered in the epidural space via a catheter, which is placed by a nurse anesthetist or an anesthesiologist. This route is often used for the administration of postoperative analgesia (see Chapter 43). Nurses who have

✳ TABLE 35-6 Factors Influencing Choice of Administration Routes

ADVANTAGES	DISADVANTAGES OR CONTRAINDICATIONS
Oral, Buccal, Sublingual Routes	
Convenient and comfortable for client	Avoided when client has alterations in gastrointestinal function (e.g., nausea, vomiting), reduced motility (after general anesthesia or bowel inflammation), and surgical resection of gastrointestinal tract.
Economical	
Easy to administer	
Often produce local or systemic effects	Gastric secretions destroy some medications. Oral administration is contraindicated in clients unable to swallow (e.g., clients with neuromuscular disorders, esophageal strictures, mouth lesions).
Rarely cause anxiety for client.	
	Oral medications sometimes irritate lining of gastrointestinal tract, discolor teeth, or have unpleasant taste.
	Unconscious or confused client is unable or unwilling to swallow or hold medication under tongue.
	Cannot administer oral medications when clients have gastric suction; are contraindicated before some tests or surgery.
Subcutaneous (Sub-Q), Intramuscular (IM), Intravenous (IV), Intradermal (ID) Routes	
Provide means of administration when oral medications are contraindicated.	Risk of introducing infection, and some medications are expensive.
	Some clients experience pain from repeated needle sticks.
More rapid absorption occurs than with topical or oral routes.	Sub-Q, IM, and ID routes avoided in clients with bleeding tendencies.
	Risk of tissue damage with Sub-Q injections.
IV infusion provides medication delivery when client is critically ill or long-term therapy is necessary. If peripheral perfusion is poor, IV route is preferred over injections.	IM and IV routes have higher absorption rates, thus placing the client at higher risk for reactions.
	Often cause considerable anxiety in many clients, especially children.
Skin	
Primarily provides local effect	Clients with skin abrasions are at risk for rapid medication absorption and systemic effects.
Painless	Medications slowly absorbed through the skin.
Limited side effects	
Transdermal	
Prolonged systemic effects with limited side effects	Leaves oily or pasty substance on skin and sometimes soils clothing.
Mucous Membranes*	
Therapeutic effects provided by local application to involved sites.	Mucous membranes are highly sensitive to some medication concentrations.
Aqueous solutions readily absorbed and capable of causing systemic effects.	Client with ruptured eardrum cannot receive irrigations.
	Insertion of rectal and vaginal medication often causes embarrassment.
Potential route of administration when oral medications are contraindicated.	Rectal suppositories contraindicated if client has had rectal surgery or if active rectal bleeding is present.
Inhalation	
Provides rapid relief for local respiratory problems.	Some local agents cause serious systemic effects.
Used for introduction of general anesthetic gases.	

*Includes eyes, ears, nose, vagina, rectum, and ostomy.

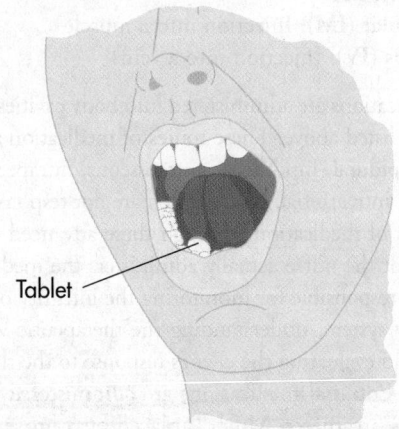

Tablet

Figure 35-4 Sublingual administration of a tablet.

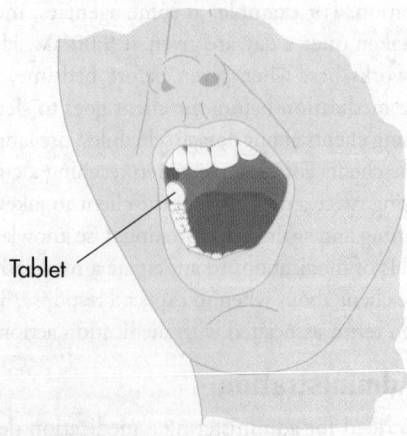

Tablet

Figure 35-5 Buccal administration of a tablet.

received advanced education in the epidural route can administer medications by continuous infusion or by a bolus dose.

Intrathecal. Nurses administer intrathecal medications through a catheter placed in the subarachnoid space or one of the ventricles of the brain. Intrathecal administration is often associated with long-term medication administration through surgically implanted catheters. In most institutions a physician usually injects medications into intrathecal catheters. However, some specially educated nurses do this as well.

Intraosseous. This method of medication administration involves the infusion of medication directly into the bone marrow. It is most commonly used in infants and toddlers who have poor access to their intravascular space. This method is most popular when an emergency arises and IV access is impossible. The physician inserts an intraosseous infusion needle into the bone, usually the tibia, for the administration of medication by the nurse.

Intraperitoneal. Medications administered into the peritoneal cavity are absorbed into the circulation. Chemotherapeutic agents, insulin, and antibiotics are administered in this fashion.

Intrapleural. An injection or chest tube is used to administer intrapleural medications directly into the pleural space. Chemotherapeutic agents are the most common medications administered via this method. Physicians also instill medications that help resolve persistent pleural effusion. This is called pleurodesis. This technique promotes adhesion between the visceral and parietal pleura.

Intraarterial. Intraarterial medications are administered directly into the arteries. Intraarterial infusions are common in clients who have arterial clots. The nurse manages a continuous infusion of clot-dissolving agents and carefully monitors the integrity of the infusion to prevent inadvertent disconnection of the system and subsequent bleeding.

Other methods of medication administration that are usually limited to physician administration are **intracardiac,** an injection of a medication directly into cardiac tissue, and **intraarticular,** an injection of a medication into a joint.

Topical Administration.
Medications applied to the skin and mucous membranes generally have local effects. Apply topical medications to the skin by painting or spreading the medication over an area, applying moist dressings, soaking body parts in a solution, or giving medicated baths. Systemic effects often occur if a client's skin is thin or broken down, if the medication concentration is high, or if contact with the skin is prolonged. A **transdermal disk** or patch (e.g., nitroglycerin, scopolamine, and estrogens) has systemic effects. The disk secures the medicated ointment to the skin. These topical applications are left in place for as little as 12 hours or as long as 7 days.

Nurses administer medications to mucous membranes in a variety of ways, by (1) directly applying a liquid or ointment (e.g., eye drops, gargling, or swabbing the throat); (2) inserting a medication into a body cavity (e.g., placing a suppository in rectum or vagina or inserting medicated packing into vagina); (3) instilling fluid into a body cavity (e.g., ear drops, nose drops, or bladder and rectal **instillation** [fluid is retained]); (4) irrigating a body cavity (e.g., flushing eye, ear, vagina, bladder, or rectum with medicated fluid [fluid is not retained]); and (5) spraying (e.g., instillation into nose and throat).

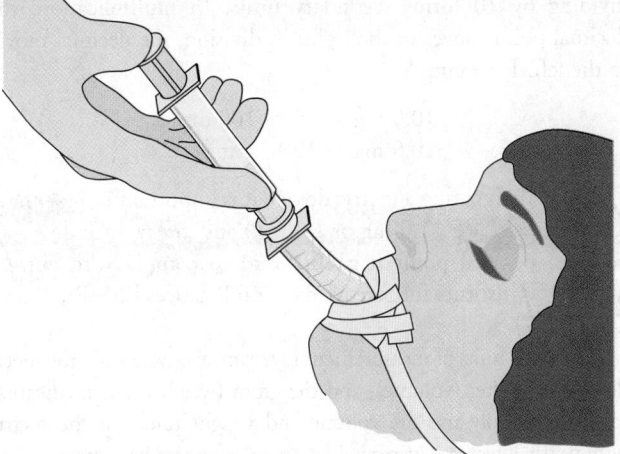

Figure 35-6 Medication instilled through an endotracheal tube.

Inhalation Route. The deeper passages of the respiratory tract provide a large surface area for medication absorption. Nurses administer inhaled medications through the nasal passages, oral passage, or endotracheal or tracheostomy tubes. Endotracheal tubes go into the client's mouth and end in the trachea (Figure 35-6), whereas tracheostomy tubes directly enter the trachea through an incision made in the neck. Medications that are administered by the **inhalation** route are readily absorbed and work rapidly because of the rich vascular alveolar capillary network present in the pulmonary tissue. Many inhaled medications have local or systemic effects.

Intraocular Route. **Intraocular** medication delivery involves inserting a medication similar to a contact lens into the client's eye. The eye medication disk has two soft outer layers that have medication enclosed in them. The nurse inserts the disk into the client's eye, much like a contact lens, and it can remain in the client's eye for up to 1 week. Pilocarpine, a medication used to treat glaucoma, is the most common medication disk.

Systems of Medication Measurement

The proper administration of a medication depends on the nurse's ability to compute medication doses accurately and measure medications correctly. Mistakes in calculating medications correctly often lead to fatal errors. The nurse is responsible for checking calculations carefully before giving a medication.

Medication therapy uses the metric, apothecary, and household systems of measurement. The apothecary system is infrequently used today. Although the U.S. Congress has not officially adopted the metric system, most health professionals in the United States use it. Health care providers usually write prescriptions to be self-administered in household measures for clients.

Metric System. As a decimal system, the **metric system** is the most logically organized. Metric units are easy to convert and compute through simple multiplication and division. Each basic unit of measurement is organized into units of 10. Multiplying or dividing by 10 forms secondary units. In multiplication, the decimal point moves to the right; in division, the decimal moves to the left. For example:

$$10.0 \text{ mg} \times 10 = 100 \text{ mg}$$
$$10.0 \text{ mg} \div 10 = 1 \text{ mg}$$

When designating a metric dosage it is important to *never* have a trailing zero (e.g., 1.0 mg or 1.0 mL) and *always* include a zero before a decimal point (e.g., 0.1 mg) to comply with current guidelines (Institute for Safe Medication Practices [ISMP], 2006a; TJC, 2007).

The basic units of measurement in the metric system are the meter (length), the liter (volume), and the gram (weight). For medication calculations only use the volume and weight units. In the metric system, use lowercase or capital letters to designate basic units:

Gram = g or Gm
Liter = l or L

Use lowercase letters for abbreviations for other units:

Milligram = mg
Milliliter = mL

A system of Latin prefixes designates subdivision of the basic units: *deci-* (1/10 or 0.1), *centi-* (1/100 or 0.01), and *milli-* (1/1000 or 0.001). Greek prefixes designate multiples of the basic units: *deka-* (10), *hecto-* (100), and *kilo-* (1000). When writing medication doses in metric units, prescribers and nurses use fractions or multiples of a unit. Convert fractions to decimals.

500 mg or 0.5 g, *not* ½ g
10 mL or 0.01 L, *not* 1/100 L

Household Measurements. Household units of measure are familiar to most people. The disadvantage of household measures is their inaccuracy. Household utensils such as teaspoons and cups often vary in size. Scales to measure pints or quarts are often not well calibrated. Household measures include drops, teaspoons, tablespoons, and cups for volume and pints and quarts for weight. Although pints and quarts are household measures, they are also used in the apothecary system. The advantage of household measurements is their convenience and familiarity. When the accuracy of a medication dose is not critical (e.g., over-the-counter medications), it is safe to use household measures. To calculate medications accurately, you need to know common equivalents of metric and household units (Table 35-7).

Solutions. The nurse uses solutions of various concentrations for injections, **irrigations**, and infusions. A **solution** is a given mass of solid substance dissolved in a known volume of fluid or a given volume of liquid dissolved in a known volume of another fluid. When a solid is dissolved in a fluid, the concentration is in units of mass per units of volume (e.g., g/L, mg/mL). A concentration of a solution can also be expressed as a percentage. A 10% solution, for example, is 10 g of solid dissolved in 100 mL of solution. A proportion also expresses concentrations. A 1/1000 solution represents a solution containing 1 g of solid in 1000 mL of liquid or 1 mL of liquid mixed with 1000 mL of another liquid.

TABLE 35-7   Equivalents of Measurement

METRIC	APOTHECARY	HOUSEHOLD
1 mL	15-16 minims	15 drops (gtt)
4-5 mL	1 fluidram	1 teaspoon (tsp)
16 mL	4 fluidrams	1 tablespoon (tbsp)
30 mL	1 fluid ounce	2 tablespoons (tbsp)
240 mL	8 fluid ounces	1 cup (c)
480 mL (approximately 500 mL)	1 pint (pt)	1 pint (pt)
960 mL (approximately 1 L)	1 quart (qt)	1 quart (qt)
3840 mL (approximately 4 L)	1 gallon (gal)	1 gallon (gal)

Nursing Knowledge Base

The Institute of Medicine (IOM) (2003) published the book *To Err Is Human: Building a Safer Health System*. This book created a new national awareness of problems within the health care system. It estimated that up to 98,000 people die in any given year from medical errors that occur in hospitals. This means that more people die from medical errors than from motor vehicle accidents, breast cancer, acquired immunodeficiency syndrome (AIDS), and workplace injuries. Medication-related errors for hospitalized clients cost roughly $2 billion annually.

Nurses play an important role in client safety, especially in the area of medication administration. The safe administration of medications is an important topic for current nursing researchers (Box 35-2). To safely administer medications to clients, nurses need to know how to calculate medication doses accurately. They also need to understand the different roles that members of the health care team play in the prescribing and administering of medications. All of the nurse's previous learning is important and is often applied to medication administration. The nursing process provides the framework for nurses to organize their thoughts and actions and is the foundation for medication administration.

Clinical Calculations

To administer medications safely, it is essential to have an understanding of basic arithmetic to calculate medication doses, mix solutions, and perform a variety of other activities. This skill is important because medications are not always dispensed in the unit of measure in which they are ordered. This occurs because medication companies package and bottle medications in standard dosages. For example, the prescriber orders 20 mg of a medication that is available only in 40-mg vials. Nurses frequently convert available units of volume and weight to desired doses. Therefore be aware of equivalents in all major measurement systems. In addition to medication administration, nurses use volume and weight conversions in a variety of other nursing activities (Box 35-3).

Conversions Within One System. Converting measurements within one system is relatively easy; simply divide or mul-

✳ BOX 35-2 — EVIDENCE-BASED PRACTICE

Reducing Distractions During Medication Administration

Evidence Summary

Many medication errors occur when nurses become distracted or lose focus during medication administration. Errors also occur when nurses fail to follow standard nursing protocols and procedures related to medication administration. Nurses experience multiple interruptions and distractions in today's health care environment. Nurses need systems in place to avoid these distractions to help avoid medication errors. In this research study, techniques to assist nurses with focusing on medication administration were used. Nurses used small checklist cards that listed the steps of medication administration. The cards were similar to checklists used by airplane pilots during the take-off and landing of airplanes. Reported medication errors decreased after 3 weeks. Then, researchers posted "Do Not Disturb" signs in medication preparation areas to help remind everyone in the hospital not to disturb nurses during the medication administration process. Following the interventions, nurses were better able to follow the hospital's medication administration procedure, and they perceived fewer distractions during medication administration.

Application to Nursing Practice

- Consistently following nursing protocols for medication administration decreases medication errors.
- Nurses who experience fewer distractions during medication administration prevent medication errors.
- Placing "Do Not Disturb" signs in medication preparation areas helps reduce distractions and errors.
- Nurses need to investigate strategies that will decrease distractions and enhance their ability to follow nursing protocols and improve their focus during medication administration.

Reference

Pape TM and others: Innovative approaches to reducing nurses' distractions during medication administration, *J Contin Educ Nurs* 36(3):108, 2005.

✳ BOX 35-3 Common Reasons for Measurement Conversions

- Converting fluid ounces to milliliters for measurement of intake and output
- Converting body weight from pounds to kilograms and vice versa
- Converting volume equivalents to calculate intravenous flow rates and prepare wound irrigation solutions, enemas, or bladder irrigations

tiply in the metric system. To change milligrams to grams, divide by 1000, moving the decimal 3 points to the left.

$$1000 \text{ mg} = 1 \text{ g}$$
$$350 \text{ mg} = 0.35 \text{ g}$$

To convert liters to milliliters, multiply by 1000 or move the decimal 3 points to the right.

$$1 \text{ L} = 1000 \text{ mL}$$
$$0.25 \text{ L} = 250 \text{ mL}$$

To convert units of measurement within the apothecary or household system, consult an equivalent table. For example, when converting fluid ounces to quarts, you first need to know that 32 ounces is the equivalent of 1 quart. To convert 8 ounces to a quart measurement, divide 8 by 32 to get the equivalent, ¼ or 0.25 quart.

Conversion Between Systems.
The nurse frequently determines the proper dose of a medication by converting weights or volumes from one system of measurement to another. Often, the nurse converts metric units to equivalent household measures for use at home. To calculate medications, it is necessary to work with units in the same measurement system. Tables of equivalent measurements are available in all health care institutions. The pharmacist is also a good resource.

Before making a conversion, compare the measurement system available with that ordered. For example, the prescriber orders Robitussin 30 mL, but the client only has tablespoons at home. To provide proper instruction to the client, the nurse converts mL to tablespoons, which requires the nurse to know the equivalent or refer to a table such as Table 35-7.

Dose Calculations.
There are many formulas used to calculate medication doses. Apply the following basic formula when preparing solid or liquid forms:

$$\frac{\text{Dose ordered}}{\text{Dose on hand}} \times \text{Amount on hand} = \text{Amount to administer}$$

The dose ordered is the amount of medication prescribed. The dose on hand is the dose (e.g., mg, units) of medication supplied by the pharmacy. The amount on hand is the basic unit or quantity of the medication that contains the dose on hand. For solid medications the amount on hand is often one capsule; the amount of liquid on hand is sometimes a milliliter or liter depending on the container. For example, a liquid medication comes in the strength of 125 mg per 5 mL. In this case 125 mg is the dose on hand, whereas 5 mL is the amount on hand. The amount to administer is the actual amount of medication the nurse will administer. Always express the amount to administer in the same unit as the amount on hand.

The following example illustrates how to apply the formula. The prescriber orders the client to receive morphine sulfate 2 mg IV. Thus the dose ordered is 2 mg. The medication is available in a vial containing 10 mg per milliliter. Thus the dose on hand is 10 mg and the amount on hand is 1 mL. The formula is applied as follows:

$$2 \text{ mg}/10 \text{ mg} \times 1 \text{ mL} = \text{Amount in milliliters to administer}$$

To simplify the $\frac{2}{10}$ fraction, divide numerator and denominator by 2:

$$\frac{1}{5} \times 1 \text{ mL} = \frac{1}{5} \text{ mL to administer}$$

Syringes are calibrated only in decimals. After converting the fraction $\frac{1}{5}$ to 0.2, accurately prepare the correct dose.

Another example demonstrates how the formula applies with solid dose forms. The prescriber orders 0.125 mg orally (PO) of digoxin. The medication is available in tablets containing 0.25 mg.

$$0.125 \text{ mg}/0.250 \text{ mg} \times 1 \text{ tablet} = \text{Number of tablets to administer}$$

The fraction $^{0.125}\!/_{0.250}$ equals $\frac{1}{2}$ or 0.5. Therefore

$$0.5 \times 1 \text{ tablet} = 0.5 \text{ or } \frac{1}{2} \text{ tablet to be administered}$$

Many tablets come with scores or indentations across the center of the tablet (Figure 35-7). A scored tablet is easy to break in half for divided doses. In some institutions pharmacists are responsible for scoring tablets. Because the potential for giving an incorrect dose is high, do not break unscored tablets.

Often, liquid medications come prepared in volumes greater than 1 mL. In applying the formula, be careful to use the correct concentration to avoid a **medication error.** For example, the order is "Erythromycin suspension 250 mg PO." The pharmacy delivers 100-mL bottles with the label stating, "5 mL contains 125 mg of erythromycin." Thus the appropriate concentration to use in this example to obtain the correct dose of medication is 125 mg in 5 mL.

$$250 \text{ mg}/125 \text{ mg} \times 5 \text{ mL} = \text{Volume to administer}$$

The fraction $^{250}\!/_{125}$ equals 2. Therefore

$$2 \times 5 \text{ mL} = 10 \text{ mL to administer}$$

Some agencies require a nurse to double-check calculations with another nurse before administering the medication, especially when the risk of administering the wrong medication dosage is high (e.g., heparin or insulin). **Always** double-check calculations or confer with another nurse or health care professional if an answer to a calculation seems unreasonable.

Pediatric Doses. Calculating children's medication doses requires caution. Children metabolize medications at different rates when compared with adults. For example, premature and newborn infants are especially vulnerable to adverse effects of medications because their liver and kidneys have not matured to full functioning levels. After the newborn period, the liver metabolizes some drugs more quickly, which often results in larger doses or more frequent administration (Hockenberry and Wilson, 2007). Other factors that influence medication dosages in children include the difficulty in evaluating the desired effect and the hydration status of the child. In most cases, the prescriber will calculate the dose for a child before ordering the medication. However, it is the nurse's responsibility to be aware of the safe dosage range for any medication administered to a child. Therefore be aware of the formulas used to calculate pediatric doses and recheck all doses before administration. Drug package inserts or medication references often list the normal ranges for pediatric doses.

Various formulas to determine appropriate medication dosages for children exist. These formulas often take the child's age, weight, body surface area, and/or the medication amount into consider-

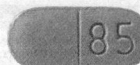

Figure 35-7 Scored medication tablet. (Courtesy Mosby's GenRx 1999.)

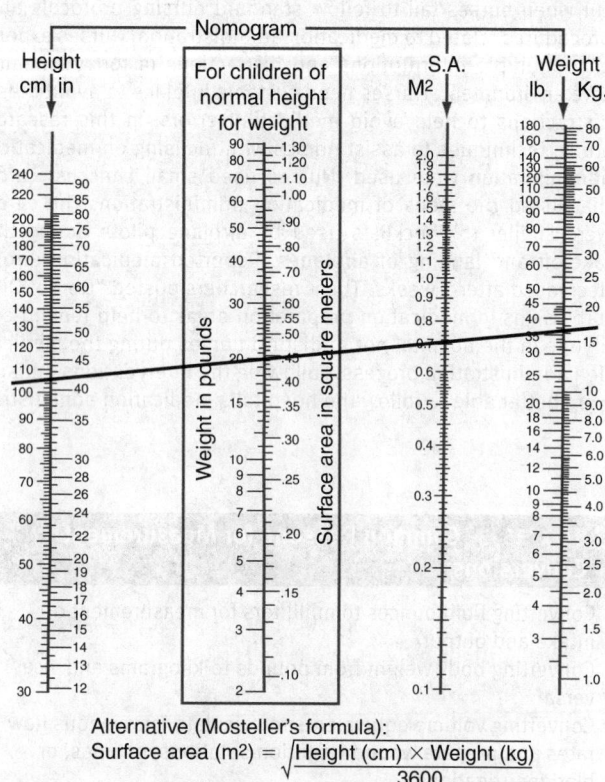

Alternative (Mosteller's formula):
$$\text{Surface area (m}^2) = \sqrt{\frac{\text{Height (cm)} \times \text{Weight (kg)}}{3600}}$$

Figure 35-8 West nomogram for estimation of surface areas in children. A straight line is drawn between height and weight. The point where the line crosses the surface area column is the estimated body surface area. (From Behrman RE and others: *Nelson textbook of pediatrics*, ed 17, Philadelphia, 2004, Saunders; modified from data of Boyd E, by West CD.)

ation. However, the most accurate method of calculating pediatric doses is based on a child's body surface area (Hockenberry and Wilson, 2007). Use Mosteller's formula or the standard nomogram (e.g., the West nomogram) to estimate a child's body surface area (Figure 35-8).

Use the formula below to calculate a pediatric dose. The formula is a ratio of the child's body surface area compared with the body surface area of an average adult (1.7 square meters, or 1.7 m²).

For example, a prescriber orders ampicillin for a child weighing 11.4 (25.08 lb) kg. The normal adult dose for ampicillin is 250 mg. The West nomogram (see Figure 35-8) shows that a child weighing 11.4 kg has a surface area of 0.51 m². Using this information, calculate the appropriate child's dose.

$$\text{Child's dose} = 0.51 \text{ m}^2/1.7 \text{ m}^2 \times 250 \text{ mg}$$

The m² units are canceled out.

Child's dose = 0.51/1.7 × 250 mg
0.51/1.7 = 0.3
Child's dose = 0.3 × 250 mg = 75 mg

An alternative method to determine dosages of medications for children involves basing the amount of medication to administer (usually in mg) on how much the child weighs (usually in kg). For example, a prescriber orders 5 mg/kg to be given to a child weighing 14 kg. Using this information, calculate the appropriate dosage based on the following calculation:

Child's dose = 5 mg/kg × 14 kg = 70 mg to be delivered

The nurse does not have sole responsibility for medication administration. The prescriber and pharmacist also have responsibility that the right medication gets to the right client. However, the nurse administering medications is accountable for calculating the correct dosage and for knowing which medications are prescribed, their therapeutic and nontherapeutic effects, and the medications' associated nursing implications. The nurse is also responsible for knowing why the client needs the medication and determining if the client requires supervision with administration and education about the medication and its effects. The nurse is also responsible for monitoring the effects of the drug after it is administered and to report any reactions to the prescriber.

Prescriber's Role

The physician, nurse practitioner, or physician's assistant prescribes medications by writing a medication order on a form in the client's medical record, in an order book, or on a legal prescription pad. Some prescribers use a desktop, laptop, or hand-held computer to enter medication orders. Prescribers must document the diagnosis, condition, or need for use for each medication ordered. Many hospitals are implementing computerized physician order entry (CPOE) to handle medication orders to decrease medication errors. In these systems, the prescriber completes all computerized fields before the order for the medication is filled, thus avoiding incomplete or illegible orders.

Sometimes a prescriber orders a medication by talking directly to the nurse or by telephone. When medications or medical treatments are ordered over the telephone, the order is called a telephone order. If the order is given verbally to the nurse, it is called a **verbal order.** When a verbal or telephone order is received, the nurse who took the order writes the complete order or enters it into a computer and then reads it back and receives confirmation from the prescriber to confirm accuracy (TJC, 2008). The nurse indicates the time and the name of the prescriber who gave the order, signs the order, and follows agency policy to indicate that the order was read back. The prescriber countersigns the order at a later time, usually within 24 hours after giving the order. Follow guidelines for taking verbal or telephone orders for medications safely (Box 35-4). Institutional policies vary regarding the personnel who can take verbal or telephone orders. Nursing students cannot take these types of medication orders. Nursing students only give newly ordered medications after a registered nurse has written and verified the order.

Common abbreviations are often used when writing orders. Abbreviations indicate dosage frequencies or times, routes of administration, and special information for giving the medication

(see Table 35-4). Medication errors frequently involve the use of abbreviations. For example, write out the complete drug name (e.g., penicillin, do not abbreviate PCN). Table 35-8 lists abbreviations that are associated with a high incidence of medication errors. Do **not** use these abbreviations when documenting medication orders or other information about medications (ISMP, 2006a; National Coordinating Council for Medication Error Reporting and Prevention [NCCMERP], 2006; TJC, 2007).

Types of Orders in Acute Care Agencies

Five common types of medication orders are based on the frequency and/or urgency of medication administration. Some conditions change the status of a client's medication orders. For example, in some agencies the client's preoperative medications are automatically discontinued, and the health care provider writes new medication orders after surgery (see Chapter 50). Agency policies that surround medication orders often vary. Nurses need to be aware of and follow these policies.

Standing Orders or Routine Medication Orders. A standing order is carried out until the prescriber cancels it by another order or until a prescribed number of days elapse. A standing order often indicates a final date or number of treatments or doses. Many institutions have policies for automatically discontinuing standing orders. The following are examples of standing orders: "Tetracycline 500 mg PO q6h" and "Decadron 10 mg daily × 5 days."

prn Orders. Sometimes the prescriber orders a medication to be given only when a client requires it. This is a prn order. Use objective and subjective assessment and discretion in determining whether or not the client needs the medication. An example is "morphine sulfate 2 mg IV q2h prn for incisional pain." This order indicates that the client needs to wait at least 2 hours between doses. When administering medications, document the assessment made and the time of medication administration. Make frequent evaluation of the effectiveness of the medication, and record findings in the appropriate record.

Single (One-Time) Orders. A prescriber will often order a medication to be given only once at a specified time. This is common for preoperative medications or medications given before diagnostic examinations, for example, "Ativan 1 mg IV on call to MRI" and "Valium 10 mg PO at 0900."

STAT Orders. A STAT order signifies that a single dose of a medication is to be given immediately and only once. STAT orders are often written for emergencies when the client's condition changes suddenly. For example, "Give Apresoline 10 mg IV STAT."

Now Orders. A now order is more specific than a one-time order and is used when a client needs a medication quickly but not right away, as in a STAT order. When receiving a now order, the nurse has up to 90 minutes to administer the medication. Only administer now medications one time. For example, "Give Vancomycin 1 g IV piggyback now."

Prescriptions. The prescriber writes **prescriptions** for clients who are to take medications outside the hospital. The prescription

Text continued on p. 703

BOX 35-4 **Recommendations to Reduce Medication Errors Associated With Verbal Medication Orders and Prescriptions (NCCMERP, 2006)**

Council Recommendations

Recommendations to Reduce Medication Errors Associated with Verbal Medication Orders and Prescriptions
    Adopted February 20, 2001
    Revised February 24, 2006

Preamble

Confusion over the similarity of drug names accounts for approximately 25% of all reports to the USP Medication Errors Reporting (MER) Program. To reduce confusion pertaining to verbal orders and to further support the Council's mission to minimize medication errors, the following recommendations have been developed.

In these recommendations, verbal orders are prescriptions or medication orders that are communicated as oral, spoken communications between senders and receivers face to face, by telephone, or by other auditory device.

Recommendations

1. Verbal communication of prescription or medication orders should be limited to urgent situations where immediate written or electronic communication is not feasible.
2. Health care organizations* should establish policies and procedures that:
   - Describe limitations or prohibitions on use of verbal orders
   - Provide a mechanism to ensure validity/authenticity of the prescriber
   - List the elements required for inclusion in a complete verbal order
   - Describe situations in which verbal orders may be used
   - List and define the individuals who may send and receive verbal orders
   - Provide guidelines for clear and effective communication of verbal orders.
3. Leaders of health care organizations should promote a culture in which it is acceptable, and strongly encouraged, for staff to question prescribers when there are any questions or disagreements about verbal orders. Questions about verbal orders should be resolved prior to the preparation, or dispensing, or administration of the medication.
4. Verbal orders for antineoplastic agents should **NOT** be permitted under any circumstances. These medications are not administered in emergency or urgent situations, and they have a narrow margin of safety.

5. Elements that should be included in a verbal order include:
   - Name of patient
   - Age and weight of patient, when appropriate
   - Drug name
   - Dosage form (e.g., tablets, capsules, inhalants)
   - Exact strength or concentration
   - Dose, frequency, and route
   - Quantity and/or duration
   - Purpose or indication (unless disclosure is considered inappropriate by the prescriber)
   - Specific instructions for use
   - Name of prescriber, and telephone number when appropriate
   - Name of individual transmitting the order, if different from the prescriber.
6. The content of verbal orders should be clearly communicated:
   - The name of the drug should be confirmed by any of the following:
     - Spelling
     - Providing both the brand and generic names of the medication
     - Providing the indication for use
   - In order to avoid confusion with spoken numbers, a dose such as 50 mg should be dictated as "fifty milligrams . . . five zero milligrams" to distinguish from "fifteen milligrams . . . one five milligrams."
   - In order to avoid confusion with drug name modifiers, such as prefixes and suffixes, additional spelling-assistance methods should be used (i.e., S as in Sam, X as in x-ray).
   - Instructions for use should be provided without abbreviations. For example, "1 tab tid" should be communicated as "Take/give one tablet three times daily."
   - Whenever possible, the receiver of the order should **write** down the complete order to enter it into a computer, then **read** it back, and receive confirmation from the individual who gave the order or test result.
7. All verbal orders should be reduced immediately to writing and signed by the individual receiving the order.
8. Verbal orders should be documented in the patient's medical record, reviewed, and countersigned by the prescriber as soon as possible.

*Health care organizations include community pharmacies, physicians' offices, hospitals, nursing homes, home care agencies, etc.

© 1998-2007 National Coordinating Council for Medication Error Reporting and Prevention. All Rights Reserved. *Permission is hereby granted to reproduce information contained herein provided that such reproduction shall not modify the text and shall include the copyright notice appearing on the pages from which it was copied.

✳ TABLE 35-8 ISMP's List of *Error-Prone Abbreviations, Symbols, and Dose Designations*

The abbreviations, symbols, and dose designations found in this table have been reported to ISMP through the USP-ISMP Medication Error Reporting Program as being frequently misinterpreted and involved in harmful medication errors. They should NEVER be used when communicating medical information. This includes internal communications, telephone/verbal prescriptions, computer-generated labels, labels for drug storage bins, medication administration records, as well as pharmacy and prescriber computer order entry screens. The Joint Commission (TJC) has established a National Patient Safety Goal that specifies that certain abbreviations must appear on an accredited organization's do-not-use list; we have highlighted these items with a double asterisk (**). However, we hope that you will consider others beyond the minimum TJC requirements. By using and promoting safe practices and by educating one another about hazards, we can better protect our patients.

ABBREVIATIONS	INTENDED MEANING	MISINTERPRETATION	CORRECTION
μg	Microgram	Mistaken as "mg"	Use "mcg"
AD, AS, AU	Right ear, left ear, each ear	Mistaken as OD, OS, OU (right eye, left eye, each eye)	Use "right ear," "left ear," or "each ear"
BT	Bedtime	Mistaken as "BID" (twice daily)	Use "bedtime"
cc	Cubic centimeters	Mistaken as "u" (units)	Use "mL"
D/C	Discharge or discontinue	Premature discontinuation of medications if D/C (intended to mean "discharge") has been misinterpreted as "discontinued" when followed by a list of discharge medications	Use "discharge" and "discontinue"
IJ	Injection	Mistaken as "IV" or "intrajugular"	Use "injection"
IN	Intranasal	Mistaken as "IM" or "IV"	Use "intranasal" or "NAS"
HS	Half-strength	Mistaken as bedtime	Use "half-strength" or "bedtime"
hs	At bedtime, hours of sleep	Mistaken as half-strength	Use "bedtime" or "half-strength"
IU**	International unit	Mistaken as IV (intravenous) or 10 (ten)	Use "units"
o.d. or OD	Once daily	Mistaken as "right eye" (OD—oculus dexter), leading to oral liquid medications administered in the eye	Use "daily"
OJ	Orange juice	Mistaken as OD or OS (right or left eye); drugs meant to be diluted in orange juice may be given in the eye	Use "orange juice"
Per os	By mouth, orally	The "os" can be mistaken as "left eye" (OS—oculus sinister)	Use "PO," "by mouth," or "orally"
q.d. or QD**	Every day	Mistaken as q.i.d., especially if the period after the "q" or the tail of the "q" is misunderstood as an "I"	Use "daily"
qhs	Nightly at bedtime	Mistaken as "qhr" or every hour	Use "nightly"
qn	Nightly or at bedtime	Mistaken as "qh" (every hour)	Use "nightly" or "at bedtime"
q.o.d. or QOD**	Every other day	Mistaken as "q.d." (daily) or "q.i.d. (four times daily) if the "o" is poorly written	Use "every other day"
q1d	Daily	Mistaken as q.i.d. (four times daily)	Use "daily"
q6PM, etc.	Every evening at 6 PM	Mistaken as every 6 hours	Use "6 PM nightly" or "6 PM daily"
SC, SQ, sub q	Subcutaneous	SC mistaken as SL (sublingual); SQ mistaken as "5 every"; the "q" in "sub q" has been mistaken as "every" (e.g., a heparin dose ordered "sub q 2 hours before surgery" misunderstood as every 2 hours before surgery)	Use "subcut" or "subcutaneously"
ss	Sliding scale (insulin) or ½ (apothecary)	Mistaken as "55"	Spell out "sliding scale;" use "one-half" or "½"
SSRI	Sliding scale regular insulin	Mistaken as selective-serotonin reuptake inhibitor	Spell out "sliding scale (insulin)"
SSI	Sliding scale insulin	Mistaken as Strong Solution of Iodine (Lugol's)	

**These abbreviations are included on TJC's "minimum list" of dangerous abbreviations, acronyms and symbols that must be included on an organization's "Do Not Use" list, effective January 1, 2004. Visit www.jointcommission.org for more information about this TJC requirement.

Permission is granted to reproduce material for internal newsletters or communications with proper attribution. Other reproduction is prohibited without written permission. Unless noted, reports were received through the USP-ISMP Medication Errors Reporting Program (MERP). Report actual and potential medication errors to the MERP via the web at www.ismp.org or by calling 1-800 FAIL-SAF(E). ISMP guarantees confidentiality of information received and respects reporters' wishes as to the level of detail included in publications.

ISMP, Institute for Safe Medication Practices.

✳ **TABLE 35-8** ISMP's List of *Error-Prone Abbreviations, Symbols, and Dose Designations*—cont'd

ABBREVIATIONS	INTENDED MEANING	MISINTERPRETATION	CORRECTION
ī/d	One daily	Mistaken as "tid"	Use "1 daily"
TIW or tiw	3 times a week	Mistaken as "3 times a day" or "twice in a week"	Use "3 times weekly"
U or u**	Unit	Mistaken as the number 0 or 4, causing a 10-fold overdose or greater (e.g., 4U seen as "40" or 4u seen as "44"); mistaken as "cc" so dose given in volume instead of units (e.g., 4u seen as 4cc)	Use "unit"

DOSE DESIGNATIONS AND OTHER INFORMATION	INTENDED MEANING	MISINTERPRETATION	CORRECTION
Trailing zero after decimal point (e.g., 1.0 mg)**	1 mg	Mistaken as 10 mg if the decimal point is not seen	Do not use trailing zeros for doses expressed in whole numbers
"Naked" decimal point (e.g., .5 mg)**	0.5 mg	Mistaken as 5 mg if the decimal point is not seen	Use zero before a decimal point when the dose is less than a whole unit
Drug name and dose run together (especially problematic for drug names that end in "l" such as Inderal40 mg; Tegretol300 mg)	Inderal 40 mg Tegretol 300 mg	Mistaken as Inderal 140 mg Mistaken as Tegretol 1300 mg	Place adequate space between the drug name, dose, and unit of measure
Numerical dose and unit of measure run together (e.g., 10mg, 100mL)	10 mg 100 mL	The "m" is sometimes mistaken as a zero or two zeros, risking a 10- to 100-fold overdose	Place adequate space between the dose and unit of measure
Abbreviations such as mg. or mL. with a period following the abbreviation	mg mL	The period is unnecessary and could be mistaken as the number 1 if written poorly	Use mg, mL, etc. without a terminal period
Large doses without properly placed commas (e.g., 100000 units; 1000000 units)	100,000 units 1,000,000 units	100000 has been mistaken as 10,000 or 1,000,000; 1000000 has been mistaken as 100,000	Use commas for dosing units at or above 1,000, or use words such as 100 "thousand" or 1 "million" to improve readability

DRUG NAME ABBREVIATIONS	INTENDED MEANING	MISINTERPRETATION	CORRECTION
ARA A	vidarabine	Mistaken as cytarabine (ARA C)	Use complete drug name
AZT	zidovudine (Retrovir)	Mistaken as azathioprine or aztreonam	Use complete drug name
CPZ	Compazine (prochlorperazine)	Mistaken as chlorpromazine	Use complete drug name
DPT	Demerol-Phenergan-Thorazine	Mistaken as diphtheria-pertussis-tetanus (vaccine)	Use complete drug name
DTO	Diluted tincture of opium, or deodorized tincture of opium (Paregoric)	Mistaken as tincture of opium	Use complete drug name

**These abbreviations are included on TJC's "minimum list" of dangerous abbreviations, acronyms and symbols that must be included on an organization's "Do Not Use" list, effective January 1, 2004. Visit www.jointcommission.org for more information about this TJC requirement.

Permission is granted to reproduce material for internal newsletters or communications with proper attribution. Other reproduction is prohibited without written permission. Unless noted, reports were received through the USP-ISMP Medication Errors Reporting Program (MERP). Report actual and potential medication errors to the MERP via the web at www.ismp.org or by calling 1-800 FAIL-SAF(E). ISMP guarantees confidentiality of information received and respects reporters' wishes as to the level of detail included in publications.

ISMP, Institute for Safe Medication Practices.

✳ **TABLE 35-8 ISMP's List of *Error-Prone Abbreviations, Symbols, and Dose Designations*—cont'd**

DRUG NAME ABBREVIATIONS	INTENDED MEANING	MISINTERPRETATION	CORRECTION
HCl	hydrochloric acid or hydrochloride	Mistaken as potassium chloride (The "H" is misinterpreted as "K")	Use complete drug name unless expressed as a salt of a drug
HCT	hydrocortisone	Mistaken as hydrochlorothiazide	Use complete drug name
HCTZ	hydrochlorothiazide	Mistaken as hydrocortisone (seen as HCT250 mg)	Use complete drug name
MgSO4**	magnesium sulfate	Mistaken as morphine sulfate	Use complete drug name
MS, MSO4**	morphine sulfate	Mistaken as magnesium sulfate	Use complete drug name
MTX	methotrexate	Mistaken as mitoxantrone	Use complete drug name
PCA	procainamide	Mistaken as patient controlled analgesia	Use complete drug name
PTU	propylthiouracil	Mistaken as mercaptopurine	Use complete drug name
T3	Tylenol with codeine No. 3	Mistaken as liothyronine	Use complete drug name
TAC	triamcinolone	Mistaken as tetracaine, Adrenalin, cocaine	Use complete drug name
TNK	TNKase	Mistaken as "TPA"	Use complete drug name
ZnSO4	zinc sulfate	Mistaken as morphine sulfate	Use complete drug name

STEMMED DRUG NAMES	INTENDED MEANING	MISINTERPRETATION	CORRECTION
"Nitro" drip	nitroglycerin infusion	Mistaken as sodium nitroprusside infusion	Use complete drug name
"Norflox"	norfloxacin	Mistaken as Norflex	Use complete drug name
"IV Vanc"	intravenous vancomycin	Mistaken as Invanz	Use complete drug name

SYMBOLS	INTENDED MEANING	MISINTERPRETATION	CORRECTION
ℨ	Dram	Symbol for dram mistaken as "3"	Use the metric system
ℳ	Minim	Symbol for minim mistaken as "mL"	
x3d	For three days	Mistaken as "3 doses"	Use "for three days"
> and <	Greater than and less than	Mistaken as opposite of intended; mistakenly use incorrect symbol; ">10" mistaken as "40"	Use "greater than" or "less than"
/ (slash mark)	Separates two doses or indicates "per"	Mistaken as the number 1 (e.g., "25 units/10 units" misread as "25 units and 110" units)	Use "per" rather than a slash mark to separate doses
@	At	Mistaken as "2"	Use "at"
&	And	Mistaken as "2"	Use "and"
+	Plus or and	Mistaken as "4"	Use "and"
°	Hour	Mistaken as a zero (e.g., q2° seen as q20)	Use "hr," "h," or "hour"

includes more detailed information than a regular order because the client needs to understand how to take the medication and when to refill the prescription if necessary. Figure 35-9 illustrates the parts of a prescription.

Pharmacist's Role

The pharmacist prepares and distributes prescribed medications. Pharmacists work with nurses, physicians, and other health care providers to evaluate the efficacy of clients' medications. The pharmacist is responsible for filling prescriptions accurately and for being sure that prescriptions are valid. The pharmacist in a health care agency rarely has to mix compounds or solutions, except in the case of intravenous solutions. Most medication companies deliver medications in a form ready for use. Dispensing the correct medication, in the proper dosage and amount, with an accurate label is the pharmacist's main task. The pharmacist also provides information about medication side effects, toxicity, interactions, and incompatibilities.

Distribution Systems

Systems for storing and distributing medications vary. Pharmacists provide the medications, but nurses distribute medications to clients. Institutions providing nursing care have a special area for stocking and dispensing medications. Special medication rooms, portable locked carts, computerized medication cabinets, and individual storage units next to clients' rooms are examples of storage areas used. Make sure that all medications are in locked containers in a room (e.g., medication room) or are under constant surveillance.

Unit Dose. The unit-dose system uses carts containing a drawer with a 24-hour supply of medications for each client. Each drawer is labeled with the name of the client in the designated room. The unit dose is the ordered dose of medication the client receives at one time. Each tablet or capsule is wrapped in a foil or paper container. At a designated time each day the pharmacist or a pharmacy technician refills the drawers in the cart with a fresh supply. The cart also contains limited amounts of prn and stock medications for special

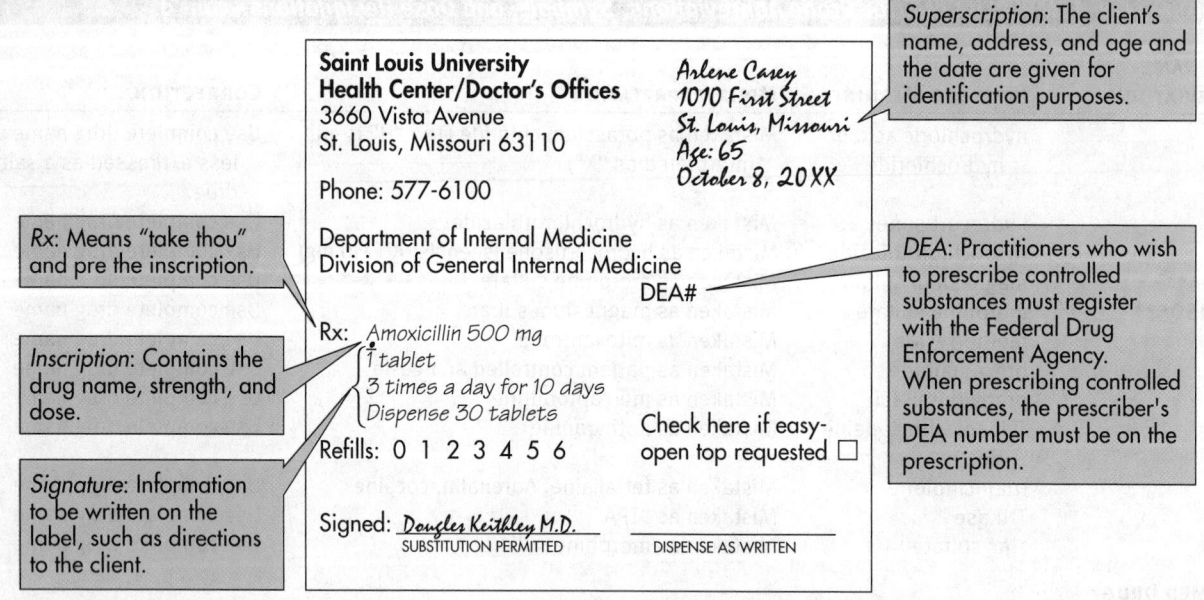

Superscription: The client's name, address, and age and the date are given for identification purposes.

**Saint Louis University
Health Center/Doctor's Offices**
3660 Vista Avenue
St. Louis, Missouri 63110

Phone: 577-6100

*Arlene Casey
1010 First Street
St. Louis, Missouri
Age: 65
October 8, 20XX*

Rx: Means "take thou" and pre the inscription.

Department of Internal Medicine
Division of General Internal Medicine
DEA#

DEA: Practitioners who wish to prescribe controlled substances must register with the Federal Drug Enforcement Agency. When prescribing controlled substances, the prescriber's DEA number must be on the prescription.

Inscription: Contains the drug name, strength, and dose.

Rx: *Amoxicillin 500 mg
1 tablet
3 times a day for 10 days
Dispense 30 tablets*

Refills: 0 1 2 3 4 5 6

Check here if easy-open top requested ☐

Signature: Information to be written on the label, such as directions to the client.

Signed: *Douglas Keithley M.D.*
SUBSTITUTION PERMITTED   DISPENSE AS WRITTEN

Figure 35-9 Example of a medication prescription. (Courtesy Saint Louis University Medical Center, St. Louis, Mo.)

situations. Controlled substances are not kept in the individual client drawer; they are kept in a larger locked drawer to keep them secure. The unit-dose system reduces the number of medication errors and saves steps in dispensing medications.

Automated Medication Dispensing Systems. Automated medication dispensing systems (AMDS) are used throughout the country (Figure 35-10). The systems within the agency are networked with each other and with other agency computer systems (e.g., computerized medical record). AMDS control the dispensing of all medications, including narcotics. Each nurse accesses the system by entering a security code. Some systems require bioidentification as well. In these systems the nurse places his or her finger on a screen to access the computer. Then the nurse selects the client's name and the client's drug profile before the AMDS will dispense a medication. In these systems the nurse is allowed to select the desired medication, dosage, and route from a list displayed on the computer screen. The system causes the drawer containing medication to open, records it, and charges it to the client. Systems that are connected to the client's computerized medical record will then record information about the medication (e.g., medication name, dose, time) as well as the nurse's name in the client's medical record. Some systems require nurses to scan bar codes to identify the client, the medication, and the nurse administering the medication before recording this information in the client's computerized medical record. AMDS often reduce the chance of medication errors (Manno, 2006).

Nurse's Role

The administration of medications to clients requires knowledge and a set of skills that are unique to the nurse. The nurse first assesses that the medication ordered is the correct medication. Do not assume that all medications that are in the client's "drawer" or pillbox are to be given to the client. Assess the client's ability to self-administer medications, determine whether a client should

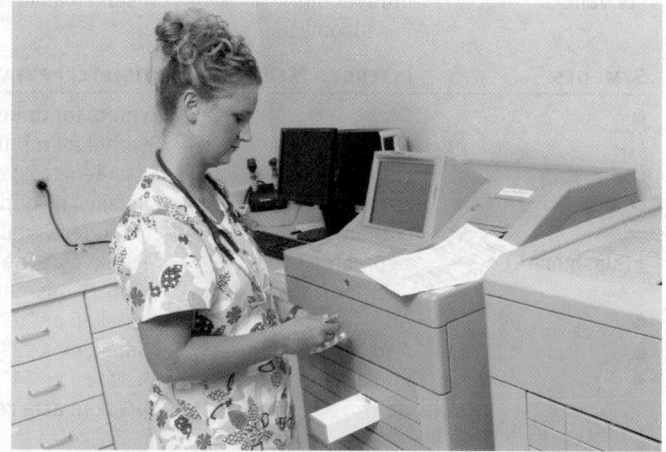

Figure 35-10 Automated medication dispensing system.

receive a medication at a given time, administer medications correctly, and monitor the effects of prescribed medications. Client and family education about proper medication administration and monitoring is an integral part of the nurse's role. Do not delegate any part of the medication administration process to assistive personnel, and use the nursing process to integrate medication therapy into care.

Medication Errors

A medication error can cause or lead to inappropriate medication use or client harm. Medication errors include inaccurate prescribing, administration of the wrong medication, giving the medication using the wrong route or time interval, and administering extra doses or failing to administer a medication. Prevention of medication errors is key. The process of administering medications has many steps and involves many members of the health care team.

✳ BOX 35-5 Steps to Take to Prevent Medication Errors

- Follow the six rights of medication administration.
- Be sure to read labels at least three times (comparing medication administration record [MAR] with label) before administering the medication.
- Use at least two client identifiers whenever administering a medication.
- Do not allow any other activity to interrupt administration of medication to a client.
- Double-check all calculations, and verify with another nurse.
- Do not interpret illegible handwriting; clarify with prescriber.
- Question unusually large or small doses.
- Document all medications as soon as they are given.
- When you have made an error, reflect on what went wrong and ask how you could have prevented the error.
- Evaluate the context or situation in which a medication error occurred. This helps to determine if nurses have the necessary resources for safe medication administration.
- When repeated medication errors occur within a work area, identify and analyze the factors that may have caused the errors and take corrective actions.
- Attend in-service programs that focus on the medications commonly administered.

Reprinted with permission of the National Coordinating Council for Medication Error Reporting and Prevention. © 2006. All Rights Reserved.

Because nurses play an essential role in the preparation and administration of medications, nurses need to be vigilant in prevention of medication errors (Box 35-5). Advances in technology have helped to decrease the occurrence of medication errors (Box 35-6).

Medication errors are related to professional practice, health care product design, or procedures and systems such as product labeling and distribution. When an error occurs, the client's safety and well-being become the top priority. The nurse assesses and examines the client's condition and notifies the physician or prescriber of the incident as soon as possible. Once the client is stable, the nurse reports the incident to the appropriate person in the institution (e.g., manager or supervisor).

When a medication error occurs, the nurse is responsible for preparing a written occurrence or incident report that usually needs to be filed within 24 hours of the error. The report includes client identification information; the location and time of the incident; an accurate, factual description of what occurred and what was done; and the signature of the nurse involved. The occurrence report is not a permanent part of the medical record and is not referred to anywhere in the record (see Chapters 23 and 26). This legally protects the health care professional and institution. Institutions use occurrence reports to track incident patterns and to initiate quality improvement programs as needed.

Report all medication errors, including those that do not cause obvious or immediate harm or near misses. It is important to feel comfortable in reporting an error and not fear repercussions from managerial staff. Even when a client suffers no harm from a medication error, the institution can still learn why the mistake occurred and what can be done to avoid similar errors in the future.

Medical errors often happen when a client is transferred to another health care agency or to a different unit within a hospital or is discharged. Therefore reconciling the list of client's

✳ BOX 35-6 Informatics and Medication Safety

Many medication errors occur when the nurse incorrectly administers medications at the client's bedside. The following innovations and advances in technology have helped reduce the number of medication errors in nursing practice:

- Networked computers allow all the client's health care providers to see a current list of ordered and discontinued medications.
- Internet and intranet access allows nurses and other health care providers to access current information about medications (e.g., indications, desired effects, adverse effects) and specific agency policies that address medication administration (e.g., how fast to administer an intravenous [IV] push medication, how to administer medications through a nasogastric tube).
- In some agencies, prescribers enter medication orders directly into a networked computer system or a personal handheld computer.
- Automated medication dispensing systems and electronic medication administration records (MARs) help with medication reconciliation, administration, and documentation (Manno, 2006; Paoletti and others, 2007).
- Bar-coding technology requires nurses to scan the medication, the client's identification bracelet, and the nurse's identification badge before administering the medication, which helps ensure the six rights of medication administration (Mills and others, 2006; Paoletti and others, 2007; Skibinski and others, 2007).

Application to Nursing Practice
- Actively participate in the selection and evaluation of advanced technologies and the creation of nursing policies and protocols used for medication administration.
- Always follow agency policies when administering medications.
- Implement agency policies when the technology cannot be used (e.g., during down time or power outages).
- Follow manufacturer's guidelines for care of electronic equipment, and report problems with technology immediately.

✳ BOX 35-7 Process for Medication Reconciliation

1. **Verify:** Obtain a current list of the client's medications.
2. **Clarify:** Make sure the list of medications, dosages, and frequencies is accurate; clarify the list with as many people as necessary (e.g., client, caregiver, health care providers, pharmacists) to ensure the list is accurate.
3. **Reconcile:** Compare new medication orders with the current list; investigate any discrepancies with the client's health care provider.
4. **Transmit:** Communicate the updated and verified list to caregivers and the client as appropriate.

Modified from Ptasinski C: Develop a medication reconciliation process, *Nurs Manage* 38(3):18, 2007.

medications during the transfer or discharge process is a National Patient Safety Goal for 2008 (TJC, 2008). Nurses play an essential role in **medication reconciliation** (Box 35-7). Whenever a nurse admits a client to any health care setting, the nurse compares the medications the client took in the previous setting (e.g., home or another nursing unit) with the client's current medication orders (Ptasinski, 2007). Whenever the client leaves that setting for another setting (e.g., skilled care facility or intensive care unit), the nurse communicates the client's current medications with the health care providers in the new setting. The nurse also reconciles the client's medications whenever the client is discharged from the agency. Many agencies have computerized or written forms to facilitate the process of medication reconciliation, an essential part of medication safety. Reconciling medications is challenging and often takes a lot of time and concentration. Eliminate distractions, and go slowly when reconciling clients' medications. Always clarify information when needed. Nurses often consult with the client, caregivers, family members, physicians, advanced practice nurses, pharmacists, and other members of the health care team when reconciling medications.

Critical Thinking

Knowledge

The nurse uses knowledge from many disciplines when administering medications to understand why the physician prescribed a particular medication for a client and how the medication will alter the client's physiology to have a therapeutic effect. For example, in physiology you learn that potassium is a major intracellular ion. When clients do not have enough potassium in their body (hypokalemia), they experience signs and symptoms, such as muscle fatigue or weakness. In some cases, severe hypokalemia is fatal due to associated dysrhythmias. Prescribed medications help to restore the client's potassium level to normal, which then relieves the signs and symptoms of hypokalemia. Knowledge about child development indicates that children often associate medication administration with a negative experience. Use principles from child development to ensure that the child cooperates with the medication experience.

Nurses administer a wide variety of medications, and new medications are constantly approved for dispensation. As a result, nurses do not always have knowledge about the medications they are asked to administer. Critical thinkers admit what they do not know and acquire the knowledge needed to safely administer unfamiliar medications. This means consulting more expert nurses, a pharmacist, the prescriber, or a medication book.

Experience

The nursing student often has limited experience with medication administration as it applies to professional practice. The clinical experience provides the student with the opportunity to use the nursing process as it applies to medication administration. As you gain experience in medication administration, psychomotor skills ("the how-to") become more refined. However, psychomotor skills represent a small part of medication administration. Client attitudes, knowledge, physical and mental status and responses make medication administration a complex experience.

Attitudes

To administer medications safely, many critical thinking skills are essential. For example, discipline is needed to take adequate time to prepare and administer medications. Nurses take the time to read their client's medical record before administering medica-

---

✳ **BOX 35-8   Case Study**

The prescriber enters an order for a medication into a computerized system. The nurse reviews the order and checks for completeness and appropriateness. The nurse questions the order if the order is vague or incomplete, the dose seems unusually low or high, or the medication seems inappropriate for the client's condition. After the nurse reviews the order, it goes to the pharmacy, where either a pharmacist or a pharmacy technician reads the order and prepares the medication. If the technician prepares the medication, the pharmacist checks the technician's work. The pharmacist also verifies that the medication is the appropriate dosage and that there are no medication interactions or medication allergies. When a medication order seems inappropriate, for example, a medication order written for 2000 mg when the proper dosage calls for 200 mg, the pharmacist asks the nurse to clarify the order from the prescriber or the pharmacist calls the prescriber directly for order clarification. When the order is appropriate, the pharmacist sends the medication to the nursing unit. The nurse receives the medication and checks the medication administration record against what the pharmacy has sent and the prescriber ordered. Before administration, the nurse performs the six rights of medication administration. The nurse uses at least two identifiers before giving the client the medication. The nurse allows the client to be the final check by reviewing the name of the medication, the dosage, and why he or she is receiving the medication.

---

tions. Carefully review the client's history, physical examination, and orders; look up medications they do not know in a medication reference book; and determine why each client is taking each of his or her prescribed medications. Every step of safe medication administration requires a disciplined attitude and a comprehensive, systematic approach. Following the same safe procedure each time medications are administered helps ensure safe medication administration.

Responsibility and accountability are other critical thinking attitudes essential to safe medication administration. Accept full accountability and responsibility for all action surrounding the administration of medications (Box 35-8). When administering medications to a client, do not assume that the medication that is ordered for the client is the correct medication or the correct dose. Be responsible for knowing that the medications ordered for clients are the correct medications and the correct doses. You are accountable for administering an ordered medication that is knowingly inappropriate for the client. Therefore be familiar with the therapeutic effect, usual dosage, anticipated changes in laboratory data, and side effects of all medications that are administered. You are also responsible for ensuring that clients who will self-administer medications have been properly informed about all aspects of self-administration. If it is determined that a client cannot safely self-administer medications, design interventions to ensure safe self-administration of medications.

Standards

Standards are those actions that ensure safe nursing practice. Standards for medication administration are set by individual health care agencies and by the nursing profession.

Institutional policy usually places limitations on the nurse's ability to administer medications in certain units of the acute care setting. Sometimes nurses are limited by certain medication routes or dosages. Most institutions have nursing procedure manuals that contain policies that define the types of medications nurses can and cannot administer. The types and dosages of medications nurses deliver often vary from unit to unit within the same facility. For example, Dilantin, a powerful medication for treating seizures, may be administered by mouth or IV push. In large dosages, Dilantin affects the rhythm of the heart. Therefore some institutions place limits on how much Dilantin nurses can give to a client on a nursing unit that does not have the ability to monitor the client's heart rate and rhythm. Not all prescribers are aware of all of the limitations and sometimes prescribe medications that nurses cannot give in a particular health care setting. Nurses need to recognize these limitations and inform the prescriber accordingly. Nurses need to take appropriate actions to ensure that clients receive medications as prescribed and within the time prescribed in the appropriate environment.

Professional standards, such as the American Nurses Association's *Nursing: Scope and Standards of Nursing Practice* (2004) (see Chapters 1 and 23), apply to the activity of medication administration. To prevent medication errors, follow the six rights of medication administration consistently every time you administer medications. Many medication errors can be linked, in some way, to an inconsistency in adhering to the six rights of medication administration. The six rights of medication administration include the following:

1. The right medication
2. The right dose
3. The right client
4. The right route
5. The right time
6. The right documentation

Right Medication. A medication order is required for every medication you administer to a client. Sometimes prescribers write orders by hand in the client's medical record. Alternatively, some agencies use computerized physician order entry (CPOE). CPOE allows the prescriber to electronically enter ordered medications, eliminating the need for written orders. Regardless of how you receive an order, compare the prescriber's written orders with the medication administration record (MAR) when the medication is initially ordered. Verify medication information whenever new MARs are written or distributed or when clients transfer from one nursing unit or health care setting to another (TJC, 2008).

Once you determine that information on the client's MAR is accurate, use the MAR to prepare and administer medications. When preparing medications from bottles or containers, compare the label of the medication container with the MAR three times: (1) before removing the container from the drawer or shelf, (2) as the amount of medication ordered is removed from the container, and (3) before returning the container to storage. Never prepare medications from unmarked containers or containers with illegible labels (TJC, 2008). With unit-dose prepackaged medications, check the label with the MAR when taking medications out of the medication dispensing system. Finally, verify all medications at the client's bedside with the

client's MAR and use at least two identifiers before giving the client any medications (TJC, 2008).

Clients who self-administer medications need to keep them in their original labeled containers, separate from other medications, to avoid confusion. Many hospitals request that all medication administration in the hospital setting be completed through nurses, rather than letting clients self-administer, to ensure that clients are not receiving double doses of medication. Because the nurse who administers the medication is responsible for any errors related to that medication, nurses administer only the medications they prepare. You cannot delegate preparation of medication to another person and then administer the medication to the client. If a client questions the medication, do not ignore these concerns. An alert client will know whether a medication is different from those received before. In most cases the client's medication order has changed; however, some client questions reveal an error. When this occurs, withhold the medication and recheck it against the prescriber's orders. If a client refuses a medication, discard it rather than returning it to the original container. Unit-dose medications can be saved if they are not opened. If a client refuses narcotics, follow proper hospital procedure by having someone else witness the "wasted" medication.

Right Dose. The unit-dose system is designed to minimize errors. When preparing a medication from a larger volume or strength than needed or when the prescriber orders a system of measurement different from what the pharmacy supplies, the chance of error increases. When performing medication calculations or conversions, have another qualified nurse check the calculated doses.

After calculating doses, prepare the medication using standard measurement devices. Use graduated cups, syringes, and scaled droppers to measure medications accurately. At home, have clients use kitchen measuring spoons rather than teaspoons and tablespoons, which vary in volume.

Only break tablets that are scored by the manufacturer. When it is necessary to break a scored tablet, make sure the break is even. Cut a scored tablet in half by using a knife-edge or a cutting device. Discard tablets that do not break evenly. Some agencies allow the nurse to save the unadministered portion of the medication tablet that remains for the next dose if the remaining medication is repackaged and labeled. Verify agency policy before administering a tablet that has been opened, cut, and repackaged. Because pill-splitting is particularly problematic in the home care setting, the Institute for Safe Medication Practices (ISMP) (2006b) has developed suggestions to help with this process. Determine if the client has the motor dexterity or visual acuity to split tablets. If at all possible, prescribers need to avoid ordering medications that will require splitting.

Often tablets are crushed and then mixed with food. Be sure to completely clean a crushing device before crushing the tablet. Remnants of previously crushed medications increase a medication's concentration or result in the client receiving a portion of an unprescribed medication. Mix crushed medications with very small amounts of food or liquid. Do not use the client's favorite foods or liquids because medications alter their taste and decrease the client's desire for them. This is especially a concern for pediatric clients.

SAFETY ALERT Nurses cannot crush all medications. Some medications, such as time-released or extended-release capsules, have special coatings to prevent the medication from being absorbed too quickly. Refer to a medication reference, such as the "Do Not Crush List" published by ISMP (2008), to ensure that the medication is safe to crush.

Right Client. Medication errors often occur because one client gets a drug intended for another client. Therefore an important step in administering medications safely is being sure that you give the medication to the right client. It is difficult to remember every client's name and face. Before giving a medication to a client, use at least two client identifiers whenever administering medications (TJC, 2008). Acceptable client identifiers include the client's name, an identification number assigned by a health care agency, or a telephone number. Do not use the client's room number as an identifier. To identify a client correctly in an acute care setting, compare the client identifiers on the MAR with the client's identification while at the client's bedside (Figure 35-11). If an identification bracelet becomes smudged or illegible or is missing, get a new one for the client. In health care settings that are not acute care settings, TJC (2008) does not require the use of armbands for identification. However, nurses still need to use a system that verifies the client's identification with at least two identifiers before administering medications.

TJC (2008) does not require clients to state their names and other identifiers when administering medications. The required identification process mandates collecting client identifiers reliably when the client is admitted to a health care agency. Once the identifiers are assigned to the client (e.g., putting identifiers on an armband and placing the armband on the client), the nurse uses the identifiers to match the client with the MAR, which lists the correct medications. Asking clients to state their full names and identification information provides a third way to verify that the nurse is giving medications to the right client.

In addition to using two identifiers, some agencies use a wireless bar code scanner to help identify the right client. This system requires the nurse to scan a personal bar code that is commonly placed on the nurse's name tag first. Then the nurse scans a bar code on the single-dose medication package. Finally, the nurse scans the client's armband. All this information is then stored in a computer for documentation purposes. This system helps eliminate medication errors because it provides another step to ensure that the right client receives the right medication.

Right Route. Always consult the prescriber if an order does not designate a route of administration. Likewise, if the specified route is not the recommended route, alert the prescriber immediately. When administering injections, precautions are necessary to ensure that the nurse gives the medications correctly. It is also important to prepare injections only from preparations designed for parenteral use. The injection of a liquid designed for oral use produces local complications, such as a sterile abscess or fatal systemic effects. Medication companies label parenteral medications for "injectable use only."

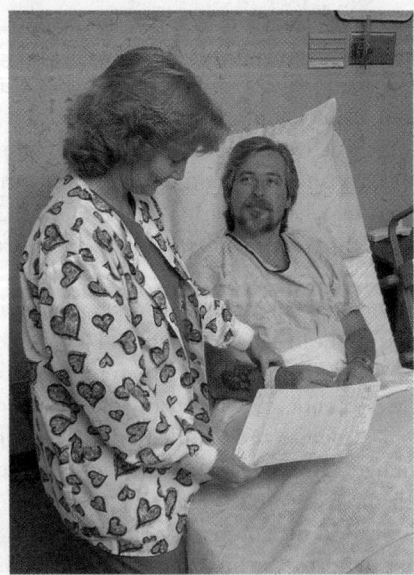

Figure 35-11 Before administering any medications, the nurse checks the client's identification and allergy bracelets. (From deWit S: *Fundamental concepts and skills for nursing*, ed 2, Philadelphia, 2005, Saunders.)

Right Time. Nurse need to know why a medication is ordered for certain times of the day and whether they are able to alter the time schedule. For example, two medications are ordered, one q8h (every 8 hours) and the other 3 times a day. Both medications are scheduled for 3 times within a 24-hour period. The prescriber intends the q8h medication to be given around-the-clock to maintain therapeutic blood levels of the medication. In contrast, the nurse needs to give the 3-times-a-day medication during the waking hours. Each agency has a recommended time schedule for medications ordered at frequent intervals. Nurses can alter these recommended times if necessary or appropriate.

The prescriber often gives specific instructions about when to administer a medication. A preoperative medication to be given "on call" means that the nurse will give the medication when the operating room staff members notify the nurse that they are coming to get the client for surgery. Give a medication ordered pc (after meals) within half an hour after a meal, when the client has a full stomach. Give a STAT medication immediately.

Give priority to medications that must act at certain times For example, nurses need to give insulin at a precise interval before a meal. Give antibiotics on time around the clock to maintain therapeutic blood levels. Give all routinely ordered medications within 60 minutes of the times ordered (30 minutes before or after the prescribed time).

Some medications require the nurse's clinical judgment in determining the proper time for administration. Administer a prn sleeping medication when the client is prepared for bed. Also use judgment when administering prn analgesics. For example, the nurse sometimes needs to obtain a STAT order from the prescriber if the client requires a medication before the prn interval has elapsed. The nurse always documents whenever the nurse calls the client's health care provider to obtain a change in a medication's order.

Before discharge in the hospital setting, evaluate a client's need for home care, especially if the client was admitted to the hospital due to a problem with medication self-administration. Clients often leave the hospital with a basic knowledge of their medications but are unable to retrieve or implement this knowledge once back home. Before clients are discharged from the hospital, evaluate whether the medications are adequate or prescribed at therapeutic levels for the client.

At home some clients have to take several medications throughout the day. Help to plan schedules based on preferred medication intervals, the medication's pharmacokinetics, and the client's daily schedule. For clients who have difficulty remembering when to take medications, make a chart that lists the times when the client will take each medication or prepare a special container to hold each timed dose.

Right Documentation. Nurses and other health care providers use accurate documentation to communicate with each other. Many medication errors result from inaccurate documentation. Therefore ensure that accurate and appropriate documentation exists before and after giving medications. Verify inaccurate documentation before giving medications.

Before administering a medication, ensure that documentation in the MAR clearly reflects the client's full name; the name of the ordered medications written out in full (no medication name abbreviations); the time the medication is to be administered; and the medication's dosage, route, and frequency. Common problems with medication orders include incomplete information, inaccurate dosage form or strength, illegible order or signature, incorrect placement of decimals leading to the wrong dosage, and nonstandard terminology (Hughes and Ortiz, 2005). If there is any question about a medication order due to its being incomplete, illegible, vague, or not understood, contact the prescribing health care provider before administering the medication. The prescribing health care provider is responsible to provide accurate, complete, and understandable medication orders. If the health care provider is unable to do this, each health care organization has a policy on who to contact when proper attention is not being given (usually a "chain of command"). The nurse is responsibile to begin this chain of command to ensure that the client receives the correct medication. The nurse is also responsible for documenting any preassessment data required of certain drugs, such as a blood pressure measurement for antihypertensive medications, or laboratory values, as in the case of Dilantin, before giving the drug.

After administering the medication, indicate which medications were given on the client's MAR per agency policy to verify that the medication was given as ordered. Record medication administration as soon as medications are given to client. Inaccurate documentation of medications, such as failing to document giving a medication or documenting an incorrect dose, leads to errors in subsequent decisions about client care. For example, errors in documentation about insulin often result in negative client outcomes. Consider the following situation: a client receives insulin before breakfast, but the nurse who gave the insulin forgot to document it. The nurse caring for the

client goes home, and the client has a new nurse for the day. The new nurse notices that the insulin is not documented and assumes that the previous nurse did not give the insulin. Therefore the new nurse gives the client another dose of insulin. About 2 hours later, the client experiences a low blood glucose level, which causes the client to have seizures. Accurate documentation would have prevented this situation from happening.

Nurses never document that they have given a medication until they have actually given it. The name of the medication, the dose, the time of administration, and the route all need to be documented on the MAR. Also document the site of any injections and the client's responses to medications, either positive or negative. Notify the client's health care provider of any negative responses to medications, and document the time, date, and name of the health care provider that was notified in the client's medical record. The efforts nurses make in ensuring the right documentation help provide safe care (Box 35-9).

Maintaining Clients' Rights. In accordance with *The Patient Care Partnership* (American Hospital Association, 2003) and because of the potential risks related to medication administration, a client has the following rights:

- To be informed of the medication's name, purpose, action, and potential undesired effects
- To refuse a medication regardless of the consequences
- To have qualified nurses or physicians assess a medication history, including allergies and use of herbals
- To be properly advised of the experimental nature of medication therapy and to give written consent for its use
- To receive labeled medications safely without discomfort in accordance with the six rights of medication administration
- To receive appropriate supportive therapy in relation to medication therapy
- To not receive unnecessary medications
- To be informed if medications are a part of a research study

Be aware of these rights, and handle all inquiries by clients and families courteously and professionally. Do not become defensive if a client refuses medication therapy, recognizing that every person of consenting age has a right to refuse medication. Nurses need to have the necessary knowledge and skill to satisfy the responsibilities of safe and effective medication administration.

✳ BOX 35-9 Nurses' Six Rights for Safe Medication Administration

1. The right to a complete and clearly written order.
2. The right to have the correct drug route and dose dispensed.
3. The right to have access to information.
4. The right to have policies on medication administration.
5. The right to administer medications safely and to identify problems in the system.
6. The right to stop, think, and be vigilant when administering medications.

From Cook MC: Nurses' six rights for safe medication administration, *Massachusetts Nurse* 69(6):8, 1999.

✳ BOX 35-10 NURSING ASSESSMENT QUESTIONS

- What prescription and nonprescription medications do you take, when do you take them, and how do you take them? Do you have a list of medications from your pharmacy or health care provider's office?
- What are your medications for?
- What side effects have you experienced?
- What have you been told to do if a side effect develops?
- Have you ever stopped taking your medications? If so, why did you stop taking them?
- What do you do to help you remember to take your medications?
- Do you have any allergies to medications or foods? If so, describe what happens when you take the medication or eat the food.
- Describe your normal eating patterns. What foods and at what times do you normally eat?
- How do your religious or cultural beliefs influence your beliefs about your medications?
- How do you pay for your medications? Do you sometimes have to stretch your budget to afford your medications or space out your medications to save money?
- What questions do you have about your medications?

The Nursing Process and Medication Administration

 Assessment

To determine the need for and potential response to medication therapy, the nurse assesses many factors. Perform a thorough assessment on all clients to help ensure safe medication administration (Box 35-10).

History. Before administering medications, obtain or review the client's medical history. A client's medical history provides indications or contraindications for medication therapy. Disease or illness places clients at risk for adverse medication effects. For example, if a client has a gastric ulcer, medications containing aspirin will increase the likelihood of bleeding. Long-term health problems (e.g., diabetes or arthritis) require specific medications. This knowledge helps the nurse anticipate the type of medications a client requires. A client's surgical history indicates use of medications. For example, after a thyroidectomy a client requires thyroid hormone replacement.

History of Allergies. Inform the other members of the health care team if the client has a history of allergies to medications and foods. Many medications have ingredients also found in food sources. For example, propofol, which is use for anesthesia and sedation contains egg lecithin and soybean oil as inactive ingredients. Therefore, clients who have an egg or soy allergy should not receive propofol (Weisner and others, 2008). Reference is from: Weisner AM and others: Implications of food allergies and intolerances on medication administration, *Orthopedics* 31(2):149, 2008. In some hospitals, clients wear identification bands listing medication and food allergies. Ensure that all allergies and the client's reactions are noted on the client's admission notes, medication records, and history and physical.

Medication Data. Assess information about each medication that the client takes, including length of time the medication has been taken, the current dosage, and whether or not the client experienced adverse effects from the medication. In addition, review medication data, including action, purpose, normal dosages, routes, side effects, and nursing implications for administration and monitoring. Often you need to consult several resources to gather needed information. Pharmacology textbooks and handbooks; electronic medication manuals available on a desktop, laptop, or handheld computer or automated medication dispensing system (AMDS); nursing journals; the *Physician's Desk Reference* (PDR); medication package inserts; and pharmacists are valuable resources. Nurses are responsible for knowing as much as possible about each medication given.

Diet History. A diet history reveals normal eating patterns and food preferences. The nurse plans the dosage schedule more effectively and teaches the client to avoid foods that interact with medications.

Client's Perceptual or Coordination Problems. For a client with perceptual fine motor or coordination limitations, self-administration is often difficult. For example, a client who takes insulin to manage blood glucose and has arthritis has difficulty manipulating a syringe. The nurse assesses the client's ability to prepare doses and take medications correctly. If the client is unable to self-administer medications, the nurse needs to assess whether family or friends will be available to assist or make a home care referral.

Client's Current Condition. The ongoing physical or mental status of a client affects whether a medication is given or how it is administered. *The nurse needs to assess a client carefully before giving any medication.* For example, check the client's blood pressure before giving an antihypertensive. A client who is nauseated is probably unable to swallow a tablet. Assessment findings also serve as a baseline in evaluating the effects of medication therapy.

Client's Attitude About Medication Use. The client's attitude about medications often reveals a level of medication dependence or drug avoidance. Some clients do not express their feelings about taking a particular medication, particularly if dependence is a problem. Observe the client's behavior for evidence of medication dependence or avoidance. Also be aware that the client's cultural beliefs about Western medicine sometimes interfere with medication compliance (Box 35-11; see Chapter 9).

Client's Knowledge and Understanding of Medication Therapy. The client's knowledge and understanding of medication therapy influence the willingness or ability to follow a medication regimen. Unless a client understands a medication's purpose, the importance of regular dosage schedules, proper administration methods, and the possible side effects, compliance is unlikely. When the client has a history of poor compliance, review resources available for purchase of medications.

Client's Learning Needs. Determine the need for instruction by assessing the client's level of knowledge about a medica-

☀ BOX 35-11   CULTURAL ASPECTS OF CARE

Influences in Medication Administration

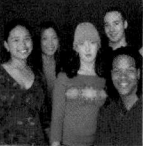

Health beliefs vary by culture and often influence how clients manage and respond to drug therapy. Significant differences in values, beliefs, and attitudes affect a client's adherence to drug therapy. For example, cultures attach different symbolic meanings to medications and drug therapy. Herbal remedies and alternative therapies are common in various cultures and ethnic groups and interfere with prescribed medications. In addition, there is often a marked difference in health beliefs between health providers and clients, which further affects a client's compliance with medical therapy. Demographic changes in both age and race are factors that affect nursing practice in medication administration. In addition to the psychosocial aspect of medication therapy, pharmacological research has shown that different ethnic and racial groups experience differences in drug response, metabolism, and side effects.

Implications for Practice

- Assess cultural beliefs, attitudes, and values when administering and teaching clients about their medications.
- Resolve conflicts between medications and cultural beliefs to achieve optimal client outcomes.
- Investigate if the client practices any alternative therapies or is taking any herbal preparations.
- Consider cultural influences on drug response, metabolism, and side effects if a client is not responding to drug therapy as expected. A change in the client's medication is sometimes necessary.

Data from Andrews MM, Boyle JS: *Transcultural concepts in nursing care*, ed 5, Philadelphia, 2007, Lippincott; and McKenry LM and others: *Mosby's pharmacology in nursing*, ed 22, St. Louis, 2006, Mosby.

tion and the resources available to take medications regularly, (see Chapter 25). It is often necessary to explain the action and purpose of the medication, expected side effects, correct administration techniques, and ways to help the client to remember the medication regimen. If a client has a newly prescribed medication, instruction will need to be more involved. Many states have Medicaid-supported programs for those that do not qualify for Medicare that assist with services similar to home care. In some states, these programs will even purchase many, if not most, medications for consumers who do not qualify for Medicare (Oklahoma Department of Human Services, 2006).

◆ Nursing Diagnosis

Assessment provides data about the client's condition, ability to self-administer medications, and medication use patterns, which determines actual or potential problems with medication therapy. Certain data are defining characteristics, which when clustered together reveal nursing diagnoses. For example, *noncompliance related to a medication regimen* is indicated when a client admits not taking prescribed medications correctly, or by evidence that a medication has not reversed symptoms as expected. The following

is a list of nursing diagnoses that may apply to clients during the administration of medications:

- Anxiety
- Ineffective health maintenance
- Health-seeking behaviors
- Deficient knowledge (medications)
- Noncompliance (medications)
- Disturbed visual sensory perception
- Impaired swallowing
- Effective therapeutic regimen management
- Ineffective therapeutic regimen management

After selecting the diagnosis, identify the related factor, which drives the selection of nursing interventions. For example, the related factors of inadequate resources versus lack of knowledge require different interventions. If the client's noncompliance is related to inadequate finances, collaborate with family members, social workers, or community agencies to help a client receive necessary medications. If the related factor is lack of knowledge, the hospital nurse will often make referrals to ensure that home care nurses follow up with the client and implement an extensive teaching plan.

◆ Planning

Always organize your care activities to ensure the safe administration of medications. Hurrying to give clients medications leads to errors. It is important to minimize distractions or interruptions when preparing and administering medications (Pape and others, 2005).

Goals and Outcomes.   Setting goals and related outcomes will help plan to use time wisely during medication administration. For example, the nurse establishes the following goal and related outcomes for a client with newly diagnosed type 2 diabetes:

Goal: The client will safely administer all ordered medications before discharge.
Outcomes:
- The client will verbalize understanding of desired effects and adverse effects of medications.
- The client will state signs, symptoms, and treatment of hypoglycemia.
- The client will be able to monitor blood glucose level to determine if medication is appropriate to take or if a low blood glucose level should be treated.
- The client will establish a daily routine that will coordinate timing of medication with mealtimes.

Setting Priorities.   Prioritize care when administering medications. Use information gathered from the client's assessment in determining which medications to give first and if it is appropriate to administer prn medications. For example, if a client is in pain, it is important to provide pain medication as soon as possible. If the client is experiencing an elevated blood pressure, administer the blood pressure medications before other medications. Nurses also prioritize when providing client education about medications. Provide the most important information about the medications first. For example, hypoglycemia is a serious side effect of insulin. The client taking insulin needs to be able to identify and treat hypoglycemia immediately, so the nurse first teaches the client about the recognition and treatment of hypoglycemia before teaching about how to administer the injection.

Collaborative Care. Collaborate with a variety of health care providers when administering medications. First, it is important to collaborate with the client's family or friends whenever possible. Family members will often reinforce the importance of medication regimens in the home setting. Nurses often collaborate with the prescriber, the pharmacist, and case managers to ensure that clients receive medications safely and that clients are able to afford their medications. Upon discharge, ensure that clients know where and how to obtain medications. Be sure that clients are able to read medication labels and printed medication teaching sheets. Some clients also need to understand how to calculate dosages and prepare complex medication regimens. Collaborate with community resources (e.g., agency on aging, public health department, medical interpreters) when clients are illiterate or have difficulty understanding medication instructions (see Chapter 25).

◆ Implementation

Health Promotion. The nurse, in promoting or maintaining the client's health, identifies factors that improve or diminish well-being. Health beliefs, personal motivations, socioeconomic factors, and habits (e.g., excessive alcohol intake) influence the client's compliance with the medication regimen. Several nursing interventions promote adherence to the medication regimen and foster independence. Teach the client and family about the benefit of a medication and the knowledge needed to take it correctly, and integrate the client's health beliefs and cultural practices into the treatment plan. Assist the client and family with establishing a medication routine that fits into the client's normal schedule. Make referrals to community resources if the client is unable to afford or cannot arrange transportation to obtain necessary medications.

Client and Family Teaching. Unless a client is properly informed about medications, he or she may take the medications incorrectly or not at all. Follow principles of client education (see Chapter 25). Provide information about the purpose of medications and their actions and effects that clients can understand. Many health care institutions offer easy-to-read leaflets on specific types of medications. Clients need to know how to take medications properly and the risks associated with failing to do so. For example, after receiving a prescription for an antibiotic, a client needs to understand the importance of taking the full prescription. Failure to do this can lead to a worsening of the condition and the development of bacteria resistant to the medication.

Nurses teach clients how to correctly administer all their medications. For example, teach a client how to accurately measure a liquid medication. Provide special education to clients who depend on daily injections (Box 35-12). The client learns to prepare and administer an injection correctly using aseptic technique.

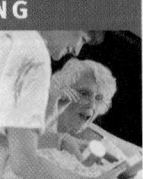

BOX 35-12 **CLIENT TEACHING**

Safe Insulin Administration

Objective
- Client will correctly administer subcutaneous insulin

Teaching Strategies
- Teach client how to determine that insulin is not out of date.
- Instruct client to keep medication in its original labeled container.
- Instruct client to keep insulin refrigerated if needed.
- Assess client's visual acuity to ensure client is able to draw up the appropriate amount of insulin, and talk client through the steps of administering subcutaneous insulin injection as the client is administering the injection.
- Demonstrate how to rotate insulin injection sites.
- Help client determine the amount of insulin required based on the results of home capillary glucose monitoring as ordered by the health care provider.
- Demonstrate how to prepare a single insulin preparation.
- Show client how to keep a daily logbook for insulin injections, including results of home capillary glucose monitoring, type and amount of insulin given, expiration date on insulin vial, time of insulin injection, and injection site used.

Evaluation
- Ask client to describe procedure used at home for determining the correct dose of insulin needed and injection site.
- Watch client prepare insulin dose based on results of capillary glucose monitoring, select injection site, and self-administer injection.
- Review information recorded in client logbook for completeness.
- If client is unable to prepare the correct amount of insulin or self-administer safely, notify the health care provider.

Teach family members or friends how to give injections in case the client becomes ill or physically unable to handle a syringe. Provide specially designed equipment such as syringes with enlarged calibrated scales or medications with labels in Braille when clients have visual alterations.

Clients need to be aware of the symptoms of medication side effects or toxicity. For example, clients taking anticoagulants learn to notify their primary care providers immediately when signs of bleeding or bruising develop. Inform family members or friends of medication side effects such as changes in behavior because they are often the first persons to recognize such effects. Clients are better able to cope with problems caused by medications if they understand how and when to act. All clients need to learn the basic guidelines for medication safety. These guidelines ensure the proper use and storage of medications in the home.

Acute Care. Clients are often hospitalized to receive expert nursing observation and documentation of responses to medications. When a nurse receives a medication order, several nursing interventions are essential for safe and effective medication administration.

※ **BOX 35-13 Components of Medication Orders**

A medication order is incomplete unless it has the following parts:

- **Client's full name:** The client's full name distinguishes the client from other persons with the same last name. In the acute care setting, clients are sometimes assigned special identification numbers (e.g., medical record number) to help distinguish clients with the same names. This number is often included on the order form.
- **Date and time that the order is written:** The day, month, year, and time need to be included. Designating the time that an order is written helps clarify when certain orders are to stop automatically. If an incident occurs involving a medication error, it is easier to document what happened when this information is available.
- **Medication name:** The prescriber orders a medication by its generic or trade name. Correct spelling is essential in preventing confusion with medications with similar spelling.
- **Dose:** The amount or strength of the medication is included.
- **Route of administration:** The prescriber uses accepted abbreviations for medication routes. Accuracy is important because some clients receive medications by more than one route.
- **Time and frequency of administration:** The nurse needs to know when to initiate medication therapy. Orders for multiple doses establish a routine schedule for medication administration.
- **Signature of physician, nurse practitioner, or physician assistant:** Signature makes the order a legal request.

Receiving Medication Orders. A medication order is required for a nurse to administer any medication. Before any other interventions, ensure that the medication order contains all of the elements in Box 35-13. If the medication order is incomplete, inform the prescriber and ensure completeness before carrying out any medication order. The prescriber gives some medication orders verbally or by telephone to the nurse. A verbal order is a medication or treatment order received by the registered nurse in the presence of the prescriber. Telephone orders are medication or treatment orders given to the nurse by the prescriber over the phone, generally after the nurse updates the prescriber about a change in the client's condition. Current National Patient Safety Goals require nurses to "read-back" verbal or telephone orders to the prescriber to ensure the correct order is obtained (TJC, 2008). The registered nurse follows institutional policy regarding the receiving, recording, and transcription of verbal and telephone orders. Generally the prescriber must sign verbal and telephone orders within 24 hours. *Nursing students are prohibited from receiving verbal and telephone orders.*

Correct Transcription and Communication of Orders. Sometimes the nurse or a designated unit secretary writes the prescriber's complete order on the appropriate medication form (e.g., the MAR) or enters the order into the client's electronic medical record. Other institutions have computerized prescribed order entry. In these systems, the prescriber enters the order directly into the computer. Computerized systems automatically transfer medication information to the MAR, the pharmacy record, and the automated dispensing system. Whether it is hand-written, printed out from a computer (Figure 35-12), or in an electronic version, the MAR includes the client's name, room, and bed number, medical record number, medical and food allergies, and other client identifiers (e.g., birth date); and medication name, dose, frequency, and route and time of administration. Each time a medication dose is prepared, the nurse refers to the MAR. The opportunity for error is reduced as the required number of transcriptions is reduced. When writing orders, be sure that medication names, dosages, and symbols are legible. Rewrite any unclear or illegible transcriptions.

A registered nurse compares the list of medications on the MAR against the original orders for accuracy and thoroughness. If an order seems incorrect or inappropriate, the nurse consults the prescriber. The nurse who gives the wrong medication or an incorrect dose assumes legally responsibility for the error. Other health care providers involved in the error are also legally responsible.

Accurate Dose Calculation and Measurement. When measuring liquid medications, use standard measuring containers. When splitting tablets, ensure the medication was scored by the manufacturer and split evenly before administering the tablet. The procedure for medication measurement is systematic to lessen the chance of error. Calculate each dose when preparing the medication, pay close attention to the process of calculation, and avoid interruptions from other people or nursing activities (Pape and others, 2005). Nurses consult with other nurses when they calculate a new or unusual dose.

Correct Administration. For safe administration, use aseptic technique and proper procedures when handling and giving medications. Verify the client's identity by using at least two client identifiers (TJC, 2008), and perform necessary assessments (e.g., assess heart rate before giving antidysrhythmic medications) before administering a medication to a client. Carefully monitor the client's response to the medication, especially when a client receives the first dose of a new medication.

Recording Medication Administration. After administering a medication, record it immediately on the appropriate record form (see Figure 35-12). **Never** chart a medication before administering it. Recording immediately after administration prevents errors. The recording of a medication includes the name of the medication, dose, route, and exact time of administration. Record the site of any injections per agency policy.

If a client refuses a medication or is undergoing tests or procedures that result in a missed dose, explain the reason the medication was not given in the nurses' notes. Some agencies require the nurse to circle the prescribed administration time on the medication record or to notify the physician when a client misses a dose. Be aware of the effects missing doses have on a client such as in hypertension or diabetes. Coordinating care with other services when testing or procedures are being completed helps ensure therapeutic control of the disease.

Restorative Care. Because of the numerous types of restorative care settings, medication administration activities vary. Clients with functional limitations often require the nurse to fully administer all medications. In the home care setting, clients usually administer their own medications. Regardless of the type of medication activity, the nurse remains responsible for instructing clients and families in medication action, administration, and side

Room: 3700-03

Saint Francis Medical Center

MEDICATION ADMINISTRATION RECORD

Patient: PDM, Pharmacy
Birth: 11/30/79   Admit: 01/01/XX
MRN: 2000403   Acct: 900015
A Doctor: Jim Smith

Age: 20 y   Ht: 5 ft 2 in   Wt: 125.2 lbs
Metric: Ht: 1 m 57 cm   Wt: 56.79 kg

Date: 01/18/XX – 01/19/XX

ADEs/Nondrug allergies: Latex – Zosyn – Amoxicillin – Insulins – Darvocet – Lugols soln. – Antihi +

Medication	0800	0900	1000	1100	1200	1300	1400	1500	1600	1700	1800	1900	2000	2100	2200	2300	2400	0100	0200	0300	0400	0500	0600	0700
P00014 Bacitracin ointment — AKA: Bacitracin ointment — Dose: Apply — STRGH: 30 gm/tube — TID — Topical: Right lower leg — For external use only — Testing			RL 10																					
P00029 Insulin/human regular — AKA: Humulin R Dose: 15 units — Strgh: 1 ml = 100 units AC Sub-Q	RL 0730																							
P00030 Fexofenadine 60 mg/psuedo 120 mg — AKA: Allegra–D Sr Tab — Dose: 1 tab STRGH: 60/120/tab — BID Oral — Auto Sub: 1 Allegra–D Tab bid — For Claritin–D 12 hr and 24 hr — Per P&T Comm			RL 10																					
P00036 Aspirin — AKA: Aspirin 325 mg Tab — Dose: 2 tab 650 mg STRGH: 325 mg/tab — Q3–4h Oral — Testing						RL 1315																		
P00039 Haloperidol tablet — AKA: Haldol 0.5 mg tab — Dose: 1 mg STRGH: 1 mg/tab — QHS Oral																								
P00035 Zolpidem — AKA: Ambien 5 mg tab — Dose: 5 mg STRGH: 5/tab — QHS PRN Oral — MR × 1 — Testing																								

Circle = Dose not given
Initials = Dose given   Page: 01 (continued)
Deltoid = R.D., L.D.
Vastus Lateralis = R.V.L., L.V.L.
Lower Abdominal = R.L.A., L.L.A.
Anterior Gluteal = R.A.G., L.A.G.
Posterior Gluteal = R.P.G., L.P.G.

Initials and signature	Initials and signature	Initials and signature
Rita Lassater RL		
Initials and signature	Initials and signature	Initials and signature
Initials and signature	Initials and signature	Initials and signature

Figure 35-12 Example of medication administration record (MAR). (Courtesy OSF Saint Francis Medical Center, Peoria, Ill.)

✳ BOX 35-14 Tips for Administering Medications to Children

Oral Medications

- Liquid forms are safer to swallow to avoid aspiration.
- Use droppers for administering liquids to infants; straws often help older children swallow pills.
- Offer juice, a soft drink, or a frozen juice bar after the child swallows a medication.
- Carbonated beverages poured over finely crushed ice reduce nausea.
- When mixing medications in other foods, use only a small amount. The child may refuse to take all of a larger mixture.
- Avoid mixing a medication with foods or liquids that the child is taking well because the child may in turn refuse them.
- A plastic, disposable syringe is the most accurate device for preparing liquid doses, especially those less than 10 mL. (Cups, teaspoons, and droppers are inaccurate.)
- When administering liquid medications, a spoon, plastic cup, or oral syringe (without needle) is useful.

Injections

- Use caution when selecting intramuscular (IM) injection sites for infants and small children. The deltoid muscle, which can be used for adults and older children, is underdeveloped in infants and small children and should not be used for them.
- Children are sometimes unpredictable and uncooperative. Make sure someone (preferably another nurse) is available to restrain a child if needed. Have the parent act as a comforter, not restrainer, if restraint is necessary.
- Always awaken a sleeping child before giving an injection.
- Distracting the child with conversation, bubbles, or a toy reduces pain perception.
- Give the injection quickly, and do not fight with the child.
- If time allows, use a eutectic mixture of local anesthetics (EMLA) cream.

✳ BOX 35-15 FOCUS ON OLDER ADULTS

- Simplify the drug therapy plan whenever possible (McKenry and others, 2006).
- Keep instructions clear and simple, and provide written material in large print (Ebersole and others, 2004).
- Assess functional status to determine if client will require assistance in taking medications (McKenry and others, 2006).
- Have client drink a little fluid *before* taking oral medications to ease swallowing, and encourage the client to drink at least 5 to 6 ounces of fluid after taking medications (Ebersole and others, 2004).
- Some older adults have a greater sensitivity to drugs, especially those that act on the central nervous system. Therefore carefully monitor clients' responses to medications, and anticipate dosage adjustments as needed (Meiner and Lueckenotte, 2006).
- If the client has difficulty swallowing a capsule or tablet:
  - Ask the physician to substitute a liquid medication if possible (Ebersole and others, 2004).
  - Have the client sit up straight and tuck the chin to decrease risk of aspiration (McKenry and others, 2006).
- Teach alternatives to medications, such as proper diet instead of vitamins and exercise instead of laxatives (Ebersole and others, 2004).
- Review medication history, including over-the-counter medications, on a frequent basis (Meiner and Lueckenotte, 2006).

---

effects. The nurse is also responsible for monitoring compliance with medication and determining the effectiveness of medications that have been prescribed.

Special Considerations for Administering Medications to Specific Age-Groups.

A client's developmental level is a factor for nurses to consider when administering medications. Knowledge of a client's developmental needs helps the nurse to anticipate responses to medication therapy.

Infants and Children. Children vary in age, weight, surface area, and the ability to absorb, metabolize, and excrete medications. Children's medication doses are lower than those of adults, so special caution is necessary when preparing medications for them. Medications are usually not prepared and packaged in standardized dose ranges for children. Preparing an ordered dose from an available amount requires careful calculation (see pp. 697 to 698).

All children require special psychological preparation before receiving medications. The child's parents are often valuable resources for determining the best way to give the child medication. Sometimes it is less traumatic for the child if a parent gives the medication and the nurse supervises. Supportive care is necessary

if a child is expected to cooperate. Explain the procedure to a child, using short words and simple language appropriate to the child's level of comprehension. Long explanations increase a child's anxiety, especially for painful procedures such as an injection. Nurses need to give medications to children even when they refuse to cooperate or resist consistently despite explanation and encouragement. If this occurs, give the medication to the child quickly and carefully (Hockenberry and Wilson, 2007). Involving the child in choices when possible usually results in greater success. For example, saying "It's time to take your tablet now. Do you want it with water or juice?" allows a child to make a choice. Do not give the child the option of not taking a medication. After giving a medication, praise the child and even offer a simple reward such as a star or token. Tips for administering medication to children are in Box 35-14.

Older Adults. Older adults also require special consideration during medication administration (Box 35-15). In addition to physiological changes of aging (Figure 35-13), behavioral and economic factors influence an older person's use of medications.

Polypharmacy. **Polypharmacy** happens when the client takes two or more medications to treat the same illness, when a client takes two or more medications from the same chemical class, when the client uses two or more medications with the same or similar actions to treat several disorders simultaneously, or when a client mixes nutritional supplements or herbal products with medications (Brager and Sloand, 2005; Ebersole and others,

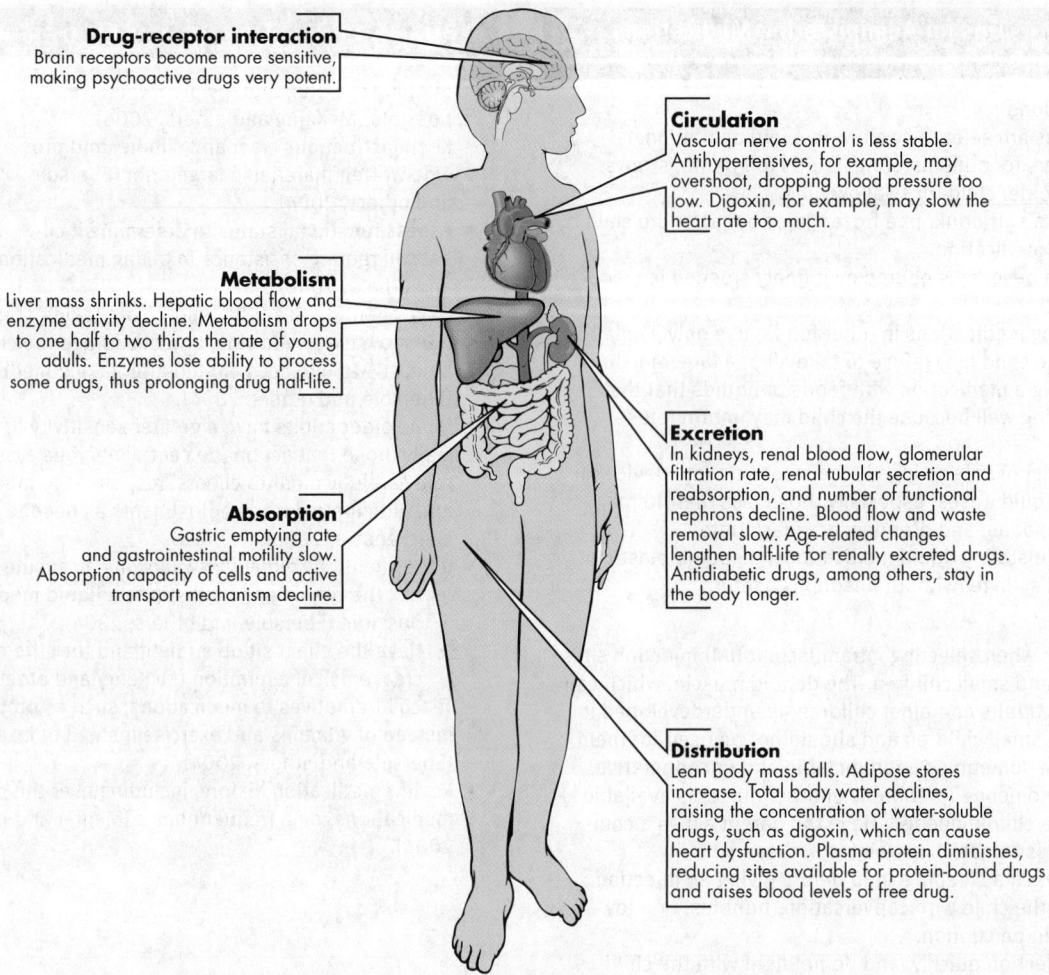

Drug-receptor interaction
Brain receptors become more sensitive, making psychoactive drugs very potent.

Circulation
Vascular nerve control is less stable. Antihypertensives, for example, may overshoot, dropping blood pressure too low. Digoxin, for example, may slow the heart rate too much.

Metabolism
Liver mass shrinks. Hepatic blood flow and enzyme activity decline. Metabolism drops to one half to two thirds the rate of young adults. Enzymes lose ability to process some drugs, thus prolonging drug half-life.

Excretion
In kidneys, renal blood flow, glomerular filtration rate, renal tubular secretion and reabsorption, and number of functional nephrons decline. Blood flow and waste removal slow. Age-related changes lengthen half-life for renally excreted drugs. Antidiabetic drugs, among others, stay in the body longer.

Absorption
Gastric emptying rate and gastrointestinal motility slow. Absorption capacity of cells and active transport mechanism decline.

Distribution
Lean body mass falls. Adipose stores increase. Total body water declines, raising the concentration of water-soluble drugs, such as digoxin, which can cause heart dysfunction. Plasma protein diminishes, reducing sites available for protein-bound drugs and raises blood levels of free drug.

Figure 35-13 Aging body and drug use. (From Lewis SM and others: *Medical-surgical nursing*, ed 6, St. Louis, 2004, Mosby.)

2004). Older adults also often experience polypharmacy when they seek relief from a variety of symptoms (e.g., pain, constipation, insomnia, and indigestion) by using over-the-counter (OTC) preparations.

Because many older adults suffer chronic health problems, polypharmacy is common in older adults. However, it is also becoming more common in children. When the client experiences polypharmacy, there is an increased risk of adverse reactions and medication interactions with other medications and food.

There are two types of polypharmacy. Rational polypharmacy happens when clients need to take several medications to treat their illnesses. This often happens in older adults. For example, many older adults take multiple medications to lower their blood pressure. Irrational polypharmacy happens when the client takes more medications than needed. There are several causes for irrational polypharmacy. Sometimes older adults have to see more than one health care provider to treat their different illnesses. When an accurate medication history is not taken and when health care providers do not communicate with each other, clients end up taking many different medications, increasing the risk of polypharmacy (Brager and Sloand, 2005).

◆Evaluation

The nurse monitors a client's response to medications on an ongoing basis. This requires knowledge of the desired effect and common side effects of each medication. A change in a client's condition is often physiologically related to health status or results from medications or both. Be alert for reactions in a client taking several medications. The goal of safe and effective medication administration involves the client's response to therapy and ability to assume responsibility for self-care.

To evaluate the effectiveness of nursing interventions when meeting established goals of care, use evaluative measures to identify if client outcomes were met. Nurses use many different evaluation measures in the context of medication administration: direct observation of behavior or response, rating scales and checklists, and oral questioning. The type of measurement used varies with the action being evaluated, the reading skill and knowledge level of the client, and the client's cognitive and psychomotor ability. The most common type of measurement that the nurse uses is a physiological measure. Examples of physiologi-

✳ TABLE 35-9 Example Evaluation for Client Goals

Goal	Expected Outcomes	Evaluative Measure With Example
Client and family understand medication therapy.	Client and family describe information about medication, dosage, schedule, purpose, and adverse effects.	Written measurement: Have client write out medication schedule for a 24-hour period. Oral questioning: Ask client to describe purpose, dosage, and adverse effects of each prescribed medication.
	Client and family identify situations that require medical intervention.	Oral questioning: Have family describe what to do when a client has adverse effects from a medication.
	Client and family demonstrate appropriate administration technique.	Direct observation: Have client demonstrate filling of an insulin syringe and self-injection.
Client safely self-administers medications.	Client follows prescribed treatment regimen.	Anecdotal notes: Have family keep log of client's adherence to therapy for 1 week.
	Client performs administration techniques correctly.	Direct observation: Observe client instill eye drops.
	Client identifies available resources for obtaining necessary medication.	Oral questioning: Ask family to identify how to contact local pharmacy or community clinic for necessary medications.

cal measures are blood pressure, heart rate, and visual acuity. Nurses also use client statements as evaluative measures. Table 35-9 contains examples of goals, expected outcomes, and corresponding evaluative measures.

Medication Administration

Medication administration is an essential part of nursing practice, which requires a sound knowledge base in order for medications to be administered safely. Nurses need to be prepared to administer medications using a variety of routes. The following sections will explain the steps involved in administering medications using various routes.

Oral Administration

The easiest and most desirable way to administer medications is by mouth (Skill 35-1). Clients usually are able to ingest or self-administer oral medications with a minimum of problems. Most tablets and capsules need to be swallowed and administered with approximately 60 to 100 mL of fluid (as allowed). There are, however, some situations that contraindicate the client's receiving medications by mouth. The primary contraindications for giving oral medications include the presence of GI alterations, the inability of a client to swallow food or fluids, and the use of gastric suction.

An important precaution to take when administering any oral preparation is to protect clients from aspiration. Aspiration occurs when food, fluid, or medication intended for gastrointestinal administration inadvertently enters the respiratory tract. The nurse protects the client from aspiration by assessing the client's ability to manage oral medications. Box 35-16 provides techniques that protect the client from aspirating. Properly positioning the client is essential in preventing aspiration. The nurse positions the client in a seated position at a 90-degree angle when administering oral

✳ BOX 35-16 Protecting the Client From Aspiration

- Determine the client's ability to swallow.
- Assess the client's cough.
- Determine the presence of a gag reflex.
- Prepare oral medications in the form that is easiest to swallow.
- Allow the client to self-administer medications if possible.
- If the client has unilateral weakness, place the medication in the stronger side of the mouth.
- Administer pills one at a time, ensuring that each medication is properly swallowed before the next one is introduced.
- Thicken regular liquids or offer fruit nectars if the client cannot tolerate thin liquids.
- Avoid straws because they decrease the control the client has over volume intake, which increases the risk of aspiration.
- Have client hold and drink from cup if possible.
- Time medications to coincide with mealtimes or when the client is well rested and awake if possible.
- Administer medications using another route if risk of aspiration is severe.

medications, if not contraindicated by a client's condition. Usually having the client slightly flex the head in a chin-down position reduces aspiration (Metheny, 2006). Use a multidisciplinary approach (e.g., speech therapist, dietitian, and occupational therapist) with clients who have difficulty swallowing (Morris, 2006). For clients with nasogastric feeding tubes, liquid medications are preferred, but nurses can crush some tablets and open some capsules to mix in a solution for administration (Box 35-17).

Topical Medication Applications

Topical medications are medications that are applied locally, most often to intact skin. They come in many forms (see Table 35-2, p. 690). They are also applied to mucous membranes.

✳ BOX 35-17

PROCEDURAL GUIDELINES

Giving Medications Through a Nasogastric Tube, Intestinal Tube, Gastrostomy Tube, or Small-Bore Feeding Tube

Delegation Considerations: The skill of giving medications through a nasogastric tube, intestinal tube, gastrostomy tube, or small-bore feeding tube cannot be delegated. The nurse instructs nursing assistive personnel in the need to report the occurrence of side effects.

Equipment: 60-mL syringe (catheter tip for large-bore tubes, Luer-Lok tip for small-bore tubes), gastric pH test strips (scale of 0.0 to 11.0 or 14.0 preferred), graduated container, water, medication to be administered, pill crusher if medication in tablet form, MAR, clean gloves.

1. Check accuracy and completeness of each medication administration record (MAR) with prescriber's written medication order. Check client's name, drug name and dosage, and route and time of administration.
2. Investigate and use alternative routes of medication administration if possible (e.g., intravenous, transdermal, rectal).
3. Avoid complicated medication regimens that frequently interrupt enteral feedings.
4. Prepare medication (see Skill 35-1, Step 7). Check label of medication with MAR three times.
5. Avoid giving elixirs or medications with a pH of less than 4.
6. Verify that the medication is compatible with the enteral feeding before administration. If the medication is incompatible with the feeding, stop the feeding 1 to 2 hours before giving medication, and restart the feeding 1 to 2 hours after the medication is given. Never add medications directly to the tube feeding.
7. Administer medications in a liquid form (suspension, elixir, or solution) when possible to prevent tube obstruction.
8. Before crushing tablets, be sure they are crushable. Buccal, sublingual, enteric-coated, or sustained-release medications cannot be crushed. Read medication labels carefully before crushing a tablet or opening a capsule.
9. Take medications to client at correct time, and perform hand hygiene.
10. Identify client by using at least two client identifiers. Compare client's name and one other identifier (e.g., hospital identification number) on identification bracelet with MAR. Ask client to state name if possible for a third identifier.
11. Compare label of medications against MAR one more time at client's bedside.
12. Explain procedure and medications to client.
13. Dissolve crushed tablets, gelatin capsules, and powders in 15 to 30 mL of warm water. Dissolve each medication separately.
14. Do not give whole or undissolved medications through the feeding tube.
15. Put on clean gloves.
16. Verify placement of any feeding tube that enters the mouth or nose using pH testing (see Chapter 44).
17. Assess gastric residual (see Chapter 44).
18. Draw up medication in syringe. Do not mix medications together.
19. Connect syringe with medication to nasogastric tube, G-tube, J-tube, or small-bore feeding tube. Do not use pigtail vent for irrigation or instillation of fluid.
20. Administer medication by either pushing the medication through the tube with the syringe or by allowing medication to flow into body freely by using gravity. Administer each medication separately.
21. Flush tube with 15 to 30 mL of warm water between each medication. Unless contraindicated, the total amount of liquid volume administered to the client is approximately 60 mL.
22. After giving all the medications, flush tube once more with 30 to 60 mL of warm water.
23. Clean area, and put supplies away.
24. Remove gloves, and perform hand hygiene.
25. Document administration of medications on MAR.
26. Continue to evaluate the client's response to medication therapy. If the desired effect is not achieved, a different medication or route of administration is probably indicated because of problems with the drug bioavailability when given the enteral route.

Modified from Jordan S and others: Administration of medicines. II. Pharmacology, *Nurs Stand* 18(3):45, 2003.

Skin Applications. Because many locally applied medications such as lotions, pastes, and ointments create systemic and local effects, apply these medications using gloves and applicators. Use sterile technique if the client has an open wound. Skin encrustation and dead tissues harbor microorganisms and block contact of medications with the tissues to be treated. Before applying medications, clean the skin thoroughly by washing the area gently with soap and water, soaking an involved site, or locally debriding tissue.

Apply each type of medication according to directions to ensure proper penetration and absorption. When applying ointments or pastes, spread the medication evenly over the involved surface and cover the area well without applying an overly thick layer. Prescribers sometimes order a gauze dressing to be applied over the medication to prevent soiling of clothes and wiping away of the medication. Lightly spread lotions and creams onto the skin's surface; rubbing often causes irritation. Apply a liniment by rubbing it gently but firmly into the skin. Dust a powder lightly to cover the affected area with a thin layer.

Some topical medications are applied in the form of a transdermal patch that remains in place for an extended amount of time (e.g., 12 hours or 7 days). Many patches are clear, which makes them difficult to see. Nurses and clients have inadvertently left old transdermal patches in place, resulting in the client receiving an overdose of the medication. Therefore carefully assess the client's skin, and be sure to remove the existing patch

Text continued on p. 723

✳ SKILL 35-1   **ADMINISTERING ORAL MEDICATIONS**

Delegation Considerations

The skill of administering medications cannot be delegated. The nurse instructs nursing assistive personnel to report potential side effects of medications to the nurse.

Equipment

- Disposable medication cups
- Glass of water, juice, or preferred liquid
- Drinking straw
- Pill-crushing or pillating device (optional)
- MAR or computer printout

STEPS	RATIONALE
1. Check accuracy and completeness of each MAR or computer printout with prescriber's original medication order. Check client's name and medication name, dosage, and route and time for administration. Recopy or re-print any portion of MAR that is difficult to read.	The order sheet is the most reliable source and only legal record of medications client is to receive. Ensures client receives the correct medications. Illegible MARs are a source of medication errors.
2. Assess for any contraindications to client receiving oral medication: Is client suffering from nausea/vomiting? Is client diagnosed with bowel inflammation or reduced peristalsis? Has client had recent GI surgery? Does client have gastric suction? Check the client's swallow, cough, and gag reflexes.	Alterations in GI function interfere with medication distribution, absorption, and excretion. Clients with GI suction do not receive benefit from oral medications because they are suctioned from the GI tract before they can be absorbed. Clients with impaired swallowing are at a risk of aspiration (Metheny, 2006).
3. Assess client's medical history, history of allergies, medication history, and diet history. List client's food and drug allergies on *each* page of the MAR, and prominently display it on the client's medical record per agency policy.	Information reflects client's need for and potential responses to medications. Information also indicates potential food and drug interactions. Communication of allergies is essential for safe, effective care.
4. Gather physical examination and laboratory data that influence medication administration (e.g., vital signs, renal and liver function laboratory findings).	Physical examination or laboratory data sometimes contraindicate medication administration. Poor liver and kidney function affects metabolism and excretion of medications (McKenry and others, 2006).

Critical Decision Point: If there are any contraindications to the client receiving oral medications, or if in doubt of the client's ability to swallow oral medications, temporarily withhold medication and inform prescriber.

5. Assess client's knowledge regarding health and medication use.	Determines client's need for medication education. Also assists in identifying client's adherence to medication therapy at home. Assessment often reveals medication use problems such as medication tolerance, noncompliance, abuse, addiction, or dependence.
6. Assess client's preferences for fluids. Maintain fluid restrictions when applicable. Determine if medication can be given with preferred fluid.	Fluids ease swallowing and facilitate absorption from the GI tract. It is necessary to maintain fluid restrictions. Some fluids interfere with absorption of medications.
7. Prepare medications:	
a. Perform hand hygiene.	Reduces transfer of microorganisms.
b. If using a medication cart, move it outside client's room.	Organization of equipment saves time and reduces error.
c. Unlock medicine drawer or cart, or log onto computerized medication dispensing system.	Medications are safeguarded when locked in cabinet, cart, or computerized medication dispensing system.
d. Prepare medication for one client at a time. Keep all pages of MARs or computer printouts for one client together, or look at only one client's medication administration computer screen.	Preventing distractions limits preparation errors (Pape and others, 2005).
e. Select correct medication from stock supply or unit-dose drawer. Compare label of medication with MAR, computer printout (see illustration), or computer screen. Check expiration date on all medication labels.	Reading labels and comparing them with the transcribed order reduces error. *This is the first accuracy check.*
f. Calculate medication dose as necessary. Double-check calculation. If needed, have another nurse verify calculations.	Double-checking reduces risk of error.
g. If preparing a controlled substance, check record for previous medication count and compare current count with supply available.	Controlled substance laws require nurses to carefully monitor and count dispensed narcotics.

Continued

✳ **SKILL 35-1**   **ADMINISTERING ORAL MEDICATIONS—CONT'D**

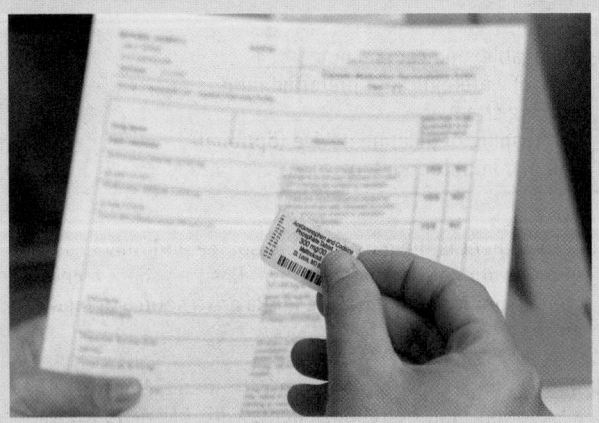

STEP 7e The nurse verifies each medication with the MAR.

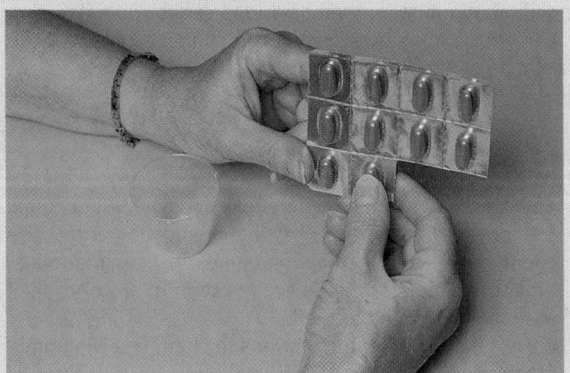

STEP 7i Place tablet into medicine cup without removing wrapper.

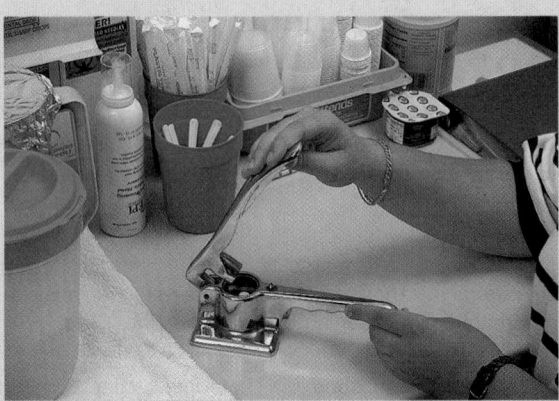

STEP 7k Pill-crushing device used to crush pills when necessary.

STEPS	RATIONALE
h. To prepare tablets or capsules from a floor stock bottle, pour required number into bottle cap and transfer medication to medication cup. Do not touch medication with fingers. Return extra tablets or capsules to bottle. Break prescored medications if needed by using a gloved hand or a clean pillating device. Identify prescored tablets by a line placed on the pill by the manufacturer that spans the center of the tablet.	Maintains clean technique required of medication administration. Cleaning the pillating (or pill-cutting) device ensures prior medications are cleaned out of device and cannot contaminate this tablet. Only split tablets that are prescored to ensure that you give accurate dose to client.
i. To prepare unit-dose tablets or capsules, place packaged tablet or capsule directly into medicine cup. Do not remove wrapper (see illustration).	Wrapper maintains cleanliness of medications and allows nurse to identify medication name and dose at client's bedside.
j. Place all tablets or capsules for client in one medicine cup, except for those requiring preadministration assessments (e.g., pulse rate or blood pressure); keep medications in their wrappers.	Keeping medications that require preadministration assessments separate from others makes it easier for the nurse to withhold medications as necessary.
k. If the client has difficulty swallowing and liquid medications are not an option, use pill-crushing device such as a mortar and pestle to grind pills (see illustration). Before using a mortar and pestle, clean them. If a pill-crushing device is not available, place tablet between two medication cups and grind with a blunt instrument. Mix ground tablet in small amount of soft food (custard or applesauce).	Large tablets are often difficult to swallow. Ground tablet mixed with palatable soft food is usually easier to swallow. Cleaning pill-crushing device ensures that contamination of medications does not occur.

✴ **SKILL 35-1**　　　　　**ADMINISTERING ORAL MEDICATIONS—CONT'D**

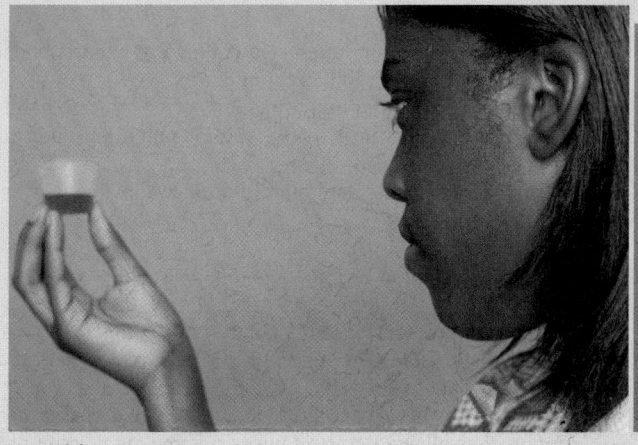
A

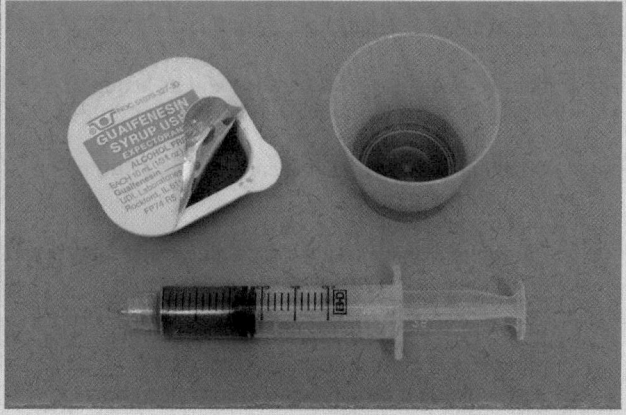
B

STEP 7l(3) A, Pour the desired volume of liquid so that base of meniscus is level with line on scale. **B,** Use needleless syringe to draw up volumes less than 10 mL.

STEPS	RATIONALE

Critical Decision Point: Not all medications can be crushed (e.g., capsules, enteric-coated drugs). Consult with pharmacist and/or the "Do Not Crush List" when in doubt. (ISMP, 2008).

STEPS	RATIONALE
l. To prepare liquids: (1) Gently shake container. If medication is in a unit-dose container with correct amount to administer, no further preparation is necessary. If medication is in a multidose bottle, remove bottle cap from container and place cap upside down.	Shaking container ensures medication is mixed before administration. Placing cap of bottle upside down prevents contamination of inside of cap.
(2) Hold multidose bottle with label against palm of hand while pouring.	Spilled liquid will not soil or fade label.
(3) Hold medication cup at eye level, and fill to desired level on scale (see illustration). Make sure scale is even with fluid level at its surface or base of meniscus, not edges. Draw up volumes of less than 10 mL in syringe without needle (see illustration).	Ensures accuracy of measurement. Use of syringe is more accurate for small doses of medication.
(4) Discard any excess liquid into sink. Wipe lip and neck of bottle with paper towel.	Prevents contamination of bottle's contents and prevents bottle cap from sticking.
(5) Administer liquid medications packaged in single-dose cups directly from the single-dose cup. Do not pour them into medicine cups.	Avoids unnecessary manipulation of dose.
m. Compare MAR, computer printout, or computer screen with prepared medication and container.	Reading labels a second time reduces error. *This is the second accuracy check.*
n. Return stock containers or unused unit-dose medications to shelf or drawer, and read label again.	*Third accuracy check.* Reading the label of medications in multiple-dose containers reduces administration errors.
o. Do not leave medications unattended.	Nurse is responsible for safekeeping of drugs.
8. Administer medications:	
a. Take medications to client at correct time, within 30 minutes before or after prescribed time.	Ensures intended therapeutic effect. Give STAT medications immediately or single-order medications at time ordered.
b. Identify client using at least two client identifiers. Compare client's name and one other identifier (e.g., hospital identification number) on MAR, computer printout, or computer screen with information on client's identification bracelet. Ask client to state name if possible for a third identifier.	Complies with TJC (2008) requirements and improves medication safety. In most acute care settings, client's name and identification number on armband and MAR are used to identify clients. Identification bracelets are made at time of client's admission and are most reliable source of identification. Client's room number is **not** an acceptable identifier.

Critical Decision Point: Replace client identification bracelets that are missing, illegible, or faded.

Continued

✳ **SKILL 35-1**   **ADMINISTERING ORAL MEDICATIONS—CONT'D**

STEPS	RATIONALE
c. Compare labels of medications with MAR at client's bedside.	Final check of medication labels against MAR at client's bedside reduces medication administration errors.
d. Explain purpose of each medication and its action to client. Allow client to ask any questions about drugs.	Client has right to be informed; questions often indicate need for teaching, nonadherence to therapy, or potential medication error.
e. Assist client to sitting or side-lying position if sitting is contraindicated.	Sitting position prevents aspiration during swallowing (Metheny, 2006).
f. Administer medications:	
(1) **For tablets:** Some clients want to hold solid medications in hand or cup before placing in mouth.	Client becomes familiar with medications by seeing each drug.
(2) Offer water or juice to help client swallow medications. Give cold carbonated water if available and not contraindicated.	Choice of fluid promotes client's comfort and helps medications enter the stomach. Carbonated water helps passage of tablet through esophagus.
(3) **For sublingual-administered medications:** Have client place medication under tongue and allow it to dissolve completely (see Figure 35-4, see p. 694). Caution client against swallowing tablet.	Medication is absorbed through blood vessels of undersurface of tongue. If swallowed, gastric juices destroy medication or the liver detoxifies it so rapidly that therapeutic blood levels are not attained.
(4) **For buccal medications:** Have client place medication in mouth against mucous membranes of the cheek until it dissolves (see Figure 35-5, see p. 694). Avoid administering liquids until buccal medication has dissolved.	Buccal medications act locally on mucosa or systemically as they are swallowed in saliva.
(5) **For powdered medications:** Mix with liquids at bedside, and give to client to drink.	When prepared in advance, powdered medications often thicken and even harden, making swallowing difficult.
(6) Caution client against chewing or swallowing lozenges.	Medication acts through slow absorption through oral mucosa, not gastric mucosa.
(7) Give effervescent powders and tablets immediately after dissolving.	Effervescence improves unpleasant taste of medication and often relieves GI problems.
g. If client is unable to hold medications, place medication cup to the lips and gently introduce each drug into the mouth, one at a time. Do not rush.	Administering single tablet or capsule eases swallowing and decreases risk of aspiration.
h. If tablet or capsule falls to the floor, discard it and repeat preparation.	Medication is contaminated when it touches floor.
i. Stay until client has completely swallowed each medication. Ask client to open mouth if uncertain whether medication has been swallowed.	Nurse is responsible for ensuring that client receives ordered dosage. If left unattended, some clients will not take dose or save medications, causing risk to health.
j. For highly acidic medications (e.g., aspirin), offer client nonfat snack (e.g., crackers) if not contraindicated by client's condition.	Reduces gastric irritation.
k. Assist client in returning to comfortable position.	Maintains client's comfort.
l. Dispose of soiled supplies, and perform hand hygiene.	Reduces transmission of microorganisms.
m. Replenish stock, such as cups and straws, return cart to medication room if used, and clean work area.	Clean and organized work space helps other staff complete duties efficiently.
9. Evaluate client's response to medications at times that correlate with the medication's onset, peak, and duration.	Evaluates medication's therapeutic benefit and detects onset of side effects or allergic reactions.
10 Ask client or family member to identify medication name and explain purpose, action, dosage schedule, and potential side effects of drug.	Determines level of knowledge gained by client and family.

Unexpected Outcomes and Related Interventions

1. Client exhibits adverse effects (side effect, toxic effect, allergic reaction).
   a. Assess for symptoms such as urticaria, rash, pruritus, rhinitis, and wheezing that indicate allergic reaction.
   b. Always notify prescriber and pharmacy when the client exhibits adverse effects.
   c. Withhold further doses, and add allergy information to client's medical record.

2. Client refuses medication.
   a. Explore reasons why client does not want medication.
   b. Educate if misunderstandings of medication therapy are apparent.
   c. Do not force client to take medication; clients have the right to refuse treatment.
   d. If client continues to refuse medication despite educational attempts, record why the drug was withheld on client's chart and notify prescriber.

Recording and Reporting
- Record administration of oral medications on computerized or paper copy of MAR immediately after administering medications. If using paper copy of MAR, nurses include their initials or signature.
- Record the reason any drug is withheld, and follow agency's policy for proper recording.
- Record and report evaluation of medication effect to prescriber if required (e.g., report urine output following administration of diuretic if ordered by prescriber).

Home Care Considerations
- Instruct clients about all aspects of medication administration, including dosage, desired effect, when to take medications, proper storage of medications, anticipated side effects, and whether to take medication with or without food, to ensure safe medication administration at home.
- Evaluate client's ability to safely self-administer medications. If unable to safely self-administer, attempt nursing interventions such as a chart or pillbox to assist in self-administration. If interventions fail and client still is unsafely able to administer medications, notify the prescriber.

before applying a new patch. Follow these guidelines to ensure safe administration of transdermal or topical medications (ISMP, 2007):

- Document where the medication was placed on the MAR.
- Whenever applying a transdermal patch, ask the client if he or she has an existing patch.
- Do not assume that a patch has fallen off or has been taken off. Assess the skin thoroughly before administering the medication.
- When taking a medication history or reconciling medications, specifically ask the client if he or she takes any medications in the forms of patches, topical creams, or any route other than the oral route.
- If the dressing or patch is difficult to see (e.g., clear), apply a noticeable label to the patch.
- Document removal of the patch or medication on the MAR.

Nasal Instillation. Clients with nasal sinus alterations sometimes receive medications by spray, drops, or tampons (Box 35-18). The most commonly administered form of nasal instillation is decongestant spray or drops, used to relieve symptoms of sinus congestion and colds. Caution clients to avoid abuse of medications because overuse leads to a rebound effect in which the nasal congestion worsens. When excess decongestant solution is swallowed, serious systemic effects also develop, especially in children. Saline drops are safer as a decongestant for children than nasal preparations that contain sympathomimetics (e.g., Afrin or Neo-Synephrine).

It is easier to have the client self-administer sprays, because the client is able to control the spray and inhale as it enters the nasal passages. For clients who use nasal sprays repeatedly, check the nares for irritation. Nasal drops are effective in treating sinus infections. Position clients to permit the medication to reach the affected sinus. Severe nosebleeds are usually treated with packing or nasal tampons, which are treated with epinephrine, to reduce blood flow. Usually a physician or advanced practice clinician places nasal tampons.

Eye Instillation. Common medications used by clients are eye drops and ointments, including over-the-counter preparations

such as artificial tears and vasoconstrictors (e.g., Visine and Murine). However, many clients receive prescribed **ophthalmic** medications for eye conditions, such as glaucoma or after cataract extraction. Many clients receiving eye medications are older adults. Age-related problems, including poor vision, hand tremors, and difficulty grasping or manipulating containers, affect the older adult's ability to self-administer eye medications. Instruct clients and family members about the proper techniques for administering eye medications (Skill 35-2). Determine the client's and family's ability to self-administer through a return demonstration of the procedure. Showing clients each step of the procedure for instilling eye drops can improve their compliance. Follow these principles when administering eye medications:

- The cornea of the eye has many pain fibers and thus is very sensitive to anything applied to it. Therefore avoid instilling any form of eye medication directly onto the cornea.
- The risk of transmitting infection from one eye to the other is high. Avoid touching the eyelids or other eye structures with eye droppers or ointment tubes.
- Use eye medication only for the client's affected eye.
- Never allow a client to use another client's eye medications.

Intraocular Administration. The nurse administers some medications intraocularly (see Skill 35-2). Medications delivered this way resemble a contact lens. Place the medication into the conjunctival sac where it remains in place for up to 1 week. Medications such as pilocarpine are administered this way. The client requires teaching about monitoring for adverse reactions to the disk. Clients also need to know how to insert and remove the disk.

Ear Instillation. Internal ear structures are very sensitive to temperature extremes. Failure to instill ear drops or irrigating fluid at room temperature causes vertigo, dizziness, or nausea. Although the structures of the outer ear are not sterile, sterile drops and solutions are used in case the eardrum is ruptured. The entrance of nonsterile solutions into middle ear structures will possibly result in infection. With ear drainage, the nurse needs to be sure the client does not have a ruptured eardrum. Never occlude or block the ear canal with the dropper or irrigating syringe. Forcing medication into an occluded ear canal creates pressure

Text continued on p. 729

✳ **BOX 35-18**   **PROCEDURAL GUIDELINES**   Video

Administering Nasal Instillations

Delegation Considerations: The skill of administration of nasal drops and ointments cannot be delegated. The nurse instructs nursing assistive personnel to report the occurrence of side effects to the nurse.

Equipment: Prepared medication with clean dropper or spray container, facial tissue, small pillow (optional), washcloth (optional), clean gloves (if client has extensive nasal drainage), medication administration record (MAR) or computer printout, penlight (to inspect nares if ointment is to be applied to a specific lesion inside the nares).

1. Check accuracy and completeness of each MAR or computer printout with prescriber's original medication order. Check client's name and medication name, dosage, route, and time for administration. Recopy any portion of MAR that is difficult to read.
2. Refer to the medical record to determine which sinus is affected if giving nasal drops.
3. Assess client's medical history (e.g., history of hypertension, heart disease, diabetes mellitus, hyperthyroidism) and for history or allergies to medications and foods. List client's food and drug allergies on each page of the MAR and prominently display them on the client's medical record per agency policy.
4. Perform hand hygiene. Using a penlight, inspect condition of nose and sinuses. Palpate sinuses for tenderness.
5. Assess client's knowledge regarding use of nasal instillations and technique for instillation and willingness to learn self-administration.
6. Prepare medication (see Skill 35-1, Steps 7a-g and m-o, pp. 719 to 721). Be sure to compare label of medication against MAR at least three times while preparing medication.
7. Take medication to client at correct time, and perform hand hygiene.
8. Identify client by using at least two client identifiers. Compare client's name and one other identifier (e.g., hospital identification number) on MAR, computer printout, or computer screen with information on client's identification bracelet. Ask client to state name if possible for a third identifier.
9. Compare MAR with medication labels at client's bedside.

10. Explain procedure to client regarding positioning and sensations to expect, such as burning or stinging of mucosa or choking sensation as medication trickles into throat.
11. Arrange supplies and medications at bedside. Apply gloves if client has nasal drainage.
12. Gently roll or shake container.
13. Instruct client to clear or blow nose gently unless contraindicated (e.g., risk of increased intracranial pressure or nosebleeds).
14. Administer nasal drops:
    a. Assist client to supine position, and position head properly.
       (1) For access to posterior pharynx, tilt client's head backward.
       (2) For access to ethmoid or sphenoid sinus, tilt head back over edge of bed or place small pillow under client's shoulder and tilt head back (see illustration).
       (3) For access to frontal and maxillary sinus, tilt head back over edge of bed or pillow with head turned toward side to be treated (see illustration).
    b. Support client's head with nondominant hand.
    c. Instruct client to breathe through mouth.
    d. Hold dropper 1 cm (½ inches) above nares, and instill prescribed number of drops toward midline of ethmoid bone.
    e. Have client remain in supine position 5 minutes.
    f. Offer facial tissue to blot runny nose, but caution client against blowing nose for several minutes.
15. Assist client to a comfortable position after medication is absorbed.
16. Dispose of soiled supplies in proper container, and perform hand hygiene.
17. Document administration of medication on MAR.
18. Observe client for onset of side effects 15 to 30 minutes after administration.
19. Ask if client is able to breathe through nose after decongestant administration. Sometimes it is necessary to have client occlude one nostril at a time and breathe deeply.
20. Evaluate client's response to medications at times that correlate with the medication's onset, peak, and duration. Evaluate client for both desired effect and adverse effects. Reinspect condition of nasal passages between the instillations.
21. Ask client to review risks of overuse of decongestants and methods for administration.
22. Have client demonstrate self-medication.

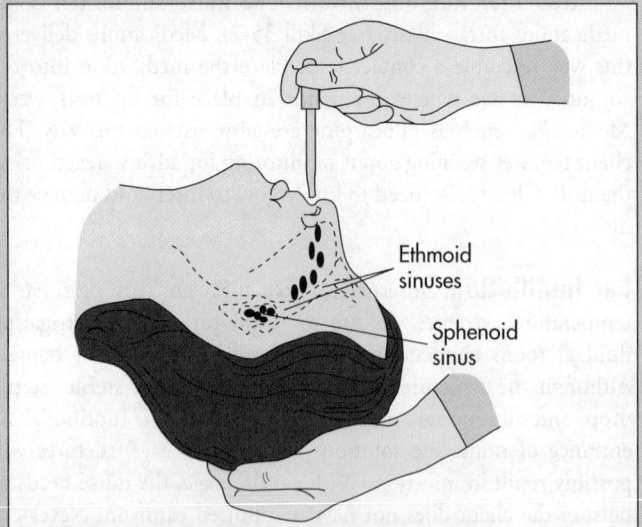

STEP 14a(2) Position for instilling nose drops into ethmoid or sphenoid sinus.

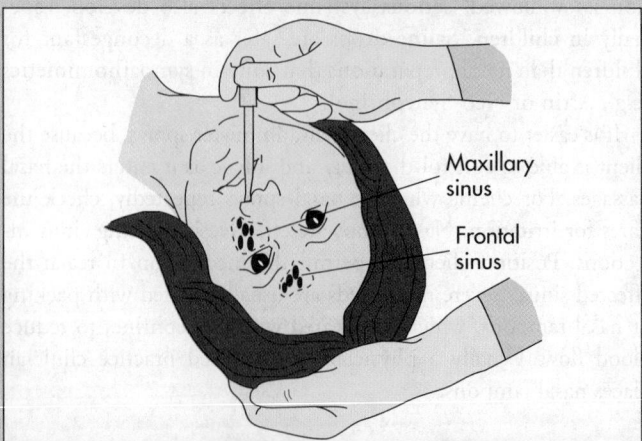

STEP 14a(3) Position for instilling nose drops into frontal and maxillary sinus.

✳ SKILL 35-2   ADMINISTERING OPHTHALMIC MEDICATIONS

Delegation Considerations

The skill of administering ophthalmic medications cannot be delegated. The nurse instructs nursing assistive personnel to report the occurrence of side effects of medications, including the potential for visual difficulty, to the nurse.

Equipment
- Medication bottle with sterile eye dropper or ointment tube or medicated intraocular disk
- Cotton ball or tissue
- Washbasin filled with warm water and washcloth if eyes have crust or drainage
- Eye patch and tape (optional)
- Clean gloves
- MAR or computer printout

STEPS	RATIONALE
1. Check accuracy and completeness of each MAR or computer printout with prescriber's medication order. Check client's name and medication name and dosage (e.g., number of drops [if a liquid] and eye [right, left, or both eyes]), and route and time of administration. Recopy or re-print any portion of MAR that is difficult to read.	The order sheet is the most reliable source and only legal record of medications client is to receive. Ensures client receives the correct medications. Illegible MARs are a source of medication errors.
2. Assess condition of external eye structures.	Provides baseline to later determine if local response to medications occurs. Also indicates need to clean eye before medication application.
3. Determine whether client has any known allergies to eye medications. Also ask if client has allergy to latex.	Protects client from risk of allergic medication response. If client has latex allergy, use nonlatex gloves.
4. Determine whether client has any symptoms of visual alterations.	Certain eye medications act to either lessen or increase these symptoms. Ensures nurse is able to recognize change in client's condition.
5. Assess client's level of consciousness and ability to follow directions.	If client becomes restless or combative during procedure, a greater risk of accidental eye injury exists.
6. Assess client's knowledge regarding medication therapy and desire to self-administer medication.	Client's level of understanding indicates need for health teaching. Motivation influences teaching approach.
7. Assess client's ability to manipulate and hold dropper.	Reflects client's ability to learn to self-administer medication.
8. Prepare medication: See Skill 35-1, Steps 7a-g and m-o, pp. 719 to 721. Be sure to check the label two times while preparing medication.	Following the same routine when preparing medications, eliminating distractions, and checking the label of the medication with transcribed order reduce error (Pape and others, 2005).
9. Take medication to client at correct time, and perform hand hygiene.	Administer medications within 30 minutes before or after prescribed time to ensure intended therapeutic effect. Give STAT medications immediately or single-order medications at time ordered. Hand hygiene reduces transmission of microorganisms.
10. Identify client using at least two client identifiers. Compare client's name and one other identifier (e.g., hospital identification number) on MAR, computer printout, or computer screen with information on client's identification bracelet. Ask client to state name if possible for a third identifier.	Complies with TJC (2008) requirements and improves medication safety. In most acute care settings, client's name and identification number on armband and MAR are used to identify clients. Identification bracelets are made at time of client's admission and are most reliable source of information. Client's room number is **not** an acceptable identifier.
11. Compare labels of medications with MAR at client's bedside.	Final check of medication labels against MAR at client's bedside reduces medication administration errors.
12. Arrange supplies at bedside; apply clean gloves. If eye drops are stored in refrigerator, allow eye drops to come to room temperature before giving eye drops.	Reduces transmission of microorganisms and follows standards to prevent accidental exposure to body fluids (Occupational Health and Safety Administration [OSHA], 2006). Warming eye drops reduces irritation to eye.
13. Gently roll container.	Ensures medication is mixed before administration. Shaking bottle causes bubbles, which makes medication administration difficult.
14. Explain procedure to client; include positioning and sensations to expect, such as burning or stinging.	Relieves anxiety about medication being instilled into eye.
15. Ask client to lie supine or sit back in chair with head slightly hyperextended.	Position provides easy access to eye for medication instillation and minimizes drainage of medication through tear duct.

Critical Decision Point: Do not hyperextend the neck of a client with cervical spine injury.

Continued

✳ **SKILL 35-2** ADMINISTERING OPHTHALMIC MEDICATIONS—CONT'D

STEPS	RATIONALE
16. If crusts or drainage are present along eyelid margins or inner canthus, gently wash away. Soak any crusts that are dried and difficult to remove by applying damp washcloth or cotton ball over eye for a few minutes. Always wipe clean from inner to outer canthus.	Crusts or drainage harbors microorganisms. Soaking allows easy removal and prevents pressure from being applied directly over eye. Cleansing from inner to outer canthus avoids entrance of microorganism into lacrimal duct.
17. Hold cotton ball or clean tissue in nondominant hand on client's cheekbone just below lower eyelid.	Cotton or tissue absorbs medication that escapes eye.
18. With tissue or cotton resting below lower lid, gently press downward with thumb or forefinger against bony orbit.	Technique exposes lower conjunctival sac. Retraction against bony orbit prevents pressure and trauma to eyeball and prevents fingers from touching eye.
19. Ask client to look at ceiling.	Action retracts sensitive cornea up and away from conjunctival sac and reduces stimulation of blink reflex.
A. Instill eye drops:	
(1) With dominant hand resting on client's forehead, hold filled medication eye dropper or ophthalmic solution approximately 1 to 2 cm (½ to ¾ inches) above conjunctival sac (see illustration).	Helps prevent accidental contact of eye dropper with eye structures, thus reducing risk of injury to eye and transfer of infection to dropper. Ophthalmic medications are sterile.
(2) Drop prescribed number of medication drops into conjunctival sac.	Conjunctival sac normally holds 1 or 2 drops. Provides even distribution of medication across eye.
(3) If client blinks or closes eye or if drops land on outer lid margins, repeat procedure.	Client obtains therapeutic effect of drug only when drops enter conjunctival sac.
(4) After instilling drops, ask client to close eye gently.	Helps to distribute medication. Squinting or squeezing of eyelids forces medication from conjunctival sac (VisionRx, 2005).
(5) When administering medications that cause systemic effects, apply gentle pressure with your finger and clean tissue on the client's nasolacrimal duct for 30 to 60 seconds.	Prevents overflow of medication into nasal and pharyngeal passages. Prevents absorption into systemic circulation.
B. Instill eye ointment:	
(1) Ask client to look at ceiling.	Action retracts sensitive cornea up and away from conjunctival sac and reduces stimulation of blink reflex.
(2) Holding ointment applicator above lower lid margin, apply thin stream of ointment evenly along inner edge of lower eyelid on conjunctiva (see illustration) from the inner canthus to outer canthus.	Distributes medication evenly across eye and lid margin.
(3) Have client close eye and rub lid lightly in circular motion with cotton ball, if rubbing is not contraindicated.	Further distributes medication without traumatizing eye.
C. Administer intraocular disk:	
(1) Application:	
a. Open package containing the disk. Gently press fingertip against the disk so that it adheres to finger. Position the convex side of the disk on fingertip (see illustration).	Allows nurse to inspect disk for damage or deformity.

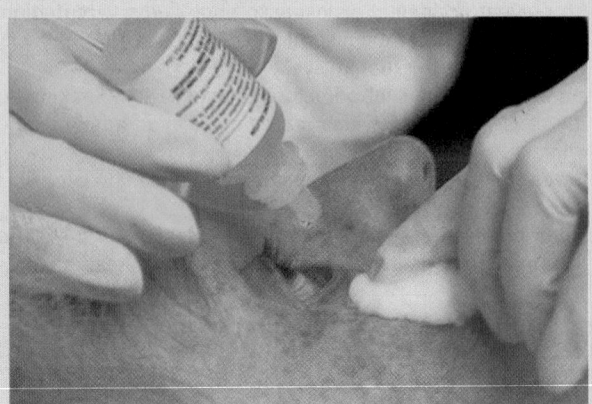

STEP 19A(1) Hold eye dropper above conjunctival sac.

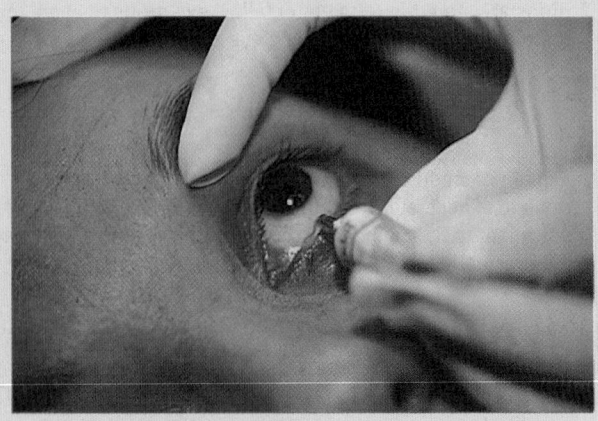

STEP 19B(2) Apply ointment along lower eyelid.

✳ SKILL 35-2 **ADMINISTERING OPHTHALMIC MEDICATIONS—CONT'D**

STEPS	RATIONALE
b. With other hand, gently pull the client's lower eyelid away from the eye. Ask client to look up.	Prepares conjunctival sac for receiving medicated disk.
c. Place the disk in the conjunctival sac, so that it floats on the sclera between the iris and lower eyelid (see illustration).	Ensures delivery of medication.
d. Pull the client's lower eyelid out and over the disk (see illustration).	Ensures accurate medication delivery.

Critical Decision Point: You should not be able to see the disk at this time. Repeat step 19C(1)d if you see the disk.

(2) Removal:	
a. Perform hand hygiene, and apply gloves.	Prevents transfer of microorganisms and follows standards for prevention of accidental exposure to body fluids (OSHA, 2006).
b. Explain procedure to client.	Relieves anxiety about manipulation of disk in eye.
c. Gently pull on the client's lower eyelid.	Exposes intraocular disk.
d. Using forefinger and thumb of opposite hand, pinch the disk and lift it out of the client's eye (see illustration).	
20. If excess medication is on eyelid, gently wipe it from inner to outer canthus.	Promotes comfort and prevents trauma to eye (VisionRx, 2005).
21. If client had eye patch, apply clean one by placing it over affected eye so entire eye is covered. Tape securely without applying pressure to eye.	Clean eye patch reduces chance of infection.

Critical Decision Point: If client receives more than one eye medication to the same eye at the same time, wait at least 5 minutes before administering the next medication to avoid interaction between medications (VisionRx, 2005).

22. If client receives eye medication to both eyes at the same time, use a different tissue or cotton ball with each eye.	Prevents cross contamination between eyes.
23. Remove gloves, dispose of soiled supplies in proper receptacle, and perform hand hygiene.	Maintains neat environment at bedside and reduces transmission of microorganisms.
24. Note client's response to instillation; ask if client felt any discomfort.	Determines if nurse performed procedure correctly and safely and if client is experiencing adverse effects of medication.
25. Observe response to medication by assessing visual changes and noting any side effects.	Evaluates effects of medication.
26. Ask client to discuss medication's purpose, action, side effects, and technique of administration.	Determines client's level of understanding.
27. Have client demonstrate self-administration of next dose.	Provides feedback regarding competency with skill.

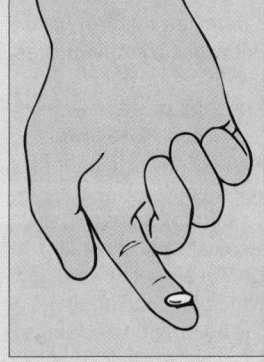

STEP 19C(1)a Gently position the convex side of the disk against fingertips.

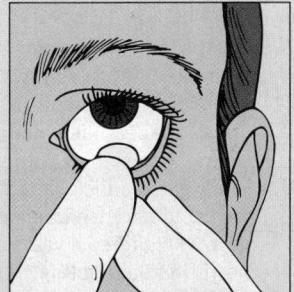

STEP 19C(1)c Place disk in the conjunctival sac between the iris and lower eyelid.

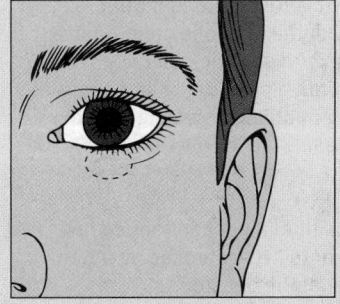

STEP 19C(1)d Gently pull lower eyelid over the disk.

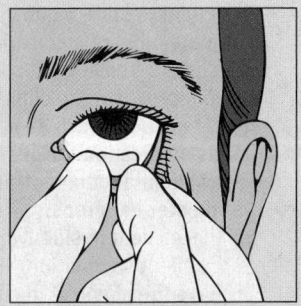

STEP 19C(2)d Carefully pinch the disk to remove it from the client's eye.

Continued

✳ **SKILL 35-2**   **ADMINISTERING OPHTHALMIC MEDICATIONS—CONT'D**

Unexpected Outcomes and Related Interventions

1. Client cannot instill drops without supervision.
   a. Reinforce teaching and allow client to self-administer drops as much as possible to enhance confidence.
   b. If client cannot self-administer drops, teach others, such as family members, to instill drops into the client's eye.
2. Client displays signs of allergic reaction (e.g., tearing, reddened sclera) or systemic response (e.g., bradycardia) to medication.
   a. Hold medication, and speak with prescriber.
   b. Follow institutional policy or guidelines for reporting of adverse or allergic reaction to medications.
   c. Add information about allergy to medical record per agency policy.

Recording and Reporting

- Record medication, concentration, number of drops, time of administration, and eye (left, right, or both) that received medication on electronic or printed MAR.
- Record appearance of eye in nurses' notes.

Home Care Considerations

- Clients with chronic health care problems need to consult with their health care provider before using over-the-counter eye medication.
- When using eye drops at home, clients should not share medications with other family members because risk of infection transmission is high.

✳ **BOX 35-19**   **PROCEDURAL GUIDELINES**

Administering Ear Medications

Delegation Considerations: Administering ear medications cannot be delegated to nursing assistive personnel (NAP). The nurse instructs NAP about potential side effects and the need to report their occurrence.

Equipment: Medication administration record (MAR), clean gloves if client has drainage from the ear; *for drops:* medication bottle with dropper, cotton-tipped applicator, cotton ball (optional); *for irrigation:* irrigating syringe, kidney-shaped basin, towel.

1. Check accuracy and completeness of each MAR or computer printout with prescriber's original medication order. Check client's name and medication name, dosage, route, and time for administration. Recopy or re-print any portion of MAR that is difficult to read.
2. Prepare medication (see Skill 35-1, Steps 7a-g and m-o). Be sure to compare the label of the medication with the MAR at least two times during medication preparation.
3. Take medication to client at correct time, and perform hand hygiene. Apply gloves if drainage is present.
4. Identify client using at least two client identifiers. Compare client's name and one other identifier (e.g., hospital identification number) on MAR, computer printout, or computer screen with information on client's identification bracelet. Ask client to state name if possible for a third identifier.
5. Compare label of medication with the MAR one more time at the client's bedside. *This is the third accuracy check.*
6. Explain procedure to client regarding positioning and sensations to expect, such as hearing bubbling or feeling water in ear as medication trickles into ear.
7. Teach client about medication.
8. **Administer ear drops:**
   a. Place client in side-lying position (if not contraindicated by client's condition) with ear to be treated facing up, or have the client sit in chair or at the bedside.
   b. Straighten ear canal by pulling auricle down and back (children less than 3 years) or upward and outward (children 4 years of age and older and adults).
   c. Instill prescribed drops holding dropper 1 cm (½ inch) above ear canal (see illustration).
   d. Ask client to remain in side-lying position 2 to 3 minutes. Apply gentle massage or pressure to tragus of ear with

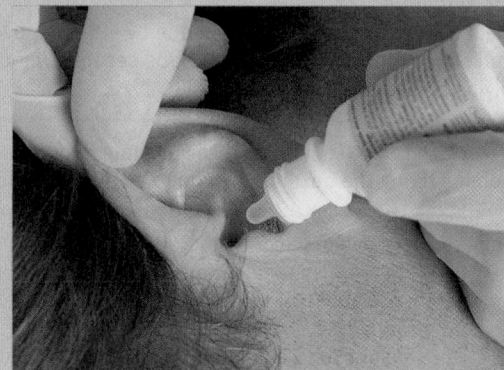

STEP 8c Placing ear drop in ear.

finger unless contraindicated due to pain.
   e. If cotton ball is needed, place cotton ball into outermost part of canal. Do not press cotton deep into canal. Remove cotton after 15 minutes.
9. **Administer Ear Irrigation:**
   a. Assess the tympanic membrane or review medical record for history of eardrum perforation, which contraindicates ear irrigation.
   b. Assist client in assuming sitting or lying position with head tilted or turned toward affected ear. Place towel under client's head and shoulder, and have client hold kidney-shaped basin under affected ear.
   c. Fill irrigating syringe with solution (approximately 50 mL).
   d. Gently grasp auricle, and straighten ear canal by pulling it down and back (children less than 3 years) or upward and outward (children 4 years of age and older and adults).
   e. Slowly instill irrigating solution by holding tip of syringe 1 cm (½ inch) above opening of ear canal. Allow fluid to drain out during instillation. Continue until canal is cleansed or all solution is used.
10. Clean the area, and put supplies away.
11. Remove gloves, and perform hand hygiene.
12. Document medication administration on MAR.
13. Evaluate client's response to the medication.

that will injure the eardrum. Box 35-19 provides guidelines for administering ear drops and ear irrigations and describes differences in straightening the ear canal for children and adults.

Vaginal Instillation.

Vaginal medications are available as suppositories, foam, jellies, or creams. Suppositories come individually packaged in foil wrappers and are sometimes stored in the refrigerator to prevent the solid, oval-shaped suppositories from melting. After a suppository is inserted into the vaginal cavity, body temperature causes it to melt and be distributed and absorbed. Foam, jellies, and creams are administered with an applicator inserter (Box 35-20). Give a suppository with a gloved hand in accordance with standard precautions (see Chapter 34). Clients often prefer administering their own vaginal medications and need privacy. After instillation of the medication, some clients wear a perineal pad to collect drainage. Because vaginal medications are often given to treat infection, discharge is usually foul smelling. Follow aseptic technique, and offer the client frequent opportunities to maintain perineal hygiene (see Chapter 39).

Rectal Instillation.

Rectal suppositories are thinner and more bullet shaped than vaginal suppositories. The rounded end prevents anal trauma during insertion. Rectal suppositories contain medications that exert local effects such as promoting defecation or systemic effects such as reducing nausea. Rectal suppositories are often stored in the refrigerator until administered.

During administration, place the unwrapped suppository past the internal anal sphincter and against the rectal mucosa (Box 35-21). Otherwise the suppository will be expelled before it is able to dissolve and be absorbed into the mucosa. With practice a nurse learns to recognize the sensation of the sphincter relaxing around the finger. Do not force the suppository into a mass of fecal material. Sometimes it is necessary to clear the rectum with a small cleansing enema before inserting a suppository.

Administering Medications by Inhalation

Medications administered with handheld inhalers are dispersed through an aerosol spray, mist, or powder that penetrates lung airways. The alveolocapillary network absorbs medications rapidly. **Metered-dose inhalers (MDIs)** and dry powder inhalers (DPIs) usually produce local effects such as bronchodilation. However, some medications create serious systemic side effects.

Clients who receive medications by inhalation frequently suffer chronic respiratory disease such as chronic asthma, emphysema, or bronchitis. Different respiratory problems require different inhaled medication. For example, clients with asthma usually receive antiinflammatory medications because asthma is primarily an inflammatory disease, whereas clients with chronic obstructive pulmonary disease (COPD) receive bronchodilators because they usually have problems with bronchoconstriction. Inhaled medications are also often described as "rescue" or "maintenance" medications. Rescue medications are short-acting medications that are taken for immediate relief of acute respiratory distress. Maintenance inhalers are used on a daily scheduled basis to prevent acute respiratory distress. The effects of maintenance inhalers start within hours of administration and last for a longer period of time

when compared with rescue inhalers. Some inhalers contain combinations of rescue and maintenance medications (Capriotti, 2005). Because clients depend on inhaled medications for disease control, they need to learn about them and ways to administer them safely (Skill 35-3).

A metered-dose inhaler delivers a measured dose of medication with each push of a canister. Chemical propellants (e.g., hydrofluorocarbons) push the medication out of the MDI. MDIs are either squeeze-and-breathe inhalers or activated by the client's breath. The squeeze-and-breathe MDI requires the client to apply approximately 5 to 10 pounds of pressure to the top of the canister to administer the medication. With this type of MDI, it is important for the nurse to assess the client's hand strength, which often diminishes with age and from the effects of chronic respiratory disease. Breath-activated MDIs release the medication when the client inhales. Release of the medication is dependent upon the strength of the client's breath on inspiration (Capriotti, 2005). Clients can use a spacer with the MDI. The spacer allows the particles of medication to slow down and break into smaller pieces, which improves the drug's absorption in the client's airway. Spacers have a facemask for infants and children under 4 years of age. Spacers are especially helpful when the client has difficulty coordinating the steps involved in self-administering inhaled medications. However, many clients, especially children, often have difficulty using spacers (Vella and Grech, 2005). When clients do not use their inhalers and spacers correctly, they do not receive the full effect of the medication. Therefore client education is essential.

DPIs hold dry, powdered medication and create an aerosol when the client inhales through a reservoir that contains a dose of the medication. DPIs require less manual dexterity, and because the device is activated with the client's breath, there is no need to coordinate puffs with inhalation. They also do not require a spacer. However, the medication inside the DPI can clump if the client is in a humid climate, and some clients cannot inspire fast enough to administer the entire dose of the medication.

One important aspect of client teaching is to help the client determine when the MDI or DPI is empty and needs to be replaced. Floating the MDI to determine how much medication is left is no longer recommended because extra propellant causes the container to float even if there is no medication left in the inhaler. Furthermore, MDIs with HFA should never be immersed (Capriotti, 2005). Some DPIs have mechanisms that indicate how many doses are left. These mechanisms are not always accurate. Therefore, to calculate how long medication in an MDI or DPI will last, divide the number of doses in the container by the number of doses the client takes per day. For example, a client is to take albuterol, a beta-adrenergic agonist bronchodilator. The ordered dose is 2 puffs 4 times a day. The canister has a total of 200 puffs. Complete the following calculations to determine how long the MDI will last:

$$2 \text{ puffs} \times 4 \text{ times a day} = 8 \text{ puffs per day}$$
$$200 \text{ puffs} \div 8 \text{ puffs per day} = 25 \text{ days}$$

The canister in this example will last 25 days. To ensure that the client does not run out of medication, teach the client to refill the medication at least 7 to 10 days before it runs out (MayoClinic.com, 2007).

Text continued on p. 735

✱ **BOX 35-20**   PROCEDURAL GUIDELINES

Administering Vaginal Medications

Delegation Considerations: The skill of administering vaginal medications cannot be delegated. The nurse instructs nursing assistive personnel to report new or increased vaginal discharge or bleeding and occurrence of potential side effects of medications.

Equipment: Vaginal cream, foam, jelly, or suppository, or irrigating solution with applicator (if required); clean gloves; towels and/or washcloth; perineal pad; drape or sheet; water-soluble lubricating jelly; medication administration record (MAR) or computer printout.

1. Check accuracy and completeness of each MAR or computer printout with prescriber's original medication order. Check client's name and medication name, form (cream or suppository), route, dosage, and time of administration.
2. Prepare medication (see Skill 35-1, Steps 7a-g, m-o, pp. 719 to 721). Compare the label of the medication with the MAR two times while preparing the medication.
3. Take medication to client at the correct time, and perform hand hygiene.
4. Identify client using at least two client identifiers. Compare client's name and one other identifier (e.g., hospital identification number) on MAR, computer printout, or computer screen with information on client's identification bracelet. Ask client to state name if possible for third identifier.
5. Compare label of medication with MAR one more time at the client's bedside.
6. Teach client about the medication. Explain procedure to client regarding positioning and sensations to expect, such as feelings of moisture or wetness in the vaginal area. Assess client's ability to manipulate applicator or suppository and to position self to insert medication. Be sure client understands the procedure if she plans to self-administer the medication.
7. Close room door or pull curtain to provide privacy.
8. Put on clean gloves.
9. Be sure there is adequate lighting to visualize vaginal opening. Inspect condition of external genitalia and vaginal canal (see Chapter 33), noting appearance of any discharge. Cleanse area with towel or washcloth if necessary

10. Assist client with lying in dorsal recumbent position.
11. Keep abdomen and lower extremities draped.
12. Administer vaginal suppository:
    a. Remove suppository from foil wrapper and apply liberal amount of sterile water-based lubricating jelly to the smooth or rounded end. Lubricate gloved index finger of dominant hand.
    b. With nondominant gloved hand, expose vaginal orifice by gently retracting labial folds.
    c. With dominant gloved hand, gently insert rounded end of suppository along posterior wall of vaginal canal entire length of finger (7.5 to 10 cm or 3 to 4 inches) to ensure equal distribution of medication along walls of vaginal cavity (see illustration).
    d. Withdraw finger, and wipe away remaining lubricant from around orifice and labia.
13. Administer cream or foam:
    a. Fill cream or foam applicator following package directions.
    b. With nondominant gloved hand, expose vaginal orifice by gently retracting labial folds.
    c. With dominant gloved hand, insert applicator approximately 5 to 7.5 cm (2 to 3 inches). Push applicator plunger to deposit medication into vagina to allows equal distribution of medication (see illustration).
    d. Withdraw applicator, and place on paper towel. Wipe off residual cream from labia or vaginal orifice.
14. Dispose of supplies, remove gloves, and perform hand hygiene.
15. Instruct client to remain on back for at least 10 minutes to allow medication to be distributed and absorbed evenly throughout vaginal cavity and not lost through orifice.
16. Document medication administration on MAR.
17. If using an applicator, wearing gloves, wash with soap and warm water, rinse, and store for future use.
18. Offer client perineal pad when she resumes ambulation.
19. Evaluate client's response to medication, and inspect appearance of discharge of vaginal canal and condition of external genitalia between applications.

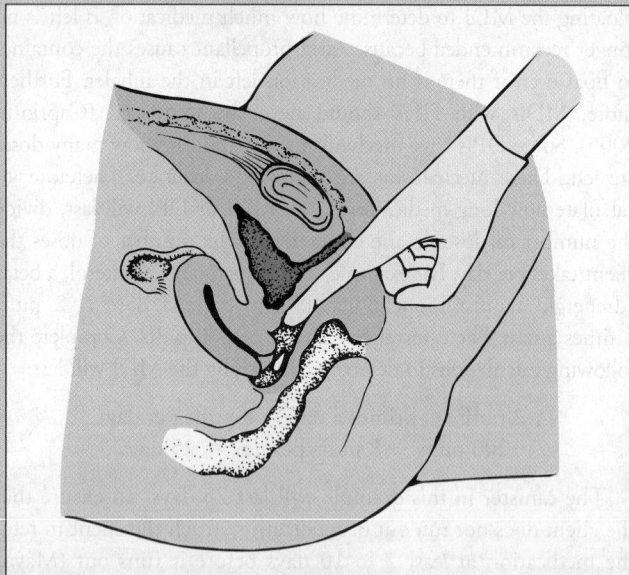

STEP 12c Insertion of suppository into the vaginal canal.

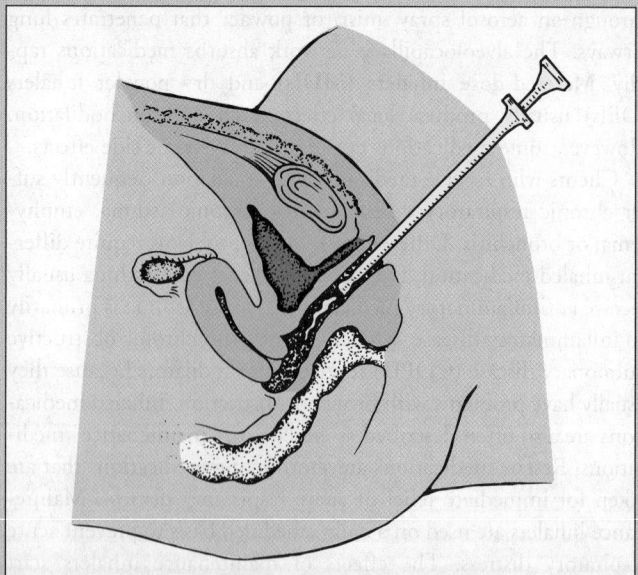

STEP 13c Instillation of medication in vaginal canal.

Administering Rectal Suppositories

Delegation Considerations: The skill of administering rectal suppositories cannot be delegated. The nurse instructs nursing assistive personnel to expect and report fecal discharge or bowel movement and to report occurrence of potential side effects of medications to the nurse

Equipment: Rectal suppository, water-soluble lubricating jelly, clean gloves, drape or sheet, tissue, medication administration record (MAR) or computer printout.

1. Check accuracy and completeness of each MAR or computer printout with prescriber's original medication order. Check client's name and medication name, dosage, route, and time of administration. Recopy or re-print any portion of MAR that is difficult to read.
2. Review medical record for history of rectal surgery or bleeding.
3. Prepare medication (see Skill 35-1, Steps 7a-g and m-o, pp. 719 to 721). Be sure to compare the label of the medication with the MAR two times during medication preparation.
4. Take medication to client at the correct time, and perform hand hygiene.
5. Identify client using at least two client identifiers. Compare client's name and one other identifier (e.g., hospital identification number) on MAR, computer printout, or computer screen with information on client's identification bracelet. Ask client to state name if possible for a third identifier.
6. Compare the label of the medication with the MAR or computer printout one more time at the client's bedside.
7. Teach client about the medication. Explain procedure to client regarding positioning and sensations to expect, such as feelings of needing to defecate. Be sure client understands the procedure if he or she is going to self-administer the medication.
8. Close room door or pull curtain to ensure privacy.
9. Put on clean gloves.
10. Assist client to the Sims' position. Keep client draped with only anal area exposed.
11. Be sure there is adequate lighting to visualize anus. Examine condition of anus externally, and palpate rectal walls as needed (see Chapter 33). Dispose of gloves in proper receptacle if soiled.
12. Apply new pair of clean gloves (if previous gloves were soiled).
13. Remove suppository from wrapper, and lubricate rounded end (see illustration) with sterile water-soluble lubricating jelly. Lubricate index finger of dominant hand with a water-soluble lubricant.
14. Ask client to take slow deep breaths through mouth and relax anal sphincter.
15. Retract buttocks with nondominant hand. Insert suppository gently through anus, past internal sphincter and against rectal wall, 10 cm (4 inches) in adults, 5 cm (2 inches) in children and infants (see illustration). Apply gentle pressure to hold buttocks together momentarily if needed to keep medication in place.
16. Withdraw finger, and wipe anal area with tissue.
17. Dispose of supplies, remove gloves, and perform hand hygiene.
18. Ask client to remain flat or on side for at least 5 minutes to prevent expulsion of suppository.
19. If suppository contains laxative or fecal softener, place call light within reach.
20. Document medication administration on MAR.
21. Observe for effects of suppository (e.g., bowel movement, relief of nausea) at times that correlate with the medication's onset, peak, and duration.

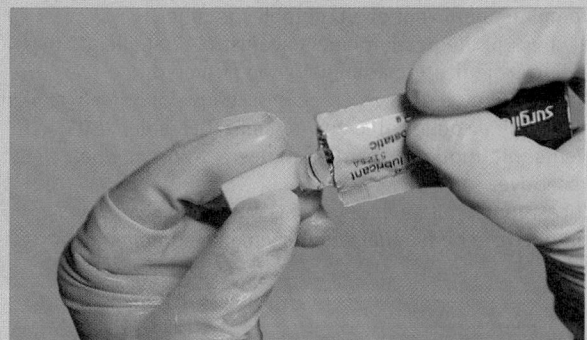

STEP 13 Remove suppository from wrapper.

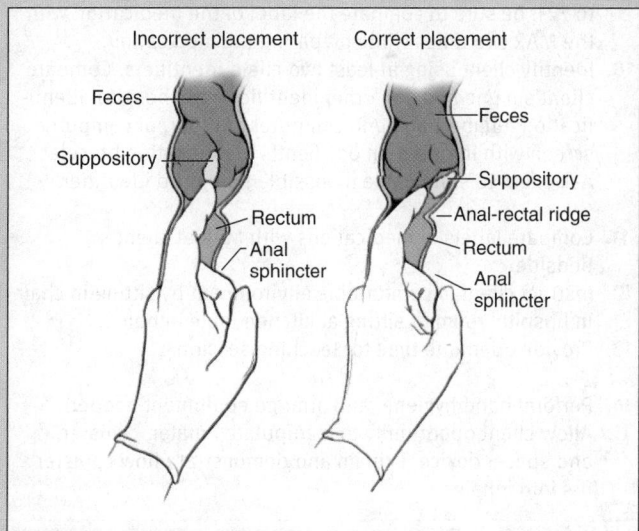

STEP 15 Inserting a rectal suppository. (From deWit S: *Fundamental concepts and skills for nursing*, ed 2, Philadelphia, 2005, Saunders.)

SKILL 35-3   USING METERED-DOSE OR DRY POWDER INHALERS   Video

Delegation Considerations

The skill of administering MDIs or DPIs and supervising clients who self-administer them cannot be delegated. The nurse instructs nursing assistive personnel to report changes in the client's respiratory status, increased coughing, or the occurrence of potential side effects.

Equipment

- MDI or DPI
- Spacer (optional with MDI)
- Facial tissues (optional)
- Washbasin or sink with warm water
- Paper towel
- MAR or computer printout

STEPS	RATIONALE
1. Check accuracy and completeness of each MAR or computer printout with prescriber's original medication order. Check client's name and medication name, dosage, route, and time for administration. Recopy or re-print any portion of MAR that is difficult to read.	The order sheet is the most reliable source and only legal record of medications client is to receive. Ensures client receives the correct medications. Illegible MARs are a source of medication errors.
2. Assess client's respiratory pattern, and auscultate breath sounds.	Establishes baseline of airway status for comparison during and after treatment.
3. If previously instructed in self-administration, assess client's technique in using inhaler.	Nurse's instruction sometimes only requires reinforcement of previous learning.
4. Assess client's ability to hold, manipulate, and depress canister or strength of inhalation.	Any impairment of grasp, ability to breathe, or coordination interferes with client's ability to use MDI or DPI correctly.
5. Assess client's *readiness* to learn: client asks questions about medication, disease, or complications; requests education in use of inhaler; is mentally alert; participates in own care.	Affects client's ability to understand explanations and actively participate in teaching process (Bastable, 2003).
6. Assess client's *ability* to learn: make sure client is not fatigued, in pain, or in respiratory distress; assess level of understanding of technical vocabulary terms.	Mental or physical limitations affect client's ability to learn and methods nurse uses for instruction (Bastable, 2003).
7. Assess client's knowledge and understanding of disease and purpose and action of prescribed medications.	Knowledge of disease is essential for client to realistically understand use of inhaler.
8. Determine medication schedule and number of inhalations prescribed for each dose.	Influences explanations nurse provides for use of inhaler.
9. Prepare medication: See Skill 35-1, Steps 7a-g, m-o, pp. 719 to 721. be sure to compare the label of the medication with the MAR two times while preparing the medication.	Following the same routine when preparing medications, eliminating distractions, and checking the label of the medication with transcribed order reduces error (Pape and others, 2005).
10. Identify client using at least two client identifiers. Compare client's name and one other identifier (e.g., hospital identification number) on MAR, computer printout, or computer screen with information on client's identification bracelet. Ask client to state name if possible for a third identifier.	Complies with TJC (2008) requirements and improves medication safety. In most acute care settings, client's name and identification number on armband and MAR are used to identify clients. Identification bracelets are made at time of client's admission and are most reliable source of information. Client's room number is **not** an acceptable identifier.
11. Compare labels of medications with MAR at client's bedside.	Final check of medication labels against MAR at client's bedside reduces medication administration errors.
12. Instruct client in comfortable environment by sitting in chair in hospital room or sitting at kitchen table in home.	Client will be more likely to remain receptive of nurse's explanations if in a comfortable environment (Bastable, 2003).
13. Provide adequate time for teaching session.	Prevents interruptions. Instruction needs to occur when client is receptive.
14. Perform hand hygiene, and arrange equipment needed.	Reduces transfer of microorganisms and saves time.
15. Allow client opportunity to manipulate inhaler, canister, and spacer device. Explain and demonstrate how canister fits into inhaler.	Client needs to be familiar with how to use equipment.

Critical Decision Point: If client is using an MDI with or without a spacer and the inhaler is new or has not been used for several days, push a "test spray" into the air. You do not need to do this for a DPI.

| 16. Explain what metered dose is, and warn client about overuse of inhaler, including medication side effects. | Client must not arbitrarily administer excessive inhalations because of risk of serious side effects. If medication is given in recommended doses, side effects are uncommon. |
| 17. Explain steps for administering squeeze-and-breathe MDI (demonstrate steps when possible):
 a. Insert MDI canister into the holder.
 b. Remove mouthpiece cover from inhaler. | Use of simple, step-by-step explanations allows client to ask questions at any point during procedure. |

⁎ **SKILL 35-3**   **USING METERED-DOSE OR DRY POWDER INHALERS—CONT'D**

STEPS	RATIONALE
c. Shake inhaler vigorously five or six times.	Ensures fine particles are aerosolized.
d. Have client take a deep breath and exhale.	Empties lungs and prepares the client's airway to receive the medication.
e. Instruct the client to position the inhaler in one of two ways.	
(1) Close mouth around MDI with opening toward back of throat (see illustration).	
(2) Position the device 2 to 4 cm (1 to 2 inches) in front of the mouth (see illustration).	Directs aerosol spray toward airway. Positioning the mouthpiece in front of mouth is the best way to deliver the medication.
f. With the inhaler properly positioned, have client hold inhaler with thumb at the mouthpiece and the index finger and middle finger at the top. This is called a three-point or lateral hand position.	MDIs work best when clients use a three-point or lateral hand position to activate canisters.
g. Instruct client to tilt head back slightly, inhale slowly and deeply through mouth for 3 to 5 seconds while depressing canister fully.	Distributes medication to airways during inhalation. Inhalation through mouth rather than nose draws medication more effectively into airways.
h. Hold breath for approximately 10 seconds.	Allows tiny drops of aerosol spray to reach deeper branches of airways.
i. Remove MDI from mouth and exhale through pursed lips.	Keeps small airways open during exhalation.
18. Explain steps to administer MDI using a spacer such as an Aerochamber (demonstrate when possible):	
a. Remove mouthpiece cover from MDI and mouthpiece of spacer. Inspect spacer for foreign objects, and ensure valve is intact if spacer has one.	Inhaler fits into end of spacer.
b. Insert MDI into end of spacer.	Spacer traps medication released from the MDI; the client then inhales the drug from the device. These devices break up and slow down the medication particles, enhancing the amount of medication received by client (Vella and Grech, 2005).
c. Shake inhaler vigorously five or six times.	Ensures fine particles are aerosolized.
d. Have client exhale completely before closing mouth around mouthpiece of the spacer. Avoid covering small exhalation slots with the lips (see illustration).	Empties lungs and prepares them for the medication.
e. Have client depress medication canister, spraying one puff into spacer.	Emits spray that allows finer particles to be inhaled. Large droplets are retained in spacer.
f. Instruct client to inhale deeply and slowly through the mouth for 3 to 5 seconds.	Maximizes amount of medication that enters the lung.
g. Have client hold breath for 10 seconds.	Ensures full medication distribution.
h. Remove MDI and spacer before exhaling.	Allows client to exhale normally.

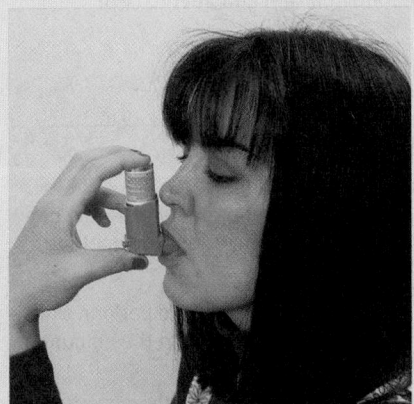

STEP 17e(1) The client opens lips and places inhaler in mouth with opening toward back of throat.

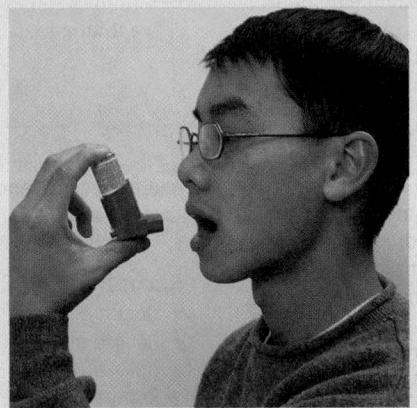

STEP 17e(2) The client positions the mouthpiece 1 to 2 inches away from the mouth. This is the best way to deliver medication.

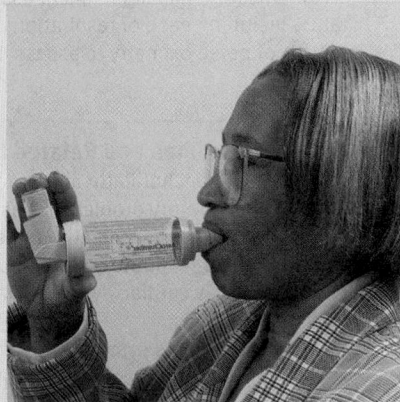

STEP 18d Have the client place mouthpiece in mouth and close lips, being careful to keep exhalation slots exposed.

✳ **SKILL 35-3   USING METERED-DOSE OR DRY POWDER INHALERS—CONT'D**

STEPS	RATIONALE
19. Explain steps to administer DPI or breath-activated MDI (demonstrate when possible):	
a. Remove cover from mouthpiece. Do not shake the inhaler.	
b. Prepare the medication as directed by manufacturer (e.g., hold inhaler upright and turn wheel to the right and then to the left until a click is heard, load medication pellet, etc.).	Primes inhaler, ensuring medication will be delivered to client (Capriotti, 2005).
c. Exhale away from inhaler before inhalation.	Prevents loss of powder.
d. Position mouthpiece between the lips.	Prevents medication from escaping through mouth.
e. Inhale deeply and forcefully through the mouth. Creates aerosol.	
f. Hold breath for 5 to 10 seconds.	Ensures full medication distribution.
20. Instruct client to wait at least 20 to 30 seconds between inhalations of the same medication and 2 to 5 minutes between inhalations or as ordered by prescriber.	Medications must be inhaled sequentially. First inhalation opens airways and reduces inflammation. Second or third inhalation penetrates deeper airways.
21. Instruct client against repeating inhalations before next scheduled dose.	Medications are prescribed at intervals during day to provide constant drug levels and minimize side effects. Beta-adrenergic MDIs are used either on an "as needed" basis or regularly every 4 to 6 hours.
22. Explain that client may feel gagging sensation in throat caused by droplets of medication on pharynx or tongue.	Results when inhalant is sprayed and inhaled incorrectly.

Critical Decision Point: If client uses a corticosteroid, have client rinse mouth out with water or salt water or brush teeth after inhalation to reduce risk of fungal infection. Also teach client to inspect oral cavity daily for redness, sores, or white patches. Report abnormal assessment findings to the client's health care provider (Capriotti, 2005).

23. Instruct client how to clean inhaler:	
a. Once a day, inhaler and cap need to be rinsed in warm running water. Inhaler needs to be completely dry before using.	Accumulation of spray around mouthpiece interferes with proper distribution during use.
b. Twice a week, the L-shaped plastic mouthpiece needs to be washed with mild dishwashing soap and warm water. Rinse and dry well before putting canister back inside mouthpiece.	Removes residual medication. Do not place inhalers holding cromolyn, nedocromil, or HFA in water.
24. Ask if client has any questions.	Clarifies misconceptions or misunderstanding.
25. Have client explain and demonstrate steps in use of inhaler.	Return demonstration provides feedback for measuring client's learning.
26. Ask client to explain medication schedule, side effects, and when to call health care provider.	Improves likelihood of adherence to therapy.
27. Ask client to calculate how many days the inhaler will last.	Helps client determine when to reorder prescription.
28. After medication has been taken, assess client's respiratory status, including ease of respirations, auscultation of lungs, and use of pulse oximetry to assess client's oxygenation status.	Determines status of breathing pattern and adequacy of ventilation.

Unexpected Outcomes and Related Interventions

1. Client needs a bronchodilator more than every 4 hours.
   a. Indicates respiratory problems; reassessment of type of medication and delivery methods needed; notify health care provider if respiratory status does not improve.
2. Client experiences cardiac dysrhythmias, especially if receiving beta-adrenergics.
   a. If client experiences symptoms with the dysrhythmias (e.g., light-headedness, syncope), withhold all further doses of medication and notify prescriber.
3. Client is not able to self-administer medication properly.
   a. Explore alternative delivery routes or methods of medication administration.

4. Client experiences paroxysms of coughing.
   a. Aerosolized particles irritate posterior pharynx. Notify prescriber. Reassess type of medication or delivery method.

Recording and Reporting
- Document skills taught and the client's ability to perform skills.
- Record medication, time of administration, and the amount of puffs on the MAR.
- Report any undesirable effects from medication.

Home Care Considerations
- Remind clients to carry their prescribed inhalers to use emergently in case of an acute asthma attack.

Administering Medications by Irrigations

Some medications irrigate or wash out a body cavity and are delivered through a stream of solution. Irrigations most commonly use sterile water, saline, or antiseptic solutions on the eye, ear, throat, vagina, and urinary tract. Use aseptic technique if there is a break in the skin or mucosa. When the cavity to be irrigated is not sterile, as in the case of the ear canal (see Box 35-19, p. 728) or vagina (see Box 35-20, p. 730), use clean technique. Irrigations cleanse an area, instill a medication, or apply hot or cold to injured tissue.

Parenteral Administration of Medications

Parenteral administration of medications is the administration of medications by injection. When medications are administered this way, it is an invasive procedure that is performed using aseptic techniques (Box 35-22). After a needle pierces the skin, there is risk of infection. Each type of injection requires certain skills to ensure that the medication reaches the proper location. The effects of a parenterally administered medication develop rapidly, depending on the rate of medication absorption. The nurse closely observes the client's response.

Equipment. A variety of syringes and needles are available, each designed to deliver a certain volume of a medication to a specific type of tissue. Use nursing judgment when determining the syringe or needle that will be most effective.

Syringes. Syringes consist of a cylindrical barrel with a tip designed to fit the hub of a hypodermic needle and a close-fitting plunger. Syringes, in general, are classified as being Luer-Lok or non–Luer-Lok. This nomenclature is based on the design of the syringe's tip. Luer-Lok syringes (Figure 35-14, A) require special needles, which are twisted onto the tip and lock themselves in place. This design prevents the inadvertent removal of the needle. Non–Luer-Lok syringes (Figure 35-14, B-D) require needles that slip onto the tip. In the clinical setting, all syringes have safety devices to prevent needle-stick injury.

The nurse fills a syringe by pulling the plunger outward while the needle tip remains immersed in the prepared solution. The nurse can touch the outside of the syringe barrel and the handle

of the plunger, but to maintain sterility, the nurse avoids letting any unsterile object touch the tip or inside of the barrel, the hub, the shaft of the plunger, or the needle (Figure 35-15).

Syringes come in a number of sizes, from 0.5 to 60 mL. It is unusual to use a syringe larger than 5 mL for an injection. A 1- to 3-mL syringe is usually adequate for a subcutaneous or intramuscular injection. A larger volume creates discomfort. Use larger syringes to administer certain intravenous medications, add medications to intravenous solutions, and irrigate wounds or drainage tubes. Syringes often come prepackaged with a needle attached. However, the nurse sometimes changes the needle based on the route of administration and size of the client.

Insulin syringes (see Figure 35-14, C and D) are available in sizes that hold 0.3 to 1 mL and are calibrated in units. Most insulin syringes are U-100s, designed to be used with U-100 strength insulin. Each milliliter of U-100 insulin contains 100 units of insulin.

The tuberculin syringe (see Figure 35-14, B) is calibrated in sixteenths of a minim and hundredths of a milliliter and has a

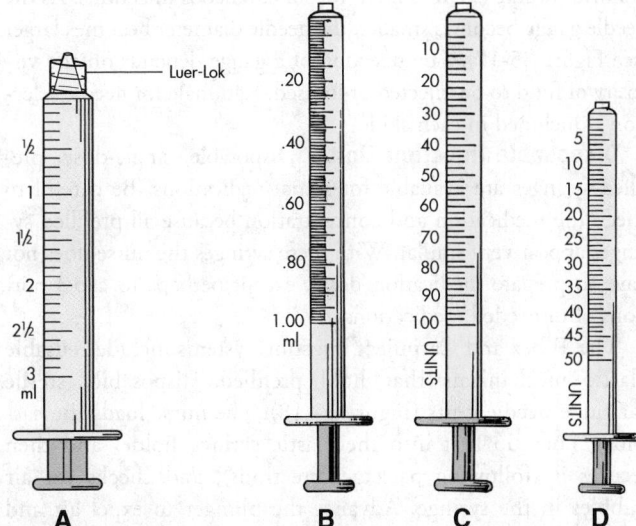

Figure 35-14 Types of syringes. **A,** Luer-Lok syringe marked in 0.1 (tenths). **B,** Tuberculin syringe marked in 0.01 (hundredths) for doses less than 1 mL. **C,** Insulin syringe marked in units (100). **D,** Insulin syringe marked in units (50).

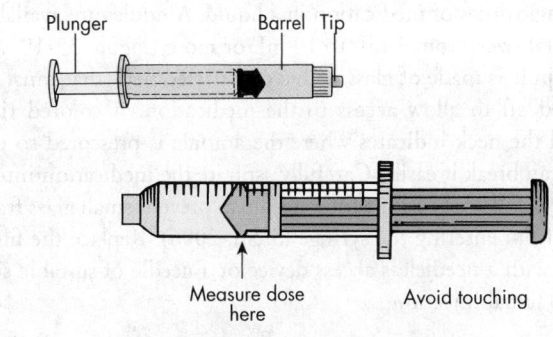

Figure 35-15 Parts of a syringe.

※ BOX 35-22 Preventing Infection During an Injection

- To prevent contamination of solution, draw medication from ampule quickly. Do not allow it to stand open.
- To prevent needle contamination, avoid letting needle touch contaminated surface (e.g., outer edges of ampule or vial, outer surface of needle cap, nurse's hands, countertop, table surface).
- To prevent syringe contamination, avoid touching length of plunger or inner part of barrel. Keep tip of syringe covered with cap or needle.
- To prepare skin, wash skin soiled with dirt, drainage, or feces with soap and water and dry. Use friction and a circular motion while cleaning with an antiseptic swab. Swab from center of site, and move outward in a 2-inch radius.

capacity of 1 mL. Use a tuberculin syringe to prepare small amounts of medications (e.g., intradermal or subcutaneous injections). A tuberculin syringe is also useful when preparing small precise doses for infants or young children.

Needles. Needles come packaged in individual sheaths to allow flexibility in choosing the right needle for a client. Some needles are preattached to standard-size syringes. Most needles are made of stainless steel, and all are disposable.

The needle has three parts: the hub, which fits onto the tip of a syringe; the shaft, which connects to the hub; and the bevel, or slanted tip (Figure 35-16). The tip of a needle, or the bevel, is always slanted. The bevel creates a narrow slit when injected into tissue. This slit quickly closes when the needle is removed to prevent leakage of medication, blood, or serum. Long beveled tips are sharper and narrower, which minimizes discomfort when entering tissue used for subcutaneous or IM injections.

Needles vary in length from ¼ to 3 inches (Figure 35-17). Choose the needle length according to the client's size and weight and the type of tissue into which the medication is to be injected. A child or slender adult generally requires a shorter needle. Use longer needles (1 to 1½ inches) for intramuscular injections and a shorter needle (⅜ to ⅝ inch) for subcutaneous injections. As the needle gauge becomes smaller, the needle diameter becomes larger (see Figure 35-17). The selection of a gauge depends on the viscosity of fluid to be injected or infused. Rationale for needle selection is included in each skill.

Disposable Injection Units. Disposable, single-dose, prefilled syringes are available for some medications. Be careful to check the medication and concentration because all prefilled syringes appear very similar. With these syringes the nurse does not have to prepare medication doses, except perhaps to expel portions of unneeded medications.

The Tubex and Carpuject injection systems include reusable plastic mechanisms that hold prefilled, disposable, sterile cartridge-needle units (Figure 35-18). The nurse loads the cartridge Luer tip first into the plastic syringe holder and then secures it (following package directions), and checks for air bubbles in the syringe. Advance the plunger to expel air and excess medication as in a regular syringe. The glass cartridge can be used with needleless systems or safety needles. After giving the medication, safely dispose of the glass cartridge in a puncture-proof and leakproof receptacle. This design reduces the risk of needle-stick injuries.

Preparing an Injection From an Ampule.
Ampules contain single doses of medication in a liquid. Ampules are available in several sizes, from 1 mL to 10 mL or more (Figure 35-19, *A*). An ampule is made of glass with a constricted neck that must be snapped off to allow access to the medication. A colored ring around the neck indicates where the ampule is prescored so the nurse can break it easily. Carefully aspirate the medication into a syringe (Skill 35-4) with a filter needle to prevent small glass fragments from entering the syringe (Stein, 2006). Replace the filter needle with a needleless access device or a needle of suitable size for the actual injection.

Preparing an Injection From a Vial.
A vial is a single-dose or multidose container with a rubber seal at the top (see Figure

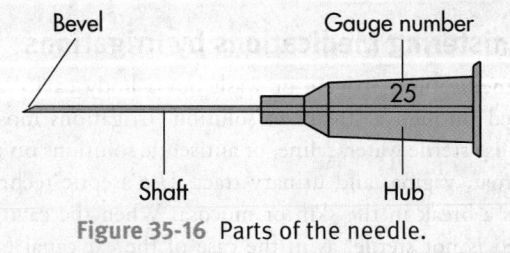

Figure 35-16 Parts of the needle.

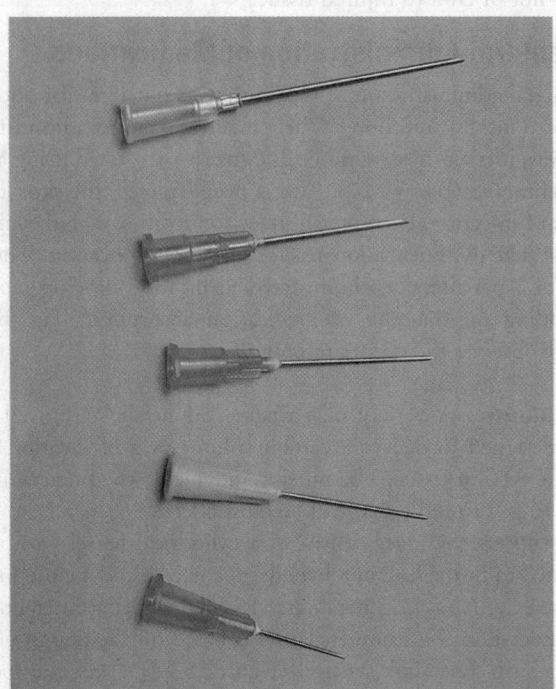

Figure 35-17 Needles. *Top to bottom:* 19 gauge, 1½-inch length; 20 gauge, 1-inch length; 21 gauge, 1-inch length; 23 gauge, 1-inch length; and 25 gauge, ⅝-inch length.

35-19, *B*). A metal cap protects the seal until it is ready for use. Vials contain liquid or dry forms of medications. Medications that are unstable in solution are packaged dry. The vial label specifies the solvent or diluent used to dissolve the medication and the amount of diluent needed to prepare a desired medication concentration. Normal saline and sterile distilled water are solutions commonly used to dissolve medications.

Unlike the ampule, the vial is a closed system, and air needs to be injected into it to permit easy withdrawal of the solution. Failure to inject air when withdrawing creates a vacuum within the vial that makes withdrawal difficult (see Skill 35-4). If concerned about drawing up parts of the rubber stopper or other particles into the syringe, use a filter needle when preparing medications from vials (Nicoll and Hesby, 2002).

To prepare a powdered medication, draw up the amount of diluent or solvent recommended on the vial's label. Then inject the diluent into the vial in the same manner as injecting air into the vial. Most powdered medications dissolve easily, but it is necessary to withdraw the needle to mix the contents thoroughly.

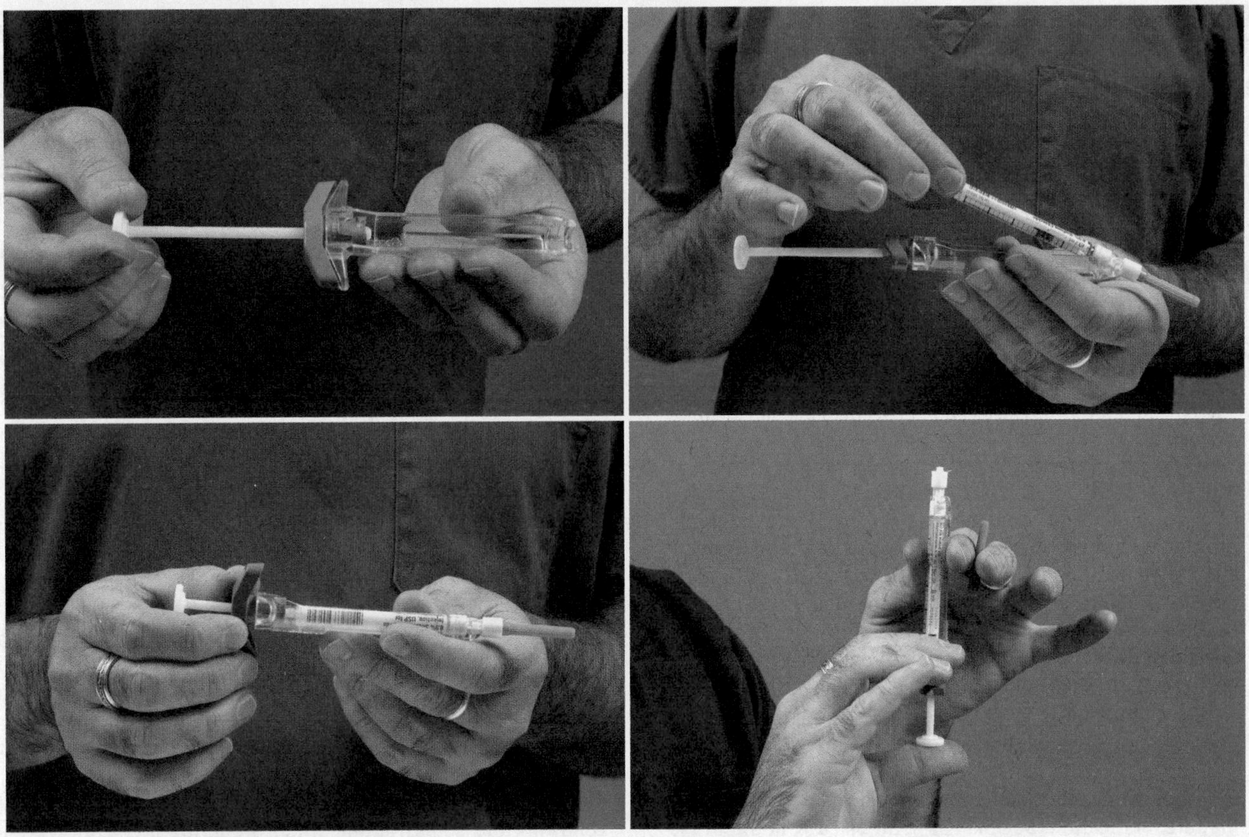

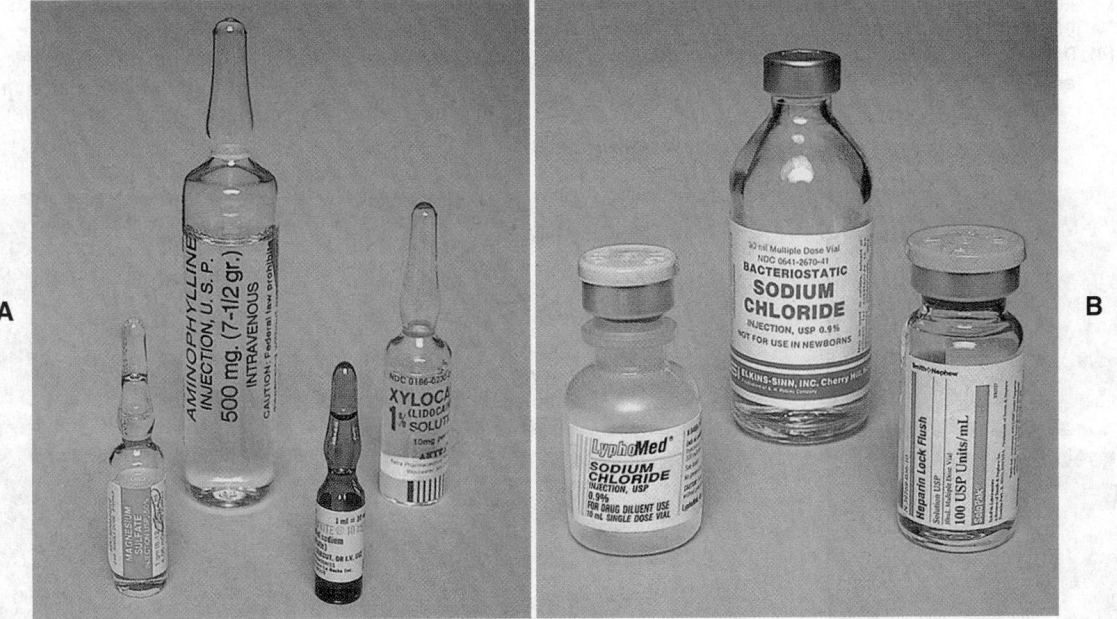

Figure 35-18 **A,** Carpuject syringe and prefilled sterile cartridge with needle. **B,** Assembling the Carpuject. **C,** The cartridge slides into the syringe barrel, turns, and locks at the needle end. The plunger then screws into the cartridge end. **D,** Expel excess medication to obtain accurate dose.

Figure 35-19 **A,** Medication in ampules. **B,** Medication in vials.

✳ **SKILL 35-4**   **PREPARING INJECTIONS**   Video

Delegation Considerations
The skill of preparing injections cannot be delegated.

Equipment
- Medication in an ampule
  - Safety syringe, needle, and filter needle
  - Small gauze pad or unopened alcohol swab
- Medication in a vial
  - Safety syringe
  - Needles:
    —Blunt tip vial access cannula (if needleless system used)
    —Filter needle (if indicated)
    —Needle for drawing up medication (if needed) and needle for injection

- Small gauze pad or alcohol swab
- Diluent (e.g., normal saline or sterile water) (if indicated)
- Both
  - Medication in vial or ampule
  - MAR or computer printout

STEPS	RATIONALE
1. Check accuracy and completeness of each MAR or computer printout with prescriber's original medication order. Check client's name and medication name, dosage, route, and time for administration. Recopy or re-print any portion of MAR that is difficult to read.	The order sheet is the most reliable source and only legal record of medications client is to receive. Ensures client receives the correct medications. Illegible MARs are a source of medication errors.
2. Review pertinent information related to medication, including action, purpose, side effects, and nursing implications.	Allows nurse to administer medication properly and to monitor client's response.
3. Assess client's body build, muscle size, and weight.	Determines type and size of syringe and needles for injection.
4. Perform hand hygiene, and assemble supplies.	Reduces transmission of microorganisms and saves nurse's time.
5. Check date of expiration for medication vial or ampule.	Medication potency increases or decreases when outdated.
6. Prepare medication: See Skill 35-1, Steps 7a-g, m-o, pp. 719 to 721. Be sure to compare the label of the medication with the MAR two times while preparing the medication.	Following the same routine when preparing medications, eliminating distractions, and checking the label of the medication with transcribed order reduce error (Pape and others, 2005).
A. Ampule preparation	
(1) Tap top of ampule lightly and quickly with finger until fluid moves from neck of ampule (see illustration).	Dislodges any fluid that collects above neck of ampule. All solution moves into lower chamber.
(2) Place small gauze pad or unopened alcohol swab just above neck of ampule (see illustration).	Placing pad around neck of ampule protects nurse's fingers from trauma as glass tip is broken off.
(3) Snap neck of ampule quickly and firmly away from hands (see illustration).	Protects nurse's fingers and face from shattering glass.
(4) Draw up medication quickly, using filter needle long enough to reach bottom of ampule.	System is open to airborne contaminants. Needle needs to be long enough to access medication for preparation. Filter needles filter out any fragments of glass (Stein, 2006).

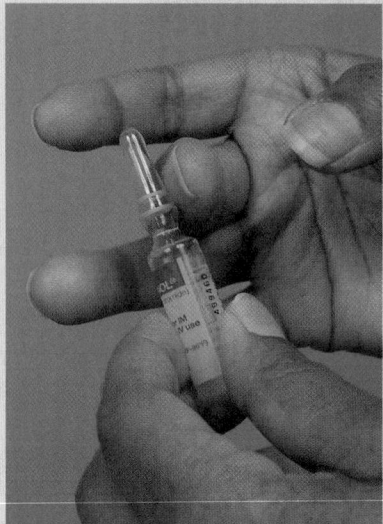

STEP 6A(1) Tapping ampule moves fluid down neck.

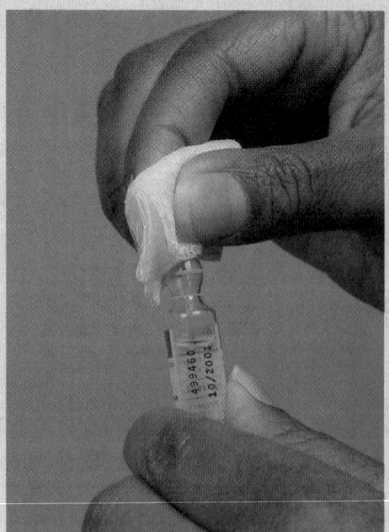

STEP 6A(2) Gauze pad placed just above neck of ampule.

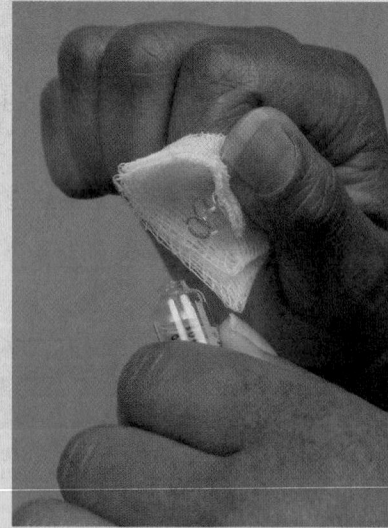

STEP 6A(3) Snapping neck away from hands.

※ **SKILL 35-4**   PREPARING INJECTIONS—CONT'D

STEPS

(5) Hold ampule upside down, or set it on a flat surface. Insert filter needle into center of ampule opening. Do not allow needle tip or shaft to touch rim of ampule.

(6) Aspirate medication into syringe by gently pulling back on plunger (see illustrations).

(7) Keep needle tip under surface of liquid. Tip ampule to bring all fluid within reach of the needle.

(8) If air bubbles are aspirated, do not expel air into ampule.

(9) To expel excess air bubbles, remove needle from ampule. Hold syringe with needle pointing up. Tap side of syringe to cause bubbles to rise toward needle. Draw back slightly on plunger, and then push plunger upward to eject air. Do not eject fluid.

(10) If syringe contains excess fluid, use sink for disposal. Hold syringe vertically with needle tip up and slanted slightly toward sink. Slowly eject excess fluid into sink. Recheck fluid level in syringe by holding it vertically.

(11) Cover needle with its safety sheath or scoop needle to recap. Replace filter needle with needle or needleless access device for injection.

B. Vial containing a solution

(1) Remove cap covering top of unused vial to expose sterile rubber seal, keeping rubber seal sterile. If a multidose vial has been used before, cap is already removed. Firmly and briskly wipe surface of rubber seal with alcohol swab, and allow it to dry.

(2) Pick up syringe, and remove needle cap or cap covering needleless vial access device (see illustration). Pull back on plunger to draw amount of air into syringe equivalent to volume of medication to be aspirated from vial.

RATIONALE

Broken rim of ampule is considered contaminated. When ampule is inverted, solution comes out if needle tip or shaft touches rim of ampule.

Withdrawal of plunger creates negative pressure within syringe barrel, which pulls fluid into syringe.

Prevents aspiration of air bubbles.

Air pressure forces fluid out of ampule and medication will be lost.

Withdrawing plunger too far will remove it from barrel. Holding syringe vertically allows fluid to settle in bottom of barrel. Pulling back on plunger allows fluid within needle to enter barrel so fluid is not expelled. Air at top of barrel and within needle is then expelled.

Medication is safely dispersed into sink. Position of needle allows medication to be expelled without flowing down needle shaft. Rechecking fluid level ensures proper dose.

Prevents contamination of needle. Filter needles cannot be used for injection.

Vial comes packaged with seal that cannot be replaced after cap removal. Not all drug manufacturers guarantee that caps of unused vials are sterile. Therefore swab seals with alcohol before preparing medication. Allowing alcohol to dry prevents needle from being coated with alcohol and mixing with medication.

Inject air first into vial to prevent buildup of negative pressure in vial when aspirating medication.

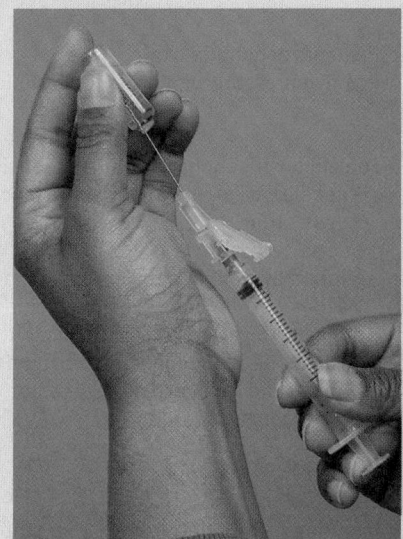
A

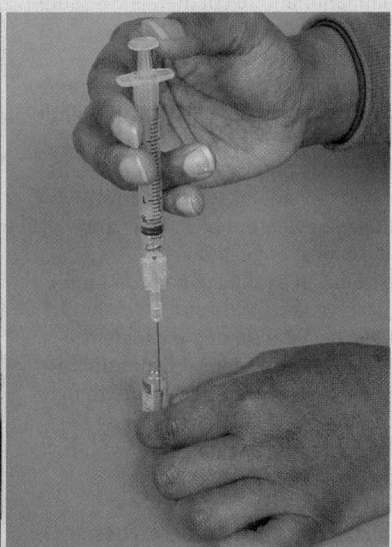
B

STEP 6A(6) A, Medication aspirated with ampule inverted. **B,** Medication aspirated with ampule on flat surface.

Continued

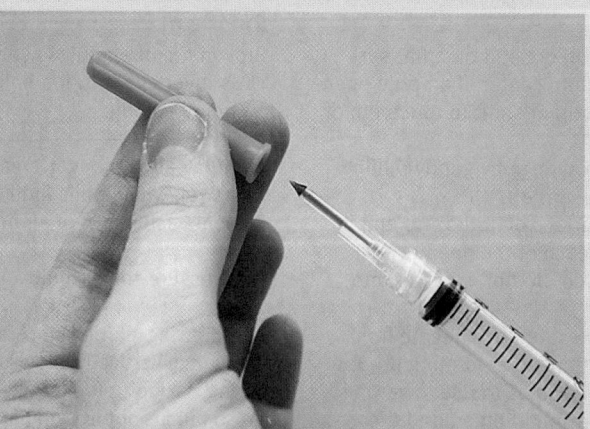

STEP 6B(2) Syringe with needleless adapter.

STEPS	RATIONALE

Critical Decision Point: Some medications and some institutions require use of a filter needle when preparing medications from a vial. Check agency policy to determine if use of filter needle is indicated (Nicoll and Hesby, 2002). If using a filter needle to aspirate the medication, it is then changed to a regular needle of suitable size to administer the medication.

(3) With vial on flat surface, insert tip of needle with beveled tip entering first through center of rubber seal. Apply pressure to tip of needle during insertion.	Center of seal is thinner and easier to penetrate. Injecting beveled tip first and using firm pressure prevent coring of rubber seal, which could enter vial or needle.
(4) Inject air into the vial's airspace, holding on to plunger. Hold plunger with firm pressure; air pressure within the vial sometimes forces the plunger backward.	Injecting air before aspirating fluid creates vacuum needed to get medication to flow into syringe. Injecting into vial's airspace prevents formation of bubbles and inaccuracy in dose.
(5) Invert vial while keeping firm hold on syringe and plunger (see illustration). Hold vial between thumb and middle fingers of nondominant hand. Grasp end of syringe barrel and plunger with thumb and forefinger of dominant hand to counteract pressure in vial.	Inverting vial allows fluid to settle in lower half of container. Position of hands prevents forceful movement of plunger and permits easy manipulation of syringe.
(6) Keep tip of needle below fluid level.	Prevents aspiration of air.
(7) Allow air pressure from the vial to fill syringe gradually with medication. If necessary, pull back slightly on plunger to obtain correct amount of solution.	Positive pressure within vial forces fluid into syringe.
(8) When desired volume is obtained, position needle into vial's airspace; tap side of syringe barrel carefully to dislodge any air bubbles. Eject any air remaining at top of syringe into vial.	Forcefully striking barrel while needle is inserted in vial will bend needle. Accumulation of air displaces medication and causes dose errors.
(9) Remove needle from vial by pulling back on barrel of syringe.	Accidentally pulling plunger rather than barrel causes plunger to separate from barrel, resulting in loss of medication.
(10) Hold syringe at eye level, at 90-degree angle, to ensure correct volume and absence of air bubbles. Remove any remaining air by tapping barrel to dislodge any air bubbles (see illustration). Draw back slightly on plunger; then push plunger upward to eject air. Do not eject fluid. Recheck volume of medication.	Holding syringe vertically allows fluid to settle in bottom of barrel. Pulling back on plunger allows fluid within needle to enter barrel so fluid is not expelled. Air at top of barrel and within needle is then expelled.
(11) If medication will be injected into client's tissue, change needle to appropriate gauge and length according to route of medication.	Inserting needle through a rubber stopper dulls beveled tip. New needle is sharper. Because no fluid is along shaft, needle will not track medication through tissues.
(12) For multidose vial, make label that includes date of mixing, concentration of medication per milliliter, and your initials.	Ensures that future doses will be prepared correctly. Some medications need to be discarded after certain number of days after mixing of vial.

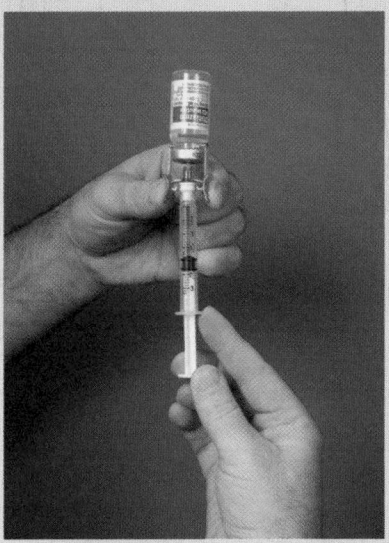

STEP 6B(5) Withdraw fluid with vial inverted.

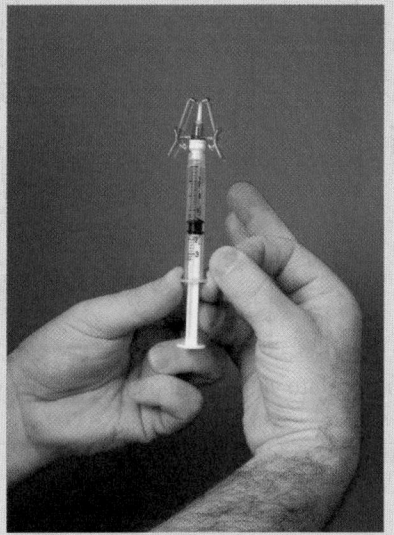

STEP 6B(10) Hold syringe upright; tap barrel to dislodge air bubbles.

STEPS	RATIONALE
C. Vial containing a powder (reconstituting medications)	
(1) Remove cap covering vial of powdered medication and cap covering vial of proper diluent. Firmly swab both seals with alcohol swab, and allow to dry.	Not all drug manufacturers guarantee that caps of unused vials are sterile. Therefore seals must be swabbed with alcohol before preparing medication. Allowing alcohol to dry prevents needle from being coated with alcohol and mixing with medication.
(2) Draw up diluent into syringe following Steps 6 B(2)-(10).	Prepares diluent for injection into vial containing powdered medication.
(3) Insert tip of needle through center of rubber seal of vial of powdered medication. Inject diluent into vial. Remove needle.	Diluent begins to dissolve and reconstitute medication.
(4) Mix medication thoroughly. Roll in palms. Do not shake.	Ensures proper dispersal of medication throughout solution. Shaking produces bubbles.
(5) Reconstituted medication in vial is ready to be drawn into new syringe. Read label carefully to determine dose after reconstitution.	Once diluent is added, concentration of medication (mg/mL) determines dose to be given.
(6) Prepare medication in syringe following Steps 6B(2)-(12).	

Critical Decision Point: Some institutions require prepared parenteral medications to be verified for accuracy by another nurse. Check institutional policies before administering medication.

---

7. Dispose of soiled supplies. Place broken ampule and/or used vials and used needle in puncture-proof and leakproof container. Clean work area, and perform hand hygiene.	Proper disposal of glass and needle prevents accidental injury to staff. Controls transmission of infection.

Unexpected Outcomes and Related Interventions

1. Air bubbles remain in syringe.
   a. Expel air from syringe, and add medication to syringe until correct dose is prepared.

2. Incorrect dose is prepared.
   a. Discard prepared dose, and prepare corrected new dose.

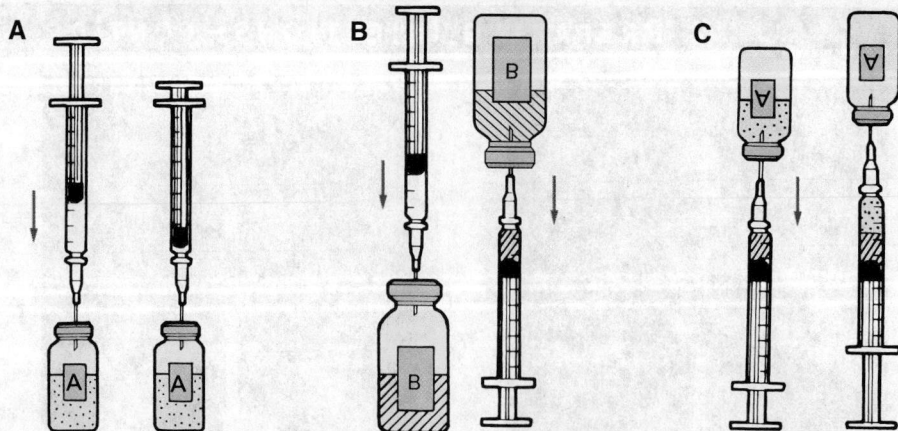

Figure 35-20 A, Injecting air into vial A. **B,** Injecting air into vial B and withdrawing dose. **C,** Withdrawing medication from vial A; medications are now mixed.

Gently rolling the vial between the hands will dissolve the powdered medication. Then reinsert the needle to draw up the dissolved medication. After mixing multidose vials, make a label that includes the date and time of mixing and the concentration of medication per milliliter. Some multidose vials require refrigeration after the contents are reconstituted.

Mixing Medications. If two medications are compatible, it is possible to mix them in one injection if the total dose is within accepted limits so that a client will not have to receive more than one injection at a time. Most nursing units have charts that list common compatible medications. If there is any uncertainty about medication compatibilities, consult a pharmacist.

Mixing Medications From a Vial and an Ampule. When mixing medication from both a vial and ampule, prepare medication from the vial first. Then, using the same syringe and filter needle, withdraw medication from the ampule. Nurses prepare the combination in this order because it is not necessary to add air to withdraw medication from an ampule.

Mixing Medications From Two Vials. The nurse applies these principles when mixing medications from two vials:

1. Do not contaminate one medication with another.
2. Ensure the final dose is accurate.
3. Maintain aseptic technique.

The nurse uses only one syringe with a needle or needleless access device attached to mix medications from two vials (Figure 35-20). Aspirate the volume of air equivalent to the first medication's dose (vial A). Inject the air into vial A, making sure the needle does not touch the solution. Withdraw the needle, aspirating air equivalent to the second medication's dose (vial B), and inject the volume of air into vial B. Immediately withdraw the medication from vial B into the syringe then insert the needle back into vial A, being careful not to push the plunger and expel the medication within the syringe into the vial. Withdraw the desired amount of medication from vial A into the syringe. After withdrawing the necessary amount, withdraw the needle and apply a new needle or needleless access device suitable for injection.

✳ BOX 35-23 Case Study

Mr. Dodds has severe insulin resistance and requires an unusually high regular insulin dosage to control his blood glucose levels. Currently he needs 250 units of regular insulin a day to maintain his blood glucose levels. The diabetes clinical nurse specialist (CNS) decides to switch Mr. Dodds from U-100 to U-500 insulin. The concentration of U-500 insulin is 500 units per 1 mL. To determine how much U-500 insulin Mr. Dodds needs, the CNS uses the following equation:

$$\frac{\text{Dose ordered}}{\text{Dose on hand}} \times \text{Amount on hand} = \text{Amount to administer}$$

The CNS then completes the following calculation:

$$\frac{250 \text{ units of insulin ordered}}{500 \text{ units of insulin on hand}} \times 1 \text{ mL} = 0.5 \text{ mL to administer}$$

Therefore the CNS teaches Mr. Dodds to prepare and administer 0.5 mL of U-500 insulin in a tuberculin syringe daily.

Insulin Preparation. Insulin is the hormone used to treat diabetes. Although inhaled insulin has recently been approved for use, it is still most commonly administered by injection. Most clients with diabetes who take insulin injections learn to administer their own injections. In the United States and Canada, health care providers usually prescribe insulin in concentrations of 100 units per milliliter of solution. This is called U-100 insulin. Insulin is also commercially available in concentrations of 500 units per milliliter of solution; it is called U-500 insulin. U-500 insulin is 5 times as strong as U-100 insulin and is used only in rare cases when clients are very resistant to insulin (American Diabetes Association [ADA], 2004).

Use the correct syringe when preparing insulin. Use a 100-unit insulin syringe to prepare U-100 insulin. Because there is no syringe currently designed to prepare U-500 insulin, many medication errors resulted with this kind of insulin. The Institute for Safe Medication Practices (2002) recommends that prescrib-

✳ TABLE 35-10 A Comparison of Insulin Preparations

Type	Onset	Peak	Duration
Rapid- and Short-Acting			
Insulin glulisine (Apidra)	15 min	1 hour	2-3 hours
Insulin lispro (Humalog)	15 min	1 hour	4 hours
Insulin aspart (NovoLog)	30 min	1-3 hours	3-5 hours
Regular insulin*	30 min-1 hour	2-4 hours	5-7 hours
Intermediate-Acting			
Isophane insulin suspension (NPH insulin, Humulin N)	3-4 hours	6-12 hours	18-28 hours
Insulin zinc suspension (Lente insulin)	1-3 hours	8-12 hours	36 hours
Long-Acting			
Extended insulin zinc suspension (Ultralente)	4-6 hours	18-24 hours	36 hours
Insulin glargine (Lantus)†	1-5 hours	Plateau	24 hours
Insulin detemir (Levemir)†	3-4 hours	"Peakless"	24 hours
Combinations			
Isophane human insulin (50%) and regular human insulin (50%) (Humulin 50/50)	30 min	3 hours	22-24 hours
Isophane human insulin (70%) and regular human insulin (30%) (Humulin 70/30, Novolin 70/30)	30 min	4-8 hours	24 hours
Insulin lispro protamine (75%) and insulin lispro (25%) (Humalog Mix 75/25)	15 min	30 min-6 hours	24 hours
Insulin aspart protamine (70%) and insulin aspart (30%) (NovoLog Mix 70/30)	15 min	1-4 hours	24 hours

*Regular insulin is the only insulin for intravenous use; intravenously, the onset of action is within 10 to 30 minutes, the peak effect is within 20 to 30 minutes, and the duration of action is between 30 and 30 minutes.

†Cannot be mixed with other insulins.

Modified from McKenry LM and others: *Mosby's pharmacology in nursing*, ed 22, St. Louis, 2006, Mosby; and Novo Nordisk: *Levemir*, 2007, www.levemir-us.com/hcp/default.asp.

ers specify units and volume (e.g., 150 units, 0.3 mL of U-500 insulin) and that nurses use tuberculin syringes to draw up the doses. Box 35-23 provides an example of how to calculate a dose of U-500 insulin.

Insulin is classified by rate of action, including rapid, short, intermediate, and long acting. Each type has a different onset, peak, and duration of action (Table 35-10). Only regular insulin can be given intravenously. Orders for insulin injections attempt to imitate the normal pattern of a client's insulin release from the pancreas. Some insulins come in a stable premixed solution (e.g., 70/30 insulin is 70% NPH and 30% regular). Clients receiving these insulins avoid the need to mix insulins. A client with diabetes sometimes requires more than one type of insulin. For example, by receiving a short-acting (regular) and an intermediate-acting (NPH) insulin, a client receives more sustained control of blood glucose levels over 24 hours.

Insulin is ordered by a specific dose at select times or by a sliding scale. A sliding scale dictates a certain dose based on the client's blood glucose level (Box 35-24). Usually, rapid or short-acting insulins are ordered for sliding scales. Before drawing up insulin doses, gently roll all cloudy insulin preparations between the palms of the hands to resuspend the insulin (ADA, 2004). Do not shake insulin vials; shaking causes bubbles to form. Bubbles take up space in the syringe and alter the dosage.

If more than one type of insulin is required to manage the client's diabetes, the nurse can mix two different types of insulin into one syringe **if** they are compatible (Box 35-25). If regular and

✳ BOX 35-24 Example of Sliding Scale Insulin Order

Give regular insulin Sub-Q:

2 units for glucose 150 to 200
4 units for glucose 201 to 275
Call for glucose greater than 275

Clinical Scenario: Before lunch, the client's blood glucose level is 201. After referring to the client's sliding scale orders, the nurse administers 4 units of insulin to the client.

American Diabetes Association. From *Diabetes Care* 27:S106-S107. Reprinted with permission from *The American Diabetes Association*.

an intermediate-acting insulin are ordered, prepare the regular insulin first to prevent the regular insulin from becoming contaminated with the intermediate-acting insulin (ADA, 2004). Use the following principles when mixing insulins (ADA, 2004; Novo Nordisk, 2007):

- Clients whose blood glucose levels are well controlled on a mixed-insulin dose need to maintain their individual routine when preparing and administering their insulin.
- Do not mix insulin with any other medications or diluents unless approved by the prescriber.
- Never mix insulin glargine (Lantus) or insulin detemir (Levemir) with other types of insulin.
- Inject rapid-acting insulins mixed with NPH, Lente, or Ultralente insulins within 15 minutes before a meal.

❋ **BOX 35-25**   PROCEDURAL GUIDELINES

Mixing Two Kinds of Insulin in One Syringe

Delegation Considerations: The skill of mixing two kinds of insulin in one syringe cannot be delegated.

Equipment: Insulin vials, insulin syringe, alcohol swabs, medication administration report (MAR) or computer printout.

1. Check accuracy and completeness of each MAR or computer printout with prescriber's original medication order. Check client's name and medication name, dosage, route, and time for administration. Recopy or re-print any portion of MAR that is difficult to read.
2. Carefully verify insulin labels; compare labels against the MAR before preparing the dose to ensure the correct type of insulin is prepared.
3. Perform hand hygiene.
4. If insulin is cloudy, roll the bottle of insulin between the hands to resuspend the insulin preparation.
5. Wipe off tops of both insulin vials with alcohol swabs.
6. Verify insulin dosages against MAR a second time.
7. If mixing rapid- or short-acting insulin with intermediate- or long-acting insulin, take insulin syringe and aspirate volume of air equivalent to the dose of insulin to be withdrawn from intermediate- or long-acting insulin first. If two intermediate- or long-acting insulins are mixed, it makes no difference which vial you prepare first.
8. Insert needle and inject air into vial of intermediate- or long-acting insulin. Do not let the tip of the needle touch the insulin.
9. Remove the syringe from the vial of intermediate- or long-acting insulin without aspirating the insulin.

10. With the same syringe, inject air, equal to the dose of insulin to be withdrawn, into the vial of rapid- or short-acting insulin. Then withdraw the correct dose into the syringe.
11. Remove the syringe from the rapid- or short-acting insulin vial after carefully removing air bubbles in the syringe to ensure correct dose.
12. After verifying insulin dosages with MAR a third time, show insulin prepared in syringe to another nurse to verify correct dosage of insulin was prepared. Then determine which point on syringe scale combined units of insulin measure by adding the number of units of both insulins together (e.g., 3 units regular + 10 units NPH = 13 units total).
13. Place the needle of the syringe back into the vial of intermediate- or long-acting insulin. Be careful not to push plunger and inject insulin in syringe into the vial.
14. Invert vial, and carefully withdraw the desired amount of insulin into the syringe.
15. Withdraw needle, and check fluid level in syringe. Keep needle of prepared syringe sheathed or capped until ready to administer medication. Show another nurse the syringe to verify correct dose was prepared.
16. Dispose of soiled supplies in proper receptacle, and perform hand hygiene.
17. Because rapid- or short-acting insulin binds with intermediate- or long-acting insulin, which reduces the action of the faster-acting insulin, administer mixture within 5 minutes of preparing it.

Modified from American Diabetes Association: Insulin administration: position statement, *Diabetes Care* 27(1S):S106, 2004.

- Do not mix short-acting and Lente insulins unless the client's blood glucose levels are currently under control with this mixture.
- Do not mix phosphate-buffered insulins (e.g., NPH) with Lente insulins.

Administering Injections

Each injection route differs based on the type of tissues the medication enters. The characteristics of the tissues influence the rate of medication absorption and thus the onset of medication action. Before injecting a medication, know the volume of the medication to administer, the medication's characteristics and viscosity, and the location of anatomical structures underlying injection sites (Skill 35-5).

If a nurse does not administer injections correctly, negative client outcomes result. Failure to select an injection site in relation to anatomical landmarks results in nerve or bone damage during needle insertion. Inability to maintain stability of the needle and syringe unit will possibly result in pain and tissue damage. If you fail to aspirate the syringe before injecting an intramuscular medication, the medication will sometimes accidentally be injected directly into an artery or vein. Injecting too large a volume of medication for the site selected causes extreme pain and results in local tissue damage.

Many clients, particularly children, fear injections. Clients with serious or chronic illness often are given several injections daily. Minimize the client's discomfort in the following ways:

- Use a sharp-beveled needle in the smallest suitable length and gauge.
- Position the client as comfortably as possible to reduce muscular tension.
- Select the proper injection site, using anatomical landmarks.
- Divert the client's attention from the injection through conversation using open-ended questioning.
- Insert the needle quickly and smoothly to minimize tissue pulling.
- Hold the syringe steady while the needle remains in tissues.
- Inject the medication slowly and steadily.

Subcutaneous Injections. Subcutaneous injections involve placing medications into the loose connective tissue under the dermis (see Skill 35-5). Because subcutaneous tissue is not as richly supplied with blood as the muscles, medication absorption is somewhat slower than with intramuscular injections. However, medications are absorbed completely if the client's circulatory status is normal. Because subcutaneous tissue contains pain receptors, the client often experiences some discomfort.

Text continued on p. 750

☀ SKILL 35-5 | ADMINISTERING INJECTIONS | Video

Delegation Considerations

The skill of administering injections cannot be delegated. The nurse instructs nursing assistive personnel to report the occurrence of potential medication side effects or any change of the client's vital signs or level of consciousness (e.g., sedation) to the nurse.

Equipment

- Proper size safety syringe and needle:
  - *Sub-Q:* syringe (1 to 3 mL) and needle (27 to 25 gauge, $^3/_8$ to $^5/_8$ inch)
  - *Sub-Q U-100 insulin:* insulin syringe (0.3, 0.5, or 1 mL) with preattached needle (28 to 31 gauge, $^5/_{16}$ to $^1/_2$ inch) (ADA, 2005)
- *IM:* syringe 2 to 3 mL for adult, 0.5 to 1 mL for infants and small children
  - —Needle, length corresponding to site of injection and age of client according to following guidelines (Nicoll and Hesby, 2002):
    - *Children:* $^5/_8$ to $1^1/_4$ inch (based on size of child)
    - *Vastus lateralis (adults):* 1 to $1^1/_2$ inch
    - *Deltoid (adults):* 1 to $1^1/_2$ inch
    - *Ventrogluteal (adults):* $1^1/_2$ inch
- *ID and Sub-Q U-500 insulin:* 1-mL tuberculin syringe with preattached 26- or 27-gauge needle
- Small gauze pad and/or alcohol swab
- Vial or ampule of medication or skin test solution
- Clean gloves
- MAR or computer printout

STEPS	RATIONALE
For All Injections	
1. Check accuracy and completeness of each MAR or computer printout with prescriber's original medication order. Check client's name and medication name, dosage, route, and time for administration. Recopy or re-print any portion of MAR that is difficult to read.	The order sheet is the most reliable source and only legal record of medications client is to receive. Ensures client receives the correct medications. Illegible MARs are a source of medication errors.
2. Assess client's medical and medication history.	Reveals need for medication.
3. Assess client's history of allergies; know substances client is allergic to and normal allergic reaction. Certain substances have similar compositions; do not administer any substance to which client is known to be allergic.	Allows for early identification of client risk. May require different medication prescription.
4. Check date of expiration for medication.	Drug potency increases or decreases when outdated.
5. Observe verbal and nonverbal responses toward receiving injection.	Injections are often painful. Some clients have anxiety, which increases pain.
6. Assess for contraindications.	
A. For subcutaneous injections	
(1) Assess for factors such as circulatory shock or reduced local tissue perfusion. Assess adequacy of client's adipose tissue.	Reduced tissue perfusion interferes with medication absorption and distribution. Physiological changes of aging or client illness often influence the amount of subcutaneous tissue a client possesses. This influences methods for administering injections.
B. For intramuscular injections	
(1) Assess for factors such as muscle atrophy, reduced blood flow, or circulatory shock.	Atrophied muscle absorbs medication poorly. Factors interfering with blood flow to muscles impair medication absorption.

Critical Decision Point: Because of documented adverse effects of IM injections, other routes of medication administration are safer. Verify that IM injection is necessary, and explore alternative medication routes if possible (Nicoll and Hesby, 2002; World Health Organization [WHO], 2005).

---

7. Aseptically prepare correct medication dose from ampule or vial (see Skill 35-4, p. 738). Check label of medication with the MAR two times while preparing medication.	Ensures that medication is sterile. Preparation techniques differ for ampule and vial. Ensures right medication is prepared for the right client.
8. Take medication to client at right time, and perform hand hygiene.	Ensures client receives effect of medication at right time and reduces transfer of microorganisms.
9. Close room curtain or door.	Provides privacy.
10. Identify client using at least two client identifiers. Compare client's name and one other identifier (e.g., hospital identification number) on MAR, computer printout, or computer screen with information on client's identification bracelet. Ask client to state name if possible for a third identifier.	Complies with TJC (2008) requirements and improves medication safety. In most acute care settings, client's name and identification number on armband and MAR are used to identify clients. Identification bracelets are made at time of client's admission and are most reliable source of identification. Client's room number is **not** an acceptable identifier.
11. Compare the label of the medication with the MAR one more time at the client's bedside.	Final check of medication labels against MAR at client's bedside reduces medication administration errors.
12. Explain steps of procedure, and tell client injection will cause a slight burning or will sting.	Helps minimize client's anxiety.
13. Apply clean gloves.	Reduces transfer of microorganisms.

Continued

✳ **SKILL 35-5**   **ADMINISTERING INJECTIONS—CONT'D**

STEPS	RATIONALE
14. Keep sheet or gown draped over body parts not requiring exposure.	Respects dignity of client while area to be injected is exposed.
15. Select appropriate injection site. Inspect skin surface over sites for bruises, inflammation, or edema.	Injection sites need to be free of abnormalities that will interfere with medication absorption. Sites used repeatedly become hardened from lipohypertrophy (increased growth in fatty tissue). Do not use an area that is bruised or has signs associated with infection.
a. *Sub-Q:* Palpate sites for masses or tenderness. Avoid these areas. For daily insulin, rotate site daily. Be sure needle is correct size by grasping skinfold at site with thumb and forefinger. Measure fold from top to bottom. Needle should be one-half length.	Sub-Q injections are sometimes mistakenly given in the muscle, especially in the abdomen and thigh sites (Annersten and Willman, 2005). Appropriate size of needle and angle of injection ensures medication is injected in the subcutaneous tissue.
b. *IM:* Note integrity and size of muscle, and palpate for tenderness or hardness. Avoid these areas. If injections are given frequently, rotate sites. Use ventrogluteal site if possible.	The ventrogluteal site is the preferred site for adults and children, including infants (Cook and Murtagh, 2006; Hockenberry and Wilson, 2007; Nicoll and Hesby, 2002; Small, 2004).
c. *ID:* Note lesions or discolorations of forearm. Select site three to four finger widths below antecubital space and a hand width above wrist. If you cannot use the forearm, inspect the upper back. If necessary, use sites for Sub-Q injections.	An ID site needs to be clear so that you can see results of skin test and interpret them correctly (Centers for Disease Control and Prevention [CDC], 2007).
16. Assist client to comfortable position:	
a. *Sub-Q:* Have client relax arm, leg, or abdomen, depending on site chosen for injection.	Relaxation of site minimizes discomfort.
b. *IM:* Position client depending on site chosen (e.g., sit or lie flat, on side, or prone).	Reduces strain on muscle and minimizes discomfort of injections.
c. *ID:* Have client extend elbow and support it and forearm on flat surface.	Stabilizes injection site for easiest accessibility.
d. Have client talk about subject of interest. Ask open-ended questions.	Distraction reduces anxiety.

Critical Decision Point: Ensure that client's position is not contraindicated by medical condition.

---

17. Relocate site using anatomical landmarks.	Injection into correct anatomical site prevents injury to nerves, bones, and blood vessels.
18. Cleanse site with an antiseptic swab. Apply swab at center of the site, and rotate outward in a circular direction for about 5 cm (2 inches) (see illustration).	Mechanical action of swab removes secretions containing microorganisms.

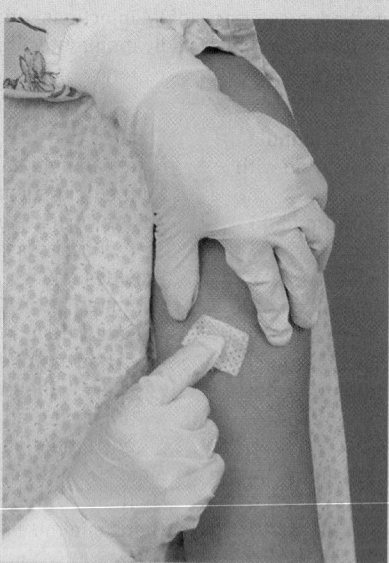

STEP 18 Cleanse site with circular motion.

✳ **SKILL 35-5**   **ADMINISTERING INJECTIONS—CONT'D**

STEPS	RATIONALE
19. Hold swab or gauze between third and fourth fingers of non-dominant hand.	Gauze or swab remains readily accessible when needle is withdrawn.
20. Remove needle cap or sheath from needle by pulling it straight off.	Preventing needle from touching sides of cap prevents contamination.
21. Hold syringe between thumb and forefinger of dominant hand	
a. *Sub-Q:* Hold as dart, palm down, or hold syringe across tops of fingertips (see illustration).	Quick, smooth injection requires proper manipulation of syringe parts.
b. *IM:* Hold as dart, palm down.	
c. *ID:* Hold bevel of needle pointing up.	With bevel up, medication is less likely to be deposited into tissues below dermis.
22. Administer injection:	
A. Subcutaneous	
(1) For average-size client, spread skin tightly across injection site or pinch skin with nondominant hand.	Needle penetrates tight skin more easily than loose skin. Pinching skin elevates subcutaneous tissue and desensitizes area.
(2) Inject needle quickly and firmly at 45- to 90-degree angle. Then release skin, if pinched.	Quick, firm insertion minimizes discomfort. (Injecting medication into compressed tissue irritates nerve fibers.) Correct angle prevents accidental injection into muscle.
(3) For obese client, pinch skin at site and inject needle at 90-degree angle below tissue fold.	Obese clients have fatty layer of tissue above subcutaneous layer.

Critical Decision Point: Piercing a blood vessel during a Sub-Q injection is very rare, so aspiration is not necessary when administering Sub-Q injections.

---

(4) Inject medication slowly (see illustration).	Minimizes discomfort.
B. Intramuscular	
(1) Position nondominant hand just below site, and pull skin approximately 2.5 to 3.5 cm down or laterally with ulnar side of hand to administer in a Z-track. Hold position until medication is injected (see Figure 35-27, p. 753).	Z-track creates zigzag path through tissues that seals needle track to avoid tracking of medication. Use Z-track for all IM injections (Nicoll and Hesby, 2002).
(2) *Option:* If client's muscle mass is small, grasp body of muscle between thumb and fingers.	Ensures that medication reaches muscle mass (Hockenberry and Wilson, 2007).

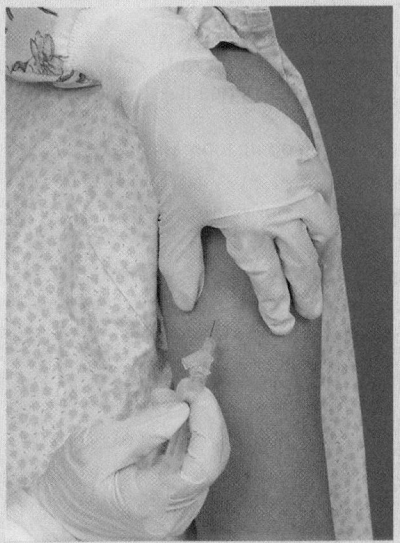

STEP 21a Hold syringe as if grasping a dart.

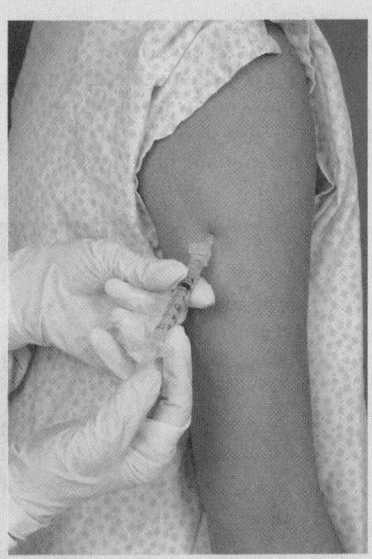

STEP 22A(4) Inject medication slowly.

Continued

✳ **SKILL 35-5**   **ADMINISTERING INJECTIONS—CONT'D**

STEPS

    (3) With dominant hand, insert needle quickly at 90-degree angle into muscle. After needle pierces skin, grasp lower end of syringe barrel with nondominant hand to stabilize syringe. Continue to hold skin tightly with nondominant hand. Move dominant hand to end of plunger. Do not move syringe.

    (4) Pull back on plunger 5 to 10 seconds. If no blood appears, inject medicine slowly, at a rate of 1 mL/10 sec.

RATIONALE

Smooth manipulation of syringe reduces discomfort from needle movement. Skin needs to remain pulled until after injecting medication to ensure Z-track administration.

Aspiration of blood into syringe indicates IV placement of needle. Slow injection rate reduces pain and tissue trauma (Nicoll and Hesby, 2002).

Critical Decision Point: If blood appears in syringe, remove needle and dispose of medication and syringe properly. Prepare another dose of medication for injection.

---

    (5) Wait 10 seconds Then smoothly and steadily withdraw needle and release skin.

  C. Intradermal

    (1) With nondominant hand, stretch skin over site with forefinger or thumb.

    (2) With needle almost against client's skin, insert it slowly with bevel up at a 5- to 15-degree angle until resistance is felt. Then advance needle through epidermis to approximately 3 mm (⅛ inch) below skin surface. You will see needle tip through skin.

    (3) Inject medication slowly. Normally, you feel resistance. If not, needle is too deep; remove and begin again. Nondominant hand can stabilize the needle during the injection.

    (4) While injecting medication, notice that small bleb approximately 6 mm (¼ inch) in diameter (resembling mosquito bite) appears on skin's surface (see illustration). Instruct client that this is a normal finding.

23. Withdraw needle while applying alcohol swab or gauze gently over site.

24. Apply gentle pressure. Do not massage site. Apply bandage if needed.

25. Assist client to comfortable position.

26. Discard uncapped needle or needle enclosed in safety shield and attached syringe into puncture-proof and leak-proof receptacle.

27. Remove gloves, and perform hand hygiene.

Allows time for medication to absorb into muscle before removing syringe rather than leaking back out through the track that the needle created (Nicoll and Hesby, 2002).

Needle pierces tight skin more easily.

Ensures needle tip is in dermis.

Slow injection minimizes discomfort at site. Dermal layer is tight and does not expand easily when solution is injected. Stabilizing the needle prevents unnecessary movements and decreases client discomfort.

Bleb indicates medication is deposited in dermis.

Support of tissue around injection site minimizes discomfort during needle withdrawal. Dry gauze minimizes client discomfort associated with alcohol on nonintact skin.

Massage often causes underlying tissue damage. Massage of ID site disperses medication into underlying tissue layers and alters test results.

Gives client sense of well-being.

Prevents injury to client and health care personnel. Recapping needles increases risk of needle-stick injury (OSHA, 2006).

Reduces transmission of microorganisms.

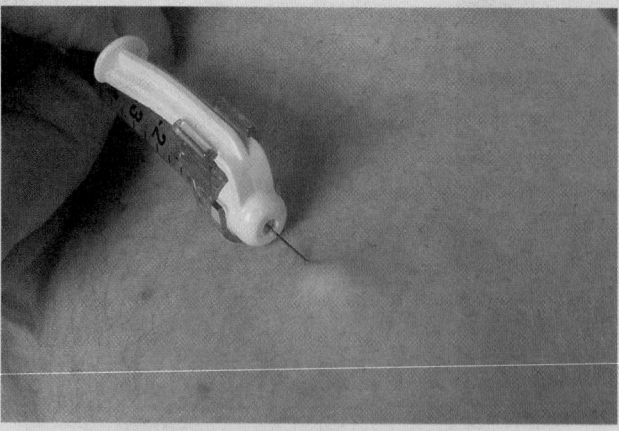

STEP 22C(4) Injection creates a small bleb.

STEPS	RATIONALE
28. Stay with client, and observe for any allergic reactions.	Dyspnea, wheezing, and circulatory collapse are signs of severe anaphylactic reaction, which is a life-threatening emergency.
29. Return to room, and ask if client feels any acute pain, burning, numbness, or tingling at injection site.	Continued discomfort often indicates injury to underlying bones or nerves.
30. Inspect site, noting any bruising or induration.	Bruising or induration indicates complication associated with injection. Document findings and notify health care provider. Provide warm compress to site.
31. Observe client's response to medication at times that correlate with the medication's onset, peak, and duration.	IM medications are rapidly absorbed. Adverse effects of parenteral medications develop rapidly. Nurse's observations determine efficacy of medication action.

Critical Decision Point: Read tuberculin test at 48 to 72 hours. Induration (hard, dense, raised area) of skin around injection site indicates positive reaction, as follows:

- 15 mm or more in clients with no known risk factors for tuberculosis (TB)
- 10 mm or more in clients who are recent immigrants; injection drug users; residents and employees of high-risk settings; mycobacteriology laboratory personnel; clients with clinical conditions placing them at high risk; children less than 4 years of age; and infants, children and adolescents exposed to high-risk adults
- 5 mm or more in clients who are human immunodeficiency virus (HIV) positive, have fibrotic changes on chest x-ray film consistent with previous TB infection, have had organ transplants, or are immunosuppressed (CDC, 2007).

32. Ask client to explain purpose and effects of medication.	Evaluates client's understanding of information taught.
33. For ID injections, use skin pencil and draw circle around perimeter of injection site. Read site within appropriate amount of time, designated by type of medication or skin test administered.	Pencil mark makes site easy to find. Results of skin testing are read at various times, based on the type of medication used or the type of skin testing completed. Refer to manufacturer's directions to determine when to read the test's results.

Unexpected Outcomes and Related Interventions

1. Raised, reddened, or hard zone (induration) forms around ID test site.
   a. Notify client's health care provider.
   b. Document sensitivity to injected allergen or positive test if tuberculin skin testing was completed.
2. Hypertrophy of skin develops from repeated Sub-Q injections.
   a. Do not use this site for future injections.
   b. Instruct client not to use site for 6 months.
3. Client develops signs and symptoms of allergy or side effects.
   a. Follow institutional policy or guidelines for appropriate response to adverse drug reactions.
   b. Notify client's health care provider immediately.
   c. Add allergy information to client's medical record.
4. Client complains of localized pain, numbness, tingling, or burning at injection site, indicating possible injury to nerve or tissues.
   a. Assess injection site.
   b. Document findings.
   c. Notify client's health care provider.

Recording and Reporting

- Chart medication dose, route, site, time, and date given on MAR immediately after giving medication per agency policy.
- Document if scheduled medication is withheld, and record the reason per agency policy.
- Report any undesirable effects from medication to prescriber.
- Record client's response to medications in nurses' notes, and report to prescriber if required.

Home Care Considerations

- Assess the client's readiness to learn before instructing in self-injections. Some clients are hesitant to administer injections to themselves, so relieve any anxiety before teaching this skill to a client.
- Some clients prefer to reuse their syringes to save costs. This practice is safe and practical if the needle is not contaminated during the preparation and administration of the injection. Teach clients to immediately recap needles after use.
- Clients can often purchase or obtain sharps boxes for home use. If this is not possible, clients can use a hard plastic bottle that they cannot see through (e.g., a fabric softener bottle or detergent bottle) to safely store syringes after use. Disposal of needles used in the home varies among communities. Check with local authorities to verify how to dispose of needles.

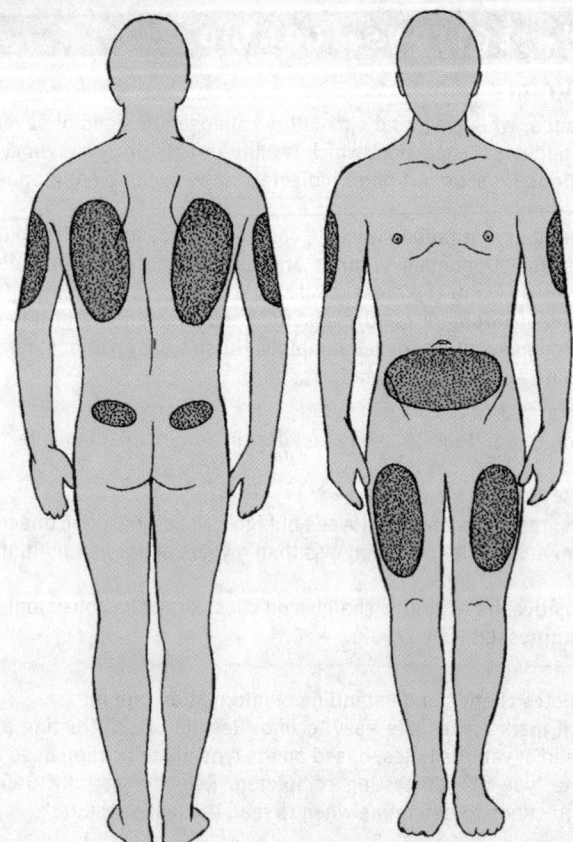

Figure 35-21 Sites recommended for subcutaneous injections.

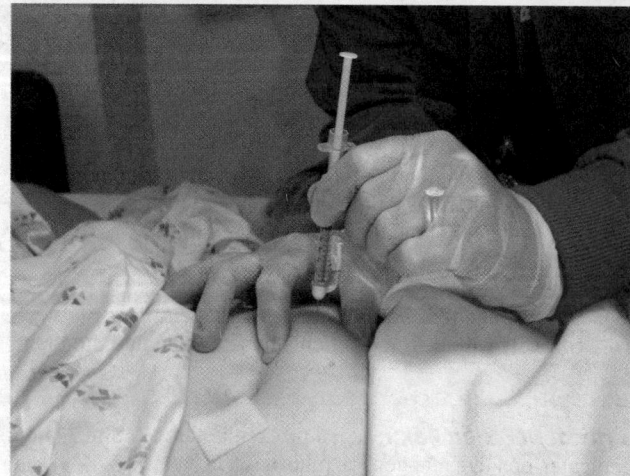

Figure 35-22 Giving Sub-Q heparin in the abdomen.

The best subcutaneous injection sites include the outer posterior aspect of the upper arms, the abdomen from below the costal margins to the iliac crests, and the anterior aspects of the thighs (Figure 35-21). The site most frequently recommended for heparin injections is the abdomen (Figure 35-22). Alternative subcutaneous sites for other medications include the scapular areas of the upper back and the upper ventral or dorsal gluteal areas. The injection site chosen needs to be free of skin lesions, bony prominences, and large underlying muscles or nerves.

The administration of low-molecular-weight heparin (LMWH) (e.g., enoxaparin) requires special considerations. When injecting the medication, use the right or left side of the abdomen at least 2 inches from the umbilicus (the client's "love handles"), pinch the injection site. Administer LMWH in its prefilled syringe with the attached needle, and do not expel the air bubble in the syringe before giving the medication (Sanofi-Aventis, 2007).

Use U-100 insulin syringes with preattached 26- to 31-gauge needles when giving U-100 insulin, and use 1-ml tuberculin syringes when giving U-500 insulin (ADA, 2005; ISMP, 2002). Recommended sites for insulin injections include the upper arm and the anterior and lateral portions of the thigh, buttocks, and abdomen. Rotating injections within the same body part (intra-site rotation) provides more consistency in the absorption of the insulin. For example, if the client receives the morning insulin in the right arm, then give the next injection in a different place in

the same arm. The injections are to be given at least an inch away from the previous site. No injection site should be used again for at least 1 month. The rate of insulin absorption varies based on the site; the abdomen has the quickest absorption, followed by the arms, thighs, and buttocks (ADA, 2004).

Only small doses (0.5 to 1 mL) of water-soluble medications are given subcutaneously because the tissue is sensitive to irritating solutions and large volumes of medications. Collection of medications within the tissues causes sterile abscesses, which appear as hardened, painful lumps under the skin.

A client's body weight indicates the depth of the subcutaneous layer. Therefore choose the needle length and angle of insertion based on the client's weight and an estimation of the amount of subcutaneous tissue (Annersten and Willman, 2005). Generally a 25-gauge ⅝-inch needle inserted at a 45-degree angle (Figure 35-23) or a ½-inch needle inserted at a 90-degree angle deposits medications into the subcutaneous tissue of a normal-size client. Some children require only a ½-inch needle. If the client is obese, the nurse often pinches the tissue and uses a needle long enough to insert through fatty tissue at the base of the skinfold. Thin clients often do not have sufficient tissue for subcutaneous injections; the upper abdomen is usually the best site in this case. To ensure a subcutaneous medication reaches the subcutaneous tissue, follow this rule: If you can grasp 2 inches (5 cm) of tissue, insert the needle at a 90-degree angle; if you can grasp 1 inch (2.5 cm) of tissue, insert the needle at a 45-degree angle (Rushing, 2004).

Intramuscular Injections. The intramuscular route provides faster medication absorption than the subcutaneous route because of a muscle's greater vascularity. However, intramuscular injections are associated with many risks. Therefore, whenever administering a medication by the IM route, first verify that the injection is justified (Nicoll and Hesby, 2002; WHO, 2005). In many cases, such as influenza and pneumonia shots, there are no other alternative sites to give the medication.

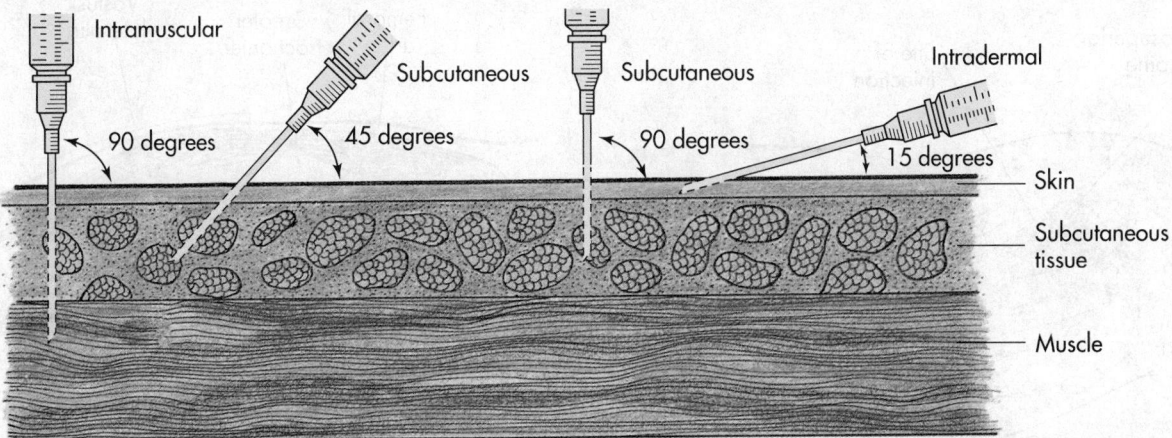

Figure 35-23 Comparison of angles of insertion for intramuscular (90 degrees), subcutaneous (45 to 90 degrees), and intradermal (15 degrees) injections.

Use a longer and heavier-gauge needle to pass through subcutaneous tissue and penetrate deep muscle tissue (see Skill 35-5). Weight and the amount of adipose tissue influence needle size selection. For example, a very obese client often requires a needle 3 inches long, whereas a thin client only requires a ½- to 1-inch needle (Nicoll and Hesby, 2002).

The angle of insertion for an intramuscular injection is 90 degrees (see Figure 35-23). Muscle is less sensitive to irritating and viscous medications. A normal, well-developed client tolerates 3 mL of medication into a larger muscle without severe muscle discomfort (Nicoll and Hesby, 2002). A larger volume of medication is unlikely to be absorbed properly. Children, older adults, and thin clients tolerate only 2 mL of an intramuscular injection. Do not give more than 1 mL to small children and older infants, and do not give more than 0.5 mL to smaller infants (Hockenberry and Wilson, 2007).

Assess the muscle before giving an injection. The muscle needs to be free of tenderness. Repeated injections in the same muscle cause severe discomfort. With the client relaxed, palpate the muscle to rule out any hardened lesions. Minimize discomfort during an injection by helping the client assume a position that will help reduce muscle strain. Other interventions, such as distraction and applying pressure to the intramuscular site decrease pain during an intramuscular injection.

Sites. When selecting an intramuscular site, consider the following: Is the area free of infection or necrosis? Are there local areas of bruising or abrasions? What is the location of underlying bones, nerves, and major blood vessels? What volume of medication is to be administered? Each site has different advantages and disadvantages (Box 35-26).

Ventrogluteal. The ventrogluteal muscle involves the gluteus medius, is situated deep and away from major nerves and blood vessels, and is a safe site for all clients because it is a large muscle that is well developed in young children, including those who do not walk, and adults (Nicoll and Hesby, 2002). Research shows that injuries such as fibrosis, nerve damage, abscess, tissue necrosis, muscle contraction, gangrene, and pain are associated with all the common IM sites *except* the ventrogluteal site. Actually, the only

BOX 35-26 Characteristics of Intramuscular Sites and Indications for Usage

Vastus Lateralis
Lacks major nerves and blood vessels
Rapid drug absorption
Site frequently used in infants (less than 12 months) receiving immunizations
Often used in older children and toddlers receiving immunizations

Ventrogluteal
A deep site, situated away from major nerves and blood vessels
Less chance of contamination in incontinent clients or infants
Easily identified by prominent bony landmarks
Preferred site for medications (e.g., antibiotics) that are larger in volume, more viscous, and irritating for adults, children, and infants

Deltoid
Easily accessible but muscle not well developed in most clients
Used for small amounts of medications
Not used in infants or children with underdeveloped muscles
Potential for injury to radial and ulnar nerves or brachial artery
Used for immunizations for toddlers, older children, and adults
Recommended site for hepatitis B vaccine and rabies injections

published case study of a complication at the ventrogluteal site reported a local reaction to the medication, which is not a complication associated with the site itself (Nicoll and Hesby, 2002).

SAFETY ALERT Research investigating complications associated with IM injection sites indicates that the ventrogluteal site is the preferred site for most injections given to adults and all children, including infants of any age (Cook and Murtagh, 2006; Hockenberry and Wilson, 2007; Nicoll and Hesby, 2002).

Locate the ventrogluteal muscle by placing the heel of the hand over the greater trochanter of the client's hip with the wrist perpendicular to the femur. Use the right hand for the left hip,

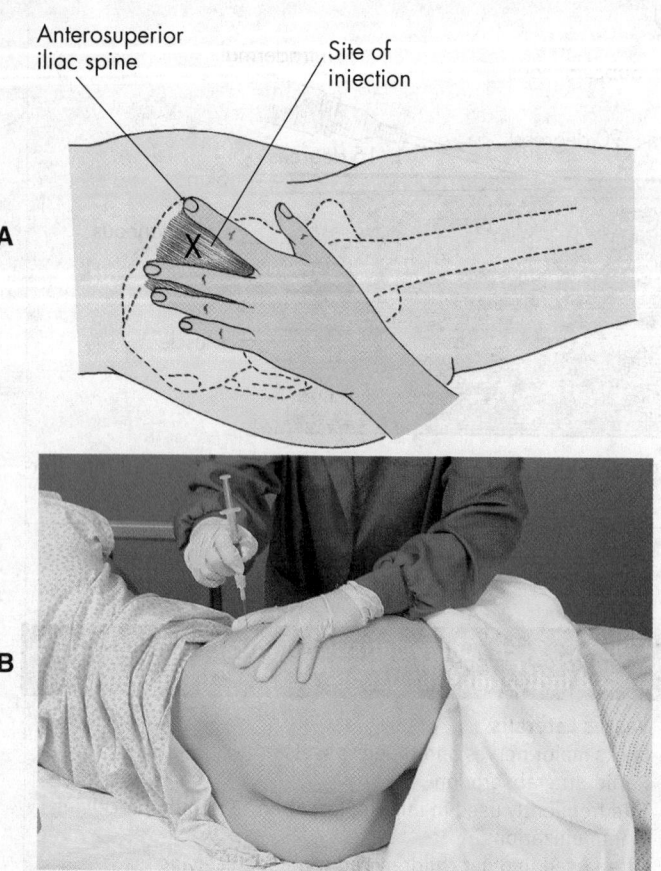

A — Anterosuperior iliac spine — Site of injection — X

B

Figure 35-24 A, Landmarks for ventrogluteal site. **B,** Giving IM injection in ventrogluteal muscle.

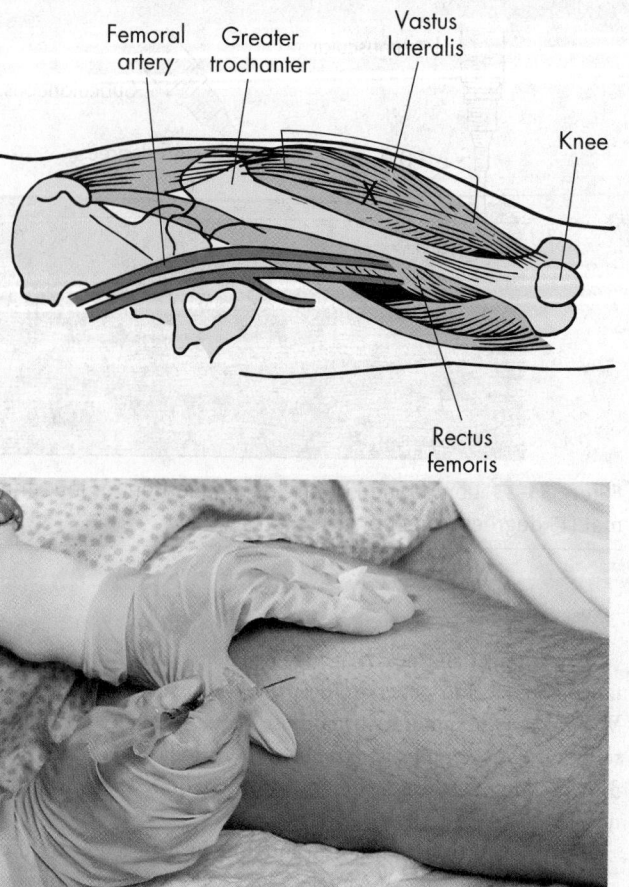

Femoral artery — Greater trochanter — Vastus lateralis — Knee — X — Rectus femoris — A

B

Figure 35-25 A, Landmarks for vastus lateralis site. **B,** Giving IM injection in vastus lateralis muscle.

and use the left hand for the client's right hip. Point the thumb toward the client's groin, the index finger toward the anterior superior iliac spine, and extend the middle finger back along the iliac crest toward the buttock. The index finger, the middle finger, and the iliac crest form a **V**-shaped triangle; the injection site is the center of the triangle (Figure 35-24, *A* and *B*). The client lies on his or her side or back. Flexing of the knee and hip helps the client relax this muscle.

Vastus Lateralis. The vastus lateralis muscle is another injection site. The muscle is thick and well developed, is located on the anterior lateral aspect of the thigh, and extends in an adult from a handbreadth above the knee to a handbreadth below the greater trochanter of the femur (Figure 35-25). Use the middle third of the muscle for injection. The width of the muscle usually extends from the midline of the thigh to the midline of the thigh's outer side. With young children or cachectic clients, it helps to grasp the body of the muscle during injection to be sure that the medication is deposited in muscle tissue. To help relax the muscle, ask the client to lie flat with the knee slightly flexed or in a sitting position. The vastus lateralis site is often used for infants, toddlers, and children receiving biologicals (e.g., immune globulins, vaccines, or toxoids) (Nicoll and Hesby, 2002).

Deltoid. Although the deltoid site is easily accessible, the muscle is not well developed in many adults. There is a potential for injury when using this site because the axillary, radial, brachial, and ulnar nerves and brachial artery lie within the upper arm along the humerus (Figure 35-26, *A*). Use this site only for small medication volumes, when giving immunizations, or when other sites are inaccessible because of dressings or casts (Nicoll and Hesby, 2002).

To locate the deltoid muscle, fully expose the client's upper arm and shoulder. Do not roll up a tight-fitting sleeve. Have the client relax the arm at the side and flex the elbow. The client may sit, stand, or lie down (Figure 35-26, *B*). Palpate the lower edge of the acromion process, which forms the base of a triangle in line with the midpoint of the lateral aspect of the upper arm. The injection site is in the center of the triangle, about 3 to 5 cm (1 to 2 inches) below the acromion process (Nicoll and Hesby, 2002). You can also locate the site by placing four fingers across the deltoid muscle, with the top finger along the acromion process. The injection site is then three finger widths below the acromion process.

Dorsogluteal. In the past, the dorsogluteal muscle was used for intramuscular injections. However, studies demonstrate that the exact location of the sciatic nerve varies from one person to another. If a needle hits a sciatic nerve, the client usually experiences adverse outcomes, including permanent or partial paralysis

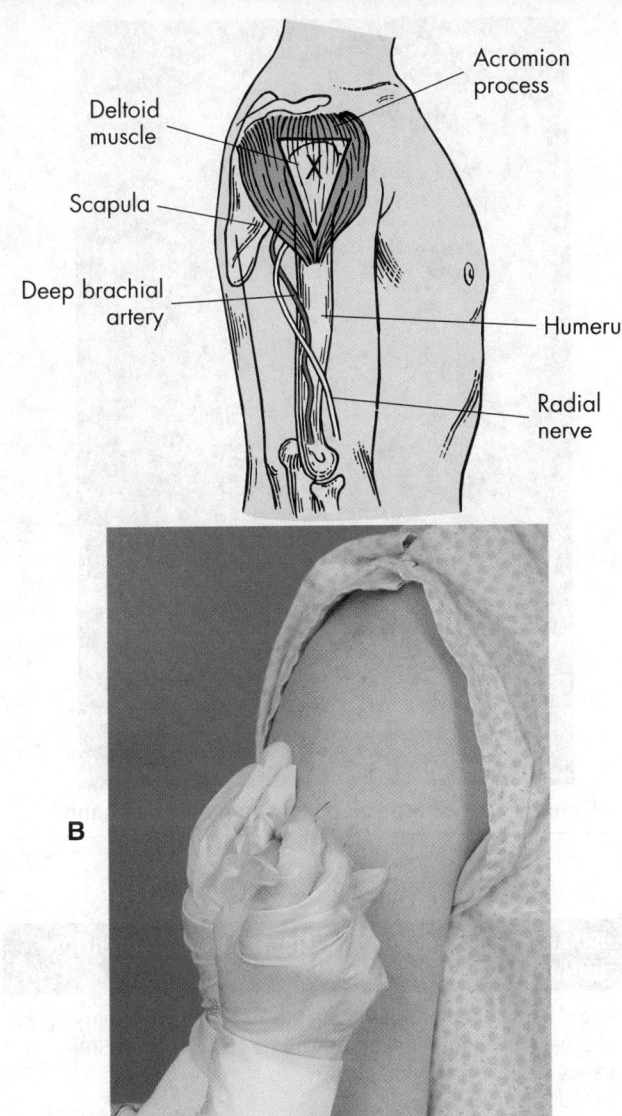

Figure 35-26 **A,** Landmarks for deltoid site. **B,** Giving IM injection in deltoid muscle.

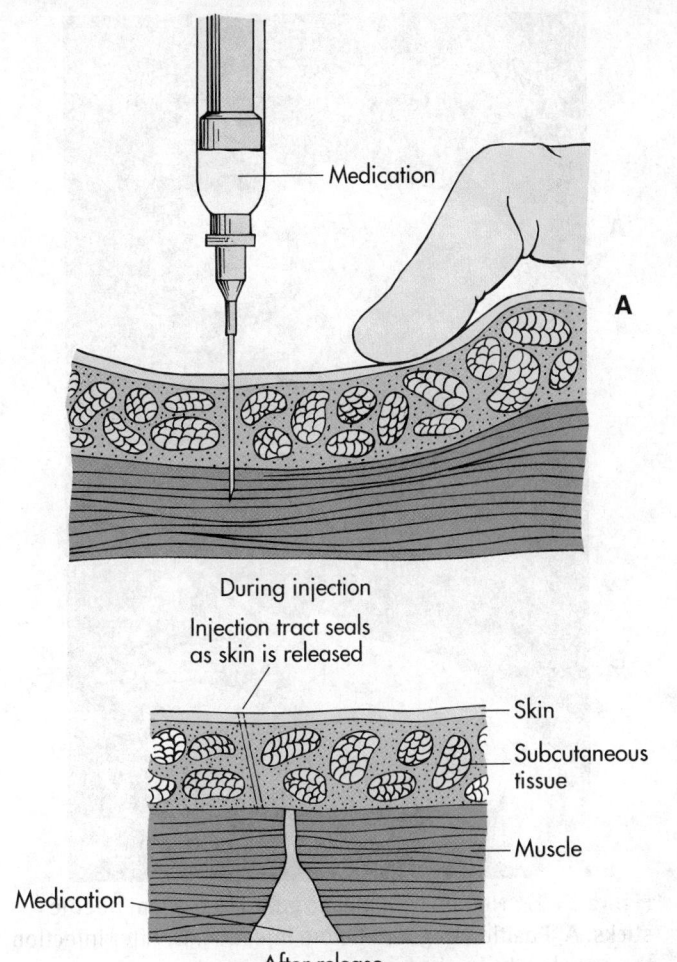

Figure 35-27 **A,** Pulling on overlying skin during IM injection moves tissue to prevent later tracking. **B,** The Z-track left after injection prevents the deposit of medication through sensitive tissue.

of the involved leg; therefore do **not** use this site (Cook and Murtagh, 2006; Nicoll and Hesby, 2002; Small, 2004).

Use of the Z-Track Method in Intramuscular Injections. It is recommended that when administering IM injections the **Z-track method** be used to minimize local skin irritation by sealing the medication in muscle tissue (Nicoll and Hesby, 2002). To use the Z-track method, put a new needle on the syringe after preparing the medication so that no solution remains on the outside needle shaft. Then select an intramuscular site, preferably in a large, deep muscle such as the ventrogluteal muscle. After preparing the site with an antiseptic swab, pull the overlying skin and subcutaneous tissues approximately 2.5 to 3.5 cm (1 to 1½ inches) laterally to the side. Holding the skin taut with the nondominant hand, inject the needle deep into the muscle and slowly inject the medication if there is no blood return on aspiration. The needle remains inserted for 10 seconds to allow the medication to disperse evenly rather than channeling back up the track of the needle. Then release the skin after withdrawing the needle.

This leaves a zigzag path that seals the needle track where tissue planes slide across each other (Figure 35-27). The medication cannot escape from the muscle tissue. Injections using this technique result in less discomfort and decrease the occurrence of lesions at the injection site (Nicoll and Hesby, 2002).

Intradermal Injections. The nurse typically gives intradermal injections for skin testing (e.g., tuberculin screening and allergy tests). Because these medications are potent, they are injected into the dermis, where blood supply is reduced and medication absorption occurs slowly. Some clients have a severe anaphylactic reaction if the medications enter the circulation too rapidly. Skin testing requires that the nurse be able to clearly see the injection sites for changes in color and tissue integrity. Intradermal sites should be lightly pigmented, free of lesions, and relatively hairless. The inner forearm and upper back are ideal locations.

Use a tuberculin or small hypodermic syringe for skin testing. The angle of insertion for an intradermal injection is 5 to 15 degrees (see Figure 35-23), and the bevel of the needle is pointed up. As you inject the medication, a small bleb resembling a mosquito bite will appear on the skin's surface (see Skill 35-5, p. 745). If a

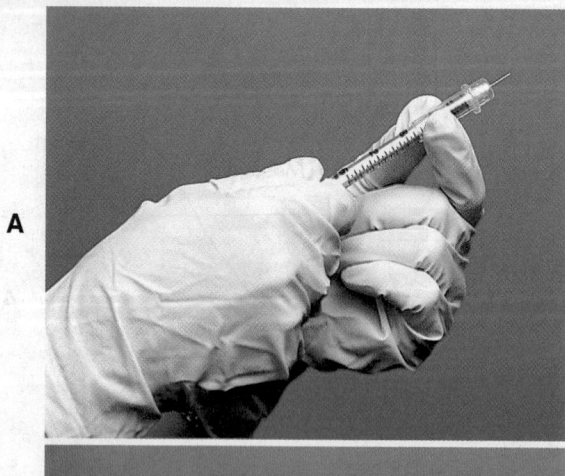

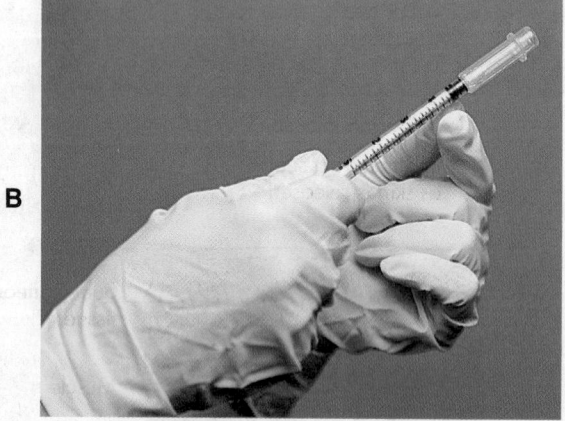

Figure 35-28 Needle with plastic guard to prevent needle sticks. **A,** Position of guard before injection. **B,** After injection the guard locks in place, covering the needle.

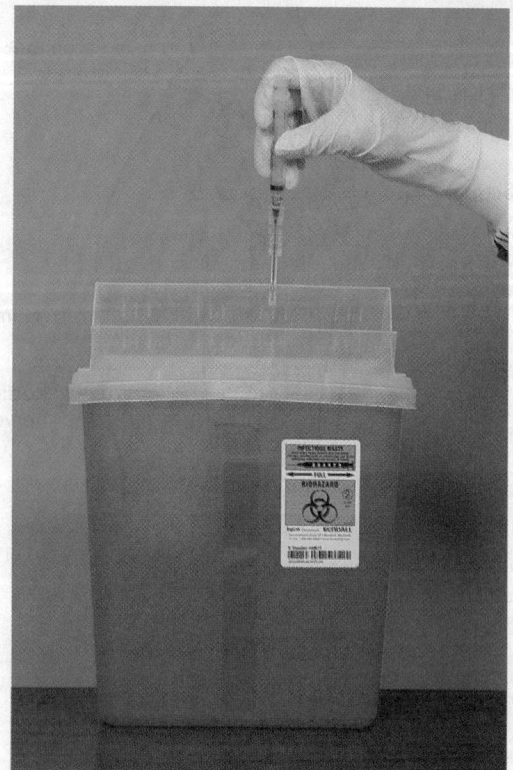

Figure 35-29 Sharps disposal using only one hand.

bleb does not appear or if the site bleeds after needle withdrawal, there is a good chance the medication entered subcutaneous tissues. In this case, test results will not be valid.

Safety in Administering Medications by Injection

Needleless Devices. Between 600,000 and 1 million accidental needle sticks and sharps injuries occur annually in health care settings (American Nurses Association [ANA], 2007). These injuries commonly occur when needles are recapped, IV lines and needles are mishandled, or needles are left at a client's bedside. Exposure to blood-borne pathogens is one of the deadliest hazards nurses are exposed to on a daily basis. The majority of needle-stick injuries are preventable with the implementation of safe needle devices. The Needlestick Safety and Prevention Act is a federal law that became effective in April, 2001. This federal law mandates the use of special needle safety devices to reduce the frequency of needle-stick injuries.

Safe syringes have a sheath or guard that covers the needle after it is withdrawn from the skin (Figure 35-28). The needle is immediately covered, eliminating the chance for a needle-stick injury. The syringe and sheath are disposed of together in a receptacle. Use "needleless" devices whenever possible to reduce the risk to health care workers of needle sticks and sharps injuries (OSHA, 2006). Always dispose of needles and other instruments consid-

BOX 35-27 Recommendations for the Prevention of Needle-Stick Injuries

- Avoid using needles when effective needleless systems or sharps with engineered sharps injury protection (SESIP) safety devices are available.
- Do not recap any needle.
- Plan safe handling and disposal of needles before beginning the procedure.
- Immediately dispose of needles, needleless systems, and SESIP into puncture-proof and leakproof sharps disposal containers.
- Maintain a sharps injury log that includes the following:
  - Type and brand of device involved in the incident
  - Location of the incident (e.g., department or work area)
  - Description of the incident
  - Maintains privacy of the employees who have had sharps injuries

Data from Occupational Safety and Health Administration: Toxic and hazardous substances: bloodborne pathogens, *Federal Register,* CFR 29, part 1910.1030, April 3, 2006, www.osha.gov/pls/oshaweb/owadisp.show_document?p_table=STANDARDS&p_id=10051.

ered "sharps" into clearly marked, appropriate containers (Figure 35-29). Containers need to be puncture proof and leakproof. Never force a needle into a full needle disposal receptacle. Never place used needles and syringes in a wastebasket, in your pocket, on a client's meal tray, or at the client's bedside. Box 35-27 summarizes the recommendations for the prevention of needle-stick injuries.

Intravenous Administration. The nurse administers medications intravenously by the following methods:

1. As mixtures within large volumes of intravenous fluids
2. By injection of a bolus or small volume of medication through an existing intravenous infusion line or intermittent venous access (heparin or saline lock)
3. By "piggyback" infusion of a solution containing the prescribed medication and a small volume of intravenous fluid through an existing intravenous line.

In all three methods the client has either an existing intravenous infusion line or an intravenous access site such as an intermittent infusion (sometimes called a heparin or saline lock). In most institutions, policies and procedures list persons who are able to give intravenous medications and the situations in which they may be given. These policies are based on the medication, capability and availability of staff, and type of monitoring equipment available.

Chapter 41 describes the technique for performing venipuncture and establishing continuous intravenous fluid infusions. Medication administration is only one reason for supplying intravenous fluids. Intravenous fluid therapy is used primarily for fluid replacement in clients unable to take oral fluids and as a means of supplying electrolytes and nutrients.

When using any method of intravenous medication administration, observe clients closely for symptoms of adverse reactions. After a medication enters the bloodstream, it begins to act immediately, and there is no way to stop its action. Thus take special care to avoid errors in dose calculation and preparation. Carefully follow the six rights of safe medication administration, double-check medication calculations with another nurse, and know the desired action and side effects of every medication you give. If the medication has an antidote, make sure it is available during administration. When administering potent medications, assess vital signs before, during, and after infusion.

Administering medications by the intravenous route has advantages. Often the nurse uses the intravenous route in emergencies when a fast-acting medication must be delivered quickly. The intravenous route is also best when it is necessary to establish constant therapeutic blood levels. Some medications are highly alkaline and irritating to muscle and subcutaneous tissue. These medications cause less discomfort when given intravenously.

SAFETY ALERT Because IV medications are immediately available to the bloodstream once they are administered, verify the prescribed rate of administration with a drug reference or a pharmacist before giving any IV medication to ensure the medication is given safely over the appropriate amount of time. Clients will experience severe adverse reactions if IV medications are administered too quickly.

Large-Volume Infusions. Of the three methods of administering intravenous medications, mixing medications in large volumes of fluids is the safest and easiest. Medications are diluted in large volumes (500 or 1000 mL) of compatible intravenous fluids such as normal saline or lactated Ringer's solution (Skill 35-6). In most institutions the pharmacist adds medications to the primary container of intravenous solution to ensure asepsis and to reduce the frequency of medication errors. Because the medication is not in a concentrated form, the risk of side effects or fatal reactions is minimal when infused over the prescribed time frame. Vitamins and potassium chloride are two types of medications commonly added to intravenous fluids. However, there is a danger with continuous infusion: if the intravenous fluid is infused too rapidly, the client is at risk for circulatory fluid overload.

Intravenous Bolus. An intravenous bolus involves introducing a concentrated dose of a medication directly into the systemic circulation (Skill 35-7, p. 759). Because a bolus requires only a small amount of fluid to deliver the medication, it is an advantage when the amount of fluid the client can take is restricted. The intravenous bolus, or "push," is the most dangerous method for administering medications because there is no time to correct errors. In addition, a bolus may cause direct irritation to the lining of blood vessels. Before administering a bolus confirm placement of the intravenous line. This involves obtaining a blood return through the intravenous catheter or needle. The inability to obtain a blood return suggests that the needle or catheter is in the client's tissues or resting against the vein wall. Never give a medication intravenously if the insertion site appears puffy or edematous or the intravenous fluid cannot flow at the proper rate. Accidental injection of a medication into the tissues around a vein causes pain, sloughing of tissues, and abscesses, depending on the medication's composition.

Determine the rate of administration of an intravenous bolus medication by the amount of medication that can be given each minute. For example, if a client is to receive 4 mL of a medication over 2 minutes, give 2 mL of the intravenous bolus medication every minute. Look up each medication to determine the recommended concentration and rate of administration. Consider the purpose for which a medication is prescribed and any potential adverse effects related to the rate or route of administration when giving a medication by intravenous push.

Text continued on p. 763

Delegation Considerations

The skill of adding medications to IV fluid containers cannot be delegated. (In some institutions only the pharmacist adds medications to primary containers of IV solutions to promote safe medication administration and ensure asepsis.)

Equipment

- Vial or ampule of prescribed medication
- Safety syringe of appropriate size (5 to 20 mL)

- Sterile needle (1 to 1½ inches, 19 to 21 gauge) with special filters if needed
- Correct diluent if indicated (e.g., sterile water, normal saline)
- Sterile IV fluid container (bag or bottle, 25 to 1000 mL in volume)
- Alcohol or antiseptic swab
- Label to attach to IV bag or bottle
- MAR or computer printout

STEPS	RATIONALE
1. Check accuracy and completeness of each MAR or computer printout with prescriber's original medication order. Check client's name and medication name, dosage, route, and time for administration. Recopy or re-print any portion of MAR that is difficult to read.	The order sheet is the most reliable source and only legal record of medications client is to receive. Ensures client receives the correct medications. Illegible MARs are a source of medication errors.
2. Assess client's medical history.	Identifies need for medication.
3. Collect information necessary to administer drug safely, including action, purpose, side effects, normal dose, time of peak onset, and nursing implications.	Allows nurse to give medication safely and to monitor client's response to therapy.
4. When adding more than one medication to IV solution, assess for compatibility of medications.	Medications often are incompatible when mixed together. Chemical reactions that occur result in clouding or crystallization of IV fluids. Check agency policy for approved medication compatibility list.
5. Assess client's systemic fluid balance, as reflected by skin hydration and turgor, body weight, pulse, and blood pressure.	Danger of continuous IV infusions is that fluids often infuse too rapidly, causing circulatory overload, especially in children and older adults (Ebersole and others, 2004; Hockenberry and Wilson, 2007).
6. Assess client's history of medication allergies.	IV administration of medications causes rapid effects. Allergic response is often immediate.
7. Perform hand hygiene.	Reduces transfer of microorganisms.
8. Assess IV insertion site for signs of infiltration or phlebitis, and assess patency of existing IV line (see Chapter 41).	An intact, properly functioning site ensures medication is given safely.
9. Assess client's understanding of purpose of medication therapy.	Reveals need for client education.
10. Prepare medication: See Skill 35-4, p. 738; use aseptic technique. Be sure to compare the label of the medication with the MAR two times while preparing the medication.	Ensures medication is sterile; preparation techniques differ for ampules and vials. Following the same routine when preparing medications, eliminating distractions, and checking the label of the medication with transcribed order reduces error (Pape and others, 2005).
11. Perform hand hygiene.	Reduces transfer of microorganisms.
12. Compare labels of medication and IV fluid bag with MAR.	Ensures right medication is injected into right IV fluid.
13. Add medication to new container (usually done in medication room or at medication cart):	
a. *Solution in a bag:* Locate medication injection port on plastic IV solution bag (port has small rubber stopper at end). Do not select port for the IV tubing insertion or air vent.	Medication injection port is self-sealing to prevent introduction of microorganisms after repeated use.
b. *Solution in a bottle:* Locate injection site on IV solution bottle, which is often covered by a metal or plastic cap.	Accidental injection of medication through main tubing port or air vent alters pressure within bottle and causes fluid leaks through air vent. Cap seals bottle to maintain its sterility.
c. Wipe off port or injection site with alcohol or antiseptic swab (see illustration).	Reduces risk of introducing microorganisms into bag during needle insertion.
d. Remove needle cap or sheath from syringe, and insert needle of syringe or needleless device through center of injection port or site; inject medication (see illustration).	Injection of needle into sides of port produces leak and leads to fluid contamination.
e. Withdraw syringe from bag or bottle.	When syringe is withdrawn, injection port self-seals, preventing introduction of microorganisms.
f. Mix medication and IV solution by holding bag or bottle and turning it gently end to end.	Allows even distribution of medication.
g. Complete medication label with client's name, name and dose of medication, date, time, and nurse's initials. Apply it to bottle or bag.	Label is easy to read during infusion of solution. Informs health care providers of contents of bag or bottle.

✳ **SKILL 35-6** **ADDING MEDICATIONS TO INTRAVENOUS FLUID CONTAINERS—CONT'D**

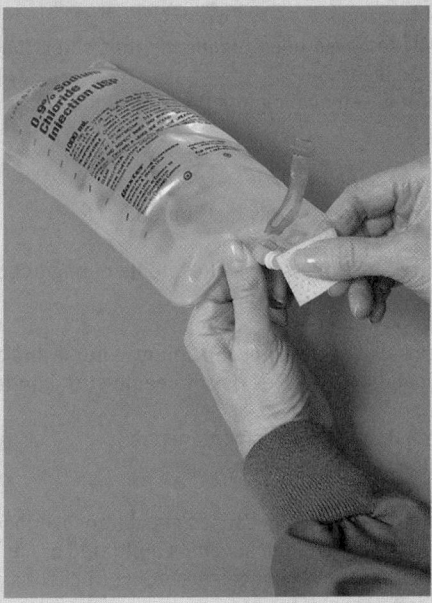

STEP 13c Cleanse injection port with antiseptic swab.

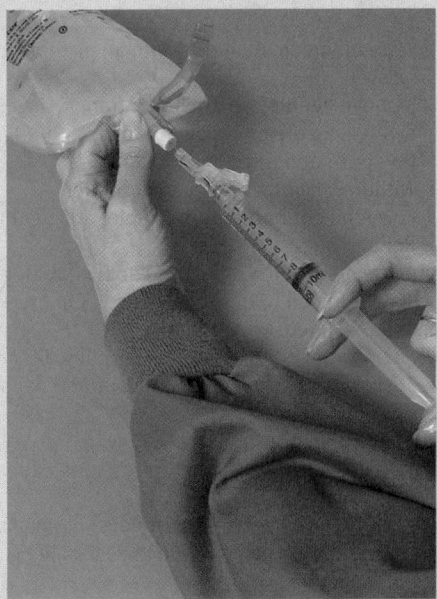

STEP 13d Inject medication through port.

STEPS

   h. If new tubing is required, spike bag or bottle with IV tubing and prime tubing.

14. Bring assembled items to client's bedside at right time.

15. Identify client using at least two client identifiers. Compare client's name and one other identifier (e.g., hospital identification number) on MAR, computer printout, or computer screen with information on client's identification bracelet. Ask client to state name if possible for a third identifier.

16. Prepare client by explaining that medication is to be given through existing IV line or one to be started. Explain that client should feel no discomfort during medication infusion. Encourage client to report symptoms of discomfort.

17. Connect new infusion tubing, or spike container with existing tubing. Regulate infusion at ordered rate (see Chapter 41).

RATIONALE

Organization reduces errors.

Complies with TJC (2008) requirements and improves medication safety. In most acute care settings, client's name and identification number on armband and MAR are used to identify clients. Identification bracelets are made at time of client's admission and are most reliable source of identification. Client's room number is **not** an acceptable identifier.

Most IV medications do not cause discomfort when diluted. However, potassium chloride is irritating. Pain at insertion site is often early indication of infiltration.

Prevents rapid infusion of fluid.

Critical Decision Point: Some medications (e.g., potassium chloride) cause serious adverse reactions, including fatal cardiac dysrhythmias. These medications need to be infused on an IV pump. Check institutional guidelines or policies indicating which IV medications require administration on an IV pump.

---

18. Add medication to existing container:

Critical Decision Point: Because there is no way to know exactly how much IV fluid is in an existing hanging IV container, there is no way to determine the exact concentration of the medication in the IV solution. Therefore add medications to **new** IV fluid containers whenever possible.

---

   a. Prepare vented IV bottle or plastic bag:
      (1) Check volume of solution remaining in bottle or bag.

      (2) Close off IV infusion clamp.

Proper minimal volume (see drug insert) is necessary to dilute medication adequately.

Prevents medication from directly entering circulation as it is injected into bag or bottle.

Continued

✳ SKILL 35-6   ADDING MEDICATIONS TO INTRAVENOUS FLUID CONTAINERS—CONT'D

STEPS	RATIONALE
(3) Wipe off medication port with an alcohol or antiseptic swab.	Mechanically removes microorganisms that enter container during needle insertion.
(4) Remove needle cap or sheath from syringe; insert syringe needle or needleless device through injection port, and inject medication.	Injection port is self-sealing and prevents fluid leaks.
(5) Withdraw syringe from bag or bottle.	Self-seals medication port.
(6) Lower bag or bottle from IV pole, and gently mix. Rehang bag.	Ensures medication is evenly distributed.
b. Complete medication label, and apply it to bag or bottle.	Informs nurses and physicians of contents of bag or bottle.
c. Regulate infusion to desired rate (see Chapter 41). Use IV pump if indicated.	Prevents rapid infusion of fluid.
19. Properly dispose of equipment and supplies. Do not cap needle of syringe. Discard specially sheathed needles as a unit with needle covered.	Proper disposal of needle prevents injury to nurse and client. Capping of needles increases risk of needle-stick injuries.
20. Perform hand hygiene.	Reduces transmission of microorganisms.
21. Observe client for signs or symptoms of medication reaction.	IV medications cause rapid effects.
22. Observe for signs and symptoms of fluid volume excess.	Rapid uncontrolled infusion causes circulatory overload.
23. Periodically return to client's room to assess IV insertion site and rate of infusion.	Over time IV site sometimes becomes infiltrated or needle malpositioned or flow rate changes according to client's position or volume left in container.
24. Observe for signs or symptoms of IV infiltration.	Infiltrated medications sometimes injure tissue.
25. Ask client to explain purpose and effects of medication therapy.	Demonstrates learning.

Unexpected Outcomes and Related Interventions

1. Client has adverse or allergic reaction to medication.
   a. Follow institutional policy or guidelines for appropriate response and reporting of adverse drug reactions.
   b. Notify client's health care provider immediately.
   c. Add allergy information to client's medical record.
2. Client develops signs of fluid volume overload (e.g., abnormal breath sounds, shortness of breath, intake greater than output).
   a. Assess client for compromised circulatory regulation.
   b. Stop IV infusion.
   c. Notify client's health care provider immediately.
3. IV site becomes swollen, warm, reddened, and tender to touch, indicating phlebitis (see Chapter 41).
   a. Stop IV infusion, and discontinue IV.
   b. Treat IV site as indicated by institutional policy.
   c. Insert new IV site if continuation of IV therapy is indicated.

4. IV site becomes cool, pale, and swollen, indicating infiltration (see Chapter 41).
   a. Some IV medications are extremely harmful to subcutaneous tissue.
   b. Provide IV extravasation care (e.g., inject phentolamine [Regitine] around the IV infiltration site) as indicated by institutional policy, or use a medication reference manual or consult a pharmacist to determine appropriate follow-up care.

Recording and Reporting

- Record solution and medication added to parenteral fluid on appropriate form.
- Report any adverse effects to client's health care provider, and document adverse effects according to institutional policy.

* **SKILL 35-7**   ADMINISTERING MEDICATIONS BY INTRAVENOUS BOLUS   Video

Delegation Considerations

The skill of administering medications by intravenous bolus cannot be delegated. The nurse instructs nursing assistive personnel to report any unexpected drug reactions, discomfort at infusion site, and any required vital signs to the nurse.

Equipment

- Watch with second hand
- MAR or computer printout
- Clean gloves
- Antiseptic swab
- Medication in vial or ampule
- Safety syringe for medication preparation
- Needleless device or sterile needle (21 to 25 gauge)
- Intravenous lock: vial of appropriate flush solution (saline most common, heparin is sometimes used; if using heparin, most common concentration is 10 to 100 units; check agency policy)

STEPS	RATIONALE
1. Check accuracy and completeness of each MAR or computer printout with prescriber's original medication order. Check client's name and medication name, dosage, route, and time for administration. Recopy or re-print any portion of MAR that is difficult to read.	The order sheet is the most reliable source and only legal record of medications client is to receive. Ensures client receives the correct medications. Illegible MARs are a source of medication errors.

Critical Decision Point: Some IV medications can only be pushed safely when the client is being continuously monitored for dysrhythmias, blood pressure changes, or other adverse effects. Therefore some medications can only be pushed in specific areas within a health care agency. Confirm institutional guidelines regarding requirements for special monitoring, and verify these requirements are available before giving medication.

STEPS	RATIONALE
2. Collect information necessary to administer medication safely, including action, purpose, side effects, normal dose, time of peak onset, how slowly to give the medication, and nursing implications, such as the need to dilute the medication or administer it through the filter.	Allows nurse to give medication safely and monitor client's response to therapy.
3. If pushing medication into an IV line, determine the compatibility of the medication with the IV fluids and any additives within the IV solution.	Intravenous medications are not always compatible with IV solution and/or additives.
4. Perform hand hygiene. Assess IV or saline (heparin) lock insertion site for signs of infiltration or phlebitis (see Chapter 41).	Confirming the placement of the IV catheter and the integrity of the surrounding tissue ensures that the medication is administered safely.
5. Check client's medical history and allergies.	Intravenous bolus delivers medication rapidly. Allergic reactions can be fatal.
6. Check date of expiration for medication vial or ampule.	Drug potency sometimes increases or decreases when medications are outdated.
7. Assess client's understanding of purpose of medication therapy.	Reveals need for client education.
8. Prepare ordered medication from vial or ampule using aseptic technique (see Skill 35-4, p. 738). Check label of medication carefully with MAR two times.	Following the same routine when preparing medications, eliminating distractions, and checking the label of the medication with transcribed order reduce error (Pape and others, 2005).

Critical Decision Point: Some IV medications require dilution before administration. Verify with agency policy. If a small amount of medication is given (e.g., less than 1 mL), dilute medication in 5 to 10 mL of normal saline or sterile water so that the medication does not collect in the "dead spaces" (e.g., Y-site injection port, IV cap) of the IV delivery system.

STEPS	RATIONALE
9. Take medication to client at correct time.	Administer medications within 30 minutes before or after prescribed time to ensure intended therapeutic effect. Give STAT medications immediately or single-order medications at the time ordered.
10. Identify client using at least two client identifiers. Compare client's name and one other identifier (e.g., hospital identification number) on MAR, computer printout, or computer screen with information on client's identification bracelet. Ask client to state name if possible for a third identifier.	Complies with TJC (2008) requirements and improves medication safety. In most acute care settings, client's name and identification number on armband and MAR are used to identify clients. Identification bracelets are made at time of client's admission and are most reliable source of identification. Client's room number is **not** an acceptable identifier.
11. Compare label of medication with MAR at client's bedside.	The *third check* of the medication label against MAR at bedside reduces medication administration errors.

Continued

✳ SKILL 35-7   ADMINISTERING MEDICATIONS BY INTRAVENOUS BOLUS—CONT'D

STEPS	RATIONALE
12. Explain procedure to client. Encourage client to report symptoms of discomfort at IV site.	Keeps client informed and involved in care. Helps identify possible infiltration early.
13. Perform hand hygiene. Apply gloves.	Reduces transmission of microorganisms. During IV bolus administration, there is a risk of blood exposure (OSHA, 2006).
14. Administer medication by IV push (existing line):	
a. Select injection port of IV tubing closest to client. Whenever possible, injection port should accept a needleless syringe. Use IV filter if required by medication reference or agency policy.	Follows provisions of the Needle Safety and Prevention Act of 2001 (OSHA, 2006).
b. Clean off injection port with antiseptic swab. Allow to dry.	Prevents introduction of microorganisms during needle insertion.
c. Connect syringe to IV line. Insert needleless tip or small-gauge needle of syringe containing prepared drug through center of injection port (see illustration).	Prevents damage to port's diaphragm and subsequent leakage.
d. Occlude IV line by pinching tubing just above injection port (see illustration). Pull back gently on syringe's plunger to aspirate blood return.	Final check that medication is being delivered into the bloodstream.

Critical Decision Point: In some cases, especially with a smaller-gauge IV needle, blood return is not always aspirated, even if IV is patent. If IV site does not show signs of infiltration, and IV fluid is infusing without difficulty, proceed with IV push.

---

e. Release tubing, and inject medication within amount of time recommended by institutional policy, pharmacist, or medication reference manual. Use watch to time administration (see illustration). Intravenous line is sometimes pinched while pushing medication and released when not pushing medication (see illustration). Allow IV fluids to infuse when not pushing medication.	Ensures safe medication infusion. Rapid injection of IV medication will possibly be fatal. Allowing IV fluids to infuse while pushing IV drug enables medications to be delivered to client at prescribed rate.

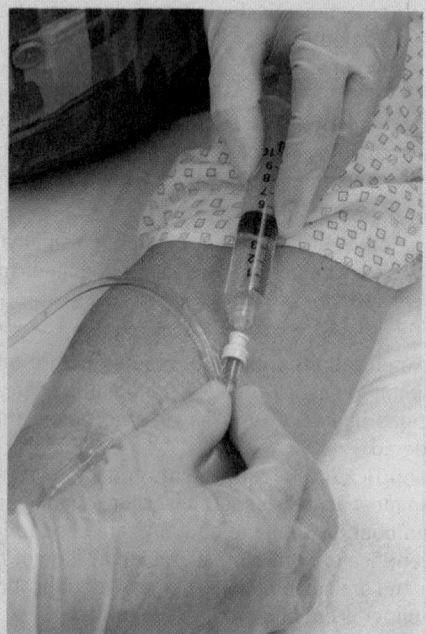

STEP 14c Connecting syringe to IV line with blunt needleless cannula tip.

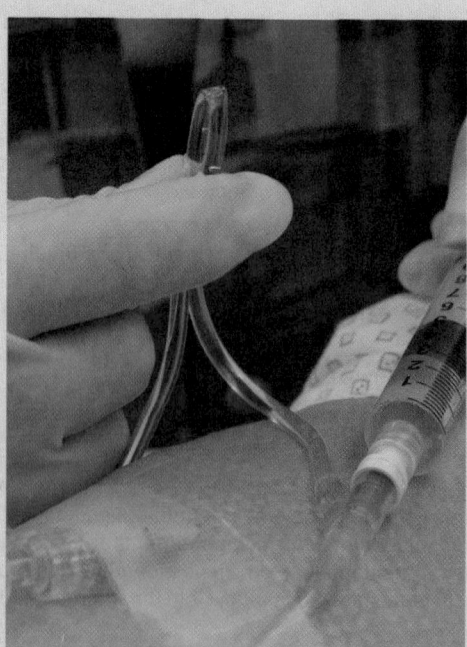

STEP 14d Intravenous line pinched above injection port for medication infusion (optional).

✳ SKILL 35-7   ADMINISTERING MEDICATIONS BY INTRAVENOUS BOLUS—CONT'D

STEPS	RATIONALE

Critical Decision Point: If IV medication is incompatible with IV fluids, stop the IV fluids, clamp the IV line, flush with 10 mL of normal saline or sterile water, give the IV bolus over the appropriate amount of time, flush with another 10 mL of normal saline or sterile water at the same rate as the medication was administered, and then restart the IV fluids at the prescribed rate. If IV that is currently hanging is a medication (e.g., ranitidine), disconnect IV and administer IV push as outlined in Step 15 to avoid giving a sudden bolus of the medication in the existing IV line to the client and to avoid creating potential risks associated with IV incompatibilities. Some IV medications and fluids cannot be stopped. Verify institutional policy regarding the temporary stopping of IV fluids or continuous IV medications. If unable to stop IV infusion, start a new IV site (see Chapter 41) and administer medication using the IV lock method.

STEPS	RATIONALE
f. After injecting medication, release tubing, withdraw syringe, and recheck fluid infusion rate.	Injection of bolus alters rate of fluid infusion. Rapid fluid infusion causes circulatory overload.
15. Administering medications by IV push (IV lock or a needleless system)	
A. Prepare flush solutions according to agency policy.	
(1) Saline flush method (preferred method):	
a. Prepare two syringes with 2 to 3 mL of normal saline (0.9%) in syringe.	Normal saline is effective in keeping IV locks patent and is compatible with a wide range of medications.
(2) Heparin flush method (traditional method):	
a. Prepare one syringe with ordered amount of heparin flush solution.	
b. Prepare two syringes with 2 to 3 mL of normal saline.	
B. Administer medication:	
(1) Clean injection port of lock with antiseptic swab.	Prevents introduction of microorganisms during needle insertion.
(2) Insert syringe containing normal saline into injection port of IV lock (see illustration).	
(3) Pull back gently on syringe plunger, and look for blood return.	Determines whether IV needle or catheter is positioned in vein.

Critical Decision Point: At times a blood return is not aspirated even though the lock is patent. If IV site does not show signs of infiltration, and IV site flushes without difficulty, proceed with IV push.

STEPS	RATIONALE
(4) Flush IV lock with normal saline by pushing slowly on plunger.	Clears IV lock of blood.

Critical Decision Point: Observe closely the area of skin above the IV catheter. Note any puffiness or swelling as the IV lock is flushed, which indicates infiltration into the vein, requiring removal of the catheter.

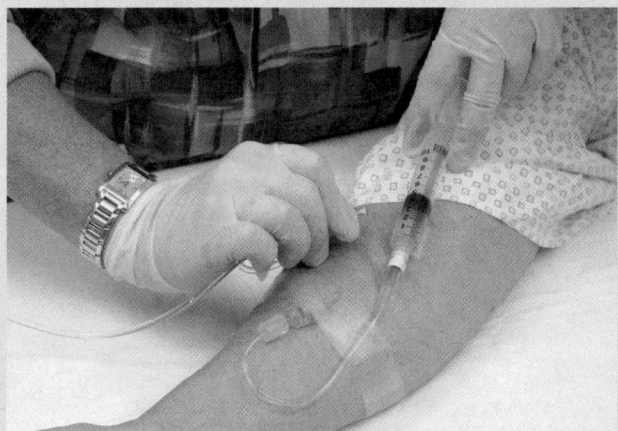

STEP 14e Using a watch to time an IV push medication.

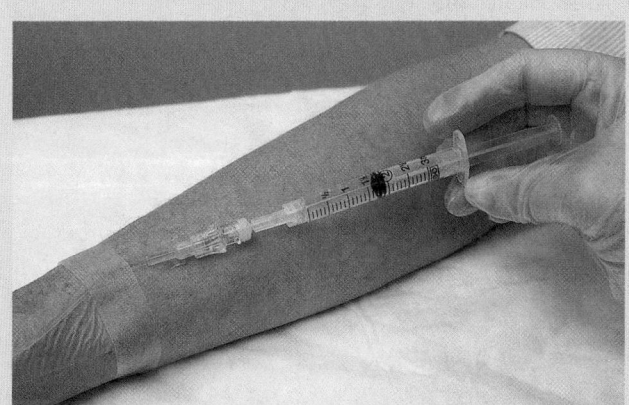

STEP 15B(2) Syringe inserted into injection port.

Continued

✳ **SKILL 35-7   ADMINISTERING MEDICATIONS BY INTRAVENOUS BOLUS—CONT'D**

STEPS	RATIONALE
(5) Remove saline-filled syringe.	
(6) Clean lock's injection port with antiseptic swab.	Prevents transmission of infection.
(7) Insert syringe containing prepared medication into injection port of IV lock.	
(8) Inject medication within amount of time recommended by institution al policy, pharmacist, or medication reference manual. Use a watch to time administration.	Rapid injection of IV medication can result in death. Following guidelines for IV push rates promotes client safety (Karch and Karch, 2003).
(9) After administering bolus, withdraw syringe.	
(10) Clean lock's injection port with antiseptic swab.	Prevents transmission of microorganisms.
(11) Attach syringe with normal saline, and inject normal saline flush at the same rate the medication was delivered.	Irrigation with saline prevents occlusion of IV access device and ensures all medication is delivered. Flushing IV site at same rate as medication ensures that any medication remaining within IV needle is delivered at the correct rate.
(12) *Heparin flush option:* Insert needle of syringe containing heparin through diaphragm. Inject heparin slowly, and remove syringe.	Maintains patency of needle by inhibiting clot formation. *SASH method: S*aline, *A*dministration of medication, *S*aline, *H*eparin.
16. Dispose of uncapped needles and syringes in puncture-proof and leakproof container.	Reduces accidental needle sticks (OSHA, 2006).
17. Remove and dispose of gloves. Perform hand hygiene.	Reduces the transmission of microorganisms.
18. Observe client closely for adverse reaction as drug is administered and for several minutes thereafter.	IV medications act rapidly.
19. Observe IV site during injection for sudden swelling.	Swelling indicates infiltration into tissues surrounding vein.
20. Assess client's status after giving medication to evaluate the effectiveness of the medication.	IV bolus medications often cause rapid changes in the client's physiological status. Some medications require careful monitoring and assessment and possibly laboratory testing (e.g., vasopressors require monitoring of blood pressure and heart rate; dilantin requires laboratory studies to determine if it is in a therapeutic level).
21. Ask client to explain medication's purposes and side effects.	Evaluates learning.

Unexpected Outcomes and Related Interventions

1. Client develops adverse reaction to medication.
   a. Stop delivering medication immediately, and follow institutional policy or guidelines for appropriate response and reporting of adverse drug reactions.
   b. Notify client's health care provider of adverse effects immediately.
   c. Add allergy information to client's medical record.
2. Intravenous site shows symptoms of infiltration or phlebitis (see Chapter 41).
   a. See related interventions in Skill 35-6, p. 756.

Recording and Reporting

- Record medication, dose, time, route, and time of administration.
- Report any adverse reactions immediately to health care provider because they could be life threatening. Client's response indicates need for additional medical therapy.
- Record client's response to medication in nurses' notes.

Volume-Controlled Infusions. Another way of administering intravenous medications is through small amounts (50 to 100 mL) of compatible intravenous fluids. The fluid is within a secondary fluid container separate from the primary fluid bag. The container connects directly to the primary intravenous line or to separate tubing that inserts into the primary line (Skill 35-8). Three types of containers are volume control administration sets (e.g., Volutrol or Pediatrol), piggyback and/or tandem set, and miniinfusors. Using volume-controlled infusions has several advantages:

- It reduces risk of rapid-dose infusion by intravenous push. Medications are diluted and infused over longer time intervals (e.g., 30 to 60 minutes).
- It allows for administration of medications (e.g., antibiotics) that are stable for a limited time in solution.
- It allows for control of intravenous fluid intake.

Piggyback. A piggyback is a small (25 to 250 mL) intravenous bag or bottle connected to a short tubing line that connects to the *upper* Y-port of a primary infusion line or to an intermittent venous access (Figure 35-30). The piggyback tubing is a microdrip or macrodrip system (see Chapter 41). The set is called a piggyback because the small bag or bottle is higher than the primary infusion bag or bottle. In the piggyback setup the main line does not infuse when the piggybacked medication is infusing. The port of the primary intravenous line contains a back-check valve that automatically stops flow of the primary infusion once the piggyback infusion flows. After the piggyback solution infuses and the solution within the tubing falls below the level of the primary infusion drip chamber, the back-check valve opens and the primary infusion again flows.

Tandem. A tandem setup is a small (25 to 100 mL) intravenous bag or bottle connected to a short tubing line to the *lower* Y-port of a primary infusion line or to an intermittent venous access. Place the tandem set at the same height as the primary infusion bag or bottle. In the tandem setup the tandem and the main line infuse simultaneously. Monitor the tandem setup closely. If the tandem setup is not immediately clamped when the medication is infused, the intravenous solution from the primary line will back up into the tandem line.

Volume-Control Administration. Volume-control administration (Volutrol, Buretrol, or Pediatrol) sets are small (50 to 150 mL) containers that attach just below the primary infusion bag or bottle. The set is attached and filled in a manner similar to that used with a regular intravenous infusion. However, the priming filling of the set is different, depending on the type of filter (floating valve or membrane) within the set. Follow package directions for priming sets (see Chapter 41).

Miniinfusion Pump. The miniinfusion pump is battery operated and allows medications to be given in very small amounts of fluid (5 to 60 mL) within controlled infusion times using standard syringes.

Intermittent Venous Access. An intermittent venous access (commonly called a heparin lock or saline lock) is an intravenous catheter with a small chamber covered by a rubber diaphragm or a specially designed cap (Figure 35-31). Special rubber-seal injec-

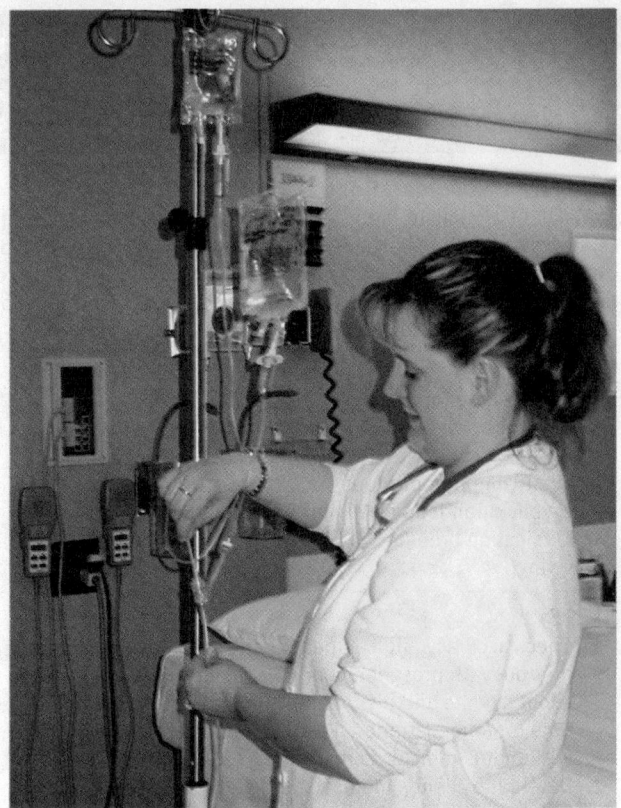

Figure 35-30 Piggyback setup.

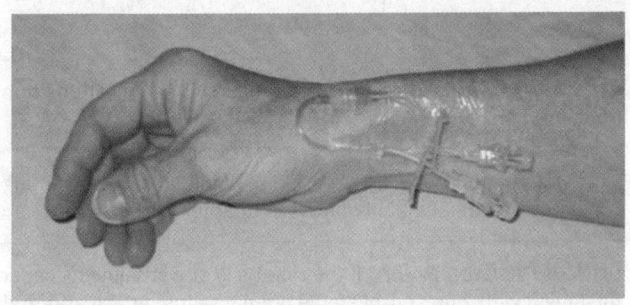

Figure 35-31 Intermittent lock covered with a rubber diaphragm.

tion caps usually accept needle safety devices (see Chapter 41). Advantages to intermittent venous access include the following:

- Cost savings resulting from the omission of continuous intravenous therapy
- Convenience to the nurse by eliminating constant monitoring of flow rates
- Increased mobility, safety, and comfort for the client

Before administering an intravenous bolus or piggyback medication, assess the patency and placement of the intravenous site. After the medication has been administered through an intermittent venous access, the access must be flushed with a solution to keep it patent. Generally, normal saline is an effective flush solution for
Text continued on p. 768

⁕ SKILL 35-8 **ADMINISTERING INTRAVENOUS MEDICATIONS BY PIGGYBACK, INTERMITTENT INTRAVENOUS INFUSION SETS, AND MINIINFUSION PUMPS**

Delegation Considerations

The skill of administering IV medications by piggyback, intermittent intravenous infusion sets, and miniinfusion pumps cannot be delegated. Instruct nursing assistive personnel about the type of unexpected medication reactions and discomfort at the infusion site to report to the nurse as soon as possible.

Equipment

- Adhesive tape (optional)
- Antiseptic swab
- IV pole
- MAR or computer printout
- Piggyback, Tandem, or Miniinfusion Pump
  - Medication prepared in 5- to 250-mL labeled infusion bag or syringe

- Short microdrip or macrodrip tubing set for piggyback (preferably with needleless system attachment)
  - Needleless device or stopcocks, preferred if available
  - Needles (21 or 23 gauge, **only** if stopcocks or other needleless methods are not available)
  - Miniinfusion pump if needed
- Volume-Control Administration Set
  - Volutrol or Buretrol
  - Infusion tubing (may have needleless system attachment)
  - Syringe (1 to 20 mL)
  - Vial or ampule of ordered medication

STEPS	RATIONALE
1. Check accuracy and completeness of each MAR or computer printout with prescriber's original medication order. Check client's name and medication name, dosage, route, and time for administration. Recopy or re-print any portion of MAR that is difficult to read.	The order sheet is the most reliable source and only legal record of medications client is to receive. Ensures client receives the correct medications. Illegible MARs are a source of medication errors.
2. Determine client's medical history.	Indicates type of appropriate IV solution used and helps ensure safe and accurate medication administration.
3. Collect information necessary to administer medication safely, including action, purpose, side effects, normal dose, time of peak onset, and nursing implications.	Allows nurse to give medication safely and to monitor client's response to therapy.
4. Assess compatibility of drug with existing IV solution.	Drugs that are incompatible with IV solutions often result in clouding or crystallization of solution in IV tubing, which will possibly harm the client.

Critical Decision Point: Never administer IV medications through tubing that is infusing blood, blood products, or parenteral nutrition solutions.

5. Assess patency of client's existing IV infusion line by noting infusion rate of main IV line (see Chapter 41).	IV line must be patent and fluids need to infuse easily for medication to reach venous circulation effectively.

Critical Decision Point: If the client's IV site is saline locked, cleanse the port with alcohol and assess the patency of the IV line by flushing it with 2 to 3 mL of sterile normal saline. Attach appropriate IV tubing to the saline lock, and administer the medication via piggyback, tandem, miniinfusion, or volume-control administration set. When the infusion is completed, disconnect the tubing, cleanse the port with alcohol, and flush the IV line with 2 to 3 mL sterile normal saline. Maintain sterility of IV tubing between intermittent infusions.

6. Perform hand hygiene. Assess IV insertion site for signs of infiltration or phlebitis: redness, pallor, swelling, tenderness on palpation.	Confirmation of placement of IV needle or catheter and integrity of surrounding tissues ensures safe medication administration.
7. Assess client's history of medication allergies.	Effects of medications develop rapidly after IV infusion. Be aware of clients at risk.
8. Assess client's understanding of purpose of medication therapy.	Reveals need for education.
9. Prepare medications from ampule or vial (see Skill 35-4, p. 738). Be sure to compare the label of the medication with the MAR two times while preparing the medication.	Following the same routine when preparing medications, eliminating distractions, and checking the label of the medication with transcribed order reduces error (Pape and others, 2005).
10. Assemble medication and supplies at bedside. Prepare client by informing client that medication will be given through IV equipment.	Allows client to understand procedure and minimizes anxiety.
11. Perform hand hygiene.	Reduces transmission of infection.

ADMINISTERING INTRAVENOUS MEDICATIONS BY PIGGYBACK, INTERMITTENT INTRAVENOUS INFUSION SETS, AND MINIINFUSION PUMPS—CONT'D

STEPS	RATIONALE
12. Identify client using at least two client identifiers. Compare client's name and one other identifier (e.g., hospital identification number) on MAR, computer printout, or computer screen with information on client's identification bracelet. Ask client to state name if possible for a third identifier.	Complies with TJC (2008) requirements and improves medication safety. In most acute care settings, client's name and identification number on armband and MAR are used to identify clients. Identification bracelets are made at time of client's admission and are most reliable source of identification. Client's room number is **not** an acceptable identifier.
13. Compare medication label with MAR at client's bedside.	*This is the third accuracy check.*
14. Explain purpose of medication and side effects to client and explain that medication is to be given through existing IV line. Encourage client to report symptoms of discomfort at site.	Keeps client informed of planned therapies. Clients who verbalize pain at the IV site help detect IV infiltrations early, lessening damage to surrounding tissues.
15. Administer infusion:	
A. Piggyback or tandem infusion	
(1) Connect infusion tubing to medication bag (see Chapter 41). Allow solution to fill tubing by opening regulator flow clamp. Once tubing is full, close clamp and cap end of tubing.	Infusion tubing needs to be filled with solution and free of air bubbles to prevent air embolus.
(2) Hang piggyback medication bag above level of primary fluid bag (use hook to lower main bag) (see illustration). Hang tandem infusion at same level as primary fluid bag.	Height of fluid bag affects rate of flow to client.
(3) Connect tubing of piggyback or tandem infusion to appropriate connector on primary infusion line:	
a. *Stopcock:* Wipe off stopcock port with alcohol swab, and connect tubing. Turn stopcock to open position.	Stopcock eliminates need for needle.
b. *Needleless system:* Wipe off needleless port, and insert tip of piggyback or tandem infusion tubing (see illustration).	Use needleless connections to prevent accidental needle-stick injuries (OSHA, 2006). Establishes route for IV medication to enter main IV line.
c. *Tubing port:* Connect sterile needle to end of piggyback or tandem infusion tubing, remove cap, cleanse injection port on main IV line, and insert needle through center of port. Secure by taping connection.	**Only** use this step if needleless system is not available. Prevents introduction of microorganisms during needle insertion.

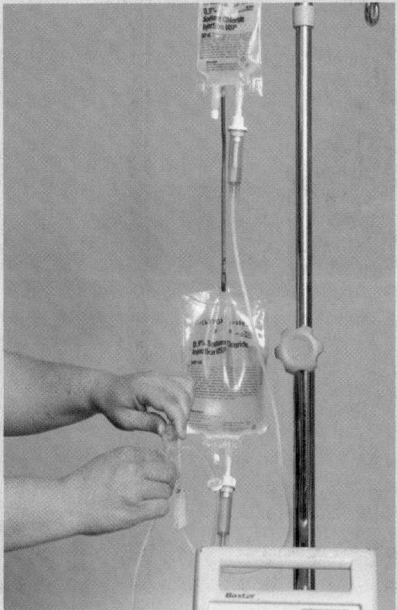

STEP 14A(2) Piggyback infusion and primary IV infusion.

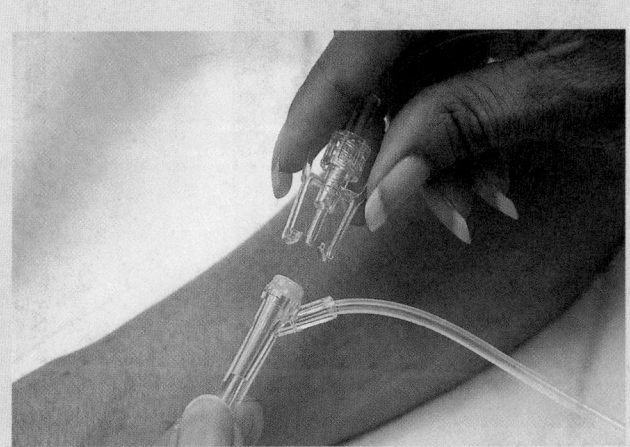

STEP 14A(3)b Needleless lever lock cannula system.

Continued

✳ **SKILL 35-8**

ADMINISTERING INTRAVENOUS MEDICATIONS BY PIGGYBACK, INTERMITTENT INTRAVENOUS INFUSION SETS, AND MINIINFUSION PUMPS—CONT'D

STEPS	RATIONALE
(4) Regulate flow rate of medication solution by adjusting regulator clamp. (Infusion times vary. Refer to medication reference or institutional policy for safe flow rate.)	Provides slow, intermittent infusion of medication and maintains therapeutic blood levels.
(5) After medication has infused, check flow regulator on primary infusion. The primary infusion automatically begins to flow after the piggyback or tandem solution is empty.	Back-check valve on piggyback stops flow of the primary infusion until second medication infuses. The tandem and primary infusions flow together until the tandem set empties. Checking flow rate ensures proper administration of IV fluids.
(6) Regulate main infusion line to desired rate, if necessary.	Infusion of piggyback sometimes interferes with the main line infusion rate.
(7) Leave IV piggyback bag and tubing in place for future medication administration, or discard in appropriate containers.	Establishment of secondary line produces route for microorganisms to enter main line. Repeated changes in tubing increase risk of infection transmission (check agency policy).
B. Volume-control administration set (e.g., Volutrol)	
(1) Fill Volutrol with desired amount of fluid (50 to 100 mL) by opening clamp between Volutrol and main IV bag (see illustration).	Small volume of fluid dilutes IV medication and reduces risk of too-rapid infusion.
(2) Close clamp, and check to be sure clamp on air vent of Volutrol chamber is open.	Prevents additional leakage of fluid into Volutrol. Air vent allows fluid in Volutrol to exit at regulated rate.
(3) Clean injection port on top of Volutrol with antiseptic swab.	Prevents introduction of microorganisms during needle insertion.
(4) Remove needle cap or sheath, and insert syringe needle through port, then inject medication (see illustrations). Gently rotate Volutrol between hands.	Rotating mixes medication with solution in Volutrol to ensure equal distribution.
(5) Regulate IV infusion rate to allow medication to infuse in time recommended by institutional policy, a pharmacist, or a medication reference manual.	For optimal therapeutic effect, medication needs to infuse in prescribed time interval.
(6) Label Volutrol with name of medication, dosage, total volume including diluent, and time of administration.	Alerts nurses to medication being infused. Prevents other medications from being added to Volutrol.

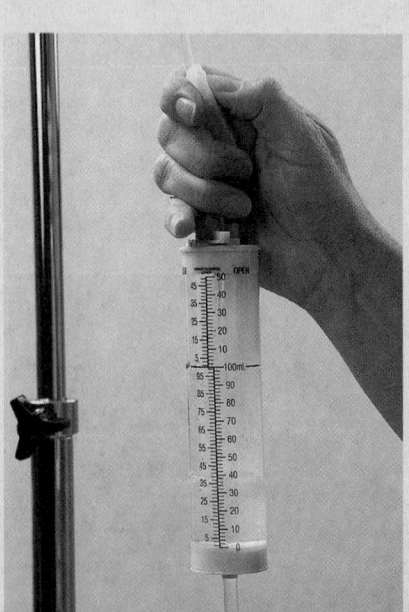

STEP 14B(1) Filling volume-control administration device.

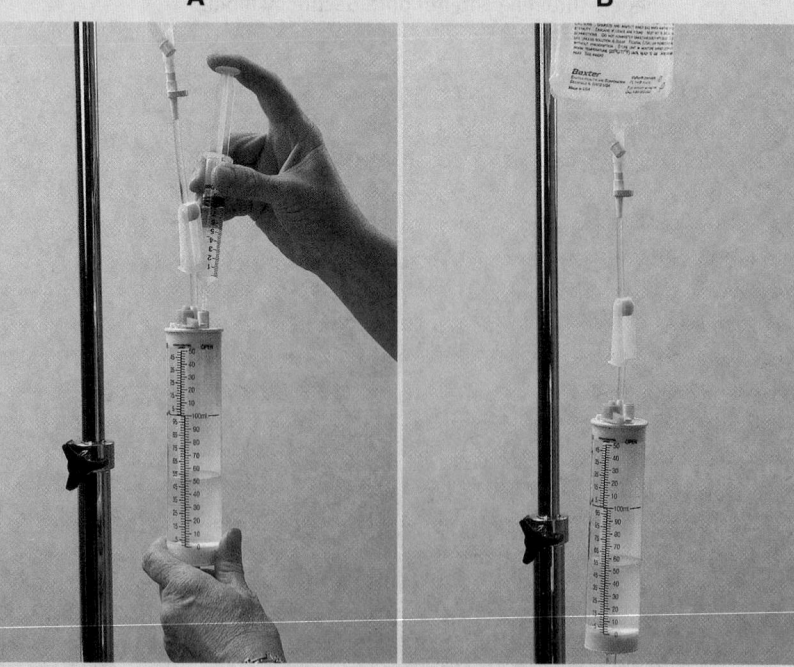

STEP 14B(4) A, Medication injected into device. **B,** Prepared device.

ADMINISTERING INTRAVENOUS MEDICATIONS BY PIGGYBACK, INTERMITTENT INTRAVENOUS INFUSION SETS, AND MINIINFUSION PUMPS—CONT'D

STEPS	RATIONALE
(7) Dispose of uncapped needle or needle enclosed in safety shield and syringe in proper container.	Prevents accidental needle sticks (OSHA, 2006).
(8) Discard supplies in appropriate container, and perform hand hygiene.	Reduces transmission of microorganisms.

C. Miniinfusion administration

STEPS	RATIONALE
(1) Connect prefilled syringe to miniinfusion tubing.	Special tubing designed to fit syringe delivers medication to main IV line.
(2) Carefully apply pressure to syringe plunger, allowing tubing to fill with medication.	Ensures that tubing is free of air bubbles to prevent air embolus.
(3) Place syringe into miniinfusor pump (follow product directions). Be sure syringe is secure (see illustration).	
(4) Connect miniinfusion tubing to main IV line.	
a. *Sto*pcock: Wipe off stopcock port with alcohol swab, and connect tubing. Turn stopcock to open position.	Stopcock reduces risk of needle-stick injuries.
b. Needleless system: Wipe off needleless port, and insert tip of miniinfusor tubing.	Needleless system reduces risk of needle-stick injuries (OSHA, 2006).
c. Tubing port: Connect sterile needle to miniinfusion tubing, remove cap, cleanse injection port on main IV line, and insert needle through center of port. Consider placing tape where IV tubing enters port to secure connection.	**Only** use this method if needleless system is not available. Cleansing reduces transmission of microorganisms.
(5) Hang infusion pump with syringe on IV pole alongside main IV bag. Set pump to deliver medication within time recommended by institutional policy, pharmacist, or medication reference manual. Press button on pump to begin infusion.	Pump automatically delivers medication at safe, constant rate based on volume in syringe. (Alarm is used if medication is delivered into heparin/saline lock.)
(6) After medication has infused, check flow regulator on primary infusion. The infusion should automatically begin to flow once the pump stops. Regulate main infusion line to desired rate as needed. (NOTE: If stopcock is used, turn off miniinfusion line.)	Maintains patency of primary IV line.

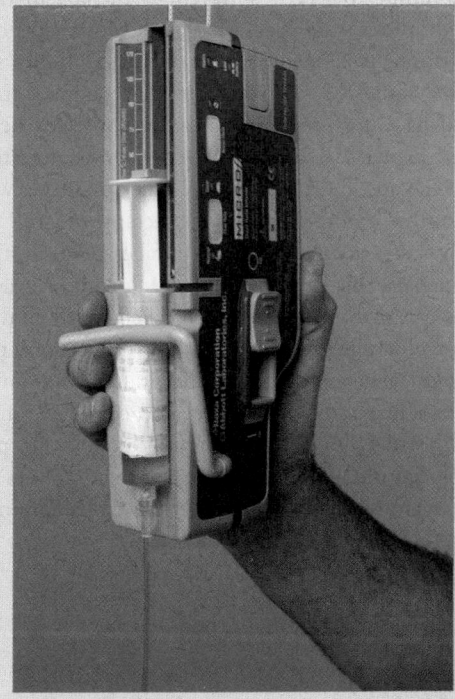

STEP 15C(3) Securing syringe into miniinfusor.

✳ **SKILL 35-8**   ADMINISTERING INTRAVENOUS MEDICATIONS BY PIGGYBACK, INTERMITTENT INTRAVENOUS INFUSION SETS, AND MINIINFUSION PUMPS—CONT'D

STEPS	RATIONALE
16. Observe client for signs of adverse reactions.	IV medications act rapidly.
17. During infusion, periodically check infusion rate and condition of IV site.	IV needs to remain patent for proper medication administration. Development of infiltration necessitates discontinuing infusion.
18. Ask client to explain purpose and side effects of medication.	Evaluates client's understanding of instruction.

Unexpected Outcomes and Related Interventions
1. Client develops adverse drug reaction.
   a. Stop medication infusion immediately.
   b. Follow institutional policy or guidelines for appropriate response and reporting of adverse drug reactions.
   c. Notify client's health care provider of adverse effects immediately.
   d. Document allergy in client's medical record.
2. Medication does not infuse over desired period.
   a. Determine reason (e.g., improper calculation of flow rate, malpositioning of IV needle at insertion site, or infiltration).
   b. Take corrective action as indicated.
3. IV site shows signs of phlebitis or infiltration (see Chapter 41).
   a. See related interventions in Skill 35-6, p. 756.

Recording and Reporting
- Record medication, dose, route, and time administered on MAR or computer printout.
- Record volume of fluid in medication bag or Volutrol on intake and output form.
- Report any adverse reactions to client's health care provider.

Home Care Considerations
- Teach client and caregiver to dispose of needles and contaminated equipment in puncture-proof containers (e.g., coffee can).
- Instruct family about community resources to obtain supplies.

peripheral catheters. Some institutions require the use of heparin. Nurses need to verify and follow the institution's policies regarding the care and maintenance of the IV site.

Administration of Intravenous Therapy in the Home. Sometimes clients are discharged from an acute care setting and continue to receive intravenous therapy in the home setting. Medications such as antibiotics, chemotherapy, total parenteral nutrition, pain medications, and blood transfusions are given in the home. Most clients who have home intravenous therapy will have a central venous catheter inserted before discharge (see Chapter 41). In addition, clients who need to receive intravenous therapy in the home have home care nurses who assist in the management of the intravenous therapy.

Carefully assess clients and their families to determine their ability to manage this therapy at home. Provide instruction on intravenous care management while the client is still in the hospital. Clients and families need to learn how to recognize problems and what to do when these problems occur. It is important for the family to recognize signs of infection and complications and to know that they need to notify the home care nurse or physician when these occur. In addition, clients and their families need information regarding maintenance of intravenous administration equipment, including the infusion pump.

✳ Key Concepts

- Learning medication classifications improves understanding of nursing implications for administering medications with similar characteristics.
- Federal medication legislation regulates the production, distribution, prescription, and administration of medications.
- All controlled substances are handled according to strict procedures that account for each medication.
- The nurse applies understanding of the physiology of medication action when timing administration, selecting routes, initiating actions to promote medication efficacy, and observing responses to medications.
- The older adult's body undergoes structural and functional changes that alter medication actions and influence the manner in which nurses provide medication therapy.
- The nurse calculates children's medication doses on the basis of body surface area or weight.
- Verify medication calculations with another nurse to ensure accuracy.
- Medications given parenterally are absorbed more quickly than medications administered by other routes.
- Each medication order needs to include the client's name, the order date, the medication name, dosage, route, time of administration, drug indication, and the prescriber's signature.
- A medication history reveals allergies, medications a client is taking, and the client's adherence to therapy.
- Use the nursing process when administering medications.
- The six rights of medication administration contribute to accurate preparation and administration of medication doses.

- The six rights of medication administration are the right medication, right dose, right client, right route, right time, and right documentation.
- Nurses need to avoid distractions and follow the same routine when preparing medications to reduce chance of making medication errors.
- Nurses administer only medications they prepare, and prepared medications are never left unattended.
- Chart medications immediately after administration.
- A nurse uses clinical judgment in determining the best time to administer prn medications.
- The nurse reports a medication error immediately.
- When preparing medications, the nurse checks the medication container label against the medication administration record or computer printout three times.
- The Z-track method for intramuscular injections protects subcutaneous tissues from irritating parenteral fluids.
- Failure to select injection sites by anatomical landmarks leads to tissue, bone, or nerve damage.

✳ Critical Thinking Exercises

You have completed the discharge teaching with Mrs. McFarland and her daughter. A few hours later, directly before she is released from the hospital, Mrs. McFarland's physician decides that she needs to be placed on two insulins (a long-acting insulin and a short-acting insulin). The short-acting insulin will have a sliding scale.

1. Before she leaves the hospital, are there any other interventions that should be implemented?

2. Because Mrs. McFarland has only been in the hospital overnight and her daughter has had little time to learn these skills, what are some concerns that you would like to see followed up in home care?

3. What are factors that often prevent clients and family members from learning in the hospital environment?

✳ NCLEX®-Style Review Questions

1. The nurse is having difficulty reading a physician's order for a medication. The nurse knows the physician is very busy and does not like to be called. The nurse should:
   1. Call a pharmacist to interpret the order
   2. Call the physician to have the order clarified
   3. Consult the unit manager to help interpret the order
   4. Ask the unit secretary to interpret the physician's handwriting

2. The client has an order for 2 tablespoons of Milk of Magnesia. The nurse converts this dose to the metric system and gives the client:
   1. 2 mL
   2. 5 mL
   3. 16 mL
   4. 30 mL

3. Most medication errors occur when the nurse:
   1. Is caring for too many clients
   2. Fails to follow routine procedures
   3. Is administering unfamiliar medications
   4. Is responsible for administering numerous medications

4. A client is to receive cephalexin (Keflex) 500 mg PO. The pharmacy has sent 250-mg tablets. The nurse gives:
   1. ½ tablet
   2. 1 tablet
   3. 1½ tablets
   4. 2 tablets

5. When identifying a new client before administering medications, the nurse asks the client to state his name. The client does not state the correct name. The nurse asks again, and the client states still another name. What is the nurse's next action?
   1. Laugh at the client, and tell him to quit "kidding."
   2. Give the medications without any further questioning.
   3. Look at the client's armband to identify the client, and disregard what the client said.
   4. Investigate the client's mental status before administering any further medications.

6. A client is transitioning from the hospital to the home environment. A home care referral is obtained. What is a priority, in relation to safe medication administration, for the discharge nurse?
   1. Set up the follow-up appointments with the physician for the client.
   2. Ensure that someone will provide housekeeping for the client at home.
   3. Ensure the home care agency is aware of medication and health teaching needs.
   4. Make sure that the client has plenty of diapers and blue pads to take home with him.

7. A nursing student takes a client's antibiotic to his room. The client asks the nursing student what it is and why he should take it. The nursing student's reply includes the following information:
   1. Only the client's physician can give this information
   2. The name of the medication and a description of its desired effect
   3. Information about medications is confidential and cannot be shared
   4. Due to limits placed on nursing students, the client will have to speak with his assigned nurse about this

8. The nurse is administering a sustained-release capsule to a new client. The client insists that he cannot swallow pills. The best course of action for the nurse is to:
   1. Ask the physician to change the order
   2. Crush the pill with a mortar and pestle
   3. Hide the capsule in a piece of solid food
   4. Open the capsule and sprinkle it over pudding

9. The nurse takes a medication to a client, and the client tells the nurse to take it away because she is not going to take it. The nurse's first action should be to:
   1. Ask the client's reason for refusal
   2. Explain that she must take the medication
   3. Take the medication away and chart the client's refusal
   4. Tell the client that her physician knows what is best for her

10. The nurse selects the route for administering medication according to:
    1. Hospital policy
    2. The prescriber's orders
    3. The type of medication ordered
    4. The client's size and muscle mass

11. A client is receiving an IV push medication. If this type of drug infiltrates into the outer tissues, the nurse will:
    1. Continue to let the IV run
    2. Apply a warm compress to infiltrated site
    3. Follow facility policy or drug manufacturer's directions
    4. Not worry about this because vesicant filtration is not a problem

12. If a client who is receiving IV fluids develops tenderness, warmth, erythema, and pain at the site, the nurse suspects:
    1. Sepsis
    2. Phlebitis
    3. Infiltration
    4. Fluid overload

36 | Complementary and Alternative Therapies

✳ OBJECTIVES

Mastery of content in this chapter will enable the student to:

- Differentiate between complementary and alternative therapies.
- Describe the clinical applications of relaxation therapies.
- Discuss the relaxation response and its effect on somatic ailments.
- Identify the principles and effectiveness of imagery, meditation, and breathwork.
- Describe the purpose and principles of biofeedback.
- Describe the methods of and the psychophysiological responses to therapeutic touch.
- Explain the scope of practice of chiropractic therapy.
- Discuss the principles and applications of acupuncture.
- Describe safe and unsafe herbal therapies.

✳ MEDIA RESOURCES ✳ KEY TERMS

 Companion CD
- NCLEX®-Style Review Questions
- Audio Glossary
- Interactive Learning Activities
- English/Spanish Glossary

evolve Website
- NCLEX®-Style Review Questions
- Audio Glossary
- English/Spanish Glossary
- Interactive Learning Activities
- Weblinks
- Audio Summaries

Acupoints, p. 780
Acupuncture, p. 780
Allopathic medicine, p. 772
Alternative therapies, p. 772
Biofeedback, p. 778
Chiropractic therapy, p. 780
Complementary therapies, p. 772
Creative visualization, p. 778
Energy flow, p. 779
Herbal therapy, p. 781
Imagery, p. 778
Integrative medical programs, p. 772

Meditation, p. 777
Meridians, p. 780
Passive relaxation, p. 776
Progressive relaxation, p. 775
Qi, p. 780
Relaxation response, p. 775
Stress response, p. 775
Therapeutic touch, p. 779
Traditional Chinese medicine (TCM), p. 780
Yin and yang, p. 780

The general health of North American people has steadily improved over the course of the last century as evidenced by lower mortality rates and increased life expectancies. Changes in science and medicine have provided the knowledge and technology to successfully alter the course of many illnesses. Despite the success of **allopathic medicine** (traditional Western medicine), many conditions such as arthritis, chronic back pain, gastrointestinal problems, allergies, headache, and insomnia have been difficult to treat, and more clients are exploring alternative methods to relieve their symptom distress. Researchers estimate that up to 75% of clients seek care from their primary care practitioners for stress, pain, and health conditions for which there are no known causes or cures (Rakel and Faass, 2006). Although allopathic medicine is quite effective in treating numerous physical ailments (e.g., bacterial infections, structural abnormalities, and acute emergencies), it is in general less effective in preventing disease, decreasing stress-induced illnesses, managing chronic disease, and caring for the emotional and spiritual needs of individuals.

The number of clients seeking unconventional treatments has risen considerably. In part this increase is due to (1) the perception that the treatments offered by the medical profession do not provide relief for a variety of common illnesses, (2) the increasing interest of clients in becoming more educated about their health and the need to take a more active role in their treatment, (3) the increased number of research articles in journals such as *Alternative Therapies in Health and Medicine* and the *Journal of Holistic Nursing,* and (4) the attraction to a holistic approach to health care that incorporates the mind, body, and spirit (Rakel and Faass, 2006).

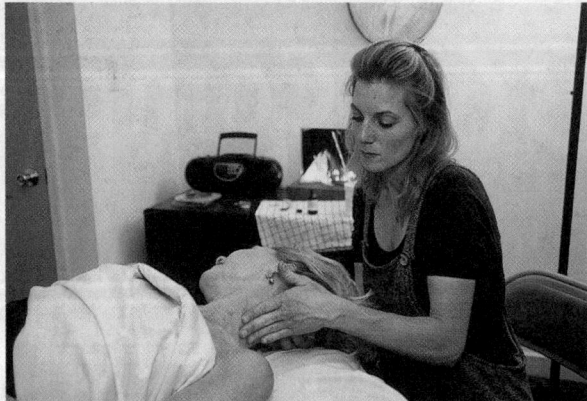

Figure 36-1 Massage therapy can be effectively used to relieve tension.

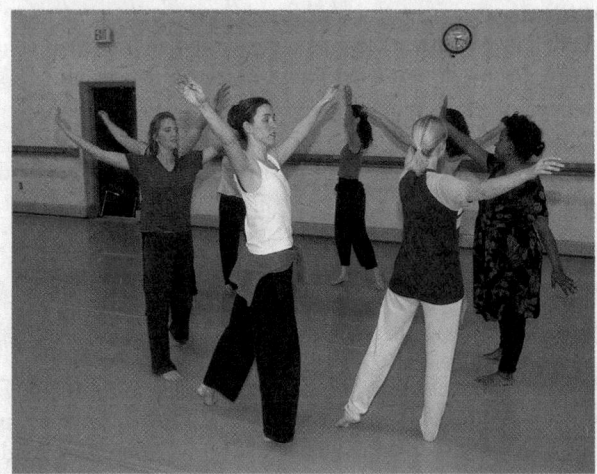

Figure 36-2 Young adults participating in dance therapy.

Complementary or Alternative Medicine Therapies in Health Care

Unconventional therapies are referred to as either complementary or alternative medicine (CAM) therapies. **Complementary therapies** are those therapies used in addition to conventional treatment recommended by the person's health care provider. As the name implies, complementary therapies complement conventional treatments. Many complementary therapies, such as therapeutic touch, contain diagnostic and therapeutic methods specific to their practice that need special training, whereas others, such as guided imagery and breathwork, are easily learned and applied. Complementary therapies also include relaxation; exercise; massage (Figure 36-1); reflexology; prayer; biofeedback; hypnotherapy; creative therapies, including art, music, or dance therapy (Figure 36-2); meditation; chiropractic therapy; osteopathy; and herbalism (Fontaine, 2005).

Alternative therapies include the same interventions as complementary therapies but frequently become the primary treatment that replaces allopathic medical care. Both complementary and alternative therapies vary in the degree to which they are compatible with allopathic medicine. For example, chiropractic and Feldenkrais (gentle body-movement therapy) practitioners frequently use diagnostic terminology and methods similar to those utilized by allopathic practitioners. They base interventions on conventional pathophysiology and anatomy but at the same time explore mind-body connections that cause or contribute to the physiological condition. Several therapies though are considered alternative because they are based on completely different philosophies and life systems than those used by allopathic medicine. Examples include Chinese medicine and acupuncture, Ayurvedic medicine, and various forms of shamanism. Some regard alternative therapies that are not supported by scientific data, such as use of shark cartilage and coffee enemas, with caution. Even the more well-established therapies have only been rigorously tested on small or otherwise limited populations, because funding for such research is limited. Table 36-1 presents types of complementary and alternative therapies.

Between one third and one half of the population in the United States uses one or more forms of CAM (Rakel and Faass, 2006). Furthermore, data from a recent survey of U.S. citizens suggest a 47.3% increase in the number of visits to alternative medicine practitioners. This exceeds the number of visits to allopathic practitioners. Because of this increased interest and use of CAM, many institutions, including mainstream medical schools, have established training programs that incorporate CAM philosophy and content into the curriculum. Some are developing **integrative medical programs** that allow health care consumers the opportunity to be treated by a team of providers consisting of

✳ TABLE 36-1 Complementary and Alternative Therapies

TYPES	DEFINITIONS
Alternative Medical Systems—Built Upon Complete Systems of Theory and Practice	
Acupuncture	A traditional Chinese method of producing analgesia or altering the function of a body system by inserting thin needles along a series of lines or channels, called meridians. Direct needle manipulation of energetic meridians influences deeper internal organs by redirecting *qi*.
Ayurveda	Traditional Hindu system of medicine practiced in India since the first century AD. A combination of remedies such as herbs, purgative, and rubbing oils treat disease.
Homeopathic medicine	System of medical treatments based on the theory that certain diseases can be cured by giving small doses of substances that in a healthy person would produce symptoms like those of the disease. Prescribed substances called remedies are made from naturally occurring plant, animal, or mineral substances.
Latin American practices	*Curanderismo* medical system, which includes a humoral model for classifying food, activity, drugs, and illnesses and a series of folk illnesses.
Native American practices	Therapies include sweating and purging, herbal remedies, and shamanic healing (healer makes contact with spirits to ask their direction in bringing healing to people).
Naturopathic medicine	System of therapeutics based on natural foods, light, warmth, massage, fresh air, regular exercise, and avoidance of medications. Recognizes inherent healing ability of the body. Treatments integrate traditional natural therapies with modern diagnostic science; includes botanical (plant) medicine.
Traditional Chinese (Asian) medicine	Set of systematic techniques and methods including acupuncture, herbal medicines, massage, acupressure, moxibustion (use of heat from burning herbs), Qigong (balancing energy flow through body movement), and Asian massage. Fundamental concepts from Taoism, Confucianism, and Buddhism.
Biologically Based Therapies—Use Substances Found in Nature, Such as Herbs, Foods, and Vitamins	
The "Zone"	Dietary program that requires eating protein, carbohydrate, and fat in a 30:40:30 ratio: 30% of calories from protein, 40% from carbohydrate, and 30% from fat. Used to balance insulin and other hormones for optimal health.
Macrobiotic diet	Predominantly a vegan diet (no animal products except fish). Initially used in the management of a variety of cancers. Emphasis placed on whole cereal grains, vegetables, and unprocessed foods.
Orthomolecular medicine (megavitamin)	Increased intake of nutrients such as vitamin C and beta-carotene. Diet treats cancer, schizophrenia, autism, and certain chronic diseases such as hypercholesterolemia and coronary artery disease.
European phytomedicines	Products developed under strict quality control in sophisticated pharmaceutical factories, packaged professionally in tablets or capsules. Examples of well-studied herbal medicines include gingko biloba, milk thistle, and bilberry. Herbs have a wide variety of uses.
Traditional Chinese herbal remedies	Over 50,000 medicinal plant species, many of which have been studied extensively. Herbs considered the backbone of medicine.
Ayurvedic herbs	Traditional Hindu system of herbs used for over 2000 years.
Manipulative and Body-Based Methods—Based on Manipulation and/or Movement of One or More Parts of the Body	
Acupressure	Therapeutic technique of applying digital pressure in a specified way on designated points on the body to relieve pain, produce analgesia, or regulate a body function.
Chiropractic medicine	System of therapy that involves manipulation of the spinal column and includes physiotherapy and diet therapy.
Feldenkrais method	Alternative therapy based on establishment of good self-image through awareness and correction of body movements. Technique integrates the understanding of the physics of the body's movement patterns with an awareness of the way people learn to move, behave, and interact.
Tai chi	Technique that incorporates breath, movement, and meditation to cleanse, strengthen, and circulate vital life energy and blood. Therapy stimulates the immune system and maintains external and internal balance.
Massage therapy	Manipulation of soft tissue through stroking, rubbing, or kneading to increase circulation, improve muscle tone, and relaxation.
Simple touch	Touching the client in appropriate and gentle ways to make connection, display acceptance, and give appreciation.
Mind-Body Interventions—Use a Variety of Techniques Designed to Enhance the Mind's Capacity to Affect Bodily Function and Symptoms	
Art therapy	Use of art to reconcile emotional conflicts, foster self-awareness, and express clients' unspoken and frequently unconscious concerns about their disease.
Biofeedback	A process providing a person with visual or auditory information about autonomic physiological functions of the body, such as muscle tension, skin temperature, and brain wave activity, through the use of instruments.

Continued

✳ **TABLE 36-1 Complementary and Alternative Therapies, cont'd**

Types	Definitions
Mind-Body Interventions—Use a Variety of Techniques Designed to Enhance the Mind's Capacity to Affect Bodily Function and Symptoms, cont'd	
Dance therapy	Intimate and powerful medium for therapy because it is a direct expression of the mind and body. Therapy treats persons with social, emotional, cognitive, or physical problems.
Breathwork	Using any of a variety of breathing patterns to relax, invigorate, or open emotional channels.
Guided imagery	Therapeutic technique for treating pathological conditions by concentrating on an image or series of images.
Meditation	Self-directed practice for relaxing the body and calming the mind using focused rhythmic breathing.
Music therapy	Uses music to address physical, psychological, cognitive, and social needs of individuals with disabilities and illnesses. Therapy improves physical movement and/or communication, develops emotional expression, evokes memories, and distracts people who are in pain.
Healing intention (prayer)	Variety of techniques used in multiple cultures that incorporate caring, compassion, love, or empathy with the target of prayer.
Psychotherapy	Treatment of emotional and mental disorders by psychological techniques.
Yoga	Discipline that focuses on the body's musculature, posture, breathing mechanisms, and consciousness. Goal of yoga is attainment of physical and mental well-being through mastery of body achieved through exercise, holding of postures, proper breathing, and meditation.
Energy Therapies—Involve the Use of Energy Fields	
	Energy therapies are of two types. *Biofield therapies* are intended to affect energy fields that purportedly surround and penetrate the human body. *Bioelectromagnetic-based therapies* involve the unconventional use of electromagnetic fields, such as pulsed fields, magnetic fields, or alternating current or direct current fields.
Reiki therapy	Therapy derived from ancient Buddhist practices in which practitioner places hands on or above a body area and transfers "universal life energy" to the client. This energy provides strength, harmony, and balance to treat health disturbances.
Therapeutic touch	Treatment involving direction of a practitioner's balanced energies in an intentional manner toward those of a client. Involves laying of practitioner's hands on or close to a client's body.

both allopathic and complementary practitioners. Furthermore, an increasing number of insurance companies are now covering costs for certain types of CAM therapies such as herbal therapy, biofeedback, chiropractic medicine, megavitamin therapy, and acupuncture (Rakel and Faass, 2006). However, this increase in insurance coverage is not proportionate to the increased use of CAM therapy. Many clients continue to pay out-of-pocket for a number of these therapies. Demographically, persons seeking CAM therapies typically include those who are professional, well educated, and from a higher socioeconomic standing.

The interest in CAM is also evident in the increased number of articles on CAM topics in respected medical journals and the development of new journals that specifically focus on complementary and alternative medicine. The Office of Alternative Medicine was established in 1992 as a part of the National Institutes of Health and then elevated to the status of the National Center for Complementary and Alternative Medicine (NCCAM) in 1998. The goals of NCCAM include facilitating the evaluation of alternative medical treatments and acting as a clearinghouse to disseminate information to the public, media, and professionals. It also funds, supports, coordinates, and conducts research and research training in the area of alternative medicine. NCCAM has organized complementary and alternative therapies into five categories that some researchers find useful (see Table 36-1). The holistic health model also reflects CAM (see Chapter 6).

Holistic nursing regards and treats the mind-body-spirit of the client. Nurses use holistic nursing interventions such as relaxation therapy, music therapy, simple touch, and healing intention (prayer). Such interventions affect the whole person (mind-body-spirit) and are effective, economical, noninvasive, nonpharmacological complements to medical care. Nurses use holistic interventions to augment standard treatments, replace interventions that are ineffective or debilitating, and promote or maintain health (Dossey, Keegan, and Guzzetta, 2005). The American Holistic Nurses Association maintains *Standards of Holistic Nursing Practice,* which defines and establishes the scope of holistic practice and describes the level of care expected from a holistic nurse (American Holistic Nurses Association, 2004).

This chapter discusses several types of complementary and alternative medicine therapies. The therapies are organized into two types. The first are nursing-accessible therapies that a nurse can begin to learn and apply in client care. The second type includes training-specific therapies, such as chiropractic therapy or acupressure, that a nurse cannot perform without additional training and/or certification. This chapter will present a description, clinical applications, and limitations of each therapy.

Nursing-Accessible Therapies

Some CAM therapies and techniques are general in nature and use natural processes (breathing, thinking and concentration, simple touch, movement, etc.) to help people feel better and cope with both acute and chronic conditions (Box 36-1). You can learn

BOX 36-1 EVIDENCE-BASED PRACTICE

Pain in Hospitalized Children

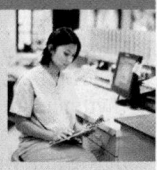

Evidence Summary
Pain is a complex phenomenon for children, involving psychological, biological, and sociological factors. The concepts of hospitalization and pain are often linked in the minds of children. Despite advances in pediatric pain management, recent studies demonstrate that many hospitalized children continue to have moderate to severe pain that is not well controlled. This literature review evaluates available evidence about the use and effectiveness of complementary therapies on children's pain experiences in hospital settings. The review includes 13 English-language research studies, all completed after 1995. The complementary and nonpharmacological therapies tested included relaxation tapes, distraction, focusing on breathing, talking with child during procedure, giving preparatory information, positive reinforcement, imagery, positioning, comforting and reassurance, touch (hand holding), hypnosis, and art therapy. Most complementary therapies successfully reduced discomfort among the children. Many times nurses did not use complementary therapies because of perceived lack of time due to heavy workloads. Methods that were commonly used included distraction and focusing on breathing. Nurses' lack of education about how to apply complementary techniques seems to be a barrier to their use of effective nonpharmacological interventions.

Application to Nursing Practice
- Children respond positively to holistic therapies to reduce the pain of hospital procedures.
- Nurses need to learn holistic techniques that aid in relieving pain in their pediatric clients. A variety of techniques are helpful and easy to learn.
- Nurses can use holistic therapies such as breathing techniques and distraction easily and quickly to alleviate the pain associated with hospital procedures especially among children.
- Nurses can teach a variety of simple and effective holistic interventions to parents of children with pain.
- Simple, effective holistic techniques will enhance the effects of analgesics to relieve pain in hospitalized children. This will result in the need for less medication.

Reference
Lassetter JH: Effectiveness of complementary therapies on the pain experience of hospitalized children, *J Holist Nurs* 24(3): 196, 2006

these kinds of techniques with minimum preparation, and you can use many of these procedures with clients as independent nursing practice (Dossey and others, 2005). Adequate assessment and the client's permission are prerequisites for implementation. Also remember that some CAM therapies alter physiological responses, making it necessary to request changes to physician-prescribed therapies, such as drug doses.

These therapies teach individuals ways in which to change their behavior to alter physical responses to stress and improve symptoms such as muscle tension, gastrointestinal discomfort, pain, or sleep disturbances. One of the principles of these therapies is that the individual becomes actively involved in the treatment. Individuals achieve better responses if they practice the techniques or exercises daily. A major principle is that the individual commits to implementing and maintaining the therapy until achieving a desired outcome.

Relaxation Therapy

People face stressful situations in everyday life that evoke the **stress response** (see Chapter 31). The mind modulates the biochemical functions of the major organ systems. Thoughts and feelings influence the production of chemicals (i.e., neurotransmitters, neurohormones, and peptides) that circulate throughout the body and convey messages via cells to various systems within the body. The stress response is a good example of the way in which systems cooperate to protect an individual from harm (see Chapter 31). Physiologically the cascade of changes associated with the stress response appears as increased heart and respiratory rates, tightened muscles, increased metabolic rate, and a general sense of foreboding, fear, nervousness, irritability, and negative mood. Other physiological responses include elevated blood pressure, dilated pupils, stronger cardiac contractions, and increased levels of blood glucose, serum cholesterol, circulating free fatty acids, and triglycerides. Although these responses prepare a person for short-term stress, the effects on the body of long-term stress sometimes include structural damage and chronic illness such as angina, tension headaches, cardiac arrhythmias, pain, ulcers, and atrophy of the immune system organs (Dossey and others, 2005).

The **relaxation response** is the state of generalized decreased cognitive, physiological, and/or behavioral arousal. Relaxation also involves arousal reduction. The process of relaxation elongates the muscle fibers, reduces the neural impulses sent to the brain, and thus decreases the activity of the brain as well as other body systems. Decreased heart and respiratory rates, blood pressure, and oxygen consumption and increased alpha brain activity and peripheral skin temperature characterize the relaxation response. The relaxation response occurs through a variety of techniques that incorporate a repetitive mental focus and the adoption of a calm, peaceful attitude (Benson, 1975). Box 36-2 lists client teaching strategies for relaxation.

Relaxation helps individuals develop cognitive skills for reducing the negative ways in which they respond to situations within their environment. Cognitive skills include the following:

- Focusing (the ability to identify, differentiate, maintain attention on, and return attention to simple stimuli for an extended period)
- Passivity (the ability to stop unnecessary goal-directed and analytic activity)
- Receptivity (the ability to tolerate and accept experiences that are uncertain, unfamiliar, or paradoxical).

The long-term goal of relaxation therapy is for persons to continually monitor themselves for indicators of tension and to consciously let go and release the tension contained in various body parts.

Progressive relaxation training teaches the individual how to effectively rest and reduce tension in the body. The person learns to detect subtle localized sensations of muscle tension in one muscle group (e.g., the forearm muscle). In addition, the individual learns to differentiate between high-intensity tension

Relaxation

Objective
- The client will demonstrate decreased anxiety and tension as a result of the relaxation intervention.

Teaching Strategies
Meditation and Rhythmic Breathing (Eliciting the Relaxation Response)
1. Provide a quiet environment.
2. Help the client get comfortable while seated or lying on back. Have client remain as still as possible, and encourage to move only if necessary to remain comfortable.
3. Instruct the client to close eyes and to hold a receptive attitude—"There is nothing more important for me to do for the next 15 minutes" or "What will be, will be."
4. Instruct client to breathe in and out slowly and deeply using the abdominal muscles, keeping the chest still.
5. At the beginning of every out-breath, have client repeat the number "one" silently in his or her mind. Continue for period of meditation.
6. Explain that when the mind wanders, bring it back to counting the out-breath without judgment.
7. Have client practice for 5, 10, 15, or 20 minutes per session. Practice daily for at least one session.

Progressive Relaxation
1. Follow Steps 1, 2, 3, and 4 of meditation and rhythmic breathing.
2. Once the client is breathing slowly and comfortably, instruct client to tighten and relax an ordered succession of muscle groups, tensing them and then relaxing them, while feeling each part relax.
3. Instruct client to tense and then relax the calves, knees, and so on.

Relaxation by Sensory Pacing
1. Follow Steps 1, 2, 3, and 4 of meditation and rhythmic breathing.
2. Instruct client to slowly repeat and finish each of the following sentences either in a low voice or to self:
   Now I am aware of seeing . . .
   Now I am aware of feeling . . .
   Now I am aware of hearing . . .
3. Instruct client to repeat and complete each sentence four times, then three times, then twice, and finally once.

Relaxing With Music
1. Provide client with a tape recorder and headset.
2. Ask client to select a favorite cassette of slow, quiet music.
3. Instruct client to get into a comfortable position (either sitting or lying down but with arms and legs uncrossed) and to close eyes and listen to the music through the headset.
4. Instruct client to imagine floating or drifting with the music while listening.

Evaluation
- Assess client's vital signs, particularly respiratory pattern.
- Ask client to describe level of tension or uneasiness felt.
- Observe client for presence of behaviors that display anxiety.

(strong fist clenching) and very subtle tension (Dossey and others, 2005). The individual then practices this activity using different muscle groups. One active progressive relaxation technique involves the use of slow, deep abdominal breathing while tightening and relaxing an ordered succession of muscle groups. When guiding a client, you may decide to begin with the muscles in the face, followed by those in the arms, hands, abdomen, legs, and feet.

Passive relaxation involves teaching the individual to relax individual muscle groups passively (i.e., without actively contracting the muscles). One passive relaxation technique incorporates slow, abdominal breathing exercises in addition to the person imagining warmth and relaxation flowing through specific muscle groups while letting go of muscle tension during expiration. Passive relaxation is useful for persons for whom the effort and energy expenditure of active muscle contracting leads to discomfort or exhaustion.

Clinical Applications of Relaxation Therapy. Relaxation techniques effectively lower heart rate and blood pressure, decrease muscle tension, improve well-being, and reduce symptom distress in persons experiencing a variety of situations (e.g., complications from medical treatment or disease or grieving the loss of a significant other) (Hui and others, 2006; Kaushik and

others, 2006). It is important to match the type of relaxation intervention to the individual's functional status, the energy expenditure of the relaxation technique, and the motivation of the individual for frequent practice.

Research shows that relaxation, alone or in combination with deep breathing, imagery, yoga (Figure 36-3), and music, reduces pain (Gustavsson and von Koch, 2006; Medlicott and Harris, 2006; Norbrink and others, 2006), reduces tension headaches (Kanji and others, 2006), and helps reduce human immunodeficiency virus (HIV) anxiety (Kempainnen and others, 2006). It also facilitates burn care (de Jong and Gambel, 2006), helps clients deal with posttraumatic stress (Stapleton and others, 2006), and even improves cognition in healthy aging adults (Galvin and others, 2006). However, better studies are needed to validate and support the effects of relaxation therapy. For example, control variables or activities that also lead to reduced physiological activity and pain level to determine if an individual's improved response is due to the relaxation therapy alone. Such variables include a healthy support network, a positive attitude including humor, and other behavioral therapies such as yoga and tai chi.

Relaxation is a valuable technique because it enables individuals to exert some control over their lives. Some experience a de-

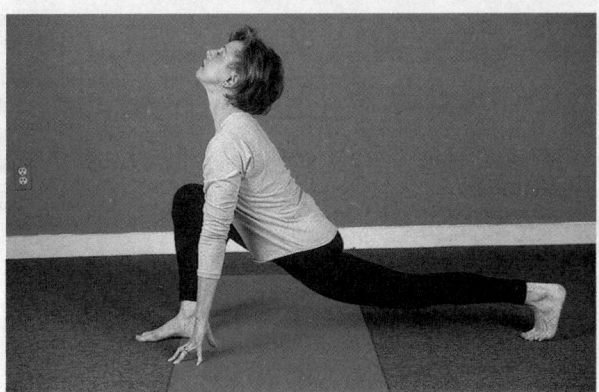

Figure 36-3 Yoga is a discipline that focuses on muscles, posture, breathing, and consciousness.

※ **BOX 36-3** Indications for Meditation

- Anxiety or tension states
- Chronic bereavement
- Chronic fatigue syndrome
- Chronic pain
- Drug abuse (alcohol or tobacco)
- Hypertension
- Irritability
- Low self-esteem or self-blame
- Mild depression
- Sleep disorders

creased feeling of helplessness and a more positive psychological state overall, which helps them to have a less negative view of their situation.

Limitations of Relaxation Therapy. Individuals undergoing relaxation training have reported fearing loss of control, feeling like they are floating, and experiencing relaxation-induced anxiety related to these feelings. During relaxation training, individuals learn to differentiate between low and high levels of muscle tension. During the first months of training sessions, when the person is learning how to focus on body sensations and tensions, there are reports of increased sensitivity in detecting muscle tension. Usually these feelings are minor and resolve as the person continues with the relaxation training. However, be aware that on occasion some relaxation techniques result in continued intensification of symptoms or the development of altogether new symptoms (Dossey and others, 2005).

An important consideration when choosing the type of relaxation technique is the physiological and psychological status of the individual. Clients with advanced disease such as cancer or acquired immunodeficiency syndrome (AIDS) often seek relaxation training to reduce their stress response. However, techniques such as active progressive relaxation training require a moderate expenditure of energy, which can increase a person's existing fatigue and limit the person's ability to complete individual relaxation sessions and practice. Therefore active progressive relaxation is not appropriate for clients with advanced disease or those who have decreased energy reserves. Passive relaxation or guided imagery is more appropriate for these individuals.

Meditation and Breathing

Meditation is any activity that limits stimulus input by directing attention to a single unchanging or repetitive stimulus (Rakel and Faass, 2006). It is a general term for a wide range of practices that involve relaxing the body and stilling the mind. The root word, *meditari,* means to consider, or to pay attention to something. Dr. Herbert Benson (1975) wrote the book *The Relaxation Response,* which drew the attention of Western health care practitioners to physical and psychological benefits of relaxation. As Benson pointed out, the components of relaxation are quite simple: (1) a

quiet space, (2) a comfortable position, (3) a receptive attitude, and (4) a focus of attention. He described meditation as a process that anyone can use to calm down, cope with stress, and, for those with spiritual inclinations, feel as one with God or the universe. Meditation requires no change in belief system and is compatible with most religious practices. Individuals or groups can practice it, and it is easy to learn. Practicing meditation does not require a teacher; many people learn the process from books or audiotapes, and it is easy to teach (Fontaine, 2005). Most meditation techniques involve slow, relaxed, deep, usually abdominal, breathing (see Box 36-2). Meditation evokes a restful state, lowers oxygen consumption, reduces respiratory and heart rates, and generates reports of reduced anxiety.

Clinical Applications of Meditation. There are many indications for meditation (Box 36-3). There is some evidence that meditation improves stress-related illnesses and breathing patterns in asthmatics and lowers blood pressure in hypertensive clients (Paul-Labrador and others, 2006; Walton and others, 2002). AIDS clients use meditation to reduce stress and anxiety (Brazier and others, 2006). Cancer clients (Zaza and others, 2005) and those suffering from depression (Brown and Gerbarg, 2005) also benefit from meditation. Battered women benefit from a meditation practice (Kane, 2006), as do those having chronic low back pain (Mehling, 2005). Meditation also increases productivity, improves mood, increases sense of identity, and lowers irritability (Dossey and others, 2005).

Considerations for the appropriateness of meditation include the degree of self-discipline of the person. Meditation is easy to learn and does not require memorization or particular procedures. It actually requires less self-discipline than most other behavioral therapies. Another consideration involves the self-reinforcing properties that meditation offers. Meditation induces a peaceful, drifting mental state that is unusually pleasurable and provides an incentive for individuals to continue.

Limitations of Meditation. Although meditation has demonstrated improvement in a variety of physiological and psychological ailments, it is contraindicated in some people. For example, a person who has a strong fear of losing control may perceive meditation as a form of mind control and thus may be resistant to learning the technique. Some individuals are also hypersensitive to meditation and require a much shorter session than the average 15- to 20-minute session.

Meditation may also increase the effects of certain drugs. For example, monitor individuals taking antihypertensive medications or thyroid-regulating, antidepressant, or antianxiety medications. Prolonged practice of meditation techniques sometimes leads to the reduced need for certain medications such as antihypertensive medications. Whatever the case, monitor individuals learning meditation closely for physiological changes with respect to their medications. Adjustment of the medication may be necessary.

Imagery

Imagery or visualization techniques use the conscious mind to create mental images to stimulate physical changes in the body, improve perceived well-being, and/or enhance self-awareness. Frequently imagery combined with some form of relaxation training facilitates the effect of the relaxation technique. Imagery is self-directed, in which individuals create their own mental images, or it is guided, during which a practitioner leads an individual through a particular scenario (Naparstek, 1995). For example, direct the client to begin slow, abdominal breathing while focusing on the rhythm of breathing. Then direct the client to visualize ocean waves coming to shore with each inspiration, then receding with each expiration. Next instruct the client to take notice of the smells, sounds, and temperatures that he or she is experiencing. As the imagery session progresses, instruct the client to visualize warmth entering the body during inspiration and tension leaving the body during expiration. Individualize imagery scenarios for each client.

Imagery often evokes powerful psychophysiological responses such as alterations in immune function (Fontaine, 2005). Many imagery techniques involve visual imagery, but they also include the auditory, proprioceptive, gustatory, and olfactory senses. An example of this involves visualizing a lemon being sliced in half and squeezing the lemon juice on the tongue. This visualization produces increased salivation as effectively as the actual event. People typically respond to their environment according to the way they perceive it, as well as by their own visualizations and expectancies. Therefore individuals learn to regulate themselves by selecting appropriate visualizations and expectations (Dossey and others, 2005).

Creative visualization is one form of self-directed imagery that is based on the principle of mind-body connectivity (i.e., every mental image leads to physical or emotional changes) (Gawain, 2002). Box 36-4 lists client teaching strategies for creative visualization.

Clinical Applications of Imagery.
Imagery has applications in a number of client populations. Imagery has been used to visualize cancer cells being destroyed by cells of the immune system (Borysenko, 1987), to control or relieve pain (Huth and others, 2004), and to achieve calmness and serenity (Borysenko, 1987). Imagery also aids in the treatment of chronic conditions such as asthma, hypertension, functional urinary disorders, menstrual and premenstrual syndromes, gastrointestinal disorders such as irritable bowel syndrome and ulcerative colitis, and rheumatoid arthritis (Dossey and others, 2005).

Limitations of Imagery.
Imagery, for the most part, is a behavioral intervention that has few side effects. However, it is probably one of the least clearly defined interventions and ranges from being highly structured to consisting of spontaneous daydreams by the individual (Rakel and Faass, 2006).

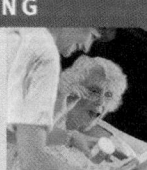

✳ BOX 36-4 **CLIENT TEACHING**

Creative Visualization

Objective
- The client will demonstrate skills in creative visualization.

Teaching Strategies
1. Set goals that the client can meet. Success achieves confidence and increased self-esteem.
2. The created image must be clear. Although it is sometimes difficult to develop a visual image, if the client views the goals of the imagery with clear thoughts and in the present tense, the client will be more successful in creating an effective image.
3. Have the client frequently visualize the image. Have the client perform this visualization during relaxing states as well as throughout the day, but particularly before bedtime or upon wakening, when the client's mind usually is more relaxed.
4. Have the client repeat encouraging statements, while focusing on the image. This alleviates any doubts about the client's ability to achieve established goals.

Evaluation
- Observe client behaviors for presence of anxiety.
- Ask client to describe if the visualization experience was helpful.
- Have client report if positive self-dialogue is used with visualization.
- Have client describe use of images of desired health habits, feelings, and desires for healing.
- Ask how the client is coping with daily stressors.

Training-Specific Therapies

Training-specific therapies are CAM treatments that nurses administer only after completing a specific course of study and training. A nurse must have a certification, degree, or license beyond the RN to administer most of these therapies. Several training-specific therapies (e.g., biofeedback and therapeutic touch) are very effective and recommended by Western health care practitioners. However, many have not been studied in a systematic way to establish their effectiveness. Many of the unproven techniques are very popular in our society and used by many persons from other cultures who live in the United States. Many have positive effects, but some have negative effects too. Some of these may also have harmful results when used in conjunction with standard Western medical therapies. Therefore you need to acquire knowledge of such treatments to effectively dialogue with clients and provide education about possible harmful interactions.

Biofeedback

Biofeedback techniques used in addition to relaxation interventions assist individuals in learning how to control specific autonomic nervous system responses. **Biofeedback** is a group of therapeutic procedures that use electronic or electromechanical instruments to measure, process, and provide information to persons about their neuromuscular and autonomic nervous system activity. The information, or feedback, is given in physical, physiological, auditory, and/or visual feedback signals. For example, clients connected to a biofeedback device hear a sound if their pulse rate or blood pressure increases out of their therapeutic zone. Practitioners help persons develop greater awareness and resulting voluntary control over their physiological responses, of which they are otherwise unaware (Rakel and Faass, 2006).

Biofeedback is an effective addition to more traditional relaxation programs because it immediately demonstrates to clients their ability to control some physiological responses. It also helps individuals to focus on and monitor specific body parts. By providing immediate feedback in terms of what stress relaxation behaviors work most effectively, it helps the client control physiological functions that are most difficult to control. Eventually the client will be able to notice positive physiological changes without the need for instrument feedback. Finally, biofeedback demonstrates to the client the relationship between thoughts, feelings, and physiological responses.

Clinical Applications of Biofeedback. Biofeedback in a variety of forms has application in numerous situations. Biofeedback has been successful in treating migraine headaches (Damen and others, 2006), other pain (Breuhl and Chung, 2006), stroke (Cirstea and others, 2006), and a variety of gastrointestinal and urinary tract disorders (Chiarioni, Salandini, and Whitehead, 2005). One of the most critical components of any behavioral program is adherence to the treatment regimen. Clients who are compliant with appointments, practice times, and goal setting and basically take responsibility for their treatment tend to be the most successful.

Limitations of Biofeedback. Although biofeedback has demonstrated effectiveness in a number of client populations, there are several precautions. During relaxation therapy and/or biofeedback sessions, repressed emotions or feelings are sometimes uncovered that clients cannot cope with by themselves. For this reason, practitioners who offer biofeedback should either be trained in more traditional psychological methods or have qualified professionals available for referral.

Therapeutic Touch

Therapeutic touch (Krieger, 1979) is a training-specific therapy that was developed by a nurse. Although the philosophical and religious assumptions of therapeutic touch are different from those of other Eastern healing modalities, therapeutic touch is similar in that it involves trained health care professionals who attempt to direct their own balanced energies in an intentional and motivated manner toward those of the client.

Therapeutic touch (TT) is a natural human potential that consists of placing the practitioner's hands either on or close to the body of a person (Figure 36-4). The process of therapeutic touch involves the practitioner scanning the body of the client and diagnosing areas of accumulated tensions. The practitioner

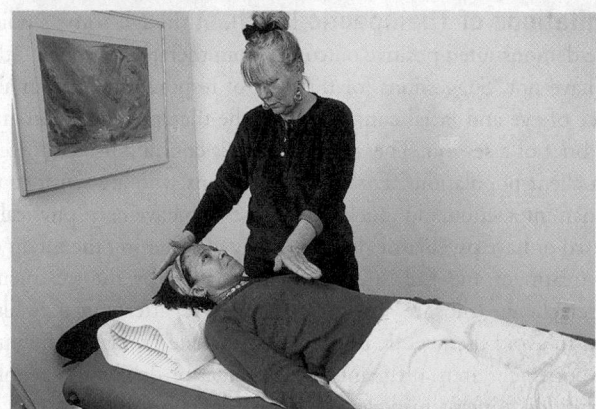

Figure 36-4 In therapeutic touch the practitioner directs the practitioner's own interpersonal energy to help or heal another.

then attempts to redirect these energies to bring the person back into energy balance similar to that of the practitioner (Krieger, 1975, 1979). TT consists of five phases: centering, assessing, unruffling, treating, and evaluating. Centering is the process whereby the practitioner becomes aware and fully present during the entire treatment. The next phase involves assessing the client, in which the practitioner moves his or her hands (roughly 2 to 6 inches from the body) in a rhythmic and symmetrical movement from the head to the toes. During this phase the practitioner notices the quality of **energy flow** and detects accumulations of energy. Clients perceive physiological indicators of energy imbalance as feelings of congestion, pressure, warmth, coolness, blockage, pulling or drawing, or static or tingling (Krieger, 1975). During the third phase, the practitioner facilitates the symmetrical and rhythmical flow of energy through the body. The practitioner performs this technique using long downward strokes over the energy field located over the entire body, either by touching the body or by maintaining the hands in a position a few inches away from the body. During the actual treatment the practitioner directs and balances the energy, attempting to rebalance the energy flow. The final phase consists of evaluating the client and reassessing the energy field. If a rebalance has occurred, the practitioner detects a more symmetrical, freely flowing energy field and greater well-being (Krieger, 1979).

Clinical Applications of Therapeutic Touch. Some of the earliest classic studies found that TT increased hemoglobin (Hb) levels in several clients (Krieger, 1975, 1979). This same positive result was found in a recent study (Movaffaghi and others, 2006). Other studies found that TT reduces anxiety levels in hospitalized clients with cardiovascular disease, reduces headache pain, and improves mood in bereaved adults (Krieger, 1975, 1979). Several research review articles support the effectiveness of TT in treating trauma recovery (Burr, 2005) and dementia (Woods and others, 2005). Completed research has shown that TT helps women with breast cancer cope with stress (Kelly and others, 2004) and reduces chemical dependency in pregnant women (Larden and others, 2004).

Limitations of Therapeutic Touch. Although some studies have demonstrated positive outcomes from therapeutic touch, others have not. Suggestions for this lack of response include an absence of eye and facial contact during the therapeutic session and too brief of a session. Therapeutic touch is contraindicated in certain client populations. For example, persons who are sensitive to human interaction and touch (e.g., those who have been physically abused or have psychiatric disorders) may misinterpret the intent of the treatment and feel threatened and anxious by the treatment. Other clients who are sensitive to energy repatterning may also need to avoid therapeutic touch. These include premature infants, newborns, children, pregnant women, older or debilitated people, or those in critical, unstable conditions (Fontaine, 2005).

Chiropractic Therapy

Chiropractic therapy, a manual healing art, was developed in 1895 in Iowa. Of the independently practicing health professions, it is the third largest in the Western world (Rakel and Faass, 2006). Chiropractors graduate from well-established preparatory programs similar to medical schools. The central belief of the chiropractic profession is spinal manipulation directed at certain joints by practitioners using their hands or an instrument. Manipulation is the forceful passive movement of a joint beyond its active limit of motion. Chiropractic therapy is a holistic therapy that does not typically use drugs or surgery.

Spinal manipulation received an endorsement from the U.S. Department of Health and Human Service's Agency for Health Care Policy and Research in 1994. The agency developed guidelines that concluded "spinal manual therapy provides relief of symptomatic discomfort as well as functional improvement." The basic principles of chiropractic therapy incorporate the idea that human beings have an innate healing potential, and the goal of this healing profession is to access this potential. Chiropractic therapy promotes both a natural diet and regular exercise as critical components for the body to function properly (Fontaine, 2005).

Clinical Applications of Chiropractic Therapy. The basic goals of chiropractic therapy focus on restoring structural and functional imbalances. Researchers believe that structure and function coexist with one another and that alterations or distortions in structure ultimately lead to abnormalities in function. One of the major structural distortions that chiropractors treat is vertebral subluxation, in which the motion of the joints decreases due to slight changes in the position of the articulating bones and subjective symptoms such as pain. A more severe form of subluxation, called fixation, exists when joint motion is restricted. Chiropractic interventions treat not only musculoskeletal abnormalities, but headaches, dysmenorrhea, blood pressure, vertigo, tinnitus, and visual disorders (Rakel and Faass, 2006).

Limitations of Chiropractic Therapy. Several diseases or joint conditions should not be treated with manipulation. If you suspect a malignancy or determine it through diagnostic testing, refer the client to a medical physician for further evaluation and treatment. Bone and joint infections also require pharmaceutical or surgical intervention, and the structural integrity of the bone may be compromised if excessive force is used. Contraindications

for chiropractic therapy include acute myelopathy, fractures, dislocations, rheumatoid arthritis, and osteoporosis.

Traditional Chinese Medicine

Traditional Chinese medicine (TCM) comprises several healing modalities, including herbs, acupuncture, moxibustion, diet, exercise, and meditation. TCM is several thousand years old and has its roots in Taoism. There are several major concepts that constitute Chinese medicine. The most important of these is the concept of **yin and yang,** which represent opposing yet complementary phenomena that exist in a state of dynamic equilibrium. Examples are night/day, hot/cold, and shady/sunny. Yin represents shade, cold, and inhibition, whereas yang represents fire, light, and excitement. Yin also represents the inner part of the body, specifically the viscera, liver, heart, spleen, lung, and kidney, whereas yang represents the outer part, specifically the bowels, stomach, and bladder. Practitioners believe that disease occurs when there is an imbalance in these two paired opposites (Fontaine, 2005).

Qi (pronounced *chi*) is defined as the vital energy of the human body. Disease is classified into three major categories: external causes, internal causes, and neither internal nor external causes (Table 36-2). Regardless of the cause, yin and yang go out of balance, thus altering the movement of *qi*. The body consists of several forms of this energy that directly influence physiological functions of the body and help to maintain homeostasis.

Channels of energy run in regular patterns through the body and over its surface. These channels, called **meridians,** are like rivers flowing through the body. An obstruction in the movement of these energy rivers is like a dam that backs up the flow in one part of the body and restricts it in others. Any obstruction and blockages or deficiencies of energy would eventually lead to disease. There have been evaluations to identify and systematize the meridians or channels through which *qi* flows. Twelve primary and eight secondary or extra channels have been identified. Located along the channels are **acupoints,** or holes through which *qi* can be influenced by the insertion of needles, a process known as **acupuncture.**

Another important component of Chinese medicine involves five elements. The five elements consist of earth, metal, water, wood, and fire. Various health phenomena are organized according to these phases and interact with each other. In Chinese medicine outward manifestations reflect the internal environment. There are two primary areas assessed in Chinese medicine: the tongue and several pulses. The color, shape, and coating of the

---

✳ **TABLE 36-2 Three Causes of Disease According to Traditional Chinese Medicine**

CAUSE OF DISEASE	INFLUENCES
External causes, or "the six evils"	Wind, cold, fire, damp, summer heat, dryness
Internal causes, or internal damage by seven effects	Joy, anger, anxiety, thought, sorrow, fear, fright
Nonexternal, noninternal causes	Dietary irregularities, excessive sexual activity, fatigue, trauma, parasites

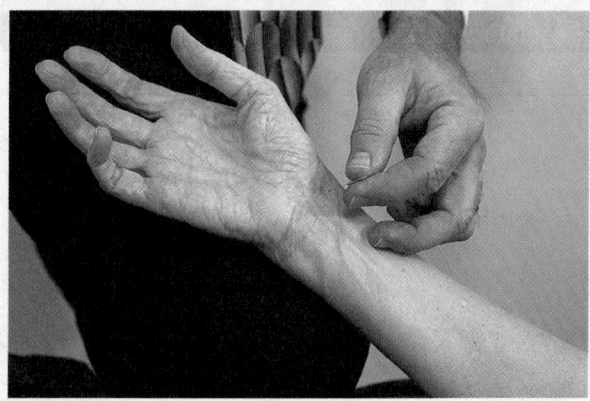

Figure 36-5 Acupuncture.

tongue reflect the general condition of the internal organs. The pulses provide information about the condition and balance of *qi,* blood, ying and yang, and the internal organs (Fontaine, 2005).

Acupuncture

Acupuncture is a method of stimulating certain points (acupoints) on the body by the insertion of special needles to modify the perception of pain, normalize physiological functions, or treat or prevent disease (Figure 36-5). Acupuncture regulates or realigns the flow of *qi*. According to Chinese traditional medicine, acupuncture needles unblock the obstruction of energy and reestablish the flow of *qi* through the meridians, thereby stimulating and activating the body's self-healing mechanism. Application of heat or weak electrical currents enhances the effects of the needles (Fontaine, 2005).

Clinical Applications of Acupuncture. Acupuncture is the primary treatment modality used by physicians of Chinese medicine. However, many allopathic physicians and health care professionals use acupuncture. Many states now have regulations and licensure requirements to practice as an acupuncturist.

The most common problems treated with acupuncture include low back pain, myofascial pain, simple and migraine headaches, sciatica, shoulder pain, tennis elbow, osteoarthritis, whiplash, and musculoskeletal sprains. Other problems that have been successfully treated include sinusitis, gastrointestinal disorders, perimenstrual symptoms, neurological disorders, chronic pulmonary diseases (including asthma), hypertension, smoking and other addictions, and clinical depression (Rakel and Faass, 2006).

Limitations of Acupuncture. Acupuncture is a safe therapy when the practitioner has the appropriate training and uses sterilized needles. Although there have been complications, they are rare if the practitioner takes appropriate steps to ensure the safety of the equipment and the client. These complications include infections resulting from inadequately sterilized needles or those that are left in place for an extended length of time, broken needles, puncture of an internal organ, bleeding, fainting, seizures, miscarriage, and posttreatment drowsiness.

Caution is necessary in the use of acupuncture in pregnant clients and those who have a history of seizures, are carriers of hepatitis, or are infected with HIV. Treatment is contraindicated in persons who have bleeding disorders, thrombocytopenia, or skin infections or who have a fear of needles. Do not use the semipermanent needles with persons who have valvular heart disease because of the increased risk of infection. Avoid electroacupuncture in persons with a pacemaker and those who have cardiac arrhythmias, epilepsy, or are pregnant (Fontaine, 2005).

Herbal Therapies

Researchers estimate that approximately 25,000 plant species are used medicinally throughout the world. It is the oldest form of medicine known to man, and archeological evidence suggests that the Neanderthals used herbal remedies 60,000 years ago. Use of **herbal therapy** gained widespread popularity in many countries as early as 3000 BC but began to decline with the development of modern scientific medicine in the early eighteenth century. However, because approximately 80% of the world's population lives in developing countries, herbal medicine is a prominent part of health care in these countries. There is renewed interest in countries whose health care is primarily allopathic medicine. There is an increase in the use of herbal medicine because of a growing concern by the general public about the complications and limitations of modern scientific medicine and consumer interest in "natural" foods (Fontaine, 2005).

The federal Food, Drug, and Cosmetic Act requires that all drugs be proven safe and effective before being sold to the public. Because herbal medicines do not undergo the same rigorous research as pharmaceuticals, the majority have not received approval for use as drugs and are not regulated by the Food and Drug Administration (FDA). For this reason manufacturers sell many herbal medicines as foods or food supplements in health food stores and through private companies. The Dietary Supplement Health and Education Act passed in 1994 allows companies to sell herbs as dietary supplements as long as there are no health claims written on their labels.

Chinese medicine herbal substances come from plants, animals, or minerals, whereas Western medicine uses herbs prepared primarily from plant materials. The active ingredients are "packaged" in tinctures or extracts, elixirs, syrups, capsules, pills, tablets, lozenges, powders, ointments or creams, drops, and suppositories. Many people tend to think that because herbs are natural plants they will not cause harm or side effects, but this is not always true. Some herbal substances contain powerful chemicals. As with any other medication, examine herbs for interaction and compatibility with other prescribed or unprescribed substances. Many herbs are also sold with claims that they can "cure" certain ailments, such as pau d'arco for curing cancer, when their efficacy has not been determined through clinical trials. Herbs are generally classified as beneficial, harmful, or neutral, in which case they have no effects on the specific ailment.

The philosophy of herbal therapy is different from that of conventional drug therapy. The goal of herbal therapy is to restore balance within the individual by facilitating the person's self-healing ability. Drug therapy, on the other hand, aims to treat specific diseases or symptoms. Herbal therapy is sometimes

✳ TABLE 36-3 Safe or Effective Herbs Determined by Non-U.S. Regulatory Authorities

COMMON NAME AND USES	EFFECTS	DRUG INTERACTIONS
Aloe	Acceleration of wound healing	Furosemide and loop diuretics
Chamomile		
Inflammatory diseases of gastrointestinal and upper respiratory tracts	Antiinflammatory	Drugs that cause drowsiness (alcohol, barbiturates, benzodiazepines, narcotics, antidepressants)
Echinacea		
Upper respiratory tract infections	Stimulant of immune system	Antirejection and other drugs that weaken immune system
Feverfew		
Wound healing	Antiinflammatory	Warfarin and blood thinners
Arthritis	Inhibition of serotonin and prostaglandins	Aspirin and ibuprofen
Garlic		
Elevated cholesterol levels	Inhibition of platelet aggregation	Warfarin and blood thinners
Hypertension		Saquinavir and other anti-HIV drugs
Ginger		
Nausea and vomiting	Antiemetic	Warfarin and blood thinners
		Aspirin and NSAIDs
Gingko biloba		
Alzheimer's disease	Memory improvement	Warfarin and blood thinners
Dementia	Increasing blood flow	Aspirin and NSAIDs
Ginseng		
Age-related diseases	Increased physical endurance	Warfarin and blood thinners
		Aspirin and NSAIDs
		MAO inhibitors
Licorice	Stomach ulcers	Corticosteroids and other immunosuppressive drugs
		Digoxin
		Antihypertensive drugs
Saw palmetto	Prevention of conversion of testosterone to dihydrotestosterone (needed for prostate cell multiplication)	Finasteride and antiandrogen drugs
Benign prostatic hyperplasia		Warfarin and blood thinners
Urinary problems		
	Minor tranquilizer	
Valerian		
Sleep disorders	Central nervous system depression	Barbiturates and other sleep medications
Restlessness		Alcohol
		Antihistamines

HIV, Human immunodeficiency virus; *NSAIDs,* nonsteroidal antiinflammatory drugs; *MAO,* monoamine oxidase.

prescribed on an individual basis with unique herbal mixtures designed for each person (Kuhn and Winston, 2001).

Clinical Applications of Herbal Therapy.
A number of herbs are safe and effective for a variety of conditions (Table 36-3). Milk thistle, for example, is effective in treating a number of liver and gallbladder conditions. It perhaps protects the liver through its antioxidant properties and by facilitating regeneration of liver cells. St. John's wort is effective as a mild antidepressant and mild sedative. Hypericin and pseudohypericin, major constituents of the drug, also have potent action against viruses.

Limitations of Herbal Therapy.
Although herbal medicines provide beneficial effects for a variety of conditions, a number of problems exist. When herbal medicines are developed, concentra-

tions of the active ingredients vary considerably. Contamination with other herbs or chemicals, including pesticides and heavy metals, also occurs. Not all companies follow strict quality control and manufacturing guidelines, which set standards for acceptable levels of pesticides, residual solvents, bacterial levels, and heavy metals. For this reason, purchase herbal medicine only from reputable manufacturers. Labels on herbal products need to contain the scientific name of the botanical, the name and address of the actual manufacturer, a batch or lot number, the date of manufacture, and the expiration date. Some herbs also contain very toxic products and cause cancer. Comfrey, for example, is used for its wound-healing properties. However, various species of comfrey contain certain pyrrolizidine alkaloids that are known to cause cancer. Comfrey has produced liver cancer in small animals. For this reason do not use comfrey internally and use only as a poultice on intact skin (Kuhn and Winston, 2001). Table 36-4 lists other unsafe herbs.

TABLE 36-4　Unsafe Herbs

COMMON NAME	EFFECTS	COMMENTS
Borage	Diuretic Expectorant	Contains toxic pyrrolizidine alkaloids
Calamus (Indian type most toxic)	Fever Digestive aid	Contains varying amounts of carcinogenic *cis*-isoasarone
Chaparral	Anticancer	No proven efficacy Induces severe liver toxicity in some cases
Coltsfoot	Antitussive	Contains carcinogenic pyrrolizidine alkaloids
Comfrey	Wound healing	Carcinogenic May induce venoocclusive disease
Ephedra *(ma huang)*	Central nervous system stimulant Bronchodilator Cardiac stimulation	Unsafe for people with hypertension, diabetes, or thyroid disease Avoid consumption with caffeine
Life root	Menstrual flow stimulant	Hepatotoxic
Pokeweed	Antirheumatic Anticancer	May be fatal in children

Despite the increased use of herbal products, there has not been an increase in reports of toxicity. Nonetheless, discourage the use of herbal products in pregnant women, nursing mothers, infants or young children, or older adults with liver or cardiovascular disease (Fontaine, 2005).

Nursing Role in Complementary and Alternative Therapies

The interest in CAM therapies has increased significantly in the past 20 years. The majority of people using and seeking information about complementary and alternative therapies are well educated and have a strong desire to actively participate in the decision making about their health care. This increased interest comes not only from health care consumers, but also allopathic physicians who have increasing concerns that current Western medicine is not meeting the needs of their clients. Many allopathic physicians do not refer their clients for CAM therapies because they are not familiar with the therapies and have had little, if any, education and training in complementary and alternative medicine. Many physicians have reservations about CAM therapies because they have not been appropriately tested in clinical trials in which other factors that influence the outcomes are strictly controlled.

In North America and the United Kingdom many professional groups are exploring the use of CAM and facilitating and monitoring research in this area. Proposals put forth by several of the these groups include assessing the need of the public for CAM therapies, incorporating CAM educational components in the curriculum for all health care programs, providing appropriate information to the public, and encouraging and facilitating communication between CAM practitioners and allopathic physicians so each will be open to the other's approaches and values. For example, if Western medicine is to accept and incorporate CAM therapies as a more integrative medical approach, practitioners of

CAM need to realize the advantages of having their therapies researched more rigorously. On the other hand, allopathic physicians and more conventional practitioners need to begin to understand the benefits of therapies that encourage active participation by their clients in preventing or managing illness rather than relying solely on surgery or drugs.

Integrative medicine, a health care strategy that is gaining popularity, involves a multiple-practitioner treatment group in which a client seeks care simultaneously from more than one type of practitioner. Clients have the option to choose the kind of practitioner they feel would benefit their particular health problem. Clients who benefit from these groups are those who have chronic health problems that have historically been difficult to treat using traditional allopathic medicine, such as fibromyalgia or chronic fatigue syndrome. This represents a pluralistic and truly complementary health care system in which both alternative and allopathic practitioners work side-by-side to improve the well-being of their clients. Although this is not reality in the majority of settings, this approach of open communication and practice between allopathic and alternative practitioners will potentially benefit a large number of clients.

The integrative medicine approach is consistent with the holistic approach nurses learn to practice. Nurses have the potential for becoming essential participants in this type of health care philosophy. Many nurses already practice the use of touch (Box 36-5). Be knowledgeable of CAM therapies to make appropriate recommendations to allopathic primary care providers about which therapies will be useful for clients. Also, provide advice to clients regarding when to seek conventional therapy or CAM therapy. For example, if a client complains of right lower abdominal pain, nausea, and vomiting, be suspicious of appendicitis and recommend assessment by an allopathic physician. However, if the client has a chronic gastrointestinal disorder and has been diagnosed with irritable bowel syndrome, the client will possibly benefit from relaxation and herbal therapy. Be aware of your state Nurse Practice Act with regard to complementary therapies, and practice only within the scope of these laws.

Receiving Therapeutic Touch

- Touch is a primal need, as necessary as food, growth, or shelter. Think of touch as a nutrient transmitted through the skin and "skin hunger" as a form of malnutrition that has reached epidemic proportions in the United States, especially among older adults (Fontaine, 2005).
- Older adults need touch as much as or more than any other age-group. However, skin hunger or poverty of touch is often acute among older adults. It is an unfortunate coincidence that older adults often have fewer family members or friends to touch them at a time when simple touch could be an enhanced form of communication when other senses are reduced (Dossey and others, 2005).
- Simple touch helps older adult clients feel more connected to and accepted by those around them and to their environment. Touch enhances self-esteem and sense of worth.
- A nurse who reacts adversely to the skin changes of older people often finds it difficult to touch an older client. The nurse's reluctance then communicates a negative message to the older adult (Dossey and others, 2005).
- A holistic nursing approach to care of older adults also includes the caregivers, who often experience poor health or have neglected their own health, encounter their own psychosocial issues as they relate to the caregiving experience, feel the effects of multiple stressors, or feel spiritual distress (Eliopoulos, 2004).

Nurses work very closely with their clients and are in the unique position of becoming familiar with the client's spiritual and cultural viewpoints. Nurses are often able to determine which CAM therapies are more appropriately aligned with these beliefs and offer recommendations accordingly.

Client interest and participation in CAM therapies is increasing. Therefore it is important for you to be knowledgeable about the multiple CAM therapies available and the use of these therapies by clients. It is important for nurses to know the current research being done in this area to provide accurate information, not only to clients, but to other health care professionals.

✳ Key Concepts

- Alternative and complementary therapies are the same, depending on whether the therapy is a primary treatment or treatment in addition to the Western medicine treatment.
- Integrative medical programs utilize a multidisciplinary (both allopathic and complementary) treatment approach providing holistic care to clients.
- The stress response is an adaptive response allowing individuals to react to stressful situations.
- A chronic stress response is often maladaptive, leading to chronic muscle tension, mood changes, and immune changes.
- Relaxation is a beneficial state characterized by lowered pulse rates, respiratory rates, blood pressure, and muscle tension and improved mood states through direct client participation.

- CAM therapies require commitment and regular involvement by the client to be most effective and have prolonged beneficial outcomes.
- CAM therapies should be appropriately chosen according to the person's functional status, belief or religious perspectives, access to health care, and insurance coverage.
- Some CAM therapies alter physiological responses such that routine medication doses need changing.
- Imagery is usually visual but also can involve the auditory, proprioceptive, gustatory, and olfactory senses.
- Many complementary and alternative therapies lack a scientific basis but are effective based on observed positive outcomes in a number of clients. Some CAM therapies have supporting research published in professional nursing journals.

✳ Critical Thinking Exercises

Margaret is a 76-year-old Catholic woman who has been diagnosed with a slow-growing renal tumor. She has been scheduled for surgery in 2 weeks. She is afraid of both the surgical procedure and the outcome. Is it cancer? Will the surgery result in a disability? Following surgery she becomes depressed.

1. What specific nursing-accessible CAM interventions can the nurse offer Margaret to prepare for the surgery and reduce her anxiety?

2. What CAM therapies will help her deal with her depression?

✳ NCLEX®-Style Review Questions

1. Nurses can educate clients about the benefits of complementary therapies. Clients with which of the following might find relief in complementary therapies?
   1. Lupus and diabetes
   2. Ulcers and hepatitis
   3. Heart disease and pancreatitis
   4. Chronic back pain and arthritis

2. Some complementary therapies, such as acupuncture, contain diagnostic and therapeutic methods specific to their field, whereas others, such as the following, are more easily learned and applied:
   1. Massage therapy
   2. Chinese medicine
   3. Relaxation response
   4. Breathwork and imagery
   5. All of the above
   6. 3 and 4 only

3. It is estimated that half of U.S. citizens use a CAM practitioner and that these visits:
   1. Exceed the visits to allopathics
   2. Are equal to visits to allopathics
   3. Are double those visits to allopathics
   4. Are slightly less than visits to allopathics

4. Holistic nursing regards and treats the:
   1. Disease, spirit, and family
   2. Desires and emotions of the client

3. Mind, body, and spirit of the client
4. Muscles, nerves, and spine disorders
5. All of the above
6. 2 and 3

5. In addition to the necessity for adequate assessment, when the nurse utilizes CAM the client's:
   1. Family must give permission
   2. Permission is a prerequisite for implementation
   3. Physician must give approval for implementation
   4. Total understanding of CAM must be documented

6. One of the principles of CAM therapies is that the individual becomes:
   1. Submissive to the practitioner
   2. Actively involved in the treatment
   3. Less competent in his or her own care
   4. A total believer in what is being taught

7. The stress response is a good example of the way in which systems:
   1. Fail and cause illness and disease
   2. Cause structural damage to the body
   3. React the same way for all individuals
   4. Protect an individual from harm

8. Clients' medications should be monitored carefully because meditation may augment the effects of certain drugs such as:
   1. Prednisone
   2. Insulin and vitamins
   3. Cough syrups and aspirin
   4. Antihypertensive and thyroid-regulating medications

9. Biofeedback techniques are frequently used in addition to relaxation interventions to assist individuals:
   1. In eating less food
   2. In controlling diabetes
   3. With AIDS in living longer
   4. In learning how to control specific autonomic nervous system responses

10. Therapeutic touch is a training-specific therapy that was developed by a(n):
    1. Nurse
    2. Physician
    3. Physical therapist
    4. Ancient Scandinavian culture

37 | Activity and Exercise

Mastery of content in this chapter will enable the student to:

- Describe the role of the musculoskeletal and nervous systems in the regulation of movement.
- Discuss physiological and pathological influences on body alignment and joint mobility.
- Describe how to maintain and use proper body mechanics.
- Describe how exercise and activity benefit physiological and psychological functioning.
- Describe the benefits of implementing an exercise program for the purpose of health promotion.
- Describe the benefits of implementing exercise and activity.
- Describe important factors to consider when planning an exercise program for clients across the life span and for those with specific chronic illnesses.

- Assess clients for impaired mobility and activity intolerance.
- Formulate nursing diagnoses for clients experiencing problems with impaired mobility and activity intolerance.
- Write a nursing care plan for a client with impaired mobility and activity intolerance.
- Describe interventions for maintaining activity tolerance and mobility.
- Evaluate the nursing care plan for maintaining activity and exercise for clients across the life span and with specific chronic illnesses.

MEDIA RESOURCES   KEY TERMS

 Companion CD
- NCLEX®-Style Review Questions
- Audio Glossary
- Interactive Learning Activities
- English/Spanish Glossary

evolve Website
- NCLEX®-Style Review Questions
- Audio Glossary
- English/Spanish Glossary
- Interactive Learning Activities
- Weblinks
- Audio Summaries

The actions of walking, turning, lifting, and carrying are essential to performing nursing care activities. Such activities require muscle exertion. Proper **body mechanics** help reduce work effort but by themselves have consistently failed to reduce musculoskeletal disorders (MSDs) among nurses (Nelson, Fragala, and Menzel, 2003). The American Nurses Association (ANA) (2003) launched a campaign to educate and advocate for the safety of nurses during the handling of their clients. Knowledge of proper body mechanics coupled with engineering solutions (e.g., mechanical lifts or friction-reducing devices) and ergonomics significantly reduce the risk of MSDs (ANA, 2003; Nelson and Baptiste, 2004).

A program of regular physical activity and **exercise** has the potential to enhance all aspects of a client's biopsychosocial and spiritual model of health (Box 37-1). This chapter provides you with knowledge of exercise and activity as they relate to health promotion, the acute phase of illness, and the restorative and continuing care of clients. Nursing strategies are included to help plan an individualized exercise and activity program for a variety of clients with specific disease entities and needs.

Scientific Knowledge Base

Regular physical activity and exercise contribute to both physical and emotional well-being (Huddleston, 2002; Konradi and Anglin, 2001). Knowing the physiology and regulation of body mechanics, exercise, and activity assists in providing individualized care.

Overview of Exercise and Activity

The coordinated efforts of the musculoskeletal and nervous systems maintain balance, **posture,** and body alignment during lifting, bending, moving, and performing **activities of daily living (ADLs).** Proper balance, posture, and body alignment help to reduce the risk of injury to the musculoskeletal system and facilitate body movements, allowing physical mobility without muscle strain and excessive use of muscle energy. Coordinated musculoskeletal activity is necessary when positioning and transferring clients. However, when the client is unable to assist in transfer, use a mechanical lift or a lift team. A lift team consists of two physically fit people, competent in lifting techniques, who use client handling equipment to perform high-risk transfers (Nelson and Baptiste, 2004).

Body Alignment. Body alignment refers to the relationship of one body part to another body part along a horizontal or vertical line. Correct alignment involves positioning so that no excessive strain is placed on clients' joints, tendons, ligaments, or muscles, thereby maintaining adequate **muscle tone** and contributing to balance.

Body Balance. Body balance occurs when a relatively low **center of gravity** is balanced over a wide, stable base of support and a vertical line falls from the center of gravity through the base of support. When the vertical line from the center of gravity does not fall through the base of support, the body loses balance. You can enhance body balance by assuming proper posture, or the body position that most favors function, requires the least muscu-

---

❊ BOX 37-1 The Gift of Exercise

The other day I was looking for a gift to give to a friend. This friend is very important to me, and I want her to be around for a long time; I want her to live a long and healthy life. I thought how great it would be if I could give her a gift that would improve the quality of her life.

So I sat down and made a list of what I would look for in this special gift:

- It would help her to be stronger, firmer, leaner, more flexible, and energetic.
- It would help lower her risk of dying from heart disease, help lower blood pressure and improve lipid profile, control blood glucose level, fight obesity, and help her to age more gracefully.
- It would help improve immune function, concentration and task performance, and the quality of sleep.
- It would help reduce stress, improve mood, enhance self-esteem, and increase optimism and confidence.
- It would help to increase self-awareness and control over choices in her life.
- It would be fun but also challenging.
- It would allow for socialization but also time alone, depending on her needs.
- It would come in all different modes and styles and adapt to various environments and weather conditions.
- Finally, it would have a good *Consumer Reports* rating, supported by scientific data from reputable sources.

After completing my list, I realized that the only gift that meets all the criteria is the gift of exercise. Have a happy and healthy life, my friend.

From Huddleston JS: Exercise. In Edelman CL, Mandle CL, editors: *Health promotion throughout the lifespan,* ed 5, St. Louis, 2002, Mosby.

---

lar work to maintain, and places the least strain on muscles, ligaments, and bones (Thibodeau and Patton, 2007). For example, raising the height of the bed when performing a procedure, such as changing a dressing, prevents bending too far at the waist and causing a shift in your base of support.

You use balance to maintain proper body alignment and posture through two simple techniques. First, widen the base of support by separating the feet to a comfortable distance. Second, increase balance by bringing the center of gravity closer to the base of support.

Coordinated Body Movement. Coordinated body movement is a result of weight, center of gravity, and balance. Weight is the force exerted on a body by gravity. When an object is lifted, the lifter must overcome the object's weight and be aware of the object's center of gravity. In symmetrical objects the center of gravity is located at the exact center of the object. The force of weight is always directed downward. An unbalanced object has its center of gravity away from the midline and falls without support. Because people are not geometrically perfect, their centers of gravity are usually at 55% to 57% of standing height and are located in the midline. Like unbalanced objects, clients who do not maintain a balance with their center of gravity are unsteady, which places them at risk for falling. You need to be able to identify these clients and intervene in order to maintain their safety.

Friction. Friction is a force that occurs in a direction to oppose movement. Reduce friction by following some basic principles. The greater the surface area of the object you are moving, the greater the friction. For example, when a client is unable to assist in moving up in bed, place the client's arms across the chest. This decreases surface area and reduces friction.

A passive or immobilized client produces greater friction to movement (see Chapter 47). When possible, use some of the client's strength and mobility when positioning and transferring the client. Explain the procedure, and tell the client when to move. For instance, you decrease friction if the client is able to bend his or her knees as you assist the client in moving up in the bed.

You can reduce friction by using an air-assisted device when performing lateral client transfers (Baptiste and others, 2006). The air-assisted devices are commercially available transfer devices that are effective solutions to reducing injury to yourself and clients. The use of the more common lift sheet also reduces friction because the client is more easily moved along the bed's surface.

Exercise and Activity.

Exercise is physical activity for the purpose of conditioning the body, improving health, maintaining fitness, or as a therapeutic measure. The exercise program chosen and individualized for a client depends heavily on the individual's **activity tolerance,** or the kind and amount of exercise or activity that the person is able to perform. Physiological, emotional, and developmental factors influence the client's activity tolerance.

An active lifestyle is important for maintaining and promoting health; it is also an essential treatment for chronic illnesses (Flood and Constance, 2002). Regular physical activity and exercise enhances functioning of all body systems, including cardiopulmonary functioning (endurance), musculoskeletal fitness (flexibility and bone integrity), weight control and maintenance (body image), and psychological well-being (Burbank and others, 2002; Gillespie, 2006).

The best program of physical activity includes a combination of exercises that produce different physiological and psychological benefits. Isotonic, isometric, and resistive isometric are three categories of exercise. They are classified according to the type of muscle contraction involved. Isotonic exercises cause muscle contraction and change in muscle length **(isotonic contraction).** Examples of isotonic exercises are walking, swimming, dance aerobics, jogging, bicycling, and moving arms and legs with light resistance. Isotonic exercises enhance circulatory and respiratory functioning; increase muscle mass, tone, and strength; and promote osteoblastic activity (activity by bone-forming cells) and thus combat osteoporosis.

Isometric exercises involve tightening or tensing of muscles without moving body parts **(isometric contraction).** Examples of isometric exercises are quadriceps set exercises and contraction of the gluteal muscles. This form of exercise is ideal for clients who are unable to tolerate increased activity. An immobilized client in bed can perform isometric exercises. The benefits are increased muscle mass, tone, and strength, thus decreasing the potential for muscle wasting; increased circulation to the involved body part; and increased osteoblastic activity.

Resistive isometric exercises are those in which the individual contracts the muscle while pushing against a stationary object or resisting the movement of an object (Hoeman, 2002). A gradual increase in the amount of resistance and length of time that the muscle contraction is held will increase muscle strength and endurance. Examples of resistive isometric exercises are push-ups and hip lifting, where a patient in a sitting position pushes with the hands against a surface such as a chair seat and raises the hips. In some long term care settings, **footboards** are placed on the end of beds for patients to push against to move up in bed. Resistive isometric exercises help promote muscle strength and provide sufficient stress against bone to promote osteoblastic activity.

Regulation of Movement

Coordinated body movement involves the integrated functioning of the skeletal, muscular, and nervous systems. Because these three systems cooperate so closely in mechanical support of the body, they are often considered as a single functional unit.

Skeletal System. Bones perform five functions in the body: support, protection, movement, mineral storage, and hematopoiesis (blood cell formation). In the discussion of body mechanics, two of these functions—support and movement—are most important (see Chapter 47). In support, bones serve as the framework and contribute to the shape, alignment, and positioning of the body parts. In movement, bones together with their joints constitute levers for muscle attachment. As muscles contract and shorten, they pull on bones, producing joint movement (Thibodeau and Patton, 2007).

Joints. An articulation, or **joint,** is the connection between bones. Each joint is classified according to its structure and degree of mobility. On the basis of connective structures, joints are classified as fibrous, cartilaginous, or synovial (Huether and McCance, 2004). **Fibrous joints** fit closely together and are fixed, permitting little, if any, movement such as the syndesmosis between the tibia and fibula. **Cartilaginous joints** have little movement but are elastic and use cartilage to unite separate body surfaces such as the synchondrosis that attaches the ribs to the costal cartilage. **Synovial joints,** or true joints, are freely movable and are the most mobile, numerous, and anatomically complex of the body's joints, such as the hinge type at the elbow.

Ligaments, Tendons, and Cartilage. Ligaments, tendons, and cartilage are structures that support the skeletal system (see Chapter 47). **Ligaments** are white, shiny, flexible bands of fibrous tissue that bind joints and connect bones and cartilage. Ligaments are elastic and aid joint flexibility and support. **Tendons** are white, glistening, fibrous bands of tissue that connect muscle to bone. **Cartilage** is nonvascular, supporting connective tissue with the flexibility of a firm, plastic material. The gristlelike nature of cartilage permits it to sustain weight and serve as a shock absorber between articulating bones.

Skeletal Muscle. When we walk, talk, run, breathe, or participate in physical activity, we do so by the contraction of skeletal muscles. There are over 600 skeletal muscles in the body. In addition to facilitating movement, these muscles determine the form and contour of our bodies. Most of our muscles span at least one joint and attach to both articulating bones. When contraction occurs, one bone is fixed while the other moves. The origin is the point of attachment that remains still; the insertion is the point that moves when the muscle contracts (Thibodeau and Patton, 2007).

Muscles Concerned With Movement. The muscles of movement are located near the skeletal region, where a lever system causes movement (Thibodeau and Patton, 2007). The lever system makes the work of moving a weight or load easier. It occurs when specific bones, such as the humerus, ulna, and radius, and the associated joints, such as the elbow, act as a lever. Thus the force applied to one end of the bone to lift a weight at another point tends to rotate the bone in the direction opposite that of the applied force. Muscles that attach to bones of leverage provide the necessary strength to move the object.

Muscles Concerned With Posture. Gravity continually pulls on parts of the body; the only way the body is held in position is for muscles to exert pull on bones in the opposite direction. Muscles accomplish this counterforce by maintaining a low level of sustained contraction. Poor posture places more work on muscles to counteract the force of gravity. This leads to fatigue and eventually interferes with bodily functions and causes deformities.

Muscle Groups. The antagonistic, synergistic, and antigravity muscle groups are coordinated by the nervous system and are responsible for maintaining posture and initiating movement. **Antagonistic muscles** bring about movement at the joint. During movement the active mover muscle contracts while its antagonist relaxes. For example, during flexion of the arm the active mover, the biceps brachii, contracts and its antagonist, the triceps brachii, relaxes. During extension of the arm the active mover, now the triceps brachii, contracts and the new antagonist, the biceps brachii, relaxes.

Synergistic muscles contract to accomplish the same movement. When the arm is flexed, the strength of the contraction of the biceps brachii is increased by contraction of the synergistic muscle, the brachialis. Thus with synergistic muscle activity there are now two active movers—the biceps brachii and the brachialis—which contract while the antagonistic muscle, the triceps brachii, relaxes.

Antigravity muscles are involved with joint stabilization. These muscles continuously oppose the effect of gravity on the body and permit a person to maintain an upright or sitting posture. In an adult the antigravity muscles are the extensors of the leg, the gluteus maximus, the quadriceps femoris, the soleus muscles, and the muscles of the back.

Skeletal muscles support posture and carry out voluntary movement. The muscles are attached to the skeleton by tendons, which provide strength and permit motion. The movement of the extremities is voluntary and requires coordination from the nervous system.

Nervous System. The nervous system regulates movement and posture. The major voluntary motor area, located in the cerebral cortex, is the precentral gyrus, or motor strip. A majority of motor fibers descend from the motor strip and cross at the level of the medulla. Thus the motor fibers from the right motor strip initiate voluntary movement for the left side of the body, and motor fibers from the left motor strip initiate voluntary movement for the right side of the body.

Transmission of the impulse from the nervous system to the musculoskeletal system is an electrochemical event and requires a neurotransmitter. Basically, neurotransmitters are chemicals (e.g., acetylcholine) that transfer the electrical impulse from the nerve across the myoneural junction to stimulate the muscle, causing movement. Movement is impaired by disorders that alter neurotransmitter production as in Parkinson's disease, transfer from the neurotransmitter to the muscle as in myasthenia gravis, or activation of muscle activity as in multiple sclerosis (Huether and McCance, 2004).

Proprioception. **Proprioception** is the awareness of the position of the body and its parts (Huether and McCance, 2004). Proprioception is monitored by proprioceptors located on nerve endings in muscles, tendons, and joints. Posture is regulated by the nervous system and requires coordination of proprioception and balance. As a person carries out ADLs, proprioceptors monitor muscle activity and body position. For example, the proprioceptors on the soles of the feet contribute to correct posture while standing or walking. In standing, pressure is continuous on the bottom of the feet. The proprioceptors monitor the pressure, communicating this information through the nervous system to the antigravity muscles. The standing person remains upright until deciding to change position. As a person walks, the proprioceptors on the bottom of the feet monitor pressure changes. Thus, when the bottom of the moving foot comes in contact with the walking surface, the individual automatically moves the stationary foot forward.

Balance. When standing, running, lifting, or performing ADLs, a person must have adequate balance. Balance is controlled by the nervous system, specifically by the cerebellum and the inner ear. The major function of the cerebellum is to coordinate all voluntary movement, particularly highly skilled movements, such as those required in skiing.

Within the inner ear are the semicircular canals, three fluid-filled structures that assist in maintaining balance. Fluid within the canals has a certain inertia, and when the head is suddenly rotated in one direction, the fluid remains stationary for a moment, whereas the canal turns with the head. This allows a person to change position suddenly without losing balance.

Principles of Transfer and Positioning Techniques

Using principles of safe client transfer and positioning during routine activities decreases work effort (Box 37-2). Teach colleagues and clients' families how to transfer or position clients properly. Teaching a client's family to transfer the client from bed to chair increases and reinforces the family's knowledge about proper transfer and position techniques.

Whether you are moving an immobilized client, assisting a client from the bed to the chair, or teaching a client to carry out ADLs efficiently, knowledge of safe client transfer and positioning is crucial. You also incorporate knowledge of physiological and pathological influences on body alignment and mobility.

Pathological Influences on Body Alignment and Mobility. Many pathological conditions affect body alignment and mobility. These conditions include congenital defects; disor-

---

✳ BOX 37-2 Principles of Safe Client Transfer and Positioning

Mechanical lifts and lift teams are essential when the client is unable to assist.

When a client is able to assist, remember the following principles:

- The wider the base of support, the greater the stability of the nurse.
- The lower the center of gravity, the greater the stability of the nurse.
- The equilibrium of an object is maintained as long as the line of gravity passes through its base of support.
- Facing the direction of movement prevents abnormal twisting of the spine.
- Dividing balanced activity between arms and legs reduces the risk of back injury.
- Leverage, rolling, turning, or pivoting requires less work than lifting.
- When friction is reduced between the object to be moved and the surface on which it is moved, less force is required to move it.

---

ders of bones, joints, and muscles; central nervous system damage; and musculoskeletal trauma.

Congenital Defects. Congenital abnormalities affect the efficiency of the musculoskeletal system in regard to alignment, balance, and appearance. Osteogenesis imperfecta is an inherited disorder that affects bone. Bones are porous, short, bowed, and deformed; as a result, children experience curvature of the spine and shortness of stature. Scoliosis is a structural curvature of the spine associated with vertebral rotation. Muscles, ligaments, and other soft tissues become shortened. Balance and mobility are affected in proportion to the severity of abnormal spinal curvatures (Hockenberry and Wilson, 2007).

Disorders of Bones, Joints, and Muscles. Osteoporosis is a well-known and well-publicized disorder of aging in which the density or mass of bone is reduced. The bone remains biochemically normal but has difficulty maintaining integrity and support. The cause is uncertain, and theories vary from hormonal imbalances to insufficient intake of nutrients (Huether and McCance, 2004).

Osteomalacia is an uncommon metabolic disease characterized by inadequate and delayed mineralization, resulting in compact and spongy bone (Lewis and others, 2007). Mineral calcification and deposition do not occur. Replaced bone consists of soft material rather than rigid bone.

Joint mobility is altered by inflammatory and noninflammatory joint diseases and articular disruption. Inflammatory joint disease (e.g., arthritis) is characterized by inflammation or destruction of the synovial membrane and articular cartilage, and by systemic signs of inflammation. Noninflammatory diseases have none of these characteristics, and the synovial fluid is normal (Huether and McCance, 2004). Joint degeneration, which can occur with inflammatory and noninflammatory disease, is marked by changes in articular cartilage combined with overgrowth of bone at the articular ends. Degenerative changes commonly affect weight-bearing joints.

Articular disruption may be as mild as a sprain or as severe as dislocation. Articular disruption involves trauma to the articular capsules, such as a tear in a sprain or a separation in a dislocation. Articular disruption usually results from trauma but can also be congenital, as with developmental dysplasia of the hip (Hockenberry and Wilson, 2007).

Central Nervous System Damage. Damage to any component of the central nervous system that regulates voluntary movement results in impaired body alignment and mobility. For example, the motor strip in the cerebrum can be damaged by trauma from a head injury. The amount of voluntary motor impairment is directly related to the amount of destruction of the motor strip. A client with a right-sided cerebral hemorrhage and damage to the right motor strip may have left-sided **hemiplegia**. However, a client with a right-sided head injury may only have cerebral edema (but not destruction) of the motor strip. With extensive physical therapy, voluntary movement may gradually return to the left side.

Musculoskeletal Trauma. Musculoskeletal trauma often results in bruises, contusions, sprains, and fractures. A fracture is a disruption of bone tissue continuity. Fractures most commonly result from direct external trauma. They also occur because of some deformity of the bone, as with pathological fractures of osteoporosis (see Chapter 47).

Nursing Knowledge Base

Application of nursing knowledge allows you to critically think about the holistic needs of clients. Nursing knowledge as it pertains to activity and exercise includes developmental changes, behavioral aspects, family and social support, cultural and ethnic origin, and environmental issues. Consider these areas of knowledge and incorporate into the plan of care whether the client is seeking health promotion, acute care, or restorative and continuing care.

Developmental Changes

Throughout the life span the body's appearance and functioning undergo change. The greatest change and impact on the maturational process occurs in childhood and old age.

Infants Through School-Age Children. The newborn infant's spine is flexed and lacks the anteroposterior curves of the adult. The first spinal curve occurs when the infant extends the neck from the prone position. As growth and stability increase, the thoracic spine straightens, and the lumbar spinal curve appears, which allows sitting and standing.

The toddler's posture is awkward because of the slight swayback and protruding abdomen. As the child walks, the legs and feet are usually far apart and the feet are slightly everted (turned outward). Toward the end of toddlerhood, posture appears less awkward, curves in the cervical and lumbar vertebrae are accentuated, and foot eversion disappears.

By the third year the body is slimmer, taller, and better balanced. Abdominal protrusion decreases, the feet are not as far apart, and the arms and legs have increased in length. The child appears more coordinated. From the third year through the beginning of adolescence, the musculoskeletal system continues to grow and develop (see Chapter 12).

Adolescence. The period of adolescence usually begins with a tremendous growth spurt. Growth is frequently uneven. As a result, the adolescent appears awkward and uncoordinated. Adolescent girls usually grow and develop earlier than boys. Hips widen, and fat deposits in the upper arms, thighs, and buttocks. The adolescent boy's changes in shape are usually a result of long-bone growth and increased muscle mass (see Chapter 12).

Young to Middle Adults. An adult with correct posture and body alignment feels good, looks good, and generally appears self-confident. The healthy adult also has the necessary musculoskeletal development and coordination to carry out ADLs (see Chapter 13). Normal changes in posture and body alignment in adulthood occur mainly in pregnant women. These changes result from the body's adaptive response to weight gain and the growing fetus. The center of gravity shifts toward the anterior. The pregnant woman leans back and is slightly swaybacked, and as a result, pregnant women often complain of back pain.

Older Adults. A progressive loss of total bone mass occurs with the older adult. Some of the possible causes of this loss include physical inactivity, hormonal changes, and increased osteoclastic activity (activity by cells responsible for bone tissue absorption). The effect of bone loss is weaker bones, causing vertebrae to be softer and long shaft bones to be less resistant to bending.

In addition, older adults may walk more slowly and appear less coordinated. They may also take smaller steps, keeping their feet closer together, which decreases the base of support. Thus body balance is unstable, and they are at greater risk for falls and injuries (see Chapter 14).

Behavioral Aspects

Clients are more likely to incorporate an exercise program into their daily lives if supported and assisted by family, friends, nurses, health care providers, and other members of the health care team. The nurse takes into consideration the client's knowledge of exercise and activity, barriers to a program of exercise and physical activity, and current exercise habits. Clients are more open to developing an exercise program when they are at a stage of readiness to change their behavior (Prochaska, Norcross, and DiClemente, 1994). Information on the benefits of regular exercise is often helpful to the client who is not at the stage of readiness to act. Clients' decisions to change behavior and include a daily exercise routine in their lives may occur gradually with repeated information individualized to clients' needs and lifestyle (Box 37-3). Once the client is at the stage of readiness, collaborate with the client to develop an exercise program that fits his or her

---

✴ BOX 37-3 General Guidelines for Initiating an Exercise Program

Five steps to beginning an exercise program:
Step 1: Assess fitness level.
- Seek approval from a health care provider to begin. Are there any limitations to consider before determining the exercises in the fitness program?
- Record baseline fitness scores such as pulse rate, how long it takes to walk 1 mile, waist circumference, and body mass index.

Step 2: Design the fitness program.
- Consider fitness goals. Make goals attainable.
- Plan a logical progression of activities (e.g., walk a mile and gradually increase the pace).
- Build the program into a daily routine.
- Plan the fitness program with creativity and different activities.

Step 3: Assemble equipment.
- Choose athletic shoes designed for the chosen exercise.
- Try equipment at a fitness center before purchasing to make sure it fits into the fitness program.
- Buy used fitness equipment.
- Try homemade equipment (e.g., half-gallon milk jugs filled with sand for weights).

Step 4: Get started.
- Start slowly, including a warm-up and cool-down period.
- Divide exercise time throughout day if time or fatigue is a barrier. Ten minutes of exercise 3 times a day instead of a single 30-minute workout may be better for some clients' schedules and medical conditions.

Step 5: Monitor progress.
- Retake fitness assessment at 6 weeks and then every 3 to 6 months.
- If losing motivation: set new goals, exercise with a friend, or incorporate new activities.

Information from Mayo Clinic Tools for Healthier Lives: *Fitness programs: ready to get started?* 2005, http://www.mayoclinic.com/health/fitness/HQ00171, accessed April 30, 2007.

---

needs and provide continued follow-up support and assistance until the exercise program becomes a daily routine.

Environmental Issues

Work Site. A common barrier for many clients is the lack of time needed to engage in a daily exercise program. Work sites can help their employees overcome the obstacle of time constraints by offering opportunities, reminders, and rewards for those committed to physical fitness (Katz and others, 2005). Reminders, such as signs, encouraging employees to use the stairs instead of elevators are useful. Rewards such as free parking or discounted parking fees are also good for employees who park in distant lots and walk.

Schools. It is increasingly clear that children are less active, resulting in an increase in childhood obesity (Harper, 2006). Schools are excellent facilitators of physical fitness and exercise. Strategies for physical activity incorporated early into a child's daily routine may provide a foundation for lifetime commitment to exercise and physical fitness.

✳ BOX 37-4   CULTURAL ASPECTS OF CARE

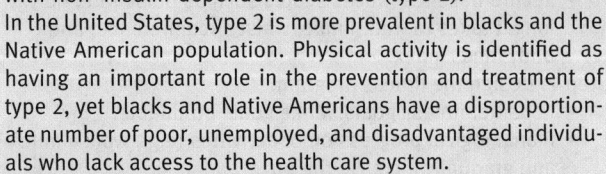

Incidence of Type 2 Dependent Diabetes Among Ethnic Groups in the United States

Studies of ethnic groups indicate that physical inactivity is one of the risk factors associated with non–insulin dependent diabetes (type 2). In the United States, type 2 is more prevalent in blacks and the Native American population. Physical activity is identified as having an important role in the prevention and treatment of type 2, yet blacks and Native Americans have a disproportionate number of poor, unemployed, and disadvantaged individuals who lack access to the health care system.

Implications for Practice

- Physical inactivity is a modifiable risk factor for the development of type 2. Prevention and treatment programs need to focus heavily on exercise and be tailored to the activity tolerance of the individual client.
- Support promotion of physical activity through formal programs in schools, churches, and government agencies within black and Native American communities.
- Incorporate motivational factors into the exercise program such as providing a healthy snack or meal for the participants and furnishing each client with a log to monitor weight loss and blood glucose levels.
- Development of an exercise/prevention program should remove potential barriers such as transportation and cost to facilitate commitment to the program.

Data from Gillespie HO: Exercise. In Edelman CL, Mandle CL, editors: *Health promotion throughout the life span*, ed 6, St. Louis, 2006, Mosby; Lee ET and others: Incidence of diabetes in American Indians of three geographic areas, *Diabetes Care* 25:49, 2002; and Rimmer JH and others: Feasibility of a health promotion intervention for a group of predominantly African American women with type 2 diabetes, *Diabetes Educ* 28(4):571, 2002.

Community. The community's support of physical fitness is instrumental in promoting the health of its members. Examples of community involvement to promote physical fitness are the provision of walking trails and track facilities in parks and physical fitness classes. Success in implementing physical fitness programs is dependent on a collaborative effort from public health agencies, parks and recreational associations, state and local government agencies, health care agencies, and the members of the community (Harper, 2006).

Cultural and Ethnic Influences

Exercise and physical fitness is beneficial to all people. When developing a physical fitness program for culturally diverse populations, consider what motivates and what is deemed appropriate and enjoyable. Also, it is important to have knowledge of what specific disease entities are associated with different cultural and ethnic origins (Box 37-4).

Family and Social Support

Social support is one motivational tool to encourage and promote exercise and physical fitness. The client can engage a friend or significant other to participate in a "buddy system" whereby they walk together each day at a specified time. This companionship provides for socialization and increases the enjoyment for some clients and thus develops a lifelong commitment to physical fitness. Parents can support their children in sports and physical activity by providing encouragement, praise, and transportation (Prochaska, Rodgers, and Sallis, 2002). In addition, parents can include their children in family outings that include such activities as bicycling or a basketball game in the neighborhood schoolyard.

Critical Thinking

Successful critical thinking requires a synthesis of knowledge, experience, information gathered from clients, critical thinking attitudes, and intellectual and professional standards. Clients' conditions are always changing. Clinical judgments require you to anticipate the information necessary, analyze the data, and make decisions regarding client care.

To understand activity tolerance and physical fitness and the impact on the client, you need to integrate knowledge from nursing and other disciplines, previous experiences, and information gathered from clients. As you begin to plan for client care, a variety of concepts need to be considered and put together to provide the best outcome for the client. Knowledge of the musculoskeletal system and health alterations that create problems for the client in the area of activity and exercise, positioning, and transfer lays the foundation for planning and decision making. The use of professional standards, such as those developed by the American College of Sports Medicine (ACSM) (1998, 2002) and the American Diabetes Association (2002), provides valuable guidelines for exercise and physical fitness. In addition, using the recommendations from the ANA (2003) reduces the risk for work-related musculoskeletal disorders (MSD).

Any acquired or congenital condition that affects the structure of the musculoskeletal or nervous system impairs to some degree activity, body alignment, or joint mobility. The impairment can be temporary, such as casting of an extremity, or permanent, as in contractures. For clients with limited **range of motion** (ROM) or mobility, the nursing care plan needs to include interventions that maintain the present level of alignment and joint mobility and increase the level of motor function.

Your experiences and critical thinking attitude affect the problem-solving approach with clients and are reevaluated with each new client. Remember that clients have the capacity for recovery in spite of the loss of some physical function. Restoration of functioning begins early in the care of clients experiencing disruption in their ability to perform self-care. Encouragement, support, commitment, and perseverance are important attitudes in critical thinking for these clients.

Perseverance is necessary when caring for clients who depend on the nurse for assistance with positioning, turning, or ambulation. Hourly responsibility for turning often becomes repetitive, and nurses often lose sight of its importance. Perseverance is especially important in delegating these activities to other personnel. Making certain that the task is performed correctly is an essential nursing function. Problems with activity and mobility are often prolonged; creativity is necessary when designing interventions for improving activity tolerance and mobility skills.

✴ BOX 37-5 NURSING ASSESSMENT QUESTIONS

Nature of the Problem
- What types of problems are you having with activities and exercise?
- Why do you think your exercise and activity are inadequate?
- Describe for me your typical daily exercise routine and activity.
- What type of exercise do you prefer?
- How long do you exercise at any given time?

Signs and Symptoms
- Do you experience muscular or joint pain during or after exercise?
- Do you experience shortness of breath during activity?
- Do you experience chest discomfort or pain during exercise or activity?

Onset and Duration
- What activities cause you to become short of breath?
- How long does it take to resume normal breathing after exercise or an activity?

Severity
- How far do you walk before the pain in your legs begins?
- On a scale of 0 to 10 (10 being the worse discomfort), rate your leg pain.
- Describe your shortness of breath as either minimal, moderate, or severe after activities and/or exercise.

Barriers to Exercise and Activity
- Do you have any chronic illnesses that affect your ability to carry out activities of daily living (ADLs) or exercise?
- Do you have any physical limitations that prevent you from exercising on a daily basis?
- Do you have access to a community walking path and exercise equipment?
- What prevents you from exercising 30 minutes each day?

Effect on Client
- Has the lack of an exercise routine affected your weight?
- Do you feel more fatigued since you have not been able to exercise on a routine basis?
- Have you noticed any increase in shortness of breath when performing activities that require little exertion?

Knowledge
- Normal activity needs for the client's developmental stage
- Normal activity patterns
- Effects of therapies on the client's activity and exercise patterns
- Physiological and emotional effects of exercise
- The influence of clients' culture on preferences for activity

Experience
- Caring for clients who require activity and exercise reconditioning
- Personal experience in beginning an exercise program

ASSESSMENT
- Assess the client's body alignment, posture, and mobility
- Identify the impact of activity and exercise on the client's overall level of health
- Assess the client's routine exercise pattern
- Observe the client's body systems' response to activity and exercise

Standards
- Apply intellectual standards such as accuracy, relevancy and specificity when obtaining data related to the client's activity and exercise status
- Apply professional standards such as those from the ACSM, ADA, and ANA

Attitudes
- Use creativity in observing the client's activity and exercise patterns
- Carry out your responsibility for collecting appropriate assessment data to assess the client's activity and exercise pattern

Figure 37-1 Critical thinking model for activity and exercise assessment.

Nursing Process

◆ Assessment

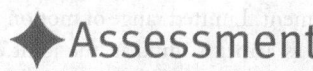

Assessment of body alignment and posture is completed with the client standing, sitting, or lying down. Use assessment to determine normal physiological changes in growth and development; deviations related to poor posture, trauma, muscle damage, or nerve dysfunction; and any learning needs of clients. In addition, provide opportunities for clients to observe their posture and obtain important information about other factors that contribute to poor alignment, such as inactivity, fatigue, malnutrition, and psychological problems. Ask questions related to the client's exercise and activity tolerance to gather important information (Box 37-5). During assessment (Figure 37-1) consider all of the elements that build toward making appropriate nursing diagnoses. The first step in assessing body alignment is to put the client at ease so that unnatural or rigid positions are not assumed. When

assessing body alignment of an immobilized or unconscious client, remove pillows from the bed if not contraindicated, and place the client in the supine position.

Standing. Assessment of the standing client includes the following: the head is erect and midline; body parts are symmetrical; the spine is straight with normal curvatures (cervical concave, thoracic convex, lumbar concave); the abdomen is comfortably tucked; the knees need to be in a straight line between the hips and ankles and slightly flexed; the feet are flat on the floor and pointed directly forward and slightly apart to maintain a wide base of support; and the arms hang comfortably at the sides (Figure 37-2). The client's center of gravity is in the midline, and the line of gravity is from the middle of the forehead to a midpoint between the feet. Laterally, the line of gravity runs vertically from the middle of the skull to the posterior third of the foot (Wilson and Giddens, 2005).

Sitting. Assessment of the client in the sitting position includes the following: the head is erect, and the neck and vertebral column

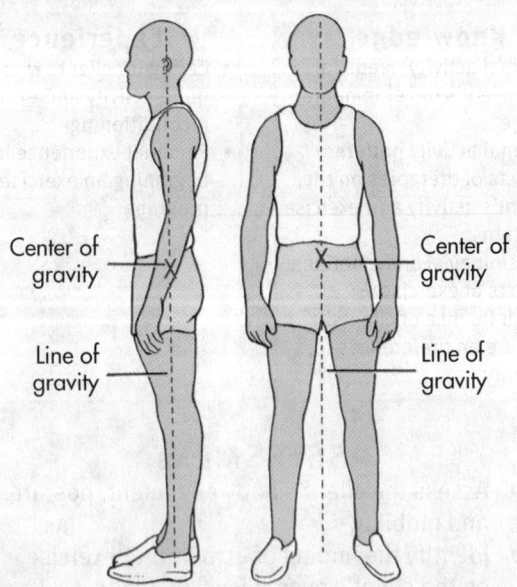

Center of gravity

Line of gravity

Center of gravity

Line of gravity

Figure 37-2 Correct body alignment when standing.

are in straight alignment; the body weight is distributed on the buttocks and thighs; the thighs are parallel and in a horizontal plane (be careful to avoid pressure on the popliteal nerve and blood supply); the feet are supported on the floor; and the forearms are supported on the armrest, in the lap, or on a table in front of the chair.

Assessment of alignment in the sitting position is particularly important for the client with muscle weakness, muscle paralysis, or nerve damage. A client with these alterations has diminished sensation in affected areas and is unable to perceive pressure or decreased circulation. Proper sitting alignment reduces the risk of musculoskeletal system damage in such a client.

Recumbent Position. Assessment of the client in the recumbent position requires that the client be placed in the lateral position with all but one pillow and all positioning supports removed from the bed. The vertebrae are in straight alignment without observable curves. This assessment provides baseline data concerning the client's body alignment.

Conditions that create a risk of damage to the musculoskeletal system when lying down include impaired mobility (e.g., traction), decreased sensation (e.g., **hemiparesis** from a stroke), impaired circulation (e.g., diabetes), and lack of voluntary muscle control (e.g., spinal cord injuries).

When a client is unable to change position voluntarily, assess the position of body parts while the client is lying down. Make sure the vertebrae are in straight alignment without any observable curves. Also check that the extremities are in alignment and not crossed over one another. The head and neck should be aligned without excessive flexion or extension.

Mobility. Assessment of mobility helps to determine the client's coordination and balance while walking, the ability to carry out ADLs, and the ability to participate in an exercise program. The assessment of **mobility** has three components: range of motion, **gait**, and exercise.

BOX 37-6 Effects of Exercise

Cardiovascular System
Increased cardiac output
Improved myocardial contraction, thereby strengthening cardiac muscle
Decreased resting heart rate
Improved venous return

Pulmonary System
Increased respiratory rate and depth followed by a quicker return to resting state
Improved alveolar ventilation
Decreased work of breathing
Improved diaphragmatic excursion

Metabolic System
Increased basal metabolic rate
Increased use of glucose and fatty acids
Increased triglyceride breakdown
Increased gastric motility
Increased production of body heat

Musculoskeletal System
Improved muscle tone
Increased joint mobility
Improved muscle tolerance to physical exercise
Possible increase in muscle mass
Reduced bone loss

Activity Tolerance
Improved tolerance
Decreased fatigue

Psychosocial Factors
Improved tolerance to stress
Reports of "feeling better"
Reports of decrease in illness (e.g., colds, influenza)

Data from Huether SE, McCance KL: *Understanding pathophysiology*, ed 3, St. Louis, 2004, Mosby; and Hoeman SP: *Rehabilitation nursing: process, application, and outcomes*, ed 3, St. Louis, 2002, Mosby.

Range of Motion. Assessing ROM is one assessment technique used to determine the degree of damage or injury to a joint (see Chapter 33). By measuring a joint's range of motion you are able to answer questions about joint stiffness, swelling, pain, limited movement, and unequal movement. Limited range of motion often indicates inflammation such as arthritis, fluid in the joint, altered nerve supply, or contractures. Increased mobility (beyond normal) of a joint may indicate connective tissue disorders, ligament tears, or possible joint fractures.

Gait. Gait is the manner or style of walking, including rhythm, cadence, and speed. Assessing gait allows the nurse to draw conclusions about balance, posture, and the ability to walk without assistance. Note conformity; a regular, smooth rhythm; symmetry in the length of leg swing; smooth swaying related to the gait phase; and a smooth, symmetrical arm swing (Wilson and Giddens, 2005).

Exercise. Exercise is physical activity for conditioning the body, improving health, maintaining fitness, or providing therapy for correcting a deformity or restoring the overall body to a maximal state of health. When a person exercises, physiological

BOX 37-7 Factors Influencing Activity Tolerance

Physiological Factors
Skeletal abnormalities
Muscular impairments
Endocrine or metabolic illnesses (e.g., diabetes mellitus, thyroid disease)
Hypoxemia
Decreased cardiac function
Decreased endurance
Impaired physical stability
Pain
Sleep pattern disturbance
Prior exercise patterns
Infectious processes and fever

Emotional Factors
Anxiety
Depression
Chemical addictions
Motivation

Developmental Factors
Age
Sex

Pregnancy
Physical growth and development of muscle and skeletal support

Modified from Monahan WJ and others: *Phipps' medical-surgical nursing: health and illness perspectives,* ed 8, St. Louis, 2007, Mosby.

BOX 37-8 NURSING DIAGNOSTIC PROCESS

Impaired Physical Mobility

Assessment Activities	Defining Characteristics
Observe client's gait.	Shuffled gait Uncoordinated gait Client reports slower walking speed
Observe client performing tasks such as feeding, dressing, or recreational activities.	Uncoordinated movements Limited fine motor coordination
Measure range of joint motion.	Reduced joint motion in lower and/or upper extremities Stiffness in joints

changes occur in body systems (Box 37-6). Determine how much the client regularly exercises.

Activity Tolerance. Activity tolerance is the kind and amount of exercise or activity a person is able to perform. Assessment of activity tolerance is necessary when planning physical activity for health promotion and for clients with acute or chronic illness. This assessment provides baseline data about the client's activity patterns and assists in determining which factors (physical, psychological, or motivational) are affecting activity tolerance. Box 37-7 lists factors affecting activity tolerance.

Client Expectations. In assessing the client's expectations concerning activity and exercise, determine the client's perception of what is normal or acceptable in regard to physical fitness. For example, one of the factors affecting physical activity is freedom from pain. If exercising is painful or tiresome to the client, compliance and commitment to the desired interventions may be lacking. Some clients are content with their present physical activity and fitness and do not perceive a need for improvement.

Nursing Diagnosis

Assessment of the client's activity tolerance, physical fitness, body alignment, and joint mobility provides clusters of data or defining characteristics to support a nursing diagnosis. You need to be ac-

curate when identifying diagnoses. For example, a client who reports being tired or weakened is potentially diagnosed as having activity intolerance or fatigue. Further review of assessed defining characteristics (e.g., abnormal heart rate or dyspnea) will possibly lead to the definitive diagnosis (activity intolerance).

When activity and exercise are problems for a client, nursing diagnoses often focus on the individual's ability to move. The diagnostic label directs nursing interventions. This requires the correct selection of the related factors. For example, activity intolerance related to excess weight gain requires very different interventions than if the related factor is prolonged bed rest. Box 37-8 provides an example of how the diagnostic process leads to accurate diagnosis selection. The following are examples of nursing diagnoses related to activity and exercise:

- Activity intolerance
- Ineffective coping
- Impaired gas exchange
- Risk for injury
- Impaired physical mobility
- Imbalanced nutrition: more than body requirements
- Acute or chronic pain

Planning

During planning synthesize information from multiple resources (Figure 37-3). Critical thinking ensures that the client's plan of care integrates all client information. Professional standards are especially important to consider when developing a plan of care. These standards often establish scientifically proven guidelines for selecting effective nursing interventions.

Concept maps are a tool to assist in the planning of care. Figure 37-4 shows the relationship between a client's medical diagnosis of congestive heart failure and the identified nursing diagnosis.

Goals and Outcomes. Once you identify the nursing diagnoses, you and the client set goals and expected outcomes to direct interventions. The plan needs to include consideration of any

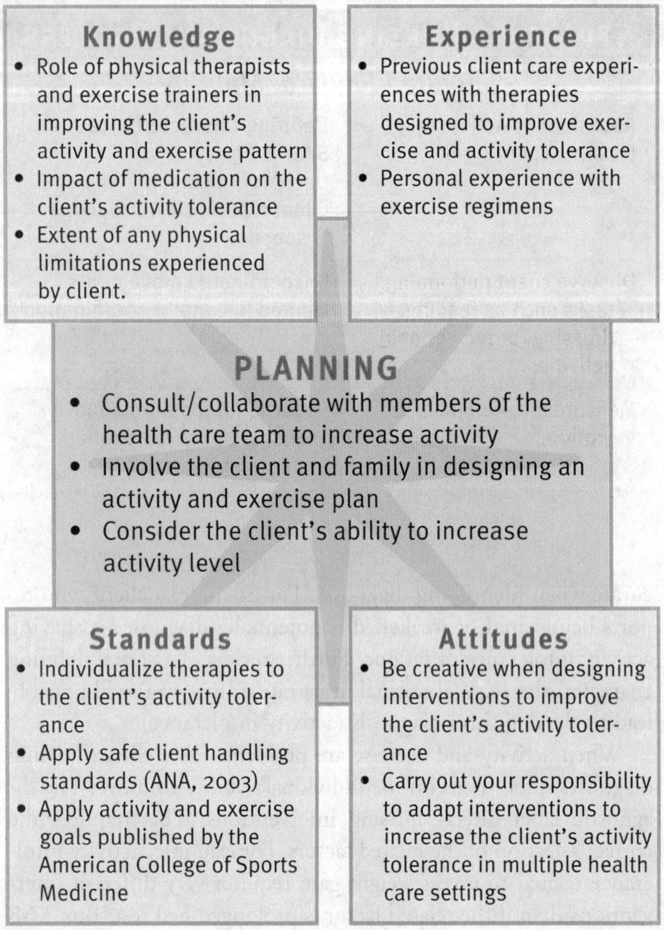

Knowledge

- Role of physical therapists and exercise trainers in improving the client's activity and exercise pattern
- Impact of medication on the client's activity tolerance
- Extent of any physical limitations experienced by client.

Experience

- Previous client care experiences with therapies designed to improve exercise and activity tolerance
- Personal experience with exercise regimens

PLANNING

- Consult/collaborate with members of the health care team to increase activity
- Involve the client and family in designing an activity and exercise plan
- Consider the client's ability to increase activity level

Standards

- Individualize therapies to the client's activity tolerance
- Apply safe client handling standards (ANA, 2003)
- Apply activity and exercise goals published by the American College of Sports Medicine

Attitudes

- Be creative when designing interventions to improve the client's activity tolerance
- Carry out your responsibility to adapt interventions to increase the client's activity tolerance in multiple health care settings

Figure 37-3 Critical thinking model for activity and exercise planning.

risks for injury to the client and preexisting health concerns. It is especially important to have knowledge of the client's home environment when planning therapies to maintain or improve activity, body alignment, and mobility. Include the client's family in the care plan. For some clients with alterations in joint mobility, family members may be the providers of care. The general goal related to exercise and activity is to improve or maintain the client's motor function and independence. The following are examples of outcomes for clients with deficits in activity and exercise (Ackley and Ladwig, 2006):

- Participates in prescribed physical activity while maintaining appropriate heart rate, blood pressure, and breathing rate
- Verbalizes an understanding of the need to gradually increase activity based on tolerance and symptoms
- Expresses understanding of balancing rest and activity

Setting Priorities. Care planning is individualized to the client, taking into consideration the client's most immediate needs. The immediacy of any problem is determined by the impact of the problem on the client's mental and physical health. Because of the many skills associated with the care of clients with activity intolerance, improper body mechanics, and/or impaired mobility, such as turning, transferring, and positioning, it is easy to over-

look the complications associated with these health alterations. Therefore be vigilant in monitoring the client and supervising assistive personnel in carrying out activities to prevent complications and potential injury.

Collaborative Care. Planning involves understanding the client's need to maintain function and independence. Collaboration with other members of the health care team, for example, physical and occupational therapists, is important for these clients. Long-term rehabilitation is sometimes necessary, and you need to begin discharge planning when a client enters the health care system. In addition, always individualize a plan of care directed at meeting the actual or potential needs of the client (see Care Plan).

◆ Implementation

Health Promotion. A sedentary lifestyle contributes to the development of health-related problems. Nurses promote health by encouraging clients to engage in a regular exercise program (Box 37-9, p. 799). A holistic approach is taken to develop and implement a plan to enhance the client's overall physical fitness. Discuss the recommendations for physical activity and fitness with the client, and a program of exercise designed in collaboration with the client.

Before starting an exercise program, clients calculate their maximum heart rate (MHR) by subtracting their current age in years from 220 and then obtain their target heart rate by taking 60% to 90% of the maximum depending upon their health care provider's recommendation. No matter what exercise prescription is implemented for the client, a warm-up and cool-down period need to be included in the program (Gillespie, 2006). The warm-up period usually lasts about 5 to 10 minutes and may include stretching, calisthenics, and/or the aerobic activity performed at a lower intensity. The warm-up activity prepares the body and decreases the potential for injury. The cool-down period follows the exercise routine and usually lasts about 5 to 10 minutes. The cool-down period allows the body to readjust gradually to baseline functioning and provides an opportunity to combine movement such as stretching with relaxation-enhancing mind-body awareness.

Many clients find it difficult to incorporate an exercise program into their daily lives because of time constraints. For these clients it is beneficial to reinforce that many ADLs are used to accumulate the recommended 30 minutes or more per day of moderate-intensity physical activity (Box 37-10, p. 800).

Other clients may benefit from a prescribed exercise and physical fitness program carefully designed to meet their needs and expectations. An exercise prescription may incorporate a combination of aerobic exercise, stretching and flexibility exercises, and resistance training. Aerobic exercise includes such activities as walking, running, bicycling, aerobic dance, jumping rope, and cross-country skiing. Recommended frequency of aerobic exercise is 3 to 5 times per week or every other day for approximately 30 minutes. Cross training is recommended for the client who prefers to exercise every day. For example, the client may run one day and do yoga the next day.

CONCEPT MAP

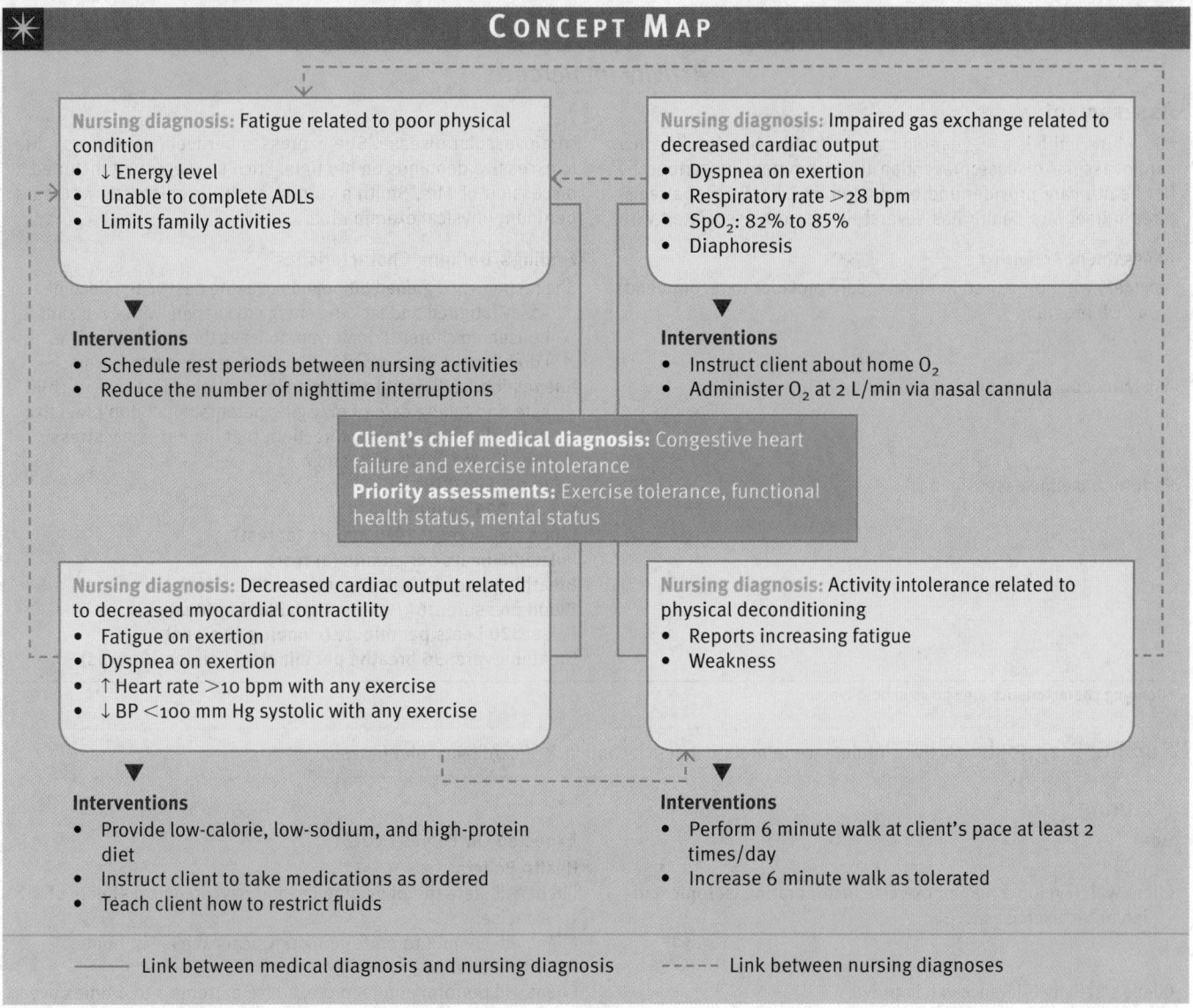

Nursing diagnosis: Fatigue related to poor physical condition
- ↓ Energy level
- Unable to complete ADLs
- Limits family activities

Interventions
- Schedule rest periods between nursing activities
- Reduce the number of nighttime interruptions

Nursing diagnosis: Impaired gas exchange related to decreased cardiac output
- Dyspnea on exertion
- Respiratory rate >28 bpm
- SpO_2: 82% to 85%
- Diaphoresis

Interventions
- Instruct client about home O_2
- Administer O_2 at 2 L/min via nasal cannula

Client's chief medical diagnosis: Congestive heart failure and exercise intolerance
Priority assessments: Exercise tolerance, functional health status, mental status

Nursing diagnosis: Decreased cardiac output related to decreased myocardial contractility
- Fatigue on exertion
- Dyspnea on exertion
- ↑ Heart rate >10 bpm with any exercise
- ↓ BP <100 mm Hg systolic with any exercise

Interventions
- Provide low-calorie, low-sodium, and high-protein diet
- Instruct client to take medications as ordered
- Teach client how to restrict fluids

Nursing diagnosis: Activity intolerance related to physical deconditioning
- Reports increasing fatigue
- Weakness

Interventions
- Perform 6 minute walk at client's pace at least 2 times/day
- Increase 6 minute walk as tolerated

——— Link between medical diagnosis and nursing diagnosis   ----- Link between nursing diagnoses

Figure 37-4 Concept map for a client with congestive heart failure and decreased activity.

Stretching and flexibility exercises include active ROM and stretch all muscle groups and joints. This form of exercise is ideal for warm-up and cool-down periods. Benefits include increased flexibility, improved circulation and posture, and an opportunity for relaxation.

Resistance training increases muscle strength and endurance and is associated with improved performance of daily activities and avoidance of injuries and disability. Formal resistance training includes weight training, but clients can obtain the same benefits by performing ADLs such as pushing a vacuum cleaner, raking leaves, shoveling snow, and kneading bread. Some clients use weight training to bulk up their muscles. However, the purpose of weight training from a health perspective is to develop tone and strength and to stimulate and maintain healthy bone (Schneider and others, 2004).

Body Mechanics. The U.S. Occupational Safety and Health Administration released federal ergonomic standards to prevent

musculoskeletal injuries in the workplace (Occupational Safety and Health Administration, 2000). Half of all back pain is associated with manual lifting tasks (Box 37-11, p. 800). The most common back injury is strain on the lumbar muscle group, which includes the muscles around the lumbar vertebrae. Injury to these areas affects the ability to bend forward, backward, and from side to side. The ability to rotate the hips and lower back is also decreased (Markusic, 2003). Body mechanics alone are not sufficient to prevent musculoskeletal injuries when positioning or transferring clients (Table 37-1, p. 801). Teaching the use of client-handling equipment in combination with proper body mechanics is more effective than either one in isolation (Nelson and Baptiste, 2004).

Manual lifting is the last resort, and it is only used when it does not involve lifting most or all of the client's weight (Nelson and Baptiste, 2004). Before lifting, assess the weight to be lifted and determine the assistance needed and the resources available. Use safe client-handling equipment in conjunction with agency lift

NURSING CARE PLAN

Activity Intolerance

Assessment

Mrs. Mary Smith is a 45-year-old housewife. She has enrolled in a cardiovascular disease prevention (CDP) program prescribed by her health care provider and conducted by Erich Sieple, a registered nurse. Mrs. Smith has several risk factors associated with cardiovascular disease. She expresses her feelings of stress due to excessive demands on her time. Erich's assessment included a discussion of Mrs. Smith's current health problem, as well as a pertinent physical examination.

Assessment Activities	Findings/Defining Characteristics*
Ask Mary what prompted her health care provider to recommend a CDP program.	She responds, "I **gained 50 pounds** over the past year. I become easily **fatigued** and lack the energy to keep up with even simple household chores. I don't want to leave the house anymore. I do not have extra money to join one of those fancy gyms."
Ask Mary about her exercise and eating habits.	She responds, "I want to exercise but with the demands of child care and taking care of my aging parents, I just don't feel like it. I feel pulled in every direction; that increases my **stress**, then I want to eat, eat, and eat!"
Perform baseline assessment.	Height: 5 feet 3 inches
	Weight: **225 pounds** (102 kg)
	Blood pressure: **152/90 mm Hg (at rest)**
	Pulse: **96 beats per minute (at rest)**
	Breathing rate: 20 breaths per minute (at rest)
	Blood pressure: **164/96 mm Hg (climbing 10 steps)**
	Pulse: **120 beats per minute (climbing 10 steps)**
	Breathing rate: **36 breaths per minute (climbing 10 steps)**

*Defining characteristics are shown in bold type.

Nursing Diagnosis: Activity intolerance related to inactivity and lack of cardiovascular fitness.

Planning

Goal	Expected Outcomes (NOC)†
	Health Beliefs
Client will develop a plan of exercise incorporating isotonic and isometric exercises.	Client will state the physiological and psychological effects of exercise.
	Client will commit to performing physical exercise at home.
	Activity Tolerance
Client's activity tolerance will improve.	Client will perform and record exercise patterns 3 to 4 times over the next 2 weeks. Client performed active exercise 4 times over last 2 weeks.
	Client's level of fatigue associated with exercise will remain the same or decrease.
	Cardiovascular Pump Effectiveness
Client's cardiopulmonary response to exercise will improve.	Client's resting diastolic blood pressure will remain below 80 mm Hg. Client's systolic blood pressure will be below 140 mm Hg. Client's resting heart rate will range between 75 and 85 beats per minute.

†Outcome classification labels from Moorhead S and others: *Nursing outcomes classification (NOC)*, ed 4, St. Louis, 2008, Mosby.

Interventions (NIC)‡

Exercise Promotion
- Instruct client about the physiological benefits of a regular exercise program.

- Develop a progressive plan of exercise with the client, such as 2 to 3 miles of brisk walking and quadriceps, bicep, and gluteal muscle isometric exercises 3 to 4 times per week.

Rationale

Physical activity and exercise protect against the development of cardiovascular disease (CVD) and decreases other risk factors associated with CVD, such as obesity, hypertension, and hyperlipidemia (Chobanian and others, 2003; Conroy and others, 2005; Padilla and others, 2005).

Cross training (combination of exercise activities) provides variety to combat boredom and increases potential for total-body conditioning (Gillespie, 2006).

‡Intervention classification labels from Bulechek GM, Butcher HK, and Dochterman JM: *Nursing interventions classification (NIC)*, ed 5, St. Louis, 2008, Mosby.

NURSING CARE PLAN

Activity Intolerance—cont'd

Interventions (NIC)‡	Rationale
Exercise Promotion	
• Instruct client to use an exercise log and to record the day, time, duration, and responses (pulse, feelings, shortness of breath, daily weight).	Keeping a log may increase adherence to exercise prescription.
• Schedule routine visits with the client for follow-up and review of exercise log, progress, and barriers.	Clients are more likely to increase physical activity and remain compliant with an exercise program if they are counseled by a health care professional (Gillespie, 2006).

‡Intervention classification labels from Bulechek GM, Butcher HK, and Dochterman JM: *Nursing interventions classification (NIC)*, ed 5, St. Louis, 2008, Mosby.

Evaluation

Nursing Actions	Client Response/Finding	Achievement of Outcome
Review client's exercise log at each visit.	"I make time to exercise because of this log. I hate missing a day and leaving a blank page; this represents failure. I want to succeed."	Client reports enjoying exercise, as well as observing some personal benefits of exercise.
	Exercise log documents activity 4 times per week.	The exercise log is facilitating adherence to the exercise prescription.
Record weight, blood pressure, and pulse.	Weight, 210 pounds. Resting heart rate remains between 80 and 85 beats per minute. Blood pressure, 146/86 mm Hg.	Improved cardiovascular effects of exercise: • Heart rate is within normal range. • Blood pressure is lower but not at expected range. Monitor blood pressure as client continues to lose weight.
Ask client if exercise is helping to lower fatigue level.	"At first, finding time to exercise was hard, but once I started feeling less tired and even less stressed, it was easy to integrate exercise into my daily activities."	Achieved improved activity tolerance with exercise.

BOX 37-9   PROCEDURAL GUIDELINES

Helping Clients to Exercise

Delegation Considerations: The skill of helping clients to exercise may be delegated. The nurse is responsible for assessing the client's ability and tolerance to exercise. In addition, the nurse teaches clients and their families how to implement exercise programs. You delegate to nursing assistive personnel (NAP) only certain activities when helping clients to exercise. These activities may include preparing the client for exercise (e.g., shoes, clothing, hygiene needs, and obtaining preexercise and postexercise vital signs). Instruct NAP to do the following:

- Notify nurse of client reports of pain before, during, or after exercise
- Notify nurse of client complaints of increased fatigue, dizziness, light-headedness when obtaining preexercise and/or postexercise vital signs
- Notify nurse of vital sign values

1. Assess for any medical limitations (e.g., weight-bearing status, untreated fracture, cardiovascular disease).
2. Know the client's mobility level before hospitalization.
3. Teach clients breathing skills to help reduce anxiety and to fully oxygenate tissues and expand lungs.
4. Assess for client's physiological and psychological limitations for learning and implementing an exercise program.
5. Assess for joint limitations, and do not force a muscle or a joint during exercise.
6. Teach client to wear comfortable shoes and clothing for exercise.
7. Let each client move at his or her own pace.
8. Observe for proper posture, body alignment, and good body mechanics during exercise.
9. Monitor vital signs before, during, and after exercise.
10. Assess for pain, shortness of breath, or a change in vital signs. If present, stop exercise.
11. Document client's progress, and provide feedback as the client exercises.

Data from Gillespie HO: Exercise. In Edelman CL, Mandle CL, editors: *Health promotion throughout the life span*, ed 6, St. Louis, 2006, Mosby; and Monahan WJ and others: *Phipps' medical-surgical nursing: health and illness perspectives*, ed 8, St. Louis, 2007, Mosby.

BOX 37-10 Incorporating Active Exercise Into Activities of Daily Living (ADLs)

Lower-Intensity ADLs
Laundry
Making the bed
Ironing
Washing dishes

Moderate-Intensity ADLs
Sweep the kitchen or sidewalk
Wash windows
Folding clothes
Vacuuming

High-Intensity ADLs
Moving furniture
Carrying boxes or heavier items up and down stairs

Hints to a Good Workout While Doing Housework
To make housework more aerobic—work faster, scrub harder
Bend your legs rather than your back
Start daily household chores with gentle stretches
Alternate cleaning activities to prevent overworking the same muscle groups

Collins A: *Getting fit: unstructured exercise,* http://www.suite101.com/lesson.cfm/18274/1552, accessed April 7, 2007.

teams to reduce the risk of injury to the client and members of the health care team (see Table 37-1).

Acute Care.
Encourage hospitalized clients to do stretching and isometric exercises, active ROM exercises, and low-intensity walking, depending on their condition. When clients cannot participate in active ROM, maintain joint mobility and prevent contractures by implementing passive ROM into the plan of care.

Musculoskeletal System.
Help maintain the musculoskeletal system during acute care by encouraging the use of stretching and isometric type of exercises. Review of the client's chart and collaboration with the health care provider alert you to any possible contraindications before initiating isometric exercises. An isometric exercise program is designed for the specific needs of a client. For example, an exercise program may include biceps and triceps isometric exercises to prepare the client for crutch walking. Instruct the client to stop the activity if pain, fatigue, or discomfort is experienced.

Generally the muscle group is tightened (contracted) for 10 seconds and then completely relaxed for several seconds (Hoeman, 2002). Repetitions are gradually increased for each muscle group until the isometric exercise is repeated 8 to 10 times. Instruct the client to perform the exercises slowly and increase repetitions as his or her physical condition improves. Muscle groups (quadriceps and gluteal) used for walking should be exercised isometrically 4 times per day until the client is ambulatory.

Joint Mobility.
The easiest intervention to maintain or improve joint mobility for clients and one that can be coordinated with other activities is the use of ROM exercises (see Chapter 47). In active ROM exercises, the client is able to move his or her joints independently. With passive ROM exercises, the nurse moves each joint in clients who are unable to perform these exer-

BOX 37-11 EVIDENCE-BASED PRACTICE

Promoting Safe Handling of Clients and Prevention of Injury to Nurses and Their Clients

Evidence Summary
Musculoskeletal disorders (MSDs) are noted as the most prevalent and debilitating occupational health hazards among nurses. Preventive interventions are needed to avert the hazards and economic burdens associated with client-handling tasks. The American Nurses Association (ANA) (2003) put forth a position statement calling for the use of assistive equipment and devices to promote a safe health care environment for nurses and their clients. The use of assistive equipment and continued use of proper body mechanics can significantly reduce the risk of musculoskeletal injuries. In addition, the Occupational Safety and Health Administration (OSHA) recommends that manual lifting of clients be minimized in all cases and eliminated when feasible. A comprehensive program initiated by the Veterans Health Administration was designed to reduce job-related musculoskeletal injuries in nurses (Nelson and others, 2003). The program included an algorithm for each major client transfer and repositioning task and the purchase of lift devices. One year after the inception of the program, preliminary data projected a cost savings of approximately $5 million over the next 9 years as a result of reduction in job-related musculoskeletal injuries. In addition, many facilities are moving toward limited lift policies (LLPs) that minimize client handling by nurses and instead use lift devices to reduce on-the-job injuries.

Application to Nursing Practice
- Know your health care facility's safety information and training concerning the transfer, positioning, and lifting of clients.
- Use recommended back safety guidelines to prevent musculoskeletal injuries.
- Use current research, standards, and guidelines regarding safe positioning and transfer of clients.
- Use "lift teams" and client-handling equipment, such as mechanical lifts, to prevent injury to yourself and the client.

Reference
Data from American Nurses Association: *Position statement on elimination of manual patient handling to prevent work-related musculoskeletal disorders,* 2003, http://www.nursing world.org/readroom/postion/workplace/pathand.htm; and Nelson A and others: Safe patient handling and movement: preventing back injury among nurses requires careful selection of the safest equipment and techniques, *Am J Nurs* 103(3):32, 2003.

cises themselves. The use of ROM exercises provide data to systematically assess and improve the client's joint mobility.

Joints that are not moved periodically are at risk for contractures, a permanent shortening of a muscle followed by the eventual shortening of associated ligaments and tendons. Over time, the joint may become fixed in one position and the client loses normal use of the joint. For the client who does not have voluntary motor control, passive ROM exercises are the exercises of choice.

The older adult has a decline in physical activity and some changes in joints that may predispose the client to problems with mobility, and joint flexibility may be limited. There are a variety

✳ TABLE 37-1 Preventing Lift Injuries in Health Care Workers

ACTION	RATIONALE
When planning to move a client, arrange for adequate help. If your institution has a lift team, use it as a resource.	A lift team is properly trained in techniques to prevent musculoskeletal injuries.
Use client-handling equipment and devices, such as height-adjustable beds, ceiling-mounted lifts, friction-reducing slide sheets, air-assisted devices (Nelson and Baptiste, 2004).	These devices help to reduce the caregiver's muscular strain during client handling.
Encourage client to assist as much as possible.	This promotes client's independence and strength while minimizing workload.
Keep back, neck, pelvis, and feet aligned. Avoid twisting.	Reduces risk of injury to lumbar vertebrae and muscle groups. Twisting increases risk of injury.
Flex knees; keep feet wide apart.	A broad base of support increases stability.
Position self close to client (or object being lifted).	Reduces horizontal reach and stress on caregiver's back.
Use arms and legs (not back).	The leg muscles are stronger, larger muscles capable of greater work without injury.
Slide client toward yourself using a pull sheet or slide board. When transferring a client onto a stretcher or bed, a slide board is more appropriate.	Sliding requires less effort than lifting. Pull sheet minimizes shearing forces, which can damage client's skin.
Person with the heaviest load coordinates efforts of team involved by counting to three.	Simultaneous lifting minimizes the load for any one lifter.
Perform manual lifting as last resort and only if it does not involve lifting most or all of a client's weight (Nelson and Baptiste, 2004).	Lifting is a high-risk activity that causes significant biochemical and postural stressors.

Markusic J: Maintain a healthy spine using good body mechanics, *Spine Universe,* 2003, http://spineuniverse.com.

✳ BOX 37-12 — FOCUS ON OLDER ADULTS

Assisting the Older Adult in Initiating and Maintaining an Exercise Program

- Encourage the sedentary older client to avoid prolonged sitting, to get up and stretch. Frequent stretching decreases joint contractures.
- Be sure that the older client maintains proper body alignment when sitting to minimize joint and muscle stress.
- Teach clients how to use stronger joints or larger muscle groups. Efficient distribution of the workload decreases joint stress and pain.
- Provide resources for planned exercise programs. Weight-bearing and resistance exercise slow further bone loss and prevent fractures in the older adult with osteoporosis (Burbank and others, 2002; Monahan and others, 2007).
- Recommend resistance- and agility-training programs. This form of exercise reduces fear of falling and increased sense of well-being in older adults (Liu-Ambrose and others, 2004).

- It is never too late to begin an exercise program (Burbank and others, 2002; Gillespie, 2006). Consult a health care provider before beginning an exercise program, particularly in the presence of heart or lung disease and other chronic illnesses.
- Exercise is extremely beneficial for older adults, but adjustments may have to be made to an exercise program for those in advanced age to prevent problems.
- When developing an exercise program for any older adult, consider not only the person's current activity level, range of motion, muscle strength and tone, and response to physical activity, but also their interests, capacities, and limitations.
- Older adults who are unable to participate in a formal exercise program are able to achieve the benefits of improved joint mobility and enhanced circulation by simply stretching and exaggerating movements during the performance of routine activities of daily living.

of recommended approaches to help older adults use proper body mechanics and prevent injury (Box 37-12).

Mechanical devices are available to place specific joints through continuous passive motion (CPM). These CPM machines are used postoperatively to place joints through a selective repetitive range of motion. You can set the machine to certain degrees of joint mobility with increasing joint mobility or flexion as the goal. The most common clients who use the CPM machine are those who have undergone some form of total joint replacement surgery.

Unless contraindicated, the nursing care plan includes exercising each joint through as nearly a full ROM as possible. Initiate passive ROM exercises as soon as the client loses the ability to

move the extremity or joint. Chapter 47 details ROM exercises for each area and illustrates the motion of each joint.

Walking. Walking increases joint mobility. Measure distances walked in feet or yards instead of charting "ambulated to nurses' station and back." In the normal walking posture the head is erect; the cervical, thoracic, and lumbar vertebrae are aligned; the hips and knees have appropriate flexion; and the arms swing freely in alternation with the legs. Illness or trauma can reduce activity tolerance, resulting in the need for assistance with walking or the use of mechanical devices such as crutches, canes, or walkers.

Helping a Client to Walk. Helping a client to walk requires preparation. Assess the client's activity tolerance, strength, coordi-

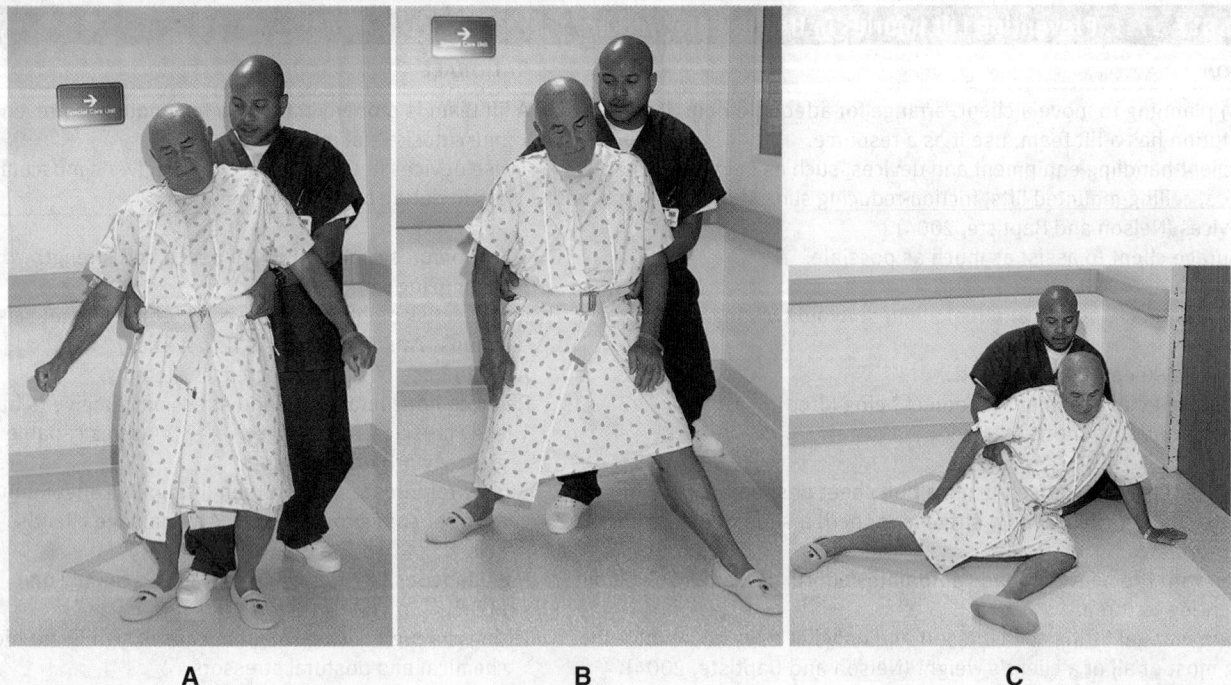

Figure 37-5 A, Stand with feet apart to provide a broad base of support. **B,** Extend one leg, and let client slide against it to the floor. **C,** Bend knees to lower body as client slides to the floor.

nation, and balance to determine the type of assistance needed. Also assess the client's orientation, and determine if there are any signs of distress, which may preclude attempts at ambulation.

Evaluate the environment for safety before ambulation; this includes the removal of obstacles, a clean and dry floor, and the identification of rest points in case the client's activity tolerance becomes less than expected or if the client becomes dizzy. Also have the client wear supportive, nonskid shoes.

Assist the client to a position of sitting at the side of the bed, and dangle for 1 to 2 minutes before standing (Dingle, 2003). Some clients experience orthostatic hypotension, a drop in blood pressure that occurs when the client changes position from a horizontal to a vertical position (Dingle, 2003; Monahan and others, 2007) (see Chapter 32). Those at higher risk are immobilized clients, those undergoing prolonged bed rest, the older adult client, and those clients with chronic illnesses such as diabetes mellitus and cardio-vascular disease (Dingle, 2003; Frederiks and others, 2003; Netea and others, 2002). Signs and symptoms of orthostatic hypotension include dizziness, light-headedness, nausea, tachycardia, pallor, and even fainting (see Chapter 32). Dangling a client before standing is an intermediate step that allows assessment of the client before changing positions to maintain safety and prevent injury to the client. In some instances you may need to obtain the client's blood pressure while he or she is sitting on the side of the bed.

Several methods are used for assisting a client with ambulation. Provide support at the waist so that the client's center of gravity remains midline. This is achieved with the use of a gait belt. A gait belt encircles the client's waist and may have handles attached for the nurse to hold while the client ambulates.

If the client has a fainting (syncope) episode or begins to fall, assume a wide base of support with one foot in front of the other,

thus supporting the client's body weight (Figure 37-5, *A*). Then extend one leg and let the client slide against the leg, and gently lower the client to the floor, protecting the client's head (Figure 37-5, *B* and *C*). Practice this technique with a friend or classmate before attempting it in a clinical setting. When the client attempts to ambulate again, proceed more slowly, monitoring for reports of dizziness, as well as the client's blood pressure before, during, and after ambulation.

Restorative and Continuing Care. Restorative and continuing care involves implementing activity and exercise strategies to assist the client in ADLs after acute care is no longer needed. Restorative and continuing care also includes activities and exercises that restore and promote optimal functioning in clients with specific chronic illnesses, such as coronary heart disease (CHD), hypertension, chronic obstructive pulmonary disease (COPD), and diabetes mellitus.

Assistive Devices for Walking. In collaboration with other health care professionals such as physical therapists, promote activity and exercise by teaching the proper use of canes, walkers, or crutches, depending on the assistive device most appropriate for the client's condition.

Walkers. Walkers are extremely light, movable devices that are about waist high and made of metal tubing (Figure 37-6). They have four widely placed, sturdy legs. The client holds the handgrips on the upper bars, takes a step, moves the walker forward, and takes another step. A walker requires a client to lift the device up and forward. In the home, many clients prefer walkers with wheels or short runners on the legs that allow them to push the walker. Instruct clients on how to use walkers safely and avoid risk of falling.

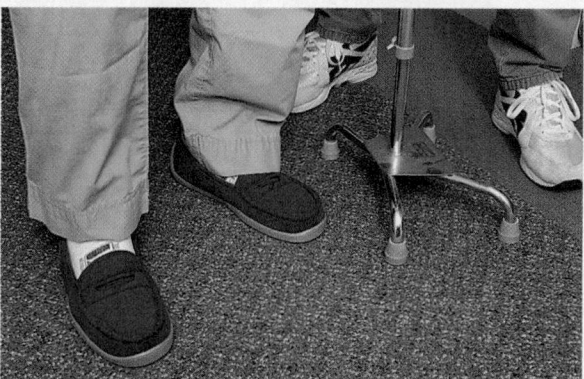

Figure 37-7 Bottom of quad cane.

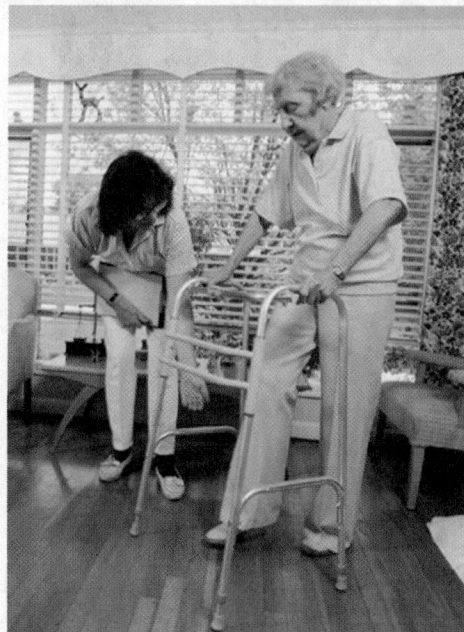

Figure 37-6 Client using a walker.

Canes. Canes are lightweight, easily movable devices and are made of wood or metal. They provide less support than a walker and are less stable. A person's cane length is equal to the distance between the greater trochanter and the floor (Hoeman, 2002). Two common types of canes are the single straight-legged cane and the quad cane. The single straight-legged cane is more common and is used to support and balance a client with decreased leg strength. Have client keep the cane on the stronger side of the body. For maximum support when walking, the client places the cane forward 15 to 25 cm (6 to 10 inches), keeping body weight on both legs. The weaker leg is moved forward to the cane so that body weight is divided between the cane and the stronger leg. The stronger leg is then advanced past the cane so that the weaker leg and the body weight are supported by the cane and weaker leg. During walking, the client continually repeats these three steps. The client needs to learn that two points of support, such as both feet or one foot and the cane, are present at all times.

The quad cane provides the most support and is used when there is partial or complete leg paralysis or some hemiplegia (Figure 37-7). You teach the same three steps that are used with the straight-legged cane to the client.

Crutches. Crutches are often needed to increase mobility. Begin crutch instruction with guidelines for safe use (Box 37-13). The use of crutches is often temporary, such as after ligament damage to the knee. However, some clients with paralysis of the lower extremities may need crutches permanently. A crutch is a wooden or metal staff. The two types of crutches are the double adjustable Lofstrand, or forearm, crutch and the axillary wooden or metal crutch. The forearm crutch has a handgrip and a metal band that fits around the client's forearm. The metal band and the handgrip are adjusted to fit the client's height. The axillary crutch has a padded curved surface at the top, which fits under the axilla. A handgrip in the form of a crossbar is held at the level of the palms to support the body. It is important to measure crutches for

the appropriate length and to teach clients how to use their crutches safely to achieve a stable gait, to ascend and descend stairs, and to rise from a sitting position.

Measuring for Crutches. The axillary crutch is the more common crutch used. Measurements include the client's height, the angle of elbow flexion, and the distance between the crutch pad and the axilla. When crutches are fitted, the length of the

---

✳ BOX 37-13   **CLIENT TEACHING**

Crutch Safety

Objective
- Client will state and demonstrate safe crutch walking.

Teaching Strategies
- Teach the client not to lean on crutches to support body weight.
- Teach client with axillary crutches about the dangers of pressure on the axillae, which occurs when leaning on the crutches to support body weight.
- Explain why client needs to use crutches that were measured for him or her.
- Show client how to routinely inspect crutch tips. Securely attach rubber tips to the crutches. When tips are worn, they need to be replaced. Rubber crutch tips increase surface friction and help prevent slipping.
- Explain that the crutch tips need to remain dry. Water decreases surface friction and increases the risk of slipping. Show client how to dry the crutch tips if they become wet; client may use paper or cloth towels.
- Show client how to inspect the structure of the crutches. Cracks in a wooden crutch decrease its ability to support weight. Bends in aluminum crutches can alter body alignment.
- Provide client with a list of medical supply companies in the community for obtaining repairs, new rubber tips, handgrips, and crutch pads.
- Instruct client to have spare crutches and tips readily available.

Evaluation
- Client states principles of crutch safety.
- Client correctly demonstrates proper use of crutches.
- Axilla will be free of pressure.

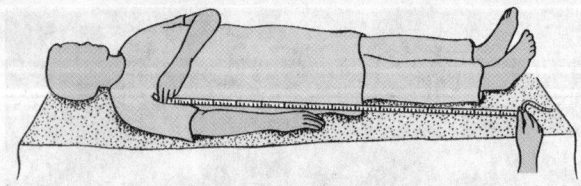

Figure 37-8 Measuring crutch length.

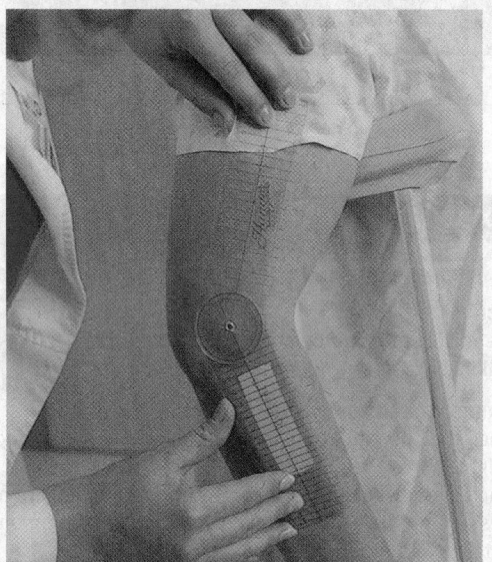

Figure 37-9 Using the goniometer to verify correct degree of elbow flexion for crutch use.

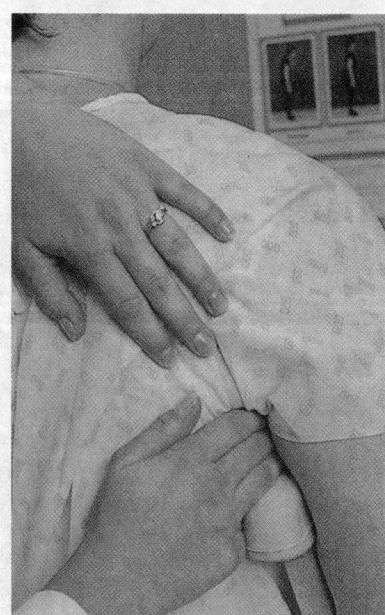

Figure 37-10 Verifying correct distance between crutch pads and axilla.

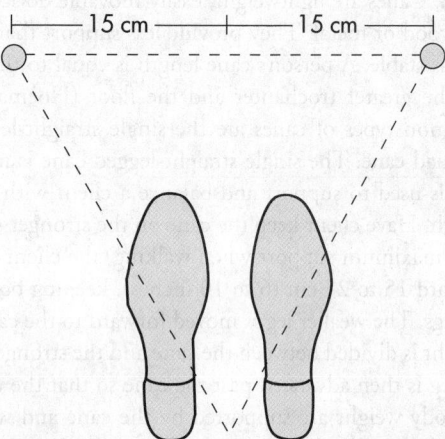

Figure 37-11 Tripod position, basic crutch stance.

crutch should be from three to four finger widths from the axilla to a point 15 cm (6 inches) lateral to the client's heel (Hoeman, 2002) (Figure 37-8).

Position the handgrips so that the axillae are not supporting the client's body weight. Pressure on the axillae increases risk to underlying nerves, which can result in partial paralysis of the arm. Determine correct position of the handgrips with the client upright, supporting weight by the handgrips with the elbows slightly flexed at 30 degrees (Hoeman, 2002). Elbow flexion may be verified with a goniometer (Figure 37-9). When you determine the height and placement of the handgrips, verify that the distance between the crutch pad and the client's axilla is three to four finger widths (Figure 37-10).

Crutch Gait. Clients assume a **crutch gait** by alternately bearing weight on one or both legs and on the crutches. Determine the gait by assessing the client's physical and functional abilities and the disease or injury that resulted in the need for crutches. This section summarizes the basic crutch stance and the four standard gaits: four-point alternating gait, three-point alternating gait, two-point gait, and swing-through gait.

The basic crutch stance is the tripod position, formed when the crutches are placed 15 cm (6 inches) in front of and 15 cm to the side of each foot (Figure 37-11). This position improves the client's balance by providing a wider base of support. The body

alignment of the client in the tripod position includes an erect head and neck, straight vertebrae, and extended hips and knees. The axillae should not bear any weight. The client assumes the tripod position before crutch walking.

Four-point alternating, or four-point, gait gives stability to the client but requires weight bearing on both legs. Each leg is moved alternately with each opposing crutch so that three points of support are on the floor at all times (Figure 37-12).

Three-point alternating, or three-point, gait requires the client to bear all of the weight on one foot. In a three-point gait, the client bears weight on both crutches and then on the uninvolved leg, repeating the sequence (Figure 37-13). The affected leg does not touch the ground during the early phase of the three-point gait. Gradually the client progresses to touchdown and full weight bearing on the affected leg.

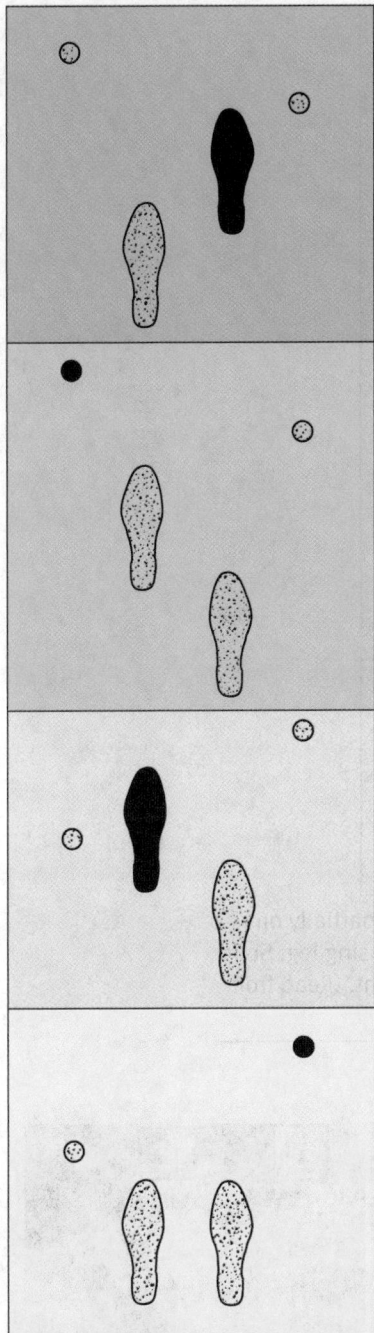

Figure 37-12 Four-point alternating gait. Solid feet and crutch tips show the order of foot and crutch tip movement in each of the four phases. (Read from bottom to top.)

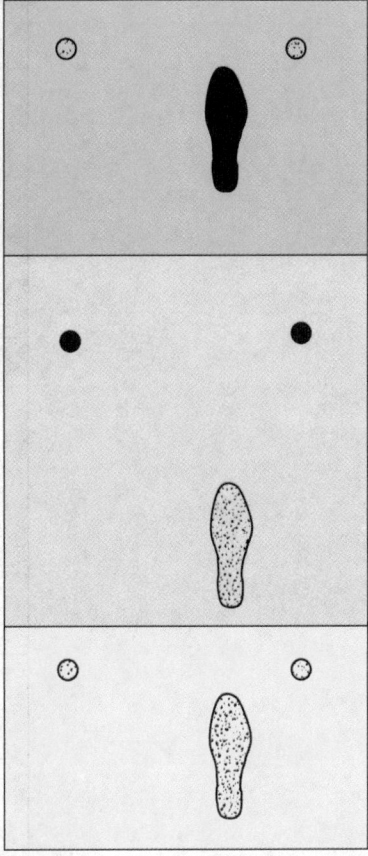

Figure 37-13 Three-point gait with weight borne on unaffected leg. Solid foot and crutch tips show weight bearing in each phase. (Read from bottom to top.)

Crutch Walking on Stairs. When ascending stairs on crutches, the client usually uses a modified three-point gait (Figure 37-15). The client stands at the bottom of the stairs and transfers body weight to the crutches. The unaffected leg is advanced between the crutches to the stairs. The client then shifts weight from the crutches to the unaffected leg. Finally, the client aligns both crutches on the stairs. The client repeats this sequence until he or she reaches the top of the stairs.

A three-phase sequence is also used to descend the stairs (Figure 37-16). The client transfers body weight to the unaffected leg. The crutches are placed on the stairs, and the client begins to transfer body weight to the crutches, moving the affected leg forward. Finally, the unaffected leg is moved to the stairs with the crutches. Again, the client repeats the sequence until reaching the bottom of the stairs.

Because in most cases clients will need to use crutches for some time, they need to be taught to use crutches on stairs before discharge. This instruction applies to all crutch-dependent clients, not only those who have stairs in their homes.

Sitting in a Chair With Crutches. As with crutch walking and crutch walking up and down stairs, the procedure for sitting in a chair involves phases and requires the client to transfer weight (Figure 37-17). First, the client gets positioned at the center front of the chair with the posterior aspect of the legs touching the chair.

The two-point gait requires at least partial weight bearing on each foot (Figure 37-14). The client moves a crutch at the same time as the opposing leg, so that the crutch movements are similar to arm motion during normal walking.

Paraplegics who wear weight-supporting braces on their legs frequently use the swing-through gait. With weight placed on the supported legs, the client places the crutches one stride in front and then swings to or through the crutches while they support the client's weight.

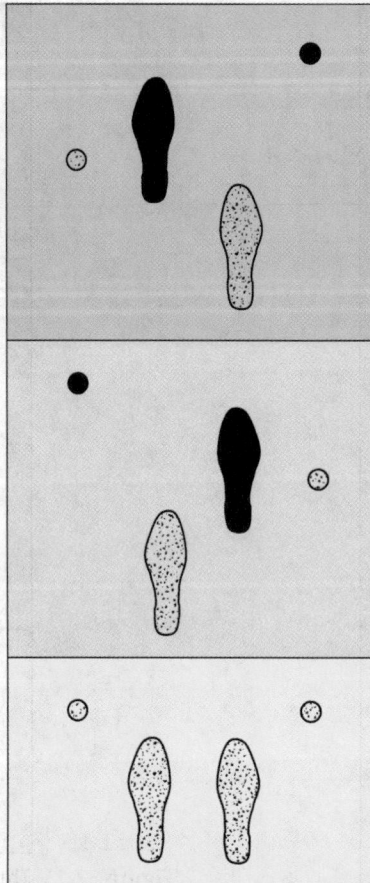

Figure 37-14 Two-point gait with weight borne partially on each foot and each crutch advancing with opposing leg. Solid areas indicate leg and crutch tips bearing weight. (Read from bottom to top.)

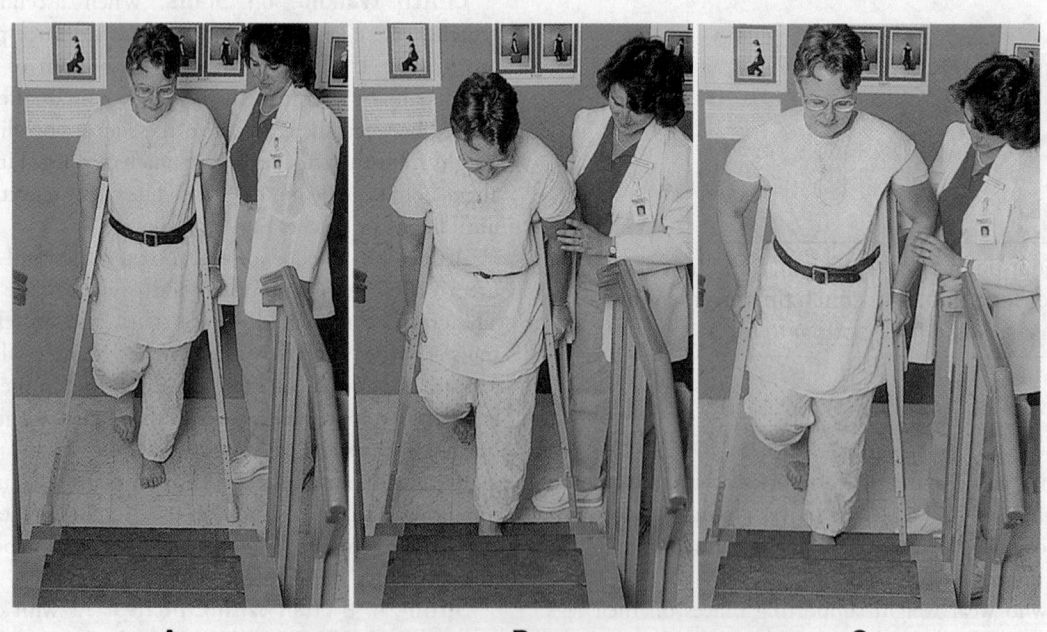

A   **B**   **C**

Figure 37-15 Ascending stairs. **A,** Weight is placed on crutch. **B,** Weight is transferred from crutches to unaffected leg on stairs. **C,** Crutches are aligned with unaffected leg on stairs.

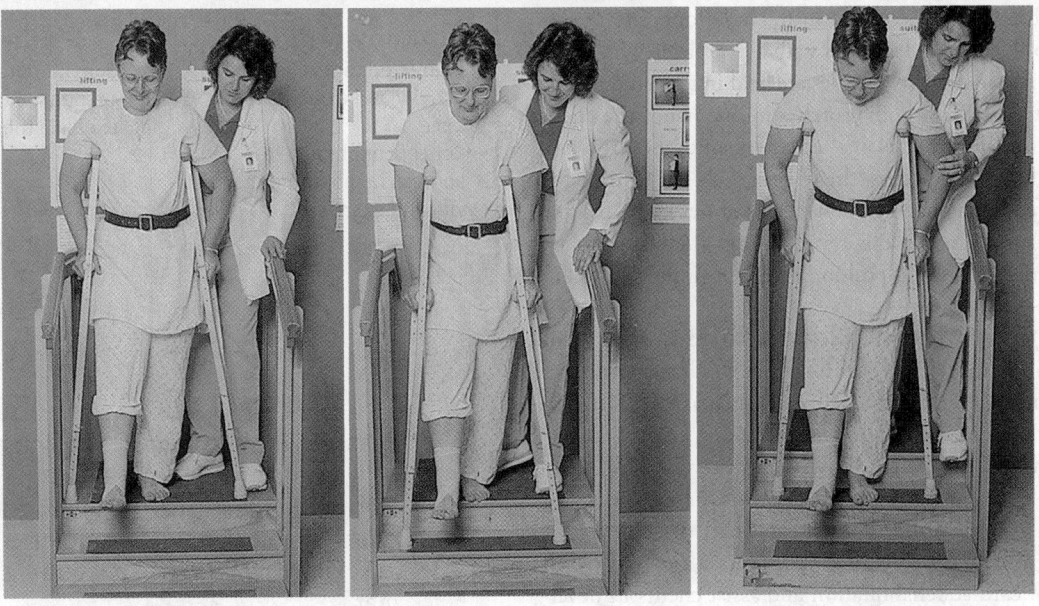

Figure 37-16 Descending stairs. **A,** Body weight is on unaffected leg. **B,** Body weight is transferred to crutches. **C,** Unaffected leg is aligned on stairs with crutches.

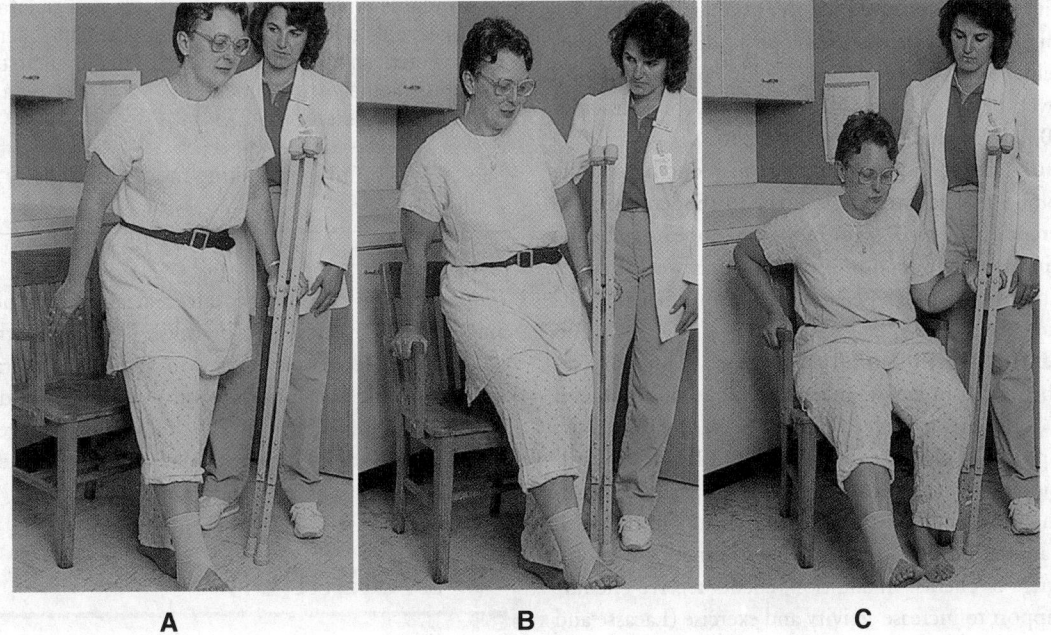

Figure 37-17 Sitting in a chair. **A,** Both crutches are held by one hand. Client transfers weight to crutches and unaffected leg. **B,** Client grasps arm of chair with free hand and begins to lower herself into chair. **C,** Client completely lowers herself into chair.

Then the client holds both crutches in the hand opposite the affected leg. If both legs are affected, as with a paraplegic who wears weight-supporting braces, the crutches are held in the hand on the client's stronger side. With both crutches in one hand, the client supports body weight on the unaffected leg and the crutches. While still holding the crutches, the client grasps the arm of the chair with the remaining hand and lowers his or her body into the chair. To stand, the procedure is reversed, and the client, when fully erect, assumes the tripod position before beginning to walk.

Restoration of Activity and Chronic Illness. Care plans are designed to increase activity and exercise in clients with specific disease conditions and chronic illnesses such as CHD, hypertension, COPD, and diabetes mellitus.

Coronary Heart Disease. Activity and exercise have been shown to play a role in secondary prevention or recurrence of CHD. Cardiac rehabilitation is an integral part of comprehensive care of clients diagnosed with CHD. Nurses are involved in many aspects of cardiac rehabilitation and assist clients in developing a program of exercise that fits their needs and level of functioning. Increased physical activity appears to benefit individuals with myocardial infarction (MI), angina pectoris, or congestive heart failure, as well as clients who have had a coronary artery bypass graft (CABG) or percutaneous transluminal coronary angioplasty (PTCA). Clients with CHD benefit from exercise and activity in terms of reduced mortality and morbidity, improved quality of life, improved left ventricular function, increased functional capacity, decreased blood lipids and apolipoproteins (protein components of lipoprotein complexes), and psychological well-being (Conroy and others, 2005; Schneider and others, 2003; Tokmakidis and Volaklis, 2003).

Hypertension. Exercise is instrumental in reducing systolic and diastolic blood pressure readings. Low- to moderate-intensity aerobic exercise (brisk walking or bicycling) appears to be the most effective in lowering blood pressure, whereas weight training and high-intensity aerobics seem to have minimal benefits (Chobanian and others, 2003; Gillespie, 2006).

Chronic Obstructive Pulmonary Disease. Pulmonary rehabilitation is beneficial in helping clients reach an optimal level of functioning. Some clients are fearful of participating in exercise because of the potential of worsening dyspnea (difficulty breathing). This aversion to physical activity sets up a progressive deconditioning in which minimal physical exertion results in dyspnea. Pulmonary rehabilitation provides a safe environment for monitoring the progress of clients. In addition, clients receive encouragement and support to increase activity and exercise (Lacasse and others, 2004; Normandin and others, 2002).

Diabetes Mellitus. Along with diet, glucose monitoring, and medication, exercise is an important component in the care of clients with diabetes mellitus. Individuals with type 1 diabetes are encouraged to exercise because it leads to improved cardiovascular fitness and psychological well-being. Instruct the diabetic with type 1 diabetes about certain risks and precautions regarding exercise. Instruction includes the need for a preexercise physical examination and precautions to monitor blood glucose level immediately before and after exercise. Also explain to clients to avoid injecting insulin into muscles that will be active during exercise, to perform low- to moderate-intensity exercises, to carry a con-

Knowledge
- Characteristics of improved activity and exercise tolerance
- Role of community resources in maintaining activity and exercise

Experience
- Consider previous client responses to activity and exercise therapies

EVALUATION
- Reassess the client for signs of improved activity and exercise tolerance
- Ask for the client's perception of activity and exercise status after interventions
- Ask if the client's expectations are being met

Standards
- Use established expected outcomes to evaluate the client's response to care (e.g., return to resting heart rate within 5 minutes) as standards for evaluation
- Apply goals published by the American College of Sports Medicine to evaluate response to exercise

Attitudes
- Use creativity in redesigning new interventions to improve the client's activity and exercise tolerance
- Demonstrate perseverance to design interventions to keep the client motivated to adhere to the activity and exercise plan

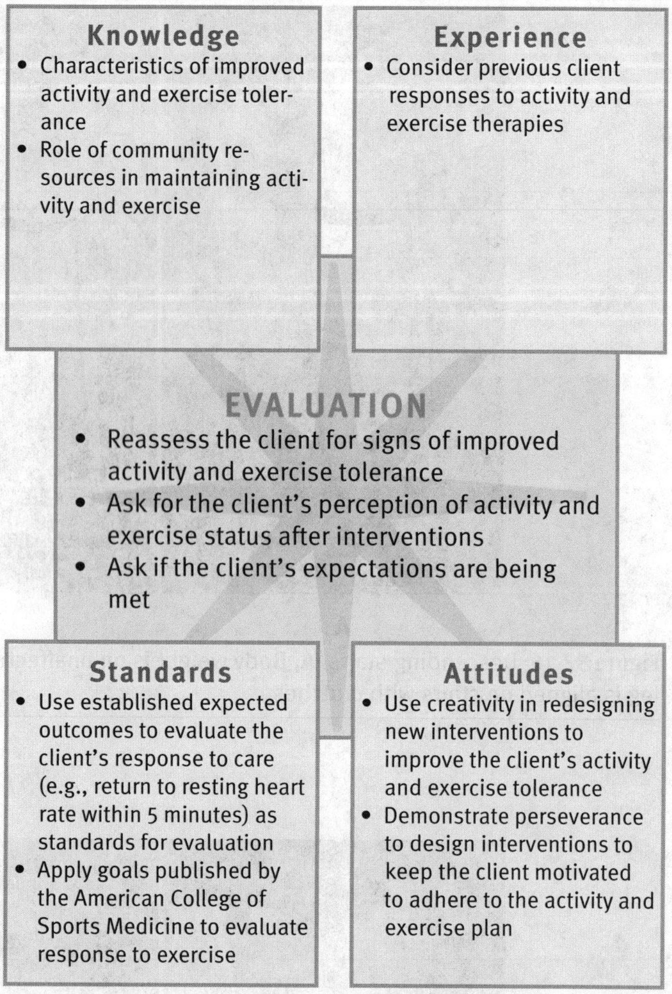

Figure 37-18 Critical thinking model for activity and exercise evaluation.

centrated form of carbohydrates (sugar packets or hard candy), and to wear a medical alert bracelet. The client with type 2 diabetes who decides to participate in a regular program of exercise should include low-intensity warm-up and cool-down exercises, aerobic exercise at 50% to 75% of maximal oxygen uptake, and exercise for 20 to 45 minutes 3 days per week (American Diabetes Association, 2002; Flood and Constance, 2002).

◆ Evaluation

Client Care. For activity and exercise, you measure the effectiveness of nursing interventions by the success of meeting the client's expected outcomes and goals of care. The client is the only one who will know the effectiveness and benefits of activity and exercise (Figure 37-18). To evaluate the effectiveness of nursing interventions to enhance activity and exercise, make comparisons with baseline measures that include pulse, blood pressure, strength, endurance, and psychological well-being. Compare actual outcomes with expected outcomes to determine the client's health status and progression. Continuous evaluation helps to determine whether new or revised therapies are needed and if new nursing diagnoses have developed.

Key Concepts

- Exercise is physical activity for the purpose of conditioning the body, improving health, and maintaining fitness, or it may be used as a therapeutic measure.
- Activity tolerance is the kind and amount of exercise or work that a person is able to perform. Physiological, emotional, and developmental factors influence the client's activity tolerance.
- The best program of physical activity includes a combination of exercises that produce different physiological and psychological benefits.
- Body mechanics are the coordinated efforts of the musculoskeletal and nervous systems as the person moves, lifts, bends, stands, sits, lies down, and completes daily activities.
- Coordinated body movement requires integrated functioning of the skeletal system, skeletal muscles, and nervous system.
- Muscles primarily associated with movement are located near the skeletal region, where movement results from leverage, which is characteristic of movements of the upper extremities.
- Coordination and regulation of muscle groups depend on muscle tone and activity of antagonistic, synergistic, and antigravity muscles.
- Balance is assisted through nervous system control in the cerebellum and inner ear function.
- Body balance is achieved when there is a wide base of support, the center of gravity falls within the base of support, and a vertical line falls from the center of gravity through the base of support.
- Developmental changes, behavioral aspects, environmental issues, cultural and ethnic origin, and family and social support influence the client's perception and motivation to engage in physical activity and exercise.
- Ability to engage in normal physical activity and exercise depends on intact and functioning nervous and musculoskeletal systems.
- Use the nursing process to provide care for clients who are experiencing or are at risk for activity intolerance and impaired physical mobility.
- After identifying nursing diagnoses, plan and implement interventions to increase activity and exercise in collaboration with the client when possible.
- Range-of-motion exercises incorporated into daily activities can include one or all of the body joints.
- Mechanical devices to promote walking include canes, walkers, and crutches.

Critical Thinking Exercises

1. Mrs. Smith (see care plan) stated, "I don't want to leave the house anymore." She also expresses feelings of overwhelming stress and excessive demands on her time.
   a. What nursing diagnostic label best reflects Mrs. Smith's health problem?
   b. What impact might these feelings have upon her initiation and maintenance of an exercise program?
   c. What interventions could you suggest to Mrs. Smith to assist in overcoming this potential barrier to exercise?

2. Mrs. Smith (see care plan) has several challenges to initiating and maintaining an exercise program.
   a. List several of these challenges. In addition, what other questions could have been helpful in eliciting other challenges for Mrs. Smith?
   b. Develop a stepwise approach for Mrs. Smith that will assist her in initiating and maintaining an exercise program, keeping in mind the challenges that Mrs. Smith faces.

3. Develop an educational component to her care plan, emphasizing the benefits of exercise.

NCLEX®-Style Review Questions

1. Mr. Stone has been on bed rest for several days. When he attempted to walk with assistance, he became dizzy and nauseated. These are most likely symptoms of which of the following?
   1. Rebound hypertension
   2. Orthostatic hypotension
   3. Dysfunctional proprioception.
   4. Central nervous system rebound hypotension

2. What are the appropriate action(s) for Mr. Stone? (Choose all that apply.)
   1. Call for assistance.
   2. Allow Mr. Stone to sit down.
   3. Take Mr. Stone's blood pressure and pulse.
   4. Continue to ambulate Mr. Stone so he begins to build up endurance.

3. Which area in the nervous system controls balance?
   1. Eye and ear
   2. Cerebrum and pons
   3. Cerebral cortex and gyrus
   4. Cerebellum and inner ear

4. When a client has a right-sided cerebral hemorrhage, what may also be present?
   1. Bilateral hemiplegia
   2. Left-sided hemiplegia
   3. Right-sided hemiplegia
   4. Degenerative hemiplegia

5. In which of the following maturational processes is the greatest change observed?
   1. Adults and elders
   2. Infants and elders
   3. Adults and infants
   4. Childhood and old age

6. Clients are more open to developing an exercise program if they are:
   1. Requested to exercise by a family member
   2. At the stage of readiness to change their behavior
   3. Diagnosed with a chronic disease such as diabetes
   4. Ordered by the health care provider to begin an exercise program

7. Which is the result of children being less physically active outside of school?
   1. An increase in obesity
   2. An increase in heart disease
   3. More computer-literate children
   4. Improved school attendance and grades

8. A principle of good body mechanics includes which of the following concepts?
   1. Keeping the knees in a locked position
   2. Bending at the waist to maintain a center of gravity
   3. Maintaining a wide base of support and bending at the knees
   4. Holding objects away from the body for improved leverage

9. A client begins to fall during ambulation. How would the nurse prevent injury to the client?
   1. Call for assistance
   2. Instruct the client to sit in the nearest chair
   3. Allow the client to fall to prevent injury to the nurse
   4. Slide the client down the nurse's body and leg to the floor

38 | Client Safety

Mastery of the content in this chapter will enable the student to:

- Describe how unmet basic physiological needs of oxygen, nutrition, temperature, and humidity threaten clients' safety.
- Discuss the purpose of the National Patient Safety Goals.
- Discuss the specific risks to safety related to developmental age.
- Identify factors to assess when it becomes necessary to physically restrain a client.
- Describe the four categories of risks in a health care agency.
- Describe assessment activities designed to identify clients' physical, psychosocial, and cognitive status as it pertains to their safety status.

- Identify nursing diagnoses associated with risks to safety.
- Develop care plans for clients whose safety is threatened.
- Describe nursing interventions specific to clients' age for reducing risk of falls, fires, poisonings, and electrical hazards.
- Describe methods to evaluate interventions designed to maintain or promote safety.

MEDIA RESOURCES

 Companion CD
- NCLEX®-Style Review Questions
- Audio Glossary
- Interactive Learning Activities
- English/Spanish Glossary

 Website
- NCLEX®-Style Review Questions
- Audio Glossary
- English/Spanish Glossary
- Interactive Learning Activities
- Weblinks
- Audio Summaries

KEY TERMS

Air pollution, p. 814
Ambularm, p. 838
Aura, p. 817
Bed-Check, p. 838
Bioterrorism, p. 814
Carbon monoxide, p. 812
Environment, p. 812
Food and Drug Administration (FDA), p. 812
Food poisoning, p. 812
Hypothermia, p. 812
Immunization, p. 813

Land pollution, p. 814
Noise pollution, p. 814
Pathogen, p. 813
Poison, p. 840
Pollutant, p. 814
Relative humidity, p. 812
Restraint, p. 829
Seizure, p. 817
Seizure precautions, p. 842
Status epilepticus, p. 845
Water pollution, p. 814

Safety, often defined as freedom from psychological and physical injury, is a basic human need that must be met. Health care, provided in a safe manner, and a safe community environment are essential for a client's survival and well-being. The nurse, incorporating critical thinking skills when using the nursing process, is responsible for assessing the client and the environment for hazards that threaten safety, as well as planning and intervening appropriately to maintain a safe environment. By doing this, the nurse is not only a provider of safe acute, restorative, and continuing care, but also an active participant in health promotion.

Scientific Knowledge Base

Environmental Safety

A client's **environment** includes all of the many physical and psychosocial factors that influence or affect the life and survival of that client. This broad definition of environment crosses the continuum of care for settings in which the nurse and client interact (e.g., the home, community center, school, clinic, hospital, and long-term care facility). Safety in health care settings reduces the incidence of illness and injury, prevents extended length of treatment and/or hospitalization, improves or maintains a client's functional status, and increases the client's sense of well-being. A safe environment gives protection to the staff as well, allowing them to function at an optimal level. A safe environment includes meeting basic needs, reducing physical hazards, reducing the transmission of pathogens, maintaining sanitation, and controlling pollution. In addition, a safe environment is one where the threat of attack from biological, chemical, or nuclear weapons is prevented or minimized.

Basic Needs. Physiological needs, including the need for sufficient oxygen, nutrition, and optimum temperature and humidity, influence a person's safety.

Oxygen. Be aware of factors in a client's environment that decrease the amount of available oxygen. A common environmental hazard in the home is an improperly functioning heating system. A furnace that is not properly vented or a car left running inside a closed garage introduces carbon monoxide into the environment. **Carbon monoxide** is a colorless, odorless, poisonous gas produced by the combustion of carbon or organic fuels. Carbon monoxide binds strongly with hemoglobin, preventing the formation of oxyhemoglobin and thus reducing the supply of oxygen delivered to tissues (see Chapter 40). Low concentrations cause nausea, dizziness, headache, and fatigue. Very high concentrations cause death after 1 to 3 minutes of exposure (National Fire Protection Association, 2006a). It is necessary to have annual inspections of heating systems, chimneys, and appliances in private homes, as well as in institutions. Carbon monoxide detectors are available for home or institutional use at a reasonable cost but are not a replacement for proper use and maintenance of fuel-burning appliances.

Nutrition. Meeting nutritional needs adequately and safely requires environmental controls and knowledge. In the home the client needs a refrigerator with a freezer compartment to keep perishable foods fresh. An adequate, clean water supply is necessary for drinking and washing fresh produce and dishes. Provisions for garbage collection are necessary to maintain sanitary conditions.

Foods that are inadequately prepared or stored, or that are subject to unsanitary conditions, increase the client's risk for infections and food poisoning (see Chapter 44). Bacterial food infections result from eating food contaminated by bacteria such as *Escherichia coli* or *Salmonella, Shigella,* or *Listeria* organisms. The ingestion of bacterial toxins produced in food causes **food poisoning;** staphylococcal and clostridial bacteria are the most common types. Although most food-borne diseases are bacterial, the hepatitis A virus is spread by fecal contamination of food, water, or milk (Nix, 2005).

For illnesses caused by bacterial contamination, the onset of symptoms is either very rapid or takes a week or longer. Clients infected with hepatitis A are most contagious during the 2-week period before onset of jaundice (Fiore, 2004). Preventive measures include thorough hand washing before handling food, adequate cooking, and proper storage and refrigeration of perishable foods.

To protect consumers, commercially processed and packaged foods are subject to **Food and Drug Administration (FDA)** regulations. The FDA is a federal agency responsible for the enforcement of federal regulations regarding the manufacture, processing, and distribution of foods, drugs, and cosmetics to protect consumers against the sale of impure or dangerous substances.

Temperature and Humidity. The comfort zone for environmental temperature varies among individuals, but the usual comfort range is between 18.3° and 23.9° C (65° and 75° F). Temperature extremes that frequently occur during the winter and summer affect not only comfort and productivity, but also safety.

Exposure to severe cold for prolonged periods causes frostbite and accidental hypothermia. Frostbite occurs when a surface area of the skin freezes as a result of exposure to extremely cold temperatures. **Hypothermia** occurs when the core body temperature is 35° C (95° F) or below (see Chapter 32). Older adults, the young, clients with cardiovascular conditions, clients who have ingested drugs or alcohol in excess, and the homeless are at high risk for hypothermia (see Chapter 32).

Exposure to extreme heat raises the core body temperature, resulting in heatstroke or heat exhaustion. Chronically ill clients, older adults, and infants are at greatest risk for injury from extreme heat. These clients need to avoid extremely hot, humid environments.

The relative humidity of the air in the environment sometimes affects the client's health and safety. **Relative humidity** is the amount of water vapor in the air compared with the maximum amount of water vapor that the air could contain at the same temperature. The comfort zone varies from person to person, but most people are comfortable when the humidity is between 60% and 70%. Increasing the environmental humidity by using a home humidifier has therapeutic benefits for clients with upper respiratory tract infections because humidity helps to liquefy pulmonary secretions and improve breathing. It is important to follow the manufacturer's directions regarding the cleaning and maintenance of home humidifiers to reduce the contamination of the water.

Physical Hazards. Physical hazards in the environment place clients at risk for accidental injury and death. According to the Centers for Disease Control and Prevention (CDC) (2006a), unintentional injures are the fifth leading cause of death for Americans of all ages. Motor vehicle accidents are the leading cause, followed by poisonings and falls. Among older adults 65 years and above, falls are the leading cause of unintentional death. Falls are the most common cause of hospital admissions for trauma for older clients. Fractures are the most serious health consequence of falls. Almost 90% of all fractures among older adults are due to falls (CDC, 2006a). You can minimize many physical hazards, especially those contributing to falls, through adequate lighting, reduction of obstacles, control of bathroom hazards, and security measures.

Lighting. Adequate lighting reduces physical hazards by illuminating areas in which a person moves and works. Outside the home, there needs to be adequate lighting on all walkways. Outdoor lighting also helps protect the home and its inhabitants from crime. Well-lighted garages, walkways, and doorways discourage intruders from entering homes or hiding in shadows.

Inside the house, halls, staircases, and individual rooms need to be adequately lighted so that residents are able to safely carry out activities of daily living. Night-lights in dark halls, bathrooms, and the rooms of children and older adults help maintain safety by reducing the risk of falls. A night-light in a guest room will help orient an overnight guest who needs to get up in the middle of the night. Make sure artificial lighting is soft and nonglaring, because glare is a major problem for older adults (Ebersole, Hess, and Luggen, 2004).

Obstacles. Injuries in the home frequently result from tripping over or coming into contact with common household objects, including doormats, small rugs on the stairs and floor, wet spots on the floor, and clutter on bedside tables, closet shelves, the top of the refrigerator, and bookshelves. The risk of falls from obstacles is present for all age-groups; however, it is greatest for older adults. Falls are usually a result of a combination of intrinsic risk factors (e.g., illness, drug therapy, or alcohol use) and extrinsic or environmental factors. In some cases an obstacle or extrinsic factor is the only cause of a fall. Intrinsic factors are difficult to modify or eliminate, but extrinsic ones are usually not.

Bathroom Hazards. Accidents such as falls, burns, and poisoning frequently occur in the bathroom. Handheld shower heads and secure, easily seen grab bars and nonslip, colored adhesive tape on the bottom of the tub are useful in reducing falls in the bathtub. An elevated toilet seat with armrests and nonslip strips on the floor in front of the toilet are also helpful (McCullagh, 2006). Lowering the thermostat setting on the water heater reduces the risk of scalding. In the medicine cabinet, medications need to be clearly marked and out of the reach of children. Child-resistant caps should be on all medication containers when there are children living in the home or visiting the home. Medication not in use or out-of-date should be flushed down the toilet.

Security. Death from fires and burns is the third leading cause of fatal home injury (Runyan and Casteel, 2004). According to the National Fire Protection Association (2006b), there were 388,500 reported home fires in the United States in 2003, resulting in 3,145 deaths and 13,650 injuries. The leading cause of fire-related death is careless smoking (Ahrens, 2003). Cooking equipment and

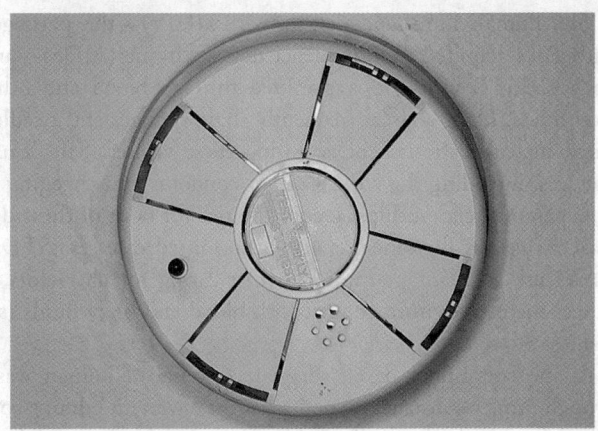

Figure 38-1 Smoke and fire detector.

appliances, particularly stoves, are the main sources for in-home fires and fire injuries. Clients should have smoke detectors (Figure 38-1), along with carbon monoxide detectors, placed strategically throughout the home. Multipurpose fire extinguishers need to be near the kitchen and any workshop areas.

Although lead has not been used in house paint or plumbing materials since the U.S. Consumer Product Safety Commission banned it in 1978, older homes continue to contain high lead levels. Soil and water systems are sometimes contaminated. Poisoning occurs from swallowing or inhaling lead. Fetuses, infants, and children are more vulnerable to lead poisoning than adults because their bodies absorb lead more easily and small children are more sensitive to the damaging effects of lead. Exposure to excessive levels of lead affects a child's growth or causes brain and kidney damage. Other health effects include impaired hearing, vomiting, headaches, appetite loss, and learning and behavioral problems (National Center for Environmental Health, 2005).

An insecure home places the client at risk for injury or burglary. Inadequate locks on doors and windows make the home susceptible to intruders. Clients need to take precautions to secure their homes. When you assess the home for safety, guide the client to evaluate doors and windows for the presence and quality of locks. Encourage clients to join block associations and work closely with law enforcement personnel to reduce crime in their neighborhoods.

Transmission of Pathogens. A **pathogen** is any microorganism capable of producing an illness. One of the most effective methods for limiting the transmission of pathogens is the medical aseptic practice of hand hygiene (see Chapter 34). Instruct clients in proper hand-hygiene techniques and to use them frequently in the home and hospital.

Immunization can also reduce, and in some cases prevent, the transmission of disease from person to person. **Immunization** is the process by which resistance to an infectious disease is produced or augmented. Individuals acquire active immunity by an injection of a small amount of attenuated (weakened) or dead organisms or modified toxins from the organism (toxoids) into the body. Passive immunity occurs when antibodies produced by other persons or animals are introduced into a person's bloodstream for protection against a pathogen.

The human immunodeficiency virus (HIV)—the pathogen that causes acquired immunodeficiency syndrome (AIDS)—and the hepatitis B virus are transmitted through blood and other body fluids. Drug abusers frequently share syringes and needles, which increases the risk of acquiring these viruses. Safe sexual practices, including the correct use of condoms and engaging in monogamous relationships, reduce the risk for both of these diseases, as well as for other sexually transmitted diseases (STDs). Nurses use standard precautions when caring for all clients to protect themselves from contact with blood and body fluids (see Chapter 34).

At the community level, adequate disposal of human waste through proper construction and repair of sewers and drains controls the transmission of disease. Insect and rodent control (e.g., spraying for mosquitoes) is also necessary to reduce the transmission of disease.

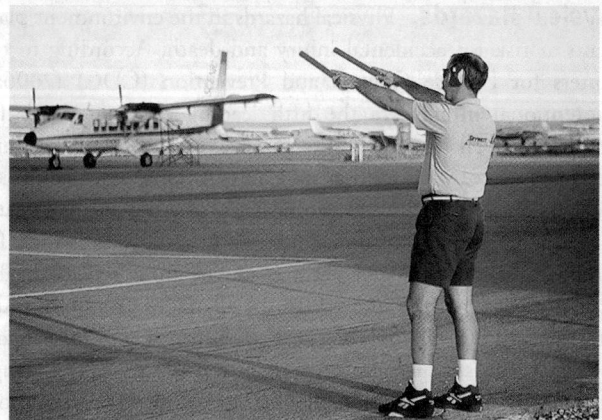

Figure 38-2 Protective device to reduce hearing loss.

Pollution. A healthy environment is free of pollution. A **pollutant** is a harmful chemical or waste material discharged into the water, soil, or air. People commonly think of pollution only in terms of air, land, or water pollution, but excessive noise is also a form of pollution that presents health risks. **Air pollution** is the contamination of the atmosphere with a harmful chemical. Prolonged exposure to air pollution increases the risk of pulmonary disease. In urban areas, industrial waste and vehicle exhaust are common contributors to air pollution. In the home, school, or workplace, cigarette smoke is the primary cause of air pollution. Improper disposal of radioactive and bioactive waste products (e.g., dioxin) can cause **land pollution.**

Water pollution is the contamination of lakes, rivers, and streams, usually by industrial pollutants. Water treatment facilities filter harmful contaminants from the water, but these systems sometimes contain flaws. If water becomes contaminated, the public should use bottled or boiled water for drinking and cooking. Flooding frequently causes damage to water treatment stations and also requires the use of bottled or boiled water.

Noise pollution occurs when the noise level in an environment becomes uncomfortable to the inhabitants of the environment. Noise levels are measured in units of sound intensity called decibels. Tolerance for noise varies from individual to individual, and an individual's health status influences tolerance. Irreversible hearing loss possibly results from constant exposure to high sound intensity. Clients working in environments with high noise levels need to wear protective devices to reduce hearing loss (Figure 38-2). Adolescents need to limit their exposure to intense noise such as that found at rock concerts.

Noise can also pollute a health care facility. The sounds of machines, people talking, intercoms, and paging systems create increased noise levels. Even when the noise level is not high enough to affect hearing acuity, it sometimes produces a syndrome called sensory overload. Sensory overload is a marked increase in the intensity of auditory and visual stimuli. It disrupts processing of information, and the client no longer perceives the environment in a meaningful way (see Chapter 49).

Terrorism. A potential environmental health threat is the possibility of a bioterrorist attack. Before 1990 and the Gulf War, the possibility of the United States coming under attack from terror-

ists groups using biological, chemical, or nuclear weapons seemed unlikely. Today, however, we are concerned about an attack by an individual or small group on one of our cities, a large sporting event, or a unit of our military forces (Jones and others, 2002). **Bioterrorism,** or the use of biological agents to create fear and threat, is the most likely form of terrorist attack to occur. Although terrorists could use any agent, health officials are most concerned with biological agents such as anthrax, smallpox, pneumonic plague, and botulism (American Medical Association, 2004). The Federal Emergency Management Agency (FEMA) and the American Red Cross provide nationwide efforts to help community members prepare for disasters of all types (FEMA, 2004). Health care facilities need to be prepared to treat mass casualties from an attack. The answer lies in the facility's emergency management plan. Such a plan details how to respond to a terrorist attack; for example, determining the agent used, determining the time and location of the attack and the affected population, obtaining and delivering supplies, and providing treatment. Nurses need to be prepared through education and training to be able to respond to an attack by taking the necessary steps to initiate an agency's emergency management plan.

Nursing Knowledge Base

In addition to being knowledgeable about the environment, nurses need to be familiar with a client's developmental level; mobility, sensory, and cognitive status; lifestyle choices; and knowledge of common safety precautions. They also need to be aware of the special risks to safety that are found in agency settings.

Risks at Developmental Stages

A client's developmental stage creates threats to safety as a result of lifestyle, mobility status, sensory impairments, and safety awareness.

Infant, Toddler, and Preschooler. Injuries are the leading cause of death in children over age 1 and cause more death and disabilities than do all diseases combined (Hockenberry and Wilson, 2007). The nature of the injury sustained is closely related to normal growth and development. For example, the inci-

dence of lead poisoning is highest in late infancy and toddlerhood because of a child's increased level of oral activity and the growing ability to explore the environment. Accidents involving children are largely preventable, but parents need to be aware of specific dangers at each stage of growth and development. Accident prevention thus requires health education for parents and the removal of dangers whenever possible.

School-Age Child. When a child enters school, the environment expands to include the school, transportation to and from school, school friends, and after-school activities. Parents, teachers, and nurses need to instruct the child in safe practices to follow at school or play. When discussing safe practices, an effective way to teach the school-age child is by using examples.

Because school-age children are participating in more activities outside their home and neighborhood environments, they are at greater risk of injury from strangers. A child needs to be warned repeatedly not to accept candy, food, gifts, or rides from strangers. In addition, a child needs to know what to do if a stranger approaches. Frequently neighborhoods have a "block home" or "safe house." In these homes the owner ensures that an adult is home during the times when children are walking to and from school. If a stranger approaches a child, the child can run to that home, and the adult will protect the child and call the proper authorities. As a nurse, you will work with school systems or neighborhoods to initiate such a system to protect children.

Sports safety is stressed in school sports, but parents and health professionals can reinforce these safety tips by insisting that children wear protective gear while participating in sports such as skateboarding and snowboarding. For example, schools provide hard batting helmets for baseball games, and parents also need to provide this equipment when children are playing baseball in their own backyards.

Bicycle-related injuries, including scooters, are a major cause of death and disability among children. Children 5 to 14 years of age account for nearly one third of bicyclists killed in traffic accidents (National Center for Injury Prevention and Control, 2002). Bikes need to be in good working order and be the proper size for the child. The child needs to learn the rules of the road and be cautioned not to engage in dangerous stunts or activities while bike riding. Children also need to wear a properly fitted helmet. Because most fatalities from bicycle accidents are related to head injuries, many states have implemented laws requiring bicycle helmets (Figure 38-3).

Adolescent. As children enter adolescence, they develop greater independence and begin to develop a sense of identity and their own values. In addition, adolescents begin to separate emotionally from their families, and peers generally have a stronger influence. The struggle toward identity causes the teenager to experience shyness, fear, and anxiety, with resulting dysfunction at home or school. In an attempt to relieve the tensions associated with physical and psychosocial changes, as well as peer pressures, some adolescents begin to act impulsively and engage in risk-taking behaviors such as smoking and using drugs. In addition to the health risks posed by nicotine and other drugs, the ingestion of drugs, including alcohol, increases the incidence of accidents such as drowning and motor vehicle accidents.

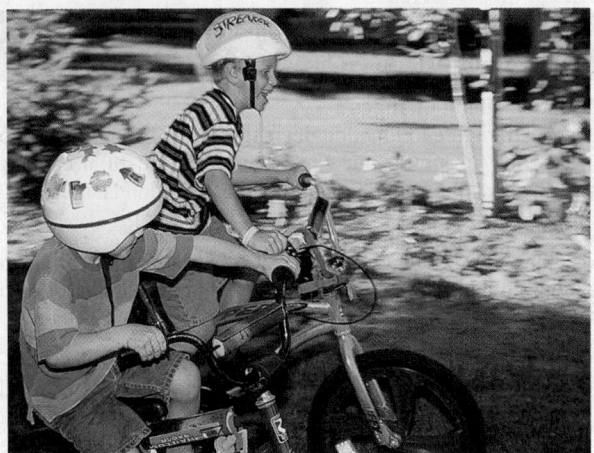

Figure 38-3 Proper bicycle safety equipment for school-age child.

When adolescents learn to drive, their environment expands and so does their potential for injury. The risk of motor vehicle accidents is higher among 16- to 19-year-old drivers than any other age-group. Teens are more likely to speed, run red lights, ride with intoxicated drivers, and drive after using alcohol and drugs. Teens also have the lowest rate of seat belt use (CDC, 2006b). The young driver needs to learn to comply with rules and regulations regarding use of a car.

> **SAFETY ALERT** Reinforce to new drivers and parents of new drivers the need to consistently wear safety belts and to never ride in a car with a driver who has been drinking. Assist parents and teen in developing a plan of action if teen is with a driver who drinks at an outing.

Because adolescence is a time when mature sexual physical characteristics develop, some adolescents begin to have physical relationships with others. They need prompt, accurate instruction about abstinence and/or safe sexual practices and birth control.

Adult. The threats to an adult's safety are frequently related to lifestyle habits. For example, the client who uses alcohol excessively is at greater risk for motor vehicle accidents. The long-term smoker has a greater risk of cardiovascular or pulmonary disease as a result of the inhalation of smoke into the lungs and the effect of nicotine on the circulatory system. Likewise, the adult experiencing a high level of stress is more likely to have an accident or illness such as headaches, gastrointestinal (GI) disorders, and infections (see Chapter 31).

Older Adult. The physiological changes that occur during the aging process increase the client's risk for falls and other types of accidents such as burns and car accidents (Box 38-1).

Older clients are more likely to fall in the bedroom, bathroom, and kitchen, and outside as a result of ice on walkways or obstacles in the garden. Inside falls most often occur while transferring from beds, chairs, and toilets; getting into or out of bathtubs; tripping over items, such as cords covered by rugs or carpets, carpet edges, or doorway thresholds; slipping on wet surfaces; and descending stairs.

• • • •

✳ BOX 38-1 Physical Assessment Findings in the Older Adult That Increase the Risk of Accidents

Musculoskeletal Changes
Muscle strength and function decrease, joints become less mobile, bones are brittle due to osteoporosis, postural changes (e.g., kyphosis) are common, and range of motion is limited.

Nervous System Changes
All voluntary or automatic reflexes slow to some extent, ability to respond to multiple stimuli decreases, and sensitivity to touch is decreased.

Sensory Changes
Peripheral vision and lens accommodation decrease, lens develops opacity (cataracts), stimuli threshold for light touch and pain increases, transmission of hot and cold impulses is delayed, and hearing is impaired as high-frequency tones become less perceptible.

Genitourinary Changes
Nocturia and occurrences of incontinence increase.

Modified from Ebersole P, Hess P, Luggen A: *Toward healthy aging*, ed 6, St. Louis, 2004, Mosby.

✳ BOX 38-2 Nine Life-Saving Patient Safety Solutions

- **Be aware of look-alike, sound-alike medication names.** Carefully review medication orders of these drugs and use the six rights of medication safety.
- **Use patient identification.** Use two forms of patient identification, such as a hospital arm band and medical record number.
- **Communication during patient handover.** Communicate critical information, provide time for health care personnel to ask and resolve questions, and involve the patient and family during the handover process.
- **Perform correct procedure at correct body site.** Mark the operative site and take a "time out" to verify correct patient, operative site, and procedure before initiating procedure.
- **Control concentrated electrolyte solutions.** Use the six rights of medication administration and follow agency protocols for these solutions.
- **Ensure medication accuracy at transitions in care.** Perform medication reconciliation at each care transition. Compare all medications a patient is taking against medical order and the patient's "home" medication list during admission, transfer, and discharge.
- **Avoid catheter and tubing misconnections.** Be meticulous in verification of catheter and tubing connections, right catheter, and right connection tubing. Label tubing and connections when patient has multiple catheters.
- **Do not reuse single-use injection devices.** Never reuse needles, injection devices, or intravenous catheters.
- **Improve hand hygiene to prevent health care–associated infections.** Perform hand hygiene before and after each patient encounter and after contact with contaminated objects (even when gloves are worn). Encourage family and visitors to perform hand hygiene before and after visits.

Courtesy WHO Collaborating Centre for Patient Safety Releases: Nine Life-Saving Patient Safety Solutions http://www.jointcommissioninternational.org/solutions, last accessed May 12, 2007.

Unfortunately, clients throughout all developmental stages are subject to abuse. Child abuse, domestic violence, and abuse of older adults are serious threats to safety. Chapters 12 through 14 discuss these topics.

Individual Risk Factors

Other risk factors posing threats to safety include lifestyle, impaired mobility, sensory or communication impairment, and lack of safety awareness.

Lifestyle. Some lifestyles increase safety risks. People who drive or operate machinery while under the influence of chemical substances (drugs or alcohol), who work at inherently dangerous jobs, or who are risk takers are at greater risk of injury. In addition, people experiencing stress, anxiety, fatigue, or alcohol or drug withdrawal, or those taking prescribed medications are sometimes more accident-prone. Because of these factors, some clients are too preoccupied to notice the source of potential accidents, such as cluttered stairs or a stop sign.

Impaired Mobility. Impaired mobility due to muscle weakness, paralysis, or poor coordination or balance is a major factor in client falls. Immobilization predisposes the client to additional physiological and emotional hazards, which in turn further restricts mobility and independence (see Chapter 37).

Sensory or Communication Impairment. Clients with visual, hearing, tactile, or communication impairment, such as aphasia or a language barrier, are at greater risk for injury. Such clients are not always able to perceive a potential danger or express their need for assistance (see Chapter 49).

Lack of Safety Awareness. Some clients are unaware of safety precautions, such as keeping medicine or poisons away from children or reading the expiration date on food products. A complete nursing assessment, including a home inspection, will help you identify the client's level of knowledge regarding home safety so that you can correct deficiencies with an individualized nursing care plan.

Risks in the Health Care Agency

Environmental safety pertains to the health care agency, as well as to the client's home and community. However, there are specific risks in health care agencies that also need to be addressed.

A landmark report published by the Institute of Medicine (IOM) in 1999 brought national attention to the serious problem of in-hospital medical errors (Kohn, Corrigan, and Donaldson, 1999). A HealthGrades report indicates that an average of 195,000 hospitalized Americans died annually in 2000, 2001, and 2002 because of potentially preventable medical errors (HealthGrades, 2005). Three types of medical errors accounted for almost 60% of the client safety incidents: infection following surgery, bed sores, and failure to diagnose and treat in time. Medication errors, also cited in these reports, can occur at any point in the medication administration process, during ordering, transcription, dispensing, and administering. The majority of errors occur during the ordering and administration stages (Agency for Healthcare Research and Quality [AHRQ], 2006). The World Health Organization and The Joint Commission (TJC) work together to enhance client safety (Box 38-2). It is essential that nurses and health care facilities build safety into processes of care and take a systems approach when taking on efforts to reduce medical errors.

Various forms of chemicals used in health care settings are a source of an environmental risk. Chemicals such as mercury (see Chapter 32) and those found in some medications, anesthetic gases, cleaning solutions, and disinfectants are potentially toxic if ingested or inhaled. Material safety data sheets (MSDSs) are available to provide detailed information about the chemical, any health hazards imposed, and precautions for safe handling and use. MSDSs all give information on the steps to take in case the material is released or spilled.

Specific risks to a client's safety within the health care environment also include falls, client-inherent accidents, procedure-related accidents, and equipment-related accidents. The nurse assesses for these four potential problem areas and, considering the developmental level of the client, takes steps to prevent or minimize accidents.

An accident necessitates the filing of an incident report, a confidential document that completely describes any client accident occurring on the premises of a health care agency (see Chapter 23). The report documents the accident, client assessment, and interventions carried out for the client. In addition to completing the incident report, you objectively document the incident in the client's medical record. Because this is a confidential document, do not mention the incident report in the medical record because this eliminates the health care agency's protective clause.

Falls.
In 2003 more than 1.8 million seniors age 65 and older were treated in emergency departments for fall-related injuries, and more than 421,000 were hospitalized (CDC, 2006a). The risk for falling is significantly higher in older clients. In addition to age, a history of previous falls, gait disturbance, balance and mobility problems, postural hypotension, sensory impairment, urinary and bladder dysfunction, and certain medical diagnostic categories (e.g., cancer and cardiovascular, neurological, and cerebrovascular diseases) increase the risk. One of the more common factors precipitating a fall is a client's attempt to get out of bed to toilet. Drug use and drug interactions are also implicated in falls. Hip fractures are among the most serious fall-related injuries. Half of older adults who suffer a hip fracture never regain their previous level of functioning, and many are unable to live independently after the injury (National Center for Injury Prevention and Control, 2002). Falls that result in injuries will possibly extend a client's length of stay in the health care environment, placing them at an even greater risk for other complications.

Client-Inherent Accidents.
Client-inherent accidents are accidents (other than falls) where the client is the primary reason for the accident. Examples of client-inherent accidents are self-inflicted cuts, injuries, and burns; ingestion or injection of foreign substances; self-mutilation or fire setting; and pinching fingers in drawers or doors.

A client-inherent accident sometimes occurs as a result of a seizure. A **seizure** is hyperexcitation and disorderly discharge of neurons in the brain leading to a sudden, violent, involuntary series of muscle contractions that is paroxysmal and episodic, as in a seizure disorder, or transient and acute, such as following a head injury. A generalized tonic-clonic, or grand mal, seizure lasts approximately 2 minutes (no longer than 5) and is characterized by a cry, loss of consciousness with falling, tonicity (rigidity), clonicity (jerking), and incontinence. During a fall, or as a result of muscle jerking, musculoskeletal injuries can occur. Before a convulsive episode, a few clients report an aura, which serves as a warning or sense that a seizure is about to occur. An **aura** is a bright light, smell, or taste. During the seizure activity the client will possibly have shallow breathing, cyanosis, and loss of bladder and bowel control. Following the seizure there is a postictal phase during which the client often has amnesia or confusion and falls into a deep sleep.

If repeated seizures occur or if a single seizure lasts longer than 5 minutes, the person needs to be taken to a medical facility immediately. Prolonged or repeated seizures indicate status epilepticus. This condition is a medical emergency and requires intensive monitoring and treatment (Epilepsy Foundation, 2006). It is important that you observe the client carefully before, during, and after the seizure so that you are able to document the episode accurately.

Procedure-Related Accidents.
Procedure-related accidents occur during therapy. They include medication and fluid administration errors, improper application of external devices, and accidents related to improper performance of procedures (e.g., Foley catheter insertion).

Nurses are able to prevent many procedure-related accidents. For example, strictly following the procedure for administering medications will prevent medication errors (see Chapter 35). Proper administration of intravenous (IV) fluids prevents fluid overload or deficit (see Chapter 41). The potential for infection is reduced when surgical asepsis is used for sterile dressing changes or any invasive procedure, such as insertion of a Foley catheter. Finally, correct use of body mechanics and transfer techniques reduces the risk of injuries when moving and lifting clients (see Chapter 47).

Equipment-Related Accidents.
Equipment-related accidents result from the malfunction, disrepair, or misuse of equipment or from an electrical hazard. To avoid rapid infusion of IV fluids, all general use and client-controlled analgesic pumps need to have free-flow protection devices. To avoid accidents, do not operate monitoring or therapy equipment without instruction. Use a checklist to assess potential electrical hazards to reduce the risk of electrical fires, electrocution, or injury from faulty equipment. In health care settings, the clinical engineering staff makes regular safety checks of equipment.

Critical Thinking

Successful critical thinking requires a synthesis of knowledge, experience, information gathered from clients, critical thinking attitudes, and intellectual and professional standards. Clinical judgments require the nurse to anticipate necessary information, analyze the data, and make decisions regarding client care. Critical thinking is an ongoing process. During assessment (Figure 38-4) you consider all critical thinking elements, as well as information about the specific client, to make appropriate nursing diagnoses.

In the case of safety the nurse integrates knowledge from nursing and other scientific disciplines, previous experiences in caring for clients who had an injury or were at risk, critical thinking attitudes

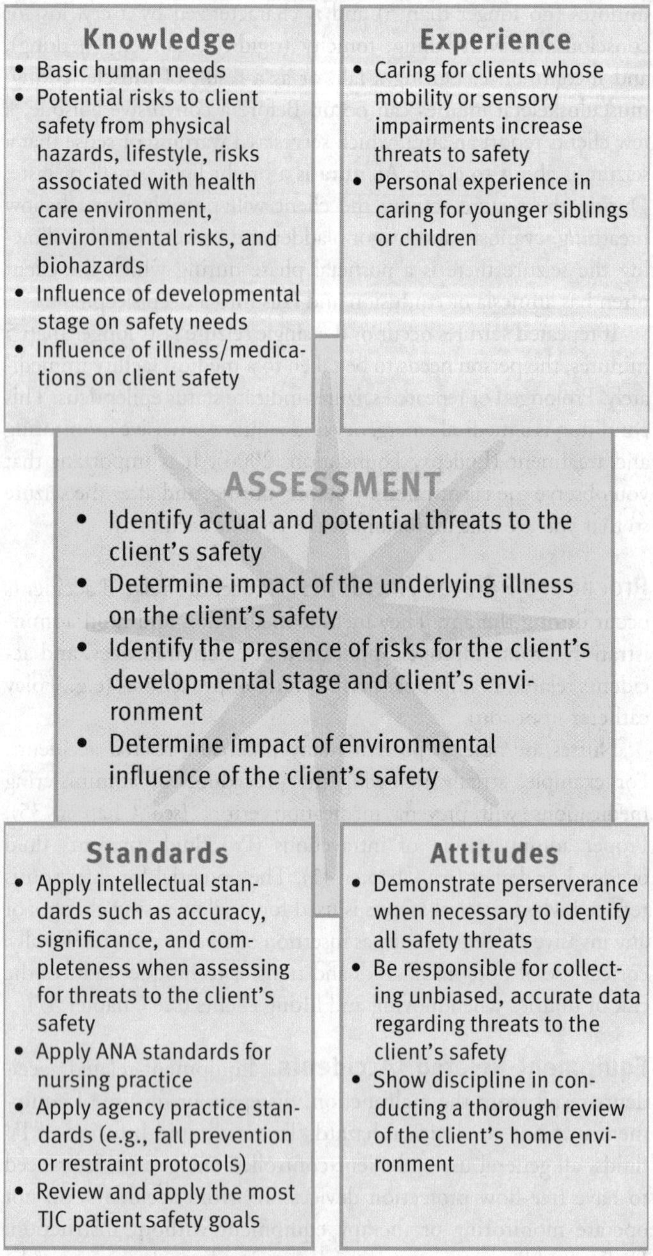

Knowledge

- Basic human needs
- Potential risks to client safety from physical hazards, lifestyle, risks associated with health care environment, environmental risks, and biohazards
- Influence of developmental stage on safety needs
- Influence of illness/medications on client safety

Experience

- Caring for clients whose mobility or sensory impairments increase threats to safety
- Personal experience in caring for younger siblings or children

ASSESSMENT

- Identify actual and potential threats to the client's safety
- Determine impact of the underlying illness on the client's safety
- Identify the presence of risks for the client's developmental stage and client's environment
- Determine impact of environmental influence of the client's safety

Standards

- Apply intellectual standards such as accuracy, significance, and completeness when assessing for threats to the client's safety
- Apply ANA standards for nursing practice
- Apply agency practice standards (e.g., fall prevention or restraint protocols)
- Review and apply the most TJC patient safety goals

Attitudes

- Demonstrate perserverance when necessary to identify all safety threats
- Be responsible for collecting unbiased, accurate data regarding threats to the client's safety
- Show discipline in conducting a thorough review of the client's home environment

Figure 38-4 Critical thinking model for safety assessment.

such as perseverance, and any standards of practice that are applicable. For example, the American Nurses Association (ANA) standards for nursing practice address the nurse's responsibility in maintaining client safety. TJC (2006) also provides standards for safety (e.g., in the administration of medications, use of restraints, and use of medical devices). You refer to all of this information and experience as you conduct a detailed assessment of a specific client. For example, while assessing a specific client's home environment, the nurse will consider knowledge regarding typical locations within the home where dangers commonly exist. If a client has a visual impairment, you will apply previous experiences in caring for clients with visual changes to anticipate how to thoroughly assess the client's needs. Critical thinking directs you to anticipate what needs to be assessed and how to make conclusions about available data.

✳ **BOX 38-3** NURSING ASSESSMENT QUESTIONS

Activity and Exercise
- Do you use any assistive devices such as a wheelchair, walker, or cane to help you move or get around? Did someone show you how to use them safely?
- Do you have any difficulty bathing? Dressing? Eating? Using the bathroom? Transferring out of the bed or chair?
- What type of exercise or physical activity do you get? How often?
- How many meals do you eat in a typical day? How do you handle meal preparation?
- Do you do your own laundry? How do you do this, and where are these appliances located?
- Do you drive an automobile? When do you normally drive? How far?
- How often do you wear a safety belt when in the car?
- Have you recently been involved in a motor vehicle accident?

Medication History
- What medications do you take?
- Has your doctor or pharmacist reviewed your medicines with you?
- Do any medications make your dizzy or light-headed?

History of Falls
- Have you ever fallen or tripped over anything in your home?
- Have you ever suffered an injury from a fall? What was it, and how did it happen?
- Did you have any symptoms right before you fell? What were they?
- What activity were you performing before the fall?

Home Maintenance and Safety
- Who does your simple home maintenance or minor home repairs?
- Who shovels your snow? Tends to your lawn?
- Do you feel safe in your home? What things in your environment make you feel unsafe?
- Do you have someone to call in case of an emergency?
- How do you feel about making modifications to your home to make it safer? Do you need help finding resources to help you do this?

Safety and the Nursing Process

◆ Assessment

To conduct a thorough client assessment, consider possible threats to the client's safety, including the client's immediate environment, as well as any individual risk factors. Ask the client specific questions related to safety (Box 38-3).

Nursing History. A nursing history includes data about the client's level of wellness to determine if any underlying conditions exist that pose threats to safety. For example, give special attention to assessing the client's gait, muscle strength and coordination, balance, and vision. Consider a review of the client's developmental status as you analyze assessment information. Also review if the client is taking any medications or undergoing any procedures that pose risks. For example, use of diuretics increases the frequency of voiding and results in the client's having to use toilet

✳ BOX 38-4 Home Hazard Assessment

Home Exterior

Are sidewalks uneven?
Are steps in good repair?
Is ice and snow removal adequate?
Do steps have securely fastened handrails?
Is there adequate lighting?
Is outdoor furniture sturdy?

Home Interior

Do all rooms, stairways, and halls have adequate, nonglare
   lighting?
Are night-lights available?
Are area rugs secured?
Does home have wooden floors?
Do nonslip floor mats cover floors where water accumulates?
Is furniture placed appropriately to permit mobility?
Is furniture sturdy enough to provide support for getting up and
   down?
Are temperature and humidity within normal range?
Are there any steps or thresholds that pose a hazard?
Are step edges clearly marked with colored tape?
Are handrails available and secure?
In homes with young children, are window guards and electrical
   outlet covers installed?
Is the poison control center number easily accessible?
Can all doors and windows with security gates and locks be
   opened from the inside without a key?

Kitchen

Are hand-washing facilities available?
Is the pilot light on for the gas stove?
Are the stovetop and oven clean?
Are the dials on the stove readable?
Are storage areas within easy reach?
Are fluids such as cleaners and bleach in original containers and
   stored properly?
In homes with young children, are safety locks on cabinets and
   corner counter protectors installed?
Is the water temperature within normal range (no greater than
   120° F)?
Are there clean areas for food storage and preparation?
Is refrigeration adequate? Are the refrigerator and freezer tem-
   peratures correct?

Bathroom

Are hand-washing facilities available?
Are there skid-proof strips or surfaces in the tub or shower?
Are bath mats secured?
Does the client need grab bars near the bathtub and toilet?
Does the client need an elevated toilet seat?
Is the medicine cabinet well lighted?
Are medications in their original containers?
Are medication containers child resistant if children live in the
   home or visit?
Has the client discarded outdated medications?

Bedroom

Are beds of adequate height to allow getting on and off easily?
Is day and night lighting adequate?
Are floor coverings nonskid?
Does the client have a telephone nearby?
Are emergency numbers visible near the telephone?

Electrical and Fire Hazards

Are smoke and carbon monoxide detectors installed?
Are the batteries for all detectors tested every month and
   changed twice a year?
Have furnaces, chimneys, and stoves been checked for proper
   ventilation?
Are extension cords in good condition and used appropriately?
Are appliances in good working order?
Are electrical appliances located away from water sources?
Is there a multipurpose fire extinguisher near the cooking area,
   and does client understand how to use it?
Are combustible items such as oil-based paints, gasoline, and
   oily rags being stored in a garage and/or basement?
Are electrical outlets overloaded?
Are flashlights available?
Is there a first aid kit available to the adult members of the
   household?
Does everyone in the family have easy access to emergency
   phone numbers?

Modified from Ebersole P, Hess P, Luggen A: *Toward healthy aging,* ed 6, St.
Louis, 2004, Mosby; and McCullagh MC: Home modification: how to help
patients make their homes safer and more accessible as their abilities
change, *Am J Nurs* 106:54, 2006.

---

facilities more often. Falls often occur with clients who have to get out of bed quickly because of urinary urgency.

Client's Home Environment. When caring for a client in the home, a home hazard assessment is necessary (Box 38-4). Walk through the home with the client, and discuss how the client normally conducts daily activities. Key areas to inspect are the bathroom, kitchen, and areas with stairs. For example, when you assess adequacy of lighting, inspect the areas where the client moves and works, such as outside walkways, steps, interior halls, and doorways. Getting a sense of the client's routines helps you recognize hazards that are not as obvious.

Assessment for risk of food infection or poisoning includes obtaining a detailed dietary assessment for the past week; conducting an examination of GI and central nervous system (CNS) function; observing for a fever; and analyzing the results of cultures of feces and vomitus. Inspect suspected food and water

sources, and assess the client's hand-washing practices. It is useful for the nurse to ask clients when they routinely wash their hands. This will then prompt a helpful discussion about the purpose and importance of hand washing.

Assessment of the environmental comfort of a client's home includes a review of when the client normally has heating and cooling systems serviced. Does the client have a functional furnace or space heater? Does the home have air conditioning or fans? You need to inform clients who use space heaters of the risk for fires.

When clients live in older homes, encourage clients to have inspections for the presence of lead in paint, dust, or soil. Because lead also comes from the solder or plumbing fixtures in a home, clients should have water from each faucet tested. Local health offices can assist a homeowner in locating a trained lead inspector who will take samples from various locations and have them analyzed at a laboratory for content of lead.

✳ **TABLE 38-1   Fall Assessment Tool**

Directions: Circle the score for the risk factor that corresponds to the client. The tool should be administered on admission, at specified intervals, and when warranted by changes in health status. Scores of 15 and higher indicate high risk, and preventive measures should be implemented.

CLIENT FACTORS	DATE ADMIT	INITIAL SCORE	DATE	REASSESSED SCORE
History of falls		15		15
Confusion		5		5
Age (over 65)		5		5
Impaired judgment		5		5
Sensory deficit		5		5
Unable to ambulate independently		5		5
Decreased level of cooperation		5		5
Increased anxiety/emotional lability		5		5
Incontinence/urgency		5		5
Cardiovascular/respiratory disease		5		5
Medications affecting blood pressure or level of consciousness		5		5
Postural hypotension with dizziness		5		5
Environmental Factors				
Attached equipment (e.g., IV pole, chest tubes)		5		5

Funk SG, Tornquist EM, Champagne MT, and Wiese RA, editors: *A fall prevention program for the acute care setting: key aspects of elder care—managing falls, incontinence, and cognitive impairment*, New York, 1992, Springer.

Health Care Environment. When the client is cared for within a health care facility, you need to determine if any hazards exist in the immediate care environment. Does the placement of equipment or furniture pose barriers when the client attempts to ambulate? Does positioning of the client's bed allow the client to reach items on a bedside table or stand? Does the client need assistance with ambulation? The nurse also collaborates with clinical engineering staff to make sure that equipment has been assessed to ensure proper function and condition.

Risk for Falls. Assessment of a client's fall risk factors is essential in determining specific needs and developing targeted interventions to prevent falls. The nurse begins by asking clients if they have had a history of falls. A fall assessment tool (Table 38-1) helps the nurse assess for potential risks before accidents and injuries result (Farmer, 2000). The illustrated tool has weighted risk factors. A client's risk of falling increases dramatically as the number of risk factors increases. Initial and daily assessment of fall risk is important in identifying clients who are at risk of falling. In many cases family members are important resources in assessing a client's fall risk. Families often are able to report on the client's level of confusion and ability to ambulate.

Risk for Medical Errors. Be alert to factors within your own environment that create conditions in which medical errors are more likely to occur. Studies have shown that overwork and fatigue cause a significant decrease in alertness and concentration, leading to errors (Trinkoff and others, 2006). It is important for nurses to be aware of these factors and to include checks and balances when working under stressful conditions. For example, to reduce the potential for a medical error, it is essential for the nurse to check the client's identification bracelet before beginning any procedure or administering a medication (see Chapter 35).

In January 2003 TJC established National Patient Safety Goals in an effort to reduce the risk of medical errors. These evidence-based recommendations require health care facilities to focus their attention on a series of specific actions. Data on the achievement of the goals will be made public each year. TJC announces new goals each year in July. The National Patient Safety Goals Hospital Program for 2008 include the following:

- Improve the accuracy of client identification.
- Improve the effectiveness of communication among caregivers.
- Improve the safety of using medications.
- Accurately and completely reconcile medications across the continuum of care.
- Reduce the risk for client harm resulting from falls.
- Reduce the risk for health care–associated infections.
- Encourage clients' active involvement in their own care as a client safety strategy.
- Reduce the risk for surgical fires.
- Reduce the risk for influenza and pneumococcal disease in institutionalized older adults.

Bioterrorist Attacks. Although the occurrence of a bioterrorist attack has been limited to the anthrax deaths following September 11, 2001, the threat is very real. Be prepared to make accurate and timely assessments in any type of setting. If an attack occurs, it will most likely involve the use of biological agents such as anthrax, botulism, smallpox, or bubonic plague. A bioterrorist attack would likely resemble a natural outbreak initially, but you will need to recognize that the microorganisms used may have been modified for increased virulence or may have resistance to antibiotics or vaccines (Jones and others, 2002). Biological attacks are either overt (announced) or covert (unannounced). Overt attacks require rapid assessment of their true occurrence, followed

✳ BOX 38-5 Biological Agent Syndromes

1. **Anthrax** (acute infectious disease caused by *Bacillus anthracis,* a spore-forming, gram-positive bacillus). Humans become infected through skin contact, ingestion, or inhalation. Person-to-person transmission of inhalational disease does not occur. Direct exposure to vesicle secretions of skin anthrax will possibly result in secondary cutaneous infection.
Clinical Features: Pulmonary: Flulike symptoms, possible brief interim improvement, within 2 to 4 days, abrupt onset of respiratory failure, shock, hemodynamic collapse and death within 24 to 36 hours. Gram-positive bacilli on blood culture tests. *Cutaneous:* Local skin involvement, common on the head, forearms, or hands; localized itching followed by a papular lesion that turns vesicular and within 2 to 6 days become a depressed black eschar. *Gastrointestinal:* Abdominal pain, nausea, vomiting, and fever after eating contaminated food (usually meat); bloody diarrhea, hematemesis; gram-positive bacilli on blood culture. Symptoms begin within 1 day to 8 weeks (average 5 days) depending on exposure route and amount of agent.

2. **Botulism** (caused by *Clostridium botulinum,* an anaerobic gram-positive bacillus that produces a potent neurotoxin). Food-borne botulism is the most common form. An airborne form of botulism is also possible.
Clinical Features: Food-borne botulism causes abdominal cramping, diarrhea, and other gastrointestinal symptoms. Both food-borne and inhalation botulism cause responsive client with absence of fever; drooping eyelids, weakened jaw clench, difficulty swallowing or speaking; blurred vision and double vision; symmetric paralysis of arms first, followed by respiratory muscles, then legs; respiratory dysfunction from respiratory muscle paraly-

sis; no sensory deficits. Neurological symptoms of food-borne botulism begin 12 to 36 hours after ingestion and 24 to 72 hours after inhalation. The disease is not transmitted from person to person.

3. **Plague** (an acute bacterial disease caused by the gram-negative bacillus *Yersinia pestis*). A bioterrorism-related outbreak may be expected to be airborne.
Clinical Features: Fever, cough, chest pain, hemoptysis within 24 hours of symptom onset, mucopurulent or watery sputum with gram-negative rods in a Gram stain test. X-ray film shows bronchopneumonia. Person-to-person transmission is possible via large aerosol droplets. Symptoms usually appear within 1 to 3 days.

4. **Smallpox** (an acute viral illness caused by the variola virus). Disease has the potential to cause severe morbidity in a non-immune population, and it can be transmitted via the airborne route. A single case of smallpox is a public health emergency.
Clinical Features: Symptoms similar to other acute viral illnesses, such as the flu. Skin lesions appear, quickly progressing from macules to papules to vesicles. Other symptoms include 2 to 4 days of fever and myalgia; rash most prominent on face and extremities (including palms and soles); rash scabs over in 1 to 2 weeks. Smallpox is transmitted by large and small respiratory droplets. Client-to-client transmission is likely from airborne and droplet exposure and by contact with skin lesions or secretions. Symptoms begin in 7 to 17 days (average 12 days).

Modified from Dire DJ: *CBRNE—Biological warfare agents,* http://www.emedicine.com/emerg/byname/cbrne—biological-warfare-agents.htm, accessed April 5, 2006.

by an appropriate response. Covert attacks become obvious only after victims present for medical care, after the incubation period has passed and clinical signs begin to appear (Jones and others, 2002). In both cases it is essential for nurses to recognize and know high-risk syndromes (Box 38-5). Acutely ill clients representing the earliest cases after a covert attack will seek care in emergency departments. Less-ill clients at the onset of an illness will possibly seek care in primary care settings.

There are basic epidemiological principles to assess whether a client's presentation of symptoms is typical of an endemic disease or is an unusual event that should raise concern. Features that alert nurses to the possibility of a bioterrorism-related outbreak include the following (Dire, 2006):

- A rapidly increasing incidence of a disease (e.g., within hours or days) in a normally healthy population
- An unusual increase in the number of people seeking care, especially with fever, respiratory, or gastrointestinal complaints
- An endemic disease rapidly emerging at an uncharacteristic time or location or in an unusual pattern
- Lower attack rates among clients who are primarily indoors, in areas with filtered or closed ventilation, compared with people who had been outdoors
- Clusters of clients arriving from a single locale
- Large numbers of rapidly fatal cases
- Any client presenting with a disease that is relatively uncommon to the geographical area and has bioterrorism potential
- Atypical clinical presentation

Nurses need to be able to recognize a biological casualty and to carry out their roles and responsibilities quickly and efficiently. Timely communication is critical for alerting both the medical and general community at large to a bioterrorist attack. Health care agencies' emergency plans will outline the predetermined departments and locations to contact in the event of an attack.

Client Expectations. Clients generally expect to be safe in their homes and health care settings. However, there are times when a client's view of what is safe does not agree with that of the nurse. For this reason, any assessment needs to include the client's understanding of his or her perception of risk factors. This is important if the nurse needs to make changes in the client's environment. Clients usually do not purposefully put themselves in jeopardy. When clients are uninformed or inexperienced, threats to their safety will occur. You will always need to consult clients on ways to reduce hazards in their environment.

◆Nursing Diagnosis

After completing an assessment of the client's safety status, review any clusters of data to determine if there are patterns suggesting that safety is threatened. Identification of defining characteristics from the data guides you in identifying appropriate nursing diagnoses. The diagnostic process requires accurate recognition of defining characteristics, as well as the related factors (Box 38-6).

BOX 38-6 NURSING DIAGNOSTIC PROCESS

Risk for Injury

Assessment Activities	Defining Characteristics
Observe client's mobility and body alignment.	Uncoordinated gait Poor posture
Ask client about visual acuity.	Reports difficulty seeing at night Reports "tripping" over rugs and furniture
Complete a home hazard appraisal.	Poorly lighted home Rooms filled with small items Excessive amount of furniture for size of room Rugs not secure

The related factor becomes the basis for selecting nursing therapies. For example, *Risk for injury related to impaired mobility* and *Risk for injury related to barriers in the home environment* require different nursing interventions. The client with altered mobility requires ambulatory aids and physical therapy. When the related factor is barriers in the home, the nurse intervenes to recommend changes that will create a safer environment. At times, multiple related factors apply. Examples of nursing diagnoses that possibly apply for clients whose safety is threatened include the following:

- Risk for imbalanced body temperature
- Impaired home maintenance
- Risk for injury
- Deficient knowledge
- Risk for poisoning
- Disturbed sensory perception
- Risk for suffocation
- Disturbed thought processes
- Risk for trauma

◆ Planning

During planning, critically synthesize information from multiple sources (Figure 38-5). Critical thinking ensures that the client's plan of care integrates all that you learned about the client, as well as the key critical thinking elements. For example, the nurse will reflect on knowledge regarding the services other disciplines (e.g., occupational therapy) provide in helping clients return to their home environments safely. Also reflect on any previous experience whereby a client benefited from safety interventions. Such experience helps you adapt approaches with a new client. Applying critical thinking attitudes such as creativity helps the nurse and client collaborate in planning interventions that are relevant and most useful, particularly when making changes in the home environment.

Goals and Outcomes. You need to plan and set goals in collaboration with the client, family, and other members of the health care team (see Care Plan, p. 825). The client who is an ac-

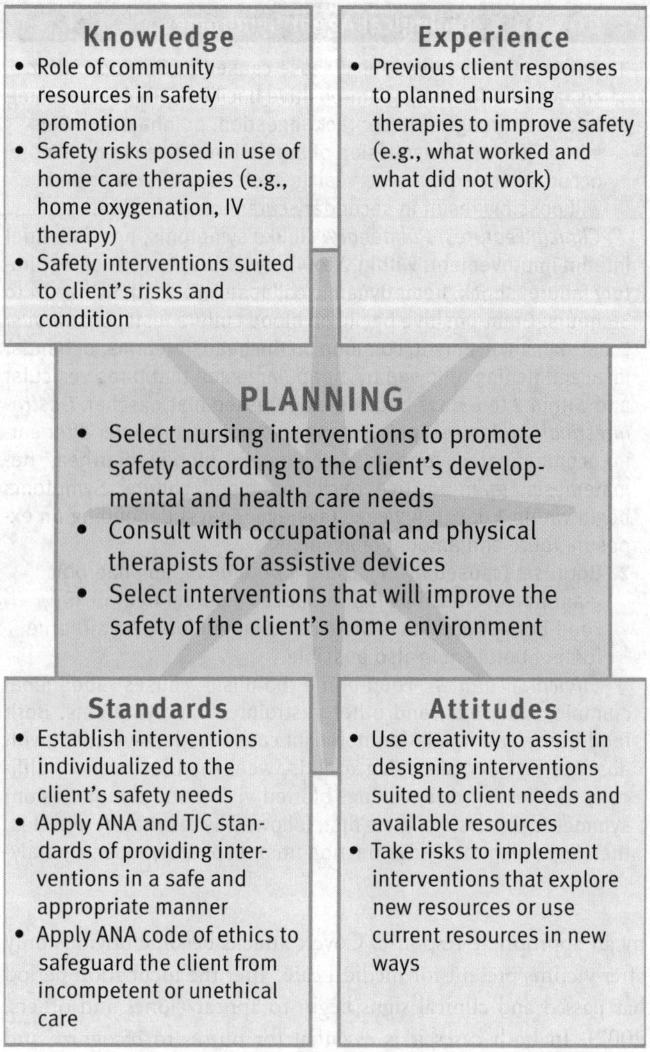

Knowledge
- Role of community resources in safety promotion
- Safety risks posed in use of home care therapies (e.g., home oxygenation, IV therapy)
- Safety interventions suited to client's risks and condition

Experience
- Previous client responses to planned nursing therapies to improve safety (e.g., what worked and what did not work)

PLANNING
- Select nursing interventions to promote safety according to the client's developmental and health care needs
- Consult with occupational and physical therapists for assistive devices
- Select interventions that will improve the safety of the client's home environment

Standards
- Establish interventions individualized to the client's safety needs
- Apply ANA and TJC standards of providing interventions in a safe and appropriate manner
- Apply ANA code of ethics to safeguard the client from incompetent or unethical care

Attitudes
- Use creativity to assist in designing interventions suited to client needs and available resources
- Take risks to implement interventions that explore new resources or use current resources in new ways

Figure 38-5 Critical thinking model for safety planning.

tive participant in reducing threats to safety becomes more alert to potential hazards. Make sure goals and outcomes are measurable and realistic, with consideration of the resources available to the client. The overall goal for a client with a threat to safety is remaining free from injury. The following are examples of expected outcomes that focus on the client's need for safety:

- Modifiable hazards will be reduced in the home environment by 100% within 1 month.
- Client does not suffer a fall or injury.
- Client identifies risks associated with visual impairment.

Setting Priorities. You prioritize nursing interventions to provide safe and efficient care. For example, the client described in the concept map (Figure 38-6) has several nursing diagnoses. The client's mobility problem is an obvious priority because of its influence on skin integrity and risk for falls. Plan individualized interventions based on the severity of risk factors and the client's developmental stage, level of health, lifestyle, and culture (Box 38-7). Planning involves an understanding of the client's need to maintain independence within physical and cognitive capabilities.

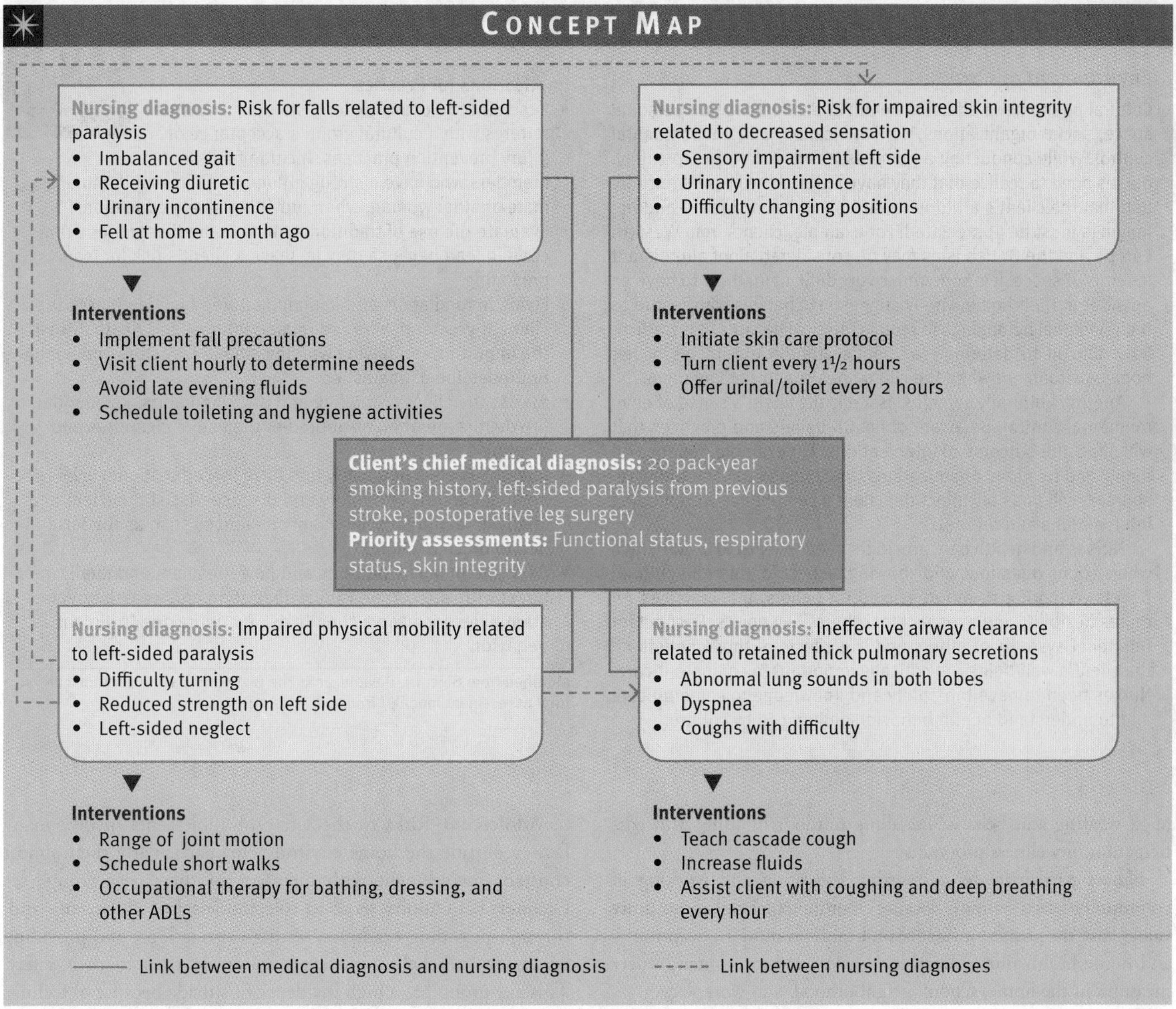

CONCEPT MAP

Nursing diagnosis: Risk for falls related to left-sided paralysis
- Imbalanced gait
- Receiving diuretic
- Urinary incontinence
- Fell at home 1 month ago

Interventions
- Implement fall precautions
- Visit client hourly to determine needs
- Avoid late evening fluids
- Schedule toileting and hygiene activities

Nursing diagnosis: Risk for impaired skin integrity related to decreased sensation
- Sensory impairment left side
- Urinary incontinence
- Difficulty changing positions

Interventions
- Initiate skin care protocol
- Turn client every 1½ hours
- Offer urinal/toilet every 2 hours

Client's chief medical diagnosis: 20 pack-year smoking history, left-sided paralysis from previous stroke, postoperative leg surgery
Priority assessments: Functional status, respiratory status, skin integrity

Nursing diagnosis: Impaired physical mobility related to left-sided paralysis
- Difficulty turning
- Reduced strength on left side
- Left-sided neglect

Interventions
- Range of joint motion
- Schedule short walks
- Occupational therapy for bathing, dressing, and other ADLs

Nursing diagnosis: Ineffective airway clearance related to retained thick pulmonary secretions
- Abnormal lung sounds in both lobes
- Dyspnea
- Coughs with difficulty

Interventions
- Teach cascade cough
- Increase fluids
- Assist client with coughing and deep breathing every hour

——— Link between medical diagnosis and nursing diagnosis   - - - - - Link between nursing diagnoses

Figure 38-6 Concept map for a client with a cerebrovascular accident 3 months ago with left-sided paralysis, 2 days postoperative after right femoral-popliteal bypass.

Collaborate to establish ways of maintaining the client's active involvement within the home and health care environment. Education of the client and family is also an important intervention to reduce safety risks over the long term.

Collaborative Care. Clients need to learn how to identify and select resources within their community that enhance safety (e.g., neighborhood block homes, local police departments, and neighbors willing to check on a client's well-being). Collaboration with the client and family and other disciplines such as social work and occupational and physical therapy become an important part of the nurse's plan of care. For example, a hospitalized client needs to go to a rehabilitation facility to gain strength and endurance before being discharged home. Make sure the client and family understand the need for resources and are willing to make changes that will promote their safety.

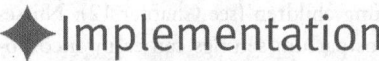Implementation

You direct nursing interventions toward maintaining the client's safety in all types of settings. Nursing measures for providing a safe environment include health promotion, developmental interventions, and environmental interventions.

Health Promotion. To promote an individual's health, it is necessary for the individual to be in a safe environment and to practice a lifestyle that minimizes risk of injury. Edelman and Mandle (2006) describe passive and active strategies aimed at health promotion. Passive strategies include public health and government legislative interventions (e.g., sanitation and clean water laws) (see Chapter 3). Active strategies are those in which the individual is actively involved through changes in lifestyle

---

✳ BOX 38-7   **CULTURAL ASPECTS OF CARE**

Environment of Care

Cultural phenomena affecting health and safety include personal space, social organizations, communication, and environmental control. While conducting a home assessment for risks to safety, nurses need to realize that they have entered the client's territory and that the client's attitude toward his or her residence and belongings must be appreciated. For example, clients from Western Europe and the British Isles may be considered aloof and distant in terms of space. It is sometimes very difficult for them to have an outsider in their home who is suggesting changes with regard to their personal belongings to reduce physical hazards. It is particularly difficult to determine a client's attitude toward his or her home environment when the client speaks another language.

Another culturally sensitive issue is the client's sense of environmental control. Be aware of health beliefs and practices that will affect the outcome of interventions. For example, reliance on family and religious organizations, as opposed to community resources, will possibly affect the client's compliance with nursing interventions and referrals.

Nurses and health care providers need to learn to be sensitive when asking questions and showing respect for different cultural beliefs. Adapting to different cultural beliefs and practices requires flexibility and a respect for others' viewpoints. Respect for the belief systems of others and the effects of those beliefs on the client's well-being are critically important to competent care. Nurses need to have the ability and knowledge to communicate and to understand health behaviors influenced by culture.

Implications for Practice

- Resistance to changing long-standing habits interferes with a cultural group's acceptance of injury prevention practices. Include family members who have a strong influence, such as a dominant male or older woman, when providing safety education.
- Evaluate the use of traditional ethnic remedies or foods that contain lead because they increase a client's risk for lead poisoning.
- Living in rural areas and in manufactured housing places the client at greater risk for fire-related injuries and death. Stress the importance of having working smoke detectors and a multipurpose fire extinguisher.
- Assess the client's smoking and drinking habits. Residential fire deaths are often attributed to the use of cigarettes and alcohol.
- Clients who live in poverty and have low educational levels are at greater risk for injury and disease. Assist the client and family in identifying community resources such as the local health office or clinic.
- Be aware of family patterns and how the client and family interact with each other. Family disruption and weak intergenerational ties increase a client's risk for injury due to violent behavior.

Modified from Giger JN, Davidhizar R: The Giger and Davidhizar transcultural assessment model, *J Transcult Nurs* 13:185, 2002.

(e.g., wearing seat belts or installing outdoor lighting) and participation in wellness programs.

Nurses participate by supporting legislation and working in community-based settings. Because environmental and community values have the greatest influence on health promotion, community and home health nurses are able to assess and recommend safety measures in the home, school, neighborhood, and workplace.

Developmental Interventions

Infant, Toddler, and Preschooler Infants, toddlers, and preschoolers depend on adults to protect them from injury. Growing children are curious and completely trusting of their environment and do not perceive themselves to be in danger. Nurses are frequently in a position to educate parents or guardians about reducing risks of injuries for young children (see Chapter 12). Nurses working in prenatal and postpartum settings can easily incorporate safety into the care plan of the childbearing family. Community health nurses are able to assess the home and show parents how to promote safety in their homes (Table 38-2). Educate parents that children under 5 years are also more susceptible to diseases such as measles, mumps, and chickenpox. Immunizations, given before the age of 2 years and at recommended intervals, protect a child from life-threatening diseases.

School-Age Child School-age children increasingly explore their environment (see Chapter 12). They have friends outside their immediate neighborhood, and they become more active in school, church, and community activities. The school-age child needs specific teaching regarding safety in school and at play. See Table 38-2 for nursing interventions to help guide the parent in providing for the safety of the school-age child.

Adolescent Risks to the safety of adolescents involve many factors outside the home environment, particularly their almost constant involvement with members of their peer group (see Chapter 12). Adults serve as role models for adolescents and, through providing examples, setting expectations, and providing education, can help adolescents minimize risks to their safety. This age-group has a high incidence of suicide because of feelings of decreased self-worth and hopelessness. Be aware of the risks posed at this time, and be prepared to teach adolescents and their parents measures to prevent accidents and injury.

Adult Risks to young and middle-age adults frequently result from lifestyle factors such as child rearing, high stress levels, inadequate nutrition, use of firearms, excessive alcohol intake, and substance abuse (see Chapter 13). In this fast-paced society there also appears to be more expression of anger, which will possibly quickly precipitate accidents (e.g., "road rage"). Adults need to have the opportunity to discuss the choices they have made in their lifestyle and the types of threats to safety that exist. Given information about threats to their well-being, some adults will make necessary modifications in lifestyle practices. Useful resources are stress management centers (see Chapter 31), employee assistance programs, and health promotion activities, which are in many communities and hospitals. In addition, neighborhood centers, community clinics, and outpatient clinics are equipped to assist adults in modifying lifestyle habits (e.g., smoking, overeating, lack of exercise, and alcoholism) that present risks to health.

Older Adult Nursing interventions for older adults reduce the risk of falls and other accidents and compensate for the physiological changes of aging (Box 38-8, p. 828). Most injuries

NURSING CARE PLAN

Risk for Injury

Assessment

Mr. Key, a visiting nurse, is seeing Ms. Cohen, an 85-year-old woman, at her home. The client is recovering from a mild stroke affecting her left side. Ms. Cohen lives alone but receives regular assistance from her daughter Peggy and son Michael, who both live within 10 miles. Mr. Key's assessment included a discussion of Ms. Cohen's health problem and how the stroke has affected her, as well as a pertinent physical examination.

Assessment Activities*	Findings/Defining Characteristics
Ask Ms. Cohen how the stroke has affected her mobility.	She responds, "**I bump into things,** and **I'm afraid I'm going to fall.**"
Conduct a home hazard assessment.	Cabinets in kitchen are **disorganized** and full of breakable items that could fall out. **Throw rugs are on floors;** bathroom **lighting is poor (40-watt bulbs); bathtub lacks safety strips or grab bars; home cluttered** with furniture and small objects.
Observe Ms. Cohen's gait and posture.	Ms. Cohen has kyphosis and has a **hesitant, uncoordinated gait.** She frequently **holds walls for support.**
Assess Ms. Cohen's muscle strength.	**Left arm and leg weaker** than right.
Assess visual acuity with corrective lenses.	Ms. Cohen has **trouble reading and seeing** familiar objects at a distance while wearing current glasses.

***Defining characteristics** are shown in bold type.*

Nursing Diagnosis: Risk for injury related to impaired mobility, decreased visual acuity, and physical environmental hazards.

Planning

Goal	Expected Outcomes (NOC)†
	Risk Control
Home will be free of hazards within 1 month.	Modifiable hazards in kitchen and hallway will be reduced in the home within 1 week. Revisions to bathroom completed in 1 month.
	Knowledge: Personal Safety
Ms. Cohen and family will be knowledgeable of potential hazards for Ms. Cohen's age-group within 1 week.	Ms. Cohen and daughter will identify risks and the steps to avoid them in the home at the conclusion of a teaching session next week.
	Fall Prevention Behavior
Ms. Cohen will express greater sense of feeling safe from falls in 1 month.	Ms. Cohen will report improved vision with the aid of new eyeglasses.
Ms. Cohen will be free of injury within 2 weeks.	Ms. Cohen will be able to safely ambulate throughout the home and perform personal care activities within 2 weeks.

†Outcome classification labels from Moorhead S and others: *Nursing outcomes classification (NOC),* ed 4, St. Louis, 2008, Mosby.

Interventions (NIC)†

Fall Prevention

Rationale

- Review findings from home hazard assessment with Ms. Cohen and daughter.

Fall risks for homebound older adults include visual disturbances, unsteady gait, and postural changes (Meiner and Leuckenotte, 2006). Home hazard evaluation will highlight extrinsic factors that lead to falls.

- Establish a list of priorities to modify, and have Ms. Cohen's son assist in installing bathroom safety devices.

Modification of environment reduces fall risk (McCullagh, 2006).

- Install lighting (75-watt bulbs, nonglare) throughout the home. Have son install blinds over kitchen windows.

With aging, the pupil loses the ability to adjust to light, causing sensitivity to glare. Glare makes it difficult to clearly see a walking path (Meiner and Lueckenotte, 2006).

- Discuss with Ms. Cohen and daughter the normal changes of aging, effects of recent stroke, associated risks for injury, and how to reduce risks.

Education regarding hazards reduces fear of falling (American Geriatrics Society, 2001).

- Encourage daughter to schedule vision testing for new prescription within 2 to 4 weeks.

Improved visual acuity reduces incidence of falls (Edelman and Mandle, 2006).

- Refer to a physical therapist to assess need for assistive devices for kyphosis, left-sided weakness, and gait.

Exercise often improves gait, balance, and flexibility. Modifying gait problems by increasing lower extremity strength reduces fall risk.

†Intervention classification labels from Bulechek GM, Butcher HK, and Dochterman JM: *Nursing interventions classification (NIC),* ed 5, St. Louis, 2008, Mosby.

Continued

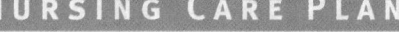

NURSING CARE PLAN

Risk for Injury—cont'd

Evaluation

Nursing Actions	Client Response/Finding	Achievement of Outcome
Ask Ms. Cohen and family to identify risks.	Ms. Cohen and daughter able to identify risks during a walk through the home and expressed a greater sense of safety as a result of changes made.	Ms. Cohen and daughter are more knowledgeable of potential hazards.
Observe environment for elimination of hazards.	Throw rugs have been removed. Lighting has increased to 75 watts except in bathroom and bedroom.	Environmental hazards have been partially reduced.
Reassess Ms. Cohen's visual acuity.	Ms. Cohen has new glasses and says she is able to read better, as well as see distant objects more clearly.	Ms. Cohen's vision has improved, enabling her to ambulate more safely.
Observe Ms. Cohen's gait and posture.	Ms. Cohen's gait remains hesitant and uncoordinated; she reports that her daughter has not had time to take her to the physical therapist.	Outcome of safe ambulation has not been totally achieved; continue to encourage Ms. Cohen and daughter to go to physical therapy appointment.

TABLE 38-2 Interventions to Promote Safety for Children and Adolescents

INTERVENTION	RATIONALE
Infants and Toddlers	
Have infants sleep on their backs or sides. Teach parents the mnemonic "back to sleep."	Sleeping on the stomach with the mouth and nose in close proximity to the mattress is associated with sudden infant death syndrome (SIDS) (Hauck and others, 2003).
Do not fill cribs with pillows, large stuffed toys, or comforters. Sheets should fit snugly.	Possibility for infants to become entwined in sheets and other bedding and suffocate.
Pacifiers should not be attached to string or ribbon and placed around a child's neck.	Reduces risk for choking.
All instructions for preparing and storing formula must be followed.	Proper formula preparation and storage prevents contamination. A formula comes in a concentrated form, or is already premixed with water and ready to use. Following directions ensures proper concentration of the formula. Undiluted formula causes fluid and electrolyte disturbances; very diluted formula will not provide sufficient nutrients.
Use large, soft toys without small parts, such as buttons.	Small parts become dislodged, and choking and aspiration will possibly occur.
Playpens with mesh sides should not be left with a side down; spaces between crib slats should be less than 2⅜ inches (6 cm) apart.	Possibility for a child's head becoming wedged in the lowered mesh side or in between crib slats, and asphyxiation may occur.
Never leave crib sides down or leave babies unattended on changing tables or in infant seats, swings, strollers, or high chairs.	Infants and toddlers roll or move and fall from changing tables or out of accessories such as infant seats or swings.
Discontinue using accessories such as infant seats, and swings when the child becomes too active, physically too big, and/ or according to the manufacturer's directions.	When physically active or too big, the child will possibly fall out of or tip over these accessories and suffer an injury.
Never leave a child alone in the bathroom, tub, or near any water source (e.g., pool).	Reduces risk for accidental drowning.
Baby-proof the home; remove small or sharp objects and toxic or poisonous substances, including plants; install safety locks on floor-level cabinets.	Babies explore their world with their hands and mouth. Choking and poisoning will possibly occur.
Remove plastic bags from the cleaners or grocery store from the home.	Reduces risk for suffocation from plastic bags.
Electrical outlets should have covers (Figure 38-7).	Reduces opportunity for crawling babies to insert objects into outlets and experience an electrical shock.

Modified from Hockenberry M, Wilson D: *Wong's nursing care of infants and children,* ed 8, St. Louis, 2007, Mosby.

✳ TABLE 38-2 Interventions to Promote Safety for Children and Adolescents—cont'd

INTERVENTION	RATIONALE
Infants and Toddlers—cont'd	
Window guards should be on all windows.	Prevents children from falling out of windows.
Install keyless locks (e.g., deadbolts) on doors above a child's reach, even when they are standing on a chair.	Prevents a toddler from leaving the house and wandering off. Death from exposure, car accidents, and drowning will possibly occur. Keyless locks allow for rapid exit in case of fire.
Children weighing less than 80 pounds or under 8 years of age should always be in an age/weight-appropriate car seat that has been installed according to the manufacturer's instructions (Figure 38-8). This includes car seats and booster seats. In cars with a passenger air bag, children under 12 should be in the back seat. All passengers should have seat belts on.	In case of a sudden stop or crash, an unrestrained child will possibly suffer severe head injuries and death.
Caregivers should learn cardiopulmonary resuscitation (CPR) and the Heimlich maneuver.	Caregivers should be prepared to intervene in acute emergencies, such as choking.
Preschoolers	
Teach children to swim at an early age, but always provide supervision near water.	Learning to swim is a useful skill that will possibly someday save a child's life. However, all children need constant supervision near water.
Teach children how to cross streets and walk in parking lots. Instruct them to never run out after a ball or toy.	Pedestrian accidents involving young children are common.
Teach children not to talk to, go with, or accept any item from a stranger.	Reduces the risk of injury and stranger abduction.
Teach children basic physical safety rules, such as proper use of safety scissors, never running with an object in their mouth or hand, and never attempting to use the stove or oven unassisted.	Risk of injury is lower if children know basic safety procedures.
Teach children not to eat items found in the street or grass.	Reduces risk for possible poisoning.
Remove doors from unused refrigerators and freezers. Instruct children not to play or hide in a car trunk or unused appliances.	If a child cannot freely exit from appliances and car trunks, asphyxiation will possibly occur.
School-Age Children	
Teach children the safe use of equipment for play and work.	The child needs to learn the safe, appropriate use of implements to avoid injury.
Teach children proper bicycle safety, including use of helmet and rules of the road.	Reduces injuries from falling off a bike or being hit by a car.
Teach children proper techniques for specific sports, as well as the need to wear proper safety gear (e.g., eyewear, mouth guards).	Using proper sports techniques, correct equipment, and protective gear prevents injuries.
Teach children not to operate electrical equipment while unsupervised.	If an electrical mishap were to occur, no one would be available to help.
Children should never have access to firearms or other weapons. All firearms should be kept in locked cabinets.	Children are often fascinated by firearms and weapons and sometimes attempt to play with them.

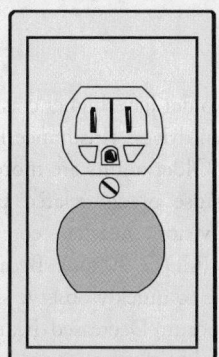

Figure 38-7 Safety covers for electrical outlets.

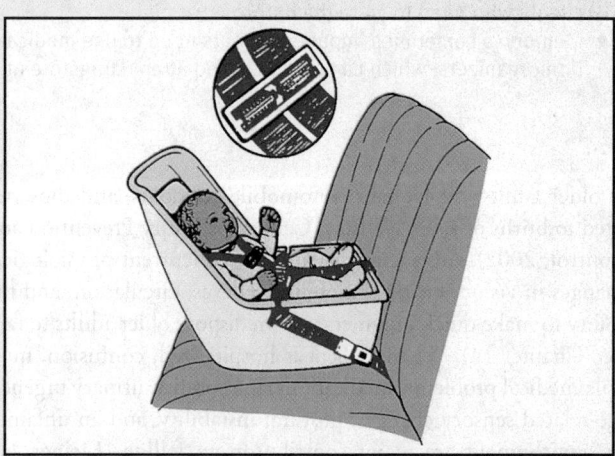

Figure 38-8 Infant car seat.

TABLE 38-2   Interventions to Promote Safety for Children and Adolescents—cont'd

INTERVENTION	RATIONALE
Adolescents	
Encourage enrollment in driver's education classes.	Many injuries in this age-group are related to motor vehicle accidents.
Provide information about the effects of using alcohol and drugs.	Adolescents are prone to risk-taking behaviors and are subject to peer pressures.
Provide sex education, emphasizing safe sex practices, including abstinence.	Many adolescents begin sexual relationships. Pregnancy and sexually transmitted diseases sometimes result.
Refer adolescents to community and school-sponsored activities.	The adolescent needs to socialize with peers, yet needs some supervision.
Encourage mentoring relationships between adults and adolescents.	Adolescents are in need of role models after whom they can pattern their behavior.
Teach them safe use of the Internet.	Avoids overuse and possible exposure to inappropriate websites.

Modified from Hockenberry M, Wilson D: *Wong's nursing care of infants and children,* ed 8, St. Louis, 2007, Mosby.

BOX 38-8   FOCUS ON OLDER ADULTS

Physiological Changes of Aging and Their Impact on Client Safety

- Older adults experience alterations in vision and hearing. Encourage yearly vision and hearing examinations and frequent cleansing of glasses and hearing aids as a means of preventing falls and burns.
- Some older adults have slowed reaction time. Teach clients safety tips for avoiding automobile accidents. Sometimes driving needs to be restricted to daylight hours or suspended.
- Range of motion, flexibility, and strength decrease. Encourage supervised exercise classes for older adults, and teach them to seek assistance with household tasks as needed. Safety features, such as grab bars in the bathroom, are often necessary.
- Reflexes are slowed, and the ability to respond to multiple stimuli is reduced. Provide adequate, meaningful stimuli but prevent sensory overload.
- Nocturia and incontinence are more frequent in older adults. Institute a regular toileting schedule for the client. A recommended frequency is every 3 hours. Give diuretics in the morning. Provide assistance, along with adequate lighting, to clients who need to go to the bathroom at night.
- Memory is sometimes impaired. Clients need to use medication organizers, which can be purchased at any drugstore at a very reasonable cost. These dispensers can be filled once a week with the proper medications to be taken at a specific time during the day.
- The family plays a significant role in the care of older adults. One in five caregivers reported providing more than 40 hours of care per week (National Alliance for Caregiving, Association for the Advancement of Retired Persons, 2004). Encourage the family to allow the older adult to remain as independent as possible and provide help only for those things that are especially stressful or depleted.
- The high prevalence of chronic conditions in older adults results in the use of a high number of prescription and over-the-counter medications. Coupled with age-related changes in pharmacokinetics, there is a greater risk of serious adverse effects. Medications typically prescribed for older adults include anticholinergics, diuretics, anxiolytic and hypnotic agents, antidepressants, antihypertensives, vasodilators, analgesics, and laxatives, all of which may themselves pose risks or may interact to increase the risk for falls. Review the client's drug profile to ensure that any of the above-noted drugs are used cautiously, and assess the client regularly for any adverse effects that increase fall risk.

---

to older adults involve falls, automobile accidents, and those related to burns or fires (National Center for Injury Prevention and Control, 2002). Advancing age and the concurrent physiological changes in vision, hearing, mobility, reflexes, circulation, and the ability to make quick judgments all predispose older adults to falls (see Chapter 14). When a client is hospitalized, confusion, multiple medical problems, medications, immobility, urinary urgency, age-related sensory changes, postural instability, and an unfamiliar environment are major contributors to falling (Meiner and Leuckenotte, 2006). Certain disease states common to older adults, such as arthritis or cerebrovascular accidents, increase chances of injury.

Drivers age 65 and older have higher crash death rates per mile driven than all but teen drivers (Insurance Institute for Highway Safety [IIHS], 2003). Older adults are more likely to have automobile accidents because of age-related physiological changes such as decreases in vision, hearing, cognitive functions, and physical impairments (CDC, 2006c). Because of this, an older adult is not always able to quickly observe situations in which an accident is likely to occur. Decreased hearing acuity alters the older client's ability to hear emergency vehicle sirens or car and truck horns. Because of decreased nervous system response, older adults are unable to react as quickly as they once could to avoid an accident. A decline in these skills accounts for the most common types of accidents, including right-of-way and turning accidents. Educate clients regarding safe driving tips (e.g., driving shorter distances or only in daylight, using side and rearview mirrors carefully, and looking behind them toward their "blind spot" before changing lanes). If hearing is a problem, have the client try to keep a window rolled down while driving or reduce the volume of the radio or CD or cassette player. Eventually, counseling is necessary to help clients make the decision of when to stop driving. At that time help locate resources in the community that provide transportation.

Burns and scalds are also more apt to occur with older people because they sometimes forget and leave hot water running or become confused when turning the dials on a stove or other heating appliance. Nursing measures for preventing burns minimize the risk from impaired vision. Hot water faucets and dials are color coded to make it easier for the adult to know what has been turned on. Recommending a reduction in temperature of the hot water heater is also very beneficial.

Older adults love to walk. Reduce pedestrian accidents for older adults and for all other age-groups by persuading people to wear reflectors on garments when walking at night; to stand on the sidewalk and not in the street when waiting to cross a street; to always cross at corners and not in the middle of the block (particularly if the street is a major one); to cross with the traffic light and not against it; and to look left, right, and left again before entering the street or crosswalk.

Environmental Interventions. Nursing interventions directed at eliminating environmental threats include general preventive measures such as meeting basic needs, reducing physical hazards, and reducing pathogen transmission.

General Preventive Measures Nurses contribute to a safer environment by helping the client meet basic needs related to oxygen, nutrition, temperature, and humidity. To ensure that oxygen availability is not threatened, recommend that the client be sure to periodically have the furnace inspected for proper functioning. To achieve a comfortable level of humidity in the home, have the client attach a humidifier to the furnace or, in the case of clients who have upper respiratory tract infections, use a room humidifier where the client sleeps. Teach basic techniques for food handling (e.g., hand washing and checking for spoilage) and preparation (e.g., keeping food refrigerated before serving) so that nutritional needs are met safely. It is also helpful to have family members label the date when leftovers are saved. Some older adults benefit from Meals on Wheels services. These services provide fresh nutritious meals to older adults who have difficulty preparing their own food. Client education for older adults or clients who enjoy outdoor activities should include ways to prevent and treat frostbite, hypothermia, heatstroke, and heat exhaustion (see Chapter 32).

Adequate lighting and security measures in and around the home, including the use of night-lights, exterior lighting, and locks on windows and doors, enable clients to reduce the risk of injury from crime. The local police department and community organizations often have safety classes available for residents to learn how to take precautions to minimize the chance of becoming involved in a crime. For example, some useful tips include always parking the car near a bright light or busy public area, carrying a whistle attached to the car keys, keeping car doors locked while driving, and always paying attention while driving to notice if anyone starts to follow the car.

To prevent the transmission of pathogens, nurses teach aseptic practices. Medical asepsis, which includes hand hygiene and environmental cleanliness, reduces the transfer of organisms (see Chapter 34). Clients and family members need to learn thorough hand hygiene (hand washing or use of hand rub) and when to use it (e.g., before and after caring for a family member, before food preparation, before preparing a medication for a family member, and after contacting any body fluids). When clients require dressing changes or the use of syringes and needles, show families how to properly dispose of contaminated items in the home. Most communities have regulations for the disposal of biohazardous waste.

Acute Care. There are a number of specific safety measures applicable to clients in the acute care environment. The nurse takes measures to help clients avoid falls, injuries from use of restraints and side rails, fires, poisoning, and electrical hazards. Special precautions are necessary to prevent injury in clients susceptible to having seizures. Radiation injuries are also a specific safety concern. Finally, be prepared to respond to the emergency of a bioterrorist attack.

Falls. Modifications in the home and health care environment will easily reduce the risk of falls (Table 38-3). Make sure a heavy or debilitated client in a bed or wheelchair or on a toilet is properly supported and secured. Side rails are necessary unless a client is able to freely and easily ambulate independently. Safety bars on toilets, locks on beds and wheelchairs, and call lights are additional safety features found in health care settings (Figures 38-9 and 38-10). Remove excess furniture and equipment, and make sure a weakened client wears rubber-soled shoes or slippers for walking or transferring. When clients use assistive aids such as canes, crutches, or walkers, it is important to routinely check the condition of rubber tips and the integrity of the aid.

To reduce the risk of injury in the home, remove all obstacles from halls and other heavily traveled areas. Necessary objects such as clocks, glasses, tissues, or medications remain on bedside tables within reach of the client but out of the reach of children. Take care to ensure that end tables are secure and have stable, straight legs. Place nonessential items in drawers to eliminate clutter. If small area rugs are used, secure them with a nonslip pad or skid-resistant adhesive strips. Make sure any carpeting on the stairs is secured with carpet tacks.

In the health care environment, frequent observations of the client at risk for falls are important to reduce the potential for injury (Meade and others, 2006). Hourly rounding by nurses significantly reduces the occurrence of client falls, as well as reducing call light usage and increasing client satisfaction (Box 38-9).

Restraints. A physical **restraint** is a human, mechanical, and/or physical device that is used with or without the client's permission to restrict his or her freedom of movement or normal access to a person's body and is not a usual part of treatment plans indicated by the person's condition or symptoms (TJC, 2006). The optimal goal for all clients is a restraint-free environment; however, clients who are at risk for injury from wandering, falls, and disruptive or agitated behavior may need restraints temporarily.

✳ TABLE 38-3 Measures to Prevent Falls by Older Adults

MEASURE	RATIONALE
Stairs	
Install treads with uniform depth of 9 inches (22.5 cm) and 9-inch risers (vertical face of steps).	When stairs are of uniform size, older adults do not have to continually adjust vision.
Install uniform-textured or plain-colored surfaces on each tread, and mark edge of tread with contrasting color.	Uniform textures or color help to decrease vertigo. Marking edge of tread provides obvious visual clue to end of stair.
Ensure proper lighting of each tread. Block sun or lightbulb glare with translucent shades or screen, or use lower-wattage or nonglare bulbs.	Older adults' vision is unable to adjust quickly to changes in lighting.
Ensure adequate headroom so that users do not have to duck to negotiate stairs.	Sudden changes in head position sometimes result in dizziness.
Remove protruding objects from staircase walls.	Decreased peripheral vision prevents client from seeing object.
Maintain outdoor walkways and stairs in good condition and free of holes, cracks, and splinters.	Decreased visual acuity prevents client from seeing any structural defect.
Handrails	
Install smooth but slip-resistant handrail at least 2 inches (5 cm) from wall.	Two-inch distance allows client to grasp handrail firmly for support.
Secure handrail firmly so that user's weight is supported, especially at bottom and top of stairway.	Older adults have greatest risk of falling at top and bottom of stairs, because center of gravity is being shifted and balance is unstable.
Install grab rails in bathroom near toilet and tub.	This enables client to have support while rising from sitting to standing position.
Floors	
Ensure that clients wear properly fitting shoes or slippers with nonskid surface.	Reduces chances of slipping.
Secure all carpeting, mats, and tile; place nonskid backing under small rugs.	Sudden slip causes dizziness and inability to regain balance.
Place bath mats or nonskid strips on bathtub or shower stall floors.	Wet surfaces increase the risk of falling.
Secure electrical cords against baseboards.	Prevents tripping.
Maintain proper illumination in areas both inside and outside where the client moves and walks.	Reduces the risk of falling due to eyestrain.
Health Care Facility	
Orientation	
Place disoriented clients in room near nurses' station.	Provides for more frequent observation by nursing staff.
Maintain close supervision of confused clients.	Confused clients often attempt to wander out of bed or room.
Show the client how to use the call light at the bedside and in bathroom, and place within easy reach.	Location and use of the call light is essential to client safety.
Place bedside tables and over-bed tables close to client.	Prevents client from searching or overreaching for items such as eyeglasses, dentures, hearing aid, or telephone.
Remove clutter from bedside tables, hallways, bathrooms, and grooming areas.	Eliminates potential hazards and promotes client independence.
Leave one side rail up and one down on the side where the oriented and ambulatory client gets out of bed.	Client uses the side rail for support when getting in and out of bed and to position self once in bed.
Transport	
Lock beds and wheelchairs when transferring a client from a bed to a wheelchair or back to bed.	Provides stability and support during transfer.
Place side rails in the up position, and secure safety straps around the client on a stretcher.	Prevents the client from rolling off the stretcher.

Modified from Chang JT and others: Interventions for the prevention of falls in older adults: systematic review with meta-analysis of randomized clinical trials, *Br Med J* 328(7441):680, 2004.

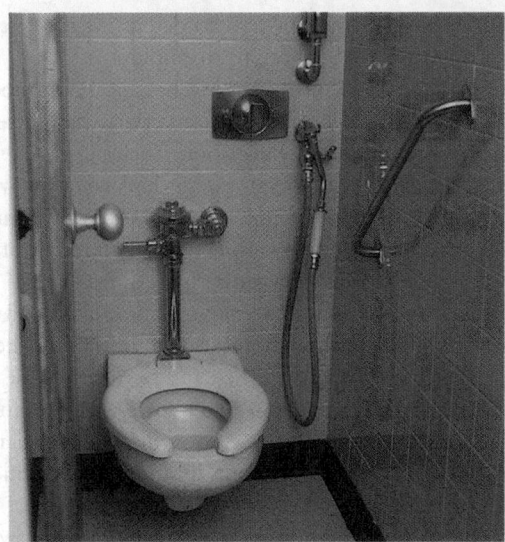

Figure 38-9 Safety bars around toilets and showers.

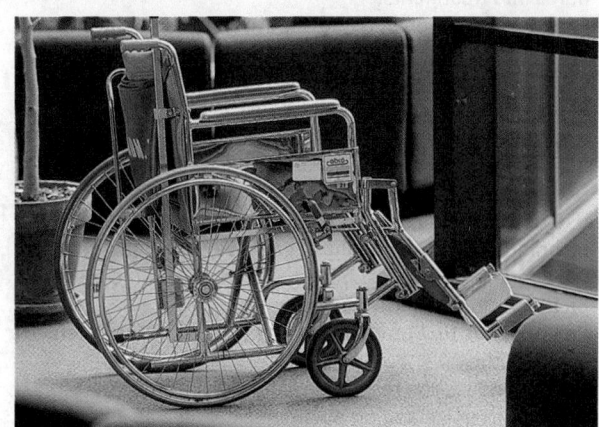

Figure 38-10 Safety locks on wheelchairs.

✳ BOX 38-9 — EVIDENCE-BASED PRACTICE

Effects of Nursing Rounds

Evidence Summary

Hospitalized clients often require assistance with basic activities of daily living such as eating, toileting, and ambulating. Clients usually communicate their needs by use of the call light. Not meeting client needs in a timely fashion decreases client satisfaction and places clients at greater risk for injury. Researchers wanted to know if ursing rounds every 1 or 2 hours would reduce call light usage, increase client satisfaction, and reduce frequency of client falls. During rounding the following items were performed for each client: pain management, toileting, positioning, and items such as call light, telephone, TV remote, bed light switch, tissue, and water placed within reach and garbage can next to bed. In addition, before leaving the room, the nurse asked, "Is there anything else I can do for you before I leave? I have time while I'm here in the room." The client was also told someone would be back in 1 (or 2) hours to round again. A 6-week nationwide quasi-experimental study was conducted on 27 nursing units in 14 hospitals. Researchers took baseline data on call light usage during the initial 2 weeks. Rounding at set intervals, including specific nursing actions, was associated with statistically significant reduced client call light usage, increased client satisfaction, and in the 1-hour rounding group, fewer client falls.

Application to Nursing Practice

• Nursing rounds performed at set intervals will positively affect client satisfaction and safety and lead to fewer distractions for staff
• The nurse's ability to meet the client's needs affects the client's perception of the quality of nursing care.
• Anticipate client needs by performing rounds, including specific actions, at 1-hour intervals.

Reference

Meade CM and others: Effects of nursing rounds on patients' call light use, satisfaction and safety, *Am J Nurs* 106(9):58, 2006.

Whenever a client is restrained, there is a natural tendency for the client to try to remove the restraint. When this occurs, client injury is common. Restrained clients easily become entangled in a restraint device in attempts to get out of the device. In some cases, death has resulted because of strangulation or asphyxiation. As a result, nursing homes and many health care facilities have banned the use of the jacket (vest) restraint because of this risk. The use of any restraint is also associated with serious complications, including pressure ulcers, constipation, pneumonia, urinary and fecal incontinence, and urinary retention (see Chapter 47). Contractures, nerve damage, and circulatory impairment are also potential hazards. In addition, restrained clients experience a loss of self-esteem, humiliation, fear, and anger.

SAFETY ALERT Routine assessment of a client in restraints is critical to prevent injury. Because of the risk of injury from restraints, regulatory agencies such as TJC and the Centers for Medicaid and Medicare Services (CMS) enforce standards for the safe use of restraints and define clients' rights and choices regarding their use. Under these guidelines, reasons for use of a physical restraint are to be clearly stated. The use of restraints must be part of the client's medical treatment, all less restrictive interventions must be tried first, other disciplines must be consulted, and supporting documentation must be provided (CMS, 2006).

The movement is for health care organizations to become restraint-free environments. Restraints do not prevent falls or injury. In fact, clients incur less severe injuries if left unrestrained (Capezuti and others, 1998; Strumpf and others, 1998). A multi-

✳ **BOX 38-10**   **Alternatives to Restraints**

- Orient clients and families to environment; explain all procedures and treatments.
- Provide companionship and supervision; use trained sitters or adjust staffing.
- Offer diversionary activities, such as music or something to hold; enlist support and input from the family.
- Assign confused or disoriented clients to rooms near the nurses' station; observe these clients frequently.
- Use calm, simple statements and physical cues as needed.
- Use de-escalation, time-out, and other verbal intervention techniques when managing aggressive behaviors.
- Provide appropriate visual and auditory stimuli (e.g., family pictures, clock, radio).
- Remove cues that promote leaving (e.g., elevators, stairs, or street clothes).
- Promote relaxation techniques and normal sleep patterns.
- Institute exercise and ambulation schedules as allowed by the client's condition; consult physical therapist for mobility and exercise programs.
- Attend to needs for toileting, food, and liquid.
- Camouflage IV lines with clothing, stockinette, or Kling dressing.
- Evaluate all medications client is receiving, and ensure effective pain management.
- Reassess physical status, and review laboratory findings.

Modified from The Joint Commission Resources: *Strategies for avoiding restraint related errors*, 2006, http://www.jcrinc.com; and Geriatric nursing resources for care of older adults: *Physical restraints*, 2006, http://www.geronurseonline.org/index.

disciplinary approach that conducts individualized assessments and develops structured treatment plans reduces the number of restraints used. It is imperative that nurses try alternative measures instead of restraints (Box 38-10). The University of Iowa Gerontological Nursing Interventions Research Center has developed a restraint use algorithm (Figure 38-11). The algorithm provides evidenced-based guidelines for how to determine if a restraint is appropriate and what interventions to employ.

The use of restraints involves a psychological adjustment for the client and family. If restraints are necessary, the nurse assists family members and clients by explaining their purpose, expected care while the client is restrained, precautions taken to avoid injury, and that the restraint is temporary and protective. Informed consent from family members is sometimes required before using restraints, as is the case in long-term care settings.

For legal purposes, know agency-specific policy and procedures for appropriate use and monitoring of restraints. The use of a restraint must be clinically justified and be a part of the client's prescribed medical treatment and plan of care. A physician's order is required, based on a face-to-face assessment of the client. The order must state the type of restraint, location, and specific client behaviors for which restraints are to be used and must have a limited time frame. These orders need to be renewed within a specific time frame according to the agency's policy. Restraints are not to be ordered prn (as needed). You must conduct ongoing assessment of clients who are restrained. Proper documentation, including the behaviors that necessitated the application of restraints, the procedure used in restraining, the condition of the body part restrained (e.g., circulation to hand), and the evaluation of the client response, is essential. Restraints must be periodically removed, and the nurse assesses the client to determine if the restraints continue to be necessary.

Skill 38-1 includes guidelines for the proper use and application of restraints. Use of restraints must meet the following objectives:

- Reduce the risk of client injury from falls.
- Prevent interruption of therapy such as traction, IV infusions, nasogastric (NG) tube feeding, or Foley catheterization.
- Prevent the confused or combative client from removing life support equipment.
- Reduce the risk of injury to others by the client.

Text continued on p. 838

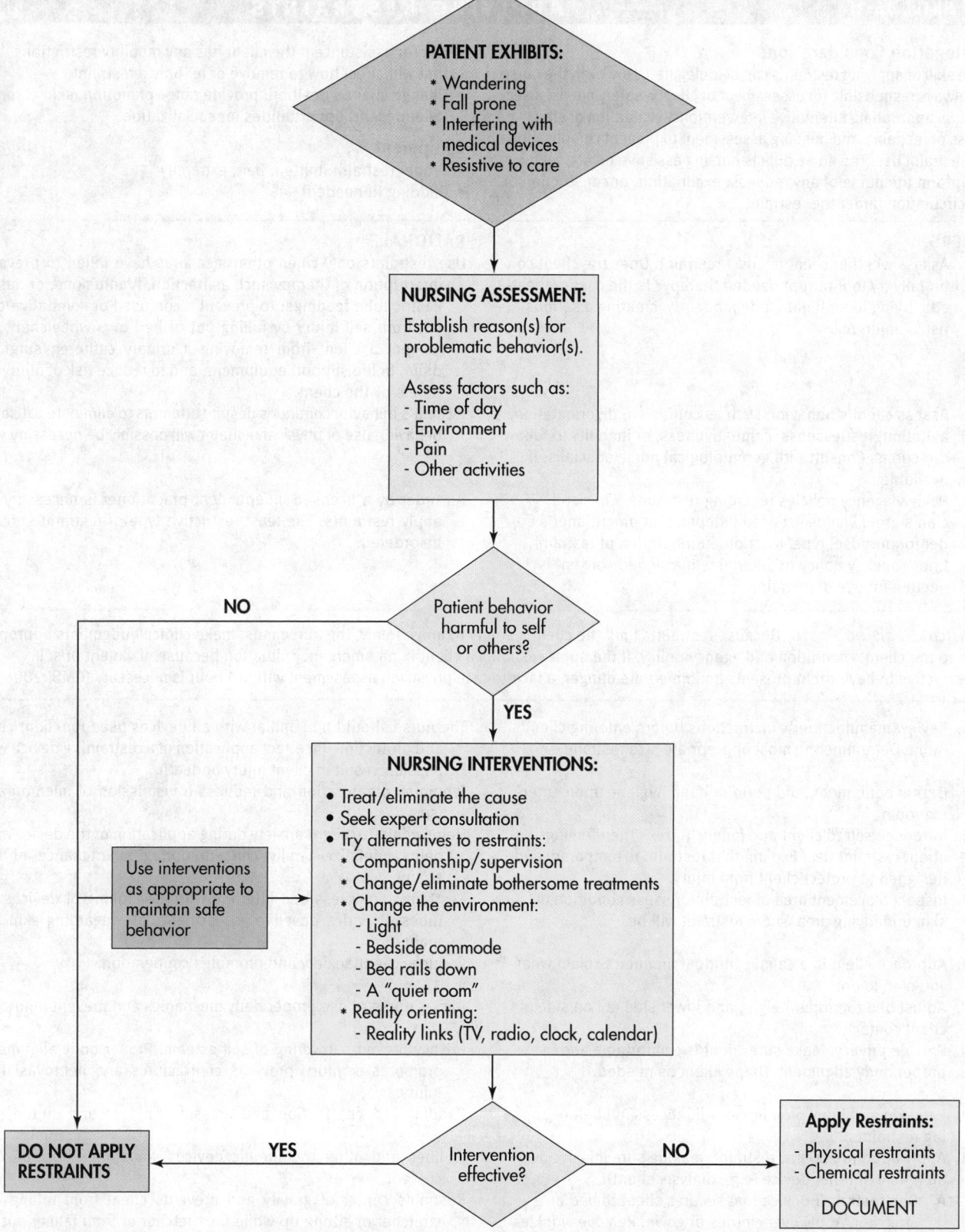

PATIENT EXHIBITS:
* Wandering
* Fall prone
* Interfering with medical devices
* Resistive to care

NURSING ASSESSMENT:

Establish reason(s) for problematic behavior(s).

Assess factors such as:
- Time of day
- Environment
- Pain
- Other activities

Patient behavior harmful to self or others?

NO

YES

Use interventions as appropriate to maintain safe behavior

NURSING INTERVENTIONS:
• Treat/eliminate the cause
• Seek expert consultation
• Try alternatives to restraints:
 * Companionship/supervision
 * Change/eliminate bothersome treatments
 * Change the environment:
  - Light
  - Bedside commode
  - Bed rails down
  - A "quiet room"
 * Reality orienting:
  - Reality links (TV, radio, clock, calendar)

DO NOT APPLY RESTRAINTS

YES

Intervention effective?

NO

Apply Restraints:
- Physical restraints
- Chemical restraints

DOCUMENT

Figure 38-11 Decision algorithm. (© The University of Iowa Gerontological Interventions Research Center Research Translation and Dissemination Core. Written 1996; revised 11/05.)

Delegation Considerations

The skill of applying restraints can be delegated. However, the nurse is always responsible for assessment of client's safety needs, selection of appropriate alternative interventions, evaluation of effectiveness of restraint, and ongoing assessment to prevent complications of restraint use. The nurse directs nursing assistive personnel to:

- Inform the nurse of any redness, excoriation, or constriction of circulation under the restraint.
- Ask for assistance if the client has any mobility restrictions that will affect how to remove or reapply a restraint.
- Change client's position; provide range of motion, skin care, toileting, and opportunities for socialization.

Equipment

- Proper restraint: mitten, belt, extremity
- Padding (if needed)

STEPS	RATIONALE
1. Assess whether client needs a restraint. Does the client continually try to interrupt needed therapy? Is the client repeatedly trying to ambulate independently, creating a serious risk of injury?	Use restraints only when other measures have failed to prevent interruption of therapy such as traction, IV infusions, or nasogastric tube feedings; to prevent a confused or combative client from self-injury by falling out of bed or a wheelchair; to prevent a client from removing a urinary catheter, surgical drain, or life support equipment; and to reduce risk of injury to others by the client.
2. Assess client's behavior, such as confusion, disorientation, agitation, restlessness, combativeness, or inability to follow directions. Consult with gerontological nurse specialist if available.	If client's behavior continues despite attempts to eliminate cause of behavior, use of physical restraint will possibly be necessary.
3. Review agency policies regarding restraints. Check physician's order versus licensed independent practitioner's order for purpose, type, location, and duration of restraint. Check agency policy to determine if a signed consent is needed for use of restraint.	An order by a licensed independent practitioner is necessary to apply restraints. The least restrictive type of restraint should be ordered.

Critical Decision Point: Because restraints limit the client's ability to move freely, the nurse must make clinical judgments appropriate to the client's condition and agency policy. If the nurse restrains a client in an emergency situation because of violent or self-destructive behavior that presents an immediate danger, a face-to-face physician assessment within 1 hour is necessary (CMS, 2006).

4. Review manufacturer's instructions before entering client's room. Determine the most appropriate size restraint.	The nurse should be familiar with all devices used for client care and protection. Incorrect application of a restraining device will possibly result in client injury or death.
5. Gather equipment, and perform hand hygiene upon entering room.	Promotes organization and reduces transmission of microorganisms.
6. Introduce self to client and family. Assess their feelings about restraint use. Explain that restraint is temporary and designed to protect client from injury.	Helps minimize client anxiety during application of the device and helps minimize family concern during maintenance of restraint.
7. Inspect placement area of restraint. Assess condition of skin underlying area where restraint will be.	Restraints compress and interfere with functioning of devices or tubes. Provides baseline assessment data regarding skin integrity.
8. Approach client in a calm, confident manner. Explain what you plan to do.	Reduces client anxiety and promotes cooperation.
9. Adjust bed to proper height, and lower side rail on side of client contact.	Allows nurse to use proper body mechanics and prevent injury.
10. Provide privacy. Make sure client is comfortable and in proper body alignment. Drape client as needed.	Privacy prevents lowering of self-esteem. Proper body alignment promotes comfort, prevents contractures and neurovascular injury.
11. Pad skin and bony prominences (if necessary) before applying restraints.	Padding reduces friction and pressure on skin and underlying tissue.
12. Apply appropriate-size restraint, making sure it is not over an IV line or other device (e.g., dialysis shunt).	IV lines and other therapeutic devices sometimes become occluded.
A. **Belt restraint:** Device that secures client to bed or stretcher. Apply over clothes or gown. Remove wrinkles from front and back of restraint while placing it around client's waist. Bring ties through slots in belt. Avoid placing belt across the chest or too tightly across the abdomen (see illustration).	Restrains center of gravity and prevents client from rolling off stretcher or sitting up while on stretcher or from falling out of bed. Tight application interferes with ventilation.

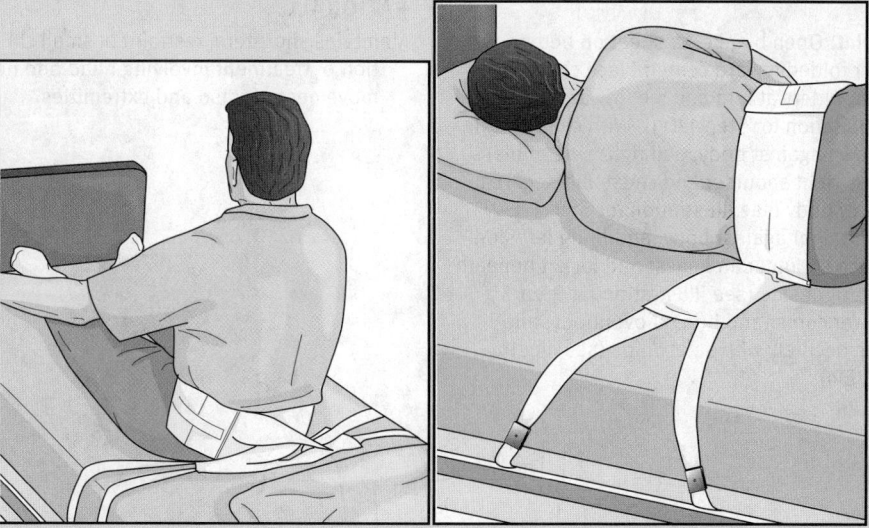

STEP 12A Belt restraint tied to the bed frame or hook under the bed and to an area that does not cause the restraint to tighten when the side rail or bed is raised or lowered. (From Sorrentino SA: *Mosby's textbook for nursing assistants,* ed 6, St. Louis, 2004, Mosby.)

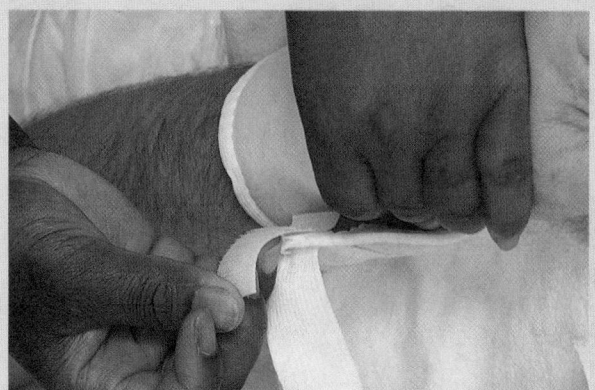

STEP 12B Extremity restraint being applied to wrist.

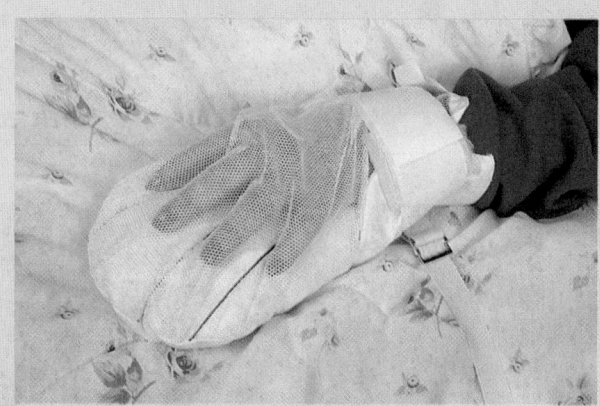

STEP 12C Mitten restraint.

STEPS	RATIONALE
B. Extremity (ankle or wrist) restraint: Restraint designed to immobilize one or all extremities. Commercially available limb restraints are composed of sheepskin or foam padding (see illustration). Wrap limb restraint around wrist or ankle with soft part toward skin and secured snugly in place by Velcro straps.	Maintains immobilization of extremity to protect client from injury from fall or accidental removal of therapeutic device (e.g., IV tube or Foley catheter). Tight application interferes with circulation.
C. Mitten restraint: Thumbless mitten device to restrain client's hands (see illustration). Place hand in mitten, being sure to bring end all the way up over the wrist.	Prevents clients from dislodging invasive equipment, removing dressings, or scratching, yet allows greater movement than a wrist restraint.
D. Elbow restraint: Piece of fabric with slots in which tongue blades are placed so that elbow joint remains rigid (see illustration).	Commonly used with infants and children to prevent elbow flexion (e.g., when an IV line is in place).

Continued

✳ **SKILL 38-1**   APPLYING RESTRAINTS—CONT'D

STEPS

E. **Mummy restraint:** Open blanket or sheet on bed or crib with one corner folded toward center. Place child on blanket with shoulders at fold and feet toward opposite corner (see illustration for Step 12E-1). With child's right arm straight down against body, pull right side of blanket firmly across right shoulder and chest and secure beneath left side of body (see illustration for Step 12E-2). Place left arm straight against body, and bring left side of blanket across shoulder and chest and lock it beneath child's body on right side (see illustration for Step 12E-3). Fold lower corner and bring it over body, and tuck or fasten it securely with safety pins (see illustration for Step 12E-4).

RATIONALE

Maintains short-term restraint of small child or infant for examination or treatment involving head and neck. Effectively controls movement of torso and extremities.

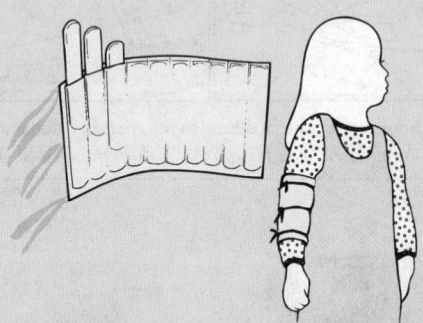

STEP 12D Elbow restraint.

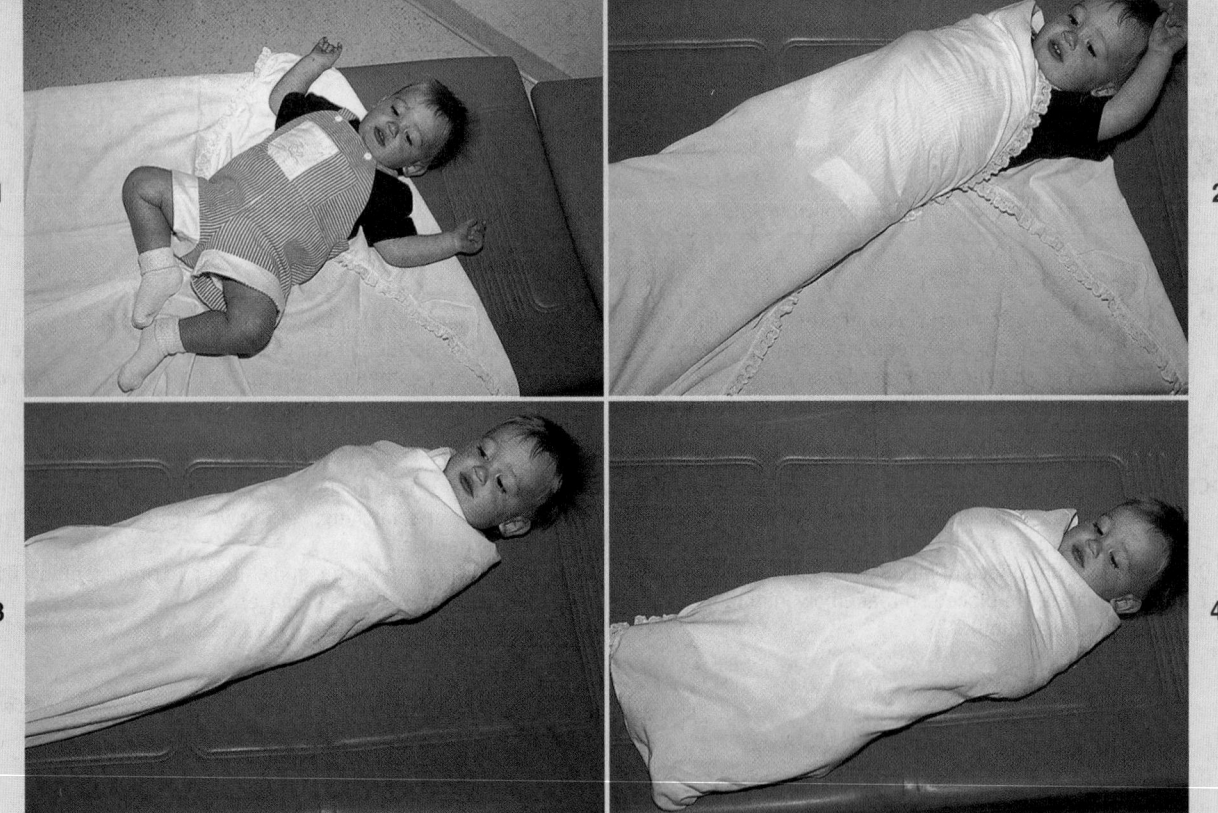

STEP 12E Mummy restraint.

STEPS

13. Attach restraints to movable part of the bed frame, which moves when the head of bed is raised or lowered (see illustration).

RATIONALE

Client will possibly be injured if restraint is secured to side rail and it is lowered.

Critical Decision Point: Do not attach end of restraint to side rails.

14. Secure restraints with a quick-release tie (see illustration). Do not tie in a knot.
15. Insert two fingers under the secured restraint (see illustration).
16. Assess proper placement of restraint, skin integrity, pulses, temperature, color, and sensation of the restrained body part at least every 2 hours (TJC, 2006) or according to agency policy.

Allows for quick release in an emergency.

A tight restraint will possibly cause constriction and impede circulation. Checking for constriction prevents neurovascular injury.

Frequent assessment prevents complications, such as suffocation, skin breakdown, and impaired circulation.

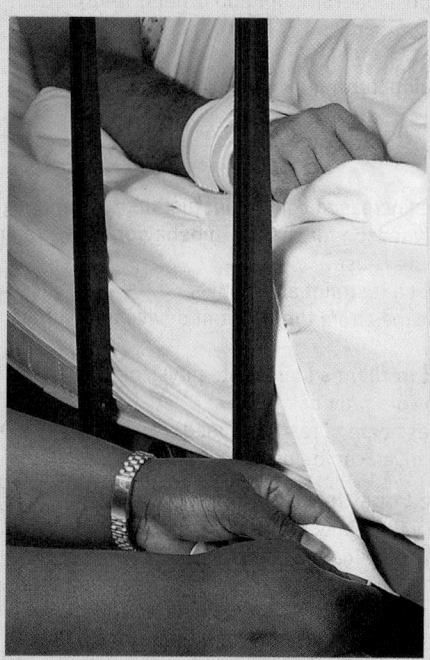

STEP 13 Tie restraint strap to bed frame or hook under bed.

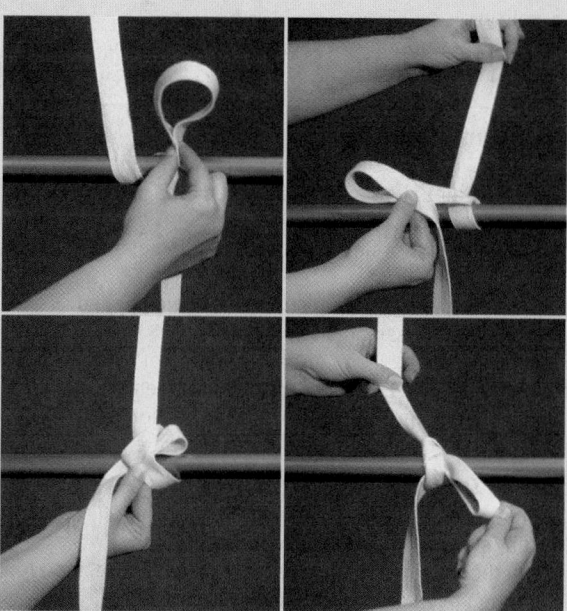

STEP 14 The Posey quick-release tie. (Courtesy JT Posey Co, Arcadia, Calif.)

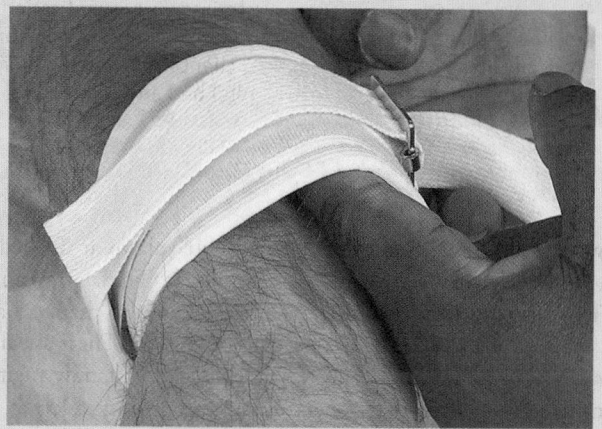

STEP 15 Place two fingers under restraint to check tightness.

Continued

SKILL 38-1   **APPLYING RESTRAINTS—CONT'D**

STEPS	RATIONALE
17. Restraints should be removed at least every 2 hours (TJC, 2006). If client is violent and noncompliant, remove one restraint at a time and/or have staff assistance while removing restraints. Do not leave client unattended at this time.	Provides opportunity to change client's position and perform full range of motion (ROM), toileting, and exercise and to provide food or fluids.
18. Secure call light or intercom system within reach.	Allows client, family, or caregiver to obtain assistance quickly.
19. Leave bed or chair with wheels locked. Bed should be in lowest position.	Locked wheels prevent bed or chair from moving if client attempts to get out. If client falls when bed is in lowest position, this will reduce the chances of injury.
20. Perform hand hygiene before leaving room.	Reduces transmission of microorganisms.
21. While restraints are in use:	
A. Inspect client for any injury, including all hazards of immobility.	Client should be free of injury and not exhibit any signs of immobility complications.
B. Observe IV catheters, urinary catheters, and drainage tubes to ensure that they are positioned correctly and that therapy remains uninterrupted.	Reinsertion is uncomfortable and increases risk of infection or interrupt therapy.
C. Frequently reassess client's need for continued use of restraint with the intent of discontinuing restraint at the earliest possible time (TJC, 2006) (see agency-specific policy).	Use of restraints is a temporary measure and discontinued as soon as possible (Strumpf and others, 1998).
D. Provide appropriate sensory stimulation, and reorient client as needed.	Use of restraints further increases disorientation.

Recording and Reporting

- Record behaviors that place client at risk for injury.
- Describe restraint alternatives attempted and client's response.
- Record client's and/or family's understanding of and consent to restraint application.
- Record type and location of restraint and time applied.
- Record time of assessments and releases.
- Document client's behavior after application of restraint.
- Document specific assessments related to orientation, oxygenation, skin integrity, circulation, and positioning.
- Describe client's response when restraints were removed.

Unexpected Outcomes and Related Interventions

1. Client has signs of impaired skin integrity.
   a. Assess skin, and provide appropriate therapy.
   b. Notify the health care provider, and reassess the need for continued use of the restraint
   c. Ensure correct application of restraint. Pad skin under a restraint, and remove restraint more frequently.
2. Client has altered neurovascular status to an extremity (cyanosis, pallor, coldness of the skin, or complaints of tingling, pain, or numbness).
   a. Remove restraint immediately, stay with the client, and notify the health care provider. Protect extremity from further injury (e.g., pressure from tubing or encumbrance, positioning).

3. Client has increased confusion, disorientation, or agitation.
   a. Identify reason for change in behavior, and attempt to eliminate cause.
   b. Attempt a restraint alternative.
4. Client escapes from the restraint device and suffers a fall or injury.
   a. Attend to client's immediate physical needs, and inform health care provider.
   b. Reassess type of restraint used, correct application, and if alternatives can be used.

Home Care Considerations

- Plan care with family. If possible, use of an Ambularm will free client from physical restraints.
- Instruct family (or other caregiver) in use of alternatives to restraints (see Box 38-10, p. 832).
- A physical restraint is a device that requires a health care provider's order. It should not be sent home with family unless the device is needed to protect client from injury. If physical restraints are necessary, you need to instruct the family (or other caregiver) in proper application, care needed while in restraints, and complications to look for. Also inform caregiver whom to contact if any abnormal findings occur.
- A client who needs to be restrained in bed should have a hospital bed and will require constant supervision in the home.

In keeping with current trends toward health promotion, improved assessment techniques and modifications of the environment are alternatives to restraints. The client can wear a device called the **Ambularm** on the leg. It signals when the leg is in a dependent position, such as over the side rail or on the floor (Figure 38-12). There are also weight-sensitive sensor mats that you can place on clients' mattresses or in the chair such as the **Bed-Check** bed exit alarm system (Figure 38-13). This device sounds an audible alarm at the bedside when pressure is released off the sensor mat. The alarm can be designed to signal at the central nurses' station so that staff are alerted quickly when a client is up and out of bed. There are also alarms that you can place on doors to alert staff or family members when a confused or disoriented client, prone to wandering, opens a door.

A less-restrictive restraint is the Posey Bed All Care Model (Figure 38-14). The bed is a soft-sided, self-contained enclosed

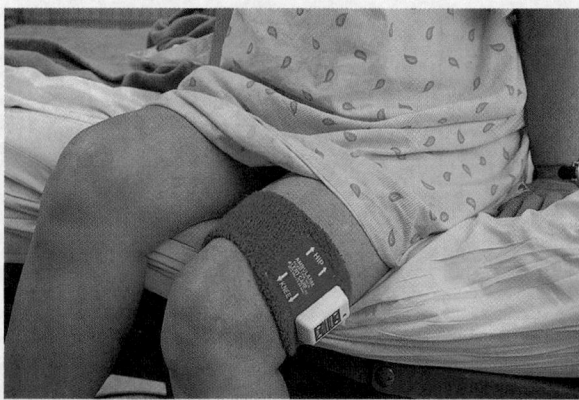

Figure 38-12 Client wearing an Ambularm device.

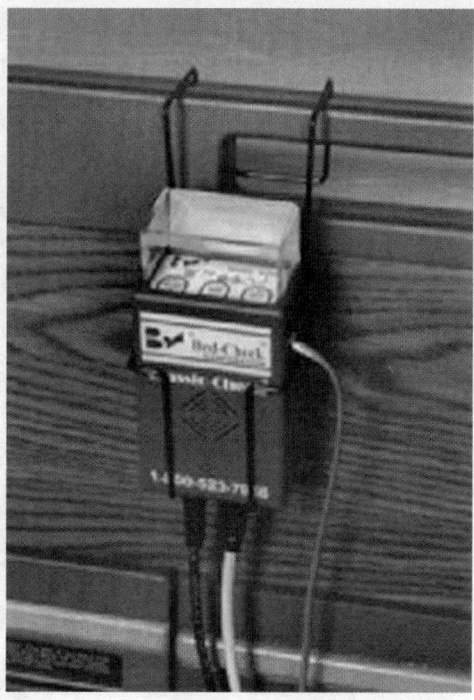

Figure 38-13 The Bed-Check bed exit alarm. (Courtesy Bed-Check Corp.)

bed that is much less restrictive than chemical or physical restraints. It allows for freedom of movement and thus reduces the side effects caused by physical restraints such as pressure ulcers and loss of dignity. A vinyl top covers the padded upper frame of the bed and the nylon-net canopy surrounds the mattress and completely encloses the client in the bed. Zippers on the four sides of the enclosure provide access to the client. The Posey Bed Enclosure works well for clients who are restless and unpredictable, cognitively impaired, and at risk for injury if they were to fall or get out of bed, such as clients on anticoagulant therapy at risk for intracranial bleed. The bed is also a safer alternative to side rails.

Side Rails. Side rails help to increase a client's mobility and/or stability when in bed or when moving from bed to chair. Side rails also help prevent the unconscious client from falling out of bed or from a stretcher (Figure 38-15). A full set of raised side rails is considered a restraint if they restrict a client's freedom of voluntary movement in and out of bed (CMS, 2006). The use of side rails alone for a disoriented client will cause more confusion and further injury. A confused client who is determined to get out of bed attempts to climb over the side rail or climbs out at the foot of the bed. Either attempt usually results in a fall or injury. Nursing interventions to reduce a client's confusion first focus on the cause of the confusion. Frequently nurses mistake a client's attempt to explore his or her environment or to self-toilet as confusion. A thorough assessment is essential. Whenever side rails are used, make sure the bed is in the lowest position possible.

SAFETY ALERT Side rails have the potential to cause entrapment of the head and body, especially in older adult clients who are frail, confused, and restless or have uncontrollable body movement (FDA, 2006). Entrapment has resulted in death, due to asphyxiation, and injuries, such as fractures and lacerations. To prevent this hazard, assess for excessive gaps and openings between the bed frame and mattress and utilize side rail netting or covers, protective padding, and/or antiskid mats to prevent the mattress from being pushed to one side.

Fires. A fire is always possible in the home or hospital. Accidental home fires typically result from smoking in bed, placing cigarettes in trashcans, grease fires, or electrical fires resulting from faulty wiring or appliances. Institutional fires typically result from an electrical or anesthetic-related fire. Although smoking is usually not allowed in the hospital setting, smoking-related fires continue to pose a significant risk due to unauthorized smoking in bed.

The interventions described here are directed toward fires occurring in health care agencies, but the same principles apply for fires in the home (Box 38-11). Homes need to be equipped with smoke and fire alarms. It is important to have a plan of action in the event of fire, including a route of exit and identification of a location where family members will meet. All clients, even young children, need to be familiar with the phrase "stop, drop and roll," which describes the actions to follow when clothing and skin are burning.

If a fire occurs in a health care agency, protect clients from immediate injury, report the exact location of the fire, and contain the fire and extinguish it if possible. All personnel are mobilized to evacuate clients. Clients who are close to the fire, regardless of its size, are at risk of injury and need to be moved to another area. If a client is receiving oxygen but not life support, discontinue the oxygen, which is combustible and will fuel an existing fire. If the client is on life support, you will need to maintain the client's respiratory status manually with a bag-valve-mask device (see Chapter 40) until the client is away from the fire. Direct ambulatory clients to walk by themselves to a safe area. In some cases, they will be able to assist in moving clients in wheelchairs. You generally move bedridden clients from the scene of a fire by a stretcher, their bed, or a wheelchair. If none of these methods is appropriate, clients need to be carried from the area. If you have to carry a client, be careful not to overextend physical limits for lifting because injury to the nurse will result in further injury to the client. If fire department personnel are on the scene, they will help evacuate the clients.

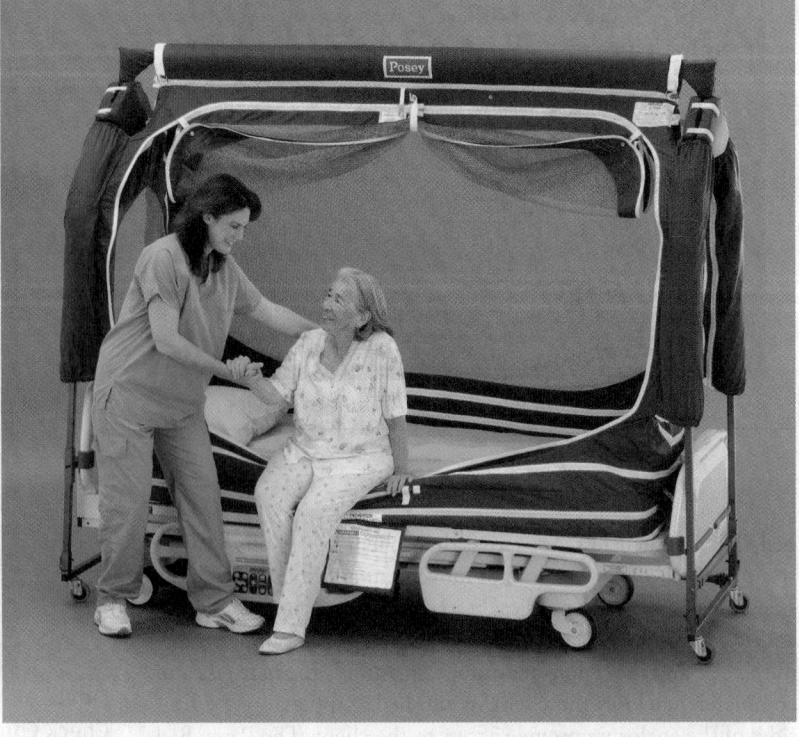

Figure 38-14 The Posey Bed All Care Model. (Courtesy JT Posey Co, Arcadia, Calif.)

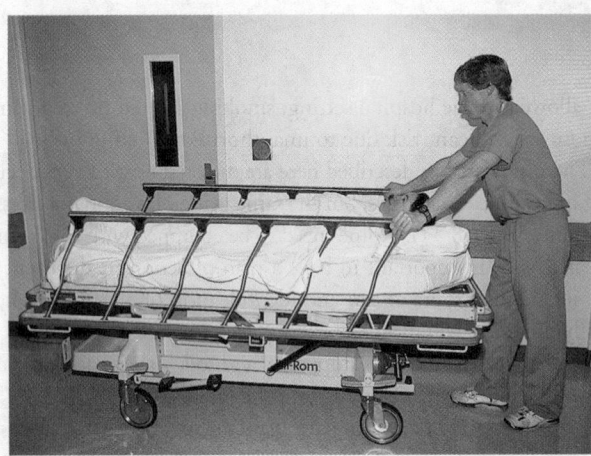

Figure 38-15 Side rails in the *up* position on a stretcher.

After a fire has been reported and clients are out of danger, nurses and other personnel take measures to contain or put out the fire, such as closing doors and windows, placing wet towels along the base of doors, turning off sources of oxygen and electrical equipment, and using a fire extinguisher. Fire extinguishers are categorized as type A, used for ordinary combustibles (e.g., wood, cloth, paper, and many plastic items); type B, used for flammable liquids (e.g., gasoline, grease, paint, and anesthetic gas); and type C, used for electrical equipment. Box 38-12 discusses the correct use of an extinguisher, and Figure 38-16 demonstrates the process as well.

The best intervention is to prevent fires. Nursing measures include complying with the agency's smoking policies and keeping combustible materials away from heat sources. Some agencies have fire doors that are held open by magnets and close auto-

---

❊ BOX 38-11 Fire Intervention Guidelines for Nurses Working in Health Care Agencies

- Keep the phone number for reporting fires visible on the telephone at all times.
- Know the agency's fire drill and evacuation plan.
- Know the location of all fire alarms, exits, extinguishers, and oxygen shut-off.
- Use the mnemonic RACE to set priorities in case of fire:
  R Rescue and remove all clients in immediate danger.
  A Activate the alarm. Always do this before attempting to extinguish even a minor fire.
  C Confine the fire by closing doors and windows and turning off oxygen and electrical equipment.
  E Extinguish the fire using an extinguisher (see Figure 38-16).

---

matically when a fire alarm sounds. It is important to keep equipment away from these doors.

Poisoning. A **poison** is any substance that impairs health or destroys life when ingested, inhaled, or otherwise absorbed by the body. Specific antidotes or treatments are available for only some types of poisons. The capacity of body tissue to recover from the poison determines the reversibility of the effect. Poisons impair the respiratory, circulatory, central nervous, hepatic, GI, and renal systems of the body.

The toddler, preschooler, young school-age child, and older adult need to be protected from accidental poisoning. Using child-resistant caps, placing medications and cleaning fluids and powders out of the reach of children, leaving potentially poisonous materials in original containers, and removing poisonous plants from the home prevent accidental ingestion of poisonous materials. Poisoning also results from swallowing miniature but-

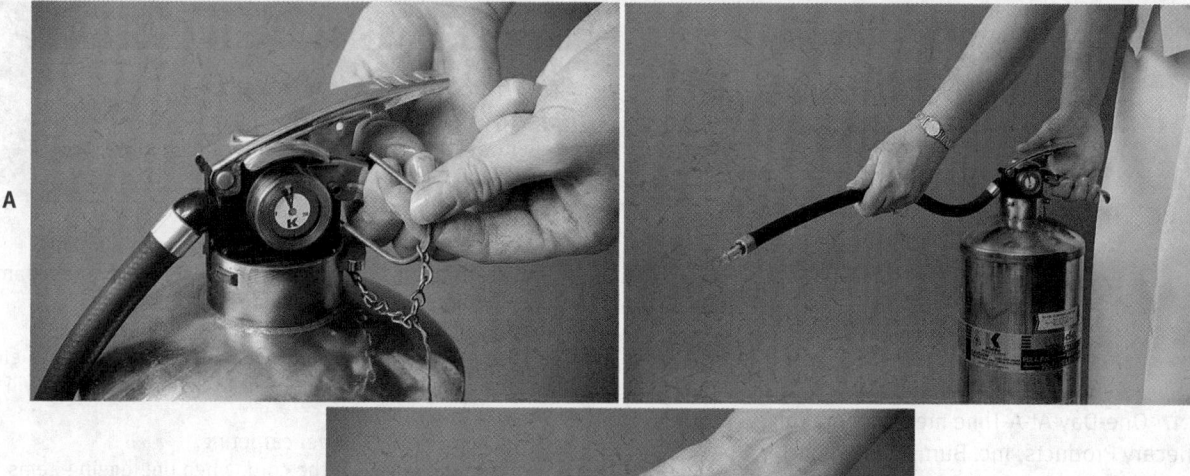

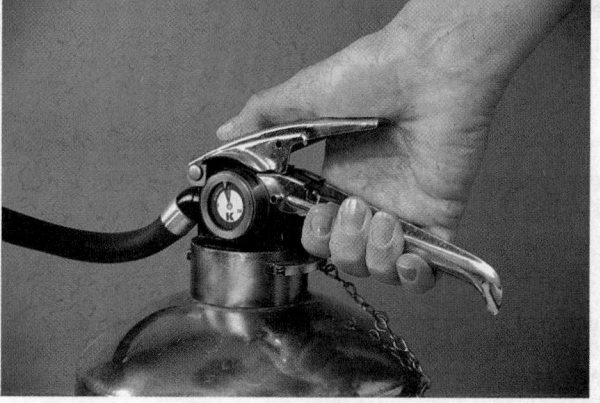

Figure 38-16 **A,** *P*ull the pin. **B,** *A*im at the base of the fire. **C,** *S*queeze the handles. *S*weep from side to side to coat the area evenly.

✳ BOX 38-12   **CLIENT TEACHING**

Correct Use of a Fire Extinguisher in the Home

Objectives
- Client will correctly place the extinguisher in the home.
- Client will describe when it is appropriate to use a home fire extinguisher.
- Client will demonstrate the correct technique when using a fire extinguisher.
- Client will state when fire extinguishers need to be replaced.

Teaching Strategies
- Discuss correct location of the extinguisher. It is recommended that one be placed on each level of the home, near an exit, in clear view, away from stoves and heating appliances, and above the reach of small children. Keep a fire extinguisher in the kitchen, near the furnace, and in the garage. Make sure clients read instructions after purchasing the extinguisher and keep them for periodic review.
- Describe the steps to take before using the extinguisher. Attempt to fight the fire only when all occupants have left the

home, the fire department has been called, the fire is confined to a small area, there is an exit route readily available, the extinguisher is the right type for the fire (see discussion in text for a description of the types of extinguishers), and the client knows how to use the extinguisher.
- Instruct the client to memorize the mnemonic PASS: *P*ull the pin to unlock handle, *A*im low at the base of the fire, *S*queeze the handles, and *S*weep the unit from side to side (see Figure 38-16).

Evaluation
- Client is able to correctly place an extinguisher in the home.
- Client correctly lists the steps to take before attempting to use an extinguisher.
- Client demonstrates correct use of the extinguisher while reciting the instructions with the mnemonic PASS.

Modified from National Safety Council: *Home fire prevention and preparedness fact sheet,* Itasca, Ill, 2002, The Council.

---

ton or disk batteries commonly found in games, cameras, calculators, and watches. In older adults, diminished eyesight and impaired memory results in accidental ingestion of poisonous substances or in accidental overdose of prescribed medications. To prevent medication errors on the part of clients in the home, recommend the use of medication organizers that are filled once

a week by the client and/or family. These organizers have the day and time on each box, so the client knows when and what to take at any given time (Figure 38-17). This is particularly useful for clients who forget whether they have taken their medications.

Also, adhere to guidelines for intervening in accidental poisoning. The poison control center phone number needs to be visible

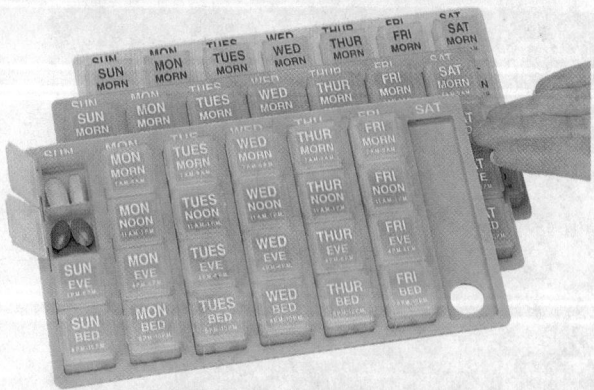

Figure 38-17 One-Day-At-A-Time medicine organizer. (Courtesy Apothecary Products, Inc, Burnsville, Minn.)

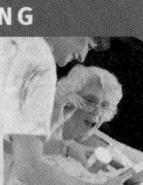

✳ BOX 38-14   CLIENT TEACHING

Prevention of Electrical Hazards

Objective
- Client will recognize electrical hazards in the home and eliminate them.

Teaching Strategies
- Discuss grounding appliances and other equipment.
- Provide examples of common hazards: frayed cords, damaged equipment, and overloaded outlets.
- Discuss guidelines to prevent electrical shocks:
  - Use extension cords only when necessary, and use electrical tape to secure the cord to the floor where it will not be stepped on.
  - Do not run wires under carpeting.
  - Grasp the plug, not the cord, when unplugging items.
  - Keep electrical items away from water.
  - Do not operate unfamiliar equipment.
  - Disconnect items before cleaning.

Evaluation
- Have client list electrical hazards existing in the home.
- Review steps the client will take to eliminate these hazards.
- Check the home after the client has had an opportunity to eliminate hazards.

✳ BOX 38-13   PROCEDURAL GUIDELINES

Interventions for Accidental Poisoning in the Home Setting

1. Assess for airway patency, breathing, and circulation (ABCs) in all clients in whom accidental poisoning is suspected.
2. Remove any visible materials from areas such as the mouth and eyes to terminate exposure.
3. Identify the type and amount of substance ingested, if possible. This helps to determine the antidote.
4. Call the poison control center before attempting any interventions. The universal phone number for poison control is (800) 222-1222.
5. If directed by a physician, give oral fluids to assist vomiting.
6. If directed, save vomitus for laboratory analysis, which will assist with further treatment.
7. Position the victim with the head to the side to prevent aspiration of vomitus, and assist in keeping the airway open.
8. Never induce vomiting in an unconscious victim or in a client experiencing convulsions, because aspiration will occur.
9. Never induce vomiting if any of the following substances have been ingested: lye, household cleaners, hair care products, grease or petroleum products, or furniture polish. Vomiting increases internal burns.
10. If instructed to take the victim to the emergency department, call an ambulance. Emergency equipment is sometimes needed en route.
11. In the case of convulsions, cessation of breathing, or unconsciousness, call 911.
12. Do not administer syrup of ipecac to induce vomiting. It has not been proven effective in preventing poisoning.

American Academy of Pediatrics: *News release—don't treat swallowed poison with syrup of ipecac*, 2004, www.aap.org/advocacy/releases/novpoison.htm.

---

on the telephone in homes with young children. In all cases of suspected poisoning, clients should call this number immediately (Box 38-13).

Electrical Hazards. Electrical equipment needs to be in good working order and grounded. The third (longer) prong in an electrical plug is the ground. Theoretically, the ground prong carries any stray electrical current back to the ground, hence its name. The other two prongs carry the power to the piece of electrical equipment. Improperly grounded or malfunctioning electrical equipment increases the risk of electrical injury and fire. Educating both the client and the family reduces the risk for electrical hazards in the home environment (Box 38-14).

If a client receives an electrical shock in a health care setting, immediately determine whether the client has a pulse. If the client has no pulse, initiate cardiopulmonary resuscitation (CPR) and notify emergency personnel (see Chapter 40). If the client has a pulse and remains alert and oriented, quickly obtain vital signs and assess the skin for signs of thermal injury. Make sure to notify the client's physician. If an electrical shock occurs in the home, follow the same procedure but have the client go to the emergency department and then notify the client's physician.

Seizures. Clients who have experienced some form of neurological injury or metabolic disturbance are at risk for a seizure. A seizure involves a hyperexcitation of neurons in the brain leading to a sudden, violent, involuntary series of contractions of a group of muscles. The client often loses consciousness. **Seizure precautions** encompass all nursing interventions to protect the client from traumatic injury, positioning for adequate ventilation and drainage of oral secretions, and providing privacy and support following the seizure (Skill 38-2).

During a seizure a client's jaw muscles become tense. Research has found that significant injury to the client's oral cavity is rare, even during the most violent seizures. Injury instead occurs from a caregiver forcing an object into the client's mouth and from the teeth biting down on a hard object. Soft objects will possibly break in the mouth during a seizure and be aspirated. The Epilepsy Foundation (2006), in its recommendations for seizure first aid,

SKILL 38-2   SEIZURE PRECAUTIONS

Delegation Considerations

The skill of seizure precautions cannot be delegated. If a seizure occurs, the nurse must constantly assess the client's airway patency, adequacy of breathing, and circulatory status. You must make clinical judgments quickly. Setting up seizure precautions and protecting clients at risk for seizures can be delegated. The nurse instructs nursing assistive personnel to:

- Notify the nurse when any seizure activity occurs.
- Protect at-risk clients from falls by assisting with ambulation and transfer.

- Never attempt to restrain a client's extremities during an actual seizure.

Equipment

- Oral airway
- Padding for side rails and headboard
- Suction machine, oral suction equipment
- Clean disposable gloves

STEPS	RATIONALE
1. Assess seizure history, noting frequency of seizures, presence of aura, and sequence of events, if known. Assess for medical and surgical conditions that will lead to seizures or exacerbate existing seizure condition. Assess medication history.	Enables the nurse to anticipate onset of seizure activity. Seizure medications must be taken as prescribed and not stopped suddenly, because this will precipitate seizure activity.
2. Inspect client's environment for potential safety hazards if risk for seizure exists: bedside stand or table, IV pole or other medical equipment.	Prevents client from sustaining injury by striking head or body on furniture or equipment.
3. Perform hand hygiene, and prepare bed with padded side rails and headboard, bed in low position, and client positioned in side-lying position when possible (see illustration).	Minimizes risks associated with seizure activity.
4. For clients with a history of seizures, an airway, suction apparatus, clean gloves, and pillows need to be visible in the hospital setting for immediate use.	Ensures prompt, organized intervention.
5. When a seizure begins, position client safely. If client is standing or sitting, guide client to floor and protect head by cradling in nurse's lap or placing a pillow under head. Clear surrounding area of furniture. If client is in bed, raise side rails, add padding, and put bed in low position.	Protects client from traumatic injury, especially head injury.
6. Provide privacy.	Embarrassment is common after a seizure, especially if others witnessed the seizure.

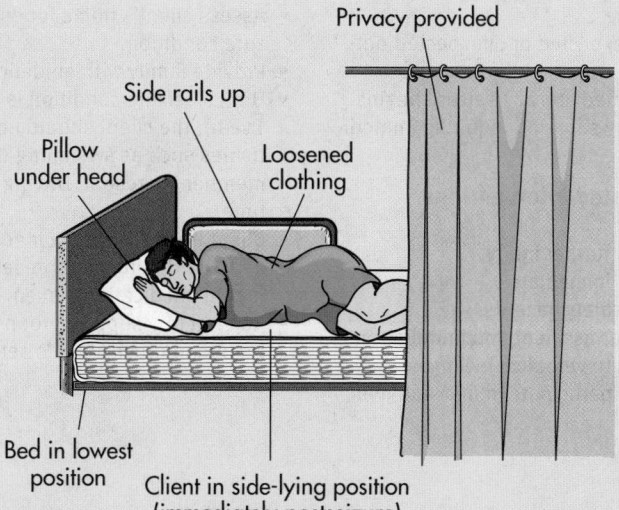

STEP 3 Provide client privacy. Put bed in lowest position with side rails up and padded. Position client in side-lying position, with pillow under head and loosened clothing.

Continued

✳ **SKILL 38-2**   **SEIZURE PRECAUTIONS—CONT'D**

STEPS

7. If possible, turn client on side, with head flexed slightly forward.
8. Do not restrain client. Loosen clothing.
9. Do not put anything into the client's mouth such as fingers, tongue depressor, or medicine.

RATIONALE

Prevents tongue and dentures from blocking the airway and promotes drainage of secretions, thus reducing risk of aspiration. Prevents musculoskeletal injury.

Critical Decision Point: Putting something in the client's mouth will possibly result in injury to the jaw, tongue, or teeth and cause stimulation of the gag reflex, causing vomiting, aspiration, and respiratory distress.

---

10. Stay with client, observing the sequence and timing of seizure activity.

Continued observation is necessary to ensure adequate ventilation during and following seizure activity. Accurate, specific observations will assist in documentation, diagnosis, and treatment of the seizure disorder.

11. After the seizure is over, explain what happened and answer client's questions. Foster an atmosphere of acceptance and respect.

Informing clients of the type of seizure activity experienced will assist them in participating knowledgeably in their care.

12. Following seizure, perform hand hygiene and assist client to position of comfort in bed with padded side rails up and bed in low position. Place call light within reach, and provide a quiet, nonstimulating environment.

Provides for continued safety. Clients are often confused and sleepy following a seizure.

Status Epilepticus

13. For a client experiencing status epilepticus, put on clean gloves and insert an oral airway when the jaw is relaxed between seizure activity. Hold airway with curved side up, insert downward until airway reaches back of throat, then rotate and follow natural curve of the tongue. Do not place fingers near or in client's mouth.

Prevents transmission of infection. Client is in continual seizure state and requires oral airway to ensure airway patency. Client will possibly inadvertently bite nurse's fingers during a seizure if nurse does not use caution.

14. Access oxygen and suction equipment. Prepare for IV insertion.

Intensive monitoring and treatment are required for this medical emergency.

15. Use pillows/pads to protect client from injuring self.

Helps avoid traumatic injury.

Recording and Reporting

- Record the timing of seizure activity and sequence of events. Record presence of aura (if any), level of consciousness, posture, color, movements of extremities, incontinence, and patterns of sleep following the seizure.
- Document client's response and expected or unexpected outcomes.
- Report to health care provider immediately as seizure begins. Status epilepticus is an emergency situation requiring immediate medical management.

Unexpected Outcomes and Related Interventions

1. Client suffers traumatic injury.
   a. Continue to protect client from further injury.
   b. Notify the health care provider immediately.
   c. Ensure environment is free of safety hazards.
2. Client verbalizes feelings of embarrassment and humiliation.
   a. Offer support, and allow client to verbalize feelings.
   b. Encourage client and family to participate in decision making and planning care.

Home Care Considerations

- Communicate with client and family to identify precipitating factors.
- Teach family to care for the client during a seizure.
- Assess client's home for environmental hazards in light of seizure condition.
- Provide family with guidelines to detect status epilepticus.
- Until a seizure condition is well controlled (usually for at least 1 year), the client should not take a tub bath or engage in activities such as swimming unless a knowledgeable family member is present. Driving may also be restricted during this time.
- Client needs to wear a medical alert bracelet or tag and have an ID card noting the presence of a seizure disorder and listing the medications taken.
- Referral to a support group or the Epilepsy Foundation will help to improve client's self-esteem and coping ability.

✳ TABLE 38-4 Postexposure Management of Bioterrorist-Related Illnesses

ILLNESS	DECONTAMINATION/EXPOSURE MANAGEMENT
Anthrax	In settings where threat of gross exposure exists, instruct clients to remove contaminated clothing and store in labeled, plastic bags. Handle clothing minimally to avoid agitation. Instruct clients to shower thoroughly with soap and water. Use standard precautions, and wear appropriate protective barriers when handling contaminated clothing or other items. Recommended postexposure prophylaxis includes the administration of IV or oral fluoroquinolones (e.g., ciprofloxacin, levofloxacin, and ofloxacin).
Botulism	Even a single case of botulism immediately raises concerns of an outbreak associated with contaminated food. The aim is to locate contaminated food and identify other persons who may have been exposed. Decontamination is not required because clients are not at risk for skin exposure or reaerosolization.
Plague	Risk for reaerosolization from contaminated clothing of exposed persons is low. In the case of gross exposure, instruct clients to remove contaminated clothing and store in labeled, plastic bags. Handle clothing minimally to avoid agitation. Instruct clients to shower thoroughly with soap and water. Use standard precautions, and wear appropriate protective barriers when handling contaminated clothing or other items. Postexposure prophylaxis is recommended for clients and health care workers. The antimicrobial agent of choice is streptomycin.
Smallpox	Client decontamination after exposure to smallpox is not indicated. Handle items potentially contaminated by infectious lesions using contact isolation precautions. Postexposure immunization with smallpox vaccine is available and effective.

Modified from Dire DJ: *CBRNE—Biological warfare agents,* 2006, http://www.emedicine.com/emerg/byname/cbrne—-biological-warfare-agents.htm.

includes avoiding the insertion of objects into the mouth. The exception is in the case of **status epilepticus,** a medical emergency whereby a person has continual seizures without interruption. An adequate airway is maintained with an oral airway. Never restrain clients experiencing a seizure. Instead, place them on seizure precautions and adequately protect them from traumatic injury.

Radiation. Radiation is a health hazard in the health care setting and the community. Radiation and radioactive materials are used in the diagnosis and treatment of clients. Hospitals have strict guidelines on the care of clients who are receiving radiation and radioactive materials. Be familiar with established agency protocols. To reduce the nurse's exposure to radiation, limit the time spent near the source, make the distance from the source as great as possible, and use shielding devices such as lead aprons. Staff working near radiation will wear devices that track the accumulative exposure to radiation.

Some communities are at risk for radiation exposure because of incorrect disposal and transportation of radioactive waste products. Community health agencies and the Environmental Protection Agency (EPA) have established specific, strict guidelines for the disposal of radioactive waste. If a radioactive leak occurs, these agencies institute measures to prevent exposure of surrounding neighborhoods, to clean up radioactive leaks as quickly as possible, and to ensure that injured parties receive prompt medical care.

Bioterrorist Attack. If a bioterrorist attack occurs, nurses working in hospital settings need to be prepared to respond and care for a sudden influx of clients. TJC (2006) requires hospitals to have an emergency management plan that addresses four phases:

- *Mitigation*—Assessment process to determine hazard vulnerability for the hospital's service area. This includes an identification of the kinds of emergency situations that are most likely to occur and their probable impact.
- *Preparedness*—Steps taken to increase a hospital's ability to manage the effects of an attack. Hospital preparedness in-

cludes creating an inventory of resources (staff to supplies) that are necessary. This includes establishing agreements with product vendors and other health care facilities to provide increased resources in the event of an attack. In addition, preparedness includes establishing primary and backup communications systems, training staff, and conducting organization-wide drills.

- *Response*—Steps taken by staff in the event of an attack. A formal response includes reporting to predetermined locations, using specific triage strategies to identify the most acutely ill, and management activities such as issuing warnings and notifications to the community. Decontamination procedures and disease reporting are also part of a hospital's response plan.
- *Recovery*—Steps taken to restore essential services and resume normal agency operations. This phase begins almost as soon as the response phase.

All hospitals must test their emergency plans twice a year. This includes implementation of planned drills. Communication is a key to any emergency management plan. If a bioterrorist attack occurs, nursing staff must know what happened, how many clients to expect, and when clients will begin to arrive so they can prepare both themselves and their facility (Steinhauer and Bauer, 2002).

Infection control practices are critical in the event of a biological attack. You need to manage all clients symptomatic with suspected or confirmed bioterrorism-related illnesses using standard precautions (see Chapter 34). For certain diseases, such as smallpox or pneumonic plague, additional precautions are necessary, such as airborne or contact isolation precautions. Although most infections associated with biological agents cannot be transmitted from client to client, in general you limit the transport and movement of clients to movement that is essential for treatment and care. An important aspect of care for clients who have a bioterrorism-related illness is postexposure management. Table 38-4 summarizes the steps to take to manage exposure to anthrax, botulism, plague, and smallpox.

◆Evaluation

You apply the components of critical thinking to the evaluation step of the nursing process (Figure 38-18). You evaluate the actual care delivered by the health care team based on the expected outcomes. If you have met the client's goals, you consider the nursing interventions effective and appropriate. If not, you determine whether new risks to the client have developed or whether previous risks remain. The client and family need to participate to find permanent ways to reduce risks to safety. The nurse continually assesses the client's and family's need for additional support services such as home care, physical therapy, counseling, and further teaching.

When you have developed a good relationship with a client and the client feels safe and secure in the relationship, as well as in the environment, the client will most likely demonstrate less anxiety and verbalize satisfaction with the surroundings. You need to determine, however, if client expectations have been met. If outcomes are not met, these are questions to ask: Are you satisfied with changes made to the environment? Do you believe that your safety is ensured? If client expectations have not been met, you reassess not only the client and the environment but also the client's expressed desires.

• • •

A safe environment is essential to promoting, maintaining, and restoring health. Incorporating critical thinking skills in the application of the nursing process, the nurse assesses the client and the environment to determine risk factors for injury; clusters risk factors; formulates a nursing diagnosis; and plans specific interventions, including client education. The expected outcomes include a safe physical environment, a client whose expectations have been met, a client who is knowledgeable about safety factors and precautions, and a client free of injury.

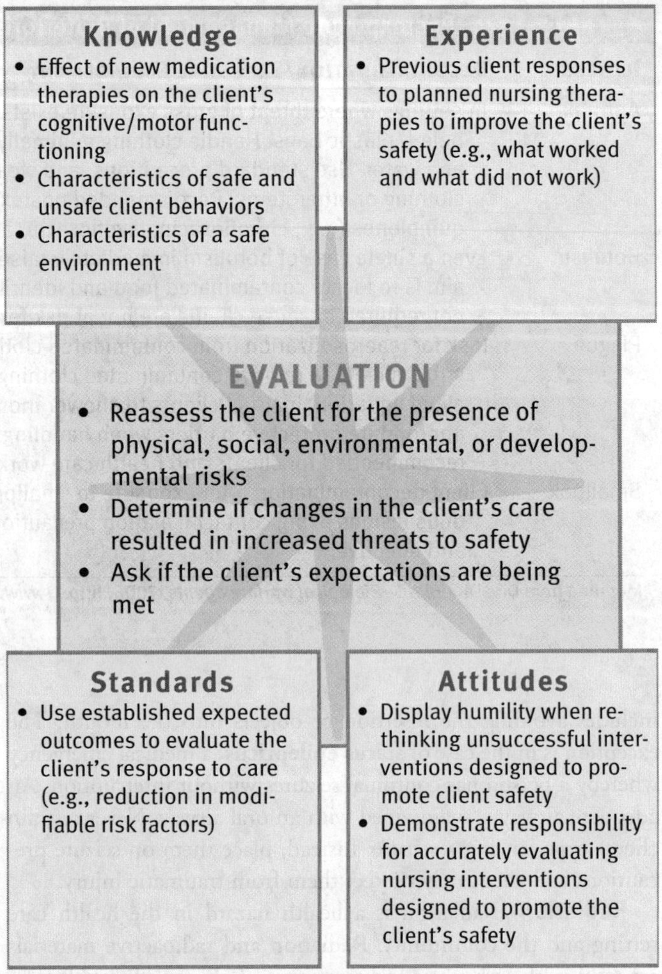

✳ Key Concepts

- In the community a safe environment means basic needs are achievable, reducing physical hazards and the transmission of pathogens, controlling pollution, and maintaining sanitation.
- In a health care agency a safe environment is one that minimizes falls, client-inherent accidents, procedure-inherent accidents, and equipment-related accidents.
- A factor that reduces atmospheric oxygen is the presence of high carbon monoxide levels, which results from an improperly functioning furnace.
- Prolonged exposure to extreme environmental temperatures causes client injury or even death.
- Reduction of physical hazards in the environment includes providing adequate lighting, decreasing clutter, and securing the home.
- Reduce the transmission of pathogens through medical and surgical asepsis, immunization, adequate food sanitation, insect and rodent control, and appropriate disposal of human waste.

Knowledge
- Effect of new medication therapies on the client's cognitive/motor functioning
- Characteristics of safe and unsafe client behaviors
- Characteristics of a safe environment

Experience
- Previous client responses to planned nursing therapies to improve the client's safety (e.g., what worked and what did not work)

EVALUATION
- Reassess the client for the presence of physical, social, environmental, or developmental risks
- Determine if changes in the client's care resulted in increased threats to safety
- Ask if the client's expectations are being met

Standards
- Use established expected outcomes to evaluate the client's response to care (e.g., reduction in modifiable risk factors)

Attitudes
- Display humility when rethinking unsuccessful interventions designed to promote client safety
- Demonstrate responsibility for accurately evaluating nursing interventions designed to promote the client's safety

Figure 38-18 Critical thinking model for safety evaluation.

- Children less than 5 years of age are at greatest risk for home accidents that result in severe injury and death.
- The school-age child is at risk for injury at home, at school, and while traveling to and from school.
- Adolescents are at risk for injury from automobile accidents, suicide, and substance abuse.
- Threats to an adult's safety are frequently associated with lifestyle habits.
- Risks for injury for older clients are directly related to the physiological changes of the aging process.
- Nursing interventions for promoting safety are individualized for developmental stage, lifestyle, and environment.
- Nursing interventions are developed to modify the environment for protection from falls, fires, poisonings, and electrical hazards.
- An emergency management plan includes the elements of mitigation, preparedness, response, and recovery.
- The nurse needs to manage all clients symptomatic with suspected or confirmed bioterrorism-related illnesses using standard precautions.

✳ Critical Thinking Exercises

While making a routine visit, Peggy, Ms. Cohen's daughter, finds Ms. Cohen at the bottom of her porch steps. Ms. Cohen is complaining of hip pain and cannot get up. Peggy calls 911. A few hours later, Ms. Cohen is hospitalized for repair of her right hip fracture.

1. List three environmental interventions to promote Ms. Cohen's safety in her room.
2. Ms. Cohen's bed has four side rails. What position would you put the rails in and why?
3. What are Ms. Cohen's intrinsic factors that make her at higher risk for falls while in the hospital?

Ms. Cohen requires IV antibiotics to be delivered postoperatively. Shortly after the first dose, she became restless and started picking at her IV.

1. What might be precipitating Ms. Cohen's behavior?
2. Why should the nurse avoid using physical restraints on Ms. Cohen?
3. List two interventions that can be utilized to prevent the use of restraints on Ms. Cohen.

Several restraint alternatives were attempted, but due to Ms. Cohen's restlessness she was successful at pulling out her IV. It becomes necessary to restrain Ms. Cohen temporarily during IV antibiotic therapy.

1. You know that a physician's or health care provider's order is required for the restraint. What are essential components of the restraint order?
2. What assessment is performed on Ms. Cohen's upper extremity while she is restrained?
3. The physician orders bilateral upper limb restraints. Your assessment of Ms. Cohen reveals that during the day only her left arm needs to be restrained in order to maintain her IV. Can you remove the right limb restraint?

✳ NCLEX®-Style Review Questions

1. The physiological changes that occur during the aging process increase the older client's risk for:
   1. Poisoning
   2. Alcoholism
   3. Falls and burns
   4. Medication errors

2. You discover an electrical fire in a client's room. Your first action would be to:
   1. Activate the fire alarm
   2. Confine the fire by closing all doors and windows
   3. Evacuate any clients or visitors in immediate danger
   4. Extinguish the fire by using the nearest fire extinguisher

3. A parent calls the pediatrician's office frantic about the bottle of cleaner that her 2-year-old son drank. Which of the following is the most important instruction you can give to this parent?
   1. Give the child milk.
   2. Give the child syrup of ipecac.
   3. Call the poison control center.
   4. Take the child to the emergency department.

4. A couple is with their adolescent daughter for a school physical. The parents tell you that they are worried about all the safety risks affecting this age. As you plan to teach the parents about these risks, you remember that adolescents are at a greater risk for injury from:
   1. Home accidents
   2. Physiological changes of aging
   3. Poisoning and child abduction
   4. Automobile accidents, suicide, and substance abuse

5. During the night shift a client is found wandering the hospital halls looking for a bathroom. The nurse's initial intervention would be to:
   1. Insert a urinary catheter
   2. Ask the physician to order a restraint
   3. Assign a staff member to stay with the client
   4. Provide scheduled toileting during the night shift

6. Lisa, a nurse assistant, is working with you during your shift. One of your clients has upper limb restraints. In delegating care of this client to the Lisa, you would tell her to:
   1. Move the client to a room closer to the nurses' station
   2. Check to see if the client can have a medication for sleep
   3. Call the physician if the client becomes more agitated with the restraint
   4. Report any signs of redness, excoriation, or constriction of circulation under the restraint

7. The family of your confused, ambulatory client insists that all four side rails be up when the client is alone. The best way to handle this situation would be to:
   1. Ask them to stay with the client at all times
   2. Inform them of the risks associated with side rail use
   3. Thank them for being conscientious and put the four rails up
   4. Provide the client a one-to-one sitter while the side rails are up

8. During your assessment of a 56-year-old man, he reports increased alcohol consumption due to stress at work. One of your expected outcomes for this client will be to:
   1. Decrease stress in his life
   2. Teach him ways to promote sleep
   3. Decrease his alcohol intake during stress
   4. Provide the client with resources for stress management classes

9. Health care workers who have direct contact with individuals suspected of being contaminated with anthrax should (select all that apply):
   1. Have the client remove clothing and place in a sealed biohazard bag
   2. Instruct client to wash hands and exposed areas with soap and water
   3. Wear an isolation gown, gloves, and high-efficiency particulate air (HEPA) mask
   4. Prepare the client for transfer to the radiology department for a chest x-ray examination

10. A child you are caring for in the hospital starts to have a grand mal seizure while playing in the playroom. What is the most important intervention you can do during this situation?
    1. Begin cardiopulmonary respiration.
    2. Restrain the child to prevent injury.
    3. Place a tongue blade over the tongue to prevent aspiration.
    4. Clear the area around the child to protect the child from injury.

39 | Hygiene

✳ OBJECTIVES

Mastery of content in this chapter will enable the student to:

- Describe factors that influence personal hygiene practices.
- Discuss the role critical thinking plays in providing hygiene.
- Conduct a comprehensive assessment of a client's total hygiene needs.
- Discuss conditions that place clients at risk for impaired skin integrity.
- Discuss factors that influence the condition of the nails and feet.
- Explain the importance of foot care for the diabetic client.

- Discuss conditions that place clients at risk for impaired oral mucous membranes.
- List common hair and scalp problems and their related interventions.
- Describe how hygiene care for the older adult client differs from that for the younger client.
- Discuss the different approaches used in maintaining a client's comfort during hygiene care.
- Successfully perform hygiene procedures for the care of the skin, perineum, feet and nails, mouth, eyes, ears, and nose.

✳ MEDIA RESOURCES   ✳ KEY TERMS

 Companion CD
- NCLEX®-Style Review Questions
- Audio Glossary
- Interactive Learning Activities
- English/Spanish Glossary

evolve Website
- NCLEX®-Style Review Questions
- Audio Glossary
- English/Spanish Glossary
- Interactive Learning Activities
- Weblinks
- Audio Summaries
- Video Clips

Acne, p. 858
Alopecia, p. 856
Apocrine, p. 858
Buccal glands, p. 851
Caries, p. 859
Cerumen, p. 857
Complete bed bath, p. 867
Cuticle, p. 851
Dermis, p. 851
Eccrine, p. 858
Edentulous, p. 859
Effleurage, p. 868

Enucleation, p. 894
Epidermis, p. 850
Gingivitis, p. 851
Halitosis, p. 856
Lunula, p. 851
Mastication, p. 851
Neuropathy, p. 856
Ophthalmologist, p. 894
Optometrist, p. 894
Partial bed bath, p. 867
Perineal care, p. 868
Stomatitis, p. 885

Personal hygiene affects client's comfort, safety, and well-being. Well people are capable of meeting their own hygiene needs. Ill or physically challenged people often require various levels of assistance. A variety of personal, social, and cultural factors influence hygiene practices. In agency or home care settings, determine a client's ability to perform self-care and provide hygienic care according to the client's needs and preferences. In addition in the home setting, help the client and family adapt hygiene techniques and approaches.

Because hygienic care requires close contact with the client, use communication skills (see Chapter 24) to promote a caring therapeutic relationship and to use the time with the client for teaching and counseling. You can integrate other nursing activities during hygiene care, including client assessment and interventions such as range-of-motion (ROM) exercises, application of dressings, or inspection and care of intravenous sites. During hygiene care, try to preserve as much of the client's independence as possible, assess client's ability to perform hygiene care, ensure privacy, convey respect, and foster the client's physical comfort.

Scientific Knowledge Base

Proper hygienic care requires an understanding of the anatomy and physiology of the integument, oral cavity, and the eyes, ears, and nose. The skin and mucosa cells exchange oxygen, nutrients, and fluids with underlying blood vessels. The cells require adequate nutrition, hydration, and circulation to resist injury and disease. Good hygiene techniques promote the normal structure and function of body tissues.

In addition, apply knowledge of pathophysiology to provide good preventive hygienic care. Learn to recognize those disease states that create changes in the integument, oral cavity, and sensory organs. For example, diabetes mellitus results in chronic vascular changes that impair healing of the skin and mucosa. In the early stages of acquired immunodeficiency syndrome (AIDS), fungal infections of the oral cavity are common. As a result of a stroke, paralysis of the trigeminal nerve (cranial nerve V) eliminates the blink reflex, causing risk of corneal drying. In the presence of conditions such as these, adapt hygiene practices to anticipate client needs and minimize any injurious effects. Integrate knowledge of anatomy, physiology, and pathophysiology during hygiene care; take this time to identify abnormalities and initiate appropriate actions to prevent further injury to sensitive tissues.

The Skin

The skin is an active organ with the functions of protection, secretion, excretion, temperature regulation, and sensation (Table 39-1). The skin has three primary layers: epidermis, dermis, and subcutaneous. The **epidermis** (outer layer) is composed of several thin layers of cells undergoing different stages of maturation. It shields underlying tissue against water loss and injury and prevents entry of disease-producing microorganisms. The innermost layer of the epidermis generates new cells to replace the dead cells that the skin's outer surface continuously sheds. Bacteria commonly reside on the outer epidermis. These resident bacteria are normal flora (see Chapter 34) that do not cause disease but instead inhibit the multiplication of disease-causing microorganisms.

✳ **TABLE 39-1 Function of the Skin and Implications for Care**

FUNCTION/DESCRIPTION	IMPLICATIONS FOR CARE
Protection Epidermis is relatively impermeable layer that prevents entrance of microorganisms. Although microorganisms reside on skin surface and in hair follicles, relative dryness of skin's surface inhibits bacterial growth. Sebum removes bacteria from hair follicles. Acidic pH of skin further retards bacterial growth.	Weakening of epidermis occurs by scraping or stripping its surface (e.g., use of dry razors, tape removal, improper turning or positioning techniques). Excessive dryness causes cracks and breaks in skin and mucosa that allow bacteria to enter. Emollients soften skin and prevent moisture loss, soaking of skin improves moisture retention, and hydration of mucosa prevents dryness. However, constant exposure of skin to moisture causes maceration or softening, which interrupts dermal integrity and promotes ulcer formation and bacterial growth. Keep bed linen and clothing dry. Misuse of soap, detergents, cosmetics, deodorant, and depilatories cause chemical irritation. Alkaline soaps neutralize the protective acid condition of skin. Cleansing of skin removes excess oil, sweat, dead skin cells, and dirt that promote bacterial growth.
Sensation Skin contains sensory organs for touch, pain, heat, cold, and pressure.	Minimize friction to avoid loss of stratum corneum, which will result in development of pressure ulcers. Smoothing linen removes sources of mechanical irritation. Remove rings from fingers to prevent accidentally injuring client's skin. Make sure bath water is not excessively hot or cold.
Temperature Regulation Radiation, evaporation, conduction, and convection control body temperature.	Factors that interfere with heat loss alter temperature control. Wet bed linen or gowns interfere with convection and conduction. Excess blankets or bed coverings interfere with heat loss through radiation and conduction. Coverings promote heat conservation.
Excretion and Secretion Sweat promotes heat loss by evaporation. Sebum lubricates skin and hair.	Perspiration and oil harbor microorganisms. Bathing removes excess body secretions, although if excessive, it causes dry skin.

The **dermis** is a thicker skin layer containing bundles of collagen and elastic fibers to support the epidermis. Nerve fibers, blood vessels, sweat glands, sebaceous glands, and hair follicles course through the dermal layers. Sebaceous glands secrete sebum, an oily, odorous fluid, into the hair follicles.

The subcutaneous tissue layer contains blood vessels, nerves, lymph, and loose connective tissue filled with fat cells. The fatty tissue is a heat insulator for the body. Subcutaneous tissue also supports upper skin layers to withstand stresses and pressure without injury. Very little subcutaneous tissue underlies the oral mucosa.

The skin often reflects a change in physical condition by alterations in color, thickness, texture, turgor, temperature, and hydration (see Chapter 33). As long as the skin remains intact and healthy, its physiological function remains optimal.

The Feet, Hands, and Nails

The feet, hands, and nails often require special attention to prevent infection. Any injury or deformity to the foot, including any growths or injuries to the overlying skin, are painful and thus interfere with a client's normal ability to walk and bear weight. The hand, in contrast to the foot, is constructed largely for manipulation rather than support.

A wide range of dexterity exists in the hand because of the wide range of movement between the thumb and fingers. Any condition that interferes with movement of the hand (e.g., superficial or deep pain or joint inflammation) impairs a client's self-help abilities.

The nails are epithelial tissues that grow from the root of the nail bed, located in the skin at the nail groove, hidden by the fold of skin called the **cuticle.** The visible part of the nail is the nail body. It has a crescent-shaped white area known as the **lunula.**

Under the nail lies a layer of epithelium called the nail bed (Figure 39-1). A normal healthy nail is transparent, smooth, and convex, with a pink nail bed and translucent white tip. Disease causes changes in the shape, thickness, and curvature of the nail (see Chapter 33).

The Oral Cavity

The oral cavity is lined with mucous membranes continuous with the skin. The oral or buccal cavity consists of the lips surrounding the opening of the mouth, the cheeks running along the sidewalls of the cavity, the tongue and its muscles, and the hard and soft palate. The oral mucosa is normally light pink and moist. The floor of the mouth and the undersurface of the tongue are richly supplied with blood vessels. Any type of ulceration or trauma results in significant bleeding. There are three pairs of salivary glands that secrete about 1 L of saliva a day. The **buccal glands** found in the mucosa lining the cheeks and mouth maintain the hygiene and comfort of oral tissues. The effects of medications, exposure to radiation, and mouth breathing impair salivary secretion in the mouth.

The teeth are the organs of chewing, or **mastication.** They are designed to cut, tear, and grind ingested food so it can be mixed with saliva and swallowed. A normal tooth consists of the crown, neck, and root (Figure 39-2). The periodontal membrane lies just below the gum margins, surrounds a tooth, and holds it firmly in place. Healthy teeth appear white, smooth, shiny, and properly aligned.

Difficulty in chewing develops when surrounding gum tissues become inflamed or infected or when teeth are lost or become loosened. Regular oral hygiene is necessary to maintain the integrity of tooth surfaces and to prevent **gingivitis,** or gum inflammation.

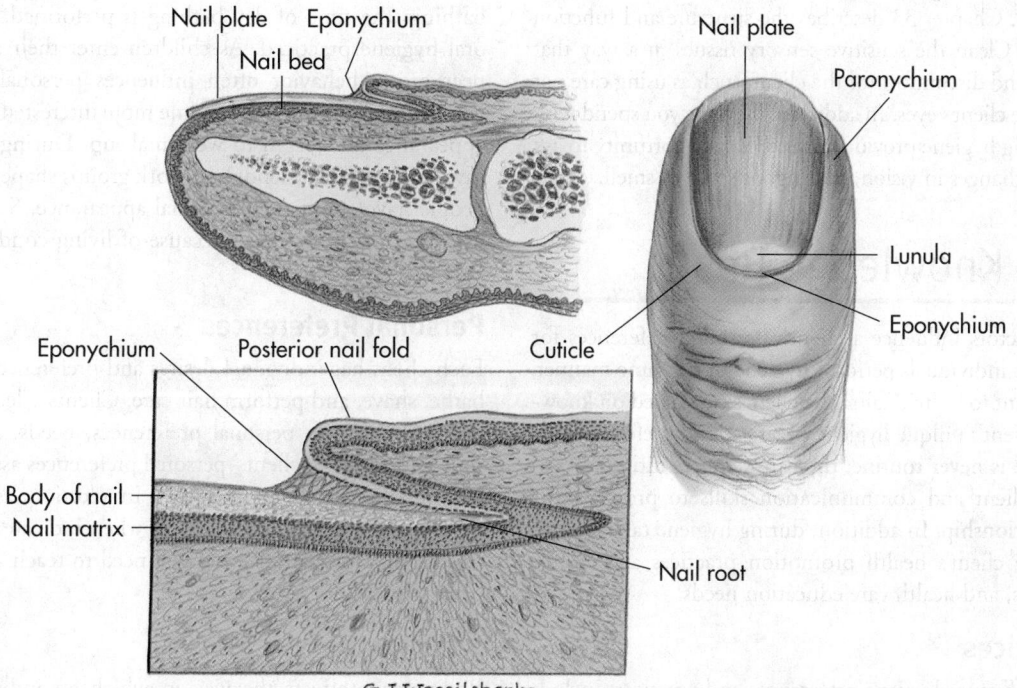

Figure 39-1 Anatomical structure of a normal nail. (From Thompson J and others: *Clinical nursing,* ed 4, St. Louis, 1997, Mosby.)

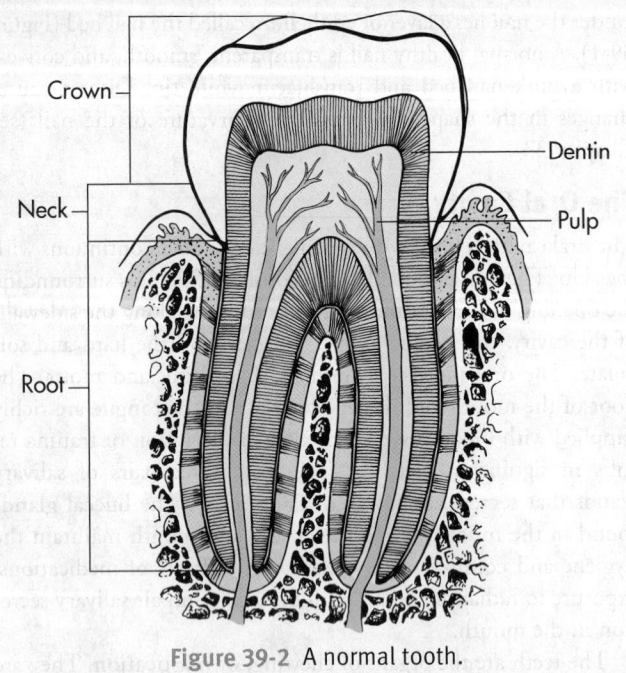

Figure 39-2 A normal tooth.

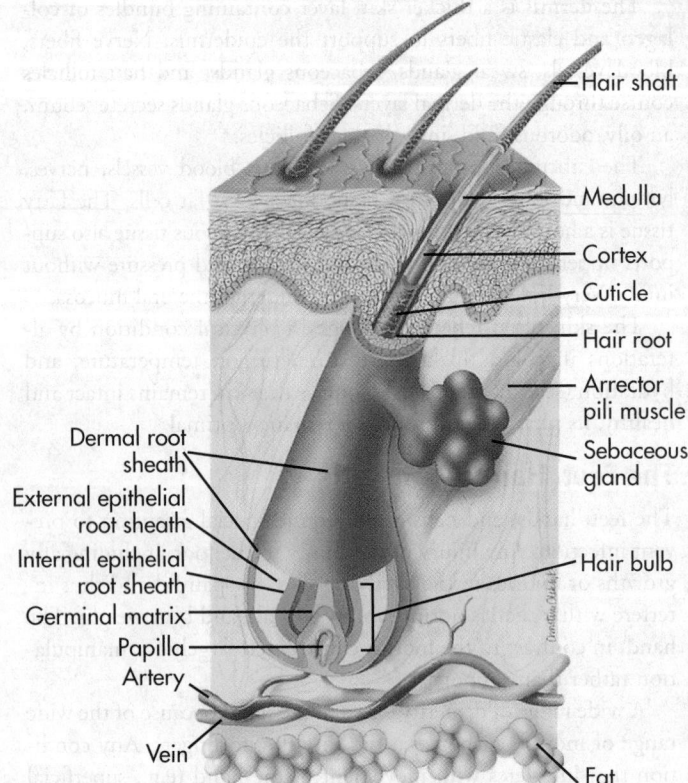

Figure 39-3 Hair follicle, relationship of a follicle and related structures to the epidermal and dermal layers of the skin. (From Thibodeau GA, Patton KT: *Anatomy and physiology,* ed 5, St. Louis, 2003, Mosby.)

The Hair

Hair growth, distribution, and pattern indicate a person's general health status. Hormonal changes, emotional and physical stress, aging, infection, and certain illnesses affect hair characteristics. The hair shaft itself is lifeless, and physiological factors do not directly affect it. However, hormonal and nutrient deficiencies of the hair follicle cause changes in its color or condition (Figure 39-3).

The Eyes, Ears, and Nose

When nurses provide hygienic care, the eyes, ears, and nose require careful attention. Chapter 33 describes the structure and function of these organs. Clean the sensitive sensory tissues in a way that prevents injury and discomfort for the client, such as using care not to get soap in the client's eyes. In addition, the time you spend with your client during hygiene provides an excellent opportunity to ask if there are any changes in vision, hearing, or sense of smell.

Nursing Knowledge Base

A number of factors influence a client's personal preferences for hygiene. No two individuals perform hygiene in the same manner, and it is important to individualize the client's care based on knowing about the client's unique hygiene practices and preferences.

Hygiene care is never routine; the care requires intimate contact with the client and communication skills to promote the therapeutic relationship. In addition, during hygiene take time to learn about the client's health promotion practices and needs, emotional needs, and health care education needs.

Social Practices

Social groups influence hygiene preferences and practices, including the type of hygienic products used and the nature and frequency of personal care. During childhood, family customs influ-

ence hygiene. This includes, for example, the frequency of bathing, the time of day bathing is performed, and the type of oral hygiene practiced. As children enter their adolescent years, peer group behavior often influences personal hygiene. Some young girls, for example, become more interested in their personal appearance and begin to wear makeup. During the adult years, involvement with friends and work groups shape the expectations people have about their personal appearance. Some older adults' hygiene practices change because of living conditions and available resources.

Personal Preferences

Each client has individual desires and preferences about when to bathe, shave, and perform hair care. Clients select different products according to personal preferences, needs, and financial resources. Knowing clients' personal preferences assists in providing individualized care for the client. In addition, assist the client in developing new hygiene practices when indicated by an illness or condition. For example, you will need to teach a client with diabetes proper foot hygiene.

Body Image

Body image affects the way in which an individual maintains hygiene. If a client is neatly groomed, consider the details of grooming when planning care and consult the client before making decisions about how to provide hygienic care. Clients who appear unkempt or uninterested in hygiene often require education about the importance of hygiene or further assessment regarding their ability to participate with daily hygiene.

A client's general appearance reflects the importance hygiene holds for that person. Body image is a person's subjective concept of his or her body, including physical appearance, structure, or function (see Chapter 27). These images change frequently. When clients undergo surgery, illness, or a change in functional status, body image changes dramatically. For this reason, take extra effort to promote the client's hygienic comfort and appearance.

Socioeconomic Status

A person's economic resources influence the type and extent of hygiene practices used. Be sensitive in considering that the client's economic status influences his or her ability to regularly maintain hygiene. When clients have the added problem of a lack of socioeconomic resources, it becomes difficult to participate and take a responsible role in health promotion activities such as basic hygiene.

When basic care items are not affordable, work to find alternatives. It is also important to learn if use of these products is a part of the social habits practiced by the client's social group. For example, not all clients choose to use deodorant or cosmetics.

Health Beliefs and Motivation

Knowledge about the importance of hygiene and its implications for a person's well-being influences hygiene practices. However, knowledge alone is not enough. Motivation is a key factor in the importance of hygiene. An internal barrier that may affect the success of hygiene practices is lack of motivation because of insufficient knowledge. Overcome this barrier by assessing the client's needs and providing appropriate information. Provide materials that discuss the health-related issues relevant to the target behavior, including the short- and long-term consequences for the client. Individuals play a critical role in the determination of their own health status, because self-care represents the dominant mode of health care in our society. Many personal decisions are made daily that shape lifestyle and the social and physical environments (Pender, Murdaugh, and Parsons, 2002).

It is important to know if a client perceives being at risk. For example, does the client perceive being at risk for dental disease, that dental disease is serious, and that brushing and flossing are effective in reducing risk? When clients recognize there is a risk and that they can take reasonable action with no negative consequence, they are more likely to be receptive to the nurse's counseling and teaching efforts.

Cultural Variables

A client's cultural beliefs and personal values influence hygiene care (Box 39-1). People from diverse cultural backgrounds follow different self-care practices (see Chapter 9). Culturally, maintaining cleanliness does not hold the same importance for some ethnic groups as it does for others (Galanti, 2004). Do not express disapproval when caring for clients whose hygienic practices are different from yours. In North America it is common to bathe or shower daily, whereas in some other cultures it is customary to completely bathe only once a week.

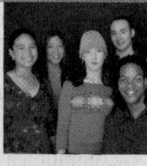

BOX 39-1 CULTURAL ASPECTS OF CARE

Hygiene Practices

Clients need a culturally competent plan for hygiene care. For some, hygiene practices are influenced by culture and are a potential source of conflict and stress in a hospital environment. Bathing, perineal hygiene, and hair care practices are sensitive issues. Hygiene is a very personal matter; clients from different cultures have different care practices and caregiver requirements.

Implications for Practice
- Maintain privacy, especially for women from cultures that value female modesty.
- Provide gender-congruent caregivers as needed or requested.
  - In some cultures touching between unrelated males and females is taboo.
  - If gender-congruent caregivers are not available, ask the family for assistance.
- Do not cut or shave hair without discussion with the client or family (Galanti, 2004).
- Some cultures (e.g., Chinese, Filipino) avoid bathing for 7 to 10 days following childbirth (Galanti, 2004).
- Some cultures (e.g., Chinese, Japanese, Koreans, Hindus) consider the top parts of the body cleaner than lower parts.
- Among Hindus and Muslims the left hand is used for cleaning, whereas the right hand is used for eating and praying.

Physical Condition

Clients with certain types of physical limitations or disabilities often lack the physical energy and dexterity to perform hygienic care. A client in traction or a cast or who has an intravenous line or other device connected to the body needs assistance with hygiene. Illnesses causing pain limit the dexterity and range of motion needed to perform certain measures. Clients still under the effects of sedation will not have the mental clarity or coordination to perform self-care. Chronic illnesses, such as cardiac disease, cancer, neurological disorders, and certain psychiatric conditions often exhaust or incapacitate a client. A weakened grasp resulting from arthritis, stroke, or muscular disorders prevents a client from using a toothbrush, washcloth, or comb.

Critical Thinking

Successful critical thinking requires synthesis of knowledge, experience, information gathered from clients, critical thinking attitudes, and intellectual and professional standards. Clinical judgments require you to anticipate the information necessary to analyze data and make decisions regarding client care. A client's condition is always changing, requiring ongoing critical thinking. During assessment, consider all elements that build toward making appropriate nursing diagnoses (Figure 39-4).

Because hygienic care is so important for a client to feel comfortable, refreshed, and renewed, avoid making hygiene care a simple routine. Instead, integrate knowledge from nursing and other disciplines, previous experiences in providing hygiene, and

Knowledge

- Anatomy and physiology of integument, oral cavity, and sense organs
- Principles of comfort and safety
- Communication principles that convey caring
- Risk factors posing hygiene problems
- Knowledge of cultural variations in hygiene

Experience

- Prior experience caring for clients requiring assistance with hygiene
- Personal hygiene practices

ASSESSMENT

- Observe the client's physical condition and integrity of integument, oral cavity, and sense organs
- Explore any developmental factors influencing the client's hygiene needs
- Note the client's self-care ability and hygiene practices
- Determine the client's cultural preferences

Standards

- Apply American Diabetes Association's practice standards for foot care
- Apply Wound Ostomy Continency Nurses (WOCN) and NPUAP guidelines on prevention and management of pressure ulcers
- Assess any skin alterations using accurate and consistent measurements

Attitudes

- Display curiosity; be thorough in assessing the condition of the client's tissues; changes may indicate signs of disease
- Display humility; hygiene care is not the same for all clients; know when to learn more about the client's preferences

Figure 39-4 Critical thinking model for hygiene assessment.

✷ BOX 39-2   NURSING ASSESSMENT QUESTIONS

Nature of Problems Related to Hygiene
- Have you noticed any skin changes or irritation?
- Is there any change in oral care requirements?
- Have you noticed a decrease in your ability to complete hygiene activities?
- Do you need assistance with any hygiene activities?

Changes in Physical Condition During Hygiene
- Do hygiene activities cause any symptoms, such as shortness of breath, pain, or fatigue?
- If you have fatigue or discomfort during hygiene, what can we do to minimize these symptoms?
- What aspects of hygiene may worsen your discomfort?

Assistance With Hygiene
- Do you need someone of the same gender or your family to assist in hygiene care?
- What aspects of personal hygiene do you feel you need to provide for yourself?
- How can I make assisting you with your hygiene easier?

information gathered from clients. The use of critical thinking attitudes, such as curiosity and humility, is necessary to design a plan of care to meet the client's hygiene needs. Use professional standards, such as those from the American Diabetes Association and skin care practices supported by the Agency for Healthcare Research and Quality (AHRQ) when planning care to meet the client's hygiene needs.

Nursing Process

◆Assessment

As you prepare to provide hygiene care, conduct a brief history to determine important areas for hygiene care (Box 39-2). This helps to focus additional areas for assessment. Nursing assessment is an ongoing process. All body regions are not completely assessed before administering hygiene; however, routinely assess the client's

condition whenever giving care. For example, during oral care inspect the condition of the teeth and oral mucosa. When a client has a repeated problem (e.g., dry skin or inflamed oral mucosa), conduct an assessment before care is administered because variations in technique are often necessary. Hygiene care is an opportunity to assess and identify findings for a variety of health care problems.

Physical Examination. While assisting a client with personal hygiene, carefully assess the integument, oral cavity structures, and the eyes, ears, and nose (see Chapter 33). Using the skills of inspection and palpation, look for alterations in the integrity and function of tissues. The assessment also reveals the type and extent of hygienic care required. Give special attention to the characteristics most influenced by hygiene measures. Is the skin intact, especially over bony prominences? Is the skin dry from too much bathing? Are there calluses of the feet that will benefit from soaking? Is there a coating of the tongue that requires frequent brushing and hydration? Over time, this assessment provides the baseline for determining whether hygienic measures maintain or improve the client's condition.

Skin. While inspecting the skin, thoroughly examine color, texture, thickness, turgor, temperature, and hydration. The skin needs to be smooth, warm, and supple with good turgor. Pay special attention to the presence and condition of any lesions (see Chapter 33). In addition, it is important to assess for dryness indicated by flaking, redness, scaling, and cracking. This is more prevalent in the winter months when the humidity is lower. Certain common skin problems affect how you administer hygiene (Table 39-2). Also give special care to assess less obvious or difficult-to-reach skin surfaces, such as under the female client's breasts, under the male client's scrotum, or around the female's perineal tissues. When you observe skin problems, explain proper skin care with the client and use the time to instruct in specific hygiene techniques.

✳ TABLE 39-2 Common Skin Problems

CHARACTERISTICS	IMPLICATIONS	INTERVENTIONS
Dry Skin		
Flaky, rough texture on exposed areas such as hands, arms, legs, or face	Skin becomes infected if epidermal layer cracks.	Bathe less frequently, and rinse body of all soap because residue left on skin can cause irritation and breakdown. Add moisture to air through use of humidifier. Increase fluid intake when skin is dry. Use moisturizing cream to aid healing. (Cream forms protective barrier and helps maintain fluid within skin.) Use cream such as Eucerin. Use creams to clean skin that is dry or allergic to soaps and detergents.
Acne		
Inflammatory, papulopustular skin eruption, usually involving bacterial breakdown of sebum; appears on face, neck, shoulders, and back	Infected material within pustule will spread if area is squeezed or picked. Permanent scarring can result.	Wash hair and skin thoroughly each day with warm water and soap to remove oil. Use cosmetics sparingly because oily cosmetics or creams accumulate in pores and tend to make condition worse. Implement dietary restrictions, if necessary. (Eliminate foods that aggravate condition from diet.) Use prescribed topical antibiotics for severe forms of acne.
Skin Rashes		
Skin eruptions that result from overexposure to sun or moisture or from allergic reaction (flat or raised, localized or systemic, pruritic or nonpruritic)	If skin is continually scratched, inflammation and infection may occur. Rashes also cause discomfort.	Wash area thoroughly, and apply antiseptic spray or lotion to prevent further itching and aid in healing process. Apply warm or cold soaks to relieve inflammation, if indicated.
Contact Dermatitis		
Inflammation of skin characterized by abrupt onset with erythema, pruritus, pain, and appearance of scaly oozing lesions (seen on face, neck, hands, forearms, and genitalia)	Dermatitis is often difficult to eliminate because person is usually in continual contact with substance causing skin reaction. Substance is often hard to identify.	Avoid causative agents (e.g., cleansers and soaps).
Abrasion		
Scraping or rubbing away of epidermis that will result in localized bleeding and later weeping of serous fluid	Infection occurs easily because of loss of protective skin layer.	Be careful not to scratch client with jewelry or fingernails. Wash abrasions with mild soap and water; dry thoroughly and gently. Observe dressing or bandage for retained moisture because it increases risk of infection.

Certain conditions place clients at risk for impaired skin integrity (Box 39-3). Be particularly alert when assessing clients with reduced sensation, vascular insufficiency, and immobility. Be sure to assess both extremities and assist in turning a client so that you can fully view a skin surface. The development of pressure ulcers is a common complication that can extend hospital stays and threaten the well-being of the long-term care client. Identifying changes in skin color and determining if these changes are normal reactive hyperemia or abnormal reactive hyperemia is important in evaluating clients' risks for pressure ulcers (see Chapter 48). When client's natural skin contains more melanin, it becomes more difficult to determine abnormal reactive hyperemia or cyanosis. When caring for clients with darkly pigmented skin, be aware of assessment techniques and skin characteristics unique to highly pigmented skin (Box 39-4).

Feet and Nails. Assessment of the feet involves a thorough examination of all skin surfaces, including areas between the toes

and over the soles of the feet. The heels, soles, and sides of the feet are prone to irritation from poorly fitting shoes. In addition, inspect the shape and size of toes and shape of the foot. The toes are normally straight and flat. The feet are in straight alignment with the ankle and tibia. Inspection of the feet for lesions includes noting areas of dryness, inflammation, or cracking.

Observe the client's gait. Painful foot disorders or decreased sensation cause limping or an unnatural gait. Ask whether the client has foot discomfort, and determine factors that aggravate the pain. Foot problems sometimes result from bone or muscular alterations or wearing poorly fitting footwear rather than skin disorders.

Assess clients with peripheral vascular disease, such as those with diabetes mellitus and other diseases that affect peripheral circulation and sensation for the adequacy of circulation to the feet (see Chapter 33). Foot ulceration is the most common single precursor to lower extremity amputations among persons with

BOX 39-3 Risk Factors for Skin Impairment

Immobilization
When restricted from moving freely, dependent body parts are exposed to pressure that reduces circulation to affected tissues. Know which clients require assistance to turn and change positions.

Reduced Sensation
Clients with paralysis, circulatory insufficiency, or local nerve damage are unable to sense an injury to the skin. During a bath assess the status of sensory nerve function by checking for pain, tactile sensation, and temperature sensation.

Nutrition and Hydration Alterations
Clients with limited caloric and protein intake develop thinner, less elastic skin, with loss of subcutaneous tissue. This results in impaired or delayed wound healing.

Secretions and Excretions on the Skin
Moisture on the skin's surface serves as a medium for bacterial growth and causes irritation, softens epidermal cells, and leads to skin maceration. Presence of perspiration, urine, watery fecal material, and wound drainage on the skin results in breakdown and infection.

Vascular Insufficiency
Inadequate arterial supply to tissues and impaired venous return decrease circulation to the extremities. Inadequate blood flow causes ischemia and breakdown. Risk of infection also exists because delivery of nutrients, oxygen, and white blood cells to injured tissues is inadequate.

External Devices
An external device applied to or around the skin exerts pressure or friction on the skin. Assess all surfaces exposed to casts, cloth restraints, bandages and dressings, tubing, or orthopedic braces.

BOX 39-4 Skin Assessment for the Client With Darkly Pigmented Intact Skin

- Assess localized skin color changes. Any of the following may occur:
  - Color darker than surrounding skin, purplish, bluish, eggplant
  - Taut
  - Shiny
  - Induration
- Assess for edema (nonpitting, swelling).
- Importance of lighting for skin assessment:
  - Use natural or halogen light.
  - Avoid fluorescent lamps, which give the skin a bluish tone.
- Assess skin temperature.
  - Use the back of your hand and fingers and, if client's condition permits, do not use gloves when doing this assessment.
  - Initially area of skin impairment feels warmer than surrounding skin.
  - Subsequently area of skin impairment feels cooler than surrounding skin.

Data from Bennet MA: Report of the Task Force on the Implications for Darkly Pigmented Intact Skin in the Prediction and Prevention of Pressure Ulcers, *Adv Wound Care* 8(6):34, 1995.

diabetes (Frykberg and others, 2006). Daily inspection and following preventive foot care are important to maintaining ulcer-free feet. Palpation of the dorsalis pedis and posterior tibial pulses indicates whether adequate blood flow is reaching peripheral tissues. Edema and changes in skin color, texture, and temperature indicate if the client requires special hygienic care. Also check persons with diabetes mellitus for **neuropathy,** degeneration of the peripheral nerves characterized by a loss of sensation. Assess the client's sensation to light touch, pinprick, and temperature (see Chapter 33).

Inspect the condition of the fingernails and toenails, looking for lesions, dryness, inflammation, or cracking (Table 39-3). The nail is surrounded by a cuticle, which slowly grows over the nail. The skin around the nail beds and cuticles remain smooth and without inflammation. Ask women whether they frequently polish their nails and use polish remover, because chemicals in these products cause excessive nail dryness. Disease changes the shape and curvature of the nails (see Chapter 33). Inflammatory lesions and fungus of the nail bed cause thickened, horny nails, which separate from the nail bed.

Oral Cavity. Inspect all areas carefully for color, hydration, texture, and lesions (see Chapter 33). Clients who do not follow regular oral hygiene practices sometimes have receding gum tissue, inflamed gums, a coated tongue, discolored teeth (particularly along gum margins), dental caries, missing teeth, and **halitosis** (bad breath). Localized pain and infection are common symptoms of a gum disease and certain tooth disorders.

Clients in acute care settings require complete oral assessment. Identification of risks for infection and other conditions identifies the type and frequency of oral care. Proper oral care reduces pneumonia in nursing home residents because it reduces the bacterial count in oral secretions, which are aspirated, causing a bacterial infection (Research update, 2002). It is especially important to examine the oral cavity of clients receiving radiation or chemotherapy. Both treatments cause reduction in the amount of saliva, and, as a result, there is drying and inflammation of the oral mucosal tissues. The nurse's assessment serves as a basis for preventive care for clients as they undergo treatment.

Hair. Before performing hair care, assess the condition of the hair and scalp. Normally the hair is clean, shiny, and untangled, and the scalp is clear of lesions. The hair of dark-skinned clients is usually thicker, drier, and curlier than that of lighter-skinned clients. Table 39-4 summarizes hair and scalp problems. In the community health and home care settings it is particularly important to inspect the hair for lice so that you can provide appropriate hygienic treatment. If you suspect pediculosis capitis (head lice), guard against self-infestations by hand washing and using gloves or tongue blades to inspect the client's hair. The loss of hair (**alopecia**) results from the effects of chemotherapy medications, hormonal changes, or improper hair care practices. Clients at risk for scalp problems are those who have experienced head trauma and those who practice poor hygiene.

Eyes, Ears, and Nose. Examine the condition and function of the eyes, ears, and nose (see Chapter 33). Normally the eyes are free of infection and irritation. The sclerae are visible anteriorly as the white portion of the eye. The conjunctivae (the lining of the eyelids) are clear, pink, and without inflammation. The eyelid margins are in close approximation with the eyeball, and the

✳ TABLE 39-3 Common Foot and Nail Problems

CHARACTERISTICS	IMPLICATIONS	INTERVENTIONS
Callus Thickened portion of epidermis consists of mass of horny, keratotic cells. Callus is usually flat, painless, and found on undersurface of foot or on palm of hand.	Local friction or pressure causes callus formation, which causes discomfort when wearing tight shoes.	Soft-sole shoes with insoles are recommended. Advise client to wear gloves when using tools or objects that create friction on palmar surfaces. Advise clients, especially with callus formation, not to self-treat but seek interventions from a podiatrist.
Corns Friction and pressure from ill-fitting or loose shoes causes keratosis. It is seen mainly on or between toes, over bony prominence. Corn is usually cone shaped, round, and raised. Soft corns are macerated.	Compresses underlying dermis, making it thin and tender. Pain is aggravated when wearing tight shoes. Tissue becomes attached to bone if allowed to grow. Client suffers alteration in gait resulting from pain.	Surgical removal is necessary, depending on severity of pain and size of corn. Avoid use of oval corn pads, which increase pressure on toes and reduce circulation. Warm water soaks soften corns before gentle rubbing with a callus file or pumice stone (consult with health care provider). Wider and softer shoes, especially shoes with a wider toe box, are helpful.
Plantar Warts Fungating lesion appears on sole of foot and is due to the papilloma virus.	Some warts are contagious. They are painful and make walking difficult.	Treatment ordered by physician often includes applications of salicylic acid, electrodesiccation (burning with electrical spark), or freezing with solid carbon dioxide.
Athlete's Foot (Tinea Pedis) Athlete's foot is fungal infection of foot; scaliness and cracking of skin occurs between toes and on soles of feet. Small blisters containing fluid appear.	Athlete's foot spreads to other body parts, especially hands. It is contagious and frequently recurs.	Make sure feet are well ventilated. Drying feet well after bathing and applying powder help prevent infection. Wearing of clean socks or stockings reduces incidence. Health care provider orders application of griseofulvin, miconazole, or tolnaftate.
Ingrown Nails Toenail or fingernail grows inward into soft tissue around nail. Ingrown nail often results from improper nail trimming.	Ingrown nails cause localized pain when pressure is applied.	Treatment is frequent hot soaks in antiseptic solution and removal of portion of nail that has grown into skin. Instruct client in proper nail-trimming techniques, and refer to podiatrist.
Foot Odors Foot odors are the result of excess perspiration, promoting microorganism growth.	Condition causes discomfort because of excess perspiration.	Frequent washing, use of foot deodorants and powders, and wearing clean footwear prevent or reduce problem.

lashes are turned outward. The lid margins are without inflammation, drainage, or lesions. The eyebrows are usually symmetrical.

Another important aspect of an eye examination is to determine if the client wears contact lenses. This is especially significant for clients who enter hospitals or other agencies unresponsive or in a confused state. To determine if a contact lens is present, stand to the side of the client's eye and observe the cornea for the presence of a soft or rigid lens. It is also important to observe the sclera to detect the presence of a contact lens that has shifted off the client's cornea. An undetected lens causes severe corneal injury when left in place too long.

Assessment of the external ear structures includes inspection of the auricle, external ear canal, and tympanic membrane. Use of an otoscope is necessary (see Chapter 33). While performing hygienic measures, look for the presence of accumulated **cerumen** or drainage in the ear canal, local inflammation, or tenderness on palpation or the client's report of pain (see Chapter 33).

Inspect the nares for signs of inflammation, discharge, lesions, edema, and deformity (see Chapter 33). The nasal mucosa is normally pink and clear and has little or no discharge. A clear, watery discharge is the result of allergies. If clients have any form of tubing exiting the nose (e.g., nasogastric), look at the nares surfaces that come in contact with the tubing for tissue sloughing, pressure areas, localized tenderness, inflammation, and bleeding.

Developmental Changes. The normal process of aging influences the condition of body tissues and structures and thus the manner in which the client performs hygienic measures. Chapter 49 addresses the changes in hearing, vision, and olfaction across the life span as a result of growth and development.

Skin. The neonate's skin is relatively immature at birth. The epidermis and dermis are loosely bound together, and the skin is very thin. Friction against the skin layers causes bruising. Handle the neonate carefully during bathing. Any break in the skin can easily result in an infection.

A toddler's skin layers are more tightly bound together. Thus the child has a greater resistance to infection and skin irritation. However, because of the child's more active play and the absence of es-

✳ TABLE 39-4   Hair and Scalp Problems

CHARACTERISTICS	IMPLICATIONS	INTERVENTIONS
Dandruff Scaling of scalp is accompanied by itching. In severe cases, dandruff is on eyebrows.	Dandruff causes person embarrassment. If dandruff enters eyes, conjunctivitis often develops.	Shampoo regularly with medicated shampoo. In severe cases, obtain health care provider's advice.
Ticks Small, gray-brown parasites burrow into skin and suck blood.	Ticks transmit several diseases to people. Most common are Rocky Mountain spotted fever, tularemia, and Lyme disease.	Do not pull ticks from skin because sucking apparatus remains and will possibly become infected. Suffocate tick by placing a drop of oil or ether on tick or covering it with petrolatum to ease removal.
Pediculosis (Lice) Tiny, grayish-white parasite insects infest mammals.		
Pediculosis Capitis (Head Lice) Parasite is on scalp attached to hair strands. Eggs look like oval particles, similar to dandruff. Bites or pustules may be observed behind ears and at hairline.	Head lice are difficult to remove and spread to furniture and other people if not treated.	Check entire scalp. Use medicated shampoo for eliminating lice. **Caution against use of products containing lindane because the ingredient is toxic and known to cause adverse reactions** (National Pediculosis Association, 2001). Repeat treatment 12 to 24 hours later. Manual removal is best option when treatment has failed. Vacuum infested areas of home.
Pediculosis Corporis (Body Lice) Parasites tend to cling to clothing, so they are not always easy to see. Body lice suck blood and lay eggs on clothing and furniture.	Client itches constantly. Scratches seen on skin become infected. Hemorrhagic spots appear on skin where lice are sucking blood.	Bathe or shower thoroughly. After skin is dried, apply recommended pediculicide lotion. After 12 to 24 hours, take another bath or shower. Bag infested clothing or linen until laundered in hot water. Vacuum rooms thoroughly, and throw away bag after completion.
Pediculosis Pubis (Crab Lice) Parasites are in pubic hair. Crab lice are grayish white with red legs.	Lice spread through bed linen, clothing, or furniture or between persons via sexual contact.	Shave hair off affected area. Cleanse as for body lice. If lice were sexually transmitted, notify partner.
Hair Loss (Alopecia) Alopecia occurs in all races. Balding patches are in periphery of hair line. Hair becomes brittle and broken.	Patches of uneven hair growth and loss alter client's appearance.	Stop hair-care practices that damage hair. The use of hair curlers, hair picks, tight braiding, and use of hot comb contribute to hair loss condition.

tablished hygienic habits, parents and caregivers need to provide thorough hygiene and to begin teaching good hygiene habits.

During adolescence the growth and maturation of the integument increases. In girls, estrogen secretion causes the skin to become soft, smooth, and thicker, with increased vascularity. In boys, male hormones produce an increased thickness of the skin with some darkening in color. Sebaceous glands become more active, predisposing adolescents to **acne. Eccrine** and **apocrine** sweat glands become fully functional during puberty. Adolescents usually begin to use antiperspirants. More frequent bathing and shampooing also become necessary to reduce body odors and eliminate oily hair. Sweating is usually more pronounced in boys.

The condition of the adult's skin depends on hygienic practices and exposure to environmental irritants. Normally the skin is elastic, well hydrated, firm, and smooth. When an adult practices frequent bathing or is exposed to an environment with low humidity, the skin becomes very dry and flaky.

As we age, the skin loses its resiliency and moisture, and sebaceous and sweat glands become less active. The epithelium thins, and elastic collagen fibers shrink, making the skin fragile and subject to bruising and breaking. These changes warrant caution when turning and repositioning older adults (Meiner and Lueckenotte, 2006). Typically the older person's skin is dry and wrinkled. Daily bathing as well as bathing with water that is too hot or soap that is harsh causes the skin to become excessively dry.

Feet and Nails. During standing, the foot provides body support and absorbs shock. With aging, the feet begin to show signs of wear and tear. This occurs earlier if a person has failed to wear comfortable, supportive footwear. The cushioning layer of fat on the soles of the feet becomes thin.

Chronic foot problems are a common part of poor foot care, improper fit of footwear, aging, or systemic disease. Older adults often have dry feet because of a decrease in sebaceous gland secretion, dehydration of epidermal cells, and poor condition of footwear. Fissures that result in itching frequently develop (Bryant and Beinlich, 1999). One of the most common problems for older adults is foot pain (Meiner and Lueckenotte, 2006). Painful feet are the result of congenital deformities, weak structure, injuries, and diseases such as diabetes, rheumatoid arthritis, or osteoarthritis. Arthritis is generally the cause for changes in the feet after age 55. Additional common problems of the feet include hammer and claw toes (flexion contractures); bunions, corns, and calluses; loss of sensation; and pathological nail conditions (Boyer, 2001).

Fungal infections occur under toenails, causing dirty yellow streaks or total discoloration. The nails also become opaque, scaly, and hypertrophied. If foot or nail problems stay unresolved, the client can easily become disabled. Apply knowledge about typical changes in the feet and nails when anticipating the client's hygiene needs.

The Mouth. At approximately 6 to 8 months of age, infants begin teething. The first permanent (secondary) teeth erupt at about 6 years of age (Hockenberry and Wilson, 2007). From adolescence, when all of the permanent teeth are in place, through middle adulthood, the teeth and gums remain healthy if a person follows good eating patterns and good dental care. Avoidance of fermentable carbohydrates and sticky sweets are central to keeping the teeth free of **caries.** Regular brushing and flossing help to prevent caries and periodontal disease.

As a person ages, there are numerous factors that result in poor oral care. These include age-related changes of the mouth, chronic disease such as diabetes, physical disabilities involving hand grasp or strength affecting the ability to perform oral care, lack of attention to oral care, and prescribed medications that have oral side effects. Aging teeth become brittle, drier, and darker in color. Teeth become uneven, jagged, and fractured; gums lose vascularity and tissue elasticity, which causes dentures to fit poorly. Often older adults are **edentulous** and wear complete or partial dentures. It is important to learn if older adults wear dentures and the condition of underlying supportive gum tissue.

Hair. Throughout life, changes in the growth, distribution, and condition of the hair influence hair hygiene. As males reach adolescence, shaving becomes a part of routine grooming. Young girls who reach puberty often begin to shave their legs and axillae. With aging, as scalp hair becomes thinner and drier, shampooing is usually performed less frequently.

The Eyes, Ears and Nose. Although much of hygiene care focuses on preventing infection and injury and maintaining function, be aware of developmental changes and risks to these special sensory organs. Although the structure of the eyes does not have marked developmental changes, altered visual acuity occurs at several points during the aging process; for example, when children start school or when clients reach middle age, there are sometimes changes in visual acuity. In addition, as clients age, they are at risk for changes in visual clarity, such as those that oc-

---

✳ BOX 39-5 Assessing a Client's Use of Sensory Aids

Eyeglasses
Purpose for wearing glasses (e.g., reading, distance, or both)
Presence of symptoms (e.g., blurred vision, photophobia, headaches, irritation)

Contact Lenses
Type of lens worn
Frequency and duration of time lenses are worn (including sleep time)
Presence of symptoms (e.g., burning, excess tearing, redness, irritation, swelling, sensitivity to light)
Techniques used by the client to cleanse, store, insert, and remove lenses
Use of eye drops or ointments
Use of emergency identification bracelet or card that warns others to remove client's lenses in case of emergency

Artificial Eye
Method used to insert and remove eye
Method for cleansing eye
Presence of symptoms (e.g., drainage, inflammation, pain involving the orbit)

Hearing Aid
Type of aid worn
Methods used to cleanse aid
Client's ability to change battery and adjust hearing aid volume

---

cur with glaucoma, and visual field losses, such as those that occur with macular degeneration or glaucoma.

Structures of the ears do not change as the client ages; however, changes in hearing acuity or balance often occur with aging. In the young child changes in hearing acuity result from foreign objects being placed in the ear; this is usually temporary and is resolved once the object is removed. Changes also result from repeated ear infections or exposure to loud music, especially when the child listens to loud music while wearing ear pods.

Older adults have changes in the structure and function of the small bones in the inner ear that affect changes in hearing acuity. Aging results in increased cerumen production, which impedes hearing acuity. In addition, there are age-related changes in the movement of fluid through the semicircular canals, and the client sometimes experiences positional dizziness or some balance problem. Although changes in the sense of smell occur at any time, they seem to be more frequent in the older adult population. It is important to remember that changes in the sense of smell also affect taste and the client's appetite.

You need to fully assess and evaluate new and acute changes in the structure and function of the eyes, ears, and nose. Timely evaluation of these changes helps to identify other illnesses or verify that they are age related.

Use of Sensory Aids. For clients who wear eyeglasses, contact lenses, artificial eyes, or hearing aids, assess client's knowledge and methods used for care and have the client describe his or her typical approach used in routine care (Box 39-5). Compare information gathered from the client with the proper care technique

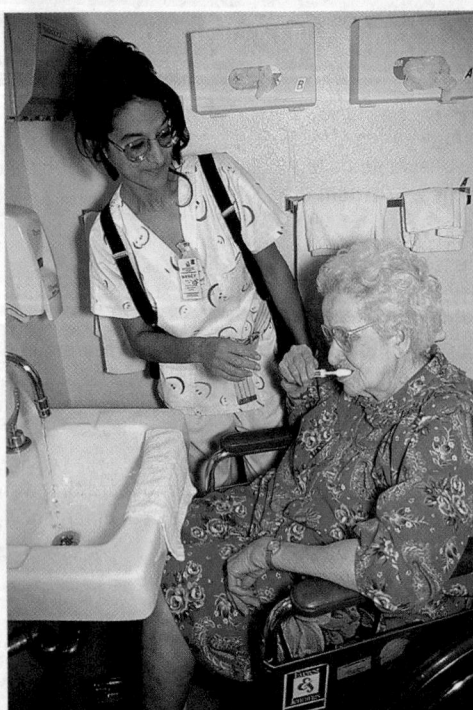

Figure 39-5 The nurse observes client brushing teeth. During such observations the nurse can determine how much assistance the client may need.

for these devices. Any difference between client practice and standard practice is an opportunity for client education.

Self-Care Ability.
Clients with physical or cognitive impairments need assistance with all or some aspects of personal hygiene. Assessment of the client's physical and cognitive status determines specifically what aspects of hygiene care can be performed independently, those that require some assistance, and those that require total assistance.

The nurse's assessment includes measurement of a client's muscle strength, flexibility and dexterity, balance, coordination, and activity tolerance necessary in performing activities such as bathing, brushing teeth, and bending over to inspect the feet (Figure 39-5). The degree of assistance needed by a client during hygienic care also depends on vision, the ability to sit without support, hand grasp strength, the range of motion in the client's extremities, or the presence of equipment, such as an intravenous (IV) line, dressings, or traction. Painful conditions of the upper extremities pose special problems. Assess self-care ability by observing clients performing activities, such as toothbrushing or combing the hair. Observe the client carefully, and note not only if the client is performing the activity correctly, but also if he or she is able to be thorough and complete the task.

When clients have self-care limitations, part of the assessment determines if family or friends are available to assist. Assess how the family will assist the client, how often they will provide this assistance, and what their feelings are about being caregivers. In addition, assess the home environment and its influence on the client's hygiene practices. Are there barriers in the home that affect the client's self-care abilities? Water faucets that are too tight

to easily adjust, bathtubs with high sides, and a bathroom too small to fit a chair in front of a sink are a few examples.

Hygiene Practices.
Assessment of hygiene practices reveals the client's preferences for grooming. For example, a client chooses to groom the hair in a certain style or chooses to trim nails in a certain way. When a client has a physical disability, special precautions are necessary to perform grooming without injury. For example, special techniques are used when trimming toenails when the client has diabetes. Asking the client to assist or show how to perform preferred grooming practices gives the client a greater sense of independence and helps to avoid causing the client any discomfort or injury.

Cultural Factors.
A client's cultural background influences hygiene needs. Culture plays a role not only in hygiene practices and preferences but also in sensitivity to personal space (see Box 39-1, p. 853 and Chapter 9). For example, some Chinese-Americans may view tasks associated with closeness and touch as being offensive or impolite, and Vietnamese-Americans feel very uneasy during a back rub. Ask a client what will make him or her feel most comfortable during a bath (Galanti, 2004). Perhaps the client prefers only a partial instead of a full bath from the nurse, with a family member completing the bathing of more private body parts. Some clients will also defer part of hygiene. If you believe hygiene is critical to prevent developing or worsening problems, such as skin breakdown, take the time to understand the client's concerns and then offer an explanation that will help the client accept your intervention.

Clients at Risk for Hygiene Problems.
There are clients who present risks that require more attentive and rigorous hygienic care (Table 39-5). These risks result from side effects of medications, a lack of knowledge, an inability to perform hygiene, or a physical condition that potentially injures the skin, integument, or other structures. For example, an immobilized client with a fever requires more frequent bathing to minimize perspiration on the skin and more frequent turning and positioning to reduce the chance of skin breakdown.

Anticipate whether a client is predisposed to any risks, and follow through with a complete assessment. For example, if a client is receiving cancer chemotherapy, there is the risk of the medication destroying normal flora in the mouth, allowing for the overgrowth of opportunistic bacteria. Therefore be more thorough and detailed during the oral examination, checking all surfaces of the tongue and mucosa. If a client is diaphoretic, provide special attention to body areas, such as beneath the woman's breasts and perineal area, to check where moisture collects and irritates skin surfaces. Anticipate problems created by these risks to provide preventive care. Assessment includes a review of the client's medical and surgical history, medications, and the specific risk factors the client is likely to have.

Special Considerations in Hygiene Assessment.
Depending on the type of hygiene needed, there are focused assessments that are important to conduct. For example, before giving foot care, assess the type of footwear a client wears. Children or young adults who frequently fail to wear socks have excess perspi-

✳ TABLE 39-5 Risk Factors for Hygiene Problems

RISKS	HYGIENE IMPLICATIONS
Oral Problems	
Clients who are unable to use upper extremities due to paralysis, weakness, or restriction (e.g., cast, dressing)	Client lacks upper extremity strength or dexterity needed to brush teeth (Lewis and others, 2007).
Dehydration, inability to take fluids or food by mouth (NPO)	Causes excess drying and fragility of mucosa; increases accumulation of secretions on tongue and gums.
Presence of nasogastric or oxygen tubes; mouth breathers	Causes drying of mucosa.
Chemotherapeutic drugs	Drugs kill rapidly multiplying cells, including normal cells lining oral cavity. Ulcers and inflammation develop.
Lozenges, cough drops, antacids, and chewable vitamins over-the-counter (OTC)	Medications contain large amounts of sugar. Repeated use increases sugar or acid content in mouth.
Radiation therapy to head and neck	Reduces salivary flow and lowers pH of saliva; leads to stomatitis and tooth decay (Lewis and others, 2007).
Oral surgery, trauma to mouth, placement of oral airway	Cause trauma to oral cavity with swelling, ulcerations, inflammation, and bleeding.
Immunosuppression; altered blood clotting	Predisposes to inflammation and bleeding gums.
Diabetes mellitus	Prone to dryness of mouth, gingivitis, periodontal disease, and loss of teeth.
Mechanical ventilation	Potential for ventilator-associated pneumonia (VAP). Use of chlorhexidine reduces the risk of VAP. Chlorhexidine is an inexpensive effective agent for reducing VAP, especially in clients who have heart surgery (Berry and others, 2007).
Skin Problems	
Immobilization	Dependent body parts are exposed to pressure from underlying surfaces. The inability to turn or change position increases risk for pressure ulcers.
Reduced sensation due to stroke, spinal cord injury, diabetes, local nerve damage	Client does not receive normal transmission of nerve impulses when applying excessive heat or cold, pressure, friction, or chemical irritants to skin.
Limited protein or caloric intake and reduced hydration (e.g., fever, burns, gastrointestinal alterations, poorly fitting dentures)	Limited caloric and protein intake predispose to impaired tissue synthesis. Skin becomes thinner, less elastic, and smoother with a loss of subcutaneous tissue. Poor wound healing results. Reduced hydration impairs skin turgor.
Excessive secretions or excretions on the skin from perspiration, urine, watery fecal material, and wound drainage	Moisture is a medium for bacterial growth and causes local skin irritation, softening of epidermal cells, and skin maceration.
Presence of external devices (e.g., cast, restraint, bandage, dressing)	Device exerts pressure or friction against skin's surface.
Vascular insufficiency	Arterial blood supply to tissues is inadequate, or venous return is impaired, causing decreased circulation to extremities. Tissue ischemia and breakdown often occur. Risk for infection is high.
Foot Problems	
Client unable to bend over or has reduced visual acuity	Client is unable to fully visualize entire surface of each foot, impairing ability to adequately assess condition of skin and nails.
Eye Care Problems	
Reduced dexterity and hand coordination	Physical limitations create inability to safely insert or remove contact lenses.

ration that promotes fungal growth. Tight or poorly fitting shoes, socks, garters, or knee-high nylon stockings cause skin irritation and interfere with circulation to the feet. Also determine whether clients wear clean footwear daily because repeated use of soiled footwear leads to infection. If the client has diabetes mellitus or other peripheral vascular disease, it is extremely important to wear the correct footwear. People with evidence of increased plantar pressure (e.g., erythema, warmth, callus, or measured pressure) use footwear that cushions and redistributes the pressure. People with bony deformities (e.g., hammertoes, prominent metatarsal

heads, and bunions) may need extrawide or extradeep shoes. People with extreme bony deformities (e.g., Charcot's foot) who cannot be accommodated with commercial therapeutic footwear may need custom-molded shoes (American Diabetes Association, [ADA], 2007).

A client's eating patterns are important to assess before oral care. The presence of any problems helps to locate abnormalities. Ask clients if any problems are noted with chewing, denture fit, or swallowing. A client may have changed the type of food in the diet as a result of chewing difficulties. The presence of an ulcer or irritation sometimes impairs chewing and causes a client to avoid eating. This is common in an older adult with poorly fitting dentures.

Client Expectations. As is the case in any nursing assessment, it is important to know what a client expects from nursing care. In regard to hygienic care, some clients simply expect to have hygiene preferences and practices applied in the health care setting. Ask questions such as "To make you most comfortable and feel at home, how can I best perform your bath and personal care?" or "How can we help you care for your teeth, nails, and hair, now that you are back home?"

Learning a client's expectations and applying them in practice is important in establishing a caring relationship. Truly individualizing hygienic care shows the nurse's respect for the client's needs. As you learn what the client expects, you incorporate this information into a plan of care.

◆Nursing Diagnosis

Assessment reveals the condition of the skin, oral cavity, and other tissues, as well as the client's need for and ability to meet personal hygiene needs. As you review all data gathered, consider previous clients you cared for, review knowledge pertaining to preexisting conditions, and then look for clusters of data suggesting a problem trend. When caring for an older adult with degenerative arthritis you observe swollen joints, weakness, and mobility limitations in the dominant hand and a generally unkempt appearance. Closer review of assessment data reveals defining characteristics of an inability to wash body parts and difficulty turning and regulating a water faucet. The nursing diagnosis of *bathing/hygiene self-care deficit* becomes part of the plan of care. Accurate selection of nursing diagnoses requires critical thinking to identify actual or potential health problems. Be thorough in assessment activities to reveal all appropriate defining characteristics so that you can make an accurate diagnosis (Box 39-6)

Whether a client has an actual alteration (e.g., impaired tissue integrity) or is at risk (e.g., risk for infection) determines the focus of nursing interventions. The client with an actual alteration requires extensive hygienic care, often more thorough than what routine hygiene involves. For example, if the client has skin breakdown, initiate care more frequently to keep skin surfaces clean and dry and to eliminate factors such as moisture or drainage that worsen the condition of the skin. Also provide care to promote healing of injured skin surfaces (see Chapter 48). If the client is at risk for a problem, take preventive measures. In the case of risk for impaired oral mucous membranes, keep the mucosa well hydrated, minimize foods irritating to tissues, and provide cleansing that soothes and reduces tissue inflammation.

The identification of related factors guides you when selecting nursing interventions. *Impaired oral mucous membrane related to malnutrition* and a diagnosis of *impaired oral mucous membrane related to chemical trauma* require very different interventions. When malnutrition is a causal factor, confer with a dietitian for appropriate dietary supplements and incorporate client education into the plan. When mucosa are injured as a result of chemotherapy, techniques for cleansing and hydrating inflamed tissues and eliminating sources of irritation will be the focus of nursing

---

✦ **BOX 39-6   NURSING DIAGNOSTIC PROCESS**

Self-Care Deficit, Bathing/Hygiene Related

Assessment Activities	Findings/Defining Characteristics
Observe client attempt to bathe self either in bed or at bathroom sink. (NOTE: Be sure positioning does not restrict potential movement.)	Client unable to wash body or body parts
Assess client's upper extremity strength, range of motion, and coordination.	Restricted upper extremity range of motion and strength coordination adequate
Ask client about level of fatigue after bathing.	Client complains of fatigue and needs to rest after bathing
Obtain vital signs after bathing.	Pulse elevated from 90 to 110 beats per minute, blood pressure stable, respirations elevated from 16 to 22 breaths per minute

---

care. Although there are many possible nursing diagnoses that apply to clients in need of hygienic care, the following list selects examples of nursing diagnoses associated with hygiene problems:

- Chronic low self-esteem
- Deficient knowledge about hygiene practices
- Fatigue
- Impaired dentition
- Impaired oral mucous membrane
- Impaired physical mobility
- Ineffective health maintenance
- Ineffective tissue perfusion
- Risk for impaired skin integrity
- Risk for infection

◆Planning

During planning synthesize information from multiple resources (Figure 39-6). Critical thinking ensures that the client's plan of care integrates all that is known about the individual client and key critical thinking elements. There are situations when clients have multiple nursing diagnoses. The concept map (Figure 39-7) shows graphically how numerous nursing diagnoses interrelate.

Previous experience with other clients is very useful in knowing how to adapt hygiene techniques for special needs. Professional standards are especially important to consider when developing a plan of care. These standards often establish evidence-based guidelines for care. For example, guidelines for diabetic foot care recommendations endorsed by the Diabetes Committee of the American Orthopedic Foot and Ankle Society 2005 identify people at risk for complications as well as preventive and treatment options (Pinzur and others, 2005).

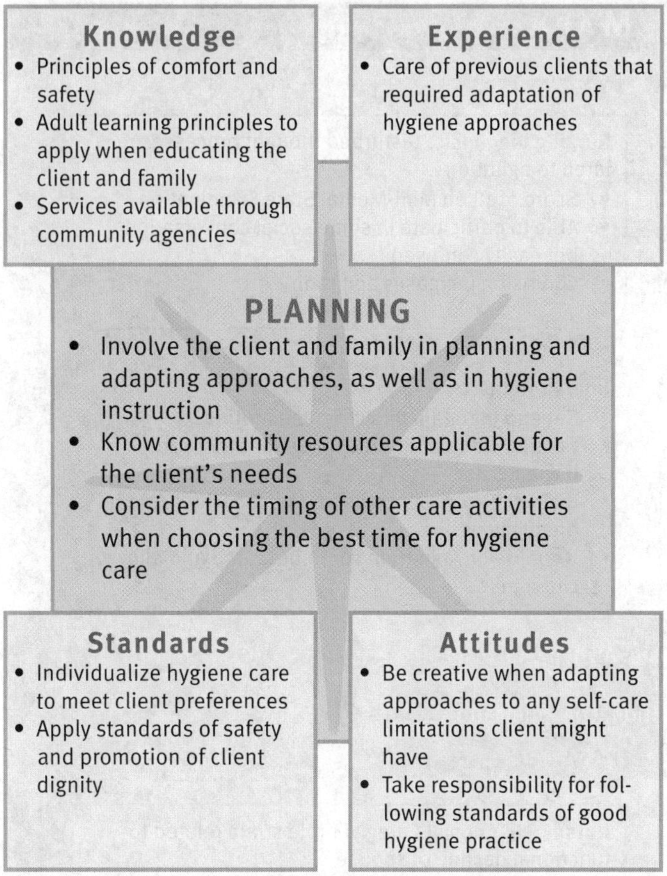

Knowledge
- Principles of comfort and safety
- Adult learning principles to apply when educating the client and family
- Services available through community agencies

Experience
- Care of previous clients that required adaptation of hygiene approaches

PLANNING
- Involve the client and family in planning and adapting approaches, as well as in hygiene instruction
- Know community resources applicable for the client's needs
- Consider the timing of other care activities when choosing the best time for hygiene care

Standards
- Individualize hygiene care to meet client preferences
- Apply standards of safety and promotion of client dignity

Attitudes
- Be creative when adapting approaches to any self-care limitations client might have
- Take responsibility for following standards of good hygiene practice

Figure 39-6 Critical thinking model for hygiene planning.

Goals and Outcomes. Partner with the client and family to identify goals and expected outcomes and develop an individualized plan of care based on the client's nursing diagnoses (see Care Plan). For example, establish goals with the client's self-care abilities and resources in mind and focus on maintaining or improving the condition of the skin and mucosa, oral mucosa, or dental hygiene. Make outcomes measurable and achievable within client limitations. In addition, work with the client to select individualized hygiene measures.

When providing for client hygiene, you will care for a variety of clients with different self-care abilities and needs. For example, the nurse and a client who has one-sided paralysis following a cerebral vascular accident develop the following goal: "Client's skin remains free of breakdown." Then establish a series of realistic individualized expected outcomes to assist the client in meeting this goal. These outcomes may include the following:

- Client's skin is clean, dry, and intact without signs of inflammation.
- Clients' skin remains elastic and well hydrated.
- Client's skin is free from areas of pressure.

Setting Priorities. The client's condition influences the plan for delivering hygiene. A seriously ill client usually needs a daily bath because body secretions accumulate. Some older clients at home require a visit from a home care aide to assist with a tub bath. Clients who are normally inactive during the day and have

skin that tends to be dry may need to bathe only twice a week. Plan for necessary assistance for clients who are weakened or possess poor coordination. For example, a partially paralyzed client who has difficulty getting out of a tub should have a tub chair, handrails, or extra personnel available for help.

Timing is also important in planning hygiene. Being interrupted in the middle of a bath to go to an x-ray examination often frustrates and embarrasses a client. Following extensive diagnostic tests (e.g., a stress test), it may be best to delay hygiene and allow a client to rest.

Collaborative Care. It is important to plan for care throughout the stay in a hospital, discharge to a rehabilitation facility, and home. When a client needs assistance as a result of a self-care limitation, the family becomes a valuable resource to the nurse. Family members usually assist with hygiene measures but often need guidance in adapting techniques to fit client limitations. Be aware of equipment and procedures used in the agency so that the client and family are knowledgeable about the care, have the skill needed to provide the care, and have access to necessary equipment. Depending on the client's limitations, some insurance plans provide staff to assist with basic hygiene needs. Explore this option with the client and family members. In addition, various community resources are necessary. For example, the nurse involved in the care of a homeless client needs to be aware of the location of clothing distribution centers for basic hygiene supplies, a shelter where bathing facilities are available, and any organization that offers free health care or reduced fees. Partner with social workers or staff in local area churches, not-for-profit organizations, and schools to be sure clients have the resources they need to maintain hygiene.

◆Implementation

Providing hygiene is a very basic part of a client's care. Caring practices help to alleviate the client's anxiety and promote comfort and relaxation while performing each hygiene measure. For example, while giving a client a bath and changing a gown, use a gentle approach in turning and repositioning. Using a soft, gentle voice while conversing with the client helps to relieve any fears or concerns. For clients suffering symptoms such as pain or nausea, administering symptom relief therapies before hygiene will better prepare the client for any procedure.

Another important part of implementation is assisting and preparing clients so that they are able to administer their own hygiene. This includes educating clients on proper hygienic techniques and connecting clients with the community resources necessary to enable them to perform hygienic care. The same clients at risk for hygiene problems are the ones in greatest need of understanding their risks, knowing the implications, and then having the information they need to make choices about when and how to perform hygiene.

Health Promotion. In primary health care settings, educate and counsel clients and families on proper hygiene techniques. A new mother needs assistance in learning how to bathe her newborn infant. An older adult needs information on the importance of regular ear care to avoid any hearing deficits resulting from ac-

CONCEPT MAP

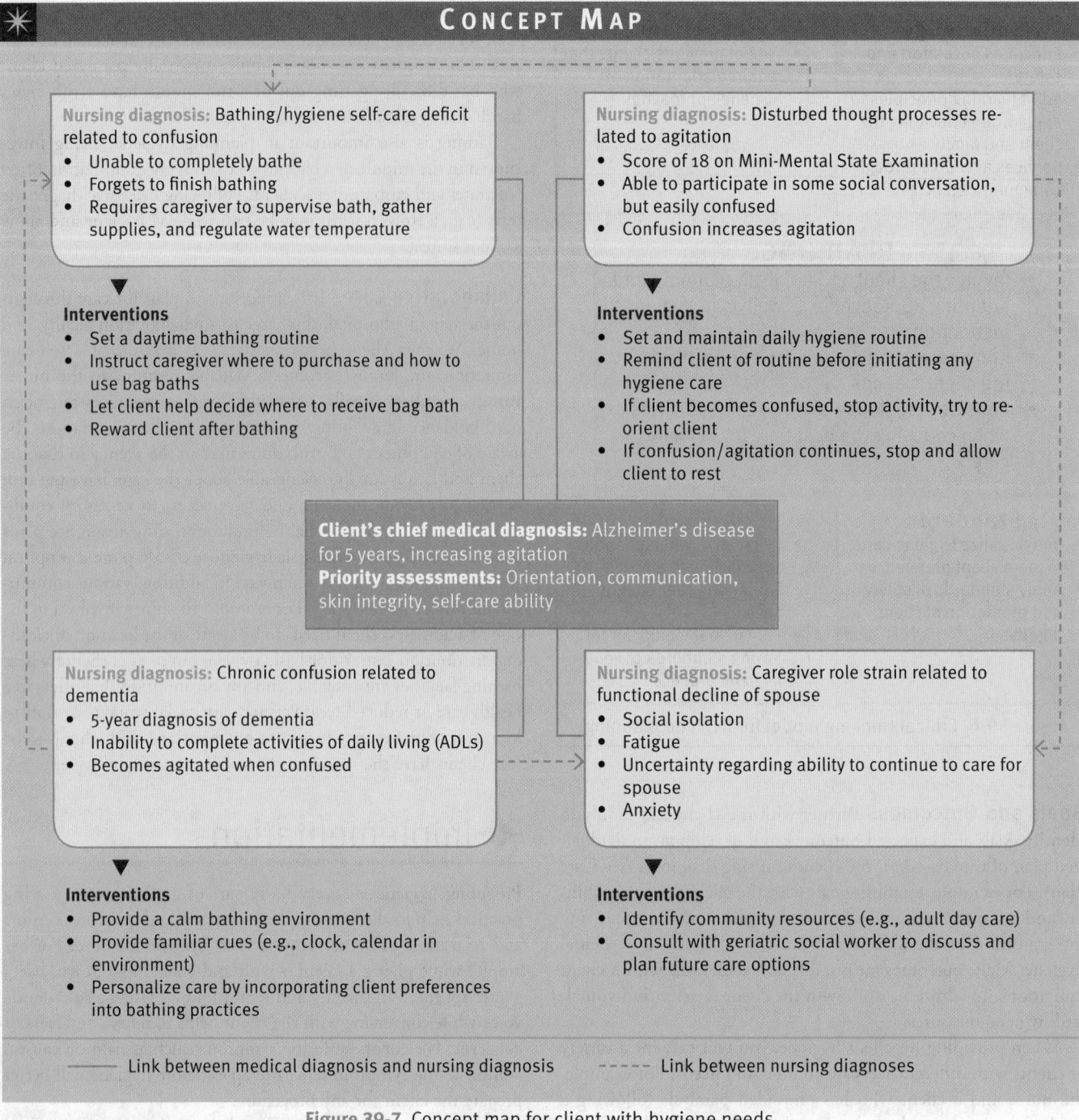

Nursing diagnosis: Bathing/hygiene self-care deficit related to confusion
- Unable to completely bathe
- Forgets to finish bathing
- Requires caregiver to supervise bath, gather supplies, and regulate water temperature

Interventions
- Set a daytime bathing routine
- Instruct caregiver where to purchase and how to use bag baths
- Let client help decide where to receive bag bath
- Reward client after bathing

Nursing diagnosis: Disturbed thought processes related to agitation
- Score of 18 on Mini-Mental State Examination
- Able to participate in some social conversation, but easily confused
- Confusion increases agitation

Interventions
- Set and maintain daily hygiene routine
- Remind client of routine before initiating any hygiene care
- If client becomes confused, stop activity, try to re-orient client
- If confusion/agitation continues, stop and allow client to rest

Client's chief medical diagnosis: Alzheimer's disease for 5 years, increasing agitation
Priority assessments: Orientation, communication, skin integrity, self-care ability

Nursing diagnosis: Chronic confusion related to dementia
- 5-year diagnosis of dementia
- Inability to complete activities of daily living (ADLs)
- Becomes agitated when confused

Nursing diagnosis: Caregiver role strain related to functional decline of spouse
- Social isolation
- Fatigue
- Uncertainty regarding ability to continue to care for spouse
- Anxiety

Interventions
- Provide a calm bathing environment
- Provide familiar cues (e.g., clock, calendar in environment)
- Personalize care by incorporating client preferences into bathing practices

Interventions
- Identify community resources (e.g., adult day care)
- Consult with geriatric social worker to discuss and plan future care options

—— Link between medical diagnosis and nursing diagnosis   - - - - Link between nursing diagnoses

Figure 39-7 Concept map for client with hygiene needs.

cumulated cerumen. The hygiene skills described throughout this chapter provide standards for excellent physical care. When assisting clients, maintain these standards and incorporate adaptations as needed to the client's lifestyle, functional status, living arrangements, and preferences. Examples of educational tips for clients about hygiene practices include:

- Make any instruction relevant. After assessing a client's knowledge, motivations, and health beliefs, provide information that relates to the client's situation and will be most useful in resolving the client's problem. For example, when offering foot care instruction to a client with diabetes mellitus, explain how the circulation to the feet can be impaired and how that poses

a risk for poor healing and infection, especially when the skin becomes cut or broken.

- Adapt instruction of any techniques to the client's personal bathing facilities. Not all clients will have the ideal situation that exists in a health care setting (e.g., easily accessible shower or a bedside table to place over a bed). Use what facilities or equipment the client has so that personal care items are easy to reach, ensure the client's safety, and make sure the client feels comfortable in performing hygiene. For example, a young mother has more room and feels that bathing an infant will be safer if she uses her kitchen sink and counter rather than her bathroom sink.

- Teach the client steps to take to avoid injury. Almost any hygienic procedure poses risks (e.g., cutting a nail too close to

NURSING CARE PLAN

Risk for Impaired Skin Integrity Related to Bathing Hygiene Self-Care Deficit

Assessment

Mrs. Edith Wyatt is a 77-year-old woman with a history of degenerative arthritis and diabetes mellitus for 3 years, She complains of pain in the joints, weakness, and mobility limitations in the dominant hand. Mrs. Wyatt is a widow with her only child, a daughter, living in a city 200 miles away. Mrs. Wyatt lives in a first-floor apartment in a retirement center. She moved in 3 weeks earlier. The nurse, Jeannette, makes the initial home visit for Mrs. Wyatt. Jeannette's assessment reveals inability to wash body parts, unkempt appearance, difficulty turning and regulating a water faucet, and limited motion of arms. Jeannette also observes that Mrs. Wyatt has a right limp. Her shoes are worn and ill fitting.

Assessment Activities	Findings/Defining Characteristics*
Ask Mrs. Wyatt what is important to her to gain from your visit.	Mrs. Wyatt wants to continue to be independent in making decisions about her care. She tells Jeannette, **"It is important for me to be able to care for myself."**
Assess client's tolerance for activity, discomfort level, cognitive ability, and musculoskeletal function.	Assess range of motion of upper extremities. She states, **"It hurts to move my arms above my head and it is hard to reach my foot."**
Assess client's bathing preferences: frequency and time of day, type of hygiene products.	Mrs. Wyatt states, **"I cannot get used to the new bathroom. The floor in the shower is slippery. I cannot reach my towels and soap."**
	Current bathroom has a shower with handgrips, levers turn up and down versus clockwise, and shower seat is available. The handles on the shower are levers versus faucets. The room also has a small closet for linens with a large countertop adjacent to the sink.
	Mrs. Wyatt's **hair is not washed or combed.**
Assess the condition of Mrs. Wyatt's feet and her knowledge about prevention and routine foot care.	Both feet are **dry** and toe **nails evenly trimmed** at end of toe. The outer aspect of the **little toe** on right foot is **reddened, tender** to touch with intact skin. Mrs. Wyatt states, "I have my doctor trim my toenails every month because of my sugar problems."

*__Defining characteristics__ are shown in bold type.

Nursing Diagnosis: Risk for impaired skin integrity related to bathing hygiene self-care deficit.

Planning

Goal	Expected Outcomes (NOC)†
	Knowledge: Illness Care
Mrs. Wyatt will verbalize preventive and routine foot care.	Mrs. Wyatt is able to accurately inspect tissue integrity of feet and toenails within 1 month.
	Mrs. Wyatt describes correct preventive foot care practices within 1 month
	Skin Integrity
Skin integrity of both feet will improve within 1 month.	Open area on right little toe will decrease or heal within 2 weeks.
	Tissue inflammation on right toe will resolve within 1 month.

†Outcome classification labels from Moorhead S and others: *Nursing outcomes classification (NOC),* ed 4, St. Louis, 2008, Mosby.

Interventions (NIC)‡
Skin Surveillance

Interventions (NIC)‡	Rationale
Review with client how to observe feet for breaks in skin and friction from shoes by using a mirror.	Injury to the diabetic foot from improper nail care, friction from poorly fitting shoes, and minor injuries to the foot increases the client's risk for infection, impaired mobility, and amputation (Strauss, Hart, and Winant, 1998).
Instruct client to observe feet for reddened areas, abrasions, blisters, and swollen areas immediately after removing shoes.	Improperly fitting shoes produce friction, redness, and swelling. Observation for these conditions immediately after removing shoes promotes timely identification of early foot problems (Bryant and Beinlich, 1999).

‡Intervention classification labels from Bulechek GM, Butcher HK, and Dochterman JM: *Nursing interventions classification (NIC),* ed 5, St. Louis, 2008, Mosby.

Continued

NURSING CARE PLAN

Risk for Impaired Skin Integrity Related to Bathing Hygiene Self-Care Deficit—cont'd

Interventions (NIC)‡	Rationale
Skin Care	
Show client how to clean and apply moisturizers and other skin care products to feet daily. Have a nurse from the retirement center provide assistance when available.	Proper foot care practices include daily cleaning and moisturizing of the feet (Boyer, 2001).
Explain that the client should see a podiatrist every 4 to 6 weeks for nail care.	Regular nail care, callus removal, and inspection of feet by a professional reduces the risk for peripheral tissue injury and subsequent immobility and morbidity (Green, Aliabaide, and Green, 2002).
Refer client to an orthotic footwear specialist.	Orthotic footwear specialist can evaluate client's walk patterns and create footwear individualized to client's walk, weight, and other individual needs. Specialized footwear can reduce the risk of impaired skin integrity of the feet.

‡Intervention classification labels from Bulechek GM, Butcher HK, and Dochterman JM: *Nursing interventions classification (NIC)*, ed 5, St. Louis, 2008, Mosby.

Evaluation

Nursing Actions	Client Response/Finding	Achievement of Outcome
Observe client's feet.	Redness and open areas are absent.	Resolution of redness and open areas are resolved.
Ask client about frequency of foot inspection.	Mrs. Wyatt states that she observes her feet daily after removing her shoes and immediately before bed.	Mrs. Wyatt reports inspecting feet daily is difficult. However, by using a mirror no new foot injuries are observed.
Observe client's foot care practice.	Mrs. Wyatt had a nurse from the retirement center wash and moisturize her feet. She was not wearing socks with her shoes. She states that she does not consistently wear socks.	Mrs. Wyatt is able to perform diabetic foot hygiene practice but is not consistent in preventative practice.
Ask client about podiatrist appointment.	Mrs. Wyatt states that she has a monthly appointment scheduled for the next 6 months for toenail trimming and care.	Mrs. Wyatt has achieved this preventative practice.

the skin, failing to adjust the water temperature of the bath, or using tap water for contact lens care). Any instruction must clearly outline safety risks.

• Reinforce infection control practices. Damage to the skin, mucosa, eyes, or other tissues creates an immediate risk for infection. Be sure the client understands the relationship between healthy and intact skin and tissues, hand hygiene practices, and the prevention of infection.

The *Healthy People 2010* initiative (see Chapter 6) includes recommendations to improve the dental health of the population of the United States. The goals for oral health are to decrease tooth loss caused by tooth decay or periodontal disease for people ages 35 to 44, reduce the number of older adults who have lost their natural teeth, reduce the prevalence of gingivitis, and reduce destructive periodontal disease among individuals ages 35 to 44 (Gadbury-Amyot and others, 2002).

Acute and Restorative Care. Nursing knowledge and skills needed for performing hygiene care are consistent across all health care settings where acute care and restorative care are provided (Box 39-7). In addition, some of the skills in this section are applicable in areas of health promotion.

In health care settings where clients receive direct nursing care, nurses provide a variety of hygiene measures. Times often change because of factors affecting the nurse's organization or scheduling of care, such as client preferences and cultural considerations, planned diagnostic and treatment procedures, the client's need for more hygiene, or the nurse's work assignment. In extended care facilities and nursing homes, the schedule for hygiene is often less frequent.

Bathing and Skin Care. Bathing and skin care are a part of total hygiene. Consider the client's normal grooming routines, including type of hygiene products used and the time of day when hygiene is routinely performed. Individualize your care based on the client's preferences. The extent of a client's bath and the methods used for bathing depend on the client's physical abilities, health problems, and the degree of hygiene required (Box 39-8).

If a client is physically dependent or cognitively impaired, increase skin assessment and provide skin care directed toward reducing the risk for skin breakdown. When bathing cognitively impaired clients there are special needs and challenges that are considered (Box 39-9).

These clients easily become afraid and use physical and verbal aggressive behaviors to avoid bathing. When family members as-

BOX 39-7 Hygiene Care Schedule in Acute and Long-Term Care Settings

Early Morning Care

Nursing personnel on the night shift provide basic hygiene to clients getting ready for breakfast, scheduled tests, or early morning surgery. "AM care" includes offering a bedpan or urinal if the client is not ambulatory, washing the client's hands and face, and assisting with oral care.

Routine Morning Care

After breakfast, assist by offering a bedpan or urinal to clients confined to bed; providing a bath or shower; providing perineal care; providing oral, foot, nail, and hair care; giving a back rub; changing the client's gown or pajamas; changing the bed linens; and straightening the client's bedside unit and room. This is often referred to as "complete AM care."

Afternoon Care

Hospitalized clients often undergo many exhausting diagnostic tests or procedures in the morning. In rehabilitation centers, clients participate in physical therapy during the morning. Afternoon hygiene care includes washing the hands and face, assisting with oral care, offering a bedpan or urinal, and straightening bed linen.

Evening, or Hour-Before-Sleep, Care

Before bedtime offer personal hygiene care that helps a client relax to promote sleep. "PM care" often includes changing soiled bed linens, gowns, or pajamas; assisting the client in washing the face and hands; providing oral hygiene; giving a back massage; and offering the bedpan or urinal to nonambulatory clients. Some clients enjoy a beverage such as juice; check diet to determine which beverages are allowed.

---

sist in bathing cognitively impaired clients, it is important to provide the family members with coaching, practice, and support (Mahoney and others, 2006).

A **complete bed bath** is an activity that is exhausting for a client. Turning during a complete bed bath and receiving back care increases oxygen consumption and demand (Verderber and Gallagher, 1994). Anticipate and assess whether clients are physically able to tolerate a complete bath. Measuring heart rate before, during, and after the bath provides a measure of the client's physical tolerance. An aging or dependent client in need of only partial hygiene or a self-sufficient bedridden client unable to reach all body parts receives a **partial bed bath.** Carefully assess to determine if clients can sufficiently bathe other body parts on their own. If either of these bath options are used, wear gloves whenever there is a risk of contacting body fluids. It is important to control environmental factors that may alter skin integrity such as moisture, heat, and external sources of pressure such as wrinkled bed linen and improperly placed drainage tubing.

When administering either a complete or partial bath, it is important to assess the condition of the skin to determine if soap is necessary or if the client requires daily bathing. Clients with excessively dry skin are predisposed to skin impairment. Using soaps that contain emollients is another option. Lubricating the skin with lotion also helps to reduce dryness.

Use the tub bath or shower to give a more thorough bath than a bed bath. Safety is of primary concern because the surface of a

---

BOX 39-8 Types of Baths

Complete bed bath: Bath administered to totally dependent client in bed (Skill 39-1).

Partial bed bath: Bed bath that consists of bathing only body parts that would cause discomfort if left unbathed, such as the hands, face, axillae, and perineal area. Partial bath also includes washing back and providing back rub. Dependent clients in need of partial hygiene or self-sufficient bedridden clients who are unable to reach all body parts receive a partial bath.

Sponge bath at the sink: Involves bathing from a bath basin or sink with the client sitting in a chair. Client is able to perform a portion of the bath independently. Assistance is needed for hard-to-reach areas.

Tub bath: Involves immersion in a tub of water that allows more thorough washing and rinsing than a bed bath. Client may still require the nurse's assistance. Some institutions have tubs equipped with lifting devices that facilitate positioning dependent clients in the tub.

Shower: Client sits or stands under a continuous stream of water. The shower provides more thorough cleaning than a bed bath but can be fatiguing.

Bed Bath/Travel Bath: Developed by Skewes (1994), the Bag Bath contains several soft, nonwoven cotton cloths that are premoistened in a solution of no-rinse surfactant cleanser and emollient. The Bed Bath offers an alternative because of the ease of use, reduced time bathing, and client comfort.

BOX 39-9 Bathing Persons With Dementia

- Provide individualized and flexible client-centered care.
  - Obtain bathing history, what works, what does not; when possible, identify client's preferences.
  - Determine what if any analgesia is needed before bathing.
  - Determine least distressing method (e.g., soaking feet in bathtub).
  - Minimize the time the client is unclothed and number of caregivers.
- Use distraction and negotiation instead of demands.
  - Create a calm bathing environment (e.g., reduce noise, set comfortable room temperature).
  - Set priorities of areas that must be bathed, others that can be "skipped."
  - If client fears water, bubble baths might help.
- Reward client after bathing.
  - Make sure goals and rewards are realistic.
  - Always give agreed reward.
- Use a person-centered approach to bathing.
  - Personalize/individualize care to each client.
  - Incorporate client preferences and habits into bathing practices.
  - Use slow, nonhurried motions.
- Use effective communication skills.
  - Use a gentle, calm voice.
- Adapt the physical environment and bathing procedure to decrease client's distress or discomfort.

Modified from Hall GR, Buckwalter KC: Evidence based protocol: bathing persons with dementia. In Titler MG, series editor: *Series on evidence-based practice for older adults,* Iowa City, 2001, The University of Iowa College of Nursing Gerontological Nursing Interventions Research Center, Research Dissemination Core, revised 2001; Hoeffer B and others: Assessing cognitively impaired nursing home residents with bathing: effects of two bathing interventions on caregiving, *Gerontologist* 46(4):524, 2006; and Rader J and others: The bathing of older adults with dementia, *Am J Nurs* 106(4):40, 2006.

tub or shower stall is slippery. In some settings a physician's order for a shower or tub bath is necessary. In some agencies, showers have a chair for clients with weakness or poor balance. Both tubs and showers need to have grab bars for clients to hold on to during entry and exit and maneuvering. Clients vary in how much help they will need. Regardless of the type of bath the client receives, use the following guidelines:

- *Provide privacy.* Close the door, or pull room curtains around the bathing area. While bathing the client, expose only the areas being bathed.
- *Maintain safety.* Keep side rails up while away from the client's bedside when clients are dependent or unconscious. NOTE: When side rails serve as a restraint, you need a health care provider's order (see agency-specific policy for restraint usage) (Chapter 38). Place the call light in the client's reach if leaving the room temporarily.
- *Maintain warmth.* Keep the room warm because the client is partially uncovered and will be easily chilled. Wet skin causes an excess loss of heat through evaporation. Control drafts, and keep windows closed. Keep client covered, only exposing the body part being washed during the bath.
- *Promote independence.* Encourage the client to participate in as much of the bathing activities as possible. Offer assistance when needed.
- *Anticipate needs.* Bring a new set of clothing and hygiene products to the bedside or bathroom.

Bag Baths. An innovative approach to the traditional bed bath was developed because of nurses' concern for clients who are predisposed to dry skin and the risk for infection (see Skill 39-1). When washbasins are not cleaned and dried completely after use, there is the risk of contamination by gram-negative organisms. Successive uses of the basin causes the client's skin to harbor more gram-negative organisms. Sheppard and Brenner (2000) tested the Bag Bath/Travel Bath, which contains a no-rinse surfactant, a humectant to trap moisture, and emollient, and found that it significantly reduced overall skin dryness, especially skin flaking and scaling. There are now several commercial body cleansing systems available that contain the same ingredients as the Bag Bath. Nurses expressed a significant overall preference for the disposable bath versus the traditional basin bath, especially for clients who are unable to bathe themselves in critical care and long-term care settings (Larson and others 2004).

Perineal Care. **Perineal care** is usually part of the complete bed bath (Skill 39-2, p. 877). Clients most in need of perineal care are those at greatest risk for acquiring an infection (e.g., uncircumcised males, clients who have indwelling urinary catheters, or clients who are recovering from rectal or genital surgery or childbirth). In addition, women who are having a menstrual period will require good perineal care. If a client is able to perform perineal self-care, encourage this independence. Sometimes you might be embarrassed about providing perineal care, particularly to clients of the opposite sex. Similarly, the client usually feels embarrassed. Do not let embarrassment cause you to overlook the client's hygiene needs. When staffing levels permit, use a gender-congruent caregiver or have a caregiver of the opposite sex present in the room during perineal care. A professional, dignified, and sensitive approach will reduce embarrassment and put the client at ease.

If a client performs self-care, various problems such as vaginal and urethral discharge, skin irritation, and unpleasant odors often go unnoticed. Be alert for complaints of burning during urination or localized soreness, excoriation, or pain in the perineum. Inspect the client's bed linen for signs of discharge. Clients most at risk for skin breakdown in the perineal area are those with urinary or fecal incontinence, rectal and perineal surgical dressings, indwelling urinary catheters, and the morbidly obese.

Back Rub. A back rub or back massage usually follows the client's bath. It promotes relaxation, relieves muscular tension, and decreases perception of pain (Piotrowski and others, 2003). Zullino and others (2005) evaluated the efficacy of massage and its effects on the physiological measures of relaxation. Their analysis showed that the long, slow, gliding strokes **(effleurage)** of a massage are associated with reduced measured anxiety, heart rate, and respiratory rate. Males seem to achieve greater reductions in systolic and diastolic blood pressure during back rub than females. Because effleurage causes an immediate rise in blood pressure and heart rate in clients who have had coronary artery bypass surgery, the researchers do not recommend the therapy for those clients within the first 48 hours of their surgery. Clients generally report that they are more comfortable following a back rub and find the experience pleasant, regardless of the length of the massage. However, a back rub of 3 minutes' duration actually enhances client comfort and relaxation and thus is very therapeutic (Zullino and others, 2005).

When providing a back rub, enhance relaxation by reducing any noise and ensuring the client is comfortable. It is important to ask whether a client would like a back rub or if the client prefers gentle instead of deep massage, because some individuals dislike physical contact. Consult the medical record for any contraindications to a massage (e.g., fractured ribs, burns of the skin, and heart surgery).

Foot and Nail Care. Incorporate foot and nail care into a person's regular hygiene routine. Routine care involves soaking to soften cuticles and layers of horny cells, thorough cleansing, drying, and proper nail trimming. The exception involves clients with diabetes mellitus who do not soak their nails because of the risk of infection. When the nurse is providing nail care, the client remains in bed or sits in a chair (Skill 39-3, p. 880). In some settings or with specific clients, such as a person with diabetes mellitus, you will need a health care provider's order to trim a client's toenails. Before implementing this procedure, check agency policy to determine if a health care provider's order is necessary.

Take time during the procedure to teach the client and family proper techniques for cleaning and nail trimming. You need to stress measures to prevent infection and promote good circulation. Clients learn to protect the feet from injury, keep the feet clean and dry, and wear footwear that fits properly. Instruct clients in the proper way to inspect all surfaces of the feet and hands for redness, lesions, dryness, or signs of infection. It is important for clients to know the appearance of any abnormalities and the importance of reporting these conditions to their caregiver (Boyer, 2001).

Text continued on p. 883

✳ **SKILL 39-1**   **BATHING A CLIENT**   Video

Delegation Considerations

The skill of bathing may be delegated. The nurse is responsible for skin and musculoskeletal assessment. The nurse informs nursing assistive personnel about:
- Not massaging reddened skin areas
- The early signs of impaired skin integrity for select clients and their situation
- Proper ways to position male and female clients with musculoskeletal limitations and indwelling Foley catheters
- Reporting changes in the client's skin to the nurse

Equipment

- Washcloths and bath towels
- Bath blanket
- Soap and soap dish
- Toiletry items (deodorant, powder, lotion, cologne)
- Toilet tissue or wipes
- Clean hospital gown or client's own pajamas or gown
- Laundry bag
- Clean gloves (when risk for contacting body fluids)
- Warm water

STEPS	RATIONALE
1. Assess client's tolerance for bathing, activity tolerance, comfort level, cognitive ability, musculoskeletal function, and presence of shortness of breath.	Determines client's ability to perform self-care and level of assistance required from nurse. Also determines type of bath to administer (e.g., tub bath, partial bed bath).

Critical Decision Point: Clients whose level of independence and mobility change frequently may require more or less assistance during bathing.

STEPS	RATIONALE
2. Assess client's visual status, ability to sit without support, hand grasp, ROM of extremities.	Determines degree of assistance needed for bathing.
3. Assess client's bathing preferences: frequency and time of day preferred for bathing, type of hygiene products, and other facts related to client preferences.	Client participates in plan of care. Promotes client's comfort and provides opportunity to include cultural or personal hygiene preferences in hygiene care.
4. Ask if client has noticed any problems or unusual marks on skin: excessive moisture, inflammation, drainage or excretions from lesions or body cavities, rashes or other skin lesions.	Provides information to direct physical assessment of skin and genitalia during bathing. Also influences selection of skin care products.
5. Assess condition of client's skin. Note the presence of dryness, indicated by flaking, redness, scaling, and cracking.	Provides a baseline for comparison over time in determining if bathing improves condition of skin.
6. Review orders for specific precautions concerning client's movement or positioning.	Prevents accidental injury to client during bathing activities. Determines level of assistance required by client.
7. Explain procedure, and ask client for suggestions on how to prepare supplies. If partial bath, ask how much of bath client wishes to complete.	Promotes client's cooperation and participation.
8. Adjust room temperature and ventilation, close room doors and windows, and draw room divider curtain.	Warm room that is free of drafts prevents rapid loss of body heat during bathing. Privacy ensures client's mental and physical comfort.
9. Prepare equipment and supplies.	Avoids interrupting procedure or leaving client unattended to retrieve missing equipment.
10. Offer client bedpan or urinal. Provide towel and washcloth.	Client will feel more comfortable after voiding. Prevents interruption of bath.
11. Perform hand hygiene. If client's skin is soiled with drainage or body secretions, apply clean gloves. Ensure client is not allergic to latex.	Reduces transmission of microorganisms.
12. Bathe client.	
A. Complete or partial bed bath	
(1) Verify that the bed is in locked position, and raise bed to your comfort level. If raised, lower side rail closest to you, and assist client in assuming comfortable position, maintaining body alignment. Bring client toward side closest to nurse.	Prevents bed from moving. Nurse does not have to reach across bed, thus minimizing strain on back muscles. Raising the height of the bed to appropriate position facilitates proper body mechanics.

Critical Decision Point: If it necessary to leave client's beside (e.g., to get additional supplies, to obtain clean water), return bed to low position and elevate side rail.

STEPS	RATIONALE
(2) Loosen top covers at foot of bed. Place bath blanket over top sheet. Fold and remove top sheet from under blanket. If possible, have client hold bath blanket while withdrawing sheet. *Optional:* Use top sheet when bath blanket is not available.	Removal of top linens prevents them from becoming soiled or moist during bath. Blanket provides warmth and privacy.

Continued

✳ **SKILL 39-1**   **BATHING A CLIENT—CONT'D**

STEPS

(3) If top sheet is to be reused, fold it for replacement later. If not, dispose in laundry bag, taking care not to allow linen to contact uniform.

(4) Remove client's gown or pajamas.

    a. If gown has snaps at sleeves, simply unsnap and remove gown without pulling on IV.

    b. If the client has a regular gown and if an extremity is injured or has reduced mobility, begin removal from *unaffected* side.

    c. If client has IV tube, remove gown from arm *without* IV first; then lower IV container or remove from pump and slide gown covering affected arm over tubing and container. Rehang IV container, and check flow rate (see illustrations).

    d. If IV pump is in use, turn pump off, clamp tubing, remove tubing from pump, proceed as in Step c. Insert tubing into pump, unclamp tubing, and turn pump on at correct rate. Observe flow rate, and regulate if necessary. **Do not disconnect tubing.**

    e. Drape client with bath blanket.

RATIONALE

Proper disposal prevents transmission of microorganisms.

Provides full exposure of body parts during bathing. Undressing unaffected side first allows easier manipulation of gown over body part with reduced ROM.

Manipulation of IV tubing and container may disrupt flow rate.

Regulation is needed to prevent improper infusion of fluids.

Critical Decision Point: If available, be sure that clients with an IV or upper extremity injury have a gown with snap or tie sleeves. Thus there is easy access to upper extremities during hygiene.

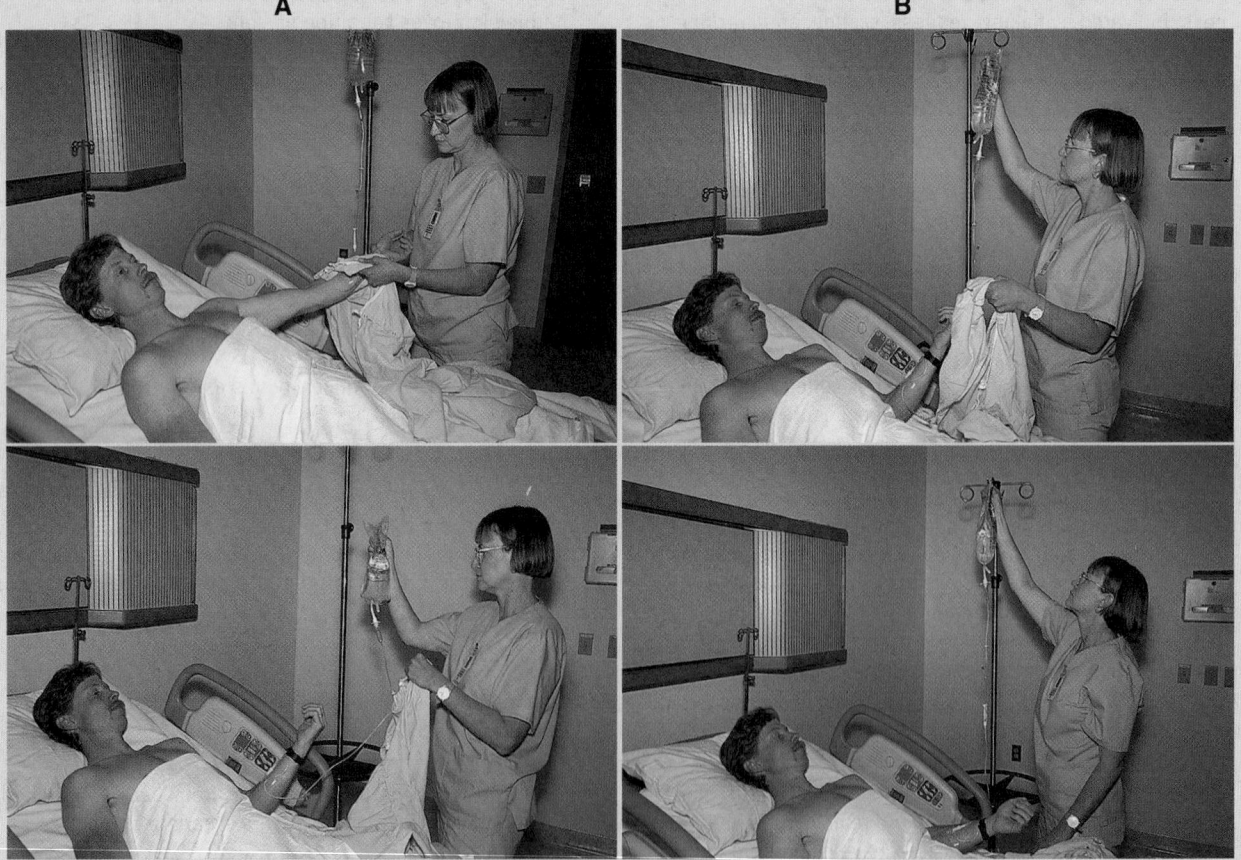

STEP 12A(4)c A, Remove client's gown. **B,** Remove IV from pole. **C,** Slide IV tubing through arm of client's gown. **D,** Rehang IV bag.

Critical Decision Point: When using an IV pump, manually adjust the IV flow rate to a keep vein open (KVO) flow and remove the IV tubing from the pump (check agency policy). When the bath is complete, reset the pump to the prescribed IV flow rate (see Chapter 41).

STEPS	RATIONALE
(5) Pull side rail up as appropriate. Fill washbasin two-thirds full with warm water. Have client place fingers in water to test temperature tolerance. Place plastic container of bath lotion in bath water to warm, if desired.	Raising side rail maintains client's safety as nurse leaves bedside. Warm water promotes comfort, relaxes muscles, and prevents unnecessary chilling. Testing temperature prevents accidental burns. Bath water warms lotion for application to client's skin.
(6) Remove pillow if allowed, and raise head of bed 30 to 45 degrees. Place bath towel under client's head. Place second bath towel over client's chest.	Removal of pillow makes it easier to wash client's ears and neck. Placement of towels prevents soiling of bed linen and bath blanket.
(7) Immerse washcloth in water, and wring thoroughly. If desired, fold washcloth around fingers of nurse's hand to form mitt (see illustration).	Mitt retains water and heat better than loosely held washcloth; keeps cold edges from brushing against client and prevents splashing.
(8) Inquire if client is wearing contact lenses. Wash client's eyes with plain warm water, and perform eye care as needed. Wash client's eyes using a different section of mitt for each eye. Move mitt from inner to outer canthus (see illustration). Soak any crusts on eyelid for 2 to 3 minutes with damp cloth before attempting removal. Dry eye thoroughly but gently.	Soap irritates eyes. Use of separate sections of mitt reduces infection transmission. Bathing eye from inner to outer canthus prevents secretions from entering nasolacrimal duct. Pressure causes internal injury.
(9) Ask if client prefers to use soap on face. Wash, rinse, and dry forehead, cheeks, nose, neck, and ears. (Men often shave at this point or after bath.)	Soap tends to dry face, which is exposed to air more than other body parts.
(10) Remove bath blanket from client's arm that is closest to nurse. Place bath towel lengthwise under arm.	Prevents soiling of bed.
(11) Bathe arm with soap and water using long, firm strokes from distal to proximal areas (fingers to axilla). Raise and support arm as needed while thoroughly washing axilla (see illustration).	Soap lowers surface tension and facilitates removal of debris and bacteria when friction is applied during washing. Long, firm strokes stimulate circulation. Movement of arm exposes axilla and exercises joint's normal ROM.
(12) Rinse and dry arm and axilla thoroughly. If client uses deodorant or talcum powder, apply it.	Alkaline residue from soap discourages growth of normal skin bacteria. Excess moisture causes skin maceration or softening. Deodorant controls body odor.
(13) Fold bath towel in half, and lay it on bed beside client. Place basin on towel. Immerse client's hand in water. Allow hand to soak for 3 to 5 minutes before washing hand and fingernails (see Skill 39-3, p. 880). Remove basin, and dry hand well.	Soaking softens cuticles and calluses of hand, loosens debris beneath nails, and enhances feeling of cleanliness. Thorough drying removes moisture from between fingers. NOTE: Do not soak if client is diabetic.

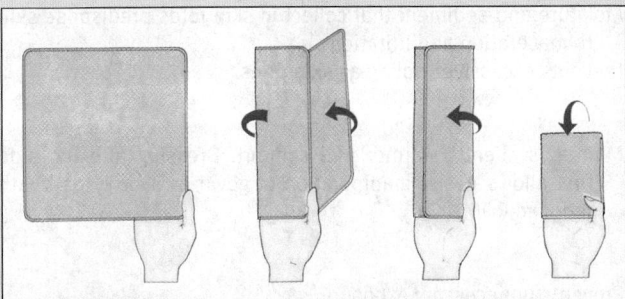

STEP 12A(7) Steps for folding washcloth to form a mitt.

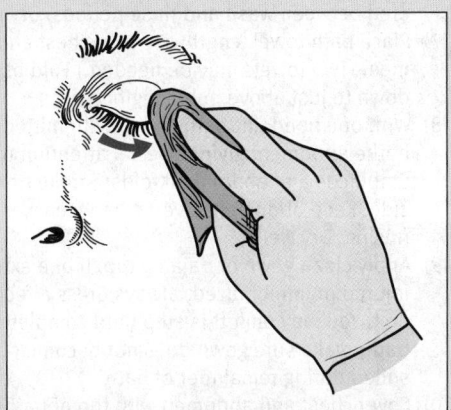

STEP 12A(8) Wash eye from inner to outer canthus.

Continued

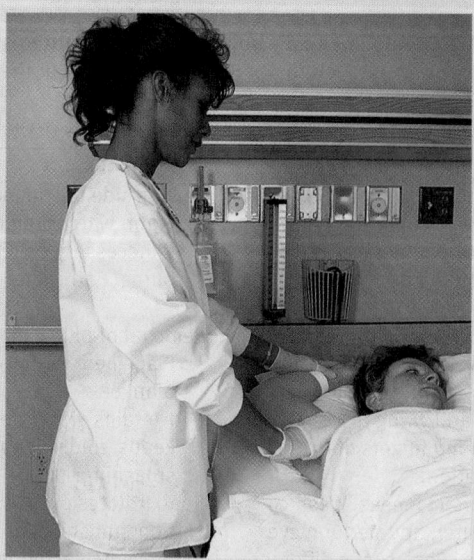

STEP 12A(11) Positioning the arm to wash the axilla.

STEPS	RATIONALE
(14) Raise side rail, and move to other side of bed. Lower side rail, and repeat Steps 10 through 13 for other arm.	
(15) Check temperature of bath water, and change water if necessary.	Warm water maintains client's comfort.

Critical Decision Point: If a client is at risk for falls, assess if full or partial side rails are needed while you obtain fresh water or other supplies. Remember, if all four side rails are elevated it is considered to be a restraint (Chapter 38). Check with agency for its rules on restraint use.

STEPS	RATIONALE
(16) Cover client's chest with bath towel, and fold bath blanket down to umbilicus. With one hand, lift edge of towel away from chest. With washcloth or mitted hand, bathe chest using long, firm strokes. Take special care to wash skin folds under female client's breasts. It is often necessary to lift breast upward while bathing underneath it. Keep client's chest covered between wash and rinse periods. Dry well.	Draping prevents unnecessary exposure of body parts. Towel maintains warmth and privacy. Secretions and dirt collect easily in areas of tight skin folds. Skin folds are susceptible to excoriation if breasts are pendulous.
(17) Place bath towel lengthwise over chest and abdomen. (Two towels may be needed.) Fold blanket down to just above pubic region.	Prevents chilling and exposure of body parts.
(18) With one hand, lift bath towel. With mitted hand, bathe abdomen, giving special attention to bathing umbilicus and abdominal folds. Stroke from side to side. Keep abdomen covered between washing and rinsing. Dry well.	Moisture and sediment that collect in skin folds predispose skin to maceration and irritation. Prevents excessive cooling as skin dries.
(19) Apply clean gown or pajama top. If one extremity is injured or immobilized, always dress affected side first. You may omit this step until completion of bath; make sure gown does not become damp or soiled during remainder of bath.	Maintains client's warmth and comfort. Dressing affected side first allows easier manipulation of gown over body part with reduced ROM.
(20) Cover chest and abdomen with top of bath blanket. Expose near leg by folding blanket toward midline. Be sure other leg and perineum are draped.	Prevents unnecessary exposure.

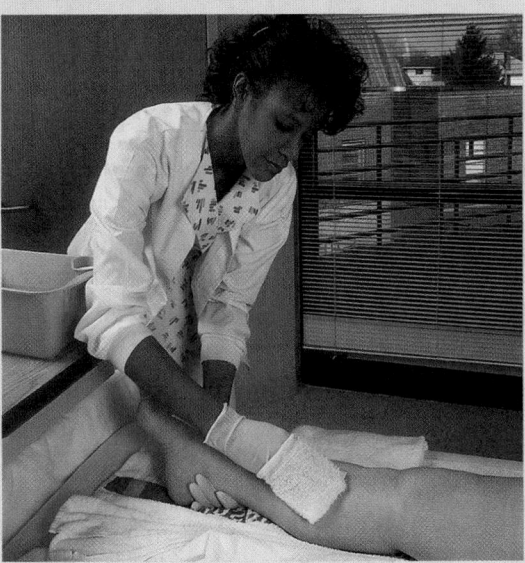

STEP 12A(22) Washing the leg.

STEPS	RATIONALE
(21) Bend client's leg at knee by positioning nurse's arm under leg. While grasping client's heel, elevate leg from mattress slightly, and slide bath towel lengthwise under leg. Ask client to hold foot still. Place bath basin on towel on bed, and secure its position next to foot to be washed.	Towel prevents soiling of bed linen. Support of joint and extremity during lifting prevents strain on musculoskeletal structures. Sudden movement by client could spill bath water. (Omit this step if client is unable to hold leg in basin.)
(22) With one hand supporting lower leg, raise it and slide basin under lifted foot. Make sure foot is firmly placed on bottom of basin. Allow foot to soak while washing leg. If client is unable to hold leg, do not immerse; simply wash with washcloth (see illustration).	Proper positioning of foot prevents pressure being applied from edge of basin against calf. Soaking softens calluses and rough skin.
(23) Unless contraindicated, use long, firm strokes in washing from ankle to knee and from knee to thigh. Dry well.	Promotes venous return.

Critical Decision Point: During the bath assess for signs of warmth, redness, swelling, tenderness, and pain in the lower extremities (Beck, 2006).

(24) Cleanse foot, making sure to bathe between toes. Clean and clip nails as per physician's orders (see Skill 39-3, p. 880). Dry well. If skin is dry, apply lotion.	Secretions and moisture are often present between toes. Lotion helps retain moisture and soften skin.

Critical Decision Point: Do not massage any reddened area on client's skin because massaging causes breaks in the skin's surface capillaries and increased risk of skin breakdown (AHCPR, 1992).

(25) Raise side rail as appropriate, and move to other side of the bed. Lower side rail, and repeat Steps 20 through 24 for other leg and foot.	
(26) Cover client with bath blanket, raise side rail according to client's need for safety, and change bath water.	Decreased bath water temperature causes chilling. Clean water reduces microorganism transmission.
(27) Lower side rail. Assist client in assuming prone or side-lying position (as applicable). Place towel lengthwise along client's side.	Exposes back and buttocks for bathing.

Continued

✳ **SKILL 39-1**   **BATHING A CLIENT—CONT'D**

STEPS	RATIONALE
(28) Keep client draped by sliding bath blanket over shoulders and thighs. Wash, rinse, and dry back from neck to buttocks using long, firm strokes. Apply clean gloves if not done previously. Pay special attention to folds of buttocks and anus. Give a back rub (see Chapter 43). Change bath water.	Maintains warmth, and prevents unnecessary exposure. Skin folds near buttocks and anus contain fecal secretions that harbor microorganisms. Changing water prevents transfer of microorganisms from anal area to genitalia.
(29) If gloves become soiled, remove, perform hand hygiene, then reapply new pair of gloves. Assist client in assuming side-lying or supine position. Cover chest and upper extremities with towel and lower extremities with bath blanket. Expose only genitalia. (If client is able to wash, covering entire body with bath blanket is preferable.) Provide perineal care (see Skill 39-2, p. 877). Pay special attention to skin folds. Apply water-repellent ointment to area exposed to moisture.	Maintains client's privacy. Clients capable of performing partial bath usually prefer to wash their own genitalia. Water-repellent ointments (e.g., A&D, Pericare) protect skin from moisture.
(30) Dispose of gloves in receptacle.	Prevents transmission of infection.
(31) Apply additional body lotion or oil as desired.	Moisturizing lotion prevents dry, chapped skin.
(32) Assist client in dressing. Comb client's hair. Some women will want to apply makeup.	Promotes client's body image.
(33) Make client's bed (see Skill 39-6, p. 900).	Provides clean environment.
(34) Remove soiled linen, and place in dirty-linen bag. Clean and replace bathing equipment. Replace call light and personal possessions. Leave room as clean and comfortable as possible.	Prevents transmission of infection. Clean environment promotes client's comfort. Keeping call light and articles of care within reach promotes client's safety.
(35) Perform hand hygiene.	Reduces transmission of microorganisms.
B. Commercial Bath Cleansing Pack	
(1) The cleansing pack contains 8 to 10 premoistened towels for cleansing (see illustrations). Warm the package contents in a microwave following package instructions.	Provides soothing heat.
(2) Use a single towel for each general body part cleansed. Follow the same order of cleansing as the total or partial bed bath.	Reduces transmission of microorganisms.
(3) Allow the skin to air dry for 30 seconds. It is permissible to lightly cover the client with a bath towel to prevent chilling.	Drying the skin with a towel removes the emollient that is left behind after the water/cleanser solution evaporates.
(4) NOTE: If there is excessive soiling (e.g., in the perineal region), use an extra cleansing pack or conventional washcloths, soap, water, and towels.	

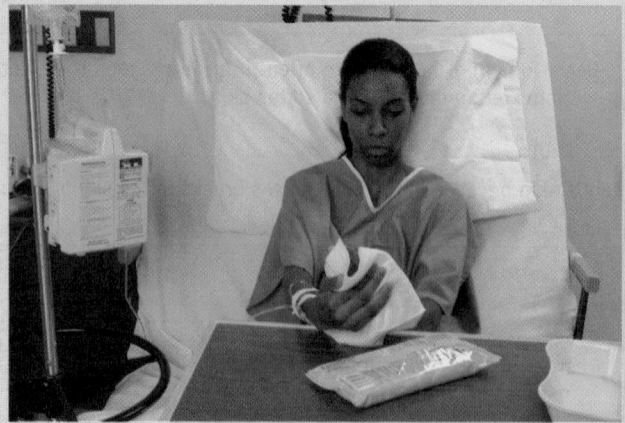
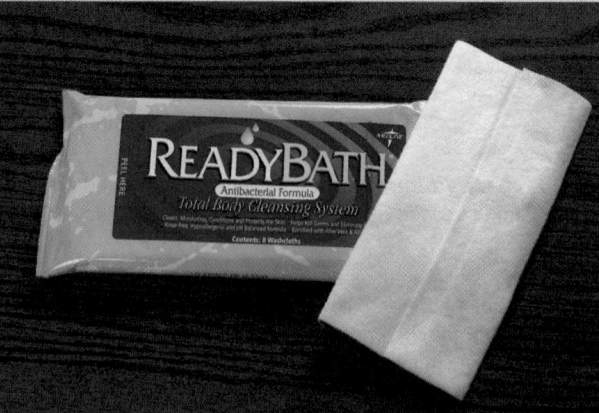

A   **B**

STEP 12B(1) Commercial bath cleansing pack. **A,** Client uses individual towels to bathe. **B,** Commercial bath cleansing pack.

☀ SKILL 39-1   **BATHING A CLIENT—CONT'D**

STEPS

C. **Tub or whirlpool bath or shower; verify with agency policy if a physician's or other health care provider's order is necessary**

   (1) Consider client's condition, and review orders for precautions concerning client's movement or positioning.

   (2) Check tub or shower for cleanliness. Use cleaning techniques outlined in agency policy. Place rubber mat on tub or shower bottom. Place disposable bath mat or towel on floor in front of tub or shower.

   (3) Collect all hygienic aids, toiletry items, and linens requested by client. Place within easy reach of tub or shower.

   (4) Assist client to bathroom if necessary. Have client wear robe and nonslip footwear to bathroom.

   (5) Demonstrate how to use call signal for assistance.

   (6) Place "occupied" sign on bathroom door.

   (7) Provide shower seat or tub chair if needed (see illustration). Fill bathtub halfway with warm water. If sensation is normal, ask client to test water, and adjust temperature if water is too warm. Explain which faucet controls hot water. If client is taking shower, turn shower on, and adjust water temperature before client enters shower stall.

   (8) Instruct client to use safety bars when getting in and out of tub or shower. Caution client against use of bath oil in tub water.

   (9) Instruct client not to remain in tub longer than 20 minutes. Check on client every 5 minutes.

  (10) Return to bathroom when client signals, and knock before entering.

  (11) For client who is unsteady, drain tub of water before client attempts to get out of it. Place bath towel over client's shoulders. Assist client in getting out of tub as needed, and assist with drying. If client is weak or unstable, have another person assist.

RATIONALE

Prevents accidental injury to client during bathing.

Cleaning prevents transmission of microorganisms. Mats prevent slipping and falling.

Placing items close at hand prevents possible falls when client reaches for equipment.

Assistance prevents accidental falls. Wearing robe and slippers prevents chilling.

Bathrooms are equipped with signaling devices in case client feels faint or weak or needs immediate assistance. Clients prefer privacy during bath, provided that it is safe to do so.

Maintains client's privacy.

Adjusting water temperature prevents accidental burns. Older adults and clients with neurological alterations (e.g., spinal cord injury) are at high risk for burns as a result of reduced sensation. Use of assistive devices facilitates bathing and minimizes physical exertion.

Prevents slipping and falling. Oil causes tub surfaces to become slippery.

Prolonged exposure to warm water causes vasodilatation and pooling of blood, leading to light-headedness or dizziness.

Provides privacy.

Prevents accidental falls. Client becomes chilled as water drains.

Critical Decision Point: Weak or unstable clients need extra assistance in getting in or out of a tub. Planning for additional personnel is essential before attempting to assist the client in or out of the tub.

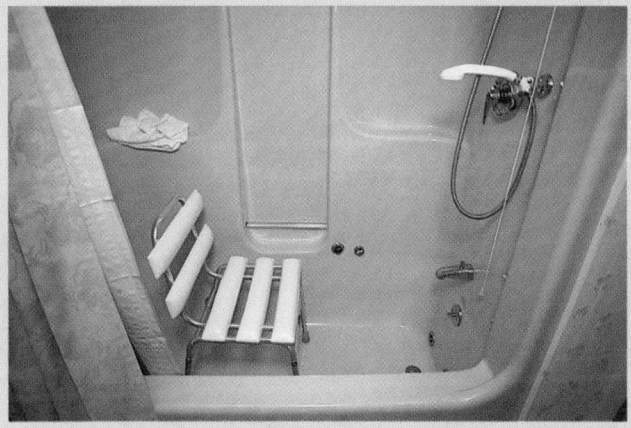

STEP 12C(7) Shower seat for client safety.

Continued

✳ **SKILL 39-1**   BATHING A CLIENT—CONT'D

STEPS

RATIONALE

(12) Assist client as needed in dressing in clean gown or pajamas, slippers, and robe. (In home setting, client will dress in regular clothing.)

Maintains warmth to prevent chilling.

(13) Assist client to room and comfortable position in bed or chair.

Maintains relaxation gained from bathing.

(14) Clean tub or shower according to agency policy. Whirlpool baths often require special cleansing. Remove soiled linen, and place in dirty-linen bag. Discard disposable equipment in proper receptacle. Place "unoccupied" sign on bathroom door. Return supplies to storage area.

Prevents transmission of infection through soiled linen and moisture.

(15) Perform hand hygiene.

Reduces transfer of microorganisms.

13. Observe skin, paying particular attention to areas that were previously soiled, reddened, or showed early signs of breakdown.

Techniques used during bathing leave skin clean and clear.

14. Observe or perform ROM during bath.

Measures joint mobility.

15. Ask client to rate level of comfort.

Evaluates success of bath in promoting client's comfort.

Unexpected Outcomes and Related Interventions

1. Areas of excessive dryness, rashes, irritation, or pressure ulcer appear on skin.
   a. Review agency skin care policy regarding special cleansing and moisturizing products.
   b. Limit frequency of complete baths.
   c. Complete pressure ulcer assessment (see Chapter 48).
   d. Institute turning and positioning measures to keep client off pressure ulcer.
   e. Obtain special bed surface if client is at risk for skin breakdown.
2. Client becomes excessively fatigued and unable to cooperate or participate in bathing.
   a. Reschedule bathing to a time when client is more rested.
   b. Clients with cardiopulmonary conditions and breathing difficulties require pillow or elevated head of bed during bathing.
   c. Notify health care provider about changes in client's fatigue level.
   d. Perform hygiene measures in stages between scheduled rest periods.

3. Client seems unusually restless or complains of discomfort.
   a. Consider analgesia before bathing.
   b. Schedule rest periods before bathing.

Recording and Reporting
- Record procedure on flow sheet if appropriate and amount of assistance, client participation.
- Record condition of skin and any significant findings (e.g., reddened areas, bruises, nevi, joint or muscle pain).
- Report evidence of alterations in skin integrity, break in suture line, or increased wound secretions to nurse in charge or health care provider.

Home Care Considerations
- Assess client's tub and shower area for the need for safety devices (e.g., grab bars).
- Assess client for the need for assistive bathing devices (e.g., shower chair, handheld shower).

✳ **SKILL 39-2**   **PERINEAL CARE**

Delegation Considerations
The skill of perineal care can be delegated. The nurse instructs nursing assistive personnel about:
- Any physical restrictions that affect proper way to position client for procedure
- Information about proper positioning of indwelling catheter during perineal care
- Informing nurse if any perineal drainage, excoriation, or rash is observed

Equipment
- Washbasin
- Soap dish with soap
- Washcloths and bath towel
- Bath blanket
- Waterproof pad or bedpan
- Toilet tissue or diaper wipes
- Clean gloves
- Additional supplies are necessary when giving perineal care other than during a bath:
  - Cotton balls or swabs
  - A solution bottle or container filled with warm water or prescribed rinsing solution
  - Waterproof bag

STEPS	RATIONALE
1. Identify clients at risk for developing infection of genitalia, urinary tract, or reproductive tract (e.g., uncircumcised male, presence of indwelling catheter, fecal incontinence).	Secretions that accumulate on surface of skin surrounding female and male genitalia act as reservoir for infection. Tissues traumatized by surgery or by presence of foreign object provide route for introduction of infectious organisms.
2. Assess client's cognitive, visual, and musculoskeletal function and activity tolerance.	Determines client's ability to perform self-care and determines level of assistance required from nurse.
3. Apply clean gloves, and assess genitalia for signs of inflammation, skin breakdown, or infection (see Chapter 33). Discard gloves. Perform hand hygiene.	Reduces infection. Determines extent of perineal care required by client.
4. Assess client's knowledge of importance of perineal hygiene.	Clients at risk for infection in perineal area are often unaware of importance of cleanliness. Reflects client's need for education.
5. Explain procedure and its purpose to client.	Helps minimize anxiety during procedure that is often embarrassing to nurse and client.
6. Prepare necessary equipment and supplies.	Used when administering a bed bath.
7. Pull curtain around client's bed, or close room door. Assemble supplies at bedside.	Maintains client's privacy and ensures orderly procedure.
8. Raise bed to comfortable working position. If raised, lower side rail, and assist client in assuming side-lying position, placing towel lengthwise along client's side and keeping client covered with bath blanket or top sheet.	Facilitates good body mechanics. Provides easy access to genitalia.

Critical Decision Point: If it necessary to leave client's beside (e.g., to get additional supplies, to obtain clean water), return bed to low position and elevate side rail as appropriate.

---

9. Apply clean gloves.	Eliminates transmission of microorganisms.
10. If fecal material is present, enclose in a fold of underpad or toilet tissue, and remove with disposable wipes or tissue. Cleanse buttocks and anus, washing front to back (see illustration). Cleanse, rinse, and dry area thoroughly. If needed, place an absorbent pad under client's buttocks. Remove and discard underpad, and replace with clean one.	Cleansing reduces transmission of microorganisms from anus to urethra or genitalia.
11. If gloves are soiled, perform hand hygiene and then apply new pair of gloves.	

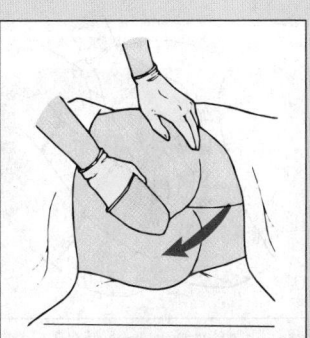

STEP 10 Cleanse buttocks from front to back.

Continued

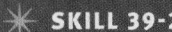

✳ **SKILL 39-2** PERINEAL CARE—CONT'D

STEPS	RATIONALE
12. Fold top bed linen down toward foot of bed, and raise client's gown above genital area. Prepare bed linen to protect client's privacy.	Exposes perineal area for easy accessibility.
a. "Diamond" drape client by placing bath blanket with one corner between client's legs, one corner pointing toward each side of bed, and one corner over client's chest. Tuck side corners around client's legs and under hips.	Prevents unnecessary exposure of body parts and maintains client's warmth and comfort during procedure.
13. Raise side rail. Fill washbasin with warm water.	Prevents client from falling. Proper water temperature prevents burns to perineum.
14. Place washbasin and toilet tissue on over-bed table. Place washcloths in basin.	Equipment placed within nurse's reach prevents accidental spills.
15. Provide perineal care.	
A. **Female perineal care**	
(1) Assist client to dorsal recumbent position.	Provides easy access to genitalia.
(2) Lower side rail, and help client flex knees and spread legs. Note restrictions or limitations in client's positioning.	Provides full exposure of female genitalia. Minimize degree of abduction in female if position causes pain because of arthritis or reduced joint mobility.
(3) Fold lower corner of bath blanket up between client's legs onto abdomen. Wash and dry client's upper thighs.	Minimizes transmission of microorganisms. Keeping client draped until procedure begins minimizes anxiety. Buildup of perineal secretions soils surrounding skin surfaces.
(4) Wash labia majora. Use nondominant hand to gently retract labia from thigh; with dominant hand, wash carefully in skin folds. Wipe in direction from perineum to rectum (front to back). Repeat on opposite side using separate section of washcloth. Rinse and dry area thoroughly.	Skin folds often contain body secretions that harbor microorganisms. Wiping from perineum to rectum (front to back) reduces chance of transmitting fecal organisms to urinary meatus.
(5) Separate labia with nondominant hand to expose urethral meatus and vaginal orifice. With dominant hand, wash downward from pubic area toward rectum in one smooth stroke (see illustration). Use separate section of cloth for each stroke. Cleanse thoroughly around labia minora, clitoris, and vaginal orifice.	Cleansing method reduces transfer of microorganisms to urinary meatus. (For menstruating women or clients with indwelling urinary catheters, use cotton balls to cleanse the meatus.)
(6) If client uses bedpan, pour warm water over perineal area. Dry perineal area thoroughly, using front-to-back method.	Rinsing removes soap and microorganisms more effectively than wiping. Retained moisture harbors microorganisms.
(7) Fold lower corner of bath blanket back between client's legs and over perineum. Assist client to lower legs and assume comfortable position. Raise side rail as appropriate.	
B. **Male perineal care**	
(1) Lower side rails, and assist client to supine position. Note restriction in mobility.	Provides full exposure of male genitalia.
(2) Fold lower corner of bath blanket up between client's legs and onto abdomen. Wash and dry client's upper thighs.	Minimizes transmission of microorganisms. Keeping client draped until procedure begins minimizes anxiety. Buildup of perineal secretions soils surrounding skin surfaces.

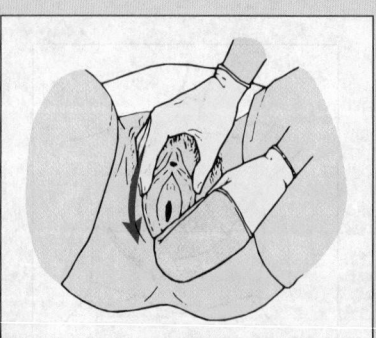

STEP 15A(5) Cleanse from perineum to rectum (front to back).

PERINEAL CARE—CONT'D

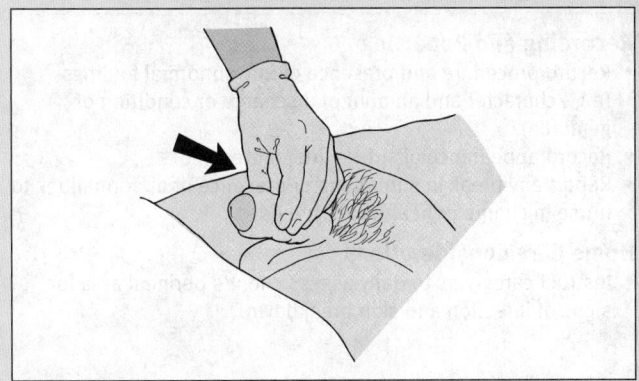

STEP 15B(3) Retract foreskin.

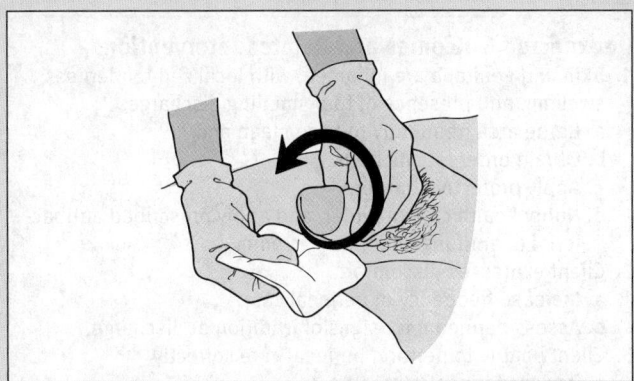

STEP 15B(4) Use circular motion to cleanse tip of penis.

STEPS	RATIONALE
(3) Gently raise penis, and place bath towel underneath. Gently grasp shaft of penis. If client is uncircumcised, retract foreskin (see illustration). If client has an erection, defer procedure until later.	Towel prevents moisture from collecting in inguinal area. Gentle but firm handling reduces chance of client having an erection. Secretions capable of harboring microorganisms collect underneath foreskin.
(4) Wash tip of penis at urethral meatus first. Using circular motion, cleanse from meatus outward (see illustration). Discard washcloth, and repeat with clean cloth until penis is clean. Rinse and dry gently.	Direction of cleansing moves from area of least contamination to area of most contamination, preventing microorganisms from entering urethra.
(5) Return foreskin to its natural position.	Tightening of foreskin around shaft of penis causes local edema and discomfort.

Critical Decision Point: Tightening of foreskin around shaft of penis can cause local edema and discomfort. After administering male perineal care, make sure the foreskin is in its natural position. This is extremely important in those clients with decreased sensation in their lower extremities.

(6) Wash shaft of penis with gentle but firm downward strokes. Pay special attention to underlying surface of penis. Rinse and dry penis thoroughly. Instruct client to spread legs apart slightly.	Vigorous massage of penis leads to erection, which will embarrass client and nurse. Underlying surface of penis often has greater accumulation of secretions. Abduction of legs provides easier access to scrotal tissues.
(7) Gently cleanse scrotum. Lift it carefully, and wash underlying skin folds. Rinse and dry.	Pressure on scrotal tissues is often painful to client. Secretions collect between skin folds.
(8) Fold bath blanket back over client's perineum, and assist client in turning to side-lying position.	Draping promotes comfort and minimizes client's anxiety. Side-lying position provides access to anal area.
16. If client has had urinary or bowel incontinence, apply thin layer of skin barrier containing petrolatum or zinc oxide over anal and perineal skin.	Protects skin from excess moisture and toxins from urine or stool
17. Remove clean gloves, dispose in proper receptacle, and perform hand hygiene.	Moisture and body secretions on gloves can harbor microorganisms.
18. Assist client in assuming a comfortable position, and cover with sheet. Raise side rails as appropriate.	Client's comfort helps to minimize stress of procedure.
19. Remove bath blanket, and dispose of all soiled bed linen. Return unused equipment to storage area.	Reduces transmission of microorganisms.
20. Inspect surface of external genitalia and surrounding skin after cleansing.	Thick secretions may cover underlying skin lesions or areas of breakdown. Evaluation determines need for additional hygiene.
21. Ask if client feels sense of cleanliness.	Evaluates client's comfort level.
22. Observe for abnormal drainage or discharge from genitalia.	Evaluates presence of infection.

Continued

✳ **SKILL 39-2**   PERINEAL CARE—CONT'D

Unexpected Outcomes and Related Interventions

1. Skin and genitalia are inflamed, with localized tenderness, swelling, and presence of foul-smelling discharge.
   a. Bathe area frequently to keep clean and dry.
   b. Obtain order for sitz bath.
   c. Apply protective barrier.
   d. Notify health care provider, and apply prescribed antibacterial or antifungal ointment/cream.
2. Client expresses discomfort.
   a. Increase frequency of perineal care.
   b. Assess perineum for signs of irritation or discharge.
3. Client unable to perform perineal care correctly.
   a. Review perineal care.
   b. Position client, and have client observe cleansing procedure.

Recording and Reporting

- Record procedure and presence of any abnormal findings (e.g., character and amount of discharge or condition of genitalia).
- Record appearance of suture line, if present.
- Report any break in suture line or presence of abnormalities to nurse in charge or health care provider.

Home Care Considerations

- Instruct caregivers to daily assess client's perineal area for signs of infection and skin breakdown.

✳ **SKILL 39-3**   PERFORMING NAIL AND FOOT CARE

Delegation Considerations

The skill of nail and foot care of clients without circulatory problems or diabetes can be delegated. If the client is diabetic, this skill cannot be delegated. The nurse instructs nursing assistive personnel about:

- Not clipping client's nails; the nurse must do this
- Any special considerations for client positioning

Equipment

- Washbasin
- Emesis basin
- Washcloth
- Bath or face towel
- Nail clippers
- Soft cuticle or nail brush
- Orangewood stick
- Emery board or nail file
- Body lotion
- Disposable bath mat
- Paper towels
- Clean gloves (only if drainage is present)

STEPS	RATIONALE
1. Inspect all surfaces of fingers, toes, feet, and nails. Pay particular attention to areas of dryness, inflammation, or cracking. Also inspect areas between toes, heels, and soles of feet.	Integrity of feet and nails determines frequency and level of hygiene required. Heels, soles, and sides of feet are prone to irritation from ill-fitting shoes.

Critical Decision Point: Client with peripheral vascular diseases or diabetes mellitus, older adults, and clients whose immune system is suppressed often require nail care from a specialist to reduce the risk of infection. During nail care the specialist will assess the condition of the client's feet. The presence of erythema, warmth, or callus formation may indicate areas of tissue damage with impending breakdown (ADA, 2007).

---

2. Assess color and temperature of toes, feet, and fingers. Assess capillary refill of nails. Palpate radial and ulnar pulse of each hand and dorsalis pedis pulse of foot; note character of pulses (see Chapter 33).	Assesses adequacy of blood flow to extremities. Circulatory alterations often change integrity of nails and increase client's chance of localized infection when break in skin integrity occurs (Bryant and Beinlich, 1999).
3. Observe client's walking gait. Have client walk down hall or walk straight line (if able).	Structural as well as painful disorders of feet cause limping or unnatural gait. These disorders are often the result of impaired circulation, improper fitting shoes, or structural foot abnormalities (e.g., bunions) (Bryant and Beinlich, 1999).
4. Ask female clients about whether they use nail polish and polish remover frequently.	Chemicals in these products cause excessive dryness.
5. Assess type of footwear worn by client: Does client wear socks? Are shoes tight or ill fitting? Does client wear garters or knee-high nylons? Is footwear clean?	Types of shoes and footwear predispose client to foot and nail problems (e.g., infection, areas of friction, ulcerations). These conditions decrease mobility and increase the risk for amputation in the diabetic client (Pinzur and others, 2005).
6. Identify client's risk for foot or nail problems: a. Older adult	Certain conditions increase likelihood of foot or nail problems. Poor vision, lack of coordination, or inability to bend over contributes to difficulty in performing foot and nail care. Normal physiological changes of aging also result in nail and foot problems (Meiner and Lueckenotte, 2006).

STEPS	RATIONALE
b. Diabetes mellitus	Vascular changes associated with diabetes mellitus reduce blood flow to peripheral tissues. Break in skin integrity places diabetic client at high risk for skin infection. Meticulous foot assessment reduces the diabetic client's risk of debilitating foot problems (Green and others, 2002; Neil, 2002).
c. Heart failure, renal disease	Both conditions increase tissue edema, particularly in dependent areas (e.g., feet). Edema reduces blood flow to neighboring tissues.
d. Cerebrovascular accident (stroke)	Presence of residual foot or leg weakness or paralysis results in altered walking patterns. Altered gait pattern causes increased friction and pressure on feet.
7. Assess type of home remedies client uses for existing foot problems:	Certain preparations or applications cause more injury to soft tissue than initial foot problem (Neil, 2002).
a. Over-the-counter liquid preparations to remove corns	Liquid preparations cause burns and ulcerations.
b. Cutting of corns or calluses with razor blade or scissors	Cutting of corns or calluses sometimes results in infection caused by break in skin integrity. The client with diabetes or any client with decreased peripheral circulation has an increased risk for infection secondary to a break in skin integrity (Green and others, 2002).
c. Use of oval corn pads	Oval pads exert pressure on toes, thereby decreasing circulation to surrounding tissues.
d. Application of adhesive tape	Skin of older adult is thin and delicate and prone to tearing when adhesive tape is removed.
8. Assess client's ability to care for nails or feet: visual alterations, fatigue, and musculoskeletal weakness.	Determines client's ability to perform self-care and degree of assistance required from nurse (Neil, 2002).
9. Assess client's knowledge of foot and nail care practices.	Determines client's need for health teaching.
10. Explain procedure to client, including fact that proper soaking requires several minutes.	Client must be willing to place fingers and feet in basins for 10 to 20 minutes. Some clients become anxious or fatigued.

Critical Decision Point: Clients with diabetes do not soak hands and feet. Soaking increases risk of infection because of maceration of the skin.

11. Obtain health care provider's order for cutting nails if agency policy requires it.	Clients with reduced circulation are more at risk for infection. Accidental cutting of skin for them increases risk for infection.
12. Perform hand hygiene. Arrange equipment on over-bed table.	Easy access to equipment prevents delays.
13. Pull curtain around bed, or close room door (if desired).	Maintaining client's privacy reduces anxiety.
14. Assist ambulatory client to sit in bedside chair. Help bed-bound client to supine position with head of bed elevated. Place disposable bath mat on floor under client's feet, or place towel on mattress.	Sitting in chair facilitates immersing feet in basin. Bath mat protects feet from exposure to soil or debris.
15. Fill washbasin with warm water. Test water temperature.	Warm water softens nails and thickened epidermal cells, reduces inflammation of skin, and promotes local circulation. Proper water temperature prevents burns.
16. Place basin on bath mat or towel, and help client place feet in basin. Place call light within client's reach.	Clients with muscular weakness or tremors often have difficulty positioning feet. Maintains client's safety.

Critical Decision Point: Soaking the feet of clients with diabetes mellitus or peripheral vascualr disease is not recommended. Soaking may lead to maceration (excessive softening of the skin), ulceration, or infection (ADA, 2001).

17. Adjust over-bed table to low position, and place it over client's lap. (Client sits in chair or lies in bed.)	Easy access prevents accidental spills.
18. Fill emesis basin with warm water, and place basin on paper towels on over-bed table.	Warm water softens nails and thickened epidermal cells.
19. Instruct client to place fingers in emesis basin and place arms in comfortable position.	Prolonged positioning causes discomfort unless normal anatomical alignment is maintained.
20. Allow client's feet and fingernails to soak for 10 to 20 minutes. Rewarm after 10 minutes.	Softening of corns, calluses, and cuticles ensures easy removal of dead cells and easy manipulation of cuticle.

Continued

※ **SKILL 39-3**   **PERFORMING NAIL AND FOOT CARE—CONT'D**

STEPS	RATIONALE
21. Clean gently under fingernails with orangewood stick or wooden end of cotton-tipped swab while fingers are immersed (see illustration). Remove emesis basin, and dry fingers thoroughly.	Orangewood stick removes debris under nails that harbors microorganisms. Thorough drying impedes fungal growth and prevents maceration of tissues.
22. Using nail clippers, clip fingernails straight across and even with tops of fingers; check agency policy (see illustration). Using a file shape nails straight across. If client has circulatory problems, do not cut nail; file the nail only.	Cutting straight across prevents splitting of nail margins and formation of sharp nail spikes that irritate lateral nail margins. Filing prevents cutting nail too close to nail bed.
23. Use a soft cuticle brush or nail brush around cuticles.	Reduces incidence of inflamed cuticles.
24. Move over-bed table away from client.	Provides easier access to feet.
25. Put on clean gloves, and scrub callused areas of feet with washcloth.	Gloves prevent transmission of fungal infection. Friction removes dead skin layers.
26. Clean gently under nails with orangewood stick. Remove feet from basin, and dry thoroughly.	Removal of debris and excess moisture reduces chances of infection.
27. Clean and trim toenails using procedures in Steps 22 and 23. Do not file corners of toenails. Check agency policy for trimming client's nails.	Shaping corners of toenails damages tissues.
28. Apply lotion to feet and hands, and assist client back to bed and into comfortable position.	Lotion lubricates dry skin by helping to retain moisture.
29. Remove clean gloves, and place in receptacle. Clean and return equipment and supplies to proper place. Dispose of soiled linen in hamper. Perform hand hygiene.	Reduces transmission of infection.
30. Inspect nails and surrounding skin surfaces after soaking and nail trimming.	Evaluates condition of skin and nails. Allows nurse to note any remaining rough nail edges.
31. Ask client to explain or demonstrate nail care.	Evaluates client's level of learning techniques.
32. Observe client's walk after toenail care.	Evaluates level of comfort and mobility achieved.
33. Record procedure and observations (e.g., breaks in skin, inflammation, ulcerations).	Documents procedure, client's response, and presence of abnormalities requiring additional therapy.
34. Report any breaks in skin or ulcerations to nurse in charge or health care provider.	These abnormalities seriously increase client's risk of infection, and caregiver needs to be observant.

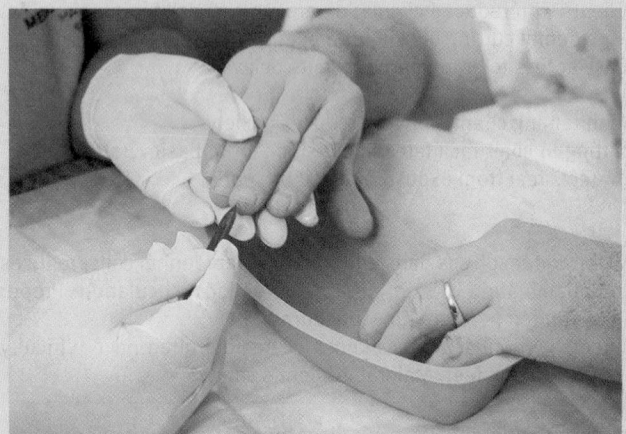

STEP 21 Clean under fingernails.

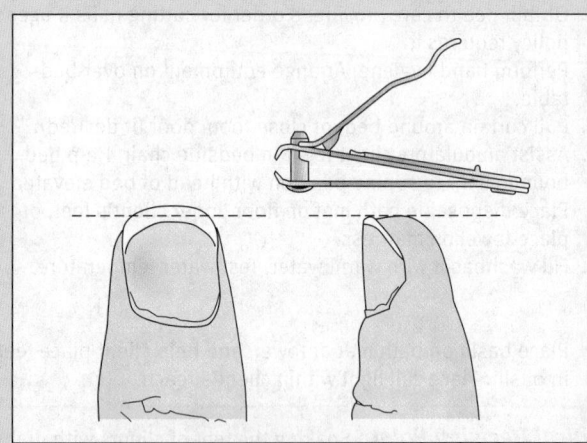

STEP 22 Use nail clippers to clip nails straight across.

Unexpected Outcomes and Related Interventions

1. Cuticles and surrounding tissues are inflamed and tender to touch.
   a. Repeated soakings are necessary to relieve inflammation and loosen layers of cells from calluses or corns.
   b. Client with peripheral vascular disease or diabetes often requires referral to a podiatrist.
   c. Evaluate need for antifungal cream.
2. Localized areas of tenderness occur on feet with calluses or corns at point of friction.
   a. Change in footwear is necessary.
   b. Refer to a podiatrist or nurse in charge.
3. Ulcer appears between toes or other pressure areas in foot.
   a. Notify physician or nurse in charge.
   b. Refer to a podiatrist or nurse certified in foot care.
   c. Increase frequency of foot assessment and hygiene.

Recording and Reporting

- Record procedure and observations (e.g., breaks in skin, inflammation, ulcerations).
- Report any breaks in skin or ulcerations to nurse in charge or physician. These are serious in client with peripheral vascular disease and illnesses in which client's circulation is impaired. Special foot care treatments are often necessary.

Home Care Considerations

- If the client has diabetes or decreased peripheral circulation, perform procedure only after consulting with a health care provider.
- Alternative therapies: moleskin applied to areas of feet that are under friction is less likely to cause pressure than corn pads; spot adhesive bandages guard against friction, but they do not have padding to protect against pressure; wrapping small pieces of lamb's wool around toes reduces irritation of soft corns between toes.
- If client is ambulatory, instruct to soak feet in bathtub. When client's mobility is limited, use a large basin or pan.

✳ **BOX 39-10 Signs of Peripheral Neuropathy or Vascular Insufficiency**

Peripheral Neuropathy
Muscle wasting of lower extremities
Absence of deep tendon reflexes
Foot deformities
Infections
Abnormal gait
Decreased or absent vibratory sensation

Vascular Insufficiency
Decreased hair growth on legs and feet
Absent or decreased pulses
Infection in the foot
Poor wound healing
Thickened nails
Shiny appearance of the skin
Blanching of the skin on elevation

Data from American Diabetes Association: Position statement on standards of medical care in diabetes 2007, *Diabetes Care* 30:S4, 2007; Pinzur MS and others: Guidelines for diabetic foot care, The Diabetes Committee of the American Orthopaedic Foot and Ankle Society, *Foot Ankle Int* 26(1):113, 2005; and Neil JA: Assessing foot care knowledge in a rural population with diabetes, *Ostomy Wound Manage* 48(1):50, 2002.

A client with diabetes mellitus or peripheral vascular disease is at risk for foot and nail problems as a result of poor peripheral blood supply to the feet (Box 39-10). In addition, sensation in the feet is often reduced. These clients are especially at risk for the development of chronic foot ulcers. These lesions typically heal very slowly and once present are difficult to treat. Over time, circulation becomes compromised enough to cause ischemia and sloughing of tissue. Although ongoing foot care helps prevent toe amputation, studies show that many clients have not learned proper care (Bryant and Beinlich, 1999).

The American Diabetes Association (ADA) (2007) identifies the following risk conditions as associated with an increased risk of amputation: peripheral neuropathy; altered biomechanics; evidence of increased pressure from callus, erythema, or hemorrhage under a callus; limited joint mobility, bony deformity, or severe nail pathological condition; peripheral vascular disease; and a history of ulcers or amputation (Pinzur and others, 2005). Observe for changes that indicate peripheral neuropathy or vascular insufficiency. Give the client information to understand how circulation directly affects the health and integrity of tissues. Advise clients to use the following guidelines in a routine foot and nail care program (ADA, 2007; Pinzur and others, 2005):

- All clients with diabetes mellitus need to receive a thorough foot examination at least once a year. People with one or more high-risk foot conditions need an evaluation more frequently. People with neuropathy need to have a visual inspection of their feet at every visit with a health care professional (ADA, 2007).
- Inspect the feet daily, including the bottoms and tops of the feet, the heels, and the areas between the toes. Use a mirror to help inspect the feet thoroughly, or ask a family member to check daily.
- Instruct client to wash feet daily in lukewarm water. Dry thoroughly, especially between the toes (Martinez and Tripp-Reimer, 2005).
- If the feet perspire, apply an unscented foot powder. Wear shoes with porous uppers.
- Always wear clean, dry socks; if necessary, change socks twice a day (Martinez and Tripp-Reimer, 2005). Never walk barefoot.
- If you notice dryness along the feet or between the toes, apply lanolin, baby oil, or even corn oil, and rub gently into the skin.
- File the toenails straight across and square; do not use scissors or clippers. Consult a podiatrist as needed.

- Do not use over-the-counter preparations to treat athlete's foot, ingrown toenails, or corn or callus removal. Consult a physician or podiatrist.
- Avoid wearing elastic stockings, knee-high hose, or constricting garters. Do not cross the legs while sitting. Both impair circulation to the lower extremities.
- Wear properly fitted shoes. The soles of shoes must be flexible and nonskid. You can use small amounts of lamb's wool between toes that rub or overlap. Shoes must be sturdy, closed in, and not restrictive to the feet. Clients with increased plantar pressure (e.g., erythema or callus) use footwear that cushions and redistributes pressure. Clients with bony deformity (e.g., bunion or Charcot's joint) need extrawide or extradeep shoes with cushioned insoles.
- Do not wear new shoes for an extended time. Wear them for short periods over several days to break them in.
- Exercise regularly to improve circulation to the lower extremities. Walk slowly and elevate, rotate, flex, and extend the feet at the ankles. Dangle the feet over the side of the bed 1 minute, and then extend both legs and hold them parallel to the bed while lying supine for 1 minute, and, finally, rest 1 minute.
- Wash minor cuts immediately, and dry them thoroughly. Use only mild antiseptics (e.g., Neosporin ointment). Avoid iodine or Mercurochrome. Contact a health care provider to treat cuts or lacerations.

Generally, any client who requires regular, thorough foot care should have a family member who is able to provide care during times when the client is incapacitated. Clients with visual difficulties, physical constraints preventing movement, or cognitive problems that impair their ability to assess the condition of the feet will need family assistance (ADA, 2007).

Oral Hygiene.
Oral hygiene helps to maintain the healthy state of the mouth, teeth, gums, and lips (Ring, 2002). Poor oral care, along with the client's overall physical condition and medications such as antihypertensives, antidepressants, and diuretics, diminishes salivary production. This in turn reduces the ability of the oral environment to help fight effects of pathogens (Box 39-11).

Brushing cleans the teeth of food particles, plaque, and bacteria. It also massages the gums and relieves discomfort resulting from unpleasant odors and tastes. Flossing further helps remove plaque and tartar from between teeth to reduce gum inflammation and infection. Complete oral hygiene enhances well-being and comfort and stimulates the appetite. Clients also benefit from a proper diet, which excludes foods promoting plaque formation and tooth decay and promotes healthy periodontal structures (Hornick, 2002). Plaque-forming foods include carbonated beverages, breads, and starches. In addition, oral hygiene immediately following a meal further reduces plaque. Assist clients in maintaining good oral hygiene by teaching the importance of correct techniques and a routine daily schedule.

Advise clients of all ages to have a dental checkup at least every 6 months. Education about common gum and tooth disorders and methods of prevention motivates clients to follow good oral hygiene practices. At times you will perform oral hygiene for weakened or disabled clients. When clients have variations in oral

---

✳ BOX 39-11   EVIDENCE-BASED PRACTICE

Oral Health
Evidence Summary

Oral care is an essential nursing intervention. A client's oral health affects his or her general level health and rate of recovery. Merely cleansing a client's teeth and tongue and dental flossing does not achieve oral health. Meticulous oral assessment and individualized interventions are needed for clients who are unable to achieve oral health. The success of oral hygiene measures is determined by salivary volume, dental plaque, and oral flora.

This study reviewed the research findings of Munro and others on oral health. Poor oral hygiene measures result in decreased salivary volume, increased dental plaque, and altered oral flora. Saliva is an essential component of the oral immune defense mechanisms. Reduced salivary production results in dry mouth and most importantly promotes dental plaque. Dental plaque serves as a reservoir for microorganisms that can cause ventilator-associated pneumonia in the critically ill client. Changes in the oral microbial flora increase the client's risk for health care–associated infections, because of the colonization of pathogens in the oropharynx. This is an especially high risk for clients on mechanical ventilation or those who are immunosuppressed. Oral hygiene is not merely "one size fits all" and should never be quickly done or omitted. Individualize oral hygiene measures to the client's needs, level of health and functional status, and illness condition.

Application to Nursing Practice

- Assess and monitor for decreased volume of saliva (e.g., dry, cracked lips, coated tongue, complaints of "dry mouth")
- Increase the frequency of oral hygiene measures if client has "dry mouth" or bad breath or develops mouth sores.
- When indicated, use an antibacterial solution, such as chlorhexidine, early in intubated clients or clients at risk for changes in the oral cavity environment.
- Observe for increasing dental plaque. To avoid dental plaque, increase the frequency of toothbrushing and use antimicrobial agents for rinsing the mouth. In clients who are unconscious or on mechanical ventilation, it is necessary to rinse the mouth and then immediately suction the oral cavity.
- Do not use foam swabs for cleansing as they are ineffective in plaque removal and do not stimulate the oral mucosa.

Reference

Munro CL and others: Oral health measurement in nursing research: state of the science, *Biol Res Nurs* 8(1):35, 2006.

---

mucosal integrity, adapt hygiene techniques to ensure thorough and effective care (Box 39-12).

Brushing and Flossing. Thorough toothbrushing at least 4 times a day (after meals and at bedtime) is basic to an effective oral hygiene program. A toothbrush needs to have a straight handle and brush small enough to reach all areas of the mouth. An even, rounded brushing surface with soft, multitufted, nylon bristles is best. Rounded soft bristles stimulate the gums without causing abrasion and bleeding. Any client who experiences decreased dexterity due to a medical condition or the aging process requires an enlarged handle on his or her toothbrush. Electronic

✳ BOX 39-12   FOCUS ON OLDER ADULTS

- Many older adults are edentulous (without teeth), and the teeth that are present are often diseased or decayed (Meiner and Lueckenotte, 2006).
- The periodontal membrane weakens, making it more prone to infection; periodontal disease predisposes the older adult to systemic infection.
- The presence of chronic illnesses (e.g., diabetes mellitus, renal insufficiency, cardiovascular diseases) increases the older adult's risk for periodontal disease (Bush and Donley, 2002).
- Dentures or partial plates do not always fit properly, causing pain and discomfort, which in turn affect digestive processes, enjoyment of food, and nutritional status.
- Weaker jaw muscles and shrinkage of the bony structure of the mouth increase the work of chewing and lead to increased fatigue when eating (Meiner and Lueckenotte, 2006).
- An age-related decline in saliva secretion and some medications (e.g., antihypertensives, diuretics, antiinflammatories, antidepressants) cause dry mouth (Meiner and Lueckenotte 2006).
- Poor nutritional status in some older adults increases the risk for and severity of dental problems (e.g., caries, periodontal disease, receding gums, tooth degeneration) (Hornick, 2002).
- Financial limitations and the belief that dentures eliminate the need for routine dental care are reasons why older adults do not seek dental care (Meiner and Lueckenotte 2006).

toothbrushes are an option, or a manual toothbrush may be adapted. One simple way to devise an enlarged brush handle is to pierce a soft rubber ball and push the brush handle through or glue a short piece of plastic tubing around the handle. Clients need to know to obtain a new toothbrush every 3 months or following a cold or strep throat to minimize growth of microorganisms on the brush surfaces.

Clients need to brush all tooth surfaces thoroughly using fluoride toothpaste. Commercially made foam rubber toothbrushes are useful for clients with sensitive gums. However, swabbing fails to cleanse teeth adequately because plaque accumulates around the base of the teeth. Use foam rubber swabs in moderation. Electric or powered toothbrushes improve the quality of care and are easier to use than manual brushes when nurses provide care for dependent clients (Brinkley and others, 2004). Electric toothbrushes are useful, but first check agency policy to determine if electric toothbrushes are permitted. Do not use lemon-glycerin sponges because they dry mucous membranes and erode teeth enamel. Moi-Stin is a salivary supplement that improves moisture and texture of the tongue and mucosa (Poland, 1987).

When teaching clients about mouth care, recommend not to share toothbrushes with family members or drink directly from a bottle of mouthwash. Cross contamination occurs easily. The use of disclosure tablets or drops to stain the plaque that collects at the gum line is useful for showing clients how effectively they brush. Many clients are able to perform their own oral care. Observe the

client to be sure he or she is using the proper techniques. The amount of assistance needed by the client when brushing the teeth will vary. When assisting with or providing oral hygiene, determine the amount of assistance needed, as well as individual oral hygiene preferences (Skill 39-4).

Flossing. Dental flossing removes plaque and tartar between teeth. Flossing involves inserting waxed or unwaxed dental floss between all tooth surfaces, one at a time. The seesaw motion used to pull floss between teeth removes plaque and tartar from tooth enamel. To prevent bleeding, use unwaxed floss on clients who are receiving chemotherapy or radiation or are on anticoagulant therapy and avoid vigorous flossing near the gum line. If toothpaste is applied to the teeth before flossing, fluoride will come in direct contact with tooth surfaces, aiding in cavity prevention. Flossing once a day is sufficient. Because it is important to clean all teeth surfaces thoroughly, do not rush to complete flossing. Placing a mirror in front of the client will help you to demonstrate the proper method for holding the floss and cleaning between the teeth. Flossing a client's teeth is not realistic or appropriate in all care settings. However, you may perform flossing more frequently in extended and rehabilitation care settings. Recent research has shown that twice daily rinsing with an essential oil–containing mouth rinse (e.g., Cool Mint Listerine Antiseptic) is an effective adjunct and at least as good as daily flossing in reducing plaque and gingivitis (Bauroth and others, 2003).

Clients With Special Needs. Some clients require special oral hygiene methods because of their level of dependence on caregivers or the presence of oral mucosa problems. Unconscious clients and those with artificial airways (e.g., endotracheal or tracheal tubes) are susceptible to drying of mucous-thickened salivary secretions because they are unable to eat or drink, frequently breathe through the mouth, and often receive oxygen therapy. The unconscious client also cannot swallow salivary secretions that accumulate in the mouth. These secretions often contain gram-negative bacteria that cause pneumonia if aspirated into the lungs. While providing hygiene to these clients, protect the client from choking and aspiration. Topical chlorhexidine is accepted for use in oral care, especially in ventilated clients. Research shows that a one-time use of chlorhexidine with oral hygiene reduces the risk for ventilator-associated pneumonia (Grap and others, 2004; Munro and others, 2006; Berry and others, 2007).

To reduce the risk of aspiration and subsequent pneumonia, the safest technique is to have two nurses provide the care. You can delegate nursing assistive personnel to participate. One nurse does the actual cleaning, and the other removes secretions with suction equipment. While cleansing the oral cavity, never use fingers to hold the client's mouth open. A human bite is highly contaminated. In some cases it is necessary to perform mouth care at least every 2 hours. Be sure to explain the steps of mouth care and the sensations the client will feel. Also tell the client when the procedure is completed (Skill 39-5).

Clients who receive chemotherapy, radiation, or nasogastric tube intubation or who have an infection of the mouth suffer from **stomatitis**. Inflammation of the oral mucosa causes oral burning, pain, and change in food tolerance. Gentle brushing and flossing are important in preventing bleeding of the gums. Advise clients to avoid alcohol and commercial mouthwash and to stop smoking. Normal saline rinses (approximately 30 mL) upon

✳ **SKILL 39-4**   **PROVIDING ORAL HYGIENE**

Delegation Considerations

The skill of brushing teeth can be delegated. The nurse instructs nursing assistive personnel to:

- Adapt procedure for the client who is at risk for aspiration. These clients include those with impaired level of consciousness, impaired swallowing, or those who are confused.
- Immediately report to the nurse excessive client coughing or choking during or after oral hygiene
- Report any bleeding of oral mucosa or gums, client report of pain, or lesions to the nurse

Equipment

- Soft-bristle toothbrush (hard toothbrushes damage enamel and gums)
- Nonabrasive fluoride toothpaste or dentifrice
- Dental floss
- Tongue depressor
- Water glass with cool water
- Normal saline or an essential-oil antiseptic mouthwash (optional; follow client's preference)
- Emesis basin
- Face towel
- Paper towels
- Clean gloves

STEPS	RATIONALE
1. Perform hand hygiene, and apply clean gloves.	Reduces transmission of microorganisms.
2. Instruct client not to bite down. Inspect integrity of lips, teeth, buccal mucosa, gums, palate, and tongue (see Chapter 33).	Determines status of client's oral cavity and extent of need for oral hygiene.
3. Identify presence of common oral problems:	Helps determine type of hygiene client requires and information client requires for self-care.
a. Dental caries—chalky white discoloration of tooth or presence of brown or black discoloration	
b. Gingivitis—inflammation of gums	
c. Periodontitis—receding gum lines, inflammation, gaps between teeth	Receding gums occur with aging, and as a result older clients require meticulous oral hygiene (Walton, Miller, and Tordecilla, 2002).
d. Halitosis—bad breath	
e. Cheilosis—cracking of lips	
f. Stomatitis—inflammation of the mouth	Clients receiving immunosuppressive chemotherapy (e.g., cancer chemotherapy, antirejection medication after organ transplant) or those clients with suppressed immune function are at risk for stomatitis (Fulton, Middleton, and McPhail, 2002).
g. Dry, cracked, coated tongue	
4. Assess client's risk for aspiration: impaired swallowing, reduced gag reflex. Remove and dispose of gloves.	Accumulation of secretions and dentifrice increase client's risk for aspiration because of reduced ability to control oral secretions.
5. Assess risk for oral hygiene problems (see Table 39-5).	Certain conditions increase likelihood of impaired oral cavity integrity and need for preventive care.
6. Remove gloves, and perform hand hygiene.	Prevents spread of microorganisms.
7. Determine client's oral hygiene practices:	Allows nurse to identify errors in technique, deficiencies in preventive oral hygiene, and client's level of knowledge regarding dental care.
a. Frequency of toothbrushing and flossing	
b. Type of toothpaste or dentifrice used	
c. Last dental visit	
d. Frequency of dental visits	
e. Type of mouthwash or moistening preparation	Lemon-glycerin preparations are often detrimental. Glycerin is an astringent that dries and shrinks mucous membranes and gums. Lemon exhausts salivary reflex and erodes tooth enamel (Poland, 1987).
8. Assess client's ability to grasp and manipulate toothbrush. (For older adult try 30-second toothbrush assessment.)	Toothbrush test assesses dexterity and strength. Determines level of assistance required.
9. Perform hand hygiene. Prepare equipment at bedside.	
10. Explain procedure to client, and discuss preferences regarding use of hygiene aids.	Some clients feel uncomfortable about having the nurse care for their basic needs. Client involvement with procedure minimizes anxiety.
11. Place paper towels on over-bed table, and arrange other equipment within easy reach.	
12. Raise bed to comfortable working position. Raise head of bed (if allowed), and lower side rail. Move client, or help client move closer. Use side-lying position if needed.	Raising bed and positioning client prevent nurse from straining muscles. Semi-Fowler's position helps prevent client from choking or aspirating.
13. Place towel over client's chest.	

✳ **SKILL 39-4**   **P R O V I D I N G   O R A L   H Y G I E N E — C O N T ' D**

STEPS	RATIONALE
14. Apply gloves.	Prevents contact with microorganisms or blood in saliva.
15. Apply toothpaste to brush, holding brush over emesis basin. Pour small amount of water over toothpaste.	Moisture aids in distribution of toothpaste over tooth surfaces.
16. Client may assist by brushing. Hold toothbrush bristles at 45-degree angle to gum line (see illustration). Be sure tips of bristles rest against and penetrate under gum line. Brush inner and outer surfaces of upper and lower teeth by brushing from gum to crown of each tooth. Clean biting surfaces of teeth by holding top of bristles parallel with teeth and brushing gently back and forth (see illustration). Brush sides of teeth by moving bristles back and forth (see illustration).	Angle allows brush to reach all tooth surfaces and to clean under gum line where plaque and tartar accumulate. Back-and-forth motion dislodges food particles caught between teeth and along chewing surfaces.
17. Have client hold brush at 45-degree angle and lightly brush over surface and sides of tongue (see illustration). Avoid initiating gag reflex.	Microorganisms collect and grow on tongue's surface and contribute to bad breath. Gagging causes aspiration of toothpaste.
18. Allow client to rinse mouth thoroughly by taking several sips of water, swishing water across all tooth surfaces, and spitting into emesis basin.	Irrigation removes food particles.
19. Allow client to gargle to rinse mouth with mouthwash as desired.	Mouthwash leaves a pleasant taste in mouth but dries mucosa after extended use if it has an alcohol base. An essential-oil antiseptic mouthwash is effective in reducing plaque and gingivitis (Bauroth and others, 2003).
20. Assist in wiping client's mouth.	Promotes sense of comfort.
21. Allow client to floss.	Reduces tartar on tooth surfaces.
22. Allow client to rinse mouth thoroughly with cool water and spit into emesis basin. Assist in wiping client's mouth.	Irrigation removes plaque and tartar from oral cavity.
23. Assist client to comfortable position, remove emesis basin and over-bed table, raise side rail as appropriate, and lower bed to original position.	Provides for client comfort and safety.
24. Wipe off over-bed table, discard soiled linen and paper towels in appropriate containers, remove soiled gloves, and return equipment to proper place.	Proper disposal of soiled equipment prevents spread of infection.
25. Perform hand hygiene.	Reduces transmission of microorganisms.
26. Ask client if any area of oral cavity feels uncomfortable or irritated.	Pain indicates more chronic problem.
27. Apply gloves, and inspect condition of oral cavity.	Determines effectiveness of hygiene and rinsing.
28. Ask client to describe proper hygiene techniques.	Evaluates client's learning.
29. Observe client brushing.	Evaluates client's ability to use correct technique.

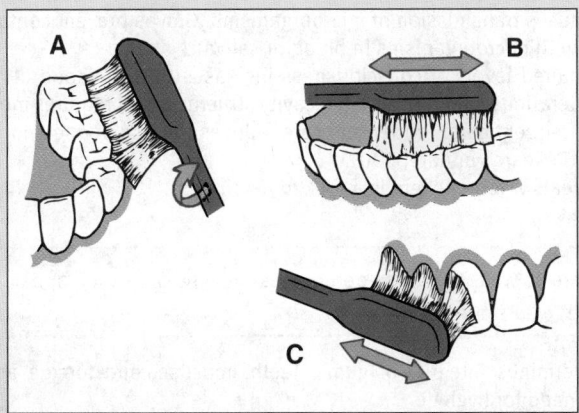

STEP 16 Direction for toothbrush placement. **A,** A 45-degree angle brushes gum line. **B,** Parallel position brushes biting surfaces. **C,** Lateral position brushes sides of teeth.

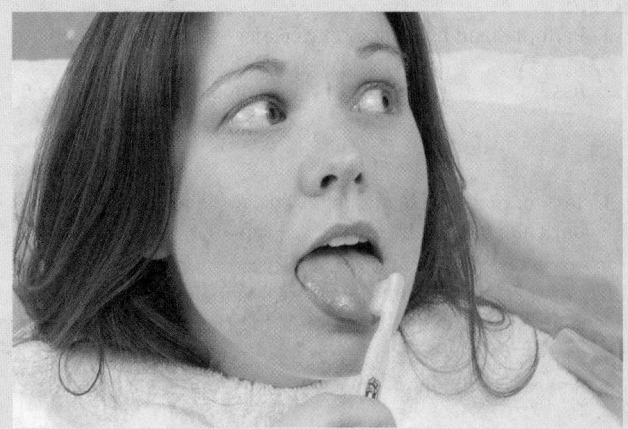

STEP 17 Assisting client with brushing.

Continued

✳ **SKILL 39-4**   **PROVIDING ORAL HYGIENE—CONT'D**

Unexpected Outcomes and Related Interventions

1. Oral mucosa is dry and inflamed.
   a. Increase frequency of oral hygiene.
   b. Increase client's hydration.
   c. Apply protectant to client's lips.
2. Gum margins are retracted from teeth, with localized areas of inflammation. Bleeding occurs around gum margins.
   a. Determine if client has underlying bleeding tendency (e.g., anticoagulant therapy).
   b. Report findings to health care provider.
   c. Use soft-bristle toothbrush.
   d. Increase frequency or oral hygiene.
3. Teeth show signs of dental caries.
   a. Refer client to dentist.
   b. Teach client oral hygiene.

Recording and Reporting

- Record procedure on flow sheet. Note condition of oral cavity in nurses' notes.
- Report bleeding or presence of lesions to nurse in charge or health care provider.

Home Care Considerations

- Teach client and caregiver to assess oral cavity daily to determine any effects of medications on the oral cavity (e.g., reddened, inflamed gums).

✳ **SKILL 39-5**   **PERFORMING MOUTH CARE FOR AN**
                  UNCONSCIOUS OR DEBILITATED CLIENT

Delegation Considerations

Brushing teeth of an unconscious or debilitated client can be delegated. The nurse must first assess client for gag reflex. The nurse informs nursing assistive personnel about:
- Proper way to position client for mouth care
- The safe use of oral suction catheter for clearing oral secretions (see Chapter 40, Skill 40-1, p. 934)
- How to recognize impaired integrity of oral mucosa
- Reporting any bleeding of mucosa or gums, painful reaction by client, or excessive coughing or choking to the nurse

Equipment

- Antiinfective solution (e.g., commercial diluted hydrogen peroxide and sodium bicarbonate solution) that loosens crusts; check agency policy

- Antibacterial solution (e.g., chlorhexidine) (requires a health care provider's order)
- Small pediatric soft-bristle toothbrush
- Tongue blade
- Face towel
- Oral airway
- Sponge toothette
- Paper towels
- Emesis basin
- Water glass with cool water
- Water-soluble lip lubricant
- Small-bulb syringe (optional)
- Suction machine equipment (optional)
- Clean gloves

STEPS	RATIONALE
1. Perform hand hygiene. Apply clean gloves.	Reduces transmission of microorganisms. Gloves prevent contact with microorganisms in blood or saliva.
2. Assess client's risk for oral hygiene problems (see Table 39-5).	Impaired levels of consciousness increases the likelihood of alterations in integrity of oral cavity structures and requires more frequent care. Proper oral care reduces the risk of pneumonia (Research update, 2002).
3. Test for presence of gag reflex by placing tongue blade on back half of client's tongue.	Reveals whether client is at risk for aspiration.

Critical Decision Point: Clients with impaired gag reflex require oral care as well. The nurse determines the type of suction apparatus needed at the bedside to protect the client's airway against aspiration.

4. Inspect condition of oral cavity (see Chapter 33).	Determines integrity of gums, teeth, mucosa, and tongue and need for hygiene.
5. Remove gloves. Perform hand hygiene.	Prevents spread of infection.
6. Explain procedure to client.	Allows debilitated client to anticipate procedure without anxiety. Unconscious client retains ability to hear.
7. Apply clean gloves.	Reduces transfer of microorganisms.
8. Place paper towels on over-bed table and arrange equipment. If needed, turn on suction machine, and connect tubing to suction catheter.	Prevents soiling of table top. Equipment prepared in advance ensures smooth, safe procedure.

✳ **SKILL 39-5** **PERFORMING MOUTH CARE FOR AN UNCONSCIOUS OR DEBILITATED CLIENT—CONT'D**

STEPS	RATIONALE
9. Pull curtain around bed, or close room door.	Provides privacy.
10. Raise bed to the appropriate height for nurse; lower head of bed, and then lower side rail.	Use of good body mechanics with bed in elevated position reduces the risk of injury to the nurse.
11. Position client close to side of bed; turn client's head toward mattress. Client can also be placed on side (Sims' position).	Turning the client's head to the side allows secretions to drain from mouth instead of collecting in back of pharynx. Prevents aspiration. Moving the client close to the side of the bed facilitates proper body mechanics during the skill.
12. Place towel under client's head and emesis basin under chin.	Prevents soiling of bed linen.
13. If client is unconscious, uncooperative, or having difficulty keeping mouth open, insert an oral airway. Insert upside down, then turn the airway sideways and then over tongue to keep teeth apart. Insert with client is relaxed. Do not use force.	Prevents client from biting down on nurse's fingers and provides access to oral cavity.

Critical Decision Point: Never place fingers into the mouth of an unconscious or debilitated client. The normal response of the client is to bite down.

14. Brush teeth with brush moistened with cleansing agent, such as chlorhexidine or diluted hydrogen peroxide and sodium bicarbonate solution. Clean chewing and inner tooth surfaces first. Clean outer tooth surfaces. Gently brush roof of mouth, gums and inside cheeks, and tongue without stimulating gag reflex. Moisten brush with water to rinse. For patients without teeth use toothette moistened in cleansing agent and then rinse (see illustration). Use bulb syringe as needed to remove rinse. Repeat rinse several times.	Brushing action removes food particles between teeth and along chewing surfaces. Rinsing helps remove secretions and moistens mucosa. Repeated rinsing removes cleansing agent, which can be irritating to mucosa. Hydrogen peroxide and sodium bicarbonate effectively remove debris, but if not diluted carefully may cause superficial burns (Munro and Grap, 2004).

Critical Decision Point: For client without teeth perform oral care using a toothette moistened in water or normal saline, which is less traumatic to mucosa or gums.

Critical Decision Point: When performing oral care on mechanically ventilated clients, the use of chlorhexidine before or immediately after intubation reduces risk of ventilator-associated pneumonia (Grap and others, 2004; Berry and others, 2007).

15. Suction oral secretions as they accumulate, if necessary.	Suction removes secretions and fluid that collect in posterior pharynx.
16. Apply thin layer of water-soluble jelly to lips (see illustration).	Water-soluble jelly lubricates lips to prevent drying and cracking.
17. Inform client that procedure is completed.	Provides meaningful stimulation to client.

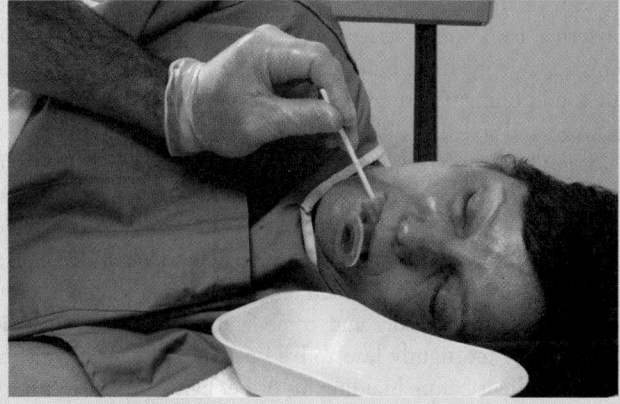

STEP 14 Use toothette for patients without teeth.

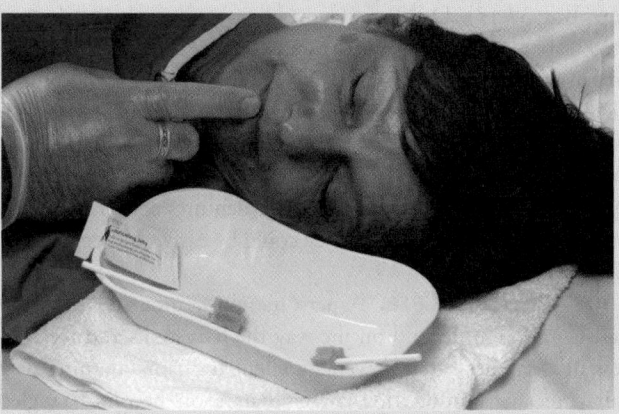

STEP 16 Application of water-soluble moisturizer to lips.

Continued

✳ SKILL 39-5

PERFORMING MOUTH CARE FOR AN UNCONSCIOUS OR DEBILITATED CLIENT—CONT'D

STEPS	RATIONALE
18. Reposition client comfortably, raise side rail as appropriate or as ordered, and return bed to original position.	Maintains client's comfort and safety. Raising all four side rails is considered a restraint, and you will need a health care provider's order.
19. Clean equipment, and return to its proper place. Place soiled linen in proper receptacle.	Proper disposal of soiled equipment prevents spread of infection.
20. Remove and discard gloves. Perform hand hygiene.	Reduces transmission of microorganisms.
21. Apply clean gloves, and inspect oral cavity.	Determines efficacy of cleansing. Once you have removed thick secretions, this will reveal any underlying inflammation or lesions.
22. Ask debilitated client if mouth feels clean.	Evaluates level of comfort.
23. Assess client's respirations on an ongoing basis.	Ensures early recognition of aspiration.

Unexpected Outcomes and Related Interventions

1. Secretions or crusts remain on oral mucosa, tongue, or gums.
   a. Increase frequency of oral hygiene.
   b. A pediatric-size toothbrush may help to provide better hygiene.
2. Localized inflammation of gums or mucosa is present.
   a. Increase frequency of oral hygiene with a soft-bristle toothbrush.
   b. Apply water-soluble moisturizing gel on oral mucosa.
   c. Chemotherapy and radiation causes stomatitis. Antiseptic mouthwashes provide relief, promote oral hygiene, and improve healing (Fulton and others, 2002).
3. Client aspirated secretions.
   a. Suction oral airway.
   b. Perform tracheal bronchial suctioning.
   c. Notify health care provider immediately.

Recording and Reporting

- Record procedure, including pertinent observations (e.g., presence of bleeding gums, dry mucosa, ulcerations, crusts on tongue).
- Report any unusual findings to nurse in charge or health care provider.

Home Care Considerations

- Irrigate cavity with bulb syringe; client can use a gravy baster.
- Give mouth care at least twice a day. Diluted hydrogen peroxide and sodium bicarbonate can effectively be used for oral care.
- Have caregivers demonstrate positioning client to prevent aspiration.

---

awaking in the morning, after each meal, and at bedtime will effectively clean the oral cavity. Client can increase the rinses to every 2 hours if necessary. Some health care providers will order a mild oral analgesic for pain control.

Clients with diabetes mellitus frequently have periodontal disease. Clients need to visit the dentist every 3 to 4 months. Handle all tissues gently with a minimum of trauma. Clients learn to follow rigid cleansing schedules, at least 4 times a day.

Denture Care. Encourage clients to clean their dentures on a regular basis to avoid gingival infection and irritation. When clients become disabled, someone must assume responsibility for denture care (Box 39-13). Dentures are the client's personal property and need to be handled with care because they are easy to break. Dentures must be removed at night to give the gums a rest and prevent bacterial buildup. To prevent warping, keep dentures covered in water when they are not worn, and always store them in an enclosed, labeled cup with the cup placed in the client's bedside stand. Discourage clients from removing their dentures and placing them on a napkin or tissue because they could be easily thrown away.

Hair and Scalp Care.
A person's appearance and feeling of well-being often depend on the way the hair looks and feels. Illness or disability often prevents a client from maintaining daily hair care. An immobilized client's hair soon becomes tangled. Some dressings leave sticky blood or antiseptic solutions on the hair. In the clinic and home care setting, nurses will encounter clients who have head lice. Proper hair care is important to the client's body image. Brushing, combing, and shampooing are basic hygiene measures for all clients.

Brushing and Combing. Frequent brushing helps to keep hair clean and distributes oil evenly along hair shafts. Combing prevents hair from tangling. Encourage the client to maintain routine hair care. However, clients with limited mobility or weakness and those who are confused require help. Clients in a hospital or extended care facility appreciate the opportunity to have their hair brushed and combed before being seen by others.

When caring for clients from different cultures, it is important to learn as much as possible from them or their family about preferred hair care practices. For example, the hair of African Americans tends to be quite dry. Use special lanolin conditioners for conditioning. Cultural preferences will also affect how hair is combed and styled.

Long hair easily becomes matted after a client is confined to bed, even for a short period. When lacerations or incisions involve the scalp, blood and topical medications also cause tangling. Frequent brushing and combing keep long hair neatly groomed. Braiding helps to avoid repeated tangles; however, clients need to unbraid hair periodically and comb it to ensure good hygiene. Braids made too tightly lead to bald patches. Obtain permission from the client before braiding his or her hair.

To brush hair, first part the hair into two sections and separate each into two more sections. It is easier to brush smaller

✳ **BOX 39-13**   **PROCEDURAL GUIDELINES**

Care of Dentures

Delegation Considerations: The skills of denture care can be delegated. The nurse instructs nursing assistive personnel to:
- Inform the nurse if there are cracks in dentures
- Inform the nurse if the client complains of oral discomfort

Equipment: Soft-bristle toothbrush or denture toothbrush, denture cleaning agent or toothpaste, denture adhesive *(optional)*, glass of water, emesis basin or sink, washcloth, clean gloves, denture cup (if dentures are to be stored after cleaning).

1. Ask client if dentures fit and if there is any gum or mucous membrane tenderness or irritation.
2. Ask client about preferences for denture care and products used. If client is unable to care for own dentures, provide this care. Clean dentures for client during routine mouth care.
3. Fill emesis basin with tepid water, or if using sink, place washcloth in bottom of sink and fill sink with an inch of water.
4. Remove dentures: If client is unable to do this independently, perform hand hygiene and apply gloves, grasp upper plate at front with thumb and index finger wrapped in gauze, and pull downward. Gently lift lower denture from jaw, and rotate one side downward to remove from client's mouth. Place dentures in emesis basin or sink.
5. Apply cleaning agent to brush, and brush surfaces of dentures (see illustration). Hold dentures close to water. Hold brush horizontally, and use back-and-forth motion to cleanse biting surfaces. Use short strokes from top of denture to biting surfaces to clean outer and inner teeth surfaces. Hold brush vertically, and use short strokes to clean inner tooth surfaces. Hold brush horizontally, and use back-and-forth motion to clean undersurface of dentures.

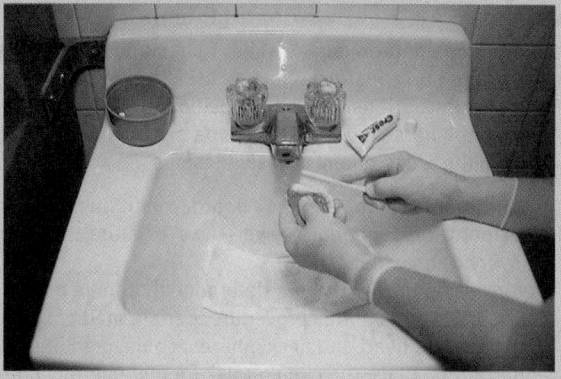

STEP 5 Brushing dentures.

6. Rinse thoroughly in tepid water.
7. Some clients use an adhesive to seal dentures in place. Apply a thin layer to undersurface before inserting.
8. If client needs assistance with insertion of dentures, moisten upper denture and press firmly to seal it in place. Then insert moistened lower denture. Ask if dentures feel comfortable.
9. Some clients prefer to have their dentures stored to give the gums a rest and to reduce risk of infection. Keeping dentures moist will prevent warping and facilitate easier insertion. Store in a secure place to prevent loss.
10. Remove and discard gloves. and perform hand hygiene.

---

sections of hair. Brushing from the scalp toward the hair ends minimizes pulling. Moistening the hair with water or alcohol frees tangles for easier combing. Never cut a client's hair without written consent.

Clients who develop head lice require special considerations in the way combing is performed. The lice are small, about the size of a sesame seed. Bright light or natural sunlight is necessary for you to see the lice. Thorough combing is recommended and is often more effective than use of pediculicidal shampoos, which are often toxic and ineffective against resistant lice. Follow these steps:

- Apply disposable gown and gloves.
- Use a grooming comb or hairbrush to remove tangles.
- Divide the client's hair in sections, and fasten off hair that is not being combed.
- Comb out from the scalp to the end of the hair (special combs are available in drug stores).
- Dip the comb in a cup of water or use a paper towel to remove lice between each passing.
- After combing, look through the hair carefully for attached lice.
- You can catch live lice with a tweezers or comb.
- Move to next section of hair after combing thoroughly.
- Instruct family to clean the comb with an old toothbrush and dental floss and boil the comb (if possible). The ideal is to discard the comb after each use, but some client's financial situations prevent the purchase of multiple combs.

- Instruct family to comb and screen for lice daily.
- Instruct family to contain client's clothes and to wash in hot water.
- Instruct family to vacuum the home and client's room, and to immediately empty vacuum bag or bagless collection device.
- Instruct caregivers in how to prevent transmission of lice:
  · Do not share any bed linens.
  · Avoid placing bare hand on client's head.
  · Immediately wash hands after providing hair care.
  · Contain all hair care products.

If a pediculicidal shampoo is ordered, instruct the client and caregiver in proper use of shampoo. These shampoos have neurological side effects. The very young and very old have increased susceptibility to the toxic effects of seizure, dizziness, headache, paresthesia, and death. Never use this type of medication on clients infected with human immunodeficiency virus (HIV), those with neurological conditions, the neonate, or clients who weigh less than 110 pounds (Zurlinden, 2003). As with any medication preparation, it is important to review and understand pertinent information. Most side effects associated with pediculicidal shampoos occurred as a result of applying too much medicated shampoo, leaving the shampoo in place too long, or repeated shampooing too soon. Many clients were overtreated because they incorrectly believed that continued itching meant that lice survived the initial treatment. They did not

✳ **BOX 39-14**   **PROCEDURAL GUIDELINES**

Shampooing Hair of Bed-Bound Client

Delegation Considerations: The skill of shampooing hair can be delegated, The nurse instructs nursing assistive personnel:
- About any precautions needed in positioning the client
- To inform the nurse if the client reports neck pain
- To inform the nurse of any new skin lesions

Equipment: Brush, comb, shampoo board, conditioner *(optional)*, hydrogen peroxide *(optional),* towels (two or more), hair dryer, basin of very warm water.

1. Before washing client's hair, determine that there are no contraindications to this procedure. Certain medical conditions, such as head and neck injuries, spinal cord injuries, and arthritis, place the client at risk for injury during shampooing because of positioning and manipulation of client's head and neck.
2. Apply gloves if needed. Inspect the hair and scalp before initiating the procedure. This determines the presence of any conditions that require the use of special shampoos or treatments (e.g., for dandruff or the removal of dried blood).
3. Place waterproof pad under client's shoulders, neck, and head (see illustration). Position client supine, with head and shoulders at top edge of bed. Place plastic trough under client's head and washbasin at end of trough. Be sure trough spout extends beyond edge of mattress.
4. Place rolled towel under client's neck and bath towel over client's shoulders.

5. Brush and comb client's hair.
6. Obtain warm water.
7. Offer client the option of holding face towel or washcloth over eyes.
8. Slowly pour water from water pitcher over hair until it is completely wet (see illustration). If hair contains matted blood, put on gloves, apply peroxide to dissolve clots, and then rinse hair with saline. Apply small amount of shampoo.
9. Work up lather with both hands. Start at hairline, and work toward back of neck. Lift head slightly with one hand to wash back of head. Shampoo sides of head. Massage scalp by applying pressure with fingertips.
10. Rinse hair with water. Make sure water drains into basin. Repeat rinsing until hair is free of soap.
11. Apply conditioner or cream rinse if requested, and rinse hair thoroughly.
12. Wrap client's head in bath towel. Dry client's face with cloth used to protect eyes. Dry off any moisture along neck or shoulders.
13. Dry client's hair and scalp. Use second towel if first becomes saturated.
14. Comb hair to remove tangles, and dry with dryer if desired.
15. Apply oil preparation or conditioning product to hair, if desired by client.
16. Assist client to comfortable position, and complete styling of hair.

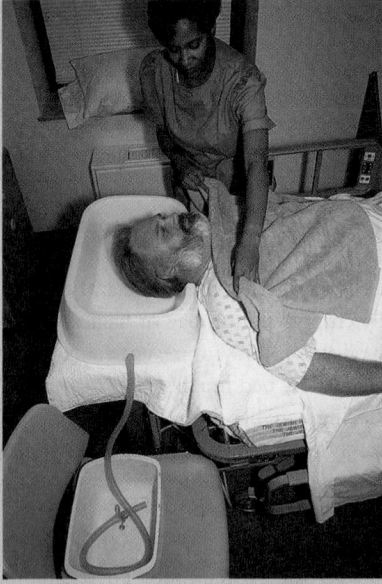

STEP 3 Pad under shoulders, neck, and head.

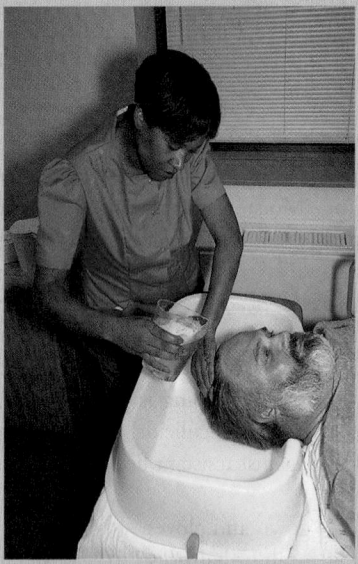

STEP 8 Pouring water over hair.

know that itching was a common side effect of the shampoo (Zurlinden, 2003).

Shampooing. Frequency of shampooing depends on a person's daily routines and the condition of the hair. Remind clients in hospitals or extended care facilities that staying in bed, excess perspiration, or treatments that leave blood or solutions in the hair require more frequent shampooing. In most agencies a physician's order is necessary for shampooing the dependent client. For dependent clients or clients with limited mobility in the

home, it is challenging to find ways to shampoo the hair without causing injury.

If the client is able to take a shower or bath, usually he or she is able to shampoo the hair without difficulty. A shower or tub chair is useful for the ambulatory, weight-bearing client who becomes tired or faint. Handheld shower nozzles allow clients to easily wash the hair in the tub or shower. Some clients allowed to sit in a chair choose to be shampooed in front of a sink or over a washbasin. However, bending is limited or contraindicated in certain conditions (e.g., eye surgery or neck injury). In these situations, teach the client and family the degree of bending allowed.

If a client is unable to sit but can be moved, transfer the client to a stretcher for transportation to a sink or shower equipped with a handheld nozzle. Long-term care facilities are commonly equipped with this option. Caution is again necessary when the client's head and neck are positioned, particularly in clients with any form of head or neck injury.

If the client is unable to sit in a chair or be transferred to a stretcher, shampoo the hair with the client in bed (Box 39-14). Position a special shampoo trough under the client's head to catch water and suds. After shampooing, clients like having their hair styled and dried. Most health care centers have portable hair dryers. Dry shampoos that reduce the need to wet the client's hair are also available but are not highly effective. These dry shampoo preparations vary, so follow the application procedures listed on the container exactly.

Shaving. Shave facial hair after the bath or shampoo. Women often prefer to shave their legs or axillae while bathing. When assisting a client, take care to avoid cutting the client with a razor blade. Clients prone to bleeding (e.g., those receiving anticoagulants or high doses of aspirin or those with low platelet counts) need to use an electric razor. Before using an electric razor, check for frayed cords or other electrical hazards. Use electric razors on only one client because of infection control considerations.

When using a razor blade for shaving, the skin must be softened to prevent pulling, scraping, or cuts. For example, placing a warm washcloth over the male client's face for a few seconds, followed by application of shaving cream or a lathering of mild soap, softens the skin. If the client is unable to shave, the nurse performs the shave. To avoid causing discomfort or razor cuts, gently pull the skin taut and use long, firm razor strokes in the direction the hair grows (Figure 39-8). Short downward strokes work best to remove hair over the upper lip or chin. A client usually explains the best way to move the razor across the skin. In the case of African Americans, facial hair tends to be curly and becomes ingrown unless shaved close to the skin.

Mustache and Beard Care. Clients with mustaches or beards require daily grooming. Keeping these areas clean is important because food particles and mucus easily collect in the hair. If the client is unable to carry out self-care, do so at the client's request. Gently comb out beards. You can trim a shaggy or unkempt mustache or beard. Do not shave off a mustache or beard without the client's consent.

Hair and Scalp Care. To best promote and restore hair and scalp health, instruct clients to keep hair clean, combed, and brushed regularly. Clients also need to know how to check for and remove parasites, such as lice (see Table 39-4). Tell clients they need to notify their primary caregiver of changes in the texture and distribution of hair, which indicates a serious systemic problem.

Care of the Eyes, Ears, and Nose. Give special attention to cleansing the eyes, ears, and nose during a routine bath and when drainage or discharge accumulates. This aspect of hygiene not only makes the client more comfortable but also improves sensory reception (see Chapter 49). Care focuses on preventing infection and maintaining normal sensory function. In addition, care of the

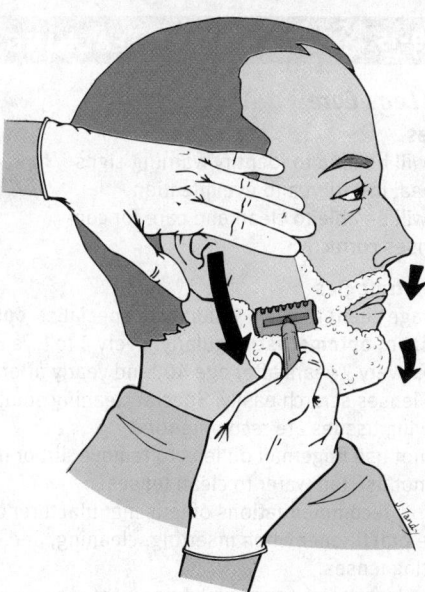

Figure 39-8 Shave in the direction of hair growth. Use longer strokes on the larger areas of the face. Use short strokes around the chin and lips. (From Sorrentino SA: *Assisting with patient care,* St. Louis, 2003, Mosby.)

eyes, ears, and nose requires approaches that consider the client's special needs.

Basic Eye Care. Cleansing the eyes simply involves washing with a clean washcloth moistened in water. Soap causes burning and irritation (see Skill 39-1, p. 869). Never apply direct pressure over the eyeball because it causes serious injury.

Unconscious clients often require more frequent eye care. When cleansing the client's eyes obtain a clean washcloth and cleanse from inner canthus to outer canthus. Use a different section of the washcloth for each eye.

Secretions collect along the lid margins and inner canthus when the blink reflex is absent or when the eye does not totally close. It is often necessary to place an eye patch over the involved eye or use paper tape to close the eye to prevent corneal drying and irritation. Give lubricating eye drops according to the health care provider's orders.

Eyeglasses. Glasses are made of hardened glass or plastic that is impact resistant to prevent shattering. Nevertheless, because of the cost, be careful when cleaning glasses, and protect them from breakage or other damage when they are not worn. Put glasses in a case in a drawer of the bedside table when not in use.

Cool water is sufficient for cleaning glass lenses. A soft cloth is best for drying to prevent scratching the lens. Paper towels scratch a lens. Plastic lenses in particular are scratched easily, and special cleansing solutions and drying tissues are available. Use whatever the client's eye care specialist recommends.

Contact Lenses. A contact lens is a small, round, transparent, and sometimes colored disk that fits directly over the cornea of the eye. Contact lenses are designed specifically to correct refractive errors of the eye or abnormalities in the cornea's shape. They are relatively easy to apply and remove.

Contact lenses are available as daily wear, extended wear, and disposable. In terms of a client's hygiene care it is important to

✳ BOX 39-15   CLIENT TEACHING

Contact Lens Care

Objectives

- Client will be able to identify warning signs of corneal irritation and eye infection.
- Client will be able to clean and care for contact lenses correctly.

Teaching Strategies

- Encourage client to see a vision care specialist (**ophthalmologist** or **optometrist**) regularly: every 3 to 5 years before age 40, every 2 years after age 40, and yearly after age 65.
- Plastic lenses scratch easily. Special cleaning solutions and drying tissues are recommended.
    - Do not use fingernail on lens to remove dirt or debris.
    - Do not use tap water to clean lenses.
    - Follow recommendations of lens manufacturer or eye care practitioner when inserting, cleaning, and disinfecting lenses.
    - Keep lens moist or wet when not worn.
    - Use fresh solution daily when storing and disinfecting lenses.
    - Thoroughly wash and rinse lens storage case on a daily basis. Clean periodically with soap or liquid detergent, rinse thoroughly with warm water, and air dry.
- Encourage client to remember the mnemonic RSVP: *R*edness, *S*ensitivity, *V*ision problems, and *P*ain. If one of these problems occurs, remove contact lenses immediately. If problems continue, contact a vision care specialist (Lewis and others, 2007).
- If lens is dropped on a hard surface, moisten finger with cleaning or wetting solution and gently touch lens to pick it up. Then clean, rinse, and disinfect lens.
- To avoid mix-up, always start with the same lens when removing or inserting lenses.
- Throw away disposable or planned replacement lenses after prescribed wearing period.

Evaluation

- Ask client to state warning signs of corneal irritation and eye infection.
- Ask client to describe methods of contact lens care that lead to infection.
- Ask client to demonstrate cleaning and storing contact lenses.

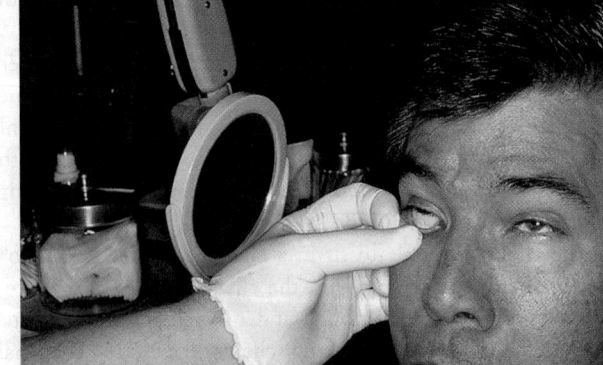

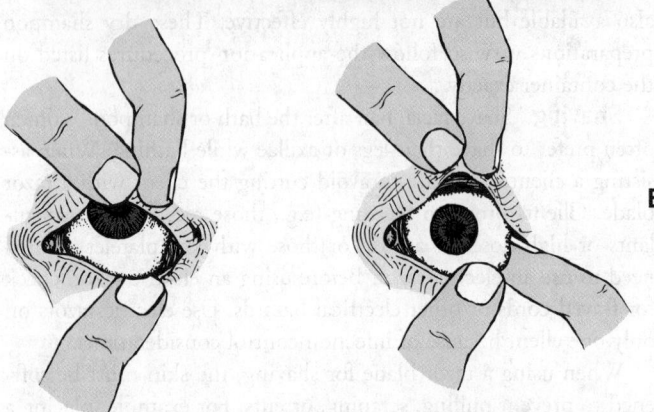

Figure 39-9 Removal of prosthetic eye.

know that all contacts must be removed periodically to prevent ocular infection and corneal ulcers or abrasions. Common infectious agents are *Pseudomonas aeruginosa* and staphylococci. Client education also includes a discussion of proper lens care techniques (Box 39-15).

Daily Wear. These lenses are removed nightly for cleaning and disinfection and replaced on an individualized schedule.

Extended Wear. These lenses are worn overnight but are removed at least weekly for cleaning and disinfection.

Disposable Wear. These lenses are removed nightly and replaced on a daily, weekly or monthly basis (American Academy of Ophthalmology, 2005). Pain, tearing, discomfort, and redness of the conjunctivae are symptoms of lens overwear. Persistence of symptoms even after lens removal is abnormal, however, and indicates serious ocular damage.

Contact lenses accumulate secretions and foreign matter. This material deteriorates and then irritates the eye, causing distorted vision and risk for infection. Once removed, clean contact lenses and thoroughly disinfect them. Caution clients to never use saliva, homemade saline, or tap water when cleaning lenses as these solutions contain microorganisms that cause serious infection.

Artificial Eyes. Clients with artificial eyes have had an **enucleation** of an entire eyeball as a result of tumor growth, severe infection, or eye trauma. Some artificial eyes are permanently implanted. Remove others for routine cleaning. Clients with artificial eyes usually prefer to care for their own eyes. Respect the client's wishes, and help by assembling needed equipment.

At times clients require assistance in prosthesis removal and cleansing. To remove an artificial eye, retract the lower eyelid and exerts slight pressure just below the eye (Figure 39-9). This action causes the artificial eye to rise from the socket because the suction holding the eye in place has been broken. You can also use a small, rubber bulb syringe or medicine dropper bulb to create a suction effect. The suction created by placing the bulb tip directly over the eye and squeezing lifts the eye from the socket.

The artificial eye is usually made of glass or plastic. Warm normal saline cleanses the prosthesis effectively. Also cleanse the edges of the eye socket and surrounding tissues with soft gauze moistened in saline or clean tap water. Report signs of infection immediately because bacteria can spread to the neighboring eye, underlying sinuses, or even underlying brain tissue. To reinsert the eye, retract the upper and lower lids and gently slip the eye into the socket, fitting it neatly under the upper eyelid. Store an artificial eye in a labeled container filled with tap water or saline.

Ear Care. Routine ear care involves cleansing the ear with the end of a moistened washcloth, rotated gently into the ear canal. When cerumen is visible, gentle, downward retraction at the entrance of the ear canal causes the wax to loosen and slip out. Instruct clients never to use sharp objects such as bobby pins or paper clips to remove ear wax. The use of such objects traumatizes the ear canal and ruptures the tympanic membrane. Avoid use of cotton-tipped applicators as well because they cause ear wax to become impacted within the canal.

Children and older adults commonly have impacted cerumen. You can usually remove excessive or impacted cerumen only by irrigation, which usually requires a health care provider's order. If a client has a history of a perforated eardrum or if you discover perforation during assessment, the procedure is contraindicated. Before irrigation first instill three drops of glycerin at bedtime to soften the wax and three drops of hydrogen peroxide twice a day to loosen the wax. Then the instillation of approximately 250 mL of warm water (37° C, or 98.6° F) into the ear canal mechanically washes away loosened wax. Cold or hot water causes nausea or vomiting.

Have the client sit or lie on his or her side with the affected ear up. Place a small curved basin under the affected ear to catch the irrigating solution. Use a Water Pik (set on No. 2 setting) or a bulb irrigating syringe to irrigate the ear canal. Make sure the tip of the syringe or Water Pik does not occlude the canal to avoid exerting pressure against the tympanic membrane. Gentle irrigation directed at the top of the canal loosens the cerumen from the sides of the canal. After the canal is clear, wipe off any moisture from the ear and inspect the canal for remaining cerumen.

Hearing Aid Care. Hearing aids are instruments made up of miniature parts working together as a system to amplify sound in a controlled manner. The aid receives normal low-intensity sound inputs and delivers them to the client's ear as louder outputs. The new class of hearing aids reduce background noise interference. Computer chips placed in the aids allow for fine adjustments to the specific client's hearing needs. Both hard-of-hearing (slight or moderate hearing loss) and deaf persons (severe or profound hearing loss) use hearing aids.

There are three popular types of hearing aids. An in-the-canal (ITC) aid (Figure 39-10, *A*) is the newest, smallest, and least visible and fits entirely in the ear canal. It has cosmetic appeal, is easy to manipulate and place in the ear, does not interfere with wearing eyeglasses or using the telephone, and the client can wear it during most physical exercise. However, it requires adequate ear diameter and depth for proper fit. It does not accommodate progressive hearing loss, and it requires manual dexterity to operate, insert, remove, and change batteries. Also, cerumen tends to plug this model more than the others.

An in-the-ear (ITE, or intraaural) aid (Figure 39-10, *B*) fits into the external auditory canal and allows for more fine tuning. It is more powerful and stronger and therefore is useful for a wider range of hearing loss than the ITC aid. It is easy to position and adjust and does not interfere with eyeglass wearing. It is, however, more noticeable than the ITC aid and is not for persons with moisture or skin problems in the ear canal.

A behind-the-ear (BTE, or postaural) aid (Figure 39-10, *C*) hooks around and behind the ear and is connected by a short,

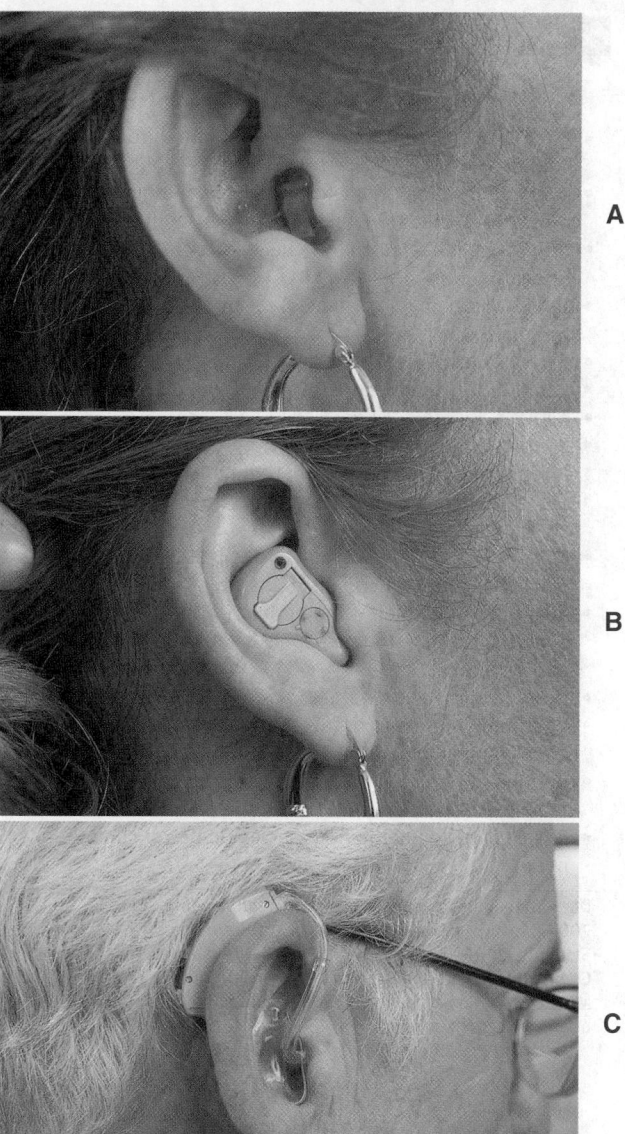

Figure 39-10 Three common types of hearing aids. **A,** Completely in canal. **B,** In the ear. **C,** Behind the ear.

clear, hollow plastic tube to an ear mold inserted into the external auditory canal. It allows for fine tuning. It is the largest of the three aids and is useful for clients with rapidly progressive hearing loss or manual dexterity difficulties or those who find partial ear occlusion intolerable. Disadvantages are that it is more visible and interferes with wearing eyeglasses and using a phone, and it is more difficult to keep in place during physical exercise. Box 39-16 reviews client education guidelines for the care and cleaning of a hearing aid.

Nasal Care. The client usually removes secretions from the nose by gently blowing into a soft tissue. Caution the client against harsh blowing that creates pressure capable of injuring the eardrum, nasal mucosa, and even sensitive eye structures. Bleeding from the nares is a sign of harsh blowing.

✳ BOX 39-16   Care and Use of Hearing Aids

- Initially wear a hearing aid 15 to 20 minutes; then gradually increase time to 10 to 12 hours.
- Once inserted, turn the aid slowly to one-third to one-half volume.
- A whistling sound indicates incorrect ear mold insertion, improper fit of aid, and buildup of earwax or fluid.
- Adjust volume to a comfortable level for talking at a distance of 1 yard.
- Do not wear aid under heat lamps or a hair dryer or in very wet, cold weather.
- Batteries last 1 week with daily wearing of 10 to 12 hours.
- Remove or disconnect battery when not in use.
- Replace ear molds every 2 or 3 years.
- Routinely check battery compartment: Is it clean? Are batteries inserted properly? Is compartment shut all the way?
- Make sure dials on hearing aid are clean and easy to rotate, creating no static during adjusting.
- Keep aid clean. See manufacturer's instructions, but aids are usually cleaned with a soft cloth.
- Avoid use of hairspray and perfume while wearing hearing aids, the residue from the spray causes aid to become oily and greasy.
- Do not submerse in water.
- Routinely check cord or tubing (depending on type of aid) for cracking, fraying, and poor connections.
- Routine follow-up with audiologist is recommended to evaluate effectiveness of current aid.
- It is easy to adjust the frequencies on newer computerized hearing aids.

Data from Ebersole P, Hess P: *Toward healthy aging*, ed 6, St. Louis, 2004, Mosby; Meiner S, Lueckenotte AG: *Gerontologic nursing*, ed 3, St. Louis, 2006, Mosby; and National Institute on Deafness and Other Communication Disorders: *Hearing aids*, Pub No. 99-4340, Bethesda, Md, 2001, National Institutes of Health, www.nidcd.nih.gov/health/hearing/hearingaid.asp.

If the client is unable to remove nasal secretions, assist by using a wet washcloth or a cotton-tipped applicator moistened in water or saline. Never insert the applicator beyond the length of the cotton tip. You can remove excessive nasal secretions by gentle suctioning.

When clients have nasogastric, feeding, or endotracheal tubes inserted through the nose, change the tape anchoring the tube at least once a day. When tape becomes moist from nasal secretions, the skin and mucosa easily becomes macerated. Friction from a tube causes tissue sloughing. After carefully removing the tape, maintain hold of the tubing and thoroughly cleanse and dry the nasal surface.

Client's Room Environment.
Attempting to make a client's room as comfortable as the home is one of the nurse's priorities. The client's room needs to be comfortable, safe, and large enough to allow the client and visitors to move about freely. Control room temperature, ventilation, noise, and odors to create a more comfortable environment. Keeping the room neat and orderly also contributes to the client's sense of well-being.

Maintaining Comfort. What makes a comfortable environment depends on the client's age, severity of illness, and level of normal daily activity. Depending on the client's age and physical condition, maintain the room temperature between 20° and 23° C (68° and 74° F). Infants, older adults, and the acutely ill often need a warmer room. However, certain ill clients benefit from cooler room temperatures to lower the body's metabolic demands.

A good ventilation system keeps stale air and odors from lingering in the room. Protect the acutely ill, infants, and older adults from drafts by ensuring they are adequately dressed and covered with a lightweight blanket.

Good ventilation also reduces lingering odors caused by draining wounds, vomitus, bowel movements, and unemptied urinals. Always empty and rinse commodes, bedpans, and urinals promptly. Room deodorizers help remove many unpleasant odors, but use them with discretion in consideration of the client's possible embarrassment. Before using room deodorizers determine that the client is not allergic to or sensitive to the deodorizer itself. Thorough hygiene measures are the best way to control body or breath odors. Most health care institutions now prohibit smoking.

Proper lighting is necessary for everyone's safety and comfort. A brightly lit room is usually stimulating, but a darkened room is best for rest and sleep. Adjust room lighting by closing or opening drapes, regulating over-bed and floor lights, and closing or opening room doors. When entering a client's room at night, refrain from abruptly turning on an overhead light unless necessary.

Room Equipment. Although there are variations across health care settings, a typical hospital room contains the following basic pieces of furniture: over-bed table, bedside stand, chairs, lamp, and bed (Figure 39-11). Long-term care and rehabilitation facilities often have similar equipment. You can adjust the over-bed table, which rolls on wheels, to various heights over the bed or a chair. The table provides ideal working space for performing procedures. It also provides a surface on which to place meal trays, toiletry items, and objects frequently used by the client. Do not place the bedpan and urinal on the over-bed table. The bedside stand is for storing the client's personal possessions and hygiene equipment. The telephone, water pitcher, and drinking cup are usually on top of the bedside stand.

Most hospital rooms contain an armless straight-backed chair or an upholstered lounge chair with arms. Straight-backed chairs are convenient when temporarily transferring the client from the bed, such as during bed making. Lounge chairs tend to be more comfortable when a client is willing and able to sit for an extended period.

Each room usually has an over-bed light and a floor or table lamp. Position movable lights that extend over the bed from the wall for easy reach, but move them aside when not in use. Additional portable lighting provides extra light during bedside procedures.

Other equipment usually found in a client's room includes a call light, a television set, a wall-mounted blood pressure gauge, oxygen and vacuum wall outlets, and personal care items. Special equipment designed for comfort or positioning clients includes foot boots (Figure 39-12), special mattresses (see Chapter 48), and bed boards. Whenever using comfort and positioning equip-

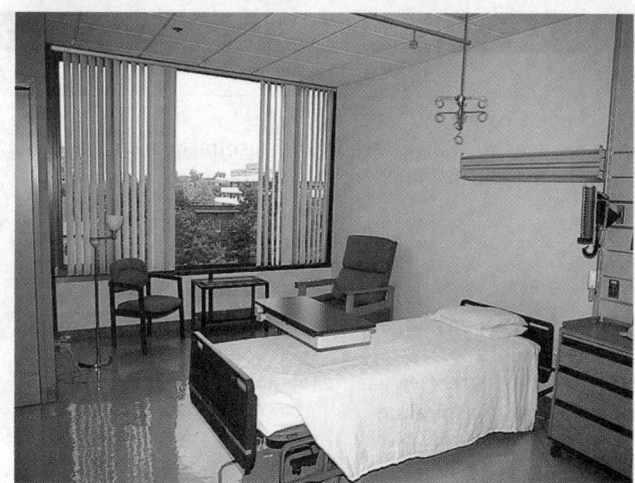

Figure 39-11 Typical hospital room.

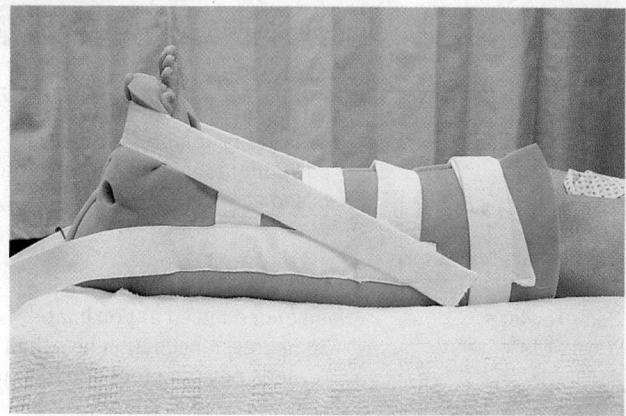

A

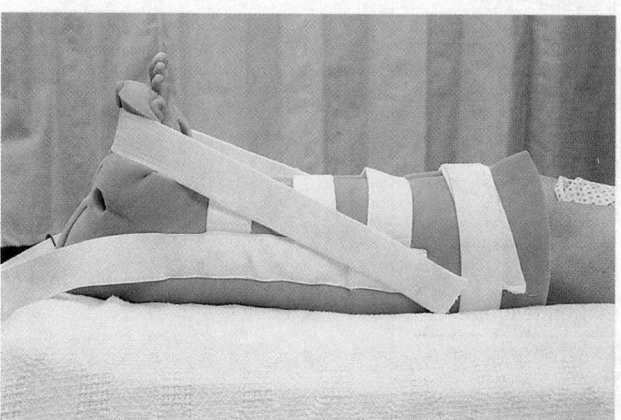

B

Figure 39-12 **A,** Foot boot. **B,** Foot boot with lower leg extension.

ment, check agency policy and manufacturer's directions before application.

Beds. Seriously ill clients often remain in bed for a long time. Because a bed is the piece of equipment used most by a hospitalized client, it is designed for comfort, safety, and adaptability for changing positions.

The typical hospital bed has a firm mattress on a metal frame that you can raise and lower horizontally. More and more hospitals are converting the standard hospital bed to one in which the mattress surface can be electronically adjusted for client comfort. Different bed positions promote client comfort, minimize symptoms, promote lung expansion, and improve access during certain procedures (Table 39-6).

You change the position of a bed usually by using electrical controls incorporated into the client's call light and in a panel on the side or foot of the bed (Figure 39-13). It is important for you to be familiar with use of the bed controls. Ease in raising and lowering a bed and in changing position of the head and foot eliminates undue musculoskeletal strain on the nurse. Instruct clients in the proper use of controls, and caution them against raising the bed to a position that causes harm.

Beds contain safety features such as locks on the wheels or casters. Lock wheels when the bed is stationary to prevent accidental movement. Side rails protect clients from accidental falls. You can remove the headboard from most beds. This is important when the medical team needs to have easy access to the head, such as during cardiopulmonary resuscitation.

Bed Making. Keep a client's bed clean and comfortable. This requires frequent inspections to be sure linen is clean, dry, and free of wrinkles. When clients are diaphoretic, have draining wounds, or are incontinent, check frequently for soiled linen.

The bed is usually made in the morning after the client's bath or while the client is bathing in a shower, sitting in a chair eating, or out of the room for procedures or tests. Throughout the day straighten linen that is loose or wrinkled. Also check the bed linen for food particles after meals and for wetness or soiling. Change any linen that becomes soiled or wet.

When changing bed linen, follow principles of medical asepsis by keeping soiled linen away from the uniform (Figure 39-14). Place soiled linen in special linen bags before discarding in a hamper. To avoid air currents, which spread microorganisms, never shake the linen. To avoid transmitting infection, do not place soiled linen on the floor. If clean linen touches the floor, immediately discard it.

During bed making, use safe client handling procedures and proper body mechanics (see Chapter 47). Always raise the bed to the appropriate height before changing linen so that you do not have to bend or stretch over the mattress. You will also move back and forth to opposite sides of the bed while applying new linen. Body mechanics and safe handling are important when turning or repositioning the client in bed.

TABLE 39-6   Common Bed Positions

POSITION	DESCRIPTION	USES
Fowler's	Head of bed raised to angle of 45 degrees or more; semi-sitting position; foot of bed may also be raised at knee	While client is eating During nasogastric tube insertion and nasotracheal suction Promotes lung expansion
Semi-Fowler's	Head of bed raised approximately 30 degrees; inclination less than Fowler's position; foot of bed may also be raised at knee	Promotes lung expansion, especially with ventilator-assisted clients Used when clients receive gastric feedings to reduce regurgitation and risk of aspiration
Trendelenburg's	Entire bed frame tilted with head of bed down	Used for postural drainage Facilitates venous return in clients with poor peripheral perfusion
Reverse Trendelenburg's	Entire bed frame tilted with foot of bed down	Used infrequently Promotes gastric emptying Prevents esophageal reflux
Flat	Entire bed frame horizontally parallel with floor	Used for clients with vertebral injuries and in cervical traction Used for clients who are hypotensive Clients usually prefer for sleeping

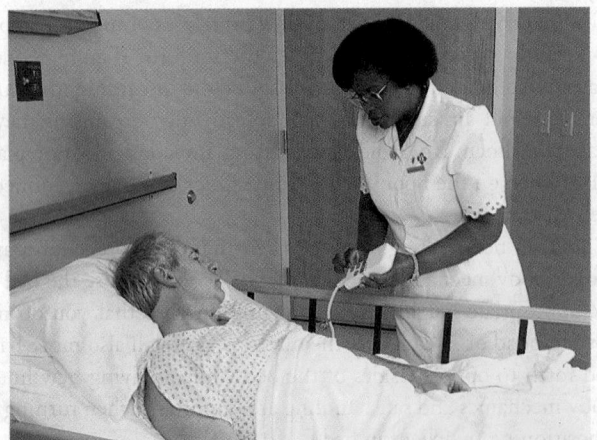

Figure 39-13 Nurse instructing client in use of call light and bed controls.

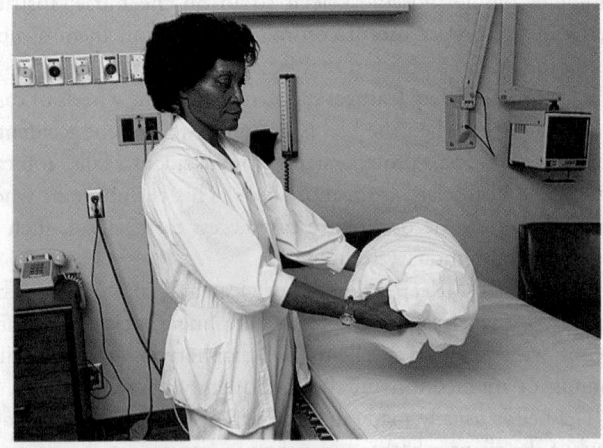

Figure 39-14 Holding linen away from the uniform prevents contact with microorganisms.

BOX 39-17

PROCEDURAL GUIDELINES

Making an Unoccupied Bed

Delegation Considerations: The skill of making an unoccupied bed can be delegated.

Equipment: Linen bag, mattress pad (change only when soiled), bottom sheet (flat or fitted), drawsheet *(optional)*, top sheet, blanket, bedspread, waterproof pads *(optional)*, pillowcases, bedside chair or table, clean gloves (if linen is soiled), washcloth, and antiseptic cleanser.

1. Determine if client has been incontinent or if excess drainage is on linen. Gloves will be necessary.
2. Assess activity orders or restrictions in mobility in planning if client can get out of bed for procedure. Assist to bedside chair or recliner.
3. Lower any side rails on both sides of bed, and raise bed to comfortable working position.
4. Remove soiled linen, and place in laundry bag. Avoid shaking or fanning linen.
5. Reposition mattress, and wipe off any moisture using a washcloth moistened in antiseptic solution. Dry thoroughly.
6. Apply all bottom linen on one side of bed before moving to opposite side.
7. Be sure fitted sheet is placed smoothly over mattress. To apply a flat unfitted sheet, allow about 25 cm (10 inches) to hang over mattress edge. Make sure lower hem of sheet lies seam down, even with bottom edge of mattress. Pull remaining top portion of sheet over top edge of mattress.
8. While standing at head of bed, miter top corner of bottom sheet (see Skill 39-6, Step 17).
9. Tuck remaining portion of unfitted sheet under mattress.
10. *Optional:* Apply drawsheet, laying center fold along middle of bed lengthwise. Smooth drawsheet over mattress, and tuck excess edge under mattress, keeping palms down.
11. Move to opposite side of bed, and spread bottom sheet smoothly over edge of mattress from head to foot of bed.
12. Apply fitted sheet smoothly over each mattress corner. For an unfitted sheet, miter top corner of bottom sheet (see Step 8), making sure corner is taut.
13. Grasp remaining edge of unfitted bottom sheet, and tuck tightly under mattress while moving from head to foot of bed. Smooth folded drawsheet over bottom sheet, and tuck under mattress, first at middle, then at top, and then at bottom.

14. If needed, apply waterproof pad over bottom sheet or drawsheet.
15. Place top sheet over bed with vertical center fold lengthwise down middle of bed. Open sheet out from head to foot, being sure top edge of sheet is even with top edge of mattress.
16. Make horizontal toe pleat: stand at foot of bed, and make fanfold in sheet 5 to 10 cm (2 to 4 inches) across bed. Pull sheet up from bottom to make fold approximately 15 cm (6 inches) from bottom edge of mattress (see illustration, Skill 39-6, Step 34).
17. Tuck in remaining portion of sheet under foot of mattress. Then place blanket over bed with top edge parallel to top edge of sheet and 15 to 20 cm (6 to 8 inches) down from edge of sheet. (*Optional:* Apply additional spread over bed.)
18. Make cuff by turning edge of top sheet down over top edge of blanket and spread.
19. Standing on one side at foot of bed, lift mattress corner slightly with one hand, and with other hand tuck top sheet, blanket, and spread under mattress. Be sure toe pleats are not pulled out.
20. Make modified mitered corner with top sheet, blanket, and spread. After making triangular fold, do not tuck tip of triangle (see illustration).
21. Go to other side of bed. Spread sheet, blanket, and spread out evenly. Make cuff with top sheet and blanket. Make modified corner at foot of bed.
22. Apply clean pillowcase.
23. Place call light within client's reach on bed rail or pillow, and return bed to height allowing for client transfer. Assist client to bed.
24. Arrange client's room. Remove and discard supplies. Perform hand hygiene.

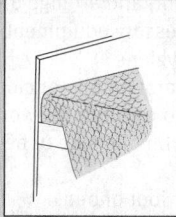

STEP 20 Modified mitered corner.

When clients are confined to bed, organize bed-making activities to conserve time and energy (Skill 39-6). The client's privacy, comfort, and safety are all important when making a bed. Using side rails to aid positioning and turning, keeping call lights within the client's reach, and maintaining the proper bed position help promote comfort and safety. After making a bed, return it to the lowest horizontal position and verify that the wheels are locked to prevent accidental falls when the client gets in and out of the bed alone.

When possible, make the bed while it is unoccupied (Box 39-17). Use judgment to determine the best time for the client to sit up in a chair while you are making the bed. When making an unoccupied bed, follow the same basic principles as for occupied bed making.

An unoccupied bed is open or closed. In an open bed, the top covers are folded back so that it is easy for a client to get into bed.

In a closed bed, the top sheet, blanket, and bedspread are drawn up to the head of the mattress and under the pillows. A closed bed is prepared in a hospital room before a new client is admitted to that room. A surgical, recovery, or postoperative bed is a modified version of the open bed. The top bed linen is arranged for easy transfer of the client from a stretcher to the bed. The top sheets and spread are not tucked or mitered at the corners. Instead, the top sheets are folded to one side or folded to the bottom third of the bed (Figure 39-16). This makes it easier to transfer the client into the bed.

Linens. In any health care agency, it is important to have an adequate supply of linen to care appropriately for clients. Many agencies have "nurse servers" either within or just outside a client's room where a daily supply of linen is stored. Because of the importance of cost control in health care, it is important to avoid bringing excess linen into a client's room. Once you bring the linen into a client's room, if unused, it must be discarded for laundering. This

SKILL 39-6   **MAKING AN OCCUPIED BED**   Video

Delegation Considerations

The skill of making an occupied bed can be delegated. The nurse reviews any precautions or activity restrictions. The nurse instructs nursing assistive personnel about:

- Looking for wound drainage, dressing material, drainage tubes, or IV tubing that becomes dislodged or is found in the linens
- What to do if client becomes fatigued

Equipment (Figure 39-15)

- Linen bag(s)
- Mattress pad (needs to be changed only when soiled)
- Bottom sheet (flat or fitted)
- Drawsheet
- Top sheet
- Blanket
- Bedspread
- Waterproof pads and/or bath blankets (optional)
- Pillowcases
- Bedside chair or table
- Clean gloves (optional)
- Towel
- Disinfectant

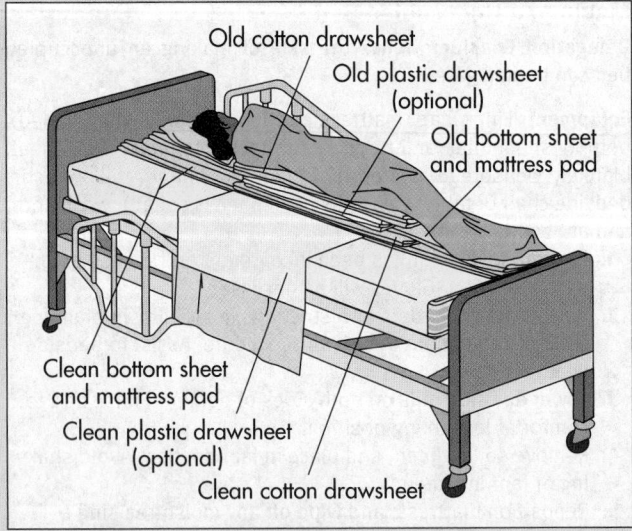

Figure 39-15 Equipment for making occupied bed

STEPS	RATIONALE
1. Assess potential for client incontinence or for excess drainage on bed linen.	Determines need for protective waterproof pads or extra bath blankets on bed.
2. Check chart for orders or specific precautions concerning movement and positioning.	Ensures client safety and use of proper body mechanics.
3. Explain procedure to the client, noting that the client will be asked to turn on side and roll over linen.	Minimizes anxiety and promotes cooperation.
4. Perform hand hygiene, and apply gloves (wear gloves only if linen is soiled or there is risk for contact with body secretions).	Reduces transmission of microorganisms.
5. Assemble equipment, and arrange on bedside chair or table. Remove unnecessary equipment such as a dietary tray or items used for hygiene.	Assembling all equipment provides for smooth procedure and assists in increasing client's comfort. Placing linen on clean surface minimizes spread of infection.
6. Draw room curtain around bed or close door.	Maintains client's privacy.
7. Adjust bed height to comfortable working position. Lower any raised side rail on one side of bed. Remove call light.	Minimizes strain on back. It is easier to remove and apply linen evenly to bed in flat position. Provides easy access to bed and linen.
8. Loosen top linen at foot of bed.	Makes linen easier to remove.
9. Remove bedspread and blanket separately. If spread and blanket are soiled, place them in linen bag. Keep soiled linen away from uniform.	Reduces transmission of microorganisms.
10. If blanket and spread are to be reused, fold them by bringing the top and bottom edges together. Fold farthest side over onto nearer bottom edge. Bring top and bottom edges together again. Place folded linen over back of chair.	Folding method facilitates replacement and minimizes wrinkles.
11. Cover client with bath blanket in the following manner: unfold bath blanket over top sheet. Ask client to hold top edge of bath blanket. If client is unable to help, tuck top of bath blanket under shoulder. Grasp top sheet under bath blanket at client's shoulders and bring sheet down to foot of bed. Remove sheet and discard in linen bag.	Bath blanket provides warmth and keeps body parts covered during linen removal.
12. With assistance from another nurse, slide mattress toward head of bed.	If mattress slides toward foot of bed when head of bed is raised, it is difficult to tuck in linen. In addition, it is uncomfortable for the client because the client's feet may be pressed against or hang over the foot of the bed.
13. Position client on the far side of the bed, turned onto side and facing away from you. Be sure side rail in front of client is up. Adjust pillow under client's head.	Turning client onto side provides space for placement of clean linen. Side rail ensures client's safety from forward falls from the bed surface and helps client in moving.

✳ SKILL 39-6   MAKING AN OCCUPIED BED—CONT'D

STEPS

14. Loosen bottom linens, moving from head to foot. With seam side down (facing the mattress), fanfold bottom sheet and drawsheet toward client—first drawsheet, then bottom sheet. Tuck edges of linen just under buttocks, back, and shoulders. Do not fanfold mattress pad if it is to be reused (see illustration).

15. Wipe off any moisture on exposed mattress with towel and appropriate disinfectant. Make sure mattress surface is dry before applying linens.

16. Apply clean linen to exposed half of bed:
    a. Place clean mattress pad on bed by folding it lengthwise with center crease in middle of bed. Fanfold top layer over mattress. (If pad is reused, simply smooth out any wrinkles.)
    b. Unfold bottom sheet lengthwise so that center crease is situated lengthwise along center of bed. Fanfold sheet's top layer toward center of bed alongside the client. Smooth bottom layer of sheet over mattress, and bring edge over closest side of mattress. Pull fitted sheet smoothly over mattress ends. Allow edge of flat unfitted sheet to hang about 25 cm (10 inches) over mattress edge. Make sure lower hem of bottom flat sheet lies seam down and even with bottom edge of mattress (see illustration).

17. Miter bottom flat sheet at head of bed:
    a. Face head of bed diagonally. Place hand away from head of bed under top corner of mattress, near mattress edge, and lift.
    b. With other hand, tuck top edge of bottom sheet smoothly under mattress so that side edges of sheet above and below mattress meet when brought together.
    c. Face side of bed and pick up top edge of sheet at approximately 45 cm (18 inches) from top of mattress (see illustration).
    d. Lift sheet, and lay it on top of mattress to form a neat triangular fold, with lower base of triangle even with mattress side edge (see illustration).
    e. Tuck lower edge of sheet, which is hanging free below the mattress, under mattress. Tuck with palms down, without pulling triangular fold (see illustration).

RATIONALE

Prepares for removal of all bottom linen simultaneously.
Provides maximum work space for placing clean linen. Later, when client turns to other side, you can remove soiled linen easily.

Reduces transmission of microorganisms.

Applying linen over bed in successive layers minimizes energy and time used in bed making.

Proper positioning of linen on one side ensures that adequate linen will be available to cover opposite side of bed. Keeping seam edges down eliminates irritation to client's skin.

Ensures secure flat sheet will not loosen easily.

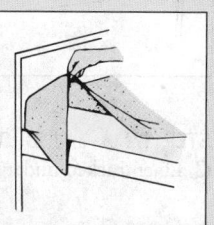
STEP 17c Top edge of sheet picked up.

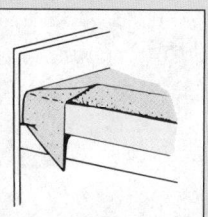
STEP 17d Sheet on top of mattress in a triangular fold.

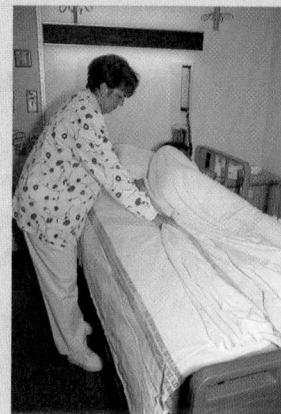
STEP 14 Old linen tucked under client.

STEP 16b Clean linen applied to bed.

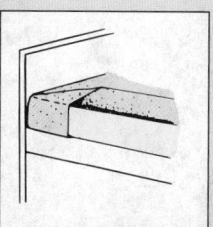
STEP 17e Lower edge of sheet tucked under mattress.

Continued

✳ **SKILL 39-6**   **MAKING AN OCCUPIED BED—CONT'D**

STEPS

    f. Hold portion of sheet covering side of mattress in place with one hand. With the other hand, pick up top of triangular linen fold and bring it down over side of mattress. Tuck this portion under mattress (see illustrations).

18. Tuck remaining portion of sheet under mattress, moving toward foot of bed. Keep linen smooth.

19. *(Optional)* Open drawsheet so that it unfolds in half. Lay centerfold along middle of bed lengthwise, and position sheet so that it will be under the client's buttocks and torso (see illustration). Fanfold top layer toward client, with edge along client's back. Smooth bottom layer out over mattress, and tuck excess edge under mattress (keep palms down).

20. Place waterproof pad over drawsheet, with centerfold against client's side. Fanfold top layer toward client.

21. Advise client that he or she will be rolling over thick layer of linens and will feel a lump. Have client roll slowly toward you, over the layers of linen. Raise side rail on working side, and go to other side of bed.

22. Lower side rail. Assist client in positioning on other side, over folds of linen. Loosen edges of soiled linen from under mattress (see illustration).

23. Remove soiled linen by folding it into a bundle or square, with soiled side turned in. Discard in linen bag. If necessary, wipe mattress with antiseptic solution, and dry mattress surface before applying new linen.

24. Pull clean, fanfolded linen smoothly over edge of mattress from head to foot of bed.

25. Assist client in rolling back into supine position. Reposition pillow.

RATIONALE

Mitered corner cannot be loosened easily even if client moves frequently in bed.

Folds of linen are source of irritation.

Drawsheet is used to lift and reposition client. Placement under client's torso distributes most of client's body weight over sheet.

Protects bed linen from being soiled.

Positions client for removal and placement of linens. Maintains client's safety and body alignment during turning.

Exposes opposite side of bed for removal of soiled linen and placement of clean linen. Makes linen easier to remove.

Reduces transmission of microorganisms.

Smooth linen will not irritate client's skin.

Maintains client's comfort.

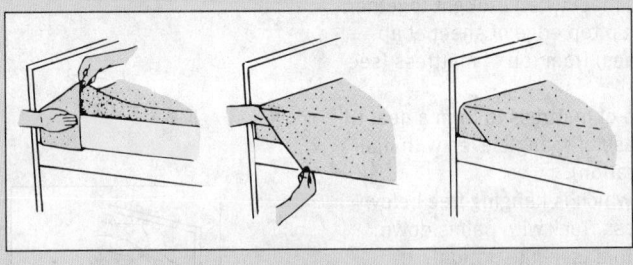

    A   **B**   **C**

STEP 17f A and **B,** Triangular fold placed over side of mattress. **C,** Linen tucked under mattress.

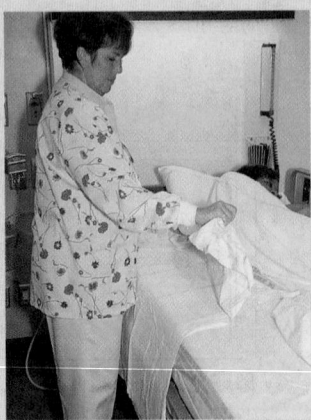

STEP 19 Optional drawsheet.

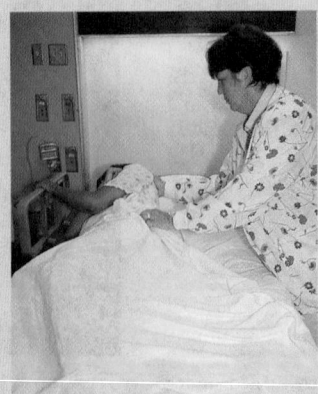

STEP 22 Assisting client in rolling over folds of linen.

STEPS	RATIONALE
26. Pull fitted sheet smoothly over mattress ends. Miter top corner of bottom sheet (see Step 17). When tucking corner, be sure that sheet is smooth and free of wrinkles.	Wrinkles and folds cause irritation to skin.
27. Facing side of bed, grasp remaining edge of bottom flat sheet. Lean back, keep back straight, and pull while tucking excess linen under mattress. Proceed from head to foot of bed. (Avoid lifting mattress during tucking to ensure fit.)	Proper use of body mechanics while tucking linen prevents injury.
28. Smooth fanfolded drawsheet out over bottom sheet. Grasp edge of sheet with palms down, lean back, and tuck sheet under mattress. Tuck from middle to top and then to bottom.	Tucking first at top or bottom will pull sheet sideways, causing poor fit.
29. Place top sheet over client with centerfold lengthwise down middle of bed. Open sheet from head to foot, and unfold over client.	Correctly positioning centerfold ensures that sheet is equally distributed over bed.
30. Ask client to hold clean top sheet, or tuck sheet around client's shoulders. Remove bath blanket and discard in linen bag.	Sheet prevents exposure of body parts. Having client hold sheet encourages client participation in care.
31. Place blanket on bed, unfolding it so that crease runs lengthwise along middle of bed. Unfold blanket to cover client. Make sure top edge is parallel with edge of top sheet and 15 to 20 cm (6 to 8 inches) from top sheet's edge.	Blanket covers client completely and provides adequate warmth.
32. Place spread over bed according to Step 31. Be sure that top edge of spread extends about 2.5 cm (1 inch) above blanket's edge. Tuck top edge of spread over and under top edge of blanket.	Gives bed neat appearance and provides extra warmth.
33. Make cuff by turning edge of top sheet down over top edge of blanket and spread.	Protects client's face from rubbing against blanket or spread.
34. Standing on one side at foot of bed, lift mattress corner slightly with one hand and tuck linens under mattress. Top sheet and blanket are tucked under together. Be sure that linens are loose enough to allow movement of client's feet. Making a horizontal toe pleat is an option (see illustration).	Makes neat-appearing bed. Pressure ulcers will develop on client's toes and heels from feet rubbing against tight-fitting bed sheets.
35. Make modified mitered corner with top sheet, blanket, and spread (see illustration in Box 39-17, Step 20, p. 899):	Ensures top covers will not loosen easily.
a. Pick up side edge of top sheet, blanket, and spread approximately 45 cm (18 inches) from foot of mattress. Lift linen to form triangular fold, and lay it on bed.	
b. Tuck lower edge of sheet, which is hanging free below mattress, under mattress. Do not pull triangular fold.	
c. Pick up triangular fold, and bring it down over mattress while holding linen in place along side of mattress. Do not tuck tip of triangle.	Secures top linen but keeps even edge of blanket and top sheet draped over mattress.
36. Raise side rail as appropriate. Make other side of bed; spread sheet, blanket, and bedspread out evenly. Fold top edge of spread over blanket and make cuff with top sheet (see Step 33); make modified mitered corner at foot of bed (see Step 35).	Correct use of side rails aids client's movement in bed.

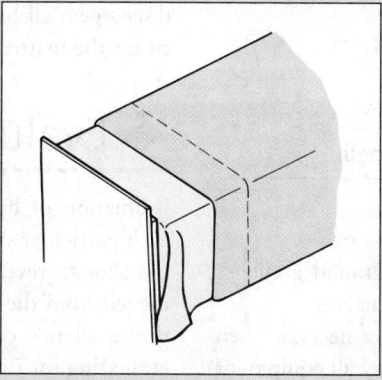

STEP 34 Optional toe pleat.

Continued

✱ SKILL 39-6   MAKING AN OCCUPIED BED—CONT'D

STEPS	RATIONALE
37. Change pillowcase:	
a. Have client raise head. While supporting neck with one hand, remove pillow. Allow client to lower head.	Support of neck muscles prevents injury during flexion and extension of neck.
b. Remove soiled case by grasping pillow at open end with one hand and pulling case back over pillow with the other hand. Discard case in linen bag.	Pillows slide out easily, thus minimizing contact with soiled linen.
c. Grasp clean pillowcase at center of closed end. Gather case, turning it inside out over the hand holding it. With the same hand, pick up middle of one end of the pillow. Pull pillowcase down over pillow with the other hand.	Eases sliding of pillowcase over pillow.
d. Be sure pillow corners fit evenly into corners of pillowcase. Place pillow under client's head.	Poorly fitting case constricts fluffing and expansion of pillow and interferes with client comfort.
38. Place call light within client's reach, and return bed to comfortable position and height.	Ensures client safety and comfort.
39. Open room curtains, and rearrange furniture. Place personal items within easy reach on over-bed table or bedside stand.	Promotes sense of well-being.
40. Discard dirty linen in hamper or chute, and perform hand hygiene.	Prevents transmission of microorganisms.
41. Ask if client feels comfortable.	Ensures bed linens are clean and smooth.
42. Inspect skin for areas of irritation.	Folds in linen cause pressure on skin.
43. Observe client for signs of fatigue, dyspnea, pain, or discomfort.	Provides you with data about client's level of activity tolerance and ability to participate in other procedures.

Unexpected Outcomes and Related Interventions
1. Client feels discomfort from linen fold.
   a. Tighten sheets.
   b. Change client's position frequently.
2. Client's skin shows signs of breakdown.
   a. Institute skin care measures to reduce risk of pressure ulcer (see Chapter 48).
   b. Change client's position frequently.

Recording and Reporting
- Making an occupied bed need not be recorded.

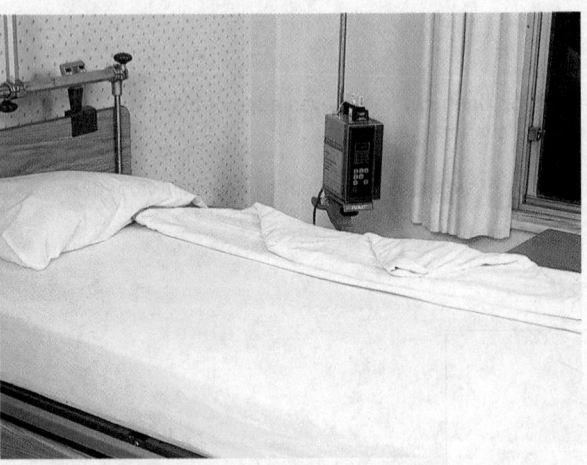

Figure 39-16 Surgical or recovery bed.

increases an agency's costs. Excess linen lying around a client's room creates clutter and obstacles for client care activities.

Before bed making, it is important to collect necessary bed linens and the client's personal items. In this way all equipment is accessible to prepare the bed and room. Linens are pressed and folded to prevent the spread of microorganisms and to make bed making easier. When fitted sheets are not available, flat sheets usually are pressed with a center crease to be placed down the center of the bed. The linens unfold easily to the sides, with creases often fitting over the mattress edge. A complete linen change is not always necessary. You can reuse the mattress pad, sheet, blanket, and bedspread for the same client if they are not wet or soiled.

Dispose of linen properly to minimize the spread of infection (see Chapter 34). Agency policies provide guidelines for the proper way to bag and dispose of soiled linen. After a client is discharged, all bed linen goes to the laundry, and housekeeping cleans the mattress and bed and applies new bed linen.

◆Evaluation

Evaluation of hygiene measures occurs both during and after each particular skill. For example, when bathing a client, inspect the skin to reveal if drainage or other soiling is effectively removed from the skin's surface. Once the bath is completed, ask if the client's comfort and relaxation have improved. When evaluating for the effectiveness of hygiene measures, observe for changes in the client's behavior. Does the client assume a more relaxed position? Is the client free of body odor? Is the client able

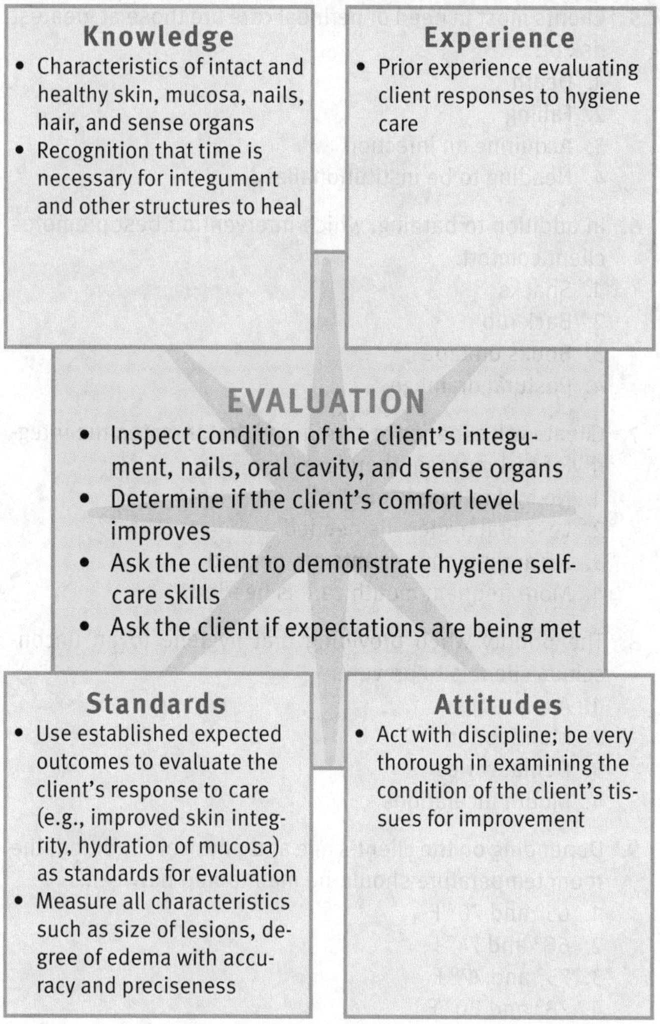

Figure 39-17 Critical thinking model for hygiene evaluation.

Knowledge
- Characteristics of intact and healthy skin, mucosa, nails, hair, and sense organs
- Recognition that time is necessary for integument and other structures to heal

Experience
- Prior experience evaluating client responses to hygiene care

EVALUATION
- Inspect condition of the client's integument, nails, oral cavity, and sense organs
- Determine if the client's comfort level improves
- Ask the client to demonstrate hygiene self-care skills
- Ask the client if expectations are being met

Standards
- Use established expected outcomes to evaluate the client's response to care (e.g., improved skin integrity, hydration of mucosa) as standards for evaluation
- Measure all characteristics such as size of lesions, degree of edema with accuracy and preciseness

Attitudes
- Act with discipline; be very thorough in examining the condition of the client's tissues for improvement

to fall asleep? Does the client's facial expression convey a sense of comfort?

Frequently it takes time for hygienic care to result in an improvement in the client's condition. The presence of oral lesions, a scalp infestation, or skin excoriation will often require repeated measures and a combination of nursing interventions. Determine if the client's condition or level of comfort improves over time and if existing therapies are effective.

Throughout evaluation consider the goals of care, and evaluate whether expected outcomes are achieved. A critical thinking approach considers all factors when evaluating the client's care (Figure 39-17). The nurse's knowledge base and experience provide important perspectives when analyzing assessment data about a client. For example, continual observation of the oral mucosa helps to determine the effectiveness of oral hygiene practices. Are previously inflamed mucosa improving? The standards for evaluation are the expected outcomes established in the planning stage of the client's care. If outcomes are not met, you will need to revise the care plan. Continue to apply critical thinking attitudes when considering all evaluation findings.

The final aspect of evaluation determines whether or not the client's expectations for hygiene were met. Ask the following ques-

tions: Do you feel your bath and back rub helped to make you comfortable? Are there ways we can do a better job with your foot care? What further measures do you think are necessary to keep your mouth clean and refreshed?

The client's expectations are important guidelines in determining client satisfaction. You need to feel comfortable in addressing the client's concerns and expectations. A caring approach will help in facilitating discussion of these issues.

✳ Key Concepts

- Assess a client's physical and cognitive ability to perform basic hygiene measures, including muscle strength, flexibility and dexterity, balance, coordination, activity tolerance, and ability to attend.
- Determine a client's ability to perform self-care, and provide hygienic care according to the client's needs and preferences.
- During hygiene, integrate other activities such as physical assessment, wound care, and range-of-motion exercises.
- While providing daily hygiene needs, use teaching and communication skills in developing a caring relationship with the client.
- Various personal, sociocultural, economic, and developmental factors influence clients' hygiene practices.
- Clients' health beliefs predict the likelihood of assuming health promotion behavior, such as the maintenance of good hygiene.
- Clients with reduced sensation, vascular insufficiency, and immobility are at greater risk for impaired skin integrity.
- For clients suffering symptoms such as pain or nausea, administering symptom relief therapies before hygiene will better prepare the client for any procedure.
- When administering oral care to unconscious clients, take measures to prevent aspiration.
- The client's room needs to be comfortable, safe, and large enough to allow the client and visitors to move about freely.
- Evaluation of hygiene care is based on the client's sense of comfort, relaxation, well-being, and understanding of hygiene techniques.

✳ Critical Thinking Exercises

Mrs. Wyatt is a 77-year-old woman being seen in the internal medicine clinic during her follow-up appointment for management of her diabetes mellitus. During the nurse's conversation with Mrs. Wyatt, the client says, "You know, the sore on my right foot is still there."

1. What type of assessment should the nurse conduct for Mrs. Wyatt?

2. What recommendations are needed for Mrs. Wyatt's foot care regimen?

Mrs. Wyatt has returned for a follow-up visit. She states, "My little toe now has an open sore, which resulted when I removed the corn pad."

3. What would you do next for Mrs. Wyatt's care?

4. Mrs. Wyatt's open area on her right toe has healed. She still seems unsure of what is required for preventative foot care. What should you teach her about preventive foot care?

✳ NCLEX®-Style Review Questions

1. Hygienic care requires close contact with the client. The nurse initially uses which of the following to promote a caring therapeutic relationship? (Choose all that apply.)
   1. Assessment skills
   2. Therapeutic touch
   3. Fundamental skills
   4. Communication skills

2. A client's personal preferences for hygiene are influenced by a number of factors. (Choose all that apply.)
   1. The nurse is in charge of the care
   2. Hygiene care is a routine procedure
   3. Hygiene has no influence on client outcomes
   4. No two individuals perform hygiene in the same manner

3. A person's body image of his or her physical appearance is affected by which concepts? (Choose all that apply.)
   1. Social
   2. Objective
   3. Subjective
   4. Developmental

4. The *Healthy People 2010* initiative included recommendations to improve:
   1. Dental health
   2. Skin care in older adults
   3. Medication management in older adults
   4. American diet by adding more carbohydrates

5. Clients most in need of perineal care are those at greatest risk of:
   1. Death
   2. Falling
   3. Acquiring an infection
   4. Needing to be institutionalized

6. In addition to bathing, which intervention best promotes client comfort:
   1. Snacks
   2. Back rub
   3. Books on tape
   4. Postural drainage

7. Clients will experience conditions that threaten the integrity of oral mucosa; therefore:
   1. No mouth care is needed
   2. Less oral hygiene is needed
   3. No antiinfective agents are needed
   4. More frequent mouth care is needed

8. The priority when providing oral hygiene to an unconscious client is to prevent:
   1. Aspiration
   2. Mouth odor
   3. Dental caries
   4. Mouth ulcerations

9. Depending on the client's age and physical condition, the room temperature should be maintained between:
   1. 65° and 70° F
   2. 68° and 74° F
   3. 75° and 77° F
   4. 78° and 80° F

10. The method for trimming nails is to:
    1. Call a foot specialist
    2. Cut the nail in a curve
    3. File the nail straight across
    4. Cut the nails to the cuticles

40 | Oxygenation

OBJECTIVES

Mastery of content in this chapter will enable the student to:

- Describe the structure and function of the cardiopulmonary system.
- Differentiate between the physiological processes of cardiac output, myocardial blood flow, and coronary artery circulation.
- Describe the relationship of cardiac output, preload, afterload, contractility, and heart rate.
- List the physiological processes of ventilation, perfusion, and exchange of respiratory gases.
- State the neural and chemical regulation of respiration.
- Discuss the effect of a client's level of health, age, lifestyle, and environment on oxygenation.

- Identify the clinical outcomes occurring as a result of disturbances in conduction, altered cardiac output, impaired valvular function, myocardial ischemia, and impaired tissue perfusion.
- Identify the clinical outcomes occurring as a result of hyperventilation, hypoventilation, and hypoxemia.
- Describe nursing care interventions to promote oxygenation in the primary care, acute care, and restorative and continuing care settings.

 MEDIA RESOURCES   KEY TERMS

 Companion CD
- NCLEX®-Style Review Questions
- Audio Glossary
- Interactive Learning Activities
- English/Spanish Glossary

evolve Website
- NCLEX®-Style Review Questions
- Audio Glossary
- English/Spanish Glossary
- Interactive Learning Activities
- Weblinks
- Audio Summaries
- Video Clips

Afterload, p. 909
Angina pectoris, p. 916
Atelectasis, p. 916
Bronchoscopy, p. 920
Cardiac index (CI), p. 908
Cardiac output, p. 908
Cardiopulmonary rehabilitation, p. 960
Cardiopulmonary resuscitation (CPR), p. 960
Chest physiotherapy (CPT), p. 930
Chest tube, p. 950
Cyanosis, p. 917
Diaphragmatic breathing, p. 963
Diffusion, p. 911
Dyspnea, p. 920

Dysrhythmias, p. 913
Electrocardiogram (ECG), p. 909
Expiration, p. 911
Hematemesis, p. 920
Hemoptysis, p. 920
Hemothorax, p. 951
Humidification, p. 930
Hyperventilation, p. 916
Hypoventilation, p. 916
Hypovolemia, p. 912
Hypoxia, p. 916
Incentive spirometry, p. 942
Inspiration, p. 911
Myocardial infarction (MI), p. 916
Myocardial ischemia, p. 916
Nasal cannula, p. 957

Nebulization, p. 930
Normal sinus rhythm (NSR), p. 909
Orthopnea, p. 920
Peak expiratory flow rate (PEFR), p. 925
Pneumothorax, p. 951
Postural drainage, p. 930
Preload, p. 909
Pursed-lip breathing, p. 963
Stroke volume, p. 909
Thoracentesis, p. 925
Ventilation, p. 910
Ventricular fibrillation, p. 913
Ventricular tachycardia, p. 913
Wheezing, p. 920

Scientific Knowledge Base

Oxygen is necessary to sustain life. The cardiac and respiratory systems supply the body's oxygen demands. Blood is oxygenated through the mechanisms of ventilation, perfusion, and transport of respiratory gases. Neural and chemical regulators control the rate and depth of respiration in response to changing tissue oxygen demands.

Cardiovascular Physiology

Cardiopulmonary physiology involves delivery of deoxygenated blood (blood high in carbon dioxide and low in oxygen) to the right side of the heart and to the pulmonary circulation and oxygenated blood (blood high in oxygen and low in carbon dioxide) from the lungs to the left side of the heart and the tissues. The cardiac system delivers oxygen, nutrients, and other substances to the tissues and removes the waste products of cellular metabolism through the vascular and other body systems (e.g., respiratory, digestive, and renal) (McCance and Huether, 2005).

Structure and Function. The right ventricle pumps blood through the pulmonary circulation. The left ventricle pumps blood through the systemic circulation (Figure 40-1). The circulatory system exchanges respiratory gases, nutrients, and waste products between the blood and the tissues.

Myocardial Pump. The pumping action of the heart is essential to oxygen delivery. The four cardiac chambers, two atria and two ventricles, fill with blood during diastole and empty during systole. Coronary artery disease (CAD) and cardiomyopathy (enlarged heart) result in decreased pumping action and a decrease in the volume of blood ejected from the ventricles (stroke volume). Hemorrhage and dehydration cause a decrease in circulating blood volume and a decrease in stroke volume.

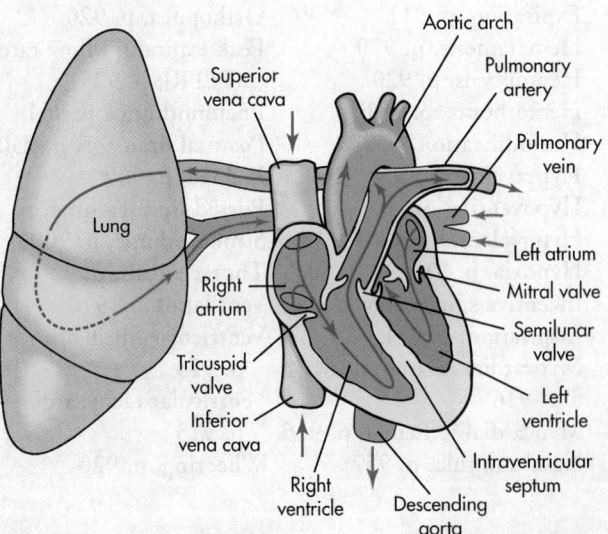

Figure 40-1 Schematic representation of blood flow through the heart. Arrows indicate direction of flow. (From Lewis SM and others: *Medical-surgical nursing: assessment and management of clinical problems,* ed 5, St. Louis, 2000, Mosby.)

Myocardial fibers have contractile properties allowing them to stretch during filling. In a healthy heart this stretch is proportionally related to the strength of contraction. As the myocardium stretches, the strength of the subsequent contraction increases; this is known as the Frank-Starling (Starling's) law of the heart. In the diseased heart, Starling's law does not apply because the stretch of the myocardium is beyond the heart's physiological limits. The subsequent contractile response results in insufficient stroke volume, and blood begins to "back up" in the pulmonary (left heart failure) or systemic circulation (right heart failure).

Myocardial Blood Flow. To maintain adequate blood flow to the pulmonary and systemic circulation, myocardial blood flow must supply sufficient oxygen and nutrients to the myocardium itself. Blood flow through the heart is unidirectional. The four heart valves ensure this forward blood flow (see Figure 40-1). During ventricular diastole the atrioventricular (mitral and tricuspid) valves open, and blood flows from the higher-pressure atria into the relaxed ventricles. This represents S_1, or the first heart sound. After ventricular filling, the systolic phase begins.

During the systolic phase semilunar (aortic and pulmonic) valves open, and blood flows from the ventricles into the aorta and pulmonary artery. Closure of aortic and pulmonic valves represents S_2, or the second heart sound. Some clients with valvular disease have backflow or regurgitation of blood through the incompetent valve, causing a murmur that you can hear on auscultation (see Chapter 33).

Coronary Artery Circulation. The coronary circulation is the branch of the systemic circulation that supplies the myocardium with oxygen and nutrients and removes waste. The coronary arteries fill during ventricular diastole (McCance and Huether, 2005). The right and left coronary arteries arise from the aorta just above and behind the aortic valve through openings called the coronary ostia (coronary openings). The left coronary artery, the most abundant blood supply, feeds the left ventricular myocardium, which is more muscular and does most of the heart's work.

Systemic Circulation. The arteries and veins of the systemic circulation deliver nutrients and oxygen to and remove waste from the tissues. Oxygenated blood flows from the left ventricle through the aorta and into large systemic arteries. These arteries branch into smaller arteries, into arterioles, and finally into the smallest vessels, the capillaries. At the capillary level the exchange of respiratory gases, nutrients, and wastes occurs, and the tissues are oxygenated. The waste products exit the capillary network through the venules that join to form veins. These veins form larger veins, which carry deoxygenated blood to the right side of the heart, where it then returns to the pulmonary circulation.

Blood Flow Regulation. The amount of blood ejected from the left ventricle each minute is the **cardiac output.** The normal cardiac output is 4 to 6 L/min in the healthy 150-pound (68-kg) adult at rest. The circulating volume of blood changes according to the oxygen and metabolic needs of the body. For example, during exercise, pregnancy, and fever, cardiac output increases, but during sleep it decreases. The following formula represents cardiac output:

$$\text{Cardiac output (CO)} = \text{Stroke volume (SV)} \times \text{Heart rate (HR)}$$

Cardiac index (CI) is a more precise measure and takes into consideration tissue perfusion and the client's body surface area

(BSA). Determine the CI by dividing the cardiac output by the BSA. The normal range is 2.5 to 4.0 L/min/m².

Stroke volume is the amount of blood ejected from the left ventricle with each contraction. The amount of blood in the left ventricle at the end of diastole (preload), the resistance to left ventricular ejection (afterload), and myocardial contractility all affect stroke volume.

Preload is the end-diastolic volume. The ventricles stretch when filling with blood. The more stretch on the ventricular muscle, the greater the contraction and the greater the stroke volume (Starling's law). In clinical situations the preload and subsequent stroke volume are manipulated by changing the amount of circulating blood volume. For example, when hemorrhage is present, fluid therapy and replacement of blood increases circulating volume and increases the preload and subsequent stroke volume and cardiac output. If volume is not replaced, preload and the subsequent cardiac output decreases.

Afterload is the resistance to left ventricular ejection. The heart must work to overcome this resistance to fully eject blood from the left ventricle. The diastolic aortic pressure is a good clinical measure of afterload. In hypertension, afterload increases, which makes cardiac workload increase. In hypertension, afterload is manipulated by reducing systemic blood pressure.

Myocardial contractility also affects stroke volume and cardiac output. Poor contraction decreases the amount of blood ejected by the ventricles. Some drugs increase the force of myocardial contraction, such as digitalis preparations, epinephrine, and sympathomimetic drugs (drugs that mimic the effects of the sympathetic nervous system). Injury to the myocardial muscle, such as an acute myocardial infarction, causes a decrease in myocardial contractility. The myocardium of the older adult is more rigid and slower, and contractility does not recover as quickly (Meiner and Leuckenotte, 2006).

Heart rate affects blood flow because of the relationship between rate and diastolic filling time. With a sustained heart rate greater than 160 beats per minute, diastolic filling time decreases, decreasing stroke volume and cardiac output. The heart rate of the older adult is slow to increase under stress (Meiner and Leuckenotte, 2006).

Conduction System. The rhythmic relaxation and contraction of the atria and ventricles depend on continuous, organized transmission of electrical impulses. The cardiac conduction system generates and transmits these impulses (Figure 40-2).

The heart's conduction system generates the impulses needed to initiate the electrical chain of events for a normal heartbeat. The autonomic nervous system influences the rate of impulse generation, as well as the speed of transmission through the conductive pathway and the strength of atrial and ventricular contractions. Sympathetic nerve fibers, which increase the rate of impulse generation and the speed of impulse transmission, innervate all parts of the atria and ventricles. The parasympathetic fibers originating from the vagus nerve decrease the rate and also innervate all parts of the atria and ventricles, as well as the sinoatrial (SA) and atrioventricular (AV) nodes (McCance and Huether, 2005).

The conduction system originates with the SA node, the "pacemaker" of the heart. The SA node is in the right atrium next to the entrance of the superior vena cava. Impulses are initiated at the SA node at an intrinsic rate between 60 and 100 beats per minute.

The electrical impulses are transmitted through the atria along intraatrial pathways to the AV node. The AV node mediates impulses between the atria and the ventricles. The intrinsic rate of the normal AV node is between 40 and 60 beats per minute. The AV node assists atrial emptying by delaying the impulse before transmitting it through the bundle of His and the ventricular Purkinje network. The intrinsic rate of the bundle of His and the ventricular Purkinje network is between 20 and 40 beats per minute.

An **electrocardiogram (ECG)** reflects the electrical activity of the conduction system. An ECG monitors the regularity and path of the electrical impulse through the conduction system; however, it does not reflect muscular work of the heart. The normal sequence on the ECG is called **normal sinus rhythm (NSR)** (Figure 40-3).

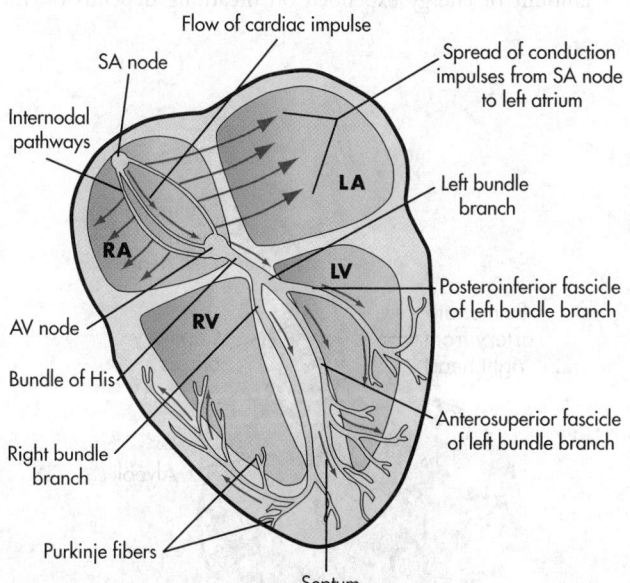

Figure 40-2 Conduction system of the heart. *LA,* Left atrium; *LV,* left ventricle; *RA,* right atrium; *RV,* right ventricle; *SA,* sinoatrial; *AV,* atrioventricular. (From Lewis SM and others: *Medical-surgical nursing: assessment and management of clinical problems,* ed 5, St. Louis, 2000, Mosby.)

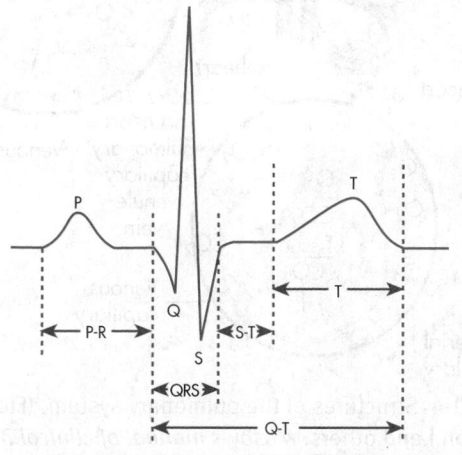

Figure 40-3 Normal ECG waveform.

NSR implies that the impulse originates at the SA node and follows the normal sequence through the conduction system. The P wave represents the electrical conduction through both atria. Atrial contraction follows the P wave. The PR interval represents the impulse travel time through the AV node, through the bundle of His, and to the Purkinje fibers. The normal length for the PR interval is 0.12 to 0.20 second. An increase in the time, greater than 0.20 second, indicates a block in the impulse transmission though the AV node, whereas a decrease, less than 0.12 second, indicates the initiation of the electrical impulse from a source other than the SA node.

The QRS complex indicates that the electrical impulse traveled through the ventricles. Normal QRS duration is 0.06 to 0.12 second. An increase in QRS duration indicates a delay in conduction time through the ventricles. Ventricular contraction usually follows the QRS complex.

The QT interval represents the time needed for ventricular depolarization and repolarization. The normal QT interval is 0.12 to 0.42 second. Changes in electrolyte values, such as hypocalcemia, or therapy with drugs such as disopyramide or amiodarone increase the QT interval. Shortening of the QT interval occurs with digitalis therapy, hyperkalemia, and hypercalcemia.

Respiratory Physiology

The exchange of respiratory gases occurs between the environment and the blood (Figure 40-4). The lung transfers oxygen from the atmosphere to the alveoli, where the oxygen is exchanged for carbon dioxide. The alveoli transfer oxygen and carbon dioxide to and from the blood through the alveolar capillary membrane. There are three steps in the process of oxygenation: ventilation, perfusion, and diffusion.

Structure and Function. Conditions or diseases that change the structure and function of the lung alter respiration. The respiratory muscles, pleural space, lungs, and alveoli (Figure 40-5) are essential for ventilation, perfusion, and exchange of respiratory gases. Gases move into and out of the lungs through pressure changes. Intrapleural pressure is negative, or less than atmospheric pressure, which is 760 mm Hg at sea level. For air to flow into the lungs, intrapleural pressure becomes more negative, setting up a pressure gradient between the atmosphere and the alveoli. The diaphragm and external intercostal muscles contract to create a negative pleural pressure and increase the size of the thorax for inspiration. Relaxation of the diaphragm and contraction of the internal intercostal muscles allow air to escape from the lungs.

Ventilation is the process of moving gases into and out of the lungs. Ventilation requires coordination of the muscular and elastic properties of the lung and thorax, as well as intact innervation. The major inspiratory muscle of respiration is the diaphragm. It is innervated by the phrenic nerve, which exits the spinal cord at the fourth cervical vertebra. Perfusion relates to the ability of the cardiovascular system to pump oxygenated blood to the tissues and return deoxygenated blood to the lungs. Last, diffusion is responsible for moving the respiratory gases from one area to another. For the exchange of respiratory gases to occur, the organs, nerves, and muscles of respiration need to be intact and the central nervous system needs to be able to regulate the respiratory cycle.

Work of Breathing. Work of breathing (WOB) is the effort required to expand and contract the lungs. In the healthy individual, breathing is quiet and accomplished with minimal effort. The amount of energy expended on breathing depends on the

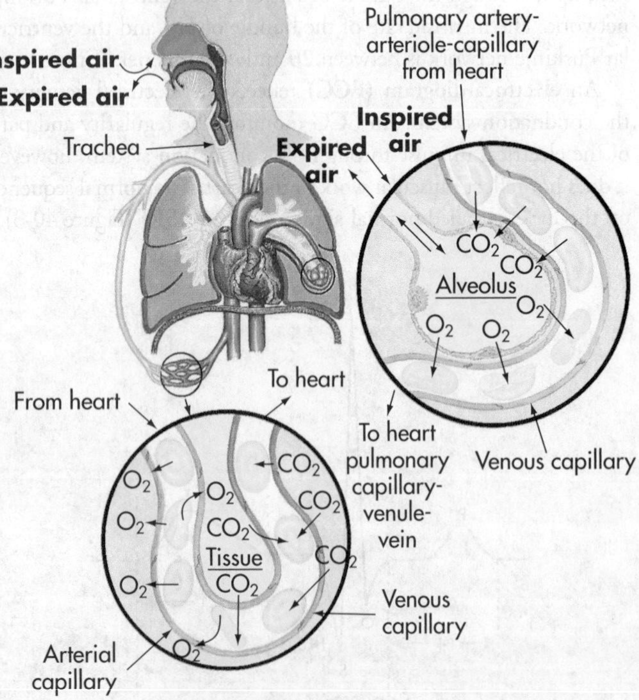

Figure 40-4 Structures of the pulmonary system. (From Thompson J and others: *Mosby's manual of clinical nursing,* ed 3, St. Louis, 1993, Mosby.)

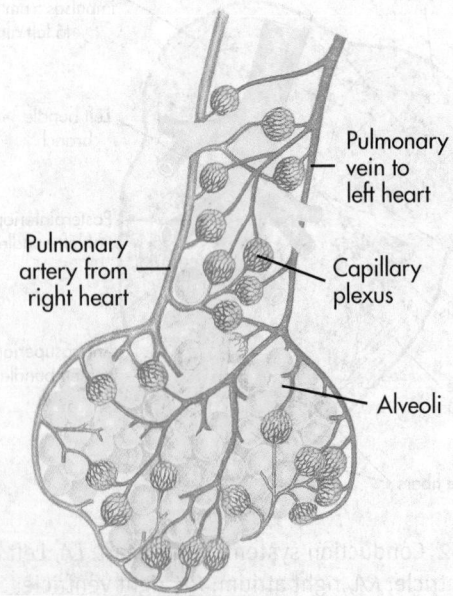

Figure 40-5 Alveoli at the terminal end of the lower airway. (From Thompson J and others: *Mosby's manual of clinical nursing,* ed 3, St. Louis, 1993, Mosby.)

rate and depth of breathing, the ease in which the lungs can be expanded (compliance), and airway resistance.

Inspiration is an active process, stimulated by chemical receptors in the aorta. **Expiration** is a passive process that depends on the elastic recoil properties of the lungs, requiring little or no muscle work. Surfactant is a chemical produced in the lungs to maintain the surface tension of the alveoli and keep them from collapsing. Clients with advanced chronic obstructive pulmonary disease (COPD) lose the elastic recoil of the lungs and thorax. As a result, the client's work of breathing increases. In addition, clients with certain pulmonary diseases have decreased surfactant production and sometimes develop atelectasis.

Accessory muscles of respiration can increase lung volume during inspiration. Clients with COPD, especially emphysema, frequently use these muscles to increase lung volume. Prolonged use of the accessory muscles does not promote effective ventilation and causes fatigue. During an assessment observe for elevation of the client's clavicles during inspiration. Elevation of the clavicles during inspiration can indicate ventilatory fatigue, air hunger, or decreased lung expansion.

Compliance is the ability of the lungs to distend or to expand in response to increased intraalveolar pressure. Compliance decreases in diseases such as pulmonary edema, interstitial and pleural fibrosis, and congenital or traumatic structural abnormalities such as kyphosis or fractured ribs.

Airway resistance is the pressure difference between the mouth and the alveoli in relation to the rate of flow of inspired gas. Airway obstruction, asthma, and tracheal edema increase airway resistance. When resistance increases, the amount of air traveling through the anatomical airways decreases.

Decreased lung compliance, increased airway resistance, and active expiration with the use of accessory muscles increase the work of breathing, resulting in increased energy expenditure. The body increases its metabolic rate, and the need for oxygen. The elimination of carbon dioxide also increases. This sequence is a vicious cycle for a client with impaired ventilation, causing further deterioration of respiratory status and the ability to oxygenate adequately.

Lung Volumes. Spirometry measures the volume of air entering or leaving the lungs. For example, the tidal volume is the amount of air exhaled in a normal breath and is assumed to equate with the amount of air inhaled with each breath. Variations in tidal volume and other lung volumes are associated with health status, such as pregnancy, exercise, obesity, or obstructive and restrictive conditions of the lungs.

Pulmonary Circulation. The primary function of the pulmonary circulation is to move blood to and from the alveolar capillary membrane for gas exchange. The pulmonary circulation is a reservoir for blood so that the lung is able to increase its blood volume without large increases in pulmonary artery or venous pressures. The pulmonary circulation also acts as a filter, removing small thrombi before they reach vital organs.

Pulmonary circulation begins at the pulmonary artery, which receives poorly oxygenated mixed venous blood from the right ventricle. Blood flow through this system depends on the pumping ability of the right ventricle. The flow continues from the pulmonary artery through the pulmonary arterioles to the pulmonary capillaries, where blood comes in contact with the alveolar capillary membrane and the exchange of respiratory gases occurs. The oxygen-rich blood then circulates through the pulmonary venules and pulmonary veins, returning to the left atrium.

Pressure and resistance within the pulmonary circulatory system is lower than that within the systemic circulatory system. The walls of the pulmonary vessels are thinner and contain less smooth muscle. The lung accepts the total cardiac output from the right ventricle and, except in cases of alveolar hypoxia or cor pulmonale, does not direct blood flow from one region to another.

Respiratory Gas Exchange. **Diffusion** is the process for the exchange of respiratory gases in the alveoli and the capillaries of the body tissues. Oxygen is transferred from the lungs to the blood, and carbon dioxide is transferred from the blood to the alveoli and exhaled. At the tissue level, oxygen is transferred from the blood to tissues, and carbon dioxide is transferred from tissues to the blood to return to the alveoli and be exhaled.

Diffusion of respiratory gases occurs at the alveolar capillary membrane. The thickness of the membrane affects the rate of diffusion. Increased thickness of the membrane impedes diffusion because gases take longer to transfer across the membrane. Clients with pulmonary edema, pulmonary infiltrates, or a pulmonary effusion have a thickened membrane, resulting in slow diffusion, slow exchange of respiratory gases, and decreased delivery of oxygen to tissues. Chronic diseases (e.g., emphysema), acute diseases (e.g., pneumothorax), and surgical processes (e.g., lobectomy) often alter the surface area of the alveolar capillary membrane.

Oxygen Transport. The oxygen transport system consists of the lungs and cardiovascular system. Delivery depends on the amount of oxygen entering the lungs (ventilation), blood flow to the lungs and tissues (perfusion), rate of diffusion, and oxygen-carrying capacity. Three things influence the capacity of the blood to carry oxygen: the amount of dissolved oxygen in the plasma, the amount of hemoglobin, and the tendency of hemoglobin to bind with oxygen. Hemoglobin, which is a carrier for oxygen and carbon dioxide, transports most oxygen (approximately 97%). The hemoglobin molecule combines with oxygen to form oxyhemoglobin. The formation of oxyhemoglobin is easily reversible, allowing hemoglobin and oxygen to dissociate, which frees oxygen to enter tissues.

Carbon Dioxide Transport. Carbon dioxide diffuses into red blood cells and is rapidly hydrated into carbonic acid (H_2CO_3). The carbonic acid then dissociates into hydrogen (H^+) and bicarbonate (HCO_3^-) ions. Hemoglobin buffers the hydrogen ion, and the HCO_3^- diffuses into the plasma (see Chapter 41). Some of the carbon dioxide in red blood cells reacts with amino acid groups, forming carbamino compounds. This reaction occurs rapidly. Reduced hemoglobin (deoxyhemoglobin) combines with carbon dioxide, and the venous blood transports the majority of carbon dioxide.

Regulation of Respiration. Regulation of respiration is necessary to ensure sufficient oxygen intake and carbon dioxide elimination to meet the body's demands (e.g., during exercise, infection, or pregnancy). Neural and chemical regulators control the process of respiration. Neural regulation includes the central nervous system control of respiratory rate, depth, and rhythm. Chemical regulation involves the influence of chemicals such as

✳ **BOX 40-1 Physiological Processes of Oxygenation**

Neural Regulation
Maintains rhythm and depth of respiration and balance between inspiration and expiration.

Cerebral Cortex
Voluntary control of respiration delivers impulses to the respiratory motor neurons by way of the spinal cord; accommodates speaking, eating, and swimming.

Medulla Oblongata
Automatic control of respiration occurs continuously.

Chemical Regulation
Maintains appropriate rate and depth of respirations based on changes in the blood's carbon dioxide (CO_2), oxygen (O_2), and hydrogen ion (H^+) concentration.

Chemoreceptors
Located in the medulla, aortic body, and carotid body. Changes in chemical content of O_2, CO_2, and H^+ stimulate chemoreceptors, which in turn stimulate neural regulators to adjust the rate and depth of ventilation to maintain normal arterial blood gas levels. Chemical regulation occurs during physical exercise and in some illnesses.

carbon dioxide and hydrogen ions on the rate and depth of respiration (Box 40-1).

Factors Affecting Oxygenation

Four factors influence adequacy of circulation, ventilation, perfusion, and transport of respiratory gases to the tissues: (1) physiological, (2) developmental, (3) lifestyle, and (4) environmental. Developmental, lifestyle, and environmental factors will be presented on pages 917 to 918.

Physiological Factors. Any condition affecting cardiopulmonary functioning directly affects the body's ability to meet oxygen demands. The general classifications of cardiac disorders include disturbances in conduction, impaired valvular function, myocardial hypoxia, cardiomyopathic conditions, and peripheral tissue hypoxia. Respiratory disorders include hyperventilation, hypoventilation, and hypoxia.

Other physiological processes affecting a client's oxygenation include alterations affecting the oxygen-carrying capacity of blood, such as the anemia; increases in the body's metabolic demands, such as pregnancy or fever and infection; and alterations affecting chest wall movement or the central nervous system.

Decreased Oxygen-Carrying Capacity. Hemoglobin carries the majority of oxygen to tissues. Anemia and inhalation of toxic substances decrease the oxygen-carrying capacity of blood by reducing the amount of available hemoglobin to transport oxygen. Anemia, a lower than normal hemoglobin level, is a result of decreased hemoglobin production, increased red blood cell destruction, and/or blood loss. Clients have fatigue, decreased activity tolerance, and increased breathlessness, as well as pallor (especially seen in the conjunctiva of the eye) and an increased heart rate.

Carbon monoxide (CO) is the most common toxic inhalant decreasing the oxygen-carrying capacity of blood. In CO toxicity, hemoglobin strongly binds with carbon monoxide, creating a functional anemia. Because of the bond's strength, carbon monoxide does not easily dissociate from hemoglobin, making hemoglobin unavailable for oxygen transport.

Decreased Inspired Oxygen Concentration. When the concentration of inspired oxygen declines, the oxygen-carrying capacity of the blood decreases. Decreases in the fraction of inspired oxygen concentration (FIO_2) are caused by an upper or lower airway obstruction limiting delivery of inspired oxygen to alveoli; decreased environmental oxygen, such as at high altitudes; or decreased inspiration, which occurs in drug overdoses.

Hypovolemia. Conditions such as shock and severe dehydration cause extracellular fluid loss and reduced circulating blood volume, or **hypovolemia**. With significant fluid loss, the body tries to adapt by increasing the heart rate and peripheral vasoconstriction to increase the volume of blood returned to the heart and, in turn, increase the cardiac output.

Increased Metabolic Rate. Increased metabolic activity increases oxygen demand. When body systems are unable to meet this demand, the level of oxygenation declines. An increased metabolic rate is normal in pregnancy, wound healing, and exercise because the body is building tissue. Most people meet the increased oxygen demand and do not display signs of oxygen deprivation. Fever increases the tissues' need for oxygen, and as a result, carbon dioxide production increases. When fever persists, the metabolic rate remains high and the body begins to break down protein stores, resulting in muscle wasting and decreased muscle mass. Respiratory muscles such as the diaphragm and intercostal muscles are also wasted.

The body attempts to adapt to the increased carbon dioxide levels by increasing the rate and depth of respiration. The client's work of breathing increases, and the client eventually displays signs and symptoms of hypoxemia. Clients with pulmonary diseases are at greater risk for hypoxemia.

Conditions Affecting Chest Wall Movement. Any condition reducing chest wall movement results in decreased ventilation. If the diaphragm does not fully descend with breathing, the volume of inspired air decreases, delivering less oxygen to the alveoli and tissues.

Pregnancy. As the fetus grows during pregnancy, the enlarging uterus pushes abdominal contents upward against the diaphragm. In the last trimester of pregnancy the inspiratory capacity declines, resulting in dyspnea on exertion and increased fatigue.

Obesity. Clients who are morbidly obese have reduced lung volumes from the heavy lower thorax and abdomen, particularly when in the recumbent and supine positions. Morbidly obese clients have a reduction in compliance as a result of encroachment of the abdomen into the chest, increased work of breathing, and decreased lung volumes. In some clients an obesity-hypoventilation syndrome develops in which oxygenation is decreased and carbon dioxide is retained. The obese client is also susceptible to pneumonia after surgery or an upper respiratory tract infection because the lungs do not fully expand and the lower lobes retain pulmonary secretions.

Musculoskeletal Abnormalities. Musculoskeletal impairments in the thoracic region reduce oxygenation. Such impairments result from abnormal structural configurations, trauma, muscular diseases, and diseases of the central nervous system. Abnormal structural configurations impairing oxygenation include those affecting the rib cage, such as pectus excavatum, and the vertebral column, such as kyphosis, lordosis, or scoliosis.

Trauma. Multiple rib fractures develop into a flail chest, a condition in which fractures cause instability in part of the chest wall. The unstable chest wall allows the lung underlying the injured area to contract on inspiration and bulge on expiration, resulting in hypoxia. Chest wall or upper abdominal incisions also decrease chest wall movement as the client uses shallow respirations to minimize chest wall movement to avoid pain. Excessive or high doses of opioids depress the respiratory center, further decreasing respiratory rate and chest wall expansion.

Neuromuscular Diseases. Neuromuscular diseases affect tissue oxygenation by decreasing the client's ability to expand and contract the chest wall. Ventilation is impaired, and atelectasis, hypercapnia, and hypoxemia occur. Myasthenia gravis, Guillain-Barré syndrome, and poliomyelitis result in hypoventilation.

Central Nervous System Alterations. Diseases or trauma involving the medulla oblongata and spinal cord result in impaired respiration. When the medulla oblongata is affected, neural regulation of respiration is damaged and abnormal breathing patterns develop. When the phrenic nerve is damaged, the diaphragm does not descend properly, thus reducing inspiratory lung volumes and causing hypoxemia. Cervical trauma at C3 to C5 usually results in paralysis of the phrenic nerve. Spinal cord trauma below the fifth cervical vertebra usually leaves the phrenic nerve intact but damages nerves that innervate the intercostal muscles, preventing anteroposterior chest expansion.

Influences of Chronic Disease. Oxygenation decreases as a direct consequence of chronic disease. It also decreases as a secondary effect, as with anemia. The physiological response to chronic hypoxemia is the development of increased red blood cells (polycythemia). This is the body's adaptive response to increase the amount of hemoglobin and increase the available oxygen-binding sites.

Alterations in Cardiac Functioning

Illnesses and conditions affecting cardiac rhythm, strength of contraction, blood flow through the chambers, myocardial blood flow, and peripheral circulation cause alterations in cardiac functioning. Older adults experience alterations in cardiac function as a result of calcification of the conduction pathways, thicker and stiffer heart valves due to lipid accumulation and fibrosis, and a decrease in the number of pacemaker cells in the SA node (Meiner and Leuckenotte, 2006).

Disturbances in Conduction. Electrical impulses that do not originate from the SA node cause conduction disturbances. These rhythm disturbances are called **dysrhythmias,** meaning a deviation from the normal sinus heart rhythm (Table 40-1). Dysrhythmias occur as a primary conduction disturbance, such as in response to ischemia, valvular abnormality, anxiety, or drug toxicity; as a result of caffeine, alcohol, or tobacco use; or as a complication of acid-base or electrolyte imbalance (see Chapter 41).

Dysrhythmias are classified by cardiac response and site of impulse origin. Cardiac response is tachycardia (greater than 100 beats per minute), bradycardia (less than 60 beats per minute), a

premature (early) beat, or a blocked (delayed or absent) beat. Tachydysrhythmias and bradydysrhythmias lower cardiac output and blood pressure. Tachydysrhythmias reduce cardiac output by decreasing diastolic filling time. Bradydysrhythmias lower cardiac output because of the decreased heart rate.

Atrial fibrillation is a common dysrhythmia, frequently seen in older adults. The electrical impulse in the atria is chaotic and originates from multiple sites. The rhythm is irregular due to the multiple pacemaker sites and the unpredictable conduction to the ventricles. The QRS complex is normal; however, it occurs at irregular intervals. Atrial fibrillation is often described as an irregularly irregular rhythm.

Abnormal impulses originating above the ventricles are supraventricular dysrhythmias. The abnormality on the waveform is the configuration and placement of the P wave. Ventricular conduction usually remains normal, and there is a normal QRS complex.

Paroxysmal supraventricular tachycardia is a sudden rapid onset of tachycardia originating above the AV node. It often begins and ends spontaneously. Sometimes excitement, fatigue, caffeine, smoking, or alcohol use precipitate paroxysmal supraventricular tachycardia. When needed, treatment includes vagal stimulation such as carotid sinus massage or Valsalva maneuver to decrease the ventricular response. Medications such as adenosine, diltiazem, digitalis, or beta-adrenergic blockers are prescribed.

Ventricular dysrhythmias represent an ectopic site of impulse formation within the ventricles. It is ectopic in that the impulse originates in the ventricle, not the SA node. The configuration of the QRS complex is usually widened and bizarre. P waves are not always present; often they are buried in the QRS complex. **Ventricular tachycardia** and **ventricular fibrillation** are life-threatening rhythms that require immediate intervention. Ventricular tachycardia is a life-threatening dysrhythmia because of the decreased cardiac output and the potential to deteriorate into ventricular fibrillation (AHA, 2003, 2005b).

Altered Cardiac Output. Failure of the myocardium to eject sufficient volume to the systemic and pulmonary circulations results in heart failure. Primary coronary artery disease, cardiomyopathy, valvular disorders, and pulmonary disease lead to myocardial pump failure.

Left-Sided Heart Failure. Left-sided heart failure is an abnormal condition characterized by decreased functioning of the left ventricle. If left ventricular failure is significant, the amount of blood ejected from the left ventricle drops greatly, resulting in decreased cardiac output. Assessment findings include fatigue, breathlessness, dizziness, and confusion as a result of tissue hypoxia from the diminished cardiac output. As the left ventricle continues to fail, blood begins to pool in the pulmonary circulation, causing pulmonary congestion. Clinical findings include crackles on auscultation, hypoxia, shortness of breath on exertion and often at rest, cough, and paroxysmal nocturnal dyspnea.

Right-Sided Heart Failure. Right-sided heart failure results from impaired functioning of the right ventricle. Right-sided heart failure more commonly results from pulmonary disease or as a result of long-term left-sided failure. The primary pathological factor in right-sided failure is elevated pulmonary vascular resistance (PVR). As the PVR continues to rise, the right ventricle

✳ **TABLE 40-1 Common Basic Cardiac Dysrhythmias**

RHYTHM CHARACTERISTICS AND ETIOLOGY	CLINICAL SIGNIFICANCE AND MANAGEMENT

Sinus Tachycardia

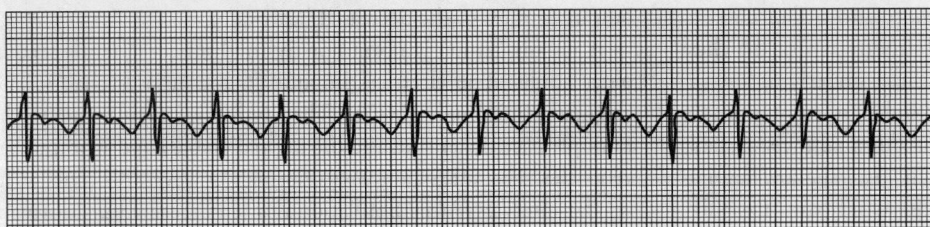

Regular rhythm, rate 100-180 beats/min (higher in infants), normal P wave, normal QRS complex

Rate increase is often normal response to exercise, emotion, or stressors such as pain, fever, pump failure, hyperthyroidism, and certain drugs (e.g., caffeine, nitrates, epinephrine, nicotine)

Some clients with heart disease are unable to increase their heart rate to meet increased oxygen demands.

Correct underlying factors; discontinue drugs producing the side effect

Sinus Bradycardia

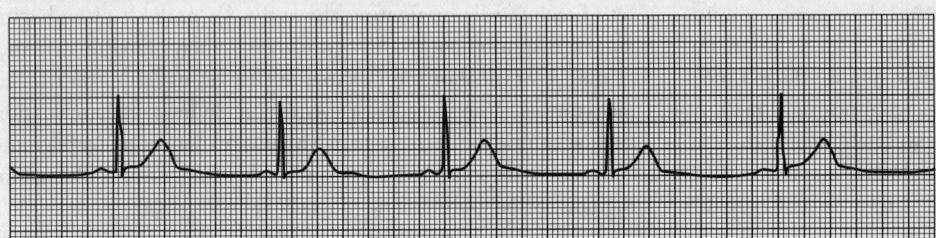

Regular rhythm, rate less than 60 beats/min, normal P wave, normal PR interval, normal QRS complex

Rate decrease is a normal response to sleep or in well-conditioned athlete; diminished blood flow to SA node, vagal stimulation, hypothyroidism, increased intracranial pressure, or pharmacological agents (e.g., digoxin, propranolol, quinidine, procainamide) sometimes cause abnormal drops in rate

No clinical significance unless associated with signs and symptoms of reduced cardiac output such as dizziness or syncope or presence of chest pain

Bradycardia with hypotension and decreased cardiac output is treated with atropine; a pacemaker is sometimes necessary

Atrial Fibrillation (A-fib)

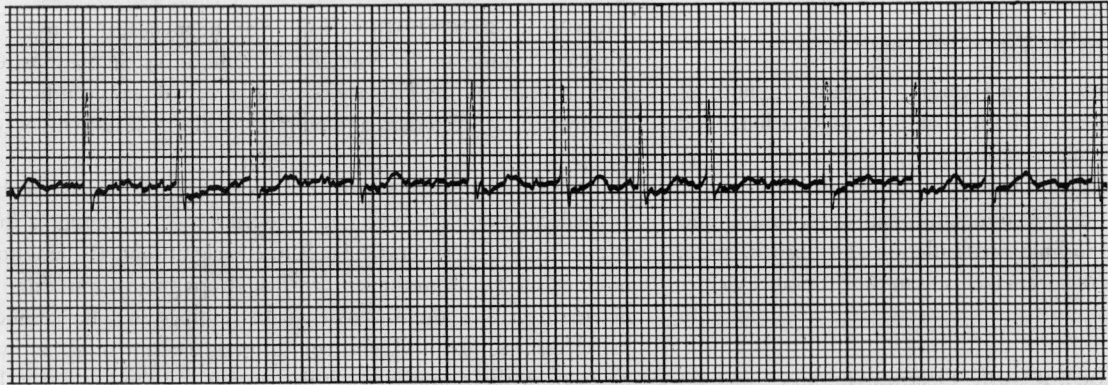

Chaotic, irregular atrial activity resulting in an irregular ventricular response. No identifiable P waves. Irregular ventricular response resulting in an irregular cardiac rate and rhythm. The conduction of the multiple atrial impulses across the AV node determines the rate.

Caused by aging, calcification of the SA node, or changes in myocardial blood supply

There is a loss of the atrial kick (portion of the cardiac output squeezed in the ventricles with a coordinated atrial contraction), pooling of blood in the atria, and development of microemboli. The client often complains of fatigue, a fluttering in the chest, or shortness of breath if the ventricular response is rapid. Commonly occurring dysrhythmia in the aging and older adult

Modified from Canobbio MM: *Cardiovascular disorders*, St. Louis, 1990, Mosby.

SA, Sinoatrial; *AV*, atrioventricular; *AED*, automated external defibrillator.

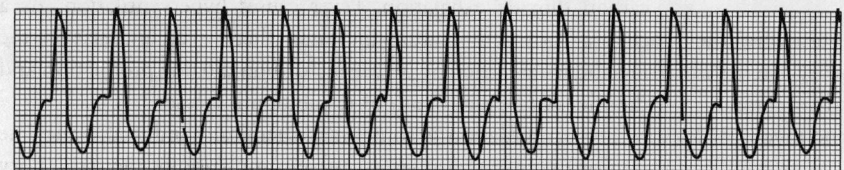

TABLE 40-1 Common Basic Cardiac Dysrhythmias—cont'd

RHYTHM CHARACTERISTICS AND ETIOLOGY	CLINICAL SIGNIFICANCE AND MANAGEMENT

Ventricular Tachycardia

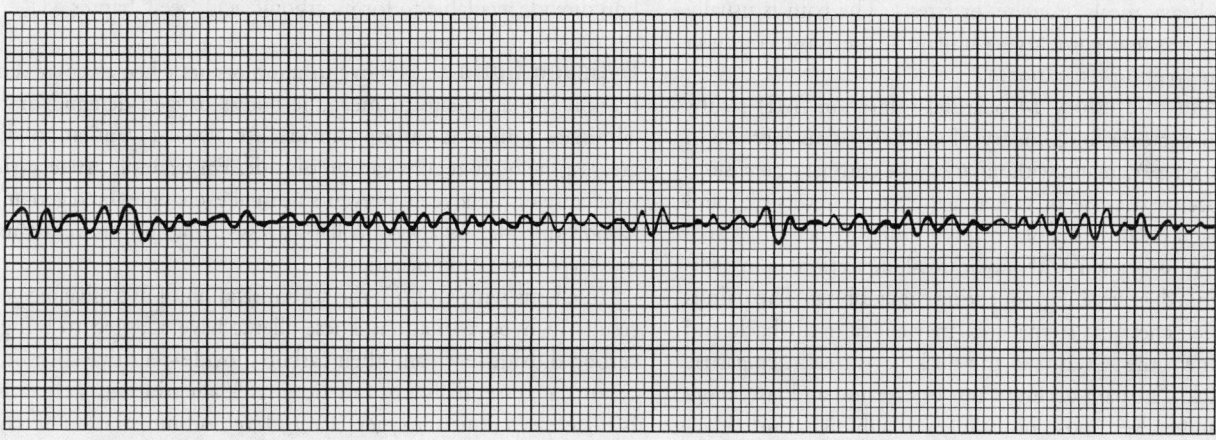

Rhythm slightly irregular, rate 100-200 beats/min, P wave absent, PR interval absent, QRS complex wide and bizarre, >0.12 second

Caused by changes in the normal pacemaker of the heart such as decrease in blood flow, ischemia, or embolus

Results in decreased cardiac output due to decreased ventricular filling time; often leads to severe hypotension and loss of pulse and consciousness

If refractory to defibrillation, amiodarone 300 mg IV followed by an additional 150 mg IV in 3-5 minutes (American Heart Association [AHA], 2005a)

Ventricular Fibrillation

Uncoordinated electrical activity. No identifiable P, QRS, or T wave

Causes include sudden cardiac death, electrical shock, acute myocardial infarction, drowning, or trauma

Acute loss of pulse and respiration. Immediate defibrillation after assessment of ABCs of CPR. Availability of AED is recommended in public and/or private places where large numbers of people gather or where people who are at high risk for heart attack live (AHA, 2003, 2005a, 2006a) (Box 40-2)

BOX 40-2 Automated External Defibrillator

- A device used to administer an electrical shock through the chest wall to the heart.
- Built-in computers assess the client's heart rhythm and determine if defibrillation is necessary.
- The automated external defibrillator (AED) delivers a shock to the client after announcing "Everyone stand back."
- Nonmedical personnel can use the AED.
- Used to strengthen the chain of survival. Every minute of a sudden cardiac arrest without defibrillation decreases the survival rate by 7% to 10% (AHA, 2003, 2005a).

generates more work, and the oxygen demand of the heart increases. As the failure continues, the amount of blood ejected from the right ventricle declines, and blood begins to "back up" in the systemic circulation. Clinically the client has weight gain, distended neck veins, hepatomegaly and splenomegaly, and dependent peripheral edema.

Impaired Valvular Function. Valvular heart disease is an acquired or congenital disorder of a cardiac valve characterized by stenosis or regurgitation of blood. When stenosis occurs, the flow of blood through the valves is obstructed. For example, when stenosis occurs in the semilunar valves (aortic and pulmonic valves), the adjacent ventricles have to work harder to move the ventricular blood volume beyond the stenotic valve. Over time the stenosis causes the ventricle to hypertrophy (enlarge), and if the condition is untreated, left- or right-sided heart failure occurs. When regurgitation occurs, there is a backflow of blood into an adjacent chamber. For example, in mitral regurgitation the mitral leaflets do not close completely. When the ventricles contract, blood escapes back into the atria, causing a murmur, or "whooshing" sound (see Chapter 33).

Myocardial Ischemia.
Myocardial ischemia results when the supply of blood to the myocardium from the coronary arteries is insufficient to meet myocardial oxygen demands. Two common manifestations of this ischemia are angina pectoris and myocardial infarction.

Angina. **Angina pectoris** is a transient imbalance between myocardial oxygen supply and demand. The condition results in chest pain that is aching, sharp, tingling, or burning, or that feels like pressure. Typically chest pain is left sided or substernal and often radiates to the left or both arms, and to the jaw, neck, and back. In some clients anginal pain does not radiate. The pain usually lasts from 1 to 15 minutes. Clients report that pain is often precipitated by activities that increase myocardial oxygen demand (e.g., eating heavy meals, exercise, or stress). The pain is usually relieved with rest and coronary vasodilators, the most common being a nitroglycerin preparation.

Myocardial Infarction. **Myocardial infarction (MI)** results from sudden decreases in coronary blood flow or an increase in myocardial oxygen demand without adequate coronary perfusion. Infarction occurs because of ischemia (which is reversible) and necrosis (which is not reversible) of myocardial tissue.

Chest pain associated with myocardial infarction in men is usually described as crushing, squeezing, or stabbing. The pain is often in the left chest and sternal area, may be felt in the back, and it radiates down the left arm to the neck, jaws, teeth, epigastric area, and back. The pain occurs at rest or exertion and lasts more than 30 minutes. Rest, position change, or sublingual nitroglycerin administration do not relieve the pain.

There is a significant difference between men and women in relation to coronary artery disease. As women get older, their risk of heart disease begins to rise (AHA, 2006c). Women's symptoms differ from men's. The most common initial symptom in women is angina, but atypical symptoms of fatigue, "indigestion," vasospasm, shortness of breath, or back or jaw pain are also present (Denke, 2001; Shaw and others, 2006). Almost twice as many women die within the first year after the first heart attack (AHA, 2006b).

Alterations in Respiratory Functioning

Illnesses and conditions affecting ventilation or oxygen transport cause alterations in respiratory functioning. The three primary alterations are hyperventilation, hypoventilation, and hypoxia.

The goal of ventilation is to produce a normal arterial carbon dioxide tension ($PaCO_2$) between 35 and 45 mm Hg and maintain a normal arterial oxygen tension (PaO_2) between 95 and 100 mm Hg. Hyperventilation and hypoventilation refer to alveolar ventilation and not to the client's respiratory rate. Arterial oxygen saturations are monitored using a noninvasive oxygen saturation monitor. The normal range is 95% to 100%. Hypoxia refers to a decrease in the amount of arterial oxygen.

Hyperventilation.
Hyperventilation is a state of ventilation in excess of that required to eliminate the carbon dioxide produced by cellular metabolism. Anxiety, infections, drugs, or an acid-base imbalance induce hyperventilation, as well as hypoxia associated with pulmonary embolus or shock. Acute anxiety leads to hyperventilation and causes loss of consciousness from excess carbon dioxide exhalation. Fever causes hyperventilation. As a client's body temperature increases, there is an increase in the metabolic rate, thereby increasing carbon dioxide production and the client's rate and depth of respiration increases.

Hyperventilation is sometimes chemically induced. Salicylate (aspirin) poisoning causes excessive stimulation of the respiratory center as the body attempts to compensate for excess carbon dioxide. Amphetamines also increase ventilation by raising carbon dioxide production. Hyperventilation also occurs as the body tries to compensate for metabolic acidosis by producing a respiratory alkalosis. For example, the client with diabetes who has gone into diabetic ketoacidosis produces large amounts of metabolic acids. The respiratory system tries to correct the acid-base balance by overbreathing. Ventilation increases to reduce the amount of carbon dioxide available to form carbonic acid (see Chapter 41).

Hypoventilation.
Hypoventilation occurs when alveolar ventilation is inadequate to meet the body's oxygen demand or to eliminate sufficient carbon dioxide. As alveolar ventilation decreases, the body retains carbon dioxide. For example, **atelectasis**, a collapse of the alveoli, prevents normal exchange of oxygen and carbon dioxide. As alveoli collapse, less of the lung is ventilated and hypoventilation occurs.

In clients with COPD, the administration of excessive oxygen results in hypoventilation. These clients have adapted to a high carbon dioxide level, and their carbon dioxide–sensitive chemoreceptors are essentially not functioning. Their stimulus to breathe is a decreased arterial oxygen (PaO_2) level. Administration of oxygen greater than 24% to 28% (1 to 3 L/min) prevents the PaO_2 from falling and obliterates the stimulus to breathe, resulting in hypoventilation. Excessive retention of carbon dioxide leads to respiratory arrest.

Signs and symptoms of hypoventilation include mental status changes, dysrhythmias, and potential cardiac arrest. Treatment requires improving tissue oxygenation, restoring ventilatory function, treating the underlying cause of the hypoventilation, and achieving acid-base balance. If untreated, the client's status will rapidly decline, leading to convulsions, unconsciousness, and death.

Hypoxia.
Hypoxia is inadequate tissue oxygenation at the cellular level. This results from a deficiency in oxygen delivery or oxygen utilization at the cellular level. Hypoxia is a life-threatening condition. Untreated, it produces cardiac dysrhythmias that will possibly result in death.

Causes of hypoxia include (1) a decreased hemoglobin level and lowered oxygen-carrying capacity of the blood; (2) a diminished concentration of inspired oxygen, which occurs at high altitudes; (3) the inability of the tissues to extract oxygen from the blood, as with cyanide poisoning; (4) decreased diffusion of oxygen from the alveoli to the blood, as in pneumonia; (5) poor tissue perfusion with oxygenated blood, as with shock; and (6) impaired ventilation, as with multiple rib fractures or chest trauma.

The clinical signs and symptoms of hypoxia include apprehension, restlessness, inability to concentrate, declining level of consciousness, dizziness, and behavioral changes. The client with hypoxia is unable to lie down and appears fatigued and agitated. Vital sign changes include an increased pulse rate and increased rate and depth of respiration. However, when caring for a client with a narcotic overdose, such as a heroin overdose, hypoventilation may occur. During early stages of hypoxia the blood pressure is elevated unless the condition is caused by shock. As the hypoxia worsens, the respiratory rate declines as a result of respiratory muscle fatigue.

Cyanosis, blue discoloration of the skin and mucous membranes caused by the presence of desaturated hemoglobin in capillaries, is a late sign of hypoxia. The presence or absence of cyanosis is not a reliable measure of oxygen status. Central cyanosis, observed in the tongue, soft palate, and conjunctiva of the eye, where blood flow is high, indicates hypoxemia. Peripheral cyanosis, seen in the extremities, nail beds, and earlobes, is often a result of vasoconstriction and stagnant blood flow.

Nursing Knowledge Base

Developmental Factors

The developmental stage of the client and the normal aging process affect tissue oxygenation.

Infants and Toddlers.
Infants and toddlers are at risk for upper respiratory tract infections as a result of frequent exposure to other children and exposure to secondhand smoke. In addition, during the teething process some infants develop nasal congestion, which encourages bacterial growth and increases the potential for respiratory tract infection. Upper respiratory tract infections are usually not dangerous, and infants or toddlers recover with little difficulty.

School-Age Children and Adolescents.
School-age children and adolescents are exposed to respiratory infections and respiratory risk factors such as secondhand smoke and cigarette smoking. A healthy child usually does not have adverse pulmonary effects from respiratory infections. A person who starts smoking in adolescence and continues to smoke into middle age, however, has an increased risk for cardiopulmonary disease and lung cancer.

Young and Middle-Age Adults.
Young and middle-age adults are exposed to multiple cardiopulmonary risk factors: an unhealthy diet, lack of exercise, stress, over-the-counter and prescription drugs not used as intended, illegal substances, and smoking. Reducing these modifiable factors decreases the client's risk for cardiac or pulmonary diseases. This is also the time when individuals establish lifelong habits and lifestyles. It is important to help your clients make good choices and informed decisions about their health care practices.

Older Adults.
The cardiac and respiratory systems undergo changes throughout the aging process (Box 40-3). The changes are associated with calcification of the heart valves, SA node, and costal cartilages. The arterial system develops atherosclerotic plaques. Osteoporosis leads to changes in the size and shape of the thorax.

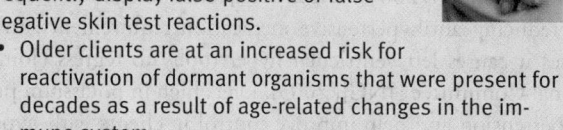

BOX 40-3 **FOCUS ON OLDER ADULTS**

Oxygenation Changes in Older Adults
- The tuberculin skin test is an unreliable indicator of tuberculosis in older clients. They frequently display false-positive or false-negative skin test reactions.
  - Older clients are at an increased risk for reactivation of dormant organisms that were present for decades as a result of age-related changes in the immune system.
  - The standard 5-TU Mantoux test is given and repeated or repeated with the 250-TU strength to create a booster effect.
  - If the older client has a positive reaction, a complete history is necessary to determine any risk factors.
- Older adults have more atypical signs and symptoms of coronary artery disease (Meiner and Leuckenotte, 2006).
- The incidence of atrial fibrillation increases with age and is the leading contributing factor for stroke in the older adult (Meiner and Leuckenotte, 2006).
- Mental status changes are often the first signs of respiratory problems and often include forgetfulness and irritability.
- Older adults do not always complain of dyspnea until it affects the activities of daily living that are important to them.
- Changes in the older adult's cough mechanism lead to retention of pulmonary secretions, airway plugging, and atelectasis if clients do not use cough suppressants with caution.

The trachea and large bronchi become enlarged from calcification of the airways. The alveoli enlarge, decreasing the surface area available for gas exchange. The number of functional cilia is reduced, causing a decrease in the effectiveness of the cough mechanism, putting the older adult at increased risk for respiratory infections (Meiner and Leuckenotte, 2006).

Lifestyle Factors

Lifestyle modifications are difficult for clients because they often have to change an enjoyable habit, such as cigarette smoking or eating certain foods. Risk factor modification is important and includes smoking cessation, weight reduction, a low-cholesterol and low-sodium diet, management of hypertension, and moderate exercise (see Chapter 6). Although it is difficult to change long-term behavior, assisting clients in acquiring healthy behaviors reduces the risk for or slows or halts the progression of cardiopulmonary diseases (Meiner and Leuckenotte, 2006).

Nutrition.
Nutrition affects cardiopulmonary function in several ways. Severe obesity decreases lung expansion, and increased body weight increases tissue oxygen demands. The malnourished client experiences respiratory muscle wasting, resulting in decreased muscle strength and respiratory excursion. Cough efficiency is reduced secondary to respiratory muscle weakness, putting the client at risk for retention of pulmonary secretions.

Clients who are morbidly obese and/or malnourished are at risk for anemia. Diets high in carbohydrates play a role in increasing the carbon dioxide load for clients with carbon dioxide retention. As carbohydrates are metabolized, an increased load of carbon dioxide is created and excreted via the lungs.

Dietary practices also influence the prevalence of cardiovascular diseases. Cardioprotective nutrition includes diets rich in fiber; whole grains; fresh fruits and vegetables; nuts; antioxidants; lean meats, fish, and chicken; and omega-3 fatty acids. In addition, potatoes and citrus fruit juices are cardioprotective in women, but not men (Albert, 2005). Dietary restriction of sodium is beneficial in reducing antihypertensive medication requirements; in some cases it causes left ventricular hypertrophy to regress (Joint National Committee [JNC], 2003). Diets high in potassium prevent hypertension and help improve control in clients with hypertension. A 2000-calorie diet high in fiber, potassium, calcium, and magnesium; made up of fruits, vegetables, and low-fat dairy foods; and low in saturated and total fat helps prevent and reduce the effects of hypertension (JNC, 2003).

Exercise. Exercise increases the body's metabolic activity and oxygen demand. The rate and depth of respiration increase, enabling the person to inhale more oxygen and exhale excess carbon dioxide. A physical exercise program has many benefits (see Chapter 37). People who exercise for 30 to 60 minutes daily have a lower pulse rate and blood pressure, decreased cholesterol level, increased blood flow, and greater oxygen extraction by working muscles. Fully conditioned people increase oxygen consumption by 10% to 20% because of increased cardiac output and increased efficiency of the myocardial muscle (JNC, 2003).

Smoking. Cigarette smoking and secondhand smoke are associated with a number of diseases, including heart disease, chronic obstructive lung disease, and lung cancer. Cigarette smoking worsens peripheral vascular and coronary artery diseases (JNC, 2003). Inhaled nicotine causes vasoconstriction of peripheral and coronary blood vessels, increasing blood pressure and decreasing blood flow to peripheral vessels. Women who take birth control pills and smoke cigarettes have an increased risk for thrombophlebitis and pulmonary emboli.

The risk of lung cancer is 10 times greater for a person who smokes than for a nonsmoker. Exposure to secondhand smoke increases the risk of lung cancer and cardiovascular disease in the nonsmoker (American Cancer Society [ACS], 2006a).

Substance Abuse. Excessive use of alcohol and other drugs impairs tissue oxygenation in two ways. First, the person who chronically abuses substances often has a poor nutritional intake. With the resultant decrease in intake of iron-rich foods, hemoglobin production declines. Second, excessive use of alcohol and certain other drugs depresses the respiratory center, reducing the rate and depth of respiration and the amount of inhaled oxygen. Substance abuse by either smoking or inhaling, such as crack cocaine or inhaling fumes from paint or glue cans, causes direct injury to lung tissue that leads to permanent lung damage.

Stress. A continuous state of stress or severe anxiety increases the body's metabolic rate and the oxygen demand. The body responds to anxiety and other stresses with an increased rate and depth of respiration. Most people adapt, but some, particularly those with chronic illnesses or acute life-threatening illnesses such as a myocardial infarction, cannot tolerate the oxygen demands associated with anxiety (see Chapter 31).

Environmental Factors

The environment also influences oxygenation. The incidence of pulmonary disease is higher in smoggy, urban areas than in rural areas. In addition, the client's workplace sometimes increases the risk for pulmonary disease. Occupational pollutants include asbestos, talcum powder, dust, and airborne fibers. For example, farm workers in dry regions of the southwestern United States are at risk for coccidioidomycosis, a fungal disease caused by inhalation of spores of the airborne bacterium *Coccidioides immitis*. Asbestosis is an occupational lung disease that develops after exposure to asbestos. The lung with asbestosis often has diffuse interstitial fibrosis, creating a restrictive lung disease. Clients exposed to asbestos are at risk for developing lung cancer, and this risk increases with exposure to tobacco smoke.

Critical Thinking

Successful critical thinking requires a synthesis of knowledge, experience, information gathered from clients, critical thinking attitudes, and intellectual and professional standards. Clinical judgments require you to anticipate information, analyze the data, and make decisions regarding your client's care. During assessment consider all elements that build toward making an appropriate nursing diagnosis (Figure 40-6).

To understand how alterations in oxygenation affect clients and the interventions necessary, you need to integrate knowledge from nursing and other disciplines, previous experiences, and information gathered from clients. Critical thinking attitudes ensure you approach client care in a methodical and logical way. The use of professional standards, such as those developed by the Agency for Healthcare Research and Quality (AHRQ), the American Cancer Society (ACS), the American Heart Association (AHA), the American Lung Association (ALA), the American Thoracic Society (ATS), and the American Nurses Association (ANA), provide valuable guidelines for care and management of your clients.

Nursing Process

◆ Assessment

Nursing assessment of cardiopulmonary functioning includes an in-depth history of the client's normal and present cardiopulmonary function, past impairments in circulatory or respiratory functioning, and measures that the client uses to optimize oxygenation. The nursing history includes a review of drug, food, and other allergies. Physical examination of the client's cardiopulmonary status reveals the extent of existing signs and symptoms. Last, a review of laboratory and diagnostic test results provides valuable assessment data.

Nursing History. The nursing history focuses on the client's ability to meet oxygen needs. The nursing history for cardiac function includes pain and characteristics of pain, dyspnea, fatigue, peripheral circulation, cardiac risk factors, and the presence

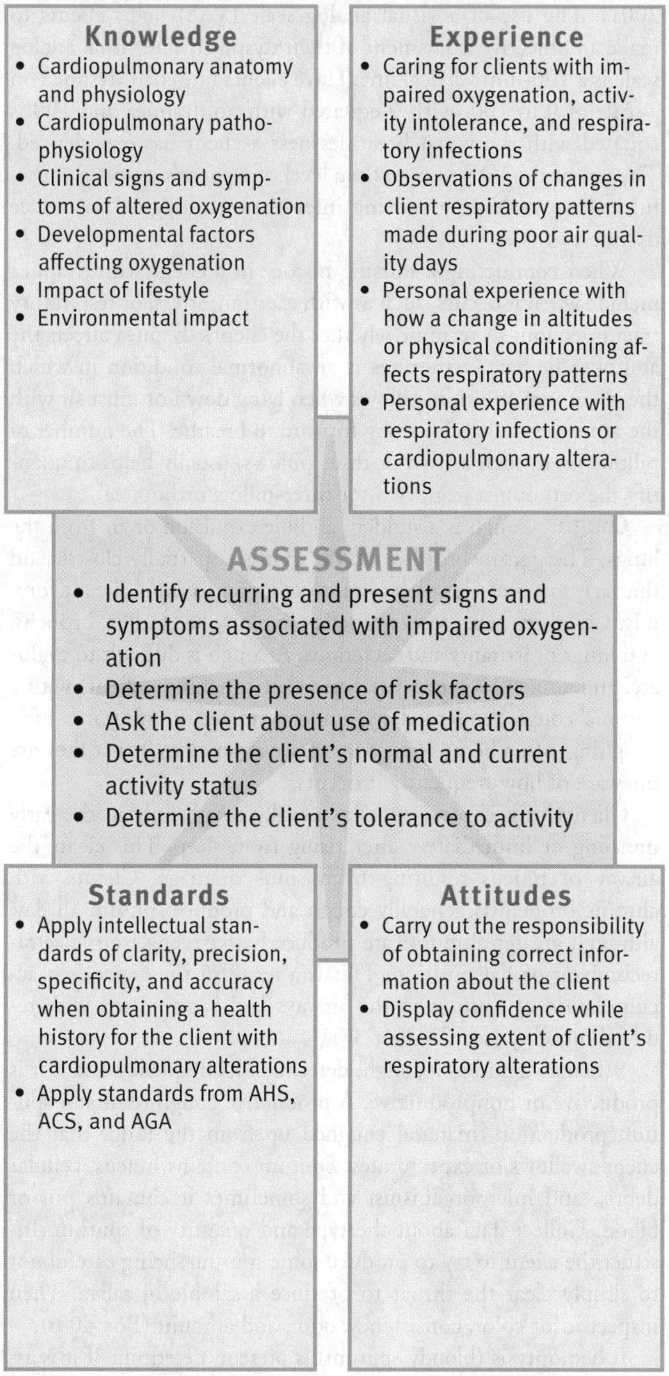

Knowledge
- Cardiopulmonary anatomy and physiology
- Cardiopulmonary pathophysiology
- Clinical signs and symptoms of altered oxygenation
- Developmental factors affecting oxygenation
- Impact of lifestyle
- Environmental impact

Experience
- Caring for clients with impaired oxygenation, activity intolerance, and respiratory infections
- Observations of changes in client respiratory patterns made during poor air quality days
- Personal experience with how a change in altitudes or physical conditioning affects respiratory patterns
- Personal experience with respiratory infections or cardiopulmonary alterations

ASSESSMENT
- Identify recurring and present signs and symptoms associated with impaired oxygenation
- Determine the presence of risk factors
- Ask the client about use of medication
- Determine the client's normal and current activity status
- Determine the client's tolerance to activity

Standards
- Apply intellectual standards of clarity, precision, specificity, and accuracy when obtaining a health history for the client with cardiopulmonary alterations
- Apply standards from AHS, ACS, and AGA

Attitudes
- Carry out the responsibility of obtaining correct information about the client
- Display confidence while assessing extent of client's respiratory alterations

Figure 40-6 Critical thinking model for oxygenation assessment.

★ **BOX 40-4** NURSING ASSESSMENT QUESTIONS

Nature of the Cardiopulmonary Problem
- What types of breathing problems are you having?
- Describe the problem you are having with your heart.
- Does it occur at a specific time of the day, during or after exercise, or all the time?

Sign and Symptoms
- How has your breathing pattern changed?
- Are you having sputum with coughing? Is this different?
- Is your sputum a different color?
- Are you having any chest pain? Does the pain occur with breathing?

Onset and Duration
- If you are having chest pain, what causes the pain and how long does it last? Is this a different type of pain?
- When did you notice your sputum change in color and amount?
- When did your coughing increase? How does this differ from your usual pattern of coughing?

Severity
- On a scale of 0 to 10, with 10 being the most severe, rate your shortness of breath.
- What helps your shortness of breath?
- On a scale of 0 to 10, with 0 being no pain and 10 the most severe pain, rate your chest pain. Is the severity of your pain different today?
- What do you do for this pain?

Predisposing Factors
- Have you been exposed to a cold or flu?
- Are you taking your prescribed medications?
- Do you smoke? Have you been exposed to secondhand smoke?
- Have you been doing any unusual exercises?

Effect of Symptoms on Client
- Do these symptoms affect your daily activities? If so how?
- What impact do these symptoms have on your: appetite, sleeping habits, activity status?

---

of past or concurrent cardiac conditions. The nursing history for respiratory function includes the presence of a cough, shortness of breath, wheezing, pain, environmental exposures, frequency of respiratory tract infections, pulmonary risk factors, past respiratory problems, current medication use, and smoking history or secondhand smoke exposure. Ask specific questions related to cardiopulmonary disease (Box 40-4).

Pain. The presence of chest pain needs an immediate thorough evaluation, including location, duration, radiation, and frequency. Cardiac pain does not occur with respiratory variations and is most often on the left side of the chest and radiates to the left arm in men. Chest pain in women is much less definitive and is often a sensation of breathlessness, jaw or back pain, nausea, and fatigue (AHA, 2006b). Pericardial pain results from inflammation of the pericardial sac, occurs on inspiration, and does not usually radiate.

Pleuritic chest pain is peripheral and radiates to the scapular regions. Inspiratory maneuvers, such as coughing, yawning, and sighing worsen pleuritic chest pain. An inflammation or infection in the pleural space often causes this, and clients usually describe it as knifelike, lasting from a minute to hours and always in association with inspiration.

Musculoskeletal pain is often present following exercise, rib trauma, and prolonged coughing episodes. Inspiration worsens this pain, and clients often confuse it with pleuritic chest pain.

Fatigue. Fatigue is a subjective sensation in which the client reports a loss of endurance. Fatigue in the client with cardiopulmonary alterations is often an early sign of a worsening of the chronic underlying process. To provide an objective measure of fatigue, ask the client to rate the fatigue on a scale of 0 to 10, with 10 being the worst level of fatigue and 0 representing no fatigue.

✳ **BOX 40-5**   **EVIDENCE-BASED PRACTICE**

The Efficacy of Exercise Training in Clients With COPD

Evidence Summary

Clients with dyspnea often have a difficult time controlling their breathing. Exercise training improves dyspnea and activity tolerance in clients with chronic obstructive pulmonary disease (COPD). This study investigated the impact of exercise training on dyspnea self-management, exercise performance, and health-related quality of life. Researchers randomly placed subjects with COPD into three groups. One group had dyspnea self-management and supervised exercise training. Dyspnea self-management included individualized education about dyspnea management strategies, a home-walking prescription, and daily logs. The other two groups received standard care. Researchers measured outcomes (symptoms) at baseline and every 2 months for a year. Clients measured their symptoms through three questionnaires: Chronic Respiratory Questionnaire (CRQ), Shortness of Breath Questionnaire, and Baseline/Transitional Dyspnea Index. The group with dyspnea self-management and supervised exercise training had improved dyspnea management and activity tolerance.

Application to Nursing Practice

- Using a routine, managed exercise program, such as walking, improves dyspnea.
- Teaching clients how to manage their shortness of breath (dyspnea) during activities helps to improve dyspnea and exercise tolerance.
- Organizing nursing care to use client's time effectively and avoid interruption helps the client manage dyspnea and reduces dyspnea-related fatigue.

Reference

Stulbarg MS and others: Exercise training improves outcomes of a dyspnea self-management program, *J Cardiopulm Rehabil* 22(2):109, 2002.

Smoking. It is important to determine clients' direct and secondary exposure to tobacco. Ask about any history of smoking; include the number of years smoked and the number of packages smoked per day. This is recorded as pack-year history. For example, if a client smoked two packs a day for 20 years, the client has a 40 pack-year history (packages per day × years smoked). Determine exposure to secondhand smoke because any form of tobacco exposure increases the client's risk for cardiopulmonary diseases.

Dyspnea. **Dyspnea** is a clinical sign of hypoxia. It is the subjective sensation of difficult or uncomfortable breathing (Box 40-5). Dyspnea is shortness of breath usually associated with exercise or excitement, but in some clients dyspnea is present without any relation to activity or exercise. Dyspnea is associated with many conditions, such as pulmonary diseases, cardiovascular diseases, neuromuscular conditions, and anemia. In addition, dyspnea occurs in the pregnant woman in the final months of pregnancy. Last, environmental factors, such as pollution, cold air, and smoking also cause or worsen dyspnea.

Dyspnea is associated with exaggerated respiratory effort, use of the accessory muscles of respiration, nasal flaring, and marked increases in the rate and depth of respirations (Jevon and Evans,

2001). The use of a visual analog scale (VAS) helps clients to make an objective assessment of their dyspnea. The visual analog scale is a 100-mm vertical line. Have clients rate their dyspnea on a scale of 0 to 100, with 0 equated with no dyspnea and 100 is equated with the worst breathlessness a client has experienced. The use of the VAS to assess the level of a client's dyspnea is useful in later evaluating nursing interventions designed to reduce dyspnea.

When conducting a nursing history in a client with dyspnea include when it occurs, such as with exertion, stress, or respiratory tract infection. Determine whether the client's dyspnea affects the ability to lie flat. **Orthopnea** is an abnormal condition in which the client uses multiple pillows when lying down or must sit with the arms elevated and leaning forward to breathe. The number of pillows used, such as two or three pillows, usually helps to quantify the orthopnea (e.g., two- or three-pillow orthopnea).

Cough. Cough is a sudden, audible expulsion of air from the lungs. The person breathes in, the glottis is partially closed, and the accessory muscles of expiration contract to expel the air forcibly. Coughing is a protective reflex to clear the trachea, bronchi, and lungs of irritants and secretions. A cough is difficult to evaluate, and almost everyone has periods of coughing. Clients with a chronic cough tend to deny, underestimate, or minimize their coughing, often because they are so accustomed to it that they are unaware of how frequently it occurs.

Clients with chronic sinusitis usually cough only in the early morning or immediately after rising from sleep. This clears the airway of mucus resulting from sinus drainage. Clients with chronic bronchitis generally cough and produce sputum all day, although greater amounts are produced after rising from a semi-recumbent or flat position. This is a result of the dependent accumulation of sputum in the airways and is associated with reduced mobility (see Chapter 37).

When a client has a cough, determine its frequency and if it is productive or nonproductive. A productive cough results in sputum production, material coughed up from the lungs that the client swallows or expectorates. Sputum contains mucus, cellular debris, and microorganisms, and sometimes it contains pus or blood. Collect data about the type and quantity of sputum. Instruct the client to try to produce some sputum, being careful not to simply clear the throat to produce a sample of saliva. Then inspect it for color, consistency, odor, and amount (Box 40-6).

If **hemoptysis** (bloody sputum) is present, determine if it is associated with coughing and bleeding from the upper respiratory tract, from sinus drainage, or from the gastrointestinal tract (**hematemesis**). Describe hemoptysis according to amount, color, and duration and whether it is mixed with sputum. When there is bloody or blood-tinged sputum, health care providers frequently perform diagnostic tests, such as examination of sputum specimens, chest x-ray examinations, **bronchoscopy**, and other x-ray studies.

Wheezing. Wheezing is a high-pitched musical sound caused by high-velocity movement of air through a narrowed airway. Wheezing is associated with asthma, acute bronchitis, or pneumonia. Wheezing occurs during inspiration, expiration, or both. Determine if there are any precipitating factors, such as respiratory infection, allergens, exercise, or stress.

Environmental or Geographical Exposures. Environmental exposure to inhaled substances is closely linked with respira-

---

BOX 40-6 Sputum Characteristics

Color
Clear
White
Yellow
Green
Brown
Red
Streaked with blood

Changes in Color
Same color throughout the day
Clearing with coughing
Progressively darker

Odor
None
Foul

Quantity
Same as usual
Increased
Decreased

Consistency
Frothy
Watery
Tenacious, thick

Presence of Blood
Occasional
Early morning
Bright or dark red
Blood tinged

---

tory disease. Investigate exposures in the client's home and workplace. The most common environmental exposures in the home are cigarette smoke, carbon monoxide, and radon. In addition, determine whether a client who is a nonsmoker is exposed to secondhand smoke.

Carbon monoxide poisoning often results from a blocked furnace flue or fireplace. The client has vague complaints of general malaise, flulike symptoms, and excessive sleepiness. Clients are particularly at risk in the late fall when they turn the heat on or begin to use the fireplace again. Radon gas, a radioactive substance, enters homes through the ground. When homes are underventilated, this gas is unable to escape and becomes trapped in the home.

Respiratory Infections. Obtain information about the client's frequency and duration of respiratory tract infections. Although everyone occasionally experiences a cold, for some people it results in bronchitis or pneumonia. On average, clients will have four colds per year. Determine if the client has had a pneumococcal or flu vaccine, and ask about any known exposure to tuberculosis and the results of the tuberculin skin test.

Determine the client's risk for human immunodeficiency virus (HIV) infection. Clients with a history of intravenous (IV) drug use and multiple unprotected sexual partners are at risk of developing HIV infection. Clients do not always display symptoms of HIV infection until they present with *Pneumocystis carinii* pneumonia (PCP) or *Mycoplasma* pneumonia. Presentation with PCP or *Mycoplasma* pneumonia indicates a significant depression of the client's immune system and progression to acquired immunodeficiency syndrome (AIDS).

Allergies. Inquire about your client's exposure to airborne allergens (e.g., pet dander or mold). The client's allergic response is often watery eyes, sneezing, runny nose, or respiratory symptoms, such as cough or wheezing. When obtaining information ask specific questions about the type of allergens, response to these allergens, and successful and unsuccessful relief measures. In addition, determine the effect of environmental air quality and secondhand smoke exposure on the client's allergy and symptoms.

Safe nursing practice also includes obtaining information about food, drug, or insect sting allergies. Collect these data on initial history and physical. However, always double-check this information with the client, especially when obtaining information about respiratory allergens.

Health Risks. Determine familial risk factors, such as a family history of lung cancer or cardiovascular disease. Documentation includes those blood relatives who had the disease and their present level of health or age at time of death. Other family risk factors include the presence of infectious diseases, particularly tuberculosis.

Medications. Another component of the nursing history describes medications the client is using. These include prescribed medications, over-the-counter medications, folk medicine, herbal medicines, alternative therapies, and illicit drugs and substances. Some of these preparations have adverse effects by themselves or because of interactions with other drugs. For example, a person using a prescribed bronchodilator drug decides to use an over-the-counter inhalant as well. Many of these contain ephedrine or *ma huang*, a natural ephedrine, which acts like epinephrine. This product reacts with the prescribed medication by potentiating or decreasing the effect of the prescribed medication. Clients taking warfarin (Coumadin) for blood thinning will prolong the prothrombin time (PT)/international normalized ratio (INR) results if they are taking gingko biloba, garlic, or ginseng with the anticoagulant. The drug interaction will possibly precipitate a life-threatening bleed.

SAFETY ALERT During history taking have clients include all over-the-counter and herbal supplements they are taking to ensure there are no medication interactions. It is sometimes necessary for a family member or friend to bring in the medication bottles.

It is important to determine if a client uses illicit drugs. Illicit drugs, particularly parenterally administered opioids, which are often diluted with talcum powder, cause pulmonary disorders resulting from the irritant effect of the powder on lung tissues.

As with all medications, assess the client's knowledge and ability to self-administer medications correctly (see Chapter 35). Of particular importance is the assessment of the client's understanding of potential side effects of the medications. Clients need to recognize adverse reactions and be aware of the dangers in combining prescribed medications with over-the-counter drugs.

Physical Examination. The physical examination includes assessment of the cardiopulmonary system (see Chapter 33). Give special consideration when assessing the older adult client because there are changes that occur with the aging process (Table 40-2). These changes affect the client's activity tolerance, level of fatigue, or cause transient changes in vital signs and are not always associated with a specific cardiopulmonary disease.

Inspection. Using inspection techniques, perform a head-to-toe observation of the client for skin and mucous membrane color, general appearance, level of consciousness, adequacy of systemic circulation, breathing patterns, and chest wall movement (Table 40-3). Investigate any abnormalities further during palpation, percussion, and auscultation.

✳ **TABLE 40-2 Assessment Findings in the Aging Cardiopulmonary System**

FUNCTION	PATHOPHYSIOLOGICAL CHANGE	KEY CLINICAL FINDINGS
Heart		
Muscle contraction	Thickening of the ventricular wall, increased collagen and decreased elastin in the heart muscle	Decreased cardiac output Diminished cardiac reserve
Blood flow	Heart valves become thicker and stiffer, more often in the mitral and aortic valves	Murmurs
Conduction system	The SA node becomes fibrotic from calcification; the number of pacemaker cells in the SA node decreases	Increased PR, QRS, and Q-T intervals, decreased amplitude of the QRS complex Irregular heart rhythm
Arterial vessel compliance	Vessels become calcified, loss of arterial distensibility, decreased elastin in the vessel walls, more tortuous vessels	Hypertension, with an increase in systolic blood pressure Fluctuation in blood pressure
Lungs		
Breathing mechanics	Decreased chest wall compliance, loss of elastic recoil Decreased respiratory muscle mass/strength	Prolonged exhalation phase Decreased vital capacity
Oxygenation	Increased ventilation/perfusion mismatch Decreased alveolar surface area Decreased carbon dioxide diffusion capacity	Decreased PaO_2 Decreased cardiac output Slightly increased $PaCO_2$
Breathing control/ breathing pattern	Decreased responsiveness of central and peripheral chemoreceptors to hypoxemia and hypercapnia	Increased respiratory rate Decreased tidal volume
Lung defense mechanisms	Decreased number of cilia Decreased IgA production and humoral and cellular immunity	Decreased airway clearance Diminished cough reflex
Sleep and breathing	Decreased respiratory drive Decreased tone of upper airway muscles	Increased risk of aspiration and respiratory infection Decreased PaO_2 Snoring, obstructive sleep apnea

SA, Sinoatrial; *PaO₂*, arterial oxygen tension; *PaCO₂*, arterial carbon dioxide tension.

Inspection includes observations of the nails for clubbing. Clubbed nails, obliteration of the normal angle between the base of the nail and the skin often occur in clients with prolonged oxygen deficiency, endocarditis, and congenital heart defects.

Observe the chest wall movement for retraction, sinking in of soft tissues of the chest between the intercostal spaces and use of accessory muscles. Also observe for paradoxical breathing, asynchronous breathing, and the client's breathing pattern. At rest, the normal adult rate is 12 to 20 regular breaths per minute. Bradypnea is less than 12 breaths per minute, and tachypnea is greater than 20 breaths per minute. Apnea is the absence of respirations. In some conditions, such as metabolic acidosis, respirations increase in both rate and depth as the client tries to "breathe off" excess carbon dioxide; this type of breathing is Kussmaul's respiration. In paradoxical breathing the chest wall contracts during inspiration and expands during exhalation. Also note the shape of the chest wall. Conditions such as emphysema, advancing age, and COPD cause the chest to assume a rounded "barrel" shape.

Palpation. Palpation of the chest provides assessment data in several areas. It documents the type and amount of thoracic excursion, elicits any areas of tenderness, and helps to identify tactile fremitus, thrills, heaves, and the cardiac point of maximal impulse (PMI). Palpation of the extremities provides data about the peripheral circulation, the presence and quality of peripheral pulses, skin temperature, color, and capillary refill (see Chapter 33).

Palpation also includes the feet and legs to determine the presence or absence of peripheral edema. Clients with alterations in their cardiac function, such as those with congestive heart failure or hypertension, often have pedal or lower extremity edema. Edema is graded from 1+ to 4+, depending on the depth of visible indentation after firm application of a finger (see Chapter 33).

Palpate the pulses in the neck and extremities to assess arterial blood flow (see Chapter 33). Use a scale of 0 (absent pulse) to 3+ (full, bounding pulse) to describe what you feel. The normal pulse is 2+, and a weak, thready pulse is 1+.

Percussion. Percussion detects the presence of abnormal fluid or air in the lungs. It also determines diaphragmatic excursion (see Chapter 33).

Auscultation. Auscultation helps identify normal and abnormal heart and lung sounds (see Chapter 33). Auscultation of the cardiovascular system includes assessment for normal S_1 and S_2 sounds, the presence of abnormal S_3 and S_4 sounds (gallops), and murmurs or rubs. Identify the location, radiation, intensity, pitch, and quality of a murmur. Auscultation also identifies any bruit over the carotid, abdominal aorta, and femoral arteries.

Auscultation of lung sounds involves listening for movement of air throughout all lung fields: anterior, posterior, and lateral. Adventitious, or abnormal, breath sounds occur with collapse of a lung segment, fluid in a lung segment, or narrowing or obstruction of an airway.

※ **TABLE 40-3** Inspection of Cardiopulmonary Status

ABNORMALITY	CAUSE
Eyes	
Xanthelasma (yellow lipid lesions on eyelids)	Hyperlipidemia
Corneal arcus (whitish opaque ring around junction of cornea and sclera)	Hyperlipidemia in young to middle adults, normal finding in older adults with arcus senilis
Pale conjunctivae	Anemia
Cyanotic conjunctivae	Hypoxemia
Petechiae on conjunctivae	Fat embolus or bacterial endocarditis
Mouth and Lips	
Cyanotic mucous membranes	Decreased oxygenation (hypoxia)
Pursed-lip breathing	Associated with chronic lung disease
Neck Veins	
Distention	Associated with right-sided heart failure
Nose	
Flaring nares	Air hunger, dyspnea
Chest	
Retractions	Increased work of breathing, dyspnea
Asymmetry	Chest wall injury
Skin	
Peripheral cyanosis	Vasoconstriction and diminished blood flow
Central cyanosis	Hypoxemia
Decreased skin turgor	Dehydration (normal finding in older adults as a result of decreased skin elasticity)
Dependent edema	Associated with right- and left-sided heart failure
Periorbital edema	Associated with kidney disease
Fingertips and Nail Beds	
Cyanosis	Decreased cardiac output or hypoxia
Splinter hemorrhages	Bacterial endocarditis
Clubbing	Chronic hypoxemia

From Potter PA, Weilitz PB: *Health assessment, pocket guide series*, ed 6, St. Louis, 2007, Mosby.

Diagnostic Tests. A variety of diagnostic tests monitor cardiopulmonary functioning. Some of these screening tests are simple blood specimens, x-ray films, or other noninvasive means. One screening mechanism is tuberculosis (TB) skin testing (Box 40-7). This is a simple test and is required for health care workers, restaurant employees, students entering schools, teachers and other school employees, correctional facility employees, prisoners, and residents of long-term care facilities (Centers for Disease Control and Prevention [CDC], 2005, 2006a and b).

In contrast, invasive diagnostic tests, such as a thoracentesis, are quite painful. Tables 40-4 through 40-6 summarize diagnostic testing used in the assessment and evaluation of the client with cardiopulmonary alterations. When reviewing results of pulmonary function studies, be aware of expected variations in clients from different cultures. These changes are due to structural variations in chest wall size in these clients (Box 40-8).

Whether a diagnostic procedure is painful depends on the client's tolerance for pain (see Chapter 43). Reduce the client's anxiety by explaining the procedure and telling the client what to expect. Be sure the client understands the importance of following instructions, such as holding the breath as requested and of not coughing during the procedure. After any procedure,

monitor the client for signs of changes in cardiopulmonary functioning, sudden shortness of breath, pain, oxygen desaturation, and anxiety.

Client Expectations. Ask clients about their priorities and what they expect from the health care visit. Identifying expectations involves clients in the decision-making process and helps them participate in their care and know what will happen to them. For example, planning a smoking cessation or weight reduction program for a client who is not ready for the change is frustrating for both the client and the nurse. Establish realistic, short-term outcomes that build to a larger goal. For example, start out by reducing the fat in the client's diet by replacing food such as whole milk with 2% milk and gradually introducing skim milk. In this example, a sudden change from whole to skim milk will most likely fail, because the change is too much. Have a plan for adding exercise to the client's lifestyle; start with a commitment to exercise once a week for 20 minutes, or have the client commit to a weight reduction plan of 5 pounds per month.

Remember that your goals and expectations do not always coincide with your client's. By addressing the client's concerns and

✱ BOX 40-7 Tuberculosis Skin Testing

- Skin testing determines whether a person is infected with *Mycobacterium tuberculosis*.
- Tuberculosis skin testing (TST) is performed by an intradermal injection of 0.1 mL of tuberculin purified protein derivative (PPD) on the inner surface of the forearm (see Chapter 35). The injection produces a pale elevation of the skin (a wheal) 6 to 10 mm in diameter. Afterward, the injection site is circled, and the client is instructed not to wash the circle off.

- Tuberculin skin tests are read between 48 to 72 hours. If the site is not read within 72 hours, the client must have another skin test.
- *Positive results:* A palpable, elevated, hardened area around the injection site, caused by edema and inflammation from the antigen-antibody reaction, measured in millimeters. (See Chapter 35 for evaluation of positive results by millimeters).
- Reddened flat areas are **not** positive reactions and are not measured.
- TST in older adults is less reliable (see Box 40-3).

✱ TABLE 40-4 Cardiopulmonary Diagnostic Blood Studies

Test and Normal Values	Interpretation
Complete Blood Count (CBC) Normal values for a CBC vary with age and gender	A CBC determines the number and type of red and white blood cells per cubic millimeter of blood.
Cardiac Enzymes Creatine kinase (CK)—a serial CK with 50% increase between two samples 3-6 hours apart, peaking 12 hours after chest pain, or a single CK elevation twofold is diagnostic for an acute myocardial infarction Male normal: 55-170 units/L Female normal: 30-135 units/L	Providers use cardiac enzymes to diagnose acute myocardial infarcts.
Cardiac Troponins Plasma cardiac troponin I <0.3 ng/mL Plasma cardiac troponin T <0.2 ng/mL	Value elevates within 12 hours of a cardiac event. Often remains elevated for 7-10 days. Often remains elevated for 10-14 days.
Myoglobin <90 mcg/L	Early index of damage to the myocardium in myocardial infarction or reinfarction. Increases within 3 hours.
Serum Electrolytes Potassium (K^+) 3.5-5 mEq/L or 3.5-5 mmol/L	Clients on diuretic therapy are at risk for hypokalemia (low potassium). Clients receiving angiotensin-converting enzyme (ACE) inhibitors are at risk for hyperkalemia (elevated potassium).
Cholesterol Fasting cholesterol 200 mg/dL	Contributing factors include sedentary lifestyle with intake of saturated fatty acids, familial hypercholesterolemia.
Low-density lipoproteins (LDLs) (bad cholesterol) 60-180 mg/dL	High LDL cholesterol (hypercholesterolemia) is caused by excessive intake of saturated fatty acids, dietary cholesterol intake, and obesity. Familial hypercholesterolemia and hyperlipidemia are also contributing factors, as well as hypothyroidism, nephrotic syndrome, and diabetes mellitus.
High-density lipoproteins (HDLs) (good cholesterol) Male: >45 mg/dL Female: >55 mg/dL	Factors such as cigarette smoking, obesity, lack of regular exercise, beta-adrenergic blocking agents, genetic disorders of HDL metabolism, hypertriglyceridemia, and type 2 diabetes cause low HDL cholesterol.
Triglycerides Male: 40-160 mg/dL Female: 35-135 mg/dL	Obesity, excessive alcohol intake, diabetes mellitus, beta-adrenergic blocking agents, and familial hypertriglyceridemia cause hypertriglyceridemia.

Pagana KD, Pagana TJ: *Mosby's diagnostic and laboratory test reference,* ed 7, St. Louis, 2005, Mosby.

✳ TABLE 40-5 Cardiac Function Diagnostic Tests

Test	Significance
Holter monitor	Portable ECG worn by the client. The test produces a continuous ECG tracing over a period of time. Clients keep a diary of activity, noting when they experience rapid heartbeats or dizziness. Evaluation of the ECG recording along with the diary provides information about the heart's electrical activity during activities of daily living.
ECG exercise stress test	ECG is monitored while the client walks on a treadmill at a specified speed and duration of time. Used to evaluate the cardiac response to physical stress. The test is not a valuable tool for evaluation of cardiac response in women due to an increased false-positive finding.
Thallium stress test	An ECG stress test with the addition of thallium-201 injected intravenously. Determines coronary blood flow changes with increased activity.
Electrophysiological study (EPS)	Invasive measure of intracardiac electrical pathways. Provides more specific information about difficult-to-treat dysrhythmias. Assesses adequacy of antidysrhythmic medication.
Echocardiography	Noninvasive measure of heart structure and heart wall motion. Graphically demonstrates overall cardiac performance.
Scintigraphy	Radionuclide angiography. Used to evaluate cardiac structure, myocardial perfusion and contractility.
Cardiac catheterization and angiography	Used to visualize cardiac chambers, valves, the great vessels, and coronary arteries. Pressures and volumes within the four chambers of the heart are also measured.

ECG, Electrocardiogram.

✳ TABLE 40-6 Ventilation and Oxygenation Diagnostic Studies

Measurement and Normal Values	Interpretation
Pulmonary Function Tests Basic ventilation studies. Pulmonary functions vary by ethnic group (see Box 40-8).	Determines the ability of the lungs to efficiently exchange oxygen and carbon dioxide. Used to differentiate pulmonary obstructive from restrictive disease.
Peak Expiratory Flow Rate (PEFR) The point of highest flow during maximal expiration. Normal is based on age and body weight.	The PEFR reflects changes in large airway sizes and is an excellent predictor of overall airway resistance in the client with asthma. Daily measurement is for early detection of asthma exacerbations.
Bronchoscopy Normal airways without masses, pus, or foreign bodies	Visual examination of the tracheobronchial tree through a narrow, flexible fiberoptic bronchoscope. Performed to obtain fluid, sputum, or biopsy samples; remove mucous plugs or foreign bodies.
Lung Scan Normal lung structure without masses	Used to identify abnormal masses by size and location. Identification of masses is used in planning therapy and treatments.
Thoracentesis Surgical perforation of the chest wall and pleural space with a needle to aspirate fluid for diagnostic or therapeutic purposes or to remove a specimen for biopsy. The procedure is performed using aseptic technique and local anesthetic. The client usually sits upright with the anterior thorax supported by pillows or an over-bed table.	Specimen of plural fluid is obtained for cytological examination. The results may indicate an infection or neoplastic disease. Identification of infection or a type of cancer is important in determining a plan of care.
Sputum Specimens Normal: negative Sputum culture and sensitivity (C and S)	Obtained to identify a specific microorganism or organism growing in the sputum. Identifies drug resistance and sensitivities.
Sputum for acid-fast bacillus (AFB)	Used to screen for the presence of AFB for detection of TB by early morning specimens on 3 consecutive days.
Sputum for cytology	Obtained to identify abnormal lung cancer. Differentiates type of cancer cells (small cell, oat cell, large cell).

TB, Tuberculosis.

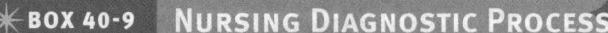

✳ BOX 40-8   CULTURAL ASPECTS OF CARE

Cultural Impact on Pulmonary Diseases

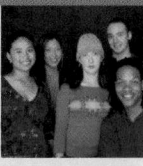

The impact of pulmonary diseases on the client and family varies between cultures. It is important to understand these variations in terms of assessing for and providing care in clients with lung diseases.

- Differences occur as a result of the variation in chest size. Whites have the largest chest volumes, followed by African Americans, Asian Americans, and Native Americans. The variations in the chest size affect the forced expiratory volume (FEV_1), forced vital capacity (FVC), and the FEV_1/FVC ratio (Meiner and Lueckenotte, 2006).
- Eighty-two percent of the reported tuberculosis (TB) cases occur in racial and ethnic minorities. Asians have the highest TB rate of any ethnic group followed by Native Hawaiian and other Pacific Islanders (CDC, 2005).
- In the minority groups born in the United States, African Americans have the highest reported rates of TB cases, followed by Hispanics (CDC, 2005).
- Female African Americans have the highest mortality rates from asthma among all ethnic/gender groups (Lewis and others, 2007).
- Whites have the highest incidences of chronic obstructive lung disease and cystic fibrosis, which is uncommon among African Americans, Hispanics, and Asian Americans (Lewis and others, 2007).

expectations, you establish a relationship that addresses other health care goals and expected outcomes. Knowing your clients' mind-set and respecting their wishes goes a long way in helping clients to make significant beneficial lifestyle changes.

◆ Nursing Diagnosis

Develop nursing diagnoses for clients with oxygenation alterations based on specific defining characteristics and the related etiology (Box 40-9). Use information gathered in the nursing assessment to identify and cluster the defining characteristics. The clustered defining characteristics support the nursing diagnosis.

Nursing diagnoses appropriate for the client with alterations in oxygenation include, but are not limited to, the following:

- Activity intolerance
- Anxiety
- Decreased cardiac output
- Fatigue
- Impaired gas exchange
- Impaired spontaneous ventilation
- Impaired verbal communication
- Ineffective airway clearance
- Ineffective breathing pattern
- Ineffective health maintenance
- Risk for imbalanced fluid volume
- Risk for infection

✳ BOX 40-9   NURSING DIAGNOSTIC PROCESS

Impaired Gas Exchange Related to Decreased Lung Expansion

Assessment Activities	Defining Characteristics
Ask client or family about client's mood, attentiveness, memory, and activity level.	Confusion Decreased activity Fatigue Irritability Restlessness Sleepiness
Observe client's respirations.	Dyspnea Nasal flaring Tachypnea Use of accessory muscles
Inspect skin and mucous membranes.	Diaphoresis Pallor
Auscultate chest.	Decreased respiratory excursion Abnormal, distant lung sounds

◆ Planning

During planning use critical thinking skills to synthesize information from multiple sources (Figure 40-7). Critical thinking ensures that your plan of care integrates individualized client needs. Professional standards are especially important to consider when developing a plan of care. These standards often establish scientifically proven guidelines for selecting effective nursing interventions.

Goals and Outcomes. Develop an individualized plan of care for each nursing diagnosis (see Care Plan). Together with your client set realistic expectations, goals, and measurable outcomes of care.

Clients with impaired oxygenation require a nursing care plan directed toward meeting actual or potential oxygenation needs. Develop individual outcomes based on client-centered goals. For example, for the goal of maintaining a patent airway select specific expected outcomes for the client, such as the following:

- Client's lungs are clear to auscultation.
- Client achieves bilateral lung expansion.
- Client coughs productively.
- Pulse oximetry (SpO_2) is maintained or improved.

Often a client with cardiopulmonary disease has multiple nursing diagnoses (Figure 40-8, p. 929). In this case identify when goals or outcomes apply to more than one diagnosis. The presence of multiple diagnoses also makes priority setting a critical activity.

Setting Priorities. The client's level of health, age, lifestyle, and environmental risks affect the level of tissue oxygenation. Clients with severe impairments in oxygenation frequently require nursing interventions in multiple areas. Consider which goal is the most important goal to achieve while the client is in

Knowledge	Experience
• Role of other health care professionals in caring for the client with impaired oxygenation • Role of community support groups in assisting the client to manage cardiopulmonary disease • Knowledge of effects of pulmonary interventions	• Previous client responses to planned nursing therapies for impaired oxygenation

PLANNING

- Select nursing interventions that promote optimal oxygenation in the primary care, acute care, or restorative and continuing care setting
- Consult with other health care professionals as needed
- Involve the client and family in designing the plan of care

Standards	Attitudes
• Individualize therapies to client's needs • Apply established pulmonary and cardiac rehabilitation guidelines • Apply established nursing care guidelines for care of the client with cardiopulmonary disease (e.g., protocols, care paths)	• Display confidence when selecting interventions • Use creativity when developing home care strategies for the client's disease management • Demonstrate responsibility and accountability when delegating care for client

Figure 40-7 Critical thinking model for oxygenation planning.

the hospital or primary care setting. For example, in an acute care setting maintaining a patent airway has a higher priority than improving the client's exercise tolerance. The need for a patent airway is an immediate need, and as the client's level of oxygen improves, activity tolerance increases. In a second example, when caring for a client who has an abdominal incision, pain control is a priority. In this situation controlling the client's pain facilitates coughing and deep breathing.

However, in a community-based or primary setting, the priority often focuses on smoking cessation, exercise, and/or diet modifications. Both you and the client need to focus on the same goal and expected outcomes. In addition to individualizing each goal, be sure the goals are realistic and attainable for the client.

Collaborative Care. The time spent with a client in any setting is limited. Therefore collaborate with family members, colleagues, and other specialists to achieve the established goals and expected outcomes. Some clients need to improve their exercise and activity tolerance; for other clients their continuing care involves participating in a community-based cardiopulmonary

rehabilitation program. Last, some clients need home physical therapy.

Collaboration with physical therapists, nutritionists, and community-based nurses is valuable for clients with congestive heart failure or chronic lung conditions. These professionals work with the client and use resources in the community to assist the client in attaining and maintaining the highest possible level of wellness. In addition, professionals help identify community resources and support systems for both the client and family in preventing and managing symptoms related to cardiopulmonary diseases.

◆Implementation

Interventions for promoting and maintaining adequate oxygenation include health promotion and prevention behaviors, positioning, and coughing techniques. Other interventions include oxygen therapy, lung inflation techniques, hydration, medication administration, and chest physiotherapy.

Health Promotion. Maintaining the client's optimal level of health is important in reducing the number and/or severity of respiratory symptoms. Prevention of respiratory infections is foremost in maintaining optimal health. Providing cardiopulmonary-related health information (Box 40-10) is an important nursing responsibility.

Vaccinations. Annual influenza vaccines are recommended for children 6 to 59 months, adults over 50, and clients with chronic illnesses. This includes clients of any age with chronic disease of the heart, lung, or kidneys; clients with diabetes; and clients with immunosuppression or severe forms of anemia. The vaccine is also recommended for people in close or frequent contact with anyone in the high-risk groups. The vaccine is effective in reducing the severity of illness and the risk of serious complications and death (CDC, 2006a).

Researchers do not fully understand the value of vaccination in immunocompromised clients. HIV-positive clients receive the flu vaccine; however, they often require a second vaccine to gain protection. Persons who should not be vaccinated include those with a known hypersensitivity to eggs or other components of the vaccine and adults with an acute febrile illness. The vaccines are formulated annually based on worldwide surveillance data.

Pneumococcal vaccine is recommended for clients at increased risk of developing pneumonia, those with chronic illnesses or immunosuppression (such as HIV/AIDS), those living in special environments such as nursing homes or the Native American population, and clients over the age of 65 (CDC, 2006a).

Healthy Lifestyle Behavior. Identification and elimination of risk factors for cardiopulmonary disease is an important part of primary care. Encourage clients to eat a healthy low-fat, high-fiber diet; monitor their cholesterol, triglyceride, high-density lipoprotein (HDL), and low-density lipoprotein (LDL) levels; reduce stress; exercise; and maintain a body weight in proportion to their height.

Elimination of cigarettes and other tobacco, reduction of pollutants, monitoring of air quality, and adequate hydration are additional healthy behaviors. Encourage clients to examine their habits and make appropriate changes.

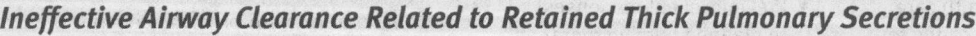

NURSING CARE PLAN

Ineffective Airway Clearance Related to Retained Thick Pulmonary Secretions

Assessment

Mr. Edwards is 75 years old; he is lying in bed talking with his wife. Ms. Kathy Allen is a junior nursing student, and she completed a respiratory assessment. Mr. Edwards continues to smoke ½ pack of cigarettes a day and does not participate in any exercise. He does not "see any reason" to increase his fluid intake. His SpO_2 ranges from 78% to 84%. He must do his self-care activities slowly. His physician has told him that if he gradually increases his exercise, drinks more fluids, and stops smoking, his respiratory status will improve. Presently he is admitted for right upper lobe pneumonia. His vital signs are temperature, 100.4° F; blood pressure, 130/90 mm Hg; pulse, 88 beats per minute; respirations, 26 breaths per minute; and SpO_2, 87%.

Assessment Activities	Findings/Defining Characteristics*
Ask Mr. Edwards how long he has had this cough.	He replies, "I have a morning **cough** every day, but this cough is different. It started about a week ago."
Ask Mr. Edwards what is different about this cough.	He replies, "My ribs are getting sore. I can't cough up anything, my **mouth** is **dry,** and I have become more **fatigued.**"
Observe Mr. Edwards's skin and mucous membranes.	**Skin and mucous membranes** are **dry**
Auscultate lung fields.	**Abnormal lung sounds** in lower lobes bilaterally.
Ask Mr. Edwards to produce a sputum sample.	Sputum is **thick,** and **discolored** yellow to yellow-green.

***Defining characteristics** are shown in bold type.

Nursing Diagnosis: Ineffective airway clearance related to retained thick pulmonary secretions.

Planning

Goal	Expected Outcomes (NOC)†
	Respiratory Status: Airway Patency
Mr. Edwards will be able to effectively clear secretions.	Lung sounds will be normal in 48 hours.
	Mr. Edwards will notice increased ease in coughing.
	Sputum will be thin and white.
	Respiratory rate will be within 20 to 24 breaths per minute in 48 hours.
Mr. Edwards will increase oral hydration.	Mr. Edwards will drink 1000 mL water every 24 hours.
	Mr. Edwards will verbalize that his mouth is not dry.

†Outcome classification labels from Moorhead S and others: *Nursing outcomes classification (NOC),* ed 4, St. Louis, 2008, Mosby.

Interventions (NIC)‡

Interventions (NIC)‡	Rationale
Airway Management	
Increase fluids to 1000 mL in 24 hours.	Fluids help to liquefy secretions and promote ease of removal (Snow and others, 2001). Fluids will relieve oral mucosa and skin dryness.
Offer fluids Mr. Edwards prefers.	
Have Mr. Edwards deep breathe and cough every 2 hours four to five times.	Retained secretions predispose client to atelectasis and pneumonia (Day and others, 2002).
Teach Mr. Edwards effective cough techniques.	Coughing techniques will help to clear the airway effectively and decrease fatigue from ineffective coughing (Snow and others, 2001).
Initiate chest physiotherapy (CPT) if there is evidence of infiltrates on chest x-ray film.	Standards for CPT include sputum production greater than 30 ml/day or infiltrates on chest x-ray film (American Association of Respiratory Care [AARC], 1991; Snow and others, 2001).

‡Intervention classification labels from Bulechek GM, Butcher HK, and Dochterman JM: *Nursing interventions classification (NIC),* ed 5, St. Louis, 2008, Mosby.

Evaluation

Nursing Actions	Client Response/Finding	Achievement of Outcome
Ask Mr. Edwards if he can deep breathe and cough.	Mr. Edwards reports it is easier to cough up his secretions.	Airway clears with coughing.
Auscultate the chest.	Mr. Edwards reports that he has not heard any rattling in his chest.	Lung sounds are normal.
Monitor respiratory rate.	Mr. Edwards says it is easer to breathe.	Rate is between 20 and 24 breaths per minute.
Assess Mr. Edwards' level of hydration.	Mucous membranes are moist.	Oral membranes are pink and moist.
Observe sputum.	Mr. Edwards states, "My sputum is thinner and white now."	Sputum is thin and white.

CONCEPT MAP

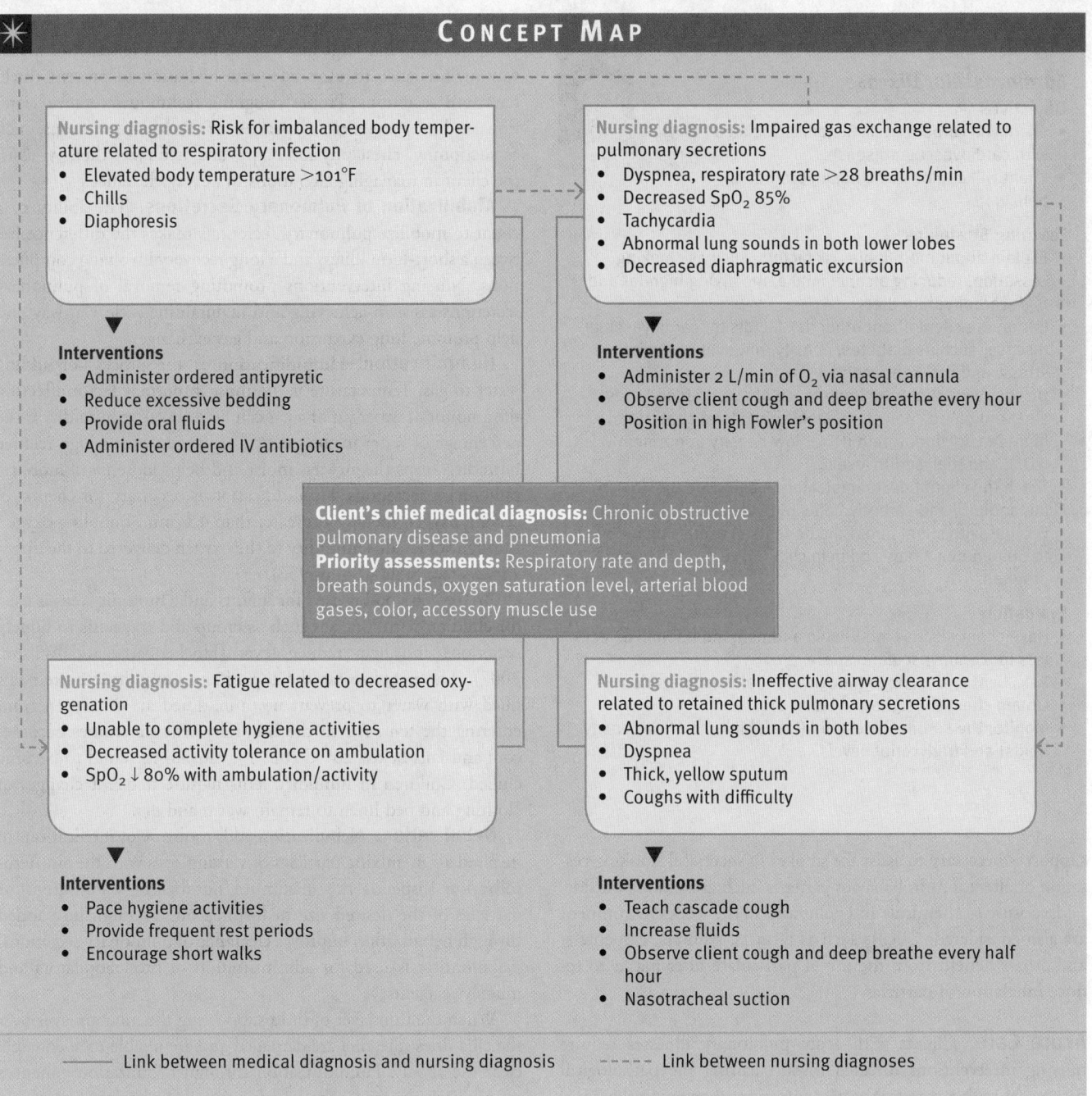

Nursing diagnosis: Risk for imbalanced body temperature related to respiratory infection
- Elevated body temperature >101°F
- Chills
- Diaphoresis

Interventions
- Administer ordered antipyretic
- Reduce excessive bedding
- Provide oral fluids
- Administer ordered IV antibiotics

Nursing diagnosis: Impaired gas exchange related to pulmonary secretions
- Dyspnea, respiratory rate >28 breaths/min
- Decreased SpO_2 85%
- Tachycardia
- Abnormal lung sounds in both lower lobes
- Decreased diaphragmatic excursion

Interventions
- Administer 2 L/min of O_2 via nasal cannula
- Observe client cough and deep breathe every hour
- Position in high Fowler's position

Client's chief medical diagnosis: Chronic obstructive pulmonary disease and pneumonia
Priority assessments: Respiratory rate and depth, breath sounds, oxygen saturation level, arterial blood gases, color, accessory muscle use

Nursing diagnosis: Fatigue related to decreased oxygenation
- Unable to complete hygiene activities
- Decreased activity tolerance on ambulation
- SpO_2 ↓ 80% with ambulation/activity

Interventions
- Pace hygiene activities
- Provide frequent rest periods
- Encourage short walks

Nursing diagnosis: Ineffective airway clearance related to retained thick pulmonary secretions
- Abnormal lung sounds in both lobes
- Dyspnea
- Thick, yellow sputum
- Coughs with difficulty

Interventions
- Teach cascade cough
- Increase fluids
- Observe client cough and deep breathe every half hour
- Nasotracheal suction

——— Link between medical diagnosis and nursing diagnosis   - - - - - Link between nursing diagnoses

Figure 40-8 Concept map for Mr. Edwards.

Exercise is a key factor in promoting and maintaining a healthy heart and lungs. Encourage clients to exercise at least 3 to 4 times a week for 30 to 60 minutes. Aerobic exercise is necessary to improve lung and heart function and strengthen muscles. Walking is an efficient way to achieve a good aerobic workout. Many shopping malls have programs allowing people to walk in the enclosed mall before the shops open. During the hot summer months teach clients to limit activities to early in the day or late in the evening, when temperatures are lower. Teach clients how to maintain adequate hydration and sodium intake, especially if they are taking diuretics.

Clients with cardiopulmonary alterations need to minimize their risk for infection, especially during the winter months. Teach clients to avoid large, crowded places; keep their mouth

and nose covered; and be sure to dress warmly, including a scarf, hat, and gloves. This is especially important during the peak of the influenza season.

Clients with known cardiac disease and those with multiple risk factors are cautioned to avoid exertion in cold weather. Shoveling snow is especially risky and often precipitates a cardiac event. Other activities, such as hanging holiday lights and decorations in the extreme cold, will possibly precipitate chest pain and bronchospasm.

Environmental Pollutants. Avoiding exposure to secondhand smoke is essential to maintaining optimal cardiopulmonary function. Most businesses and restaurants now ban smoking or have separate areas designated as smoking areas. If clients are exposed to secondhand smoke in their home environments, counseling and

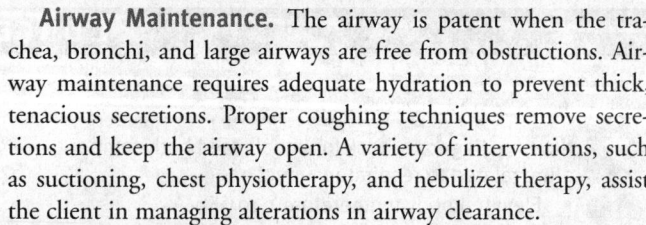

> ✳ **BOX 40-10**   **CLIENT TEACHING**
>
> ### Cardiovascular Disease
>
> **Objectives**
> - Client will verbalize risk factors associated with cardiovascular disease.
> - Client will demonstrate health promotion behaviors.
>
> **Teaching Strategies**
> - Explain about modifiable risk factors, such as smoking cessation, reducing alcohol intake, modifying high-fat and high-carbohydrate diets.
> - Inform the client about other risk factors for cardiovascular disease, such as diabetes, obesity, physical inactivity, stress, and oral contraceptives.
> - Discuss with client the importance of regular blood pressure and blood cholesterol monitoring: total cholesterol, high-density lipoprotein (HDL), low-density lipoprotein (LDL), and triglyceride levels.
> - Teach the client how to implement a balanced diet low in fat, sodium, and carbohydrates. Provide sample menus.
> - Discuss with client about the benefits of exercising for 30 to 60 minutes a day, and help client develop an exercise program.
>
> **Evaluation**
> - Have client discuss modifiable and nonmodifiable risk factors for cardiovascular disease.
> - Ask client to describe strategies for balanced nutrition.
> - Obtain client's weight and blood pressure.
> - Monitor the serum cholesterol (total, high- and low-density lipids) and triglyceride levels.

support is necessary to assist the smoker in successful smoking cessation or alterations in behavior patterns, such as smoking outside.

Exposure to chemicals and pollutants in the work environment are also considered. Clients such as farmers, painters, carpenters, and others benefit from the use of particulate filter masks to reduce inhalation of particles.

Acute Care. Clients with acute pulmonary illnesses require nursing interventions directed toward halting the pathological process, as with a respiratory tract infection; shortening the duration and severity of the illness, such as hospitalization with pneumonia; and preventing complications from the illness or treatments, such as hospital-acquired infection resulting from invasive procedures.

Dyspnea Management. Dyspnea is difficult to measure and treat. Treatments are individualized for each client, and more than one therapy is usually implemented. Treat the underlying process causing dyspnea, then add additional therapies (e.g., pharmacological measures, oxygen therapy, physical techniques, and psychosocial techniques). Pharmacological agents include bronchodilators, inhaled steroids, mucolytics, and low-dose antianxiety medications. Oxygen therapy reduces dyspnea associated with exercise. Physical techniques, such as cardiopulmonary reconditioning (e.g., exercise, breathing techniques, and cough control), help reduce dyspnea. Last, relaxation techniques, biofeedback, and meditation help reduce dyspnea.

Airway Maintenance. The airway is patent when the trachea, bronchi, and large airways are free from obstructions. Airway maintenance requires adequate hydration to prevent thick, tenacious secretions. Proper coughing techniques remove secretions and keep the airway open. A variety of interventions, such as suctioning, chest physiotherapy, and nebulizer therapy, assist the client in managing alterations in airway clearance.

Mobilization of Pulmonary Secretions. The ability of a client to mobilize pulmonary secretions makes the difference between a short-term illness and a long recovery involving complications. Nursing interventions promoting removal of pulmonary secretions assist in achieving and maintaining a clear airway and help promote lung expansion and gas exchange.

Humidification. **Humidification** is the process of adding water to gas. Temperature is the most important factor affecting the amount of water vapor a gas can hold. Relative humidity is the percentage of water in the gas. Air or oxygen with a high relative humidity keeps the airways moist and helps loosen and mobilize pulmonary secretions. Humidification is necessary for clients receiving oxygen therapy at greater than 4 L/min. Bubbling oxygen through water adds humidity to the oxygen delivered to the upper airways (see Skill 40-4, p. 956).

An oxygen hood is used for infants and a humidity tent is used for children with illnesses such as croup and tracheitis to liquefy secretions and help reduce fever (Hockenberry and Wilson, 2007). The nebulizer at the top of the humidity tent remains filled with water to prevent nonhumidified air or oxygen from entering the tent. Air in the humidity tent sometimes becomes cool and falls below 20° C (68° F), causing the child to become chilled. Children in humidity tents require frequent changes of clothing and bed linen to remain warm and dry.

Nebulization. **Nebulization** adds moisture or medications to inspired air by mixing particles of varying sizes with the air. Aerosolization suspends the maximum number of water drops or particles of the desired size in inspired air. The moisture added through nebulization improves clearance of pulmonary secretions. Nebulization is used for administration of bronchodilators and mucolytic agents.

When the thin layer of fluid supporting the mucous layer over the cilia dries, the cilia are damaged and are unable to adequately clear the airway. Humidification through nebulization enhances mucociliary clearance, the body's natural mechanism for removing mucus and cellular debris from the respiratory tract.

Chest Physiotherapy. **Chest physiotherapy** (CPT) is a group of therapies used to mobilize pulmonary secretions. These therapies include postural drainage, chest percussion, and vibration (Oermann and others, 2000). Chest physiotherapy is followed by productive coughing and suctioning of the client who has a decreased ability to cough. Chest physiotherapy is recommended for clients who produce greater than 30 mL of sputum per day or have evidence of atelectasis by chest x-ray examination. This procedure is safe for infants and young children; however, at times conditions and diseases unique to children contraindicate this procedure. Chest physiotherapy is for a select group of clients. Box 40-11 describes the guidelines to determine if CPT is indicated for the client.

Postural drainage is a component of pulmonary hygiene; it consists of drainage, positioning, and turning and is sometimes

✳ BOX 40-11 Guidelines for Chest Physiotherapy

Base nursing care and selection of chest physiotherapy (CPT) skills on specific assessment findings. The following guidelines help in physical assessment and subsequent decision making:

- Know the client's normal range of vital signs. Conditions such as atelectasis and pneumonia requiring CPT affect vital signs. The degree of change is related to the level of hypoxia, overall cardiopulmonary status, and tolerance to activity.
- Conduct a respiratory assessment to confirm need for chest physiotherapy: sputum production; effectiveness of cough; history of pulmonary problems successfully relieved with CPT; abnormal lung sounds; documented conditions, such as atelectasis, pneumonia, and changes in oxygenation status (AARC, 1991).
- Know the client's medications. Certain medications, particularly diuretics and antihypertensives, cause fluid and hemodynamic changes, which decreases the client's tolerance to the positional changes of postural drainage. Steroid medications increase the client's risk of pathological rib fractures and often contraindicate rib shaking.
- Know the client's medical history. Certain conditions, such as increased intracranial pressure, spinal cord injuries, active hemorrhage, pulmonary embolism, thoracic trauma or surgery, and abdominal aneurysm resection, contraindicate the positional changes of postural drainage. In addition, underlying physical conditions contraindicate specific positions, such as Trendelenburg's (AARC, 1991).
- Know the client's level of cognitive function. Participation in controlled coughing techniques requires the client to follow instructions.
- Be aware of the client's exercise tolerance. CPT maneuvers are fatiguing. When the client is not used to physical activity, initial tolerance to the maneuvers is often decreased. However, with gradual increases in activity and planned CPT, client tolerance for the procedure improves.

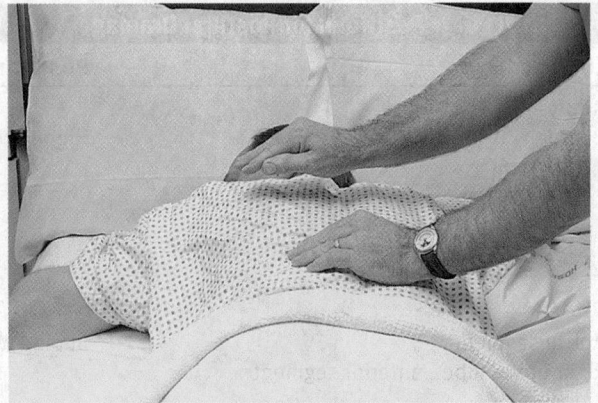

Figure 40-9 Chest wall percussion, alternating hand clapping against the client's chest wall.

accompanied by chest percussion and vibration (AARC, 1991). It improves secretion clearance and oxygenation. Positioning includes most lung segments (Table 40-7) and helps to drain secretions from specific segments of the lungs and bronchi into the trachea. Some clients do not require postural drainage of all lung segments, and clinical assessment is crucial in identifying specific lung segments requiring postural drainage. For example, clients with left lower lobe atelectasis require postural drainage of only the affected region, whereas a child with cystic fibrosis often requires postural drainage of all lung segments.

Chest percussion involves striking the chest wall over the area being drained. Position the hand so that the fingers and thumb touch and cup the hands. Percussion on the surface of the chest wall sends waves of varying amplitude and frequency through the chest, changing the consistency and location of the sputum. Perform chest percussion by striking the chest wall alternately with cupped hands (Figure 40-9). Perform percussion over a single layer of clothing, not over buttons, snaps, or zippers. The single layer of clothing prevents slapping the client's skin. Thicker or multiple layers of material dampen the vibrations.

Percussion is contraindicated in clients with bleeding disorders, osteoporosis, or fractured ribs. Take caution to percuss the lung fields and not the scapular regions, or trauma will possibly occur to the skin and underlying musculoskeletal structures.

Vibration is a fine, shaking pressure applied to the chest wall only during expiration. This technique increases the velocity and turbulence of exhaled air, facilitating secretion removal. Vibration increases the exhalation of trapped air and shakes mucus loose and induces a cough.

Suctioning Techniques. Suctioning is necessary when the client is unable to clear respiratory secretions from the airways. Suctioning techniques include oropharyngeal and nasopharyngeal suctioning, orotracheal and nasotracheal suctioning, and suctioning an artificial airway.

In most cases use sterile technique for suctioning because the oropharynx and trachea are considered sterile. The mouth is considered clean, and therefore you suction oral secretions after suctioning of the oropharynx and trachea. In the home setting a "clean" versus "sterile" technique is used because the client is not exposed to pathogens common to health care settings (AARC, 1999).

Each type of suctioning requires the use of a rounded-tipped catheter with a number of side holes at the distal end of the catheter. Client assessment determines the frequency of suctioning. When you auscultate secretions, and other methods to remove airway secretions have failed, suctioning is indicated (AARC, 2004). Too-frequent suctioning puts the client at risk for development of hypoxemia, hypotension, arrhythmias, and possible trauma to the mucosa of the lungs (Day and others, 2002).

Oropharyngeal and Nasopharyngeal Suctioning. Oropharyngeal or nasopharyngeal suctioning is used when the client is able to cough effectively but is unable to clear secretions by expectorating or swallowing. Apply suction after the client has coughed (Skill 40-1). As the amount of pulmonary secretions is reduced and the client is less fatigued, the client is then able to expectorate or swallow the mucus and suctioning is no longer necessary.

Orotracheal and Nasotracheal Suctioning. Orotracheal or nasotracheal suctioning is necessary when the client with pulmonary secretions is unable to manage secretions by coughing and does not have an artificial airway present (see Skill 40-1, p. 934). A catheter is passed through the mouth or nose into the trachea. The nose is the preferred route because stimulation of the gag reflex is minimal. The procedure is similar to nasopharyngeal

Text continued on p. 940

✳ TABLE 40-7 Positions for Postural Drainage

LUNG SEGMENT	POSITION OF CLIENT
Adult	
Bilateral	High-Fowler's position
Apical segments Right upper lobe—anterior segment	Supine with head of bed elevated 15 to 30 degrees
Left upper lobe—anterior segment	Supine with head elevated
Right upper lobe—posterior segment	Side lying with right side of chest elevated on pillows
Left upper lobe—posterior segment	Side lying with left side of chest elevated on pillows
Right middle lobe—anterior segment	Three-fourths supine position with dependent lung in Trendelenburg's position
Right middle lobe—posterior segment	Prone with thorax and abdomen elevated
Both lower lobes—anterior segments	Supine in Trendelenburg's position

✳ **TABLE 40-7** Positions for Postural Drainage—cont'd

LUNG SEGMENT	POSITION OF CLIENT
Adult—cont'd	
Left lower lobe—lateral segment	Left lateral in Trendelenburg's position

Right lower lobe—lateral segment	Right side-lying in Trendelenburg's position

Right lower lobe—posterior segment	Prone in Trendelenburg's position with abdomen and thorax elevated

Both lower lobes—posterior segments	Prone in Trendelenburg's position with abdomen and thorax elevated

Child	
Bilateral—apical segments	Sitting on nurse's lap, leaning slightly forward, flexed over pillow

Bilateral—middle anterior segments	Sitting on nurse's lap, leaning against nurse

Bilateral lobes— anterior segments	Lying supine on nurse's lap, back supported with pillow

✳ **SKILL 40-1**   **S U C T I O N I N G**   `Video`

Delegation Considerations

The skill of nasotracheal suctioning and suctioning a new artificial airway cannot be delegated. The skill of oropharyngeal suctioning can be delegated. When a client has an established tracheostomy and when you determine that the client is stable, you can delegate suctioning a tracheostomy. The nurse instructs nursing assistive personnel about:

- Unique modifications of the skill, such as the need to reapply any supplemental oxygen equipment following the procedure
- Reporting any change in client's respiratory status, secretion color or volume, or unresolved coughing or gagging
- Reporting any change in client's color, vital signs, or complaints of pain

Equipment

- Appropriate-size suction catheter (smallest diameter that will remove secretions effectively) or Yankauer catheter (oral suction). Catheter's outer diameter should not exceed half of internal diameter of an artificial airway (Moore, 2003)
- Nasal or oral airway (if indicated)
- Oropharyngeal suctioning: clean gloves
- Two sterile gloves or one sterile and one clean disposable glove, or one disposable (refer to technique)
- Clean towel or paper drape
- Portable or wall suction
- Mask or face shield
- Connecting tube (6 feet)
- Small Y adapter (if catheter does not have a suction-control port)
- Pulse oximeter
- Stethoscope
- Water-soluble lubricant
- Sterile basin
- Sterile normal saline solution or water (about 100 mL)

STEPS	RATIONALE
1. Assess for signs and symptoms of upper and lower airway obstruction requiring nasotracheal or orotracheal suctioning: abnormal respiratory rate, adventitious sounds, nasal secretions, gurgling, drooling, restlessness, gastric secretions or vomitus in mouth, and coughing without clearing secretions from airway.	Physical signs and symptoms result from decreased oxygen to tissues, as well as pooling of secretions in upper and lower airways. Complete assessment before and following the suction procedure (AARC, 2004; Moore, 2003).
2. Assess signs and symptoms associated with hypoxia and hypercapnia: decreased SpO_2, increased pulse and blood pressure, increased respiratory rate, apprehension, anxiety, decreased ability to concentrate, lethargy, decreased level of consciousness (especially acute), increased fatigue, dizziness, behavioral changes (especially irritability), dysrhythmias, pallor, and cyanosis.	Physical signs and symptoms resulting from decreased oxygen to tissues indicate need for suctioning (AARC, 2004).
3. Assess for risk factors for upper or lower airway obstruction.	
a. Pulmonary disease: chronic obstructive pulmonary disease, pulmonary infection.	Increases client's risk for retaining pulmonary secretions. Clients with pulmonary infections are prone to increased secretions that are thicker and sometimes more difficult to expectorate.
b. Changes in level of consciousness	Impairs client's ability to cough independently or follow instructions to cough and clear airway.
c. Fluid balance	Fluid overload increases amount of secretions. Dehydration promotes thicker secretions.
d. Lack of humidity	The environment influences secretion formation and gas exchange, necessitating airway suctioning when client cannot clear secretions effectively.
e. Decreased cough or gag reflex	Increases client's risk for aspiration and subsequent pulmonary infection.
f. Anatomy	Abnormal anatomy or head and neck trauma impairs normal drainage of secretions. For example, nasal swelling, a deviated septum, or facial fractures may impair nasal drainage. Tumors in or around the lower airway impair secretion removal by occluding or externally compressing the lumen of the airway.
4. Identify contraindications to **nasotracheal suctioning**: occluded nasal passages; nasal bleeding, epiglottitis, or croup; acute head, facial, or neck injury or surgery, coagulopathy, or bleeding disorder; irritable airway or laryngospasm or bronchospasm; gastric surgery with high anastomosis; myocardial infarction (AARC, 2004).	These conditions are **contraindicated because the passage of a catheter through the nasal route** causes trauma to existing facial trauma or surgery, increases nasal bleeding, or causes severe bleeding in the presence of bleeding disorders. In the presence of epiglottitis, croup, laryngospasm, or irritable airway, the entrance of a suction catheter via the nasal route causes intractable coughing, hypoxemia, and severe bronchospasm necessitating emergency intubation or tracheostomy (Moore, 2003).

✳ SKILL 40-1   **SUCTIONING—CONT'D**

STEPS

5. Obtain sputum microbiology data.

6. Assess client's understanding of procedure.
7. Explain to client how procedure will help clear airway and relieve breathing problems and that temporary coughing, sneezing, gagging, or shortness of breath is normal. Encourage client to cough out secretions. Practice coughing, if able. Splint surgical incisions, if necessary.

8. Explain importance of and encourage coughing during procedure.
9. Assist client with assuming position comfortable for nurse and client (usually semi-Fowler's or sitting upright with head hyperextended, unless contraindicated).

10. Place pulse oximeter on client's finger. Take reading, and leave pulse oximeter in place.

11. Place towel across client's chest.

12. Perform hand hygiene, and apply face shield if splashing is likely.
13. Connect one end of connecting tubing to suction machine, and place other end in convenient location near client. Turn suction device on and set vacuum regulator to appropriate negative pressure (120 to 150 mm Hg) (AARC, 2004).

14. If indicated, increase supplemental oxygen therapy to 100% or as ordered by physician. Encourage client to deep breathe.

15. Preparation for all types of suctioning.
    A. Open appropriate suction kit or catheter, using aseptic technique. If sterile drape is available, place it across client's chest or on the over-bed table. Do not allow the suction catheter to touch any nonsterile surfaces.
    B. Unwrap or open sterile basin, and place on bedside table. Fill basin or cup with approximately 100 mL of sterile normal saline solution or water (see illustration).
    C. Check that suction is functioning properly by suctioning a small amount of water from basin.

RATIONALE

Certain bacteria are easier to transmit or require isolation because of virulence or antibiotic resistance.
Reveals need for client instruction and encourages cooperation.
Encourages cooperation and minimizes risks, anxiety, and pain.

Facilitates secretion removal and reduces frequency and duration of future suctioning.
Reduces stimulation of gag reflex, promotes client comfort and secretion drainage, and prevents aspiration. Position lessens strain on nurse's back. Hyperextension facilitates insertion of catheter into trachea.
Provides baseline SpO_2 to determine client's response to suctioning.
Reduces transmission of microorganisms by protecting gown from secretions.
Reduces transmission of microorganisms.

Excessive negative pressure damages nasal pharyngeal and tracheal mucosa and induces greater hypoxia. Negative pressures should not exceed 150 mm Hg because higher pressure increases risk for airway trauma, hypoxemia, and atelectasis (AARC, 2004).
Hyperoxygenation provides some protection from suction-induced decline in oxygenation. Hyperoxygenation is most effective in the presence of hyperinflation, such as encouraging the client to deep breathe or increase ventilator tidal volume settings (Bourgault and others, 2006; Moore, 2003).

Prepares catheter and prevents transmission of microorganisms. Provides sterile surface on which to lay suction catheter between passes, if needed.

Solution used to flush catheter.

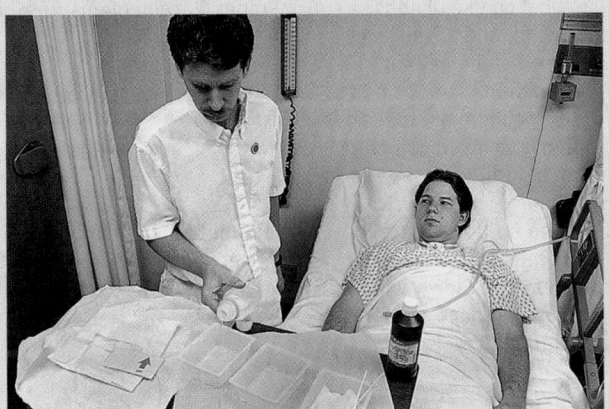

STEP 15b Pouring sterile saline into basin.

Continued

✳ **SKILL 40-1**   **SUCTIONING—CONT'D**

STEPS	RATIONALE
16. Suction airway.	
A. Oropharyngeal suctioning	
(1) Apply clean disposable glove to dominant hand.	Suction of oral cavity does not require sterile glove use.
(2) Remove oxygen mask if present. Oral cannula remains in place (if present).	Allows access to client's mouth.

Critical Decision Point: Be prepared to quickly reapply oxygen mask if SpO₂ falls or respiratory distress develops during or at the end of suctioning.

STEPS	RATIONALE
(3) Insert catheter into client's mouth. With suction applied, move catheter around mouth, including pharynx and gum line, until secretions are cleared.	If catheter does not have a suction control to apply intermittent suction, take care not to allow suction tip to invaginate oral mucosal surfaces with continuous suction (Moore, 2003).
(4) Encourage client to cough, and repeat suctioning if needed. Replace oxygen mask if used.	Coughing moves secretions from lower to upper airways into mouth.
(5) Suction water from basin through catheter until catheter is cleared of secretions.	Clearing secretions before they dry reduces probability of transmission of microorganisms and enhances delivery of preset suction pressures.
(6) Place catheter in a clean, dry area for reuse with suction turned off or within client's reach, with suction on, if client is capable of suctioning self.	Facilitates prompt removal of airway secretions when suctioning is necessary in the future.
B. Nasopharyngeal and nasotracheal suctioning	
(1) Open lubricant. Squeeze small amount onto open sterile catheter package without touching package.	Prepares lubricant while maintaining sterility. Water-soluble lubricant helps to avoid lipid aspiration pneumonia. Excessive lubricant occludes catheter.
(2) Apply sterile glove to each hand, or apply nonsterile glove to nondominant hand and sterile glove to dominant hand.	Reduces transmission of microorganisms and allows nurse to maintain sterility of suction catheter.

Critical Decision Point: In selected settings, such as the home or long-term care facility, or with clients with an established tracheostomy who do not have an airway infection, use a clean technique (AARC, 1999).

STEPS	RATIONALE
(3) Pick up suction catheter with dominant hand without touching nonsterile surfaces. Pick up connecting tubing with nondominant hand. Secure catheter to tubing.	Maintains catheter sterility. Connects catheter to suction.
(4) Check that the equipment is functioning properly by suctioning small amount of normal saline solution from basin.	Ensures equipment function; lubricates catheter and tubing.
(5) Lightly coat distal 6 to 8 cm (2 to 3 inches) of catheter with water-soluble lubricant.	Lubricates catheter for easier insertion.
(6) Remove oxygen delivery device, if applicable, with nondominant hand. Without applying suction and using dominant thumb and forefinger, gently insert catheter into naris during inhalation.	Application of suction pressure while introducing catheter into nasopharyngeal tissues increases risk of damage to mucosa. When advanced into trachea, suction could damage mucosa and increase risk of hypoxia.
(7) *Nasopharyngeal:* Follow natural course of naris; slightly slant catheter downward, and advance to back of pharynx. In adults insert catheter about 16 cm (6 to 7 inches); in older children, 8 to 12 cm (3 to 5 inches); in infants and young children, 4 to 8 cm (2 to 3 inches). Rule of thumb is to insert catheter distance from tip of nose (or mouth) to base of earlobe.	Proper placement ensures removal of pharyngeal secretions.
(a) Apply intermittent suction for up to 10 to 15 seconds by placing and releasing nondominant thumb over catheter vent. Slowly withdraw catheter while rotating it back and forth between thumb and forefinger.	Intermittent suction up to 15 seconds safely removes pharyngeal secretions (AARC, 2004). Suction time greater than 15 seconds increases risk for suction-induced hypoxemia (Oh and Seo, 2003).

STEPS

(8) *Nasotracheal:* Follow natural course of naris, and advance catheter slightly slanted and downward to just above entrance into trachea. Allow client to take a breath. Quickly insert catheter about 16 to 20 cm (6 to 8 inches in adult) into trachea (see illustration). Client will begin to cough. NOTE: In older children advance 14 to 20 cm (5½ to 8 inches); in young children and infants, 8 to 14 cm (3 to 5½ inches).

RATIONALE

Ensures catheter will be inserted into trachea with minimum stress to client.

Critical Decision Point: Insert catheter during client inhalation, especially if inserting catheter into trachea because epiglottis is open. **Do not insert during swallowing,** or catheter will most likely enter esophagus. **Never** apply suction during insertion. Client should cough. If client gags or becomes nauseated, catheter is most likely in esophagus and needs to be removed.

(a) *Positioning option for nasotracheal suctioning:* In some instances turning client's head to right helps suction the left mainstem bronchus; turning head to left helps suction the right mainstem bronchus. If you feel resistance after insertion of catheter to maximum recommended distance, catheter has probably hit carina. Pull catheter back 1 cm before applying suction.

Turning the client's head to the side elevates the bronchial passage on the opposite side and facilitates passage of the catheter.

Critical Decision Point: Use nasal approach, and perform tracheal suctioning before pharyngeal suctioning whenever possible. The mouth and pharynx contain more bacteria than the trachea does. If copious oral secretions are present before beginning the procedure, suction mouth with oral suction device.

(b) Apply intermittent suction for up to 10 to 15 seconds by placing and releasing nondominant thumb over vent of catheter and slowly withdrawing catheter while rotating it back and forth between dominant thumb and forefinger. Encourage client to cough. Replace oxygen device, if applicable.

Intermittent suction and rotation of catheter prevent injury to mucosa. If catheter "grabs" mucosa, remove thumb to release suction. Suctioning longer than 10 seconds causes cardiopulmonary compromise, usually from hypoxemia or vagal overload.

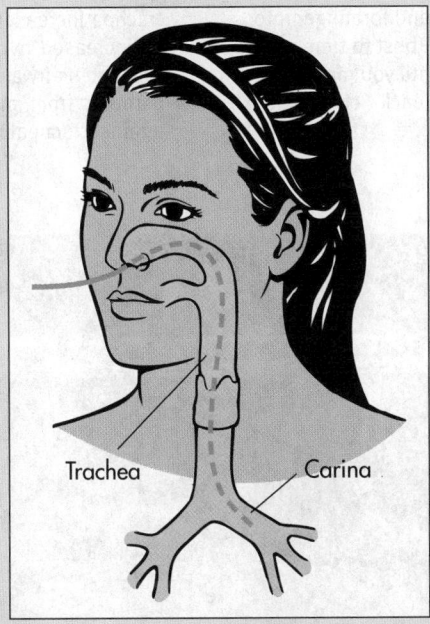

STEP 16B(8) Distance of insertion of nasotracheal catheter.

Continued

✳ **SKILL 40-1**   **SUCTIONING—CONT'D**

Critical Decision Point: If ordered to monitor client's vital signs and oxygen saturation during procedure, note whether there is a change of 20 beats per minute (either increase or decrease) or if pulse oximetry falls below 90% or 5% from baseline (Akgul and Akyolcu, 2002).

STEPS

(9) Rinse catheter and connecting tubing with normal saline or water until cleared.

(10) Assess for need to repeat suctioning procedure. Do not perform more than two passes with catheter. Allow at least 1 minute between suction passes for ventilation and oxygenation (AARC, 2004). Ask client to deep breathe and cough, or preoxygenate with 100% supplemental oxygen.

C. **Performing Artificial Airway (Tracheostomy or Endotracheal Tube) Suctioning**

(1) Apply face shield.

(2) Apply one sterile glove to each hand, or apply non-sterile glove to nondominant hand and sterile glove to dominant hand.

(3) Pick up suction catheter with dominant hand without touching nonsterile surfaces. Pick up connecting tubing with nondominant hand. Secure catheter to tubing.

(4) Check that equipment is functioning properly by suctioning small amount of saline from basin.

(5) Hyperinflate and/or hyperoxygenate client before suctioning, using manual resuscitation Ambu-bag connected to oxygen source or sigh mechanism on mechanical ventilator. Some mechanical ventilators have a button that when pushed delivers 100% oxygen for a few minutes and then resets to the previous value.

(6) If client is receiving mechanical ventilation, open swivel adapter, or if necessary remove oxygen or humidity delivery device with nondominant hand.

(7) Without applying suction, gently but quickly insert catheter using dominant thumb and forefinger into artificial airway (see illustration) (best to time catheter insertion with inspiration) until you meet resistance or client coughs; then pull back 1 cm (½ inch).

RATIONALE

Removes secretions from catheter. Secretions that remain in suction catheter or connecting tubing decrease suctioning efficiency.

Observe for alterations in cardiopulmonary status. Suctioning induces hypoxemia, dysrhythmias, laryngospasm, and bronchospasm (AARC, 2004). Deep breathing or preoxygenation hyperventilates and reoxygenates alveoli and reduces the risk for suction-induced hypoxemia (Bourgault and others, 2006). Repeated passes clear the airway of excessive secretions but also remove oxygen and will possibly induce laryngospasm.

Reduces transmission of microorganisms.

Reduces transmission of microorganisms and allows nurse to maintain sterility of suction catheter.

Maintains catheter sterility. Establishes suction.

Ensures equipment function; lubricates catheter and tubing.

Hyperinflation decreases the risk for atelectasis caused by negative pressure of suctioning (Moore, 2003). Preoxygenation converts large proportion of resident lung gas to 100% oxygen to offset amount used in metabolic consumption while ventilator or oxygenation is interrupted, as well as to offset volume lost during suction procedure (Bourgault and others, 2006; Day and others 2002; Oh and Seo, 2003).

Exposes artificial airway.

Application of suction pressure while introducing catheter into trachea increases risk of damage to tracheal mucosa, as well as increased hypoxia related to removal of entrained oxygen present in airways. Pulling back stimulates cough and removes catheter from mucosal wall so that catheter is not resting against tracheal mucosa during suctioning.

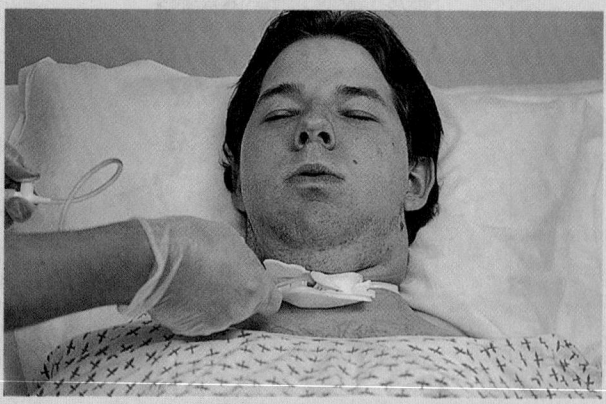

STEP 16C(7) Suctioning tracheostomy.

✳ **SKILL 40-1**   **SUCTIONING—CONT'D**

Critical Decision Point: If unable to insert catheter past the end of the ET tube, the catheter is probably caught in the Murphy eye (i.e., side hole at the distal end of the ET tube that allows for collateral airflow in the event of main stem intubation). If this happens, rotate the catheter to reposition it away from the Murphy eye, or withdraw it slightly and reinsert with the next inhalation. Usually the catheter meets resistance at the carina. One indication that the catheter is at the carina is acute onset of coughing because the carina contains many cough receptors. Pull the catheter back 1 cm (½ inch).

STEPS

(8) Apply intermittent suction by placing and releasing nondominant thumb over vent of catheter; slowly withdraw catheter while rotating it back and forth between dominant thumb and forefinger. Encourage client to cough. Watch for respiratory distress.

RATIONALE

Intermittent suction and rotation of catheter prevent injury to tracheal mucosal lining. If catheter "grabs" mucosa, remove thumb to release suction.

Critical Decision Point: If client develops respiratory distress during the suction procedure, immediately withdraw catheter and supply additional oxygen and breaths as needed. You can administer oxygen directly through the catheter in an emergency. Disconnect suction and attach oxygen at prescribed flow rate through the catheter.

(9) If client is receiving mechanical ventilation, close swivel adapter or replace oxygen delivery device.

Reestablishes the artificial airway.

(10) Encourage client to deep breathe, if able. Some clients respond well to several manual breaths from the mechanical ventilator or Ambu-bag.

Reoxygenates and expands alveoli. Suctioning sometimes causes hypoxemia and atelectasis.

(11) Rinse catheter and connecting tubing with normal saline until clear. Use continuous suction.

Removes catheter secretions. Secretions left in tubing decrease suction and provide environment for microorganism growth. Secretions left in connecting tube decrease suctioning efficiency.

(12) Assess client's cardiopulmonary status for secretion clearance and complications. Repeat Steps 16C(6) through 16C(12) once or twice more to clear secretions. Allow adequate time (at least 1 full minute) between suction passes for ventilation and hyperoxygenation. Perform nasopharyngeal and oropharyngeal suctioning (Steps 16A, 16B). After performing nasopharyngeal and oropharyngeal suctioning, catheter is contaminated; do not reinsert into ET or tracheostomy tube.

Suctioning sometimes induces dysrhythmias, hypoxia, and bronchospasm and impairs cerebral circulation or adversely affects hemodynamics (AARC, 2004; Akgul and Akyolcu, 2002; Kerr and others, 1999). Repeated passes with suction catheter clear airway of excessive secretions and promote improved oxygenation.

Upper airway is "clean," and lower airway is "sterile." Therefore you can use the same catheter to suction from sterile to clean areas, but not from clean to sterile areas.

17. Complete procedure.
    A. Disconnect catheter from connecting tubing. Roll catheter around fingers of dominant hand. Pull glove off inside out so that catheter remains in glove. Pull off other glove over first glove in same way to contain contaminants. Discard into appropriate receptacle. Turn off suction device.

Reduces transmission of microorganisms. Do not touch clean equipment with contaminated gloves.

    B. Remove towel and place in laundry, or remove drape and discard in appropriate receptacle.
    C. Reposition client as indicated by condition. Reapply clean gloves for client's personal care (e.g., oral hygiene).

Proper positioning based on client's condition promotes comfort, encourages secretion drainage, and reduces risk of aspiration.

    D. If indicated, readjust oxygen to original level.

Helps client's blood oxygen level return to baseline.

Critical Decision Point: Readjust the client's oxygen to avoid increased risk of oxygen toxicity and absorption atelectasis from prolonged administration of high concentrations of oxygen and increased carbon dioxide retention in clients with chronic obstructive lung diseases (Day and others, 2002).

    E. Discard remainder of normal saline into appropriate receptacle. If basin is disposable, discard into appropriate receptacle. If basin is reusable, rinse and place in soiled utility room.

Solution is contaminated.

    F. Remove and discard face shield, and perform hand hygiene.

Reduces transmission of microorganisms.

    G. Place unopened suction kit on suction machine table or at head of bed according to institution preference.

Provides for immediate access of suction catheter and equipment in the event of an emergency or for the next suctioning procedure.

Continued

✳ **SKILL 40-1**   **SUCTIONING—CONT'D**

STEPS

18. Compare client's vital signs and SpO$_2$ saturation before and after suctioning.

19. Ask client if breathing is easier and if congestion is decreased.

20. Auscultate lungs for change in adventitious lung sounds.

21. Observe airway secretions.

RATIONALE

Provides objective data about any physiological effects of suctioning.

Provides subjective confirmation that airway obstruction is relieved with suctioning procedure.

Provides objective information about any improvement in lung sounds.

Provides data to document presence or absence of respiratory tract infection.

Unexpected Outcomes and Related Interventions

1. Client's respiratory status worsens
   a. Limit length of suctioning.
   b. Determine need for more frequent suctioning, possibly of shorter duration.
   c. Notify physician.
2. Bloody secretions
   a. Determine amount of suction pressure used. Decrease if necessary.
   b. Evaluate suctioning frequency.
   c. Provide more frequent oral hygiene.
3. Unable to pass suction catheter through first naris attempted
   a. Try other naris or oral route.
   b. Insert nasal airway, especially if suctioning through client naris frequently.
   c. Guide catheter along naris floor to avoid turbinates.
   d. If obstruction is mucus, apply suction to relieve obstruction, but do not apply suction to mucosa. If you think the obstruction is a blood clot, consult health care provider.
   e. Increase lubrication of catheter.
4. Paroxysms of coughing develop
   a. Administer supplemental oxygen.
   b. Allow client to rest between passes of suction catheter.
   c. Consult physician or health care provider regarding need for inhaled bronchodilators or topical anesthetics.

5. No secretions obtained
   a. Evaluate client's fluid status; increase fluids as appropriate.
   b. Assess for signs of infection.
   c. Determine need for chest physiotherapy.
   d. Assess adequacy of humidification on oxygen delivery device.

Recording and Reporting

- Record the amount, consistency, color, and odor of secretions and client's response to procedure; document client's presuctioning and postsuctioning cardiopulmonary status.

Home Care Considerations

- It is necessary to adhere to best practices for infection control while weighing cost-effectiveness in the presence of a chronic situation. If the client has an established tracheostomy or requires long-term nasotracheal suctioning and infection is not present, clean suction technique is appropriate (AARC, 1999).
- Teach client and family how to practice infection-control measures when emptying the secretion jar. These secretions are emptied in the toilet but have a splash risk. Instruct caregiver to apply mask (shield if available) and gloves and bring the secretion jar as close to the toilet bowel as possible to decrease the risk of splash.

---

suctioning, but the catheter tip is moved farther into the client's trachea. The entire procedure from catheter passage to its removal is done quickly, lasting no longer than 15 seconds (AARC, 2004). Unless in respiratory distress, allow the client to rest between passes of the catheter. If the client is using supplemental oxygen, replace the oxygen cannula or mask during rest periods.

Tracheal Suctioning. Tracheal suctioning occurs through an artificial airway, such as an endotracheal tube or tracheostomy tube. Make sure the suction catheter is no greater than half the size of the internal diameter of the artificial airway (Moore, 2003). Secretion removal should be as atraumatic as possible. To avoid trauma to the mucosa of the lung, never apply suction pressure while inserting the catheter. Once it is inserted, maintain suction pressure between 120 and 150 mm Hg (AARC, 2004). Apply suction intermittently while withdrawing the catheter. Rotating the catheter will enhance removal of secretions that have adhered to the sides of the endotracheal tube. Apply a mask and goggles, and wear a barrier gown to prevent splashes with body fluids.

The practice of normal saline instillation (NSI) into artificial airways to improve secretion removal is inconclusive. Clinical

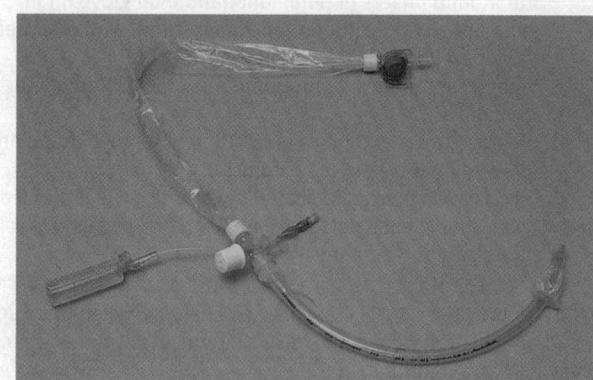

Figure 40-10 Ballard tracheal care, closed suction.

studies comparing the results of suctioning following NSI with standard suctioning have not shown any clinical or significant results (Akgul and Akyolcu, 2002; Moore, 2003). There are anecdotal results supporting the theory that NSI stimulates the client to cough and as a result the airway secretions are loosened and

BOX 40-12

PROCEDURAL GUIDELINES

Closed (In-Line) Suction Catheter

Delegation Considerations: The skill of airway suction with a closed (in-line) suction catheter cannot be routinely delegated. In special situation, such as suctioning a permanent tracheostomy, you may delegate this procedure. The nurse is responsible for the cardiopulmonary assessment and evaluation of the client. The nurse instructs nursing assistive personnel about:

- Any individualized aspects of client care that pertain to suctioning (e.g., position, duration of suction, pressure settings)
- The expected quality, quantity, and color of secretions and to inform the nurse immediately if there are changes
- Client's anticipated response to suction and to immediately report to the nurse changes in vital signs, complaints of pain, shortness of breath, confusion, or increased restlessness

Equipment: Closed system or in-line suction catheter; suction machine, 6 feet of connecting tubing, two clean gloves (optional), face shield

1. Perform assessment as in Skill 40-1, p. 934.
2. Explain the procedure to the client and the importance of coughing during the suctioning procedure.
3. Assist client with assuming a position of comfort for both client and nurse, usually semi-or high-Fowler's position. Place towel across the client's chest.
4. Perform hand hygiene, apply face shield and gloves, and attach suction.
   a. In some settings a respiratory therapist attaches the catheter to the ventilator circuit. If catheter is not already in place, open closed suction catheter package using aseptic technique, attach catheter to ventilator circuit by removing swivel adapter and placing catheter apparatus on endotracheal or tracheostomy tube. Connect Y on ventilator circuit to closed suction catheter with flex tubing (see Figure 40-10).
   b. Connect one end of connecting tubing to suction machine, and connect other to the end of a closed system or in-line suction catheter, if not already done. Turn suction device on, and set vacuum regulator to appropriate negative pressure (see manufacturer's directions).
5. Hyperinflate and/or hyperoxygenate client with Ambu-bag or manual breathing mechanism on mechanical ventilator according to institution protocol and clinical status (usually 100% oxygen).
6. Unlock suction-control mechanism if required by manufacturer. Open saline port, and attach saline syringe or vial.

7. Pick up suction catheter enclosed in plastic sleeve with dominant hand. If client requires normal saline, advance catheter 2 to 3 cm (1 to 1½ inches) and squeeze vial or push syringe with other hand to release 5 to 10 mL of normal saline during inspiratory cycle.

Critical Decision Point The use of normal saline instillation with closed in-line suction catheters is not appropriate for all clients and needs further investigation. Normal saline instillation in conjunction with endotracheal tube suctioning leads to the dispersion of microorganisms into the lower respiratory tract (Fretag and others, 2003; Sole and others, 2002).

8. Insert catheter, use a repeating maneuver of pushing catheter and sliding (or pulling) plastic sleeve back between thumb and forefinger until you feel resistance or client coughs.
9. Encourage client to cough, and apply suction by squeezing on suction-control mechanism while withdrawing catheter. It is difficult to apply intermittent pulses of suction and nearly impossible to rotate the catheter compared with a standard catheter. Be sure to withdraw catheter completely into plastic sheath so it does not obstruct airflow.
10. Reassess cardiopulmonary status, including pulse oximetry, to determine need for subsequent suctioning or complications. Repeat Steps 5 through 9 one to two more times to clear secretions. Allow adequate time (at least 1 full minute) between suction passes for ventilation and reoxygenation.
11. When airway is clear, withdraw catheter completely into sheath. Be sure that colored indicator line on catheter is visible in the sheath. Squeeze vial or push syringe while applying suction to rinse inner lumen of catheter. Use at least 5 to 10 mL of saline to rinse the catheter until it is clear of retained secretions, which cause bacterial growth and increase the risk of infection (Fretag and others, 2003). Lock suction mechanism, if applicable, and turn off suction.
12. If client requires oral or nasal suctioning, perform Skill 40-1, p. 934 with separate standard suction catheter.
13. Reposition client.
14. Remove gloves and face shield and discard into appropriate receptacle, and perform hand hygiene.
15. Compare client's respiratory assessments before and after suctioning and observe airway secretions.

---

dislodged. However, the practice of NSI has the potential of causing detrimental effects, such as decreased heart rate and hypotension, and, as a result, there is an adverse effect on the client's oxygen status (Moore, 2003).

The two current methods of suctioning are the open and closed methods. Open suctioning involves a sterile catheter that is opened at the time of suctioning. Wear sterile gloves during the suction procedure. Closed suctioning involves a multiple-use suction catheter that is encased in a plastic sheath (Figure 40-10). Closed suctioning is most often used on clients who require mechanical ventilation to support their respiratory efforts, because it permits continuous delivery of oxygen while suction is performed, thus reducing the risk of oxygen desaturation. Although

sterile gloves are not used in this procedure, nonsterile gloves are recommended to prevent contact with splashes from body fluids (Box 40-12).

Artificial Airways. An artificial airway is for clients with decreased level of consciousness or airway obstruction and aids in removal of tracheobronchial secretions.

Oral Airway. The oral airway, the simplest type of artificial airway, prevents obstruction of the trachea by displacement of the tongue into the oropharynx (Figure 40-11). The oral airway extends from the teeth to the oropharynx, maintaining the tongue in the normal position. Use the correct-size airway. Determine the proper oral airway size by measuring the distance from the corner of the mouth to the angle of the jaw just below the ear. The length

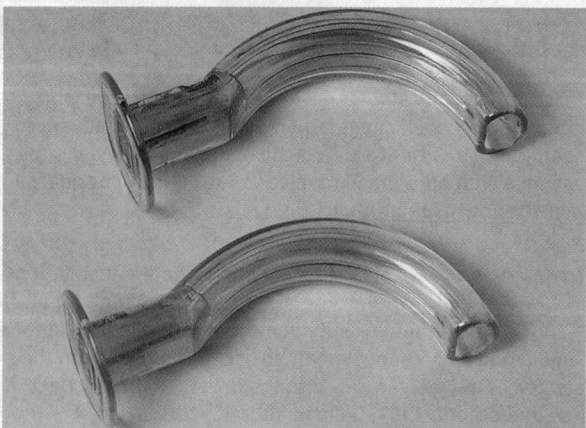

Figure 40-11 Artificial oral airways.

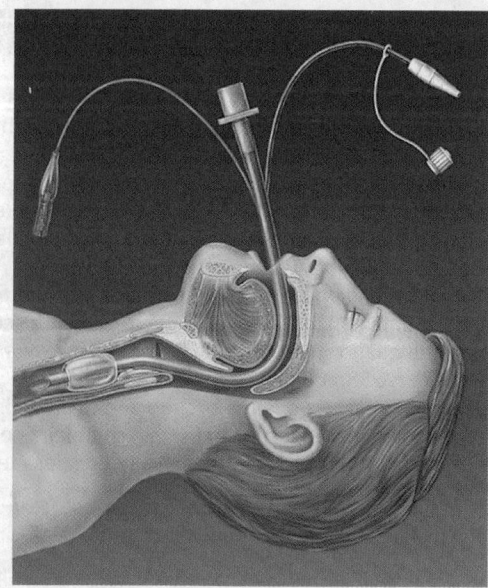

Figure 40-12 Endotracheal tube inserted into trachea with cuff inflated.

is equal to the distance from the flange of the airway to the tip. If the airway is too small, the tongue does not stay in the anterior portion of the mouth; if the airway is too large, it forces the tongue toward the epiglottis and obstructs the airway.

Insert the airway by turning the curve of the airway toward the cheek and placing it over the tongue. When the airway is in the oropharynx, turn it so that the opening points downward. Correctly placed, the airway moves the tongue forward away from the oropharynx and the flange, the flat portion of the airway, rests against the client's teeth. Incorrect insertion merely forces the tongue back into the oropharynx.

Endotracheal and Tracheal Airway. The presence of an artificial airway places the client at high risk for infection and airway injury. Use sterile technique in caring for and maintaining an artificial airway to prevent health care–associated infections (HAIs). Artificial airways need to stay in the correct position to prevent airway damage (Skill 40-2).

Endotracheal tubes (ETs) are short-term artificial airways to administer mechanical ventilation, relieve upper airway obstruction, protect against aspiration, or clear secretions. An ET tube is inserted by a physician or specially trained provider. The tube is passed through the client's mouth, past the pharynx, and into the trachea (Figure 40-12). ETs are generally removed within 14 days; however, they are sometimes used for a longer period of time if the client is showing progress toward weaning from mechanical ventilation and extubation.

If the client requires long-term assistance from an artificial airway, a tracheostomy is considered. A surgical incision is made into the trachea, and a short artificial airway (a tracheostomy tube) is inserted.

Maintenance and Promotion of Lung Expansion. Nursing interventions to maintain or promote lung expansion include noninvasive techniques, such as positioning and incentive spirometry. Invasive procedures, such as chest tube insertion and management, assist in restoring lung expansion.

Positioning. The healthy, completely mobile person maintains adequate ventilation and oxygenation by frequent position

changes during daily activities. However, when a person's illness or injury restricts mobility, there is an increased risk for respiratory impairment. Frequent changes of position are simple and cost-effective methods for reducing stasis of pulmonary secretions and decreased chest wall expansion, both of which increase the risk of pneumonia.

The 45-degree semi-Fowler's position is the most effective position. This position uses gravity to assist in lung expansion and reduces pressure from the abdomen on the diaphragm. When the client is in this position, be sure that the client does not slide down in bed, which will possibly reduce lung expansion. A client with unilateral lung disease, such as pneumothorax, atelectasis, pneumonia, thoracotomy, and multiple trauma affecting one lung, should be positioned in a manner to promote perfusion of the healthy lung and improve oxygenation. In most cases the client is positioned with the "good lung" down. In the presence of pulmonary abscess or hemorrhage, position the client with the affected lung down to prevent drainage toward the healthy lung.

Incentive Spirometry. **Incentive spirometry** encourages voluntary deep breathing by providing visual feedback to clients about inspiratory volume. Incentive spirometry promotes deep breathing and prevents or treats atelectasis in the postoperative client. There is solid evidence to support the use of lung expansion with incentive spirometry in preventing postoperative pulmonary complications following abdominal surgery (Lawrence and others, 2006).

Flow-oriented incentive spirometers consist of one or more plastic chambers that contain freely moving colored balls. The client inhales slowly and with an even flow to elevate the balls and to keep them floating as long as possible to ensure a maximally sustained inhalation.

Text continued on p. 950

SKILL 40-2   CARE OF AN ARTIFICIAL AIRWAY   Video

Delegation Considerations

The skill of care of an artificial airway cannot be delegated. In some settings you can delegate the care for clients who have well-established tracheostomy tubes. It is the responsibility of the nurse to assess and ensure that proper artificial airway care is provided. The nurse instructs nursing assistive personnel to:

- Report to nurse any changes in client's respiratory status, level of consciousness, confusion, pain
- Inform the nurse immediately if the tracheostomy tube inadvertently becomes dislodged when ties are changed
- Report unexpected drainage or secretions from tracheostomy

Equipment

- Stethoscope
- Endotracheal tube care
  - Towel
  - ET and oropharyngeal suction equipment
  - 1- to 1½-inch adhesive or waterproof tape (not paper tape) or commercial ET holder (follow manufacturer's instructions for securing) (check agency policy)
  - Clean gloves (two pairs)
  - Adhesive remover swab or acetone on a cotton ball
  - Mouth care supplies (e.g., toothbrush, anti-bacterial mouthwash or toothpaste, sponge toothette)
- Face cleanser (e.g., wet washcloth, towel, soap, shaving supplies)
- Clean 2 × 2 gauze
- Tincture of benzoin or liquid adhesive
- Face shield (if indicated)
- Tracheostomy care
  - Towel
  - Tracheostomy suction supplies
  - Sterile tracheostomy care kit, if available, or three sterile 4 × 4 gauze pads
  - Sterile cotton-tipped applicators
  - Sterile tracheostomy dressing (precut and sewn surgical dressing)
  - Sterile basin
  - Small sterile brush (or disposable cannula)
  - Tracheostomy ties (e.g., twill tape, manufactured tracheostomy ties, Velcro tracheostomy ties)
  - Normal saline (NS)
  - Scissors
  - Sterile gloves (two)
  - Face shield, if indicated

STEPS	RATIONALE
1. Perform pulmonary assessment.	
a. Auscultate lung sounds.	Provides baseline information.
b. Assess patency of airway and condition of surrounding tissues.	Determines need for airway care and identifies potential pressure sites from airway devices.
c. Note type and size of tube, movement of tube, cuff size.	Movement of tube predisposes client to tracheal trauma or tube dislodgment and indicates the need for another size airway. Cuff size indicates the amount of air needed to properly inflate cuff. An underinflated cuff increases client's risk for aspiration.
2. Explain procedure to client and family.	Reinforces information given to client and family and provides opportunity to ask additional questions.
3. Position client. Clients usually prefer to be lying down. A client with a long-term well-established tracheostomy may be seated.	Provides access to site and facilitates completion of the procedure.
4. Place towel across client's chest.	Reduces transmission of microorganisms and protects linens and bedclothes.
5. Perform hand hygiene. Apply face shield (if needed).	Reduces transmission of microorganisms.
6. Perform airway care.	
A. Endotracheal Tube Care	
(1) Observe for signs and symptoms of need to perform care of the artificial airway:	
(a) Soiled or loose tape in artificial airway holder	A client with an artificial airway is at increased risk due to an inability or difficulty controlling secretions and due to pressure points of the artificial airway.
(b) Skin irritation or pressure sores on nares, lip, or corner of mouth	Pressure from the artificial airway causes irritation and skin breakdown.
(c) Unstable tube	
(d) Excessive secretions	
(2) Identify factors that increase risk of complications from ET tubes:	Tube moving up and down trachea disposes client to tracheal trauma or dislodgment. Underinflated cuff offers no protection from aspiration. Overinflated cuff causes tracheal mucosa injury (Hess, 2005).
(a) Type and size of tube	
(b) Movement of tube up and down trachea	
(c) Cuff size	
(d) Duration of placement	

Continued

✳ **SKILL 40-2**   **CARE OF AN ARTIFICIAL AIRWAY—CONT'D**

STEPS	RATIONALE
(3) Suction endotracheal tube (see Skill 40-1, p. 934).	Removes secretions. Diminishes client's need to cough during procedure.

Critical Decision Point: An oral airway is always immediately accessible in the event that the client bites down and obstructs the ET tube.

STEPS	RATIONALE
(a) Instruct client not to bite or move ET tube with tongue or pull on tubing; removal of tape is often uncomfortable.	Prepares client for procedure and what to expect.
(b) Leave Yankauer suction catheter connected to suction source.	Prepares for oropharyngeal suctioning.
(4) Prepare method to secure endotracheal tube (check agency policy).	
(a) **Tape method:** Cut piece of tape long enough to go completely around client's head from naris to naris plus 15 cm (6 inches): Adult, about 30 to 60 cm (1 to 2 feet). Lay adhesive side up on bedside table. Cut and lay 8 to 16 cm (3 to 6 inches) of tape, adhesive sides together, in center of long strip to prevent tape from sticking to hair. Smaller strip of tape covers area between ears around back of head.	Adhesive tape needs to be placed around head from cheek to cheek below ears. Avoid over ears because this results in a pressure sore.
(b) **Commercially available endotracheal tube holder:** Open package per manufacturer's instructions. Set device aside with the head guard in place and the Velcro strips open.	
(5) Apply gloves, and instruct assistant to apply gloves and hold ET tube firmly at clients' lips. Note the number marking on the ET tube at the gum line.	Reduces transmission of microorganisms. Maintains proper tube position and prevents accidental extubation.
(6) Remove old tape or device.	Provides access to underlying skin for assessment and hygiene.
(a) **Tape:** Carefully remove tape from ET tube and client's face. If tape is difficult to remove, moisten with water or adhesive tape remover. Discard tape in appropriate receptacle if nearby.	
(b) **Commercially available device:** Remove Velcro strips from ET tube, and remove ET tube holder from client.	Devices are latex free, fast, and convenient. Because they do not require tape, they are easy to apply in the presence of facial hair and reduce the risk for skin irritation. The Velcro strips secure the ET tube in place.
(7) Remove excess secretions or adhesive left on client's face.	Promotes hygiene. Retained adhesive causes damage to skin and makes it difficult for the new tape to adhere.
(8) Remove oral airway or bite block if present.	Provides access and complete observation of client's oral cavity.

Critical Decision Point: Do not remove oral airway if client is actively biting. Wait until tape or device is partially or completely secured to ET tube.

STEPS	RATIONALE
(9) With another nurse assisting, brush mucosa, gums and teeth with toothbrush or toothette dipped in mouthwash or toothpaste. Suction orally as needed. Moisten brush with water to rinse. Repeat suctioning.	Provides oral hygiene and allows for observation of any pressure ulcers. Assistance during oral hygiene ensures accumulated secretions are suctioned, preventing aspiration.
(10) Note "cm" ET tube marking at lips or gums. With help of assistant, move ET tube to opposite side or center of mouth. Do not change tube depth.	Prevents pressure sore formation at sides of client's mouth. Ensures correct position of tube and allows for quick visual of displaced tube.
(11) Repeat oral cleaning as in Step (9) on opposite side of mouth.	Removes secretions from mouth and oropharynx.
(12) Clean face and neck with soapy washcloth; rinse and dry. Shave male client as necessary.	Moisture and beard growth prevent adhesive tape adherence.
(13) Use small amount of skin protectant or liquid adhesive on clean 2 × 2 gauze and dot on upper lip (oral ET tube) or across nose (nasal ET tube) and cheeks to ear. Allow tincture to dry completely.	Protects and makes skin more receptive to tape.

✳ **SKILL 40-2**   **CARE OF AN ARTIFICIAL AIRWAY—CONT'D**

STEPS	RATIONALE
(14) Secure ET tube.	
(a) **Tape Method**	
[1] Slip tape under client's head and neck, adhesive side up. Take care not to twist tape or catch hair. Do not allow tape to stick to itself. It helps to stick tape gently to tongue blade, which serves as a guide as tape is passed behind the client's head. Center tape so that double-faced tape extends around back of neck from ear to ear.	Positions tape to secure ET tube in proper position.
[2] On one side of face, secure tape from ear to naris (nasal ET tube) or edge of mouth (oral ET tube). Tear remaining tape in half lengthwise, forming two pieces that are ½- to ¾-inch wide. Secure bottom half of tape across upper lip (oral ET tube) or across top of nose (nasal ET tube) (see illustration, *A*). Wrap top half of tape around tube (see illustration, *B*). Tape encircles the tube at least two times for security.	Secures tape to face. Using top tape to wrap prevents downward drag on ET tube.
[3] Gently pull other side of tape firmly to pick up slack, and secure to remaining side of face (see illustration). Have assistant release hold when tube is secure. You need an assistant to help reinsert oral airway.	Secures tape to face and tube. ET tube should be at same depth at the lips. Check earlier assessment for verification of tube depth in centimeters.
(b) **Commercially Available Device**	
[1] Place ET tube through the opening designed to secure the ET tube. Be sure that the pilot balloon to the ET tube is accessible.	Commercially available holders have a slit in the front of the holder designed to secure the ET tube

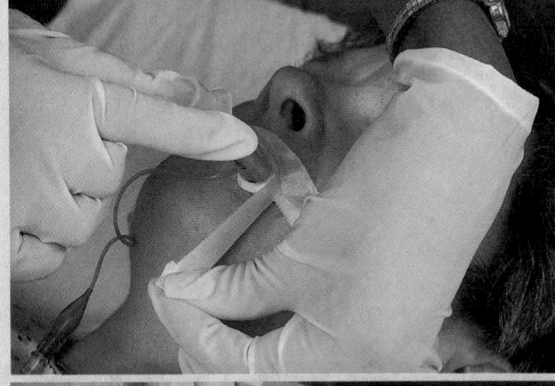

A

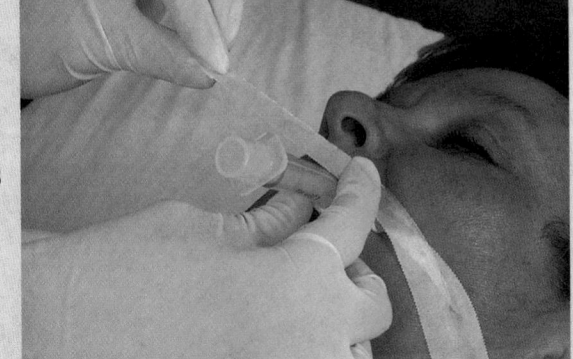

B

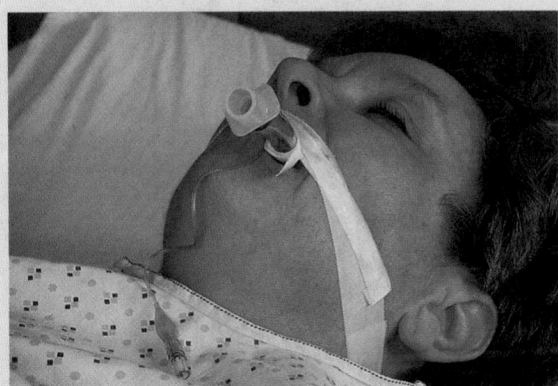

STEP 6A(14)(a)[2] A, Securing bottom half of tape across client's upper lip. **B,** Securing top half of tape around tube.

STEP 6A(14)(a)[3] Tape securing ET tube.

Continued

✳ SKILL 40-2   CARE OF AN ARTIFICIAL AIRWAY—CONT'D

STEPS	RATIONALE
[2] Place Velcro strips of ET holder under the client at the occipital region of the head.	
[3] Verify that the ET tube is at the established position using the lip or gum line marker as a guide.	Ensures that the ET tube remains at the correct depth as determined during assessment.
[4] Secure the Velcro strips at the base of the client's head. Leave 1 cm (½ inch) slack in the strips.	
[5] Verify that the tube is secure, it does not move forward from the client's mouth or backward down into the client's throat, and there are no pressure areas on the oral mucosa or the occipital region of the head. (see illustration).	The tube needs to be secure so that the position of the tube remains at the correct depth.
(15) Clean oral airway in warm soapy water, and rinse well. Shake excess water from oral airway.	Promotes hygiene. Reduces transmission of microorganisms.
(16) For unconscious client, reinsert oral airway without pushing tongue into oropharynx.	Prevents client from biting ET tube and allows access for oropharyngeal suctioning. An oral airway in a conscious, cooperative client causes excessive gagging and pressure ulcers to the mouth and tongue.

B. Tracheostomy Care

(1) Observe for signs and symptoms of need to perform tracheostomy care: (a) Soiled/loose ties or dressing (b) Nonstable tube (c) Excessive secretions	A client with a tracheostomy tube is at increased risk due to loss of natural airway protection of the upper airway.
(2) Suction tracheostomy (see Skill 40-1, p. 934). Before removing gloves, remove soiled tracheostomy dressing and discard in glove with coiled catheter.	Removes secretions so as not to occlude outer cannula while inner cannula is removed. Reduces need for client to cough. Prevents aspiration of retained secretions. Disposal method contains microorganisms.
(3) Prepare equipment. (a) Open two packages of cotton-tipped swabs, and pour NS onto the swabs. (b) Open tracheostomy kit. (c) Unwrap sterile basin, and pour about 2 cm (¾ inch) of normal saline into it.	Preparation and organization of equipment allows completion of tracheostomy care procedure efficiently and then reconnection of client to oxygen source in a timely manner. A tracheostomy tube has multiple components (see illustration). Some of these components might be used during tracheostomy care.

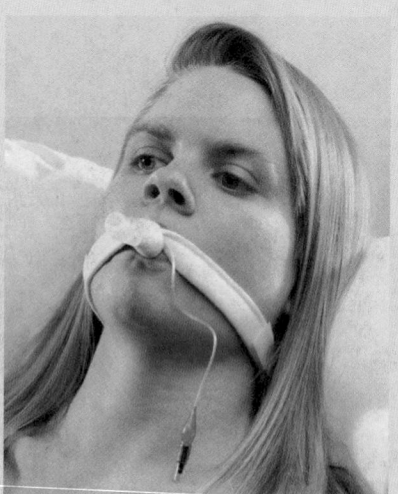

STEP 6A(14)(b)[5] Endotracheal tube holder in place. (Courtesy Dale Medical Products, Plainesville, Mass.)

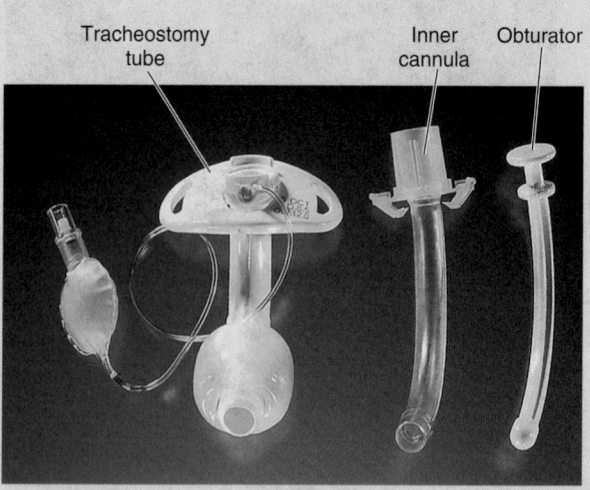

Tracheostomy tube   Inner cannula   Obturator

STEP 6B(3)(b) Tracheostomy tube. (Courtesy Mallinckrodt Inc. Shiley Tracheostomy Products, St. Louis, Mo.)

STEPS	RATIONALE
(d) Open small sterile brush package, and place aseptically into sterile basin.	
(e) Do not recap NS.	
(4) Apply sterile gloves. Keep dominant hand sterile throughout procedure.	Reduces transmission of microorganisms.
(5) Remove oxygen source. Apply oxygen source loosely over tracheostomy if client desaturates during procedure.	Helps reduce amount of desaturation.

Critical Decision Point: It is important to stabilize the tracheostomy tube at all times during tracheostomy care to prevent injury and unnecessary discomfort.

(6) Tracheostomy with **inner cannula** care	
(a) While touching only the outer aspect of the tube, unlock and remove the inner cannula with nondominant hand. Drop inner cannula into normal saline basin.	Removes inner cannula for cleaning. Hydrogen peroxide loosens secretions from inner cannula.
(b) Place tracheostomy collar or T tube and ventilator oxygen source over or near outer cannula. (NOTE: T tube and ventilator oxygen devices cannot be attached to all outer cannulas when inner cannula is removed.)	Maintains supply of oxygen to client.
(c) To prevent oxygen desaturation in affected clients, quickly pick up inner cannula and use small brush to remove secretions inside and outside cannula (see illustration).	Tracheostomy brush provides mechanical force to remove thick or dried secretions.
(d) Hold inner cannula over basin, and rinse with NS, using nondominant hand to pour.	Removes secretions and hydrogen peroxide from inner cannula.
(e) Replace inner cannula, (see illustration) and secure "locking" mechanism. Reapply ventilator or oxygen sources.	
(7) **Disposable inner cannula** care	
(a) Remove cannula from manufacturer's packaging.	
(b) While touching only the outer aspect of the tube, withdraw inner cannula and replace with new cannula. Lock into position.	
(c) Dispose of contaminated cannula in appropriate receptacle, and apply oxygen source. Prevents unnecessary oxygen desaturation.	

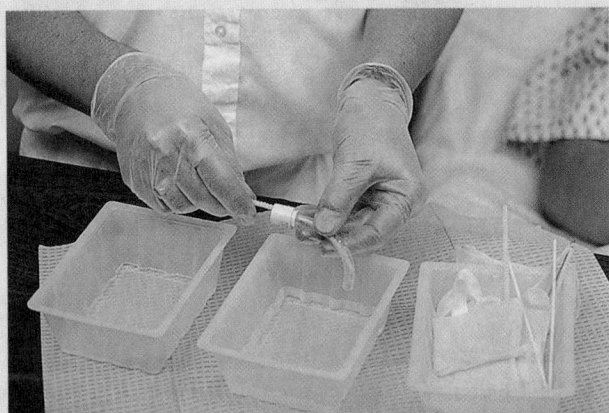

STEP 6B(6)(c) Cleaning the tracheostomy inner cannula.

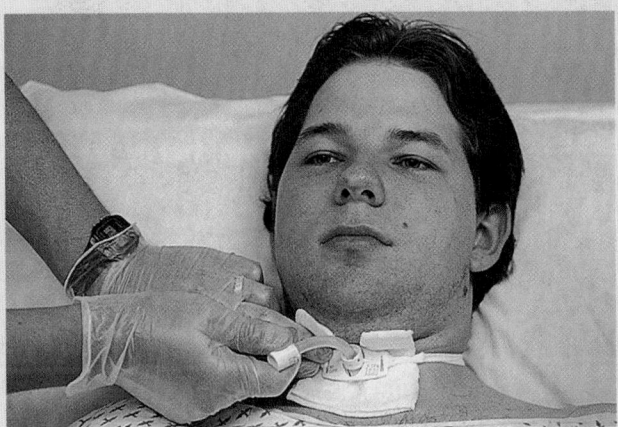

STEP 6B(6)(e) Reinserting the inner cannula.

Continued

✳ **SKILL 40-2**   CARE OF AN ARTIFICIAL AIRWAY—CONT'D

STEPS

(8) Using sterile swabs dipped in sterile normal saline and 4 × 4 gauze, clean exposed outer cannula surfaces and stoma under faceplate, extending 5 to 10 cm (2 to 4 inches) in all directions from stoma (see illustration). Clean in circular motion from stoma site outward, using dominant hand to handle sterile supplies.

(9) Using NS-prepared cotton-tipped swabs and 4 × 4 gauze, clean the tracheostomy tube and skin surfaces.

(10) Using dry 4 × 4 gauze, pat lightly at skin and exposed outer cannula surfaces.

(11) Secure tracheostomy.

(a) **Tracheostomy tie method**

[1] Instruct assistant, if available, to hold tracheostomy tube securely in place while ties are cut.

RATIONALE

Aseptically removes secretions from stoma site. Unless there are excessive tracheal secretions or drainage from the stoma, cleansing 1 or 2 times a day is sufficient (Lewarski, 2005).

Rinses hydrogen peroxide from surfaces, preventing possible irritation.

Dry surfaces prohibit formation of moist environment from growth of microorganisms and skin excoriation.

Promotes hygiene, reduces transmission of microorganisms, and secures tracheostomy tube.

Critical Decision Point: Assistant must not release hold on tracheostomy tube until new ties are firmly tied to reduce risk of accidental extubation. If no assistant is present, do not cut old ties until new ties are in place and securely tied.

---

[2] Cut length of twill tape long enough to go around client's neck two times, about 60 to 75 cm (24 to 30 inches) for an adult. Cut ends on a diagonal.

Cutting ends of tie on a diagonal aids in inserting tie through eyelet.

Critical Decision Point: Keep tracheostomy obturator at bedside with a fresh tracheostomy to facilitate reinsertion of the outer cannula, if dislodged. Keep an additional tracheostomy tube of the same size and shape on hand for emergency replacement (Seay and others, 2002).

---

[3] Take prepared tie and insert one end of tie through faceplate eyelet, and pull ends even (see illustration).

[4] Slide both ends of tie behind head and around neck to other eyelet, and insert one tie through second eyelet.

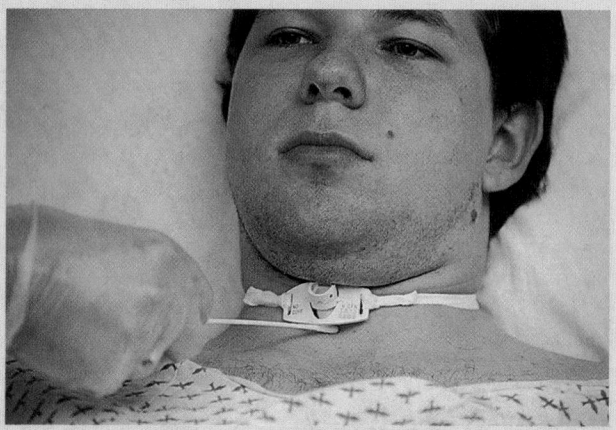

STEP 6B(8) Cleansing around stoma.

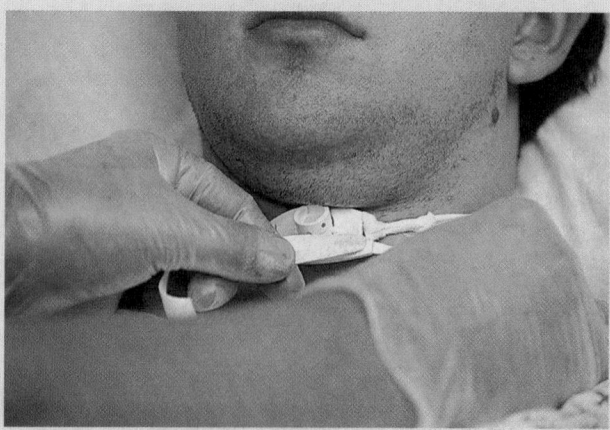

STEP 6B(11)(a)[3] Replacing tracheostomy ties when an assistant is not available. Do not remove old tracheostomy ties until new ones are secure.

✳ **SKILL 40-2**   CARE OF AN ARTIFICIAL AIRWAY—CONT'D

STEPS	RATIONALE
[5] Pull snugly.	Secures tracheostomy tube in place.
[6] Tie ends securely in double square knot, allowing space for only one finger in tie.	One-finger slack prevents ties from being too tight when tracheostomy dressing is in place.
(b) **Tracheostomy tube holder method** (see illustration)	
[1] While wearing gloves, maintain a secure hold on the tracheostomy tube. You can do this with an assistant or, when an assistant is not available, by leaving the old tracheostomy tube holder in place until the new device is secure.	Prevents accidental displacement of tube.
[2] Align strap under client's neck. Be sure that the Velcro attachments are positioned on either side of the tracheostomy tube.	
[3] Place narrow end of the ties under and through the faceplate eyelets. Pull ends even, and secure with the Velcro closures.	
[4] Verify that there is space for only one loose or two snug finger width(s) under neck strap.	Prevents skin necrosis.
(12) Insert fresh tracheostomy dressing under clean ties and faceplate (see illustration).	Absorbs drainage. Dressing prevents pressure on clavicle heads.
(13) Position client comfortably, and assess respiratory status.	Promotes comfort. Some clients require post–tracheostomy care suctioning.
7. Replace any oxygen delivery devices.	Maintains oxygen therapy.
8. Remove and discard gloves. Perform hand hygiene.	Prevents transmission of microorganisms.
9. Compare respiratory assessments before and after procedure.	Identifies any changes in presence and quality of breath sounds after procedure.
10. Observe depth and position of tubes.	Verifies that position of tube is correct.
11. Evaluate security of tape or commercial ET or tracheostomy tube holder by tugging at tube.	Artificial airway should not move. Client may cough.
12. Evaluate skin around mouth and oral mucosa (ET tube) and tracheostomy stoma for drainage, pressure, and signs of irritation.	Skin breakdown and/or irritation should not be present.

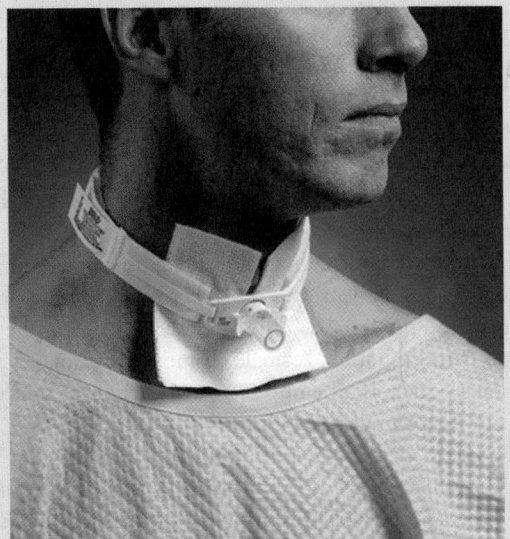

STEP 6B(11)(b)[4] Tracheostomy tube holder in place. (Courtesy Dale Medical Products, Plainesville, Mass.)

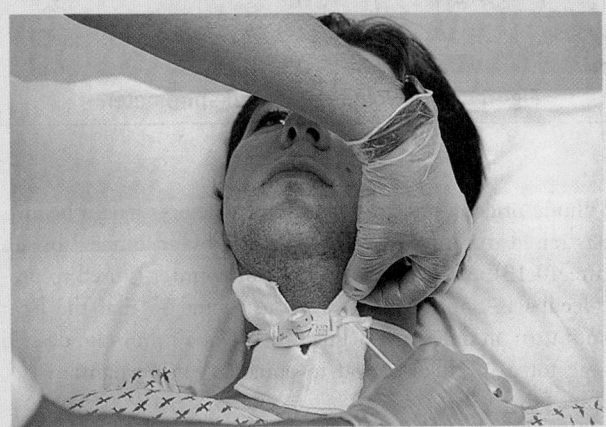

STEP 6B(12) Applying tracheostomy dressing.

Continued

✳ SKILL 40-2   CARE OF AN ARTIFICIAL AIRWAY—CONT'D

Unexpected Outcomes and Related Interventions

1. Artificial airway accidentally is displaced or falls out (Seay and others, 2002).
   a. Call for assistance.
   b. Maintain patent airway:
      (1) Obtain replacement tracheostomy tube.
      (2) Verify that cuff on new tube is completely deflated.
      (3) Using obturator, insert new tube and secure tube.
   c. Observe vital signs and signs of respiratory distress.
2. Hard, reddened areas with or without excessive or foul-smelling secretions are observed.
   a. Indicates infection. Notify physician or health care provider.
   b. Increase frequency of tube care.
   c. Remove inner cannula, if applicable, for cleaning and suctioning.
3. Tube is not secure, and artificial airway moves in or out or client coughs it out.
   a. Assess client's respiratory status, and observe for the presence of mucus plugs.
   b. Adjust or apply new ties.

4. Breakdown, pressure areas, or stomatitis (tracheostomy tube) are observed.
   a. Increase frequency of tube care.
   b. Make sure skin areas are clean and dry.

Recording and Reporting

- Record respiratory assessments before and after care.
- Record ET tube care: depth of ET tube, frequency and extent of care, client tolerance, and any complications related to presence of the tube.
- Record tracheostomy care: type and size of tracheostomy tube, frequency and extent of care, client tolerance, and any complications related to presence of the tube.

Home Care Considerations (Tracheostomy Only)

- Instruct caregivers in how to obtain supplies.
- Instruct caregivers in signs and symptoms of respiratory distress, tube dysfunction, respiratory and stoma infections.

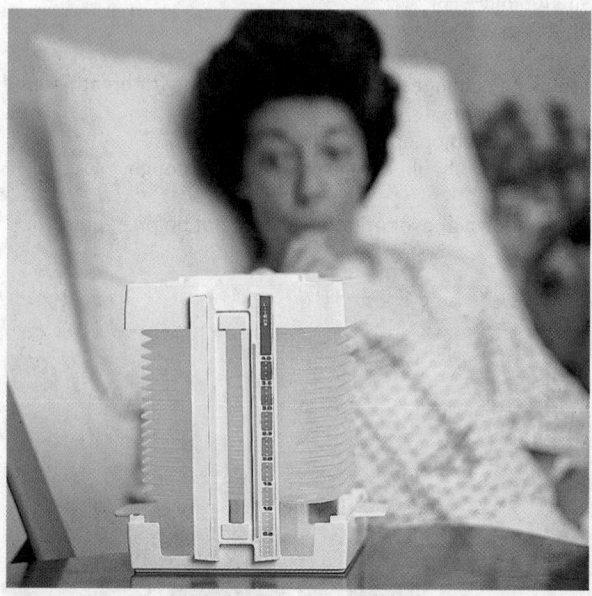

Figure 40-13 Volume-oriented spirometer.

Volume-oriented incentive spirometry devices have a bellows that is raised to a predetermined volume by an inhaled breath (Figure 40-13). An achievement light or counter is used to provide feedback. Some devices are constructed so that the light will not turn on unless the bellows is held at a minimum desired volume for a specified period to enhance lung expansion (see Chapter 50).

Incentive spirometry encourages clients to use visual feedback to maximally inflate their lungs and to sustain that inflation (Basoglu and others, 2005). A postoperative inspiratory capacity one half to three fourths of the preoperative volume is acceptable because of postoperative pain. Administration of pain medica-

tions before incentive spirometry will help the client achieve deep breathing by reducing pain and splinting (Pullen, 2003).

Chest Tubes.   A **chest tube** is a catheter inserted through the thorax to remove air and fluids from the pleural space, to prevent air or fluid from reentering the pleural space, or to reestablish normal intrapleural and intrapulmonic pressures (Roman and Mercado, 2006) (Figure 40-14). There are a variety of chest tubes available. In addition to the usual disposable waterless system, the traditional reusable glass three-bottle systems are still used. The newest system available is the mobile chest drain and the dry chest drainage system.

Mobile systems rely on gravity, not suction, for drainage. In selected clients these mobile drains reduce the length of time needed for the chest tube, improve ambulation, and decrease the length of time in the hospital (Carroll, 2005). Nonventilated clients and clients who had thoracoscopic lung surgery or minimally invasive cardiac surgery do well with these mobile chest drains. These devices are lighter and smaller, and thus the client is able to move more easily. As a result, this reduces the risks of deep vein thrombosis and pulmonary embolism.

The simplest closed drainage system is the use of a single chamber. The chamber serves as a collector and a water seal. During normal respiration the fluid will ascend with inspiration and descend with expiration. A single chamber is for smaller amounts of drainage, such as an empyema—a collection of infected fluid or pus in the pleural space.

The use of two chambers permits the liquid to flow into the collection chamber as air flows into the water-sealed chamber. Fluctuations in the water-seal tube are still anticipated. Use of two chambers allows for more accurate measurement of chest drainage and is used when larger amounts of drainage are expected.

When a volume of air or fluid needs to be evacuated with controlled suction, all three chambers are used. Mark the suction control with centimeter readings to adjust the amount of suc-

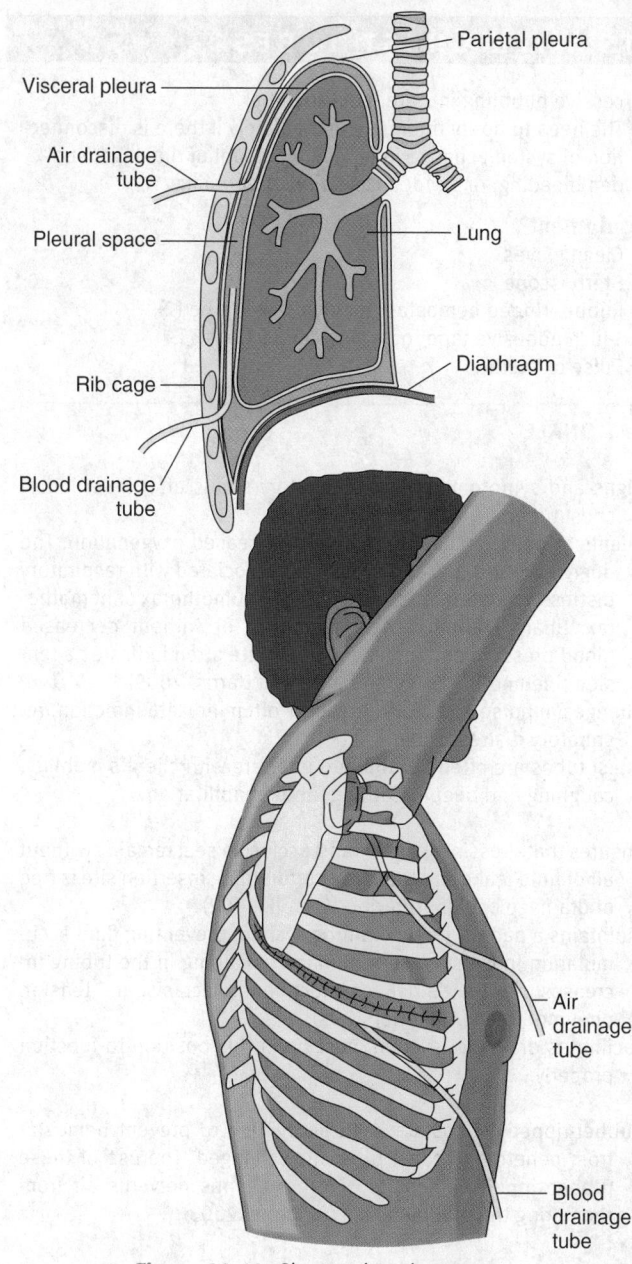

Figure 40-14 Chest tube placement.

tion. Usually 15 to 20 cm of water is used for adults (Roman and Mercado, 2006). This means that the chamber is filled with sterile water to the 15- or 20-cm water level.

A new dry chest drainage system does not use water in the suction chamber. An automatic control valve (ACV) is located inside the regulator and continuously balances the force of the suction with the atmospheres. As a result, the ACV responds to and adjusts to changes in client air leaks and fluctuations in suction source vacuum to deliver accurate suction. Set pressure between −10 cm H_2O and −40 cm H_2O (Roman and Mercado, 2006).

Regardless of the system used, the principles of client management are the same (Carroll, 2002). Chest tubes are common after chest surgery and chest trauma and for pneumothorax or hemothorax to promote lung reexpansion (Skill 40-3).

A **pneumothorax** is a collection of air in the pleural space. The loss of negative intrapleural pressure causes the lung to col-

lapse. There are a variety of mechanisms for a pneumothorax. Sometimes it occurs spontaneously or as a result of chest trauma, such as a stabbing or the chest striking the steering wheel in an automobile accident. A pneumothorax may result from the rupture of an emphysematous bleb on the surface of the lung (a large bulla resulting from the destruction caused by emphysema) or from an invasive procedure, such as insertion of a subclavian IV line.

A client with a pneumothorax usually feels pain as atmospheric air irritates the parietal pleura. The pain is sharp and pleuritic and worsens on inspiration. Dyspnea is common and worsens as the size of the pneumothorax increases.

A **hemothorax** is an accumulation of blood and fluid in the pleural cavity between the parietal and visceral pleurae, usually as a result of trauma. It produces a counterpressure and prevents the lung from full expansion. A rupture of small blood vessels from inflammatory processes, such as pneumonia or tuberculosis, can cause a hemothorax. In addition to pain and dyspnea, signs and symptoms of shock develop if blood loss is severe.

Special Considerations. Clamping a chest tube is contraindicated when ambulating or transporting the client. Clamping the chest tube will possibly result in a tension pneumothorax. Air pressure builds in the pleural space, collapsing the lung and creating a life-threatening event.

Handle the chest drainage unit carefully and maintain the drainage device below the client's chest. If the tubing disconnects from the drainage unit, instruct the client to exhale as much as possible and to cough. This maneuver rids the pleural space of as much air as possible. Temporarily reestablish a water seal by immersing the open end of the chest tube into a container of sterile water (Roman and Mercado, 2006).

Removal of chest tubes requires client preparation. Clients report sensations during chest tube removal. The most frequent sensations include burning, pain, and a pulling sensation.

Maintenance and Promotion of Oxygenation. Promotion of lung expansion, mobilization of secretions, and maintenance of a patent airway assists the client in meeting oxygenation needs. Some clients, however, also require oxygen therapy to keep a healthy level of tissue oxygenation.

Oxygen Therapy. Oxygen therapy is cheap, widely available, and used in a variety of settings to relieve or prevent tissue hypoxia (Thomson and others, 2002). The goal of oxygen therapy is to prevent or relieve hypoxia. Oxygen is not a substitute for other treatment, however, and is used only when indicated. Oxygen is a medication. It has dangerous side effects, such as atelectasis or oxygen toxicity (Thomson and others, 2002). As with any medication, the dosage or concentration of oxygen is continuously monitored. Routinely check the physician's orders to verify that the client is receiving the prescribed oxygen concentration. The six rights of medication administration also pertain to oxygen administration (see Chapter 35).

Safety Precautions. Oxygen is a highly combustible gas. Although it does not spontaneously burn or cause an explosion, it can easily cause a fire in a client's room if it contacts a spark from an open flame or electrical equipment. With increasing use of home oxygen therapy, clients and health care professionals need to be aware of the dangers of combustion. Chapter 38 describes steps to take in case of fire.

Text continued on p. 957

✳ **SKILL 40-3** **CARE OF CLIENTS WITH CHEST TUBES**

Delegation Considerations

The skill of care of clients with chest tubes cannot be delegated. Nursing assistive personnel (NAP) provide supportive care to clients with chest tubes. The nurse instructs NAP about:

- How to properly position the client to facilitate chest tube drainage and optimal function of the system
- How to safely ambulate and transfer client with chest drainage
- The appropriate setup of drainage equipment for the type of system to be used
- The need to immediately inform the nurse of any changes in vital signs, chest pain, or sudden shortness of breath, or excessive bubbling in water-seal chamber
- The need to notify the nurse immediately if there is disconnection of system, change in type and amount of drainage, sudden bleeding, or sudden cessation of bubbling.

Equipment

- Clean gloves
- Stethoscope
- Rubber-tipped hemostats for each chest tube (2)
- 1-inch adhesive tape for taping connections
- Pulse oximeter

STEPS	RATIONALE
1. Perform hand hygiene, and assess client.	
a. *Pulmonary status:* Assess respirations, presence of chest pain, breath sounds over affected lung area.	Signs and symptoms reflect respiratory status after insertion of chest tube.
b. Signs and symptoms of increased respiratory distress and/or chest pain are decreased breath sounds over the affected and nonaffected lungs, marked cyanosis, asymmetrical chest movements, presence of subcutaneous emphysema around tube insertion site or neck, hypotension, and tachycardia (Carroll, 2002).	Clients in need of chest tubes have decreased oxygenation. The degree of the signs and symptoms associated with respiratory distress is related to the size of the pneumothorax or hemothorax. Sharp stabbing chest pain with or without decreased blood pressure and increased heart rate often indicates a tension pneumothorax (Leigh-Smith and Harris, 2005).
c. Vital signs and SpO_2.	Changes in pulse and blood pressure often indicate infection, respiratory distress, pain.
d. If possible, ask client to rate level of comfort on a scale of 0 to 10.	Chest tubes are often painful and interfere with client's mobility, coughing and deep breathing, and rehabilitation.
2. Observe:	
a. Chest tube dressing and site surrounding tube insertion. Apply clean gloves if drainage is present.	Ensures that dressing is intact and occlusive seal remains without air or fluid leaks and that area surrounding insertion site is free of drainage or skin irritation (Carroll, 2002).
b. Tubing for kinks, dependent loops, or clots.	Maintains a patent, freely draining system, preventing fluid accumulation in chest cavity. Drainage remaining in the tubing increases the client's risk for infection, atelectasis, and tension pneumothorax (Allibone, 2003).
c. Chest drainage system remains upright and below level of tube insertion. Note amount of drainage in system (see illustration).	Facilitates drainage; system must be in this position to function properly.
3. Provide two rubber-tipped hemostats or approved clamps for each chest tube, attached to top of client's bed with adhesive tape. Chest tubes are only clamped under specific circumstances per physician order or nursing policy and procedure:	Rubber-tipped hemostats have a covering to prevent hemostat from penetrating chest tube once changed. The use of these rubber-tipped hemostats or other clamps prevents air from reentering the pleural space (Allibone, 2003).
a. To assess air leak	
b. To quickly empty or change disposable systems; performed by a nurse who has received education in the procedure	
c. If there is an accidental disconnection of drainage tubing from the drainage collection device or damage to the device	
d. To assess if client is ready to have chest tube removed (which is done by physician's order)	

Critical Decision Point: If a chest tube is ever clamped, assess client for signs and symptoms of tension pneumothorax.

---

4. Position client.	Permits optimal drainage of fluid and/or air.
a. Semi-Fowler's position to evacuate air (pneumothorax)	Air rises to highest point in chest. Pneumothorax tubes are usually placed on anterior aspect at midclavicular line, second or third intercostal space.
b. High-Fowler's position to drain fluid (hemothorax, effusion)	Permits optimal drainage of fluid. Posterior tubes are placed on midaxillary line, eighth or ninth intercostal space.

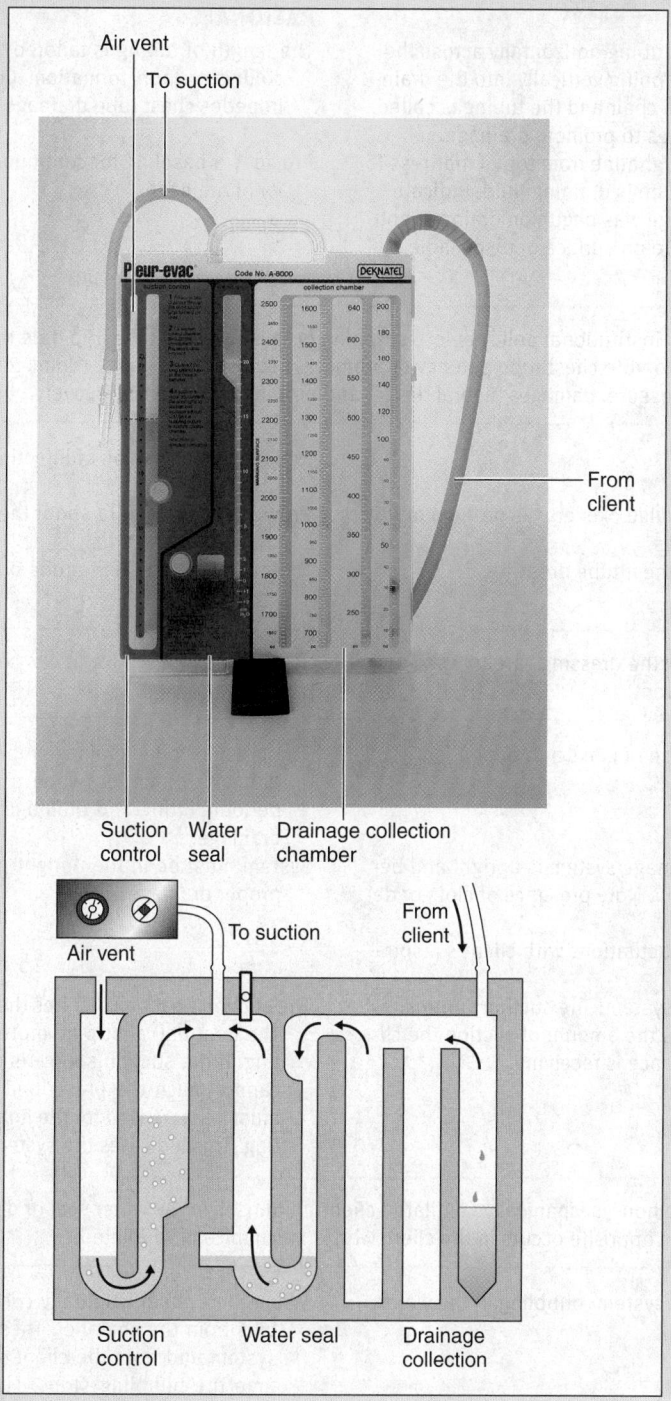

STEP 2c *Top,* The Pleur-Evac drainage system, a commercial three-bottle chest drainage device. *Bottom,* Schematic of the drainage device.

STEPS	RATIONALE
5. Be sure tube connection between chest and drainage tube is intact and taped.	Secures chest tube to drainage system and reduces risk of air leak causing breaks in airtight system.
a. Determine that water-seal vent is not occluded.	Permits displaced air to pass into atmosphere.
b. Be sure suction-control chamber vent is not occluded when using suction. Waterless systems have relief valves without caps.	Provides safety factor of releasing excess negative pressure into atmosphere. Too little suction prevents lung reexpansion and increases client risk for infection, atelectasis, and tension pneumothorax. Too much suction damages the lung tissue and perpetuates existing air leaks (Allibone, 2003).

Continued

✳ **SKILL 40-3**   **CARE OF CLIENTS WITH CHEST TUBES—CONT'D**

STEPS	RATIONALE
6. Avoid excess tubing; lay the tubing horizontally across the client bed or chair before dropping vertically into the drainage bottle. If the client is in a chair and the tubing is coiled, lift the tubing every 15 minutes to promote drainage.	The length of tubing is tailored to each client to avoid excessive coiling or loop formation. Coiled, looped, or clotted tubing impedes chest tube drainage (Allibone, 2003).
7. Adjust tubing to hang in straight line from top of mattress to drainage chamber. If chest tube is draining fluid, indicate time (e.g., 0900) that drainage was begun on drainage bottle's adhesive tape or on write-on surface of disposable commercial system.	Provides a baseline for continuous assessment of type and quality of drainage.

Critical Decision Point: Check institutional policy before stripping or milking chest tubes. To date there is no evidence to support manipulation of chest tubes to promote chest tube patency or promote mediastinal drainage (Holm, 2007). Chest tube stripping increases negative intrathoracic pressure, damages pleural tissue, and prolongs the client's recovery.

8. Perform hand hygiene.	Reduces transmission of infection.
9. Evaluation	
a. Monitor vital signs and pulse oximetry as ordered or if client's condition changes.	Provides ongoing data about the client's level of oxygenation.
b. Observe appearance of chest tube dressing.	Drainage is often due to tube occlusion, causing drainage to exit around tube.

Critical Decision Point: Check the dressing carefully because it needs to remain occlusive. It can come loose from the skin, although this is not readily apparent.

c. Observe that tubing is free of kinks and dependent loops.	Straight and coiled drainage tube positions are optimal for pleural drainage. However, when a dependent loop is unavoidable, periodic lifting and drainage of the tube will promote pleural drainage.
d. Verify that the chest drainage system is upright and below level of tube insertion. Note presence of clots or debris in tubing.	System must be in the upright position to function and facilitate proper drainage.
e. Observe water seal for fluctuations with client's inspiration and expiration.	
(1) Observe waterless system: The suction control (float ball) indicates the amount of suction the client's intrapleural space is receiving.	The suction float ball dictates the amount of suction in the system. The float ball allows no more suction than dictated by its setting. If the suction source is set too low, the suction float ball cannot reach the prescribed setting. In this case the suction must be increased for the float ball to reach the prescribed setting. This indicates the system is properly functioning.

Critical Decision Point: In the non–mechanically ventilated client, fluid rises in the water seal or diagnostic indicator with inspiration and falls with expiration. The opposite occurs in the client who is mechanically ventilated.

(2) Observe water seal system: bubbling in the water seal chamber.	When the system is initially connected to the client, expect bubbles from the chamber. These are from the air present in the system and from the client's intrapleural space. After a short time the bubbling stops. Fluid continues to fluctuate in the water seal on inspiration and expiration until the lung reexpands or the system is occluded.
(3) Observe water-seal system: bubbling in the suction-control chamber (when using suction).	Suction-control chamber has constant gentle bubbling. Tubing remains free of obstruction and the suction source is turned to appropriate setting.
f. Observe type of fluid, and measure fluid drainage: Note color and amount of drainage, client's vital signs, and skin color.	
(1) *In the adult:* less than 50 to 200 mL/hr immediately after surgery in a mediastinal chest tube; approximately 500 mL in first 24 hours.	Dark-red drainage is expected only in the postoperative period, turning serous with time.

CARE OF CLIENTS WITH CHEST TUBES—CONT'D

STEPS

(2) Between 100 and 300 mL of fluid drain in pleural chest tube in an adult during first 3 hours after insertion. This rate will decrease after 2 hours; expect 500 to 1000 mL in first 24 hours. Drainage is grossly bloody during first several hours after surgery and then changes to serous. Remember that a sudden gush of drainage is often retained blood and not active bleeding. This increase in drainage often results from client position changes.

RATIONALE

Reexpansion of lungs forces drainage into the tube. Coughing also causes large gushes of drainage or air.

Report excessive amounts and/or continued presence of frank, bloody drainage the first several hours after surgery to the health care provider, along with client's vital signs and respiratory status.

Critical Decision Point: Inform the health care provider if drainage suddenly increases or if there is more than 100 mL/hr of bloody drainage (except for the first 3 hours postoperatively) (Allibone, 2003).

---

g. Observe client for decreased respiratory distress and chest pain, auscultate lung sounds over affected lung area, and monitor SpO_2.

Normally breath sounds are equal. Decreased breath sounds on the affected side indicate that air or fluid has reaccumulated in the pleural space. Increasing respiratory distress, decreased breath sounds, cyanosis, and asymmetrical chest wall motion along with declining vital signs sometimes indicate a tension pneumothorax and must be reported immediately to the client's health care provider (Carroll, 2002).

h. Ask client to evaluate pain on a level of 0 to 10.

Indicates the need for medication for pain.

Unexpected Outcomes and Related Interventions

1. Continuous bubbling is observed in water-sealed chamber, indicating leak between client and water seal.
   a. Assess all connections between client and drainage system, and tighten any loose connections (Cerfolio, 2005).
   b. Cross-clamp chest tube close to client's chest. If bubbling stops, air leak is inside client's thorax or at chest tube insertion site. Unclamp tube, and notify physician immediately. Reinforce chest dressing. Leaving chest tube clamped causes a tension pneumothorax and mediastinal shift.
   c. Gradually move clamps down drainage tubing away from client and toward drainage chamber, moving one clamp at a time. When bubbling stops, leak is in section of tubing or connection distal to the clamp. Replace tubing or secure connection, and release clamp.
   d. When an air leak is located, prepare to change drainage system. Physician or certified provider will change system.
2. Tension pneumothorax is present.
   a. Determine that chest tubes are not clamped, kinked, or occluded. *Obstructed chest tubes trap air in intrapleural space when air leak originates within client and can cause a tension pneumothorax.*
   b. Notify client's health care provider immediately.
   c. Prepare immediately for another chest tube insertion; obtain a flutter (Heimlich) valve or large-gauge needle for short-term emergency release of air in intrapleural space; have emergency equipment (e.g., oxygen, code cart) near client.

Recording and Reporting

- Record patency of chest tube; presence, type, and amount of drainage; presence of fluctuations; client's vital signs; chest dressing status, amount of suction and/or water seal; and level of comfort.

Home Care Considerations

- Some clients with chronic conditions (e.g., uncomplicated pneumothorax, effusions, empyema) requiring a chest tube are discharged home with smaller mobile chest drains. These systems do not have a suction-control chamber and use a mechanical one-way valve instead of a water-seal chamber (Carroll, 2002, 2005).
- Instruct client in how to ambulate and remain active with a home chest tube drainage system
- Provide client with information as to when to contact health care professionals regarding changes in health status or drainage system (e.g., chest pain, breathlessness, change in drainage).

✳ **SKILL 40-4**   # APPLYING A NASAL CANNULA OR OXYGEN MASK   `Video`

Delegation Considerations

The skill of applying a nasal cannula or oxygen mask can be delegated. However, the nurse is responsible for assessing the client and providing safe and accurate oxygen therapy, including adjustment of oxygen flow rate and evaluation of client response. The nurse directs nursing assistive personnel to inform by:

- Clarifying the correct placement and positioning of delivery device
- Instructing personnel to report to nurse if the client has an increased rate of breathing, decreased level of consciousness, or increased confusion and pain
- Having personnel provide skin care around client's ears and nose

Equipment

- Oxygen delivery device as ordered by client's health care provider
- Oxygen tubing
- Humidifier, if indicated
- Sterile water for humidification, if indicated
- Oxygen source
- Oxygen flow meter
- Appropriate room signs

STEPS	RATIONALE
1. Inspect client for signs and symptoms associated with hypoxia and presence of airway secretions.	Left untreated, hypoxia produces cardiac dysrhythmias and death. Presence of airway secretions decreases effectiveness of oxygen delivery.

Critical Decision Point: Clients with sudden changes in their vital signs, level of consciousness, or behavior are often experiencing profound hypoxia. Clients who demonstrate subtle changes over time have worsening of a chronic or existing condition or a new medical condition (Jevon and Evans, 2001).

2. Obtain client's most recent SpO_2 or arterial blood gas (ABG) values.	Provides objective baseline data to use to compare outcome of oxygen therapy.
3. Explain to client and family what happens during the procedure and purpose of oxygen therapy.	Decreases client's anxiety, which reduces oxygen consumption and increases client cooperation.
4. Perform hand hygiene.	Reduces transmission of infection.
5. Attach nasal cannula or mask to oxygen tubing, and attach to humidified oxygen source adjusted to prescribed flow rate (see illustration).	Prevents drying of nasal and oral mucous membranes and airway secretions.
6. Place tips of cannula into client's nares, and adjust elastic headband or plastic slide until cannula fits snugly and comfortably (see illustration). If using an oxygen mask, adjust elastic headband until mask fits comfortably over client's face and mouth.	Directs flow of oxygen into client's upper respiratory tract. Client is more likely to keep cannula or face mask in place if it fits comfortably.

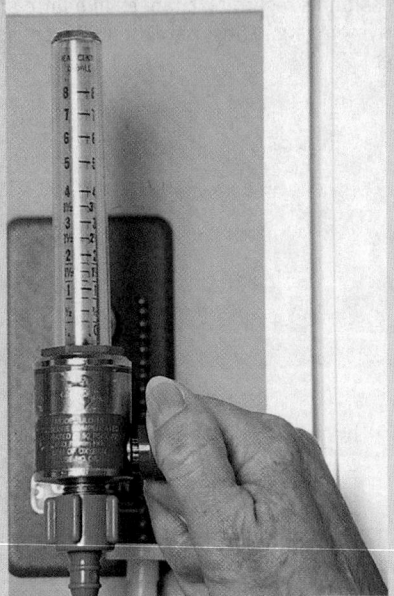

STEP 5 Adjusting flowmeter to prescribed oxygen flow rate.

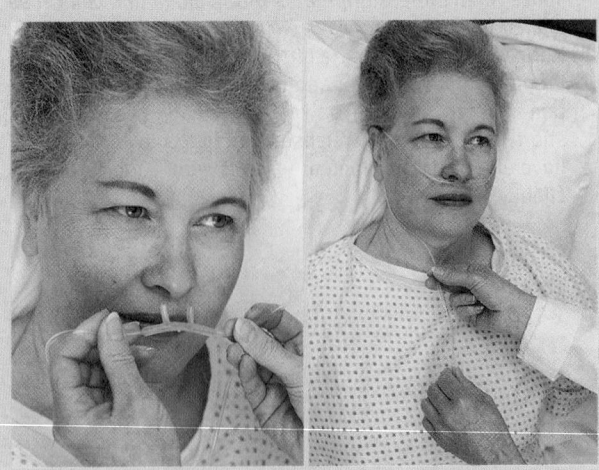

STEP 6 Applying nasal cannula and adjusting fit to client comfort.

✳ SKILL 40-4 APPLYING A NASAL CANNULA OR OXYGEN MASK—CONT'D

STEPS

7. Maintain sufficient slack on oxygen tubing, and secure to client's clothes.
8. Check cannula at least every 8 hours or with changes in client's cardiopulmonary status. Keep humidification jar filled at all times.
9. Observe client's nares and superior surface of both ears for skin breakdown.
10. Check oxygen flow rate and physician's orders at least every 8 hours or with changes in client's cardiopulmonary status.
11. Perform hand hygiene.
12. Inspect client for relief of symptoms associated with hypoxia.

RATIONALE

Allows client to turn head without removing oxygen mask or dislodging cannula and reduces pressure on tips of nares.
Ensures patency of cannula and oxygen flow. Prevents inhalation of dehumidified oxygen.

Oxygen therapy causes drying of nasal mucosa. Pressure on ears from cannula tubing or elastic causes skin irritation.
Ensures delivery of prescribed oxygen flow rate and patency of cannula.
Reduces transmission of microorganisms.
Indicates that hypoxia is corrected or reduced.

Unexpected Outcomes and Related Interventions

1. Worsening respiratory status
   a. Check that oxygen delivery device is patent, not kinked, and attached to the oxygen flowmeter.
   b. Check oxygen level set on flowmeter; determine if delivered amount is consistent with physician's order.
   c. If not using wall oxygen, determine if the oxygen source contains enough oxygen to deliver the prescribed oxygen amount.
   d. Notify physician.
2. Dry nasal and upper airway mucosa
   a. If oxygen flow rate is greater than 4 L/min, determine the need for humidification.
   b. Assess the client's fluid status, and increase fluids if appropriate.
   c. Provide frequent oral care.
   d. Obtain physician's or other health care provider's order for use of sterile nasal saline intermittently.

4. Skin breakdown over the ears
   a. Adjust tightness of elastic strap to looser level.
   b. Provide good hygiene and skin care around the ears.
   c. Use soft, woven 4 × 4s as nonabrasive pad between elastic and ears.
   d. Reposition elastic strap frequently.

Recording and Reporting

- Record oxygen delivery device and liter flow in medical record; document client and family education.
- Report oxygen delivery device, liter flow, and response to changes in therapy to oncoming shift.

SAFETY ALERT Oxygen in high concentrations has a great combustion potential and readily fuels fire.

Promote oxygen safety by the following measures:

- Oxygen is a medication and adjusted only with a health care provider's order.
- Place an "Oxygen in Use" sign on the client's door and in the client's room. If using oxygen at home, place a sign on the door of the house.
- Keep oxygen delivery systems 10 feet from any open flames. Oxygen supports combustion; however, it will not explode.
- No smoking should be allowed on the premises.
- When using oxygen cylinders, secure them so that they will not fall over. Store oxygen cylinders upright, chained, or in appropriate holders.
- Determine that all electrical equipment in the room is functioning correctly and is properly grounded (see Chapter 38). An electrical spark in the presence of oxygen can result in a serious fire.
- Check the oxygen level of portable tanks before transporting a client to ensure that there is enough oxygen in the tank.

Supply of Oxygen. Oxygen is supplied to the client's bedside either by oxygen tanks or through a permanent wall-piped system.

Oxygen tanks are transported on wide-based carriers that allow the tank to be placed upright at the bedside. Regulators control the amount of oxygen delivered. One common type is an upright flowmeter with a flow adjustment valve at the top. A second type is a cylinder indicator with a flow adjustment handle. In the home setting, oxygen therapy is also supplied in a variety of methods, including refillable cylinders (Cuvelier and others, 2002).

In the hospital or home, oxygen tanks are delivered with the regulator in place. In the hospital the respiratory care department usually connects the regulator to the oxygen source. Home care vendors are usually responsible for connecting the oxygen tank to the regulator for home use.

Methods of Oxygen Delivery. The nasal cannula and oxygen masks are the most common devices to deliver oxygen to a client.

Nasal Cannula. A **nasal cannula** is a simple, comfortable device used for oxygen delivery (Skill 40-4). The two cannulas, about 1.5 cm (½ inch) long, protrude from the center of a disposable tube and are inserted into the nares. Oxygen is delivered via the cannulas with a flow rate of up to 6 L/min. Flow rates greater than 4 L/min are not often used because of the drying effect on the mucosa and the relatively little increase in delivered oxygen concentration. Know what flow rate produces a given percentage of inspired oxygen concentration (FIO_2) (Table 40-8). Also be alert

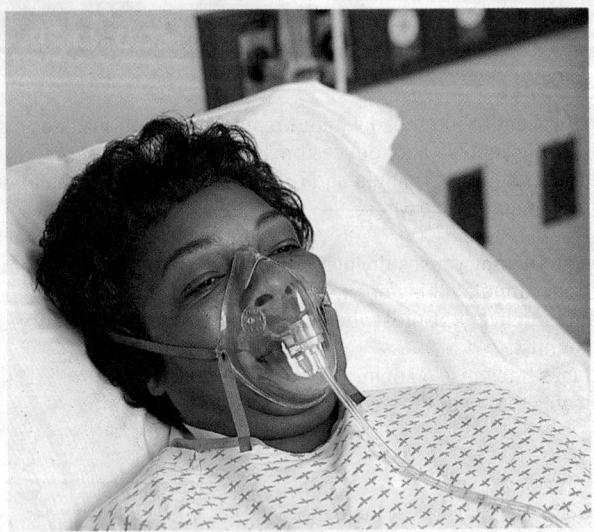

Figure 40-15 Simple face mask.

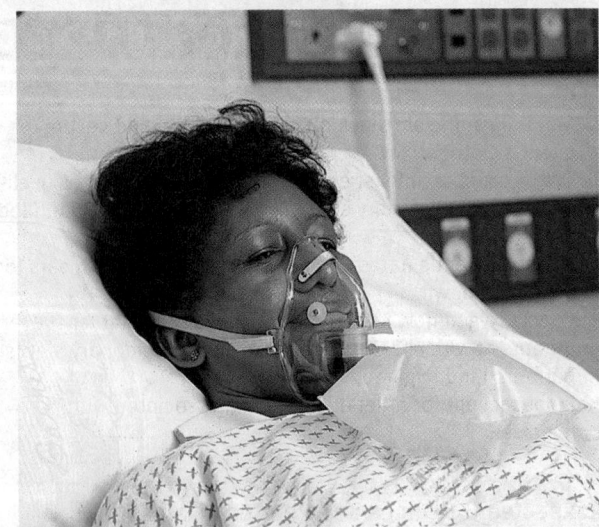

Figure 40-16 Plastic face mask with reservoir bag.

✳ TABLE 40-8   Approximate FIO₂ With Different Oxygen Delivery Devices

Oxygen Delivery Device	FIO₂ Delivered	Advantages	Disadvantages
Nasal cannula	1 L/min: 24% 2 L/min: 28% 3 L/min: 32% 4 L/min: 36% 5 L/min: 40% 6 L/min: 44%	Safe and simple Easily tolerated Delivers low concentrations while allowing the client to eat, speak, and drink Does not impede eating or talking Inexpensive, disposable	Unable to use with nasal obstruction Drying to mucous membranes Can dislodge easily Causes skin irritation or breakdown Client's breathing pattern will affect exact FIO₂
Simple face mask	5-6 L/min: 40% 6-7 L/min: 50% 7-8 L/min: 60% >8 L/min: 60%	Assists in providing humidified oxygen	Exact FIO₂ level is difficult to estimate Requires high FIO₂ levels to prevent rebreathing of carbon dioxide Client inhales room air through the side holes in the mask
Venturi mask	4 L/min: 24%-28% 8 L/min: 35%-40% 12 L/min: 50%-60%	Controls the amount of specified oxygen concentration; delivers percentage of FIO₂ from 24% to 60% Does not dry mucous membranes Delivers humidity with oxygen concentration	Hot and confining, increased levels of humidification irritate skin A specific flow rate is necessary to deliver a specific FIO₂, and the FIO₂ can decrease if the mask does not fit properly Interferes with eating and talking

FIO₂, Fraction of inspired oxygen concentration.

for skin breakdown over the ears and in the nares from too tight an application of the nasal cannula.

Oxygen Masks. An oxygen mask is a device used to administer oxygen, humidity, or heated humidity. It fits snugly over the mouth and nose and is secured in place with a strap. There are two primary types of oxygen masks: those delivering low concentrations of oxygen and those delivering high concentrations.

The simple face mask (Figure 40-15) is used for short-term oxygen therapy. It fits loosely and delivers oxygen concentrations from 30% to 60%. The mask is contraindicated for clients with carbon dioxide retention because retention can be worsened.

A plastic face mask with a reservoir bag (Figure 40-16) and a Venturi mask (Figure 40-17) are capable of delivering higher con-

centrations of oxygen. When used as a nonrebreather, the plastic face mask with a reservoir bag delivers from 60% to 95% oxygen with a flow rate of 6 to 10 L/min. This oxygen mask maintains a high-concentration oxygen supply in the reservoir bag. Frequently inspect the reservoir bag to make sure it is inflated. If it is deflated, the client is breathing large amounts of exhaled carbon dioxide.

The Venturi mask (see Figure 40-17) delivers oxygen concentrations of 24% to 60% with oxygen flow rates of 4 to 12 L/min, depending on the flow-control meter selected (see Table 40-8).

Home Oxygen Therapy. Indications for home oxygen therapy include an arterial partial pressure (PaO_2) of 55 mm Hg or less or an arterial oxygen saturation (SaO_2) of 88% or less on room air at rest, on exertion, or with exercise. Home oxygen

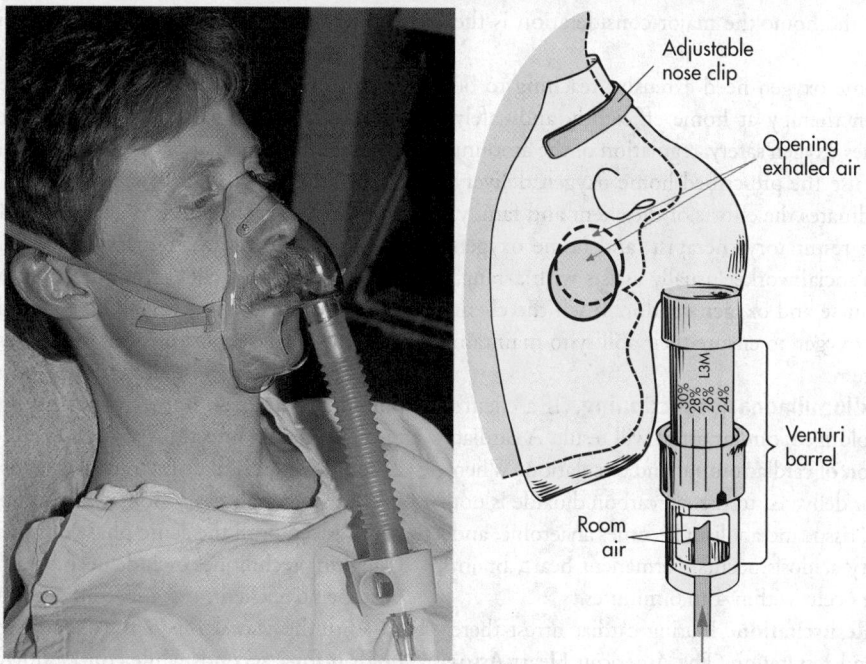

Figure 40-17 Venturi mask.

✳ TABLE 40-9 Home Oxygen Systems

PRIMARY USE	ADVANTAGES	DISADVANTAGES
Compressed Gas Cylinders Intermittent therapy, such as for exercise or sleep only	100% oxygen stored in steel or aluminum cylinders; relatively inexpensive, no loss of gas during storage, relatively portable, delivery of up to 15 L/min; does not require electrical source; smaller tanks available.	Bulky and heavy; frequent refilling necessary with continuous use; client must know how to read regulator and must understand when to call supplier; portable cylinders weigh 15 pounds.
Liquid Oxygen Systems System of choice for high-volume users and active clients	100% oxygen; more oxygen occupies a smaller space; client carries convenient ambulatory units refilled at home as a shoulder bag, backpack, or wheeled luggage cart; delivery of up to 6 L/min; client can safely refill ambulatory units from larger reservoir; quiet and easy operation; does not require electricity for operation; requires relatively fewer deliveries of oxygen.	Evaporates, especially in warmer temperatures and when not in use; potential for connections to freeze together or form frost at connections if tight connection not maintained during filling; costly in setup and delivery fees.
Oxygen Concentrators Cost-effective for clients requiring low-flow continuous oxygen and clients with limited mobility inside or outside the home	Inexpensive, fixed monthly costs; most units with delivery of up to 4 or 5 L/min; good choice for people who do not leave their homes frequently; no cylinders or tanks to refill.	Oxygen concentration decreases as liter flow increases (usually 85% to 90%); power supply needed; increased electric costs; is not an ambulatory unit, therefore requires a second system for portability; requires regular maintenance and backup system.

Data from Findeisen M: Long-term oxygen therapy in the home, *Home Healthc Nurse* 19(11):692, 2001; and Petty TL: *Guide to prescribing home oxygen: home oxygen options,* 2004, National Lung Health Education Program, http://www.nlhep.org/resources/Prescrb-Hm-Oxygen/home-oxygen-options-4.html, accessed November 18, 2006.

therapy is administered via nasal cannula or face mask (e.g., simple reservoir) (Petty, 2004). When a client has a permanent tracheostomy, a T tube or tracheostomy collar is used.

Home oxygen therapy has beneficial effect for clients with chronic cardiopulmonary diseases (Snow and others, 2001). This therapy improves clients' exercise tolerance and fatigue levels and

in some situations assists in the management of dyspnea (Fujimoto and others, 2002).

Three types of oxygen are used: compressed oxygen, liquid oxygen, and oxygen concentrators. The advantages and disadvantages (Table 40-9) of each type are assessed, along with the client's needs and community resources, before placing a certain delivery system in the home. In the home the major consideration is the oxygen delivery source.

Clients requiring home oxygen need extensive teaching to be able to continue oxygen therapy at home efficiently and safely (Skill 40-5). This includes oxygen safety, regulation of the amount of oxygen, and how to use the prescribed home oxygen delivery system. The nurse coordinates the efforts of the client and family, home care nurse, home respiratory therapist, and home oxygen equipment vendor. The social worker usually assists with arranging for the home care nurse and oxygen vendor. Teach the client and family about home oxygen to ensure their ability to maintain the oxygen delivery system.

Restoration of Cardiopulmonary Functioning. If a client's hypoxia is severe and prolonged, cardiac arrest will result. A cardiac arrest is a sudden cessation of cardiac output and circulation. When this occurs, oxygen is not delivered to tissues, carbon dioxide is not transported from tissues, tissue metabolism becomes anaerobic, and metabolic and respiratory acidosis occurs. Permanent heart, brain, and other tissue damage occur within 4 to 6 minutes.

Cardiopulmonary Resuscitation. During cardiac arrest there is an absence of pulse and respiration. The American Heart Association continues to research cardiac arrest treatment and outcomes. The 2005 Consensus Conference reviewed current information and developed the *2005 AHA Guidelines for Cardiopulmonary Resuscitation (CPR) and Emergency Cardiac Care (ECC),* thus simplifying the basic life support (BLS) steps (AHA, 2005a, 2005b).

The "ABCs" of **cardiopulmonary resuscitation** are to establish an Airway, initiate Breathing, and maintain Circulation. When you cannot establish an airway, reassess for proper head position and airway obstruction. There is no clinical benefit to cardiac compressions if an airway is not established. The purpose of CPR is to circulate oxygenated blood to the brain to prevent permanent tissue damage (AHA, 2005a).

Restorative and Continuing Care. Restorative and continuing care emphasize cardiopulmonary reconditioning as a structured rehabilitation program. **Cardiopulmonary rehabilitation** helps the client to achieve and maintain an optimal level of health through controlled physical exercise, nutrition counseling, relaxation and stress management techniques, and prescribed medications and oxygen. As physical reconditioning occurs, the client's complaints of dyspnea, chest pain, fatigue, and activity intolerance decrease. In addition, client's anxiety, depression, or somatic concerns often decrease. The client and the rehabilitation team define goals of rehabilitation.

Hydration. Maintenance of adequate systemic hydration keeps mucociliary clearance normal. In clients with adequate hydration, pulmonary secretions are thin, white, watery, and easily removable with minimal coughing. Excessive coughing to clear thick, tenacious secretions is fatiguing and energy depleting. The best way to maintain thin secretions is to provide a fluid intake of 1500 to 2000 mL/day unless contraindicated by cardiac status. The color, consistency, and ease of secretion expectoration determine adequacy of hydration.

Coughing Techniques. Coughing is effective for maintaining a patent airway. Coughing permits the client to remove secretions from both the upper and lower airways. The normal series of events in the cough mechanism are deep inhalation, closure of the glottis, active contraction of the expiratory muscles, and glottis opening. Deep inhalation increases the lung volume and airway diameter, allowing the air to pass through partially obstructing mucous plugs or other foreign matter. Contraction of the expiratory muscles against the closed glottis causes a high intrathoracic pressure to develop. When the glottis opens, a large flow of air is expelled at a high speed, providing momentum for mucus to move to the upper airways, where the client can expectorate or swallow it.

Evaluate the effectiveness of coughing by sputum expectoration, the client's report of swallowed sputum, or clearing of adventitious sounds by auscultation. Encourage clients with chronic pulmonary diseases, upper respiratory tract infections, and lower respiratory tract infections to deep breathe and cough at least every 2 hours while awake. Encourage clients with a large amount of sputum to cough every hour while awake and every 2 to 3 hours while asleep until the acute phase of mucus production has ended. Coughing techniques include deep breathing and coughing for the postoperative client, cascade, huff, and quad coughing.

With the *cascade cough,* the client takes a slow, deep breath and holds it for 2 seconds while contracting expiratory muscles. Then the client opens the mouth and performs a series of coughs throughout exhalation, thereby coughing at progressively lowered lung volumes. This technique promotes airway clearance and a patent airway in clients with large volumes of sputum.

The *huff cough* stimulates a natural cough reflex and is generally effective only for clearing central airways. While exhaling, the client opens the glottis by saying the word *huff.* With practice the client inhales more air and is able to progress to the cascade cough.

The *quad cough* technique is for clients without abdominal muscle control, such as those with spinal cord injuries. While the client breathes out with a maximal expiratory effort, the client or nurse pushes inward and upward on the abdominal muscles toward the diaphragm, causing the cough.

Respiratory Muscle Training. Respiratory muscle training improves muscle strength and endurance, resulting in improved activity tolerance. Respiratory muscle training prevents respiratory failure in clients with COPD.

One method for respiratory muscle training is the incentive spirometer resistive breathing device (ISRBD). Clients achieve resistive breathing by placing a resistive breathing device into a volume-dependent incentive spirometer. Clients achieve muscle training when they use the ISRBD on a scheduled routine (e.g., twice a day for 15 minutes or 4 times a day for 15 minutes).

Breathing Exercises. Breathing exercises include techniques to improve ventilation and oxygenation. The three basic techniques are deep breathing and coughing exercises, pursed-lip breathing, and diaphragmatic breathing. Deep breathing and coughing exercises are routine interventions for postoperative clients (see Chapter 50).

Pursed-Lip Breathing. **Pursed-lip breathing** involves deep inspiration and prolonged expiration through pursed lips to prevent alveolar collapse. While sitting up, instruct the client to take a deep breath and to exhale slowly through pursed lips, as if blowing through a straw. Have the client blow through a straw into a glass of water to learn the technique. Clients need to gain control

☀ SKILL 40-5

USING HOME OXYGEN EQUIPMENT

Delegation Considerations
The skill of using home oxygen equipment cannot be delegated. The nurse directs nursing assistive personnel about:
- The unique needs of the client (e.g., amount of assistance in applying nasal cannula or mask) and any assistance needed in filling liquid canisters
- The type of equipment the client should have in the home and the oxygen flow rate

- Immediately reporting to the nurse increased rate of breathing, decreased level of consciousness, increased confusion, and pain

Equipment
- Nasal cannula equipment (see Skill 40-4, p. 956)
- Oxygen tubing
- Home oxygen delivery system with appropriate equipment

STEPS	RATIONALE
1. While client is still in the hospital, determine client's or family's ability to use oxygen equipment correctly. In the home setting reassess for appropriate use of equipment.	Physical or cognitive impairments necessitate instructing family member or significant other how to operate home oxygen equipment. Ongoing assessment enables nurse to determine specific components of skill that client or family can easily complete.
2. Assess home environment for adequate electrical service if oxygen concentrator is ordered.	Oxygen concentrators require electricity to work. Continuous oxygen therapy must not be interrupted.
3. Assess client's and family's ability to observe for signs and symptoms of hypoxia: apprehension, anxiety, decreased ability to concentrate, decreased level of consciousness, increased fatigue, dizziness, behavioral changes, increased pulse, increased respiratory rate, pallor, or cyanosis of the mucous membranes.	Hypoxia occurs at home despite use of oxygen therapy. Worsening of client's physical condition or another underlying condition, such as a change in the respiratory status, can cause hypoxia.
4. Determine appropriate resources in the community for equipment and assistance, including maintenance and repair services, and medical equipment supplier.	Ensures readily available assistance for clients with home oxygen systems.
5. In case there is a power failure, determine appropriate backup systems when using compressor. Have a spare oxygen tank available.	Many municipalities require that clients with home oxygen equipment notify emergency medical service (EMS) before bringing the equipment home. When there is a power outage, EMS calls the home, and in some cases the home is on a priority list for power restoration.
6. Perform hand hygiene.	Reduces transmission of infection.
7. Place oxygen delivery system in a clutter-free environment that is well ventilated; away from walls, drapes, bedding, combustible materials; and at least 8 feet from heat source.	Prevents injury from improper placement of oxygen equipment.
8. Demonstrate each step for preparation and completion of oxygen therapy.	Teaches psychomotor skill and enables client to ask questions.
a. Compressed oxygen system	
(1) Turn cylinder valve counterclockwise two or three turns with wrench. Store wrench with oxygen tank.	Turns on oxygen. Keeps wrench available.
(2) Check cylinders by reading amount on pressure gauge (see illustration).	Verifies adequate oxygen supply for client use.

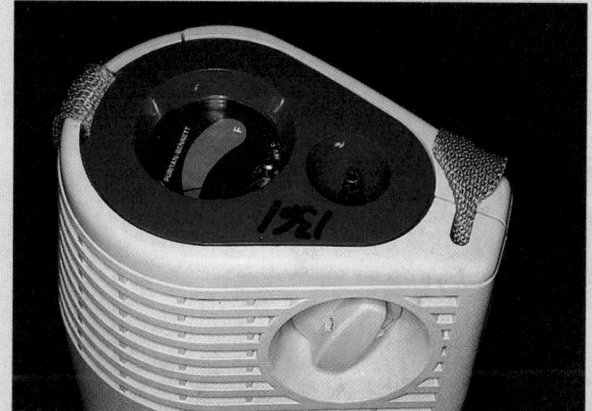

STEP 8a(2) Verify the oxygen level by reading the gauge on top of the canister.

Continued

✳ **SKILL 40-5**   **USING HOME OXYGEN EQUIPMENT—CONT'D**

STEPS

b. Oxygen concentrator system
   (1) Plug concentrator into appropriate outlet.
   (2) Turn on power switch
   (3) Alarm will sound for a few seconds.

c. Refilling oxygen tank
   (1) Wipe both filling connectors with a clean, dry, lint-free cloth.
   (2) Turn off flow selector of ambulatory unit.
   (3) Attach ambulatory unit to stationary reservoir by inserting adapter from ambulatory tank into adapter of stationary reservoir.
   (4) Open fill valve on ambulatory tank, and apply firm pressure to top of stationary reservoir (see illustration). Stay with unit while it is filling. You will hear a loud hissing noise. Tank fills in about 2 minutes.
   (5) Disengage ambulatory unit from stationary reservoir when hissing noise changes and vapor cloud begins to form from stationary unit.
   (6) Wipe both filling connectors with clean, dry, lint-free cloth.

RATIONALE

Provides power source.
Starts concentrator motor.
Alarm turns off when desired pressure inside concentrator is reached.

Removes dust and moisture from system.

Prevents leaking of oxygen during filling process. If oxygen leaks during filling process, connection between ambulatory tank and reservoir will ice up and stick together.

Overfilling causes ambulatory unit to malfunction due to high pressure in tank.

Ice sometimes forms during filling. Removes moisture from oxygen system.

Critical Decision Point: If ambulatory unit does not separate easily, valves from reservoir and ambulatory unit may be frozen together. Wait until valves warm to disengage (about 5 to 10 minutes). Do not touch any frosted areas because contact with skin causes skin damage from frostbite.

---

 9. Connect oxygen delivery device to oxygen system.
10. Adjust to prescribed flow rate (L/min).
11. Place oxygen delivery device on client.
12. Perform hand hygiene.
13. Instruct client and family not to change oxygen flow rate.
14. Guide the client and family as they perform each step. Provide written material for reinforcement and review.

Connects oxygen source to delivery system.
Ensures appropriate oxygen prescription.
Delivers oxygen to client.
Reduces transmission of microorganisms.

Allows nurse to correct for errors in technique and discuss their implications.

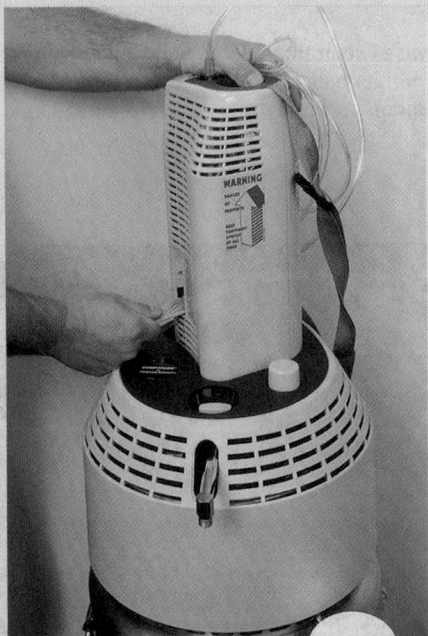

STEP 8c(4) Open fill valve on ambulatory tank while applying firm pressure to top of ambulatory unit.

✳ *SKILL 40-5*   **USING HOME OXYGEN EQUIPMENT—CONT'D**

STEPS	RATIONALE
15. Instruct client and family to notify physician if signs or symptoms of hypoxia or respiratory tract infection (e.g., fever, increased sputum, change in color of sputum, odor) occur.	Respiratory tract infections increase oxygen demand and affect oxygen transfer from lungs to blood. Can create severe exacerbation of client's pulmonary disease.
16. Discuss emergency plan for power loss, natural disaster, and acute respiratory distress. Have client or family/caregiver call 911 and notify physician or health care provider and home care agency.	Ensures appropriate response and prevents worsening of client's condition.
17. Instruct client in safe home oxygen practices, including not allowing smoking in the house, keeping oxygen tanks away from open flame, and storing tanks upright.	Ensures safe use of oxygen in the home and prevents injury to client and family.
18. Monitor oxygen delivery rate.	Determines if client is using oxygen at prescribed rate.
19. Ask client and family about ease or problems associated with home oxygen.	Determines ability of client and family to deal with stressors associated with home oxygen use.
20. Ask client and family to state safety guidelines, emergency precautions, and emergency plan.	Determines client's knowledge of what to do if power fails, there is a failure in equipment, or client's status worsens.

Unexpected Outcomes and Related Interventions

1. Client reports no oxygen flow.
   a. Check tank pressure gauge. If level of oxygen is low, refill tank if portable, or provide alternate source of oxygen, such as concentrator or H cylinder.
   b. Notify home oxygen supplier of need for refill.
   c. Reassure client and family.
2. Unable to fill portable liquid oxygen from main source.
   a. Check to see that portable tank is connected correctly.
   b. Determine if valve is frozen.
   c. Contact home oxygen supplier for service visit.
   d. Provide alternate oxygen source if necessary.

Recording and Reporting

- Record the teaching plan, the client's and family's ability to safely use the home oxygen equipment; report the type of home oxygen equipment to be used, the client's and family's understanding of how to use the equipment, knowledge of safety guidelines and unexpected outcomes, and ability to return demonstrate proper use of the oxygen delivery device.

---

of the exhalation phase so that it is longer than inhalation. The client is usually able to perfect this technique by counting the inhalation time and gradually increasing the count during exhalation. In studies using pulse oximetry as a feedback tool, clients are able to demonstrate an increase in their arterial oxygen saturation during pursed-lip breathing.

Diaphragmatic Breathing. **Diaphragmatic breathing** is more difficult and requires the client to relax intercostal and accessory respiratory muscles while taking deep inspirations. The client concentrates on expanding the diaphragm during controlled inspiration and learns to place one hand flat below the breastbone above the waist and the other hand 2 to 3 cm below the first hand. Ask the client to inhale while the lower hand moves outward during inspiration. The client observes for inward movement as the diaphragm ascends. The client practices these exercises initially in the supine position and then while sitting and standing. The exercise is often used with the pursed-lip breathing technique.

Diaphragmatic breathing is also useful for clients with pulmonary disease, for postoperative clients, and for women in labor to promote relaxation and provide pain control. The exercise improves efficiency of breathing by decreasing air trapping and reducing the work of breathing.

 Evaluation

Evaluate nursing interventions and therapies by comparing the client's progress with the goals and expected outcomes of the nursing care plan (Figure 40-18). Client expectations evaluate the care from the client's perspective.

Ask the client about his or her degree of breathlessness. Ask the client to rate breathlessness on a scale of 0 to 10, with 0 being no shortness of breath and 10 being severe shortness of breath. Ask the client what interventions help reduce dyspnea.

Evaluation of arterial blood gas levels, pulmonary function tests, vital signs, ECG tracings, and physical assessment data provide objective measurement of the success of therapies and treatments. When nursing measures directed to improve oxygenation are unsuccessful, do not hesitate to notify the physician about a client's deteriorating oxygenation status. Prompt notification helps avoid an emergency situation or even the need for CPR. Compare outcomes with expected outcomes to determine the client's health status. Continuous evaluation helps to determine whether new or revised therapies are required and if new nursing diagnoses have developed and require a new plan of care.

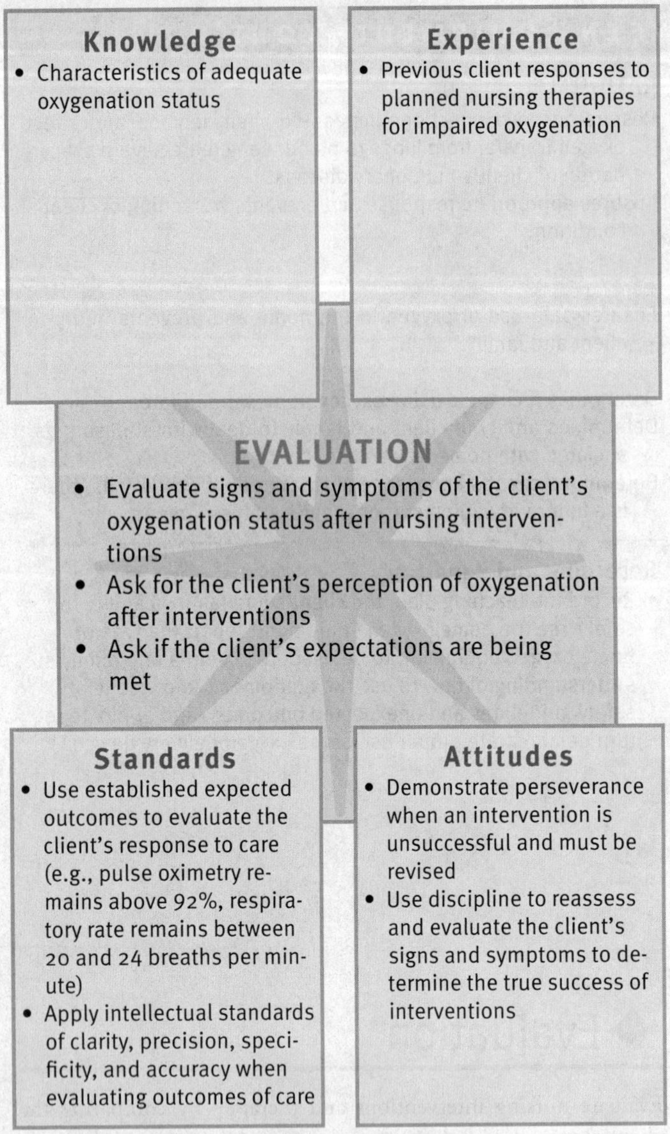

Knowledge
- Characteristics of adequate oxygenation status

Experience
- Previous client responses to planned nursing therapies for impaired oxygenation

EVALUATION
- Evaluate signs and symptoms of the client's oxygenation status after nursing interventions
- Ask for the client's perception of oxygenation after interventions
- Ask if the client's expectations are being met

Standards
- Use established expected outcomes to evaluate the client's response to care (e.g., pulse oximetry remains above 92%, respiratory rate remains between 20 and 24 breaths per minute)
- Apply intellectual standards of clarity, precision, specificity, and accuracy when evaluating outcomes of care

Attitudes
- Demonstrate perseverance when an intervention is unsuccessful and must be revised
- Use discipline to reassess and evaluate the client's signs and symptoms to determine the true success of interventions

Figure 40-18 Critical thinking model for oxygenation evaluation.

Key Concepts
- The primary function of the heart is to deliver deoxygenated blood to the lungs for oxygenation and to deliver oxygen and nutrients to the tissues.
- Preload, afterload, contractility, and heart rate alter cardiac output.
- Cardiac dysrhythmias are classified by cardiac activity and site of impulse origin.
- The primary function of the lungs is to transfer oxygen from the atmosphere into the alveoli and to transfer carbon dioxide out of the body as a waste product.
- Ventilation is the process of providing adequate oxygenation from the alveoli to the blood.
- Changes in intrapleural and intraalveolar pressures and lung volumes cause the process of inspiration (active process) and expiration (passive process).

- Decreased hemoglobin levels alter the client's ability to transport oxygen.
- Impaired chest wall movement reduces the level of tissue oxygenation.
- Hyperventilation is a respiratory rate greater than that required to maintain normal levels of carbon dioxide.
- Hypoventilation causes carbon dioxide retention.
- Hypoxia occurs if the amount of oxygen delivered to tissues is too low.
- The nursing history and assessment includes information about the client's cough, dyspnea, fatigue, wheezing, chest pain, environmental exposures, respiratory infection, cardiopulmonary risk factors, and use of medications.
- Diagnostic and laboratory tests complete the database for a client with decreased oxygenation.
- Breathing exercises improve ventilation, oxygenation, and sensations of dyspnea.
- Chest physiotherapy includes postural drainage, percussion, and vibration to mobilize pulmonary secretions.
- Coughing and suctioning techniques help maintain a patent airway.
- Nasal cannulas and oxygen masks deliver oxygen therapy, which improves the levels of tissue oxygenation.

Critical Thinking Exercises

Mr. Edwards is placed on a Venturi mask at an oxygen concentration of 24%. He now has abnormal lung sounds in the left base as well as both upper lobes. His vital signs are now temperature, 102.4° F; blood pressure, 140/92 mm Hg; pulse, 90 beats per minute; respirations, 28 breaths per minute; and SpO_2, 82%. He cannot lie flat, and it is difficult for him to speak.

1. What does the new finding of abnormal lung sounds in left base indicate?
2. How does this affect Mr. Edwards's ability to oxygenate?
3. Would you increase Mr. Edwards's percentage of oxygen?
4. List at least two interventions or nursing activities that you need to implement now based on the information above.

Mr. Edwards's health care provider obtains another chest x-ray film and arterial blood gas levels. His chest x-ray film indicates that both upper lobes and the left lower lobe have infiltrates and his pneumonia is worsening. The arterial blood gas levels indicate a worsening respiratory acidosis (see Chapter 41). His PaO_2 is 55 mm Hg, $PaCO_2$ is 65 mm Hg, pH is 7.3, and SpO_2 is 80%.

1. What else do you need to know about Mr. Edwards's blood gas levels?
2. He is hypoxic (PaO_2 55 mm Hg, SpO_2 80%). What assessment would you expect to find? What assessments would indicate a worsening of his oxygenation status?

Mr. Edwards's condition worsened, and he spent 5 days in an intensive care unit (ICU) and 2 weeks in a transitional care unit. He is being discharged on home oxygen therapy. His discharge plan includes an outpatient rehabilitation program to begin 1 month after discharge.

1. What do you need to do to prepare Mr. and Mrs. Edwards for home oxygen therapy?

✳ NCLEX®-Style Review Questions

1. A person who starts smoking in adolescence and continues to smoke into middle age has an increased risk for:
   1. Alcoholism
   2. Obesity and diabetes
   3. Stress-related illnesses
   4. Cardiopulmonary disease and lung cancer

2. Symptoms associated with anemia include (choose all that apply):
   1. Increased breathlessness
   2. Decreased breathlessness
   3. Increased activity tolerance
   4. Decreased activity tolerance

3. Carbon monoxide is a toxic inhalant that decreases the oxygen-carrying capacity of blood by:
   1. Forming a weak bond with hemoglobin
   2. Forming a strong bond with hemoglobin
   3. Forming a weak bond with carbamino compounds
   4. Forming a strong bond with carbamino compounds

4. Conditions such as shock and severe dehydration resulting from extracellular fluid loss and reduced circulating blood volume cause:
   1. Hypoxia
   2. Hypovolemia
   3. Hypervolemia
   4. Uncontrolled bleeding

5. Fever increases the tissues' need for oxygen, and as a result:
   1. Metabolic demands decrease
   2. Blood glucose stores stabilize
   3. Carbon dioxide production increases
   4. Carbon dioxide production decreases

6. Left-sided heart failure causes:
   1. Increased cardiac output
   2. Lowered cardiac pressures
   3. Decreased functioning of the left atrium
   4. Decreased functioning of the left ventricle

7. Cyanosis, the blue discoloration of the skin and mucous membranes caused by the presence of desaturated hemoglobin in capillaries, is a(n):
   1. Late sign of hypoxia
   2. Early sign of hypoxia
   3. Non–life-threatening event
   4. Reliable measure of oxygenation status

8. A simple and cost-effective method for reducing the risks of stasis of pulmonary secretions and decreased chest wall expansion is:
   1. Antiinfectives
   2. Chest physiotherapy
   3. Oxygen humidification
   4. Frequent change of position

9. Which of the following assessments indicate that the client needs airway suctioning? (Choose all that apply.)
   1. Thick sputum
   2. Thin, watery sputum
   3. Decreased coughing ability
   4. Secretions that clear with coughing
   5. Abnormal lung sounds only in left lower lobe

10. Clients with chest tubes are at risk for tension pneumothorax. Some of the symptoms of a tension pneumothorax include (choose all that apply):
    1. Increased heart rate
    2. Decreased heart rate
    3. Increased respiratory rate
    4. Increased blood pressure
    5. Decreased blood pressure
    6. Asymmetrical chest wall movement

41 | Fluid, Electrolyte, and Acid-Base Balance

✴ OBJECTIVES

Mastery of content in this chapter will enable the student to:

- Describe the distribution, composition, movement, and regulation of body fluids.
- Describe the regulation and movement of major electrolytes.
- Describe the processes involved in acid-base balance.
- Describe common disturbances in fluid, electrolyte, and acid-base balances.
- Identify factors that affect normal fluid, electrolyte, and acid-base balances.
- Discuss clinical assessments for determining fluid, electrolyte, and acid-base imbalances.
- Describe laboratory studies performed for fluid, electrolyte, and acid-base imbalances.

- List and discuss nursing interventions for clients with fluid, electrolyte, and acid-base imbalances.
- Discuss purpose and procedure for initiation and maintenance of intravenous therapy.
- Calculate an intravenous flow rate.
- Measure and record fluid intake and output.
- Demonstrate how to change intravenous solutions, tubing, and dressings and how to discontinue an infusion.
- Discuss the complications of intravenous therapy.
- Discuss the procedure for initiating a blood transfusion and interventions to manage a transfusion reaction.

✴ MEDIA RESOURCES   ✴ KEY TERMS

 Companion CD
- NCLEX®-Style Review Questions
- Audio Glossary
- Interactive Learning Activities
- English/Spanish Glossary

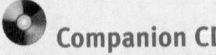 **Website**
- NCLEX®-Style Review Questions
- Audio Glossary
- English/Spanish Glossary
- Interactive Learning Activities
- Weblinks
- Audio Summaries
- Video Clips

Acidosis, p. 971
Active transport, p. 969
Aldosterone, p. 970
Alkalosis, p. 971
Angiotensin, p. 970
Anion gap, p. 977
Anions, p. 967
Antidiuretic hormone (ADH), p. 969
Arterial blood gas (ABG), p. 974
Atrial natriuretic peptide (ANP), p. 970
Autologous transfusion, p. 1022
Buffer, p. 971
Cations, p. 967
Colloid osmotic pressure, p. 968
Colloids, p. 991
Concentration gradient, p. 968
Crystalloids, p. 991
Dehydration, p. 969
Diffusion, p. 968
Edema, p. 968

Electrolytes, p. 967
Erythema, p. 1021
Extracellular fluids, p. 967
Filtration, p. 968
Fluid volume deficit (FVD), p. 978
Fluid volume excess (FVE), p. 991
Hemolysis, p. 1022
Homeostasis, p. 969
Hydrostatic pressure, p. 968
Hypernatremia, p. 972
Hypertonic, p. 968
Hypokalemia, p. 972
Hyponatremia, p. 972
Hypotonic, p. 968
Hypovolemia, p. 969
Infiltration, p. 1012
Infusion pumps, p. 1006
Insensible water loss, p. 970
Interstitial fluid, p. 967
Intracellular fluids, p. 967
Intravascular fluid, p. 967
Ions, p. 967

Isotonic, p. 968
Metabolic acidosis, p. 977
Metabolic alkalosis, p. 977
Milliequivalents per liter (mEq/L), p. 967
Oncotic pressure, p. 968
Osmolality, p. 968
Osmolarity, p. 968
Osmols, p. 968
Osmoreceptors, p. 969
Osmosis, p. 967
Osmotic pressure, p. 968
Phlebitis, p. 1021
Respiratory acidosis, p. 977
Respiratory alkalosis, p. 977
Sensible water loss, p. 970
Solute, p. 967
Solution, p. 967
Solvent, p. 967
Transcellular fluid, p. 967
Transfusion reaction, p. 1021
Vascular access devices (VADs), p. 991
Venipuncture, p. 1005

Fluid, electrolyte, and acid-base balances within the body maintain health and function in all body systems. These balances are maintained by the intake and output of water and electrolytes, their distribution in the body, and regulated by the renal and pulmonary systems. The body maintains fluid and electrolyte balance despite variations in intake and loss. Physical, behavioral, and environmental factors affect the body's ability to regulate fluid, electrolyte, and acid base balances. Imbalances result from illnesses, altered fluid intake, or prolonged episodes of vomiting or diarrhea. Acid-base balance is necessary for many physiological processes. Imbalances alter respiration, metabolism, and cardiovascular, renal, and central nervous system function. Your knowledge and understanding of the mechanisms that contribute to fluid, electrolyte, and acid-base imbalances are essential (Monahan and others, 2007).

Scientific Knowledge Base

Water balance is the balance between water intake and water output. Water is the largest single component of the body; 60% of the average adult's weight is fluid. The proportion of water is lower in women, obese, and older adults, but higher in children (Davidhizar and others, 2004). A series of mechanisms that are responsive to alterations in intake and loss control and regulate total body water. Fluid imbalance is evaluated based on the amount of sodium lost or gained in relationship to water. A healthy, active, well-oriented adult usually maintains normal fluid, electrolyte, and acid-base balances because of the body's adaptive physiological mechanisms.

Distribution of Body Fluids

Body fluids are distributed into two distinct compartments, one containing **intracellular fluids** and the other **extracellular fluids.** Intracellular fluid (ICF) comprises all fluid within the cells of the body, about 42% of total body weight. In adults, approximately two thirds of the total body water, or approximately 28 L in the average male and 20 L in the average female, is ICF (Casey, 2004).

Extracellular fluid (ECF) is all the fluid outside a cell, which is divided into three smaller compartments: **interstitial fluid, intravascular fluid,** and **transcellular fluid.** Extracellular fluid makes up about 17% of total body weight, or one third of the total body water. Interstitial fluid, which contains lymph, is the fluid between the cells and outside the blood vessels. Intravascular fluid is blood plasma found in the vascular system. Transcellular fluid is fluid separated from other fluids by a cellular barrier and consists of cerebrospinal, pleural, gastrointestinal (GI), intraocular, peritoneal, and synovial fluids (Elgart, 2004). Loss of transcellular fluid can produce fluid and electrolyte disturbance.

Composition of Body Fluids

As water moves through the compartments of the body, it contains substances that are sometimes called minerals or salts but are technically known as **electrolytes** (Christensen and Kockrow, 2003). An electrolyte is an element or compound that, when dissolved or dissociated in water or another solvent, separates into **ions** that are electrically charged. Positively charged electrolytes

TABLE 41-1 Electrolyte Distribution in Body Fluid	
ELECTROLYTES	**EXTRACELLULAR**
Sodium (Na^+)	135-145 mEq/L
Potassium (K^+)	3.5-5.0 mEq/L
Ionized Calcium (Ca^{2+})	4.5-5.5 mg/dl
Bicarbonate (HCO_3^-)	22-26 (arterial) mEq/L
	24-30 (venous) mEq/L
Chloride (Cl^-)	95-105 mEq/L
Magnesium (Mg^{2+})	1.5-2.5 mEq/L
Phosphate (PO_4^{3-})	2.8-4.5 mg/dl

are **cations** (e.g., sodium [Na^+], potassium [K^+], calcium [Ca^{2+}]). Negatively charged electrolytes are **anions** (e.g., chloride [Cl^-], bicarbonate [HCO_3^-], sulfate [SO_4^-]). It is essential for health that fluid volume and electrolyte accumulations remain equal in all compartments. Table 41-1 presents the distribution of electrolytes in body fluids.

Electrolytes are vital to body functions. The value **milliequivalents per liter (mEq/L)** represents the number of grams of the specific electrolyte (**solute**) dissolved in a liter of plasma (**solution**). Sugar dissolved in tea is an example of sugar as a solute. Crystalloids are solutes comprised of salts and large molecule colloids that do not easily dissolve. The solution in which a solute is dissolved is called a **solvent** (Chernecky, Macklin, and Murphy-Ende, 2006). In the sugar and tea example, the tea is the solvent. In the body, water is the solvent and the solutes are electrolytes, oxygen, carbon dioxide, glucose, and proteins.

Minerals are ingested as compounds and are constituents of all body tissues and fluids. Minerals maintain physiological processes. Minerals also act as catalysts in nerve response, muscle contraction, and metabolism of nutrients in foods. In addition, they regulate electrolyte balance and hormone production and strengthen skeletal structures. Examples of minerals are iron and zinc.

Movement of Body Fluids

Each body compartment is separated by a cell wall and capillary membrane. Fluids and electrolytes constantly shift from compartment to compartment to facilitate body processes such as tissue oxygenation, acid-base balance, and urine formation. Because cell membranes separating the body fluid compartments are selectively permeable, water passes through them easily. However, most ions and molecules pass through them more slowly. The larger the ion molecule, the more slowly it passes through the membranes. Fluids and solutes move across these membranes by four processes: osmosis, diffusion, filtration, and active transport.

Osmosis. Osmosis involves the movement of a pure solvent, such as water, across a semipermeable membrane from an area of lesser solute concentration to an area of greater solute concentration. Osmosis attempts to equalize concentrations of molecules (ions) on both sides of the membrane (Figure 41-1). The membrane is permeable to the solvent, but is impermeable to the solute. The rate of osmosis depends on the concentration of the solutes in the solution, the temperature of the solution, the electrical charges of the solutes, and the differences between the os-

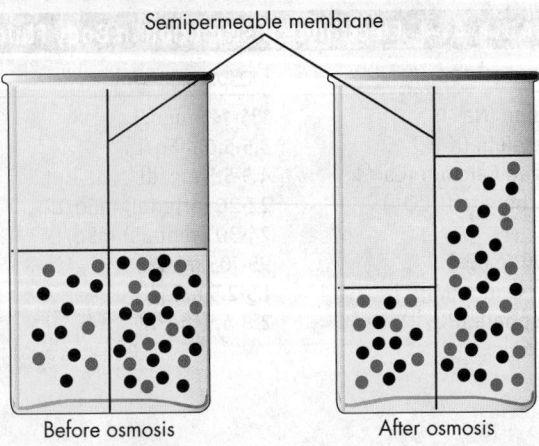

Figure 41-1 Osmosis through a semipermeable membrane. (From Lewis SL and others: *Medical-surgical nursing: assessment and management of clinical problems*, ed 7, St. Louis, 2007, Mosby.)

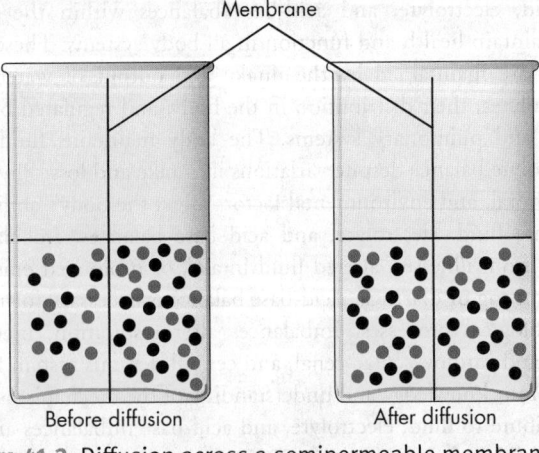

Figure 41-2 Diffusion across a semipermeable membrane. (From Lewis SL and others: *Medical-surgical nursing: assessment and management of clinical problems*, ed 7, St. Louis, 2007, Mosby.)

motic pressures exerted by the solutions. The concentration of a solution is measured in **osmols**, which reflects the amount of a substance in solution in the form of molecules, ions, or both. For example, boiling a hot dog is an example of osmosis. The concentration of molecules inside the hot dog is greater than in water. The water passes through the hot dog skin, which is a semipermeable membrane, in an attempt to equalize the number of molecules on both sides of the membrane. Finally, when the hot dog can no longer hold anymore water, the skin, or semipermeable membrane, ruptures (Christensen and Kockrow, 2003).

Osmotic pressure is the drawing power of water and depends on the number of molecules in solution. A solution with a high solute concentration has a high osmotic pressure and draws water toward itself. If the concentration of the solute is greater on one side of the semipermeable membrane, the rate of osmosis is quicker, and a more rapid transfer of solvent occurs across the membrane. This continues until reaching an equilibrium. The osmotic pressure of a solution is its **osmolality**, which is expressed in osmols, or milliosmols per kilogram (mOsm/kg) of the solution. The normal serum osmolality is 275 to 295 mOsm/kg. Osmolality is the measure used to evaluate serum and urine in clinical practice and reflects the total solute concentration in a fluid compartment. Changes in extracellular osmolality results in changes in both ECF and ICF volume. **Osmolarity** is another term that describes the concentration of solutions, reflects the number of molecules in a liter of solution, and is measured in milliosmoles per liter (mOsm/L).

Solutions are classified as **hypertonic, isotonic,** or **hypotonic.** A solution with the same osmolarity as blood plasma is isotonic, indicating that the solutions on both sides of the semipermeable membrane are equal in concentration. Isotonic solutions such as normal saline, 0.9% sodium chloride, expand the body's fluid volume without causing a fluid shift from one compartment to another. A hypertonic solution (a solution of higher osmotic pressure), such as 3% sodium chloride, pulls fluid from cells, causing them to shrink. Hypotonic solution (a solution of lower osmotic pressure), such as 0.45% sodium chloride, moves fluid into the

cells, causing them to enlarge. Each of these actions occurs through osmosis, which is a passive process.

Plasma proteins, especially albumin, a serum protein naturally produced by the body, affect the osmotic pressure of blood. Albumin exerts **colloid osmotic** or **oncotic pressure,** which tends to keep fluid in the intravascular compartment by pulling water from the interstitial space back into the capillaries (vascular compartment) (Chernecky and others, 2006).

Diffusion. **Diffusion** is the random movement of a solute (gas or solid) in a solution across a semipermeable membrane from an area of higher concentration to an area of lower concentration (Figure 41-2). The result is an even distribution of the solute in a solution. For example, when you pour a small amount of cream into a cup of black coffee, the cream left unmixed will diffuse through the whole cup of coffee (Chernecky and others, 2006). The rate of diffusion is affected by molecule size, concentration, and temperature of a solution. The larger the molecule and cooler the solution, the slower the rate of diffusion. A physiological example is the movement of oxygen and carbon dioxide between the alveoli and blood vessels in the lungs. The difference between the two concentrations is known as a **concentration gradient.**

Filtration. **Filtration** is the process by which water and diffusible substances move together across a membrane, in response to fluid pressure, moving from an area of higher pressure to one of lower pressure. This process is active in capillary beds, where **hydrostatic pressure** differences determine the movement of water (Figure 41-3). When there is increased hydrostatic pressure on the venous side of the capillary bed, as occurs in congestive heart failure (CHF), there is a reversal in the normal movement of water from the interstitial space into the intravascular space by filtration. This results in an accumulation of excess fluid in the interstitial space, known as **edema.** Hydrostatic pressure causes the movement of fluids from an area of higher pressure to an area of lower pressure. At the arterial end of the capillary, the hydrostatic pressure is greater than the colloid osmotic pressure, causing fluid

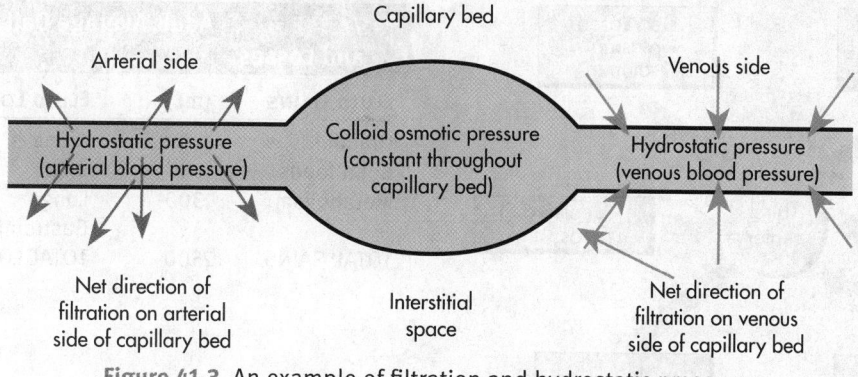

Figure 41-3 An example of filtration and hydrostatic pressure.

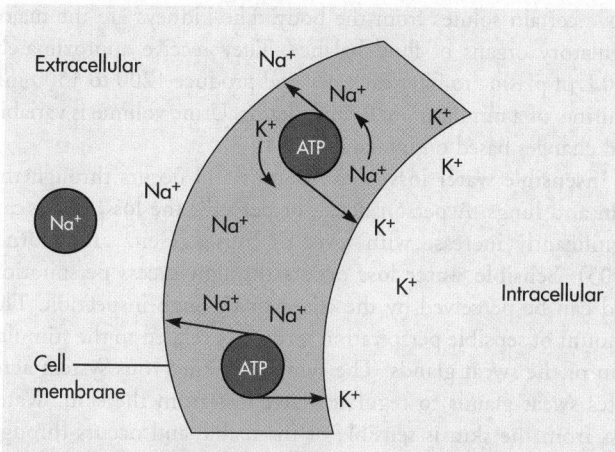

Figure 41-4 The sodium-potassium pump. As sodium diffuses into the cell and potassium out of the cell, active transport delivers sodium back to the extracellular compartment and potassium to the intracellular compartment. (From Lewis SL and others: *Medical-surgical nursing: assessment and management of clinical problems,* ed 7, St. Louis, 2007, Mosby.)

and diffusible solutes to move out of the capillary into the interstitial space. At the venous end, the colloid osmotic pressure, or pull, is greater than the hydrostatic pressure, and fluids and some solutes move into the capillary from the interstitial space. The excess fluid and solutes that remain in the interstitial space return to the intravascular compartment via the lymph channels.

Active Transport. Unlike diffusion, osmosis, and filtration, **active transport** requires metabolic activity and expenditure of energy to move substances across cell membranes. This allows cells to admit larger molecules than they would otherwise be able to admit or to move molecules from areas of lesser concentration to areas of greater concentration "uphill" (Figure 41-4). Examples of active transport are the sodium-potassium-ATPase pump. Sodium is pumped out of the cell and potassium is pumped in, against the concentration gradient. This process keeps a higher concentration of potassium in the ICF and a higher concentration of sodium in the ECF.

Active transport is enhanced by carrier molecules within a cell that bind themselves to incoming molecules. There is a specified carrier molecule for each substance. For example, glucose enters cells after it binds with the transport vehicle insulin. Active transport is the mechanism by which cells absorb glucose and other substances to carry out metabolism.

Regulation of Body Fluids

Fluid intake, hormonal controls, and fluid output regulate body fluids. This physiological balance is termed **homeostasis** (Heitz and Horne, 2005). In health, the body responds to disturbances in fluids and electrolytes to prevent and repair damage.

Fluid Intake. The thirst mechanism primarily regulates fluid intake. The thirst-control center is located within the hypothalamus in the brain. Thirst is the conscious desire for water and is one of the major factors that determines fluid intake (Chernecky and others, 2006). The **osmoreceptors** continually monitor the serum osmotic pressure, and when osmolality increases, the hypothalamus is stimulated. Eating potato chips is an example; the salt on the chips increases the osmotic pressure of the body fluids and stimulates the thirst mechanism (Monahan and others, 2007). Increased plasma osmolality occurs with any condition that interferes with the oral ingestion of fluids, or it can occur with the intake of hypertonic fluids. The hypothalamus is also stimulated when excess fluid is lost, and **hypovolemia** occurs, as in excessive vomiting and hemorrhage. Figure 41-5 illustrates other stimuli that affect the sensation of thirst.

The average adult's intake is about 2200 to 2700 mL per day; oral intake accounts for 1100 to 1400 mL, solid foods about 800 to 1000 mL, and oxidative metabolism 300 mL daily (Heitz and Horne, 2005). Water oxidation (oxidative metabolism) is the byproduct of cellular metabolism of ingested solid foods. Fluid intake requires an alert state. Infants, clients with neurological or psychological problems, and some older adults who are unable to perceive or respond to the thirst mechanism are at risk for **dehydration** (Grandjean and others, 2003).

Hormonal Regulation. Hormones such as antidiuretic hormone, the renin-angiotensin-aldosterone mechanism, and atrial natriuretic peptide (NAP) regulate fluid intake through various mechanisms. **Antidiuretic hormone (ADH)** is stored in the posterior pituitary gland and is released in response to changes in

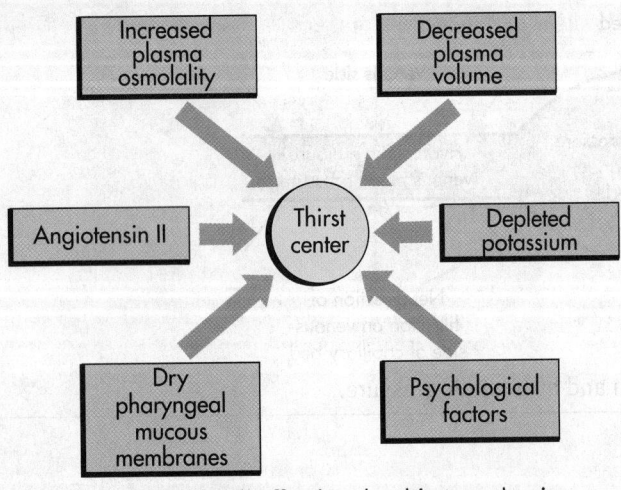

Figure 41-5 Stimuli affecting the thirst mechanism.

TABLE 41-2		Adult Average Daily Fluid Gains and Losses	
FLUID GAINS	**(mL)**	**FLUID LOSSES**	**(mL)**
Oral fluids	1200	Kidneys	1500
Solid foods	1000	Skin	300
Metabolism	300	Lungs	500
		Gastrointestinal	200
TOTAL GAINS	2500	TOTAL LOSSES	2500

blood osmolarity. Pain, stress, circulating blood volume, and some drugs affect ADH production and release in the body. ADH prevents diuresis, thus causing the body to save water. An increase in osmolarity stimulates the osmoreceptors in the hypothalamus to release the hormone ADH. The ADH works directly on the renal tubules and collecting ducts to make them more permeable to water. This in turn causes water to return to the systemic circulation, which dilutes the blood and decreases its osmolarity. As the body attempts to compensate, there will be a temporary decrease in urinary output. When the blood becomes diluted, the osmoreceptors stop the release of ADH and urinary output is restored.

Changes in renal perfusion initiate the renin-angiotensin-aldosterone mechanism. Renin, a proteolytic enzyme secreted by the kidneys, responds to decreased renal perfusion secondary to a decrease in extracellular volume. Renin acts to produce **angiotensin** I, which causes some vasoconstriction. However, angiotensin I almost immediately becomes reduced by an enzyme that converts angiotension I into angiotensin II. Angiotensin II then causes massive selective vasoconstriction of many blood vessels and relocates and increases the blood flow to the kidney, improving renal perfusion. Angiotensin II also stimulates the release of aldosterone when the sodium concentration is low.

The adrenal cortex releases **aldosterone** in response to increased plasma potassium levels or as a part of the renin-angiotensin-aldosterone mechanism to counteract hypovolemia. Aldosterone acts on the distal portion of the renal tubule to increase the reabsorption (saving) of sodium and the secretion and excretion of potassium and hydrogen. Because sodium retention leads to water retention, the release of aldosterone acts as a volume regulator (Heitz and Horne, 2005). The overall effect of the renin-angiotensin-aldosterone mechanism is sodium and water retention, leading to restoration of blood volume (Chernecky and others, 2006).

Atrial natriuretic peptide (ANP) plays a critical role in the balance of fluid and electrolytes and the maintenance of vascular tone. ANP is a hormone secreted from atrial cells of the heart in response to atrial stretching and an increase in circulating blood volume. ANP acts as a diuretic that causes sodium loss and inhibits the thirst mechanism. Monitoring ANP has therapeutic potential (Scotland, Ahluwalia, and Hobbs, 2005).

Fluid Output Regulation. Fluid output occurs through four organs of water loss: the kidneys, skin, lungs, and the GI tract. There is a small amount of obligatory fluid loss necessary to remove certain solutes from the body. The kidneys are the major regulatory organs of fluid balance. They receive approximately 180 L of plasma to filter each day and produce 1200 to 1500 mL of urine, or a minimum of 0.5 mL/kg/hr. Urine volume is variable and changes based on intake (Table 41-2).

Insensible water loss is continuous and occurs through the skin and lungs. A person does not perceive the loss, but it can significantly increase with fever or burns (Heitz and Horne, 2005). **Sensible water loss** occurs through excess perspiration and can be perceived by the client or through inspection. The amount of sensible perspiration is directly related to the stimulation of the sweat glands. The sympathetic nervous system activates sweat glands to regulate water loss from the skin. Water loss from the skin is sensible or insensible and occurs through diffusion or perspiration. An average of 500 to 600 mL of sensible and insensible fluid is lost via the skin each day (Heitz and Horne, 2005).

The second type of insensible loss is through the lungs, which expire about 500 mL of water daily. This insensible water loss increases in response to changes in respiratory rate and depth. In addition, devices for administering oxygen increase insensible water loss from the lungs.

The GI tract plays a vital role in fluid regulation. Approximately 3 to 6 L of isotonic fluid moves into the gastrointestinal tract and then returns again to the extracellular fluid. Under normal conditions, the average adult loses only 200 mL of the 3 to 6 L each day through feces. However, in the presence of a disease process, for example, diarrhea, the GI tract becomes a site of large fluid losses. This loss significantly affects maintenance of normal fluid regulation.

Regulation of Electrolytes

Cations. Major cations within the body fluids include sodium (Na^+), potassium (K^+), calcium (Ca^{2+}), and magnesium (Mg^{2+}). Cations interchange when one cation leaves the cell and is replaced by another. This occurs because cells tend to maintain electrical neutrality.

Sodium Regulation. Sodium is the most abundant cation (90%) in ECF. Sodium ions are the major contributors to maintaining water balance through their effect on serum osmolality, nerve impulse transmission, regulation of acid-base balance, and participation in cellular chemical reactions (McCance and Huether, 2005). Sodium intake is regulated by dietary intake and aldosterone secretion. The normal extracellular sodium concentration is 135 to 145 mEq/L.

Potassium Regulation. Potassium is the major electrolyte and principal cation in the intracellular compartment (Monahan and others, 2007). It regulates many metabolic activities and is necessary for glycogen deposits in the liver and skeletal muscle, transmission and conduction of nerve impulses, normal cardiac conduction, and skeletal and smooth muscle contraction (McCance and Huether, 2005). A relatively small amount (approximately 2%) of potassium is located within the ECF (Heitz and Horne, 2005). The normal range for serum potassium concentrations is 3.5 to 5 mEq/L. Dietary intake and renal excretion regulate potassium. The body conserves potassium poorly, so any condition that increases urine output decreases the serum potassium concentration.

Calcium Regulation. Calcium is stored in bone, plasma, and body cells. Ninety-nine percent of calcium is located in bone, and only 1% is in ECF. Approximately 50% of calcium in the plasma binds to protein, primarily albumin, and 40% is free ionized calcium. The remaining small percentage combines with nonprotein anions such as phosphate, citrate, and carbonate (Heitz and Horne, 2005). Normal serum ionized calcium is 4.5 to 5.5 mg/dL. Normal total calcium is 8.5 to 10.5 mg/dL. Calcium is necessary for bone and teeth formation, blood clotting, hormone secretion, cell membrane integrity, cardiac conduction, transmission of nerve impulses, and muscle contraction.

Magnesium Regulation. Magnesium is essential for enzyme activities, neurochemical activities, and cardiac and skeletal muscle excitability. Plasma concentrations of magnesium range from 1.5 to 2.5 mEq/L. Serum magnesium is regulated by dietary intake, renal mechanisms, and actions of the parathyroid hormone (PTH). About 50% to 60% of body magnesium is contained within the bone, and only 1% is contained within the ECF compartment; the remainder is located inside the cell (Monahan and others, 2007).

Anions. The three major anions of body fluids are chloride (Cl^-), bicarbonate (HCO_3^-), and phosphate (PO_4^{3-}) ions.

Chloride Regulation. Chloride is the major anion in ECF. The transport of chloride follows sodium. Normal concentrations of chloride range from 95 to 105 mEq/L. Serum chloride is regulated by dietary intake and the kidneys. A person with normal renal function who has a high chloride intake will excrete a higher amount of urine chloride.

Bicarbonate Regulation. Bicarbonate is the major chemical base buffer within the body. The bicarbonate ion is found in both ECF and ICF. The bicarbonate ion is an essential component of the carbonic acid–bicarbonate buffering system essential to acid-base balance. The kidneys regulate bicarbonate. Normal arterial bicarbonate levels range between 22 and 26 mEq/L; normal venous bicarbonate (carbon dioxide content) is 24 to 30 mEq/L.

Phosphorus-Phosphate Regulation. Nearly all the phosphorus in the body exists in the form of phosphate (PO_4^{3-}), and the terms *phosphorus* and *phosphate* often are used interchangeably (Heitz and Horne, 2005). Phosphate is a buffer anion found primarily in ICF, with a small amount found in ECF. It assists in acid-base regulation. Phosphate and calcium help to develop and maintain bones and teeth. Calcium and phosphate are inversely proportional; if one rises, the other falls. Phosphate also promotes normal neuromuscular action and participates in carbohydrate metabolism. Phosphate is normally absorbed through the GI tract. It is regulated by dietary intake, renal excretion, intestinal absorption, and PTH. The normal serum level is 2.8 to 4.5 mg/dL.

Regulation of Acid-Base Balance

For optimal functioning of the cells, metabolic processes maintain a steady balance between acids and bases. Body metabolism produces acids that are continuously buffered by body systems. These buffering systems neutralize acids and bases and include the lungs and kidneys. A **buffer** is a substance or a group of substances that can absorb or release H^+ to correct an acid-base imbalance. Arterial pH is an indirect measurement of the hydrogen ion (H^+) concentration. For example, the greater the concentration of H^+, the more acidic the solution and the lower the pH; the lower the concentration of H^+ ions, the more alkaline the solution and the higher the pH. The pH is also a reflection of the balance between carbon dioxide (CO_2), which is regulated by the lungs, and bicarbonate (HCO_3^-), a base regulated by the kidneys (Heitz and Horne, 2005). Acid-base balance exists when the rate at which the body produces acids or bases equals the rate at which acids or bases are excreted. This balance results in a stable concentration of hydrogen ions (H^+) in body fluids that is expressed as the pH value. Normal hydrogen ion level is necessary to maintain cell membrane integrity and the speed of cellular enzymatic actions. The pH is a scale for measuring the acidity or alkalinity of a fluid. A pH value of 7 is neutral, below 7 is acid, and above 7 is alkaline. Normal values in arterial blood range from 7.35 to 7.45. The three general types of acid-base regulators in the body are chemical (the carbonic acid–base buffer system), biological (the absorption and release of hydrogen ions by cells), and physiological buffering systems (the lungs and kidneys).

Chemical Regulation. The largest chemical buffer in ECF is the carbonic acid and bicarbonate buffer system (Figure 41-6), expressed as the following:

$$CO_2 + H_2O \leftrightarrow H_2CO_3 \leftrightarrow H^+ + HCO_3^-$$

$$\text{Carbon dioxide} + \text{Water} \leftrightarrow \text{Carbonic acid}$$
$$\leftrightarrow \text{Hydrogen ion} + \text{Bicarbonate}$$

The carbonic acid–bicarbonate buffer system is the first buffering system to react to change in the pH of ECF, and it reacts within seconds. The previous equation demonstrates how hydrogen ions (H^+) and carbon dioxide (CO_2) concentrations are directly related. Whenever carbon dioxide increases, there is an increase in hydrogen ions produced, and whenever hydrogen ions are produced, there is more carbon dioxide produced (Ignatavicius and Workman, 2005). As the ECF becomes more acidic, the pH decreases, producing **acidosis.** As the ECF receives more base substances, the pH rises, producing **alkalosis.** The lungs primarily control the excretion of carbon dioxide resulting from metabolism. The kidneys control excretion of hydrogen and bicarbonate ions.

Biological Regulation. Biological buffering occurs when hydrogen ions are absorbed or released by cells. Biological buffering occurs after chemical buffering. The hydrogen ion has a positive charge and must be exchanged with another positively

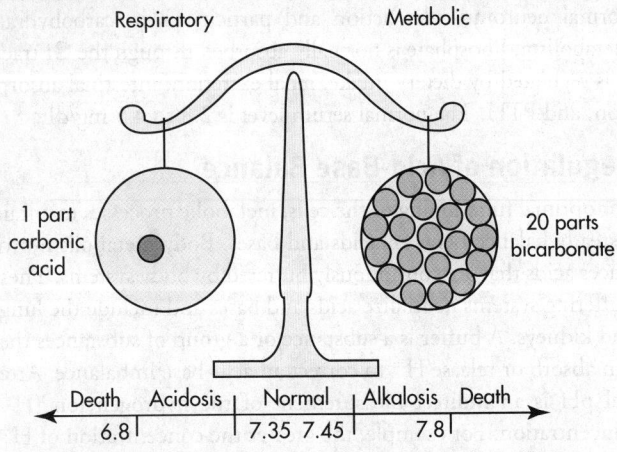

Figure 41-6 Carbonic acid–bicarbonate ratio and pH.

charged ion, frequently potassium (K^+). In conditions producing excess acid, a hydrogen ion enters the cell and a potassium ion leaves the cell and enters the ECF, thus causing an elevated serum potassium level. An example is the release of fatty acids that occurs with diabetic ketoacidosis and starvation. A second biological buffer is the hemoglobin-oxyhemoglobin system. Carbon dioxide diffuses into the red blood cell (RBC) and forms carbonic acid. The carbonic acid dissociates into hydrogen and bicarbonate ions. The hydrogen ions attach to hemoglobin, and the bicarbonate ion becomes available for buffering by exchanging with extracellular chloride (Chernecky and others, 2006).

Another biological buffer is the chloride shift within RBCs. When blood is oxygenated in the lungs, bicarbonate diffuses into the cells and chloride travels from the hemoglobin to the plasma to maintain electrical neutrality. The reverse occurs when carbon dioxide moves into the red cells in tissue capillary beds. This process is referred to as the chloride shift and is a reciprocal exchange between these anions (Brashers, 2006).

Physiological Regulation. The two physiological buffers in the body are the lungs and the kidneys.

However, when there is preexisting lung or kidney disease, the diseased system is no longer effective for physiological regulation. The lungs adapt rapidly to an acid-base imbalance, acting to return the pH to normal before the action of the biological buffers. Ordinarily, increased levels of hydrogen ions and carbon dioxide stimulate respiration. When there is an alteration in hydrogen ion concentration, the lungs react to correct the imbalance by altering the rate and depth of respiration. For example, with metabolic acidosis respirations increase, resulting in a greater amount of exhaled carbon dioxide, which results in a decreased acidic level. With metabolic alkalosis the lungs retain carbon dioxide by decreasing respirations, thereby increasing the acidic level (Monahan and others, 2007).

The kidneys take from a few hours to several days to regulate acid-base imbalances. In response to acid-base imbalance the kidneys increase or decrease bicarbonate production. They reabsorb bicarbonate in cases of acid excess and excrete it in cases of acid deficit. In addition, the kidneys use a phosphate ion (PO_4^{3-}) to excrete hydrogen ions by forming phosphoric acid (H_3PO_4). Fi-

nally, the kidneys use the ammonia mechanism to regulate acid-base balance. In this mechanism certain amino acids within the renal tubules chemically change into ammonia (NH_3^-), which in the presence of hydrogen ions forms ammonium (NH_4), which is excreted in the urine, hence releasing hydrogen ions from the body (Monahan and others, 2007).

Disturbances in Electrolyte, Fluid, and Acid-Base Balances

Disturbances in electrolyte, fluid, or acid-base balance seldom occur alone and disrupt normal body processes or homeostasis. When there is a loss of body fluids because of burns, illnesses, or trauma, the client is also at risk for electrolyte imbalance (Table 41-3). In addition, electrolyte imbalance may occur from vomiting, diarrhea, or a client's inability to communicate fluid needs; resulting in acid-base disturbances. Trauma, disease, and medications all contribute to alterations in fluid, electrolyte, and acid-base balance.

Electrolyte Imbalances

Sodium Imbalances. **Hyponatremia** is a lower-than-normal concentration of sodium in the blood (serum), which can occur with a net sodium loss or net water excess (see Table 41-3). It occurs frequently in seriously ill clients. Clinical indicators and treatment depend on the cause of hyponatremia and whether it is associated with a normal, decreased, or increased ECF volume (Heitz and Horne, 2005). Usually there is a loss of sodium without a loss of fluid, resulting in a decrease in the osmolality of ECF. As the sodium loss continues, the body continues to preserve the blood and interstitial (tissue) volume. As a result, the sodium in ECF becomes diluted.

Hypernatremia is a greater-than-normal concentration of sodium in ECF that can be caused by excess water loss or an overall sodium excess (see Table 41-3). When the cause of hypernatremia is increased aldosterone secretion, sodium is retained and potassium is excreted. When hypernatremia occurs, the body conserves as much water as possible through renal reabsorption.

Potassium Imbalances. **Hypokalemia** is one of the most common electrolyte imbalances, in which an inadequate amount of potassium circulates in ECF (see Table 41-3). When severe, hypokalemia affects cardiac conduction and function. Because the normal amount of serum potassium is so small, there is little tolerance for fluctuations. The most common cause of hypokalemia is vomiting and the use of potassium-wasting diuretics.

Hyperkalemia is a greater-than-normal amount of potassium in the blood. Severe hyperkalemia produces marked cardiac conduction abnormalities (see Table 41-3). The primary cause of hyperkalemia is renal failure, because any decrease in renal function diminishes the amount of potassium the kidney can excrete.

Calcium Imbalances. **Hypocalcemia** represents a drop in total serum and/or ionized calcium. It results from illness, which directly affects the thyroid and parathyroid glands (see Table 41-3). Another cause is renal insufficiency (in which the kidneys' inability to excrete phosphorus causes the phosphorus level to rise and the calcium level to decline). Signs and symptoms are often related to diminished function of the neuromuscular and cardiac systems.

Hypercalcemia is an increase in the total serum concentration of calcium and/or ionized calcium. Hypercalcemia is frequently a symptom of an underlying disease such as hyperpara-

✳ TABLE 41-3 Electrolyte Imbalances

IMBALANCE AND RELATED CAUSES	SIGNS AND SYMPTOMS
Hyponatremia GI losses: vomiting, diarrhea, NG suction Renal loss: kidney disease resulting in salt wasting; diuretics; adrenal insufficiency Skin loss: excessive perspiration; burns Psychogenic polydipsia Syndrome of inappropriate ADH (SIADH)	*Physical examination:* apprehension, personality change, postural hypotension, postural dizziness, abdominal cramping, nausea and vomiting, diarrhea, tachycardia, dry mucous membranes, convulsions and coma *Laboratory findings:* serum sodium level **below** 135 mEq/L, serum osmolality 280 mOsm/kg, and urine specific gravity **below** 1.010 (if not caused by SIADH)
Hypernatremia Excess salt intake: ingestion of large amounts of concentrated salt solutions; iatrogenic administration of hypertonic saline solution parenterally Excess aldosterone secretion Diabetes insipidus Increased sensible and insensible water loss Water deprivation	*Physical examination:* extreme thirst, dry and flushed skin, dry and sticky tongue and mucous membranes, postural hypotension, fever, agitation, convulsions, restlessness, and irritability *Laboratory findings:* serum sodium levels **above** 145 mEq/L, serum osmolality 300 mOsm/kg, and urine specific gravity 1.030 (if not caused by diabetes insipidus)
Hypokalemia Use of potassium-wasting diuretics Diarrhea, vomiting, or other GI losses Alkalosis Excess aldosterone secretion Polyuria Extreme sweating Excessive use of potassium-free intravenous (IV) solutions Treatment of diabetic ketoacidosis with insulin	*Physical examination:* weakness and fatigue, muscle weakness, nausea and vomiting, intestinal distention, decreased bowel sounds, decreased deep tendon reflexes, ventricular dysrhythmias, paresthesias and weak, irregular pulse *Laboratory findings:* serum potassium level **below** 3.5 mEq/L and electrocardiogram (ECG) abnormalities: flattened T wave; ST segment depression; U wave; potentiated digoxin effects (e.g., ventricular dysrhythmias)*
Hyperkalemia Renal failure Fluid volume deficit Massive cellular damage such as from burns and trauma Iatrogenic administration of large amounts of potassium intravenously Adrenal insufficiency Acidosis, especially diabetic ketoacidosis Rapid infusion of stored blood Use of potassium-sparing diuretics Ingestion of K$^+$ salt substitutes	*Physical examination:* anxiety, dysrhythmias, paresthesia, weakness, abdominal cramps, and diarrhea *Laboratory findings:* serum potassium level **above** 5.0 mEq/L and ECG abnormalities: peaked T wave and widened QRS complex (bradycardia, heart block, dysrhythmias); eventually QRS pattern widens and cardiac arrest occurs*
Hypocalcemia Rapid administration of blood transfusions containing citrate Hypoalbuminemia Hypoparathyroidism Vitamin D deficiency Pancreatitis Alkalosis Chronic renal failure Chronic alcoholism	*Physical examination:* numbness and tingling of fingers and circumoral (around mouth) region, hyperactive reflexes, positive Trousseau's sign (carpopedal spasm with hypoxia), positive Chvostek's sign (contraction of facial muscles when facial nerve is tapped), tetany, muscle cramps, and pathological fractures (chronic hypocalcemia) *Laboratory findings:* serum ionized calcium level **below** 4.5 mEq/L or total serum calcium **below** 8.5 mg/dL and ECG abnormalities: ventricular tachycardia

*Data from Heitz UE, Horne MM: *Mosby's pocket guide series: fluid, electrolyte, and acid-base balance,* ed 5, St. Louis, 2005, Mosby.

GI, Gastrointestinal; *NG,* nasogastric; *ADH,* antidiuretic hormone; *AV,* atrioventricular.

Continued

✳ TABLE 41-3 Electrolyte Imbalances—cont'd

IMBALANCE AND RELATED CAUSES	SIGNS AND SYMPTOMS
Hypercalcemia Hyperparathyroidism Osteometastasis Paget's disease Osteoporosis Prolonged immobilization Acidosis Thiazide diuretics	*Physical examination:* anorexia, nausea and vomiting, weakness, hypoactive reflexes, lethargy, flank pain (from kidney stones), decreased level of consciousness, personality changes, and cardiac arrest *Laboratory findings:* serum ionized calcium level **above** 5.5 mEq/L or total serum calcium level **above** 10.5 mg/dL; x-ray examination showing generalized osteoporosis, widespread bone cavitation, radiopaque urinary stones; and elevated blood urea nitrogen (BUN) level 25 mg/100 mL and elevated creatinine level 1.5 mg/100 mL caused by fluid volume deficit (FVD) or renal damage caused by urolithiasis; ECG abnormalities: heart block
Hypomagnesemia Inadequate intake: malnutrition and alcoholism Inadequate absorption or loss: diarrhea, vomiting, nasogastric drainage, fistulas, diseases of small intestine Excessive loss resulting from thiazide diuretics Aldosterone excess Polyuria	*Physical examination:* muscular tremors, hyperactive deep tendon reflexes, confusion and disorientation, tachycardia, hypertension, dysrhythmias, and positive Chvostek's sign and Trousseau's sign *Laboratory findings:* serum magnesium level **below** 1.5 mEq/L
Hypermagnesemia Renal failure Excess oral or parenteral intake of magnesium	*Physical examination:* acute elevations in magnesium levels: hypoactive deep tendon reflexes, decreased depth and rate of respirations, hypotension, and flushing *Laboratory findings:* serum magnesium level **above** 2.5 mEq/L; ECG abnormalities: prolonged QT interval, AV block

*Data from Heitz UE, Horne MM: *Mosby's pocket guide series: fluid, electrolyte, and acid-base balance,* ed 5, St. Louis, 2005, Mosby.

GI, Gastrointestinal; *NG,* nasogastric; *ADH,* antidiuretic hormone; *AV,* atrioventricular.

---

thyroidism or neoplasm, resulting in excess bone reabsorption with release of calcium. Bone loss of calcium also results from prolonged immobilization.

Magnesium Imbalances. Hypomagnesemia, a drop in serum magnesium, occurs with malnutrition and with malabsorption disorders (see Table 41-3). Signs and symptoms are directly related to neuromuscular excitability and appear very similar to hypocalcemia.

Hypermagnesemia is an increase in serum magnesium levels, which depresses skeletal muscles and nerve function. Most frequently it is the result of excess magnesium intake in a client with renal insufficiency. The depression of acetylcholine leads to a sedative effect, which can lead to bradycardia, electrocardiogram (ECG) changes, cardiac arrhythmias, and decreased respiratory rate and depth (Monahan and others, 2007).

Chloride Imbalances. Hypochloremia occurs when the serum chloride level falls below normal. Chloride imbalance is usually associated with sodium imbalance. Vomiting or excessive nasogastric or fistula drainage results in hypochloremia because of the loss of hydrochloric acid. The use of loop and thiazide diuretics also results in increased chloride loss as sodium is excreted. When serum chloride levels fall, metabolic alkalosis results as the body adapts by increasing reabsorption of the bicarbonate ion to maintain electrical neutrality.

Hyperchloremia occurs when the serum chloride level rises above normal, which usually occurs when the serum bicarbonate value falls or sodium level rises. Hypochloremia and hyperchloremia rarely occur as a single disease process but are commonly associated with acid-base imbalance. There is no unique set of symptoms associated with these ion alterations.

Fluid Disturbances. Fluid imbalance usually occurs because illness or injury disturbs the body's ability to maintain homeostasis. Therapeutic measures such as medication administration cause fluid disturbances (Table 41-4). The two basic types of fluid imbalances are isotonic and osmolar. Isotonic deficit and excess exist when water and electrolytes are gained or lost in equal proportions but osmolality remains unchanged. In contrast, osmolar imbalances are losses or excesses of only water that affect the concentration (osmolality) of the serum.

Acid-Base Balance. Chemical balance in the body is regulated by acidity or alkalinity, which is measured by a pH value. Acid-base balance is regulated in the body by the ability to maintain the arterial pH between 7.35 and 7.45. **Arterial blood gas (ABG)** analysis is the most effective way to evaluate acid-base balance and oxygenation. Deviation from a normal value will indicate that the client is experiencing an acid-base imbalance. Mea-

✳ TABLE 41-4 Fluid Disturbances

IMBALANCE AND RELATED CAUSES	SIGNS AND SYMPTOMS
Isotonic Imbalances	
FLUID VOLUME DEFICIT (FVD)—WATER AND ELECTROLYTES LOST IN EQUAL OR ISOTONIC PROPORTIONS	
GI Losses: such as diarrhea, vomiting, or drainage from fistulas or tubes Loss of plasma or whole blood, such as with burns or hemorrhage Excessive perspiration Fever Decreased oral intake of fluids Confusion or depression Use of diuretics	*Physical examination:* postural hypotension, tachycardia, dry mucous membranes, poor skin turgor, thirst, confusion, rapid weight loss, slow vein filling, flat neck veins, lethargy, oliguria (<30 mL/hr), weak pulse *Laboratory findings:* urine specific gravity >1.030, increased hematocrit level >50%, and increased BUN level >25 mg/100 mL (hemoconcentration)
FLUID VOLUME EXCESS (FVE)—WATER AND SODIUM RETAINED IN ISOTONIC PROPORTIONS	
Congestive heart failure Renal failure Cirrhosis of the liver Increased serum aldosterone and steroid levels Excessive sodium intake or administration	*Physical examination:* rapid weight gain, edema (especially in dependent areas), hypertension, polyuria (if renal mechanisms are normal), neck vein distention, increased blood and venous pressure, crackles in lungs, confusion *Laboratory findings:* decreased hematocrit level <38% and decreased BUN level <10 mg/100 mL (hemodilution)
Osmolar Imbalances	
HYPEROSMOLAR IMBALANCE—DEHYDRATION	
Diabetes insipidus Interruption of neurologically driven thirst drive Diabetic ketoacidosis Osmotic diuresis Administration of hypertonic parenteral fluids or tube feeding formulas	*Physical examination:* dry and sticky mucous membranes, flushed and dry skin, thirst, elevated body temperature, irritability, convulsions, coma *Laboratory findings:* increased serum sodium level >145 mEq/L and increased serum osmolality >295 mOsm/kg
HYPOOSMOLAR IMBALANCE—WATER EXCESS	
Syndrome of inappropriate of antidiuretic hormone (SIADH) Excess water intake	*Physical examination:* decreased level of consciousness, convulsions, coma *Laboratory findings:* decreased serum sodium level <135 mEq/L and decreased serum osmolality <280 mOsm/kg

GI, Gastrointestinal; *BUN*, blood urea nitrogen.

surement of ABGs involves analysis of six components: pH, $PaCO_2$, PaO_2, oxygen saturation, base excess, and (HCO_3^-).

pH. The pH measures hydrogen ion (H^+) concentration in the body fluids. Even a slight change is potentially life threatening. An increase in concentration of H^+ makes a solution more acidic; a decrease makes the solution more alkaline. Normal arterial blood pH is 7.35 to 7.45 (acidic is less than 7.35, and alkalotic is greater than 7.45).

$PaCO_2$. $PaCO_2$ is the partial pressure of carbon dioxide in arterial blood and is a reflection of the depth of pulmonary ventilation. The normal range is 35 to 45 mm Hg. Hyperventilation occurs when the $PaCO_2$ is less than 35 mm Hg. As rate and depth of respiration increase, more carbon dioxide is exhaled and the carbon dioxide concentration decreases. Hypoventilation occurs when the $PaCO_2$ is more than 45 mm Hg. As rate and depth of respiration decrease, less carbon dioxide is exhaled and more is retained, increasing the concentration of carbon dioxide.

PaO_2. PaO_2 is the partial pressure of oxygen in arterial blood. Normal range for PaO_2 is 80 to 100 mm Hg. It has no primary role in acid-base regulation when it is within normal limits. A PaO_2 less than 60 mm Hg leads to anaerobic metabolism, resulting in lactic acid production and metabolic acidosis. There is a normal decline in PaO_2 in older adults (Reuben and others, 2005). Hyperventilation also causes a decrease in PaO_2, resulting in respiratory alkalosis (Heitz and Horne, 2005).

Oxygen Saturation. Saturation is the point at which hemoglobin is saturated by oxygen (O_2). Normal range is 95% to 99%. When a client is hypoxic and uses up readily available oxygen, the oxygen reserve (oxygen attached to hemoglobin) is drawn upon to provide oxygen to the tissues (Ignatavicius and Workman, 2005). Changes in temperature, pH, and $PaCO_2$ affect oxygen. When the PaO_2 falls below 60 mm Hg, there is a large drop in saturation (Heitz and Horne, 2005).

Base Excess. Base excess is the amount of blood buffer (hemoglobin and bicarbonate) that exists. The normal range is ±2 mEq/L. A high value indicates alkalosis and can result from the ingestion of large amounts of sodium bicarbonate solutions (some antacids), citrate excess from rapid blood transfusions, or intravenous (IV) infusion of sodium bicarbonate to correct ketoacidosis. A low value indicates acidosis and is usually the result of

---

✳ **TABLE 41-5 Acid-Base Imbalances**

IMBALANCE AND RELATED CAUSES	SIGNS AND SYMPTOMS
Respiratory Acidosis	
HYPOVENTILATION RESULTING FROM PRIMARY RESPIRATORY PROBLEMS	
Atelectasis (obstruction of small airways often caused by retained mucus) Pneumonia Cystic fibrosis Respiratory failure Airway obstruction Chest wall injury	*Physical examination:* confusion, dizziness, lethargy, headache, ventricular dysrhythmias, warm and flushed skin, muscular twitching, convulsions, and coma *Laboratory findings:* arterial blood gas alterations: pH <7.35, PaCO$_2$ >45 mm Hg, PaO$_2$ <80 mm Hg, and bicarbonate level normal (if uncompensated) or >26 mEq/L (if compensated)
HYPOVENTILATION RESULTING FROM FACTORS OUTSIDE OF THE RESPIRATORY SYSTEM	
Drug overdose with a respiratory depressant Paralysis of respiratory muscles caused by various neurological alterations Head injury Obesity	
Respiratory Alkalosis	
HYPERVENTILATION RESULTING FROM PRIMARY RESPIRATORY PROBLEMS	
Asthma Pneumonia Inappropriate mechanical ventilator settings	*Physical examination:* dizziness, confusion, dysrhythmias, tachypnea, numbness and tingling of extremities, convulsions, and coma *Laboratory findings:* arterial blood gas alterations: pH >7.45, PaCO$_2$ <35 mm Hg, PaO$_2$ normal, and bicarbonate level normal (if short lived or uncompensated) or <22 mEq/L (if compensated)
HYPERVENTILATION RESULTING FROM FACTORS OUTSIDE OF THE RESPIRATORY SYSTEM	
Anxiety Hypermetabolic states (fever, exercise) Disorders of the central nervous system (head injuries, infections) Salicylate overdose	
Metabolic Acidosis	
HIGH ANION GAP	
Starvation	*Physical examination:* headache, lethargy, confusion, dysrhythmias, tachypnea with deep respirations, abdominal cramps, and flushed skin
Diabetic ketoacidosis Renal failure Lactic acidosis from heavy exercise	*Laboratory findings:* arterial blood gas alterations: pH <7.35, PaCO$_2$ normal (if uncompensated) or <35 mm Hg (if compensated), PaO$_2$ normal or increased (with rapid, deep respirations), bicarbonate level <22 mEq/L, and oxygen saturation normal
Use of drugs (e.g., methanol, ethanol, formic acid, paraldehyde, aspirin)	
NORMAL ANION GAP	
Renal tubular acidosis Diarrhea	
Metabolic Alkalosis	
Excessive vomiting Prolonged gastric suctioning Hypokalemia or hypercalcemia Excess aldosterone Use of drugs (steroids, sodium bicarbonate, diuretics)	*Physical examination:* dizziness, dysrhythmias, numbness and tingling of fingers, toes, and circumoral region; muscle cramps, tetany *Laboratory findings:* arterial blood gas alterations: pH >7.45, PaCO$_2$ normal (if uncompensated) or >45 mm Hg (if compensated), PaO$_2$ normal, and bicarbonate level >26 mEq/L

✳ TABLE 41-6 Anion Gap

ANION GAP TYPE	VALUES	CAUSES
Normal anion gap	12 ($\pm$2) mEq/L	Diarrhea, renal tubular acidosis, or pancreatic fistula causing a direct loss of (HCO_3^-); addition of chloride-containing acids
Increased anion gap	>14 mEq/L	Lactic acidosis, uremia, diabetic ketoacidosis (DKA), or salicylate and methanol toxicity, resulting in accumulation of nonvolatile acids with decrease in (HCO_3^-)

From Adams BD and others: The anion gap does not accurately screen for lactic acidosis in emergency clients, *Emerg Med J* 23:179, 2006; and Heitz UE, Horne MM: *Mosby's pocket guide series: fluid, electrolyte, and acid-base balance,* ed 5, St. Louis, 2005, Mosby.

---

the elimination of too many bicarbonate ions. An example is diarrhea, where the increased intestinal motility that accompanies diarrhea forces the bicarbonate-containing fluid to be lost instead of being absorbed (Ignatavicius and Workman, 2005).

Bicarbonate. Serum bicarbonate (HCO_3^-) is the major renal component of acid-base balance. The kidneys excrete and retain HCO_3^- to maintain a normal acid-base environment. It is the principal buffer of the extracellular fluids of the body, and once bicarbonate is in the ECF, it is maintained at a concentration of 20 times that of the fluid concentration of carbonic acid (Ignatavicius and Workman, 2005). The normal range is 22 to 26 mEq/L. Less than 22 mEq/L usually indicates metabolic acidosis, greater than 26 mEq/L indicates metabolic alkalosis.

Types of Acid-Base Imbalances. Acid-base imbalances are either respiratory or metabolic depending on their underlying cause. The body corrects acid-base imbalances through the process of compensation. The four primary types of acid-base imbalance are respiratory acidosis, respiratory alkalosis, metabolic acidosis, and metabolic alkalosis (Table 41-5).

Respiratory Acidosis. **Respiratory acidosis** is a combination of increased arterial carbon dioxide concentration ($PaCO_2$), excess carbonic acid (H_2CO_3), and an increased hydrogen ion concentration (pH less than 7.35). Respiratory acidosis is the result of hypoventilation. With respiratory acidosis, the cerebrospinal fluid and brain cells become acidic, causing neurological changes. Hypoxemia occurs because of respiratory depression, resulting in further neurological impairment. Electrolyte changes such as hyperkalemia and hypercalcemia may accompany acidosis. To compensate for the acidosis, the kidneys conserve bicarbonate and release hydrogen ions in the urine. The kidneys are slow to compensate, and this process may take 24 hours.

Respiratory Alkalosis. **Respiratory alkalosis** is marked by a decreased $PaCO_2$ and increased pH (greater than 7.45). Like respiratory acidosis, respiratory alkalosis begins outside the respiratory system (e.g., anxiety with hyperventilation) or within the respiratory system (e.g., initial phase of an asthma attack). The body does not usually compensate for respiratory alkalosis because the pH returns to normal before the kidneys can respond.

Metabolic Acidosis. **Metabolic acidosis** results because of the high acid content of the blood, which also causes a loss of sodium bicarbonate, the alkaline half of the carbonate buffer system, resulting in a bicarbonate deficit (Chernecky and others, 2006). Severe diarrhea or renal disease causes metabolic acidosis. In an attempt to identify the cause of metabolic acidosis, an analysis of serum electrolytes to detect an anion gap may be helpful. An **anion gap** reflects unmeasurable anions present in plasma.

Calculate an anion gap by subtracting the sum of chloride and bicarbonate from the amount of plasma sodium concentration (Table 41-6) (Heitz and Horne, 2005). Compensation for metabolic acidosis is an increased CO_2 excretion by the lungs with an increase in rate and depth of respiration.

Metabolic Alkalosis. **Metabolic alkalosis** is the result of the heavy loss of acid from the body or an increase in levels of bicarbonate. The most common causes are vomiting and gastric suction. Other causes include the overcorrection of metabolic acidosis, potassium deficiency, hyperaldosteronism, and the use of thiazide therapy that causes an increase in renal excretion of acid (Monahan and others, 2007). Compensation occurs with a decrease in respiratory rate and, if there is no underlying kidney disease, renal loss of bicarbonate.

Nursing Knowledge Base

Fluid and electrolyte imbalances potentially affect any client. Infants, severely ill adults, disoriented or immobile clients, and older adults are frequently at greater risk because of their inability to respond independently to the early warnings of an impending problem (Davidhizar and others, 2004; Elgart, 2004; Grandjean and others, 2003). Over time, the body's adaptive compensatory mechanisms can no longer maintain fluid and electrolyte or acid-base balance adequately, and the client's health becomes compromised. The severity and long-term effects on the client's health will influence a client's ability to return to a state of optimal functioning. Prolonged or severe compromises may lead to irreversible chronic health problems that will change the lifestyle of the client and also impact family and friends (Table 41-7).

Critical Thinking

Successful critical thinking requires a synthesis of knowledge, experience, information gathered from clients, critical thinking attitudes, and intellectual and professional standards. Clinical judgments require you to anticipate the information necessary to analyze the data and to make decisions regarding client care. Clients' conditions are always changing. During assessment (Figure 41-7) consider all critical thinking elements, as well as data about the specific client, to develop appropriate nursing diagnoses.

In the case of fluid, electrolyte, and acid-base balance, it is necessary to integrate knowledge of physiology, pathophysiology, and pharmacology, as well as previous experiences and information gathered from clients. Critical analysis of data enables an

✳ TABLE 41-7 Risk Factors for Fluid, Electrolyte, and Acid-Base Imbalances

Age	Very young; very old
Gender	Women
Environment	Diet; exercise; hot weather and sweating
Chronic diseases	Cancer; cardiovascular disease, such as congestive heart failure; endocrine disease such as Cushing's disease and diabetes mellitus; malnutrition; chronic obstructive pulmonary disease; renal disease
Trauma	Crush injuries; head injuries; burns
Therapies	Diuretics; steroids; intravenous (IV) therapy; total parenteral nutrition (TPN)
Gastrointestinal losses	Gastroenteritis; nasogastric suctioning; fistulas

understanding of how fluid, electrolyte, and acid-base imbalances affect the client and family. In addition, your use of critical thinking attitudes such as accountability, discipline, and integrity aids in correctly identifying diagnoses and then planning successful interventions. The use of professional standards, such as those developed by the clinical laboratory for electrolyte values, provides valuable guidelines for comprehensive assessment.

Nursing Process

Assessment

It is essential to understand the importance of fluid, electrolyte, and acid-base balances in maintaining homeostasis. By gathering assessment data through a history and physical examination and using critical thinking skills, nurses identify clients at risk, which leads to the development of appropriate nursing diagnoses. Ask specific, focused questions related to fluid and electrolyte balance (Box 41-1).

Nursing History. Assessment begins with a client history, which is designed to reveal any risk factors or preexisting conditions that may cause or contribute to a disturbance of fluid, electrolyte, and acid-base balances. Explore with the client any factors that may contribute to a disturbance, and integrate the information with knowledge of fluid volume regulation, electrolyte concentration, and acid-base regulation.

Age. Age should be one of your first assessment considerations. An infant's proportion of total body water (70% to 80% total body weight) is greater that that of children or adults. Infants and young children have greater water needs and are more vulnerable to fluid volume alterations. Infants are not protected from fluid loss because they ingest and excrete a relatively greater daily water volume than adults as a result of immature kidneys (Hockenberry and Wilson, 2007). Therefore infants are at greater risk for **fluid volume deficits (FVDs)** and hyperosmolar imbalance because body water loss is proportionally greater per kilogram of weight.

Children ages 2 through 12 have less stable regulatory responses to imbalance, and in childhood illnesses they tend to

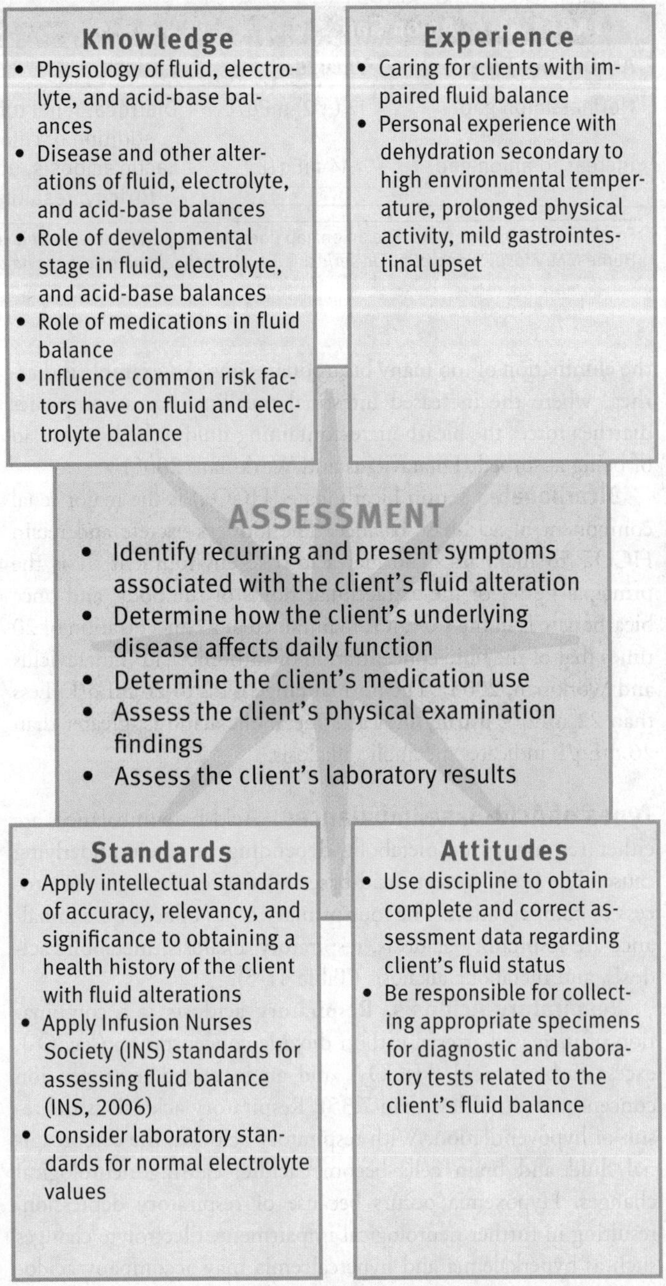

Knowledge
- Physiology of fluid, electrolyte, and acid-base balances
- Disease and other alterations of fluid, electrolyte, and acid-base balances
- Role of developmental stage in fluid, electrolyte, and acid-base balances
- Role of medications in fluid balance
- Influence common risk factors have on fluid and electrolyte balance

Experience
- Caring for clients with impaired fluid balance
- Personal experience with dehydration secondary to high environmental temperature, prolonged physical activity, mild gastrointestinal upset

ASSESSMENT
- Identify recurring and present symptoms associated with the client's fluid alteration
- Determine how the client's underlying disease affects daily function
- Determine the client's medication use
- Assess the client's physical examination findings
- Assess the client's laboratory results

Standards
- Apply intellectual standards of accuracy, relevancy, and significance to obtaining a health history of the client with fluid alterations
- Apply Infusion Nurses Society (INS) standards for assessing fluid balance (INS, 2006)
- Consider laboratory standards for normal electrolyte values

Attitudes
- Use discipline to obtain complete and correct assessment data regarding client's fluid status
- Be responsible for collecting appropriate specimens for diagnostic and laboratory tests related to the client's fluid balance

Figure 41-7 Critical thinking model for fluid, electrolyte, and acid-base balances assessment.

operate within a more narrow range with less tolerance for severe fluid and electrolyte imbalance. Children frequently respond to illnesses with fevers of higher temperatures and longer duration than those of adults (Hockenberry and Wilson, 2007). At any age, fever in childhood increases the rate of insensible water loss. Adolescents have increased metabolic processes and increased water production because of the rapid changes that occur in the anatomical and physiological process. Changes in fluid balance are greater in adolescent girls because of hormonal changes associated with the menstrual cycle.

Older adults experience a number of age-related changes that affect fluid, electrolyte, and acid-base balances. They have a decreased thirst sensation, which affects their oral intake of fluids (Grandjean and others, 2003). The kidneys have a decrease in

BOX 41-1 NURSING ASSESSMENT QUESTIONS

Nature of the Problem
- Are you currently under the care of a health care provider for management of any ongoing health problems such as kidney, heart disease, endocrine disease, or blood pressure problems?
- Describe any new-onset problems such as vomiting, diarrhea, or surgical procedure.
- Are you on any regular medications such as salt substitutes, antacids, diuretics, antihypertensives, or calcium or potassium supplements?

Signs and Symptoms
- In the past several weeks, have you lost or gained any weight without trying?
- Do you feel thirsty, have a dry mouth or skin, or notice a lack of tears?
- Have you noticed a change in your urine output: decreased volume, dark color, or concentrated appearance?
- Have you had any recent problems with vomiting or diarrhea? If so, for how long?
- Are you experiencing any problems with swelling of your hands, feet, ankles, or lower legs?
- Do you have problems breathing when you lie down at night?
- Have you noticed any dizziness, weakness, cramps, or unusual sensations such as tingling?

Severity
- How many times a day do you go to the bathroom to urinate?
- Do you continue to feel thirsty no matter how much fluid you drink?
- Are you experiencing these symptoms more at night than in the morning?
- Are you having difficulty concentrating or feeling confused?
- How does this compare with what is normal or usual for you?

Predisposing Factors
- How much do you usually drink every day? What type of fluids do you drink?
- Describe your normal diet. Do you frequently eat processed, canned, or frozen foods? Do you use a salt substitute?
- Are you following any weight loss program?
- Have you had any recent changes in taste or appetite?

Effect on Client
- How have these symptoms affected you?
- Are you losing sleep, feeling irritable, or having difficulty performing your usual daily tasks?

Prior Medical History

Acute Illness. Recent surgery, head and chest trauma, shock, and second- or third-degree burns are conditions that place clients at high risk for fluid, electrolyte, and acid-base alterations. Clients continue to be at risk during the acute phase until the underlying process is resolved. For example, the stress response of surgery causes fluid-balance changes in the second to fifth postoperative day, when aldosterone, glucocorticoids, and ADH are increasingly secreted, causing sodium and chloride retention, potassium excretion, and decreased urinary output (Monahan and others, 2007).

Surgery. The more extensive the surgery and fluid loss during the procedure, the greater the body's response to the surgical trauma. In addition, after surgery clients exhibit many acid-base changes. The client who is reluctant to breathe deeply and cough may develop respiratory acidosis due to retained $PaCO_2$. The client with nasogastric suction may develop metabolic alkalosis due to the loss of gastric acid, fluids, and electrolytes.

Burns. The greater the body surface burned, the greater the fluid loss. The burned client loses body fluids by one of five routes. First, plasma leaves the intravascular space and becomes trapped edema. This is also called the plasma-to-interstitial fluid shift. It is accompanied by a loss of serum proteins. Second, plasma and interstitial fluids are lost as burn exudate. Third, water vapor and heat are lost in proportion to the amount of skin that is burned. Fourth, blood leaks from damaged capillaries, adding to the intravascular fluid volume loss. Finally, sodium and water shift into the cells, further compromising extracellular fluid volume (Monahan and others, 2007).

Respiratory Disorders. Many alterations in respiratory function predispose the client to respiratory acidosis. For example, changes involved in pneumonia and sedative overdose interfere with the elimination of carbon dioxide. Pneumonia causes pulmonary congestion, which leads to CO_2 retention from hypoventilation. Carbon dioxide is retained during hypoventilation. As the carbon dioxide continues to build up in the bloodstream, the body's compensatory mechanisms can no longer adapt and the pH decreases. Similarly, hyperventilation that occurs with conditions such as fever or anxiety causes the client to experience respiratory alkalosis by blowing off too much carbon dioxide with the increased respiratory rate.

Head Injury. Head injury can result in cerebral edema. Occasionally this edema creates pressure on the pituitary gland, altering ADH secretion. The first alteration is diabetes insipidus, which occurs when too little ADH is secreted and the client excretes large volumes of diluted urine with a low specific gravity. The second alteration is the syndrome of inappropriate antidiuretic hormone (SIADH), in which there is continued excess secretion of ADH. This results in water intoxication characterized by fluid volume expansion and hyponatremia and hypotonicity of fluids as a result of high urine osmolality and low serum osmolality (Monahan and others, 2007).

Chronic Illness. Chronic disease (e.g., cancer, CHF, or renal disease) comprises a variety of conditions that create fluid, electrolyte, and acid-base imbalances. In the presence of chronic disease an understanding of the normal course of such conditions is needed to determine how fluid, electrolyte, and acid-base status may be affected. In addition, it is valuable to know the current treatment regimen and duration of the disease.

glomerular filtration rate and in the number of filtering nephrons (Burke and Laramie, 2004). These changes often cause sodium depletion or overload in the older adult who may be unable to maintain homeostasis, causing a more severe imbalance. In addition, older adults are at risk for decreased excretion of medications, which leads to imbalances causing metabolic or respiratory acidosis, FVD, hyperosmolar imbalance, hyponatremia, and hypernatremia (Heitz and Horne, 2005). The changes in lung function that accompany aging lead to respiratory acidosis and the inability to compensate for metabolic acidosis. Therefore the older adult with any condition that involves renal function, fluid and electrolyte balance, or plasma volume and osmolality is more likely to experience serious consequences (Monahan and others, 2007).

Cancer. The variety of fluid and electrolyte imbalances that are observed in a client with cancer depends on the type and progression of the cancer and treatment regimen. All electrolyte imbalances can occur with cancer and are caused by anatomical distortion and functional impairment from tumor growth and tumor-caused metabolic and endocrine abnormality. In addition, clients with cancer are at risk for fluid and electrolyte imbalances due to the side effects (e.g., diarrhea and anorexia) of chemotherapy and radiation therapy.

Cardiovascular Disease. Cardiovascular disease may result in a diminished cardiac output, which reduces kidney perfusion, causing the client to experience a decrease in urinary output. The client will retain sodium and water, resulting in circulatory overload, and run the risk of developing pulmonary edema. Fluid and electrolyte imbalances associated with heart disease may be controlled with medications and fluid and sodium restrictions. The goal of fluid reduction is to decrease the workload of the left ventricle by reducing excess circulating fluid volume.

Renal Disorders. Kidney disease alters fluid and electrolyte balance by causing an abnormal retention of sodium, chloride, potassium, and water in the extracellular compartment. The plasma levels of metabolic waste products such as blood urea nitrogen (BUN) and creatinine are elevated because the kidneys are unable to filter and excrete the waste products of cellular metabolism. Metabolic acidosis results when hydrogen ions are retained due to decreased renal function. Because of impaired renal function, the usual renal compensatory mechanisms such as bicarbonate reabsorption are not available, so the body loses ability to restore normal acid-base balance (Monahan and others, 2007).

The severity of fluid and electrolyte imbalance is proportional to the degree of renal failure. Occasionally, acute renal failure–induced shock or a decrease in extracellular fluid may be reversible. Although chronic renal failure is progressive, successful treatment is possible with dietary control of protein and salt intake, diuretic medications, fluid restrictions, and dialysis.

Gastrointestinal Disturbances. Gastroenteritis and nasogastric suctioning result in a loss of fluid, potassium, and chloride ions. Hydrogen ions are also lost, causing a disturbance in acid-base balance. Timely education of infant and child caregivers is necessary to prevent dehydration when the infant or child is experiencing diarrhea (Hockenberry and Wilson, 2007). Gastrointestinal fistulas can also result in a loss of potassium, resulting in an increased risk for hypokalemia. The loss of potassium increases the risk for acid-base disturbances.

• • •

Regardless of the presence of any disease process, it is essential to determine how long the client has suffered from that disease and the type of treatment currently employed. In addition to chronic health problems, it is important to gather a history of new-onset acute illnesses with symptoms of diarrhea or vomiting and conditions such as colostomy, nasogastric suctioning, or intestinal drainage. Any condition that results in the loss of GI fluids predisposes the client to dehydration and a variety of electrolyte disturbances.

Environmental Factors. Assess information related to environmental factors in the client history. Clients who have participated in vigorous exercise or have been exposed to temperature extremes may have clinical signs of fluid and electrolyte alterations. Exposure to environmental temperatures exceeding 28° to 30° C (82.4° to 86° F) results in excessive sweating with weight loss. A body weight loss over 7% decreases the ability of the cooling mechanism to conserve water. Loss of fluid from sweating varies and can reach a maximal rate of 2 L/hr (Ignatavicius and Workman, 2005). Inadequate fluid replacement leads to fluid volume disturbances.

Diet. A client's current dietary history is an important component of the assessment. Dietary intake of fluids, salt, potassium, calcium, magnesium, and necessary carbohydrates, fats, and protein maintains normal fluid, electrolyte, and acid-base homeostasis. Recent changes in appetite or the ability to chew and swallow affects nutritional status and fluid hydration. When nutritional intake is inadequate, the body tries to preserve its protein stores by breaking down glycogen and fat stores. When excess free fatty acids are released, metabolic acidosis can occur because the liver converts free fatty acids to ketones, a strong acid. After those resources are depleted, the body begins to destroy protein stores. Serum protein levels drop below normal and hypoalbuminemia results. Hypoalbuminemia causes the serum colloid osmotic pressure to decrease. Fluid shifts from the circulating blood volume and enters the interstitial fluid space in the peritoneal cavity, causing edema. In addition, dieting can lead to acidosis, because rapid water loss can lead to osmolar fluid imbalance.

Lifestyle. Be sure to include lifestyle factors in the client history. If there are preexisting medical risks, such as a history of smoking or alcohol consumption, they can further impair the client's ability to adapt to fluid, electrolyte, and acid-base alterations. For example, the excess use of alcohol and tobacco can cause respiratory depression, which can result in respiratory acidosis and an alteration in adequate fluid and electrolyte balance.

Medication. Another important category to include in the client assessment is a history of medication use (Box 41-2). If the assessment reveals a medication that is likely to cause an electrolyte or acid-base imbalance, closely assess laboratory values. Include assessment of the client's knowledge of side effects and adherence to medication schedules, understanding of potential side effects of over-the-counter medications on fluid, electrolyte, and

---

BOX 41-2 Medications That Cause Fluid, Electrolyte, and Acid-Base Disturbances

- **Diuretics:** Metabolic alkalosis, hyperkalemia, and hypokalemia
- **Steroids:** Metabolic alkalosis
- **Potassium supplements:** Gastrointestinal disturbances, including intestinal and gastric ulcers and diarrhea
- **Respiratory center depressants (e.g., opioid analgesics):** Decreased rate and depth of respirations, resulting in respiratory acidosis
- **Antibiotics:** Nephrotoxicity (e.g., vancomycin, methicillin, aminoglycosides); hyperkalemia and/or hypernatremia (e.g., azlocillin, carbenicillin, piperacillin, ticarcillin, Unasyn)*
- **Calcium carbonate (Tums):** Mild metabolic alkalosis with nausea and vomiting*
- **Magnesium hydroxide (Milk of Magnesia):** Hypokalemia*
- **Nonsteroidal antiinflammatory drugs:** Nephrotoxicity

*Data from McKenry LM and others: *Mosby's pharmacology in nursing,* ed 22, St. Louis, 2006, Mosby.

acid-base balances in the assessment and history (Monahan and others, 2007).

Physical Assessment. A thorough physical examination (see Chapter 33) is necessary, because fluid and electrolyte imbalances or acid-base disturbances can affect all body systems. Data obtained during the physical assessment validates and extends the information collected through the client history. For example, an examination of the oral cavity reveals signs of dehydration when the client is experiencing a fluid deficit. Table 41-8 summarizes

possible physical findings for clients with fluid, electrolyte, and acid-base imbalances.

Daily Weights and Fluid Intake and Output Measurement. Measuring and recording all liquid intake and output (I&O) during a 24-hour period is an important part of the client's assessment database for fluid and electrolyte balance. Recognition of trends in the I&O is important (e.g., a gradually decreasing urine output can indicate that the body is trying to adapt to an FVD or hyperosmolar fluid imbalance). Accurate assessment of fluid status, including I&O, identifies both clients

---

✳ **TABLE 41-8 Physical and Behavioral Nursing Assessment for Fluid, Electrolyte, and Acid-Base Imbalances**

Assessment	Imbalance
Weight Changes	
2%-5% loss	Mild fluid volume deficit (FVD)*
5%-8% loss	Moderate FVD*
8%-15% loss	Severe FVD*
>15% loss	Death*
2% gain	Mild fluid volume excess (FVE)
5%-8% gain	Moderate to severe FVE
Head	
History:	
Headache	FVD,* metabolic or respiratory acidosis, metabolic alkalosis
Dizziness	FVD,* respiratory acidosis or alkalosis, hyponatremia
Observation:	
Irritability	Metabolic or respiratory alkalosis, hyperosmolar imbalance, hypernatremia, hypokalemia
Lethargy	FVD,* metabolic acidosis or alkalosis, respiratory acidosis, hypercalcemia
Confusion, disorientation	FVD,* hypomagnesemia, metabolic acidosis, hypokalemia
Eyes	
History:	
Blurred vision	FVE
Inspection:	
Sunken, dry conjunctivae, decreased or absent tearing	FVD
Periorbital edema, papilledema	FVE
Throat and Mouth	
Inspection:	
Sticky, dry mucosa, dry cracked lips, decreased salivation, longitudinal tongue furrows	FVD, hypernatremia
Cardiovascular System	
Inspection:	
Flat neck veins	FVD
Distended neck veins	FVE
Dependent body parts: legs, sacrum, back	FVD*
Slow venous filling	
Palpation:	
Edema: dependent body parts: (legs, sacrum, back)	FVE*
Dysrhythmias (also noted as ECG changes)	Metabolic acidosis, respiratory alkalosis and acidosis, potassium imbalance, hypomagnesemia
Increased pulse rate	Metabolic alkalosis, respiratory acidosis, hyponatremia, FVD, FVE, hypomagnesemia
Decreased pulse rate	Metabolic alkalosis, hypokalemia
Weak pulse	FVD, hypokalemia
Decreased capillary filling	FVD
Bounding pulse	FVE

*Data from Heitz UE, Horne MM: *Mosby's pocket guide series: fluid, electrolyte, and acid base balance,* ed 5, St. Louis, 2005, Mosby.
ECG, Electrocardiogram.

Continued

⬥ TABLE 41-8 Physical and Behavioral Nursing Assessment for Fluid, Electrolyte, and Acid-Base Imbalances—cont'd

ASSESSMENT	IMBALANCE
Cardiovascular System—cont'd	
Auscultation:	
Blood pressure (BP) low or with orthostatic changes	FVD, hyponatremia, hyperkalemia, hypermagnesemia
Third heart sound (except in young children)	FVE
Hypertension	FVE
Respiratory System	
Inspection:	
Increased rate	FVE, respiratory alkalosis, metabolic acidosis
Dyspnea	FVE
Auscultation:	
Crackles	FVE
Gastrointestinal System	
History:	
Anorexia	Metabolic acidosis
Abdominal cramps	Metabolic acidosis
Inspection:	
Sunken abdomen	FVD
Distended abdomen	Third-space syndrome
Vomiting	FVD, hypercalcemia, hyponatremia, hypochloremia, metabolic alkalosis
Diarrhea	Hyponatremia, metabolic acidosis
Auscultation:	
Loud "growling" sounds from hyperperistalsis with diarrhea, or no sounds from hypoperistalsis	FVD, hypokalemia
Renal System	
Inspection:	
Oliguria or anuria	FVD, FVE
Diuresis (if kidneys are normal)	FVE
Increased urine specific gravity	FVD
Neuromuscular System	
Inspection:	
Numbness, tingling	Metabolic alkalosis, hypocalcemia, potassium imbalances
Muscle cramps, tetany	Hypocalcemia, metabolic or respiratory alkalosis
Coma	Hyperosmolar or hypoosmolar imbalances, hyponatremia
Tremors	Respiratory acidosis, hypomagnesemia
Palpation:	
Hypotonicity	Hypokalemia, hypercalcemia*
Hypertonicity	Hypocalcemia, hypomagnesemia, metabolic alkalosis
Skin	
Body temperature:	
Increased	Hypernatremia, hyperosmolar imbalance, metabolic acidosis
Decreased	FVD
Inspection:	
Dry, flushed	FVD, hypernatremia, metabolic acidosis
Palpation:	
Inelastic skin turgor, cold, clammy skin	FVD

*Data from Heitz UE, Horne MM: *Mosby's pocket guide series: fluid, electrolyte, and acid base balance*, ed 5, St. Louis, 2005, Mosby.
ECG, Electrocardiogram.

✳ BOX 41-3   EVIDENCE-BASED PRACTICE

Determining Adequate Oral Intake for Older Adults
Evidence Summary
It is essential for health care providers to prevent dehydration and the associated problems of confusion, infection, and mortality in older adults. One approach is to determine adequate oral intake and maintain hydration. The purpose of this study was to provide clinical validation of methods to provide older adults adequate hydration. Researchers audited 318 charts and used a rating scheme to evaluate the strength of the clinical evidence. Results indicated that fluid management consists of both acute and ongoing management of oral intake. Nurses can evaluate hydration management by monitoring 24-hour intake, urine color, and urine specific gravity checks.

Application to Nursing Practice
• Initial assessment of hydration status should include physiological measures, including urine specific gravity, urine color, 24-hour intake/output, patterns of fluid intake, and treatments.

• Risk of underhydration assesses potential degree of hydration. Evaluate acute losses such as vomiting, medical issues such as diabetes or malnutrition, medications such as diuretics, age greater than 85 years, cognitive level, and functional status.
• Acute management requires close monitoring of high-risk clients, implementing intake and output measurement, and providing additional fluids.
• Ongoing management consists of daily fluid goals, comparing current intake with physiological needs, and provision of fluids.
• Documentation is more accurate when alert and oriented clients participate in fluid management.

Reference
Mentes JC: Hydration management. In Titler M, editor: *Series on evidence-based practice for older adults,* Iowa City, 2004, University of Iowa Gerontological Nursing Interventions Research Center.

---

at risk and clients who are experiencing fluid, electrolyte, and acid-base disturbances. Weigh clients with fluid and electrolyte alterations daily. Daily weights are the single most important indicator of fluid status (Heitz and Horne, 2005). Each kilogram (2.2 pounds) of weight gained or lost is equal to 1 L of fluid retained or lost. These fluid gains or losses indicate changes in total body fluid volume, not changes in a specific compartment of the body. Obtain a weight at the same time each day with the same scale after the client voids. Calibrate the scale each day or routinely. The client should wear the same clothes or clothes that weigh the same; if using a bed scale, use the same number of sheets on the scale with each weighing. Determining I&O is an important component in assessing daily fluid balance (Box 41-3).

For clients in health care settings, I&O measurement is a nursing assessment routinely used for clients following a procedure, clients whose conditions are unstable, clients who are febrile, clients on fluid restriction, and clients who are receiving diuretic or IV therapy. Nurses measure I&O for any client with chronic cardiopulmonary or renal illnesses and clients whose health status has deteriorated or has become unstable.

Oral intake includes all liquids taken by mouth, (e.g., gelatin, ice cream, soup, juice, and water), through nasogastric or jejunostomy feeding tubes (see Chapter 44), IV fluids (including continuous infusions and intermittent IV piggybacks), and blood or its components. Occasionally clients receive a specific amount of a liquid medication every 1 to 2 hours. A client receiving tube feedings may receive numerous liquid medications, and water may be used to flush the tube before and/or after medications. Over a 24-hour period, these liquids can amount to significant intake and should always be recorded on the I&O record. Liquid output includes urine, diarrhea, vomitus, gastric suction, and drainage from postsurgical wounds or other tubes (see Chapter 50).

Instruct ambulatory clients to save their urine in a calibrated insert, which attaches to the rim of the toilet bowl (Figure 41-8). Record urinary output after each trip to the bathroom. When a

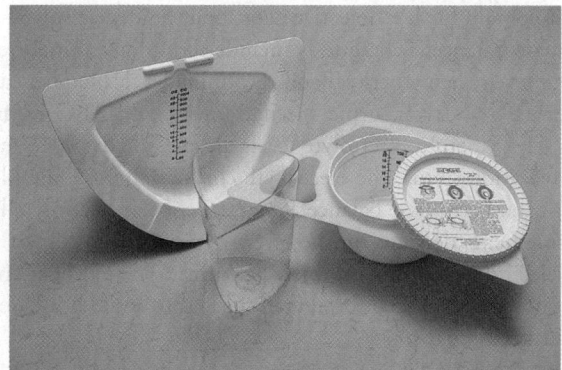

A

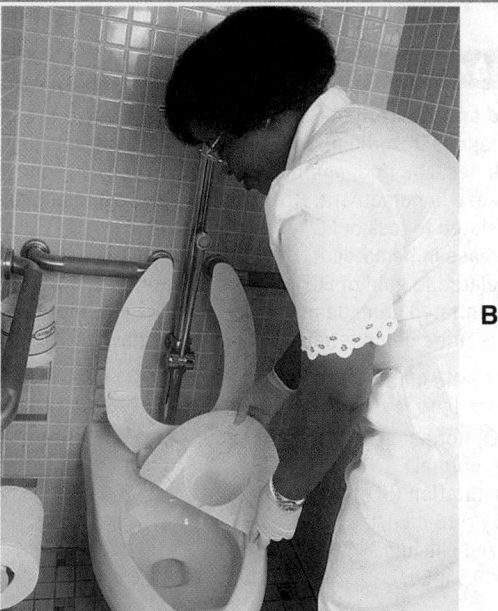

B

Figure 41-8 A, Graduated measuring containers. *Clockwise from far left:* "hat" receptacle, specipan, and graduated measuring container. **B,** Emptying collected urine.

client has an indwelling Foley catheter, drainage tube, or suction, that output is recorded (e.g., at the end of each nursing shift or every hour) as the client's condition requires. Cooperation from the client and family is essential to maintaining accurate I&O measurements. It is important for the client to have good vision and motor skills to perform assessments. Teach the client and family the purpose of the measurements and either to notify the nurse to empty any container with voided fluid or how to measure and empty the container themselves. Clients with basic literacy problems will not be able to calculate I&O totals easily.

In the hospital, forms for recording I&O are available attached to the bedside chart or room door (Figure 41-9). Calculate the 24-hour total as directed by agency policy. Delegate measurement of I&O recording to nursing assistive personnel (NAP) with competent skills in measurement and calculation. Estimation of I&O is not acceptable. NAP must report findings to the responsible registered nurse (RN) or licensed practical nurse/licensed vocational nurse (LPN/LVN). Recording I&O is essential for an accurate database. This information helps maintain an ongoing evaluation of the client's hydration status to prevent severe imbalances.

Laboratory Studies. Review the client's laboratory test results to obtain further objective data about fluid, electrolyte, and acid-base balances. These tests include serum and urinary electrolyte levels, hematocrit, blood creatinine level, blood urea nitrogen (BUN) levels, urine specific gravity, and ABG readings (Box 41-4). Serum electrolyte levels are measured to determine the hydration status, the electrolyte concentration of the blood plasma, and acid-base balance. The frequency of electrolyte level measurements depends on the severity of the client's illness. Serum electrolyte tests are routinely performed on any client entering a hospital to screen for alterations and to serve as a baseline for future comparisons.

Client Expectations. Often the client's fluid, electrolyte, or acid-base disturbance is so serious that it prevents a review of client expectations. However, if a client is alert enough to discuss care, a review of expectations may reveal short-term needs (e.g., provision of comfort from nausea) or long-term needs (e.g., understanding how to prevent alterations from occurring in the future). The client must be able to understand the implications of fluid, electrolyte, or acid-base changes to be able to express expectations of care. Strengthen the client's trust through a competent response to sudden changes in condition and through communication with clients and/or family members.

Nursing Diagnosis

When caring for clients with suspected fluid, electrolyte, and acid-base imbalances, it is particularly important to use critical thinking to formulate nursing diagnoses. The assessment data that establish the risk for or the actual presence of a nursing diagnosis in these areas may be subtle, and patterns and trends emerge only when there has been astute assessment. Multiple body systems may be involved; careful clustering of defining characteristics will lead to selection of the appropriate diagnoses (Box 41-5).

In addition to the accurate clustering of assessment data, an important part of formulating nursing diagnoses is identifying the relevant causative or related factor. You will choose interventions that treat or modify the related factor in order for the diagnosis to be resolved. For example, *Deficient fluid volume related to loss of gastrointestinal fluids from vomiting* will require therapies that manage the clients' emesis and restore fluid volume by way of intravenous therapy. In contrast, the diagnosis of *Deficient fluid volume related to elevated body temperature* will require therapies to lower the client's body temperature and to

---

✳ BOX 41-4 Laboratory Data for Fluid, Electrolyte, and Acid-Base Imbalances

Fluid and Electrolytes
Alterations in sodium, potassium, magnesium, calcium, phosphates, chloride, and bicarbonate (venous CO_2 concentrations)
Increase in hematocrit, BUN, sodium, and osmolality in serum (related to loss of ECF or gain of solutes)
Decrease in hematocrit, BUN, sodium, and osmolality in serum (related to gain of ECF or loss of solutes)
Concentrated urine demonstrated by urine specific gravity >1.030
Dilute urine demonstrated by a specific gravity >1.010

Metabolic Alkalosis
pH >7.45
$PaCO_2$ normal or >45 mm Hg if lungs are compensating
PaO_2 normal
O_2 saturation (SO_2) normal
HCO_3^- >26 mEq/L
Ionized calcium <4.5 mg/dL
K^+ <3.5 mEq/L

Metabolic Acidosis
pH <7.35
$PaCO_2$ normal or <35 mm Hg if lungs are compensating
PaO_2 normal

O_2 saturation (SaO_2) normal
HCO_3^- <22 mEq/L
K^+ >5.0 mEq/L

Respiratory Alkalosis
pH >7.45
$PaCO_2$ <35 mm Hg
PaO_2 normal
O_2 saturation (SaO_2) normal
HCO_3^- <22 mEq/L
Ionized calcium <4.5 mg/dL
K^+ <3.5 mEq/L

Respiratory Acidosis
pH <7.35
$PaCO_2$ >45 mm Hg
PaO_2 normal or <80 mm Hg, depending on cause of acidosis
SaO_2 normal or <95%, depending on cause of acidosis
HCO_3^- normal if early respiratory acidosis or >26 mEq/L if kidneys are compensating
K^+ >5.0 mEq/L

BUN, Blood urea nitrogen; *ECF,* extracellular fluid.

Patient Name_____ ☐Male ☐Female

Date of Birth_____ Age_____

Patient Label

GRAPHIC/DAILY CARE RECORD
Side I
Deaconess Hospital, Inc.

Temperature Legend: r = rectal   ax = axillary   T.M. = tympanic

		Date:																							
Hospital/Post Op d																									

Temp C° / F°: 40.5/105, 40.0/104, 39.4/103, 38.8/102, 38.3/101, 37.7/100, 37.2/99, 37.0/98.6, 36.6/98, 36.1/97

Times: 0001 0400 0800 1200 1600 2000 (repeated across 4 date columns)

Pulse

Resp

BP — Standing / Sitting / Lying

Other B/P's — Time

Intake	0600	1400	2200	0600	1400	2200	0600	1400	2200	0600	1400	2200
PO												
IV												
Tube Fdg												
Blood Products												

8 hr Total

Output: Voided / Catheter / GI Contents / Stools

8 hr Total

Initials

24 hr TOTALS:	Intake	Output	Balance	Intake	Output	Balance	Intake	Output	Balance	Intake	Output	Balance

Diet:

% eaten:	Breakfast	Lunch	Dinner	Breakfast	Lunch	Dinner	Breakfast	Lunch	Dinner	Breakfast	Lunch	Dinner

ht:_____ weight_____ kg   weight_____ kg   weight_____ kg   weight_____ kg

Name/Status	Initials	Name/Status	Initials	Name/Status	Initials	Name/Status	Initials

F-4226* (10-03)

Figure 41-9 Daily care record. (Courtesy Deaconess Hospital, Evansville, Ind.)

Continued

Patient Name_____ ☐Male ☐Female

Date of Birth_____ Age_____

Patient Label

GRAPHIC/DAILY CARE RECORD

Side 2

Deaconess Hospital, Inc.

	Time/Initials	Date:	Time/Initials	Date:	Time/Initials	Date:	Time/Initials	Date:
Fluid Restriction								
Pulse Oximetry (state if done on room air or liter flow/% of oxygen)								
Respiratory Treatments (coach, suction, etc.)								
Circulatory Treatments TED's, K-pad, Antithrombic pump								
Wound Care Bacitracin, H_2O_2, heat lamp, drsg chg, etc.								
Oral Care toothettes, etc.								
Hygiene/ Skin Care type of bath, etc.								
Activity BRP, BR, turns, dangle, HOB elevated, reverse Trendelenburg, ABD pillow, etc.								

Name/Status	Initials	Name/Status	Initials	Name/Status	Initials	Name/Status	Initials

F- 4226*   (10-03)

Figure 41-9, cont'd Daily care record. (Courtesy Deaconess Hospital, Evansville, Ind.)

✳ BOX 41-5 **NURSING DIAGNOSTIC PROCESS**

Deficient Fluid Volume Related to Loss of Gastrointestinal Fluids via Vomiting

Assessment Activities	Defining Characteristics
Assess blood pressure and pulse.	Client is hypotensive with increased heart rate.
Obtain daily weight measurements.	Client experiences sudden weight loss.
Observe volume of urine output, and measure intake and specific gravity.	Decreased volume of output in comparison to intake; increased urine specific gravity is present.
Palpate skin turgor.	Inelastic skin turgor noted.
Ask if client is thirsty or weak.	Client verbalizes thirst and weakness.
Inspect mucous membranes for degree of moisture.	Dry mucous membranes are noted.

replace lost body fluids through oral fluid replacement or possibly intravenous therapy.

Possible nursing diagnoses for clients with fluid, electrolyte, and acid-base alterations may include the following:

- Decreased cardiac output
- Acute confusion
- Deficient fluid volume
- Excess fluid volume
- Impaired gas exchange
- Risk for injury
- Deficient knowledge regarding disease management
- Impaired oral mucous membrane
- Impaired skin integrity
- Ineffective tissue perfusion

◆ Planning

During the planning process use critical thinking to synthesize information from multiple resources (Figure 41-10) . Ensure that the client's plan of care integrates both scientific and nursing knowledge, as well as all the knowledge that you collected about the individual client.

Goals and Outcomes. Establish an individual client plan of care for each nursing diagnoses (see Care Plan). You also develop mutually established client goals for care during planning. Goals need to be individualized and realistic with measurable outcomes. For example, the following related outcomes may be established for the goal "The client will achieve normal hydration status at discharge":

- The client will be free of complications associated with the IV device throughout the duration of IV therapy.
- The client will demonstrate moist mucous membranes, balanced I&O measurements, and stable daily weights within 48 hours.
- The client will have serum electrolytes within the normal range within 48 hours.

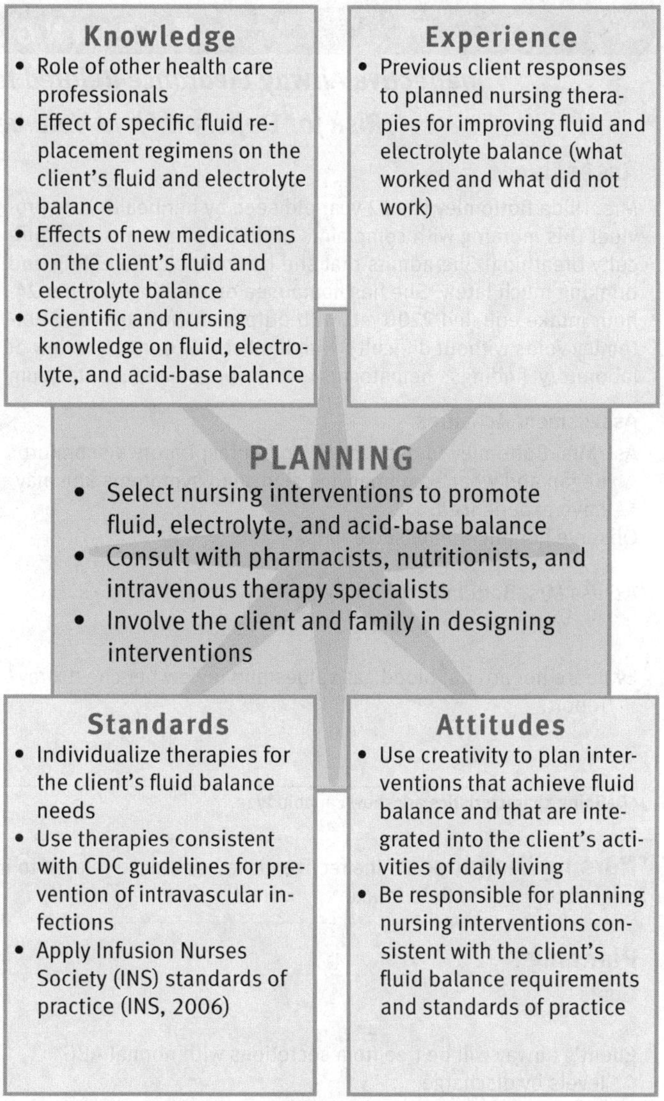

Knowledge
- Role of other health care professionals
- Effect of specific fluid replacement regimens on the client's fluid and electrolyte balance
- Effects of new medications on the client's fluid and electrolyte balance
- Scientific and nursing knowledge on fluid, electrolyte, and acid-base balance

Experience
- Previous client responses to planned nursing therapies for improving fluid and electrolyte balance (what worked and what did not work)

PLANNING
- Select nursing interventions to promote fluid, electrolyte, and acid-base balance
- Consult with pharmacists, nutritionists, and intravenous therapy specialists
- Involve the client and family in designing interventions

Standards
- Individualize therapies for the client's fluid balance needs
- Use therapies consistent with CDC guidelines for prevention of intravascular infections
- Apply Infusion Nurses Society (INS) standards of practice (INS, 2006)

Attitudes
- Use creativity to plan interventions that achieve fluid balance and that are integrated into the client's activities of daily living
- Be responsible for planning nursing interventions consistent with the client's fluid balance requirements and standards of practice

Figure 41-10 Critical thinking model for fluid, electrolyte, and acid-base balances planning.

Setting Priorities. The client's clinical condition determines which of the diagnoses takes the greatest priority. Many nursing diagnoses in the area of fluid, electrolyte, and acid-base balances are of highest priority, because the consequences for the client can be serious or even life threatening. For example, in the concept map (Figure 41-11, p. 990) for the client with gastroenteritis and dehydration, the occurrence of nausea and diarrhea has created a serious problem of deficient fluid volume. In this situation, intervention is necessary to help resolve the client's nausea and diarrhea. If these priorities are unmet, the client's fluid imbalance will likely worsen.

Consultation with the client's health care provider assists in setting realistic time frames for the goals of care, particularly when the client's physiological status is unstable. Collaboration during planning with the client and family and other members of the interdisciplinary health care team such as IV therapy and pharmacy assists in achieving client outcomes. The family can be helpful in identifying approaches for being successful with therapies (e.g., ways to increase fluid intake). Incorporate client preferences and resources into the plan of care. Administration of medications IV and/or oxygen

NURSING CARE PLAN

Ineffective Airway Clearance Related to Increased Mucus From Airway Infection
Risk for Deficient Fluid Volume Related to Reduced Fluid Intake

Assessment

Mrs. Hilda Bottomley is a 72-year-old seen by her health care provider this morning with complaints of flulike symptoms and difficulty breathing. She admits that she has not felt like eating and drinking much lately. She has no nausea or vomiting, but her 24-hour intake equaled 2200 mL, with output of 1800 mL. Mrs. Bottomley voids without difficulty, with light yellow urine. A review of laboratory findings: hematocrit 43% (hypovolemia); potassium 4.0 mEq/L, and sodium 140 mEq/L. After an outpatient chest x-ray examination, Mrs. Bottomley has been admitted for respiratory toileting and IV antibiotic and fluid therapy. The health care provider orders O_2 at 4 L/min with humidification, respiratory treatments, fluids by mouth and IV, pulse oximetry, and activity with assistance.

Assessment Activities

Ask Mrs. Bottomley to describe when her respiratory discomfort began and what accompanying signs and symptoms she may have experienced.

Observe her pulmonary secretions.

Assess Mrs. Bottomley's vital signs.

Evaluate her arterial blood gas values and review her chest x-ray report.

Findings/Defining Characteristics*

She states that she became congested about 2 weeks ago and has chills, feels weak, **is not interested in eating,** and aches all over.

Mrs. Bottomley has **difficulty coughing** and at times produces **thick and yellowish-greenish sputum.**

Mrs. Bottomley's **temperature is 38.3° C (101° F);** her respiratory rate is 28 breaths per minute, with **rhonchi breath sounds** present bilaterally. Other vital signs are within normal limits.

Mrs. Bottomley's arterial blood gas results indicate a mild respiratory acidosis, and the chest x-ray film reveals a left lower lobe pneumonia. Arterial blood gas analysis: pH, 7.33; PaO_2, 95 mm Hg; $PaCO_2$, 48 mm Hg, HCO_3^-, 23 mEq/L.

*__Defining characteristics__ are shown in bold type.

Nursing Diagnoses: Ineffective airway clearance related to increased mucus from airway infection. Risk for deficient fluid volume related to reduced fluid intake

Planning

Goals

Client's airway will be free from secretions with normal ABG levels by discharge.

Client's fluid volume will remain within normal limits throughout hospital stay.

Expected Outcomes (NOC)†

Respiratory Status: Airway Patency
Breath sounds will be clear on auscultation.
Mucus will become thin and clear in 48 hours.
ABG levels will be within normal limits in 24 hours.
Respiratory rate will be within normal limits with activity in 24 hours.

Fluid Balance
Urine output will equal intake of approximately 1500 mL.
Daily weights will not vary ±2 pounds.
Mucous membranes will remain moist.
Vital signs will remain within normal limits.

†Outcome classification labels from Moorhead S and others: *Nursing outcomes classification (NOC),* ed 4, St. Louis, 2008, Mosby.

Interventions‡ (NIC)

Airway Management

- Schedule coughing and deep breathing exercises every 2 hours while awake.
- Administer chest physiotherapy every 4 hours while awake to affected regions of the lung.

- Ambulate client once every 8 hours and encourage client to get out of bed and into chair often.

Rationale

Cough control exercises and deep breathing promote pulmonary secretion clearance (Pruitt, 2006).

Chest physiotherapy, breathing exercises, cough techniques, along with ambulating the client, promote airway clearance (Booker, 2005).

Mobility promotes air exchange and position change prevents settling of secretions in lung tissue.

‡Intervention classification labels from Bulechek GM, Butcher HK, and Dochterman JM: *Nursing interventions classification (NIC),* ed 5, St. Louis, 2008, Mosby.

Continued

NURSING CARE PLAN

Ineffective Airway Clearance Related to Increased Mucus From Airway Infection

Risk for Deficient Fluid Volume Related to Reduced Fluid Intake—cont'd

Interventions‡ (NIC)	Rationale
Fluid Management	
• Provide client with an additional 16 ounces of noncaffeinated oral fluids every 8 hours. • Administer IV therapy, as prescribed.	Increased fluid intake helps to liquefy pulmonary secretions and in turn facilitate productive coughing (Davidhizar and others, 2004).

‡Intervention classification labels from Bulechek GM, Butcher HK, and Dochterman JM: *Nursing interventions classification (NIC)*, ed 5, St. Louis, 2008, Mosby.

Evaluation

Nursing Actions	Client Response/Finding	Achievement of Outcome
Monitor ABG levels, vital signs, I&O, daily weight, and O_2 saturation levels. Assess mucous membranes.	Arterial blood gas analysis: pH 7.36, PaO_2 95, $PaCO_2$ 38. Mucous membranes are moist.	24 mEq/L. Vital signs and O_2 saturation are within normal range. Intake 2100 ml, output 2000 mL. Mrs. Bottomley's acid-base balance has returned to normal. Her I&O measurements are balanced. Daily weight remained stable. She is able to walk down the hall without respiratory discomfort. Mrs. Bottomley states she is drinking more fluids. She no longer experiences chills and a fever.
Auscultate breath sounds.	Mrs. Bottomley's breath sounds are clear bilaterally on inspiration and expiration.	Mrs. Bottomley is able to breathe without discomfort.
Evaluate effectiveness of coughing and deep breathing exercises.	Mrs. Bottomley demonstrated three deep breaths followed by coughing and said she no longer coughs up sputum.	Mrs. Bottomley is free of sputum production.

therapy, and hemodynamic assessment cannot be delegated to NAP. When the client is stable, daily weights, intake and output, and direct physical care can be delegated to NAP.

Collaborative Care. Begin discharge planning early for those clients with acute fluid and electrolyte disturbances. In the hospital the needs of the client and family are anticipated, and collaboration with the other members of the health care team ensures that care can continue in the home or long-term care setting with few disruptions. Therapeutic regimens established in one setting should continue through completion at the next setting. For example, for the client who is discharged on IV therapy, the knowledge and skills of the family member or friend who is to assume caregiving responsibilities must be assessed and a referral to home IV therapy should be instituted as soon as possible. Close collaboration with members of the health care team, such as the health care provider, dietitian, and pharmacist, is essential to ensure client outcomes. The dietitian can be a valuable resource in recommending food sources to either increase or reduce intake of certain electrolytes. Chapter 44 describes various therapeutic diets (e.g., low sodium). The pharmacist can assist in identifying medications or combinations of medications likely to cause electrolyte or acid-base disturbances. Furthermore, the pharmacist can offer information regarding client education on side effects to anticipate for prescribed drugs. The health care provider will direct the treatment of any fluid, electrolyte, or acid-base alteration.

Implementation

Health Promotion. Health promotion activities focus primarily on client education. Clients and caregivers need to recognize risk factors for development of imbalances and implement appropriate preventive measures. For example, parents of infants need to understand that GI losses can quickly lead to serious imbalances; therefore when vomiting or diarrhea occur in the infant, the parent needs to recognize the risk and promptly seek health care to restore normal balance. Even the healthy adult is at risk for developing imbalances when subjected to elevated environmental temperatures. Advise active adults to supplement fluid loss from perspiration by increasing oral fluids such as water, maintaining adequate environmental ventilation, and refraining from excessive activity during times of excess environmental heat. Sometimes it is difficult to separate the effects of age-related changes from changes associated with disease processes. For example, any older adult who has a chronic condition involving renal or respiratory function is more likely to suffer serious consequences when an acute disease process occurs (Monahan and others, 2007).

All clients with chronic health alterations are at risk for developing changes in their fluid, electrolyte, and acid-base balances. They need to understand their own risk factors and the measures to be taken to avoid imbalances. For example, clients with renal

CONCEPT MAP

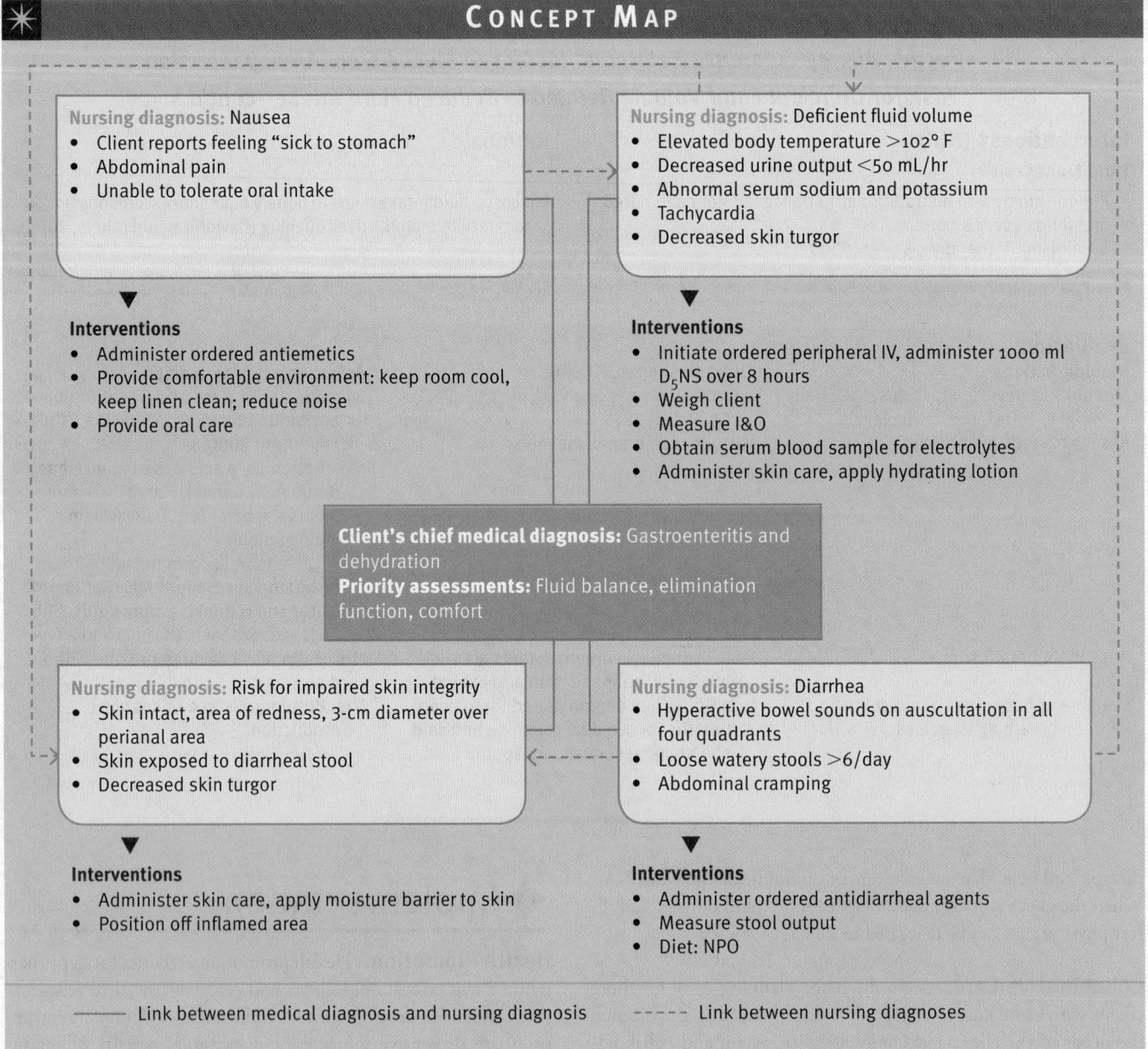

Nursing diagnosis: Nausea
- Client reports feeling "sick to stomach"
- Abdominal pain
- Unable to tolerate oral intake

Interventions
- Administer ordered antiemetics
- Provide comfortable environment: keep room cool, keep linen clean; reduce noise
- Provide oral care

Nursing diagnosis: Deficient fluid volume
- Elevated body temperature >102° F
- Decreased urine output <50 mL/hr
- Abnormal serum sodium and potassium
- Tachycardia
- Decreased skin turgor

Interventions
- Initiate ordered peripheral IV, administer 1000 ml D$_5$NS over 8 hours
- Weigh client
- Measure I&O
- Obtain serum blood sample for electrolytes
- Administer skin care, apply hydrating lotion

Client's chief medical diagnosis: Gastroenteritis and dehydration
Priority assessments: Fluid balance, elimination function, comfort

Nursing diagnosis: Risk for impaired skin integrity
- Skin intact, area of redness, 3-cm diameter over perianal area
- Skin exposed to diarrheal stool
- Decreased skin turgor

Interventions
- Administer skin care, apply moisture barrier to skin
- Position off inflamed area

Nursing diagnosis: Diarrhea
- Hyperactive bowel sounds on auscultation in all four quadrants
- Loose watery stools >6/day
- Abdominal cramping

Interventions
- Administer ordered antidiarrheal agents
- Measure stool output
- Diet: NPO

——— Link between medical diagnosis and nursing diagnosis   - - - - - Link between nursing diagnoses

Figure 41-11 Concept map for a client with gastroenteritis and dehydration.

failure need to avoid excess intake of fluid, sodium, potassium, and phosphorus. Through diet education these clients learn the types of foods to avoid and the suitable volume of fluid they are permitted daily (see Chapter 44). Make clients with chronic diseases aware of early signs and symptoms of fluid, electrolyte, and acid-base imbalances. For example, a client with heart disease should learn to obtain an accurate body weight each day at the approximate same time and to inform the health care provider of significant changes of weight from one day to another.

Acute Care. Although fluid, electrolyte, and/or acid-base imbalances occur in all settings, there are now more demanding expectations due to the changes in the acute care delivery system. Today, management of the client's complex medical care is completed in a shorter span of time while there are expectations to perform more difficult technological skills.

Enteral Replacement of Fluids. Oral replacement of fluids and electrolytes is appropriate as long as the client is not so physiologically unstable that oral fluids cannot be replaced rapidly. Oral replacement of fluids is contraindicated when the client is vomiting, has a mechanical obstruction of the GI tract, is at risk for aspiration, or has impaired swallowing. Clients unable to tolerate solid foods may still be able to ingest fluids. Strategies to encourage fluid intake include offering small sips of fluid frequently, popsicles, and ice chips. Ice chips are included in I&O measurements, as one-half the volume of the ice chips. For example, if a client ingests 240 mL of ice chips, the amount of I&O recorded would be 120 mL.

When replacing fluids by mouth in a client with a fluid deficit, it is important to choose fluids with adequate calories and electrolyte content (e.g., fruit juices, gelatin, and replacements such as Pedialyte and Gastrolyte). However, it is important to remember that liquids containing lactose, caffeine, or low sodium content may not be appropriate when the client has diarrhea.

A feeding tube is appropriate when the client's GI tract is healthy but the client cannot ingest fluids (e.g., after oral surgery or with impaired swallowing). Options for administering fluids include gastrostomy or jejunostomy instillations or infusions through small-bore nasogastric feeding tubes (see Chapter 44).

Restriction of Fluids. Clients who retain fluids and have **fluid volume excess (FVE)** require restricted fluid intake. Fluid restriction is often difficult for clients, particularly if they take medications that dry the oral mucous membranes or if they are mouth breathers, experiencing a sensation of thirst. Explain the reason fluids are restricted and ensure the client knows the amount of fluid permitted orally and understands that ice chips, gelatin, and ice cream are fluids. Help the client to decide the amount of fluid to drink with each meal, between meals, before bed, and with medications. It is important to allow clients to choose preferred fluids, unless contraindicated. Frequently clients on fluid restriction can swallow a number of pills with as little as 1 ounce (30 mL) of liquid.

In acute care settings, fluid restrictions usually allot half the total oral fluids between 7 AM and 3 PM, the period when clients are more active, receive two meals, and take most of their oral medications. Offer the remainder of the fluids during the evening and night shifts. Clients on fluid restriction require frequent mouth care to moisten mucous membranes, decrease the chance of mucosal drying and cracking, and maintain comfort (see Chapter 39).

Parenteral Replacement of Fluids and Electrolytes. Fluid and electrolytes may be replaced through infusion of fluids directly into the bloodstream rather than via the digestive system. Parenteral replacement includes total parenteral nutrition (TPN), IV fluid and electrolyte therapy (**crystalloids**), and blood and blood component (**colloids**) administration.

Practice standard precautions when administering parenteral fluids (see Chapter 34) to minimize the risk to health care workers for exposure to the human immunodeficiency virus (HIV), the cause of acquired immunodeficiency syndrome (AIDS), hepatitis B virus (HBV), and other infectious diseases. Understand the policy and procedure for parenteral infusions at each institution.

Total Parenteral Nutrition. Total parenteral nutrition is a nutritionally adequate hypertonic solution consisting of glucose, other nutrients, and electrolytes administered through an indwelling or central IV catheter, which may be inserted peripherally, percutaneously, implanted, or tunneled. Chapter 44 reviews principles and guidelines for TPN administration, which is used as an intervention in severe cases of malnutrition, when the GI tract is nonfunctional.

Intravenous Therapy (Crystalloids). The goal of IV fluid administration is to correct or prevent fluid and electrolyte disturbances. It allows for direct access to the vascular system, permitting the continuous infusion of fluids over a period of time. Intravenous fluid therapy must be continuously regulated because of ongoing changes in the client's fluid and electrolyte balance. When clients require IV fluid administration, knowledge of the correct ordered solution, the equipment needed, the procedures required to initiate an infusion, how to regulate the infusion rate and maintain the system, how to identify and correct problems,

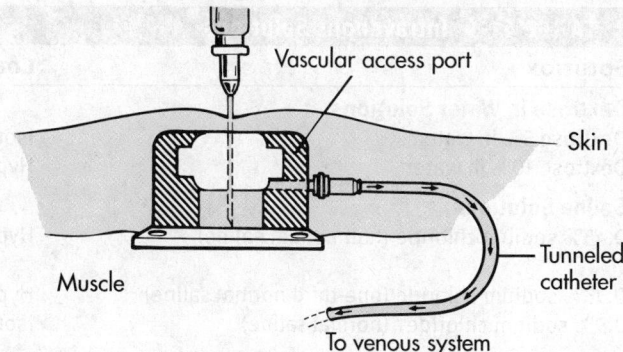

Figure 41-12 Example of an implantable vascular access device.

and how to discontinue the infusion are necessary for safe and appropriate therapy.

Vascular Access Devices. Vascular access devices (VADs) are catheters, cannulas, or infusion ports designed for repeated access to the vascular system. Peripherally placed cannulas are for short-term use (e.g., fluid restoration postoperatively and short-term antibiotic administration). Devices such as central line catheters, peripherally inserted central venous catheters (PICCs), and implanted ports (Figure 41-12) are for long-term use. These devices are more effective than peripherally placed catheters for administering medications and solutions that are irritating to veins. The use of central venous catheters and implanted infusion ports requires education in the care of these devices.

Types of Solutions. Many prepared IV solutions are available for use (Table 41-9). Intravenous solutions fall into the following categories: isotonic, hypotonic, and hypertonic. Isotonic solutions are those that have the same effective osmolality as body fluids and are the most common solution. Hypotonic solutions are those that have an effective osmolality less than body fluids. Hypertonic solutions are those that have an effective osmolality greater than body fluids (Heitz and Horne, 2005).

In general, isotonic fluids are indicated for extracellular volume replacement (e.g., FVD after prolonged vomiting). The decision to use a hypotonic or hypertonic solution is based on the client's specific fluid and electrolyte imbalance. For example, the client with a hypertonic fluid imbalance will generally receive a hypotonic solution to dilute the ECF and rehydrate the cells. Administer all IV fluids carefully, especially hypertonic solutions, because these pull fluid into the vascular space by osmosis, resulting in an increased vascular volume that can lead to pulmonary edema, particularly in clients with heart or renal failure. It is common to add additives such as vitamins and potassium chloride (KCl) to IV solutions.

SAFETY ALERT *Under no circumstances should potassium chloride (KCl) be given IV push. A direct IV infusion of KCl may be fatal.* A health care provider's order is necessary if an IV is to have additives added; for example, Bottle 1: 1000 mL $D_5\frac{1}{2}$ NS with 20 mEq KCl at 125 mL/hr.

Clients with normal renal function who are receiving nothing by mouth should have potassium added to IV solutions. The body cannot conserve potassium, and even when the serum level falls, the kidneys continue to excrete potassium. If there is no

✳ TABLE 41-9 Intravenous Solutions

SOLUTION	CONCENTRATION	OTHER NAMES
Dextrose in Water Solutions		
Dextrose 5% in water*	Isotonic	D_5W
Dextrose 10% in water	Hypertonic	$D_{10}W$
Saline Solutions		
0.45% sodium chloride (half normal saline)	Hypotonic	½ NS
		0.45% NS
0.33% sodium chloride (one-third normal saline)	Hypotonic	⅓ NS
0.9% sodium chloride† (normal saline)	Isotonic	NS
		0.9% NS
		0.9% NaCl
3%-5% sodium chloride	Hypertonic	3%-5% NS
		3%-5% NaCl
Dextrose in Saline Solutions		
Dextrose 5% in 0.9% sodium chloride	Hypertonic	$D_5$0.9% NaCl
		$D_5$0.9% NS
		D_5NS
Dextrose 5% in 0.45% NaCl sodium chloride	Hypertonic	$D_5$0.45% NaCl
		$D_5$0.45% NS
		D_5½ NS
Multiple Electrolyte Solutions		
Lactated Ringer's‡	Isotonic	LR
Dextrose 5% in lactated Ringer's	Hypertonic	D_5LR

*Dextrose is quickly metabolized, leaving free water to be distributed evenly in all fluid compartments (Heitz and Horne, 2005).
†Although it is isotonic because the total concentration of electrolytes equals plasma concentration, it contains 154 mEq of both sodium and chloride, which is a higher concentration of these electrolytes than is found in the plasma, which can cause fluid volume excess (Heitz and Horne, 2005).
‡Contains sodium, potassium, calcium, chloride, and lactate.

potassium intake orally or parenterally, hypokalemia develops quickly. Conversely, verify that the client has adequate kidney function and urine output before administering an IV solution containing potassium, which may result in hyperkalemia.

Equipment. Correct selection and preparation of IV equipment assists in safe and quick placement of an IV line. Because fluids infuse directly into the bloodstream, sterile technique is necessary. Organize all equipment at the bedside for an efficient insertion. Intravenous equipment includes needles or cannulas, tourniquet, gloves, dressings, solution containers, various types of tubing, and IV pumps or volume control devices. Intravenous cannulas are available in a variety of gauges, such as the commonly used 22 gauge. The larger the gauge, the smaller the diameter of the cannula. These cannulas are plastic tubing, threaded over a needle. Once the needle is inserted into the vein, the needle is withdrawn, leaving the cannula in place. There are devices designed to reduce the risk of needlestick injury and promote client safety when connecting, accessing, or removing IV equipment (Figure 41-13). Needleless systems use recessed needles or allow for connections without using needles.

Injectable medications such as antibiotics may be added to a small IV solution bag and "piggybacked" as a secondary set into the primary line or as a primary intermittent infusion to be administered over a 30- to 60-minute period (see Chapter 35). The type and amount of solution depends on the medication added

and the client's physiological status. Nurses use different types of tubing to administer medications or IV fluids. A solution given rapidly needs to be infused with macrodrip tubing, which delivers large drops (standard drop size is 10 or 15 gtt/mL depending on the manufacturer) so that the prescribed rate of infusion can be maintained. In contrast, microdrip tubing provides a standard drop size of 60 gtt/mL. Microdrip tubing allows for precise regulation of IV fluids even at slow rates. In addition, clients may require IV extension tubing to increase mobility, decrease manipulation and potential contamination at the insertion site, or to facilitate changes in position.

SAFETY ALERT Use intravenous pumps or volume control devices with children, with clients with renal or cardiac failure, with medications that require precise rates, or with critically ill clients to ensure prescribed infusion rate and to prevent uncontrolled fluid administration.

Initiating the Intravenous Line. After you collect the equipment at the bedside, prepare to insert the IV line by assessing the client for a venipuncture site (Skill 41-1). Common IV puncture sites include the hand and the arm (Figure 41-14). The use of the foot for an IV site is common with children but is avoided in the adult because of the danger of thrombophlebitis (Intravenous Nurses Society [INS], 2006). As you assess the client for potential venipuncture sites, consider conditions and contraindications that exclude certain sites. For example, because very young children and older adults have fragile veins, avoid sites that

Text continued on p. 1005

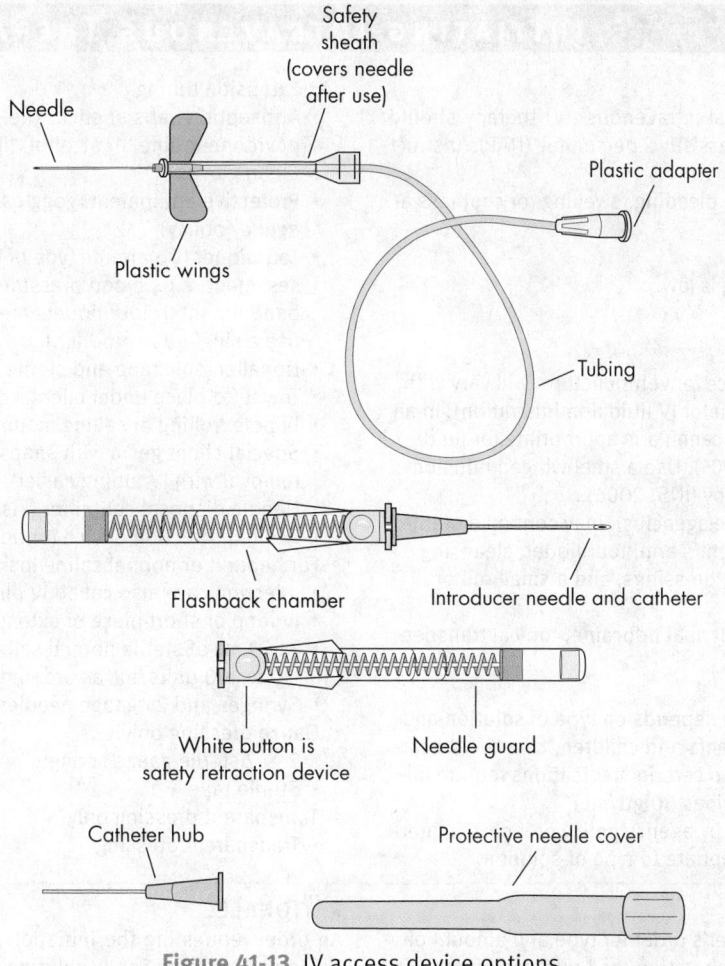

Figure 41-13 IV access device options.

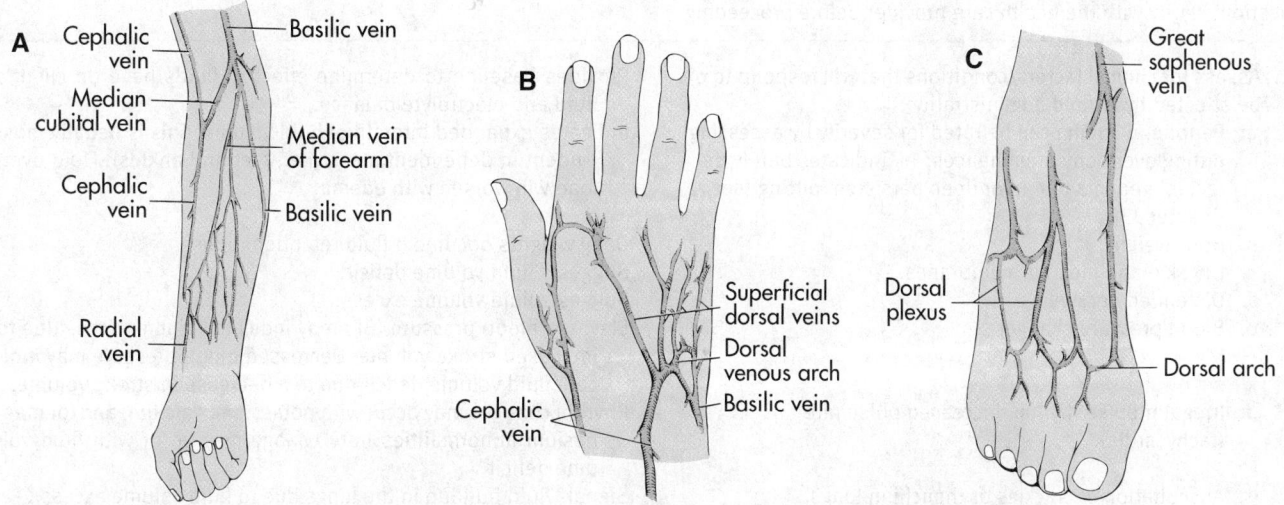

Figure 41-14 Common IV sites. **A,** Inner arm. **B,** Dorsal surface of hand. **C,** Dorsal surface of foot (used only for children).

SKILL 41-1   INITIATING INTRAVENOUS THERAPY

Delegation Considerations

The skill of initiating peripheral intravenous (IV) therapy should not be delegated to nursing assistive personnel (NAP). Instruct NAP to report the following:

- Client complains of burning, bleeding, swelling, or coolness at the cannula insertion site.
- IV dressing becomes wet.
- Volume of fluid in the IV bag is low.

Equipment

- Correct IV solution
- Proper IV safety access device for venipuncture (will vary with client's body size and reason for IV fluid administration). In an adult a peripheral 22-gauge cannula is appropriate for fluid maintenance (Rosenthal, 2005). Use a steel-winged infusion set only for short-term therapy (INS, 2006).
- IV start kit (available in some agencies): may contain a sterile drape to place under the client's arm, tourniquet, cleansing and antiseptic preparations, dressings, and a small roll of sterile tape
- Local anesthetic (e.g., intradermal lidocaine, topical transdermal anesthetic)
- For IV fluid infusion
  - Administration set (choice depends on type of solution and rate of administration; infants and children, clients with cardiac and renal disease, and certain medications require microdrip tubing, which provides 60 gtt/mL)
  - 0.22-mm filter (if required by agency policy or if particulate matter is likely; size appropriate to type of solution)
- Extension tubing
- Antiseptic swabs or sticks (i.e., chlorhexidine gluconate, povidone-iodine, or alcohol) (INS, 2006)
- Clean gloves
- Protective equipment: goggles, mask (optional, check agency policy)
- Tourniquet (Determine type of tourniquet based on client assessment, e.g., blood pressure cuff [older adult], rubber band [infants]. Tourniquets are a source of contamination; use a single-use product.)
- Nonallergenic tape and sterile tape
- Towel (to place under client's hand or arm)
- IV pole, rolling or ceiling mounted
- Special client gown with snaps at shoulder seams (makes removal with IV tubing easier), if available
- Needle disposal container (also called sharps container)
- IV site protection device (optional)
- For heparin or normal saline lock
  - Injection cap (also called IV plug, PRN adapter, INT)
  - IV loop or short piece of extension tubing, if necessary
  - 1 to 3 mL of sterile normal saline or heparin flush solution (10 to 100 units/mL as ordered or per agency protocol)
  - Syringes and 25-gauge needles
- Gauze dressing only
  - 2 × 2 sterile gauze sponge
  - Sterile tape
- Transparent dressing only
  - Transparent dressing

STEPS	RATIONALE
1. Review health care provider's order for type and amount of IV fluid, rate of fluid administration, and purpose of infusion. Follows six rights for administration of medications (see Chapter 35).	An order requesting the initiation of a peripheral IV access and administration of an IV solution must be made by a health care provider before the initiation of this therapy.

Critical Decision Point: Health care providers do not write orders to "initiate peripheral access" or "perform venipuncture." "Start IV" may be written, followed by the exact IV therapy order. The order to perform venipuncture is implied. If the order is confusing or in question, clarify with the health care provider before proceeding.

2. Assess for clinical factors/conditions that will respond to or be affected by IV fluid administration:	Provides baseline to determine effect IV fluids have on client's fluid and electrolyte balance.
a. Peripheral edema can be rated for severity by assessing pitting over bony prominences; 1+ indicates barely detectable edema to 4+ for deep persistent pitting (see Chapter 33).	Indicates expanded interstitial fluid volume. This is usually most evident in dependent areas (i.e., feet and ankles). Fluid overload will worsen with edema.
b. Body weight.	Daily weights document fluid retention or loss.
c. Dry skin and mucous membranes.	Suggests fluid volume deficit.
d. Distended neck veins.	Suggests fluid volume excess.
e. Blood pressure changes.	Elevated blood pressure (BP) may indicate volume excess due to increased stroke volume. Decreased blood pressure may indicate fluid volume deficit due to a decrease in stroke volume.
f. Irregular pulse rhythm; increased pulse rate (tachycardia).	Rhythm changes may occur with potassium, calcium, and/or magnesium abnormalities; rate change may occur with fluid volume deficit.
g. Auscultation of crackles or rhonchi in lungs.	Signals fluid buildup in the lungs due to fluid volume excess.
h. Inelastic skin turgor (after pinching, fails to return to normal position within 3 seconds).	With fluid volume deficit, the pinched skin stays elevated for several seconds. This is called "tenting." *This is a less reliable indicator for older adult clients because their skin has lost elasticity naturally due to aging* (Burke and Laramie, 2004).

✳ **SKILL 41-1**   **INITIATING INTRAVENOUS THERAPY—CONT'D**

STEPS	RATIONALE
i. Anorexia, nausea, and vomiting.	May occur with acute fluid volume deficit or fluid volume excess.
j. Thirst.	Symptomatic of fluid volume deficit.
k. Decreased urine output.	During dehydration, kidneys restore fluid balance by reducing urine production. Average daily adult urine output is 1500 mL; urine output of less than 400 mL/24 hr (oliguria) signals the retention of metabolic wastes (Heitz and Horne, 2005).
l. Behavioral changes (i.e., confusion, restlessness).	Occurs with fluid volume deficit or acid-base imbalance.
m. Decreased capillary refill.	Indicates poor tissue perfusion.
3. Assess client's previous or perceived experience with IV therapy and arm placement preference.	Determines level of emotional support and instruction necessary. If client is hypersensitive to venipunctures, use a local anesthetic.
4. Obtain information from drug reference books or pharmacist about composition of IV fluids, purposes of administration, potential incompatibilities, and side effects for monitoring guidelines.	This allows detection of an inadvisable IV fluid order and helps to determine priority assessments.
5. Determine if client is to undergo any planned surgeries or is to receive blood infusion later.	Allows anticipation and placement of large-gauge cannula for fluid infusion and avoids placement in an area that will interfere with medical procedures.
6. Assess for the following risk factors: child or older adult; presence of heart failure or renal failure; skin lesions; infection; low platelet count; or receiving anticoagulants.	Older adults develop fluid imbalances more rapidly because they have a proportionately larger extracellular fluid volume, persons with heart failure cannot adapt to sudden increases in vascular volume, and persons with renal failure cannot eliminate excess extracellular fluid. Skin lesions or infection influence choice of access site. Low platelets or use of anticoagulants increase client's risk for bleeding from IV site and seepage of blood from puncture site.
7. Assess laboratory data and client's history of allergies to iodine, adhesive, or latex.	Assesses need for IV therapy and client's risk for allergies.
8. Explain to client and family the procedure, its purpose, and what is expected of client. Explain what sensations client is to expect.	Cognitive and sensory information decreases anxiety and helps promote cooperation.
9. Assist client to comfortable sitting or supine position. Be positioned at a level position with client. Provide adequate lighting.	Promotes comfort and relaxation for client. Provides proper body mechanics for nurse. Aids in successful vein location.
10. Check client's identification using two identifiers.	Ensures right client receives right intravenous fluid.
11. Perform hand hygiene. Organize equipment on clean, clutter-free bedside stand or over-bed table.	Reduces transmission of infection and risk of accidents.
12. Change client's gown to the more easily removed gown with snaps at the shoulder, if available.	Use of a special IV gown facilitates safe removal of the gown once the IV has been inserted.
13. Open sterile packages using sterile aseptic technique (see Chapter 34).	Maintains sterility of equipment and reduces spread of microorganisms.
14. Prepare IV tubing and solution.	
a. Check IV solution, using six rights of medication administration (see Chapter 35). Make sure prescribed additives, such as potassium and vitamins, have been added. Check solution for color, clarity, and expiration date. Check bag for leaks, which is best if done before reaching the bedside.	IV solutions are medications. Carefully check to reduce risk of error. Do not use solutions that are discolored, contain particles, or are expired. Leaky bags present an opportunity for infection and must not be used.
b. Open infusion set, maintaining sterility of both ends of tubing. Many sets allow for priming of tubing without removal of cap end.	Prevents microorganisms from entering infusion equipment and bloodstream.
c. Place roller clamp (see illustration) about 2 to 5 cm (1 to 2 inches) below drip chamber, and move roller clamp to "off" position (see illustrations).	Close proximity of roller clamp to drip chamber allows more accurate regulation of flow rate. Moving clamp to "off" prevents accidental spillage of IV fluid when inserting tubing into bag.
d. Remove protective sheath over IV tubing port on plastic IV solution bag (see illustration).	Provides access for insertion of infusion tubing into solution.
e. Insert infusion set into fluid bag or bottle: Remove protector cap from tubing insertion spike, not touching spike, and insert spike into opening of IV bag (see illustration). Cleanse rubber stopper on glass-bottled solution with antiseptic, and insert spike into black rubber stopper of IV bottle.	Flat surface on the top of bottled solution may contain contaminants, whereas opening to plastic bag is recessed. Prevents contamination of bottled solution during insertion of spike.

Continued

✳ **SKILL 41-1**   **INITIATING INTRAVENOUS THERAPY—CONT'D**

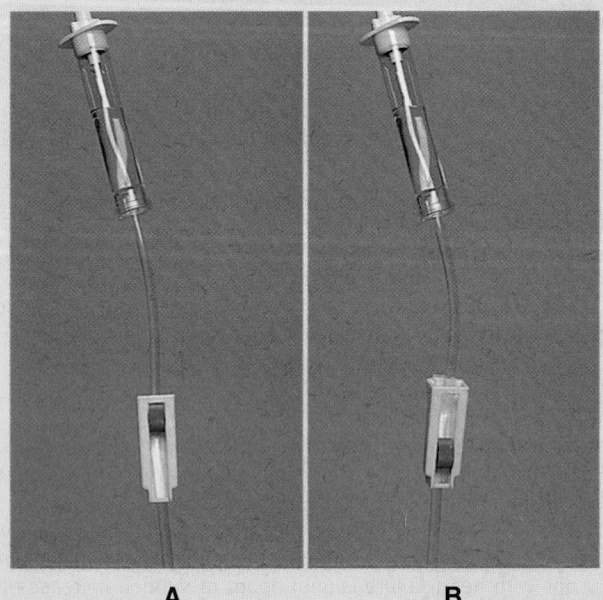

STEP 14c **A,** Roller clamp in open position. **B,** Roller clamp in closed position.

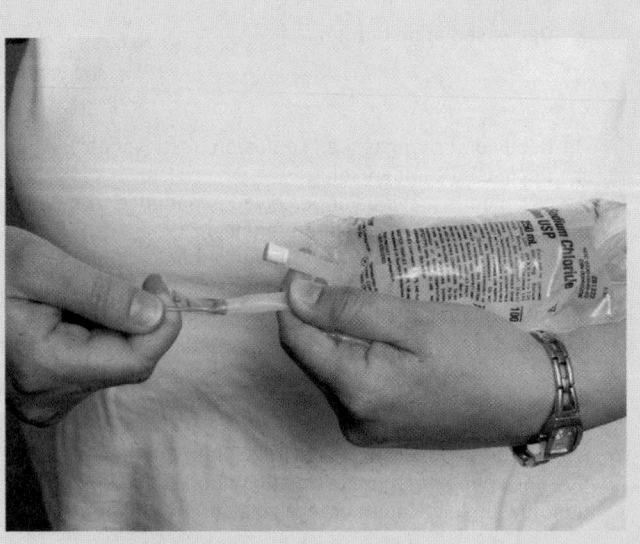

STEP 14d Remove protective covering from IV solution.

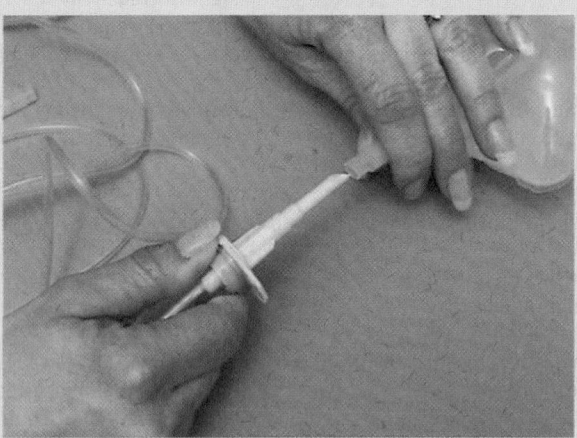

STEP 14e Inserting spike into IV bag.

STEPS	RATIONALE

Critical Decision Point: Do not touch spike. It is sterile. If contamination occurs (e.g., spike is accidentally dropped on the floor), then discard IV tubing and obtain a new one.

STEPS	RATIONALE
f. Prime infusion tubing by filling with IV solution: Compress the drip chamber and release, allowing it to fill one-third to one-half full (see illustration).	Ensures tubing is cleared of air before connection with IV site. Creates suction effect; fluid enters drip chamber to prevent air from entering tubing.
g. Remove protector cap on end of tubing (some tubing can be primed without removal), and slowly open roller clamp to allow fluid to travel from drip chamber through tubing to needle adapter. Return roller clamp to "off" position after priming tubing (filled with IV fluid).	Slow fill of tubing decreases turbulence and chance of bubble formation. Removes air from tubing and permits tubing to fill with solution. Closing the clamp prevents accidental loss of fluid.

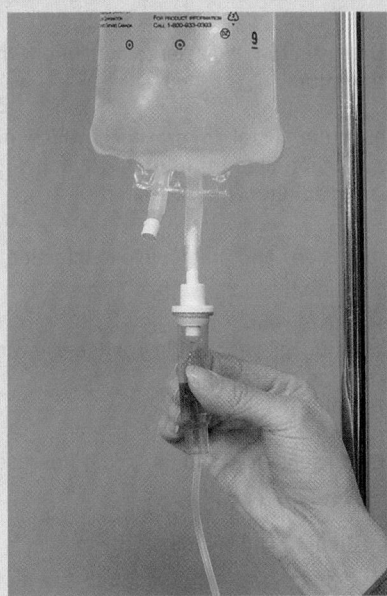

STEP 14f Squeezing drip chamber to fill with fluid.

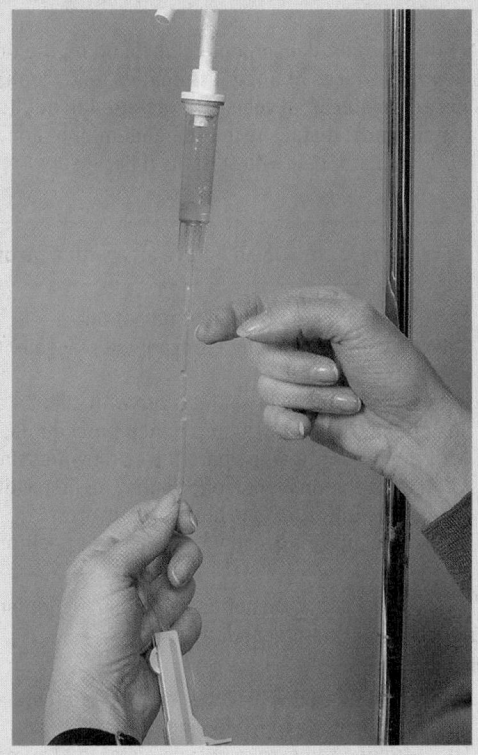

STEP 14h Removing air bubbles from tubing.

STEPS	RATIONALE
h. Be certain tubing is clear of air and air bubbles by tapping IV tubing where air bubbles are located. Check entire length of tubing to ensure that all air bubbles are removed (see illustration). If using multiple-port tubing, turn port upside down, and tap to fill and remove air. *Optional:* Add an extension tubing to IV tubing to allow for more length, enabling client to move freely while keeping IV line stable.	Tapping causes air bubbles to rise up to drip chamber. Large air bubbles may act as emboli.
i. Replace cap protector on end of infusion tubing.	Maintains system sterility.
15. *Optional:* Prepare heparin or normal saline lock for infusion:	Maintains system sterility.
a. If a loop or short extension tubing is needed because of awkward IV site placement, use sterile technique to connect the IV plug to the loop or short extension tubing. Inject 1 to 3 mL normal saline through the plug and through the loop or short extension tubing before connecting it to IV site.	Removes air to prevent introduction into the vein. Do the same with the saline plug.
16. Apply clean gloves. Eye protection and mask may be worn (see agency policy) if splash or spray of blood is possible.	Decreases exposure to blood-borne organisms (Centers for Disease Control and Prevention [CDC], 2002; INS, 2006) and prevents spraying of blood on nurse's mucous membranes.
17. Identify accessible vein for IV cannula. Apply tourniquet 4 to 6 inches (10 to 15 cm) above the proposed insertion site. Do not apply tourniquet too tightly to avoid injury or bruising the skin. Check for presence of radial pulse. You may apply tourniquet on top of a thin layer of clothing such as a gown sleeve, to protect fragile skin or excess hair. It may become necessary to remove tourniquet and move lower down arm. *Optional:* Apply blood pressure cuff instead of tourniquet. Inflate to a level just below client's normal diastolic pressure. Maintain inflation at that pressure until venipuncture is completed.	Tourniquet impedes venous return but should not occlude arterial flow. If vein cannot be found in the hand or lower arm, move up to the antecubital fossa. Use of BP cuff creates less trauma to skin.

Continued

✳ **SKILL 41-1**   **INITIATING INTRAVENOUS THERAPY—CONT'D**

STEPS	RATIONALE
18. Select the vein for IV insertion. Veins found on the dorsal and ventral surfaces of upper extremities (e.g., cephalic, basilic, and metacarpal veins) are preferred in adults.	Ensures adequate vein that is easier to puncture with needle and less likely to rupture.
a. Use the most distal site in the nondominant arm, if possible. Clip arm hair with scissors if necessary.	Perform venipuncture distal to proximal, which increases the availability of other sites for future IV therapy. Hair impedes venipuncture or adherence of dressing.

Critical Decision Point: Do not shave area with a razor. Shaving may cause microabrasions and predispose to infection (INS, 2006).

STEPS	RATIONALE
b. Avoid areas that are painful to palpation.	May indicate inflamed vein.
c. Select a vein large enough for cannula placement.	Prevents interruption of venous flow while allowing adequate blood flow around the cannula.
d. Choose a site that will not interfere with client's activities of daily living (ADLs) or planned procedures.	Keeps client as mobile as possible.
e. With the index finger, palpate the vein by pressing downward. Note the resilient, soft, bouncy feeling while releasing the pressure (see illustration).	Fingertip is more sensitive and is better for assessing vein condition.
f. If possible, place extremity in dependent position.	Permits venous dilation and visibility.

Critical Decision Point: **Do not use** vigorous friction and multiple tapping to dilate vein. This may cause hematoma and/or venous constriction especially in older adults.

STEPS	RATIONALE
g. Select well-dilated vein. Other methods to foster venous distention include the following:	Increases the volume of blood in the vein at the venipuncture site.
(1) Stroking the extremity from distal to proximal below the proposed venipuncture site.	Promotes venous filling.
(2) Applying warmth to the extremity for several minutes, for example, with a warm washcloth.	Increases blood supply and fosters venous dilation.
h. Avoid sites distal to previous venipuncture site, sclerosed or hardened cordlike veins, infiltrate site or phlebotic vessels, bruised areas, and areas of venous valves or bifurcation.	Such sites can cause infiltration of newly placed IV cannula and excessive vessel damage. Antecubital fossa area is used for blood draws; also limits mobility.
i. Avoid fragile dorsal veins in older adult clients and vessels in an extremity with compromised circulation (e.g., in cases of mastectomy, dialysis graft, or paralysis).	Venous alterations can increase risk of complications (e.g., infiltration and decreased cannula dwell time).
19. Release tourniquet temporarily and carefully. *Optional:* At this point of the procedure there is the option of applying a local anesthetic to site. Monitor client for allergic reaction. A local anesthetic is preferred by clients (Brown, 2003).	Restores blood flow while preparing for venipuncture.
20. Place connection of infusion set or IV plug nearby, maintaining sterility of system.	Permits smooth, quick connection of cannula to IV system.

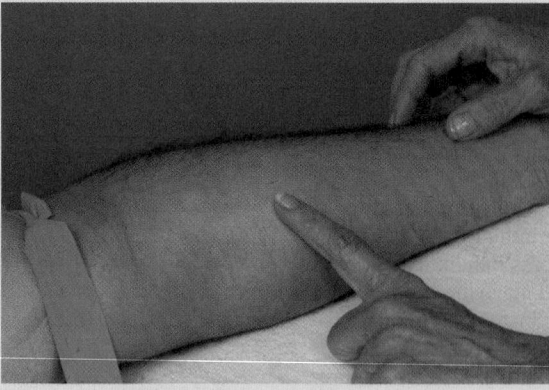

STEP 18e Palpate vein for resilience.

✳ SKILL 41-1   INITIATING INTRAVENOUS THERAPY—CONT'D

STEPS

21. If area of insertion appears to need cleansing, use soap and water first. Use antiseptic swab to cleanse insertion site using friction in a horizontal plane, then a vertical plane (see illustration) followed with a circular motion (middle to outward); allow antiseptic to dry completely. Refrain from touching the cleansed site unless using sterile technique.

22. Reapply tourniquet 10 to 12 cm (4 to 6 inches) above anticipated insertion site. Check presence of distal pulse.

23. Perform venipuncture. Anchor vein by placing thumb over vein, and gently tighten the skin distal to the site 1½ to 2 inches (4 to 5 cm) (see illustration). Warn client of a sharp, quick stick.

   a. *ONC cannula with safety device:* Insert with the bevel up at 10- to 30-degree angle slightly distal to actual site of venipuncture in the direction of the vein (see illustration).

   b. *Winged needle:* Hold needle at 10- to 30-degree angle with bevel up, slightly distal to actual site of venipuncture.

RATIONALE

Mechanical friction in this pattern allows penetration of the antiseptic solution into the cracks and fissures of the epidermal layer of the skin (Rosenthal, 2003).

Antiseptic solutions should be allowed to air-dry completely to effectively reduce microbial counts (INS, 2006). If antiseptic agents are used in combination, allow each to air-dry separately. Chlorhexidine 2% preparation is preferred (CDC, 2002; Hindley, 2004).

If fingers touch cleansed area, the site will need to be prepped again.

Diminished arterial flow prevents venous filling. The pressure of the tourniquet should cause the vein to dilate.

Stabilizes vein for needle insertion.

Places needle at a 10- to 30-degree angle to the vein. When vein is punctured, risk of puncturing posterior vein wall is reduced. Superficial veins require a smaller angle. Deeper veins require a greater angle.

Critical Decision Point: Each cannula should be used only once for each insertion attempt.

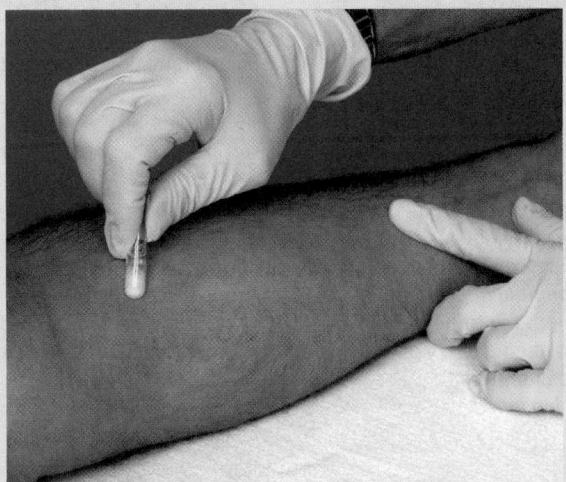

STEP 21 Cleansing site with chlorhexidine.

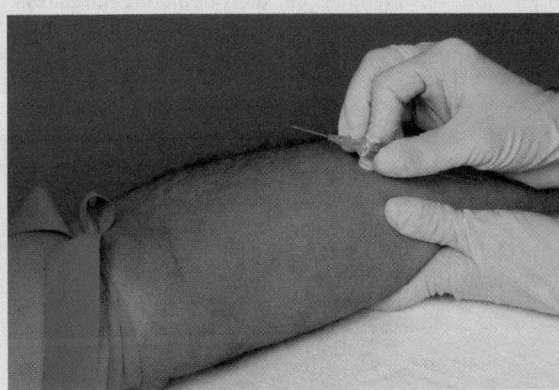

STEP 23 Stabilize vein below insertion site.

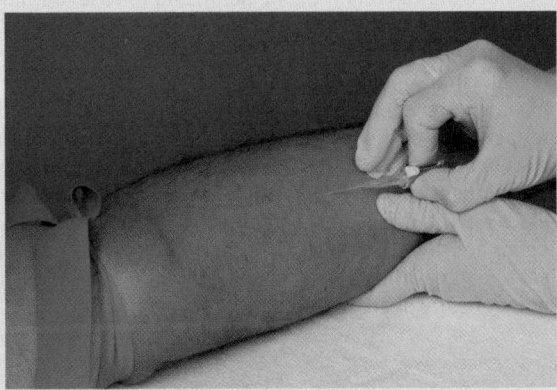

STEP 23a Puncture skin with ONC catheter at 10- to 30-degree angle.

Continued

✳ **SKILL 41-1**   **INITIATING INTRAVENOUS THERAPY—CONT'D**

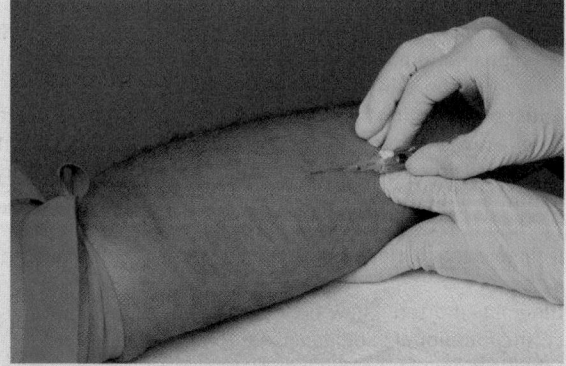

A

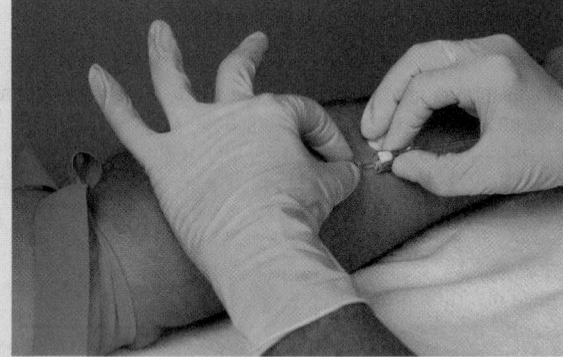

B

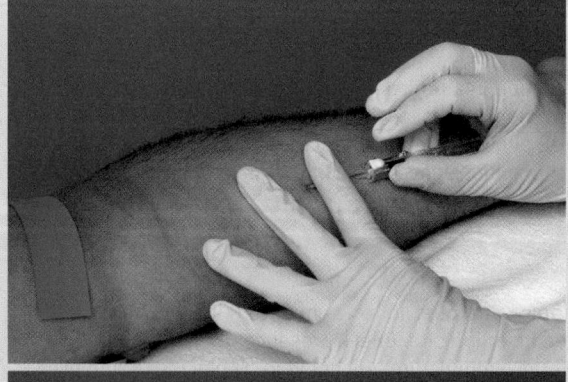

A

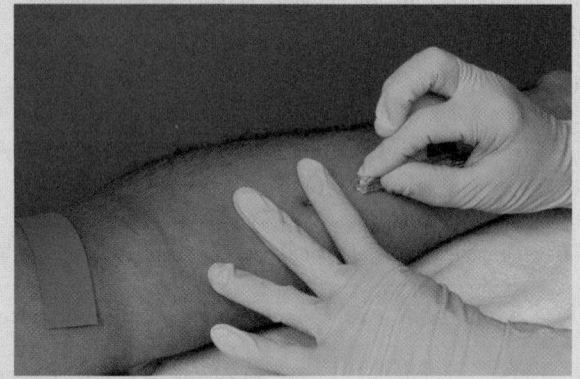

B

STEP 24 A, Look for blood return in flashback chamber. **B,** Advance catheter into vein.

STEP 25 A, Apply pressure above insertion site with middle finger of nondominant hand. **B,** Retract the stylet by pressing safety tab.

STEPS

24. Observe for blood return through flashback cannula or tubing of winged needle, indicating that needle has entered vein (see illustration). Lower cannula/winged needle until almost flush with skin. *(Advance cannula approximately ¼ inch into vein, and then loosen stylet).* Continue to hold skin taut, and advance cannula/winged needle into vein until hub rests at venipuncture site (see illustration). *Do not reinsert the stylet once it is loosened.*

RATIONALE

Increased venous pressure from tourniquet increases backflow of blood into cannula or tubing.

Allows for full penetration of the vein wall, placement of the cannula in the vein's inner lumen, and advancement of the cannula off the stylet. Reduces risk of introduction of infectious microorganisms along cannula.

Reinsertion of stylet can cause cannula shearing and potential cannula embolization.

Critical Decision Point: No more than two attempts at inserting an IV should be made by a single nurse (INS, 2006).

---

25. Stabilize the cannula with one hand, and release tourniquet with other. Apply gentle pressure with the middle finger of nondominant hand 1¼ inches (3 cm) above insertion site (see illustration, *A*). Keep cannula stable with index finger. In many safety devices the stylet retracts automatically, or retract stylet by pressing safety tab (see illustration, *B*).A click indicates the device is locked over the stylet. (NOTE: Techniques will vary with each IV device.) Remove the stylet. Place directly into sharps container.

26. *Continuous infusion:* Quickly connect end of infusion tubing set to end of ONC cannula (see illustration). Do not touch point of entry of adapter.

Permits venous flow, reduces backflow of blood, and allows connection with administration set with minimal blood loss. Prevents transmission of infection.

Prompt connection of infusion set maintains patency of vein and prevents exposure to blood. Maintains sterility.

SKILL 41-1 ✲ **INITIATING INTRAVENOUS THERAPY—CONT'D**

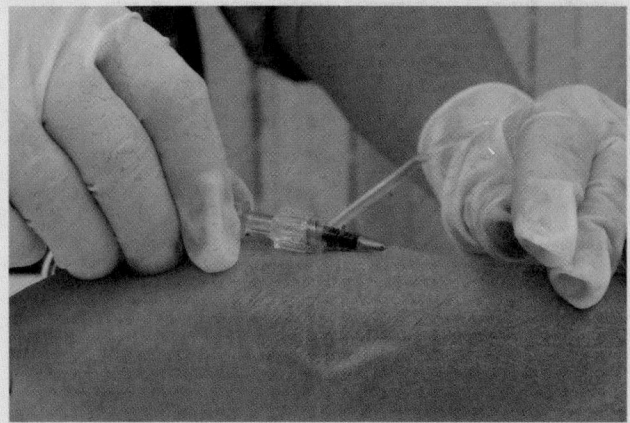

STEP 26 Connect end of IV tubing to catheter tubing. Secure connector.

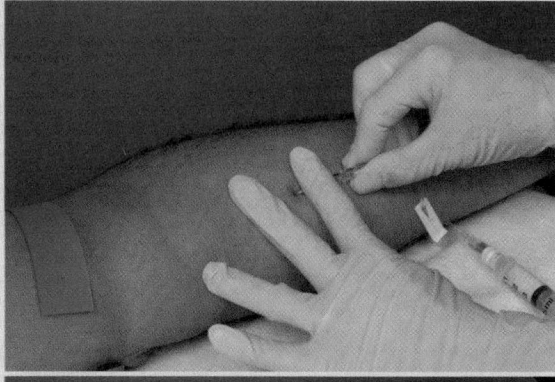

A

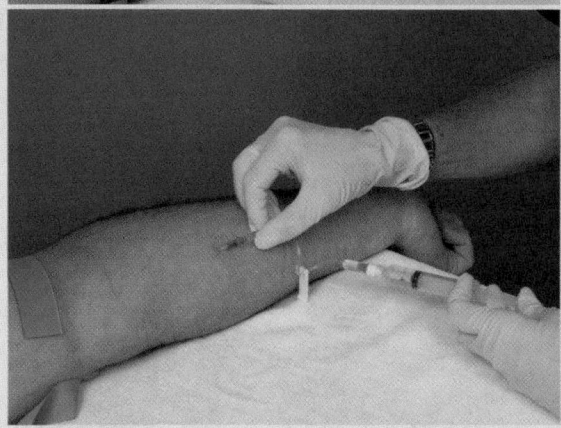

B

STEP 27 A, Connecting end of saline lock. **B,** Flush injection cap slowly.

STEPS

27. *Intermittent infusion:* Quickly connect adapter of heparin lock to hub of ONC cannula (see illustration, *A*). Clean hub of heparin lock with alcohol. Insert prefilled syringe containing flush solution into injection cap (see illustration, *B*). Flush injection cap slowly with flush solution. Use positive flow adapter, or withdraw the syringe while still flushing.
28. *Continuous infusion:* Begin infusion by slowly opening the clamp of the IV tubing.

RATIONALE

"Positive pressure flushing" allows fluid to create positive pressure in the cannula and prevents reflux of blood during flushing (Fulcher and Frazier, 2007).

Initiates flow of fluid through IV cannula, preventing clotting of device.

Critical Decision Point: Be sure to calculate rate (see Skill 41-2) so as not to infuse IV solution too rapidly or too slowly.

---

29. Secure cannula (procedures can differ; follow agency policy).
    a. *Transparent dressing:* Secure cannula with nondominant hand while preparing to apply dressing.
    b. *Sterile gauze dressing:* Place narrow piece (½ inch) of tape under cannula hub with sticky side up, and crisscross tape over cannula hub to make a chevron (see illustrations) or place strip of tape directly over hub. Do not apply tape around arm. Place tape only on the cannula, *never* over the insertion site.
30. Apply sterile dressing over site. (Procedures can differ; follow agency policy.)
    a. **Transparent dressing**
       (1) Remove adherent backing. Apply one edge of dressing, and then gently smooth remaining dressing over IV site, leaving connection between IV tubing and cannula hub uncovered. Remove outer covering and smooth dressing gently over site (see illustration).

Prevents accidental dislodgment of cannula.

Prevents accidental removal of cannula from vein. Prevents back-and-forth motion, which can irritate the vein and introduce microorganisms on the skin into the vein.

Occlusive dressing protects site from bacterial contamination. Connection between administration set and hub needs to be uncovered to facilitate changing the tubing if necessary. The Centers for Disease Control and Prevention (CDC) (2002) no longer recommends application of antimicrobial ointment to cannula site.

Continued

✳ **SKILL 41-1** **INITIATING INTRAVENOUS THERAPY—CONT'D**

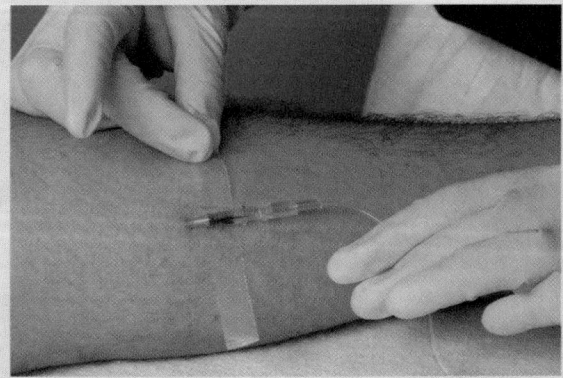 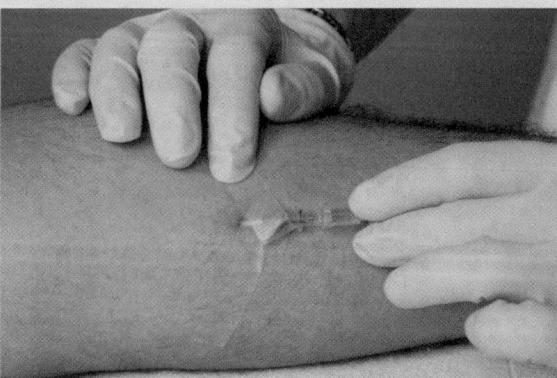

STEP 29b A, Place tape under catheter hub. **B,** Crisscross ends of tape over hub to form a chevron (applied before gauze dressing).

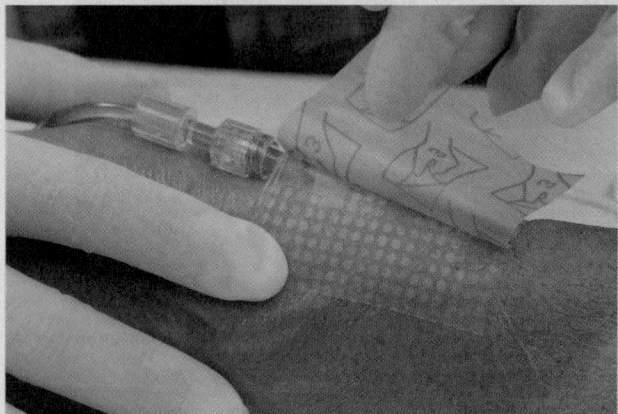

STEP 30a(1) Apply transparent dressing.

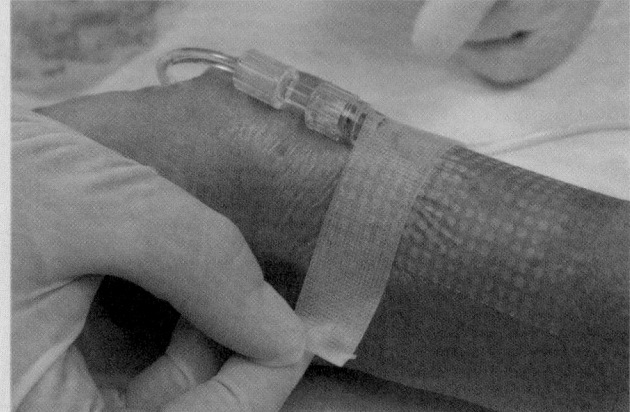

STEP 30a(2) *Option:* Place tape over transparent dressing. (NOTE: Some clinicians only use dressing to cover and secure site.)

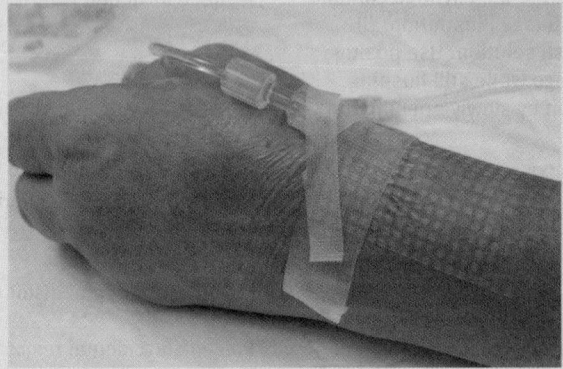

STEP 30a(3) Apply chevron over tape.

STEPS

   (2)   Apply a 1-inch piece of transparent tape from end of hub of cannula to insertion site, over transparent dressing (see illustration).

   (3)   Apply chevron to infusion tubing, and place only over tape, not the transparent dressing (see illustration), or use strip of tape to simply secure tubings just above connection.

RATIONALE

✳ SKILL 41-1   INITIATING INTRAVENOUS THERAPY—CONT'D

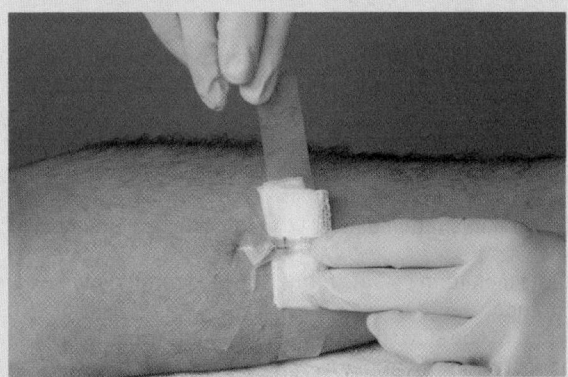

STEP 30b(1) Fold 2 × 2 gauze in half, cover with 1-inch tape, and place under catheter hub.

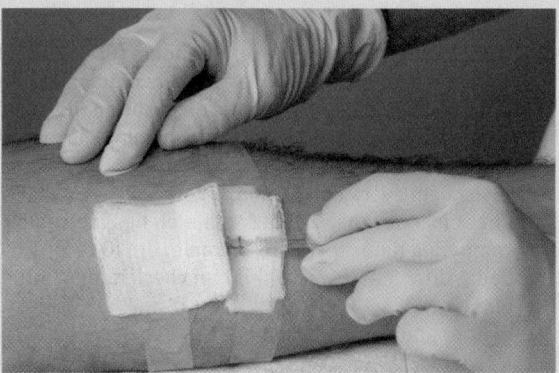

STEP 30b(2) Apply 2 × 2 gauze over insertion site.

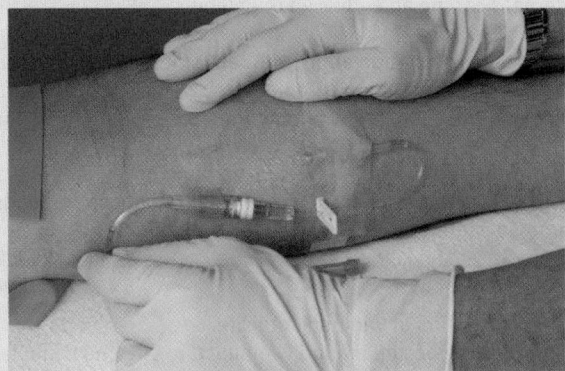

STEP 31 Loop and secure tubing.

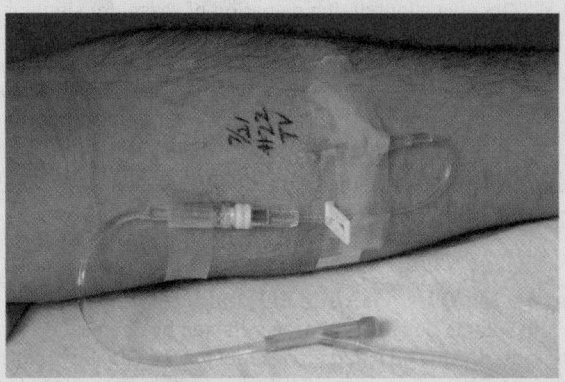

STEP 33 Label IV dressing.

STEPS

b. **Sterile gauze dressing**
   (1) Fold a 2 × 2 gauze in half, and cover with a 1-inch-wide tape extending about an inch from each side. Place under the tubing/cannula hub junction (see illustration).

   (2) Place a gauze pad over insertion site and cannula hub (see illustration). Secure all edges with tape. Do not cover connection between IV tubing and cannula hub.

31. Loop tubing alongside the arm, and place a second piece of tape directly over the tape covering the transparent dressing or over the padded 2 × 2 (see illustration).
32. For IV fluid administration, recheck flow rate to correct drops per minute (see Skill 41-2) or connect to electronic infusion device (EID) as per agency policy.
33. Write date and time of IV placement, cannula, gauge size and length, and nurse's initials on dressing or dressing label (see illustration).
34. Dispose of stylet or other sharps in appropriate sharps container. Discard supplies. Remove gloves, and perform hand hygiene.
35. Instruct client in how to move or turn without pulling on IV cannula.

RATIONALE

Gauze pad elevates hub off skin to prevent pressure area. Securing loop of tubing reduces risk of dislodging cannula should the IV tubing get pulled (i.e., the loop would come apart before the cannula dislodges). Tape on top of tape makes it easier to access hub/tubing junction.

Taping prevents client from pulling tubing.

Manipulation of cannula during dressing application may alter flow rate. Maintains correct rate of flow for IV solution. Flow can fluctuate, so it must be checked at intervals for accuracy.

Provides immediate access to data as to when IV was inserted and when site rotation is needed.

Reduces transmission of microorganisms and protects staff from infection and injury.

Prevents accidental dislodgment of cannula.

Continued

SKILL 41-1 INITIATING INTRAVENOUS THERAPY—CONT'D

STEPS

36. Change peripheral IV access every 72 hours (CDC, 2002; INS, 2006) or per health care provider's orders or immediately upon suspected contamination or complication (INS, 2006).
37. When solution has less than 100 ml remaining, have next solution available at client's bedside.
38. Observe client every 1 to 2 hours.
    a. Check if correct amount of IV solution has infused by comparing time tape on IV container or EID record.
    b. Count drip rate (if gravity drip), or check rate on infusion pump.
    c. Check patency of IV cannula.

RATIONALE

Incidence of complications may be higher when peripheral IV is allowed to remain in a vein over 72 hours (INS, 2006).

Subsequent container provides continuation of IV without interruption and risk of occlusion from empty container.

Correct administration of fluid volume prevents fluid imbalance.

Accurate monitoring of rate further ensures correct volume administration.
Flow rate will be slowed or stopped if cannula is partially occluded or obstructed.

Critical Decision Point: If IV is positional, fluid will run less slowly or stop depending on position of client's arm. Instruct client to position arm to maintain flow; if this continues, IV may have to be restarted in another site.

    d. Observe client during palpation of vessel for signs of discomfort.
    e. Inspect insertion site, note skin color (e.g., redness, pallor). Inspect for presence of swelling, infiltration (Table 41-10), and phlebitis (Table 41-11). Palpate temperature of skin above dressing.
39. Evaluate client's response to therapy (i.e., measure intake and output [I&O], weights, vital signs).

Tenderness can be an early sign of phlebitis.

Redness or inflammation along with tenderness and warmth indicate vein inflammation or phlebitis. Swelling above insertion site and cool temperature may indicate infiltration of fluids into tissues.
IV fluids and additives are given to maintain or restore fluid and electrolyte balance. Early recognition of complications leads to prompt treatment.

Unexpected Outcomes and Related Interventions

1. Fluid volume deficit (FVD) as manifested by decreased urine output, dry mucous membranes, decreased capillary refill, a disparity in central and peripheral pulses, hypotension, tachycardia, shock.
   a. Notify health care provider; requires readjustment of infusion rate.
2. Fluid volume excess (FVE) as manifested by crackles in the lungs, shortness of breath, edema
   a. Reduce IV flow rate if symptoms appear, and notify health care provider.
3. Electrolyte imbalances manifested by abnormal serum electrolyte levels, changes in mental status, vital signs, and alterations in cardiac and neuromuscular function.
   a. Notify health care provider. Additives in IV or type of IV fluid may be adjusted.
4. Infiltration at site as indicated by swelling and possible pitting edema, pallor, coolness, pain at insertion site, and possible decrease in flow rate (see Table 41-9).
   a. Stop infusion, and discontinue IV (see Skill 41-3, p. 1013). Elevate affected extremity. Restart new IV if continued therapy is necessary.
   b. Document degree of infiltration and nursing intervention.
5. Phlebitis is indicated by pain, increased skin temperature, erythema along path of vein (see Table 41-10).
   a. Stop infusion, and discontinue IV (see Skill 41-3, p. 1013). Restart new IV if continued therapy is necessary.
   b. Place moist warm compress over area of phlebitis.
   c. Document degree of phlebitis and nursing interventions per agency policy and procedure.
6. Bleeding occurs at venipuncture site.
   a. If bleeding occurs around venipuncture site and cannula is within vein, apply gauze dressing over site. Be aware that if you use gauze dressing, it must be removed to accurately assess insertion site.
   b. Blood on the dressing can result when the administration set becomes disconnected from the hub of the cannula. When blood appears on the dressing, verify that the system is intact, and change the dressing.

Recording and Reporting

- Record in the notes the number of attempts for insertion, type of infusion, insertion site by vessel, flow rate, size and type of cannula, and when infusion was begun. Use a parenteral therapy flow sheet if available.
- If using an EID, document type and rate of infusion.
- Record client's response to IV fluid, amount infused, and integrity and patency of system according to agency policy (usually done hourly for vulnerable populations).
- Report the following to oncoming staff: type of infusion, flow rate, status of venipuncture site, amount of fluid remaining in present solution, expected time to hang subsequent infusion, and any side effects.
- Report to health care provider any adverse reactions.

Home Care Considerations

- Ensure that the client is able and willing to self-administer IV therapy or that there is a reliable caregiver to provide IV therapy at home.
- Instruct client and primary caregiver about procedures related to IV therapy, including hand hygiene and aseptic technique while handling syringes and other supplies.

✴ **SKILL 41-1**   **INITIATING INTRAVENOUS THERAPY—CONT'D**

- Teach primary caregiver to apply pressure with sterile gauze if cannula falls out and, if client is on anticoagulant therapy, to tape several pieces of sterile gauze in place for at least 20 minutes with pressure or until bleeding stops.
- Teach client and primary caregiver to protect IV site during hand hygiene or during bathing to avoid getting it wet. If using an EID, do not plug or unplug around water. For showering, protect the IV site and dressing from getting wet by covering completely with plastic.

- Teach client and family to accurately monitor I&O using measuring devices.
- Ensure that all sharps and equipment contaminated by blood are disposed of in puncture-resistant containers with lids. Some suppliers will provide sharps containers for needle disposal. Teach client and family to dispose of any open and sheathed needles into sharps container. All sharps containers must be stored in safe area away from children.

✴ **TABLE 41-10**   **Infiltration Scale**

GRADE	CLINICAL CRITERIA
0	No symptoms
1	Skin blanched
	Edema, <1 inch in any direction
	Cool to touch
	With or without pain
2	Skin blanched
	Edema 1-6 inches in any direction
	Cool to touch
	With or without pain
3	Skin blanched, translucent
	Gross edema >6 inches in any direction
	Cool to touch
	Mild-moderate pain
	Possible numbness
4	Skin blanched, translucent
	Skin tight, leaking
	Skin discolored, bruised, swollen
	Gross edema >6 inches in any direction
	Deep pitting tissue edema
	Circulatory impairment
	Moderate to severe pain
	Infiltration of any amount of blood product, irritant, or vesicant

From Infusion Nurses Society: Infusion nursing standards of practice, *J Intraven Nurs* 29(1S): S60, 2006.

✴ **TABLE 41-11**   **Phlebitis Scale**

GRADE	CLINICAL CRITERIA
0	No symptoms
1	Erythema at access site with or without pain
2	Pain at access site with erythema and/or edema
3	Pain at access site with erythema and/or edema
	Streak formation
	Palpable venous cord
4	Pain at access site with erythema and/or edema
	Streak formation
	Palpable venous cord >1 inch in length
	Purulent drainage

From Infusion Nurses Society: Infusion nursing standards of practice, *J Intraven Nurs* 29(1S): S59, 2006.

---

are easily moved or bumped such as the dorsal surface of the hand (Rosenthal, 2005) (Box 41-6).

Venipuncture is contraindicated in a site that has signs of infection, infiltration, or thrombosis. An infected site is red, tender, swollen, and possibly warm to the touch. Exudate may be present. An infected site is not used because of the danger of introducing bacteria from the skin surface into the bloodstream. Avoid using an extremity with a vascular (dialysis) graft/fistula or on the same side as a mastectomy. Initially, place IV lines at the most distal point when possible. Using a distal site first allows for the use of proximal sites later if the client needs a venipuncture site change (Hadaway and Millam, 2005).

A **venipuncture** is a technique in which a vein is punctured through the skin by a sharp rigid stylet (e.g., butterfly needle or metal needle), a stylet partially covered with a plastic cannula (over-the-needle cannula [ONC]), or a needle attached to a syringe. Peripheral and central cannulas placed into a central vein such as the subclavian vein and superior vena cava deliver large volumes of fluids and TPN for long-term infusions or to administer irritating medications. Nurses require specialized knowledge and education to place PICCs; however, some central line cannulas require insertion by physicians or advanced practice nurses. Both types of cannulas require close monitoring and maintenance. When veins are fragile or collapse, venipuncture is extremely difficult, but the intervention may be life-saving. Experienced practitioners should perform venipuncture for difficult clients such as older adults. Guidelines in Box 41-6 are for correct placement in older adults. The general purposes of venipuncture are to collect a blood specimen, to instill a medication, to start an IV infusion, or to inject a radiopaque or radioactive tracer for special examinations. Skill 41-1 describes venipuncture for IV fluid infusion and incorporates INS (2006) standards of practice.

Regulating the Infusion Flow Rate. After initiating the IV infusion and checking the line for patency, regulate the rate of infusion according to the health care provider's orders (Skill 41-2). An infusion rate that is too slow can lead to further cardiovascular and circulatory collapse in a client who is dehydrated, in shock, or critically ill. In addition, an IV infusion that is running too slowly is at increased risk of becoming clotted. An infusion rate that is too rapid can cause fluid overload, resulting in cardiovascular, kidney, and neurological complications in vulnerable clients (e.g., older adults or clients with preexisting heart and renal disease).

✴ BOX 41-6 FOCUS ON OLDER ADULTS

Protection of Skin and Veins

- Use the smallest gauge cannula or needle possible (e.g., 22 to 24 gauge). Veins are very fragile, and a smaller gauge allows better blood flow to provide increased hemodilution of the IV fluids or medications (Schelper, 2003).
- Avoid the back of the hand, which may compromise the client's need for independence and mobility.
- Impaired skin integrity leads to susceptibility of tearing, difficulty detecting complications, and venous sclerosis.
- Avoid placement of IV in veins that are easily bumped because there is less subcutaneous support tissue.
- If the client has fragile skin and veins, use minimal or no tourniquet pressure.
- After applying tourniquet, venous pressure rises rapidly, the vein is overstretched, and puncture with even a thin needle can rupture the wall of vein (Hadaway and Milam, 2005).
- If using a tourniquet, place it over the client's sleeve to decrease shearing of fragile skin.
- With loss of supportive tissue, veins tend to lie more superficially; lower insertion angle for venipuncture to 5 to 15 degrees (Coulter, 2004; INS, 2006; Rosenthal, 2005).
- If the client has lost subcutaneous tissue, the veins lose stability and will roll away from the needle. To stabilize the vein, apply traction to the skin below the projected insertion site.
- Secure the device with mesh dressing or securement device for protection (Coulter, 2004).
- Nutritional deficiencies promote fluid to migrate into tissues surrounding vessels, making IV access more difficult.
- Multiple medication usage (e.g., anticoagulants, antibiotics, and steroids) increases the likelihood of fragile, transparent skin that bruises and bleeds easily.
- Dehydration related to a lower percentage of body weight as water, diminished thirst mechanism, and social factors of bladder control contribute to difficult IV access (Grandjean and others, 2003; Rosenthal, 2005; Toth, 2002).

Calculate IV infusion rates to prevent too-slow or too-rapid administration of the IV fluids. There are numerous methods to ensure an accurate hourly infusion rate for IV therapy. Adjust fluids that run by gravity through the use of a flow control/regulator clamp. Fluids infused by an electronic infusion device (EID) or IV volume controller are regulated by a mechanical mechanism set at the prescribed rate. When used correctly, these devices maintain flow rates, cannula patency, and prevent an unexpected bolus of IV

infusion. Regardless of the device in use, the client requires close monitoring to verify the correct infusion of the IV solution and to detect and prevent complications.

Electronic **infusion pumps** are necessary when administering small hourly volumes (e.g., less than 20 mL/hr) and for clients who are at risk for volume overload such as neonatal, pediatric, and geriatric clients. In addition, when infusing high volumes of IV fluids (more than 150 mL/hr) to clients with impaired renal clearance, older adults, or pediatric clients, or when infusing drugs or IV fluids that require specific hourly volumes, electronic infusion devices permit accurate infusion. Electronic infusion pumps deliver the infusion via positive pressure. A rate controller used on gravity infusions regulates the infusion, but unlike the electronic pump, is affected by many mechanical and client factors. Recent advances in infusion technology have resulted in a variety of devices available for use to ensure accurate delivery.

Many devices have operating and programming capabilities that allow for single- and multiple-solution infusions at different rates. A variety of detectors and alarms respond to air in IV lines, completion of infusion, high and low pressure, low battery power, occlusion, and the inability to deliver at a preset rate.

SAFETY ALERT An anti–free flow safeguard (preventing bolus infusion in the event of machine malfunction or when tubing is removed from machine) is an important element of an electronic infusion device and is required. Check the manufacturer's instructions for specific device features.

Patency of the IV cannula means that there are no clots at the tip of the cannula and that the cannula is not against the vein wall. A blocked cannula affects the rate of infusion of the IV fluids. IV flow rates can also be affected by infiltration, a knot or kink in the tubing, the height of the solution, a restrictive IV dressing, and the position of the client's extremity. One method to assess patency is by lowering the IV container below the level of the IV insertion site and observing for a blood return, however, this method does not confirm patency. If no blood return occurs and fluid does not flow easily from the drip chamber when the roller clamp is opened, assess for potential causes: a too-tight IV dressing may be impeding the flow, a clot may be occluding the cannula of the IV, or the cannula tip may be occluded against the wall of the vein. Inspect the tubing and area around the insertion site for anything that could obstruct the flow of IV fluids. A knot or kink in the tubing decreases the flow rate. Occasionally the tubing kinks under a dressing, which requires removal of the dressing to locate the problem. The flow rate frequently resumes after straightening the tubing. The client may lie or sit on the tubing, which may cause an occlusion. The height of the IV container can also affect flow rates. Raising the container usually increases the rate because of increased hydrostatic pressure.

Text continued on p. 1011

✳ **SKILL 41-2**   **REGULATING INTRAVENOUS FLOW RATE**   [Video]

Delegation Considerations

The skill of regulating intravenous flow rate should not be delegated to nursing assistive personnel (NAP). Instruct NAP to report the following:

- Client complaints of burning, bleeding, swelling, coolness at the cannula insertion site.
- Electronic infusion device (EID) alarm signals.
- Fluid container is almost empty.

Equipment

- Watch with second hand
- Calculator or paper and pen/pencil
- Tape
- Label
- IV regulating device (EID, volume control device [optional])

STEPS	RATIONALE
1. Check client's medical record for order of solution and additives. Follow six rights of medication administration (see Chapter 35). Usual order includes name of solution, additives or medications (if included), and time over which each liter is to infuse or an hourly infusion rate or volume in specified time period. Occasionally, an IV order calls for 1 L to keep vein open (KVO).	IV fluids are medications. The six rights prevent medication administration error.
2. Perform hand hygiene. Observe for patency of IV line and cannula.	For fluid to infuse at proper rate, IV line and cannula must be free of kinks and thrombi.
3. Assess client's knowledge of how positioning of the IV site affects flow rate.	Fosters client participation in maintaining most effective position of arm with IV equipment. Position or setting of control clamp or infusion device rate should be set by nurse or health care provider.
4. Inspect IV site and verify with client how venipuncture site feels; determine if there is pain or burning. Palpate site for tenderness.	Pain or burning may be early indication of phlebitis. Includes client in decision making.
5. Have paper and pencil or calculator to calculate flow rate.	Use mathematical calculations to obtain correct rate.

6. Know calibration (drop factor) in drops per milliliter (gtt/mL) of infusion set currently in use:
Microdrip: 60 gtt/mL
Macrodrip: Abbott: 15 gtt/mL
                Travenol: 10 gtt/mL
                McGaw: 15 gtt/mL
	Use microdrip tubing, also called pediatric tubing, when infusing small or very precise volumes. There are different commercial parenteral administration sets for macrodrip tubing. Use macrodrip tubing to infuse large quantities or fast rates.

7. Review how long each liter of fluid should run. Calculate mL/hr (hourly rate) by dividing volume by hours, for example: $$mL/hr = \frac{total\ infusion\ (mL)}{hours\ of\ infusion}$$ 1000 mL/8 hr = 125 mL/hr or if 3 L is ordered for 24 hours 3000 mL/24 hr = 125 mL/hr	Provides even infusion of fluid over prescribed hourly rate.

Critical Decision Point: It is common for health care providers to write an abbreviated IV order such as "D_5W with 20 mEq KCl 125 mL/hr continuous." This order implies that the IV should be maintained at this rate until order has been written for IV to be discontinued.

STEPS	RATIONALE

8. Select one of the following formulas to calculate minute flow rate (drops/min) based on drop factor of infusion set:
   a. mL/hr/60 min = mL/min and
      Drop factor × mL/min = drops/min
      Or
   b. mL/hr × drop factor/60 min = drops/min
      Using formula b above, calculate minute flow rate
        for bottle 1:1000 mL with 20 mEq KCl
      Microdrip:
      125 mL/hr × 60 gtt/mL = 7500 gtt/hr
      7500 gtt ÷ 60 minutes = 125 gtt/min
      Macrodrip:
      125 mL/hr × 15 gtt/mL = 1875 gtt/hr
      1875 gtt ÷ 60 minutes = 31-32 gtt/min
	Formulas compute correct flow rate over a minute.
	
	When using microdrip, mL/hr always equals gtt/min.
	
	Volume is multiplied by drop factor, and the product is divided by time (in minutes).

Continued

✳ **SKILL 41-2**   **REGULATING INTRAVENOUS FLOW RATE—CONT'D**

STEPS

9. Place marked adhesive tape or commercial fluid indicator tape on IV container next to volume markings (see illustration).

RATIONALE

Time taping IV bags provides visual clues as to whether fluids are being administered over correct period of time. Time tapes should be used for all IV infusions, including those on therapies infused via EIDs.

Critical Decision Point: On IV bags made of polyvinylchloride (PVC) avoid drawing directly with felt-tip pens or permanent markers because ink could leach into solution (Hadaway and Millam, 2005).

---

10. Regulate flow rate manually by counting drops in drip chamber for 1 minute by watch, then adjust roller clamp to increase or decrease rate of infusion (see illustration).

11. Set up and regulate infusion gravity controller or EID pump.

   a. Consult manufacturer's directions for setup of the infusion. Place electronic eye over drip chamber (see illustration). If a gravity controller is used, ensure that IV container is 36 inches above the IV site.

   b. Insert IV tubing into chamber of control mechanism (see manufacturer's directions) (see illustration).

Regulate to prescribed rate.

IV controller works by gravity.

Most electronic infusion pumps use positive pressure to infuse.

Critical Decision Point: Special infusion tubing is required for some pumps Electronic pump tubing is designed to prevent free flow of fluid when tubing is removed from device. Check agency equipment and associated policies.

---

   c. Select required drops per minute or volume per hour, close door to control chamber, turn on power button, and press start button (see illustrations).

   d. Open drip regulator completely while EID is in use.

   e. Monitor infusion rate and IV site for infiltration according to agency policy. Check rate of infusion by comparing volume in the container with the calculated amount that should have been infused even when EID is used.

   f. Assess patency of system when alarm signals.

Ensures the pump freely regulates infusion rate.

Infusion controllers or pumps are not infallible and do not replace frequent, accurate evaluation. Infusion pumps may continue to infuse IV fluids after an infiltration has begun.

Alarm on infusion pump can be triggered by empty solution container, tubing obstruction, closed drip regulator, infiltration, thrombus formation, air in the tubing, and/or low battery.

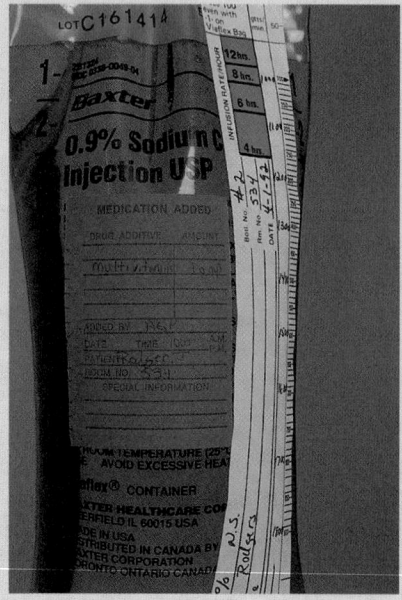

STEP 9 IV fluid bag with time tape.

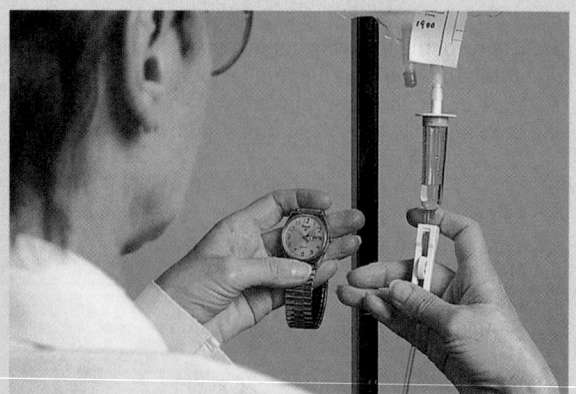

STEP 10 Counting IV drip rate.

SKILL 41-2   REGULATING INTRAVENOUS FLOW RATE—CONT'D

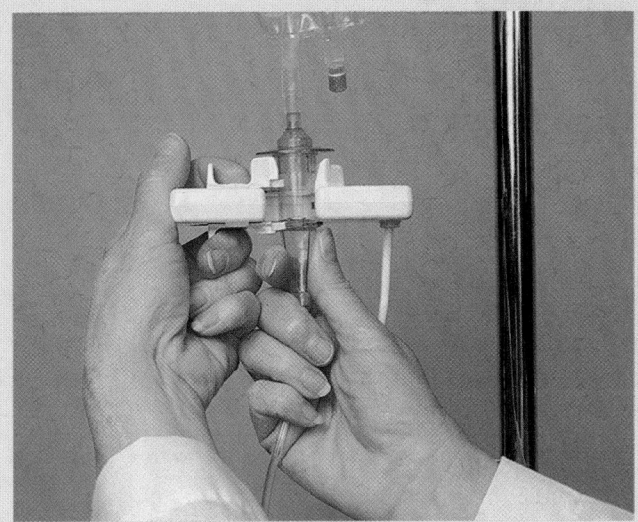

STEP 11a Electronic eye placed over drip chamber.

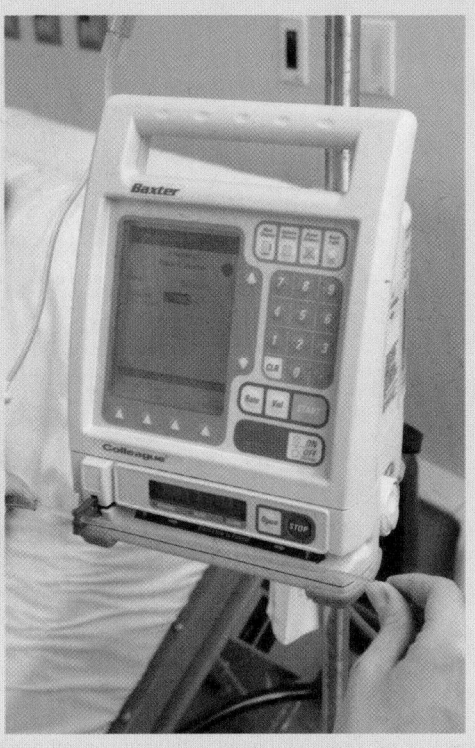

STEP 11b Insert IV tubing into chamber of controller.

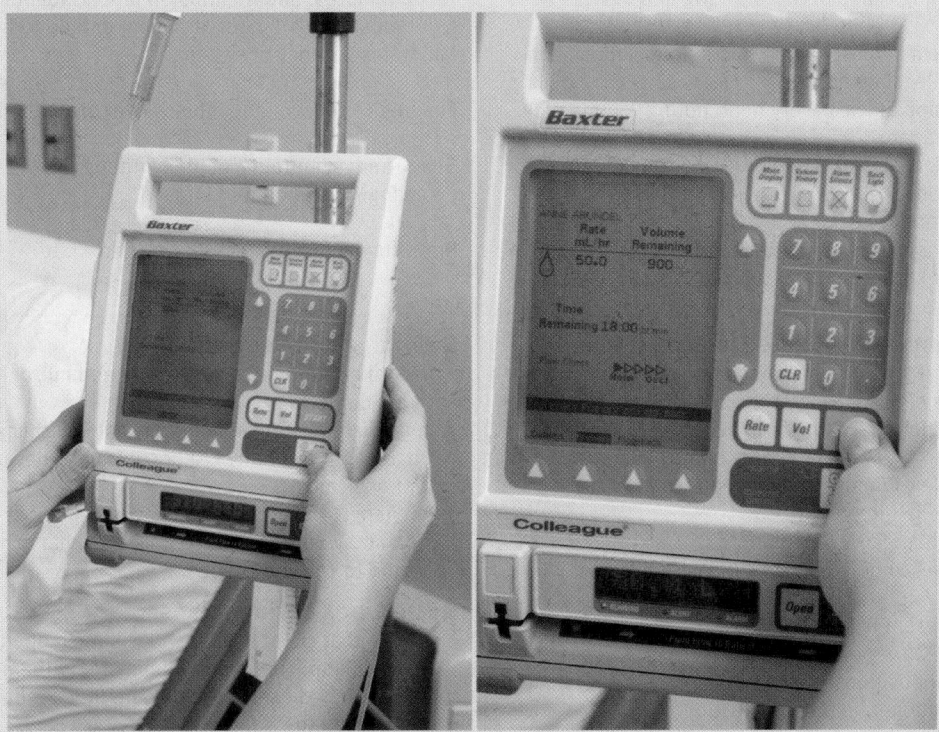

STEP 11c Select rate and volume to be infused and press start button.

Continued

⁕ **SKILL 41-2**   REGULATING INTRAVENOUS FLOW RATE—CONT'D

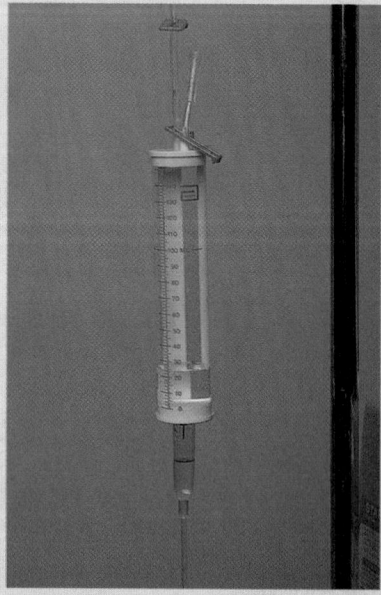

STEP 12a Volume control device.

STEPS	RATIONALE
12. Follow this procedure for gravity volume control device:	
a. Place volume control device (see illustration) between IV bag and insertion spike of infusion set using aseptic technique.	Delivers small volume, but must be refilled as it becomes low.
b. Place no more than 2 hours' allotment of fluid into device by opening clamp between IV bag and device.	Provides a safeguard if the system cannot be checked in exactly 60 minutes. Should infusion rate accidentally increase, allows at most only a 2-hour allotment of fluid to infuse.
c. Assess system at least hourly; add fluid to volume control device. Regulate flow rate.	Maintains patency of system.
13. Monitor IV infusion at least every hour, noting volume of IV fluid infused and rate.	Ensures correct volume infuses over prescribed time period.
14. Observe client for signs of overhydration or dehydration to determine response to therapy and restoration of fluid and electrolyte balance.	Signs and symptoms of dehydration or overhydration warrant changing rate of fluid infused.
15. Evaluate for signs of infiltration, inflammation at site, clot in cannula, kink or knot in infusion tubing.	Prevents decrease or cessation of flow rate.

Unexpected Outcomes and Related Interventions

1. Sudden infusion of large volume of solution occurs with client having symptoms of dyspnea, crackles in the lung, and increased urine output, indicating fluid overload.
   a. Slow infusion to KVO rate and notify health care provider immediately. New IV orders will be required.
   b. Client may require diuretics.
   c. Place client in high-Fowler's position.
2. IV fluid container is completed with subsequent loss of IV line patency.
   a. Discontinue present IV, and restart IV.
3. The IV infusion is slower than ordered.
   a. Check client for positional change that might affect rate, height of IV container, tubing obstruction.
   b. An infiltration may be developing at IV site. Check condition of site.
   c. If volume infused is deficient, consult health care provider for new order to provide necessary fluid volume.

Recording and Reporting

- Record rate of infusion, gtt/min, and mL/hr in notes or parenteral fluid form.
- Immediately record in notes any ordered changes in IV fluid rates.
- Document use of any EID or controlling device and number on that device.
- At change of shift or when leaving on break, report rate of infusion and volume left in container to charge nurse or staff assigned to care for client.

Home Care Considerations

- Ensure that client is able and willing to operate the infusion pump (if applicable) and administer IV therapy. If client is unable to provide self-care, be sure that a reliable caregiver is available in the home.
- Ensure EID is functioning properly before use with client.
- If gravity administration is used, teach client and primary caregiver to time drops per minute using watch with second hand.
- Ensure that client's electrical outlets are functioning properly.

The position of an extremity, particularly at the wrist or elbow, can decrease flow rates. Occasionally the use of an arm board helps to keep the joint extended (Figure 41-15). Caution must be used in applying arm boards because they restrict movement. The arm board helps to protect the IV site and tubing. Sometimes it is more comfortable for the client to have an infusion started in a new location rather than relying upon a site that causes problems. Before discontinuing the current infusion, choose another site and start the infusion to verify that the client has other accessible veins.

Children, older adults, clients with severe head trauma, and clients susceptible to volume overload must be protected from sudden increases in infusion volumes by using an infusion device to regulate flow. It is necessary to understand that when you open certain IV controller devices, the IV fluid will infuse rapidly. An excessive amount of solution infuses if not controlled. Sudden increases can occur accidentally. For example, a restless client may loosen the roller clamp with a sudden movement and thus increase the flow rate, or the flow rate may be accidentally changed

by gravity influence. A sudden increase in IV infusion rate causes a rapid increase in vascular volume, which can make the client critically ill or even cause death. Volume control devices, such as a Volutrol burette, prevent sudden excessive increases in the volume of IV solution infused.

Maintaining the System. After placing the IV line and regulating the flow rate, maintain the system. Agency policy regulates the maintenance of IV lines. Line maintenance involves (1) keeping the system sterile; (2) changing solutions, tubing, and site dressings; and (3) assisting the client with self-care activities so as to not disrupt the system.

An important component of client care is maintaining the integrity of an IV to prevent infection. The potential sites for contamination of an intravascular device are shown in Figure 41-16. The client's microflora and contamination by insertion are initially controlled for in the procedure for IV insertion. However, other factors are controlled through the conscientious use of infection control principles (Hindley, 2004). This begins with the use of thorough hand hygiene before and after handling any component of the IV system.

Always maintain the integrity of an IV system. Never disconnect tubing because it becomes tangled or it might seem more convenient in positioning or moving a client or applying a gown. If a client needs more room to maneuver, add extension tubing to an IV line. However, keep the use of extension tubing to a minimum, because each connection of tubing provides opportunity for contamination. Stopcocks for connecting more than one solution to a single IV site are sources of contamination and should be avoided (Centers for Disease Control and Prevention [CDC], 2002; INS, 2006). Whenever disconnecting an IV line from a stopcock, plug the port with a sterile cap. Do not allow a port to remain exposed to air, which will cause contamination. A new administration set should be exchanged with the subsequent fluid change. Intravenous tubing also contains injection ports through which adapters can be inserted for medication administration.

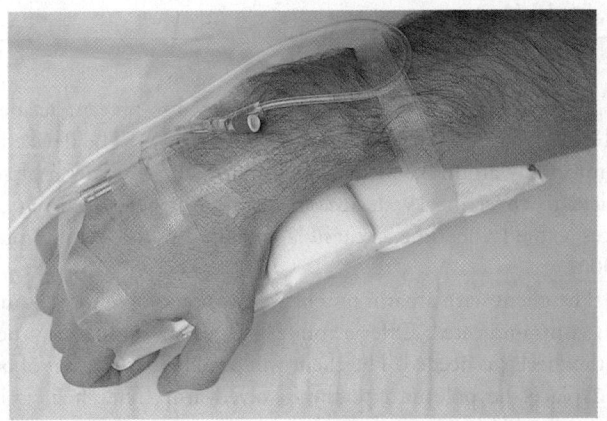

Figure 41-15 IV arm board and cover.

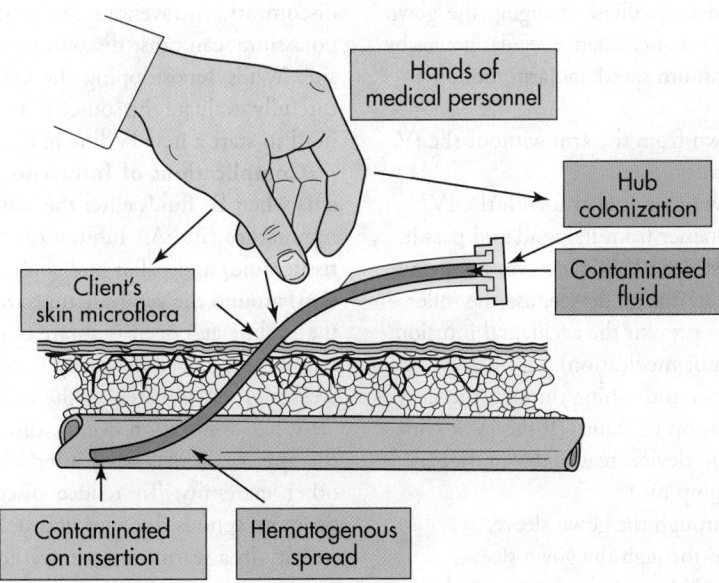

Figure 41-16 Potential sites for contamination of an intravascular device.

Cleanse an injection port thoroughly with 70% alcohol, chlorhexidine, or povidone-iodine solution before accessing the system (INS, 2006).

Clients receiving IV therapy over several days will require periodic changes of solutions. It is important to organize tasks so that you can change solutions before a thrombus forms in a cannula. The Centers for Disease Control and Prevention (CDC) (2002) has no recommendation for the hang time of IV fluids. Skill 41-3 reviews steps for changing IV solutions.

Intravenous tubing administration sets can remain sterile for 72 hours (CDC, 2002; INS, 2006). The CDC (2002) recommends changing tubing no more frequently than every 72 hours. The INS (2006) recommends 72-hour intervals for continuous tubing changes, adding that more frequent changes may occur if the tubing has been compromised or has become contaminated. The exception is tubing containing blood, TPN, blood products, and lipid emulsions, which are more likely to promote bacterial growth. Agency policy may require more frequent tubing changes (e.g., every 24 hours). Whenever possible, schedule tubing changes when it is time to hang a new IV container to promote aseptic technique. To prevent entry of bacteria into the bloodstream, maintain sterility during tubing and solution changes.

The dressings over IV sites reduce the entrance of bacteria into the insertion site. The two forms of dressings are transparent and gauze. Transparent dressings reliably secure the IV device, allow continuous visual inspection of the IV site, become less easily soiled or moistened, and require less frequent changes than standard gauze (CDC, 2002; Hindley, 2004). Change gauze dressing every 48 hours (INS, 2006). Either form of dressing must be changed when the IV device is removed or replaced or when the dressing becomes damp, loosened, or soiled (INS, 2006). Agency policy may require IV dressings to be routinely changed within a certain time frame (e.g., 48 to 72 hours) (Skill 41-4, p. 1019).

To prevent the accidental disruption of an IV system, the client may need assistance with hygiene, comfort measures, meals, and ambulation. Because a client with an infusion in the arm finds it difficult to meet hygiene needs, assistance is needed with bathing and changing gowns. It helps to use a gown specifically made with snaps along the top sleeve seam to facilitate changing the gown without disturbing the venipuncture site. Change regular gowns by following these six steps for maximum speed and arm mobility:

1. Remove the sleeve of the gown from the arm without the IV, maintaining the client's privacy.
2. Remove the sleeve of the gown from the arm with the IV.
3. Remove the IV solution container from its stand and pass it and the tubing through the sleeve. (If this involves removing the tubing from an electronic infusion device, use the roller clamp to slow the infusion to prevent the accidental infusion of a large volume of solution or medication).
4. Place the IV solution container and tubing through the sleeve of the clean gown and hang it on its stand. (If the IV is connected to a electronic infusion device, reassemble and open the roller clamp. Turn the pump on.)
5. Place the arm with the IV through the gown sleeve.
6. Place the arm without the IV through the gown sleeve. (Breaking the integrity of an IV line to change a gown leads to contamination.)

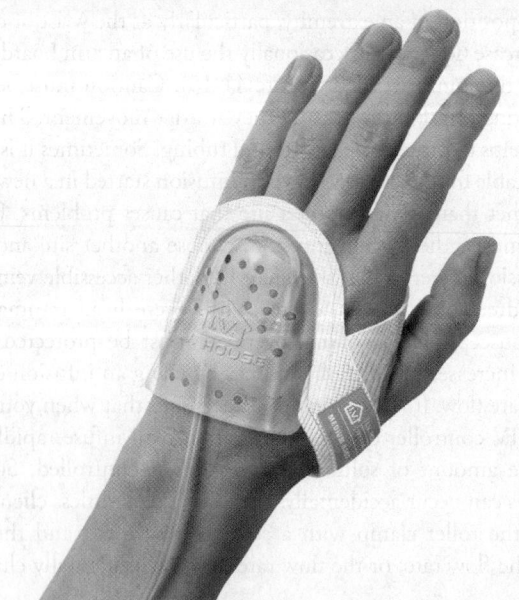

Figure 41-17 IV House Protective Device. (Courtesy IV House, St. Louis, Mo.)

There are now protective devices designed to prevent accidental dislodgment of an IV cannula (Figure 41-17). The device fits comfortably around a client's hand or arm and provides a plastic shield to cover the IV device. Mechanical catheter-securing devices extend the time a cannula remains in the vein (Smith, 2006).

The client with an arm or a hand infusion is able to walk, unless contraindicated. Offer a rolling IV pole (a standard IV pole with wheels) as needed. The client will need help to get out of bed and place the pole next to the involved arm. The client is instructed to hold on to the pole with the involved hand and to push it while walking. Check the equipment to ensure that the IV container is at the proper height, that there is no tension on the tubing, and that the flow rate is correct. Instruct the client to report any blood in the tubing, a stoppage in the flow, or increased discomfort. Intravenous medications, especially antibiotics and potassium, can cause discomfort and burning sensations at the IV site. While repositioning the extremity may relieve discomfort, carefully evaluate the source of discomfort. There still may be the need to start a new IV line in a larger vein.

Complications of Intravenous Therapy. An **infiltration** occurs when IV fluids enter the subcutaneous tissue around the venipuncture site. An infiltration causes swelling (from increased tissue fluid) and pallor and coolness (caused by decreased circulation) around the venipuncture site. Fluid may be flowing through the IV line at a decreased rate or may have stopped flowing. Pain may be present and usually results from tissue edema. Pain increases proportionally as the infiltration progresses.

When infiltration occurs, discontinue the infusion and, if IV therapy is still necessary, insert a new cannula into a vein in another extremity. To reduce discomfort, raise the extremity to promote venous drainage and decrease edema. Wrapping the extremity in a warm, moist towel for 20 minutes promotes venous return, increases circulation, and reduces pain and edema. Heat therapy can be repeated three to four times during the day.

✳ **SKILL 41-3** **MAINTENANCE OF INTRAVENOUS SYSTEM**

Delegation Considerations

The skill of changing an intravenous solution and tubing and discontinuing a peripheral IV cannula cannot be delegated to nursing assistive personnel (NAP). Delegate NAP to collect supplies, assist with comfort measures, and distract the client during the procedure. Instruct the NAP to report the following:
- When the IV container is near completion
- If there is any bleeding after the cannula has been removed

Equipment
- Changing IV solution and tubing (continuous infusion)
  - Bottle/bag of IV solution as ordered by health care provider
  - Time tape
  - Infusion tubing and tubing label
  - Filter (size appropriate to solution) and extension tubing (if necessary)
- Changing IV solution and tubing (intermittent saline/heparin lock)
  - Syringe filled with normal saline or heparin flush solution (check agency policy)
  - 2 × 2 gauze pads (optional)
  - Label
  - Clean gloves
  - Loop of extension tubing, inspection cap
  - Antiseptic swab or stick (e.g., chlorhexidine, povidone-iodine, alcohol)
- Discontinuation of peripheral intravenous access
  - Clean gloves
  - Antiseptic swabs
  - Sterile 2 × 2 gauze or 4 × 4 gauze sponge
  - Tape

STEPS	RATIONALE
1. Assemble equipment, and position client to make IV site accessible.	Keeps procedure organized.
2. Determine client's/family member's understanding of need for IV therapy.	Reveals need for client instruction.
3. Explain to client/family member each procedure, its purpose, and what is expected of client.	Promotes cooperation and lessens anxiety or uncertainty.
4. **Change intravenous solution**	
a. Check health care provider's order for type of fluid and infusion rate. Follow the six rights of medication administration.	Ensures that correct solution will be used. Prevents medication error.
b. If order is written for keep vein open (KVO) or to keep open (TKO), note date and time when solution was last changed.	A hang time is no longer recommended by the Centers for Disease Control and Prevention (CDC) (2002) to ensure sterility of solutions in bag or bottle. Refer to agency policy.
c. Determine the compatibility of all IV fluids and additives by consulting appropriate literature or the pharmacy.	Incompatibilities may lead to precipitate formation and can cause physical, chemical, and therapeutic client changes.
d. Determine if current IV access is patent by carefully adjusting the roller clamp to see an increase in flow rate then regulating back to ordered rate. *Lowering IV container below level of IV site for presence of blood return (retrograde) is an unreliable indicator*. Assess swelling, coolness to touch, or tenderness around IV site.	If patency is not verified, a new IV access site may be needed. Notify health care provider. When there is no obstruction, flow rate will increase as roller clamp is adjusted. Indications of infiltration.

Critical Decision Point: If flow rate does not increase when clamp is adjusted open, systematically check the IV system starting at the IV site up to the IV container for catheter and dressing integrity, tubing kinks, secure connections, inadvertent clamps, tubing puncture, tubing spike communicated with IV container, and distance between IV site and IV container for adequate gravity.

e. Have next solution prepared and accessible at least 1 hour before needed. Check that solution is correct and properly labeled. Check solution expiration date. Observe for precipitate, discoloration, and leakage.	Adequate planning reduces risk of thrombus formation in vein caused by disruption of flow with empty IV container. Checking prevents medication error.
f. Check client's identification by checking identification band and asking client to state name and birth date.	Ensures correct solution is administered to correct client.
g. Prepare to change solution when less than 25 to 50 mL of fluid remains in container.	Prevents air from entering tubing and vein from clotting from lack of flow. IV containers contain an estimated 5% overfill to compensate for priming of tubing and subsequent container changes.
h. Be sure drip chamber is at least half full.	Provides fluid to vein while bag is changed.
i. Perform hand hygiene.	Reduces transmission of microorganisms.
j. Prepare new solution for changing. If using plastic bag, remove protective cover from IV tubing port. If using glass bottle, remove metal cap and metal and rubber disks.	Permits quick, smooth, and organized change from old to new solution.
k. Move roller clamp to stop flow rate on existing infusion. Turn off EID, remove tubing.	Prevents solution remaining in drip chamber from emptying while changing solutions.

Continued

✳ **SKILL 41-3**   **MAINTENANCE OF INTRAVENOUS SYSTEM—CONT'D**

STEPS	RATIONALE
l. Remove old IV fluid container from IV pole.	Brings work to eye level. Prevents fluid from pouring out when spike is removed.
m. Quickly remove spike from old solution container and, without touching tip, insert spike into new container.	Reduces risk of solution in drip chamber running dry and maintains sterility.

Critical Decision Point: If spike is contaminated, a new IV tubing set is required. Sterile IV tubing may be used for 72 hours unless compromised.

n. Hang new container of solution.	Position allows gravity to assist with delivery of fluid into drip chamber.
o. Check for air in tubing. If bubbles form, they can be removed by closing the roller clamp below the bubbles, stretching the tubing downward, and tapping the tubing with the finger (bubbles rise in the fluid to the drip chamber) (see illustration). For larger amounts of air, remove using a needleless syringe: swab port with alcohol, allow to dry, insert needleless syringe into port below the air, and aspirate the air into the syringe.	Reduces risk of air embolus. Use of an air-eliminating filter also reduces this risk.
p. Make sure drip chamber is one-third to one-half full. If the drip chamber is too full, pinch off tubing below the drip chamber, invert container, squeeze the drip chamber (see illustration), release tubing, and hang bag.	Reduces risk of air entering tubing. If chamber is completely filled, the drip rate cannot be observed and rate cannot be accurately regulated.
q. Insert tubing into EID and restart pump or regulate flow to prescribed rate.	Maintains measures to restore fluid balance and deliver IV fluid as ordered.
r. Place time label on side of container, and label with the time hung, the time of anticipated completion, and appropriate intervals. If using polyvinylchloride (PVC) containers, mark only on the label and not the container.	Provides visual comparison of volume infused compared with prescribed rate of infusion. Ink may leach into PVC containers.
s. Observe client for signs of overhydration or dehydration.	Provides ongoing evaluation of client's fluid and electrolyte status.
t. Periodically check infusion rate.	Prevents improper fluid infusion.

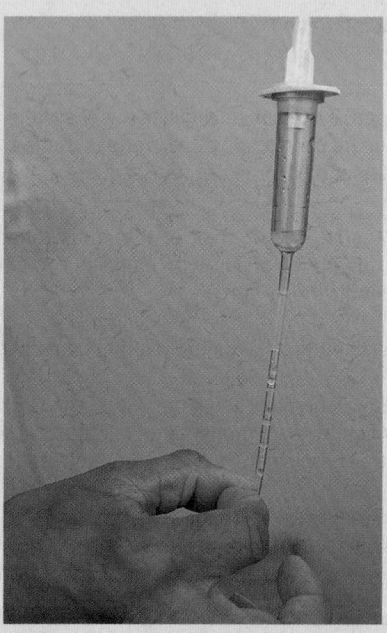

STEP 4o Tap tubing to cause air bubbles to rise up to drip chamber.

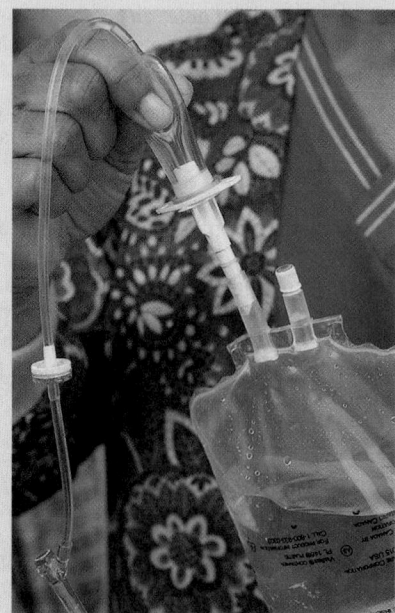

STEP 4p Squeeze drip chamber to remove a portion of fluid. Be sure to leave chamber one-third to one-half full.

STEPS	RATIONALE
5. **Changing infusion tubing**	
a. Determine when new infusion set is needed:	
(1) Agency policy will indicate frequency of routine change for IV administration sets and heparin/saline flushes.	CDC (2002) and INS (2006) recommend tubing change no more often than 72-hour intervals or whenever tubing has been compromised.
(2) Puncture of infusion tubing requires immediate change.	Punctured tubing results in fluid leakage and bacterial contamination.
(3) Contamination of tubing requires immediate change.	Contamination of tubing allows entry of pathogens into client's bloodstream.
(4) Occlusions in tubing following infusion of packed red cells, whole blood, albumin, or other blood components, or administration of incompatible mixtures requires an immediate change.	Whole blood or blood component products can occlude or partially occlude tubing because viscous solutions adhere to walls of tubing and decrease the size of lumen.
b. Perform hand hygiene.	Reduces transmission of microorganisms.
c. Open new infusion set, keeping protective coverings over infusion spike and connector site for cannula. Secure all connections.	Provides ready access to new infusion set and maintains sterility of infusion set.
d. Apply clean gloves.	Reduces risk of exposure to HIV, hepatitis, and other blood-borne pathogens (CDC, 2002).
e. If cannula hub is not visible, remove IV dressing as directed in Skill 41-4, p. 1019. Do not remove tape securing cannula to skin.	Cannula hub must be accessible to provide smooth transition when removing old and inserting new tubing.
f. **Continuous infusion**	
(1) Move roller clamp on new IV tubing to "off" position.	Prevents spillage of solution after container is spiked.
(2) Slow rate of infusion by regulating drip rate on old tubing. Be sure rate is at KVO rate.	Prevents complete infusion of solution remaining in tubing, which results in increased risk of occlusion of IV cannula.
(3) Compress drip chamber of old tubing, and fill chamber.	Provides surplus of fluid in drip chamber so there is enough fluid to maintain IV patency while changing tubing.
(4) Remove IV solution container from IV pole.	Brings work to eye level.
(5) Invert container, and remove old tubing from container: keep spike sterile until new tubing connected. *Optional:* Tape old drip chamber to IV pole without contaminating spike.	Allows fluid to continue to flow through IV cannula while new tubing is prepared.
(6) Place insertion spike of new tubing into old solution container opening, and hang solution container on IV pole.	Permits flow of fluid from solution into new infusion tubing.

Critical Decision Point: If spike becomes contaminated, a new IV tubing set is required.

(7) Compress and release drip chamber on new tubing; slowly fill drip chamber one-third to one-half full (see Skill 41-1, Step 14f).	Allows drip chamber to fill and promotes rapid, smooth flow of solution through new tubing.
(8) Slowly open roller clamp, remove protective cap from adapter (if necessary), and flush new tubing with solution. Stop infusion. Replace cap. Place end of adapter near client's IV site.	Removes air from tubing and replaces it with fluid. Position equipment for quick smooth connection of new tubing. Reduces air in tubing by priming slowly instead of allowing a wide-open flow.
(9) Turn roller clamp on old tubing to "off" position.	Prevents spillage of fluid as tubing is removed from cannula.
g. **Saline/heparin lock**	
(1) If a loop or short extension tubing is needed because of an awkward IV site placement, use sterile technique to connect the new injection cap to the loop or tubing.	Prevents transmission of infection.
(2) Swab injection cap with antiseptic swab. Insert syringe with 1 to 3 mL saline or heparin flush solution, and inject through the injection cap into the loop or short extension tubing (see illustration).	Removes air to prevent introduction into the vein.
h. *Optional:* Place 2 × 2 gauze under cannula hub.	Prevents tubing from accidentally contacting skin and collects blood that may leak from cannula hub.

※ **SKILL 41-3**   **MAINTENANCE OF INTRAVENOUS SYSTEM—CONT'D**

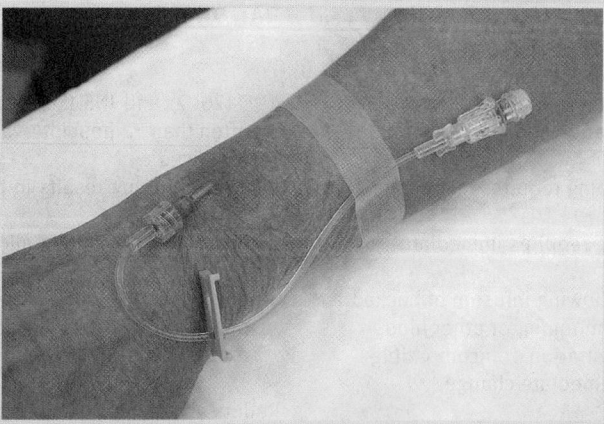

STEP 5g(2) IV cannula connected to saline lock extension tube.

A   B

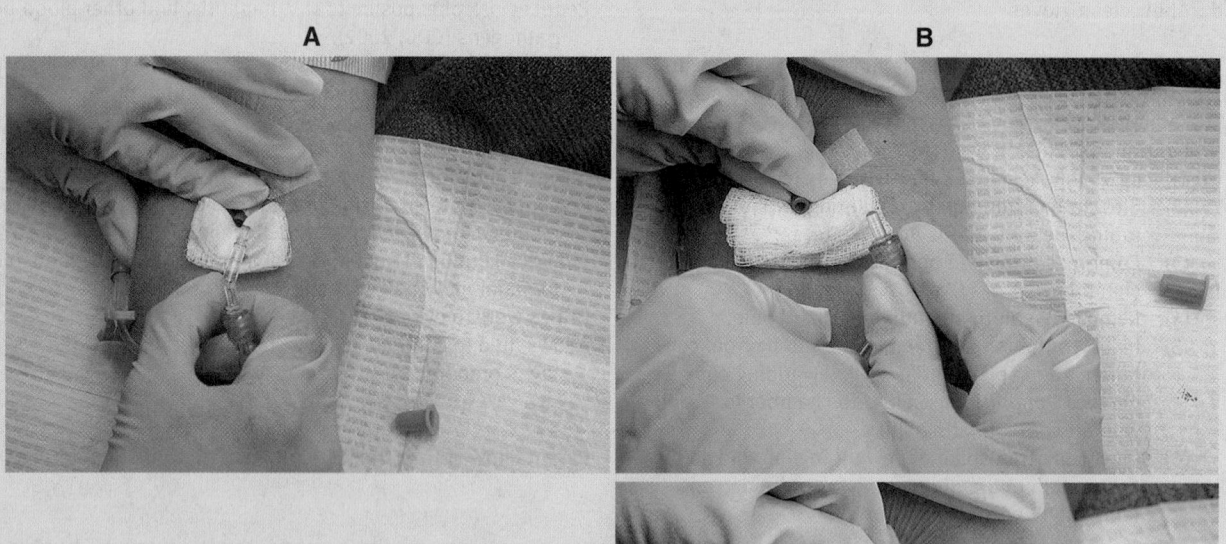

STEP 5i A, Maintain stability of catheter hub while removing
old tubing. **B,** Connect new infusion tubing. **C,** Be sure connection at hub is secure.

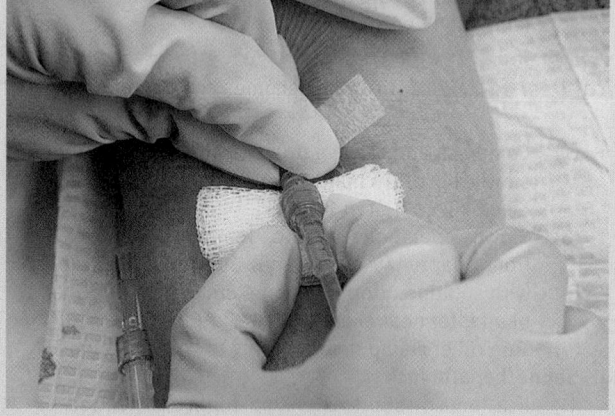

C

STEPS

   i. Stabilize cannula hub, and apply pressure over vein just
above cannula tip (at least 1½ inches above insertion
site). Gently disconnect old tubing from cannula hub,
and quickly insert adapter of new tubing into cannula
hub (see illustrations).

RATIONALE

Allows smooth transition from old to new tubing, minimizing time
system is open to infection.

✳ **SKILL 41-3** MAINTENANCE OF INTRAVENOUS SYSTEM—CONT'D

STEPS	RATIONALE
j. For continuous infusion, open roller clamp on new tubing, allowing solution to run rapidly for 30 to 60 seconds, then regulate IV drip according to health care provider's orders, and monitor rate hourly. *Optional:* Connect new tubing to electronic infusion device (EID) and regulate.	Ensures patency of cannula and maintenance of venous access.
k. Attach a piece of tape or a preprinted label with date and time of tubing change onto tubing below the drip chamber.	Provides reference to determine next time for tubing change.
l. Form a loop of tubing, and secure it to client's arm with a strip of tape.	Avoids accidental pulling against site and cannula movement.
m. If necessary, apply new dressing (see Skill 41-4, p. 1019).	Reduces transmission of microorganisms.
6. **Discontinuing peripheral IV access**	
a. Observe IV site for signs and symptoms of infection, infiltration, or phlebitis.	Findings will determine if therapy is needed following cannula removal.
b. Review health care provider's order for discontinuation of IV.	Order required for discontinuation of IV therapy. The order for cannula removal may be implied.
c. Explain to client that burning sensation might be felt when catheter is removed. Explain that affected extremity must be held still and how long procedure will take (about 5 minutes or less).	Prepares client to cooperate during procedure.
d. Perform hand hygiene. Apply clean gloves.	Reduces transmission of microorganisms.
e. Turn IV tubing roller clamp to "off" position or turn EID off and then turn roller clamp to "off" position.	Prevents spillage of IV fluid.
f. Remove IV site dressing, stabilizing IV device (see Skill 41-4). Then remove tape securing cannula.	Exposes cannula with minimal discomfort.
g. Hold cannula, and clean site with antimicrobial swab. Allow to dry completely.	Removes secretions around skin puncture site.
h. Place clean sterile gauze over venipuncture site, apply light pressure and remove cannula by pulling straight away from insertion site in a slow, steady motion (see illustration). Keep the cannula parallel to the skin during withdrawal. Do not raise or lift catheter before it is completely out of the vein. Inspect catheter for intactness after removal.	Dry pad causes less irritation to the puncture site. Prevents damage to client's vein; determines if catheter tip is intact. Tips of catheter can break off, causing an embolus, and emergency situation. Notify health care provider if tip is broken. Removal technique avoids trauma to vein or hematoma formation.
i. Keep gauze in place, and apply continuous pressure to site for 2 to 3 minutes.	Controls bleeding and hematoma formation. Contraction is enhanced by pressure to site for at least 2 to 3 minutes (INS, 2006).

Critical Decision Point: If client has received anticoagulants (e.g., low-dose aspirin, warfarin sodium [Coumadin], heparin) or has a low platelet count, apply steady pressure for 5 to 10 minutes and assess bleeding.

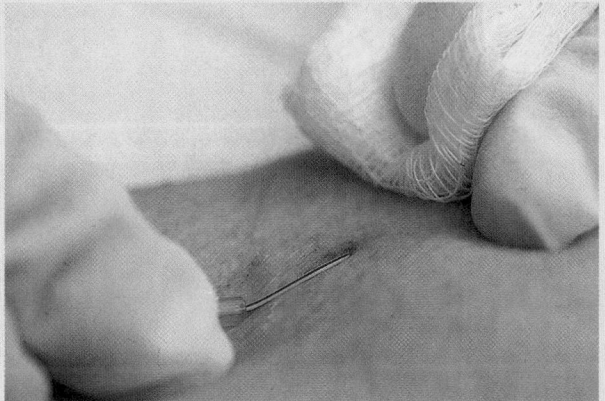

STEP 6h IV catheter is removed slowly, keeping catheter parallel to vein.

Continued

✳ **SKILL 41-3**   **MAINTENANCE OF INTRAVENOUS SYSTEM—CONT'D**

STEPS

    j. Apply clean folded gauze dressing over insertion site, and secure with tape.

    k. Discard all used supplies, remove gloves, and perform hand hygiene.

    l. Continue to inspect site for redness, edema, and tenderness for 48 hours.

RATIONALE

Maintains pressure to prevent bleeding and reduces bacterial entry into puncture site.

Reduces transmission of microorganisms.

Detects postinfusion phlebitis (INS, 2006).

Unexpected Outcomes and Related Interventions

1. Flow rate is incorrect; client receives too little or too much fluid.
   a. Readjust infusion rate to ordered rate.
   b. Evaluate client for adverse effects; notify health care provider.
   c. Determine and correct the cause of the incorrect flow rate.
   d. Use EID when accurate flow rate is critical.
   e. Notify health care provider if client's anticipated infusion is 100 to 200 mL less than or greater than expected (check agency policy).
2. Decreased or absent flow of IV fluid is indicated by a decreased rate.
   a. Assess IV infusion system for patency.
   b. Recalibrate drip rate on new tubing.
   c. Assess IV site for infiltration.
3. Venipuncture site is inflamed and/or has purulent drainage.
   a. Remove IV, and notify health care provider. Blood cultures may be ordered.
   b. Cover site if drainage present.
   c. If area infected, initiate appropriate wound care protocol (see Chapter 48).
4. Catheter tip is missing after withdrawal.
   a. Apply tourniquet high on the extremity to restrict mobility of catheter embolus.
   b. Immediately notify health care provider.

Recording and Reporting

- Record amount and type of fluid infused and amount and type of new fluid according to agency policy. A special flow sheet may be used for parenteral fluids.
- Record changing of tubing and solution on client's record.
- Record the time peripheral IV was discontinued. Include site assessment information and status of catheter including gauge, length, and catheter tip integrity.
- Report that IV was discontinued and any significant complications.

Home Care Considerations

- Ensure that client is able and willing to self-manage IV therapy (including changing IV solutions) or that there is a reliable caregiver or support person at home to provide IV care.
- Instruct client or primary caregiver in procedure for performing an IV solution and tubing change.
- Instruct client or primary caregiver to notify health care provider if bleeding or drainage is noted at insertion site or if pain or tenderness is experienced. Postinfusion phlebitis may occur 48 to 96 hours after catheter removal.

Delegation Considerations

The skill of changing a peripheral intravenous dressing should not be delegated to nursing assistive personnel (NAP). NAP may be delegated the task of collecting supplies, assisting with comfort measures, and distracting the client during the procedure. Instruct NAP to report the following:

- If client complains of moistness or loosening of an IV dressing

Equipment

- Antiseptic swab sticks
- Adhesive remover (if needed)
- Skin protectant swab
- Clean gloves
- Mask and gown *(optional)*
- Strips of nonallergenic tape
- IV catheter safety device (if needed)
- For gauze dressing
  - Sterile 2 × 2 gauze pad
- For transparent dressing
  - Sterile transparent dressing

STEPS	RATIONALE
1. Determine when dressing was last changed. Many institutions require the date and time written on the dressing and date the device was first placed.	Provides information regarding length of time present dressing has been in place.
2. Perform hand hygiene. Observe present dressing for moisture and intactness.	Moisture is a medium for bacterial growth and renders dressing contaminated.
3. Observe IV system for proper functioning or complications: current flow rate, presence of kinks in infusion tubing or IV catheter. Palpate the skin around the cannula site through the intact dressing for inflammation or subjective complaints of pain or burning.	Unexplained decrease in flow rate requires investigating placement and patency of the IV cannula. Pain can be associated with both phlebitis and infiltration.
4. Assess client's body temperature.	Elevated temperature may be related to infection at IV site.
5. Assess client's understanding of need for continued IV infusion.	Determines need for client instruction.
6. Explain procedure and purpose to client and family. Explain that affected extremity must be held still and how long procedure will take.	Decreases anxiety, promotes cooperation, and gives client time frame around which personal activities can be planned.
7. Apply clean gloves.	Reduces transmission of microorganisms. Infections related to IV therapy are most often caused by catheter hub contamination, so careful technique must be used throughout the dressing change. Gloves reduce the risk of exposure to HIV, hepatitis, and other blood-borne viruses or bacteria.
8. Remove tape, gauze, and/or transparent dressing from old dressing one layer at a time by pulling toward the insertion site, leaving tape that secures IV cannula in place. Be cautious if cannula tubing becomes tangled between two layers of dressing. When removing transparent dressing, hold cannula hub and tubing with nondominant hand.	Prevents accidental displacement of cannula.
9. Observe insertion site for signs and/or symptoms of infection: tenderness, redness, swelling, and exudate.	Inflammation indicates phlebitis. Swelling indicates infiltration, with fluid infusing into surrounding tissues. These signs require removal of IV cannula.
10. If complication exists or if ordered by health care provider, discontinue infusion (see Skill 41-3, p. 1013).	
11. If IV is infusing properly, gently remove tape securing cannula. Stabilize cannula with one hand. Use adhesive remover to cleanse skin and remove adhesive residue, if needed.	Exposes venipuncture site. Stabilization prevents accidental displacement of cannula. Adhesive residue decreases ability of new tape to adhere securely to skin.

Critical Decision Point: Keep one finger over cannula at all times until dressing is applied.

12. Cleanse insertion site with antiseptic swab using friction. Use the first swab in a horizontal plane, cleansing the skin from side to side. Apply the second swab on a vertical plane, up and down. Apply the final swab in a circular pattern moving outward from the insertion site (see illustration). Allow each swab to dry completely.	Mechanical friction in this pattern allows penetration of the antiseptic solution into the cracks and fissures of the epidermal layer of the skin (Hadaway and Milam, 2005). Allow antiseptic solutions to air-dry completely to effectively reduce microbial counts (INS, 2006). If antiseptic agents are used in combination, allow each to air-dry separately.

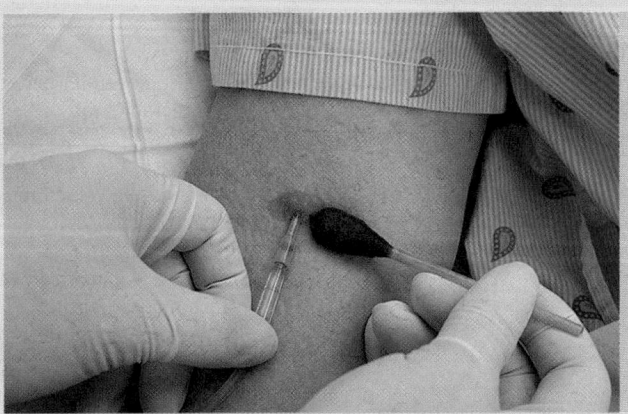

STEP 12 Cleanse peripheral insertion site.

STEPS	RATIONALE
13. *Optional:* Apply skin protectant solution to the area where the tape or dressing will be applied. Allow to dry.	Coats the skin with protective solution to maintain skin integrity, prevent irritation from the adhesion, and promote adherence of dressing.
14. Tape or secure catheter.	
a. Transparent dressing: As directed in Skill 41-1, Step 29a, p. 1001, secure cannula with nondominant hand.	Prevents catheter dislodgment.
b. Gauze dressing: As directed in Skill 41-1, Step 29b, p. 1003, apply chevron or strip of tape to stabilize catheter.	Secures cannula. Inspection of the insertion site is essential.

Critical Decision Point: Do not tape over connection of access tubing or port to IV catheter.

STEPS	RATIONALE
15. Apply sterile dressing over site	
a. Transparent dressing (see Skill 41-1, Step 30a[1]-[3], pp. 1001 to 1002).	Secures catheter and provides tight dressing seal.
	Access to cannula hub is needed for access to change tubing and in emergencies.
b. Gauze dressing (see Skill 41-1, Step 30b[1]-[2]).	Gauze prevents pressure of cannula hub against skin. Securing loop of tubing reduces risk of dislodging catheter from accidental pull.
	Gauze dressing must be occlusive to prevent air flow (Hindley, 2004; Rosenthal, 2003).
16. Remove and discard gloves.	Reduces transmission of microorganisms.
17. *Optional:* Apply a protective device if client is active and uses hand freely.	Reduces the risk of phlebitis and infiltration from mechanical motion.
18. Anchor IV tubing with additional pieces of tape if necessary. When using transparent dressing, avoid placing tape over dressing.	Prevents accidental displacement of IV cannula.
19. Place date and time of dressing change and size and gauge of cannula directly on dressing.	Provides information about dressing change.
20. Discard equipment, and perform hand hygiene.	Reduces transmission of microorganisms.
21. Ensure flow rate is accurate.	Validates that IV is patent and functioning correctly. Manipulation of cannula and tubing may affect rate of infusion.
22. Monitor client's body temperature.	Elevated temperature indicates an infection that may be associated with bacterial contamination of the venipuncture site.

✳ **SKILL 41-4**   **CHANGING A PERIPHERAL INTRAVE**

Unexpected Outcomes and Related Interventions

1. IV cannula becomes infiltrated, as evidenced by decreased flow rate or edema, pallor, or decreased temperature around insertion site.
   a. Stop infusion, and discontinue IV (see Skill 41-3, p. 1013).
   b. Restart new IV in other extremity if continued therapy is necessary.
   c. Elevate affected extremity.
2. Phlebitis is present, as evidenced by erythema and tenderness along vein pathway.
   a. Stop infusion, and discontinue IV (see Skill 41-3).
   b. Restart new IV in other extremity if continued therapy is necessary.
3. IV cannula is accidentally removed.
   a. Restart IV if continued therapy is needed.
4. Client has an elevated temperature.
   a. Notify health care provider. IV may be removed and restarted.
   b. Client will be evaluated for source of infection.

5. Insertion
   has prese
   ture site.
   a. Notify
      dered
   b. Disco
   c. Antib
      bloo

Recordi
- Record
  used.
  ture s
- Repor
  chang
  system.
- Report any complications to health ca

Phlebitis is an inflammation of the vein. Selected risk factors for phlebitis include the type of cannula material, chemical irritation of additives and drugs given intravenously (e.g., antibiotics), and the anatomical position of the cannula. Signs and symptoms may include pain, edema, **erythema,** and increased skin temperature over the vein, and, in some instances, redness traveling along the path of the vein (INS, 2006). Dehydration may also be a contributing factor because of the increase in blood viscosity.

When phlebitis develops, discontinue the IV line and insert a new line in another vein. Warm, moist heat on the site of phlebitis offers some relief to the client (see Chapter 48). Phlebitis can be dangerous, because blood clots (thrombophlebitis) can form and in some cases may result in emboli. This may result in permanent damage to veins, as well as resulting in extended agency care. You prevent phlebitis by the routine removal and rotation of IV sites. The CDC recommends replacing peripheral venous cannulas and rotating sites at least every 72 hours (CDC, 2002; INS, 2006; Rosenthal, 2003). In contrast, studies suggest that peripheral cannulas in children do not need to be rotated on a specified time frame (CDC, 2002).

Another complication of IV therapy is fluid volume excess, which occurs when the client has received a too-rapid administration of IV solutions. Assessment findings include shortness of breath, crackles in the lungs, and tachycardia. If these clinical signs are present, slow the rate of IV infusion, notify the health care provider, raise the head of the bed, and monitor vital signs.

Bleeding can occur around the venipuncture site during the infusion or through the cannula or tubing if these become inadvertently disconnected. Bleeding is common in clients who have received heparin or who have a bleeding disorder (e.g., hemophilia or thrombocytopenia). If bleeding occurs around the venipuncture site and the cannula is within the vein, apply a pressure dressing over the site to control the bleeding. Bleeding from a vein is usually a slow, continuous seepage and is not serious.

Discontinuing Intravenous Infusions. Discontinuing an infusion is necessary after the prescribed amount of fluid has been infused, when an infiltration occurs, if phlebitis is present, or if the infusion cannula develops a thrombus at its tip. Skill 41-3, p. 1013, outlines the steps of discontinuation of an infusion in detail.

Blood Replacement (Colloids). Blood replacement or transfusion is the IV administration of whole blood or a component such as plasma, packed RBCs, or platelets. The objectives for blood transfusions include (1) increasing circulating blood volume after surgery, trauma, or hemorrhage; (2) increasing the number of RBCs and maintaining hemoglobin levels in clients with severe anemia; and (3) providing selected cellular components as replacement therapy (e.g., clotting factors, platelets, albumin).

Blood Groups and Types. The most important grouping for transfusion purposes is the ABO system, which includes A, B, O, and AB blood types. The determination of blood groups is based on the presence or absence of A and B red cell antigens. Individuals with A antigens, B antigens, or no antigens belong to groups A, B, and O, respectively. The individual with A and B antigens has AB blood.

Individuals with type A blood naturally produce anti-B antibodies in their plasma. Similarly, type B individuals naturally produce anti-A antibodies. A type O individual has neither type A nor type B antigen and thus is considered a universal blood donor. A type AB individual produces neither antibody, which is why a type AB individual can be a universal recipient and receive any type of blood. In the event blood that is mismatched with the client's blood is transfused, a **transfusion reaction** occurs. The transfusion reaction is an antigen-antibody reaction and can range from a mild response to severe anaphylactic shock, which can be life threatening (Davis, Hui, and Quested, 2006).

Another consideration when matching for blood transfusions is the Rh factor, which is an antigenic substance in the erythrocytes of most people. A person with the factor is Rh positive, and a person without it is Rh negative.

Autologous Transfusion. Autologous transfusion (autotransfusion) is the collection and reinfusion of a client's own blood. The blood for an autologous transfusion can be obtained by preoperative donation up to 5 weeks before the planned surgery (e.g., heart, orthopedic, plastic, or gynecological). The client can donate 1 to 5 units of blood depending on the type of surgery and the ability of the client to maintain an acceptable hematocrit. The blood will be tested for HIV and HBV. An autologous transfusion can also be obtained during perioperative blood salvage (e.g., during vascular and orthopedic surgery, organ transplant surgery, and traumatic injuries) and reinfused during the surgery. Blood can also be salvaged postoperatively from mediastinal and chest-tube drainage and after joint and spinal surgery. Autologous transfusions are safer for the client because they decrease the risk of complications such as mismatched blood and exposure to blood-borne infectious agents.

Blood Transfusions. Transfusing blood or blood components is a nursing procedure. Nurses complete thorough client assessment before, during, and after the transfusion and for regulation of the transfusion. Assessment is critical because of the risk of allergic reactions. If the client has an IV line in place, assess the venipuncture site for signs of infection, infiltration and patency. Determine the gauge of the IV cannula. A large cannula such as an 18- or 19-gauge is preferred because blood is more viscous than IV fluids, although smaller gauge sizes will accommodate transfusions. However, a catheter no smaller than a 20-gauge should be used (Hadaway and Millam, 2005). The tubing for blood administration has an in-line filter (Figure 41-18). Prime the tubing with 0.9% normal saline to prevent **hemolysis,** or breakdown of RBCs.

Pretransfusion assessment also includes obtaining information from the client and establishing whether the client knows the reason for the blood transfusion and whether the client has ever had a previous transfusion or transfusion reaction. A client who has had a transfusion reaction is usually at no greater risk for a reaction with a subsequent transfusion. However, the client may be anxious about the transfusion, requiring nursing intervention. Before beginning a transfusion, explain the procedure and instruct the client to report any side effects (e.g., chills, dizziness, or fever) once the transfusion begins. Ensure that the client has signed an informed consent. Clients with certain cultural backgrounds may require different assessment techniques or may abstain from blood transfusions (Box 41-7).

Because of the danger of transfusion reactions, it is very important to use specific precautions in administering blood or blood products. Obtain the client's baseline vital signs before the transfusion begins. This data will determine when changes in vital signs occur, which can indicate the development of a transfusion reaction. To ensure that the right client receives the correct type of blood or blood product, follow a thorough procedure to check the identity of the blood products, the client, and the compatibility of the blood and the client. Although not involved in the blood labeling process, nurses are responsible for determining that the blood delivered to the client corresponds to the client's blood type listed in the medical record. Together, two registered nurses or one registered nurse and a licensed practical nurse (see agency policy) must check the label on the blood product against the client's identification number, blood group, and complete name. If even a minor discrepancy exists, the blood should not be given and the blood bank should be notified immediately. This detailed system of checking blood and blood products assists in preventing infusion errors (Short, 2006).

Initiation of a transfusion begins slowly to allow for the early detection of a transfusion reaction. Maintain the infusion rate,

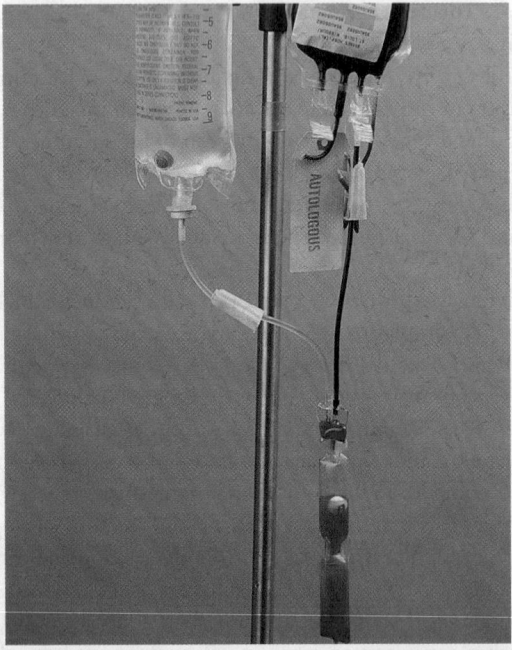

Figure 41-18 Tubing for blood administration has an in-line filter.

✳ BOX 41-7   CULTURAL ASPECTS OF CARE

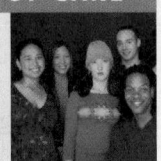

Preinfusion Assessments

When a client's natural skin contains more melanin, it becomes more difficult to determine color changes. Early assessment for IV complications such as phlebitis and infiltration may not be easily detected.

Clients within certain cultural backgrounds have fear related to the donor process for blood.

Clients with certain religious or personal beliefs may abstain from receiving blood transfusions and/or medications.

Implications for Practice
- Establish communication. Understand value of family elders and whom to speak with about IV procedures.
- Assess clients individually to determine their acceptance of or abstinence from therapeutic regimens.
- Appreciate clients' choice related to their therapy.
- Although some clients will abstain from receiving whole blood or packed red blood cells, there are other blood products or alternatives that they will accept.

Modified from Rudnicke C: Transfusion alternatives, *J Infus Nurs* 26(3):29, 2003.

IV, Intravenous.

monitor for side effects, assess vital signs, and promptly record all findings. It is important to stay with the client during the first 15 minutes, the time when a reaction is most likely to occur. After that initial time period, continue to monitor the client and obtain vital signs periodically during the transfusion as directed by agency policy. If a transfusion reaction is anticipated or suspected, obtain vital signs more frequently (Table 41-12).

The rate of transfusion is usually specified in the health care provider's orders. Ideally a unit of whole blood or packed RBCs is transfused in 2 hours. This time can be lengthened to 4 hours if

the client is at risk for FVE. Beyond 4 hours there is a risk for bacterial contamination of the blood (Davis and others, 2006).

When clients have a severe blood loss such as with hemorrhage, they may receive rapid transfusions through a central venous catheter. A blood-warming device is often necessary, because the tip of the central venous cannula lies in the superior vena cava, above the right atrium. Rapid administration of cold blood can result in cardiac dysrhythmia (Burgess, 2006).

Transfusion Reactions. A transfusion reaction is a systemic response by the body to incompatible blood. Causes include red

✳ TABLE 41-12 Acute Transfusion Reactions

REACTION	CAUSE	CLINICAL MANIFESTATIONS	MANAGEMENT	PREVENTION
Acute hemolytic	Infusion of ABO-incompatible whole blood, RBCs, or components containing 10 ml or more of RBCs Antibodies in the recipient's plasma attach to antigens on transfused RBCs, causing RBC destruction	Chills, fever, low back pain, flushing, tachycardia, tachypnea, hypotension, vascular collapse, hemoglobinuria, hemoglobinemia, bleeding, acute renal failure, shock, cardiac arrest, death	Stop transfusion. Treat shock, if present. Obtain blood samples for serological testing slowly to avoid hemolysis during the draw. Send urine specimen to the laboratory. Maintain BP with IV colloid solutions. Give diuretics as prescribed to maintain urine flow. Insert indwelling catheter or measure voided amounts to monitor hourly urine output. Dialysis may be required if renal failure occurs. Do not transfuse additional RBC-containing components until transfusion service has provided newly crossmatched units.	Meticulously verify and document client identification from sample collection to component infusion.
Febrile, nonhemolytic (most common)	Sensitization to donor white blood cells, platelets, or plasma proteins	Sudden chills and fever (rise in temperature of greater than 1° C), headache, flushing, anxiety, muscle pain	Stop transfusion. Give antipyretics as prescribed—avoid aspirin in thrombocytopenic clients. **Safety Alert. Do not restart transfusion.**	Consider leukocyte-poor blood products (filtered, washed, or frozen).
Mild allergic	Sensitivity to foreign plasma proteins	Flushing, itching, urticaria (hives)	Give antihistamine as directed. If symptoms are mild and transient, transfusion may be restarted slowly. **Safety Alert. Do not restart transfusion if fever or pulmonary symptoms develop.**	Treat prophylactically with antihistamines.
Anaphylactic	Infusion of IgA proteins to IgA-deficient recipient who has developed IgA antibody	Anxiety, urticaria, wheezing, progressing to cyanosis, shock, possible cardiac arrest	Stop transfusion. Initiate CPR, if indicated. Have epinephrine ready for injection (0.4 mL of a 1:1000 solution subcutaneously or 0.1 mL of 1:1000 solution diluted to 10 mL with saline for IV use). **Safety Alert. Do not restart transfusion.**	Transfuse extensively washed RBC products, from which all plasma has been removed. Alternately, use blood from IgA-deficient donor.

Data from Brecher M, editor: *AABB technical manual*, ed 15, Bethesda, Md, 2005, AABB; and Goodnough LT: Risks of blood transfusions, *Anesthesiol Clin North Am* 23(2):241, 2005.

ABO, Blood group consisting of groups A, AB, B, and O; *RBCs*, red blood cells; *BP*, blood pressure; *IV*, intravenous; *IgA*, immunoglobulin A; *CPR*, cardiopulmonary resuscitation.

Continued

✳ **TABLE 41-12   Acute Transfusion Reactions—cont'd**

REACTION	CAUSE	CLINICAL MANIFESTATIONS	MANAGEMENT	PREVENTION
Circulatory overload	Fluid administered faster than the circulation can accommodate	Cough, dyspnea, pulmonary congestion (rales), headache, hypertension, tachycardia, distended neck veins	Place client upright with feet in dependent position. Administer prescribed diuretics, oxygen, morphine. Phlebotomy may be indicated.	Adjust transfusion volume and flow rate based on client size and clinical status. Have transfusion service divide unit into smaller aliquots for better spacing of fluid input.
Sepsis	Transfusion of contaminated blood components	Rapid onset of chills, high fever, vomiting, diarrhea, and marked hypotension and shock	Obtain culture of client's blood, and send bag with remaining blood to transfusion service for further study. Treat septicemia as directed—antibiotics, IV fluids, vasopressors, steroids.	Collect, process, store, and transfuse blood products according to blood banking standards and infuse within 4 hours of starting time.

Data from Brecher M, editor: *AABB technical manual,* ed 15, Bethesda, Md, 2005, AABB; and Goodnough LT: Risks of blood transfusions, *Anesthesiol Clin North Am* 23(2):241, 2005.
ABO, Blood group consisting of groups A, AB, B, and O; *RBCs,* red blood cells; *BP,* blood pressure; *IV,* intravenous; *IgA,* immunoglobulin A; *CPR,* cardiopulmonary resuscitation.

cell incompatibility or allergic sensitivity to the components of the transfused blood or to the potassium or citrate preservative in the blood. Blood transfusion can also result in the transmission of infectious disease. Several types of acute reactions can result from blood transfusions (see Table 41-12).

A second category of reactions includes diseases transmitted by infected blood donors who are asymptomatic. Diseases transmitted through transfusions are malaria, hepatitis, and AIDS. Because all units of blood collected must undergo serological testing and screening for HIV and HBV, the risk of acquiring bloodborne infections from blood transfusions is reduced.

Circulatory overload is a risk when a client receives massive whole blood or packed RBC transfusions for massive hemorrhagic shock or when a client with normal blood volume receives blood. Clients particularly at risk for circulatory overload are older adults and those with cardiopulmonary diseases. Blood transfusion reactions are life threatening, but prompt intervention can maintain the client's physiological stability. Follow these guidelines when a reaction develops:

SAFETY ALERT   If a blood reaction is suspected, *stop the transfusion immediately.*

- Keep the IV line open by "piggybacking" 0.9% normal saline directly into the IV line and running the saline.
- Do not turn off the blood and simply turn on the 0.9% normal saline that is connected to the Y-tubing infusion set. This would cause blood remaining in the Y tubing to infuse into the client. Even a small amount of mismatched blood can cause a major reaction.
- Immediately notify the health care provider.
- Remain with the client, observing signs and symptoms and monitoring vital signs as often as every 5 minutes.

- Prepare to administer emergency drugs such as antihistamines, vasopressors, fluids, and steroids per health care provider order or protocol.
- Prepare to perform cardiopulmonary resuscitation.
- Obtain a urine specimen, and send it to the laboratory to determine presence of hemoglobin as a result of RBC hemolysis.
- Save the blood container, tubing, attached labels, and transfusion record and return to the laboratory.

Interventions for Acid-Base Imbalances.   Nursing interventions to promote acid-base balance support prescribed medical therapies and aim at reversing the existing acid-base imbalance. Such imbalances can be life threatening and require rapid correction. It is essential to maintain a functional IV line and frequently check the health care provider's orders for new medications or fluids. Give prescribed drugs, such as insulin or sodium bicarbonate, and fluid and electrolyte replacement promptly. Chapter 40 reviews appropriate therapies for clients with respiratory acidosis. In addition, monitor clients closely for changes in acid-base balance. Clients with acid-base disturbances usually require repeated ABG analysis. This procedure provides arterial blood samples for analysis of hydrogen ion concentration.

Arterial Blood Gases.   Determination of ABG levels requires the removal of a sample of blood from an artery for laboratory testing to assess the client's acid-base status and the adequacy of ventilation and oxygenation. A qualified RN or other health care provider draws arterial blood from a peripheral artery (usually the radial) or from an existing arterial line (see agency policy). Before the arterial blood draw, ensure that the client has an ulnar pulse, to prevent loss of blood flow to the hand if the radial artery is damaged. After obtaining the specimen, take care to prevent air from entering the syringe because this will affect the blood gas analysis. To reduce oxygen metabolism of cells, submerge the syringe in crushed ice and transport it immediately to the laboratory. After the ABG puncture, apply pressure to the puncture site for at least 5 minutes to reduce the risk of hematoma formation. Reassess the radial pulse after removing the pressure.

Restorative Care. After experiencing acute alterations in fluid, electrolyte, or acid-base balance, clients often require ongoing maintenance to prevent a recurrence of health alterations. Older adults and the chronically ill require special considerations to prevent complications from developing (see Box 41-6, p. 1006).

Home Intravenous Therapy. Intravenous therapy often continues in the home setting for clients requiring long-term hydration, parenteral nutrition, or long-term medication administration. A home IV therapy nurse will work closely with the client to ensure that a sterile IV system is maintained and that complications can be avoided or recognized promptly. Box 41-8 summarizes client education guidelines for home IV therapy.

Nutritional Support. Most clients who have had electrolyte disorders or metabolic acid-base disturbances require ongoing nutritional support. Depending on the type of disorder, fluid or food intake may be encouraged or restricted (see Chapter 44). If clients are still responsible for meal preparation, they should learn to understand nutritional content of foods and to read the labels of commercially prepared foods.

Medication Safety. Numerous medications and over-the-counter (OTC) drugs contain components or create potential side effects that can alter fluid and electrolyte balance. Clients with chronic disease who are receiving multiple medications and those with renal or liver disorders are at significant risk for alterations in fluid and electrolyte status. Once clients return to a restorative care setting, whether in the home, long-term care, or a nursing home, drug safety becomes very important. Client and family education is essential to providing information regarding potential drug interactions and what side effects they cause. Review all medications with clients, and encourage them to consult with their local pharmacist, especially if they try a new over-the-counter medication.

◆ Evaluation

Evaluate the effectiveness of interventions using the goals established during the planning process of maintaining and restoring fluid, electrolyte, and acid-base balance. The evaluation of a client's clinical status is especially important if an acute fluid and electrolyte or acid-base disturbance exists. Data about the client's condition can change very quickly, and it is important to recognize the signs and symptoms of impending problems by integrating the client's presenting risk factors, clinical status, the effects of the present treatment regimen, and the potential causative agent. Knowledge about the health alterations, the effects of medications and fluids, and the client's presenting clinical status aid in evaluation (Figure 41-19).

Perform evaluative measures to determine if changes have occurred from the last client assessment. For example, if the assessment of a client's hypokalemia is showing signs of improvement, the physical signs and symptoms of hypokalemia should begin to

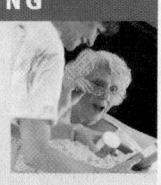

BOX 41-8   **CLIENT TEACHING**

Home Intravenous Therapy
Objective
- The client and/or primary caregiver will demonstrate understanding and competence with IV therapy for safe delivery in the home setting.

Teaching Strategies
- Explain the importance of IV therapy in maintaining hydration and access for the delivery of medications.
- Emphasize the risks involved when the IV system is not kept sterile.
- Be sure the client and/or primary caregiver is able to manipulate the required equipment.
- Instruct in aseptic technique and hand hygiene in the handling of all IV equipment.
- Instruct in how to change IV solutions, tubing, and dressing when they become soiled or dislodged. (NOTE: The home care nurse may be able to visit frequently enough to perform scheduled tubing and dressing changes.)
- Instruct in procedures for safe disposal, in appropriate containers, of all sharps and IV materials exposed to blood.
- Instruct about signs and symptoms of infiltration, phlebitis, and infection and reporting symptoms immediately.
- Instruct client and/or primary caregiver to report if the infusion slows or stops or if blood is seen in the tubing.
- Teach client with caregiver's assistance how to ambulate, perform hygiene, and participate in other activities of daily living without dislodging or disconnecting cannula and tubing.

Evaluation
- Ask client and caregiver why it is necessary to maintain hydration and IV access for the delivery of medications.
- Ask what to do if IV stops.
- Ask client and caregiver to describe signs and symptoms of complications and the action they should take.
- Observe the client or caregiver changing the IV container, tubing, and dressing.
- Observe the client ambulating and participating in activities of daily living to see how he or she protects and manipulates the IV cannula and apparatus.

IV, Intravenous.

disappear or lessen in intensity. The client's heart rhythm becomes more regular, and normal bowel function returns.

For clients with less acute alterations, evaluation likely occurs over a longer period of time. In this situation the evaluation may be more focused on behavioral changes (e.g., the client's ability to follow dietary restrictions and medication schedules). The family's ability to anticipate alterations and prevent problems from recurring is also an important element of evaluation.

The client's level of progress determines whether the plan of care needs to continue or needs revision. If goals are not met, consultation with a health care provider to discuss additional methods such as increasing the frequency of an intervention (e.g., provide more fluids to a dehydrated client), introducing a new therapy (e.g., initiate insertion of an IV), or discontinuing a particular therapy may be necessary to improve client outcomes.

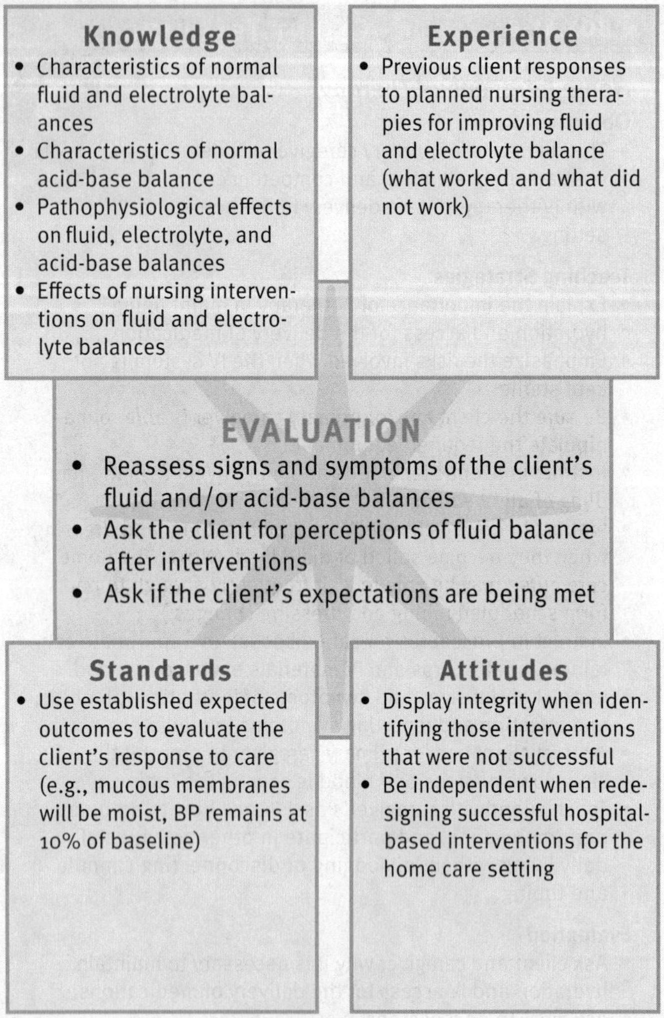

Knowledge

- Characteristics of normal fluid and electrolyte balances
- Characteristics of normal acid-base balance
- Pathophysiological effects on fluid, electrolyte, and acid-base balances
- Effects of nursing interventions on fluid and electrolyte balances

Experience

- Previous client responses to planned nursing therapies for improving fluid and electrolyte balance (what worked and what did not work)

EVALUATION

- Reassess signs and symptoms of the client's fluid and/or acid-base balances
- Ask the client for perceptions of fluid balance after interventions
- Ask if the client's expectations are being met

Standards

- Use established expected outcomes to evaluate the client's response to care (e.g., mucous membranes will be moist, BP remains at 10% of baseline)

Attitudes

- Display integrity when identifying those interventions that were not successful
- Be independent when redesigning successful hospital-based interventions for the home care setting

Figure 41-19 Critical thinking model for fluid, electrolyte, and acid-base balances evaluation.

Once outcomes have been met, the nursing diagnosis is resolved and focus can be centered on other priorities.

Review with the client success in meeting the client's expectations of care. "Tell me if I have helped you feel more comfortable" is a question that might be raised if the client's expectations revolve around comfort and symptom management. If the client's concerns involve having a better understanding of a chronic problem, focus the evaluation on the client's satisfaction with educational offerings. Often the client's level of satisfaction with care also depends on success in involving family and friends. If the client has concerns about returning home or to a different care setting, it is important to evaluate if the client feels prepared for the transition from acute care. If established outcomes are not achieved, it is important to explore the reasons that contributed to why the planned outcomes were not reached. Modification of the care plan occurs after this evaluation. Questions that might be asked if outcomes are not achieved may include the following:

- "Do you understand what food and fluids you are permitted to consume?"
- "Are you measuring your intake and output daily and keeping a record?"

- "Are you losing fluid other than through urination, such as frequent loose stools?"
- "Are you taking any unprescribed over-the-counter drugs or herbal preparations?"

✳ Key Concepts

- Body fluids consisting of electrolytes, cells, and water are distributed in ECF and ICF compartments.
- Fluid intake, output, and hormonal regulation regulate body fluids.
- Volume disturbances include isotonic and osmolar deficits and excesses.
- Dietary intake and hormonal controls regulate electrolyte levels.
- Acid-base imbalances are buffered by chemical, biological, and physiological buffering, especially the lungs and kidneys.
- Chronic and serious illnesses increase the risk of fluid, electrolyte, and acid-base imbalances.
- Clients who are very young or very old are at greater risk for fluid, electrolyte, and acid-base imbalances.
- Treatment for electrolyte disturbances include dietary and pharmacological interventions.
- Acid-base balance depends on the hydrogen ion concentration in the blood.
- The body's chemical buffering system responds first to acid-base abnormalities.
- Osmolar imbalances and FVD can be corrected by enteral or parenteral administration of fluid.
- Common complications of IV therapy include infiltration, phlebitis, infection, FVE, and bleeding at the infusion site.
- Blood transfusions are given to replace fluid volume loss from hemorrhage, to treat anemia, or to replace coagulation factors.
- Blood transfusions can be donor, autologous, or obtained through perioperative salvage.
- Administration of blood or blood products requires a specific procedure for correct identification of client and blood product and responding to transfusion reactions quickly.
- In addition to transfusion reactions, the risks of transfusion also include hyperkalemia, hypocalcemia, FVE, and infection.
- Respiratory acidosis is characterized by increased carbon dioxide and hydrogen ion concentrations.
- Respiratory alkalosis is characterized by decreased carbon dioxide and hydrogen ion concentrations.
- Metabolic acidosis is characterized by a decrease in bicarbonate level and increase in hydrogen ion concentration.
- Metabolic alkalosis is characterized by an increase in bicarbonate level and decrease in hydrogen ion concentration.
- The goals of therapy for acid-base imbalances are to treat the underlying illness and to restore the arterial pH to normal.

✳ Critical Thinking Exercises

Mrs. Hilda Bottomley is a 72-year-old seen by her health care provider this morning with complaints of flulike symptoms and difficulty breathing. Her vital signs are normal except for an elevated temperature of 37.8° C (101° F). She has decreased skin turgor but moist mucous membranes. Respirations are 28 breaths per minute with rhonchi heard bilaterally. Arterial blood gas analysis: pH, 7.33; PaO_2, 95 mm Hg; $PaCO_2$, 48 mm Hg; HCO_3^-, 23 mEq/L.

1. Which laboratory findings would you expect based on her complaints? What interventions would you expect the health care provider to order?

2. What does Mrs. Bottomley's arterial blood gas (ABG) analysis indicate? Why would the health care provider order a chest x-ray examination? If left untreated, could this problem become life threatening?

3. Mrs. Bottomley's intravenous (IV) fluid order is 1000 mL 0.9% normal saline with 20 mEq KCl to run over 8 hours. What IV tubing should be used to administer these fluids in terms of drop size? Calculate the drops per minute using macrotubing. What assessments are necessary before these IV fluids are initiated?

NCLEX®-Style Review Questions

1. A client is admitted to the hospital with a history of vomiting for 2 days and diminished oral intake. Arterial blood gas levels on admission are pH, 7.30; $PaCO_2$, 36 mm Hg; PaO_2, 92 mm Hg; and HCO_3^-, 18. You understand that the client's acid-base imbalance is:
   1. Metabolic acidosis
   2. Metabolic alkalosis
   3. Respiratory acidosis
   4. Respiratory alkalosis

2. A client with a cardiac history is taking a potassium-wasting diuretic (furosemide) and is seen in the emergency department for complaints of weakness. You expect to evaluate which laboratory values?
   1. Albumin and protein
   2. Sodium and chloride
   3. Hemoglobin and hematocrit
   4. Potassium and blood glucose

3. The following four clients are all at risk for fluid volume excess. Which of the clients do you see **first**?
   1. An 88-year-old with a fractured femur scheduled for surgery
   2. A 65-year-old recently diagnosed with congestive heart failure
   3. A 50-year-old with second-degree burns on the ankles and feet
   4. A 20-year-old with a 5-year history of type 1 diabetes mellitus

4. A client has the following blood gas levels: pH, 7.52; $PaCO_2$, 28 mm Hg; PaO_2, 92 mm Hg; HCO_3^-, 17 mEq/L. You would expect the health care provider to order:
   1. Oxygen at 3 L/min via nasal cannula
   2. Sodium bicarbonate 1 amp every 12 hours
   3. Potassium chloride 20 mEq in ½ normal saline
   4. Deep breathing exercises to ease respiratory effort

5. You assess four clients. Which client is at greatest risk for the development of hypocalcemia?
   1. 56-year-old with acute renal failure
   2. 40-year-old with systemic lupus erythematosus
   3. 28-year-old who has just undergone a total thyroidectomy
   4. 65-year-old with hypertension taking beta-adrenergic blockers

6. Which of the following activity(ies) can be successfully delegated to nursing assistive personnel? (Choose all that apply.)
   1. Measuring intake and output
   2. Preparing IV tubing for systematic change
   3. Reporting an IV container that is low in fluid
   4. Discontinuing an IV per health care provider's orders

7. Many factors are initially controlled for in the IV insertion procedure. Place the following steps for IV insertion in the correct order:
   1. Perform hand hygiene.
   2. Open and prepare infusion set.
   3. Assess client experience with IV therapy.
   4. Select appropriate vein, and insert cannula.
   5. Ensure the six rights of medication administration.
   6. Assess for risk factors, such as age or platelet count.
   7. Carefully check the health care provider's order for the IV therapy.

8. Assessment of IV fluid infiltration includes (choose all that apply):
   1. Edema and pain
   2. Streak formation
   3. Pain and erythema
   4. Pallor and coolness
   5. Numbness and pain

9. Clinical assessment of dehydration would be confirmed if you identified (select all the apply):
   1. A 1-pound weight loss
   2. Engorged neck vessels
   3. Dry mucous membranes
   4. Full bounding radial pulse

42 | Sleep

OBJECTIVES

Mastery of content in this chapter will enable the student to:

- Explain the effect the 24-hour sleep-wake cycle has on biological function.
- Discuss mechanisms that regulate sleep.
- Describe the stages of a normal sleep cycle.
- Explain the functions of sleep.
- Compare and contrast the sleep requirements of different age-groups.
- Identify factors that normally promote and disrupt sleep.

- Discuss characteristics of common sleep disorders.
- Conduct a sleep history for a client.
- Identify nursing diagnoses appropriate for clients with sleep alterations.
- Identify nursing interventions designed to promote normal sleep cycles for clients of all ages.
- Describe ways to evaluate sleep therapies.

MEDIA RESOURCES KEY TERMS

 Companion CD
- NCLEX®-Style Review Questions
- Audio Glossary
- Interactive Learning Activities
- English/Spanish Glossary

evolve **Website**
- NCLEX®-Style Review Questions
- Audio Glossary
- English/Spanish Glossary
- Interactive Learning Activities
- Weblinks
- Audio Summaries

Biological clocks, p. 1029
Cataplexy, p. 1034
Circadian rhythm, p. 1029
Excessive daytime sleepiness (EDS), p. 1033
Hypersomnolence, p. 1032
Hypnotics, p. 1048
Insomnia, p. 1033
Narcolepsy, p. 1034
Nocturia, p. 1032
Nonrapid eye movement (NREM) sleep, p. 1029

Polysomnogram, p. 1033
Rapid eye movement (REM) sleep, p. 1029
Rest, p. 1034
Sedatives, p. 1048
Sleep, p. 1029
Sleep apnea, p. 1033
Sleep deprivation, p. 1034
Sleep hygiene, p. 1033

Proper rest and sleep are as important to good health as good nutrition and adequate exercise. Individuals need different amounts of sleep and rest. Physical and emotional health depends on the ability to fulfill these basic human needs. Without proper amounts of rest and sleep, the ability to concentrate, make judgments, and participate in daily activities decreases and irritability increases.

Identifying and treating clients' sleep pattern disturbances is an important goal. To help clients, you need to understand the nature of sleep, the factors influencing it, and clients' sleep habits. Clients require an individualized approach based on their personal habits and pattern of sleep, as well as the particular problem influencing sleep. Nursing interventions are often effective in resolving short- and long-term sleep disturbances.

Sleep provides healing and restoration (McCance and Huether, 2006). Achieving the best possible sleep quality is important for the promotion of good health as well as the recovery from illness. Ill clients often require more sleep and rest than healthy clients. However, the nature of illness often prevents some clients from getting adequate rest and sleep. The environment of a hospital or long-term care facility and the activities of health care personnel make sleep difficult. Some clients have preexisting sleep disturbances and other clients develop sleep problems as a result of illness or hospitalization.

Scientific Knowledge Base

Physiology of Sleep

Sleep is a cyclical physiological process that alternates with longer periods of wakefulness. The sleep-wake cycle influences and regulates physiological function and behavioral responses.

Circadian Rhythms.
People experience cyclical rhythms as part of their everyday life. The most familiar rhythm is the 24-hour, day-night cycle known as the diurnal or **circadian rhythm** (derived from Latin: *circa,* "about," and *dies,* "day"). Circadian rhythms influence the pattern of major biological and behavioral functions. The predictable changing of body temperature, heart rate, blood pressure, hormone secretion, sensory acuity, and mood depend on the maintenance of the 24-hour circadian cycle (Izac, 2006).

Factors such as light, temperature, social activities, and work routines affect circadian rhythms and daily sleep-wake cycles. All persons have **biological clocks** that synchronize their sleep cycles. This explains why some people fall asleep at 8 PM, whereas others go to bed at midnight or early in the morning. Different people also function best at different times of the day.

Hospitals or extended care facilities usually do not adapt care to an individual's sleep-wake cycle preferences. Typical hospital routines interrupt sleep or prevent clients from falling asleep at their usual time. A person has a poor quality of sleep if his or her sleep-wake cycle changes significantly. Reversals in the sleep-wake cycle such as falling asleep during the day (or vice versa for people who work nights) often indicates a serious illness.

The biological rhythm of sleep frequently becomes synchronized with other body functions. Changes in body temperature, for example, correlate with sleep patterns. Normally, body temperature peaks in the afternoon, decreases gradually, and then drops sharply after a person falls asleep. When the sleep-wake cycle becomes disrupted (e.g., by working rotating shifts), other physiological functions usually change as well. For example, the person experiences a decreased appetite and loses weight. Anxiety, restlessness, irritability, and impaired judgment are other common symptoms of sleep cycle disturbances. Failure to maintain the individual's usual sleep-wake cycle negatively influences the client's overall health.

Sleep Regulation.
Sleep involves a sequence of physiological states maintained by highly integrated central nervous system (CNS) activity. This is associated with changes in the peripheral nervous, endocrine, cardiovascular, respiratory, and muscular systems (McCance and Huether, 2006). Specific physiological responses and patterns of brain activity identify each sequence. Instruments such as the electroencephalogram (EEG), which measures electrical activity in the cerebral cortex, the electromyogram (EMG), which measures muscle tone, and the electrooculogram (EOG), which measures eye movements, provide information about some structural physiological aspects of sleep.

Current theory suggests that sleep is an active multiphase process. The major sleep center in the body is the hypothalamus. The hypothalamus secretes hypocreatins (orexins) that promote wakefulness and rapid eye movement sleep. Prostaglandin D_2, L-tryptophan, and growth factors control sleep (McCance and Huether, 2006).

Researchers believe the ascending reticular activating system (RAS) located in the upper brain stem to contain special cells that maintain alertness and wakefulness. The RAS receives visual, auditory, pain, and tactile sensory stimuli. Activity from the cerebral cortex (e.g., emotions or thought processes) also stimulates the RAS. Arousal, wakefulness, and maintenance of consciousness results from neurons in the RAS that release catecholamines such as norepinephrine (Izac, 2006).

Researchers hypothesize that the release of serotonin from specialized cells in the raphe nuclei sleep system of the pons and medulla produces sleep. This area of the brain is also called the bulbar synchronizing region (BSR). Whether a person remains awake or falls asleep depends on a balance of impulses received from higher centers (e.g., thoughts), peripheral sensory receptors (e.g., sound or light stimuli), and the limbic system (emotions) (Figure 42-1). As people try to fall asleep, they close their eyes and assume relaxed positions. Stimuli to the RAS decline. If the room is dark and quiet, activation of the RAS further declines. At some point the BSR takes over, causing sleep.

Stages of Sleep.
Different brain-wave, muscle, and eye activity are associated with different stages of sleep (Izac, 2006). Normal sleep involves two phases: **nonrapid eye movement (NREM) sleep** and **rapid eye movement (REM) sleep** (Box 42-1). During NREM a sleeper progresses through four stages during a typical 90-minute sleep cycle. The quality of sleep from stage 1 through stage 4 becomes increasingly deep. Lighter sleep is characteristic of stages 1 and 2, and a person is more easily arousable. Stages 3 and 4 involve a deeper sleep, called slow-wave sleep. Rapid eye movement sleep is the phase at the end of each sleep cycle. Different factors promote or interfere with various stages of the sleep

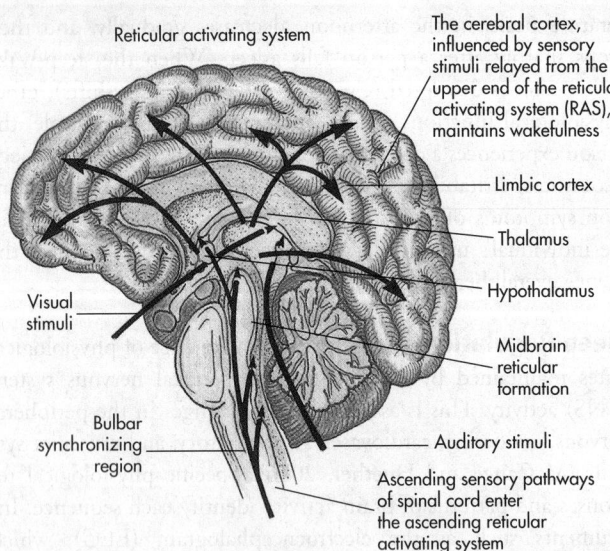

Reticular activating system

The cerebral cortex, influenced by sensory stimuli relayed from the upper end of the reticular activating system (RAS), maintains wakefulness

Limbic cortex

Thalamus

Hypothalamus

Visual stimuli

Midbrain reticular formation

Bulbar synchronizing region

Auditory stimuli

Ascending sensory pathways of spinal cord enter the ascending reticular activating system

Figure 42-1 RAS and BSR control sensory input, intermittently activating and suppressing the brain's higher centers to control sleep and wakefulness.

cycle. Choose therapies that foster sleep and eliminate factors that disrupt it.

Sleep Cycle. The normal sleep pattern for an adult begins with a presleep period during which the person is aware only of a gradually developing sleepiness. This period normally lasts 10 to 30 minutes, but if a person has difficulty falling asleep, it will last an hour or more.

Once asleep, the person usually passes through four to five complete sleep cycles per night, each consisting of four stages of NREM sleep and a period of REM sleep (McCance and Huether, 2006). Each cycle lasts approximately 90 to 100 minutes. The cyclical pattern usually progresses from stage 1 through stage 4 of NREM, followed by a reversal from stage 4 to 3 to 2, ending with a period of REM sleep (Figure 42-2). A person usually reaches REM sleep about 90 minutes into the sleep cycle. Seventy-five to eighty percent of sleep time is spent in NREM sleep.

With each successive cycle, stages 3 and 4 shorten, and the period of REM lengthens. REM sleep lasts up to 60 minutes during the last sleep cycle. Not all people progress consistently through the stages of sleep. For example, a sleeper moves back and forth for short intervals between NREM stages 2, 3, and 4 before entering REM stage. The amount of time spent in each stage varies over the life span. Newborns and children spend more time in deep sleep. With aging, sleep becomes more fragmented and a person spends more time in lighter stages (National Sleep Foundation, 2003). Shifts from stage to stage of sleep tend to accompany body movements. Shifts to light sleep or wakefulness tend to occur suddenly, whereas shifts to deep sleep tend to be gradual (Izac, 2006). The number of sleep cycles depends on the total amount of time that the person spends sleeping.

Functions of Sleep

The purpose of sleep remains unclear. Sleep contributes to physiological and psychological restoration. NREM sleep contributes to body tissue restoration (McCance and Huether,

BOX 42-1   Stages of the Sleep Cycle

Stage 1: NREM
Includes lightest level of sleep.
Stage lasts a few minutes.
Decreased physiological activity begins with gradual fall in vital signs and metabolism.
Sensory stimuli such as noise easily arouses person.
Awakened, person feels as though daydreaming has occurred.

Stage 2: NREM
Period of sound sleep.
Relaxation progresses.
Arousal remains relatively easy.
Stage lasts 10 to 20 minutes.
Body functions continue to slow.

Stage 3: NREM
Involves initial stages of deep sleep.
Sleeper is difficult to arouse and rarely moves.
Muscles are completely relaxed.
Vital signs decline but remain regular.
Stage lasts 15 to 30 minutes.

Stage 4: NREM
Deepest stage of sleep.
Very difficult to arouse sleeper.
If sleep loss has occurred, sleeper will spend considerable portion of night in this stage.
Vital signs are significantly lower than during waking hours.
Stage lasts approximately 15 to 30 minutes.
Sleepwalking and enuresis (bed-wetting) sometimes occur.

REM Sleep
Vivid, full-color dreaming occurs.
Less vivid dreaming occurs in other stages.
Stage usually begins about 90 minutes after sleep has begun.
Typified by autonomic response of rapidly moving eyes, fluctuating heart and respiratory rates, and increased or fluctuating blood pressure.
Loss of skeletal muscle tone occurs.
Gastric secretions increase.
Very difficult to arouse sleeper.
Duration of REM sleep increases with each cycle and averages 20 minutes.

NREM, Nonrapid eye movement; *REM,* rapid eye movement.

2006). During NREM sleep, biological functions slow. A healthy adult's normal heart rate throughout the day averages 70 to 80 beats per minute or less if the individual is in excellent physical condition. However, during sleep the heart rate falls to 60 beats per minute or less. This means that the heart beats 10 to 20 fewer times in each minute during sleep or 60 to 120 fewer times in each hour. Clearly, restful sleep is beneficial in preserving cardiac function. Other biological functions decreased during sleep are respirations, blood pressure, and muscle tone (McCance and Huether, 2006).

The body needs sleep to routinely restore biological processes. During deep slow-wave (NREM stage 4) sleep, the body releases human growth hormone for the repair and renewal of epithelial and specialized cells such as brain cells (Jones, 2005). Protein synthesis and cell division for renewal of tissues such as the skin, bone marrow, gastric mucosa, or brain occur during rest and

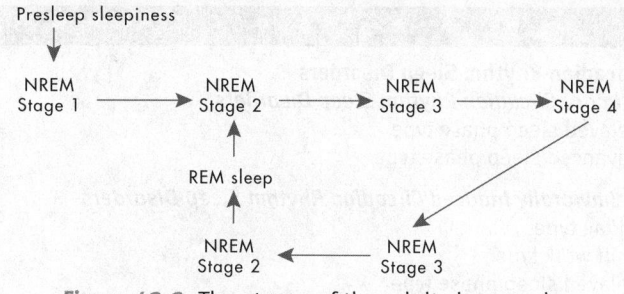

Figure 42-2 The stages of the adult sleep cycle.

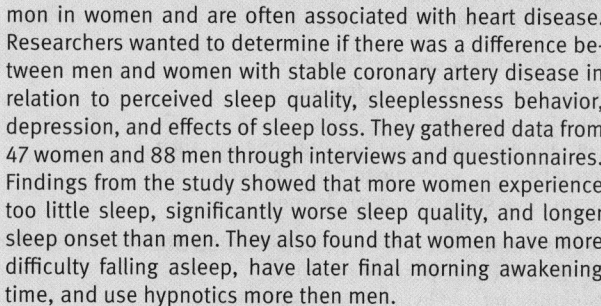

BOX 42-2   **EVIDENCE-BASED PRACTICE**

Sleep Disorders in Clients With Coronary Artery Disease
Evidence Summary
Prior research shows a relationship between heart disease, sleep, and the occurrence of sleep disorders. Sleep problems are more common in women and are often associated with heart disease. Researchers wanted to determine if there was a difference between men and women with stable coronary artery disease in relation to perceived sleep quality, sleeplessness behavior, depression, and effects of sleep loss. They gathered data from 47 women and 88 men through interviews and questionnaires. Findings from the study showed that more women experience too little sleep, significantly worse sleep quality, and longer sleep onset than men. They also found that women have more difficulty falling asleep, have later final morning awakening time, and use hypnotics more then men.

Application to Nursing Practice
- Be aware that there are differences in sleep problems between women and men with coronary artery disease.
- During assessment of health problems, be sure to ask questions related to sleep quality and sleep patterns.
- If the client indicates a problem with sleep, do a thorough sleep history.
- Reinforce teaching on good sleep hygiene habits.
- Encourage clients to notify their health care provider if they begin to experience sleep problems.

Edell-Gustafson U and others: A gender perspective on sleeplessness behavior, effects of sleep loss, and coping resources in patients with stable coronary artery disease, *Heart Lung* 35(2):75, 2006.

sleep. NREM sleep is especially important in children, who experience more stage 4 sleep.

Another theory about the purpose of sleep is that the body conserves energy during sleep. The skeletal muscles relax progressively, and the absence of muscular contraction preserves chemical energy for cellular processes. Lowering of the basal metabolic rate further conserves the body's energy supply (Izac, 2006).

REM sleep is necessary for brain tissue restoration and appears to be important for cognitive restoration (Buysse, 2005). REM sleep is associated with changes in cerebral blood flow, increased cortical activity, increased oxygen consumption, and epinephrine release. This association assists with memory storage and learning (McCance and Huether, 2006). During sleep, the brain filters stored information about the day's activities.

The benefits of sleep on behavior often go unnoticed until a person develops a problem resulting from sleep deprivation. A loss of REM sleep leads to feelings of confusion and suspicion. Various body functions (e.g., mood, motor performance, memory, and equilibrium) are altered when prolonged sleep loss occurs (National Sleep Foundation, 2002a). Changes in the natural and cellular immune function also occur with moderate to severe sleep deprivation (Buysse, 2005). Research estimates that traffic, home, and work-related accidents caused by falling asleep cost billions of dollars a year in the United States due to lost productivity, health care costs, and accidents (Irwin and others, 2006).

Dreams. Although dreams occur during both NREM and REM sleep, the dreams of REM sleep are more vivid and elaborate and some believe they are functionally important to learning, memory processing, and adaptation to stress (Stickgold, 2005). REM dreams progress in content throughout the night from dreams about current events to emotional dreams of childhood or the past. Personality influences the quality of dreams; for example, a creative person has elaborate and complex dreams, while a depressed person dreams of helplessness.

Most people dream about immediate concerns such as an argument with a spouse or worries over work. Sometimes a person is unaware of fears represented in bizarre dreams. Clinical psychologists try to analyze the symbolic nature of dreams as part of a client's psychotherapy. The ability to describe a dream and interpret its significance sometimes helps resolve personal concerns or fears.

Another theory suggests that dreams erase certain fantasies or nonsensical memories. Because most people forget their dreams, few have dream recall or do not believe they dream at all. To remember a dream, a person has to consciously think about it on awakening. People who recall dreams vividly usually awake just after a period of REM sleep.

Physical Illness

Any illness that causes pain, physical discomfort, or mood problems, such as anxiety or depression, often results in sleep problems. Persons with such alterations frequently have trouble falling or staying asleep. Illnesses also force clients to sleep in unfamiliar positions. For example, it is difficult for a client with an arm or leg in traction to get in a comfortable position.

Respiratory disease often interferes with sleep. Clients with chronic lung disease such as emphysema are short of breath and frequently cannot sleep without two or three pillows to raise their heads. Asthma, bronchitis, and allergic rhinitis alter the rhythm of breathing and disturb sleep. A person with a common cold has nasal congestion, sinus drainage, and a sore throat, which impair breathing and the ability to relax.

Connections between heart disease, sleep, and sleep disorders exist (Box 42-2). Sleep-related breathing disorders are linked to increased incidence of nocturnal angina (chest pain), increased heart rate, electrocardiogram changes, high blood pressure, and risk of heart diseases and stroke (McCance and Huether, 2006). Hypertension often causes early morning awakening and fatigue. Hypothyroidism decreases stage 4 sleep, whereas hyperthyroidism causes persons to take more time to fall asleep. Last, research

---

⁕ BOX 42-3 **Classification of Select Sleep Disorders**

Insomnias
Adjustment sleep disorder (acute insomnia)
Inadequate sleep hygiene
Paradoxical insomnia
Insomnia due to mental disorder
Behavioral insomnia of childhood
Idiopathic insomnia
Insomnia due to medical condition

Sleep-Related Breathing Disorder
Central Sleep Apnea Syndromes
Primary central sleep apnea
Central sleep apnea due to a drug or substance
Central sleep apnea due to a medical condition
Obstructive sleep apnea syndromes

Hypersomnias Not Due to a Sleep-Related Breathing Disorder
Narcolepsy (four specified types)
Menstrual-related hypersomnia
Idiopathic hypersomnia with long sleep time
Behaviorally induced insufficient sleep syndrome
Hypersomnia due to a medical condition

Parasomnias
Disorders of Arousal
Sleepwalking
Sleep terrors

Parasomnias Usually Associated With REM Sleep
Nightmare disorder
REM sleep behavior disorder
Sleep paralysis

Other Parasomnias
Sleep-related groaning
Sleep-related hallucinations
Sleep-related eating disorder
Sleep-related enuresis (bed-wetting)

Circadian Rhythm Sleep Disorders
Primary Circadian Rhythm Sleep Disorders
Delayed sleep phase type
Advanced sleep phase type

Behaviorally Induced Circadian Rhythm Sleep Disorders
Jet lag type
Shift work type
Delayed sleep phase type
Drug or substance use

Sleep-Related Movement Disorders
Restless leg syndrome
Periodic limb movements
Sleep-related leg cramps
Sleep-related bruxism (teeth grinding)

Isolated Symptoms, Apparently Normal Variants, and Unresolved Issues
Long sleeper
Short sleeper
Snoring
Sleep talking
Benign sleep myoclonus of infancy

Other Sleep Disorders
Physiological (organic) sleep disorders
Environmental sleep disorder
Sleep disorder not due to a substance or physiological condition

---

Data from American Academy of Sleep Medicine: International classes of diseases and international classification of sleep disorders. In Thorpy M: Classification of sleep disorders. In Kryger M and others, editors: *Principles and practice of sleep medicine*, ed 5, Philadelphia, 2005, Saunders.

REM, Rapid eye movement.

---

identifies an increased risk of sudden cardiac death in the first hours after wakening.

Nocturia, or urination during the night, disrupts sleep and the sleep cycle. This condition is most common in older people with reduced bladder tone or persons with cardiac disease, diabetes, urethritis, or prostatic disease. After a person awakens repeatedly to urinate, returning to sleep is difficult.

Older adults often experience restless legs syndrome (RLS), which occurs before sleep onset. People experience recurrent, rhythmical movements of the feet and legs. Clients feel an itching sensation deep in the muscles. Relief comes only from moving the legs, which prevents relaxation and subsequent sleep. RLS is sometimes a relatively benign condition depending on how severely sleep is disrupted. Primary restless legs syndrome is a central nervous system disorder. Researchers associate secondary RLS with lower levels of iron, pregnancy, and uremia (National Heart, Lung, and Blood Institute, 2000).

Persons with peptic ulcer disease often awaken in the middle of the night. Research showing a relationship between gastric acid secretion and stages of sleep are conflicting. One consistent find-

ing is that persons with duodenal ulcers fail to suppress acid secretion in the first 2 hours of sleep (Orr, 2005).

Sleep Disorders

Sleep disorders are conditions that, if untreated, generally cause disturbed nighttime sleep that results in one of three problems: insomnia, abnormal movements or sensation during sleep or when awakening at night, or excessive daytime sleepiness (Malow, 2005). Many adults in the United States have significant sleep problems from inadequacies in either the quantity or quality of their nighttime sleep and experience **hypersomnolence** on a daily basis (National Sleep Foundation, 2002a). The American Academy of Sleep Medicine developed the International Classification of Sleep Disorders version 2 (ICSD-2), which classifies sleep disorders into eight major categories (Box 42-3).

The insomnias are primary disorders related to difficulty falling asleep. Individuals with sleep-related breathing disorders have disordered respirations during sleep. Hypersomnia not due to sleep-related breathing disorders is a group of disorders that is not caused by disturbed circadian rhythms or nocturnal sleep. The circadian rhythm sleep disorders are caused by a misalignment between the timing of sleep and what the individual desires or what the societal norm is. The parasomnias are undesirable behaviors that occur usually during sleep. Sleep and wake disturbances are associated with many medical and psychiatric sleep disorders, including psychiatric, neurological, or other medical disorders. In sleep-related movement disorders, the person experiences simple stereotyped movements that disturb sleep. The category of isolated symptoms, apparently normal variants, and unresolved issues includes sleep-related symptoms that fall between normal and abnormal sleep. The other sleep disorders category contains sleep problems that do not fit into other categories.

Sleep laboratory studies diagnose a sleep disorder (Buysse, 2005). A **polysomnogram** involves the use of EEG, EMG, and EOG to monitor stages of sleep and wakefulness during nighttime sleep. The Multiple Sleep Latency Test (MSLT) provides objective information about sleepiness and selected aspects of sleep structure by measuring eye movements, muscle-tone changes, and brain electrical activity during at least four napping opportunities spread throughout the day. The MSLT takes 8 to 10 hours to complete. Clients wear an Actigraph device on the wrist to measure sleep-wake patterns over an extended period of time. Actigraphy data provides information on sleep time, sleep efficiency, number and duration of awakenings, and levels of activity and rest (Buysse, 2005).

Insomnia. Insomnia is a symptom clients experience when they have chronic difficulty falling asleep, frequent awakenings from sleep, and/or a short sleep or nonrestorative sleep (Edinger and Means, 2005). It is the most common sleep-related complaint. The insomniac complains of excessive daytime sleepiness, as well as insufficient quantity and quality of sleep. Frequently, however, the client gets more sleep than he or she realizes. Insomnia often signals an underlying physical or psychological disorder. Insomnia occurs more frequently in women and is the most common sleep problem for women.

People experience transient insomnia as a result of situational stresses such as family, work, or school problems; jet lag; illness; or loss of a loved one. Insomnia sometimes recurs, but between episodes the client is able to sleep well. However, a temporary case of insomnia due to a stressful situation will possibly lead to chronic difficulty in obtaining sufficient sleep, perhaps due to the worry and anxiety that develops about obtaining adequate sleep.

Insomnia is often associated with poor **sleep hygiene,** or practices the client associates with sleep. If the condition continues, the fear of not being able to sleep is enough to cause wakefulness. During the day, persons with chronic insomnia feel sleepy, fatigued, depressed, and anxious. Treatment is symptomatic, including improved sleep hygiene measures, biofeedback, cognitive techniques, and relaxation techniques. Behavioral and cognitive therapies have few adverse effects and show evidence of sustained improvement in sleep over a 6-month period (Morin and others, 2007).

Sleep Apnea. Sleep apnea is a disorder characterized by the lack of airflow through the nose and mouth for periods of 10 seconds or longer during sleep. There are three types of sleep apnea: central, obstructive, and mixed apnea. The most common form is obstructive sleep apnea (OSA). Research estimates that 12 to 18 million people in the United States meet the diagnostic criteria for OSA (Holman, 2005). OSA affects 10% to 15% of middle-age adults (Groth, 2005). Obesity, smoking, alcohol, and a positive family history of OSA greatly increase the risk of developing the problem (Redline, 2005). Many think OSA affects middle-age men more frequently, particularly when they are obese (Groth, 2005). However, obstructive sleep apnea is also common in postmenopausal women, as well as younger women and children (Mendez and Olson, 2006a).

OSA occurs when muscles or structures of the oral cavity or throat relax during sleep. The upper airway becomes partially or completely blocked, diminishing nasal airflow (hypopnea) or stopping it (apnea) for as long as 30 seconds (Guilleminault and Bassiri, 2005). The person still attempts to breathe because chest and abdominal movement continue, which often results in loud snoring and snorting sounds. When breathing is partially or completely diminished, each successive diaphragmatic movement becomes stronger until the obstruction is relieved. Structural abnormalities such as a deviated septum, nasal polyps, certain jaw configurations, or enlarged tonsils predispose a client to obstructive apnea. The effort to breathe during sleep results in arousals from deep sleep often to the stage 2 cycle. In severe cases, hundreds of hypopnea/apnea episodes occur every hour, resulting in severe interference with deep sleep.

Excessive daytime sleepiness (EDS) and fatigue are the most common complaints of people with OSA (Holman, 2005). Persons with severe OSA often report taking daytime naps and experience a disruption in their daily activities because of sleepiness (National Sleep Foundation, 2002b). Feelings of sleepiness are usually most intense waking up, or right before going to sleep, and about 12 hours after the midsleep period. EDS often results in impaired waking function, poor work or school performance, accidents while driving or using equipment, and behavioral or emotional problems.

Obstructive apnea causes a serious decline in arterial oxygen saturation level. Clients are at risk for cardiac dysrhythmias, right heart failure, pulmonary hypertension, angina attacks, stroke, and hypertension. Sleep apnea contributes to high blood pressure and increased risk for heart attack and stroke (National Sleep Foundation, 2002b).

Central sleep apnea (CSA) involves dysfunction in the brain's respiratory control center. The impulse to breathe temporarily fails, and nasal airflow and chest wall movement cease. The oxygen saturation of the blood falls. The condition is common in clients with brain stem injury, muscular dystrophy, and encephalitis and people who breathe normally during the day. Less than 10% of sleep apnea is predominantly central in origin. People with CSA tend to awaken during sleep and therefore complain of insomnia and excessive daytime sleepiness. Mild and intermittent snoring is also present.

Clients with sleep apnea rarely achieve deep sleep. In addition to complaints of excessive daytime sleepiness, sleep attacks, fatigue, morning headaches, irritability, depression, difficulty concentrating, and decreased sex drive are common (White, 2005). OSA affects marital relationships, interactions within and outside the family, and is an embarrassment to the client (Reishtein and others, 2006). Treatment includes therapy for underlying cardiac or respiratory complications and emotional problems that occur as a result of the symptoms of this disorder.

Narcolepsy. **Narcolepsy** is a dysfunction of mechanisms that regulate the sleep and wake states. Excessive daytime sleepiness is the most common complaint associated with this disorder. During the day a person suddenly feels an overwhelming wave of sleepiness and falls asleep; REM sleep occurs within 15 minutes of falling asleep. **Cataplexy,** or sudden muscle weakness during intense emotions such as anger, sadness, or laughter, occurs at any time during the day. If the cataplectic attack is severe, the client loses voluntary muscle control and falls to the floor. A person with narcolepsy often has vivid dreams that occur as the person is falling asleep. These dreams are difficult to distinguish from reality. Sleep paralysis, or the feeling of being unable to move or talk just before waking or falling asleep, is another symptom (Guilleminault and Fromberz, 2005). Some studies show a genetic link for narcolepsy (Mignot, 2005).

A person with narcolepsy has the problem of falling asleep uncontrollably at inappropriate times. When individuals do not understand this disorder, a sleep attack is easily mistaken for laziness, lack of interest in activities, or drunkenness. Typically, the symptoms first begin to appear in adolescence and are often confused with the excessive daytime sleepiness that commonly occurs in teens. Narcoleptics are treated with stimulants that often only partially increase wakefulness and reduce sleep attacks. They are also treated with antidepressant medications that suppress cataplexy and the other REM-related symptoms. Brief daytime naps no longer than 20 minutes help reduce subjective feelings of sleepiness. Drugs classified as wakefulness-promoting agents, such as modafinil, are available to treat narcolepsy. Other management methods that help are following a regular exercise program, avoiding shifts in sleep, strategically timed daytime naps if possible, and eating light meals high in protein, practicing deep breathing, chewing gum, and taking vitamins (Guilleminault and Fromberz, 2005). Clients with narcolepsy need to avoid factors that increase drowsiness (e.g., alcohol, heavy meals, exhausting activities, long-distance driving, and long periods of sitting in hot, stuffy rooms).

Sleep Deprivation. **Sleep deprivation** is a problem many clients experience as a result of the dyssomnia. Causes include illness (e.g., fever, difficulty breathing, or pain), emotional stress, medications, environmental disturbances (e.g., frequent nursing care), and variability in the timing of sleep due to shift work. Physicians and nurses are particularly prone to sleep deprivation due to long work schedules and rotating shifts.

Hospitalization, especially in intensive care units (ICUs), makes clients particularly vulnerable to the extrinsic and circadian sleep disorders that cause the "ICU syndrome of sleep deprivation" (Dines-Kalinowski, 2002; Honkus, 2003). Constant environmental stimuli within the ICU, such as strange noises from equipment, the frequent monitoring and care given by nurses, and ever-present lights, confuse clients. Repeated environmental stimuli and the client's poor physical status lead to sleep deprivation (Olson and others, 2001).

BOX 42-4 Sleep Deprivation Symptoms

Physiological Symptoms	Psychological Symptoms
Ptosis, blurred vision	Confusion and disorientation
Fine motor clumsiness	Increased sensitivity to pain
Decreased reflexes	Irritable, withdrawn, apathetic
Slowed response time	Agitation
Decreased reasoning and judgment	Hyperactivity
Decreased auditory and visual alertness	Decreased motivation
Cardiac arrhythmias	Excessive sleepiness

A person's response to sleep deprivation is highly variable. Clients experience a variety of physiological and psychological symptoms (Box 42-4). The severity of symptoms is often related to the duration of sleep deprivation. The most effective treatment for sleep deprivation is elimination or correction of factors that disrupt the sleep pattern. Nurses play an important role in identifying treatable sleep deprivation problems.

Parasomnias. The parasomnias are sleep problems that are more common in children than in adults. Some have hypothesized that sudden infant death syndrome (SIDS) is thought to be related to apnea, hypoxia, and cardiac arrhythmias caused by abnormalities in the autonomic nervous system that are manifested during sleep (Verrier and Josephson, 2005). Currently the American Academy of Pediatrics recommends that parents place apparently healthy infants in the supine position during sleep because of an association between the prone position and the occurrence of SIDS (Levy Raydo and Reu-Donlon, 2005).

Parasomnias that occur among older children include somnambulism (sleepwalking), night terrors, nightmares, nocturnal enuresis (bed-wetting), body rocking, and bruxism (tooth grinding). When adults have these problems, it often indicates more serious disorders. Specific treatment for these disorders varies. However, in all cases it is important to support clients and maintain their safety.

Nursing Knowledge Base

Sleep and Rest

When people are at **rest** they usually feel mentally relaxed, free from anxiety, and physically calm. Rest does not imply inactivity, although everyone often thinks of it as settling down in a comfortable chair or lying in bed. When people are at rest they are in a state of mental, physical, and spiritual activity that leaves them feeling refreshed, rejuvenated, and ready to resume the activities of the day. People have their own habits for obtaining rest and can find ways to adjust to new environments or conditions that affect the ability to rest. People gain rest from reading a book, practicing a relaxation exercise, listening to music, taking a long walk, or sitting quietly.

Illness and unfamiliar health care routines easily affect the usual rest and sleep patterns of persons entering a hospital or other health care facility. Nurses frequently care for clients on bed rest in a variety of health care settings. This treatment confines clients to bed to reduce physical and psychological demands on the body. However, these people do not necessarily feel rested. Some still have emotional worries that prevent complete relaxation. For example, concern over physical limitations or a fear of being unable to return to their usual lifestyle causes such clients to feel stressed and unable to relax. You must always be aware of the client's need for rest. A lack of rest for long periods causes illness or worsening of existing illness.

Normal Sleep Requirements and Patterns

Sleep duration and quality vary among persons of all age-groups. For example, one person feels adequately rested with 4 hours of sleep, whereas another requires 10 hours.

Neonates. The neonate up to the age of 3 months averages about 16 hours of sleep a day, sleeping almost constantly during the first week. The sleep cycle is generally 40 to 50 minutes with wakening occurring after one to two sleep cycles. Approximately 50% of this sleep is REM sleep, which stimulates the higher brain centers. This is essential for development because the neonate is not awake long enough for significant external stimulation.

Infants. Infants usually develop a nighttime pattern of sleep by 3 months of age. The infant normally takes several naps during the day but usually sleeps an average of 8 to 10 hours during the night for a total daily sleep time of 15 hours. About 30% of sleep time is in the REM cycle. Awakening commonly occurs early in the morning, although it is not unusual for an infant to awaken during the night.

Toddlers. By the age of 2, children usually sleep through the night and take daily naps. Total sleep averages 12 hours a day. After 3 years of age, children often give up daytime naps (Hockenberry and Wilson, 2006). It is common for toddlers to awaken during the night. The percentage of REM sleep continues to fall. During this period toddlers may be unwilling to go to bed at night due to a need for autonomy or a fear of separation from their parents.

Preschoolers. On average a preschooler sleeps about 12 hours a night (about 20% is REM). By the age of 5, the preschooler rarely takes daytime naps except in cultures where a siesta is the custom (Hockenberry and Wilson, 2006). The preschooler usually has difficulty relaxing or quieting down after long, active days and has problems with bedtime fears, waking during the night, or nightmares. Partial wakening followed by normal return to sleep is frequent (Hockenberry and Wilson, 2006). In the waking period the child exhibits brief crying, walking around, unintelligible speech, sleepwalking, or bed-wetting.

School-Age Children. The amount of sleep needed varies during the school years. A 6-year-old averages 11 to 12 hours of sleep nightly, whereas an 11-year-old sleeps about 9 to 10 hours (Hockenberry and Wilson, 2006). The 6- or 7-year-old will usually go to bed with some encouragement or by doing quiet activities. The older child often resists sleeping because of an unawareness of fatigue or a need to be independent.

Adolescents. On average, teenagers get about 7½ hours of sleep per night. The typical adolescent is subject to a number of changes such as school demands, after-school social activities, and part-time jobs that reduce the time spent sleeping (National Sleep Foundation, 2006a). This shortened sleep time often results in EDS. Reduced performance in school, vulnerability to accidents, behavior and mood problems, and increased use of alcohol are often the result of EDS due to insufficient sleep (Spilsbury and others, 2004; Walsh and others, 2005).

Young Adults. Most young adults average 6 to 8½ hours of sleep a night. Approximately 20% of sleep time is REM sleep, which remains consistent throughout life. It is common for the stresses of jobs, family relationships, and social activities frequently to lead to insomnia and the use of medication for sleep. Daytime sleepiness contributes to an increased number of accidents, decreased productivity, and interpersonal problems in this age-group. Pregnancy increases the need for sleep and rest. Insomnia, periodic limb movements, restless leg syndrome, and sleep-disordered breathing are common problems during the third trimester of pregnancy (Wolfson and Lee, 2005).

Middle Adults. During middle adulthood the total time spent sleeping at night begins to decline. The amount of stage 4 sleep begins to fall, a decline that continues with advancing age. Insomnia is particularly common, probably because of the changes and stresses of middle age. Anxiety, depression, or certain physical illnesses cause sleep disturbances. Women experiencing menopausal symptoms often experience insomnia.

Older Adults. Complaints of sleeping difficulties increase with age. More than 50% of adults 65 years or older report problems with sleep (Hoffman, 2003). Episodes of REM sleep tend to shorten. There is a progressive decrease in stages 3 and 4 NREM sleep; some older adults have almost no stage 4, or deep sleep. An older adult awakens more often during the night, and it takes more time for an older adult to fall asleep. The tendency to nap seems to increase progressively with age because of the frequent awakenings experienced at night.

The presence of chronic illness often results in sleep disturbances for the older adult. For example, an older adult with arthritis frequently has difficulty sleeping because of painful joints. Changes in sleep pattern are often due to changes in the CNS that affect the regulation of sleep. Sensory impairment reduces an older person's sensitivity to time cues that maintain circadian rhythms.

Factors Affecting Sleep

A number of factors affect the quantity and quality of sleep. Often a single factor is not the only cause for a sleep problem. Physiological, psychological, and environmental factors frequently alter the quality and quantity of sleep.

Drugs and Substances. Sleepiness, insomnia, and fatigue often result as a direct effect of commonly prescribed medications (Box 42-5). These medications alter sleep and weaken daytime alertness, which is problematic for individuals (Schweitzer, 2005). Medications prescribed for sleep often cause more problems than

✳ BOX 42-5 Drugs and Their Effect on Sleep

Hypnotics
Interfere with reaching deeper sleep stages
Provide only temporary (1 week) increase in quantity of sleep
Eventually cause "hangover" during day; excess drowsiness, confusion, decreased energy
Sometimes worsens sleep apnea in older adults

Antidepressants and Stimulants
Suppress REM sleep
Decrease total sleep time

Alcohol
Speeds onset of sleep
Reduces REM sleep
Awakens person during night and causes difficulty returning to sleep

Caffeine
Prevents person from falling asleep
Causes person to awaken during night
Interferes with REM sleep

Diuretics
Nighttime awakenings caused by nocturia

Beta-Adrenergic Blockers
Cause nightmares
Cause insomnia
Cause awakening from sleep

Benzodiazepines
Alter REM sleep
Increase sleep time
Increase daytime sleepiness

Narcotics
Suppress REM sleep
Cause increased daytime drowsiness

Anticonvulsants
Decrease REM sleep time
Causes daytime drowsiness

REM, Rapid eye movement.

---

benefits. Older adults take a variety of drugs to control or treat chronic illness, and the combined effects of several drugs seriously disrupt sleep. One substance that promotes sleep in many people is L-tryptophan, a natural protein found in foods such as milk, cheese, and meats.

Lifestyle. A person's daily routine influences sleep patterns. An individual working a rotating shift (e.g., 2 weeks of days followed by a week of nights) often has difficulty adjusting to the altered sleep schedule. For example, the body's internal clock is set at 11 PM, but the work schedule forces sleep at 9 AM instead. The individual is able to sleep only 3 or 4 hours because the body's clock perceives that it is time to be awake and active. Difficulties with maintaining alertness during work time results in decreased and even hazardous performance. After several weeks of working a night shift a person's biological clock usually does adjust. Other alterations in routines that disrupt sleep patterns include performing unaccustomed heavy work, engaging in late-night social activities, and changing evening mealtime.

Usual Sleep Patterns. In the past century the amount of sleep obtained nightly by U.S. citizens has decreased over 20% (National Sleep Foundation, 2003), indicating that many Americans are sleep deprived and experience excessive sleepiness during the day. Sleepiness becomes pathological when it occurs at times when individuals need or want to be awake. People who experience temporary sleep deprivation as a result of an active social evening or lengthened work schedule usually feel sleepy the next day. However, they are able to overcome these feelings even though they have difficulty performing tasks and remaining attentive. Chronic lack of sleep is much more serious than temporary sleep deprivation and causes serious alterations in the ability to perform daily functions. Sleepiness tends to be most difficult to overcome during sedentary (inactive) tasks. For example, single-vehicle accidents related to a driver falling asleep at the wheel

occur most often between 2 AM and 5 AM due to the sleepiness that occurs when people are awake during what is their normal period of sleep (Sitzman, 2005).

Emotional Stress. Worry over personal problems or a situation frequently disrupts sleep. Emotional stress causes a person to be tense and often leads to frustration when sleep does not occur. Stress also causes a person to try too hard to fall asleep, to awaken frequently during the sleep cycle, or to oversleep. Continued stress causes poor sleep habits.

Older clients frequently experience losses that lead to emotional stress such as retirement, physical impairment, or the death of a loved one. Older adults and other individuals who experience depressive mood problems experience delays in falling asleep, earlier appearance of REM sleep, frequent awakening, increased total bed time, feelings of sleeping poorly, and early awakening (National Sleep Foundation, 2006b).

Environment. The physical environment in which a person sleeps significantly influences the ability to fall and remain sleep. Good ventilation is essential for restful sleep. The size, firmness, and position of the bed affect the quality of sleep. If a person usually sleeps with another individual, sleeping alone often causes wakefulness. On the other hand, sleeping with a restless or snoring bed partner disrupts sleep.

In hospitals and other inpatient facilities, noise creates a problem for clients. Noise in hospitals is usually new or strange and is often loud. Thus clients wake easily. This problem is greatest the first night of hospitalization, when clients often experience increased total wake time, increased awakenings, and decreased REM sleep and total sleep time. People-induced noises (e.g., nursing activities) are sources of increased sound levels. Intensive care units are sources for high noise levels due to staff, monitor alarms, and equipment. Close proximity of clients, noise from confused and ill clients, the ringing of alarm systems and telephones, and disturbances caused by emergencies make the environment unpleasant. Noise causes hearing loss, delayed healing, impaired immune function, and increased blood pressure, heart rate, and stress (Cmiel and others, 2004).

Light levels affect the ability to fall asleep. Some clients prefer a dark room, whereas others, such as children or older adults, prefer keeping a soft light on during sleep. Clients also have trouble sleeping based on the temperature of a room. A room that is too warm or too cold often causes a client to become restless.

Exercise and Fatigue. A person who is moderately fatigued usually achieves restful sleep, especially if the fatigue is the result of enjoyable work or exercise. Exercising 2 hours or more before bedtime allows the body to cool down and maintains a state of fatigue that promotes relaxation. However, excess fatigue resulting from exhausting or stressful work makes falling asleep difficult. This is a common problem for grade school children and adolescents.

Food and Caloric Intake. Following good eating habits is important for proper sleep. Eating a large, heavy, and/or spicy meal at night often results in indigestion that interferes with sleep. Caffeine, alcohol, and nicotine consumed in the evening produce insomnia. Coffee, tea, cola, and chocolate contain caffeine and xanthines that cause sleeplessness. A drastic reduction or avoidance of these substances is an important strategy that people can use to improve sleep. Some food allergies cause insomnia. In infants, a milk allergy sometimes causes nighttime waking and crying or colic.

Weight loss or weight gain influences sleep patterns. Weight gain contributes to obstructive sleep apnea because of increased size of the soft tissue structures in the upper airway (Schwab and others, 2005). Weight loss causes insomnia and decreased amounts of sleep (Benca and Schenck, 2005). Certain sleep disorders are the result of the semistarvation diets popular in a weight-conscious society.

Critical Thinking

Successful critical thinking requires a synthesis of knowledge, including information gathered from clients, experience, critical thinking attitudes, and intellectual and professional standards. Clinical judgments require you to anticipate the information necessary, analyze the data, and make decisions regarding client care. You adapt critical thinking to the changing needs of the client. During assessment (Figure 42-3), consider all elements to make appropriate nursing diagnoses.

In the case of sleep, you will integrate knowledge from nursing and disciplines such as pharmacology and psychology. Personal experience with a sleep problem, as well as experience with clients, will prepare you to know effective forms of sleep therapies. You will need the use of critical thinking attitudes such as perseverance, confidence, and discipline to complete a comprehensive assessment and to develop a plan of care to provide successful management of the sleep problem. The use of professional standards, such as the *Nursing Scope and Standards of Practice* (American Nurses Association, 2004) and "Evaluating Excessive Sleepi-

Knowledge
- Sleep cycle physiology
- Pathophysiology and clinical signs of sleep disturbances
- Factors that potentially affect a person's ability to sleep
- Pharmacological agents' effects on sleep
- A normal sleep pattern

Experience
- Caring for clients with chronic sleep problems
- Caring for clients experiencing acute sleep disturbances in a health care setting
- Personal experience with acute or chronic sleep disruption

ASSESSMENT
- Determine the client's current sleep pattern
- Review factors affecting the client's sleep
- Evaluate the client's response to sleep disturbance
- Evaluate the client's developmental level
- Explore the client's approaches to improve sleep

Standards
- Apply intellectual standards (e.g., clarity, accuracy, completeness) when gathering a sleep history
- Apply *Standards of Clinical Practice*
- Apply "Nursing Standard-of-Practice Protocol for Sleep Disturbances in Elderly Patients" (Foreman and Wykle, 1995)

Attitudes
- Display perseverance in exploring causes and possible solutions to long-term sleep problems
- Use creativity in assessment to reveal a more thorough picture of the client's sleep problem
- Explore the client's thought about possible causes of the problem

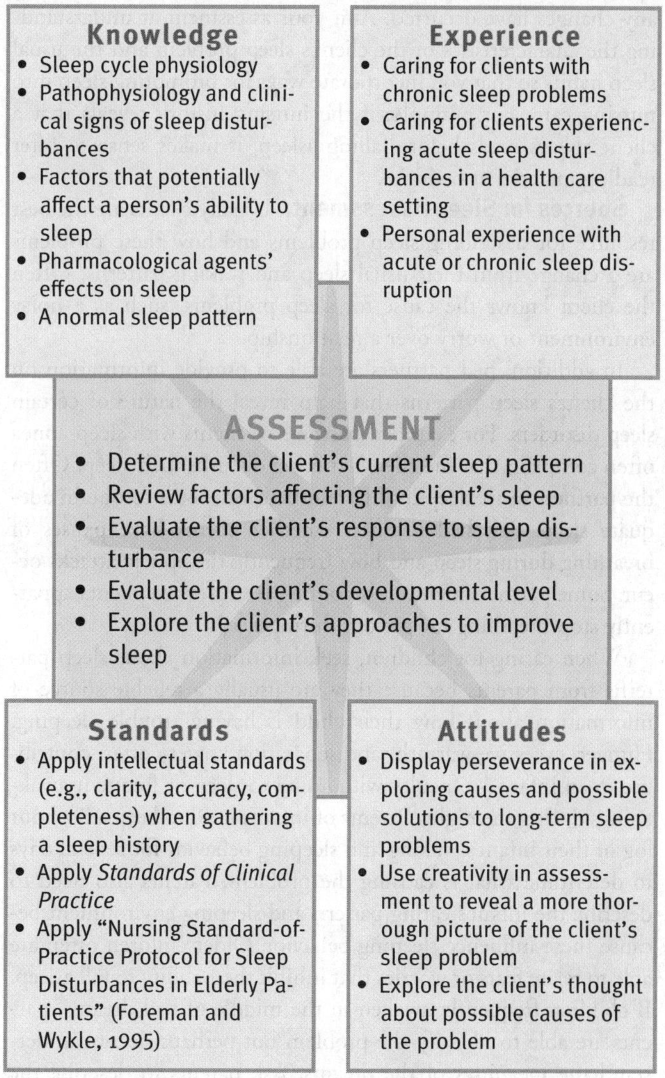

Figure 42-3 Critical thinking model for sleep assessment.

ness in the Older Adult" (National Guideline Clearinghouse, 2006), provides valuable guidelines to assess and address the needs of clients with sleep disorders.

Nursing Process

 Assessment

Assess clients' sleep patterns by using the nursing history to gather information about factors that usually influence sleep. Sleep is a subjective experience. Only the client is able to report whether or not it is sufficient and restful. If the client is satisfied with the quantity and quality of sleep received, you will consider it normal and the nursing history is brief. If a client admits to or suspects a sleep problem, you will need a detailed history.

Sleep Assessment. Most persons are able to provide a reasonably accurate estimate of their sleep patterns, particularly if any changes have occurred. Aim your assessment at understanding the characteristics of the client's sleep problem and the usual sleep habits so that you incorporate ways for promoting sleep into nursing care. For example, if the nursing history reveals that a client always reads before falling asleep, it makes sense to offer reading material at bedtime.

Sources for Sleep Assessment. Usually clients are the best resource for describing sleep problems and how these problems are a change from their usual sleep and waking patterns. Often the client knows the cause for sleep problems, such as a noisy environment or worry over a relationship.

In addition, bed partners are able to provide information on the client's sleep patterns that help reveal the nature of certain sleep disorders. For example, partners of clients with sleep apnea often complain that the client's snoring disturbs their sleep. Often the partners must sleep in different beds or rooms to obtain adequate sleep. Ask bed partners whether clients have pauses of breathing during sleep and how frequently the apneic attacks occur. Some partners mention becoming fearful when clients apparently stop breathing for periods during sleep.

When caring for children, seek information about sleep patterns from parents because they are usually a reliable source of information about how their child is having trouble sleeping. Hunger, excessive warmth, and separation anxiety often contribute to an infant's difficulty with going to sleep or frequent awakenings during the night. Parents of infants need to keep a 24-hour log of their infant's waking and sleeping behavior for several days to determine what is causing the problem. Parents also need to describe the infant's eating pattern and sleeping environment because these influence sleeping behavior. Older children often are able to relate fears or worries that inhibit their ability to fall asleep. If children frequently awaken in the middle of bad dreams, parents are able to identify the problem but perhaps do not understand the meanings of the dreams. Ask parents to describe the typical behavior patterns that foster or impair sleep. For example, excessive stimulation from active play or visiting friends will predictably impair sleep. With chronic sleep problems, parents need to relate the duration of the problem, its progression, and children's responses.

Tools for Assessment of Sleep. Subjective reports of sleep are reliable and valid measures of sleep according to researchers (Lashley, 2004). One effective, brief method for assessing sleep quality is the use of a visual analog scale (Lashley, 2004). Draw a straight horizontal line 100 mm (4 inches) long. Opposing statements such as "best night's sleep" and "worst night's sleep" are at opposite ends of the line. Ask clients to place a mark on the horizontal line at the point corresponding to their perceptions of the previous night's sleep. Then measure the distances of the mark along the line in millimeters, and it offers a numerical value for satisfaction with sleep. Use the scale repeatedly to show change over time. Such a scale is useful to assess an individual client, not to compare clients.

Another brief subjective method to assess sleep is a numeric scale with a 0 to 10 sleep rating (Lashley, 2004). Ask individuals to separately rate their quantity and quality of sleep on the scale. Instruct clients to indicate with a number between 0 and 10 their sleep quantity then their quality of sleep with 0 being the worst sleep and 10 being the best sleep.

Sleep History. When a client reports having adequate sleep, a sleep history is usually brief. A determination of usual bedtime, normal bedtime rituals, preferred environment for sleeping, and what time the client usually rises gives you information for planning care conducive to sleep. When suspecting a sleep problem, assess the quality and characteristics of sleep in greater depth by asking the client to describe the sleep problem. This includes recent changes in sleep pattern, sleep symptoms experienced during waking hours, use of sleep and other prescribed or over-the-counter medications, diet and intake of substances such as caffeine or alcohol that influence sleep, and recent life events that have affected the client's mental and emotional status.

Description of Sleeping Problems. Conduct a more detailed history when a client has a sleep problem. This ensures therapeutic care is appropriately provided. Open-ended questions help a client to describe a problem more fully. A general description of the problem followed by more focused questions usually reveals specific characteristics that are useful in planning therapies. To begin, you need to understand the nature of the sleep problem, its signs and symptoms, its onset and duration, its severity, any predisposing factors or causes, and the overall effect on the client. Ask specific questions related to the sleep problem (Box 42-6).

Proper questioning helps to determine the type of sleep disturbance and the nature of the problem. Box 42-7 gives examples of additional questions for you to ask the client when you suspect specific sleep disorders. The questions assist in selecting specific sleep therapies and the best time for implementation.

As an adjunct to the sleep history, have the client and bed partner keep a sleep-wake log for 1 to 4 weeks (Lashley, 2004). The client completes the sleep-wake log daily to provide information on day-to-day variations in sleep-wake patterns over extended periods. Entries in the log often include 24-hour information about various waking and sleeping health behaviors such as physical activities, mealtimes, type and amount of intake (alcohol and caffeine), time and length of daytime naps, evening and bedtime routines, the time the client tries to fall asleep, nighttime awakenings, and the time of morning awakening. A partner helps record the estimated times the client falls asleep or awakens. Although the log is helpful, the client has to be motivated to participate in its completion.

Usual Sleep Pattern. Normal sleep is difficult to define because individuals vary in perception of adequate quantity and quality of sleep. It is important, however, to have clients describe their usual sleep pattern to determine the significance of the changes caused by a sleep disorder. Knowing a client's usual, preferred sleep pattern allows a nurse to try to match sleeping conditions in a health care setting with those in the home. Ask the following questions to determine a client's sleep pattern:

1. What time do you usually get in bed each night?
2. What time do you usually fall asleep? Do you do anything special to help you fall asleep?
3. How many times do you awaken during the night? Why?
4. What time do you typically wake up in the morning?
5. What is the average number of hours you sleep each night?

Compare client data with the predominant pattern usually found for other clients of the same age. Based on this comparison, you begin to assess for identifiable patterns such as insomnia.

✳ BOX 42-6   NURSING ASSESSMENT QUESTIONS

Nature of the Problem

What type of problem are you having with your sleep?

Why do you think your sleep is inadequate?

Describe for me a recent typical night's sleep. How is this sleep different from what you are used to?

Signs and Symptoms

Do you have difficulty falling asleep, staying asleep, or waking up?

Have you been told that you snore loudly?

Do you have headaches when awakening? Does your child awaken from nightmares?

Onset and Duration

When did you notice the problem?

How long has this problem lasted?

Severity

How long does it take you to fall asleep?

How often during the week do you have trouble falling asleep?

How many hours of sleep a night did you get this week?

How does this compare to what is usual for you?

What do you do when you awaken during the night or too early in the morning?

Predisposing Factors

What do you do just before you go to bed?

Have you recently had any changes at work or at home?

How is your mood, and have you noticed any changes recently?

What medications or recreational drugs do you take on a regular basis?

Are you taking any new prescription or over-the-counter medications?

Do you eat food (spicy or greasy foods) or drink substances (alcohol or caffeinated beverages) that interfere with your sleep?

Do you have a physical illness that interferes with your sleep?

Does anyone in your family have a history of sleep problems?

Effect on Client

How has the loss of sleep affected you?

Do you feel excessively sleepy, irritable, or have trouble concentrating during waking hours?

Do you have trouble staying awake or have you fallen asleep at inappropriate times, for example, while driving, sitting quietly in a meeting, or watching TV?

✳ BOX 42-7   Questions to Ask to Assess for Specific Sleep Disorders

Insomnia

How easily do you fall asleep?

Do you fall asleep and have difficulty staying asleep? How many times do you awaken?

What time do you awaken in the morning? What causes you to awaken early?

What do you do to prepare for sleep? To improve your sleep?

What do you think about as you try to fall asleep?

How often do you have trouble sleeping?

Sleep Apnea

Do you snore loudly? Or does anyone else in your family snore loudly?

Has anyone ever told you that you often stop breathing for short periods during sleep? (Spouse or bed partner/roommate may report this.)

Do you experience headaches after awakening?

Do you have difficulty staying awake during the day?

Narcolepsy

Do you fall asleep at inopportune times? (Friends or relatives may report this.)

Do you have episodes of losing muscle control or falling to the floor?

Have you ever had the feeling of being unable to move or talk just before waking or falling asleep?

Do you have vivid, lifelike dreams when going to sleep or waking up?

Clients with sleep problems frequently show patterns drastically different from their usual one, or sometimes the change is relatively minor. Hospitalized clients usually need or want more sleep as a result of illness. However, some require less sleep because they are less active. Some clients who are ill think that it is important to try to sleep more than what is usual for them, eventually making sleeping difficult.

Physical and Psychological Illness. Determine whether the client has any preexisting health problems that interfere with sleep. A history of psychiatric problems also makes a difference. For example, a bipolar or manic-depressive client sleeps more when depressed than when manic. A depressed client often experiences an inadequate amount of fragmented sleep. Chronic diseases such as chronic obstructive pulmonary disease and painful disor-

ders such as arthritis interfere with sleep. Also assess the client's medication history, including a description of over-the-counter and prescribed drugs. If a client takes medications to aid sleep, gather information about the type and amount of medication that the client uses. Also assess the client's daily caffeine intake.

If the client has recently had surgery, expect the client to experience some disturbance in sleep. Clients usually awaken frequently during the first night after surgery and receive little deep or REM sleep. Depending on the type of surgery, it takes several days to months for a normal sleep cycle to return.

Current Life Events. In your assessment, learn whether the client is experiencing any changes in lifestyle that disrupt sleep. A person's occupation often offers a clue to the nature of the sleep problem. Changes in job responsibilities, rotating shifts, or long hours contribute to a sleep disturbance. Questions about social activities, recent travel, or mealtime schedules help clarify the sleep assessment.

Emotional and Mental Status. The client's emotions and mental status affect the ability to sleep. For example, if the client is experiencing anxiety, emotional stress related to illness, or situational crises such as loss of job or a loved one, insomnia is often experienced. Clients with psychiatric disorders may need mild sedation for adequate rest. Assess the effectiveness of any medication and its effect on daytime function.

Bedtime Routines. Ask clients what they do to prepare for sleep. For example, the client may drink a glass of milk, take a sleeping pill, eat a snack, or watch television. Assess habits that are beneficial compared with those that disturb sleep. For example, watching television promotes sleep for one person, whereas watching TV stimulates another to stay awake. Sometimes pointing out that a particular habit is interfering with sleep helps clients to find ways to change or eliminate habits that are disrupting sleep.

Pay special attention to a child's bedtime rituals. The parents need to report whether it is necessary, for example, to read the child a bedtime story, rock the child to sleep, or engage in quiet play. Some young children need a special blanket or stuffed animal when going to sleep.

Bedtime Environment. During assessment, ask the client to describe preferred bedroom conditions. These include preferences for lighting in the room, music or television in the background, or needing to have the door open versus closed. In addition, some children require the company of a parent to fall asleep. In a health care environment there are environmental distractions that often interfere with sleep such as a roommate's television, an electronic monitor in the hallway, a noisy nurses' station, or another client who cries out at night. Identify factors to reduce or control the environment.

Behaviors of Sleep Deprivation. Some clients are unaware of how their sleep problems are affecting their behavior. Observe for behaviors such as irritability, disorientation (similar to a drunken state), frequent yawning, and slurred speech. If sleep deprivation has lasted a long time, psychotic behavior such as delusions and paranoia sometimes develop. For example, a client reports seeing strange objects or colors in the room. Or the client acts afraid when the nurse enters the room.

Client Expectations. A poor night's sleep for a client often starts a vicious cycle of anticipatory anxiety. The client fears that sleep will again be disturbed while trying harder and harder to sleep (Attarian, 2000). Use a skilled and caring approach to assess the client's sleep needs. A caring nurse individualizes care for each client's need. Always ask clients what they expect regarding sleep. This includes asking about the interventions they currently use and how successful the interventions are. Also ask clients which other interventions they prefer and how to implement them. It is important to understand clients' expectations regarding their sleep pattern. When clients ask for assistance because of sleep disturbances, they typically expect a nurse to respond promptly to assist them in improving their quantity and quality of sleep.

◆ Nursing Diagnosis

Review your assessment data looking for clusters of data that include defining characteristics for a sleep pattern disturbance. If you identify a sleep pattern disturbance, specify the condition. By specifying the nature of a sleep disturbance, you are able to design more effective interventions. For example, you choose different therapies for clients with insomnia who are unable to fall asleep than for those with sleep apnea. Box 42-8 demonstrates how to use nursing assessment activities to identify and cluster defining characteristics to make an accurate nursing diagnosis.

Assessment also identifies the related factor or probable cause of the sleep disturbance, such as a noisy environment or a high

BOX 42-8   NURSING DIAGNOSTIC PROCESS
Insomnia

Assessment Activities	Defining Characteristics
Ask client to explain nature of sleep problem.	Client reports difficulty in falling asleep, taking up to 1 hour. Client reports awakening two to three times nightly with difficulty returning to sleep.
Observe client's behavior, and ask spouse if client is experiencing behavior changes.	Client admits to not feeling well rested. Spouse describes times when client was lethargic and irritable.
Determine if client has had recent lifestyle changes.	Spouse reports client recently lost job, is concerned about finding new position.

intake of caffeinated beverages in the evening. These causes become the focus of interventions for minimizing or eliminating the problem. For example, if a client is experiencing insomnia as a result of a noisy health care environment, offer some basic recommendations for helping sleep such as controlling the noise of hospital equipment, reducing interruptions, or keeping doors closed. If the insomnia is related to worry over a threatened marital separation, introduce coping strategies and create an environment for sleep. If you incorrectly define the probable cause or related factors, the client will not benefit from care.

Sleep problems affect clients in other ways. For example, you will find that a client with sleep apnea has problems with a spouse who is tired and frustrated over the client's snoring. In addition, the spouse is concerned that the client is breathing improperly and thus is in danger. The nursing diagnosis of *compromised family coping* indicates that you need to provide support to the client and spouse so that they understand sleep apnea and obtain the medical treatment needed. Examples of nursing diagnoses for clients with sleep problems include the following:

- Anxiety
- Ineffective breathing pattern
- Acute confusion
- Compromised family coping
- Ineffective coping
- Fatigue
- Ineffective protection
- Insomnia
- Disturbed sensory perception
- Sleep deprivation

◆ Planning

Goals and Outcomes. During planning you again synthesize information from multiple resources in order to develop an individualized plan of care (Figure 42-4) (see Care Plan). Professional standards are especially important to consider in developing a care plan. These standards often offer scientifically proven guidelines

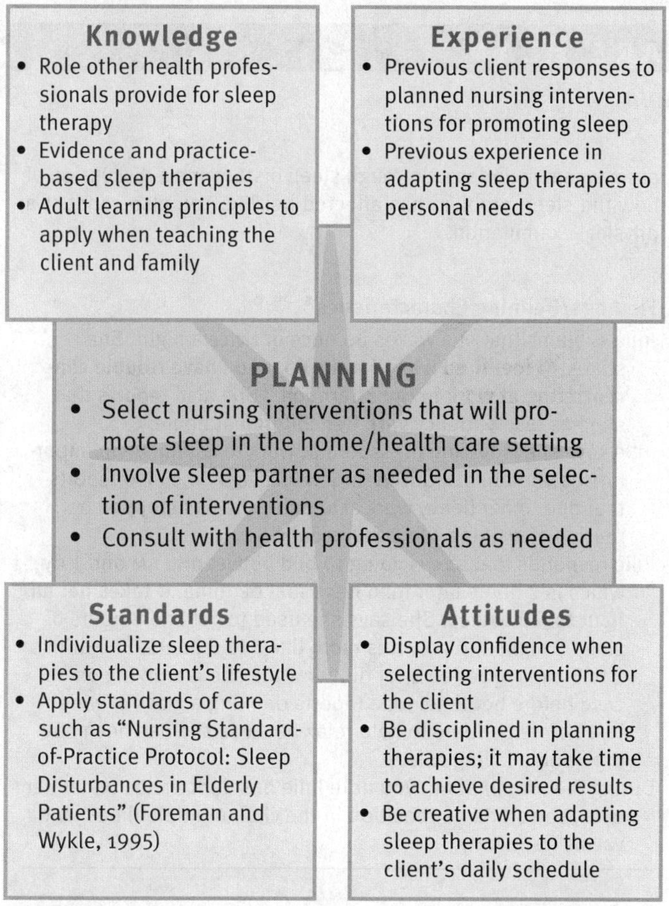

Knowledge
- Role other health profes-sionals provide for sleep therapy
- Evidence and practice-based sleep therapies
- Adult learning principles to apply when teaching the client and family

Experience
- Previous client responses to planned nursing interven-tions for promoting sleep
- Previous experience in adapting sleep therapies to personal needs

PLANNING
- Select nursing interventions that will pro-mote sleep in the home/health care setting
- Involve sleep partner as needed in the selec-tion of interventions
- Consult with health professionals as needed

Standards
- Individualize sleep thera-pies to the client's lifestyle
- Apply standards of care such as "Nursing Standard-of-Practice Protocol: Sleep Disturbances in Elderly Patients" (Foreman and Wykle, 1995)

Attitudes
- Display confidence when selecting interventions for the client
- Be disciplined in planning therapies; it may take time to achieve desired results
- Be creative when adapting sleep therapies to the client's daily schedule

Figure 42-4 Critical thinking model for sleep planning.

for effective nursing interventions. For example, the National Guideline Clearinghouse (2006) guideline titled "Evaluating Excessive Sleepiness in the Older Adult" recommends individualized nursing interventions that maintain and support an older adult's normal sleep pattern and bedtime ritual. It is important for a plan of care for sleep promotion to include strategies appropriate to the client's sleep routines, living environment, and lifestyle.

As you plan care for the client with sleep disturbances, creation of a concept map is another method for developing holistic client-centered care (Figure 42-5, p. 1044). Create the map after identifying relevant nursing diagnoses from the assessment database. In this example, the nursing diagnoses are linked to the client's medical diagnosis of depression following the death of the spouse. The concept map shows the relationships between the nursing diagnoses *complicated grieving, insomnia,* and *impaired social interaction.* This approach to planning care assists the nurse in recognizing relationships between planned interventions. For this client, interventions and successful outcomes for one nursing diagnosis affect the resolution of another nursing diagnosis.

When developing goals and outcomes, it is important for the nurse and client to collaborate. As a result, you will be more likely to set realistic goals and measurable outcomes. An effective plan includes outcomes established over a realistic time frame that focus on the goal of improving the quantity and quality of sleep in the home. Often family members are very helpful in contributing

to the plan. A sleep promotion plan frequently requires many weeks to accomplish. The following is an example of a goal with client outcomes:

Goal: The client will control environmental sources disrupting sleep within 1 month.
Outcomes:
- Client will identify factors in the immediate home environ-ment that disrupt sleep in 2 weeks.
- Client will report having a discussion with family members about environmental barriers to sleep in 2 weeks.
- Client will report changes made in the bedroom to promote sleep within 4 weeks.
- Client will report having fewer than two awakenings per night within 4 weeks.

Setting Priorities. Work with the client to establish the priority outcomes and interventions for the client. Frequently sleep disturbances are the result of other health problems. For example, when physical symptoms are interfering with sleep, management of the symptoms is your first priority. Once symptoms are relieved, then focus on sleep therapies. Clients are a helpful resource in determining which interventions hold priority. For example, once clients understand the factors that disrupt sleep, they make choices in the types of changes they would like to make in their lifestyle or sleeping environment.

Collaborative Care. Partner closely with the client and significant others to ensure that any therapies, such as a change in the sleep schedule or changes to the bedroom environment, are realistic and achievable. In a health care setting, plan treatments or routines so that the client is able to rest. For example, in the intensive care unit, use available electronic monitors to track trends in vital signs without awakening a client each hour. Other staff members need to be aware of the care plan so that they can cluster activities at certain times to reduce awakenings. In a nursing home the focus of the plan involves better planning of rest periods around the activities of the other residents. Oftentimes roommates have very different schedules.

The nature of the sleep disturbance determines whether referrals to additional health care providers are necessary. For example, if a sleep problem is related to a situational crisis or emotional problem, refer the client to a psychiatric clinical nurse specialist or clinical psychologist for counseling. When chronic insomnia is the problem, a medical referral or referral to a sleep center is beneficial. If the nurse works in an inpatient setting and the client needs a referral for continued care after discharge, offering information about the sleep problem will be useful to the home care nurse. The success of sleep therapy depends on an approach that fits the client's lifestyle and the nature of the sleep disorder.

◆Implementation

Nursing interventions designed to improve the quality of a person's rest and sleep are largely focused on health promotion. Clients need adequate sleep and rest to maintain active and produc-

NURSING CARE PLAN

Insomnia

Assessment

Julie Arnold, a 42-year-old attorney, is the first client of the morning at the neighborhood health clinic where you work. When you ask her how she is doing, she tells you she is having difficulty sleeping. Julie is married and has two school-age children. Julie's assessment includes a thorough sleep history and a discussion of how the sleep problem has affected her life. You also conduct a physical examination.

Assessment Activities	Findings/Defining Characteristics*
Ask Julie to explain the nature of her sleep problem.	Julie explains that she wakes up once or twice a night. She states, **"I feel tired when I wake up, and I have trouble concentrating at work in the afternoon."** She also **reports** that **she has less patience with her children** at home.
Ask Julie if there have been any recent changes in her life.	Julie says she is feeling pressured at work to complete an important case that she started on 2 weeks ago. She also reports that due to her heavy work schedule, she has **stopped** her **routine of walking 1 to 2 miles daily.**
Ask Julie to describe her bedtime routine.	Julie responds that she is going to bed between 12 AM and 1 AM, which is 2 hours later than her usual bedtime. **It takes her an hour to fall asleep.** She says she used to get 7 to 8 hours of sleep a night and now **it is more like 5 to 6 hours.** She drinks 2 to 3 cups of coffee after dinner while she is working on her case before bedtime. Julie reports drinking a glass of wine just before bedtime to help relax because she has been having trouble falling asleep.
Assess Julie for physical signs of sleep problems.	During the examination, you note Julie has dark circles under her eyes, she shifts her position in the chair multiple times, and yawns frequently.

*__Defining characteristics__ are shown in bold type.

Nursing Diagnosis: Insomnia related to psychological stress from job pressures.

Planning

Goal	Expected Outcomes (NOC)†
	Sleep
Client will achieve an improved sense of adequate sleep within 4 weeks.	Client will report waking up less frequently during the night and feeling rested within 4 weeks.
	Client will verbalize adherence to a regular bedtime routine within 4 weeks.
Client will achieve a more normal sleep pattern within 4 weeks.	Client will fall asleep within 30 minutes of going to bed within 4 weeks.
	Client will report sleeping 7 hours nightly within 4 weeks.

†Outcome classification labels from Moorhead S and others: *Nursing outcomes classification (NOC)*, ed 4, St. Louis, 2008, Mosby.

Interventions (NIC)‡

Sleep Enhancement

Interventions	Rationale
Encourage client to establish a bedtime routine and a regular sleep pattern.	Maintaining a consistent schedule helps induce sleep (National Guideline Clearinghouse, 2006).
Instruct client to avoid caffeine, nicotine, and alcohol before bedtime.	Caffeine and nicotine are stimulants and cause difficulty in falling asleep. Alcohol lightens and fragments sleep (National Guideline Clearinghouse, 2006).
Assist client in identifying ways to eliminate stressful concerns about work before bedtime (e.g., taking time before actual sleep time to read a light novel).	Excess worry and intense activities before bedtime will stimulate client and prevent sleep (Robinson and others, 2005).
Adjust environment; have client control noise, temperature, and light in the bedroom.	This develops an environment conducive to sleep (Morin and others, 2007).

‡Intervention classification labels from Bulechek GM, Butcher HK, and Dochterman JM: *Nursing interventions classification (NIC)*, ed 5, St. Louis, 2008, Mosby.

NURSING CARE PLAN

Insomnia—cont'd

Interventions (NIC)‡

Exercise Promotion
Encourage client to begin walking routinely during the day, but not 2 to 3 hours before bedtime.

Relaxation Therapy
Instruct client in how to perform muscle relaxation before bedtime; include demonstration.

Rationale

Regular exercise increases activity levels and improves sleep quality. Exercise just before bedtime is a stimulant that prevents sleep (Hoffman, 2003).

Relaxation therapy helps reduce anxiety, which interferes with sleep (Richardson, 2003).

‡Intervention classification labels from Bulechek GM, Butcher HK, and Dochterman JM: *Nursing interventions classification (NIC),* ed 5, St. Louis, 2008, Mosby.

Evaluation

Nursing Actions	Client Response/Finding	Achievement of Outcome
Ask Julie if she is able to fall asleep and stay asleep.	Julie responds, "It usually takes me 15 to 20 minutes to fall asleep, and I woke up once for only two nights last week."	Julie reports she falls asleep within 30 minutes and wakes up less frequently during the night.
Ask Julie to describe her waking behaviors at work and home during the day.	Julie responds that she has completed her case at work and feels less pressure. She has restarted her walking routine and is better able to cope with her children. She is able to concentrate at work more.	Julie reports feeling more rested.
Observe Julie's waking nonverbal expressions and behavior.	Julie sits in the chair without shifting position. She does not yawn during the conversation. The dark circles under her eyes are almost gone.	Julie reports she is sleeping an average of 7 hours a night.

tive lifestyles. During times of illness, rest and sleep promotion are important for recovery. Nursing care in an acute care, restorative care, or continuing care setting differs from that provided in a client's home. The primary differences are in the environment and the nurse's ability to support normal rest and sleep habits. The client's age also influences the types of therapies that are most effective. Box 42-9 (p. 1045) provides principles for promoting sleep in older clients.

Health Promotion. In community health and home settings help clients develop behaviors conducive to rest and relaxation. To develop good sleep habits at home, clients and their bed partners need to learn techniques that promote sleep and conditions that interfere with sleep (Morin, 2005) (Box 42-10, p. 1045). Parents also learn how to promote good sleep habits for their children. Clients benefit most from instructions based on information about their homes and lifestyles such as what type of activities will promote sleep in a third-shift worker or how to make the home environment more conducive to sleep. Similarly, they will more likely apply information that is useful and valued.

Environmental Controls. All clients require a sleeping environment with a comfortable room temperature and proper ventilation, minimal sources of noise, a comfortable bed, and proper lighting (Bulechek and others, 2008). Children and adults vary more in regard to comfortable room temperature. Instruct parents to position cribs away from open windows or drafts and to cover

the infant with a light, warm blanket. Older adults often require extra blankets or covers.

Eliminate distracting noise so that the bedroom is as quiet as possible. In the home the television, telephone, or the intermittent chiming of a clock often disrupts a client's sleep. The family becomes an important part of the nurse's approach to reduce noise in the home, especially if there are several family members, all with different schedules for going to sleep. It is also important to remember that some clients sleep with familiar inside noises, such as the hum of a fan. Commercial products that produce a soothing noise such as ocean waves or rainfall create a soothing environment for sleep.

A bed and mattress needs to provide support and comfortable firmness. Bed boards placed under mattresses add support. Sometimes extra pillows are important to help a person position comfortably in bed. The position of the bed in the room also makes a difference for some clients.

Clients vary in regard to the amount of light that they prefer at night. Infants and older adults sleep best in softly lit rooms. Light should not shine directly on their eyes. Small table lamps prevent total darkness. For older adults light reduces the chance of confusion and prevents falls while walking to the bathroom. If streetlights shine through windows or when clients nap during the day, heavy shades, drapes, or slatted blinds are helpful.

Promoting Bedtime Routines. Bedtime routines relax clients in preparation for sleep (Bulechek and others, 2008). It is always

CONCEPT MAP

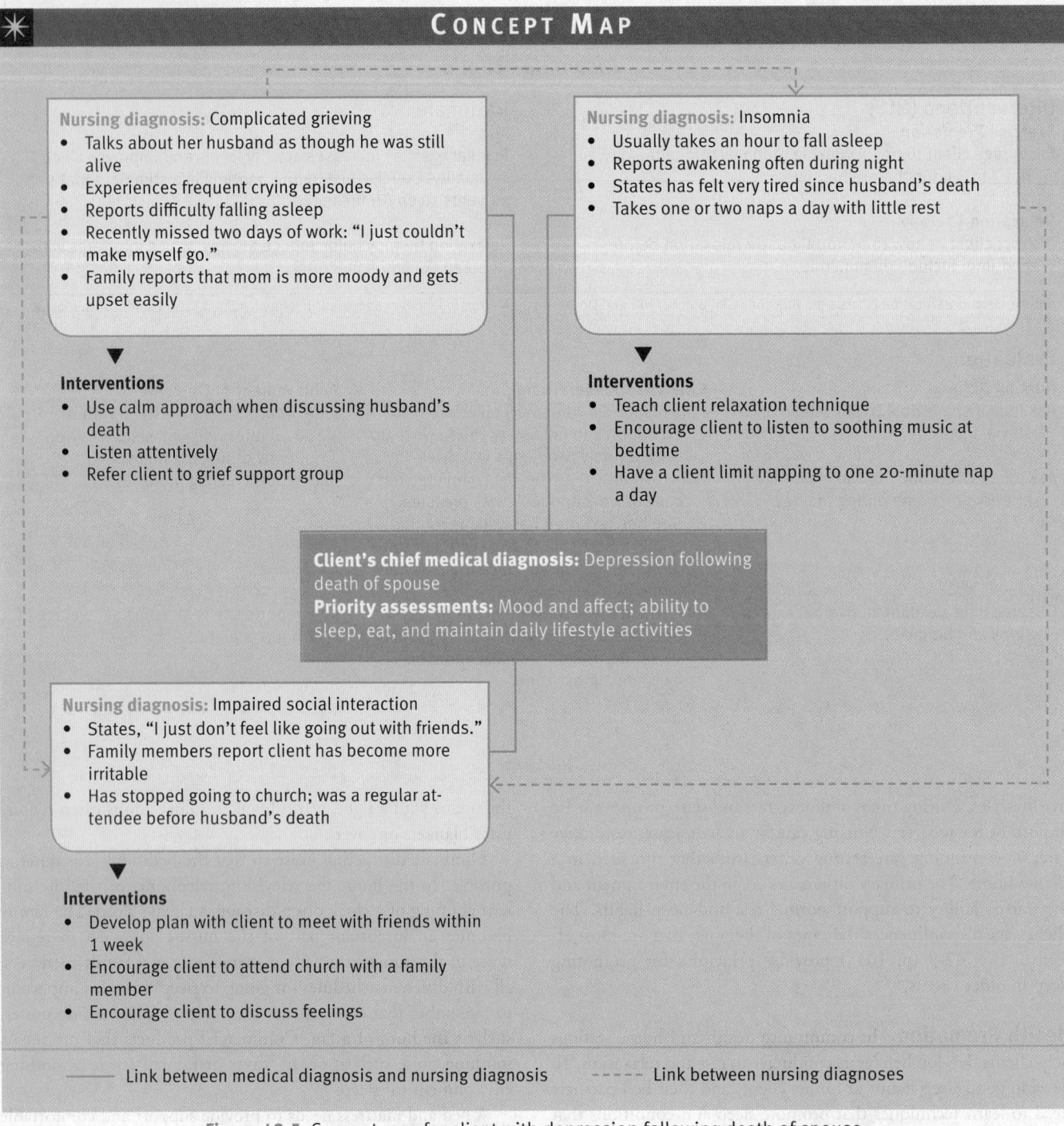

Nursing diagnosis: Complicated grieving
- Talks about her husband as though he was still alive
- Experiences frequent crying episodes
- Reports difficulty falling asleep
- Recently missed two days of work: "I just couldn't make myself go."
- Family reports that mom is more moody and gets upset easily

Interventions
- Use calm approach when discussing husband's death
- Listen attentively
- Refer client to grief support group

Nursing diagnosis: Insomnia
- Usually takes an hour to fall asleep
- Reports awakening often during night
- States has felt very tired since husband's death
- Takes one or two naps a day with little rest

Interventions
- Teach client relaxation technique
- Encourage client to listen to soothing music at bedtime
- Have a client limit napping to one 20-minute nap a day

Client's chief medical diagnosis: Depression following death of spouse
Priority assessments: Mood and affect; ability to sleep, eat, and maintain daily lifestyle activities

Nursing diagnosis: Impaired social interaction
- States, "I just don't feel like going out with friends."
- Family members report client has become more irritable
- Has stopped going to church; was a regular attendee before husband's death

Interventions
- Develop plan with client to meet with friends within 1 week
- Encourage client to attend church with a family member
- Encourage client to discuss feelings

——— Link between medical diagnosis and nursing diagnosis   - - - - Link between nursing diagnoses

Figure 42-5 Concept map for client with depression following death of spouse.

important for persons to go to sleep when they feel fatigued or sleepy. Going to bed while fully awake and thinking about other things often causes insomnia and interferes with the bed as a stimulus for sleep. Newborns and infants sleep through so much of the day that a specific routine is hardly necessary. However, quieting activities, such as holding them snugly in blankets, singing or talking softly, and gentle rocking, help infants fall asleep.

A bedtime routine (e.g., same hour for bedtime, snack, or quiet activity) used consistently helps young children avoid delaying sleep. Parents need to reinforce patterns of preparing for

bedtime. Quiet activities such as reading stories, coloring, allowing children to sit in a parent's lap while listening to music or listening to a prayer are routines that are often associated with preparing for bed.

Adults need to avoid excessive mental stimulation just before bedtime. Reading a light novel, watching an enjoyable television program, or listening to music helps a person relax. Relaxation exercises such as slow, deep breathing for 1 or 2 minutes relieve tension and prepare the body for rest (see Chapter 43). Guided imagery and praying also promote sleep for some clients.

✳ BOX 42-9   FOCUS ON OLDER ADULTS

Promoting Sleep

Sleep-Wake Pattern

- Maintain a regular bedtime and wake-up schedule (National Guideline Clearinghouse, 2006).
- Eliminate naps unless they are a routine part of the schedule.
- If naps are taken, limit to 20 minutes or less twice a day.
- Go to bed when sleepy.
- Use warm bath and relaxation techniques (Meiner and Lueckenotte, 2006).
- If unable to sleep in 15 to 30 minutes, get out of bed.

Environment

- Sleep where you sleep best.
- Keep noise to minimum; use soft music to mask noise if necessary.
- Use night-light, and keep path to bathroom free of obstacles.
- Set room temperature to preference; use socks to promote warmth.
- Listen to relaxing music (Hoffman, 2003).

Medications

- Use sedatives and hypnotics as last resort and then only short term if absolutely necessary (Maur, 2005).
- Adjust medications being taken for other conditions, and assess for drug interactions that may cause insomnia or excessive daytime sleepiness (EDS).

Diet

- Limit alcohol, caffeine, and nicotine in late afternoon and evening (National Guideline Clearinghouse, 2006).
- Consume carbohydrates or milk as a light snack before bedtime (Meiner and Lueckenotte, 2006).
- Decrease fluids 2 to 4 hours before sleep (Meiner and Lueckenotte, 2006).

Physiological/Illness Factors

- Elevate head of bed, and provide extra pillows as preferred.
- Use analgesics 30 minutes before bed to ease aches and pains.
- Use therapeutics to control symptoms of chronic conditions as prescribed (Maur, 2005).

✳ BOX 42-10   CLIENT TEACHING

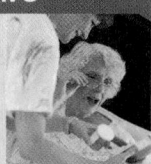

Sleep Hygiene Habits

Objective

- Client will follow proper sleep hygiene habits at home.

Teaching Strategies

- Instruct client to try to exercise daily, preferably in morning or afternoon, and to avoid vigorous exercise in the evening within 2 hours of bedtime.
- Caution client against sleeping long hours during weekends or holidays to prevent disturbance of normal sleep-wake cycle.
- Explain that if possible, not to use the bedroom for intensive studying, snacking, TV watching, or other nonsleep activity, besides sex.
- Explain that client needs to try to avoid worrisome thinking when going to bed and to use relaxation exercises.
- Advise to get out of bed and do some quiet activity until feeling sleepy enough to go back to bed if client does not fall asleep within 30 minutes of going to bed.
- Recommend client limit caffeine to morning coffee and limit alcohol intake (more than 1 to 2 drinks a day interrupts sleep cycle).
- Ask client to examine environment. Instruct that use of earplugs and eyeshades may be helpful.
- Instruct client to avoid heavy meals for 3 hours before bedtime; a light snack may help.

Evaluation

- Have client complete sleep-wake log for 1 week, and compare it with previous sleep-wake log.
- Ask client to periodically complete visual analog or sleep rating scale for perceptions of quality of sleep.

At home discourage clients from trying to finish office work or resolve family problems before bedtime. The bedroom is not a place to work, and clients need to always associate it with sleep. Working toward a consistent time for sleep and wakening helps most clients gain a healthy sleep pattern and strengthens the rhythm of the sleep-wake cycle.

Promoting Safety. For any client prone to confusion or falls, safety is critical. A small night-light assists the client in orienting to the room environment before going to the bathroom. Beds set lower to the floor lessen the chance of a person falling when first standing. Instruct clients to remove clutter and throw rugs from the path used to walk from the bed to the bathroom. If a client needs assistance in ambulating from a bed to the bathroom, place a small bell at the bedside to call family members. Sleepwalkers are unaware of their surroundings and are slow to react, increasing

the risk of falls. Do not startle sleepwalkers but instead gently awaken them and lead them back to bed.

Infants' beds need to be safe. To reduce the chance of suffocation, do not place pillows, stuffed toys, or the ends of loose blankets in cribs. Loose-fitting plastic mattress covers are dangerous because infants will pull them over their faces and suffocate. Parents usually place infants on their back to prevent suffocation.

Promoting Comfort. People fall asleep only after feeling comfortable and relaxed (Bulechek and others, 2008). Minor irritants often keep clients awake. Soft cotton nightclothes keep infants or small children warm and comfortable. Instruct clients to wear loose-fitting nightwear. An extra blanket is sometimes all that is necessary to prevent a person from feeling chilled and being unable to fall asleep. Clients need to void before retiring so they are not kept awake by a full bladder.

Establishing Periods of Rest and Sleep. In the home it helps to encourage clients to stay physically active during the day so that they are more likely to sleep at night. Increasing daytime activity lessens problems with falling asleep.

In the home setting the nurse frequently cares for clients with chronic debilitating disease. The nursing care plan includes having clients set aside afternoons for rest to promote optimal health. The nurse helps adjust medication schedules, instructs clients to

---

✳ BOX 42-11   CULTURAL ASPECTS OF CARE

Co-sleeping

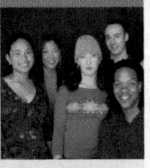

Practices and patterns of sleep and rest vary among cultures. Culture and biology influence the development of sleep problems in children. Sleep patterns, bedtime routines, sleep aids, and sleep arrangements are a component of the cultural practices related to the use of space and interaction distances. Traditionally experts recommend having infants and children sleep in their own beds. Co-sleeping, where infants and children sleep with their parents, is a culturally preferred habit. Co-sleeping is more common in nonindustrialized countries. This practice is also common in the United States with Asian and African American families. Health care personnel in the United States discourage this practice because of safety issues even though research does not show that the practice is unsafe. American culture promotes independence in childhood. Co-sleeping does not promote this independence, and thus health care workers discourage it. As a nurse, be culturally sensitive when discussing co-sleeping practices with parents and developing sleeping plans for children. The type of bed for a child will also vary. Some Native American tribes use a cradle board for infants, whereas American Samoan infants sleep on a pandanus mat covered with a blanket. These approaches lessen the child's anxiety and create a strong sense of security.

Implications for Practice

- Complete a thorough sleep assessment of the child and family.
- Discuss the risks of co-sleeping with parents. During the discussion remain culturally sensitive and respectful of the parents' views.
- Co-sleeping affects the infant's normal sleep pattern by decreasing slow wave sleep and increasing the number of nighttime arousals.
- Co-sleeping has been linked to increased risk of sudden infant death syndrome (SIDS) under certain conditions such as parental smoking and alcohol or drug use.
- Instruct parents that practice co-sleeping to avoid using alcohol or drugs that impair arousal. Decreased arousal prevents the parents from awakening if the child is having problems.
- Co-sleeping should occur only with parents and not another adult or child.
- Encourage the parents to use light sleeping clothes, to keep the room temperature comfortable, and to not bundle the child tightly or in too many clothes.

Data from Andrews MM, Boyle JS: *Transcultural concepts in nursing care*, ed 4, Philadelphia, 2003, Lippincott; Davis KF and others: Sleep in infants and young children. I. Normal sleep, *J Pediatr Health Care* 18(2):65, 2004; Giger JN, Davidhizar RE: *Transcultural nursing: assessment and intervention*, ed 4, St. Louis, 2004, Mosby; and Jenni OG, O'Connor BB: Children's sleep: an interplay between culture and biology, *Pediatrics* 115(1):204, 2005.

regularly void before rest periods, and suggests unplugging the telephone so that rest periods are uninterrupted.

Stress Reduction. The inability to sleep because of emotional stress also makes a person feel irritable and tense. When clients feel emotionally upset, encourage them to try not to force sleep. Otherwise, insomnia frequently develops, and soon bed-

time is associated with the inability to relax. Encourage a client who has difficulty falling asleep to get up and pursue a relaxing activity, such as sewing or reading, rather than staying in bed and thinking about sleep.

Preschoolers have bedtime fears (fear of the dark or strange noises), awaken during the night, or have nightmares. After nightmares, the parent enters the child's room immediately and talks to the child briefly about fears to provide a cooling-down period. One approach is to comfort children and leave them in their own beds so that their fears are not used as excuses to delay bedtime. Keeping a light on in the room will also help some children. Cultural tradition causes families to approach sleep practices differently (Box 42-11). A nurse respects those that differ from traditional recommendations.

Bedtime Snacks. Some persons enjoy bedtime snacks, whereas others cannot sleep after eating. A dairy product snack such as warm milk or cocoa that contains L-tryptophan is often helpful in promoting sleep. A full meal before bedtime often causes gastrointestinal upset and interferes with the ability to fall asleep.

Encourage clients not to drink or ingest caffeine before bedtime. Coffee, tea, cola, and chocolate act as stimulants, causing a person to stay awake or awaken throughout the night. Coffee, tea, colas, and alcohol act as diuretics and cause a person to awaken in the night to void (National Guideline Clearinghouse, 2006).

Infants require special measures to minimize nighttime awakenings for feeding. It is common for children to have a need for middle-of-the-night bottle-feeding or breast-feeding. Hockenberry and Wilson (2006) recommend offering the last feeding as late as possible. Tell parents not to give infants bottles in bed.

Pharmacological Approaches. Melatonin is a neurohormone produced in the brain that helps control circadian rhythms and promote sleep (Scheer and others, 2005). It is a popular nutritional supplement to aid sleep. The recommended dosage is 0.3 to 1 mg taken 2 hours before bedtime. Older adults who have decreased levels of melatonin find melatonin more beneficial as a sleep aid (Scheer and others, 2005). There are several other herbal products that assist in sleep. Valerian is effective in mild insomnia. It effects release of neurotransmitters and produces very mild sedation (Buysse and others, 2005). Kava helps promote sleep in clients who have sleep problems related to anxiety. Kava needs to be used cautiously because of its potential toxic effects on the liver (Morin and others, 2007). Chamomile, passionflower, lemon balm, and lavender are other herbal products that have mild sedative effects (Elliott, 2001). Caution clients about the dosage and use of herbal compounds because the U.S. Food and Drug Administration (FDA) does not regulate them. Herbal compounds may create interactions with prescribed medication, and clients need to avoid using these together (Meiner and Lueckenotte, 2006) (see Chapter 35).

The use of nonprescription sleeping medications is not advisable. Clients need to learn the risks of such drugs. Over the long term, these drugs lead to further sleep disruption even when they initially seemed to be effective. Caution older adults about using over-the-counter antihistamines because of their long duration of action that can cause confusion, constipation, urinary retention, and increased risk of falls (Nagel and others, 2003). Help clients use behavioral and proper sleep hygiene measures to establish sleep patterns that do not require the use of drugs.

BOX 42-12 Control of Noise in the Hospital

- Close doors to clients' room when possible.
- Keep doors to work areas on unit closed when in use.
- Reduce volume of nearby telephone and paging equipment.
- Wear rubber-soled shoes. Avoid clogs.
- Turn off bedside oxygen and other equipment that is not in use.
- Turn down alarms and beeps on bedside monitoring equipment.
- Turn off room TV and radio unless client prefers soft music.
- Avoid abrupt loud noise such as flushing a toilet or moving a bed.
- Keep necessary conversations at low levels, particularly at night.
- Conduct conversations and reports in a private area away from client rooms.

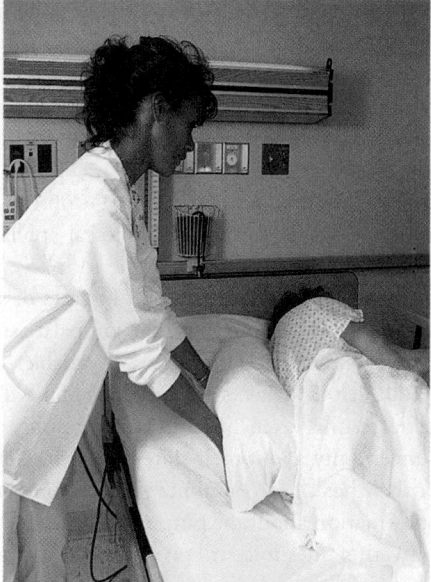

Figure 42-6 Positioning client for sleep.

Acute Care. Clients in an acute care setting have their normal rest and sleep routine disrupted, which generally leads to sleep problems. In this setting the nursing interventions focus on controlling factors in the environment that disrupt sleep, relieving physiological or psychological disruptions to sleep, and providing for uninterrupted rest and sleep periods for the client. The "Evaluating Excessive Sleepiness in the Older Adult" practice guideline is based on the principle that nurses have to individualize an effective strategy based on client needs and that sleep medications are a last-resort intervention (National Guideline Clearinghouse, 2006).

Environmental Controls. In a hospital the nurse controls the environment in several ways. Close the curtains between clients in semiprivate rooms. Dim lights on a hospital nursing unit at night. One of the biggest problems for clients in the hospital is noise. Important ways to reduce noise are to conduct conversations and reports in a private area away from client rooms and to keep necessary conversations to a minimum, especially at night (Cmiel and others, 2004). Additional ways to control noise in the hospital are listed in Box 42-12.

Promoting Comfort. Compared with beds at home, hospital beds are often harder and of a different height, length, or width. Keeping beds clean and dry and in a comfortable position helps clients relax. Some clients suffer painful illnesses requiring special comfort measures such as application of dry or moist heat, use of supportive dressings or splints, and proper positioning before retiring (Figure 42-6).

Establishing Periods of Rest and Sleep. In a hospital or extended care setting it is difficult to provide clients with the time needed to rest and sleep. However, you need to plan care to avoid awakening clients for nonessential tasks. Do this by scheduling assessments, treatments, procedures, and routines for times when clients are awake. For example, if a client's physical condition has been stable, avoid awakening the client to check vital signs. Allowing clients to determine the timing and methods of delivery of basic care measures will promote rest. Do not give baths and routine hygiene measures during the night for nursing convenience. Draw blood samples at a time when the client is awake. Unless maintaining a drug's therapeutic blood level is essential, give medications during waking hours. Work with the radiology department and other support services to schedule diagnostic stud-

ies and therapies at intervals that allow clients time for rest. Always try to provide the client with 2 to 3 hours of uninterrupted sleep during the night (Cmiel and others, 2004).

When the client's condition demands more frequent monitoring, plan activities to allow extended rest periods. A nurse instructs assistive personnel in the coordination of client care to reduce client disturbances. This means planning activities so that instead of a nurse or other personnel returning to the room every few minutes, the client has up to an hour or more to rest quietly. For example, if a client needs frequent dressing changes, is receiving intravenous therapy, and has drainage tubes from several sites, do not make a separate trip into the room to check each problem. Instead use a single visit to change the dressing, regulate the intravenous system, and empty the drainage tubes. Become the client's advocate for promoting optimal sleep. This means becoming a gatekeeper by postponing or rescheduling visits by family, asking consultants to reschedule visits, or questioning the frequency of certain procedures.

Promoting Safety. Clients with obstructive sleep apnea are at risk for complications while in the hospital. Surgery and anesthesia disrupt normal sleep patterns in clients. Postoperatively these clients reach deep levels of REM sleep. This deep sleep causes muscle relaxation that leads to obstructive sleep apnea (Cullen, 2001). Reducing the risk of postoperative complications for clients with obstructive sleep apnea is a safety concern (The Joint Commission, 2007). Clients with OSA who are given opioid analgesics after surgery have an increased risk of developing airway obstruction because the medications suppress normal arousal mechanisms (Cullen, 2001). Monitor the client's airway, respiratory rate, depth, and breath sounds frequently after surgery.

Recommend lifestyle changes to clients with OSA that include sleep hygiene, alcohol moderation, quitting smoking, and a weight-loss program for clients experiencing obstructive sleep apnea. (Mendez and Olson, 2006b). Teach the client to prevent sleeping in the supine position by wearing a fanny pack or tight shirt with a tennis ball on the back or elevating the head of the bed 30 to 45 degrees (Holman, 2005).

One of the most effective therapies is use of a nasal continuous positive airway pressure (CPAP) device at night, which requires a client to wear a mask over the nose. A mask delivers room air at a high pressure. The air pressure prevents airway collapse. The CPAP device is portable and effective particularly for obstructive apnea. Another treatment option is the use of an oral appliance. These appliances advance the mandible or tongue to relieve pharyngeal obstruction (Mendez and Olson, 2006b). In cases of severe sleep apnea the tonsils, uvula, or portions of the soft palate are surgically removed. Success with surgical procedures is variable.

Stress Reduction. Clients who are hospitalized for extensive diagnostic testing often have difficulty resting or sleeping because of uncertainty about their state of health. Giving clients control over their health care minimizes uncertainty and anxiety. Providing information about the purpose of procedures and routines and answering questions will give clients the peace of mind needed to rest or fall asleep. A nurse on the night shift needs to take time to sit and talk with clients unable to sleep. This helps to determine the factors keeping clients awake. Back rubs also help clients relax more thoroughly. If a sedative is indicated, confer with the physician to be sure that the lowest dosage is used initially. Discontinuing a sedative as soon as possible prevents a dependence that seriously disrupts the normal sleep cycle. Older adults' metabolism of drugs is slow, making them more vulnerable to the side effects of sedatives, hypnotics, antianxiety drugs, or analgesics.

Restorative or Continuing Care. The nursing interventions implemented in the acute care setting are also used in the restorative or continuing care environment. Controlling the environment, especially noise, establishing periods of rest and sleep, and promoting comfort are important considerations. Nursing interventions related to stress reduction and controlling physiological disturbances are also implemented in these settings. Helping a client achieve restful sleep in this environment sometimes takes a period of time.

Promoting Comfort. Providing for personal hygiene improves a client's sense of comfort. A warm bath or shower before bedtime is relaxing. Offer clients restricted to bed the opportunity to void and wash their face and hands. Toothbrushing and care of dentures also help to prepare the client for sleep. Position the client to support dependent body parts and protect pressure points. Offer a massage to aid in muscle relaxation just before the client goes to sleep (Robinson and others, 2005) (see Chapter 43).

Controlling Physiological Disturbances. For clients with physical illness, the nurse helps control symptoms that disrupt sleep. For example, a client with respiratory abnormalities sleeps with two pillows or in a semisitting position to ease the effort to breathe. The client benefits from taking prescribed bronchodilators before sleep to prevent airway obstruction. A client with a hiatal hernia also needs special care. After meals the client often experiences a burning sensation as a result of gastric reflux. To prevent sleep disturbances, have the client eat a small meal several hours before bedtime and sleep in a semisitting position. Clients with pain, nausea, or other recurrent symptoms receive any symp-tom-relieving medication timed so that the drug takes effect at bedtime. Remove or change any irritants against the client's skin such as moist dressings or drainage tubes.

Pharmacological Approaches. The liberal use of drugs to manage insomnia is quite common in American culture. Central nervous system stimulants such as amphetamines, caffeine, nicotine, terbutaline, theophylline, and pemoline need to be used sparingly and under medical management (McKenry and Salerno, 2003). In addition, withdrawal from CNS depressants such as alcohol, barbiturates, tricyclic antidepressants (amitriptyline, imipramine, and doxepin), and triazolam cause insomnia. You will need to manage these carefully.

Medications that induce sleep are called **hypnotics. Sedatives** are medications that produce a calming or soothing effect (McKenry and Salerno, 2003). Hypnotics and sedatives as sleep medications will help if used correctly. A client who takes sleep medications needs to know about their proper use, as well as the risks and possible side effects. However, long-term use of anti-anxiety, sedative, or hypnotic agents will disrupt sleep and lead to more serious problems. The Food and Drug Administration has mandated that the product labels of all sleep medications contain new safety information related to the potential adverse effects of severe allergic reactions, severe facial swelling, and complex sleep behaviors such as sleep-driving, making phone calls, and preparing and eating food while asleep (FDA, 2007).

One group of drugs considered to be relatively safe is the benzodiazepines. The benzodiazepines cause relaxation, antianxiety, and hypnotic effects by facilitating the action of neurons in the CNS that suppress responsiveness to stimulation, thereby decreasing levels of arousal (Mendelson, 2005). These medications do not cause general CNS depression as sedatives or hypnotics do and have a lower potential for abuse. Physicians prescribe this group of drugs because antianxiety effects occur at safe, nontoxic doses. In the older adult, short-acting benzodiazepines such as temazepam and triazolam are used before long-acting drugs, and the drug should not be used for more than 10 days in a row in any 30-day period (McHenry and Salerno, 2003).

Use the benzodiazepines cautiously with children under 12 years of age. These medications are contraindicated in infants less than 6 months. Pregnant clients need to avoid benzodiazepines because their use is associated with risk of congenital anomalies. Nursing mothers do not receive the drugs because they are excreted in breast milk. Initial doses are small, and increments are added gradually, based on client response, for a limited period of time. Warn clients not to take more than the prescribed dose, especially if the medication seems to become less effective after initial use. If older clients who were recently continent, ambulatory, and alert become incontinent, confused, and/or demonstrate impaired mobility, the use of benzodiazepines needs to be considered as a possible cause.

Regular use of any sleep medication often leads to tolerance and withdrawal. Rebound insomnia is a problem after stopping the medication. Immediately administering a sleeping medication when a hospitalized client complains of being unable to sleep will do the client more harm than good. Consider alternative approaches to promote sleep. Routine monitoring of client response to sleeping medications is important.

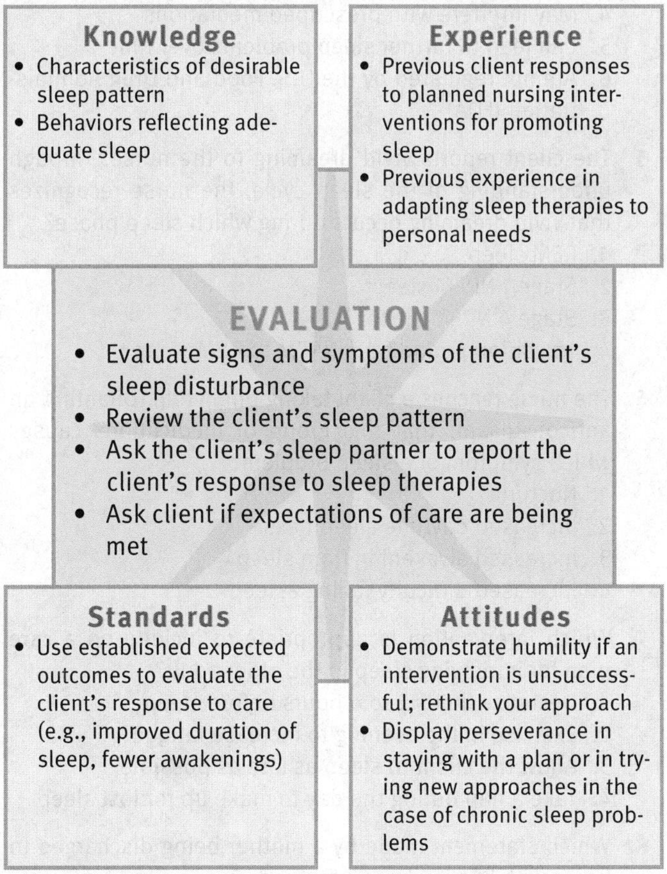

Knowledge
- Characteristics of desirable sleep pattern
- Behaviors reflecting adequate sleep

Experience
- Previous client responses to planned nursing interventions for promoting sleep
- Previous experience in adapting sleep therapies to personal needs

EVALUATION
- Evaluate signs and symptoms of the client's sleep disturbance
- Review the client's sleep pattern
- Ask the client's sleep partner to report the client's response to sleep therapies
- Ask client if expectations of care are being met

Standards
- Use established expected outcomes to evaluate the client's response to care (e.g., improved duration of sleep, fewer awakenings)

Attitudes
- Demonstrate humility if an intervention is unsuccessful; rethink your approach
- Display perseverance in staying with a plan or in trying new approaches in the case of chronic sleep problems

Figure 42-7 Critical thinking model for sleep evaluation.

◆Evaluation

With regard to problems with sleep, the client is the source for evaluating outcomes. Each client has a unique need for sleep and rest. The client is the only who will know if sleep problems are improved and which interventions or therapies are most successful in promoting sleep (Figure 42-7). To evaluate the effectiveness of nursing interventions, make comparisons with baseline sleep assessment data to evaluate if sleep has improved.

Determine whether expected outcomes have been met. Use evaluative measures shortly after a therapy has been tried (e.g., observing whether a client falls asleep after reducing noise and darkening a room). Use other evaluative measures after a client awakens from sleep (e.g., asking a client to describe the number of awakenings during the previous night). The client and bed partner usually provide accurate evaluative information. Over longer periods, use assessment tools such as the visual analog scale or sleep rating scale to determine whether sleep has progressively improved or changed.

Also evaluate the level of understanding that clients or family members gain after receiving instruction in sleep habits. You measure compliance with these practices during a home visit, when you are able to observe the environment. When expected outcomes are not met, revise the nursing measures or expected outcomes based on the client's needs or preferences. When outcomes are not met, ask questions such as "Do you feel as though you slept better when you exercised?" or "Do you feel rested when you wake up?"

If a nurse has successfully developed a good relationship with a client and has developed a therapeutic plan of care, subtle behaviors often indicate the level of the client's satisfaction. Note the absence of signs of sleep problems, such as lethargy or frequent yawning or position changes, in the client. It is important to ask the client if his or her sleep needs have been met. For example, ask the client, "Are you feeling more rested?" or "Can you tell me if you feel we have done all we can to help improve your sleep?" If the client's expectations have not been met, you will need to spend more time trying to understand the client's needs and preferences. Working closely with the client and bed partner will enable you to redefine those expectations that will be realistically met within the limits of the client's condition and treatment. You are effective in promoting rest and sleep if the client's goals and expectations are met.

✶ Key Concepts
- Sleep provides physiological and psychological restoration.
- The 24-hour sleep-wake cycle is a circadian rhythm that influences physiological function and behavior.
- The control and regulation of sleep depends on a balance between regulators within the central nervous system.
- During a typical night's sleep a person passes through four to five complete sleep cycles. Each sleep cycle contains three NREM stages of sleep and a period of REM sleep.
- The most common type of sleep disorder is insomnia.
- The hectic pace of a person's lifestyle, emotional and psychological stress, and alcohol ingestion frequently disrupt the sleep pattern.
- If a client's sleep is adequate, the nurse assesses the client's usual bedtime, normal bedtime ritual, the preferred environment for sleeping, and usual preferred rising time.
- When a client has a sleep problem, the nurse conducts a complete sleep history. Diagnosing sleep problems depends on identifying factors that impair sleep.
- When planning interventions to promote sleep, the nurse considers the usual characteristics of the client's home environment and normal lifestyle.
- A regular bedtime routine of relaxing activities prepares a person physically and mentally for sleep.
- An environment with a darkened room, reduced noise, comfortable bed, and good ventilation promotes sleep.
- Important nursing interventions for promoting sleep in the hospitalized client are establishing periods for uninterrupted sleep and rest and controlling noise levels.
- Pain or other disease symptom control is essential to promoting the ability to sleep.
- Long-term use of sleeping pills often leads to difficulty in initiating and maintaining sleep.

Critical Thinking Exercises

Julie returns to the neighborhood health clinic with her husband, David, for a follow-up visit. Julie tells you that since she started her sleep hygiene plan she feels more rested but is still having some problems sleeping because of her husband's loud snoring. Besides Julie's report of David's snoring, you note that he is overweight.

1. Based on Julie's report of David's snoring, what additional assessment data should you gather from David?

2. Based on David's reported symptoms, what problem do you suspect he might have? What action do you take at this time?

3. What recommendations do you give David to improve his sleeping?

Julie and David tell you that they are concerned about their 15-year-old daughter. Her grades in school are getting worse, and she says she is always tired.

4. What do you need to know about their daughter's sleep patterns?

5. List at least four suggestions for Julie and David to use to improve their daughter's sleep patterns.

NCLEX®-Style Review Questions

1. The nurse is gathering a sleep history from a client who is being evaluated for obstructive sleep apnea. What common symptom will the client most likely report? (Select all that apply)
   1. Headache
   2. Early wakening
   3. Impaired reasoning
   4. Excessive daytime sleepiness

2. The nurse incorporates what priority nursing intervention into a plan of care to promote sleep for a hospitalized client?
   1. Have client follow hospital routines.
   2. Avoid awakening client for nonessential tasks.
   3. Give prescribed sleeping medications at dinner.
   4. Turn television on low to late-night programming.

3. Older adults are cautioned about the use of nonprescription sleeping medications because these medications can:
   1. Cause headaches and nausea
   2. Be expensive and difficult to obtain
   3. Cause severe depression and anxiety
   4. Lead to further sleep disruption even when they initially seemed to be effective

4. The nurse is providing health teaching for a client using herbal compounds such as valerian for sleep. What points need to be included? (Choose all that apply.)
   1. Can cause urinary retention
   2. Should not be used indefinitely
   3. May cause diarrhea and anxiety
   4. May interfere with prescribed mediations
   5. Can lead to further sleep problems over time
   6. Are not regulated by the U.S. Food and Drug Administration (FDA)

5. The client reports vivid dreaming to the nurse. Through understanding of the sleep cycle, the nurse recognizes that vivid dreaming occurs during which sleep phase?
   1. REM sleep
   2. Stage 1 NREM sleep
   3. Stage 4 NREM sleep
   4. Transition period from NREM to REM sleep

6. The nurse teaches a client taking phenytoin (Dilantin), an anticonvulsant, that this group of medications causes which symptom of a sleep problem?
   1. Nocturia
   2. Increased daytime sleepiness
   3. Increased awakening from sleep
   4. Increased difficulty falling asleep

7. Which intervention is appropriate to include on a care plan for improving sleep in the older adult?
   1. Decrease fluids 2 to 4 hours before sleep
   2. Exercise in the evening to increase fatigue
   3. Allow the client to sleep as late as possible
   4. Take a nap during the day to make up for lost sleep

8. Which statement made by a mother being discharged to home with her newborn infant indicates a need for further teaching?
   1. "I won't put the baby to bed with a bottle."
   2. "For the first few weeks, we are putting the cradle in our room."
   3. "My grandmother told me that babies sleep better on their stomachs."
   4. "I know I will have to get up during the night to feed the baby when he wakes up."

9. The nurse is developing a plan of care for a client experiencing narcolepsy. Which intervention is appropriate to include on the plan?
   1. Instruct the client to increase carbohydrates in the diet.
   2. Have client limit fluid intake 2 hours before bedtime.
   3. Preserve energy by limiting exercise to morning hours.
   4. Encourage client to take one or two 20-minute naps during the day.

10. What nursing measure promotes sleep in school-age children?
   1. Encourage evening exercise.
   2. Encourage television viewing.
   3. Make sure the room is dark and quiet.
   4. Encourage quiet activities before bedtime.

43 | Pain Management

✳ OBJECTIVES

Mastery of content in this chapter will enable the student to:

- Discuss common misconceptions about pain.
- Describe the physiology of pain.
- Identify components of the pain experience.
- Explain how the physiology of pain relates to selecting interventions for pain relief.
- Describe the components of pain assessment.
- Perform an assessment of a client experiencing pain.
- Explain how cultural factors influence the pain experience.

- Describe guidelines for selecting and individualizing pain interventions.
- Explain various pharmacological approaches to treating pain.
- Describe applications for use of nonpharmacological pain interventions.
- Discuss nursing implications for administering analgesics.
- Identify barriers to effective pain management.
- Evaluate a client's response to pain interventions.

✳ MEDIA RESOURCES ✳ KEY TERMS

Companion CD
- NCLEX®-Style Review Questions
- Audio Glossary
- Interactive Learning Activities
- English/Spanish Glossary

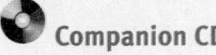 **Website**
- NCLEX®-Style Review Questions
- Audio Glossary
- English/Spanish Glossary
- Interactive Learning Activities
- Weblinks
- Audio Summaries

Acupressure, p. 1073
Acute pain, p. 1055
Addiction, p. 1081
Adjuvants/coanalgesics, p. 1073
Analgesics, p. 1073
Biofeedback, p. 1071
Breakthrough pain, p. 1080
Chronic pain, p. 1055
Cutaneous stimulation, p. 1071
Drug tolerance, p. 1081
Epidural analgesia, p. 1077
Epidural space, p. 1077
Guided imagery, p. 1071
Idiopathic pain, p. 1056
Local anesthesia, p. 1077
Modulation, p. 1053
Neurotransmitters, p. 1052
Nociceptor, p. 1052
Opioids, p. 1073

Pain, p. 1052
Pain threshold, p. 1054
Pain tolerance, p. 1055
Patient-controlled analgesia (PCA), p. 1076
Perception, p. 1053
Perineural infusion, p. 1077
Physical dependence, p. 1081
Placebos, p. 1081
Prostaglandins, p. 1052
Pruritus, p. 1078
Pseudoaddiction, p. 1055
Pseudotolerance, p. 1081
Regional anesthesia, p. 1077
Relaxation, p. 1071
Transcutaneous electrical nerve stimulation (TENS), p. 1073
Transduction, p. 1052
Transmission, p. 1052

Everyone has experienced some type or degree of **pain**. Although pain is the most common reason people seek health care, it is not well understood. A person in pain feels distress or suffering and seeks relief. However, you as the nurse cannot see or feel the client's pain. Pain is purely subjective; no two persons experience pain in the same way, and no two painful events create identical responses or feelings in a person. The International Association for the Study of Pain (IASP) (1979) defined pain as "an unpleasant, subjective sensory *and* emotional experience associated with actual or potential tissue damage, or described in terms of such damage." Thus physical pain can cause psychological pain and vise versa.

Congress declared 2000 through 2010 the Decade of Pain Control and Research, yet pain continues to be a leading public health problem in the United States (American Pain Foundation, 2005). Providing pain relief is a basic human right and is in the Pain Care Bill of Rights (American Pain Foundation, 2001). The American Bar Association (2000) declared pain relief a basic legal right. Nurses are legally and ethically responsible for managing pain and relieving suffering.

When caring for clients in pain consider the nurse-client relationship, compassion, and respect (Ferrell, 2005). Caring for clients in pain requires recognition that their pain can and should be relieved (Ferrell, 2005). Clients in pain are certain of their pain, whereas their caregivers are uncertain because pain cannot be objectively measured. Providing nursing care to clients suffering pain is not simply "doing for," rather it is making a commitment to "be with" the client (Ferrell, 2005). Effective communication among the client, family, and professional caregivers is essential if you are to achieve adequate pain management (Kimberlin and others, 2004; Manias and others, 2005). You show respect for a client in pain when you accept McCaffery's definition of pain (1979): "Pain is whatever the experiencing person says it is, existing whenever he says it does." Effective pain management improves quality of life, reduces physical discomfort, promotes earlier mobilization and return to work, results in fewer hospital/clinic visits, and shortens hospital stays, thus reducing health care costs.

Scientific Knowledge Base

Historically pain has been an integral component of the human experience. Traditionally pain was simply a symptom of an illness or condition. However, we now consider pain to be a separate disease.

Nature of Pain

The pain experience is complex, involving physical, emotional and cognitive components. Pain is subjective and highly individualized. The stimulus for pain is physical and/or mental in nature. Pain is exhausting and demands a person's energy. It interferes with personal relationships and influences the meaning of life (Davis, 2002). You cannot objectively measure pain, such as with a blood test. Only the client knows whether pain is present and what the experience is like. It is not the responsibility of clients to prove that they are in pain, it is the nurse's responsibility to accept clients' report of pain (American Pain Society [APS], 2003).

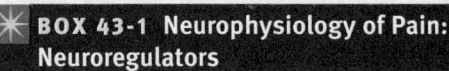

BOX 43-1   Neurophysiology of Pain: Neuroregulators

Neurotransmitters (Excitatory)
Substance P
Found in the pain neurons of the dorsal horn (excitatory peptide)
Needed to transmit pain impulses from the periphery to higher brain centers
Causes vasodilation and edema

Serotonin
Released from the brain stem and dorsal horn to inhibit pain transmission

Prostaglandins
Generated from the breakdown of phospholipids in cell membranes
Thought to increase sensitivity to pain

Bradykinin
Released from plasma that leaks from surrounding blood vessels at the site of tissue injury
Binds to receptors on peripheral nerves, increasing pain stimuli
Binds to cells that cause the chain reaction producing prostaglandins

Neuromodulators (Inhibitory)
Are the body's natural supply of morphine-like substances
Activated by stress and pain
Located within the brain, spinal cord, and gastrointestinal tract
Cause analgesia when they attach to opiate receptors in the brain
Present in higher levels in people who have less pain than others with a similar injury

Physiology of Pain

There are four physiological processes of nociceptive (normal) pain: transduction, transmission, perception, and modulation (McCaffery and Pasero, 1999). A client in pain cannot discriminate among the processes. However, understanding each process will help you recognize factors that cause pain, symptoms that accompany pain, and the rationale for selected therapies.

Thermal, chemical, or mechanical stimuli usually cause pain. The energy of these stimuli is converted to electrical energy. This energy conversion is **transduction.** Transduction begins in the periphery when a pain-producing stimulus sends an impulse across a sensory peripheral pain nerve fiber (**nociceptor**), initiating an action potential. Once transduction is complete, **transmission** of the pain impulse begins.

Cellular damage caused by thermal, mechanical, or chemical stimuli results in the release of excitatory **neurotransmitters** such as **prostaglandins,** bradykinin, potassium, histamine, and substance P (Box 43-1). These pain-sensitizing substances surround the pain fibers in the extracellular fluid, spreading the pain message and causing an inflammatory response (Renn and Dorsey, 2005). The pain fiber enters the spinal cord via the dorsal horn and travels one of several routes until ending within the gray matter of the spinal cord. At the dorsal horn substance P is released, causing a synaptic transmission from the afferent (sensory) peripheral nerve to spinothalamic tract nerves, which cross to the opposite side (Wall and Melzack, 1999) (Figure 43-1).

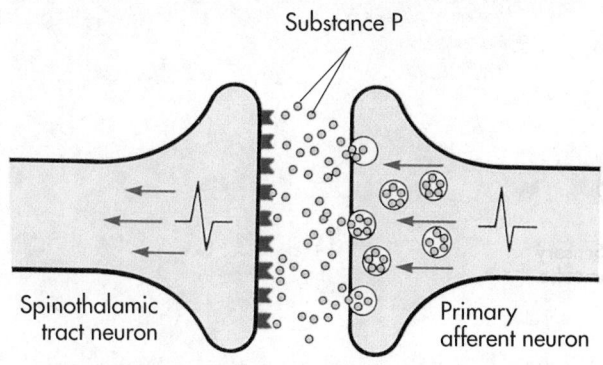

Figure 43-1 Substance P and other neurotransmitters are released from primary afferent fibers that terminate in the dorsal horn of the spinal cord. (From Paice J: Unraveling the mystery of pain, *Oncol Nurs Forum* 18[5]:843, 1991.)

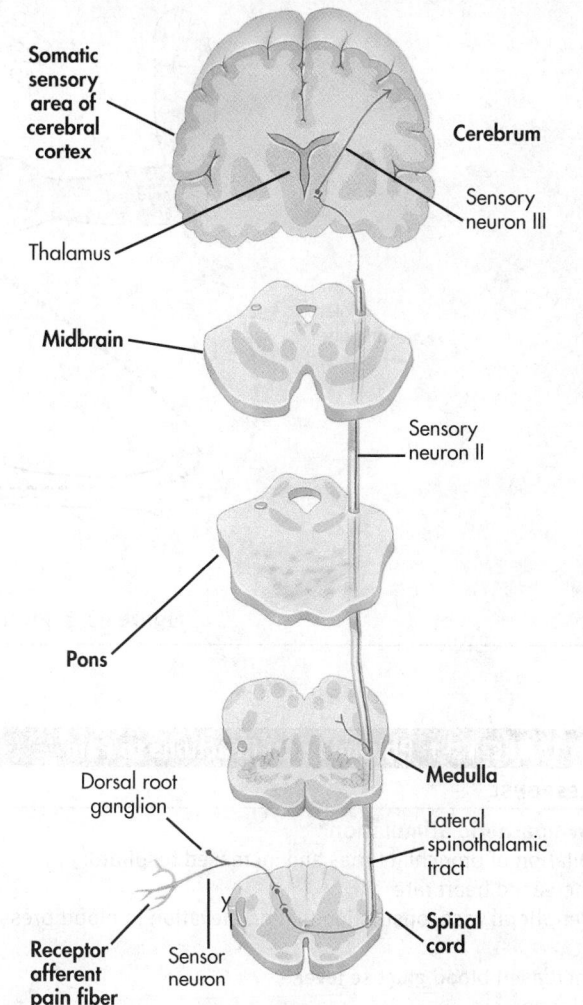

Figure 43-2 Spinothalamic pathway that conducts pain stimuli to the brain.

Nerve impulses resulting from the painful stimulus travel along afferent (sensory) peripheral nerve fibers. Two types of peripheral nerve fibers conduct painful stimuli: the fast, myelinated A-delta fibers and the very small, slow, unmyelinated C fibers. The A fibers send sharp, localized, and distinct sensations that localize the source of the pain and detect its intensity. The C fibers relay impulses that are poorly localized, burning, and persistent (Wall and Melzack, 1999). For example, after stepping on a nail, a person initially feels a sharp, localized pain, which is a result of A-fiber transmission. Within a few seconds, the pain becomes more diffuse and widespread, until the whole foot aches because of C-fiber innervation.

Along the spinothalamic tract, pain impulses travel up the spinal cord. Figure 43-2 shows the normal pain reception pathway. After the pain impulse ascends the spinal cord, the thalamus transmits information to higher centers in the brain, including the reticular formation, limbic system, somatosensory cortex, and association cortex. Once a pain stimulus reaches the cerebral cortex, the brain interprets the quality of the pain and processes information from past experience, knowledge, and cultural associations in the perception of the pain (McCaffery and Pasero, 1999). **Perception** is the point at which a person is aware of pain. The somatosensory cortex identifies the location and intensity of pain, and the association cortex, primarily the limbic system, determines how we feel about the pain. There is no single pain center.

As a person becomes aware of pain, a complex reaction unfolds. Psychological and cognitive factors interact with neurophysiological ones in the perception of pain. Perception gives awareness and meaning to pain so that a person then reacts. The reaction to pain is the physiological and behavioral responses that occur after an individual perceives pain. Recently *N*-methyl-D-aspartate (NMDA) receptors have been implicated in pain perception (Arbuck and others, 2004).

Once the brain perceives pain, there is a release of inhibitory neurotransmitters (see Box 43-1) such as endogenous opioids (endorphins and enkephalins), serotonin (5HT), norepinephrine, and gamma aminobutyric acid (GABA), which work to hinder the transmission of pain and help produce an analgesic effect

(McCaffery and Pasero, 1999). This inhibition of the pain impulse is the fourth phase of the nociceptive process known as **modulation.**

A protective reflex response also occurs with pain reception (Figure 43-3). A-delta fibers send sensory impulses to the spinal cord, where they synapse with spinal motor neurons. The motor impulses travel via a reflex arc along efferent (motor) nerve fibers back to a peripheral muscle near the site of stimulation, thus bypassing the brain. Contraction of the muscle leads to a protective withdrawal from the source of pain. For example, when you accidentally touch a hot iron, you feel a burning sensation, but the hand also reflexively withdraws from the iron's surface. This reflex is usually absent, below the injury, in clients with spinal cord injuries. However, spinal cord–injured clients still experience pain above the level of injury (Finnerup and Jensen, 2004).

Gate-Control Theory of Pain. Melzack and Wall's gate-control theory (1965) was the first to suggest that pain has emotional and cognitive components in addition to a physical sensation. They also suggested that gating mechanisms located along the central nervous system can regulate or even block pain impulses.

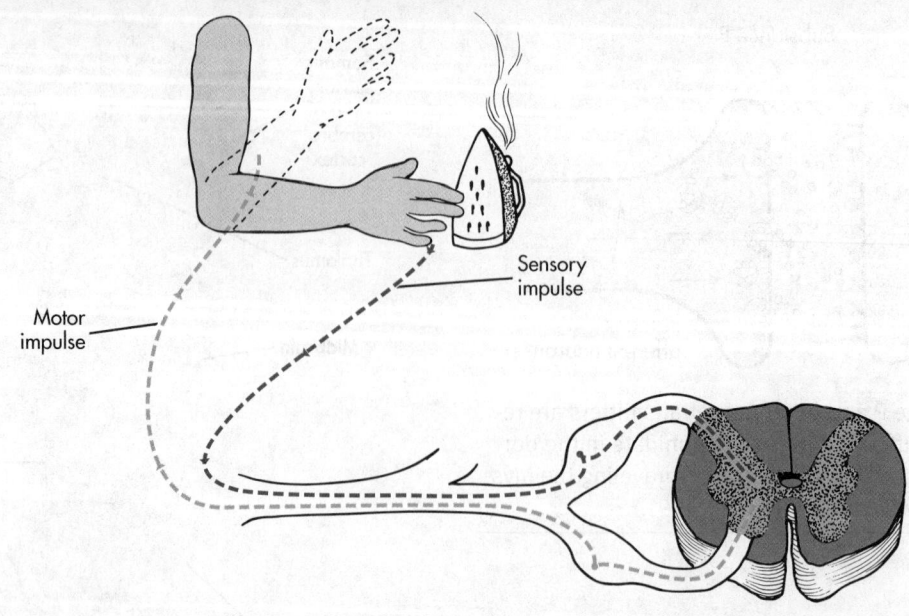

Motor
impulse

Sensory
impulse

Figure 43-3 Protective reflex to pain stimulus.

✳ **TABLE 43-1   Physiological Reactions to Pain**

RESPONSE	CAUSE OR EFFECT
Sympathetic Stimulation*	
Dilation of bronchial tubes and increased respiratory rate	Provides increased oxygen intake
Increased heart rate	Provides increased oxygen transport
Peripheral vasoconstriction (pallor, elevation in blood pressure)	Elevates blood pressure with shift of blood supply from periphery and viscera to skeletal muscles and brain
Increased blood glucose level	Provides additional energy
Diaphoresis	Controls body temperature during stress
Increased muscle tension	Prepares muscles for action
Dilation of pupils	Affords better vision
Decreased gastrointestinal motility	Frees energy for more immediate activity
Parasympathetic Stimulation†	
Pallor	Causes blood supply to shift away from periphery
Muscle tension	Results from fatigue
Decreased heart rate and blood pressure	Results from vagal stimulation
Rapid, irregular breathing	Causes body defenses to fail under prolonged stress of pain

*Pain of low to moderate intensity and superficial pain.
†Severe or deep pain.

The theory suggests that pain impulses pass through when a gate is open and are blocked when a gate is closed. Closing the gate is the basis for nonpharmacological pain-relief interventions. By understanding what influences these gates (physiology, emotional and cognitive processes), you will gain a useful conceptual framework for pain management. For example, stress, exercise, and other factors increase the release of endorphins, raising an individual's **pain threshold** (the point at which a person feels pain). Because the amount of circulating substances varies with every individual, the response to pain will be different.

Physiological Responses. As pain impulses ascend the spinal cord toward the brain stem and thalamus, the autonomic nervous system becomes stimulated as part of the stress response. Pain of low to moderate intensity and superficial pain elicit the fight-or-flight reaction of the general adaptation syndrome (see Chapter 31). Stimulation of the sympathetic branch of the autonomic nervous system results in physiological responses (Table 43-1). If the pain is continuous, severe, or deep, typically involving the visceral organs (e.g., with a myocardial infarction or colic from gallbladder or renal stones), the parasympathetic nervous system goes into action. Sustained physiological responses to pain sometimes seriously harm individuals. Except in cases of severe traumatic pain, which sends a person into shock, most people reach a level of adaptation in which physical signs return to normal. Thus clients in pain will *not* always have changes in their vital signs. Changes in vital signs are more often indicative of problems other than pain.

Behavioral Responses. If left untreated or unrelieved, pain significantly alters the quality of a person's life. Pain interferes with every aspect of a person's life, which helps explain why the management of pain is such a challenge. Pain threatens physical and psychological well-being. Some clients choose not to report pain if they believe their pain inconveniences others or if it signals loss of self-control. Some clients will endure severe pain without assistance. Encourage your clients to accept pain-relieving measures so that they remain active and continue to maintain nutritional intake. In contrast, other clients seek relief before pain occurs, having learned that pain is easier to prevent than to treat. A client's ability to tolerate pain significantly influences your perceptions of the degree of the client's discomfort. Clients who have a low **pain tolerance** (level of pain a person is willing to put up with) are sometimes inaccurately perceived as whiners. Teach clients the importance of reporting their pain sooner rather than later.

Body movements and facial expressions indicating pain include clenching the teeth, holding the painful part, bent posture, and grimaces. Some clients cry or moan, are restless, or make frequent requests of a nurse. You will soon learn to recognize patterns of behavior that reflect pain. This becomes especially important in clients who are unable to report their pain, such as the cognitively impaired. However, lack of pain expression does not necessarily mean that the client is not experiencing pain (McCaffery and Pasero, 1999).

Types of Pain

Pain is categorized by duration (acute or chronic) or by pathologic condition (e.g., cancer or neuropathic).

Acute/Transient Pain.
Acute pain is protective, has an identifiable cause, is of short duration, and has limited tissue damage and emotional response. Acute pain eventually resolves with or without treatment after a damaged area heals. Because acute pain has a predictable ending (healing) and an identifiable cause, this usually results in a willingness by health team members to treat acute pain aggressively. It is important to realize that unrelieved acute pain can progress to chronic pain (Cousins and Power, 2003; Kehlet and others, 2006).

Acute pain seriously threatens a client's recovery by resulting in prolonged hospitalization, increased risks of complications from immobility (see Chapter 37), and delayed rehabilitation. Physical or psychological progress is delayed as long as acute pain persists, because the client focuses all energy on pain relief. Efforts aimed at teaching and motivating the client toward self-care are often hampered until the pain is successfully managed. Complete pain relief is not always achievable, but reducing pain to a tolerable level is realistic. Thus a primary nursing goal is to provide pain relief that allows clients to participate in their recovery.

Chronic/Persistent Pain.
An important difference between chronic pain and acute pain is that chronic pain is not protective and thus serves no purpose. **Chronic pain** lasts longer than anticipated, does *not* always have an identifiable cause, and leads to great personal suffering. Chronic pain is noncancerous or cancerous. Examples of chronic noncancer pain include arthritis, low back pain, myofascial pain, headache, and peripheral neuropathy. Chronic noncancer pains are usually non–life threatening. Some-

times an injured area has healed long ago, yet the pain is ongoing and does not respond to treatment.

The possible unknown cause of noncancer pain, combined with the unrelenting pain and uncertainty of its duration, frustrates the client, frequently leading to psychological depression and perhaps suicide. Chronic noncancer pain is a major cause of psychological and physical disability, leading to problems such as loss of a job, inability to perform simple daily activities, sexual dysfunction, and social isolation from family and friends.

The person with chronic noncancer pain often does not show obvious symptoms and does not adapt to the pain; rather, the person seems to suffer more with time because of physical and mental exhaustion. Associated symptoms of chronic noncancer pain include fatigue, insomnia, anorexia, weight loss, apathy, hopelessness, and anger. Chronic noncancer pain creates the insecurity of never knowing how one will feel from day to day. If there is no objective evidence to confirm the existence of pain (a subjective experience) the "burden of proof" lies with the client (Shaw, 2006). Health care workers are usually less willing to treat chronic noncancer pain with opioids, although a recent policy statement (APS, 2002) supports the use of opioids for noncancer pain. In addition, the American Society of Anesthesiologists (1997) developed "Practice Guidelines for Chronic Pain Management," which includes the use of opioids. Often a person with chronic noncancer pain who "doctor shops" is labeled a drug seeker, when they are actually seeking pain relief. This is **pseudoaddiction.** Nurses need to discourage clients from having multiple health care providers for treating pain and refer them to pain experts. Pain centers offer a holistic approach to chronic pain using nonpharmacological as well as pharmacological strategies for pain management.

Chronic Episodic Pain.
Pain that occurs sporadically over an extended duration of time is episodic pain. Pain episodes last for hours, days, or weeks. Examples are migraine headaches and pain related to sickle cell disease (Gruener and Lande, 2006).

Cancer Pain.
Not all clients with cancer experience pain. But for those who do, the Agency for Healthcare Research and Quality (AHRQ), formerly the Agency for Health Care Policy and Research (AHCPR), reports that up to 90% are able to have their pain managed with relatively simple means (Jacox and others, 1994). Some clients with cancer experience acute and/or chronic pain. The pain is sometimes nociceptive and/or neuropathic. Cancer pain is usually due to tumor progression and its related pathological process, invasive procedures, toxicities of treatment, infection, and physical limitations. The client senses pain at the actual site of the tumor or distant to the site, which is referred pain. Assess any new report of pain by a client with existing pain. Although the need for treatment of cancer pain has improved, the issue of undertreatment continues. Approximately 70% to 90% of clients with advanced cancer experience pain. Sixty percent of these report moderate to severe pain (Maxwell and others, 2005).

Pain by Inferred Pathological Process.
Identifying the cause of pain is the first step in successfully treating pain. Nociceptive pain includes somatic (musculoskeletal) and visceral (internal organ) pain. Neuropathic pain arises from abnormal or damaged pain nerves (Table 43-2). Each of these pathological

---

✳ **TABLE 43-2 Classification of Pain by Inferred Pathology**

NOCICEPTIVE PAIN	NEUROPATHIC PAIN
I. *Nociceptive pain:* Normal processing of stimuli that damages normal tissues or has the potential to do so if prolonged; usually responsive to nonopioids and/or opioids.	II. *Neuropathic pain:* Abnormal processing of sensory input by the peripheral or central nervous system; treatment usually includes adjuvant analgesics.
A. Somatic pain: Comes from bone, joint, muscle, skin, or connective tissue. It is usually aching or throbbing in quality and is well localized.	A. Centrally generated pain
B. Visceral pain: Arises from visceral organs, such as the gastrointestinal tract and pancreas. Categories include the following:	1. Deafferentation pain: Injury to either the peripheral or central nervous system. *Examples:* Phantom pain reflects injury to the peripheral nervous system; burning pain below the level of a spinal cord lesion reflects injury to the central nervous system.
1. Tumor involvement of the organ capsule that causes aching and fairly well localized pain	2. Sympathetically maintained pain: Associated with dysregulation of the autonomic nervous system. *Examples:* pain associated with reflex sympathetic dystrophy/causalgia (complex regional pain syndrome, type I, type II).
2. Obstruction of hollow viscus, which causes intermittent cramping and poorly localized pain	B. Peripherally generated pain
	1. Painful polyneuropathies: Client feels pain along the distribution of many peripheral nerves. *Examples:* diabetic neuropathy, alcohol-nutritional neuropathy, and Guillain-Barré syndrome.
	2. Painful mononeuropathies: Usually associated with a known peripheral nerve injury, and pain is felt at least partly along the distribution of the damaged nerve. *Examples:* nerve root compression, nerve entrapment, trigeminal neuralgia.

Modified from McCaffery M, Pasero C: *Pain: clinical manual,* ed 2, St. Louis, 1999, Mosby; data from Max MB, Portenoy RK: Methodological challenges for clinical trials of cancer pain treatments. In Chapman CR, Foley KM, editors: *Current and emerging issues in cancer pain: research and practice,* New York, 1993, Raven Press; and Portenoy RK: Neuropathic pain. In Portenoy RK, Kanner RM, editors: *Pain management: theory and practice,* Philadelphia, 1996, FA Davis.

---

processes has distinct pain characteristics. The pain assessment section discusses these further.

Idiopathic Pain. Because not all pain has an identifiable cause, a third category is necessary: idiopathic pain. **Idiopathic pain** is chronic pain in the absence of an identifiable physical or psychological cause or pain perceived as excessive for the extent of an organic pathological condition. An example of idiopathic pain is complex regional pain syndrome (CRPS). It is hoped that future technology will identify the cause or causes, thus leading to a more effective treatment.

Nursing Knowledge Base

Nursing knowledge of pain mechanisms and interventions continues to grow through nursing research. This section explores factors that influence the pain experience.

Knowledge, Attitudes, and Beliefs

The attitude of health care personnel affects pain management. Unless clients have objective signs of pain, some nurses do not believe they are uncomfortable. The traditional medical model of illness causes these attitudes about pain. This model suggests that physical problems result from physical causes. Thus pain is a physical response to organic dysfunction. When there is no obvious source of pain (e.g., the client with chronic low back pain or

✳ **BOX 43-2 Common Biases and Misconceptions About Pain**

The following statements are *false:*

- Drug abusers and alcoholics overreact to discomforts.
- Clients with minor illnesses have less pain than those with severe physical alteration.
- Administering analgesics regularly will lead to drug addiction.
- The amount of tissue damage in an injury accurately indicates pain intensity.
- Health care personnel are the best authorities on the nature of a client's pain.
- Psychogenic pain is not real.
- Chronic pain is psychological.
- Clients should expect to have pain in a hospital.
- Clients who cannot speak do not feel pain.

neuropathies), health care providers sometimes stereotype pain sufferers as malingerers, complainers, or difficult clients.

McCaffery and others (2000) studied nurses' attitudes regarding pain management and found that a nurse's personal opinion about a client's report of pain affects pain assessment and titration of opioid doses. Puntillo and others (2003), when comparing nurse and client pain intensity scores, found 50% or less agreement across disease conditions examined. Wilson and McSherry (2006) found that specialist nurses tended to infer lower levels of

✳ TABLE 43-3 Pain in Infants

MISCONCEPTION	CORRECTION
Infants cannot feel pain.	Infants have the anatomical and functional requirements for pain processing by mid to late gestation.
Infants are less sensitive to pain than older children and adults.	Term neonates have the same sensitivity to pain as older infants and children. Preterm neonates have a greater sensitivity to pain than term neonates or older children.
Infants cannot express pain.	Although infants cannot verbalize pain, they respond with behavioral cues and physiological indicators that are observable.
Infants must learn about pain from previous painful experiences.	Pain requires no prior experience; infants do not need to learn it from earlier painful experience. Pain occurs with the first insult.
Pain cannot be accurately assessed in infants.	Behavioral cues (i.e., facial expressions, cry, body movements) and physiological indicators of pain can be reliably and validly assessed either alone or in combination. The most valid approach is facial expression (Craig, 1998). A composite pain measure can also be used (Stevens, 1998).
Infants cannot remember pain.	Early exposure to noxious stimuli sometimes has an effect on the infant's future responses to painful events (Grunau and others, 1994; Taddio and others, 1997).
You cannot safely give analgesics and anesthetics to infants and neonates because of their immature capacity to metabolize and eliminate drugs and their sensitivity to opioid-induced respiratory depression.	Infants older than 1 month of age metabolize drugs in the same manner as older infants and children. Careful selection of the agent, dosage, administration route and time, and frequent monitoring for desired and undesired effects, and drug titration and weaning minimize the adverse effects of opioids and nonopioids for pain management in neonates (Stevens, 1998).

Modified from McCaffery M, Pasero C: *Pain: clinical manual,* ed 2, St. Louis, 1999, Mosby.

physical pain than general nurses when given client vignettes. Thus nurses' assessment of clients' pain intensity does not always match clients' report of pain intensity.

Nurses' assumptions about clients in pain seriously limits their ability to offer pain relief. Unfortunately, biases based on culture, education, and experience influence everyone. Too often, nurses allow misconceptions about pain (Box 43-2) to affect their willingness to intervene. Many nurses avoid acknowledging a client's pain because of their own fear and denial. Nurses may not believe a client's report of pain if they do not "look" like they are in pain. You are entitled to your personal beliefs; however, you must *accept* a client's report of pain and act according to professional guidelines, standards, position statements, policies and procedures, and evidence-based research findings.

To help a client gain pain relief, view the experience through the client's eyes. Acknowledging personal prejudices or misconceptions helps you address the client's problem more professionally. When you become an active, knowledgeable observer of a client in pain, you will more objectively analyze the pain experience. The client makes the diagnosis that pain is present, and you apply techniques and skills that ultimately give relief.

Factors Influencing Pain

Pain is complex, involving physiological, social, spiritual, psychological, and cultural influences. Thus each individual's pain experience is different. Consider all factors that affect the client in pain. This is necessary to ensure a holistic approach to the assessment and care of the client.

Physiological Factors

Age. Age influences pain, particularly in infants and older adults. Developmental differences found between these age-groups influence how children and older adults react to pain. Young children

have trouble understanding pain and the procedures nurses administer that cause pain. Young children who have not developed full vocabularies have difficulty verbally describing and expressing pain to parents or caregivers. Toddlers and preschoolers are unable to recall explanations about pain or associate pain with experiences that occur in various situations. With these developmental considerations in mind, you need to adapt approaches for assessing a child's pain (including what to ask and the behaviors to observe for) and how to prepare a child for a painful medical procedure (Table 43-3).

Pain is not an inevitable part of aging. However, older adults have a greater likelihood of developing pathological conditions, which are accompanied by pain (Herr, 2002a; Kelly, 2003). Once an older client suffers pain, there can be serious impairment of functional status. Pain has the potential to reduce mobility, activities of daily living (ADLs), social activities outside the home, and activity tolerance. The presence of pain in an older adult requires aggressive assessment, diagnosis, and management (Box 43-3).

The ability of older clients to interpret pain is complicated. They often suffer from multiple diseases with vague symptoms that often affect similar parts of the body. You need to make detailed assessments when there is more than one source of pain, (Herr, 2002b). Different diseases sometimes cause similar symptoms. For example, chest pain does not always indicate a heart attack; it is possibly a symptom of arthritis of the spine or of an abdominal disorder. Not all older adults experience cognitive impairment. However, when older adults experience confusion, recalling pain experiences and providing detailed explanations are difficult. There are misconceptions about pain management in the very young and in older adults that you need to address before you are able to adequately intervene for a client (Table 43-4).

Fatigue. Fatigue heightens the perception of pain and decreases coping abilities. If fatigue occurs along with sleeplessness,

BOX 43-3 — FOCUS ON OLDER ADULTS

Factors Influencing Pain in Older Adults

- With aging there is a decrease in muscle mass, an increase in body fat, and a decrease in percentage of body water. This increases concentration of water-soluble drugs such as morphine. Also, the volume of distribution for fat-soluble drugs such as fentanyl increases (Lehne, 2005).
- Older adults frequently eat poorly, resulting in low serum albumin levels. Many drugs are highly protein bound. In the presence of low serum albumin, more free drug (active form) is available, thus increasing the risk for side and/or toxic effects (Lehne, 2005).

- A decline of liver and renal function is a natural occurrence with aging. This results in reduced metabolism and excretion of drugs. Hence, older adults often experience a greater peak effect and longer duration of analgesics (Kelly, 2003).
- Age-related changes in the skin such as thinning and loss of elasticity affect the absorption rate of topical analgesics.

TABLE 43-4 Misconceptions About Pain in Older Adults

MISCONCEPTION	CORRECTION
Pain is a natural outcome of growing old.	Older adults are at greater risk (as much as twofold) than younger adults for many painful conditions, However, pain is not an inevitable result of aging.
Pain perception, or sensitivity, decreases with age.	This assumption is unsafe. Although there is evidence that emotional suffering specifically related to pain is possibly less in older than in younger clients, no scientific basis exists for the claim that a decrease in perception of pain occurs with age or that age dulls sensitivity to pain.
If the older client does not report pain, he or she does not have pain.	Older clients commonly underreport pain. Reasons include expecting to have pain with increasing age; not wanting to alarm loved ones; being fearful of losing their independence; not wanting to distract, anger, or bother caregivers; and believing caregivers know they have pain and are doing all they can to relieve it. The absence of a report of pain does not mean the absence of pain.
If an older client appears to be occupied, asleep, or otherwise distracted from pain, he or she does not have pain.	Older clients often believe it is unacceptable to show pain and have learned to use a variety of ways to cope with it instead (e.g., many clients use distraction successfully for short periods of time). Sleeping may be a coping strategy, or it may indicate exhaustion, not pain relief. Assumptions about the presence or absence of pain cannot be made solely on the basis of a client's behavior.
The potential side effects of opioids make them too dangerous to use to relieve pain in older adults.	Opioids are safe to use in older adults. Although the opioid-naive older adult may be more sensitive to opioids, this does not justify withholding the use of them in pain management. Slow titration prevents potentially dangerous opioid-induced side effects. Regular, frequent monitoring and assessment of the client's response is necessary. Adjust dose and interval between doses when you detect side effects. If necessary, you administer an opioid antagonist drug to reverse clinically significant respiratory depression
Clients with Alzheimer's disease and other cognitive impairments do not feel pain, and their reports of pain are most likely invalid.	No evidence exists that cognitively impaired older adults experience less pain or that their reports of pain are less valid than those of individuals with intact cognitive function. It is probable that clients with dementia or other deficits of cognition suffer significant unrelieved pain and discomfort. Assessment of pain in these clients is challenging but possible. The best approach is to accept the client's report of pain and treat the pain as it would be treated in an individual with intact cognitive function.
Older clients report more pain as they age.	Even though older clients experience a higher incidence of painful conditions, such as arthritis, osteoporosis, peripheral vascular disease, and cancer, than younger clients, studies have shown that they underreport pain. Many older adult clients grew up valuing the ability to "grin and bear it," and, unfortunately, the "Just Say No" to drugs campaign has heavily influenced them.

Modified from McCaffery M, Pasero C: *Pain: clinical manual,* ed 2, St. Louis, 1999, Mosby; data from Butler RN, Gastel B: Care of the aged: perspectives on pain and discomfort. In Turk DC, Melzack R, editors: *The handbook of pain assessment,* New York, 1992, Guilford Press; Melzack R, Wall D: *Handbook of pain management,* London, 2003, Churchill Livingstone; and American Geriatrics Society: The management of persistent pain in older persons, *J Am Geriatr Soc* 50(S6):205, 2002.

the perception of pain is even greater. Pain is often experienced less after a restful sleep than at the end of a long day.

Genes. Research on healthy human subjects suggests that genetic information passed on by parents possibly increases or decreases the person's sensitivity to pain. Genetic makeup possibly determines a person's pain threshold or pain tolerance.

Neurological Function. A client's neurological function influences the pain experience. Any factor that interrupts or influences normal pain reception or perception (e.g., spinal cord injury, peripheral neuropathy, or neurological disease) affects the client's awareness of and response to pain. Some pharmacological agents (analgesics, sedatives, and anesthetics) influence pain perception and response and thus require preventive nursing care.

Social Factors

Attention. The degree to which a client focuses attention on pain influences pain perception. Increased attention is associated with increased pain, whereas distraction is associated with a diminished pain response (Carroll and Seers, 1998). This concept is one that nurses apply in various pain-relief interventions such as relaxation, guided imagery, and massage. By focusing clients' attention and concentration on other stimuli, their awareness of pain declines.

Previous Experience. Each person learns from painful experiences. Prior experience does not mean that a person will accept pain more easily in the future. Previous frequent episodes of pain without relief or bouts of severe pain cause anxiety or even fear to recur. In contrast, if a person has had repeated experiences with the same type of pain but the pain has been successfully relieved, it becomes easier to interpret the pain sensation. As a result, the client is better prepared to take necessary actions to relieve the pain.

When a client has no experience with a painful condition, the first perception of it can impair the ability to cope. For example, after abdominal surgery it is common for a client to experience severe incisional pain for several days. Unless the client is aware of this, the onset of pain will seem like a serious complication. Rather than participate actively in postoperative breathing exercises (see Chapter 50), the client will lie immobile in bed and maintain shallow breathing because of fear that something has gone wrong. In the anticipatory phase of the pain experience, you need to prepare the client with a clear explanation of the type of pain to expect and methods to reduce it. This usually results in a reduced perception of pain.

Family and Social Support. People in pain often depend on family members or close friends for support, assistance, or protection. Although pain still exists, the presence of family or friends can often make the pain experience less stressful. The presence of parents is especially important for children experiencing pain.

Spiritual Factors.
Spirituality stretches beyond religion and includes an active searching for meaning to situations in which one finds oneself. Spiritual questions include "Why has this happened to me?" "Why am I suffering?" Spiritual pain goes beyond what we can see. "Why has God done this to me?" "Is this suffering teaching me something?" Other spiritual concerns include loss of independence and becoming a burden to family (Otis-Green and oth-

ers, 2002). Spiritual assessment tools such as the FICA (Faith and belief, Importance, Community, and Address/Action in care) are available (Maxwell and others, 2005). It is important for you to express to the client that he or she matters. Consider requesting a clergy consult for a client with chronic pain. Recall that pain is an experience that has physical *and* emotional components. Thus providing interventions designed to treat both aspects is essential for the best possible pain management.

Psychological Factors

Anxiety. The degree and quality of pain perceived by a client are related to the meaning of pain. The relationship between pain and anxiety is complex. Anxiety often increases the perception of pain, but pain also causes feelings of anxiety. It is difficult to separate the two sensations. Wall and Melzack (1999) reported that painful stimuli activate the portion of the limbic system believed to control emotion, particularly anxiety. The limbic system processes the emotional reaction to pain, aggravating or relieving it.

Critically ill or injured clients, who often perceive a lack of control over their environment and care, have high anxiety levels. This anxiety leads to serious pain management problems. Pharmacological and nonpharmacological approaches to the management of anxiety are appropriate; however, anxiolytic medications are not a substitute for analgesia.

Coping Style. Coping style influences the ability to deal with pain. Persons with internal loci of control perceive themselves as having control over events in their life and the outcomes, such as pain (Gil, 1990). In contrast, persons with external loci of control perceive other factors in their life, such as nurses, are responsible for the outcome of events. This concept is applied in the use of patient-controlled analgesia (PCA). Clients who are able to self-administer small doses of intravenous (IV) pain medication during an acute episode successfully achieve pain control more quickly than those who rely on nurses to administer intermittent doses of pain medications.

It is important to understand a client's coping resources during a painful experience. These resources, such as communicating with a supportive family, exercise, or praying, can be used in your plan of care to support the client and offer a degree of pain relief.

Cultural Factors

Meaning of Pain. The meaning that a person associates with pain affects the experience of pain and how one adapts to it. This is often closely associated with the person's cultural background. A person will perceive pain differently if it suggests a threat, loss, punishment, or challenge. For example, a woman in labor will perceive pain differently than a woman with a history of cancer who is experiencing a new pain and fearing recurrence. The degree and quality of pain perceived by a client are related to the meaning of pain.

Ethnicity. Cultural beliefs and values affect how individuals cope with pain. Individuals learn what is expected and accepted by their culture, including how to react to pain (Davidhizar and Giger, 2004; Lasch, 2002). Health care providers often mistakenly assume that everyone responds to pain in the same way. There are different meanings and attitudes associated with pain across various cultural groups. An understanding of the cultural

✳ BOX 43-4   CULTURAL ASPECTS OF CARE

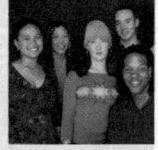

Assessing Pain in Culturally Diverse Clients

Pain is a biopsychosocial phenomenon. Culture shapes the experience of pain, its expression, pain behaviors, or coping responses. Culture also affects lay remedies, help-seeking activities, and receptivity to medical treatment. Recent evidence suggests that undertreatment of clients who belong to a minority culture is due to differences in staff perception of clients' pain intensity, which is possibly related to the ethnicity of the clinician. It is important to note that there are differences within cultural and ethnic groups as well as between them. Increasingly nurses care for clients with pain from a variety of cultures; thus it is important for nurses to develop strategies to assess and manage pain in culturally diverse clients.

Implications for Practice

- Use culturally appropriate assessment tools to assess pain, such as tools written in the client's native language.
- Recognize variations in affective response to pain. Some clients are stoic and less expressive of their pain, whereas others are emotive and more likely to verbalize pain.
- Be sensitive to variations in communication styles. Some cultures feel nonverbal expression of pain is sufficient to describe the pain experience, whereas others assume that if pain medication is appropriate the nurse will bring it; thus asking is inappropriate.
- Understand that expression of pain is unacceptable within certain cultures. Asking for assistance may be seen as a lack of respect. Others consider acknowledging pain a sign of weakness.
- The meaning of pain varies between cultures. Pain is personal and is related to religious beliefs. Some cultures consider suffering a part of life and to be endured to enter heaven.
- Use knowledge of biological variations of pain. Significant differences in drug metabolism, dosing requirements, therapeutic response, and adverse effects occur in racial and ethnic groups. But recall that a wide range of responses is possible within a cultural group and you need to assess each client individually.
- Develop personal awareness of values and beliefs that may affect responses to pain.
- Encourage individuals to tell their pain stories (narratives as therapy, empathy builders, advocacy, and windows into meaning of pain).

Data from Davidhizar R, Giger J: A review of the literature on care of clients in pain who are culturally diverse, *Int Nurs Rev* 51(1):47, 2004; and Lasch K: Culture and pain, 2002, http://www.iasp-pain.org/PCU02-5.html/.

meaning of pain helps you to design culturally sensitive care for people with pain.

Culture affects pain expression. Some cultures believe it is natural to be demonstrative about pain. Others tend to be more introverted. In addition, it is also important to know to what extent a member of a particular culture has assimilated into American society. For example, if several generations of a Hispanic cli-

ent's family have lived in the United States, the influence of the Spanish culture may be limited, whereas newly immigrated clients still embrace their cultural norms.

As a nurse, explore the impact of cultural differences on the client's pain experience, and make adjustments to the plan of care (Box 43-4). Work with the client and family to facilitate communication about the assessment and management of pain. Find a culturally appropriate assessment tool, and communicate use of that tool to other health care providers.

Critical Thinking

Successful critical thinking requires a synthesis of knowledge, experience, information gathered from clients, critical thinking attitudes, and intellectual and professional standards. Clinical judgments require that you anticipate what information you need, analyze the data, and make decisions regarding client care. A client's condition or situation is always changing. During assessment consider all critical thinking elements that build toward making appropriate nursing diagnoses.

Knowledge of pain physiology and the many factors that influence pain help you manage the client's pain. Previous experience in caring for clients with pain sharpens your assessment skills and ability to choose effective therapies. Critical thinking attitudes and intellectual standards ensure the aggressive assessment, creative planning, and thorough evaluation needed to obtain an acceptable level of client pain relief. Successful pain management does not necessarily mean pain elimination, but rather attainment of a mutually agreed-upon pain-relief goal that allows clients to control their pain instead of the pain controlling them.

Nursing Process and Pain

Nurses need to approach pain management systematically to understand and treat a client's pain. Successful management of pain depends on establishing a relationship of trust between health care providers, client, and family. Pain management extends beyond pain relief, encompassing the client's quality of life and ability to work productively, to enjoy recreation, and to function normally in the family and society (Jacox and others, 1994).

Several clinical guidelines are available for managing pain in specific disorders. Guidelines are available through the American Pain Society (APS) on the management of pain in the primary care setting, management of sickle cell pain, cancer pain in adults and children, and pain in osteoarthritis, rheumatoid arthritis, and juvenile chronic arthritis. In addition, the National Guideline Clearing House (www.guideline.gov) posts a variety of pain management guidelines, including ones on acute, spinal, chest, low back, cancer, heel, and pancreatic pain.

◆ Assessment

The American Nurses Association (ANA) (2005) believes that pain assessment and management is within the scope of every nurse's practice. Thus the ANA offers a certification examination in pain management to staff nurses (http://www.aspmn.org/certification/index.htm/).

Because pain is not static but dynamic, it is necessary to monitor pain on a regular basis along with other vital signs. Some institutions treat pain as the fifth vital sign. It is important for you to understand that pain assessment is *not* simply a number. Relying solely on a number is unsafe (Vila and others, 2005). Although pain assessment is a nursing function, unlicensed staff members also need to screen for pain (Schulman-Green and others, 2005). When an unlicensed staff member believes a client is having pain, he or she has the responsibility to inform the nurse immediately so that the nurse is able to make a confirming assessment.

The ability to establish a nursing diagnosis, decide on appropriate interventions, and evaluate the client's response (outcomes) to interventions depends on the fundamental activity of a factual, timely, accurate pain assessment (Figure 43-4). The core of this complex activity is the exploration of the pain experience through the eyes of the client. A variety of tools are available for assessing the client's pain. There are tools for assessing nociceptive pain and also neuropathic pain (Jensen and others, 2006). This chapter focuses on nociceptive pain scales. The goal in using these tools is to identify how much pain exists without interfering with client function and not to identify how much pain the client tolerates.

AHRQ has established specific guidelines for assessing clients with acute and cancer pain. The focus is on planning successful pain management interventions before the client has pain. Because it involves a collaborative approach, the AHRQ pain treatment flow chart (Figure 43-5) offers a useful conceptual approach to the control of acute pain. Clients need to understand that informed reporting of pain is valuable and necessary if the health care team is to manage pain effectively.

When assessing pain, be sensitive to the client's level of discomfort. In addition, ask the client what level will allow him or her to function. For example, when caring for a client with pain you ask, "What level of pain will allow you to walk the hall?" The client answers that he or she is able to walk when pain is at a level 2 pain (on a scale of 0 to 10, with 0 being no pain and 10 being worst pain imaginable). You then focus efforts on getting the pain decreased to that level. If pain is acute or severe, it is unlikely that the client will be able to provide a detailed description of the entire experience. During an episode of acute pain you primarily assess the location, severity, and quality of the pain. Collect a more detailed acute pain assessment when the client is more comfortable (Kim, 2002). For clients with chronic pain a thorough pain assessment includes affective, cognitive, behavioral, spiritual, and social dimensions (St. Marie, 2002). In the home care setting, family members become the assessors of pain. Using the ABCs of pain management is an effective way to manage pain (Box 43-5).

Always be aware of possible errors in pain assessment (Box 43-6). Using the right tools and methods helps you to avoid errors and ensures that you choose the right pain interventions. Failure of clinicians to assess a client's pain, accept the findings, and treat the report of pain is a common cause of unrelieved pain and suffering (McCaffery and Pasero, 1999).

Client's Expression of Pain.

A client's self-report of pain is the single most reliable indicator of the existence and intensity of pain (AHCPR, 1992; APS, 2003). Pain is individualistic. Many

Knowledge
- Physiology of pain
- Factors that potentially increase or decrease responses to pain
- Pathophysiology of conditions causing pain
- Awareness of biases affecting pain assessment and treatment
- Cultural variations in how pain is expressed
- Knowledge of nonverbal communication

Experience
- Caring for clients with acute, chronic, and cancer pain
- Caring for clients who experienced pain as a result of a health care therapy
- Personal experience with pain

ASSESSMENT
- Determine the client's perspective of pain including history of pain; its meaning; and physical, emotional, and social effects
- Measure objectively the characteristics of the client's pain
- Review potential factors affecting the client's pain
- Identify medical comorbidities (e.g., diabetes, cancer, etc.)

Standards
- Refer to AHRQ guidelines for acute pain management
- Refer to clinical guidelines of APS and ASPMN
- Apply intellectual standards (e.g., clarity, specificity, accuracy, and completeness) when gathering assessment
- Apply relevance when letting the client explore the pain experience

Attitudes
- Persevere in exploring causes and possible solutions for chronic pain
- Display confidence when assessing pain to relieve the client's anxiety
- Display integrity and fairness to prevent prejudice from affecting assessment

Figure 43-4 Critical thinking model for pain assessment.

clients fail to report or discuss discomfort; at the same time, many nurses believe that clients will report pain if they have it. In addition, if clients sense that you doubt that pain exists, they will share little information about their pain experience or will minimize their report. It is imperative that you establish a caring therapeutic relationship that allows for open communication about pain. Simple measures such as sitting when talking to clients about pain lets them know that you are sincerely concerned about their pain.

Clients unable to communicate effectively often require special attention during assessment. Children, persons who are developmentally delayed, clients who are psychotic, the critically ill, clients with dementia, and clients who do not speak English all require different approaches. Herr and others (2006a, 2006b) examined

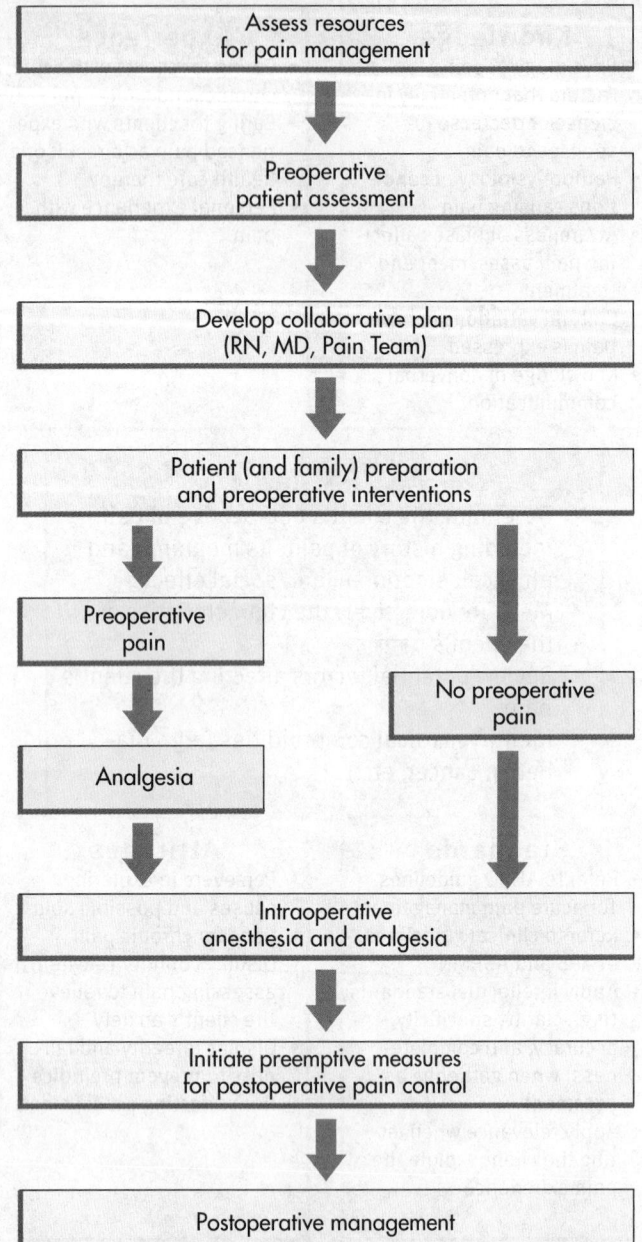

Figure 43-5 Pain treatment flow chart: preoperative and intraoperative phases. (From Agency for Health Care Policy and Research, Acute Pain Management Guideline Panel: *Acute pain management: operative or medical procedures and trauma,* Clinical Practice Guideline, AHCPR Pub No. 92-0032, Rockville, Md, 1992, Agency for Health Care Policy and Research, Public Health Service, U.S. Department of Health and Human Services; and Jacox A and others: *Management of cancer pain,* Clinical Practice Guideline No. 9, AHCPR Pub No. 94-0592, Rockville, Md, 1994, Agency for Health Care Policy and Research, Public Health Service, U.S. Department of Health and Human Services.)

✳ BOX 43-5 Routine Clinical Approach to Pain Assessment and Management: ABCDE

A **Ask** about pain regularly. *A*ssess pain systematically.
B **Believe** the client and family in their report of pain and what relieves it.
C **Choose** pain control options appropriate for the client, family, and setting.
D **Deliver** interventions in a timely, logical, and coordinated fashion.
E **Empower** clients and their families. Enable them to control their course to the greatest extent possible.

From Jacox A and others: *Management of cancer pain,* Clinical Practice Guideline No. 9, AHCPR Publication No. 94-0592, Rockville, Md, 1994, Agency for Health Care Policy and Research, Public Health Service, U.S. Department of Health and Human Services.

✳ BOX 43-6 Possible Sources for Error in Pain Assessment

- Bias, which causes nurses to consistently overestimate or underestimate the pain that clients experience
- Vague or unclear assessment questions, which lead to unreliable assessment data
- Use of pain assessment tools that have not been proven reliable and valid with identical clients
- Clients who do not always provide complete, relevant, and accurate pain information
- Cognitively impaired older clients who are unable to use pain scales

---

various pain behavior assessment tools used with cognitively impaired clients. Although no one tool had sufficient reliability and validity, there are clinical practice recommendations (Box 43-7). However, it is important to understand that "the number obtained when using a pain-behavior scale is a pain-behavior score, not a pain-intensity rating" (Pasero and McCaffery, 2005). These tools identify the presence of pain, but do not determine the intensity of pain.

Cognitively impaired clients might require simple assessment approaches involving close observation of behavior changes, especially with movement. A critically ill client who has a clouded sensorium or the presence of nasogastric tubes or artificial airways requires you to ask specific questions that the client is able to answer with a nod of the head or by writing out a response. If the client speaks a different language, pain assessment will be difficult. A family member or interpreter is often necessary.

Characteristics of Pain. Assessment of common characteristics of pain helps you form an understanding of the type of pain, its pattern, and types of interventions that bring relief. Use of instruments to quantify the extent and degree of pain depends on a client being sufficiently cognitively alert to be able to understand your instructions.

Onset and Duration. Ask questions to determine the onset, duration, and sequence of pain. When did the pain begin? How

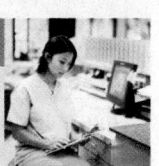

BOX 43-7   EVIDENCE-BASED PRACTICE

Pain Assessment in the Nonverbal Client

Evidence Summary

An appointed task force of the American Society for Pain Management Nursing (ASPMN) developed this position statement and clinical practice recommendations.

No single assessment strategy, such as interpretation of behaviors, pathology, or estimates of pain by others, is sufficient by itself in determining the presence of pain in a nonverbal client.

Application to Nursing Practice

- Recommended assessment considerations:
  - Attempt a self-report of pain using simple yes/no response or vocalizations.
  - Explain why self-report cannot be used.
  - Search for potential causes of pain.
  - Assume pain is present (APP) after ruling out other problems (infection, constipation) that cause pain.
  - Identify pathological conditions or procedures that cause pain.
  - Observe client behaviors and list behaviors (e.g., facial expressions, vocalizations, body movements, changes in interactions or mental status) that indicate pain. These will vary depending on client's developmental level.
  - Ask family members, parents, caregivers for a surrogate report.
- Use behavioral pain assessment tool.
  - Use reliable and valid tools to ensure use of appropriate criteria in the pain assessment.

- Appropriate scale determined client by client, no one scale should be required for all specific groups of clients.
- Vital signs are not sensitive indicators for the presence of pain.
- Attempt an analgesic trial.
  - Choose analgesic, dose, and titration based on estimated intensity of pain.
  - For mild to moderate pain, give nonopioid analgesics around-the-clock.
  - After 24 hours, reassess. If behaviors improve, assume pain was the cause.
  - If behaviors persist, consider giving a single, low-dose short-acting opioid (e.g., hydrocodone, oxycodone, morphine). Observe effect.
  - If behaviors continue, titrate dose upward by 25% to 50% and observe effect.
  - Continue to titrate up until a therapeutic effect or bothersome adverse effects occur, or if there is no benefit.
  - If behaviors continue after a reasonable analgesic trial, explore other potential causes.
  - For severe pain, it may be appropriate to start the analgesic trial with an opioid.

Reference

Herr K and others: Pain assessment in the nonverbal patient: position statement with clinical practice recommendations *Pain Manag Nurs* 7(2):44, 2006a.

long has it lasted? Does it occur at the same time each day? How often does it recur?

Location. To assess pain location, ask the client to tell or to point to all areas of discomfort. Do not assume that pain will always occur in the same location. When describing pain location, use anatomical landmarks and descriptive terminology. The statement "Pain is localized in the upper right abdominal quadrant" is more specific than "The client states the pain is in the abdomen." Pain, classified by location, is superficial or cutaneous, deep or visceral, referred, or radiating (Table 43-5).

Intensity. One of the most subjective and therefore most useful characteristics for the reporting of pain is its severity, or intensity. A variety of pain scales are available for clients to communicate their pain intensity. Examples of pain intensity scales include the verbal descriptor scale (VDS), the numerical rating scale (NRS), and the visual analog scale (VAS) (Figure 43-6). When using the NRS a report of 0 to 3 indicates mild pain, 4 to 6 moderate pain, and 7 to 10 severe pain, considered a pain emergency (Miaskowski, 2005). These scales work best when assessing pain intensity before and after therapeutic interventions. Many of these scales are available in several languages to aid nurses when an interpreter or family is not present (McCaffery and Pasero, 1999). In addition to the current pain level, also ask what rating to give the average pain and the worst pain over the past 24 hours.

Although different clients prefer different pain scales, it is important for you to select and consistently use the same scale with a specific client. You do not use a pain scale to compare the pain of one client to that of another client.

Assessing pain intensity in children requires special techniques. Children's verbal statements are most important (Hockenberry and Wilson, 2007). Young children do not always know what the word *pain* means, and therefore assessment requires you to use words such as *owie, boo-boo,* or *hurt*. There are some unique tools available to measure pain intensity in children. Beyer and others (1992) developed the "Oucher." Photographs of the face of a child (in increasing levels of discomfort) cue children into understanding what pain is and its severity. A child merely points to the face, thus simplifying the task of describing the pain. There are also ethnic versions of the tool (Figure 43-7). Wong and Baker (1988) developed the FACES scale to assess pain in verbal children (Figure 43-8, p. 1065). The scale consists of six cartoon faces ranging from a smiling face ("no hurt") to increasingly less happy faces, to a final sad, tearful face ("hurts worst"). Children as young as 3 years of age are able to use the scale. There are a variety of tools available for assessing pain in neonates, infants, nonverbal toddlers, and children with cognitive impairment.

Quality. Because there is no common or specific pain vocabulary in general use, the words a client chooses to describe pain vary. Clients of American descent often use *hurt* and *ache* to describe their pain, reserving the word *pain* for severe discomfort. Always use words other than *pain* to obtain an accurate report. For example, you say, "Tell me what your discomfort feels like." The client will likely describe the pain as crushing, throbbing,

✳ TABLE 43-5 Classification of Pain by Location

LOCATION	CHARACTERISTICS	EXAMPLES OF CAUSES
Superficial or Cutaneous Pain resulting from stimulation of skin	Pain is of short duration and is localized. It usually is a sharp sensation.	Needle stick; small cut or laceration
Deep or Visceral Pain resulting from stimulation of internal organs	Pain is diffuse and radiates in several directions. Duration varies, but it usually lasts longer than superficial pain. Pain is sharp, dull, or unique to organ involved.	Crushing sensation (e.g., angina pectoris); burning sensation (e.g., gastric ulcer)
Referred Common phenomenon in visceral pain because many organs themselves have no pain receptors; entrance of sensory neurons from affected organ into same spinal cord segment as neurons from areas where individual feels pain; perception of pain is in unaffected areas	Pain is in part of body separate from source of pain and assumes any characteristic.	Myocardial infarction, which causes referred pain to the jaw, left arm, and left shoulder; kidney stones, which refer pain to groin
Radiating Sensation of pain extending from initial site of injury to another body part	Pain feels as though it travels down or along body part. It is intermittent or constant.	Low back pain from ruptured intravertebral disk accompanied by pain radiating down leg from sciatic nerve irritation

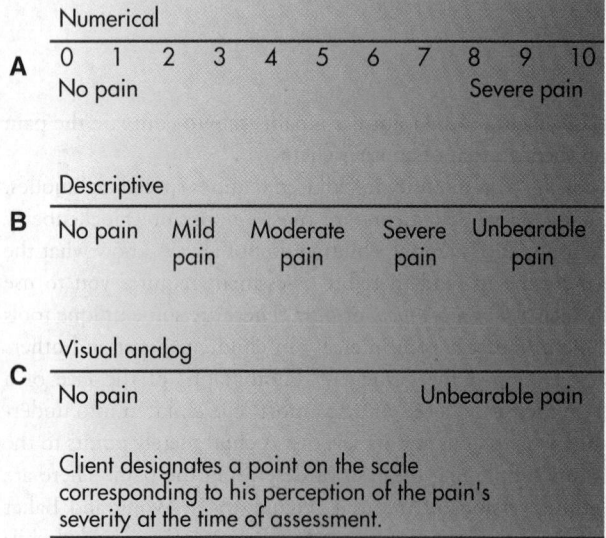

Figure 43-6 Sample pain scales. **A,** Numerical. **B,** Verbal descriptive. **C,** Visual analog.

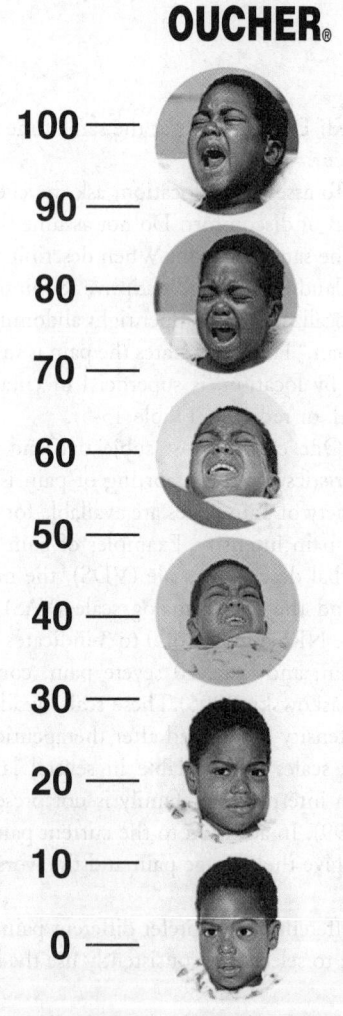

Figure 43-7 African American version of the Oucher pain scale. (Copyright Denyes, Villarrael, 1990.)

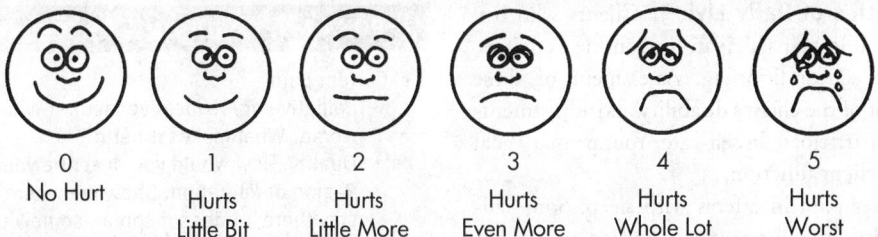

Brief word instructions: Point to each face using the words to describe the pain intensity. Ask the child to choose face that best describes own pain and record the appropriate number.

Figure 43-8 Wong-Baker FACES Pain Rating Scale. (From Hockenberry MJ, Wilson D, Winkelstein ML: *Wong's essentials of pediatric nursing,* ed 7, St. Louis, 2005, Mosby.)

sharp, or dull. Although a list of descriptive terms is available, it is more accurate to have clients describe the pain in their own words whenever possible.

There is some consistency in the way people describe certain types of pain. The pain associated with a myocardial infarction is often described as crushing or viselike, whereas the pain of a surgical incision is often described as dull, aching, and throbbing, indicating nociceptive pain. Neuropathic pain is usually burning, shooting, or electric-like (Williams, 2006). When the client's descriptions fit the pattern forming in the assessment, you are then able to make a clearer analysis of the nature and type of pain. This will lead to more appropriate pain management because you treat nociceptive and neuropathic pain differently.

Pain Pattern. Various factors affect the pattern of pain. It helps to assess specific events or conditions that precipitate or aggravate pain. Ask the client to describe activities that cause pain, such as physical movement or food. Also ask the client to demonstrate actions that cause a painful response, such as coughing or turning a certain way. For example, with a ruptured intravertebral disk, the low back pain usually radiates down the leg to the foot and bending over or lifting objects aggravates it. Asking the client if there is a particular time of day the pain is worse, or if the pain is intermittent, constant, or a combination helps you to plan interventions to prevent pain from occurring or worsening.

Relief Measures. It is useful to know whether a client has an effective way of relieving pain, such as changing position, using ritualistic behavior (pacing, rocking, or rubbing), eating, meditation, prayer, or applying heat or cold to the painful site. The client's methods often work best for you, too. Clients gain trust from knowing that you are willing to try their relief measures. Clients also gain a sense of control over the pain instead of the pain controlling them. Assessment of relieving factors also includes identification of practitioners (e.g., internist, orthopedist, acupuncturist, chiropractor, or dentist) whose services the client has used.

Contributing Symptoms. There are some symptoms (depression, anxiety, fatigue, sedation, anorexia, sleep disruption, spiritual distress, and guilt) that cause worsening of pain. You need to assess for these associated symptoms and evaluate their effects on the client's pain perception. Reporting and treating associated symptoms contributes to successful pain management.

Effects of Pain on the Client. Pain alters a person's lifestyle and affects psychological well-being. Chronic/persistent pain causes suffering, loss of control, loneliness, disabilities, exhaus-

---

> ### ✳ BOX 43-8 Behavioral Indicators of Effects of Pain
>
> **Vocalizations**
> Moaning
> Crying
> Gasping
> Grunting
>
> **Facial Expressions**
> Grimace
> Clenched teeth
> Wrinkled forehead
> Tightly closed or widely
>   opened eyes or mouth
> Lip biting
>
> **Body Movement**
> Restlessness
> Immobilization
> Muscle tension
>
> Increased hand and finger
>   movements
> Pacing activities
> Rhythmic or rubbing motions
> Protective movement of body
>   parts
> Grabbing or holding a body
>   part
>
> **Social Interaction**
> Avoidance of conversation
> Focus only on activities for
>   pain relief
> Avoidance of social contacts
> Reduced attention span
> Reduced interaction with
>   environment

---

tion, and impaired quality of life throughout the client's existence. By recognizing the effects pain has on clients, you will better understand the client's experience and provide the best pain management. When a client is in pain, you need to conduct a focused physical and neurological examination and observe for nonverbal responses to pain (e.g., posturing or guarding a painful area). Examine the painful area to see if palpation or manipulation of the site increases pain (Jacox and others, 1994).

Behavioral Effects. When a client has pain, assess verbalization, vocal response, facial and body movements, and social interaction. A verbal report of pain is a vital part of assessment. You need to be willing to listen and understand. Many clients are unable to communicate their pain. An infant or a client who is unconscious, disoriented or confused, aphasic, or who speaks a foreign language is unable to explain the pain experience. In these cases it is especially important for you to be alert for behaviors that indicate pain (Box 43-8).

The nonverbal expression of pain either supports or contradicts other information about pain. If a woman in labor reports that her labor pains are occurring more frequently, and if she begins to massage her abdomen more often, this confirms her report. If a client reports severe abdominal pain but continues to grasp the chest, a more detailed assessment is necessary.

Influence on Activities of Daily Living. Clients who live with daily pain are less able to participate in routine activities, which leads to physical deconditioning. Assessment of these changes reveals the extent of the client's disability and adjustments necessary to help clients participate in self-care. Your primary goal as a nurse is to improve client function.

Ask the client whether pain interferes with sleep. Some clients experience difficulty in falling asleep and/or in staying asleep. The pain awakens the client during the night and creates difficulty in falling back to sleep. Consider giving medications or trying nonpharmacological interventions to promote sleep (see Chapter 42).

Depending on the location of the pain, some clients have difficulty independently performing ADLs. For example, some pain restricts mobility to the point that the client is no longer able to bathe in a bathtub. Clients with severe arthritis find it painful to grasp eating utensils or lower themselves to a toilet seat. Assess the client's need for assistance with self-care activities, and collaborate with members of the health care team (e.g., physical therapy and occupational therapy). Also consider the need for family members or friends to assist the client with basic hygiene.

Pain sometimes impairs the ability to maintain normal sexual relations. Include in your assessment the extent to which pain affects the client's sexual activity. It also helps to learn whether a client is physically unable to participate or if pain reduces the desire for sexual intercourse.

Pain can seriously threaten a person's ability to work. The more physical activity required in a job, the greater the risk of discomfort when the pain is associated with movement. Pain related to emotional stress increases in individuals whose jobs involve stressful decision making. Assess the work that clients do and their abilities to function in their jobs. Assess the daily chores of homemakers in the same manner as the duties involved in jobs outside the home. Also assess whether it is necessary for clients to stop activity occasionally because of pain, and then help clients select ways of minimizing or controlling the pain so that they are able to remain productive.

It is also important to include an assessment of the effect of pain on social activities. The pain may be so debilitating that the client becomes too exhausted to socialize. Identify the client's normal social activities, the extent to which they have been disrupted, and the client's wish to participate.

Client Expectations. The public often views pain as a part of life. Some clients experience pain for many hours or days before seeking health care assistance. They often expect and even accept a certain amount of pain while being hospitalized. Asking the client about the pain level that is tolerable is the first step in encouraging the client to regain control. Assessing previous pain experiences and effective home interventions provides a foundation on which you can build. Clients expect nurses to accept their reports of pain and be prompt in meeting their pain needs.

✦Nursing Diagnosis

You make an accurate diagnosis only after you have performed a complete assessment (Box 43-9). The development of an accurate nursing diagnosis for a client in pain results from thorough data

---

✦ BOX 43-9 NURSING ASSESSMENT QUESTIONS

- Current pain
  - *Palliative* or *Provocative* factors: What makes your pain worse? What makes it better?
  - *Quality:* How would you describe your pain?
  - *Region* or *Radiation:* Show me where you hurt. Does it stay there, or does it spread somewhere else?
  - *Severity:* On a scale of 0 to 10, how bad is your pain now?
  - What is the worst pain you have had in the past 24 hours?
  - What is the average pain you have had in the past 24 hours?
  - *Timing:* Is your pain constant, intermittent, or both?
  - *U:* Effect of pain on you: What does your pain prevent you from doing that you would like to do?
- Do you have any allergies?
- What medications are you taking now, including herbs?
- What have you done to try to relieve the pain?
- What medications have you tried in the past that worked to stop a pain?
- Have you ever used recreational drugs or alcohol to alleviate pain?
- Have you ever been diagnosed with a gastrointestinal bleed, kidney or liver disorder?
- Do you have any medical conditions for which you are being treated?
- Who do you live with, and how do they help you when you have pain?

---

collection and analysis (Box 43-10). Careful assessment will reveal the presence or potential for pain. In addition, examine the client's history for recent procedures or preexisting painful conditions.

The nursing diagnosis focuses on the specific nature of the pain to help you identify the most useful types of interventions for alleviating pain and improving the client's function. *Acute pain related to physical trauma* and *acute pain related to natural childbirth processes* require very different nursing interventions. Accurate identification of related factors is necessary to choosing appropriate nursing interventions. For example, interventions for *acute pain related to physical trauma* require pharmacological intervention, whereas you manage *acute pain related to natural childbirth processes* more appropriately with nonpharmacological interventions such as controlled breathing techniques.

Your assessment may direct you to diagnoses other than that of *acute* or *chronic pain.* The extent to which pain affects a client's function and general state of health determines whether other nursing diagnoses are relevant. For example, your assessment reveals that a client suffers from pain of the hands and shoulders as a result of crippling arthritis that the client has had for over 3 years. As a result, the client is unable to remove or fasten necessary items of clothing. The nursing diagnoses for this client are *dressing/grooming self-care deficit* and *chronic pain.* The diagnosis of *self-care deficit* requires involvement by members of the health care team to provide the client with assistive devices for performing self-care. Examples of other diagnoses that are applicable to clients experiencing pain include the following:

- Anxiety
- Fatigue

BOX 43-10 NURSING DIAGNOSTIC PROCESS

Chronic Pain

Assessment Activities	Defining Characteristics
Have client describe pain intensity.	Pain is constant; client verbally reports 5 out of 10
Assess onset and location of pain.	Present for 7 months in lower lumbar area
Observe client behaviors.	Grimaces and grunts with movement, rubs flanks frequently; reduced movement
Assess effect of pain on activities of daily living (ADLs).	Appetite poor; gets little sleep; difficulty dressing
Review medical history.	Previous trauma; effectiveness of past pain control measures

- Hopelessness
- Impaired physical mobility
- Imbalanced nutrition: less than body requirements
- Powerlessness
- Chronic low self-esteem
- Insomnia
- Impaired social interaction
- Spiritual distress

Planning

The planning step of the nursing process requires you to synthesize information from multiple resources. Critical thinking ensures that the client's plan of care (see Care Plan) integrates all that you know about the individual client, as well as key critical thinking elements (Figure 43-9). Professional standards are especially important to consider when you develop a plan of care. These standards often establish scientifically proven guidelines for selecting effective nursing interventions. Professional standards of care regarding pain management are available as agency policies or through professional organizations such as the American Society for Pain Management Nursing (ASPMN).

Another effective method for planning care is a concept map. Clients who are in pain frequently have interrelated problems. As one problem gets worse, other aspects of the client's level of health also change. The concept map assists you in relating how the nursing diagnoses are interrelated with each other and linked to the client's medical diagnosis. Using the example here, as you plan care for the client with rheumatoid arthritis, note the relationships between *acute pain, impaired physical mobility, self-care deficit,* and *fatigue* (Figure 43-10). Identifying these relationships assists you in developing a holistic and client-centered plan of care.

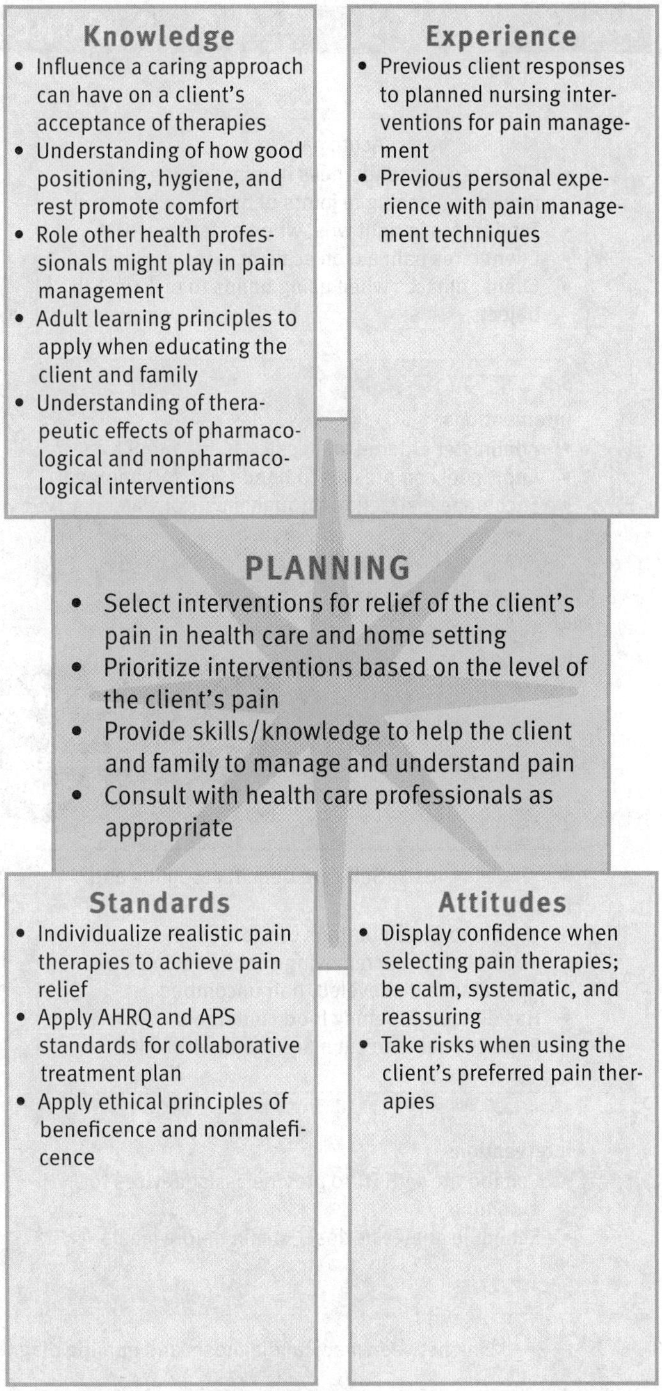

Goals and Outcomes. When managing clients' pain, your goals of care should promote the client's optimal function. Determine, along with the client, what the pain has prevented the client

Knowledge
- Influence a caring approach can have on a client's acceptance of therapies
- Understanding of how good positioning, hygiene, and rest promote comfort
- Role other health professionals might play in pain management
- Adult learning principles to apply when educating the client and family
- Understanding of therapeutic effects of pharmacological and nonpharmacological interventions

Experience
- Previous client responses to planned nursing interventions for pain management
- Previous personal experience with pain management techniques

PLANNING
- Select interventions for relief of the client's pain in health care and home setting
- Prioritize interventions based on the level of the client's pain
- Provide skills/knowledge to help the client and family to manage and understand pain
- Consult with health care professionals as appropriate

Standards
- Individualize realistic pain therapies to achieve pain relief
- Apply AHRQ and APS standards for collaborative treatment plan
- Apply ethical principles of beneficence and nonmaleficence

Attitudes
- Display confidence when selecting pain therapies; be calm, systematic, and reassuring
- Take risks when using the client's preferred pain therapies

Figure 43-9 Critical thinking model for pain management.

from doing. Then decide on a mutually acceptable level of pain that allows return of function. An indication of a plan's success is determined through attainment of goals and outcomes. For example, in the case of the goal of "the client will achieve a satisfactory level of pain relief within 24 hours," the following are possible outcomes:

- Reports that pain is a 3 or less on a scale of 0 to 10
- Identifies factors that intensify pain
- Uses pain-relief measures safely
- Level of discomfort will not interfere with ADL activities

CONCEPT MAP

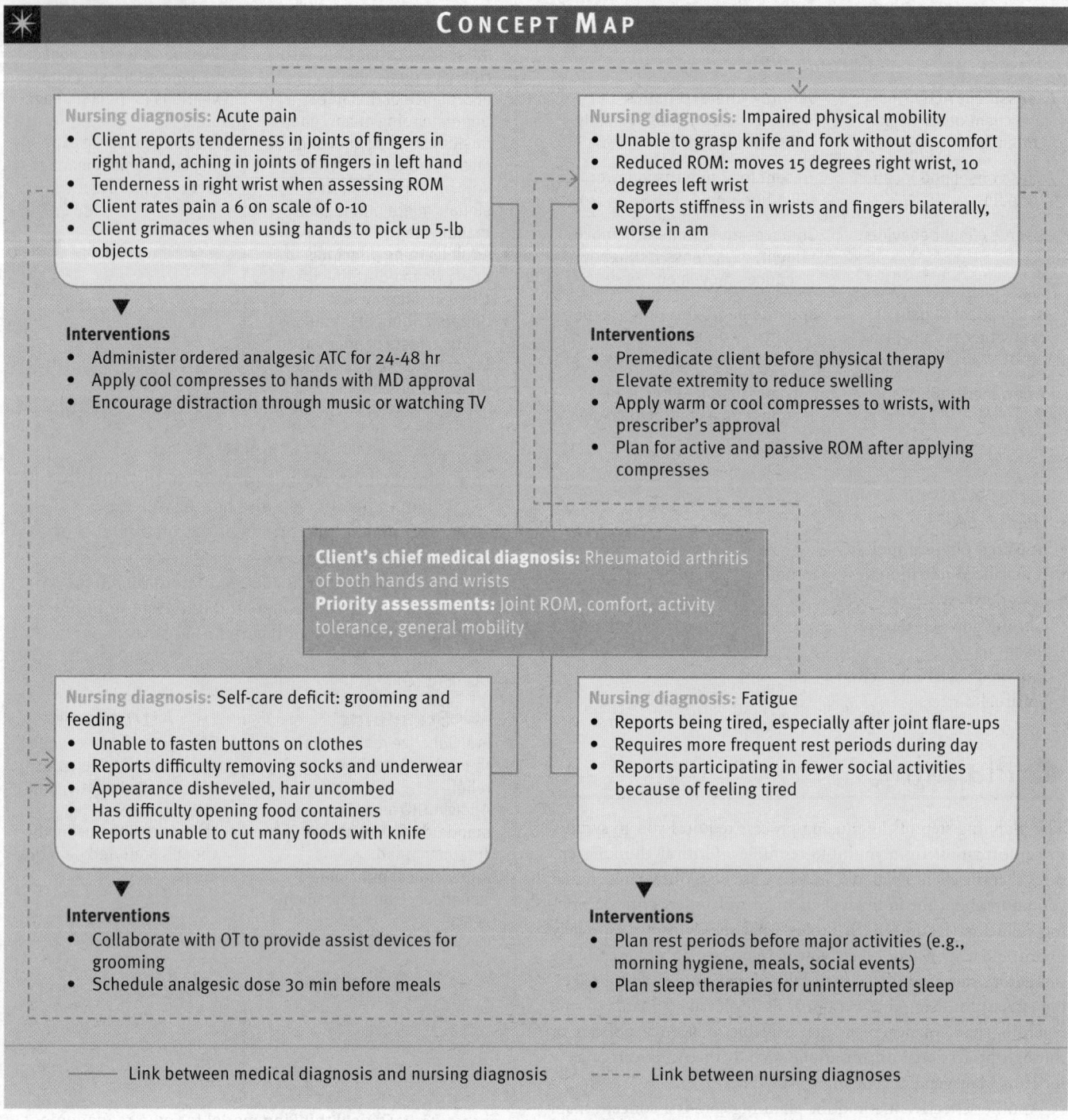

Nursing diagnosis: Acute pain
- Client reports tenderness in joints of fingers in right hand, aching in joints of fingers in left hand
- Tenderness in right wrist when assessing ROM
- Client rates pain a 6 on scale of 0-10
- Client grimaces when using hands to pick up 5-lb objects

Interventions
- Administer ordered analgesic ATC for 24-48 hr
- Apply cool compresses to hands with MD approval
- Encourage distraction through music or watching TV

Nursing diagnosis: Impaired physical mobility
- Unable to grasp knife and fork without discomfort
- Reduced ROM: moves 15 degrees right wrist, 10 degrees left wrist
- Reports stiffness in wrists and fingers bilaterally, worse in am

Interventions
- Premedicate client before physical therapy
- Elevate extremity to reduce swelling
- Apply warm or cool compresses to wrists, with prescriber's approval
- Plan for active and passive ROM after applying compresses

Client's chief medical diagnosis: Rheumatoid arthritis of both hands and wrists
Priority assessments: Joint ROM, comfort, activity tolerance, general mobility

Nursing diagnosis: Self-care deficit: grooming and feeding
- Unable to fasten buttons on clothes
- Reports difficulty removing socks and underwear
- Appearance disheveled, hair uncombed
- Has difficulty opening food containers
- Reports unable to cut many foods with knife

Interventions
- Collaborate with OT to provide assist devices for grooming
- Schedule analgesic dose 30 min before meals

Nursing diagnosis: Fatigue
- Reports being tired, especially after joint flare-ups
- Requires more frequent rest periods during day
- Reports participating in fewer social activities because of feeling tired

Interventions
- Plan rest periods before major activities (e.g., morning hygiene, meals, social events)
- Plan sleep therapies for uninterrupted sleep

——— Link between medical diagnosis and nursing diagnosis   - - - - Link between nursing diagnoses

Figure 43-10 Concept map for client with pain related to chronic joint inflammation.

Setting Priorities. When setting priorities in pain management, consider the type of pain the client is experiencing and the effects pain has on various body functions. Partner with the client in selection of interventions appropriate for the nature and effects of pain. For example, if a client has had acute pain but an analgesic has brought relief, center your attention on how the pain is influencing activity, appetite, and sleep. In contrast, when a client's pain continues to be severe, preventing you from implementing other interventions, immediate pain relief is the obvious priority. Your priorities will change as the client's pain experience changes.

Collaborative Care. A comprehensive plan includes a variety of resources for pain control. Resources available include nurse specialists, doctors of pharmacology (PharmDs), physical therapists, occupational therapists, and clergy. An oncology nurse specialist is very familiar with pharmacological and nonpharmacological interventions that are most effective for chronic/persistent pain. Doctors of pharmacology are knowledgeable about pharmacological treatments of pain. Physical therapists plan exercises that strengthen muscle groups and lessen pain in affected areas through exercises that reduce muscle tension. Occupational therapists may devise splints to support painful body parts. Clergy

NURSING CARE PLAN

Acute Pain

Assessment

Mrs. Mays, 75 years old, was diagnosed with a cancerous tumor in her left lung 2 months ago. She also has a history of osteoarthritis. After chemotherapy and radiation therapy she was taking ibuprofen 200 mg on an as-needed (prn) basis. Until today she was able to clean her home and climb the stairs to her bedroom without diffi-culty. She also maintained her body weight and slept well through the night. However, she is now admitted to the hospital with uncon-trollable chest pain and possible pneumonia. Her husband is with her. The nurse begins a patient-controlled analgesia (PCA) of mor-phine 0.5 mg demand dose with a 10-minute lockout.

Assessment Activities	Findings/Defining Characteristics*
Ask Mrs. Mays what she did at home to control her pain.	Her **pain escalated** from a 3 to a 10, so she doubled her medica-tion and went to bed, but this did not help.
Ask Mrs. Mays what her pain intensity is now.	On a scale of 0 to 10, **she reports a 9.**
Ask Mrs. Mays what her pain has prevented her from doing.	She responds that she is **unable to complete her own hygiene activities, sleep, or eat well.**
Observe Mrs. Mays's nonverbal behavior.	She is **restless, unable to stay focused,** and remains very still; **muscles tense and frowning** during the history taking.
Ask Mrs. Mays her pain intensity goal (out of 10).	She says that a pain intensity of 5 out of 10 helps her function better right now. A goal of 3 is preferable.

*__Defining characteristics__ are shown in bold type.

Nursing Diagnosis: Acute pain related to abrupt onset of inflammation.

Planning

Goal	Expected Outcomes (NOC)†
	Pain Control
Client will obtain a tolerable level of pain before discharge.	Client will report pain at stated goal or below.
	Client uses PCA device appropriately.
	Pain: Disruptive Effects
Client will actively participate in ADLs.	Mrs. Mays will report sleeping for 5 to 6 hours without interrup-tion from pain.
	She will complete her own hygiene with minimal assistance.
	She will walk the hallway with her husband every 4 hours for 15 minutes.
	Medication Response
Mrs. Mays will not experience unmanageable opioid side effects.	Mrs. Mays will report having a normal bowel movement every other day.

†Outcome classification labels from Moorhead S and others: *Nursing outcomes classification (NOC)*, ed 4, St. Louis, 2008, Mosby.

Interventions (NIC)‡
Pain Management

	Rationale
• Begin PCA at ordered dose. Explain to client and spouse how to use the PCA. Emphasize the importance of only the client pushing the button, not the husband.	Acute cancer pain rated a 7 (or more) out of 10 requires immedi-ate-release opioid. Discouraging the husband from pushing the button will prevent unnecessary doses and reduce poten-tial toxic effects of the opioid. Client needs to be awake to perceive the pain and push the button (Pasero, 2003).
• Monitor IV PCA morphine use. Explain to client and spouse the action of the medication, potential side effects, and the importance of reporting unrelieved pain.	Pain is easier to prevent than to treat. Side effects are usually transient, except for constipation. Calculating 24-hour dose of opioid helps determine appropriate oral dose (Pasero, 2003).
• Have clients select nonpharmacological interventions that have relieved pain in the past (e.g., distraction, music, sim-ple relaxation therapy) or that are acceptable to them.	Rehabilitative approaches augment pharmacological therapy and help clients regain impaired physical functioning, as well as manage life changes, anxiety, and depression (Gruener and Lande, 2006).
• Teach spouse how to perform slow-stroke back massage.	Slow-stroke back massage is easy to do, takes a brief time, and induces relaxation (Snyder and Wieland, 2003).

‡Intervention classification labels from Bulechek GM, Butcher HK, and Dochterman JM: *Nursing interventions classification (NIC)*, ed 5, St. Louis, 2008, Mosby.

Continued

NURSING CARE PLAN

Acute Pain—cont'd

Evaluation

Nursing Actions	Client Response/Finding	Achievement of Outcome
Ask Mrs. Mays if she attained her pain relief goal most of the time.	She responds, "My pain usually runs around a 3, except when I start walking."	Mrs. Mays reports an acceptable level of pain. Instruct her to push her button before ambulating.
Observe Mrs. Mays performing ADLs, walking, and during sleep.	She is dressed for breakfast, walking the hallway every 4 hours with her husband. The night nurse's notes indicate she slept through the night.	Ability to perform ADLs and sleep has improved. Continue to monitor.
Observe Mrs. Mays as she ambulates the hallway.	Mrs. Mays successfully ambulated the hallway with her husband twice during the shift with minimal increase in pain intensity.	Improved pain control increased her activity, a nonverbal indicator of pain. Continue to monitor.
Ask Mr. Mays if he was able to give his wife a back rub.	He reported that she did not want a back rub but preferred to have her feet rubbed, which he was happy to do. "She said it made her feel more relaxed."	Nonpharmacological intervention successful, but needs changing from back rub to foot rub in the nursing care plan.
Ask Mrs. Mays when was the last time she had a bowel movement and its consistency.	She has not had a bowel movement in 3 days (since starting the morphine PCA).	Assess her abdomen for bowel sounds and distention and for return of flatus. Consult with primary health care provider about starting a stimulant laxative once intestinal obstruction is ruled out (St. Marie, 2002).
Observe Mrs. Mays for excessive drowsiness.	Mrs. Mays is awake and alert during conversations and interacts frequently with her husband.	Sedation, an indicator of too much opioid, is not identified. Continue to monitor.

members help clients resolve spiritual pain. It is important to involve the family in the plan of care because they often administer care in the home after discharge. If the pain management plan is not successful in achieving the identified pain relief goal, talk with the primary health care provider about changing the plan. Pain expert consultation is sometimes necessary.

Implementation

Pain therapy requires an individualized approach, perhaps more so than any other client problem. The nurse, client, and oftentimes the family are partners in using pain-control measures. Nurses administer and monitor interventions ordered by primary health care providers (HCPs) for pain relief and independently use pain-relief measures that complement those prescribed by a primary HCP. Generally you try the least invasive or safest therapy first along with previously used successful client remedies. If there is doubt about a medical therapy, consult with the primary HCP.

Heightened public awareness and increased political pressure are improving adult and pediatric pain management. Researchers are refining methods for managing children's acute or chronic pain and exploring new modalities (Brislin and Rose, 2005; Schechter and others, 2003).

Health Promotion. Clients are better prepared to handle almost any situation when they understand it. The experience of pain is no exception. However, clients with moderate to severe pain are not always able to participate in the decision-making process until the pain is controlled to a tolerable level. Once you accomplish this, you are able to begin teaching.

Because pain affects a person's physical and mental functioning, holistic health approaches are important interventions for maintaining a person's wellness. Holistic health is an ongoing state of wellness that involves taking care of the physical self, expressing emotions appropriately and effectively, using the mind constructively, being creatively involved with others, and becoming aware of higher levels of consciousness (American Holistic Health Association, 1999). The concept of holistic health parallels the values of nursing in maintaining the integrity of the whole person.

The role of clients is to actively participate in their own well-being. Common holistic health approaches include wellness education, regular exercise, rest, attention to good hygiene practices and nutrition, and management of interpersonal relationships. When a person develops pain, there are nonpharmacological as well as pharmacological strategies for you to offer. Several of the nonpharmacological interventions do not need an order, but are nurse initiated.

Nonpharmacological Pain-Relief Interventions. A number of nonpharmacological interventions are available that lessen pain; however, they are to be used *with* and not in place of pharmacological measures (Gruener and Lande, 2006; McCaffery and Pasero, 1999). Nonpharmacological interventions include cognitive-behavioral and physical approaches. The goals of cognitive-behavioral interventions are to change clients' perceptions of pain, to alter pain behavior, and to provide clients with a greater sense of control. Distraction, prayer, relaxation, guided imagery, music, and **biofeedback** are examples. Physical approaches have the goal of providing pain relief, correcting physical dysfunction, altering physiological responses, and reducing fears associated with pain-related immobility. Chiropractic therapy and acupuncture/acupressure therapy are examples (see Chapter 36). Complementary and alternative medicine (CAM) therapies such as therapeutic touch are also available. The AHCPR guidelines for acute pain management (1992) cite non-pharmacological interventions to be appropriate for clients who meet the following criteria:

- Find such interventions appealing
- Express anxiety or fear
- Will possibly benefit from avoiding or reducing drug therapy
- Are likely to experience and need to cope with a prolonged interval of postoperative pain
- Have incomplete pain relief after use of pharmacological interventions

Relaxation and Guided Imagery. Clients are able to alter affective-motivational and cognitive pain perception through relaxation and **guided imagery. Relaxation** is mental and physical freedom from tension or stress that provides individuals a sense of self-control. You are able to use relaxation techniques at any phase of health or illness. Physiological and behavioral changes associated with relaxation include the following: decreased pulse, blood pressure, and respirations; heightened global awareness; decreased oxygen consumption; a sense of peace; and decreased muscle tension and metabolic rate. Relaxation techniques include meditation, yoga, Zen, guided imagery, and progressive relaxation exercises (see Chapter 36). For effective relaxation, teach techniques only when the client is not distracted by acute discomfort. Chapter 36 offers several relaxation exercise approaches. Sometimes you will need to use a combination of these techniques to achieve optimal pain relief. With practice the client will soon be able to perform relaxation exercises independently.

Distraction. The reticular activating system inhibits painful stimuli if a person receives sufficient or excessive sensory input. With sufficient sensory stimuli, a person is able to ignore or become unaware of pain. Persons who are bored or in isolation have only their pain to think about and thus perceive it more acutely. Distraction directs a client's attention to something other than pain and thus reduces the awareness of pain. There is one disadvantage. If it works, HCPs or family members will question the existence or severity of the pain. Distraction works best for short, intense pain lasting a few minutes, such as during an invasive procedure or while waiting for an analgesic to work. Use activities enjoyed by the client that will act as distractions. These might include singing, praying, or describing pictures aloud, listening to music, and playing games. You will use most distractions in a hospital, home, or long-term care facility.

Music. Music treats acute or chronic pain, stress, anxiety, and depression (Siedlecki, 2006). Music diverts the person's attention away from the pain and creates a relaxation response. You are able to use music creatively in many clinical situations. Clients can per-

form (play an instrument or sing a song) or listen to music. Music therapy uses all kinds of music. It is important to let the clients select the type of music preferred. Music produces an altered state of consciousness through sound, silence, space, and time. The client has to listen to it for at least 15 minutes for it to be therapeutic (Gerdner, 2001). The use of earphones helps clients concentrate on the music uninterrupted, by increasing the volume, while also avoiding annoying other clients or staff.

Cutaneous Stimulation. Stimulation of the skin helps relieve pain. A massage, warm bath, ice bag, and transcutaneous electrical nerve stimulation (TENS) stimulate the skin to reduce pain perception (When your pain, 2002). How **cutaneous stimulation** works is unclear. One suggestion is that it causes release of endorphins, thus blocking the transmission of painful stimuli. The gate-control theory suggests that cutaneous stimulation activates larger, faster-transmitting A-beta sensory nerve fibers. This closes the gate, thus decreasing pain transmission through small-diameter C fibers (Melzack and Wall, 1965).

Cutaneous stimulation gives clients and families some control over pain symptoms and treatment in the home. The proper use of cutaneous stimulation helps reduce muscle tension that increases pain. When using cutaneous stimulation, eliminate sources of environmental noise, help the client to assume a comfortable position, and explain the purpose of the therapy. Do not use cutaneous stimulation directly on sensitive skin areas (e.g., burns, bruises, skin rashes, inflammation, and underlying bone fractures).

Massage is effective for producing physical and mental relaxation, reducing pain, and enhancing the effectiveness of pain medication. Massaging the back, shoulders, hands, and/or feet for 3 to 5 minutes relaxes muscles and promotes sleep and comfort. Cassileth and Vickers (2004) reported a 50% reduction in pain, fatigue, stress/anxiety, nausea, and depression in clients with cancer who systematically used massage therapy. Massages communicate caring and are easy for family members or other health care personnel to learn (Box 43-11).

Cold and heat applications (see Chapter 48) relieve pain and promote healing. The selection of heat versus cold interventions varies with clients' conditions (McCarberg and O'Connor, 2004). For example, moist heat helps to relieve the pain from a tension headache, and cold applications reduce the acute pain from inflamed joints. When using any form of heat or cold application, instruct the client to avoid injury to the skin by checking the temperature and avoiding direct application of cold or heat to the skin. Especially at risk are clients with spinal cord or other neurological disorders, older adults, and confused clients.

Cold therapies are particularly effective for pain relief. Ice massage involves the use of a large ice cube or a small paper cup filled with water and frozen (water rises out of the cup as it freezes to create a smooth surface of ice for massage). A nurse or the client applies the ice with firm pressure to the skin, followed by a slow, steady, circular massage over the area. You apply cold near the pain site, on the opposite side of the body corresponding to the pain site, or on a site located between the brain and the pain site. Each client responds differently to the site of application. Application near the actual site of pain tends to work best. A client feels cold, burning, and aching sensations and numbness. When numbness occurs, remove the ice for usually 5 to 10 minutes. Cold is particularly effective for tooth or mouth pain when you

✳ **BOX 43-11**   **PROCEDURAL GUIDELINES**

Massage

Delegation Considerations: It is the nurse's responsibility to assess for any possible contraindication or client response to massage. The skill of administering a massage may be delegated to nursing assistive personnel (NAP). The nurse directs NAP by:

- Instructing NAP as to which body parts to massage, the importance of not massaging reddened skin areas, and clarifying the early signs of impaired skin integrity for select clients and their situation.
- Instructing NAP to report changes in the client's skin to the nurse.

Equipment: Bath towel, moisturizing lotion, bath towel or blanket.
1. Assist client with assuming a comfortable position.
2. Dim room lights and/or turn on soft music according to client preference.
3. Perform hand hygiene. Place container of lotion in warm water.
4. Adjust or remove client's bed clothing.
5. Place small amount of warmed lotion in hands.

Critical Decision Point: Do not give back or neck massages to clients who have had neck or spinal trauma and/or surgery without an order by their primary health care provider.

6. Massage each body part at least 10 minutes.
   a. *Back:* Beginning at sacral area, massage in a circular motion (see illustration) while moving upward from buttocks to shoulders. Use a firm smooth stroke over the scapula. Continue in one smooth stroke to upper arms and laterally along sides of back down to iliac crests. Use long, gliding strokes along muscles of spine (see illustrations). Knead any muscles that feel tense or tight. Knead skin by gently grasping tissue between thumb and fingers. Knead upward along one side of the spine from buttocks to shoulders around nape of neck. Knead or stroke downward toward sacrum. Repeat along other side of the back.

   b. *Neck:* Support the neck at the hairline with one hand, and massage up with a gliding stroke. Knead muscles on one side. Switch hands to support neck, and knead other side. Stretch the neck slightly, with one hand at the top and the other at the bottom.
   c. *Arms:* Use a gliding stroke to massage from the client's wrist or forearm. With thumb and forefinger of both hands, knead muscles from forearm to shoulder. Continue kneading biceps, deltoid, and triceps muscles. Finish with gliding strokes from the wrists to the shoulder.
   d. *Hands:* Slowly open the client's palm; glide fingers over the palmar surface. Use thumbs to apply friction to the palm and move thumbs in a circular motion; stretch the palm outward. Massage each finger using a corkscrew-like motion from base of finger to the tip. Gently knead each muscle in the client's fingers. Glide hands smoothly from fingertips to wrists. Repeat for other hand.
   e. *Feet:* Gently massage the top and bottom of each foot. Using gliding motion, massage from heel to toe. Gently massage the dorsal surface of the foot and each toe. Repeat for other foot.

Critical Decision Point: Do not massage client's legs or calf muscles because there is a risk of dislodging a vascular clot.

5. Wipe excess lotion off client's back, neck, or extremity. If necessary, retie gown or assist with pajamas, and assist client to comfortable position.
6. Ask client to rate level of pain. Note any areas of muscle pain or tension.

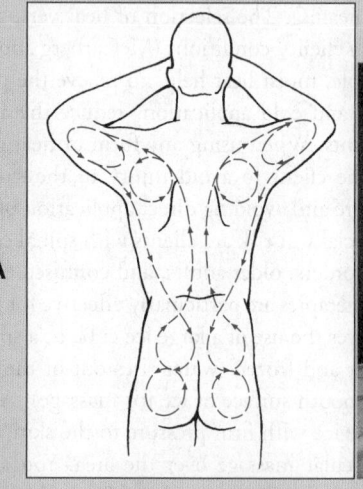
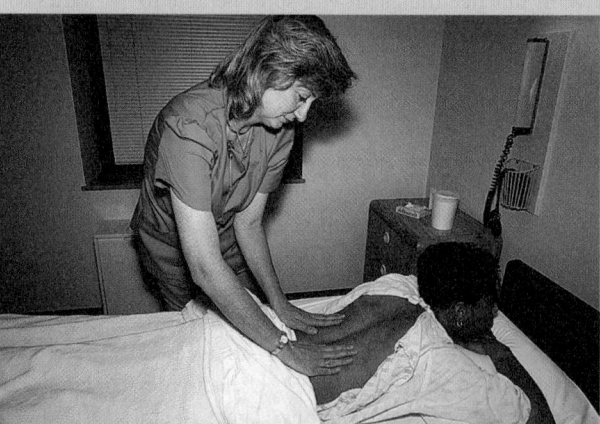

STEP 6a A, Back massage pattern. **B,** Nurse massages muscles along spine.

❋ BOX 43-12 Controlling Painful Stimuli in the Client's Environment

- Tighten and smooth wrinkled bed linen.
- Reposition tubing on which client is lying.
- Loosen constricting bandages (unless specifically applied as a pressure dressing).
- Change wet dressings and linens.
- Position client in anatomical alignment according to client's preference or requirements.
- Check temperature of hot or cold applications, including bathwater.
- Lift client in bed—do not pull.
- Position client correctly on bedpan.
- Avoid exposing skin or mucous membranes to irritants (e.g., urine, stool, wound drainage).
- Keep clients clean, dry, and turned if needed. Use urinary incontinence pads if indicated.
- Prevent urinary retention by keeping Foley catheters patent and free flowing, while also monitoring urinary output.
- Prevent constipation with fluids, diet, exercise, and stimulant laxatives if needed.

place the ice on the web of the hand between the thumb and index finger. This point on the hand is an **acupressure** point that apparently influences nerve pathways to the face and head. Cold applications are also effective before invasive needle punctures.

Heat application is more effective for some clients. You can use heating pads or warm compresses, but teach clients to check the temperature of the compress and not to lie on the heating element because burning will possibly occur. Commercial pillows that can be warmed in the microwave and that contour to the body are also available.

Another form of cutaneous stimulation is **transcutaneous electrical nerve stimulation** (TENS), involving stimulation of the skin with a mild electrical current passed through external electrodes (Melzack and Wall, 2003). The therapy requires a primary HCP order. The TENS unit consists of a battery-powered transmitter, lead wires, and electrodes. You place the electrodes directly over or near the site of pain. Remove any hair or skin preparations before attaching the electrodes. The client turns the transmitter on when feeling pain. This creates a buzzing or tingling sensation. The client may adjust the intensity and quality of skin stimulation. The tingling sensation can be applied until pain relief occurs. TENS is effective for postsurgical and procedural pain control.

Herbals. Although herbals have not been sufficiently studied to recommend for pain relief, many clients self-medicate using herbals such as echinacea, ginseng, ginkgo biloba, and garlic supplements (Wirth and others, 2005). Herbals could have an interaction with prescribed analgesics; thus ask the client to report all substances taken to relieve pain (Yoon and Schaffer, 2006) (see Chapter 36).

Reducing Pain Perception. One simple way to promote comfort is by removing or preventing painful stimuli (Box 43-12). This is especially important for clients who are immobilized or have difficulty expressing themselves. For example, you have a client who becomes constipated, and who suffers from distention and abdominal cramping. As the nurse, you intervene

to ensure that the normal elimination process continues: increasing fluids, ambulating the client, and/or requesting stool softeners or laxatives. Another example involves reducing pain perception in the way you perform procedures. Always consider the client's condition, aspects of the procedure that are uncomfortable, and techniques to avoid causing pain. In a client with severe arthritic knee pain, who has severe discomfort during any extreme flexion of the knee, take precautions before walking the client to the bathroom. Make sure that an elevated toilet seat is available. Then the client will be able to sit and rise with minimal discomfort.

Acute Care

Acute Pain Management. Nurses care for clients who have acute pain due to invasive procedures (e.g., surgery or endoscopy) or trauma. The AHCPR (1992) established a pain treatment flow chart (Figure 43-11) for treatment of postoperative pain and pain from medical procedures and trauma. This systematic approach ensures quick response on the part of caregivers to client discomfort. The key to success is ongoing evaluation of interventions: Does the client feel relief? Are there any unacceptable side effects from the medications? It is the responsibility of the health care team to collaborate to find the combination of therapy that works best for a client.

Pharmacological Pain-Relief Interventions. Many pharmacological agents are available that provide pain relief. You must administer all analgesics using guidelines from The Joint Commission's National Patient Safety Goals (2007). A nurse's judgment in the use and management of analgesics helps ensure the best pain relief possible. The ideal analgesic has yet to be developed.

Analgesics. **Analgesics** are the most common and effective method of pain relief. However, primary HCPs and nurses still tend to undertreat clients because of incorrect drug information, concerns about addiction, anxiety over errors in using opioid analgesics, and administration of excessive medication. Nurses need to understand the drugs available for pain relief and their pharmacological effects.

There are three types of analgesics: (1) nonopioids, including acetaminophen and nonsteroidal antiinflammatory drugs (NSAIDs); (2) **opioids** (traditionally called narcotics); and (3) **adjuvants/coanalgesics,** a variety of medications that enhance analgesics or have analgesic properties that were originally unknown.

Acetaminophen (Tylenol) has no antiinflammatory or antiplatelet effects. It works peripherally and centrally, but its action is unknown. Its major adverse effect is hepatotoxicity. It is in a variety of over-the-counter (OTC) cold, flu, and allergy remedies. The maximum 24-hour dose is 4 g (the same dose limitation for aspirin). It is often combined with opioids (e.g., Percocet, Vicodin, Lortab, and Ultracet) because it reduces the dose of opioid needed to achieve successful pain control. You treat overdoses of acetaminophen with acetylcysteine (Mucomyst).

Nonselective NSAIDs, such as aspirin and ibuprofen, provide relief for mild to moderate acute intermittent pain, such as the pain associated with a headache or muscle strain. Treatment of mild to moderate postoperative pain begins with an NSAID unless contraindicated (AHCPR, 1992). NSAIDs are thought to act by inhibiting the synthesis of prostaglandins (Williams, 2005) and thus the cellular responses to inflammation. Most NSAIDs act on peripheral nerve receptors to reduce transmission of pain

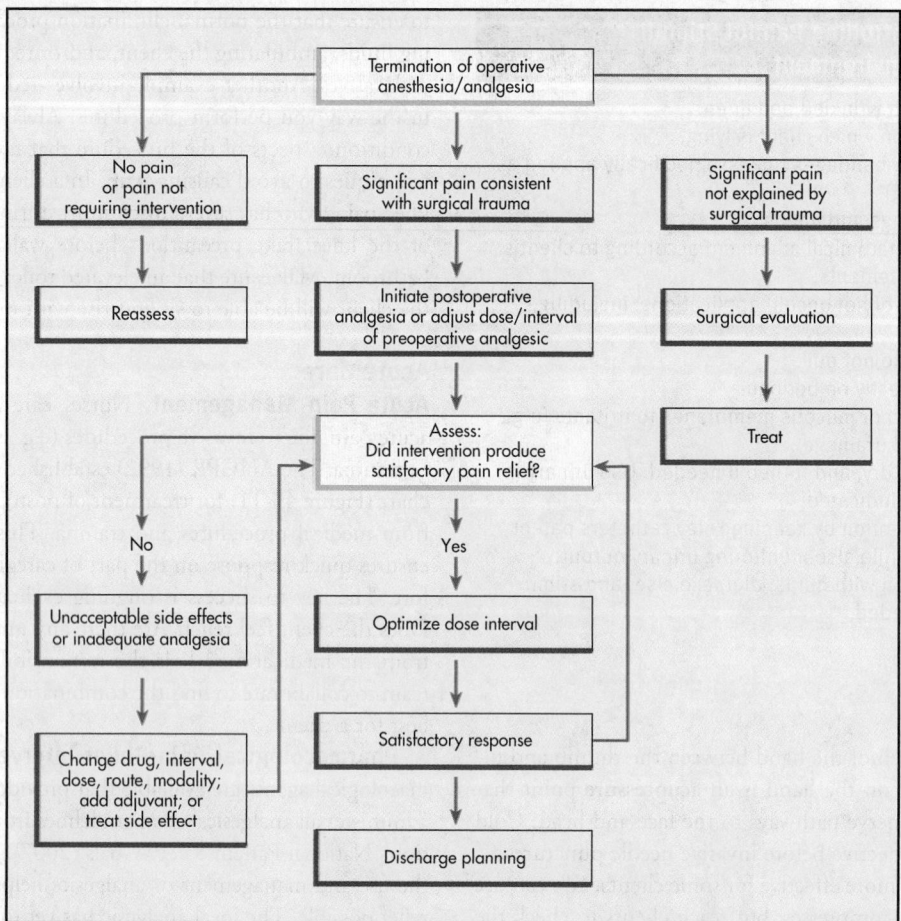

Figure 43-11 Pain treatment flow chart: postoperative phase. (From Agency for Health Care Policy and Research, Acute Pain Management Guideline Panel: *Acute pain management: operative or medical procedures and trauma,* Clinical Practice Guideline, AHCPR Pub No. 92-0032, Rockville, Md, 1992, Agency for Health Care Policy and Research, Public Health Service, U.S. Department of Health and Human Services.)

stimuli. Unlike opioids, NSAIDs do not depress the central nervous system, nor do they interfere with bowel or bladder function (AHCPR, 1992). Chronic NSAID use in the older client, though, is associated with more frequent adverse effects (gastrointestinal bleeding and renal insufficiency) and should be avoided. Mild to moderate musculoskeletal pain in older adults is effectively managed with the nonopioid acetaminophen (American Geriatrics Society [AGS], 2002).

Nonselective NSAIDs have been found to be safe when taken for short periods of time. Selective COX-2 inhibitors have caused heart attack and stroke and have been withdrawn from the market. Celebrex is the only selective COX-2 inhibitor currently available; however, it should not be used in clients with a sulfa allergy. Some clients with asthma or allergy to aspirin are also allergic to other NSAIDs (Williams, 2005). Some NSAIDs are available OTC; thus advise clients to discuss the use of OTC NSAIDs to manage pain with their primary HCP (D'Arcy, 2006).

Opioid or opioid-like analgesics are generally prescribed for moderate to severe pain. These analgesics act on higher centers of the brain and spinal cord by binding with opiate receptors to modify perception of pain. A rare adverse effect of opioids in opioid-naive clients is respiratory depression (Wheeler and others, 2002). Respiratory depression is only clinically significant if there is a decrease in

the rate *and* depth of respirations from the client's baseline assessment (McCaffery and Pasero, 1999). Clients who are breathing deeply rarely have clinical respiratory depression. It is important to note that another adverse effect of opioids, sedation, *always* occurs before respiratory depression. Thus closely monitor for sedation in opioid-naive clients (Pasero and McCaffery, 2002).

If a client experiences respiratory depression, you administer naloxone (0.4 mg diluted with 9 mL of saline) intravenous push (IVP) at a rate of 0.5 mL every 2 minutes until the respiratory rate is greater than 8 breaths per minute with good depth. Too fast an administration will reverse the analgesic effect and possibly cause pulmonary edema (APS, 2002). Reassess clients who receive naloxone every 15 minutes for 2 hours following drug administration because of the risk of renarcotization and the return of respiratory depression.

Additional adverse effects of opioids include nausea, vomiting, constipation, itching, urinary retention, myoclonus, and altered mental processes (Ersek and others, 2004). Except for constipation, these side effects usually stop once the client receives an opioid around-the-clock (ATC) for 4 to 10 days. You consider clients opioid-naive up until this point and opioid-tolerant after about a week of ATC opioid dosing. One way to maximize pain relief while potentially decreasing drug use is to administer analge-

---

✳ BOX 43-13 Nursing Principles for Administering Analgesics

Know the Client's Previous Response to Analgesics

Determine whether the client has allergies.

Know whether client is at risk for using NSAIDs (e.g., history of GI bleeding or renal insufficiency) or opioids (e.g., history of obstructive or central sleep apnea).

Identify previous doses and routes of analgesic administration to avoid undertreatment.

Determine whether client obtained relief.

Ask whether a nonopioid was as effective as an opioid.

Select Proper Medications When More Than One Is Ordered

Use nonopioid analgesics or opioid combination drugs for mild to moderate pain.

You can give opioids with nonopioids.

In older adults, avoid combinations of opioids.

Fentanyl patches, morphine, or hydromorphone are the opioids of choice for long-term management of severe pain.

Intravenous medications act more quickly and can relieve severe, acute pain within 1 hour, whereas oral medication may take as long as 2 hours to relieve pain.

Know to avoid intramuscular analgesics, especially in older adults.

Use an opioid with a nonopioid analgesic for severe pain because such combinations treat pain peripherally and centrally.

For chronic pain, give sustained-release oral formulations around-the-clock (ATC).

Know the Accurate Dosage

Recall that 4 g is considered the maximum 24-hour dose for acetaminophen and acetylsalicylic acid (ASA); 3200 mg for ibuprofen.

Adjust doses, as appropriate, for children and older clients.

Large doses of opioids are acceptable in opioid-tolerant clients, but not opioid-naive clients.

When titrating opioids, it is important to titrate to effect or to uncontrollable side effects.

Assess the Right Time and Interval for Administration

Administer analgesics as soon as pain occurs and before it increases in severity.

An ATC administration schedule is usually best.

Give analgesics before pain-producing procedures or activities.

Know the average duration of action for a drug and the time of administration so that the peak effect occurs when the pain is most intense.

Use extended-release opioid formulations to treat chronic pain.

Avoid abrupt stopping of opioids in clients who are opioid-tolerant.

Modified from McCaffery M, Pasero C: *Pain: clinical manual*, ed 2, St. Louis, 1999.

GI, Gastrointestinal; *NSAIDs*, nonsteroidal antiinflammatory drugs.

---

sics on an ATC basis rather than on a prn basis. Paice and others (2005) found that clients receiving ATC opioids reported lower pain intensity scores than clients receiving prn opioids. The American Pain Society (2003) states that if you anticipate pain for the majority of the day you should consider ATC administration.

The American Geriatrics Society (AGS) (2002) feels that opioids are probably not used enough with older persons. The AGS suggests a "start low" (dose) and "go slow" (upward dose titration) philosophy. Furthermore, the AGS discourages the use of meperidine or propoxyphene in elders (AGS, 2002; Fick and others, 2003; Willens, 2006). Meperidine is not recommended as an analgesic at any age because of its toxic metabolite, normeperidine, which can cause seizures (APS, 2003; Eksterowicz, 2003; Latta and others, 2002).

The proper use of analgesics requires careful assessment and critical thinking in the application of pharmacological principles and logic (Box 43-13). A person's response to an analgesic is highly individualized. An NSAID is sometimes as effective as or more effective than an opioid for some clients if the pain is due to inflammation. An orally administered analgesic usually has a longer onset and duration of action than an injectable form. In addition, controlled- or extended-release opioid formulations (MS Contin, OxyContin, Kadian, Avinza, and methadone) are available for administration every 8 to 12 hours ATC. Physicians should not order these long-acting formulations prn.

You need to know the comparative potencies of analgesics in oral and injectable form. In addition, know the route of administration most effective for a client so that you achieve controlled, sustained pain relief. If nurses on succeeding shifts choose different routes for the same doses, the client will not receive the same level of analgesia, and pain control will be poor. Equianalgesic charts, charts converting one opioid to another or parenteral

forms of opioids (e.g., morphine to hydromorphone) to oral forms (or visa versa), are available on most nursing units or by contacting pharmacy staff. Experimentally, researchers are mixing opioids in gels and applying topically to open painful wounds (Drew and Peltier, 2005; Shukla and others, 2005).

Before administering opioids it is important to consider the client's situation, including current treatments, diseases/conditions, and/or organ (kidneys/liver) function. Opioid doses often need adjusting up or down according to client circumstances. Situations requiring special considerations include breast-feeding mothers, clients on dialysis, those with neurological or respiratory conditions, and clients with recent abdominal surgery.

The Joint Commission (2007) requires health care agencies to have range order policies in place to help guide nurses in selecting the most appropriate dose of a medication. "Range orders are medication orders in which the dose varies over a prescribed range depending on the situation or the patient's status" (Manworren, 2006). An example is "Administer 5 to 10 mg morphine sulfate IVP for acute pain." Such an order is dangerous when there are no real clinical guidelines to use for selecting the exact dose. Range orders give nurses the flexibility needed to treat clients' pain in a timely way while allowing for differences in client response to pain and to analgesia. Range orders should, for example, take into consideration the client's age, pain intensity, and comorbidities; avoid frequency ranges; and prescribe a maximum dose that is at least two times but not more than four times the minimum dose in the range (Pasero, Manworren, and McCaffery, 2007). For additional examples of clinical guidelines to use for range orders, see Manworren (2006) and ASPMN (2004) position statements on range orders.

Adjuvants/coanalgesics are drugs originally developed to treat conditions other than pain but have been shown to have analgesic properties. For example, tricyclic antidepressants (e.g., nortriptyline) and anticonvulsants (e.g., gabapenti [Neurontin]) successfully treat neuropathic pain (Gordon and Love, 2004), as does infusional lidocaine (Ferrini and Paice, 2004). Corticosteroids relieve pain associated with inflammation and bone metastasis. Other examples of adjuvants are bisphosphonates and calcitonin given for bone pain (Jacox and others, 1994).

Sedatives, antianxiety agents, and muscle relaxants have *no* analgesic effect; however, they *can* cause drowsiness and impaired coordination, judgment, and mental alertness and contribute to respiratory depression. It is important to avoid solely attributing these adverse effects to the opioid. You need to conduct a thorough reassessment.

Patient-Controlled Analgesia. When clients depend on nurses for prn analgesia, an erratic cycle of alternating pain and analgesia often occurs. The client feels pain and asks for medication, but you must first assess the client and then prepare the medication. Under this circumstance, analgesia finally occurs in about an hour, but pain relief may last only 30 minutes. Then gradually the client again feels discomfort, and the cycle begins again. The client is constantly going in and out of analgesic therapeutic range.

A drug delivery system called **patient-controlled analgesia (PCA)** is a safe method for pain management that many clients prefer. It is a drug delivery system that allows clients to self-administer opioids (morphine, hydromorphone, and fentanyl) with minimal risk of overdose. The goal is to maintain a constant plasma level of analgesic to avoid the problems of prn dosing. Systemic PCA traditionally involves IV or subcutaneous drug administration; however, oral PCA systems are currently under study. PCAs are portable infusion pumps (usually computerized), containing a chamber for a syringe or bag that delivers a small, preset dose of opioid (Figure 43-12). To receive a demand dose, the client pushes a button attached to the PCA device. Systems

are designed to deliver a specified number of doses every 1 to 4 hours (depending on the pump) given every 5 to 15 minutes (programmable) to avoid overdoses (APS, 2003). Most pumps have locked safety systems that prevent tampering by clients or family members and are generally safe to be managed in the home. For clients with cancer pain, a low-dose continuous infusion (basal rate) of 0.5 to 1 mg/hr may be programmed to deliver a steady dose of continuous medication. New *disposable* infusion pumps are currently under investigation.

There are many benefits to PCA use. The client gains control over pain, and pain relief does not depend on nurse availability. Clients also have access to medication when they need it. This decreases anxiety and leads to decreased medication use. Small doses of medications are delivered at short intervals, stabilizing serum drug concentrations for sustained pain relief.

Client preparation and teaching is critical to the safe and effective use of PCA devices (Box 43-14). Clients need to understand the PCA and be physically able to locate and press the button to deliver the dose. Be sure to instruct family members not to "hit the button" for the client. However, Authorized Agent Controlled Analgesia (AACA) guidelines, *authorizing* a family member or nurse to administer the analgesic, are available (Wuhrman and others, 2006).

Check the IV line and PCA device regularly to ensure proper functioning. Even though clients control administration of analgesics, programmable PCA errors do occur. In opioid-naive clients, do not increase demand or basal dose *and* shorten the interval time simultaneously because this will increase the risk for oversedation and respiratory depression. Document drug dosages, and track any waste of medications according to agency policy (Pasero, 2003)

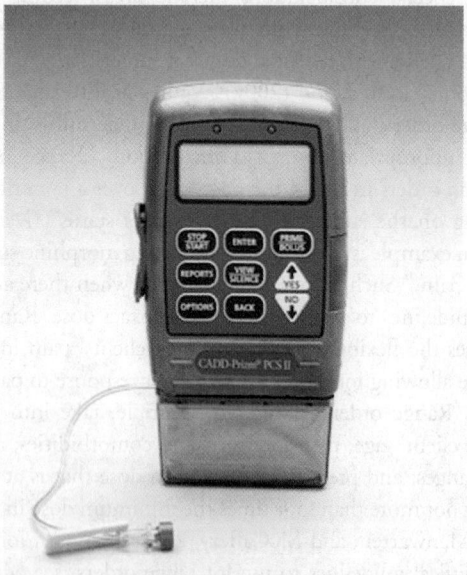

Figure 43-12 Patient-controlled analgesia pump with cassette. (Courtesy Smiths Medical MD, Inc, St. Paul, Minn.)

✱ **BOX 43-14** **CLIENT TEACHING**

Preparation for Patient-Controlled Analgesia
Objectives
- Client will be able to explain purpose of PCA in managing pain.
- Client will use the PCA device correctly.
- Client achieves pain control.

Teaching Strategies
- Teach the use of PCA before any procedure so that clients understand how to use it after awakening from anesthesia or sedation. Reinforce as needed.
- Instruct client in the purpose of PCA, emphasizing that the client controls medication delivery.
- Explain that the pump prevents the risk of overdose.
- Tell family members or friends to not operate the PCA device for the client.
- Have the client demonstrate use of the PCA delivery button.

Evaluation
- Ask client to tell you the purpose of the PCA device.
- Observe the client administering a dose.
- Evaluate the severity of the client's pain 15 to 20 minutes after use of the PCA device.

PCA, Patient-controlled analgesia.

SAFETY ALERT PCA basal doses are *not* recommended for opioid-naive clients following surgery because of the possibility for respiratory depression.

The first controlled analgesia device for oral medications, Medication on Demand [MOD] recently became available. This device allows clients access to their own oral prn mediations, including opioids and other analgesics, antiemetics, and anxiolytics, at the bedside (Medication on Demand, 2006).

Perineural Local Anesthetic Infusion. You are able to manage pain for a variety of inpatient and outpatient adult and pediatric surgical procedures with **perineural infusion** pumps (e.g., Breg, On-Q, and disposable units under investigation). An unsutured catheter from a surgical wound placed near a nerve or groups of nerves connects to a pump containing a local anesthetic (bupivacaine or ropivacaine). The pump is set as a demand or continuous mode, usually left in place for 48 hours. The client learns how to discontinue the pump at home and to bring the catheter to the next primary HCP visit. Some clients still need oral analgesics, but this often reduces the total dose (Pasero, 2004).

Topical Analgesics. Topical analgesics such as ELA-Max/LMX and EMLA (eutectic mixture of local anesthetics) are available for children. You apply EMLA via a disk or thick cream to the skin 30 to 60 minutes before minor procedures (e.g., IV start) or anesthetic infiltration of soft tissue. Do not place EMLA around eyes, the tympanic membrane, or over large skin surfaces.

The Lidoderm patch is a topical analgesic effective for cutaneous neuropathic pain in adults. Place three patches, cut to size, on and around the pain site using a 12-hour on, 12-hour off schedule to avoid lidocaine toxicity. Other topical analgesics include ketoprofen patch and capsaicin lotion.

Local and Regional Anesthetics. **Local anesthesia** is the local infiltration of an anesthetic medication to induce loss of sensation to a body part. Primary HCPs frequently use local anesthesia during brief surgical procedures such as removal of a skin lesion or suturing a wound. Apply local anesthetics topically on skin and mucous membranes or inject subcutaneously or intradermally to anesthetize a body part. The drugs produce temporary loss of sensation by inhibiting nerve conduction. Local anesthetics also block motor and autonomic functions, depending on the amount used and the location and depth of an injection. Smaller sensory nerve fibers are more sensitive to local anesthetics than are large motor fibers. As a result, the client loses sensation before losing motor function, and conversely, motor activity returns before sensation.

Local anesthetics cause side effects, depending on their absorption into the circulation. Itching or burning of the skin or a localized rash is common after topical applications. Application to vascular mucous membranes increases the chance of systemic effects, such as a change in heart rate.

Regional anesthesia is the injection of a local anesthetic to block a group of sensory nerve fibers. Tissues are anesthetized layer by layer, as the surgeon or anesthesia provider introduces the agent into deeper structures of the body. Kinds of regional anesthesia include epidural anesthesia, pudendal blocks, and spinal anesthesia. **Epidural analgesia** is common for the treatment of acute postoperative pain, labor and delivery pain, and chronic cancer pain (Roman and Cabaj, 2005). It permits control or re-duction of severe pain and reduces the client's overall opioid requirement; thus minimizing adverse effects. Epidural analgesia is short or long term, depending on the client's condition and life expectancy.

The HCP administers epidural analgesia into the spinal **epidural space** (Figure 43-13). The primary HCP inserts a blunt-tip needle into the level of the vertebral interspace nearest to the area requiring analgesia. When the needle reaches the space, this allows solutions to be freely injected and for small catheters to be passed into it. Once a catheter is advanced into the epidural space and the needle is removed, the remainder of the catheter is secured with a dressing and taped along the back of the client. If the catheter is only temporary, it is connected to tubing positioned along the spine and over the client's shoulder. The end of the catheter is then placed on the client's chest for the nurse's access. Epidural analgesia is anesthesiology or nurse controlled, depending on agency policy. Some clients are given control of the demand dose, known as patient-controlled epidural analgesia (PCEA).

Nursing Implications. You are responsible for providing emotional support to clients receiving local or regional anesthesia by explaining the insertion technique and warning clients that they will temporarily lose sensory function within minutes of injection. In the case of regional anesthesia, motor and autonomic (bowel and bladder control) function are also quickly lost. It is common for clients to fear paralysis because epidural and spinal injections come close to the spinal cord. To reassure the client, explain that numbness, tingling, and coldness are common. Catheter insertion is painful unless the primary HCP first numbs the injection site. Prepare clients for such discomfort. Before a client receives an analgesic, check for allergies. Also check to be sure the drugs (Duramorph and Sublimaze) administered via the epidural catheter are free of potentially neurotoxic substances such as preservatives and additives (Roman and Cabaj, 2005). Assess vital signs to monitor systemic effects.

After administration of a local anesthetic, protect the client from injury until full sensory and motor function return. Clients are at risk for injuring the anesthetized body part without knowing it. For example, after an injection into a joint, warn the client

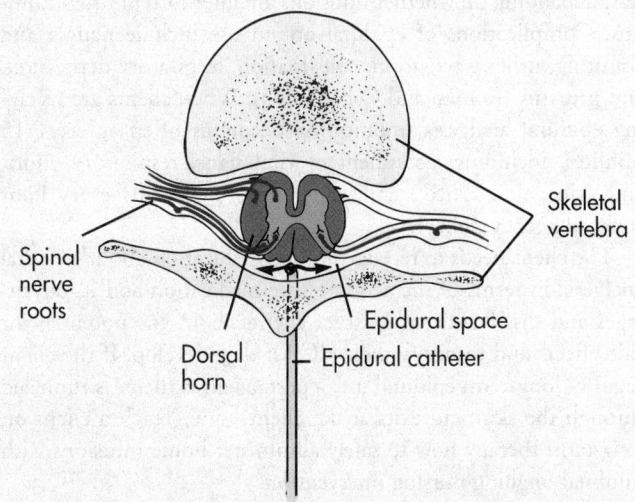

Figure 43-13 Anatomical drawing of epidural space.

✳ **TABLE 43-6 Nursing Care for Clients With Epidural Infusions**

GOAL	ACTIONS
Prevent catheter displacement.	Secure catheter (if not connected to implanted reservoir) carefully to outside skin.
Maintain catheter function.	Check external dressing around catheter site for dampness or discharge. (Leak of cerebrospinal fluid may develop.)
	Use transparent dressing to secure catheter and to aid inspection.
	Inspect catheter for breaks.
Prevent infection.	Use strict aseptic technique when caring for catheter (see Chapter 34).
	Do not routinely change dressing over site.
	Change infusion tubing every 24 hours.
Monitor for respiratory depression.	Monitor vital signs, especially respirations, per policy.
	Use pulse oximetry and apnea monitoring.
Prevent undesirable complications.	Assess for pruritus (itching) and nausea and vomiting.
	Administer antiemetics as ordered.
Maintain urinary and bowel function.	Monitor intake and output.
	Assess for bladder and bowel distention.
	Assess for discomfort, frequency, and urgency.

to avoid using the joint until function returns. For clients with topical anesthesia, avoid applying heat or cold to numb areas. After spinal anesthesia the client stays in bed until sensory and motor function return. Assist the client during the first attempt at getting out of bed.

When managing epidural infusions, connect the catheter to an infusion pump, a port, or reservoir, or cap it off for bolus injections. To reduce the risk of accidental epidural injection of drugs intended for IV use, clearly label the catheter "epidural catheter." Always administer continuous infusions through electronic infusion devices for proper control. Because of the catheter location, use surgical asepsis to prevent a serious and potentially fatal infection. Notify primary HCPs immediately of any signs or symptoms of infection or pain at the insertion site. Thorough hygiene is necessary during nursing procedures to keep the catheter system clean and dry.

Nursing implications for managing epidural analgesia are numerous (Table 43-6). Avoid supplemental doses of opioids or sedative/hypnotics because of possible additive central nervous system adverse effects. Monitoring for effects of medications differs, depending on whether infusions are intermittent or continuous. Complications of epidural opioid use include nausea and vomiting, urinary retention, constipation, respiratory depression, and **pruritus** (Roman and Cabaj, 2005). When clients are receiving epidural analgesia, monitoring occurs as often as every 15 minutes, including assessment of vital signs, respiratory effort, and skin color. Once stabilized, monitoring occurs every hour (refer to agency policy).

The client needs to receive thorough education about epidural analgesia in terms of the action of the medication and its advantages and disadvantages. Instruct clients about the potential for side effects and to notify their HCP if they develop. If the client requires long-term epidural use, a permanent catheter is tunneled through the skin and exits at the client's side. Teach a client on long-term therapy how to safely administer home infusions with minimal ongoing nursing intervention.

Invasive Interventions for Pain Relief. When severe pain persists despite medical treatment, invasive interventions available

for consideration include intrathecal implantable pumps or injections, spinal cord stimulators, deep brain stimulation, neuroablative procedures (cordotomy, rhizotomy, thalamotomy), trigger point injections, radiofrequency ablation, cryoablation, intradiscal electrothermal (IDET) annuloplasty, vertebroplasty, intraspinal medications (opioids, steroids, local anesthetics, alpha agonists), and others. It is not acceptable to tell a client with severe unrelieved pain that there is "nothing more that we can do for you." Clients with pain unresponsive to medications need consultation with a pain expert.

Procedure Pain Management. The Thunder Project II (Puntillo and others, 2001) identified several procedures causing pain in critical care clients: turning, wound drain removal, tracheal suctioning, femoral catheter removal, placement of a central line, and changing of nonburn wound dressings.

Premedicating clients before painful procedures allows clients to cooperate more fully and reduces the experience of pain. Clients with abdominal pain who present in the emergency department need pain medication *before* an extensive physical examination and diagnostic procedures to attain more accurate data (APS, 2003). In addition, the American Society of Anesthesiologists (Practice Guidelines, 2004) recommends premedicating clients before surgery as part of a multimodal analgesic pain management program.

Chronic Noncancer and Cancer Pain Management. Cancer pain is either chronic or acute. The AHCPR released clinical practice guidelines for cancer pain management (Jacox and others, 1994). The guidelines treat cancer pain in a more comprehensive and aggressive manner. Similarly, they provide clients and families more options for pain relief. Figure 43-14 is a flow chart depicting cancer pain management from assessment to various treatment options. The best choice of treatment often changes as the client's condition and the characteristics of pain change. You can use nonpharmacological interventions with pharmacological interventions.

Various medications and routes of administration provide relief for clients with cancer pain. Long-acting or controlled-release medications have been very successful in managing all types of

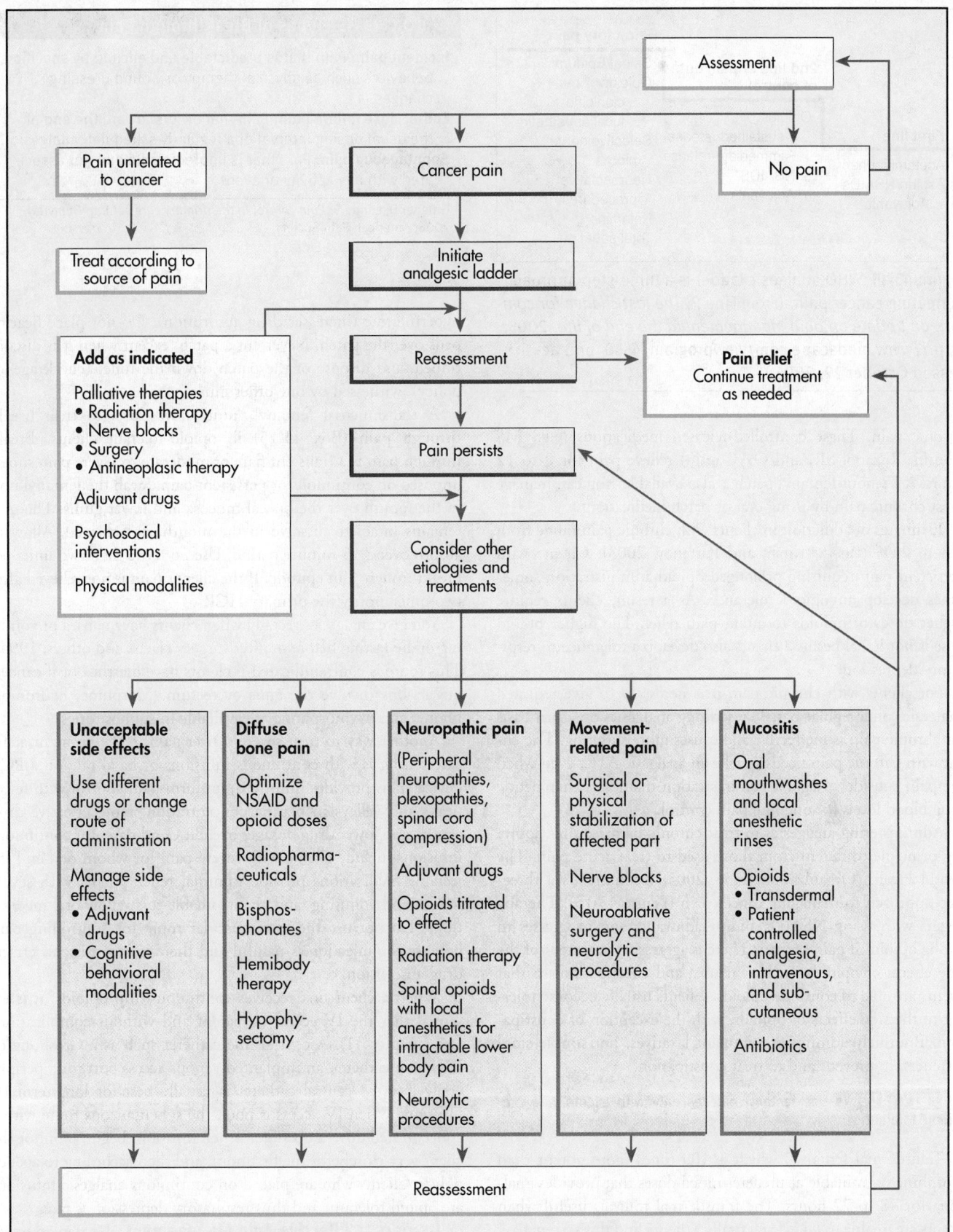

Figure 43-14 Flow chart: continuing pain management in clients with cancer. (From Jacox A and others: *Management of cancer pain*, Clinical Practice Guideline No. 9, AHCPR Pub No. 94-0592, Rockville, Md, 1994, Agency for Health Care Policy and Research, Public Health Service, U.S. Department of Health and Human Services.)

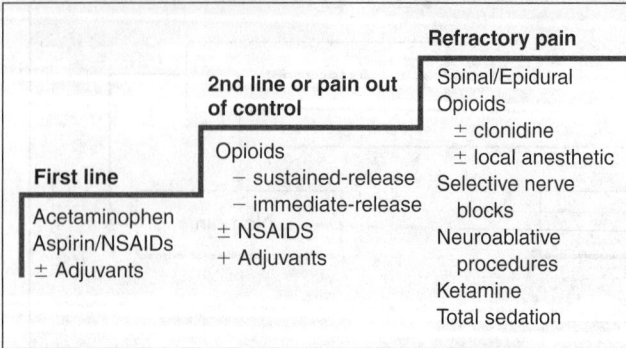

Figure 43-15 WHO analgesic ladder is a three-step approach in treating cancer pain. (From Fine P: *The last chance for comfort: an update on pain management at the end of life,* 2005, http://www.medscape.com/viewprogram/4550_pnt, accessed October 22, 2005.)

chronic pain. These controlled-released medications (e.g., MS Contin, Roxanol SR, and OxyContin) relieve pain for 8 to 12 hours. A 72-hour fentanyl patch is also available. You can manage most chronic pain by using oral or patch medications.

Estimates of addiction in clients with chronic pain range from 1% to 24% (Passik, Kirsh, and Portenoy, 2003). Clients with persistent pain requiring prolonged opioid administration sometimes develop an opioid tolerance. As a result, clients require higher doses of opioids to attain pain relief. The higher opioid dose is not lethal because clients also develop a tolerance to respiratory depression.

For clients with chronic pain it is necessary to give required analgesics on a regular basis. Prescribing analgesics on a prn basis for chronic pain is ineffective and causes more suffering. The client with chronic pain needs to take an analgesic ATC, even when the pain subsides. Regular administration maintains therapeutic drug blood levels for ongoing pain control.

Administering analgesics to treat chronic pain requires applying principles different from those used to treat acute pain. The World Health Organization (Fine, 2005) recommends a three-step approach to managing cancer pain (Figure 43-15). Therapy begins with using NSAIDs and/or adjuvants and progresses to strong opioids if pain persists. There is aggressive treatment of the side effects of opioids, such as nausea and constipation, so that clients are able to continue opioids. Clients usually become tolerant to the side effects of opioids, with the exception of constipation. Routinely administer stimulant laxatives, not simple stool softeners, to prevent and to treat constipation.

SAFETY ALERT Use fentanyl patches **only** with clients who are opioid tolerant.

Transdermal fentanyl, which is 100 times more potent than morphine, is available at predetermined doses that provides analgesia for 48 to 72 hours. The transdermal route is useful when clients are unable to take drugs orally. Clients find this system easy to use because it allows for continuous opioid administration without needles or pumps. Self-adhesive patches release the medication slowly over time, achieving effective analgesia. Transdermal fentanyl is not for adult clients who weigh less than 100 pounds (too little subcutaneous tissue for absorption) or who are

✳ BOX 43-15 Types of Breakthrough Pain

Incident pain: Pain that is predictable and elicited by specific behaviors such as physical therapy or wound dressing changes
End-of-dose failure pain: Pain that occurs toward the end of the usual dosing interval of a regularly scheduled analgesic
Spontaneous pain: Pain that is unpredictable and not associated with any activity or event

Gruener D, Lande S: *Pain control in the primary care setting*, Glenview, Ill, 2006, American Pain Society.

hyperthermic (increases drug absorption). Do not place heating pads over the patch. Never cut a patch, except when it is discontinued, and dispose of the patch down the toilet (check agency policy), witnessed by one other nurse.

A transmucosal fentanyl "unit" now exists to treat **breakthrough pain** (Box 43-15) in opioid-tolerant clients. Breakthrough pain is a transient flare of moderate to severe pain superimposed on continuous or persistent pain. Swab the fentanyl unit in the mouth over the buccal mucosa and lower gums. The unit remains intact to dissolve in the mouth, not chewed, Allow to absorb over a 15-minute period. Use no more than two units per breakthrough pain episode. If the client's pain is not relieved after two units, notify the primary HCP.

You give analgesics rectally when clients have nausea or vomiting or are fasting before or after surgery (Jacox and others, 1994). This route is contraindicated if clients have diarrhea or if cancerous lesions involve the anus or rectum. Morphine, hydromorphone, and oxymorphone are available in suppositories.

Another way to treat severe cancer pain in the home or acute care setting is with continuous infusions or basal rate on a PCA device. This provides improved, uniform pain control with fewer peaks and valleys in plasma concentration, more effective drug action, and lower drug dosages overall. Candidates for continuous infusions include clients with severe pain for whom oral and injectable medications provide minimal relief, clients with severe nausea and vomiting, and clients unable to swallow oral medications. Do not use the intramuscular route for controlling pain because the injection is painful and there is inconsistent, erratic drug absorption.

When a client first receives continuous-drip opioids, it is essential that the IV access be patent and without complications (see Chapter 41). A central line catheter such as a Groshong or Hickman catheter, an implanted venous access port, or a peripherally inserted central catheter is usually best for long-term IV infusion. When IV access is poor, the subcutaneous route with a concentrated dose is possible. When infusions begin, monitor the client very closely for the first hour, and then according to agency policy. Clients who are placed on continuous analgesic infusions are opioid tolerant, and thus respiratory depression is rare.

Barriers to Effective Pain Management. Barriers to effective pain management are complex, involving the client, health care provider, and health care system (Box 43-16). Many health care providers and clients fear addiction when long-term opioid use is prescribed to manage pain, though this fear is often inappropriate. Because of this concern, HCPs require opioid agree-

✳ BOX 43-16 Barriers to Effective Pain Management

Client Barriers
Fear of addiction
Worry about side effects
Fear of tolerance (won't be there when I need it)
Take too many pills already
Fear of injections
Concern about not being a "good" client
Don't want to worry family and friends
May need more tests
Need to suffer to be cured
Pain is for past indiscretions
Inadequate education
Reluctance to discuss pain
Pain is inevitable
Pain is part of aging
Fear of disease progression
Primary health care providers and nurses are doing all that they can
Just forget to take analgesics
Fear of distracting primary health care providers from treating illness
Primary health care providers have more important or ill clients to see
Suffering in silence is noble and expected

Health Care Provider Barriers
Inadequate pain assessment
Concern with addiction
Opiophobia, fear of opioids
Fear of legal repercussions
No visible cause of pain
Clients must learn to live with pain
Reluctance to deal with side effects of analgesics
Not believing client's report of pain
Fear of giving a dose that will kill the client
Primary health care provider time constraints
Inadequate reimbursement
Belief that opioids "mask" symptoms
Belief that pain is part of aging
Overestimation of rates of respiratory depression

Health Care System Barriers
Concern with creating "addicts"
Ability to fill prescriptions
Absolute dollar restriction on amount reimbursed for prescriptions
Mail order pharmacy restrictions
Nurse practitioners and physician assistants not used efficiently
Extensive documentation requirements
Poor pain policies and procedures regarding pain management
Lack of money
Inadequate access to pain clinics
Poor understanding of economic impact of unrelieved pain

---

ments and random urine testing from clients who require long-term opioid therapy. Evidence of the effectiveness of agreements, however, is lacking, and there are ethical concerns about using them on all clients who require long-term opioid therapy (Arnold and others, 2006). This raises the question as to whether agreements protect clients or health care providers.

There is a difference between **physical dependence, addiction,** and **drug tolerance** (Box 43-17). You need to clarify the differences to clients and other HCPs. Experiencing a physical dependency does not imply addiction, and drug tolerance in and of itself is not the same as addiction. That is not to say that addiction does not occur or that true addicts should not be treated for pain. "Patients with addictive disease and pain have the right to be treated with dignity, respect, and the same quality of pain assessment and management as all other patients" (ASPMN Position Statement, 2002). Nurses and other HCPs need to avoid labeling clients as "drug seeking" because this term is poorly defined. If you are concerned that a client is abusing opioids, voice your concerns to the client and notify the primary HCP, explaining the reasons for your unease.

Mehta and Langford (2006) have published recommendations for the management of acute pain in clients dependent on opioids, who are not necessarily addicted. A study (Morgan, 2006) of addicts with pain revealed that they did not feel respected by nurses who cared for them. These drug abusers also learned presentation (try to be nice and thank the nurse) and self-management strategies (do not get angry or make waves) to obtain pain relief.

Placebos. Placebos are medications or procedures that produce positive or negative effects in clients. These effects are not related to the placebo's specific physical or chemical properties

✳ BOX 43-17 Definitions Related to the Use of Opioids in Pain Treatment

Approved by the Boards of Directors of the American Academy of Pain Medicine, the American Pain Society, and the American Society of Addiction Medicine, February 2001.

Physical Dependence
A state of adaptation that is manifested by a drug class specific withdrawal syndrome produced by abrupt cessation, rapid dose reduction, decreasing blood level of the drug, and/or administration of an antagonist.

Drug Tolerance
A state of adaptation in which exposure to a drug induces changes that result in a diminution of one or more of the drug's effects over time.

Addiction
A primary, chronic, neurobiologic disease, with genetic, psychosocial, and environmental factors influencing its development and manifestations. Addictive behaviors include one or more of the following: impaired control over drug use, compulsive use, continued use despite harm, and craving.

Pseudoaddiction
Client behaviors (drug seeking) that occur when pain is undertreated.

Pseudotolerance
Need to increase opioid dose for reasons other than opioid tolerance: progression of disease, onset of new disorder, increased physical activity, lack of adherence, change in opioid formulation, drug-drug interaction, drug-food interaction (Wall and Melzack, 1999).

(Coggins and others, 2004). Professional organizations discourage the use of placebos to treat pain. It is considered unethical and deceitful to administer placebos (Coggins and others, 2004; Grace, 2006; McCaffery and Arnstein, 2006; Sullivan, 2005). Placebo use jeopardizes the trust between clients and HCPs. If a placebo is ordered, you must question the order and ask, "Why?" Many health care agencies have policies that limit the use of placebos to research only.

Restorative and Continuing Care

Pain Clinics, Palliative Care, and Hospices. Because of the implementation of The Joint Commission pain standard and the designation of the years 2000 to 2010 as the Decade of Pain Control and Research, health professionals have recognized pain as a significant health problem. There has been an increased growth of pain centers, palliative care departments, and hospices designed to manage pain and suffering. A comprehensive pain center treats persons on an inpatient or outpatient basis. Staff members representing all health care disciplines, such as nursing, medicine, physical therapy, pastoral care, and dietetics, work with clients to find the most effective pain-relief measures. A comprehensive clinic provides not only diverse therapy but also research into new treatments and training for professionals.

Many hospitals are developing palliative care departments to assist clients and their family members in successfully managing their diseases (Morrison and others, 2005). Learning to live life fully with an incurable condition is the goal of palliative care (see Chapter 30). It is essential to give clients and their family members ongoing assistance in managing their pain at home (Schumacher and others, 2002). The National Patient Safety Goal 2E (TJC, 2006) recommends standardizing communication when a client transfers into, out of, and within the medical system. Teaching pain management during discharge is often a part of agency protocol.

Hospices are programs for care of clients at the end of life (see Chapter 30). Clients at the end of life emphasize quality of life over quantity (Douglass and others, 2004). Hospice helps terminally ill clients continue to live at home in comfort and privacy. Pain control is a priority for hospices. Clients receive the dosage and form of analgesics that provide pain relief (Whitecar and others, 2004). Under the guidance of hospice nurses, families learn to monitor clients' symptoms and become the primary caregivers. A hospice client may become hospitalized in the event of a brief, acute care crisis or family problem.

Hospice programs help nurses overcome their fears of contributing to a client's death when administering large doses of opioids. The American Nurses Association (ANA) supports aggressive treatment of pain and suffering even if it hastens a client's death (ANA Code of Ethics, 2002). Recent research suggests that moderate opioid dose increases in terminally ill clients at the end of life does not hasten death (Vitetta, Kenner, and Sali, 2005). It is the client's disease that is killing the client, not the opioid.

◆Evaluation

Evaluation of pain is one of many nursing responsibilities that require effective critical thinking (Figure 43-16). The client's behavioral responses to pain-relief interventions are not always obvi-

Knowledge
- Characteristics of an improved level of comfort for a client

Experience
- Previous client responses to pain relief measures

EVALUATION
- Reassess signs and symptoms of the client's pain response; the severity and characteristics of pain and the client's self-report
- Evaluate the family and friends' observation of the client's response to therapies
- Evaluate impact of pain on physical and social functioning

Standards
- Use established expected outcomes to evaluate the client's response to care (e.g., reduced pain severity)
- Apply AHRQ guidelines for chronic pain evaluation
- Determine if the client's expectations are met

Attitudes
- Apply humility; rethink your approach; if pain continues, confer with other clinicians
- Be responsible and accountable when care is ineffective; the client's rights must be maintained

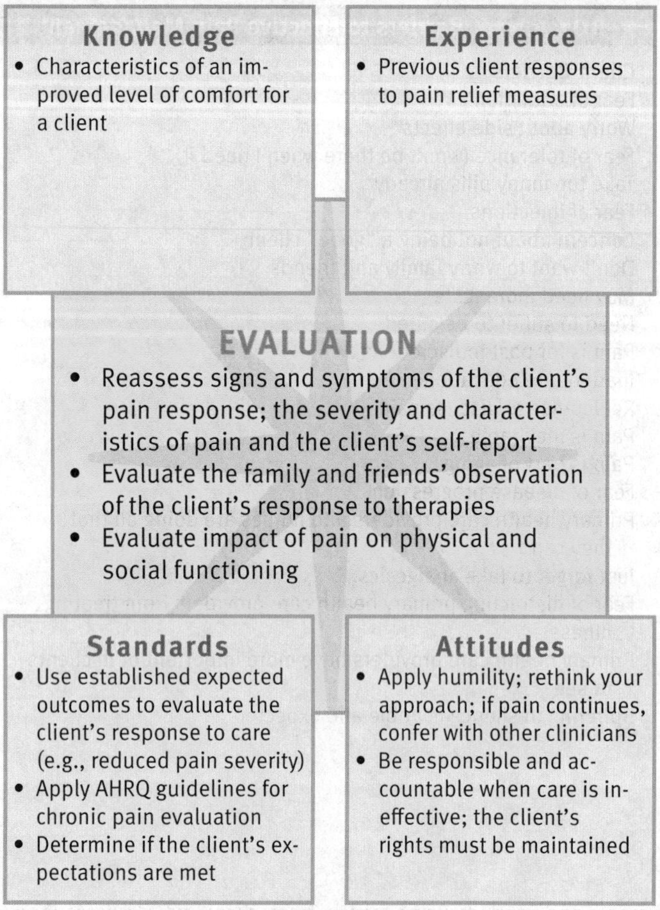

Figure 43-16 Critical thinking model for pain management evaluation.

ous. Evaluating the effectiveness of a pain intervention requires you to evaluate the client after an appropriate period of time. For instance, oral medications usually peak in about 1 hour; whereas IVP medications peak in 15 to 30 minutes. Ask the client if the medication alleviated the pain when it is peaking. Do not expect the client to volunteer the information. Evaluate psychological as well as physiological responses to pain. "Do you ever wonder why you are having this pain?" Or, "Does your pain ever cause you to get depressed or angry?" This is especially important in the home care setting.

If you evaluate that a client continues to have discomfort after an intervention, use a new approach. For example, if an analgesic provides only partial relief, add relaxation exercises or guided-imagery exercises. You also consult with the primary HCP about increasing the dosage, decreasing the interval between doses, or trying different analgesics.

Evaluate the client's perceptions of the effectiveness of interventions. The client helps to decide the best times to attempt a treatment. In essence, the client is the best judge of whether an intervention works. Also evaluate tolerance to therapy and the overall relief obtained. If an intervention aggravates discomfort, stop it immediately and seek an alternative. Time and patience are necessary to maximize the effectiveness of pain management.

✳ **BOX 43-18 Nurse–Primary Health Care Provider Pain Communication**

1. Identify primary health care provider by name.
2. Give your name.
3. State the general nature of the call.
4. Identify the client by name and diagnosis.
5. State the pain management goal: rating and activities.
6. Summarize the current pain rating and effect of pain on activities.
7. List the current analgesic doses and relevant side effects.
8. Identify nonpharmacological strategies used.
9. Suggest a solution (on the basis of a clinical practice guideline, if possible).

Modified from McCaffery M, Pasero C: *Pain: clinical manual*, ed 2, St. Louis, 1999, Mosby.

Evaluate the entire pain experience to determine interventions that are most effective and times for administration.

The client, if able, is the best resource for evaluating the effectiveness of pain-relief measures. You need to continually assess whether the character of the client's pain changes and whether individual interventions are effective. The family often is another valuable resource, particularly in the case of the client with pain who is not able to express discomfort. You are successful in treating pain when the client's expectations of pain relief are met. Use evaluative criteria in determining the outcome of pain-relief interventions.

Effective communication of a client's assessment of pain and his or her response to intervention is facilitated by accurate and thorough documentation. This communication needs to happen from nurse to nurse, shift to shift, and nurse to other HCPs. It is the professional responsibility of the nurse caring for the client to report what has been effective for managing the client's pain. A variety of tools such as a pain flow sheet or diary will help centralize information about pain management. The client expects you to be sensitive to his or her pain and to be attentive in attempts to manage that pain. Effectively communicating with primary HCPs (Box 43-18) will assist you in achieving optimal pain relief for clients.

✳ Key Concepts

- Pain is a purely subjective physical and psychosocial experience.
- Misconceptions about pain often result in doubt about the degree of the client's suffering and unwillingness to provide relief.
- Knowledge of the nociceptive pain processes of the pain experience—transmission, transduction, perception, and modulation—provides guidelines for selecting pain-relief measures.
- An interaction of psychological and cognitive factors affects pain perception.
- A person's cultural background influences the meaning of pain and how it is expressed.
- It is common for older clients not to report pain.
- Clients who are in chronic pain are unlikely to show behavioral changes.

- The difference between acute and chronic pain involves the concept of harm. Acute pain is protective, thus preventing harm; chronic pain is no longer protective.
- Do not collect an in-depth pain history when the client is experiencing severe discomfort.
- Pain causes physical signs and symptoms similar to the signs and symptoms of other diseases.
- Individualize pain interventions by collaborating closely with the client, using assessment findings, and trying a variety of interventions.
- Eliminating sources of painful stimuli is a basic nursing measure for promoting comfort.
- Using a regular schedule for analgesic administration is more effective than an as-needed schedule in controlling pain.
- Sedation is an adverse effect of opioids that always precedes respiratory depression (which is rare).
- A patient-controlled analgesia device gives clients pain control with low risk of overdose.
- While caring for a client who receives local anesthesia, protect the client from injury.
- Nursing implications for administering epidural analgesia include preventing infection and monitoring closely for respiratory depression.
- Addiction rarely occurs in clients who take opioids to relieve pain.
- The goal of pain management is to anticipate and prevent pain rather than treat it.
- Pain evaluation includes measurement of the changing character of pain, the client's response to interventions, and the client's perceptions of a therapy's effectiveness.

✳ Critical Thinking Exercises

After three doses (0.5 mg each) of morphine from the PCA, Mrs. Mays started vomiting and stated she was feeling "out of her head." She rated her chest pain as a 3 out of 10. She is breathing comfortably on 2 L of nasal canula oxygen, and her lung sounds are clear to auscultation. Her husband is very concerned and anxious about his wife and wants the morphine stopped so that she will not get "addicted."

1. What does the nurse tell Mr. and Mrs. Mays about the adverse effects of morphine?

2. What recommendation would the nurse make to the physician with regards to the dose of morphine and why?

3. What laboratory reports are important for the nurse to evaluate before recommending any analgesics?

✳ NCLEX®-Style Review Questions

1. Which of the following signs or symptoms in an opioid-naive client is of greatest concern to the nurse when assessing the client 1 hour after administering an opioid?
   1. Oxygen saturation of 95%
   2. Difficulty arousing the client
   3. Respiratory rate of 10 breaths per minute
   4. Pain intensity rating of 5 on a scale of 0 to 10

2. A physician writes the following order on an opioid-naive client who returned from the operating room following a total hip replacement. "Fentanyl patch 100 mcg, change every 3 days." Based on this order the nurse takes the following action:
   1. Call the physician, and question the order
   2. Apply the patch the third postoperative day
   3. Apply the patch as soon as the client reports pain
   4. Place the patch as close to the hip dressing as possible

3. A client is being discharged home on an ATC opioid for chronic back pain. Because of this order, which class of medication does the nurse request an order for?
   1. Stool softener
   2. Stimulant laxative
   3. H_2 receptor blocker
   4. Proton pump inhibitor

4. An intern new to the service writes an order for OxyContin SR 10 mg PO q12 hours prn. Which part of the order does the nurse question?
   1. The drug
   2. The time
   3. The dose
   4. The route
   5. The interval

5. After returning from vacation, the nurse notices that her client has been receiving Percocet (5/325), two tablets PO every 3 hours for the past 3 days. What is the nurse most concerned about?
   1. The client's level of pain
   2. The potential for addiction
   3. The amount of daily acetaminophen
   4. The risk for gastrointestinal bleeding

6. A client with chronic low back pain who was receiving an opioid ATC for the past year decided to abruptly stop the medication for fear of addiction. He is now experiencing shaking chills, abdominal cramps, and joint pain. The nurse recognizes that this client is experiencing symptoms of:
   1. Addiction
   2. Tolerance
   3. Pseudoaddiction
   4. Physical dependence

7. After having received 0.2 mg of naloxone IVP, a client's respiratory rate and depth are within normal limits. The nurse now plans to implement the following action:
   1. Discontinue all ordered opioids
   2. Close the room door to allow the client to recover
   3. Administer the remaining naloxone over 4 minutes
   4. Assess client's vital signs every 15 minutes for 2 hours

8. Which one of the following instructions is crucial for the nurse to give to both family members and the client who is about to be started on a PCA of morphine?
   1. Only the client should push the button.
   2. Do not use the PCA until the pain is severe.
   3. The PCA prevents overdoses from occurring.
   4. Notify the nurse when the button is pushed.

9. A client with a history of a stoke that left her confused and unable to communicate has returned from interventional radiology following placement of a gastrostomy tube. The physician's order reads as follows: "Vicodin 1 tab, per tube, q4 hours, prn." Which action by the nurse is most appropriate?
   1. No action is required by the nurse because the order is appropriate.
   2. Request to have the ordered changed to ATC for the first 48 hours.
   3. Ask for a change of medication to Demerol 50 mg IVP, q3 hours, prn.
   4. Begin the Vicodin when the client shows nonverbal symptoms of pain.

44 | Nutrition

✳ OBJECTIVES

Mastery of content in this chapter will enable the student to:

- Explain the importance of a balance between energy intake and energy requirements.
- List the end products of carbohydrate, protein, and fat metabolism.
- Explain the significance of saturated, unsaturated, and polyunsaturated fats.
- Describe the food guide pyramid and the healthy eating index and discuss their value in planning meals for good nutrition.
- List the current dietary guidelines for the general population.
- Explain the variance in nutritional requirements throughout growth and development.
- Discuss the major methods of nutritional assessment.
- Identify three major nutritional problems, and describe clients at risk.

- Establish a plan of care to meet the nutritional needs of the client.
- Describe the procedure for initiating and maintaining tube feedings.
- Describe the methods to avoid complications of tube feedings.
- Describe the methods for avoiding complications of parenteral nutrition.
- Discuss medical nutrition therapy in relation to three medical conditions.
- Discuss diet counseling and client teaching in relation to client expectations.

✳ MEDIA RESOURCES   ✳ KEY TERMS

 Companion CD

- NCLEX®-Style Review Questions
- Audio Glossary
- Interactive Learning Activities
- English/Spanish Glossary

 Website

- NCLEX®-Style Review Questions
- Audio Glossary
- English/Spanish Glossary
- Interactive Learning Activities
- Weblinks
- Audio Summaries
- Video Clips

Amino acid, p. 1087
Anabolism, p. 1089
Anorexia, p. 1108
Anorexia nervosa, p. 1093
Anthropometry, p. 1098
Basal metabolic rate (BMR), p. 1086
Body mass index (BMI), p. 1098
Bulimia nervosa, p. 1093
Carbohydrates, p. 1086
Catabolism, p. 1089
Chyme, p. 1088
Daily values, p. 1090
Dietary reference intakes (DRIs), p. 1090
Dispensable amino acids, p. 1087
Dysphagia, p. 1101
Enteral nutrition (EN), p. 1111
Enzymes, p. 1088
Fat-soluble vitamins, p. 1088
Fatty acids, p. 1087

Fiber, p. 1087
Gluconeogenesis, p. 1090
Glycogenesis, p. 1090
Glycogenolysis, p. 1090
Hypervitaminosis, p. 1088
Ideal body weight (IBW), p. 1098
Indispensable amino acids, p. 1087
Ketones, p. 1090
Kilocalorie (kcal), p. 1086
Lipid emulsions, p. 1121
Lipids, p. 1087
Macrominerals, p. 1088
Malabsorption, p. 1126
Malnutrition, p. 1097
Medical nutrition therapy (MNT), p. 1126
Metabolism, p. 1089
Minerals, p. 1088
Monounsaturated (fatty acids), p. 1087

Nitrogen balance, p. 1087
Nutrient density, p. 1086
Nutrients, p. 1086
Parenteral nutrition (PN), p. 1121
Peristalsis, p. 1088
Polyunsaturated (fatty acids), p. 1087
Resting energy expenditure (REE), p. 1086
Saccharides, p. 1087
Saturated (fatty acids), p. 1087
Simple carbohydrates, p. 1087
Trace element, p. 1088
Triglycerides, p. 1087
Unsaturated (fatty acids), p. 1087
Vegetarianism, p. 1094
Vitamins, p. 1087
Water-soluble vitamins, p. 1088

Food provides sustenance and also holds symbolic meaning. The giving or taking of food is part of ceremonies, social gatherings, holiday traditions, religious events, the celebration of birth, and the mourning of death. The difficulty of the decision to withdraw food in a terminal illness, even in the form of intravenous (IV) nutrients, is a testament to the symbolic power of food and feeding.

Florence Nightingale understood the importance of nutrition, stressing the nurse's role in the science and art of feeding during the mid-1800s (Dossey, 1999). Since then, the nurse's role in nutrition and diet therapy has changed. Medical nutrition therapy (MNT) uses nutritional therapy and counseling to manage diseases (American Dietetic Association, 2006). In some illnesses, such as type 1 diabetes mellitus or mild hypertension, diet therapy is often the major treatment for disease control (American Diabetes Association, 2006; American Heart Association, 2006). Other conditions, such as severe inflammatory bowel disease, require specialized nutrition support such as enteral nutrition (EN) or parenteral nutrition (PN). Standards now exist that clearly designate the standard of care for promotion of optimal nutrition in all health care clients (American Heart Association, 2006; Kushi and others, 2006).

In 1997 the U.S. Department of Health and Human Services (USDHHS) and the Public Health Service (PHS) began a consensus process, establishing nutritional goals and objectives for *Healthy People 2010: National Health Promotion and Disease Prevention Objectives*. *Healthy People 2010* is the contribution of the United States to the World Health Organization's (WHO's) "Health for All" strategy. The report defines national goals to be met to increase the proportion of Americans who live long, healthy lives (Box 44-1). *Healthy People 2010* continues the objectives initiated in *Healthy People 2000* with an overall goal to promote health and reduce chronic disease related to diet and weight. All nutrition-related objectives include baseline data, from which progress is measured. The challenge remains to motivate consumers to put these dietary recommendations into practice. Many objectives of *Healthy People 2010* show positive indicators, including decrease in fat consumption and death rates from coronary heart disease. An increase in overall life expectancy has also occurred; however, obesity remains problematic. Health professionals play a key role in promoting healthy dietary practices.

✴ BOX 44-1 Examples of Nutrition Objectives for *Healthy People 2010*

Weight and Growth
Increase proportion of adults who are at a healthy weight (BMI 18.5 to 24.9)
Reduce obesity in adults by 15%
Reduce obesity in children (6 to 11) and adolescents (12 to 19) by 15%
Reduce growth retardation in low-income children under 5 years of age

Food and Nutrient Consumption
Decrease fat intake to less than 30% daily intake and saturated fat intake to less than 10% of total calories daily
Increase vegetable and fruit intake to five daily servings in 75% of people
Increase grain products intake to six daily servings in 50% of people
Meet calcium DRI in 75% of people
Reduce sodium daily intake to no more than 2400 mg in 65% of people

Iron Deficiency and Anemia
Reduce prevalence of iron deficiency in children and childbearing women
Reduce prevalence of anemia in pregnant women in third trimester to 20%

Schools, Work Sites, and Nutrition Counseling
Increase proportion of school-age children whose intake of meals and snacks at school contribute to good overall dietary quality
Increase work-site nutrition education and weight management program offerings
Offer nutrition assessment and individualized planning at primary care sites

Food Security
Increase food security to 94% of households

Data from U.S. Department of Health and Human Services: *Healthy people 2010*, 2002, http://www.healthypeople.gov.

Scientific Knowledge Base

Nutrients: The Biochemical Units of Nutrition

The body requires fuel to provide energy for cellular metabolism and repair, organ function, growth, and body movement. The **basal metabolic rate** (BMR) is the energy needed to maintain life-sustaining activities (breathing, circulation, heart rate, and temperature) for a specific period of time at rest. Factors such as age, body mass, gender, fever, starvation, menstruation, illness, injury, infection, activity level, or thyroid function affect energy requirements. The **resting energy expenditure** (REE), or resting metabolic rate, is the amount of energy an individual needs to consume over a 24-hour period for the body to maintain all its internal working activities while at rest. Factors that affect metabolism include illness, pregnancy, lactation, and activity level. In hospitals, providers measure energy requirements by measuring oxygen consumption, carbon dioxide production, and nitrogen excretion by means of a metabolic chart.

In general, when energy requirements are completely met by **kilocalorie** (kcal) intake in food, weight does not change. When the kilocalories ingested exceed a person's energy demands, the individual gains weight. If the kilocalories ingested fail to meet a person's energy requirements, the individual loses weight.

Nutrients are the elements necessary for body processes and function. Energy needs are met from a variety of nutrients: carbohydrates, proteins, fats, water, vitamins, and minerals. Foods are sometimes described according to their **nutrient density**, the proportion of essential nutrients to the number of kilocalories. High-nutrient-density foods, such as fruits and vegetables, provide a large number of nutrients in relationship to kilocalories. Low-nutrient-density foods, such as alcohol or sugar, are high in kilocalories but are nutrient poor.

Carbohydrates. **Carbohydrates** are the main source of energy in the diet. Each gram of carbohydrate produces 4 kcal and serves as the main source of fuel (glucose) for the brain, skeletal muscles during exercise, erythrocyte and leukocyte production, and cell function of the renal medulla. People obtain carbohydrates primarily from plant foods, except for lactose (milk sugar). Carbohydrates are classified according to their carbohydrate units, or **saccharides.**

Monosaccharides such as glucose (dextrose) or fructose cannot be broken down into a more basic carbohydrate unit. Disaccharides such as sucrose, lactose, and maltose are made up of two monosaccharides and water. Both monosaccharides and disaccharides are classified as **simple carbohydrates** and are found primarily in sugars. Polysaccharides such as glycogen are made up of many carbohydrate units and are complex carbohydrates. They are insoluble in water and are digested to varying degrees. Starches are polysaccharides.

The body is unable to digest some polysaccharides because humans do not have enzymes capable of breaking them down. **Fiber** has received attention as a dietary factor in disease prevention and treatment and prevention of diarrhea in tube-fed clients (Rolandelli and others, 2005). Insoluble fibers are not digestible and include cellulose, hemicellulose, and lignin. Soluble fibers include pectin, guar gum, and mucilage.

Proteins. Proteins provide a source of energy (4 kcal/g) and they are essential for synthesis (building) of body tissue in growth, maintenance, and repair. Collagen, hormones, enzymes, immune cells, DNA, and RNA are all made of protein. In addition, blood clotting, fluid regulation, and acid-base balance require proteins. These proteins transport nutrients and many drugs in the blood.

The simplest form of protein is the **amino acid.** The body does not synthesize **indispensable amino acids,** so these need to be provided in the diet. Examples of indispensable amino acids are histidine, lysine, and phenylalanine. The body synthesizes **dispensable amino acids.** Examples of amino acids synthesized in the body are alanine, asparagine, and glutamic acid. Amino acids can be linked together. Albumin and insulin are simple proteins because they contain only amino acids or their derivatives. The combination of a simple protein with a nonprotein substance produces a complex protein, such as lipoprotein, formed by a combination of a lipid and a simple protein.

A complete protein, also called a high-quality protein, contains all essential amino acids in sufficient quantity to support growth and maintain nitrogen balance. Examples of foods that contain complete proteins are fish, chicken, soybeans, turkey, and cheese. Ingestion of proteins is not primary for meeting energy needs but is most important for continued positive nitrogen balance. Incomplete proteins do not have one or more of the nine indispensable amino acids and include cereals, legumes (beans, peas), and vegetables. Complementary proteins are pairs of incomplete proteins that when combined supply the total amount of protein provided by complete protein sources.

Nitrogen balance is achieved when the intake and output of nitrogen are equal. When the intake of nitrogen is greater than the output, the body is in positive nitrogen balance. Positive nitrogen balance is required for growth, normal pregnancy, maintenance of lean muscle mass and vital organs, and wound healing. The body uses nitrogen retained for building, repair, and replacement of body tissues. Negative nitrogen balance occurs when the body loses more nitrogen than the body gains, for example, with infection, sepsis, burns, fever, starvation, head injury, and trauma. The increased nitrogen loss is the result of body-tissue destruction or loss of nitrogen-containing body fluids. Nutrition during this period needs to provide nutrients to put clients into positive balance for healing.

Protein provides energy, but because of protein's essential role in growth, maintenance, and repair, a diet needs to provide adequate kilocalories from nonprotein sources. When there is sufficient carbohydrate in the diet to meet the energy needs of the body, protein is spared as an energy source.

Fats. Fats (**lipids**) are the most calorie-dense nutrient, providing 9 kcal/g. Fats are composed of triglycerides and fatty acids. **Triglycerides** circulate in the blood and are made up of three fatty acids attached to a glycerol. **Fatty acids** are composed of chains of carbon and hydrogen atoms with an acid group on one end of the chain and a methyl group at the other. Fatty acids can be **saturated,** in which each carbon in the chain has two attached hydrogen atoms, or **unsaturated,** in which an unequal number of hydrogen atoms are attached and the carbon atoms attach to each other with a double bond. **Monounsaturated** fatty acids have one double bond, whereas **polyunsaturated** fatty acids have two or more double carbon bonds. The various types of fatty acids have significance for health and the incidence of disease and are referred to in dietary guidelines.

Fatty acids are also classified as essential or nonessential. Linoleic acid, an unsaturated fatty acid, is the only essential fatty acid in humans. Linolenic acid and arachidonic acid (also unsaturated fatty acids) are important for metabolic processes but are manufactured by the body when linoleic acid is available. Deficiency occurs when fat intake falls below 10% of daily nutrition. Most animal fats have high proportions of saturated fatty acids, whereas vegetable fats have higher amounts of unsaturated and polyunsaturated fatty acids.

Water. Water is a critical component of the body because cell function depends on a fluid environment. Water makes up 60% to 70% of total body weight. The percent of total body water is greater for lean people than obese people because muscle contains more water than any other tissue except blood. Infants have the greatest percentage of total body water, and older people have the least. When deprived of water, a person will not survive for more than a few days.

An individual meets fluid needs by drinking liquids and eating solid foods high in water content, such as fresh fruits and vegetables. Water is also produced during digestion when food is oxidized. In a healthy individual, fluid intake from all sources equals fluid output through elimination, respiration, and sweating (see Chapters 41 and 45). An ill person has an increased need for fluid (e.g., with fever or gastrointestinal [GI] losses). By contrast, an ill person also has a decreased ability to excrete fluid (e.g., with cardiopulmonary or renal disease), which often leads to the need for fluid restriction.

Vitamins. Vitamins are organic substances present in small amounts in foods that are essential to normal metabolism. Vitamins are chemicals used as catalysts in biochemical reactions. When there is enough of any specific vitamin to meet the catalytic demands, the rest of the vitamin supply acts as a free chemical and is often toxic to the body. Certain vitamins are currently of interest in their role as antioxidants. These vitamins neutralize substances called free radicals, which produce oxidative damage to body cells and tissues. Researchers think that oxidative damage increases a person's risk for various cancers. These vitamins include beta-carotene and vitamins A, C, and E (Nix, 2005).

The body is unable to synthesize vitamins in the required amounts and depends on dietary intake. Vitamin content is usually highest in fresh foods that are used quickly after minimal exposure to heat, air, or water. Vitamins are classified as fat soluble and water soluble.

Fat-Soluble Vitamins. The **fat-soluble vitamins** (A, D, E, and K) are stored in the fatty compartments of the body. With the exception of vitamin D, these vitamins are provided through dietary intake. **Hypervitaminosis** of fat-soluble vitamins results from megadoses (intentional or unintentional) of supplemental vitamins, excessive amounts in fortified food, and large intake of fish oils.

Water-Soluble Vitamins. The **water-soluble vitamins** are vitamin C and the B complex (which is eight vitamins). The body does not store water-soluble vitamins, so these need to be provided in the daily food intake. Water-soluble vitamins are absorbed easily from the gastrointestinal tract. Although water-soluble vitamins are not stored, toxicity can still occur.

Minerals. **Minerals** are inorganic elements essential to the body as catalysts in biochemical reactions. Minerals are classified as **macrominerals** when the daily requirement is 100 mg or more and microminerals or **trace elements** when less than 100 mg is needed daily. Selenium is a trace element that also has antioxidant properties. Silicon, vanadium, nickel, tin, cadmium, arsenic, aluminum, and boron play an unidentified role in nutrition. Arsenic, aluminum, and cadmium have toxic effects.

Anatomy and Physiology of the Digestive System

Digestion. Digestion of food is the mechanical breakdown that results from chewing, churning, and mixing with fluid and chemical reactions where food is reduced to its simplest form. Each part of the GI system has an important digestive or absorptive function (Figure 44-1). **Enzymes** are the proteinlike substances that act as catalysts to speed up chemical reactions. Enzymes are an essential part of the chemistry of digestion.

Most enzymes have one specific function. Each enzyme works best at a specific pH. For example, the enzyme amylase in the saliva breaks down starches into sugars. The secretions of the GI tract have very different pH levels. For example, saliva is relatively neutral, gastric juice is highly acidic, and the secretions of the small intestine are alkaline.

The mechanical, chemical, and hormonal activities of digestion are interdependent. Enzyme activity depends on the mechanical breakdown of food to increase its surface area for chemical action. Hormones regulate the flow of digestive secretions needed for enzyme supply. Physical, chemical, and hormonal factors regulate the secretion of digestive juices and the motility of the GI tract. Nerve stimulation from the parasympathetic nervous system (e.g., the vagus nerve) increases gastrointestinal tract action.

Digestion begins in the mouth, where chewing mechanically breaks down food. The food is mixed with saliva, which contains ptyalin (salivary amylase), an enzyme that acts on cooked starch to begin its conversion to maltose. The longer an individual chews food, the more starch digestion occurs in the mouth. Proteins and fats are broken down physically but remain unchanged chemically because enzymes in the mouth do not react with these nutrients. Chewing reduces food particles to a size suitable for swallowing, and saliva provides lubrication to further ease swallowing of the food. The epiglottis is a flap of skin that closes over the trachea as a person swallows to prevent aspiration. Swallowed food enters the esophagus, and wavelike muscular contractions (**peristalsis**) move the food to the base of the esophagus, above the cardiac sphincter. Pressure from a bolus of food at the cardiac sphincter causes it to relax, allowing the food to enter the fundus, or uppermost portion, of the stomach.

The stomach's chief cells secrete pepsinogen, and the pyloric glands secrete gastrin, a hormone that triggers parietal cells to secrete hydrochloric acid (HCl). The parietal cells also secrete HCl as well as intrinsic factor (IF), which is necessary for absorption of vitamin B_{12} in the ileum. HCl turns pepsinogen into pepsin, a protein-splitting enzyme. The body produces gastric lipase and amylase to begin fat and starch digestion, respectively. A thick layer of mucus protects the lining of the stomach from autodigestion. Alcohol and aspirin are two substances directly absorbed through the lining of the stomach. The stomach acts as a reservoir where food remains for approximately 3 hours, with a range of 1 to 7 hours.

Food leaves the antrum, or distal stomach, through the pyloric sphincter and enters the duodenum. Food is now an acidic, liquefied mass called **chyme.** Chyme flows into the duodenum and is quickly mixed with bile, intestinal juices, and pancreatic secretions. The small intestine secretes the hormones secretin and cholecystokinin (CCK). Secretin activates release of bicarbonate from the pancreas, raising the pH of chyme. CCK inhibits further gastrin secretion and initiates release of additional digestive enzymes from the pancreas and gallbladder.

Bile is manufactured in the liver and stored in the gallbladder. Bile acts as a detergent, because it emulsifies fat to permit enzyme action while suspending fatty acids in solution. Pancreatic secretions contain six enzymes: amylase to digest starch; lipase to break down emulsified fats; and trypsin, elastase, chymotrypsin, and carboxypeptidase to break down proteins.

Peristalsis continues in the small intestine, mixing the secretions with chyme. The mixture becomes increasingly alkaline, inhibiting the action of the gastric enzymes and promoting the action of the duodenal secretions. Epithelial cells in the small intestinal villi secrete enzymes to facilitate digestion. These include sucrase, lactase, maltase, lipase, and peptidase. The major portion of digestion occurs in the small intestine, producing glucose, fructose, and galactose from carbohydrates; amino acids and dipeptides from proteins; and fatty acids, glycerides, and glycerol from lipids. Peristalsis usually takes approximately 5 hours to pass food through the small intestine.

Absorption. The small intestine is the primary absorption site for nutrients. It is lined with fingerlike projections called villi. Villi increase the surface area available for absorption. The body absorbs nutrients by means of passive diffusion, osmosis, active transport, and pinocytosis (Table 44-1, p. 1090)

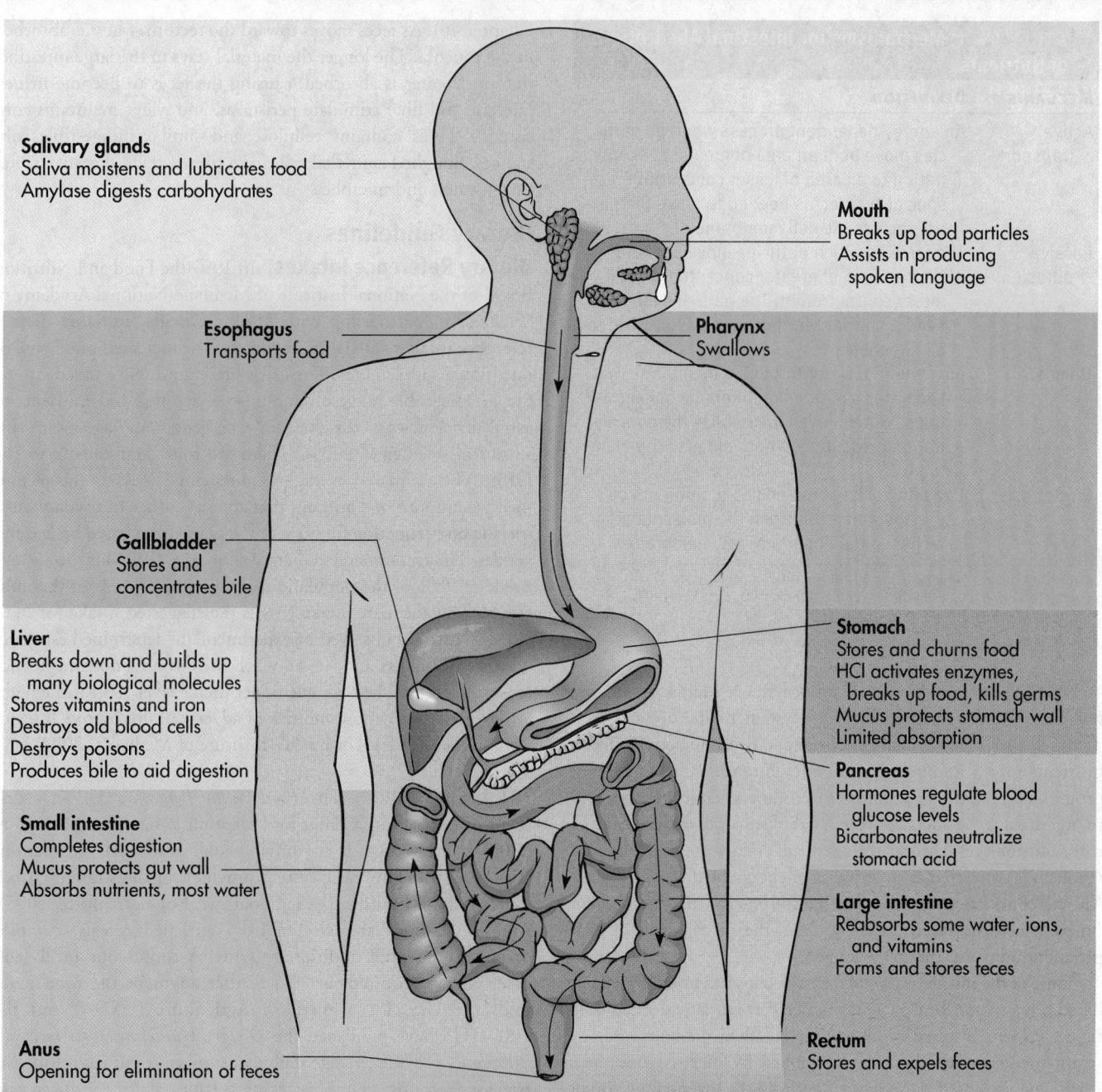

Salivary glands
Saliva moistens and lubricates food
Amylase digests carbohydrates

Mouth
Breaks up food particles
Assists in producing
spoken language

Esophagus
Transports food

Pharynx
Swallows

Gallbladder
Stores and
concentrates bile

Liver
Breaks down and builds up
many biological molecules
Stores vitamins and iron
Destroys old blood cells
Destroys poisons
Produces bile to aid digestion

Small intestine
Completes digestion
Mucus protects gut wall
Absorbs nutrients, most water

Stomach
Stores and churns food
HCl activates enzymes,
breaks up food, kills germs
Mucus protects stomach wall
Limited absorption

Pancreas
Hormones regulate blood
glucose levels
Bicarbonates neutralize
stomach acid

Large intestine
Reabsorbs some water, ions,
and vitamins
Forms and stores feces

Anus
Opening for elimination of feces

Rectum
Stores and expels feces

Figure 44-1 Summary of digestive system anatomy/organ function. (From Rolin Graphics.)

Carbohydrates, protein, minerals, and water-soluble vitamins are absorbed by in the small intestine, processed in the liver, and released into the portal vein circulation. Fatty acids are absorbed in the lymphatic circulatory systems through lacteal ducts at the center of each microvilli in the small intestine.

The majority of water is absorbed in the intestine. Approximately 8.5 L of GI secretions and 1.5 L of oral intake is managed daily within the GI tract. The small intestine reabsorbs 9.5 L, and the colon absorbs approximately 0.4 L. The remaining 0.1 L is eliminated in feces. In addition in the colon, electrolytes and minerals are absorbed, and bacteria synthesize vitamin K and some B complex vitamins. Finally, feces are formed for elimination.

Metabolism and Storage of Nutrients. **Metabolism** refers to all the biochemical reactions within the cells of the body. Metabolic processes are anabolic (building) or catabolic (breaking down). **Anabolism** is the building of more complex biochemical substances by synthesis of nutrients. Anabolism occurs when an individual adds lean muscle through diet and exercise. Amino acids are anabolized into tissues, hormones, and enzymes. Normal metabolism and anabolism are physiologically possible when the body is in positive nitrogen balance. **Catabolism** is the breakdown of biochemical substances into simpler substances and occurs during physiological states of negative nitrogen balance. Starvation is an example of catabolism, when wasting of body tissues occurs.

✴ **TABLE 44-1   Mechanisms for Intestinal Absorption of Nutrients**

MECHANISM	DEFINITION
Active transport	An energy-dependent process whereby particles move from an area of greater concentration to an area of lesser concentration. A special "carrier" is needed to move the particle across the cell membrane.
Passive diffusion	The force by which particles move outward from an area of greater concentration to lesser concentration. The particles do not need a special "carrier" to move outward in all directions.
Osmosis	Movement of water through a membrane that separates solutions of different concentrations. Water moves to equalize the concentration pressures on both sides of the membrane.
Pinocytosis	Engulfing of large molecules of nutrients by the absorbing cell when the molecule attaches to the absorbing cell membrane.

Data from Nix S: *Williams' basic nutrition and diet therapy*, ed 12, St. Louis, 2005, Mosby; and Williams SD, Schlenker ED: *Essentials of nutrition and diet therapy*, ed 8, St. Louis, 2003, Mosby.

Nutrients absorbed in the intestines, including water, are transported through the circulatory system to the body tissues. Through the chemical changes of metabolism, the body converts nutrients into a number of required substances. Carbohydrates, protein, and fat are metabolized to produce chemical energy and to maintain a balance between anabolism and catabolism. To carry out the body's work, the chemical energy produced by metabolism is converted to other types of energy by different tissues. Muscle contraction involves mechanical energy, nervous system function involves electrical energy, and the mechanisms of heat production involve thermal energy.

Some of the nutrients required by the body are stored in tissues. The body's major form of reserve energy is fat, stored as adipose tissue. Protein is stored in muscle mass. When the body's energy requirements exceed the energy supplied by ingested nutrients, stored energy is used. Monoglycerides from the digested portion of fats are converted to glucose by gluconeogenesis. Amino acids are also converted to fat and stored or catabolized into energy through gluconeogenesis. All body cells except red blood cells and neurons oxidize fatty acids into **ketones** for energy when dietary carbohydrates (glucose) are not adequate. Glycogen, synthesized from glucose, provides energy during brief periods of fasting (e.g., during sleep). Glycogen is stored in small reserves in liver and muscle tissue. Nutrient metabolism consists of three main processes:

1. Catabolism of glycogen into glucose, carbon dioxide, and water (**glycogenolysis**)
2. Anabolism of glucose into glycogen for storage (**glycogenesis**)
3. Catabolism of amino acids and glycerol into glucose for energy (**gluconeogenesis**)

Elimination. Chyme moves by peristaltic action through the ileocecal valve into the large intestine, where it becomes feces (see

Chapter 46). As feces moves toward the rectum, water is absorbed in the mucosa. The longer the material stays in the large intestine, the more water is absorbed, causing the feces to become firmer. Exercise and fiber stimulate peristalsis, and water maintains consistency. Feces contains cellulose and similar indigestible substances, sloughed epithelial cells from the GI tract, digestive secretions, water, and microbes.

Dietary Guidelines

Dietary Reference Intakes. In 1997 the Food and Nutrition Board of the National Institute of Medicine/National Academy of Sciences, in partnership with Health Canada, initiated **dietary reference intakes (DRIs)** in response to the increased public use of nutritional supplements. The DRIs present evidence-based criteria for an acceptable range of amounts of vitamins and nutrients to avoid deficiencies or toxicities for each gender and age-group (Institute of Medicine, 2005). There are four components to the DRIs. The estimated average requirement (EAR) is the recommended amount of a nutrient that appears sufficient to maintain a specific body function for 50% of the population based on age and gender. The recommended dietary allowance (RDA) is the average needs of 98% of the population, not the exact needs of the individual. The adequate intake (AI) is the suggested intake for individuals based on observed or experimentally determined estimates of nutrient intakes and is used when there is not enough evidence to set the RDA. The tolerable upper intake level (UL) is the highest level that likely poses no risk of adverse health events. It is not a recommended level of intake (Institute of Medicine, 2002).

Food Guidelines. The *Food Guide Pyramid,* (U.S. Department of Agriculture Center for Nutrition Policy and Promotion, 2005) is a basic guide for buying food and meal preparations (Figure 44-2). This basic system provides for diets ranging from 1600 to 2800 kcal/day (U.S. Department of Agriculture, 2005). Additional foods are selected from enriched cereals, complex carbohydrates, and additional grains to round out meals and meet energy requirements. To further augment the food pyramid, the U.S. Department of Agriculture (USDA) and the USDHHS have published the *Dietary Guidelines for Americans 2005* and provide average daily consumption guidelines for the five food groups: grains, vegetables, fruits, dairy products, and meats (Box 44-2, p. 1092). These guidelines are for Americans over the age of 2. You need to make sure to consider the food preferences of different racial and ethnic groups, vegetarians, and others when planning diets.

Daily Values. The Food and Drug Administration (FDA) created **daily values** for food labels in response to the 1990 Nutrition Labeling and Education Act (NLEA). The FDA first established two sets of reference values. The referenced daily intakes (RDIs) are the first set, comprising protein, vitamins, and minerals based upon the RDA. The daily reference values (DRVs) make up the second set and consist of nutrients such as total fat, saturated fat, cholesterol, carbohydrates, fiber, sodium, and potassium. Combined, both sets make up the daily values used on food labels (USFDA, 1999). Daily values did not replace RDAs but provided a separate, more understandable format for the public. Daily values are based on percentages of a diet consisting of 2000 kcal/day.

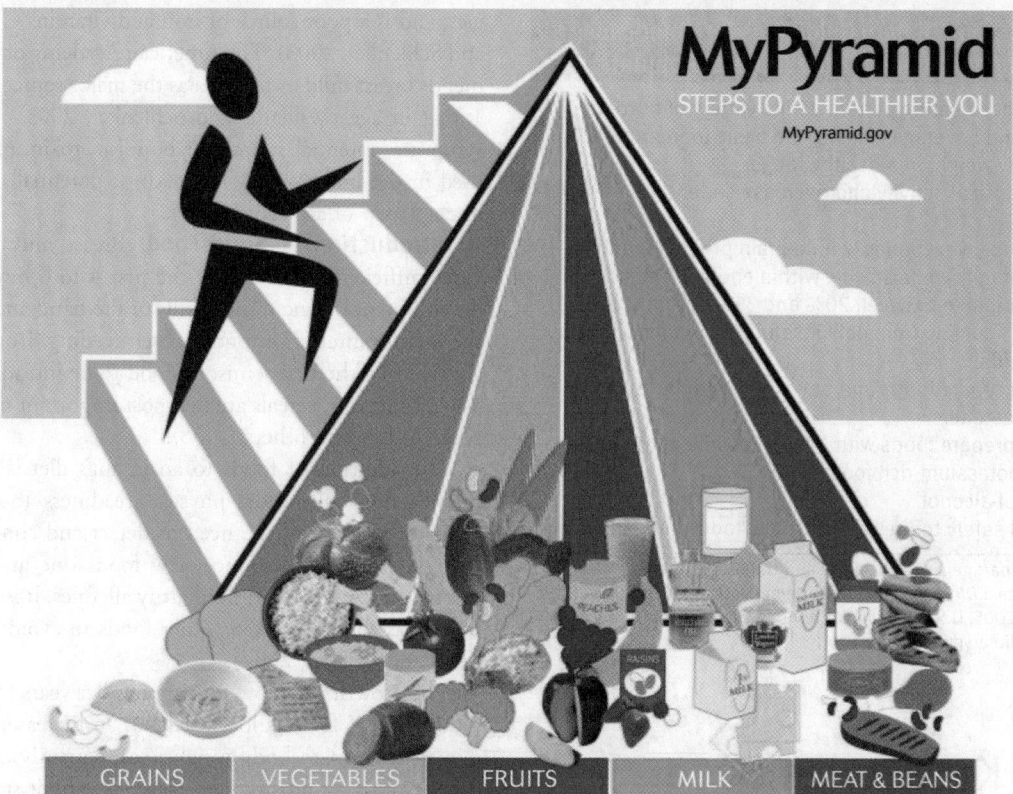

MyPyramid
STEPS TO A HEALTHIER YOU
MyPyramid.gov

GRAINS	VEGETABLES	FRUITS	MILK	MEAT & BEANS

GRAINS	VEGETABLES	FRUITS	MILK	MEAT & BEANS
Make half your grains whole	Vary your veggies	Focus on fruits	Get your calcium-rich foods	Go lean with protein
Eat at least 3 oz. of whole-grain cereals, breads, crackers, rice, or pasta every day	Eat more dark-green veggies like broccoli, spinach, and other dark leafy greens	Eat a variety of fruit	Go low-fat or fat-free when you choose milk, yogurt, and other milk products	Choose low-fat or lean meats and poultry
		Choose fresh, frozen, canned, or dried fruit		Bake it, broil it, or grill it
1 oz. is about 1 slice of bread, about 1 cup of breakfast cereal, or ½ cup of cooked rice, cereal, or pasta	Eat more orange vegetables like carrots and sweetpotatoes	Go easy on fruit juices	If you don't or can't consume milk, choose lactose-free products or other calcium sources such as fortified foods and beverages	Vary your protein routine — choose more fish, beans, peas, nuts, and seeds
	Eat more dry beans and peas like pinto beans, kidney beans, and lentils			

For a 2,000-calorie diet, you need the amounts below from each food group. To find the amounts that are right for you, go to MyPyramid.gov.

Eat 6 oz. every day	Eat 2½ cups every day	Eat 2 cups every day	Get 3 cups every day; for kids aged 2 to 8, it's 2	Eat 5½ oz. every day

Find your balance between food and physical activity
- Be sure to stay within your daily calorie needs.
- Be physically active for at least 30 minutes most days of the week.
- About 60 minutes a day of physical activity may be needed to prevent weight gain.
- For sustaining weight loss, at least 60 to 90 minutes a day of physical activity may be required.
- Children and teenagers should be physically active for 60 minutes every day, or most days.

Know the limits on fats, sugars, and salt (sodium)
- Make most of your fat sources from fish, nuts, and vegetable oils.
- Limit solid fats like butter, margarine, shortening, and lard, as well as foods that contain these.
- Check the Nutrition Facts label to keep saturated fats, trans fats, and sodium low.
- Choose food and beverages low in added sugars. Added sugars contribute calories with few, if any, nutrients.

MyPyramid.gov
STEPS TO A HEALTHIER YOU

U.S. Department of Agriculture
Center for Nutrition Policy and Promotion
April 2005
CNPP-15

USDA

Figure 44-2 Sample food guide pyramid for adults. (From U.S. Department of Agriculture Center for Nutrition Policy and Promotion, *USDA's food guide pyramid,* April 2005, http://www.MyPyramid.gov.)

BOX 44-2 2005 Dietary Guidelines for Americans: Key Recommendations for the General Population

- Adopt a balanced eating pattern with a variety of nutrient-dense food and beverages among the basic food groups.
- Maintain body weight in a healthy range.
- Encourage physical activity and decrease sedentary activities.
- Encourage fruits, vegetables, whole-grain products, and fat-free or low-fat milk while staying within energy needs.
- Keep total fat intake between 20% and 35% of total calories with most fats coming from polyunsaturated or monounsaturated fatty acids.
- Choose and prepare foods and beverages with little added sugars or sweeteners.
- Choose and prepare foods with little salt while at the same time eating potassium-rich foods.
- Limit intake of alcohol.
- Practice food safety to prevent microbial food-borne illness.

Data from U.S. Department of Agriculture and U.S. Department of Health and Human Services: *Dietary guidelines for Americans 2005,* ed 6, Washington, DC, 2005, U.S. Government Printing Office, http://www.healthierus.gov/dietaryguidelines.

Nursing Knowledge Base

Nutrition During Human Growth and Development

Infants Through School-Age. Infancy is marked by rapid growth and high protein, vitamin, mineral, and energy requirements. The average birth weight of an American baby is 3.2 to 3.4 kg (7 to 7½ pounds). The infant usually doubles birth weight at 4 to 5 months and triples it at 1 year. Infants need an energy intake of approximately 108 kcal/kg of body weight in the first half of infancy and 98 kcal/kg in the second half (USDA, 2005). Commercial formulas and human breast milk both provide approximately 20 kcal/oz. A full-term newborn is able to digest and absorb simple carbohydrates, proteins, and a moderate amount of emulsified fat. Infants need about 100 to 120 mL/kg/day of fluid because a large portion of total body weight is water.

Breast-Feeding. The American Academy of Pediatrics (2005) strongly supports breast-feeding. There are multiple benefits of breast-feeding to both infant and mother. These benefits include reduced food allergies and intolerances; fewer infant infections; easier digestion; convenient, always correct temperature, available, and fresh; economical, because it is less expensive than formula; and increased time for mother and infant interaction (Williams and Schlenker, 2003).

Formula. Infant formulas contain the approximate nutrient composition of human milk. Protein in the formula is typically whey, soy, cow's milk base, casein hydrolysate, or elemental amino acids. The American Academy of Pediatrics set standards for the level of nutrients in infant formulas. Use of soy protein–based formulas has increased in recent years (Williams and Schlenker, 2003).

Infants should not have regular cow's milk during the first year of life. It causes gastrointestinal bleeding, is too concentrated for the infant's kidneys to manage, increases the risk of milk product aller-

gies, and is a poor source of iron and vitamins C and E (Williams and Schlenker, 2003). The American Academy of Pediatrics recommends breast milk or formula as the major source of food for up to 1 year in age (Williams and Schlenker, 2003). Honey and corn syrup are potential sources of botulism toxin and should not be used in the infant's diet. The toxin is potentially fatal in children under 1 year of age (Nix, 2005).

Introduction to Solid Food. Breast milk or formula provides sufficient nutrition for the first 4 to 6 months of life. The development of fine motor skills of the hand and fingers parallels the infant's interest in food and self-feeding. Iron-fortified cereals are typically the first semisolid food to be introduced. For infants 4 to 11 months, cereals are the most important nonmilk source of protein (Fox and others, 2006).

The addition of foods to an infant's diet is governed by the infant's nutrient needs, physical readiness to handle different forms of foods, and the need to detect and control allergic reactions. Caregivers introduce new foods one at a time, approximately 4 to 7 days apart to identify allergies. It is best to introduce new foods before milk or other foods to avoid satiety (Hockenberry and Wilson, 2007).

The growth rate slows during toddler years (1 to 3 years). The toddler needs fewer kilocalories but an increased amount of protein in relation to body weight; consequently appetite often decreases at 18 months of age. Toddlers exhibit strong food preferences and become picky eaters. Small frequent meals consisting of breakfast, lunch, and dinner with three interspersed high nutrient-density snacks help improve nutritional intake (Hockenberry and Wilson, 2007). Calcium and phosphorus are important for healthy bone growth.

Toddlers who consume more than 24 ounces of milk daily in place of other foods sometimes develop milk anemia, because milk is a poor source of iron. Toddlers need to drink whole milk until the age of 2 years to make sure there is adequate intake of fatty acids necessary for brain and neurological development. Certain foods such as hot dogs, candy, nuts, grapes, raw vegetables, and popcorn have been implicated in choking deaths and need to be avoided. Preschoolers' (3 to 5 years) dietary requirements are similar to toddlers. They consume slightly more than toddlers, and nutrient density is more important than quantity.

School-age children, 6 to 12 years old, grow at a slower and steadier rate, with a gradual decline in energy requirements per unit of body weight. Despite better appetites and more varied food intake, you need to assess school-age children's diets carefully for adequate protein and vitamins A and C. School-age children often fail to eat a proper breakfast and have unsupervised intake at school. High fat, sugar, and salt result from too-liberal intake of snack foods. There is a consistent decrease in physical activity level and increase in consumption of high-calorie readily available food, leading to an increase in childhood obesity (Edwards, 2005).

In the last 20 years the prevalence of overweight children ages 6 to 11 years has doubled and the prevalence of overweight adolescents has tripled, leading to a total of 25 million children who are overweight or nearly overweight (Mayo Clinic Staff, 2006; National Center for Chronic Disease Prevention and Health Promotion, 2007). A combination of factors contributes to the problem, including a diet rich in high-calorie foods, inactivity, genetic predisposition, use of food as a coping mechanism for stress or boredom, and family and social factors (Mayo Clinic Staff, 2006). Childhood obesity contributes to medical problems related to the cardiovascular system, endocrine system, and mental health (American Academy of Pediatrics, 2003). Prevention of childhood obesity is critical because of the long-term effects. Family education is an important component of decreasing the prevalence of this problem. Promote healthy food choices and eating in moderation along with increased physical activity.

Adolescents. During adolescence, physiological age is a better guide to nutritional needs than chronological age. Energy needs increase to meet greater metabolic demands of growth. Daily requirement of protein also increases. Calcium is essential for the rapid bone growth of adolescence, and girls need a continuous source of iron to replace menstrual losses. Boys also need adequate iron for muscle development. Iodine supports increased thyroid activity, and use of iodized table salt ensures availability. B complex vitamins are necessary to support heightened metabolic activity.

Many factors other than nutritional needs influence the adolescent's diet. This includes concern about body image and appearance, desire for independence, eating at fast-food restaurants, peer pressure, and fad diets. Nutritional deficiencies often occur in adolescent girls as a result of dieting and use of oral contraceptives. The adolescent boy's diet is often inadequate in total kilocalories, protein, iron, folic acid, B vitamins, and iodine. Snacks provide approximately 25% of the teenager's total dietary intake. Fast food is common and adds extra salt, fat, and kilocalories. Skipping meals or eating meals with wrong choices of snacks contributes to nutrient deficiency and obesity (Hockenberry and Wilson, 2007).

Fortified foods (nutrients added) are important sources of vitamins and minerals. Snack food from the dairy and fruit and vegetable groups are good choices. To counter obesity, increasing physical activity is often more important than curbing intake. The onset of eating disorders such as **anorexia nervosa** or **bulimia nervosa** often occurs during adolescence. Recognition of eating disorders is essential for early intervention (Box 44-3).

Sports and regular moderate-to-intense exercise necessitate dietary modification to meet increased energy needs for adolescents. Carbohydrates, both simple and complex, are the main source of energy, providing 55% to 60% of total daily kilocalories. Protein needs increase to 1.0 to 1.5 g/kg/day. Fat needs are not increased. Adequate hydration is very important for all athletes. They need to ingest water before and after exercise to prevent dehydration, especially in hot, humid environments. Vitamin and mineral supplements are not required, but intake of iron-rich foods is required to prevent anemia.

Parents have more influence on the adolescent diet than they believe. Effective strategies include limiting the amount of unhealthy food choices kept at home and enhancing the appearance and taste of healthy foods. Making healthy food choices more convenient at home and at fast-food restaurants, as well as discouraging eating while watching television, are ways to promote healthy eating in adolescents (Befort and others, 2006).

Pregnancy occurring within 4 years of menarche places the mother and fetus at risk because of anatomical and physiological immaturity. Malnutrition at the time of conception increases risk to the adolescent and her fetus. Most teenage girls do not want to

---

⁕ BOX 44-3 Potential Assessment for Eating Disorders

Anorexia Nervosa

A. Refusal to maintain body weight over a minimal normal weight for age and height (e.g., weight loss leading to maintenance of body weight less than 85% of IBW) or failure to make expected weight gain during period of growth, leading to body weight less than 85% of that expected.

B. Intense fear of gaining weight or becoming fat, although underweight.

C. Disturbance in the way in which one's body weight, size, or shape is experienced (e.g., the person claims to "feel fat" even when emaciated, believes that one area of the body is "too fat" even when obviously underweight).

D. In females, absence of at least three consecutive menstrual cycles when otherwise expected to occur (primary or secondary amenorrhea). A woman is considered to have amenorrhea if her periods occur only following hormone (e.g., estrogen) administration.

Bulimia Nervosa

A. Recurrent episodes of binge eating (rapid consumption of a large amount of food in a discrete period of time).

B. A feeling of lack of control over eating behavior during the eating binges.

C. The person regularly engages in self-induced vomiting, use of laxatives or diuretics, strict dieting or fasting, or vigorous exercise in order to prevent weight gain.

D. A minimum average of two binge eating episodes a week for at least 3 months.

Reprinted with permission from the *Diagnostic and Statistical Manual of Mental Disorders*, Fourth Edition, Text Revision, (Copyright 2000). American Psychiatric Association.

---

gain weight. Counseling related to nutritional needs of pregnancy is often difficult, and teens tolerate suggestions better than rigid directions. The diet of pregnant adolescents is often deficient in calcium, iron, and vitamins A and C. Prenatal vitamin and mineral supplements are recommended.

Young and Middle Adults. The demands for most nutrients are reduced as the growth period ends. Mature adults need nutrients for energy, maintenance, and repair. Energy needs usually decline over the years. Obesity becomes a problem due to decreased physical exercise, dining out more often, and increased ability to afford more luxury foods. Adult women who use oral contraceptives often need extra vitamins. Iron and calcium intake continues to be important.

Maintaining good oral health is significant throughout adulthood. Poor oral hygiene and periodontal disease are potential risk factors for systemic diseases such as bacteremia, endocarditis, cardiopulmonary disease, diabetes mellitus, and adverse outcomes in pregnancy (Hornick, 2002).

Pregnancy. Poor nutrition during pregnancy causes low birth weight in infants and decreases chances of survival. Generally the fetus's needs are met at the expense of the mother. However, if nutrient sources are not available, both suffer. The nutritional status of the mother at the time of conception is important. Significant aspects of fetal growth and development often occur before the mother suspects the pregnancy. The energy requirements of pregnancy are related to the mother's body weight and activity. The quality of nutrition during pregnancy is important, and food intake in the first trimester includes balanced portions of essential nutrients with emphasis on quality. Protein intake throughout pregnancy needs to increase to 60 g daily. Calcium intake is especially critical in the third trimester, when fetal bones are mineralized. Iron needs to be supplemented to provide for increased maternal blood volume, for fetal blood storage, and for blood loss during delivery.

Folic acid intake is particularly important for DNA synthesis and the growth of red blood cells. Inadequate intake will possibly lead to fetal neural tube defects, anencephaly, or maternal megaloblastic anemia (Williams and Schlenker, 2003). It is now recommended that women of child-bearing age consume 400 mcg of folic acid daily increasing to 600 mcg daily during pregnancy. In 1998 the FDA began requiring that grain products be fortified with folic acid. Prenatal care usually includes vitamin and mineral supplementation to ensure daily intakes; however, pregnant women should not take additional supplements beyond prescribed amounts.

Lactation. The lactating woman needs 500 kcal/day above the usual allowance because the production of milk increases energy requirements. Protein requirements during lactation are greater than the protein requirement during pregnancy. The need for calcium remains the same as during pregnancy. There is an increased need for vitamins A and C. Daily intake of water-soluble vitamins (B and C) is necessary to ensure adequate levels in breast milk. Fluid intake needs to be adequate but not excessive. Caffeine, alcohol, and drugs are excreted in breast milk and should be avoided. Tobacco use decreases milk production (Food and Nutrition Board, 1992).

Older Adults. Adults 65 years and older have a decreased need for energy as metabolic rate slows with age. However, vitamin and mineral requirements remain unchanged from middle adulthood. Numerous factors influence the nutritional status of the older adult. Income is significant because living on a fixed income often reduces the amount of money available to buy food (Box 44-4). Health is another important influence. The older adult is often on a therapeutic diet or has difficulty eating because of physical symptoms, lack of teeth, or dentures or is at risk for drug-nutrient interactions (Table 44-2). Caution older adults to avoid grapefruit and grapefruit juice because these will decrease absorption of many drugs. Thirst sensation diminishes, leading to inadequate fluid intake or dehydration (see Chapter 41). Symptoms of dehydration in older adults include confusion, weakness, hot dry skin, furrowed tongue, rapid pulse, and high urinary sodium. Some older adults avoid meats because of cost or because they are difficult to chew. Cream soups and meat-based vegetable soups are nutrient-dense sources of protein. Cheese, eggs, and peanut butter are also useful high-protein alternatives. Milk continues to be an important food for older women and men who need adequate calcium to protect against osteoporosis (a decrease of bone mass density). After age 70, osteoporosis equally affects men and women (Williams and Schlenker, 2003). Screening and treatment are necessary for both older men and women. The diet of older adults needs to contain choices from all food groups and often requires a vitamin and mineral supplement.

✳ BOX 44-4   FOCUS ON OLDER ADULTS

Factors Affecting Nutritional Status

- Age-related gastrointestinal changes that affect digestion of food and maintenance of nutrition include changes in the teeth and gums, reduced saliva production, atrophy of oral mucosal epithelial cells, increased taste threshold, decreased thirst sensation, reduced gag reflex, and decreased esophageal and colonic peristalsis (Linton and Lach, 2006).
- The presence of chronic illnesses (e.g., diabetes mellitus, end-stage renal disease, cancer) often affects nutrition intake (Furman, 2006).
- Malnutrition in older adults has multiple causes, such as income, educational level, physical functional level to meet activities of daily living (ADLs), loss, dependency, loneliness, and transportation (DiMaria-Ghalili and Amella, 2005).
- Adverse effects of medications cause problems such as anorexia, xerostomia, early satiety, and impaired smell and taste perception (Linton and Lach, 2006).
- Factors affecting nutrient needs: calcium, vitamin D, or phosphorus for basic metabolic demand (BMD). B_{12} may not be synthesized because of lack of intrinsic factor in terminal ileum, decreased lean muscle mass, lower basic energy expenditure (BEE) (Meiner and Lueckenotte, 2006).
- Cognitive impairments such as delirium, dementia, and depression affect ability to obtain, prepare, and eat healthy foods (Linton and Lach, 2006).

The USDHHS's Administration on Aging (AOA) requires states to provide nutritional screening services to older adult clients who benefit from home-delivered or congregate meal services. Reports of findings are sent to AOA. An estimated 5% to 10% of community-dwelling older adults suffer from food inadequacies within any 6-month period (Furman, 2006). Undernourishment of older adults often results in health problems that lead to admission to acute care hospitals or long-term care facilities.

SAFETY ALERT Homebound older adults with chronic illness have additional nutritional risks. Frequently this group lives alone with little or no social or financial resources to assist in obtaining or preparing nutritionally sound meals. Increased nutritional screening by the nurse results in early recognition of potential nutritional deficiencies and needed treatment of these deficiencies (Chen and others, 2005).

Alternative Food Patterns

Long before the FDA issued recommended allowances and guidelines, many people followed special patterns of food intake based on religion (Table 44-3, p. 1096), cultural background (Box 44-5, p. 1097), ethics, health beliefs, personal preference, or concern for the efficient use of land to produce food. Such special diets are not necessarily more or less nutritious than diets based on the food pyramid or other nutritional guidelines, because good nutrition depends on a balanced intake of all required nutrients. Nurses care for clients who have a variety of food intake patterns.

Vegetarian Diet. A common alternative dietary pattern is the vegetarian diet. **Vegetarianism** is the consumption of a diet

✳ TABLE 44-2 Sample of Drug-Nutrient Interactions*

DRUG	EFFECT
Analgesic	
Acetaminophen	Decreased drug absorption with food; overdose associated with liver failure
Aspirin	Absorbed directly through stomach; decreased drug absorption with food; decreased folic acid, vitamins C and K, and iron absorption
Antacid	
Aluminum hydroxide	Decreased phosphate absorption
Sodium bicarbonate	Decreased folic acid absorption
Antiarrhythmic	
Amiodarone	Taste alteration
Digitalis	Anorexia, decreased renal clearance in older persons
Antibiotic	
Penicillins	Decreased drug absorption with food, taste alteration
Cephalosporin	Decreased vitamin K
Rifampin	Decreased vitamin B_6, niacin, vitamin D
Tetracycline	Decreased drug absorption with milk and antacids, decreased nutrient absorption of calcium, riboflavin, vitamin C due to binding
Trimethoprim/sulfamethoxazole	Decreased folic acid
Anticoagulant	
Coumarin	Acts as antagonist to vitamin K
Anticonvulsant	
Carbamazepine	Increased drug absorption with food
Phenytoin	Decreased calcium absorption; decreased vitamins D and K and folic acid; taste alteration; decreased drug absorption with food
Antidepressant	
Amitriptyline	Appetite stimulant
Clomipramine	Taste alteration, appetite stimulant
Fluoxetine (selective serotonin reuptake inhibitors [SSRIs])	Taste alteration, anorexia
Antihypertensive	
Captopril	Taste alteration, anorexia
Hydralazine	Enhanced drug absorption with food, decreased vitamin B_6
Labetalol	Taste alteration (weight gain for all beta-blockers)
Methyldopa	Decreased vitamin B_{12}, folic acid, iron
Antiinflammatory	
All steroids	Increased appetite and weight, increased folic acid, decreased calcium (osteoporosis with long-term use), promotes gluconeogenesis of protein
Antiparkinson	
Levodopa	Taste alteration, decreased vitamin B_6 and drug absorption with food
Antipsychotic	
Chlorpromazine	Increased appetite
Thiothixene	Decreased riboflavin, increased need
Bronchodilator	
Albuterol sulfate	Appetite stimulant
Theophylline	Anorexia
Cholesterol Lowering	
Cholestyramine	Decreased fat-soluble vitamins (A, D, E, K); vitamin B_{12}; iron
Diuretic	
Furosemide	Decreased drug absorption with food
Spironolactone	Increased drug absorption with food
Thiazides	Decreased magnesium, zinc, and potassium

Data from McKenry LM, Salerno E: *Mosby's pharmacology in nursing*, ed 21 revised, St. Louis, 2003, Mosby; and *Nutrient-drug interactions*, 2006, http://www.faqs.org/nutrition/Met-Obe/Nutrient-Drug-Interactions.html, accessed December 12, 2006.
*Not intended to be an exhaustive or all-inclusive list. Always check pharmacology references before administering medications.

Continued

✳ TABLE 44-2 Sample of Drug-Nutrient Interactions*—cont'd

DRUG	EFFECT
Laxative	
Mineral oil	Decreased absorption of fat-soluble vitamins (A, D, E, K), carotene
Platelet Aggregate Inhibitor	
Dipyridamole	Decreased drug absorption with food
Potassium Replacement	
Potassium chloride	Decreased vitamin B_{12}
Tranquilizer	
Benzodiazepines	Increased appetite

Data from McKenry LM, Salerno E: *Mosby's pharmacology in nursing,* ed 21 revised, St. Louis, 2003, Mosby; and *Nutrient-drug interactions,* 2006, http://www.faqs.org/nutrition/Met-Obe/Nutrient-Drug-Interactions.html, accessed December 12, 2006.
*Not intended to be an exhaustive or all-inclusive list. Always check pharmacology references before administering medications.

✳ TABLE 44-3 Religious Dietary Restrictions

ISLAM	CHRISTIANITY	HINDUISM	JUDAISM	CHURCH OF JESUS CHRIST OF LATTER-DAY SAINTS (MORMONS)	SEVENTH-DAY ADVENTISTS CHURCH
Pork	Minimal or no alcohol	All meats	Pork	Alcohol	Pork
Alcohol	Holy day observances may restrict meat	Alcohol	Predatory fowl	Tobacco	Shellfish
Caffeine			Shellfish (eat only fish with scales)	Caffeine	Alcohol
Ramadan fasting sunrise to sunset for month			Rare meats	Limit meat	Coffee, tea
Ritualized methods of animal slaughter required for meat ingestion			Blood (blood sausage, etc.)		Vegetarian or ovolactovegetarian diets encouraged
			Mixing of milk or dairy products with meat dishes		
			Must adhere to kosher food preparation methods		
			24 hr of fasting on Yom Kippur, a day of atonement		
			No leavened bread eaten during Passover (8 days)		
			No cooking on the Sabbath (Saturday)		

consisting predominantly of plant foods. Some vegetarians are ovolactovegetarian (avoid meat, fish, and poultry but eat eggs and milk), lactovegetarians (drink milk but avoid eggs), or vegans (consume only plant foods). Vegan, Zen macrobiotic (eat primarily brown rice, other grains, and herb teas), and fruitarian (eat only fruit, nuts, honey, and olive oil) diets are nutrient poor and frequently result in malnutrition. Knowledge related to complementary use of complete and incomplete proteins is necessary. Children who follow a vegetarian diet are especially at risk for protein and vitamin deficiencies, such as vitamin B_{12}.

Critical Thinking

Successful critical thinking requires a synthesis of knowledge, experience, information collected from clients, critical thinking attitudes, and intellectual and professional standards. Clinical judg-

ments require you to anticipate the required information, analyze the data, and make decisions regarding client care. Critical thinking is a dynamic process. During assessment (Figure 44-3) consider all elements that build toward making appropriate nursing diagnoses.

Integrate knowledge from nursing and other disciplines, previous experiences, and information gathered from clients and families regarding customary food preferences, as well as recent dietary history. Use of professional standards, such as the DRIs, the USDA's food guide pyramid, dietary guidelines, and *Healthy People 2010* objectives provide guidelines to assess and maintain the clients' nutritional status. Other professional standards by the American Heart Association (2006), the American Diabetes Association (ADA) (2006), The American Cancer Society (Kushi and others, 2006), and the American Society for Parenteral and Enteral Nutrition (ASPEN) (2001) are available. These standards are evidence based and are regularly updated for optimal client care.

✳ BOX 44-5   CULTURAL ASPECTS OF CARE

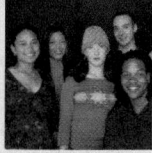

Nutrition

Food patterns developed as a child, habits, and culture interact to influence food intake. Culture also influences the meaning of food not related to nutrition. Eating is associated with sentiments and feelings such as "good" and "bad." For example, children are often rewarded for "being good" with a treat such as candy. They then associate candy with "being good."

The incidence of lactose intolerance around the world occurs from high to low in the following ethnic or racial groups: Asian-Pacific, African and African American, Native American, Mexican American, Middle Eastern, and whites. This condition affects nutrient absorption, and calcium deficiency results. Calcium is necessary for maintaining bone mass density.

The theory of hot and cold foods predominates in many cultures. The origin appears to be from Hippocratic beliefs concerning health and the four humors. Arabs were keepers of this knowledge during the Dark Ages and later influenced the Spanish to adopt this belief system in the later Middle Ages. The foundation of the theory is keeping harmony with nature by balancing "cold," "hot," "wet," and "dry." Some cultures believe hot is warmth, strength, and reassurance, whereas cold is menacing and weak. Classification has nothing to do with spiciness but is a symbolic representation of temperature.

Implications for Practice

- Identify the meaning that certain types of food have for each client.
- Lactose and other food intolerances unique to specific cultures require diet adaptation to meet nutrient, mineral, and vitamin daily intake requirements.
- When clients use hot and cold foods as part of their cultural health practices, dietary modifications are necessary. Hot foods include rice, grain cereals, alcohol, beef, lamb, chili peppers, chocolate, cheese, temperate zone fruits, eggs, peas, goat's milk, cornhusks, oils, onions, pork, radishes, and tamales. By contrast, cold foods are beans, citrus fruits, tropical fruits, dairy products, most vegetables, honey, raisins, chicken, fish, and goat.
    - In some cultures specific conditions require hot foods. Menstruation, cancer, pneumonia, earache, colds, paralysis, headache, and rheumatism are cold illnesses requiring hot foods.
    - Other conditions, such as pregnancy, fever, infections, diarrhea, rashes, ulcers, liver problems, constipation, kidney problems, and sore throats are hot conditions requiring cold foods.

Modified from Giger JN, Davidhizar RE: *Transcultural nursing: assessment and intervention,* ed 3, St. Louis, 2004, Mosby.

Knowledge

- Normal nutrition parameters
- Anatomy and physiology of gastrointestinal system
- Cultural influences on nutrition
- Developmental factors affecting nutrition
- Effects of medications on nutrition

Experience

- Caring for clients with altered nutrition
- Observation of nutritional practices of friends and family
- Personal assessment of nutritional practices

ASSESSMENT

- Identify the signs and symptoms associated with altered nutrition
- Gather data from clients regarding nutritional practices
- Determine client's nutritional energy needs (REE × activity or illness factor)
- Obtain client's dietary history

Standards

- Apply intellectual standards of accuracy, completeness, and significance when obtaining a health history for clients with altered nutrition
- Compare gathered data with established nutritional standards, (e.g., dietary reference intake, food pyramid, *Healthy People 2010,* and healthy eating index)

Attitudes

- Be open minded about the client's nutritional practices when obtaining nutritional assessment
- Display confidence when collecting data related to culture, socioeconomic status, physical functioning, dietary restrictions, and personal preferences as necessary to a complete nutritional assessment

Figure 44-3 Critical thinking model for nutrition assessment.

Nursing Process and Nutrition

As the nurse, you are in an excellent position to recognize signs of poor nutrition and to take steps to initiate change. Close contact with clients and their families enables you to make observations about physical status, food intake, food preferences, weight changes, and response to therapy.

◆ Assessment

Early recognition of malnourished or at-risk clients has a strong positive influence on both short- and long-term health outcomes. Studies have identified 40% to 55% of adult hospitalized clients as being either malnourished or at risk for malnutrition (Mason, 2006). Clients who are malnourished on admission are at greater risk of life-threatening complications during hospitalization such as arrhythmia, sepsis, or hemorrhage (Covinsky, 2002). Assessment of nutritional status is essential due to the common need of all human beings for nutrients, energy, and fluids.

Screening. Nutrition screening is part of an initial assessment. Screening a client is a quick method of identifying **malnutrition** or risk of malnutrition (ASPEN, 2002). Nutritional screening tools need to gather data based on four main principles: What is the condition now? Is the condition stable? Will the condition get worse? and Will the disease process accelerate nutritional deterioration? (Kondrup and others, 2003). These tools typically include objective measures such as height, weight, weight change, primary diagnosis, and the presence of other comorbidities (ASPEN, 2002). Using a single objective measure alone is ineffective in predicting risk of nutritional problems (Sarhill and others, 2003). Combine multiple objective measures with subjective measures related to nutrition to adequately screen for nutritional problems. Identification of risk factors such as unintentional weight loss, presence of a modified diet, or the presence of altered nutritional impact symptoms (i.e., nausea, vomiting, diarrhea, and constipation) require nutritional consultation.

Several standardized nutrition screening tools are available for use in the outpatient setting. The Subjective Global Assessment (SGA) is a validated clinical method that uses the client history, weight, and physical assessment data to evaluate nutritional status (National Guideline Clearinghouse, 2006). SGA is a simple, inexpensive technique that is able to predict nutrition-related complications. The Mini Nutritional Assessment (MNA) (Figure 44-4) was developed to use for screening older adults in home care programs, nursing homes, and hospitals. The tool has 18 items that are divided into screening and assessment. If the client scores 11 or less on the screening portion, the health care provider completes the assessment portion (Kondrup and others, 2003). A total score of less than 17 indicates protein-energy malnutrition (Guigoz and others, 1996; Guigoz and Vellas, 1999).

Assess clients for malnutrition when a condition that interferes with the ability to ingest, digest, or absorb adequate nutrients exists (Figure 44-5, p. 1100). When possible use standardized tools to assess nutrition risks. Congenital anomalies and surgical revisions of the gastrointestinal tract interfere with normal function. Clients fed only by intravenous infusion of 5% or 10% dextrose are at risk for nutritional deficiencies. The presence of chronic disease or increased metabolic requirements are risk factors for development of nutritional problems. Infants and older adults are at greatest risk.

Anthropometry. **Anthropometry** is a measurement system of the size and makeup of the body. Height and weight are obtained for each client on hospital admission or entry into any health care setting. If you are not able to measure height with the client standing, position the client lying flat in bed as straight as possible, arms folded on the chest, and measure the client lengthwise. Serial measures of weight over time provide more useful information than one measurement. The client needs to be weighed at the same time each day, on the same scale, and with the same clothing or linen. Compare height and weight to standards for height-weight relationships. An **ideal body weight** (IBW) provides an estimate of what a person should weigh. Weight gain usually reflects fluid shifts. One pint or 500 mL of fluid equals 1 pound. Document any recent weight changes. For example, for a client with renal failure or congestive heart failure a weight increase of 2 pounds in 24 hours is significant, because it usually indicates that the client has retained a liter (1000 mL) of fluid.

Other anthropometric measurements that help in identifying nutritional problems include the ratio of height to wrist circumference, mid-upper arm circumference (MAC), triceps skin fold (TSF), and mid-upper arm muscle circumference (MAMC). Significant variation results unless the examiner is skilled and has

proper equipment. Compare values for MAC, TSF, and MAMC to standards, and calculate them as a percentage of the standard. Changes in values for an individual over time are of greater significance than isolated measurements (Nix, 2005).

Body mass index (BMI) measures weight corrected for height and serves as an alternative to traditional height-weight relationships. Calculate BMI by dividing the client's weight in kilograms by height in meters squared: Weight (kg) divided by Height^2 (m^2). For example, a client who weighs 75 kg (165 pounds) and is 1.8 m (5 feet 9 inches) tall has a BMI of 23.15 ($75 \div 1.8^2 = 23.15$). A client is considered overweight if the BMI is 25 to 30. A BMI of greater than 30 is defined as obesity and places a client at higher medical risk of coronary heart disease, some cancers, diabetes mellitus, and hypertension. Other factors such as lack of access to healthy food and inadequate health care also contribute to the development of these problems (Williams and Schlenker, 2003).

Laboratory and Biochemical Tests. No single laboratory or biochemical test is diagnostic for malnutrition. Factors that frequently alter test results include fluid balance, liver function, kidney function, and the presence of disease. Common laboratory tests used to study nutritional status include measures of plasma proteins such as albumin, transferrin, prealbumin, retinol binding protein, total iron-binding capacity, and hemoglobin. After feeding, the response time for changes in these proteins ranges from hours to weeks. The metabolic half-life of albumin is 21 days, transferrin is 8 days, prealbumin is 2 days, and retinol binding protein is 12 hours. This range demonstrates why albumin level, for example, is not an accurate short-term indicator of serum protein status (Pagana and Pagana, 2005). Factors that affect serum albumin levels include hydration; hemorrhage; renal or hepatic disease; large amounts of drainage from wounds, drains, burns, or the gastrointestinal tract; steroid administration; exogenous albumin infusions; age; and trauma, burns, stress, or surgery. In summary, albumin level is a better indicator for chronic illnesses, whereas prealbumin level is preferred for acute conditions.

Nitrogen balance is important to establishing serum protein status (see the discussion of protein in this chapter). Calculate nitrogen balance by dividing 6.25 into the total grams of protein ingested in a day (24 hours). Measure the output of nitrogen through laboratory analysis of a 24-hour urinary urea nitrogen (UUN). For clients with diarrhea or fistula drainage, estimate a further addition of 2 to 4 g of nitrogen output. Nitrogen balance is found by subtracting the nitrogen output from the nitrogen intake. A positive 2- to 3-g nitrogen balance is necessary for anabolism. By contrast, negative nitrogen balance is present when catabolic states exist.

Dietary History and Health History. In addition to the general nursing history, use data from a more specific diet history to assess the client's actual or potential needs. Box 44-6 (p. 1101) lists some specific assessment questions to ask in the dietary history. The diet history focuses on the client's habitual intake of foods and liquids, as well as information about preferences, allergies, and other relevant areas, such as the client's ability to obtain food. Gather information about the client's illness/activity level to determine energy needs and compare food intake. Your nursing

Text continued on p. 1101

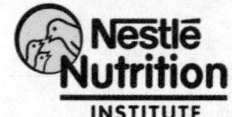

Mini Nutritional Assessment
MNA®

Last name:	First name:	Sex:	Date:

Age:	Weight, kg:	Height, cm:	I.D. Number:

Complete the screen by filling in the boxes with the appropriate numbers.
Add the numbers for the screen. If score is 11 or less, continue with the assessment to gain a Malnutrition Indicator Score.

Screening

A Has food intake declined over the past 3 months due to loss of appetite, digestive problems, chewing or swallowing difficulties?
0 = severe loss of appetite
1 = moderate loss of appetite
2 = no loss of appetite ☐

B Weight loss during the last 3 months
0 = weight loss greater than 3 kg (6.6 lbs)
1 = does not know
2 = weight loss between 1 and 3 kg (2.2 and 6.6 lbs)
3 = no weight loss ☐

C Mobility
0 = bed or chair bound
1 = able to get out of bed/chair but does not go out
2 = goes out ☐

D Has suffered psychological stress or acute disease in the past 3 months
0 = yes   2 = no ☐

E Neuropsychological problems
0 = severe dementia or depression
1 = mild dementia
2 = no psychological problems ☐

F Body Mass Index (BMI) (weight in kg) / (height in m²)
0 = BMI less than 19
1 = BMI 19 to less than 21
2 = BMI 21 to less than 23
3 = BMI 23 or greater ☐

Screening score (subtotal max. 14 points) ☐☐
12 points or greater   Normal – not at risk – no need to complete assessment
11 points or below   Possible malnutrition – continue assessment

Assessment

G Lives independently (not in a nursing home or hospital)
0 = no   1 = yes ☐

H Takes more than 3 prescription drugs per day
0 = yes   1 = no ☐

I Pressure sores or skin ulcers
0 = yes   1 = no ☐

Ref. Vellas B, Villars H, Abellan G, et al. Overview of the MNA® - Its History and Challenges. J Nut Health Aging 2006;10:456-465.
Rubenstein LZ, Harker JO, Salva A, Guigoz Y, Vellas B. Screening for Undernutrition in Geriatric Practice:Developing the Short-Fom Mini Nutritional Assessment (MNA-SF). J. Geront 2001;56A: M366-377.
Guigoz Y. The Mini-Nutritional Assessment (MNA®) Review of the Literature - What does it tell us? J Nutr Health Aging 2006; 10:466-487.

© Nestlé, 1994, Revision 2006. N67200 12/99 10M

For more information : www.mna-elderly.com

J How many full meals does the patient eat daily?
0 = 1 meal
1 = 2 meals
2 = 3 meals ☐

K Selected consumption markers for protein intake
• At least one serving of dairy products (milk, cheese, yogurt) per day   yes ☐ no ☐
• Two or more servings of legumes or eggs per week   yes ☐ no ☐
• Meat, fish or poultry every day   yes ☐ no ☐
0.0 = if 0 or 1 yes
0.5 = if 2 yes
1.0 = if 3 yes ☐.☐

L Consumes two or more servings of fruits or vegetables per day?
0 = no   1 = yes ☐

M How much fluid (water, juice, coffee, tea, milk…) is consumed per day?
0.0 = less than 3 cups
0.5 = 3 to 5 cups
1.0 = more than 5 cups ☐.☐

N Mode of feeding
0 = unable to eat without assistance
1 = self-fed with some difficulty
2 = self-fed without any problem ☐

O Self view of nutritional status
0 = views self as being malnourished
1 = is uncertain of nutritional state
2 = views self as having no nutritional problem ☐

P In comparison with other people of the same age, how does the patient consider his/her health status?
0.0 = not as good
0.5 = does not know
1.0 = as good
2.0 = better ☐.☐

Q Mid-arm circumference (MAC) in cm
0.0 = MAC less than 21
0.5 = MAC 21 to 22
1.0 = MAC 22 or greater ☐.☐

R Calf circumference (CC) in cm
0 = CC less than 31   1 = CC 31 or greater ☐

Assessment (max. 16 points) ☐☐.☐

Screening score ☐☐

Total Assessment (max. 30 points) ☐☐.☐

Malnutrition Indicator Score

17 to 23.5 points   at risk of malnutrition ☐

Less than 17 points   malnourished ☐

Figure 44-4 Mini Nutritional Assessment (MNA). (Reprinted with permission by Nestlé Nutrition.)

Nutrition Risk Assessment

Name _____ Adm date _____ Rm _____ Assess type _____

DOB _____ Age _____ Sex: M F Advance directive _____ Physician _____

Diagnosis _____

Ht (in) _____ Wt (lb) _____ Wt (kg) _____ Usual body wt range _____ BMI _____

BEE _____ Activity factor _____ Injury factor _____ Total cal _____ Total protein _____ g (_____ g/kg)

Total fluids _____ cc (_____ cc/kg) Fluid restriction _____

Diet order _____ Food allergies/sensitivities _____

Supplement/snacks _____ Cultural/religious preferences _____

Risk Factor	No/Low Risk (0 pts)	Moderate Risk (1 pt)	High Risk (3 pts)	MDS Ref	Pts	Comments
Weight status; loss or gain	BMI 19-27 No weight change	<5% wt change in 30 days; <7.5% within 90 days; or <10% within 6 mo	BMI <19 or >27 ≥5% wt change in 30 days; ≥7.5% in 90 days; or ≥10% within 6 mo	J, K, E		
Oral/nutrition intake; food	Intake meets 76-100% of estimated needs	Intake meets 26-75% of estimated needs	Intake meets ≤25% of estimated needs	AC, J, K		
Oral/nutrition intake; fluids	Consumes 1,500-2,000 cc/day	Consumes 1,000-1,499 cc/day	Consumes < 1,000 cc/day	AC, J, K		
Medications; nutrition-related	0-1 drugs/day	2-4 drugs/day	5 or more drugs/day	O		
Relevant conditions and diagnoses	HTN, DM, heart disease, or other controlled diseases/ conditions	Anemia, infection, CVA (recent), fracture, UTI, alcohol abuse, drug abuse, COPD, edema, surgery (recent), osteoporosis, hx of GI bleed, food intolerances and allergies, poor circulation, constipation, diarrhea, GERD, anorexia, Parkinson's	Cancer (advanced), septicemia, liver failure, dialysis, ESRD, Alzheimer's, dementia, depression, dehydration, dysphagia, radiation/chemo, active GI bleed, chronic nausea, vomiting, ostomy, gastrectomy, fecal impaction, uncontrolled diseases or conditions	E, H, I, J, M, P		
Physical and mental functioning	Ambulatory, alert, able to feed self, no chewing or swallowing problems	Out of bed w/assistance, motor agitation (tremors, wandering), limited feeding assistance, supervision while eating, chewing or swallowing problems, teeth in poor repair, ill-fitting dentures or refusal to wear dentures, edentulous, taste and sensory changes, unable to communicate needs	Bedridden, inactive, total dependence, extensive or total assistance or dependence while eating, aspirates, tube feeding, TPN, mouth pain	A, B, E, G, L, P		
Lab values	Albumin and other nutrition-related lab values WNL	Albumin 3.0-3.4 g/dL, 1-2 other nutrition-related labs abnormal	Albumin less than 3.0 g/dL, 3-5 other nutrition-related labs abnormal	P		
Skin conditions	Skin intact	Stage I/II pressure ulcers or skin tears not healing, hx of pressure ulcers, stasis ulcer, fecal incontinence	Stage III/IV pressure ulcers or multiple impaired areas	M		

Overall Risk Category: 0-2 points: NO/LOW RISK 3-7 points: MODERATE RISK ≥8 points: HIGH RISK

Total Points: _____   Overall Risk Category: _____

Signature: _____ Date: _____

© 1999, The American Dietetic Association. May be reproduced for clinical purposes.

Figure 44-5 Nutrition Risk Assessment (NRA). (Reprinted with permission by Consultant Dietitians in Health Care Facilities Practice Group of the American Dietetic Association.)

※ **BOX 44-6** NURSING ASSESSMENT QUESTIONS

Dietary Intake and Food Preferences
- What type of food do you like?
- How many meals a day do you eat?
- What times do you normally eat meals and snacks?
- What are the portion sizes that you eat at each meal?
- Are you on a special diet because of a medical problem?
- Do you have any diet restrictions because of your religion or culture?
- Who prepares the food?
- Who purchases the food?
- How do you cook your food (e.g., fried, broiled, baked, grilled)?

Unpleasant Symptoms
- What foods cause indigestion, gas, or heartburn?
- Does this occur each time you have the food?
- What relieves the symptoms?

Allergies
- Are you allergic to any foods?
- What types of problems do you have with these foods?
- How are these food allergies treated (e.g., EpiPen, oral antihistamines)?

Taste, Chewing, and Swallowing
- Have you noticed any changes in taste?
- Did these changes occur with medications or following an illness?
- Do you wear dentures? Are the dentures comfortable?
- Do you have any mouth pain or sores (e.g., cold sore, canker sores)?
- Do you have difficulty swallowing?
- Do you cough or gag when you swallow?

Appetite and Weight
- Have you had a change in appetite?
- Have you noticed a change in your weight?
- Was this change an anticipated change (e.g., were you on a weight reduction diet)?

Use of Medications
- What medications do you take?
- Do you take any over-the-counter medications that your doctor does not prescribe?
- Do you take any nutritional or herbal supplements?

※ **BOX 44-7** Causes of Dysphagia

Myogenic
Myasthenia gravis
Aging
Muscular dystrophy
Polymyositis

Neurogenic
Stroke
Cerebral palsy
Guillain-Barré syndrome
Multiple sclerosis
Amyotrophic lateral sclerosis (Lou Gehrig disease)
Diabetic neuropathy
Parkinson's disease

Obstructive
Benign peptic stricture
Lower esophageal ring
Candidiasis
Head and neck cancer
Inflammatory masses
Trauma/surgical resection
Anterior mediastinal masses
Cervical spondylosis

Other
Gastrointestinal or esophageal resection
Rheumatologic disorders
Connective tissue disorders
Vagotomy

areas to evaluate the client's nutritional status. The clinical signs of nutritional status (Table 44-4) serve as guidelines for observation during physical assessment.

Dysphagia. Dysphagia refers to difficulty when swallowing. Causes of dysphagia include neurogenic, myogenic, and obstructive problems (Box 44-7). The complications of dysphagia vary, including aspiration pneumonia, dehydration, decreased nutritional status, and weight loss. Dysphagia leads to disability or decreased functional status, increased length of stay and cost of care, increased likelihood of discharge to institutionalized care, and increased mortality (Ashley and others, 2006).

Be aware of warning signs for dysphagia. Signs of dysphagia include cough during eating; change in voice tone or quality after swallowing; abnormal movements of the mouth, tongue, or lips; and slow, weak, imprecise, or uncoordinated speech. Abnormal gag, delayed swallowing, incomplete oral clearance or pocketing, regurgitation, pharyngeal pooling, delayed or absent trigger of swallow, and inability to speak consistently are other signs of dysphagia. Clients with dysphagia often do not show overt signs such as coughing when food enters the airway. "Silent aspiration" is aspiration that occurs without a cough and occurs in clients with neurological problems that lead to decreased sensation (Nowlin, 2006). Silent aspiration accounts for most of the 40% to 70% of aspiration in clients with dysphagia following stroke (Kwon and others, 2006).

Dysphagia often leads to an inadequate amount of food intake, which possibly results in malnutrition. Frequently clients with dysphagia become frustrated with eating and show changes in skinfold thickness and albumin. Adjustment to new dietary restrictions during the rehabilitation period affects intake for long periods of time. Malnutrition significantly slows down recovery (Bending, 2001; Perry and Love, 2001). Early screening with a formal dysphagia screening protocol significantly decreases the risk of aspiration pneumonia in clients (Hinchey and others, 2005; Kwon and others, 2006).

Dysphagia screening quickly identifies problems with swallowing and helps nurses initiate referrals for more in-depth assessment (Skill 44-1). An early and ongoing assessment of clients with swallowing difficulties increases quality of care and decreases

assessment of nutrition includes health status; age; cultural background (see Box 44-5); religious food patterns (see Table 44-3); socioeconomic status; personal food preferences; psychological factors; use of alcohol or illegal drugs; use of vitamin, mineral, or herbal supplements; prescription or over-the-counter (OTC) drugs (see Table 44-2); and the client's general nutrition knowledge (Williams and Schlenker, 2003).

In outpatient settings the client keeps a 3- to 7-day food diary. This allows you to calculate nutritional intake and to compare it with DRIs to see if the client's dietary habits are adequate. Use food-frequency questionnaires to establish patterns over time.

Physical Examination. The physical examination is one of the most important aspects of a nutritional assessment. Because improper nutrition affects all body systems, observe for malnutrition during physical assessment (see Chapter 33). Complete the general physical assessment of body systems and recheck relevant

Text continued on p. 1104

✳ TABLE 44-4 Physical Signs of Nutritional Status

BODY AREA	SIGNS OF GOOD NUTRITION	SIGNS OF POOR NUTRITION
General appearance	Alert: responsive	Listless, apathetic, cachectic
Weight	Weight normal for height, age, body build	Obesity (usually 10% above IBW) or underweight (special concern for underweight)
Posture	Erect posture; straight arms and legs	Sagging shoulders; sunken chest; humped back
Muscles	Well-developed, firm; good tone; some fat under skin	Flaccid, poor tone, underdeveloped tone; "wasted" appearance; impaired ability to walk properly
Nervous system control	Good attention span; not irritable or restless; normal reflexes; psychological stability	Inattention; irritability; confusion; burning and tingling of hands and feet (paresthesia); loss of position and vibratory sense; weakness and tenderness of muscles (may result in inability to walk); decrease or loss of ankle and knee reflexes; absent vibratory sense
Gastrointestinal function	Good appetite and digestion; normal regular elimination; no palpable organs or masses	Anorexia; indigestion; constipation or diarrhea; liver or spleen enlargement
Cardiovascular function	Normal heart rate and rhythm; lack of murmurs; normal blood pressure for age	Rapid heart rate (above 100 beats/min), enlarged heart; abnormal rhythm; elevated blood pressure
General vitality	Endurance; energy; sleeps well; vigorous	Easily fatigued; no energy; falls asleep easily; tired and apathetic
Hair	Shiny, lustrous; firm; not easily plucked; healthy scalp	Stringy, dull, brittle, dry, thin, and sparse, depigmented; easily plucked
Skin (general)	Smooth and slightly moist skin with good color	Rough, dry, scaly, pale, pigmented, irritated; bruises; petechiae; subcutaneous fat loss
Face and neck	Uniform color; smooth, pink, healthy appearance; not swollen	Greasy, discolored, scaly, swollen; dark skin over cheeks and under eyes; lumpiness or flakiness of skin around nose and mouth
Lips	Smooth; good color; moist; not chapped or swollen	Dry, scaly, swollen; redness and swelling (cheilosis); angular lesions at corners of mouth; fissures or scars (stomatitis)
Mouth, oral membranes	Reddish pink mucous membranes in oral cavity	Swollen, boggy oral mucous membranes
Gums	Good pink color; healthy and red; no swelling or bleeding	Spongy gums that bleed easily; marginal redness, inflammation; receding
Tongue	Good pink or deep reddish color; no swelling; smooth, presence of surface papillae; lack of lesions	Swelling, scarlet and raw; magenta, beefiness (glossitis); hyperemic and hypertrophic papillae; atrophic papillae
Teeth	No cavities; no pain; bright, straight; no crowding; well-shaped jaw; clean with no discoloration	Unfilled caries; missing teeth; worn surfaces; mottled (fluorosis), malpositioned
Eyes	Bright, clear, shiny; no sores at corner of membranes; eyelids; moist and healthy pink; prominent blood vessels or lack of mound of tissue or sclera; no fatigue circles beneath eyes	Eye membranes pale (pale conjunctivas); redness of membrane (conjunctival injection); dryness; signs of infection; Bitot's spots; redness and fissuring of eyelid corners (angular palpebritis); dryness of eye membrane (conjunctival xerosis); dull appearance of cornea (corneal xerosis); soft cornea (keratomalacia)
Neck (glands)	No enlargement	Thyroid or lymph node enlargement
Nails	Firm, pink	Spoon shape (koilonychia); brittleness; ridges
Legs, feet	No tenderness, weakness, or swelling; good color	Edema; tender calf; tingling; weakness
Skeleton	No malformations	Bowlegs; knock-knees; chest deformity at diaphragm; prominent scapulae and ribs

From Nix S: *Williams' basic nutrition and diet therapy,* ed 12, St. Louis, 2005, Mosby.
IBW, Ideal body weight.

✳ **SKILL 44-1** | **ASPIRATION PRECAUTIONS**

Delegation Considerations

The assessment of a client's risk for aspiration and determination of positioning cannot be delegated. Nursing assistive personnel (NAP) may feed clients after receiving instructions in aspiration precautions. Instruct NAP to:

- Position client appropriately to decrease aspiration risk
- Report any onset of coughing, gagging, or pocketing of food

Equipment

- Chair or electric bed (to allow client to sit upright)
- Thickening agents as needed (rice, cereal, yogurt, gelatin, commercial thickening agent)
- Tongue blade
- Penlight

STEPS	RATIONALE
1. Perform nutritional screening.	Clients at risk for aspiration from dysphagia often alter their eating patterns or choose foods that do not provide adequate nutrition (Perry and McLaren, 2003).
2. Assess clients who are at increased risk of aspiration for signs and symptoms of dysphagia (e.g., cough, pharyngeal pooling, change in voice after swallowing).	Clients at risk include those who have neurological or neuromuscular diseases and those who have had trauma to or surgical procedures of the oral cavity or throat.
3. Observe client during mealtime for signs of dysphagia, and allow client to attempt to feed self. Observe client eat various consistencies of foods and liquids. Note at end of meal if client becomes tired.	Helps detect abnormal eating patterns such as frequent clearing of throat or prolonged eating time. Fatigue increases risk of aspiration.
4. Ask client about any difficulties with chewing or swallowing various textures of food.	Certain types of food are more easily aspirated than others.
5. Report signs and symptoms of dysphagia to the health care provider.	Signs or symptoms associated with aspiration indicate the need for further evaluation of swallowing by a radiologist or speech language pathologist, such as a fluoroscopic swallow study (Ashley and others, 2006).
6. Place identification on client's chart or Kardex indicating that dysphagia is present.	Identifying client as having dysphagia alerts the health care team to the problem to help the team develop and implement an individualized plan of care (Nowlin, 2006).
7. Explain to client why you are observing him or her while he or she eats.	Increases client cooperation.
8. Perform hand hygiene.	Reduces transmission of microorganisms.
9. Using penlight and tongue blade, gently inspect mouth for pockets of food.	Pockets of food in the mouth often indicate difficulty swallowing.
10. Elevate head of client's bed so that hips are flexed at a 90-degree angle and head is flexed slightly forward, or help client to same position in a chair.	Reduces risk of aspiration (Metheny, 2004).
11. Observe client consume various consistencies of foods and liquids.	Referral to a dietitian is appropriate if a client has difficulty with a particular consistency.
12. Add thickener to thin liquids to create the consistency of mashed potatoes, or serve client pureed foods.	Thin liquids such as water and fruit juice are difficult to control in the mouth and are more easily aspirated (Ashley and others, 2006; Metheny, 2004).
13. Place ½ to 1 teaspoon of food on unaffected side of the mouth, allowing utensil to touch the mouth or tongue.	Provides client with tactile cues to begin eating.
14. Place hand on throat to gently palpate swallowing event as it occurs. Swallowing twice is often necessary to clear the pharynx.	Helps evaluate swallowing effort.

15. Provide verbal coaching while feeding client and positive reinforcement to client.
  a. Open your mouth.
  b. Feel the food in your mouth.
  c. Chew and taste the food.
  d. Raise your tongue to the roof of your mouth.
  e. Think about swallowing.
  f. Close your mouth and swallow.
  g. Swallow again.
  h. Cough to clear airway.
	Verbal cueing keeps client focused on swallowing. Positive reinforcement enhances client's confidence in ability to swallow.

16. Observe for coughing, choking, gagging, and drooling of food; suction airway as necessary.	These are indications that suggest dysphagia and risk for aspiration.
17. Provide rest periods as necessary during meal to avoid rushed or forced feeding.	Avoiding fatigue decreases the risk of aspiration (Metheny, 2004).
18. Ask client to remain sitting upright for at least 30 minutes after the meal.	Reduces the risk of gastroesophageal reflux, which causes aspiration (Nowlin, 2006).

Continued

✳ **SKILL 44-1**   **ASPIRATION PRECAUTIONS—CONT'D**

STEPS

19. Help client to perform hand hygiene and perform mouth care.

20. Return client's tray to appropriate place, and perform hand hygiene.

21. Observe client's ability to ingest foods of various textures and thickness.

22. Monitor client's food and fluid intake.

23. Weigh client weekly at the same time on the same scale.

24. Observe client's oral cavity after meal to detect pockets of food.

RATIONALE

Mouth care after meals helps prevent dental caries and reduces colonization of bacteria, which reduces the risk of pneumonia (Nowlin, 2006).

Reduces spread of microorganisms.

Indicates whether aspiration risk is increased with thin liquids.

Client needs to avoid certain types and textures of food that are difficult to swallow.

Determines if weight is stable and reflects adequate caloric level.

Determines client's ability to swallow.

Unexpected Outcomes and Related Interventions

1. Client coughs, gags, complains of food "stuck in throat," or has pockets of food in mouth.
   a. Client may require a swallowing evaluation.
   b. Initiate consultation with a speech therapist for swallowing exercises and techniques to improve swallowing and reduce risk of aspiration.
   c. Notify health care provider and speech pathologist of any symptoms that occurred during meal and which foods caused the symptoms.
2. Client avoids certain textures of food.
   a. Change consistency and texture of food.

3. Client experiences weight loss.
   a. Discuss findings with health care provider, speech pathologist, and/or registered dietitian.

Recording and Reporting

• Document the following in the client's chart: client's tolerance of various food textures, amount of assistance required, position during meal, absence or presence of any symptoms of dysphagia, and amount eaten.

• Report any coughing, gagging, choking, or swallowing difficulties to nurse in charge or health care provider.

✦ **BOX 44-8   NURSING DIAGNOSTIC PROCESS**

Imbalanced Nutrition: More Than Body Requirements

Assessment Activities	Defining Characteristics
Body mass index (BMI)	BMI = 37
Obtain height and weight	52-year-old man Height: 5 feet 11 inches Weight: 270 pounds (122.5 kg)
Obtain 24-hour food and fluid history	Lack of satiety High fat and carbohydrate intake, three to four beers per day Fluid intake is coke and juice, all high caloric
Physical assessment	Short of breath on walking Large abdomen Blood pressure: 155/85 mm Hg Pulse: 102 beats per minute Respirations: 32 breaths per minute
Laboratory values	Cholesterol and triglycerides elevated; all others within normal limits (WNL)
Medication	None
Social	Wife and family eat out 2 or 3 times a week

incidence of aspiration pneumonia (Perry and McLaren, 2003; Runions and others, 2004). A number of screening tools are available. The Registered Dietitian Dysphagia Screening Tool includes medical record review; observation of a client at a meal for change in voice quality, posture, and head control; percentage of meal consumed; eating time; drooling of liquids and solids; cough during/after a swallow; facial or tongue weakness; difficulty with secretions; pocketing; and presence of voluntary and dry cough (Brody and others, 2000). Screening tools such as the Burke Dysphagia Screening Test and the Standardized Swallowing Assessment were validated in clients with dysphagia (Perry and Love, 2001). These tools evaluate holding, leakage, coughing, choking, breathlessness, and quality of voice. The tools are for multidisciplinary use by nurses, dietitians, health care providers, and speech language pathologists (Brody and others 2000; Daniels and others, 2000; Perry and Love, 2001).

◆ Nursing Diagnosis

Assessment data lead to actual or potential nutrition problems (Box 44-8). A problem frequently occurs when overall intake is significantly decreased or increased or when one or more nutrients are not ingested, completely digested, or completely absorbed. Nursing diagnoses are related to either the actual nutrition problems (e.g., inadequate intake) or problems that place the client at risk for nutritional deficiencies, such as oral trauma, severe burns, or infections.

Select a nursing diagnostic statement based on defining characteristics present in the assessment database. Be sure to select the appropriate related factor for the nursing diagnosis. The following are examples of nursing diagnoses that apply to clients with nutritional problems:

- Risk for aspiration
- Constipation
- Diarrhea
- Health-seeking behaviors (nutrition)
- Deficient knowledge (nutrition)
- Imbalanced nutrition: less than body requirements
- Imbalanced nutrition: more than body requirements
- Risk for imbalanced nutrition: more than body requirements
- Readiness for enhanced nutrition
- Feeding self-care deficit

◆Planning

Planning to maintain optimal nutritional status requires a higher level of care than simply correction of nutritional problems. Synthesis of client information from multiple sources is necessary to devising an individualized approach of care that is relevant to the client's needs (Figure 44-6). Critical thinking application is the best way to ensure that all data sources are considered in developing a client's plan of care. The identification of clients at risk for nutritional problems results in a care plan that prevents or minimizes nutritional problems (see Care Plan). Referring to professional standards for nutrition is especially important during this step, because published standards are based on scientific findings.

In addition, there are also clinical situations in which clients have multiple related problems. The concept map in Figure 44-7 shows the relationship of nursing diagnoses in a client with myasthenia gravis.

Goals and Outcomes. Goals and outcomes and priorities of care reflect the client's physiological, therapeutic, and individualized needs. Nutritional education and counseling are important for all clients to prevent disease and promote health. Clients on therapeutic diets need to understand the implications of the diet and how the diet helps to control their illness. Be aware of factors that influence a client's food intake. For example, in one study, clients with congestive heart failure identified that decreased hunger, diet restrictions, fatigue, shortness of breath, anxiety, and sadness influenced their food intake (Lennie and others, 2006).

Individualized planning cannot be overemphasized. For example, it is important to explore clients' feelings about their weight and food and to help them set realistic and achievable goals (Daniels, 2006). Mutually planned goals negotiated between the client, registered dietitian, and nurse ensure success. For this type of client an overall goal is "Client will achieve appropriate BMI height-weight range or within 10% of IBW." The following outcomes assist in achievement of the goal:

- Client's daily nutritional intake meets the minimal DRIs.
- Client's daily fat nutritional fat intake is less than 30%.
- Client removes sugared beverages from diet.

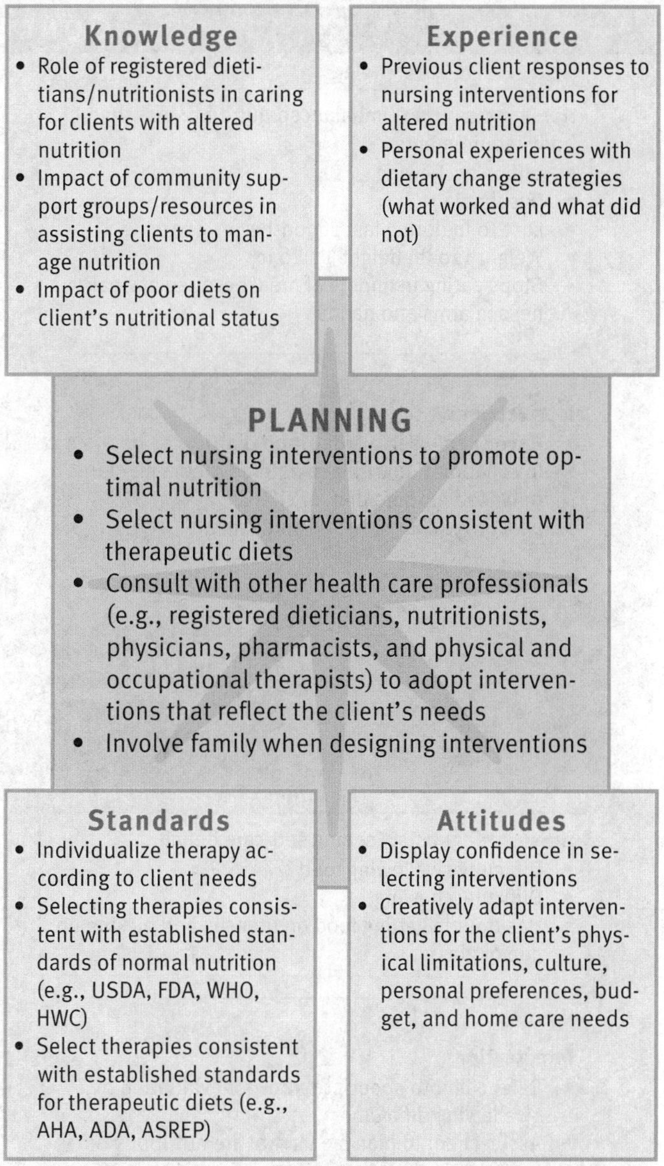

Knowledge
- Role of registered dietitians/nutritionists in caring for clients with altered nutrition
- Impact of community support groups/resources in assisting clients to manage nutrition
- Impact of poor diets on client's nutritional status

Experience
- Previous client responses to nursing interventions for altered nutrition
- Personal experiences with dietary change strategies (what worked and what did not)

PLANNING
- Select nursing interventions to promote optimal nutrition
- Select nursing interventions consistent with therapeutic diets
- Consult with other health care professionals (e.g., registered dieticians, nutritionists, physicians, pharmacists, and physical and occupational therapists) to adopt interventions that reflect the client's needs
- Involve family when designing interventions

Standards
- Individualize therapy according to client needs
- Selecting therapies consistent with established standards of normal nutrition (e.g., USDA, FDA, WHO, HWC)
- Select therapies consistent with established standards for therapeutic diets (e.g., AHA, ADA, ASREP)

Attitudes
- Display confidence in selecting interventions
- Creatively adapt interventions for the client's physical limitations, culture, personal preferences, budget, and home care needs

Figure 44-6 Critical thinking model for nutrition evaluation.

- Client refrains from eating unhealthy foods between meals and after dinner.
- Client loses at least ½ to 1 pound per week.

Meeting nutritional goals requires multidisciplinary input. Knowledge of each discipline's role in provision of nutrition support is necessary to maximizing nutritional outcomes. For example, collaboration with a registered dietitian helps develop appropriate nutrition treatment plans. Calorie counts are frequently ordered and assistance is necessary in obtaining accurate data. An effective plan of care requires accurate exchange of information between disciplines.

Setting Priorities. The identification of clients at risk for nutritional problems results in timely interventions to prevent or minimize nutritional problems. Although changes in the client's weight are often gradual, a priority is to improve nutritional intake.

During acute illness or surgery the intake of food is often altered in the perioperative period. The priority of care is to provide

CONCEPT MAP

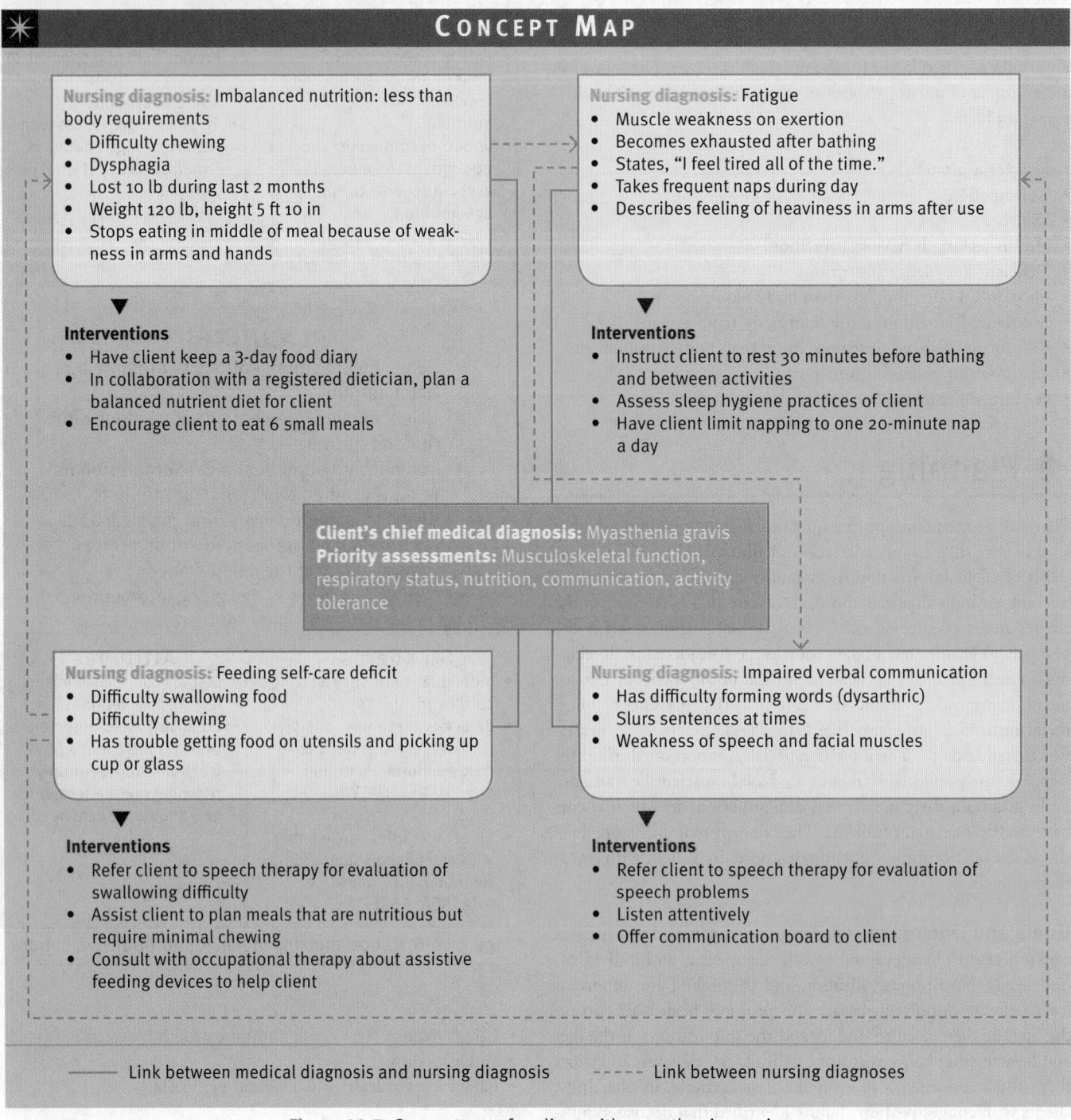

Nursing diagnosis: Imbalanced nutrition: less than body requirements
- Difficulty chewing
- Dysphagia
- Lost 10 lb during last 2 months
- Weight 120 lb, height 5 ft 10 in
- Stops eating in middle of meal because of weakness in arms and hands

Interventions
- Have client keep a 3-day food diary
- In collaboration with a registered dietician, plan a balanced nutrient diet for client
- Encourage client to eat 6 small meals

Nursing diagnosis: Fatigue
- Muscle weakness on exertion
- Becomes exhausted after bathing
- States, "I feel tired all of the time."
- Takes frequent naps during day
- Describes feeling of heaviness in arms after use

Interventions
- Instruct client to rest 30 minutes before bathing and between activities
- Assess sleep hygiene practices of client
- Have client limit napping to one 20-minute nap a day

Client's chief medical diagnosis: Myasthenia gravis
Priority assessments: Musculoskeletal function, respiratory status, nutrition, communication, activity tolerance

Nursing diagnosis: Feeding self-care deficit
- Difficulty swallowing food
- Difficulty chewing
- Has trouble getting food on utensils and picking up cup or glass

Interventions
- Refer client to speech therapy for evaluation of swallowing difficulty
- Assist client to plan meals that are nutritious but require minimal chewing
- Consult with occupational therapy about assistive feeding devices to help client

Nursing diagnosis: Impaired verbal communication
- Has difficulty forming words (dysarthric)
- Slurs sentences at times
- Weakness of speech and facial muscles

Interventions
- Refer client to speech therapy for evaluation of speech problems
- Listen attentively
- Offer communication board to client

——— Link between medical diagnosis and nursing diagnosis   ----- Link between nursing diagnoses

Figure 44-7 Concept map for client with myasthenia gravis.

optimal preoperative nutrition support in clients with malnutrition. The priority for the resumption of food intake postoperatively is dependent upon the return of bowel function, the extent of the surgical procedure, and the presence of any complications (see Chapter 50). For example, when clients have oral and throat surgery, they chew and swallow food in the presence of excision sites, sutures, or otherwise manipulated tissue. The priority of care is to first provide comfort and pain control. Then address nutritional priorities and plan care to maintain nutrition that does not cause pain or injury to the healing tissues.

The client and family must collaborate with the nurse in the planning of care and setting of priorities. This is important because food preferences, food purchases, and preparation involve the entire family. The plan of care will not succeed without their commitment to, involvement in, and understanding of the nutritional priorities.

Collaborative Care. The care of the client often extends beyond the acute hospital setting, requiring collaboration among the members of the health care team. It is important that discharge

NURSING CARE PLAN

Imbalanced Nutrition: Less Than Body Requirements

Assessment

Ms. Maria Steiner, a nurse practitioner in a senior citizens' center, is seeing Mrs. Cooper, who is 68 years old and has a history of congestive heart failure. Recently Mrs. Cooper noticed a weight loss (15%). Three months have passed since Mrs. Cooper started taking sertraline for depression related to the loss of her husband 6 months ago. Mrs. Cooper was also referred for counseling 3 months ago for help with grief and depression through a local senior service agency. When Maria inquired as to her financial situation, Mrs. Cooper responded that it was tight living on a small pension and Social Security, but she was able to manage.

Assessment Activities	Findings/Defining Characteristics*
Ask Mrs. Cooper about her food intake during the last 2 days.	She responds that she drinks some juice in the morning and two or three cups of coffee. In addition, she often has a sandwich in the late afternoon. **"I'm just not interested in food. It has no taste."**
Ask Mrs. Cooper about social interaction.	Mrs. Cooper **complains of loneliness** and said she **does not get out much**, although her psychologist recommended more socializing. Her friends at church call her to come back to meetings, but she is just not ready. She says she **tires easily.**
Weigh client, and assess posture.	Her **weight is 20% below her IBW** and her **BMI is 17.** This weight loss has happened over the past 6 months, and she has **lost 24 pounds.** **Stooped posture**
Observe Mrs. Cooper for signs of poor nutrition.	**Hair loss** **Dry scaling skin** **Pale conjunctivae** and mucous membranes
Palpate muscles and extremities.	2+ bilateral pitting ankle edema **Generalized poor muscle tone**

***Defining characteristics** are shown in bold type.

Nursing Diagnosis: Imbalanced nutrition: less than body requirements related to a decreased ability to ingest food as a result of depression.

Planning

Goals	Expected Outcomes (NOC)†
	Weight Gain Behavior
Mrs. Cooper will progressively gain weight.	Mrs. Cooper will gain 1 to 2 pounds per month until goal of 130 pounds is reached.
	Nutritional Status
Mrs. Cooper will consume adequate nourishment each day.	Mrs. Cooper will ingest 1900 kcal/day, including 50 g of protein per day.
	Nutritional Status: Biochemical Measures
Mrs. Cooper will exhibit no signs of malnutrition.	Physical assessment findings will be within normal limits. Laboratory values will be within normal limits.

†Outcome classification labels from Moorhead S and others: *Nursing outcomes classification (NOC),* ed 4, St. Louis, 2008, Mosby.

Interventions (NIC)‡

Nutritional Counseling

- Coordinate plan of care with health care provider, psychologist, Mrs. Cooper, and registered dietitian.
- Individualize menu plans.

- Teach Mrs. Cooper about the food pyramid.

Nutritional Monitoring

- Monitor Mrs. Cooper monthly for weight gain, anemia, serum albumin level, and total lymphocyte count (TLC).

- Perform physical assessment of hair, eyes, mouth, skin, and muscle tone.

Rationale

Successful nutrition care planning is a multidisciplinary approach throughout the continuum of care (Chen and others, 2001).
Encourages the client to eat by incorporating her food preferences into the meal plans.
USDA (2005) and *Healthy People 2010* recommendations for food selections provide optimal nutrition (USDA, 2002).

Weight gain should be slow and progressive. Serum albumin of 4.0 g/100 mL and TLC 1500/mm^3 are within normal limits (Williams and Schlenker, 2003).
Provides progressive monitoring for improved nutritional status.

‡Intervention classification labels from Bulechek GM, Butcher HK, and Dochterman JM: *Nursing interventions classification (NIC),* ed 5, St. Louis, 2008, Mosby.

Continued

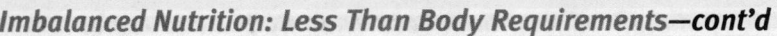

NURSING CARE PLAN

Imbalanced Nutrition: Less Than Body Requirements—cont'd

Interventions (NIC)‡	Rationale
Nutritional Management	
• Encourage client to eat small meals and to increase dietary intake and to help offset anorexia secondary to sertraline.	Sertraline is a selective serotonin reuptake inhibitor (SSRI) antidepressant medication, which causes diminished taste and anorexia. Frequent small meals helps to reduce anorexia-associated weight loss.
• Encourage fluid intake.	Older adults need eight 8-ounce (240 mL) glasses per day of fluid from beverage and food sources. Concentrating intake in morning and early afternoon is acceptable to prevent nocturia (Meiner and Lueckenotte, 2006).
• Encourage fiber intake.	Deters constipation, enhancing appetite.
• Encourage Mrs. Cooper to eat lunch at the senior center 5 times per week.	Eating with others encourages good nutrition and promotes socialization with peers (Callen and Wells, 2003; Furman, 2006).

‡Intervention classification labels from Bulechek GM, Butcher HK, and Dochterman JM: *Nursing interventions classification (NIC)*, ed 5, St. Louis, 2008, Mosby.

Evaluation

Nursing Actions	Client Response/Finding	Achievement of Outcome
Ask Mrs. Cooper to keep a food diary for 3 days.	Food diary reflects that she ate her main meal at the senior center, has fruit and bran flakes for breakfast, and in the evening either has soup or a sandwich with fruit.	Mrs. Cooper is selecting more nutritionally rich foods, consistent with current guidelines.
Observe client's appearance.	Skin is less pale, hair appears to be in better condition and styled. Ankle edema is present, but less than 1+.	Mrs. Cooper has improved physical parameters of nutrition, still needs follow-up.
Weigh client.	Weight gain of 4 pounds in 4 weeks.	Weight gain is steady; client is still below ideal body weight.
Ask client about appetite and energy level.	Mrs. Cooper responds that on days she eats at the senior center her appetite seems better and she "wants to do more things." She notes that weekends are very lonely.	Weekday support for nutritional status appears effective, needs to increase client's activity status and nutritional intake during weekends.

planning extends nutritional interventions as clients return to their homes or extended care facilities. Speech therapists work with clients with dysphagia. Enteral tube feedings are often administered into the stomach or intestines via a tube inserted through the nose or a percutaneous access (see Skill 44-2, p. 1113, and Skill 44-3, p. 1118). These enteral feedings supplement the clients' oral nutritional intake in the home, acute care, extended care, or rehabilitation setting when they cannot meet their nutritional needs by mouth. Regardless of the setting, the registered dietitian monitors the client's nutritional status and intake and makes recommendations for changes, based primarily upon data documented in the client's medical record. Registered dietitians are expert in choice of enteral formulas and dietary modifications required for specific disease states.

When PN, a solution consisting of glucose, amino acids, lipids, minerals, electrolytes, trace elements, and vitamins, is necessary, clients receive it through an indwelling peripheral or central venous catheter (see Chapter 41). The pharmacist is an expert who reviews medications to identify drug-nutrient interactions. Pharmacists are also experts in preparing mixtures of total parenteral nutrition (TPN).

When clients have difficulty feeding themselves, occupational therapists work with clients and families to identify assistive devices. Devices such as utensils with large handles and plates with elevated sides assist a client with self-feeding. A speech therapist assists a client with swallowing exercises and techniques to reduce the risk of aspiration. Occupational therapists also help clients maintain function in the home setting by rearranging food preparation areas in an effort to maximize the client's functional capacity.

Implementation

Ill or debilitated clients often have poor appetites. **Anorexia** has many causes (e.g., pain or deficiency in certain vitamins and minerals). You need to help clients to understand the factors that cause anorexia and use creative approaches to stimulate appetite. Clients worried about families, finances, employment, or illnesses are often not able to eat an adequate diet. Both physiological stress due to illness and emotional stress influence dietary need and intake. Medications frequently interfere with taste, cause nausea, interfere with absorption, or affect metabolism (see Table 44-2).

✳ TABLE 44-5 Food Safety

Food-borne Disease	Organism	Food Source	Symptoms*
Botulism	C. botulinum	Improperly home-canned foods, smoked and salted fish, ham, sausage, shellfish	Symptoms are varied from mild discomfort to death in 24 hours, initially nausea and dizziness, progressing to motor (respiratory) paralysis
Escherichia coli	Escherichia E. coli 0157:H7	Undercooked meat (ground beef)	Severe cramps, nausea, vomiting, diarrhea (may be bloody), renal failure. Appears 1-8 days after eating, lasts 1-7 days
Listeriosis	Listeria L. monocytogenes	Soft cheese, meat (hot dogs, pate, lunch meats), unpasteurized milk, poultry, seafood	Severe diarrhea, fever, headache, pneumonia, meningitis, endocarditis. Appears 3-21 days after infection
Perfringens enteritis	Clostridium C. perfringens	Cooked meats, meat dishes held at room or warm temperature	Mild diarrhea, vomiting. Appears 8-24 hours after eating, lasts 1-2 days
Salmonellosis	Salmonella S. typhi S. paratyphi	Milk, custards, egg dishes, salad dressings, sandwich fillings, polluted shellfish	Mild to severe diarrhea, cramps, vomiting. Appears 12 to 24 hours after ingestion, lasts 1-7 days
Shigellosis	Shigella S. dysenteriae	Milk, milk products, seafood, salads	Mild diarrhea to fatal dysentery. Appears 7-36 hours after ingestion; lasts 3-14 days.
Staphylococcus	Staphylococcus S. aureus	Custards, cream fillings, processed meats, ham, cheese, ice cream, potato salad, sauces, casseroles	Severe abdominal cramps, pain, vomiting, diarrhea, perspiration, headache, fever, prostration. Appears 1-6 hours after ingestion, lasts 1-2 days

From Nix S: *Williams' basic nutrition and diet therapy,* ed 12, St. Louis, 2005, Mosby.
*Symptoms are generally most severe for youngest and oldest age-groups.

Health Promotion. As the nurse, you are in a key position to educate clients about healthy diet choices and good nutrition. Incorporating knowledge of nutrition into lifestyle serves as prevention against the development of many diseases. Outpatient and community-based settings are optimal locations for nursing assessment of nutritional practices and status. Early identification of potential or actual problems is the best way to avoid more serious problems. Similarly, in other health care settings, clients with nutritional problems such as obesity often require assistance in menu planning and compliance strategies. Your role as educator includes educating families and providing information about community resources. Telephone numbers of a dietitian or nurse for follow-up questions are always a part of counseling.

Meal planning takes into account the family's budget and different preferences of family members. Choose specific foods on the basis of the dietary prescription and food groups. For families on limited budgets, use substitutes. For example, bean or cheese dishes often replace meat in a meal, and evaporated milk or dry skim milk is used for cooking. Have clients modify the method of preparation when it is necessary to minimize certain substances. Baking rather than frying reduces fat intake, and clients can use lemon juice or spices to add flavor to low-sodium diets.

Planning menus a week in advance has several benefits. It helps ensure good nutrition or compliance with a specific diet and helps the family stay within the allotted budget. Nurses or registered dietitians need to check menus for content. Often a simple tip is helpful in meal planning, such as avoiding grocery shopping when hungry, which can lead to spur-of-the-moment purchases of more expensive or less nutritional foods that are not included in meal plans. The USDA (2006) provides sample weekly meal-planning services for a range of sample budgets accessible on the USDA website.

SAFETY ALERT Food safety is an important public health issue. Food-borne bacteria can occur from improper food cleansing, preparation, or poor hygiene practices of food workers. Health care professionals not only need to be aware of the factors related to food safety but also should provide client education to reduce the risks for food-borne illnesses (Table 44-5, Box 44-9).

Acute Care. The nutritional care of acutely ill clients requires the nurse to consider a variety of factors that influence nutritional intake. Ill or debilitated clients frequently have poor appetites. In addition, diagnostic testing and procedures in the acute care setting is another disruptive influence on intake. Frequently as preparation for or immediately following a diagnostic procedure the client is to receive nothing by mouth (NPO). Frequently the mealtimes in a health care setting are interrupted, or the client is too fatigued or uncomfortable to eat. It is important that the nurse continuously assess the client's nutritional status and adopt interventions that promote normal intake, digestion, and metabolism of nutrients. Clients who are NPO and receive only standard IV fluids for more than 4 to 7 days are at nutritional risk.

Advancing Diets. Acute and chronic conditions affect the client's immune system and nutritional status. Clients with decreased immune function (e.g., due to cancer, human immunodeficiency virus/acquired immunodeficiency syndrome [HIV/AIDS], or organ transplants) require special diets that decease their exposure to microorganisms and are higher in selected nutrients. Table 44-6 gives an overview of the immune system, the malnutrition impact, and what nutrients are beneficial. In addition, clients who are ill, who have had surgical procedures, or who were NPO for a period of time have specialized dietary needs. Health care providers order a gradual progression of dietary intake or therapeutic diet to manage clients' illness. Box 44-10 lists common therapeutic diets.

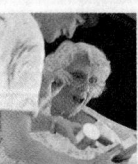

BOX 44-9 CLIENT TEACHING

Food Safety

Objectives
- Client is able to verbalize measures to protect from food-borne illness.
- Client understands the primary types of food-borne illness and how they are transmitted.
- Client does not experience food-borne illness.

Teaching Strategies
- Explain that food safety is an important public health issue. Populations particularly at risk are older and younger persons, as well as immunosuppressed individuals.
- Instruct clients in the following:
  - Wash hands with warm, soapy water before touching or eating food.
  - Use a food thermometer to verify meat, poultry, and fish are cooked properly.
  - Wash fresh fruits and vegetables thoroughly.
- Do not eat raw meats or unpasteurized milk.
- Do not buy or eat food that has passed the expiration date.
- Keep foods properly refrigerated at 40° F and frozen at 0° F.
- Wash dishes and cutting boards with hot soapy water.
- Do not save leftovers for more than 2 days in refrigerator.
- Wash dishrags, towels, and sponges regularly, or use paper towels.
- Clean the inside of refrigerator and microwave regularly to prevent microbial growth.

Evaluation
- Ask client to verbalize measures to prevent food-borne illnesses.
- Observe the client at home for safe practices, if making home visit.

TABLE 44-6 Nutrition and the Immune System

Immune/Physiological Component	Malnutrition Effect	Vital Nutrient
Antibodies	Decreased amount	Protein, vitamins A, C, B_{12}, B_6, folic acid, thiamin, biotin, riboflavin, niacin
GI tract	Translocation of bacteria to systemic bodily areas	Arginine, glutamine, omega-3 fatty acids
Granulocytes and macrocytes	Longer time for phagocytosis kill time and lymphocyte activation	Protein, vitamins A, C, B_{12}, B_6, folic acid, thiamin, riboflavin, niacin, zinc, iron
Mucus	Flat microvilli in GI tract, decreased antibody secretion	Vitamins B_{12}, B_6, C, biotin
Skin	Integrity compromised, density reduced, wound healing slowed	Protein, vitamins A, B_{12}, C, niacin, copper, zinc
T-lymphocytes	Depressed T-cell distribution	Protein, arginine, iron, zinc, omega-3 fatty acids, vitamins A, B_{12}, B_6, folic acid, thiamin, riboflavin, niacin, pantothenic acid

Modified from Grodner M, Long S, DeYoung S: *Foundations and clinical applications of nutrition: a nursing approach*, ed 3, St. Louis, 2004, Mosby. *GI,* Gastrointestinal.

Promoting Appetite. Providing an environment that promotes nutritional intake includes keeping the client's environment free of odors, providing oral hygiene as needed to remove unpleasant tastes, and maintaining client comfort. In addition, certain medications affect dietary intake and nutrient use. For example, medications such as insulin, glucocorticoids, and thyroid hormones affect metabolism. Other medications, such as antifungal agents, frequently affect taste. Some of the psychotropic medications affect appetite, cause nausea, and also alter taste. The nurse and dietitian help the client to select foods that reduce the altered taste sensations or nausea. In other situations medications need to be changed. Assessing clients for the need for pharmacological agents to stimulate appetite such as cyproheptadine (Periactin), megestrol (Megace), or dronabinol (Marinol) or to manage symptoms that interfere with nutrition requires health care provider consultation.

Mealtime is usually a social activity. When clients experience anorexia, encourage other nurses or care providers to converse and engage the client in a conversation. Mealtime is also an excellent

opportunity for client education. Instruct the client about any therapeutic diets, medications, energy conservation measures, or adaptive devices to assist the client in independently feeding.

Assisting Clients With Oral Feeding. When clients need assistance with eating, it important to protect the client's safety, independence, and dignity. Assess the client's risk of aspiration (see Skill 44-1, p. 1103). Clients at high risk for aspiration are those clients with decreased level of alertness, decreased gag and/or cough reflexes, and clients who have difficulty managing saliva (see assessment section of this chapter).

Clients with dysphagia are at risk for aspiration and need more assistance with feeding and swallowing. A speech language pathologist identifies clients at risk and provides recommendations for therapy (Perry and Love, 2001). Provide a 30-minute rest period before eating (Metheny, 2004). Position the client in an upright, seated position in a chair, or raise the head of the bed to 90 degrees. Have the client slightly flex the head to a chin-down position to help prevent aspiration. If the client has unilateral weakness, teach the client and caregiver to place food in the stronger side of the

BOX 44-10 Diet Progression and Therapeutic Diets

Clear Liquid
Broth, bouillon, coffee, tea, carbonated beverages, clear fruit juices, gelatin, Popsicles.

Full Liquid
As above with addition of smooth-textured dairy products (e.g., ice cream), custards, refined cooked cereals, vegetable juice, pureed vegetables, all fruit juices.

Pureed
All of above with addition of scrambled eggs; pureed meats, vegetables, and fruits; mashed potatoes and gravy.

Mechanical Soft
All of above with addition of ground or finely diced meats, flaked fish, cottage cheese, cheese, rice, potatoes, pancakes, light breads, cooked vegetables, cooked or canned fruits, bananas, soups, peanut butter.

Soft/Low Residue
Addition of low-fiber, easily digested foods, such as pastas, casseroles, moist tender meats, and canned cooked fruits and vegetables. Desserts, cakes, and cookies without nuts or coconut.

High Fiber
Addition of fresh uncooked fruits, steamed vegetables, bran, oatmeal, and dried fruits.

Low Sodium
4-g (no added salt), 2-g, 1-g, or 500-mg sodium diets. These diets vary from no added salt to severe sodium restriction (500-mg sodium diet) that requires selective food purchases.

Low Cholesterol
300 mg/day cholesterol, in keeping with American Heart Association guidelines for serum lipid reduction.

Diabetic
Recommended food exchanges by the American Diabetic Association. Usually the caloric recommendations are around 1800 calories. The diet needs to include a balanced intake of carbohydrates, fats, and proteins. Caloric recommendations vary to accommodate the client's metabolic demands.

Regular
No restrictions, unless specified.

---

mouth. Determine the viscosity of foods that the client tolerates best through the use of trials of different consistencies of foods and fluids. Thicker fluids are generally easier to swallow. The American Dietetic Association published the National Dysphagia Diet Task Force's (NDDTF's) National Dysphagia Diet in 2002 to provide uniformity of diets provided to clients with dysphagia (NDDTF, 2002). There are four levels of diet: dysphagia puree, dysphagia mechanically altered, dysphagia advanced, and regular. The four levels of liquid include thin liquids (low viscosity), nectarlike liquids (medium viscosity), honeylike liquids (viscosity of honey), and spoon-thick liquids (viscosity of pudding) (NDDTF, 2002).

Feed the client with dysphagia slowly, providing smaller-size bites, and allow the client to chew thoroughly and swallow the bite before taking another. More frequent chewing and swallowing assessments throughout the meal are necessary. Allow the client time to empty the mouth after each spoonful, matching the speed of feeding to the client's readiness. If the client begins to cough or choke, remove the food immediately (Nowlin, 2006).

Provide opportunities for clients to direct the order in which they want to eat the food items, as well as how fast they wish to eat. Determine the client's food preferences, and, unless contraindicated, try to have these items included on the client's dietary tray. If the client requests the food to be warmer or cooler, try to meet this need. These seem like small acts, but they go a long way in maintaining the client's sense of independence.

Clients with visual deficits also need special assistance. Clients with decreased vision are able to independently feed themselves when they are given adequate information. Identify the food location on the plate as if it were a clock (e.g., meat at 9 o'clock and vegetable at 3 o'clock). Tell the client where the beverages are located in relation to the plate. Be sure other care providers set the meal tray and plate in the same manner. Clients with impaired vision, as well as those clients with decreased motor skill, are more independent during mealtimes with the use of large-handled adaptive utensils. These are easier to grip and manipulate.

Enteral Tube Feeding. Enteral nutrition (EN) is nutrients given in the GI tract. Enteral nutrition is the preferred method of meeting nutritional needs if the client's GI tract is functioning by providing physiological, safe, and economical nutritional support. Enterally fed clients receive formula via nasogastric, jejunal, or gastric tubes. Clients with a low risk of gastric reflux receive gastric feedings; however, if there is a risk of gastric reflux, which leads to aspiration, jejunal feeding is preferred. Box 44-11 lists indications for tube feeding. Enteral tube feedings can be easily given in the home setting by either the nurse or the family. The nurse inserts the enteral tube, and verification of tube placement by x-ray examination needs to occur before the client receives the first enteral feeding (Skill 44-2).

Enteral formulas are usually one of four types. Polymeric (1 to 2 kcal/mL) include milk-based blenderized foods prepared by hospital dietary staff or in the client home. The polymeric classification also includes commercially prepared whole nutrient formulas. For this type of formula to be effective, the client's gastrointestinal tract needs to be able to absorb whole nutrients. The second type, modular formulas (3.8 to 4 kcal/mL), are single macronutrient (e.g., protein, glucose, polymers, or lipids) preparations and are not nutritionally complete. This type of formula is added to other foods for meeting the client's individual nutritional needs. The third type, elemental formulas (1.0 to 3.0 kcal/mL), contain predigested nutrients that are easier for a partially dysfunctional gastrointestinal tract to absorb. The last type are the specialty formulas (1 to 2 kcal/mL) that are designed to meet specific nutritional needs in certain illness (e.g., liver failure, pulmonary disease, or HIV infection).

Tube feedings are typically started at full strength at slow rates (see Skill 44-3, p. 1118, and Box 44-12, p. 1117). Increase the hourly rate every 8 to 12 hours if no signs of intolerance appear (high gastric residuals, nausea, cramping, vomiting, and diarrhea). Studies have demonstrated a beneficial effect of enteral feedings compared with parenteral nutrition. Feeding by the enteral route reduces sepsis, minimizes the hypermetabolic response to trauma, and maintains intestinal structure and function (ASPEN, 2002; Cirgin Ellett, 2006). Enteral nutrition is successful within 24 to 48 hours after surgery or trauma to provide fluids, electrolytes,

✳ BOX 44-11 Indications for Enteral and Parenteral Nutrition

Enteral Nutrition
Cancer
Head and neck
Upper GI

Critical Illness/Trauma
Neurological and Muscular Disorders
Brain neoplasm
Cerebrovascular accident
Dementia
Myopathy
Parkinson's disease

Gastrointestinal Disorders
Enterocutaneous fistula
Inflammatory bowel disease
Mild pancreatitis

Respiratory Failure With Prolonged Intubation
Inadequate Oral Intake
Anorexia nervosa
Difficulty chewing, swallowing
Severe depression

Parenteral Nutrition
Nonfunctional GI Tract
Massive small bowel resection/GI surgery/massive GI bleed
Paralytic ileus
Intestinal obstruction
Trauma to abdomen, head, or neck
Severe malabsorption
Intolerance to enteral feeding (established by trial)
Chemotherapy, radiation therapy, bone marrow transplantation

Extended Bowel Rest
Enterocutaneous fistula
Inflammatory bowel disease exacerbation
Severe diarrhea
Moderate to severe pancreatitis

Preoperative TPN
Preoperative bowel rest
Treatment for comorbid severe malnutrition in clients with non-functional GI tracts
Severely catabolic clients when GI tract nonusable for more than 4 to 5 days

GI, Gastrointestinal; *TPN*, total parenteral nutrition.

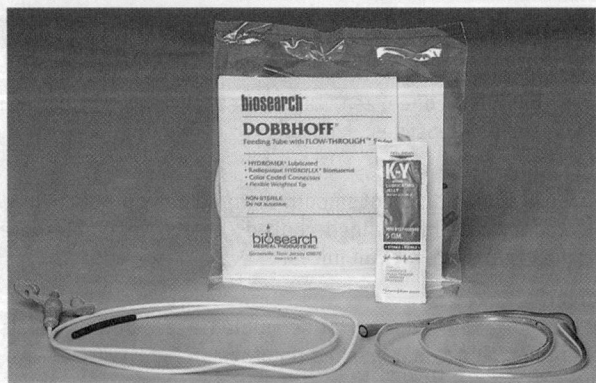

Figure 44-8 Enteral tubes, small bore.

Some of the common conditions that increase the risk of aspiration include coughing, nasotracheal suctioning, an artificial airway, decreased level of consciousness, and lying flat. Prokinetic medications such as metoclopramide, erythromycin, or cisapride, promote gastric emptying and decrease the risk of aspiration (Cirgin Ellett, 2006; Metheny, 2006). Keep the head of the bed elevated 30 degree or higher, and measure gastric residual volumes (GRVs) (Metheny, 2006). Measure the GRV every 4 to 6 hours in clients receiving continuous feedings and immediately before the feeding in clients receiving intermittent feedings (Metheny, 2006). The following recommendations are made regarding gastric residual volumes: (1) stop feedings immediately if aspiration occurs; (2) withhold feedings and reassess client tolerance to feedings if GRV is over 200 mL for two successive measurements; and (3) routinely evaluate the client for aspiration, and use nursing measures to reduce the risk of aspiration if GRV is greater than 200 mL (Metheny, 2006).

Enteral Access Tubes. When the client is unable to ingest food but is still able to digest and absorb nutrients, enteral tube feeding is indicated. Feeding tubes are inserted through the nose (nasogastric or nasointestinal), surgically (gastrostomy or jejunostomy), or endoscopically (percutaneous endoscopic gastrostomy or jejunostomy [PEG or PEJ]). If enteral nutrition therapy is for less than 4 weeks total, nasogastric or nasojejunal feeding tubes may be used. Surgical or endoscopically placed tubes are preferred for long-term feeding (more than 4 weeks) to reduce the discomfort of a nasal tube and to provide a more secure, reliable access (Rolandelli and others, 2005). Clients with gastroparesis (decreased or absent innervation to the stomach that results in delayed gastric emptying) or esophageal reflux or with a history of aspiration pneumonia are some types of clients that require placement of tubes beyond the stomach into the intestine (Cirgin Ellett, 2006; Metheny and others, 2002).

Nursing research investigated the problems associated with nasoenteric tube placement, type of feeding instilled, rate of feeding, and complications associated with tube feeding. Most settings use small-bore feeding tubes because they create less discomfort for the client (Figure 44-8). For the adult, most of these tubes are 8 to 12 Fr and 36 to 44 inches long. A stylet is often used during insertion of a small-bore tube to stiffen it. The stylet is removed when the correct position of the feeding tube is confirmed. Skill 44-3 (p. 1118) describes the procedure for initiating beginning nasogastric, gastrostomy, and jejunostomy enteral feedings.

and nutritional support. Gastric ileus prevents nasogastric feedings from being given. Nasointestinal or jejunal tubes allow successful postpyloric feeding, because formula is placed directly into the small intestine or jejunum or beyond the pyloric sphincter of the stomach (ASPEN, 2002).

A serious complication associated with enteral feedings is aspiration of formula into the tracheobronchial tree. Aspiration of enteral formula into the lungs irritates the bronchial mucosa, resulting in decreased blood supply to affected pulmonary tissue (Metheny and others, 2002). This leads to necrotizing infection, pneumonia, and potential abscess formation. The high glucose content of a feeding serves as a bacterial medium for growth, promoting infection. Acute respiratory distress syndrome (ARDS) is also an outcome frequently associated with pulmonary aspiration.

Text continued on p. 1122

SKILL 44-2   INSERTING A SMALL-BORE NASOENTERIC TUBE FOR ENTERAL FEEDINGS

 Video

Delegation Considerations

The skill of inserting a small-bore nasoenteric tube cannot be delegated. Nursing assistive personnel are able to assist with client positioning during the procedure.

Equipment

- Nasogastric or nasointestinal tube (8 to 12 Fr) with guide wire or stylet
- Stethoscope
- 60-mL or larger Luer-Lok or catheter-tip syringe
- Hypoallergenic tape and tincture of benzoin or tube fixation device
- pH indicator strip (scale 0.0 to 14.0)
- Glass of water and straw
- Emesis basin
- Towel
- Facial tissues
- Clean gloves
- Suction equipment in case of aspiration
- Penlight to check placement in nasopharynx
- Tongue blade

STEPS	RATIONALE
1. Assess client for the need for enteral tube feeding: NPO or insufficient intake for more than 5 days, functional GI tract, unable to ingest sufficient nutrients.	Identifying clients who need tube feedings before they become nutritionally depleted helps to prevent complications related to malnutrition.
2. Review client's medical history for nasal problems (e.g., nosebleeds, oral facial surgery, facial trauma, past history of aspiration, or anticoagulation therapy).	Nasoenteric tubes are contraindicated in clients with recent nasal surgery, facial traumas, or nosebleeds, and those receiving anticoagulation therapy. This includes clients with surgical procedures requiring a transsphenoid approach used to remove pituitary tumors, because there is a risk for improper tube placement (Metheny, 2002).
3. Assess client's mental status.	Alert client is better able to cooperate with tube insertion. If vomiting occurs, an alert client will usually expectorate vomitus, which helps reduce the risk of aspiration.
4. Review health care provider's order for type of tube and enteral feeding schedule.	Procedure and tube feedings require a health care provider's order.
5. Perform hand hygiene. Assess patency of nares. Have client close each nostril alternately and breathe. Examine each naris for patency and skin breakdown.	Evaluates nares for patency. Nares are often obstructed or irritated, or septal defect is present.
6. Assess for gag reflex. Place tongue blade in client's mouth, touching uvula to induce a gag response.	Identifies ability to swallow and determines if there is a risk for aspiration.

Critical Decision Point: Clients with impaired level of consciousness often have impaired gag reflex; their risk of aspiration is increased during this type of procedure and subsequent tube feedings.

7. Auscultate abdomen for bowel sounds	Absence of bowel sounds indicates decreased or absent peristalsis and increased risk for aspiration and/or abdominal distention.
8. Explain procedure to client and how to communicate during intubation by raising index finger to indicate gagging or discomfort.	Reduces anxiety and helps client to assist in insertion.
9. Stand on same side of bed as naris for insertion, and assist client to high-Fowler's position unless contraindicated. Place pillow behind head and shoulders.	Allows easier manipulation of tube. Fowler's position reduces risk of aspiration and promotes effective swallowing.
10. Place bath towel over chest. Keep facial tissues within reach.	Prevents soiling of gown. Insertion of tube frequently produces tearing.
11. Determine length of tube to be inserted and mark with tape: a. *Traditional method:* Measure distance from tip of nose to earlobe to xiphoid process of sternum (see illustration).	Length approximates distance from nose to stomach in 98% of clients. For duodenal or jejunal placement, an additional 20 to 30 cm is required.
12. Prepare nasogastric or nasointestinal tube for intubation: NOTE: Do not ice plastic tubes.	Tubes becomes stiff and inflexible, causing trauma to mucous membranes.
a. Inject 10 mL of water from 30-mL or larger Luer-Lok or catheter-tip syringe into the tube.	Aids in guide wire or stylet insertion.
b. Make certain that guide wire is securely positioned against weighted tip and that both Luer-Lok connections are snugly fitted together.	Promotes smooth passage of tube into GI tract. Improperly positioned stylet induces serious trauma.
13. Cut tape 10 cm (4 inches) long, or prepare tube fixation device.	Anchors tubing following insertion.

Continued

✳ **SKILL 44-2**   **INSERTING A SMALL-BORE NASOENTERIC TUBE FOR ENTERAL FEEDINGS—CONT'D**

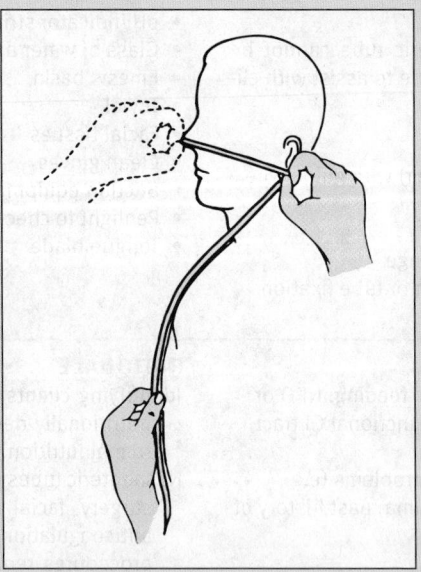

STEP 11a Determine length of tube to be inserted.

STEPS	RATIONALE
14. Apply clean gloves.	Reduces transmission of microorganisms (Matlow and others, 2006).
15. Dip tube with surface lubricant into glass of water.	Activates lubricant to facilitate passage of tube into naris to GI tract.
16. Insert tube through nostril to back of throat (posterior nasopharynx). Aim back and down toward ear.	Natural contour facilitates passage of tube into GI tract and reduces gagging by client.
17. Have client flex head toward chest after tube has passed through nasopharynx.	Closes off glottis and reduces risk of tube entering trachea.

Critical Decision Point: Encourage client to swallow by giving small sips of water or ice chips when possible. Advance tube as client swallows. Rotate tube 180 degrees while inserting.

18. Emphasize need to mouth breathe and swallow during the procedure.	Helps facilitate passage of tube and alleviates client's fears during the procedure.
19. When tip of tube reaches the carina (about 25 cm [10 inches] in an adult), stop, hold end of tube near ear and listen for air exchange from the distal portion of the tube.	If you hear air, the tube is possibly in the respiratory tract; remove tube and start over. **Never** use this step for tube verification (Metheny and Meert, 2004).
20. Advance tube each time client swallows until desired length has been passed.	Reduces discomfort and trauma to client.

Critical Decision Point: Do not force tube. If you meet resistance or client starts to cough, choke, or become cyanotic, stop advancing the tube and pull tube back.

21. Check for position of tube in back of throat with penlight and tongue blade.	Tube may be coiled, kinked, or entering trachea.
22. Perform measurement of gastric pH to verify placement of tube (see Box 44-12, p. 1117) by obtaining gastric aspirate.	Properly obtained pH of 0 to 4 is a good indication of gastric placement (Metheny, 2006).

Critical Decision Point: Auscultation is not a reliable method for verification of tube placement because a tube inadvertently placed in the lungs, pharynx, or esophagus also transmits a sound similar to that of air entering the stomach (Metheny and Meert, 2004; Metheny and Titler, 2001; Serna and McCarthy, 2006).

※ **SKILL 44-2**

INSERTING A SMALL-BORE NASOENTERIC TUBE FOR ENTERAL FEEDINGS—CONT'D

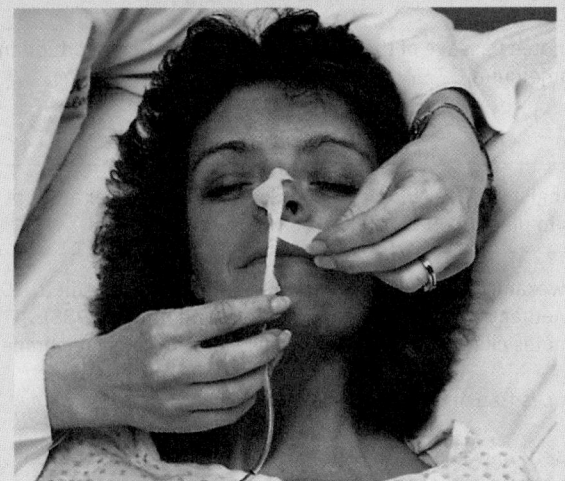

STEP 23a(3) Wrapping tape to anchor nasoenteral tube.

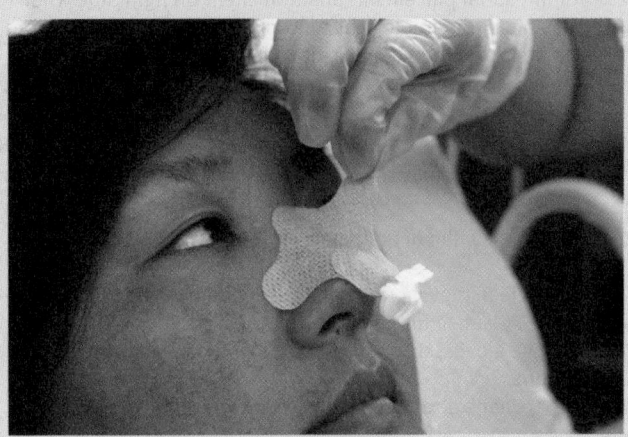

STEP 23b(1) Applying patch to bridge of nose.

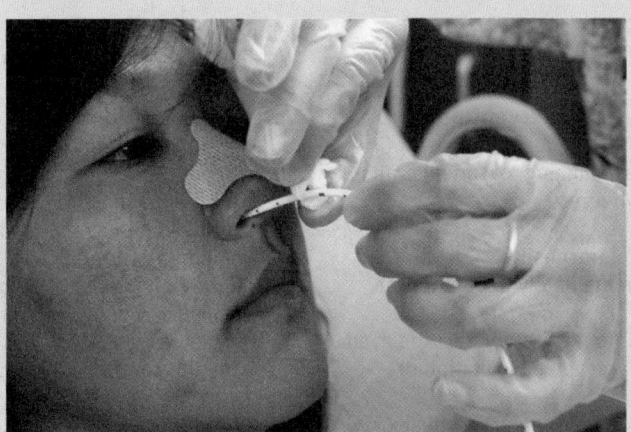

STEP 23b(2) Slip connector around feeding tube.

STEPS	RATIONALE
23. After gastric aspirates are obtained, anchor tube to nose and avoid pressure on nares. Mark exit site with indelible ink. Select one of the following options.	A properly secured tube allows the client more mobility and prevents trauma to nasal mucosa.
a. Apply tape	
(1) Apply tincture of benzoin or other skin adhesive on tip of client's nose and tube, and allow it to become "tacky."	Helps tape adhere better. Protects skin.
(2) Remove gloves, and split one end of tape lengthwise 5 cm (2 inches).	
(3) Place the intact end of tape over bridge of client's nose. Wrap each of the 5-cm strips around tube as it exits nose (see illustration).	Securing tape to nares prevents tissue necrosis.
b. Apply tube fixation device using shaped adhesive patch.	Secures tube and reduces friction on naris.
(1) Apply wide end of patch to bridge of nose (see illustration).	
(2) Slip connector around tube as it exits nose (see illustration).	
24. Fasten end of nasogastric tube to client's gown using a piece of tape. Do not use safety pins to fasten the tube to the gown.	Reduces traction on the naris if tube moves. Safety pins become unfastened and possibly cause injury to the client.

Continued

✳ SKILL 44-2 **INSERTING A SMALL-BORE NASOENTERIC TUBE FOR ENTERAL FEEDINGS—CONT'D**

STEPS	RATIONALE
25. For intestinal placement, position client on right side when possible until radiological confirmation of correct placement has been verified. Remove gloves, perform hand hygiene, and assist client to a comfortable position.	Promotes passage of the tube into the small intestine (duodenum or jejunum).

Critical Decision Point: Leave guide wire or stylet in place until a radiologist verifies correct position by x-ray film. Never attempt to reinsert partially or fully removed guide wire or stylet while feeding tube is in place.

STEPS	RATIONALE
25. Obtain x-ray film of abdomen.	X-ray examination verifies placement of tube (Cirgen Ellett, 2006; Metheny and Meert, 2004; Metheny and others, 1988).
26. Apply clean gloves, and administer oral hygiene (see Chapter 39). Cleanse tubing at nostril.	Promotes client comfort and integrity of oral mucous membranes.
27. Remove gloves, dispose of equipment, and perform hand hygiene.	Reduces transmission of microorganisms.
28. Inspect naris and oropharynx for any irritation after insertion.	If insertion was difficult, irritation of naris or oropharynx possibly occurred.
29. Ask if client feels comfortable.	Evaluates client's level of comfort.
30. Observe client for any difficulty breathing, coughing, or gagging.	Malposition of the tube causes these symptoms.
31. Auscultate lung sounds.	Abnormal lung sounds are an early sign of aspiration.
32. Confirm x-ray results.	Verifies position of tube before initiating enteral feeding.

Unexpected Outcomes and Related Interventions

1. Aspiration of stomach contents into the respiratory tract (immediate response), evidenced by coughing, dyspnea, cyanosis, auscultation of crackles or wheezes
   a. Position client on side.
   b. Suction nasotracheally and oral tracheally.
   c. Consult health care provider immediately to order chest x-ray examination.
2. Aspiration of stomach contents into respiratory tract (delayed response), evidenced by dyspnea, fever, auscultation of crackles or wheezes
   a. Consult health care provider to obtain order for chest x-ray film.
   b. Prepare for possible initiation of antibiotics.
3. Displacement of feeding tube to another site (e.g., from duodenum to stomach, mark at exit site if tube is moved); possibly occurs when client coughs or vomits
   a. Aspirate GI contents and measure pH (Metheny and Meert, 2004).
   b. Remove displaced tube, and insert and verify placement of new tube.
   c. If there is a question of aspiration, obtain chest x-ray film.

4. Clogging of feeding tube
   a. Aspirate gastric contents to assess patency of tube.
   b. Irrigate tube.
   c. If tube remains clogged after attempts to restore patency, notify health care provider and prepare for possible insertion of new tube.
5. Irritation of naris or nasal mucosa
   a. Provide hygiene, and remove and replace tape.
   b. Consider removing tube and inserting into other naris (health care provider order required).

Recording and Reporting

- Record and report type and size of tube placed, location of distal tip of tube, client's tolerance of procedure, pH value, and confirmation of tube position by x-ray examination.
- If client develops signs of aspiration, notify health care provider immediately.

✳ BOX 44-12   PROCEDURAL GUIDELINES

Obtaining Gastrointestinal Aspirate for pH Measurement, Large-Bore and Small-Bore Feeding Tubes: Intermittent and Continuous Feeding

Delegation Considerations: The skill of measuring pH in gastrointestinal (GI) aspirate is not delegated to nursing assistive personnel.

Equipment: Cone-tipped or Asepto syringe, pH test paper (scale of 1 to 14), paper towel, small medication cup, clean gloves.

1. Perform measures to verify placement of tube:
   a. For intermittently fed clients, test placement immediately before feeding (usually a period of at least 4 hours will have elapsed since previous feeding). More frequent checking has been associated with increased clogging of small-bore tubes. To avoid clogging, flush tube with 30 mL water after aspirating for the residual volume (Edwards and Metheny, 2000).
   b. For continuously tube-fed clients, test placement every 4 to 6 hours (Metheny, 2006). If the client is tolerating the feedings without incident and other indicators of correct location are present (the mark on the tube at the exit site has remained in its original position and the most recent x-ray films confirm tube's correct position), it is reasonable to continue feedings. **If risk of tube displacement is high and the tube has moved, consider the need for an x-ray film to verify placement** (Metheny and Meert, 2004). Plan pH testing at times when feeding may be withheld (e.g., during diagnostic testing, chest physical therapy, or to avoid medication interaction).
   c. Wait at least 1 hour after medication administration by tube or mouth.
2. Perform hand hygiene and apply clean gloves.

3. Draw up 30 mL of air into syringe, then attach to end of feeding tube. Flush tube with 30 mL of air before attempting to aspirate fluid. It will likely be more difficult to aspirate fluid from the small intestine than from the stomach. Repositioning the client from side to side will be helpful. More than one bolus of air through the tube is necessary in some cases. Burst of air aids in aspirating fluid more easily (Metheny and others, 1993).
4. Draw back on syringe, and obtain 5 to 10 mL of gastric aspirate. Observe appearance of aspirate (see illustration Step 4A).
   Gently mix aspirate in syringe. Then expel a few drops into a clean medicine cup. Dip the pH strip into the fluid, or apply a few drops of the fluid to the strip (see illustration Step 4B). Compare the color of the strip with the color on the chart provided by the manufacturer (Metheny and others, 1998b).
   a. Gastric fluid from client who has fasted for at least 4 hours usually has pH range of 1 to 4 (Metheny and others, 1998a).
   b. Fluid from nasointestinal tube of fasting client usually has pH greater than 6 (Metheny and others, 1989).
   c. Client with continuous tube feeding often has pH of 5 or higher.
   d. pH of pleural fluid from tracheobronchial tree is generally greater than 6.
5. Remove gloves, and discard supplies. Perform hand hygiene.

Critical Decision Point: If after repeated attempts it is not possible to aspirate fluid from a tube that was originally established by x-ray examination to be in desired position, and (a) there are no risk factors for tube dislocation, (b) there is no change in external marked tube length, and (c) client is not experiencing difficulty, assume tube is correctly placed (Metheny and Meert, 2004; Metheny and others, 2005).

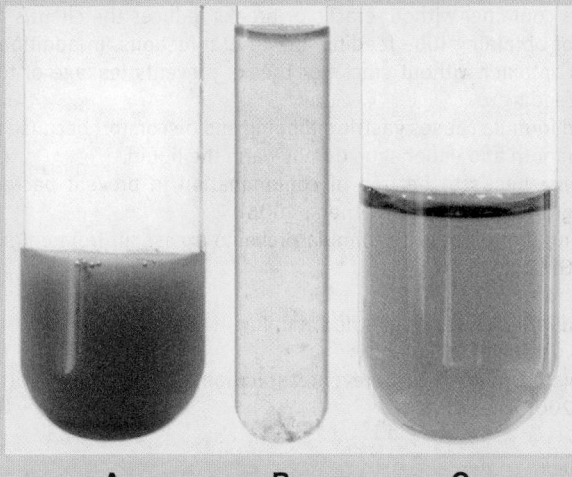

STEP 4A Gastrointestinal contents. **A,** Stomach. **B,** Stomach. **C,** Intestinal (Courtesy Dr. Norma Metheny, Professor, St. Louis University School of Nursing.)

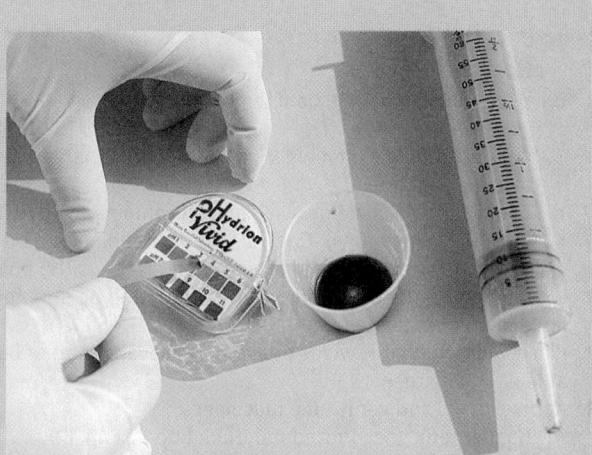

STEP 4B Comparing pH strip with color chart.

✳ **SKILL 44-3**   ADMINISTERING ENTERAL FEEDINGS VIA NASOENTERIC, GASTROSTOMY, OR JEJUNOSTOMY TUBES

Delegation Considerations

Administration of enteral tube feeding via a nasoenteric, gastrostomy, or jejunostomy tube is a procedure that can be delegated to nursing assistive personnel (NAP) after the tube placement is verified by the nurse. The nurse is responsible for client assessment. The nurse directs the NAP to:

- Elevate the head of the client's bed at a minimum of 30 degrees or sit the client up in bed or a chair
- Infuse the feeding slowly
- Report any difficulty infusing the feeding or any discomfort voiced by the client

Equipment

- Disposable feeding bag and tubing or ready-to-hang system
- 30-mL or larger Luer-Lok or catheter-tip syringe
- Stethoscope
- pH indicator strip (scale 0.0 to 14 preferred)
- Infusion pump (required for continuous or intestinal feedings): use pump designed for tube feedings
- Prescribed enteral feedings
- Clean gloves
- Equipment to obtain blood glucose by finger stick

STEPS	RATIONALE
1. Assess client's need for enteral tube feedings: impaired swallowing, decreased level of consciousness, head or neck surgery, facial trauma, surgeries of upper alimentary canal.	Identify clients who need tube feedings before they become nutritionally depleted.
2. Evaluate client's nutritional status (see Table 44-4, p. 1102). Obtain baseline weight and laboratory values. Assess client for fluid volume excess or deficit, electrolyte abnormalities, and metabolic abnormalities such as hyperglycemia.	Enteral feedings are to restore or maintain a client's nutritional status. Provides objective data to measure effectiveness of feedings.
3. Verify health care provider's order for formula, rate, route, and frequency. Laboratory data and bedside assessments, such as finger-stick blood glucose measurement, are also ordered by the health care provider.	Tube feedings, laboratory tests, and bedside tests must be ordered by health care provider.
4. For feeding tubes placed through the abdominal wall, assess tube site for breakdown, irritation, or drainage.	Infection, pressure from tube, or drainage of gastric secretions causes skin breakdown.
5. Explain procedure to client.	Well-informed client is more cooperative and at ease.
6. Perform hand hygiene.	Reduces transmission of microorganisms.
7. Auscultate for bowel sounds before feeding.	Absent bowel sounds indicate decreased ability of GI tract to digest or absorb nutrients.
8. Prepare feeding container to administer formula: 　a. Check expiration date on formula and integrity of container.	Tube feedings administered within the designated shelf life from a container without cracks or breaks reduces the client's risk of obtaining tube feeding–borne GI infections. In addition, a container without cracks or breaks prevents leakage of tube feeding.
b. Have tube feeding at room temperature.	Cold formula causes gastric cramping and discomfort because the mouth and esophagus do not warm the liquid.
c. Connect tubing to container as needed or prepare ready-to-hang container.	Tubing needs to be free of contamination to prevent bacterial growth (Matlow and others, 2006).
d. Shake formula container well, and fill container with formula (see illustration). Open stopcock on tubing and fill with formula to remove air. Hang on intravenous (IV) pole.	Filling the tubing with formula prevents excess air from entering GI tract.
9. For intermittent feeding have syringe ready, and be sure formula is at room temperature.	Cold formula causes gastric cramping.
10. Place client in high-Fowler's position, or elevate head of bed at least 30 degrees.	Elevated head helps prevent aspiration (Serna and McCarthy, 2006).
11. Apply gloves, and verify tube placement: 　A. **Nasoenteric** (see Procedural Guideline Box 44-12). 　B. **Gastrostomy tube:** Attach syringe, and aspirate 5 to 10 mL of gastric secretions; observe their appearance, and check pH.	Gastric fluid of client who has fasted for at least 4 hours usually has a pH of 1 to 4, especially when client is not receiving a gastric-acid inhibitor. Continuous administration of tube feedings elevates pH (Metheny and Meert, 2004; Metheny and Titler, 2001).
C. **Jejunostomy tube:** Aspirate intestinal secretions, observe their appearance, and check pH.	Presence of intestinal fluid indicates that the end of the tube is in the small intestine. Generally the intestinal residual is very small (≤10 mL) (Metheny and others, 2005). If fluid tests acidic on pH test, looks like gastric fluid, or the residual volume is large (>10 mL), displacement of the tube into the stomach has possibly occurred.

✳ SKILL 44-3   ADMINISTERING ENTERAL FEEDINGS VIA NASOENTERIC, GASTROSTOMY, OR JEJUNOSTOMY TUBES—CONT'D

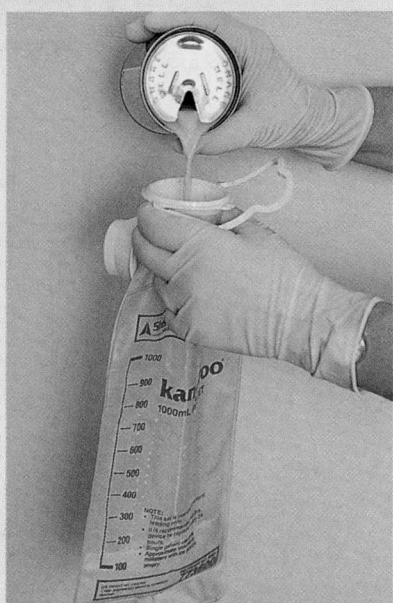

STEP 8d Pour formula into feeding container.

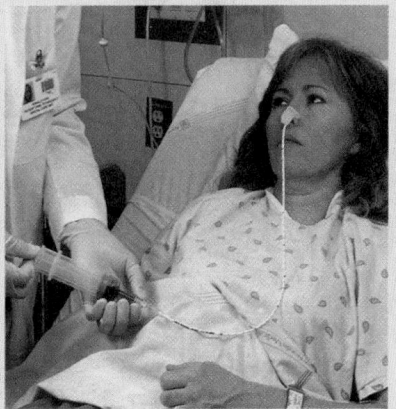

STEP 12b Check for gastric residual (small-bore tube).

STEPS	RATIONALE

Critical Decision Point: Auscultation is no longer considered a reliable method for verification of placement of tube because a tube inadvertently placed in lungs, pharynx, or esophagus transmits sound similar to that of air entering stomach (Metheny and Meert, 2004; Metheny and others, 1990a, 1990b; Serna and McCarthy, 2006).

STEPS	RATIONALE

12. Check for gastric residual.
  a. Draw up 30 mL of air with syringe. Connect to end of feeding tube. Flush tube with air.
  b. Pull back evenly to aspirate gastric contents (see illustration).
  c. Return aspirated contents to stomach unless the volume exceeds 200 mL (check agency policy).
	Gastric residual volume indicates if gastric emptying is delayed. Delayed gastric emptying is a concern if 200 mL or more remains in the client's stomach (Metheny, 2006). Return of aspirate prevents fluid and electrolyte imbalance.

13. Flush tubing with 30 mL water.	Ensures tube is clear and patent.
14. Initiate feeding:	Usually clients receive enteral feedings continuously to ensure proper absorption. However, clients often receive initial feedings by bolus to assess client's tolerance to formula. See Box 44-13, p. 1123, for guidelines to advance enteral feedings.
A. Syringe or intermittent feeding (1) Pinch proximal end of the feeding tube.	Prevents excessive air from entering client's stomach/intestine or leaking of contents.
(2) Remove plunger from syringe, and attach barrel of syringe to end of tube.	
(3) Fill syringe with measured amount of formula (see illustration). Release tube, and hold syringe high enough to allow it to empty gradually by gravity; refill; repeat until prescribed amount has been delivered to the client.	Height of syringe allows for safe, slow, gravity drainage of formula This gradual emptying of tube feeding by gravity reduces risk of abdominal discomfort, vomiting, or diarrhea induced by bolus or too-rapid infusion of tube feedings.
(4) If feeding bag is used, hang feeding bag on an IV pole (see illustration). Allow bag to empty gradually over 30 to 60 minutes by setting rate by adjusting roller clamp on tubing or placing on a feeding pump.	

Continued

✳ **SKILL 44-3**   **ADMINISTERING ENTERAL FEEDINGS VIA NASOENTERIC, GASTROSTOMY, OR JEJUNOSTOMY TUBES—CONT'D**

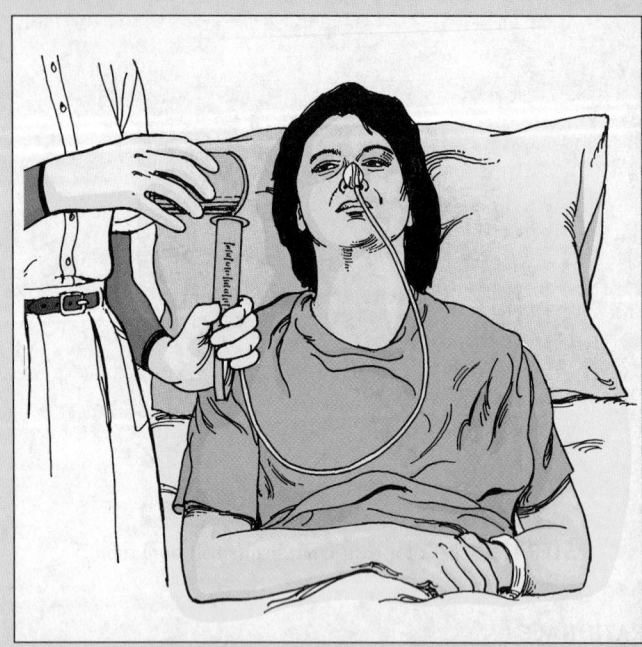

STEP 14A(3) Fill syringe with formula.

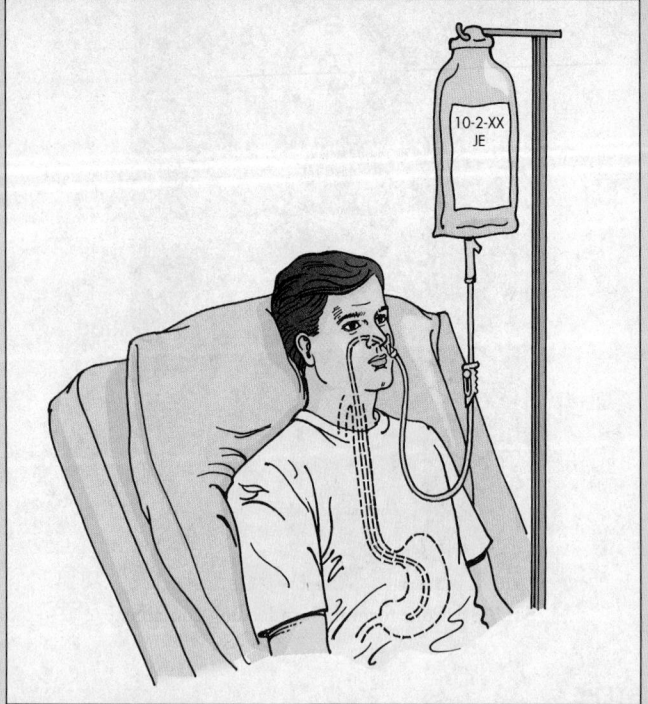

STEP 14A(4) Administer feeding.

STEPS	RATIONALE
B. Continuous-drip method	
(1) Connect distal end of tubing to the proximal end of the feeding tube.	Continuous feeding method is designed to deliver prescribed hourly rate of feeding. This method reduces risk of abdominal discomfort.
(2) Connect tubing through infusion pump and set rate (see illustration).	The use of an infusion pump delivers continuous feeding at a steady rate and pressure. Pump alarms for increased resistance.
15. Advance tube feeding gradually (Box 44-13, p. 1123).	Tube feedings are advanced gradually to prevent diarrhea and gastric intolerance to formula.

Critical Decision Point: Tube feedings are infused by feeding pumps and not by an IV pump.

16. Administer water via feeding tube as ordered with or between feedings.	Products vary in amount of water, and additional water is often needed to meet the free water requirement of 30 to 35 mL/kg/day (Thomas, 2001).
17. Following intermittent infusion or at end of continuous infusion, flush feeding tubing with 30 mL of water. Repeat every 4 to 6 hours. Remove gloves, or perform hand hygiene.	Maintains patency of feeding tube and provides client with a source of water to help maintain fluid and electrolyte balance.

Critical Decision Point: It is often necessary to consult with a dietitian to recommend a total free water requirement per day. This avoids the potential of fluid overload.

18. When tube feedings are not being administered, cap or clamp the proximal end of the feeding tube.	Prevents air from entering stomach between feedings.
19. Rinse bag and tubing with warm water whenever feedings are interrupted.	Rinsing bag and tubing with warm water clears old tube feedings and reduces bacterial growth.
20. Change bag and use a new administration set every 24 hours.	Reduces client's exposure to bacterial growth occurring in bag and tubing.

✳ **SKILL 44-3** | **ADMINISTERING ENTERAL FEEDINGS VIA NASOENTERIC, GASTROSTOMY, OR JEJUNOSTOMY TUBES—CONT'D**

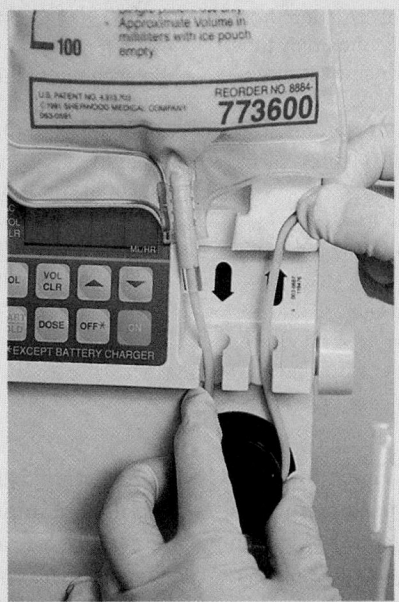

STEP 14B(3) Connect tubing through infusion pump.

STEPS	RATIONALE
21. Measure amount of aspirate (residual) every 4 to 6 hours.	Evaluates tolerance of tube feeding.
22. Monitor finger-stick blood glucose every 6 hours until maximum administration rate is reached and maintained for 24 hours.	Alerts nurse to client's tolerance of glucose. Glucose testing is often continued if blood glucose levels are elevated.
23. Monitor intake and output every 8 hours, and calculate daily totals every 24 hours.	Intake and output are indications of fluid balance or fluid volume excess or deficit.
24. Weigh client daily until maximum administration rate is reached and maintained for 24 hours; then weigh client 3 times per week at the same time using the same scale.	Weight gain is indicator of improved nutritional status; however, sudden gain of more than 2 pounds in 24 hours usually indicates fluid retention.
25. Monitor laboratory values.	Improving laboratory values (e.g., albumin, transferrin, and prealbumin) indicate an improved nutritional status.
26. Observe client's respiratory status.	Change in respiratory status (e.g., increased rate, declining SpO_2) may indicate aspiration of tube feeding.
27. Auscultate bowel sounds.	Assesses gastric peristalsis.
28. For tubes placed through the abdominal wall, inspect insertion site for signs of impaired skin integrity.	Enteral tubes often cause pressure and excoriation at the insertion site. In addition, gastric secretions also cause irritation to the skin.

Unexpected Outcomes and Related Interventions
(in addition to those in Skill 44-1, p. 1103)
1. Gastric residual exceeds 200 mL (see agency policy).
    a. Hold feeding.
    b. Notify health care provider.
    c. Maintain client in semi-Fowler's or at least have head of bed elevated 30 degrees.
    d. Recheck residual in 1 hour.
2. Client develops diarrhea 3 times or more in 24 hours.
    a. Notify health care provider.
    b. Confer with dietitian.
    c. Institute skin care measures.
    d. Consider change in antibiotics, only for clients receiving antibiotics.

3. Client develops nausea and vomiting.
    a. Notify health care provider.
    b. Check patency of tube.
    c. Aspirate for residual.
4. Client vomits and aspirates formula when gastric emptying is delayed or formula is administered too rapidly and produces vomiting.
    a. Position client in side-lying position.
    b. Suction airway.
    c. Notify health care provider.
    d. Obtain chest x-ray film.
5. Skin around gastrostomy/jejunostomy site breaks down.
    a. Institute skin care practices.
    b. Use pressure-relief measures around tube.
    c. Provide appropriate wound care (see Chapter 48).
    d. Auscultate for bowel sounds.

Continued

✳ SKILL 44-3   ADMINISTERING ENTERAL FEEDINGS VIA NASOENTERIC, GASTROSTOMY, OR JEJUNOSTOMY TUBES—CONT'D

6. Drainage (signs of hemorrhage, infection, or obstruction) from the abdominal insertion site of gastrostomy/jejunostomy tube.
  a. Notify health care provider; describe and document the type of drainage.
  b. For purulent drainage anticipate the need for cultures.
  c. Place a dry drain-gauze around the site, and change every shift and prn.

Recording and Reporting
- Record amount and type of feeding. Client's response to tube feeding, patency of tube, condition of skin at tube site for tubes placed in abdominal wall, and any side effects.
- Report client's tolerance and adverse effects.

Home Care Considerations
- Teach client or primary caregiver how to determine correct placement of feeding tube.
- Inform client or primary caregiver of signs associated with pulmonary aspiration, delayed gastric emptying.
- Reinforce signs and symptoms associated with feeding tube complications and when to call health care provider.
- Teach client or primary caregiver how to do skin care around the gastrostomy or jejunostomy tube and the signs and symptoms of infection at the insertion site.

Historically, nurses verified feeding tube placement by injecting air through the tube while auscultating the stomach for a gurgling or bubbling sound or asking the client to speak (Metheny and others, 1998b). These methods have a high degree of inaccuracy. Rolandelli and others (2005) report that clients were able to speak despite placement of feeding tubes in the lung. Auscultation has repeatedly been shown to be ineffective in detecting tubes accidentally placed in the lung (Metheny and others, 1998a). Further, it is not effective in distinguishing between gastric and intestinal placement for feeding tubes (Metheny, 2006; Metheny and Meert, 2004; Metheny and others, 1999). Thus the nurse must suspect tube displacement in clients at risk and use meticulous assessment skills.

At present the most reliable method for verification of placement of small-bore feeding tubes is x-ray examination (Box 44-14). The measurement of pH of secretions withdrawn from the feeding tube helps to differentiate the location of the tube (see Box 44-12, p. 1117). For accurate pH measurements, 30 mL of air is injected into the tube before measurement. Flushing the tube with air clears out formula, medications, or flush solutions. Only 5 to 10 mL of gastric fluid is needed for pH testing. The pH of gastric aspirate typically ranges between 0 and 4. A client who takes acid-inhibitor medications will usually have an acidic pH value ranging from 4.0 (after 4 hours of fasting) to 6.0 (with continuous EN infusion). By contrast, intestinal aspirate has a pH of 7.8 to 8.0. You will need more precise indicators to help differentiate the source of tube feeding aspirate (Cirgin Ellett, 2006; Metheny and Meert, 2004).

The addition of blue food coloring to enteral formula to assist with the detection of formula aspirated into the lung, presumably by staining the tracheobronchial secretions, is no longer used. The FDA issued a public health advisory reporting an association between use of Blue No. 1 food coloring and client deaths (USFDA, 2003). Research has determined that the absence of blue-stained tracheobronchial secretions does not rule out pulmonary aspiration (Metheny, Aud, and Wunderlich, 1999).

Table 44-7 outlines major complications of enteral nutrition. Of special note, severely malnourished clients are at risk for electrolyte disturbances from refeeding syndrome as cations such as potassium, magnesium, and phosphate move intracellularly during EN or PN therapy.

Parenteral Nutrition. **Parenteral nutrition (PN)** is a form of specialized nutrition support in which nutrients are provided intravenously. Safe administration of this form of nutrition depends on appropriate assessment of nutrition needs, meticulous management of the central venous catheter (CVC), and careful monitoring to prevent or treat metabolic complications. Parenteral nutrition is administered in a variety of settings, including the client's home. Regardless of the setting, adhere to principles of asepsis and infusion management to ensure safe nutrition support.

Clients who are unable to digest or absorb enteral nutrition benefit from PN. Clients in highly stressed physiological states such as sepsis, head injury, or burns are candidates for PN therapy (see Box 44-11, p. 1112).

Clinical and laboratory monitoring by a multidisciplinary team is required throughout PN therapy. The need for continued PN is consistently reevaluated. The goal to move toward use of the GI tract is constant (ASPEN, 2002). Disuse of the GI tract has been associated with villus atrophy and generalized cell shrinkage. Translocation of bacteria from the local gut to systemic regions has been noted in relation to GI cell shrinkage, resulting in gram-negative septicemia.

Lipid emulsions provide supplemental kilocalories and prevent essential fatty acid deficiencies. Administer these emulsions through a separate peripheral line, through the central line by Y-connector tubing (see Chapter 41), or as an admixture to the PN solution. The addition of lipid emulsion to the PN solution is called a 3-in-1 admixture. The client receives this over a 24-hour period. Do not use the admixture if you observe oil droplets or an oil or creamy layer on the surface of the admixture. This observation indicates that the emulsion has broken into large lipid droplets that cause fat emboli if administered. Lipid emulsions are white and opaque. Take care to avoid confusing enteral formula with parenteral lipids.

Initiating PN. Clients with short-term nutritional needs often receive intravenous solutions of less than 10% dextrose via a peripheral vein in combination with amino acids and lipids. Peripheral solutions are not as caloricly dense as TPN solutions and therefore are usually temporary. Parenteral nutrition with greater than 10% dextrose requires a CVC that a physician places into a high-flow central vein such as the superior vena cava under sterile conditions (see Chapter 41). If you are using a CVC that has multiple lumens,

✳ BOX 44-13 Advancing the Rate of Tube Feeding

Protocols for advancing tube feedings are commonly institution specific. Most of these protocols are untested for validity. There does not appear to be a benefit to slow initiation of enteral nutrition over days. Most clients are able to tolerate feeding 2 to 3 days post initiation (ASPEN, 2002; Parrish and McCray, 2003). Do not dilute formulas with water; this increases the risk of bacterial contamination (ASPEN, 2002).

Intermittent
1. Start formula at full strength for isotonic formulas (300 to 400 mOsm) or at ordered concentration.
2. Infuse bolus of formula over at least 20 to 30 minutes via syringe or feeding container.
3. Begin feedings with no more than 150 to 250 mL at one time. Increase by 50 mL per feeding per day to achieve needed volume and calories in four to six feedings (Parrish and McCray, 2003).

Continuous
1. Start formula at full strength for isotonic formulas (300 to 400 mOsm) or at ordered concentration.
2. Begin infusion rate at designated rate.
3. Advance rate slowly (e.g., 30 to 60 mL/hr every 8 to 12 hours) to target rate if tolerated (tolerance indicated by absence of nausea and diarrhea, and low gastric residuals) (Parrish and McCray, 2003).

use a port that is exclusively dedicated for the TPN. Label the port for TPN, and do not infuse other solutions or medications through the port (National Guideline Clearinghouse, 2003). Nurses with special training insert peripherally inserted central catheters (PICCs) that are started in a vein of the forearm and threaded into the subclavian or superior vena cava vein.

After catheter placement, wait to flush and use the catheter until the position is radiographically confirmed. The physician secures the CVC with a securement device and covers the site with a sterile dressing. A PICC is usually stabilized with sterile strips of tape and a sterile dressing. A chest x-ray examination identifies any complications.

Before beginning any parenteral nutrition infusion, verify the health care provider's order and inspect the solution for particulate matter or a break in the lipid emulsion. Always use an infusion pump. An initial rate of 40 to 60 mL/hr is recommended. The rate is gradually increased until the client's complete nutrition needs are supplied. Clients receiving PN at home frequently administer the entire daily solution over 12 hours at night. This allows the client to disconnect from the infusion each morning, flush the central line, and have independent mobility during the day. Home PN therapy often interferes with clients' normal activities, causing a poorer quality of life (Winkler, 2005).

Preventing Complications. Complications of PN include catheter-related problems and metabolic alterations (Table 44-8). Pneumothorax results from a puncture insult to the pulmonary system and results in accumulation of air in the pleural cavity with subsequent collapse of the lung and impaired breathing. Pneumothorax is usually accompanied by symptoms of sudden sharp chest pain, dyspnea, and coughing. In relation to PN, pneumothorax most often occurs during CVC placement. Monitor client for the first 24 hours for signs and symptoms of pulmonary distress.

✳ BOX 44-14 EVIDENCE-BASED PRACTICE

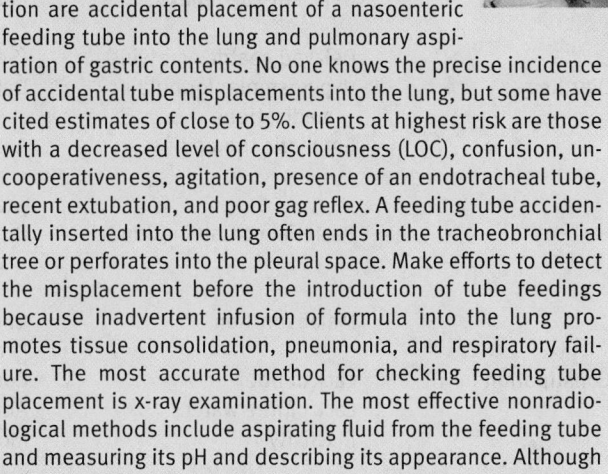

Accuracy in Determining Placement of Feeding Tubes
Evidence Summary
Two possible adverse outcomes of enteral nutrition are accidental placement of a nasoenteric feeding tube into the lung and pulmonary aspiration of gastric contents. No one knows the precise incidence of accidental tube misplacements into the lung, but some have cited estimates of close to 5%. Clients at highest risk are those with a decreased level of consciousness (LOC), confusion, uncooperativeness, agitation, presence of an endotracheal tube, recent extubation, and poor gag reflex. A feeding tube accidentally inserted into the lung often ends in the tracheobronchial tree or perforates into the pleural space. Make efforts to detect the misplacement before the introduction of tube feedings because inadvertent infusion of formula into the lung promotes tissue consolidation, pneumonia, and respiratory failure. The most accurate method for checking feeding tube placement is x-ray examination. The most effective nonradiological methods include aspirating fluid from the feeding tube and measuring its pH and describing its appearance. Although observing for respiratory distress is helpful in alert clients (especially when firm large-diameter tubes are used), it is of little benefit in those who have a decreased LOC and when small-bore tubes are used. Risk factors for pulmonary aspiration in tube-fed clients include feeding into the stomach when gastric atony is present (resulting in high gastric residual volumes), poor gag reflexes, mechanical ventilation, and flat positioning in bed. Bedside methods used to detect pulmonary aspiration are not well defined.

Application to Nursing Practice
- X-ray verification of feeding tube placement is the most reliable method available to confirm correct feeding tube location and is required in most acute care facilities when small-bore tubes are initially inserted.
- When the x-ray method is not feasible, the next best method involves testing the feeding tube aspirate's pH and observing its appearance. A properly obtained pH of 0 to 4 is a good indication of gastric placement; a pH of 6 or higher likely indicates placement in the lung, intestine, or even the stomach when gastric pH is unusually high. Intestinal fluid is usually bile-stained (dark golden yellow); in contrast, gastric fluid is usually grassy green, off-white to tan, or clear and colorless.
- Do not use the auscultatory method to determine tube location.

References
Metheny N, Aud M, Ignatavicius D: Detection of improperly placed feeding tubes, *J Healthc Risk Manage* 18(3):37, 1998; Metheny NA, Aud MA, Wunderlich RJ: A survey of bedside methods used to detect pulmonary aspiration of enteral formula in intubated tube-fed patients, *Am J Crit Care* 8(3):160, 1999; Metheny NA, Meert KL: Monitoring feeding tube placement, *Nutr Clin Pract* 19(5):487, 2004; and Metheny NA: Preventing respiratory complications of tube feedings: evidence-based practice, *Am J Crit Care* 15(4):360, 2006.

✳ TABLE 44-7 Enteral Tube Feeding Complications

PROBLEM	POSSIBLE CAUSE	INTERVENTION*
Pulmonary aspiration	Regurgitation of formula	Verify tube placement. Elevate head of bed 30 to 45 degrees during feedings and for 2 hours afterward.
	Feeding tube displaced	Reposition tube, and verify tube placement.
	Deficient gag reflex	Reassess for return of normal gag reflex; until then place client on aspiration precautions and place client in semi-Fowler's position.
	Delayed gastric emptying	(See delayed gastric emptying below.)
Diarrhea	Hyperosmolar formula or medications	Deliver formula continuously, lower rate, dilute, or change to isotonic EN.
	Antibiotic therapy	Antibiotics destroy normal intestinal flora; consult with a health care provider to consider changing medication; treat symptoms with antidiarrheal agents; culture stool for *Clostridium difficile*.
	Bacterial contamination	Do not hang formula longer than 4-8 hours in bag, wash bag out well when refilling, change tube feeding bags and tubing q24h, and use aseptic practices. Check expiration dates.
	Malabsorption	Check for pancreatic insufficiency; use low-fat, lactose-free formula, and continuous feedings.
Constipation	Lack of fiber	Consult with a dietitian to select a formula containing fiber.
	Lack of free water	Add water as needed as flushes.*
	Inactivity	Monitor client's ability to ambulate; collaborate with health care provider and/or physical therapist for activity order.
Tube occlusion	Pulverized medications given per tube	Irrigate with 30 mL water before and after each medication per tube.* Dilute crushed medications if not liquid. Avoid crushed medications, if liquid available.
	Sedimentation of formula	Shake cans well before administering (read label).
	Reaction of incompatible medications or formula	Read pharmacological information on compatibility of drugs and formula.
Tube displacement	Coughing, vomiting	Replace tube, and confirm placement before restarting tube feeding.
	Not taped securely	With placement verification, check that tape is secure (nasoenteric).
Abdominal cramping, nausea/vomiting	High osmolality of formula	Suggest an isotonic formula or dilution of current formula to health care provider.
	Rapid increase in rate/volume	Lower rate of delivery to increase tolerance. Maintain head of bed at least 30 degrees.
	Lactose intolerance	Suggest use of lactose-free formula.
	Intestinal obstruction	Stop feeding with GI obstruction.
	High-fat formula used	Use greater proportion of carbohydrate.
	Cold formula used	Warm formula to room temperature.
Delayed gastric emptying	Diabetic gastroparesis	Consult with health care provider regarding medication for increasing gastric motility.
	Serious illnesses	Consult health care provider regarding advancing tube to intestinal placement.
	Inactivity	Monitor medications and pathological conditions that affect GI motility.
Serum electrolyte imbalance	Excess GI losses	Monitor serum electrolyte levels daily.
	Dehydration	Provide free water as per dietitian recommendation.
	Presence of disease states such as cirrhosis, renal insufficiency, heart failure, or diabetes mellitus	Know of links with specific pathological conditions.
Fluid overload	Refeeding syndrome in malnutrition	Restrict fluids if necessary, and use either a specialized formula or a diluted enteral formula at first.
	Excess free water or diluted (hypotonic) formula	Monitor levels of serum proteins and electrolytes. Use a more concentrated formula with fluid volume excess without risk of refeeding syndrome.
Hyperosmolar dehydration	Hypertonic formula with insufficient free water	Slow rate of delivery, dilute, or change to isotonic formula.

*Check first for fluid-restricted conditions that would affect volume of water given.
EN, Enteral nutrition; *GI*, gastrointestinal.

✳ TABLE 44-8 Metabolic Complications of Parenteral Nutrition (PN)

PROBLEM	SIGNS/SYMPTOMS	INTERVENTION
Electrolyte imbalance	Monitor Na, Ca, K, Cl, PO_4, Mg, and CO_2 levels	See Chapter 41 for signs of deficiency/toxicity. Check TPN for supplemental electrolyte levels. Notify health care provider of imbalances.
Hypercapnia	Increased oxygen consumption, increased CO_2, respiratory quotient >1.0, minute ventilation	To prevent; ventilator-dependent clients are at risk; provide 30% to 60% of energy requirements as fat per health care provider's order.
Hypoglycemia	Diaphoresis, shakiness, confusion, loss of consciousness	To prevent; do not abruptly discontinue TPN but taper rate down to within 10% of infusion rate 1 to 2 hours before stopping. If you suspect hypoglycemia, test blood glucose, administer IV bolus of 50% dextrose or glucagon per order or protocol if necessary.
Hyperglycemia	Thirst, headache, lethargy, increased urination	Monitor blood glucose level daily until stable, then as ordered or prn. TPN is initiated slowly and tapered up to maximal infusion rate. Additional insulin may be required during therapy if problem persists (or if client has diabetes mellitus).
Hyperglycemic hyperosmolar nonketotic dehydration/coma (HHNC)	Hyperglycemia (>500 mg/dl), glycosuria, serum osmolarity >350 mOsm/L, confusion, azotemia, headache, severe signs of dehydration (see Chapter 41), hypernatremia, metabolic acidosis, convulsions, coma	To prevent; monitor blood glucose, BUN, serum osmolarity, glucose in urine, and fluid losses; administer insulin as ordered; replace fluids as ordered; maintain consistent infusion rate; and provide 30% of daily energy needs as fat. Clients at risk are hypermetabolic, receiving steroids, older adults diagnosed with diabetes, have impaired renal or pancreatic function, or are septic.

TPN, Total parenteral nutrition; *IV*, intravenous; *BUN*, blood urea nitrogen.

An air embolus possibly occurs during insertion of the catheter or when changing the tubing or cap. Having the client perform a Valsalva maneuver (holding the breath and "bearing down") while assuming a left lateral decubitus position helps prevent air embolus. The increased venous pressure created by the maneuver prevents air from entering the bloodstream during catheter insertion. Maintaining integrity of the closed intravenous system also helps prevent air embolus.

Catheter occlusion is present when there is sluggish or no flow through the catheter. Temporarily stop the infusion, and flush with saline or heparin per protocol or orders. If this is unsuccessful, attempt to aspirate a clot. If still unsuccessful, follow the institution's protocol for use of thrombolytic agent (e.g., urokinase).

Suspect catheter sepsis if the client develops fever, chills, glucose intolerance and has a positive blood culture. To avoid infection, change the TPN infusion tubing every 24 hours. Do not hang a single container of PN for more than 24 hours or lipids more than 12 hours. During CVC dressing changes, always use a sterile mask and gloves and assess insertion sites for signs and symptoms of infection (see Chapter 41). Change the CVC dressing per institution policy and anytime it becomes wet or contaminated. Use either alcohol or an alcoholic solution of chlorhexidine gluconate to clean the injection port or catheter hub before and after each time it is used (National Guideline Clearinghouse, 2003). In some instances you will use an in-line 0.22-μm filter to remove bacteria.

The PN solution contains most of the major electrolytes, vitamins, and minerals. Clients also need supplemental vitamin K as ordered throughout therapy. Vitamin K is synthesized by microflora found in the jejunum and ileum with normal use of the GI tract; however, because PN circumvents GI use, clients need to receive exogenous vitamin K.

Electrolyte and mineral imbalances often occur. Administration of concentrated glucose is accompanied by increases in endogenous insulin production, which causes cations (potassium, magnesium, and phosphorus) to move intracellularly. In malnourished or cachectic clients the resulting low serum (extracellular) levels of electrolytes and edema causes cardiac dysrhythmias, congestive heart failure, respiratory distress, convulsions, coma, or death. This is called refeeding syndrome.

Too-rapid administration of hypertonic dextrose can result in an osmotic diuresis and dehydration (see Chapter 41). If an infusion falls behind schedule, the nurse should not increase the rate in an attempt to catch up. Sudden discontinuation of the solution can cause hypoglycemia. Usually, 10% dextrose is infused when PN solution is suddenly discontinued. Clients with diabetes are more at risk.

The goal is to move clients from PN to EN and/or oral feeding. Once clients are meeting one third to one half of their kilocalorie needs per day, PN is usually decreased to half the original volume. EN feedings are then increased to meet needs. When 75% of daily energy needs are consistently met with tube feeding, PN is discontinued. Clients who make the transition from PN to oral feedings typically have early satiety and decreased appetite. Parenteral nutrition is gradually decreased in response to increased oral intake. If oral intake is inadequate, small frequent meals are helpful. Calorie/protein counts are recommended when clients begin taking soft foods. When 75% of needs are being met by reliable dietary intake, PN therapy is usually discontinued.

Restorative and Continuing Care. Clients discharged from a hospital with diet prescriptions often need dietary education to plan meals that meet specific therapeutic requirements. Restorative care includes both immediate postsurgical care and routine medical care and therefore includes hospitalized and home care clients. The following sections address nutritional interventions for some common disease states.

Medical Nutrition Therapy. Optimal nutrition is important in health and illness, but the specific dietary intake pattern that results in optimal nutrition is modified for clients with particular diseases. **Medical nutrition therapy** (MNT) is the use of specific nutritional therapies to treat an illness, injury, or condition. MNT is necessary to assist the body's ability to metabolize certain nutrients, correct nutritional deficiencies related to the disease, and eliminate foods that may exacerbate disease symptoms. This section provides a summary of MNT for a variety of diseases.

Gastrointestinal Diseases. Peptic ulcers are controlled with regular meals and medications such as histamine receptor antagonists that block secretion of hydrochloric acid. Marshall and Warren first identified *Helicobacter pylori* in 1984. *H. Pylori* is a bacteria that causes peptic ulcers and is confirmed by laboratory tests. It is treated with antibiotics that control the bacterial infection. Stress and overproduction of gastric HCl also contribute to peptic ulcer disease. Encourage clients to avoid foods that increase stomach acidity and pain, such as caffeine, decaffeinated coffee, frequent milk intake, citric acid juices, and certain seasonings (hot chili peppers, chili powder, black pepper). Discourage smoking, alcohol, aspirin, and nonsteroidal antiinflammatory drugs (NSAIDs). Teach clients to avoid eating large quantities of food and to eat three regular meals without snacks especially at bedtime (Nix, 2005).

Inflammatory bowel disease includes Crohn's disease and idiopathic ulcerative colitis. Treatment of acute inflammatory bowel disease includes elemental diets (formula with the nutrients in their simplest form ready for absorption) or parenteral nutrition when symptoms such as diarrhea and weight loss are prevalent. In the chronic stage of the disease, a regular highly nourishing diet is appropriate. Vitamins and iron supplements are often required to correct or prevent anemia. Clients manage irritable bowel syndrome by increasing fiber, reducing fat, avoiding large meals, and avoiding lactose or sorbitol-containing foods for susceptible individuals.

The treatment of **malabsorption** syndromes, such as celiac disease, includes a gluten-free diet. Gluten is present in wheat, rye, barley, and oats. Short-bowel syndrome results from extensive resection of bowel after which clients suffer from malabsorption due to lack of intestinal surface area. These clients require lifetime feeding with either elemental enteral formulas or parenteral nutrition.

Diverticulitis is a condition that results from an inflammation of diverticula, which are abnormal but common pouchlike herniations that occur in the bowel lining. This condition is nutritionally treated with a moderate- or low-residue diet until the infection subsides. Afterward, a high-fiber diet is generally prescribed for chronic diverticula problems.

Diabetes Mellitus. Type 1 diabetes mellitus (DM) requires both insulin and dietary restrictions for optimal control, beginning with diagnosis (ADA, 2006). By contrast, clients control type 2 diabetes mellitus initially with exercise and diet therapy. If these measures prove ineffective, it is common to add oral medications. Insulin injections often follow if type 2 diabetes worsens or fails to respond to these initial interventions.

Individualize the diet according to the client's age, build, weight, and activity level. Maintaining carbohydrate intake is the key in diabetes management. A diet that includes carbohydrates from fruits, vegetables, whole grains, legumes, and low-fat milk is recommended (ADA, 2006). Carbohydrate intake for men is 60 to 75 g per meal, and for women 45 to 60 g is recommended (Watts and Anselmo, 2006). Limit saturated fat to less than 7% of the total calories and cholesterol intake to less than 200 mg/day. Also recommended are a variety of foods containing fiber. Clients are able to substitute sucrose-containing foods for carbohydrates but need to make sure to avoid excess energy intake. The ADA (2006) also states that sugar alcohols and nonnutritive sweeteners are able to be eaten as long as the recommended daily intake levels are followed.

The goal of MNT treatment is to have glycemic levels that are normal or as close to normal as safely possible, lipid and lipoprotein profiles that decrease the risk of microvascular (e.g., renal and eye disease) and cardiovascular, neurological, and peripheral vascular complications, and blood pressure in the normal or near-normal range (ADA, 2006). Be aware of signs and symptoms of hypoglycemia and hyperglycemia.

Cardiovascular Diseases. The American Heart Association's (AHA's) dietary guidelines (2006) are intended to reduce risk factors for the development of hypertension and coronary artery disease. Dietary therapy for reducing the risk of cardiovascular disease includes balancing calorie intake with exercise to maintain a healthy body weight; eating a diet high in fruits, vegetables, and whole grain high fiber foods; eating fish at least 2 times per week; and limiting food and beverages that are high in added sugar and salt. The AHA guidelines (2006) also recommend limiting saturated fat to less than 7%, trans fat to less than 1%, and cholesterol to less than 300 mg/day. To accomplish this goal, clients choose lean meats and vegetables, use fat-free dairy products, and limit intake of fats (Olendzki and others, 2006).

Cancer and Cancer Treatment. Malignant cells compete with normal cells for nutrients, increasing the metabolic needs of the client. Most cancer treatments cause nutritional problems. Clients with cancer often complain of anorexia, nausea, vomiting, and taste distortions. The goal of nutrition therapy is to meet the increased metabolic needs of the client (Nix, 2005). Malnutrition in cancer is associated with increased morbidity and mortality. Enhanced nutritional status often improves the client's quality of life.

Radiation therapy destroys rapidly dividing malignant cells; however, other normal rapidly dividing cells, such as the epithelial lining of the GI tract, are often affected. Radiation therapy causes anorexia, stomatitis, severe diarrhea, strictures of the intestine, and pain. Radiation treatment of the head and neck region causes taste and smell disturbances, decreased salivation, and dysphagia. Nutrition management of the client with cancer focuses on maximizing intake of nutrients and fluids. Individualize diet choices to the client's needs, symptoms, and situation (Nix, 2005). The nurse uses creative approaches to manage alterations in taste and smell. For example, clients with altered taste often prefer chilled foods or foods that are spicy. Encourage clients to eat small frequent meals and snacks that are nutritious and easy to digest.

Human Immunodeficiency Virus/Acquired Immunodeficiency Syndrome. Clients with HIV/AIDS typically experience body wasting and severe weight loss. The wasting is related to anorexia, stomatitis, oral thrush infection, nausea, or recurrent vomiting, all resulting in inadequate intake. Factors associated with weight loss and malnutrition include severe diarrhea, GI malabsorption, and altered metabolism of nutrients. Systemic infection results in hypermetabolism from cytokine elevation. Often the medications taken to treat HIV infection cause side effects that alter nutritional status.

Restorative care of malnutrition resulting from AIDS focuses upon maximizing kilocalories and nutrients. Diagnose and address each cause of nutritional depletion in the care plan. Individually tailored nutrition support progresses in stages from oral, to enteral, and lastly to parenteral. Good hand hygiene and food safety are essential because of the client's reduced resistance to infection. For example, minimization of exposure to *Cryptosporidium* in drinking water, lakes, or swimming pools is important. Small, frequent, nutrient-dense meals that limit fatty foods and overly sweet foods are easier to tolerate. Clients benefit from eating cold foods, and drier or saltier foods with fluid in between (Nix, 2005).

Evaluation

Care plans need to reflect achievable goals and outcomes. You need to evaluate outcomes of nursing actions and be alert for signs that goals are being met. Allow adequate time to test each nursing approach to a problem. Multidisciplinary collaboration remains essential in provision of nutrition support.

Measure the effectiveness of nutritional interventions by evaluating the client's expected outcomes and goals of care (Figure 44-9). Nutrition therapy does not always produce rapid results. Ongoing comparisons need to be made with baseline measures of weight, serum albumin or prealbumin, and protein and kilocalorie intake. If you do not observe gradual weight gain or if weight loss continues, evaluate the dietary EN prescription and determine if the client is experiencing any adverse effects from medications that are affecting the client's nutritional status. Changes in condition also indicate a need to change the nutritional plan of care. Consult multidisciplinary members of the health care team in an effort to better individualize the client's plan of care. The client is an active participant whenever possible. In the end, the client's ability to incorporate dietary changes into his or her lifestyle with the least amount of stress or disruption ensures that outcome measures are successfully met. When expected outcomes are not met, revise the nursing measures or expected outcomes based on the client's needs or preferences. When outcomes are not met, ask questions such as "Have you had a change in appetite?" "Have you noticed a change in your weight?" "How much would you like to weigh?" or "Have you changed your exercise pattern?"

Clients expect competent and accurate care. If ongoing nutritional therapies are not resulting in successful outcomes, clients expect nurses to recognize this fact and alter the plan of care accordingly. Expectations and health care values held by nurses frequently differ from those held by clients. Successful interventions and outcomes depend on recognition of this concept in addition to nursing knowledge and skill. Working closely with the client enables you to redefine those expectations that are realistically met within the limits of the client's conditions and treatment as well as their dietary preferences and cultural beliefs.

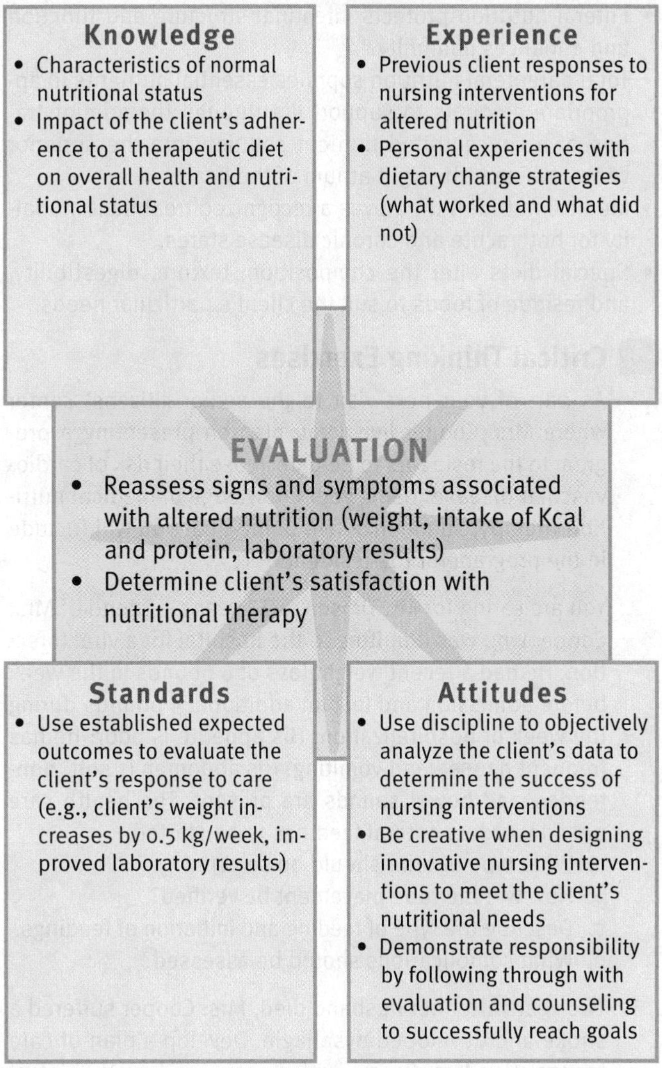

Knowledge
- Characteristics of normal nutritional status
- Impact of the client's adherence to a therapeutic diet on overall health and nutritional status

Experience
- Previous client responses to nursing interventions for altered nutrition
- Personal experiences with dietary change strategies (what worked and what did not)

EVALUATION
- Reassess signs and symptoms associated with altered nutrition (weight, intake of Kcal and protein, laboratory results)
- Determine client's satisfaction with nutritional therapy

Standards
- Use established expected outcomes to evaluate the client's response to care (e.g., client's weight increases by 0.5 kg/week, improved laboratory results)

Attitudes
- Use discipline to objectively analyze the client's data to determine the success of nursing interventions
- Be creative when designing innovative nursing interventions to meet the client's nutritional needs
- Demonstrate responsibility by following through with evaluation and counseling to successfully reach goals

Figure 44-9 Critical thinking model for nutrition evaluation.

✳ Key Concepts

- Ingestion of a diet balanced with carbohydrates, fats, proteins, vitamin, and minerals provides the essential nutrients to carry out the body's normal physiological functioning throughout the life span.
- Through digestion, food is broken down into its simplest form for absorption. Digestion and absorption occur mainly in the small intestine.
- Dietary reference intakes provide a range of values that address the needs of both groups (estimated average requirement) and individuals (adequate intakes, recommended dietary allowances, and tolerable upper intake level).
- Guidelines for dietary change recommend reduced fat, saturated fat, sodium, refined sugar, and cholesterol and increased intake of complex carbohydrates and fiber.
- Because improper nutrition affects all body systems, nutritional assessment includes a review of total physical assessment.
- Tube feedings are for clients who are unable to ingest food but are able to digest and absorb food.

- Enteral nutrition protects intestinal structure and function and enhances immunity.
- Total parenteral nutrition supplies essential nutrients in appropriate amounts to support life through the administration of a concentrated nutrient solution into the superior vena cava near the right atrium of the heart.
- Medical nutrition therapy is a recognized treatment modality for both acute and chronic disease states.
- Special diets alter the composition, texture, digestibility, and residue of foods to suit the client's particular needs.

✳ Critical Thinking Exercises

1. As part of your next visit to the senior citizens' center where Mrs. Cooper lives, you plan on presenting a program to the residents to help decrease their risk of cardiovascular disease. Using your knowledge of medical nutrition therapy, summarize five points that you will include in the program for the residents.

2. You are caring for Mr. Timson, a 72-year-old friend of Mrs. Cooper who was admitted to the hospital for a viral infection. He had a recent weight loss of 6 pounds in the week before admission and lost an additional 4 pounds during the week of hospitalization. His appetite is poor; he has frequent nausea and vomiting. His abdomen is soft, nontender, and bowel sounds are present. The health care provider orders enteral feedings to be started.
   a. What type of tube should be selected?
   b. How will the tube placement be verified?
   c. Describe the type of feeding and initiation of feedings.
   d. What complications should be assessed?

3. Two years after her husband died, Mrs. Cooper suffered a stroke and developed dysphagia. Develop a plan of care for assisting Mrs. Cooper with meals to reduce the risk of aspiration.

✳ NCLEX®-Style Review Questions

1. You are teaching a client about healthy nutrition. You recognize that the client understands the teaching when he states:
   1. I need to stop eating red meat
   2. I will increase the servings of fruit juice to four a day
   3. I will make sure that I eat a balanced diet and exercise regularly
   4. I will not eat so many dark green vegetables and eat more yellow vegetables

2. As a nurse, you teach a client who has had surgery to increase which nutrient to help with tissue repair?
   1. Fat
   2. Protein
   3. Vitamin
   4. Carbohydrate

3. You are caring for a client experiencing dysphagia. Which interventions will help decrease the risk of aspiration during feeding? (Choose all that apply.)
   1. Sit the client upright in a chair.
   2. Give liquids at the end of the meal.

3. Place food in the strong side of the mouth.
4. Provide thin foods to make it easier to swallow.
5. Feed the client slowly, allowing time to chew and swallow.
6. Encourage client to lie down to rest for 30 minutes after eating.

4. The nurse suspects that the client receiving PN through a CVC has an air embolus. What action does the nurse need to take first?
   1. Raise the head of the bed to 90 degrees.
   2. Turn client to left lateral decubitus position.
   3. Notify the health care provider immediately.
   4. Have the client perform the Valsalva maneuver.

5. Which action is initially taken by the nurse to verify correct position of a newly placed small-bore feeding tube?
   1. Place an order for x-ray examination to check position.
   2. Confirm the distal mark on the feeding tube after taping.
   3. Test the pH of the gastric contents, and observe the color.
   4. Auscultate over the gastric area as air is injected into the tube.

6. The catheter of the client receiving PN becomes occluded. Order the steps for caring for the occluded catheter in the order in which you would perform them.
   1. Attempt to aspirate a clot.
   2. Temporarily stop the infusion.
   3. Flush line with saline or heparin.
   4. Use a thrombolytic agent if ordered or per protocol.

7. Based on knowledge of peptic ulcer disease (PUD), the nurse anticipates the presence of which bacteria when reviewing the laboratory data for a client suspected of having PUD?
   1. *Micrococcus*
   2. *Staphylococcus*
   3. *Corynebacterium*
   4. *Helicobacter pylori*

8. You are assessing a client receiving enteral feedings via a small-bore nasointestinal tube. Which assessment findings need further intervention?
   1. Gastric pH of 6.0 during placement check
   2. Weight gain of 1 pound over the course of a week
   3. Active bowel sounds in the four abdominal quadrants
   4. Gastric residual aspirate of 300 mL for the second consecutive time

9. The home care nurse is seeing the following clients. Which client is at greatest risk for experiencing inadequate nutrition?
   1. A 55-year-old obese man recently diagnosed with diabetes mellitus
   2. A recently widowed 76-year-old woman recovering from a mild stroke
   3. A 22-year-old mother with a 3-year-old toddler who had tonsillectomy surgery
   4. A 46-year-old man recovering at home following coronary artery bypass surgery

45 | Urinary Elimination

OBJECTIVES

Mastery of content in this chapter will enable the student to:

- Describe the process of urination.
- Identify factors that commonly influence urinary elimination.
- Compare and contrast common alterations in urinary elimination.
- Obtain a nursing history for a client with urinary elimination problems.
- Identify nursing diagnoses appropriate for clients with alterations in urinary elimination.
- Obtain urine specimens.
- Describe characteristics of normal and abnormal urine.

- Describe the nursing implications of common diagnostic tests of the urinary system.
- Discuss nursing measures to promote normal micturition and reduce episodes of incontinence.
- Insert a urinary catheter.
- Discuss nursing measures to reduce urinary tract infection.
- Irrigate a urinary catheter.
- Identify two modalities of renal replacement therapy.

MEDIA RESOURCES KEY TERMS

 Companion CD
- NCLEX®-Style Review Questions
- Audio Glossary
- Interactive Learning Activities
- English/Spanish Glossary

 Website
- NCLEX®-Style Review Questions
- Audio Glossary
- English/Spanish Glossary
- Interactive Learning Activities
- Weblinks
- Audio Summaries
- Video Clips
- Nursing Skills Online

Anuria, p. 1133
Bacteremia, p. 1134
Bacteriuria, p. 1134
Catheterization, p. 1151
Cystitis, p. 1134
Diuresis, p. 1133
Dysuria, p. 1134
Erythropoietin, p. 1130
Hematuria, p. 1134
Ketonuria, p. 1141
Meatus, p. 1138
Micturition, p. 1131
Nephron, p. 1130
Nephrostomy, p. 1134
Nocturia, p. 1133
Nocturnal enuresis, p. 1135
Oliguria, p. 1133
Pelvic floor exercises (PFEs) (Kegel exercises), p. 1170

Polyuria, p. 1133
Proteinuria, p. 1130
Pyelonephritis, p. 1134
Reflex incontinence, p. 1132
Renal calculus, p. 1131
Renal replacement therapies, p. 1132
Renin, p. 1130
Residual urine, p. 1135
Specific gravity, p. 1140
Stoma, p. 1133
Uremic syndrome, p. 1132
Urinalysis, p. 1140
Urinary diversion, p. 1133
Urinary frequency, p. 1135
Urinary incontinence (UI), p. 1134
Urinary retention, p. 1133
Urosepsis, p. 1134

Normal elimination of urinary wastes is a basic function most people take for granted. When the urinary system fails to function properly, eventually all organ systems are affected. Clients with alterations in urinary elimination may also suffer emotionally from body image changes. The nurse needs to understand the reasons for urinary elimination problems, find acceptable solutions, and provide understanding and sensitivity to all clients' needs.

Scientific Knowledge Base

Urinary elimination depends on the function of the kidneys, ureters, bladder, and urethra. Kidneys remove wastes from the blood to form urine. Ureters transport urine from the kidneys to the bladder. The bladder holds urine until the urge to urinate develops. Urine leaves the body through the urethra. All organs of the urinary system must be intact and functional for successful removal of urinary wastes (Figure 45-1).

Kidney

The kidneys lie on either side of the vertebral column behind the peritoneum and against deep muscles of the back. Normally the left kidney is higher than the right because of the anatomical position of the liver.

Kidneys filter waste products of metabolism that collect in the blood. The blood reaches each kidney by a renal (kidney) artery that branches from the abdominal aorta. Approximately 20% to 25% of the cardiac output circulates each minute through the kidneys. The **nephron**, the functional unit of the kidney, forms the urine. The nephron is composed of the glomerulus, Bowman's capsule, proximal convoluted tubule, loop of Henle, distal tubule, and collecting duct (Figure 45-2).

A cluster of blood vessels forms the capillary network of the glomerulus, which is the initial site of filtration of the blood and the beginning of urine formation. The glomerular capillaries permit filtration of water, glucose, amino acids, urea, creatinine, and major electrolytes into Bowman's capsule. Large proteins and blood cells do not normally filter through the glomerulus. The presence of large proteins in the urine (**proteinuria**) is a sign of glomerular injury. The glomerulus filters approximately 125 mL of filtrate per minute.

Not all the glomerular filtrate is excreted as urine. About 99% of the filtrate is reabsorbed into the plasma, with the remaining 1% excreted as urine (Copstead and Banasik, 2005). The kidneys play a key role in fluid and electrolyte balance (see Chapter 41). Although output does depend on intake, the normal adult urine output is 1500 to 1600 mL/day. An output of less than 30 mL/hr indicates possible renal alterations.

The kidneys produce several substances vital to production of red blood cells (RBCs), blood pressure, and bone mineralization. The kidneys are responsible for maintaining a normal RBC volume by producing **erythropoietin.** Erythropoietin functions within the bone marrow to stimulate red blood cell production and maturation and prolongs the life of mature RBCs (Copstead and Banasik, 2005). Clients with chronic alterations in kidney function cannot produce sufficient quantities of this hormone; therefore they are prone to anemia.

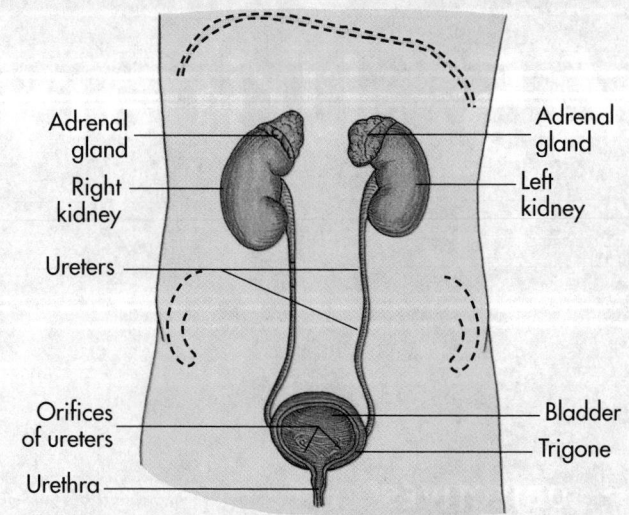

Figure 45-1 Organs of the urinary system.

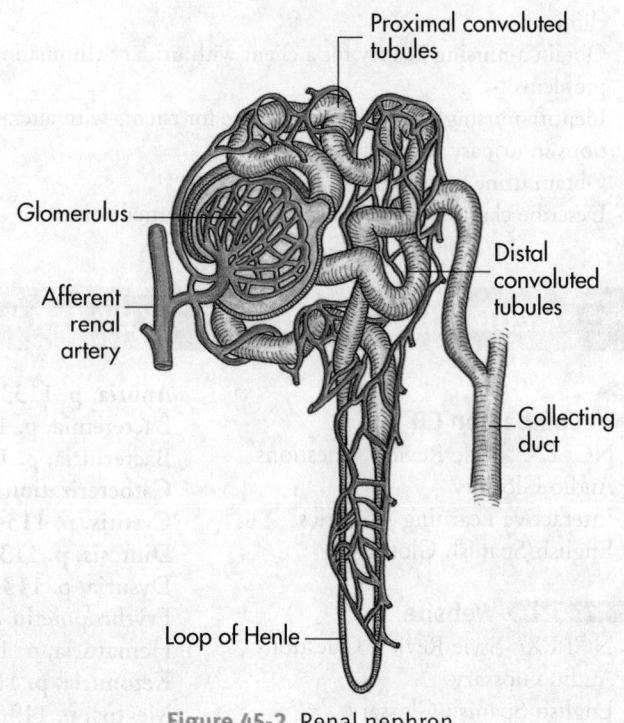

Figure 45-2 Renal nephron.

Renal hormones affect blood pressure regulation in several ways. In times of renal ischemia (decreased blood supply), **renin** is released from juxtaglomerular cells (Figure 45-3). Renin functions as an enzyme to convert angiotensinogen (a substance synthesized by the liver) into angiotensin I. Angiotensin I is converted to angiotensin II in the lungs. Angiotensin II causes vasoconstriction and stimulates aldosterone release from the adrenal cortex. Aldosterone causes retention of water, which increases blood volume. The kidneys also produce prostaglandin E_2 and prostacyclin, which help maintain renal blood flow through vaso-

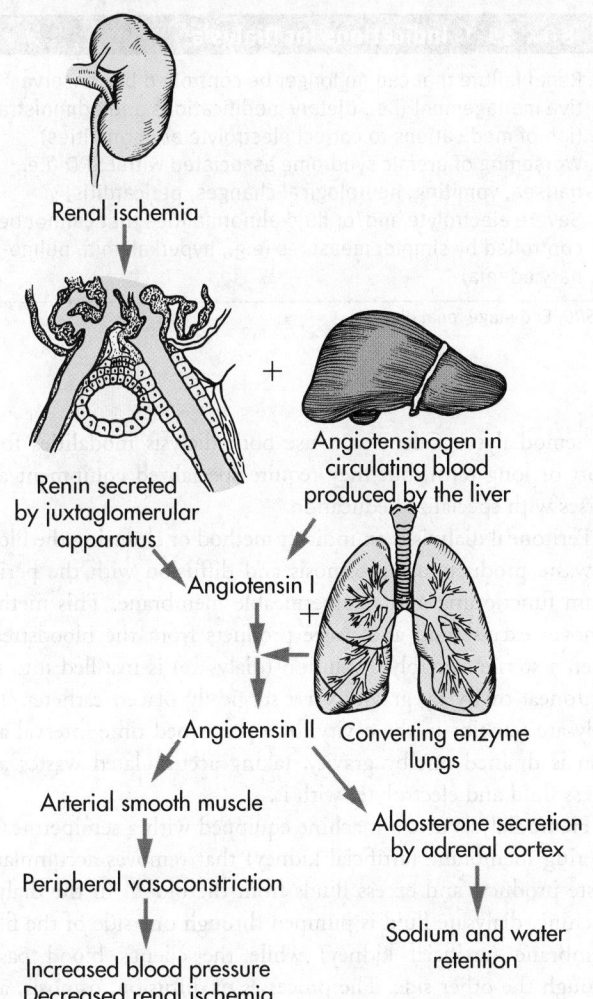

Figure 45-3 Physiological effects of renin-angiotensin mechanism.

dilation. These mechanisms increase arterial blood pressure and renal blood flow (Copstead and Banasik, 2005).

The kidneys affect calcium and phosphate regulation by producing a substance that converts vitamin D into its active form. Clients with chronic alterations in kidney function do not make sufficient amounts of the active vitamin D. They are prone to develop renal bone disease resulting from the demineralization of bone caused by impaired calcium absorption.

Ureters

The ureters are tubular structures that enter the urinary bladder. Urine draining from the ureters to the bladder is usually sterile.

Peristaltic waves cause the urine to enter the bladder in spurts rather than steadily. The ureters enter obliquely through the posterior bladder wall. This arrangement normally prevents the reflux of urine from the bladder into the ureters during the act of **micturition** by the compression of the ureter at the ureterovesical junction (the juncture of the ureters with the bladder). An obstruction within a ureter, such as a kidney stone (**renal calculus**), results in strong peristaltic waves that attempt to move the ob-

struction into the bladder. These strong peristaltic waves result in pain often referred to as renal colic.

Bladder

The urinary bladder is a hollow, distensible, muscular organ that stores and excretes urine. When empty, the bladder lies in the pelvic cavity behind the symphysis pubis. In men the bladder lies against the anterior wall of the rectum and in women it rests against the anterior walls of the uterus and vagina.

The bladder expands as it becomes filled with urine. Pressure within the bladder is usually low, even when partly full, a factor that protects against infection. When the bladder is full, it expands and extends above the symphysis pubis. A greatly distended bladder may reach the level of the umbilicus. In a pregnant woman the developing fetus pushes against the bladder, reducing the bladder's capacity and causing a feeling of fullness. This effect is more likely to occur in the first and third trimesters.

The trigone (a smooth triangular area on the inner surface of the bladder) is at the base of the bladder. An opening exists at each of the trigone's three angles. Two are for the ureters, and one is for the urethra.

Urethra

Urine travels from the bladder through the urethra and passes outside of the body through the urethral meatus. Normally the turbulent flow of urine through the urethra washes it free of bacteria. Mucous membrane lines the urethra, and urethral glands secrete mucus into the urethral canal. Thick layers of smooth muscle surround the urethra. In addition, the urethra descends through a layer of skeletal muscles called the pelvic floor muscles. When these muscles are contracted, it is possible to prevent urine flow through the urethra (Copstead and Banasik, 2005).

In women the urethra is approximately 4 to 6.5 cm (1½ to 2½ inches) long. The external urethral sphincter, located about halfway down the urethra, permits voluntary flow of urine. The short length of the urethra predisposes women and girls to infection. It is easy for bacteria to enter the urethra from the perineal area. In men the urethra, which is both a urinary canal and a passageway for cells and secretions from reproductive organs, is about 20 cm (8 inches) long. The male urethra has three sections: the prostatic urethra, the membranous urethra, and the penile urethra.

Act of Urination

Several brain structures influence bladder function, including the cerebral cortex, thalamus, hypothalamus, and brain stem. Together they may inhibit the urge to void or allow voiding. Normal voiding involves contraction of the bladder and coordinated relaxation of the urethral sphincter and pelvic floor muscles.

The bladder normally holds as much as 600 mL of urine. However, individuals are able to sense the desire to urinate when the bladder contains a smaller amount of urine (150 to 200 mL in an adult and 50 to 100 mL in a child). As the volume increases, the bladder walls stretch, sending sensory impulses to the micturition center in the sacral spinal cord. Impulses from the micturition center respond to or ignore this urge, thus making urination under voluntary control. If the person chooses not to void, the external urinary sphincter remains contracted, inhibiting the micturition reflex. However, when a person is ready to void, the external sphincter relaxes, the micturition reflex stimulates the detrusor muscle to contract, and efficient emptying of the bladder occurs. When a bladder is overfull, bladder pressure exceeds sphincter pressure and involuntary leakage of urine can occur.

Damage to the spinal cord above the sacral region causes loss of voluntary control of urination, but the micturition reflex pathway often remains intact, allowing urination to occur without sensation of the need to void. This condition is called a **reflex incontinence.** If a chronic obstruction such as prostate enlargement hinders bladder emptying, over time the micturition reflex changes, causing bladder overactivity, and can cause the bladder to not completely empty.

Factors Influencing Urination. Many factors influence the volume and quality of urine and the client's ability to urinate. Some pathophysiological conditions are acute and reversible (urinary tract infection), whereas others are chronic and irreversible (slow, progressive development of renal dysfunction). Sociocultural factors, psychological factors, fluid balance, and surgical and diagnostic procedures affect urine and urination in several ways. In addition, medications, including anesthesia, interfere with both the production and characteristics of urine and affect the act of urination.

Disease Conditions. Disease processes that affect urine elimination affect renal function (changes in urine volume or quality), the act of urine elimination, or both. Conditions that affect urine volume and quality are generally categorized as prerenal, renal, or postrenal in origin.

Decreased blood flow to and through the kidney (prerenal), disease conditions of the renal tissue (renal), or obstruction in the lower urinary tract that prevents urine flow from the kidneys (postrenal) sometimes alter renal function. Conditions of the lower urinary tract, including narrowing of the urethra, altered innervation of the bladder, or weakened pelvic and/or perineal muscles also affect urinary elimination.

Many diseases and conditions affect the ability to micturate. Diabetes mellitus and multiple sclerosis cause changes in nerve functions that can lead to possible loss of bladder tone, reduced sensation of bladder fullness, or inability to inhibit bladder contractions. Older men often suffer from benign prostatic hyperplasia (BPH), which makes them prone to urinary retention and incontinence. Some clients with cognitive impairments, such as Alzheimer's disease, lose the ability to sense a full bladder or are unable to recall the procedure for voiding. Diseases that slow or hinder physical activity interfere with the ability to void. Degenerative joint disease and Parkinsonism are examples of conditions that make it difficult to reach and use toilet facilities.

Diseases that cause irreversible damage to kidney tissue result in end-stage renal disease (ESRD). Eventually the client has symptoms resulting from **uremic syndrome.** An increase in nitrogenous wastes in the blood, marked fluid and electrolyte abnormalities, nausea, vomiting, headache, coma, and convulsions characterize this syndrome. As the uremic symptoms worsen, aggressive treatment is indicated for survival (Box 45-1). These treatments are **renal replacement therapies.**

Dialysis and organ transplantation are two methods of renal replacement. Dialysis takes one of two forms, peritoneal dialysis

✳ BOX 45-1 Indications for Dialysis
• Renal failure that can no longer be controlled by conservative management (i.e., dietary modifications and administration of medications to correct electrolyte abnormalities)
• Worsening of uremic syndrome associated with ESRD (i.e., nausea, vomiting, neurological changes, pericarditis)
• Severe electrolyte and/or fluid abnormalities that cannot be controlled by simpler measures (e.g., hyperkalemia, pulmonary edema)

ESRD, End-stage renal disease.

or hemodialysis. Clients can use both dialysis modalities for a short or long term, but they require specialized equipment and nurses with specialized education.

Peritoneal dialysis is an indirect method of cleansing the blood of waste products using osmosis and diffusion with the peritoneum functioning as a semipermeable membrane. This method removes excess fluid and waste products from the bloodstream when a sterile electrolyte solution (dialysate) is instilled into the peritoneal cavity by gravity via a surgically placed catheter. The dialysate remains in the cavity for a prescribed time interval and then is drained out by gravity, taking accumulated wastes and excess fluid and electrolytes with it.

Hemodialysis uses a machine equipped with a semipermeable filtering membrane (artificial kidney) that removes accumulated waste products and excess fluids from the blood. In the dialysis machine, dialysate fluid is pumped through one side of the filter membrane (artificial kidney) while the client's blood passes through the other side. The processes of diffusion, osmosis, and ultrafiltration cleanse the client's blood. Then the blood returns through a specially placed vascular access device (Gore-Tex graft, arteriovenous fistula, or hemodialysis catheter).

Organ transplantation is the replacement of the client's diseased kidneys with a healthy one from a living or cadaver donor of compatible blood and tissue type. The new organ is surgically implanted into the abdomen. Special medications (immunosuppressives) are administered for life to prevent the body from rejecting the transplanted organ. Unlike the other treatments, successful organ transplantation offers the client the potential for restoration of normal kidney function.

Sociocultural Factors. The degree of privacy needed for urination varies with cultural norms. North Americans expect toilet facilities to be private, whereas some European cultures accept communal toilet facilities. Social expectations (e.g., school recesses) influence the time of urination.

Psychological Factors. Anxiety and emotional stress cause a sense of urgency and increased frequency of urination. Anxiety often prevents a person from being able to urinate completely; as a result, the urge to void returns shortly after voiding. Emotional tension makes it difficult to relax abdominal and perineal muscles. Attempting to void in a public restroom sometimes results in a temporary inability to void. Privacy and adequate time to urinate are usually important to most people.

Fluid Balance. The kidneys primarily maintain the balance between retention and excretion of fluids (see Chapter 41). If fluids and the concentration of electrolytes and solutes are in equilibrium, an increase in fluid intake causes an increase in urine production. This amount varies with food and fluid intake. The volume of urine formed at night is about half of the volume formed during the day, because both intake and metabolism decline. **Nocturia** (awakening to void one or more times at night) is often a sign of renal alteration. In a healthy person the intake of water in food and fluids balances the output of water in urine, feces, and insensible losses in perspiration and respiration. An excessive output of urine is **polyuria**. A urine output that is decreased despite normal intake is called **oliguria**. Oliguria often occurs when fluid losses through other means increases (perspiration, diarrhea, or vomiting). It also occurs in early kidney disease. Oftentimes in severe kidney disease no urine is produced (**anuria**).

Ingestion of certain fluids directly affects urine production and excretion. Coffee, tea, cocoa, and cola drinks that contain caffeine promote increased urine formation (**diuresis**). Alcohol inhibits the release of antidiuretic hormone (ADH), also resulting in increased water loss in urine.

Febrile conditions affect urine production. The client with excessive perspiration loses a large amount of fluids through insensible water loss, which decreases urine production. Fever causes an increase in body metabolism and accumulation of body wastes. Although urine volume is reduced, it is highly concentrated.

Surgical Procedures. The stress of surgery initially triggers the general adaptation syndrome (see Chapter 31). The surgical client usually has altered fluid balance before surgery as a result of the disease process or preoperative fasting, which further reduces urine output. The stress response releases an increased amount of ADH, which increases water reabsorption. Stress also elevates the level of aldosterone, causing retention of sodium and water. Both of these substances reduce urine output in an effort to maintain circulatory fluid volume.

Anesthetics and narcotic analgesics slow the glomerular filtration rate, reducing urine output. These pharmacological agents also impair sensory and motor impulses traveling between the bladder, spinal cord, and brain. Clients are often unable to sense bladder fullness and are unable to initiate or inhibit micturition. Spinal anesthetics, in particular, create the risk of urinary retention because of an inability to sense the need to void and a possible inability of the bladder muscles and urethral sphincters to respond (Lewis and others, 2007).

Surgery of lower abdominal and pelvic structures sometimes impairs urination because of local trauma to surrounding tissues. After returning from surgery involving the ureters, bladder, and urethra, clients routinely have urinary catheters.

Medications. Diuretics prevent reabsorption of water and certain electrolytes to increase urine output. The use of anticholinergics (e.g., atropine) or antihistamines (e.g., diphenhydramine) often causes urinary retention. Some medications change the color of urine. Phenazopyridine (Pyridium) colors the urine a bright orange to rust; amitriptyline causes a green or blue discoloration, whereas levodopa discolors the urine to brown or black. Cancer chemotherapy drugs also color the urine and are often toxic to the kidneys or the bladder. Clients with impaired kidney function require dosage adjustments in medications excreted by the kidneys.

Diagnostic Examination. Examination of the urinary system influences micturition. Some procedures, such as an intrave-

nous pyelogram, require the client to limit fluids before the test. A restriction in fluid intake commonly lowers urine output. Diagnostic examinations (e.g., cystoscopy) involving direct visualization of urinary structures cause localized edema of the urethral passageway and spasm of the bladder sphincter. Post procedure the client may have difficulty voiding or have red or pink urine because of trauma to the urethral or bladder mucosa.

Alterations in Urinary Elimination. Most clients with urinary problems are unable to store urine or to fully empty the bladder. These disturbances result from impaired bladder function, obstruction to urine outflow, or inability to voluntarily control micturition.

Some clients may have permanent or temporary changes in the normal pathway of urinary excretion. The surgical formation of a **urinary diversion** temporarily or permanently bypasses the bladder and urethra as the exit routes for urine. Permanent urinary diversions are often necessary in the client with cancer of the bladder. The client with a urinary diversion has a **stoma** (artificial opening) on the abdomen to drain urine. The client with a urinary diversion has many special needs because urine drains to the outside through a stoma.

Urinary Retention. **Urinary retention** is an accumulation of urine resulting from an inability of the bladder to empty properly. Normally urine production slowly fills the bladder and prevents activation of stretch receptors until it distends to a certain level of stretch. The micturition reflex occurs, and the bladder empties. In urinary retention the bladder is unable to respond to the micturition reflex and thus is unable to empty. Urine continues to collect in the bladder, stretching its walls and causing feelings of pressure, discomfort, tenderness over the symphysis pubis, restlessness, and diaphoresis (sweating).

As retention progresses, retention with overflow develops. Pressure in the bladder builds to a point where the external urethral sphincter is unable to hold back urine. The sphincter temporarily opens to allow a small volume of urine (25 to 60 mL) to escape. As urine exits, the bladder pressure falls enough to allow the sphincter to regain control and close. With retention the client may void small amounts of urine 2 or 3 times an hour with no real relief of discomfort or may continually dribble urine. Be aware of the volume and frequency of voiding to assess this condition in the client. Assess the abdomen for evidence of bladder distention and tenderness.

In acute retention key signs are bladder distention and absence of urine output over several hours. The client under the influence of anesthetics or analgesics often feels only pressure, but the alert client has severe pain as the bladder distends beyond its normal capacity. In severe urinary retention the bladder holds as much as 2000 to 3000 mL of urine. Retention occurs as a result of urethral obstruction, surgical or childbirth trauma, alterations in motor and sensory innervation of the bladder, medication side effects, or anxiety.

Urinary Tract Infections. Urinary tract infections (UTIs) are responsible for more than 8.3 million health care provider visits a year (Mehnert-Kay, 2005). They are the most common health care–associated infection (HAI) in the United States, accounting for 40% of all HAIs (Foxman, 2002). Many urinary HAIs result from catheterization or surgical manipulation. Although several different microorganisms cause UTIs, *Escherichia coli* remains the most common causative pathogen, responsible for 75% to 95% of uncomplicated infections (Mehnert-Kay, 2005). **Bacteriuria** (bacteria in the urine) leads to the spread of organisms into the kidneys and possibly leads to **bacteremia** or **urosepsis** (bacteria in the bloodstream) (Lewis and others, 2007). Microorganisms commonly enter the urinary tract through the ascending urethral route. Bacteria inhabit the distal urethra and external genitalia in men and women, and the vagina in women. Organisms enter the urethral meatus easily and travel up the inner mucosal lining to the bladder. Women are more susceptible to infection because of a short urethra and the proximity of the anus to the urethral meatus. In men, prostatic secretions containing an antibacterial substance and the length of the urethra reduce the susceptibility to UTIs. However, men are at increased risk for infection-related renal disease. Older adults and clients with progressive underlying disease or decreased immunity are also at increased risk.

In a healthy person with good bladder function, organisms are flushed out during voiding. Residual (retained) urine in the bladder becomes more alkaline and is an ideal site for microorganism growth. Any condition resulting in urinary retention, such as a kinked, obstructed, or clamped catheter, increases the risk of a bladder infection.

Poor perineal hygiene is another cause of UTIs in women. Inadequate hand washing, failure to wipe from front to back after voiding or defecating, and frequent sexual intercourse predispose women to infection.

Clients with lower UTIs have pain or burning during urination (**dysuria**) as urine flows over inflamed tissues. Fever, chills, nausea, vomiting, and malaise develop as the infection worsens. An irritated bladder (**cystitis**) causes a frequent and urgent sensation of the need to void. Irritation to bladder and urethral mucosa results in blood-tinged urine (**hematuria**). The urine appears concentrated and cloudy because of the presence of white blood cells (WBCs) or bacteria. If infection spreads to the upper urinary tract (kidneys—**pyelonephritis**), flank pain, tenderness, fever, and chills are common.

Another common cause of infection is the introduction of instruments into the urinary tract. For example, the introduction of a catheter through the urethra provides a direct route for microorganisms. With an indwelling bladder catheter, bacteria ascend along the outside of the catheter on the urethral wall or travel up the catheter's lumen. Local irritation to the urethra or bladder predisposes tissues to bacterial invasion.

Urinary Incontinence. Urinary incontinence (UI) is the involuntary leakage of urine that is sufficient to be a problem (Mauk, 2005). It is either temporary or permanent. Leakage of urine is continuous or intermittent. Urinary incontinence related to urinary causes is called either stress or urge urinary incontinence (Palmer and Newman, 2007). Some clients may have a mixed form of incontinence that has features of both stress and urge urinary incontinence. Table 45-5 in a later section of this chapter describes the types of UI, their symptoms, and treatment interventions.

Incontinence often develops in people of every age; however, it is more common in older adults (Newman and Palmer, 2003). It is estimated that 15% to 30% of adult women experience UI. It is present in as many as 50% of nursing home residents and in 30%

of adults living at home (Mauk, 2005). Incontinence can impair body image and often leads to a loss of independence. Clothing becomes wet with urine, and the accompanying odor adds to embarrassment. As a result, clients with this problem often avoid social activities. Clients often fail to discuss this condition with health care providers or nurses, and as a result urinary incontinence is underreported and undertreated. Resources for information about continence care, client education, and treatment are available at the following websites: the Society for Urological Nurses and Associates (http://www.suna.org), the National Association for Continence (http://www.nafc.org) and the Simon Foundation (http://www.simonfoundation.org).

Older adults sometimes have special problems with incontinence because of physical limitations and environmental barriers. Older persons with restricted mobility have greater chances of being incontinent because of their inability to reach toilet facilities in time. Low-set chairs and beds raised well above the floor are obstacles for older adults who must get up to reach a toilet. Some clients often lack the energy to walk very far at one time. The toilet is sometimes too far away for clients with urge incontinence. Older clients who have difficulty undoing buttons or manipulating zippers face another obstacle.

Continued episodes of incontinence create the potential for skin breakdown. The character of urine changes when it remains in contact with skin, causing skin breakdown. The immobilized client with frequent incontinence is especially at risk for pressure ulcers (see Chapter 47). Additional health care and client education resources are available at the websites for the American Geriatrics Society (http://www.americangeriatrics.org) or the American Urogynecologic Society (http://www.augs.org).

Urinary Diversions. Some clients have a urinary stoma to divert the flow of urine from the kidneys directly to the abdominal surface for several reasons (e.g., trauma, cancer of the bladder, radiation injury to the bladder, fistulas, or chronic cystitis). Such a urinary diversion is either temporary or permanent (Figure 45-4).

The ileal loop or conduit involves separating a loop of intestinal ileum with its blood supply intact. The ureters are implanted into the isolated segment of ileum. The remaining ileum is reconnected to the rest of the digestive tract. The ileal segment is then used as a conduit for continuous urine drainage or fashioned into a continent reservoir (Copstead and Banasik, 2005). The client with an incontinent urinary diversion (ileal conduit) wears a stomal pouch continuously because there is no sphincter control for regulation of urine flow. Local irritation and skin breakdown occurs when urine comes in contact with the skin for long periods.

The continent pouch provides urinary storage in a leakproof pouch. The portion of the ileum connected to the abdominal wall acts as a continent nipple, requiring intermittent catheterization for emptying. The disadvantage of either an ileal conduit or reservoir is that if urine outflow is obstructed, irreversible damage to the kidneys occurs secondary to chronic infections or hydronephrosis.

Some clients have a need for urinary drainage directly from one or both kidneys. In this case a tube placed directly into the renal pelvis. This procedure is called a **nephrostomy.**

Any urinary diversion poses threats to a client's body image. The client must learn to manage the diversion, and those who do not have a continent urinary diversion must wear an artificial

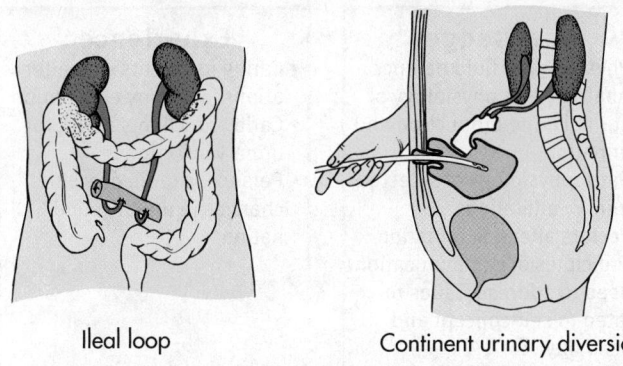

Ileal loop   Continent urinary diversion

Figure 45-4 Types of urinary diversions.

device to collect urine. However, most clients are able to wear normal clothing, engage in physical activity, travel, and have sexual relations.

Clients with a urinary diversion need a referral to an ostomy nurse (a nurse with specialized education in this area). This specialist is a valuable resource for assisting the client with matters pertaining to all aspects of care. The ostomy nurse will often meet with the client before surgery. Also, refer the client to the United Ostomy Associations of America (http://www.uoaa.org). This organization provides information about support groups to enhance coping and adaptation to lifestyle and body-image changes.

Nursing Knowledge Base

Urinary elimination is a basic function and is usually a private process. Many clients need physiological and psychological assistance from the nurse. Whether the client has an actual or potential urinary problem, be sensitive to the client's elimination needs. You will need knowledge of concepts beyond the anatomy and physiology of the urinary system to give appropriate care. In addition, you need to understand and apply knowledge about infection control principles, hygiene measures, growth and development, and psychosocial influences.

Infection Control and Hygiene

The urinary tract is sterile. Use infection control principles to help prevent the development and spread of urinary tract infections, as well as to treat existing infections. *E. coli,* a common bacteria found in feces, causes many UTIs. Infection can occur in any location of the urinary tract. Apply knowledge of medical and surgical asepsis when providing care involving the urinary tract or external genitalia (see Chapter 34). Any invasive procedure of the urinary tract, such as catheterization, requires sterile technique. Procedures such as perineal care or examination of the genitalia require medical asepsis, including proper hand hygiene.

Growth and Development

Growth and development factors determine the client's ability to control the act of urination during the life span. Infants and young children cannot effectively concentrate urine. Their urine appears light yellow or clear. In relation to their small body size,

infants and children excrete large volumes of urine. For example, a 6-month-old infant who weighs 6 to 8 kg (13 to 18 pounds) excretes 400 to 500 mL of urine daily.

As the neurological system matures, a toddler of 2 to 3 years is able to associate the sensations of bladder filling and urination. A child must be able to recognize the feeling of bladder fullness, to hold urine for 1 to 2 hours, and to communicate the sense of urgency. Many toddlers are then able to control the external sphincter, and toilet training begins. The young child needs parents' understanding, patience, and consistency. Daytime control of urination is easier to accomplish than nighttime control and occurs earlier in the child's development, usually by 2 to 3 years of age. Some children do not gain full control until age 4 or 5. Occasional daytime accidents or **nocturnal enuresis** (nighttime voiding without awakening) sometimes continue until age 5 (see Chapter 12).

During pregnancy urinary frequency is common, and susceptibility to urinary tract infection increases. Temporary or permanent changes resulting from repeated deliveries or hormonal changes often result in decreased perineal muscle tone, leading to urgency and stress incontinence (see Chapter 14).

Aging often impairs micturition. In men, prostate enlargement usually begins during the 40s and continues throughout life, resulting in urinary frequency and possible urinary retention. In women, changes in the urethral mucosa associated with loss of estrogen during and after menopause contribute to increased susceptibility to UTIs (Palmer and Newman, 2007).

Changes in kidney and bladder function also occur with aging. The kidney's ability to concentrate urine declines. The older adult often experiences nocturia. The bladder loses muscle tone and capacity decreases, resulting in increased **urinary frequency.** Because the bladder cannot contract effectively, an older adult often retains urine in the bladder after voiding (**residual urine**). These changes increase the risk for bacterial growth and development of UTIs.

Muscle Tone

Weak abdominal and pelvic floor muscles impair the ability of the urinary sphincter to maintain tone during increased abdominal pressure. Poor control of micturition or incontinence results from muscle wasting caused by prolonged immobility, muscle damage during vaginal childbirth, muscle atrophy secondary to menopause, or other traumatic damage to pelvic nerves and muscles.

Psychosocial Considerations

Remember that urinary elimination problems result in alterations of self-concept and sexuality. Self-concept, which includes body image, self-esteem, roles, and identity, develops over a life span. Because the penis is an organ for both urination and for sex, urinary dysfunction often greatly affects a man's self concept.

Gender influences positioning for urination: males stand, whereas females sit. Place clients in a position of comfort. Some men who cannot stand to urinate become overly distressed. In addition, gender differences also affect risk factors associated with urinary alterations. Men are at risk for urinary incontinence and have greater psychological distress related to UI (Gray, 2003). If a client prefers privacy, try to prevent interruptions as the client voids. Treat all clients with understanding and acceptance. Make sure your approach to a client's elimination needs consider personal, social, and gender habits.

Cultural Considerations

Culture influences the choice of appropriate nursing interventions. In some cultures the embarrassment related to urinary elimination problems is so great that many clients, especially women, refuse to seek treatment (Gray, 2003). In some cultures the client prefers to squat over a receptacle rather than sit on one. Culture dictates when and where it is appropriate to urinate. Culture also determines whether it is proper for a male to care for the urinary needs of a female or if gender-congruent care is needed (see Chapter 9).

Critical Thinking

Successful critical thinking requires synthesis of knowledge, experience, information gathered from clients, critical thinking attitudes, and intellectual and professional standards. Clinical judgments require you to collect necessary information, analyze the data, and anticipate and make decisions regarding client care.

During assessment consider all elements that build toward making appropriate nursing diagnoses. In the case of urinary elimination, integrate knowledge from nursing and other disciplines, previous experiences, and information gathered from clients to understand the process of urinary elimination and the impact on the client and family. As a result, you will be able to identify the unique impact of these problems on the client and family.

In addition, use critical thinking attitudes such as perseverance to find a plan of care to provide successful management of urinary elimination problems. Professional standards provide valuable directions for management.

When planning and implementing care for the client with alterations in urinary elimination, also use standards developed by professional organizations such as the International Continence Society, (ICS) American Nurses Association (ANA), and the United Ostomy Associations of America as a guide for individualized client care.

Nursing Process and Alterations in Urinary Function

◆Assessment

To identify a urinary elimination problem and gather data for a care plan, use scientific and nursing knowledge, conduct a nursing history, perform a physical assessment, assess the client's urine, and review information from diagnostic tests and examinations. Use critical thinking to synthesize this information as assessment proceeds (Figure 45-5). Adequate assessment results in the formulation of nursing diagnoses appropriate for alterations in urinary elimination. When assessing for problems with urinary elimina-

Knowledge
- Physiology of fluid balance
- Anatomy and physiology of normal urine production and urination
- Pathophysiology of selected urinary alterations
- Factors affecting urination
- Principles of communication used to address issues related to self-concept and sexuality

Experience
- Caring for clients with alterations in urinary elimination
- Caring for clients at risk for urinary infection
- Personal experience with changes in urinary elimination

ASSESSMENT
- Gather nursing history for the client's urination pattern, symptoms, and factors affecting urination
- Conduct physical assessment of the client's body systems potentially affected by urinary change
- Assess characteristics of urine
- Assess the client's perception of urinary problems as it affects self-concept and sexuality
- Gather relevant laboratory and diagnostic test data

Standards
- Maintain the client's privacy and dignity
- Apply intellectual standards to ensure client history and assessment are complete and in depth
- Apply professional standards of care from professional organizations such as ANA, International Continence Society (ICS), United Ostomy Associations of America

Attitudes
- Display humility in recognizing limitations in knowledge
- Establish trust with the client to reveal full picture of this potentially sensitive area of assessment

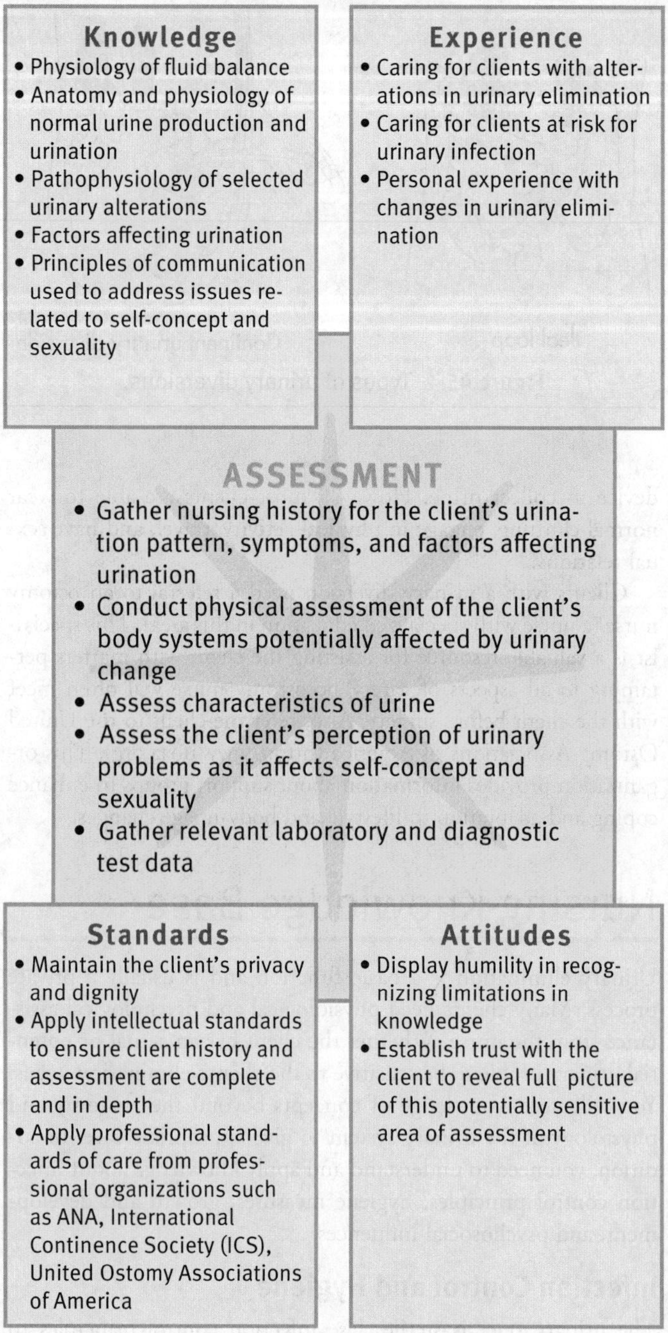

Figure 45-5 Critical thinking model for urinary elimination assessment.

tion, be aware of the impact of the client's culture and language in the assessment process (Box 45-2).

Nursing History. The nursing history includes a review of the client's elimination patterns and symptoms of urinary alterations and an assessment of other factors that are possibly affecting the ability to urinate normally. Use questions to help direct the client to focus on specific urinary problems (Box 45-3).

Pattern of Urination. Ask the client about daily voiding patterns, including frequency and times of day, normal volume at each voiding, and any recent changes. Frequency varies among individuals and varies with intake and other types of fluid losses.

✳ BOX 45-2 CULTURAL ASPECTS OF CARE

Urinary Elimination

Urine elimination is a personal, private activity that individuals do not share with others. When clients have needs related to urine elimination, be aware of the intrusive nature of intervention. In addition, other characteristics of the client, such 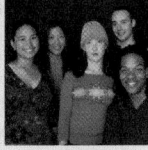 as culture, also affect care. Although you cannot be knowledgeable about every culture's impact on client care, it is important to be open to and respect practices different from your own.

Implications for Practice

- In communicating with clients when English is a second language use simple and clear sentences. Remember, speaking louder or more slowly does not always help. Learn at least a few important words in the client's language to allow for future interchanges. In some situations an interpreter is needed.
- Provide written materials, if available, in client's primary language. If not, then provide the English version. Some clients are able to read better than they understand the spoken word. Time to review the information also increases understanding.
- In some cultures intimate contact between genders is forbidden outside marriage. Urological care, whether involving questions or contact, is usually considered intimate care. Gender-congruent caregivers are assigned to a client from these cultures (e.g., Muslim culture).
- Cultures view disease differently. It is important to understand how the culture views the cause and treatment of the condition and how traditional Western medicine may or may not fit with that understanding.
- Cultures allow for varying involvement of the client's family in the client's care. This source of strength is important to the health of the client, and family must be included in the plan of care.
- Cultural influences may affect the willingness of the client to seek care.

Data from Chang MK, Harden JT: Meeting the challenge of the new millennium: caring for culturally diverse patients, *Urol Nurs* 22(6):372, 2002; and Gray ML: Gender, race, and culture in research on UI, *Am J Nurs* 103(3 suppl):20, 2003.

✳ BOX 45-3 NURSING ASSESSMENT QUESTIONS

Nature of the Problem
- What type of problems are you having with urination?
- Describe a recent day and or night when you were having urinary problems.
- Has this pattern remained constant, or do you have different patterns on different days/nights?

Signs and Symptoms
- Do you have urgency—feeling as though you have to void immediately?
- Do you ever lose some urine when you cough or sneeze?
- Does leakage occur at other times?

Onset and Duration
- When did you first notice a problem?
- How long has this problem lasted?

Severity
- How many times a day or night do you void or have leakage?
- How does this pattern compare with the pattern you last remember?
- What do you do when the symptoms occur?

Predisposing Factors
- Have you ever had a vaginal birth? More than once?
- Do you notice what you are doing at the time of urinary incidents?
- Do your symptoms increase after eating or drinking food with caffeine or alcohol?
- What medications do you routinely take, and have any recently changed?
- Do have a physical illness that may interfere with your usual urinary pattern?

Effect on Client
- How have these symptoms affected your life?
- Have you had to change any of your usual activities?
- Have you sought any health care assistance with this problem?

The common times for urination are on awakening, after meals, and before bedtime. Most people void an average of 5 or more times a day. Some clients who void frequently during the night may have renal disease, prostate enlargement, or cardiac disease. Information about the pattern of urination establishes a baseline for comparison.

Symptoms of Urinary Alterations. Certain symptoms specific to urinary alterations may occur in more than one type of disorder. During assessment ask the client about any symptoms related to urination (Table 45-1). Also assess whether the client is aware of conditions or factors that precipitate or aggravate symptoms. Likewise, it is important to determine what the client does when any of these symptoms occur.

Factors Affecting Urination. Summarize factors in the client's history that normally affect urination such as age, environmental factors, medication history, psychological factors, muscle tone, fluid balance, current surgical or diagnostic procedures, and presence of disease conditions. Be alert to individual needs related to normal changes of aging that predispose older adults to certain elimination problems (Box 45-4). Consider the bowel elimination pattern, because constipation often interferes with normal urine elimination. Evaluate environmental barriers in the home or health care setting. Such aids as elevated toilet seats, grab bars, or a portable commode are often necessary.

Note the presence of an indwelling catheter. An indwelling catheter places a client at risk for infection, catheter blockage, or skin care problems (Getliffe, 2003). Monitor fluid balance through regular intake and output (I&O) measurements (see Chapter 41). Clients with a urinary diversion sometimes need special assistance to maintain adequate urine elimination and skin care integrity.

Physical Assessment. A physical examination (see Chapter 33) provides you with data to determine the presence and severity of urinary elimination problems. The primary structures to assess include the skin and mucosal membranes, kidneys, bladder, and urethral meatus.

✳ TABLE 45-1 Common Types of Urinary Alterations

SYMPTOMS	DESCRIPTIONS	CAUSES OR ASSOCIATED FACTORS
Urgency	Feeling of need to void immediately	Full bladder, bladder irritation or inflammation from infection, overactive bladder, psychological stress
Dysuria	Painful or difficult urination	Bladder inflammation, trauma or inflammation of urethral sphincter
Frequency	Voiding at frequent intervals (<2 hr)	Increased fluid intake, bladder inflammation, increased pressure on bladder (pregnancy), diuretic therapy
Hesitancy	Difficulty initiating urination	Prostate enlargement, anxiety, urethral edema
Polyuria	Voiding large amounts of urine	Excess fluid intake, diabetes mellitus or insipidus, use of diuretics, postobstructive diuresis
Oliguria	Diminished urinary output relative to intake (usually 400 mL/24 hr)	Dehydration, renal failure, UTI, increased ADH secretion, congestive heart failure
Nocturia	Voiding one or more times at night	Excessive fluid intake before bed (especially coffee or alcohol), renal disease, aging process, prostate enlargement
Dribbling	Leakage of urine despite voluntary control of urination	Stress incontinence, overflow from urinary retention (e.g., from BPH)
Incontinence	Involuntary loss of urine	Multiple factors: unstable urethra, loss of pelvic muscle tone, fecal impaction, neurological impairment, overactive bladder
Hematuria	Blood in the urine	Neoplasms of the kidney or bladder, glomerular disease, infection of kidney or bladder, trauma to urinary structures, calculi, bleeding disorders
Retention	Accumulation of urine in the bladder, with inability of bladder to empty fully	Urethral obstruction (stricture), decreased sensory activity, neurogenic bladder, prostate enlargement, postanesthesia effects, side effects of medications (e.g., anticholinergics, opioid narcotics)
Residual urine	Volume of urine remaining after voiding (>100 mL)	Inflammation or irritation of bladder mucosa from infection, neurogenic bladder, prostate enlargement, trauma, or inflammation of urethra

ADH, Antidiuretic hormone; *BPH*, benign prostatic hyperplasia; *UTI*, urinary tract infection.

✳ BOX 45-4   FOCUS ON OLDER ADULTS

Promoting Urinary Health

- High-quality nursing care is essential in care of the older adult. When older adults become dependent on others for personal care, maintenance of their urinary health falls into the domain of nursing practice (Specht, 2005).
- Dilute urine discourages bacterial growth, so encourage older adults to increase their fluid intake to at least six to eight glasses a day, unless medically contraindicated (Gray and Krissovich, 2003).
- Make fluids, such as cranberry juice, available as part of the client's fluid intake. Cranberry juice discourages bacterial adherence to the bladder wall (Gray, 2002; Lynch, 2004).
- Restricting fluid intake does not decrease urinary incontinence severity or frequency. However, transient restriction, 2 hours before sleep, combined with nocturnal toileting diminished the severity of UI (Gray and Krissovich, 2003).
- Do not use indwelling catheters routinely in older adults. If one is necessary, use it no longer than necessary. The risk of infection increases dramatically for catheterized clients (Fernandez and Griffiths, 2006).
- Note that incontinence is not a normal part of aging, and make efforts to assess incontinence and provide interventions to promote return to continence (Specht, 2005).

Skin and Mucosal Membranes. Observe the condition of the skin and mucosal membranes. Problems with urinary elimination are frequently associated with fluid and electrolyte disturbances. By assessing skin turgor and the oral mucosa you gather data about the client's hydration status. Urinary incontinence increases the risk for skin breakdown. Observe the perineum for rashes, blistering, irritation, and breakdown.

Kidneys. Nurses with advanced examination skills learn to palpate the kidneys during abdominal examination. The kidneys' position, shape, and size reveal problems such as tumors, whereas tenderness indicates inflammation. Auscultation is sometimes performed to detect the presence of a renal artery bruit (sound resulting from turbulent blood flow through a narrowed artery).

Bladder. In adults the bladder rests below the symphysis pubis. When the bladder is distended, it rises above the symphysis pubis at the midline of the abdomen and often extends to just below the umbilicus. On inspection you may note a swelling or convex curvature of the lower abdomen. Gently palpate the lower abdomen. The partially filled bladder normally feels smooth and rounded. Gentle palpation on a distended bladder causes the client to feel the urge to urinate, tenderness, or even pain. Percussion of a full bladder yields a dull percussion note.

Urethral Meatus. Observe the urinary **meatus** for any discharge, inflammation, and lesions. To examine the female, a dorsal recumbent position provides full exposure of the genitalia. While wearing clean gloves, retract the labial folds to see the urethral meatus. Normally the meatus is pink and appears as a small slitlike opening below the clitoris and above the vaginal orifice. Normally there is no discharge from the meatus; if present, obtain specimens of urethral discharge before the client voids.

Women with vaginal infections are susceptible to UTIs because it is easy for the drainage to travel to the urethral meatus. Older women may have vaginitis as a result of estrogen deficiency. Inspect the vaginal orifice carefully for signs of inflammation, and describe any drainage.

A man's urethral meatus is normally a small opening at the tip of the penis. Inspect the meatus for discharge, inflammation, and lesions. It is necessary to retract the foreskin in uncircumcised men to see the meatus. Wear clean gloves when retracting the foreskin. Be sure to replace the foreskin after the examination is complete.

Assessment of Urine. Assessment of urine involves measuring the client's fluid intake and output and observing characteristics of the client's urine.

Intake and Output. Assess the client's average daily fluid intake. If you need an accurate measurement of fluid intake from the client who is at home, ask the client to estimate his or her intake by showing a measurement on a commonly used glass or cup.

In a health care setting measure a client's fluid intake either when the health care provider orders I&O measurements or when you need a more precise measurement (see Chapter 41). A change in urine volume is a significant indicator of fluid alterations or kidney disease. While caring for the client, use a graduated receptacle to measure urinary output from a bedpan or urinal after each voiding. Special receptacles (urimeters) attach between indwelling catheters and drainage bags and are a convenient means of accurately measuring urine volume. A urimeter holds 100 to 200 mL of urine. After measuring urine from a urimeter, drain the cylinder into the urinary drainage bag or into a receptacle for disposal. Urimeters are indicated when precise hourly measurements of urine are necessary.

When you measure urine from a drainage bag, the use of a separate plastic graduated measuring receptacle obtains a more precise measurement of urine output (Figure 45-6). Each client needs to have a graduated receptacle for his or her exclusive use to prevent potential cross contamination.

Report any extreme increase or decrease in volume. An hourly output of less than 30 mL for more than 2 hours is cause for concern. Similarly, you need to report consistently high volumes of urine (polyuria), over 2000 to 2500 mL daily.

Characteristics of Urine. Inspect the client's urine for color, clarity, and odor.

Color. Normal urine ranges from a pale, straw color to amber, depending on its concentration. Urine is usually more concentrated in the morning or with fluid volume deficits. As the person drinks more fluids, urine becomes less concentrated.

Bleeding from the kidneys or ureters causes urine to become dark red; bleeding from the bladder or urethra causes a bright red urine. Various medications and foods also change urine color. For example, Pyridium, a urinary analgesic, colors the urine bright orange. Eating beets, rhubarb, or blackberries causes red urine. Special dyes used in intravenous diagnostic studies eventually discolor urine. Dark amber urine is the result of high concentrations of bilirubin caused by liver dysfunction. Document and report any abnormal color or sediment, especially if the cause is unknown.

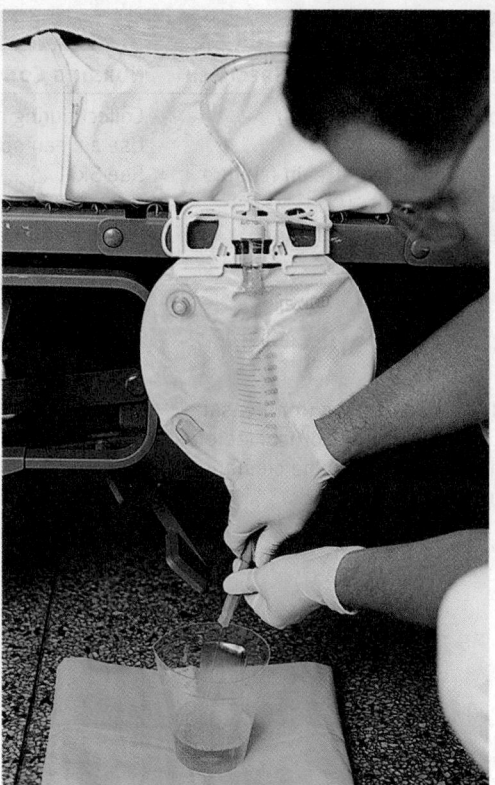

Figure 45-6 Urine drainage bag.

Clarity. Normal urine appears transparent at voiding. Urine that stands in a container becomes cloudy. Freshly voided urine in clients with renal disease will appear cloudy or foamy because of high protein concentrations. Urine also appears thick and cloudy as a result of bacteria and white blood cells.

Odor. Urine has a characteristic odor. The more concentrated the urine, the stronger the odor. Stagnant urine has an ammonia odor, which is common in clients who are repeatedly incontinent. A sweet or fruity odor occurs from acetone or acetoacetic acid (by-products of incomplete fat metabolism) seen with diabetes mellitus or starvation.

Urine Testing. Nurses often collect urine specimens for laboratory testing. The type of test determines the method of collection. Label all specimens with the client's name, date, and time of collection. Transport specimens to the laboratory in a timely fashion to ensure accuracy of test results. Agency infection control policies require the adherence to standard precautions by all personnel during specimen handling (see Chapter 34).

Specimen Collection. The nurse collects random, clean-voided or midstream, sterile, and timed specimens (Table 45-2). The method of collection varies based on the client's developmental level and the type of specimen ordered.

Urine Collection in Children. Specimen collection from infants and children is often difficult. Adolescents and school-age children are usually able to cooperate, although some will be embarrassed. Preschool children and toddlers have difficulty voiding on request. It often helps to offer the child fluids 30 minutes before requesting a specimen. You need to use terms for urination

✳ TABLE 45-2 Urine Testing

COLLECTION TYPE/USE OF SPECIMEN	NURSING CONSIDERATIONS
Random (routine urinalysis)	Collect during normal voiding, from an indwelling catheter or urinary diversion collection bag. Use a clean specimen cup.
Clean-voided or midstream (culture and sensitivity)	See Skill 45-1. Use a sterile specimen cup.
Sterile specimen (culture and sensitivity)	If the client has an indwelling catheter, collect a sterile specimen by using aseptic technique through the special sampling port (Figure 45-7) found on the side of the catheter. Clamp the tubing below the port, allowing fresh, uncontaminated urine to collect in the tube. After wiping the port with an antimicrobial swab, insert a sterile syringe hub and withdraw at least 3 to 5 mL of urine (check agency policy). Using sterile aseptic technique, transfer the urine to a sterile container (see Chapter 34).
Timed urine specimens (for measuring levels of adrenocortical steroids or hormones, creatinine clearance, or protein quantity tests)	Time required may be 2-, 12-, or 24-hour collections. The timed period begins after the client urinates and ends with a final voiding at the end of the time period. The client voids into a clean receptacle, and the urine is transferred to the special collection container, which often contains special preservatives. Each specimen must be free of feces and toilet tissue. Missed specimens make the whole collection inaccurate. Check with agency policy and the laboratory for specific instructions.

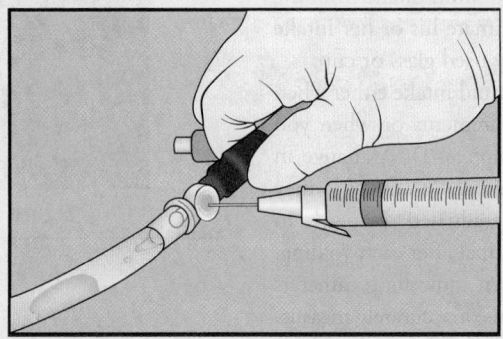

Figure 45-7 Urine specimen collection: aspiration from a collection port in drainage tubing of an indwelling catheter (needleless technique).

that the child is able understand. A young child is often reluctant to void in unfamiliar receptacles. A potty chair or specimen hat placed under the toilet seat is usually effective. You will need to use special collection devices for infants or toddlers who are not toilet trained. You can attach clear plastic, single-use bags with self-adhering material over the child's urethral meatus. Do not obtain specimens by squeezing urine from the diaper material because the results will be inaccurate.

Common Urine Tests

Urinalysis. The laboratory performs a **urinalysis** on a specimen obtained by any of the previously described methods. Table 45-3 lists normal values for a urinalysis. Examine the specimen as soon as possible, preferably within 2 hours. Make sure it is the first voided specimen in the morning to ensure a uniform concentration of constituents. For a quick screening perform certain portions of the urinalysis with special reagent strips. You dip the strips into the urine and then observe for a color change in the time interval designated on the package (Figure 45-8).

Specific Gravity. The **specific gravity** is the weight or degree of concentration of a substance compared with an equal volume

of water. Pour a urine specimen into a special clean, dry cylinder. The weighted urinometer is suspended in the cylinder of urine. The concentration of dissolved substances in the urine aids in determination of a client's fluid balance. This measurement is always part of a complete urinalysis. Nurses in critical care units are often responsible for doing periodic measurements of urine specific gravity.

If questions regarding the accuracy of specific gravity measurements arise, obtain a urine osmolality test. Although both tests measure urine concentration, the osmolality test is more accurate because it measures the total number of particles in a solution (see Chapter 41).

Urine Culture. A urine culture requires a sterile or clean-voided sample of urine. It takes approximately 24 to 48 hours before the laboratory can report findings of bacterial growth. While awaiting results, a broad-spectrum antibiotic is sometimes ordered as soon as a culture has been obtained. The test for sensitivity determines which specific antibiotics are effective. The results (sensitivities) of a urine culture may show that another antibiotic would be more effective. In this case a new antibiotic is ordered.

TABLE 45-3 Routine Urinalysis

MEASUREMENT AND NORMAL VALUE	INTERPRETATION
pH (4.6-8.0)	pH of urine will indicate acid-base balance. An acid pH helps protect against bacterial growth. Urine that stands for several hours becomes alkaline.
Protein (none or up to 8 mg/100 mL)	Normally protein is not present in urine. It is common in renal disease because damage to glomeruli or tubules allows protein to enter urine.
Glucose (none)	Clients with diabetes mellitus often have glucose in urine as a result of inability of tubules to reabsorb high glucose concentrations (>180 mg/100 mL). Ingestion of high concentrations of glucose causes some glucose to appear in urine of healthy persons.
Ketones (none)	Clients whose diabetes mellitus is poorly controlled experience breakdown of fatty acids. End products of fat metabolism are ketones. Some clients with dehydration, starvation, or excessive aspirin usage also have **ketonuria.**
Blood	A positive test for occult blood occurs when intact erythrocytes, hemoglobin, or myoglobin is present. In women, blood in a routine urine specimen may be a result of contamination with menstrual fluid.
Specific gravity (1.0053-1.030)	Specific gravity measures concentration of particles in urine. High specific gravity reflects concentrated urine, and low specific gravity reflects diluted urine. Dehydration, reduced renal blood flow, and increased ADH secretion elevate specific gravity. Overhydration, early renal disease, and inadequate ADH secretion reduce specific gravity.
Microscopic Examination	
RBCs (up to 2)	Damage to glomeruli or tubules allows RBCs to enter the urine. Trauma, disease, or surgery of the lower urinary tract also causes blood to be present.
WBCs (0-4 per low-power field)	Greater numbers indicate urinary tract infection.
Bacteria (none)	Bacteria indicate urinary tract infection. (Client do not always have symptoms.)
Casts (none)	Casts are cylindrical bodies whose shapes take on likeness of objects within the renal tubule. Types include hyaline, WBCs, RBCs, granular cells, and epithelial cells. Their increased presence is always an abnormal finding and indicates renal alterations.
Crystals (none)	Crystals are result of food metabolism. Excess crystals such as uric acid or calcium phosphate result in renal stone formation.

Data from Pagana KD, Pagana TJ: *Mosby's diagnostic and laboratory test reference,* ed 8, St. Louis, 2007, Mosby.
ADH, Antidiuretic hormone; *RBCs,* red blood cells; *WBCs,* white blood cells.

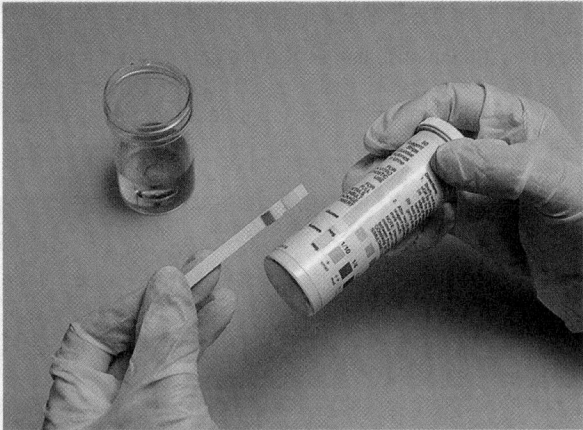

Figure 45-8 Checking results of a chemical reagent strip dipped in urine.

✳ **SKILL 45-1**   **COLLECTING MIDSTREAM (CLEAN-VOIDED) URINE SPECIMEN**

Delegation Considerations

The skill of collecting midstream (clean-voided) urine specimens can be delegated. If appropriate, you can instruct an alert client who is physically able to collect the specimen. It is the nurse's responsibility to ensure that this specimen is obtained correctly and in a timely manner. Be aware of agency policy regarding specimen collection. The nurse instructs nursing assistive personnel to:

- Inform the nurse when the specimen was obtained
- Inform the nurse if client is unable to initiate a stream or has pain or burning on urination
- Inform the nurse if the collected specimen is dark, bloody, or cloudy, is odorous, or contains mucus

Equipment

- Soap or cleansing solution, washcloth, and towel
- Commercial kit for clean-voided specimen or individual supplies as listed
  - Sterile cotton balls or sterile 2 × 2 or 4 × 4 gauze pads
  - Antiseptic solution (e.g., chlorhexidine or povidone-iodine); check for client allergy; if allergic, provide an alternative
  - Sterile water or sterile saline
- Sterile specimen collection cup or jar
- Sterile and clean gloves
- Bedpan, bedside commode, or specimen hat
- Completed specimen label
- Completed laboratory requisition form

STEPS	RATIONALE
1. Assess voiding status of client.	
a. When client last voided	Indicates bladder fullness.
b. Level of awareness or developmental stage	Reveals client's ability to cooperate during procedure.
c. Mobility, balance, and physical limitations	Determines level of assistance in acquiring specimen.
2. Assess client's understanding of purpose of test and method of collection.	Information allows you to clarify misunderstandings and promotes client cooperation.
3. Provide fluids to drink ½ hour before collection unless contraindicated (i.e., fluid restriction) if client does not feel urge to void.	Improves likelihood of client being able to void.
4. Explain procedure to client:	Helps client understand the procedure.
a. Reason midstream specimen is necessary	
b. Ways for client and family to assist	
c. Ways to obtain specimen free of feces	Feces change characteristics of urine and cause abnormal values.
d. Use visual aids (if applicable) to explain procedure	Illustrations demonstrating midstream collection techniques help to clarify a complex procedure, especially with clients for whom English is a second language.
5. Identify client, and perform hand hygiene.	Ensures accuracy of specimen identification. Decreases likelihood of transfer of microorganisms.
6. Provide privacy for client by closing door or bed curtain.	Privacy allows client to relax and produce specimen more quickly.
7. Give client or family members cleansing towelette, soap, washcloth, and towel to cleanse perineal area, or assist client as needed.	Client often prefers to wash own perineal area. Cleansing prevents contamination of specimen as urine passes from urethra.
8. Assist client who cannot ambulate onto bedpan. Raise head of bed.	Provides easy access to perineal area to collect specimen. Semisitting position may ease voiding.
9. Using surgical asepsis, open sterile kit (see illustration), or prepare sterile supplies.	Sterile technique is essential to maintaining sterility of equipment and specimen.

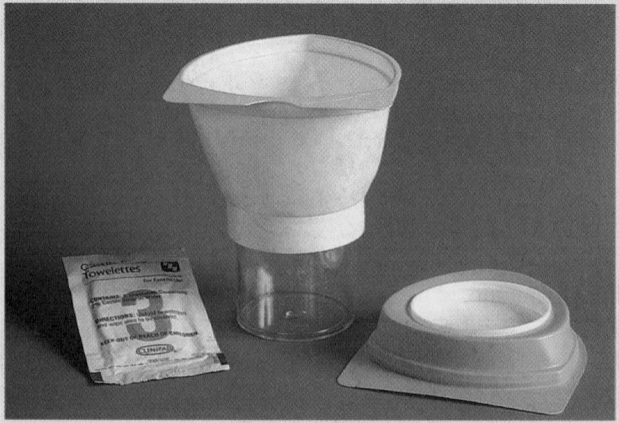

STEP 9 Commercial midstream urine collection kit.

✳ SKILL 45-1 COLLECTING MIDSTREAM (CLEAN-VOIDED) URINE SPECIMEN—CONT'D

STEPS	RATIONALE
10. Apply sterile gloves after opening sterile specimen cup, placing cap with sterile inside surface up, and do not touch inside of container or cap (see Chapter 34).	Sterile gloves prevent introduction of microorganisms from nurse's hands to specimen. Contaminated specimen is most frequent reason for inaccurate reporting of urine cultures and sensitivities.
11. Pour antiseptic solution over cotton balls or gauze pads unless kit contains prepared gauze pads in antiseptic solution.	Cotton balls or gauze pads will be used to further cleanse the perineum.
12. Perform urine collection by assisting or allowing client to independently cleanse perineum and collect specimen: A. **Female**	

Critical Decision Point: If client is menstruating, record this information on laboratory requisition form.

(1) Spread labia with thumb and forefinger of nondominant hand.	Provides access to urethral meatus.
(2) Cleanse area with cotton ball or gauze, moving from front (above urethral orifice) to back (toward anus). Using a fresh swab each time, repeat front-to-back motion three times (begin with left side, then right side, then center) (see illustration).	Cleanse from area of least contamination to area of greatest contamination to decrease bacterial levels.
(3) If agency policy indicates, rinse area with sterile water, and dry with dry cotton ball or gauze.	Prevents contamination of specimen with antiseptic solution.
(4) While continuing to hold labia apart, have client initiate stream. After client achieves a stream, pass container into stream and collect 30 to 60 mL (see illustration).	Initial stream flushes out microorganisms that accumulate at urethral meatus and prevents transfer into specimen.
B. **Male**	
(1) Hold penis with one hand, and using circular motion and antiseptic swab, cleanse end of penis, moving from center to outside (see illustration). In uncircumcised men, retract the foreskin before cleansing.	Cleanse from area of least contamination to area of greatest contamination to decrease bacterial levels.
(2) If agency procedure indicates, rinse area with sterile water, and dry with cotton or gauze.	Prevents contamination of specimen with antiseptic solution.
(3) After client has initiated urine stream, pass specimen collection container into stream, and collect 30 to 60 mL (see illustration).	Initial stream flushes out microorganisms that accumulate at urethral meatus and prevents transfer into specimen.

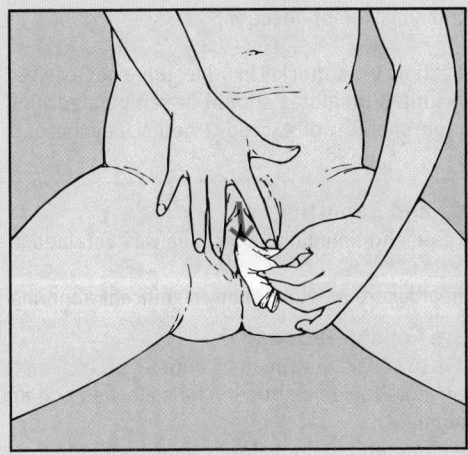

STEP 12A(2) Cleansing technique (female).

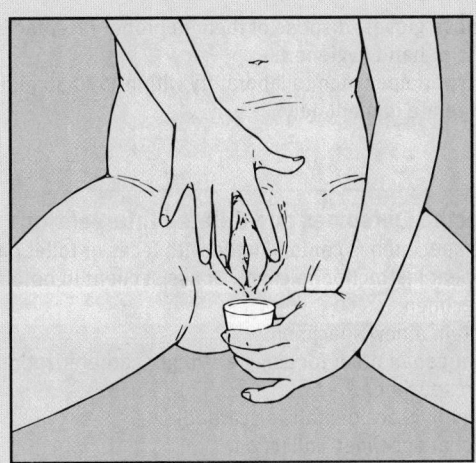

STEP 12A(4) Specimen collection (female).

Continued

✳ **SKILL 45-1** **COLLECTING MIDSTREAM (CLEAN-VOIDED) URINE SPECIMEN—CONT'D**

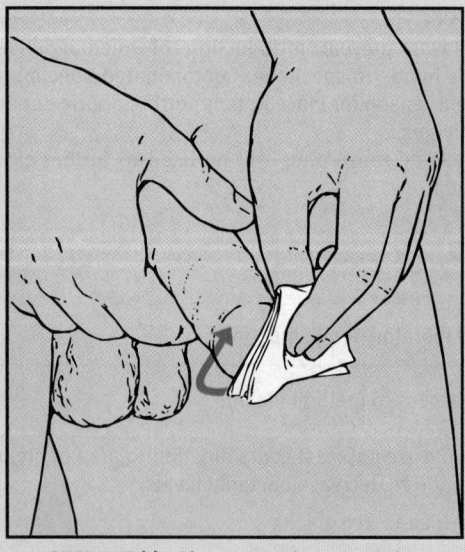

STEP 12B(1) Cleansing technique (male).

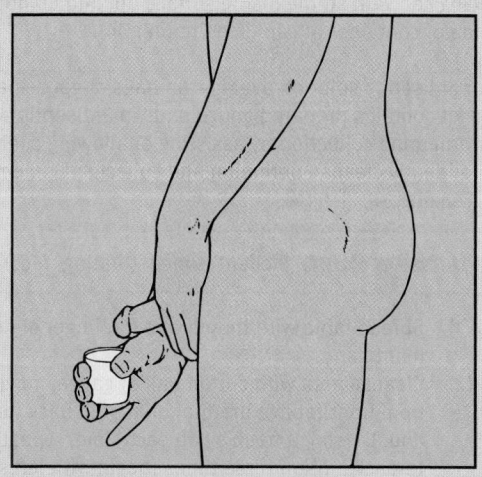

STEP 12B(3) Specimen collection (male).

STEPS	RATIONALE
13. Remove specimen container before flow of urine stops and before releasing labia or penis. Client finishes voiding in bedpan or toilet.	Prevents contamination of specimen with skin flora.

Critical Decision Point: If foreskin was retracted for specimen collection, replace it over the glans. If foreskin is not replaced, swelling and constriction will occur, causing pain and possible obstruction to urine flow.

STEPS	RATIONALE
14. Replace cap securely on specimen container (touch outside only).	Retains sterility of inside of container and prevents spillage of urine.
15. Cleanse any urine from exterior surface of container, and place in a plastic specimen bag as required by agency.	Prevents transfer of microorganisms to others.
16. Remove and empty bedpan (if applicable), and assist client to comfortable position.	Promotes relaxing environment.
17. Label specimen, and attach laboratory requisition.	Prevents inaccurate identification and minimizes errors in diagnosis or treatment.
18. Remove gloves, dispose of them in proper receptacle, and perform hand hygiene.	Reduces transmission of infection.
19. Transport specimen to laboratory within 15 to 30 minutes, or refrigerate immediately.	Because bacteria grow quickly in urine, urine not received by laboratory within 30 minutes should be refrigerated. However, refrigeration should not exceed 2 hours (Pagana and Pagana, 2007).

Unexpected Outcomes and Related Interventions

1. Urine specimen is contaminated with feces or toilet paper.
   a. Repeat instruction to client, or assist client in obtaining specimen.
   b. Obtain a new specimen.
   c. Request an order for using a straight catheterization to obtain specimen.
2. Specimen is accidentally discarded.
   a. Repeat specimen collection.

Recording and Reporting

- Record date and time urine specimen was obtained in nurses' notes.
- Notify health care provider of any significant abnormalities.

Home Care Considerations

- If client is to collect specimen as outpatient, a clean technique may be used. Provide instruction for collection and appropriate equipment.
- Provide information about storing specimen until time for delivery to physician's office or hospital laboratory.

NURSING CARE PLAN
Stress Urinary Incontinence

Assessment

Mrs. Kay, the nurse, is seeing Mrs. Grayson, a 55-year-old woman, for symptoms of urinary incontinence. Mrs. Grayson is postmenopausal, has a history of three vaginal births, and is "overweight." She lives with her husband, and her three grown children live nearby. Mrs. Grayson works as a secretary for a local social service

agency. She confided to her gynecological practitioner that uncontrollable urine leakage has affected her life. Mrs. Kay's assessment included a discussion of Mrs. Grayson's current health status with emphasis on her urinary concerns.

Assessment Activities	Findings/Defining Characteristics*
Ask Mrs. Grayson about the effects of her urinary symptoms on her daily life.	She responds, "I find myself being embarrassed and frustrated for **losing control**. If my bladder is a little full, I **dribble** easily just picking something up or when I'm on my way to the bathroom. I'm afraid to laugh any more, because that is another time I **leak urine**. At work I try to avoid being close to my co-workers because I am afraid I might have an odor."
Ask her what she has been doing about her condition.	She states that she has been wearing "one of those little pads" all the time now.
Ask Mrs. Grayson about any other effects that her leakage has caused.	Mrs. Grayson begins to cry and states, "You know, I don't even like to go out to the movies or a party anymore. It is safer to stay home. I have problems being intimate with my husband because of leaking. We used to go to dancing occasionally, but we don't do that anymore."
Observe Mrs. Grayson's behavior.	Mrs. Grayson appears anxious and is slowly pacing the floor.
Take a focused nursing history addressing urinary leakage and other lower urinary tract symptoms.	Mrs. Grayson's report of **urine leakage upon physical exertion, sneezing, and laughing** increases the likelihood of a diagnosis of stress incontinence. Her risk factors for this condition include a **history of three pregnancies**, being **postmenopausal**, and being **overweight**. The history will help define the proper interventions.

*__Defining characteristics__ are shown in bold type.

Nursing Diagnosis: Stress urinary incontinence related to weakened pelvic musculature.

Planning

Goals	Expected Outcomes (NOC)†
	Urinary Continence
Mrs. Grayson will have reduced episodes of urine leakage (incontinence) between voidings within 1 month.	Client will report less than two episodes of incontinence following initiation of a pattern of pelvic muscle strengthening exercises (Kegel). Client will state increased comfort.
	Urinary Elimination
Mrs. Grayson will achieve and maintain an optimum urinary elimination pattern within 1 month.	Client will remain free of urinary tract infection. Client will demonstrate ability to start and stop urinary stream with no leaking between voidings. Client will void greater than 150 mL each time.

†Outcome classification labels from Moorhead S and others: *Nursing outcomes classification (NOC)*, ed 4, St. Louis, 2008, Mosby.

Interventions (NIC)‡

Urinary Incontinence Care
• Have client complete a 3-day 24-hour log of urination.

Rationale

The bladder log provides objective verification of urine elimination pattern and patterns of urine leakage and provides a baseline for evaluation of effectiveness of management plans (Lewis and others, 2007; Wyman, 2003).

A bladder log also demonstrates pattern of voiding that indicates more serious urinary problems related to urinary tract infections or other renal diseases (Lewis and others, 2007).

‡Intervention classification labels from Bulechek GM, Butcher HK, and Dochterman JM: *Nursing interventions classifications (NIC)*, ed 5, St. Louis, 2008, Mosby.

Continued

NURSING CARE PLAN

Stress Urinary Incontinence—cont'd

Interventions (NIC)‡	Rationale
Urinary Incontinence Care—cont'd	

• Assist client in supportive measures to reduce intraabdominal pressure by
  • Losing weight
  • Avoiding heavy lifting
• Refer to urinary continence specialist, if needed.
	These measures reduce intraabdominal pressure and bladder pressure that increase leakage.

Pelvic Muscle Exercise	
• Work with client to establish a program of pelvic muscle exercises that will increase bladder control. Instruct Mrs. Grayson to tighten, then relax, the ring of muscle around the urethra and anus, as if trying to prevent urination. Instruct her to work up to a total of 15 (3 sets of 5) contractions a day, ultimately holding the contraction for 10 seconds each, resting 10 seconds between each contraction and resting 30 seconds between sets (Doughty, 2006).	Pelvic muscle rehabilitation alleviates or even cures stress incontinence for many women. Noticeable change will probably take 4 weeks, and maximum effect may take 6 weeks (Specht, 2005).

‡Intervention classification labels from Bulechek GM, Butcher HK, and Dochterman JM: *Nursing interventions classifications (NIC)*, ed 5, St. Louis, 2008, Mosby.

Evaluation

Nursing Actions	Client Response/Finding	Achievement of Outcomes
Ask Mrs. Grayson about degree of continence since starting pelvic muscle exercises	She responds, "I'm dry most of the time now, and when I do leak it's only a few drops."	Mrs. Grayson reports increasing success with bladder control. She is satisfied that with time her success will be complete. Mrs. Grayson has had no symptoms of a urinary tract infection and states that she is voiding larger amounts than she used to.

Conversely, the client with stress incontinence often has a long-term goal that is dependent on weeks of pelvic floor muscle exercise to achieve urinary control: "Client will achieve full urinary continence within 8 weeks after start of exercise program (Kegel)." Make sure goals are reasonably achievable and relevant to the client's situation.

Setting Priorities. Urinary elimination is a personal and intimate activity. Establish a relationship with the client that allows discussion and intervention. While you are collaborating with the client, the client's priorities will become apparent and the client should develop an understanding of all the goals.

In the case when a client has multiple nursing diagnoses (Figure 45-10), it becomes important for the nurse to recognize the primary health problem and its influence on other problems. In the example of the client with chronic confusion, the resultant incontinence creates several risks. Focusing on the management of incontinence helps resolve more than one nursing diagnosis. Although physical care needs appear to have higher priority, the psychological needs related to self-esteem or sexuality are sometimes a higher priority for the client. Attention to the client's perceived needs is the most satisfactory and successful approach to accomplishing all the goals. Reinforcement of good health habits that are already followed improves compliance with the care plan.

Collaborative Care. The plan of care incorporates health promotion activities and therapeutic interventions individualized to the client's needs. Consider the client's home environment and normal elimination routines when planning therapies. The plan of care requires collaboration among several health care disciplines, the client, and the client's family. For example, a nurse specialist in urinary continence teaches pelvic floor exercises, while a physical therapist designs an exercise plan to increase overall strength and endurance so the client will be able to ambulate to the bathroom. In addition, a health care provider prescribes medication to reduce troublesome symptoms, while a nurse provides teaching for clients at risk for urinary problems. Explore the need for home care services, and make the appropriate referrals. The family will probably need to alter the home environment to make it easier and safer for the client to use the bathroom. The client's plan requires multiple interventions.

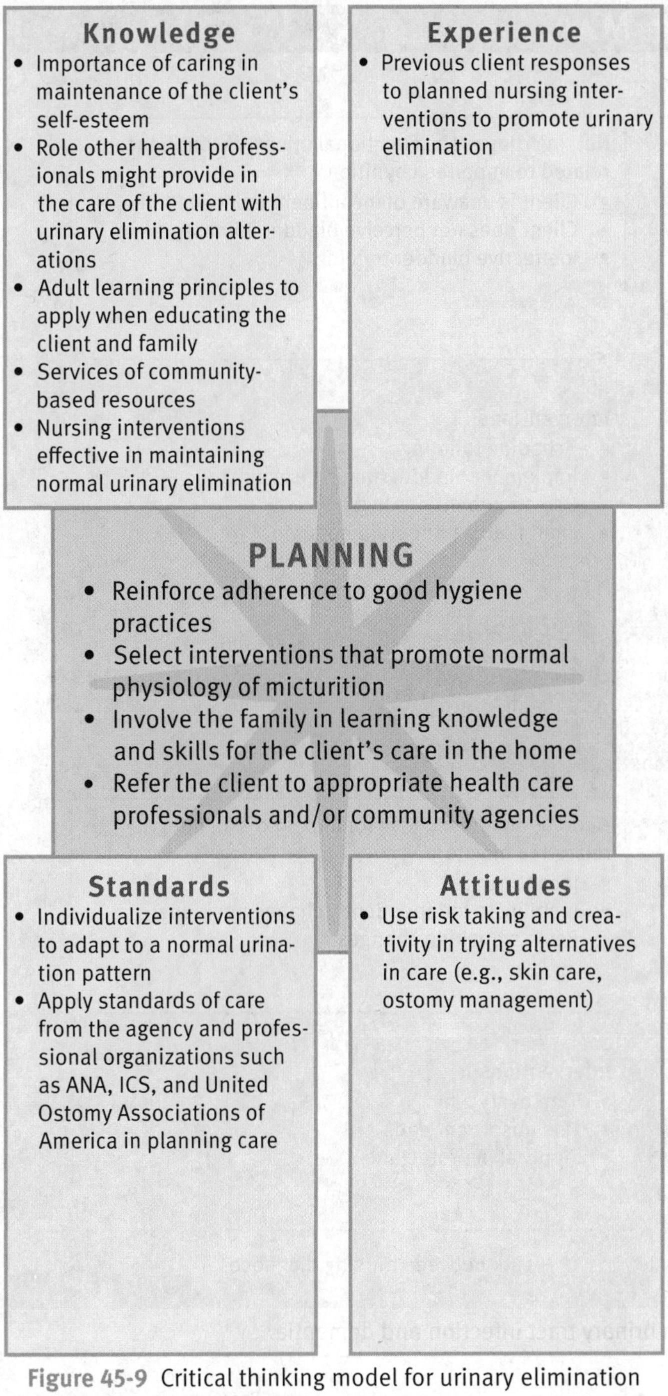

Knowledge	Experience
• Importance of caring in maintenance of the client's self-esteem • Role other health professionals might provide in the care of the client with urinary elimination alterations • Adult learning principles to apply when educating the client and family • Services of community-based resources • Nursing interventions effective in maintaining normal urinary elimination	• Previous client responses to planned nursing interventions to promote urinary elimination

PLANNING

- Reinforce adherence to good hygiene practices
- Select interventions that promote normal physiology of micturition
- Involve the family in learning knowledge and skills for the client's care in the home
- Refer the client to appropriate health care professionals and/or community agencies

Standards	Attitudes
• Individualize interventions to adapt to a normal urination pattern • Apply standards of care from the agency and professional organizations such as ANA, ICS, and United Ostomy Associations of America in planning care	• Use risk taking and creativity in trying alternatives in care (e.g., skin care, ostomy management)

Figure 45-9 Critical thinking model for urinary elimination planning.

◆ Implementation

Implementation is the action phase of the nursing process. Complete independent and collaborative interventions to assist the client in achieving the desired outcomes and goals. The independent activities are those in which nurses use their own judgment. An example of this is teaching self-care activities to the client. Collaborative activities are those prescribed by the health care provider and carried out by the nurse, such as medication administration.

Health Promotion. Health promotion assists the client in understanding and participating in self-care practices to preserve and protect healthy urinary system function. You can achieve this focus using several means.

Client Education. Success of therapies aimed at eliminating or minimizing urinary elimination problems depends in part on successful client education (Box 45-6). Although many clients need to learn about all aspects of urinary elimination, first focus the teaching on the client's specific elimination problems. For example, clients who practice poor hygiene benefit most from learning about normal sterility of the urinary tract and how frequent hand washing and proper perineal hygiene reduce the risks for infection. Clients also learn the significance of symptoms of urinary alterations so they can initiate early preventive health care.

You can easily incorporate teaching when giving nursing care. For example, a good time to discuss the benefits of increasing fluid intake is while giving fluids with medications or meals. Often you will be more successful in teaching about perineal hygiene while giving a bath or performing catheter care.

Promoting Normal Micturition. Maintaining normal urinary elimination helps to prevent many urination problems. Many nursing measures promote normal voiding in clients at risk for urination difficulties and in clients with established urination problems. Some of these measures are independent nursing interventions.

Stimulating Micturition Reflex. The client's ability to void depends on feeling the urge to urinate, being able to control the urethral sphincter, and being able to relax during voiding. Help a client learn to relax and stimulate the reflex to void by assisting the client in assuming the normal position for voiding. A woman is better able to void in a squatting or sitting position. If the client is unable to use toilet facilities, position the client in a squatting position on a bedpan (see Chapter 46) or bedside commode. A man voids more easily in the standing position. If the man cannot reach toilet facilities, have him stand at the bedside and void into a urinal (a metal or plastic receptacle for urine) (Figure 45-11). At times it will be necessary for one or more nurses to assist a man with standing.

Other measures that promote relaxation and the ability to void include sensory stimuli. The sound of running water helps many clients void through the power of suggestion. Stroking the inner aspect of the thigh stimulates sensory nerves and promotes the micturition reflex. You can also pour warm water over the client's perineum and create the sensation to urinate. If you need to measure urine output, first measure the volume of water you pour over the perineal area.

Maintaining Elimination Habits. Many clients follow routines to promote normal voiding. In a hospital or long-term care facility health care routines often conflict with those of clients. Integrating clients' habits into the care plan fosters normal voiding and will assist in preventing problems related to urination.

Maintaining Adequate Fluid Intake. A simple method of promoting normal micturition is maintaining good fluid intake. A client with normal renal function and who does not have heart or kidney disease needs to drink 2000 to 2500 mL of fluid daily. However, an average daily intake of 1200 to 1500 mL of fluids is usually adequate unless the client has a history of urinary tract infection.

CONCEPT MAP

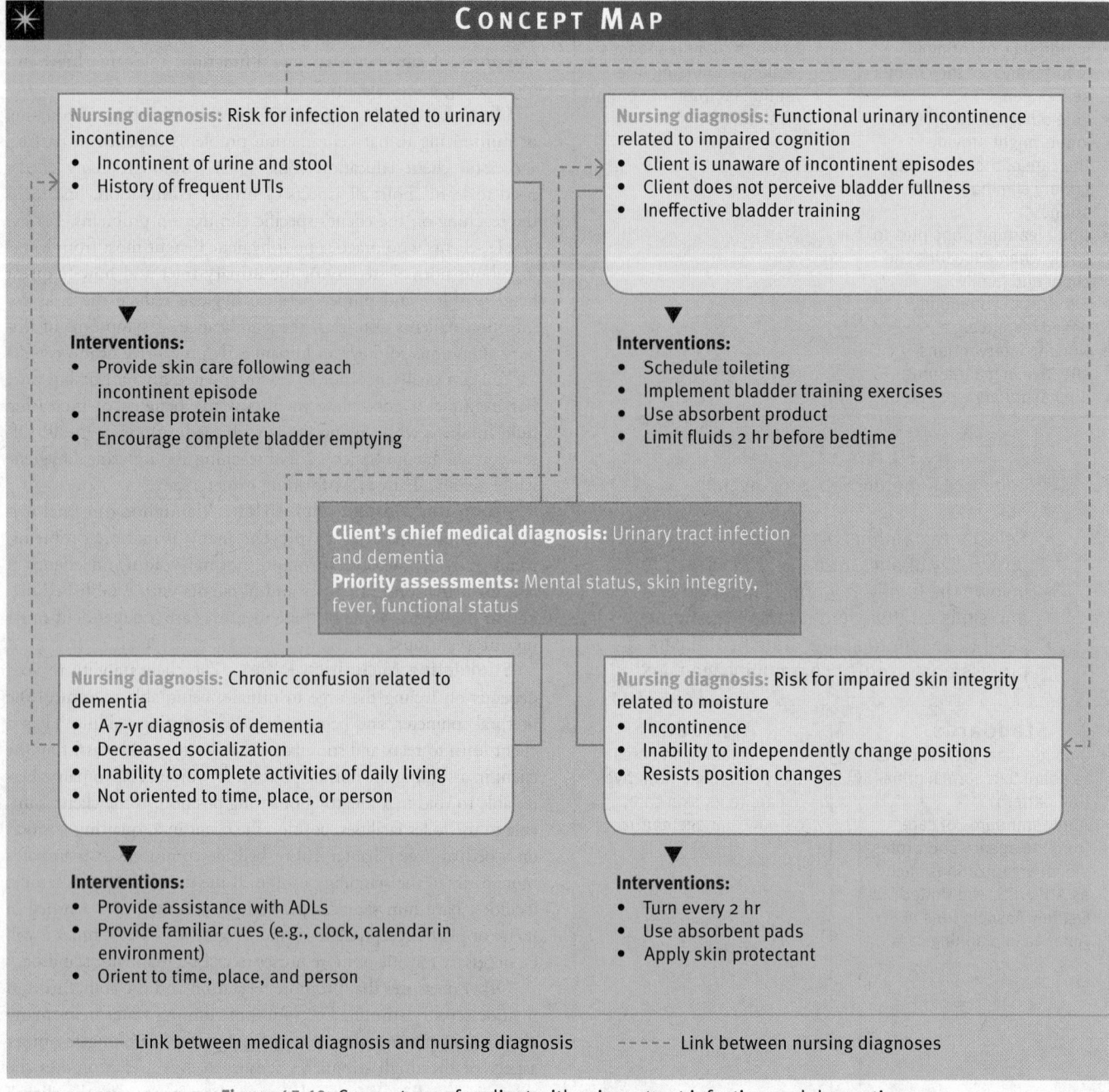

Nursing diagnosis: Risk for infection related to urinary incontinence
- Incontinent of urine and stool
- History of frequent UTIs

Interventions:
- Provide skin care following each incontinent episode
- Increase protein intake
- Encourage complete bladder emptying

Nursing diagnosis: Functional urinary incontinence related to impaired cognition
- Client is unaware of incontinent episodes
- Client does not perceive bladder fullness
- Ineffective bladder training

Interventions:
- Schedule toileting
- Implement bladder training exercises
- Use absorbent product
- Limit fluids 2 hr before bedtime

Client's chief medical diagnosis: Urinary tract infection and dementia
Priority assessments: Mental status, skin integrity, fever, functional status

Nursing diagnosis: Chronic confusion related to dementia
- A 7-yr diagnosis of dementia
- Decreased socialization
- Inability to complete activities of daily living
- Not oriented to time, place, or person

Interventions:
- Provide assistance with ADLs
- Provide familiar cues (e.g., clock, calendar in environment)
- Orient to time, place, and person

Nursing diagnosis: Risk for impaired skin integrity related to moisture
- Incontinence
- Inability to independently change positions
- Resists position changes

Interventions:
- Turn every 2 hr
- Use absorbent pads
- Apply skin protectant

——— Link between medical diagnosis and nursing diagnosis   - - - - - Link between nursing diagnoses

Figure 45-10 Concept map for client with urinary tract infection and dementia.

When clients increase fluid intake, this helps flush out solutes or particles that collect in the urinary system. Because some clients are unwilling to drink 2500 mL of water daily, encourage fluids that the client prefers. Many vegetables and fruits also have a high fluid content. At home it helps to set a schedule for drinking fluids (e.g., with meals or medications). To minimize nocturia, avoid fluids 2 hours before bedtime.

Promoting Complete Bladder Emptying. Under normal conditions a small amount of the client's urine remains in the bladder after voiding (residual urine). Encouraging clients to wait until urine stops flowing or to attempt to void again (double-voiding) can improve bladder emptying (Table 45-5).

Preventing Infection. One of the most important considerations for a client with urinary alterations is the need to prevent infection of the urinary system. Good perineal hygiene that includes cleansing the urethral meatus after each voiding or bowel movement is essential. A daily fluid intake of 2000 to 2500 mL dilutes urine, promotes regular micturition, and flushes the urethra of microorganisms.

Acidifying Urine. Urine is normally acidic and tends to inhibit growth of microorganisms. Meats, eggs, whole-grain breads, cranberries, and prunes increase urine acidity. In addition, cranberry juice decreases bacterial adherence to the bladder wall (Gray, 2002).

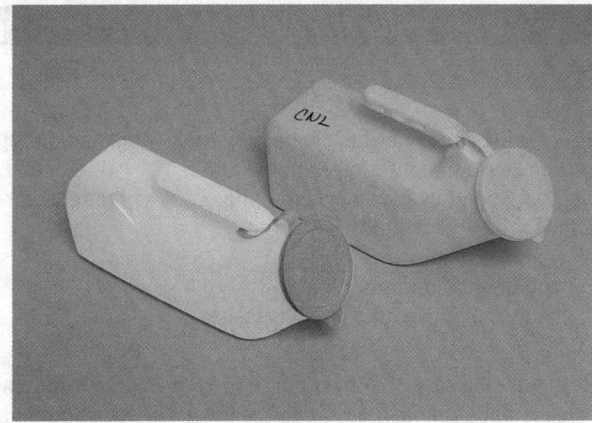

✦ **BOX 45-6** **CLIENT TEACHING**

Urinary Elimination Problems Related to Urinary Sphincter Dysfunction

Objectives
- Client will achieve continence through increased sphincter control.

Teaching Strategies
- Have client attempt to tighten urinary sphincter during urination to feel the sensations associated with urinary sphincter contraction.
- Teach client progressive use of pelvic floor exercises (PFEs) (Kegel exercises).
- Provide written instructions and/or audiotape for reinforcement of technique.
- Have client sit or stand without tensing muscles of legs, buttocks, or abdomen.
  - Have client contract and relax circumvaginal muscles and urinary and anal sphincters for 3 to 4 seconds and repeat in quick succession.
  - Have client repeat these cycles for 10 times, 5 times a day with 30-second rest in between. Gradually increase to 3 sets of 5 contractions of 10 seconds with a 10-second rest between. Rest 30 seconds between sets.
  - For maintenance, have client do 1 to 2 sets per week. Client should contract pelvic muscles and sphincters before sneezing, coughing, or lifting.
  - Maintain optimum strength through practicing hard contractions.
- Teach and monitor use of a voiding record.

Evaluation
- Ask client and caregiver about voiding record to identify changes in patterns of urinary elimination.
- Ask client and caregiver about degree of satisfaction related to control achieved in urinary elimination.
- Ask client and caregiver about selection and usage of incontinence control devices.

Teaching strategies modified from Mauk KL: Conservative therapy for urinary incontinence can help older adults, *Nursing* 35(8):20, 2005; and Doughty DB: *Urinary and fecal incontinence: current management concepts,* ed 3, St. Louis, 2006, Mosby.

Figure 45-11 Types of male urinals.

by a partition or room divider. Young children are often unable to void in the presence of persons other than their parents.

When possible, encourage the continued use of special measures that the client uses to void. Some clients are able to relax and void more easily while reading or listening to music. Having a cup or glass of fluids also promotes urination.

Medications. Drug therapy given alone or with other therapies often helps problems of incontinence or retention. The bladder is innervated by the parasympathetic nervous system. Drugs that block the muscarinic receptors suppress bladder contractions and reduce incontinence caused by bladder irritation. Examples of these drugs include solifenacin (Vesicare) and oxybutynin chloride (Ditropan). These medications can cause constipation, dry mouth, and skin irritation (Lehne, 2007). Irritants present in the urine such as caffeine or alcohol may cause uncontrolled bladder contractions and should be avoided for some clients.

When the bladder empties, the detrusor muscle contracts in response to parasympathetic stimulation. Incomplete bladder emptying results from impaired innervation or weakness of the detrusor muscle. The client experiences retention and possible overflow incontinence. Cholinergic drugs increase contraction of the bladder and improve emptying. Bethanechol (Urecholine) stimulates parasympathetic nerves to increase bladder wall contraction and relax the sphincter. You can administer bethanechol by subcutaneous or oral routes. Cholinergic drugs often cause diarrhea as a side effect (Lehne, 2007).

The dribbling or overflow incontinence seen in men with prostatic enlargement can be treated with an alpha₁-adrenergic blocker, such as tamsulosin (Flomax). Tamsulosin is given orally and relaxes prostatic smooth muscle, thus relieving obstructive symptoms. This drug has few side effects and does not cause transient hypotension as other alpha-adrenergic blockers do (Lehne, 2007).

Catheterization. Catheterization of the bladder involves introducing a latex or plastic tube through the urethra and into the bladder. The catheter provides a continuous flow of urine in clients unable to control micturition or those with obstructions. It also provides a means of assessing urine output in hemodynamically unstable clients. Because bladder catheterization carries the risk of UTI, blockage, and trauma to the urethra, it is prefer-

Acute Care

Maintaining Elimination Habits. Clients usually require time to void. Requesting a urine specimen on demand does not contribute to relaxation and normal voiding habits. Give clients at least 30 minutes to provide a specimen. Clients normally void upon awakening or before meals, so offer the opportunity to use toilet facilities then. Also important is the need to respond to and anticipate clients' urges to urinate. For example, many falls in the older adult are related to the urge to urinate. Anticipate the need, and provide for scheduled bathroom visits to help reduce the fall risk in these client.

Many clients need privacy for voiding. If the client cannot reach the bathroom and uses a bedside commode or bedpan, make sure that the bedside curtain is closed. Clients who are debilitated and live at home often prefer using a bedside commode screened

✳ TABLE 45-5   Urinary Incontinence and Treatment Options

TYPE	SIGNS AND SYMPTOMS	INTERVENTIONS
Functional		

Loss of urine caused by factors outside the urinary tract that interfere with the ability to respond in a socially appropriate way to the urge to void
Relevant factors:
  Environmental barriers
  Sensory, cognitive, and mobility issues
	Urge to void that causes loss of urine before reaching appropriate receptacle	Clothing modifications
		Environmental alterations
		Scheduled toileting
		Absorbent products

Stress		
Involuntary leakage of urine during increased abdominal pressure in the absence of bladder muscle contraction	Loss of urine with increased intraabdominal pressure (coughing, laughing, sneezing, or lifting with a full bladder)	Pelvic floor exercises (Kegel) Surgical interventions Biofeedback Electrical stimulation Absorbent products
Urge		
Involuntary passage of urine after a strong sense of urgency to void	Urinary urgency, often with frequency (more often than every 2 hours); bladder spasm or contraction	Antimuscarinic agents Behavioral interventions Biofeedback Bladder retraining Pelvic floor exercises Lifestyle modifications (smoking cessation, weight loss and fluid modifications) Absorbent products
Mixed		
Combination of urge urinary incontinence and stress urinary incontinence signs and symptoms	Combination of urge and stress symptoms	Main treatments usually based on the symptoms that are most bothersome to client
Reflex		
Involuntary loss of urine at intervals without sensation of urge to void Relevant factors: Spinal cord dysfunction—loss of cerebral awareness or impairment of reflex arc	Lack of urge to void, unawareness of bladder filling, reflex emptying when certain volume reached	Intermittent catheterization Condom catheter (male) Credé's method

Modified from Palmer MH, Newman DK: Urinary incontinence and estrogen, *Am J Nurs* 107(3):35, 2007; Doughty DB: *Urinary and fecal incontinence: current management concepts*, ed 3, St. Louis, 2006, Mosby; and Wyman JF: Treatment of urinary incontinence in men and older women, *Am J Nurs* 103(3 suppl):26, 2003.

able to rely on other measures for either specimen collection or management of incontinence (Getliffe, 2003).

Types of Catheterization. Intermittent and indwelling retention catheterizations are the two forms of catheter insertion. With the intermittent technique you introduce a straight single-use catheter (Figure 45-12, *A*) long enough to drain the bladder (5 to 10 minutes). When the bladder is empty, you immediately withdraw the catheter. You can repeat intermittent catheterization as necessary, but each catheter insertion increases risk of trauma and infection. An indwelling or Foley catheter (Figure 45-12, *B*) remains in place for a longer period of time until a client is able to void voluntarily or continuous accurate measurements are no longer necessary (Box 45-7).

The straight single-use catheter has a single lumen with a small opening about 1.3 cm (½ inch) from the tip. Urine drains from the tip, through the lumen, and to a receptacle. An indwelling Foley catheter has a small inflatable balloon that encircles the catheter just above the tip. When inflated, the balloon rests against the bladder outlet to anchor the catheter in place. The

indwelling retention catheter often has two or three lumens within the body of the catheter (see Figure 45-12, *B*). One lumen drains urine through the catheter to a collecting tube. A second lumen carries sterile water to and from the balloon when it is inflated or deflated. A third (optional) lumen is sometimes used to instill fluids or medications into the bladder. It is easy to determine the number of lumens by the number of drainage and injection ports at the catheter's end.

A second type of intermittent catheter has a curved tip. A Coudé catheter is used on male clients who may have enlarged prostates that partly obstruct the urethra. The Coudé catheter is less traumatic during insertion because it is stiffer and easier to control than the straight-tip catheter.

Catheters come in many diameters to fit the size of a client's urethral canal. Box 45-8 provides suggestions on how to make appropriate decisions regarding catheter selection.

Catheter Insertion. Urethral catheterization requires a health care provider's order. You must use strict aseptic technique (see Chapter 34). Organizing equipment before the procedure

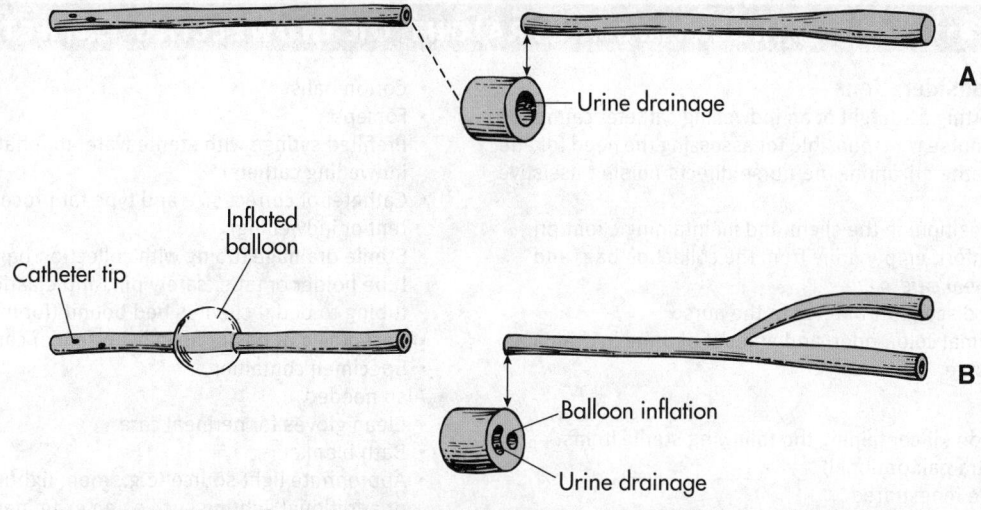

Figure 45-12 Types of urinary catheters. **A**, Straight catheter. **B**, Indwelling (Foley).

BOX 45-7 Indications for Catheterization

Intermittent Catheterization
Relief of discomfort of bladder distention, provision of decompression
Obtaining sterile urine specimen when clean-catch specimen is unobtainable
Assessment of residual urine after urination
Long-term management of clients with spinal cord injuries, neuromuscular degeneration, or incompetent bladders

Short-Term Indwelling Catheterization
Obstruction to urine outflow (e.g., prostate enlargement)
Surgical repair of bladder, urethra, and surrounding structures
Prevention of urethral obstruction from blood clots after genitourinary surgery
Measurement of urinary output in critically ill clients
Continuous or intermittent bladder irrigations

Long-Term Indwelling Catheterization
Severe urinary retention with recurrent episodes of UTI
Skin rashes, ulcers, or wounds irritated by contact with urine
Terminal illness when bed linen changes are painful for client

UTI, Urinary tract infection.

BOX 45-8 Guidelines for Appropriate Catheter Selection

- The catheter size should be determined by the size of the client's urethral canal. When the French system is used, the larger the gauge number, the larger the catheter size. Generally, children require an 8 to 10 Fr, women require a 14 to 16 Fr, and men require a 16 to 18 Fr (Gray and others, 2006). To prevent trauma, the smallest effective catheter size is preferred. Larger sizes than 18 Fr create discomfort, increase risk of blockage, and lead to UTI, urethral irritation, and erosion (Gray and others, 2006)
- The expected duration of the catheterization will determine the catheter material selection.
  - Plastic catheters are suitable only for intermittent use due to their inflexibility.
  - Latex catheters are recommended for use up to 3 weeks. Be aware of allergies.
  - Pure silicon or Teflon catheters are best suited for long-term use (2 to 3 months) because of less encrustation at the urethral meatus (Parkin and Keeley, 2003).
- Balloon size is important in selecting an indwelling catheter. Balloon sizes range from 3 mL (pediatric) to large postoperative volumes (75 mL). In adults the 5-mL and 30-mL sizes are the most common: The 5-mL size allows for optimal drainage, whereas the 30-mL size is used after prostatectomies to provide hemostasis of the prostatic bed (Gray and others, 2006).
- Use only sterile water to inflate the balloon because saline will crystallize, resulting in incomplete deflation of the balloon at the time of removal.
- If leakage occurs around the catheter, a change in lumen size or use of antispasmodic medication is necessary.

prevents interruptions. The steps for inserting indwelling and single-use straight catheters are basically the same. The difference lies in the procedure taken to inflate the indwelling catheter balloon and secure the catheter. Skill 45-2 lists steps for performing female and male urethral catheterization.

Closed Drainage Systems. After inserting an indwelling catheter, maintain a closed urinary drainage system to minimize the risk of infection. Urinary drainage bags are plastic and hold about 1000 to 1500 mL of urine. The bag hangs on the bed frame or wheelchair without touching the floor. Never hang the bag on the bed rail because it can be accidentally raised above the level of the bladder. In clients with indwelling catheters you can obtain specimens without opening the drainage system using a special port in the tubing (see Figure 45-7).

When the client ambulates, the nurse or client carries the bag below the client's waist. Never raise the drainage bag above the level of the client's bladder. Urine in the bag and tubing becomes a medium for bacteria, and infection is likely to develop if urine flows back into the bladder.

Most drainage bags contain an antireflux valve to prevent urine in the bag from reentering the drainage tubing and contaminating

Text continued on p. 1161

★ SKILL 45-2   **INSERTING A STRAIGHT OR INDWELLING CATHETER**

Delegation Considerations

The skill of inserting a straight or an indwelling catheter cannot be delegated. The nurse is responsible for assessing the need for and evaluation of catheterization. The nurse directs nursing assistive personnel to:

- Assist with positioning the client and maintaining client privacy and comfort, empty urine from the collection bag, and provide perineal care
- Report client discomfort or fever to the nurse
- Report abnormal color, odor, and amount of urine in drainage bag to the nurse

Equipment

- Catheterization kit containing the following sterile items:
  - Gloves (extra pair optional)
  - Drapes, one fenestrated
  - Lubricant
  - Antiseptic cleansing solution
- Cotton balls
- Forceps
- Prefilled syringe with sterile water to inflate the balloon of indwelling catheter
- Catheter of correct size and type for procedure (i.e., intermittent or indwelling)
- Sterile drainage tubing with collection bag and multipurpose tube holder or tape, safety pin, and elastic band for securing tubing to bed if client is bed bound (for indwelling catheter)
- Receptacle or basin (usually bottom of catheterization tray)
- Specimen container
- Also needed
  - Clean gloves for perineal care
  - Bath blanket
  - Appropriate light source (e.g., room lighting may be adapted or additional lighting such as an examination lamp)

STEPS	RATIONALE
1. Review client's medical record, including health care provider's order and nurses' notes.	Determines purpose of inserting catheter: preparation for surgery, urinary irrigations, collection of sterile specimens, or measurement of residual urine. Assess for previous catheterization, including catheter size, response of client, and time of last catheterization.
2. Assess status of client:	
a. Ask client when last voided, or check I&O flow sheet, or palpate bladder.	Determine time of last voiding or potential for bladder fullness.
b. Level of awareness or developmental stage.	Reveals the client's ability to cooperate and level of explanation needed.
c. Mobility and physical limitations of client.	Affect way the nurse positions client.
d. Client's gender and age.	In general, catheter size 8 to 10 Fr is used for children, whereas 14 to 16 Fr is recommended for most clients. Men often need a slightly larger size than women, but the smallest functional size will provide client comfort (Wong and Hooton, 2005).
e. Perform hand hygiene. Apply clean gloves. Inspect perineum for erythema, drainage, and odor. Remove gloves following inspection and perform hand hygiene.	Reduces infection. Determines condition of the perineum.
f. Note any pathological condition that will impair passage of catheter (e.g., enlarged prostate in men).	Obstruction prevents passage of catheter through urethra into the bladder. Often requires use of Coudé catheter.
g. Allergies.	Procedure risks exposure to antiseptic, tape, latex, and lubricant. Betadine allergies are common; if the client is unaware of allergy, ask if allergic to shellfish.
3. Assess client's knowledge of the purpose for catheterization.	Reveals need for client instruction.
4. Explain procedure to client.	Promotes cooperation.
5. Arrange for extra nursing personnel to assist as necessary.	Some clients are unable to assume positioning for procedure.
6. Perform hand hygiene.	Reduces transmission of microorganisms.
7. Close curtain or door.	Offers privacy, reduces embarrassment, and aids in relaxation during procedure.
8. Raise bed to appropriate working height.	Promotes use of proper body mechanics.
9. Facing client, stand on left side of bed if right-handed (on right side of bed if left-handed). Clear the bedside table, and arrange equipment.	Successful catheter insertion requires nurse to assume comfortable position with all equipment easily accessible.
10. If side rails are in use, raise side rail on opposite side of bed, and put side rail down on working side.	Promotes client safety.
11. Place waterproof pad under client.	Prevents soiling of bed linen.
12. Position client.	Proper positioning provides good visualization of perineal structures and increases successful insertion with minimal trauma (Smith, 2006).
A. **Female client**	
(1) Assist to dorsal recumbent position (supine with knees flexed). Ask client to relax thighs so you can rotate the hips.	Support legs with pillows to reduce muscle tension and promote comfort.

✳ **SKILL 45-2**   **INSERTING A STRAIGHT OR INDWELLING CATHETER—CONT'D**

STEPS	RATIONALE
(2) Position female client in side-lying (Sims') position with upper leg flexed at hip if unable to assume dorsal recumbent position.	This alternate position is used if client cannot abduct leg at hip joint (e.g., if client has arthritic joints). Also, this position is more comfortable for client. Support client with pillows if necessary to maintain position.
B. Male client	
(1) Assist to supine position with thighs slightly abducted.	Comfortable position for client that aids in visualization.
13. Drape client.	
A. Female client (see illustration)	
(1) Drape with bath blanket. Place blanket diamond fashion over client, with one corner at client's midsection, side corners over each thigh and abdomen, and last corner over perineum.	Avoids unnecessary exposure of body parts and maintains client's comfort.
B. Male client (see illustration)	
(1) Drape upper trunk with bath blanket, and cover lower extremities with bed sheets, exposing only genitalia.	Avoids unnecessary exposure of body parts and maintains client's comfort.
14. Wearing disposable gloves, wash perineal area with soap and water as needed; dry thoroughly. Remove and discard gloves; perform hand hygiene.	Reduces microorganisms near urethral meatus and allows further opportunity to visualize perineum and landmarks.
15. Position light source to illuminate perineal area. (Have an assistant hold flashlight if necessary).	Permits accurate identification and good visualization of urethral meatus.
16. Open package containing drainage system; place drainage bag over edge of bottom bed frame, and bring drainage tube up between side rails and mattress.	Positions system equipment for eventual attachment.

Critical Decision Point: This step is necessary only when an indwelling catheter is to be inserted and drainage system is not part of the catheterization kit.

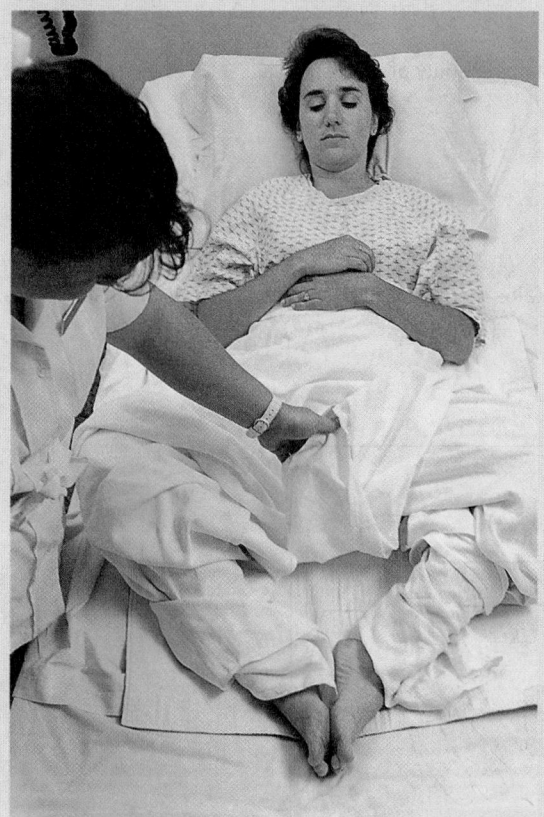

STEP 13A Draping technique (female).

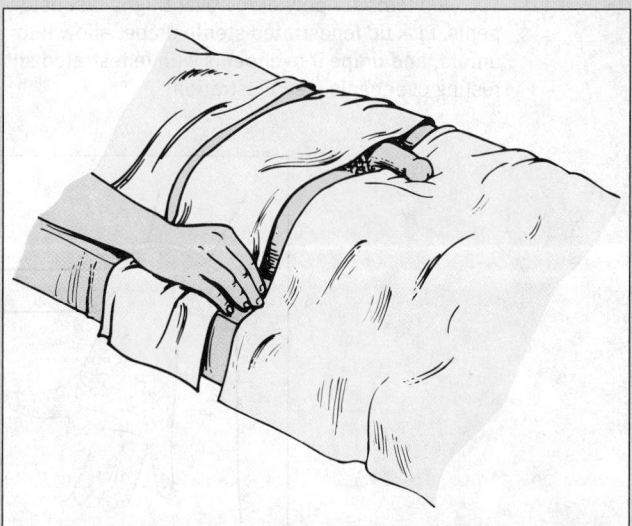

STEP 13B Draping technique (male).

Continued

✳ **SKILL 45-2**   **INSERTING A STRAIGHT OR INDWELLING CATHETER—CONT'D**

STEPS

17. Open catheterization kit according to directions, keeping bottom of container sterile.

18. Place plastic bag that contained kit within reach of work area to use as a waterproof bag to dispose of used supplies.
19. Apply sterile gloves (see Chapter 34).

RATIONALE

Prevents transmission of microorganisms from table or work area to sterile supplies. The materials in the kit are arranged in sequence of use.

Allows nurse to handle sterile supplies without contamination.

Critical Decision Point: If underpad is first item in kit, place pad plastic side down under client, touching only the edges so as to maintain sterility. Then apply sterile gloves.

---

20. Organize supplies on sterile field. Open inner sterile package containing catheter. Pour sterile antiseptic solution into correct compartment containing sterile cotton balls. Open packet containing lubricant. Remove specimen container (lid should be placed loosely on top) and prefilled syringe from collection compartment of tray, and set them aside on sterile field. Do not open pretest balloon.

21. Generously lubricate 2.5 to 5 cm (1 to 2 inches) of catheter for women and 12.5 to 17.7 cm (5 to 7 inches) for men.

Maintains principles of surgical asepsis and organizes work area.
NOTE: Pretesting of balloon is no longer recommended because catheters are pretested during manufacturing and inflation may distort the balloon, leading to increased trauma (Smith, 2006).

Prevents urethral trauma. Inflamed tissue is more susceptible to infection (Haberstich, 2002).

Critical Decision Point: Some catheters will have a plastic sheath over the catheter that you have to remove before lubrication. In some cases the health care provider will order the use of a lubricant containing a local anesthetic.

---

22. Apply sterile drape:
    A. **Female client**
       (1) Allow top edge of drape to form a cuff over both gloved hands. Place drape down on bed between client's thighs. Slip cuffed edge just under buttocks, taking care not to touch contaminated surface with gloves. If using Sims' position (side-lying), take extra precautions to cover rectal area with a sterile drape.
       (2) Pick up fenestrated sterile drape, and allow it to unfold without touching an unsterile object. Apply drape over perineum, exposing labia and being sure not to touch contaminated surface.
    B. **Male client:** There are two methods for draping depending on preferences.
       (1) *First method:* Apply drape over thighs and under penis without completely opening fenestrated drape.
       (2) *Second method:* Apply drape over thighs just below penis. Pick up fenestrated sterile drape, allow it to unfold, and drape it over penis with fenestrated slit resting over penis (see illustration).

Outer surface of drape covering hands remains sterile. Sterile drape against sterile gloves is sterile. If using Sims' position, the rectal drape prevents cross contamination (Smith, 2006).

Maintains sterility of work surface.

Maintains sterility of work surface while only exposing penis.

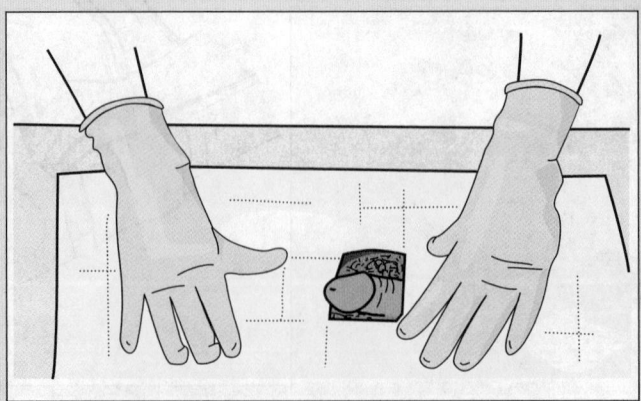

STEP 22B(2) Draping male with fenestrated drape.

✳ **SKILL 45-2** **INSERTING A STRAIGHT OR INDWELLING CATHETER—CONT'D**

STEPS

23. Place sterile tray and contents on sterile drape. Open specimen container. Actual positioning of sterile tray will depend on client size and positioning. This method works best with flexible, average-size clients.

24. Cleanse urethral meatus:
   A. Female client
   (1) With nondominant hand, carefully retract labia to fully expose urethral meatus. Maintain position of nondominant hand throughout procedure.

RATIONALE

Provides easy access to supplies during catheter insertion.

Maintains aseptic technique during procedure.

Provides full visualization of urethral meatus. Full retraction prevents contamination of urethral meatus during cleansing.

Critical Decision Point: Closure of labia during cleansing requires that the cleansing procedure be repeated because the area has become contaminated.

---

   (2) Using forceps in sterile dominant hand, pick up cotton ball saturated with antiseptic solution and clean perineal area, wiping from front to back from clitoris toward anus. Using a new cotton ball for each area, wipe along the far labial fold, near labial fold, and directly over center of urethral meatus (see illustration).

   B. Male client
   (1) If client is not circumcised, retract foreskin with nondominant hand. Grasp penis at shaft just below glans. Retract urethral meatus between thumb and forefinger. Maintain nondominant hand in this position throughout procedure.
   (2) With dominant hand, pick up cotton ball with forceps and clean penis. Move in a circular motion from urethral meatus down to base of glans. Repeat cleansing three more times, using a clean cotton ball each time (see illustration).

Cleansing reduces number of microorganism at urethral meatus. Use of a new cotton ball for each wipe prevents transfer of microorganisms. Cleansing for each of the three areas proceeds from area of least contamination to that of most contamination. Dominant hand remains sterile.

Retraction of foreskin provides full visualization of meatus and allows for adequate cleansing. Cleansing reduces number of microorganisms. Accidental release of foreskin or dropping of penis during cleansing requires repetition of process because area has become contaminated.
Reduces number of microorganisms at urethral meatus and moves from area of least to most contamination. Dominant hand remains sterile.

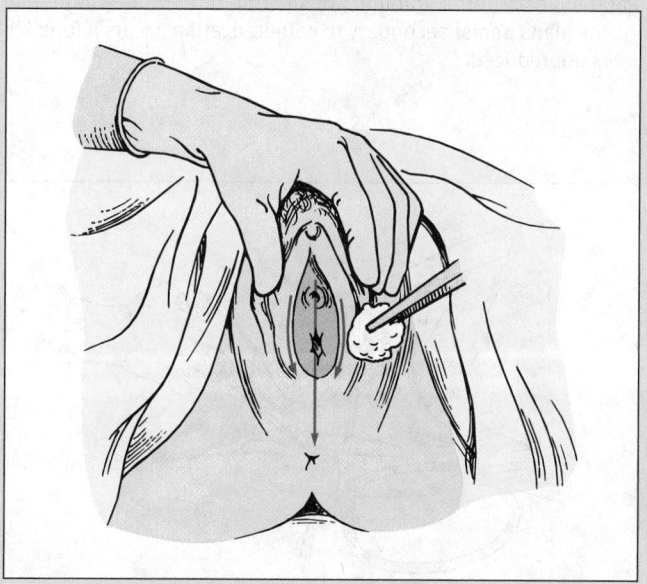

STEP 24A(2) Cleansing technique (female).

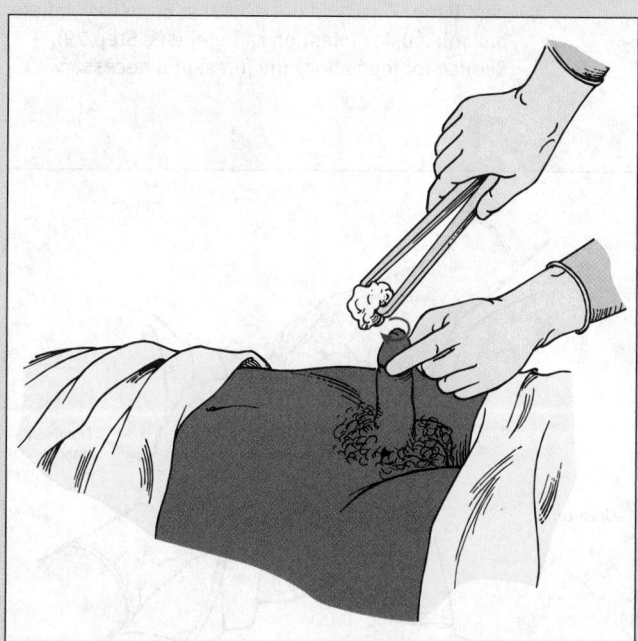

STEP 24B(2) Cleansing technique (male).

Continued

SKILL 45-2   INSERTING A STRAIGHT OR INDWELLING CATHETER—CONT'D

STEPS	RATIONALE
25. Pick up catheter with gloved dominant hand 7.5 to 10 cm (3 to 4 inches) from catheter tip. Hold end of catheter loosely coiled in palm of dominant hand. (*Optional:* May grasp catheter with forceps.)	Prevents soiling of client and bed with draining urine. Place distal end of catheter in urine tray receptacle if straight catheterization is ordered.
26. Insert catheter:	
A. Female client	
(1) Ask client to bear down gently as if to void, and slowly insert catheter through urethral meatus (see illustration).	Relaxation of external sphincter aids in insertion of catheter.
(2) Advance catheter a total of 5 to 7.5 cm (2 to 3 inches) in adult or **until urine flows out of catheter's end.** When urine appears, advance catheter another 2.5 to 5 cm (1 to 2 inches). **Do not use force to insert a catheter.**	Female urethra is short. Appearance of urine indicates that catheter tip is in bladder or lower urethra. Advancement of catheter ensures bladder placement.

Critical Decision Point: If no urine appears, check if catheter is in vagina. If misplaced, leave catheter in vagina as landmark indicating where not to insert, and insert another sterile catheter.

(3) Release labia, and hold catheter securely with nondominant hand. Slowly inflate balloon if using retention catheter (see illustrations) (see Step 29).	Bladder or sphincter contraction will cause accidental expulsion of catheter.
B. Male client	
(1) Lift penis to position perpendicular to client's body, and apply light traction (see illustration).	Straightens urethral canal to ease catheter insertion.
(2) Ask client to bear down as if to void, and slowly insert catheter through urethral meatus.	Relaxation of external sphincter aids in insertion of catheter.
(3) Advance catheter 17 to 22.5 cm (7 to 9 inches) in adult **or until urine flows out catheter's end.** If you feel resistance, withdraw catheter; do not force it through urethra. When urine appears, advance catheter another 2.5 to 5 cm (1 to 2 inches) (see illustration). **Do not use force to insert a catheter.**	The adult male urethra is long. It is normal to meet resistance at the prostatic sphincter. When resistance is met, hold catheter firmly against sphincter without forcing catheter. After a few seconds, the sphincter relaxes, and the catheter is advanced. Appearance of urine indicates catheter tip is in bladder or urethra. Advancement of the catheter to the bifurcation ensures proper placement (Daneshgari and others, 2002).
(4) Lower penis, and hold catheter securely in nondominant hand. Place end of catheter in urine tray. Inflate balloon if using retention catheter (see Step 29).	Bladder or urethral contraction can accidentally expel catheter. Collection of urine prevents soiling and provides output measurement.
(5) Reduce (or reposition) the foreskin if necessary.	Paraphimosis (retraction and constriction of the foreskin behind the glans penis) secondary to catheterization occurs if foreskin is not reduced.

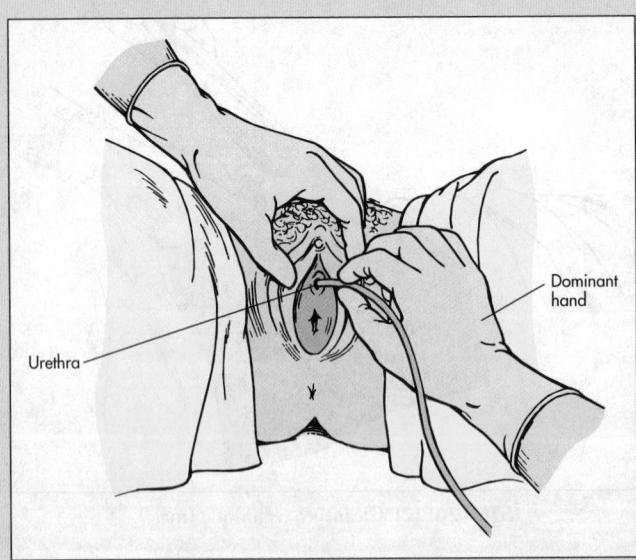

STEP 26A(1) Inserting the catheter.

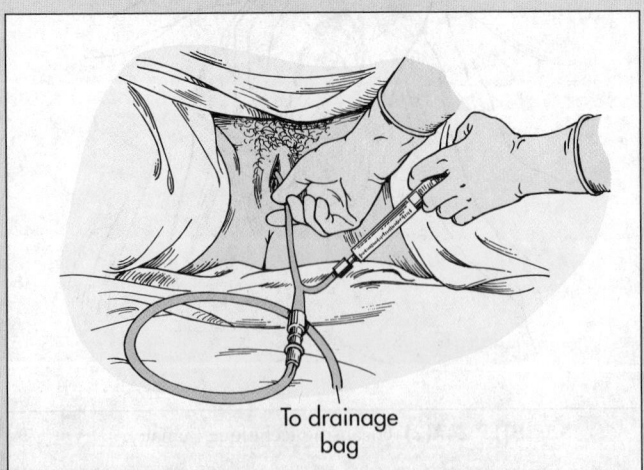

STEP 26A(3) Inflating the balloon (indwelling catheter)

✳ SKILL 45-2	INSERTING A STRAIGHT OR INDWELLING CATHETER—CONT'D

STEPS

27. Collect urine specimen as needed. Fill specimen cup or jar to desired level (20 to 30 mL) by holding end of catheter in dominant hand over cup.
28. Allow bladder to empty fully (about 800 to 1000 mL) unless agency policy restricts maximal volume of urine to drain with each catheterization. Check policy before beginning catheterization. If a restriction is in place, the range is often 800 to 1000 mL.

RATIONALE

Allows nurse to obtain sterile specimen for culture analysis.

As always, the nurse needs to monitor the client's condition, and if the vital signs change or bleeding occurs, temporarily stop the flow of urine and continue when the client's condition demands it. Retained urine serves as a reservoir for growth of microorganisms (Smith, 2006).

Critical Decision Point: If inserting a straight, single-use catheter, withdraw it slowly but smoothly until it is removed.

---

29. Inflate balloon fully per manufacturer's recommendation, and then release catheter with nondominant hand and pull gently (see illustration).

Inflation of balloon anchors catheter tip in place above the bladder outlet to prevent removal of the catheter. Note size of balloon on catheter. Most commonly a 5-mL balloon is used, but health care providers will order a 30-mL balloon in some cases. A prefilled syringe is often included with the kit. A 5-mL balloon should be inflated with the supplied amount (10 mL) to allow symmetrical expansion (Smith, 2006).

Critical Decision Point: If you notice resistance to inflation or if client complains of pain, the balloon is not entirely in the bladder. Stop inflation, aspirate the fluid injected into the balloon, and advance the catheter a little more before attempting to inflate the balloon again.

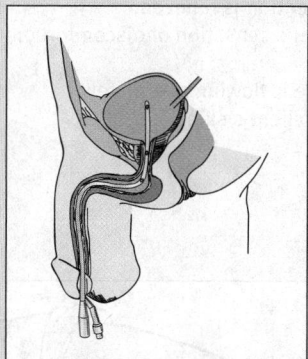

STEP 26B(3) Male anatomy with correct catheter insertion to the bifurcation of the drainage and balloon inflation port.

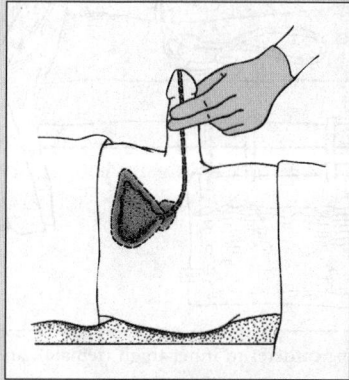

STEP 26B(1) Position penis perpendicular to body for catheter insertion.

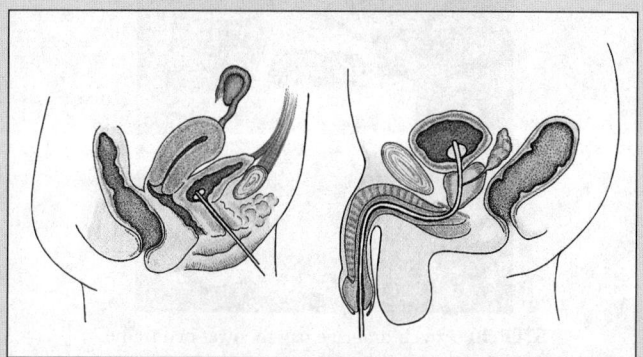

STEP 29 Placement of inflated balloon in bladder.

Continued

✳ **SKILL 45-2** **INSERTING A STRAIGHT OR INDWELLING CATHETER—CONT'D**

STEPS	RATIONALE
30. Attach end of retention catheter to collecting tube of drainage system. Make sure drainage bag is below level of bladder; attach bag to bed frame; do not place bag on side rails of bed (see illustration).	Drainage bag above level of bladder will allow urine in tubing to reflux back into bladder, increasing possibility of infection.
31. Anchor catheter:	
A. Female client	
(1) Secure catheter tubing to inner thigh with strip of nonallergenic tape (or multipurpose tube holders with a Velcro strap). Allow for slack so movement of thigh does not create tension on catheter (see illustration).	Anchoring catheter to inner thigh reduces pressure on urethra, thus reducing possibility of tissue injury (Smith, 2006)
B. Male client	
(1) Secure catheter tubing to top of thigh or lower abdomen (with penis directed toward chest). Allow slack in catheter so movement does not create tension on catheter (see illustration).	Anchoring catheter to lower abdomen reduces pressure on urethra at junction of penis and scrotum, thus reducing possibility of tissue injury.

Critical Decision Point: Be sure there are no obstructions in tubing. Coil excess tubing on bed, and fasten it to the bottom sheet with clip from kit or use rubber band and safety pin.

STEPS	RATIONALE
32. Assist client to comfortable position. Wash and dry perineal area as needed.	Maintains comfort and security.
33. Dispose of equipment, drapes, and urine in proper receptacles and remove gloves.	Reduces transmission of microorganisms.
34. Perform hand hygiene.	Reduces transmission of microorganisms.
35. Palpate bladder.	Determines if distention is relieved.
36. Ask about client's comfort.	Determines if client's sensation of discomfort or fullness has been relieved.
37. Observe character and amount of urine in drainage system.	Determines if urine is flowing adequately.
38. Determine that there is no urine leaking from catheter or tubing connections.	Prevents injury to client's skin.

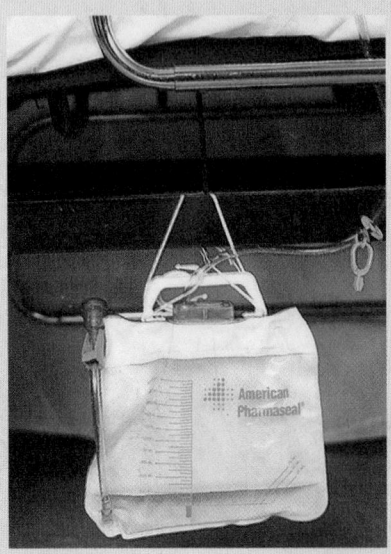

STEP 30 Attach drainage bag to lower bed frame.

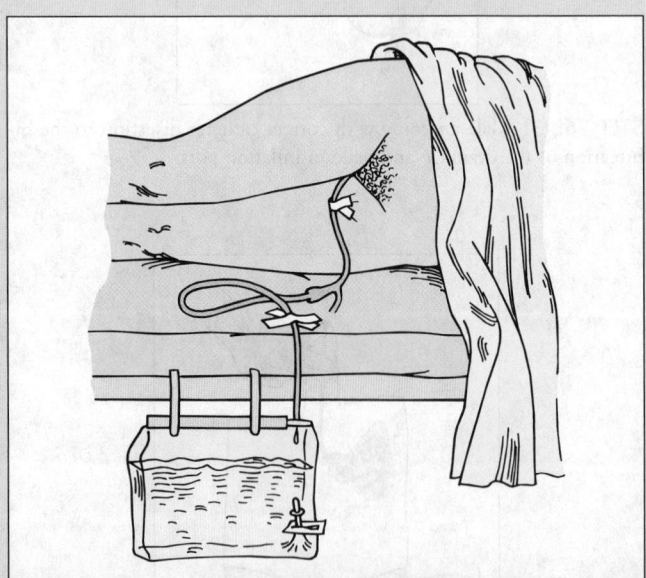

STEP 31A(1) Tape catheter to inner thigh (female), and coil extra tubing on bed and attach to sheet.

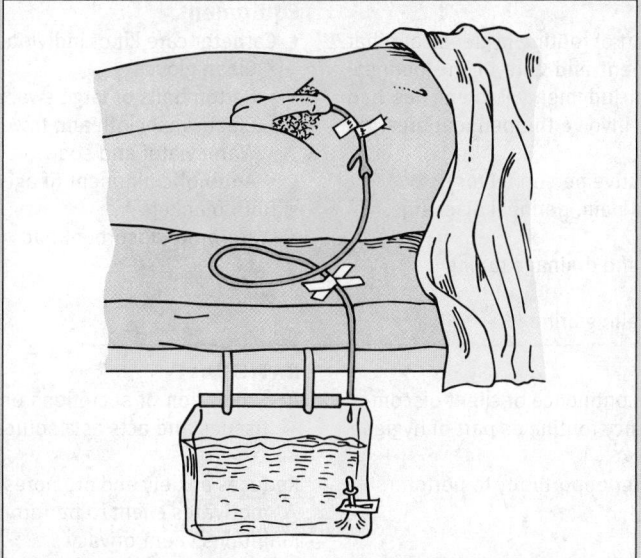

STEP 31B(1) Tape catheter to lower abdomen (male), and coil extra tubing on bed and attach to sheet.

Unexpected Outcomes and Related Interventions

1. Urethral or perineal irritation is present.
   a. Observe for catheter leaking; replace if necessary.
   b. Assess that indwelling catheter is anchored properly.
   c. Perform perineal hygiene and catheter care more frequently.
2. Client has fever and/or odor is present, or client experiences small frequent voiding, burning or bleeding on voiding.
   a. Obtain clean-voided urine specimen.
   b. Notify health care provider.
3. Client experiences urinary retention and is unable to void after you remove the catheter.
   a. Provide adequate fluid intake, and ensure client privacy.
   b. If client unable to void 6 to 8 hours following catheter removal, notify health care provider.

Recording and Reporting

- Report and record type and size of catheter inserted, amount of fluid used to inflate the balloon, characteristics of urine, amount of urine, reasons for catheterization, specimen collection if appropriate, and client's response to procedure and teaching concepts.
- Initiate I&O record.
- If catheter is definitely in bladder and no urine is produced within an hour, immediately report absence of urine to health care provider.

Home Care Considerations

- Clients at home often use a leg bag during the day and switch to a large-volume bag at night so sleep will be uninterrupted.
- Clients who catheterize themselves at home frequently use a clean technique.

the client's bladder. A spigot at the base of the bag provides a means for emptying the bag. The spigot always needs to be clamped, except during emptying, and tucked into the protective pouch on the side of the bag (see agency policy). To keep the drainage system patent check for kinks or bends in the tubing, avoid positioning the client on the drainage tubing, and observe for clots or sediment that occlude the drainage tubing.

Routine Catheter Care. Clients with indwelling catheters have a number of special care needs. Direct nursing measures at preventing infection and maintaining unobstructed flow of urine through the catheter drainage system

Perineal Hygiene. Buildup of secretions or encrustation at the catheter insertion site is a source of irritation and potential infection. Nurses provide perineal hygiene (see Chapter 39) at

least 3 times daily or as needed for a client with a retention catheter. Soap and water are effective in reducing the number of organisms around the urethra. Accidentally advancing the catheter up into the bladder during cleansing increases the risk of introducing bacteria into the bladder.

Catheter Care. In addition to routine perineal hygiene, many institutions recommend that clients with catheters receive special care 3 times a day and after defecation or bowel incontinence to help minimize discomfort and infection (Skill 45-3).

Fluid Intake. All clients with catheters should have a daily intake of 2000 to 2500 mL if permitted. Clients can do this through oral intake or intravenous infusion. A high fluid intake produces a large volume of urine that flushes the bladder and keeps catheter tubing free of sediment.

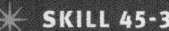

SKILL 45-3   INDWELLING CATHETER CARE

Delegation Considerations

The skill of perineal care is often part of routine hygiene care that can be delegated. Proper assessment and care of the perineal area will need professional clinical judgment. If client has had trauma or surgical procedures that involve the perineal area, do not delegate this care.

The nurse instructs nursing assistive personnel to:

- Report client discomfort, perineal pain, perineal discharge, perineal rash, and/or odor
- Report condition of the catheter and drainage tubing (e.g., leaks, encrustations)
- Report any discolored or foul-smelling urine

Equipment

- Catheter care kit or individual supplies
  - Clean gloves
  - Cotton balls or large swabs
  - Clean washcloth and towel
  - Warm water and soap
  - Antibiotic ointment (if agency policy)
- Bath blanket
- Waterproof absorbent pad

STEPS	RATIONALE
1. Assess for episode of bowel incontinence or client discomfort, or provide care as per agency routine as part of hygiene measures (see Chapter 39).	Accumulation of secretions or feces causes irritation to perineal tissues and acts as a source of bacterial growth.
2. Explain procedure to client. Offer opportunity to perform self-care to able client.	Reduces anxiety and promotes cooperation. Embarrassment often motivates client to perform own hygiene.
3. Close door or bedside curtain.	Maintains client privacy.
4. Perform hand hygiene.	Reduces transmission of infection.
5. Position client:	Ensures easy access and visualization of perineal tissues.
A. Female	
(1) Dorsal recumbent position	
B. Male	
(1) Supine or Fowler's position	
6. Place waterproof pad under client.	Protects bed linens from soiling.
7. Drape bath blanket on client so that only perineal area is exposed.	Prevents unnecessary exposure of body parts.
8. Apply clean gloves.	
9. Remove anchor device to free catheter tubing.	
10. With nondominant hand:	
A. Female	
(1) Gently retract labia to fully expose urethral meatus and catheter insertion site, maintaining position of hand throughout procedure.	Provides full visualization of urethral meatus. Full retraction of labia prevents contamination of meatus during cleansing.
B. Male	
(1) Retract foreskin if not circumscribed, and hold penis at shaft just below glans, maintaining position throughout procedure.	Retraction of foreskin provides full visualization of urethral meatus.

Critical Decision Point: Accidental closure of labia or dropping of penis during cleansing requires procedure to be repeated.

11. Assess urethral meatus and surrounding tissue for inflammation, swelling, and discharge. Note amount, color, odor, and consistency of discharge. Ask client if any burning or discomfort is felt.	Determines presence of local infection and status of hygiene.
12. Cleanse perineal tissue:	
A. Female	
(1) Use clean cloth, soap, and water. Cleanse around urethral meatus and catheter. Cleaning from pubis toward anus, clean labia minora. Use a clean side of cloth for each wipe. Finally clean around anus. Dry each area well.	Reduces the number of microorganisms at urethral meatus. Use of clean cloth prevents transfer of microorganisms.
B. Male	
(1) While spreading urethral meatus, cleanse around catheter first, and then wipe in circular motion around meatus and glans.	Cleansing moves from area of least to most contamination.
13. Reassess urethral meatus for discharge.	Determines if cleansing is complete.

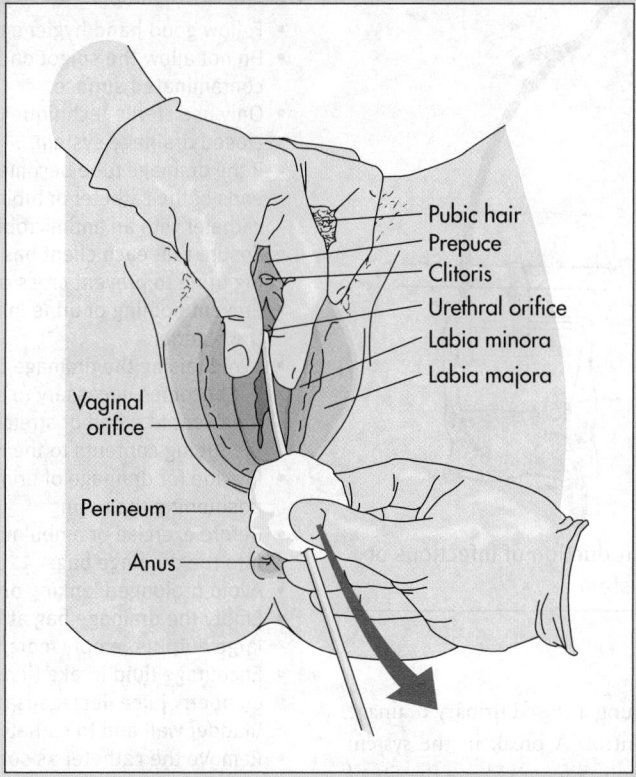

STEP 14 Cleansing the catheter during catheter care. (From Sorrentino S: *Mosby's textbook for nursing assistants,* St. Louis, 2004, Mosby).

STEPS	RATIONALE
14. While stabilizing the catheter with nondominant hand, cleanse length of the catheter from meatus to tubing in a circular motion. Follow agency guidelines (see illustration).	Reduces presence of secretions, drainage, and bacteria on exterior of catheter surface.
15. In male client reduce (or reposition) the foreskin after care.	
16. Reanchor catheter tubing.	
17. Place client in a safe, comfortable position.	Promotes comfort.
18. Dispose of contaminated supplies, remove gloves, and perform hand hygiene.	Prevents spread of infection.

Unexpected Outcomes and Related Interventions

1. Urethral discharge
   a. Increase frequency of indwelling catheter care.
   b. Apply topical antibiotic ointment per agency policy.
   c. Notify health care provider.
2. Accidental catheter dislodgment
   a. Notify health care provider.
   b. Assess for urethral trauma.
   c. Monitor urine output.

Recording and Reporting

- Report and record presence and characteristics of drainage, condition of perineal tissue, and any discomfort reported by client.
- If infection is suspected, report findings to health care provider.

Home Care Considerations

- If client is discharged with indwelling catheter, teach the client and family catheter care and signs and symptoms to report to nurse or health care provider.

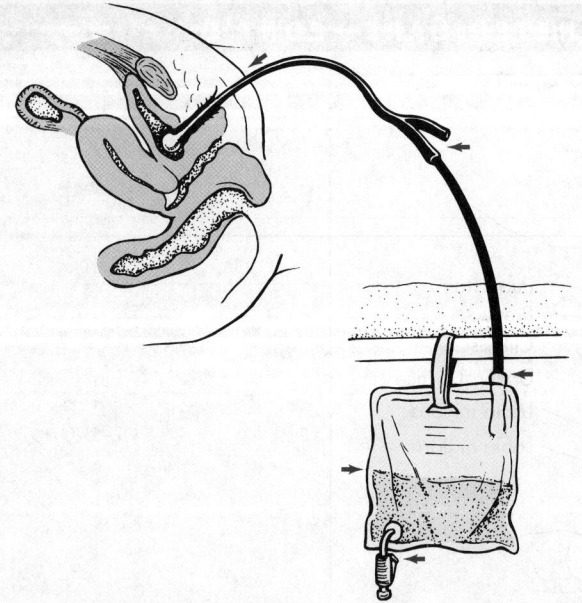

Figure 45-13 Potential sites for introduction of infectious organisms into a urinary drainage system.

✳ BOX 45-9 Tips for Preventing Infection in Clients With Catheters

- Follow good hand hygiene techniques (see Chapter 34).
- Do not allow the spigot on the drainage system to touch a contaminated surface.
- Only use sterile technique to collect specimens from a closed drainage system.
- If the drainage tube becomes disconnected, do not touch the ends of the catheter or tubing. Wipe the end of the tubing and catheter with an antimicrobial solution before reconnecting.
- Ensure that each client has a separate receptacle for measuring urine to prevent cross contamination.
- Prevent pooling of urine in the tubing and reflux of urine into the bladder.
- Avoid raising the drainage bag above the level of the bladder.
- If it becomes necessary to raise the bag during transfer of the client to a bed or stretcher, clamp the tubing or empty the tubing contents to the drainage bag first.
- Provide for drainage of urine from the tubing to the bag by positioning the tubing.
- Before exercise or ambulation drain all urine from the tubing into the drainage bag.
- Avoid prolonged kinking or clamping of the tubing.
- Empty the drainage bag at least every 8 hours. If you note large outputs, empty more frequently.
- Encourage fluid intake (if not contraindicated). Inclusion of cranberry juice decreases the adherence of bacteria to the bladder wall and to catheter lumen (Gray, 2002).
- Remove the catheter as soon as clinically necessary (Fernandez and Griffiths, 2006).
- Tape or secure the catheter appropriately for the client (see Skill 45-2, p. 1154).
- Perform routine perineal hygiene per agency policy and after defecation or bowel incontinence (see Skill 45-3, p. 1162).

Preventing Infection. Maintaining a closed urinary drainage system is important in infection control. A break in the system leads to introduction of microorganisms. Sites at risk are the site of catheter insertion, the drainage bag, the spigot, the tube junction, and the junction of the tube and the bag (Figure 45-13).

In addition, monitor the patency of the system to prevent pooling of urine within the tubing. Urine in the drainage bag is an excellent medium for microorganism growth. Bacteria will possibly travel up drainage tubing to grow in pools of urine. If this urine flows back into the client's bladder, an infection is more to develop (Parkin and Keeley, 2003). Many urine drainage systems are equipped with an antireflux valve. Suggestions for ways to prevent infections in clients with catheters are provided in Box 45-9.

Catheter Irrigations and Instillations. To maintain the patency of indwelling urinary catheters, it sometimes becomes necessary to irrigate or flush a catheter. Blood, pus, or sediment can collect within tubing and result in bladder distention and the buildup of stagnant urine. Instillation of a sterile solution ordered by the health care provider clears the tubing of accumulated material. For clients with bladder infections, a health care provider often orders antiseptic or antibiotic bladder irrigations to wash out the bladder or treat local infection. In both irrigations, follow sterile aseptic technique.

Before performing irrigation, assess the catheter for blockage. If the amount of urine in the drainage bag is less than the client's intake or less than the output during the previous shift, expect some blockage. If urine does not drain freely, milk the tubing. You milk the tube by squeezing then releasing the drainage tube starting from the client to the drainage bag so a clot or sediment will not be forced back into the catheter.

Maintenance of a closed system is recommended during intermittent irrigations or instillations. This technique is effective for irrigating a partially blocked catheter or for bladder instillations. One method of closed bladder irrigation system provides for frequent intermittent irrigations or continuous irrigation without disruption of the sterile catheter system through use of a three-way catheter (Skill 45-4). This method is used most often in clients who have had genitourinary surgery and are at risk for blood clots and mucus fragments occluding the catheter. The other method involves accessing the closed drainage system to instill bladder irrigations (see Skill 45-4). This method is often used for unanticipated irrigation or for intermittent instillations.

Removal of Indwelling Catheter. When removing an indwelling catheter, promote normal bladder function and prevent trauma to the urethra.

Removing a catheter requires a clean, disposable towel; a trash receptacle; and a sterile syringe the same size as the volume of solution within the catheter's inflated balloon. Perform hand hygiene and put on clean gloves before removing the catheter. The end of each catheter contains a label that denotes the volume of solution (5 to 30 mL) within the balloon. If a different volume was used, you will probably find a notation on the client record.

Position the client in the same position as during catheterization. Some institutions recommend collecting a sterile urine specimen at this time or sending the catheter tip for culture and sensitivity tests. After removing the tape, place the towel between a female client's thighs or over a male client's thighs. Insert the syringe into the balloon injection port. Most ports are self-sealing and require that only the tip of the syringe be inserted. Slowly withdraw all of the solution to deflate the balloon totally. If a portion of the solution remains, the partially inflated balloon will traumatize the urethral canal as the catheter is removed. After deflation explain that the client will feel a burning sensation as the catheter is withdrawn. Then pull the catheter out smoothly and slowly.

It is normal for the client to experience some dysuria, especially if the catheter has been in place several days or weeks. Until the bladder regains full tone, some clients also experience frequency of urination or urinary retention.

Assess the client's urinary function by noting the first voiding after catheter removal and documenting the time and amount of voiding for the next 24 hours. If amounts are small, frequent assessment of bladder for distention is necessary. If 6 to 8 hours have elapsed without voiding or the client experiences discomfort, it often becomes necessary to reinsert the catheter.

Alternatives to Urethral Catheterization. To avoid the risks associated with urethral catheters, there are two alternatives for urinary drainage.

Suprapubic Catheterization. Suprapubic catheterization involves surgical placement of a catheter through the abdominal wall above the symphysis pubis and into the urinary bladder. The health care provider performs the procedure under local or general anesthesia. The catheter is anchored in place with sutures, a commercially prepared ring seal, or both. Urine drains into a urinary drainage bag. Maintenance of the tubing and drainage bag is the same as for an indwelling catheter. Studies comparing the use of this method of urinary drainage with indwelling catheters have shown mixed results. Infection rates may be slightly lower; however, long-term complications are similar (Doughty, 2006). Sediment, clots, or the abdominal wall itself can block the suprapubic catheter. Adequate fluid intake will help to minimize risk of blockage by increasing urine flow. The suprapubic catheter must remain patent at all times. Monitor the client's I&O carefully, monitor the urine characteristics, and observe for signs of infection (e.g., fever and chills). Also administer skin care around the insertion site. This method may be used in men and women.

Condom Catheter. The second alternative to catheterization is the condom catheter (Box 45-10, p. 1169), which is suitable for incontinent or comatose men who still have complete and spontaneous bladder emptying. The condom is a soft, pliable, latex sheath that slips over the penis. Clients wear it only at night or continuously, depending on the client's needs. There are three general methods of securing the condom catheter. One method uses a strip of elastic tape or rubber that encircles the top of the condom to secure it in place. Another type uses a self-adhesive condom sheath. The third method uses an inflatable ring within the condom to secure placement. Take care to ensure that whatever type or size is used, blood supply to the penis is not impaired. Never use standard adhesive tape to secure a condom catheter because it does not expand with change in penis size and is painful to remove.

The end of the condom is attached to plastic drainage tubing and a bag that you attach to the side of the bed or strap to the client's leg. The condom catheter itself poses little risk of urinary tract infection. Infections usually result from buildup of secretions around the urethra, trauma to the urethral meatus, or buildup of pressure in the outflow tubing.

If the condom catheter is made of opaque material, remove the condom catheter daily to check for skin irritation. Some new condom catheters are more transparent, and you are able to observe the skin through them more easily. With each catheter change clean the urethral meatus and penis thoroughly. Check the drainage tubing often for patency.

For a man with a retracted penis, maintaining a conventional condom catheter often proves difficult. Special devices are available to help alleviate this problem (Figure 45-14, p. 1170). Consult the manufacturer's guidelines for product application.

There are no collection devices for women as effective as the condom catheter is for men, so frequently the only devices used are pads and protective clothing. To maintain dignity, do not refer to pads and protective clothing as adult diapers and change them frequently to control odor. Only use these products temporarily to minimize or prevent episodes of incontinence while treatment is ongoing. Monitor clients frequently, and give good skin care to prevent irritation caused by urine. Some manufacturers have developed a female urinal (Figure 45-15, p. 1170); however, their ease of use may be an issue.

Text continued on p. 1170

Delegation Considerations

The skill of closed catheter irrigation or instillation cannot be delegated. The nurse is responsible for assessing the need for irrigation. Catheter irrigation is usually done in clients with complications such as urinary tract infections or postsurgically after prostatectomy. The nurse directs nursing assistive personnel caring for the client to:

- Report client complaints of pain, discomfort, or fever
- Report the presence of clots in the output or a change in output

Equipment

- Closed intermittent method for irrigation or instillation
  - Sterile irrigation or instillation solution at room temperature (unless otherwise ordered)
  - Sterile graduated container

- Sterile 30- to 50-mL irrigation or cone syringe (used to instill irrigant into catheter)
- Antiseptic swab
- Clamp for catheter or tubing
- Closed continuous method
  - Sterile irrigation solution at room temperature (unless otherwise ordered)
  - Irrigation tubing and clamp (with or without a Y connector) (Clamp regulates irrigation flow rate. Y connector allows intravenous [IV] or irrigant bags to be connected to tubing.)
  - IV pole
  - Antiseptic swab
  - Y connector (optional) (used to connect irrigation tubing to double-lumen catheter).
  - Bath blanket

STEPS	RATIONALE
1. Assess client's record to determine:	
a. Purpose of bladder irrigation	Allows nurse to anticipate observations to make (e.g., blood or mucus in urine)
b. Prescriber's order for type and amount of irrigant (e.g., saline)	Order required to initiate therapy. Ensures that correct medication or solution and amount will be administered. Amount of solution used to flush system may be a nurse judgment or indicated by prescriber or institution policy. Frequency of irrigation is based on need of client (e.g., client who has just had prostate gland surgery may require continuous irrigation for 24 hours).
c. Type of irrigation: continuous or intermittent	Allows nurse to select proper equipment. In continuous irrigation, clamp regulates slow, steady flow into bladder. Because outflow should correspond to regulated drip, patency of catheter must be checked frequently to prevent distension of bladder. For intermittent irrigation, flow from irrigating solution is clamped for a specified time, and designated amount of irrigating solution is allowed to flush into the bladder. Intermittent irrigation requires close observation of catheter patency between irrigations.
d. Type of catheter used. (NOTE: Appropriate catheter should be inserted during the original catheterization.)	Indicates if it is necessary to break into closed system for irrigation.
(1) Single lumen (single use) for open intermittent irrigation only	
(2) Double lumen (one lumen to inflate balloon, one to allow outflow of urine)	
(3) Triple lumen (one lumen to inflate balloon, one to instill irrigation solution, one to allow outflow of urine)	
2. Assess the following:	
a. Color of urine and presence of mucus, clots, or sediment	Indicates if client is bleeding or sloughing tissue and determines necessity for increasing irrigation rates with continuous irrigations or increasing frequency with intermittent irrigations.
b. Palpate bladder.	Determines if urine is draining freely from bladder.
c. Existing closed irrigation system	
(1) Note if fluid entering bladder and fluid draining from bladder are in approximate proportions.	Determines presence of bladder distention.
(2) Determine that drainage tubing is not kinked, clamped off incorrectly, or looped below bladder level.	Determines if system is obstructed. You would expect more output than fluid instilled because of urine production.
(3) Note amount of fluid remaining in existing irrigating solution container.	Allows nurse to anticipate hanging of new irrigation bag.
3. Review I&O record.	Determines baseline for prior urine output measures. All clients with continuous bladder irrigations should have I&O measurements (see Chapter 41).
4. Assess client for presence of bladder spasms and discomfort.	Reveals need for bladder irrigation.
5. Assess client's knowledge regarding purpose of performing catheter irrigations.	Reveals need for client instruction.

✳ SKILL 45-4   CLOSED CATHETER IRRIGATION—CONT'D

STEPS	RATIONALE
6. Perform hand hygiene, and apply clean gloves for closed methods.	Prevents transmission of microorganisms.
7. Provide privacy by pulling bed curtains closed. Fold back covers so that catheter is exposed. Cover client's upper torso with bath blanket.	Promotes client comfort and provides easy access to the catheter.
8. Position client in dorsal recumbent or supine position.	Promotes flow of irrigating solution into bladder.
9. Closed intermittent irrigation or instillation with double-lumen catheter:	
a. Prepare prescribed sterile solution in sterile graduated cup.	Ensures that irrigation or instillation fluid remains sterile.
b. Clamp indwelling retention catheter just below the specimen port.	Occlusion of catheter provides resistance against which the nurse can forcefully instill irrigant into catheter.
c. Draw sterile solution into syringe using aseptic technique.	Ensures sterility of irrigation fluid.

Critical Decision Point: Avoid cold solution as irrigant or instillation because it will result in bladder spasm and discomfort.

d. Apply gloves, and cleanse injection port with antiseptic swab (same port used for specimen collection).	Reduces transmission of infection.
e. Insert hub of syringe through port at 30-degree angle toward bladder using needleless or blunt-needle syringe system.	Ensures that hub enters lumen of catheter and flow is directed into bladder.
f. Slowly inject fluid into catheter and bladder.	Slow, continuous pressure dislodges clots and sediment without traumatizing bladder wall.

Critical Decision Point: If catheter does not irrigate easily, the tip of the catheter is incorrectly placed in the urethra and not in the bladder. Use slow pressure when injecting fluid. Too much pressure will traumatize the urethral or bladder wall.

g. Withdraw syringe, remove clamp, and allow solution to drain into drainage bag. If an instillation, keep catheter clamped to allow solution to remain in bladder for ordered time.	Allows drainage by gravity.

Critical Decision Point: If solution is to remain in bladder, do not forget to unclamp tubing at the end of the instillation period.

10. Closed continuous irrigation (see illustration):	
a. Apply gloves, and using aseptic technique, insert spike of sterile irrigation tubing into bag of sterile irrigating solution.	Prevents entrance of microorganisms.
b. Close clamp on tubing, and hang bag of solution on IV pole.	
c. Open clamp, and allow solution to flow through tubing, keeping end of tubing sterile. Close clamp.	Removes air from tubing.
d. Use aseptic technique to wipe off irrigation port of triple-lumen catheter, or attach sterile Y connector to double-lumen catheter and then attach to irrigation tubing.	Third lumen or Y connector provides means for irrigation solution to enter bladder. System must remain sterile.
e. Be sure that drainage bag and tubing are securely connected to drainage port of triple-lumen catheter or other arm of Y connector.	Ensures that urine and irrigation solution will drain from bladder without leaking.
f. For continuous drainage, calculate drip rate and adjust clamp on irrigation tubing accordingly. Be sure that clamp on drainage tubing is open, and check volume of drainage in drainage bag. Make sure drainage tubing is patent, and avoid kinks.	Ensures continuous, even irrigation of catheter system. Prevents accumulation of solution in bladder, which will cause bladder distention and possible injury.
g. For intermittent flow, clamp tubing on drainage system, open clamp on irrigation tubing, and allow prescribed amount of fluid to enter bladder (100 mL is normal for adults). Close irrigation clamp, and then open drainage tubing clamp. (*Optional:* Leave clamp closed for 20 to 30 minutes if ordered. See previous Critical Decision Point.)	Fluid instills through catheter into bladder, flushing system. Fluid drains out after irrigation is completed.
11. When procedure completed, dispose of contaminated supplies, remove gloves, and perform hand hygiene.	Prevents spread of infection.

Continued

✳ **SKILL 45-4**   **CLOSED CATHETER IRRIGATION—CONT'D**

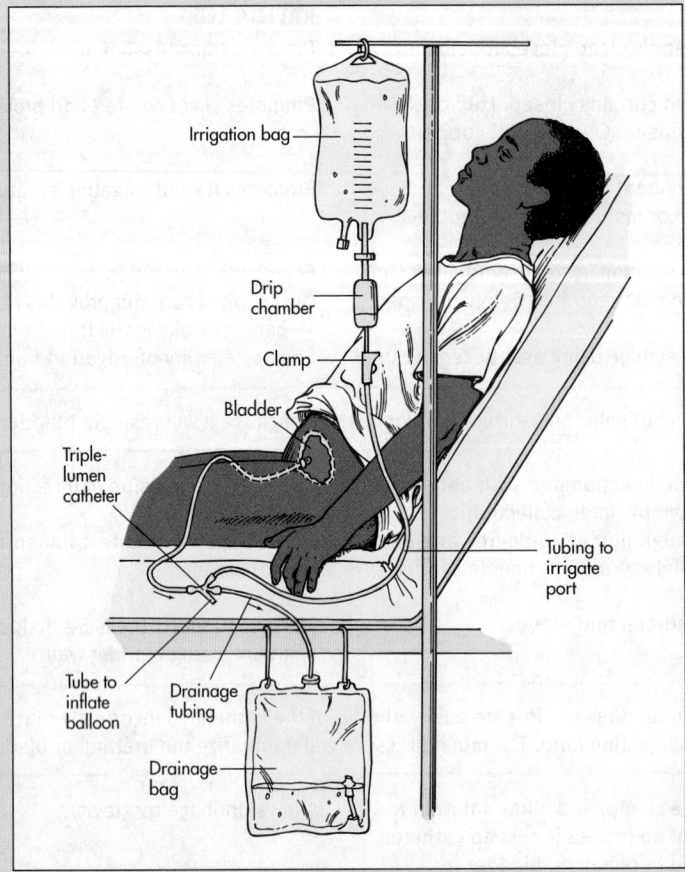

STEP 10 Closed continuous bladder irrigation.

STEPS	**RATIONALE**
12. Calculate amount of irrigation or instillation fluid, and subtract from total output.	Determines accurate urinary output.
13. Assess characteristics of output: viscosity, color, and presence of matter (e.g., sediment, clots, blood).	Evaluates results of irrigation or instillation.

Unexpected Outcomes and Related Interventions

1. Irrigant or instillation solution does not return, or continuous solution is not flowing at prescribed rate, which indicates possible occlusion of catheter.
   a. Examine tubing for kinks, clots, or urine sediment.
   b. Notify health care provider if irrigant or instillation is retained, client complains of pain, or bladder is distended.
2. Cloudy or foul urine, fever
   a. Monitor fever.
   b. Notify health care provider.
   c. Obtain sterile urine specimen if ordered by health care provider.
3. Increase in bladder spasms; indicates occlusion of catheter with foreign object (e.g., blood clot)
   a. Notify health care provider.
   b. Will possibly be instructed to perform intermittent irrigations until clots clear.

Recording and Reporting

- Record type and amount of irrigation solution used, amount returned as drainage, and the character of drainage.
- Record and report any findings such as complaints of bladder spasms, inability to instill fluid into bladder, and/or presence of blood clots.

Home Care Considerations

- If client is discharged with indwelling catheter and requires bladder irrigations, instruct the client and/or the family on proper care.
- Because irrigation or instillation carries a risk of contamination, assess the level of understanding of surgical asepsis by the client and family and provide appropriate instruction. The client and family will need guidelines for the skill and for conditions requiring a call to the health care provider.

✳ BOX 45-10　　　　　　　**PROCEDURAL GUIDELINES**

Condom Catheter

Delegation Considerations: The skill of applying a condom catheter can be delegated. The nurse is responsible for assessing the condition of the penis over time. The nurse directs the nursing assistive personnel to:
- Report any signs of skin irritation or swelling of tissues

Equipment: Condom catheter (may come with self-adhesive or elastic adhesive), collection bag, basin with warm water, towel and washcloth, clean gloves, scissors.

1. Verify health care provider's order.
2. Perform hand hygiene.
3. Assess urinary elimination patterns, client's ability to voluntarily urinate, and continence.
4. Assess mental status of client so you can implement appropriate teaching related to condom care.
5. Assess condition of penis and scrotum.
6. Assess client's knowledge of the purpose of the condom catheter.
7. Explain procedure to client.
8. Raise bed to working height, and raise far upper side rail.
9. Using sheet, drape client so only genitals are exposed.
10. Prepare condom catheter and drainage system (see manufacturer's directions).
11. Apply gloves, and provide perineal care.
    a. If needed, clip hair at base of penile shaft.
12. Apply skin prep to penile shaft, and allow to dry.
13. Holding penis in nondominant hand, apply condom by rolling smoothly onto penis. NOTE: Leave a 2.5- to 5-cm (1- to 2-inch) space between tip of penis and end of catheter (see illustration).
14. Secure condom catheter:
    a. If using elastic adhesive, wrap the strip of adhesive over the condom to secure it in place by using a spiral technique (see illustration). NOTE: Never use adhesive tape.
    b. For self-adhesive catheter, follow manufacturer's directions.
15. Attach catheter to drainage bag, and attach drainage bag to lower bed frame or leg bag (see illustration).
16. Make client comfortable.
17. Observe urinary drainage, drainage tube patency, condition of penis, and tape placement.

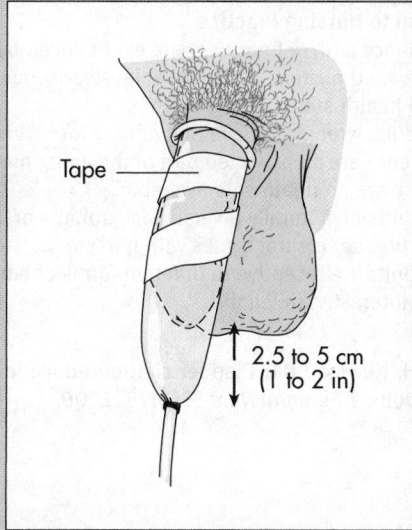

Tape

2.5 to 5 cm
(1 to 2 in)

STEPS 13 and 14A Distance between end of penis and tip of catheter. Elastic tape is applied in spiral fashion to secure the condom catheter to the penis.

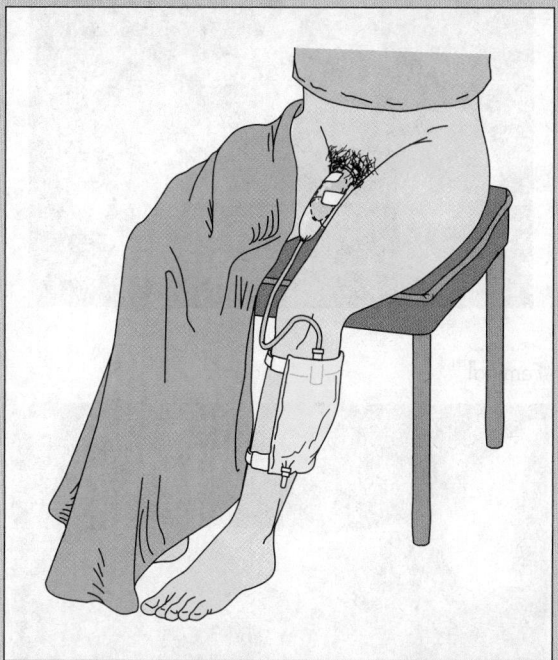

STEP 15 Attach condom catheter tubing to leg bag.

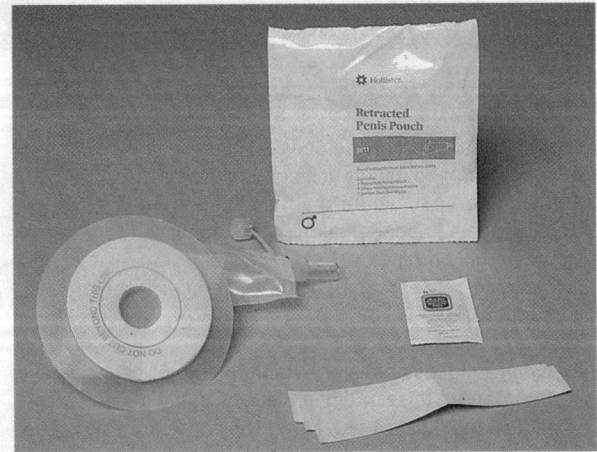

Figure 45-14 Retracted penis pouch external urinary device.

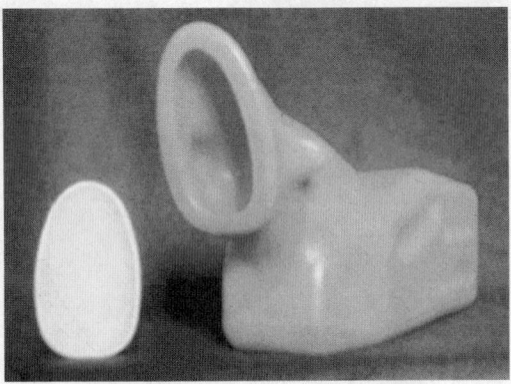

Feminal™

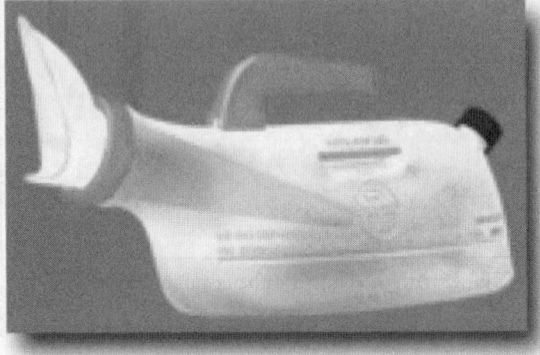

URSEC™

Figure 45-15 Types of female urinals. (Feminal courtesy Bruce Medical, Waltham, Mass; URSEC, Providence Spillproof Container, courtesy Allegro Medical, Providence, RI.)

Restorative Care. Some clients regain normal urinary voiding function through special activities such as bladder retraining, habit training, or cognitive therapy (Box 45-11). In some cases self-catheterization may be used to restore a measure of control to the client.

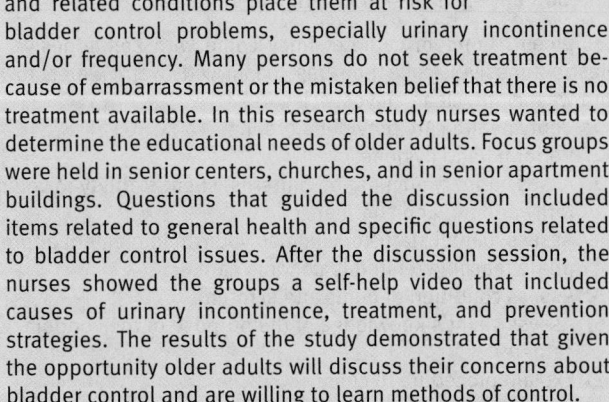

✳ BOX 45-11   EVIDENCE-BASED PRACTICE

Bladder Control: Educational Needs of Older Adults

Evidence Summary

The majority of older adults have bladder control, but changes due to aging, chronic diseases, and related conditions place them at risk for bladder control problems, especially urinary incontinence and/or frequency. Many persons do not seek treatment because of embarrassment or the mistaken belief that there is no treatment available. In this research study nurses wanted to determine the educational needs of older adults. Focus groups were held in senior centers, churches, and in senior apartment buildings. Questions that guided the discussion included items related to general health and specific questions related to bladder control issues. After the discussion session, the nurses showed the groups a self-help video that included causes of urinary incontinence, treatment, and prevention strategies. The results of the study demonstrated that given the opportunity older adults will discuss their concerns about bladder control and are willing to learn methods of control.

   Although the participants in the focus groups were mainly active older adults in an urban setting, the information gathered was helpful as a starting point for designing educational programs for that population. The participant groups included both men and women and were diverse in ethnicity and race.

Application to Nursing Practice
- Incontinence and/or frequency are experienced by adults of all ages, ethnicities, educational levels, economic status, and health status.
- Many adults wrongly believe that urinary incontinence and/or frequency are an expected part of the aging process and that there are no treatments available.
- Older adults of culturally diverse backgrounds are willing to discuss bladder control issues with nurses.
- Older adults are receptive to different forms of education and are interested in learning.

Reference

Palmer MH, Newman DK: Bladder control: educational needs of older adults, *J Gerontol Nurs* 32(1):28, 2006.

Strengthening Pelvic Floor Muscles. Clients who have stress or urge urinary incontinence may benefit from **pelvic floor exercises (PFEs).** Pelvic floor exercises, also known as Kegel exercises, improve the strength of pelvic floor muscles and consist of repetitive contractions of muscle groups (Thompson and Smith, 2002). These exercises have demonstrated effectiveness in treating stress incontinence, overactive bladders, and mixed cause of urinary incontinence (Sampselle, 2003). A client begins these exercises during voiding to learn the technique. They are then practiced at nonvoiding times. Improvement is usually gradual. Clients need to be alert and motivated to perform the exercises. The client needs to continue to use these exercises to maintain effectiveness (see Box 45-6, p. 1151). These exercises are noninvasive and carry a low risk of adverse effects.

Bladder Retraining. The goal of bladder retraining is to reduce the voiding frequency and perhaps to increase the bladder capacity (Doughty, 2006). This method is a specific program for clients with urge urinary incontinence related to overactive bladder. Ultimately the overall goal of this retraining is to restore a normal pattern of voiding by teaching clients to ignore the frequent urge and suppress it. Initially clients keep a bladder diary or log noting times, volumes, fluid intake, and any other related symptoms. This provides a baseline for comparison during the retraining. For bladder retraining to be successful, clients must be alert and physically able to follow a training program.

Assess the client's current pattern of urination. This information allows the nurse to plan a program that often takes 2 weeks or more to learn. Although clients may start the program in the hospital or in rehabilitation, they may need to continue it in an extended care facility or at home. Generally the client is asked to suppress urination for each voiding and increase time by increments of 15 minutes every week. The goal is to void every 3 to 4 hours in volumes of 240 to 500 mL. If the client has an underlying UTI, treat this at the same time.

As part of restorative and rehabilitative care, clients with different types of incontinence may benefit from specific measures that address particular continence issues. These guidelines help the client control factors that affect the number of incontinence episodes.

For clients with stress urinary incontinence the following measures may help the client to gain control over urination:

- Learning exercises to strengthen the pelvic floor (see Box 45-6)
- Initiating a toileting schedule on awakening, at least every 2 hours during the day and evening, before getting into bed, and every 4 hours at night (individualizing time frame as needed)
- Avoid an overfilled bladder because this increases chances of incontinence related to increased bladder pressure
- Minimizing tea, coffee, other caffeine drinks, and alcohol
- Taking prescribed diuretic medication early in the morning
- Following a weight-control program if obesity is a problem causing increased abdominal pressure

Habit Training. A client with functional incontinence benefits from habit training, which helps clients improve voluntary control over urination. The client establishes a flexible toileting schedule based on the client's pattern. Have the client establish the pattern by documenting episodes of incontinence and then scheduling voiding opportunities just before the urge time interval. The goal is to keep the client dry. Help the client to the bathroom before the urge usually occurs. Time fluids and medications to prevent interference with the toileting schedule. Clients with moderate or severe mental or physical dysfunction benefit. When combined with positive reinforcement to reward successful voiding, this approach is also called prompted voiding.

Self-Catheterization. Some clients with chronic disorders such as spinal cord injury learn to perform self-catheterization. The client must be able to physically manipulate equipment and assume a position for successful catheterization. The nurse teaches the client the structures of the urinary tract, clean versus sterile technique, the importance of adequate fluid intake, and the frequency of self-catheterization. Generally, the goal is to have clients perform self-catheterization 4 to 6 times a day with volumes of 400 to 500 mL, but be sure to individualize the schedule.

Maintenance of Skin Integrity. The normal acidity of urine is irritating to skin. Urine allowed to remain in contact with the skin becomes alkaline, causing encrustations or precipitates to collect on the skin, fostering breakdown. Washing with mild soap and warm water is the best way to remove urine from skin. Body lotion keeps skin moisturized, and petroleum-based ointments provide a barrier to the urine. Clients who wet their clothing need to receive partial baths and dry clothing after voiding. Continuous exposure of the perineal area or skin around an ostomy leads to gradual maceration and excoriation (see Chapter 48) requiring special care.

When the skin becomes irritated or inflamed, often the health care provider will prescribe a cream or spray containing steroids (e.g., Kenalog) to reduce inflammation. If fungal growth develops, the antifungal drug nystatin (Mycostatin), available in cream or powder, is effective.

Promotion of Comfort. Clients with urinary alterations become uncomfortable as a result of the symptoms of urinary problems. Frequent or unpredictable voiding, dysuria, and painful distention are sources of discomfort.

The incontinent client gains comfort from having clean, dry clothing. When stress incontinence is the problem, a protective pad offers protection against soiling. Wet clothing adheres to the skin and can cause rubbing and irritation.

Urinary analgesics that act on the urethral and bladder mucosa relieve dysuria (e.g., phenazopyridine [Pyridium]). Often you will combine this drug with sulfonamide antibiotics in preparations such as Azo-Gantanol and Azo-Gantrisin. Clients taking drugs with phenazopyridine need to be aware that their urine will be orange. They must drink large amounts of fluids to prevent toxicity from the sulfonamides and to maintain optimal flow through the urinary system (Lehne, 2007).

If the client has local discomfort from an inflamed urethra, a warm sitz bath will provide pain relief. The warm water soothes inflamed tissues near the urethral meatus by improving blood supply. The client is often relaxed after a sitz bath, so voiding occurs easily. Clients cannot relieve pain of distention unless they are able to empty the bladder. Interventions that stimulate micturition or intermittent catheterization may be the only sources of pain relief.

 Evaluation

The client is the best source of evaluation of outcomes and responses to nursing care (Figure 45-16). However, the nurse will also evaluate the effectiveness of nursing interventions through comparisons with the outcome goals. Evaluate for changes in the client's voiding pattern and continued presence of urinary tract alteration. Actual outcomes are compared with expected outcomes to determine success or partial success in achieving those outcomes. If the client has had problems with frequency, ask, "Tell me, how frequently are you voiding now?" If the problem had been urgency, ask, "Do you continue to have the feeling of urgency every time you void?" or "Have the symptoms of urgency decreased since you changed your caffeine intake?" Evaluation of an intervention that may take weeks to accomplish, such as pelvic

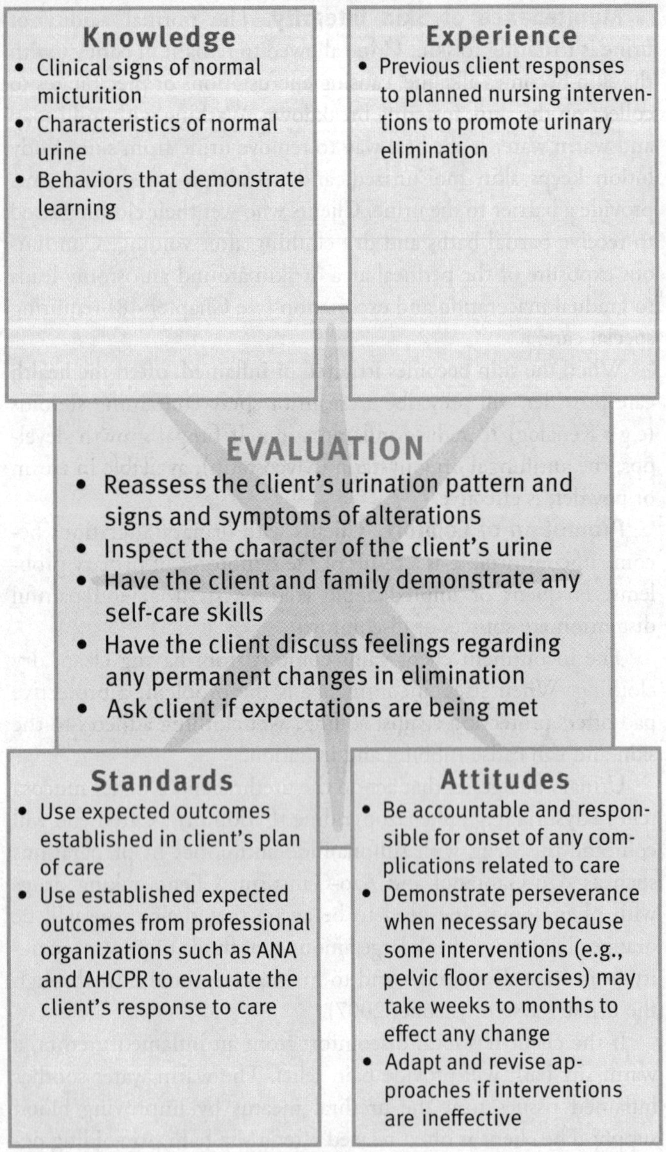

Knowledge

- Clinical signs of normal micturition
- Characteristics of normal urine
- Behaviors that demonstrate learning

Experience

- Previous client responses to planned nursing interventions to promote urinary elimination

EVALUATION

- Reassess the client's urination pattern and signs and symptoms of alterations
- Inspect the character of the client's urine
- Have the client and family demonstrate any self-care skills
- Have the client discuss feelings regarding any permanent changes in elimination
- Ask client if expectations are being met

Standards

- Use expected outcomes established in client's plan of care
- Use established expected outcomes from professional organizations such as ANA and AHCPR to evaluate the client's response to care

Attitudes

- Be accountable and responsible for onset of any complications related to care
- Demonstrate perseverance when necessary because some interventions (e.g., pelvic floor exercises) may take weeks to months to effect any change
- Adapt and revise approaches if interventions are ineffective

Figure 45-16 Critical thinking model for urinary elimination evaluation.

floor exercises, will require follow-up beyond the hospital or rehabilitation facility. Specific information about how well an intervention has met the need will determine if you need to revise the plan of care. Continuous evaluation allows the nurse to determine whether any new symptoms or nursing diagnoses have developed. Assist the client in redefining goals when impairment in function is not likely to be altered as completely as the client might like.

Key Concepts

- Voluntary control from higher brain centers and involuntary control from the spinal cord influence the act of micturition or voiding.
- Symptoms common to urinary disturbances include frequency, urgency, dysuria, polyuria, oliguria, incontinence, and difficulty in starting the urinary stream.

- When collected properly, a clean-voided urine specimen does not contain bacteria from the urethral meatus.
- Methods of promoting the micturition reflex assist clients in sensing the urge to urinate and controlling urethral sphincter relaxation.
- An increased fluid intake results in increased diluted urine formation that reduces the risk of urinary tract infections.
- An indwelling urinary catheter remains in the bladder for an extended period, making the risk of infection greater than with intermittent catheterization.
- Catheter irrigation becomes necessary when the catheter becomes occluded with sediment or blood clots.
- A catheter drainage system should be a closed system positioned to allow free drainage of urine by gravity.
- Incontinence is classified as functional, overflow, stress, urge, or total. Each type has specific nursing interventions.
- Follow specific guidelines for catheter selection so that the catheter does not cause harm.

Critical Thinking Exercises

Mrs. Grayson is a 55-year-old woman who has had problems with stress incontinence for the past 2 years. She has not spoken to anyone about her problems because she is embarrassed. She finally confides to her health care practitioner that the problem is causing her to avoid social situations and she would like help to regain urinary control. Mrs. Grayson weighs 200 pounds, and her height is 5 feet 1 inch. She has been referred to a continence specialist. A plan of care was devised after a thorough assessment of her urinary pattern and symptoms.

1. She has recently begun Kegel exercises to attempt improvement in her urinary control. She does not feel any difference occurring with the episodes. She has been attempting to deal with the problem by using an absorbent pad in her underwear, but she feels as though everyone knows her problem.
   a. What additional teaching does she need?
   b. What other measures will help her regain control of her urinary elimination?

Two months after your first encounter with Mrs. Grayson, she has been seen by her primary health care provider for burning on urination with increased frequency and urgency. She has also noticed some blood in her urine for a week, but she was hoping it would go away.

2. a. What diagnostic studies will assist in a diagnosis?
   b. What measures will assist in reducing her symptoms?

Although the Kegel exercises have helped Mrs. Grayson to regain urinary control most of the time, and she has eliminated caffeinated liquids from her diet, she is not satisfied with her current state of urinary control.

3. Mrs. Grayson has decided on a more permanent solution to her stress incontinence. She opts for a minimally invasive procedure that will provide support for the urethra (tension-free vaginal tape [TVT]). She will be going home with an indwelling catheter. She asks how to care for the catheter while she is home. She does not want another urinary tract infection.
   a. What do you tell her about measures at home to remain infection free?

❋ NCLEX®-Style Review Questions

1. A female client reports that she is experiencing burning on urination, frequency, and urgency. The nurse notes that a clean-voided urine specimen is markedly cloudy. The probable cause of these symptoms and findings is:
   1. Cystitis
   2. Hemorrhage
   3. Incontinence
   4. A renal stone

2. The urine appears concentrated and cloudy because of the presence of white blood cells or _____.

3. Elimination changes that result from obstruction to the flow of urine in the urinary collecting system may cause which of the following? (Choose all that apply.)
   1. Blood clots
   2. Dehydration
   3. Renal damage
   4. Urinary retention
   5. Urinary tract infection

4. Health care–acquired UTIs are often related to poor hand washing and:
   1. Poor urinary output
   2. Poor perineal hygiene
   3. Urinary drainage bags
   4. Improper catheter care

5. Some medications change the color of urine. Pyridium colors the urine:
   1. Blue
   2. Brown
   3. Yellow
   4. Bright orange to rust

6. To minimize nocturia, clients should avoid fluids:
   1. After lunch
   2. In the late afternoon
   3. 2 hours before bedtime
   4. 4 hours before bedtime

7. Maintaining a Foley catheter drainage bag in the dependent position prevents:
   1. Urinary reflux
   2. Urinary retention
   3. Reflex incontinence
   4. Urinary incontinence

8. When applying a condom catheter, it is important to secure the catheter on the penile shaft in such a manner that the catheter is:
   1. Tight and draining well
   2. Dependent and draining well
   3. Secured with adhesive tape applied in a circular pattern
   4. Snug and secure, but does not cause constriction to blood flow

9. After a transurethral prostatectomy a client returns to his room with a triple-lumen indwelling catheter and continuous bladder irrigation. The irrigation is normal saline at 150 mL/hr. The nurse empties the drainage bag for a total of 2520 mL after an 8-hour period. How much of the total is urine output? _____

10. A client undergoes a kidney ultrasound examination. The nurse providing postprocedure care remembers:
    1. That there are no special precautions
    2. To assess each urine specimen for blood for 24 hours
    3. To save all urine in a radiation-safe container for 12 hours
    4. Limit contact with the client to 10 minutes each hour for 6 hours

46 | Bowel Elimination

OBJECTIVES

Mastery of content in this chapter will enable the student to:

- Discuss the role of gastrointestinal organs in digestion and elimination.
- Describe three functions of the large intestine.
- Explain the physiological aspects of normal defecation.
- Discuss psychological and physiological factors that influence the elimination process.
- Describe common physiological alterations in elimination.
- Assess a client's elimination pattern.
- List nursing diagnoses related to alterations in elimination.

- Describe nursing implications for common diagnostic examinations of the gastrointestinal tract.
- List nursing interventions that promote normal elimination.
- List nursing interventions included in bowel training.
- Discuss nursing care measures required for clients with a bowel diversion.
- Utilize critical thinking in the provision of care to clients with alterations in bowel elimination.

MEDIA RESOURCES   KEY TERMS

Companion CD
- NCLEX®-Style Review Questions
- Audio Glossary
- Interactive Learning Activities
- English/Spanish Glossary

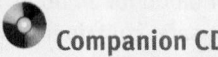 **Website**
- NCLEX®-Style Review Questions
- Audio Glossary
- English/Spanish Glossary
- Interactive Learning Activities
- Weblinks
- Audio Summaries
- Video Clips
- Nursing Skills Online

Bolus, p. 1175
Bowel training, p. 1216
Cathartics, p. 1178
Chyme, p. 1175
Clostridium difficile, p. 1180
Colitis, p. 1178
Colostomy, p. 1181
Constipation, p. 1179
Crohn's disease, p. 1178
Defecation, p. 1176
Diarrhea, p. 1179
Effluent, p. 1203
Endoscopy, p. 1178
Enema, p. 1197
Excoriation, p. 1203
Fecal occult blood testing
   (FOBT), p. 1188

Fiber, p. 1177
Flatulence, p. 1181
Hemorrhoids, p. 1181
Ileostomy, p. 1181
Impaction, p. 1179
Incontinence, p. 1180
Lactose intolerant, p. 1177
Laxatives, p. 1178
Masticate, p. 1175
Paralytic ileus, p. 1178
Peristalsis, p. 1175
Polyps, p. 1181
Segmentation, p. 1175
Stoma, p. 1181
Valsalva maneuver, p. 1176
Wound ostomy continence
   nurse (WOCN), p. 1210

Regular elimination of bowel waste products is essential for normal body functioning. Alterations in elimination are often early signs or symptoms of problems within either the gastrointestinal or other body systems. Because bowel function depends on the balance of several factors, elimination patterns and habits vary among individuals.

Understanding normal elimination and factors that promote, impede, or cause alterations in elimination help manage clients' elimination problems. Supportive nursing care respects the client's privacy and emotional needs. Measures designed to promote normal elimination also need to minimize discomfort for the client.

Scientific Knowledge Base

The gastrointestinal (GI) tract is a series of hollow mucous membrane–lined muscular organs. The purposes of these organs are to absorb fluid and nutrients, prepare food for absorption and use by the body's cells, and provide for temporary storage of feces (Figure 46-1). The volume of fluids absorbed by the GI tract is high, making fluid and electrolyte balance a key function of the GI system. In addition to ingested fluids and foods, the GI tract also receives secretions from the gallbladder and pancreas.

Mouth

Digestion begins in the mouth and ends in the small intestine. The mouth mechanically and chemically breaks down nutrients into a usable size and form. The teeth **masticate** food, breaking it down into a size suitable for swallowing. Saliva, produced by the salivary glands in the mouth, dilutes and softens the food in the mouth for easier swallowing.

Esophagus

As food enters the upper esophagus, it passes through the upper esophageal sphincter, a circular muscle that prevents air from entering the esophagus and food from refluxing into the throat. The **bolus** of food travels down the esophagus and is pushed along by **peristalsis**, which propels food through the length of the GI tract.

As food moves down the esophagus, it reaches the cardiac or lower esophageal sphincter, which lies between the esophagus and the upper end of the stomach. The sphincter prevents reflux of stomach contents back into the esophagus.

Stomach

The stomach performs three tasks: storing swallowed food and liquid; mixing of food, liquid, and digestive juices; and emptying its contents into the small intestine. The stomach produces and secretes hydrochloric acid (HCl), mucus, the enzyme pepsin, and the intrinsic factor. Pepsin and HCl facilitate the digestion of protein. Mucus protects the stomach mucosa from acidity and enzyme activity. The intrinsic factor is essential for the absorption of vitamin B_{12}.

Small Intestine

Segmentation and peristaltic movement in the small intestine facilitate both digestion and absorption (Figure 46-2). **Chyme** mixes with digestive juices (e.g., bile and amylase). Reabsorption in the

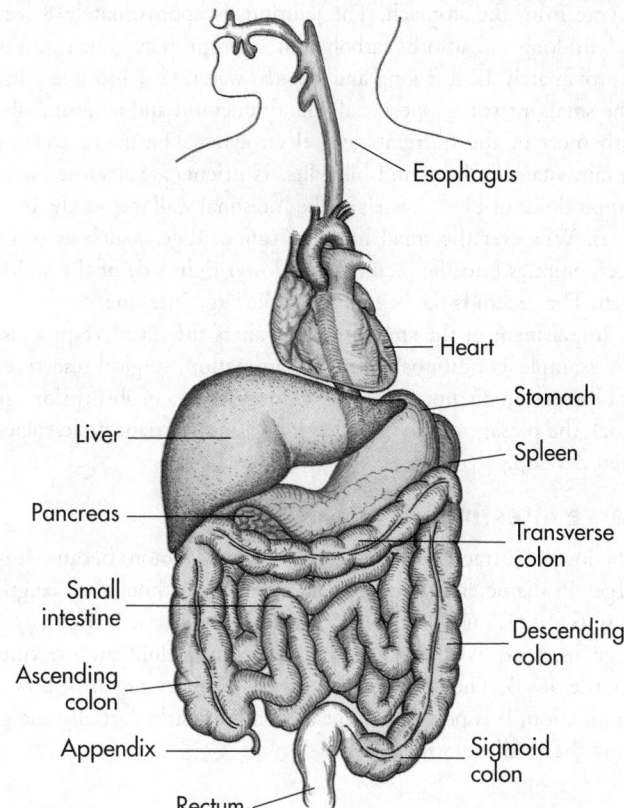

Figure 46-1 Organs of the gastrointestinal tract (with the heart as a reference point).

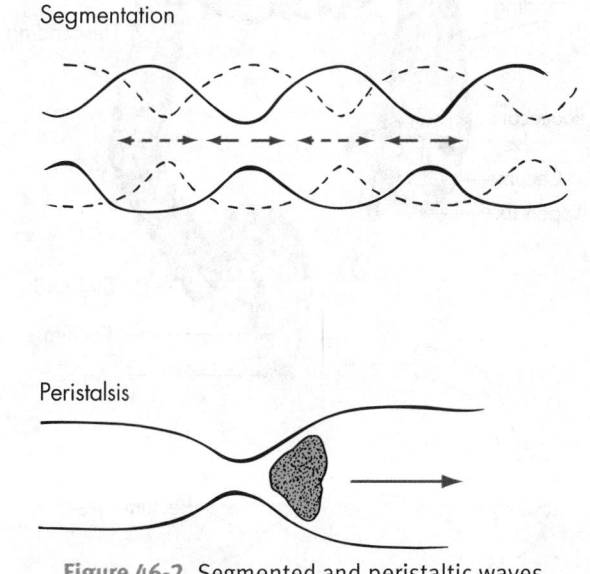

Figure 46-2 Segmented and peristaltic waves.

small intestine is so efficient that by the time the chyme reaches the end of the small intestine, it is pastelike in consistency.

The small intestine has three sections: the duodenum, the jejunum, and the ileum. The duodenum is approximately 8 to 11 inches (20 to 28 cm) long and continues to process the chyme from the stomach. The jejunum is approximately 8 feet (2.5 m) long and absorbs carbohydrates and proteins. The ileum is approximately 12 feet long and absorbs water, fats, and bile salts. The small intestines, specifically the duodenum and jejunum, absorb most of the nutrients and electrolytes. The ileum absorbs certain vitamins, iron, and bile salts. Nutrients are absorbed into lymph fluids or blood vessels in the intestinal wall (across the mucosa). Whatever the small intestine cannot digest, such as plant fiber, empties into the cecum at the lower right side of the abdomen. The cecum is the beginning of the large intestine.

Impairment of the small intestine alters the digestive process. For example, conditions such as inflammation, surgical resection, or obstruction disrupt peristalsis, reduce the area of absorption, or block the passage of chyme. Electrolyte and nutrient deficiencies then develop.

Large Intestine

The lower GI tract is called the *large intestine* (colon) because it is larger in diameter than the small intestine. Although its length (5 to 6 feet [1.5 to 1.8 m]) is much shorter, it is much wider. The large intestine is divided into the cecum, colon, and rectum (Figure 46-3). The large intestine is the primary organ of bowel elimination. It is positioned like a question mark, partially encircling the small intestine.

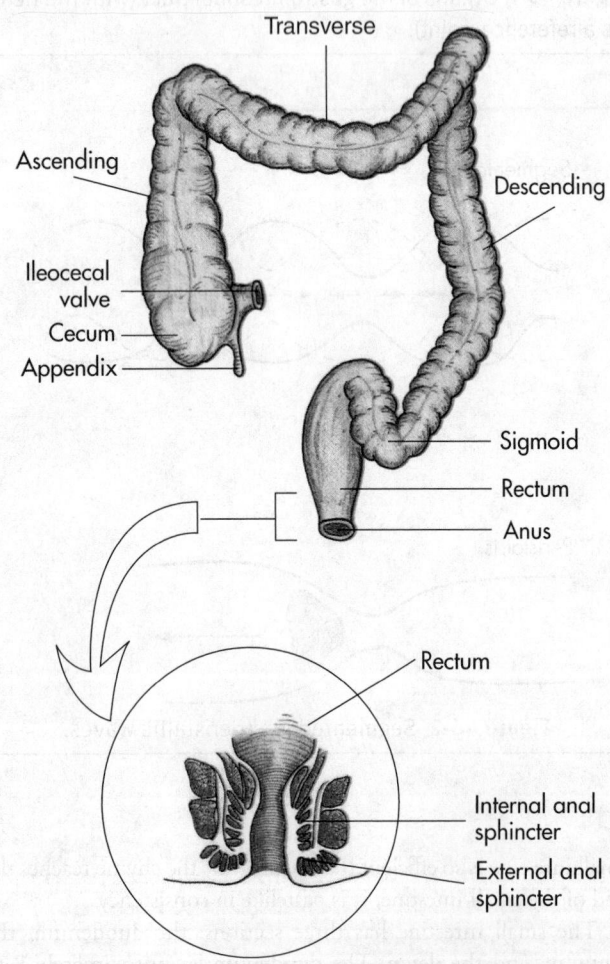

Figure 46-3 Divisions of the large intestine.

Chyme enters the large intestine by waves of peristalsis through the ileocecal valve, a circular muscular layer that prevents regurgitation. The colon is divided into the ascending, transverse, descending, and sigmoid colons. The colon's muscular tissue allows it to accommodate and eliminate large quantities of waste and gas (flatus). The colon has three functions: absorption, secretion, and elimination. The large intestine absorbs water, sodium, and chloride from the digested food that has passed from the small intestine. Healthy adults absorb more than a gallon of water and an ounce of salt from the colon every 4 hours. The amount of water absorbed from chyme depends on the speed at which colonic contents move. Chyme is normally a soft, formed mass. If peristalsis is abnormally fast, there is less time for water to be absorbed and the stool will be watery. If peristaltic contractions slow down, water continues to be absorbed and a hard mass of stool forms, resulting in constipation.

The secretory function of the colon aids in electrolyte balance. Bicarbonate is secreted in exchange for chloride. The colon excretes about 4 to 9 mEq of potassium daily. Serious alterations in colon function (e.g., diarrhea) cause severe electrolyte disturbances.

Slow peristaltic contractions move contents through the colon. Intestinal content is the main stimulus for contraction. Mass peristalsis pushes undigested food toward the rectum. These mass movements occur only three or four times daily, with the strongest during the hour after mealtime.

The rectum is the final portion of the large intestine. Here, bacteria convert fecal matter into its final form. Normally the rectum is empty of waste products (feces) until just before defecation. The rectum contains vertical and transverse folds of tissue that help to temporarily hold fecal contents during **defecation.** Each fold contains an artery and vein that can become distended from pressure during straining. This distention often results in hemorrhoid formation.

Anus

The body expels feces and flatus from the rectum through the anal canal and anus. Contraction and relaxation of the internal and external sphincters, innervated by sympathetic and parasympathetic stimuli, aid in the control of defecation. The anal canal is richly supplied with sensory nerves that help to control continence.

Defecation

The physiological factors critical to bowel function and **defecation** include normal GI tract function, sensory awareness of rectal distention and rectal contents, voluntary sphincter control, and adequate rectal capacity and compliance (Doughty, 2006). Normal defecation begins with movement in the left colon, moving stool toward the anus. When stool reaches the rectum, the distention causes relaxation of the internal sphincter, and an awareness of the need to defecate. At the time of defecation, the external sphincter relaxes and abdominal muscles contract, increasing intrarectal pressure and forcing the stool out (Doughty, 2006). Pressure can be exerted to expel feces through a voluntary contraction of the abdominal muscles while maintaining forced expiration against a closed airway. This is the **Valsalva maneuver,** which assists in stool passage. Clients with cardiovascular disease, glaucoma, increased intracranial pressure, or a new surgical wound are at greater risk, such as cardiac irregularities and elevated blood pressure, with this maneuver and need to avoid straining to pass the stool. Normal defecation is painless, resulting in passage of soft, formed stool.

Nursing Knowledge Base

Factors Affecting Bowel Elimination

Many factors influence the process of bowel elimination. Knowledge of these factors will assist in anticipating measures required to maintain a normal elimination pattern.

Age. Developmental changes affecting elimination occur throughout life. An infant has a small stomach capacity and less secretion of digestive enzymes. Food passes quickly through an infant's intestinal tract because of rapid peristalsis. The infant is unable to control defecation because of a lack of neuromuscular development. This development usually does not take place until 2 to 3 years of age.

Systemic changes in the function of digestion and absorption of nutrients result from changes in older clients' cardiovascular and neurological systems, rather than their gastrointestinal system. For example, arteriosclerosis causes decreased mesenteric blood flow, thus decreasing absorption from the small intestine (Meiner and Lueckenotte, 2006). In addition, there is a decrease in peristalsis, and esophageal emptying slows. Older adults often experience changes in the GI system that impair digestion and elimination (Table 46-1).

Older adults also loose muscle tone in the perineal floor and anal sphincter. Although the integrity of the external sphincter remains intact, older adults often have difficulty controlling bowel evacuation and are at risk for incontinence. In addition, there is a slowing of nerve impulses to the anal region, and some individuals become less aware of the need to defecate and as a result develop irregular bowel movements and are at risk for constipation, especially residents in long-term care facilities (Bosshard and others, 2004).

Diet. Regular daily food intake helps maintain a regular pattern of peristalsis in the colon. **Fiber,** the nondigestible residue in the diet, provides the bulk of fecal material. Bulk-forming foods, such as whole grains, fresh fruits, and vegetables, help flush the fats and waste products from the body with more efficiency. The bowel walls stretch, creating peristalsis and initiating the defecation reflex. By stimulating peristalsis, bulk foods pass quickly through the intestines, keeping the stool soft. Ingestion of a high-fiber diet improves the likelihood of a normal elimination pattern if other factors are normal. When there is no fiber to transport waste matter through the colon, it increases the risk for polyps (Miskovitz and Betancourt, 2005).

Gas-producing foods such as onions, cauliflower, and beans also stimulate peristalsis. The gas formed distends intestinal walls and increases colon motility. Some spicy foods increase peristalsis but also cause indigestion and watery stools.

Food intolerance is not an allergy, but a particular food that causes the body distress within a few hours of ingestion. The result is diarrhea, cramps, or flatulence. For example, people who drink cow's milk who have these symptoms are not allergic to milk. They lack the enzyme needed to digest the milk sugar lactose and are **lactose intolerant** (Miskovitz and Betancourt, 2005).

Fluid Intake. An inadequate fluid intake or disturbances resulting in fluid loss (such as vomiting) affect the character of feces. Fluid liquefies intestinal contents, easing its passage through the

---

✳ TABLE 46-1 Normal Age-Related Changes in the Gastrointestinal Tract

PORTION OF GASTROINTESTINAL TRACT	FUNCTIONAL OR PHYSIOLOGICAL CHANGE	CAUSES
Mouth	Decreased chewing and decreased salivation, including oral dryness	Degeneration of cells, medications.
Esophagus	Reduced motility, especially in lower third	Degeneration of neural cells.
Stomach	Decrease in:	
	Acid secretions	Degeneration of gastric mucosa. Alkaline gastric medium contributes to malabsorption of iron. Although digestive enzymes are decreased, enough remain available for digestion.
	Motor activity	Delayed gastric emptying, causing fewer hunger contractions.
	Mucosal thickness	Loss of parietal cells also leads to loss of intrinsic factor, which is necessary for vitamin B_{12} absorption.
Small intestine	Decreased nutrient absorption	Fewer absorbing cells.
Large intestine	Increase in pouches on the weakened intestinal wall called diverticulosis	Weakened musculature. Does not significantly affect absorption.
	Constipation	Decreased peristalsis.
	Missed defecation signal	Duller nerve sensations.
	Increasing risk for fecal incontinence	
Liver	Size decreased	Reduced storage capacity and ability to synthesize protein and metabolize medications.

Data from Meiner S, Lueckenotte AG: *Gerontologic nursing,* ed 3, St. Louis, 2006, Mosby.

colon. Reduced fluid intake slows passage of food through the intestine and results in hardening of stool contents. Unless there is a medical contraindication, an adult needs to drink six to eight glasses (1500 to 2000 mL) of noncaffeinated fluid daily. An increase in fluid intake with the use of fruit juices softens stool and increases peristalsis. Poor fluid intake increases the risk of constipation due to reabsorption of fluid in the colon, resulting in hard, dry stools (Wilson, 2005).

Physical Activity. Physical activity promotes peristalsis, whereas immobilization depresses peristalsis. Encourage early ambulation as illness begins to resolve or as soon as possible after surgery to promote maintenance of peristalsis and normal elimination. Maintaining tone of skeletal muscles used during defecation is important. Weakened abdominal and pelvic floor muscles impair the ability to increase intraabdominal pressure and to control the external sphincter. Muscle tone is sometimes weakened or lost as a result of long-term illness or neurological disease that impairs nerve transmission. As a result of these changes in the abdominal and pelvic floor muscles, there is an increased risk for constipation.

Psychological Factors. Prolonged emotional stress impairs the function of almost all body systems (see Chapter 31). During emotional stress the digestive process is accelerated, and peristalsis is increased. Side effects of increased peristalsis are diarrhea and gaseous distention. A number of diseases of the GI tract are associated with stress. These include ulcerative **colitis,** irritable bowel syndrome, certain gastric and duodenal ulcers, and **Crohn's disease.** If a person becomes depressed, the autonomic nervous system slows impulses and peristalsis decreases, resulting in constipation.

Personal Habits. Personal elimination habits influence bowel function. Most people benefit from being able to use their own toilet facilities at a time that is most effective and convenient for them. A busy work schedule sometimes prevents the individual from responding appropriately to the urge to defecate, disrupting regular habits and causing possible alterations such as constipation. Individuals need to recognize the best time for elimination.

Chronically ill and hospitalized clients are not always able to maintain privacy during defecation. In a hospital or extended care setting, clients sometimes share bathroom facilities with a roommate with different hygienic habits. In addition, chronic illness limits a client's balance, activity tolerance, or physical activity and requires the use of a bedpan or bedside commode. The sights, sounds, and odors associated with sharing toilet facilities or using bedpans are often embarrassing. This embarrassment may prompt clients to ignore the urge to defecate, which begins a vicious cycle of constipation and discomfort.

Position During Defecation. Squatting is the normal position during defecation. Modern toilets facilitate this posture, allowing the person to lean forward, exert intraabdominal pressure, and contract the thigh muscles. For the client immobilized in bed, defecation is often difficult. In a supine position it is impossible to contract the muscles used during defecation. If the client's condition permits, raise the head of the bed; this assists the client to a more normal sitting position on a bedpan, enhancing the ability to defecate.

Pain. Normally the act of defecation is painless. However, a number of conditions result in discomfort, such as hemorrhoids, rectal surgery, rectal fistulas, and abdominal surgery. In these instances the client often suppresses the urge to defecate to avoid pain, and thus develops constipation.

Pregnancy. As pregnancy advances, the size of the fetus increases and pressure is exerted on the rectum. A temporary obstruction created by the fetus impairs passage of feces. Slowing of peristalsis during the third trimester often leads to constipation. A pregnant woman's frequent straining during defecation or delivery results in formation of permanent hemorrhoids.

Surgery and Anesthesia. General anesthetic agents used during surgery cause temporary cessation of peristalsis (see Chapter 50). Inhaled anesthetic agents block parasympathetic impulses to the intestinal musculature. The anesthetic's action slows or stops peristaltic waves. The client who receives local or regional anesthesia is less at risk for elimination alterations because this often affects bowel activity minimally or not at all.

Any surgery that involves direct manipulation of the bowel temporarily stops peristalsis. This condition, called **paralytic ileus,** usually lasts about 24 to 48 hours. If the client remains inactive or is unable to eat after surgery, return of normal bowel function is further delayed.

Medications. Some medications have certain expected actions on the bowel; for example, there are medications to promote defecation or control diarrhea. In addition, medications prescribed for acute and chronic conditions often have secondary effects on the client's bowel elimination patterns (Table 46-2).

Laxatives and **cathartics** soften the stool and promote peristalsis. Although similar, laxatives are milder in action than cathartics. When used correctly, laxatives and cathartics safely maintain normal elimination patterns. However, chronic use of cathartics causes the large intestine to lose muscle tone and become less responsive to stimulation by laxatives. Laxative overuse also causes serious diarrhea that leads to dehydration and electrolyte depletion. Mineral oil, a common laxative, decreases fat-soluble vitamin absorption. Laxatives often influence the efficacy of other medications by altering the transit time (i.e., the time the medication remains in the GI tract and is available for absorption).

Diagnostic Tests. Diagnostic examinations involving visualization of GI structures often require a prescribed bowel preparation (e.g., medications, cathartics, and/or enemas) to ensure that the bowel is empty. In addition, the client is not allowed to eat or drink after midnight of the day preceding examinations such as a colonoscopy, **endoscopy,** or other testing that requires visualization of the lower GI tract. Following the diagnostic procedure, there are often changes in elimination, such as increased gas or loose stools, until the client resumes a normal eating pattern.

✳ TABLE 46-2 Medications and the Gastrointestinal System

MEDICATIONS	ACTION
Dicyclomine HCl (Bentyl)	Suppresses peristalsis and decreases gastric emptying.
Opioid analgesics	Slow peristalsis and segmental contractions, often resulting in constipation (McKenry, Tessier, and Hogan, 2006).
Anticholinergic drugs, such as atropine or glycopyrrolate (Robinul)	Inhibit gastric acid secretion and depress GI motility (McKenry and others, 2006). Although useful in treating hyperactive bowel disorders, anticholinergics cause constipation.
Antibiotics	Produce diarrhea by disrupting the normal bacterial flora in the GI tract. An increase in the use of fluoroquinolones in recent years has provided a selective advantage for the epidemic of *C. difficile* (Todd, 2006).
Nonsteroidal antiinflammatory drugs	Causes gastrointestinal irritation that increases the incidence of bleeding with serious consequences to older adults (McKenry and others, 2006).
Aspirin	A prostaglandin inhibitor, it interferes with the formation and production of protective mucus and causes GI bleeding (McKenry and others, 2006).
Histamine$_2$ (H$_2$) antagonists	Suppress the secretion of hydrochloric acid and interferes with the digestion of some foods.
Iron	Causes discoloration of the stool (black), nausea, vomiting, constipation (diarrhea is less commonly reported), and abdominal cramps (McKenry and others, 2006).

Common Bowel Elimination Problems

Caring for clients who have or are at risk for elimination problems because of emotional stress (anxiety or depression), physiological changes in the GI tract such as surgical alteration of intestinal structures, inflammatory diseases, prescribed therapy, or disorders impairing defecation is common in the practice of nursing.

Constipation.

Constipation is a symptom, not a disease (Box 46-1). Improper diet, reduced fluid intake, lack of exercise, and certain medications can cause constipation. The signs of constipation usually include infrequent bowel movements (less than every 3 days), difficulty passing stools, excessive straining, inability to defecate at will, and hard feces (Eberhardie, 2003). When intestinal motility slows, the fecal mass becomes exposed over time to the intestinal walls and most of the fecal water content is absorbed. Little water is left to soften and lubricate the stool. Passage of a dry, hard stool causes rectal pain (Figure 46-4) (Stressman, 2003).

Constipation is a significant health hazard. Straining during defecation causes problems to the client with recent abdominal, gynecological, or rectal surgery. The effort to pass a stool can cause sutures to separate, reopening the wound. In addition, clients with histories of cardiovascular disease, diseases causing elevated intraocular pressure (glaucoma), and increased intracranial pressure need to prevent constipation and avoid using the Valsalva maneuver.

Impaction.

Fecal **impaction** results from unrelieved constipation. It is a collection of hardened feces, wedged in the rectum that a person cannot expel. In cases of severe impaction, the mass extends up into the sigmoid colon. Clients who are debilitated, confused, or unconscious are most at risk for impaction. They are too weak or unaware of the need to defecate, or they are dehydrated so that the stool becomes too hard and dry to pass.

An obvious sign of impaction is the inability to pass a stool for several days, despite the repeated urge to defecate. When a continuous oozing of diarrhea stool occurs, suspect impaction. The

✳ BOX 46-1 Common Causes of Constipation

- Irregular bowel habits and ignoring the urge to defecate.
- Chronic illnesses (e.g., Parkinson's disease, multiple sclerosis, rheumatoid arthritis, chronic bowel diseases, depression, diabetic neuropathy, eating disorders) (Eberhardie, 2003; Richmond, 2003).
- Low-fiber diet high in animal fats (e.g., meats, dairy products, eggs). Also, low fluid intake slows peristalsis (Eberhardie, 2003).
- Anxiety, depression, cognitive impairment (Eberhardie, 2003).
- Lengthy bed rest or lack of regular exercise.
- Laxative misuse (Eberhardie, 2003).
- Older adults experience slowed peristalsis, loss of abdominal muscle elasticity, and reduced intestinal mucus secretion. Older adults often eat low-fiber foods (Stanley and others, 2005).
- Neurological conditions that block nerve impulses to the colon (e.g., spinal cord injury, tumor).
- Organic illnesses such as hypothyroidism, hypocalcemia, or hypokalemia (Richmond, 2003).
- Medications such as anticholinergics, antispasmodics, anticonvulsants, antidepressants, antihistamines, antihypertensives, antiparkinsonism drugs, bile acid sequestrants, diuretics, antacids, iron supplements, calcium supplements, and opioids slow colonic action (Stressman, 2003).

liquid portion of feces located higher in the colon seeps around the impacted mass. Loss of appetite (anorexia), nausea and/or vomiting, abdominal distention and cramping, and rectal pain often accompany the condition. If you suspect an impaction, gently perform a digital examination of the rectum and palpate for the impacted mass.

Diarrhea.

Diarrhea is an increase in the number of stools and the passage of liquid, unformed feces. It is associated with disorders affecting digestion, absorption, and secretion in the GI tract. Intestinal contents pass through the small and large intestine too

The Bristol Stool Form Scale

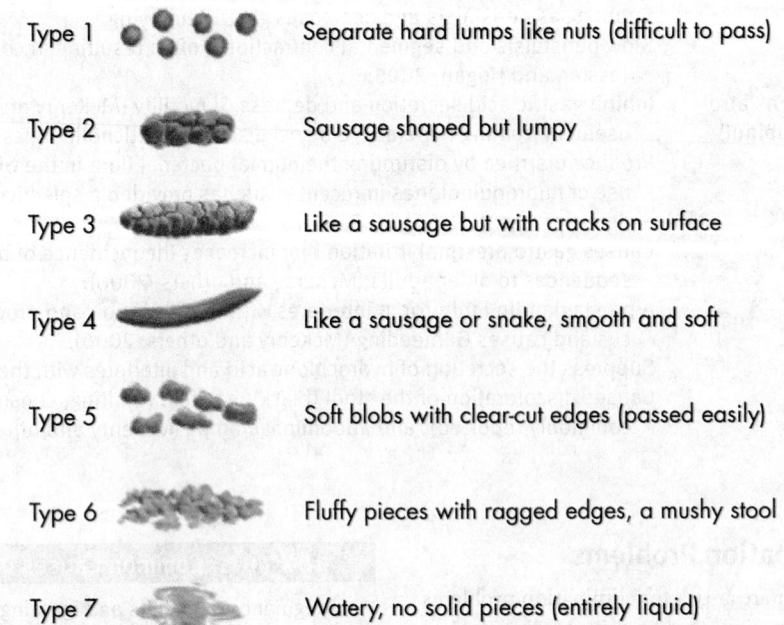

Type 1   Separate hard lumps like nuts (difficult to pass)

Type 2   Sausage shaped but lumpy

Type 3   Like a sausage but with cracks on surface

Type 4   Like a sausage or snake, smooth and soft

Type 5   Soft blobs with clear-cut edges (passed easily)

Type 6   Fluffy pieces with ragged edges, a mushy stool

Type 7   Watery, no solid pieces (entirely liquid)

Figure 46-4 Bristol stool form scale. (Used with permission. *Bristol Stool Form Guideline,* http://www.aboutconstipation.org/bristol.html, accessed July 31, 2006.)

quickly to allow for the usual absorption of fluid and nutrients. Irritation within the colon results in an increased mucus secretion. As a result, feces become watery and the client is unable to control the urge to defecate. Normally an anal bag is safe and effective in long-term treatment of home, hospice, or hospitalized bedridden clients with fecal incontinence. Fecal incontinence is expensive and a potentially dangerous condition in terms of contamination and risk of skin ulceration. Anatomical characteristics and physiological motility of the pelvic floor have hampered the development of suitable disposable containers that can be applied directly to the anus (Palmieri, Benuzzi, and Bellini, 2005).

Excess loss of colonic fluid results in serious fluid and electrolyte or acid-base imbalances. Infants and older adults are particularly susceptible to associated complications (see Chapter 41). Because repeated passage of diarrhea stools also exposes the skin of the perineum and buttocks to irritating intestinal contents, meticulous skin care and containment of fecal drainage is necessary to prevent skin breakdown (see Chapter 48).

Many conditions cause diarrhea. Antibiotic use via any route of administration alters the normal flora in the gastrointestinal tract (Bartlett, 2002). Clients receiving enteral nutrition are also at risk for diarrhea, which is possibly due to the GI response. Interventions to prevent diarrhea include the following: administer canned formulas at room temperature, follow strict sanitation when preparing the formula, increase the rate slowly, administer the volume at a rate tolerable to your client, or if using a hypertonic solution, give the initial feeding at half strength and gradually increase the volume to allow the client to adjust to a hypertonic solution. Consult a dietitian when diarrhea occurs (Tabloski, 2006). Food allergies and intolerances increase peristalsis and

cause diarrhea. Surgeries or diagnostic testing of the lower gastrointestinal tract also cause diarrhea. The aims of treatment are to remove precipitating conditions and to slow peristalsis.

Another common causative agent of diarrhea is *Clostridium difficile* (*C. difficile*), in which symptoms range from mild diarrhea to severe colitis. *C. difficile* infection is acquired in one of two ways, by factors that cause an overgrowth of *C. difficile* and by contact with the *C. difficile* organism. Antibiotics (cephalosporins, ampicillin, amoxicillin, and clindamycin [Harris, 2006]), chemotherapy, and invasive bowel procedures such as surgery or colonoscopy disrupt normal bowel flora and cause an overgrowth of *C. difficile*. Some clients acquire the organism from a health care worker's hands or direct contact with the environmental surfaces contaminated with *C. difficile*. Poor hand hygiene and erratic disinfection practices result in the transmission of *C. difficile* (Todd, 2006). The most common diagnostic test for the bacteria is the enzyme-linked immunosorbent assay (ELISA) test. It detects *C. difficile* A and B in the stool. Two to three stool specimens are required for this test (Harris, 2006).

Communicable food-borne pathogens also cause diarrhea. Simple hand washing following the use of the bathroom, before and after preparing foods, and cleaning and storing fresh produce and meats greatly reduces the risk of food-borne illnesses. When diarrhea is the result of a food-borne virus, the goal is usually to rid the gastrointestinal system of the pathogen, rather than to slow peristalsis.

Incontinence. Fecal **incontinence** is the inability to control passage of feces and gas from the anus. Incontinence harms a client's body image (see Chapter 27). In many situations the client is mentally alert but physically unable to avoid defecation. The embarrassment of soiling clothes often leads to social isolation. Physical conditions that impair anal sphincter function or control cause incontinence. Incontinence occurs in a variety of settings. Conditions that create frequent, loose, large-volume, watery stools also predispose to incontinence. Using an anal bag or a bowel management system, such as Zassi bowel management system, helps to prevent perineal skin breakdown.

Flatulence. As gas accumulates in the lumen of the intestines, the bowel wall stretches and distends (**flatulence**). It is a common cause of abdominal fullness, pain, and cramping. Normally, intestinal gas escapes through the mouth (belching) or the anus (passing of flatus). However, if there is a reduction in intestinal motility resulting from opiates, general anesthetics, abdominal surgery, or immobilization, flatulence becomes severe enough to cause abdominal distention and severe sharp pain.

Hemorrhoids. **Hemorrhoids** are dilated, engorged veins in the lining of the rectum. They are either external or internal. External hemorrhoids are clearly visible as protrusions of skin. If the underlying vein is hardened, there is usually a purplish discoloration (thrombosis). This causes increased pain and often needs to be excised. Internal hemorrhoids have an outer mucous membrane. Increased venous pressure from straining at defecation, pregnancy, heart failure, and chronic liver disease cause hemorrhoids.

Bowel Diversions

Certain diseases cause conditions that prevent normal passage of feces through the rectum. The treatment for these disorders results in the need for a temporary or permanent artificial opening (**stoma**) in the abdominal wall. Surgical openings are created in the ileum (**ileostomy**) or colon (**colostomy**) with the ends of the intestine brought through the abdominal wall to create the stoma.

The standard bowel diversion creates a stoma, or the client has reconstructive bowel surgery that uses the native sphincter for bowel continence. The reconstructive surgery includes a continent stoma procedure, or the ileoanal pouch anastomosis, which is described later in the chapter.

Ostomies. The location of an ostomy determines the consistency of stool. An ileostomy bypasses the entire large intestine. As a result, stools are frequent and liquid. The same is true for a colostomy of the ascending colon. A colostomy of the transverse colon generally results in a more solid, formed stool. The sigmoid colostomy releases near-normal stool. The client's medical problem and general condition determine the location of a colostomy. There are three types of colostomy construction: loop colostomy, end colostomy, and double-barrel colostomy.

Loop Colostomy. A loop colostomy is usually performed in a medical emergency when health care providers anticipate closure of the colostomy. These are usually temporary large stomas constructed in the transverse colon (Figure 46-5, A-D). The surgeon pulls a loop of bowel onto the abdomen (Figure 46-5, E). An external supporting device such as a plastic rod, bridge (Figure 46-5, C and D), or rubber catheter is temporarily placed under the bowel loop to keep it from slipping back (Figure 46-5, A). The surgeon then opens the bowel and sutures it to the skin of the

abdomen (Figure 46-5, F). A communicating wall remains between the proximal and distal bowel. The loop ostomy has two openings through the one stoma (Figure 46-5, D and G). The proximal end drains stool, whereas the distal portion drains mucus. Within 7 to 10 days the surgeon removes the external supporting device.

End Colostomy. The end colostomy consists of one stoma formed from the proximal end of the bowel with the distal portion of the GI tract either removed or sewn closed (called Hartmann's pouch) and left in the abdominal cavity. For many clients, end colostomies are a result of surgical treatment of colorectal cancer. In such cases the rectum is usually removed. Clients with diverticulitis who are treated surgically often have a temporary end colostomy with a Hartmann's pouch (Figure 46-6).

Double-Barrel Colostomy. Unlike the loop colostomy, the bowel is surgically severed in a double-barrel colostomy (Figure 46-7, A), and the two ends are brought out onto the abdomen (Figure 46-7, B). The double-barrel colostomy consists of two distinct stomas: the proximal functioning stoma and the distal nonfunctioning stoma.

Alternative Procedures

Ileoanal Pouch Anastomosis. The ileoanal pouch anastomosis is a surgical procedure that is used in clients who need to have a colectomy for treatment of ulcerative colitis or familial **polyps** (Beitz, 2004). In this procedure the provider removes the colon, creates a pouch from the end of the small intestine, and attaches the pouch to the client's anus (Figure 46-8). This pouch provides for the collection of waste material, which is similar to the rectum. The client is continent of stool because stool is evacuated via the anus. When the ileal pouch is created, the client has a temporary ileostomy to allow the anastomosis to heal.

Kock Continent Ileostomy. The Kock continent ileostomy is created using the client's small intestine, detubularizing its cylindrical shape and creating a spherical reservoir (Beitz, 2004). This procedure is occasionally used in the treatment of ulcerative colitis. The pouch has a continent stoma, a nipple type of valve that is drained with an external catheter, which the client places intermittently in the stoma (Figure 46-9).

Macedo-Malone Antegrade Continence Enema. The Macedo-Malone antegrade continence enema (MACE) procedure was developed to improve continence in clients with fecal soiling associated with neuropathic or structural abnormalities of the anal sphincter. This procedure isolates a 3-cm flap on the left colon. A Foley catheter placed on the surface of the flap creates a tubular passage. This produces a continence valve mechanism. The distal end of the tube is made into a V shape to the skin flap (Figure 46-10). Enema administration begins 7 to 10 days postoperatively. Clients receive enemas daily with the volume varying from 250 to 800 mL and taking 45 to 60 minutes to administer. Colonic evacuation occurs within 30 to 60 minutes (Calado and others, 2005).

Psychological Considerations. A stoma causes serious body image changes, particularly if it is permanent. Clients who have had stoma surgery face a variety of anxieties and concerns, from learning how to manage their stoma to coping with conflicts of self-esteem and body image. Provide emotional support preoperatively and postoperatively (Barr, 2004). Clients often perceive a stoma as invasive and disfiguring. However, a well-placed stoma does not usually interfere with the client's activities and is concealed with clothing

Text continued on p. 1185

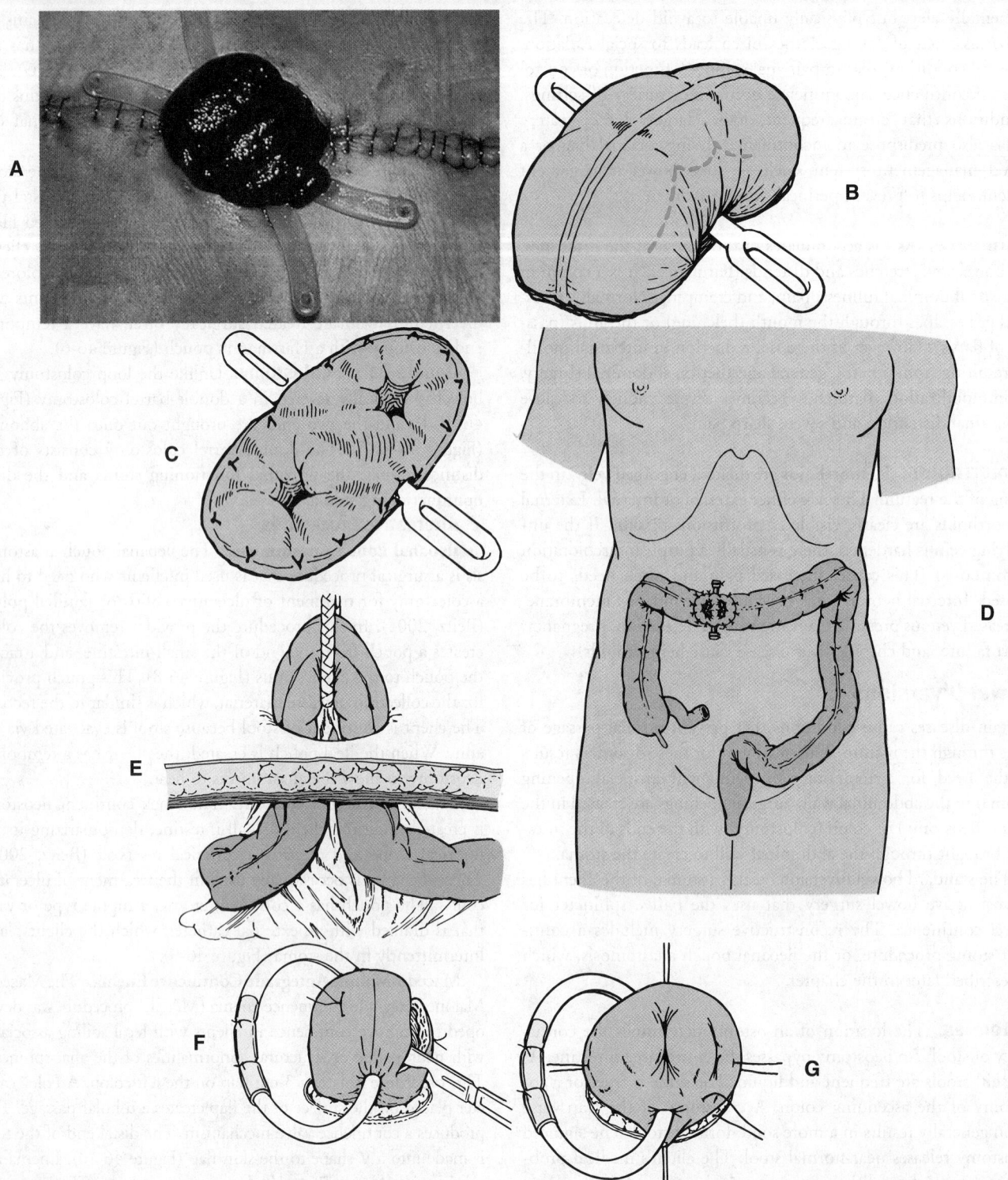

Figure 46-5 A, Transverse loop colostomy supported by a loop ostomy bridge. **A** and **B,** Abdominal view of loop colostomy in transverse colon. **C,** Loop colostomy construction is much the same as construction of loop ileostomy. Stoma is created with longitudinal incision through sacculations in colon. **D,** Loop colostomy matured. **E,** Loop ostomy construction, loop of bowel exteriorized. **F,** Support device placed to maintain position of bowel on abdominal surface. Distal bowel of ileum is incised, mesentery. Stitch placed to designate proximal bowel. **G,** Loop ileostomy matured with protruding functional limb. (**A,** Permission to use and/or reproduce this copyrighted photo has been granted by the owner, Hollister, Incorporated; **B** to **G** from Hampton BG, Bryant RA: *Ostomies and continent diversions: nursing management,* St. Louis, 1992, Mosby.)

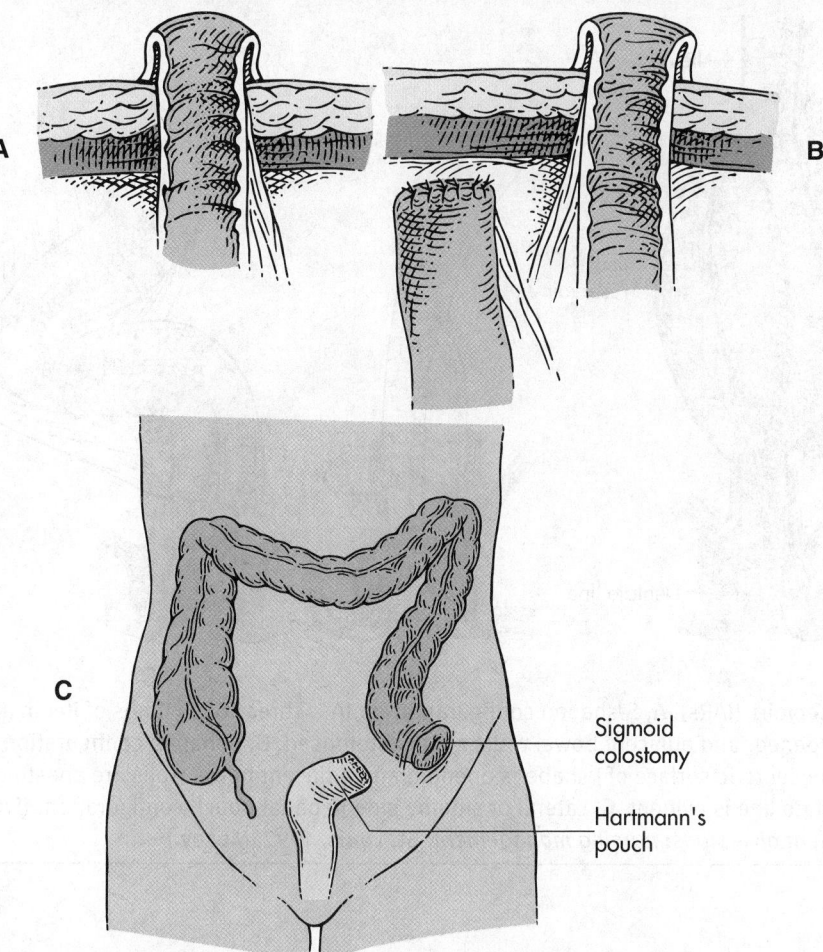

Figure 46-6 End colostomy. **A,** Cross-sectional view of end stoma. **B,** Cross-sectional view of end stoma with distal bowel over-sewn and secured to anterior peritoneum at stoma site. **C,** Sigmoid colostomy. Distal bowel is oversewn and left in place to create Hartmann's pouch. (From Hampton BG, Bryant RA: *Ostomies and continent diversions: nursing management,* St. Louis, 1992, Mosby.)

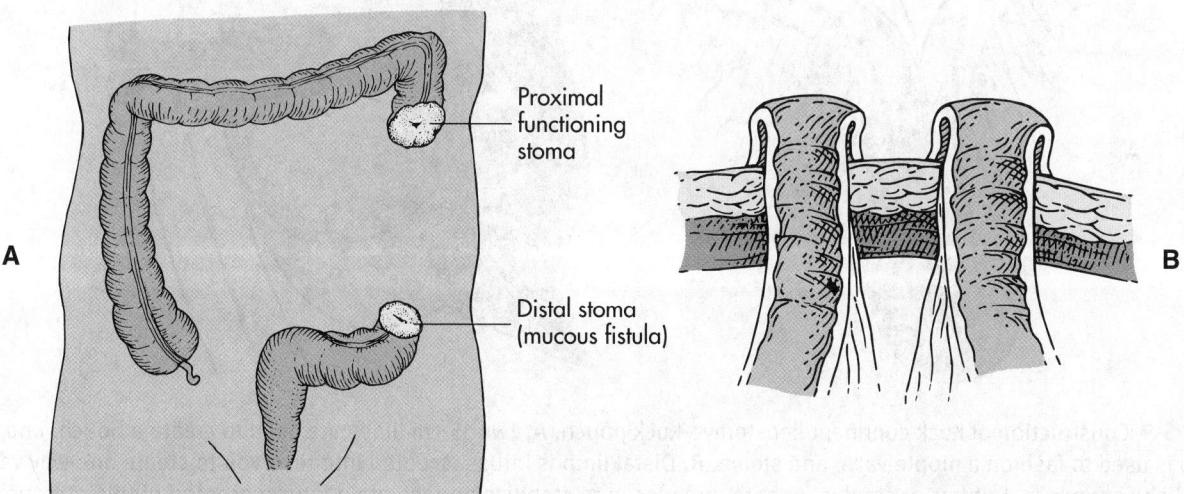

Figure 46-7 Double-barrel colostomy. **A,** Double-barrel colostomy in the descending colon. **B,** Cross-sectional view of double-barrel stoma. (From Hampton BG, Bryant RA: *Ostomies and continent diversions: nursing management,* St. Louis, 1992, Mosby.)

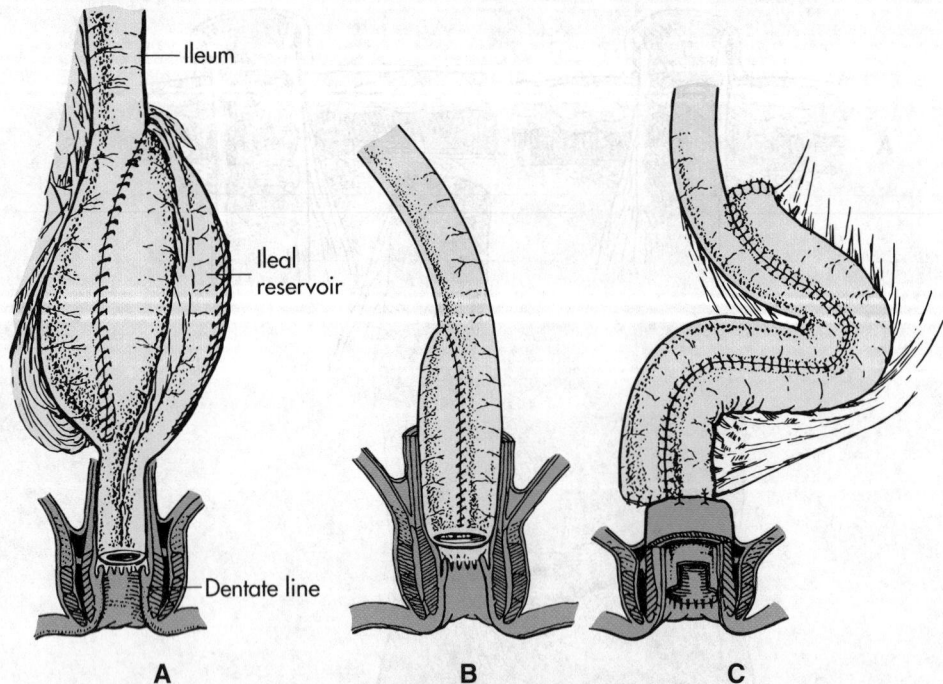

Figure 46-8 Ileoanal reservoirs (IARs). **A,** S-shaped configuration for IAR. Three 10-cm limbs of ileum are used, antimesenteric surface of each limb is opened, and adjacent bowel walls are anastomosed. **B,** J-shaped configuration for IAR. Distal ileum is aligned in J shape, antimesenteric surface of J shape is opened, and adjacent bowel walls are anastomosed. Side-to-end anastomosis of bowel to dentate line is evident. **C,** Lateral or side-by-side ileoanal pouch configuration. (From Hampton BG, Bryant RA: *Ostomies and continent diversions: nursing management,* St. Louis, 1992, Mosby.)

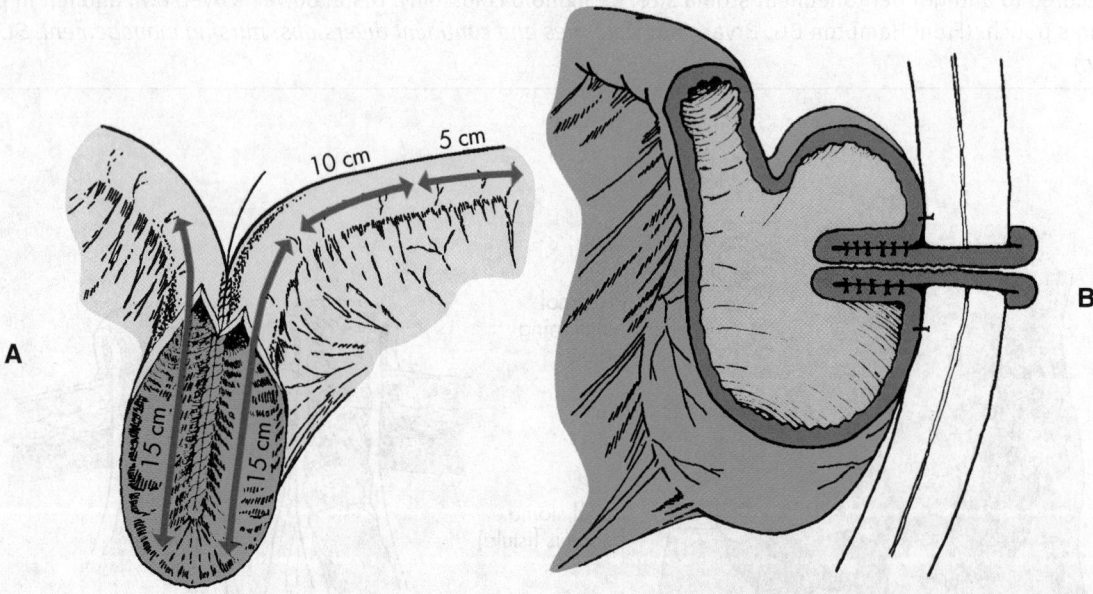

Figure 46-9 Construction of Kock continent ileostomy—Kock pouch. **A,** Two 15-cm limbs are used to create a pouch, and one 15-cm limb is used to fashion a nipple valve and stoma. **B,** Distal limb is intussuscepted into reservoir to create one-way valve and accomplish continence. Sutures or staples, or both, are placed to stabilize and maintain intussuscepted nipple. Anterior surface of reservoir is anchored to anterior peritoneal wall. (From Hampton BG, Bryant RA: *Ostomies and continent diversions: nursing management,* St. Louis, 1992, Mosby.)

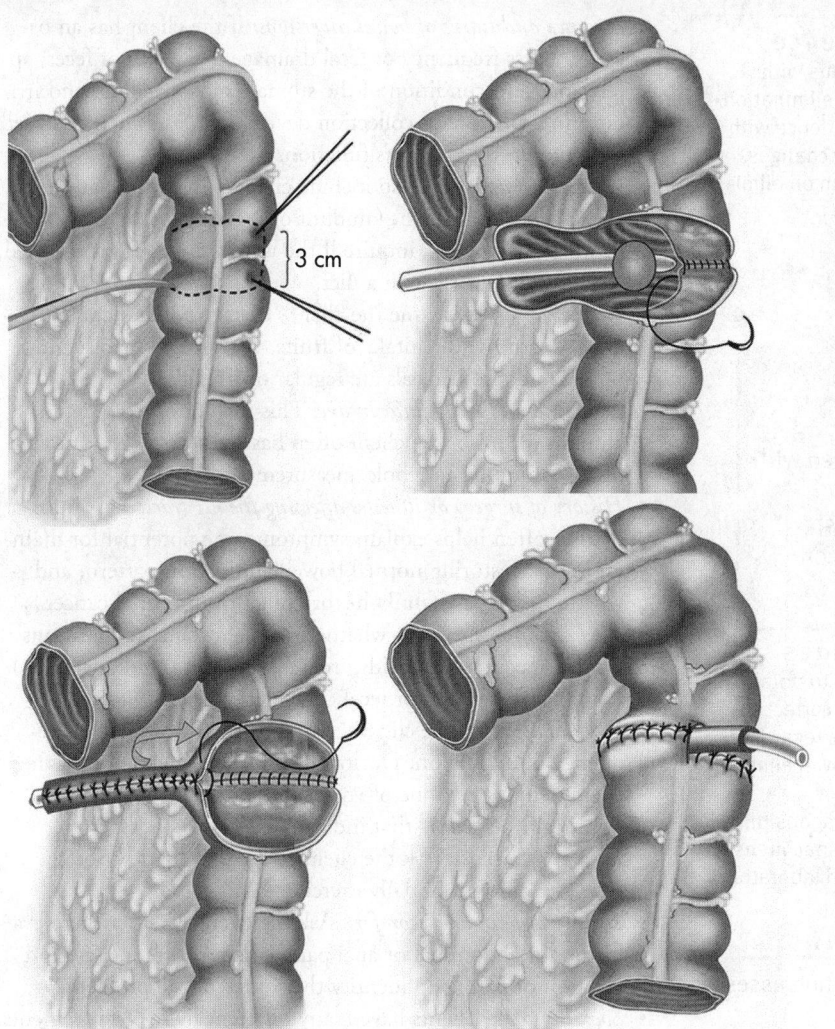

Figure 46-10 Macedo-Malone antegrade continence enema procedure. Surgical techniques A, B, C, D. (Used with permission. From Calado A and others: The Macedo-Malone antegrade continence enema procedure: early experience. *J Urol* 173:1340, 2005.)

(Banks and Razor, 2003). Nonetheless, even though clothing conceals the ostomy, the client feels different. Many clients have difficulty maintaining or initiating normal sexual relations (see Chapter 28). Important factors affecting the client's reactions is the character of fecal secretions and the ability to control them. Foul odors, spillage, or leakage of liquid stools and inability to regulate bowel movements give the client a loss of self-esteem. Refer your client to ostomy support groups such as the United Ostomy Association or the National Foundation for Ileitis and Colitis.

Critical Thinking

Successful critical thinking requires a synthesis of knowledge, experience, information gathered from clients, critical thinking attitudes, and intellectual and professional standards. Clinical judgments require you to anticipate the information necessary, analyze the data, and make decisions regarding client care. During assessment (Figure 46-11) consider all critical thinking elements that build toward making appropriate diagnoses.

In the case of bowel elimination, integrate the knowledge from nursing and other disciplines to understand the client's response to bowel elimination alterations. Your experience in caring for clients

with elimination alterations will better enable you to provide an appropriate plan of care. Use critical thinking attitudes such as fairness, confidence, and discipline when listening to and exploring the client's nursing history. Apply relevant standards of practice, such as wound care standards, when selecting nursing measures.

Nursing Process and Bowel Elimination

◆Assessment

Assessment for bowel elimination patterns and abnormalities includes a nursing history, a physical assessment of the abdomen, inspection of fecal characteristics, and a review of relevant test results. In addition, determine the client's medical history pattern and types of fluid and food intake, chewing ability, medications, and recent illnesses and/or stressors.

Nursing History. The nursing history provides a review of the client's usual bowel pattern and habits. What a client describes as

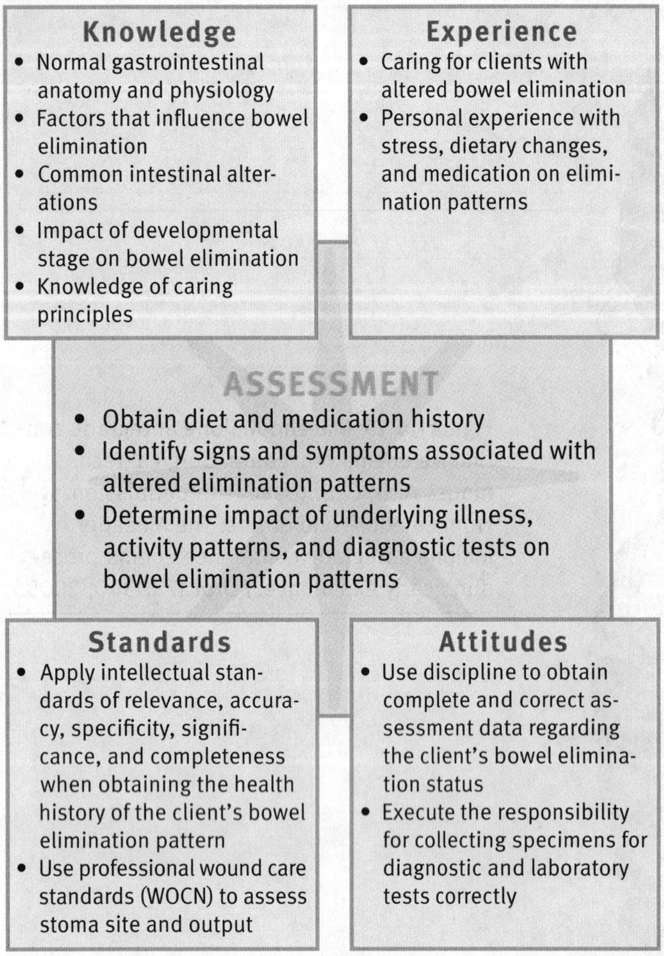

Knowledge
- Normal gastrointestinal anatomy and physiology
- Factors that influence bowel elimination
- Common intestinal alterations
- Impact of developmental stage on bowel elimination
- Knowledge of caring principles

Experience
- Caring for clients with altered bowel elimination
- Personal experience with stress, dietary changes, and medication on elimination patterns

ASSESSMENT
- Obtain diet and medication history
- Identify signs and symptoms associated with altered elimination patterns
- Determine impact of underlying illness, activity patterns, and diagnostic tests on bowel elimination patterns

Standards
- Apply intellectual standards of relevance, accuracy, specificity, significance, and completeness when obtaining the health history of the client's bowel elimination pattern
- Use professional wound care standards (WOCN) to assess stoma site and output

Attitudes
- Use discipline to obtain complete and correct assessment data regarding the client's bowel elimination status
- Execute the responsibility for collecting specimens for diagnostic and laboratory tests correctly

Figure 46-11 Critical thinking model for elimination assessment.

normal or abnormal is often different from factors and conditions that tend to promote normal elimination. Identifying normal and abnormal patterns, habits, and the client's perception of normal and abnormal in regard to bowel elimination allows for the determination of the client's problems. You can organize much of the nursing history around the factors that affect elimination (Jarvis, 2004):

- *Determination of the usual elimination pattern:* Include frequency and time of day. Having the client or caregiver complete a bowel elimination diary will assist accurate assessment of a client's current bowel elimination pattern.
- *Client's description of usual stool characteristics:* Determines whether the stool is normally watery or formed, soft or hard, the typical color, and the presence of blood. Ask the client to describe the usual shape of the stool and the number of stools per day.
- *Identification of routines followed to promote normal elimination:* Examples are drinking hot liquids, eating specific foods, or taking time to defecate during a certain part of the day.
- *Assessment of the use of artificial aids at home:* Assess whether the client uses enemas, laxatives, or bulk-forming food additives before having a bowel movement. Ask how often client used them.

- *Presence and status of bowel diversions:* If the client has an ostomy, assess frequency of fecal drainage, character of feces, appearance and condition of the stoma (color, swelling, and irritation), type of fecal collection device used, and methods used to maintain the ostomy's function.
- *Changes in appetite:* Also include changes in eating patterns and a change in weight (amount of loss or gain). If a change of weight is present, inquire if the weight change was planned, such as weight loss with a diet.
- *Diet history:* Determine the client's dietary preferences for a day. Determine the intake of fruits, vegetables, cereals, and breads and also if meals are regular or irregular.
- *Description of daily fluid intake:* This includes the type and amount of fluid. The client often has to estimate the amount using common household measurements.
- *History of surgery or illnesses affecting the GI tract:* This information often helps explain symptoms, the potential for maintaining or restoring normal bowel elimination pattern, and whether there is a family history of gastrointestinal cancer.
- *Medication history:* Ask whether the client takes medications (such as laxatives, antacids, iron supplements, and analgesics) that alter defecation or fecal characteristics.
- *Emotional state:* The client's emotions significantly alter frequency of defecation. During assessment, observation of the client's emotions, tone of voice, and mannerisms will reveal significant behaviors that indicate stress.
- *History of exercise:* Ask the client to specifically describe the type and amount of daily exercise.
- *History of pain or discomfort:* Ask the client whether there is a history of abdominal or anal pain. The type, frequency, and location of pain help identify the source of the problem.
- *Social history:* Clients have many different living arrangements. Where clients live affects their toileting habits. If the client is sharing living quarters, how many bathrooms are there? Do clients have their own bathroom, or do they need to share and thus adjust the time they use the bathroom to accommodate others? If clients live alone, are they capable of ambulating to the toilet safely? If the client is not independent in bowel management, determine who assists the client and how.
- *Mobility and dexterity:* The client's mobility and dexterity need to be evaluated to determine if the client needs assistive devices or help from personnel.

Box 46-2 summarizes types of assessment questions to use for gathering a detailed nursing history.

Physical Assessment. Conduct a physical assessment of body systems and functions likely to be influenced by the presence of elimination problems (see Chapter 33).

Mouth. Inspect the client's teeth, tongue, and gums. Poor dentition or poorly fitting dentures influence the ability to chew. Sores in the mouth make eating not only difficult, but also painful.

Abdomen. Inspect all four abdominal quadrants for contour, shape, symmetry, and skin color. Inspection also includes noting masses, peristaltic waves, scars, venous patterns, stomas, and lesions. Normally, peristaltic waves are not visible. However, observable peristalsis is often a sign of intestinal obstruction.

BOX 46-2 NURSING ASSESSMENT QUESTIONS

Signs and Symptoms

Nausea or Vomiting: Onset, Duration, Associated Symptoms, Character, Exposures
- When did the nausea/vomiting start?
- Is it related to particular stimuli (odors, after eating specific food)?
- How does the emesis look (mucous type, bloody or coffee grounds, color, or undigested food)?
- Do you have other symptoms such as dizziness, headaches, abdominal pain, or weight loss?
- Do you have family members who are experiencing the same symptoms?

Indigestion: Onset, Character, Location, Associated Symptoms, Alleviating Factors
- Is the indigestion related to meals, types or quantity of food, time of day or night?
- Does the discomfort from indigestion radiate to the shoulders or arms?
- Do you feel bloated after eating?
- Do you have any other symptoms (vomiting, headaches, diarrhea, belching, flatulence, heartburn or pain)?
- Does the indigestion respond to antacids or other self-care measures?

Diarrhea: Onset, Duration, Character, Associated Symptoms, Alleviating Factors, Exposure
- When did the diarrhea start? Was it gradual or sudden?
- How many stools per day? Is it watery or explosive? What is the color and consistency?
- Have you had fever, chills, weight loss, or abdominal pain?

- Have you taken antibiotics recently?
- Have you been under undue stress?
- What have you done to alleviate the diarrhea, and was it successful?
- Have you been out of the country recently?

Constipation: Onset, Character, Symptoms, Alleviating Factors
- When was your last bowel movement? How many per week?
- Has constipation been a recent occurrence or a long-standing problem?
- Describe your bowel movements.
- Do you have to strain to have a bowel movement?
- Do you have abdominal or rectal pain when you have a bowel movement?
- Do you feel as though your bowel movement was incomplete?
- Have you had a recent change in your diet or fluid intake?
- Do you use stool softeners, laxatives, or enemas?
- Is it necessary to manually remove the bowel movements?

Medical History
- Have you had any previous history of gastrointestinal problems? If yes, explain.
- Have you had abdominal surgery or trauma?
- Do you have a history of major illnesses such as cancer, arthritis, respiratory disease (steroid use), kidney disease, or cardiac disease?

Effect on the Client
- How have these symptoms affected you?
- Have these symptoms caused you to miss work or social engagements?

Abdominal distention appears as an overall outward protuberance of the abdomen. Intestinal gas, large tumors, or fluid in the peritoneal cavity causes distention. A distended abdomen feels tight, like a drum, and the skin appears taut, as if stretched.

Auscultate the abdomen with the stethoscope to assess bowel sounds in each quadrant (see Chapter 33). Normal bowel sounds occur every 5 to 15 seconds and last a second to several seconds. During auscultation, note the character and frequency of bowel sounds. You hear an increase in pitch or a tinkling sound with abdominal distention. Absent (no auscultated bowel sounds) or hypoactive sounds (less than five sounds per minute) occur with paralytic ileus, such as after abdominal surgery. High-pitched and hyperactive bowel sounds (35 or more sounds per minute) occur with small intestine obstruction and inflammatory disorders.

Gently palpate the abdomen for masses or areas of tenderness. It is important for the client to relax. Tensing abdominal muscles interferes with palpating underlying organs or masses.

Percussion detects lesions, fluid, or gas within the abdomen. Familiarity with the five percussion notes also permits identification of underlying abdominal structures. Gas or flatulence creates a tympanic note. Masses, tumors, and fluid are dull to percussion.

Rectum. Inspect the area around the anus for lesions, discoloration, inflammation, and hemorrhoids. Carefully record abnormalities.

Laboratory Tests. Laboratory and diagnostic examinations yield useful information concerning elimination problems (Table 46-3). Laboratory analysis of fecal contents will detect pathological conditions such as tumors, bleeding, and infection.

Fecal Specimens. The nurse is directly responsible for ensuring that specimens are accurately obtained, properly labeled in appropriate containers, and transported to the laboratory on time. Institutions provide special containers for fecal specimens. Some tests require that you place specimens in chemical preservatives.

Use medical aseptic technique during collection of stool specimens (see Chapter 34). Because about 25% of the solid portion of a stool is bacteria from the colon, wear clean gloves when handling specimens.

Hand hygiene is necessary for anyone who comes in contact with the specimen. Often the client is able to obtain the specimen if properly instructed. Explain that you cannot mix feces with urine or water. For this reason, have the client defecate into a clean, dry bedpan or place a special container under the toilet seat.

Tests performed by the laboratory for occult (microscopic) blood in the stool and stool cultures require only a small sample. Collect about an inch of formed stool or 15 to 30 mL of liquid diarrhea stool. Tests for measuring the output of fecal fat require a 3- to 5-day collection of stool. You need to save all fecal material throughout the test period.

After obtaining a specimen, label and tightly seal the container and complete all laboratory requisition forms. Then record speci-

✳ TABLE 46-3 Laboratory and Diagnostic Tests for Bowel Function

MEASUREMENT AND NORMAL VALUES	INTERPRETATION
Laboratory Tests	
• Total bilirubin: 0.1-1.0 mg/dL	• Increased in hepatobiliary diseases, obstructions in bile duct, certain anemias, and following transfusion reactions.
• Alkaline phosphatase: 30-85 ImU/mL	• Elevated in obstructive hepatobiliary diseases, hepatobiliary carcinomas, bone tumors, healing fractures.
• Amylase: 56-190 international units/L	• Elevated in abnormalities of the pancreas, such as inflammation or tumors, cholecystitis, necrotic bowel, and diabetic ketoacidosis.
• Carcinoembryonic antigen (CEA): <5 ng/mL	• Elevated in the presence of cancer or inflammation of the GI tract or hepatobiliary organs.
Direct Visualization	
• Endoscopy, colonoscopy	• Routine examination, such as a colonoscopy, is recommended for people after 50 years of age. Normally the GI tract is free of polyps, tumors, inflammation, ulcers, hernias, obstruction, and ulcerations. If a lesion such as a polyp is identified, the health care provider removes the growth or a portion of the growth and sends it to pathology for analysis. If bleeding is present, the health care provider usually attempts to stop the bleeding at the source. In some cases the identification of an abnormality indicates the need for follow-up surgery for the client.
Indirect Visualization	
• X-ray film with contrast medium	• The x-ray film identifies the presence of abnormalities in the GI tract. A series of x-ray films allow for indirect visualization of the entire tract. The presence of tumors, ulcerations, inflammation, or other abnormalities indicates the need for further diagnostic testing and medical or surgical intervention.

From Pagana KD, Pagana TJ: *Mosby's diagnostic and laboratory test reference,* ed 7, St. Louis, 2005, Mosby.
GI, Gastrointestinal.

men collections in the client's medical record. It is important to avoid delays in sending specimens to the laboratory. Some tests such as measurement for ova and parasites require the stool to be warm. When stool specimens remain at room temperature, bacteriological changes that alter test results occur.

A common laboratory test that clients can perform at home or nurses perform at the client's bedside is **fecal occult blood testing (FOBT)**, or guaiac test, which measures microscopic amounts of blood in feces (Box 46-3). It is useful as a diagnostic screening tool for colon cancer (Box 46-4). The noninvasive FOBT is one of five colorectal cancer screening regimens recommended by the American Cancer Society. There are three types of FOBT available to date. They include the most commonly used guaiac fecal occult blood test (gFOBT), the immunochemical fecal occult blood test (iFOBT), and the stool deoxyribonucleic acid (DNA) test (Greenwald, 2005). One positive gFOBT result does not confirm GI bleeding. You need to repeat the test at least three times while the client refrains from ingesting foods and medications that cause false-positive results. For example, red meat, poultry, fish, and some raw vegetables are food sources, and vitamin C, aspirin, and nonsteroidal antiinflammatory drugs are medications that can cause false-positive results (Beckman Coulter, Inc, 2003). Clients who are receiving anticoagulants or who have a bleeding disorder or a GI disorder known to cause bleeding (e.g., intestinal tumors, bowel inflammation, or ulcerations) need a regular screening for fecal occult blood.

Fecal Characteristics. Inspection of fecal characteristics (Table 46-4) reveals information about the nature of elimination alterations. Several factors influence each characteristic. Knowing whether there have been any recent changes is a key to assessment.

The client will best provide this information during the nursing history.

Diagnostic Examinations. A variety of radiological and diagnostic tests are used with the client experiencing altered bowel elimination (Box 46-5). GI structures are visualized by direct or indirect approaches. Many facilities use conscious sedation during these procedures. The most common type of drugs used to achieve moderate sedation include benzodiazepines and opiates. It is essential to understand the safety precautions involved concerning this form of anesthesia. In many institutions special training is required. A crash cart must be present at the bedside, and you must monitor the client continuously with pulse oximetry and frequent vital signs, usually every 15 minutes during and immediately following the procedure (check agency policy).

Client Expectations. Clients expect you to answer all of their questions regarding diagnostic tests and the preparation for those tests. Clients will be concerned about discomfort and exposure of their more personal areas. Nonetheless, bowel problems are often devastating for the client and their families. Fecal incontinence in older people, most commonly caused by overflow leakage as a result of constipation, often means the breakdown of care at home, causing older people to be admitted to a residential facility (Wilson, 2005). Some older clients who fail to recognize their elimination needs will need monitoring for elimination patterns so that negative consequences will not occur. It is important to remember that each client has a unique situation and a perception of what is "right" for them. In the area of bowel elimination the

BOX 46-3

The Guaiac Fecal Occult Blood Test (gFOBT)

Delegation Considerations: This skill can be delegated. The nurse, however, assesses for significance of findings.

Equipment: Hemoccult test paper, Hemoccult developer, and wooden applicator (see illustration below).

1. Explain purpose of the test and ways for the client to assist. Client can collect own specimen if possible.
2. Perform hand hygiene.
3. Apply clean disposable gloves.
4. Use tip of wooden applicator to obtain a small portion of a stool specimen. Be sure that specimen is free of tissue paper.
5. Perform Hemoccult slide test.
   a. Open flap of slide, and, using the wooden applicator, thinly smear stool in the first box of the guaiac paper. Apply a second fecal specimen from a different portion of the stool to the slide's second box (see illustration).
   b. Close slide cover, and turn the packet over to the reverse side (see illustration). After waiting 3 to 5 minutes, open cardboard flap and apply two drops of developing solution on each smear.
   c. Interpret the color of the guaiac paper within 60 seconds. A blue color indicates a positive guaiac, or presence of fecal occult blood.
   d. After determining if the client's specimen is positive or negative, apply one drop of developer to the quality control section and interpret within 10 seconds.
   e. Dispose of test slide in proper receptacle.
6. Wrap wooden applicator in paper towel, remove gloves, and discard in proper receptacle.
7. Perform hand hygiene.
8. Record results of test; note any unusual fecal characteristics.

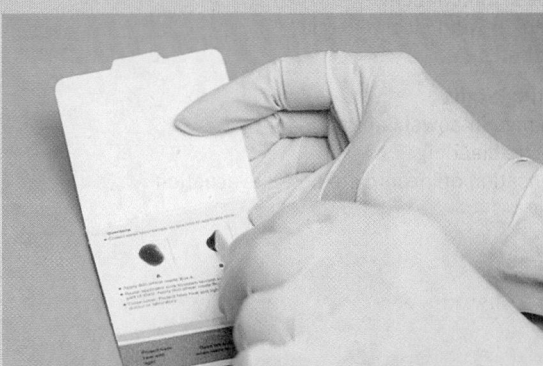

STEP 5a Application of fecal specimen on guaiac paper.

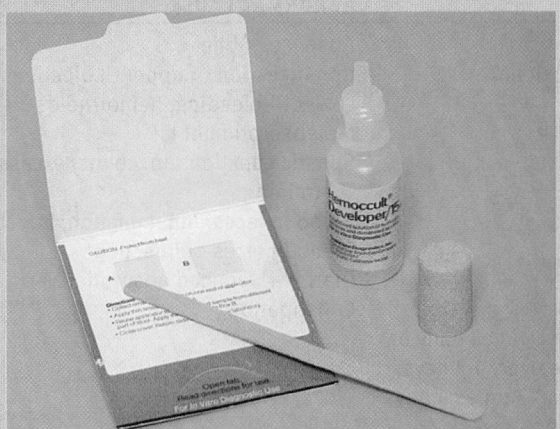

Equipment for performing fecal occult blood testing.

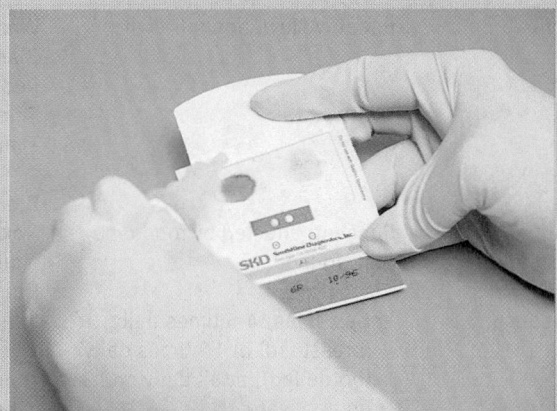

STEP 5b Application of Hemoccult developing solution on the guaiac paper on the reverse side of the test kit.

---

client will expect a knowledgeable nurse who is able to teach the client methods of promoting and maintaining a normal bowel elimination pattern. Consider the client's cultural practices and preferences, because clients of different cultures can have various expectations as well (Box 46-6).

◆ Nursing Diagnosis

The nursing assessment of the client's bowel function reveals data that indicate an actual or potential elimination problem or a problem resulting from elimination alterations. In the examples discussed in the Care Plan on p. 1193, a client with cancer devel-

ops constipation as a result of activity intolerance and imbalanced nutrition. Both of these conditions are a result of the client's pain. Examples of diagnoses that apply to clients with elimination problems include the following:

- Bowel incontinence
- Constipation
- Risk for constipation
- Perceived constipation
- Diarrhea
- Toileting self-care deficit

Associated problems, such as body-image changes or skin breakdown, require interventions unrelated to bowel function

BOX 46-4 Screening for Colon Cancer

Risk Factors
- Age: over 50 years of age
- Family history: colorectal cancer
- Personal history of colorectal cancer, colorectal polyps, chronic inflammatory bowel disease (IBD), including ulcerative colitis and Crohn's disease
- Ethnic background: Jews of Eastern European descent
- Race: African Americans
- Diet: high intake of animal fats and low in fruits and vegetables
- Obesity and inactivity
- Smoking and alcohol intake
- Diabetes

Warning Signs
- Change in bowel habits
- Rectal bleeding
- Sensation of incomplete bowel evacuation

American Cancer Society Colorectal Cancer Screening Guidelines
Beginning at age 50, men and women who are at average risk for developing colorectal cancer need to have one of the five screening options below:
- A fecal occult blood test or fecal immunochemical test every year **OR**
- Flexible sigmoidoscopy every 5 years **OR**
- A gFOBT or iFOBT every year plus flexible sigmoidoscopy every 5 years **OR** (Of these first three options, the combination of gFOBT or iFOBT every year plus flexible sigmoidoscopy every 5 years is preferable.)
- Double contrast barium enema every 5 years **OR**
- Colonoscopy every 10 years

From The American Cancer Society: *Detailed guide: colon and rectum cancer: revised 02/22/2007*, http://www.cancer.org/docroot/CRI_2_4_3X_Can_colon_and_rectum_cancer, accessed April 28, 2007, and http://www.cancer.org/docroot/CRI_2_4_2X_What_are_the_Risk_factors_for_colorectal_cancer?, accessed April 28, 2007.

gFOBT, Guaiac fecal occult blood test; *iFOBT,* immunochemical fecal occult blood test.

TABLE 46-4 Fecal Characteristics

CHARACTERISTIC	NORMAL	ABNORMAL	ABNORMAL CAUSE
Color	Infant: yellow; adult: brown	White or clay	Absence of bile
		Black or tarry (melena)	Iron ingestion or upper GI bleeding
		Red	Lower GI bleeding, hemorrhoids
		Pale with fat	Malabsorption of fat
		Translucent mucus	Spastic constipation, colitis, excessive straining
		Bloody mucus	Blood in feces, inflammation, infection
Odor	Pungent; affected by food type	Noxious change	Blood in feces or infection
Consistency	Soft, formed	Liquid	Diarrhea, reduced absorption
		Hard	Constipation
Frequency	*Varies:* Infant 4-6 times daily (breast-fed) or 1-3 times daily (bottle-fed); adult daily or 2-3 times a week	Infant more than 6 times daily or less than once every 1-2 days; adult more than 3 times a day or less than once a week	
Amount	150 g/day (adult)		Hypomotility or hypermotility
Shape	Resembles diameter of rectum	Narrow, pencil shaped	Obstruction, rapid peristalsis
Constituents	Undigested food, dead bacteria, fat, bile pigment, cells lining intestinal mucosa, water	Blood, pus, foreign bodies, mucus, worms	Internal bleeding, infection, swallowed objects, irritation, inflammation
		Excess fat	Malabsorption syndrome, enteritis, pancreatic disease, surgical resection of intestine

GI, Gastrointestinal.

✳ BOX 46-5   Radiological and Diagnostic Tests

Plain Film of Abdomen/Kidneys, Ureter, Bladder
A simple x-ray film of the abdomen requiring no preparation.

Upper GI/Barium Swallow
An x-ray examination using an opaque contrast medium (barium) to examine the structure and motility of the upper GI tract, including pharynx, esophagus, and stomach.

Client must be allowed nothing by mouth (NPO) after midnight the night before the examination.

Client needs to remove all jewelry or other metallic objects.

After the test, client needs to increase fluids to facilitate passage of barium.

Upper Endoscopy
An endoscopic examination of the upper GI tract allowing more direct visualization through a lighted fiber-optic tube that contains a lens, forceps, and brushes for biopsy.

Preparation is similar to that of the upper GI.

Light sedation is required.

Barium Enema
An x-ray examination using an opaque contrast medium to examine the lower GI tract.

Preparation includes NPO after midnight, a bowel prep such as magnesium citrate, and in some instances enemas to empty out any remaining stool particles.

Ultrasound
A technique that uses high-frequency sound waves to echo off body organs, creating a picture.

Preparation depends on the organ to be visualized and includes NPO or no preparation.

Colonoscopy
An endoscopic examination of the entire colon with the use of colonoscope inserted into the rectum.

Preparation is similar to that of barium enema: clear liquids the day before and then some form of bowel cleanser, such as GoLytely. Enemas until clear are also common.

Light sedation is required.

Flexible Sigmoidoscopy
An examination of the interior of the sigmoid colon through the use of a flexible or rigid lighted tube.

Preparation is similar to that of a barium enema or colonoscopy.

Light sedation is required.

Computerized Tomography Scan
An x-ray examination of the body from many angles utilizing a scanner analyzed by a computer.

Preparation is usually NPO.

The client needs to lie very still. If claustrophobia is a problem, use light sedation.

Magnetic Resonance Imaging
A noninvasive examination that uses magnet and radio waves to produce a picture of the inside of the body.

Preparation is NPO 4 to 6 hours before examination.

No metallic objects are allowed in the room, including metal objects on clothes.

Enteroclysis
Introduction of contrast material to jejunum, allowing entire small intestine to be studied.

Preparation is 24 hours of clear liquid diet and colon cleansing, such as GoLytely or enemas until clear.

GI, Gastrointestinal.

✳ BOX 46-6   CULTURAL ASPECTS OF CARE

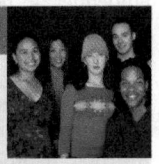

African Americans have the highest incidence of colon cancer among United States racial and ethnic groups. Some disparities are due to access to health care and socioeconomic differences. This study found that colon cancer incidence varies geographically and is related to socioeconomic status factors that include education and number of available health care providers.

Implications for Practice
- Lack of routine visits to a primary care provider is one of the strongest predictors for inadequate colorectal cancer screening and advanced stage at presentation.
- The positive relationship of socioeconomic status with digestive cancers reflects a lifestyle in which individuals have a dietary intake with higher levels of nutrients such as fats and lower levels of fruits and vegetables, known to be an associated risk for colon cancer.

- Lifestyle factors such as physical activity have a significant impact on colon cancer incidence and stage of diagnosis.
- Even residing in counties with higher levels of education and white collar employment, African Americans were more likely to have higher distant colon cancer disease rates than the white population.
- Patterns of distant colon cancer among African Americans are not completely explained by socioeconomic status factors alone. Therefore cultural or genetic factors also come into play.

Shipp M and others: Population-based study of the variation in colon cancer incidence in Alabama: relationship to socioeconomic status indicators and physician density, *South Med J* 98(11):1076, 2005.

BOX 46-7   NURSING DIAGNOSTIC PROCESS

Diarrhea Related to Food Intolerance

Assessment Activities	Defining Characteristics
Ask client to describe recent food intake.	Client reveals in a 24-hour dietary recall that he consumed many lactose products: 2% milk, pudding, and ice cream.
Auscultate bowel sounds.	Bowel sounds are hyperactive and audible without a stethoscope.
Assess frequency and consistency of stools.	Client reports eight liquid stools in the past 24 hours.
Have client describe pain, cramping, or any associated factors.	Pain is colicky in nature, spasmodic, and has a sense of urgency with each stool.

impairment. Ability to identify the correct diagnosis depends not only on the thoroughness of assessment, but also on recognition of defining characteristics and factors that impair elimination (Box 46-7). Determine the client's risk, and institute measures to ensure maintenance of normal bowel function.

✦Planning

During the planning of care synthesize information from multiple resources (Figure 46-12). Critical thinking ensures that the plan of care integrates all you know about the client and the clinical problem. Rely on professional standards. The guidelines on incontinence assist in protecting the client's skin, promoting continence, and reducing the embarrassment associated with incontinence. In addition, the Agency for Health Care Policy and Research (AHCPR), now the Agency for Healthcare Research and Quality (AHRQ), guidelines on reduction of pressure ulcers also assist in developing care for clients with bowel incontinence (see Chapter 48).

Goals and Outcomes. You and the client establish goals and outcomes by incorporating the client's elimination habits or routines as much as possible and reinforcing those routines that promote health (see Care Plan). In addition, also consider pre-existing health concerns. For example, if the client is at risk for the worsening of heart failure, you need to individualize an outcome of increased fluid intake to the client's cardiac function and ability to safely handle the increased fluid. In another example, if the client's bowel habits caused the elimination problem, help the client learn new ones. The overall goal of returning the client to a normal bowel elimination pattern includes the following outcomes:

- Client sets regular defecation habits.
- Client is able to list proper fluid and food intake needed to achieve bowel elimination.
- Client implements a regular exercise program.
- Client reports daily passage of soft, formed brown stool.
- Client does not report any discomfort associated with defecation.

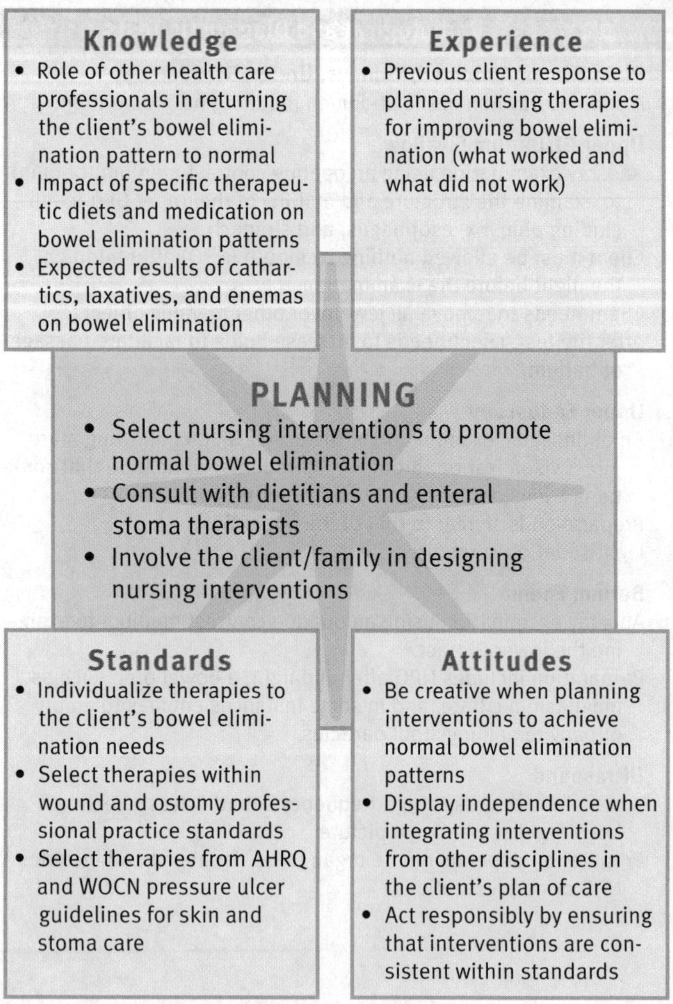

Knowledge
- Role of other health care professionals in returning the client's bowel elimination pattern to normal
- Impact of specific therapeutic diets and medication on bowel elimination patterns
- Expected results of cathartics, laxatives, and enemas on bowel elimination

Experience
- Previous client response to planned nursing therapies for improving bowel elimination (what worked and what did not work)

PLANNING
- Select nursing interventions to promote normal bowel elimination
- Consult with dietitians and enteral stoma therapists
- Involve the client/family in designing nursing interventions

Standards
- Individualize therapies to the client's bowel elimination needs
- Select therapies within wound and ostomy professional practice standards
- Select therapies from AHRQ and WOCN pressure ulcer guidelines for skin and stoma care

Attitudes
- Be creative when planning interventions to achieve normal bowel elimination patterns
- Display independence when integrating interventions from other disciplines in the client's plan of care
- Act responsibly by ensuring that interventions are consistent within standards

Figure 46-12 Critical thinking model for elimination planning.

Setting Priorities. Defecation patterns vary among individuals. For this reason, the nurse and client must work together closely to plan effective interventions. Clients often have multiple diagnoses. The concept map (Figure 46-13) shows an example of how the nursing diagnosis of constipation is related to three other diagnoses and their respective interventions. What is a realistic time frame to establish a normal defecation pattern for one client is sometimes very different for another. In the client with a new ostomy resulting from newly diagnosed cancer, the priority of coping with cancer and its treatment precede the client's need to independently manage the bowel diversion. In addition, when a bowel diversion is necessary, coping with the changes in body image often become a high priority for both the client and family.

Collaborative Care. When clients are disabled or debilitated by illness, it is necessary to include the family in the plan of care. In some situations the family members can have the same ineffective elimination habits as the client. Thus client and family teaching is an important part of the care plan. Other health team members such as dietitians and wound ostomy continence nurses (WOCNs) are often valuable resources. When clients require

NURSING CARE PLAN

Constipation Related to Opiate-Containing Pain Medication and Decreased Fiber Intake

Assessment

Javier, a home care nurse, is visiting Larry at his home on one of the local cattle ranches. Larry lives 20 miles from town. He is 22 years old and had surgery 6 days ago for repair of a badly broken right leg, from being thrown from a horse. Larry also tells Javier that he "just doesn't feel good." His past history includes pneumonia at age 12 and a traumatic injury to the abdomen. The injury required emergency surgery after being struck by a bull's horns last summer.

Assessment Activities	Findings/Defining Characteristics*
Ask Larry about his recent bowel elimination patterns over the last 5 days.	Larry tells Javier that he **has not had a bowel movement since he left the hospital 4 days ago,** and that he feels like his **abdomen is tight and sore.**
Review client's medication.	Percocet for pain. Larry says he is taking one tablet every 6 hours, up to three a day.
Review dietary intake over last day.	Diet included eggs, bacon, and toast for breakfast, soup for lunch, and chicken, rice, and corn for dinner. He drinks about six cups of coffee each day, no water but will drink a Coke.
Ask about any nausea or vomiting.	No feelings of nausea.
Auscultate client's abdomen.	**Decreased bowel sounds** are auscultated throughout all four abdominal quadrants.
Palpate abdomen.	While Javier is palpating Larry's abdomen, Larry tells Javier, **"It really hurts."**
	On palpation, **left lower quadrant is tender and firm.**

*Defining characteristics are shown in bold type.

Nursing Diagnosis: Constipation related to opiate-containing pain medication and decreased fiber intake.

Planning

Goals	Expected Outcomes (NOC)†
	Bowel Elimination
Larry will establish normal defecation.	Larry will report passage of soft, formed stool without straining in next 24 hours.
	Nutritional Status: Food and Fluid Intake
Larry will make changes to his diet to prevent constipation.	Larry will drink at least 1500 mL of fluid over the next 8 hours. Larry will increase the fiber content of his diet.

†Outcome classification labels from Moorhead S and others: *Nursing outcomes classification (NOC),* ed 4, St. Louis, 2008, Mosby.

Interventions (NIC)‡	Rationale
Constipation/Impaction Management	
• Encourage fluid intake of appropriate fluids, fruit juice, and water.	At least 1500 mL fluid intake daily is necessary to prevent hard, dry stool.
• Encourage activity within the limits of client's mobility regimen.	Even minimal activity (such as leg lifts) increases peristalsis.
• Instruct Larry to add 20 g/day of wheat bran to diet.	Bran along with physical activity prevents constipation (Bosshard and others, 2004).
• Provide laxative or stool softeners as ordered.	Medications soften the stool and prevent straining (McKenry and others, 2006).
• Provide privacy.	Clients need to feel relaxed when moving bowels.

‡Intervention classification label from Bulechek GM, Butcher HK, and Dochterman JM: *Nursing interventions classification (NIC),* ed 5, St. Louis, 2008, Mosby.

Continued

NURSING CARE PLAN

Constipation Related to Opiate-Containing Pain Medication and Decreased Fiber Intake—cont'd

Evaluation

Nursing Actions	Client Response/Finding	Achievement of Outcome
Ask Larry to identify foods high in fiber.	Able to state appropriate foods. Review of 24-hour diet diary shows Larry is selecting high-fiber, low-fat foods.	Larry is making excellent progress in introducing high-fiber and low-fat foods into his diet.
Ask Larry about physical activity.	Larry states that he has not changed his activity pattern.	Larry did not increase activity pattern and needs to continue to work on this intervention.
Observe Larry's subsequent stool for characteristics such as consistency and color.	Stools are now every 24 to 48 hours. Larry does not "feel regular." Abdomen is soft and nondistended. Stools are formed and hard, and Larry does report straining.	Larry did not achieve passage of regular, formed stool.

CONCEPT MAP

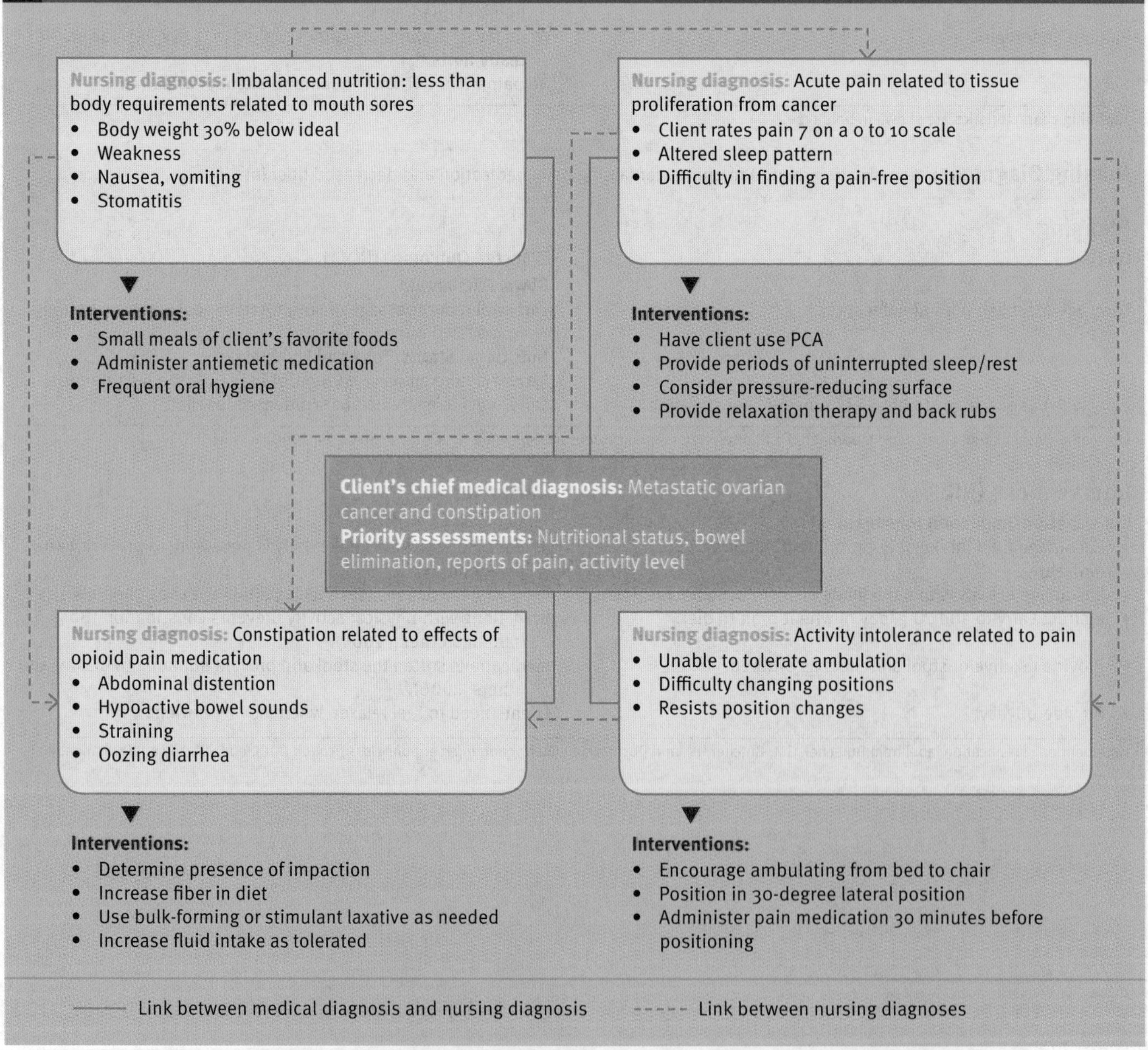

Nursing diagnosis: Imbalanced nutrition: less than body requirements related to mouth sores
- Body weight 30% below ideal
- Weakness
- Nausea, vomiting
- Stomatitis

▼

Interventions:
- Small meals of client's favorite foods
- Administer antiemetic medication
- Frequent oral hygiene

Nursing diagnosis: Acute pain related to tissue proliferation from cancer
- Client rates pain 7 on a 0 to 10 scale
- Altered sleep pattern
- Difficulty in finding a pain-free position

▼

Interventions:
- Have client use PCA
- Provide periods of uninterrupted sleep/rest
- Consider pressure-reducing surface
- Provide relaxation therapy and back rubs

Client's chief medical diagnosis: Metastatic ovarian cancer and constipation
Priority assessments: Nutritional status, bowel elimination, reports of pain, activity level

Nursing diagnosis: Constipation related to effects of opioid pain medication
- Abdominal distention
- Hypoactive bowel sounds
- Straining
- Oozing diarrhea

▼

Interventions:
- Determine presence of impaction
- Increase fiber in diet
- Use bulk-forming or stimulant laxative as needed
- Increase fluid intake as tolerated

Nursing diagnosis: Activity intolerance related to pain
- Unable to tolerate ambulation
- Difficulty changing positions
- Resists position changes

▼

Interventions:
- Encourage ambulating from bed to chair
- Position in 30-degree lateral position
- Administer pain medication 30 minutes before positioning

——— Link between medical diagnosis and nursing diagnosis   - - - - - Link between nursing diagnoses

Figure 46-13 Concept map for client with ovarian cancer with bone metastases and constipation.

surgical intervention, it is important to coordinate activities of the multidisciplinary health care team.

The client with alterations in bowel elimination will require intervention from many members of the health care team. Certain tasks, such as assisting clients onto the bedpan or bedside commode, are appropriate to delegate to assistive personnel. It will be important to remind the assistant to report any abnormal findings or difficulties encountered during the elimination process. Many of the diagnostic tests for evaluation of the gastrointestinal system will be performed by nonnursing personnel. Maintain ongoing communication with these caregivers to ensure that you address the client's needs, wants, and concerns.

✦ Implementation

Success of planned nursing interventions depends on improving the clients' and family members' understanding of bowel elimination. In the home, hospital, or long-term care facility, clients are capable of learning effective bowel habits.

Teach the client and family about proper diet, adequate fluid intake, and factors that stimulate or slow peristalsis, such as emotional stress. This is often best done during the client's mealtime. The client also needs to learn the importance of establishing regular bowel routines and regular exercise and taking appropriate measures when elimination problems develop.

Health Promotion. One of the most important habits to teach regarding bowel habits is to take time for defecation. To establish regular bowel habits, a client needs to know when the urge to defecate normally occurs. Advise the client to begin establishing a routine during a time when defecation is most likely to occur, usually an hour after a meal. Many evidenced-based interventions are available to reduce the risk of constipation (Box 46-8). If a client is restricted to bed or requires assistance in ambulating, offer a bedpan or help the client reach the bathroom in a timely manner.

Many clients have established routines for defecation. In a hospital or long-term care facility, make certain that treatment routines do not interfere with the client's routine. It is important to provide privacy. When clients forced to use a bedpan share rooms with other persons, pull the curtain around the area so that clients are able to relax, knowing that interruptions will not occur. Always place the call light within the client's reach. Close bathroom doors, although you may stand close in case the client needs assistance.

Promotion of Normal Defecation. To help clients evacuate bowel contents normally and without discomfort, a number of interventions stimulate the defecation reflex, affect the character of feces, or increase peristalsis.

Sitting Position. Assist clients who have difficulty sitting because of muscular weakness and mobility problems. Regular toilets are too low for clients unable to lower themselves to a sitting position because of joint- or muscle-wasting diseases. Clients can purchase elevated toilet seats for the home. With such a seat, the client needs less effort to sit or stand.

Positioning on Bedpan. Clients restricted to bed need to use bedpans for defecation. Women use bedpans to pass both urine and

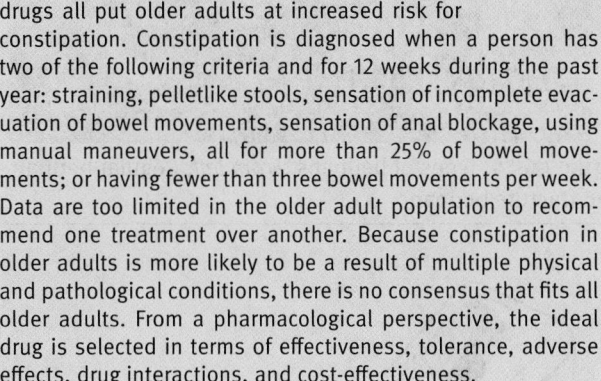

✳ BOX 46-8   EVIDENCE-BASED PRACTICE

Treatment of Chronic Constipation in Older Adults

Evidence Summary

The combined effect of decreased activity, change in diet, multiple diseases, and multiple drugs all put older adults at increased risk for constipation. Constipation is diagnosed when a person has two of the following criteria and for 12 weeks during the past year: straining, pelletlike stools, sensation of incomplete evacuation of bowel movements, sensation of anal blockage, using manual maneuvers, all for more than 25% of bowel movements; or having fewer than three bowel movements per week. Data are too limited in the older adult population to recommend one treatment over another. Because constipation in older adults is more likely to be a result of multiple physical and pathological conditions, there is no consensus that fits all older adults. From a pharmacological perspective, the ideal drug is selected in terms of effectiveness, tolerance, adverse effects, drug interactions, and cost-effectiveness.

Application to Nursing Practice

- When possible, replace a medication causing constipation with a substitute.
- Encourage elders to increase physical activity when feasible.
- Give attention to the potential risk of fluid overload in older adult clients with congestive heart failure or renal failure.
- Encourage fiber intake of 20 g/day of wheat bran to start. Observe for bloating and flatulence in older adults.
- Stool softeners are no longer recommended for constipation.
- Fiber and bulk-forming laxatives are the first step in treating constipation in older adults.
- Osmotic laxatives are effective in the treatment of constipation in older adults because they are well tolerated and have no known interactions with other drugs.
- Stimulant laxatives are more effective than placebo, but concern remains regarding their adverse effects on older adults.
- Older adults who have mobility problems often need enemas to avoid an impaction. The tap water enema is the safest for regular use. Glycerol suppositories trigger the defecatory reflex and are sometimes useful in treating older adults.

Reference

Bosshard W and others: The treatment of chronic constipation in elderly people: an update, *Drugs Aging* 21(14):911, 2004.

feces, whereas men use bedpans only for defecation. Sitting on a bedpan is extremely uncomfortable. Help position clients comfortably. Two types of bedpans are available (Figure 46-14). The regular bedpan, made of hard plastic, has a curved smooth upper end and a sharp-edged lower end and is about 5 cm (2 inches) deep. A fracture pan, designed for clients with lower extremity fractures, has a shallow upper end about 1.3 cm (½ inch) deep. The shallow end of the pan fits under the buttocks toward the sacrum, with the deeper end which has a handle, goes just under the upper thighs. The pan needs to be high enough so that feces enter the pan.

When positioning a client, it is important to prevent muscle strain and discomfort. Never try to lift a client onto a bedpan.

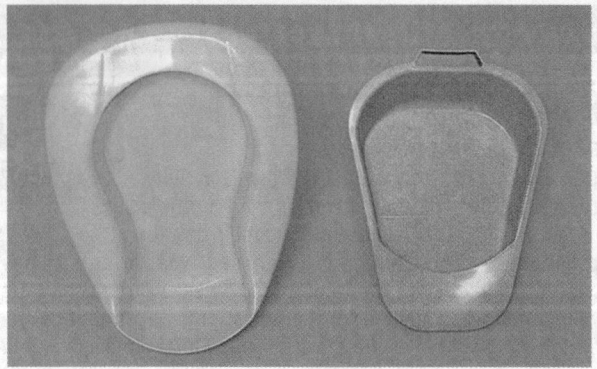

Figure 46-14 Types of bedpans. *From left,* Regular bedpan and fracture bedpan.

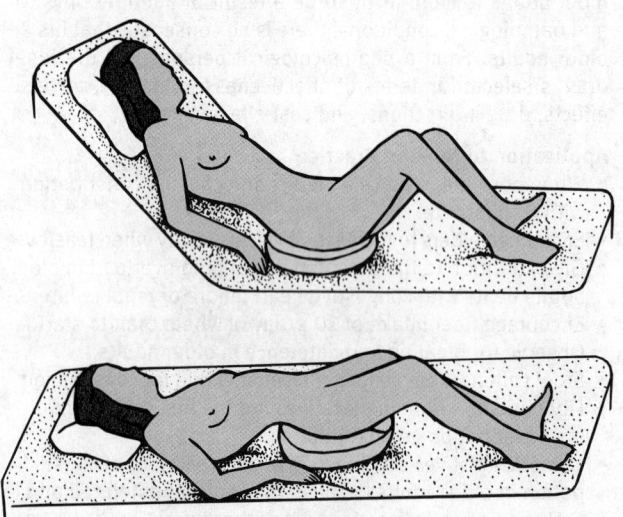

Figure 46-15 Positions on a bedpan. *Top,* Proper position reduces client's back strain. *Bottom,* Improper positioning of client.

Never place a client on a bedpan and then leave with the bed flat unless activity restrictions demand it. If the bed is flat, the hips remain hyperextended.

Figure 46-15 shows proper and improper positions on bedpans. The best method for bedpan placement is to first be sure the client is positioned high in bed. Then raise the client's head about 30 degrees, to prevent hyperextension of the back and to provide support to the upper torso. The client then raises the hips by bending the knees and lifting the hips upward. Place a hand palm up under the client's sacrum, resting the elbow on the mattress and using it as a lever to help in lifting, while slipping the pan under the client. Clients who have had abdominal surgery are hesitant to exert strain on suture lines and often have difficulty positioning on a pan. Always wear gloves when handling a bedpan.

If the client is immobile or it is unsafe to allow the client to exert such effort, the client remains flat and rolls onto the bedpan by using the following steps:

1. Lower the head of the bed flat, and assist the client in rolling onto one side, backside toward the nurse.

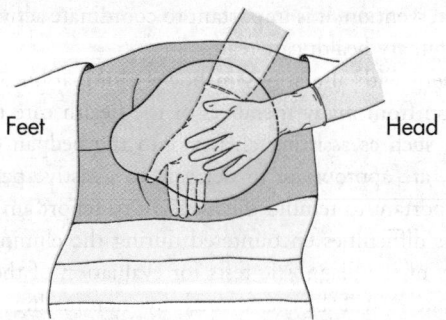

Figure 46-16 Positioning an immobilized client on a bedpan.

2. Apply a little powder to back and buttocks to prevent skin from sticking to the pan.
3. Place the bedpan firmly against the buttocks, down into the mattress with the open rim toward the client's feet (Figure 46-16).
4. Keeping one hand against the bedpan, place the other around the client's far hip. Ask the client to roll back onto the pan, flat in bed. Do not shove the pan under the client.
5. With the client positioned comfortably, raise the head of the bed 30 degrees.
6. Place a rolled towel or small pillow under the lumbar curve of the client's back for added comfort.
7. Raise the knee gatch or ask the client to bend the knees to assume a squatting position. Do not raise the knee gatch if contraindicated.

Privacy. Maintain the client's privacy during bowel elimination. This is especially important for a client using a bedpan. The call light and a supply of toilet paper need to be within easy reach. When the client finishes, respond to the call signal immediately and remove the pan. The client often requires assistance with wiping. To remove the pan, ask the client to roll off to the side or raise the hips. Hold the pan steady to avoid spilling. Avoid pulling or shoving the pan from under the client's hips because this will pull the client's skin and cause tissue injury such as shearing (see Chapter 48). After removing the pan, clean the anal and perineal areas while wearing gloves.

After assessing the stool, immediately empty the bedpan's contents into the toilet or in a special receptacle in the utility room. A spray faucet attached to most toilets allows for the ability to rinse the bedpan thoroughly. The client uses the same bedpan each time. Lastly, document the characteristics of the feces.

Offer the bedpan often. Clients may accidentally soil bedclothes if forced to wait. Many clients try to avoid using a bedpan because it is embarrassing and uncomfortable. They often try to get to the bathroom even though their conditions prohibit ambulation. Warn clients about the risk of falls or accidents.

Acute Care. With any acute illness the GI system may become affected. Changes in the client's fluid status, mobility patterns, nutrition, and sleep cycle affect regular bowel habits. Surgical interventions on the GI tract obviously affect bowel elimination. However, surgery on other systems, such as the musculoskeletal and cardiovascular systems, sometimes affects the client's bowel elimination patterns. Remain sensitive to the client's elimination needs, and intervene to assist the client in maintaining as normal bowel elimination habits as possible.

Medications. Some medications initiate and facilitate bowel elimination. Cathartics, laxatives, and occasionally an enema are used to control constipation, whereas antidiarrheal preparations assist the client in resolving diarrhea. All of these medications are available over-the-counter; stronger preparations are available through prescriptions. Clients need to be cautioned not to use these over-the-counter medications on a prolonged basis without consulting their health care provider.

> **SAFETY ALERT** Excessive use of laxatives, enemas, and/or bulk-forming agents increases the client's risk for diarrhea and abnormal bowel elimination. Excessive use of these agents destroys the client's normal defecation reflex. In addition, the client will develop altered absorption of nutrients, fluid and electrolyte imbalances, and generalized weakness. In chronically ill or older adult clients the frequent need to use toilet facilities and weakness often result in an increased risk for falls and other injuries.

Cathartics and Laxatives. Often a client is unable to defecate normally because of pain, constipation, or impaction. Cathartics and laxatives have the short-term action of emptying the bowel. They are prescribed for bowel evacuation for clients undergoing GI tests and abdominal surgery. Although the terms *cathartic* and *laxative* are often used interchangeably, cathartics have a stronger effect on the intestines. Five types of laxatives and cathartics are available (Table 46-5).

Cathartics and laxatives are available in oral, tablet, and powder suppository dosage forms (see Chapter 35). Although the oral route is most commonly used, cathartics that come prepared as suppositories are more effective because of their stimulant effect on the rectal mucosa. Cathartic suppositories such as bisacodyl (Dulcolax) act within 30 minutes. Older adults often get a strong sudden urge to defecate with Dulcolax.

Antidiarrheal Agents. For clients with diarrhea, frequent passage of liquid stools becomes a problem. Many clients use over-the-counter agents, such as Imodium, to relieve common diarrhea. However, the most effective antidiarrheal agents are prescriptive opiates such as codeine phosphate, opium tincture (paregoric), and diphenoxylate (Lomotil). Antidiarrheal opiate agents decrease intestinal muscle tone to slow passage of feces. Opiates inhibit peristaltic waves that move feces forward, but they also increase segmental contractions that mix intestinal contents. As a result, the intestinal walls absorb more water. Use antidiarrheal agents with caution because opiates are habit forming.

Enemas. An **enema** is the instillation of a solution into the rectum and sigmoid colon. The primary reason for an enema is to promote defecation by stimulating peristalsis. The volume of fluid instilled breaks up the fecal mass, stretches the rectal wall, and initiates the defecation reflex. Enemas are also a vehicle for medications that exert a local effect on rectal mucosa. The most common use for an enema is temporary relief of constipation. Other indications include removing impacted feces, emptying the bowel before diagnostic tests or surgery, and beginning a program of bowel training.

Cleansing Enemas. Cleansing enemas promote the complete evacuation of feces from the colon. They act by stimulating peristalsis through the infusion of a large volume of solution or through local irritation of the colon's mucosa. Cleansing enemas include tap water, normal saline, soapsuds solution, and low-volume hypertonic saline. Each solution has a different osmotic effect, influencing the movement of fluids between the colon and interstitial spaces beyond the intestinal wall. Infants and children should receive only normal saline because they are at risk for fluid imbalance.

Tap Water. Tap water is hypotonic and exerts a lower osmotic pressure than fluid in interstitial spaces. After infusion into the colon, tap water escapes from the bowel lumen into interstitial spaces. The net movement of water is low. The infused volume stimulates defecation before large amounts of water leave the bowel. Do not repeat tap water enemas because water toxicity or circulatory overload will develop if the body absorbs large amounts of water.

Normal Saline. Physiologically normal saline is the safest solution to use because it exerts the same osmotic pressure as fluids in interstitial spaces surrounding the bowel. The volume of infused saline stimulates peristalsis. Giving saline enemas does not create the danger of excess fluid absorption.

Hypertonic Solutions. Hypertonic solutions infused into the bowel exert osmotic pressure that pulls fluids out of interstitial spaces. The colon fills with fluid, and the resultant distention promotes defecation. Clients unable to tolerate large volumes of fluid benefit most from this type of enema, which is, by design, low volume. This type of enema is contraindicated in clients who are dehydrated and young infants. A hypertonic solution of 120 to 180 mL (4 to 6 ounces) is usually effective. The commercially prepared Fleet Enema is the most common.

Soapsuds. You can add soapsuds to tap water or saline to create the effect of intestinal irritation to stimulate peristalsis. Only pure castile soap is safe, and it comes in a liquid form included in most soapsuds enema kits. Harsh soaps or detergents cause serious bowel inflammation.

The health care provider sometimes orders a high or low cleansing enema. The terms *high* and *low* refer to the height from which, and hence the pressure with which, the fluid is delivered. High enemas cleanse the entire colon. After the enema is infused, ask the client to turn from the left lateral to the dorsal recumbent, over to the right lateral position. The position change ensures that fluid reaches the large intestine. A low enema cleanses only the rectum and sigmoid colon.

Oil Retention. Oil-retention enemas lubricate the rectum and colon. The feces absorb the oil and become softer and easier to pass. To enhance action of the oil, the client retains the enema for several hours if possible.

Other Types of Enemas. Carminative enemas provide relief from gaseous distention. They improve the ability to pass flatus. An example of a carminative enema is MGW solution, which contains 30 mL of magnesium, 60 mL of glycerin, and 90 mL of water.

Medicated enemas contain drugs. An example is sodium polystyrene sulfonate (Kayexalate), used to treat clients with dangerously high serum potassium levels. This drug contains a resin that exchanges sodium ions for potassium ions in the large intestine. Another medicated enema is neomycin solution, an antibiotic used to reduce bacteria in the colon before bowel surgery.

Enema Administration. Enemas are available in commercially packaged, disposable units or with reusable equipment

✳ **TABLE 46-5   Common Types of Laxatives and Cathartics**

Agent/Brand Name	Action	Indications	Risks
Bulk Forming Methylcellulose (Cologel, Hydrolose) Psyllium (Metamucil, Naturacil) Polycarbophil calcium (Mitrolan)	High-fiber content absorbs water and increases solid intestinal bulk. Agents stretch intestinal wall to stimulate peristalsis. Absorbs water and increases solid intestinal bulk.	Agents are least irritating, most natural, and safest cathartics. Agents are drugs of choice for chronic constipation (e.g., pregnancy, low-residue diet). Also relieves mild diarrhea. If treating diarrhea, administer less water.	Agents cause obstruction if not mixed with at least 240 mL of water or juice and swallowed quickly. Caution is necessary with bulk-forming laxatives that also contain stimulants. Agents are not for clients whom large fluid intake is contraindicated. Follow each dose with 8 ounces water.
Emollient or Wetting Docusate sodium (Colace, Disonate) Docusate calcium (Surfak) Docusate potassium (Dialose)	Stool softeners are detergents that lower surface tension of feces, allowing water and fat to penetrate. They increase secretion of water by intestine.	Agents are for short-term therapy to relieve straining on defecation (e.g., hemorrhoids, perianal surgery, pregnancy, recovery from myocardial infarction).	Agents are of little value for treatment of chronic constipation.
Saline Magnesium citrate or citrate of magnesia (Citroma) Magnesium hydroxide (Milk of Magnesia) Sodium phosphate (Fleet Phospho-Soda, Fleet Enema)	Agents contain salt preparation not absorbed by intestines. Osmotic effect increases pressure in bowel to act as stimulant for peristalsis. Agents also lubricate feces.	Agents are only for acute emptying of bowel (e.g., endoscopic examination, suspected poisoning, acute constipation).	Agents are not for long-term management of constipation. Agents are not for clients with kidney dysfunction (toxic buildup of magnesium). Phosphate salts are not for clients on fluid restriction.
Stimulant Cathartics Bisacodyl (Dulcolax) Castor oil (Neoloid, Purge) Casanthranol (Dialose Plus, Peri-Colace) Danthron (Modane Bulk) Phenolphthalein (Doxidan, Correctol, Ex-Lax)	Agents irritate intestinal mucosa to increase motility. Agents decrease absorption in small bowel and colon. Phenolphthalein and danthron cause pink or red urine.	Agents prepare bowel for diagnostic procedures.	Agents cause severe cramping. Agents are not for long-term use. Chronic use causes fluid and electrolyte imbalances. Agents are not for clients who are pregnant or breast-feeding.
Lubricants Mineral oil (Haley's M-O, Petrogalar Plain)	Agents coat fecal contents, allowing easier passage of stool. Agents reduce water absorption in colon.	Agents prevent straining on defecation (e.g., hemorrhoids, perianal surgery).	Agents decrease absorption of fat-soluble vitamins (A, D, E, and K). Agents cause dangerous form of pneumonia if aspirated into lungs. When taken with emollients, mineral oil increases risk for fat emboli.

BOX 46-9 PROCEDURAL GUIDELINES

Digital Removal of Stool

Delegation considerations: The procedure of digital removal of stool cannot be delegated.

Equipment: Clean gloves, stethoscope, water-soluble anesthetic lubricant (check agency policy on type of lubricant), bedpan, towel, washcloth, soap and water, and bedpan.

1. Verify medical history of impaction and client's last bowel movement.
2. Perform hand hygiene. Observe for abdominal distention, and auscultate abdomen.
3. Explain the procedure to the client.
4. Obtain baseline vital signs before the procedure.
5. Position the client on the left side with knees flexed and back toward you.
6. Pull curtains around bed . Drape the trunk and lower extremities with a bath blanket, and place a waterproof pad under the buttocks. Place a bedpan next to the client.
7. Apply gloves, and lubricate the index and middle fingers of your dominant hand with anesthetic lubricating jelly.
8. Instruct client to take slow deep breaths, and gently and gradually insert the gloved index finger and feel the anal sphincter relax around the finger. Then insert middle finger into the rectum and advance the finger slowly along the rectal wall toward the umbilicus.
9. Gently loosen the fecal mass by moving fingers in a scissors motions to fragment fecal mass. Work the finger into the hardened mass.
10. Work the feces downward toward the end of the rectum. Remove small pieces at a time, and discard into bedpan.
11. Periodically assess the client's vital signs and look for signs of fatigue.

Critical Decision Point: Stop the procedure if the heart rate drops significantly or the rhythm changes.

12. Continue to remove feces, and allow the client to rest at intervals.
13. After completion, wash and dry the buttocks and anal area.
14. Remove bedpan, and dispose of feces. Remove gloves by turning them inside out, and then discard.
15. Assist client to toilet or clean bedpan if urge to defecate develops.
16. Perform hand hygiene. Record results of removal of impaction by describing fecal characteristics.
17. Assess client's vital signs, and determine client's level of comfort. Auscultate bowel sounds, and gently palpate abdomen.
18. Observe for rectal bleeding, diarrhea, changes from baseline vital signs, and increasing pain or abdominal distention.

prepared before use. Sterile technique is unnecessary because the colon normally contains bacteria. However, wear gloves to prevent the transmission of fecal microorganisms.

Explain the procedure, including the position to assume, precautions to take to avoid discomfort, and the length of time necessary to retain the solution before defecation. If the client is to receive the enema at home, explain the procedure to a family member.

Often the health care provider orders "enemas till clear." This means that the enema is repeated until the client passes fluid that is clear and contains no fecal material. It is often necessary to give as many as three enemas, but caution the client against using more than three. Excess enema use seriously depletes fluids and electrolytes. If the enema fails to return a clear solution after three times (check agency policy) or if the client seems to not be tolerating the rigors of repeated enemas, notify the health care provider.

Giving an enema to a client who is unable to contract the external sphincter will pose difficulties. Give the enema with the client positioned on the bedpan. Giving the enema with the client

sitting on the toilet is unsafe because the curved rectal tubing will scrape the rectal wall. Skill 46-1 outlines the steps for an enema administration.

Digital Removal of Stool. For clients with an impaction, the fecal mass is sometimes too large for the client to pass voluntarily. If enemas fail, break up the fecal mass with the fingers and remove it in sections. This is a last resort in the management of severe constipation and practiced when all other methods have failed (Kyle and Prynn, 2004). The procedure is very uncomfortable for the client. Excess rectal manipulation can cause irritation to the mucosa, bleeding, and stimulation of the vagus nerve, which results in a reflex slowing of the heart rate. Because of the procedure's potential complications, a health care provider's order is necessary to remove a fecal impaction (Box 46-9).

Inserting and Maintaining a Nasogastric Tube. A client's condition or situation sometimes requires special interventions to decompress the GI tract. Such conditions include surgery (see Chapter 50), infections of the GI tract, trauma to the GI tract, and conditions in which peristalsis is absent.

Text continued on p. 1203

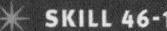 **SKILL 46-1**   ADMINISTERING A CLEANSING ENEMA

Delegation Considerations

The skill of administering an enema can be delegated. It is the nurse's responsibility to assess client for specific considerations such as need for alternative positioning, comfort, and stable vital signs before procedure. Instruct nursing assistive personnel about:

- Proper way to position clients who have mobility restrictions, such as those clients with arthritis or severe fatigue.
- How to position clients who also have therapeutic equipment present, such as drains, intravenous catheters, or traction.
- Specific signs and symptoms of client's intolerance to the procedure and when to stop it. For example, these signs and symptoms include abdominal pain more than a pressure sensation, abdominal cramping, abdominal distention, or rectal bleeding.

Equipment

- Clean gloves
- Water-soluble lubricant
- Waterproof, absorbent pads
- Bath blanket

- Toilet tissue
- Bedpan, bedside commode, or access to toilet
- Washbasin, washcloths, towel, and soap
- Intravenous (IV) pole
- Enema bag administration
  - Enema container
  - Tubing and clamp (if not already attached to container)
  - Appropriate-size rectal tube:
    - *Adult:* 22 to 30 Fr
    - *Child:* 12 to 18 Fr
  - Correct volume of warmed solution:
    - *Adult:* 750 to 1000 mL
    - *Child:*
      - 150 to 250 mL, infant
      - 250 to 350 mL, toddler
      - 300 to 500 mL, school-age child
      - 500 to 750 mL, adolescent
- Prepackaged enema
- Prepackaged enema container with rectal tip

STEPS	RATIONALE
1. Assess status of client: last bowel movement, normal bowel patterns, hemorrhoids, mobility, external sphincter control, and abdominal pain.	Determines factors indicating need for enema and influencing the type of enema used.
2. Assess for presence of increased intracranial pressure, glaucoma, or recent rectal or prostate surgery.	Conditions contraindicate use of enemas.
3. Check client's medical record to clarify the rationale for the enema.	Determines purpose of enema administration: preparation for special procedure or relief of constipation.
4. Review health care provider's order for enema.	Order by health care provider is required. Determines number and type of enema to give.
5. Inspect for abdominal distension, and auscultate for bowel sounds.	Establishes baseline for determining effectiveness of enema.
6. Determine client's level of understanding of purpose of enema.	Allows time to plan for appropriate teaching measures.
7. Correctly identify client, and explain procedure.	Information promotes client cooperation and reduces anxiety.
8. Collect appropriate equipment, and arrange at beside.	Ensures smooth procedure.
9. Assemble enema bag with appropriate solution and rectal tube.	
10. Perform hand hygiene, and apply gloves.	Reduces transmission of microorganisms.
11. Provide privacy by closing curtains around bed or closing door.	Reduces embarrassment for client.
12. Raise bed to appropriate working height: raise side rail on client's left.	Promotes good body mechanics and client safety.
13. Assist client into left side-lying (Sims') position with right knee flexed. You can also place children in dorsal recumbent position.	Allows enema solution to flow downward by gravity along natural curve of sigmoid colon and rectum, thus improving retention of solution.

Critical Decision Point: If you suspect client has poor sphincter control, position client in dorsal recumbent position on bedpan. Clients with poor sphincter control have difficulty retaining enema solution. Administering an enema with client sitting on toilet is unsafe because curved rectal tubing can abrade rectal wall.

14. Place waterproof pad under hips and buttocks.	Prevents soiling of linen.
15. Cover client with bath blanket, exposing only rectal area, clearly visualizing anus.	Provides warmth, reduces exposure of body parts, and allows client to feel more relaxed and comfortable.
16. Place bedpan or commode in easily accessible position. If client will be expelling contents in toilet, ensure that toilet is free. (If client will be getting up to bathroom to expel enema, place client's slippers and bathrobe in easily accessible position.)	Used in case client is unable to retain enema solution.

✳ **SKILL 46-1**   **ADMINISTERING A CLEANSING ENEMA—CONT'D**

STEPS	RATIONALE
17. Administer enema: **A. Enema bag**	
(1) Add warmed solution to enema bag: warm tap water as it flows from faucet; place saline container in basin of hot water before adding saline to enema bag; check temperature of solution by pouring small amount of solution over inner wrist.	Hot water burns intestinal mucosa. Cold water causes abdominal cramping and is difficult to retain.
(2) Raise container, release clamp, and allow solution to flow long enough to fill tubing.	Removes air from tubing.
(3) Reclamp tubing.	Prevents further loss of solution.
(4) Lubricate 6 to 8 cm (2½ to 3 inches) of tip of rectal tube with lubricating jelly.	Allows smooth insertion of rectal tube without risk of irritation or trauma to mucosa.
(5) Gently separate buttocks, and locate anus. Instruct client to relax by breathing out slowly through mouth.	Breathing out promotes relaxation of external anal sphincter.

(6) Insert tip of rectal tube slowly by pointing tip in direction of client's umbilicus (see illustration). Length of insertion varies:
    Adult: 7.5 to 10 cm (3 to 4 inches)
    Adolescent: 7.5 to 10 cm (3 to 4 inches)
    Child: 5 to 7.5 cm (2 to 3 inches)
    Infant: 2.5 to 3.75 cm (1 to 1½ inches)
	Careful insertion prevents trauma to rectal mucosa from accidental lodging of tube against rectal wall. Insertion beyond proper limit causes bowel perforation.

Critical Decision Point: If pain occurs or resistance is felt at any time during procedure, stop and confer with physician.

---

(7) Hold tubing in rectum constantly until end of fluid instillation.	Bowel contraction causes expulsion of rectal tube.
(8) Open regulating clamp, and allow solution to enter slowly with container at client's hip level.	Rapid instillation stimulates evacuation of rectal tube.

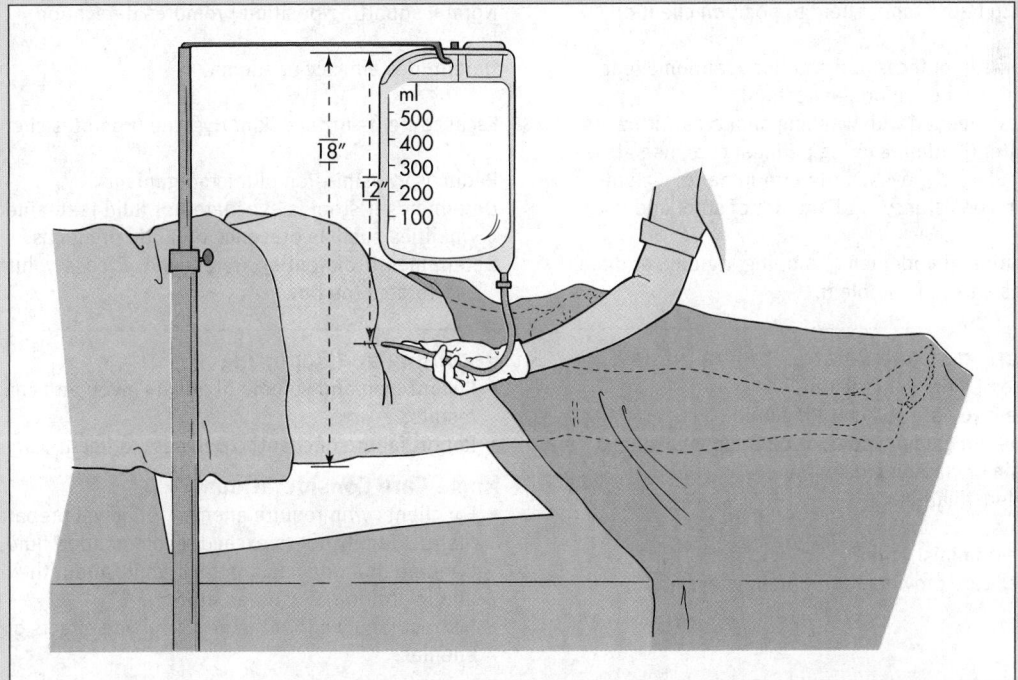

STEP 17A(6) Insertion of a rectal tube into rectum.

Continued

✳ SKILL 46-1   **ADMINISTERING A CLEANSING ENEMA—CONT'D**

STEPS	RATIONALE
(9) Raise height of enema container slowly to appropriate level above anus: 30 to 45 cm (12 to 18 inches) for high enema, 30 cm (12 inches) for regular enema, 7.5 cm (3 inches) for low enema (see illustration for Step 17A[6]). Instillation time varies with the volume of solution administered.	Allows for continuous, slow instillation of solution. Raising container too high causes rapid instillation and possible painful distention of colon. High pressure causes rupture of bowel in infant.
(10) Lower container or clamp tubing if client complains of cramping or if fluid escapes around rectal tube.	Temporary cessation of instillation prevents cramping, which prevents client from retaining all fluid, altering effectiveness of enema.
(11) Clamp tubing after all solution is instilled.	Prevents air from entering rectum.
B. Prepackaged disposable container	
(1) Remove plastic cap from rectal tip. Tip is already lubricated, but you can apply more jelly as needed.	Lubrication provides for smooth insertion of rectal tube without causing rectal irritation or trauma.
(2) Gently separate buttocks, and locate rectum. Instruct client to relax by breathing out slowly through mouth.	Breathing out promotes relaxation of external rectal sphincter.
(3) Insert tip of bottle gently into rectum: *Adult:* 7.5 to 10 cm (3 to 4 inches) *Adolescent:* 7.5 to 10 cm (3 to 4 inches) *Child:* 5 to 7.5 cm (2 to 3 inches) *Infant:* 2.5 to 3.75 cm (1 to 1½ inches)	Gentle insertion prevents trauma to rectal mucosa.
(4) Squeeze bottle until all of solution has entered rectum and colon. Instruct client to retain solution until the urge to defecate occurs, usually 2 to 5 minutes.	Hypertonic solutions require only small volumes to stimulate defecation.
18. Place layers of toilet tissue around tube at anus, and gently withdraw rectal tube.	Provides client's comfort and cleanliness.
19. Explain to client that feeling of distention is normal. Ask client to retain solution as long as possible while lying quietly in bed. (For infant or young child, gently hold buttocks together for a few minutes.)	Solution distends bowel. Length of retention varies with type of enema and client's ability to contract rectal sphincter. Longer retention promotes more effective stimulation of peristalsis and defecation.
20. Discard enema container and tubing in proper receptacle, or rinse out thoroughly with warm soap and water if reusing container.	Reduces transmission and growth of microorganisms.
21. Assist client to bathroom, or help to position client on bedpan.	Normal squatting position promotes defecation.
22. Observe character of feces and solution (caution client against flushing toilet before inspection).	Determines efficacy of enema.
23. Assist client as needed with washing anal area with warm soap and water (if administering perineal care, use gloves).	Fecal contents irritate skin. Hygiene promotes client's comfort.
24. Remove and discard gloves, and perform hand hygiene.	Reduces transmission of microorganisms.
25. Inspect color, consistency, and amount of stool and fluid passed.	Determines if stool is evacuated or fluid is retained. Note abnormalities such as presence of blood or mucus.
26. Assess condition of abdomen; cramping, rigidity, or distention indicates a serious problem.	Determines if distention is relieved. Excess volume distends or perforates the bowel.

Unexpected Outcomes and Related Interventions

1. Abdomen becomes rigid and distended.
   a. Stop enema if you are still instilling fluid.
   b. Notify the health care provider, and obtain vital signs.
2. Abdominal pain or cramping develops.
   a. Slow rate of instillation.
3. Bleeding occurs.
   a. Stop enema administration.
   b. Notify health care provider, and obtain vital signs.

Recording and Reporting

- Record type and volume of enema given and characteristics of results.
- Report failure of client to defecate to health care provider.

Home Care Considerations

- For clients who require enemas for bowel preparation at home, instruct family not to exceed recommended fluid volume levels or number of enemas. Instruct family about the need for slow administration of warmed fluid.
- Instruct family about the negative side effects of tap water enemas.

TABLE 46-6 Purposes of Nasogastric Intubation

PURPOSE	DESCRIPTION	TYPE OF TUBE
Decompression	Removal of secretions and gaseous substances from gastrointestinal tract; prevention or relief of abdominal distention	Salem sump, Levin, Miller-Abbott
Enteral feeding (see Chapter 44)	Instillation of liquid nutritional supplements or feedings into stomach for clients unable to swallow fluid	Duo, Dobhoff, Levin
Compression	Internal application of pressure by means of inflated balloon to prevent internal esophageal or gastrointestinal hemorrhage	Sengstaken-Blakemore
Lavage	Irrigation of stomach in cases of active bleeding, poisoning, or gastric dilation	Levin, Ewald, Salem sump

A nasogastric (NG) tube is a pliable hollow tube that you insert through the client's nasopharynx into the stomach. Nasogastric intubation has several purposes (Table 46-6). There are two main categories of nasogastric tubes: Fine- or small-bore tubes and large-bore tubes. Large-bore tubes, 12 Fr and above, are usually used for gastric decompression or removal of gastric secretions (Phillips, 2006). Small-bore tubes are frequently used for medication administration and enteral feedings (see Chapter 44 for enteral feedings) (Metheny and others, 2005).

The Levin and Salem sump tubes are the most common for stomach decompression. The Levin tube is a single-lumen tube with holes near the tip. You can connect it to a drainage bag or to an intermittent suction device to drain stomach secretions.

The Salem sump tube is preferable for stomach decompression. The tube has two lumina: one for removal of gastric contents and one to provide an air vent. A blue "pigtail" is the air vent that connects with the second lumen. When the sump tube's main lumen is connected to suction, the air vent permits free, continuous drainage of secretions. Never clamp off the air vent, connect it to suction, or use it for irrigation.

Nasogastric tube insertion does not require sterile technique. Simply use clean technique. The procedure is uncomfortable. The client experiences a burning sensation as the tube passes through the sensitive nasal mucosa. When the tube reaches the back of the pharynx, the client sometimes begins to gag. Help the client relax to make tube insertion easier. Some institutions allow you to use Xylocaine jelly when inserting the tube because it increases client comfort during the procedure (Skill 46-2).

One of the greatest problems in caring for a client with an NG tube is maintaining comfort. The tube is a constant irritation to nasal mucosa. Assess the condition of the nares and mucosa for inflammation and **excoriation.** The tape or fixation device used to anchor the tube often becomes soiled. Change it every day to lessen irritation. Frequent lubrication of the nares also minimizes excoriation. With one nares occluded, the client may breathe through the mouth. Frequent mouth care (at least every 2 hours) helps minimize dehydration. A glass of cool water for rinsing is useful, but the client who is allowed nothing by mouth (NPO) should not swallow the water. The client will frequently complain of a sore throat. An ice bag applied externally to the throat helps. Gargling with topical Xylocaine jelly and/or lozenges helps as well, if ordered by the health care provider.

After you insert the tube, maintain its patency. The tip of the tubing sometimes rests against the stomach wall, or the tube may

become blocked with thick secretions. Therefore regular irrigation is necessary. Flushing the tube with normal saline by way of a catheter-tipped syringe clears blockage within the tube. If an NG tube continues to drain improperly after irrigation, reposition it by advancing or withdrawing it slightly. Any change in tube position requires verification of placement of the tube in the client's GI tract.

The NG tube sometimes causes distention. The presence of the tube causes many clients to swallow large volumes of air. Channels of gastric secretions also form along the walls of the stomach and bypass the suction holes. Turning the client regularly helps to collapse the channels and promotes emptying of stomach contents.

Continuing and Restorative Care. For a client to recover and return home or to an extended care facility, regular elimination patterns need to begin. When clients have a colostomy, they need to learn to care for the ostomy. Other clients require bowel retraining. It is important to remember that you initiate ostomy care and bowel retraining in the acute care settings. However, because these are long-term care needs, these activities are usually completed in restorative care settings.

Care of Ostomies. Clients with temporary or permanent bowel diversions have unique elimination needs. Persons with an ostomy wear a pouch or appliance to collect effluent from the stomas (Hyland, 2002). The stool discharged from an ostomy is called **effluent,** and that term will be used throughout this section. These clients need to use meticulous skin care to prevent liquid stool from irritating the skin around the stoma.

Irrigating a Colostomy. Although this practice is not as common as it once was, some clients need to learn to irrigate their left-sided colostomies in order to regulate colon emptying. Other clients do not want to spend the additional 60 to 90 minutes in the bathroom every day, so they empty their pouch as necessary (Hyland, 2002). Only a colostomy can be irrigated.

Use specific equipment for irrigating a colostomy. **Never** use an enema set to irrigate a colostomy. Use a special cone-tipped irrigator (Figure 46-17, p. 1210). This device prevents bowel penetration and backflow of the irrigating solution. Clients usually sit on the toilet and place an irrigating sleeve over the stoma. The end of this sleeve extends into the bowl of the commode. The health care provider orders the amount and type of solution. For adults, the amount ranges from 500 to 700 mL of tap water. The solution is instilled slowly through the lubricated cone tip. Irrigation usually takes 5 to 10 minutes. The client then removes the

Text continued on p. 1210

SKILL 46-2   **INSERTING AND MAINTAINING A NASOGASTRIC TUBE FOR GASTRIC DECOMPRESSION**

Delegation Considerations

The skill of inserting and maintaining a nasogastric (NG) tube cannot be delegated. Instruct nursing assistive personnel to:

- Measure and record the drainage
- Provide oral and nasal hygiene
- Perform selected comfort measures
- Correctly anchor NG tube to client's gown after changing gown or repositioning client

Equipment

- Inserting large-bore tube
  - 14 or 16 Fr NG tube (smaller lumens are not used for decompression in adults because they must be able to remove thick secretions)
  - Water-soluble lubricating jelly
  - Clean gloves
  - pH test strips (measure gastric aspirate acidity)
  - Tongue blade
  - Flashlight
  - Emesis basin
- Asepto bulb or catheter-tipped syringe
- Normal saline
- 1 inch (2.5 cm)–wide hypoallergenic tape or commercial fixation device.
- Tincture of benzoin (optional)
- Safety pin and rubber band
- Clamp, or suction machine or pressure gauge if wall suction is used
- Towel, facial tissues
- Glass of water with straw
- Irrigating NG tube
  - Asepto bulb or catheter-tipped syringe
  - Normal saline and basin
  - Clean gloves
- Discontinuing NG tube
  - Towel, facial tissue
  - Clean gloves
  - Soap and water

STEPS	RATIONALE
1. Perform hand hygiene.	Reduces transmission of organisms.
2. Inspect condition of client's nasal and oral cavity.	Baseline condition of nasal and oral cavity determines need for special nursing measures for oral hygiene after tube placement.
3. Ask if client has had history of nasal surgery, and note if deviated nasal septum is present.	Nurse should insert tube into **uninvolved** nasal passage. Procedure may be contraindicated if surgery is recent.
4. Auscultate for bowel sounds. Palpate client's abdomen for distention, pain, and rigidity.	Baseline determination of level of abdominal distention later serves as comparison once tube is inserted. In the presence of diminished or absent bowel sounds, auscultate each quadrant for 5 minutes (Seidel and others, 2006).
5. Assess client's level of consciousness and ability to follow instructions.	Determines client's ability to assist in procedure.

Critical Decision Point: If client is confused, disoriented, or unable to follow commands, obtain assistance from another staff member to insert the tube.

6. Determine if client has had an NG tube insertion in the past and which naris was used.	Previous experience complements any explanations.
7. Check medical record for health care provider's order, type of NG tube to be placed, and whether tube is to be attached to suction.	Procedure requires health care provider's order. Adequate decompression depends on NG suction.
8. Prepare equipment at the bedside. Cut a piece of tape about 4 inches (10 cm) long, and split one end in half to form a V, or have NG tube fixator device available.	Ensures well-organized procedure. Tape or fixator device will be used to hold the tube in place after insertion.
9. Identify client, and explain procedure.	Identification prevents error of placing tube in wrong client. Explanation gains client's cooperation and lessens possibility that client will remove tube.
10. Position client in high-Fowler's position with pillows behind head and shoulders. Raise bed to a horizontal level comfortable for the nurse.	Promotes client's ability to swallow during procedure. Positioning of bed prevents strain on nurse.
11. Have client blow nose. Place bath towel over client's chest; give facial tissues to client. Place emesis basin within reach.	Removes existing nasal secretions. Prevents soiling of client's gown. Tube insertion through nasal passages may cause tearing and coughing with increased salivation.
12. Pull curtain around the bed, or close room door.	Provides privacy.
13. Stand on client's right side if right-handed, left side if left-handed.	Allows easiest manipulation of tubing.
14. Apply clean gloves.	Reduces transmission of microorganisms.
15. Instruct client to relax and breathe normally while occluding one naris. Then repeat this action for other naris. Select nostril with greater air flow.	Tube passes more easily through naris that is more patent. Ensures tube insertion does not obstruct nasal air flow.

✴ **SKILL 46-2**

INSERTING AND MAINTAINING A NASOGASTRIC TUBE FOR GASTRIC DECOMPRESSION—CONT'D

STEPS

16. Measure distance to insert tube:

    a. *Traditional method*: Measure distance from tip of nose to earlobe to xiphoid process (see illustrations).
    b. *Hanson method*: First mark 50-cm point on tube, and then do traditional measurement. Tube insertion should be to midway point between 50 cm (20 inches) and traditional mark.

17. Mark length of tube to be inserted with small piece of tape placed so it can easily be removed.
18. Curve 10 to 15 cm (4 to 6 inches) of end of tube tightly around index finger, then release.
19. Lubricate 7.5 to 10 cm (3 to 4 inches) of end of tube with water-soluble lubricating jelly.
20. Alert client that procedure is to begin.
21. Initially instruct client to extend neck back against pillow (see illustration); insert tube gently and slowly through naris, aiming end of tube downward.

RATIONALE

Approximates distance from naris to stomach. Tube should extend from naris to stomach; distance varies with each client.

Marks amount of tube to be inserted from nares to stomach.

Curving tube tip aids insertion and decreases stiffness of tube.

Minimizes friction against nasal mucosa and aids insertion of tube. Water-soluble lubricant is less toxic than oil based if aspirated.

Decreases client anxiety and increases client cooperation.

Facilitates initial passage of tube through naris and maintains clear airway for open naris.

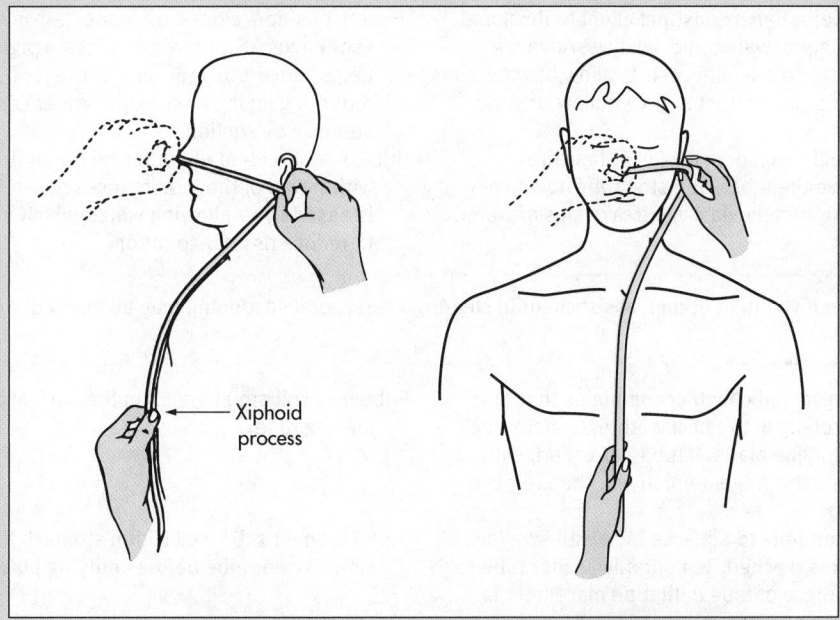

Xiphoid process

STEP 16a Technique for measuring distance to insert NG tube.

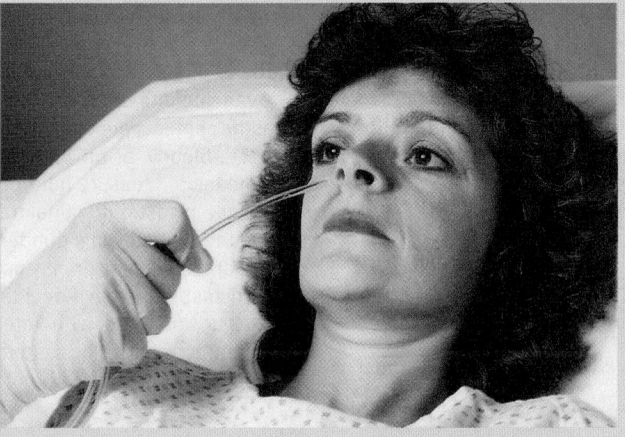

STEP 21 Insert NG tube with curved end pointing downward.

Continued

✳ **SKILL 46-2**   **INSERTING AND MAINTAINING A NASOGASTRIC TUBE FOR GASTRIC DECOMPRESSION—CONT'D**

STEPS	RATIONALE
22. Continue to pass tube along floor of nasal passage, aiming downward toward client's ear. If resistance is met, apply gentle downward pressure to advance tube. (Do not force past resistance.)	Minimizes discomfort of tube rubbing against upper nasal turbinates. Resistance is caused by posterior nasopharynx. Downward pressure helps tube curl around corner of nasopharynx.
23. If resistance is met, try to rotate the tube and see if it advances. If still resistant, withdraw tube, allow client to rest, relubricate tube, and insert into other naris.	Forcing against resistance can cause trauma to mucosa. Helps relieve client's anxiety.

Critical Decision Point: If unable to insert tube in either naris, stop procedure and notify health care provider.

---

24. Continue insertion of tube until just past nasopharynx by gently rotating tube toward opposite nostril, and then pass tube just above oropharynx.	Helps prevent coiling of tube in oropharynx.
a. Stop tube advancement, allow client to relax, and provide tissues.	Relieves client's anxiety; tearing is natural response to mucosal irritation, and excessive salivation may occur because of oral stimulation.
b. Explain to client that next step requires that client swallow. Give client glass of water unless contraindicated.	Slipping of water aids passage of NG tube into esophagus.
25. With tube just above oropharynx, instruct client to flex head forward, take a small sip of water, and swallow. Advance tube 2.5 to 5 cm (1 to 2 inches) with each swallow of water. If client is not allowed fluids, instruct to dry swallow or suck air through straw.	Flexed position closes off upper airway to trachea and opens esophagus. Swallowing closes epiglottis over trachea and helps move the tube into the esophagus. Swallowing water reduces gagging or choking. Water can be removed later from stomach by suction.
26. If client begins to cough, gag, or choke, withdraw tube slightly (do not remove the tube), and stop tube advancement. Instruct client to breathe easily and take sips of water.	Tube may accidentally enter larynx and produce coughing, and withdrawal of the tube reduces risk of laryngeal entry. Gagging is eased by swallowing water, which must be given cautiously to reduce risk of aspiration.

Critical Decision Point: If vomiting occurs, assist client in clearing airway; oral suctioning may be needed. Do not proceed until airway is cleared.

---

27. If client continues to gag and cough or complains that tube feels as though it is coiling in the back of throat, check back of oropharynx using tongue blade. If tube has coiled, withdraw it until the tip is back in the oropharynx. Then reinsert with client swallowing.	Tube may coil around itself in the back of the throat and stimulate the gag reflex.
28. After client relaxes, continue to advance tube with swallowing until tape or mark is reached. Temporarily anchor tube to client's cheek with a piece of tape until tube placement is checked.	Tip of tube must be well within stomach for adequate decompression. Anchor tube before verifying placement.
29. Verify tube placement. Check agency policy for preferred methods for checking NG tube placement.	
a. Ask client to talk.	Inability to speak can indicate that tube is through client's vocal cords into the lungs.
b. Inspect posterior pharynx for presence of coiled tube.	Tube is pliable and can coil up in back of pharynx instead of advancing into esophagus.
c. Attach Asepto or catheter-tipped syringe to end of tube, and aspirate gently back on syringe to obtain gastric contents, observing color (see illustration).	Gastric contents are usually cloudy and green, but may be off-white, tan, bloody, or brown in color. Aspiration of contents provides means to measure fluid pH and thus determine tube tip placement in gastrointestinal tract. Other common aspirate colors include the following: duodenal placement (yellow or bile stained), esophagus (may or may not have saliva-appearing aspirate).
d. Measure pH of aspirate with color-coded pH paper with range of whole numbers from 1 to 11 (see illustration).	Gastric aspirates have decidedly acidic pH values, preferably 4 or less, compared with intestinal aspirates, which are usually greater than 4, or respiratory secretions, which are usually greater than 5.5 (Metheny and Titler, 2001).

✳ **SKILL 46-2** # INSERTING AND MAINTAINING A NASOGASTRIC TUBE FOR GASTRIC DECOMPRESSION—CONT'D

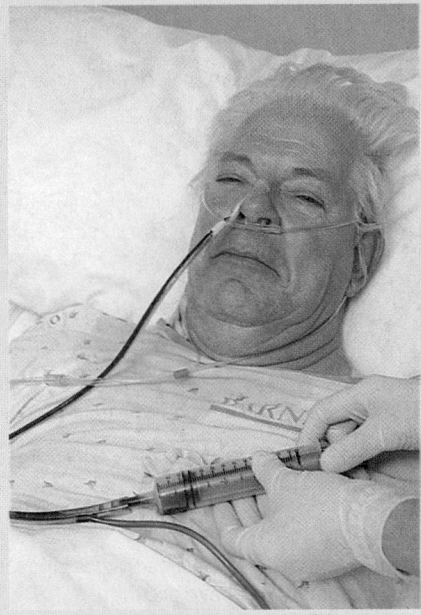

STEP 29c Aspiration of gastric contents.

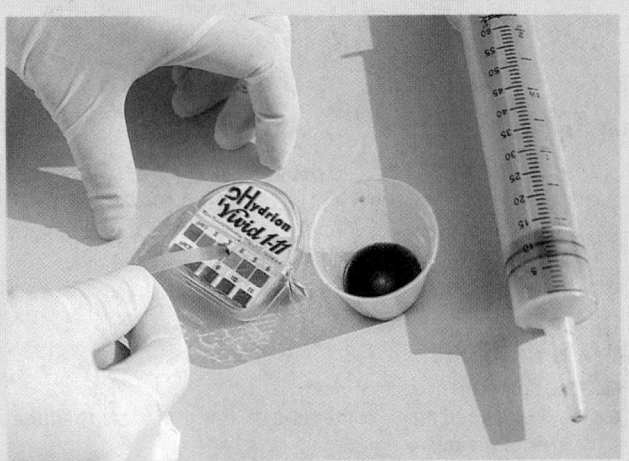

STEP 29d Checking pH of gastric aspirate.

STEPS	RATIONALE
Critical Decision Point: Be sure to use gastric (Gastrocult) pH test and not Hemoccult test.	

STEPS	RATIONALE
e. Have ordered x-ray examination performed of chest/abdomen.	X-ray film is best verification of initial placement of the tube (Metheny and Titler, 2001).
f. If tube is not in stomach, advance another 2.5 to 5 cm (1 to 2 inches) and repeat Steps 29a-e to check tube position.	Tube must be in stomach to provide decompression.

Critical Decision Point: Insufflating air into tube and listening with a stethoscope is not a reliable method to determine tube placement. In studies with feeding tubes, tubes inadvertently placed in lungs, intestines, or esophagus can transmit sounds similar to that of air entering the stomach (Metheny and others, 1998a, 1998b).

STEPS	RATIONALE
30. Anchoring tube:	
a. After tube is properly inserted and positioned, either clamp end or connect it to drainage bag or suction source.	Drainage bag is used for gravity drainage. Intermittent suction, low suction, is most effective for decompression. Client going to the operating room often has tube clamped.
b. Tape tube to nose; avoid putting pressure on nares.	Prevents tissue necrosis. Tape anchors tube securely.
(1) Apply small amount of tincture of benzoin to lower end of nose, and allow to dry *(optional).*	
(2) Apply tape to nose, leaving split ends free. Be sure top end of tape over nose is secure.	Benzoin prevents loosening of tape if client perspires.
(3) Carefully wrap two split ends of tape around tube (see illustration).	
(4) Alternative: Apply tube fixation device using shaped adhesive patch (see illustration).	
c. Fasten end of NG tube to client's gown by looping rubber band around tube in slip knot. Pin rubber band to gown (provides slack for movement).	Reduces pressure on the nares if tube moves.
31. Unless health care provider orders otherwise, head of bed should be elevated 30 degrees.	Helps prevent esophageal reflux and minimizes irritation of tube against posterior pharynx.

Continued

✳ SKILL 46-2

INSERTING AND MAINTAINING A NASOGASTRIC TUBE FOR GASTRIC DECOMPRESSION—CONT'D

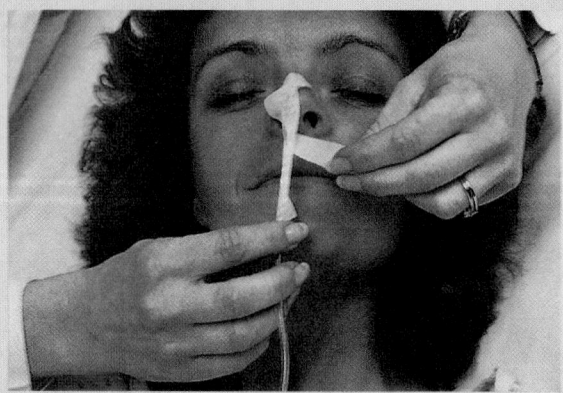

STEP 30b(3) Tape is crossed over and around NG tube.

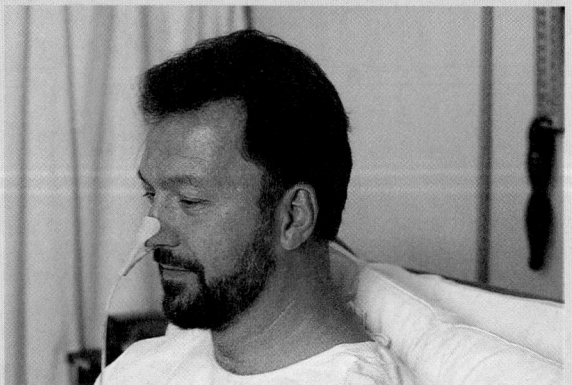

STEP 30b(4) Client with tube fixation device.

STEPS	RATIONALE
32. Once placement is confirmed:	
a. Place a red mark on the tube to indicate where the tube exits the nose.	The mark or tube length is to be used as a guide to indicate whether displacement may have occurred.
b. Measuring the tube length from nares to connector as an alternative method.	
c. Document the tube length in the client record.	
33. Remove gloves, and perform hand hygiene.	Reduces transmission of microorganisms.
34. Tube irrigation:	
a. Perform hand hygiene, and apply gloves.	Reduces transmission of microorganisms.
b. Check for tube placement in stomach (see Step 29). Reconnect NG tube to connecting tube.	Prevents accidental entrance of irrigating solution into lungs.
c. Draw up 30 mL of normal saline into Asepto or catheter-tipped syringe.	Use of saline minimizes loss of electrolytes from stomach fluids.
d. Clamp NG tube. Disconnect from connection tubing and lay end of connection tubing on towel.	Reduces soiling of client's gown and bed linen.
e. Insert tip of irrigating syringe into end of NG tube. Remove clamp. Hold syringe with tip pointed at floor and inject saline slowly and evenly. Do not force solution.	Position of syringe prevents introduction of air into vent tubing, which could cause gastric distention. Solution introduced under pressure can cause gastric trauma.

Critical Decision Point: Do not introduce saline through blue colored "pigtail" air vent of Salem sump tube.

f. If resistance occurs, check for kinks in tubing. Turn client onto left side. Repeated resistance should be reported to the health care provider.	Tip of tube may lie against stomach lining. Repositioning on left side may dislodge tube away from the stomach lining. Buildup of secretions will cause distention.
g. After instilling saline, immediately aspirate or pull back slowly on syringe to withdraw fluid. If amount aspirated is greater than amount instilled, record the difference as output. If amount aspirated is less than amount instilled, record the difference as intake.	Irrigation clears tubing, so stomach should remain empty. Fluid remaining in stomach is measured as intake.
h. Reconnect NG tube to drainage or suction. (If solution does not return, repeat irrigation.)	Reestablishes drainage collection; may repeat irrigation or repositioning of tube until NG tube drains properly.
i. Remove gloves, and perform hand hygiene.	Reduces transmission of microorganisms.
35. Observe amount and character of contents draining from NG tube. Ask if client feels nauseated.	Determines if tube is decompressing stomach of contents.
36. Palpate client's abdomen periodically, noting any distention, pain, and rigidity, and auscultate for the presence of bowel sounds. Turn off suction while auscultating.	Determines success of abdominal decompression and the return of peristalsis. The sound of the suction apparatus may be transmitted to abdomen and be misinterpreted as bowel sounds.
37. Inspect condition of nares and nose.	Evaluates onset of skin and tissue irritation.
38. Observe position of tubing.	Determines if tension is being applied to nasal structures.
39. Ask if client feels sore throat or irritation in pharynx.	Evaluates level of client's discomfort.

✷ SKILL 46-2 ### INSERTING AND MAINTAINING A NASOGASTRIC TUBE FOR GASTRIC DECOMPRESSION—CONT'D

STEPS	RATIONALE
40. Discontinuation of NG tube:	
a. Verify order to discontinue NG tube.	Health care provider's order required for procedure.

Critical Decision Point: Immediately prior to removing the nasogastric tube verify the presence of bowel sounds.

---

b. Explain procedure to client, and reassure that removal is less distressing than insertion.	Minimizes anxiety and increases cooperation. Tube passes out smoothly.
c. Perform hand hygiene, and apply clean gloves.	Reduces transmission of microorganisms.
d. Turn off suction, and disconnect NG tube from drainage bag or suction. Remove tape or fixation device from bridge of nose, and unpin tube from gown.	Have tube free of connections before removal.
e. Stand on client's right side if right-handed, left side if left-handed.	Allows easiest manipulation of tube.
f. Hand the client facial tissue; place clean towel across chest. Instruct client to take and hold a deep breath.	Client may wish to blow nose after tube is removed. Towel may keep gown from getting soiled. Airway will be temporarily obstructed during tube removal.
g. Clamp or kink tubing securely, and then pull tube out steadily and smoothly into towel held in other hand while client holds breath.	Clamping prevents tube contents from draining into oropharynx. Reduces trauma to mucosa and minimizes client's discomfort. Towel covers tube, which can be an unpleasant sight. Holding breath helps to prevent aspiration.
h. Measure amount of drainage, and note character of content. Dispose of tube and drainage equipment into proper container.	Provides accurate measure of fluid output. Reduces transfer of microorganisms.
i. Clean nares, and provide mouth care.	Promotes comfort.
j. Position client comfortably, and explain procedure for drinking fluids, if not contraindicated.	Depends on health care provider's order. Sometimes clients are allowed nothing by mouth (NPO) for up to 24 hours. When fluids are allowed, the order usually begins with a small amount of ice chips each hour and increase as client is able to tolerate more.
41. Clean equipment, and return to proper place. Place soiled linen in utility room or proper receptacle.	Proper disposal of equipment prevents spread of microorganisms and ensures proper exchange procedures.
42. Remove gloves, and perform hand hygiene.	Reduces transmission of microorganisms.
43. After tube removal, ascultate client's bowel sounds and periodically check for abdominal distention.	Confirms peristalsis has returned.

Unexpected Outcomes and Related Interventions

1. Client's abdomen becomes distended and/or painful.
   a. Assess patency of tube, and irrigate as needed.
2. Client complains of sore throat from dry, irritated mucous membranes.
   a. Increase frequency of oral hygiene.
   b. Ask health care provider if client may suck on ice chips, throat lozenges.
3. Client develops irritation of skin around nares.
   a. Provide skin care to nares.
   b. Retape so tube does not press against nares.
   c. Consider switching tube to other naris.
4. Client develops signs of pulmonary aspiration: fever, shortness of breath, pulmonary congestion.
   a. Perform respiratory assessment.
   b. Notify health care provider.
   c. Obtain chest x-ray film as ordered.

Recording and Reporting

- Record in nurses' notes time and type of NG tube inserted, client's tolerance of procedure, confirmation of placement, character of gastric contents, pH value, whether tube is clamped or connected to drainage device, and amount of suction applied.
- Record in nurses' notes and/or flow sheet amount and character of contents draining from NG tube every shift, unless ordered more frequently by health care provider.
- Record in nurse's notes time and date that NG tube was removed, client's tolerance of procedure, and client's status following procedure.

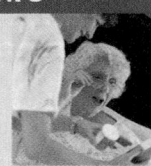

Figure 46-17 Ostomy irrigation cone inserted into stoma.

BOX 46-10   CLIENT TEACHING

The Client With an Ostomy
Objective
• Client/caregiver will be able to demonstrate changing an ostomy pouch.

Teaching Strategies
• Provide a comprehensive list of the products needed to care for the ostomy.
• Provide client/caregiver with supplies to last 1 to 2 weeks and the contact number and location of nearest medical supply store.
• Show client/caregiver the step-by-step approach for changing an ostomy pouch.
• Provide at least one opportunity for client/caregiver to change the ostomy pouch while client is in the hospital.
• Set up visits from a community stoma care nurse or home care nurse, and provide contact numbers.
• Provide detailed discharge instructions for skin care, driving, lifting, resuming exercise, and when to contact the health care provider.

Evaluation
• Observe client/caregiver change ostomy pouch.
• Ask client/caregiver to state signs of stoma irritation and how to relieve it.
• Ask client/caregiver about expected output from stoma and when to call the health care provider.

Cronin E: Best practice in discharging patients with a stoma, *Nursing Times* 101(47):67, 2005

cone tip and waits 30 to 45 minutes for the solution and feces to drain out of the irrigation sleeve. Once the drainage stops, the client applies a stoma cap or a pouch. If a client chooses to irrigate the colostomy, you individualize the time of irrigation to the client's lifestyle.

Pouching Ostomies. Ostomies require a pouch to collect fecal material. An effective pouching system protects the skin, contains fecal material, remains odor free, and is comfortable and inconspicuous. A person wearing a pouch needs to feel secure in participating in any activity.

Many pouching systems are available. To ensure that a pouch fits well and meets the client's needs, consider the location of the ostomy, type and size of the stoma, type and amount of ostomy drainage, size and contour of the abdomen, condition of the skin around the stoma, physical activities of the client, client's personal preference, age and dexterity, and cost of equipment. A **wound ostomy continence nurse (WOCN)** is a nurse specially educated to care for ostomy clients; the WOCN collaborates with staff nurses to be sure the client uses the correct pouching system. For example, referral to a WOCN is appropriate when planning the care of a client who has a high-output ostomy that requires a pouch modification.

A pouching system consists of a pouch and skin barrier. Some pouching systems, such as Squibb-ConvaTec, Hollister, Coloplast, and Smith & Nephew, are attached to the client's skin from the product's adhesive surface, whereas other pouching systems, such as VIP, are nonadhesive systems. Pouches come in one- and two-piece systems that are disposable or reusable. Some pouches have the opening precut by the manufacturer; others require the stoma opening to be custom cut to the client's specific stoma size.

Skin barriers include wafers, pastes, powders, and liquid film applied to the skin around the stoma. Some wafer skin barriers are permanently attached to the ostomy pouch. These are called one-piece pouch systems. In a two-piece system, the client can detach the pouch from the skin barrier for emptying or changing. This allows the skin barrier to remain around the client's stoma for several days, thus minimizing the chance of skin damage from too-frequent removal of the skin barrier from the peristomal skin. When using a two-piece pouching system, it is important to remember that the skin barrier and pouch need to be the same corresponding size and from the same manufacturer. A pouch from one manufacturer will not fit correctly on a skin barrier from another manufacturer. Be sure to use an ostomy pouch made for collecting fecal matter (colostomy or ileostomy) and not one for collecting urine.

It is important to measure the stoma size carefully when selecting and cutting out the opening on the wafer skin barrier. A good skin barrier protects the skin, prevents irritation from repeated removal of the pouch, and is comfortable for the client to wear. Skill 46-3 describes steps for applying a pouching system.

Clients with new stomas often feel vulnerable when they leave the hospital. To provide a smooth transition from hospital to home, offer help for the client and family caregivers (Cronin, 2005). Client teaching achieves a smooth transition to home for a client with a new ostomy (Box 46-10).

Nutritional Considerations for Clients With Ostomies. Nutritional therapy is important for clients with ostomies. During the first weeks after surgery, many health care providers recommend low-fiber diets, particularly for clients with ileostomies, because the small bowel requires time to adapt to the diversion. Low-fiber foods include bread, noodles, rice, cream cheese, eggs (not fried), strained fruit juices, lean meats, fish, and poultry. As ostomies heal, clients are able to eat almost any food. High-fiber foods such as fresh fruits and vegetables help ensure a more solid stool needed to achieve success at irrigation. Clients need to avoid blockage. The stoma's surgical construction affects the likelihood of blockage.

Text continued on p. 1216

✳ **SKILL 46-3**   **POUCHING AN OSTOMY**

Delegation Considerations

The skill of pouching an ostomy, especially a newly established ostomy cannot be delegated. Pouching of an established ostomy can be delegated. Inform nursing assistive personnel about:

- Appropriate pouch and skin barrier
- The signs of stoma and peristomal skin changes to report to a registered professional nurse
- Monitoring and reporting characteristics and volume of ostomy output and reporting changes in volume and/or consistency for further assessment

Equipment (Figure 46-18)

- Clear drainable colostomy/ileostomy pouch in correct size for two-piece system or custom cut-to-fit one-piece type with attached skin barrier
- Pouch closure device, such as clamp
- Ostomy measuring guide
- Adhesive remover (optional)
- Clean gloves
- Ostomy deodorant
- Gauze pads and washcloths
- Towel or disposable waterproof barrier
- Basin with warm tap water
- Scissors/pen
- Skin barrier if not attached to pouching system
- Stoma paste or Stomahesive (optional)
- Tape or ostomy belt (optional)
- Stethoscope

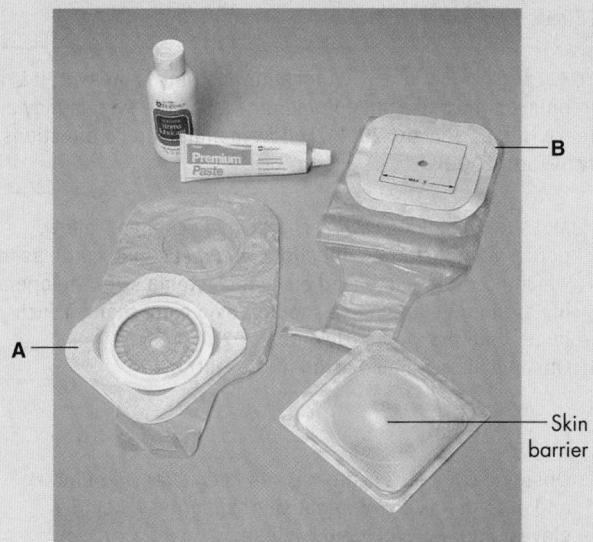

Figure 46-18 Ostomy pouches and skin barriers. **A,** Two-piece detachable system. (NOTE: Skin barrier would need to be custom cut according to stoma size.) The pouch opening is already precut by the manufacturer to fit the size of the flange on the skin barrier. **B,** One-piece pouch with skin barrier attached. (Permission to use and/or reproduce this copyrighted photo has been granted by the owner, Hollister Incorporated.)

STEPS	RATIONALE
1. Perform hand hygiene, and auscultate for bowel sounds.	Documents presence of peristalsis.
2. Apply gloves, and observe skin barrier and pouch for leakage and length of time in place. NOTE: Depending on type of pouching system used (such as with an opaque pouch), the nurse may have to remove the pouch to fully observe the stoma. Clear pouches permit the viewing of the stoma without their removal.	Indicates need for different type of pouch or sealant. Routine observation allows for early detection of potential problems (Thompson, 2000). Leaking may indicate need for a different pouch or sealant.

Critical Decision Point: Intact skin barriers with no evidence of leakage do not need to be changed daily and remain in place for 3 to 7 days (Erwin-Toth, 2001; Ignatavicius and Workman, 2006).

3. Observe stoma for color, swelling, trauma, and healing; stoma is normally moist and reddish-pink. Assess type of stoma. Stoma is flush with the skin or a budlike protrusion on the abdomen (see illustration for a normal bud stoma).	Stoma characteristics are one of the factors to consider when selecting an appropriate pouching system (Wound, Ostomy and Continence Nurses Society, 2005).

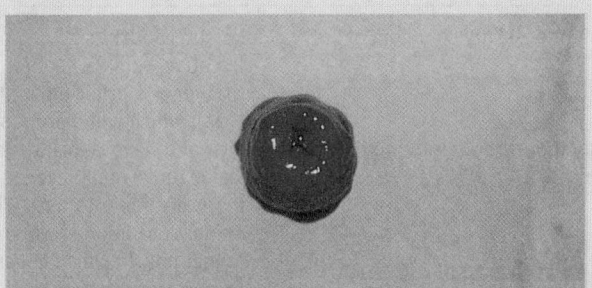

STEP 3 Bud stoma. (Permission to use and/or reproduce this copyrighted photo has been granted by the owner, Hollister Incorporated.)

POUCHING AN OSTOMY—CONT'D

STEPS	RATIONALE

Critical Decision Point: When a new ostomy is present, it is important to measure the stoma with each pouching system change to determine correct size of equipment because the system may need modifications as the stoma size changes (Wound, Ostomy and Continence Nurses Society, 2005). Follow manufacturer's directions and measuring guide to determine correct size for pouching system (Erwin-Toth, 2000).

STEPS	RATIONALE
4. Measure the stoma with each pouching change. Follow pouch manufacturer's directions and measuring guide as to which pouch to use based on client's stoma size. The opening around the appliance should be no more than 1/16 inch larger than the stoma (Hyland, 2002).	Determines correct size equipment, preventing trauma to stoma. Too large an opening will permit fecal drainage to ooze from under the appliance, causing skin irritation. Too small an opening causes the appliance to cut into the stoma (Hyland, 2002).
5. Observe abdominal incision (if present).	Relationship of abdominal incision to stoma determines proper placement of pouch. The presence of pressure areas from the pouching system may require a different system (Wound, Ostomy and Continence Nurses Society, 2005).
6. Observe effluent from stoma, and keep a record of intake and output. Ask client about skin tenderness. Remove gloves, and perform hand hygiene.	Effluent from stoma is caustic, and if it comes in contact with the sensitive peristomal skin, the risk of skin breakdown increases (Hyland, 2002).
7. When assessing skin for irritation, check that pouching system is not leaking.	Leaking indicates the need for a different type of pouch or sealant.
8. Check existing bag for gas accumulation.	If excessive gas accumulation is present, determine the need for the client to switch to a pouch with a vent or filter (Wound, Ostomy and Continence Nurses Society, 2004a).

Critical Decision Point: Because of stoma and abdominal characteristics, some clients need their ostomy pouching system to curve outward to avoid leakage (Thompson, 2000).

STEPS	RATIONALE
9. Assess abdomen for best type of pouching system to use. Consider the following: a. Contour and peristomal plane b. Presence of scars, incisions c. Location and type of stoma	Determines pouching system selection and need for other equipment. For a stoma to have an adequate seal with an ostomy appliance, the stoma needs to be placed within the abdominal rectus muscle, away from abdominal creases and folds, away from the bony understructures, and surrounded by at least 2 inches of smooth surface on all sides (Banks and Razor, 2003).
10. Select appropriate pouching system option: a. One-piece pouch with skin barrier already attached b. Precut pouch and skin barrier	Proper selection of pouch ensures good fit without leakage of effluent.
c. Two-piece pouch system, which consists of pouch that detaches from skin barrier and remains around client's stoma for several days.	Two-piece pouches give client choice of using either an open-ended or closed-ended pouch. This is because the client is able to remove the pouch from the skin barrier to empty effluent. For some people, accessory products such as karaya paste or careful use of a pouch belt will enhance the seal and prevent leakage (Erwin-Toth, 2001).

Critical Decision Point: If client has a large volume of liquid stool from an ileostomy, consider using a "high-output" pouch that will contain the volume of effluent and reduce the frequency of pouch emptying.

STEPS	RATIONALE
11. To minimize skin irritation, avoid unnecessary changing of entire pouching system.	Make sure pouches are emptied when one-third to one-half full, because weight of contents will dislodge skin seal and ostomy drainage is irritating to the skin. Also, pouches collect flatus (gas), which will disrupt skin seal if it is not expelled.
12. Assess the client's self-care ability to further determine the best type of pouching system to use.	Clients who have difficulty using their hands or who have limited vision find a one-piece system or a precut pouch and skin barrier more desirable to use. Clients who have mobility problems or spinal cord injuries will benefit by using equipment that has a longer pouch, which is easier to empty independently when sitting (Erwin-Toth, 2003; Thompson, 2000). For clients who prefer being able to keep the skin barrier in place for several days and changing just the pouch, the two-piece system is desirable.

✳ **SKILL 46-3** POUCHING AN OSTOMY—CONT'D

STEPS	RATIONALE
13. After skin barrier and pouch removal, assess skin around stoma, noting scars, folds, skin breakdown, and peristomal suture line, if present. Keep pouch loosely attached to stoma to collect any drainage while changing the system. Remove gloves, and perform hand hygiene.	Determines need for barrier paste to increase adherence of pouch to skin or to fill in irregularities.

Critical Decision Point: If the skin around the stoma is discolored, weeping, itchy, or sore, refer the client to an ostomy specialist (Hyland, 2002).

STEPS	RATIONALE
14. Determine client's emotional response and knowledge and understanding of an ostomy and its care.	Assists in determining how much client is able to participate in care and need for teaching and information clarification.
15. Explain procedure to client; encourage client's interaction and questions.	Lessens anxiety and promotes client's participation.
16. Change pouch when client is comfortable; before a meal is better.	Avoids increased peristalsis and chance of evacuation during pouch change.
17. Perform hand hygiene. Assemble equipment, and close room curtains or door.	Reduces infection transmission. Optimizes use of time; conserves client's and nurse's energy. Provides privacy.
18. Position client either standing or supine, and drape. If seated, position either on or in front of the toilet. Apply clean gloves.	When client is supine, fewer wrinkles allow for ease of application of pouching system; maintains client's dignity.
19. Place towel or disposable waterproof barrier under the client.	Protects bed linen.

Critical Decision Point: If portions of the skin barrier remain, use an adhesive remover to gently remove them. Improper removal of barrier will irritate skin, cause skin tears, and result in poor adhering of the new pouch.

STEPS	RATIONALE
20. If not done in Step 2, completely remove used pouch and skin barrier gently by pushing the skin away from the barrier. When necessary, use an adhesive remover to facilitate removal of the skin barrier.	Reduces trauma; jerking irritates the skin and causes tears.
21. Cleanse peristomal skin gently with warm tap water using gauze pads or clean washcloth; do not scrub the skin; dry completely by patting the skin with gauze or towel.	Avoid use of soap because it leaves a residue on the skin that interferes with pouch adhesion to the skin. Skin must be dry; pouch does not adhere to wet skin. If blood appears on the gauze pad, do not be alarmed; the stoma, if rubbed, will ooze some blood from the cleaning process. The stoma's surface is a highly vascular mucous membrane. Bleeding into the pouch is abnormal (Wound, Ostomy and Continence Nurses Society, 2004b).

Critical Decision Point: Adhesive remover should not be routinely used. However, adhesive removers may be necessary when the client's skin tears easily or there is a buildup of sticky residue over the peristomal skin. When adhesive removers are used, follow up with washing the skin with water and a mild soap to remove the oily coating on the skin from the adhesive remover (Wound, Ostomy and Continence Nurses Society, 2004a).

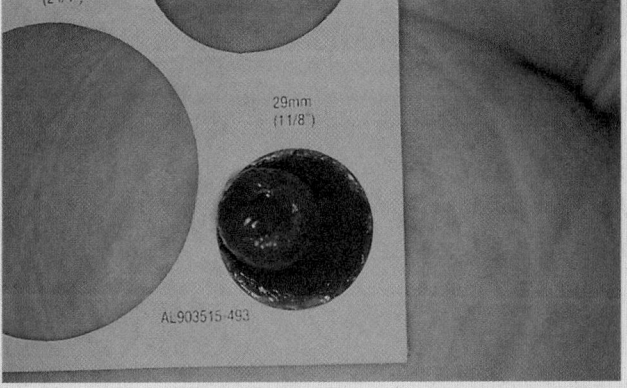

STEP 22 Measuring a stoma.

Continued

✳ **SKILL 46-3**   **POUCHING AN OSTOMY—CONT'D**

STEPS	RATIONALE
22. Measure the stoma for correct size of pouching system needed, using the manufacturer's measuring guide (see illustration).	Ensures accuracy in determining correct pouch size needed. Stoma shrinks and does not reach usual size for 6 to 8 weeks (Thompson, 2000).
23. Prepare selected pouch. With a custom cut-to-fit pouch, use an ostomy guide to cut opening on the pouch $\frac{1}{16}$ inch larger than stoma before removing backing (Hyland, 2002). Prepare pouch by removing backing from barrier and adhesive (see illustration). With ileostomy, apply thin circle of barrier paste around opening in pouch; allow to dry.	The paste facilitates seal and protects skin. Size of pouch opening keeps drainage off skin and lessens risk of damage to stoma during peristalsis or activity. Change pouch and skin barrier whenever leaking. You can also change it before or after tub bath or shower. Stool is alkaline, and this irritates the skin; fecal bacteria often colonize on the skin and increase risk of infection.
24. Apply the skin barrier and pouch. If creases next to stoma occur, use barrier paste to fill in; let dry 1 to 2 minutes.	Paste creates a flatter surface for pouch placement.

Critical Decision Point: If client has surgical incision near stoma, you will have to trim the skin barrier to fit.

A. For one-piece pouching system: (1) Use skin sealant wipes on skin directly under adhesive skin barrier or pouch; allow to dry. Press the adhesive backing of the pouch and/or skin barrier smoothly against the skin, starting from the bottom and working up and around the sides.	Ensures smooth, wrinkle-free seal. Be aware of any irritated or open areas because the skin sealant wipes often contain alcohol (Wound, Ostomy and Continence Nurses Society, 2004a).
(2) Hold pouch by barrier, center over stoma, and press down gently on barrier; bottom of pouch should point toward client's knees (see illustration).	A different positioning of the pouch is sometimes necessary to allow better gravity flow. For example, a client confined to bed needs to have a pouch positioned horizontally over the side of the abdomen (Thompson, 2000).
(3) Maintain gentle finger pressure around the barrier for 1 to 2 minutes.	Gentle pressure and body heat assist the adhesion.
B. For two-piece pouching system: (1) Apply flange (barrier with adhesive) as in steps above for one-piece system (see illustration). Then snap on pouch, and maintain finger pressure.	Creates wrinkle-free, secure seal; decreases irritation from the adhesive on skin.
C. For both pouching systems, gently tug on the pouch in a downward direction.	Determines if the pouch is securely attached.
25. Gently press on the pectin or karaya flange to facilitate adhesion.	A pectin, karaya, or synthetic skin barrier adds to security of keeping the pouch system attached securely (Erwin-Toth, 2001). Some clients prefer a belt attached to the pouch for extra security.

Critical Decision Point: If the client chooses to wear a belt, be sure belt is not too tight by placing two fingers between belt and client's skin.

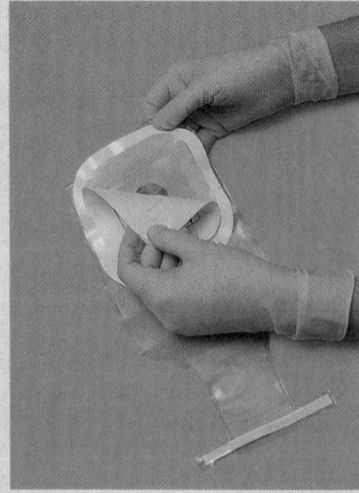

STEP 23 Preparing an ostomy pouch.

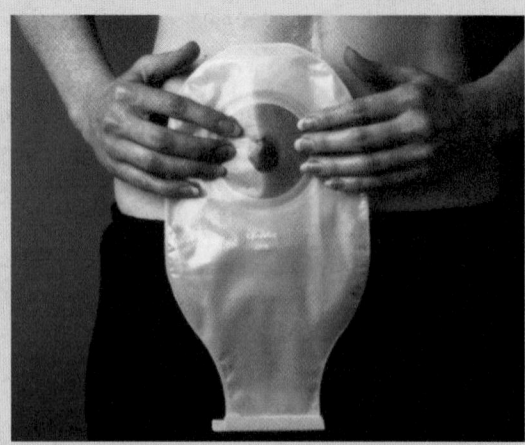

STEP 24(A)2 Applying a one-piece pouch. (Courtesy ConvaTec, Princeton, NJ.)

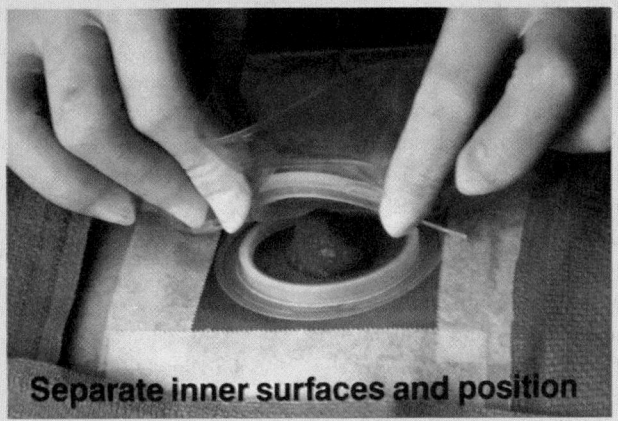

Separate inner surfaces and position

STEP 24(B)1 Application of barrier-paste flange. (Courtesy ConvaTec, Princeton, NJ.)

STEPS	RATIONALE
26. Although many ostomy pouches are odor-proof, some nurses and clients like to put a small amount of ostomy deodorant into the pouch. Do not use "home remedies," such as aspirin, to control ostomy odor.	Aspirin or other substances harm the stoma.

Critical Decision Point: Never add aspirin to an ostomy pouch. It will cause stoma bleeding.

STEPS	RATIONALE
27. Fold bottom of drainable open-ended pouches up once, and close using a closure device such as a clamp (or follow manufacturer's instructions for closure).	Maintains secure seal to prevent leaking.
28. Properly dispose of old pouch and soiled equipment. Consider spraying deodorant in room if needed.	Lessens odors in room.
29. Remove gloves, and perform hand hygiene.	Reduces transmission of microorganisms.
30. Ask if client feels discomfort around stoma.	Determines presence of skin irritation.
31. Observe condition of skin barrier and adhesive.	Determines presence of leaks.
32. Auscultate bowel sounds, and observe characteristics of stool.	Determines status of peristalsis and bowel elimination.
33. Observe client's nonverbal behaviors while applying the pouch. Ask if client has any questions about pouching.	Indicates emotional response to stoma and readiness for teaching. Determines level of understanding of procedure.

Unexpected Outcomes and Related Interventions.

1. Client experiences damage to peristomal skin.
   a. Assess for and report to health care provider for treatment:
      (1) Mechanical damage due to inappropriate skin care, incorrect tape removal
      (2) Chemical damage due to waste coming into contact with peristomal skin, skin reaction to adhesive
      (3) Damage due to a fungal infection (candidiasis), usually caused by persistent moisture on peristomal skin
2. Stoma becomes necrotic as manifested by purple or black color, dry instead of moist, failure to bleed, or there is tissue sloughing.
   a. Assess circulation to stoma.
   b. Observe for excessive edema or tension on bowel suture line (if present).
   c. Immediately report this finding to the health care provider.

Recording and Reporting

- Record type of pouch and skin barrier applied; amount and appearance of stool, texture, condition of peristomal skin, and sutures.
- Report any of the following to the nurse and/or health care provider:
  - Abnormal appearance of stoma, suture line, peristomal skin, character of output, absence of bowel sounds
  - No flatus in 24 to 36 hours and no stool by third day
- Document abdominal distention and excessive tenderness, nature of bowel sounds.
- Record client's level of participation and need for teaching.

Home Care Considerations

- Evaluate the client's home toileting facilities. This includes presence of adequate toileting facilities, flushable toilet, and number and location of toilets.
- Caution the client that most ostomy pouches and barriers cannot be flushed down the toilet; they clog the system. Dispose of used ostomy pouch according to local sanitation regulations.

Clients with an ileostomy need to eat slowly and chew food completely. Drinking 10 to 12 glasses of water daily (unless contraindicated) also prevents blockage. High-fiber foods that cause problems include stringy meats, mushrooms, popcorn, fruits such as cherries, and some seafood such as shrimp and crab. Clients with ostomies often benefit from avoiding foods that cause gas and odor, including broccoli, cauliflower, dried beans, and Brussels sprouts.

Bowel Training. The client with incontinence is unable to maintain bowel control. A **bowel training** program helps some clients to defecate normally, especially those who still have some neuromuscular control.

The training program involves setting up a daily routine. By attempting to defecate at the same time each day and using measures that promote defecation, the client gains control of bowel reflexes. The program requires time, patience, and consistency. The health care provider determines the client's physical readiness and ability to benefit from bowel training. A successful program includes the following:

- Assessing the normal elimination pattern and recording times when the client is incontinent
- Incorporating principles of gerontological nursing when providing bowel retraining programs for the older adult client (Box 46-11)
- Choosing a time in the client's pattern to initiate defecation-control measures
- Giving stool softeners orally every day or a cathartic suppository at least half an hour before the selected defecation time (lower colon needs to be free of stool so that suppository contacts intestinal mucosa)
- Offering a hot drink (hot tea) or fruit juice (prune juice) (or whatever fluids normally stimulate peristalsis for the client) before the defecation time
- Assisting the client to the toilet at the designated time
- Avoiding medications, such as analgesics, that increase constipation
- Providing privacy and setting a time limit for defecation (15 to 20 minutes)
- Instructing the client to lean forward at the hips while sitting on the toilet, to apply manual pressure with the hands over the abdomen, and to bear down but not strain to stimulate colon emptying
- Not criticizing or conveying frustration if the client is unable to defecate
- Maintaining normal exercise within the client's physical ability

Maintenance of Proper Fluid and Food Intake. In choosing a diet for promoting normal elimination, consider the frequency of defecation, characteristics of feces, and types of foods that impair or promote defecation. The client with frequent constipation or impaction requires an increased intake of high-fiber foods and more fluids. However, the client needs to realize that diet therapy provides only long-term relief of elimination problems and does not give immediate relief from problems such as constipation.

When diarrhea is a problem, recommend foods with low fiber content and discourage foods that typically cause gastric upset or abdominal cramping. Diarrhea caused by illness is sometimes debilitating. If the client cannot tolerate foods or liquids orally,

---

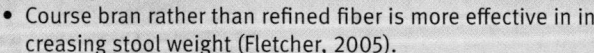

✷ BOX 46-11   **FOCUS ON OLDER ADULTS**

Bowel Retraining

- Constipation is a common complaint in older clients. Among clients older than 65 years, constipation is present in up to 30% of outpatients, 41% of inpatients, and 80% of nursing home residents (Fletcher, 2005).
- Course bran rather than refined fiber is more effective in increasing stool weight (Fletcher, 2005).
- A minimum of 1500 mL of fluid per day reduces the risk of constipation, with increased fluid needs during summer months and those on diuretics with stable cardiovascular status (Fletcher, 2005).
- If holding drinking cups is a problem, consider using lighter plastic cups and filling half full, refilling frequently (Wilson, 2005).
- Fruit juices increase fiber content as well as intake (Wilson, 2005).
- Encourage regular exercise. Even maintaining an erect posture in an immobile client reduces the risk of constipation (Fletcher, 2005).
- Clients need to feel at ease during elimination. Lack of privacy leads the client to ignore the urge to defecate.
- Review all medications with the health care provider to provide substitute medications that are less likely to cause constipation whenever possible (Bosshard and others, 2004).
- Use of behavioral intervention such as habit training provides relief of constipation. Have clients sit on the toilet about 30 minutes after a meal, whether or not they feel the urge to defecate (Wilson, 2005).

GI, Gastrointestinal.

---

intravenous therapy (with potassium supplements) is necessary. The client returns to a normal diet slowly, often beginning with fluids. Excessively hot or cold fluids stimulate peristalsis, causing abdominal cramps and further diarrhea. As the tolerance to liquids improves, the client is able to eat solid foods.

Promotion of Regular Exercise. A daily exercise program helps prevent elimination problems. Walking, riding a stationary bicycle, or swimming stimulates peristalsis. Clients who are sedentary at work are most in need of regular exercise.

For a client temporarily immobilized, attempt ambulation as soon as possible. If the condition permits, assist a postoperative client in walking to a chair on the evening of the day of surgery. Have the client walk farther each day.

Some clients have difficulty passing stool because of weak abdominal and pelvic floor muscles. Exercises help bedridden clients using a bedpan. The client practices the exercises as follows:

- Lie supine; tighten the abdominal muscles as though pushing them to the floor. Hold them tight to the count of three; relax. Repeat 5 to 10 times as tolerated.
- Flex and contract the thigh muscles by raising one knee slowly toward the chest. Repeat for each leg at least five times, and increase frequency as tolerated.

Hemorrhoids. Pain results when hemorrhoid tissues are directly irritated. The primary goal for the client with hemorrhoids is to have soft-formed, painless bowel movements. Proper diet, fluids, and regular exercise improve the likelihood of stools being soft. If the client becomes constipated, passage of hard stools causes bleeding and irritation. Local heat provides temporary relief to swollen hemorrhoids. A sitz bath is the most effective means of heat application (see Chapter 48).

Maintenance of Skin Integrity. The client with diarrhea or fecal incontinence is at risk for skin breakdown when fecal contents remain on the skin. The same problem exists for the client with an ostomy that drains liquid stool. Liquid stool is usually acidic and contains digestive enzymes. Irritation from repeated wiping with toilet tissue aggravates skin breakdown. Bathing the skin after soiling helps, but sometimes it results in more breakdown unless the client dries the skin thoroughly.

When caring for a client who is debilitated, incontinent, and unable to ask for assistance, check often for defecation. You can protect the anal areas with petrolatum, zinc oxide, or another ointment that holds moisture in the skin, preventing drying and cracking. Yeast infections of the skin often develop easily. Several powdered antifungal agents are effective against yeast. Do not use baby powder or cornstarch because they have no medical properties and they frequently cake on the skin and become difficult to remove.

◆ Evaluation

The effectiveness of care depends on success in meeting the expected outcomes of self-care. Optimally the client will be able to have regular, pain-free defecation of soft-formed stools. In order to evaluate the expected client outcomes, it is necessary to ask questions such as: Is the client able to demonstrate the information gained regarding establishment of a normal elimination pattern? Is the client able to demonstrate the skills learned, such as ostomy protocols and skin protection? Is the client able to accomplish normal defecation by manipulating natural components of daily living such as diet, fluid intake, and exercise? Does the client use minimal artificial means of defecation such as enemas and laxatives? The client is the only one who is able to determine if the bowel elimination problems have been relieved and which therapies were the most effective (Figure 46-19).

If the nurse has been successful in establishing a therapeutic relationship with the client, the client will feel comfortable in discussing the intimate details often associated with bowel elimination. The client will not be embarrassed as the nurse assists the client with elimination needs. The client will relate a feeling of comfort and freedom from pain as elimination needs are met within the limits of the client's condition and treatment.

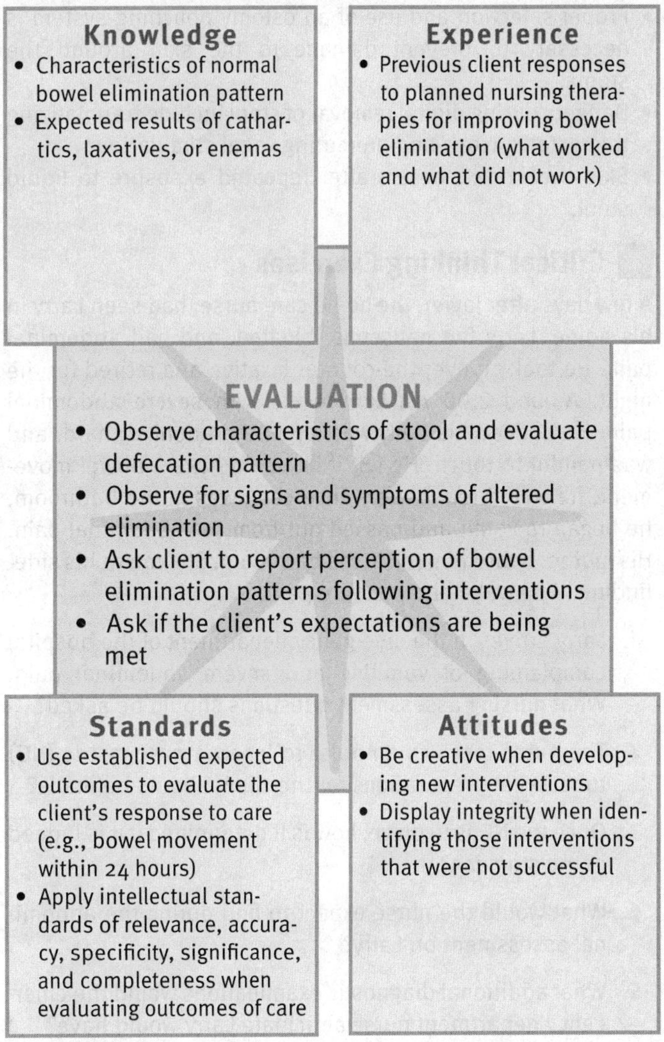

✳ Key Concepts

- Mechanical breakdown of food elements, gastrointestinal motility, and selective absorption and secretion of substances by the large intestine influence the character of feces.
- Food high in fiber content and an increased fluid intake keep feces soft.
- Ongoing use of cathartics, laxatives, and enemas affects and delays normal defecation reflexes.
- Vagal stimulation, which slows the heart rate, occurs during straining while defecating, taking rectal temperatures, enemas, and digital removal of impacted stool.

Knowledge
- Characteristics of normal bowel elimination pattern
- Expected results of cathartics, laxatives, or enemas

Experience
- Previous client responses to planned nursing therapies for improving bowel elimination (what worked and what did not work)

EVALUATION
- Observe characteristics of stool and evaluate defecation pattern
- Observe for signs and symptoms of altered elimination
- Ask client to report perception of bowel elimination patterns following interventions
- Ask if the client's expectations are being met

Standards
- Use established expected outcomes to evaluate the client's response to care (e.g., bowel movement within 24 hours)
- Apply intellectual standards of relevance, accuracy, specificity, significance, and completeness when evaluating outcomes of care

Attitudes
- Be creative when developing new interventions
- Display integrity when identifying those interventions that were not successful

Figure 46-19 Critical thinking model for elimination evaluation.

- The greatest danger from diarrhea is development of fluid and electrolyte imbalance.
- The location of an ostomy influences consistency of the stool.
- Focus assessment of elimination patterns on bowel habits, factors that normally influence defecation, recent changes in elimination, and a physical examination.
- Indirect and direct visualization of the lower gastrointestinal tract requires cleansing of the bowel before the procedure.
- Consider frequency of defecation, fecal characteristics, and effect of foods on gastrointestinal function when selecting a diet promoting normal elimination.
- Proper positioning on a bedpan allows the client to assume a position similar to squatting without experiencing muscle strain.
- Nasogastric intubation decompresses the gastric contents by removing secretions and gaseous products from the gastrointestinal tract.
- The purposes of gastric decompression are to keep the gastrointestinal tract free of secretions, reduce nausea and gas, and decrease the risk of vomiting and aspiration.

- Proper selection and use of an ostomy pouching system is necessary to prevent damage to the skin around the stoma.
- Dangers during digital removal of stool include traumatizing the rectal mucosa and promoting vagal stimulation.
- Skin breakdown occurs after repeated exposure to liquid stool.

✳ Critical Thinking Exercises

A few days after Javier, the home care nurse, had seen Larry in his home, Larry felt nauseous, bloated, and had abdominal pain. He took an over-the-counter laxative and retired for the night. Around 2:00 AM Larry woke with severe abdominal pain. He noticed his belly was larger than normal, hard, and was painful to touch. He felt if he could have a bowel movement, he would feel better. Once Larry was in the bathroom, he began to vomit and passed out from the abdominal pain. His mother heard him fall in the bathroom. She ran to his side, finding him awake but in severe pain.

1. Larry arrives in the emergency department of the hospital complaining of vomiting and severe abdominal pain. What nursing assessment questions should be asked?

2. The nurse receives an order to insert a nasogastric (NG) tube. What preparations for the client should be made?

3. Once the NG is in place, how is it determined if it is indeed in the stomach?

4. What would the nurse expect to find during the abdominal assessment on Larry?

5. What additional diagnostic examinations would the emergency department nurse anticipate Larry would have?

✳ NCLEX®-Style Review Questions

1. Most nutrients and electrolytes are absorbed in the:
   1. Colon
   2. Stomach
   3. Esophagus
   4. Small intestine

2. During the nursing assessment the client reveals that he has diarrhea and cramping every time he has ice cream. He attributes this to the cold nature of the food. However, the nurse begins to suspect that these symptoms might be associated with:
   1. Food allergy
   2. Irritable bowel
   3. Lactose intolerance
   4. Increased peristalsis

3. In assessing a 55-year-old client who is in the clinic for a routine physical, instruct the client about the need to obtain a stool specimen for guaiac fecal occult blood testing (gFOBT):
   1. If client reports rectal bleeding
   2. When there is a family history of polyps
   3. As part of a routine examination for colon cancer
   4. If a palpable mass is detected on digital examination

4. Which of the following medications listed in a client's medication history may cause gastrointestinal bleeding? (Choose all that apply.)
   1. Aspirin
   2. Cathartics
   3. Antidiarrheal opiate agents
   4. Nonsteroidal antiinflammatory drugs

5. Diarrhea that occurs with a fecal impaction is the result of:
   1. A clear liquid diet
   2. Irritation of the intestinal mucosa
   3. Inability of the client to form a stool
   4. Seepage of stool around the impaction

6. A cleaning enema is ordered for a 55-year-old client before intestinal surgery. The maximum amount of fluid given is:
   1. 150 to 200 mL
   2. 200 to 400 mL
   3. 400 to 750 mL
   4. 750 to 1000 mL

7. During the enema the client begins to complain of pain. The nurse notes blood in the return fluid and rectal bleeding. The nurse's actions are to:
   1. Stop the instillation
   2. Slow down the rate of instillation
   3. Tell the client to breathe slowly and relax
   4. Stop the instillation and obtain vital signs

8. Number the steps to irrigating a nasogastric tube in correct order:
   1. Slowly aspirate the syringe.
   2. Reconnect the NG tube to suction.
   3. Clamp and disconnect the NG tube.
   4. Perform hand hygiene, and apply clean gloves.
   5. Insert tip of syringe into NG tube, and slowly inject 30 mL saline.

9. List the correct order in which to apply an ostomy pouch:
   1. Remove the used pouch and skin barrier.
   2. Perform hand hygiene, and apply clean gloves.
   3. Assess the stoma for color, swelling, and healing.
   4. Gently cleanse the peristomal skin with warm tap water.
   5. Apply nonallergenic tape around the pectin skin barrier.
   6. Cut an opening on the pouch $1/16$ inch larger than the stoma.
   7. Press the adhesive backing of the pouch smoothly against the skin.

10. A nurse specially educated to care for ostomy clients is a (an):
    1. GI therapist
    2. Nurse practitioner
    3. Ostomy practitioner
    4. Wound ostomy continence nurse

47 | Mobility and Immobility

✳ OBJECTIVES

Mastery of content in this chapter will enable the student to:

- Describe the functions of the musculoskeletal (skeleton, skeletal muscles) and nervous systems in the regulation of movement.
- Discuss physiological and pathological influences on body alignment and joint mobility.
- Identify changes in physiological and psychosocial function associated with mobility and immobility.
- Assess for correct and impaired body alignment and mobility.
- Formulate appropriate nursing diagnoses for impaired body alignment and mobility.
- Develop individualized nursing care plans for clients with impaired body alignment and mobility.
- Discuss the importance of no-lift policies for the client and health care provider.
- Describe equipment needed for safe client handling and movement.
- Compare and contrast active and passive range-of-motion exercises.
- Evaluate the nursing plan for maintaining body alignment and mobility.

✳ MEDIA RESOURCES   ✳ KEY TERMS

Companion CD
- NCLEX®-Style Review Questions
- Audio Glossary
- Interactive Learning Activities
- English/Spanish Glossary

 Website
- NCLEX®-Style Review Questions
- Audio Glossary
- English/Spanish Glossary
- Interactive Learning Activities
- Weblinks
- Audio Summaries
- Video Clips
- Nursing Skills Online

Activity tolerance, p. 1236
Anthropometric measurements, p. 1238
Atelectasis, p. 1226
Bed rest, p. 1225
Body alignment, p. 1220
Body mechanics, p. 1220
Cartilage, p. 1222
Cartilaginous joint, p. 1221
Chest physiotherapy (CPT), p. 1247
Concentric tension, p. 1222
Disuse osteoporosis, p. 1227
Eccentric tension, p. 1222
Embolus, p. 1238
Exercise, p. 1236
Fibrous joint, p. 1221
Flat bones, p. 1220
Footdrop, p. 1228
Fractures, p. 1221
Friction, p. 1220
Gait, p. 1236
Gait belt, p. 1275

Hemiparesis, p. 1275
Hemiplegia, p. 1275
Hypostatic pneumonia, p. 1226
Immobility, p. 1225
Instrumental activities of daily living (IADLs), p. 1261
Irregular bones, p. 1220
Isometric contraction, p. 1222
Isotonic contraction, p. 1222
Joint contracture, p. 1228
Joints, p. 1221
Leverage, p. 1223
Ligaments, p. 1222
Logroll, p. 1257
Long bones, p. 1220
Mobility, p. 1220
Muscle atrophy, p. 1224
Muscle tone, p. 1223

Negative nitrogen balance, p. 1225
Neurotransmitters, p. 1223
Orthostatic hypotension, p. 1227
Osteoporosis, p. 1227
Pathological fractures, p. 1221
Posture, p. 1223
Pressure ulcer, p. 1228
Range of motion (ROM), p. 1230
Renal calculi, p. 1228
Short bones, p. 1220
Synostotic joint, p. 1221
Synovial joint, p. 1221
Tendons, p. 1222
Thrombus, p. 1227
Trapeze bar, p. 1251
Trochanter roll, p. 1251
Unossified, p. 1222
Urinary stasis, p. 1228

Movement is one of the visible aspects of human life and contributes to self-worth and well-being. People use **mobility** for many purposes (e.g., expression of emotions or satisfaction of basic needs with nonverbal gestures). Mobility is also used to show self-defense, perform activities of daily living (ADLs), and participate in recreational activities. Many functions of the body depend upon mobility. To maintain optimal physical mobility and functioning, the body's musculoskeletal and nervous systems need to be intact.

Clinical nursing practice related to mobility and immobility requires the incorporation of nursing knowledge and skills to provide competent care. Knowing the movements and functions of muscles in maintaining posture and movement and implementing evidence-based knowledge about safe client handling are essential to protecting the safety of both the client and the nurse.

Scientific Knowledge Base

Nature of Movement

Movement is a complex process that requires coordination between the musculoskeletal and nervous systems. **Body mechanics** is a term used to describe the coordinated efforts of the musculoskeletal and nervous systems. Although nurses need to understand the physics surrounding body mechanics, lifting techniques historically used in nursing practice that emphasize body mechanics often cause debilitating injuries to nursing and other health care staff (de Castro and others, 2006). Today, nurses use information about body alignment, balance, gravity, and friction when implementing nursing interventions such as positioning clients, determining the risk of client falls, and selecting the safest way to move or transfer clients.

Alignment and Balance. The terms *body alignment* and *posture* are similar and refer to the positioning of the joints, tendons, ligaments, and muscles while standing, sitting, and lying. **Body alignment** means that the individual's center of gravity is stable. Correct body alignment reduces strain on musculoskeletal structures, aids in maintaining adequate muscle tone, promotes comfort, and contributes to balance and conservation of energy. Without balance control, the center of gravity is displaced, thus creating a risk for falls and subsequent injuries. Balance is enhanced by keeping the body's center of gravity low with a wide base of support and maintaining correct body posture.

Individuals require balance for maintaining a static position (e.g., sitting) and for moving (e.g., walking). Disease, injury, pain, physical development (e.g., age), and life changes (e.g., pregnancy) compromise the ability to remain balanced. Medications that cause dizziness and prolonged immobility also affect balance. Impaired balance is a major threat to physical safety and contributes to a fear of falling and self-imposed restrictions on activity.

SAFETY ALERT The Surgeon General of the United States noted that falls represent the largest threat to bone health and functional independence of older individuals. For those over the age of 60, falls usually occur for a variety of reasons: problems with balance, mobility, vision, lower extremity weakness, and/or changes in blood pressure or circulation. Often an acute illness (e.g., infection, fever, dehydration, or arrhythmia), a new medication, or an environmental stress (e.g., standing or walking on an unsafe surface or poor lighting) compound these problems. Health care providers need to take an active role in preventing falls and fractures by assessing older adults and identifying those at greatest risk for injury (U.S. Department of Health and Human Services [USDHHS], 2004).

Gravity and Friction. Weight is the force exerted on a body by gravity. The force of weight is always directed downward, which is why an unbalanced object falls. Unsteady clients fall if their centers of gravity become unbalanced because of the gravitational pull on their weight.

To lift safely, the lifter has to overcome the weight of the object and know its center of gravity. In symmetrical inanimate objects the center of gravity is at the exact center of the object. People, however, are not geometrically perfect; their centers of gravity are usually at 55% to 57% of standing height and are in the midline, which is why only using principles of body mechanics in lifting clients often leads to injury of the nurse or health care professional.

Friction is a force that occurs in a direction to oppose movement. Nurses reduce friction by following some basic principles. The greater the surface area of the object that is moved, the greater the friction. A larger object produces greater resistance to movement. To decrease surface area and reduce friction when clients are unable to assist with moving up in bed, nurses use an ergonomic assistive device, such as a full body sling. It mechanically lifts the client off the surface of the bed, thereby preventing friction, tearing, or shearing of the client's delicate skin, and protects the nurse and other staff from injury (Nelson and others, 2003a).

Physiology and Regulation of Movement

Skeletal System. The skeleton provides attachments for muscles and ligaments and provides the leverage necessary for movement. Thus the skeleton is the body's supporting framework and is made up of four types of bones: long, short, flat, and irregular. **Long bones** contribute to height (e.g., the femur, fibula, and tibia in the leg) and length (e.g., the phalanges of the fingers and toes). **Short bones** (e.g., the carpal bones in the foot and the patella in the knee) occur in clusters and, when combined with ligaments and cartilage, permit movement of the extremities. **Flat bones,** such as some bones in the skull and the ribs in the thorax, provide structural contour. **Irregular bones** make up the vertebral column and some bones of the skull, such as the mandible.

Bones are further characterized by firmness, rigidity, and elasticity. Firmness results from inorganic salts, such as calcium and phosphate that are in the bone matrix. Firmness is related to the bone's rigidity, which is necessary to keep long bones straight, and enables bones to withstand weight bearing. In addition, bones have a degree of elasticity and skeletal flexibility that change with age. For example, the newborn has a large amount of cartilage and is highly flexible but is unable to support weight. The toddler's bones are more pliable than those of an older person and are better able to withstand falls. Older adults, especially women, are more susceptible to bone loss (resorption) and osteoporosis, which increase the risk of fractures.

The skeletal system has several functions. It protects vital organs (e.g., the skull around the brain and the ribs around the heart and lungs), and aids in calcium regulation. Bones store calcium

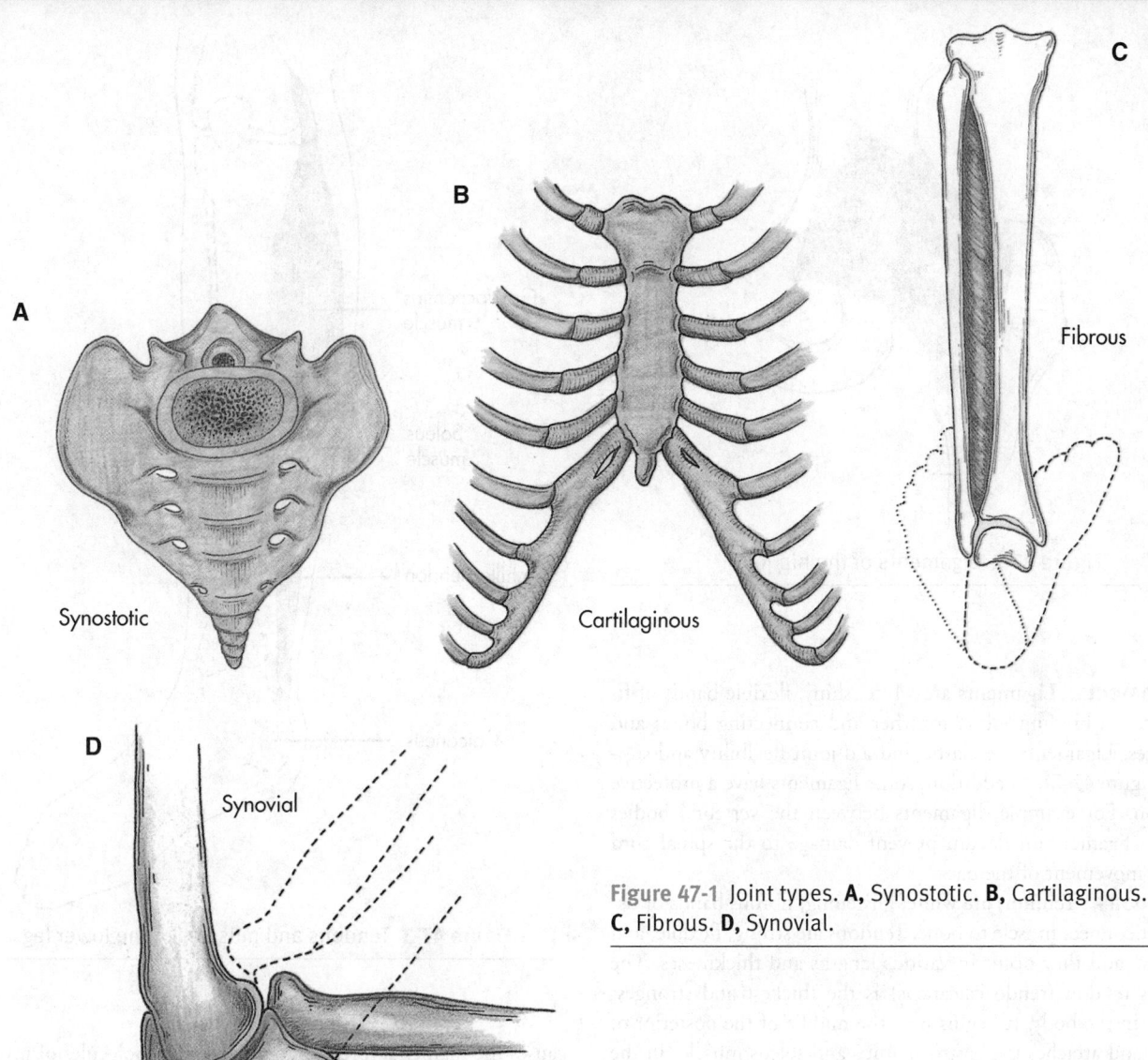

Figure 47-1 Joint types. **A,** Synostotic. **B,** Cartilaginous. **C,** Fibrous. **D,** Synovial.

and release it into the circulation as needed. Clients with decreased calcium regulation and metabolism are at risk for developing osteoporosis and **pathological fractures** (fractures caused by weakened bone tissue). In addition, the internal structure of long bones contains bone marrow, participates in red blood cell (RBC) production, and acts as a reservoir for blood. Clients with altered bone marrow function or diminished RBC production are usually weakened and fatigue easily, which decreases their mobility and places them at risk of falling.

Joints. **Joints** are the connections between bones. Each joint is classified according to its structure and degree of mobility. There are four classifications of joints: synostotic, cartilaginous, fibrous, and synovial.

The **synostotic joint** refers to bones jointed by bones. No movement is associated with this type of joint, and the bony tissue that forms between the bones provides strength and stability. The classic example of this type of joint is the skull, where fusion of the joint occurs later in life (Figure 47-1, *A*).

In the **cartilaginous joint,** or synchondrosis joint, cartilage unites bony components. This type of joint allows for bone growth while providing stability. When bone growth is complete, the joints ossify. The first sternocostal joint is an example of a synchondrosis joint (Figure 47-1, *B*).

The **fibrous joint,** or syndesmosis joint, is a joint in which a ligament or membrane unites two bony surfaces. The fibers of ligaments are flexible and stretch, permitting a limited amount of movement. The paired bones of the lower leg (tibia and fibula) are syndesmotic joints (Copstead-Kirkhorn and Banasik, 2005) (Figure 47-1, *C*).

The **synovial joint,** or true joint, is a freely movable joint in which contiguous bony surfaces are covered by articular cartilage and connected by ligaments lined with a synovial membrane. Joining of the humeral radius and ulna by cartilage and ligaments forms a pivotal joint (Figure 47-1, *D*). Other types of synovial joints are the ball-and-socket joints, such as the hip joint, and the hinge joints, such as the interphalangeal joints of the fingers.

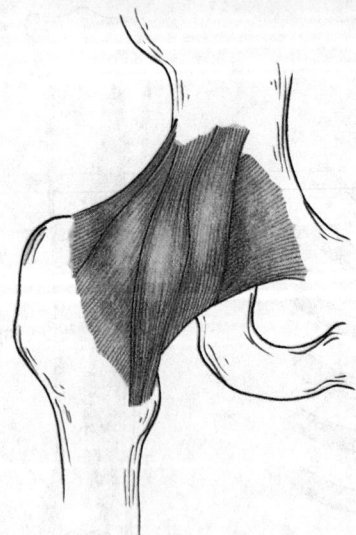

Figure 47-2 Ligaments of the hip joint.

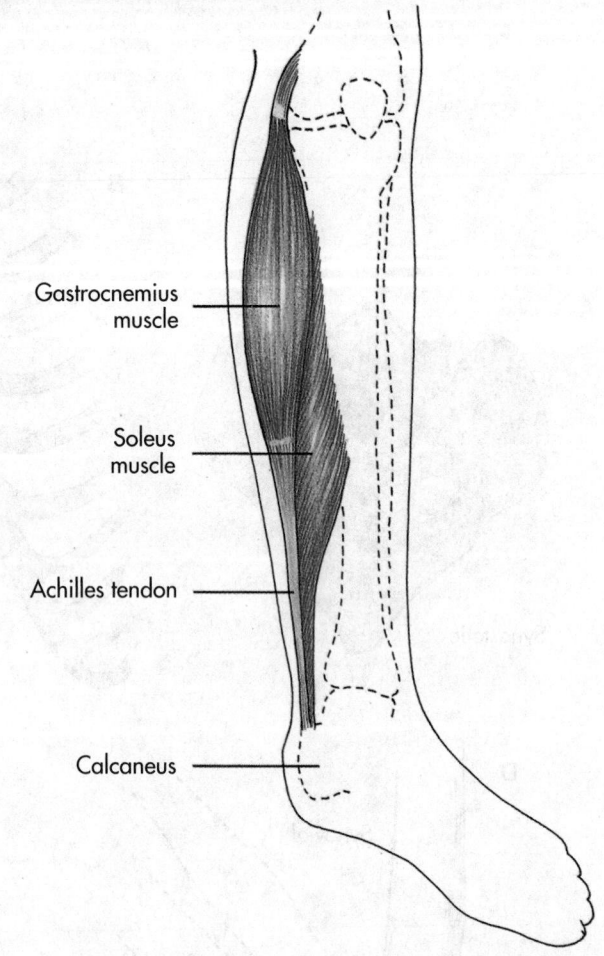

Figure 47-3 Tendons and muscles of the lower leg.

Ligaments. **Ligaments** are white, shiny, flexible bands of fibrous tissue binding joints together and connecting bones and cartilages. Ligaments are elastic and aid joint flexibility and support (Figure 47-2). In addition, some ligaments have a protective function. For example, ligaments between the vertebral bodies and the ligamentum flavum prevent damage to the spinal cord during movement of the back.

Tendons. **Tendons** are white, glistening, fibrous bands of tissue that connect muscle to bone. Tendons are strong, flexible, and inelastic, and they occur in various lengths and thicknesses. The Achilles tendon (tendo calcaneus) is the thickest and strongest tendon in the body. It begins near the middle of the posterior of the leg and attaches the gastrocnemius and soleus muscles in the calf to the calcaneal bone in the back of the foot (Figure 47-3).

Cartilage. **Cartilage** is nonvascular, supporting connective tissue located chiefly in the joints and thorax, trachea, larynx, nose, and ear. The fetus has a large amount of temporary cartilage, which is replaced by bone developed during infancy. Permanent cartilage is **unossified** (not hardened) except in advanced age and diseases such as osteoarthritis.

Joints, ligaments, tendons, and cartilage permit strength and flexibility of the skeleton. Strength enables the skeletal system to support the body. A person's flexibility is demonstrated through range of motion (ROM). However, strength and flexibility do not result entirely from these four structures. Adequate skeletal muscle is also necessary.

Skeletal Muscle. Movement of bones and joints involves active processes that are carefully integrated to achieve coordination. Skeletal muscles, because of their ability to contract and relax, are the working elements of movement. Anatomical structure and attachment to the skeleton enhance contractile elements of the skeletal muscle.

Muscles are made of fibers that contract when stimulated by an electrochemical impulse that travels from the nerve to the muscle across the neuromuscular junction. The electrochemical impulse causes the filaments (predominantly protein molecules of myosin and actin) within the fiber to slide past each other, with the filaments changing length.

Muscle contractions are categorized by functional purpose: moving, resisting, or stabilizing body parts. In **concentric tension**, increased muscle contraction causes muscle shortening resulting in movement, such as when a client uses an overhead trapeze to pull up in bed. **Eccentric tension** helps control the speed and direction of movement. In the example of the overhead trapeze, the client slowly lowers to the bed. The lowering is controlled when the antagonistic muscles lengthen. Concentric and eccentric muscle actions are necessary for active movement and are therefore referred to as dynamic or **isotonic contraction.** **Isometric contraction** (static contraction) causes an increase in muscle tension or muscle work but no shortening or active movement of the muscle (e.g., instructing the client in tightening and relaxing a muscle group, as in quadriceps set exercises or pelvic floor exercises). Voluntary movement is a combination of isotonic and isometric contractions.

Although isometric contractions do not result in muscle shortening, energy expenditure increases. This type of muscle work is comparable to having a car in neutral with the driver continually depressing the accelerator and racing the engine. The driver is not going anywhere but expends a large amount of energy. It is important to understand the energy expenditure (increased respiratory rate and increased work on the heart) associated with isometric exercises because they are sometimes contraindicated in certain clients' illnesses (e.g., myocardial infarction or chronic obstructive pulmonary disease).

Muscle Movement and Posture. Muscles that attach to bones of leverage provide necessary strength to move an object. **Leverage** is an inducing or compelling force and occurs when specific bones, such as the humerus, ulna, and radius, and the associated joint, such as the elbow, act together as a lever. Force is applied to one end of the bone to lift a weight as another point rotates the bone in the opposite direction.

Muscles associated primarily with maintaining posture are short and featherlike in appearance because they converge obliquely at a common tendon. Muscles of the lower extremities, trunk, neck, and back are concerned primarily with **posture** (the position of the body in relation to the surrounding space). These muscle groups work together to stabilize and support body weight, and they allow an individual to maintain a sitting or standing posture.

Muscle Regulation of Posture and Movement. Posture and movement depend on the skeleton and the shape and development of skeletal muscles. They also contribute to musculoskeletal function and often reflect personality, discomfort, and mood. For example, a person with a dramatic personality gestures with the hands, a person who is fatigued or depressed may slouch, and a person with abdominal pain may curl into a fetal-like position.

Coordination and regulation of different muscle groups depend on muscle tone and activity of antagonistic, synergistic, and antigravity muscles (see Chapter 37). **Muscle tone,** or tonus, is the normal state of balanced muscle tension. The body achieves tension by alternating contraction and relaxation without active movement of neighboring fibers of a specific muscle group. Muscle tone helps maintain functional positions such as sitting or standing without excess muscle fatigue and is maintained through continual use of muscles. ADLs require muscle action and help maintain muscle tone. When a client is immobile or on prolonged bed rest, activity level, activity tolerance, and muscle tone decrease.

Nervous System. The nervous system regulates movement and posture. The precentral gyrus, or motor strip, is the major voluntary motor area and is in the cerebral cortex. A majority of motor fibers descend from the motor strip and cross at the level of the medulla. Thus the motor fibers from the right motor strip initiate voluntary movement for the left side of the body, and motor fibers from the left motor strip initiate voluntary movement for the right side of the body.

During voluntary movement, impulses descend from the motor strip to the spinal cord. An impulse exits the spinal cord through efferent motor nerves and travels through the nerves. Through a complex process, **neurotransmitters,** or chemicals such as acetylcholine, transfer electric impulses from the nerve across the neuromuscular junction to the muscle. The neurotransmitter reaches a muscle and stimulates it, causing movement. Movement is impaired by disorders that alter neurotransmitter production, transfer of impulses from the nerve to the muscle, or activation of muscle activity. Parkinsonism is an example of such a disorder (see Chapter 37).

Pathological Influences on Mobility

Many pathological conditions affect mobility. Although a complete description of each is beyond the scope of this chapter, an overview of four pathological influences are presented.

Postural Abnormalities. Congenital or acquired postural abnormalities affect the efficiency of the musculoskeletal system, as well as body alignment, balance, and appearance. During assessment, observe body alignment and ROM (see Chapter 37). Postural abnormalities can cause pain, impair alignment or mobility, or both. Knowledge about the characteristics, causes, and treatment of common postural abnormalities is necessary for lifting, transfer, and positioning (Table 47-1). Some postural abnormalities limit ROM. Nurses intervene to maintain maximum ROM in unaffected joints and then design interventions to strengthen affected muscles and joints, improve the client's posture, and adequately use affected and unaffected muscle groups. Referral to and/or collaboration with a physical therapist enhances the nurse's interventions for a client with a postural abnormality.

Impaired Muscle Development. Injury and disease lead to numerous alterations in musculoskeletal function. The muscular dystrophies, for example, are a group of familial disorders that cause degeneration of skeletal muscle fibers. They are the most prevalent of the muscle diseases in childhood. Clients with muscular dystrophy experience progressive, symmetrical weakness and wasting of skeletal muscle groups, with increasing disability and deformity (McCance and Huether, 2005).

Damage to the Central Nervous System. Damage to any component of the central nervous system that regulates voluntary movement results in impaired body alignment, balance, and mobility. Trauma from a head injury, ischemia from a stroke or brain attack (cerebrovascular accident [CVA]), or bacterial infection like meningitis can damage the cerebellum or the motor strip in the cerebral cortex. Damage to the cerebellum causes problems with balance, and motor impairment is directly related to the amount of destruction of the motor strip. For example, a person with a right-sided cerebral hemorrhage with necrosis will have destruction of the right motor strip that results in left-sided hemiplegia. Trauma to the spinal cord also impairs mobility. For example, a complete transection of the spinal cord results in a bilateral loss of voluntary motor control below the level of the trauma because motor fibers are cut.

Direct Trauma to the Musculoskeletal System. Direct trauma to the musculoskeletal system results in bruises, contusions, sprains, and fractures. A fracture is a disruption of bone tissue continuity. Fractures most commonly result from direct external trauma, but they also occur as a consequence of some deformity of the bone (e.g., pathological fractures of osteoporosis, Paget's disease, or osteogenesis imperfecta). Young children are usually able to form new bone more easily than adults and, as a result, have few complications after a fracture. Treatment often includes positioning the fractured bone in proper alignment and immobilizing it to promote healing and restore function. Even

✳ **TABLE 47-1 Postural Abnormalities**

Abnormality	Description	Cause	Possible Treatments*
Torticollis	Inclining of head to affected side, in which sternocleidomastoid muscle is contracted	Congenital or acquired condition	Surgery, heat, support, or immobilization, depending on cause and severity, gentle ROM
Lordosis	Exaggeration of anterior convex curve of lumbar spine	Congenital condition Temporary condition (e.g., pregnancy)	Spine-stretching exercises (based on cause)
Kyphosis	Increased convexity in curvature of thoracic spine	Congenital condition Rickets, osteoporosis Tuberculosis of spine	Spine-stretching exercises, sleeping without pillows, using bed board, bracing, spinal fusion (based on cause and severity)
Scoliosis	Lateral "S"- or "C"-shaped spinal column with vertebral rotation, unequal heights of hips and shoulders	Sometimes is a consequence of numerous congenital, connective tissue, and neuromuscular disorders	Approximately half of children with scoliosis will require surgery Nonsurgical treatment is with braces and exercises
Congenital hip dysplasia	Hip instability with limited abduction of hips and, occasionally, adduction contractures (head of femur does not articulate with acetabulum because of abnormal shallowness of acetabulum)	Congenital condition (more common with breech deliveries)	Maintenance of continuous abduction of thigh so that head of femur presses into center of acetabulum Abduction splints, casting, surgery
Knock-knee (genu valgum)	Legs curved inward so that knees come together as person walks	Congenital condition Rickets	Knee braces, surgery if not corrected by growth
Bowlegs (genu varum)	One or both legs bent outward at knee, which is normal until 2 to 3 years of age	Congenital condition Rickets	Slowing rate of curving if not corrected by growth With rickets, increase of vitamin D, calcium, and phosphorus intake to normal ranges
Clubfoot	95%: medial deviation and plantar flexion of foot (equinovarus) 5%: lateral deviation and dorsiflexion (calcaneovalgus)	Congenital condition	Casts, splints such as Denis Browne splint, and surgery (based on degree and rigidity of deformity)
Footdrop	Inability to dorsiflex and invert foot because of peroneal nerve damage	Congenital condition Trauma Improper position of immobilized client	None (cannot be corrected) Prevention through physical therapy Bracing with ankle-foot orthotic (AFO)
Pigeon toes	Internal rotation of forefoot or entire foot, common in infants	Congenital condition Habit	Growth, wearing reversed shoes

Data from McCance KL, Huether SE: *Pathophysiology: the biologic basis for disease in adults and children*, ed 5, St. Louis, 2005, Mosby.

ROM, Range of motion.

*Severity of condition and cause will dictate treatment, which is individualized to the client's needs.

this temporary immobilization results in some **muscle atrophy,** loss of muscle tone, and joint stiffness.

Nursing Knowledge Base

Fully understanding movement and mobility requires more than an overview of movement and the physiology and regulation of movement by the musculoskeletal and nervous systems. You need to be knowledgeable about how to apply these scientific principles in the clinical setting to determine the safest way to move clients and to understand the effect of immobility on the physiological, psychosocial, and developmental aspects of client care.

Safe Client Handling

Nurses are exposed to the hazards related to lifting and transferring clients in many settings, such as inpatient nursing units, long-term care facilities, and the operating room (de Castro and others, 2006). Manually lifting and transferring clients contributes to the high incidence of work-related musculoskeletal problems and back injuries in nurses and other health care staff (Nelson and Baptiste, 2006). Current evidence shows that many nurses frequently transfer to different positions and leave the profession due to work-related injuries (de Castro and others, 2006). Implementing evidence-based interventions and programs (e.g., lift teams) reduces the number of work-related injuries, which improves the health of the nurse and reduces indirect costs to the health care agency (e.g., workers' compensation and replacing injured workers).

Today many states have laws that mandate safe client handling in health care agencies. Health care agencies are implementing comprehensive safe-client-handling programs in all parts of the United States. Comprehensive safe-client-handling programs include the following elements: an ergonomics assessment protocol for health care environments, client assessment criteria, algorithms for client handling and movement, special equipment kept in convenient locations to help transfer clients, back injury resource nurses, an "after-action review" that allows the health care team to apply knowledge about safe client moving in different settings, and a no-lift policy (Nelson and others, 2006).

Mobility-Immobility

To determine how to move clients safely, assess the clients' ability to move. Mobility refers to a person's ability to move about freely, and **immobility** refers to the inability to do so. Some clients can be mobile or immobile, whereas others experience varying degrees of partial immobility. Think of mobility as a continuum, with mobility on one end, immobility on the other, and varying degrees of partial immobility in between the end points. Some clients move back and forth between mobility and immobility, but for others, immobility is absolute and continues indefinitely. The terms *bed rest* and *impaired physical mobility* are frequently used when discussing clients on the mobility-immobility continuum.

Bed rest is an intervention that restricts clients to bed for therapeutic reasons. Nurses and health care providers most often prescribe this intervention. Bed rest has many different interpretations among health care professionals. Clients with a wide variety of conditions are placed on bed rest. The duration of bed rest depends on the illness or injury and the client's prior state of health (Box 47-1).

NANDA International (NANDA-I) defines *impaired physical mobility* as a limitation in independent, purposeful physical movement of the body or one or more extremities (Ackley and Ladwig, 2006). Alterations in the client's level of physical mobility often result from prescribed restriction of movement in the form of bed rest, physical restriction of movement because of external devices (e.g., a cast or skeletal traction), voluntary restriction of movement, or impairment of motor or skeletal function.

The effects of muscular deconditioning associated with lack of physical activity are often apparent in a matter of days. This cluster of symptoms is often referred to as the "hazards of immobility." The individual of average weight and height and without a chronic illness on bed rest loses muscle strength from baseline levels at a rate of 3% a day. Immobility also is associated with cardiovascular, skeletal, and other organ changes. The term *disuse atrophy* describes the tendency of cells and tissue to reduce in size and function in response to prolonged inactivity resulting from bed rest, trauma, casting, or local nerve damage (Copstead-Kirkhorn and Banasik, 2005).

In a classic study, Deitrick and others (1948) found that young healthy men put on bed rest had physiological problems. Periods of immobility or prolonged bed rest cause major physiological, psychological, and social effects. These effects are gradual or immediate and vary from client to client. The greater the extent and

> ### ✳ BOX 47-1 General Objectives of Bed Rest
> - Reducing physical activity and the oxygen needs of the body
> - Reducing pain, including postoperative pain or after acute injury to the lower back
> - Allowing ill or debilitated clients to rest
> - Allowing exhausted clients the opportunity for uninterrupted rest

the longer the duration of immobility, the more pronounced the consequences. The client with complete mobility restrictions is continually at risk for the hazards of immobility.

Systemic Effects. All body systems work more efficiently with some form of movement. Exercise has positive outcomes for all major systems of the body. When there is an alteration in mobility, each body system is at risk for impairment. The severity of the impairment depends on the client's overall health, degree and length of immobility, and age. For example, older adults with chronic illnesses develop pronounced effects of immobility more quickly than do younger clients with the same immobility problem.

Metabolic Changes. Changes in mobility alter endocrine metabolism, calcium resorption, and functioning of the gastrointestinal system. The endocrine system, made up of hormone-secreting glands, maintains and regulates vital functions such as (1) response to stress and injury, (2) growth and development, (3) reproduction, (4) maintenance of the internal environment, and (5) energy production, utilization, and storage.

When injury or stress occurs, the endocrine system triggers a series of responses aimed at maintaining blood pressure and preserving life. The endocrine system is important in maintaining homeostasis. Tissues and cells live in an internal environment that the endocrine system helps regulate through maintenance of sodium, potassium, water, and acid-base balance. The endocrine system also regulates energy metabolism. Thyroid hormone increases the basal metabolic rate (BMR), and energy becomes available to cells through the integrated action of gastrointestinal and pancreatic hormones (Copstead-Kirkhorn and Banasik, 2005).

Immobility disrupts normal metabolic functioning: decreasing the metabolic rate; altering the metabolism of carbohydrates, fats, and proteins; causing fluid, electrolyte, and calcium imbalances; and causing gastrointestinal disturbances such as decreased appetite and slowing of peristalsis. However, in the presence of an infectious process, immobilized clients often have an increased BMR as a result of fever or wound healing because these increase cellular oxygen requirements (Copstead-Kirkhorn and Banasik, 2005).

A deficiency in calories and protein is characteristic of clients with a decreased appetite secondary to immobility. The body is constantly synthesizing proteins and breaking them down into amino acids to form other proteins (see Chapter 41). When the client is immobile, the client's body often excretes more nitrogen (the end product of amino acid breakdown) than it ingests in proteins, resulting in **negative nitrogen balance** (Figure 47-4).

Weight loss, decreased muscle mass, and weakness result from tissue catabolism (tissue breakdown) (Copstead-Kirkhorn and Banasik, 2005).

Another metabolic change associated with immobility is calcium resorption (loss) from bones. Immobility causes the release of calcium into the circulation. Normally the kidneys excrete the excess calcium. However, if the kidneys are unable to respond appropriately, hypercalcemia results. Pathological fractures occur if calcium reabsorption continues as the client remains on bed rest or continues to be immobile. (Copstead-Kirkhorn and Banasik, 2005).

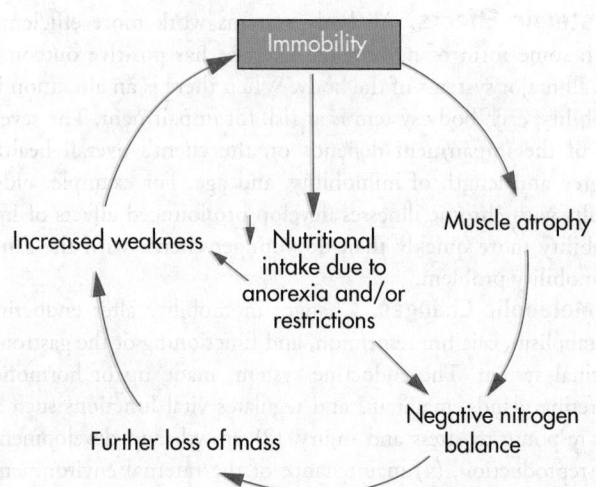

Figure 47-4 Factors contributing to negative nitrogen balance associated with immobility. (From Gröer MW, Shekleton ME: *Basic pathophysiology: a holistic approach,* ed 3, St. Louis, 1989, Mosby.)

Impairments of gastrointestinal functioning due to decreased mobility vary. Difficulty in passing stools (constipation) is a common symptom, although pseudodiarrhea often results from a fecal impaction (accumulation of hardened feces). Be aware that this finding is not normal diarrhea, but rather liquid stool passing around the area of impaction (see Chapter 46). Left untreated, fecal impaction results in a mechanical bowel obstruction that partially or completely occludes the intestinal lumen, blocking normal propulsion of liquid and gas. The resulting fluid in the intestine produces distention and increases intraluminal pressure. Over time, intestinal function becomes depressed, dehydration occurs, absorption ceases, and fluid and electrolyte disturbances worsen.

Respiratory Changes. Regular aerobic exercise enhances respiratory functioning. Lack of movement and exercise places clients at higher risk for respiratory complications. Clients who are immobile are at high risk for developing pulmonary complications. The most common respiratory complications are **atelectasis** (collapse of alveoli) and **hypostatic pneumonia** (inflammation of the lung from stasis or pooling of secretions). Both decrease oxygenation and prolong recovery and add to the client's discomfort (Black and Hawks, 2005). In atelectasis, secretions block a bronchiole or a bronchus, and the distal lung tissue (alveoli) collapses as the existing air is absorbed, producing hypoventilation. The site of the blockage affects the severity of atelectasis. Sometimes an entire lung lobe or a whole lung collapses. At some point in the development of these complications, there is a proportional decline in the client's ability to cough productively. Ultimately the distribution of mucus in the bronchi increases, particularly when the client is in the supine, prone, or lateral position (Figure 47-5). Mucus accumulates in the dependent regions of the airways (Figure 47-6). Hypostatic pneumonia frequently results because mucus is an excellent place for bacteria to grow.

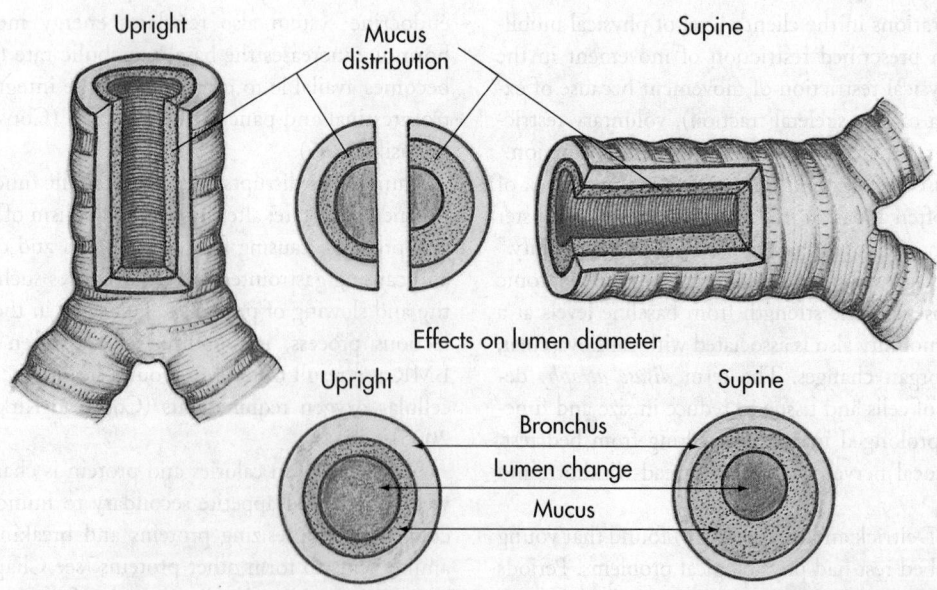

Figure 47-5 Effect of recumbency and gravity on distribution of respiratory tract and diameter of bronchiolar lumen. (From Gröer MW, Shekleton ME: *Basic pathophysiology: a holistic approach,* ed 3, St. Louis, 1989, Mosby.)

Cardiovascular Changes. Immobilization also affects the cardiovascular system. The three major changes are orthostatic hypotension, increased cardiac workload, and thrombus formation.

Orthostatic hypotension is an increase in heart rate of more than 15% and a drop of 15 mm Hg or more in systolic blood pressure, or a drop of 10 mm Hg or more in diastolic blood pressure when the client changes from the supine to standing position (Copstead-Kirkhorn and Banasik, 2005). In the immobilized client, decreased circulating fluid volume, pooling of blood in the lower extremities, and decreased autonomic response occur. These factors result in decreased venous return, followed by a decrease in cardiac output, which is reflected by a decline in blood pressure (McCance and Heuther, 2005). These are especially evident in the older adult client.

As the workload of the heart increases, so does its oxygen consumption. The heart therefore works harder and less efficiently during periods of prolonged rest. As immobilization increases, cardiac output falls, further decreasing cardiac efficiency and increasing workload.

Clients who are immobile are also at risk for thrombus formation. A **thrombus** is an accumulation of platelets, fibrin, clotting factors, and the cellular elements of the blood attached to the interior wall of a vein or artery, which sometimes occludes the lumen of the vessel (Figure 47-7). There are three factors that contribute to venous thrombus formation: (1) damage to the vessel wall (e.g., injury during surgical procedures), (2) alterations of blood flow (e.g., slow blood flow in calf veins associated with bed rest), and (3) alterations in blood constituents (e.g., a change in clotting factors or increased platelet activity). These three factors are often referred to as Virchow's triad (Copstead-Kirkhorn and Banasik, 2005).

Musculoskeletal Changes. The effects of immobility on the musculoskeletal system include permanent or temporary impairment or permanent disability. Restricted mobility sometimes results in loss of endurance, strength, and muscle mass and decreased stability and balance. Other effects of restricted mobility affecting the skeletal system are impaired calcium metabolism and impaired joint mobility.

Muscle Effects. Because of protein breakdown, the client loses lean body mass. The reduced muscle mass is unable to sustain activity without increased fatigue. If immobility continues and the client does not exercise, there is further loss of muscle mass. Muscle weakness always occurs with immobility, and prolonged immobility often leads to disuse atrophy. Muscle atrophy is a widely observed response to illness, decreased ADLs, and immobilization. Loss of endurance, decreased muscle mass and strength, and joint instability (see Skeletal Effects) put clients at risk for falls (see Chapter 37).

Skeletal Effects. Immobilization causes two skeletal changes: impaired calcium metabolism and joint abnormalities. Because immobilization results in bone resorption, the bone tissue is less dense or is atrophied, and **disuse osteoporosis** results. When disuse osteoporosis occurs, the client is at risk for pathological fractures.

Osteoporosis is a major health concern in this country. The first Surgeon General's report on the topic of bone health stated that one in two Americans over 50 years of age will be at risk for fractures related to osteoporosis by the year 2020 (USDHHS, 2004). Furthermore, the National Osteoporosis Foundation (2007) reports that 44 million Americans (55% of those over the age of 50) either have osteoporosis or are at risk for developing osteoporosis. About 80% of people who have osteoporosis are female. Although primary osteoporosis is different in origin from

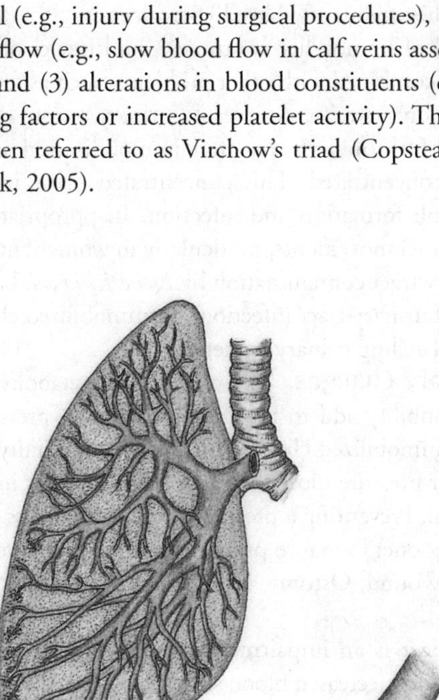

Figure 47-6 Pooling of secretions in dependent regions of the lungs in the supine position.

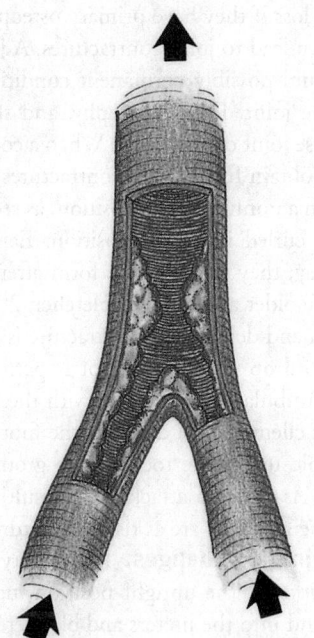

Figure 47-7 Thrombus formation in a vessel.

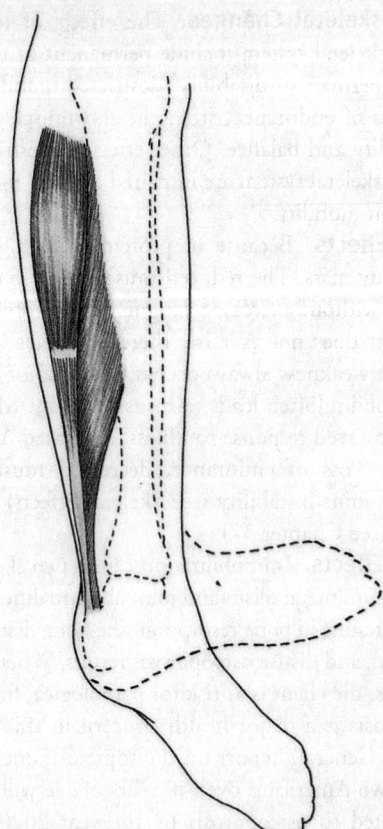

Figure 47-8 Footdrop. Ankle is fixed in a plantar flexion. Normally the ankle is able to flex *(dotted line),* which eases walking.

the osteoporosis that results from immobility, it is imperative for nurses to recognize that immobilized clients are at high risk for accelerated bone loss if they have primary osteoporosis.

Immobility can lead to joint contractures. A **joint contracture** is an abnormal and possibly permanent condition characterized by fixation of the joint. Disuse, atrophy, and shortening of the muscle fibers cause joint contractures. When a contracture occurs, the joint cannot obtain full ROM. Contractures sometimes leave a joint or joints in a nonfunctional position, as seen in clients who are permanently curled in a fetal position. Early prevention of contractures is key; they can begin to form after only 8 hours of immobility in the older adult client (Fletcher, 2005).

One common and debilitating contracture is footdrop (Figure 47-8). When **footdrop** occurs, the foot is permanently fixed in plantar flexion. Ambulation is difficult with the foot in this position, because the client cannot dorsiflex the foot. The client with footdrop is unable to lift the toes off the ground. Clients who have suffered CVAs or brain attacks with resulting right- or left-sided paralysis (hemiplegia) are at risk for footdrop.

Urinary Elimination Changes. Immobility alters the client's urinary elimination. In the upright position, urine flows out of the renal pelvis and into the ureters and bladder because of gravitational forces. When the client is recumbent or flat, the kidneys and the ureters move toward a more level plane. Urine formed by the kidney needs to enter the bladder unaided by gravity. Because the peristaltic contractions of the ureters are insufficient to over-

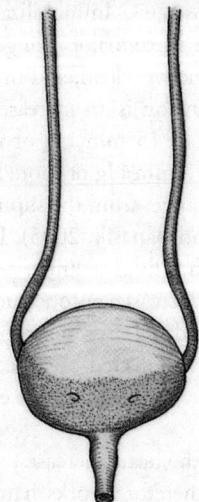

Figure 47-9 Stasis of urine with reflux to ureters.

come gravity, the renal pelvis fills before urine enters the ureters (Figure 47-9). This condition is called **urinary stasis** and increases the risk of urinary tract infection and renal calculi (see Chapter 45). **Renal calculi** are calcium stones that lodge in the renal pelvis or pass through the ureters. Immobilized clients are at risk for calculi because they frequently have hypercalcemia.

As the period of immobility continues, fluid intake often diminishes. When combined with other problems, such as fever, the risk for dehydration increases. As a result, urinary output declines on or about the fifth or sixth day after immobilization and the urine becomes concentrated. This concentrated urine increases the risk for calculi formation and infection. Inappropriate perineal care after bowel movements, particularly in women, increases the risk of urinary tract contamination by *Escherichia coli* bacteria. Another cause of urinary tract infections in immobilized clients is the use of an indwelling urinary catheter.

Integumentary Changes. The changes in metabolism that accompany immobility add to the harmful effect of pressure on the skin in the immobilized client. This makes immobility a major risk factor for pressure ulcers Any break in the skin's integrity is difficult to heal. Preventing a pressure ulcer is much less expensive than treating one; therefore preventive nursing interventions are imperative (Wound, Ostomy and Continence Nurses Society [WOCN], 2003).

A **pressure ulcer** is an impairment of the skin as a result of prolonged ischemia (decreased blood supply) in tissues (see Chapter 48). The ulcer is characterized initially by inflammation and usually forms over a bony prominence. Ischemia develops when the pressure on the skin is greater than the pressure inside the small peripheral blood vessels supplying blood to the skin.

Tissue metabolism depends on the supply of oxygen and nutrients and the elimination of metabolic wastes from the blood. Pressure affects cellular metabolism by decreasing or totally eliminating tissue circulation. When a client lies in bed or sits in a chair, the weight of the body is on bony prominences. The longer the pressure is applied, the longer the period of ischemia and therefore the greater the risk of skin breakdown. The older adult client is especially at risk. For example, an older adult client who is immobilized on a backboard following a trauma can develop skin breakdown within 3 hours (Fletcher, 2005).

SAFETY ALERT Implement a comprehensive skin care program to prevent skin breakdown in all clients, from neonates to older adults. Effective skin care programs include accurate and consistent assessment and documentation as well as interventions to protect the skin (e.g., turn the client at least every 2 hours and use mechanical devices like lifts when needed to move the client) (Butler, 2006).

Psychosocial Effects. Immobilization often leads to emotional and behavioral responses, sensory alterations, and changes in coping. When normal, healthy, young men, who were part of a National Aeronautics and Space Administration (NASA) study, were on bed rest for several weeks, they exhibited signs of sensory deprivation: altered sleep patterns and significant increases in anxiety, hostility, and depression (Fletcher, 2005). Every client responds to immobility differently.

Behavioral changes resulting from immobilization vary widely. Common behavioral changes include hostility, giddiness, fear, and anxiety. Long-term immobility or bed rest also frequently affects coping and creates sleep-wake alterations because of changes in routine or the environment. The immobilized client often becomes depressed because of changes in role and self-concept (see Chapter 27). Depression is an affective disorder characterized by exaggerated feelings of sadness, melancholy, dejection, worthlessness, emptiness, and hopelessness out of proportion to reality. Depression results from worrying about present and future levels of health, finances, and family needs. Because immobilization removes the client from a daily routine, he or she has more time to worry about disability. Worrying quickly increases the client's depression, causing withdrawal. Withdrawn clients often do not want to participate in their own care.

Developmental Changes. Developmental changes tend to be associated with immobility in the very young and in older adults. The immobilized young or middle-age adult who has been healthy experiences few, if any, developmental changes. However, there are exceptions. For example, a mother with complications following birth has to go onto bed rest and as a result cannot interact with her newborn as expected.

Infants, Toddlers, and Preschoolers. The newborn infant's spine is flexed and lacks the anteroposterior curves of the adult (see Chapter 12). As the baby grows, musculoskeletal development permits support of weight for standing and walking. Posture is awkward because the head and upper trunk are carried forward. Because body weight is not evenly distributed along a line of gravity, posture is off balance, and falls occur often. The infant, toddler, or preschooler is usually immobilized because of trauma or the need to correct a congenital skeletal abnormality. Prolonged immobilization delays the child's gross motor skills, intellectual development, or musculoskeletal development.

Adolescents. The adolescence stage usually begins with a tremendous increase in growth (see Chapter 12). Growth is frequently uneven. Prolonged immobilization alters adolescent growth patterns. In addition, adolescents who experience immobility often are behind peers in gaining independence and accomplishing certain skills, such as obtaining a driver's license. Social isolation is a concern for this age-group when immobilization occurs.

BOX 47-2 FOCUS ON OLDER ADULTS

Hazards of Immobility in Hospitalized Older Adults

For many elders, admission to the hospital often results in functional decline despite the treatment for which they were admitted. Some older adults have problems related to mobility and quickly regress to a dependent state. Rapid intervention of an interdisciplinary health team is necessary to maintain mobility and functional capacity.

Usual aging is associated with decreased muscle strength and aerobic capacity. Placing clients on bed rest without sufficient ambulation leads to loss of mobility and functional decline. Immobility causes weakness, fatigue, and an increased risk for falls. It results in shallow breathing, which often leads to pneumonia, and inadequate turning or repositioning results in skin breakdown and pressure ulcers.

A nutritional assessment needs to be included in the plan of care for the older adult client experiencing immobility. Hospitalization often affects the nutritional status of the older adult. Anorexia and insufficient assistance with eating leads to malnutrition, which contributes to the problems associated with immobility.

Finally, multiple interruptions and noise in the environment impair sleep, causing fatigue, depression, and confusion. Clients require adequate rest to remain mobile. Nurses need to implement interventions to ensure that the older adult client is able to rest without interruptions to maintain or improve the older adult's mobility.

Modified from Ebersole P and others: *Geriatric nursing and healthy aging*, ed 2, St. Louis, 2005, Mosby.

Adults. An adult who has correct posture and body alignment feels good, looks good, and generally appears self-confident. The healthy adult also has the necessary musculoskeletal development and coordination to carry out ADLs (see Chapter 13). When periods of prolonged immobility occur, all physiological systems are at risk. In addition, the role of the adult often changes with regard to the family or social structure. Some adults lose their jobs, which affects their self-concept (see Chapter 27).

Older Adults. A progressive loss of total bone mass occurs with the older adult. Some of the possible causes of this loss include decreased physical activity, hormonal changes, and bone resorption. The effect of bone loss is weaker bones. Older adults often walk more slowly, take smaller steps, and appear less coordinated. Prescribed medications alter their sense of balance or affect their blood pressure when they change position too quickly, increasing their risk for falls and injuries (see Chapter 14). The outcomes of a fall include not only possible injury, but also hospitalization, loss of independence, and psychological effects.

Older adults often experience functional status changes secondary to hospitalization and altered mobility status (Box 47-2). Immobilization of older adults increases their physical dependence on others and accelerates functional losses. For some older adults their immobilization results from a degenerative disease, neurological trauma, or chronic illness. For others, it occurs gradually and progressively, and for others—especially those who have had a stroke—immobilization is sudden. When providing

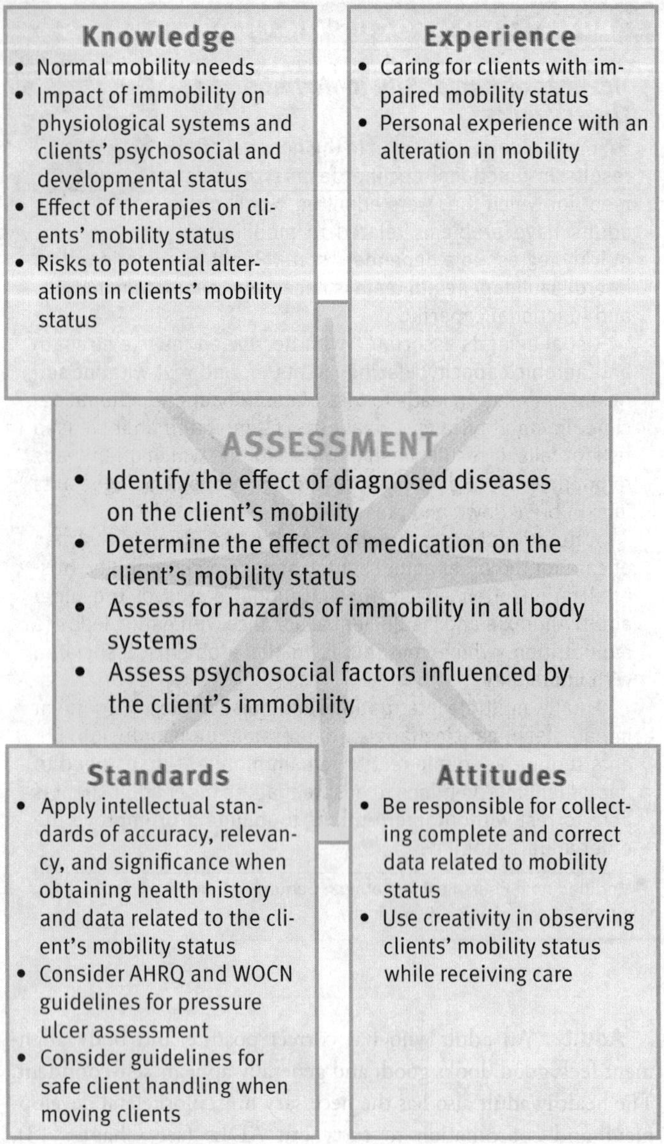

Knowledge
- Normal mobility needs
- Impact of immobility on physiological systems and clients' psychosocial and developmental status
- Effect of therapies on clients' mobility status
- Risks to potential alterations in clients' mobility status

Experience
- Caring for clients with impaired mobility status
- Personal experience with an alteration in mobility

ASSESSMENT
- Identify the effect of diagnosed diseases on the client's mobility
- Determine the effect of medication on the client's mobility status
- Assess for hazards of immobility in all body systems
- Assess psychosocial factors influenced by the client's immobility

Standards
- Apply intellectual standards of accuracy, relevancy, and significance when obtaining health history and data related to the client's mobility status
- Consider AHRQ and WOCN guidelines for pressure ulcer assessment
- Consider guidelines for safe client handling when moving clients

Attitudes
- Be responsible for collecting complete and correct data related to mobility status
- Use creativity in observing clients' mobility status while receiving care

Figure 47-10 Critical thinking model for immobility assessment.

BOX 47-3   NURSING ASSESSMENT QUESTIONS

Mobility
- Describe any changes you have noticed in your ability to walk and take care of yourself on a daily basis.
- Have you experienced any stiffness, swelling, pain, or difficulty with moving? If so, describe how you felt.
- Describe what activity you do in a normal day. Has this recently changed?

Immobility
- How have your appetite and diet changed since you have been having problems moving around?
- Describe what you eat in a normal day.
- Are you feeling short of breath or dizzy?
- Have you noticed any places on your skin that are reddened or have any open sores?
- Describe any changes you have noticed in urinating and/or in having bowel movements.

addition, the use of critical thinking attitudes such as creativity are necessary to devise a plan to provide successful interventions for immobility. Professional standards such as those developed by the Agency for Healthcare Research and Quality (AHRQ) and the Wound, Ostomy and Continence Nurses Society (WOCN) and intellectual standards such as accuracy provide valuable guides for mobility management (Figure 47-10). In addition, many agencies have standards for practice related to transferring clients and to fall and pressure ulcer prevention.

Nursing Process for Impaired Body Alignment and Mobility

Apply the nursing process and use a critical thinking approach to develop individualized care plans for clients with preexisting mobility impairments and for those who are at risk for immobility. Design a care plan that improves the client's functional status, promotes self-care, maintains psychological well-being, and reduces the hazards of immobility.

◆ Assessment

Nursing assessment of the client includes aspects of both mobility and immobility. Usually the nurse assesses and asks questions about both areas during physical examination (Box 47-3).

Mobility. Assessment of client mobility focuses on ROM, gait, exercise and activity tolerance, and body alignment. When unsure of the client's abilities, begin assessment of mobility with the client in the most supportive position and move to higher levels of mobility according to the client's tolerance. Generally the assessment of movement starts while the client is lying, then proceeds to assessing sitting positions in bed, transfers to chair, and finally while walking. This helps to protect the client's safety.

Range of Motion. Range of motion (ROM) is the maximum amount of movement available at a joint in one of the three

nursing care for an older adult, nurses encourage the client to perform as many self-care activities as possible, thereby maintaining the highest level of mobility. Sometimes nurses inadvertently contribute to a client's immobility by providing unnecessary help with activities such as bathing and transferring.

Critical Thinking

Critical thinking requires the combination of knowledge, experiences, client data, critical thinking attitudes, and intellectual and professional standards. The needs of the immobile client are multiple and complex. After conducting a thorough assessment, the nurse identifies appropriate nursing diagnoses and implements effective nursing care.

To understand the impact of immobility on the client and family, integrate knowledge from nursing and other disciplines, previous experiences, and information gathered from clients. In

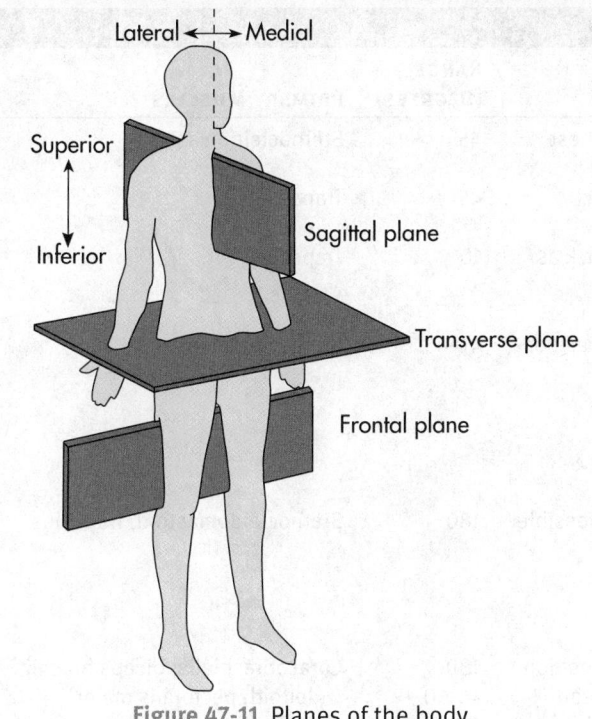

Figure 47-11 Planes of the body.

planes of the body: sagittal, frontal, or transverse (Figure 47-11). The sagittal plane is a line that passes through the body from front to back, dividing the body into a left and a right side. The frontal plane passes through the body from side to side and divides the body into front and back. The transverse plane is a horizontal line that divides the body into upper and lower portions.

Ligaments, muscles, and the nature of the joint limit joint mobility in each of the planes. However, some joint movements are specific to each plane. In the sagittal plane, movements are flexion and extension (e.g., fingers and elbows), dorsiflexion and plantar flexion (feet), and extension (e.g., hip). In the frontal plane, movements are abduction and adduction (e.g., arms and legs) and eversion and inversion (feet). In the transverse plane, movements are pronation and supination (hands) and internal and external rotation (hips).

When assessing ROM, ask questions about and physically examine the client for stiffness, swelling, pain, limited movement, and unequal movement. Chapter 33 describes specific techniques for measuring the degrees of motion in a joint. Assessment of ROM is important as a baseline measure to compare and evaluate whether loss in joint mobility has occurred. Clients whose mobility is restricted require ROM to reduce the hazards of immobility. Therefore assess the type of ROM exercise a client is able to perform. ROM exercises are active (the client moves all joints through their ROM unassisted), passive (the client is unable to move independently, and the nurse moves each joint through its ROM), or somewhere in between (Table 47-2). With a weak client, for example, provide support while the client performs most of the movement. Some clients are able to move some joints actively, whereas the nurse passively moves others. First assess the client's ability to engage in active ROM exercises and the need for assistance, teaching, or reinforcement. In general, exercises need

to be as active as health and mobility allow. Contractures develop in joints not moved periodically through their full ROM. Assessment data from clients with limited joint movements vary based on the area affected.

Neck. A flexion contracture of the neck is a serious disability because the client's neck is permanently flexed with the chin close to or actually touching the chest. Assessment reveals altered body alignment, changes in the visual field, and decreased level of independent functioning.

Shoulder. One feature of the shoulder that sets it apart from other joints in the body is that the strongest muscle controlling it, the deltoid, is in complete elongation in the normal position. No other muscle exerts its full strength when in complete elongation. Clients with limited movement in the shoulder have difficulty moving their arms.

Elbow. The elbow functions optimally at an angle of about 90 degrees. An elbow fixed in full extension is disabling and limits the client's independence.

Forearm. Most functions of the hand are best carried out with the forearm in moderate pronation. When the forearm is fixed in a position of full supination, the client's use of the hand is limited.

Wrist. The primary function of the wrist is to place the hand in slight dorsiflexion, the position of functioning. When the wrist is fixed in even a slightly flexed position, the grasp is weakened.

Fingers and Thumb. The ROM in the fingers and thumb enables the client to perform ADLs and activities requiring fine motor skills, such as carpentry, needlework, drawing, and painting. The functional position of the fingers and thumb is slight flexion of the thumb in opposition to the fingers.

Hip. Because the lower extremities are concerned chiefly with locomotion and weight bearing, stability of the hip joint is more important than its mobility. For example, if one hip has no mobility but is fixed in a neutral position and fully extended, it is possible to walk without a significant limp. However, contractures often fix the hip in positions of deformity. Excessive abduction makes the affected leg appear too short, whereas excessive adduction makes the affected leg appear too long. In either case the client has limited locomotion and walks with an obvious limp. Internal and external rotation contractures cause an abnormal and unbalanced gait.

Knee. A primary function of the knee is stability, which is achieved by ROM, ligaments, and muscles. However, the knees cannot remain stable under weight-bearing conditions unless there is adequate quadriceps power to maintain the knee in full extension. An immobile knee joint results in serious disability. The degree of disability depends on the position in which the knee is stiffened. If the knee is fixed in full extension, the person needs to sit with the leg out in front. When the knee is flexed, the person limps while walking. The greater the flexion, the greater the limp.

Ankle and Foot. Without full ROM of the ankle, there will be gait deviations. If the joint is not stable, the person will fall. When the person relaxes as in sleep or coma, the foot relaxes and assumes a position of plantar flexion. As a result, the foot becomes fixed in plantar flexion (footdrop), which impairs the ability to walk.

Toes. Excessive flexion of the toes results in clawing. When this is a permanent deformity, the foot is unable to rest flat on the floor and the client is unable to walk properly. Flexion contractures are the most common foot deformity associated with reduced joint mobility.

✳ **TABLE 47-2** Range-of-Motion Exercises

Body Part	Type of Joint	Type of Movement	Range (Degrees)	Primary Muscles
Neck, cervical spine	Pivotal	*Flexion:* Bring chin to rest on chest	45	Sternocleidomastoid
		Extension: Return head to erect position	45	Trapezius
		Hyperextension: Bend head back as far as possible	10	Trapezius
		Lateral flexion: Tilt head as far as possible toward each shoulder	40-45	Sternocleidomastoid
		Rotation: Turn head as far as possible in circular movement	180	Sternocleidomastoid, trapezius
Shoulder	Ball and socket	*Flexion:* Raise arm from side position forward to position above head	180 45-60	Coracobrachialis, biceps brachii, deltoid, pectoralis major
		Extension: Return arm to position at side of body	180	Latissimus dorsi, teres major, triceps brachii
		Hyperextension: Move arm behind body, keeping elbow straight	45-60	Latissimus dorsi, teres major, deltoid
		Abduction: Raise arm to side to position above head with palm away from head	180	Deltoid, supraspinatus
		Adduction: Lower arm sideways and across body as far as possible	320	Pectoralis major

✳ **TABLE 47-2   Range-of-Motion Exercises—cont'd**

Body Part	Type of Joint	Type of Movement	Range (Degrees)	Primary Muscles
Shoulder, cont'd	Ball and socket, cont'd	*Internal rotation:* With elbow flexed, rotate shoulder by moving arm until thumb is turned inward and toward back	90	Pectoralis major, latissimus dorsi, teres major, subscapularis
		External rotation: With elbow flexed, move arm until thumb is upward and lateral to head	90	Infraspinatus, teres major, deltoid
		Circumduction: Move arm in full circle (Circumduction is combination of all movements of ball-and-socket joint.)	360	Deltoid, coracobrachialis, latissimus dorsi, teres major
Elbow	Hinge	*Flexion:* Bend elbow so that lower arm moves toward its shoulder joint and hand is level with shoulder	150	Biceps brachii, brachialis, brachioradialis
		Extension: Straighten elbow by lowering hand	150	Triceps brachii
Forearm	Pivotal	*Supination:* Turn lower arm and hand so that palm is up	70-90	Supinator, biceps brachii
		Pronation: Turn lower arm so that palm is down	70-90	Pronator teres, pronator quadratus
Wrist	Condyloid	*Flexion:* Move palm toward inner aspect of forearm	80-90	Flexor carpi ulnaris, flexor carpi radialis
		Extension: Move fingers and hand posterior to midline	80-90	Extensor carpi radialis brevis, extensor carpi radialis longus, extensor carpi ulnaris
		Hyperextension: Bring dorsal surface of hand back as far as possible	80-90	Extensor carpi radialis brevis, extensor carpi radialis longus, extensor carpi ulnaris
		Abduction: Place hand with palm down and extend wrist laterally toward fifth finger.	Up to 30	Flexor carpi radialis, extensor carpi radialis brevis, extensor carpi radialis longus
		Adduction: Place hand with palm down and extend wrist medially toward thumb	30-50	Flexor carpi ulnaris, extensor carpi ulnaris

Continued

✳ **TABLE 47-2   Range-of-Motion Exercises—cont'd**

Body Part	Type of Joint	Type of Movement	Range (Degrees)	Primary Muscles
Fingers	Condyloid hinge	*Flexion:* Make fist	90	Lumbricales, interosseus volaris, interosseus dorsalis
		Extension: Straighten fingers	90	Extensor digiti quinti proprius, extensor digitorum communis, extensor indicis proprius
		Hyperextension: Bend fingers back as far as possible	30-60	
		Abduction: Spread fingers apart	30	Interosseus dorsalis
		Adduction: Bring fingers together	30	Interosseus volaris
Thumb	Saddle	*Flexion:* Move thumb across palmar surface of hand	90	Flexor pollicis brevis
		Extension: Move thumb straight away from hand	90	Extensor pollicis longus, extensor pollicis brevis
		Abduction: Extend thumb laterally (usually done when placing fingers in abduction and adduction)	30	Abductor pollicis brevis
		Adduction: Move thumb back toward hand	30	Adductor pollicis obliquus, adductor pollicis transversus
		Opposition: Touch thumb to each finger of same hand		Opponens pollicis, opponens digiti minimi
Hip	Ball and socket	*Flexion:* Move leg forward and up	90-120	Psoas major, iliacus, sartorius
		Extension: Move back beside other leg	90-120	Gluteus maximus, semitendinosus, semimembranosus
		Hyperextension: Move leg behind body	30-50	Gluteus maximus, semitendinosus, semimembranosus

✳ **TABLE 47-2   Range-of-Motion Exercises—cont'd**

Body Part	Type of Joint	Type of Movement	Range (Degrees)	Primary Muscles
Hip, cont'd	Ball and socket, cont'd	*Abduction:* Move leg laterally away from body	30-50	Gluteus medius, gluteus minimus
		Adduction: Move leg back toward medial position and beyond if possible	30-50	Adductor longus, adductor brevis, adductor magnus
		Internal rotation: Turn foot and leg toward other leg	90	Gluteus medius, gluteus minimus, tensor fasciae latae
		External rotation: Turn foot and leg away from other leg	90	Obturatorius internus, obturatorius externus
		Circumduction: Move leg in circle		Psoas major, gluteus maximus, gluteus medius, adductor magnus
Knee	Hinge	*Flexion:* Bring heel back toward back of thigh	120-130	Biceps femoris, semitendinosus, semimembranosus, sartorius
		Extension: Return leg to floor	120-130	Rectus femoris, vastus lateralis, vastus medialis, vastus intermedius
Ankle	Hinge	*Dorsal flexion:* Move foot so that toes are pointed upward	20-30	Tibialis anterior
		Plantar flexion: Move foot so that toes are pointed downward	45-50	Gastrocnemius, soleus

Continued

✳ TABLE 47-2 Range-of-Motion Exercises—cont'd

Body Part	Type of Joint	Type of Movement	Range (Degrees)	Primary Muscles
Foot	Gliding	*Inversion:* Turn sole of foot medially	10 or less	Tibialis anterior, tibialis posterior
		Eversion: Turn sole of foot laterally	10 or less	Peroneus longus, peroneus brevis
Toes	Condyloid	*Flexion:* Curl toes downward	30-60	Flexor digitorum, lumbricalis pedis, flexor hallucis brevis
		Extension: Straighten toes	30-60	Extensor digitorum longus, extensor digitorum brevis, extensor hallucis longus
		Abduction: Spread toes apart	15 or less	Abductor hallucis, interosseus dorsalis
		Adduction: Bring toes together	15 or less	Adductor hallucis, interosseus plantaris

Gait. The term **gait** describes a particular manner or style of walking. The gait cycle begins with the heel strike of one leg and continues to the heel strike of the other leg. Assessing a client's gait allows you to draw conclusions about balance, posture, safety, and ability to walk without assistance. The mechanics of human gait involve coordination of the skeletal, neurological, and muscular systems of the human body.

Exercise and Activity Tolerance. **Exercise** is physical activity for conditioning the body, improving health, and maintaining fitness. Nurses use it as therapy to correct a deformity or restore the overall body to a maximal state of health. When a person exercises, physiological changes occur in body systems (see Chapter 37).

Assessment of the client's energy level includes the physiological effects of exercise and activity tolerance. **Activity tolerance** is the type and amount of exercise or work that a person is able to perform. Assessment of activity tolerance is necessary when planning activity such as walking, ROM exercises, or ADLs. Activity tolerance assessment includes data from physiological, emotional, and developmental domains (see Chapter 37). This assessment is applicable in all clinical settings.

As activity begins, monitor clients for symptoms such as dyspnea, fatigue, chest pain, and/or a change in vital signs. The weak or debilitated client is unable to sustain even slight changes in activity because of the increased demand for energy. Seemingly simple tasks such as eating and moving in bed often result in extreme fatigue. When the client experiences decreased activity tolerance, carefully assess how much time the client needs to recover. Decreasing recovery time indicates improving activity tolerance.

People who are depressed, worried, or anxious are frequently unable to tolerate exercise. Depressed clients tend to withdraw rather than participate. Clients who worry or who are frequently anxious expend a tremendous amount of mental energy and often report feeling fatigued. Because of this, they also experience physical and emotional exhaustion.

Developmental changes also affect activity tolerance. As the infant enters the toddler stage, the activity level increases, and the need for sleep declines. The child entering preschool or primary grades expends mental energy in learning and often requires more rest after school or before strenuous play. The adolescent going through puberty requires more rest because much of the body's energy is expended for growth and hormone changes (see Chapter 42).

Changes still occur through the adult years, but many of these changes are related to work and lifestyle choices. Pregnancy causes fluctuations in a woman's energy tolerance, especially during the first and third trimesters, when she experiences increased fatigue. Hormonal changes and fetal development use body energy, and the woman is sometimes unable or unmotivated to carry out physical activities. During the last trimester, fetal development consumes a great deal of the mother's energy, and the size and location of the fetus limits the ability to take a deep breath, resulting in less oxygen being available for physical activities.

As the person grows older, activity tolerance changes. Muscle mass is reduced, and posture and the composition of bones change. There are often changes in the cardiorespiratory system, such as decreased maximum heart rate and decreased lung compliance that affect the intensity of exercise. As age progresses, some older individuals still exercise but will do so at a reduced intensity. The more inactive a client is, the more pronounced these activity changes are.

Body Alignment. Perform assessment of body alignment with the client standing, sitting, or lying down. This assessment has the following objectives:

• Determining normal physiological changes in body alignment resulting from growth and development for each individual client

- Identifying deviations in body alignment caused by incorrect posture
- Providing opportunities for clients to observe their posture
- Identifying learning needs of clients for maintaining correct body alignment
- Identifying trauma, muscle damage, or nerve dysfunction
- Obtaining information concerning other factors that contribute to incorrect alignment, such as fatigue, malnutrition, and psychological problems

The first step in assessing body alignment is to put clients at ease so that they do not assume unnatural or rigid positions. When assessing the body alignment of an immobilized or unconscious client, remove pillows and positioning supports from the bed and place the client in the supine position.

Standing. Characteristics of correct body alignment for the standing client include the following:

1. The head is erect and midline.
2. When observed posteriorly, the shoulders and hips are straight and parallel.
3. When observed posteriorly, the vertebral column is straight.
4. When the client is observed laterally, the head is erect and the spinal curves are aligned in a reversed **S** pattern. The cervical vertebrae are anteriorly convex, the thoracic vertebrae are posteriorly convex, and the lumbar vertebrae are anteriorly convex.
5. When observed laterally, the abdomen is comfortably tucked in and the knees and ankles are slightly flexed. The person appears comfortable and does not seem conscious of the flexion of knees or ankles.
6. The arms hang comfortably at the sides.
7. The feet are slightly apart to achieve a base of support, and the toes are pointed forward.
8. When viewing the client from behind, the center of gravity is in the midline, and the line of gravity is from the middle of the forehead to a midpoint between the feet. Laterally the line of gravity runs vertically from the middle of the skull to the posterior third of the foot (Figure 47-12).

Sitting. Characteristics of correct alignment of the sitting client include the following:

1. The head is erect, and the neck and vertebral column are in straight alignment.
2. The body weight is evenly distributed on the buttocks and thighs.
3. The thighs are parallel and in a horizontal plane.
4. Both feet are supported on the floor (Figure 47-13), and the ankles are comfortably flexed. With clients of short stature, use a footstool to ensure the ankles are comfortably flexed.
5. A 2.5- to 5-cm (1- to 2-inch) space is maintained between the edge of the seat and the popliteal space on the posterior surface of the knee. This space ensures that there is no pressure on the popliteal artery or nerve to decrease circulation or impair nerve function.
6. The client's forearms are supported on the armrest, in the lap, or on a table in front of the chair.

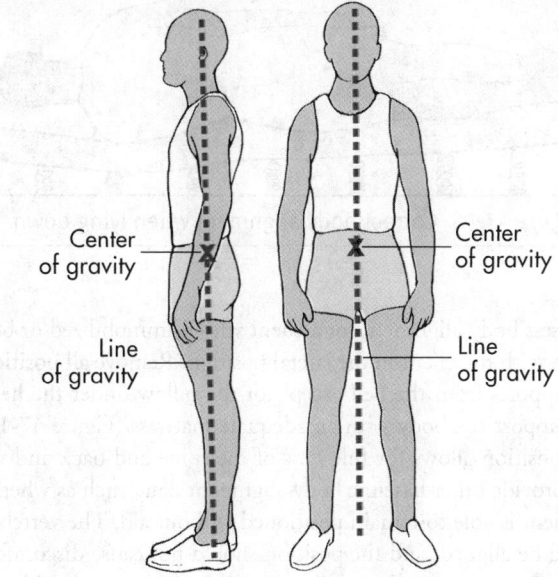

Figure 47-12 Correct body alignment when standing.

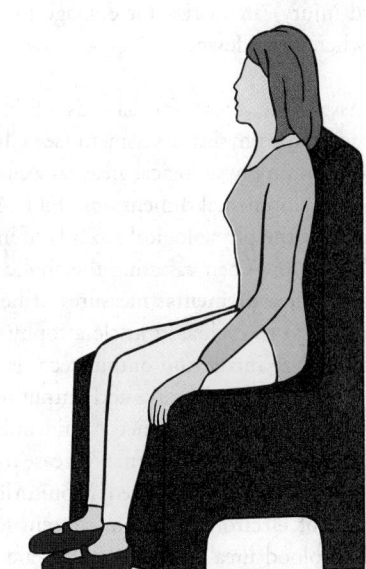

Figure 47-13 Correct body alignment when sitting.

It is particularly important to assess alignment when sitting if the client has muscle weakness, muscle paralysis, or nerve damage. Clients who have these problems have diminished sensation in the affected area and are unable to perceive pressure or decreased circulation. Proper alignment while sitting reduces the risk of musculoskeletal system damage in such a client. The client with severe respiratory disease sometimes assumes a posture of leaning on the table in front of the chair in an attempt to breathe more easily. This is called orthopnea.

Lying. People who are conscious have voluntary muscle control and normal perception of pressure. As a result, they usually assume a position of comfort when lying down. Because their ROM, sensation, and circulation are within normal limits, they change positions when they perceive muscle strain and decreased circulation.

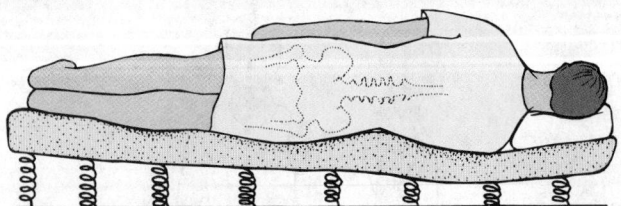

Figure 47-14 Correct body alignment when lying down.

Assess body alignment for a client who is immobilized or bed-ridden with the client in the lateral position. Remove all positioning supports from the bed except for the pillow under the head, and support the body with an adequate mattress (Figure 47-14). This position allows for full view of the spine and back and will help provide other baseline body alignment data, such as whether the client is able to remain positioned without aid. The vertebrae should be aligned, and the position should not cause discomfort. Clients with impaired mobility (e.g., traction or arthritis), decreased sensation (e.g., hemiparesis following a CVA), impaired circulation (e.g., diabetes), and lack of voluntary muscle control (e.g., spinal cord injury) are at risk for damage to the musculoskeletal system when lying down.

Immobility. Assess the client for hazards of immobility by performing a head-to-toe physical assessment (see Chapter 33). In addition, focus on certain physiological areas, as well as the client's psychosocial and developmental dimensions. Table 47-3 summarizes how to assess for the physiological hazards of immobility.

Metabolic System. When assessing metabolic functioning, use **anthropometric measurements** (measures of height, weight, and skinfold thickness) to evaluate muscle atrophy (see Chapter 33). In addition, analyze intake and output records for fluid balance. Does intake equal output? Intake and output measurements assist the nurse in determining whether a fluid imbalance exists (see Chapter 41). Dehydration and edema increase the rate of skin breakdown in a client who is immobilized. Monitoring laboratory data such as levels of electrolytes, serum protein (albumin and total protein), and blood urea nitrogen (BUN) aid the nurse in determining metabolic functioning.

Monitoring food intake and elimination patterns and assessing wound healing help to determine altered gastrointestinal functioning and potential metabolic problems. If the client has a wound, the rate of healing indicates how well nutrients are delivered to tissues. Normal progression of healing indicates that metabolic needs of injured tissues are being met. Anorexia occurs commonly in clients who are immobilized. Assess the client's food intake before the meal tray is removed to determine the amount eaten. Assess the client's dietary patterns and food preferences at the onset of immobilization to help prevent nutritional imbalances (see Chapter 44).

Respiratory System. Perform a respiratory assessment at least every 2 hours for clients with restricted activity. Inspect chest wall movements during the full inspiratory-expiratory cycle. If a client has an atelectatic area, chest movement is often asymmetrical. Auscultate the entire lung region to identify diminished breath sounds, crackles, or wheezes. Focus auscultation on the dependent lung fields because pulmonary secretions tend to collect in these lower regions.

Cardiovascular System. Cardiovascular nursing assessment of the client who is immobilized includes blood pressure monitoring, evaluation of apical and peripheral pulses, and observation for signs of venous stasis (e.g., edema and delayed wound healing).

Although not all clients will experience orthostatic hypotension, nurses monitor clients' vital signs during the first few attempts at sitting or standing (see Chapter 32). Move the client gradually during position changes, and monitor the client closely for dizziness while assessing orthostatic blood pressures. The longer the period of immobility, the greater the risk of hypotension when the client stands (Copstead-Kirkhorn and Banasik, 2005).

Also assesses apical and peripheral pulses. Lying down increases cardiac workload and results in an increased pulse rate. In some clients, particularly older adults, the heart does not tolerate the increased workload, and a form of cardiac failure develops. A third heart sound, heard at the apex, is an early indication of congestive heart failure. Monitoring peripheral pulses allows the nurse to evaluate the heart's ability to pump blood. Immediately document and report the absence of a peripheral pulse in the lower extremities to the client's health care provider, especially if the pulse was previously present.

Edema sometimes develops in clients who have had injury or whose heart is unable to handle the increased workload of bed rest. Because edema moves to dependent body regions, assessment of the client experiencing immobility includes the sacrum, legs, and feet. If the heart is unable to tolerate the increased workload, peripheral body regions, such as the hands, feet, nose, and earlobes, will be colder than central body regions. Because deep vein thrombosis (DVT) is a hazard of immobility, assess the venous system. A dislodged venous thrombus, called an **embolus**, will possibly travel through the circulatory system to the lungs and impair circulation and oxygenation. Venous emboli that travel to the lungs are sometimes life threatening. More than 90% of all pulmonary emboli begin in the deep veins of the lower extremities (Copstead-Kirkhorn and Banasik, 2005).

To assess for a deep vein thrombosis, remove the client's elastic stockings and/or sequential compression devices (SCDs) every 8 hours and observe the calves for redness, warmth, and tenderness. Homans' sign, or calf pain on dorsiflexion of the foot, was once used as an indicator of a DVT; however, there is disagreement on its continued use for assessing for DVT. This is because some investigators believe that vigorous dorsiflexion will possibly dislodge the thrombus if there is one present. Measure bilateral calf circumference, and record it daily as an alternative assessment for DVT. To do this, mark a point on each calf 10 cm down from the midpatella. Measure the circumference each day using the mark for placement of the tape measure. Unilateral increases in calf circumference are an early indication of thrombosis. Because DVTs also occur in the thigh, take thigh measurements daily if the client is prone to thrombosis.

Musculoskeletal System. Major musculoskeletal abnormalities to identify during nursing assessment include decreased muscle tone and strength, loss of muscle mass, and contractures. The anthropometric measurements described previously indicate losses in muscle tone and muscle mass.

Early assessment of ROM is important because it establishes a baseline against which later measurements can be compared to

✳ TABLE 47-3 Assessment of the Physiological Hazards of Immobility

SYSTEM	ASSESSMENT TECHNIQUES	ABNORMAL FINDINGS
Metabolic	Inspection	Slowed wound healing, abnormal laboratory data
	Inspection	Muscle atrophy
	Anthropometric measurements (mid-upper arm circumference, triceps skinfold measurement)	Decreased amount of subcutaneous fat
	Palpation	Generalized edema
Respiratory	Inspection	Asymmetrical chest wall movement, dyspnea, increased respiratory rate
	Auscultation	Crackles, wheezes
Cardiovascular	Auscultation	Orthostatic hypotension
	Auscultation, palpation	Increased heart rate, third heart sound, weak peripheral pulses, peripheral edema
Musculoskeletal	Inspection, palpation	Decreased ROM, erythema, increased diameter in calf or thigh
	Palpation	Joint contracture
	Inspection	Activity intolerance, muscle atrophy, joint contracture
Skin	Inspection, palpation	Break in skin integrity
Elimination	Inspection	Decreased urine output, cloudy or concentrated urine, decreased frequency of bowel movements
	Palpation	Distended bladder and abdomen
	Auscultation	Decreased bowel sounds

ROM, Range of motion.

evaluate whether a loss in joint mobility has occurred. Measure ROM with a goniometer (see Chapter 37, Figure 37-9, p. 804).

Physical assessment cannot identify disuse osteoporosis. However, clients on prolonged bed rest, postmenopausal women, clients taking steroids, and persons with increased serum and urine calcium levels have a greater risk for bone demineralization. Consider the risk of disuse osteoporosis when planning nursing interventions. Although some falls result in injury, other falls occur because of pathological fractures secondary to osteoporosis.

Integumentary System. Continually assess the client's skin for breakdown and color changes such as pallor or redness. Consistently use a standardized tool, such as the Braden Scale. This identifies clients with a high risk for impaired skin integrity or early changes in the condition of clients' skin. Early identification allows for early intervention. Observe the skin often during routine care (e.g., when the client is turned, during hygiene measures, and when providing for elimination needs). At a minimum, skin assessment occurs every 2 hours (see Chapter 48).

Elimination System. Evaluate the client's elimination status on each shift, and evaluate total intake and output every 24 hours. Compare the amounts over time. Determine that the client is receiving the correct amount and type of fluids orally or parenterally (see Chapter 45). Inadequate intake and output or fluid and electrolyte imbalances increase the risk for renal system impairment, ranging from recurrent infections to kidney failure. Dehydration also increases the risk for skin breakdown, thrombus formation, respiratory infections, and constipation.

Assessment of elimination status includes the adequacy of dietary choices, bowel sounds, and the frequency and consistency of bowel movements (see Chapter 46). Accurate assessment enables the nurse to intervene before constipation and fecal impaction occur.

Psychosocial Assessment. Many alterations in physiological, sociocultural, and developmental functioning are related to immobility. Often, these problems are interrelated, and it is imperative that nursing care focus on all dimensions. Often the focus of immobility is on the easily visible physical problems, such as skin impairment, but do not overlook the psychosocial and developmental aspects of immobility.

Abrupt changes in personality often have a physiological cause, such as surgery, a medication reaction, a pulmonary embolus, or an acute infection. For example, compromised older clients have confusion as their primary symptom with an acute urinary tract infection or fever. Identifying confusion is an important component of the nurse's assessment. Acute confusion in older adults is not normal; a thorough nursing assessment is the priority (Ebersole and others, 2005).

Common reactions to immobilization include boredom and feelings of isolation, depression, and anger. Observe for changes in a client's emotional status, and listen carefully to family if they report emotional changes. Examples of change that indicate psychosocial concerns are a cooperative client who becomes less cooperative or an independent client who asks for more help than is necessary. The nurse investigates reasons for such alterations. Identifying how the client usually copes with loss is vital (see Chapters 30 and 31). A change in mobility status, whether permanent or not, causes a grief reaction. Families are a key resource for information about behavior changes.

Identify and correct unexplained changes in the sleep-wake cycle. Nurses can prevent or minimize most stimuli that interrupt the sleep-wake cycle (e.g., nursing activities, a noisy environment, or discomfort). Some medications such as analgesics, sleeping pills, or cardiovascular drugs also cause sleep disturbances (see Chapter 42).

Because psychosocial changes usually occur gradually, observe the client's behavior on a daily basis. If behavioral changes occur, determine the cause(s) and evaluate the changes. Identifying the cause helps you to design appropriate nursing interventions.

Developmental Assessment. Include a developmental assessment of clients who are immobilized. When caring for a young child, determine whether the child is able to meet developmental tasks and is progressing normally. The child's development sometimes regresses or slows because of immobilization. Design nursing interventions that maintain normal development and provide physical and psychosocial stimuli after identifying a child's developmental needs, and assure the parents that developmental delays are usually temporary.

Immobilization of a family member changes the family's functioning. The family's response to this change often leads to problems, stress, and anxieties. Children seeing parents who are immobile sometimes have difficulty understanding what is occurring and have difficulty coping.

Immobility has a significant effect on the older adult's levels of health, independence, and functional status. Nursing assessment enables the nurse to determine the older client's ability to meet needs independently and to adapt to developmental changes such as declining physical functioning and altered family and peer relationships. A decline in developmental functioning needs prompt investigation to determine why the change occurred and interventions that can return the client to an optimal level of functioning as soon as possible. Activities that reduce immobility and promote participation in ADLs are vital to preventing functional decline (Kawamoto and others, 2006). Assessment also includes the client's home and community to identify factors that are risks to the client's mobility and safety (see Chapter 38).

◆Nursing Diagnosis

A client who is experiencing an alteration in mobility often has one or more nursing diagnoses. The two diagnoses most directly related to mobility problems are *impaired physical mobility* and *risk for disuse syndrome*. The diagnosis of *impaired physical mobility* applies to the client who has some limitation but is not completely immobile. The diagnosis of *risk for disuse syndrome* applies to the client who is immobile and at risk for multisystem problems because of inactivity. Beyond these diagnoses, the list of potential diagnoses is extensive, because immobility affects multiple body systems. Other possible nursing diagnoses include the following:

- Ineffective airway clearance
- Ineffective individual coping
- Risk for injury
- Impaired skin integrity
- Insomnia
- Social isolation
- Impaired urinary elimination

Assessment reveals clusters of data that indicate whether a client is at risk or if an actual problem exists. The clusters of data include defining characteristics that support the diagnostic label and probable cause of the diagnosis. Locating the probable cause of the diagnosis (based on assessment data) is important to planning client-centered goals and subsequent nursing interventions that will best help the client.

Impaired physical mobility related to reluctance to initiate movement requires slightly different interventions than *impaired physi-*

✳ BOX 47-4 NURSING DIAGNOSTIC PROCESS

Impaired Physical Mobility Related to Left Shoulder Pain

Assessment Activities	Defining Characteristics
Measure ROM during exercises of extremities.	Client has limited ROM in left shoulder. Client has impaired coordination while attempting to perform ROM with left shoulder.
Observe client use left shoulder in ADLs.	Client is reluctant to attempt movement with left shoulder.
Ask client about perception of pain.	Client complains of sharp pain in shoulder.
Ask client about endurance and activity tolerance.	Client reports decreased muscle strength in left shoulder.

ROM, Range of motion; *ADLs,* activities of daily living.

---

cal mobility related to pain in the left shoulder. Thus it is critical that nursing assessment activities identify and cluster defining characteristics that ultimately support the nursing diagnosis selected (Box 47-4). The diagnosis related to reluctance to initiate movement requires interventions aimed at keeping the client as mobile as possible and encouraging the client to do self-care and ROM. The diagnosis related to pain requires the nurse to assist the client with comfort measures so that the client is then willing and more able to move. In both situations the nurse explains how activity enhances healthy body functioning.

Often the physiological dimension is the major focus of nursing care for clients with impaired mobility. Thus the psychosocial and developmental dimensions are neglected. Yet all dimensions are important to health. During immobilization some clients experience decreased social interaction and stimuli. These clients frequently use the nurse's call bell to request minor physical attention when their real need is greater socialization. Nursing diagnoses for health needs in developmental areas reflect changes from the client's normal activities. Immobility leads to a developmental crisis if the client is unable to resolve problems and continue to mature.

Immobility also leads to complications such as pulmonary emboli or pneumonia. If these conditions develop, collaborate with the health care provider or nurse practitioner for prescribed therapy to intervene. Be alert for and prevent these potential complications when possible.

◆Planning

During planning the nurse synthesizes information from resources such as knowledge of the role of respiratory and physical therapy, standards such as skin care guidelines from the AHRQ and WOCN, protocols for clients at risk for falls, attitudes such as creativity and perseverance, and past experiences with immobilized clients (Figure 47-15). Critical thinking ensures that the client's plan of care integrates all that you know about the individual, as well as key critical thinking elements. Professional

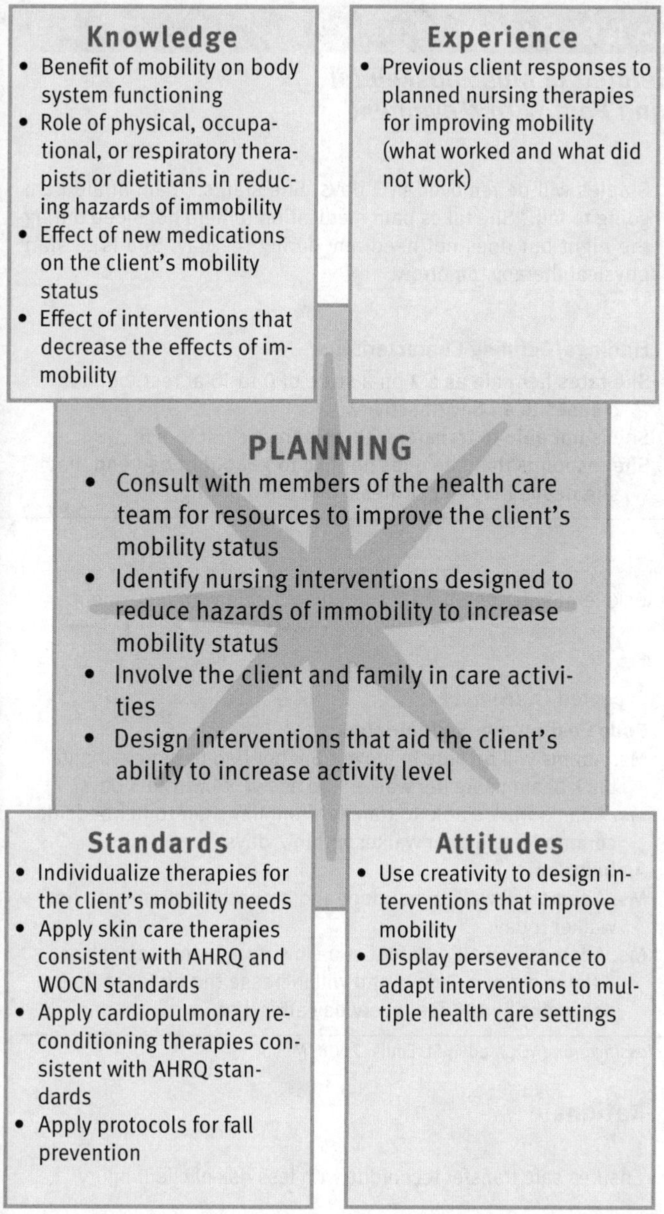

Knowledge
- Benefit of mobility on body system functioning
- Role of physical, occupational, or respiratory therapists or dietitians in reducing hazards of immobility
- Effect of new medications on the client's mobility status
- Effect of interventions that decrease the effects of immobility

Experience
- Previous client responses to planned nursing therapies for improving mobility (what worked and what did not work)

PLANNING
- Consult with members of the health care team for resources to improve the client's mobility status
- Identify nursing interventions designed to reduce hazards of immobility to increase mobility status
- Involve the client and family in care activities
- Design interventions that aid the client's ability to increase activity level

Standards
- Individualize therapies for the client's mobility needs
- Apply skin care therapies consistent with AHRQ and WOCN standards
- Apply cardiopulmonary reconditioning therapies consistent with AHRQ standards
- Apply protocols for fall prevention

Attitudes
- Use creativity to design interventions that improve mobility
- Display perseverance to adapt interventions to multiple health care settings

Figure 47-15 Critical thinking model for immobility planning.

standards are especially important to consider when you develop a plan of care. These standards often establish scientifically proven guidelines for selecting effective nursing interventions.

Goals and Outcomes. Develop an individualized plan of care for each nursing diagnosis (see Care Plan). Set realistic expectations for care, and include the client and family when possible. Set goals that are individualized, realistic, and measurable. The goals focus on preventing problems or risks to body alignment and mobility.

Develop goals and expected outcomes to assist the client in achieving his or her highest level of mobility and reducing the hazards of immobility. For example, a client who has left-sided paralysis following a stroke has two long-term goals. The first, directed toward improved mobility, is "Client uses walker to ambulate safely in the home." A parallel goal directed toward the hazards of immobility is "Client's skin remains intact." Both of these goals

are essential to restoring maximal mobility for this client. Because there is impaired sensation, both the client and caregivers need to be aware of the client's need to have the skin free of pressure. Expected outcomes for the second goal include the following:

- Client's skin color and temperature return to normal baseline within 20 minutes of position change.
- Client changes position at least every 2 hours.

Setting Priorities. The effect problems have on the client's mental and physical health determines the immediacy of any problem. Set priorities when planning care to ensure immediate needs are met first. This is particularly important when clients have multiple diagnoses (Figure 47-16). Plan therapies according to severity of risks to the client, and individualize the plan according to the client's developmental stage, level of health, and lifestyle.

It is especially important in priority setting to make sure you do not overlook potential complications. Many times actual problems such as pressure ulcers and disuse syndrome are addressed only after they develop. Therefore monitor the client often, reinforcing prevention techniques to both the client and other caregivers and supervising nursing assistive personnel in carrying out activities aimed at preventing complications of impaired mobility.

Collaborative Care. Care of the client experiencing alterations in mobility requires a team approach. Nurses often delegate some interventions to nursing assistive personnel. Nursing assistive personnel can encourage the client to do leg exercises, use the incentive spirometer, and cough and deep breathe (see Chapter 40). They may turn and position clients, and apply elastic stockings. They can also assist the nurse with measurements of leg circumferences and height and weight.

Collaborate with other health care team members such as physical or occupational therapists when considering mobility needs. For example, physical therapists are a resource for planning ROM or strengthening exercises, and occupational therapists are a resource for planning ADLs that clients need to modify or relearn. Wound care specialists and respiratory therapists are often involved in client care, especially with clients who are experiencing complications related to their immobility. Consult a registered dietitian when the client is experiencing nutritional problems, and refer the client to a mental health advanced practice nurse, licensed social worker, or psychologist to assist with coping or other psychosocial issues.

Discharge planning begins when a client enters the health care system. In anticipation of the client's discharge from an institution, make appropriate referrals or consult a case manager or a discharge planner to ensure the client's needs will be met at home. Consider the client's home environment when planning therapies to maintain or improve body alignment and mobility. Referrals to home care or outpatient therapy are often needed.

Implementation

Health Promotion. Health promotion activities include a variety of interventions that include education, prevention, and early detection. Examples of health promotion activities that address

NURSING CARE PLAN

Impaired Physical Mobility Related to Musculoskeletal Impairment From Surgery and Pain With Movement

Assessment

Ms. Barbara Adams, an 84-year-old client, is admitted to a skilled care unit for rehabilitation after a total hip replacement (THR) for osteoarthritis. She has a history of smoking and hypertension. She experiences "aches" and "stiffness" in her joints, especially in her knees and fingers. The wound is clean, dry, and intact.

Staples will be removed in 2 days. She states, "I am afraid I am going to fall." She takes pain medication to help her sleep during the night but does not need any during the day. She is to start physical therapy tomorrow.

Assessment Activities

Assess Ms. Adams' pain level.

Assess Ms. Adams' ability to transfer.
Ask Ms. Adams how her surgery has affected her mobility.

Findings/Defining Characteristics*

She **rates her pain as a 2** on a scale of 0 to 10 at rest, but it **increases to an 8** with activity.
She is **not able to transfer** with help from chair to bed.
She responds that she **does not** like to **get out of bed** and that she **needs help to get dressed** in the morning.

*__Defining characteristics__ are shown in bold type.

Nursing Diagnosis: Impaired physical mobility related to musculoskeletal impairment from surgery and pain with movement.

Planning

Goals

Ms. Adams will be able to transfer with assistive device by discharge.

Ms. Adams will walk 1000 feet using her walker by discharge.

Expected Outcomes†

Body Positioning: Self-Initiated
Ms. Adams will be able to move from her bed to her chair and back again using her walker and assist ×1 within 3 days.
Ms. Adams will be able to transfer from her chair to her bedside commode using her walker within 7 days.

Ambulation
Ms. Adams will walk to her door and around her room with her walker today.
Ms. Adams will walk 100 feet at a slow pace using her walker 3 times a day in 2 days and will increase the distance that she walks by 100 feet every day after that.

---

†Outcome classification labels from Moorhead S and others: *Nursing outcomes classification (NOC)*, ed 4, St. Louis, 2008, Mosby.

Interventions‡

Exercise Therapy: Ambulation
Consult with physical therapist on selection of transfer technique.
Instruct Ms. Adams on safe transfer and ambulation techniques in an environment with few distractions. Provide written materials that reinforce verbal instructions.
Establish realistic increments for transferring and increasing distance for ambulation.

Pain Management
Use nonpharmacological techniques (e.g., guided imagery) before, after, and if possible, during painful activities.

Encourage Ms. Adams to use adequate pain medication.

Rationale

Ensures safe transfer technique with less risk of client injury.

Providing instruction in a quiet environment and giving written instructions in large, easy-to-read print enhances learning in the older client (Mamaril, 2006).
Gradually increasing physical activity and setting realistic goals for ambulation encourages activity in older adults (Yen, 2005).

Guided imagery can decrease pain and increase mobility in older women with osteoarthritis who are experiencing mobility difficulties (Baird and Sands, 2004).
Aggressive pain management is needed following surgery to decrease the effects of pain and increase mobility in the older adult client (Rakel and Herr, 2004).

---

‡Intervention classification labels from Bulechek GM, Butcher HK, and Dochterman JM: *Nursing interventions classification (NIC)*, ed 5, St. Louis, 2008, Mosby.

NURSING CARE PLAN

Impaired Physical Mobility Related to Musculoskeletal Impairment From Surgery and Pain With Movement—*cont'd*

Evaluation

Nursing Actions	Client Response/Finding	Achievement of Outcome
Ask Ms. Adams if her mobility has improved postoperatively. Observe client transfer from bed to chair. Assess Ms. Adams as she walks in the hall; measure how far she walks.	Ms. Adams is able to transfer from the chair to the bed using her walker and stand-by assistance of nurse. Ms. Adams is able to walk 400 feet in the hall with her walker.	Ms. Adams has achieved goal of transferring with walker and assistance. Activity level is improving. Continue interventions, and continue to encourage ambulation.

CONCEPT MAP

Nursing diagnosis: Impaired physical mobility
- Unable to change positions
- No independent range of motion
- Unable to move voluntarily

Interventions
- Obtain appropriate assistive devices to enhance mobility
- Position client in an upright position 3 times a day to minimize cardiovascular deconditioning
- Refer to physical and occupational therapy

Nursing diagnosis: Risk for impaired skin integrity
- Urine and bowel incontinence
- Unable to perceive pressure
- Unable to assist with position changes
- Loss of 20 lb since the injury

Interventions
- Assess the skin frequently
- Turn and reposition every 1 to 2 hours
- Use appropriate skin barrier to limit effects of incontinence on skin

Client's chief medical diagnosis: Acute spinal cord injury at C7, quadriplegia
Priority assessments: Skin condition, body alignment, feelings about paralysis

Nursing diagnosis: Anxiety
- Restless
- Unable to concentrate
- Altered sleeping patterns

Interventions
- Teach relaxation breathing
- Assess for risk for suicide
- Provide a positive, safe environment

Nursing diagnosis: Ineffective denial
- Refuses to look at himself
- Does not acknowledge injury
- Refuses to participate in care

Interventions
- Develop therapeutic relationship with client
- Allow client to make choices about treatment when possible
- Refer client to commmunity resources (e.g., support groups)

——— Link between medical diagnosis and nursing diagnosis   - - - - - Link between nursing diagnoses

Figure 47-16 Concept map for client with acute spinal cord injury at C7 and quadriplegia.

mobility and immobility include prevention of work-related injury, fall prevention measures, exercise, and early detection of scoliosis.

Prevention of Work-Related Musculoskeletal Injuries. The rate of work-related injuries in health care settings has increased in recent years. In 2004 there were 8.7 cases per 100 full-time workers who experienced occupational injury and illness compared with 5 cases per 100 for private industry overall. The rate for nursing homes was 10.1 per 100 workers (U.S. Department of Labor [USDL], 2005). The majority of these injuries occurred as a result of overexertion, which resulted in back injuries and other musculoskeletal problems. Back injuries are often the direct result of improper lifting and bending. The most common back injury is strain on the lumbar muscle group, which includes the muscles around the lumbar vertebrae. Injury to these areas affects the ability to bend forward, backward, and from side to side and limits the ability to rotate the hips and lower back. Research has demonstrated that ergonomic programs in health care facilities reduce costs, injuries to employees, and missed work days. These programs also enhance recruitment, retention, and satisfaction of employees (Siddharthan and others, 2005).

Nurses and other health care staff are especially at risk for injury to lumbar muscles when lifting, transferring, or positioning immobilized clients. Therefore be aware of agency policies and protocols that protect staff and clients from injury. When lifting, assess the weight you will lift and determine the assistance you will need (Figure 47-17). Current evidence supports that using mechanical or other ergonomic assistive devices is the safest way to reposition and lift clients who are unable to do these activities themselves (Box 47-5). Many agencies have developed special client lift teams and have instituted a no-lift policy.

Musculoskeletal injuries among health care workers are not only related to lifting and transferring clients. Nurses spend time in many activities bending and twisting, which also cause injury. Examples of such activities include lifting objects; pushing beds; and bathing, feeding, dressing, and undressing clients (Nelson, and others, 2003a). Therefore, in addition to knowing how to move clients safely, nurses also need to apply concepts related to body mechanics in the workplace. Before beginning a task, know your individual capabilities for activities such as lifting and moving objects. If providing care (e.g., bathing) to a client, consider the condition of the client and whether or not the client can assist you. When you cannot safely complete a task (e.g., moving a bed from one room to another), assess the number of people you will need to help you and do not start until the task can be completed safely to prevent injury to you, the other members of the health care team, and the client. Follow these steps to prevent injury:

1. Keep the weight to be lifted as close to the body as possible; this action places the object in the same plane as the lifter and close to the center of gravity for balance.
2. Bend at the knees; this helps to maintain the center of gravity and uses the stronger leg muscles to do the lifting (Figure 47-18).
3. Tighten abdominal muscles and tuck the pelvis; this provides balance and helps protect the back.
4. Maintain the trunk erect and knees bent so that multiple muscle groups work together in a coordinated manner (see Chapter 37); do not allow the trunk to twist.

✳ BOX 47-5 **EVIDENCE-BASED PRACTICE**

Evaluation of Devices for Transferring Clients

Evidence Summary
This study compared seven lateral transfer devices with the traditional drawsheet method in a variety of acute care nursing units. Caregivers, who were mostly nurses, were given surveys after they used a transfer device to rank the device's comfort, ease of use, perceived injury risk, time efficiency, and client safety. Caregivers rated the air-assisted devices higher than all the other devices when performing a lateral transfer, and the traditional drawsheet method performed poorly when compared with the other devices.

Application to Nursing Practice
- Health care agencies need to provide devices to reduce the risk of injury associated with lateral transfers.
- Nurses need to stop using the traditional drawsheet method when transferring clients.
- Use assistive devices, preferably air-assisted devices, when performing lateral transfers.
- New devices to transfer clients are being developed; take an active role in the evaluation of these devices whenever possible.

Reference
Baptiste A and others: Friction-reducing devices for lateral patient transfers, *AAOHN J* 54(4):173, 2006.

Exercise. Although many diseases and physical problems cause or contribute to immobility, it is important to remember that exercise programs enhance feelings of well-being and improve endurance, strength, and health. Exercise reduces the risk of many health problems such as cardiovascular disease, diabetes, and osteoporosis. Help the chronically ill to overcome barriers to physical activity. For example, if a client has a below-the-knee amputation, suggest activities, such as lifting soup cans, that capitalize on the client's strengths and abilities. Encourage hospitalized clients to do stretching, ROM, and light walking within the limits of their condition (see Chapter 37).

Nurses contribute to promoting health for many clients by encouraging or starting managed exercise programs. Exercise is a key prescription for health promotion of all clients regardless of their age. In older adults, routine exercise or activity helps maintain ROM, functional mobility, and improves balance (Ebersole and others, 2004). Take cultural preferences into consideration when helping clients design exercise plans (Box 47-6).

Bone Health in Clients With Osteoporosis. Clients at risk for or diagnosed with osteoporosis have special health promotion needs. Encourage clients at risk to be screened for osteoporosis, and assess their diet for calcium and vitamin D intake. Clients who have a lactose intolerance need dietary teaching about alternative sources of calcium.

For clients diagnosed with osteoporosis, early evaluation, consultation, and referral with health care providers, dietitians, and physical therapists are important interventions, especially when they become immobilized. For the client with osteoporosis the goal is to maintain independence with activities of daily living.

Assessment Criteria and Care Plan for Safe Patient Handling and Movement

I. Patient's Level of Assistance:
_____ Independent— Patient performs task safely, with or without staff assistance, with or without assistive devices.
_____ Partial Assist—Patient requires no more help than stand-by, cueing, or coaxing, or caregiver is required to lift no more than 35 lbs. of a patient's weight.
_____ Dependent—Patient requires nurse to lift more than 35 lbs. of the patient's weight, or is unpredictable in the amount of assistance offered. In this case assistive devices should be used.

An assessment should be made prior to each task if the patient has varying level of ability to assist due to medical reasons, fatigue, medications, etc. When in doubt, assume the patient cannot assist with the transfer/repositioning.

II. Weight Bearing Capability
_____ Full
_____ Partial
_____ None

III. Bi-Lateral Upper Extremity Strength
_____ Yes
_____ No

IV. Patient's level of cooperation and comprehension:
_____ Cooperative — may need prompting; able to follow simple commands.
_____ Unpredictable or varies (patient whose behavior changes frequently should be considered as "unpredictable"), not cooperative, or unable to follow simple commands.

V. Weight: _____ Height: _____
Body Mass Index (BMI) [needed if patient's weight is over 300][1]:_____
If BMI exceeds 50, institute Bariatric Algorithms

The presence of the following conditions are likely to affect the transfer/repositioning process and should be considered when identifying equipment and technique needed to move the patient.

VI. Check applicable conditions likely to affect transfer/repositioning techniques.

_____ Hip/Knee/Shoulder Replacements _____ Respiratory/Cardiac Compromise _____ Fractures
_____ History of Falls _____ Wounds Affecting Transfer/Positioning _____ Splints/Traction
_____ Paralysis/Paresis _____ Amputation _____ Severe Osteoporosis
_____ Unstable Spine _____ Urinary/Fecal Stoma _____ Severe Pain/Discomfort
_____ Severe Edema _____ Contractures/Spasms _____ Postural Hypotension
_____ Very Fragile Skin _____ Tubes (IV, Chest, etc.)

Comments:_____
_____
_____

VII. Care Plan:

Algorithm	Task	Equipment/ Assistive Device	# Staff
1	Transfer To and From: Bed to Chair, Chair To Toilet, Chair to Chair, or Car to Chair		
2	Lateral Transfer To and From: Bed to Stretcher, Trolley		
3	Transfer To and From: Chair to Stretcher, or Chair to Exam Table		
4	Reposition in Bed: Side-to-Side, Up in Bed		
5	Reposition in Chair: Wheelchair and Dependency Chair		
6	Transfer Patient Up from the Floor		
Bariatric 1	Bariatric Transfer To and From: Bed to Chair, Chair to Toilet, or Chair to Chair		
Bariatric 2	Bariatric Lateral Transfer To and From: Bed to Stretcher or Trolley		
Bariatric 3	Bariatric Reposition in Bed: Side-to-Side, Up in Bed		
Bariatric 4	Bariatric Reposition in Chair: Wheelchair, Chair or Dependency Chair		
Bariatric 5	Patient Handling Tasks Requiring Access to Body Parts (Limb, Abdominal Mass, Gluteal Area)		
Bariatric 6	Bariatric Transporting (Stretcher)		
Bariatric 7	Bariatric Toileting Tasks		

Sling Type: Seated_____   Seated (Amputation)_____   Standing_____   Supine_____   Ambulation_____   Limb Support_____

Sling Size: _____

Signature: _____   **Date:** _____

[1]If patient's weight is over 300 pounds, the BMI is needed. For Online BMI table and calculator see:
http://www.nhlbi.nih.gov/guidelines/obesity/bmi_tbl.htm

Figure 47-17 Assessment criteria and care plan for safe client handling and movement. (From Nelson A: *Safe patient handling and movement algorithms,* 2006, VISN8 Patient Safety Center, http://www.visn8.med.va.gov/patientsafetycenter/ safePtHandling/default.asp.)

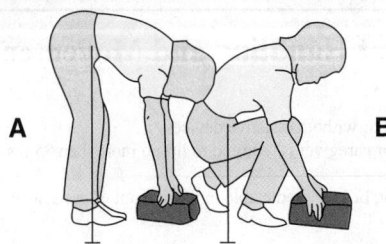

Figure 47-18 Incorrect **(A)** and correct **(B)** body position for lifting.

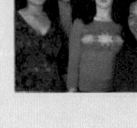

✳ BOX 47-6 **CULTURAL ASPECTS OF CARE**

Activity and Exercise

There are many activities specifically linked to culture, such as time orientation, health care practices, health promotion, nutrition, religion, family systems, and death. Less attention has been given to the impact of culture on mobility. However, cultural influences have an important role in exercise and physical activity.

Culture influences preferences for activity and exercise. Certain cultures discourage involvement in organized recreational physical activities such as basketball, running, and aerobics. Ethnic dancing is an effective activity that is acceptable in Korean countries. Other cultures emphasize exercise in terms of activities of daily living such as walking, gardening, and prayer/meditation. As an example, people from Bangladesh often view prayer as a structured form of exercise, whereas many Muslims value participation in community activities and consider walking to the mosque a part of their weekly exercise regimen.

A sedentary lifestyle puts a client at risk for being overweight. Children from many cultures who live in the United States are becoming more sedentary. The number of obese children is especially increasing in Hispanic and Native American populations. One researcher found that older Hispanic women only participated in exercise classes that were required when they were in school. They believed that doing housework and caring for their families met their exercise needs.

Implications for Practice
- Evaluate patterns of daily living and culturally prescribed activities before suggesting specific forms of exercise to clients.
- Help clients plan physical activities that are culturally acceptable.
- Exercise programs need to be flexible and accommodate family and community responsibilities of the culture.
- Encourage culturally specific and individually tailored interventions to facilitate commitment to exercise.
- Educate clients of all ages on the importance of exercise in preserving health, and correct any misconceptions.

Data from Andrews M, Boyle J: *Transcultural concepts in nursing care,* ed 4, Philadelphia, 2002, Lippincott, Williams & Wilkins; Cromwell SL, Berg JA: Lifelong physical activity patterns of sedentary Mexican American women, *Geriatr Nurs* 27(4):209, 2006; Lim K and others: Aging, health and physical activity in Korean Americans, *Geriatr Nurs* 28(2):112, 2007; Reifsnider E and others: Factors related to overweight and risk for overweight status among low-income Hispanic children, *J Pediatr Nurs* 21(3):86, 2006; and Shin Y and others: A tailored program for the promotion of physical exercise among Korean adults with chronic diseases, *Appl Nurs Res* 19(2):88, 2006.

✳ BOX 47-7 **CLIENT TEACHING**

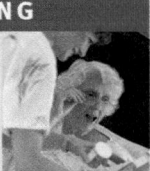

Clients With Osteoporosis

Objective
- Client will verbalize strategies to prevent or limit the severity of osteoporosis.

Teaching Strategies
- Instruct client and/or caregiver in common risk factors and how to modify lifestyle (e.g., smoking, caffeine, alcohol, hormone replacement as recommended by health care provider).
- Teach client and/or caregiver the current recommended dietary allowances for calcium, and review foods high in calcium (e.g., milk fortified with vitamin D, leafy green vegetables, yogurt, and cheese).
- Instruct clients and/or caregiver in appropriate types of weight-bearing exercises as recommended by health care provider or physical therapist to prevent injury or fractures.
- Teach client and/or caregiver about safety, fall prevention, and strategies to create a safe home environment (e.g., remove scatter rugs; ensure hallways, steps, and rooms are well lit).
- Instruct client and/or caregiver in self-administration of prescribed medication used to treat osteoporosis.
- Promote positive self-image in client by providing realistic yet optimistic and positive feedback about changes in appearance and mobility.

Evaluation
- Client and/or caregiver verbalize strategies to modify lifestyle such as stopping smoking, reducing caffeine or alcohol intake, or increasing dietary calcium.
- Client and/or caregiver verbalize foods high in calcium and vitamin D.
- Client and/or caregiver verbalize appropriate weight-bearing exercises and plan times for exercise.
- Client and/or caregiver verbalize safety strategies to prevent falls.
- Client and/or caregiver verbalize appropriate knowledge about medications.
- Client and/or caregiver express positive but realistic feedback regarding effects of disease.

Assistive ambulatory devices, adaptive clothing, and safety bars assist the client with maintaining independence. Client teaching needs to focus on limiting the severity of the disease through diet and activity (Box 47-7).

Acute Care. Clients in acute care settings who experience altered physical mobility usually have some problems associated with the hazards of immobility, such as impaired respiratory status, orthostatic hypotension, and impaired skin integrity. Therefore design nursing interventions to reduce the impact of immobility on body systems and to prepare the client for the restorative phase of care.

Metabolic System. Because the body needs protein to repair injured tissue and rebuild depleted protein stores, give the immobilized client a high-protein, high-calorie diet. A high-calorie intake provides sufficient fuel to meet metabolic needs and to replace subcutaneous tissue. Also ensure that the client is taking vitamin B and C supplements when necessary. Supplementation with vitamin C is necessary to replace protein stores, and vitamin B complex is needed for skin integrity and wound healing.

If the client is unable to eat, nutrition must be provided parenterally or enterally. Total parenteral nutrition refers to delivery of nutritional supplements through a central or peripheral intravenous catheter. Enteral feedings include delivery through a nasogastric, gastrostomy, or jejunostomy tube of high-protein, high-calorie solutions with complete requirements of vitamins, minerals, and electrolytes (see Chapter 44).

Respiratory System. Nursing interventions that support the respiratory system are needed in the client who is immobile for many reasons. First, clients experiencing immobility need to frequently reexpand their lungs to maintain the lungs' elastic recoil property. In addition, secretions accumulate in the dependent areas of the lungs. Finally, clients who are immobilized or who are on prolonged bed rest often become weak. If weakness progresses, the cough reflex gradually becomes inefficient. All these factors put the client at risk of developing pneumonia. The stasis of secretions in the lungs is life threatening for an immobilized client.

There are a variety of nursing interventions to expand the lungs, to dislodge and mobilize stagnant secretions, and to clear the lungs. All these interventions help reduce the risk of pneumonia. Prevention begins with assessment. Assess the client's respiratory status per agency policy. Assessment findings that indicate pneumonia include productive cough with greenish-yellow sputum; fever; pain on breathing; and crackles, wheezes, and dyspnea. It is essential to implement pulmonary interventions in all clients, even those who do not have pneumonia.

Encourage the client to deep breathe and cough every 1 to 2 hours. Teach alert clients to deep breathe or yawn every hour or to use an incentive spirometer (see Chapter 40). Instruct the client to take in three deep breaths and cough with the third exhalation. This technique produces a more forceful, productive cough without excessive fatigue. These respiratory interventions will aid alveolar expansion and prevent atelectasis. Coughing reduces the stasis of pulmonary secretions. Unconscious clients with artificial airways cannot always effectively cough on their own. Nurses expand the chest and lungs in these clients by using an Ambu-bag and clear secretions by suctioning the airway when needed (see Chapter 40).

Chest physiotherapy (CPT) (percussion and positioning) is another effective method for preventing pneumonia and keeping the airway clear. CPT helps the client drain secretions from specific segments of the bronchi and lungs into the trachea so that the client is able to cough and expel the secretions. Respiratory assessment findings identify areas of the lungs requiring CPT (see Chapter 40). A respiratory therapist often provides CPT.

If the client needs to wear abdominal binders, remove them every 2 hours to allow the client to breathe deeply. Assess binders for correct positioning, and adjust them as necessary to prevent interference with respirations. Often clients will wear the binder only when ambulating. Specific health care provider instructions for the use of binders vary (Chapter 48).

Ensure that clients who are immobile take in a minimum of 2000 ml of fluid a day, if not contraindicated, to help keep mucociliary clearance normal. Expect pulmonary secretions to be easily removed with coughing and appear thin, watery, and clear. Without adequate hydration, pulmonary secretions become thick and tenacious and difficult to remove. Offering fluids on a regularly timed schedule also benefits in helping with bowel and urine elimination and aids in maintaining circulation and skin integrity.

Cardiovascular System. The effects of bed rest or immobilization on the cardiovascular system include orthostatic hypotension, increased cardiac workload, and thrombus formation. Design nursing therapies to minimize or prevent these alterations.

Reducing Orthostatic Hypotension. When clients who have been on bed rest or who have been immobile arise to a sitting or standing position, they often experience orthostatic hypotension. Clients who have orthostatic hypotension have an increased pulse rate, a decreased pulse pressure, and a drop in blood pressure. If symptoms become severe enough, the client can faint (Copstead-Kirkhorn and Banasik, 2005). To prevent injury, nurses implement interventions that reduce or eliminate the effects of orthostatic hypotension. Mobilize the client as soon as the physical condition allows, even if this only involves dangling at the bedside or moving to a chair. This activity maintains muscle tone and increases venous return. Isometric exercises, those activities that involve muscle tension without muscle shortening, do not have any beneficial effect on preventing orthostatic hypotension but will improve activity tolerance. When getting an immobile client up for the first time, assess the situation using a safe-client-handling algorithm (Nelson, 2003b). This is a precautionary step that will protect the nurse and client from injury and will also allow the client to do as much of the transfer as possible.

Reducing Cardiac Workload. The nurse designs interventions to reduce cardiac workload, which is increased by immobility. A primary intervention is to discourage the client from using the Valsalva maneuver. When using this maneuver, such as while straining during defecation or moving up in bed, the client holds his or her breath, which increases intrathoracic pressure. This decreases venous return and cardiac output. When the strain is released, venous return and cardiac output immediately increase and systolic blood pressure and pulse pressure rise. These pressure changes produce a reflex bradycardia and possible decrease in blood pressure that can result in sudden cardiac death in clients with heart disease. Teach the client to breathe out while moving side-to-side or up in bed.

Preventing Thrombus Formation. The most cost-effective way to address the deep vein thrombosis (DVT) problem is through an aggressive program of prophylaxis. It begins with identification of clients at risk and continues throughout the clients' immobilization. This is clearly a collaborative role between nurses and health care providers. Use the nursing assessment to identify risk factors. Many interventions will reduce the risk of thrombus formation in the immobilized client. Leg, foot, and ankle exercises; regularly providing fluids; position changes; and client teaching need to begin when the client becomes immobile. Give preoperative clients this information before surgery, and get them out of bed as soon as possible (see Chapter 50). Other interventions such as medications, intermittent pneumatic compression (IPC), and SCDs require a health care provider's order.

Heparin and low-molecular-weight heparin (LMWH) are the most widely used drugs in the prophylaxis of DVT. Common

BOX 47-8   PROCEDURAL GUIDELINES

Application of Sequential Compression Device Stockings

Delegation Considerations: The skill of applying sequential compression devices (SCDs) can be delegated. The nurse is responsible for assessing circulation in the extremities. Instruct nursing assistive personnel to:
- Notify nurse if client complains of pain in leg
- Notify nurse if discoloration develops in extremities

Equipment: Tape measure, sequential stockings, stockinette, hygiene supplies

1. Assess client for need for sequential compression stockings. In some agencies, an order is required. Perform hand hygiene.
2. Obtain baseline assessment data about client's lower extremities (e.g., circulation, pulse, and skin integrity) before initiating sequential compression stockings.
3. Perform hand hygiene. Provide hygiene to lower extremities if needed.
4. Measure client for proper-size stocking by measuring around the largest part of the client's thigh. Review manufacturer's directions regarding measuring for proper fit.
5. Place a protective stockinette over the client's leg.
6. Wrap the stocking around the leg, starting at the ankle, with the opening over the patella (see illustration).

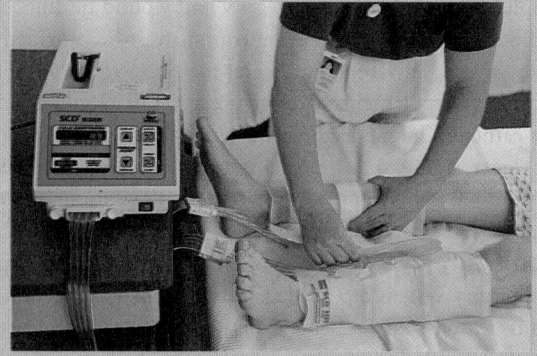

STEP 6 Application of sequential stocking.

7. Attach the stockings to the insufflators, and verify that the intermittent pressure is between 35 and 45 mm Hg.
8. Perform hand hygiene, and record date and time of stocking application and stocking length and size in nurses' notes.
9. Record condition of skin and circulatory assessment.
10. Monitor skin integrity and circulation to client's lower extremities as ordered or according to manufacturer's guidelines.

---

dosage for heparin therapy for DVT prophylaxis is 5000 units given subcutaneously 2 hours before surgery and repeated every 8 to 12 hours until the client is fully mobile or discharged. Heparin is an anticoagulant, and it suppresses clot formation. Common dosage of Lovenox (LMWH) in the prophylaxis of DVTs is 30 to 40 mg subcutaneously 2 hours before surgery and continued throughout the postoperative period. Because bleeding is a potential side effect of these medications, continually assess the client for signs of bleeding, such as hematuria, bruising, guaiac-positive stools, and bleeding gums.

SCDs and IPCs consist of sleeves or stockings made of fabric or plastic that are wrapped around the leg and secured with Velcro (Box 47-8). Once they are applied, connect the sleeves to a pump that alternately inflates and deflates the stocking around the leg. A typical cycle is inflation for 10 to 15 seconds and deflation for 45 to 60 seconds. Inflation pressures average 40 mm Hg. Use of SCD/IPCs on the legs decreases venous stasis by increasing venous return through the deep veins of the legs. For optimal results, begin use of SCD/IPCs as soon as possible and maintain it until the client becomes fully ambulatory.

Elastic stockings (sometimes called thromboembolic device [TED] hose) also aid in maintaining external pressure on the muscles of the lower extremities and thus promote venous return (Box 47-9). To obtain the correct size, measure the client's calf, thigh, and leg length accurately. When considering applying graded compression stockings, first assess the client's suitability for wearing them. Do not apply the stockings if the client has a local condition affecting the leg (e.g., any skin lesion, gangrenous condition, or recent vein ligation), because application compromises circulation. Apply the stockings properly, and remove and reapply them at least twice a day. Be sure to assess circulation at

the toes to ensure the TEDs are not too tight. In addition, the stockings always need to be clean and dry. If a client needs TEDs for a prolonged period of time, it is helpful to have an extra pair available for the client. That way, when one pair needs to be cleaned, another pair is available for the client to wear.

Proper positioning reduces the client's risk of thrombus formation because compression of the leg veins is minimized. Therefore, when positioning clients, use caution to prevent pressure on the posterior knee and deep veins in the lower extremities. Teach clients to avoid the following: crossing the legs, sitting for prolonged periods of time, wearing clothing that constricts the legs or waist, putting pillows under the knees, and massaging the legs.

ROM exercises reduce the risk of contractures and aid in preventing thrombi. Activity causes contraction of the skeletal muscles, which in turn exerts pressure on the veins to promote venous return, thereby reducing venous stasis. Specific exercises that help prevent thrombophlebitis are ankle pumps, foot circles, and knee flexion. Ankle pumps, sometimes called calf pumps, include alternating plantar flexion and dorsiflexion. Foot circles require the client to rotate the ankle. Encourage clients to make the letters of the alphabet with their feet every 1 to 2 hours. Knee flexion involves alternately extending and flexing the knee. These exercises are sometimes referred to as antiembolic exercises and need to be done hourly while awake.

Report suspected DVTs immediately to the client's health care provider. Elevate the leg, but avoid pressure on the thrombus. Instruct the family, client, and all health care personnel not to massage the area because of the danger of dislodging the thrombus.

Musculoskeletal System. The client who is immobilized needs to do some exercise to prevent excessive muscle atrophy and joint contractures. If the client is unable to move part or all of the

Application of TED Hose

Delegation Considerations: The skill of applying TED hose can be delegated. The nurse is responsible for assessing circulation to the lower extremities. Instruct nursing assistive personnel to:
• Notify nurse if client develops leg pain or discoloration

Equipment: Tape measure, TED hose, hygiene supplies

1. Assess the need for elastic stockings and condition of the client's skin.
2. Observe for conditions that contraindicate use of stockings.
3. Perform hand hygiene. Provide hygiene to lower extremities if needed.
4. Use tape measure to measure client's legs to determine proper stocking size (measure according to manufacturer's directions). Elastic stockings come in two lengths: knee length and thigh length.
5. Apply stockings:
   a. Turn elastic stocking inside out up to the heel. Place one hand into sock, holding heel. Pull top of sock with the other hand inside out over foot of sock.
   b. Place client's toes into foot of elastic stocking, making sure that sock is smooth (see illustration).
   c. Slide remaining portion of sock over client's foot, being sure that the toes are covered. Make sure the foot fits into the toe and heel position of the sock (see illustration).
   d. Slide top of sock up over client's calf until sock is completely extended. Be sure sock is smooth and no ridges or wrinkles are present, particularly behind the knee (see illustration).
6. Instruct client not to roll socks partially down.
7. Record date and time of stocking application and stocking length and size in nurses' notes.
8. Record condition of skin and circulatory assessment.

TED, Thromboembolic device.

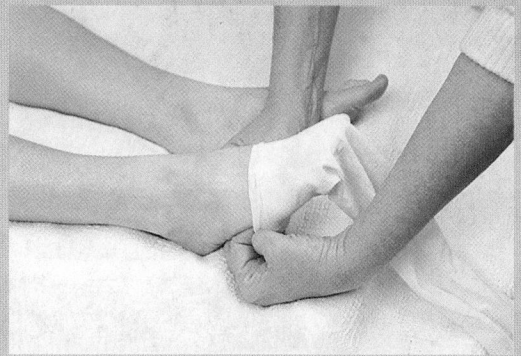

STEP 5b

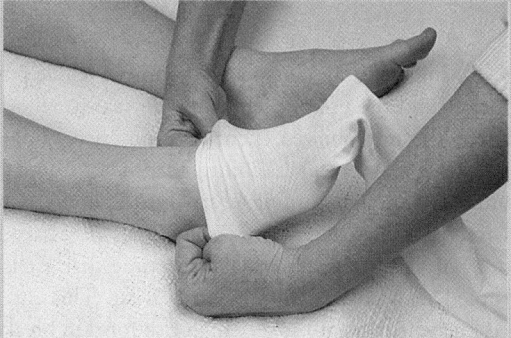

STEP 5c

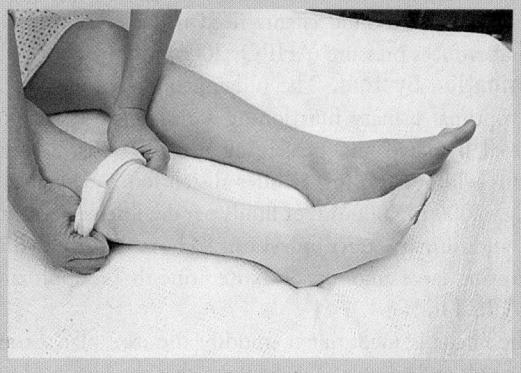

STEP 5d

body, perform passive ROM exercises for all immobilized joints while bathing the client and at least 2 or 3 more times a day. If one extremity is paralyzed, teach the client to put each joint independently through its ROM. Clients on bed rest need to have active ROM exercises incorporated into their daily schedules. Teach clients to integrate exercises during ADLs. Some orthopedic conditions require more frequent passive ROM exercises to restore the injured joint's function after surgery. Clients with such conditions need to use automatic equipment (continuous passive motion [CPM]) for passive ROM exercises (Figure 47-19). The CPM machine moves an extremity to a prescribed angle for a prescribed period. This is beneficial when the client must gradually increase the degree and duration of flexion and extension. Researchers are currently investigating new uses for CPM. In one study, clients who

had a CVA and who received CPM therapy to their affected shoulder had better joint stability when compared with clients who received traditional ROM exercises (Lynch and others, 2005).

Active ROM exercises also maintain function of the musculoskeletal system. Encourage clients to participate in active ROM, and establish an individualized progressive exercise program when possible (Shin and others, 2006). A progressive exercise program gradually increases the client's physical activity to reverse the deconditioning associated with immobility. Progressive exercise programs are successful in clients with musculoskeletal, neurological, cardiopulmonary, renal, and other chronic diseases.

Integumentary System. The major risk to the skin from restricted mobility is the formation of pressure ulcers. Early identification of high-risk clients helps prevent pressure ulcers (see

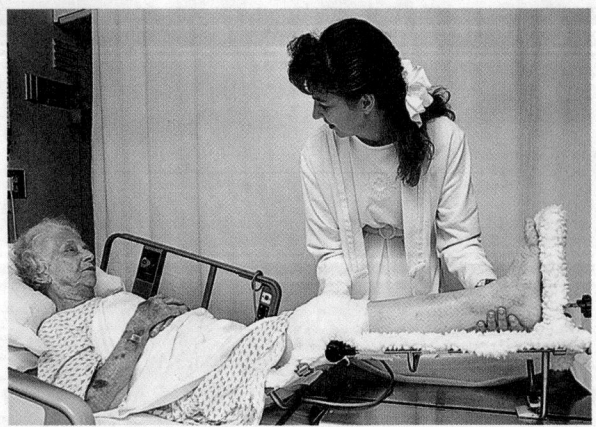

Figure 47-19 Continuous passive range-of-motion machine.

Chapter 48). Interventions aimed at prevention include positioning, skin care, and the use of therapeutic devices to relieve pressure. Change the immobilized client's position according to the client's activity level, perceptual ability, treatment protocols, and daily routines. Although turning every 1 to 2 hours is recommended for preventing ulcers, it is sometimes necessary to use devices for relieving pressure. Usually the time that a client sits uninterrupted in a chair is limited to 1 hour. This interval is shortened in clients who are at very high risk for skin breakdown. Reposition clients frequently because uninterrupted pressure will cause skin breakdown. Teach clients to shift their weight every 15 minutes. Chair-bound clients need to have a device for the chair that reduces pressure (AHRQ, 2003).

Elimination System. The nursing interventions for maintaining optimal urinary functioning are directed at keeping the client well hydrated and preventing urinary stasis, calculi, and infections without causing bladder distention. Adequate hydration (e.g., 2000 to 3000 mL of fluids per day) helps prevent renal calculi and urinary tract infections. The well-hydrated client needs to void large amounts of dilute urine that is approximately equal to fluid intake.

If the client is incontinent, modify the care plan to include toileting aids and a hygiene schedule so that the increased urinary output does not cause skin breakdown. To prevent bladder distention, assess the frequency and amount of urinary output. A client who continually dribbles urine and whose bladder is distended possibly has reflex incontinence. If the immobilized client does not have voluntary control of bladder elimination, bladder retraining is necessary. If the client experiences bladder distention, the nurse may need to insert a straight catheter or an indwelling Foley catheter (see Chapter 45).

Also record the frequency and consistency of bowel movements. Provide a diet rich in fluids, fruits, vegetables, and fiber to facilitate normal peristalsis. If a client is unable to maintain regular bowel patterns, stool softeners, cathartics, or enemas are sometimes necessary (see Chapter 46).

Psychosocial Changes. Use assessment data to identify effects of prolonged immobilization. People who have a tendency toward depression or mood swings are at greater risk for developing psychosocial effects during bed rest or immobilization. There are many nursing interventions to meet the client's psychosocial needs. Anticipate changes in the client's psychosocial status, and provide routine and informal socialization. Observe the client's ability to cope with restricted mobility. In institutional health care settings, schedule nursing care activities between 10:00 PM and 7:00 AM to minimize interruptions of sleep. For example, the nurse administers medications and assesses vital signs at the time when the client is turned or receives special skin care. If the nursing care plan is not improving coping patterns, consult a clinical nurse specialist, counselor, social worker, spiritual adviser, or other health care professional. Incorporate their recommendations into the care plan.

Nurses provide stimuli to maintain a client's orientation. Plan nursing activities so that the client is able to talk and interact with staff. If possible, place the client in a room with others who are mobile and interactive. If a private room is required, ask staff members to visit throughout the shift to provide meaningful interaction. A daily newspaper helps the client keep track of events and time. Bedside conversations at appropriate moments familiarize the client with nursing activities, meals, and visiting hours. Books help occupy the client when he or she is alone. The client can participate in craft activities. Radio, television, and videotapes provide stimulation and help pass the time.

Involve clients in their care whenever possible. For example, encourage the client to determine when the bed should be made. Some clients rest better during the night when fresh sheets are put on in the evening rather than in the morning. The client needs to provide as much self-care as possible. Keep hygiene and grooming articles within easy reach. Encourage clients to wear their glasses or artificial teeth and to shave or apply makeup. These are activities people use to maintain their body images, thus improving the client's outlook.

Developmental Changes. Ideally, immobilized clients continue normal development. Nursing interventions can help. Nursing care needs to provide mental and physical stimulation, particularly for a young child. Incorporate play activities into the care plan. Completing puzzles, for example, helps a child to develop fine motor skills, and reading helps the child to develop cognitively. Encourage parents to stay with a child who is hospitalized. Place a child who is immobilized with children of the same age who are not immobilized, unless a contagious disease is present. Allow the child to participate in nursing interventions such as dressing changes, cast care, and care of traction. The nurse needs to recognize significant changes from normal behavioral patterns and consult with a pediatric clinical nurse specialist, counselor, or other health care professional.

Restricted mobility of older clients presents unique nursing problems. Older clients who are frail or have chronic illnesses are often at increased risk for the psychosocial hazards of immobility. Maintaining a calendar and clock with a large dial, conversing about current events and family members, and encouraging visits from significant others reduce the risk of social isolation. Spending time in the room talking and listening to the client will also help reduce the risk of social isolation.

Nursing care needs to encourage older immobilized clients to perform as many ADLs as independently as possible. Clients need to continue to perform personal grooming if they did so before their mobility was restricted. This type of activity preserves the client's dignity and gives the client a sense of accomplishment.

Positioning Techniques. Clients with impaired nervous, skeletal, or muscular system functioning and increased weakness and fatigability often require help from the nurse to attain proper body alignment while in bed or sitting. Several positioning devices are available for maintaining good body alignment for clients. Pillows are positioning aids and are sometimes readily available. Before using a pillow, determine whether it is the proper size. A thick pillow under the client's head increases cervical flexion. A thin pillow under body prominences will not protect skin and tissue from damage caused by pressure. When additional pillows are unavailable or if they are an improper size, use folded sheets, blankets, or towels as positioning aids.

Apply positioning boots, or high-top tennis shoes on client's feet to prevent footdrop by maintaining the feet in dorsiflexion. A more common technique is the use of high-top tennis shoes or an ankle-foot orthotic (AFO) to help maintain dorsiflexion. Clients who wear tennis shoes or AFOs usually have a schedule they follow (e.g., 2 hours on, 2 hours off).

A **trochanter roll** prevents external rotation of the hips when the client is in a supine position. To form a trochanter roll, fold a cotton bath blanket lengthwise to a width that will extend from the greater trochanter of the femur to the lower border of the popliteal space (Figure 47-20). The nurse places the blanket under the buttocks and then rolls it counterclockwise until the thigh is in neutral position or in inward rotation. When the hip is aligned correctly, the patella faces directly upward. Use sandbags in place of or in addition to trochanter rolls. Sandbags are sand-filled plastic tubes or bags that are shaped to body contours. They immobilize an extremity or maintain body alignment.

Hand rolls maintain the thumb in slight adduction and in opposition to the fingers. A hand roll maintains the hand, thumb, and fingers in a functional position. Evaluate the hand roll to make sure that the hand is indeed in a functional position. Hand rolls are most often used with clients whose arms are paralyzed or who are unconscious. Do not use rolled washcloths as hand rolls, because they do not keep the thumb well abducted, especially in clients who have a spastic paralysis. Hand-wrist splints are individually molded for the client to maintain proper alignment of the thumb (slight adduction) and the wrist (slight dorsiflexion). Use splints only on the client for whom the splint was made, and follow the splint schedule (e.g., wear for 2 hours, remove for 2 hours).

The **trapeze bar** is a triangular device that hangs down from a securely fastened overhead bar that is attached to the bed frame. It allows the client to pull with the upper extremities to raise the trunk off the bed, to assist in transfer from bed to wheelchair, or to perform upper arm exercises (Figure 47-21). It increases independence, maintains upper body strength, and decreases the shearing action from sliding across or up and down in bed.

Although each procedure for positioning has specific guidelines, there are some universal steps the nurse follows for clients who require positioning assistance (Skill 47-1). Following the guidelines reduces the risk of injury to the musculoskeletal system when the client is sitting or lying. When joints are unsupported, their alignment is impaired. Likewise, if joints are not positioned in a slightly flexed position, their mobility is decreased. During positioning, also assess for pressure points (see Figure 48-12, p. 1294). When actual or potential pressure areas exist, nursing interventions involve re-

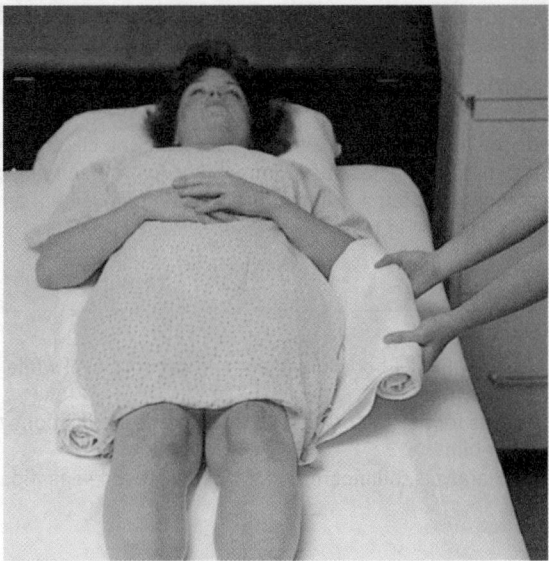

Figure 47-20 Trochanter roll.

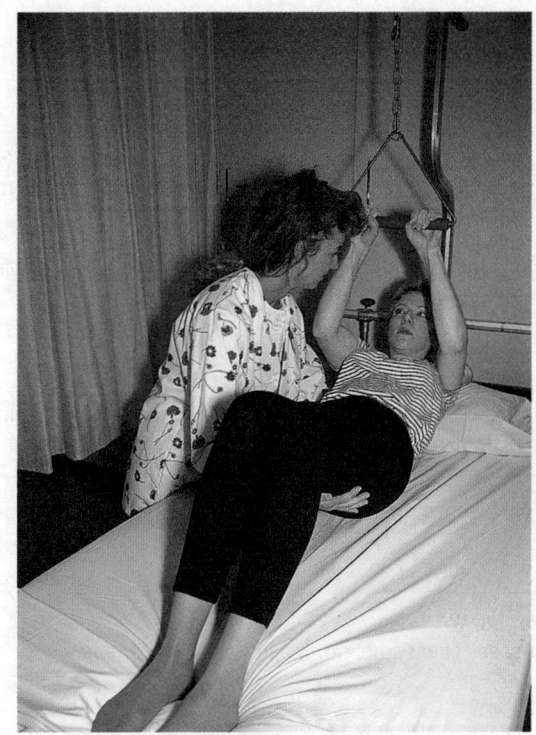

Figure 47-21 Client using a trapeze bar.

moval of the pressure, thus decreasing the risk for development of pressure ulcers and further trauma to the musculoskeletal system. In these clients use the 30-degree lateral position.

Supported Fowler's Position. In the supported Fowler's position, the head of the bed is elevated 45 to 60 degrees and the client's knees are slightly elevated without pressure to restrict circulation in the lower legs. The client's illness and overall condition influence the angle of head and knee elevation and the length of

Text continued on p. 1259

※ **SKILL 47-1**   **MOVING AND POSITIONING CLIENTS IN BED**

Delegation Considerations

The skill of moving and positioning clients in bed can be delegated. The nurse is responsible for assessing the client's level of comfort and for any hazards of immobility. Instruct nursing assistive personnel about any limitations affecting movement and positioning of client in bed.

Equipment

- Pillows
- Ankle-foot orthotic or high-top tennis shoes
- Trochanter roll
- Sandbag
- Hand rolls
- Side rails
- Appropriate safe-client-handling assistive device

STEPS	RATIONALE
1. Assess client's body alignment and comfort level while client is lying down.	Provides baseline data for later comparisons. Determines ways to improve position and alignment.
2. Assess for risk factors that contribute to complications of immobility:	Increased risk factors require more frequent repositioning.
a. Paralysis, hemiparesis, and/or decreased sensation	Paralysis impairs movement; muscle tone changes; sensation is often affected. Because of difficulty in moving and poor awareness of involved body part, client is unable to protect and position body part for self (Black and Hawks, 2005).
b. Impaired mobility from traction, arthritis, or other contributing disease processes	Impaired mobility often results in decreased ROM.
c. Impaired circulation	Decreased circulation predisposes client to pressure sores.
d. Age: very young, older adults	Premature and young infants require frequent turning because their skin is fragile. Normal physiological changes associated with aging predispose older adults to greater risks for developing complications of immobility (Butler, 2006; Ebersole and others, 2005).
e. Level of consciousness and mental status.	Comatose or semicomatose clients are unable to verbalize areas of skin pressure, increasing the risk for skin breakdown.
3. Refer to appropriate algorithm for repositioning client (see Figure 47-22, p. 1260). Assess client's physical ability to help with moving and positioning:	Enables nurse to use client's mobility and strength; encouraging client to help promotes independence (Nelson and others, 2003b).
a. Age	Older adult client will move more slowly with less strength.
b. Ability to understand instructions and cooperate with nursing staff	Determines need for special aids or devices.
	Clients with dementia or altered levels of consciousness do not always understand instructions and are sometimes unable to help.

Critical Decision Point: If you are uncertain about the client's ability to cooperate with the transfer, assume that the client will not participate in transfer or repositioning (Nelson, 2003b).

c. Disease process	Cardiopulmonary disease often requires client to have head of bed elevated.
d. Strength, coordination	Determines amount of assistance provided by client during position change.
e. ROM	Limited ROM contraindicates certain positions.
4. Assess client's height, weight, and body shape.	Devices used for safe client handling have different weight restrictions; bariatric clients require special beds, lifts, wheelchairs, and toileting and bathing equipment (Nelson, 2003b).
5. Assess health care provider's orders. Clarify whether any positions are contraindicated because of client's condition (e.g., spinal cord injury; respiratory difficulties; joint replacement, certain neurological conditions).	Placing client in an inappropriate position causes injury.
6. Perform hand hygiene.	Reduces transfer of microorganisms.
7. Assess for the presence of tubes, incisions, drains, and equipment (e.g., traction).	Will alter positioning procedure and affect client's ability to independently change positions.
8. Assess ability and motivation of client, family members, and primary caregiver to participate in moving and positioning client in bed in anticipation of discharge to home.	Determines ability of client and caregivers to assist with positioning.
9. Raise level of bed to comfortable working height, and get extra help if needed.	Raises level of work to your center of gravity and provides for client's and your safety.

✳ **SKILL 47-1**   **MOVING AND POSITIONING CLIENTS IN BED—CONT'D**

STEPS	RATIONALE
10. Explain procedure to client and what client is expected to do during procedure.	Decreases anxiety and increases client cooperation.
11. Position client flat in bed if tolerated.	Repositioning from a flat position decreases friction and possible shear on client's skin.

Critical Decision Point: Before flattening bed, account for all tubing, drains, and equipment to prevent dislodgment or tipping if caught in mattress or bed frame as bed is lowered.

---

12. Position client in bed.	
A. Move client up in bed	
(1) Put bed flat or in Trendelenburg's position with the side rail down.	Use of gravity helps prevent injury. Putting side rail down reduces muscle strain.
(2) Place height of bed at level appropriate for all staff.	Putting bed at elbow level reduces staff's muscle strain.
(3) For client able to move self without assistance:	
a. Instruct client to move self.	Caregiver assistance is not needed (Nelson, 2003b).
b. Offer positioning aid if needed.	Will help with positioning; not all clients need aid.
(4) For client partially able to move self:	
a. Ask appropriate number of staff to help with task. For clients less than 200 pounds, two to three caregivers are needed; for clients greater than 200 pounds, at least three caregivers are needed.	Moving a client up in bed is **not** a one-person task. Ensure that appropriate staff are available to help before progressing to prevent injury (Nelson, 2003b).
b. Select appropriate friction-reducing device (e.g., friction-reducing slide sheet).	Enhances staff safety (Nelson and Baptiste, 2006).
c. Encourage client to assist using positioning aid if possible.	Reduces workload of nurse.
d. Use friction-reducing device per manufacturer's guidelines with appropriate number of help, and move client up in bed. Instruct client to flex the knees and push on the count of three if the client is able to help.	Many friction-reducing devices are available. Following manufacturer's guidelines ensures safe and effective use of equipment.
(5) For client unable to assist:	
a. Ask appropriate number of staff to help with repositioning; at least two caregivers are needed.	Moving a client up in bed is **not** a one-person task. Ensure that appropriate staff are available to help before progressing to prevent injury (Nelson and others, 2003b).
b. Select appropriate safe-client-handling device (e.g., full-body sling, friction-reducing device).	Safe-client-handling equipment is necessary when clients are unable to assist with repositioning.
c. Use friction-reducing device or full-body sling per manufacturer's guidelines with appropriate number of staff, and move client up in bed.	Many devices and slings are available. Following manufacturer's guidelines ensures safe and effective use of equipment.
B. Position client in supported Fowler's position (see illustration)	
(1) Elevate head of bed 45 to 60 degrees.	Increases comfort, improves ventilation, and increases client's opportunity to socialize or relax.
(2) Rest head against mattress or on small pillow.	Prevents flexion contractures of cervical vertebrae.
(3) Use pillows to support arms and hands if client does not have voluntary control or use of hands and arms.	Prevents shoulder dislocation from effect of downward pull of unsupported arms, promotes circulation by preventing venous pooling, and prevents flexion contractures of arms and wrists.
(4) Position pillow at lower back.	Supports lumbar vertebrae and decreases flexion of vertebrae.

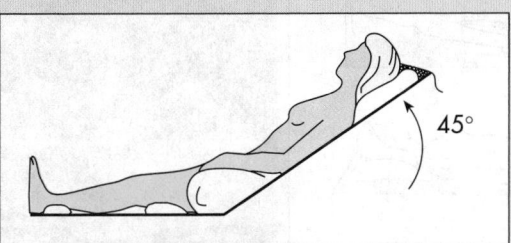

STEP 12B Supported Fowler's position.

Continued

✳ SKILL 47-1   MOVING AND POSITIONING CLIENTS IN BED—CONT'D

STEPS	RATIONALE
(5) Place small pillow under thigh.	Prevents hyperextension of knee and occlusion of popliteal artery caused by pressure from body weight.
(6) Position patient's heel in heel boots or other heel pressure relief devices.	Heel pressure relief devices are more effective than pillows for consistently reducing pressure from the mattress on the heels. When pillows are used they must be repositioned each time the patient moves. (Walsh and Plonczynski, 2007).

Critical Decision Point: A foot cradle may also be used in patients with poor peripheral circulation as a means of reducing pressure on the tips of a patients toes.

C. Position client with hemiplegia in supported Fowler's position	
(1) Elevate head of bed 45 to 60 degrees.	Increases comfort, improves ventilation, and increases client's opportunity to relax.
(2) Position client in sitting position as straight as possible.	Counteracts tendency to slump toward affected side. Improves ventilation and cardiac output; decreases intracranial pressure. Improves client's ability to swallow and helps to prevent aspiration of food, liquids, and gastric secretions.
(3) Position head on small pillow with chin slightly forward. If client is totally unable to control head movement, avoid hyperextension of the neck.	Prevents hyperextension of neck. Too many pillows under head cause or worsen neck flexion contracture.

Critical Decision Point: If the client has a paralyzed extremity, provide support for involved arm and hand on over-bed table in front of client. Place arm away from client's side, and support elbow with pillow.
• Position *flaccid* hand in normal resting position with wrist slightly extended, arches of hand maintained, and fingers partially flexed; use section of rubber ball cut in half; clasp client's hands together.
• Position *spastic* hand with wrist in neutral position or slightly extended; extend fingers with palm down, or leave them in relaxed position palm up. At times it is difficult to position spastic hands without the use of specially made splints for the client.

(4) Flex knees and hips by using pillow or folded blanket under knees.	Ensures proper alignment. Flexion prevents prolonged hyperextension, which will possibly impair joint mobility.
(5) Support feet in dorsiflexion with ankle-foot orthotic or high-top tennis shoes.	Prevents footdrop. Stimulation of ball of foot by firm surface has tendency to increase muscle tone in client with extensor spasticity of lower extremity.
D. Position client in supine position	
(1) Be sure client is comfortable on back with head of bed flat.	Some clients' physical conditions will not tolerate supine position.
(2) Place small rolled towel under lumbar area of back.	Provides support for lumbar spine.
(3) Place pillow under upper shoulders, neck, or head.	Maintains correct alignment and prevents flexion contractures of cervical vertebrae.
(4) Place trochanter rolls or sandbags parallel to lateral surface of client's thighs.	Reduces external rotation of hip.
(5) Place small pillow or roll under ankle to elevate heels (see illustration for Step 12B).	Reduces pressure on heels, helping to prevent pressure sores.

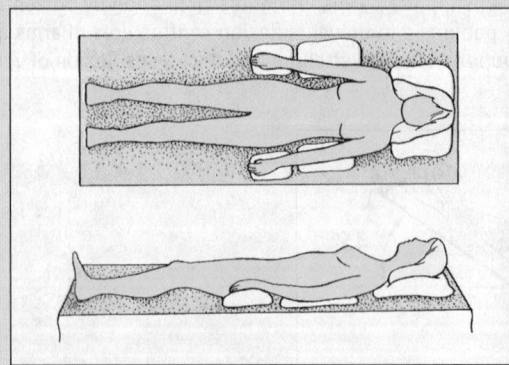
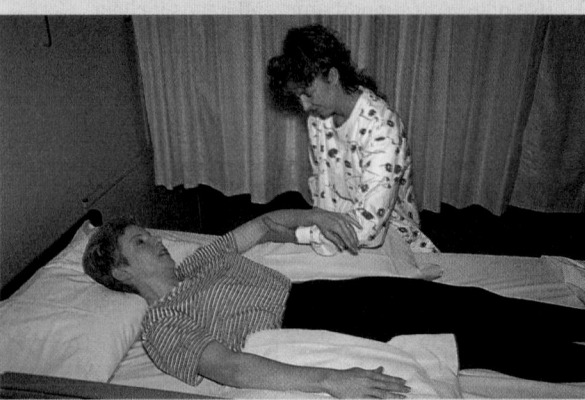

STEP 12D(8) Supine position with pillows in place.

✳ SKILL 47-1 MOVING AND POSITIONING CLIENTS IN BED—CONT'D

STEPS	RATIONALE
(6) Place firm pillows against bottom of client's feet (if available).	Maintains dorsiflexion and prevents footdrop.
(7) Place foot splints or high-top sneakers on client's feet if ordered.	Maintains feet in dorsiflexion. Prevents footdrop.
(8) Place pillows under pronated forearms, keeping upper arms parallel to client's body (see illustrations).	Reduces internal rotation of shoulder and prevents extension of elbows. Maintains correct body alignment.
(9) Place hand rolls in client's hands. Consider physical therapy referral for use of hand splints.	Reduces extension of fingers and abduction of thumb. Maintains thumb slightly adducted and in opposition to fingers.
E. Position client with hemiplegia in supine position	
(1) Place head of bed flat.	Necessary for positioning in supine position.
(2) Place folded towel or small pillow under shoulder or affected side.	Decreases possibility of pain, joint contracture, and subluxation. Maintains mobility in muscles around shoulder to permit normal movement patterns.
(3) Keep affected arm away from body with elbow extended and palm up. (Alternative is to place arm out to side, with elbow bent and hand toward head of bed.)	Maintains mobility in arm, joints, and shoulder to permit normal movement patterns. (Alternative position counteracts limitation of ability of arm to rotate outward at shoulder [external rotation]. External rotation needs to be present to raise arm overhead without pain.)

Critical Decision Point: Position affected hand in one of the recommended positions for flaccid or spastic hand.

---

(4) Place folded towel under hip of involved side.	Diminishes effect of spasticity in entire leg by controlling hip position.
(5) Flex affected knee 30 degrees by supporting it on pillow or folded blanket.	Slight flexion breaks up abnormal extension pattern of leg. Extensor spasticity is most severe when client is supine.
(6) Support feet with soft pillows at right angle to leg.	Maintains foot in dorsiflexion and prevents footdrop. Pillows prevent stimulation to ball of foot by hard surface, which has tendency to increase muscle tone in client with extensor spasticity of lower extremity.
F. Position client in prone position	
(1) Determine need for assistance from other caregivers.	At least two or three caregivers may be necessary to safely position client in prone position, especially if client is unable to assist or is obese.
(2) With client supine, roll client over arm positioned close to body, with elbow straight and hand under hip. Position on abdomen in center of bed.	Positions client correctly so alignment can be maintained.
(3) Turn client's head to one side, and support head with small pillow (see illustration).	Reduces flexion or hyperextension of cervical vertebrae.
(4) Place small pillow under client's abdomen below level of diaphragm (see illustration).	Reduces pressure on breasts of some female clients and decreases hyperextension of lumbar vertebrae and strain on lower back.
(5) Support arms in flexed position level at shoulders.	Maintains proper body alignment. Support reduces risk of joint dislocation.

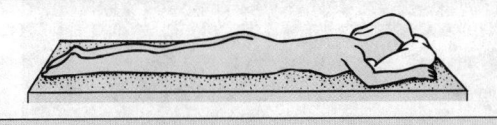

STEP 12F(3) Prone position, head supported with pillow.

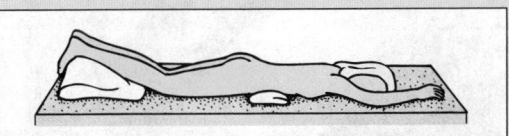

STEP 12F(4) Prone position, pillow under client's abdomen and feet.

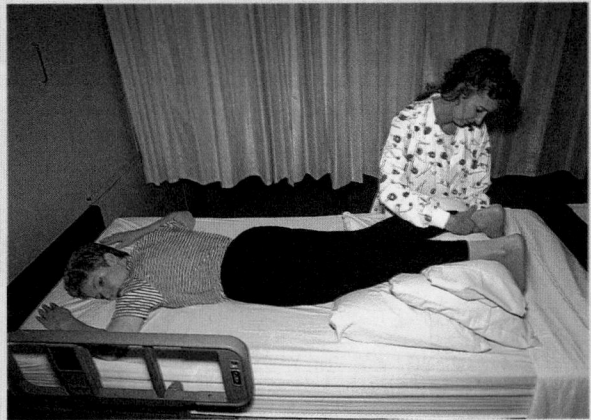

STEP 12F(6) Prone position.

Continued

✳ SKILL 47-1   MOVING AND POSITIONING CLIENTS IN BED—CONT'D

STEPS	RATIONALE
(6) Support lower legs with pillows to elevate toes (see illustration).	Prevents footdrop. Reduces external rotation of hips. Eliminates mattress pressure on toes.
G. Position client with hemiplegia in prone position	
(1) Determine need for friction-reducing device or full-body sling and number of people needed to help with repositioning.	At least two or three caregivers will be needed; friction-reducing device or full-body sling reduces chance of injury and skin tears or pressure ulcers (Nelson, 2003b).
(2) Move client toward unaffected side using assistance and safe-client-handling equipment following manufacturer's guidelines.	Creates room for proper client alignment in center of bed when client rolls onto abdomen.
(3) Roll client onto side.	
(4) Place pillow on client's abdomen.	Prevents sagging of abdomen when client rolls over; decreases hyperextension of lumbar vertebrae and strain on lower back.
(5) Roll client onto abdomen by positioning involved arm close to client's body, with elbow straight and hand under hip. Roll client carefully over arm.	Prevents injury to affected side.
(6) Turn head toward involved side.	Promotes development of neck and trunk extension, which is necessary for standing and walking.
(7) Position involved arm out to side, with elbow bent, hand toward head of bed, and fingers extended (if possible).	Counteracts limitation of arm's ability to rotate outward at shoulder (external rotation). External rotation needs to be present to raise arm over head without pain.
(8) Flex knees slightly by placing pillow under legs from knees to ankles.	Flexion prevents prolonged hyperextension, which impairs joint mobility.
(9) Keep feet at right angle to legs by using pillow high enough to keep toes off mattress.	Maintains feet in dorsiflexion.
H. Position client in lateral (side-lying) position	
(1) Obtain assistance from at least one or two other people.	Skill requires at least two to three people. Reduces risk for caregiver injury and promotes client's comfort.
(2) Lower head of bed completely or as low as client is able to tolerate.	Provides position of comfort for client and removes pressure from bony prominences on back and buttocks.
(3) Position client to side of bed. Use friction-reducing device or mechanical lift per manufacturer's guidelines if client cannot assist with rolling or is obese.	Provides room for client to turn to side. Use of safe-client-handling equipment reduces workload of caregivers and enhances safety (deCastro and others, 2006).
(4) Prepare to turn client onto side. Flex client's knee that will not be next to mattress. Place one hand on client's hip and one hand on client's shoulder.	Positioning will set up leverage for easy turning.
(5) Roll client onto the side opposite of the flexed knee.	Decreases trauma to tissues. In addition, client is positioned so leverage on hip makes turning easy.
(6) Place pillow under client's head and neck.	Maintains alignment. Reduces lateral neck flexion. Decreases strain on sternocleidomastoid muscle.
(7) Bring shoulder blade forward.	Prevents client's weight from resting directly on shoulder joint.
(8) Position both arms in slightly flexed position. Upper arm is supported by pillow level with shoulder; other arm, by mattress.	Decreases internal rotation and adduction of shoulder. Supports both arms in slightly flexed position.

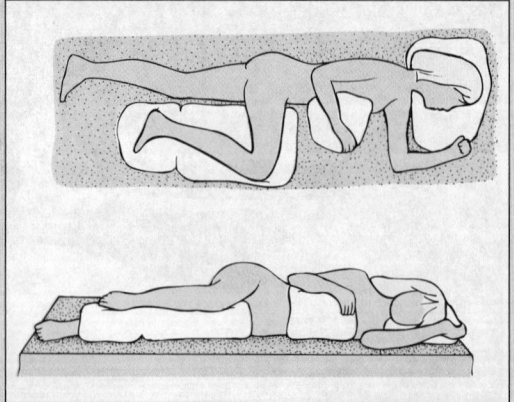
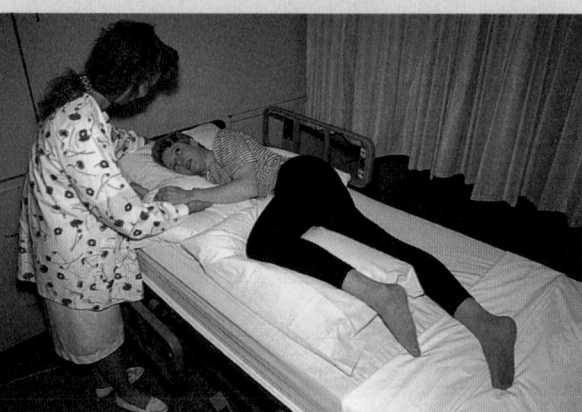

STEP 12H(10) Side-lying position with pillows in place.

✳ SKILL 47-1 **MOVING AND POSITIONING CLIENTS IN BED—CONT'D**

STEPS	RATIONALE
(9) Place tuck-back pillow behind client's back. (Make by folding pillow lengthwise. Smooth area is slightly tucked under client's back.)	Provides support to maintain client on side.
(10) Place pillow under semiflexed upper leg level at hip from groin to foot (see illustrations).	Maintains leg in correct alignment. Prevents pressure on bony prominence.
(11) Place ankle-foot orthotic on client's feet.	Maintains dorsiflexion of feet. Prevents footdrop.
I. Position client in Sims' (semiprone) position	
(1) Obtain assistance from at least one or two other people.	Skill requires at least two to three people. Reduces risk for caregiver injury and promotes client's comfort.
(2) Lower head of bed completely.	Provides for proper body alignment while client is lying down.
(3) Be sure client is comfortable in supine position.	Prepares client for position. Client is rolled partially onto abdomen.
(4) Position client in lateral position, with dependent arm straight along client's body and with client lying partially on abdomen.	
(5) Carefully lift client's dependent shoulder, and bring arm back behind client.	
(6) Place small pillow under client's head.	
(7) Place pillow under flexed upper arm, supporting arm level with shoulder.	Maintains proper alignment and prevents lateral neck flexion. Prevents internal rotation of shoulder. Maintains alignment.
(8) Place pillow under flexed upper leg, supporting leg level with hip.	Prevents internal rotation of hip and adduction of leg. Flexion prevents hyperextension of leg. Reduces mattress pressure on knees and ankles.
(9) Place ankle orthotic shoe or sandbags parallel to plantar surface of foot (see illustration).	Maintains foot in dorsiflexion. Prevents footdrop.
J. Logrolling the client	

Critical Decision Point: Supervise and aid personnel when there is a health care provider's order to **logroll** a client. Clients who have suffered from spinal cord injury or are recovering from neck, back, or spinal surgery often need to keep the spinal column in straight alignment to prevent further injury.

---

(1) Obtain assistance from at least two or three other people.	At least three to four people are needed to perform this skill safely.
(2) Place pillow between client's knees.	Prevents tension on the spinal column and adduction of the hip.
(3) Cross client's arms on chest.	Prevents injury to arms.
(4) Position two nurses or other staff members on side of bed to which the client will be turned. Position third nurse or staff member on the other side of bed (see illustration). If needed, four nurses are used; fourth nurse stands on same side as third nurse.	Distributes weight equally between nurses.
(5) Fanfold or roll the drawsheet or pull sheet.	Provides strong handles in order to grip the drawsheet or pull sheet without slipping.

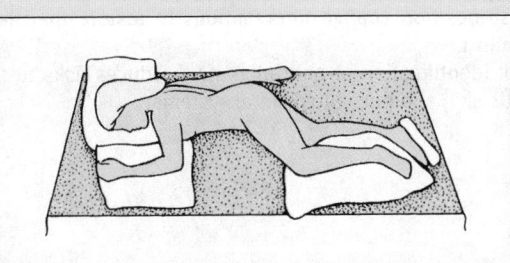

STEP 12I(9) Sims' (semiprone) position with pillows and sandbags in place.

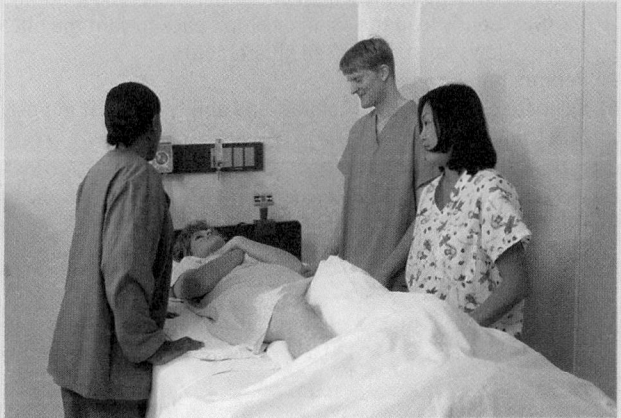

STEP 12J(4) Position nurses on each side of client.

Continued

✳ **SKILL 47-1**   MOVING AND POSITIONING CLIENTS IN BED—CONT'D

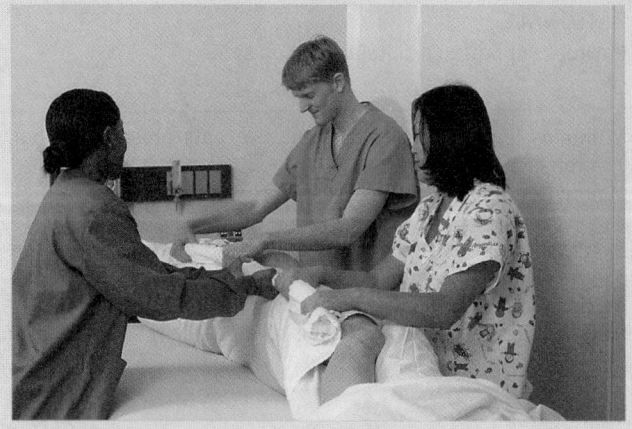

STEP 12J(6) Move client as a unit, maintaining proper alignment.

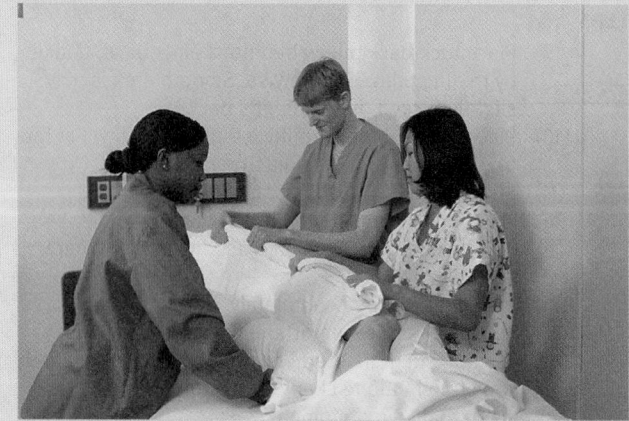

STEP 12J(7) Place pillows along client's back for support.

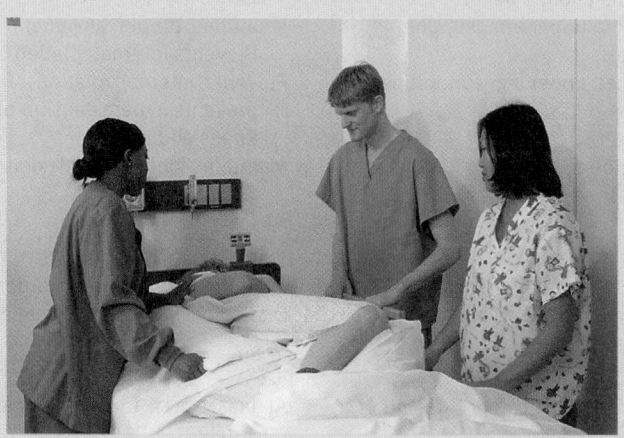

STEP 12J(8) Gently lean client as a unit against pillows.

STEPS	RATIONALE
(6) Move the client as one unit in a smooth, continuous motion on the count of three (see illustration).	This maintains proper alignment by moving all body parts at the same time, preventing tension or twisting of the spinal column.
(7) Nurse on the opposite side of the bed places pillows along the length of the client (see illustration).	Pillows keep client aligned.
(8) Gently lean the client as a unit back toward the pillows for support (see illustration).	Ensures continued straight alignment of spinal column, preventing injury.
13. Perform hand hygiene.	Reduces transmission of microorganisms.
14. Evaluate client's level of comfort and ability to assist in position change.	Clients with reduced activity tolerance and increased levels of pain often find position changes very fatiguing and will need post–position change interventions to restore their level of comfort.
15. Following each position change, evaluate client's body alignment, positioning, and presence of any pressure areas.	Prompt identification of poor alignment reduces risks to the client's skin and musculoskeletal systems.

✳ SKILL 47-1   MOVING AND POSITIONING CLIENTS IN BED—CONT'D

Unexpected Outcomes and Related Interventions

1. Joint contractures develop or worsen.
   a. Consult physical and/or occupational therapy.
   b. Ensure activity and ROM orders are consistently implemented.
2. Skin shows areas of erythema and breakdown.
   a. Increase frequency of turning and repositioning; place turning schedule above client's bed.
   b. Consult skin care team.
   c. Implement other activites per agency's skin care policy or protocol (e.g., more frequent assessments, consult dietitian, place client on pressure-relieving mattress).
3. Client avoids moving.
   a. Administer pain medications as ordered by a health care provider to ensure client's comfort before moving if client is in pain, and allow pain medication to take effect before proceeding.
   b. Provide client education about benefits of moving.

Recording and Reporting

- Document repositioning or turn and observations during procedure (e.g., condition of skin, joint movement, client's ability to assist with positioning) in nurses' notes.
- Report observations at change of shift.

Home Care Considerations

- Teach family how to use safe-client-handling equipment if necessary.
- Teach client and family about the signs of skin breakdown and the importance of safety during positioning for clients with decreased sensation.

---

time that the client needs to remain in the supported Fowler's position. Supports need to permit flexion of the hips and knees and proper alignment of the normal curves in the cervical, thoracic, and lumbar vertebrae. The following are common trouble areas for the client in the supported Fowler's position:

- Increased cervical flexion because the pillow at the head is too thick and the head thrusts forward
- Extension of the knees, allowing the client to slide to the foot of the bed
- Pressure on the posterior aspect of the knees, decreasing circulation to the feet
- External rotation of the hips
- Arms hanging unsupported at the client's sides
- Unsupported feet or pressure on the heels
- Unprotected pressure points at the sacrum and heels
- Increased shearing force on the back and heels when the head of the bed is raised greater than 60 degrees

Supine Position. Clients in the supine position rest on their backs. In the supine position the relationship of body parts is essentially the same as in good standing alignment except that the body is in the horizontal plane. Use pillows, trochanter rolls, and hand rolls or arm splints to increase comfort and reduce injury to the skin or musculoskeletal system. The mattress needs to be firm enough to support the cervical, thoracic, and lumbar vertebrae. Shoulders are supported, and the elbows are slightly flexed to control shoulder rotation. A foot support prevents footdrop and maintains proper alignment. The following are some common trouble areas for clients in the supine position:

- Pillow at the head that is too thick, increasing cervical flexion
- Head flat on the mattress
- Shoulders unsupported and internally rotated
- Elbows extended
- Thumb not in opposition to the fingers
- Hips externally rotated
- Unsupported feet

- Unprotected pressure points at the occipital region of the head, vertebrae, coccyx, elbows, and heels

Prone Position. The client in the prone position lies face or chest down. Often the client's head is turned to the side, but if a pillow is under the head, it needs to be thin enough to prevent cervical flexion or extension and maintain alignment of the lumbar spine. Placing a pillow under the lower leg permits dorsiflexion of the ankles and some knee flexion, which promotes relaxation. If a pillow is unavailable, the ankles need to be in dorsiflexion over the end of the mattress. Although the prone position is seldom used in practice, consider this as an alternative especially in clients who normally sleep in this position. The prone position also may have some benefits in clients with acute respiratory distress syndrome and acute lung injury (Marklew, 2006). Specialty beds that safely position acutely ill clients in the prone position are available. Assess for and correct any of the following potential trouble points with clients in the prone position:

- Neck hyperextension
- Hyperextension of the lumbar spine
- Plantar flexion of the ankles
- Unprotected pressure points at the chin, elbows, hips, knees, and toes

Side-Lying Position. In the side-lying (or lateral) position the client rests on the side with the major portion of body weight on the dependent hip and shoulder. A 30-degree lateral position is recommended for clients at risk for pressure ulcers (see Chapter 48) (AHRQ, 2003). Trunk alignment needs to be the same as in standing. The client needs to maintain the structural curves of the spine, the head needs to be supported in line with the midline of the trunk, and rotation of the spine needs to be avoided. The following trouble points are common in the side-lying position:

- Lateral flexion of the neck
- Spinal curves out of normal alignment

- Shoulder and hip joints internally rotated, adducted, or unsupported
- Lack of support for the feet
- Lack of protection for pressure points at the ear, shoulder, anterior iliac spine, trochanter, and ankles
- Excessive lateral flexion of the spine if the client has large hips and a pillow is not placed superior to the hips at the waist

Sims' Position. Sims' position differs from the side-lying position in the distribution of the client's weight. In Sims' position, the client places the weight on the anterior ileum, humerus, and clavicle. Trouble points common in Sims' position include the following:

- Lateral flexion of the neck
- Internal rotation, adduction, or lack of support to the shoulders and hips
- Lack of support for the feet
- Lack of protection for pressure points at the ileum, humerus, clavicle, knees, and ankles

Transfer Techniques. Nurses often provide care for immobilized clients whose position must be changed, who must be moved up in bed, or who must be transferred from a bed to a chair or from a bed to a stretcher. As noted earlier, body mechanics alone do not protect the nurse from injury to the musculoskeletal system when moving, lifting, or transferring clients. Although nurses use many transfer techniques, knowledge of ergonomics and safe client handling is crucial in maintaining caregiver and client safety.

Assess every situation that involves client handling and movement to minimize risk of injury. After completing the assessment, nurses use an algorithm (Figure 47-22) to guide decisions about safe client handling (Nelson, 2006). Use the client's strength when lifting, transferring, or moving when possible. Involving the client has the added bonus of increasing participation in self-care, thus promoting a sense of accomplishment. In addition to handling clients safely, nurses need to assume an active role in their workplaces to ensure that a culture of safety exists and that appropriate client-handling equipment is readily available (Waters and others, 2007).

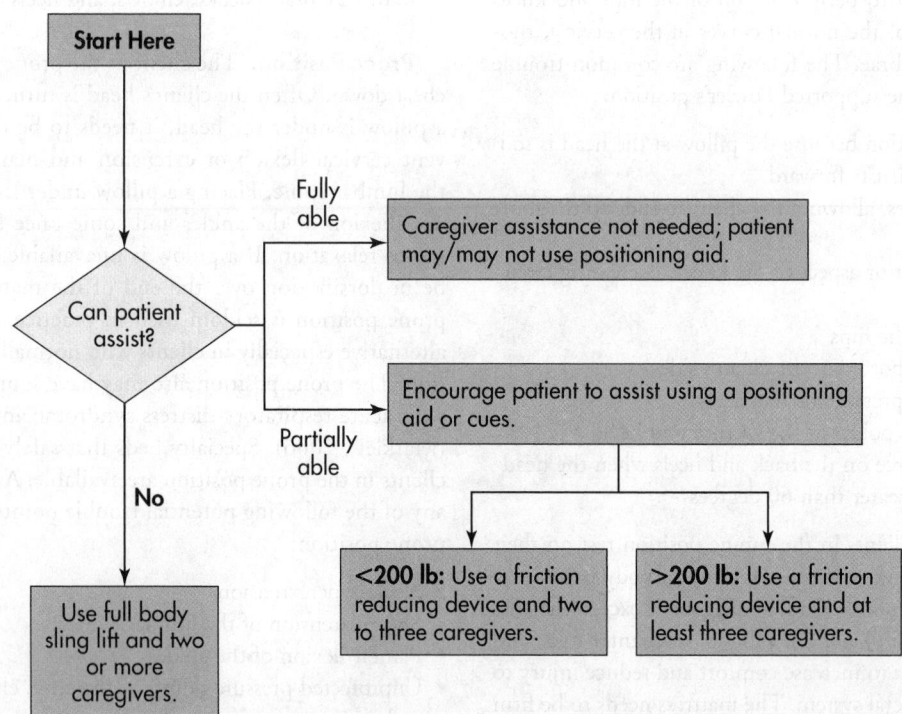

- This is not a one-person task: DO NOT PULL FROM HEAD OF BED.
- When pulling a patient up in bed, the bed should be flat or in a Trendelenburg position (when tolerated) to aid in gravity, with the side rail down.
- For patients with stage III or IV pressure ulcers, care should be taken to avoid shearing force.
- The height of the bed should be appropriate for staff safety (at the elbows).
- If the patient can assist when repositioning "up in bed," ask the patient to flex the knees and push on the count of three.
- During any patient handling task, if the caregiver is required to lift more than 35 lb of a patient's weight, then the patient should be considered to be fully dependent and assistive devices should be used.

Figure 47-22 Algorithm used to reposition client in the bed. (From: Nelson A: *Safe patient handling and movement algorithms,* 2006, VISN8 Patient Safety Center, http://www.visn8.med.va.gov/patientsafetycenter/safePtHandling/default.asp.)

Moving Clients. A safe transfer is the first priority. Clients require various levels of assistance to move up in bed, move to the side-lying position, or sit up at the side of the bed. For example, a young, healthy woman needs only a little support as she sits at the side of the bed for the first time after childbirth, whereas an older man needs help from two or more nurses to do the same task one day after abdominal surgery.

Always ask the client to help to the fullest extent possible. To determine what the client is able to do alone and how many people are needed to help move the client in bed, assess the client to determine whether the illness contradicts exertion (e.g., cardiovascular disease). Next, determine whether the client comprehends what is expected. For example, a client recently medicated for postoperative pain is too lethargic to understand instruction; thus to ensure safety, two nurses are necessary to move the client. Then determine the comfort level of the client. It is important to evaluate your personal strength and knowledge of the procedure. Finally, determine whether the client is too heavy or immobile for you to move the client alone (Nelson and others, 2003b). Through the use of assessment tools and client movement algorithms, you determine the safest method by which to move the client. Skills 47-1 (p. 1252) and 47-2 (p. 1265) describe the steps commonly used in moving clients in bed and transferring them to a sitting position at the side of the bed.

Transferring a Client From a Bed to a Chair. Refer to an algorithm when transferring a client from a bed to a chair (Figure 47-23, p. 1262). Before beginning, move obstacles out of the way to prepare the environment and ensure that enough help is available. If a caregiver needs to lift more than 35 pounds, use assistive devices for the transfer (Figure 47-24, pp. 1263-1264). Explain the procedure to the client before the transfer. Place the chair next to the bed with the chair back in the same plane as the head of the bed.

Next, determine if the client can bear weight. If the client can bear weight fully, stand near the client during the transfer as needed for safety reasons. If the client can only partially bear weight and is cooperative, the transfer requires one caregiver. The nurse either stands and pivots the client into the chair using a gait or transfer belt or uses a powered standing-assist lift. Two caregivers and a full body sling are needed for transferring uncooperative clients who can bear partial weight and for clients who cannot bear weight and are either uncooperative or do not have upper body strength. A seated transfer aid, such as a friction-reducing lateral-assist device, is used with or without a gait belt for clients who cannot bear weight but who are cooperative and have sufficient upper body strength to complete the transfer. If a seated transfer aid is used, the chair needs to have arms that are able to be removed or moved out of the way. Transfer clients who have partial weight bearing toward their stronger side (Baptiste and others, 2006; Nelson, 2003b).

Transferring a Client From a Bed to a Stretcher. To transfer a client from a bed to a stretcher, first consult an appropriate algorithm (Figure 47-25, p. 1264). Determine if the client is able to assist in the procedure. For clients who can complete the transfer independently, allow them to move to the stretcher on their own and stand by to ensure a safe transfer. Determine the client's weight if the client can assist partially or cannot assist at all. Use a friction-reducing device for clients who weigh less than 200 pounds. If the client weighs 200 pounds or more, use a friction-

reducing device and three caregivers. Before moving the client, place the stretcher and the bed side by side to allow the client to transfer quickly and easily using the friction-reducing device.

Use caution when the client has or is suspected of having spinal cord trauma. If you have to move the client, place a transfer board under the client to maintain spinal alignment before transferring the client to a stretcher. Prepare the client for the transfer, and ask for help when possible (e.g., by folding the arms over the chest). Make sure the environment is free from obstacles, and remove unnecessary equipment from the bed.

Restorative and Continuing Care. The goal of restorative care for the client who is immobile is to maximize functional mobility and independence and reduce residual functional deficits such as impaired gait and decreased endurance. The focus in restorative care is not only on ADLs that relate to physical self-care, but also on **instrumental activities of daily living (IADLs)**. IADLs are activities that are necessary to be independent in society beyond eating, grooming, transferring, and toileting and include such skills as shopping, preparing meals, banking, and taking medications.

The nurse uses many of the same interventions as described in the health promotion and acute care sections, but the emphasis is on working collaboratively with clients and their significant others and with other health care professionals to facilitate the client's return to maximal functional ability in both ADLs and IADLs.

Intensive specialized therapy such as occupational or physical therapy is common. The client, if in an institution, will likely go to the therapy department 2 to 3 times a day. The nurse's role is to work collaboratively with these professionals and reinforce exercises and teaching. For example, after a stroke or brain attack, a client will likely receive gait training from a physical therapist, speech rehabilitation from a speech therapist, and help from an occupational therapist on food preparation or other household chores. The therapy is not always able to restore total functional health, but it often helps the client adapt to the mobility limitations or complications. Equipment frequently used to help clients adapt to mobility limitations include walkers, canes, wheelchairs, and assistive devices such as toilet seat extenders, reaching sticks, special silverware, and clothing with Velcro closures.

Range-of-Motion Exercises. To ensure adequate joint mobility, teach the client about ROM exercises. Walking also increases joint mobility. Clients with restricted mobility are unable to perform some or all ROM exercises independently. Provide ROM exercises to maintain maximum joint mobility. To ensure that clients routinely receive ROM exercises, schedule them at specific times, perhaps with another nursing activity, such as during the client's bath. This enables the nurse to systematically reassess mobility while improving the client's ROM. In addition, bathing usually requires that extremities and joints are put through complete ROM.

Unless contraindicated, the care plan includes moving the client's extremities through the fullest ROM possible. ROM exercises are active, passive, or somewhere in between. With a weak client, for example, the nurse supports an extremity while the client performs the movement. Some clients are able to move some joints actively, whereas the nurse passively moves others. In general, exercises need to be as active as health and mobility allow.

Text continued on p. 1274

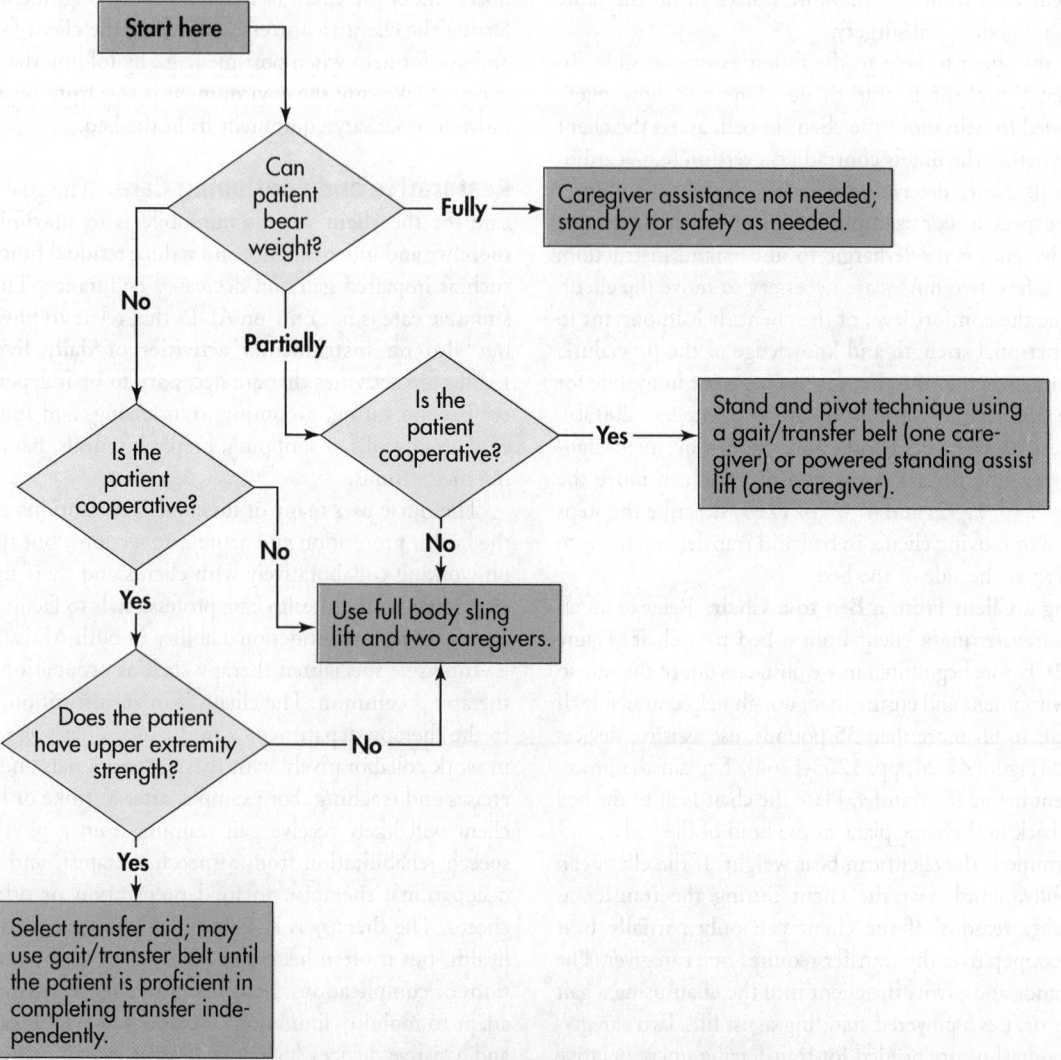

Start here

Can patient bear weight? — **Fully** → Caregiver assistance not needed; stand by for safety as needed.

No

Partially

Is the patient cooperative? — **Yes** → Stand and pivot technique using a gait/transfer belt (one caregiver) or powered standing assist lift (one caregiver).

Is the patient cooperative?

No

Yes

No

Use full body sling lift and two caregivers.

Does the patient have upper extremity strength? — **No**

Yes

Select transfer aid; may use gait/transfer belt until the patient is proficient in completing transfer independently.

- For seated transfer aid, must have chair with arms that recess or are removable.
- For full body sling lift, select a lift that was specifically designed to access a patient from the car (if the car is the starting or ending destination).
- If patient has partial weight-bearing capacity, transfer toward stronger side.
- Toileting slings are available for toileting.
- Mesh slings are available for bathing.
- During any patient transferring task, if any caregiver is required to lift more than 35 lb of a patient's weight, then the patient should be considered to be fully dependent and assistive devices should be used for the transfer.

Figure 47-23 Algorithm used to transfer client to and from the bed to chair, chair to toilet, chair to chair, or car to chair. (From Nelson A: *Safe patient handling and movement algorithms*, 2006, VISN8 Patient Safety Center, http://www.visn8.med.va.gov/patientsafetycenter/SafePtHandling/default.asp.)

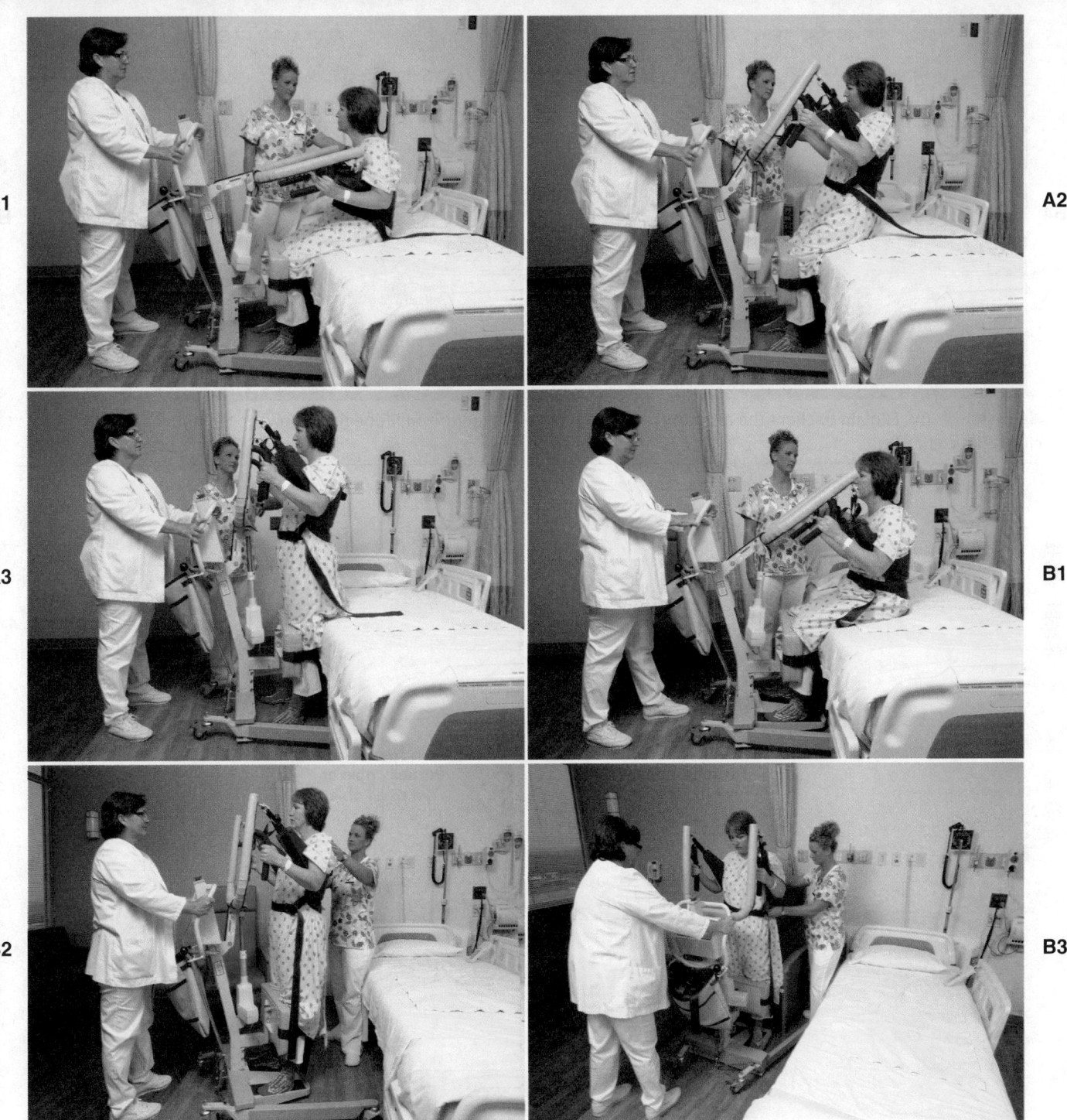

Figure 47-24 **A1,** Ensure safety straps are secured appropriately when using motorized lift to help client move to standing position. **A2,** Client grasps handles as nurse enables motorized lift. **A3,** Client is in standing position with feet on floor and is ready to ambulate to chair with nurses' help. **B1,** When client is unable to walk, secure safety straps, and use platform of motorized lift. **B2,** Client in upright position. **B3,** Position client in front of chair.

Continued

B4   B5

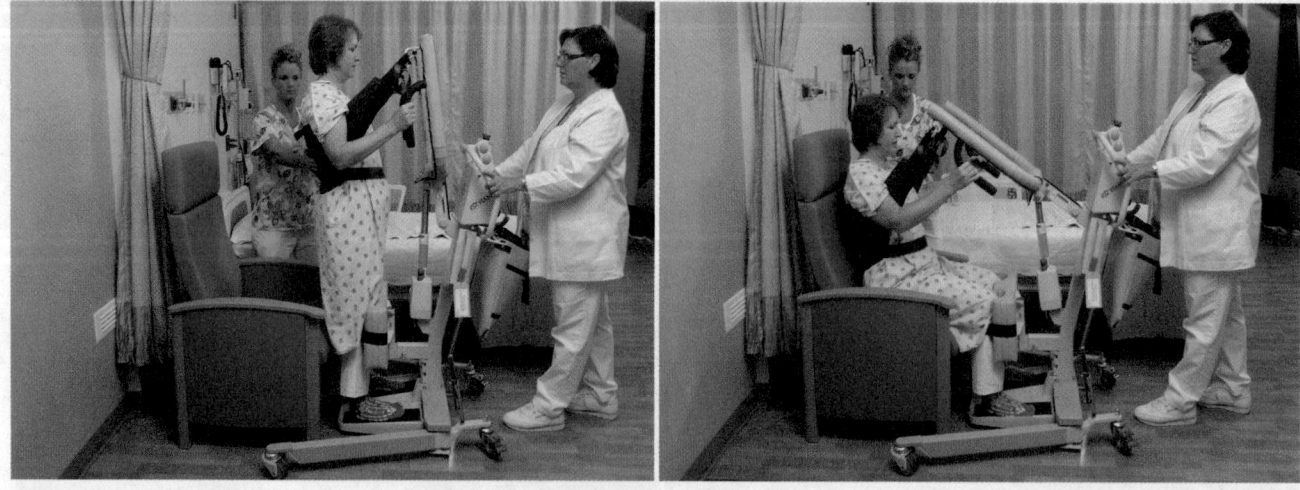

Figure 47-24 B4, Explain to client the need to hold on to handles as motorized lift begins to lower client into chair. **B5,** Guide client into chair.

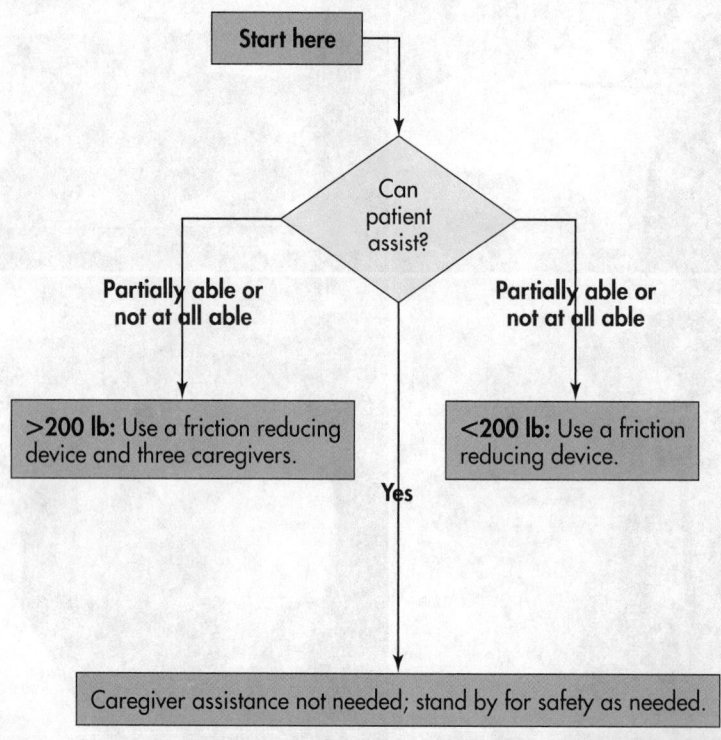

Figure 47-25 Algorithm used to complete lateral transfer to and from bed to stretcher, trolley. (From Nelson A: *Safe patient handling and movement algorithms,* 2006, VISN8 Patient Safety Center, http://www.visn8.med.va.gov/patientsafetycenter/SafePtHandling/default.asp.)

✳ SKILL 47-2   USING SAFE AND EFFECTIVE TRANSFER TECHNIQUES

Delegation Considerations
The skill of effective transfer techniques can be delegated. Clients who are transferred for the first time after prolonged bed rest, extensive surgery, critical illness, or spinal cord trauma usually require supervision by the nurse. Advise nursing assistive personnel:
- To follow safe client handling policies when moving clients
- About client limitations that affect safe transfer techniques

Equipment
- Transfer belt, sling, or friction-reducing device (as needed), nonskid shoes, bath blankets, and pillows
- Wheelchair: Position chair at 45-degree angle to bed, lock brakes, remove footrests, lock bed brakes
- Stretcher: Position next to bed, lock brakes on stretcher and on bed
- Mechanical/hydraulic lift: Use frame, canvas strips or chains, and hammock or sling

STEPS	RATIONALE
1. Assess the client for the following:	Provides information relative to the client's abilities, physical status, ability to comprehend, and the number of individuals needed to provide safe transferring.
a. Muscle strength (legs and upper arms)	Immobile clients have decreased muscle strength, tone, and mass. Affects ability to bear weight or raise body.
b. Joint mobility and contracture formation	Immobility or inflammatory processes (e.g., arthritis) sometimes lead to contracture formation and impaired joint mobility.
c. Paralysis or paresis (spastic or flaccid)	Client with central nervous system damage often has bilateral paralysis (requiring transfer by swivel bar, sliding bar, friction-reducing device, or mechanical [Hoyer] lift) or unilateral paralysis (belt transfer) to "best" side. Weakness (paresis) requires stabilization of knee while transferring. Flaccid arm needs to be supported with sling during transfer.
d. Orthostatic hypotension	Determines risk of fainting or falling during transfer.
e. Activity tolerance	Determines ability of client to assist with transfer.
f. Level of comfort	Pain reduces client's motivation and ability to be mobile. Pain relief before transfer enhances client participation.
g. Vital signs	Vital sign changes such as increased pulse and respiration indicate activity intolerance (see Chapter 32).

2. Assess client's sensory status:
  a. Adequacy of central and peripheral vision
  b. Adequacy of hearing
  c. Loss of peripheral sensation
	Visual field loss decreases client's perception and ability to see in direction of transfer. Peripheral sensation loss decreases proprioception. Clients with visual and hearing losses need transfer techniques adapted to deficits.

Critical Decision Point: Some clients with hemiplegia "neglect" one side of the body (inattention to or unawareness of one side of body or environment), which distorts perception of the visual field.

3. Assess client's cognitive status.	Determines client's ability to follow directions and learn transfer techniques.

4. Assess client's level of motivation:
  a. Is client eager or unwilling to be mobile?
  b. Does client avoid activity and offer excuses?
	Altered psychological states (e.g., depression, dementia) reduce client's desire to engage in activity.

5. Refer to appropriate safe client handling algorithm, and assess previous mode of transfer (if applicable).	Determines mode of transfer and assistance required to provide continuity.
6. Assess client's specific risk of falling when transferred.	Certain conditions (e.g., neuromuscular deficits, motor weakness, calcium loss from long bones, cognitive and visual dysfunction, altered balance) increase risk of injury and influence number of caregivers and equipment needed for procedure.
7. Perform hand hygiene, and ensure bed's brakes are locked.	Reduces transmission of microorganisms and promotes client safety.
8. Explain procedure to client and what client is expected to do during the procedure.	Decreases anxiety, increasing client participation.
9. Determine number of people needed to assist with transfer; do not start procedure until all required caregivers are available.	Ensures safe client transfer.

Continued

✳ **SKILL 47-2** **USING SAFE AND EFFECTIVE TRANSFER TECHNIQUES—CONT'D**

STEPS	RATIONALE

10. Transfer client.
   A. **Assist cooperative client who can partially bear weight to sitting position with bed at waist level**

Critical Decision Point: If client can bear weight and move to a sitting position independently, allow client to move to sitting position on own and stand by and offer assistance (Nelson and Baptiste, 2006).

---

(1) Place client in supine position. Use assistance of additional caregiver if necessary.	Allows assessment of client's body alignment and indicates need for additional care, such as suctioning or hygiene needs.
(2) Face head of bed at a 45-degree angle, and remove pillows.	Proper positioning reduces twisting of your body when moving the client. Pillows cause interference when the client is sitting up in bed.
(3) Place feet apart with foot nearer bed behind other foot, continuing at a 45-degree angle to the head of the bed.	Improves balance and allows transfer of body weight as client is sitting up in bed.
(4) Place hand farther from client under shoulders, supporting client's head and cervical vertebrae.	Maintains alignment of head and cervical vertebrae and allows for even lifting of client's upper trunk.
(5) Place other hand on bed surface.	Provides support and balance.
(6) Raise client to sitting position by shifting weight from front to back leg.	Improves balance, overcomes inertia, and transfers weight in direction in which client is moved.
(7) Push against bed using arm that is on bed surface.	Divides activity between arms and legs and protects back from strain. Bracing one hand against mattress and pushing against it as client is lifted transfers part of weight from back muscles through arm onto mattress.

B. **Assist cooperative client who can partially bear weight to sitting position on side of bed with bed in low position**

(1) Turn client to side, using assistance of another caregiver if necessary; client needs to face nurse on side of bed that client will be sitting (see illustration).	Decreases amount of work needed to raise client to sitting position.
(2) Raise head of bed 30 degrees.	Prepares client to move to side of bed and protects from falling.
(3) Stand opposite client's hips. Turn diagonally so you face client and far corner of foot of bed.	Places your center of gravity nearer client. Reduces twisting of your body because you are facing direction of movement.

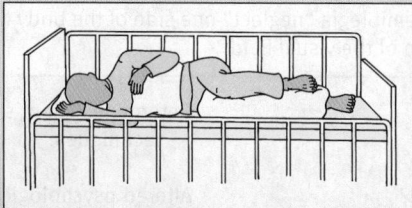

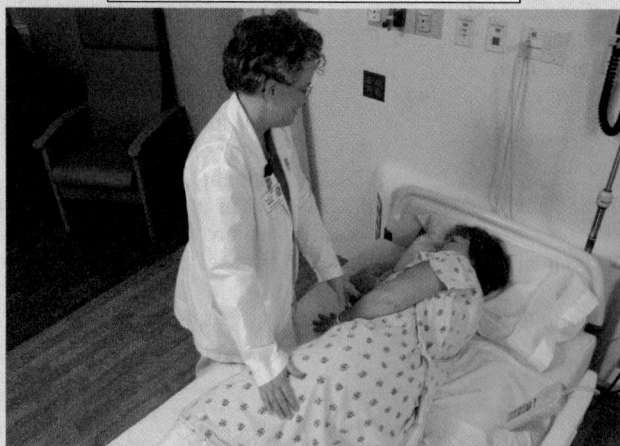

STEP 10B(1) Side-lying position.

☀ SKILL 47-2 **USING SAFE AND EFFECTIVE TRANSFER TECHNIQUES—CONT'D**

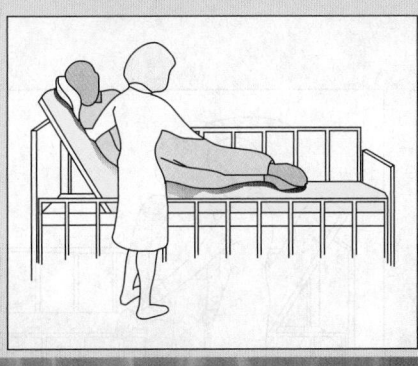

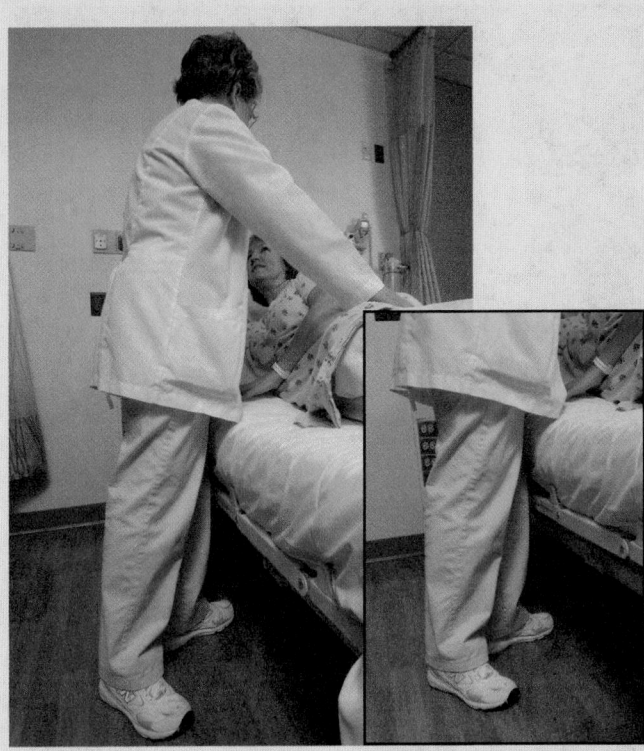

STEP 10B(4) Proper foot placement.

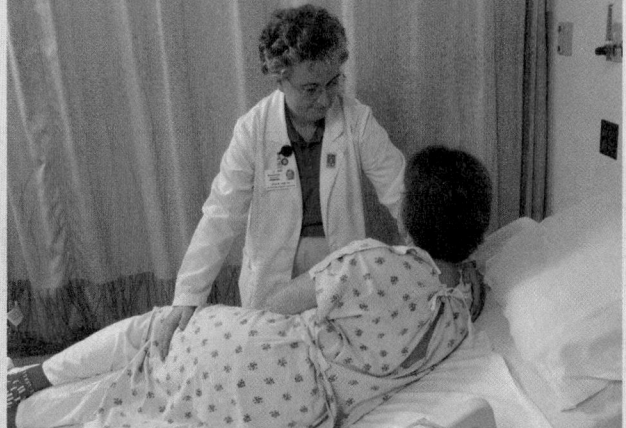

STEP 10B(6) Nurse places arm over client's thighs.

STEPS	RATIONALE
(4) Place feet apart with foot closer to head of bed in front of other foot (see illustration).	Increases balance and allows you to transfer weight as you bring client to a sitting position on side of bed.
(5) Place arm nearer head of bed under client's shoulders, supporting head and neck.	Maintains alignment of head and neck as you bring client to sitting position.
(6) Place other arm over client's thighs (see illustration).	Supports hip and prevents client from falling backward during procedure.
(7) Move client's lower legs and feet over side of bed. Pivot toward rear leg, allowing client's upper legs to swing downward.	Decreases friction and resistance. Weight of client's legs when off bed allows gravity to lower legs, and weight of legs assists in pulling upper body in sitting position.
(8) At same time, shift weight to rear leg and elevate client (see illustration).	Reduces client risk for falling. Some immobilized clients experience light-headedness or dizziness when assuming a sitting position.

C. Transfer cooperative client who is partially weight bearing from bed to chair with bed in low position (see algorithm, Figure 47-23, p. 1262)

Critical Decision Point: Allow client to transfer independently if able to fully bear weight. Stand by as needed to promote safe transfer (Nelson, 2003b).

(1) Assist client to sitting position on side of bed. Have chair in position at 45-degree angle to bed.	Positions chair within easy access for transfer.

Continued

✳ **SKILL 47-2**   USING SAFE AND EFFECTIVE TRANSFER TECHNIQUES—CONT'D

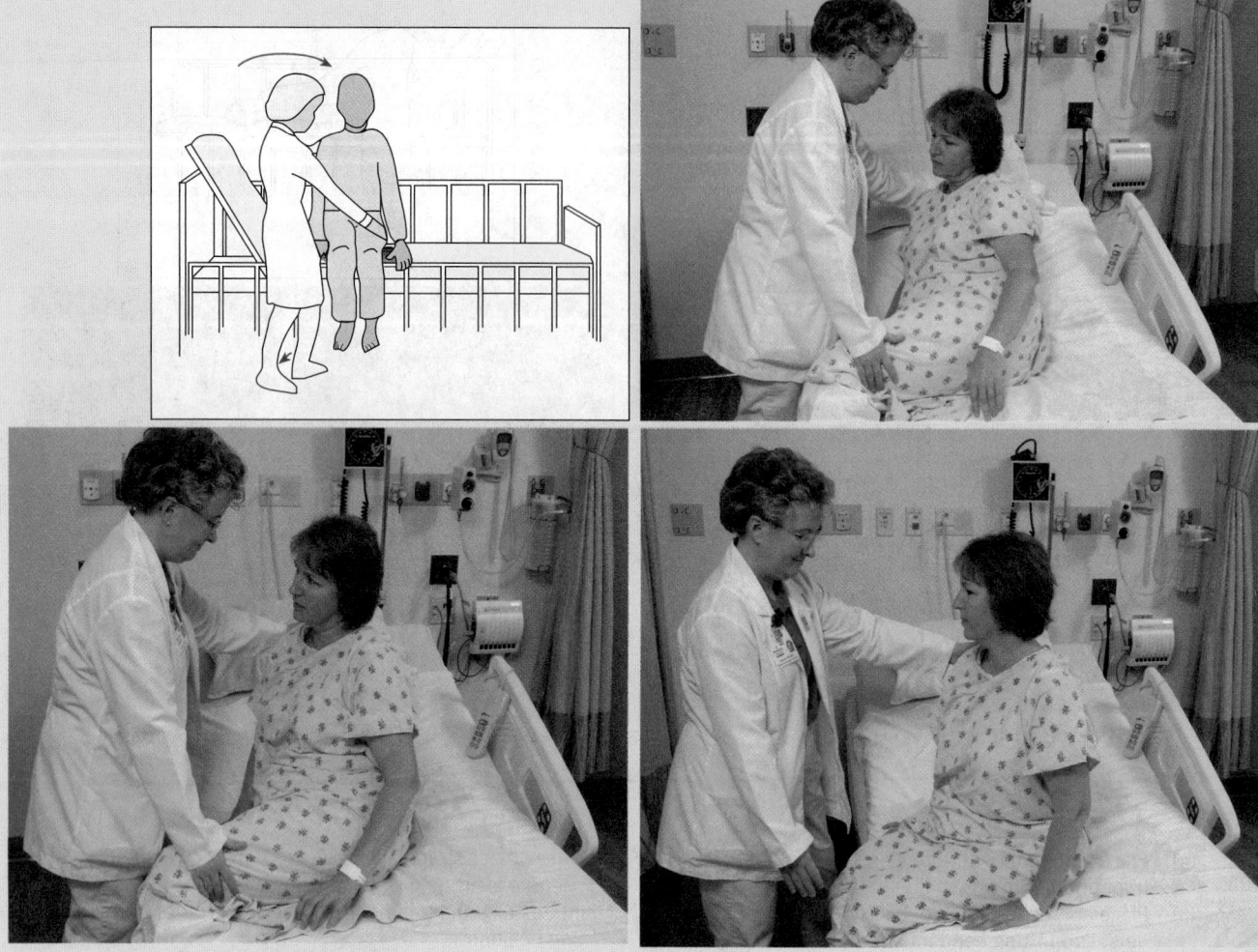

STEP 10B(8) A, Nurse guides client to sitting position. **B,** Nurse shifts weight to rear leg as client raises to sitting position. **C,** Nurse ensures client is steady when sitting upright.

STEPS	RATIONALE
(2) Apply transfer or gait belt.	Belt maintains stability of client during transfer. Client's arm needs to be in sling if flaccid paralysis is present.

Critical Decision Point: If client is overweight or nurse determines that use of transfer belt is not safe, move client from bed to wheel chair using powered standing-assist lift following manufacturer's guidelines (Nelson, 2003b).

---

(3) Ensure that client has stable nonskid shoes. Weight-bearing or strong leg is forward, with weak foot back.	Nonskid soles decrease risk of slipping during transfer. Always have client wear shoes during transfer; bare feet increase risk of falls. Client will stand on stronger, or weight-bearing, leg.
(4) Spread feet apart.	Ensures balance with wide base of support.

✳ **SKILL 47-2**   **USING SAFE AND EFFECTIVE TRANSFER TECHNIQUES—CONT'D**

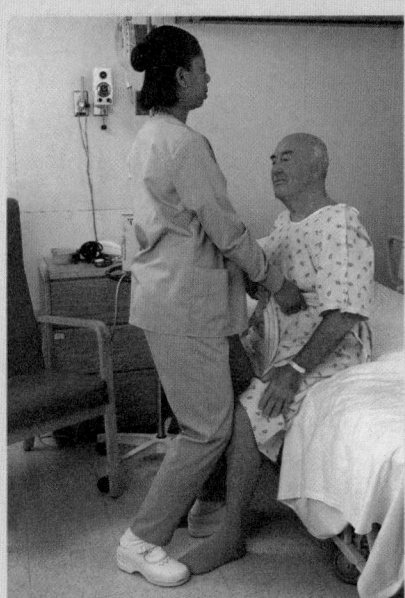

STEP 10C(5) Nurse flexes hips and knees, aligning knees with client's knees.

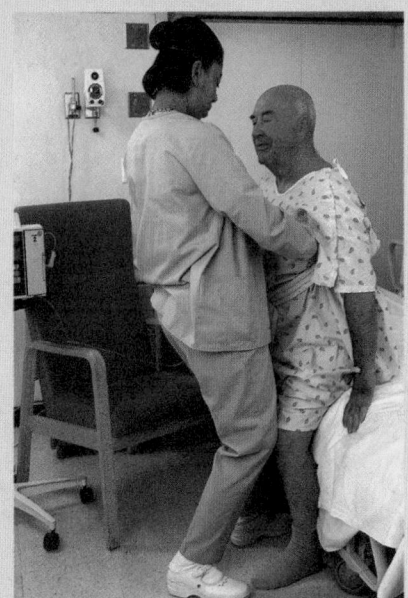

STEP 10C(7) Nurse rocks client to standing position.

STEPS	RATIONALE
(5) Flex hips and knees, aligning knees with client's knees (see illustration).	Flexion of knees and hips lowers the center of gravity to object to be raised; aligning knees with client's allows for stabilization of knees when client stands.
(6) Grasp transfer belt from underneath.	Grasp transfer at client's side to provide movement of client at center of gravity. Never lift clients with upper extremity paralysis or paresis by or under arms.
(7) Rock client up to standing position on count of three while straightening hips and legs and keeping knees slightly flexed (see illustration). Unless contraindicated, instruct client to use hands to push up.	Rocking motion gives client's body momentum and requires less muscular effort to lift client.
(8) Maintain stability of client's weak or paralyzed leg with knee.	Clients often maintain the ability to stand in paralyzed or weak limb with support of knee to stabilize.
(9) Pivot on foot farther from chair.	Maintains support of client while allowing adequate space for client to move.
(10) Instruct client to use armrests on chair for support, and ease into chair (see illustration).	Increases client stability.
(11) Flex hips and knees while lowering client into chair (see illustration).	Prevents injury to nurse from poor body mechanics.
D. Transfer cooperative client who cannot bear weight but who has upper extremity strength from bed to chair with bed in low position (see algorithm, Figure 47-23, p. 1262)	

Critical Decision Point: Verify that clients with spinal cord injuries are stabilized before transfer. Only experienced care providers should attempt to move these clients. If client is too weak, use motorized lift (see Figure 47-24, pp. 1263-1264).

(1) Remove arms from chair, or move them out of the way.	Allows client to slide from bed to chair.
(2) Assist client to sitting position on side of bed. Have chair in position at 45-degree angle to bed. Apply transfer or gait belt until client is able to transfer independently with ease.	Prepares client for transfer. Gait belt is used if needed to guide client during transfer.
(3) Using seated transfer aid, have client use upper body to slide from bed to chair. Follow manufacturer's directions for use of the transfer aid (see illustration).	Moves client safely into the chair (Nelson, 2003b).

Continued

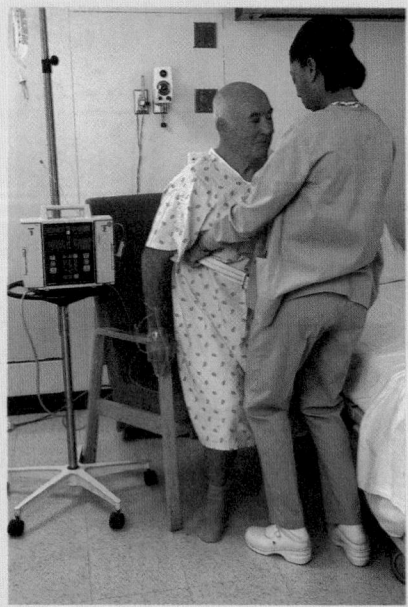

STEP 10C(10) Client uses armrests for support.

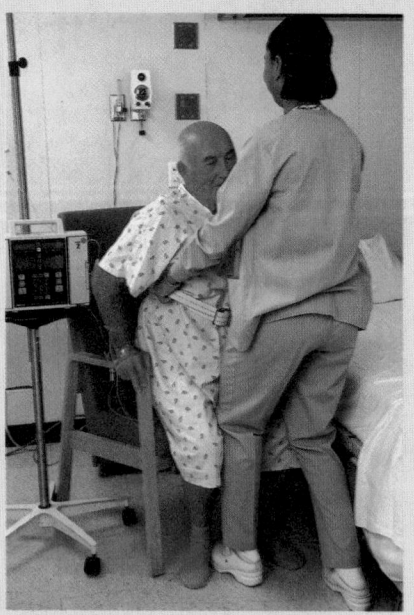

STEP 10C(11) Nurse eases client into chair.

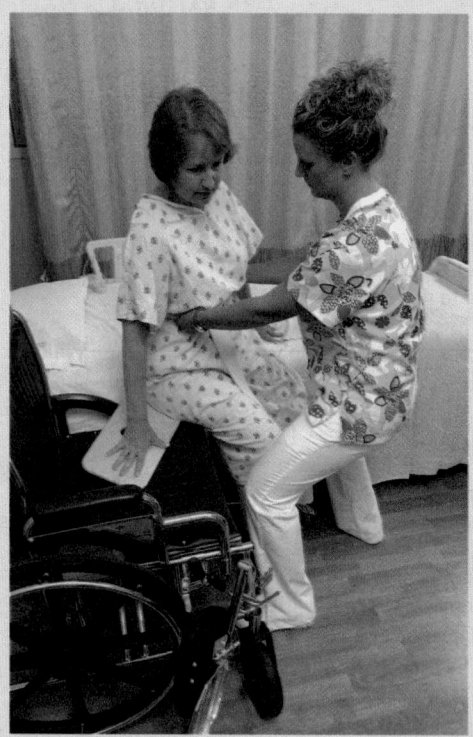

STEP 10D(3) Using friction-reducing device to transfer client from the bed to the chair.

✳ **SKILL 47-2** **USING SAFE AND EFFECTIVE TRANSFER TECHNIQUES—CONT'D**

STEPS	RATIONALE
E. **Use mechanical lift and full-body sling to transfer unco-operative client who can bear partial weight or client who cannot bear weight and is either uncooperative or does not have upper body strength into chair** (see algorithm, Figure 47-23, p. 1262)	

Critical Decision Point: This skill requires two caregivers. Do not start the skill until both caregivers are present and ready to assist the client (Nelson, 2003b).

(1) Position lift properly at bedside.	Ensures safe elevation of client off bed. (Before using lift, be thoroughly familiar with its operation.)
(2) Position chair near bed, and allow adequate space to maneuver lift.	Prepares environment for safe use of lift and subsequent transfer.
(3) Raise bed to high position with mattress flat. Lower side rail.	Maintains nurses' alignment during transfer.
(4) Roll client to side.	Allows positioning of client on mechanical/hydraulic sling.
(5) Place sling under client. Place lower edge under client's knees (wide piece) and upper edge under client's shoulders (narrow piece).	Places sling under client's center of gravity and greatest portion of body weight.
(6) Roll client to opposite side and pull body sling through.	Completes positioning of client on mechanical/hydraulic sling.
(7) Roll client supine onto canvas seat.	Sling needs to extend from shoulders to knees (hammock) to support client's body weight equally.
(8) Remove client's glasses, if appropriate.	Swivel bar is close to client's head and will possibly break eyeglasses.
(9) If using a transportable Hoyer lift, place lift's horseshoe-shaped base under side of bed (on side with chair).	Positions lift efficiently and promotes smooth transfer.
(10) Lower upper horizontal bar to sling level following manufacturer's directions. Some lifts require valve to be locked.	Positions lift close to client. Locking valve prevents injury to client.
(11) Attach hooks on strap to holes in sling. Short straps hook to top holes of sling; longer straps hook to bottom of sling.	Secures hydraulic lift to sling.
(12) Elevate head of bed.	Positions client in sitting position.
(13) Fold client's arms over chest.	Prevents injury to paralyzed arms.
(14) Use lift to raise client off bed (see illustration).	Positions client in sitting position.
(15) Move lift to chair.	Moves client from bed to chair.
(16) Position client, and lower slowly into chair following manufacturer's guidelines (see illustration).	Places client safely into chair.

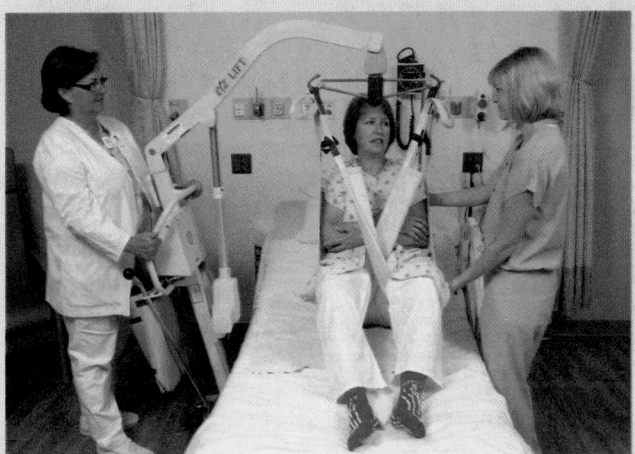

STEP 10E(14) Use mechanical lift to raise the client off the bed.

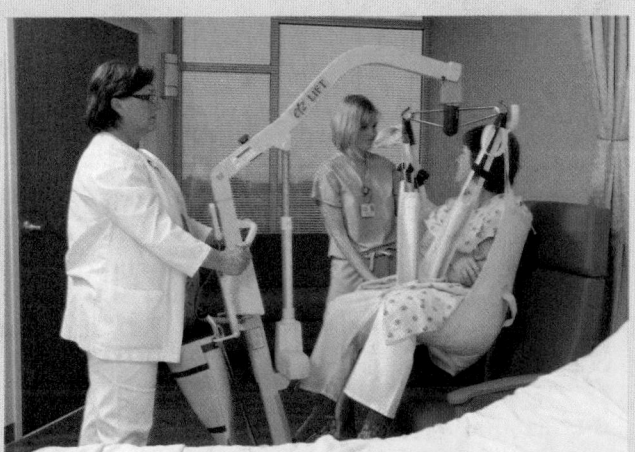

STEP 10E(16) Use mechanical lift to lower client into chair.

Continued

✳ **SKILL 47-2**   **USING SAFE AND EFFECTIVE TRANSFER TECHNIQUES—CONT'D**

STEPS	RATIONALE
(17) Remove straps and mechanical/hydraulic lift.	Prevents damage to skin and underlying tissues from canvas or hooks.
(18) Check client's sitting alignment and correct if necessary.	Prevents injury from poor posture.
F. Transfer client from bed to stretcher (bed at stretcher level) (see algorithm, Figure 47-25, p. 1264)	

Critical Decision Point: Allow client to transfer to stretcher independently if possible. Only proceed with this skill if client is unable to move to stretcher on own (Nelson, 2003b).

---

(1) Place bed flat, and position at same level as stretcher. Ensure bed brakes are locked.	Bed and stretcher need to be at same level to allow client to slide from bed to stretcher.
(2) Lower side rails. Two caregivers stand on the side where the stretcher will be while third caregiver stands on the other side.	Minimizes caregivers' stretching. Prevents client from falling out of bed and promotes safety.
(3) Two caregivers help client roll onto side toward one caregiver.	Positions client for friction-reducing lateral transfer device.
(4) Caregivers work together to position friction-reducing device properly under client's back following manufacturer's guidelines (see illustrations).	Client needs to be placed on transfer device properly to allow safe transfer.

A

B

C

D

STEP 10F(4) A, Two caregivers position sliding board under client. **B,** Two caregivers place air-assisted device under client. **C,** Client rolls to opposite side while other caregiver unrolls air-assisted device. **D,** Secure safety straps.

※ **SKILL 47-2**   **USING SAFE AND EFFECTIVE TRANSFER TECHNIQUES—CONT'D**

STEPS

(5)   Roll stretcher along the side of the bed. Lock wheels of stretcher once it is in place. Instruct the client not to move.

(6)   All three caregivers place feet widely apart with one slightly in front of the other, and grasp the friction-reducing device.

(7)   On the count of three, caregivers pull the client from the bed onto the stretcher using the friction-reducing device and shifting weight from front foot to back foot (see illustration).

(8)   Put up side rail of stretcher on side where caregivers are, then roll stretcher away from side of bed and put side rails up on that side.

(9)   Cover client with sheet or blanket.

RATIONALE

Positions stretcher in correct position for transfer and prevents client from falling out of bed.

Prepares for transfer. Wide base of support allows nurse to shift weight and minimizes back strain.

Transfers client smoothly and efficiently to the stretcher.

Side rails prevent client from falling off stretcher.

Promotes comfort and preserves client dignity.

A

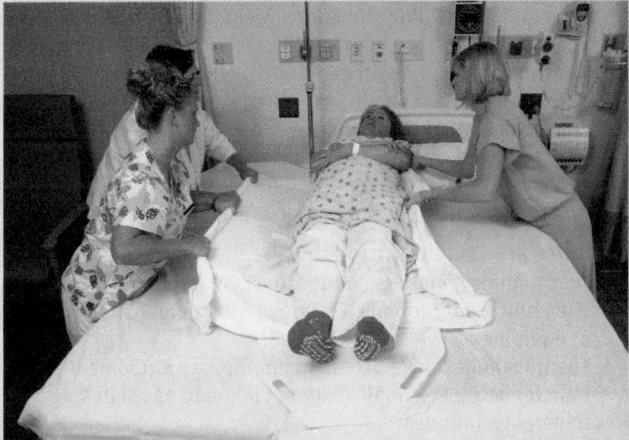

B

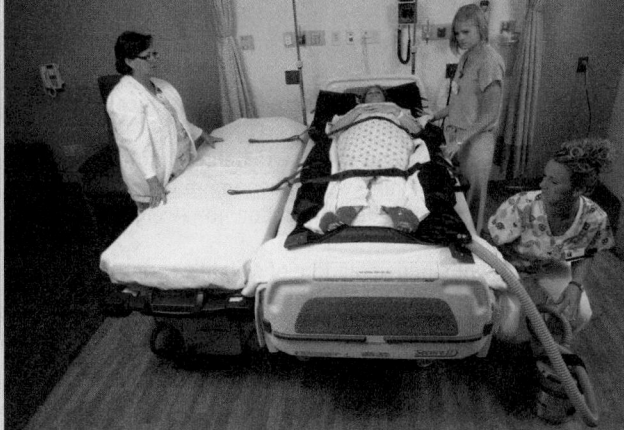

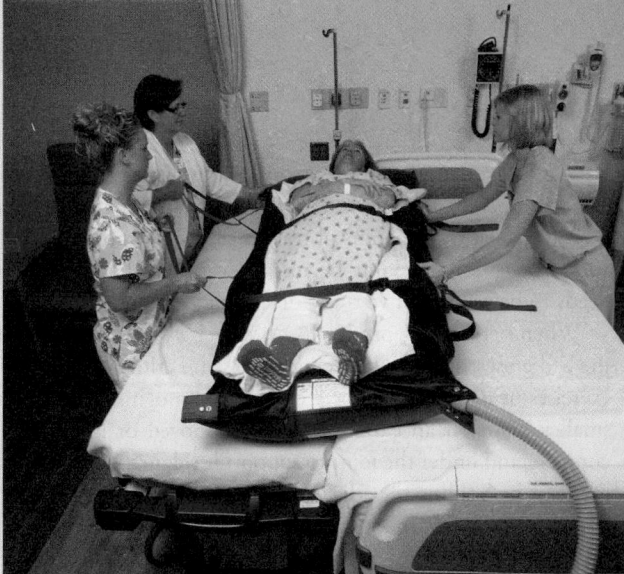

C

STEP 10F(7) A, Transfer of client from bed to stretcher using sliding board. **B,** Inflating air-assisted transfer device. **C,** Transfer of client using air-assisted transfer device.

Continued

✳ SKILL 47-2   USING SAFE AND EFFECTIVE TRANSFER TECHNIQUES—CONT'D

STEPS	RATIONALE
11. Perform hand hygiene.	Reduces transmission of microorganisms.
12. With each transfer evaluate client's tolerance and level of fatigue and comfort. Praise the client's progress, effort, or performance.	Increased activity often results in symptoms associated with activity intolerance (e.g., increased pulse, changes in blood pressure, increased respirations, and decreased level of comfort). Some clients find transfer very fatiguing and will need posttransfer interventions to restore their level of comfort. Continue encouragement provides incentives for client cooperation and participation in care.
13. Following each transfer, evaluate client's body alignment.	Prompt identification of poor alignment reduces risks to the client's skin and musculoskeletal systems.

Unexpected Outcomes and Related Interventions

1. Client sustains injury on transfer.
   a. Provide appropriate care to client (e.g., apply cool compress, place appropriate dressing on skin tear)
   b. Evaluate incident that caused injury (e.g., assessment inadequate, change in client status, improper use of equipment) and change next transfer techniques to prevent injury.
   c. Complete occurrence report according to institution policy.
2. Client is too weak to transfer.
   a. Physical impairments require increased assistance from nursing personnel.
   b. Increase bed activity and exercise to heighten tolerance.
3. Client who needs to be non–weight bearing (e.g., following hip fracture) continues to bear weight on non–weight-bearing limb.
   a. Reassess client's understanding of weight-bearing status.
   b. Reinforce information and provide client education as needed.
4. Client transfers well on some occasions, poorly on others.
   a. Assess client for fatigue or pain before transfer
   b. Allow client to rest or medicate for pain before transferring if indicated.
5. Localized areas of erythema develop that do not disappear quickly.
   a. Implement evidence-based care of pressure sores (see Chapter 48).

Recording and Reporting

- Record procedure, including pertinent observations: weakness, ability to follow directions, weight-bearing ability, balance, ability to pivot, number of personnel needed to assist, and amount of assistance (muscle strength) required in nurses' notes.
- Report any unusual occurrence to nurse in charge. Report transfer ability and assistance needed to next shift or other caregivers. Report progress or remission to rehabilitation staff (physical therapist or occupational therapist).

Home Care Considerations

- Teach family members about safe client handling and how to use equipment properly. Observe return demonstration of use of equipment.
- Ensure families have access to appropriate equipment (e.g., transfer belts, mechanical lifts) at home to assist in safe transfer techniques.

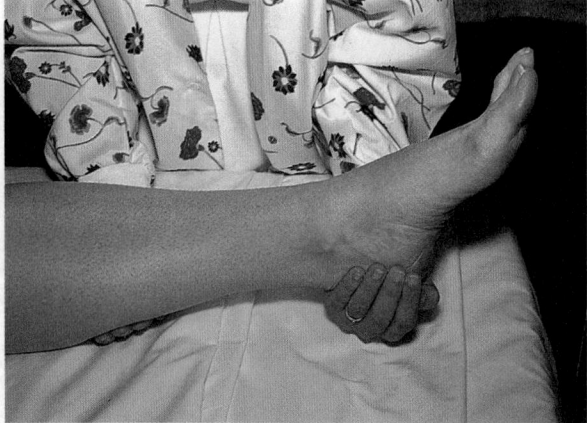

Figure 47-26 Using a cupped hand to support a joint.

Passive ROM exercises begin as soon as the client's ability to move the extremity or joint is lost. Carry out movements slowly and smoothly, just to the point of resistance; ROM should not cause pain. Never force a joint beyond its capacity. Each movement needs to be repeated five times during the session.

When performing passive ROM exercises, stand at the side of the bed closest to the joint being exercised. Perform passive ROM exercises using a head-to-toe sequence and moving from larger to smaller joints. If an extremity is to be moved or lifted, place a cupped hand under the joint to support it (Figure 47-26), support the joint by holding the adjacent distal and proximal areas (Figure 47-27), or support the joint with one hand and cradle the distal portion of the extremity with the remaining arm (Figure 47-28). See Table 47-2, p. 1232, for detailed ROM and illustrated motion for each joint. Appropriate ROM exercises are based on the client and the affected joint. For example, when caring for a client with limited shoulder mobility, you need to provide support devices for the shoulder, such as slings when the client is standing or sitting or pillows when the client is in bed. Correctly positioning the

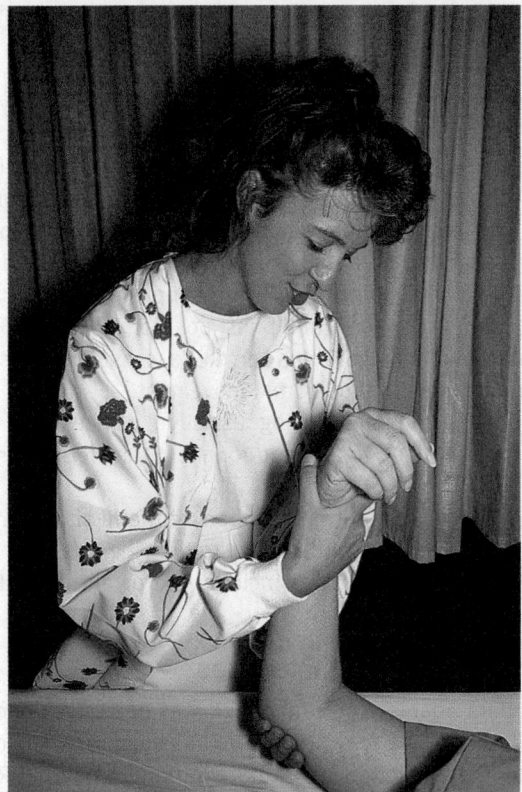

Figure 47-27 Supporting the joint by holding the distal and proximal areas adjacent to the joint.

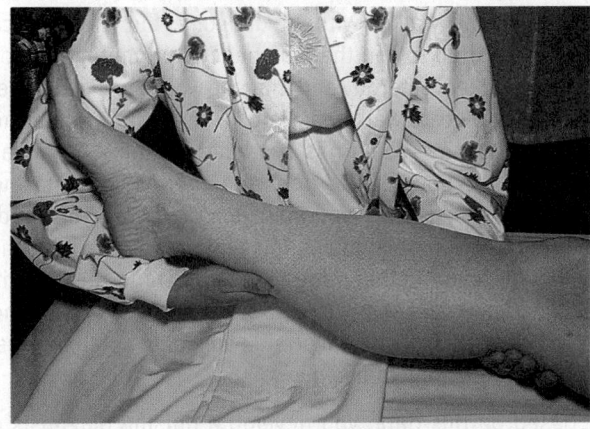

Figure 47-28 Cradling the distal portion of an extremity.

shoulder prevents pain, joint dislocation, and further changes in body alignment.

Walking. When a client has a limited ability to walk, assess the client's activity tolerance, tolerance to the upright position (orthostatic hypotension), strength, presence of pain, coordination, and balance to determine the amount of assistance needed. Explain how far the client should try to walk, who is going to help, when the walk will take place, and why walking is important. In addition, determine with the client how much independence the client can assume.

Check the environment to be sure that there are no obstacles in the client's path. Clear chairs, over-bed tables, and wheelchairs out of the way so that the client has ample room to walk safely. Before starting, establish rest points in case activity tolerance is less than estimated or the client becomes dizzy. For example, place a chair in the hall for the client to rest if needed. A nurse who does not have a lot of strength and who is unable to ambulate a client alone needs to request help and ensure the client has an assistive device such as a walker (see Chapter 37). The two nurses stand on either side of the client, and each holds one side of the gait belt.

Provide support at the waist by using a **gait belt** so that the client's center of gravity remains midline. While walking, the client should not lean to one side because this alters the center of gravity, distorts balance, and increases the risk of falling. Return a client who at any point appears unsteady or complains of dizziness to a nearby bed or chair. If the client faints or begins to fall, assume a wide base of support with one foot in front of the other, thus supporting the body weight. Then gently lower the client to the floor, protecting the head. Although lowering a client to the floor is not difficult, the nursing student needs to practice this technique with a friend or classmate before attempting it in a clinical setting.

Clients with **hemiplegia** (one-sided paralysis) or **hemiparesis** (one-sided weakness) often need assistance with walking. Always stand on the client's affected side, and support the client by using a gait belt. Providing support by holding the client's arm is incorrect because the nurse cannot easily support the client's weight to lower the client to the floor if the client faints or falls. In addition, if the client falls with the nurse holding an arm, a shoulder joint may be dislocated.

◆ Evaluation

To evaluate outcomes and response to nursing care, compare the client's actual outcomes with the outcomes selected during planning, such as the client's ability to maintain or improve body alignment, joint mobility, walking, moving, or transferring. Evaluate the effectiveness of specific interventions designed to promote body alignment, improve mobility, and protect the client from the hazards of immobility. Evaluate the client's and family's understanding of all teaching provided as well (Figure 47-29). The continuous nature of evaluation allows you to determine whether new or revised therapies are required and if new nursing diagnoses have developed. When outcomes are not met, consider asking the following questions:

- Tell me why you have been unable to increase your activity as we had planned.
- What activities are you having trouble completing right now?
- Tell me how you feel about not being able to dress yourself and make your own meals.
- What exercises do you find most helpful?
- What goals for your activity would you like to set now?

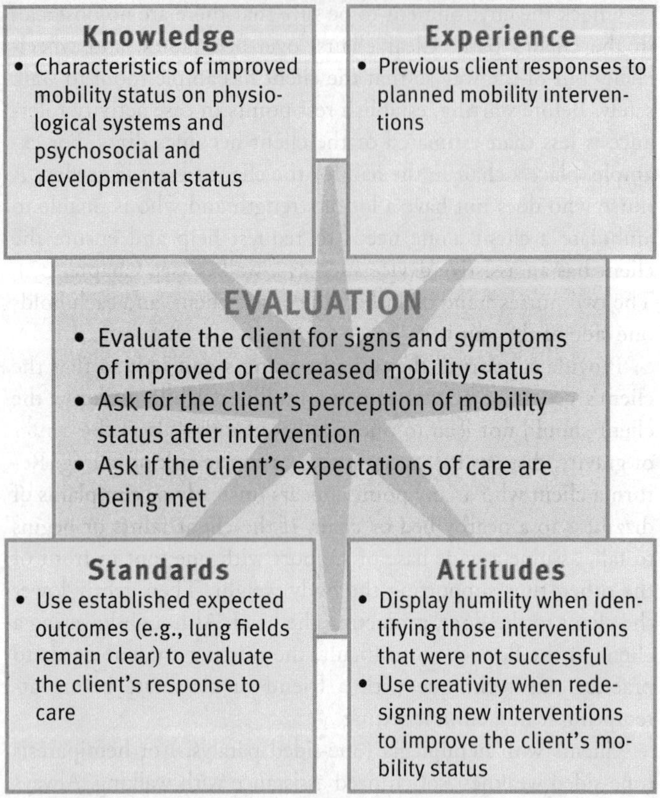

Knowledge	Experience
• Characteristics of improved mobility status on physiological systems and psychosocial and developmental status	• Previous client responses to planned mobility interventions

EVALUATION

- Evaluate the client for signs and symptoms of improved or decreased mobility status
- Ask for the client's perception of mobility status after intervention
- Ask if the client's expectations of care are being met

Standards	Attitudes
• Use established expected outcomes (e.g., lung fields remain clear) to evaluate the client's response to care	• Display humility when identifying those interventions that were not successful • Use creativity when redesigning new interventions to improve the client's mobility status

Figure 47-29 Critical thinking model for immobility evaluation.

Key Concepts

- Body mechanics are the coordinated efforts of the musculoskeletal and nervous systems as the person moves, lifts, bends, stands, sits, lies down, and completes daily activities.
- Findings from evidence-based nursing research about safe client handling prevents injuries to nurses and clients when moving and transferring clients.
- The skeletal system provides bony support structure for movement, attachment of ligaments and muscles, protection of vital organs, some of the regulation of calcium, and production of red blood cells.
- The nervous system provides initiation and voluntary control of movement.
- Coordination and regulation of muscle groups depend on muscle tone; activity of antagonistic, synergistic, and antigravity muscles; and neural input to muscles.
- Body alignment is the condition of joints, tendons, ligaments, and muscles in various body positions.
- Balance occurs when there is a wide base of support, the center of gravity falls within the base of support, and a vertical line falls from the center of gravity through the base of support.
- Developmental stages influence body alignment and mobility; the greatest impact of physiological changes on the musculoskeletal system is observed in children and older adults.
- The risk of disabilities related to immobilization depends on the extent and duration of immobilization and the client's overall level of health.

- Immobility sometimes results from illness or trauma or is prescribed for therapeutic reasons.
- Immobility presents hazards in the physiological, psychological, and developmental dimensions.
- The nursing process and critical thinking assist in providing care for clients who are experiencing or are at risk for the adverse effects of impaired body alignment and immobility.
- Clients with impaired body alignment require nursing interventions to maintain them in the supported Fowler's, supine, prone, side-lying, and Sims' positions.
- Client movement algorithms serve as assessment tools and guide safe client handling and movement.
- Appropriate friction-reducing assistive devices and mechanical lifts need to be used for client transfers when applicable.
- No-lift policies benefit all members of the health care system: clients, nurses, and administration.
- Range-of-motion exercises include one or all of the body joints.

Critical Thinking Exercises

Ms. Barbara Adams, 84 years of age, has been a resident on the skilled care unit for a week. She has been receiving rehabilitation therapy following a total hip replacement (THR) for osteoarthritis. The staples to her incision were removed 5 days ago, and the incision continues to show signs of healing (e.g., no swelling, redness, warmth, or drainage). Although Ms. Adams is progressing with her therapy, she still is able to walk only 400 feet in the hallway with her walker. She was initially able to use the walker without difficulty, but the physical therapist reported to you that she needed prompting on how to use the walker yesterday and that she was very discouraged about her inability to walk unassisted. The certified nurses aid tells you that Ms. Adams has not been finishing her meals over the past 2 days due to poor appetite. As you enter her room today, she states, "Go away. I am tired of all this, and I just want to stay in bed today." You explore why she feels this way. You discover that she does not understand the benefits of being mobile, and she is unable to describe how to use her walker. She states, "I still am afraid I am going to fall because I keep forgetting how to use my walker."

1. Based on this data, you develop a nursing diagnosis of deficient knowledge (use of walker and effects of mobility) related to lack of recall. Identify one goal, two expected outcomes, and three related nursing interventions with rationale that will help her meet the identified goal and outcomes.

2. You finish teaching Ms. Adams about the hazards of immobility, and you begin your morning assessment. As you are assessing her skin, you notice that she has a 2-cm reddened area on her coccyx. The skin in this area is intact, and you find no other reddened areas anywhere else.
   a. How would you document this finding?
   b. What risk factors contribute to this finding?
   c. What will you do next?

3. You convince Ms. Adams to get out of bed and sit in her chair for 30 minutes. Describe the decision-making process you will use to determine the safest way to transfer her. Include essential assessment data you will need before transferring her into her chair.

✳ NCLEX®-Style Review Questions

1. Which of the following laboratory values would you expect in a client experiencing prolonged immobility?
   1. Calcium 11.5 mg/dL
   2. Sodium 142 mmol/L
   3. Hemoglobin 14.6 g/dL
   4. Potassium 4.2 mmol/L

2. A client has been on bed rest for several days. The client stands, and the nurse notes that the client's systolic pressure drops 20 mm Hg. Which of the following should the nurse document in the medical record?
   1. Rebound hypotension
   2. Positional hypotension
   3. Orthostatic hypotension
   4. Central venous hypotension

3. The nurse puts elastic stockings on a client following major abdominal surgery. The nurse teaches the client that the stockings are used after a surgical procedure to:
   1. Prevent varicose veins
   2. Prevent muscular atrophy
   3. Ensure joint mobility and prevent contractures
   4. Facilitate the return of venous blood to the heart

4. You are caring for a client who has osteoporosis. The nurse is teaching her about ways to prevent fractures. Which of the following client statements reflects a need for further education?
   1. "I usually go swimming with my family at the YMCA 3 times a week."
   2. "I need to ask my doctor if I need to have a bone mineral density check this year."
   3. "If I don't drink milk at dinner, I will eat broccoli or cabbage to get the calcium that I need in my diet."
   4. "The more frequently I walk, the more likely I will be to fall and break my leg. I think I will get a wheelchair so I don't have to walk any more."

5. The client at greatest risk for developing adverse effects of immobility is a:
   1. 3-year-old child with a fractured femur
   2. 78-year-old man in traction for a broken hip
   3. 48-year-old woman following a thyroidectomy
   4. 38-year-old woman undergoing a hysterectomy

6. A client who was in a car accident and broke his femur has been immobilized for 5 days. When the nurse gets this client out of bed for the first time, a nursing diagnosis related to the safety of this client will be:
   1. Pain
   2. Impaired skin integrity
   3. Altered tissue perfusion
   4. Risk for activity intolerance

7. A client had a left-sided cerebral vascular accident 3 days ago and is receiving 5000 units of heparin subcutaneously every 12 hours to prevent thrombophlebitis. The client is receiving enteral feedings through a small-bore nasogastric tube because of dysphagia. Which of the following symptoms requires the nurse to call the health care provider immediately?
   1. Hematuria
   2. Unilateral neglect
   3. Limited ROM in the right hip
   4. Coughing up moderate amount clear, thin sputum

8. A home care nurse is preparing the home for a client who is going home following a left hip replacement. The client is cooperative and can partially bear weight. What should the nurse order from the home medical supply company to help the client move from the bed to the chair?
   1. A trapeze bar
   2. A small transfer board
   3. A powered standing-assist device
   4. An ankle foot orthotic (AFO) for the affected foot

9. The nurse is caring for a client who has right-sided weakness. The nurse needs to help the client walk. What should the nurse do while walking with the client?
   1. Hold the client's left hand while walking
   2. Hold the client's right hand while walking
   3. Put a gait belt on the client and provide support on the left side
   4. Put a gait belt on the client and provide support on the right side

10. Before transferring a client from the bed to a stretcher, which assessment data does the nurse need to gather? (Choose all that apply.)
    1. The client's weight
    2. How cooperative the client is
    3. The client's nutritional status
    4. The presence of intravenous (IV) tubes

48 | Skin Integrity and Wound Care

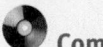

Skin, the body's largest organ, constitutes 15% of the total adult body weight (Wysocki, 2007). It is a protective barrier against disease-causing organisms, a sensory organ for pain, temperature, and touch, and it synthesizes vitamin D. Injury to the skin poses risks to safety and triggers a complex healing response. One of the nurse's most important responsibilities is to monitor skin integrity and to plan, implement, and assess interventions to maintain skin integrity. Knowing normal wound healing helps in identifying conditions requiring nursing intervention.

Scientific Knowledge Base

Skin

The skin has two layers: the epidermis and the dermis (Figure 48-1). These two layers are separated by a membrane, often referred to as the dermal-epidermal junction. The epidermis, or the top layer, has several layers. The stratum corneum is the thin, outermost layer of the epidermis. It consists of flattened, dead, keratinized cells. The cells originate from the innermost epidermal layer, commonly called the basal layer. Cells in the basal layer divide, proliferate, and migrate toward the epidermal surface. After cells reach the stratum corneum, they flatten and die. This constant movement ensures replacement of surface cells sloughed during normal desquamation or shedding. The thin stratum corneum protects underlying cells and tissues from dehydration and prevents entrance of certain chemical agents. The stratum corneum allows evaporation of water from the skin and permits absorption of certain topical medications.

The dermis, the inner layer of the skin, provides tensile strength, mechanical support, and protection to the underlying muscles, bones, and organs. It differs from the epidermis in that it contains mostly connective tissue and few skin cells. **Collagen** (a tough, fibrous protein), blood vessels, and nerves are in the dermal layer. Fibroblasts, which are responsible for collagen formation, are the only distinctive cell type within the dermis.

Understanding skin structure helps you to maintain skin integrity and promote wound healing. Intact skin protects the client from chemical and mechanical injury. When the skin is injured, the epidermis functions to resurface the wound and restore the barrier against invading organisms while the dermis responds to restore the structural integrity (collagen) and the physical properties of the skin. Age alters skin characteristics and makes skin more vulnerable to damage. Box 48-1 provides a summary of the changes in aging skin.

Pressure Ulcers

Pressure ulcer, pressure sore, decubitus ulcer, and *bedsore* are terms used to describe impaired skin integrity related to unrelieved, prolonged pressure. The most current terminology is **pressure ulcer** (Figure 48-2), which is consistent with the recommendations of the pressure ulcer guidelines written by the Wound, Ostomy and Continence Nurses Society (WOCN) (2003). A pressure ulcer is localized injury to the skin and other underlying tissue, usually over a body prominence, as a result of pressure or pressure in combination with shear and/or friction. A number of

---

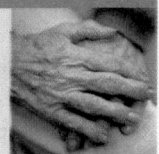

✳ BOX 48-1   FOCUS ON OLDER ADULTS

Skin-Associated Issues

- Age-related changes, such as reduced skin elasticity, decreased collagen, and thinning of underlying muscle and tissues, cause the older adult's skin to be easily torn in response to mechanical trauma, especially shearing forces (Wysocki, 2007).
- Concomitant medical conditions and polypharmacy, which is common in the older adult, are factors that interfere with wound healing.
- The attachment between the epidermis and dermis becomes flattened in older adults, allowing the skin to be easily torn in response to mechanical trauma (e.g., tape removal).
- Aging causes a diminished inflammatory response, resulting in slow epithelialization and wound healing (Doughty and Sparks-Defriese, 2007).
- The hypodermis decreases in size with age. Older clients have little subcutaneous padding over bony prominences, so they are more prone to skin breakdown (Wysocki, 2007).
- Reduced nutritional intake, commonly seen in older adults, increases risk for pressure ulcer development and impaired wound healing (Posthauer and Thomas, 2004).

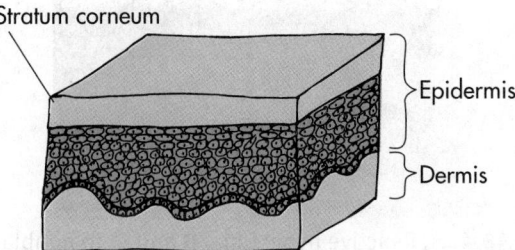

Figure 48-1 Layers of skin. (From Pires M, Muller A: Detection and management of early tissue pressure indicators: a pictorial essay, *Progressions* 3[3]:3, 1991.)

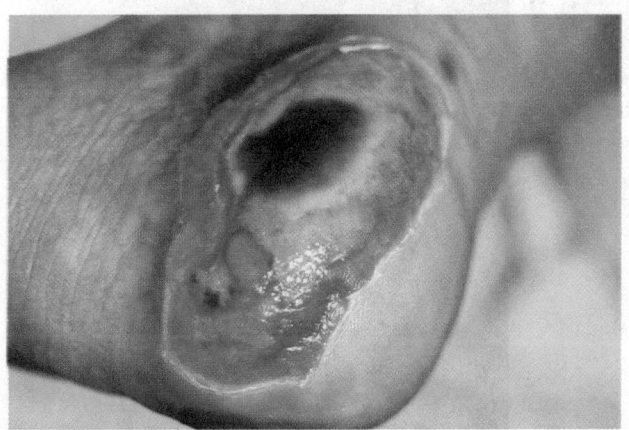

Figure 48-2 Pressure ulcer with tissue necrosis.

contributing factors are also associated with pressure ulcers; the significance of these factors is yet to be elucidated (National Pressure Ulcer Advisory Panel [NPUAP], 2007a). Any client experiencing decreased mobility, decreased sensory perception, fecal or urinary incontinence, and/or poor nutrition is at risk for pressure ulcer development.

There are many factors contributing to the formation of a pressure ulcer. Pressure is the major cause in pressure ulcer formation. Tissues receive oxygen and nutrients and eliminates metabolic wastes via the blood. Any factor that interferes with blood flow in turn interferes with cellular metabolism and the function or life of the cells. Prolonged, intense pressure affects cellular metabolism by decreasing or obliterating blood flow, resulting in tissue ischemia and ultimately tissue death.

Pathogenesis of Pressure Ulcers.
Pressure is the major element in the cause of pressure ulcers. Three pressure-related factors contribute to pressure ulcer development: (1) pressure intensity, (2) pressure duration, and (3) tissue tolerance.

Pressure Intensity. A classic research study identified capillary closing pressure as the minimal amount of pressure required to collapse a capillary (e.g., when the pressure exceeds the normal capillary pressure range of 15 to 32 mm Hg) (Burton and Yamada, 1951). Therefore, if the pressure applied over a capillary exceeds the normal capillary pressure, and the vessel is occluded for a prolonged period of time, **tissue ischemia** can occur. If the client has reduced sensation and cannot respond to the discomfort of the ischemia, tissue ischemia and tissue death result.

The clinical presentation of obstructed blood flow occurs when evaluating areas of pressure. After a period of tissue ischemia, if the pressure is relieved and the blood flow returns, the skin turns red. The effect of this redness is vasodilation (blood vessel expansion), called hyperemia (redness) (Figure 48-3, *A*). Evaluate the area of hyperemia by pressing a finger over the af-

fected area. If the area blanches (turns lighter in color), (Figure 48-3, *B*) and the erythema returns when you remove your finger, the hyperemia is transient and is an attempt to overcome the ischemic episode, thus called blanching hyperemia (Pieper, 2007). If, however, the erythematous area does not blanch (nonblanching erythema) (Figure 48-4) when you apply pressure, deep tissue damage is probable.

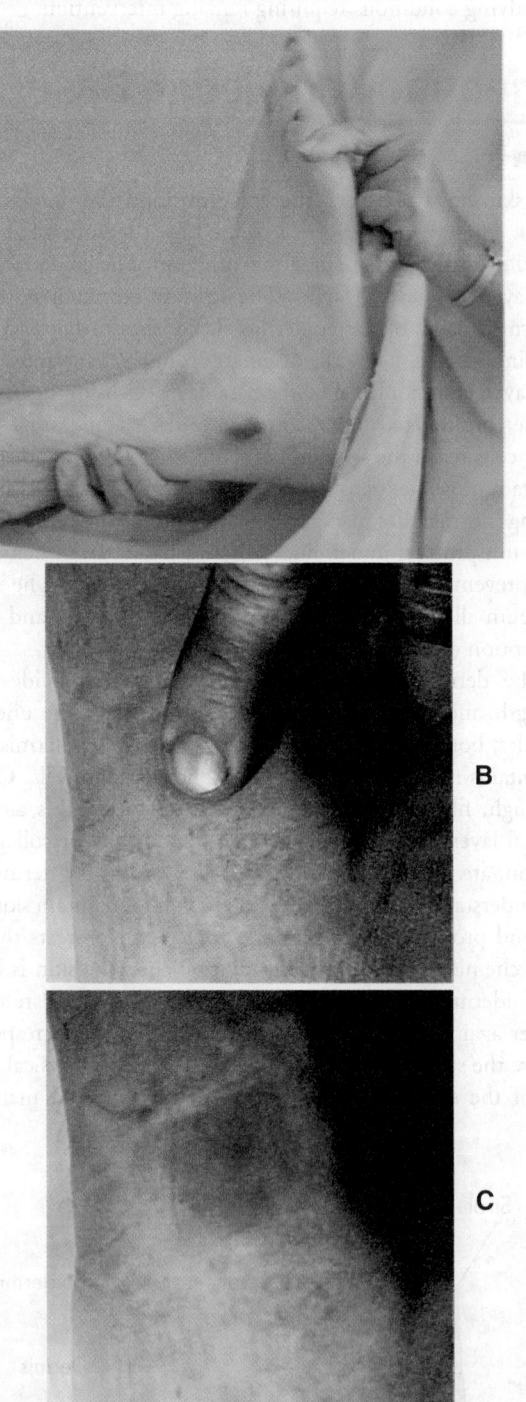

Figure 48-4 **A,** Reactive hyperemia. **B** and **C,** In nonblanching erythema the area is much darker than the surrounding skin and does not blanch with fingertip pressure. (From Pires M, Muller A: Detection and management of early tissue pressure indicators: a pictorial essay, *Progressions* 3[3]:3, 1991.)

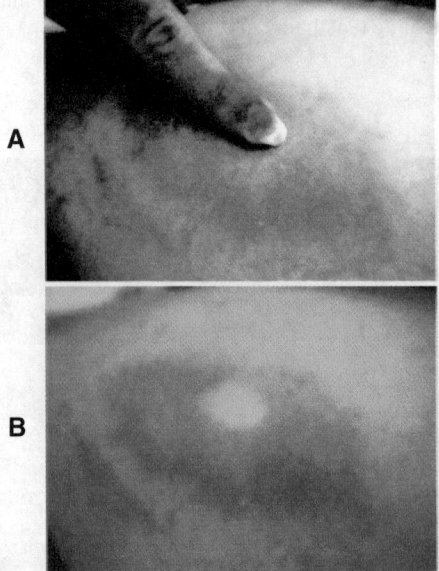

Figure 48-3 **A,** Reactive hyperemia. **B,** Blanches with fingertip pressure, blanching erythema.

Blanching occurs when the normal red tones of the light-skinned client are absent. Blanching does not occur in clients with darkly pigmented skin. The Task Force on the Implications for Darkly Pigmented Intact Skin in the Prediction and Prevention of Pressure Ulcers (Bennett, 1995) defined **darkly pigmented skin** as skin that "remains unchanged (does not blanch) when pressure is applied over a bony prominence, irrespective of the client's race or ethnicity." Characteristics of intact dark skin that alert nurses to the potential for pressure ulcers are in Box 48-2.

Pressure Duration. There are two considerations related to the duration of pressure. Low pressures over a prolonged time period cause tissue damage, as well as high-intensity pressure over a short period of time. Extended pressure occludes blood flow and nutrients and contributes to cell death (Pieper, 2007). Clinical implications of pressure duration include evaluating the amount of pressure (checking skin for reactive hyperemia) and determining the amount of time that a client tolerates pressure (checking to be sure after relieving pressure that the affected area blanches).

Tissue Tolerance. The ability of tissue to endure pressure depends upon the integrity of the tissue and the supporting structures. The extrinsic factors of shear, friction, and moisture affect the ability of the skin to tolerate pressure: the greater degree to which the factors of shear, friction, and moisture are present, the more susceptible the skin will be to damage from pressure. The second factor related to tissue tolerance pertains to the ability of the underlying skin structures (blood vessels, collagen) to assist in redistributing pressure. Systemic factors such as poor nutrition, increased aging, and low blood pressure affect the tissue's tolerance to externally applied pressure.

Risk Factors for Pressure Ulcer Development. A variety of factors predispose a client to pressure ulcer formation. These factors are often directly related to disease, such as decreased level of consciousness, related to the after-effects of trauma, the presence of a cast, or secondary to an illness, such as decreased sensation following a cerebrovascular accident.

✳ BOX 48-2 Characteristics of Dark Skin at Risk for Skin Breakdown

Assessment Issues
Natural or halogen light source best for assessing skin
Avoid fluorescent light source, because it casts a bluish hue, making accurate assessment difficult

Color
Appears darker than surrounding skin
Has purplish/bluish hue

Temperature
Initial warmth when compared with surrounding skin
Later coolness as tissue is devitalized

Touch	Appearance
Indurated	Taut
Edema	Shiny
Soft, boggy	Scaly

Modified from Bennett MA: Report of the Task Force on the Implications for Darkly Pigmented Intact Skin in the Prediction and Prevention of Pressure Ulcers, *Adv Wound Care* 8(6):34, 1995.

Impaired Sensory Perception. Clients with altered sensory perception for pain and pressure are more at risk for impaired skin integrity than clients with normal sensation. Clients with impaired sensory perception of pain and pressure are unable to feel when a portion of their body senses increased, prolonged pressure or pain. Thus the client without the ability to feel or sense that there is pain or pressure is at risk for the development of pressure ulcers.

Impaired Mobility. Clients unable to independently change positions are at risk for pressure ulcer development. For example, clients with spinal cord injuries have decreased or absent motor and sensory impairment and are unable to reposition off bony prominences.

Alteration in Level of Consciousness. Clients who are confused or disoriented, or who have changing levels of consciousness, are unable to protect themselves from pressure ulcer development. Clients who are confused or disoriented are sometimes able to feel pressure but are not always able to understand how to relieve it or communicate their discomfort. Clients in a coma cannot perceive pressure and are unable to move voluntarily to relieve pressure.

Shear. Shear is the force exerted parallel to skin resulting from both gravity pushing down on the body and resistance (friction) between the client and a surface (Pieper, 2007). For example, shear force occurs when the head of the bed is elevated and the sliding of the skeleton starts but the skin is fixed because of friction with the bed (Figure 48-5). In addition, shear force also occurs when transferring a client from bed to stretcher and the client's skin is pulled across the bed. When shear is present, the skin and subcutaneous layers adhere to the surface of the bed, and the layers of muscle and the bones slide in the direction of body movement. The underlying tissue capillaries are stretched and angulated by the shear force. As a result, necrosis occurs deep within the tissue layers. The tissue damage occurs deep in the tissues, causing undermining of the dermis.

Friction. The force of two surfaces moving across one another, such as the mechanical force exerted when skin is dragged across a coarse surface such as bed linens is called **friction** (WOCN, 2003). Unlike shear injuries, friction injuries affect the epidermis or top layer of the skin. The denuded skin appears red and painful and is sometimes referred to as a "sheet burn." A friction injury occurs in clients who are restless, in those who have uncontrollable movements, such as spastic conditions, and in

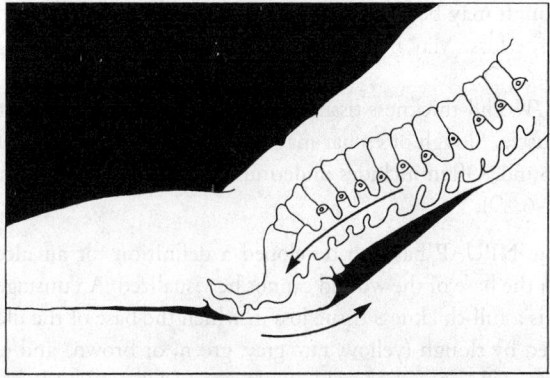

Figure 48-5 As you elevate the head of the bed, the skeleton slides down while the skin stays fixed, resulting in shearing.

those whose skin is dragged rather than lifted from the bed surface during position changes.

Moisture. The presence and duration of moisture on the skin increases the risk of ulcer formation. Moisture reduces the skin's resistance to other physical factors such as pressure and/or shear force. Prolonged moisture softens skin, making it more susceptible to damage. Immobilized clients, who are unable to perform their own hygiene needs, depend on the nurse to keep the skin dry and intact. Skin moisture originates from wound drainage, excessive perspiration, and fecal or urinary incontinence.

Classification of Pressure Ulcers

You need to assess pressure ulcers at regular intervals using systematic parameters to evaluate wound healing, plan appropriate interventions, and evaluate progress. Assessment includes depth of tissue involvement (staging), type and approximate percentage of tissue in wound bed, wound dimensions, exudate description, and condition of surrounding skin.

One method for assessment of a pressure ulcer is the use of a staging system. Staging systems for pressure ulcers are based on describing the depth of tissue destroyed. Accurate staging requires knowledge of the skin layers, and a major drawback of a staging system is that you cannot stage an ulcer covered with necrotic tissue because the necrotic tissue is covering the depth of the ulcer. The necrotic tissue must be debrided or removed to expose the wound base to allow for assessment.

The National Pressure Ulcer Advisory Panel (NPUAP) (2007a) has advanced a four-stage classification system. Pressure ulcer staging describes the pressure ulcer depth at the point of assessment. Thus once you have staged the pressure ulcer, this stage endures even as the pressure ulcer heals. Pressure ulcers do not progress from a stage III to a stage I, rather a stage III ulcer demonstrating signs of healing is described as a healing stage III pressure ulcer (Nix, 2007).

Stage I: Intact skin with nonblanchable redness of a localized area, usually over a bony prominence. Darkly pigmented skin may not have visible blanching; its color may differ from surrounding area (Figure 48-6, *A*).

Stage II: Partial-thickness skin loss involving epidermis, dermis, or both. The ulcer is superficial and presents clinically as an abrasion, blister, or shallow crater (Figure 48-6, *B*).

Stage III: Full-thickness tissue loss. Subcutaneous fat may be visible, but bone, tendon, or muscle are not exposed. Slough may be present but does not obscure the depth of tissue loss. May include undermining and tunneling (Figure 48-6, *C*).

Stage IV: Full-thickness tissue loss with exposed bone, tendon, or muscle. Slough or eschar may be present on some parts of the wound. Often includes undermining and tunneling (Figure 48-6, *D*).

The NPUAP has also developed a definition for an ulcer in which the base of the wound cannot be visualized. An unstageable ulcer is a full-thickness tissue loss in which the base of the ulcer is covered by slough (yellow, tan, gray, green, or brown) and/or eschar (tan, brown, or black) in the wound bed. Until enough slough and/or eschar is removed to expose the base of the wound,

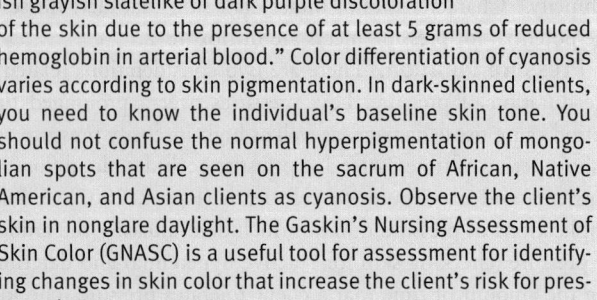

✳ BOX 48-3   CULTURAL ASPECTS OF CARE

Skin Color Impact

Detecting cyanosis and other changes in skin color in clients is an important clinical skill. However, this detection becomes a challenge in dark-skinned clients. Cyanosis is "a slightly bluish grayish slatelike or dark purple discoloration of the skin due to the presence of at least 5 grams of reduced hemoglobin in arterial blood." Color differentiation of cyanosis varies according to skin pigmentation. In dark-skinned clients, you need to know the individual's baseline skin tone. You should not confuse the normal hyperpigmentation of mongolian spots that are seen on the sacrum of African, Native American, and Asian clients as cyanosis. Observe the client's skin in nonglare daylight. The Gaskin's Nursing Assessment of Skin Color (GNASC) is a useful tool for assessment for identifying changes in skin color that increase the client's risk for pressure ulcers.

Implications for Practice

- Cyanosis is difficult but possible to detect in the dark-skinned client.
- Be aware of situations that produce changes in skin tone, such as inadequate lighting.
- Examine body sites with the least melanin, such as under the arm, for underlying color identification.
- Evaluate pigmented skin for color-specific changes in skin tone.

Modified from Gaskin FC: Detection of cyanosis in the person with dark skin, *J Natl Black Nurses Assoc* 1:52, 1986; and Henderson CT and others: Draft definition of stage I pressure ulcers: inclusion of persons with darkly pigmented skin, *Adv Wound Care* 10(5):16, 1997

the true depth and therefore the stage cannot be determined (NPUAP, 2007a).

In addition, Bennett (1995) suggests that when assessing clients with darkly pigmented skin, proper lighting is important to accurately assess the skin (see Box 48-2). Either natural light or a halogen light is recommended. This prevents the blue tones that fluorescent light sources produce on darkly pigmented skin, which interferes with accurate assessment. Additional aspects of assessing dark skin are in Box 48-3.

For a wound with nonviable tissue, you will need to assess the type of tissue in the wound base, because this information will be used to plan appropriate interventions. The assessment of tissue type includes the amount (percentage) and appearance (color) of viable and nonviable tissue. **Granulation tissue** is red moist tissue composed of new blood vessels, the presence of which indicates progression toward healing. Soft yellow or white tissue is characteristic of **slough** (stringy substance attached to wound bed), and you will need to remove this before the wound is able to heal. Black or brown necrotic tissue is **eschar,** which you will also need to remove before healing can proceed.

The measurement of the size of the wound provides overall changes in size, which is an indicator for wound healing progress (Nix, 2007). Use disposable wound-measuring devices to obtain measurement of width and length. Measure depth by using a cotton-tipped applicator in the wound bed.

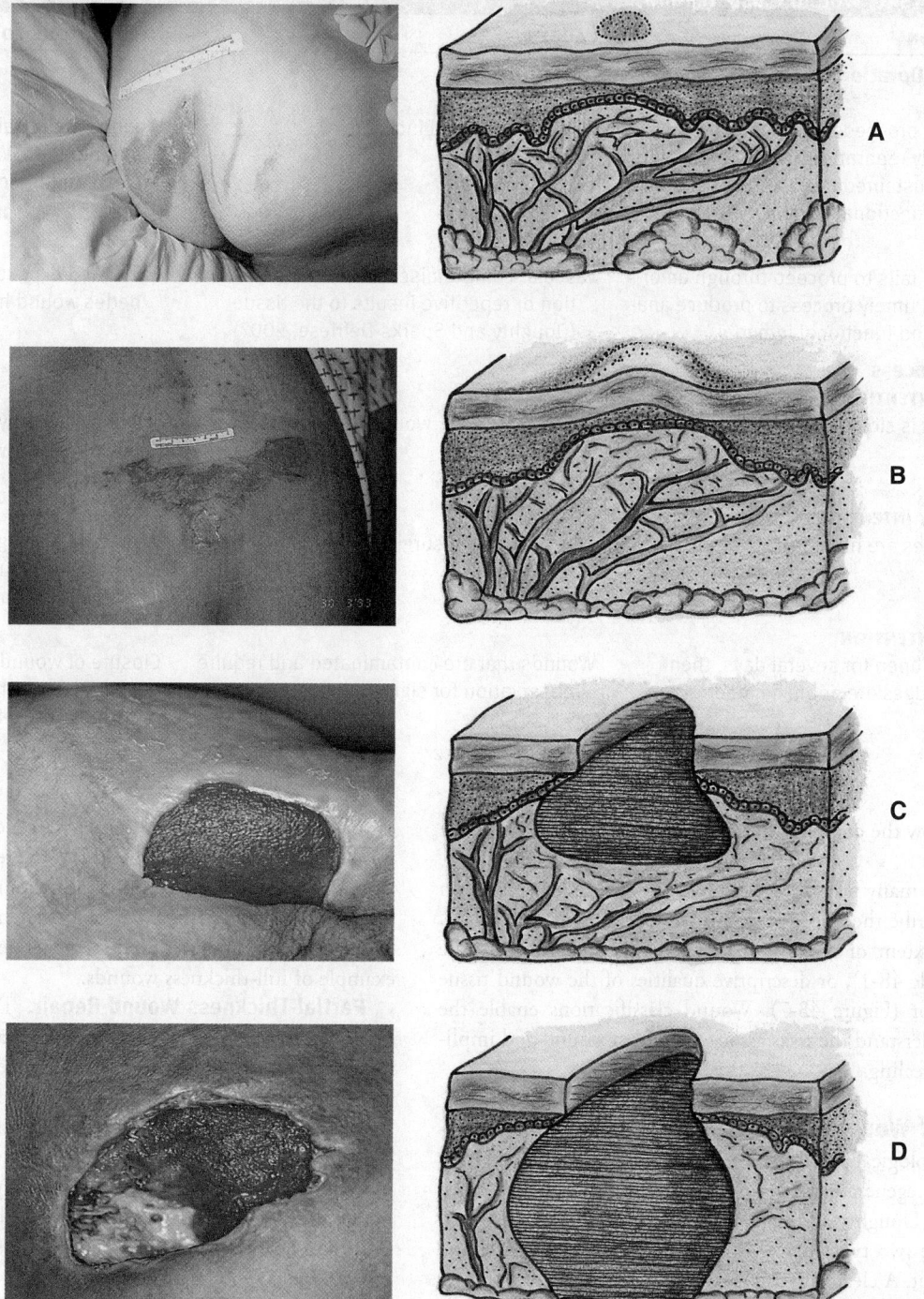

Figure 48-6 Diagram of stages. **A,** Stage I pressure ulcer. **B,** Stage II pressure ulcer. **C,** Stage III pressure ulcer. **D,** Stage IV pressure ulcer. (Courtesy Laurel Wiersma, RN, MSN, Clinical Nurse Specialist, Barnes-Jewish Hospital, St. Louis, Mo.)

Wound **exudate** describes the amount, color, consistency, and odor of wound drainage and is part of the wound assessment. Excessive exudate indicates the presence of infection. Finally, evaluate the condition of the skin surrounding the wound for redness, warmth, maceration, or edema (swelling). The presence of any of these factors on the skin surrounding the wound is indicative of wound deterioration.

Wound Classifications

A **wound** is a disruption of the integrity and function of tissues in the body (Baharestani, 2004). It is imperative for the nurse to know that *all wounds are not created equal.* Understanding the etiology of a wound is important, because the treatment for the wound varies depending on the underlying disease process. Some treatments are even harmful to certain wounds, so the nurse always

---

✳ **TABLE 48-1 Wound Classification**

DESCRIPTION	CAUSES	IMPLICATIONS FOR HEALING
Onset and Duration		
ACUTE Wound that proceeds through an orderly and timely reparative process that results in sustained restoration of anatomical and functional integrity	Trauma, a surgical incision	Wounds are usually easily cleaned and repaired. Wound edges are clean and intact.
CHRONIC Wound that fails to proceed through an orderly and timely process to produce anatomical and functional integrity	Vascular compromise, chronic inflammation or repetitive insults to the tissue (Doughty and Sparks-Defriese, 2007)	Continued exposure to insult impedes wound healing.
Healing Process		
PRIMARY INTENTION Wound that is closed	Surgical incision, wound that is sutured or stapled	Healing occurs by epithelialization; heals quickly with minimal scar formation.
SECONDARY INTENTION Wound edges are not approximated	Pressure ulcers, surgical wounds that have tissue loss	Wound heals by granulation tissue formation, wound contraction, and epithelialization.
TERTIARY INTENTION Wound left open for several days, then wound edges are approximated	Wounds that are contaminated and require observation for signs of inflammation	Closure of wound is delayed until risk of infection is resolved (Doughty and Sparks-Defriese, 2007).

needs to know the complete history, including the etiology of the wound.

There are many ways to classify wounds. Wound classification systems describe the status of skin integrity, cause of the wound, severity or extent of tissue injury or damage, cleanliness of the wound (Table 48-1), or descriptive qualities of the wound tissue such as color (Figure 48-7). Wound classifications enable the nurse to understand the risks associated with a wound and implications for healing.

Process of Wound Healing. Wound healing involves integrated physiological processes. The tissue layers involved and their capacity for regeneration determine the mechanism for repair for any wound (Doughty and Sparks-Defriese, 2007).

There are two types of wounds: those with loss of tissue and those without. A clean surgical incision is an example of a wound with little tissue loss. The surgical wound heals by **primary intention.** The skin edges are **approximated,** or closed, and the risk of infection is low. Healing occurs quickly, with minimal scar formation, as long as infection and secondary breakdown is prevented (Doughty and Sparks-Defriese, 2007). In contrast, a wound involving loss of tissue, such as a burn, pressure ulcer, or severe laceration, heals by **secondary intention.** The wound is left open until it becomes filled by scar tissue. It takes longer for a wound to heal by secondary intention, and thus the chance of infection is greater. If scarring from secondary intention is severe, there is often permanent loss of tissue function (Figure 48-8).

Wound Repair. Partial-thickness wounds are shallow wounds involving loss of the epidermis (top layer) and possibly partial loss

of the dermis. These wounds heal by regeneration because epidermis regenerates. An example of this is the repair of a clean surgical wound or an abrasion. Full-thickness wounds extending into the dermis (involving both layers of tissue) heal by scar formation because deeper structures do not regenerate. Pressure ulcers are an example of full-thickness wounds.

Partial-Thickness Wound Repair. There are three components involved in the healing process of a partial-thickness wound: inflammatory response, epithelial proliferation (reproduction) and migration, and reestablishment of the epidermal layers.

Tissue trauma causes the *inflammatory response*, which in turn causes redness and swelling to the area with a moderate amount of serous exudate. This response is generally limited to the first 24 hours after wounding. The epithelial cells begin to regenerate, providing new cells to replace the lost cells. This *epithelial proliferation and migration* starts at both the wound edges and the epidermal cells lining the epidermal appendages, allowing for quick resurfacing. Epithelial cells begin to migrate across the wound bed soon after the wound occurs. A wound left open to air can resurface within 6 to 7 days, whereas a wound that is kept moist can resurface in 4 days. The difference in the healing rate is related to the fact that epidermal cells only migrate across a moist surface. In a dry wound the cells migrate down into a moist level before migration can occur (Doughty and Sparks-Defriese, 2007). New epithelium is only a few cells thick and must undergo *reestablishment of the epidermal layers*. The cells slowly reestablish normal thickness and appear as dry, pink tissue.

Full-Thickness Wound Repair. The three phases involved in the healing process of a full-thickness wound are inflammatory, proliferative, and remodeling.

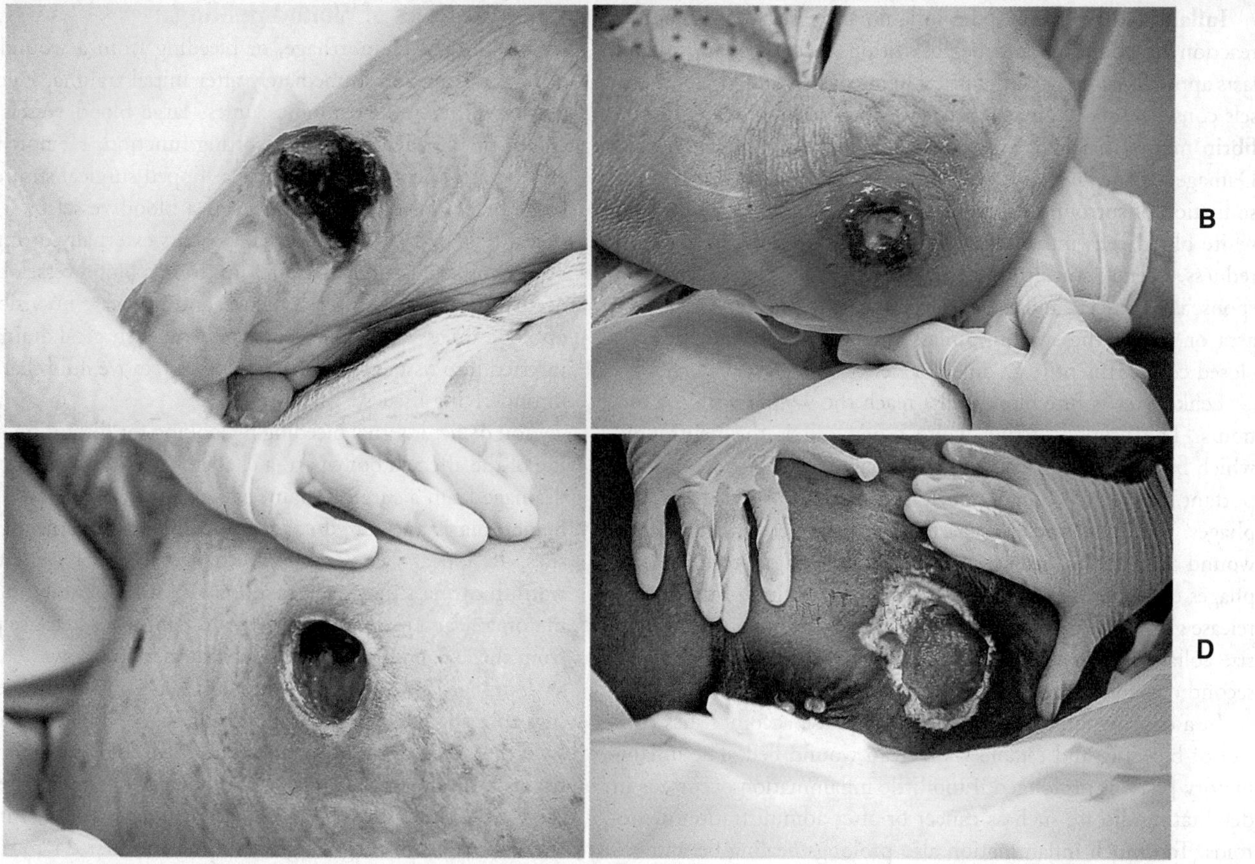

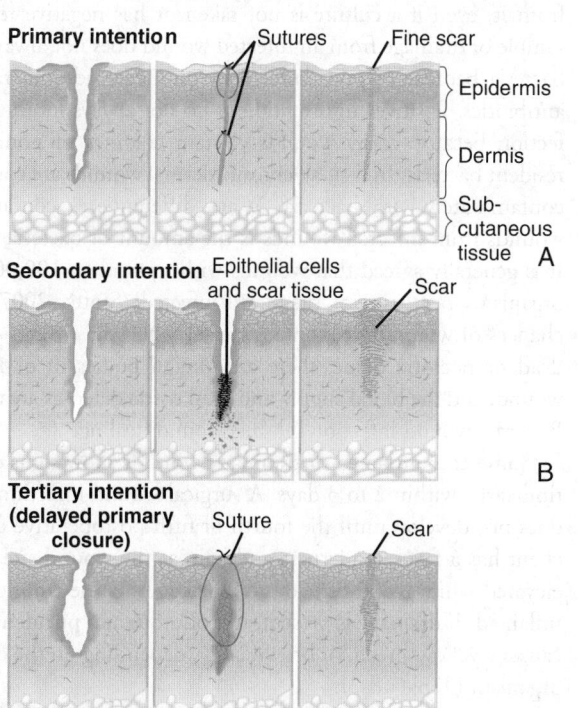

Figure 48-7 Wounds classified by color assessment. **A,** Black wound. **B,** Yellow wound. **C,** Red wound. **D,** Mixed-color wound. (Courtesy Scott Health Care—A Molnlyche Company, Philadelphia, Pa.)

Figure 48-8 A, Wound healing by primary intention such as a surgical incision. Wound healing edges are pulled together and approximated with sutures or staples, and healing occurs by connective tissue deposition. **B,** Wound healing by secondary intention. Wound edges are not approximated, and healing occurs by granulation tissue formation and contraction of the wound edges. (Used with permission: Bryant RA, Nix DP, editors: *Acute and chronic wounds: nursing management,* ed 3, St. Louis, 2007, Mosby.)

Inflammatory Phase. The inflammation stage is the body's reaction to wounding and begins within minutes of injury and lasts approximately 3 days. During **hemostasis,** injured blood vessels constrict, and platelets gather to stop bleeding. Clots form a **fibrin** matrix that later provides a framework for cellular repair. Damaged tissue and mast cells secrete histamine, resulting in vasodilation of surrounding capillaries and exudation of serum and white blood cells into damaged tissues. This results in localized redness, edema, warmth, and throbbing. The inflammatory response is beneficial, and there is no value in attempting to cool the area or reduce the swelling unless the swelling occurs within a closed compartment (e.g., ankle or neck).

Leukocytes (white blood cells) reach the wound within a few hours. The primary acting white blood cell is the neutrophil, which begins to ingest bacteria and small debris. The second important leukocyte is the monocyte, which transforms into macrophages. The macrophages are the "garbage cells" that clean a wound of bacteria, dead cells, and debris by phagocytosis. Macrophages continue the process of clearing the wound of debris and release growth factors that attract fibroblasts, the cells that synthesize collagen (connective tissue). Collagen appears as early as the second day and is the main component of scar tissue.

In a clean wound the inflammatory phase accomplishes control of bleeding and establishes a clean wound bed. The inflammatory phase is prolonged if too little inflammation occurs, as in debilitating disease such as cancer or after administration of steroids. Too much inflammation also prolongs healing because arriving cells compete for available nutrients. An example is a wound infection in which the increased metabolic energy requirements present in an infected wound compete for the available calorie intake.

Proliferative Phase. With the appearance of new blood vessels as reconstruction progresses, the proliferative phase begins and lasts from 3 to 24 days. The main activities during this phase are the filling of the wound with granulation tissue, contraction of the wound, and the resurfacing of the wound by **epithelialization.** Fibroblasts are present in this phase and are the cells that synthesize collagen, providing the matrix for granulation. Collagen mixes with the granulation tissue, and this matrix will support the reepithelialization. Collagen provides strength and structural integrity to a wound. During this period the wound contracts to reduce the area that requires healing. Last, the epithelial cells migrate from the wound edges to resurface. In a clean wound the proliferative phase accomplishes the following: the vascular bed is reestablished (granulation tissue), the area is filled with replacement tissue (collagen, contraction, and granulation tissue), and the surface is repaired (epithelialization). Impairment of healing during this stage usually results from systemic factors such as age, anemia, hypoproteinemia, and zinc deficiency.

Remodeling. Maturation, the final stage of healing, sometimes takes place for more than a year, depending on the depth and extent of the wound. The collagen scar continues to reorganize and gain strength for several months. However, a healed wound usually does not have the tensile strength of the tissue it replaces. Collagen fibers undergo remodeling or reorganization before assuming their normal appearance. Usually scar tissue contains fewer pigmented cells (melanocytes) and has a lighter color than normal skin.

Complications of Wound Healing

Hemorrhage. **Hemorrhage,** or bleeding from a wound site, is normal during and immediately after initial trauma. Hemostasis occurs within several minutes unless large blood vessels are involved or the client has poor clotting function. Hemorrhage occurring after hemostasis indicates a slipped surgical suture, a dislodged clot, infection, or erosion of a blood vessel by a foreign object (e.g., a drain). Hemorrhage occurs externally or internally. For example, if a surgical suture slips from a blood vessel, bleeding occurs internally within the tissues, and there are no visible signs of blood unless a surgical drain is present. A surgical drain may be inserted into tissues beneath a wound to remove fluid that collects in underlying tissues.

You detect internal bleeding by looking for distention or swelling of the affected body part, a change in the type and amount of drainage from a surgical drain, or signs of hypovolemic shock. A **hematoma** is a localized collection of blood underneath the tissues. It appears as a swelling, change in color, sensation, or warmth or mass that often takes on a bluish discoloration. A hematoma near a major artery or vein is dangerous because pressure from the expanding hematoma obstructs blood flow.

External hemorrhaging is obvious. The nurse observes dressings covering the wound for bloody drainage. If bleeding is extensive, the dressing soon becomes saturated, and frequently blood drains from under the dressing and pools beneath the client. Observe all wounds closely, particularly surgical wounds, in which the risk of hemorrhage is great during the first 24 to 48 hours after surgery or injury.

Infection. Wound infection is the second most common health care–associated infection (nosocomial) (see Chapter 34). According to the Centers for Disease Control and Prevention (CDC) (2001), a wound is infected if purulent material drains from it, even if a culture is not taken or has negative results. A sample of drainage from an infected wound does not always reveal bacteria because of poor culture technique or administration of antibiotics. Positive culture findings do not always indicate an infection because many wounds contain colonies of noninfective resident bacteria. In fact, all chronic dermal wounds are considered contaminated with bacteria. What differentiates contaminated wounds from infected wounds is the amount of bacteria present. It is generally agreed that wounds with more than 100,000 (10^5) organisms per gram of tissue are infected (Stotts, 2007b). The chances of wound infection are greater when the wound contains dead or necrotic tissue, there are foreign bodies in or near the wound, and the blood supply and local tissue defenses are reduced. Bacterial wound infection inhibits wound healing.

Some contaminated or traumatic wounds show signs of infection early, within 2 to 3 days. A surgical wound infection usually does not develop until the fourth or fifth postoperative day. The client has a fever, tenderness and pain at the wound site, and an elevated white blood cell count. The edges of the wound appear inflamed. If drainage is present, it is odorous and **purulent,** which causes a yellow, green, or brown color, depending on the causative organism (Table 48-2).

Dehiscence. When a wound fails to heal properly, the layers of skin and tissue separate. This most commonly occurs before collagen formation (3 to 11 days after injury). **Dehiscence** is the partial or total separation of wound layers. A client who is at risk

✳ **TABLE 48-2** Types of Wound Drainage

TYPE	APPEARANCE
Serous	Clear, watery plasma
Purulent	Thick, yellow, green, tan, or brown
Serosanguineous	Pale, red, watery: mixture of clear and red fluid
Sanguineous	Bright red: indicates active bleeding

✳ **BOX 48-4** Risk for Skin Breakdown From Body Fluids

Low Risk
Saliva
Serosanguineous drainage

Moderate Risk
Bile
Stool
Urine
Ascitic fluid
Purulent exudate

High Risk
Gastric drainage
Pancreatic drainage

towels soaked in sterile saline over the extruding tissues to reduce chances of bacterial invasion and drying of the tissues. If the organs protrude through the wound, blood supply to the tissues is compromised. Do not allow the client anything by mouth (NPO), observe the client for signs and symptoms of shock, and prepare the client for emergency surgery.

Fistulas. A **fistula** is an abnormal passage between two organs or between an organ and the outside of the body. Most fistulas form as a result of poor wound healing or as a complication of disease, such as Crohn's disease. Trauma, infection, radiation exposure, and diseases such as cancer will prevent tissue layers from closing properly and allow the fistula tract to form. Fistulas increase the risk of infection and fluid and electrolyte imbalances from fluid loss. Chronic drainage of fluids through a fistula also predisposes a person to skin breakdown (Box 48-4).

Nursing Knowledge Base

Prediction and Prevention of Pressure Ulcers

A major aspect of nursing care is the maintenance of skin integrity. Consistent, planned skin care interventions are critical to ensuring high quality in care. Nurses constantly observe their clients' skin for breaks or impaired skin integrity. Impaired skin integrity occurs from prolonged pressure, irritation of the skin, and/or immobility, leading to the development of pressure ulcers. A pressure ulcer is a localized injury to the skin and/or underlying tissue, usually over a bony prominence, as a result of pressure or pressure in combination with shear and/or friction (NPUAP, 2007a).

Risk Assessment. There are several instruments for assessing clients who are at risk for developing a pressure ulcer. By identifying at-risk clients, you are able to put interventions into place and spare clients with little risk for pressure ulcer development the unnecessary and sometimes costly preventive treatments and the related risk of complications. Prevention and treatment of pressure ulcers are major nursing priorities. The incidence of pressure ulcers in a facility or agency is an important indicator of quality of care. There is evidence that a program of prevention guided by risk assessment simultaneously reduces the institutional incidence of pressure ulcers by as much as 60% and brings down the costs of prevention at the same time (Braden, 2001). Several assessment risk scales (Bergstrom and others, 1987; Norton, McLaren, and

for poor wound healing (e.g., poor nutritional status, infection, or obesity) is at risk for dehiscence. However, obese clients have a higher risk because of the constant strain placed on their wounds and the poor healing qualities of fat tissue (Camden, 2007). Dehiscence involves abdominal surgical wounds and occurs after a sudden strain, such as coughing, vomiting, or sitting up in bed. Clients often report feeling as though something has given way. When there is an increase in serosanguineous drainage from a wound, be alert for the potential for dehiscence. A strategy to prevent dehiscence is to use a folded thin blanket or pillow placed over an abdominal wound when the client is coughing. This provides a splint to the area, supporting the healing tissue when coughing increases the intraabdominal pressure.

Evisceration. With total separation of wound layers, **evisceration** (protrusion of visceral organs through a wound opening) sometimes occurs. The condition is an emergency that requires surgical repair. When evisceration occurs, the nurse places sterile

✳ TABLE 48-3 Norton Scale

PHYSICAL CONDITION		MENTAL CONDITION		ACTIVITY		MOBILITY		CONTINENCE	
Good	4	Alert	4	Ambulating	4	Full	4	Not	4
Fair	3	Apathetic	3	Walks with help	3	Slightly limited	3	Occasional	3
Poor	2	Confused	2	Chairbound	2	Limited	2	Usually	2
Very bad	1	Stuporous	1	Bedridden	1	Very limited, immobile	1	Double	1
TOTAL		TOTAL		TOTAL		TOTAL		TOTAL	

GRAND TOTAL

A score of 14 or less indicates risk of pressure ulcer development.

Data from Wound, Ostomy and Continence Nurses Society, *Guideline for prevention and management of pressure ulcers*, WOCN Clinical Practice Guidelines Series, Glenview, Ill, 2003, The Society.

✳ TABLE 48-4 Braden Scale for Predicting Pressure Ulcer Risk

Client's Name _____ Evaluator's Name _____ Date of Assessment _____

Sensory Perception

Ability to respond meaningfully to pressure-related discomfort

1. Completely limited	2. Very limited	3. Slightly limited	4. No impairment
Unresponsive (does not moan, flinch, or grasp) to painful stimuli due to diminished level of consciousness or sedation. OR Limited ability to feel pain over most of body surface.	Responds only to painful stimuli. Cannot communicate discomfort except by moaning or restlessness. OR Has a sensory impairment which limits the ability to feel pain or discomfort over ½ of body.	Responds to verbal commands, but cannot always communicate discomfort or need to be turned. OR Has some sensory impairment that limits ability to feel pain or discomfort in 1 or 2 extremities.	Responds to verbal commands. Has no sensory deficit that would limit ability to feel or voice pain or discomfort.

Moisture

Degree to which skin is exposed to moisture

1. Constantly moist	2. Moist	3. Occasionally moist	4. Rarely moist
Skin is kept moist almost constantly by perspiration, urine, etc. Dampness is detected every time client is moved or turned.	Skin is often, but not always, moist. Linen must be changed at least once a shift.	Skin is occasionally moist, requiring an extra linen change approximately once a day.	Skin is usually dry. Linen only requires changing at routine intervals.

Activity

Degree of physical activity

1. Bedfast	2. Chairfast	3. Walks occasionally	4. Walks frequently
Confined to bed.	Ability to walk severely limited or nonexistent. Cannot bear own weight and/or must be assisted into chair or wheelchair.	Walks occasionally during day, but for very short distances, with or without assistance. Spends majority of each shift in bed or chair.	Walks outside the room at least twice a day and inside room at least once every 2 hours during waking hours.

Mobility

Ability to change and control body position

1. Completely immobile	2. Very limited	3. Slightly limited	4. No limitations
Does not make even slight changes in body or extremity position without assistance.	Makes occasional slight changes in body or extremity position but unable to make frequent or significant changes independently.	Makes frequent though slight changes in body or extremity position independently.	Makes major and frequent changes in position without assistance.

Copyright 1988. Used with permission of Barbara Braden, PhD, RN, Professor, Creighton University School of Nursing, Omaha, Nebraska, and Nancy Bergstrom, Professor, University of Texas-Houston, School of Nursing, Houston, Texas, http://www.bradenscale.com.

※ **TABLE 48-4 Braden Scale for Predicting Pressure Ulcer Risk—cont'd**

Client's Name _____   Evaluator's Name _____   Date of Assessment _____

Nutrition

Usual food intake pattern	1. Very poor	2. Probably inadequate	3. Adequate	4. Excellent
	Never eats a complete meal. Rarely eats more than $1\frac{1}{3}$ of any food offered. Eats 2 servings or less of protein (meat or dairy products) per day. Takes fluids poorly. Does not take a liquid dietary supplement. OR Is NPO and/or maintained on clear liquids or IVs for more than 5 days.	Rarely eats a complete meal and generally eats only about $1\frac{1}{2}$ of any food offered. Protein intake includes only 3 servings of meat or dairy products per day. Occasionally will take a dietary supplement. OR Receives less than optimum amount of liquid diet or tube feeding.	Eats over half of most meals. Eats a total of 4 servings of protein (meat, dairy products) each day. Occasionally will refuse a meal, but will usually take a supplement if offered. OR Is on a tube feeding or total parenteral nutrition regimen that probably meets most of nutritional needs.	Eats most of every meal. Never refuses a meal. Usually eats a total of 4 or more servings of meat and dairy products. Occasionally eats between meals. Does not require supplementation.

Friction and Shear

	1. Problem	2. Potential problem	3. No apparent problem	
	Requires moderate to maximum assistance in moving. Complete lifting without sliding against sheets is impossible. Frequently slides down in bed or chair, requiring frequent repositioning with maximum assistance. Spasticity, contractures, or agitation leads to almost constant friction.	Moves feebly or requires minimum assistance. During a move skin probably slides to some extent against sheets, chair, restraints, or other devices. Maintains relatively good position in chair or bed most of the time but occasionally slides down.	Moves in bed and in chair independently and has sufficient muscle strength to lift up completely during move. Maintains good position in bed or chair at all times.	
			TOTAL SCORE	

Copyright 1988. Used with permission of Barbara Braden, PhD, RN, Professor, Creighton University School of Nursing, Omaha, Nebraska, and Nancy Bergstrom, Professor, University of Texas-Houston, School of Nursing, Houston, Texas, http://www.bradenscale.com.

Exon-Smith, 1962) developed by nurses enable systematic risk assessment of clients. The Norton Scale and the Braden Scale are in the WOCN guidelines (2003) as being valid tools to use for pressure ulcer risk assessment. Each tool has five or six risk factors that are ranked by number. Obtain the client's risk assessment score by adding the individual numbers given for each risk factor. Interpretation of the meaning of the numerical score differs with each scale.

Norton Scale. The first scale reported in the literature is the Norton Scale (Norton and others, 1962) (Table 48-3). It scores five risk factors: physical condition, mental condition, activity, mobility, and incontinence. The total score ranges from 5 to 20; a lower score indicates a higher risk for pressure ulcer development (WOCN, 2003).

Braden Scale. The Braden Scale (Table 48-4) was developed based on risk factors in a nursing home population (Bergstrom and others, 1987). The Braden Scale is composed of six subscales: sensory perception, moisture, activity, mobility, nutrition, and friction and shear. The total score ranges from 6 to 23; a lower

total score indicates a higher risk for pressure ulcer development (Braden and Bergstrom, 1989). The cutoff score for onset of pressure ulcer risk with the Braden Scale in the general adult population is 18 (Ayello and Braden, 2002). Researchers have suggested a cutoff score of 18 for black and Latino clients with darkly pigmented skin (Lyder and others, 2001). The Braden Scale is highly reliable when used to identify clients at greatest risk for pressure ulcers (Bergstrom and others, 1987; Braden and Bergstrom, 1994). The Braden Scale is the most commonly used assessment scale for pressure ulcer risk.

Prevention. The prevention of pressure ulcers is a priority in caring for clients and is not limited to clients with restrictions in mobility. Impaired skin integrity is not usually a problem in healthy, immobilized individuals but is a serious and potentially devastating problem in ill or debilitated clients (WOCN, 2003).

Economic Consequences of Pressure Ulcers. Pressure ulcers are a continual problem in acute and restorative care settings. When considering pressure ulcers, prevalence is defined as the number of clients with at least one pressure ulcer who exist in a client population at a given point in time (WOCN, 2004). More than 1 million individuals develop pressure ulcers each year (WOCN, 2003). Pressure ulcers usually develop within the first 2 weeks of hospitalization (Longemo and others, 1989). There is a lack of clarity about the prevalence of pressure ulcers among persons being cared for in the home without supervision or assistance of professionals (Agency for Health Care Research and Policy [AHCPR], 1994). In the home care setting, some have reported prevalence rates to be 9.12%, and approximately 30% were at risk for new pressure ulcers (Ferrell and others, 2000).

When a pressure ulcer occurs, the length of stay in a hospital and the overall cost of health care increases (AHCPR, 1994). The actual cost of treatment is difficult to estimate. About 1.6 million clients each year in acute care settings develop pressure ulcers, representing a cost of $2.2 to $3.6 billion to the U.S. health care system (Pieper, 2007). Although treatment of pressure ulcers is more costly than prevention (Richardson, Gardner, and Frantz, 1998), the preventive measures themselves are expensive. Extra equipment, such as special beds and mattresses, and increased nursing time are necessary to administer these measures. When an ulcer develops, mean hospital costs ($37,288 versus $13,924) and

length of stay (30.4 versus 12.8 days) have been shown to increase (Allman and others, 1999).

Factors Influencing Pressure Ulcer Formation and Wound Healing

Impaired skin integrity resulting in pressure ulcers is primarily the result of pressure. However, additional factors increase the client's risk for pressure ulcer development and poor wound healing. In addition to shear force, friction, and moisture, other factors influence pressure ulcer formation, including nutrition, tissue perfusion, infection, age, and wound healing.

Nutrition. For clients weakened or debilitated by illness, nutritional therapy is especially important. A client who has undergone surgery (see Chapter 50) and is well nourished still requires at least 1500 kcal/day for nutritional maintenance. Alternatives such as enteral feedings (see Chapter 44) and parenteral nutrition (see Chapter 41) are available for clients unable to maintain normal food intake.

Normal wound healing requires proper nutrition (Table 48-5). Deficiencies in any of the nutrients result in impaired or delayed healing (Stotts, 2007a). Physiological processes of wound healing

✳ **TABLE 48-5** Role of Selected Nutrients in Wound Healing

NUTRIENT	ROLE IN HEALING	RECOMMENDATIONS	SOURCES
Calories	Fuel for cell energy "Protein protection"	35-40 kcal/kg/day, or enough to maintain positive nitrogen balance	
Protein	Fibroplasia, angiogenesis, collagen formation and wound remodeling, immune function	1.0-1.5 g/kg/day, or enough to maintain positive nitrogen balance	Poultry, fish, eggs, beef
Vitamin C (ascorbic acid)	Collagen synthesis, capillary wall integrity, fibroblast function, immunologic function, antioxidant	100-1000 mg/day Need long time to develop clinical scurvy from vitamin C deficiency Low toxicity	Citrus fruits, tomatoes, potatoes, fortified fruit juices
Vitamin A	Epithelialization, wound closure, inflammatory response, angiogenesis, collagen formation Can reverse steroid effects on skin and delayed healing	1600-2000 retinol equivalents per day Supplement if deficient 20,000 units × 10 days	Green leafy vegetables (spinach), broccoli, carrots, sweet potatoes, liver
Vitamin E	No known role in wound healing, antioxidant	None	Fish, oysters, liver, dark meat, eggs, legumes
Zinc	Collagen formation, protein synthesis, cell membrane and host defenses	15-30 mg Correct deficiencies No improvement in wound healing with supplementation unless zinc deficient Use with caution—large doses can be toxic May inhibit copper metabolism and impair immune function	Vegetables, meats, legumes
Fluid	Essential fluid environment for all cell function	30-35 mL/kg/day Increase by another 10-15 mL/kg if client is on an air-fluidized bed	Use noncaffeine, nonalcoholic fluids without sugar Water is best—6-8 glasses/day

Modified from Ayello EA, Thomas DR, Litchford MA: Nutritional aspects of wound healing, *Home Healthc Nurse* 17(11):719, 1999; and Stotts NA: Nutritional assessment and support. In Bryant RA, Nix DP, editors: *Acute and chronic wounds: current management concepts*, ed 3, St. Louis, 2007a, Mosby.

depend on the availability of protein, vitamins (especially A and C), and the trace minerals zinc and copper. Collagen is a protein formed from amino acids acquired by fibroblasts from protein ingested in food. Vitamin C is necessary for synthesis of collagen. Vitamin A reduces the negative effects of steroids on wound healing. Trace elements are also necessary; zinc is necessary for epithelialization and collagen synthesis, and copper is necessary for collagen fiber linking.

Calories provide the material needed to support the cellular activity of wound healing. Protein needs are especially increased. A balanced intake of various nutrients is critical to support wound healing. A balanced diet should include protein, fat, carbohydrates, vitamins, and minerals.

Serum proteins are biochemical indicators of malnutrition (Stotts, 2007a). Serum albumin is probably the most frequently measured of these laboratory parameters. Albumin alone is not sensitive to rapid changes in nutritional status. Transferrin also evaluates protein status, but alone it does not determine malnutrition. The best measure of nutritional status is prealbumin, because it reflects not only what the client has ingested but also what the body has absorbed, digested, and metabolized (Stotts, 2007a).

Tissue Perfusion. Oxygen fuels the cellular functions essential to the healing process; therefore the ability to perfuse the tissues with adequate amounts of oxygenated blood is critical to wound healing (Doughty and Sparks-Defriese, 2007). Clients with shock or peripheral vascular diseases, such as diabetes, are at risk for poor tissue perfusion due to poor circulation. Oxygen requirements depend upon the phase of wound healing; for instance, chronic tissue hypoxia is associated with impaired collagen synthesis and reduced tissue resistance to infection.

Infection. Wound infection prolongs the inflammatory phase, delays collagen synthesis, prevents epithelialization, and increases the production of proinflammatory cytokines, which leads to additional tissue destruction (Stotts, 2007b). Indications that a wound infection is present include the presence of pus; change in odor, volume, or character of wound drainage; redness in the surrounding tissue; fever; or pain.

Age. Increased age affects all phases of wound healing. A decrease in the functioning of the macrophage leads to a delayed inflammatory response, delayed collagen synthesis, and slower epithelialization.

Psychosocial Impact of Wounds. The psychosocial impact of wounds on the physiological process of healing is unknown. The client's psychological response to any wound is part of the nurse's assessment. Body image changes often impose a great stress on the client's adaptive mechanisms. In addition, body image changes influence self-concept (see Chapter 27) and sexuality (see Chapter 28). Make sure the client's personal and social resources for adaptation are a part of the assessment. Factors that affect the client's perception of the wound include the presence of scars, drains (drains are often necessary for weeks or even months after certain procedures), odor from drainage, and temporary or permanent prosthetic devices.

Critical Thinking

Successful critical thinking requires a synthesis of knowledge, experience, information gathered from clients, critical thinking attitudes, and intellectual and professional standards. Clinical judgments require the nurse to anticipate the information necessary, analyze the data, and make decisions regarding client care. Critical thinking is always changing. During assessment (Figure 48-9) consider all elements that build toward making appropriate nursing diagnoses.

When caring for clients who have impaired skin integrity and chronic wounds, integrate knowledge from nursing and other disciplines, previous experiences, and information gathered from clients to understand the risk to skin integrity and wound healing. Knowledge of normal musculoskeletal physiology, the pathogenesis of pressure ulcers, normal wound healing, and the pathophysiology of underlying diseases enables you to have a scientific basis for care. The WOCN (2003) has guidelines for assessment

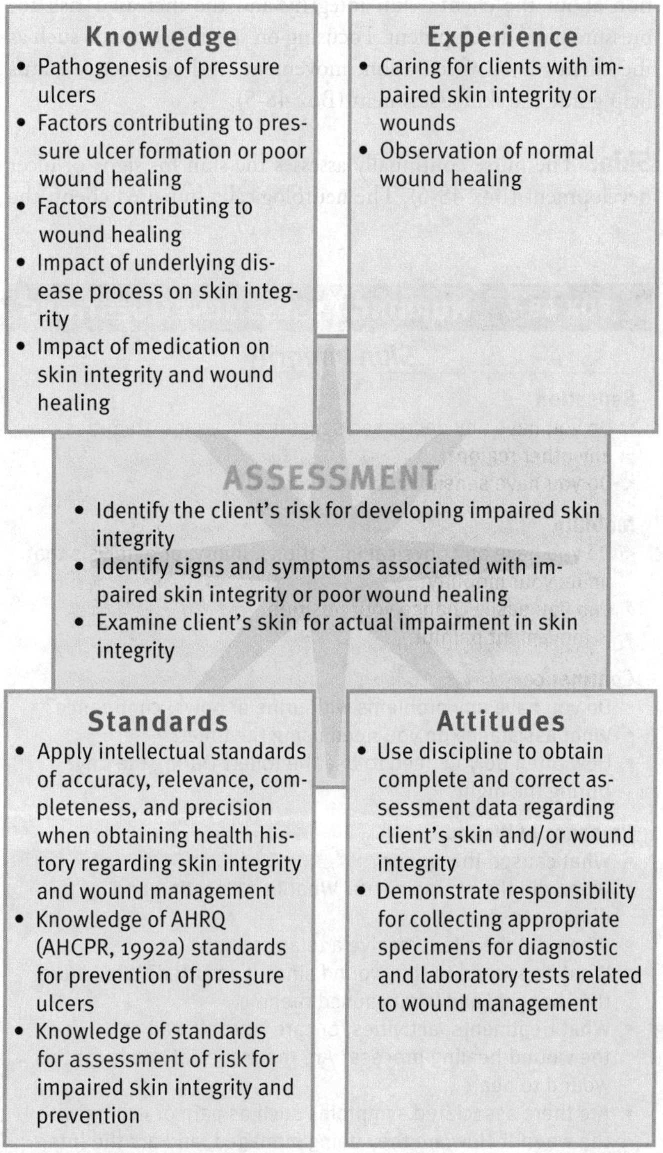

Figure 48-9 Critical thinking model for skin integrity and wound care assessment.

of risk for impaired skin integrity, prevention measures, and interventions to promote wound healing, as well as other standards of practice, which you should use in planning care. Past experience with clients at risk for impaired skin integrity or with clients with wounds increases the experiential knowledge base helping you to identify interventions. Finally, you need to be disciplined during assessment to obtain comprehensive and correct assessment data. You also need to be creative. Because chronic wounds are difficult to heal, be diligent in evaluating nursing interventions and determining which interventions are effective and which need modification.

Nursing Process

◆Assessment

Baseline and continual assessment data provide critical information about the client's skin integrity and the increased risk for pressure ulcer development. Focusing on specific elements such as the client's level of sensation, movement, and continence status help guide the skin assessment (Box 48-5).

Skin. The nurse continually assesses the skin for signs of ulcer development (Box 48-6). The neurologically impaired client; the chronically ill client in long-term care; the client with diminished mental status; and the intensive care unit (ICU), oncology, hospice, or orthopedic client have increased potential for developing pressure ulcers.

Assessment for tissue pressure damage includes visual and tactile inspection of the skin. You perform baseline assessment to determine the client's normal skin characteristics and any actual or potential areas of breakdown. You need to individualize assessment characteristics of a client's skin, depending on the client's skin tone (Bennett, 1995; Henderson and others, 1997). Assessment characteristics of darkly pigmented skin are in Boxes 48-2, p. 1281 and 48-3, p. 1282.

Pay particular attention to areas located over bony prominences or under casts, traction, splints, braces, collars, or other orthopedic devices. The frequency of pressure checks depends on the schedule of appliance application and the skin's response to the external pressure (Figure 48-10).

When you note hyperemia, document the location, size, and color and reassesses the area after 1 hour (Figure 48-11, *A*). When you suspect **abnormal reactive hyperemia**, outline the affected area with a marker to make reassessment easier. These signs are early indicators of impaired skin integrity, but damage to the

---

 BOX 48-5   NURSING ASSESSMENT QUESTIONS

Skin Integrity

Sensation
- Do you have any decreased sensation in your extremities or any other region?
- Do you have sensitivity to heat or cold?

Mobility
- Do you have any physical limitations, injury, or paralysis that limits your mobility?
- Can you easily change your position?
- Is movement painful?

Continence
- Do you have any problems with urine or bowel continence?
- What assistance do you need using the toilet?
- How often do you need to use the toilet? During the day? During the night?

Presence of Wound
- What caused the wound?
- When did the wound occur? What is its location and dimensions?
- When did the client receive a tetanus shot?
- What happened to this wound since it occurred? What were the changes, and what caused them?
- What treatments, activities, or care have slowed or helped the wound-healing process? Are there special needs for this wound to heal?
- Are there associated symptoms such as pain or itching with the wound? How are they being managed, and are the interventions effective?
- What is the goal for the client, wound, and healing?

BOX 48-6   PROCEDURAL GUIDELINES

Skin Assessment

Delegation considerations: Skin assessment for skin integrity or the presence of skin breakdown cannot be delegated. The nurse instructs nursing assistive personnel to report:
- Any changes in the client's skin to the nurse immediately
- Client's exposure to body fluids (e.g., urine, feces, wound drainage, gastric secretions)

Equipment: skin assessment documentation record (check agency policy)

1. Observe pressure points. Compression of these areas for prolonged periods of time by bony prominences or external sources cause tissue ischemia and cell death (WOCN, 2003).
   a. Bony prominences—heels, ankles, knees, hips, sacral area, ischial area, spinal area, shoulders, and elbows (see Figure 48-12)
   b. Cast edges, area next to nasogastric tubes, drainage tubes, or oxygen tubing
2. When you find reddened areas, gently press the area with a gloved finger to assess the ability of the tissue to blanch. If the area does not blanch, suspect tissue injury.
3. Check perineal area for signs of reddened, irritated skin. Perineal skin is at high risk for skin breakdown in the client with fecal and/or urinary incontinence.
4. Observe underlying skin areas where tape, tubing, casts, or splints are in contact with skin.
5. Note previous areas of skin breakdown, check for any breaks in the skin integrity, or note nonblanching erythema in this area. Areas of previous skin breakdown do not heal to the same strength as intact noninjured skin; therefore these areas are at higher risk of skin breakdown.
6. Determine if potential or actual skin breakdown is present, and institute appropriate preventive or treatment protocols.
7. Record findings and the preventive or treatment protocols initiated as per agency policy.

underlying tissue is sometimes more progressive (Figure 48-11, *B*). Tactile assessment enables you to use palpation to acquire further data about **induration** and the damage to the skin and underlying tissues.

Gently palpate the reddened tissue, observing for blanching with return to normal skin tones in clients with light-toned skin. In addition, palpate for induration, noting the size in millimeters or centimeters of the induration around the injured area. Also use palpation to note changes in temperature of the surrounding skin and tissues.

Use visual and tactile inspection over the body areas most frequently at risk for pressure ulcer development (Figure 48-12). For example, when a client lies in bed or sits in a chair, he or she places body weight heavily on certain bony prominences. Body surfaces subjected to the greatest weight or pressure are at greatest risk for pressure ulcer formation.

Pressure Ulcers. Because pressure ulcers have multiple etiological factors, assessment for pressure ulcer risk (Skill 48-1) includes several important factors. These include using an appropriate predictive measure and assessing the client's mobility, nutrition, presence of body fluids, and comfort level.

Predictive Measures. On admission to acute care and rehabilitation hospitals, nursing homes, home care programs, and other health care facilities, assess individuals for risk of pressure ulcer development (WOCN, 2003). Perform pressure ulcer risk assessment systematically (WOCN, 2003). Use an assessment tool, such as the Norton or Braden scale, which measures the risk for developing a pressure ulcer (see Tables 48-3, p. 1288, and 48-4, p. 1288). The interpretation of the meaning of the total numerical scores differs with each risk assessment scale. Lower numerical score on the Braden Scale or the Norton Scale indicate that a client is at high risk for skin breakdown. A benefit of the predictive instruments is to increase the nurse's early detection of clients at greatest risk for ulcer development. Once you identify

these clients, you institute the appropriate interventions to maintain skin integrity. Perform reassessment for pressure ulcer risk on a scheduled basis. Once you identify that a client is at risk for developing pressure ulcers, implement prevention strategies (WOCN, 2003).

Mobility. Assessment includes documenting the level of mobility and the potential effects of impaired mobility on skin integrity. Documenting assessment of mobility also includes obtaining data regarding the quality of muscle tone and strength. For example, determine whether the client is able to lift weight off of the sacral area and roll the body to a side-lying position. Some clients have adequate range of motion (ROM) to move independently into a more protective position. Finally, note the client's activity tolerance (see Chapter 37).

You must assess mobility as part of baseline data. If the client has some degree of independence in mobility, reinforce the frequency of position changes and measures to relieve pressure. The frequency of position changes is based on ongoing skin assessment, and you revise it as data change. Be meticulous when assessing pressure sites.

Nutritional Status. An assessment of the client's nutritional status is an integral part of the initial assessment data for clients at risk for impaired skin integrity and wounds (Stotts, 2007a). Malnutrition is a major risk factor for pressure ulcer development

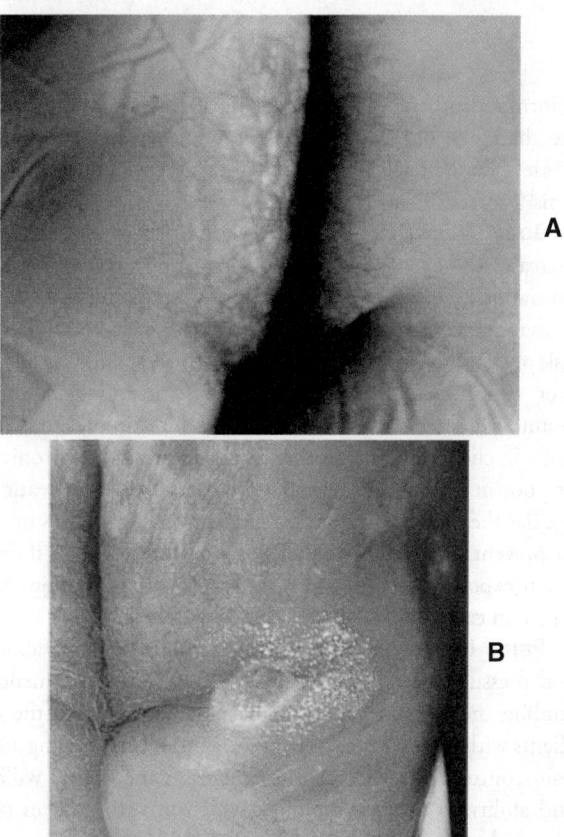

A

B

Figure 48-11 A, Hyperemia on ischial tuberosity. **B,** Ulcer. (From Pires M, Muller A: Decision and management of early tissue pressure indicators: a pictorial essay, *Progressions* 3[3]:3, 1991.)

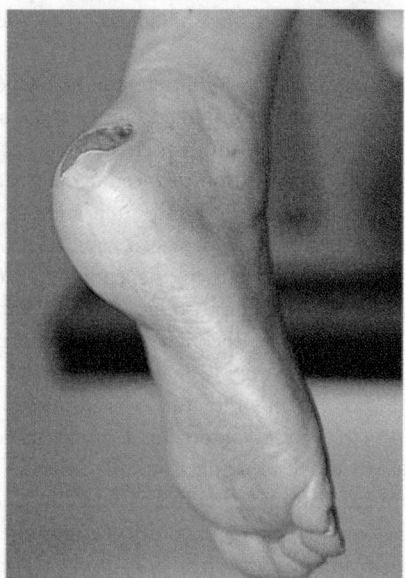

Figure 48-10 Formation of pressure ulcer on heel resulting from external pressure from mattress of bed.

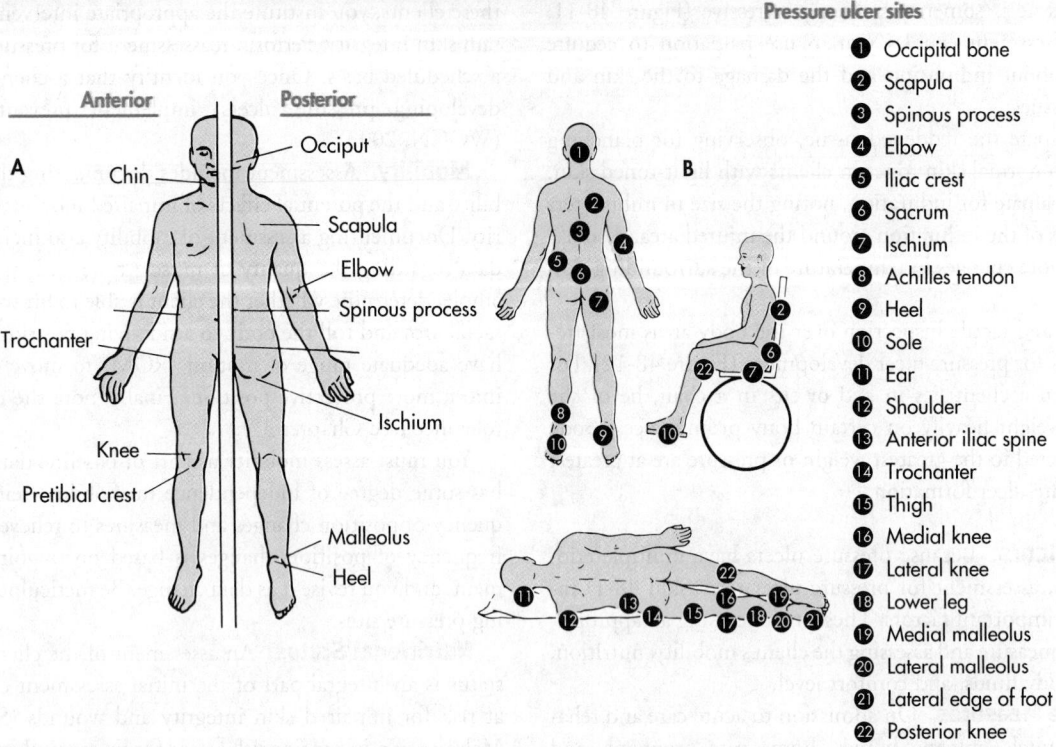

Figure 48-12 **A,** Bony prominences most frequently underlying pressure ulcer. **B,** Pressure ulcer sites. (Modified from Trelease CC: Developing standards for wound care, *Ostomy Wound Manage* 20:46, 1988.)

(Horn and others, 2002). A loss of 5% of usual weight, weight less than 90% of ideal body weight, or a decrease of 10 pounds in a brief period are all signs of actual or potential nutritional problems (Stotts, 2007a).

Body Fluids. Continual exposure of the skin to body fluids increases the client's risk for skin breakdown and pressure ulcer formation (see Box 48-4). Some body fluids, such as saliva and serosanguineous drainage, are not as caustic to the skin and the risk of skin breakdown from exposure to these fluids is low. However, exposure to urine, bile, stool, ascitic fluid, and purulent wound exudates carries a moderate risk for skin breakdown, especially in clients who have other risk factors, such as chronic illness or poor nutrition. Last, exposure to gastric and pancreatic drainage has the highest risk for skin breakdown. Again, it is important to prevent and reduce the client's exposure to body fluids, and when exposure occurs, you need to provide meticulous hygiene and skin care.

Pain. Until recently, there has been little research about pain and pressure ulcers. The WOCN (2003) has recommended including the assessment and management of pain in the care of clients with pressure ulcers (Krasner, 2001). Maintaining adequate pain control and client comfort increases the client's willingness and ability to increase mobility, which in turn reduces pressure ulcer risk.

Wounds. The nurse often assesses wounds under two conditions: at the time of injury before treatment and after therapy, when the wound is relatively stable. Each condition requires the nurse to make different observations and to take different actions. Regardless of the setting, it is important that you initially obtain information regarding the cause and history of the wound (see Box 48-5).

Emergency Setting. You will see wounds in any setting, including clinic, emergency department, youth camps, or your own backyard. The type of wound determines the criteria for inspection. For example, you need not inspect for signs of internal bleeding after an abrasion but should do so in the event of a puncture wound.

When you judge a client's condition to be stable because of the presence of spontaneous breathing, a clear airway, and a strong carotid pulse (see Chapter 40), inspect the wound for bleeding. An **abrasion** is superficial with little bleeding and is considered a partial-thickness wound. The wound often appears "weepy" because of plasma leakage from damaged capillaries. A **laceration** sometimes bleeds more profusely, depending on the wound's depth and location. For example, minor scalp lacerations tend to bleed profusely because of the rich blood supply to the scalp. Lacerations greater than 5 cm (2 inches) long or 2.5 cm (1 inch) deep cause serious bleeding. **Puncture** wounds bleed in relation to the depth and size of the wound; for example, a nail puncture does not cause as much bleeding as a knife wound. The primary dangers of puncture wounds are internal bleeding and infection.

Inspect the wound for foreign bodies or contaminant material. Most traumatic wounds are dirty. Soil, broken glass, shreds of cloth, and foreign substances clinging to penetrating objects sometimes become embedded in the wound.

★ SKILL 48-1 ASSESSMENT FOR RISK FOR PRESSURE ULCER DEVELOPMENT

Delegation Considerations

The skill of assessment of clients for risk of pressure ulcers cannot be delegated. The nurse directs nursing assistive personnel to:

- Report any changes to the client's skin, such as redness, blistering, abrasion, or cuts, to the nurse for further nursing assessment
- Keep the client's skin dry and provide hygiene following incontinence of urine or stool or exposure to other body fluids
- Reposition the client according to the frequency established on the nursing care plan or agency policy
- Avoid trauma to the client's skin from tape, pressure, friction, or shear

Equipment

- Risk assessment tool, Braden Scale (used in this skill) or Norton Scale
- Documentation record

STEPS	RATIONALE
1. Identify at-risk individuals needing prevention and the specific factors placing them at risk.	Determines factors that increase the client's risk for developing pressure ulcers (Braden, 2001).
a. Use a validated risk assessment tool such as the Braden Scale.	Ensures consistent, reliable, comparable assessments (WOCN, 2003).
b. Assess the client upon admission to acute care, rehabilitation hospitals, nursing homes, home care programs, and other health care facilities.	Provides a baseline assessment.
c. Inspect the condition of the client's skin at least once a day (see Box 48-6, p. 1292), and examine all bony prominences, noting skin integrity. (Check agency policy for reassessment, and reassess at periodic intervals.) If you notice redness or discoloration, use thumb to gently palpate area of redness. The discoloration often varies from pink to deep red.	Routine skin assessments will identify changes in client's pressure ulcer risk. Nonblanchable erythema or discoloration in the client's skin is an early indicator of skin injury (Pieper, 2007).

Critical Decision Point: In dark-skinned clients the discoloration appears as a deepening of the normal ethnic color (see Boxes 48-2 and 48-3). Darkly pigmented skin does not always show direct changes in color (Bennett, 1995; NPUAP, 1998).

d. Observe all assistive devices, such as braces or casts, and medical equipment, such as nasogastric tubes and catheters, for pressure points.	Presence of medical equipment has the potential to cause pressure and skin breakdown to sensitive regions, such as the nares, ears, over bony prominences, and other pressure areas.
2. Determine the client's ability to respond meaningfully to pressure-related discomfort (sensory perception).	Client with complete or partial limited ability to respond to pressure-related discomfort cannot communicate discomfort, has a limitation in the ability to feel pain, and thus is at risk for developing pressure ulcers.
3. Assess the degree to which the client's skin is exposed to moisture.	A person whose skin is exposed to excessive moisture has an increased risk of developing skin breakdown (Pieper, 2007).
4. Evaluate the client's activity level.	The client who is bedfast, chairfast, or only walks occasionally is at risk for developing pressure areas because of the degree of physical inactivity (WOCN, 2003).
a. Determine the client's ability to change and control body position (mobility).	Potential for friction and shear increases when the client is completely dependent on others for position change.
b. Determine client's preferred positions.	Weight of body is on certain bony prominences, and the client will resist repositioning off these areas.
5. Assess the client's usual food intake pattern (nutrition).	A client who never eats a complete meal or rarely eats a complete meal is at risk for pressure ulcer formation.
a. Review weight pattern and nutritional laboratory values (see Box 48-12, p. 1312).	Decreased nutrition status is linked with pressure ulcer formation and poor wound healing (WOCN, 2003).
b. Complete fluid intake assessment.	Fluid imbalance, either dehydration or edema, increases the client's risk for pressure ulcers (Stotts, 2007a).
6. Evaluate the presence of friction and/or shear.	The client who has a problem in moving, requires maximum assistance in moving, or slides against sheets when moved is at an increased risk of skin damage (Pieper, 2007).
7. Document the risk assessment. (NOTE: Numerical values in steps 2 through 6 refer to the Braden Scale.)	The documentation will provide a baseline for comparison of increased or decreased risk for development of pressure ulcers and allow planning of interventions.
a. As the Braden Scale scores become lower, predicted risk becomes higher.	Scores: 15 to 18, at risk 13 to 14, moderate risk 10 to 12, high risk 9 or below, very high risk

Continued

✳ **SKILL 48-1 ASSESSMENT FOR RISK FOR PRESSURE ULCER DEVELOPMENT—CONT'D**

STEPS	RATIONALE
b. Link the risk assessment to preventive protocols.	Protocols will target problem areas to assist in prevention of skin breakdown.
c. Institute at-risk interventions (score of 15 to 18). Consider instituting frequent turning, protection of client's heels, use of a pressure-redistribution surface, and managing moisture.	Decreases the risk of skin breakdown.
d. Institute moderate-risk interventions (score of 13 to 14). Consider a protocol of frequent turning, protect client's heels, provide a pressure-redistribution surface, provide foam wedges for 30-degree lateral positioning, and manage moisture, shear, and friction.	Decreases the increased risk of skin breakdown with appropriate interventions.
e. Institute high-risk interventions (score of 10 to 12). Consider a protocol that increases the frequency of turning, supplements turning with small shifts in position, facilitates maximal remobilization, protects the client's heels, provides a pressure-redistribution surface, provides foam wedges for 30-degree lateral positioning, and manages moisture, friction, and shear. If needed, institute nutritional interventions to reduce risk of pressure ulcer development.	Addresses the factors that contribute to skin breakdown and plans for interventions to address the causative factors (Pieper, 2007).
f. Institute very-high-risk interventions (score of 9 or below). Consider a protocol that incorporates the points for high-risk clients plus uses a pressure-redistribution surface if the client has intractable pain, severe pain exacerbated by turning.	Plans interventions to decrease the effects of immobility, decreased sensory perception, moisture, friction, shear, decreased activity, and nutritional issues in a high-risk individual.
8. Provide education to client and family regarding pressure ulcer risk and prevention.	Assists clients and family in understanding the interventions designed to reduce pressure ulcer risk.
9. Evaluate measures to reduce pressure ulcer development	
a. Observe client's skin for areas at risk.	Determines over time client's response to risk redistribution interventions.
b. Observe tolerance of client for positioning.	Frequent change in position further reduces client's risk for pressure ulcer development.
c. Monitor the success of a toileting program or other measures to reduce the frequency of incontinence of urine or stool.	Determines timeliness of a toileting program or schedule to assist the client in meeting elimination needs.
d. Evaluate nutrition laboratory values.	Determines the success of nutritional supplements in improving nutritional status.

Unexpected Outcomes and Related Interventions

1. Skin does not blanch when firmly pressed, has purple discoloration, or has significant color change.
   a. Reassess frequency of turning schedule.
   b. Implement agency's skin care protocols.
   c. Consider use of pressure-redistribution surface to reduce pressure ulcer risk.

Recording and Reporting

- Record client's risk score.
- Record appearance of skin under pressure.

- Describe position, turning intervals, pressure-redistribution devices, and other prevention strategies.
- Report any need for additional consultations for the high-risk client.

Home Care Considerations

- Instruct caregiver in the use of the 30-degree lateral position. This position prolongs the time between position changes, resulting in fewer sleep interruptions for client and caregiver.
- Individualize pressure-redistribution maneuvers for client needs and home environment. Provide family with resources for hospital equipment.

TABLE 48-6 Assessment of Abnormal Healing in Primary and Secondary Intention Wounds

PRIMARY INTENTION WOUNDS	SECONDARY INTENTION WOUNDS
Incision line poorly approximated	Pale or fragile granulation tissue, granulation tissue bed is excessively dry or moist
Drainage present more than 3 days after closure	Exudate present
Inflammation decreased in first 3-5 days after injury	Necrotic or slough tissue present in wound base
No epithelialization of wound edges by day 4	Epithelialization not continuous
No healing ridge by day 9	Fruity, earthy, or putrid odor present
	Presence of fistula(s), tunneling, undermining

Modified from Stotts NA, Cavanaugh CE: Assessing the client with a wound, *Home Healthc Nurse* 17(1):27, 1999.

The size of the wound is the next step in assessment. A deep laceration requires suturing. A large, open wound may expose bone or tissue that needs to be protected.

When the injury is a result of trauma from a dirty penetrating object, determine when the client last received a tetanus toxoid injection. Tetanus bacteria reside in soil and in the gut of humans and animals. A tetanus antitoxin injection is necessary if the client has not had one within 5 years.

Stable Setting. When the client's condition is stabilized (e.g., after surgery or treatment), assess the wound to determine progress toward healing. If the wound is covered by a dressing and the health care provider has not ordered it changed, do not directly inspect the wound unless you suspect serious complications. In such a situation, inspect only the dressing and any external drains. If the health care provider prefers to change the dressing, the health care provider will assess the wound at least daily. When removing dressings, take care to avoid accidental removal or displacement of underlying drains. Because removal of dressings is painful, it often helps to give an analgesic at least 30 minutes before exposing a wound.

Wound Appearance. Observe whether wound edges are closed. A surgical incision healing by primary intention should have clean, well-approximated edges. Crusts often form along the wound edges from exudate. A puncture wound is usually a small, circular wound with the edges coming together toward the center. If a wound is open, the wound edges are separated, and you inspect the condition of tissue at the wound base. Also look for complications such as dehiscence and evisceration. The outer edges of a wound normally appear inflamed for the first 2 to 3 days, but this slowly disappears. Within 7 to 10 days a normally healing wound resurfaces with epithelial cells, and edges close. Table 48-6 lists assessment characteristics for abnormal wound healing in primary and secondary wounds. If infection develops, the area directly surrounding the wound becomes brightly inflamed and swollen.

Skin discoloration usually results from bruising of interstitial tissues or hematoma formation. Blood collecting beneath the skin first takes on a bluish or purplish appearance. Gradually, as the clotted blood is broken down, shades of brown and yellow appear.

Character of Wound Drainage. Note the amount, color, odor, and consistency of drainage. The amount of drainage depends on the location and extent of the wound. For example, drainage is minimal after a simple appendectomy. In contrast,

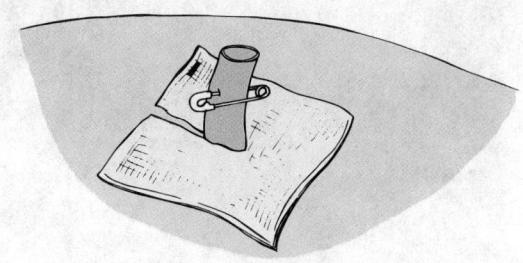

Figure 48-13 Penrose drain.

wound drainage is moderate for 1 to 2 days after drainage of a large abscess. When you need an accurate measurement of the amount of drainage within a dressing, weigh the dressing and compare it with the weight of the same dressing when clean and dry. The general rule is that 1 g of drainage equals 1 mL of volume of drainage. Another method of quantifying wound drainage is to chart the number of dressings used and the frequency of change. An increase or decrease in the number or frequency of dressings will indicate a relative increase or decrease in wound drainage. The color and consistency of drainage vary depending on the components. Types of drainage include the following: **serous, sanguineous, serosanguineous,** and purulent (see Table 48-2). If the drainage has a pungent or strong odor, you should suspect an infection. Describe the wound's appearance according to characteristics observed. An example of accurate recording follows:

> Abdominal incision is 5 cm in width, in RLQ (right lower quadrant); edges well approximated without inflammation or exudate. 1.2-cm diameter circle of serous drainage present on one 4 × 4 gauze changed every 8 hours.

Drains. The health care provider inserts a drain into or near a surgical wound if there is a large amount of drainage. Some drains are sutured in place. Exercise caution when changing the dressing around drains that are not sutured in place to prevent accidental removal. A Penrose drain lies under a dressing; at the time of placement a pin or clip is placed through the drain to prevent it from slipping farther into a wound (Figure 48-13). It is usually the health care provider's responsibility to pull or advance the drain as drainage decreases to permit healing deep within the drain site.

Assess the number of drains, drain placement, character of drainage, and condition of collecting equipment. First observe vac or Jackson-Pratt (Figure 48-14) exert a constant low pressure as long as the suction device (bladder or bag) is fully compressed. These types of drainage devices are often referred to as self-suction. When the evacuator device is unable to maintain a vacuum on its own, notify the surgeon, who will then order a secondary vacuum system (such as wall suction). If fluid accumulates within the tissues, wound healing will not progress at an optimal rate, and this increases the risk of infection.

Wound Closures. Surgical wounds are closed with staples, sutures, or wound closures. A frequent skin closure is the stainless-steel staple. The staple provides more strength than nylon or silk sutures and tends to cause less irritation to tissue. Look for irritation around staple or suture sites and note whether closures are intact. Nurses often count sutures when the health care provider has removed a portion of them. Normally for the first 2 to 3 days after surgery the skin around sutures or staples is edematous. Continued swelling indicates that the closures are too tight. The skin can be cut by overly tight suture material, leading to wound separation. Sutures that are too tight are a common cause of wound dehiscence. Early suture removal reduces formation of defects along the suture line and minimizes chances of unattractive scar formation.

Dermabond is a tissue adhesive that forms a strong bond across apposed wound edges, allowing normal healing to occur below. It can be used to replace small sutures for incisional repair. A vial containing the Dermabond solution is used to apply the product to approximated tissue. The wound edges are held together until the solution dries, providing an adhesive closure. Although generally used for small superficial lacerations, some surgeons use it on larger wounds where subcutaneous sutures are needed (Bruns and Worthington, 2000).

Palpation of Wound. When inspecting a wound, observe swelling or separation of wound edges. While wearing gloves, lightly press the wound edges, detecting localized areas of tenderness or drainage collection. If pressure causes fluid to be expressed, note the character of the drainage. The client is normally sensitive to palpation of wound edges. Extreme tenderness indicates infection.

Wound Cultures. If you detect purulent or suspicious-looking drainage, obtaining a specimen of the drainage for culture may be necessary (see Chapter 34). Never collect a wound culture sample from old drainage. Resident colonies of bacteria from the skin grow within exudate and are not always the true causative organisms of a wound infection. Clean a wound first with normal saline to remove skin flora. Aerobic organisms grow in superficial wounds exposed to the air, and anaerobic organisms tend to grow within body cavities. Use a different method of specimen collection for each type of organism as per agency policy (Box 48-7).

Gram stains are often performed as well. This test often allows the health care provider to order appropriate treatment earlier than when only cultures are done. No additional specimens are usually required. The microbiology laboratory needs only to be notified to perform the additional test.

The gold standard of wound culture is tissue biopsy. A health care provider or wound care specialist with special training obtains the biopsy (Stotts, 2007b).

Client Expectations. When clients have an acute surgical or traumatic wound, the wound will sometimes heal promptly and

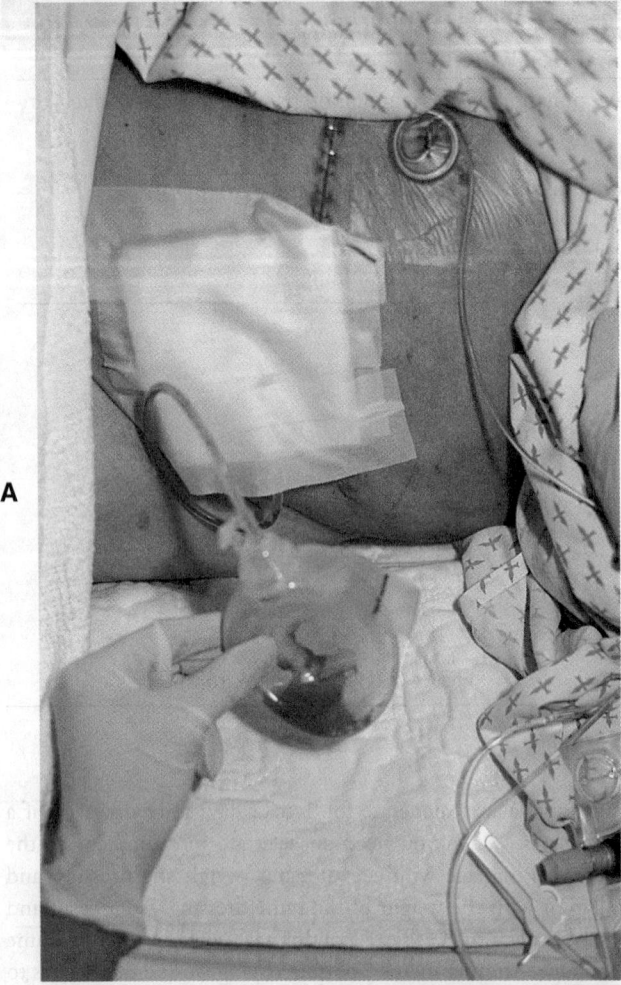

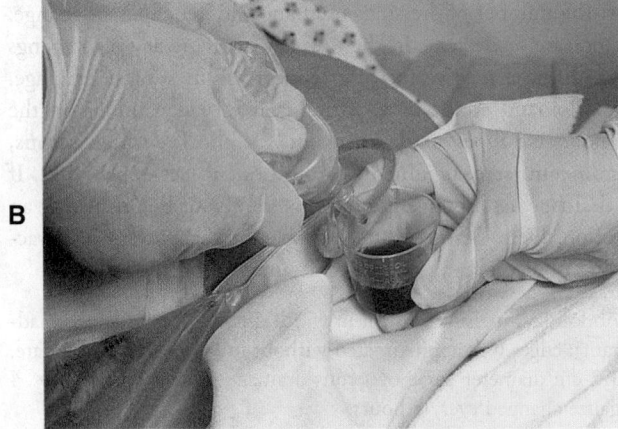

Figure 48-14 Jackson-Pratt drainage device. **A,** Drainage tubes and reservoir. **B,** Emptying drainage reservoir.

the security of the drain and its location with respect to the wound. Next note the character of drainage. If there is a collecting device, measure the drainage volume. Because a drainage system needs to be patent, look for drainage flow through the tubing, as well as around the tubing. A sudden decrease in drainage through the tubing may indicate a blocked drain, and you need to notify the health care provider. When a drain is connected to suction, assess the system to be sure that the pressure ordered is being exerted. Evacuator units such as a Hemo-

✳ **BOX 48-7 Recommendations for Standardized Techniques for Wound Cultures***

Needle Aspiration Procedure
• Clean intact skin with a disinfectant solution. Allow to dry.
• Use a 10-mL disposable syringe with a 22-gauge needle, pulling 0.5 mL of air into the syringe.
• Insert the needle through intact skin next to the wound, applying suction to the 10-mL mark.
• Move the needle back and forward at different angles for two to four explorations.
• Remove the needle and expel the excess air, and cap and prepare the syringe for the laboratory (Stotts, 2007b).

Quantitative Swab Procedure
• Clean the wound surface with a nonantiseptic solution.
• Use a sterile swab from a culturette tube (Figure 48-15).
• Moisten the swab with normal saline.
• Rotate the swab in 1 cm^2 of clean tissue in the open wound. Apply pressure to the swab to elicit tissue fluid (Stotts, 2007b). Insert the tip of the swab into the appropriate sterile container, label, and transport to the laboratory.

Modified from Stotts NA: Wound infection: diagnosis and management. In Bryant RA, Nix DP, editors: *Acute and chronic wounds: current management concepts,* ed 3, St. Louis, 2007, Mosby.

*Check agency policy to determine need to obtain health care provider order.

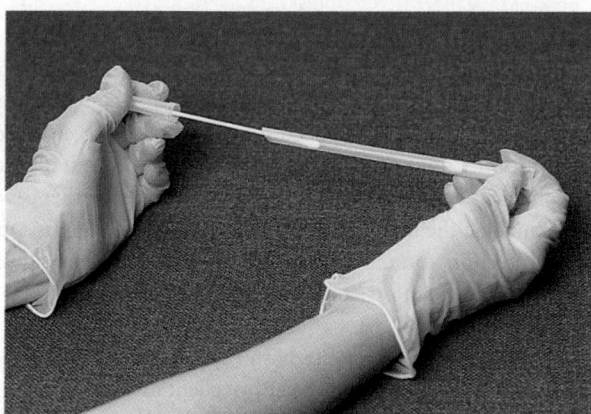

Figure 48-15 Wound culturette tube.

without complications. However, when pressure ulcers or chronic wounds are present, the course of treatment is lengthy and costly. Because the client and family need to be involved with wound care management, it is important to know the client's expectations. A client who has realistic goals and is informed about the length of time for wound healing is more likely to adhere to the specific therapies designed to promote wound healing and prevent further skin breakdown.

◆Nursing Diagnosis

Assessment reveals clusters of data to indicate whether an actual or a risk for *impaired skin integrity* exists. In addition, the assessment data sometimes support more than one diagnostic label. For example, a postoperative client has purulent drainage from a surgical wound and reports tenderness around the area of the wound. These

✳ **BOX 48-8 NURSING DIAGNOSTIC PROCESS**

Impaired Skin Integrity Related to Infection

Assessment Activities	Defining Characteristics
Inspect surface of skin.	Presence of wound, break in skin integrity
	Yellow, foul-smelling drainage from wound
	Edges of wound red and warm, not approximated
	Sutures remain in place
Inspect wound for signs of healing.	Brown-red drainage 5 days after surgery
	Edges of wound not approximated
Obtain client's temperature, heart rate, white blood cell count, and serum albumin level	Client is febrile, heart rate is 125 beats per minute, leukocyte (white blood cell) count is 12,000/mm^3, serum albumin is less than 3.5 mg/100 mL

data support a nursing diagnosis of *impaired skin integrity related to a contaminated wound* (Box 48-8). After completing an assessment of the client's wound, the nurse identifies nursing diagnoses that will direct supportive and preventive care. There are multiple nursing diagnoses associated with impaired skin integrity and wounds:

• Risk for infection
• Imbalanced nutrition: less than body requirements
• Acute or chronic pain
• Impaired physical mobility
• Impaired skin integrity
• Risk for impaired skin integrity
• Ineffective tissue perfusion
• Impaired tissue integrity

Some clients are at risk for poor wound healing because of previously defined factors that impair healing. Thus even though the client's wound appears normal, the nurse identifies nursing diagnoses, such as *impaired nutrition* or *ineffective tissue perfusion,* that direct nursing care toward support of wound repair.

The nature of a wound can cause problems unrelated to wound healing. Alteration in comfort and impaired mobility are problems that have implications for the client's eventual recovery. For example, a large abdominal incision causes enough pain to interfere with the client's ability to turn in bed effectively.

◆Planning

After identifying nursing diagnoses, you develop a plan of care for the client who has actual or is at risk for impaired skin integrity. During planning synthesize information from multiple resources (Figure 48-16). Critical thinking ensures that the client's plan of care integrates all that you know about the individual, as well as key critical thinking elements. Professional standards are especially important to consider when you develop a plan of care.

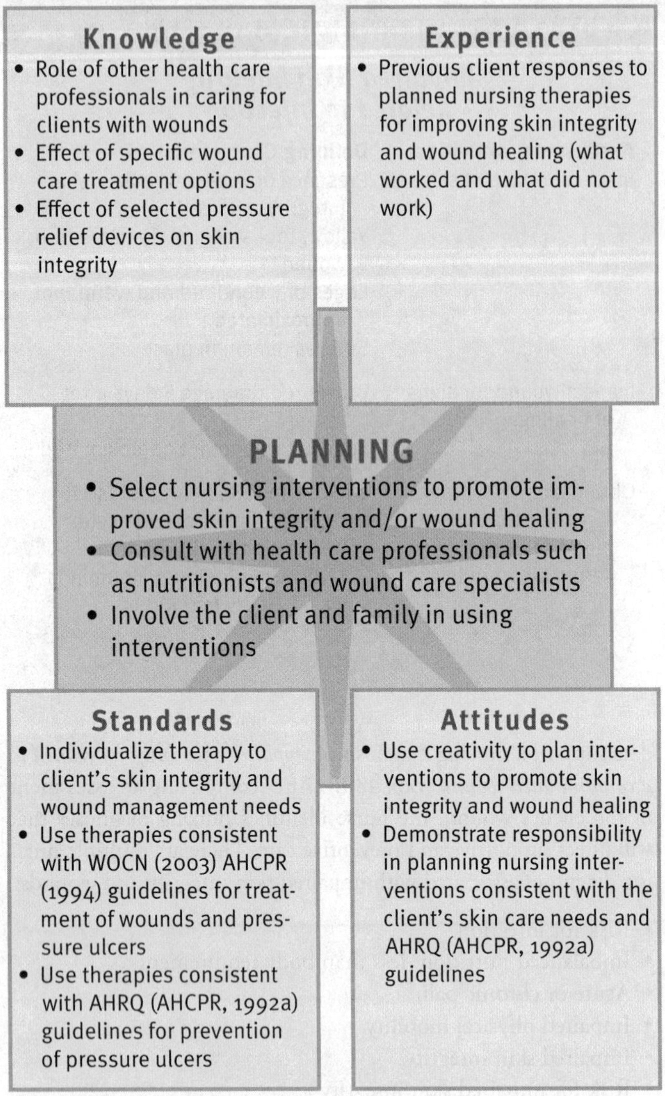

Knowledge

- Role of other health care professionals in caring for clients with wounds
- Effect of specific wound care treatment options
- Effect of selected pressure relief devices on skin integrity

Experience

- Previous client responses to planned nursing therapies for improving skin integrity and wound healing (what worked and what did not work)

PLANNING

- Select nursing interventions to promote improved skin integrity and/or wound healing
- Consult with health care professionals such as nutritionists and wound care specialists
- Involve the client and family in using interventions

Standards

- Individualize therapy to client's skin integrity and wound management needs
- Use therapies consistent with WOCN (2003) AHCPR (1994) guidelines for treatment of wounds and pressure ulcers
- Use therapies consistent with AHRQ (AHCPR, 1992a) guidelines for prevention of pressure ulcers

Attitudes

- Use creativity to plan interventions to promote skin integrity and wound healing
- Demonstrate responsibility in planning nursing interventions consistent with the client's skin care needs and AHRQ (AHCPR, 1992a) guidelines

Figure 48-16 Critical thinking model for skin integrity and wound care planning.

Clients who have large or chronic wounds have multiple nursing care needs. For example, consider the following scenario:

A nurse is caring for Mrs. Kathy Crane, a 65-year-old woman with a 30-year history of diabetes mellitus. She currently takes insulin. Her diabetes is poorly controlled due to her inability to adhere to a 1600-calorie diet. She is 70 pounds overweight. For the last 10 years she has reported decreased sensation to her lower extremities. She does not practice good foot care; she cuts her own toenails and goes barefoot. She was admitted to the hospital for elective repair of an abdominal aneurysm. The surgery went well, but postoperatively Mrs. Crane had difficulty ambulating and performing coughing and deep breathing exercises. On her second postoperative day she developed a postoperative pneumonia, which required intravenous antibiotics. During the course of her pneumonia, Mrs. Crane refused to walk, she became incontinent of urine and stool, and she complained about position changes. After her position was changed, she would reposition herself on her back. Two weeks after her surgery Mrs. Crane developed a large draining sacral wound, which is now 6 cm in diameter and is a stage IV pressure ulcer. In addition, she has a smaller, stage III ulcer on her left heel. Skin

assessment also reveals areas of prolonged redness over pressure points, especially on the right heel and over both hips.

When planning for care for Mrs. Crane, a concept map helps to individualize care for this client who has multiple health problems and related nursing diagnoses (Figure 48-17). This map assists you in using critical thinking skills to organize complex client assessment data and related nursing diagnoses with the client's chief medical diagnosis. As you identify linkages between the nursing diagnoses and the chief medical diagnosis, the concept map also links potential interventions with the client's health care needs.

Goals and Outcomes. Nursing care is based on the client's identified needs and priorities. You establish goals and expected outcomes, and from the goals you plan interventions according to the risk for pressure ulcers or the type and severity of the wound and the presence of any complications, such as infection, poor nutrition, peripheral vascular diseases, or immunosuppression, that can affect wound healing (see Care Plan).

A goal frequently identified when working with a client with a wound is to see wound improvement within a 2-week period. The outcomes of this goal will possibly include the following:

- Higher percentage of granulation tissue in the wound base
- No further skin breakdown in any body location
- An increase in the caloric intake by 10%

These outcomes are reasonable if the overall goal for the client is to heal the ulcer. Plan therapies according to the severity and type of wound and the presence of any complicating conditions (e.g., infection, poor nutrition, immunosuppression, and diabetes) that will affect wound healing. Other goals of care for clients with wounds include the following: promoting wound hemostasis, preventing infection, promoting wound healing, maintaining skin integrity, gaining comfort, and health promotion.

Setting Priorities. You establish nursing care priorities in wound care based on the comprehensive client assessment and goal and established outcomes. These priorities also depend on whether the client's condition is stable or emergent. An acute wound needs immediate intervention, whereas in the presence of a chronic, stable wound, the client's hygiene needs have a greater priority. When there is a risk for pressure ulcer development, preventive interventions, such as skin care practices, elimination of shear, and positioning, are high priorities. Promotion of wound healing is a major nursing priority, and the type of wound care administered depends on the type, size, and location of the wound and overall treatment goals.

Other client factors to consider when establishing priorities include client preferences, daily activities, and family factors. These factors are important regardless of the setting for health care. The priorities of care may not vary from outpatient, home, acute care, or restorative care settings.

Collaborative Care. With early discharge from health care settings, it is important to consider the client's plan for discharge. Anticipating the client's discharge wound care needs and related equipment and resources, such as referral to a home care agency or outpatient wound care clinic, assist not only in improving wound healing but also improve the client's level of indepen-

CONCEPT MAP

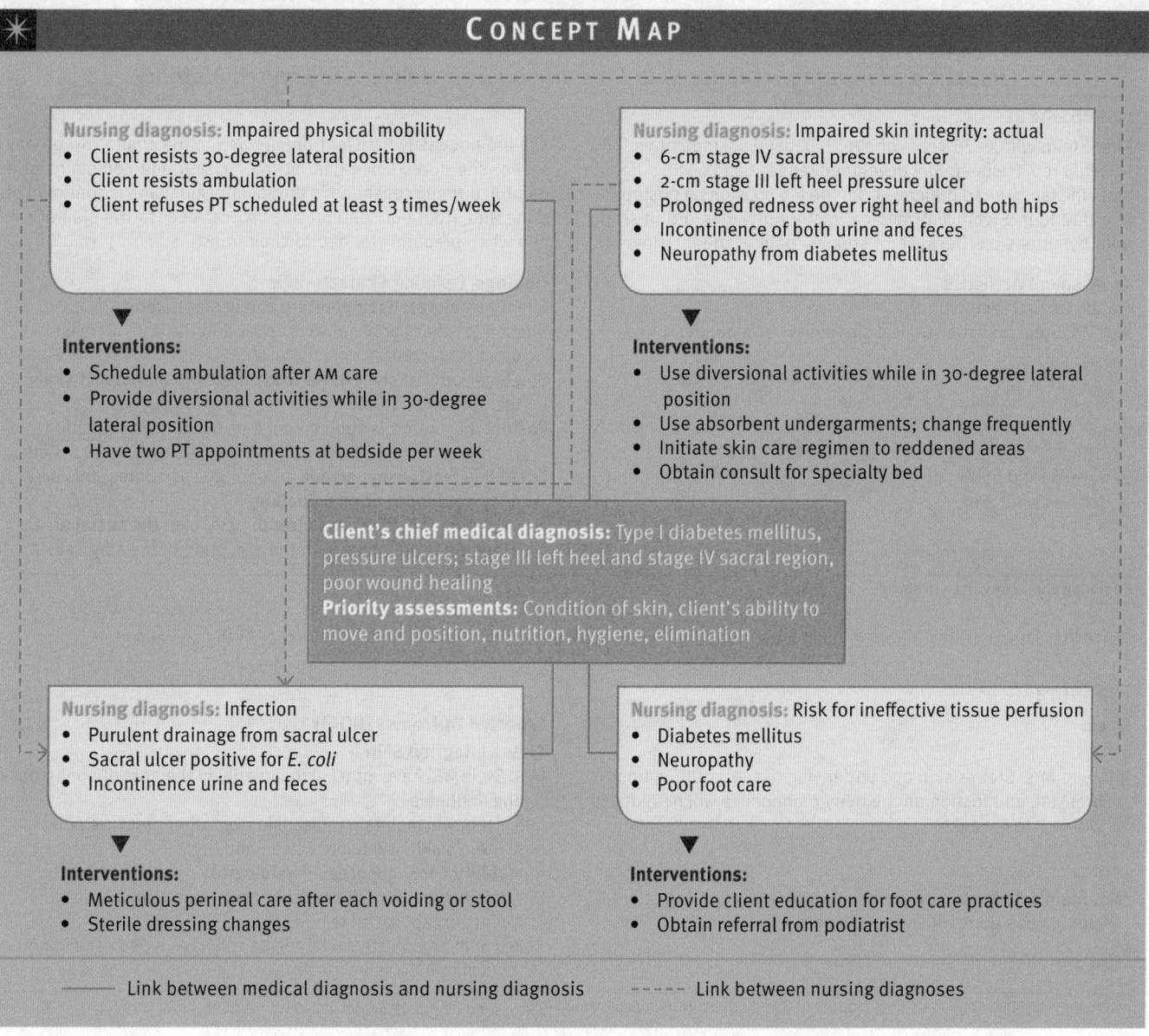

Nursing diagnosis: Impaired physical mobility
- Client resists 30-degree lateral position
- Client resists ambulation
- Client refuses PT scheduled at least 3 times/week

Interventions:
- Schedule ambulation after AM care
- Provide diversional activities while in 30-degree lateral position
- Have two PT appointments at bedside per week

Nursing diagnosis: Impaired skin integrity: actual
- 6-cm stage IV sacral pressure ulcer
- 2-cm stage III left heel pressure ulcer
- Prolonged redness over right heel and both hips
- Incontinence of both urine and feces
- Neuropathy from diabetes mellitus

Interventions:
- Use diversional activities while in 30-degree lateral position
- Use absorbent undergarments; change frequently
- Initiate skin care regimen to reddened areas
- Obtain consult for specialty bed

Client's chief medical diagnosis: Type I diabetes mellitus, pressure ulcers; stage III left heel and stage IV sacral region, poor wound healing
Priority assessments: Condition of skin, client's ability to move and position, nutrition, hygiene, elimination

Nursing diagnosis: Infection
- Purulent drainage from sacral ulcer
- Sacral ulcer positive for *E. coli*
- Incontinence urine and feces

Interventions:
- Meticulous perineal care after each voiding or stool
- Sterile dressing changes

Nursing diagnosis: Risk for ineffective tissue perfusion
- Diabetes mellitus
- Neuropathy
- Poor foot care

Interventions:
- Provide client education for foot care practices
- Obtain referral from podiatrist

——— Link between medical diagnosis and nursing diagnosis   - - - - Link between nursing diagnoses

Figure 48-17 Concept map for client with a chronic wound.

dence. Clients and their families often need to continue the objectives of wound management after discharge (Box 48-9). You need to consider the ability of the caregiver and the amount of time needed to change a particular dressing when selecting a dressing for the client to use after discharge. For example, in the home setting, some caregivers choose more expensive dressing materials to reduce the frequency of dressing changes (WOCN, 2003). The nurse and client work together to establish ways of maintaining client involvement in nursing care and to promote wound healing whether the client is in the hospital or home.

◆Implementation

Health Promotion. Perhaps the most effective intervention for problems with skin integrity and wound care is prevention. Prompt identification of high-risk clients and their risk factors aids in prevention of pressure ulcers.

Prevention of Pressure Ulcers. When the client is immobile, the major risk to the skin is the formation of pressure ulcers. Nursing interventions focus on prevention. The first step in prevention is to assess the client's risk factors for pressure ulcer development. Plan on reducing or eliminating the identified risk factors.

Early identification of clients at risk and their risk factors aids the nurse in preventing pressure ulcers. Prevention minimizes the impact that risk factors or contributing factors have on pressure ulcer development. Table 48-7 provides some universal preventive measures. Three major areas of nursing interventions for prevention of pressure ulcers are (1) skin care, which includes hygiene and skin care; (2) mechanical loading and support devices, which include proper positioning and the use of therapeutic surfaces; and (3) education (WOCN, 2003).

Topical Skin Care. You need to perform frequent skin assessment (see Box 48-6, p. 1292) at a minimum on a once-a-day basis. However, high-risk clients will have more frequent skin assessments, such as every shift. In addition, you ensure that the

NURSING CARE PLAN

Impaired Skin Integrity Related to Pressure on Sacral Area and Limited Mobility

Assessment

Mrs. Stein, who is 76 years of age, is 7 days postoperative for a total hip replacement. She developed redness and oozing of foul-smelling tan-colored drainage from the hip incision on postoperative day four. Significant medical history includes arthritis and mild hypertension. Because of surgical pain at the incision site, she did not easily transfer from her bed to the chair. Now on day seven, she notes some pain at the incision and complains of a painful, burning sensation in the sacral region. She is continent of urine and stool but continues to "scoot" over to the side of the bed when preparing for bed-to-chair transfers.

Assessment Activities	Findings/Defining Characteristics*
Obtain an oral temperature.	Client has **elevated temperature** and is diaphoretic.
Ask Ms. Stein how the surgical site limits her mobility.	She relates that her hip always aches and the pain increases upon movement.
	She tells you that she prefers to keep the hip immobile to keep the pain level down.
	Position of comfort is supine, and Mrs. Stein resists position changes.
Perform a total body skin assessment, paying special attention to the sacral area.	Client has **reactive hyperemia** around the sacral area; this **area does not blanch upon palpation.**
	There is a **partial-thickness ulcer directly over the sacral area.**
	No other areas are open, with the exception of the surgical site.

*Defining characteristics are shown in bold type.

Nursing Diagnosis: Impaired skin integrity related to pressure and friction on the bony prominence in the sacral region.

Planning

Goals	Expected Outcomes (NOC)†
	Tissue Integrity: Skin
Injury to Mrs. Stein's skin and underlying tissue resulting from pressure and friction on the bony prominence will be reduced within 2 to 4 weeks.	Mrs. Stein will have intact skin integrity in the area of nonblanching erythema.
	Mrs. Stein will maintain intact skin over other pressure points.
	Mrs. Stein's skin will remain clean and dry.
	Immobility Consequences: Physiological
Mrs. Stein's ability to tolerate position changes and correctly change positions will improve within 2 to 4 weeks.	Reactive hyperemia will be within normal limits in all pressure points except sacral region.
	Reactive hyperemia in sacral region will have a decrease in nonblanchable pressure areas.

†Outcome classification labels from Moorhead S and others: *Nursing outcomes classification (NOC),* ed 4, St. Louis, 2008, Mosby.

Interventions (NIC)‡	Rationale
Pressure Management	
• Reposition Mrs. Stein every 90 minutes. Offer pain medication at least 20 minutes before position change. When Mrs. Stein transfers from bed to chair, remind her not to slide over sheets but to pick up pelvis and relocate from one position to another. Be careful not to slide Mrs. Stein on the sheets.	Repositioning removes pressure and allows normal hyperemic response. Frequency of turning is based on initial assessment (Pieper, 2007; WOCN, 2003). Sliding the client's skin on the sheets will cause friction and deteriorate the involved area.
• Elevate the head of the bed no more than 30 degrees.	The higher the head of the bed is elevated, the more likely that shearing forces will be present, adding to pain and deterioration of the skin loss in the sacral area (WOCN, 2003).
Pressure Ulcer Care	
• Keep skin dry and clean; avoid rubbing area.	Moisture softens the skin and causes a break in the skin integrity. Rubbing an area of nonblanching erythema will cause further tissue damage (WOCN, 2003).
• Use a moisture barrier ointment over the ulcer at least 3 times a day to decrease friction and to provide moisture to the open tissue.	An ointment will cover the area, providing the base of the ulcer with moisture, which will encourage healing. The ointment will prevent the sheets from rubbing on the area, thus decreasing the friction (Bryant and Clark, 2007).

‡Intervention classification labels from Bulechek GM, Butcher HK, and Dochterman JM: *Nursing interventions classification (NIC),* ed 5, St. Louis, 2008, Mosby.

NURSING CARE PLAN

Impaired Skin Integrity Related to Pressure on Sacral Area and Limited Mobility—cont'd

Evaluation

Nursing Actions	Client Response/Findings	Achievement of Outcome
Perform a daily total body skin assessment. Chart results.	No new skin breakdown noted.	No other areas of pain or discomfort are reported.
	Decreased redness at the sacral area.	Decreased pain at the sacral site is reported.
Palpate the reddened area over the sacrum.	Sacral area begins to show signs of normal reactive hyperemia blanching following palpation.	Sacral region is improving; no break in epidermis.
	Other pressure points have normal reactive hyperemia and blanching.	Other pressure points remain intact.

✳ BOX 48-9 Home Care Recommendations

Ulcer/Wound Assessment

Assessment and documentation of a pressure ulcer needs to occur at least weekly, unless there is evidence of deterioration, in which case the nurse will need to reassess both the pressure ulcer and the client's overall management immediately. In the home setting, this will require the assistance of the client and family because weekly assessment is not always feasible.

Psychosocial Assessment and Management

- Assess the client's resources (e.g., availability and skill of caregivers, finances, equipment). A successful treatment program requires adequate caregiver and equipment resources.
- Evaluate caregivers for their ability to comprehend and implement the treatment requirements.
- Also evaluate caregivers for their level of strength and endurance.
- Consider economic factors, because they often limit the supply and availability of equipment, as well as opportunities to relieve caregivers.
- Use an approach that focuses upon the psychosocial and physical factors affecting wound care (Teare and Barrett, 2002).

Ulcer Care Dressings

- Consider caregiver time when selecting a dressing.
- In the home setting, some caregivers choose more expensive dressing materials to reduce the frequency of dressing changes.

Infection Control

- Clean dressings are sometimes used in the home setting.
- Clean dressings, as opposed to sterile ones, are recommended for home use until research demonstrates otherwise. This recommendation is in keeping with principles regarding nosocomial infections and with past success of clean urinary catheterization in the home setting, and it takes into account the expense of sterile dressings and the dexterity required for application. The caregiver can use the "no-touch" technique for dressing changes. This technique is a method of changing surface dressings without touching the wound or the surface of any dressing that might be in contact with the wound. Adherent dressings should be grasped by the corner and removed slowly, whereas gauze dressings can be pinched in the center and lifted off.
- Disposal of contaminated dressings in the home should be done in a manner consistent with local regulations. The Environmental Protection Agency recommends placing soiled dressings in securely fastened plastic bags before adding them to other household trash. Local regulations vary, however, and home care agencies and clients need to follow procedures that are consistent with local laws.

Modified from Agency for Health Care Policy and Research, Panel for the Treatment of Pressure Ulcers in Adults: *Treatment of pressure ulcers,* Clinical Practice Guideline No. 15, AHCPR Pub No. 95-0653, Rockville, Md, 1994, Agency for Health Care Policy and Research, Public Health Service, U.S. Department of Health and Human Services.

✳ TABLE 48-7 A Quick Guide to Pressure Ulcer Prevention

RISK FACTOR	NURSING INTERVENTIONS
Decreased sensory perception	Assess pressure points for signs of nonblanching reactive hyperemia.
	Provide pressure-redistribution surface.
Moisture	Assess need for incontinence management.
	Following each incontinent episode, cleanse area with no-rinse perineal cleanser and protect skin with a moisture barrier ointment.
Friction and shear	Reposition client using a drawsheet and lifting off surface.
	Provide a trapeze to facilitate movement.
	Position client at a 30-degree lateral turn and limit head elevation to 30 degrees.
Decreased activity/mobility	Establish and post individualized turning schedule.
Poor nutrition	Provide adequate nutritional and fluid intake; assist with intake as necessary.
	Consult dietitian for nutritional evaluation.

client's skin is clean and dry. Assessment and skin hygiene are two initial defenses for preventing skin breakdown.

When you clean the skin, avoid soaps and hot water. Use cleansers with nonionic surfactants that are gentle to the skin (WOCN, 2003). There are many types of products available for skin care, and you need to match their use to the specific needs of the client.

After you cleanse the skin and make sure it is completely dry, apply moisturizer to keep the epidermis well lubricated but not oversaturated.

Make an effort to control, contain, or correct incontinence, perspiration, or wound drainage (Bryant and Clark, 2007). Clinicians find the Agency for Health Care Research and Policy (AHCPR) guidelines on urinary incontinence (1992b) helpful (see Chapter 45). Clients who have fecal incontinence and who are also receiving enteral tube feeding provide a management challenge. When clients have an incontinent episode, gently cleanse the area, dry, and apply a thick layer of moisture barrier to the exposed areas. A moisture barrier protects the skin from excessive moisture and bacteria found in the urine or stool.

It is helpful to use the expertise of an advanced practice nurse with a focus on wound care or management of incontinence while caring for at-risk clients. Methods for controlling or containing incontinence vary. You can treat urinary incontinence with behavioral techniques, medication, and surgery. Behavioral techniques help clients learn ways to control their bladder and sphincter muscles. Two examples are bladder training and habit training, which is also called timed voiding.

Consider using absorbent pads and garments only after trying the above measures. Although controversial, absorbent products, such as absorptive underpads and garments, are sometimes part of the treatment plan for an incontinent client. Use only products that wick moisture away from the client's skin (Bryant and Clark, 2007; WOCN, 2003). Use underpads with caution because some of these pads do not wick the drainage away from the client's skin and will cause skin damage.

Positioning. Positioning interventions reduce pressure and **shearing force** to the skin. Elevating the head of the bed to 30 degrees or less will decrease the chance of pressure ulcer development from shearing forces (WOCN, 2003). Change the immobilized client's position according to activity level, perceptual ability, and daily routines (Braden, 2001). Therefore a standard turning interval of 1½ to 2 hours does not always prevent pressure ulcer development in some clients. Clients need repositioning at least every 2 hours on a schedule. When repositioning, use positioning devices to protect bony prominences (WOCN, 2003). The WOCN guidelines (2003) recommend a 30-degree lateral position (Figure 48-18). The 30-degree lateral position should prevent positioning directly over the bony prominence. To prevent shear and friction injuries, use a transfer device to lift rather than drag the client when changing positions (Chapter 47).

> **SAFETY ALERT** Incorrect positioning of an immobile client will possibly create a shearing injury. When repositioning the client, place a transfer sliding board under the client's body. Obtain assistance for repositioning, and with at least one other caregiver, use the board to slide the client up and toward the new position. Dragging the client on bed sheets will place the client at high risk for shearing and friction injuries.

Some clients are able to sit in a chair. Make sure to limit the amount of time clients sit to 2 hours or less. Again, individualize the exact time, but do not allow the client to sit for a period longer than the recommended time that was calculated during assessment. Thus if the interval is every 1½ hours, the client should remain in a sitting position for less than 1½ hours. In the sitting position the pressure on the ischial tuberosities is greater than in the supine position. In addition, teach a client at risk for skin breakdown in a sitting position to shift weight every 15 minutes (WOCN, 2003). Shifting weight provides short-term relief on the ischial tuberosities. Also have the client sit on foam, gel, or an air cushion to redistribute weight away from the ischial areas. Rigid and donut-shaped cushions are contraindicated because they reduce blood supply to the area, resulting in wider areas of ischemia (WOCN, 2003).

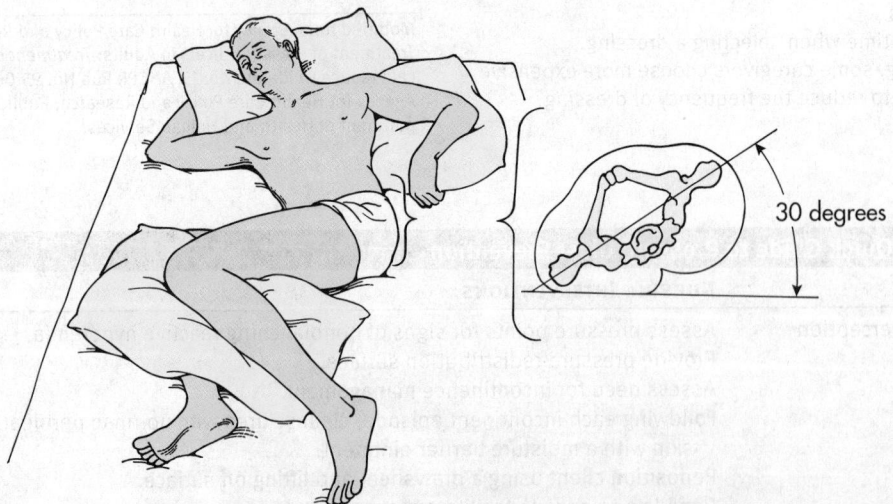

Figure 48-18 Thirty-degree lateral position at which pressure points are avoided. (From Pieper B: Mechanical forces: pressure, shear, and friction. In Bryant RA, Nix DP, editors: *Acute and chronic wounds: current management concepts,* ed 3, St. Louis, 2007, Mosby.)

After repositioning the client, reassess the skin. Identifying characteristics that indicate early signs of tissue ischemia in darkly pigmented skin are in Boxes 48-2, p. 1281, and 48-3, p. 1282. For clients with light-toned skin, observe for **normal reactive hyperemia** and blanching. Never massage the reddened areas. Massaging reddened areas increases breaks in the capillaries in the underlying tissues and increases the risk of injury to underlying tissue and pressure ulcer formation (AHCPR, 1992a).

Support Surfaces (Therapeutic Beds and Mattresses). A support surface is a specialized device for pressure redistribution designed for management of tissue loads, microclimate, and/or other therapeutic functions (i.e., mattresses, integrated bed system, mattress replacement, overlay or seat cushion, or seat cushion overlay) (NPUAP, 2007b). There are a variety of support surfaces, including specialty beds and mattresses that reduce the hazards of immobility to the skin and musculoskeletal system. However, none eliminates the need for meticulous nursing care. No single device eliminates the effects of pressure on the skin.

When selecting support surfaces, thoroughly assess the client's needs. Knowledge about support surface characteristics (Table 48-8) assists the nurse in clinical decision making. In selecting a support surface, know the client's risks, as well as the purpose for the support surface; a flow chart is often helpful (Figure 48-19).

Teach clients and families the reason for and proper use of the beds or mattresses (Box 48-10). Some common errors with support surfaces are placing the wrong side of the support surface toward the client, not plugging powered support surfaces into the electrical source, not turning on the power source for powered support surfaces, failing to do "hand checks" for some support surfaces, and improperly inflating some support surfaces. When used correctly, these support services assist in reducing pressure ulcers in clients at risk.

Acute Care

Management of Pressure Ulcers. Treatment of clients with pressure ulcers requires a holistic approach that uses the expertise of several multidisciplinary health care professionals (WOCN, 2003). In addition to the nurse, the health care provider, physical therapist, occupational therapist, nutritionist, and pharmacist are involved. Aspects of pressure ulcer treatment include local care of the wound and supportive measures such as adequate nutrients and redistribution of pressure (Skill 48-2, p. 1308).

When treating a pressure ulcer, reassess the wound for location, stage, size, tissue type and amount, exudate, and surrounding skin condition (Nix, 2007). Acute wounds require close monitoring (every 8 hours.) Sometimes chronic wound assessment occurs less frequently. Depending upon the topical manage-

✳ TABLE 48-8 Support Surfaces

Categories and Definitions	Mechanism of Action	Indications	Examples of Manufacturers' and Product Names
Low-Air-Loss Available in a mattress placed directly on the existing bed frame or an overlay placed directly on top of an existing surface	Pressure redistribution Provides a flow of air to assist in managing the heat and humidity of the skin	Prevention or treatment of skin breakdown	Hill Rom/Flexiair Kinetic Concepts, Inc/First Step Select Crown Therapeutics/Select Air Mattress
Nonpowered Any support surface not requiring or using external sources of energy for operation. Examples: foam, interconnected air-filled cells	Pressure redistribution Air moves to and from cells as body position changes	Prevention or treatment of skin breakdown	Crown Therapeutics RoHo Dry Flotation Mattress Gaymar Industries/Sof-Care
Air-Fluidized Beds Surfaces that change load distribution properties when powered and when client is in contact with the surface	Provides pressure redistribution via a fluidlike medium created by forcing air through beads as characterized by immersion and envelopment	Prevention or treatment of skin breakdown May also be used to protect newly flapped or grafted surgical sites and for clients with excessive moisture	Kinetic Concepts, Inc/FluidAir Hill Rom/Clinitron
Lateral Rotation Provides passive motion to promote mobilization of respiratory secretions and provides low-air-loss therapy	A feature of a support surface that provides rotation about a longitudinal axis as characterized by degree of client turn, duration, and frequency	Treatment and prevention of pulmonary complications associated with immobility	Hill Rom/Total Care Sport Kinetic Concepts, Inc/TriaDyne

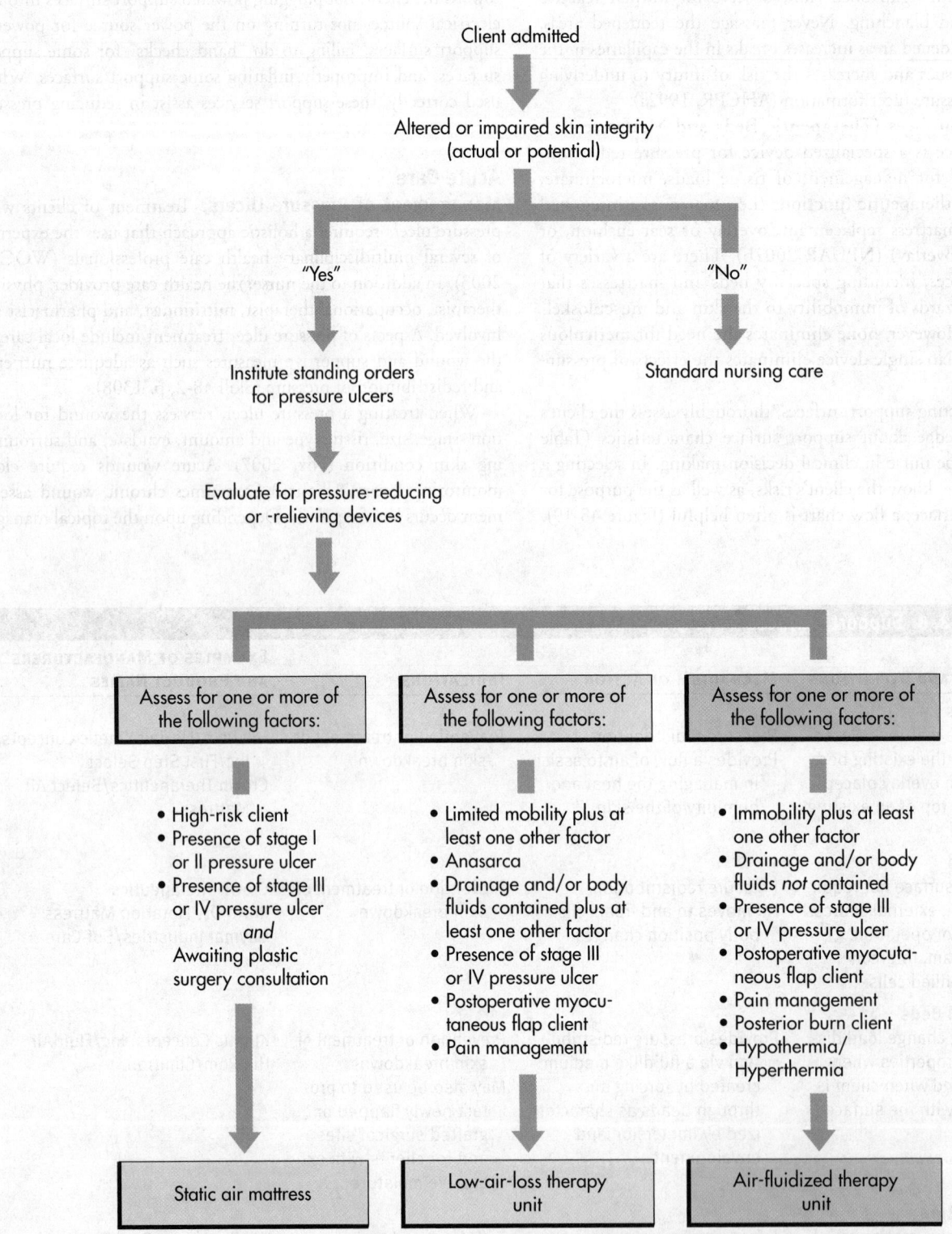

Client admitted

↓

Altered or impaired skin integrity
(actual or potential)

"Yes" ← → "No"

| Institute standing orders for pressure ulcers | Standard nursing care |

↓

Evaluate for pressure-reducing
or -relieving devices

↓

| Assess for one or more of the following factors: | Assess for one or more of the following factors: | Assess for one or more of the following factors: |

- High-risk client
- Presence of stage I or II pressure ulcer
- Presence of stage III or IV pressure ulcer *and* Awaiting plastic surgery consultation

- Limited mobility plus at least one other factor
- Anasarca
- Drainage and/or body fluids contained plus at least one other factor
- Presence of stage III or IV pressure ulcer
- Postoperative myocutaneous flap client
- Pain management

- Immobility plus at least one other factor
- Drainage and/or body fluids *not* contained
- Presence of stage III or IV pressure ulcer
- Postoperative myocutaneous flap client
- Pain management
- Posterior burn client
- Hypothermia/ Hyperthermia

↓

| Static air mattress | Low-air-loss therapy unit | Air-fluidized therapy unit |

Figure 48-19 Flow diagram for ordering specialty beds. (Modified from Thomas C: Specialty beds: decision-making made easy, *Ostomy Wound Manage* 23:51, 1989.)

BOX 48-10   **CLIENT TEACHING**

Pressure-Redistribution Surfaces

Objective
- Client and family will describe understanding of the purposes and basic operations of the pressure-redistribution surfaces.

Teaching Strategies
- Explain the reasons for the pressure-redistribution surface.
- Explain proper body mechanics while using the pressure-redistribution surface.
- Educate the use and care of the pressure-redistribution surface.
- Explain additional pressure-redistribution measures.

Evaluation
- Client and family will state basic purposes for the pressure-redistribution surface.
- Client and family will be able to describe the function of the pressure-redistribution surface.
- Client and family will be able to demonstrate proper use of the pressure-redistribution surface.

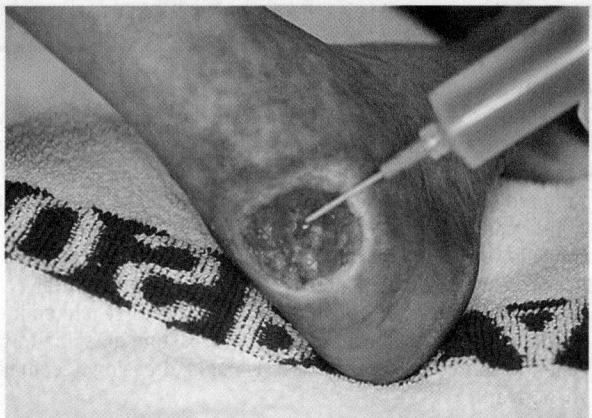

Figure 48-20 Wound irrigation.

ment system, evaluate the wound with every dressing change, usually not more than one time per day.

The use and documentation of a systematic approach to the assessment of the actual pressure ulcers leads to better decision making and optimum outcomes (Nix, 2007). There are several healing and documentation tools you can use to document wound assessments over time. Using a tool helps link assessment to outcomes so that an evaluation of the plan of care follows objective criteria (Nix, 2007). For example, the Pressure Ulcer Status Tool (PSST) (Bates-Jensen, 1995) addresses 15 wound characteristics. You score individual items and sum them, providing an overall indication of wound status. The scoring assists in evaluating whether the goals of the wound management are effective.

Wound Management. Maintenance of a physiological local wound environment is the goal of effective wound management (Rolstad and Ovington, 2007). In order to maintain a healthy wound environment, you need to address the following principles: prevent and manage infection, cleanse the wound, remove nonviable tissue, manage exudate, maintain the wound in a moist environment, and protect the wound.

A wound will not move through the phases of wound healing if the wound is infected. Prevention of wound infection includes wound cleansing and removal of nonviable tissue. You clean pressure ulcers only with noncytotoxic wound cleansers, such as normal saline or commercial wound cleansers. Noncytotoxic cleansers will not damage or kill fibroblasts and healing tissue (Rolstad and Ovington, 2007). Some commonly used cytotoxic solutions are Dakin's solution (sodium hypochlorite solution), acetic acid, povidone-iodine, and hydrogen peroxide. These are not used in clean, granulating wounds.

Irrigation is a common method of delivering the wound-cleansing solution to the wound. Studies have shown that there is an optimal effective range of irrigation pressures that ensure ade-

quate removal of bacteria (Rodeheaver, 2001). One method to ensure an irrigation pressure within the correct range is to use a 19-gauge needle or an angiocatheter and a 35-mL syringe that delivers saline to a pressure ulcer at 8 psi (Figure 48-20).

Debridement is the removal of nonviable, necrotic tissue. Removal of necrotic tissue is necessary to rid the ulcer of a source of infection, to enable visualization of the wound bed, and to provide a clean base necessary for healing. However, a dry necrotic heel pressure ulcer is an exception. According to the WOCN guidelines (2003), "stable, dry, black eschar on heels should not be debrided if they are non-tender, nonfluctuant, nonerythematous and nonsuppurative."

The method of debridement will depend on which is most appropriate to the client's condition and care goals (WOCN, 2003). It is important to remember that during the debridement process some normal wound observations to make include an increase in wound exudate, odor, and size. You will need to assess and prevent or effectively manage pain that occurs with debridement (WOCN, 2003).

Methods of debridement include mechanical, autolytic, chemical, and sharp/surgical. One method of mechanical debridement is the use of wet-to-dry saline gauze dressings. Place moistened gauze into the wound and allow the dressing to dry thoroughly before "pulling" the gauze that has adhered to the tissue out of the pressure ulcer. This is a nonselective method of debridement because devitalized and viable tissue are both removed, and thus it is not used routinely. Never use this method in a clean, granulating wound. Other methods of mechanical debridement are wound irrigation (high-pressure irrigation and pulsatile high-pressure lavage) and whirlpool treatments (Ramundo, 2007).

Autolytic debridement uses synthetic dressings over a wound to allow the eschar to be self-digested by the action of enzymes that are present in wound fluids (WOCN, 2003). You accomplish this by using dressings that support moisture at the wound surface. If the wound base is dry, use a dressing that will add moisture; if there is excessive exudate, use a dressing that absorbs the excessive moisture while maintaining moisture at the wound bed. Some examples of these dressings are transparent film dressings and hydrocolloid dressings.

Delegation Considerations

The skill of treatment of pressure ulcers cannot be delegated. In some practice settings you can delegate *nonsterile* dressing application for chronic, established wounds where a nurse has evaluated and designated the protocol. The *assessment* of the wound remains within the scope of the nurse even if the dressing change is delegated. Instruct nursing assistive personnel to:

- Report changes in skin integrity to the nurse immediately
- Report pain, fever, or wound drainage to the nurse immediately
- Report any potential contamination to existing dressing (e.g., client incontinence or other bodily fluids, dressing becomes dislodged)

Equipment

- Clean gloves
- Plastic bag for dressing disposal
- Measuring device
- Cotton-tipped applicators
- Topical cleansing agent
- Dressing of choice (see Table 48-9, p. 1313)
- Hypoallergenic tape (if needed)
- Documentation record
- Scale for assessing wound healing
- Sterile gloves (check agency policy)

STEPS	RATIONALE
1. Assess client's level of comfort using a scale of 0 to 10 and need for pain medication.	Clients tolerate dressing change procedure better if pain is controlled.
2. Determine if client has allergies to topical agents.	Topical agents cause localized skin reactions.
3. Review order for topical agent or dressing and location.	Ensures that you administer proper medication and treatment.
4. Close room door or bedside curtains. Position client to allow dressing removal.	Provides privacy and ensures that area is accessible for dressing change.
5. Perform hand hygiene, and apply clean gloves. Remove dressing, and place in plastic bag.	Reduces transmission of microorganisms and prevents accidental exposure to body fluids.
6. Assess pressure ulcer(s). All pressure ulcers need individual assessments (see illustration).	Consistent assessment will provide the basis for evaluating wound progress (Nix, 2007).
a. Note color, type, and percentage of tissue present in the wound base.	The tissue type will assist in the choice of dressing.
b. Measure width and length of the ulcer(s). Determine width by measuring the dimension from left to right, and the length from top to bottom (see illustration).	Ulcer size will change as healing progresses, and therefore the longest and widest areas of the wound will change over time. Measuring the width and length by measuring consistent areas will provide a consistent measurement (Nix, 2007).
c. Measure depth of pressure ulcer using sterile cotton-tipped applicator or other device that will allow measurement of wound depth (see illustration).	Depth measure is important for determining wound volume. Although surface area adequately represents tissue loss in stage II ulcers, volume more adequately represents tissue loss in stage III and IV wounds.
d. Measure depth of undermining using a cotton-tipped applicator and gently probing under skin edges (see illustration).	Undermining represents the loss of the underlying tissue (subcutaneous and muscle) to a greater extent than the skin. Undermining indicates progressive tissue loss and needs to be accommodated with an appropriate dressing.

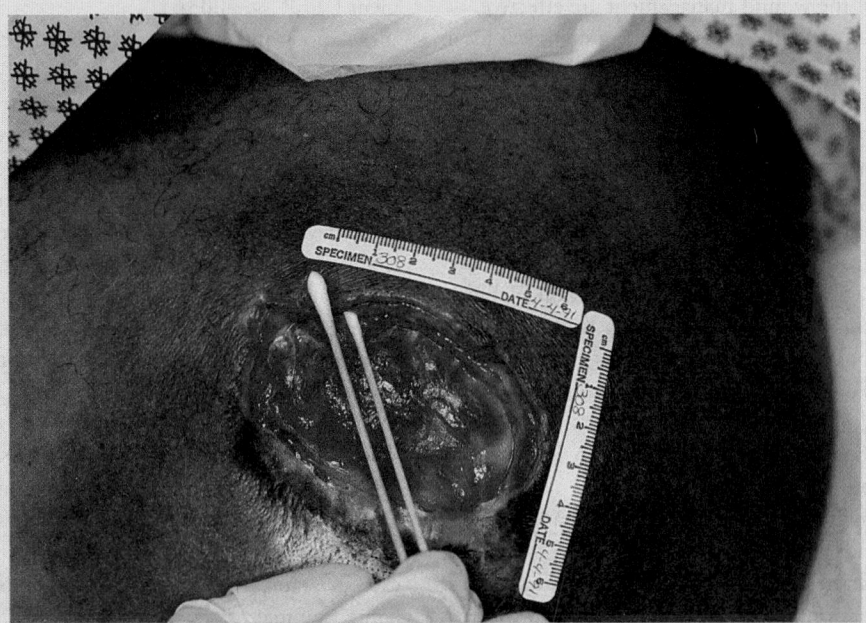

STEP 6 Measuring wound depth. (Steps b [use of centimeter ruler], c [use of cotton-tipped applicator], and d [use of cotton-tipped applicator to measure undermining.])

TREATING PRESSURE ULCERS—CONT'D

STEPS	RATIONALE
7. Assess the periwound skin; check for maceration, redness, denuded area.	Deterioration of the skin around a wound indicates infection, excessive wound exudate, or skin stripping from adhesive removal.
8. Change to sterile gloves (check agency policy).	Aseptic technique needs to be maintained during cleansing and application of dressings. Refer to institutional policy regarding use of clean or sterile gloves.
9. Cleanse ulcer thoroughly with normal saline or cleansing agent. Cleanse with irrigating syringe for deep ulcers.	Removes wound debris.
10. Check client's identification using two identifiers.	Ensures right client receives correct topical agent.

11. Apply topical agents, as prescribed:

   A. Enzymes

(1) Apply thin, even layer of ointment over necrotic areas of ulcer only. Do not apply enzyme to surrounding skin. Check manufacturer's direction for frequency of application.	Thin layer absorbs and acts more effectively than thick layer. Excess medication irritates surrounding skin (Rolstad and Ovington, 2007). Some enzymes cause burning, paresthesia, and dermatitis to surrounding skin.
(2) Apply gauze dressing directly over ulcer.	Protects wound. Prevents bacteria from entering wound.
(3) Tape securely in place.	Keeps dressing in place.

   B. Hydrogel

(1) Cover surface of ulcer with hydrogel using applicator or gloved hand.	Provides maintenance of a moist wound environment.
(2) Apply dry gauze, hydrocolloid, or transparent film dressing over wound, and adhere to intact skin.	Covers wound base, maintaining hydrogel wound interface.

   C. Calcium alginate

(1) Pack wound with alginate using applicator or gloved hand.	Provides maintenance of wound moisture while absorbing excess drainage.
(2) Apply dry gauze or foam over alginate. Tape in place.	Holds alginate against wound surface.

STEPS	RATIONALE
12. Remove gloves, and dispose of soiled supplies. Perform hand hygiene.	Reduces transmission of microorganisms.
13. Assess the pressure ulcer at each dressing change or sooner if the wound or client's condition deteriorates (Nix, 2007). Utilize the agency's tool for wound assessment.	Not all clients with wounds will demonstrate quick wound healing because of other health care issues. The wound assessment will provide a report of wound healing progress or the lack of healing.
14. Compare wound assessment to the identified plan of care, and if the wound is not progressing toward healing as indicated by an increase in size, increased presence of pain, foul-smelling drainage, or increase in devitalized tissue, discuss findings with the health care team.	Ensures an appropriate plan for wound care is in place.

Critical Decision Point: A clean pressure ulcer should show evidence of some healing within 2 to 4 weeks. Do *not* use the pressure ulcer staging system to measure pressure ulcer healing. System measures depth of wound, not healing (WOCN, 2003).

---

15. Complete wound documentation required for one of the wound assessment instruments per agency's protocol.	Provides comparison of assessments over time to determine progress toward wound healing.

Unexpected Outcomes and Related Interventions

1. Skin surrounding ulcer becomes macerated.
   a. Reduce exposure of surrounding skin to topical agents and moisture.
   b. Consider the use of a liquid skin barrier on periwound skin.
2. Ulcer becomes deeper with increased drainage.
   a. Notify health care provider for possible change in pressure ulcer status.
   b. Obtain necessary wound cultures.
   c. Obtain additional consults (e.g., wound care specialist).

Recording and Reporting

- Record assessment of ulcer in client's record.
- Describe type of topical agent used, dressing applied, and client's response.
- Report any deterioration in ulcer appearance.

Home Care Considerations

- Cost is often a factor. Some clients have more time than financial resources. Some choose a less expensive treatment option such as dressing material, especially if there is no third-party reimbursement.
- Clients need to dispose of contaminated dressings in the home in a manner consistent with local regulations (WOCN, 2003).
- Discuss need for home pressure-redistribution surface or bed.

A moist environment will support the movement of epithelial cells and facilitate wound closure. A wound that has excessive wound exudate (drainage) provides an environment that supports bacterial growth, macerates the periwound skin, and slows the healing process. If excessive wound exudate is present, evaluate the volume, consistency, and odor of the drainage to determine if signs and symptoms of infection are present.

You can accomplish chemical debridement with the use of a topical enzyme preparation, Dakin's solution, or sterile maggots. Topical enzymes induce changes in the substrate resulting in the breakdown of necrotic tissue (Ramundo, 2007). Depending on the type of enzyme used, the preparation either digests or dissolves the tissue. These preparations require a health care provider's order. Dakin's solution breaks down and loosens dead tissue in a wound. Apply the solution to a gauze, packing into the wound. Sterile maggots are used in a wound because it is thought that they ingest the dead tissue.

Surgical debridement is the removal of devitalized tissue by using a scalpel, scissors, or other sharp instrument. Health care providers and, in some states, trained advanced practice nurses perform surgical debridement of a pressure ulcer. Nurses should check the Nurse Practice Act for their state to see if surgical debridement is a nursing function. It is the quickest method of debridement. It is usually indicated when the client has signs of cellulitis or sepsis.

Remember, the wound will not heal unless the contributory factors are controlled or eliminated. Therefore it is critically important for you to address the causative factors (e.g., shear, friction, pressure, and moisture), or it is unlikely that the wound will heal despite topical therapy (Rolstad and Ovington, 2007).

The treatment plan will need to be altered as the ulcer heals. For example, in the management of a necrotic wound, a transparent film dressing is used initially to autolytically debride (liquefy the tissue using the body's own moisture) the wound. Once the wound is cleansed of necrotic tissue, you will discontinue the transparent film dressing and, based upon the wound base characteristics, choose a new dressing. A wound with excessive drainage will require a dressing with a high absorptive capacity. Continued reassessment is key to supporting the wound as it moves through the phases of wound healing.

Growth Factors. Growth factors regulate most of the key actions of cells during wound healing. Through extensive studies of the molecular regulation of healing, researchers now better understand the role of various growth factors. Topical growth factors regulate the healing of chronic wounds (Schultz, 2007). Growth factors involved in wound healing include epidermal growth factor, platelet-derived growth factor, fibroblast growth factor, and transforming growth factor. The nurse is often responsible for the use of this treatment modality. Teaching the client or significant other about the use of growth factors is also the nurse's responsibility. The nurse teaches the use of the medication, wound care, and the prevention of wound breakdown and recurrence.

Education. Education of the client and caregivers is an important nursing function (Rolstad and Ovington, 2007). There are a variety of educational tools, including videotapes and written materials, for you to use when teaching clients and caregivers/family to prevent and treat pressure ulcers. Written materials are available on a variety of topics, including dressing changes;

there are also guides for measuring wounds and charts for positioning clients. AHCPR (1992a, 1994) has booklets for clients on pressure ulcer prevention and treatment that are helpful when teaching clients and their caregivers/family. These booklets are available in English and in Spanish. Individualize your teaching for each client, especially with older clients.

Understanding and assessment of the experience of the client and support person are also important dimensions in the treatment of people with pressure ulcers (WOCN, 2003). Clinicians are only just now exploring through research the caregiver's perspective of the concerns and issues faced by frail older spouses caring for their loved ones with pressure ulcers. You need to plan interventions to meet the identified psychosocial needs of clients and their support persons (WOCN, 2003).

Nutritional Status. Nutritional assessment and support of the client with a wound is based upon the appreciation that nutrition is fundamental to normal cellular integrity and tissue repair (Stotts, 2007a). Early intervention is necessary to correct inadequate nutrition and to support healing. The Joint Commission (2007) recommends nutritional assessment within 24 hours of admission. Reassessments reflect changes in status and effects of interventions (Stotts, 2007a). Box 48-11 defines parameters for clinically significant malnutrition (AHCPR, 1994). Assess the client's mouth and skin for signs of nutritional deficiencies (see Chapter 44). Give vitamin and mineral supplements if you suspect or know of any deficiencies.

✳ BOX 48-11 AHCPR Recommendations for Nutritional Assessment and Management of Pressure Ulcers

Assessment of Clinically Significant Malnutrition
Serum albumin is less than 3.5 mg/100 mL.
Total lymphocyte count is less than 1800/mm³.
Body weight has decreased more than 15%.

Interventions
- Ensure adequate dietary intake to prevent malnutrition to the extent that this is compatible with the individual's wishes and ideal body weight.
  - Maintain serum albumin greater than 3.5 mg/100 mL.
  - Maintain total lymphocyte count greater than 1800/mm³.
- Perform an abbreviated nutritional assessment, as defined by the Nutritional Screening Initiative, at least every 3 months for individuals who are unable to take food by mouth or who experience an involuntary change in weight.
- Encourage dietary intake or supplementation if an individual with a pressure ulcer is malnourished. If dietary intake continues to be inadequate, impractical, or impossible, use nutritional support (usually tube feeding) to place the client into positive nitrogen balance (approximately 30 to 35 calories/kg/day and 1.25 to 1.50 g of protein/kg/day) according to the goals of care.
- Give vitamin and mineral supplements if you suspect or confirm deficiencies.

Modified from Agency for Health Care Policy and Research, Panel for Treatment of Pressure Ulcers in Adults: *Treatment of pressure ulcers,* Clinical Practice Guideline No. 15, AHCPR Pub No. 95-0653, Rockville, Md, 1994, Agency for Health Care Policy and Research, Public Health Service, U.S. Department of Health and Human Services.

AHCPR, Agency for Health Care Policy and Research.

Protein Status. Clients with a potential for or actual decreased serum albumin levels or poor protein intake need a nutritional evaluation to ensure proper caloric intake (AHCPR, 1994). A client can lose as much as 50 g of protein per day from an open, weeping pressure ulcer. Although the recommended intake of protein for adults is 0.8 g/kg/day, a higher intake of protein up to 1.8 g/kg/day is necessary for healing. Increased protein intake helps rebuild epidermal tissue. Increased caloric intake helps replace subcutaneous tissue. Vitamin C promotes collagen synthesis, capillary wall integrity, fibroblast function, and immunological function.

Hemoglobin. A low hemoglobin level decreases delivery of oxygen to the tissues and leads to further ischemia. When possible, maintain hemoglobin at 12 g/100 mL.

First Aid for Wounds. In an emergency setting use first aid measures for wound care. Under stable conditions a variety of interventions ensure wound healing. When a client suffers a traumatic wound, first aid interventions include stabilizing cardiopulmonary function (see Chapter 40), promoting hemostasis, cleansing the wound, and protecting the wound from further injury.

Hemostasis. After assessing the type and extent of the wound, control bleeding by applying direct pressure on the wound with a sterile or clean dressing, such as a washcloth. After bleeding subsides, an adhesive bandage or gauze dressing taped over the laceration allows skin edges to close and a blood clot to form. If a dressing becomes saturated with blood, add another layer of dressing, continue to apply pressure, and elevate the affected part. Avoid further disruption of skin layers. Serious lacerations need to be sutured by a health care provider. Pressure dressings used during the first 24 to 48 hours after trauma help maintain hemostasis.

Normally, allow a puncture wound to bleed to remove dirt and other contaminants, such as saliva from a dog bite. When a penetrating object, such as a knife blade, is present, **do not remove the object**. The presence of the object provides pressure and controls some bleeding. Removal causes massive, uncontrolled bleeding. Except for skull injuries, apply pressure around the penetrating object, but not on it, and transport the client to an emergency facility.

Cleansing. The process of cleansing a wound involves selecting both an appropriate cleansing solution and using a mechanical means of delivering that solution without causing injury to the healing wound tissue (WOCN, 2003). Gentle cleansing of a wound removes contaminants that serve as sources of infection. However, vigorous cleaning using a method with too much mechanical force causes bleeding or further injury. For abrasions, minor lacerations, and small puncture wounds, first rinse the wound with normal saline, and lightly cover the area with a dressing. When a laceration is bleeding profusely, only brush away surface contaminants and concentrate on hemostasis until the client can be cared for in a clinic or hospital.

According to the WOCN guidelines (2003), normal saline is the preferred cleansing agent. It is physiologically neutral and will not harm tissue. Gentle cleansing with normal saline and the application of moist saline dressings are often used in healing wounds. Use saline to maintain the moist surface needed to promote the development and migration of epithelial tissue. Wet-to-dry saline dressings are only for debriding wounds. Never use them in a clean, granulating wound.

Protection. Regardless of whether bleeding has stopped, protect the wound from further injury by applying sterile or clean dressings and immobilizing the body part. A light dressing applied over minor wounds prevents entrance of microorganisms.

Dressings. The more extensive the wound, the larger the dressing required. In the home a clean towel or diaper is often the best secondary dressing. A bulky dressing applied with pressure minimizes movement of underlying tissues and helps immobilize the entire body part. A bandage or cloth wrapped around a penetrating object should immobilize it adequately.

There are alternative dressings to cover and protect certain types of wounds such as large wounds, wounds with drainage tubes or suction catheters in the wound, wounds that need frequent changing, and fistulas. For these wounds, pouches or special wound collection systems cover the wound and collect the wound drainage. Some of these devices have a plastic door on the front of the wound pouch, allowing you to change the wound packing without removing the wound pouch from the skin.

The use of dressings requires an understanding of wound healing. A variety of dressing materials are commercially available. The correct dressing selection facilitates wound healing (Rolstad and Ovington, 2007). The dressing type depends on the assessment of the wound and the phase of wound healing. When you identify the objectives for the wound care, the dressing choice becomes clear. A wound that requires infection management requires a different set of dressings than a wound requiring the removal of nonviable tissue.

For surgical wounds that heal by primary intention, it is common to remove dressings as soon as drainage stops. In contrast, when dressing a wound healing by secondary intention, the dressing material becomes a means for providing moisture to the wound or assisting in debridement.

Purposes of Dressings. A dressing serves several purposes:

- Protects a wound from microorganism contamination
- Aids in hemostasis
- Promotes healing by absorbing drainage and debriding a wound
- Supports or splints the wound site
- Protects the client from seeing the wound (if perceived as unpleasant)
- Promotes thermal insulation of the wound surface
- Provides a moist environment

When the skin is broken, a dressing helps reduce exposure to microorganisms. However, when wound drainage is minimal, the healing process forms a natural fibrin seal that eliminates the need for a dressing. Wounds with extensive tissue loss always need a dressing.

Pressure dressings promote hemostasis. Applied with elastic bandages, a pressure dressing exerts localized downward pressure over an actual or potential bleeding site. A pressure dressing eliminates dead space in underlying tissues so that wound healing progresses normally. Check pressure dressings to be sure that they do not interfere with circulation to a body part. Assess skin color, pulses in distal extremities, the client's comfort, and changes in sensation. Pressure dressings are not routinely removed.

A primary function of a dressing on a healing wound is to absorb drainage. Most traditional surgical dressings have three layers: a contact or primary layer, an absorbent layer, and an outer protective or secondary layer. The contact dressing covers the incision and part of the adjacent skin. Fibrin, blood products, and debris adhere to the contact dressing's surface. A problem occurs if the wound drainage dries, causing the dressing to stick to the suture line. Improper removal of the dressing causes disruption of the healing epidermal surface. If the dressing is sticking to the surgical incision, lightly moisten the dressing with saline solution. This will cause the dressing to become saturated, loosening it from the incisional area, and preventing trauma to the incisional area during removal.

The dressing technique will vary depending on the goal of the treatment plan for the wound. For example, if the goal is to maintain a moist environment for a clean granulating wound, it is important to not let the saline-moistened gauze dressing dry and stick to the healing wound. This is in direct contrast to the dressing technique that you use if the goal of care is to mechanically debride the wound using a saline wet-to-dry dressing. When wounds require debriding, such as a necrotic wound, you use a wet-to-dry dressing technique. You place the moist dressing (contact dressing) into the wound and allow it to dry. The contact dressing debrides necrotic tissue and debris. In this case the contact dressing is allowed to dry so that it sticks to underlying tissue, and debridement occurs during removal.

Dressings applied to a draining wound require frequent changing to prevent microorganism growth and skin breakdown. Bacteria grow readily in the dark, warm, moist environment under a dressing. Skin surfaces become macerated and irritated. Minimize periwound skin breakdown by keeping the skin clean and dry and reducing the use of tape.

The absorbent dressing layer serves as a reservoir for additional secretions. The wicking action of woven gauze dressings pulls excess drainage into the dressing and away from the wound. The final outer layer of a dressing helps prevent bacteria and other external contaminants from reaching the wound surface. Usually the outer dressing is made of a thicker dressing material. You apply adhesives to this layer to secure the dressings.

A dressing needs to support a moist wound environment if the wound is healing by secondary intention. A moist wound base facilitates the movement of epithelialization, thus allowing the wound to resurface as quickly as possible.

Types of Dressings. Dressings vary by type of material and mode of application (wet or dry) (Skill 48-3). They need to be easy to apply, comfortable, and made of materials that promote wound healing. The WOCN guidelines (2003) are helpful when selecting dressings based on the goal of wound treatment (Box 48-12). To avoid causing damage to the periwound skin, it is important that the dressing technique you use to treat pressure ulcers and other wounds is not excessively moist (Box 48-13).

Pressure ulcers require dressings. The type of dressing is usually based on the stage of the pressure ulcer and the objective of the dressing (Table 48-9). Before placing a dressing on a pressure ulcer, it is important that you know the stage of the pressure ulcer, the goal of the dressing, and principles of wound care.

BOX 48-13 EVIDENCE-BASED PRACTICE

Moisture-Associated Skin Damage From Dressings
Evidence Summary
Wound management and wound healing are critical to clients at risk for pressure ulcers, with pressure ulcers, and with other chronic wounds. The advances in wound healing document the benefit of a moist wound environment and the accepted practice of moist wound healing. A moist wound environment has the potential to damage the wound edges (periwound skin). This damage is maceration; the tissues of the periwound skin soften, and the connective fibers are damaged. This condition is also classified as moisture-associated skin damage (MASD). This study reviewed the existing literature to evaluate the effect of moist wound healing on the periwound skin. Although further research is needed to identify and evaluate the best strategy for managing existing periwound maceration, there are some clinical applications that may help prevent or manage MASD.

Application to Nursing Practice
- Use of a skin protectant (no-sting film barrier, petrolatum-based or zinc-based protectant) helps to prevent periwound skin maceration.
- Dressing selection needs to be individualized to the type of wound and wound-healing goals.
- Selection of topical prescriptions such as BCT ointment (Xenaderm) helps to manage moisture-associated damage to periwound skin.
- Use of negative pressure wound therapy (NPWT) may reduce the risk of periwound maceration by reducing local edema and exudates in the periwound tissue.

Reference
Gray M, Weir D: Prevention and treatment of moisture-associated skin damage (maceration) in the periwound skin, *J WOCN* 34(2): 153, 2007.

BOX 48-12 WOCN Dressing Recommendations
- Use a dressing that will continuously provide a moist environment. Wet-to-dry dressings are only for debridement and are not continuously moist saline dressings.
- Perform wound care using topical dressings as determined by a thorough assessment. No specific studies have proven an optimal dressing type for pressure ulcers
- Choose a dressing that keeps the surrounding intact (periulcer) skin dry while keeping the ulcer bed moist.
- Choose a dressing that controls exudate but does not desiccate the ulcer bed.
- Consider caregiver time, ease of use, availability, and cost when selecting a dressing.
- Eliminate wound dead space by loosely filling all cavities with dressing material.

Modified from Wound, Ostomy and Continence Nurses Society, *Guideline for prevention and management of pressure ulcers*, WOCN Clinical Practice Guidelines Series, Glenview, Ill, 2003, The Society.
WOCN, Wound, Ostomy and Continence Nurses Society.

✳ TABLE 48-9 Dressings by Pressure Ulcer Stage

Pressure Ulcer Stage	Pressure Ulcer Status	Dressing	Comments*	Expected Change	Adjuvants
I	Intact	None	Allows visual assessment.	Resolves slowly without epidermal loss over 7-14 days.	Turning schedule. Support hydration. Nutritional support.
		Transparent Dressing	Protects from shear. Do not use in the presence of excessive moisture.		
		Hydrocolloid	Does not always allow visual assessment.		Pressure-redistribution surface or chair cushion.
II	Clean	Composite film	Limits shear.	Heals through reepithelialization.	See previous stage.
		Hydrocolloid	Change when seal of dressing breaks; maximal wear time is 7 days.		Manage incontinence.
		Hydrogel	Provides a moist environment.		
III	Clean	Hydrocolloid	See stage II.	Heals through granulation and reepithelialization.	See previous stages. Evaluate pressure-redistribution needs.
		Hydrogel covered with foam dressing	Apply over wound to protect and absorb moisture.		
		Calcium alginate	Use when there is significant exudate. Cover with secondary dressing.		
		Gauze	Use with normal saline or other prescribed solutio; unfold to make contact with wound.		
		Growth factors	Use with gauze per manufacturer's instructions.		These products are very expensive; follow manufacturer's directions for storage and application.
IV	Clean	Hydrogel	See stage III, clean.	Heals through granulation and reepithelialization.	Surgical consult is often necessary for closure. See stages I, II, and III.
		Calcium alginate	See stage III, clean.		
		Gauze	See stage III, clean. Fill all dead space with gauze.		
		Growth factors	Use with gauze.		
	Unstageable: wound covered with eschar	Adherent film	Will facilitate softening of eschar.	Eschar will lift at edges as healing progresses.	See previous stages. Surgical consult is sometimes considered for debridement.
		Gauze plus ordered solution	Will deliver solution and wick wound drainage.		
		Enzymes	Will facilitate debridement.	Eschar will soften.	
		None	Rarely, if eschar is dry and intact, no dressing is used, allowing the eschar to act as physiological cover.		

*As with all occlusive dressings, wound should *not* be clinically infected.

✳ **SKILL 48-3** APPLYING DRY AND MOIST DRESSINGS

Delegation Considerations

The skill of applying dry and moist dressings to the new acute wound cannot be delegated. In some settings, aspects of wound care such as changing of dressings using *clean* technique for chronic wounds are delegated. The *assessment* of the wound remains within the scope of the nurse even if the dressing change is delegated. The nurse instructs nursing assistive personnel to:

- Report pain, fever, bleeding, or wound drainage to the nurse immediately
- Report any potential contamination to existing dressing (e.g., client incontinence or other bodily fluids, dressing becomes dislodged)

Equipment

- Sterile gloves
- Variety of gauze dressings and pads
- Irrigation kit
- Cleansing solution
- Sterile solution
- Clean, disposable gloves
- Tape, ties, or bandage as needed
- Waterproof pad and bag
- Extra gauze dressings, or topper dressing (ABD pads)
- Montgomery ties; elastic net

STEPS	RATIONALE
1. Perform hand hygiene. Obtain information about size and location of wound.	Reduces transmission of microorganisms. Helps to plan for proper type and amount of supplies needed. Alerts you when assistance is needed to hold dressings in place.
2. Assess client's level of comfort.	Removal of dry dressing is painful; some clients require pain medication.
3. Review orders for dressing change procedure.	Indicates type of dressing or applications to use.
4. Explain procedure to client, and instruct client not to touch wound area or sterile supplies.	Decreases anxiety. Sudden, unexpected movement on client's part will result in contamination of wound and supplies.
5. Close room or cubicle curtains and windows.	Provides privacy and reduces airborne microorganisms.
6. Position client comfortably, and drape with bath blanket to expose only wound site.	Provides access to wound, yet minimizes unnecessary exposure.
7. Place disposable bag within reach of work area. Fold top of bag to make cuff (see illustration).	Ensures easy disposal of soiled dressings. Prevents soiling of bag's outer surface.
8. Apply face mask and protective eyewear, if splashing occurs.	Reduces transmission of pathogens to exposed tissues. Protects nurse from splashes.

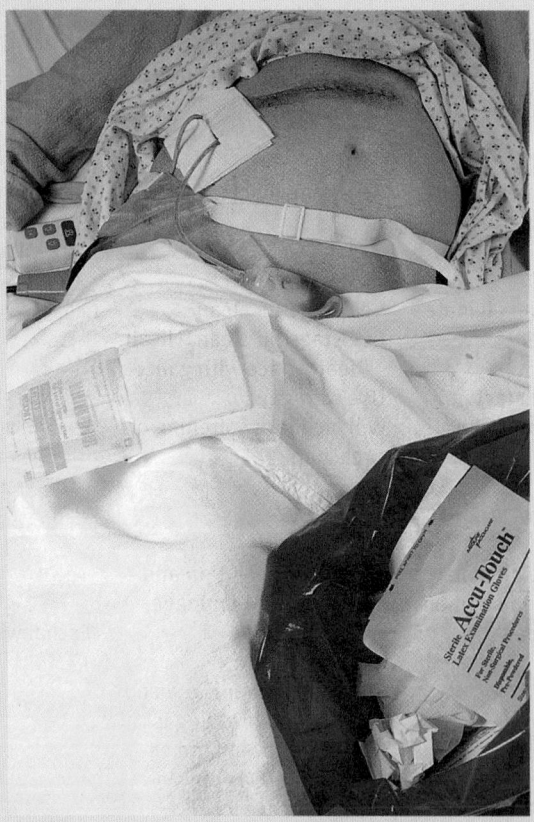

STEP 7 Disposable waterproof bag placed near dressing site.

SKILL 48-3 **APPLYING DRY AND MOIST DRESSINGS—CONT'D**

STEPS	RATIONALE
9. Put on clean, disposable gloves, and remove tape, bandage, or ties.	Prevents transmission of infectious organisms from soiled dressings to hands.
10. Remove tape: pull parallel to skin toward dressing; remove remaining adhesive from skin.	Pulling tape toward dressing reduces stress on suture line or wound edges.
11. With gloved hand carefully remove gauze dressings one layer at a time, taking care not to dislodge drains or tubes.	Appearance of drainage is sometimes upsetting to client. Removal of one layer at a time reduces the chance of accidental removal of underlying drains.
a. If dressing sticks on a wet-to-dry dressing, do not moisten it; instead gently free dressing, and alert client of potential discomfort.	Wet-to-dry dressing should debride wound (Ramundo, 2007). Do not wet the dressing to remove it. It is supposed to be dry so that it removes necrotic tissue from the wound.
b. If dressing sticks on a dry dressing, moisten with saline and then remove.	Prevents tearing of wound edges.

Critical Decision Point: Never use a wet-to-dry dressing in a clean granulating wound. Use only for debridement (Ramundo, 2007).

12. Observe character and amount of drainage on dressing and appearance of wound.	Provides estimate of drainage amount and assessment of wound's condition.
13. Fold dressings with drainage contained inside, and remove gloves inside out. With small dressings, remove gloves inside out over dressing (see illustration). Dispose of gloves and soiled dressings in disposable bag. Perform hand hygiene.	Reduces transmission of microorganisms. Prevents contact of hands with material on gloves.
14. Open sterile dressing tray or individually wrapped sterile supplies. Place on bedside table (see illustration).	Sterile dressings remain sterile while on or within sterile surface. Preparation of supplies prevents break in technique during dressing change.
15. If ordered, cleanse or irrigate wound:	Removes drainage containing microorganisms.
a. Pour ordered solution into sterile irrigation container.	
b. Apply clean gloves. Place waterproof pad under client. Using syringe, gently allow solution to flow over wound.	
c. Continue until the irrigation flow is clear.	
d. Dry surrounding skin.	
e. Some commercial cleansers come in a spray bottle. Spray the wound to loosen the debris.	
16. Apply dressing:	
A. **Dry dressing**	
(1) Apply sterile gloves.	Allows handling of sterile supplies without contamination.
(2) Inspect wound for appearance, drains, drainage, and integrity.	Indicates status of wound healing.
(3) Cleanse wound with solution:	
a. Clean from least-contaminated area to most-contaminated area.	Prevents contamination of previously cleaned area.
(4) Dry area.	Provides protection and absorption of wound drainage.
(5) Apply sterile dry dressing covering wound.	Protects wound from external environment.
(6) Apply topper dressing if indicated.	Topper dressing (e.g., ABD) prevents strike through of wound drainage and provides a surface to tape the dressing in place.

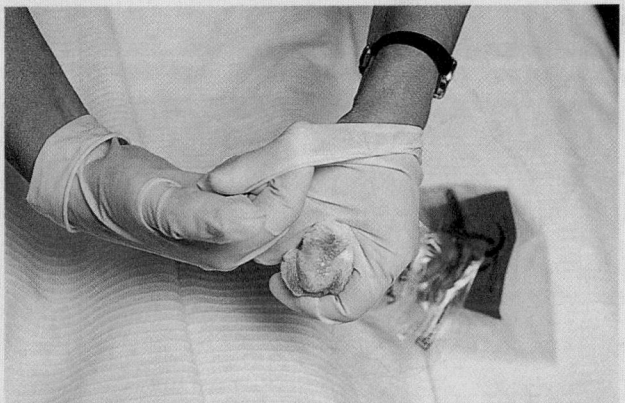

STEP 13 Removal of disposable gloves over contaminated dressing.

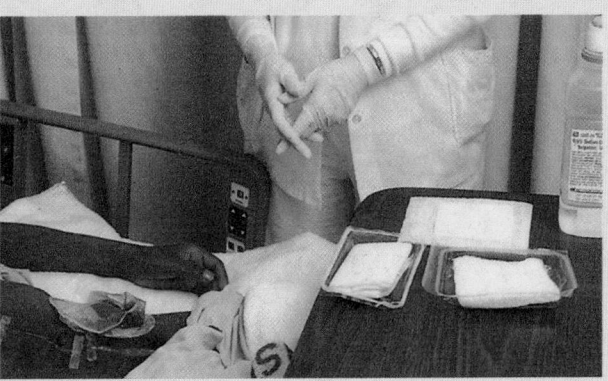

STEP 14 Sterile dressing equipment.

Continued

✳ **SKILL 48-3**   **APPLYING DRY AND MOIST DRESSINGS—CONT'D**

STEPS	RATIONALE
B. Moist dressing	
(1) Apply sterile gloves.	Allows handling of sterile supplies without contamination.
(2) Assess appearance of surrounding skin (see illustration).	Surrounding skin assessment provides an evaluation of wound management.
(3) Cleanse wound base with normal saline or commercially prepared wound cleanser. Assess wound base.	Cleansing removes wound debris for adequate assessment.
(4) Moisten gauze with prescribed solution. Gently wring out excess solution. Unfold.	Gauze needs to be moist to allow for absorption of wound debris.
(5) Apply gauze as a single layer directly onto the wound surface. If wound is deep, gently pack dressing into wound base by hand or forceps until all wound surfaces are in contact with the gauze. If tunneling is present, use a cotton-tipped applicator to place gauze into tunneled area. Be sure gauze does not touch the surrounding skin (see illustration).	Inner gauze needs to be moist, not dripping wet, to absorb drainage and adhere to debris. Excessively moist dressings result in moisture-associated skin damage (maceration) in the periwound skin (Gray and Weir, 2007). The wound needs to be loosely packed to facilitate wicking of drainage into absorbent outer layer of dressing.
(6) Cover with sterile dry gauze and topper dressing.	Topper dressing prevents strike through of wound drainage and provides a surface to tape the dressing in place.

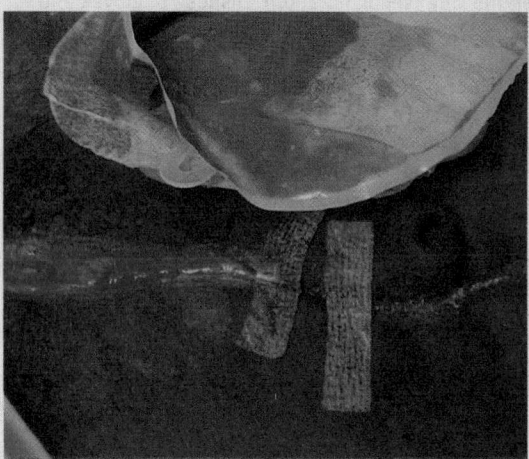

STEP 16B(3) Exposure of wound facilitates assessment of wound and surrounding skin.

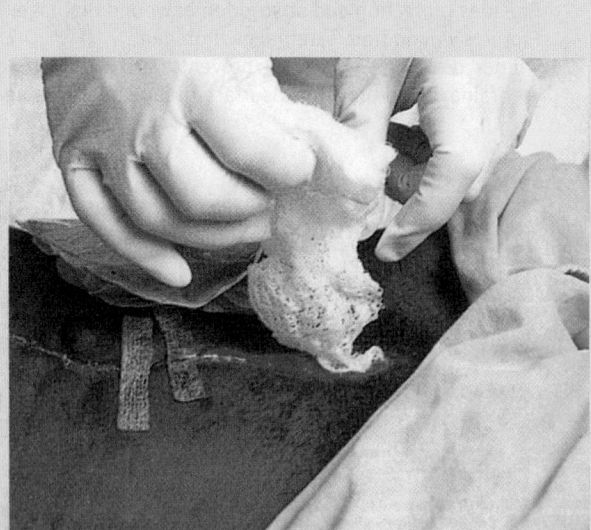
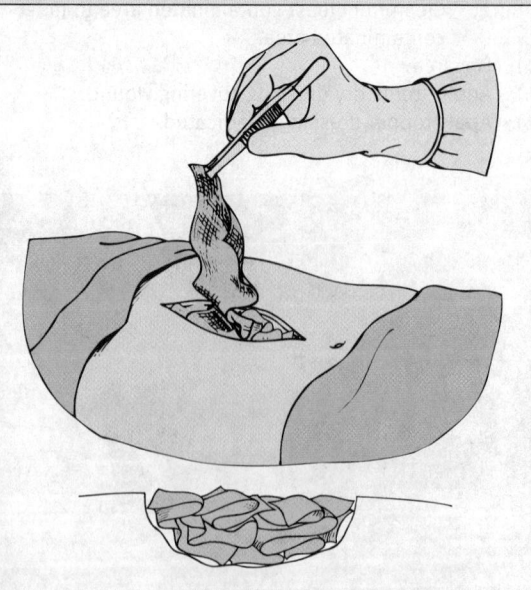

STEP 16B(5) Packing wound with single layer of gauze.

※ **SKILL 48-3**   **APPLYING DRY AND MOIST DRESSINGS—CONT'D**

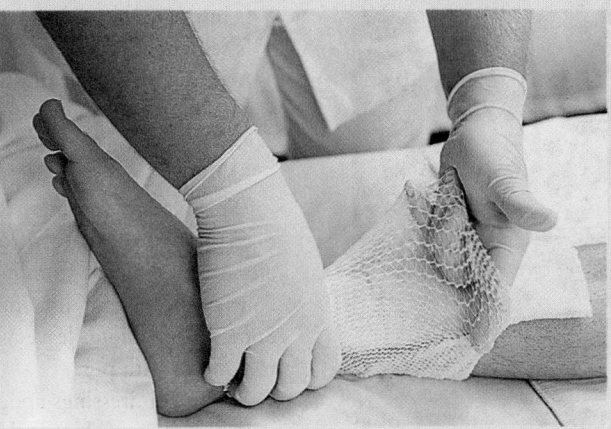

STEP 17c Elastic net securing a lower extremity dressing.

STEPS

17. Secure dressing.
  a. Tape: Apply nonallergenic tape to secure dressing in place.

  b. Montgomery ties (see Figure 48-25, p. 1324)
    (1) Expose adhesive surface of tape on end of each tie.
    (2) Place ties on opposites of dressing.
    (3) Place adhesive directly on skin, or use skin barrier.

    (4) Secure dressing by lacing ties across it.
  c. For dressings on an extremity, secure dressing with rolled gauze or an elastic net (see illustration).
18. Remove gloves, and dispose of in bag. Remove any mask or eyewear.
19. Write date and time dressing applied on tape in ink (not marker).
20. Dispose of supplies, and perform hand hygiene.
21. Assist client to comfortable position.

RATIONALE

The goal for securing a dressing is to keep the dressing in place and intact without causing damage to underlying and surrounding skin.

Skin barrier (Stomahesive) protects intact skin from stretch and tension of adhesive tape.

Prevents slipping of dressing.

Reduces transmission of infection.

Reduces transmission of infection.
Promotes client's sense of well being. Enhances comfort.

Unexpected Outcomes and Related Interventions
1. Wound appears inflamed, tender, with or without drainage.
  a. Monitor client for signs of infection (e.g., increased temperature, white blood cell count).
  b. Obtain wound culture.
  c. Notify health care provider.
2. Wound drainage increases.
  a. Increase frequency of dressing changes.
  b. Notify health care provider, who may consider drain placement to facilitate wound drainage.
3. Wound bleeds during dressing change.
  a. Observe color. If drainage is bright red and excessive, you will need to apply pressure.
  b. Inspect along dressing and underneath client to determine amount of bleeding.
  c. Obtain vital signs as needed.
  d. Notify health care provider.
4. Client reports a sensation that "something has given way under the dressing."
  a. Observe wound for increased drainage or separation of sutures.
  b. Protect wound. Cover with sterile moist dressing.
  c. Instruct client to lie still.
  d. Notify health care provider.

Recording and Reporting
• Report brisk, bright red bleeding or evidence of wound dehiscence or evisceration to health care provider immediately.
• Report wound and periwound tissue appearance, color, and tissue type and presence and characteristics of exudate, type and amount of dressings used, and tolerance of client to procedure.
• Record client's level of comfort.

Home Care Considerations
• More expensive specialty dressings are sometimes used, because they decrease the frequency of dressing changes.
• Clean dressings may also be used in the home setting.
• Clients need to dispose of contaminated dressings in the home in a manner consistent with local regulations.

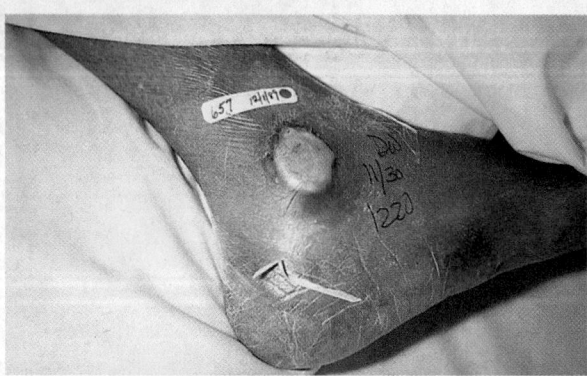

Figure 48-21 Transparent film dressing.

Gauze sponges are the oldest and most common dressing. They are absorbent and are especially useful in wounds to wick away the wound exudate. Gauze is available in different textures and in various lengths and sizes; the 4 × 4 is the most common size. Gauze can be saturated with solutions and used to cleanse and pack a wound. When used to pack a wound, the gauze is saturated with the solution (usually normal saline), wrung out, unfolded, and lightly packed into the wound. The purpose of this type of dressing is to provide moisture to the wound, yet to allow wound drainage to be wicked into the gauze pad. Unfolding the dressing allows easier wicking action.

Use nonadherent gauze dressings such as Telfa over clean wounds with little or no drainage. Telfa gauze has a shiny, nonadherent surface that does not stick to incisions or wound openings but allows drainage to pass through to the gauze topper.

Another type of dressing is a self-adhesive, transparent film. This type of dressing traps the wound's moisture over the wound, providing a moist environment (Figure 48-21). The transparent film dressing is ideal for small, superficial wounds such as partial-thickness wounds or to protect high-risk skin. Use a film dressing as a secondary dressing, as well as for autolytic debridement of small wounds. It has the following advantages:

- Adheres to undamaged skin
- Serves as a barrier to external fluids and bacteria but still allows the wound surface to "breathe," because oxygen passes through the transparent dressing
- Promotes a moist environment that speeds epithelial cell growth
- Can be removed without damaging underlying tissues
- Permits viewing the wound
- Does not require a secondary dressing

Hydrocolloid dressings are dressings with complex formulations of colloids, elastomeric, and adhesive components. These dressings are adhesive and occlusive. The wound contact layer of this dressing forms a gel as fluid is absorbed and maintains a moist healing environment. Hydrocolloids support healing in clean granulating wounds and autolytically debride necrotic wounds; they are available in a variety of sizes and shapes. This type of dressing has the following functions:

- Absorbs drainage through the use of exudate absorbers in the dressing

- Maintains wound moisture
- Slowly liquefies necrotic debris
- Is impermeable to bacteria and other contaminants
- Is self-adhesive and molds well
- Acts as a preventive dressing for high-risk friction areas
- May be left in place for 3 to 5 days, minimizing skin trauma and disruption of healing

This type of dressing is most useful on shallow to moderately deep dermal ulcers. Hydrocolloid dressings cannot absorb the amount of drainage from heavily draining wounds, and some are contraindicated for use in full-thickness and infected wounds. Some hydrocolloids leave a residue in the wound bed that is easy to confuse with pus.

Hydrogel dressings are gauze or sheet dressings impregnated with water- or glycerin-based amorphous gel. This type of dressing hydrates wounds and absorbs some smaller amounts of exudate. Hydrogel dressings are for partial-thickness and full-thickness wounds, deep wounds with some exudate, necrotic wounds, burns, and radiation-damaged skin. They are very useful in painful wounds, because they are very soothing to the client and do not adhere to the wound bed and thus cause little trauma during dressing removal. A disadvantage is that some hydrogels require a secondary dressing and you must take care to prevent periwound maceration. Hydrogels come in a sheet dressing or in a tube, so you are able to squirt the gel directly into the wound base.

Hydrogel has the following advantages:

- Is soothing and reduces pain in the wound
- Provides a moist environment
- Debrides the wound (by softening the necrotic tissue)
- Does not adhere to the wound base and is easy to remove

There are many other types of dressings available. Foam dressings and alginate dressings are for wounds with large amounts of exudate and for wounds that need packing. Foam dressings are also used around drainage tubes to absorb drainage. Calcium alginate dressings are manufactured from seaweed and come in sheet and rope form. The alginate forms a soft gel when it comes in contact with wound fluid. These highly absorbent dressings are for infected wounds and do not cause trauma when removed from the wound. **Do not use these in dry wounds, and they require a secondary dressing.** Several manufacturers produce composite dressings. These dressings combine two different dressing types into one dressing. Research is ongoing regarding what type of dressing is best for what type of wound.

Changing Dressings. To prepare for changing a dressing, you need to know the type of dressing, the presence of underlying drains or tubing, and the type of supplies needed for wound care. Poor preparation causes a break in aseptic technique (see Chapter 34) or accidental dislodging of a drain. Your judgment in modifying a dressing change procedure is important during wound care, particularly if the character of a wound changes. Notifying the health care provider of any change is essential.

The health care provider's order for changing a dressing indicates the dressing type, the frequency of changing, and any solutions or ointments to be applied to the wound. An order to "reinforce dressing prn" (add dressings without removing the original one) is common right after surgery, when the health care provider does not want accidental disruption of the suture line or bleeding. The medical or operating room record usually indicates whether drains are present and from what body cavity they drain. After the first dressing change, describe the location of drains and the type of dressing materials and solutions to use in the client's care plan. The CDC (2001) recommends the following during the dressing change procedure:

- Assessment of the skin beneath the tape
- Performing thorough hand hygiene before and after wound care
- Wearing sterile gloves before directly touching an open or fresh wound (see Chapter 34)
- Removing or changing dressings over closed wounds when they become wet or if the client has signs or symptoms of infection and as ordered

There is a growing body of literature about sterile versus clean dressings. The WOCN guidelines (2003) recommend using clean dressings and gloves on pressure ulcers. For surgical wounds, preliminary research indicates no difference in the healing rate of wounds when clean rather than sterile dressing change technique is used.

To prepare a client for a dressing change, do the following:

- Administer required analgesics so that peak effects occur during the dressing change
- Describe steps of the procedure to lessen client anxiety
- Gather all supplies required for the dressing change
- Recognize normal signs of healing
- Answer questions about the procedure or the wound

Often it is necessary to teach clients how to change dressings in preparation for home care. In this situation you need to demonstrate dressing changes to the client and family and then provide an opportunity for the client or family member to practice. Usually in this situation wound healing has progressed to the point that risks of complications such as dehiscence or evisceration are minimal. The client needs to be able to change a dressing independently or with assistance from a family member before discharge. The AHCPR guidelines (1994) state that "clean dressing may also be used in the home setting for pressure ulcers. Disposal of contaminated dressings in the home should be done in a manner consistent with local regulations." Skill 48-3 outlines the steps for changing dry and moist dressings.

Packing a Wound. The first step in packing a wound is to assess the size, depth, and shape of the wound. These wound characteristics are important in determining the size and type of dressing used to pack a wound. The dressing needs to be flexible and in contact with all of the wound surface. Make sure that the type of material used to pack the wound is appropriate. There are many new dressing materials, such as alginates, that are also used to pack wounds. If gauze is the appropriate dressing material, saturate the gauze with the ordered solution, wring it out, unfold it and lightly pack it into the wound. The entire wound surface needs to be in contact with part of the moist gauze dressing (see Skill 48-3). As stated in the WOCN guidelines (2003), "keep the

periwound skin dry while maintaining a moist wound base" and when using a dressing "eliminate dead space by loosely filling all cavities." Dead space is space in the wound that is not filled with a dressing. Dead space allows wound debris to accumulate in that area, causing complications.

It is important to remember not to pack the wound too tightly. Overpacking the wound causes pressure on the tissue in the wound bed. Pack the wound only until the packing material reaches the surface of the wound; there should never be so much packing material in the wound that it extends higher than the wound surface. Wound packing that overlaps onto the wound edges causes maceration of the tissue surrounding the wound. It also prevents the proper healing and closing of the wound.

A treatment modality for wounds is negative pressure wound therapy (NPWT) or vacuum-assisted closure (one brand name is V.A.C.). The **Vacuum Assisted Closure (V.A.C.)** is a device that assists in wound closure by applying localized negative pressure to draw the edges of a wound together (Figure 48-22, *A, B*). NPWT supports wound healing by evacuating wound fluids, stimulating granulation tissue formation, reducing the bacterial burden of a wound, and maintaining a moist wound environment (Frantz and others, 2007) (Figure 48-23). There are recent modifications of the V.A.C. V.A.C. Instill allows intermittent instillation of fluids into the wound, especially those wounds not responding to traditional NPWT (Jerome, 2007).

NPWT is used for treating acute and chronic wounds (Skill 48-4). The schedule for changing NPWT dressings varies depending upon the type of wound and amount of drainage. Wear time for the dressing is anywhere from 24 hours to 5 days (Frantz and others, 2007). As the wound heals, the wound base granulation tissue will line the surface of the wound. The wound has a stippled or granulated appearance. The surface area of the wound sometimes increases or decreases depending on wound location and the amount of drainage removed by the NPWT system. The NPWT is also used to enhance the take of split-thickness skin grafts. It is placed over the graft intraoperatively, decreasing the ability of the graft to shift and evacuating fluids that build up under the graft (Frantz and others, 2007).

Securing Dressings. Use tape, ties, or a secondary dressing and cloth binders to secure a dressing over a wound site. The choice of anchoring depends on the wound size and location, the presence of drainage, the frequency of dressing changes, and the client's level of activity.

Most often, strips of tape are used to secure dressings if the client is not allergic to tape. Nonallergenic paper and plastic tapes minimize skin reactions. Common adhesive tape adheres well to the skin's surface, whereas elastic adhesive tape compresses closely around pressure bandages and permits more movement of a body part. Skin sensitive to adhesive tape becomes severely inflamed and denuded and in some cases even sloughs when the tape is removed. It is important to assess skin under tape at each dressing change.

Tape is available in various widths such as ½, 1, 2, and 3 inches. Choose the size that sufficiently secures the dressing. For example, a large abdominal wound dressing needs to remain secure over a large area despite frequent stress from movement, respiratory effort, and possibly abdominal distention. Strips of

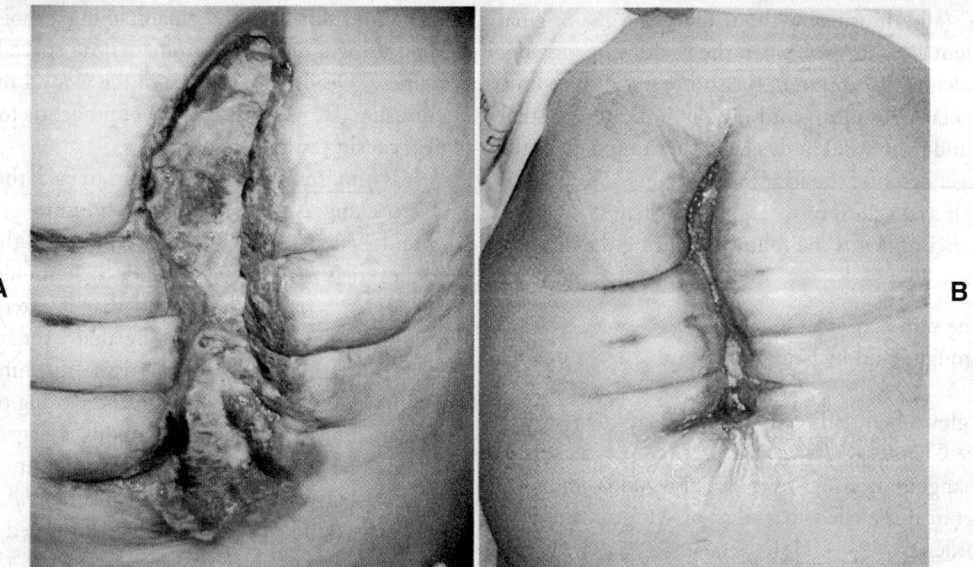

Figure 48-22 A, Dehisced wound before wound V.A.C. therapy. **B,** Dehisced wound after wound V.A.C. therapy. (Courtesy Kinetic Concepts, Inc [KCI], San Antonio, Tex.)

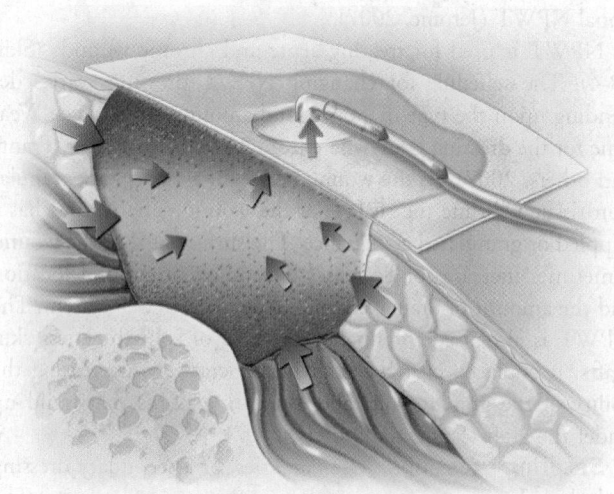

Figure 48-23 V.A.C. system using negative pressure to remove fluid from area surrounding the wound, reducing edema and improving circulation to the area. (Courtesy Kinetic Concepts, Inc [KCI], San Antonio, Tex.)

3-inch adhesive better stabilize such a large dressing so that it does not continually slip off. When applying tape, ensure that it adheres to several inches of skin on both sides of the dressing and that it is placed across the middle of the dressing. When securing the dressing, press the tape gently, exerting pressure away from the wound. This way, tension occurs in both directions away from the wound, minimizing skin distortion and irritation. Never apply tape over irritated or broken skin. Some nurses protect the skin beneath the tape with a skin sealant product.

To remove tape safely, loosen the tape ends and gently pull the outer end parallel with the skin surface toward the wound. Apply light traction to the skin away from the wound as the tape is loosened and removed. Adhesive remover also loosens the tape from the skin. The traction minimizes pulling of the skin. If tape covers an area of hair growth, the client experiences less discomfort if you pull the tape in the direction of hair growth.

Text continued on p. 1324

✳ SKILL 48-4 IMPLEMENTATION OF NEGATIVE PRESSURE WOUND THERAPY [Video]

Delegation Considerations

The assessment for and placement of Vacuum Assisted Closure (V.A.C.) cannot be delegated. The nurse instructs nursing assistive personnel to:

- Report to the nurse any change in client's temperature, level of comfort
- Change in the pressure in the NPWT unit
- Any change in the integrity of the dressing

Equipment

- NPWT unit (e.g., V.A.C.) (requires health care provider order) (Figure 48-24)
- V.A.C. foam dressing and transparent dressing
- Tubing for connection between NPWT unit and dressing
- Gloves, clean and sterile
- Scissors (sterile)
- Skin prep/skin barrier
- Moist washcloth
- Plastic trash bag
- Linen bag
- Stethoscope
- Protective gown, mask, goggles if risk of splashing wound drainage

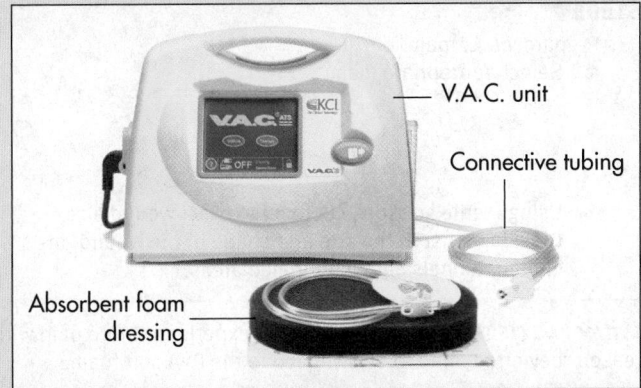

Figure 48-24 V.A.C. unit. *Top to bottom:* V.A.C. unit itself, connective tubing to go between V.A.C. unit and V.A.C. dressing, absorbent foam dressing. (Courtesy Kinetic Concepts, Inc [KCI], San Antonio, Tex.)

STEPS	RATIONALE
1. Perform hand hygiene. Assemble supplies.	Reduces transmission of microorganisms. Organizes procedure.
2. Position client comfortably, and drape to expose only wound site. Instruct client not to touch wound or sterile supplies. Administer ordered analgesic 30 minutes before dressing change.	Maintaining client comfort assists in completing skill smoothly. Draping provides access to wound while minimizing unnecessary exposure.
3. Place disposable waterproof bag within reach of work area with top folded to make a cuff.	Facilitates safe disposal of soiled dressings.
4. Keep system in a "de vac" mode for 30 to 45 minutes before changing dressing.	Found to loosen foam dressing for easier, less painful removal (Price and others, 2006).
5. When NPWT is in place, push therapy on/off button.	
a. Keeping tube connectors with NPWT unit, disconnect tubes from each other to drain fluids into canister.	Deactivates therapy and allows for proper drainage of fluid in drainage tubing.
b. Before lowering, tighten clamp on canister tube.	
6. Gently stretch transparent film horizontally, and slowly pull away from the skin.	Reduces stress on suture line or wound edges and reduces irritation and discomfort.
7. Remove old dressing, observing appearance and drainage on dressing. Use caution to avoid tension on any drains that are present. Discard dressing, and remove gloves. Perform hand hygiene.	Determines dressings needed for replacement. Avoids accidental removal of drains because they are sometimes sutured in place.
8. Apply sterile or clean gloves. Irrigate the wound with normal saline or other solution ordered by the health care provider. Blot to dry.	Irrigation removes wound debris.

Critical Decision Point: When drainage looks purulent, or there is change in amount or color, or it has a foul odor, obtain wound cultures even when they are not ordered for that particular dressing change (Chua and others, 2000; Jerome, 2007).

9. Measure wound as ordered: at baseline, first dressing change, weekly, and discharge from therapy.	Objectively documents wound healing process in response to negative pressure, wound therapy (Nix, 2007).
10. Apply skin protectant/barrier film to skin around wound.	Maintains air-tight seal needed for NPWT and protects periwound skin from maceration.
11. Remove and discard gloves. Perform hand hygiene.	Reduces transmission of microorganisms.
12. Depending on the type of wound, apply sterile gloves or new clean gloves.	Fresh sterile wounds require sterile gloves. Chronic wounds require clean technique. However, do not use the same gloves to remove old dressing because cross contamination will occur.

Continued

✳ **SKILL 48-4** **IMPLEMENTATION OF NEGATIVE PRESSURE WOUND THERAPY—CONT'D**

STEPS	RATIONALE
13. Prepare V.A.C. foam. a. Select appropriate foam.	Black, polyurethane (PU) foam has larger pores and is most effective in stimulating granulation tissue and **wound contraction**. White, polyvinyl alcohol (PVA) soft foam is denser with smaller pores and is used when the growth of granulation tissue needs to be restricted (Frantz and others, 2007; KCI, 2004).
b. Using sterile scissors, cut foam to exact wound size. Dressing must fit the size and shape of the wound, including tunnels and undermined areas.	

Critical Decision Point: Some clients experience more pain with the black foam because of excessive wound contraction. For this reason they often need to be switched to the PVA soft foam.

14. Gently place foam in wound; be sure that the foam is in contact with entire wound base and margins and tunneled and undermined areas (see illustration Step 14, *A*).	Maintains negative pressure to entire wound.
15. Apply wrinkle-free transparent dressing over foam and 3 to 5 cm of surrounding healthy skin. Secure tubing to the unit (see illustration Step 14, *B* and *C*).	Ensures that the wound is properly covered and helps achieve a negative pressure seal (Box 48-14). Connects the negative pressure from the NPWT unit to the wound foam.

Critical Decision Point: Consider using the V.A.C. Instill in wounds not responding to NPWT. However, this is contraindicated in untreated osteomyelitis, nonenteric and unexplored fistulas, and necrotic tissue with eschar (Jerome, 2007).

16. Secure tubing to transparent film, aligning drainage holes to ensure an occlusive seal (see illustration Step 14, *C*). Do not apply tension to drape and tubing.	Excessive tension compresses foam dressing and impedes wound healing. Excessive tension also produces a shear force on periwound area (KCI, 2004).
17. Secure tubing several centimeters away from the dressing.	Prevents pull on the primary dressing, which causes leaks in the negative pressure system (Chua and others, 2000; KCI, 2004).

STEP 14 Dressing application. **A,** Properly sized foam to cover wound (Step 12). **B,** Wrinkle-free transparent dressing applied over foam (Step 15). **C,** Secure tubing to the foam and transparent dressing (Step 16). (Courtesy Kinetic Concepts, Inc [KCI], San Antonio, Tex.)

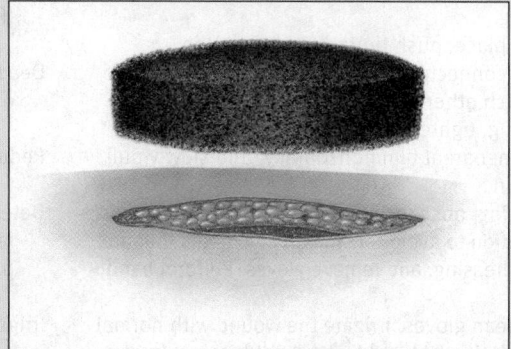

A

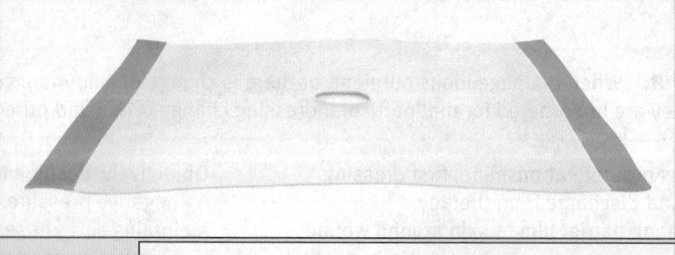

B

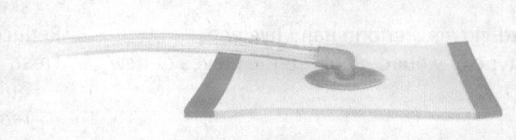

C

✳ SKILL 48-4 IMPLEMENTATION OF NEGATIVE PRESSURE WOUND THERAPY—CONT'D

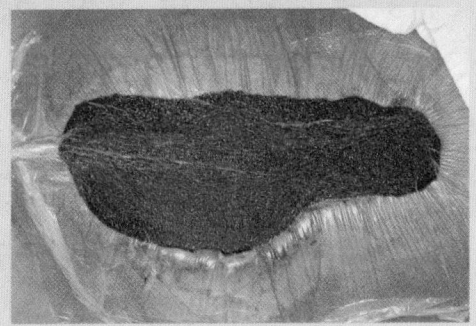

STEP 18 Foam, transparent dressing, and tubing secured over existing wound. (Courtesy Kinetic Concepts, Inc [KCI], San Antonio, Tex.)

STEPS	RATIONALE
18. Once you have completely covered the wound (see illustration), connect the tubing from the dressing to the tubing from the canister and NPWT unit.	Intermittent or continuous negative pressure can be administered at 50 to 175 mm Hg, according to health care provider order and client comfort. The average is 125 mm Hg (Frantz and others, 2007).

18.
a. Remove canister from sterile packaging, and push into V.A.C. unit until you hear a click. **NOTE: An alarm will sound if the canister is not properly engaged.**
b. Connect the dressing tubing to the canister tubing. Make sure both clamps are open.
c. Place V.A.C. unit on a level surface or hang from the foot of the bed. **NOTE: The V.A.C. unit will alarm and deactivate therapy if the unit is tilted beyond 45 degrees.**
d. Press in green-lit power button, and set pressure as ordered.

19. Discard old dressing materials; remove gloves, and perform hand hygiene.	Reduces transmission of microorganisms.
20. Inspect NPWT system to verify that negative pressure is achieved.	Negative pressure is achieved when there is an airtight seal.

20.
a. Verify that display screen reads THERAPY ON.
b. Be sure clamps are open and tubing is patent.
c. Identify air leaks by listening with stethoscope or by moving hand around edges of wound while applying light pressure.
d. If a leak is present, use strips of transparent film to patch areas.

21. Compare wound with baseline wound assessment.	Provides objective documentation of wound healing.
22. Verify airtight dressing seal and proper negative pressure.	In order to achieve prescribed vacuum level, the wound must be covered with an airtight seal. This airtight seal and the negative pressure promote wound drainage, circulation, and healing.

Unexpected Outcomes and Related Interventions

1. Wound appears inflamed and tender, drainage has increased, and an odor is present.
   a. Notify health care provider.
   b. Obtain wound culture.
   c. Increase frequency of dressing changes.
2. Client reports increase in pain.
   a. If using black foam, switch to the PVA foam product.
   b. Client sometimes needs more analgesic support when NPWT is initiated.
   c. Reduce negative pressure.
3. Negative pressure seal has broken.
   a. Take preventive measures: Shave hair around wound, avoid wrinkles in transparent dressing, and avoid use of adhesive remover because it leaves residue that hinders film adherence.
   b. Reinforce with transparent dressing strips.

Recording and Reporting

- Record appearance of wound, color, characteristics of any drainage, presence of wound healing augmentation.
- Record pressure setting of NPWT.
- Record date and time of dressing change.
- Report brisk, bright bleeding, evidence of poor wound healing, and possible wound infection.

Home Care Considerations

- Clients can use NPWT in the home safely. Some clients need clinic visits or home care nursing visits to monitor wound healing.
- Provide resources to client for supplies for NPWT.
- Instruct family and caregiver regarding proper disposal of contaminated product.

✳ BOX 48-14 Maintaining an Airtight Seal

To avoid wound desiccation, the wound needs to stay sealed once therapy is initiated. Problem seal areas include wounds around joints and near the sacrum. The following points will assist in maintaining an airtight seal:

- Shave hair around wound.
- Cut transparent film to extend 3 to 5 cm beyond wound parameter.
- Avoid wrinkles in transparent film.
- Patch leaks with transparent film.
- Use multiple small strips of transparent film to hold dressing in place before covering dressing with large piece of transparent film.
- Avoid adhesive remover because it leaves a residue that hinders film adherence.

From Chua PC and others: Vacuum-assisted wound closure, *Am J Nurs* 100(12):45, 2000.

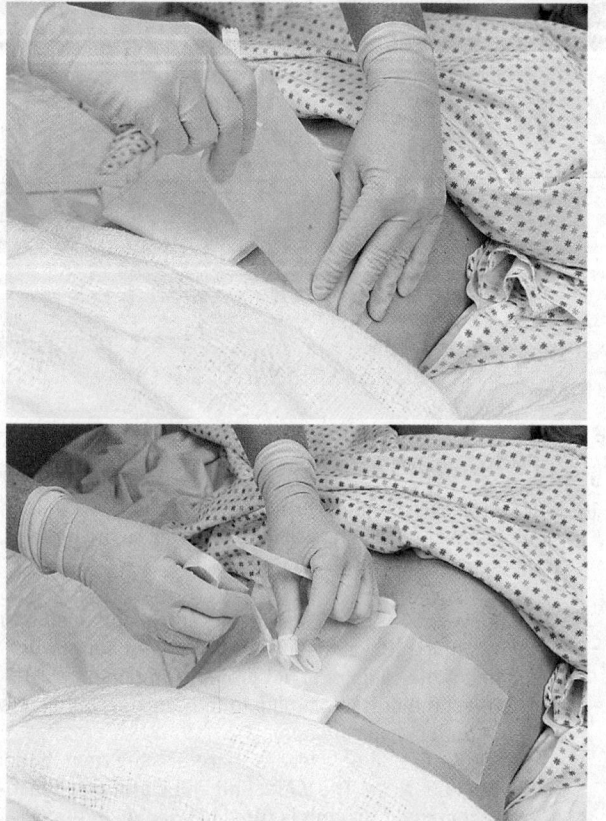

Figure 48-25 Montgomery ties. **A,** Each tie is placed at side of dressing. **B,** Securing ties encloses dressing.

To avoid repeated removal of tape from sensitive skin, you secure dressings with pairs of reusable Montgomery ties (Figure 48-25). Each section consists of a long strip; half contains an adhesive backing to apply to the skin, and the other half folds back and contains a cloth tie or a safety pin and rubber band combination that you fasten across a dressing and untie at dressing changes. A large, bulky dressing often requires two or more sets of Montgomery ties. Another method to protect the surrounding skin on wounds that need frequent dressing changes is to place strips of hydrocolloid dressings on either side of the wound edges, cover the wound with a dressing, and then apply the tape to the hydrocolloid dressing. To provide even support to a wound and immobilize a body part, apply elastic gauze or cloth bandages and binders over a dressing.

Comfort Measures. A wound is often painful, depending on the extent of tissue injury. Use several techniques to minimize discomfort during wound care. Careful removal of tape, gentle cleansing of wound edges, and careful manipulation of dressings and drains minimize stress on sensitive tissues. Careful turning and positioning also reduce strain on a wound. Administration of analgesic medications 30 to 60 minutes before dressing changes (depending on a drug's time of peak action) also reduces discomfort.

Cleansing Skin and Drain Sites. Although a moderate amount of wound exudate promotes epithelial cell growth, some health care providers will order cleansing of a wound or drain site if a dressing does not properly absorb drainage or if an open drain deposits drainage onto the skin. Wound cleansing requires good hand hygiene and aseptic techniques (see Chapter 34). You will sometimes use irrigation to remove debris from a wound.

Basic Skin Cleansing. Cleanse surgical or traumatic wounds by applying noncytotoxic solutions with sterile gauze or by irrigation. The following three principles are important when cleansing an incision or the area surrounding a drain:

1. Cleanse in a direction from the least contaminated area, such as from the wound or incision to the surrounding skin (Figure 48-26) or from an isolated drain site to the surrounding skin (Figure 48-27).

2. Use gentle friction when applying solutions locally to the skin.
3. When irrigating, allow the solution to flow from the least to most contaminated area (see Skill 48-5).

After applying a solution to sterile gauze, cleanse away from the wound. Never use the same piece of gauze to cleanse across an incision or wound twice.

Drain sites are a source of contamination because moist drainage harbors microorganisms. If a wound has a dry incisional area and a moist drain site, cleansing moves from the incisional area toward the drain. Use two separate swabs or gauze pads, one to cleanse from the top of the incision toward the drain and one to cleanse from the bottom of the incision toward the drain. To cleanse the area of an isolated drain site, clean around the drain, moving in circular rotations outward from a point closest to the drain. In this situation the skin near the site is more contaminated than the site itself. To cleanse circular wounds, use the same technique as in cleansing around a drain.

Irrigations. Irrigations are a special way of cleansing wounds. You use an irrigating syringe to flush the area with a constant low-pressure flow of solution. The gentle washing action of the irrigation cleanses a wound of exudate and debris. Irrigations are particularly useful for open, deep wounds; wounds involving an inaccessible body part, such as the ear canal; or when cleansing sensitive body parts, such as the conjunctival lining of the eye.

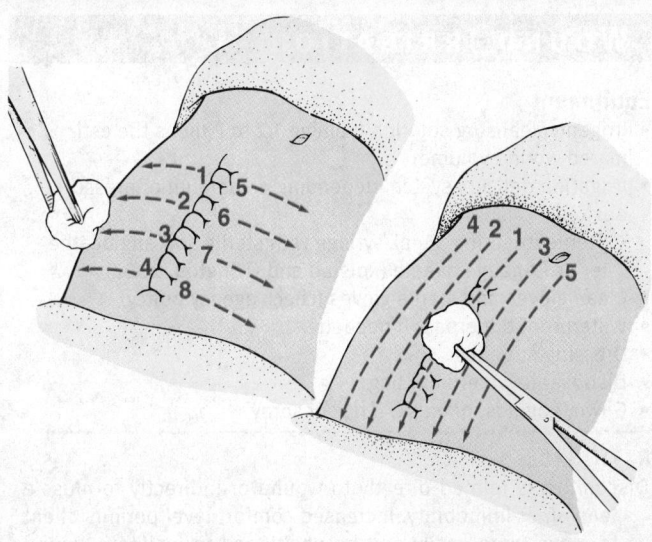

Figure 48-26 Methods for cleansing a wound site.

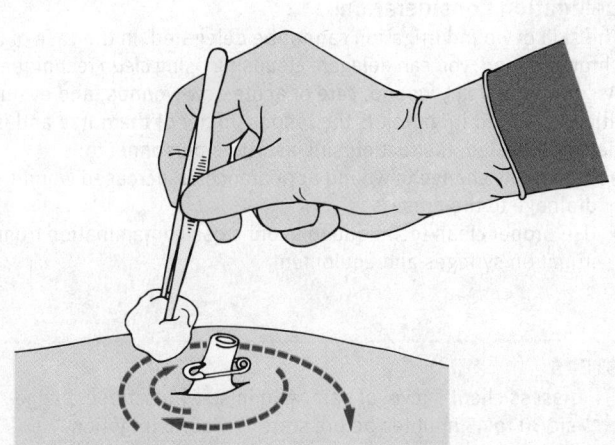

Figure 48-27 Cleansing a drain site.

Wound Irrigations. Irrigation of an open wound requires sterile technique. Use a 35-mL syringe with a 19-gauge needle (Rolstad and Ovington, 2007) to deliver the solution. This irrigation system has a safe pressure and will not damage healing wound tissue. It is important to never occlude a wound opening with a syringe, because this results in the introduction of irrigating fluid into a closed space. The pressure of the fluid causes tissue damage and discomfort. Always irrigate a wound with the syringe tip over but not in the drainage site. Make sure fluid flows directly into the wound and not over a contaminated area before entering the wound. Skill 48-5 lists steps for wound irrigation.

Suture Care. A surgeon closes a wound by bringing the wound edges as close together as possible to reduce scar formation. Proper wound closure involves minimal trauma and tension to tissues with control of bleeding.

Sutures are threads or metal used to sew body tissues together (Figure 48-28). The client's history of wound healing, the site of surgery, the tissues involved, and the purpose of the sutures determine the suture material you will use. For example, if the client has had repeated surgery for an abdominal hernia, the health care provider will possibly choose wire sutures to provide greater strength for wound closure. In contrast, a small laceration of the face calls for the use of very fine Dacron (polyester) sutures to minimize scar formation.

Sutures are available in a variety of materials, including silk, steel, cotton, linen, wire, nylon, and Dacron. Sutures come with or without sharp surgical needles attached. Steel staples are a common type of outer skin closure that cause less trauma to tissues than sutures, while providing extra strength. It is also common to see wounds closed with tape closures such as Steri-Strips applied over the wound to keep the edges closed.

Sutures are placed within tissue layers in deep wounds and superficially as the final means for wound closure. Deep sutures are usually an absorbable material that will disappear over time. Sutures are foreign bodies and thus are capable of causing local inflammation. The surgeon tries to minimize tissue injury by using the finest suture possible and the smallest number necessary.

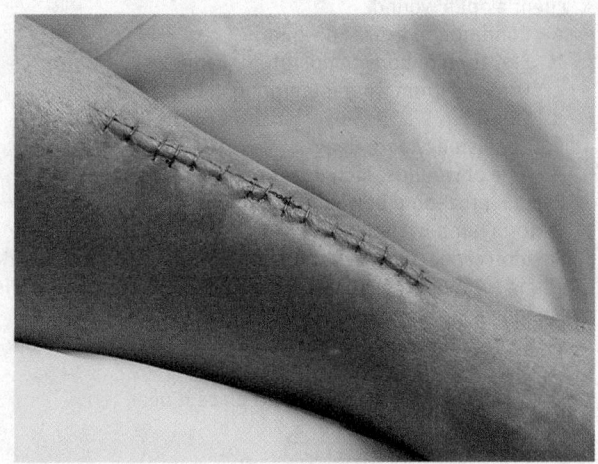

Figure 48-28 Incision closed with metal staples.

Policies vary within institutions as to who is able to remove sutures. If it is appropriate that the nurse remove them, a health care provider's order is required. An order for suture removal is not written until the health care provider believes that the wound has closed (usually in 7 days). Special scissors with curved cutting tips or special staple removers slide under the skin closures for suture removal (Figure 48-29, p. 1328). The health care provider usually specifies the number of sutures or staples to remove. If the suture line appears to be healing in certain locations better than in others, some health care providers choose to have only some sutures removed (e.g., every other one).

To remove staples, simply insert the tips of the staple remover under each wire staple. While slowly closing the ends of the staple remover together, you squeeze the center of the staple with the tips, freeing the staple from the skin (see Figure 48-29).

To remove sutures, first check the type of suturing used (Figure 48-30, p. 1328). With intermittent suturing, the surgeon ties each individual suture made in the skin. Continuous suturing, as the

✳ **SKILL 48-5** **PERFORMING WOUND IRRIGATION**

Delegation Considerations

The skill of wound irrigation cannot be delegated. In the case of a chronic wound, you can delegate cleansing using *clean* technique. Assessment of any wound, care of acute new wounds, and evaluation of wound irrigation is the responsibility of the nurse and is never delegated. Instruct nursing assistive personnel to:

- Report any change in wound appearance or increased wound drainage to the nurse
- Use proper clean technique to avoid cross contamination from irrigation syringes and equipment

Equipment

- Irrigant/cleansing solution (volume 1.2 to 2 times the estimated wound volume)
- Irrigation delivery system depending on amount of pressure desired:
  - Sterile irrigation 35-mL syringe with sterile soft angiocatheter or 19-gauge needle (Rolstad and Ovington, 2007)
- Clean gloves and sterile gloves (check agency policy)
- Waterproof underpad, if needed
- Dressing supplies
- Disposable waterproof bag
- Gown, goggles, or mask, if risk of spray

STEPS	RATIONALE
1. Assess client's level of pain. Administer prescribed analgesic 30 to 45 minutes before starting wound irrigation procedure.	Discomfort is related directly to wound or indirectly to muscle tension or immobility. Increased comfort level permits client to move more easily and be positioned to facilitate wound irrigation.
2. Review medical record for health care provider's prescription for irrigation of open wound and type of solution to be used.	Open wound irrigation requires medical order, including type of solution to use.
3. Assess recent recording of signs and symptoms related to client's open wound.	Data provide a baseline to indicate change in condition of wound (Nix, 2007).
a. Condition of skin and wound	
b. Elevation of body temperature	Indicates response to infection.
c. Drainage from wound (amount, color)	Amount will decrease as healing takes place.
d. Odor	Strong odor indicates infectious process.
e. Consistency of drainage	Leukocytes produce thick drainage.
f. Size of wounds, including depth, length, and width	Determines stage of healing.
4. Explain procedure of wound irrigation and cleansing.	Information will reduce client's anxiety.
5. Perform hand hygiene.	Reduces transmission of microorganisms.
6. Position client comfortably to permit gravitational flow of irrigating solution through wound and into collection receptacle. Position client so that wound is vertical to collection basin.	Directing solution from top to bottom of wound and from clean to contaminated area prevents further infection.
7. Warm irrigation solution to approximate body temperature.	Warmed solution increases comfort and reduces vascular constriction response in tissues.
8. Form cuff on waterproof bag and place it near bed.	Cuffing helps to maintain large opening, thereby permitting placement of contaminated dressing without touching refuse bag itself.
9. Close room door or bed curtains.	Maintains privacy.
10. Apply gown, mask or goggles if needed.	Protects nurse from splashes or sprays of blood and body fluids.
11. Put on clean gloves, and remove soiled dressing and discard in waterproof bag. Discard gloves.	Reduces transmission of microorganisms.
12. Prepare equipment; open sterile supplies.	
13. Put on sterile gloves. (Check agency policy)	
14. To irrigate wound with wide opening:	
a. Fill 35-mL syringe with irrigation solution.	Flushing wound helps remove debris and facilitates healing by secondary intention.
b. Attach 19-gauge needle or angiocatheter (see Figure 48-20, p. 1307).	Provides ideal pressure for cleansing and removal of debris.
c. Hold syringe tip 2.5 cm (1 inch) above upper end of wound and over area being cleansed.	Prevents syringe contamination. Careful placement of the syringe prevents unsafe pressure of the flowing solution.
d. Using continuous pressure, flush wound; repeat steps 14 a, b, and c until solution draining into basin is clear.	Clear solution indicates that you have removed all debris.
15. To irrigate deep wound with very small opening:	
a. Attach soft angiocatheter to filled irrigating syringe.	Catheter permits direct flow of irrigant into wound. Expect wound to take longer to empty when opening is small.
b. Lubricate tip of catheter with irrigating solution; then gently insert tip of catheter and pull out about 1 cm (½ inch).	Removes tip from fragile inner wall of wound.

★ **SKILL 48-5** **PERFORMING WOUND IRRIGATION—CONT'D**

STEPS

  c. Using slow, continuous pressure, flush wound.
    CAUTION: Splashing sometimes occurs during this step.
  d. Pinch off catheter just below syringe while keeping catheter in place.
  e. Remove and refill syringe. Reconnect to catheter, and repeat until solution draining into basin is clear.

RATIONALE

Cleanses all wound surfaces.

Avoids contamination of sterile solution.

Critical Decision Point: Consider culturing a wound if it has a foul, purulent odor; inflammation surrounds the wound; a nondraining wound begins to drain; or client is febrile.

---

16. Obtain cultures, if needed, after cleansing with nonbacteriostatic saline.

The WOCN guidelines (2003) suggest obtaining a quantitative culture if you suspect high levels of bacteria in a wound exhibiting clinical signs of infection. Although tissue biopsy is considered the gold standard to confirm infection, quantitative swab cultures are a reasonable alternative.

17. Dry wound edges with gauze.

Prevents maceration of surrounding tissue caused by excess moisture.

18. Apply appropriate dressing (see Skills 48-2, p. 1308, and 48-3, p. 1314).

Maintains protective barrier and healing environment for wound.

19. Remove gloves and, if worn, mask, goggles, and gown.

Prevents transfer of microorganisms.

20. Dispose of equipment and soiled supplies. Perform hand hygiene.

Reduces transmission of microorganisms.

21. Assist client to comfortable position.
22. Assess type of tissue in the wound bed.

Identifies wound-healing progress and determines type of wound cleansing needed.

23. Inspect dressing periodically.

Determines client's response to wound irrigation and need to modify plan of care.

24. Evaluate skin integrity.

Determines if extension of wound has occurred.

25. Observe client for signs of discomfort.

Client's pain should not increase as a result of wound irrigation.

26. Observe for presence of retained irrigant.

Retained irrigant is a medium for bacterial growth and subsequent infection.

Unexpected Outcomes and Related Interventions

1. Wound does not appear to heal.
  a. Obtain wound culture.
  b. Notify health care provider, who may change dressing and or irrigation frequency.
2. Wound drainage increases.
  a. Apply more absorbent gauze.
  b. Increase the frequency of irrigation.

Recording and Reporting

- Record wound irrigation and client response on progress notes.
- Immediately report any evidence of fresh bleeding, sharp increase in pain, retention of irrigant, or signs of shock to attending health care provider.
- At change of shift, report expected and unexpected outcomes that have actually occurred.

Home Care Considerations

- Teach client and caregiver how to make normal saline, especially if cost is an issue. You make normal saline by using 8 teaspoons of salt in 1 gallon of distilled water (Fellows and Cresodina, 2006).

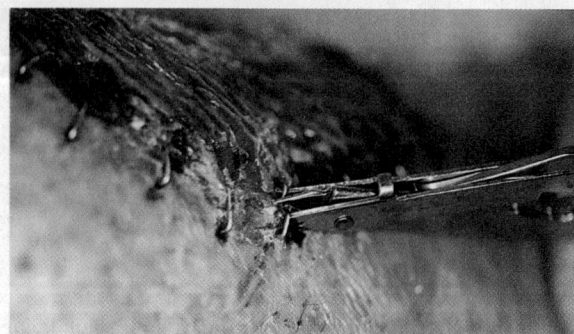

Figure 48-29 Staple remover.

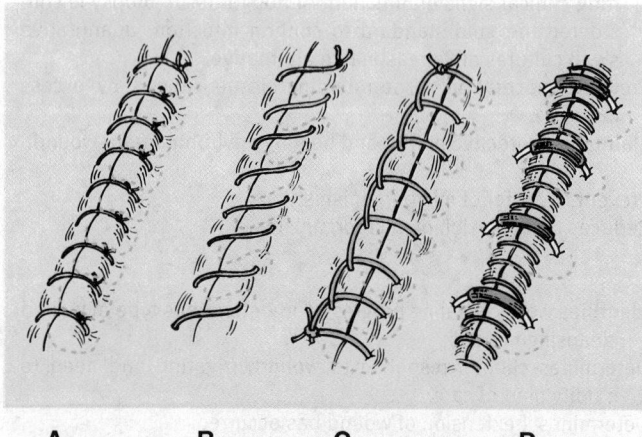

A   B   C   D

Figure 48-30 Examples of suturing methods. **A,** Intermittent. **B,** Continuous. **C,** Blanket continuous. **D,** Retention.

name implies, is a series of sutures with only two knots, one at the beginning and one at the end of the suture line. Retention sutures are placed more deeply than skin sutures, and nurses may or may not remove them, depending on agency policy. The manner in which the suture crosses and penetrates the skin determines the method for removal. *Never pull the visible portion of a suture through underlying tissue.* Sutures on the skin's surface harbor microorganisms and debris. The portion of the suture beneath the skin is sterile. Pulling the contaminated portion of the suture through tissues will possibly lead to infection. The nurse clips suture materials as close to the skin edge on one side as possible and pulls the suture through from the other side (Figure 48-31).

Drainage Evacuation. When drainage interferes with healing, you achieve drainage evacuation by using either a drain alone or a drainage tube with continuous suction. You may apply special skin barriers, including hydrocolloid dressings, similar to those used with ostomies (see Chapter 46), around drain sites. The skin barriers are soft material applied to the skin with adhesive. Drainage flows on the barrier but not directly on the skin. **Drainage evacuators** (Figure 48-32) are convenient, portable units that connect to tubular drains lying within a wound bed and exert a safe, constant, low-pressure vacuum to remove and collect drainage. Ensure that suction is

exerted and that connection points between the evacuator and tubing are intact. The evacuator collects drainage. Assess for volume and character every shift and as needed. When the evacuator fills, measure output by emptying the contents into a graduated cylinder and immediately reset the evacuator to apply suction.

Bandages and Binders. A simple gauze dressing is often not enough to immobilize or provide support to a wound. Binders and bandages applied over or around dressings provide extra protection and therapeutic benefits by the following:

1. Creating pressure over a body part (e.g., an elastic pressure bandage applied over an arterial puncture site)
2. Immobilizing a body part (e.g., an elastic bandage applied around a sprained ankle)
3. Supporting a wound (e.g., an abdominal binder applied over a large abdominal incision and dressing)
4. Reducing or preventing edema (e.g., a pressure bandage applied to lower leg)
5. Securing a splint (e.g., a bandage applied around hand splints for correction of deformities)
6. Securing dressings (e.g., elastic webbing applied around leg dressings after a vein stripping)

Bandages are available in rolls of various widths and materials, including gauze, elasticized knit, elastic webbing, flannel, and muslin. Gauze bandages are lightweight and inexpensive, mold easily around contours of the body, and permit air circulation to prevent skin maceration. Elastic bandages conform well to body parts but are also for exerting pressure.

Binders are bandages that are made of large pieces of material to fit a specific body part. Most binders are made of elastic or cotton. An abdominal binder and a breast binder are examples.

Principles for Applying Bandages and Binders. Correctly applied bandages and binders do not cause injury to underlying and nearby body parts or create discomfort for the client. For example, a chest binder should not be so tight as to restrict chest wall expansion. Before applying a bandage or binder, the nurse's responsibilities include the following:

- Inspecting the skin for abrasions, edema, discoloration, or exposed wound edges
- Covering exposed wounds or open abrasions with a sterile dressing
- Assessing the condition of underlying dressings and changing if soiled
- Assessing the skin of underlying areas that will be distal to the bandage for signs of circulatory impairment (coolness, pallor or cyanosis, diminished or absent pulses, swelling, numbness, and tingling) to provide a means for comparing changes in circulation after bandage application

After applying a bandage, the nurse assesses, documents, and immediately reports changes in circulation, skin integrity, comfort level, and body function (e.g., ventilation or movement). The nurse who applies a bandage loosens or readjusts it as necessary. The nurse needs a health care provider's order before loosening or removing a bandage applied by a health care provider. The nurse explains to the client that any bandage or binder feels relatively

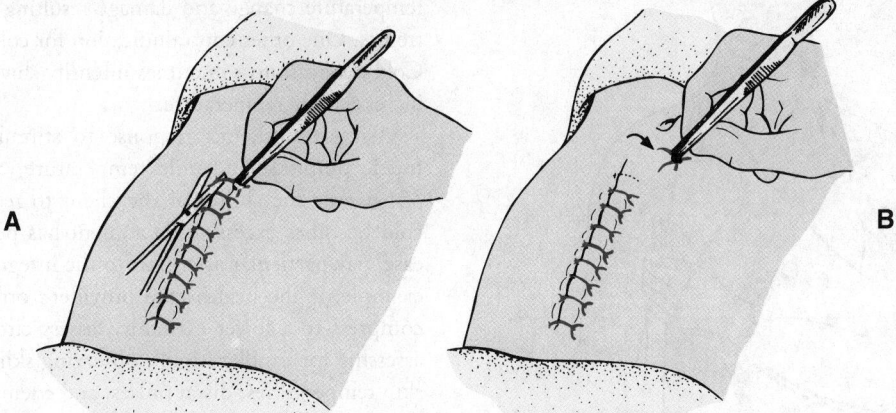

Figure 48-31 Removal of intermittent suture. **A,** Cut the suture as close to the skin as possible, away from the knot. **B,** Remove the suture and never pull the contaminated stitch through the tissues.

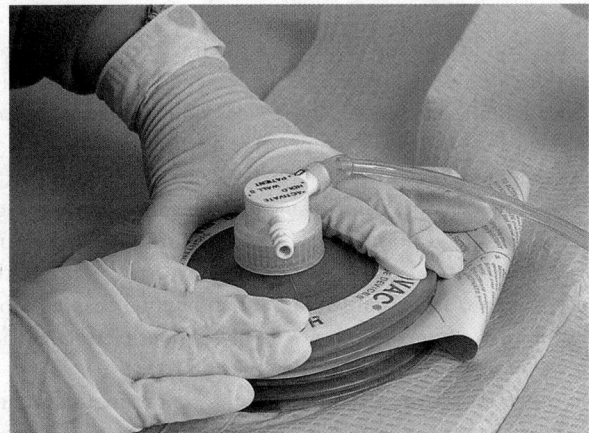

Figure 48-32 Setting the suction on a drainage evacuator. 1. With the drainage port open, the level on the diaphragm is raised. 2. Push straight down on the lever to lower the diaphragm. 3. Closure of the port prevents escape of air and creates vacuum pressure.

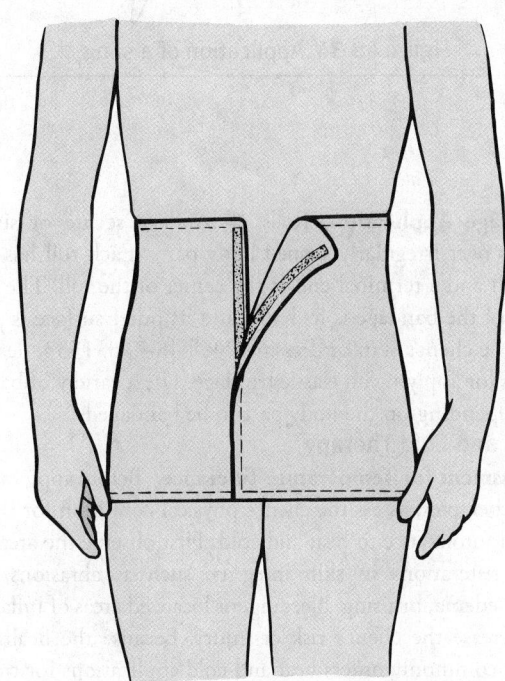

Figure 48-33 Securing an abdominal binder with Velcro.

firm or tight. Carefully assess a bandage to be sure that it is properly applied and is providing therapeutic benefit, and replace any soiled bandages.

Binder Application. Binders are especially designed for the body part to be supported. The most common type of binder is the abdominal binder (Skill 48-6). Well-fitting bras are now replacing breast binders. Both provide support after breast surgery or exert pressure to reduce lactation in a woman after childbirth.

Abdominal Binders. An abdominal binder supports large abdominal incisions that are vulnerable to tension or stress as the client moves or coughs (Figure 48-33). Secure an abdominal binder with safety pins, Velcro strips, or metal stays.

Slings. Slings support arms with muscular sprains or fractures. A commercially manufactured sling consists of a long sleeve that extends above the elbow, with a strap that fits around the neck. In

the home, clients can use a large triangular piece of cloth. The client sits or lies supine during sling application (Figure 48-34). Instruct the client to bend the affected arm, bringing the forearm straight across the chest. The open sling fits under the client's arm and over the chest, with the base of the triangle under the wrist and the triangle's point at the client's elbow. One end of the sling fits around the back of the client's neck. Bring the other end up and over the affected arm while supporting the extremity. Tie the two ends at the side of the neck so that the knot does not press against the cervical spine. The loose material at the elbow is folded evenly around the elbow and pinned. Always support the lower arm and hand at a level above the elbow to prevent the formation of dependent edema.

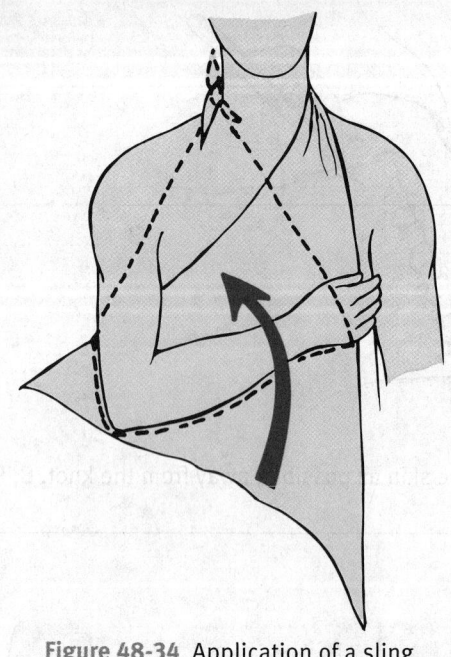

Figure 48-34 Application of a sling.

Bandage Application. Rolls of bandage secure or support dressings over irregularly shaped body parts. Each roll has a free outer end and a terminal end at the center of the roll. The rolled portion of the bandage is its body, and its outer surface is placed against the client's skin or dressing. Skill 48-7, p. 1333, describes the steps for applying an elastic bandage. Use a variety of bandage turns, depending on the body part to be bandaged.

Heat and Cold Therapy

Assessment for Temperature Tolerance. Before applying heat or cold therapies, assess the client's physical condition for signs of potential intolerance to heat and cold. First observe the area to be treated. Alterations in skin integrity, such as abrasions, open wounds, edema, bruising, bleeding, or localized areas of inflammation, increase the client's risk of injury. Because the health care provider commonly orders heat and cold applications for traumatized areas, the baseline skin assessment provides a guide for evaluating skin changes that will possibly occur during therapy.

Assessment includes identification of conditions that contraindicate heat or cold therapy. Do not cover an active area of bleeding by a warm application because bleeding will continue. Warm applications are contraindicated when the client has an acute, localized inflammation such as appendicitis because the heat will cause the appendix to rupture. If a client has cardiovascular problems, it is unwise to apply heat to large portions of the body because the resulting massive vasodilation will disrupt blood supply to vital organs.

Cold is contraindicated if the site of injury is already edematous. Cold further retards circulation to the area and prevents absorption of the interstitial fluid. If the client has impaired circulation (e.g., arteriosclerosis), cold further reduces blood supply to the affected area. Cold therapy is also contraindicated in the presence of neuropathy, because the client is unable to perceive

temperature change and damage resulting from temperature extremes. One other contraindication for cold therapy is shivering. Cold applications sometimes intensify shivering and dangerously increase body temperature.

Assess the client's response to stimuli. Sensation to light touch, pinprick, and mild temperature variations (see Chapter 33) reveals the ability of the client to recognize when heat or cold becomes excessive. If a client has peripheral vascular disease, pay particular attention to the integrity of extremities. For example, if the health care provider's order is to apply a cold compress to a lower extremity, assess circulation to the leg by assessing for capillary refill, observing skin color, and palpating skin temperatures, distal pulses, and edematous areas. If signs of circulatory inadequacy are present, it is important for you to question the order.

Level of consciousness influences the ability to perceive heat, cold, and pain. If a client is confused or unresponsive, the nurse needs to make frequent observations of skin integrity after therapy begins.

Also assess the condition of equipment being used. Check electrical equipment for cracked cords, frayed wires, damaged insulation, and exposed heating components. Make sure equipment containing circulating fluids does not have leaks. Check equipment for evenness of temperature distribution.

Local application of heat and cold to an injured body part is sometimes therapeutic. Before using these therapies, however, you need to understand normal body responses to local temperature variations, assess the integrity of the body part, determine the client's ability to sense temperature variations, and ensure proper operation of equipment. You are legally responsible for safe administration of heat and cold applications.

Bodily Responses to Heat and Cold. Exposure to heat and cold causes systemic and local responses. Systemic responses occur through heat-loss mechanisms (sweating and vasodilation) or mechanisms promoting heat conservation (vasoconstriction and piloerection) and heat production (shivering) (see Chapter 33). Local responses to heat and cold occur through stimulation of temperature-sensitive nerve endings within the skin. This stimulation sends impulses from the periphery to the hypothalamus, which becomes aware of local temperature sensations and triggers adaptive responses for maintenance of normal body temperature. If alterations occur along temperature sensation pathways, the reception and eventual perception of stimuli will be altered.

The body is able to tolerate wide variations in temperature. The normal temperature of the skin's surface is 34° C (93.2° F), but temperature receptors usually adapt quickly to local temperatures between 15° and 45° C (59° and 113° F). Pain develops when local temperatures exceed this range. Excessive heat causes a burning sensation. Cold produces a numbing sensation before pain.

The body's adaptive ability creates the major problem in protecting clients from injury resulting from temperature extremes. A person initially feels an extreme change in temperature but within a short time hardly notices it. This is dangerous because a person insensitive to heat and cold extremes can suffer serious tissue injury. You need to recognize clients most at risk for injuries from heat and cold applications (Table 48-10, p. 1334).

Text continued on p. 1334

✳ **SKILL 48-6**   **APPLYING AN ABDOMINAL BINDER**

Delegation Considerations

The skill of applying an abdominal binder can be delegated. The nurse is responsible for wound assessment, the evaluation of wound care interventions, and assessment of the client's ability to breathe deeply, cough effectively, and move independently; of skin for irritation/abrasion; of incision/wound and dressing; and of comfort level before a binder or sling is applied for the first time. Instruct nursing assistive personnel to:

- Immediately notify the nurse of any change in client's respiratory status
- Report any increase in wound drainage to the nurse
- Report any changes in skin integrity under or adjacent to the binder to the nurse
- Remove the binder at prescribed intervals

Equipment

- Gloves, if wound drainage is present
- Abdominal binder:
  - Correct size cloth/elastic straight binder
  - Safety pins (unless Velcro closure or metal fasteners are attached): six to eight safety pins are usually adequate for abdominal binders

STEPS	RATIONALE
1. Observe client with need for support of abdomen. Observe ability to breathe deeply and cough effectively.	Baseline assessment determines client's ability to breathe and cough. Impaired ventilation of lung leads to alveolar atelectasis and inadequate arterial oxygenation.
2. Review medical record if medical prescription for binder is required and reasons for application.	Application of supportive binders is based on nursing judgment. In some situations, health care provider input is required.
3. Inspect skin for actual or potential alterations in integrity. Observe for irritation, abrasion, skin surfaces that rub against each other, or allergic response to adhesive tape used to secure dressing.	Actual impairments in skin integrity sometimes worsen with application of a binder. Binders sometimes cause pressure and excoriation.
4. Inspect any surgical dressing.	Dressing replacement or reinforcement precedes application of any binder.
5. Assess client's comfort level, using analog scale of 0 to 10 (see Chapter 43) and noting any objective signs and symptoms.	Data will determine effectiveness of binder placement.

Critical Decision Point: Expect client in moderate-to-severe pain to have diaphoresis, tachycardia, and elevated blood pressure.

6. Gather necessary data regarding size of client and appropriate binder.	Ensures proper fit of binder.
7. Explain procedure to client.	Promotes client's understanding and cooperation.
8. Teach skill to client or significant other.	Reduces anxiety and ensures continuity of care after discharge.
9. Perform hand hygiene, and apply gloves (if likely to contact wound drainage).	Reduces transmission of microorganisms.
10. Close curtains or room door.	Maintains client's comfort and dignity.
11. Apply binder.	
A. **Abdominal binder**	
(1) Position client in supine position with head slightly elevated and knees slightly flexed.	Minimizes muscular tension on abdominal organs.
(2) Fanfold far side of binder toward midline of binder.	Reduces time client remains in uncomfortable position.
(3) Instruct and help client to roll away from nurse toward raised side rail while firmly supporting abdominal incision and dressing with hands.	Reduces pain and discomfort.
(4) Place fanfolded ends of binder under client.	Permits placement and centering of binder with minimal discomfort.
(5) Instruct or assist client in rolling over folded ends.	
(6) Unfold and stretch ends out smoothly on far side of bed.	Maintains skin integrity and comfort.
(7) Instruct client to roll back into supine position.	Facilitates chest expansion and adequate wound support when binder is closed.
(8) Adjust binder so that supine client is centered over binder using symphysis pubis and costal margins as lower and upper landmarks.	Centers support from binder over abdominal structures, which reduces incidence of decreased lung expansion.

Continued

✳ **SKILL 48-6**   APPLYING AN ABDOMINAL BINDER—CONT'D

STEPS	RATIONALE

Critical Decision Point: Cover any exposed areas of an incision or wound with sterile dressing.

STEPS	RATIONALE
(9) Close binder. Pull one end of binder over center of client's abdomen. While maintaining tension on that end of binder, pull opposite end of binder over center and secure with Velcro closure tabs, metal fasteners, or horizontally placed safety pins (see Figure 48-33, p. 1329).	Provides continuous wound support and comfort.
12. Assess client's comfort level.	Helps determine effectiveness of binder placement.
13. Adjust binder as necessary.	Promotes comfort and chest expansion.
14. Remove gloves, and perform hand hygiene.	Reduces transmission of microorganisms.
15. Observe site for skin integrity, circulation, and characteristics of the wound. (Periodically remove binder and surgical dressing to assess wound characteristics.)	Determines that binder has not resulted in complication to skin, wound, or underlying organs.
16. Assess comfort level of client, using analog scale of 0 to 10 and noting any objective signs and symptoms.	Binders should not increase discomfort.
17. Assess client's ability to ventilate properly, including deep breathing and coughing.	Identifies any impaired ventilation and potential pulmonary complications.
18. Identify client's need for assistance with activities such as hair combing, dressing, and ambulating.	Mobility of upper extremities is often limited, depending on severity and location of incision.

Unexpected Outcomes and Related Interventions
1. Client's pain increases.
   a. Remove binder and assess wound.
   b. Reapply binder using less pressure.
2. Client's respiratory rate decreases.
   a. Remove binder.
   b. Encourage client to cough and deep breathe.
   c. Reapply binder using less pressure.
3. Client develops impaired skin integrity under the binder.
   a. Remove binder.
   b. Initiate skin care measure to heal affected site.

Recording and Reporting
- Report any skin irritation to nurse at between-shift report.
- Record application of binder, condition of skin, circulation, integrity of dressing, and client's comfort level.
- Report ineffective lung expansion to health care provider immediately.

Home Care Considerations
- Abdominal binders are washable and are placed over a line to dry.
- Instruct caregiver to avoid excessive pressure with binder application.

✳ **SKILL 48-7** APPLYING AN ELASTIC BANDAGE

Delegation Considerations

The skill of applying an elastic bandage can be delegated. The nurse is responsible for wound assessment and the evaluation of the wound. In addition, the nurse is responsible for assessing for adequate circulation to the extremity distal to the elastic bandage. Instruct nursing assistive personnel to do the following:

- Any restrictions that the client has (e.g., unable to independently raise leg or independently roll over)
- Report any change in the skin color of the client's injured extremity
- Report any increases in client's pain

Equipment

- Correct width and number of bandages
- Safety pins, clips, or adhesive tape
- Clean gloves, if wound drainage is present

STEPS	RATIONALE
1. Review medical record for specific orders related to application of elastic bandage. Note area to be covered, type of bandage required, frequency of change, and previous response to treatment.	Specific prescriptions sometimes direct procedure, including factors such as extent of application (e.g., toe to knee, toe to groin) and duration of treatment.
2. Perform hand hygiene, and apply gloves if needed. Inspect skin for alterations in integrity as indicated by abrasions, discoloration, chafing, or edema. (Look carefully at bony prominences.)	Altered skin integrity contraindicates the use of elastic bandages.
3. Inspect surgical dressing if present. Remove gloves, and perform hand hygiene.	Surgical dressing replacement or reinforcement precedes application of any bandage. Reduces transmission of microorganisms.
4. Observe adequacy of circulation (distal to bandage) by noting surface temperature, skin color, and sensation in body parts to be wrapped.	Comparison of area before and after application of bandage is necessary to ensure continued adequate circulation. Impairment of circulation will possibly result in coolness to touch when compared with opposite side of body, cyanosis or pallor of skin, diminished or absent pulses, edema or localized pooling, and numbness or tingling of part.
5. Identify client's and primary caregiver's present knowledge level of skill if bandaging will be continued at home.	Ensures that planning and teaching are individualized.
6. Explain procedure to client.	Increased knowledge promotes cooperation and reduces anxiety.
7. Teach skill to client or significant other.	Reduces anxiety and ensures continuity of care after discharge.
8. Perform hand hygiene, and apply gloves if drainage is present.	Reduces transmission of microorganisms.
9. Close room door or curtains.	Maintains client's comfort and dignity.
10. Help client to assume comfortable, anatomically correct position.	Maintains alignment. Prevents musculoskeletal deformity.

Critical Decision Point: Apply bandages to lower extremities before client sits or stands. Elevate dependent extremities for 20 minutes before bandage application to enhance venous return.

11. Hold roll of elastic bandage in dominant hand, and use other hand to lightly hold beginning of bandage at distal body part. Continue transferring roll to dominant hand as bandage is wrapped.	Maintains appropriate and consistent bandage tension.

Critical Decision Point: Toes or fingertips need to be visible for follow-up circulatory assessment.

12. Apply bandage from distal point toward proximal boundary using variety of turns to cover various shapes of body parts. A spiral dressing is often used to cover cylindrical body parts such as wrist or upper arms. Bandage in an ascending motion, overlapping the previous bandage by one-half or two-thirds width of bandage. Use a figure-eight dressing to cover joint because the snug fit provides excellent immobilization. *To apply:* Overlap turns, alternately ascending and descending over bandaged part; each turn crossing previous one to form figure eight.	Bandage is applied in manner that conforms evenly to body part and promotes venous return.
13. Unroll and very slightly stretch bandage.	Maintains uniform bandage tension.

Continued

※ SKILL 48-7   APPLYING AN ELASTIC BANDAGE—CONT'D

STEPS	RATIONALE
14. Overlap turns by one-half to two-thirds width of bandage roll.	Prevents uneven bandage tension and circulatory impairment.
15. Secure first bandage with clip or tape before applying additional rolls.	
a. Apply additional rolls without leaving any skin surface uncovered. Secure last bandage applied.	Prevents wrinkling or loose ends.
16. Remove gloves if worn, and perform hand hygiene	Reduces transmission of microorganisms.
17. Assess distal circulation when bandage application is complete and at least twice during 8-hour period.	Early detection and management of circulatory impairment ensures healthy neurovascular status.
a. Observe skin color for pallor or cyanosis.	
b. Palpate skin for warmth.	
c. Palpate pulses, and compare bilaterally.	
d. Ask if client is aware of pain, numbness, tingling, or other discomfort.	Neurovascular changes indicate impaired venous return.
e. Observe mobility of extremity.	Determines if bandage is too tight, which restricts movement, or determines if joint immobility is attained.
18. Have client demonstrate bandage application.	Return demonstration documents learning.

Unexpected Outcomes and Related Interventions

1. Impaired circulation distal to elastic bandage
   a. Release bandage.
   b. Palpate extremity and assess pulse, temperature, and capillary refill.
   c. Reapply dressing with less pressure.
2. Break in skin under elastic bandage
   a. Remove bandage.
   b. Reapply bandage with less pressure.
3. Client unable to perform dressing change
   a. Reinstruct client or family caregiver on bandage application.
   b. Observe client or family caregiver apply bandage.

Recording and Reporting

- Document condition of wound, integrity of dressing, application of bandage, circulation, and client's comfort level.
- Report any changes in neurological or circulatory status to nurse in charge or health care provider.

Home Care Considerations

- Instruct client or caregiver not to make bandages too tight, which interferes with circulation.
- Elastic bandages that reduce swelling are best applied to the feet in the morning, before getting out of bed.
- Always remove an elastic bandage daily and inspect skin beneath it.

※ TABLE 48-10 Conditions That Increase Risk of Injury From Heat and Cold Application

CONDITION	RISK FACTORS
Very young clients or older clients	Thinner skin layers in children increase risk of burns. Older clients have reduced sensitivity to pain.
Open wounds, broken skin, stomas	Subcutaneous and visceral tissues are more sensitive to temperature variations. They also contain no temperature and fewer pain receptors.
Areas of edema or scar formation	Reduced sensation to temperature stimuli occurs because of thickening of skin layers from fluid buildup or scar formation.
Peripheral vascular disease (e.g., diabetes, arteriosclerosis)	Body's extremities are less sensitive to temperature and pain stimuli because of circulatory impairment and local tissue injury. Cold application further compromises blood flow.
Confusion or unconsciousness	Perception of sensory or painful stimuli is reduced.
Spinal cord injury	Alterations in nerve pathways prevent reception of sensory or painful stimuli.
Abscessed tooth or appendix	Infection is highly localized. Application of heat causes rupture with spread of microorganisms systemically.

Local Effects of Heat and Cold. Heat and cold stimuli create different physiological responses. The choice of heat or cold therapy depends on local responses desired for wound healing (Table 48-11).

Effects of Heat Application. Heat generally is quite therapeutic, improving blood flow to an injured part. If heat is applied for 1 hour or more, however, the body will reduce blood flow by a reflex vasoconstriction to control heat loss from the area. Periodic removal and reapplication of local heat restores vasodilation. Continuous exposure to heat damages epithelial cells, causing redness, localized tenderness, and even blistering.

Effects of Cold Application. The application of cold initially diminishes swelling and pain. Prolonged exposure of the skin to cold results in a reflex vasodilation. The cells' inability to receive

✳ TABLE 48-11 Therapeutic Effects of Heat and Cold Applications

PHYSIOLOGICAL RESPONSE	THERAPEUTIC BENEFIT	EXAMPLES OF CONDITIONS TREATED
Heat		
Vasodilation	Improves blood flow to injured body part; promotes delivery of nutrients and removal of wastes; lessens venous congestion in injured tissues	Open wounds; rectal surgery; episiotomy; painful hemorrhoids; muscle tension; vaginal inflammation; wound debridement
Reduced blood viscosity	Improves delivery of leukocytes and antibiotics to wound site	
Reduced muscle tension	Promotes muscle relaxation and reduces pain from spasm or stiffness	
Increased tissue metabolism	Increases blood flow; provides local warmth	
Increased capillary permeability	Promotes movement of waste products and nutrients	
Cold		
Vasoconstriction	Reduces blood flow to injured body part, preventing edema formation; reduces inflammation	Direct trauma (sprains, strains, fractures, muscle spasms); superficial laceration or puncture wound; minor burn; suspected malignancy in area of injury or pain; injections; arthritis and joint trauma
Local anesthesia	Reduces localized pain	
Reduced cell metabolism	Reduces oxygen needs of tissues	
Increased blood viscosity	Promotes blood coagulation at injury site	
Decreased muscle tension	Relieves pain	

adequate blood flow and nutrients results in tissue ischemia. The skin initially takes on a reddened appearance, followed by a bluish purple mottling with numbness and a burning type of pain. The skin's tissues freeze from exposure to extreme cold.

Factors Influencing Heat and Cold Tolerance. The body's response to heat and cold therapies depends on the following factors:

- A person is better able to tolerate short exposure to temperature extremes.
- Exposed skin layers and certain areas of the skin are more sensitive to temperature variations. These include the neck, inner aspect of the wrist and forearm, and perineal region. The foot and palm of the hand are less sensitive.
- The body responds best to minor temperature adjustments. If a body part is cool and a hot stimulus touches the skin, the response is greater than if the skin were already warm.
- A person has less tolerance to temperature changes to which a large area of the body is exposed.
- Tolerance to temperature variations changes with age. Clients who are very young or old are most sensitive to heat and cold.
- If a client's physical condition reduces the reception or perception of sensory stimuli, tolerance to temperature extremes is high, but the risk of injury is also high.
- Uneven temperature distribution suggests that the equipment is functioning improperly.

SAFETY ALERT Before application of heat or cold therapy the client needs to understand its purpose, the symptoms of temperature exposure, and precautions taken to prevent injury. Box 48-15 provides methods for the safe application of heat and cold therapy.

Application of Heat and Cold Therapies. A prerequisite to using any heat or cold application is a health care provider's order,

✳ BOX 48-15 Safety Suggestions for Applying Heat or Cold Therapy

- *Do* explain to the client sensations to be felt during the procedure.
- *Do* instruct the client to report changes in sensation or discomfort immediately.
- *Do* provide a timer, clock, or watch so that the client can help the nurse time the application.
- *Do* keep the call light within the client's reach.
- *Do* refer to the institution's policy and procedure manual for safe temperatures.
- *Do not* allow the client to adjust temperature settings.
- *Do not* allow the client to move an application or place hands on the wound site.
- *Do not* place the client in a position that prevents movement away from the temperature source.
- *Do not* leave unattended a client who is unable to sense temperature changes or move from the temperature source.

which includes the body site to be treated and the type, frequency, and duration of application. Consult the agency's procedure manual for correct temperatures to use.

Choice of Moist or Dry. You can administer heat and cold applications in dry or moist forms. The type of wound or injury, the location of the body part, and the presence of drainage or inflammation are factors to consider in selecting dry or moist applications. Box 48-16 summarizes advantages and disadvantages of both.

Warm, Moist Compresses. For open wounds, sterile, warm, moist compresses improve circulation, relieve edema, and promote consolidation of pus and drainage. A compress is a piece of

✴ BOX 48-16 Choice of Dry or Moist Applications

Advantages
Moist Applications
Moist application reduces drying of skin and softens wound exudate.
Moist compresses conform well to most body areas.
Moist heat penetrates deeply into tissue layers.
Warm moist heat does not promote sweating and insensible fluid loss.

Dry Applications
Dry heat has less risk of burns to skin than moist applications.
Dry application does not cause skin maceration.
Dry heat retains temperature longer because evaporation does not occur.

Disadvantages
Moist Applications
Prolonged exposure causes maceration of skin.
Moist heat will cool rapidly because of moisture evaporation.
Moist heat creates greater risk for burns to skin because moisture conducts heat.

Dry Applications
Dry heat increases body fluid loss through sweating.
Dry applications do not penetrate deep into tissues.
Dry heat causes increased drying of skin.

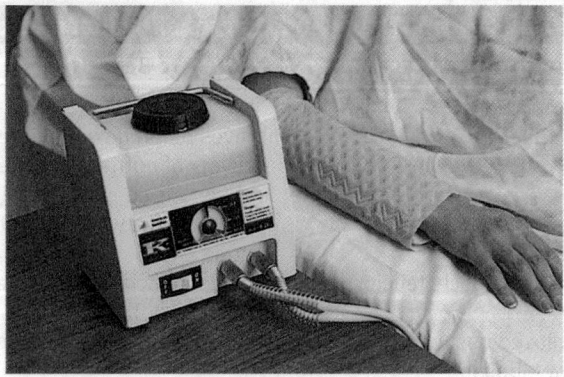

Figure 48-35 Aquathermia pad.

gauze dressing moistened in a prescribed warmed solution. A pack is a larger cloth or dressing applied to a larger body area.

Heat from warm compresses dissipates quickly. To maintain a constant temperature, you need to change the compress often or apply a warm aquathermic pad or waterproof heating pad over the compress. Because moisture conducts heat, any device's temperature setting should be lower for a moist compress than for a dry application. You can also use a layer of plastic wrap or a dry towel to insulate the compress and retain heat. Moist heat promotes vasodilation and evaporation of heat from the skin's surface. For this reason, a client will possibly feel chilly. Always try to control drafts within the room and keep the client covered with a blanket or robe. Skill 48-8 describes the steps for applying a warm, moist compress.

Warm Soaks. Immersion of a body part in a warmed solution promotes circulation, lessens edema, increases muscle relaxation, and provides a means to debride wounds and apply medicated solution. Sometimes a soak is also accompanied by wrapping the body part in dressings and saturating them with the warmed solution.

Position the client comfortably, place waterproof pads under the area to be treated, and heat the solution to about 40.5° to 43° C (105° to 110° F). After immersing the body part, cover the container and extremity with a towel to reduce heat loss. It is usually necessary to remove the cooled solution and add heated solution after about 10 minutes. The problem is to keep the solution at a constant temperature. Never add a hotter solution while the body part remains immersed. After any soak, dry the body part thoroughly to prevent maceration.

Sitz Baths. The client who has had rectal surgery, an episiotomy during childbirth, painful hemorrhoids, or vaginal inflammation will benefit from a sitz bath, a bath in which only the pelvic area is immersed in warm or in some situations cool fluid. The client sits in a special tub or chair or in a basin that fits on the toilet seat so that the legs and feet remain out of the water. Immersing the entire body causes widespread vasodilation and nullifies the effect of local heat application to the pelvic area.

The desired temperature for a sitz bath depends on whether the purpose is to promote relaxation or to clean a wound. It is often necessary to add warm or cool water during the procedure, which normally lasts 20 minutes, to maintain a constant temperature. Agency procedure manuals recommend safe water temperatures. A disposable sitz basin contains an attachment resembling an enema bag that allows gradual introduction of additional water.

Prevent overexposure of the client by draping bath blankets around the client's shoulders and thighs and controlling drafts. The client should be able to sit in the basin or tub with feet flat on the floor and without pressure on the sacrum or thighs. Because exposure of a large portion of the body to heat causes extensive vasodilation, assess the pulse and facial color and ask whether the client feels light-headed or nauseated.

Aquathermia (Water-Flow) Pads. A popular device in health care institutions is the aquathermia pad, or water-flow pad (Figure 48-35), used for treating muscle sprains and areas of mild inflammation or edema. The aquathermia unit consists of a waterproof plastic or rubber pad connected by two hoses to an electrical control unit that has a heating element and motor.

Distilled water circulates through hollowed channels within the pad to the control unit where water is heated or cooled (depending on temperature setting). Some pads have an absorbent surface to apply moist heat. The units are safer than conventional heating pads. However, you still need to check for equipment malfunctions. You fix the temperature setting by inserting a plastic key into the temperature regulator. In many institutions the central supply room sets the regulators to the recommended temperature (40.5° to 43° C [105° to 110° F]). If the distilled water in the unit runs low, simply fill the reservoir two-thirds full. Never add plain tap water, because it will leave mineral deposits in the unit.

To avoid burning the client's skin, do not place the pad directly on it. A thin towel or pillow case fits easily over the heating pad. Tape, ties, or a gauze roll holds the pad in place. Do not use pins, because they will possibly cause a leak. Check the client's skin often for signs of burning. An application should last only

✳ **SKILL 48-8**   **APPLYING A WARM, MOIST COMPRESS TO AN OPEN WOUND**

Delegation Considerations

The skill of applying a warm, moist compress to an open wound can be delegated. The nurse is responsible for wound assessment and evaluation of wound care interventions. Instruct nursing assistive personnel to:

- Maintain proper temperature of application during duration of treatment.
- Keep application in place for only the length of time specified in health care provider's orders.
- Notify the nurse when treatment is complete so that the nurse can make an evaluation of client's response.

Equipment

- Prescribed solution warmed to appropriate temperature
- Sterile gauze dressings or commercially prepared compresses
- Sterile container for solution
- Dry bath towel
- Clean gloves
- Sterile gloves
- Waterproof pad
- Ties or tape
- Aquathermia or heating pad (optional)
- Bath blanket

STEPS	RATIONALE
1. Refer to health care provider's order for type of compress, location and duration of application, desired temperature, and institutional policies regarding temperature of compress.	Ensures safe and correct application.
2. Refer to medical record to identify any systemic contraindications to heat application.	Heat causes vasodilation, which aggravates active bleeding. Heat applied to localized area of acute inflammation or tumor will possibly cause rupture or activate cell growth.
3. Perform hand hygiene.	Reduces transmission of microorganisms.
4. Inspect condition of exposed skin and wound where you will apply compress.	Provides baseline to determine changes in skin during heat application.
5. Assess client's extremities for sensitivity to temperature and pain by measuring light touch, pinprick, and temperature sensation.	Clients insensitive to heat or cold sensations need close monitoring during treatment.

Critical Decision Point: Clients with diabetes mellitus, victims of stroke, and clients with peripheral neuropathy or who have very thin or damaged skin are particularly at risk for thermal injury.

6. Assemble equipment and supplies.	Organization of supplies prevents unnecessary delays in the procedure.
7. Explain steps of procedure and purpose to client. Describe sensations to be felt, such as decreasing warmth and wetness. Explain precautions to prevent burning.	Minimizes client's anxiety and promotes cooperation during the procedure.
8. Close door and bedside curtains.	Decreases drafts, thus decreasing the transmission of microorganisms. Provides for client privacy.
9. Assist client in assuming comfortable position in proper body alignment, and place waterproof pad under area you will treat.	Compress remains in place for several minutes. Limited mobility in uncomfortable position causes muscular stress. Pad prevents soiling of bed linen.
10. Expose body part you will treat with compress, and drape client with bath blanket.	Prevents unnecessary cooling and exposure of body part.

11. Prepare compress:
  a. Pour solution into sterile container.
  b. If using portable heating source, warm solution. Commercially prepared compresses remain under infrared lamp until just before use. Open sterile packages, and drop gauze into container to become immersed in solution. NOTE: You must test the temperature by applying sterile solution to your forearm (without contaminating solution).
  c. Adjust temperature of aquathermia pad (if needed).
	Ensures orderly procedure.
	Compresses must retain warmth for therapeutic benefit.

12. Apply clean gloves. Remove any existing dressing covering wound. Dispose of gloves and dressings in proper receptacle.	Reduces transmission of microorganisms.
13. Assess condition of wound and surrounding skin. Inflamed wound appears reddened, but surrounding skin is less red in color.	Provides baseline to determine skin changes following compress application.

Critical Decision Point: If skin surrounding wound is reddened, application may be contraindicated.

Continued

✳ SKILL 48-8   APPLYING A WARM, MOIST COMPRESS TO AN OPEN WOUND—CONT'D

STEPS	RATIONALE
14. Apply sterile gloves.	Allows nurse to manipulate sterile dressing and touch open wound.
15. Pick up one layer of immersed gauze, wring out any excess solution, and apply it lightly to open wound.	Excess moisture macerates skin and increases risks of burns and infection. Skin is sensitive to sudden change in temperature.
16. In a few seconds, lift edge of gauze to assess for redness.	Increased redness indicates burn.
17. If client tolerates compress, pack gauze snugly against the wound. Be sure to cover all wound surfaces with the warm compress.	Packing of compress prevents rapid cooling from underlying air currents.
18. Cover moist compress with dry sterile dressing and bath towel. If necessary, pin or tie in place. Remove sterile gloves.	Dry sterile dressing will prevent transfer of microorganisms to wound via capillary action caused by moist compress. Towel insulates compress to prevent heat loss.
19. *Optional:* Apply aquathermia or waterproof heating pad over towel. Keep it in place for desired duration of application.	Provides constant temperature to compress.
20. If you are not using an aquathermia pad to maintain temperature of application, change warm compress using sterile technique every 5 minutes or as ordered during duration of therapy.	Prevents cooling and maintains therapeutic benefit of compress.
21. After prescribed time, apply clean gloves and remove pad, towel, and compress. Reassess wound and condition of skin, and replace dry sterile dressing as ordered.	Continued exposure to moisture will macerate skin. Prevents entrance of microorganisms into wound site.
22. Assist client to preferred comfortable position.	Maintains client's comfort.
23. Dispose of equipment and soiled compress. Perform hand hygiene.	Reduces transmission of microorganisms.
24. Inspect affected area covered by compress and heating pad every 5 to 10 minutes.	Assists in determining effects of application.
25. Ask every 5 to 10 minutes if client notices any unusual burning sensation not felt before application.	It is often difficult to assess burn merely by color changes if wound is inflamed or drainage is present.
26. Have client explain and demonstrate application.	Evaluates client's understanding of and ability to perform procedure.

Unexpected Outcomes and Related Interventions

1. Client's wound remains the same.
   a. Report to health care provider.
   b. Evaluate the continued use of warm compress.
2. Client's skin is broken, erythematous, and warm to the touch.
   a. Verify that correct temperature of compress is maintained.
   b. Institute skin care practices.

Recording and Reporting

- Record type, location, and duration of application. Note solution and temperature.
- Describe condition of wound and skin before and after treatment, as well as client's response to therapy.

- Describe any instructions given and client's ability to explain and perform procedure.
- Report unusual findings to nurse in charge or health care provider.

Home Care Considerations

- When necessary, assess availability of primary caregivers to assist clients in application of compress, their understanding of purpose of procedure, and their willingness to comply with procedure and not leave client with compress in place beyond prescribed time limit.
- Assess physical environment to determine existence of adequate facilities to prepare warm compress and provide for sterile technique.

---

20 to 30 minutes. Do not allow a client to lie on a pad. Pressure against a mattress prevents normal heat dissipation. If you are applying the pad to a region of the back, have the client lie prone or on one side.

Commercial Hot Packs. Commercially prepared, disposable hot packs apply warm, dry heat to an injured area. The chemicals mix and release heat when you strike, knead, or squeeze the pack. Package directions recommend the time for heat application.

Cold, Moist, and Dry Compresses. The procedure for applying cold, moist compresses is the same as that for warm compresses. Apply cold compresses for 20 minutes at a temperature of 15° C

(59° F) to relieve inflammation and swelling. You can use clean or sterile compresses.

There are commercially prepared cold packs that are similar to the disposable hot packs for dry applications. They come in various shapes and sizes to fit different body parts. When using cold compresses, observe for adverse reactions such as burning or numbness, mottling of the skin, redness, extreme paleness, and a bluish skin discoloration.

Cold Soaks. The procedure for preparing cold soaks and immersing a body part is the same as for warm soaks. The desired temperature for a 20-minute cold soak is 15° C (59° F). Control drafts and use outer coverings to protect the client from chilling. It is often necessary to add cold water during the procedure to maintain a constant temperature.

Ice Bags or Collars. For a client who has a muscle sprain, localized hemorrhage, or hematoma or who has undergone dental surgery, an ice bag is ideal to prevent edema formation, control bleeding, and anesthetize the body part. Proper use of the bag requires the following steps:

1. Fill the bag with water, secure the cap, invert to check for leaks, and pour out the water.
2. Fill the bag two-thirds full with crushed ice so you are able to easily mold the bag over a body part.
3. Release any air from the bag by squeezing its sides before securing the cap, because excess air interferes with conduction of cold.
4. Wipe off excess moisture.
5. Cover the bag with a flannel cover, towel, or pillow case.
6. Apply the bag to the injury site for 30 minutes; you can reapply the bag in an hour.

◆Evaluation

You evaluate nursing interventions for reducing and treating pressure ulcers by determining the client's response to nursing therapies and by determining whether the client achieved each goal. To evaluate outcomes and responses to care, you measure the effectiveness of interventions. The optimal outcomes are to prevent injury to the skin and tissues, reduce injury to the skin and underlying tissues, and restore skin integrity.

Because each client has different risk factors for impaired skin integrity, you need to individualize nursing interventions. Clients with minimal mobility impairments or relatively stable health status need only a few measures. You evaluate nursing interventions for reducing and treating pressure ulcers by determining the client's response to nursing therapies and by determining whether the client achieved each goal (Figure 48-36).

Clients with impaired skin integrity need assessment on an ongoing basis for factors that contribute to skin breakdown. This includes a comprehensive skin assessment and a wound assessment using a validated risk assessment tool. Assessment provides the foundation for the plan of care and is critical for monitoring the effectiveness of the plan (Nix, 2007).

It is important to include the client and the caregiver in the assessment process. Determine what they know about the formation of impaired skin integrity, and develop a plan of care to provide education. Chronic wounds such as pressure ulcers take time to heal, and it is likely that the client will be in the home setting with the pressure ulcer.

If the identified outcomes are not met for a client with impaired skin integrity, questions to ask include the following:

• Was the etiology of the skin impairment addressed? Were the pressure, friction, shear, and moisture components identified, and did the plan of care decrease the contribution of each of these components?

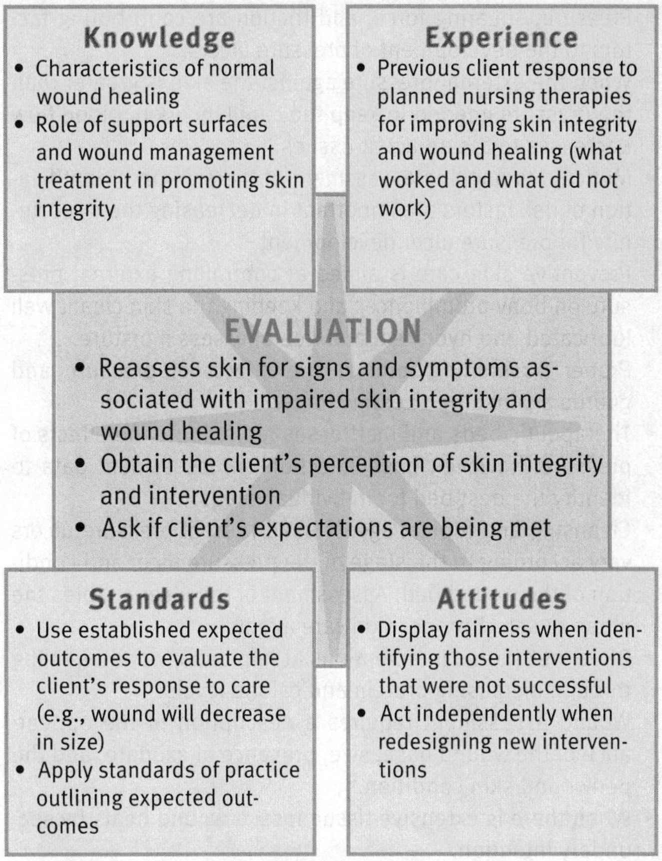

Figure 48-36 Critical thinking model for skin integrity and wound care evaluation.

• Was wound healing supported by providing the wound base with a moist protected environment?
• Were issues such as nutrition assessed and a plan of care developed that provided the client with the calories to support healing?

Finally, evaluate the need for additional referrals to other experts in pressure ulcers, such as nurses certified in wound care when indicated. Care of the client with a pressure ulcer requires a multidisciplinary team approach.

✷ Key Concepts

• Pressure ulcers contribute to client discomfort and decreased functional status, increase the length of stay in acute and extended care settings, and increase cost of care.
• Wound assessment scales help measure improvement of a healing pressure ulcer; do not use the staging systems for wound depth for this purpose.
• Evaluate all clients for risk factors that contribute to development of impaired skin integrity.
• Alterations in mobility, sensory perception, level of consciousness, and nutrition and the presence of moisture increase the risk for pressure ulcer development.
• The risk of impaired skin integrity related to immobilization depends on the extent and duration of immobilization.

- Pressure, shearing force, and friction are contributing factors to the development of pressure ulcers.
- When the external pressure against the skin is greater than the pressure needed to keep the capillary open, blood flow decreases to the adjacent tissues.
- Meticulous ongoing assessment of the skin and identification of risk factors are important in decreasing the opportunity for pressure ulcer development.
- Preventive skin care is aimed at controlling external pressure on bony prominences and keeping the skin clean, well lubricated and hydrated, and free of excess moisture.
- Proper positioning reduces the effects of pressure and guards against the shearing force.
- Therapeutic beds and mattresses redistribute the effects of pressure; however, base selection on assessment data to identify the best bed for individual needs.
- Cleansing and topical agents used to treat pressure ulcers vary according to the stage of the pressure ulcer and condition of the wound bed. Assessment of the ulcer enables the nurse to select proper skin care agents.
- Direct nutritional interventions at improving wound healing through increasing protein and calorie levels.
- Wound assessment requires a description of the appearance of the wound base, size, presence of exudate, and the periwound skin condition.
- When there is extensive tissue loss, a wound heals by secondary intention.
- The chances of wound infection are greater when the wound contains dead or necrotic tissue, when foreign bodies lie on or near the wound, and when the blood supply and tissue defenses are reduced.
- The principles of wound first aid include control of bleeding, cleansing, and protection.
- The layers of a dry dressing absorb drainage and prevent entrance of bacteria.
- A moist environment supports wound healing.
- The wet-to-dry dressing mechanically removes dead tissue and wound exudate to debride the wound.
- When cleansing wounds or drain sites, clean from the least to most contaminated area, away from wound edges.
- Apply a bandage or binder in a manner that does not impair circulation or irritate the skin.
- An acute sprain, closed fracture, or bruise responds best to cold applications.

✳ Critical Thinking Exercises

Mrs. Stein, who is 76 years of age, is 7 days postoperative for a total hip replacement. She developed redness and oozing of foul-smelling tan-colored drainage from the hip incision on postoperative day four. Significant medical history includes arthritis and mild hypertension. Because of surgical pain at the incision site, she did not easily transfer from her bed to the chair. Now on day seven, she notes some pain at the incision and complains of a painful, burning sensation in the sacral region. She is continent of urine and stool but continues to "scoot" over the to side of the bed when preparing for bed-to-chair transfers.

1. The staples from the surgical incision were removed by the health care provider, and an order was written for moist saline gauze dressing to the area 3 times a day. When the dressing is removed, what are the critical factors to assess?

2. A head-to-toe skin assessment is done per institutional policy on a daily basis. At the most recent assessment, redness was noted over the sacral area, and upon direct examination a small area of denuded tissue was noted. The involved area has minimal depth and a red moist base. How would you describe the impairment in skin integrity in your charting?

3. What will you include in your plan of care to address the impairment in skin integrity in the sacral area?

4. Mrs. Stein will be discharged tomorrow. What issues must be assessed regarding her care before discharge? Describe why those issues are of importance.

✳ NCLEX®-Style Review Questions

1. When repositioning an immobile client, the nurse notices redness over a bony prominence. When the area is assessed, the red spot blanches with fingertip touch, indicating:
   1. A local skin infection requiring antibiotics
   2. This client has sensitive skin and requires special bed linen
   3. A stage III pressure ulcer needing the appropriate dressing
   4. Reactive hyperemia, a reaction that causes the blood vessels to dilate in the injured area

2. This type of pressure ulcer has an observable pressure-related alteration of intact skin whose indicators, compared with an adjacent or opposite area on the body, may include changes in one or more of the following: skin temperature (warmth or coolness), tissue consistency (firm or beefy feel), and/or sensation (pain, itching).
   1. Stage I
   2. Stage II
   3. Stage III
   4. Stage IV

3. When obtaining a wound culture to determine the presence of a wound infection, the specimen should to be taken from the:
   1. Necrotic tissue
   2. Wound drainage
   3. Drainage on the dressing
   4. Wound after it has first been cleansed with normal saline

4. Postoperatively the client with a closed abdominal wound reports a sudden "pop" after coughing. When the nurse examines the surgical wound site, the sutures are open and pieces of small bowel are noted at the bottom of the now opened wound. The correct intervention would be to:
   1. Allow the area to be exposed to air until all drainage has stopped
   2. Place several cold packs over the areas, protecting the skin around the wound
   3. Cover the areas with sterile saline-soaked towels and immediately notify the surgical team; this is likely to indicate a wound evisceration
   4. Cover the area with sterile gauze, place a tight binder over the areas, and ask the client to remain in bed for 30 minutes because this is a minor opening in the surgical wound and should reseal quickly

5. Serous drainage from a wound is defined as:
   1. Fresh bleeding
   2. Thick and yellow
   3. Clear, watery plasma
   4. Beige to brown and foul smelling

6. For a client who has a muscle sprain, localized hemorrhage, or hematoma, what wound care product helps prevent edema formation, control bleeding, and anesthetize the body part?
   1. Binder
   2. Ice bag
   3. Elastic bandage
   4. Absorptive diaper

7. Interventions to manage a client who is experiencing fecal and urinary incontinence include:
   1. Keeping the buttocks exposed to air at all times
   2. Use of a large absorbent diaper, changing when saturated
   3. Utilization of an incontinence cleanser, followed by application of a moisture barrier ointment
   4. Frequent cleansing, application of an ointment, and covering the areas with a thick absorbent towel

8. The best description of a hydrocolloid dressing is:
   1. A seaweed derivative that is highly absorptive
   2. Premoistened gauze, placed over a granulating wound
   3. A debriding enzyme that is used to remove necrotic tissue
   4. A dressing that forms a gel that interacts with the wound surface

9. A binder placed around a surgical client with a new abdominal wound is indicated for:
   1. Collection of wound drainage
   2. Reduction of abdominal swelling
   3. Reduction of stress on the abdominal incision
   4. Stimulation of peristalsis (return of bowel function) from direct pressure

10. Application of a warm compress is indicated:
    1. To relieve edema
    2. For a client who is shivering
    3. To improve blood flow to an injured part
    4. To protect bony prominences from pressure ulcers

49 | Sensory Alterations

✳ OBJECTIVES

Mastery of content in this chapter will enable the student to:

- Differentiate among the processes of reception, perception, and reaction to sensory stimuli.
- Discuss the relationship of sensory function to an individual's level of wellness.
- Discuss common causes and effects of sensory alterations.
- Discuss common sensory changes that normally occur with aging.
- Identify factors to assess in determining a client's sensory status.

- Identify nursing diagnoses relevant to clients with sensory alterations.
- Develop a plan of care for clients with sensory deficits.
- List interventions for preventing sensory deprivation and controlling sensory overload.
- Describe conditions in the health care agency or client's home that you can adjust to promote meaningful sensory stimulation.
- Discuss ways to maintain a safe environment for clients with sensory deficits.

✳ MEDIA RESOURCES   ✳ KEY TERMS

 Companion CD
- NCLEX®-Style Review Questions
- Audio Glossary
- Interactive Learning Activities
- English/Spanish Glossary

evolve Website
- NCLEX®-Style Review Questions
- Audio Glossary
- English/Spanish Glossary
- Interactive Learning Activities
- Weblinks
- Audio Summaries

Aphasia, p. 1350
Auditory, p. 1343
Conductive hearing loss, p. 1357
Delusions, p. 1349
Expressive aphasia, p. 1350
Gustatory, p. 1343
Hyperesthesia, p. 1357
Illusions, p. 1349
Kinesthetic, p. 1343
Olfactory, p. 1343

Otolaryngologist, p. 1348
Ototoxic, p. 1351
Proprioceptive, p. 1346
Receptive aphasia, p. 1350
Refractive error, p. 1355
Sensory deficit, p. 1344
Sensory deprivation, p. 1345
Sensory overload, p. 1345
Stereognosis, p. 1343
Strabismus, p. 1355
Tactile, p. 1343

Imagine the world without sight, hearing, or the ability to feel objects or sense aromas around you. Human beings rely on a variety of sensory stimuli to give meaning and order to events occurring in their environment. The senses form the perceptual base of our world (Ebersole and others, 2005). Stimulation comes from many sources in and outside the body, particularly through the senses of sight (visual), hearing (**auditory**), touch (**tactile**), smell (**olfactory**), and taste (**gustatory**). The body also has a **kinesthetic** sense that enables a person to be aware of the position and movement of body parts without seeing them. **Stereognosis** is a sense that allows a person to recognize an object's size, shape, and texture. The ability to speak is not a sense, but it is similar in that some clients lose the ability to interact meaningfully with other human beings. Meaningful stimuli allow a person to learn about the environment and are necessary for healthy functioning and normal development. When sensory function is altered, the person's ability to relate to and function within the environment changes drastically.

Many clients seeking health care have preexisting sensory alterations. Others develop sensory alterations as a result of medical treatment (e.g., hearing loss from antibiotic use or hearing or visual loss from brain tumor removal) or hospitalization. The health care environment is a place of unfamiliar sights, sounds, and smells, as well as minimal contact with family and friends. If clients feel depersonalized and are unable to receive meaningful stimuli, serious sensory alterations develop.

As a nurse, you need to meet the needs of clients with existing sensory alterations and recognize clients most at risk for developing sensory problems. You will help clients who have partial or complete loss of a major sense to find alternative ways to function safely within their environment.

Scientific Knowledge Base

Normal Sensation

Normally the nervous system continually receives thousands of bits of information from sensory nerve organs, relays the information through appropriate channels, and integrates the information into a meaningful response. Sensory stimuli reach the sensory organs to elicit an immediate reaction or present information to the brain to be stored for future use. The nervous system must be intact for sensory stimuli to reach appropriate brain centers and for the individual to perceive the sensation. After interpreting the significance of a sensation, the person is then able to react to the stimulus. Table 49-1 summarizes normal hearing and vision.

Reception, perception, and reaction are the three components of any sensory experience (see Chapter 43). Reception begins with stimulation of a nerve cell called a receptor, which is usually for only one type of stimulus, such as light, touch, or sound. In the case of special senses, the receptors are grouped close together or located in specialized organs, such as the taste buds of the tongue or the retina of the eye. When a nerve impulse is created, it travels along pathways to the spinal cord or directly to the brain. For example, sound waves stimulate hair cell receptors within the organ of Corti, which causes impulses to travel along the eighth cranial nerve to the acoustic area of the temporal lobe. Sensory nerve pathways usually cross over to send stimuli to opposite sides of the brain. The actual perception or awareness of unique sensations depends on the receiving region of the cerebral cortex, where specialized brain cells interpret the quality and nature of sensory stimuli. When the person becomes conscious of the stimuli and receives the information, perception takes place. Perception in-

---

✳ TABLE 49-1 Normal Hearing and Vision

FUNCTION	ANATOMY AND PHYSIOLOGY
The Ear	
Transmits to the brain an accurate pattern of all sounds received from the environment, the relative intensity of these sounds, and the direction from which they originate	Two ears provide stereophonic hearing to judge sound direction.
	The external ear canal shelters the eardrum and maintains relatively constant temperature and humidity to maintain elasticity.
	The middle ear is an air-containing space between the eardrum and oval window. It contains three small bones (ossicles).
	The eardrum and ossicles transfer sound to the fluid-filled inner ear.
	Movement of the stapes in the oval window creates vibrations in the fluid that bathes the membranous labyrinth, which contains the end organs of hearing and balance.
	The union of the vestibular (balance) and cochlear (hearing) portions of the labyrinth explains the combination of hearing and balance symptoms that occur with inner ear disorders.
	Vibration of the eardrum transmits through the bony ossicles. Vibrations at the oval window transmit in perilymph within the inner ear to stimulate hair cells that send impulses along the eighth cranial nerve to the brain.
The Eye	
Transmits to the brain an accurate pattern of light reflected from solid objects in the environment and transformed into color and hue	Light rays enter the convex cornea and begin to converge.
	Fine adjustment of light rays occurs as they pass through the pupil and through the lens.
	Change in the shape of the lens focuses light on the retina.
	The retina has a pigmented layer of cells to enhance visual acuity.
	The sensory retina contains the rods and cones—photoreceptor cells sensitive to stimulation from light.
	Photoreceptor cells send electrical potentials by way of the optic nerve to the brain.

✳ BOX 49-1 Common Sensory Deficits

Visual Deficits

Presbyopia: A gradual decline in the ability of the lens to accommodate or to focus on close objects. Individual is unable to see near objects clearly.

Cataract: Cloudy or opaque areas in part of the lens or the entire lens that interfere with passage of light through the lens, causing problems with glare and blurred vision. Cataracts usually develop gradually, without pain, redness, or tearing in the eye.

Dry eyes: Result when tear glands produce too few tears resulting in itching, burning, or even reduced vision.

Glaucoma: A slowly progressive increase in intraocular pressure that causes progressive pressure against the optic nerve, resulting in peripheral visual loss, decreased visual acuity with difficulty adapting to darkness, and a halo effect around lights, if left untreated.

Diabetic retinopathy: Pathological changes occur in the blood vessels of the retina, resulting in decreased vision or vision loss due to hemorrhage and macular edema.

Macular degeneration: Condition in which the macula (specialized portion of the retina responsible for central vision) loses its ability to function efficiently. First signs include blurring of reading matter, distortion or loss of central vision, and distortion of vertical lines.

Hearing Deficits

Presbycusis: A common progressive hearing disorder in older adults.

Cerumen accumulation: Buildup of earwax in the external auditory canal. Cerumen becomes hard and collects in the canal and causes a conduction deafness.

Balance Deficit

Dizziness and disequilibrium: Common condition in older adulthood, usually resulting from vestibular dysfunction. Frequently a change in position of the head precipitates an episode of vertigo or disequilibrium.

Taste Deficit

Xerostomia: Decrease in salivary production that leads to thicker mucus and a dry mouth. Often interferes with the ability to eat and leads to appetite and nutritional problems.

Neurological Deficits

Peripheral neuropathy: Disorder of the peripheral nervous system, characterized by symptoms that include numbness and tingling of the affected area and stumbling gait.

Stroke: Cerebrovascular accident caused by clot, hemorrhage, or emboli disrupting blood flow to the brain. Creates altered proprioception with marked incoordination and imbalance. Loss of sensation and motor function in extremities controlled by the affected area of the brain also occurs. A stroke affecting the left hemisphere of the brain results in symptoms on the right side such as difficulty with speech. A stroke on the right hemisphere will have symptoms on the left side, which includes visual spatial alterations such as loss of half of a visual field or inattention and neglect, especially to the left side.

cludes integration and interpretation of the stimuli based on the person's experiences. A person's level of consciousness influences perception and interpretation of stimuli. Any factors lowering consciousness impair sensory perception. If sensation is incomplete, such as blurred vision, or if past experience is inadequate for understanding stimuli such as pain, the person will possibly react inappropriately to the sensory stimulus.

It is impossible to react to all stimuli entering the nervous system. The brain prevents sensory bombardment by discarding or storing sensory information. A person will usually react to stimuli that are most meaningful or significant at the time. After continued reception of the same stimulus, however, a person stops responding and the sensory experience goes unnoticed. For example, a person concentrating on reading a good book is not aware of background music. This adaptability phenomenon occurs with most sensory stimuli except for those of pain.

The balance between sensory stimuli entering the brain and those actually reaching a person's conscious awareness maintains a person's well-being. If an individual attempts to react to every stimulus within the environment or if there is insufficient variety and quality of stimuli, sensory alterations will occur.

Sensory Alterations

The most common types of sensory alterations are sensory deficits, sensory deprivation, and sensory overload. When a client suffers from more than one sensory alteration, the ability to function and relate effectively within the environment is seriously impaired.

Sensory Deficits. A deficit in the normal function of sensory reception and perception is a **sensory deficit.** A person loses a sense of self with impaired senses. Initially a person withdraws by avoiding communication or socialization with others in an attempt to cope with the sensory loss. It becomes difficult for the person to interact safely with the environment until he or she learns new skills. When a deficit develops gradually or when considerable time has passed since the onset of an acute sensory loss, the person learns to rely on unaffected senses. Some senses may even become more acute to compensate for an alteration. For example, a blind client often develops an acute sense of hearing.

Clients with sensory deficits often change behavior in adaptive or maladaptive ways. For example, one client with a hearing impairment turns the unaffected ear toward the speaker to hear better, whereas another client avoids other people because he or she is embarrassed about not being able to understand their speech. Box 49-1 summarizes common sensory deficits and their influence on those affected.

Sensory Deprivation. The reticular activating system in the brain stem mediates all sensory stimuli to the cerebral cortex, so even in deep sleep, clients are able to receive stimuli. Sensory stimulation must be of sufficient quality and quantity to maintain a person's awareness. In health care settings, meaningful touch is limited, environments lack sensory stimulatory properties, meals are dull and bland, and bath times are unpleasant and distressing experiences (MacDonald, 2002). When a person experiences an

✳ BOX 49-2 Effects of Sensory Deprivation

Cognitive
Reduced capacity to learn
Inability to think or problem solve
Poor task performance
Disorientation
Bizarre thinking
Increased need for socialization, altered mechanisms of attention

Affective
Boredom
Restlessness
Increased anxiety
Emotional lability
Panic
Increased need for physical stimulation

Perceptual
Changes in visual/motor coordination
Reduced color perception
Less tactile accuracy
Changes in ability to perceive size and shape
Changes in spatial and time judgment

Modified from Ebersole P and others: *Toward healthy aging: human needs and nursing response*, ed 6, St. Louis, 2004, Mosby.

inadequate quality or quantity of stimulation, such as monotonous or meaningless stimuli, **sensory deprivation** occurs. Three types of sensory deprivation are reduced sensory input (sensory deficit from visual or hearing loss), elimination of patterns or meaning from input (e.g., exposure to strange environments), and restrictive environments (e.g., bed rest) that produce monotony and boredom (Ebersole and others, 2005).

There are many effects of sensory deprivation (Box 49-2). In adults the symptoms of sensory deprivation are similar to psychological illness, confusion, symptoms of severe electrolyte imbalance, or the influence of psychotropic drugs. Therefore always be aware of the client's existing sensory function and the quality of stimuli within the environment.

Sensory Overload. When a person receives multiple sensory stimuli and cannot perceptually disregard or selectively ignore some stimuli, **sensory overload** occurs. Excessive sensory stimulation prevents the brain from appropriately responding to or ignoring certain stimuli. Because of the multitude of stimuli leading to overload, the person no longer perceives the environment in a way that makes sense. Overload prevents meaningful response by the brain; the client's thoughts race, attention scatters in many directions, and anxiety and restlessness occur. As a result, overload causes a state similar to that produced by sensory deprivation. However, in contrast to deprivation, overload is individualized. The amount of stimuli necessary for healthy function varies with each individual. Persons are often subject to environmental overload more at one time than at another. A person's tolerance to sensory overload varies by level of fatigue, attitude, and emotional and physical well-being.

The acutely ill client easily falls victim to sensory overload. The client in constant pain or who undergoes frequent monitoring of

vital signs or who has irritation from drainage tubes is at risk. Multiple stimuli combine to cause overload even if the nurse offers a comforting word or provides a gentle back rub. Some clients do not benefit from nursing intervention because their attention and energy are focused on more stressful stimuli. Another example is the client who is hospitalized in an intensive care unit (ICU), where the activity is constant. Lights are always on. Clients can hear sounds from monitoring equipment, staff conversations, equipment alarms, and the activities of people entering the unit. Even at night, an ICU is very noisy.

It is easy to confuse the behavioral changes associated with sensory overload with mood swings or simple disorientation. Look for symptoms such as racing thoughts, scattered attention, restlessness, and anxiety. Clients in ICUs sometimes resort to constantly fingering tubes and dressings. Constant reorientation and control of excessive stimuli become an important part of the client's care.

Nursing Knowledge Base

Factors Affecting Sensory Function

Many factors influence the capacity to receive or perceive stimuli. All are conditions or situations that you as the nurse will try to manage when delivering care.

Age. Infants and children are at risk for visual and hearing impairment because of a number of genetic, prenatal, and postnatal conditions. A concern with high-risk neonates is that early, intense visual and auditory stimulation could adversely affect visual and auditory pathways and alter the developmental course of other sensory organs (Hockenberry and Wilson 2007). Visual changes during adulthood include presbyopia and the need for glasses for reading. These changes usually occur from ages 40 to 50. Also, the cornea, which assists with light refraction to the retina, becomes flatter and thicker. These aging changes lead to astigmatism. Pigment is lost from the iris, and collagen fibers build up in the anterior chamber, which increases the risk of glaucoma by decreasing the reabsorption of intraocular fluid. Other normal visual changes associated with aging include reduced visual fields, increased glare sensitivity, impaired night vision, reduced depth perception, and reduced color discrimination.

Hearing changes begin at the age of 30. Changes associated with aging include decreased hearing acuity, speech intelligibility, and pitch discrimination. Low-pitched sounds are easiest to hear, but it is difficult to hear conversation over background noise. It is also difficult to discriminate the consonants (z, t, f, g) and high-frequency sounds (s, sh, ph, k). Vowels that have a low pitch are easiest to hear. Speech sounds are distorted, and there is a delayed reception and reaction to speech. A concern with normal age-related sensory changes is that older adults with a deficit are sometimes inappropriately diagnosed with dementia (Ebersole and others, 2005). It is common to confuse abnormal changes due to eye and ear pathological conditions with normal age-related sensory changes (Crews and Campbell, 2004).

Gustatory and olfactory changes begin around age 50 and include a decrease in the number of taste buds and a decrease in the number of sensory cells in the nasal lining. Reduced taste discrimination and reduced sensitivity to odors are common.

Proprioceptive changes common after age 60 include increased difficulty with balance, spatial orientation, and coordination. Older adults cannot avoid obstacles as quickly, and the automatic response to protect and brace oneself when falling is slower. Older adults experience tactile changes, including declining sensitivity to pain, pressure, and temperature secondary to peripheral vascular disease and neuropathies.

Meaningful Stimuli. Meaningful stimuli reduce the incidence of sensory deprivation. In the home, meaningful stimuli include pets, music, television, pictures of family members, and a calendar and clock. The same stimuli need to be present in a nursing center. In a health care setting the nurse notes whether clients have roommates or visitors. The presence of others offers positive stimulation. However, a roommate who constantly watches television, persistently tries to talk, or continuously keeps lights on will contribute to sensory overload. The presence or absence of meaningful stimuli influences alertness and the ability to participate in care.

Amount of Stimuli. Excessive stimuli in an environment causes sensory overload. The frequency of observations and procedures performed in an acute health care setting are often stressful. If the client is in pain, has many tubes and dressings, or is restricted by cast or traction, overstimulation can be a problem. A room that is near repetitive or loud noises (e.g., an elevator, stairwell, or nurses' station) will also contribute to sensory overload.

Social Interaction. The amount and quality of social contact with supportive family members and significant others influence sensory function. The absence of visitors during hospitalization or residency in an extended care facility influences the degree of isolation a client feels. This is a common problem in hospital intensive care settings, where visitation is often restricted. The ability to discuss concerns with loved ones is an important coping mechanism for most people. Therefore the absence of meaningful conversation will result in feelings of isolation, loneliness, anxiety, and depression for the client. Often, this is not apparent until behavioral changes occur.

Environmental Factors. A person's occupation places him or her at risk for hearing, visual, and peripheral nerve alterations. Individuals who have occupations involving exposure to high noise levels (e.g., factory or airport workers) are at risk for noise-induced hearing loss and need to be screened for hearing impairments. Hazardous noise is common in work settings as well as recreational activities. Noisy recreational activities that weaken hearing ability include target shooting and hunting, woodworking, and listening to loud music. Individuals who have occupations involving risk of exposure to chemicals or flying objects (e.g., welders) are at risk for eye injuries and need to be screened for visual impairments. Sports activities and consumer fireworks also place individuals at risk for visual alterations. Occupations that involve repetitive wrist or finger movements (e.g., heavy assembly line work) cause pressure on the median nerve, resulting in carpal tunnel syndrome. Carpal tun-

---

✴ BOX 49-3   CULTURAL ASPECTS OF CARE

Disparities in Sensory Alteration

- Whites have a higher incidence of hearing impairment than African Americans or Asian Americans (Smith and Wilbur, 2004).
- Native American children suffer from otitis media at a disproportionately higher rate than other ethnic groups (National Institute on Deafness and Other Communication Disorders, 2005).
- Glaucoma is almost 3 times as common in African Americans as in white Americans (National Eye Institute, 2004).
- Hispanic Americans have an increased incidence of diabetic retinopathy (Smith and Wilbur, 2004).
- Whites have a higher incidence of macular degeneration than Hispanic Americans, African Americans, and Asian Americans (Smith and Wilbur, 2004).

---

nel syndrome alters tactile sensation and is one of the most common industrial or work-related injuries. Clients at risk for carpal tunnel need to be carefully assessed for numbness, tingling, weakness, and pain.

A hospitalized client is sometimes at risk for sensory alterations due to exposure to environmental stimuli or a change in sensory input. Clients who are immobilized by bed rest or physical impediments (e.g., casts or traction) or who have chronic disability are unable to experience all of the normal sensations of free movement. Another group at risk includes clients isolated in a health care setting or at home due to conditions such as active tuberculosis (see Chapter 34). These clients often stay in private rooms and are unable to enjoy normal interactions with visitors.

Cultural Factors. Certain sensory alterations occur more commonly in select ethnic groups. Analysis of data from a recent study showed that Aleuts, Eskimos, and Native Americans have more than 3 times the rate of simultaneous hearing impairment and visual impairment relative to Asian/Pacific Islander Americans. Researchers do not know why these groups have significantly higher rates of hearing impairment and visual impairment, but it is possibly because of limited health care access or in combination with increased risks of auditory disorders and angle-closure glaucoma (Caban and others, 2005). Box 49-3 summarizes additional sensory alterations that are associated with a client's cultural heritage.

Critical Thinking

Successful critical thinking requires a synthesis of knowledge and information gathered from clients, experience, critical thinking attitudes, and intellectual and professional standards. Clinical judgments require you to anticipate the information necessary, analyze the data, and make decisions regarding client care. Clients' conditions are always changing. During assessment (Figure 49-1) you must consider all critical thinking elements that build toward making appropriate nursing diagnoses. In the case of sensory alterations you need to integrate knowledge of the pathophysiology of sensory deficits, factors that affect sensory function,

Knowledge
- Pathophysiology of specific sensory deficit
- Factors that potentially may alter sensory function
- Effects of sensory deprivation/overload
- Communication principles used to interact with clients having sensory deficits

Experience
- Caring for clients with sudden and long-term sensory alterations
- Personal experience with temporary or permanent sensory deficit

ASSESSMENT
- Client's health promotion practices
- Nursing history regarding extent of risks for and existing sensory deficits
- Review of potential factors that may affect the client's sensory function
- Extent of lifestyle and self-care alterations
- Determine the client's expectations regarding sensory alterations

Standards
- Apply intellectual standards of clarity, precision, accuracy, and depth when assessing the client's sensory function
- Standards of care from American Academy of Ophthalmology and American Speech-Language-Hearing Association

Attitudes
- Show confidence in your ability to provide a safe level of care
- Use curiosity to clarify and explore the nature of signs and symptoms to rule out causes other than sensory change

Figure 49-1 Critical thinking model for sensory alterations assessment.

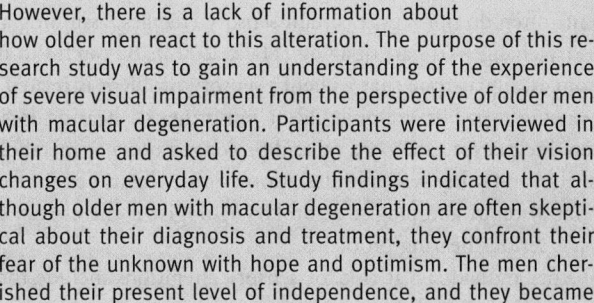

★ BOX 49-4 **EVIDENCE-BASED PRACTICE**

Promoting Quality Care in Older Men With Severe Visual Impairment

Evidence Summary

Severe visual impairment caused by macular degeneration is common in many older adults. However, there is a lack of information about how older men react to this alteration. The purpose of this research study was to gain an understanding of the experience of severe visual impairment from the perspective of older men with macular degeneration. Participants were interviewed in their home and asked to describe the effect of their vision changes on everyday life. Study findings indicated that although older men with macular degeneration are often skeptical about their diagnosis and treatment, they confront their fear of the unknown with hope and optimism. The men cherished their present level of independence, and they became creative in developing strategies to overcome their problems.

Application to Nursing Practice
- Assess for the presence of social networks and supportive relationships.
- Complete a thorough health history and physical assessment to identify health problems that complicate life with visual impairment.
- Encourage clients to discuss what goals are important to them.
- Provide factual information about the disease, and answer questions truthfully.
- Assist with identification of creative strategies to promote self-care.
- Explore the client's ability to cope with the loss of vision and encourage expression of feelings (e.g., denial, anger, hopelessness).

Reference
Moore LW, Miller M: Older men's experiences of living with severe visual impairment, *J Adv Nurs* 43(1):10, 2003.

and therapeutic communication principles. This knowledge positions you to conduct appropriate assessments, anticipate what to recognize when a client describes a sensory problem and to make judgments of any abnormalities. For example, knowing the typical symptoms of a cataract helps you to recognize the pattern of visual changes a client with a cataract will report.

Previous experiences in caring for clients with sensory deficits enable nurses to recognize limitations in function in each new client and how limitations will affect the client's ability to carry out daily activities. For example, after caring for a client with a hearing impairment, you will be able to conduct a more effective assessment of the next client by using approaches that promote the client's ability to hear your questions.

Critical thinking attitudes and standards, when applied during assessment, ensure a thorough and accurate database from which to make decisions. For example, perseverance is necessary to learn details about how visual changes influence a client's ability to socialize. Standards of care and practice, such as those from the American Academy of Ophthalmology and the American Speech-Language-Hearing Association, provide criteria for screening

sensory problems and for establishing standards for competent, safe, effective care and practice. Using critical thinking, you can conduct a thorough assessment and then plan, implement, and evaluate care that will enable the client to function safely and effectively (Box 49-4).

Nursing Process

 Assessment

When assessing clients with or at risk for sensory alterations, it is important for you to first consider any pathophysiology of existing deficits, as well as all of the factors influencing sensory function, to anticipate how to approach a given client's assessment. For example, if the client has a hearing disorder, adjust your communication style and then focus the assessment on relevant criteria related to hearing deficits. Collect a history that also assesses the client's current sensory status and the degree to which a sensory deficit affects the client's lifestyle, psychosocial adjustment, developmental status, self-care ability, health promotion habits, and safety. Also focus the assessment on the quality and quantity of stimuli within the client's environment.

Persons at Risk. Older adults are a high-risk group because of normal physiological changes involving sensory organs. Older clients often do not report certain sensory changes, assuming any sensory change is a part of aging (Halle, 2002). Be careful to not automatically assume that a client's sensory problem is related to advancing age. For example, adult sensorineural hearing loss is often due to exposure to excess and prolonged noise or metabolic, vascular, and other systemic alterations. Some clients benefit from a referral to an audiologist or **otolaryngologist** if the assessment reveals serious hearing problems.

Other individuals at risk for sensory alterations include those living in a confined environment such as a nursing home. Although most quality nursing homes or centers offer meaningful stimulation through group activities, environmental design, and mealtime gatherings, there are exceptions. The individual who is confined to a wheelchair, suffers from poor hearing and/or vision, has decreased energy, and avoids contact with others is at significant risk for sensory deprivation. If the environment creates monotony, the individual is less able to learn and to think. Acutely ill clients are also at risk because of an unfamiliar and unresponsive environment. This does not mean that all hospitalized clients have sensory alterations. However, you will need to carefully assess those clients subjected to continued sensory stimulation (e.g., ICU settings, long-term hospitalization, or multiple therapies). Assess the client's environment, within both the health care setting and the home, looking for factors that pose risks or that need adjustment to provide safety and more stimulation.

Sensory Alterations History. The nursing history includes assessment of the nature and characteristics of sensory alterations or any problem related to an alteration (Box 49-5). When taking the sensory alterations history, you need to consider the ethnic or cultural background of the client because certain alterations are higher in some cultural groups.

During the history it is useful to assess the client's self-rating for a sensory deficit. You can simply say, "Rate your hearing as excellent, good, fair, poor, or bad." Then, based on the client's self-rating, explore the client's perception of a sensory loss more fully. This provides an in-depth look at how the sensory loss influences the client's quality of life. In the case of hearing problems, a screening tool developed by Ventry and Weinstein effectively identifies clients needing audiological intervention. The screening version of the Hearing Handicap Inventory for the Elderly (HHIE-S) is a 5-minute, 10-item questionnaire developed to assess how the individual perceives the social and emotional effects of hearing loss. Persons who perceive their hearing loss to be a problem are more likely to have further testing and accept the need for a hearing aid. The higher the HHIE-S score, the greater the handicapping effect of a hearing impairment (Demers, 2004).

A nursing history also reveals any recent changes in a client's behavior. Frequently friends or family are the best resources for this information because the client is often unaware of any change. It

---

⚹ BOX 49-5   NURSING ASSESSMENT QUESTIONS

Nature of the Problem
- What type of problem are you having with your vision/hearing?
- What have you tried to correct the vision/hearing difficulty?
- Do you use any devices to improve your vision/hearing?

Signs and Symptoms
- Ask a client with visual alterations: Do you require books with large print, or those on audiotape? Are you able to prepare a meal or write a check?
- Ask a client with hearing alterations: What types of sounds or tones do you have difficulty hearing? Do people tell you that they have to "shout" for you to hear them? Do you have a ringing, crackling, or buzzing in you ears?
- Is there pain: sharp, dull, burning, itching?
- Have you noticed any redness, swelling, or drainage? Any signs of infection?

Onset and Duration
- When did you notice the problem? How long has this problem lasted?
- Does it come and go, or is it constant?

Predisposing Factors
- How do you practice eye/ear hygiene?
- Do you work or participate in any activities that have the potential for vision/hearing injury? If so, how do you protect your hearing and vision?
- Do you have a family history of cataracts, glaucoma, macular degeneration, or hearing loss?
- When was your last vision/hearing examination?

Effect on Client
- What effect has your vision/hearing problem had on your work, family, or social life?
- Have changes in your vision/hearing affected your feelings of independence?
- How does your vision/hearing problem make you feel about yourself?
- Do you have problems with routine care of glasses, contact lenses, or hearing aids?

---

is also important to remember that many adults are sensitive about admitting losses and hesitate to share information. Ask the family the following questions:

- Has your family member shown any recent mood swings (e.g., outbursts of anger, nervousness, fear, or irritability)?
- Have you noticed the family member avoiding social activities?

Mental Status. Mental status assessment is an important part of any evaluation of sensory function (Box 49-6). Observation of the client during history taking, during the physical examination, and during nursing care provides valuable data for evaluation of a client's mental status. Assessment of mental status is valuable when you suspect sensory deprivation or overload. Observation of the client provides data that reveal key client behaviors. Observe the client's physical appearance and behavior, measure cognitive ability, and assess the client's emotional status. The Mini-Mental State Examination (MMSE) is an example of a tool that you can *formally* use to measure disorientation, altered conceptualization

✳ **BOX 49-6 Assessment of Mental Status**

Physical Appearance and Behavior
Motor activity, posture, facial expression, hygiene

Cognitive Ability
Level of consciousness, abstract reasoning, calculation, attention, judgment
Ability to carry on conversation, ability to read, write, and copy figure
Recent and remote memory

Emotional Stability
Agitation, euphoria, irritability, hopelessness, or wide mood swings
Auditory, visual, or tactile hallucinations, **illusions, delusions**

and abstract thinking, and change in problem-solving abilities (see Chapter 33). For example, a client with severe sensory deprivation is not always able to carry on a conversation, remain attentive, or display recent or past memory. A recent study using the MMSE found that near-vision impairment was associated with cognitive decline in older Mexican-Americans (Reyes-Ortiz and others, 2005). An important step toward preventing cognition-related disability is education by nurses about disease process, available services, and assistive devices.

Physical Assessment. To identify sensory deficits and their severity, assess vision, hearing, olfaction, taste, and the ability to discriminate light touch, temperature, pain, and position. Chapter 33 describes assessment techniques in detail. Table 49-2 summarizes additional assessment techniques for identifying sensory deficits. In all examples you will gather more accurate data if the examination room is private, quiet, and comfortable for the client. In addition, rely on personal observation of the client to detect sensory alterations. Ebersole and Hess (2004) identified useful initial screening observations, which include does the client seem inattentive to others, respond with inappropriate anger when spoken to, believe people are talking about him or her, answer questions inappropriately, have trouble following clear directions, and have monotonous voice quality and speak unusually loud or soft.

The typical physical tests used to screen for hearing impairment rely on an examiner's whispered voice or a tuning fork. The Welch-Allyn audioscope is very effective for measuring hearing acuity. The handheld instrument includes an ear speculum that you place within the external ear canal. The examiner views the tympanic membrane to ensure that cerumen is not blocking the canal. You initiate a series of varying tones at random intervals by pressing a button the audioscope. The instrument is highly sensitive to detecting hearing loss.

Ability to Perform Self-Care. Assess clients' functional abilities in their home environment or health care setting, including feeding, dressing, grooming, and toileting activities. For example, assess whether a client with altered vision is able to find items on a meal tray and is able to read directions on a prescription. Also determine a visually impaired client's ability to perform daily routines such as reading bills and writing checks, differentiating

money denominations, and driving a vehicle at night. If a client seems sensorially deprived, does he or she show concern for grooming? Does a client's loss of balance prevent rising from a toilet seat safely? Can the client recovering from a stroke manipulate buttons or zippers for dressing? If a sensory alteration impairs a client's functional ability, providing resources within the home is a necessary part of discharge planning.

Health Promotion Habits. It is important to assess the daily routines clients follow to maintain sensory function. What type of eye and ear care is a part of the client's daily hygiene? For those individuals who participate in sports (e.g., racquetball) or recreational activities (e.g., motorcycle riding) or who work in a setting where ear or eye injury is a possibility (e.g., chemical exposure, welding, glass or stone polishing, or constant exposure to loud noise), determine if clients wear safety glasses or hearing protective devices (HPDs). Do clients who use assistive devices such as eyeglasses, contact lenses, or hearing aids know how to provide daily care (see Chapter 39)? Do clients use the devices, and are they in proper working order?

It is also important to assess the client's compliance with routine health screening. When was the last time the client had an eye examination or hearing evaluation? For adults, routine screening of visual and hearing function is imperative to detect problems early. This is especially true in the case of glaucoma, which if undetected will lead to permanent visual loss. Recommended screening guidelines usually occur on the basis of age. When a client begins to show a hearing deficit, incorporate routine screening in regular examinations.

Environmental Hazards. Clients with sensory alterations are at risk for injury if their living environments are unsafe. For example, a client with reduced vision cannot see potential hazards clearly. A client with proprioceptive problems often loses balance easily. The condition of the home, the rooms, and the front and back entrances are problematic to the client with sensory alterations. Assess the clients' home for common hazards, including the following:

- Uneven, cracked walkways leading to front/back door
- Doormats with slippery backing
- Extension and phone cords in the main route of walking traffic
- Loose area rugs and runners placed over carpeting
- Bathrooms without shower or tub grab bars
- Water faucets unmarked to designate hot and cold
- Bathroom floor with slippery surface
- Absence of smoke detectors in rooms
- Unlit stairways, lack of handrails
- Cluttered floors, furniture, including footstools
- Kitchen equipment (e.g., ranges, irons, toasters) with hard-to-read settings

In the hospital environment, caregivers often forget to rearrange furniture and equipment to keep paths from the bed and chair to the bathroom and entrance clear. Walking into a client's room and looking for safety hazards is a useful exercise:

- Is the call light within easy, safe reach?
- Are intravenous (IV) poles on wheels and easy to move?

✳ **TABLE 49-2 Assessment of Sensory Function**

ASSESSMENT ACTIVITIES	BEHAVIOR INDICATING DEFICIT (CHILDREN)	BEHAVIOR INDICATING DEFICIT (ADULTS)
Vision Ask client to read newspaper, magazine, or lettering on menu. Ask client to identify colors on color chart or crayons. Observe clients performing ADLs.	Self-stimulation, including eye rubbing, body rocking, sniffing or smelling, arm twirling; hitching (using legs to propel while in sitting position) instead of crawling	Poor coordination, squinting, under-reaching or overreaching for objects, persistent repositioning of objects, impaired night vision, accidental falls
Hearing Assess client's hearing acuity (see Chapter 33) and history of tinnitus. Observe client conversing with others. Inspect ear canal for hardened cerumen. Observe client behaviors in a group.	Frightened when unfamiliar people approach, no reflex or purposeful response to sounds, failure to be awakened by loud noise, slow or absent development of speech, greater response to movement than to sound, avoidance of social interaction with other children	Blank looks, decreased attention span, lack of reaction to loud noises, increased volume of speech, positioning of head toward sound, smiling and nodding of head in approval when someone speaks, use of other means of communication such as lipreading or writing, complaints of ringing in ears
Touch Check client's ability to discriminate between sharp and dull stimuli. Assess whether client is able to distinguish objects (coin or safety pin) in the hand with eyes closed. Ask whether client feels unusual sensations.	Inability to perform developmental tasks related to grasping objects or drawing, repeated injury from handling of harmful objects (e.g., hot stove, sharp knife)	Clumsiness, overreaction or underreaction to painful stimulus, failure to respond when touched, avoidance of touch, sensation of pins and needles, numbness. Unable to identify object placed in hand
Smell Have client close eyes and identify several nonirritating odors (e.g., coffee, vanilla).	Difficult to assess until child is 6 or 7 years old, difficulty discriminating noxious odors	Failure to react to noxious or strong odor, increased body odor, decreased sensitivity to odors
Taste Ask client to sample and distinguish different tastes (e.g., lemon, sugar, salt). (Have client drink or sip water and wait 1 minute between each taste.)	Inability to tell whether food is salty or sweet, possible ingestion of strange-tasting things	Change in appetite, excessive use of seasoning and sugar, complaints about taste of food, weight change

ADLs, Activities of daily living.

- Are footstools in the middle of the room?
- Are suction machines, IV pumps, or drainage bags positioned so that a client can rise from a bed or chair easily?

An additional problem faced by the visually impaired is the inability to read medication labels and syringe gauges. Ask the client to read a label to determine if the client is able to read the dosage and frequency. If a client has a hearing impairment, check to see whether the sounds of a doorbell, telephone, smoke alarm, and alarm clock are easy to discriminate.

Communication Methods. To understand the nature of a communication problem, you need to know whether a client has trouble speaking, understanding, naming, reading, or writing. Clients with existing sensory deficits often develop alternative ways of communicating. To interact with the client and to promote interaction with others (Figure 49-2), understand the client's method of communication. Vision becomes almost a primary sense for the hearing impaired.

Visually impaired clients are unable to observe facial expressions and other nonverbal behaviors that clarify the content of spoken communication. Instead, they rely on voice tones and inflections to detect the emotional tone of communication. Clients with visual deficits often learn to read Braille. Clients with **aphasia** are often unable to produce or understand language. **Expressive aphasia**, a motor type of aphasia, is the inability to name common objects or to express simple ideas in words or writing. For example, a client understands a question but is unable to express an answer. Sensory or **receptive aphasia** is the inability to understand written or spoken language. The client may be able to express words but is unable to understand questions or comments of others. Global aphasia is the inability to understand language or communicate orally.

The temporary or permanent loss of the ability to speak is extremely traumatic to an individual. Assess a client's alternative communication method and whether it causes anxiety in the client. Clients who have undergone laryngectomies often write notes, use communication boards or laptop computers, speak

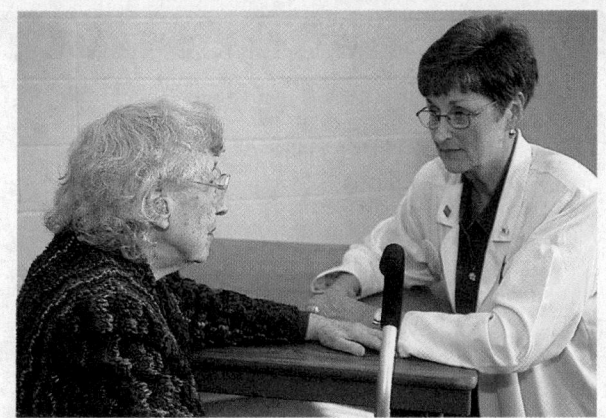

Figure 49-2 Nurse sits at eye level so that client with hearing impairment can communicate.

✳ BOX 49-7 NURSING DIAGNOSTIC PROCESS ◆

Risk for Injury Related to Visual Impairment From Cataract Formation

Assessment Activities	Defining Characteristics
Assess client's visual acuity.	Has reduced ability to see objects clearly. Needs brighter light to read. Has trouble distinguishing edges of stairs.
Visit home setting, and inspect for any hazards that will pose risks to client.	Lighting in rooms, hallways, and stairwells is very dim. Carpet in living room is old, and edges are curled up. Steps lead up to front entrance of home.
Review medical record from clinic visit.	Client has been diagnosed as having senile cataracts in both eyes.

---

with mechanical vibrators, or use esophageal speech. Clients with endotracheal or tracheostomy tubes have a temporary loss of speech. Most use a notepad to write their questions and requests. However, some clients become incapacitated and unable to write messages. Determine whether the client has developed a sign language system or symbols to communicate needs.

Social Support. Assess if a client lives alone and whether family or friends frequently visit. It is important to assess the client's social skills and level of satisfaction with the support given by family and friends. Is the client satisfied with the support available? Is the client able to solve problems with family members? Does the family offer the support needed when the client requires assistance as a result of a sensory loss? The long-term effects of sensory alterations influence family dynamics and a client's willingness to remain active in society.

Use of Assistive Devices. Assess the use of assistive devices (e.g., use of a hearing aid or glasses) and the sensory effects for the client. This includes learning how often the client uses the devices daily, the client's or family caregiver's method for cleaning, and the client's knowledge of what to do when a problem develops. When you identify that the client has an assistive device, it is important to remember that just because the individual has the assistive device, it does not mean that it works or that the client uses it or benefits from it (McConnell, 2002).

Other Factors Affecting Perception. Always remember that factors other than sensory deprivation or overload cause impaired perception (e.g., medications or pain). Be sure to assess the client's medication history, which includes prescribed and over-the-counter medications and herbal products. Also gather information regarding the frequency, dose, method of administration, and last time these medications were taken. Some antibiotics (e.g., streptomycin, gentamicin, and tobramycin) are **ototoxic** and permanently damage the auditory nerve; chloramphenicol sometimes irritates the optic nerve. Opioid analgesics, sedatives, and antidepressant medications often alter the perception of stimuli. Conduct a thorough pain assessment (see Chapter 43)

when you suspect pain is causing perceptual problems. Also assess the use of caffeine and other remedies.

Client Expectations. When conducting an assessment, review the client's expectations. Many clients have a definite plan as to how they want their care delivered. Some clients expect caregivers to recognize and appropriately manage and adjust their environment to meet their sensory needs. This includes assisting the individual client in learning and adapting to a changed lifestyle based on the specific sensory impairment. Determine from clients exactly what they expect to achieve and what interventions have been helpful in the past in the management of any limitation. Always remember that clients with sensory alterations have strengthened their other senses and expect caregivers to anticipate their needs (e.g., for safety and security).

◆ Nursing Diagnosis

After assessment, review all available data and look critically for patterns and trends suggestive of a health problem relating to sensory alterations (Box 49-7). For example, a client's advanced age, apathy, inattentiveness during conversations, and self-rating of hearing as "poor" are all defining characteristics for the nursing diagnosis of *disturbed sensory perception: auditory.* Validate findings to ensure accuracy of the diagnosis. For example, the diagnosis of *disturbed thought processes* could mistakenly be made if you do not confirm the client's hearing deficit and perception of poor hearing.

Determine the factor that likely causes the client's health problem. In the previous example impacted cerumen is the cause of the client's hearing alteration. The etiology or related factor of a nursing diagnosis is a condition that nursing interventions can affect. The etiology needs to be accurate; otherwise, nursing therapies will be ineffective. For a client with impacted cerumen, regular irrigations of the ear canal have the potential for improving auditory perception (Barnett, 2007). In contrast, if the client's auditory alteration is related to hearing loss from nerve deafness, then nursing interventions for alternative communication methods are necessary.

CONCEPT MAP

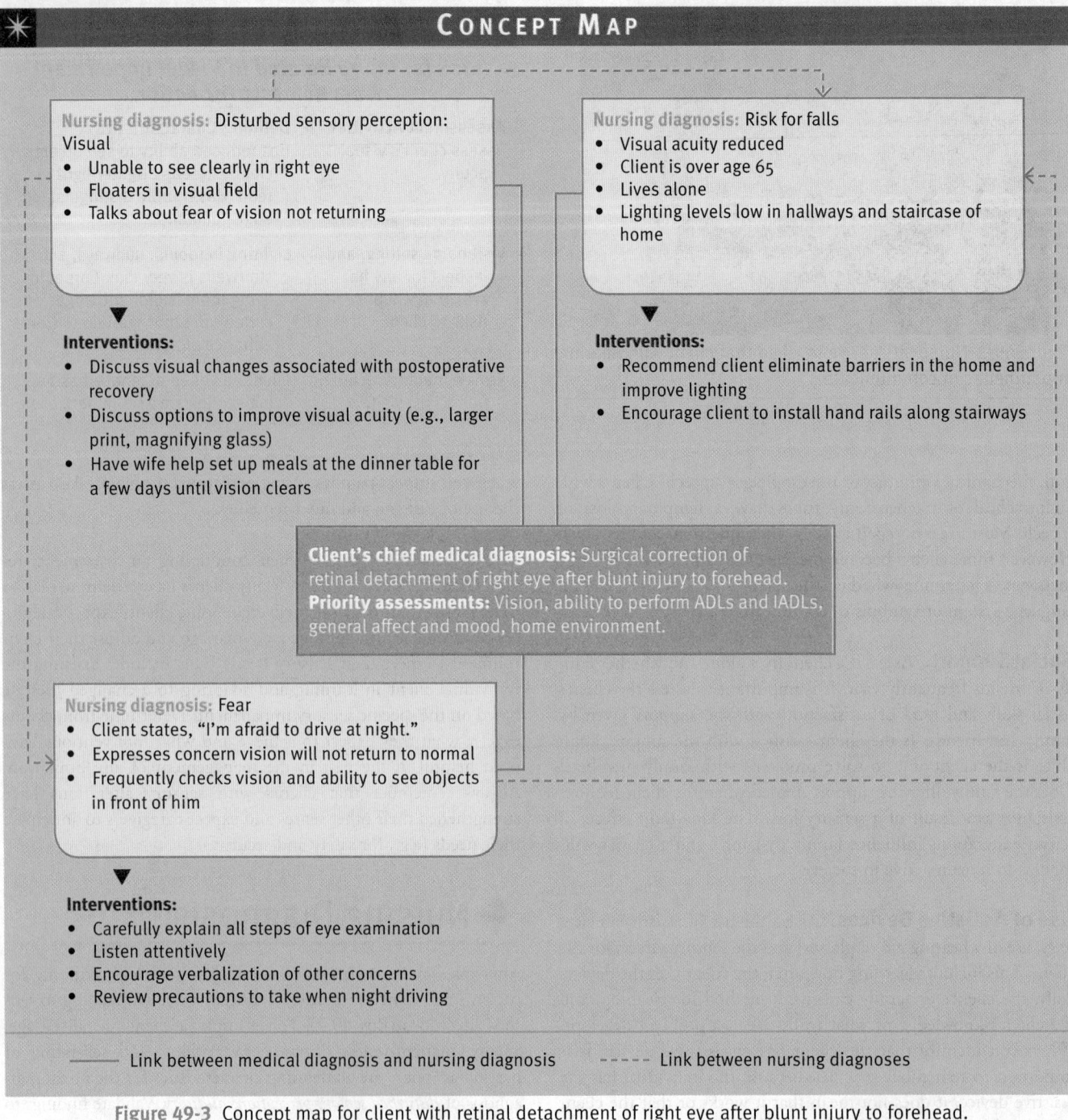

Nursing diagnosis: Disturbed sensory perception: Visual
- Unable to see clearly in right eye
- Floaters in visual field
- Talks about fear of vision not returning

Interventions:
- Discuss visual changes associated with postoperative recovery
- Discuss options to improve visual acuity (e.g., larger print, magnifying glass)
- Have wife help set up meals at the dinner table for a few days until vision clears

Nursing diagnosis: Risk for falls
- Visual acuity reduced
- Client is over age 65
- Lives alone
- Lighting levels low in hallways and staircase of home

Interventions:
- Recommend client eliminate barriers in the home and improve lighting
- Encourage client to install hand rails along stairways

Client's chief medical diagnosis: Surgical correction of retinal detachment of right eye after blunt injury to forehead.
Priority assessments: Vision, ability to perform ADLs and IADLs, general affect and mood, home environment.

Nursing diagnosis: Fear
- Client states, "I'm afraid to drive at night."
- Expresses concern vision will not return to normal
- Frequently checks vision and ability to see objects in front of him

Interventions:
- Carefully explain all steps of eye examination
- Listen attentively
- Encourage verbalization of other concerns
- Review precautions to take when night driving

——— Link between medical diagnosis and nursing diagnosis   - - - - - Link between nursing diagnoses

Figure 49-3 Concept map for client with retinal detachment of right eye after blunt injury to forehead.

Some clients also have health care problems for which sensory alteration is the etiology, such as with the diagnosis of *risk for injury.* Select nursing diagnoses by recognizing the way that sensory alterations affect a client's ability to function (e.g., self-care deficit). In addition, most clients present themselves to health care professionals with multiple diagnoses (Figure 49-3). In the example of the concept map, a client with retinal detachment has the nursing diagnosis of *disturbed sensory perception: visual,* as well as *fear* and *risk for falls.* The diagnosis of altered sensory perception is an etiology for both fear and risk for falls. Furthermore, fear occurs as a response to a perceived risk of falling. You need to recognize patterns of data that reveal health problems created by

the client's sensory alteration. Examples of nursing diagnoses that apply to clients with sensory alterations include the following:

- Risk-prone health behavior
- Impaired verbal communication
- Risk for injury
- Impaired physical mobility
- Self-care deficit: bathing/hygiene, dressing/grooming, toileting
- Situational low self-esteem
- Disturbed sensory perception
- Social isolation
- Disturbed thought processes

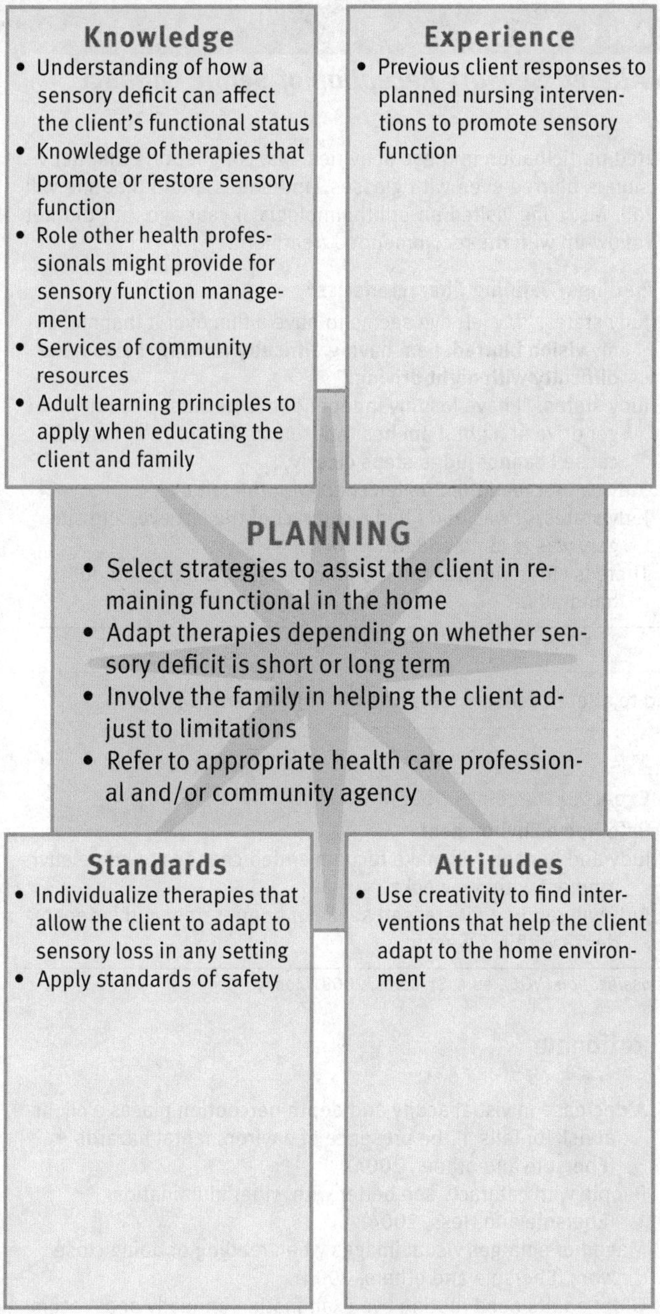

Knowledge	Experience
• Understanding of how a sensory deficit can affect the client's functional status • Knowledge of therapies that promote or restore sensory function • Role other health professionals might provide for sensory function management • Services of community resources • Adult learning principles to apply when educating the client and family	• Previous client responses to planned nursing interventions to promote sensory function

PLANNING

• Select strategies to assist the client in remaining functional in the home
• Adapt therapies depending on whether sensory deficit is short or long term
• Involve the family in helping the client adjust to limitations
• Refer to appropriate health care professional and/or community agency

Standards	Attitudes
• Individualize therapies that allow the client to adapt to sensory loss in any setting • Apply standards of safety	• Use creativity to find interventions that help the client adapt to the home environment

Figure 49-4 Critical thinking model for sensory alterations planning.

◆ Planning

During planning you again synthesize information from multiple resources (Figure 49-4). Reflect on knowledge gained from the assessment and knowledge of how sensory deficits affect normal functioning. In this way you will be able to recognize the extent of the client's deficit and know the type of interventions most likely to be helpful. Also consider the role that health professionals play in planning care and the available community resources that will be useful. Previous experience in caring for clients with sensory alterations will be invaluable. Caring for a client, for example, with a visual loss will assist you in knowing how to plan

nursing approaches that ensure the client's safety while maximizing the client's independence.

When applying critical thinking to planning care, professional standards are particularly useful. These standards, in the form of clinical pathways or evidence-based treatment protocols, for example, often recommend scientifically proven interventions for the client's condition. For example, clients who have visual deficits and are hospitalized are often placed on a fall prevention protocol that will incorporate research-based precautions to ensure client safety.

Goals and Outcomes. During planning, develop an individualized plan of care for each nursing diagnosis (see Care Plan). Partner with the client to develop a realistic plan that incorporates what you know about the client's sensory problems and the extent to which the client can maintain or improve sensory function. Goals and outcomes need to be realistic and measurable. A goal of care for a client with an actual or potential sensory alteration is "The client will achieve improvement in hearing acuity within 2 weeks." Associated outcomes for this goal will possibly include the following:

• The client will report using communication techniques for improved reception of messages within 2 weeks.
• The client will successfully demonstrate technique for cleansing hearing aid within 1 week.
• Client and family will be observed using proper communication skills to send and receive messages.
• Client will self-report improved hearing acuity.

Setting Priorities. You need to set priorities of care with regard to the type and extent of sensory alteration that affects a client. For example, a client who enters the emergency department after experiencing eye trauma, has priorities of reducing anxiety and preventing further injury to the eye. In contrast, a client who is being discharged from an outpatient surgery department following cataract removal has the priority of learning about any self-care restrictions. However, safety is always a top priority. The client also helps prioritize aspects of care. For example, a client wishes to learn ways to communicate more effectively or to participate in favorite hobbies given his or her limitation.

Some sensory alterations are short term (e.g., a client suffering sensory/perceptual alterations as a result of sensory overload in an ICU). Appropriate interventions are thus likely to be temporary (e.g., frequent reorientation or introduction of intimate and pleasant stimuli such as a back rub). Sensory alterations such as permanent visual loss require long-term goals of care for clients to adapt. However, clients who have sensory alterations at the time of entering a health care setting are usually most informed about how to adapt interventions to their lifestyles. The blind in particular need to control whatever part of their care they can. Sometimes it becomes necessary for the client to make major changes in self-care activities, communication, and socialization.

Collaborative Care. When developing a plan of care, consider all resources available to clients. The family plays a key role in providing meaningful stimulation and learning ways to help the client adjust to any limitations. You may also refer the client

NURSING CARE PLAN

Disturbed Sensory Perception: Visual, Related to Altered Sensory Reception of Senile Cataract

Assessment

Judy Long is a 70-year-old retired widow who resides in a two-story home with her son. She complains to the community health nurse of increased difficulty with night driving and blurry vision. She enjoys reading and sewing; however, her reduced vision has lim- ited participation in these activities. Ms. Long reports that her vi- sion is blurred even with glasses, and she is afraid that she will fall. Ms. Long visited an ophthalmologist 1 year ago, but did not follow-up with the recommended treatment.

Assessment Activities	Findings/Defining Characteristics*
Ask Judy to describe her vision changes.	Judy states, "My left eye seems to have a film over it that makes my **vision blurred.** I am having **difficulty reading.** I also have **difficulty with night driving."**
Ask Judy to describe any life changes that have occurred since the change in vision.	Judy states, "I have lost my independence because I can no lon- ger drive at night. **I am hesitant to use the stairs at home be- cause I cannot judge steps clearly."**
Assess Judy's visual acuity.	Judy cannot read the Snellen chart with the left eye.
Ask Judy the results of the visit to the ophthalmologist.	Judy states, "I was told I had a cataract of the left eye, and sur- gery was recommended."
Conduct a home hazard assessment.	There is clutter in the home, dim lighting, and stairs without handrails.

*Defining characteristics are shown in bold type.

Nursing Diagnosis: Disturbed sensory perception: visual, related to altered sensory reception of senile cataract.

Planning

Goal	Expected Outcomes (NOC)†
	Safe Home Environment
Judy will maintain independence in a safe home environment.	Judy and her son will make recommended changes to home envi- ronment within 4 weeks.
	Judy will report an increased sense of home safety and indepen- dence within 4 weeks.

†Outcome classification labels from Moorhead S and others: *Nursing outcomes classification (NOC),* ed 4, St. Louis, 2008, Mosby.

Interventions (NIC)‡	Rationale
Environmental Management	
• Teach Judy and her son methods to improve environmental safety such as installation of handrails along stairs, securing carpeting, removal of throw rugs, and painting of stairs.	A decrease in visual acuity and depth perception places a client at risk for falls in the presence of environmental hazards (Ebersole and others, 2004).
• Teach Judy to use a light over the shoulder for reading and sewing.	People with cataracts see better with wider illumination (Ebersole and Hess, 2004).
• Explain use of a pocket magnifier, and offer list of locations where Judy can purchase one.	Magnifier enlarges visual images when reading or doing close work (Ebersole and others, 2004).
• Have Judy make appointment with ophthalmologist within the next 4 weeks.	Older adults need routine eye examination annually or as recom- mended (American Academy of Ophthalmology, 2004).
Emotional Support	
• Encourage Judy to express feelings regarding loss of vision and lifestyle changes.	Visual impairment often leads to functional disabilities that have adverse effects on quality of life (Houde and Huff, 2003).

‡Intervention classification labels from Bulechek GM, Butcher HK, and Dochterman JM: *Nursing interventions classification (NIC),* ed 5, St. Louis, 2008, Mosby.

Evaluation

Nursing Actions	Client Response/Finding	Achievement of Outcome
Ask Judy to describe the changes made in the home to reduce environmental hazards.	Judy responds that she has removed the clutter and placed handrails at the entry- way. She has also placed lighting behind her chair, and there are 100-watt lights in the living room.	Judy reports feeling safer walking the stairs and moving about in her home. The home hazards have been reduced.
During a home visit, observe the home en- vironment for safety hazards		
Observe Judy's verbal and nonverbal re- sponses to the lifestyle adaptations.	Judy says, "I feel safer with walking in my home."	

NURSING CARE PLAN

Disturbed Sensory Perception: Visual, Related to Altered Sensory Reception of Senile Cataract—cont'd

Evaluation, cont'd

Nursing Actions	Client Response/Finding	Achievement of Outcome
As Judy uses magnifier, have her read a medication label. Ask Judy if she is able to maintain a degree of independence with the environmental and lifestyle modifications.	Judy is able to read name of medication and dosage correctly. Judy states, "I am more independent at home, and until surgery I do not mind someone driving for me."	Visual acuity has not been further compromised. Judy has attained some degree of independence.

to other health care professionals. Early referrals to occupational or speech therapists, for example, will speed a client's recovery. If a client has a major loss of sensory function and is also unable to manage medical needs such as medication self-administration or dressing changes, referral to home care is an option. There are also numerous community-based resources (e.g., local chapter of the Society for the Blind and Visually Impaired, and the Area Agency on Aging). Try to arrange a volunteer to visit a client, or have printed materials made available that describe ways to cope with sensory problems.

◆Implementation

Nursing interventions involve the client and family so that the client is able to maintain a safe, pleasant, and stimulating sensory environment. The most effective interventions enable the client with sensory alterations to function safely with existing deficits and to continue a normal lifestyle. Clients can learn to adjust to sensory impairments at any age with the proper support and resources. Use measures to maintain a client's sensory function at the highest level possible.

Health Promotion. Good sensory function begins with prevention. When a client seeks health care, take the opportunity to provide education on interventions that reduce the risk for sensory losses. Also provide education on recommended visual and hearing guidelines.

 Screening. An estimated 150 million people suffer from blinding eye diseases (Boyd-Monk, 2007). Preventable blindness is a worldwide health issue. Therefore prevention of visual impairment begins with children and requires appropriate screening. Three recommended interventions are (1) screening for rubella or syphilis in women who are considering pregnancy; (2) advocating adequate prenatal care to prevent premature birth (with the danger of exposure of the infant to excessive oxygen); and (3) periodic screening of all children, especially newborns through preschoolers, for congenital blindness and visual impairment caused by refractive errors and **strabismus.**

Visual impairments are common during childhood. The most common visual problem is a **refractive error** such as nearsightedness. The nurse's role is one of detection, education, and referral. Parents need to know the signs of visual impairment (e.g., failure to react to light and reduced eye contact from the infant). Instruct parents to report these signs to their health care provider immedi-

ately. Vision screening of school-age children and adolescents will help detect problems early. The school nurse is usually responsible for vision testing.

Hearing impairment is one of the most common disabilities in the United States. An estimated 28 million people in the United States are deaf or hard of hearing (U.S. Department of Health and Human Services, 2004). Children at risk include those with a family history of childhood hearing impairment, perinatal infection (rubella, herpes, or cytomegalovirus), low birth weight, chronic ear infection, and Down syndrome. Advise pregnant women of the importance of early prenatal care, avoidance of ototoxic drugs, and testing for syphilis or rubella.

Children with chronic middle ear infections, a common cause of impaired hearing, need to receive periodic auditory testing. Warn parents of the risks and to seek medical care when the child has symptoms of earache or respiratory infection.

In the United States, glaucoma is the second leading cause of blindness in the general population and the primary cause of blindness in African Americans. If left undetected and untreated, glaucoma leads to permanent visual loss. The American Academy of Ophthalmology (2004) recommends a regular medical eye examination with measurement of intraocular pressure every 2 years for those over 40 years old. Examinations need to occur every 1 to 2 years if there is a family history of glaucoma or if the client is of African ancestry, has had a serious eye injury in the past, is taking steroid medications, or is over 65 years of age.

Because aging is associated with degenerative changes in the ear, clients over age 40 should have a routine hearing assessment as part of their annual physical examination (Barnett, 2007). Once a client reports a hearing loss, regular testing also becomes necessary. In addition, a client who works or lives in a high-noise-level environment should have an annual screening. Occupational health nurses play a key role in the assessment of the auditory system and the initiation of prompt referrals. The early identification and treatment of problems will make certain a more active and healthy population of older adults.

 Preventive Safety. Trauma is a common cause of blindness in children. Penetrating injury from propulsive objects such as firecrackers, slingshots, or rocks or from penetrating wounds from sticks, scissors, or toy weapons are just a few examples. Parents and children require counseling on ways to avoid eye trauma, such as avoiding use of toys with long pointed projections and instructing children not to walk or run while carrying pointed objects. You can find safety equipment in most sports shops and large department stores.

Adults are at risk for eye injury while playing sports and working in jobs involving exposure to chemicals or flying objects. The Occupational Safety and Health Administration (OSHA) (2004) has guidelines for workplace safety. Employers are required to have employees wear eye goggles and/or use equipment such as HPDs to reduce the risk of injury. *Healthy People 2010* (U.S. Department of Health and Human Services, 2000) has identified goals that include the use of HPDs to minimize or prevent hearing loss in workers, as well as children. Occupational health nurses play a key role in reinforcing the use of protective devices. In addition, nurses need to routinely assess clients for noise exposure and participate in providing hearing conservation classes for teachers, students, and clients.

Another means of prevention involves regular immunization of children against diseases capable of causing hearing loss (e.g., rubella, mumps, and measles). Nurses who work in physicians' or other health care providers' offices, schools, and community clinics need to reinforce the importance of early and timely immunization. Advise pregnant women to seek early prenatal care and to undergo testing for syphilis and rubella. In all populations, use caution when administering drugs that are ototoxic.

Use of Assistive Devices. Clients who wear corrective contact lenses, eyeglasses, or hearing aids need to make sure they are clean, accessible, and functional (see Chapter 39). It is helpful to have a family member or friend also know how to clean an assistive aid (Box 49-8). It is critical for contact lens wearers to frequently clean lenses (see Chapter 39) and to use the appropriate solutions for cleaning and disinfection. Contact lens wearers are subject to serious eye infections, caused by infrequent lens disinfection, contamination of lens storage cases or contact lens solutions, and use of homemade saline. Swimming while wearing lenses also creates a serious risk of infection. Reinforce proper lens care in any health maintenance discussion.

The older adult is often reluctant to use a hearing aid. Reasons cited most often include cost, appearance, insufficient knowledge about hearing aids, amplification of competing noise, and unrealistic expectations. For the older adult, neuromuscular changes such as stiff fingers, enlarged joints, and decreased sensory perception also make the handling and care of a hearing aid difficult (Smith and Wilbur, 2004). Fortunately, today there are a wide variety of aids that not only successfully enhance a person's hearing, but also are cosmetically acceptable and useful for persons with manual dexterity issues. Chapter 39 summarizes the types of hearing aids available and tips for proper care and use.

Acknowledging a need to improve hearing is a person's first step. Give clients useful information on the benefits of hearing aid use. A person who sees the need for good hearing will likely be influenced to wear hearing aids (Sommer and Sommer, 2002). It is also important to have a significant other available to assist with hearing aid adjustment. Federal regulations require medical clearance from a physician before an individual can purchase a hearing aid. Hearing aids are contraindicated for the following conditions: visible congenital or traumatic deformity of the ear, active drainage in the last 90 days, sudden or progressive hearing loss within the last 90 days, acute or chronic dizziness, unilateral sudden hearing loss within the last 90 days, visible cerumen accumulation or a foreign body in the ear canal, pain or discomfort in the ear, or an audiometric air-bone gap of 15 decibels or greater. A nurs-

---

BOX 49-8 | CLIENT TEACHING

Troubleshooting Hearing Aid Malfunction

Objectives
- Client and family member will identify source of malfunction in hearing aid.
- Client and family member will demonstrate hearing aid care.

Teaching Strategies
- Show client and family member locations on hearing aid device where damage (e.g., cracks, fraying) is likely to occur: ear mold or case, earphone, dials, cord, and connection plugs.
- Demonstrate battery replacement: Have extra set of unused batteries available.
- Review method to check volume: Turn dial to maximum gain, and then check. Is voice clear?
- Consult manufacturer's directions for specific care measures for cleaning battery case and ear mold.
- Review factors to report to hearing aid laboratory: static, distortion of sound, poor volume quality.

Evaluation
- Have client and family member describe types of common malfunctions with hearing aid.
- Have client and family demonstrate battery removal and cleaning.

---

ing assessment will detect the first seven of these conditions during a physical examination. Refer the client to an otolaryngologist for further counseling (Ebersole and others, 2004).

Promoting Meaningful Stimulation. Life becomes more enriching and satisfying when meaningful and pleasant stimuli exist within the environment. There are many ways for you to help clients adjust to their environment so that it becomes more stimulating. You do this best by considering the normal physiological changes that accompany sensory deficits.

Vision. As a result of the normal changes of aging, the pupil's ability to adjust to light diminishes. As a result, older adults are often very sensitive to glare. You can suggest ways for the client to minimize glare by selecting satin and nongloss finishes for walls and countertops in the home and choosing sheer curtains, tinted windows, or adjustable shades to reduce outdoor light. Wearing sunglasses outside obviously reduces the glare of direct sunlight.

The ability to read is important to everyone. Therefore allow clients to use their glasses whenever possible (e.g., during procedures and client instruction). Clients with reduced visual acuity often need more than corrective lenses. A pocket magnifier will help a client read most printed material. Telescopic lens eyeglasses are smaller, easier to focus, and have a greater range. There are also books and other publications available in larger print. If a client has a legal or other important document he or she wishes to read, standard copying machines have enlarging capabilities. There are now closed-circuit television magnifying units that enlarge written characters up to 45 times (Ebersole and Hess, 2004).

With aging, a person experiences a change in color perception. Perception of the colors blue, violet, and green usually declines.

Brighter colors such as red, orange, and yellow are easier to see. Offer suggestions of ways to decorate a room and paint hallways or stairwells so that the client is able to make differentiations in surfaces and objects in a room.

Hearing. To maximize residual hearing function, work closely with the client to suggest ways to modify the environment. Clients can amplify telephones and televisions. Alarm clocks that shake the bed or signaling devices, such as a flashing light on a phone, allow the hearing impaired greater independence. An innovative way to enrich the lives of the hearing impaired is recorded music. Some clients with severe hearing loss are able to hear music recorded in the low-frequency sound cycles.

One way to help an individual with a hearing loss is to ensure that the problem is not impacted cerumen. With aging, cerumen thickens and builds up in the ear canal. Excessive cerumen occluding the ear canal causes **conductive hearing loss.** Irrigation of the canal with 2 to 3 ounces of tepid water in a 60-mL syringe (see Chapter 39) will remove cerumen and significantly improve the client's hearing ability (Barnett, 2007).

Taste and Smell. You can easily promote the sense of taste by using measures to enhance remaining taste perception. Good oral hygiene keeps the taste buds well hydrated. Well seasoned, differently textured food eaten separately heightens taste perception. Flavored vinegar or lemon juice adds tartness to food. Always ask the client what foods are most appealing. Improvement in taste perception improves food intake and appetite as well.

Stimulation of the sense of smell with aromas such as brewed coffee, cooked garlic, and baked bread heightens taste sensation. The client needs to avoid blending or mixing foods, because these actions make it difficult to identify tastes. Older persons need to chew food thoroughly to allow more food to contact remaining taste buds.

You improve smell by strengthening pleasant olfactory stimulation. Make a client's environment more pleasant with smells such as cologne, mild room deodorizers, fragrant flowers, and sachets. The removal of unpleasant odors (e.g., bedpans or soiled dressings) will also improve the quality of a client's environment.

Touch. Clients with reduced tactile sensation usually have the impairment over a limited portion of their bodies. Providing touch therapy stimulates existing function. If the client is willing to be touched, hair brushing and combing, a back rub, and touching of the arms or shoulders are ways of increasing tactile contact. When sensation is reduced, a firm pressure is often necessary for the client to feel the nurse's hand. Turning and repositioning will also improve the quality of tactile sensation. When performing invasive procedures, it is important to use touch by holding the client's hands, and keeping them warm and dry.

If a client is overly sensitive to tactile stimuli (**hyperesthesia**), minimize irritating stimuli. Keeping bed linens loose to minimize direct contact with the client and protecting the skin from exposure to irritants are helpful measures. If the client has numbness and tingling or pain in the hands, as with carpal tunnel syndrome, have clients wear special wrist splints to dorsiflex the wrist to relieve the nerve pressure. For those clients who use computers, there are special keyboards and wrist pads available to decrease the pressure on the median nerve and aid in relief of pain and promote healing.

Establishing Safe Environments. When sensory function becomes impaired, individuals become less secure within their home and workplace. Security is necessary for a person to feel

independent. Make recommendations for improving safety within a client's living environment without restricting his or her independence. During a home visit or while completing an examination in the clinic, offer several useful suggestions for home safety. The nature of the actual or potential sensory loss determines the safety precautions taken.

Adaptations for Visual Loss. When a client experiences a decrease in visual acuity, peripheral vision, adaptation to the dark, or depth perception, safety is a concern. With reduced peripheral vision a client cannot see panoramically, because the outer visual field is less discrete. With reduced depth perception a person is unable to judge how far away objects are located. This is a special danger when a person attempts to walk down stairs or over uneven surfaces.

SAFETY ALERT To create a safe environment, begin by looking at the results of the home environment assessment (see Chapter 38).

Driving is a particular safety hazard for older adults with visual alterations. Reduced peripheral vision prevents a driver from seeing a car in an adjacent lane. A sensitivity to glare creates a problem for driving at night with headlights. Vision is a primary consideration for safety, but there are other factors as well. In the case of older adults, decreased reaction time, reduced hearing, and decreased strength in the legs and arms will further compromise driving skills. Some safety tips to share with those who continue to drive include the following: drive in familiar areas, do not drive during rush hour, avoid interstate highways for local drives, drive defensively, use rear-view and side-view mirrors when changing lanes, avoid driving at dusk or night, go slow but not too slow, keep the car in good working condition, and carry a portable or preprogrammed cellular phone.

The presence of visual alterations makes it difficult for a person to conduct normal activities of living within the home. Because of reduced depth perception, clients can trip on throw rugs, runners, or the edge of stairs. Keep all flooring in good repair. Advise the client to use low-pile carpeting. Thresholds between rooms need to be level with the floor. Remove clutter to ensure clear pathways for walking. Arrange furniture so that a client can move about easily without fear of tripping or running into objects. Make sure any stairwell has a securely fastened banister or handrail extending the full length of the stairs.

Front and back entrances to the home, work areas, and stairwells need to be properly lighted. Light fixtures need high-wattage bulbs with wider illumination. A light switch should be located at the top and bottom of stairwells. It is also important to be sure lighting on the stairs does not cast shadows. Be sure the client is able to clearly see the edge of each step, especially the first and last. When possible have clients replace steps inside and outside the home with ramps.

An added consideration for the visually impaired is to administer eye medications safely. For conditions such as glaucoma, clients need to closely adhere to regular medication schedules. Labels on medication containers need to be in large print. Make sure a friend or spouse is familiar with dosage schedules in case a client is unable to self-administer a medication. The visually impaired often have difficulty manipulating eye droppers.

Adaptations for Reduced Hearing. Clients hear important environmental sounds (e.g., doorbells and alarm clocks) best if they are amplified or changed to a lower-pitched, buzzerlike sound. Sound lamps that respond with light to sounds such as doorbells, burglar alarms, smoke detectors, and babies crying are also available. Family members or anyone who calls the client regularly need to learn to let the phone ring for a longer period. There are amplified receivers for telephones and telephone communications devices (TCDs) that use a computer and printer to transfer words over the telephone for the hearing impaired. Both sender and receiver need to have the special device to complete a call.

Adaptations for Reduced Olfaction. The client with a reduced sensitivity to odors is often unable to smell leaking gas, a smoldering cigarette, fire, or spoiled food. Advise clients to use smoke detectors and to take precautions such as checking ashtrays or placing cigarette butts in water. Also, advise clients to check food package dates and to inspect the appearance of food. Leftovers need to be kept in labeled containers with the preparation date. Pilot gas flames need to be checked visually.

Adaptations for Reduced Tactile Sensation. When clients have reduced sensation in their extremities, they are at risk for injury from exposure to temperature extremes. Always caution these clients on the use of water bottles or heating pads (see Chapter 48). The temperature setting on the home water heater should be no higher than 48.8° C (120° F). If a client also has a visual impairment, it is important to be sure that water faucets are clearly marked "hot" and "cold," or use color codes (i.e., red for hot and blue for cold).

Communication. A sensory deficit often causes a person to feel isolated because of an inability to communicate with others. It is important for individuals to be able to interact with people around them. The nature of the sensory loss influences the methods and styles of communication that nurses use during interactions with clients (Box 49-9). You can also teach communication methods to family members and significant others. For clients with visual deficits or blindness, speak normally, not from a distance, and be sure to have sufficient lighting.

The client with a hearing impairment is often able to speak normally. To more clearly hear what a person communicates, family and friends need to learn to move away from background noise, rephrase rather than repeat sentences, be positive, and have patience. In a group setting it is better to form a semicircle in front of the client so that the client can see who is speaking next; this helps foster group involvement. On the other hand, some deaf clients have serious speech alterations. Some clients use sign language or lipreading, wear special hearing aids, write with a pad and pencil, or learn to use a computer for communication. Special communication boards that contain common terms (e.g., *pain, bathroom, dizzy,* or *walk*) used in nursing care help clients express their needs.

Client instruction is one aspect of communication. There are teaching booklets available in large print for clients with visual loss. The client who is blind often requires more frequent and detailed verbal descriptions of information. This is particularly true if there are no instructional booklets written in Braille. The visually impaired can also learn by listening to audiotapes or the sound portion of a televised teaching session. Clients with hearing impairment often benefit from written instructional materials and visual teaching aids (e.g., posters and graphs). Demonstrations by the nurse are very useful. Hospitals are required to make professional interpreters available to read sign language of deaf clients.

✳ BOX 49-9 Communication Methods

Clients With Aphasia

Listen to the client, and wait for the client to communicate.

Do not shout or speak loudly (hearing loss is not the problem).

If the client has problems with comprehension, use simple, short questions and facial gestures to give additional clues.

Speak of things familiar and of interest to the client.

If the client has problems speaking, ask questions that require simple yes or no answers or blinking of the eyes. Offer pictures or a communication board so that the client can point.

Give the client time to understand; be calm and patient; do not pressure or tire the client.

Avoid patronizing and childish phrases.

Clients With an Artificial Airway

Use pictures, objects, or word cards so that the client can point.

Offer a pad and pencil or Magic Slate for the client to write messages.

Do not shout or speak loudly.

Give the client time to write messages, because these clients become easily fatigued.

Provide an artificial voice box (vibrator) for the client with a laryngectomy to use to speak.

Clients With Hearing Impairment

Get the client's attention. Do not startle the client when entering the room. Do not approach a client from behind. Be sure the client knows you wish to speak.

Face the client, and stand or sit on the same level. Be sure your face and lips are illuminated to promote lipreading. Keep hands away from mouth.

Be sure clients keep eyeglasses clean so that they are able to see your gestures and face.

If the client wears a hearing aid, make sure it is in place and working.

Speak slowly, and articulate clearly. Older adults often take longer to process verbal messages.

Use a normal tone of voice and inflections of speech. Do not speak with something in your mouth.

When you are not understood, rephrase rather than repeat the conversation.

Use visible expressions. Speak with your hands, your face, and your eyes.

Do not shout. Loud sounds are usually higher pitched and often impede hearing by accentuating vowel sounds and concealing consonants. If you need to raise your voice, speak in lower tones.

Talk toward the client's best or normal ear.

Use written information to enhance the spoken word.

Do not restrict a deaf client's hands. Never have IV lines in both of the client's hands if the preferred method of communication is sign language.

Avoid eating, chewing, or smoking while speaking.

Avoid speaking from another room or while walking away.

Acute Care. When clients enter acute care settings for therapeutic management of sensory deficits or as a result of traumatic injury, use different approaches to maximize sensory function existing at the time. Safety again is an obvious priority until the client's sensory status is either stabilized or improved. For example, clients with sensory deficits have a high risk for falls in the acute care environment. It also becomes very important to know the extent of any existing sensory impairment before the acute episode of illness so that you are able to reinforce what the client already knows about self-care or plan for more instruction before and following discharge.

Orientation to the Environment. The client with recent sensory impairment requires a complete orientation to the immediate environment. Provide reorientation to the institutional environment by ensuring that name tags on uniforms are visible, addressing the client by name, explaining where the client is (especially if clients are transported to different areas for treatment), and using conversational cues to time or location. Reduce the tendency for clients to become confused by offering short and simple, repeated explanations and reassurance. Encourage family members and visitors to help orient clients to the hospital surroundings.

Clients with serious visual impairment need to feel comfortable in knowing the boundaries of the immediate environment. Normally we see physical boundaries within a room. The blind or severely visually impaired often touch the boundaries or objects to gain a sense of their surroundings. The client needs to walk through a room and feel the walls to establish a sense of direction. Help clients by explaining objects within the room, such as furniture or equipment. It takes time for the client to absorb a room's arrangement. The client often needs to reorient again, with you explaining the location of key items (e.g., call light, telephone, and chair). Remember to approach a blind client from the front to avoid startling him or her.

It is important to keep all objects in the same position and place. After an object is moved even a short distance, it no longer exists for a blind person. Simply moving a chair aside will create a safety hazard. Ask the client if any item needs to be arranged to make ambulation easier. Traffic patterns need to be clear and use of furniture with sharp edges avoided. The client who is blind always needs extra time to perform any task. The client needs a detailed description of how to perform an activity and will move slowly to remain safe.

Bedridden clients are at risk for sensory deprivation. Normally movement gives an awareness of the self through vestibular and tactile stimulation. Movement patterns influence a person's sensory perception. The limited movement of bed rest changes how a person interprets the environment; surroundings seem different, and objects seem to assume shapes different from normal. A person who is on bed rest requires routine stimulation through range-of-motion exercises, positioning, and participation in self-care activities (as appropriate). Comfort measures such as washing the face and hands and providing back rubs improve the quality of stimulation and lessen the chance of sensory deprivation. Planning time to talk with clients is also essential. Explain unfamiliar environmental noises and sensations. A calm, unhurried approach during contact with a client gives you quality time to help reorient and familiarize the client with care activities. The client who is well enough to read will benefit from a variety of reading material.

Communication. The most common language disorder following a stroke is aphasia. As a result of a disruption in blood flow to the brain, the speech center becomes damaged, altering a person's ability to either use or understand spoken words. Depending on the type of aphasia, the inability to communicate is often frustrating and frightening (see Box 49-9). Initially you need to establish very basic communication and recognize that aphasia does not indicate intellectual impairment or degeneration of personality. Explain situations and treatments that are pertinent to the client because he or she is able to understand the speaker's words. Because a stroke often causes partial or complete paralysis of one side of the client's body, an aphasic client will need special assistive devices. There are communication boards that have been developed for several levels of disability. Sensitive pressure switches, activated by the touch of an ear, nose, or chin, control electronic communication boards (Ebersole and Hess, 2005). Clients who have had a stroke usually acquire referrals to speech therapists to develop appropriate rehabilitation plans.

In acute care hospitals or long-term care facilities, nurses often care for clients with artificial airways (see Chapter 40). For example, an endotracheal tube is inserted into the oropharynx and down through the vocal cords of the larynx into the upper bronchus. The placement of the tube prevents a client from speaking. In this case the nurse uses special communication methods to facilitate the client's ability to express needs (see Box 49-9). The client is sometimes completely alert and able to hear and see the nurse normally. Giving the client time to convey any needs or requests is very important. Use creative communication techniques (e.g., a communication board or a laptop computer) to foster and strengthen the client's interactions with health care personnel, family, and friends.

Controlling Sensory Stimuli. Control excessive stimuli for clients at risk for sensory overload. Clients need time for rest and freedom from stress caused by frequent monitoring and repeated tests. You can reduce sensory overload by organizing the client's plan of care. Combining activities such as dressing changes, bathing, and vital sign measurement in one visit prevents the client from becoming overly fatigued. The client also needs scheduled time for rest and quiet. Planning for rest periods often requires cooperation from family, visitors, and health care colleagues. Coordination with laboratory and radiology departments will help minimize the number of interruptions for procedures the client must undergo. A creative solution to decrease excessive environmental stimuli that prevents restful, healing sleep is to institute "quiet time" in the ICU. Quiet time means dimming the lights throughout the unit, closing the shades, and shutting the doors. It also includes repositioning clients, giving back massages, and offering clients earplugs. Data collected from one hospital that implemented "quiet time" suggested that "quiet time" in the ICU had a positive impact on quality, safety, customer satisfaction (clients, families, and staff), and cost (Ruggierro and Dziedzic, 2004).

When clients experience sensory overload or deprivation, the resultant behavior is difficult for family or friends to accept. Encourage the family not to argue with or contradict the confused client, but to calmly explain location, identity, and time of day.

Engaging the client in a normal discussion about familiar topics will assist in reorientation. Prearranging tests and procedures with departments reduces the amount of time needed for tests and examinations. Anticipating client needs such as voiding helps reduce uncomfortable stimuli.

Try to control extraneous noise in and around the client's room. It is often necessary to ask a roommate to lower the volume on a television or to move the client to a quieter room. Keep equipment noise to a minimum. Turn off bedside equipment not in use, such as suction and oxygen equipment. Avoid making abrupt loud noises, such as dropping objects or causing the overbed table to suddenly adjust to the lowest level. Nursing staff should also try to control laughter or conversation at the nurses' station. Allow clients to close their room doors.

When the client leaves an acute care setting for the home environment, communicate with colleagues in the home care setting about the interventions that helped the client adapt to sensory problems. Similarly, report any information describing the client's existing sensory deficits. You achieve continuity of care when the client has to make only minimal changes in the home setting.

Safety Measures. The client with recent visual impairment often requires help with walking. The presence of an eye patch, frequently instilled eye drops, or the swelling of eyelid structures following surgery are just a few factors that cause a client to need more assistance than usual. A sighted guide will give confidence to the visually impaired and ensure safe mobility. Ebersole and others (2005) list three suggestions for a sighted guide:

1. Ask the blind client if he or she wants a "sighted guide." If assistance is accepted, offer an elbow or arm. Instruct the client to grasp your arm just above the elbow. If necessary, physically assist the person by guiding his or her hand to your arm or elbow (Figure 49-5).
2. Go one-half step ahead and slightly to the side of the blind person. The shoulder of the person needs to be directly behind your shoulder. If the person is frail, place the hand on your forearm.
3. Relax and walk at a comfortable pace. Warn the client when you approach doorways or narrow spaces.

While walking with the client, describe the course of movement and ensure that obstacles have been removed. Never leave a client with a visual impairment standing alone in an unfamiliar area. For clients who undergo eye surgery, it is important to teach family members techniques for assisting with ambulation.

A visually impaired client who spends considerable time in bed needs to have a call light nearby. Place necessary objects in front of the client to prevent falls caused by reaching over the bedside. Appropriate use of side rails is also an option (see Chapter 38).

Nurses often rely on clients in health care settings to report unusual sounds, such as a suction apparatus running improperly or an IV pump alarm. However, the client with a hearing loss does not always hear such sounds and thus requires more frequent visits by the nurse. The client will also benefit from learning to use vision to discover sources of danger. Never restrict both arms of deaf or hearing-impaired clients (e.g., with restraints or IV lines), because they need their hands to communicate. Face the client when speaking, use simple sentences, and speak more slowly and in a normal

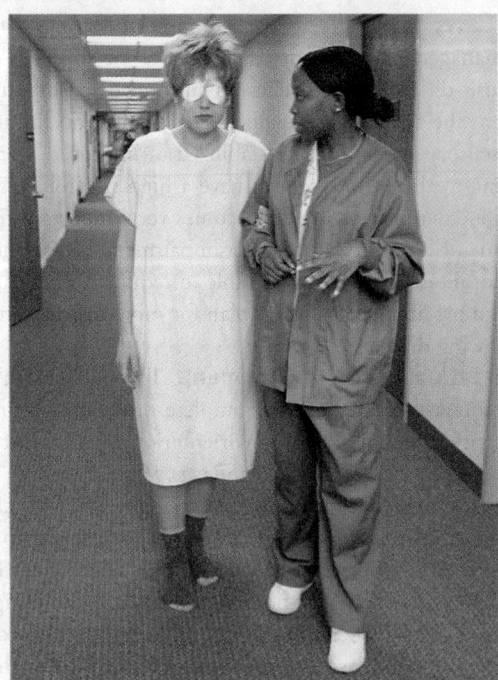

Figure 49-5 Nurse assists in the ambulation of a client wearing eye patches.

volume (McConnell, 2002). It is wise to note on the intercom button and a client's chart if the client is deaf and/or blind. A client lacking the ability to speak cannot call out for assistance. Clients should have message boards or the call light close at hand.

Clients with reduced tactile sensation risk injury when their conditions confine them to bed, because they are unable to sense pressure on bony prominences or the need to change position. These clients rely on nurses for timely repositioning, moving tubes or devices the client is lying on, and turning to avoid skin breakdown. When a client is less able to sense temperature variations, use extra caution in applying heat and cold therapies (see Chapter 48) and preparing bathwater. You need to check the condition of the client's skin frequently.

Restorative and Continuing Care
Maintaining Healthy Lifestyles. After a client has experienced a sensory loss, it becomes important to understand the implications of the loss and to make the adjustments needed to continue a normal lifestyle. Sensory impairments need not prevent a person from leading an active, rewarding life. Many of the interventions applicable to health promotion, such as adapting the home environment, are useful after a client leaves an acute care setting.

Understanding Sensory Loss. Clients who have experienced a recent loss need to understand how to adapt so that their living environments are safe and appropriately stimulating. All family members need to understand the way that a client's sensory impairment affects normal daily activities. Family and friends will be more supportive when they understand sensory deficits and the types of elements that worsen or lessen sensory problems. For example, family and friends need to learn how to communicate with someone who has a hearing loss. There are resources within a community

✳ BOX 49-10 **FOCUS ON OLDER ADULTS**

Principles for Reducing Loneliness

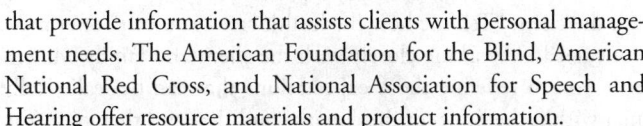

- Spend time with a person in silence or conversation.
- Use physical contact—holding a hand, embracing a shoulder—to convey caring.
- Help recommend alterations in living arrangements if physical isolation is a factor.
- Assist older adults in keeping contact with people important to them.
- Help obtain information about mutual help groups.
- Arrange for security escort services as needed.
- Bring a pet that is easy to care for into the home.
- Link a person with religious organizations attuned to the social needs of older adults.

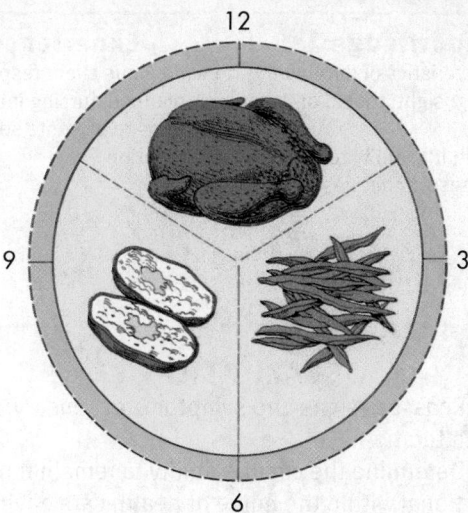

Figure 49-6 Location of food using clock as frame of reference.

that provide information that assists clients with personal management needs. The American Foundation for the Blind, American National Red Cross, and National Association for Speech and Hearing offer resource materials and product information.

Socialization. The ability to communicate is gratifying. It tests our intellect, opens opportunities, and allows us to exchange the feelings we have about others. When sensory alterations hinder interactions, a person feels ineffective and loses self-esteem. If clients feel socially unaccepted, they will perceive sensory losses as seriously impairing their quality of life.

Interacting with others becomes a burden for many clients with sensory alterations. Many clients lose the motivation to engage in social situations, resulting in a deep sense of loneliness. Use therapies to reduce loneliness, particularly in older adults (Box 49-10). These principles support the *Healthy People 2010* objective to increase life satisfaction among all people with disabilities. In addition, family members need to learn to focus on a person's ability to interact rather than on the person's disability. Do not assume, for example, that a person who is hard of hearing does not wish to speak. A blind person can still enjoy a walk through a park with a companion describing the sights around them.

Promoting Self-Care. The ability to perform self-care is essential for self-esteem. Frequently, family members and nurses believe that sensorially impaired persons require assistance, when in fact they are able to help themselves. There are useful guidelines to assist clients with visual or tactile impairment so that they are able to continue self-care activities. In the case of eating meals, arrange food on the plate and condiments, salad, or drinks according to numbers on the face of a clock (Figure 49-6). It is easy for the visually impaired client to become oriented to the items after the nurse or family member explains each item's location.

The client with visual problems needs assistance in reaching toilet facilities safely. Safety bars need to be installed near the toilet. It is often helpful to have the bar a different color than the wall for easier visibility. Never place towels on a safety bar because they will interfere with a person's grasp. Toilet paper needs to be within easy reach. Sharply contrasting colors within the room will assist the partially sighted and promote functional independence. General principles for promoting self-care in older adults also include the

following: use warm incandescent lighting, and control glare by using shades and blinds (Ebersole and others, 2005).

If touch is diminished, the client can dress more easily with zippers or Velcro strips, pullover sweaters or blouses, and elasticized waists. If a client has partial paralysis and reduced sensation, the client dresses the affected side first. Encourage family members responsible for selecting clothing for visually impaired clients to follow the client's preferences. Any sensory impairment has a significant influence on body image, and it is important for the client to feel well groomed and attractive. Some clients need assistance with basic grooming such as brushing, combing, and shampooing hair. Others need assistance with medication administration, clothing identification, and learning to manage routine procedures such as blood pressure and glucose monitoring. An assortment of low-vision devices are now available. It is important for you to make appropriate referrals to allow the client to maintain a maximum degree of independence.

Clients with proprioceptive problems often lose their balance easily. Make sure bathrooms have nonskid surfaces in the tub and shower. Install grab bars either vertically or horizontally in tubs and showers, depending on how the client is able to grasp or hold onto the bar. Instruct family members to supervise ambulation and sitting, make frequent checks to prevent falls, and caution the client against leaning forward.

◆ Evaluation

It is important to evaluate whether care measures maintain or improve a client's ability to interact and function within the environment. The client is the source for evaluating outcomes. The client is the only one who will know if his or her sensory abilities are improved and which specific interventions or therapies are most successful in facilitating a change in the client's performance (Figure 49-7). To evaluate the effectiveness of nursing interventions, use critical thinking and make comparisons with the base-

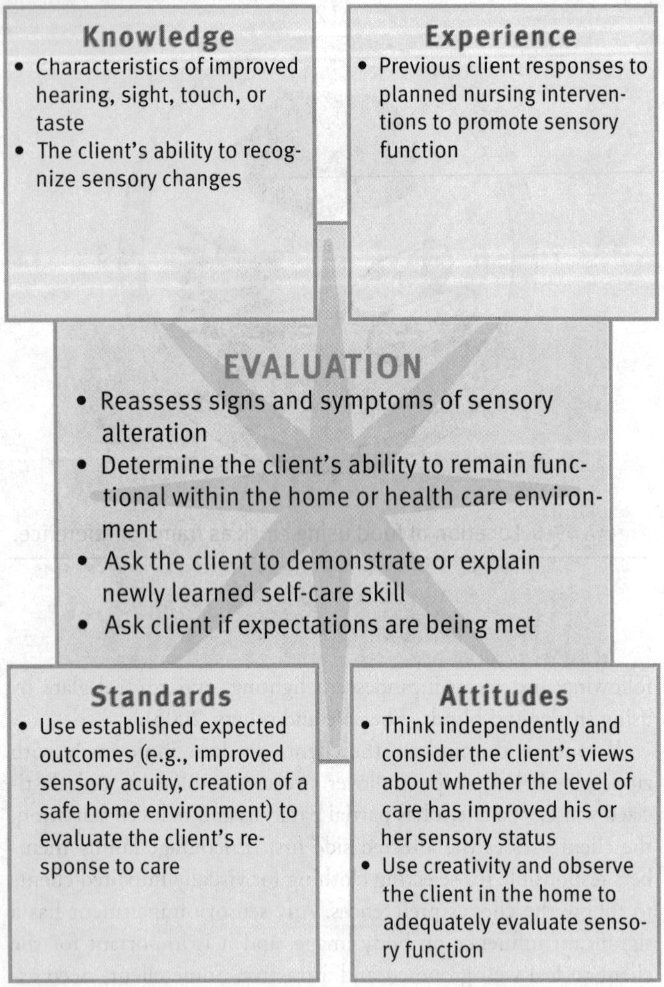

Knowledge
- Characteristics of improved hearing, sight, touch, or taste
- The client's ability to recognize sensory changes

Experience
- Previous client responses to planned nursing interventions to promote sensory function

EVALUATION
- Reassess signs and symptoms of sensory alteration
- Determine the client's ability to remain functional within the home or health care environment
- Ask the client to demonstrate or explain newly learned self-care skill
- Ask client if expectations are being met

Standards
- Use established expected outcomes (e.g., improved sensory acuity, creation of a safe home environment) to evaluate the client's response to care

Attitudes
- Think independently and consider the client's views about whether the level of care has improved his or her sensory status
- Use creativity and observe the client in the home to adequately evaluate sensory function

Figure 49-7 Critical thinking model for sensory alterations evaluation.

line sensory assessment data to evaluate if sensory alterations have changed.

It is your responsibility to determine if expected outcomes have been met. For example, use evaluative data to determine whether care measures improve or at least maintain a client's ability to interact and function within the environment. The nature of a client's sensory alterations influences how you evaluate the outcome of care. For example, use proper communication techniques with a client with a hearing deficit, and then evaluate whether the client has gained the ability to hear or interact more effectively. When expected outcomes have not been achieved, there will be a need to change interventions or alter the client's environment. If outcomes are not met, it is important to ask questions such as "How are you feeling emotionally?" "Do you feel you are at risk for injury?"

If you have directed nursing care at improving or maintaining sensory acuity, evaluate the integrity of the sensory organs and the client's ability to perceive stimuli. Evaluate any interventions designed to relieve problems associated with sensory alterations on the basis of the client's ability to function normally without injury. When you directly or indirectly (through education) alter the client's environment, direct evaluation at observing whether

the client makes environmental changes. When designing client teaching to improve a client's sensory function, it is important to determine whether the client is following recommended therapies and meeting mutually set goals. Asking the client to explain or demonstrate self-care skills is an effective evaluative measure. It is often necessary to reinforce previous instruction if learning has not taken place. If outcomes are not met, these are questions to ask: "How often do you wear your hearing aids/corrective lenses?" "Are you able to participate in a small group discussion?" "Are you able to read the newspaper without squinting?"

If you have successfully developed a good relationship with a client and have a therapeutic plan of care, subtle behaviors often indicate the level of the client's satisfaction. You may notice that the client responds appropriately, such as by smiling. However, it is important for you to ask the client if his or her sensory needs have been met. For example, ask the client, "Can you tell me if you feel we have done all we can do to help improve your ability to hear?" If the client's expectations have not been met, ask the client "Tell me how the health care team can better meet your needs." Working closely with the client and family will enable you to redefine those expectations that can be realistically met within the limits of the client's condition and therapies. You have been effective when the client's goals and expectations have been met.

✳ Key Concepts

- Sensory reception involves the stimulation of sensory nerve fibers and the transmission of impulses to higher centers within the brain.
- When sensory function is impaired, the sense of self is impaired and affects one's ability to socialize.
- Sensory deprivation results from an inadequate quality or quantity of sensory stimuli.
- Aging results in a gradual decline of acuity in all senses.
- Clients who are older, immobilized, or confined in isolated environments are at risk for sensory alterations.
- Assessment of a client's health promotion habits helps to reveal risks for sensory impairment.
- An older adult often will not admit to a sensory loss.
- An assessment of hazards in the environment requires the nurse to tour living areas in the home and to look for conditions that increase the chances of injury such as falls.
- The plan of care for clients with sensory alterations needs to include participation by family members. The extent of support from family members and significant others will influence the quality of sensory experiences.
- Clients with sensory deficits develop alternative ways of communicating that rely on other senses.
- Care of clients at risk for sensory deprivation includes introducing meaningful and pleasant stimuli for all senses.
- To prevent sensory overload, control stimuli and orient the client to the environment.
- Clients with artificial airways are able to communicate effectively with communication boards, laptop computers, and written messages.

✳ Critical Thinking Exercises

One month has passed since Judy made an informed decision to have cataract surgery. Postoperatively she reported improved vision and ability to participate in activities of daily living. Today the community health nurse visits, and Judy reports shortness of breath with activity. After the nurse consults with Judy's physician, Judy is admitted to the emergency department with a diagnosis of heart failure exacerbation.

1. Three days after being admitted to the hospital, Judy reports less shortness of breath; however, she is restless and fatigued. She is on a cardiac monitor and continues to receive oxygen. The staff nurse reports that Judy has slept very little since her admission. Her semi-private room is directly across from a busy central nurses' station, and she frequently calls out for assistance.
   a. Discuss factors that put Judy at risk for sensory overload.
   b. What nursing interventions should the nurse implement to promote sleep for Judy?

2. Judy was released from the hospital in good health 1 week after admission. Following the recommendation of her health care provider, she regularly attends a heart failure support group. She has asked you to speak with the heart failure support group regarding age-related visual changes, as well as signs and symptoms that may indicate problems. What information will you share with this group to promote healthy vision?

3. Hearing impairments related to aging are numerous; therefore, while presenting an education session to older adults, what nursing approaches can you implement to strengthen communication?

✳ NCLEX®-Style Review Questions

1. Jason has been on contact isolation for 4 days because of a gastrointestinal infection. He has had few visitors and has had few opportunities to leave his room. His ambulation is also still limited. Nursing measures to reduce sensory deprivation include: (Choose all that apply.)
   1. Arranging for Jason to have a roommate
   2. Turning off the lights and closing the room drapes
   3. Arranging for peacefulness and frequent rest periods
   4. Assisting Jason to a chair or bringing a flower into the room
   5. Sitting down, speaking, touching, and listening to Jason's feelings and perceptions

2. The home care nurse is providing instructions to a nursing assistant regarding care of an older client with visual loss. The nurse is considering normal age-related visual changes by telling the nurse assistant that clients with visual loss:
   1. Have improved visual acuity with fluorescent lighting
   2. Are able to live independently in restricted environments

   3. Have reduced adaptation to the dark; however, peripheral vision is unchanged
   4. Often use colored tape to distinguish settings on electrical appliances and to highlight the edge of stairs

3. Ms. Douglas is a 72-year-old client with bilateral hearing loss. She wears a hearing aid in her left ear. Which of the following approaches best facilitate communication?
   1. Speak directly into the client's left ear.
   2. Approach the client from behind, and speak frequently.
   3. Face the client when speaking; speak slower and in a normal volume.
   4. Face the client when speaking; use a louder than normal tone of voice.

4. The nurse is caring for an older client with glaucoma. While developing a discharge plan, which of the priority interventions will enable the client to function safely with existing deficits and continue a normal lifestyle?
   1. Encourage the client's family to visit the client once a month.
   2. Suggest to the client that he or she consider moving to a long-term care facility.
   3. Say nothing because it is most appropriate that the client identify personal interventions to compensate for a sensory alteration.
   4. Work closely with the client to identify ways to modify his or her home environment, and as appropriate, refer to community-based resources.

5. Rita Spezio is 74-year-old client who has returned to the nursing home following surgical removal of bilateral cataracts. She reports feeling a little uncertain about walking by herself. Which of the following approaches should a nurse use to assist the client with ambulation?
   1. Walk one-half step behind the client and slightly to the side of the client.
   2. If the client requires assistance, place your hand around the client's waist.
   3. Allow the client to stand alone in unfamiliar areas to encourage confidence building.
   4. Have the client grasp your arm just above the elbow, and walk at a comfortable pace, warning the client when you approach obstacles.

6. Because hearing impairment is one of the most common disabilities among children, a nursing intervention is to teach parents, schoolteachers, and children to:
   1. Avoid activities in which crowds and loud noises occur
   2. Delay childhood immunizations until hearing can be verified
   3. Prophylactically administer antibiotics to reduce the incidence of infections
   4. Take precautions when involved in activities associated with high-intensity noises

7. The nurse is conducting discharge teaching for a client with diminished tactile sensation. Which of the following statements by the client would indicate that teaching was ineffective?
   1. "I am at risk for injury from temperature extremes."
   2. "I may be able to dress more easily with zippers or pullover sweaters."
   3. "A home care referral may help me to achieve a maximum degree of independence."
   4. "I have right-sided partial paralysis and reduced sensation, so I should dress the left side of my body first."

8. The nurse has completed an assessment of a 67-year-old female client who comes to the clinic for the first time. During the examination the client's temperature was 99.6° F, heart rate 80 beats per minute, respiratory rate 18 breaths per minute, and blood pressure 142/84 mm Hg. The client displayed inattention as the nurse asked questions. At one point, the client seemed to shout answers to questions about her diet. However, as the nurse spoke, the client consistently smiled and nodded in agreement. The nurse's assessment indicates:
   1. A visual deficit
   2. Client is normal
   3. A hearing deficit
   4. Sensory overload

9. A nursing history of the nature and characteristics of a visual loss includes assessment of the nature of the problem. An example of an assessment question targeted to assess the nature of a sensory problem is:
   1. How do you practice eye hygiene?
   2. When did you notice the problem?
   3. At what age did you notice the visual change?
   4. What have you tried to correct the vision difficulty?

10. Mr. Grayson has a history of a hearing deficit. He comes to the medicine clinic for a routine checkup. He now reports having difficulty seeing distant objects clearly. His wife died 2 years ago, and he admits to feeling lonely much of the time. Interventions the nurse might use to reduce loneliness, include: (Choose all that apply.)
    1. Reassuring the client that loneliness is a normal part of aging
    2. Keeping your distance while talking to avoid overstimulating client
    3. Providing information about local social groups in the client's neighborhood
    4. Recommending the client consider making living arrangements that will put him closer to family or friends

50 | Care of Surgical Clients

![star graphic]

✳ OBJECTIVES

Mastery of content in this chapter will enable the student to:
- Explain the concept of perioperative nursing care.
- Differentiate between classifications of surgery and types of anesthesia.
- List assessment data for the surgical client.
- Demonstrate postoperative exercises: diaphragmatic breathing, coughing, incentive spirometer use, turning, and leg exercises.
- Design a preoperative teaching plan.
- Prepare a client for surgery.
- Explain the nurse's role in the operating room.
- Describe the rationale for nursing interventions designed to prevent postoperative complications.
- Explain the differences and similarities in caring for ambulatory versus inpatient surgical clients.

✳ MEDIA RESOURCES   ✳ KEY TERMS

Companion CD
- NCLEX®-Style Review Questions
- Audio Glossary
- Interactive Learning Activities
- English/Spanish Glossary

 Website
- NCLEX®-Style Review Questions
- Audio Glossary
- English/Spanish Glossary
- Interactive Learning Activities
- Weblinks
- Audio Summaries

Perioperative nursing care is nursing care given before (preoperative), during (intraoperative), and after surgery (postoperative). It takes place in hospitals, in surgical centers attached to hospitals, in freestanding surgical centers, or in health care providers' offices. Perioperative nursing is a fast-paced, changing, and challenging field. It is based on the nurse's understanding of several important principles, including the following:

- High-quality and client safety–focused care
- Multidisciplinary teamwork
- Effective therapeutic communication and collaboration with the client, the client's family, and the surgical team
- Effective and efficient assessment and intervention in all phases of surgery
- Advocacy for the client and the client's family
- Understanding of cost containment

A nurse needs to practice strict surgical asepsis, thoroughly document care, and emphasize client safety in all phases of care. Effective teaching and discharge planning prevent or minimize complications and ensure quality outcomes. The nursing process provides a basis for perioperative nursing, with the nurse individualizing strategies throughout the perioperative period so that the client has a smooth course from admission into the health care system through convalescence. Continuity of care is stressed in the perioperative model.

Care of the client having surgery has shifted from hospital-based convalescence to home-based convalescence, with much responsibility shifting to the client and/or family. As the length of hospital stay decreases, the educational needs of the client undergoing a surgical procedure increase. Clients return home with complex medical/surgical conditions that require both education and follow-up. Proper client education is essential to ensuring positive surgical outcomes

History of Surgical Nursing

It was not until the twentieth century that the discipline of surgery progressed as a science. Surgery gave physicians the means to treat conditions that were difficult or impossible to manage only by pure medicine. Early surgeons had little knowledge of the principles of asepsis, and anesthesia techniques were primitive and unsafe. The discovery of anesthesia in the 1840s revolutionized surgery. Anesthesia provided for the combination of analgesia, muscle relaxation, and amnesia, which allowed the surgical procedure time to be extended. The value of hand washing in the 1800s, along with the development of the germ theory (Pasteur), triggered the study of aseptic technique, which reduced postoperative infections and mortality.

Nursing played a major role in disease prevention, beginning with Florence Nightingale's belief that the environment was a key factor in disease prevention. Nurses working in the first operating rooms (ORs) cleaned the rooms and equipment, performed technical tasks such as obtaining supplies, and often went with clients to the surgical ward to deliver nursing care.

In 1956 the **Association of Operating Room Nurses (AORN)** was formed to gain knowledge of surgical principles and explore methods to improve nursing care of surgical clients. The organiza-

tion developed standards of nursing practice that outlined the scope of responsibility of the perioperative nurse. AORN was the first nursing organization to develop structure, process, and outcome standards as defined by the American Nurses Association (ANA). Current standards of perioperative nursing include (1) administrative practice, (2) clinical practice, (3) professional performance, (4) quality improvement, and (5) client outcomes (AORN, 2006). The AORN has changed its name to the Association of periOperative Registered Nurses; however, AORN is still its acronym. The organization is a driving force for the practice of perioperative nursing.

Ambulatory Surgery

During the 1970s, the advent of **ambulatory surgery** centers (ASCs), also referred to as outpatient surgery, short-stay surgery, or same-day surgery, changed the perioperative process. Centers providing these services are hospital based or freestanding surgical centers. Starting in 1982, Medicare began paying for surgeries performed in ASCs, and now over half of all surgical procedures occur on an outpatient basis. These procedures include ophthalmic, gastroenterological, gynecological, eye-ear-nose-throat, orthopedic, cosmetic/restorative, and general procedures (Federated Ambulatory Surgery Association, 2006). Many clients are discharged the day of surgery upon reversal of the anesthetic agent. One-day surgery, in which the client is admitted the day of surgery and observed overnight (23-hour admission), also occurs.

There are distinct benefits for the client who has ambulatory surgery. Anesthetic drugs that metabolize rapidly with few aftereffects allow shorter operative times and faster recovery time. Ambulatory surgery also offers cost savings by eliminating the need for hospital stays. This reduces the possibility of acquiring health care–associated infections, which occur when normal skin flora changes with hospitalization and clients become colonized with bacteria found in the hospital setting. Many abdominal procedures such as tumor biopsies and gallbladder removal (**cholecystectomy**) are now done using **laparoscopic** procedures. Laparoscopic surgery involves the use of minimally invasive techniques such as small incisions for performance of the surgery as opposed to a large incision required for an open surgery. Because of the small incision, a laparoscopic cholecystectomy involves only a few hours to a 24-hour hospital stay and a recovery period of a week. By contrast, a traditional open cholecystectomy involves a large abdominal incision. Clients require a 3- to 5-day hospitalization and at least a 4-week recovery period. Thus many surgeons use laparoscopic procedures instead of traditional surgical procedures, thereby decreasing the length of surgery, hospitalization, and associated costs.

Scientific Knowledge Base

Classification of Surgery

The types of surgical procedures are classified according to seriousness, urgency, and purpose (Table 50-1). Some procedures fall into more than one classification. For example, surgical removal of a disfiguring scar is minor in seriousness, elective in urgency, and reconstructive in purpose. Frequently the classes overlap. An urgent procedure is also major in seriousness. Sometimes the same

TABLE 50-1   Classification for Surgical Procedures

TYPE	DESCRIPTION	EXAMPLE
Seriousness		
Major	Involves extensive reconstruction or alteration in body parts; poses great risks to well-being	Coronary artery bypass, colon resection, removal of larynx, resection of lung lobe
Minor	Involves minimal alteration in body parts; often designed to correct deformities; involves minimal risks compared with major procedures	Cataract extraction, facial plastic surgery, tooth extraction
Urgency		
Elective	Performed on basis of client's choice; is not essential and is not always necessary for health	Bunionectomy, facial plastic surgery, hernia repair, breast reconstruction
Urgent	Necessary for client's health, often prevents additional problems from developing (e.g., tissue destruction or impaired organ function); not necessarily emergency	Excision of cancerous tumor, removal of gallbladder for stones, vascular repair for obstructed artery (e.g., coronary artery bypass)
Emergency	Must be done immediately to save life or preserve function of body part	Repair of perforated appendix, repair of traumatic amputation, control of internal hemorrhaging
Purpose		
Diagnostic	Surgical exploration that allows health care providers to confirm diagnosis; often involves removal of tissue for further diagnostic testing	Exploratory laparotomy (incision into peritoneal cavity to inspect abdominal organs), breast mass biopsy
Ablative	Excision or removal of diseased body part	Amputation, removal of appendix, cholecystectomy
Palliative	Relieves or reduces intensity of disease symptoms; will not produce cure	Colostomy, debridement of necrotic tissue, resection of nerve roots
Reconstructive/Restorative	Restores function or appearance to traumatized or malfunctioning tissues	Internal fixation of fractures, scar revision
Procurement for transplant	Removal of organs and/or tissues from a person pronounced brain dead for transplantation into another person	Kidney, heart, or liver transplant
Constructive	Restores function lost or reduced as result of congenital anomalies	Repair of cleft palate, closure of atrial septal defect in heart
Cosmetic	Performed to improve personal appearance	Blepharoplasty to correct eyelid deformities; rhinoplasty to reshape nose

TABLE 50-2   Physical Status (PS) Classification of the American Society of Anesthesiologists

CLASS	DESCRIPTION	CHARACTERISTICS
P1	A normal healthy client	No physiological, biological, organic disturbance
P2	A client with a mild systemic disease	Cardiovascular (CV) disease with minimal restriction on activity
P3	A client with a severe systemic disease	Hypertension (HTN), obesity, diabetes mellitus (DM)
P4	A client with a severe systemic disease that is a constant threat to life	CV or pulmonary disease that limits activity; severe diabetes with systemic complications; history of myocardial infarction (MI), angina pectoris, or poorly controlled HTN
P5	A **moribund** client who is not expected to survive without the operation	Severe cardiac, pulmonary, renal, hepatic, or endocrine dysfunction
P6	A client declared brain dead whose organs are being removed for donor purpose	Clients may have a wide variety of dysfunctions that are being managed to optimize blood flow to the heart and organs (e.g., aggressive fluid replacement and blood pressure medications)

Modified from Physical Status (PS) Classification is reprinted with permission of the American Society of Anesthesiologists, 520 N. Northwest Highway, Park Ridge, Illinois, 60068-2573, http://www.asahq.org/clinical/physicalstatus.htm, 2008.

operation is performed for different reasons on different clients. For example, a gastrectomy may be performed as an emergency procedure to resect a bleeding ulcer or as an urgent procedure to remove a cancerous growth. The classification indicates to the nurse the level of care a client requires.

The American Society of Anesthesiologists (ASA) assigns classification based on a client's physiological condition independent of the proposed surgical procedure (Table 50-2). Anesthesia involves risks even in healthy clients, but certain clients are at higher risk, including those who are volume depleted or who have poor cardiac function (Rothrock, 2007). ASA physical status class 1 and 2 and also stable class 3 are now acceptable for ambulatory surgery. Classes 4 and 5 require inpatient surgery.

Nursing Knowledge Base

Nurses have made significant contributions in showing the benefit preoperative education and preparation has in promoting positive client outcomes following surgery. Structured preoperative teaching that includes the AORN standards (2002d) and return demonstration of postoperative exercises has improved outcomes such as pain severity, pulmonary function, length of stay, and clients' level of anxiety.

There is also significant evidence-based knowledge available for proper wound care interventions. Nursing research has contributed to our knowledge of the characteristics of wound healing and the types of applications most likely to be beneficial. Chapter 48 describes in detail a variety of interventions used to treat wounds, including surgical wounds.

Within the operating room setting, nursing knowledge has improved the standards for infection control and client safety. For example, nurses can now perform surgical hand scrubs, a skill beyond the scope of this textbook, without the use of brushes as a result of research that has shown the efficacy of alcohol-based hand antiseptics in reducing bacteria on the skin (Hobson and others, 1998; Larson and others, 1990). Evidence-based practice changes within the OR improve the quality of care for surgical clients and ultimately improve client outcomes.

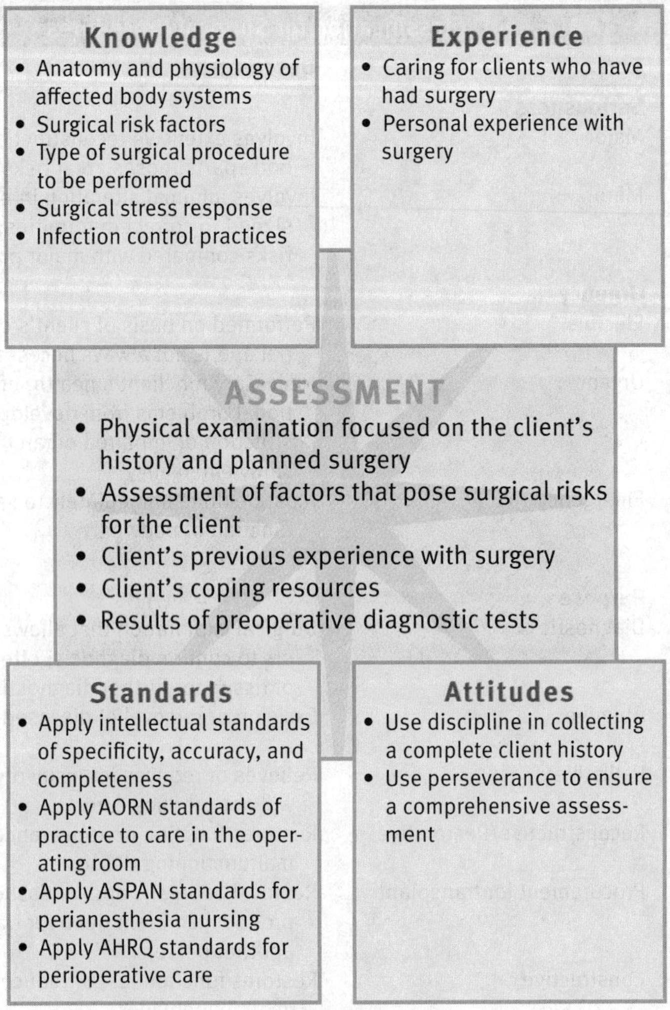

Critical Thinking

Successful critical thinking synthesizes knowledge, information gathered from clients, previous experience, critical thinking attitudes, and intellectual and professional standards. Clinical judgments require you as a nurse to anticipate the necessary information, analyze the data, and make decisions about client care. A client's condition is always changing. During assessment (Figure 50-1) consider all of the elements that build toward making appropriate nursing diagnoses.

In the case of caring for the perioperative client, integrate knowledge from anatomy and physiology, pathophysiology, and the surgical stress response, along with previous experiences in caring for surgical clients. Apply this knowledge along with information gathered from the client as you make clinical decisions for the client's care. The use of critical thinking attitudes ensures that a plan of care is comprehensive and incorporates principles for successful perioperative care (e.g., airway management, infection control, pain management, and discharge planning). The use of professional standards as developed by the Agency for Health Care Research and Quality (AHRQ), AORN, the **American Society of PeriAnesthesia Nurses (ASPAN)**, and the **American Society of Anesthesiologists (ASA)** provide valuable guidelines for perioperative management and evaluation of process and outcomes (http://www.ahrq.gov, http://www.aorn.org, http://www.aspan.org, http://www.asahq.org). However, review these guidelines within the context of new emerging evidence-based practice,

Figure 50-1 Critical thinking model for surgical client assessment.

agency policies, and the scope of practice of the state in which you practice.

The Nursing Process in the Preoperative Surgical Phase

Clients having surgery enter the health care setting in different stages of health. A client may enter the hospital or ambulatory surgical center on a predetermined day feeling relatively healthy and prepared to face elective surgery. In contrast, a person in a motor vehicle crash may face emergency surgery with no time to prepare. The ability to establish rapport and maintain a professional relationship with the client is an essential component of the preoperative phase. Nurses must do this quickly, but compassionately and effectively.

Clients have a variety of tests and procedures to confirm or rule out alterations requiring surgery. Most testing occurs before the day of surgery. Usually clients scheduled for ambulatory surgery have tests done several days before surgery. Testing done the day of surgery is usually limited to such tests as glucose monitoring for the client with diabetes. Nurses need to be familiar with the tests, their purposes, and how to monitor results.

The client meets many health care personnel, including surgeons, nurse anesthetists, anesthesiologists, surgical technologists, and nurses. All play a role in the client's care and recovery. Family members attempt to provide support through their presence but face many of the same stressors as the client. You need to effectively communicate with the client and family because the nurse-client relationship is the foundation of care (see Chapter 24). Assess the client's physical, emotional, and spiritual well-being and cultural heritage; recognize the degree of surgical risk; coordinate diagnostic tests; identify nursing diagnoses and nursing interventions; and establish outcomes in collaboration with the client and the client's family. Communicate pertinent data and the plan of care to the surgical team members.

◆Assessment

The aim of the assessment of the client before surgery is to establish the client's normal preoperative function to prevent and minimize possible postoperative complications. Ambulatory and same-day surgical programs offer challenges in gathering a complete assessment in a limited time. A multidisciplinary team approach is essential. Clients are admitted only hours before the surgical event, so it is important for you to organize and verify data obtained preoperatively and implement a perioperative plan of care. This occurs not only in ASCs, but also with clients who will require a hospital stay. It has become common practice for clients to be admitted the day of surgery, even for such major procedures as open heart surgery or craniotomy.

The majority of assessments begin before admission for surgery—in the health care provider's office, preadmission clinic, anesthesia clinic, or by telephone. Some clients answer a self-report inventory. Other times a health care provider performs a physical examination or orders laboratory tests. Before surgery, nurses begin teaching, answer questions, and begin paperwork. This streamlines the care required by the client on the day of surgery. In the immediate preoperative period, assess the client's understanding of previous teaching.

So as not to waste time duplicating information from the preoperative examination, focus on key measurements for all body systems to ensure that no one overlooked any obvious problems. Also, make sure the client understands the education previously provided. Even though the surgeon will screen the client before scheduling surgery, preoperative assessment occasionally reveals an abnormality that delays or cancels surgery. For example, consider an infection in a client with a cough and low-grade fever on admission, and notify the surgeon immediately.

Nursing History. You will conduct an initial interview to collect a client history similar to that described in Chapter 33. If a client is unable to relate all of the necessary information, rely on family members as resources.

Medical History. A review of the client's medical history includes past illnesses and surgeries and the primary reason for seeking medical care. The client's current medical record and medical records from past hospitalizations are excellent sources of data. Preexisting illnesses influence the choice of anesthetic agents

used, as well as the client's ability to tolerate surgery and reach full recovery (Table 50-3). Screen clients having ambulatory surgery for medical conditions that increase the risk for complications during or after surgery. For example, a client who has a history of congestive heart failure (CHF) may experience a further decline in cardiac function both intraoperatively and postoperatively. Interventions for the client with CHF in the preoperative period include beta-blocker medications (Mukjerjee and Eagle, 2003), intravenous (IV) fluids infused at a slower rate, or administration of a diuretic after blood transfusions. Box 50-1 highlights a focused assessment for the client with a cardiac history.

The history of previous surgery influences the level of physical care required after an upcoming surgical procedure. For example, a client who has had a previous thoracotomy for resection of a lung tumor has a greater risk for postoperative pulmonary complications than a client with normal lungs.

Risk Factors. Various conditions and factors increase a person's risk in surgery. Knowledge of risk factors enables you to take necessary precautions in planning care.

Age. Very young and old clients are at risk during surgery because of immature or declining physiological status. Mortality rates are higher in very young and very old surgical clients. During surgery, nurses and health care providers are especially concerned with maintaining an infant's normal body temperature. The infant has an underdeveloped shivering reflex, and often wide temperature variations occur. Anesthesia adds to the risk because anesthetics often cause vasodilation and heat loss.

During surgery an infant has difficulty maintaining a normal circulatory blood volume. An infant has considerably less total blood volume than an older child or an adult. Even a small amount of blood loss is serious. A reduced circulatory volume makes it difficult for the infant to respond to increased oxygen demands during surgery. In addition, the infant is highly susceptible to complications associated with dehydration. However, if blood or fluids are replaced too quickly, overhydration may occur. Other unique aspects of a child's surgical care include airway management, management of temperature alterations, and treatment of emergence delirium or delayed emergence from anesthesia.

With advancing age, clients have less physical capacity to adapt to the stress of surgery because of deterioration in certain body functions. Despite the risk, the majority of clients undergoing surgery are older adults. Table 50-4 summarizes physiological factors that place older clients at risk during surgery.

Nutrition. Normal tissue repair and resistance to infection depend on adequate nutrients. Surgery intensifies this need. After surgery a client requires at least 1500 kcal/day to maintain energy reserves. Increased protein, vitamins A and C, and zinc facilitate wound healing (see Chapters 44 and 48). A client who is malnourished is prone to poor tolerance to anesthesia, negative nitrogen balance from lack of protein, delayed blood-clotting mechanisms, infection, poor wound healing, and the potential for multiple organ failure. Many hospitalized clients display some degree of malnutrition. If a client has elective surgery, attempt to correct nutritional imbalances before surgery. However, if a client who is malnourished must undergo an emergency procedure, efforts to restore nutrients occur after surgery.

TABLE 50-3   Medical Conditions That Increase the Risks of Surgery

Type of Condition	Reason for Risk
Bleeding disorders (thrombocytopenia, hemophilia)	Increase risk of hemorrhaging during and after surgery.
Diabetes mellitus	Increases susceptibility to infection and impairs wound healing from altered glucose metabolism and associated circulatory impairment (Furnary, 2003). Stress of surgery often causes increases in blood glucose levels.
Heart disease (recent myocardial infarction, dysrhythmias, congestive heart failure) and peripheral vascular disease	Stress of surgery causes increased demands on myocardium to maintain cardiac output. General anesthetic agents depress cardiac function.
Obstructive sleep apnea	Administration of opioids increases risk of airway obstruction postoperatively. Clients will desaturate as revealed by drop in O_2 saturation by pulse oximetry.
Upper respiratory infection	Increases risk of respiratory complications during anesthesia (e.g., pneumonia and spasm of laryngeal muscles).
Liver disease	Alters metabolism and elimination of drugs administered during surgery and impairs wound healing and clotting time because of alterations in protein metabolism.
Fever	Predisposes client to fluid and electrolyte imbalances and may indicate underlying infection.
Chronic respiratory disease (emphysema, bronchitis, asthma)	Reduces client's means to compensate for acid-base alterations (see Chapter 41). Anesthetic agents reduce respiratory function, increasing risk for severe hypoventilation.
Immunological disorders (leukemia, acquired immunodeficiency syndrome [AIDS], bone marrow depression, and use of chemotherapeutic drugs or immunosuppressive agents)	Increases risk of infection and delayed wound healing after surgery.
Abuse of street drugs	Persons abusing drugs sometimes have underlying disease (HIV, hepatitis) that affects healing.
Chronic pain	Regular use of pain medications often results in higher tolerance. Increased doses of analgesics are sometimes necessary to achieve postoperative pain control.

HIV, Human immunodeficiency virus.

BOX 50-1   NURSING ASSESSMENT QUESTIONS

Nature of the Problem
- Do you have a history of heart attack, heart failure, angina (chest pain), irregular heartbeat, or valve disease?
- What medications are you taking?
- Have you had any recent medical testing on your heart, for example, cardiac catheterization or echocardiogram?

Signs and Symptoms
- Are you having any chest pain?
- How do you sleep at night (position, use of pillows, awakened with chest pain)?
- Do you have any swelling of your feet?
- Are you short of breath or having any difficulty breathing?

Onset and Duration
- How often do you have chest pain, when does it start, how long does it last, what alleviates it?
- When do your feet swell (all the time, end of the day, only after a busy day)?
- When do you become short of breath?

Severity
- On a scale of 0 to 10 (zero is no pain and ten the worst pain), what number do you give your chest pain?
- Describe your usual activity level. Can you climb stairs; can you do housework?
- Are you performing any regular exercise? What exercise?

Predisposing Factors
- Have you changed your activity level, sleep amount, diet, or fluid intake recently?
- Are you taking any herbal or over-the-counter medications?

Effect on Client
- How are you feeling about your upcoming surgery? Has it affected your symptoms?
- Are you having any additional stress currently?

✳ **TABLE 50-4 Physiological Factors That Place the Older Adult at Risk During Surgery**

ALTERATIONS	RISKS	NURSING IMPLICATIONS
Cardiovascular System		
Degenerative change in myocardium and valves	Reduced cardiac reserve.	Assess baseline vital signs. Recognize the longer time period required for heart rate to return to normal following stress on the heart, and evaluate the occurrence of tachycardia accordingly (Eliopoulos, 2004).
Rigidity of arterial walls and reduction in sympathetic and parasympathetic innervation to heart	Alterations predispose client to postoperative hemorrhage and rise in systolic and diastolic blood pressure.	Maintain adequate fluid balance to minimize stress to the heart. Ensure blood pressure level is adequate to meet circulatory demands.
Increase in calcium and cholesterol deposits within small arteries; thickened arterial walls	Predispose client to clot formation in lower extremities.	Instruct client in techniques for performing leg exercises and proper turning. Apply elastic stockings, sequential compression devices (SCDs). Administer anticoagulants as prescribed by health care provider. Provide education regarding effects, side effects, and dietary considerations.
Integumentary System		
Decreased subcutaneous tissue and increased fragility of skin	Prone to pressure ulcers and skin tears.	Assess skin every 4 hours; pad all bony prominences during surgery. Turn or reposition at least every 2 hours.
Pulmonary System		
Rib cage stiffened and reduced in size	Reduced vital capacity.	Instruct client in proper technique for coughing, deep breathing, and use of spirometer.
Reduced range of movement in diaphragm	Residual capacity (volume of air is left in lung after normal breath) increases, reducing amount of new air brought into lungs with each inspiration.	When possible, have client ambulate and sit in chair frequently.
Stiffened lung tissue and enlarged air spaces	Alteration reduces blood oxygenation.	Obtain baseline oxygen saturation; measure as indicated throughout perioperative period.
Renal System		
Reduced blood flow to kidneys	Increased risk of shock when blood loss occurs.	For clients hospitalized before surgery, determine baseline urinary output for 24 hours.
Reduced glomerular filtration rate and excretory times	Limits ability to eliminate drugs or toxic substances.	Assess for adverse response to drugs.
Reduced bladder capacity	Voiding frequency increases, and larger amount of urine stays in bladder after voiding. Sensation of need to void often does not occur until bladder is filled.	Instruct client to notify nurse immediately when sensation of bladder fullness develops. Keep call light and bedpan within easy reach. Toilet every 2 hours or more frequently if indicated.
Neurological System		
Sensory losses, including reduced tactile sense and increased pain tolerance	Decreased ability to respond to early warning signs of surgical complications.	Inspect bony prominences for signs of pressure that client is unable to sense. Orient client to surrounding environment. Observe for nonverbal signs of pain.
Decreased reaction time	Confusion after anesthesia.	Allow adequate time to respond, process information, and perform tasks. Institute fall precautions.
Metabolic System		
Lower basal metabolic rate	Reduced total oxygen consumption.	Ensure adequate nutritional intake when diet is resumed, but avoid intake of excess calories.
Reduced number of red blood cells and hemoglobin levels	Ability to carry adequate oxygen to tissues is reduced.	Administer necessary blood products. Monitor blood test results and oxygen saturation.
Change in total amounts of body potassium and water volume	Greater risk for fluid or electrolyte imbalance occurs.	Monitor electrolyte levels, and supplement as necessary. Cardiac monitoring (telemetry) as needed.
Impaired thermoregulatory mechanisms	Cold operating rooms; exposure of body parts during procedure, IV fluids, medications.	Ensure careful, close monitoring of client temperature; provide warm blankets; monitor cardiac function; warm IV fluids.

Obesity. Obesity increases surgical risk by reducing ventilatory and cardiac function. Obstructive sleep apnea, hypertension, coronary artery disease, diabetes mellitus, and congestive heart failure are common in the **bariatric** (obese) population. Embolus, **atelectasis,** and pneumonia are also more frequent postoperative complications in the client who is obese. The client often has difficulty resuming normal physical activity after surgery and is susceptible to poor wound healing and wound infection because of the structure of fatty tissue, which contains a poor blood supply. This slows delivery of essential nutrients, antibodies, and enzymes needed for wound healing (see Chapter 48). It is often difficult to close the surgical wound of a client who is obese because of the thick adipose layer; thus the client is at risk for dehiscence (opening of the suture line) and evisceration (abdominal contents protruding through surgical incision).

Obstructive Sleep Apnea. Obstructive sleep apnea (OSA) is a syndrome of periodic, partial or complete obstruction of the upper airway during sleep. It often results in sleep-associated oxygen desaturation (see Chapter 42). OSA increases the risk of perioperative complications. Assess for a history of diagnosed OSA and use of continuous positive airway pressure (CPAP), noninvasive positive pressure ventilation (NIPPV), or apnea monitoring. Instruct clients with diagnosed OSA using CPAP or NIPPV to bring their machine to the hospital or ambulatory surgery center. However, many clients with OSA are undiagnosed. Therefore, to assess for risk of OSA, ask focused questions to the client and family regarding snoring, apnea during sleep, frequent arousals during sleep, morning headaches, daytime somnolence, and chronic fatigue (ASA, 2006; Blouin and Magro, 2005).

Immunocompromise. For the client with cancer, bone marrow alterations can occur and increase the risk of infection. In addition, radiation therapy is sometimes given preoperatively to reduce the size of the cancerous tumor so that it can be removed surgically. Radiation has some unavoidable effects on normal tissue, such as excess thinning of skin layers, destruction of collagen, and impaired vascularization of tissue. Ideally, the surgeon waits to perform surgery 4 to 6 weeks after completion of radiation treatments. Otherwise, the client may face serious wound-healing problems. Also, chemotherapeutic drugs used for cancer treatment, immunosuppressive medications used to prevent rejection after organ transplantation, and steroids used to treat a variety of inflammatory conditions increase the risk for infection.

Fluid and Electrolyte Imbalance. The body responds to surgery as a form of trauma. Severe protein breakdown causes a negative nitrogen balance (see Chapter 44), and an elevation in blood glucose level occurs. Both of these effects decrease tissue healing and increase the risk of infection. As a result of the adrenocortical stress response, the body retains sodium and water and loses potassium within the first 2 to 5 days after surgery. The severity of the stress response influences the degree of fluid and electrolyte imbalance. More extensive surgery will result in a greater stress response. A client who is hypovolemic or who has serious preoperative electrolyte alterations is at significant risk during and after surgery. For example, an excess or depletion of potassium increases the chance of dysrhythmia during or after surgery. If the client has preexisting diabetes mellitus or renal, gastrointestinal, or cardiovascular abnormalities, the risk of fluid and electrolyte alterations is even greater.

Pregnancy. The perioperative plan of care addresses not one, but two clients: the mother and the developing fetus. The pregnant client has surgery only on an emergent or urgent basis. Because all major systems of the mother are affected during pregnancy, the risk for operative complications are increased. For example, cardiac output significantly increases to accommodate the increase in metabolic rate. Gastrointestinal motility decreases. Fibrinogen levels increase, so pregnant clients are more susceptible to the development of deep vein thrombosis due to increased coagulability. Hemoglobin and hematocrit levels decrease, mostly as a result of the effects of hemodilution (increased circulating volume). The white blood cell (WBC) count increases when the woman is near term and postpartum without the presence of infection. General anesthesia is administered with caution because of the increased risk of fetal death and preterm labor. Psychological considerations for mother and family are essential.

Perceptions and Knowledge Regarding Surgery.
A client's past experience with surgery influences physical and psychological responses to a procedure. Assess the client's previous experiences with surgery as a foundation for teaching, addressing fears, and clarifying concerns. Ask the client to discuss the previous type of surgery, level of discomfort, extent of disability, and overall level of care required. Address any complications that the client experienced. It is also important to assess clients for motion sickness and nausea and vomiting with previous surgeries (Gan, 2002; Tramer, 2001). These factors increase the risk for aspiration. Prior anesthesia records are a useful source of information if other previous problems occurred. This information helps you anticipate the client's preoperative and postoperative needs.

The surgical experience affects the family unit as a whole, as well as the client. Therefore prepare both the client and the family for the surgical experience. Understanding of a client's and family's knowledge, expectations, and perceptions allows you to plan teaching and to provide individualized emotional support measures.

Each client brings fears to the surgical setting. Some are due to past hospital experiences, warnings from friends and family, or lack of knowledge. Assess the client's understanding of the planned surgery, its implications, and planned postoperative activities. Ask questions such as "Tell me what you think will happen before and after surgery" or "Explain what you know about surgery." Nurses face ethical dilemmas when clients are misinformed or unaware of the reason for surgery. Confer with the surgeon if the client has an inaccurate perception or knowledge of the surgical procedure before the client is sent to the surgical suite. Also, determine whether the health care provider explained routine preoperative and postoperative procedures, and assess the client's readiness and willingness to learn. When a client is well prepared and knows what to expect, reinforce the client's knowledge.

Medication History.
If a client regularly uses prescription or over-the-counter medications, the surgeon or anesthesia provider may temporarily discontinue the drugs before surgery or adjust the dosages. Certain medications have special implica-

✴ TABLE 50-5 Drugs With Special Implications for the Surgical Client

DRUG CLASS	EFFECTS DURING SURGERY
Antibiotics	Antibiotics potentiate (enhance action of) anesthetic agents. If taken within 2 weeks before surgery, aminoglycosides (gentamicin, tobramycin, neomycin) may cause mild respiratory depression from depressed neuromuscular transmission.
Antidysrhythmics	Antidysrhythmics (e.g., beta blockers such as metoprolol [Lopressor]) can reduce cardiac contractility and impair cardiac conduction during anesthesia.
Anticoagulants	Anticoagulants, such as warfarin (Coumadin), alter normal clotting factors and thus increase risk of hemorrhaging. Discontinued at least 48 hours before surgery. Aspirin is a commonly used medication that alters clotting mechanisms.
Anticonvulsants	Long-term use of certain anticonvulsants (e.g., phenytoin [Dilantin] and phenobarbital) alters metabolism of anesthetic agents.
Antihypertensives	Antihypertensives, such as beta blockers and calcium channel blockers, interact with anesthetic agents to cause bradycardia, hypotension, and impaired circulation. They inhibit synthesis and storage of norepinephrine in sympathetic nerve endings.
Corticosteroids	With prolonged use, corticosteroids, such as prednisone, cause adrenal atrophy, which reduces the body's ability to withstand stress. Before and during surgery, dosages are often temporarily increased.
Insulin	Clients' need for insulin changes after surgery. Stress response and intravenous (IV) administration of glucose solutions often increase dosage requirements after surgery. Decreased nutritional intake often decreases dosage requirements.
Diuretics	Diuretics such as furosemide (Lasix) potentiate electrolyte imbalances (particularly potassium) after surgery.
Nonsteroidal antiinflammatory drugs (NSAIDs)	NSAIDs (e.g., ibuprofen) inhibit platelet aggregation and prolong bleeding time, increasing susceptibility to postoperative bleeding.
Herbal therapies: ginger, gingko, ginseng	These herbal therapies have the ability to affect platelet activity and increase susceptibility to postoperative bleeding. Ginseng is reported to increase hypoglycemia with insulin therapy.

tions for the surgical client, creating greater risks for complications (Table 50-5). Instruct clients to ask the health care provider if they need to take usual medications the morning of surgery. Also, ask clients if they take any herbal preparations, because many clients do not view herbs as medications and often omit them from their medication history (see Chapter 36). Certain herbs interfere with the action of other medications (consult the pharmacist). For hospitalized clients, prescription drugs taken preoperatively are automatically discontinued postoperatively unless the health care provider reorders them. The use of a medication reconciliation process (see Chapter 35) is common practice to ensure that at the time of a client's discharge all home medications are reviewed and there is an accurate and current medication list for the client.

Allergies. Assess for allergies to drugs that clients receive during the perioperative period. In addition, assess for latex, food, and contact allergies (e.g., to tape, ointments, or solutions). For clients with known latex allergies, the surgical center provides a latex-free environment. Some clients are too young or have not had any exposure to drugs; hence they do not know if they have allergies. The type of allergic response is very important to assess. Allergies are not the same as unpleasant side effects. For example, the client states that codeine causes nausea (a side effect) or hypotension and confusion (an allergy). When asking a client about allergies, realize that the term *allergy* is confusing for some clients. Asking a client if he or she has ever "had a problem with a medication or substance" is a helpful approach to questioning. Ensure

that you list the client's allergies appropriately in the client's chart and/or the hospital computer system, as well as any other places designated by institutional policy, such as an allergy band.

Smoking Habits. The client who smokes is at greater risk for postoperative pulmonary complications than a client who does not. The chronic smoker already has an increased amount and thickness of mucous secretions in the lungs. General anesthetics increase airway irritation and stimulate pulmonary secretions, which the airways retain as a result of reduction in ciliary activity during anesthesia. After surgery the client who smokes has greater difficulty clearing the airways of mucous secretions and needs emphasis on the importance of postoperative deep breathing and coughing (see Chapter 40).

Alcohol Ingestion and Substance Use and Abuse. Habitual use of alcohol and illegal drugs predisposes the client to adverse reactions to anesthetic agents. Some clients also experience a cross-tolerance to anesthetic agents, necessitating higher-than-normal doses. In addition, the health care provider may need to increase postoperative dosages of analgesics. Clients with a history of excessive alcohol ingestion are often malnourished, which delays wound healing. These clients are also at risk for liver disease, portal hypertension, and esophageal varices (predisposing the client to bleeding disorders). The client who habitually uses alcohol and is required to remain in the hospital longer than 24 hours is also at risk for acute alcohol withdrawal and its more severe form, delirium tremens (DTs).

Support Sources. It is important to determine the extent of the client's support from family members or friends. Because family does not always mean blood relations, it is best to have the client identify his or her source of support. The client usually cannot immediately assume the same level of physical activity enjoyed before surgery. With ambulatory surgery, clients and families assume responsibility for postoperative care. The family is an important resource for the client with physical limitations and provides the emotional support needed to motivate the client to return to a previous state of health. Sometimes the family will remember preoperative and postoperative teaching better. With older adults having ambulatory surgery, note that it is important to establish preoperatively that the client will receive a postdischarge phone call as a check on recovery progress. Because some older adult clients are unable to hear the phone or reach the phone due to decreased mobility after surgery, identify if a family member will be staying with the client to answer the phone. Another option is an arrangement for the family member to call the surgery center the next day to ensure proper follow-up (Mamaril, 2006).

Ask if family members or friends are able to provide support. Some clients want someone else present when you provide instructions or explanations. Encourage family presence when feasible, especially for clients in the ambulatory setting. Often a family member becomes the client's coach, offering valuable support during the postoperative period, when the client's participation in care is vital.

Occupation. Surgery sometimes results in physical alterations that prevent a person from returning to work. Assess the client's occupational history to anticipate the possible effects of surgery on recovery and eventual work performance. Explain any restrictions before a client returns to work, such as lifting, use of the extremities, or climbing stairs. When a client is unable to return to a job, refer the client to a social worker and/or occupational therapist for job-training programs or to help the client seek economic assistance.

Preoperative Pain Assessment. Surgical manipulation of tissues, treatments, and positioning on the operating room table may result in postoperative pain for the client. Pain is a very personal experience and requires an individualized plan of care. Preoperatively, conduct a comprehensive pain assessment, including the client's and family's expectations for pain management following surgery. Ask clients to describe their perceived tolerance to pain, past experiences, and interventions used. Begin education regarding pain management as soon as possible (Barnes, 2001). Preoperative assessment should include the use of a pain instrument to rate the presence and severity of pain (see Chapter 43). Several instruments for both pediatric and adult clients have shown reliability and validity (Summers, 2001). Frequent pain assessments are necessary to alert nurses to treat the pain and assess the adequacy (outcome) of pain interventions.

Review of Emotional Health. Surgery is psychologically stressful. Clients are often anxious about the surgery and its implications and feel they are powerless over their situation. Family members may perceive the client's surgery as a disruption of their lifestyle. Hospitalization and the recovery period at home are sometimes lengthy. The family is usually concerned about the client returning to a normal, productive life. When the client has chronic illness, the family is either fearful that surgery will result in further disability or hopeful that it will improve their lifestyle. To understand the impact of surgery on a client's and family's emotional health, assess the client's feelings about surgery, self-concept, body image, and coping resources.

It is difficult to assess clients' feelings thoroughly when ambulatory surgery is scheduled because you have less time to establish a relationship with the client. Costa (2001) found that clients having ambulatory surgery expressed three key concerns: fear, knowledge, and caregivers' presence. Clients needed to discuss their feelings, to have adequate preoperative teaching, and to know they mattered as an individual. You can address these concerns initially with the client during a home visit or on the telephone before surgery. In a hospital room, choose a time for discussion after completing admitting procedures or diagnostic tests. Explain that it is normal to have fears and concerns. The client's ability to share feelings partially depends on your willingness to listen, be supportive, and clarify misconceptions.

If the client feels powerless, attempt to determine the reason. The medical diagnosis often causes concern about dependence and loss of physical or mental function. The thought of being "put to sleep" under anesthesia sometimes creates concern about loss of control. Many clients feel the need to retain the power to make decisions about treatment. Assure clients of their right to ask questions and seek information.

A client may be angry about the need for surgery. Surgery may occur at a time when it is inconvenient or potentially disruptive. Some clients express anger and anxiety by verbally attacking the nurse or health care providers. Other manifestations of anger and anxiety include being argumentative or overly demanding, refusing to cooperate, or criticizing the nurse's efforts to provide care.

Self-Concept. Clients with a positive self-concept are more likely to approach surgical experiences appropriately. Assess self-concept by asking clients to identify personal strengths and weaknesses (see Chapter 27). Clients who are quick to criticize or scorn personal characteristics may have little self-regard or may be testing your opinion of their characters. Poor self-concept hinders the ability to adapt to the stress of surgery and aggravates feelings of guilt or inadequacy.

Body Image. Surgical removal of any diseased body part often leaves permanent disfigurement, alteration in body function, or concern over mutilation. Loss of certain body functions (e.g., with a colostomy or amputation) may compound a client's fears. Assess for body image alterations that clients perceive will result from surgery. Individuals will respond differently depending on their culture, age, self-concept, and self-esteem (see Chapter 27).

Often surgery changes the physical or psychological aspects of clients' sexuality. Excision of breast tissue, an ostomy, hysterectomy, or removal of the prostate gland affect clients' perceptions of their sexuality. Augustus (2002) found that African American women delayed having hysterectomies because of the negative sexuality connotations associated with hysterectomy. Surgery such as hernia repair or cataract extraction forces clients to temporarily refrain from sexual intercourse until they return to normal physical activity.

Encourage clients to express concerns about their sexuality. The client facing even temporary sexual dysfunction requires understanding and support. Hold discussions about the client's sexuality with the client's sexual partner so that the partner will gain a shared understanding of how to cope with limitations in sexual function (see Chapter 28).

Coping Resources. Assessment of feelings and self-concept reveals whether the client is able to cope with the stress of surgery. The physiological effects of stress are well documented. Activation of the endocrine system results in the release of hormones and catecholamines, which increases blood pressure, heart rate, and respiration. Platelet aggregation also occurs, along with many other physiological responses. Be aware of these responses, and assist with stress management (see Chapter 31).

Ask the client about past stress management and behaviors that helped resolve any tension or nervousness. When reviewing the client's coping resources, ask the client about specific family members and friends who may provide support. Once identified, include these individuals in any client teaching and interventions to manage stress and anxiety.

Culture.

Culture is a system of beliefs developed over time and passed on through many generations. Clients come from diverse cultural, ethnic, and religious backgrounds. These backgrounds affect the way each client perceives and reacts to the surgical experience. If you do not acknowledge and plan for cultural, ethnic, and religious differences in the perioperative plan of care, you may not achieve desired surgical outcomes. Therefore the acquisition of knowledge regarding a client's cultural and ethnic heritage assists you in caring for the perioperative client. Although it is important to recognize and plan for differences based on culture, it is also necessary to recognize that members of the same culture are individuals and do not always hold these shared beliefs. Box 50-2 highlights cultural care aspects in the perioperative period.

Client Expectations.

Individualize each plan of care for each client, including the client's expectations. Does the client expect full pain relief or simply to have his or her pain reduced? Does the client expect to be independent immediately after surgery, or does he or she expect to be fully dependent on the nurse or family? These are only a few of the questions that you need to ask to establish a plan of care that matches the client's needs and expectations.

Physical Examination.

Conduct a partial or complete physical examination, depending on the amount of time available and the client's preoperative condition. Chapter 33 describes physical assessment techniques. Assessment focuses on findings related to the client's medical history and on body systems that the surgery is likely to affect. The nursing assessment complements the surgeon's and anesthesia provider's physical examination (Barnes, 2002).

General Survey. Observe the client's general appearance. Gestures and body movements may reflect weakness caused by illness. Asses the client for a malnourished appearance. Height, body weight, and history of recent weight loss are important indicators of nutritional status.

Preoperative vital signs, including blood pressure while sitting and standing, provide important baseline data with which to

BOX 50-2 **CULTURAL ASPECTS OF CARE**

Providing Culturally Sensitive Care for the Client Having Surgery

Providing clients of various cultures, religious groups, and countries with individualized education and perioperative nursing care is challenging. The use of a wide variety of resources within a health care agency, in the literature, and from the Internet helps nurses to provide culturally sensitive care.

Implications for Practice
- Preoperative assessment needs to include a cultural assessment with questions such as primary language spoken, feelings regarding surgery and pain, pain management, expectations, support system, and feelings toward self-care with postoperative implications (e.g., Does client relate to concept of pain? Does client have feelings about gender of caregiver? Does client follow custom giving family members control over decisions?).
- Use professional interpreters to communicate with non–English-speaking clients.
- Use pictures or phrase cards with various languages to communicate and assess the non–English-speaking client regarding pain, comfort, temperature, etc.
- Provide preoperative and postoperative educational materials in a variety of languages.

Modified from De Ruiter HP, Larsen KE: Developing a transcultural client care web site, *J Transcult Nurs* 13(1):61, 2002.

compare alterations that occur during and after surgery. Some institutions request that you obtain blood pressure in both arms for comparison. Anxiety and fear commonly cause elevations in heart rate and blood pressure. Preoperative assessment of vital signs is also important to rule out fluid and electrolyte abnormalities (see Chapter 41).

An elevated temperature before surgery is a cause for concern. If the client has an underlying infection, the surgeon may choose to postpone surgery until the infection has been treated. An elevated body temperature increases the risk of fluid and electrolyte imbalance after surgery. Notify the surgeon immediately if the client has an elevated temperature.

Head and Neck. The condition of oral mucous membranes is one indicator of the level of hydration. Inspect the soft palate and nasal sinuses. Sinus drainage is indicative of respiratory or sinus infection. Inspect the jugular veins for distention. Excess fluid within the circulatory system or failure of the heart to contract efficiently leads to jugular vein distention and reveals a risk for cardiovascular complications during surgery.

During the examination of the oral mucosa, identify any loose or capped teeth because they can become dislodged during endotracheal intubation. Note dentures so they can be removed before surgery especially if the client will receive general anesthesia.

Integument. Carefully inspect the skin, especially over bony prominences, such as the heels, elbows, sacrum, and scapula. During surgery a client often lies in a fixed position for several hours. As a result, the client has an increased risk for pressure ulcers (see Chapter 48). Chronic use of steroids also increases the client's

✳ TABLE 50-6   Diagnostic Screening for Surgical Clients

MEASUREMENT AND NORMAL VALUES	INTERPRETATION

Complete blood count (CBC)
  RBC: Men: 4.7-6.1 million/mm³
    Women: 4.2-5.4 million/mm³
  Hgb: Men: 14-18 g/100 mL
    Women: 12-16 g/100 mL
  Hct: Men: 42%-52%; *Women:* 37%-47%
  WBC: Adults and children >2 yr: 5000-10,000/mm³
	Peripheral venous sample of blood may reveal infection, low blood volume, and potential for oxygenation problems. Surgeon may order blood replacement.

Serum electrolytes
  Sodium (Na): 136-145 mEq/L
  Potassium (K): 3.5-5.0 mEq/L
  Chloride (Cl): 98-106 mEq/L
  Bicarbonate : 21-28 mEq/L
	Peripheral venous sample of blood may reveal significant fluid and electrolyte imbalances preoperatively. Attention is given to Na, K, and Cl levels. IV fluid replacement may be indicated preoperatively.

Coagulation studies
  PT: 11-12.5 seconds
  INR: 0.76-1.27
  APTT: 30-40 seconds
  Platelets: 150,000-400,000/mm³
	Prothrombin time (PT), international normalized ratio (INR), activated partial thromboplastin time (APTT), and platelet counts reveal clotting ability of blood. Reveals clients at risk for bleeding tendencies and thrombus formation.

Serum creatinine
  Men: 0.6-1.2 mg/100 mL
  Women: 0.5-1.1 mg/100 mL
	Ability of kidneys to excrete creatinine, by-product of muscle metabolism, indicates renal function. Elevated level can indicate renal failure.

Blood urea nitrogen (BUN) 10-20 mg/100 mL	Ability of kidneys to excrete urea and nitrogen indicates renal function. BUN becomes elevated if client is dehydrated. Preoperative IV fluid replacement is often necessary.
Glucose *Fasting:* 70-105 mg/100 mL	Finger stick or peripheral blood sample. Clients often require treatment of low or high levels preoperatively and postoperatively.

Modified from Pagana KD, Pagana TJ: *Mosby's diagnostic and laboratory test reference*, ed 8, St. Louis, 2007, Mosby.

RBC, Red blood cell; *Hgb,* hemoglobin; *Hct,* hematocrit; *WBC,* white blood cell.

---

susceptibility to skin tears. The overall condition of the skin also reveals the client's level of hydration. An older adult is at high risk for alteration in skin integrity from positioning (pressure forces) and sliding on the operating room table (shearing forces).

Thorax and Lungs. Assessment of the client's breathing pattern and chest excursion measures ventilatory capacity. A decline in ventilatory function places the client at risk for respiratory complications. Auscultation of breath sounds will indicate whether the client has pulmonary congestion or narrowing of airways. Existing atelectasis or moisture in the airways will be aggravated during surgery. Serious pulmonary congestion usually results in postponement of the surgery. Certain anesthetics cause laryngeal muscle spasm. If you auscultate wheezing in the airways preoperatively, the client is at risk for further airway narrowing during surgery and after extubation (removal of the endotracheal tube); therefore notify health care providers of these findings.

Heart and Vascular System. Assess the character of the apical pulse, and listen to heart sounds. Assess peripheral pulses, capillary refill, and the color and temperature of extremities. If peripheral pulses are not palpable, use a Doppler instrument for assessment of their presence. Acceptable capillary refill occurs in less than 2 seconds. Measurement of capillary refill and assessment of peripheral pulses are particularly important for the client having vascular surgery or for a client who has casts or constricting bandages applied to the extremities after surgery (see Chapter 33).

Abdomen. Assess the abdomen for size, shape, symmetry, and presence of distention. Ask whether the client has regular bowel movements, and inquire about the color and consistency of stools. Auscultate bowel sounds.

Neurological Status. Preoperative assessment of neurological status is imperative for all clients receiving general anesthesia. The baseline neurological status assists with the assessment of ascent from anesthesia. During the health history and physical assessment, observe the client's level of orientation, alertness, and mood, noting whether the client answers questions appropriately and is able to recall recent and past events. A client who will have surgery for neurological disease (e.g., brain tumor or aneurysm) sometimes demonstrates an impaired level of consciousness or altered behavior.

If the client is scheduled for spinal anesthesia, preoperative assessment of gross motor function and strength is important. Spinal anesthesia causes temporary paralysis of the lower extremities (see Chapter 43). Be aware of a client entering surgery with weakness or impaired mobility of the lower extremities and communicate this to the perioperative team so care providers will not become alarmed when full motor function does not return as the spinal anesthetic wears off.

Diagnostic Screening. Preoperatively the surgeon orders diagnostic tests to screen for preexisting abnormalities. The client's history and physical assessment determine the ordered tests. The surgical procedure determines tests as well. For procedures where blood loss is expected (e.g., hip and knee replacements), a type and crossmatch would be indicated preoperatively in case the client needs a blood transfusion during surgery. The surgeon designates the number of blood units to have available during surgery. Table 50-6 gives the purpose and normal values for common blood tests. If diagnostic tests reveal severe problems, the surgeon will probably cancel surgery until the condition stabilizes. You are responsible for the preparation of clients for diagnostic studies and for coordinating completion of the tests. Review diagnostic results as they become available and alert health care providers to findings, and assist with planning appropriate therapy.

If a client is over the age of 40 or has heart disease, the health care provider often orders a chest x-ray examination or an electrocardiogram (ECG). The chest x-ray is an examination of the condition of the heart and lungs. An ECG measures the heart's electrical activity to determine whether the heart rate, rhythm, and other factors are normal.

Pulmonary function testing and occasionally arterial blood gas analysis are often performed on clients with preexisting lung disease. Blood glucose levels are measured preoperatively when clients have diabetes.

Autologous infusions are an option for some clients who choose to donate their own blood before surgery to reduce the risk of transfusion-related infections and transfusion reactions (see Chapter 41). The client makes the donation several weeks before the scheduled surgery. The client who does self-donation sometimes exhibits a lower hemoglobin and hematocrit level on the day of surgery. Autotransfusion via the use of a cell-saver device in surgery is possible if health care providers are anticipating large blood loss (e.g., open heart surgery). The cell saver, although expensive, returns washed red blood cells to the client and decreases the risk of transfusion reactions and blood-related infections by using the client's own blood (Rothrock, 2007).

◆Nursing Diagnosis

Cluster patterns of defining characteristics gathered during assessment to identify nursing diagnoses for the surgical client (Box 50-3). The client with preexisting health problems is likely to have a variety of risk diagnoses. For example, a client with preexisting bronchitis who has abnormal breath sounds and a productive cough will be at risk for *ineffective airway clearance*. The nature of the surgery and the client's health status provide defining characteristics for a number of nursing diagnoses. For example, a client who undergoes a surgical procedure is at risk for developing infection at the surgical site, at the IV site, or in the bloodstream (sepsis). A diagnosis of *risk for infection* will require your attention from admission through recovery.

The related factors for each diagnosis establish directions for nursing care that will be provided during one or all surgical phases. For example, the diagnosis of *risk for infection related to an invasive procedure* will require different interventions than if the related factor is *inadequate immune response*. Preoperative nursing

---

BOX 50-3 NURSING DIAGNOSTIC PROCESS

Fear Related to Knowledge Deficit and Previous Surgical Experience

Assessment Activities	Defining Characteristics
Ask client to describe previous surgical experiences.	Apprehension over anesthesia and postoperative pain
Ask client about preoperative education/preparation before admission.	Fear of the unknown, of having complications
	Unaware of preoperative testing
Observe client's nonverbal behavior.	Increased tension
Assess vital signs.	Increased heart rate, increased blood pressure

---

diagnoses allow you to take precautions and actions so that care provided during the intraoperative and postoperative phases is consistent with the client's needs.

Nursing diagnoses made preoperatively will also focus on the potential risks a client may face after surgery. Preventive care is essential so that you can manage the surgical client effectively. The following are some common nursing diagnoses relevant to the client having surgery:

- Ineffective airway clearance
- Anxiety
- Fear
- Risk for deficient fluid volume
- Risk for perioperative-positioning injury
- Deficient knowledge (specify)
- Impaired physical mobility
- Nausea
- Acute pain
- Delayed surgical recovery

◆Planning

During planning, synthesize information from multiple resources (Figure 50-2). For example, knowledge pertaining to adult learning principles, coupled with the client's unique needs, will ensure a well-designed **preoperative teaching** plan. Critical thinking ensures that the client's plan of care integrates knowledge, previous experiences, and established standards of care. Previous experience in caring for surgical clients helps you to anticipate how to approach client care (e.g., complications to prevent and anticipate and methods to reduce anxiety). Professional standards are especially important to consider when developing a plan of care. These standards often establish scientifically proven guidelines for selecting effective nursing interventions. Develop an individualized plan of care for each nursing diagnosis (see Care Plan). The nurse and client set realistic expectations for care.

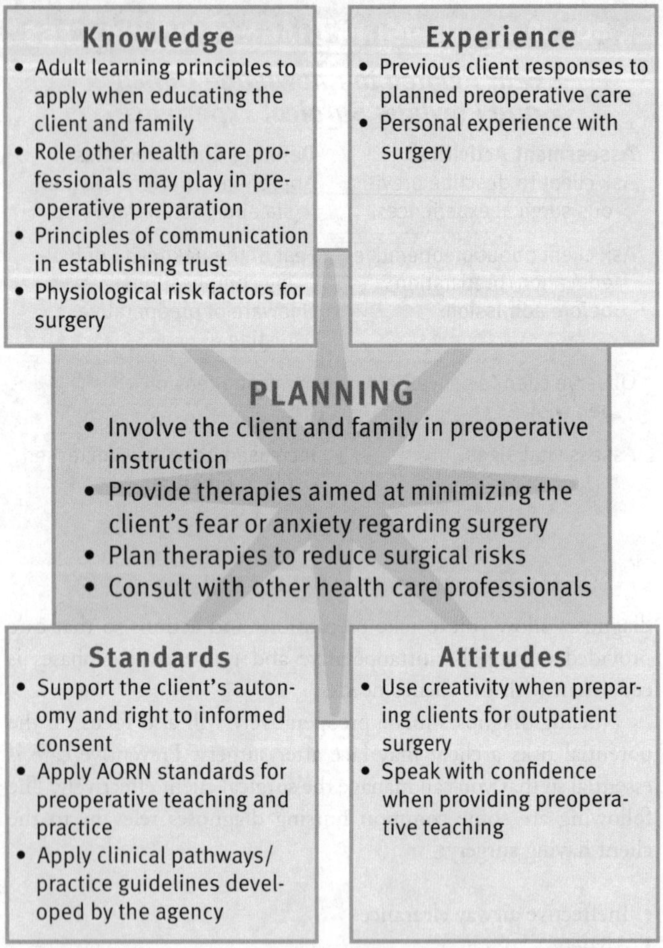

Knowledge
- Adult learning principles to apply when educating the client and family
- Role other health care professionals may play in preoperative preparation
- Principles of communication in establishing trust
- Physiological risk factors for surgery

Experience
- Previous client responses to planned preoperative care
- Personal experience with surgery

PLANNING
- Involve the client and family in preoperative instruction
- Provide therapies aimed at minimizing the client's fear or anxiety regarding surgery
- Plan therapies to reduce surgical risks
- Consult with other health care professionals

Standards
- Support the client's autonomy and right to informed consent
- Apply AORN standards for preoperative teaching and practice
- Apply clinical pathways/ practice guidelines developed by the agency

Attitudes
- Use creativity when preparing clients for outpatient surgery
- Speak with confidence when providing preoperative teaching

Figure 50-2 Critical thinking model for surgical client planning.

Successful planning requires the involvement of the surgical client and family in establishing the plan of care. Early involvement of the client when developing the surgical care plan minimizes surgical risks and postoperative complications. A client informed about the surgical experience is less likely to be fearful and is able to participate in the postoperative recovery phase so that outcomes are met. Establish diagnosis, interventions, and outcomes to ensure recovery or maintenance of the preoperative state.

Goals and Outcomes. Base the preoperative care plan on individualized nursing diagnoses. Review and modify the plan during the intraoperative and postoperative periods. Outcomes established for each goal of care provide measurable behavioral evidence to gauge the client's progress toward meeting stated goals.

As an example, the goal "Client is able to verbalize significance of postoperative exercises" will be measured through the following expected outcomes:

- Client verbalizes prevention of lung congestion and pneumonia as reasons for deep breathing and coughing exercises and incentive spirometer.
- Client verbalizes promotion of blood flow to prevent leg clots as reason for postoperative leg exercises and ambulation.

- Client verbalizes rationale for early ambulation as it improves lung function, assists with return of bowel function, and promotes recovery.

Setting Priorities. Using clinical judgment, prioritize nursing diagnoses and interventions based on the assessed unique needs of each client. Clients requiring emergent surgery often experience changes in their physiological status that require you to reprioritize quickly. For example, if a client's blood pressure begins to drop, hemodynamic stabilization becomes a priority over education and stress management. Ensure the approach to each client is thorough and reflects an understanding of the implications of the client's age, physical and psychological health, educational level, cultural and religious practices, and stated and/ or written wishes concerning advance medical directives.

Collaborative Care. For clients having ambulatory surgery and clients admitted the day of their scheduled surgery, preoperative planning occurs days before admission to the hospital or surgical center. Frequently, preoperative education begins in the health care provider's office, continues during the scheduled preadmission testing visit, and is reinforced by the nurse the day of admission. Preoperative instruction gives the client time to think about the surgical experience, make necessary physical preparations (e.g., altering diet or discontinuing medication use), and ask questions about postoperative procedures. The client having ambulatory surgery usually returns home on the day of surgery. Thus well-planned preoperative care ensures that the client is well informed and able to be an active participant during recovery. The family or spouse also plays an active supportive role for the client.

◆Implementation

Preoperative nursing interventions provide the client with a complete understanding of the surgery and prepare the client physically and psychologically for surgical intervention.

Informed Consent. Surgery cannot be legally or ethically performed until a client understands the need for a procedure, the steps involved, risks, expected results, and alternative treatments. Chapter 23 discusses in detail the nurse's responsibilities for **informed consent**. It is the surgeon's responsibility to explain the procedure and obtain the informed consent. After the client completes the consent form, place it in the medical record. The record goes to the operating room with the client.

Health Promotion. Health promotion activities during the preoperative phase focus on health maintenance, prevention of complications, and support of possible rehabilitation needs postoperatively.

Preoperative Teaching. Client education is an important aspect of the client's surgical experience (see Chapter 25). Provided in a systematic and structured format with teaching and learning principles, preoperative teaching regarding a client's expected postoperative course has a positive influence on the client's recovery. Preadmission nurses call clients up to 1 week before surgery to clarify questions and reinforce explanations. Preoperative

NURSING CARE PLAN

Deficient Knowledge Regarding Preoperative and Postoperative Care Requirements Related to Lack of Exposure to Information

Assessment

Mrs. Campana is an 80-year-old client scheduled to be admitted in 5 days for elective bowel resection. You are the nurse in the ASC assigned to prepare Mrs. Campana for surgery. During your initial discussion with Mrs. Campana, you assess that she is alert and oriented. Mrs. Campana states she has severely reduced visual acuity but is able to hear your questions clearly. Mrs. Campana has had previous surgery. She lives alone and has a daughter who will be coming in town the day of surgery and will stay with her 2 weeks after surgery.

Assessment Activities	Findings/Defining Characteristics*
Ask Mrs. Campana what she has been told regarding her surgery.	She states her surgeon explained the procedure with a drawing of the bowel and the location of the part to be removed.
Ask Mrs. Campana what she understands about preoperative preparation and what to expect postoperatively.	She verbalizes understanding of medicines to take the morning of surgery, her diet before surgery and when to stop eating, and whom to call for questions. She is unable to explain what to expect postoperatively.
Assess Mrs. Campana's fears about surgery.	**Mrs. Campana appears slightly anxious. She states, "I am afraid I will die during my surgery."**

*****Defining characteristics** are shown in bold type.

Nursing Diagnosis: Deficient knowledge regarding preoperative and postoperative care requirements related to lack of exposure to information.

Planning

Goals	Expected Outcomes (NOC)†
	Knowledge: Treatment Procedures
Mrs. Campana will understand the postoperative routines of surgical care by day before surgery.	Mrs. Campana will be able to describe importance of postoperative exercises by morning of surgery.
	Mrs. Campana will be able to describe the schedule for activity and nutritional management following surgery by day 1 postoperatively.
Mrs. Campana will participate actively in postoperative recovery activities by postoperative day 1.	Mrs. Campana will successfully perform postoperative exercises (turning, coughing, deep breathing [TCDB], diaphragmatic breathing [DB], incentive spirometer [IS], and leg exercises) by morning of surgery.

†Outcome classification labels from Moorhead S and others: *Nursing outcomes classification (NOC)*, ed 4, St. Louis, 2008, Mosby.

Interventions (NIC)‡	Rationale
Preoperative Teaching	
• Before admission to the hospital, provide Mrs. Campana with audiotape program that explains preoperative and postoperative routines. Supply instruction booklet designed for clients with visual impairments. Make a follow-up call to client and daughter encouraging them to ask questions and voice concerns. Document education provided.	Preadmission education often results in less teaching time and better performance of exercises on admission. Education has a beneficial effect in reducing postoperative anxiety (American College of Surgeons, 2006).
• On admission to hospital, demonstrate to Mrs. Campana and daughter the performance of postoperative exercises and how to get out of bed with assistance.	Demonstration is an effective method to reinforce instruction.
• Explain sensations to expect postoperatively (e.g., incisional pain, IV, nasogastric tube, wound care).	Reduces client anxiety.
• Have Mrs. Campana provide return demonstration of postoperative exercises before surgery.	Assesses learning and provides opportunity to reinforce instruction.
• Correct any unrealistic expectations Mrs. Campana or daughter have regarding surgery.	Unrealistic expectations, when unmet, contribute to client's anxiety. Psychological preparation for surgery reduces anxiety (American College of Surgeons, 2006; Lee and others, 1998).

‡Intervention classification labels from Bulechek GM, Butcher HK, and Dochterman JM: *Nursing interventions classification (NIC)*, ed 5, St. Louis, 2008, Mosby.

Continued

NURSING CARE PLAN

Deficient Knowledge Regarding Preoperative and Postoperative Care Requirements Related to Lack of Exposure to Information—cont'd

Evaluation

Nursing Actions	Client Response/Finding	Achievement of Outcome
Ask Mrs. Campana to describe typical monitoring and care activities following surgery. Document evaluation of her understanding.	She is able to verbalize typical monitoring and care following surgery. She states the booklet and audiotape were both helpful.	Mrs. Campana has a good understanding of the typical postoperative course.
Observe Mrs. Campana's demonstration of postoperative exercises.	She correctly demonstrates leg exercises and TCDB but is having difficulty with IS use.	Mrs. Campana demonstrates most of postoperative exercises, but needs further teaching and practice on IS use.
Explore with Mrs. Campana and daughter if they have any remaining fears or concerns.	Both Mrs. Campana and her daughter deny any fears or concerns at the present time.	Informational and psychological needs of Mrs. Campana and her daughter have been met.

information and instructions include telephone calls, mailings from the health care provider's office or hospital, preoperative teaching guidelines and checklists, or the use of videotapes or websites. The American College of Surgeons developed a client education website titled *Partners in Surgical Care,* which provides a supplement to the surgeon's teaching (American College of Surgeons, 2006). Education throughout the perioperative period is essential. Lee and others (1998) conducted postdischarge surveys of 206 clients hospitalized over a 6-week period. Results from this study indicated that continuity of care was enhanced if clients received education before, during, and after discharge. They found that half of the clients requested additional education. Therefore it seems ideal to attempt perioperative education before admission, during the hospital stay, and after discharge. Including family members in perioperative preparation is advisable. Often a family member is the coach for postoperative exercises when the client returns from surgery. If anxious relatives do not understand routine postoperative events, it is likely that their anxiety will heighten the client's fears and concerns. Perioperative preparation of family members before surgery helps to minimize anxiety and misunderstanding.

Provide clients with information about sensations typically experienced after surgery. Preparatory information helps clients anticipate the steps of a procedure and thus helps them form realistic images of the surgical experience. For example, in the operating room the anesthesia provider applies ointment to clients' eyes to prevent corneal damage. Warning clients about sensations of blurred vision will reduce their anxiety on awakening from surgery. Other sensations to describe include the expected pain at the surgical site, the tightness of dressings, dryness of the mouth, and the sensation of a sore throat resulting from an endotracheal tube.

Anxiety and fear are barriers to learning, and both emotions heighten as surgery approaches. If the client is capable of and receptive to learning, present information in a logical sequence, beginning with preoperative events and advancing to intraoperative and postoperative routines. The ANA and AORN (2002d) have established the following standards to demonstrate client understanding of the surgical experience.

Client Cites Reasons for Preoperative Instructions and Exercises. Given a rationale for preoperative and postoperative procedures, the client is better prepared to participate in care. Every preoperative teaching program includes explanation and demonstration of postoperative exercises: diaphragmatic breathing, incentive spirometry, coughing, turning, and leg exercises. These exercises help to prevent postoperative complications (Skill 50-1).

If the client needs elastic stockings or **sequential (pneumatic) compression devices,** teaching about the purposes and nursing care required following application is necessary (see Chapter 47).

After you explain each exercise, demonstrate it for the client. Guide the client through each exercise. For example, assess whether the client is sitting properly, and help the client place the hands in the proper position during breathing. Then allow the client time for independent practice, and return later to evaluate effectiveness before surgery.

Client States the Time of Surgery. Tell the client and family the approximate time that surgery will begin and when they should arrive to the hospital or ASC. The surgeon will inform the client and family of the anticipated length of surgery. Unanticipated delays occur for many reasons. Make the family aware that delays occur for various reasons and do not necessarily indicate a problem.

Client States the Postoperative Unit and Location of the Family During Surgery and Recovery. The unit to which the client is admitted before surgery is often different from the postoperative unit. The family needs to know where the client will be after surgery. Also explain where the family can wait and where the surgeon will attempt to find family members after surgery. Many institutions have implemented programs in which the circulating nurse gives periodic reports to the family in the waiting room for surgeries that are expected to be prolonged. If the client will be taken to a special unit, it helps to orient the client and family members to the unit's environment before surgery.

Client Discusses Anticipated Postoperative Monitoring and Therapies. The client and family need to know about postoperative events. If they understand the frequency of postoperative vital sign monitoring before surgery occurs, they will be less apprehensive when nurses measure vital signs. You also explain

Text continued on p. 1386

✳ SKILL 50-1   DEMONSTRATING POSTOPERATIVE EXERCISES   Video

Delegation Considerations

Do not delegate the skill of demonstrating postoperative exercises to nursing assistive personnel (NAP). Direct NAP to:

- Encourage clients to practice exercises regularly following instruction
- Inform the nurse if client is unwilling to perform these exercises

Equipment

- Pillow or wrapped blanket (used to splint surgical incision during coughing)
- Incentive spirometer

STEPS	RATIONALE
1. Assess client's risk for postoperative respiratory complications. Review medical history to identify presence of chronic pulmonary conditions (e.g., emphysema, asthma), any condition that affects chest wall movement, history of smoking, and presence of reduced hemoglobin.	During general anesthesia the lungs are not fully inflated during surgery and the cough reflex is suppressed, so mucus collects within airway passages. After surgery, client may have reduced lung volume and require greater efforts to cough and deep breathe; inadequate lung expansion can lead to atelectasis and pneumonia. Previous chronic lung conditions increase clients' risk for developing respiratory complications. Smoking damages ciliary clearance and increases mucus secretion. Reduced hemoglobin level leads to inadequate oxygenation.
2. Assess ability to cough and deep breathe by having client take deep breath, and observe movement of shoulders and chest wall. Measure chest excursion during deep breath. Ask client to cough after taking deep breath.	Reveals maximum potential for chest expansion and ability to cough forcefully; serves as baseline to measure ability to perform exercises after surgery.
3. Assess risk for postoperative thrombus formation (e.g., older clients, those with active cancer, and clients immobilized for more than 3 days). Observe for localized tenderness along the distribution of the venous system, swollen calf or thigh, calf swelling more than 3 cm compared with asymptomatic leg, pitting edema in symptomatic leg, and collateral superficial veins. If any of these signs are present, notify the health care provider.	Venous stasis, hypercoagulability, and vein trauma exist simultaneously for thrombus formation to occur (Lewis and others, 2007). After general anesthesia, circulation slows, and when rate of blood flow slows, there is greater tendency for clot formation. Immobilization results in decreased muscular contraction in lower extremities, which promotes venous stasis.

Critical Decision Point: If any of the signs of thrombus formation are present, notify the health care provider immediately.

4. Assess client's ability to move independently while in bed.	Determines existence of any mobility restrictions.
5. Explain postoperative exercises to client, including importance to recovery and physiological benefits.	Information allows client to understand significance of exercises and can motivate learning. Persons tend to learn new skills when they know the benefits they will gain.

6. Demonstrate exercises.
  A. Diaphragmatic breathing
  (1) Assist client to comfortable sitting position on side of bed or in chair or standing position.
	Upright position facilitates diaphragmatic excursion.

(2) Stand or sit facing client.	Allows client to observe breathing exercise.
(3) Instruct client to place palms of hands across from each other, down and along lower borders of anterior rib cage. Place tips of third fingers lightly together (see illustration). Demonstrate for client.	Position of hands allows client to feel movement of chest and abdomen as diaphragm descends and lungs expand.

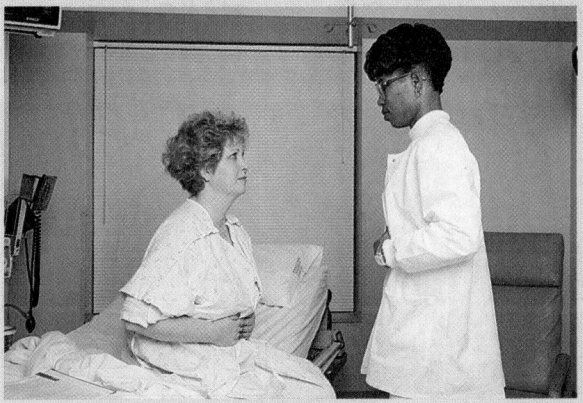

STEP 6A(3) Client learns how to feel proper abdominal breathing.

Continued

✳ **SKILL 50-1**   **DEMONSTRATING POSTOPERATIVE EXERCISES—CONT'D**

STEPS	RATIONALE
(4) Have client take slow, deep breaths, inhaling through nose, and push abdomen against hands. Tell client to feel middle fingers separate during inhalation. Demonstrate.	Taking slow, deep breaths prevents panting or hyperventilation. Inhaling through nose warms, humidifies, and filters air.
(5) Explain that client will feel normal downward movement of diaphragm during inspiration. Explain that abdominal organs descend and chest wall expands.	Explanation and demonstration focus on normal ventilatory movement of chest wall. Client develops understanding of how diaphragmatic breathing feels.
(6) Avoid using chest and shoulders while inhaling, and instruct client in same manner.	Using auxiliary chest and shoulder muscles increases useless energy expenditure.
(7) Have client hold slow, deep breath for count of three and then slowly exhale through mouth as if blowing out a candle (pursed lips). Tell client middle fingertips will touch as chest wall contracts.	Allows for gradual expulsion of all air.
(8) Repeat breathing exercise three to five times.	Allows client to observe slow, rhythmic breathing pattern. Repetition of exercise reinforces learning.
(9) Instruct client to take 10 slow, deep breaths every hour while awake during postoperative period until mobile.	Regular deep breathing prevents postoperative complications such as atelectasis and pneumonia.
B. Incentive spirometry (IS)	
(1) Perform hand hygiene.	Reduces transmission of microorganisms.
(2) Instruct client to assume semi-Fowler's or high-Fowler's position.	Promotes optimal lung expansion during respiratory maneuver.
(3) For the bariatric client, consider the reverse Trendelenburg's position.	Bariatric clients are often able to move their diaphragm better in the reverse Trendelenburg's position better than in a Fowler's position.
(4) Either set or indicate to client on the IS device scale the volume level to be attained with each breath.	Establishes goal to volume level necessary for lung expansion. Package insert helps determine target based on client height and age (Pruitt, 2006).
(5) Demonstrate to client how to place mouthpiece of IS so that lips completely cover mouthpiece (see illustration).	Demonstration is reliable technique for teaching psychomotor skill and enables client to ask questions.
(6) Instruct client to inhale slowly and maintain constant flow through unit, attempting to reach goal volume. When client reaches maximal inspiration, have client hold breath for 3 to 5 seconds (see illustration) and then exhale slowly (Pruitt, 2006). Ensure number of breaths does not exceed 10 to 12 per session.	Maintains maximal inspiration and reduces risk of progressive collapse of individual alveoli. Slow breath prevents or minimizes pain from sudden pressure changes in chest.

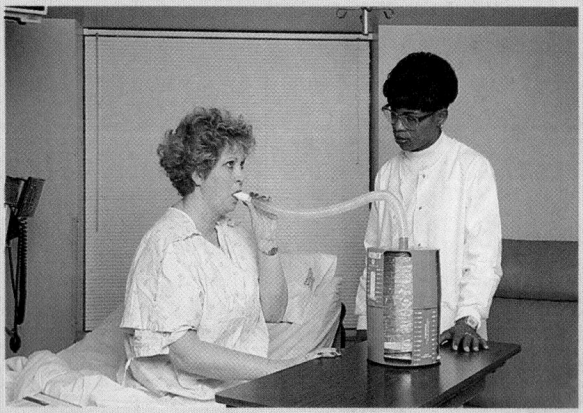

STEP 6B(5) Client inhales using incentive spirometer.

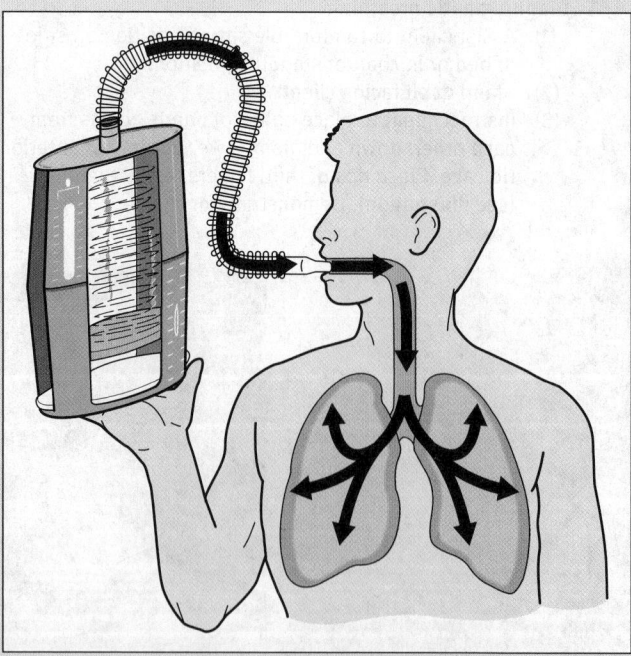

STEP 6B(6) Incentive spirometer increases flow of air into lungs.

✳ **SKILL 50-1**   **DEMONSTRATING POSTOPERATIVE EXERCISES—CONT'D**

STEPS	RATIONALE
(7) Instruct client to breathe normally for short period between the 10 breaths on IS.	Prevents hyperventilation and fatigue.
(8) Have client repeat maneuver until goals are achieved.	Ensures correct use of spirometer.
(9) Have client end with two coughs after end of 10 IS breaths.	The cough will assist with lung secretion mobilization (Pruitt, 2006).
(10) Perform hand hygiene.	Reduces transmission of microorganisms.

C. Controlled coughing

(1) Explain importance of maintaining upright position.	Position facilitates diaphragm excursion and enhances thorax expansion.
(2) Demonstrate coughing. Take two slow, deep breaths, inhaling through nose and exhaling through mouth.	Deep breaths expand lungs fully so that air moves behind mucus and facilitates effects of coughing.
(3) Inhale deeply third time, and hold breath to count of three. Cough fully for two or three consecutive coughs without inhaling between coughs. (Tell client to push all air out of lungs.)	Consecutive coughs help remove mucus more effectively and completely than one forceful cough.

Critical Decision Point: Coughing is often contraindicated after brain, spinal, head, neck, or eye surgery.

---

(4) Caution client against just clearing throat instead of coughing. Explain that coughing will not cause injury to incision when done correctly.	Clearing throat does not remove mucus from deep in airways. Postoperative incisional pain makes it harder for the client to cough effectively.
(5) If surgical incision will be abdominal or thoracic, teach client to place one hand over incisional area and other hand on top of first. During breathing and coughing exercises, client presses gently against incisional area to splint or support it. Pillow over incision is optional (see illustration).	Surgical incision cuts through muscles, tissues, and nerve endings. Deep breathing and coughing exercises place additional stress on suture line and cause discomfort. Splinting incision with hands provides firm support and reduces incisional pulling. (Some clients prefer to have pillow to place over incision.)
(6) Client continues to practice coughing exercises, splinting imaginary incision. Instruct client to cough two to three times every 2 hours while awake.	Stress value of deep coughing with splinting to effectively expectorate mucus with less discomfort.
(7) Instruct client to examine sputum for consistency, odor, amount, and color changes.	Sputum characteristics indicate presence of pulmonary complication, such as pneumonia.

D. Turning

(1) Instruct client to assume supine position and move to side of bed if permitted by surgery. Have client move by bending knees and pressing heels against the mattress to raise and move buttocks (see illustration). Top side rails on both sides of bed should be in up position.	Positioning begins on side of bed so that turning to other side will not cause client to roll toward bed's edge.
(2) Instruct client to place right hand over incisional area to splint it.	Supports and minimizes pulling on suture line during turning.

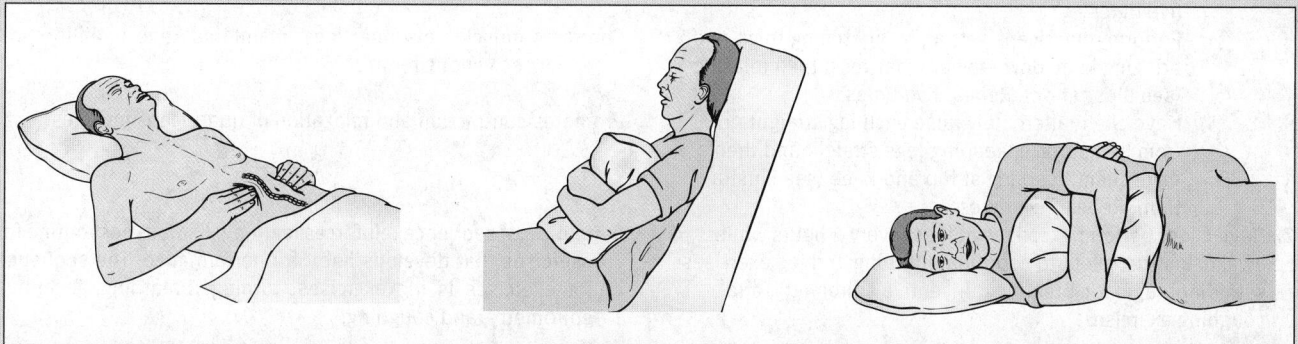

STEP 6C(5) Techniques for splinting incision. (From Lewis S and others: *Medical-surgical nursing: assessment and management of clinical problems*, ed 7, St. Louis, 2007, Mosby.)

Continued

✳ **SKILL 50-1**   **DEMONSTRATING POSTOPERATIVE EXERCISES—CONT'D**

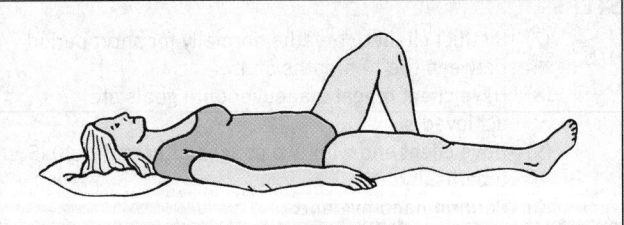

STEP 6D(1) Buttocks lift.

STEP 6D(3) Leg position for turning.

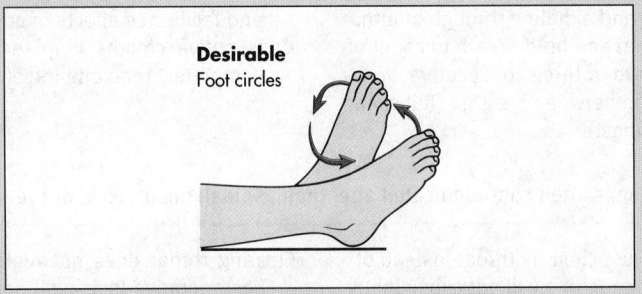

Desirable
Foot circles

STEP 6E(2) Foot circles. (From Lewis S and others: *Medical-surgical nursing: assessment and management of clinical problems,* ed 7, St. Louis, 2007, Mosby.)

STEPS	RATIONALE
(3) Instruct client to keep right leg straight and flex left knee up (see illustration). If back or vascular surgery was performed, client will need to logroll or will require assistance with turning.	Straight leg stabilizes client's position. Flexed left leg shifts weight for easier turning.
(4) Have client grab right side rail with left hand, pull toward right, and roll onto right side.	Pulling toward side rail reduces effort needed for turning.
(5) Instruct client to turn every 2 hours while awake.	Reduces risk of vascular and pulmonary complications.
E. **Leg exercises**	
(1) Have client assume supine position in bed. Demonstrate leg exercises by performing passive range-of-motion exercises and simultaneously explaining exercise.	Provides normal anatomical position of lower extremities. Depending on the surgical procedure and client status, some of these leg exercises may be contraindicated.
(2) Rotate each ankle in complete circle. Instruct client to draw imaginary circles with big toe (see illustration). Repeat five times.	Leg exercises maintain joint mobility and promote venous return to prevent thrombi.
(3) Alternate dorsiflexion and plantar flexion of both feet. Direct client to feel calf muscles contract and relax alternately (see illustrations *A* and *B*). Repeat five times.	Stretches and contracts gastrocnemius muscles.
(4) Perform quadriceps setting by tightening thigh and bringing knee down toward mattress, then relaxing (see illustration). Repeat five times.	Contracts muscles of upper legs, maintains knee mobility, and enhances venous return.
(5) Have client alternately raise each leg straight up from bed surface, keeping legs straight and then have client bend leg at hip and knee (see illustration). Repeat five times.	Promotes contraction and relaxation of quadriceps muscles.
7. Have client perform exercises at least every 2 hours while awake. Instruct client to coordinate turning and leg exercises with diaphragmatic breathing, incentive spirometry, and coughing exercises.	Repetition of sequence reinforces learning. Establishes routine for exercises that develops habit for performance. The sequence for exercises is leg exercises, turning, breathing, incentive spirometry, and coughing.

✳ **SKILL 50-1**   **DEMONSTRATING POSTOPERATIVE EXERCISES—CONT'D**

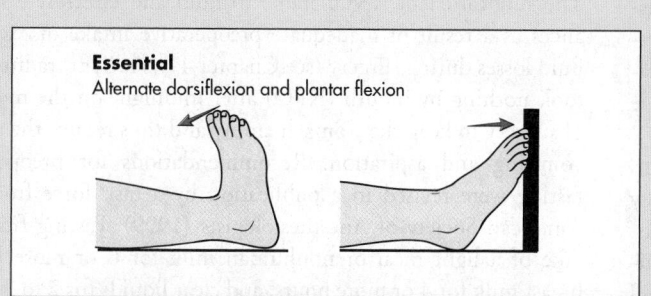

A

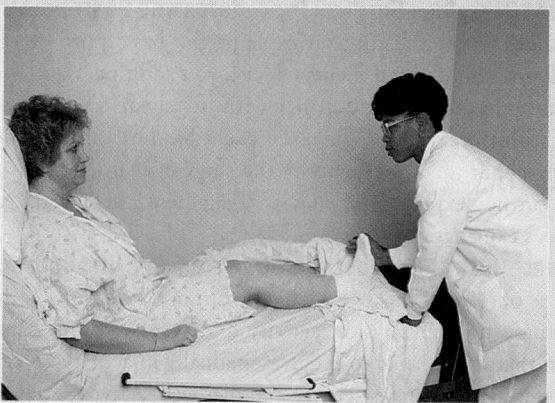

B

STEP 6E(3) A, Alternate dorsiflexion and plantar flexion. (From Lewis S and others: *Medical-surgical nursing: assessment and management of clinical problems,* ed 7, St. Louis, 2007, Mosby.) **B,** Client pushes feet to perform plantar flexion.

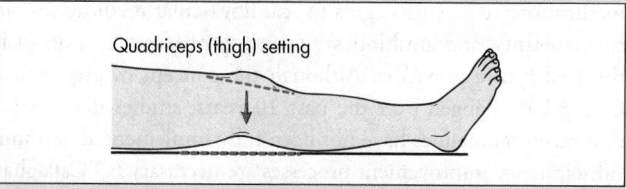

STEP 6E(4) Quadriceps (thigh) setting. (From Lewis S and others: *Medical-surgical nursing: assessment and management of clinical problems,* ed 7, St. Louis, 2007, Mosby.)

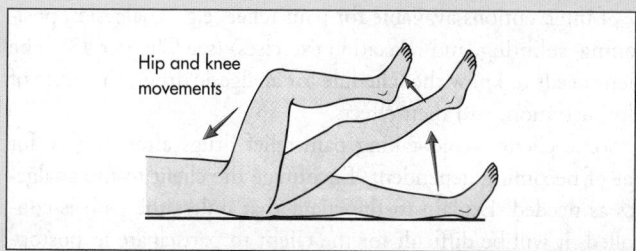

STEP 6E(5) Hip and knee movements. (From Lewis S and others: *Medical-surgical nursing: assessment and management of clinical problems,* ed 7, St. Louis, 2007, Mosby.)

STEPS	RATIONALE
8. Observe and document client's ability to perform all five exercises independently.	Ensures that client has learned correct technique. Documentation of client's response to education provides data for instructional follow-up.

Unexpected Outcomes and Related Interventions

1. Client is unable to perform exercises correctly preoperatively.
   a. Assess for the presence of anxiety, pain, and fatigue.
   b. Teach client stress reduction techniques and/or pain management strategies.
   c. Repeat teaching using more demonstration or redemonstration at time when family or friends are present.
2. Client is unwilling to perform exercises postoperatively because of incisional pain of thorax or abdomen (deep breathing, coughing, and turning) or because of surgery involving lower abdomen, groin, buttocks, or legs (leg exercises, turning).
   a. Instruct client to ask for pain medication 30 minutes before performing postoperative exercise or to use patient-controlled analgesia (PCA) immediately before exercising.
   b. Report to surgeon or pain team inadequate pain relief and need to change analgesic or increase dose.

Recording and Reporting

- Record exercises demonstrated and whether client is able to perform them independently.
- Report any problems client has in completing exercises to nurse assigned to client on next shift for follow-up.

Home Care Considerations

- Incorporate teaching of family members to assist client with implementation of postoperative exercises at home.

whether the client is likely to have IV lines, monitoring lines, dressings, or drainage tubes or will require ventilator support.

Client Describes Surgical Procedures and Postoperative Treatment. After the surgeon explains the basic purpose of a surgical procedure, some clients will ask you additional questions to clarify information. First clarify with the client what was discussed with the surgeon. When the client has little or no understanding about the surgery, notify the surgeon that the client requires further explanation. You can augment the health care provider's explanations.

Client Describes Postoperative Activity Resumption. The type of surgery clients undergo determines how quickly they can resume normal physical activity and regular eating habits. Explain that it is normal to progress gradually in activity and eating. If the client tolerates activity and diet well, activity levels will progress more quickly.

Client Verbalizes Pain-Relief Measures. Pain is one of the surgical client's fears. The family is also concerned for the client's comfort. Pain after surgery is expected. Inform the client and family of interventions available for pain relief (e.g., analgesics, positioning, splinting, and relaxation exercises) (see Chapter 43). The client needs to know the schedule for analgesic drugs, the route of administration, and their effects.

Some clients avoid taking pain-relief drugs after surgery for fear of becoming dependent. Encourage the client to use analgesics as needed. Explain to the client that unless the pain is controlled, it will be difficult for the client to participate in postoperative therapy. Encourage the client to take pain medications at regular intervals. Closely assess client's pain level, tolerance to activity, and response to pain-relieving interventions. When pain is not regularly addressed, it becomes excruciating, and an analgesic often will not provide relief at the dose ordered. Teach clients who will have patient-controlled analgesia (PCA) how to push the button, the need to push the button when beginning to feel discomfort, and that use of the PCA will not cause overmedication (see Chapter 43). Also explain to the client the length of time that it takes for the drug to begin working. Information from preoperative pain assessment will be helpful when teaching about pain-relief measures. Explore pain reporting and expectations regarding pain management based on a client's cultural beliefs.

Client Expresses Feelings Regarding Surgery. Some clients feel like part of an assembly line during the preoperative phase. Frequent visits by staff, diagnostic testing, and physical preparation for surgery consume time, and the client has few opportunities to reflect on the experience. Recognize the client as a unique individual. The client and family need time to express feelings about surgery. The client's level of anxiety influences the frequency of discussions. While delivering routine care, encourage expression of concerns. The family may wish to discuss concerns without the client so that their fears will not frighten the client and vice versa. The establishment of a trusting and therapeutic relationship with the client and family allows this to happen.

Acute Care. Acute care activities in the preoperative phase focus on interventions to physically prepare the client for surgery.

Physical Preparation. The degree of preoperative physical preparation depends on the client's health status, the planned

surgery, and the surgeon's preferences. A seriously ill client receives more supportive care in the form of medications, IV fluid therapy, and monitoring than the client facing a minor elective procedure.

Maintenance of Normal Fluid and Electrolyte Balance. The surgical client is vulnerable to fluid and electrolyte imbalances as a result of inadequate preoperative intake or excessive fluid losses during surgery (see Chapter 41). A client traditionally took nothing by mouth (NPO) after midnight on the morning of surgery to keep the stomach empty and thus reduce the risk of vomiting and aspiration. Recommendations for preoperative fasting were revised in a publication by a task force from the American Society of Anesthesiologists (1999). Fasting from intake of a light meal or nonhuman milk for 6 or more hours, breast milk for 4 or more hours, and clear liquids for 2 to 3 hours before elective procedures requiring general anesthesia, regional anesthesia, or sedation is now recommended.

Agencies vary as to the extent these guidelines have been adopted. Remove fluids and solid foods from the client's bedside, and post a sign over the bed to alert hospital personnel and family members about fasting restrictions. Some clients take specific medications (e.g., anticoagulants, cardiovascular medications, anticonvulsants, and antibiotics) with a sip of water as ordered by the health care providers. Although the concept of preoperative fasting has changed over the past 10 years, studies demonstrate that recent guidelines have not been fully implemented and multidisciplinary improvement processes are necessary (O'Callaghan, 2002).

A client who is at home the evening before surgery needs to understand the importance of the specific fasting period that is ordered. Allow the client to rinse the mouth with water or mouthwash and brush the teeth immediately before surgery as long as the client does not swallow water. Notify the surgeon and anesthesia provider if the client eats or drinks during the fasting period.

During surgery, normal mechanisms for controlling fluid and electrolyte balance, including respiration, digestion, circulation, and elimination, are disturbed. Extensive losses of blood and other body fluids sometimes occurs. The surgical stress response aggravates any fluid and electrolyte imbalance. Preoperatively, the client is encouraged to eat foods high in protein, with sufficient carbohydrates, fat, and vitamins. If a client cannot eat because of gastrointestinal alterations or impairments in consciousness, you will probably start an IV route for fluid replacement. The health care provider assesses serum electrolyte levels to determine the type of IV fluids and electrolyte additives to administer. Clients with severe nutritional imbalances sometimes require supplements with concentrated protein and glucose (see Chapter 44).

Reduction of Risk of Surgical Wound Infection. The risk of developing a surgical wound infection is determined by the amount and type of microorganisms contaminating a wound, susceptibility of the host, and the surgical wound itself. All three factors interact to cause infection. Antibiotics may be ordered in the preoperative period. A reduction in wound infection rates occurs when an antibiotic is present in sufficient concentrations at the wound site before incision (Polk and Christmas, 2000). The surgeon will order a specific time before surgery for the oral antibiotic to be taken or IV antibiotic to be administered.

The skin is a favorite site for microorganisms to grow and multiply. Without proper skin preparation, the risk of postoperative wound infection is high. Many surgeons have clients bathe or shower the evening before surgery. Some health care providers request clients to bathe or shower more than once, whereas others may have clients use an antibacterial soap to cleanse the proposed operative site. Depending on the surgical procedure, some clients shower the morning of surgery. If the surgical procedure involves the head, neck, or upper chest area, the client may also be required to shampoo the hair. Cleansing and trimming of fingernails and toenails is sometimes necessary.

The need for hair removal depends on the amount of hair, location of the incision, and surgical procedure planned (AORN, 2002c). Hair removal can damage and cause breaks in the client's skin, which allows for the entry of microorganisms. If required, perform hair removal, preferably with a clipper or shaver, as close to the time of surgery as possible. Short hospital stays reduce the chance of a health care–associated infection. Clients can acquire respiratory, urinary tract, and wound infections during hospitalization. This is one advantage to having ambulatory surgical procedures, because the client usually returns home after surgery.

Prevention of Bowel and Bladder Incontinence. Some clients receive a bowel preparation (e.g., a cathartic or enema) if the surgery involves the lower gastrointestinal system or lower abdominal organs. Manipulation of portions of the gastrointestinal tract during surgery results in absence of peristalsis for 24 hours and sometimes longer. Enemas and cathartics, such as GoLytely, cleanse the gastrointestinal tract to prevent intraoperative incontinence and postoperative constipation. An empty bowel reduces risk of injury to the intestines and minimizes contamination of the operative wound if a portion of the bowel is incised or opened accidentally or if colon surgery is planned. The surgeon's order will read "give enemas until clear." This means that you administer enemas until the enema return contains no solid fecal material (see Chapter 46). Too many enemas given over a short time can cause serious fluid and electrolyte imbalances. Most agencies limit the number of enemas (usually three) a nurse may administer successively. Recheck potassium level after completing bowel preparation.

Promotion of Rest and Comfort. Rest is essential for normal healing. Anxiety about the impending surgery can easily interfere with the ability to relax or sleep. The underlying condition requiring surgery is often painful, further impairing rest. Attempt to make the client's environment quiet and comfortable. The health care provider may order a sedative-hypnotic or anxiolytic agent for the night before surgery. Sedative-hypnotics (e.g., temazepam [Restoril]) affect and promote sleep. Anxiolytic agents (e.g., alprazolam [Xanax]) act on the cerebral cortex and limbic system to relieve anxiety.

Preparation on the Day of Surgery.
Nurses complete several routine procedures before releasing clients for surgery.

Hygiene. Basic hygiene measures provide additional comfort before surgery. If the hospitalized client is unwilling to take a complete bath, a partial bath is refreshing and removes irritating secretions or drainage from the skin. Because the client cannot wear personal nightwear to the operating room because it is restrictive and can be a flammable hazard, provide a clean hospital gown. If the client has been NPO the last several hours, the cli-

ent's mouth is often very dry. Offer the client mouthwash and toothpaste, again cautioning the client not to swallow water.

Hair and Cosmetics. During surgery with the client under general anesthesia, the client's head is positioned to introduce an endotracheal tube into the airway (see Chapter 40). This procedure may involve manipulation of the client's hair and scalp. To avoid injury ask the client to remove hairpins or clips before leaving for surgery. Electrocautery is frequently used during surgery. Hairpins and clips can become an exit source for the electricity and cause burns. Remove hairpieces or wigs as well. Braid long hair. The client applies a disposable hat before entering the operating room.

During and after surgery the anesthesia provider and nurse assess skin and mucous membranes to determine the client's level of oxygenation and circulation. Therefore remove all makeup (lipstick, powder, blush, nail polish) to expose normal skin and nail coloring. Pulse oximetry records accurate measurements through most nail polish colors, but removal is still considered good practice. Also remove contact lenses, false eyelashes, and eye makeup. Give the client's glasses to the family immediately before the client enters the operating room.

Removal of Prostheses. It is easy for any type of prosthetic device to become lost or damaged during surgery. The client needs to remove all prostheses, including partial or complete dentures, artificial limbs, artificial eyes, and hearing aids. If a client has a brace or splint, check with the health care provider to determine whether it should remain with the client.

For many clients it is embarrassing to remove dentures, wigs, or other devices that enhance personal appearance. Always offer privacy as the client removes personal items. Clients are sometimes allowed to keep personal items until they reach the preoperative area. Place dentures in special containers labeled with the client's name and other identification required by the agency, for safekeeping to prevent loss or breakage. In many agencies you will document an inventory of all prosthetic devices or personal items and have them locked away for safekeeping according to policy. It is also common practice for nurses to give prostheses to family members or to keep the devices at the client's bedside. Document these actions in the nursing notes, surgical checklist, or per agency policy.

Safeguarding Valuables. If a client has any valuables, give them to family members or secure them for safekeeping. Many hospitals require clients to sign a release to free the institution of responsibility for lost valuables. Valuables are usually stored and locked in a designated location. Often clients are reluctant to remove wedding rings or religious medals. A wedding band can be taped in place but this is not the preferred practice. If there is a risk that the client will experience swelling of the hand or fingers (mastectomy, hand surgery, fluid shifts), remove the band. Many hospitals allow clients to pin religious medals to their gowns, although the risk of loss increases. For safety as discussed above with risk of burns, remove other metal items such as piercings. Document the location of valuables per hospital policy.

Preparing the Bowel and Bladder. Some clients require an enema or cathartic the morning of surgery to ensure that the colon is empty. If so, give it at least an hour before the client will leave, allowing time for the client to defecate without rushing. Instruct the client to void just before leaving for the operating room and before giving preoperative medications. An empty bladder reduces discomfort during the procedure and reduces the risk of incontinence during surgery. If the client is unable to void, record this information on the preoperative checklist. An indwelling or straight urinary catheter may be placed if the surgery is long or the incision is in the lower abdomen.

Vital Signs. The nurse measures a final preoperative set of vital signs. The anesthesia provider uses these values as a baseline for intraoperative vital signs. If preoperative vital signs are abnormal, surgery may need to be postponed. Notify the health care providers of any abnormalities before sending the client to surgery.

Documentation. Before the client goes to the operating room, check the contents of the medical record to be sure that pertinent laboratory results are present. Check consent forms for accuracy of information. A preoperative checklist (Figure 50-3) provides guidelines for ensuring completion of nursing interventions. Check the nurses' notes to be sure that documentation of care is current. This is especially important if the hospitalized client experienced unpredicted problems the night before surgery. Send a current medication administration record to the operating room.

BARNES JEWISH Hospital
BJC HealthCare™
SURGICAL/PROCEDURE CHECKLIST
Complete this side for inpatients & outpatients having any invasive procedure

Please check (✔) the appropriate box (☐) and fill in the blank(s) as needed.

ADDRESSOGRAPH

Date of Procedure: _____ Type of Procedure: _____

Off Floor Reports printed and placed in chart: ☐ Yes ☐ No ☐ N/A: _____

ITEM	Yes/Initials	NA	COMMENT	Date
Face sheet in chart				
Consent to Surgery or Other Procedure signed			☐ To be signed in treatment area.	
SPECIALTY Consent signed			☐ To be signed in treatment area. (Specify)	
Transfusion consent signed				
ID Band on				
Allergies Noted: ☐ Armband ☐ Front of Chart ☐ Medication Record				
Height & Weight documented				
Dentures, eyeglasses, contact lenses, nail polish, hairpins, prosthesis, jewelry removed				
Surgical/Procedural skin prep done				
Patient in hospital gown/pajamas				
Patient has been NPO since: _____				
Voided or catheterized				
Vital Signs taken and documented				
Patient is on Isolation			(Specify)	
History & physical in chart				
Lab work in chart (Printed Off Floor reports)				
Urinalysis in chart				
EKG in chart				
Chest X-ray (done if ordered)				
Change in condition/VS reported to:				
Valuables/Inventory checklist done				
Pre-Operative meds given:				
Addressograph plate in chart				
Patient transferred to Surgical/Procedure area in HIS				
Mode of travel: ☐ Amb ☐ W/C ☐ Stretcher ☐ Bed				
Operative Site Marked			☐ Site to be marked in holding area	
Case Cancelled				

Family contact during surgery:

Name: _____ Location: _____ Phone: _____

INITIALS	SIGNATURES	INITIALS	SIGNATURES

BJ 2-3343-465 V15 (07/03) Page 1 of 2 TAB: TREATMENT

DO NOT WRITE BELOW THIS LINE

BJ 2-3343-465

Figure 50-3 Preoperative checklist. (Courtesy Barnes-Jewish Hospital, St. Louis.)

CHAPTER 11
References

Baltes PB, Kunzmann U: The two faces of wisdom: Wisdom as a general theory of knowledge and judgment about excellence in mind and virtue vs. wisdom as everyday realization in people and products, *Hum Dev* 47:290, 2004.

Berger KS: *The developing person: through the life span,* ed 6, New York, 2005, Worth Publishers.

Berk L: *Child development,* ed 6, Boston, 2003, Allyn & Bacon.

Crain W: *Theories of development: concepts and applications,* ed 3, Englewood Cliffs, NJ, 1992, Prentice Hall.

Elder GH, Shanahan MJ: The life course and human development. In Damon W, Lerner R, editors: *Handbook of child psychology,* ed 6, New York, 2006, Wiley.

Erikson E: *Childhood and society,* New York, 1963, Norton.

Gesell A: *Studies in child development,* New York, 1948, Harper.

Hockenberry MJ, Wilson D: *Wong's nursing care of infants and children,* ed 8, St. Louis, 2007, Mosby.

Kagan J, Fox NA: Biology, culture, and temperamental biases. In Damon W, Lerner R, editors: *Handbook of child psychology,* ed 6, New York, 2006, Wiley.

Kohlberg L. *The philosophy of moral development: moral stages and the idea of justice,* San Francisco, 1981, Harper & Row.

LoBiondo-Wood G, Haber J: *Nursing research: methods and critical appraisal for evidence-based practice,* ed 6, St. Louis, 2006, Mosby.

Santrock JW: *Life-span development,* ed 9, San Francisco, 2004, McGraw-Hill.

Singer DG, Revenson TA: *A Piaget primer: how a child thinks,* New York, 1996, Penguin Books.

Taffell R: Values you teach your child by age five, *Parents,* p 118, December 2002.

Research Reference

Ugarriza DN: Elderly women's explanation of depression, *J Gerontol Nurs* 28(5):22, 2002.

CHAPTER 12
References

American Heart Association: Dietary recommendations for children and adolescents: a guide for practitioners: consensus statement for the American Heart Association, *Circulation,* 112:2061, 2005.

Ball J, Bindler R: *Child health nursing: partnering with children and families,* Upper Saddle River, NJ, 2006, Pearson Prentice Hall.

Behrman R, Kliegman R, Jenson H: *Nelson textbook of pediatrics,* Philadelphia, 2000, Saunders.

Berger K: *The developing person: through the life span,* New York, 2005, Worth.

Deering C, Cody D: Communicating with children and adolescents, *Am J Nurs* 102(3):34, 2002.

Erikson EH: *Childhood and society,* ed 2, New York, 1963, Norton.

Erikson EH: *Identity: youth and crises,* New York, 1968, Norton.

Galanti G: *Caring for patients from different cultures,* ed 3, Philadelphia, 2004, University of Pennsylvania Press.

Hilton J: Folic acid intake of young women, *J Obstet Gynecol Neonatal Nurse* 31(2):172, 2002.

Hockenberry M, Wilson D: *Wong's nursing care of infants and children,* ed 8, St. Louis, 2007, Mosby.

Kinservik M, Friedhoff M: Control issues in toilet training, *Pediatr Nurs* 26(3):267, 2000.

Kohlberg L: Development of moral character and moral ideology. In Hoffman ML, Hoffman LNW, editors: *Review of child development research,* vol 1, New York, 1964, Russell Sage Foundation.

Murray S, McKinney E: *Foundations of maternal-newborn nursing,* ed 4, St. Louis, 2006, Saunders.

Piaget J: *The origins of intelligence in children,* New York, 1952, International Universities Press.

Santrock J: *Life-span development,* ed 9, New York, 2007, McGraw Hill.

U.S. Department of Agriculture, Center for Nutrition Policy and Promotion, *MyPyramid for kids,* Washington, DC, 2005, The Department, http://www.cnpp.usda.gov/MyPyramidforKids.htm, accessed March 3, 2007.

U.S. Department of Health and Human Services: *Healthy People 2010: with understanding and improving health and objectives for improving health,* ed 2, Washington, DC, 2000, U.S. Government Printing Office.

U.S. Department of Health and Human Services, Administration on Children, Youth, and Family: *Child maltreatment 2002,* Washington, DC, 2004, The Department.

Research References

Askin D: Complication in the transition from fetal to neonatal life, *J Obstet Gynecol Neonatal Nurs* 31(3):318, 2002.

Gill S: The little things: perceptions of breastfeeding support, *J Obstet Gynecol Neonatal Nurs* 30(4):401, 2001.

Popovich D: Sexuality in early childhood: pediatric nurses' attitudes, knowledge, and clinical practice, *Pediatr Nurs* 26(5):484, 2000.

CHAPTER 13
References

AFL-CIO: *Working women fast facts,* 2004, http://www.aflcio.org/issues/factsstats/upload/women.pdf.

American Academy of Pediatrics: Technical report: coparent or second-parent adoption by same-sex parents, *Pediatrics* 109(2):341, 2002, http://www.aap.org/policy/020008t.html.

Diekelmann J: The young adult: the choice is health or illness, *Am J Nurs* 76:1276, 1976.

Edelman C, Mandle C: *Health promotion throughout the life span,* ed 5, St. Louis, 2002, Mosby.

Erickson E: *Childhood society,* ed 2, New York, 1963, WW Norton.

Erickson E: *The lifecycle completed: a review,* New York, 1982, WW Norton.

Fortinash K, Holoday Worret, P: *Psychiatric mental health nursing,* ed 3, St. Louis, 2004, Mosby.

Gilligan C: *In a different voice,* Cambridge, Mass, 1993, Harvard University Press.

Havighurst R: Successful aging. In Williams RH, Tibbits C, Donahue W, editors: *Process of aging,* vol 1, New York, 1972, Atherton.

Huether S, McCance K: *Understanding pathophysiology,* ed 3, St. Louis, 2004, Mosby.

Levinson D and others: *The seasons of a man's life,* New York, 1978, Knopf.

Lowdermilk D, Perry S: *Maternity nursing,* ed 6, St. Louis, 2003, Mosby.

Masters W, Johnson V: *Human sexual response,* Boston, 1970, Little, Brown.

Stanhope M, Lancaster J: *Community and public health nursing,* ed 6, St. Louis, 2004, Mosby.

U.S. Census Bureau: *U.S. interim projections by age, sex, race, and Hispanic origin,* March 2004, http://www.census.gov/ipc/www/usinterimproj.

U.S. Census Bureau: *Income, poverty and health insurance coverage in the United States, 2005,* August 2006, http://www.census.gov/prod/2006pubs/p60-231.pdf .

U.S. Department of Commerce, Census Bureau: *Resident population estimates of the United States by age and sex,* 2000, http://eire.census.gov/popest/archives/national/nation2/intfile2-1.txt.

U.S. Department of Health and Human Services, Centers for Disease Control and Prevention: Trends in reportable sexually transmitted diseases in the United States, 2004, 2004, http://www.cdc.gov/std/stats/04pdf/trends2004.pdf.

U.S. Department of Health and Human Services, Public Health Service: Deaths: leading causes for 2002, *Natl Vital Stat Rep* 53(17), Hyattsville, Md, 2005, Centers for Disease Control and Prevention, National Center for Health Statistics, http://www.cdc.gov/nchs/data/nvsr/nvsr53/nvsr53_17.pdf.

U.S. Department of Health and Human Services, Centers for Disease Control and Prevention: State-specific prevalence of obesity among adults—United States, 2005, *MMWR* 55(36):985, 2006.

U.S. Department of Labor, Bureau of Labor Statistics: *Tomorrow's jobs,* 2005.

U.S. Department of Labor, Women's Bureau: *Older women workers, ages 55 and over,* Washington, DC, 2006, U.S. Department of Labor, http://www.dol.gov/wb/factsheets/Qf-olderworkers55.htm.

Woman Employed Institute: *Facts about working women,* 2004, http://www.womenemployed.org/docs/Facts%20about%20Working%20Women.pdf#search=%22Facts%20on%20women%20workers%22.

Research References

Campbell DA and others: A randomized control trial of continuous support in labor by a lay doula, *J Obstet Gynecol Neonatal Nurs* 35(4):456, 2006.

Dunn S and others: The relationship between vulnerability factors and breastfeeding outcome, *J Obstet Gynecol Neonatal Nurs* 35(1):87, 2006.

Fager JH, Melnyk B: The effectiveness of intervention studies to decrease alcohol use in college undergraduate students: an integrative analysis, *J Nurs Scholarsh* 1(2):102, 2004.

Hung C: Predictors of postpartum women's health status, *J Nurs Scholarsh* 36(4):345, 2004.

McManus A and others: Lesbian experiences and needs during childbirth: guidance for health care providers, *J Obstet Gynecol Neonatal Nurs* 35(1):13, 2006.

Santacroce SJ, Lee YL: Uncertainty, posttraumatic stress, and health behavior in young adult childhood cancer survivors, *Nurs Res* 55(4):259, 2006.

Sauls DJ: Dimensions of professional labor support for intrapartum practice, *J Nurs Scholarsh* 38(1):36, 2006.

Wang CY, Chan SMA: Culturally tailored diabetes education program for Chinese Americans, *Nurs Res* 54(5):347, 2005.

CHAPTER 14
References

Administration on Aging: *A profile of older Americans: 2005,* 2005, http://www.aoa.gov/PROF/statistics/profile/2005/2.asp.

Administration on Aging: *A statistical profile of older Americans aged 65+,* 2006, http://www.aoa.gov/PRESS/fact/pdf/Attachment_1304.pdf.

Amella EJ: Mealtime difficulties. In Mezey M, Fulmer T, Abraham I, Editors: *Geriatric nursing protocols for best practice,* ed 2, New York, 2003, Springer.

Amella EJ: Presentation of illness in older adults, *Am J Nurs* 104(10):40, 2004.

American Association of Retired Persons: *A profile of older Americans: 2004,* 2004, http://assets.aarp.org/rgcenter/general/profile_2004.

American Cancer Society: *Cancer facts and figures,* 2006, http://www.cancer.org.

American Geriatrics Society Panel on Persistent Pain in Older Persons: The management of persistent pain in older persons, *J Am Geriatr Soc* 50(6 suppl):S205, 2002.

Atkinson PJ: Intimacy and sexuality. In Meiner S, Lueckenotte A, editors: *Gerontologic nursing,* ed 3, St. Louis, 2006, Mosby.

Beers MH: *The Merck manual of geriatrics,* ed 3, Whitehouse Station, NJ, 2000, Merck.

Beers MH: *The Merck manual of geriatrics,* ed 3, Whitehouse Station, NJ, 2005, Merck, http://www.merck.com/mrkshared/mmg/sec11/ch85/ch85a.jsp.

Bolla L, Fille C, Palmer R: Office diagnosis of the four major types of dementia, *Geriatrics* 55(1):34, 2000.

Centers for Disease Control and Prevention: *Healthy aging: preventing disease and improving quality of life among older Americans 2003, at a glance,* 2003, Department of Health and Human Services.

Centers for Disease Control and Prevention: *National vital statistics report, death: leading causes for 2002,* 2005, http:www.cdc.gov/nchs/data/nvsr/nvsr53_17.pdf.

Centers for Disease Control and Prevention: Web-based injury statistics query and reporting system (WISQARS), 2006, National Center for Injury Prevention and Control, Centers for Disease Control and Prevention, http://www.cdc.gov/wisqars.

Cummings E, Henry W: *Growing old: the process of disengagement,* New York, 1961, Basic Books.

Davidhizar R, Eshlernan J, Moody M: Health promotion for aging adults, *Geriatr Nurs* 23(1):28, 2002.

Day C: Validation therapy: a review of the literature, *J Gerontol Nurs* 23(4):29, 1997.

Dowling-Castronovo A, Bradway C: Urinary incontinence. In Mezey M, Fulmer T, Abraham I, editors: *Geriatric nursing protocols for best practice,* ed 2, New York, 2003, Springer.

Ebersole P, Hess P, Luggen, A: *Toward healthy aging: human needs and nursing response,* ed 6, St. Louis, 2004, Mosby.

Ebersole P and others: *Gerontological nursing and healthy aging,* ed 2, St. Louis, 2005, Mosby.

Flaherty E, Fulmer T, Mezey M, Editors: *Geriatric nursing review syllabus: a core curriculum in advanced practice geriatric nursing,* New York, 2003, American Geriatrics Society.

Foreman M and others: Assessing cognitive function. In Mezey M, Fulmer T, Abraham I, Editors: *Geriatric nursing protocols for best practice,* ed 2, New York, 2003, Springer.

Friedman S: Loss and end-of-life issues. In Meiner S, Lueckenotte A, editors: *Gerontolgic nursing,* ed 3, St. Louis, 2006, Mosby.

Hammerlein A, Derendorf H, Lowenthal DT: Pharmacokinetic and pharmacodynamic changes in the elderly: clinical implications, *Clin Pharmacokinet* 35(1):49, 1998.

Havighurst RJ, Neugarten BL, Tobin SS: Disengagement, personality and life satisfaction in the later years. In Hansen P, editor: *Age with a future,* Copenhagen, 1963, Munksgoasrd.

Herr K: Chronic pain: challenges and assessment strategies, *J Gerontol Nurs* 28(1):20, 2002.

Kanapaux W: Homosexual seniors face stigma, *Geriatric Times* 4(6), 2003.

Krevesic DM, Mezey M: Assessment of function. In Mezey M, Fulmer T, Abraham I, Editors: *Geriatric nursing protocols for best practice,* ed 2, New York, 2003, Springer.

Meiner SE, Lueckenotte AG: Overview of gerontologic nursing. In Meiner SE, Lueckenotte AG, editors: *Gerontolgic nursing,* ed 3, St. Louis, 2006, Mosby.

Murphy SL: Deaths: final data for 1998, *Natl Vital Stat Rep* 48(11), Hyattsville, Md, 2000, National Center for Health Statistics Trends in Health and Aging: *Prevalence of selected chronic conditions by age, sex, race/ethnicity: United States, 1997-2004,* NHIS (NHIC04). http://www.cdc.gov/nchs/agingact.htm, accessed on January 12, 2007.

National Osteoporosis Foundation: *Fast facts,* 2006, http://www.nof.org/osteoporosis/diseasefacts.htm.

Neugarten B: *Personality in middle and late life,* New York, 1964, Atherton.

Rantz M, Popejoy L, Zwygart-Stauffacher M: *The new nursing homes: a 20-minute way to find great long-term care,* Minneapolis, 2001, Fairview Press.

Regan S, Fowler C: Influenza: past, present, and future, *J Gerontol Nurs* 28(11):31, 2002.

Resnick B: Health promotion and illness/disability prevention. In Meiner S, Lueckenotte A, editors: *Gerontolgic nursing,* ed 3, St. Louis, 2006, Mosby.

Reuben DB and others: *Geriatrics at your fingertips,* ed 7, New York, 2005, The American Geriatrics Society.

The Joint Commission: *National patient safety goals,* 2007, http://www.jointcommission.org/PatientSafety/, 2006, accessed January 31, 2007.

Tideiksaar R: *Falls in older people: prevention and management,* ed 3, Baltimore, 1998, Health Professions Press.

U. S. Census Bureau: *65+ in the United States: 2005,* 2005, http://www.census.gov/prod/2006pubs/p23-209.pdf.

U.S. Department of Health and Human Services, Public Health Service: *Healthy People 2010,* 2000, http://www.healthypeople.gov.

Research References

Naylor MD and others: Cognitively impaired older adults: from hospital to home, *Am J Nurs* 105(2):52, 2005.

Resnick B: Health promotion practices of older adults: testing an individualized approach, *J Clin Nurs* 12(1):46, 2003.

Wang, KL, Hermann C: Pilot study to test the effectiveness of healing touch on agitation in people with dementia, *Geriatr Nurs* 27(1):34, 2006.

CHAPTER 15
References

American Nurses Association: *Nursing's social policy statement,* Washington, DC, 2003, The Association.

Benner P: *From novice to expert: excellence and power in clinical nursing practice,* Menlo Park, Calif, 1984, Addison-Wesley.

Bilinski H: The mentored journal, *Nurs Educ* 27(1):37, 2002.

Chaffee J: *Thinking critically,* ed 7, Boston, 2002, Houghton Mifflin.

Facione N, Facione P: Externalizing the critical thinking in knowledge development and clinical judgment, *Nurs Outlook* 44:129, 1996.

Ferrario CG: Developing nurses' critical thinking skills with concept mapping, *JNSD,* 20(6):261-267, 2004.

Glaser E: *An experiment in the development of critical thinking,* New York, 1941, Bureau of Publications, Teachers College, Columbia University.

Hill C: Integrating clinical experiences into the concept mapping process, *Nurse Educ* 31(1):36, 2006.

Kataoka-Yahiro M, Saylor C: A critical thinking model for nursing judgment, *J Nurs Educ* 33(8):351, 1994.

Kessler PD, Lund CH: Reflective journaling: developing an online journal for distance education, *Nurse Educ* 29(1):20, 2004.

Miller M, Malcolm N: Critical thinking in the nursing curriculum, *Nurs Health Care* 11:67, 1990.

Paul RW: The art of redesigning instruction. In Willsen J, Blinker AJA, editors: *Critical thinking: how to prepare students for a rapidly changing world,* Santa Rosa, Calif, 1993, Foundation for Critical Thinking.

Paul RW, Heaslip P: Critical thinking and intuitive nursing practice, *J Adv Nurs* 22:40, 1995.

Perry W: *Forms of intellectual and ethical development in the college years: a scheme,* New York, 1979, Holt, Rinehart, & Winston.

Schuster PM: *Concept mapping: a critical thinking approach to care planning,* St. Louis, 2003, Mosby.

Watson G, Glaser E: *Watson-Glaser critical thinking appraisal manual,* New York, 1980, MacMillan.

Research References

Di Vito-Thomas P: Nursing student stories on learning how to think like a nurse, *Nurse Educ* 30(3):133, 2005.

Facione P: *Critical thinking: a statement of expert consensus for purposes of educational assessment and instruction. The Delphi report: research findings and recommendations prepared for the American Philosophical Association*, ERIC Doc No. ED 315-423, Washington, DC, 1990, ERIC.

Roche JP: A pilot study of teaching clinical decision making with the clinical educator model, *J Nurs Educ* 41(8):365, 2002.

Settersten L, Lauver DR: Critical thinking, perceived health status, and participation in health behaviors, *Nurs Res* 53(1):11, 2004.

Smith Higuchi KA, Donald JG: Thinking processes used by nurses in clinical decision making, *J Nurs Educ* 41(4):145, 2002.

Tanner C and others: The phenomenology of knowing the patient, *Image J Nurs Sch* 25:273, 1993.

White AH: Clinical decision making among fourth year nursing students: an interpretive study *J Nurs Educ* 42(3):113, 2003.

CHAPTER 16
References

Agency for Health Care Policy and Research, Acute Pain Management Guideline Panel: *Acute pain management: operative or medical procedures and trauma*, Clinical Practice Guideline, AHCPR Pub No. 92-0032, Rockville, Md, 1992, Agency for Health Care Policy and Research, Public Health Service, U.S. Department of Health and Human Services.

American Nurses Association: *Nursing's social policy statement*, ed 2, Washington, DC, 2003, The Association.

Benner P, Wrubel J: *The primacy of caring*, Menlo Park, Calif, 1989, Addison-Wesley.

Carpenito-Moyet LJ: *Nursing diagnosis: application to clinical practice*, ed 11, Philadelphia, 2005, Lippincott, Williams & Wilkins.

Gordon M: *Manual of nursing diagnoses: 1991-1992*, St. Louis, 1991, Mosby.

Gordon M: *Nursing diagnosis: process and application*, ed 3, St. Louis, 1994, Mosby.

HIPAAdvisory: OCR guidance explaining significant aspects of the privacy rule, http://www.hipaadvisory.com/regs/finalprivacymod/guidance.htm, accessed August 2006.

King M, Shell R: Teaching and evaluating critical thinking with concept maps, *Nurse Educ* 27(5):214, 2002.

Lunney M: Helping nurses use NANDA, NOC, and NIC: novice to expert, *J Nurs Adm*, 36(3):118, 2006.

Pender NJ: *Health promotion and nursing practice*, ed 3, Stamford, Conn, 1996, Appleton & Lange.

Seidel HM and others: *Mosby's guide to physical examination*, ed 5, St. Louis, 2003, Mosby.

U.S. Department of Health and Human Services, Office for Civil Rights—HIPAA: *Summary of HIPAA privacy rule*, http://www.hhs.gov/ocr/hipaa/, accessed July 23, 2006.

Research References

Hinck SM and others: Student learning with concept mapping of care plans in community-based education, *J Prof Nurs* 22(1):23, 2006.

Potter P and others: Understanding the cognitive work of nursing in the acute care environment, *J Nurs Adm* 35(7/8):327, 2005.

CHAPTER 17
References

American Nurses Association: *Model nurse practice act*, Washington, DC, 1955, The Association.

American Nurses Association: *Standards of nursing practice*, Washington, DC, 1973, The Association.

American Nurses Association: *Nursing: a social policy statement*, Washington, DC, 1980, The Association.

American Nurses Association: *Scope of nursing practice*, Washington, DC, 1987, The Association.

American Nurses Association: *Nursing's social policy statement*, ed 2, Washington, DC, 2003, The Association.

Carpenito-Moyet LJ: *Nursing diagnoses: application to clinical practice*, ed 11, Philadelphia, 2005, Lippincott, Williams & Wilkins.

Dochterman JM, Jones DA: *Unifying nursing languages: the harmonization of NANDA, NIC, NOC*, Washington, DC, 2003, American Nurses Association.

Ferrario CG: Developing nurses' critical thinking skills with concept mapping, *J Nurses Staff Dev* 20(6):261, 2004.

Fry VS: The creative approach to nursing, *Am J Nurs* 53:301, 1953.

Kim MJ, McFarland GK, McLean AM, editors: *Classification of nursing diagnoses: proceedings of the fifth conference (NANDA)*, St. Louis, 1984, Mosby.

Lunney M: Accuracy of nurses' diagnoses: foundation of NANDA, NIC, and NOC, *Nurs Diagn* 9(2):83, 1998.

McFarland GK, McFarlane EA: *Nursing diagnosis and intervention: planning for patient care*, St. Louis, 1989, Mosby.

Mueller A, Johnston M, Bligh D: Joining mind mapping and care planning to enhance student critical thinking and achieve holistic nursing care, *Nurs Diagn* 13(1):24, 2002.

NANDA International: *NANDA-I nursing diagnoses: definitions and classification, 2007-2008*, Philadelphia, 2007, NANDA International.

Schuster PM: *Concept mapping: a critical thinking approach to care planning*, St. Louis, 2003, Mosby.

Wieck KL: Diagnostic language consistency among multicultural English-speaking nurses, *Nurs Diagn* 7(2):70, 1996.

Research References

Hinck SM and others: Student learning with concept mapping of care plans in community based education, *J Prof Nurs* 22(1):23, 2006.

Hsu L, Hsieh S: Concept maps as an assessment tool in a nursing course, *J Prof Nurs* 21(3):141, 2005.

CHAPTER 18
References

Bryant RA, Nix DP: *Acute and chronic wounds: nursing management*, ed 3, St. Louis, 2007, Mosby.

Bulechek GM, Butcher HK, Dochterman JM: *Nursing interventions classification (NIC)*, ed 5, St. Louis, 2008, Mosby.

Carpenito-Moyet LJ: *Nursing diagnosis: application to clinical practice*, ed 11, Philadelphia, 2005, Lippincott, Williams & Wilkins.

Fontana D: *Managing Time*, Leicester, 1993, The British Psychological Society.

Gordon M: *Nursing diagnosis: process and application*, ed 3, St. Louis, 1994, Mosby.

Iowa Intervention Project: The NIC taxonomy structure, *Image J Nurs Sch* 25:1816, 1993.

King M, Shell R: Teaching and evaluating critical thinking with concept maps, *Nurse Educ* 27(5):214, 2002.

McCaffery M, Pasero C: *Pain: clinical manual*, ed 2, St. Louis, 1999, Mosby.

McCloskey JC, Bulechek GM: Standardizing the language for nursing treatments: an overview of the issues, *Nurs Outlook* 42:56, 1994.

Moody LE and others: Electronic health records documentation in nursing, *Comput Nurs* 22(6):337, 2004.

Moorhead S and others: *Nursing outcomes classification*, ed 4, St. Louis, 2008, Mosby.

NANDA International: *NANDA-I nursing diagnoses: definitions and classification 2007-2008*, Philadelphia, 2007, NANDA International.

Nursing and Midwifery Council: *Code of professional conduct*, London, 2002, Nursing and Midwifery Council.

Schuster PM: *Concept mapping: a critical thinking approach to care planning*, St. Louis, 2003, Mosby.

White L: *Documentation and the nursing process*, Clifton Park, NY, 2003, Delmar Learning.

Research References

Agency for Health Care Policy and Research, Panel for Treatment of Pressure Ulcers in Adults: *Treatment of pressure ulcers*, Clinical Practice Guideline No. 15, AHCPR Pub No. 95-0653, Rockville, Md, 1994, Agency for Health Care Policy and Research, Public Health Service, U.S. Department of Health and Human Services.

Hendry C, Walker A: Priority setting in clinical nursing practice: literature review, *J Adv Nurs* 47(4):427, 2004.

Potter P and others: Understanding the cognitive work of nursing in the acute care environment, *J Nurs Adm* 35(7/8):327, 2005.

CHAPTER 19
References

American Nurses Association: *Principles for delegation*, http://nursingworld.org/staffing/lawsuit/PrinciplesDelegation.pdf, accessed October 15, 2006.

Bulechek GM, Butcher HK, Dochterman JM: *Nursing interventions classification (NIC)*, ed 5, St. Louis, 2008, Mosby.

Gerontological Nursing Interventions Research Center: *Evidence-based guidelines,* University of Iowa, http://www.nursing.uiowa.edu/centers/gnirc/protocols.htm, accessed September 25, 2006.

National Guideline Clearinghouse: *Clinical practice guidelines,* Agency for Healthcare Research and Quality, http://www.guideline.gov, accessed September 25, 2006.

Redman BK: *The practice of patient education,* ed 10, St. Louis, 2005, Mosby.

Snyder M: *Independent nursing interventions,* New York, 2000, John Wiley & Sons.

Trossman S: Getting a clearer picture on delegation, *Am Nurs Today* 1(1):54, 2006.

Research References

Benner P: *From novice to expert,* Menlo Park, Calif, 1984, Addison-Wesley.

Di Vito-Thomas P: Nursing student stories on learning how to think like a nurse, *Nurse Educ* 30(3):133, 2005.

Potter P, Grant E: Understanding RN and unlicensed assistive personnel working relationships in designing care delivery strategies, *J Nurs Adm* 34(1):19, 2004.

CHAPTER 20
References

Bower JO: Designing and implementing a patient safety program for the OR, *AORN J,* 76(3):452, 2002.

Brown S: The performance improvement decision, *Nurs Manage* 37(4):16, 2006.

Donabedian A: Methods for deriving criteria for assessing the quality of medical care. *Med Care Rev* 37(7):653,1980.

Given BA, Sherwood PR: Nursing-sensitive patient outcomes—a white paper, *Oncol Nurs Forum* 32(4):773, 2005.

Institute of Medicine: *Definition of quality of care,* 2002, http://www.iom.edu/iom.

Moorhead S and others: *Nursing outcomes classification (NOC),* ed 4, St. Louis, 2008, Mosby.

The Joint Commission: *2007 Comprehensive accreditation manual for hospitals: the official handbook (CAMH),* vol 1, Standards, Chicago, 2007, The Joint Commission.

CHAPTER 21
References

American Nurses Association: Position statement on registered nurse utilization of assistive personnel, *Am Nurse* 25(2):7, 1995.

American Nurses Association (ANA), National Council of State Boards of Nursing (NCSBN): *Joint statement on delegation,* 2006, http://www.ncsbn.org/pdfs/Joint_statement.pdf.

American Nurses Credentialing Center: *ANCC magnet recognition program,* 2006, http://www.nursingworld.org/ancc/magnet/index.html.

American Nurses Credentialing Center: *Forces of magnetism,* 2007, http://www.nursecredentialing.org.magnet/forces.html.

Anders RL, Hawkins JA: *Mosby's nursing leadership and management online,* St. Louis, 2006, Mosby.

Batcheller J and others: A practice model for patient safety: the value of the experienced registered nurse, *J Nurs Adm* 34(4):200, 2004.

Bolton LB, Goodenough A: A magnet nursing service approach to nursing's role in quality management, *Nurs Adm Q* 27(4):344, 2003.

Case B: Delegation skills: critical-thinking strategies you can apply to the challenges of delegating, *Greater Chicago/Wisconsin/Indiana Advances for Nurses* 19(July 19), 2004.

Case Management Society of America: *About us: definition of case management,* 2006, http://www.cmsa.org/Default.aspx?tabid=104.

Curtis E, Nicholl H: Delegation: a key function of nursing, *Nurs Manage* 11(4):26, 2004.

Gardner DB: Ten lessons in collaboration, *Online J Issues Nurs* 10(1), Manuscript 1, 2005, http://www.nursingworld.org/ojin/topic26/tpc26_1.htm.

Hambleton JM: Fostering respectful collaboration through communication, *Pa Nurse* 60(4):10, 2005.

Hicks F: Collective action. In Yoder-Wise PS, editor: *Leading and managing in nursing,* ed 3, St. Louis, 2003, Mosby.

Keeling B and others: Appropriate delegation, *Am J Nurs* 100(12):24, 2000.

Kuntz KR: Life care plans provide a pathway to improved outcomes, *J Spec Pediatr Nurs* 10(3):143, 2005.

Marriner Tomey A: *Guide to nursing management and leadership,* ed 7, St. Louis, 2004, Mosby.

National Council of State Boards of Nursing: *Delegation: concepts and decision-making process,* Chicago, 1995, The Council.

National Council of State Boards of Nursing: *The five rights of delegation,* Chicago, 1997, The Council.

National Council of State Boards of Nursing: *Working with others: a position paper,* Chicago, 2005, The Council.

Pinkerton SE: Nurses executives: Who are they; what do they do; and what challenges do they face? In McCloskey JC, Grace HK, editors: *Current issues in nursing,* ed 6, St. Louis, 2001, Mosby.

Ritter-Teitel J: The impact of restructuring on professional nursing practice. *J Nurs Adm* 32(1):31, 2002.

Tiedeman ME, Lookinland S: Traditional models of care delivery: what have we leaned? *J Nurs Adm* 34(6): 291, 2004.

Wywialowski E: *Managing client care,* ed 3, St. Louis, 2004, Mosby.

Research References

Avitall B: Nurse telemanagement improved outcomes and reduced cost of care more than home nurse visits in chronic heart failure, *ACP J Club* 139(2):35, 2003.

Hendry C, Walker A: Priority setting in clinical nursing practice: literature review, *J Adv Nurs* 47(4):427, 2004.

Kramer M, Schmalenberg C: Development and evaluation of Essentials of Magnetism tool, *J Nurs Adm* 34(7/8):365, 2004.

Schmalenberg C and others: Securing collegial/collaborative nurse-physician relationship, part I, *J Nurs Adm* 35(10):450, 2005.

Tschannen D: The effect of individual characteristics on perceptions of collaboration in the work environment, *Medsurg Nurs* 13(5):312, 2004.

Ulrich BT and others: How RNs view the work environment: results of a national survey of registered nurses, *J Nurs Adm* 33(9):389, 2005.

CHAPTER 22
References

American Nurses Association: *Code of ethics for nurses with interpretive statements,* 2001, http://www.nursingworld.org/ethics/code/protected_nwcoe303.htm.

Beauchamp T, Childress J: *Principles of biomedical ethics,* ed 4, New York, 2001, Oxford University Press.

Boyer JR, Nelson JL: A comment on Fry's "The role of caring in a theory of nursing ethics," *Hypatia* 5(3):153, 1990.

Bureau of Health Professions: *Projected supply, demand, and shortages of registered nurses: 2000-2020,* 2002, http://newsroom.hrsa.gov/NewsBriefs/2002/nurse-shortagereport.htm.

Burke MM, Laramie JA: *Primary care of the older adult: a multidisciplinary approach,* St. Louis, 2003, Mosby.

Curtin L: The ethical handling of ethical issues. In *Journal for Respiratory Care and Sleep Medicine,* June 22, 2004, Thomson Gale.

Dressler L: *Consensus through conversation: how to achieve high-commitment decisions,* San Francisco, 2006, Barrett-Koehler.

Fallowfield L: *The quality of life: the missing measurement in health care,* London, 1990, Souvenir Press.

Henry J. Kaiser Family Foundation: *The uninsured and their access to healthcare,* 2005, http://www.kff.org/uninsured/1420-07.cfm.

Kohn LT, Corrigan JM, Donaldson MS, editors: *To err is human,* Washington, DC, 2000, National Academy Press.

Leininger M: *Caring: an essential human need,* Detroit, 1988, Wayne State University Press.

Levine M, Ganz P: Beyond the development of quality-of-life instruments: where do we go from here? *J Clin Oncol* 20(9):2215, 2002.

Maslow A: *New knowledge in human values,* New York, 1977, Harper & Row.

Merriam Webster online dictionary, 2006, http://www.m-w.com/dictionary/futile.

Miller MA, Babcock, DE: *Critical thinking applied to nursing,* St. Louis, 1996, Mosby.

Noddings N: *Caring: a feminist approach to ethics and moral education,* Berkeley, 1984, University of California Press.

Pellegrino ED: The caring ethic: the relation of physician to patient. In Bishop AH, Scudder JR, editors: *Caring, curing, coping: nurse, physician, and patient relations,* Birmingham, 1985, University of Alabama Press.

Pottinger A, Perivolaris A, Howes D: The end of life. In Srivaastava RH, editor: *Guide to clinical cultural competence,* Toronto, 2007, Canada.

Renwick GW, Rhinesmith SH: *An exercise in cultural analysis for managers,* Chicago, 1995, Intercultural Press.

Rokeach M: *The nature of human values,* New York, 1973, Free Press.

Shannon SE: The roots of interdisciplinary conflict around ethical issues, *Crit Care Nurs Clin North Am* 9(1):13, 1997.

Sherwin S: *No longer patient: feminist ethics and health care*, Philadelphia, 1993, Temple University Press.

United Network for Organ Sharing (UNOS), 2006, http://www.unos.org/.

U.S. Department of Health and Human Services, Office for Civil Rights: *HIPAA medical privacy, national standards to protect the privacy of personal health information*, 2006, http://www.hhs.gov/ocr/hipaa/.

Watson J, editor: *Applying art and science of human caring*, New York, 1994, National League of Nursing Press.

Wexler A: *Mapping fate: a memoir of family, risk, and genetic research*, New York, 1996, Times Books.

Wolf SM, editor: *Feminism and bioethics*, New York, 1996, Oxford University Press.

Zoloth L: Learning a practice of uncertainty: clinical ethics and the nurse. In Cowen PS, Moorhead S, editors: *Current issues in nursing*, ed 7, St. Louis, 2006, Mosby.

Research References

Borry P, Schotsmans P, Dierickx K: Evidence-based medicine and its role in ethical decision-making, *J Eval Clin Pract* 12(3):306, 2006.

Crawley LM and others: Strategies for culturally effective end-of-life care, *Ann Intern Med* 136:673, 2002.

Volker DL: Control and end of life care: does ethnicity matter? *Am J Hosp Palliat Care* 22(6):442, 2005.

CHAPTER 23
References

American Nurses Association: *Nursing: scope and standards of practice*, Silver Spring, Md, 2004, The Association, http://www.Nursesbooks.org.

Ashley RC: The second element of negligence, *Crit Care Nurse* 24(1):68, 2004.

Austin S: Ladies of the jury, I present the nursing documentation, *Nursing* 36(1):56, 2006.

Benko LB: Ratio fight goes national, *Modern Healthc* 34(24):23, 2004.

Black HC: *Black's law dictionary*, ed 7, St. Paul, Minn, 2004, West Publishing.

Blair P: Determine your scope of practice, *Nurs Manage* 34(4):20, 2003.

Blumenreich G: The doctrine of corporate liability, *AANA J* 73(4):253, 2005.

Bross W: Healthcare issues: patient self determination acts and informed consent, *Ala Nurse* 32(4):9, 2006.

Burns J and others: Do-not-resuscitate order after 25 years, *Crit Care Med* 31(5):1543, 2003.

Cady R: Nurse executive's legal primer, *JONAS Healthc Law Ethics Regul* 7(1):10, 2005.

Centers for Disease Control and Prevention, http://www.CDC.gov/.

Centers for Medicare and Medicaid Services, 2004, U.S. Department of Health and Human Services, http://www.cms.hhs.gov/.

Dalinis P: Informed consent and decisional capacity, *J Hosp Palliat Nurs* 7(1):52, 2005.

Erickson J, Millar S: Caring for patients while respecting their privacy: renewing our commitment, *Online J Issues Nurs* 10(2), 2005, http://www.nursingworld.org/ojin/topic27/tpc27_1htm.

Ersek M: The continuing challenge of assisted death, *J Hosp Palliat Nurs* 6(1): 46, 2004.

Follin S, editor: *Nurses Legal Handbook*, ed 5, Philadelphia, 2004, Lippincott Williams & Wilkins.

Guido G: *Legal and ethical issues in nursing*, ed 4, Upper Saddle River, NJ, 2006, Prentice Hall.

Harman L: HIPAA: a few years later, *Online J Issues Nurs* 10(2), 2005, http://www.nursingworld.org/ojin/topic27/tpc27_2.htm.

Kane-Urrabazo C: Said another way: our obligation to float, *Nurs Forum* 41(2):95, 2006.

Kleen, K. Restraint regulation: the tie that binds, *Nurs Manage* 35(11):36, 2004.

Kohn L, Corrigan J, Donaldson M, editor: *To err is human: building a safer health system*, 2000, Committee on Quality of Health Care in America, Institute of Medicine, http://www.nap.edu/books/0309068371/html/.

Mental Health Parity Act, 1996, U.S. Department of Labor, http://www.dol.gov/dol/topic/health-plans/mental.htm.

Mrayyan M, Huber D: The nurse's role in changing health policy related to patient safety, *JONAS Healthc Law Ethics Regul* 5(1):13, 2003.

National Council State Boards of Nursing: *Working with others: a position paper*, 2005, http://www.ncsbn.org/pdfs/Working_with_Others.pdf.

Occupational Safety and Health Administration, U.S. Department of Labor, http://www.osha.gov.

Orentlicher D, Callahan C: Feeding tubes, slippery slopes, and physician-assisted suicide, *The J Leg Med* 25:389, 2004.

Sloan A: A landmark decision for nurses: *Sullivan v. Edward Hospital, Virginia Nurses Today* 12(2):5, 2004.

The Joint Commission: *Comprehensive accreditation manual for hospitals: the official handbook (CAMH)*, Chicago, 2008, The Joint Commission.

The Joint Commission International Center for Patient Safety, 2007, http://www.jcipatientsafety.org, accessed January 19, 2007.

United Network for Organ Sharing, http://www.unos.org/.

Research References

Rogers AE and others: The working hours of hospital staff nurses and patient safety, *Health Aff* 23(4):202, 2004.

Statutes

Americans With Disabilities Act (ADA), 42 USC §§121.010-12213 (1990).

California Assembly Bill 394 (AB394), http://www.leginfo.ca.gov/pub/99-00/bill/asm/ab_0351-0400/ab_394_bill_19991010_chaptered.pdf.

Emergency Medical Treatment and Active Labor Act (EMTALA), 42 USC §1395 (dd) (1986).

Federal Nursing Home Reform Act from the Omnibus Budget Reconciliation Act of 1987.

Good Samaritan Act, IL Compiled Statutes (745 ILCS 49/) (1997).

Health Insurance Portability and Accountability Act of 1996 (HIPAA), Public Law No. 104 (1996).

Medical Patient Rights Act, IL Compiled Statutes (410 ILCS 50) (1994).

Mental Health Parity Act of 1996, 29 USC §1885 (1996).

National Organ Transplant Act, Public Law 98-507 (1984).

New York DNR Statute, NY Public Health Laws §2962 (1988).

Oregon Death With Dignity Act, Ore Rev Stat §§127.800-127.897 (1994).

Patient Self-Determination Act, 42 CFR 417 (1991).

State of Illinois: 225 Illinois Compiled Statutes 2002, 65/1-65/49 Inclusive, *Nursing and Advanced Practice Nursing Act*, Dept of Financial and Professional Regulation, Division of Professional Regulation, 2005.

Uniform Anatomical Gift Act (1987).

Uniform Determination of Death Act (1980).

Cases

Barber v Time Magazine, 159 SW2d 291 (1942).

Bouvia v Superior Court, 225 Cal Rptr 297 (1986).

Bragdon v Abbott, 524 U.S. 624 (1998).

Compassion in Dying v Washington, 79 F3d 790 (9th Cir 1997).

Cruzan v Director Missouri Department of Health, 497 U.S. 261 (1990).

Darling v Charleston Community Memorial Hospital, 33 Ill 2d 326 (IL 1965).

Quill v Vacco, 80 F3d 716 (2nd Cir 1997).

Roe v Wade, 410 U.S. 113 (1973).

Spires v Hospital Corporation of America, 28 U.S.C. §1391(b) Kansas (2006), http://www.kansas.com/multimedia/kansas/archive/pdfs/041106spireshca.pdf.

Washington v Glucksberg, 521 U.S. 702 (1997).

Webster v Reproductive Health Services, 492 U.S. 490 (1989).

Wendland v Wendland, 28 P.3d 151 (California 2001).

Winkelman v Beloit Memorial Hospital, 484 NW2d 211 (W 1992).

YG v Jewish Hospital, 795 SW2d 488 (Mo App 1990).

CHAPTER 24
References

Arnold E, Boggs KU: *Interpersonal relationships: professional communication skills for nurses*, ed 4, St. Louis, 2003, Saunders.

Balzer Riley J: *Communication in nursing*, ed 5, St. Louis, 2004, Mosby.

Beebe SA, Beebe SJ, Redmond MV: *Interpersonal communication: relating to others*, ed 4, Boston, 2005, Allyn & Bacon.

Berry P, Mascia J, Steinman BA: Vision and hearing loss in older adults: "Double trouble," *Care Manage J* 5(1):35, 2004.

Chitty KK: *Professional nursing concepts and challenges*, ed 4, St. Louis, 2005, Saunders.

Doenges ME, Moorhouse MF, Murr AC: *Nursing diagnosis manual: planning, individualizing, and documenting client care*, Philadelphia, 2005, FA Davis.

Gleeson M, Timmins F: Touch: a fundamental aspect of communication with older people experiencing dementia, *Nurs Older People* 16(2):18, 2004.

Gravely S: When your patient speaks Spanish—and you don't, *RN* 64(5):65, 2001.

McCaffrey R, Fowler NL: Qigong practice: a pathway to health and healing, *Holist Nurs Pract* 17(2):110, 2003.

Paul R: The art of redesigning instruction. In Willsen J, Blinker AJA, editors: *Critical thinking: how to prepare students for a rapidly changing world,* Santa Rosa, Calif, 1993, Foundation for Critical Thinking.

Stanhope M, Lancaster J: *Community and public health nursing,* ed 6, St. Louis, 2004, Mosby.

Stuart GW, Laraia MT: *Principles and practice of psychiatric nursing,* ed 8, St. Louis, 2005, Mosby.

Sully P, Dallas J: *Essential communication skills for nursing,* St. Louis, 2005, Mosby.

Tavarnier SS: An evidence-based conceptual analysis of presence, *Holist Nurs Pract* 20(3):152, 2006.

The Joint Commission: *Sentinel event statistics—March 31, 2006,* http://www.jointcommission.org/SentinelEvents/Statistics/.

Townsend M: *Psychiatric mental health nursing: concepts of care,* Philadelphia, 2003, FA Davis.

Watson J: *Nursing: human science and health care,* Norwalk, Conn, 1985, Appleton-Century-Crofts.

Research References

American Association of Critical Care Nurses: AACN standards for establishing and sustaining healthy work environments: a journey to excellence, *Am J Crit Care* 14(3):187, 2005.

Apker J and others: Collaboration, credibility, compassion, and coordination: professional nurse communication skill set in health care team interactions, *J Prof Nurs* 22(3):180, 2006.

Cutilli CC: Do your patients understand? Providing culturally congruent patient education, *Orthop Nurs* 25(3):218, 2005.

Feldman-Stewart D, Brundage M, Tishelman C: A conceptual framework for patient-professional communication: an application to the cancer context, *Psychooncology* 14(10):801, 2005.

Goldfarb R, Pietro MJ: Support systems: older adults with neurogenic communication disorders, *J Ambul Care Manage* 27(4):356, 2004.

Grover S: Shaping effective communication skills and therapeutic relationships at work: the foundation of collaboration, *AAOHN J* 53(4):177, 2005.

Hemsley B and others: Nursing the patient with severe communication impairment, *J Adv Nurs* 35(6):827, 2001.

Hoffman JM and others: Effect of communication disability on satisfaction with health care: a survey of Medicare beneficiaries, *Am J Speech Lang Pathol* 14(3):221, 2005.

Iezzoni LI and others: Communicating about health care: observations from persons who are deaf or hard of hearing, *Ann Intern Med* 140(5):356, 2004.

Lane MR: Arts in health care: a new paradigm for holistic nursing practice, *J Holist Nurs* 24(1):70, 2006.

Lehna C: Interpreter services in pediatric nursing, *Pediatr Nurs* 31(4):292, 2005.

McCabe C: Nurse-patient communication: an exploration of patients' experiences, *J Clin Nurs* 13(1):41, 2004.

Nilsson K, Larsson US: Conceptions of gender: a study of female and male head nurses' statements, *J Nurs Manage* 13(2):179, 2005.

Rudan VT: The best of both worlds: a consideration of gender in team building, *J Nurs Adm* 33(3):179, 2003.

Seed A: Crossing the boundaries: experience of neophyte nurses, *J Adv Nurs* 21(6):1136, 1995.

Shattell M, Hogan B: Facilitating communication: how to truly understand what patients mean, *J Psychosoc Nurs Ment Health Serv* 43(10):29, 2005.

Sheldon LK, Barrett R, Ellington L: Difficult communication in nursing, *J Nurs Scholarsh* 38(2):141, 2006.

Stefanek M, McDonald PG, Hess SA: Religion, spirituality, and cancer: current status and methodological challenges, *Psychooncology* 14(6):450, 2005.

Triola N: Dialogue and discourse: are we having the right conversations? *Crit Care Nurse* 26(1):60, 2006.

Vannorsdall T and others: The relation between nonessential touch and children's distress during lumbar punctures, *Child Health Care* 33(4):299, 2004.

Williams AM, Irurita VF: Emotional comfort: the patient's perspective of a therapeutic context, *Int J Nurs Stud* 43(4):405, 2006.

Williams K, Kemper S, Hummert L: Enhancing communication with older adults: overcoming elderspeak, *J Gerontol Nurs* 30(10):17, 2004.

CHAPTER 25
References

American Hospital Association: *The patient care partnership: understanding expectations, rights, and responsibilities,* 2003, http://www.aha.org/aha/issues/Communicating-With-Patients/pt-care-partnership.html.

American Nurses Association: *Position statement on promotion and disease prevention,* 1997, http://www.nursingworld.org/readroom/position/social/scprmo.htm.

Bandura A: *Self-efficacy: the exercise of control,* New York, 1997, WH Freeman.

Bandura A: Social cognitive theory: an agentic perspective, *Annu Rev Psychol* 52:1, 2001.

Bastable SB: *Nurse as educator: principles of teaching and learning for nursing practice,* Sudbury, Mass, 2003, Jones & Bartlett.

Bastable SB: *Essentials of patient education,* Sudbury, Mass, 2006, Jones & Bartlett.

Black JM: Assessing learning preferences, *Plast Surg Nurs* 24(2):68, 2004.

Bloom BS, editor: Taxonomy of educational objectives, *Cognitive domain,* vol 1, New York, 1956, Longman.

Bulechek GM, Butcher HK, Dochterman JM: *Nursing interventions classification (NIC),* ed 5, St. Louis, 2008, Mosby.

Cutilli CC: Do your patients understand? Determining your patients' health literacy skills, *Orthop Nurs* 24(5):372, 2005.

Cutilli CC: Do your patients understand? Providing culturally congruent patient education, *Orthop Nurs* 25(3):218, 2006.

Dreger V, Trembeck T: Optimize patient health by treating literacy and language barriers, *AORN J* 75(2):280, 2002.

Edelman CL, Mandle CL: *Health promotion throughout the life span,* ed 6, St. Louis, 2006, Mosby.

Falvo DR: *Effective patient education: a guide to increased compliance,* ed 3, Sudbury, Mass, 2004, Jones & Bartlett.

Felder R: *Learning styles,* 2006, http://www.ncsu.edu/felder-public/Learning_Styles.html.

Hockenberry M, Wilson D: *Wong's nursing care of infants and children,* ed 8, St. Louis, 2007, Mosby.

Krathwohl DR and others: *Taxonomy of educational objectives: the classification of educational goals, handbook II, affective domain,* New York, 1964, David McKay.

Kuiken S, Seiffert D: Thinking outside the box! Enhance patient education by using shared medical appointments, *Plast Surg Nurs* 25(4):191, 2005.

Mauk KL: Reaching and teaching older adults, *Nursing* 36(2):17, 2006.

Mika VS and others: The ABCs of health literacy, *Fam Community Health* 28(4):351, 2005.

Minerd J: *Health information goes over the heads of many U.S. adults,* 2006, http://www.medpagetoday.com/tbprint.cfm?tbid=4069.

Moorhead S and others: *Nursing outcomes classification (NOC),* ed 4, St. Louis, 2008, Mosby.

Osborne H: Health literacy from a to z: practical ways to communicate your health message, Boston, 2005, Jones & Bartlett.

Redman BK: The ethics of self-management preparation for chronic illness, *Nurs Ethics* 12(4):360, 2005.

Redman BK: *The practice of patient education,* ed 10, St. Louis, 2007, Mosby.

Saarmann L, Daugherty J, Riegel B: Teaching staff a brief cognitive-behavioral intervention, *Medsurg Nurs* 11(3):144, 2002.

Stephenson PL: Before the teaching begins: managing patient anxiety prior to providing education, *Clin J Oncol Nurs* 10(2):241, 2006.

The Joint Commission: *Joint Commission 2006 requirements related to the provision of culturally and linguistically appropriate health care,* 2006, http://www.jointcommission.org/NR/rdonlyres/1401C2EF-62F0-4715-B28A-7CE7F0F20E2D/0/hlc_jc_stds.pdf.

The Joint Commission: *The Joint Commission's new speak up program urges patients to "Know Your Rights,"* Oakbrook Terrace, Ill, 2007, The Commission, http://www.jointcommission.org.

The Joint Commission: *"What did the doctor say?": improving health literacy to protect patient safety,* 2007, http://www.jointcommission.org.

Wingard R: Patient education and the nursing process: meeting the patient's needs, *Nephrol Nurs J* 32(2):211, 2005.

Research References

Behar-Horenstein LS and others: Improving patient care through patient-family education programs, *Hosp Top* 83(1):21, 2005.

Bonner S and others: An individualized intervention to improve asthma management among urban Latino and African-American families, *J Asthma* 39(2):167, 2002.

Jack L and others: Understanding the environmental issues in diabetes self management education research: a re-examination of 8 studies in community-based settings, *Ann Intern Med* 140(11):964, 2004.

Kutner M and others: *The health literacy of America's adults: results from the 2003 National Assessment of Adult Literacy* (NCES 2006-483), Washington, DC, 2006, U.S. Department of Education, National Center for Education Statistics, http://nces.ed.gov/pubs2006/2006483.pdf.

Kutzleb J, Reiner D: The impact of nurse-directed patient education on quality of life and functional capacity in people with heart failure, *J Am Acad Nurse Pract* 18(3):116, 2006.

Noble Walker S and others: Determinants of older rural women's activity and eating, *West J Nurs Res* 28(4):449, 2006.

Oermann M and others: Clinic visit and waiting: patient education and satisfaction, *Medsurg Nurs* 11(5):247, 2002.

Oliva G and others: A university and community-based organization collaboration to build capacity to develop, implement, and evaluate an innovative HIV prevention intervention for an urban African American population, *AIDS Educ Prev* 17(4):300, 2005.

Sousa VD, Zauszniewski: Toward a theory of diabetes self-care management, *Journal of Theory Construction and Testing* 9(2):61, 2005/2006.

Speros C: Health literacy: concept analysis, *J Adv Nurs* 50(6):633, 2005.

Steven D and others: Knowledge, attitudes, beliefs and practices regarding breast and cervical cancer screening in selected ethnocultural groups in northwestern Ontario, *Oncol Nurs Forum* 31(2):305, 2004.

Strut J and others: Complex intervention development for diabetes self-management, *J Adv Nurs* 54(3):293, 2006.

Wendell I and others: Group diabetes patient education: a model for use in a continuing care retirement community, *J Gerontol Nurs* 29(2):37, 2003.

Wilson FL and others: Literacy, readability and cultural barriers: critical factors to consider when educating older African Americans about anticoagulation therapy, *J Clin Nurs* 12(2):275, 2003.

CHAPTER 26
References

American Nurses Association: *Scope and standards of nursing informatics practice,* Washington, DC, 2001, American Nurses Publishing.

Ammenwerth E and others: Nursing process documentation systems in clinical routine—prerequisites and experiences, *Int J Med Inf* 64(2-3):187, 2001.

Bailey J: Nursing specialty: what is nursing informatics? *Pa Nurse,* p. 25, March 2006.

Boroughs DS: Documentation in the long-term care setting, *J Nurs Adm* 29(12):46, 1999.

Dorenfest S: Defining CPOE, *ADVANCE Health Inform Exec* 7(3):33, 2003.

Frank-Stromborg M, Ganschow JR: How HIPAA will change your practice, *Nursing* 32(9):54, 2002.

Fratto M: Control the keys to the kingdom, *Network Computing* 13(18):36, 2002.

Gordon M: *Manual of nursing diagnosis,* ed 10, St. Louis, 2002, Mosby.

Healthcare Information and Management Systems Society: *EHR definition, attributes, and essential requirements,* version 1.1, September 24, 2003, http://himss.org/content/files/ehattributes070703.pdf, accessed July 21, 2007.

Healthcare Information and Management Systems Society: *The electronic health record,* http://himss.org/ASP/topics_her.asp, accessed July 21, 2007.

Hebda T and others: *Handbook of informatics for nurses and health care professionals,* ed 3, Upper Saddle River, NJ, 2005, Pearson Prentice Hall.

Institute of Medicine: *Crossing the quality chasm: a new health system for the twenty-first century,* Washington, DC, 2001, National Academies Press.

Iyer PW, Camp NH: *Nursing documentation: a nursing process approach,* St. Louis, 1999, Mosby.

Korst LM: Nursing documentation time during implementation of an electronic medical record, *J Nurs Adm* 33(1):24, 2003.

Lawson NA, Orr JM, Klar DS: The HIPAA privacy rule: an overview of compliance initiatives and requirements—the privacy rule contains a maze of mandates and exceptions requiring that entities covered by HIPAA need the best of health care counsel, *Defense Counsel J* 70(1):127, 2003.

Mosby's surefire documentation: how, what, and when nurses need to document, ed 2, St. Louis, 2006, Mosby.

National Coordination Office for Computing, Information, and Communications: *High performance computing and communications FY 1997 implementation plan,* Washington, DC, 1996, U.S. Government Printing Office, http://www.ccic.gov/pubs/imp97/136.html.

Nurses Service Organization, 2006, http://www.nso.com/newsletter/features/common.php.

Pew Health Commission: *Recreating health profession practice for a new century: fourth report of the Pew Health Professions Commission,* San Francisco, 1998, University of California.

The Joint Commission: *2007 Comprehensive accreditation for home care,* Chicago, 2006, The Joint Commission.

U.S. Department of Health and Human Services: *HHS fact sheet: protecting the privacy of patients' health information,* May 9, 2001, http://www.hhs.gov/news.

Wenzel GR: Creating an interactive interdisciplinary electronic assessment, *Comput Inform Nurs* 20(6):251, 2002.

Williams S: Computerized documentation of case management from diagnosis to outcomes: *Nurs Case Manag* 3(6), 1998.

Yocum RF: Documenting for quality patient care, *Nursing* 32(8):58, 2002.

Research Reference

Currell R, Urquhart C: Nursng record systems: effects on nursing practice and health care outcomes, *Cochrane Library* 2006(4):CD002099.

CHAPTER 27
References

Bulechek GM, Butcher HK, Dochterman JM: *Nursing interventions classification (NIC),* ed 5, St. Louis, 2008, Mosby.

Ebersole P and others: *Gerontological nursing and healthy aging,* ed 2, St. Louis, 2005, Mosby.

Erikson E: *Childhood and society,* ed 2, New York, 1963, WW Norton.

Moorhead S and others: *Nursing outcomes classification (NOC),* ed 4, St. Louis, 2008, Mosby.

NANDA International: *NANDA-I nursing diagnoses: definitions and classifications,* 2007-2008, Philadelphia, 2007, NANDA International.

Rosenberg M: *Society and the adolescent self-image,* Princeton, NJ, 1965, Princeton University Press.

Stuart GW, Laraia MT: *Principles and practice of psychiatric nursing,* ed 8, St. Louis, 2005, Mosby.

Research References

Birndorf S and others: High self-esteem among adolescents: longitudinal trends, sex differences, and protective factors, *J Adolesc Health* 37:194, 2005.

Collins A, Smyer MA: The resilience of self-esteem in late adulthood: *J Aging Health* 17(4):471, 2005

Folse VN and others: Detecting suicide risk in adolescents and adults in an emergency department: a pilot study, *J Psychosoc Nurs Ment Health Serv* 44(3):23, 2006.

Kelly AM and others: Adolescent girls with high body satisfaction: who are they and what can they teach us? *J Adolesc Health* 37:391, 2005.

Parker JS, Benson, MJ: Parent-adolescent relations and adolescent functioning: self-esteem, substance abuse, and delinquency, *Adolescence* 39(155):519, 2004.

Phares V and others: Race/ethnicity and self-esteem in families of adolescents, *Child and Family Behavior Therapy* 27(3):13, 2005.

Robins RW and others: Global self-esteem across the life span, *Psychol Aging* 17(3):423, 2002.

Ruiz SY and others: Predictors of self-esteem for Mexican American and European American youths: a reexamination of the influence of parenting, *J Fam Psychol* 16(1):70, 2002.

Salazar LF and others: Self-esteem and theoretical mediators of safer sex among African American female adolescents: implications for sexual risk reduction interventions, *Health Educ Behav* 32(3):413, 2005.

Sterk CE and others: Self-esteem and at risk women: determinants and relevance to sexual and HIV-related risk behaviors, *Women Health* 40(4):75, 2004.

Trzesniewski KH and others: Low self-esteem during adolescence predicts poor health, criminal behavior, limited economic prospects during adulthood, *Develop Psychol* 42(2):381, 2006.

Twenge JM, Crocker J: Race and self-esteem: meta-analyses comparing whites, blacks, Hispanics, Asians, and American Indians, *Psychol Bull* 128(3):371, 2002.

Van Baarsen B: Theories on coping with loss: the impact of social support and self-esteem on adjustment to emotional and social loneliness following a partner's death in later life, *J Gerontol* 57(1):S33, 2002.

Voorhees CC and others: Early predictors of daily smoking in young women: the National Heart, Lung, and Blood Institute growth and health study, *Prev Med* 34:616, 2002.

Wilburn VR, Smith DE: Stress, self-esteem, and suicidal ideation in late adolescents, *Adolescence* 40(157):33, 2005.

White MA and others: Racial/ethnic differences in weight concerns: protective and risk factors for the development of eating disorders and obesity among adolescent females, *Eat Weight Disord* 8:20, 2003.

CHAPTER 28
References

Andrews G: *Women's sexual health,* ed 3, St. Louis, 2005, Elsevier.

Annon JS: The PLISSIT model: a proposed conceptual scheme for the behavioral treatment of sexual problems, *J Sex Educ Ther* (2):1, 1976.

Bulechek GM, Butcher HK, Dochterman JM: *Nursing interventions classification (NIC),* ed 5, St. Louis, 2008, Mosby.

Centers for Disease Control and Prevention: *Chlamydia—CDC fact sheet,* 2006a, http://www.cdc.gov/std/chlamydia/STDFact-Chlamydia.htm.

Centers for Disease Control and Prevention: HPV vaccine questions and answers, 2006b, http://www.cdc.gov/std/hpv/hpv-vaccine.pdf.

Centers for Disease Control and Prevention: Youth risk behavior surveillance—2005, *MMWR Morb Mortal Wkly Rep* 55(SS-5)1, 2006c, http://www.cdc.gov/mmwr/PDF/SS/SS5505.pdf.

Crumlish B: Sexual counselling by cardiac nurses for patients following an MI, *Br J Nurs* 13(12):710, 2004

DeLamaster J, Friedrich WN: Human sexual development, *J Sex Res* 39(1):10, 2002.

Dobranowski Dixon K, Dixon PN: The PLISSIT model: care and management of patients' psychosexual needs following radical surgery, *Lippincott's Case Manag* 11(2):101, 2006.

Edelman CL, Mandle CL: *Health promotion throughout the life span,* ed 6, St. Louis, 2006, Mosby.

Hockenberry MJ, Wilson D: *Wong's nursing care of infants and children,* ed 8, St. Louis, 2007, Mosby.

King BM: *Human sexuality today,* ed 5, Upper Saddle River, NJ, 2005, Pearson Prentice Hall.

McCarthy BW, Bodnar LE: The equity model of sexuality: navigating and negotiating the similarities and differences between men and women in sexual behaviour, roles and values, *Sexual and Relationship Therapy* 20(2):225, 2005.

Meiner S, Lueckenotte A: *Gerontologic nursing,* ed 3, St. Louis, 2006, Mosby.

Metcalfe T: Sexual health: meeting adolescents' needs, *Nurs Stand* 18(46):40, 2004.

Moorhead S and others: *Nursing outcomes classification (NOC),* ed 4, St. Louis, 2008, Mosby.

Murray SS, McKinney ES: *Foundations of maternal-newborn nursing,* ed 4, St. Louis, 2006, Saunders.

Nusbaum MRH, Hamilton CD: The proactive sexual health history, *Am Fam Physician* 66(9):1705, 2002.

Nusbaum MRH and others: Chronic illness and sexual functioning, *Am Fam Physician* 67(2):347, 2003.

Nusbaum MRH and others: Sexual health in aging men and women: addressing the physiologic and psychological sexual changes that occur with age, *Geriatrics* 60(9):18, 2005.

Price D: A developmental perspective of treatment for sexually vulnerable youth, *Sexual Addiction and Compulsivity* 10(4):225, 2003.

Running A, Berndt A: *Management guidelines for nurse practitioners working in family practice,* Philadelphia, 2003, FA Davis.

Stanhope M, Lancaster J: *Community and public health nursing,* ed 6, St. Louis, 2004, Mosby.

Stausmire J: Sexuality at the end of life, *Am J Hosp Palliat Care* 21(1):33, 2004.

Steinke EE: Intimacy needs and chronic illness: strategies for sexual counseling and self-management, *J Gerontol Nurs* 31(10):40, 2005.

Stuart GW, Laraia MT: *Principles and practice of psychiatric nursing,* ed 8, St. Louis, 2005, Mosby.

Townley Bakewell R, Volker DL: Sexual dysfunction related to the treatment of young women with breast cancer, *Clin J Oncol Nurs* 9(6):697, 2005.

U.S. Department of Health and Human Services: *Healthy People 2010: understanding and improving health,* ed 2,. Washington, DC, 2000, U.S. Government Printing Office, http://www.healthypeople.gov/Document/html/uih/uih_bw/uih_4.htm#sex.

World Health Organization: What constitutes sexual health? *Progress in Reproductive Health Research* 67:2, 2004, http://www.who.int/reproductive-health/hrp/progress/67.pdf.

Research References

Adimora AA, Schoenbach VJ: Social context, sexual networks, and racial disparities in rates of sexually transmitted infections, *Social Context and Social Networks* 191(suppl 1):S115, 2005.

Amy NK and others: Barriers to routine gynecological cancer screening for white and African-American obese women, *Int J Obes* 30(1):147, 2006.

Burt J and others: Radical prostatectomy: men's experiences and postoperative needs, *Clin Nurs* 14(7):883, 2005.

Farmer D and others: Psychosocial correlates of mammography screening in older African American women, *Oncol Nurs Forum* 34(1):117, 2007.

Galbraith ME and others: Prostate cancer survivors' and partners' self-reports of health-related quality of life, treatment symptoms, and marital satisfaction 2.5-5.5 years after treatment, *Oncol Nurs Forum* 32(2):E30, 2005.

Heck JE and others: Health care access among individuals involved in same-sex relationships, *Am J Public Health* 96(6):1111, 2006.

Juon HS and others: Predictors of regular Pap smears among Korean-American women, *Prev Med* 37(6):585, 2003.

Kristofferzon ML and others: Coping, social support and quality of life over time after myocardial infarction, *J Adv Nurs* 52(2):113, 2005.

Matin M, LeBaron S: Attitudes toward cervical cancer screening among Muslim women: a pilot study, *Women Health* 39(3):63, 2004.

Morrison-Beedy D and others: HIV risk behaviors and testing rates in adolescent girls: evidence to guide clinical practice, *Pediatr Nurs* 31(6):508, 2005.

Ott MA and others: Greater expectations: adolescents' positive motivations for sex, *Perspect Sex Reprod Health* 38(2):84, 2006.

Plowden KO: To screen or not to screen: factors influencing the decision to participate in prostate cancer screening among urban African-American men, *Urol Nurs* 26(6):477, 2006.

Shah M and others: Hispanic acculturation and utilization of cervical cancer screening in the US, *Prev Med* 42(2):146, 2006.

Whyte J: Sexual assertiveness in low-income African American women: unwanted sex, survival and HIV risk, *J Community Health Nurs* 23(4):235, 2006.

Zambrana RE and others: Latinas and HIV/AIDS risk factors: implications for harm reduction strategies, *Am J Public Health* 94(7):1152, 2004.

CHAPTER 29
References

Adegbola M: Spirituality and quality of life in chronic illness, *J Theory Construction Testing* 10(2):42, 2006.

American Nurses Association: *Code of ethics for nurses with interpretive statements,* 2001, http://www.nursingworld.org/ethics/code/protected_nwcoe303.htm.

Bash A: Spirituality: the emperor's new clothes? *J Clin Nurs* 13(1):11, 2004.

Benner DG: *Baker encyclopedia of psychology,* Grand Rapids, Mich, 1985, Baker Book House.

Benner P: *From novice to expert,* Menlo Park, Calif, 1984, Addison-Wesley.

Bennett MP, Lengacher C: Humor and laughter may influence health. II. Complementary therapies and humor in a clinical population, *eCAM* 3(2):187, 2006.

Boyd AS, Wilmoth MC: An innovative community-based intervention for African American women with breast cancer: the Witness Project, *Health Soc Work* 31(1):77, 2006.

Bulechek GM, Butcher HK, Dochterman JM: *Nursing interventions classification (NIC),* ed 5, St. Louis, 2008, Mosby.

Davis C: Empathy and transcendence, *Topi Geriatr Rehab* 19(4):265, 2003.

Delgado C: A discussion of the concept of spirituality, *Nurs Sci Q* 18(2):157, 2005.

Ebersole P and others: *Toward healthy aging: human needs and nursing response,* ed 6, St. Louis, 2004, Mosby.

Edelman CL, Mandle CL: *Health promotion throughout the life span,* ed 6, St. Louis, 2006, Mosby.

Elkins M, Cavendish R: Developing a plan for pediatric spiritual care, *Holist Nurs Pract* 18(4):179, 2004.

Friedemann M and others: Nursing the spirit: the Framework of Systemic Organization, *J Adv Nurs* 39(4):325, 2002.

Gray J: Measuring spirituality: conceptual and methodological considerations, *Journal of Theory Construction and Testing* 10(2):58, 2006.

Hoare J: The best medicine, *Nurs Stand* 19(14-16):18, 2004.

Hollins S: Spirituality and religion: exploring the relationship, *Nurs Manage* 12(6):22, 2005.

Hungelmann J and others: Focus on spiritual well-being: harmonious interconnectedness of mind-body-spirit—use of the JAREL spiritual well-being scale, *Geriatr Nurs* 17(6):262, 1996.

Jackson C: Healing ourselves, healing others: first in a series, *Holist Nurs Pract* 18(2):67, 2004.

James D: What emergency department staff need to know about near-death experiences, *Top Emerg Med* 26(1):29, 2004.

Kelly J: Spirituality as a coping mechanism, *Dimens Crit Care Nurs* 23(4):162, 2004.

Krebs K: Complementary healthcare practices: the spiritual aspect of caring—an integral part of health and healing, *Gastroenterol Nurs* 26(5):212, 2003.

LaPierre LL: JCACHO safeguards spiritual care, *Holist Nurs Pract* 17(4):219, 2003.

MacDonald: A chuckle a day keeps the doctor away: therapeutic humor and laughter, *J Psychosoc Nurs Ment Health Serv* 42(3):18, 2004.

Mauk KL, Schmidt NK: *Spiritual care in nursing practice,* Philadelphia, 2004, Lippincott, Williams & Wilkins.

Mazanec P, Tyler MK: Cultural considerations in end-of-life care: how ethnicity, age, and spirituality affect decisions when death is imminent, *Home Healthc Nurse* 22(5):317, 2004.

McEvoy M: Culture and spirituality as an integrated concept in pediatric care, *MCN Am J Matern Child Nurs* 28(1):39, 2003.

McSherry W, Ross L: Dilemmas of spiritual assessment: considerations for nursing practice, *J Adv Nurs* 38(5):479, 2002.

Moorhead S and others: *Nursing outcomes classification (NOC)*, ed 4, St. Louis, 2008, Mosby.

Miner-Williams D: Putting a puzzle together: making spirituality meaningful for nursing using an evolving theoretical framework, *J Clin Nurs* 15(7):811, 2006.

NANDA International: *NANDA-I nursing diagnoses: definitions and classification 2007-2008*, Philadelphia, 2007, The Association.

Newlin K and others: African-American spirituality: a concept analysis, *ANS Adv Nurs Sci* 25(2):57, 2002.

Perdue B and others: Assessing spirituality in mentally ill African Americans, *ABNF J* 17(2):78, 2006.

Perry DJ: Self-transcendence: Lonergan's key to integration of nursing theory, research, and practice, *Nurs Philos* 5(1):67, 2004.

Skalla KA, McCoy P: Spiritual assessment of patients with cancer: the moral authority, vocational, aesthetic, social and transcendent model, *Oncol Nurs Forum* 33(4):745, 2006.

Smith AR: Using the synergy model to provide spiritual nursing care in critical care settings, *Crit Care Nurse* 26(4):41, 2006.

Smith J, McSherry W: Spirituality and child development: a concept analysis, *J Adv Nurs* 45(3):307, 2004.

Smith-Stoner M: End-of-life needs of patients who practice Tibetan Buddhism, *J Hosp Palliat Nurs* 7(4):228, 2005.

Tanyi R: Towards clarification of the meaning of spirituality, *J Adv Nurs* 39(5):500, 2002.

Taylor EJ: *Spiritual care: nursing theory, research, and practice*, Upper Saddle River, NJ, 2002, Prentice Hall.

Villagomeza LR: Spiritual distress in adult cancer patients, *Holist Nurs Pract* 19(6):285, 2005.

Wright LM: *Spirituality, suffering, and illness: ideas for healing*, Philadelphia, 2005, FA Davis Co.

Young C, Koopsen C: *Spirituality, health, and healing*, Thorofare, NJ, 2005, SLACK Inc.

Research References

Aaron KF and others: African American church participation and health care practices, *J Gen Intern Med* 18(11):908, 2003.

Antall G, Kresevic D: The use of guided imagery to manage pain in an elderly orthopaedic population, *Orthop Nurs* 23(5):335, 2004.

Banks-Wallace J, Parks L: It's all sacred: African American women's perspectives on spirituality, *Issues Ment Health Nurs* 25(1):25, 2004.

Barry LC and others, Identification strategies used to cope with chronic pain in older persons receiving primary care from a veterans affairs medical center, *J Am Geriatr Soc* 52(6):950, 2004.

Brazier A and others: Evaluating a yogic breathing and meditation intervention for individuals living with HIV/AIDS, *Am J Health Promot* 20(3):192, 2006.

Buckley J, Herth K: Fostering hope in terminally ill patients, *Nurs Stand* 19(10):33, 2004.

Campesino M, Schwartz GE: Spirituality among Latinas/os: implications of culture in conceptualization and measurement, ANS *Adv Nurs Sci* 29(1):69, 2006.

Cavendish R and others: Patients' perceptions of spirituality and the nurse as a spiritual care provider, *Holist Nurs Pract* 20(1):41, 2006.

Chiu L and others: An integrative review of the concept of spirituality in the health sciences, *West J Nurs Res* 26(4):405, 2004.

Figueroa LR and others: The influence of spirituality on health care–seeking behaviors among African Americans, *ABNF J* 17(2):82, 2006.

Fisch MJ and others: Assessment of quality of life in outpatients with advanced cancer: the accuracy of clinician estimations and the relevance of spiritual well-being—a Hoosier Oncology Group study, *J Clin Oncol* 21(14):2754, 2003.

Gibson LM, Hendricks CS: Integrative review of spirituality in African American breast cancer survivors, *ABNF J* 7(2):67, 2006.

Grant D: Spiritual interventions: how, when, and why nurses use them, *Holist Nurs Pract* 18(1):36, 2004.

Grey M and others: Preliminary testing of a program to prevent type 2 diabetes among high-risk youth, *J Sch Health* 74(1):10, 2004.

Grimsley LP: Spirituality and quality of life in HIV-positive persons, *J Cult Divers* 13(2):113, 2006.

Hammermeister J and others: Gender differences in spiritual well-being: are females more spiritually-well than males? *American Journal of Health Studies* 20(2):80, 2005.

Holstad MKM and others: Factors associated with adherence to antiretroviral therapy, *J Assoc Nurses AIDS Care* 17(2):14, 2006.

Hsieh C and others: Positive psychological measure: constructing and evaluating the reliability and validity of a Chinese humor scale applicable to professional nursing, *J Nurs Res* 13(3):206, 2005.

Koenig HG and others: Religion, spirituality, and health in medically ill hospitalized older patients, *J Am Geriatr Soc* 52:554, 2004.

Lindberg DA: Integrative review of research related to meditation, spirituality, and the elderly, *Geriatr Nurs* 26(6):372, 2005.

Lohne V, Severinsson E: Hope during the first months after acute spinal cord injury, *J Adv Nurs* 47(3):279, 2004.

McEwen M: Spiritual nursing care: state of the art, *Holist Nurs Pract* 19(4):161, 2005.

McSherry and others: Meaning of spirituality: implications for nursing practice, *J Clin Nurs* 13(8):934, 2004.

Narayanasamy A: Spiritual coping mechanisms in chronic illness: a qualitative study, *J Clin Nurs* 13(1):116, 2004.

Narayanasamy A and others: Responses to the spiritual needs of older people, *J Adv Nurs* 48(1):6, 2004.

Peters L, Sellick K: Quality of life of cancer patients receiving inpatient and home-based palliative care, *J Adv Nurs* 53(5):524, 2006.

Pincharoen S, Congdon JG: Spirituality and health in older Thai persons in the United States, *West J Nurs Res* 25(1):93, 2003.

Spurlock WR: Spiritual well-being and caregiver burden in Alzheimer's caregivers, *Geriatr Nurs* 26(3):154, 2005.

Taylor EJ: Spiritual needs of patients with cancer and family caregivers, *Cancer Nurs* 26(4):260, 2003.

Villagomeza LR: Mending broken hearts: the role of spirituality in cardiac illness: a research synthesis, 1991-2004, *Holist Nurs Pract* 20(4):169, 2006.

CHAPTER 30
References

Aging With Dignity: *Five wishes*, 2005, http://www.agingwithdignity.org.

Amella E, Lawrence J, Gresle S: Tube feeding: prolonging life or death in vulnerable populations? *Mortality* 10(1):69, 2005.

American Medical Association: *Autopsy: life's final chapter*, 2004, http://www.ama-assn.org/ama/pub/category/7635.html#7.

Barbus AJ: The dying person's bill of rights, *Am J Nurs* 75:99, 1975.

Blum C: "Till death do us part?": the nurse's role in the care of the dead historical perspective—1850-2004, *Geriatr Nurs* 27(1):58, 2006.

Bowlby J: *Attachment and loss*, vol 3, Loss, sadness, and depression, New York, 1980, Basic Books.

Bulechek GM, Butcher HK, Dochterman JM: *Nursing interventions classification (NIC)*, ed 5, St. Louis, 2008, Mosby.

Carroll-Johnson R, Gorman L, Bush N: *Psychosocial nursing care along the cancer continuum*, ed 2, Pittsburg Pa, 2006, Oncology Nurses Society.

Chochinov HM: Dignity-conserving care—a new model for palliative care: helping the patient feel valued, *JAMA* 287(17):2253, 2002.

Clements P: Grief: promoting adaptive coping after loss and death, *J Psychosoc Nurs Ment Health Serv* 41(7):6, 2003.

Clements P and others: Cultural perspectives of death, grief, and bereavement, *J Psychosoc Nurs Ment Health Serv* 41(7):18, 2003.

Corless I: Bereavement. In Ferrell B, Coyle N, editors, *Textbook of palliative nursing*, New York, 2006, Oxford University Press.

Craib I: Fear, death and sociology, *Mortality* 8(3):285, 2003.

Dahlin C: Oral complications at the end-of-life, *Am J Nurs* 104(7):40, 2004.

Derby S, O'Mahony S: Elderly patients. In Ferrell B, Coyle N, editors, *Textbook of palliative nursing*, New York, 2006, Oxford University Press.

Doka K: Ethics, end-of-life decisions and grief, *Mortality* 10(1):83, 2005.

Douglass A, Maxwell T, Whitecar P: Principles of palliative care medicine. I. Patient assessment, *Adv Studies Med* 4(1):15, 2004.

Dying person's bill of rights, http://www.learningplaceonline.com/stages/together/dying-rights.htm.

Emanuel L, VonGunten C, Ferris F: *The education in palliative and end of life care [EPEC] curriculum: the EPEC project*, Chicago, 2003, Northwestern University.

End-of-Life Nursing Education Consortium: *Graduate curriculum faculty guide*, Philadelphia, 2003, City of Hope National Medical Center and American Association of Colleges of Nursing.

Ersek M: Artificial nutrition and hydration: clinical issues, *J Hosp Palliat Nurs* 5(4):231, 2003.

Ferrell B, Coyle N: *Textbook of palliative nursing*, ed 2, New York, 2006, Oxford University Press.

Green A: A person-centered approach to palliative care nursing, *J Hosp Palliat Nurs* 8(5):304, 2006.

Herr K, Bjoro K, Decker S: Pain assessment in the nonverbal patient: position statement with clinical practice recommendations, *J Pain Symptom Manage* 31(2):170, 2006.

Holloway K: Passed on: African American mourning stories: a memorial, Durham, NC, 2002, Duke University Press.

Hooyman N, Kramer B: *Living through loss: interventions across the lifespan*, New York, 2006, Columbia University Press.

Hospice Foundation of America: *Services,* 2004, http://www.hospicefoundation.org/hospiceInfo/services.asp.

Kemp C: Cultural issues in palliative care, *Semin Oncol Nurs* 21(1):44, 2005.

Kemp C, Bhungalia S: Culture and the end-of-life: a review of major world religions, *J Hosp Palliat Nurs* 4(4):235, 2002.

Kemp C, Chang B: Culture and the end-of-life: Chinese, *J Hosp Palliat Nurs* 4(3):173, 2002.

Kristjanson L, Aoun S: Palliative care for families: remembering the hidden patients, *Can J Psychiatry* 49:359, 2004.

Kübler-Ross E: *On death and dying,* New York, 1969, Macmillan.

Lentz J: Daily baths: torment or comfort at the end-of-life, *J Hosp Palliat Nurs* 5(1):34, 2003.

Matzo M, Sherman D: *Palliative care nursing: quality care to the end-of-life,* New York, 2006, Springer.

Matzo M and others: Strategies for teaching loss, grief and bereavement, *Nurse Educ* 28(2):71, 2003.

Mok E, Chiu P: Nurse-patient relationships in palliative care, *J Adv Nurs* 48(5):475, 2004.

Moorhead S and others: *Nursing outcomes classification (NOC),* ed 4, St. Louis, 2008, Mosby.

Myers G: Restoration or transformation? Choosing ritual strategies for end-of-life care, *Mortality* 8(4):372, 2003.

O'Gorman M: Spiritual care at the end-of-life, *Crit Care Nurs Clin North Am* 14(2):171, 2002.

Paice J, Fine P: Pain at the end-of-life. In Ferrell B, Coyle N, editors, *Textbook of palliative nursing,* New York, 2006, Oxford University Press.

Pitorak E: Care at the time of death, *Am J Nurs* 103(7):42, 2003.

Scanlon C: Ethical concerns in end-of-life care, *Am J Nurs* 103(1):48, 2003.

Stanley K: The healing power of presence: a respite from the fear of abandonment, *Oncol Nurs Forum,* 20(6):935, 2002.

Stroebe M, Schut H: The dual process model of coping with bereavement: rationale and description, *Death Stud* 23:197, 1999.

Stroebe M, Schut H: Complicated grief: a conceptual analysis of the field, *Omega* 52(1):53, 2006.

Stroebe W, Schut J, Stroebe M: Grief work, disclosure and counseling: do they help the bereaved? *Clin Psychol Rev* 25(4):395, 2005.

Talerico K: Aging matters: addressing issues related to geropsychiatry and the well-bring of older adults, *J Psychosoc Nurs Ment Health Serv* 41(7):12, 2006.

Virani R, Sofer D: Improving the quality of end-of-life care, *Am J Nurs* 2003(5):52, 2003.

Wayman L, Gaydos H: Self-transcending through suffering, *J Hosp Palliat Nurs* 7(5):263, 2005.

Weiner J, Roth J: Avoiding iatrogenic harm to patient and family while discussing goals of care near the end-of-life, *J Palliat Med* 9(2):451, 2006.

Whitecar P, Maxwell T, Douglass A: Principles of palliative care medicine. II. Pain and symptom management, *Adv Studies Med* 4(2):88, 2004.

Worden JW: G*rief counseling and grief therapy,* New York, 1982, Springer.

World Health Organization: *Palliative care,* 2003, http://www.who.int/hiv/topics/palliative/palliative care.

Wortman C, Silver R: The myths of coping with loss, *J Consult Clin Psychol* 57(3):349, 1989.

Research References

Allchin L: Caring for the dying: nursing student perspectives. *J Hosp Palliat Nurs* 8(2):112, 2006.

Arnaert A, Filteau M, Sourial R: Stroke patients in the acute care phase: the role of hope in healing, *Holist Nurs Pract* 20(3):137, 2006.

Briggs L, Colvin E: The nurse's role in end-of-life decision making for patients and families, *Geriatr Nurs* 23(6):302, 2002.

Buckley J, Herth K: Fostering hope in terminally ill patients, *Nurs Stand* 19(10):33, 2004.

Carnelly KB and others: The time course of grief reactions to spousal loss: evidence from a national probability sample, *J Pers Soc Psychol* 91(3):476, 2006.

Cohen S, Doyle W, Baum A: Socioeconomic status is associated with stress hormones, *Psychosom Med* 68:414, 2006.

Coyle N: The hard work of living in the face of death, *J Pain Symptom Manage* 32(3):266, 2006.

Davis B and others: Family stress and advance directives, *J Hosp Palliat Nurs* 7(4):219, 2005.

Enes S, de Vries K: A survey of ethical issues experienced by nurses caring for terminally ill elderly people, *Nurs Ethics* 11(2):150, 2004.

Frattaroli J: Experimental disclosure and its moderators: a meta-analysis. *Psychol Bull* 132(6):823, 2006.

Harstäde C, Andershed B: Good palliative care: how and where? The patients' opinions, *J Hosp Palliat Nurs* 6(1):27, 2004.

Holland JM, Currier JM, Neimeyer RA: Meaning reconstruction in the first two years of bereavement: the role of sense-making and benefit-finding, *Omega* 53(3):165, 2006.

Holmberg L: Communication in action between family caregivers and a palliative home care team, *J Hosp Palliat Nurs* 8(5):276, 2006.

Kolcaba K and others: Efficacy of hand massage for enhancing the comfort of hospice patients, *J Hosp Palliat Nurs* 6(2):91, 2004.

Maciejewski PK and others:). An empirical examination of the stage theory of grief, *JAMA* 297:716, 2007.

Maercker A and others: Prediction of complicated grief by positive and negative themes in narratives, *J Clin Psychol* 54(8):1117, 1998.

Matheis E, Tulsky D, Matheis R: The relation between spirituality and quality of life among individuals with spinal cord injury, *Rehabil Psychol* 51(3):265, 2006.

Mathews LL: Hardiness and grief in a sample of bereaved college students, *Death Stud* 31(3):183, 2007.

McSteen K, Peden-McAlpine C: The role of the nurse as advocate in ethically difficult care situations with dying patients, *J Hosp Palliat Nurs* 8(5):259, 2006.

Miller S and others: Does receipt of hospice care in nursing homes improve the management of pain at the end-of-life? *J Am Geriatr Soc* 50(3):507, 2002.

Ong AD and others: Psychological resilience, positive emotions and successful adaptation to stress in later life, *J Pers Soc Psychol* 91(4):730, 2006.

Onrust S and others: Predictors of psychological adjustment after bereavement, *Int Psychogeriatr* 14(1):1, 2006.

Prigerson HG, Maciejewski PK: A call for sound empirical testing and evaluation of criteria for complicated grief proposed for DSM-V, *Omega* 52(1):9, 2005.

Saldiner A, Cain A: Deromanticizing anticipated death: denial, disbelief and disconnection in bereaved spouses, *J Psychosoc Oncol* 22(3):69, 2004.

CHAPTER 31
References

Ackley BJ, Ladwig GB: *Nursing diagnosis handbook: a guide to planning care,* ed 7, St. Louis, 2006, Mosby.

Aguilera DC: *Crisis intervention: theory and methodology,* ed 8, St. Louis, 1998, Mosby.

American Nurses Association: *Statement on the scope and standards of psychiatric–mental health nursing practice,* Washington, DC, 2000, The Association.

American Psychiatric Association: *Diagnostic and statistical manual of mental disorders,* ed 4, text revision, Washington, DC, 2000, The Association.

Bulechek GM, Butcher HK, Dochterman JM: *Nursing interventions classification (NIC),* ed 5, St. Louis, 2008, Mosby.

Gulanick M and others: *Nursing care plans: nursing diagnosis and intervention,* ed 5, St. Louis, 2003, Mosby.

Hyer LA, Sohnle SJ: *Trauma among older people,* Ann Arbor, Mich, 2001, Taylor & Francis.

Lewis SM, Heitkemper MM, Dirksen SR: *Medical surgical nursing,* ed 6, St. Louis, 2004, Mosby.

Monat A, Lazarus RS, Reevy, G: *The Praeger handbook on stress and coping,* Westport, Conn, 2007, Praeger.

Moorhead S and others: *Nursing outcomes classification (NOC),* ed 4, St. Louis, 2008, Mosby.

Neuman B, Fawcett J, editors: *The Neuman Systems Model,* ed 4, Upper Saddle River, NJ, 2002, Prentice Hall.

Page GG, Lindsey AM: Stress response. In Carrieri-Kohlman V and others, editors: *Pathophysiological phenomena in nursing: human responses to illness,* St. Louis, 2003, Saunders.

Pender NJ, Murdaugh C, Parsons MA: *Health promotion in nursing practice,* ed 5, Upper Saddle River, NJ, 2006, Howorth Press.

Varcarolis EM, Carson VB, Shoemaker NC: *Foundations of psychiatric mental health nursing: a clinical approach,* ed 5, St. Louis, 2006, Saunders.

Research References

Chen JL and others: Cultural variations in children's coping behaviour, TV viewing time, and family functioning, *Int Nurs Rev* 52:186, 2005.

Gaugler JE and others: Family involvement in nursing homes: effects on stress and well-being, *Aging Ment Health* 8(1):65, 2004.

CHAPTER 32
References

Bulechek GM, Butcher HK, Dochterman JM: *Nursing interventions classification (NIC),* ed 5, St. Louis, 2008, Mosby.

Ebersole P and others: *Toward healthy aging: human needs and nursing response*, ed 6, St. Louis, 2004, Mosby.

Environmental Protection Agency: *What should I do if I have a mercury spill?* Updated May 21, 2007, http://www.epa.gov/epaoswer/hazwaste/mercury/spills.htm, accessed June 23, 2007.

Evans D and others: *Vital signs: a systematic review*, London, 2004, Joanna Briggs Institute for Evidence Based Nursing and Midwifery.

Grap MJ: Pulse oximetry, *Crit Care Nurse* 22(3):69, 2002.

Guyton AC, Hall JE: *Textbook of medical physiology*, ed 9, Philadelphia, 2000, Saunders.

Henker R, Carlson KK: Fever, *Adv Crit Care* 18(1):76, 2007.

Hockenberry MJ, Wilson D: *Wong's nursing care of infants and children*, ed 8, St. Louis, 2007, Mosby.

Holtzclaw BJ: *Use of thermoregulatory principles in patient care: fever management*, Glendale, Calif, 2003, CINAHL Information Systems, http://www.cinahl.com/cgi-bin/ojcishowdoc.cgi?vol05.htm.

Jones H and others: Reactivity of ambulatory blood pressure to physical activity varies with time of day, *Hypertension* 37(4):778, 2006.

Moorhead S and others: *Nursing outcomes classification (NOC)*, ed 4, St. Louis, 2008, Mosby.

National High Blood Pressure Education Program (NHBPEP); National Heart, Lung, and Blood Institute; National Institutes of Health: The seventh report of the Joint National Committee on Detection, Evaluation, and Treatment of High Blood Pressure, *JAMA* 289(19):2560, 2003.

Pickering TG: Self-monitoring of blood pressure. In White WB: *Blood pressure monitoring in cardiovascular medicine and therapeutics*, Totowa, NJ, 2001, Humana Press.

Redon J: The normal circadian pattern of blood pressure: implications for treatment. *Int J Clin Pract* 58 (suppl 145):3, 2004.

Research References

Jones DW and others: Measuring blood pressure accurately, *JAMA* 289(8):1027, 2003.

Maxton, FJ, Justin L, Gilles D: Estimating core temperature in infants and children after cardiac surgery: a comparison of six methods, *J Adv Nurs* 45(2):214, 2004.

Potter P and others: Evaluation of chemical dot thermometers for measuring body temperature of orally intubated patients, *Am J Crit Care* 12(5):403, 2003.

Schell K and others: Clinical comparison of automatic, noninvasive measurements of blood pressure in the forearm and upper arm with the patient supine or with the head of the bed raised 45 degrees: a follow-up study, *Am J Crit Care* 15(2):196, 2006.

Sidberry GK and others: Comparison of temple temperatures with rectal temperatures in children under two years of age, *Clin Pediatr* 41:405, 2002.

Thomas SA and others: A review of nursing research on blood pressure, *J Nurs Scholarsh* 34(4):313, 2002.

CHAPTER 33
References

American Cancer Society: *Cancer facts and figures 2007*, Atlanta, 2007, The Society.

American Psychiatric Association: *Diagnostic and statistical manual of mental disorders*, ed 4, text revision, Washington, DC, 2000, The Association.

Barkauskas VH and others: *Health and physical assessment*, ed 3, St. Louis, 2002, Mosby.

Caulker-Burnett I: Primary care screening for substance abuse, *Nurse Pract* 19(6):42, 1994.

Chin J, editor: *Control of communicable diseases manual*, Washington, DC, 2000, American Public Health Association.

Crowther J, McCourt K: Get the edge on deep vein thrombosis, *Nurs Manage* 35(1):22, 2004.

Day MW: Recognizing and management: DVT-deep vein thrombosis, *Nursing* 33(5):36, 2003.

Ebersole P and others: *Toward healthy aging: human needs and nursing response*, ed 6, St. Louis, 2004, Mosby.

Frakes MA, Evans T: TB: your vigilance is vital, *RN* 67(11):30, 2004.

Friedman L and others: *Source book of substance abuse and addiction*, Baltimore, 1996, Williams & Wilkins.

Fulmer T: Elder abuse and neglect assessment, *J Gerontol Nurs* 29(1):8, 2003.

Galanti G: *Caring for patients from different cultures*, ed 3, Philadelphia, 2004, University of Pennsylvania Press.

Graham A and others: *Principles of addiction medicine*, ed 3, Chevy Chase, Md, 2003, American Society of Addiction Medicine.

Gray-Vickrey P: What's behind acute delirium? *Nursing Made Incredibly Easy!* 3(1):20, 2005.

Guide to clinical preventive services, AHRQ Publication No. 05-0570, Agency for Healthcare Research and Quality, Rockville, Md, 2005, http://www.ahrp.gov/clinic/pocketgd.htm.

Guinto C H and others: Evaluation of dedicated stethoscopes as a potential source of nosocomial pathogens, *Am J Infect Control* 30(8):499, 2002.

Hardy M: What can you do about your patient's dry skin? *J Gerontol Nurs* 22(5):10, 1996.

Hayes JL: Are you assessing for melanoma? *RN* 66(2):36, 2003.

Hockenberry MJ, Wilson P: *Wong's nursing care of infants and children*, ed 8, St. Louis, 2007, Mosby.

Holcomb S: Boning up on osteoporosis, *Nursing Made Incredibly Easy!* 3(2):7, 2005.

Kovach K: Intimate partner violence, *RN* 67(8):38, 2004.

Lewis C: Osteoporosis: a man's issue, *Prepared Foods* 172(1):99, 2003.

McKenry L and others: *Mosby's pharmacology in nursing*, ed 22, St. Louis, 2006, Mosby.

Meiner SE, Lueckenotte A: *Gerontologic nursing*, ed 3, St. Louis, 2006, Mosby.

Metropolitan Life Insurance Company, *Statistical bulletin*, New York, 2000, Metropolitan.

Moore MC: *Pocket guide to nutritional assessment and care*, ed 5, St. Louis, 2005, Mosby.

National Pediculosis Association: *Child care provider's guide to controlling head lice*, http://www.headlice.org.

Quinn MJ: Undue influence and elder abuse: recognition and intervention strategies, *Geriatr Nurs* 23(1):11, 2002.

Seidel HM and others: *Mosby's guide to physical examination*, ed 6, St. Louis, 2006, Mosby.

Smith DE, Seymour RB: *Clinician's guide to substance abuse*, New York, 2001, McGraw-Hill.

Stuart G, Laraia M: *Principles and practice of psychiatric nursing*, ed 8, St. Louis, 2005, Mosby.

Talbot L, Curtis L: The challenges of assessing skin indicators in people of color, *Home Healthc Nurse* 14(3):167, 1996.

Thompson JM and others: *Mosby's clinical nursing*, ed 5, St. Louis, 2001, Mosby.

Truscott W: The role of PPE in contact transfer, *Infection Control Today* 9(10):18, 2005.

U.S. Department of Agriculture, Center for Nutrition Policy and Promotion, 2005, http://www.mypyramid.gov.

U.S. Preventative Services Task Force: Screening for osteoporosis in postmenopausal women: recommendations and rationale, *Am J Nurse* 103(1):73, 2003.

Widlitz M, Marin D: Substance abuse in older adults: an overview *Geriatrics* 57(12):29, 2002.

Research References

Folstein MF, Folstein S, McHugh PR: Mini-mental state: a practical method for grading the cognitive state of patients for the clinician, *J Psychiatr Res* 12:82, 1975.

Kahn RL and others: Brief objective measures for the determination of mental status of the aged, *Am J Psychiatry* 117:326, 1960.

CHAPTER 34
References

Association of PeriOperative Nurses: *Standards, recommended practices, and guidelines*, Denver, 2005, The Association.

Boyce JM, Pittet D: HICPAC/SHEA/APIC/IDSA Hand Hygiene Task Force and the CDC Healthcare Control Practices Advisory Committee draft guidelines for hand hygiene in healthcare settings, 2001.

Bulechek GM, Butcher HK, Dochterman JM: *Nursing interventions classification (NIC)*, ed 5, St. Louis, 2008, Mosby.

Burns E: *Aging and the immune system*, Milwaukee, Wis, 2001, Healthlink, College of Wisconsin.

Centers for Disease Control and Prevention, Hospital Infection Control Practices Advisory Committee: Recommendations for preventing the spread of vancomycin resistance, *Am J Infect Control* 23(2):87, 1995.

Centers for Disease Control and Prevention: *Guidelines for the Prevention and Transmission of hepatitis B, hepatitis C and human immunodeficiency virus in health care personnel*, Washington, DC, Centers for Disease Control and Prevention, 2001.

Centers for Disease Control and Prevention, Hospital Infection Control Practices Advisory Committee: *Draft: Guidelines for prevention of health care-associated pneumonia*, 2002a, http://www.cdc.gov.

Centers for Disease Control and Prevention, Hospital Infection Control Practices Advisory Committee: *Guideline for hand hygiene in health-care settings,* 2002b, http://www.cdc.gov.

Centers for Disease Control and Prevention: *Guideline for preventing the transmission of* Mycobacterium tuberculosis *in health-care facilities,* Washington, DC, 2005a, Centers for Disease Control and Prevention.

Centers for Disease Control and Prevention: *Updated U.S. Public Health Service guidelines for the management of occupational exposures to HIV and recommendations for post exposure prophylaxis,* Washington, DC, 2005b, Centers for Disease Control and Prevention.

Centers for Disease Control and Prevention: *Draft guideline for isolation precautions: preventing transmission of infectious agents in healthcare settings—recommendations to the Healthcare Infection Control Practices Advisory Committee (HICPAC),* Washington, DC, 2006a, Centers for Disease Control and Prevention.

Centers for Disease Control and Prevention: *Management of multidrug-resistant organisms in healthcare settings,* 2006b, Centers for Disease Control and Prevention.

Cipriano P: Save a life—wash your hands, *American Nurse Today* 2(1):10, 2007 http://www.AmericanNurseToday.com.

Fauerbach L: Risk factors for infection transmission. In Carrico R, editor: *APIC text of infection control and epidemiology,* Washington, DC, 2005, Association for Professionals in Infection Control and Epidemiology.

Gantz NM: Geriatric infections. In Carrico R, editor: *APIC text of infection control and epidemiology,* Washington, DC, 2005, Association for Professionals in Infection Control and Epidemiology.

Griffith CJ and others: Environmental surface cleanliness and the potential for contamination during hand washing, *Am J Infect Control* 31(2):93, 2003.

Harrison WA and others: Bacterial transfer and cross contamination potential associated with paper-towel dispensing, *Am J Infect Control* 31(7):387, 2003.

Larson E: APIC guideline for hand washing and hand antisepsis in health-care settings. In *APIC infection control and applied epidemiology: principles and practice,* St. Louis, 2005, Mosby.

Lesser KJ, Paiusi IC, Leips J: Naturally occurring genetic variation in the age-specific immune response of *Drosophila melanogaster, Aging Cell* 5(4):293, 2006.

Meiner S, Lueckenotte AG: *Gerontologic nursing,* ed 3, St. Louis, 2006, Mosby.

Moorhead S and others: *Nursing outcomes classification (NOC),* ed 4, St. Louis, 2008, Mosby.

Occupational Safety and Health Administration: Respiratory protection standard, *Federal Register* 60:3036, 1995.

Occupational Safety and Health Administration: Needlestick Safety and Prevention Act, Public Law 106-430 (2001).

Occupational Safety and Health Administration: Enforcement procedures for the occupational exposure to bloodborne injury final rule, *Federal Register* 66:5318, 2001.

Occupational Safety and Health Administration: Occupational Safety and Health Act of 2001, 2001, 2005, http://www.cdc.gov.

Pagana KD, Pagana TJ: *Diagnostic testing and nursing implications: a case study approach,* ed 7, St. Louis, 2005, Mosby.

Ritter H: Microbiology/laboratory diagnostics. In Carrico R, editor: *APIC text of infection control and epidemiology,* Washington, DC, 2005, Association for Professionals in Infection Control and Epidemiology.

Rutala W, Weber DJ: Centers for Disease Control and Prevention, Hospital Infection Control Practices Advisory Committee: *Guideline for disinfection and sterilization in healthcare facilities,* 2005, http://www.cdc.gov.

The Joint Commission, *National patient safety goals,* 2008, http://www.jointcommission.org/Patient Safety/NationalPatientSafetyGoals/, 2007, accessed February 13, 2008.

Tweeten SM. General principles of epidemiology. In Carrico R, editor: *APIC text of infection control and epidemiology,* Washington, DC, 2005, Association for Professionals in Infection Control and Epidemiology.

Research References

Gupta A and others: Outbreak of extended-spectrum-beta-lactamase-producing *Klebsiella pneumoniae* in a neonatal intensive care unit linked to artificial nails, *Infect Control Hosp Epidemiol* 25(3):210, 2004.

Hedderwick SA and others: Pathogenic organisms associated with artificial fingernails worn by healthcare workers, *Infect Control Hosp Epidemiol* 21(8):505, 2000.

Potter P and others: Evaluation of chemical dot thermometers for measuring body temperature of orally intubated patients, *Am J Crit Care* 12(5):403, 2003.

CHAPTER 35
References

American Diabetes Association: Insulin administration: position statement, *Diabetes Care* 27(1S):S106, 2004.

American Diabetes Association: Insulin delivery, *Diabetes Forecast* 58(1):RG16, 2005.

American Hospital Association: *The patient care partnership,* 2003, http://www.hospitalconnect.com/aha/ptcommunication/partnership/index.html.

American Nurses Association: *Nursing: scope and standards of practice,* Silver Springs, Md, 2004, The Association.

American Nurses Association: *Needlestick injury,* 2007, http://www.nursingworld.org/readroom/fsneedle.htm.

Andrews MM, Boyle JS: *Transcultural concepts in nursing care,* ed 5, Philadelphia, 2007, Lippincott.

Bastable S: *Nurse as educator: principles of teaching and learning for nursing practice,* Sudbury, Mass, 2003, Jones & Bartlett.

Brager R, Sloand E: The spectrum of polypharmacy, *Nurs Pract* 30(6):44, 2005.

Capriotti T: Changes in inhaler devices for asthma and COPD, *Medsurg Nurs* 14(3):185, 2005.

Centers for Disease Control and Prevention: TB elimination, 2007, http://www.cdc.gov.tb.

Ebersole P and others: *Toward healthy aging: human needs and nursing response,* ed 6, St. Louis, 2004, Mosby.

Hockenberry MJ, Wilson D: *Wong's nursing care of infants and children,* ed 8, St. Louis, 2007, Mosby.

Hughes R, Ortiz E: Medication errors: why they happen, and how they can be prevented, *Am J Nurs* 105(3 suppl):14, 2005.

Institute of Medicine: Report brief, to err is human: building a safer health system, 2003, http://iom.edu/CMS/8089/5575/4117.aspx.

Institute for Safe Medication Practices: *ISMP medication safety alert!* 2002, http://www.ismp.org/Newsletters/acutecare/articles/A1Q02Action.asp.

Institute for Safe Medication Practices: ISMP list of error-prone abbreviations, symbols, and dose designations, 2006a, http://www.ismp.org/tools/errorprone-abbreviations.pdf.

Institute of Safe Medication Practices (ISMP): *Oral dosage forms that should not be crushed,* 2008, http://www.ismp.org/Tools/DoNotCrush.pdf.

Institute for Safe Medication Practices: *Preventing errors with tablet splitting,* 2006b, http://www.accessdata.fda.gov/scripts/cdrh/cfdocs/psn/transcript.cfm?show=54#7.

Institute for Safe Medication Practices: Patches: what you can't see can harm patients, *Nurse Advise-ERR* 5(4):1, 2007.

Jordan S and others: Administration of medicines. II. Pharmacology, *Nurs Stand* 18(3):45, 2003.

Karch AM, Karch FE: Not so fast! *Am J Nurs* 103(8):71, 2003.

Manno MS: Preventing adverse drug events, *Nursing* 36(3):56, 2006.

MayoClinic.com: *Asthma,* 2007, http://www.mayoclinic.com/health/asthma.

McKenry LM and others: *Mosby's pharmacology in nursing,* ed 22, St. Louis, 2006, Mosby.

Meiner S, Lueckenotte A: *Gerontologic nursing,* ed 3, St. Louis, 2006, Mosby.

Morris H: Managing dysphagia in older people, *Primary Health Care* 16(6):34, 2006.

National Coordinating Council for Medication Error Reporting and Prevention: *Council recommendations: recommendations to reduce medication errors associated with verbal medication orders and prescriptions,* 2006, http://www.nccmerp.org/council/council2001-02-20.html?USP_Print=true&frame=lowerfrm.

Novo Nordisk: *Levimir,* 2007, http://www.levemir-us.com/hcp/default.asp.

Occupational Safety and Health Administration: Toxic and hazardous substances: bloodborne pathogens, *Federal Register,* CFR 29, part 1910.1030, April 3, 2006, www.osha.gov/pls/oshaweb/owadisp.show_document?p_table=STANDARDS&p_id=10051.

Oklahoma Department of Human Services: Advantage program services, 2006, http://www1.okdhs.org/en/library/policy/oac317/035/17/0003000.htm.

Ptasinski C: Develop a medication reconciliation process, *Nurs Manage* 38(3):18, 2007.

Rushing J: How to administer a subcutaneous infection, *Nursing* 34(6):32, 2004.

Sanofi-Aventis: A 6-step Guide for the Self-Administration of Lovenox®, 2007 http://www.lovenox.com/hcp/dosingAdministration/lovenoxSelfAdministration.aspx

The Joint Commission: *National patient safety goals,* 2008, http://www.jointcommission.org/PatientSafety/NationalPatientSafetyGoals/.

U.S. Food and Drug Administration: *MedWatch,* 2007, http://www.fda.gov/medwatch/.

VisionRx: *Encyclopedia: eye drops,* 2005, http://www.visionrx.com/library/enc/enc_eyedrops.asp.

Weisner AM and others: Implications of food allergies and intolerances on medication administration, *Orthopedics* 31(2):149, 2008

Research References

Annersten M, Willman A: Performing subcutaneous injections; a literature review, *Worldviews Evid Based Nurs* 2(3):122, 2005.

Cook IF, Murtagh J: Ventrogluteal area—a suitable site for intramuscular vaccination of infants and toddlers, *Vaccine* 24(13):2403, 2006.

Metheny NA: Preventing aspiration in older adults with dysphagia, *Medsurg Nurs* 15(2):110, 2006.

Mills PD and others: Improving the bar-coded administration system at the Department of Veteran Affairs, *Am J Health Syst Pharm* 63:1442, 2006.

Nicoll LH, Hesby A: Intramuscular injection: an integrative research review and guideline for evidence-based practice, *Appl Nurs Res* 16(2):149, 2002.

Paoletti RD and others: Using bar-code technology and medication observation methodology for safer medication administration, *Am J Health Syst Pharm* 64:536, 2007.

Pape TM and others: Innovative approaches to reducing nurses' distractions during medication administration, *J Cont Educ Nurs* 36(3):108, 2005.

Skibinski KA and others: Effects of technological interventions on the safety of a medication-use system, *Am J Health Syst Pharm* 64:90, 2007.

Small SP: Preventing sciatic nerve injury from intramuscular injections: literature review, *J Adv Nurs* 47(3):287, 2004.

Stein HG: Glass ampules and filter needles: an example of implementing the sixth "R" in medication administration, *Medsurg Nurs* 15(5):290, 2006.

Vella C, Grech V: Assessment of use of spacer devices for inhaled drug delivery to asthmatic children, *Pediatr Allergy Immunol* 16:258, 2005.

World Health Organization: *Report of the global injection safety and infection control meeting*, 2005, http://www.who.int/injection_safety/en/.

CHAPTER 36
References

American Holistic Nurses Association: *Standards of holistic nursing practice*, Flagstaff, Ariz, 2004, The Association.

Benson H: *The relaxation response*, New York, 1975, Avon.

Borysenko J: *Minding the body, mending the mind*, New York 1987, Bantam.

Dossey B, Keegan L, Guzzetta C: *Holistic nursing: a handbook for practice*, ed 4, Gaithersburg, Md, 2005, Aspen.

Eliopoulos C: *Gerontological nursing*, ed 6, Philadelphia, 2004, Lippincott, Williams & Wilkins.

Fontaine K: *Healing practices: alternative therapies for nursing*, ed 2, Upper Saddle River, NJ, 2005, Prentice Hall.

Gawain S: *Creative visualization*, ed 25, New York, 2002, New World Library.

Krieger D: Therapeutic touch: the imprimatur of nursing, *Am J Nurs* 75:784, 1975.

Krieger D: Searching for evidence of physiological change, *Am J Nurs* 79:660, 1979.

Kuhn M, Winston D: *Herbal therapy and supplements: a scientific and traditional approach*, New York, 2001, Lippincott, Williams & Wilkins.

Naparstek B: *Staying well with guided imagery*, New York, 1995, Warner.

Rakel DP, Faass N: *Complementary medicine in clinical practice*, Sudbury, Mass, 2006, Jones & Bartlett.

Research References

Brazier A and others: Evaluating a yogic breathing and meditation intervention for individuals living with HIV/AIDS, *Am J Health Promot* 20(3):192, 2006.

Breuhl S, Chung OY: Psychological and behavioral aspects of complex regional pain syndrome management, *Clin J Pain* 22(5):430, 2006.

Brown RP, Gerbarg PL: Sudarshan Kriya Yogic breathing in the treatment of stress, anxiety, and depression. II. Clinical applications and guidelines, *J Altern Complement Med* 11(4):711, 2005.

Chiarioni G, Salandini L, Whitehead WE: Biofeedback benefits only patients with outlet dysfunction, not patients with isolated slow transit constipation, *Gastroenterology* 129(1):86, 2005.

Cirstea CM and others: Feedback and cognition in arm motor skill reacquisition after stroke, *Stroke* 37(5):1237, 2006.

Damen L and others: Prophylactic treatment of migraine in children. I. A systematic review of non-pharmacological trials, *Cephalalgia* 26(4):373, 2006.

de Jong AE, Gambel C: Use of a simple relaxation technique in burn care: literature review, *J Adv Nurs* 54(6):710, 2006.

Galvin JA and others: The relaxation response: reducing stress and improving cognition in healthy aging adults, *Complement Ther Clin Pract* 12(3):186, 2006.

Gustavsson C, von Koch L: Applied relaxation in the treatment of long-lasting neck pain: a randomized controlled pilot study, *J Rehabil Med* 38(2):100, 2006.

Hui PN and others: An evaluation of two behavioral rehabilitation programs, qigong versus progressive relaxation, in improving the quality of life in cardiac patients, *J Altern Complement Med* 12(4):351, 2006.

Huth M and others: Imagery reduces children's post-operative pain. *Pain* 110 (1-2):439, 2004.

Kane KE: The phenomenology of meditation for female survivors of intimate partner violence, *Violence Against Women* 12(5):501, 2006.

Kanji N and others: Autogenic training for tension type headaches: a systematic review of controlled trials, *Complement Ther Med* 14(2):144, 2006.

Kaushik RM and others: Effects of mental relaxation and slow breathing in essential hypertension, *Complement Ther Med* 14(2):120, 2006.

Kempainnen JK and others: Strategies for self-management of HIV-related anxiety, *AIDS Care* 18(6):597, 2006.

Larden CN and others: Efficacy of therapeutic touch in treating pregnant inpatients who have a chemical dependency, *J Holist Nurs* 22(4):320,2004.

Lassetter JH: Effectiveness of complementary therapies on the pain experience of hospitalized children, *J Holist Nurs* 24(3):196, 2006.

Medlicott MS, Harris SR: A systematic review of the effectiveness of exercise, manual therapy, electrotherapy, relaxation training, and biofeedback in the management of temporomandibular disorder, *Phys Ther* 86(7):910, 2006.

Mehling WE and others: Randomized, controlled trial of breath therapy for patients with chronic low-back pain, *Altern Ther Health Med* 11(4):44, 2005.

Movaffaghi Z and others: Effects of therapeutic touch on blood hemoglobin and hematocrit level, *J Holist Nurs* 24(1):41, 2006.

Norbrink Budh C and others: A comprehensive pain management programme comprising educational, cognitive and behavioural interventions for neuropathic pain following spinal cord injury, *J Rehabil Med* 38(3):172, 2006.

Paul-Labrador M and others: Effects of a randomized controlled trial of transcendental meditation on components of the metabolic syndrome in subjects with coronary heart disease, *Arch Intern Med* 166(11):1218, 2006.

Stapleton JA and others: Effects of three PTSD treatments on anger and guilt: exposure therapy, eye movement desensitization and reprocessing, and relaxation training, *J Trauma Stress* 19(1):19, 2006.

Walton KG and others: Psychosocial stress and cardiovascular disease. II. Effectiveness of the transcendental meditation program in treatment and prevention, *Behav Med* 28(3):106, 2002.

Zaza C and others: Coping with cancer: what do patients do, *J Psychosoc Oncol* 23(1):5, 2005.

CHAPTER 37
References

Ackley BJ, Ladwig GB: *Nursing diagnosis handbook: a guide to planning care*, ed 7, St. Louis, 2006, Mosby.

American College of Sports Medicine Position Stand: The recommended quantity and quality of exercise for developing and maintaining cardiorespiratory and muscular fitness, and flexibility in healthy adults, *Med Sci Sports Exerc* 30(6):975, 1998.

American College of Sports Medicine: *Position stand on fitness: the recommended quantity and quality of exercise for developing and maintaining cardiorespiratory and muscular fitness, and flexibility in healthy adults*, 2002, Fifty Plus Fitness Association, http://www.50plus.org/Libraryitems/1_5positionstandonfitness.htm, accessed June, 2006.

American Diabetes Association: Diabetes and exercise: position statement, *Diabetes Care* 25(suppl 1):S64, 2002.

American Nurses Association: *Position statement on elimination of manual patient handling to prevent work-related musculoskeletal disorders*, 2003, http://www.nursingworld.org/readroom/postion/workplace/pathand.htm.

Bulechek GM, Butcher HK, Dochterman JM: *Nursing interventions classification (NIC)*, ed 5, St. Louis, 2008, Mosby.

Burbank PM and others: Exercise and older adults: changing behavior with the transtheoretical model, *Orthop Nurs* 21(4):51, 2002.

Chobanian AV and others: Seventh report of the joint national committee on prevention, detection, evaluation, and treatment of high blood pressure, *Hypertension* 42(6):1206, 2003.

Collins A: *Getting fit: unstructured exercise*, http://www.suite101.com/lesson.cfm/18274/1552, accessed April 7, 2007.

Dingle M: Role of dangling when moving from supine to standing position, *Br J Nurs* 12(6):346, 2003.

Flood L, Constance A: Diabetes and exercise safety, *Am J Nurs* 102(6):47, 2002.

Frederiks C and others: Evaluation of skills and knowledge on orthostatic blood pressure measurements in elderly patients, *Age Aging* 31(3):211, 2003.

Gillespie HO: Exercise. In Edelman CL, Mandle CL, editors: *Health promotion throughout the life span*, ed 6, St. Louis, 2006, Mosby.

Harper MG: Childhood obesity: strategies for prevention, *Fam Community Health* 29(4):288, 2006.

Hockenberry M, Wilson D: *Nursing care of infants and children*, ed 8, St. Louis, 2007, Mosby.

Hoeman SP: *Rehabilitation nursing: process, application, and outcomes*, ed 3, St. Louis, 2002, Mosby.

Huddleston JS: Exercise. In Edelman CL, Mandle CL, editors: *Health promotion throughout the life span,* ed 5, St. Louis, 2002, Mosby.

Huether SE, McCance KL: *Understanding pathophysiology,* ed 3, St. Louis, 2004, Mosby.

Katz DL and others: Public health strategies for preventing and controlling overweight and obesity in school and worksite settings: a report on recommendations of the Task Force on Community Preventive Services, *MMWR Recomm Rep* 54(RR-10):1, 2005.

Konradi DB, Anglin LT: Moderate-intensity exercise for our patients, for ourselves, *Orthop Nurs* 20(1):47, 2001.

Lewis SL and others: *Medical-surgical nursing assessment and management of clinical problems,* ed 7, St. Louis, 2007, Mosby.

Markusic J: *Maintain a healthy spine using good body mechanics,* 2003, Spine Universe, http://spineuniverse.com.

Mayo Clinic Tools for Healthier Lives: *Fitness programs: ready to get started?* 2005, http://www.mayoclinic.com/health/fitness/HQ00171.

Monahan F and others: *Phipps' medical-surgical nursing: health and illness perspectives,* ed 8, St. Louis, 2007, Mosby.

Moorhead S and others: *Nursing outcomes classification (NOC),* ed 4, St. Louis, 2008, Mosby.

Nelson A, Baptiste A: Evidence-based practices for safe patient handling and movement, *Online J Issues Nurs* 9(3), 2004.

Nelson A, Fragala, G, Menzel, N: Myths and facts about back injuries in nursing, *Am J Nurs* 103(2):4, 2003.

Nelson A and others: Safe patient handling and movement: preventing back injury among nurses requires careful selection of the safest equipment and techniques, *Am J Nurs* 103(3):32, 2003.

Occupational Safety and Health Administration: *Ergonomics standard regulatory text,* 2000, http://www.osha-slc.gov/ergonomics-standard/regulatory/regtext.html.

Prochaska JO, Norcross JC, DiClemente CC: *Changing for good,* New York, 1994, William Morrow.

Thibodeau GA, Patton KT: *Anatomy and physiology,* ed 6, St. Louis, 2007, Mosby.

Wechsler H and others: Childhood obesity, *The State Education Standard,* p 4, December, 2004.

Wilson SF, Giddens JF: *Health assessment for nursing practice,* ed 3, St. Louis, 2005, Mosby.

Research References

Baptiste A and others: Friction-reducing devices for lateral patient transfers: a clinical evaluation, *AAOHN J* 54(4):173, 2006.

Conroy MB and others: Past physical activity, current physical activity, and risk of coronary heart disease, *Med Science Sports Exerc* 37(8):1251, 2005.

Lacasse Y and others: Pulmonary rehabilitation for chronic obstructive pulmonary disease, *Cochrane Review* 3, 2004.

Lee ET and others: Incidence of diabetes in American Indians of three geographic areas, *Diabetes Care* 25:49, 2002.

Liu-Ambrose T and others: Resistance and agility training reduce fall risk in women aged 75 to 85 with low bone mass: a 6-month randomized, controlled trial, *J Am Geriatr Soc* 52:657, 2004.

Neatea R and others: Body position and blood pressure measurement in patients with diabetes mellitus, *J Intern Med* 251:393, 2002.

Normandin EA and others: An evaluation of two approaches to exercise conditioning in pulmonary rehabilitation, *Chest* 121(4):1085, 2002.

Padilla J and others: Accumulation of physical activity reduces blood pressure in pre- and hypertension, *Med Science Sports Exerc* 37(8):1264, 2005.

Prochaska JJ, Rodgers MW, Sallis JF: Association of parent and peer support with adolescent physical activity, *Res Q Exerc Sport* 73(2):206, 2002.

Rimmer JH and others: Feasibility of a health promotion intervention for a group of predominantly African American women with type 2 diabetes, *Diabetes Educ* 28(4):571, 2002.

Schneider JK and others: Exercise training program for older adults, *J Gerontol Nurs* 29:21, 2003.

Schneider JK and others: Promoting exercise behavior in older adults, *J Gerontol Nurs* 30(4):45, 2004.

Tokmakidis SP, Volaklis KA: Training and detraining effects of a combined-strength and aerobic exercise program on blood lipids in patients with coronary artery disease, *J Cardiopulm Rehabil* 23(3):193, 2003.

CHAPTER 38
References

Agency for Healthcare Research and Quality: *Reducing and preventing adverse drug events to decrease hospital costs,* 2006, http://www.ahrq.gov/qual/aderia/aderia.htm.

Ahrens M: *The U.S. fire problem overview report: leading causes and other patterns and trends,* Quincy Mass, 2003, NFPA.

American Academy of Pediatrics: *News release: don't treat swallowed poison with syrup of ipecac,* 2004, http://www.aap.org/advocacy/releases/novpoison.htm.

American Geriatrics Society Panel on Falls Prevention: Guideline for the prevention of falls in older persons, *J Am Geriatr Soc* 49(5):664, 2001.

American Medical Association: *Bioterrorism: frequently asked questions,* 2004, http://www.ama.assn.org/ama/pub/category/6667.html.

Bulechek GM, Butcher HK, Dochterman JM: *Nursing interventions classification (NIC),* ed 5, St. Louis, 2008, Mosby.

Centers for Disease Control and Prevention: *Older adult drivers: fact sheet,* 2006a, http://www.cdc.gov/ncipc/factsheets/older.htm.

Centers for Disease Control and Prevention: *Teen drivers: fact sheet,* 2006b, http://www.cdc.gov/ncipc/factsheets/teenmvh.htm.

Centers for Disease Control and Prevention: *Web based injury statistics query and reporting system (WISQARS),* 2006c, http://www.cdc.gov/ncipc/wisqars.

Dire DJ: *CBRNE—Biological warfare agents,* 2006, http://www.emedicine.com/emerg/byname/cbrne—biological-warfare-agents.htm.

Ebersole P, Hess P, Luggen A: *Toward healthy aging: human needs and nursing response,* ed 6, St. Louis, 2004, Mosby.

Edelman CL, Mandle CL: *Health promotion throughout the life span,* ed 6, St. Louis, 2006, Mosby.

Epilepsy Foundation: *First aid for generalized tonic clonic (grand mal) seizures,* 2006, http://www.epilepsyfoundation.org/answerplace/medical/firstaid/firstaidkeys.cfm.

Farmer B: *Try this: best practices in nursing care to older adults,* New York, 2000, The Hartford Institute for Geriatric Nursing, New York University.

Federal Emergency Management Agency: *Your family disaster plan,* 2004, http://www.fema.gov/rrr/famplan/shtm.

Funk SG and others: *A fall prevention program for the acute care setting: key aspects of elder care—managing falls, incontinence, and cognitive impairments,* New York, 1992, Springer.

Geriatric nursing resources for care of older adults: *Physical restraints,* 2006, http://www.geronurseonline.org/index.

Giger JN, Davidhizar R: The Giger and Davidhizar transcultural assessment model, *J Transcult Nurs* 13(3):185, 2002.

Hauck C and others: The contribution of prone sleeping position to racial disparity in SIDS: the Chicago Infant Mortality Study, *Pediatrics* 110(4):772, 2003.

HealthGrades, Inc: *HealthGrades quality study: second annual patient safety in American hospitals report,* New York, 2005, Sterling.

Hockenberry M, Wilson D: *Wong's nursing care of infants and children,* ed 8, St. Louis, 2007, Mosby.

Insurance Institute for Highway Safety: *Fatality facts, older people,* 2003, http://www.highwaysafety.org/safetyfacts/fatalityfacts/olderpeople.htm.

Jones J and others: Future challenges in preparing for and responding to bioterrorism events, *Emerg Med Clin North Am* 20(2):501, 2002, Centers for Disease Control and Prevention.

Kohn LT, Corrigan JM, Donaldson MS, editors: *To err is human: building a safer health system,* Washington, DC, 1999, Institute of Medicine, National Academy Press, Committee on Quality of Healthcare in America.

McCullagh MC: Home modification: How to help patients make their homes safer and more accessible as their abilities change, *Am J Nurs* 106(10):54, 2006.

Meiner S, Lueckenotte A: *Gerontologic nursing,* ed 3, St. Louis, 2006, Mosby.

Moorhead S and others: *Nursing outcomes classification (NOC),* ed 4, St. Louis, 2008, Mosby.

National Center for Environmental Health, Division of Emergency and Environmental Health Services, Centers for Disease Control and Prevention: *Childhood lead poisoning,* May 2005, http://www.cdc.gov/nceh/publications/factsheets/childleadpoisoning.pdf.

National Center for Injury Prevention and Control, Centers for Disease Control and Prevention: *Injury Fact Book 2001-2002,* Atlanta, 2002, Centers for Disease Control and Prevention.

National Fire Protection Association: *Carbon monoxide poisoning,* 2006a, http://www.nfpa.org/itemDetail.html.

National Fire Protection Association: *Home fire statistics,* 2006b, http://www.nfpa.org/itemDetail.

National Safety Council: *Home fire protection and preparedness fact sheet,* Itasca, Ill, 2002, The Council.

Nix S: *Williams' basic nutrition and diet therapy,* ed 12, St. Louis, 2005, Mosby.

Runyan SW, Casteel C, editors: *The state of home safety in America: facts about unintentional injuries in the home,* ed 2, Washington, DC, 2004, Home Safety Council.

Sorrentino SA: *Mosby's textbook for nursing assistants,* ed 6, St. Louis, 2004, Mosby.

Steinhauer R, Bauer J: The emergency management plan, *RN* 65(6):40, 2002.

Strumpf N and others: *Restraint free care: individualized approaches for frail elders,* New York, 1998, Springer.

The Joint Commission: *Comprehensive accreditation manual for hospitals: the official handbook,* Oakbrook Terrace, Ill, 2007, The Joint Commission.

The Joint Commission: *National patient safety goals, 2007,* http://www.jointcommission.org/PatientSafety/NationalPatientSafetyGoals/08_npsg_facts.html.

The Joint Commission Resources: *Strategies for avoiding restraint related errors,* 2006, http://www.jcrinc.com.

Research References

Capezuti E and others: The relationship between physical restraint removal and falls and injuries among nursing home residents, *J Gerontol A Biol Sci Med Sci* 53A:M47, 1998.

Chang JT and others: Interventions for the prevention of falls in older adults: systematic review with meta-analysis of randomized clinical trials, *Br Med J* 328(7441):680, 2004.

Fiore AE: Hepatitis A transmitted by food, *Clin Infect Dis* 38:705, 2004.

Ledford L, Mentals J: *Restraints: a research-based protocol,* Iowa City, Iowa, 1998, University of Iowa Gerontological Nursing Interventions Research Center.

Meade CM and others: Effects of nursing rounds on patients' call light use, satisfaction and safety, *Am J Nurs* 106(9):58, 2006.

Trinkoff A and others: How long and how much are nurses working? *Am J Nurs* 106(4):60, 2006.

CHAPTER 39
References

Agency for Health Care Policy and Research: *Pressure ulcers in adults: prediction and prevention,* Pub Nos. 92-0047, 92-0050, Rockville, Md, 1992, U.S. Department of Health and Human Services, Public Health Service.

American Academy of Ophthalmology: *Contact lenses,* 2005, http://www.nlm.nih.gov/medlineplus/eyewear.

American Diabetes Association: Position statement on standards of medical care in diabetes 2007, *Diabetes Care* 30:S4, 2007.

American Diabetes Association: Preventive foot care in people with diabetes, *Diabetes Care* 21(suppl 1):S56, 2001.

Beck DM: Venous thromboembolism (VTE) prophylaxis: implications for medical-surgical nurses, *Medsurg Nurs* 15(5):282, 2006.

Bennet MA: Report of the Task Force on the Implications for Darkly Pigmented Intact Skin in the Prediction and Prevention of Pressure Ulcers, *Adv Wound Care* 8(6):34, 1995.

Berry AM and others: Systematic literature review of oral hygiene practices for intensive care patients receiving mechanical ventilation, *Am J Crit Care* 16(6):552, 2007.

Brinkley C and others: Survey of oral care practices in U.S. intensive care units, *Am J Infect Control* 32(6):161, 2004.

Bryant JL, Beinlich NR: Foot care: focus on the elderly, *Orthop Nurs* 18(6):53, 1999.

Bulechek GM, Butcher HK, Dochterman JM: *Nursing interventions classification (NIC),* ed 5, St. Louis, 2008, Mosby.

Bush BC, Donley TG: A model for dental hygiene education concerning the relationship between periodontal health and systemic health, *Educ Health* 15(1):19, 2002.

Ebersole P, Hess P: *Toward healthy aging: human needs and nursing response,* ed 6, St. Louis, 2004, Mosby.

Fulton JS, Middleton GJ, McPhail JT: Management of oral complications, *Semin Oncol Nurs* 18:28, 2002.

Galanti GA: Caring for patients from different cultures, ed 3, Philadelphia, 2004, University of Pennsylvania Press.

Green MF, Aliabaide Z, Green BT: Diabetic foot: evaluation and management, *South Med J* 95(1):95, 2002.

Hockenberry ML, Wilson D: *Wong's nursing care of infants and children,* ed 8, St. Louis, 2007, Mosby.

Lewis SL and others: *Medical surgical nursing: assessment and management of clinical problems,* ed 7, St. Louis, 2007, Mosby.

Martinez N, Tripp-Reimer T: Diabetes nurse educators' prioritized elder foot care behaviors, *Diabetes Educ* 31(6):858, 2005.

Meiner S, Lueckenotte AG: *Gerontologic nursing,* ed 3, St. Louis, 2006, Mosby.

Moorhead S and others: *Nursing outcomes classification (NOC),* ed 4, St. Louis, 2008, Mosby.

National Institute on Deafness and Other Communication Disorders: *Hearing aids,* Pub No. 99-4340, Bethesda, Md, 2001, National Institutes of Health, http://www.nidcd.nih.gov/health/hearing/hearingaid.asp.

National Pediculosis Association: *Child care provider's guide to controlling head lice,* 2001, http://www.headlice.org.

Pender N, Murdaugh C, Parsons M: *Health promotion in nursing practice,* Upper Saddle River, NJ, 2002, Pearson Education.

Poland JM: Comparing Moi-Stin to lemon glycerin swabs, *Am J Nurs* 87:422, 1987.

Research update: oral care prevents pneumonia in nursing homes, *Aust Nurs J* 9(11):18, 2002.

Skewes SM: No more bed baths!, *RN* 57:30, 1994.

Verderber A, Gallagher KJ: Effects of bathing, passive range-of-motion exercises, and turning on oxygen consumption in healthy men and women, *Am J Crit Care* 3:374, 1994.

Walton JC, Miller J, Tordecilla L: Elder oral assessment and care, *ORL Head Neck Nurs* 202:12, 2002.

Zurlinden J: Drug news: new warnings for Lindane Shampoo and Lotion, *Nurs Spectr-Midwestern Ed* 40(6):10, 2003.

Research References

Bauroth K and others: The efficacy of an essential oil antiseptic mouthwash vs. dental flossing in controlling interproximal gingivitis: a comparative study, *J Am Dental Assoc* 134(3):359, 2003.

Boyer L: News from NNGF: home care nurse's thoughts on dry skin and foot care in the older person, *World Council of Enterostomal Therapists Journal* 21(1):9, 2001.

Bryant J L, Beinlich NR: Foot care: focus on the elderly, *Orthop Nurs* 18(6):53, 1999.

Frykberg R and others: Diabetic foot disorders: a clinical practice guideline, *J Foot Ankle Surg* 45(5): S2, 2006.

Gadbury-Amyot CC and others: Prioritization of the National Dental Hygiene Research Agenda, *J Dent Hyg* 76(2):157, 2002.

Grap MJ and others: Duration of action of a single, early oral application of chlorhexidine on oral microbial flora in mechanically ventilated patients: a pilot study, *Heart Lung* 33(2):83, 2004.

Hall GR, Buckwalter KC: *Evidence-based protocol: bathing persons with dementia.* In Titler MG, series editor: Series on evidence-based practice for older adults, Iowa City, 1995, The University of Iowa College of Nursing Gerontological Nursing Interventions Research Center, Research Dissemination Core, revised 2001.

Hoeffer B: Assisting cognitively impaired nursing home residents with bathing: effects of two bathing interventions on caregiving, *Gerontologist* 46(4):524, 2006.

Hornick B: Diet and nutrition implications for oral health, *J Dent Hyg* 76(1):67, 2002.

Larson E and others: Comparison of traditional and disposable bed baths in critically ill patients, *Am J Crit Care* 13(3):235, 2004.

Mahoney EK and others: Challenges to intervention implementation lessons learned in the Bathing Persons With Alzheimer's Disease at Home Study, *Nurs Res* 55(2 suppl):S10, 2006.

Munro CL, Grap MJ. Oral health and care in the intensive care unit: state of the science, *Am J Crit Care,* 13(1):25, 2004.

Munro CL and others: Oral health measurement in nursing research: state of the science, *Biol Res Nurs* 8(1):35, 2006.

Neil JA: Assessing foot care knowledge in a rural population with diabetes, *Ostomy Wound Manage* 48(1):50, 2002

Pinzur MS and others: Guidelines for diabetic foot care, The Diabetes Committee of the American Orthopaedic Foot and Ankle Society, *Foot Ankle Int* 26(1):113, 2005.

Piotrowski M and others: Massage as an adjuvant therapy in the management of acute postoperative pain: a preliminary study. *J Am Coll Surg* 197(6):1037, 2003.

Rader J and others: The bathing of older adults with dementia, *Am J Nurs* 106(4):40, 2006.

Ring T: Trends in dental hygiene education, *Access* 16(7):16, 2002.

Sheppard CM, Brenner PS: The effects of bathing and skin care practices on skin quality and satisfaction with an innovative product. *J Gerontol Nurs* 26(10):36, 2000.

Strauss MB: Hart JD, Winant DM: Preventive foot care: a user-friendly system for patients and physicians, *Postgrad Med* 103(5):233, 1998.

Zullino DF and others: Local back massage with an automated massage chair: several muscle and psychophysiologic relaxing properties, *J Altern Complement Med* 11(6):1103, 2005.

CHAPTER 40
References

Albert NM: We are what we eat: women and diet for cardiovascular health, *J Cardiovasc Nurs* 20:451, 2005.

Allibone L: Nursing management of chest drains, *Nurs Stand* 17(22):45, 2003.

American Association of Respiratory Care: AARC clinical practice guideline, nasotracheal suction—2004 revision and update, *Respir Care* 49:1080, 2004.

American Association of Respiratory Care: AARC clinical practice guideline, suctioning of the patient in the home, *Respir Care* 44:99, 1999, http://www.rcjournal.com/cpgs/pdf/01.99.99.pdf, accessed June 29, 2007.

American Association of Respiratory Care: AARC clinical practice guideline, postural drainage therapy, *Respir Care* 36:1418, 1991, accessed June 29, 2007.

American Cancer Society: *Second hand smoke—what is it?* Atlanta, 2006a, The Society, http://www.cancer.org/docroot/PED/content/PED_10_2X_Secondhand_Smoke-Clean_Indoor_Air.asp, accessed June 29, 2007.

American Cancer Society: *Cancer prevention and early detection facts and figures 2006*, Atlanta, 2006b, The Society, http://www.cancer.org/docroot/STT/content/STT_1x_Cancer_Prevention_and_Early_Detection_Facts__Figures_2006.asp, accessed June 29, 2007.

American Heart Association: *CPR and AEDs*, 2003, http://www.AHA.org.

American Heart Association: 2005 American Heart Association guidelines for cardiopulmonary resuscitation and emergency cardiovascular care, *Circulation* 112(suppl I):IV-1, 2005a.

American Heart Association: Part 3, overview of CPR, *Circulation* 112 (suppl I): IV-12, 2005b.

American Heart Association: Community lay rescuer automated external defibrillator programs, *Circulation* 113:1260, 2006a.

American Heart Association: *Women and coronary heart disease*, 2006b, The Association, http://www.americanheart.org/presenter.jhtml?identifier=2859, accessed June 29, 2007.

American Heart Association: *Women, heart disease and stroke*, 2006c, The Association, http://www.americanheart.org/presenter.jhtml?identifier=4786, accessed June 29, 2007.

Bulechek GM, Butcher HK, Dochterman JM: *Nursing interventions classification (NIC)*, ed 5, St. Louis, 2008, Mosby.

Canobbio MM: *Cardiovascular disorders*, St. Louis, 1990, Mosby.

Carroll P: A guide to mobile chest drains, *RN* 65(5):56, 2002.

Carroll P: Keeping up with mobile chest drains, *RN* 68(10):26, 2005.

Centers for Disease Control and Prevention: *Targeted tuberculin testing and interpreting tuberculin skin test results*, Atlanta, April 2005, Centers for Disease Control and Prevention.

Centers for Disease Control and Prevention: *Adult immunization schedule 2006-2007, National Immunization Program*, Atlanta, 2006a, Centers for Disease Control and Prevention, http://www.cdc.gov/nip/recs/adult-schedule.htm#print, accessed June 29, 2007.

Centers for Disease Control and Prevention: *Tuberculin Skin Testing*, 2006b, Atlanta, Centers for Disease Control and Prevention, Division of TB Elimination, http://www.phppo.cdc.gov/tb/pubs/tbfactsheets/skintesting.pdf, accessed June 29, 2007.

Cerfolio RJ: Recent advances in the treatment of air leaks, *Curr Opin Pulm Med* 11:319, 2005.

Findeisen M: Long-term oxygen therapy in the home, *Home Healthc Nurse* 19(11):692, 2001.

Fujimoto K and others: Benefits of oxygen therapy on exercise performance and pulmonary hemodynamics in patients with COPD and mild hypoxemia, *Chest* 122(2):457, 2002.

Granger BB, Miller CM: Acute coronary syndrome: putting the new guidelines to work, *Nursing* 31(11):36, 2001.

Halm M: To strip or not to strip: physiological effects of chest tube manipulation. *Am J Crit Care* 16(6):609, 2007.

Hess DR: Tracheostomy tubes and related appliances, *Respir Care* 50:497, 2005.

Hockenberry MJ, Wilson D: *Wong's nursing care of infants and children*, ed 8, St. Louis, 2007, Mosby.

Jevon P, Evans B: Assessment of a breathless patient, *Nurs Stand* 15(16):48, 2001.

Leigh-Smith S, Harris T: Tension pneumothorax: time for a re-think? *Emerg Med J* 22:8, 2005.

Lewarski JS: Long-term care of the patient with a tracheostomy, *Respir Care* 50:534, 2005.

Lewis SL and others: *Medical-surgical nursing: assessment and management of clinical problems*, ed 7, St. Louis, 2007, Mosby.

McCance KL, Huether SE: *Pathophysiology: the biologic basis for disease in adults and children*, ed 5, St. Louis, 2005, Mosby.

Meiner S and Lueckenotte AG: *Gerontologic nursing*, ed 3, St. Louis, 2006, Mosby.

Moore, T: Suctioning techniques for the removal of respiratory secretions, *Nurs Stand* 18(9):47, 2003.

Moorhead S and others: *Nursing outcomes classification (NOC)*, ed 4, St. Louis, 2008, Mosby.

Pagana KD, Pagana TJ: *Mosby's diagnostic and laboratory test reference*, ed 7, St. Louis, 2005, Mosby.

Petty TL: Guide to prescribing home oxygen: home oxygen options, 2004, National Lung Health Education Program, http://www.nlhep.org/resources/Prescrb-Hm-Oxygen/home-oxygen-options-4.html, accessed November 18, 2006.

Potter PA, Weilitz PB: *Health assessment pocket guide series*, ed 6, St. Louis, 2007, Mosby.

Pullen RL: Teaching bedside incentive spirometry, *Nursing* 33(8):24, 2003.

Roman M, Mercado D: Review of chest tube use, *Medsurg Nurs* 15(1):41, 2006.

Seay SJ and others: Tracheostomy emergencies: correcting accidental decannulation or displaced tracheostomy tube, *Am J Nurs* 102:59, 2002.

Thomson A and others: Oxygen therapy in acute medical care: the potential dangers of hyperoxia need to be recognised, *Br Med J* 324(7351):1406, 2002.

Research References

Akgul S, Akyolcu N: Effects of normal saline on endotracheal suctioning, *J Clin Nurs* 11(6): 826, 2002.

Basoglu O and others: The efficacy of incentive spirometry in patients with COPD, *Respirology* 10:349, 2005.

Bourgault AM and others: Effects of endotracheal tube suctioning on arterial oxygen tension and heart rate variability, *Biol Res Nurs* 7:268, 2006.

Cuvelier A and others: Refillable oxygen cylinders may be an alternative for ambulatory oxygen therapy in COPD, *Chest* 122(2):451, 2002.

Day T and others: Tracheal suctioning: an exploration of nurses' knowledge and competence in acute and high dependency ward areas, *J Adv Nurs* 39(1):35, 2002.

Denke MA: Primary prevention of heart disease in women, *Curr Atheroscler Rep* 3(2):136, 2001.

Fretag CC and others: Prolonged application of closed in-line suction catheters increase microbial colonization of lower respiratory tract bacterial growth on catheter surface, *Infection* 31(1):31, 2003.

Kerr ME and others: Effect of endotracheal suctioning on cerebral oxygen in traumatic brain injured patients, *Crit Care Med* 27(2):2776, 1999.

Lawrence VA and others: Strategies to reduce postoperative pulmonary complications after noncardiothoracic surgery: systematic review for the American college of physicians, *Ann Intern Med* 144:596, 2006.

Oerman CM and others: Validation of an instrument measuring patient satisfaction with chest physiotherapy techniques in cystic fibrosis, *Chest* 118:92, 2000.

Oh H, Seo W: A meta-analysis of the effects of various interventions in preventing endotracheal suction–induced hypoxemia, *J Clin Nurs* 12:912, 2003.

Shaw LJ and others: The economic burden of angina in women with suspected ischemic heart disease, *Circulation* 114:894, 2006.

Sole ML and others: Bacterial growth in secretions on suction equipment of orally intubated patients: a pilot study, *Am J Crit Care* 11(2):41, 2002.

Snow V and others: The evidence base for management of acute exacerbations of COPD: clinical practice guideline, part I, *Chest* 119(4):1185, 2001.

Stulbarg MS and others: Exercise training improves outcomes of a dyspnea self-management program, *J Cardiopulm Rehabil* 22(2):109, 2002.

The Joint National Committee on Prevention, Detection, Evaluation and Treatment of High Blood Pressure: *The sixth report of the Joint National Committee on Prevention, Detection, Evaluation and Treatment of High Blood Pressure (JNC VII)*, Bethesda, Md, 2003, U.S. Department of Health and Human Services, National Heart, Lung, and Blood Institute, http://www.nhlbi.nih.gov/guidelines/hypertension/express.pdf, accessed November 2006.

CHAPTER 41
References

Brashers V: *Clinical applications of pathophysiology: an evidence-based practice approach*, ed 3, St. Louis, 2006, Mosby.

Brecher M, editor: *AABB technical manual*, ed 15, Bethesda, Md, 2005, AABB.

Brown J: Using lidocaine for peripheral IV insertions: patients' preferences and pain experiences, *MEDSURG Nurs* 12(2):100, 2003.

Bulechek GM, Butcher HK, Dochterman JM: *Nursing interventions classification (NIC)*, ed 5, St. Louis, 2008, Mosby.

Burgess R: Blood transfusion in A&E, *Emerg Nurs* 13(10): 21, 2006.

Burke MM, Laramie JA: *Primary care of the older adult: a multidisciplinary approach*, St. Louis, 2004, Mosby.

Casey G: Oedema: causes, physiology and nursing management, *Nurs Stand* 18(51):45, 2004.

Centers for Disease Control and Prevention: Guidelines for the prevention of intravascular cannula-related infections, *MMWR Morb Mortal Wkly Rep* 51 (RR-10), 2002.

Chernecky C, Macklin D, Murphy-Ende K: *Saunders' nursing survival guide: fluid and electrolytes*, ed 2, Philadelphia, 2006, Saunders.

Christensen B, Kockrow E: *Foundations of nursing*, ed 4, St. Louis, 2003, Mosby.

Coulter K: The older adult patient. In Macklin D, Chernecky C: *Real world survival nursing guide IV therapy*, St. Louis, 2004, Saunders.

Davidhizar R and others: A review of the literature on how important water is to the world's elderly population, *Int Nurs Rev* 51:160, 2004.

Davis K, Hui C, Quested B: Transfusing safely: a 2006 guide for nurses, *Am J Nurs* 13(6):4, 2006.

Elgart H: Assessment of fluid and electrolytes, *AACN Clin Issues* 15(4):607, 2004.

Fulcher E, Frazier M: *Introduction to intravenous therapy for health professionals*, St. Louis, 2007, Saunders.

Goodnough LT: Risks of blood transfusions, *Anesthesiol Clin North Am* 23(2):241, 2005.

Grandjean AC and others: Hydration: issues for the 21st century, *Nutr Rev* 61(8):264, 2003.

Hadaway M, Milam D: On the road to successful IV starts, *Nursing* 35(S):22, 2005.

Heitz UE, Horne MM: *Mosby's pocket guide series: fluid, electrolyte, and acid-base balance*, ed 5, St. Louis, 2005, Mosby.

Hindley G: Infection control in peripheral cannulae, *Nurs Stand* 18(27):39, 2004.

Hockenberry M and Wilson D: *Wong's essentials of pediatric nursing*, ed 8, St. Louis, 2007, Mosby.

Ignatavicius D, Workman MJ: *Medical-surgical nursing*, ed 5, Philadelphia, 2005, Saunders.

Infusion Nurses Society: Infusion nursing standards of practice, *J Intraven Nurs* 29(1S):S1-S90, 2006.

Lewis SL and others: *Medical-surgical nursing: assessment and management of clinical problems*, ed 7, St. Louis, 2007, Mosby.

McCance KL, Huether SE: *Pathophysiology: the biologic basis for disease in adults and children*, ed 5, St. Louis, 2005, Mosby.

McKenry LM and others: *Mosby's pharmacology in nursing*, ed 22, St. Louis, 2006, Mosby.

Monahan F and others: *Phipps' medical-surgical nursing: health and illness perspectives*, ed 8, St. Louis, 2007, Mosby.

Moorhead S and others: *Nursing outcomes classification (NOC)*, ed 4, St. Louis, 2008, Mosby.

Pruitt B: Help your patient combat postoperative atelectasis, *Nursing* 36(5):64, 2006.

Reuben DB and others: *2005 Geriatrics at your fingertips*, ed 7, Malden, Mass, 2005, Blackwell.

Rosenthal K: Pinpointing intravascular site infections, *Nurs Manage* 34(6):38, 2003.

Rosenthal K: Tailor your IV insertion techniques to special populations, *Nursing* 35(5):37, 2005.

Rudnicke C: Transfusion alternatives, *J Infus Nurs* 26(3):29, 2003.

Schelper R: The aging venous system, *Journal of Vascular Access Devices* 7(1):8, 2003.

Scotland R, Ahluwalia A, Hobbs A: C-type natriuretic peptide in vascular physiology and disease, *Pharmacol Ther* 105(2):85, 2005.

Short R: Poor checks for bedside blood transfusion put patients at risk, *Br Med J* 332(7551):1771, 2006.

Research References

Adams BD and others: The anion gap does not accurately screen for lactic acidosis in emergency patients, *Emerg Med J* 23:179, 2006.

Mentes JC: *Hydration management*. In Titler M, editor. Series on evidence-based practice for older adults, Iowa City, 2004, The University of Iowa College of Nursing Gerontological Nursing Interventions Research Center.

Smith B: Peripheral intravenous catheter dwell times: a comparison of three securement methods for implementation of a 96-hours scheduled change protocol, *J Infus Nurs* 29(1):17, 2006.

Toth L: Monitoring infusion therapy in patients residing in long-term care facilities, *Journal of Vascular Access Devices* 7(1):34, 2002.

CHAPTER 42
References

American Academy of Sleep Medicine: International classes of diseases and international classification of sleep disorders. In Thorpy M: Classification of sleep disorders. In Kryger M and others, editors: *Principles and practice of sleep medicine*, ed 5, Philadelphia, 2005, Saunders.

American Nurses Association: *Nursing scope and standards of practice*, Washington, DC, 2004, The Association.

Andrews MM, Boyle JS: *Transcultural concepts in nursing care*, ed 4, Philadelphia, 2003, Lippincott.

Attarian HP: Helping patients who say they cannot sleep: practical ways to evaluate and treat insomnia, *Postgrad Med* 107(3):127, 2000.

Bulechek GM, Butcher HK, Dochterman JM: *Nursing interventions classification (NIC)*, ed 5, St. Louis, 2008, Mosby.

Benca RM, Schneck CH: Sleep and eating disorders. In Kruger MH and others: *Principles and practice of sleep medicine*, ed 4, St. Louis, 2005, Saunders.

Buysse DJ: Diagnosis and assessment of sleep and circadian rhythm disorders, *J Psychiatr Pract* 11(2):102, 2005.

Buysse DJ and others: Clinical pharmacology of other drugs used as hypnotics. In Kryger MH, Roth T, Dement WC, editors: *Principles and practice of sleep medicine*, ed 4, Philadelphia, 2005, Saunders.

Cmiel CA and others: Noise control: a nursing team's approach to sleep promotion, *Am J Nurs* 104(2):40, 2004.

Cullen DF: Obstructive sleep apnea and postoperative analgesia: a potentially dangerous combination, *J Clin Anesth* 13:83, 2001.

Davis KF and others: Sleep in infants and young children. I. Normal sleep, *J Pediatr Health Care* 18(2):65, 2004.

D'Cruz OF, Vaughn BV: Parasomnias: an update, *Semin Pediatr Neurol* 8(4):251, 2001.

Dines-Kalinowski CM: Promoting sleep in the ICU, *Nursing* 32(2):326, 2002.

Edinger JD, Means MK: Overview of insomnia: epidemiology, differential diagnosis, and assessment. In Kryger MH, Roth T, Dement WC, editors: *Principles and practice of sleep medicine*, ed 4, Philadelphia, 2005, Saunders.

Elliott AC: Primary care assessment and management of sleep disorders, *J Am Acad Nurse Pract* 13(9):409, 2001.

Giger JN, Davidhizar RE: *Transcultural nursing: assessment and intervention*, ed 4, St. Louis, 2004, Mosby.

Groth M: Sleep apnea in the elderly, *Clin Geriatr Med* 21:701, 2005.

Guilleminault C, Bassiri A: Clinical features and evaluation of obstructive apnea. In Kryger MH, Roth T, Dement WC, editors, *Principles and practice of sleep medicine*, ed 4, Philadelphia, 2005, Saunders.

Guilleminault C, Fromberz S: Narcolepsy: diagnosis and management. In Kryger MH, Roth T, Dement WC, editors, *Principles and practice of sleep medicine*, ed 4, Philadelphia, 2005, Saunders.

Hockenberry MJ, Wilson D: *Wong's nursing care of infants and children*, ed 8, St. Louis, 2007, Mosby.

Hoffman S: Sleep in the older adult: implications for nurses, *Geriatr Nurs* 24(4):210, 2003.

Holman ML: Obstructive sleep apnea syndrome: implications for primary care, *Nurs Pract* 30(9):38, 2005.

Honkus VL: Sleep deprivation in critical care units, *Crit Care Nurse* 26(3):179, 2003.

Izac SM: Basic anatomy and physiology of sleep, *Am J Electroneurodiagnostic Technol* 46:18, 2006.

Jenni OG, O'Connor BB: Children's sleep: an interplay between culture and biology, *Pediatrics* 115(1):204, 2005.

Jones B: Basic mechanisms of sleep-wake states. In Kryger MH, Roth T, Dement WC, editors: *Principles and practice of sleep medicine*, ed 4, Philadelphia, 2005, Saunders.

Lashley F: Measuring sleep. In Frank-Stromborg M, Olsen SJ, editors: *Instruments for clinical-healthcare research*, ed 3, Boston, 2004, Jones & Bartlett.

Levy Raydo LJ, Reu-Donlon CM: Putting babies "back to sleep": can we do better? *Neonatal Network* 24(6):9, 2005.

Malow BA: Approach to the patient with disordered sleep. In Kryger MH, Roth T, Dement WC, editors: *Principles and practice of sleep medicine*, ed 4, Philadelphia, 2005, Saunders.

Maur KL: Promoting sound sleep habits in older adults, *Nursing* 35(2):22, 2005.

McCance KL, Huether SE: *Pathophysiology: the biologic basis for disease in adults and children*, ed 5, St. Louis, 2006, Mosby.

McKenry LM, Salerno E: *Mosby's pharmacology in nursing*, ed 21, St. Louis, 2003, Mosby.

Meiner SE, Lueckenotte AG: *Gerontologic nursing*, ed 3, St. Louis, 2006, Mosby.

Mendelson WB: Hypnotic medications: basic mechanisms and mechanisms of action and pharmacologic effects. In Kryger MH, Roth T, Dement WC, editors: *Principles and practice of sleep medicine*, ed 4, Philadelphia, 2005, Saunders.

Mendez JL, Olson EJ: Obstructive sleep apnea syndrome. I. Identifying the problem, *J Respir Dis* 27(4):144, 2006a.

Mendez JL, Olson EJ: Obstructive sleep apnea syndrome. II. Reviewing the treatment options, *J Respir Dis* 27(5):222, 2006b.

Mignot E: Narcolepsy: pharmacology, pathophysiology, and genetics. In Kryger MH, Roth T, Dement WC, editors: *Principles and practice of sleep medicine*, ed 4, Philadelphia, 2005, Saunders.

Moorhead S and others: *Nursing outcomes classification (NOC)*, ed 4, St. Louis, 2008, Mosby.

Morin AK and others: Therapeutic options for sleep-maintenance and sleep-onset insomnia, *Pharmacotherapy* 27(1):89, 2007.

Morin CM. Psychological and behavioral treatments for primary insomnia. In Kryger MH, Roth T, Dement WC, editors: *Principles and practice of sleep medicine*, ed 4, Philadelphia, 2005, Saunders.

Nagel U and others: Sleep promotion in hospitalized elders, *Med Surg Nurs* 12(5):279, 2003.

National Guideline Clearinghouse: *Evaluating excessive sleepiness in the older adult,* 2006, http://www.guideline.gov.

National Heart, Lung, and Blood Institute Working Group on Restless Leg Syndrome: Restless leg syndrome: detection and management in primary care, *Am Fam Physician* 61(1):108, 2000.

National Sleep Foundation: *The ABCs of ZZZs,* Washington, DC, 2002a, The Foundation.

National Sleep Foundation: *Sleep apnea,* Washington, DC, 2002b, The Foundation.

National Sleep Foundation: *The nature of sleep,* 2003, http://www.sleepfoundation.org/publications/nos.html#1.

National Sleep Foundation: *How sleep changes,* 2006a, http://www.sleepfoundation.org/hottopics/index.php?secid=12&id=183.

National Sleep Foundation: *2006 sleep in America poll highlights and key findings,* 2006b, http://sleepfoundation.org.

Orr WC: Gastrointestinal physiology. In Kryger MH, Roth T, Dement WC, editors: *Principles and practice of sleep medicine,* ed 4, Philadelphia, 2005, Saunders.

Redline S: Genetics of obstructive sleep apnea. In Kryger MH, Roth T, Dement WC, editors: *Principles and practice of sleep medicine,* ed 4, Philadelphia, 2005, Saunders.

Robinson SB and others: The sh-h-h-h project: nonpharmacological interventions, *Holist Nurs Pract* 19(6):263, 2005.

Scheer FA and others: Melatonin in the regulation of sleep and circadian rhythms. In Kryger MH, Roth T, Dement WC, editors: *Principles and practice of sleep medicine,* ed 4, Philadelphia, 2005, Saunders.

Schwab PJ and others: Anatomy and physiology of upper airway obstruction. In Kruger MH and others: *Principles and practice of sleep medicine,* ed 4, St. Louis, 2005, Saunders.

Schweitzer PK: Drugs that disturb sleep and wakefulness. In Kryger MH, Roth T, Dement WC, editors: *Principles and practice of sleep medicine,* ed 4, Philadelphia, 2005, Saunders.

Sitzman K: Avoid sleepiness while driving, *Home Healthc Nurs* 23(4):260, 2005.

Stickgold R: Why we dream. In Kryger MH, Roth T, Dement WC, editors: *Principles and practice of sleep medicine,* ed 4, Philadelphia, 2005, Saunders.

The Joint Commission: *News release: Joint Commission seeks input on potential national patient safety goals,* http://www.jointcommission.org/NewReleases/, accessed January 22, 2007.

U.S. Food and Drug Administration: *FDA News: FDA requests label change for all sleep disorders drug products,* http://www.fda.gov/bbs/topics/NEWS/2007/NEW01587.html, retrieved March 26, 2007.

Verrier RL, Josephson ME: Cardiac arrhythmogenesis during sleep: mechanisms, diagnosis, and therapy. In Kryger MH, Roth T, Dement WC, editors: *Principles and practice of sleep medicine,* ed 4, Philadelphia, 2005, Saunders.

Walsh JK and others: Sleep medicine, public policy and public health. In Kryger MH, Roth T, Dement WC, editors: *Principles and practice of sleep medicine,* ed 4, Philadelphia, 2005, Saunders.

White DP: Central sleep apnea. In Kryger MH, Roth T, Dement WC, editors: *Principles and practice of sleep medicine,* ed 4, Philadelphia, 2005, Saunders.

Wolfson AR, Lee KP: Pregnancy and the postpartum period. In Kryger MH, Roth T, Dement WC, editors: *Principles and practice of sleep medicine,* ed 4, Philadelphia, 2005, Saunders.

Research References

Edell-Gustafsson U and others: A gender perspective on sleeplessness behavior, effects of sleep loss, and coping resources in patients with stable coronary artery disease, *Heart Lung* 35(2):75, 2006.

Irwin MR and others: Comparative meta-analysis of behavioral interventions for insomnia and their efficacy in middle-aged adults and in older adults 55+ years of age, *Health Psych* 25(1):3, 2006.

Olson DM and others: Quiet time: a nursing intervention to promote sleep in neurocritical care units, *Am J Crit Care* 10(2):74, 2001.

Reishtein JL and others: Sleepiness and relationships in obstructive sleep apnea, *Issues Ment Health Nurs* 27:319, 2006.

Richardson S: Effects of relaxation and imagery on the sleep of critically ill adults, *Dimens Crit Care Nurs* 22(4):182, 2003.

Spilsbury JC and others: Sleep behavior in an urban U.S. sample of school aged children, *Arch Pediatr Adolesc Med* 58:988, 2004.

CHAPTER 43
References

Agency for Health Care Policy and Research, Acute Pain Management Guideline Panel: *Acute pain management: operative or medical procedures and trauma,* Clinical Practice Guideline, AHCPR Pub No. 92-0032, Rockville, Md, 1992, Agency for Health Care Policy and Research, Public Health Service, U.S. Department of Health and Human Services.

American Bar Association: *Commission on legal problems of the elderly: report to the house of delegates,* 2000, http://www.abanet.org.

American Geriatrics Society: The management of persistent pain in older persons, *J Am Geriatr Soc* 50(S6):205, 2002.

American Holistic Health Association: *Wellness from within: the first step,* Anaheim, Calif, 1999, The Association.

American Nurses Association: *Code of ethics with interpretive statements,* Silver Spring, Md, 2002, The Association.

American Nurses Association: *Pain management nursing: scope and standards of practice,* Silver Spring, Md, 2005, The Association.

American Pain Foundation: *Pain care bill of rights,* 2001, http://www.painfoundation.org/www.painfoundation.org.

American Pain Foundation: *Pain facts,* 2005, http://www.painfoundation.org/www.painfoundation.org.

American Pain Society: *The use of opioids for the treatment of chronic pain,* Glenview, Ill, 2002, The Society, http://www.ampainsoc.org/advocacy/opioids.htm.

American Pain Society: *Principles of analgesic use in the treatment of acute and cancer pain,* ed 5, Glenview, Ill, 2003, The Society.

American Society of Anesthesiologists: Practice guidelines for chronic pain management, *Anesthesiology* 86:995, 1997.

Arbuck D and others: *Effective opioid therapies across the spectrum of chronic pain,* 2004, http://www.medscape.com/viewprogram/3080_pnt.

Arnold R and others: Opioid contracts in chronic nonmalignant pain management: objectives and uncertainties, *Am J Med* 119(4):292, 2006.

ASPMN Position statement on pain management in patients with addictive disease, Pensacola, Fla, 2002, http://www.asmpn.org/Organization/documents/AddictiveDisease.pdf.

ASPMN position statement on the use of "as needed" range orders for opioid analgesics in the management of acute pain, Pensacola, Fla, 2004, http://www.asmpn.org/pdfs/As%20Needed%20Range%20Orders.pdf/.

Brislin R, Rose J: Pediatric acute pain management, *Anesthesiol Clin North Am* 23(4):789, 2005.

Bulechek GM, Butcher HK, Dochterman JM: *Nursing interventions classification (NIC),* ed 5, St. Louis, 2008, Mosby.

Butler RN, Gastel B: Care of the aged: perspectives on pain and discomfort. In Turk DC, Melzack R, editors: *The handbook of pain assessment,* New York, 1992, Guilford Press.

Carroll D, Seers K: Relaxation for the relief of chronic pain: a systematic review, *J Adv Nurs* 27(3):1, 1998.

Coggins C and others: *Position statement on use of placebos in pain management,* 2004, http://www.aspmn.org/Use%20of%20Placebos.pdf/.

Cousins M, Power I: Acute and postoperative pain. In Melzack R, Wall P, editors: *Handbook of pain management,* New York, 2003, Churchill Livingstone.

Craig KD: The facial display of pain in infants and children. In Finley GA, McGrath PJ editors: Measurement of pain in infants and children, *Prog Pain Res Manage* 10:103, 1998.

D'Arcy Y: Hot topics in pain management: using NSAIDs safely, *Nursing* 35(2):22, 2006.

Davidhizar R, Giger J: A review of the literature on care of clients in pain who are culturally diverse, *Int Nurs Rev* 51(1):47, 2004.

Douglass AB and others: Principles of palliative care medicine. I. Patient assessment, *Adv Stud Med* 4(1):15, 2004.

Drew D, Peltier C: Topical morphine provides pain relief for open wounds, *Pain Man SIG Newsletter* 15(3):5, 2005.

Eksterowicz N: Meperidine—using evidence-based rationale, *ASPMN Pathways* 12(1):4, 2003.

Ersek M and others: The cognitive effects of opioids, *Pain Manag Nurs* 5(2):75, 2004.

Ferrell B: Ethical perspectives on pain and suffering, *Pain Manag Nurs* 6(3):83, 2005.

Ferrini R., Paice J: How to initiate and monitor infusional lidocaine for severe and/or neuropathic pain, *J Support Oncol* 2(1):91, 2004.

Fick D and others: *Updating the Beers criteria for potentially inappropriate medication use in older adults: results of a U.S. consensus panel of experts* 163(22):2716, 2003.

Fine P: *The last chance for comfort: an update on pain management at the end of life,* 2005, http://www.medscape.com/viewprogram/4550_pnt, accessed October 22, 2005.

Finnerup N, Jensen R: Spinal cord injury pain—mechanisms and treatment, *Eur J Neurol* 11(2):73, 2004.

Gil K: Psychologic aspects of acute pain, *Anesthesiol Rep* 2(2):246, 1990.

Gordon D: Nonopioid and adjuvant analgesics in chronic pain management: strategy for effective use, *Nurs Clin North Am* 38(3):447, 2003.

Gordon D, Love G: Pharmacologic management of neuropathic pain, *Pain Manag Nurs* 5(4, S1):19, 2004.

Grace P: The clinical use of placebos, *Am J Nurs* 106(20):58, 2006.

Gruener D, Lande S: *Pain control in the primary care setting*, Glenview, Ill, 2006, American Pain Society.

Herr K: Chronic pain: challenges and assessment strategies, *J Gerontol Nurs* 28(1):20, 2002a.

Herr K: Chronic pain in the older patient: management strategies, *J Gerontol Nurs* 28(2):28, 2002b.

Herr K and others: Pain assessment in the nonverbal patient: position statement with clinical practice recommendations, *Pain Manag Nurs* 7(2):44, 2006a.

Herr K and others: Tools for assessment of pain in nonverbal older adults with dementia: a state-of-the-science review, *J Pain Symptom Manage* 31(2):170, 2006b.

Hockenberry MJ and Wilson D: *Wong's nursing care of infants and children,* ed 8, St. Louis, 2007, Mosby.

International Association for the Study of Pain, Subcommittee on Taxonomy: Pain terms: a list with definitions and notes on usage, *Pain* 6:249, 1979.

Jacox A and others: *Management of cancer pain,* Clinical Practice Guideline No. 9, AHCPR Pub No. 94-0592, Rockville, Md, 1994, Agency for Health Care Policy and Research, Public Health Service, U.S. Department of Health and Human Services.

Kehlet H and others: Persistent postsurgical pain: Risk factors and prevention, *Lancet* 367(9522):1618, 2006.

Kelly A: *Geriatric pain assessment: self-directed learning module,* Pensacola, Fla, 2003, American Society for Pain Management Nursing.

Lasch K: Culture and pain, 2002, http://www.iasp-pain.org/PCU02-5.html/.

Latta K and others: Meperidine: a critical review, *Am J Ther* 9(1):53, 2002.

Lehne R: *Pharmacology for nursing care,* ed 6, Philadelphia, 2005, Saunders.

Manworren R: A call to action to protect range orders, *Am J Nurs* 106(7):65, 2006.

Max MB, Portenoy RK: Methodological challenges for clinical trials of cancer pain treatments. In Chapman CR, Foley KM, editors: *Current and emerging issues in cancer pain: research and practice,* New York, 1993, Raven Press.

Maxwell T and others: *Palliative and end-of-life pain management: self-directed learning module,* Pensacola, Fla, 2005, American Society for Pain Management Nursing.

McCaffery M: *Nursing management of the patient with pain,* ed 2, Philadelphia, 1979, Lippincott.

McCaffery M, Arnstein P: The debate over placebos in pain management, *Am J Nurs* 106(2):62, 2006.

McCaffery M, Pasero C: *Pain: clinical manual,* ed 2, St. Louis, 1999, Mosby.

McCarberg B, O'Connor A: A new look at heat treatment for pain disorders, part I, *APS Bulletin* 14(6):4, 2004.

Medication on Demand, Avancen, 2006, http://www.avancen.com.

Mehta V, Langford R: Acute pain management for opioid dependent patients, *Anaesthesia* 61(3):269, 2006.

Melzack R, Wall D: *Handbook of pain management,* London, 2003, Churchill Livingstone.

Melzack R, Wall PD: Pain mechanisms: a new theory, *Science* 150:971, 1965.

Miaskowski C: The next step to improving cancer pain management, *Pain Manag Nurs* 6(1):1, 2005.

Moorhead S and others: *Nursing outcomes classification (NOC),* ed 4, St. Louis, 2008, Mosby.

Morrison R, and others: The growth of palliative care programs in United States hospitals, *J Palliat Med* 8(6):1127, 2005.

Otis-Green S and others: An integrated psychosocial model for cancer pain management, *Cancer Pract* 10(S1):58, 2002.

Paice J: Unraveling the mystery of pain, *Oncol Nurs Forum* 18(5):843, 1991.

Pasero C: *Intravenous patient-controlled analgesia for acute pain management: self-directed learning module,* Pensacola, Fla, 2003, American Society for Pain Management Nursing.

Pasero C: Perineural local anesthetic infusion, *Am J Nurs* 104(7):89, 2004.

Pasero C, McCaffery M: Monitoring sedation, *Am J Nurs* 102(2):67, 2002.

Pasero C, McCaffery M: No self-report means no pain-intensity rating, *Am J Nurs* 205(10):50, 2005.

Pasero C, Manwarren RC, McCaffery M: Pain control: IV opioid range orders for acute pain management, *Am J Nurs* 107(2)52-59, 2007.

Passik S, Kirsh K, Portenoy R: Substance abuse issues in palliative care. In Berger A, Portenoy R, Weissman D, editors: *Principles and practice of palliative care and supportive oncology,* Philadelphia, 2003, Lippincott, Williams & Wilkins.

Portenoy RK: Neuropathic pain. In Portenoy RK, Kanner RM, editors: *Pain management: theory and practice,* Philadelphia, 1996, FA Davis.

Practice guidelines for acute pain management in the perioperative setting, *Anesthesiology* 100(6):1573, 2004.

Renn C, Dorsey S: The physiology and processing of pain: a review, *AACN Clin Issues* 16(3):277, 2005.

Roman M, Cabaj T: Epidural analgesia, *Medsurg Nurs* 14(4):257, 2005.

Schechter N and others: *Pain in infants, children, and adolescents.* Baltimore, 2003, Lippincott, Williams & Wilkins.

Schulman-Green D and others: Unlicensed staff members' experiences with patients' pain on an inpatient oncology unit: implications for redesigning the care delivery system, *Cancer Nurs* 28(5):340, 2005.

Shaw S: Nursing and supporting patients with chronic pain, *Nurs Stand* 20(19):60, 2006.

Snyder M, Weland, J: Complementary and alternative therapies: what is their place in the management of chronic pain? *Nurs Clin North Am* 38(3):495, 2003.

St. Marie B: *Core curriculum for pain management nursing.* Philadelphia, 2002, Saunders.

Sullivan M: APS position statement on the use of placebos in pain management, *J Pain* 6(4):215, 2005.

The Joint Commission: *National patient safety goals,* 2007, http://www.jointcommission.org/PatientSafety/NationalPatientSafetyGoals/07_npsg_facts.html, 2006.

Vila H and others: The efficacy and safety of pain management before and after implementation of hospital-wide pain management standards: is patient safety compromised by treatment based solely on numerical pain ratings? *Anesth Analg* 101(2):474, 2005.

Wall P, Melzack R: *Textbook of pain,* ed 4, London, 1999, Churchill Livingstone.

When your pain flares up: easy, proven techniques for managing chronic pain, Minneapolis, 2002, Fairview Press.

Whitecar P and others: Principles of palliative care medicine. II. Pain and symptom management, *Adv Stud Med* 4(2):88, 2004.

Willens J: Consumer group urges food and drug administration to ban drug Darvon, *Pain Manag Nurs* 7(2); 43, 2006.

Williams G: Determining the appropriate use of COX-2 inhibitors in pain management, *Clin Advisor* 9, 2005.

Williams H: Assessing, diagnosing and managing neuropathic pain, *Nurs Times* 102(16):22, 2006.

Wirth J and others: Use of herbal therapies to relieve pain: a review of efficacy and adverse effects, *Pain Manag Nurs* 6(4):145, 2005.

Wong DL, Baker CM: Pain in children: comparison of assessment scales, *Okla Nurse* 33(1):8, 1988.

Wuhrman E and others: *Authorized and unauthorized ("PCA by PROXY") dosing of analgesic infusion pumps,* 2006, http://www.aspmn.org/organization/documents/PCAbyProxy-final-ew_004.pdf.

Yoon S, Schaffer S: Herbal, prescribed, and over-the-counter drug use in older women: prevalence of drug interactions, *Geriatr Nurs* 27(2):118, 2006.

Research References

Beyer JE and others: The creation, validation, and continuing development of the Oucher: a measure of pain intensity in children, *J Pediatr Nurs* 7(5):335, 1992.

Cassileth B, Vickers A: Massage therapy for symptom control: outcome study at a major cancer center, *J Pain Symptom Manag* 28(3):244, 2004.

Davis G: Barriers to managing chronic pain of older adults with arthritis, *J Nurs Scholarsh* 34(2):121, 2002.

Gerdner L. *Evidence-based protocol: individualized music,* Iowa City, 2001, The University of Iowa Gerontological Nursing Interventions Research Center, Research Dissemination Core.

Grunau RVE and others: Early pain experience, child and family factors, as precursors of somatization: a prospective study of extremely premature and full-term children, *Pain* 56:353, 1994.

Jensen M and others: The validity of the neuropathic pain scale for assessing diabetic neuropathic pain in a clinical trial, *Clin J Pain* 22(1):97, 2006.

Kim MK: Analgesia for children with acute abdominal pain, *Acad Emerg Med* 9(4):281, 2002.

Kimberlin C and others: Cancer patient and caregiver experiences: communication and pain management, *J Pain Symptom Manage* 28(2):566, 2004.

Manias E and others: Nurses' strategies for managing pain in the postoperative setting, *Pain Manag Nurs* 6(1):18, 2005.

McCaffery M and others: Nurses' personal opinion about patients' pain and their effect on recorded assessments and titration of opioid doses, *Pain Manag Nurs* 1(3):79, 2000.

McCaffery M and others: On the meaning of "drug seeking," *Pain Manag Nurs* 6(4):122, 2005.

Morgan B: Knowing how to play the game: hospitalized substance abusers' strategies for obtaining pain relief, *Pan Manag Nurs* 7(1):31, 2006.

Paice J and others: Efficacy and safety of scheduled dosing of opioid analgesics: a quality improvement study, *J Pain* 6(10):639, 2005.

Puntillo K and others: Patients' perceptions and responses to procedural pain: results from Thunder Project II, *Am J Crit Care* 10(4):238, 2001.

Puntillo K and others: Accuracy of emergency nurses in assessment of patients' pain, *Pain Manag Nurs* 4(4):171, 2003.

Schumacher K and others: Putting cancer pain management regimens into practice at home, *J Pain Symptom Manage* 23(5):369, 2002.

Shukla D and others: Pain in acute and chronic wounds: a descriptive study, *Ostomy Wound Manage* 51(11):47, 2005.

Siedlecki S: Effect of music on power, pain, depression and disability, *J Adv Nurs* 54(5):553, 2006.

Stevens B: Composite measures of pain. In Finley GA, McGrath PJ editors: Measurement of pain in infants and children, *Prog Pain Res Manage* 10:161, 1998.

Taddio A and others: Neonatal circumcision and pain response during routine vaccination 4 to 6 months later, *Lancet* 349:599, 1997.

Vitetta L, Kenner D, Sali A: Sedation and analgesia-prescribing patterns in terminally ill patients at the end of life, *Am J Hosp Palliat Care* 22(6):465, 2005.

Wheeler M and others: Adverse events associated with postoperative opioid analgesia: a systemic review, *J Pain* 3(3):159, 2002.

Wilson B, McSherry W: A study of nurses' inferences of patients' physical pain, *J Clin Nurs* 15(4):459, 2006.

CHAPTER 44
References

American Academy of Pediatrics: Policy statement: prevention of pediatric overweight and obesity, *Pediatrics* 112(2):424, 2003.

American Academy of Pediatrics: Policy statement: breastfeeding and the use of human milk, *Pediatrics* 115(2):496, 2005.

American Diabetes Association: Position statement: nutrition recommendations and interventions for diabetes—2006, *Diabetes Care* 29(9):2140, 2006.

American Dietetic Association: Position of the American Dietetic Association: food and nutrition misinformation, *J Am Diet Assoc* 106(4):601, 2006.

American Heart Association: AHA scientific statement: diet and lifestyle recommendations revision 2006, *Circulation* 114:82, 2006.

American Psychiatric Association: *Diagnostic and statistical manual of mental disorders,* ed 4, text revision, Washington, DC, 2000, The Association.

American Society for Parenteral and Enteral Nutrition: Standards of practice, nutrition support nurse, *Nutr Clin Pract* 16(1):56, 2001.

American Society for Parenteral and Enteral Nutrition: Guidelines for the use of parenteral and enteral nutrition in adult and pediatric patients, *J Parenter Enteral Nutr* 26(1):1SA, 2002.

Ashley J and others: Speech, language, and swallowing disorders in the older adult, *Clin Geriatr Med* 22:291, 2006.

Bending A: Meeting the challenges of managing dysphagia, *Community Nurse* 7(1):13, 2001.

Brody RR and others: Role of registered dietitians in dysphagia screening, *J Am Diet Assoc* 100(9):1029, 2000.

Bulechek GM, Butcher HK, Dochterman JM: *Nursing interventions classification (NIC),* ed 5, St. Louis, 2008, Mosby.

Chen CC and others: A concept analysis of malnutrition in the elderly, *J Adv Nurs* 36(1):131, 2001.

Covinsky KE: Malnutrition and bad outcomes, *J Gen Intern Med* 17(12):956, 2002.

Daniels J: Obesity: America's epidemic, *Am J Nurs* 106(1):40, 2006.

DiMaria-Ghalili RA, Amella E: Nutrition in older adults, *Am J Nurs* 105(3):40, 2005.

Dossey B: *Florence Nightingale: mystic, visionary, and healer,* Philadelphia, 1999, Springhouse.

Edwards B: Childhood obesity: a school-based approach to increase nutritional knowledge and activity levels, *Nurs Clin North Am* 40:661, 2005.

Edwards S, Metheny N: Measurement of gastric residual volume: state of the science, *Medsurg Nurs* 9(3):125, 2000.

Food and Nutrition Board: *Nutrition during pregnancy and lactation: an implementation guide,* Washington, DC, 1992, National Academy Press.

Furman EF: Undernutrition in older adults across the continuum of care: nutritional assessment, barriers, and interventions, *J Gerontol Nurs* 32(1):22, 2006.

Giger JN, Davidhizar RE: *Transcultural nursing: assessment and intervention,* ed 3, St. Louis, 2004, Mosby.

Grodner M, Long S, DeYoung S: *Foundations and clinical applications of nutrition: a nursing approach,* ed 3, St. Louis, 2004, Mosby.

Hockenberry MJ, Wilson D: *Wong's nursing care of infants and children,* ed 8, St. Louis, 2007, Mosby.

Hornick B: Diet and nutrition implications for oral health, *J Dent Hyg* 76(1):67, 2002.

Institute of Medicine: *Dietary reference intakes: frequently asked questions (FAQs),* 2005, http://www.iom.edu/CMS/3788/4574/13063.aspx?printfriendly=true, accessed October 10, 2006.

Kondrup J and others: ESPEN guidelines for nutrition screening 2002, *Clin Nutr* 22(4):415, 2003.

Kushi LH and others: American Cancer Society guidelines on nutrition and physical activity for cancer prevention: reducing the risk of cancer with health food choices and physical activity, CA *Cancer J Clin* 56:254, 2006.

Linton AD, Lach HW: *Matteson and McConnell's gerontological nursing: concepts and practice,* ed 3, St. Louis, 2006, Saunders.

Mason P: Undernutrition in hospital: causes and consequences, *Hosp Pharm* 13:353, 2006.

Mayo Clinic Staff: *Childhood obesity,* 2006, http://www.mayoclinic.com/health/childhood-obesity/DS00698, accessed July 10, 2007.

McKenry LM, Salerno E: *Mosby's pharmacology in nursing,* ed 21 revised, St. Louis, 2003, Mosby.

Meiner SE, Lueckenotte AG: *Gerontologic nursing,* ed 3, St. Louis, 2006, Mosby.

Metheny NA: Preventing aspiration in older adults with dysphagia, *Try This: Best Practices in Nursing Care to Older Adults,* issue 20, 2004, http://www.hartfordign.org.

Moorhead S and others: *Nursing outcomes classification (NOC),* ed 4, St. Louis, 2008, Mosby.

National Center for Chronic Disease Prevention and Health Promotion: *Health topics: childhood overweight,* 2007, http://www.cdc.gov/HealthyYouth/overweight/index.htm, accessed July 10, 2007.

National Dysphagia Diet Task Force: *National Dysphagia Diet: standardization for optimal care,* Chicago, 2002, American Dietetic Association.

National Guideline Clearinghouse: *Infection control: prevention of healthcare–associated infection in primary and community care,* 2003, http://www.guideline.gov/summary/summary.aspx?doc_id=5069&nbr=003553&string=Prevention+AND+healthcare-associated+AND+infection, accessed December 19, 2006.

National Guideline Clearinghouse: *Nutrition assessment: adults guideline,* 2006, http://www.guideline.gov/summary/summary.aspx?ss=15&doc_id=3625&nbr=002851&string=nutrition+AND+assessment, accessed December 14, 2006.

Nix S: *Williams' basic nutrition and diet therapy,* ed 12, St. Louis, 2005, Mosby.

Nowlin A: The dysphagia dilemma: how you can help, *RN* 69(6):44, 2006.

Nutrient-drug interactions, 2006, http://www.faqs.org/nutrition/Met-Obe/Nutrient-Drug-Interactions.html, accessed December 12, 2006.

Olendzki B and others: Nutritional assessment and counseling for prevention and treatment of cardiovascular disease, *Am Fam Physician* 73(2):257, 2006.

Pagana KD, Pagana TJ: *Mosby's diagnostic and laboratory test reference,* ed 7, St. Louis, 2005, Mosby.

Parrish C, McCray S: Enteral feedings: dispelling myths, *Pract Gastroenterol* 9:33, 2003.

Perry L, McLaren S: Implementing evidence-based guidelines for nutrition support in acute stroke, *Evid Based Nurs* 6:68, 2003b, http://www.evidencebasednursing.com

Rolandelli RH and others: *Clinical nutrition: enteral feeding and tube feeding,* Philadelphia, 2005, Saunders.

Serna ED, McCarthy MS: Heads up to prevent aspiration during enteral feeding, *Nursing* 36(1):76, 2006.

Thomas DF: A complete primer on enteral feeding, *Annals of Long-Term Care: Clinical Care and Aging* 9(1):41, 2001.

U.S. Department of Agriculture: *Shopping, cooking, and meal planning,* 2006, http://www.nutrition.gov/index.php?mode=subject&subject=ng_cooking&d_subject=shopping,%20Cooking_ampersand_Meal20%Planning.

U.S. Department of Agriculture Center for Nutrition Policy and Promotion: *USDA's food guide pyramid,* 2005, http://www.MyPyramid.gov.

U.S. Department of Agriculture and U.S. Department of Health and Human Services: *Dietary guidelines for Americans 2005,* ed 6, Washington, DC, 2005, U.S. Government Printing Office, http://www.healthierus.gov/dietaryguidelines.

U.S. Department of Health and Human Services: *Healthy people 2010,* 2002, http://www.health.gov/healthypeople.

U.S. Food and Drug Administration: *The food label,* 1999, http://vm.cfsan.fda.gov/~dms/fdnewlab.htmL.

U.S. Food and Drug Administration: *FDA public health advisory: reports of blue discoloration and death in patients receiving enteral feedings tinted with the dye FD&C Blue No. 1,* Washington, DC, 2003, U.S. Food and Drug Administration.

Watts SA, Anselmo J: Nutrition for diabetes: all in a day's work, *Nursing* 36(6):46, 2006.

Williams SD, Schlenker ED: *Essentials of nutrition and diet therapy,* ed 8, St. Louis, 2003, Mosby.

Research References

Befort C and others: Fruit, vegetable and fat intake among non-Hispanic black and non-Hispanic white adolescents: associations with home availability and food consumption settings, *J Am Diet Assoc* 106(3):367, 2006.

Brown B and others: Comparison of an institutional nutrition screen with four validated nutrition screening tools, *Top Clin Nutr* 21(2):122, 2006.

Callen BL, Wells TJ: Views of community-dwelling, old-old people on barriers and aids to nutritional health, *J Nurs Scholarsh* 35(3):257, 2003.

Chen CC and others: Dynamics of nutritional health in a community sample of American elders, *Adv Nurs Sci* 28(4):376, 2005.

Cirgin Ellett ML: Important facts about intestinal feeding tube placement, *Gastroenterol Nurs* 29(2):112, 2006.

Daniels S and others: Clinical predictors of dysphagia and aspiration risk: outcome measure in acute stroke patients, *Arch Phys Med Rehabil* 81:1030, 2000.

Fox MK and others: Sources of energy and nutrients in the diets of infants and toddlers, *J Am Diet Assoc* 106(suppl 1):S28e1, 2006.

Guigoz Y, Vellas B: The Mini Nutritional Assessment (MNA) for grading the nutritional state of elderly patients: presentation of the MNA, history and validation, *Nestle Nutr Workshop Ser Clin Perform Programme* 1:3, 1999.

Guigoz YB and others: Assessing the nutritional status of the elderly: the Mini Nutritional Assessment as part of the geriatric evaluation, *Nutr Rev* 54(1 pt 2):S59, 1996.

Hinchey JA and others: Formal dysphagia screening protocols prevent pneumonia, *Stroke* 36:1972, 2005

Kwon HM and others: The pneumonia score: a simple grading scale for prediction of pneumonia after acute stroke, *Am J Infect Control* 34(2):64, 2006.

Lennie TA and others: Factors influencing food intake in patients with heart failure: a comparison with healthy elders, *J Cardiovasc Nurs* 21(2):123, 2006.

Matlow A and others: Enteral tube hub as a reservoir for the transmissible enteric bacteria, *Am J Infect Control* 34(3):131, 2006.

Metheny NA: Inadvertent intracranial nasogastric tube placement, *Am J Nurs* 102(8):25, 2002.

Metheny NA: Preventing respiratory complications of tube feedings: evidence-based practice, *Am J Crit Care* 15(4):360, 2006.

Metheny N, Aud M, Ignatavicius D: Detection of improperly placed feeding tubes, *J Health Risk Manage* 18(3):37, 1998.

Metheny N, Aud MA, Wunderlich RJ: A survey of bedside methods used to detect pulmonary aspiration of enteral formula in intubated tube-fed patients, *Am J Crit Care* 8(3):160, 1999.

Metheny NA, Meert KL: Monitoring feeding tube placement, *Nutr Clin Pract* 19(5):487, 2004.

Metheny N, Titler, M: Assessing placement of feeding tubes, *Am J Nurs* 101(5):36, 2001.

Metheny N and others: Measures to test placement of nasogastric and nasointestinal feeding tubes: a review, *Nurse Res* 37:324, 1988.

Metheny N and others: Effectiveness of pH measurement in predicting feeding tube placement, *Nurse Res* 38(5):262, 1989.

Metheny N and others: Detection of inadvertent respiratory placement of small-bore feeding tubes: a report of 10 cases, *Heart Lung* 19(6):631, 1990a.

Metheny N and others: Effectiveness of the auscultatory method in predicting feeding tube location, *Nurse Res* 39(5):262, 1990b.

Metheny N and others: How to aspirate fluid from small bore feeding tubes, *Am J Nurs* 93(5):86, 1993.

Metheny N and others: pH, color, and feeding tubes, *RN* 61(1):277, 1998a.

Metheny N and others: Testing feeding tube placement: auscultation vs. pH method, *Am J Nurs* 98:37, 1998b.

Metheny N and others: pH and concentrations of bilirubin in feeding tube aspirates as predictors of tube placement, *Nurs Res* 48(4):189, 1999.

Metheny N and others: Pepsin as a marker for pulmonary aspiration, *Am J Crit Care* 11(2):150, 2002.

Metheny NA and others: Effect of feeding-tube properties on residual volumes measurements in tube-fed patients, *JPEN* 29(3):192, 2005a.

Metheny NA and others: Indicators of tube site during feedings, *J Neuroscience Nurs* 37(6):320, 2005b.

Perry L, Love C: Screening for dysphagia and aspiration in acute stroke: a systematic review, *Dysphagia* 16:7, 2001.

Perry L, McLaren S: Eating difficulties after stroke, *J Adv Nurs* 44(4):360, 2003b.

Runions S and others: Practice on an acute stroke unit after implementation of a decision-making algorithm for dietary management of dysphagia, *J Neuroscience Nurs* 36(4):200, 2004.

Sarhill N and others: Evaluation of nutritional status in advanced metastatic cancer, *Support Care Cancer* 11(10): 652, 2003.

Winkler MF: Quality of life in adult home parenteral nutrition patients, *JPEN J Parenter Enteral Nutr* 29(3):162, 2005.

CHAPTER 45
References

Ackley BJ, Ladwig GB: *Nursing diagnosis handbook: a guide to planning care*, ed 6, St. Louis, 2004, Mosby.

Bulechek GM, Butcher HK, Dochterman JM: *Nursing interventions classification (NIC)*, ed 5, St. Louis, 2008, Mosby.

Chang MK, Harden JT: Meeting the challenge of the new millennium: caring for culturally diverse patients, *Urol Nurs* 22(6):372, 2002.

Copstead LE, Banasik JL: *Pathophysiology*, ed 3, St. Louis, 2005, Saunders, p 1130.

Daneshgari F and others: Evidence-based multidisciplinary practice: improving the safety and standards of male bladder catheterization, *MedSurg Nurs* 11(5):236, 2002.

Doughty DB: *Urinary and fecal incontinence: current management concepts*, ed 3, St. Louis, 2006, Mosby.

Foxman B: Epidemiology of urinary tract infections: incidence, morbidity, and economic costs, *Am J Med* 113(1A):5S, 2002.

Gray M and others: Expert review: best practices in managing the indwelling catheter. *Perspectives*, special edition sponsored by Dale Medical Products, Burlington, Vt, 2006, Saxe Healthcare Communications.

Haberstich NJ: Protecting catheterized patients from infection, *Nurs Residential Care* 4(10):482, 2002

Lehne RA: *Pharmacology for nursing care*, ed 6, St. Louis, 2007, Saunders.

Lewis SM and others: *Medical-surgical nursing: assessment and management of clinical problems*, ed 7, St. Louis, 2007, Mosby.

Lynch D: Cranberry for prevention of urinary tract infections, *Am Family Physician*, 70(11):2175-7, 2004

Malarkey LM, McMorrow ME: *Saunders' nursing guide to laboratory and diagnostic tests*, St. Louis, 2005, Saunders.

Mauk KL: Conservative therapy for urinary incontinence can help older adults, *Nursing 2005*, 35(8): 20, 2005.

Mehnert-Kay S: Diagnosis and management of uncomplicated urinary tract infection. *Am Family Physician* 72(3) 451-6, 2005

Moorhead S and others: *Nursing outcomes classification (NOC)*, ed 4, St. Louis, 2008, Mosby.

Pagana KD, Pagana TJ: *Mosby's diagnostic and laboratory reference* ed 8, St. Louis, 2007, Mosby

Palmer MH, Newman DK: Urinary incontinence and estrogen, *Am J Nurs* 107(3):35, 2007.

Smith JM: Current concepts in catheter management. In Doughty DB: *Urinary and fecal incontinence: current management concepts*, ed 3, St. Louis, 2006, Mosby.

Specht JKP: Nine myths of incontinence in older adults, *Am J Nurs* 105(6):58, 2005.

Thompson DL, Smith DA: Continence nursing: a whole person approach, *Holist Nurs Pract* 16(2):14, 2002.

Research References

Fernandez RS, Griffiths RD: Duration of short-term indwelling catheters: a systematic review of the evidence, *J Wound Ostomy Continence Nurs* 33(2):145, 2006.

Getliffe K: Managing recurrent urinary catheter blockage: problems, promises, and practicalities, *J Wound Ostomy Continence Nurs* 30(3):146, 2003.

Gray M: Are cranberry juice or cranberry products effective in the prevention or management of urinary tract infection? *J Wound Ostomy Continence Nurs* 29(3):122, 2002.

Gray M, Krissovich M: Does fluid intake influence the risk for urinary incontinence, urinary tract infection, and bladder cancer? *J Wound Ostomy Continence Nurs* 30(3):126, 2003.

Gray ML: Gender, race, and culture in research on UI, *Am J Nurs* 103(3 suppl):20, 2003.

Newman DK, Palmer MH: State of the science on urinary incontinence: executive summary, *Am J Nurs* 103(3 suppl):4, 2003.

Palmer MK, Newman DK: Bladder control: educational needs of older adults, *J Gerontol Nurs* 32(1):28, 2006.

Parkin J, Keeley FX: Indwelling catheter–associated urinary tract infections, *Br J Community Nurs* 8(4):166, 2003.

Sampselle CM: Behavioral interventions in young and middle-age women, *Am J Nurs* 103(3 suppl):9, 2003.

Wong S, Hooton TM: *Guideline for prevention of catheter-associated urinary tract infections*, updated April 1, 2005, Centers for Disease Control and Prevention, http://www.cdc.gov/ncidod/dhqp/gl_catheter_assoc.html, accessed May 25, 2007.

Wyman JF: Treatment of urinary incontinence in men and older women, *Am J Nurs* 103(3 suppl):26, 2003.

CHAPTER 46
References

The American Cancer Society: *Detailed guide: colon and rectum cancer: revised 02/22/2007,* http://www.cancer.org/docroot/CRI_2_4_3X_Can_colon_and_rectum_cancer, accessed April 28, 2007, and http://www.cancer.org/docroot/CRI_2_4_2X_What_are_the_Risk_factors_for_colorectal_cancer?, accessed April 28, 2007.

Banks N, Razor B: Preoperative stoma site assessment and marking: trained RNs can improve ostomy outcomes, *Am J Nurs* 103(3):64A, 2003.

Beckman Coulter, Inc: Hemoccult: physicians' #1 choice in fecal occult blood testing (package insert), Fullerton, Calif, 2003.

Bulechek GM, Butcher HK, Dochterman JM: *Nursing interventions classification (NIC),* ed 5, St. Louis, 2008, Mosby.

Cronin E: Best practice in discharging patients with a stoma, *Nurs Times* 101(47):67, 2005.

Doughty D: *Urinary and fecal incontinence nursing,* ed 3, St. Louis, 2006, Mosby.

Eberhardie C: Constipation: identifying the problem, *Nurs Older People* 15(9):22, 2003.

Erwin-Toth P: Ostomies and fistulas: prevention and management of peristomal skin complications, *Adv Skin Wound Care* 13(4):125, 2000.

Erwin-Toth P: Caring for a stoma is more than skin deep, *Nursing* 31(5):36, 2001.

Erwin-Toth P: Ostomy pearls, *Adv Skin Wound Care* 16(3):1, 2003.

Fletcher K: Elimination: geriatric self-learning module, *Medsurg Nurs* 14(2):127, 2005.

Harris H: *C. difficile* attack of the killer diarrhea, *Nursing Made Incredibly Easy* 4(3):12, 2006.

Hyland J: Basics of ostomies, *Gastroenterol Nurs* 25(6):241, 2002.

Ignatavicius D, Workman L: *Medical-surgical nursing: critical thinking for collaborative care,* ed 5, St. Louis, 2006, Saunders.

Jarvis C: *Physical exam and health assessment,* ed 4, St. Louis, 2004, Saunders.

Kyle G, Prynn P: An evidence-based procedure for the digital removal of faeces, *Nurs Times* 100(48):71, 2004.

McKenry L, Tessier E, Hogan MA: *Mosby's pharmacology in nursing,* ed 22, St. Louis, 2006, Mosby.

Meiner S, Lueckenotte AG: *Gerontologic nursing,* ed 3, St. Louis, 2006, Mosby.

Miskovitz P, Betancourt M: *The doctor's guide to gastrointestinal health,* Hoboken, NJ, 2005, John Wiley & Sons.

Moorhead S and others: *Nursing outcomes classification (NOC),* ed 4, St. Louis, 2008, Mosby.

Pagana KD, Pagana TJ: *Mosby's diagnostic and laboratory test reference,* ed 7, St. Louis, 2005, Mosby.

Richmond J: Prevention of constipation through risk management, *Nurs Stand* 17(16):39, 2003.

Seidel Hm and others: *Mosby's guide to physical examination,* ed 6, St. Louis, 2006, Mosby.

Stanley M and others: *Gerontological nursing: promoting successful aging with older adults,* ed 7, Philadelphia, 2005, FA Davis.

Tabloski P: *Gerontological nursing,* Upper Saddle River, NJ, 2006, Pearson Prentice Hall.

Thompson J: A practical ostomy guide, part I, *RN* 63(11):61, 2000.

Todd B: *Clostridium difficile:* familiar pathogen, changing epidemiology, *Am J Nurs* 106(5):33, 2006.

Wilson L: Understanding bowel problems in older people, part I. *Nurs Older People* 17(8):19, 2005.

Research References

Barr E: Assessment and management of stomal complications: a framework for clinical decision making, *Ostomy Wound Manage* 50(9):50, 2004.

Bartlett JG: Antibiotic-associated diarrhea, *N Engl J Med* 3(5):334, 2002.

Beitz J: Continent diversions: the new gold standards of ileoanal reservoir and neobladder, *Ostomy Wound Manage* 50(9):26, 2004.

Bosshard W and others: The treatment of chronic constipation in elderly people: an update, *Drugs Aging* 21(14):911, 2004.

Calado A and others: The Macedo-Malone antegrade continence enema procedure: early experience, *J Urol* 173:1340, 2005.

Greenwald B: A comparison of three stool tests for colorectal cancer, *Medsurg Nurs* 14(5):292, 2005.

Metheny NA, Titler MG: Assessing placement of feeding tubes, *Am J Nurs* 101(5):36, 2001.

Metheny NA and others: Testing feeding tube placement auscultation vs. pH method, *Am J Nurs* 98(5):37, 1998a.

Metheny NA and others: pH, color, and feeding tubes, *RN* 61(1):25, 1998b.

Metheny NA and others: Effect of feeding-tube properties on residual volume measurements in tube-fed patients, *J Parenter Enteral Nutr* 29(3):192, 2005.

Palmieri B, Benuzzi G, Bellini N: The anal bag: a modern approach to fecal incontinence management, *Ostomy Wound Manage* 51(12):44, 2005.

Phillips N: Nasogastric tubes: an historical context, *Medsurg Nurs* 15(2):84, 2006.

Shipp M and others: Population-based study of the variation in colon cancer incidence in Alabama: relationship to socioeconomic status indicators and physician density, *South Med J* 98(11):1076, 2005.

Stressman M: Biofeedback: its role in the treatment of chronic constipation, *Gastroenterol Nurs* 26(6):251, 2003.

Wound Ostomy and Continence Nurses Society: *Basic ostomy skin care: a guide for patients and healthcare workers,* Glenview, Ill, 2004a, The Society.

Wound Ostomy and Continence Nurses Society. *Peristomal skin complications: best practice for clinicians,* Glenview, Ill, 2004b, The Society.

Wound Ostomy and Continence Nurses Society. *Stoma complications: best practice for clinicians,* Glenview, Ill, 2005, The Society.

CHAPTER 47
References

Ackley B, Ladwig G: *Nursing diagnosis handbook: a guide to planning care,* ed 7, St. Louis, 2006, Mosby.

Andrews M, Boyle J: *Transcultural concepts in nursing care,* ed 5, Philadelphia, 2007, Lippincott, Williams & Wilkins.

Black J, Hawks J: *Medical-surgical nursing: clinical management for positive outcomes,* ed 7, Philadelphia, 2005, Saunders.

Bulechek GM, Butcher HK, Dochterman JM: *Nursing interventions classification (NIC),* ed 5, St. Louis, 2008, Mosby.

Butler CT: Pediatric skin care: guidelines for assessment, prevention and treatment, *Pediatr Nurs* 32(5):443, 2006.

Copstead-Kirkhorn LC, Banasik J: *Pathophysiology,* ed 3, 2005, Saunders.

deCastro AB and others: Prioritizing safe patient handling, *J Nurs Adm* 36(7/8):363, 2006.

Ebersole P and others: *Toward healthy aging: human needs and nursing response,* ed 6, 2004, Mosby.

Ebersole P and others: *Gerontological nursing and healthy aging,* ed 2, St. Louis, 2005, Mosby.

Fletcher K: Immobility: geriatric self-learning module, *Medsurg Nurs* 14(1):35, 2005.

Mamaril ME: Nursing considerations in the geriatric surgical patient: the perioperative continuum of care, *Nurs Clin North Am* 41(2):313, 2006.

McCance KL, Huether SE: *Pathophysiology: the biologic basis for disease in adults and children,* ed 5, St. Louis, 2005, Mosby.

Moorhead S and others: *Nursing outcomes classification (NOC),* ed 4, St. Louis, 2008, Mosby.

National Osteoporosis Foundation: *Fast facts,* Washington, DC, 2007, The Foundation, http://www.nof.org/osteoporosis/diseasefacts.htm.

Nelson A: *Safe patient handling and movement algorithms,* 2006, VISN8 Patient Safety Center, http://www.visn8.med.va.gov/patientsafetycenter/safePtHandling/default.asp.)

Nelson A and others: Myths and facts about back injuries in nursing, *Am J Nurs* 103(2):32, 2003a.

Nelson A and others: Safe patient handling movement, *Am J Nurs* 103(3):32, 2003b.

U.S. Department of Health and Human Services: *Bone health and osteoporosis: a report of the surgeon general,* 2004, http://www.hhs.gov/surgeongeneral/library/bonehealth/Executive_Summary.html#MessageFromTommyGThompson.

U.S. Department of Labor: *Career guide to industries: health care,* 2005, http://www.bls.gov/oco/cg/cgs035.htm#conditions.

Waters TR and others: Patient handling tasks with high risk for musculoskeletal disorders in critical care, *Crit Care Nurs Clin North Am* 19:131, 2007.

Wound, Ostomy and Continence Nurses Society: *Guideline for prevention and management of pressure ulcers,* WOCN Clinical Practice Guidelines Series, Glenview, Ill, 2003, The Society.

Yen PK: Physical activity—the "new" nutrition guideline, *Geriatr Nurs* 26(6):341, 2005.

Research References

Agency for Healthcare Research and Quality: *Pressure ulcer prevention and treatment,* 2003, http://hstat.nlm.nih.gov/hq/Hquest/screen/TextBrowse/t/1049658066834/s/40521.

Baird AL, Sands L: A pilot study of the effectiveness of guided imagery with progressive muscle relaxation to reduce chronic pain and mobility difficulties of osteoarthritis, *Pain Manag Nurs* 5(3):97, 2004.

Baptiste A and others: Friction-reducing devices for lateral patient transfers, *AAOHN J* 54(4):173, 2006.

Cromwell SL, Berg JA: Lifelong physical activity patterns of sedentary Mexican American women, *Geriatr Nurs* 27(4):209, 2006.

Deitrick JE and others: Effects of immobilization upon various metabolic and physiological functions of normal men, *Am J Med* 4:3, 1948.

Kawamoto R and others: Predictors of functional status in Japanese community-dwelling older persons during a 2-year follow up, *Geriatr Gerontol Int* 6(2):116, 2006.

Lim K and others: Aging, health and physical activity in Korean Americans, *Geriatr Nurs* 28(2):112, 2007.

Lynch D and others: Continuous passive motion improves shoulder joint integrity following stroke, *Clin Rehabil* 19(6):594, 2005.

Marklew A: Body positioning and its effect on oxygenation: a literature review, *Nurs Crit Care* 11(1):16, 2006.

Nelson A, Baptiste AS: Evidence-based practices for safe patient handling and movement, *Orthop Nurs* 25(6):366, 2006.

Rakel B, Herr K: Assessment and treatment of postoperative pain in older adults, *J Perianesth Nurs* 19(3):194, 2004.

Reifsnider E and others: Factors related to overweight and risk for overweight status among low-income Hispanic children, *J Pediatr Nurs* 21(3):86, 2006.

Shin Y and others: A tailored program for the promotion of physical exercise among Korean adults with chronic diseases, *Appl Nurs Res* 19(2):88, 2006.

Siddharthan K and others: A business case for patient care ergonomic interventions, *Nurs Admin Q* 29(1):63, 2005

CHAPTER 48
References

Agency for Health Care Policy and Research, Panel for the Prediction and Prevention of Pressure Ulcers in Adults: *Pressure ulcers in adults: prediction and prevention,* Clinical Practice Guideline No. 3, AHCPR Pub No. 92-0047, Rockville, Md, 1992a, Agency for Health Care Policy and Research, Public Health Service, U.S. Department of Health and Human Services.

Agency for Health Care Policy and Research, Panel for Urinary Incontinence Guideline: *Urinary incontinence in adults,* Clinical Practice Guideline, AHCPR Pub No. 92-0038, Rockville, Md, 1992b, Agency for Health Care Policy and Research, Public Health Service, U.S. Department of Health and Human Services.

Agency for Health Care Policy and Research, Panel for Treatment of Pressure Ulcers in Adults: *Treatment of pressure ulcers,* Clinical Practice Guideline No. 15, AHCPR Pub No. 95-0653, Rockville, Md, 1994, Agency for Health Care Policy and Research, Public Health Service, U.S. Department of Health and Human Services.

Ayello EA, Braden B: How and why to do pressure ulcer risk assessment, *Adv Skin Wound Care* 15(13):125, 2002.

Ayello EA, Thomas DR, Litchford MA: Nutritional aspects of wound healing, *Home Healthc Nurse* 17(11):719, 1999

Bates-Jensen BM: Toward an intelligent wound assessment system, *Ostomy Wound Manage* 41(suppl 7A):80S,1995.

Bennett MA: Report of the Task Force on the Implications for Darkly Pigmented Intact Skin in the Prediction and Prevention of Pressure Ulcers, *Adv Wound Care* 8(6):34, 1995.

Braden BJ: Risk assessment in pressure ulcer prevention. In Krasner DL, Rodeheaver GT, Sibbald RG, editors: *Chronic wound care: a clinical source book for healthcare professionals,* Wayne, Pa, 2001, HMP Communications.

Bryant RA, editor: *Acute and chronic wounds: nursing management,* ed 2, St. Louis, 2000, Mosby.

Bulechek GM, Butcher HK, Dochterman JM: *Nursing interventions classification (NIC),* ed 5, St. Louis, 2008, Mosby.

Byrant RA, Clark RAF. Skin pathology and types of damage. In Bryant RA, Nix DP, editors: *Acute and chronic wounds: current management concepts,* ed 3, St. Louis, 2007, Mosby.

Camden SG: Skin care needs of the obese patient. In Bryant RA, Nix DP, editors: *Acute and chronic wounds: current management concepts,* ed 3, St. Louis, 2007, Mosby.

Centers for Disease Control and Prevention: Feeding back surveillance data to prevent hospital acquired infections, *Emerg Infect Dis* 7(2):295, 2001.

Chua PC and others: Vacuum-assisted wound closure, *Am J Nurs* 100(12):45, 2000.

Doughty DB, Sparks-Defriese B: Wound-healing physiology. In Bryant RA, Nix DP, editors: *Acute and chronic wounds: current management concepts,* ed 3, St. Louis, 2007, Mosby.

Fellows J, Cresodina L. Home prepared saline: a safe, cost effective alternative for wound cleansing in home care. *J Wound Ostomy Continence Nurs* 33(6):606, 2006.

Frantz RA and others. Device and technology in wound care. In Bryant RA, Nix DP, editors: *Acute and chronic wounds: current management concepts,* ed 3, St. Louis, 2007, Mosby.

Gaskin FC: Detection of cyanosis in the person with dark skin, *J Natl Black Nurses Assoc* 1:52, 1986.

Henderson CT and others: Draft definition of stage I pressure ulcers: inclusion of persons with darkly pigmented skin, *Adv Wound Care* 10(5):16, 1997.

Horn SD and others: Description of the national pressure ulcer long-term care study, *J Am Geriatr Soc* 50(11):1816, 2002.

Jerome D: Advances in negative pressure wound therapy: The V.A.C. Instill, *J Wound Ostomy Continence Nurs* 34(2):191, 2007.

Langemo DK and others. Incidence of pressure sores in acute care, rehabilitation, extended care, home health and hospice in one locale, *Decubitus* 2(2):42, 1989

KCI USA: The V.A.C.: vacuum assisted closure—guidelines for use, physician and caregiver reference manual. Product information, San Antonio, Tex, 1999.

Krasner D: Caring for the person experiencing chronic pain. In Krasner DL, Rodeheaver GT, Sibbald RG, editors: *Chronic wound care: a clinical source book for healthcare professionals,* Wayne, Pa, 2001, HMP Communications.

Moorhead S and others: *Nursing outcomes classification (NOC),* ed 4, St. Louis, 2008, Mosby.

National Pressure Ulcer Advisory Panel: *Position statement on stage I assessment in darkly pigmented skin,* 1998, http://www.NPUAP.org/position4/htm.

National Pressure Ulcer Advisory Panel. Pressure ulcer definitions, 2007a, http://www.npuap.org/documents/NPUAP2007_PU_Def_and_Descriptions.pdf.

National Pressure Ulcer Advisory Panel. *Terms and definitions related to support surfaces,* 2007b, http://www.npuap.org/pdf/NPUAP_S3I_TD.pdf.

Nix D: Patient assessment and evaluation of healing. In Bryant RA, Nix DP, editors: *Acute and chronic wounds: current management concepts,* ed 3, St. Louis, 2007, Mosby.

Norton D, McLaren R, Exon-Smith AN: *An investigation of geriatric nursing problems in hospital,* Edinburgh, 1962, Churchill Livingstone.

Pieper B: Mechanical forces: pressure, shear and friction. In Bryant RA, Nix DP, editors: *Acute and chronic wounds: current management concepts,* ed 3, St. Louis, 2007, Mosby.

Pires M, Muller A: Detection and management of early tissue pressure indicators: a pictorial essay, *Progressions* 3(3):3, 1991.

Posthauer ME, Thomas DR: Nutrition and wound care. In Baranoski S, Ayello EA, editors: *Wound care essentials: practice principles,* Philadelphia, 2004, Lippincott, Williams & Wilkins.

Ramundo JM: Wound debridement. In Bryant RA, Nix DP: *Acute and chronic wounds: current management concepts,* ed 3, St. Louis, 2007, Mosby.

Richardson GM, Gardner S, Frantz RA: Nursing assessment: impact on type and cost of interventions to prevent pressure ulcers, *J Wound Ostomy Continence Nurs* 25(6):1273, 1998.

Rodeheaver GT: Wound cleansing, wound irrigation, wound disinfection. In Krasner DL, Rodeheaver GT, Sibbald RG, editors: *Chronic wound care: a clinical source book for healthcare professionals,* Wayne, Pa, 2001, HMP Communications.

Rolstad BS, Ovington L: Principles of wound management. In Bryant RA, Nix DP, editors: *Acute and chronic wounds: current management concepts,* ed 3, St. Louis, 2007, Mosby.

Schultz G. Molecular regulation of wound healing. In Bryant RA, Nix DP, editors: *Acute and chronic wounds: current management concepts,* ed 3, St. Louis, 2007, Mosby.

Stotts NA: Nutritional assessment and support. In Bryant RA, Nix DP, editors: *Acute and chronic wounds: current management concepts,* ed 3, St. Louis, 2007a, Mosby.

Stotts NA: Wound infection: diagnosis and management. In Bryant RA, Nix DP, editors: *Acute and chronic wounds: current management concepts,* ed 3, St. Louis, 2007b, Mosby.

Stotts NA, Cavanaugh CE: Assessing the patient with a wound, *Home Healthc Nurse* 17(1):27, 1999.

Teare J, Barrett C: Using a quality of life assessment in wound care, *Nurs Stand* 17(6):67, 2002.

The Joint Commission: *Comprehensive accreditation manual for hospitals: the official handbook (CAMH),* Chicago, 2007, The Joint Commission.

Thomas C: Specialty beds: decision-making made easy, *Ostomy Wound Manage* 23:51, 1989.

Trelease CC: Developing standards for wound care, *Ostomy Wound Manage* 20:46, 1988.

Wound, Ostomy and Continence Nurses Society, *Guideline for prevention and management of pressure ulcers,* WOCN Clinical Practice Guidelines Series, Glenview, Ill, 2003, The Society.

Wound, Ostomy and Continence Nurses Society, *Prevalence and incidence: a toolkit for clinicians,* Glenview, Ill, 2004, The Society.

Wysocki AB: Anatomy and physiology of skin and soft tissue. In Bryant RA Nix DP, editors: *Acute and chronic wounds: current management concepts,* ed 3, St. Louis, 2007, Mosby.

Research References

Allman RM and others: Pressure ulcers, hospital complications, and disease severity: impact on hospital costs and length of stay, *Adv Wound Care* 12(1):22, 1999.

Baharestani MM: The lived experience of wives caring for their frail, homebound, elderly husbands with pressure ulcers, *Adv Wound Care* 7(3):40, 1994.

Braden BJ, Bergstrom N: Clinical utility of the Braden Scale for predicting pressure sore risk, *Decubitus* 2(3):50,1989.

Braden BJ, Bergstrom N: Predictive validity of the Braden Scale for pressure sore risk in a nursing home population, *Res Nurs Health* 17(6):459, 1994.

Bergstrom N and others: The Braden Scale for predicting pressure sore risk, *Nurs Res* 36(4):205, 1987.

Bruns TB, Worthington JM: Using tissue adhesive for wound repair: a practical guide to Dermabond, *Am Fam Physician* 61(5)1383, 2000.

Burton AC, Yamada S: Relation between blood pressure and flow in the human forearm, *J Appl Physiol*, 4(5):329, 1951.

Ferrell BA and others: Pressure ulcers among patients admitted to home care, *J Am Geriatr Soc* 48(9):1042, 2000.

Gray M; Weir D: Prevention and treatment of moisture-associated skin damage (maceration) in the periwound skin, *J Wound Ostomy Continence Nurs* 34(2):153, 2007.

Lyder CH and others: Quality of care for hospitalized Medicare patients at risk for pressure ulcers, *Arch Intern Med* 161(12):1549, 2001.

CHAPTER 49
References

American Academy of Ophthalmology: *Comprehensive adult medical eye evaluation*, San Francisco, 2004, The Academy.

Barnett TO: Problems of the ear. In Monahan F and others: *Phipps' medical-surgical nursing: health and illness perspectives*, ed 8, St. Louis, 2007, Mosby.

Boyd-Monk HG: Problems of the eye. In Phipps WJ and others: *Medical-surgical nursing: health and illness perspectives*, ed 8, St. Louis, 2007, Mosby.

Bulechek GM, Butcher HK, Dochterman JM: *Nursing interventions classification (NIC)*, ed 5, St. Louis, 2008, Mosby.

Demers K: Hearing screening, *Medsurg Nurs* 13(3):202, 2004.

Ebersole P and others: *Toward healthy aging: human needs and nursing response*, ed 6, St. Louis, 2004, Mosby.

Ebersole P and others: *Gerontological nursing and healthy aging*, ed 2, St. Louis, 2005, Mosby.

Halle C: Achieve new vision screening objectives, *Nurse Pract* 27(3):15, 2002.

Hockenberry MJ, Wilson D: *Wong's nursing care of infants and children*, ed 8, St. Louis, 2007, Mosby.

Houde SC, Huff MA: Age related vision loss in older adults: a challenge for gerontological nurses, *J Gerontol Nurs* 29(4):25, 2003.

MacDonald C: Back to the real sensory world our "care" has taken away, *J Dementia Care* 10(1):33, 2002.

McConnell EA: How to converse with a hearing impaired patient, *Nursing* 32(8):20, 2002.

Moorhead S and others: *Nursing outcomes classification (NOC)*, ed 4, St. Louis, 2008, Mosby.

National Eye Institute: *Vision loss from eye diseases will increase as Americans age*, 2004, http://www.nei.nih.gov.

National Institute on Deafness and Other Communication Disorders: *Healthy Hearing 2010: where are we now*, 2005, http://www.nidcd.nih.gov.

Occupational Safety and Health Administration: *Eye protection for the workplace*, 2004, U.S. Department of Labor, http://www.osha.gov.

Ruggiero C, Dziedzic L: Promoting a healing environment: quiet time in the intensive care unit, *Jt Comm J Qual Saf* 30(8):465, 2004.

Smith SC, Wilbur ME: Nursing management: visual and auditory problems. In Lewis SM and others: *Medical-surgical nursing: assessment and management of clinical problems*, ed 6, St. Louis, 2004, Mosby.

Sommer S, Sommer S: When your patient is hearing impaired, *RN* 65(12):28, 2002.

U.S. Department of Health and Human Services: *Healthy People 2010: understanding and improving health*, Washington, DC, 2000, Jones & Bartlett.

U.S. Department of Health and Human Services: *Progress review: vision and hearing*, 2004, http://www.healthypeople.gov.

Research References

Caban A and others: Prevalence of concurrent hearing and visual impairment in U.S. adults: the national health interview survey, 1997-2002, *Am J Public Health* 95(11):1940, 2005.

Crews JE, Campbell VA: Vision impairment and hearing loss among community-dwelling older Americans: implications for health and functioning, *Am J Public Health* 94(5):823, 2004.

Moore LW, Miller M: Older men's experiences of living with severe visual impairment, *J Adv Nurs* 43(1):10, 2003.

Reyes-Ortiz C and others: Near vision impairment predicts cognitive decline: data from the Hispanic established populations for epidemiologic studies of the elderly, *J Am Geriatr Soc* 53(4):681, 2005.

CHAPTER 50
References

Agency for Health Care Policy and Research: *Acute pain management: operative or medical procedures and trauma*, Clinical Practice Guideline, AHCPR Pub No. 92-0032, Rockville, Md, 1992, Public Health Service, U.S. Department of Health and Human Services, http://www.ahrq.gov.

Aldrete JA: Modifications to the post anesthesia score for use in ambulatory surgery, *J Perianesth Nurs* 13(3):148, 1998.

Aldrete JA, Kroulik D: A post-anesthetic recovery score, *Anesth Analg* 49:924, 1970.

American Association of Nurse Anesthetists: *AANA latex protocol*, Park Ridge, Ill, 2001, The Association, http://www.aana.com/resources, accessed October 2007.

American College of Surgeons: *Patient education: partners in surgical care*, 2006, http://www.facs.org/patienteducation/index.html.

American Society of Anesthesiologists: Practice guidelines for the perioperative management of patients with obstructive sleep apnea: a report by the American Society of Anesthesiologists Task Force on Perioperative Management of Patients With Obstructive Sleep Apnea, *Anesthesiology* 104:1081, 2006.

American Society of PeriAnesthesia Nurses: *Standards of perianesthesia nursing practice*, Cherry Hill, NJ, 2002, The Society.

American Society of PeriAnesthesia Nurses: *Standards of perianesthesia nursing practice*, 2006, http://www.aspan.org.

Association of Operating Room Nurses: Recommended practices for managing the patient receiving moderate sedation/analgesia, *AORN J* 75(3):642, 2002b.

Association of Operating Room Nurses: Recommended practices for skin preparation of patients, *AORN J* 75(1):184, 2002c.

Association of Operating Room Nurses: *Standards, recommended practices, and guidelines*, Denver, 2002d, The Association.

Association of periOperative Registered Nurses, 2006, http://www.aorn.org.

Barnes S: Pain management: what do patients need to know and when do they need to know it? *J Perianesth Nurs* 16(2):107, 2001.

Barnes S: Patient preparation: the physical assessment, *J Perianesth Nurs* 17(1):46, 2002.

Blouin MB, Magro S: How to handle the risks of obstructive sleep apnea, *Outpatient Surgery*, December 2005.

Bulechek GM, Butcher HK, Dochterman JM: *Nursing interventions classification (NIC)*, ed 5, St. Louis, 2008, Mosby.

De Ruiter HP, Larsen KE: Developing a transcultural patient care web site, *J Transcult Nurs* 13(1):61, 2002.

Eliopoulos C: *Gerontologic nursing*, ed 6, Philadelphia, 2004, Lippincott.

Federated Ambulatory Surgery Association/Foundation for Ambulatory Surgery in America: *Most common outpatient procedures*, 2006, http://www.fasa.org.

Lewis S and others: *Medical-surgical nursing: assessment and management of clinical problems*, ed 7, St. Louis, 2007, Mosby.

Malignant Hyperthermia Association of the United States: *Managing malignant hypertension: clinical update*, online brochure, http://www.mhaus.org, accessed October 2006.

Mamaril ME: Nursing consideration in geriatric surgical patient: the perioperative continuum of care, *Nurs Clin North Am* 41:313, 2006.

Meiner SE, Lueckenotte AG: *Gerontologic nursing*, ed 3, St. Louis, 2006, Mosby.

Moorhead S and others: *Nursing outcomes classification (NOC)*, ed 4, St. Louis, 2008, Mosby.

Mukherjee D, Eagle KA: Perioperative cardiac assessment for noncardiac surgery, *Circulation* 107: 2771, 2003.

Pagana KD, Pagana TJ: *Mosby's diagnostic and laboratory test reference*, ed 8, St. Louis, 2007, Mosby.

Polk HC, Christmas AB: Prophylactic antibiotics in surgery and surgical wound infections, *Am Surg* 66(2):105, 2000.

Pruitt B: Help your patient combat postoperative atelectasis, *Nursing* 36(5):64, 2006.

Rothrock JC: *Alexander's care of the patient in surgery*, ed 13, St. Louis, 2007, Mosby.

Steelman VM, Titler MG: *Evidence-based protocol: latex precautions*, Iowa City, 2001, The University of Iowa Gerontological Nursing Interventions Research Center, Research Dissemination Core.

Sullivan EE: Preoperative holding areas, *J Perianesth Nurs* 15(5):353, 2000.

The Joint Commission: *2007 National patient safety goals,* 2006, http://www.jointcommission.org.

Research References

American Society of Anesthesiologists Task Force on Preoperative Fasting: Practice guidelines for preoperative fasting and the use of pharmacologic agents to reduce the risk of pulmonary aspiration: application to healthy patients undergoing elective procedures, *Anesthesiology* 90(3):896, 1999.

Apfelbaum JL and others: Eliminating intensive postoperative care in same-day surgery patients using short-acting anesthetics, *Anesthesiology* 97(1):66, 2002.

Aragon D: Evaluation of nursing work effort and perceptions about blood glucose testing in tight glycemic control, *Am J Crit Care* 15(4):370, 2006.

Augustus CE: Beliefs and perceptions of African American women who have had hysterectomy, *J Transcult Nurs* 13(4):296, 2002.

Costa MJ: The lived perioperative experience of ambulatory surgery patients, *AORN J* 74(6):874, 2001.

Fredman B and others: Fast-track eligibility of geriatric patients undergoing short urologic procedures, *Anesth Analg* 94:560, 2002.

Furnary AP and others: Continuous insulin infusion reduces mortality in patients with diabetes undergoing coronary artery bypass grafting, *J Thorac Cardiovasc Surg* 125(5):1007, 2003.

Gan TJ: Postoperative nausea and vomiting: can it be eliminated? *JAMA* 287(10):1233, 2002.

Gupta A and others: Postoperative analgesia after radical retropubic prostatectomy: a double-blind comparison between low thoracic epidural and patient-controlled intravenous analgesia, *Anesth* 105(4):784, 2006.

Hansdottir V and others: Thoracic epidural versus intravenous patient-controlled analgesia after cardiac surgery: a randomized controlled trial on length of hospital stay and patient-perceived quality of recovery, *Anesth* 104(1):142, 2006.

Haycock C and others: Implementing evidence-based practice findings to decrease postoperative sternal wound infections following open heart surgery, *J Cardiovasc Nurs* 20(5):299, 2005.

Hobson DW and others: Development and evaluation of a new alcohol-based surgical hand scrub formulation with persistent antimicrobial characteristics and brushless application, *Am J Infect Control* 26:507, 1998.

Larson EL and others: Alcohol for surgical scrubbing? *Infect Control Hosp Epidemiol* 11:139, 1990.

Lee N and others: A survey of patient education postdischarge, *J Nurs Care Qual* 13(1):63, 1998.

Madsen D and others: Listening to bowel sounds: an evidence-based practice project, *Am J Nurs* 105(12):40, 2005.

O'Callaghan N: Pre-operative fasting, *Nurs Stand* 16(36):33, 2002.

Pieper B and others: Bariatric surgery: patient incision care and discharge concerns, *Ostomy Wound Manage* 52(6):48, 2006.

Summers S: Evidence-based practice. II. Reliability and validity of selected acute pain instruments, *J Perianesth Nurs* 16(1):35, 2001.

Taqi A and others: Thoracic epidural analgesia facilitates the restoration of bowel function and dietary intake in patients undergoing laparoscopic colon resection using a traditional, nonaccelerated, perioperative care program, *Surg Endosc* 21(2):247, 2007.

Taylor BE and others: Efficacy and safety of an insulin infusion protocol in a surgical ICU, *J Am Coll Surg* 202(1):1, 2006.

Tramer MR: A rational approach to the control of postoperative nausea and vomiting: evidence from systematic reviews. II. Recommendations for prevention and treatment, and research agenda, *Acta Anaesthesiol Scand* 45:14, 2001.

Van Den Berghe G and others: Intensive insulin therapy in critically ill patients, *N Engl J Med* 345: 1359, 2001.

Zerr KJ and others: Glucose control lowers the risk of wound infection in diabetics after open heart operations, *Ann Thorac Surg* 63:356, 1997.

NCLEX®-Style Review Question Answer Key

CHAPTER 1
1. 4
2. 3
3. 4
4. 2
5. 3
6. 4
7. 4
8. 1

CHAPTER 2
1. 3
2. 4
3. 2, 4
4. 2, 4
5. 2, 3, 4
6. 1, 2
7. 1

CHAPTER 3
1. 4
2. 1, 2
3. 1, 2, 3, 4
4. 4
5. 5
6. 2
7. 1
8. 2
9. 1, 2, 3, 4
10. 3

CHAPTER 4
1. 4
2. 3
3. 2
4. 4
5. 3
6. 3
7. 2
8. 2
9. 1
10. 4

CHAPTER 5
1. 2
2. 2
3. 1
4. 4
5. 4, 1, 5, 3, 2
6. 4
7. 3
8. 1

CHAPTER 6
1. 2
2. 1
3. 3
4. 2
5. 4
6. 4
7. 1
8. 2
9. 4
10. 4

CHAPTER 7
1. 4
2. 1
3. 1, 2, 3
4. 3
5. 3, 5
6. 4

CHAPTER 8
1. 4
2. 4
3. 2
4. 4
5. 3
6. 1
7. 4
8. 3
9. 2

CHAPTER 9
1. 4
2. 2
3. 4
4. 4
5. 2
6. 1
7. 3
8. 4
9. 3

CHAPTER 10
1. 3
2. 2
3. 4
4. 2
5. 1
6. 4
7. 2

CHAPTER 11
1. 4
2. 1
3. 2
4. 2
5. 4
6. 2
7. 2
8. 3
9. 2
10. 3

CHAPTER 12
1. 1
2. 4
3. 3
4. 3
5. 3
6. 4
7. 3
8. 1
9. 2

CHAPTER 13
1. 2
2. 3
3. 3
4. 4
5. 1
6. 4
7. 3
8. 4

CHAPTER 14
1. 4
2. 3
3. 2
4. 4
5. 4
6. 3
7. 2
8. 2
9. 3

CHAPTER 15
1. 2
2. 1
3. 3
4. 3
5. 3
6. 2
7. 3

CHAPTER 16
1. 4
2. 4
3. 4
4. 1
5. 4
6. 3
7. 1, 2, 3
8. 1, 3, 5

CHAPTER 17

1. 3
2. 4
3. 4
4. 4
5. 2
6. 1
7. 3
8. 4
9. 4
10. 1, 2

CHAPTER 18

1. 2, 3
2. 1
3. 1, 2
4. 4
5. 4
6. 4
7. 1, 5
8. 4

CHAPTER 19

1. 3
2. 2
3. 1
4. 2
5. 1
6. 3
7. 1, 2, 3, 4, 5

CHAPTER 20

1. 3
2. 2, 4
3. 4
4. 4
5. 2
6. 1, 2

CHAPTER 21

1. 2, 3, 4, 5
2. 4
3. 3
4. 4
5. 3
6. 1
7. 3
8. 2
9. 4
10. 4

CHAPTER 22

1. 4
2. 3
3. 2
4. 1
5. 4
6. 1
7. 2
8. 3
9. 2

CHAPTER 23

1. 2, 3, 4, 5
2. 3, 4
3. 3
4. 2
5. 3
6. 2
7. 3
8. 1, 4
9. 3
10. 1, 2, 3, 4, 5

CHAPTER 24

1. 2
2. 3
3. 1
4. 3
5. 4
6. 2
7. 1
8. 3
9. 2, 3, 4
10. 3

CHAPTER 25

1. 4
2. 2
3. 2
4. 3
5. 3
6. 1
7. 1
8. 4
9. 2
10. 2

CHAPTER 26

1. 4
2. 3
3. 4
4. 3
5. 2
6. 4
7. Repositioned client on right side. Encouraged client to use PCA device. (P) The pain increases every time I try to turn on my left side. (S) Acute pain related to tissue injury from surgical incision. (A) Left lower abdominal surgical incision, 3 inches in length, closed, sutures intact, no drainage. Pain noted on mild palpation. (O)
8. 2

CHAPTER 27

1. 4
2. 1
3. 2
4. 3
5. 3
6. 4
7. 2
8. 2
9. 1, 2, 3, 4

CHAPTER 28

1. 2
2. 3
3. 3
4. 2
5. 2
6. 1, 2, 3
7. 4
8. 1
9. 2
10. 2

CHAPTER 29

1. 2
2. 2
3. 1
4. 4
5. 2
6. 1, 5
7. 3
8. 1, 2, 5

CHAPTER 30

1. 1
2. 2
3. 3
4. 2
5. 4
6. 4
7. 6, 2, 5, 3, 1, 4, 7, 8
8. 2
9. 3
10. 2

CHAPTER 31

1. 3
2. 4
3. 1
4. 3
5. 1
6. 2
7. 4
8. 4
9. 4
10. 2

CHAPTER 32

1. 3
2. 1, 5, 2, 4, 3
3. 3
4. 3
5. 1, 2, 6, 7, 8
6. T, RR
7. Tympanic—the client has an oxygen mask on, which would rule out an oral temperature. The client has a fractured right arm and a left antecubital IV, which would make an axillary temperature more difficult to obtain. The client has multiple fractures, which would make a rectal temperature difficult and uncomfortable. A temporal temperature would not be appropriate because of the laceration on her forehead.
8. 6
9. 3
10. 1, 2, 3, 4

CHAPTER 33

1. 1
2. 3
3. 4
4. 3
5. 3
6. 3
7. 3
8. 4
9. 4
10. 2, 4, 3, 1
11. 3
12. 4
13. 4
14. 4

CHAPTER 34

1. 2
2. 1
3. 1
4. 1
5. 4
6. 3
7. 4
8. 3
9. 2
10. 1

CHAPTER 35

1. 2
2. 4
3. 2
4. 4
5. 3
6. 3
7. 2
8. 1
9. 3
10. 2
11. 3
12. 2

CHAPTER 36

1. 4
2. 6
3. 1
4. 3
5. 2
6. 2
7. 4
8. 4
9. 4
10. 1

CHAPTER 37

1. 2
2. 1, 2, 3
3. 4
4. 2
5. 4
6. 2
7. 1
8. 3
9. 4

CHAPTER 38

1. 3
2. 3
3. 3
4. 4
5. 4
6. 4
7. 2
8. 4
9. 1
10. 4

CHAPTER 39

1. 1, 3, 4
2. 4
3. 1, 2, 3, 4
4. 1
5. 3
6. 2
7. 4
8. 1
9. 2
10. 3

CHAPTER 40

1. 4
2. 1, 4
3. 2
4. 2
5. 3
6. 4
7. 1
8. 4
9. 1, 3, 5
10. 2, 3, 5, 6

CHAPTER 41

1. 1
2. 4
3. 2
4. 4
5. 1
6. 1, 3
7. 7, 5, 3, 6, 1, 2, 4
8. 1, 4
9. 3

CHAPTER 42

1. 1, 4
2. 2
3. 4
4. 4, 5, 6
5. 1
6. 2
7. 1
8. 3
9. 4
10. 4

CHAPTER 43

1. 2
2. 1
3. 2
4. 2
5. 3
6. 4
7. 4
8. 1
9. 2

CHAPTER 44

1. 3
2. 2
3. 1, 3, 5
4. 2
5. 1
6. 2, 3, 1, 4
7. 4
8. 4
9. 2

CHAPTER 45

1. 1
2. Bacteria
3. 3, 4, 5
4. 4
5. 4
6. 3
7. 1
8. 4
9. 1320 mL urine for the 8-hour period
10. 1

CHAPTER 46

1. 4
2. 3
3. 3
4. 1, 4
5. 4
6. 4
7. 4
8. 4, 3, 5, 1, 2
9. 2, 1, 3, 4, 6, 5, 7
10. 4

CHAPTER 47

1. 1
2. 3
3. 4
4. 4
5. 2
6. 4
7. 1
8. 2
9. 4
10. 1, 2, 4

CHAPTER 48

1. 4
2. 1
3. 4
4. 3
5. 3
6. 2
7. 3
8. 4
9. 3
10. 3

CHAPTER 49

1. 4, 5
2. 4
3. 3
4. 4
5. 4
6. 4
7. 4
8. 3
9. 4
10. 3, 4

CHAPTER 50

1. 3
2. 4
3. 1
4. 1
5. 3
6. 4
7. 4
8. 2
9. 2
10. 4

Index

Page numbers followed by *f* denote figures; *t*, tables; and
b, boxes.

Special Features

Client Teaching

Concept Maps

Nursing Care Plans